ASHP® Injectable Drug Information™

ASHP®
Injectable Drug Information™

A Comprehensive Guide
to Compatibility and Stability

2021

Published under the Editorial Authority of ASHP®

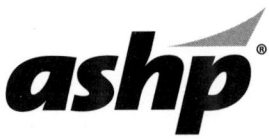

Published under the editorial authority of ASHP®. Any correspondence regarding this publication should be sent to the publisher, American Society of Health-System Pharmacists, 4500 East-West Highway, Suite 900, Bethesda, MD 20814, attn: ASHP Injectable Drug Information or to publications@ashp.org.

The nature of drug information and its applications is constantly evolving because of ongoing research and clinical experience and is often subject to professional judgment and interpretation by the practitioner due to the uniqueness of each clinical situation and patient. While care has been taken to ensure the accuracy of the information presented, the reader is advised that the authors, editors, contributors, reviewers, and publisher cannot be responsible for the continued currency of the information, for any errors or omissions, and/or any consequences arising from the use of this information in a clinical setting.

Any reader of this work is cautioned that ASHP makes no representation, guarantee, or warranty, express or implied, as to the accuracy and appropriateness of the information contained in this work and specifically disclaims any liability to any party for the accuracy and/or completeness of the material contained in the work or for any damages arising out of the use or non-use of any of the information contained in this work.

Because of the dynamic nature of drug information, readers also are advised that decisions regarding drug use and patient care must be based on the independent judgment of the clinician, changing information about a drug (e.g., as represented in the literature), and changing professional practices.

Vice President, Publishing Office: Daniel J. Cobaugh, PharmD, DABAT, FAACT

Assistant Editor for Injectables: Lisa M. Kohoutek, PharmD, BCPS

Project Manager: Elizabeth P. Shannon, BS

Production Services/Printing: Sheridan

Cover Design: DeVall Advertising

Cover Art: iStock-913469346

Page Design: David Wade

ISBN: 978-1-58528-658-4 (hardcover)
ISBN: 978-1-58528-685-0 (adobe pdf)
ISBN: 978-1-58528-690-4 (ePub)
DOI: 10.37573/9781585286850

10 9 8 7 6 5 4 3 2 1

TABLE OF CONTENTS

DOI: 10.37573/9781585286850.fm

PREFACE

ASHP® Injectable Drug Information™ 2021 is a collection of compatibility and stability information on parenteral drug products and is the most recent contribution to this continuing series. With its publication, all previous editions are considered out of date.

One of the core focuses of ASHP as a professional and scientific society has been its long history of publishing internationally recognized, authoritative sources of drug information. Beginning with publication of the Society's ground-breaking work the *American Hospital Formulary Service®* (*AHFS®*; now *AHFS Drug Information®*) in 1959 and continuing with the definitive works the *Parenteral Drug Information Guide™* in 1974, the *Handbook on Injectable Drugs®* in 1977, and the *Medication Teaching Manual®* (now *AHFS Patient Medication Information™*) in 1978, ASHP has consistently set the standard for objective drug information focused on safe and effective drug therapy. For more than 75 years, ASHP has been at the forefront of efforts to improve medication use and patient safety. Publication of *ASHP® Injectable Drug Information™* 2021 is an important component of those efforts. With the 2021 edition of *ASHP® Injectable Drug Information™*, ASHP marks 49 years of publishing such an invaluable resource on parenteral medications.

First published in 1977 as a key outgrowth of pharmaceutics research and pharmacy practice at the US Public Health Service and National Institutes of Health (NIH), the *Handbook on Injectable Drugs®* has a long legacy of translating pharmaceutics research into an essential resource for practical patient-care applications. Lawrence A. Trissel, who served as co-author of ASHP's first resource on injectable drugs—the *Parenteral Drug Information Guide™*, established this legacy by serving as the distinguished author of the *Handbook on Injectable Drugs®* for the first 17 editions. ASHP and the profession as a whole remain grateful to Mr. Trissel for his contribution to the pharmaceutics literature and his unyielding dedication to the science of stability and compatibility information on parenteral products.

With the publication of the *Mirror to Hospital Pharmacy* in 1964, ASHP paved the way for a transition from nursing-driven to pharmacy-led sterile compounding services and has remained an industry leader for both advocacy and best practices related to parenteral medications. The mission of ASHP's reference publications on compatibility and stability of parenteral products has always been to facilitate the use of the vast body of pharmaceutics research on parenteral medications in a way that could enable those who prescribe, prepare, and administer injectable drugs to more fully apply this information to the benefit of patients. With increasingly complex drug therapy regimens, an abundance of new drug and drug formulation approvals, and ever-present drug shortage issues, pharmaceutics research has important implications for patient care in the inpatient, specialty pharmacy, and home infusion settings. Recent examples of inappropriate compounding practices involving parenteral medications have resulted in increased sterile compounding regulation and have reinforced the importance of adherence to sterile compounding standards, implementation of best practices in the preparation and administration of parenteral drug products (commercially available or extemporaneously compounded), and application of principles and findings of pharmaceutics research to patient care. For additional information on sterile compounding, ASHP's Resource Center can be consulted (**www.ashp.org/sterilecompounding**).

Beginning with the 18th edition, the *Handbook on Injectable Drugs®* became an integral component of ASHP's *AHFS®* resource collection of authoritative drug information. Applying its expansive drug information and informatics expertise, ASHP's focus with the subsequent editions has been on the continuing addition and revision of new and existing drug monographs as well as important database enhancements to this indispensable authority on parenteral drugs. *ASHP® Injectable Drug Information™* 2021, which was begun to provide a single standardized source of the primary research on the stability, compatibilities, and incompatibilities of injectable drugs, continues to be the most widely recognized "Gold Standard" for such information.

ASHP® Injectable Drug Information™ 2021 includes 18 new monographs, bringing the total in this edition to 406 monographs on parenteral drugs available in the United States and in other countries. In addition, more than 500 revisions to existing monographs (affecting nearly 60% of the existing monographs) have been accomplished to update information on stability, compatibility, and safety (e.g., Food and Drug Administration [FDA] MedWatch alerts) and to provide more specific referencing of manufacturer information and other enhancements to the more than 24,100 compatibility pairs contained in *ASHP® Injectable Drug Information™* 2021. The information cited throughout the text has been compiled from 3603 references, including 195 new to this edition. Because information from pharmaceutical manufacturers had not been uniquely cited until the 18th edition, the number of unique references supporting *ASHP® Injectable Drug Information™* 2021 information actually greatly exceeds this number. While primary,

DOI: 10.37573/9781585286850.fm

peer-reviewed literature remains a major source of compatibility and stability information, ongoing efforts are underway to provide increased specificity of references to the pharmaceutics research of drug manufacturers. Other relevant information and pertinent study details supplied by corresponding authors of the published literature also have been incorporated when available.

In addition to the noted enhancements to the 2021 print edition of *ASHP® Injectable Drug Information™* 2021, the regularly updated online edition features linked monographs to *Extended Stability for Parenteral Drugs*, forming a single, comprehensive resource on injectable drug information. This extended stability information is specifically designed for use in home infusion and other infusion practices, providing critical stability data to support realistic and cost-effective compounding and patient delivery schedules. *ASHP® Injectable Drug Information™* 2021 also will soon be available as an ebook in a variety of formats (e.g., PDF, EPUB, full-text HTML).

Regular updates, FDA MedWatch alerts and other guidances, and wall-chart custom views of compatibility information continue to be available for digital versions.

For proper use of this reference work, the reader must review "How to Use *ASHP® Injectable Drug Information™*," which immediately follows this Preface. This section will acquaint the user of *ASHP® Injectable Drug Information™* with its organization, content, structure, summarization strategy, interpretation of the information presented, and limitations of the published literature upon which this reference text is based. Without a good working knowledge of these points, *ASHP® Injectable Drug Information™* 2021 may not be used to its best advantage or even interpreted correctly.

USERS GUIDE

HOW TO USE *ASHP® INJECTABLE DRUG INFORMATION™*

What Is *ASHP® Injectable Drug Information™*?

ASHP® Injectable Drug Information™ is a collection of summaries of information from the published literature on the pharmaceutics of parenteral medications as applied to the clinical setting. *ASHP® Injectable Drug Information™* is constructed from information derived from 3603 references with the information presented in the standardized structure described below. The purpose of this reference text is to facilitate the use of this clinical pharmaceutics research by knowledgeable health care professionals for the benefit of patients. The summary information from published research is supplemented with information from the labeling of each product and from other references.

The information base summarized in *ASHP® Injectable Drug Information™* is large and highly complex, requiring thoughtful consideration for proper use. This reference text is not, nor should it be considered, elementary in nature or a primer. A single quick glance in a table is not adequate for proper interpretation of this highly complex information base. Proper interpretation includes the obvious need to consider and evaluate all relevant research information and results. Additionally, information on the formulation components (e.g., excipients), product attributes (especially pH), and the known stability behaviors of each parenteral drug, as well as the clinical situation of the patient, must be included in a thoughtful, reasoned evaluation of clinical pharmaceutics questions. Stability and sterility both must be considered in the assignment of beyond-use dates.

Who Should Use *ASHP® Injectable Drug Information™*?

ASHP® Injectable Drug Information™ is designed for use as a professional reference and guide to the literature on the clinical pharmaceutics of parenteral medications. The intended audience consists of knowledgeable healthcare professionals, particularly pharmacists, who are well versed in the formulation and clinical use of parenteral medications and who have the highly specialized knowledge base, training, and skill set necessary to interpret and apply the information. Practitioners who are not well versed in the formulation, essential properties, and clinical application of paren-

teral drugs should seek the assistance of more knowledgeable and experienced healthcare professionals to ensure patient safety.

Users of *ASHP® Injectable Drug Information™* must recognize that no reference work, including this one, can substitute for adequate decision-making by healthcare professionals. Proper clinical decisions must be made after considering all aspects of the patient's condition and needs, with particular attention to the special demands imposed by parenteral medications. *ASHP® Injectable Drug Information™* cannot make decisions for its users. However, in knowledgeable hands, it is a valuable tool for the proper use of parenteral medications.

Organization of *ASHP® Injectable Drug Information™*

ASHP® Injectable Drug Information™ has been organized as a collection of monographs on each of the drugs. The monographs are arranged alphabetically by nonproprietary (generic) name. The nonproprietary names of the drugs are the United States Adopted Names (USAN) and other official names for drugs as described in the *USP Dictionary of USAN and International Drug Names*. Also included are some of the trade (proprietary, brand) names and manufacturers of the drug products; this listing is not necessarily comprehensive and should not be considered an endorsement of any product or manufacturer.

All of the information included in *ASHP® Injectable Drug Information™* is referenced so that those who wish to study the original sources may find them. Efforts are ongoing to provide increased specificity of references to product labeling as individually cited references to the labeling for a drug product, including the proprietary name (if available), manufacturer, and revision date of the prescribing information; this will facilitate location of specific labeling that has been used as a reference. In addition, the full list of the *AHFS®* Pharmacologic-Therapeutic Classification© system and specific classification numbers within each individual monograph have been included to facilitate the location of therapeutic information on the drugs.

The monographs have been divided into the subheadings described below:

Products—lists many of the sizes, strengths, volumes, and forms in which the drug is supplied, along with other components of the formulation. Instructions for reconstitution (when applicable) are included in this section.

DOI: 10.37573/9781585286850.fm

The products described do not necessarily comprise a comprehensive list of all available products. Rather, some common representative products are described. Furthermore, dosage forms, sizes, and container configurations of parenteral products may undergo important changes during the lifespan of this edition of *ASHP® Injectable Drug Information™*.

Following the product descriptions, the pH of the drug products, the osmotic value(s) of the drug and/or dilutions (when available), and other product information such as the sodium content and definition of units are presented.

Practitioners have not always recognized the value and importance of incorporating product formulation information into the thought process that leads to their decision on handling drug compatibility and stability questions. Excipients used in the formulation of commercially available products may vary among manufacturers and can influence drug compatibility and stability; specific product labeling should be consulted for additional formulation details. Consideration of the product information and formulation components, as well as the properties and attributes of the products (especially pH), is essential to proper interpretation of the information presented in *ASHP® Injectable Drug Information™*.

Administration—includes route(s) by which the drug can be given, rates of administration (when applicable), and other related administration details.

The administration information is a condensation derived principally from product labeling. For complete information, including dosage information sufficient for prescribing, the reader should refer to product labeling and therapeutically comprehensive references, such as the *AHFS® Drug Information®*.

Stability—describes the drug's stability and storage requirements. The storage condition terminology of *The United States Pharmacopeia*, 42nd ed., is used in *ASHP® Injectable Drug Information™*.

The United States Pharmacopeia defines controlled room temperature as a temperature that encompasses the usual and customary working environment of 20–25°C and that results in a mean kinetic temperature no greater than 25°C.[17] Temperature excursions between 15–30°C that are experienced in pharmacies, hospitals, warehouses, and during shipping are permitted.[17] Transient temperature elevations up to 40°C also are permitted provided that they do not persist beyond 24 hours and that the mean kinetic temperature does not exceed 25°C.[17] In contrast, room (ambient) temperature is defined simply as a temperature prevailing in a working environment.[17]

Protection from excessive heat is often required; excessive heat is defined as any temperature above 40°C.[17] Similarly, protection from freezing may be required for products that are subject to loss of strength or potency or to destructive alteration of their characteristics, in addition to the risk of container breakage, upon exposure to freezing temperatures.[17]

Some products may require storage at a cool temperature, which is defined as any temperature between 8–15°C, or a cold temperature, which is defined as any temperature not exceeding 8°C.[17] A refrigerator is defined as a cold place in which the temperature is controlled between 2–8°C.[17] A freezer refers to a place in which the temperature is controlled between -25 and -10°C.[17] Some products may have a recommended storage condition below -20°C, and in such cases, the temperature should be controlled to within 10°C of -20°C.[17]

In addition to storage requirements, aspects of drug stability related to pH, freezing, and exposure to light are presented in this section. Also presented is information on repackaging of the drugs or their dilutions in container/closure systems other than the original package (e.g., prefilling into syringes or in ambulatory pump reservoirs). Sorption and filtration characteristics of the drugs are provided as well when this information is available. The information is derived principally from the primary published research literature and is supplemented with information from other sources when available.

Compatibility Information—tabulates the compatibility results of the drug about which the monograph is written with infusion solutions and other drugs based on published reports from the primary research as well as the product labeling. The various entries are listed alphabetically by solution or drug name; the information is completely cross-referenced among the monographs.

Four types of tables are utilized to present the available information, depending on the kind of test being reported. The first type is for information on the compatibility of a drug in various infusion solutions and is depicted in **Table 1**. The second type of table presents information on two or more drugs in intravenous solutions and is shown in **Table 2**. The third type of table is used for tests of two or more drugs in syringes and is shown in **Table 3**. The fourth table format is used for reports of simulated or actual injection into Y-sites and manifolds of administration sets and is shown in **Table 4**.

Many published articles, especially older ones, do not include all of the information necessary to complete the tables. However, the tables have been completed as fully as possible from the original articles; in some cases, editorial staff have supplemented the published information based on direct communication with the authors of the published research.

Table 1. Solution Compatibility

Monograph drug name

Solution	Mfr	Mfr	Conc/L or %	Remarks	Ref	C/I
(1)	(2)	(3)	(4)	(5)	(6)	(7)

1. Solution in which the test was conducted.
2. Manufacturer of the solution.
3. Manufacturer of the drug about which the monograph is written.
4. Concentration of the drug about which the monograph is written. (See *The Listing of Concentration*.)
5. Description of the results of the test.
6. Reference to the original source of the information.
7. Designation of the compatibility (C) or incompatibility (I) of the test result according to conventional guidelines.

Table 2. Additive Compatibility

Monograph drug name

Drug	Mfr	Conc/L or %	Mfr	Conc/L or %	Test Soln	Remarks	Ref	C/I
(1)	(2)	(3)	(4)	(5)	(6)	(7)	(8)	(9)

1. Monograph title for the test drug.
2. Manufacturer of the test drug.
3. Concentration of the test drug.
4. Manufacturer of the drug about which the monograph is written.
5. Concentration of the drug about which the monograph is written. (See *The Listing of Concentration*.) Infusion solution in which the test was conducted.
6. Description of the results of the test.
7. Reference to the original source of the information.
8. Designation of the compatibility (C) or incompatibility (I) of the test result according to conventional guidelines.

Table 3. Drugs in Syringe Compatibility

Monograph drug name

Drug (in syringe)	Mfr	Amt	Mfr	Amt	Remarks	Ref	C/I
(1)	(2)	(3)	(4)	(5)	(6)	(7)	(8)

1. Monograph title for the test drug.
2. Manufacturer of the test drug.
3. Actual amount of the test drug
4. Manufacturer of the drug about which the monograph is written.
5. Actual amount of the drug about which the monograph is written.
6. Description of the results of the test.
7. Reference to the original source of the information.
8. Designation of the compatibility (C) or incompatibility (I) of the test result according to conventional guidelines.

Table 4. Y-Site Injection Compatibility (1:1 Mixture)

Monograph drug name

Drug	Mfr	Conc	Mfr	Conc	Remarks	Ref	C/I
(1)	(2)	(3)	(4)	(5)	(6)	(7)	(8)

1. Monograph title for the test drug
2. Manufacturer of the test drug.
3. Concentration of the test drug prior to mixing at the Y-site.
4. Manufacturer of the drug about which the monograph is written.
5. Concentration of the drug about which the monograph is written prior to mixing at the Y-site.
6. Description of the results of the test.
7. Reference to the original source of the information.
8. Designation of the compatibility (C) or incompatibility (I) of the test result according to conventional guidelines.

Additional Compatibility Information—provides additional information and discussions of compatibility presented largely in narrative form.

Other Information—contains any relevant auxiliary information concerning the drug that does not fall into the previous categories.

The Listing of Concentration

The concentrations of all admixtures in intravenous solutions in the tables (Table 1 and Table 2) generally have been indicated in terms of concentration per liter (L) to facilitate comparison of the various studies. In some cases, this may result in amounts of the drug that are greater or lesser than those normally administered (as when the recommended dose is tested in 100 mL of vehicle), but the listings do accurately reflect the actual concentrations tested, expressed in standardized terms. Concentration may be expressed as a percentage for certain drugs or solutions (e.g., dextran, hetastarch, mannitol, fat emulsion) to reflect the style commonly used to express concentration for these products.

For studies involving syringes, the amounts actually used are indicated. The volumes are also listed if available.

For studies of actual or simulated Y-site injection of drugs, the concentrations are cited in terms of concentration per mL of each drug solution prior to mixing at the Y-site. Most published research reports have presented the drug concentrations in this manner, and *ASHP® Injectable Drug Information*™ follows this convention. For those few published reports that presented the drug concentrations after mixing at the Y-site, the concentrations have been recalculated to be consistent with the more common presentation style to maintain the consistency of presentation in *ASHP® Injectable Drug Information*™. Note that the Y-Site Injection Compatibility table is designed with the assumption of a 1:1 mixture of the subject drug and infusion solution or admixture. For citations reporting other than a 1:1 mixture, the actual amounts tested are specifically noted.

Designating Compatibility or Incompatibility

Each summary of a published research report appearing in the Compatibility Information tables bears a compatibility indicator (*C*, *I*, or *?*). A report receives a designation of *C* when the study results indicate that compatibility of the test samples existed under the test conditions. If the study determined an incompatibility existed under the test conditions, then an *I* designation is assigned for the *ASHP® Injectable Drug Information*™ entry for that study result. A designation of *?* indicates that the test result does not clearly fit either the compatibility or incompatibility definition. Specific standardized guidelines are used to assign these compatibility designations and are described below. The citation is designated as a report of *compatibility* when results of the original article indicated one or more of the following criteria were met:

1. Physical or visual compatibility of the combination was reported (no visible or electronically detected indication of particulate formation, haze, precipitation, color change, or gas evolution).

2. Stability of the components for at least 24 hours in an admixture under the specified conditions was reported (decomposition of 10% or less).

3. Stability of the components for the entire test period, although in some cases it was less than 24 hours, was reported (time periods less than 24 hours have been noted).

The citation is designated as a report of *incompatibility* when the results of the original article indicated either or both of the following criteria were met:

1. A physical or visual incompatibility was reported (visible or electronically detected particulate formation, haze, precipitation, color change, or gas evolution).

2. Greater than 10% decomposition of one or more components in 24 hours or less under the specified

conditions was reported (time periods of less than 24 hours have been noted in the table).

Reports of test results that do not clearly fit into the compatibility or incompatibility definitions cannot be designated as either. These are indicated with a *question mark*.

Although these criteria have become the conventional definitions of compatibility and incompatibility, the reader should recognize that the criteria may need to be tempered with professional judgment. Inflexible adherence to the compatibility designations should be avoided. Instead, they should be used as aids in the exercising of professional judgment.

Therapeutic incompatibilities or other drug interactions are not within the scope of *ASHP® Injectable Drug Information*™ and are therefore not addressed. Therapeutically comprehensive references and the product labeling should be consulted for such information.

Interpreting Compatibility Information in ASHP® Injectable Drug Information™

As mentioned above, the body of information summarized in *ASHP® Injectable Drug Information*™ is large and complicated. With the possible exception of a report of immediate gross precipitation, it usually takes some degree of thoughtful consideration and judgment to properly evaluate and appropriately act on the research results that are summarized in this book.

Nowhere is the need for judgment more obvious than when apparently contradictory information appears in two or more published reports. The body of literature in drug-drug and drug-solution compatibility is replete with apparently contradictory results. Except for study results that have been documented later to be incorrect, the conflicting information has been included in *ASHP® Injectable Drug Information*™ to provide practitioners with all of the information for their consideration. The conflicting information will be readily apparent to the reader because of the content of the Remarks section as well as the *C*, *I*, and *?* designations following each citation.

Many or most of the apparently conflicting citations may be the result of differing conditions or materials used in the studies. A variety of factors that can influence the compatibility and stability of drugs must be considered in evaluating such conflicting results, and absolute statements are often difficult or impossible to make. Differences in concentrations, buffering systems, preservatives, vehicles, temperatures, and order of mixing all may play a role. By reviewing a variety of reports, the user of *ASHP® Injectable Drug Information*™ is better able to exercise professional judgment with regard to compatibility and stability.

The reader must guard against misinterpretation of research results, which may lead to inappropriate assumptions of compatibility and stability. As an example, a finding of precipitate formation two hours after two drugs are mixed does not imply nor should it be interpreted to mean that the combination is compatible until that time point, when a sudden precipitation occurs. Rather, it should be interpreted to mean that precipitation occurred at some point between mixing and the first observation point at two hours. Such a result would lead to a designation of incompatibility in *ASHP® Injectable Drug Information*™.

Precipitation reports can be particularly troublesome for practitioners to deal with because of the variability of the time frames in which they may occur. Apart from combinations that repeatedly result in immediate precipitation, the formation of a precipitate can be unpredictable to some degree. Numerous examples of variable precipitation time frames can be found in the literature, including paclitaxel, etoposide, and sulfamethoxazole-trimethoprim (co-trimoxazole) in infusion solutions and calcium and phosphates precipitation in parenteral nutrition mixtures (e.g., TNAs, TPNs). Differing drug concentrations also can play a role in creating variability in results. A good example of this occurs with co-administered vancomycin hydrochloride and beta-lactam antibiotics. Users of the information in *ASHP® Injectable Drug Information*™ must always be aware that a marginally incompatible combination might exhibit precipitation earlier or later than that reported in the literature. In many such cases, the precipitation is ultimately going to occur, it is just the timing that is in question. This is of particular importance for precipitate formation because of the potential for serious adverse clinical consequences, including death, that have occurred. Certainly, users of *ASHP® Injectable Drug Information*™ information should always keep in mind and anticipate the possibility of precipitation and its clinical ramifications. Furthermore, all injections and infusions should be inspected for particulate matter and discoloration prior to administration. If found, such injections and solutions should be discarded.

In addition, many research reports cite test solutions or concentrations that may not be appropriate for clinical use. An example would be a report of a drug's stability in unsterile water. Although the *ASHP® Injectable Drug Information*™ summary will accurately reflect the test solutions and conditions that existed in a study, it is certainly inappropriate to misinterpret a stability report like this as being an authorization to use the product clinically. In such cases, the researchers may have used the clinically inappropriate diluent to evaluate the drug's stability for extrapolation to a more suitable vehicle that is similar, or they may not have recognized that the diluent is clinically unsuitable. In either event, it is incumbent on the practitioner in the clinical setting to use professional judgment to apply the information in an appropriate manner and recognize what is not acceptable clinically.

Further, it should be noted that many of the citations designated incompatible are not absolute. While a particular admixture may incur more than 10% decomposition within 24 hours, the combination may be useful for a shorter time period. The concept of "utility time" or the time to 10% decomposition may be useful in these cases. Unfortunately, such information is often not available. Included in the Remarks columns of the tables are the amount of decomposition, the time period involved, and the temperature at which the study was conducted when this information is available.

Users of *ASHP® Injectable Drug Information™* should always keep in mind that the information contained in this reference text must be used as a tool and a guide to the research that has been conducted and published. It is not a replacement for thoughtfully considered professional judgment. It falls to the practitioner to interpret the information in light of the clinical situation, including the patient's needs and status. What is certain is that relying solely on the *C* or *I* designation without the application of professional judgment is inappropriate.

Limitations of the Literature

In addition to conflicting information, many of the published articles have provided only partial evaluations, not looking at all aspects of a drug's stability and compatibility. This is not surprising considering the complexity, difficulty, and costs of conducting such research. There are, in fact, articles that do provide evaluations of both physical stability/compatibility and chemical stability. But some are devoted only to physical issues, while others examine only chemical stability. Although a finding of precipitation, haze, or other physical effects may constitute an incompatibility (unless transient), the lack of such changes does not rule out chemical deterioration. In some cases, drugs initially designated as compatible because of a lack of visual change were later shown to undergo chemical decomposition. Similarly, the determination of chemical stability does not rule out the presence of unacceptable levels of particulates and/or turbidity in the combination. In a classic case, the drugs leucovorin calcium and fluorouracil were determined to be chemically stable for extended periods by stability-indicating HPLC assays in several studies, but years later, repeated episodes of filter clogging led to the discovery of unacceptable quantities of particulates in combinations of these drugs. The reader must always bear in mind these possibilities when only partial information is available.

And, finally, contemporary practitioners have come to expect that the analytical methods used in reports on the chemical stability of drugs will be validated, stability-indicating methods. However, many early studies used methods that were not demonstrated to be stability indicating.

Biological drugs (therapeutic proteins [e.g., enzymes, monoclonal antibodies, immune globulins]) are particularly sensitive to environmental factors and undergo more complex and numerous degradation pathways than classical drugs.[3207][3208][3212] In addition to physicochemical instability issues similar to those observed with classical drugs (e.g., precipitation, decomposition), such proteins are subject to other stability issues (e.g., protein conformation, biologic activity) that must be considered.[3207][3208][3209][3212] Therefore, a single analytic method that only assesses protein concentration is insufficient to determine stability of biological products.[3209][3210] Interpretation of the results of compatibility and stability studies of such proteins poses a challenge because both analytic methods and meaningful acceptance criteria should be specific to the biologic; official compendial standards (e.g., *The United States Pharmacopeia* monographs and analytic methods) should be consulted when available.[3206][3209][3212] Although many experts agree that multiple complementary methods should be used to assess the physical and chemical stability as well as assessment of biologic activity, no clear guideline or recommendation for in-use stability studies for therapeutic proteins is available.[3208][3210][3211][3212]

Literature Search for Updating ASHP® Injectable Drug Information™

To gather the bulk of the published compatibility and stability information for updating *ASHP® Injectable Drug Information™*, a literature search is performed using the *International Pharmaceutical Abstracts™ (IPA™)* database and PubMed. By using key terms (e.g., stability), a listing of candidate articles for inclusion in *ASHP® Injectable Drug Information™* is generated. From this list, relevant articles are critically evaluated and prioritized for inclusion. As a supplement to this automated literature searching, a manual search of the references of the articles is also conducted, and any articles not included previously are similarly evaluated for inclusion. In addition, pharmaceutical manufacturers may be contacted for additional in-house (unpublished) data.

ABBREVIATIONS

AA	Amino acids (percentage specified)
D	Dextrose solution (percentage unspecified)
D5LR	Dextrose 5% in Ringer's injection, lactated
D5R	Dextrose 5% in Ringer's injection
D-S	Dextrose-saline combinations
D2.5½S	Dextrose 2.5% in sodium chloride 0.45%
D2.5S	Dextrose 2.5% in sodium chloride 0.9%
D5¼S	Dextrose 5% in sodium chloride 0.225%
D5½S	Dextrose 5% in sodium chloride 0.45%
D5S	Dextrose 5% in sodium chloride 0.9%
D10S	Dextrose 10% in sodium chloride 0.9%
D5W	Dextrose 5%
D10W	Dextrose 10%
IM	Isolyte M
IP	Isolyte P
IS10	Invert sugar 10%
I.U.[a]	International unit(s)
LR	Ringer's injection, lactated
NM	Normosol M
NR	Normosol R
NRD5W	Normosol R in dextrose 5%
NS	Sodium chloride 0.9%
R	Ringer's injections
REF	Refrigeration
RT	Room temperature
S	Saline solution (percentage unspecified)
½S	Sodium chloride 0.45%
SL	Sodium lactate (1/6) M
TNA	Total nutrient admixture (3-in-1)
TPN	Total parenteral nutrition (2-in-1)
W	Sterile water for injection

[a] It is well accepted that "IU" is not a preferred abbreviation for international units. There is some difference of opinion among medication safety stakeholders on whether such units should be referred to simply as "units" or as "International Units." Throughout the text of this reference, we generally have used the term international units to describe such units; however, because of space limitations within the columns of the Compatibility Information tables, the term international units has been abbreviated as I.U. where necessary.

MANUFACTURER AND COMPENDIUM ABBREVIATIONS

AB	Abbott
ABV	AbbVie
ABX	Abraxis
ACA	Acacia
ACC	American Critical Care
ACD	Accord Healthcare
ACH	Achaogen
ACT	Actavis
AD	Adria
AFT	AFT
AGT	Aguettant
AH	Allen & Hanburys
AHP	Ascot Hospital Pharmaceuticals
AKN	Akorn
ALL	Allergan
ALP	Alpharma
ALT	Altana Pharma
ALV	Alveda Pharma
ALZ	Alza
AM	ASTA Medica
AMA	AMAG
AMB	Amneal Biosciences
AMD	Amdipharm
AMG	Amgen
AMP	Amphastar
AMR	American Regent
AMS	Amerisource
AND	Andromaco
ANT	Antigen
AP	Asta-Pharma
APC	Apothecon
APN	Aspen
APO	Apotex
APP	American Pharmaceutical Partners
APR	Aspri
APT	Aspen Triton
AQ	American Quinine
AR	Armour
ARC	American Red Cross
ARD	Ardeapharm
ARR	Arrow
AS	Arnar-Stone
ASC	Ascot
ASP	Astellas Pharma
AST	Astra

ASZ	AstraZeneca		CEL	Celgene
AT	Alpha Therapeutic		CEN	Centocor
AUB	Aurobindo		CER	Cerenex
AUR	Auromedics		CET	Cetus
AVD	Avadel Legacy Pharmaceuticals		CH	Lab. Choay Societe Anonyme
AVE	Aventis		CHI	Chiron
AVG	Alvogen		CHS	Chiesi
AW	Asta Werke		CHU	Chugai
AY	Ayerst		CI	Ciba
AZV	Laboratórios Azevedos		CIS	CIS US
BA	Baxter		CL	Clintec
BB	B & B Pharmaceuticals		CLA	Claris Lifesciences
BAN	Banyu Pharmaceuticals		CLN	Clinigen
BAY	Bayer		CMB	Cumberland
BC	Bencard		CMP	CMP Pharma
BCT	BioCryst Pharmaceuticals		CN	Connaught
BD	Becton Dickinson		CNF	Centrafarm
BE	Beecham		CO	Cole
BED	Bedford		COM	CommScope
BEH	Behring		COR	COR Therapeutics
BEL	R. Bellon		COV	Covis
BFM	Bieffe Medital		CP	Continental Pharma
BI	Boehringer Ingelheim		CPP	CP Pharmaceuticals
BIO	Bioniche Pharma		CPR	Cooper
BK	Berk		CR	Critikon
BKN	Baker Norton		CRC	Caraco
BM	Boehringer Mannheim		CSL	CSL Ltd.
BMS	Bristol-Myers Squibb		CTI	Cell Therapeutics Inc.
BN	Breon		CU	Cutter
BP	British Pharmacopoeia		CUB	Cubist
BPC	British Pharmaceutical Codex[b]		CUP	Cura Pharmaceuticals
BPI	BPI Labs		CUR	Curomed
BR	Bristol		CY	Cyanamid
BRD	Bracco Diagnostics		DAK	Dakota
BRK	Breckenridge		DB	David Bull Laboratories
BRN	B. Braun		DCC	Dupont Critical Care
BRT	Britianna		DGL	Douglas
BT	Boots		DI	Dista
BTK	Biotika		DIA	Diamant
BV	Ben Venue		DM	Dome
BW	Burroughs Wellcome		DME	Dupont Merck Pharma
BX	Berlex		DMX	Dumex
BXT	Baxalta		DRA	Dr. Rentschler Arzneimittel
CA	Calmic		DRT	Durata Therapeutics
CAD	Cadence Pharmaceuticals		DRX	Draxis
CAR	Cardinal Health		DU	DuPont
CBH	CSL Behring		DUR	Dura
CDM	CDM Lavoisier		DW	Delta West
CE	Carlo Erba		EA	Eaton

EBE	Ebewe		HC	Hillcross
ECL	Éclat		HE	Hengrui Medicine Co.
EGL	Eagle		HEL	Helsinn
EI	Eisai		HER	Heritage
ELN	Elan		HIK	Hikma
EN	Endo		HMR	Hoechst Marion Roussel
ENZ	Enzon		HO	Hoechst-Roussel
ERF	Erfa		HOS	Hospira
ERM	Erempharma		HQS	HQ Specialty Pharma
ES	Elkins-Sinn		HR	Horner
ESL	ESI Lederle		HRN	Heron
ESP	ESP Pharma		HY	Hyland
EST	Esteve		ICI	ICI Pharmaceuticals
EV	Evans		ICN	ICN Pharmaceuticals
EX	Essex		IMM	Immunex
EXL	Exela		IMS	IMS Ltd.
FA	Farmitalia		IN	Intra
FAC	Facta Farmaceutical		INT	Intermune
FAN	Fandre Laboratories		IV	Ives
FAU	Faulding		IVX	Ivex
FC	Frosst & Cie		IX	Invenex
FED	Federa		JAZ	Jazz
FER	Ferring		JC	Janssen-Cilag
FI	Fisons		JHP	JHP Pharmaceuticals
FOR	Forest Laboratories		JJ	Johnson & Johnson
FP	Faro Pharma		JN	Janssen
FRE	Fresenius		JP	Jones Pharma
FRK	Fresenius Kabi		KA	Kabi
FUJ	Fujisawa		KED	Kedrion
GEI	Geistich Pharma		KEY	Key Pharmaceuticals
GEM	Geneva-Marsam		KN	Knoll
GEN	Genentech		KP	Kabi Pharmacia
GG	Geigy		KV	Kabi-Vitrum
GH	Generic Health		KY	Kyowa
GIL	Gilead		LA	Lagap
GIU	Giulini		LE	Lederle
GL	Glaxo		LEM	Lemmon
GLT	Generics Limited		LEO	Leo Laboratories
GNS	Gensia-Sicor		LFB	Laboratoire Français du Fractionnement et des Biotechnologies
GO	Goedecke			
GRI	Grifols		LI	Lilly
GRP	Gruppo		LIF	Lifeshield
GRU	Grunenthal		LJ	La Jolla
GSK	GlaxoSmithKline		LME	Laboratoire Meram
GVA	Geneva		LUN	Lundbeck
GW	Glaxo Wellcome		LY	Lyphomed
GZ	Genzyme		LZ	Labaz Laboratories
HAE	Haemonetics		MA	Mallinckrodt
HB	Hoechst-Biotika		MAC	Maco Pharma

MAR	Marsam		OR	Organon
MAY	Mayne Pharma		ORC	Orchid
MB	May & Baker		ORP	Orphan Medical
MCD	Merck Chibret Dohme		ORT	Ortho
MDI	Medimmune		OTS	Otsuka
MDX	Medex		OVA	Ovation
MDZ	Medicianz		PAD	Paddock
ME	Merck		PAL	Paladin
MEL	Melinta Therapeutics		PAN	Panpharma Laboratory
MER	Merus Labs		PAR	Par
MG	McGaw		PB	Pohl-Boskamp
MGI	MGI Pharma		PD	Parke-Davis
MI	Miles		PE	Pentagone
MIL	Millimed		PF	Pfizer
MJ	Mead Johnson		PFM	Pfrimmer
MM	Merrimack		PH	Pharmacia
MMD	Marion Merrell Dow		PHC	Pharmachemie
MMT	Meridian Medical Technologies		PHM	Pharmacosmos
MN	McNeil		PHS	Pharmascience
MON	Monarch		PHT	Pharma-Tek
MRD	Merrell-Dow		PHU	Pharmacia & Upjohn
MRN	Merrell-National		PHX	Phoenix
MSD	Merck Sharp & Dohme		PNN	Pantheon
MTN	Marathon		PNT	Parenta
MUN	Mundi Pharma		PO	Poulenc
MY	Maney		PP	Pharmaceutical Partners
MYL	Mylan		PPC	Pharmaceutical Partners of Canada
MYR	Mayrhofer Pharmazeutika		PPR	Premier Pro Rx
NA	National		PR	Pasadena Research
NAB	Nabi		PRF	Pierre Fabre
NAP	NAPP Pharmaceuticals		PRK	Parkfields
NCI	National Cancer Institute		PRM	Premier
NE	Norwich-Eaton		PRP	Premier Pro
NIN	Ningbo Team		PTK	Paratek
NF	National Formulary[b]		PX	Pharmax
NO	Nordic		QI	Qilu
NOP	Novopharm		QLM	Qualimed Labs
NOV	Novo Pharm		QU	Quad
NVA	Novartis		RB	Robins
NVN	Novo Nordisk		RBP	Ribosepharm
NVP	Nova Plus		RC	Roche
NVX	Novex Pharma		REN	Renaudin
NYC	Nycomed		RI	Riker
OCT	Octapharma		RKB	Reckitt & Benckhiser
OHM	Ohmeda		RKC	Reckitt & Colman
OM	Omega		ROR	Rorer
OMJ	OMJ Pharmaceuticals		ROX	Roxane
OMN	Ortho-McNeil		RP	Rhone-Poulenc
ON	Orion		RPR	Rhone-Poulenc Rorer

RR	Roerig
RS	Roussel
RU	Rugby
SA	Sankyo
SAA	Sanofi Aventis
SAG	Sageant
SAN	Sanofi
SB	Sintetica Bioren
SC	Schering
SCI	Scios
SCN	Schein
SCS	SCS Pharmaceuticals
SE	Searle
SEQ	Sequus
SER	Servier
SGS	SangStat
SGT	Sagent
SHI	Shionogi
SIA	Siam Pharmaceutical
SIC	Sicor
SIG	Sigma Tau
SKB	SmithKline Beecham
SKF	Smith Kline & French
SM	Smith
SMX	SteriMax
SN	Smith + Nephew
SO	SoloPak
SP	Spectrum Pharmaceuticals
SQ	Squibb
SRB	Serb
SS	Sanofi-Synthelabo
ST	Sterilab
STP	Sterop
STR	Sterling
STS	Steris
STU	Stuart
SUN	Sun
SV	Savage
SW	Sanofi Winthrop
SX	Sabex
SY	Syntex
SYN	Synergen
SYO	Synthelabo
SZ	Sandoz
TAK	Takeda
TAL	Talon Therapeutics
TAP	TAP Holdings
TAR	Targanta Therapeutics
TAY	Taylor

TE	Teva
TEC	Teclapharm
TEL	Teligent
TES	Tesaro
TET	Tetraphase
TL	Tillotts
TMC	The Medicines Company
TO	Torigian
TR	Travenol
UCB	UCB
UP	Upjohn
USB	US Bioscience
USP	United States Pharmacopeia[b]
USV	USV Pharmaceuticals
UT	United Therapeutics
VHA	VHA Plus
VI	Vitarine
VIC	Vicuron Pharmaceuticals
VT	Vitrum
WAS	Wasserman
WAT	Watson
WAY	Wyeth-Ayerst
WB	Winthrop-Breon
WC	Warner-Chilcott
WED	Weddel
WEL	Wellcome
WI	Winthrop
WG	WG Critical Care
WL	Warner Lambert
WOC	Wockhardt
WW	Westward
WY	Wyeth
XGN	X-Gen
XU	Xudong Pharmaceutical Co.
YAM	Yamanouchi
ZEN	Zeneca
ZLB	ZLB Biopharma
ZNS	Zeneus Pharma
ZY	ZyGenerics
ZYD	Zydus

[b] While reference to a compendium does not indicate the specific manufacturer of a product, it does help to indicate the formulation that was used in the test.

REFERENCES

For a list of references cited in the text of this monograph, search the monograph titled References.

AHFS® Pharmacologic-Therapeutic Classification©

AHFS CLASSIFICATION

4:00 - Antihistamine Drugs

4:04 - First Generation Antihistamines
4:04.04 - Ethanolamine Derivatives*
4:04.08 - Ethylenediamine Derivatives*
4:04.12 - Phenothiazine Derivatives*
4:04.16 - Piperazine Derivatives*
4:04.20 - Propylamine Derivatives*
4:04.92 - Miscellaneous Derivatives*

4:08 - Second Generation Antihistamines

4:92 - Other Antihistamines*

8:00 - Anti-infective Agents

8:08 - Anthelmintics

8:12 - Antibacterials
8:12.02 - Aminoglycosides
8:12.06 - Cephalosporins
  8:12.06.04 - First Generation Cephalosporins
  8:12.06.08 - Second Generation Cephalosporins
  8:12.06.12 - Third Generation Cephalosporins
  8:12.06.16 - Fourth Generation Cephalosporins
  8:12.06.20 - Fifth Generation Cephalosporins
  8:12.06.28 - Siderophore Cephalosporins
8:12.07 - Miscellaneous β-Lactams
  8:12.07.04 - Carbacephems*
  8:12.07.08 - Carbapenems
  8:12.07.12 - Cephamycins
  8:12.07.16 - Monobactams
8:12.08 - Chloramphenicol
8:12.12 - Macrolides
  8:12.12.04 - Erythromycins
  8:12.12.12 - Ketolides*
  8:12.12.92 - Other Macrolides
8:12.16 - Penicillins
  8:12.16.04 - Natural Penicillins
  8:12.16.08 - Aminopenicillins
  8:12.16.12 - Penicillinase-resistant Penicillins
  8:12.16.16 - Extended-spectrum Penicillins
8:12.18 - Quinolones
8:12.20 - Sulfonamides
8:12.24 - Tetracyclines
  8:12.24.04 - Aminomethylcyclines
  8:12.24.08 - Fluorocyclines
  8:12.24.12 - Glycylcyclines
8:12.28 - Antibacterials, Miscellaneous
  8:12.28.04 - Aminocyclitols*
  8:12.28.08 - Bacitracins
  8:12.28.12 - Cyclic Lipopeptides
  8:12.28.16 - Glycopeptides
  8:12.28.20 - Lincomycins
  8:12.28.24 - Oxazolidinones
  8:12.28.26 - Pleuromutilins
  8:12.28.28 - Polymyxins
  8:12.28.30 - Rifamycins
  8:12.28.32 - Streptogramins
  8:12.28.92 - Other Miscellaneous Antibacterials*

8:14 - Antifungals
8:14.04 - Allylamines
8:14.08 - Azoles
8:14.16 - Echinocandins
8:14.28 - Polyenes
8:14.32 - Pyrimidines
8:14.92 - Antifungals, Miscellaneous

8:16 - Antimycobacterials
8:16.04 - Antituberculosis Agents
8:16.92 - Antimycobacterials, Miscellaneous

8:18 - Antivirals
8:18.04 - Adamantanes
8:18.08 - Antiretrovirals
  8:18.08.04 - HIV Entry and Fusion Inhibitors
  8:18.08.08 - HIV Protease Inhibitors
  8:18.08.12 - HIV Integrase Inhibitors
  8:18.08.16 - HIV Nonnucleoside Reverse Transcriptase Inhibitors
  8:18.08.20 - HIV Nucleoside and Nucleotide Reverse Transcriptase Inhibitors
  8:18.08.92 - Antiretrovirals, Miscellaneous*
8:18.20 - Interferons
8:18.24 - Monoclonal Antibodies
8:18.28 - Neuraminidase Inhibitors
8:18.32 - Nucleosides and Nucleotides
8:18.40 - HCV Antivirals
  8:18.40.04 - HCV Cyclophilin Inhibitors*
  8:18.40.08 - HCV Entry Inhibitors*
  8:18.40.16 - HCV Polymerase Inhibitors
  8:18.40.20 - HCV Protease Inhibitors
  8:18.40.24 - HCV Replication Complex Inhibitors
  8:18.40.92 - HCV Antivirals, Miscellaneous*
8:18.92 - Antivirals, Miscellaneous

8:30 - Antiprotozoals
8:30.04 - Amebicides
8:30.08 - Antimalarials
8:30.92 - Antiprotozoals, Miscellaneous

8:36 - Urinary Anti-infectives

8:92 - Anti-infectives, Miscellaneous*

10:00 - Antineoplastic Agents

12:00 - Autonomic Drugs

12:04 - Parasympathomimetic (Cholinergic) Agents

12:08 - Anticholinergic Agents
12:08.04 - Antiparkinsonian Agents*
12:08.08 - Antimuscarinics/Antispasmodics

12:12 - Sympathomimetic (Adrenergic) Agents
12:12.04 - α-Adrenergic Agonists
12:12.08 - β-Adrenergic Agonists
  12:12.08.04 - Nonselective β-Adrenergic Agonists
    12:12.08.08 - Selective β1-Adrenergic Agonists
    12:12.08.12 - Selective β2-Adrenergic Agonists
12:12.12 - α- and β-Adrenergic Agonists

12:16 - Sympatholytic (Adrenergic Blocking) Agents
12:16.04 - α-Adrenergic Blocking Agents
  12:16.04.04 - Nonselective α-Adrenergic Blocking Agents
  12:16.04.08 - Nonselective α1-Adrenergic Blocking Agents*
  12:16.04.12 - Selective α1-Adrenergic Blocking Agents
12:16.08 - β-Adrenergic Blocking Agents*
  12:16.08.04 - Nonselective β-Adrenergic Blocking Agents*
  12:16.08.08 - Selective β-Adrenergic Blocking Agents*

12:20 - Skeletal Muscle Relaxants
12:20.04 - Centrally Acting Skeletal Muscle Relaxants
12:20.08 - Direct-acting Skeletal Muscle Relaxants
12:20.12 - GABA-derivative Skeletal Muscle Relaxants
12:20.20 - Neuromuscular Blocking Agents
12:20.92 - Skeletal Muscle Relaxants, Miscellaneous

12:92 - Autonomic Drugs, Miscellaneous

16:00 - Blood Derivatives

DOI: 10.37573/9781585286850.fm

Abciximab
AHFS 20:12.18

Products

Abciximab is available as a 2-mg/mL solution, which also contains sodium phosphate 0.01 M, sodium chloride 0.15 M, and polysorbate 80 0.001% in water for injection.[3278]

pH

7.2.[3278]

Trade Name(s)

ReoPro

Administration

Abciximab is administered by direct intravenous injection followed by continuous intravenous infusion using a controlled infusion device after dilution in sodium chloride 0.9% or dextrose 5%.[3278]

Stability

The clear, colorless injection in intact vials should be stored under refrigeration and protected from freezing.[3278] The vials should not be shaken.[3278] No incompatibilities with glass bottles or PVC containers and sets have been observed.[3278]

Although refrigerated storage is required, the manufacturer has stated that the drug may be stored at room temperature for 8 days.[2745]

Filtration

The manufacturer recommends filtration through a low protein-binding 0.2- or 5-μm syringe filter during preparation of an intravenous infusion or using a 0.2- or 0.22-μm inline filter during its administration.[3278] The manufacturer also recommends using a low protein-binding 0.2- or 5-μm syringe filter for bolus doses.[3278]

Compatibility Information

Y-Site Injection Compatibility (1:1 Mixture)

Abciximab

Test Drug	Mfr	Conc	Mfr	Conc	Remarks	Ref	C/I
Adenosine	FUJ	3 mg/mL	LI	36 mcg/mL[a]	Visually compatible for 12 hr at 23°C	2374	C
Argatroban	GSK	1 mg/mL[a b c]	LI	36 mcg/mL[a b c]	Physically compatible with no loss of argatroban in 4 hr at 23°C. Abciximab not tested	2630	C
Atropine sulfate	AMR	0.4 mg/mL	LI	36 mcg/mL[a]	Visually compatible for 12 hr at 23°C	2374	C
Bivalirudin	TMC	5 mg/mL[a]	CEN	10 mcg/mL[a]	Physically compatible for 4 hr at 23°C	2373	C
Cangrelor tetrasodium	TMC	1 mg/mL[b]		10 mcg/mL[b]	Physically compatible for 4 hr	3243	C
Diphenhydramine HCl	ES	25 mg/mL	LI	36 mcg/mL[a]	Visually compatible for 12 hr at 23°C	2374	C
Fentanyl citrate	AB	50 mcg/mL	LI	36 mcg/mL[a]	Visually compatible for 12 hr at 23°C	2374	C
Metoprolol tartrate	AB	1 mg/mL	LI	36 mcg/mL[a]	Visually compatible for 12 hr at 23°C	2374	C
Midazolam HCl	BED	2 mg/mL	LI	36 mcg/mL[a]	Visually compatible for 12 hr at 23°C	2374	C

[a] Tested in dextrose 5%.

[b] Tested in sodium chloride 0.9%.

[c] Mixed argatroban:abciximab 1:1 and 4:1.

DOI: 10.37573/9781585286850.001

Acetaminophen
AHFS 28:08.92
Paracetamol

Products

Acetaminophen injection is available in 100-mL glass vials containing 1 g of acetaminophen.[2840] Each 100 mL of the injection solution also contains mannitol 3.85 g, cysteine hydrochloride monohydrate 25 mg, and dibasic sodium phosphate anhydrous 10.4 mg.[2840] Hydrochloric acid and/or sodium hydroxide are used to adjust the pH.[2840]

pH

Approximately 5.5.[2840]

Tonicity

Acetaminophen injection is isotonic.[2840]

Osmolality

The osmolality of acetaminophen 10-mg/mL injection was determined to be approximately 290 mOsm/kg.[2840]

Trade Name(s)

Ofirmev

Administration

For acetaminophen doses of 1 g, the dose should be administered by inserting a vented intravenous infusion set directly into the septum of the 100-mL glass vial.[2840]

For acetaminophen doses less than 1 g, the manufacturer recommends withdrawing the appropriate dose of acetaminophen 10-mg/mL injection from the intact, sealed, glass vial and transferring the measured dose to an empty sterile container (e.g., glass bottle, plastic intravenous container, syringe), employing aseptic technique.[2840] The manufacturer states that the entire 100-mL vial is not intended for use in patients weighing less than 50 kg.[2840] Volumes less than 60 mL (e.g., pediatric doses) should be placed in syringes and administered over 15 minutes using a syringe pump.[2840]

Acetaminophen injection should be administered by intravenous infusion over 15 minutes.[2840]

Stability

Acetaminophen injection is a clear, colorless solution.[2840] Intact containers should be stored at controlled room temperature and should not be refrigerated nor frozen.[2840]

The vials are for single use; any unused portions should be discarded.[2840] Once penetration of the vacuum seal of the glass vial has occurred or the solution has been transferred to another container, the manufacturer states that acetaminophen injection should be administered within 6 hours.[2840]

Syringes

To assess stability in syringes, acetaminophen 10-mg/mL injection was withdrawn from the original glass vial in volumes of 10, 25, and 50 mL, which were repackaged undiluted in 10-, 30-, and 60-mL propylene syringes, respectively, to be stored at 23 to 25°C.[2845] After 84 hours, no physical changes were detected in acetaminophen injection by visual assessment, and the injection retained greater than 90% of the mean initial concentration regardless of storage container.[2845] Sterility, however, was not assessed.[2845]

Compatibility Information

Solution Compatibility

Acetaminophen

Test Soln Name	Mfr	Mfr	Conc/L or %	Remarks	Ref	C/I
Dextrose 5%	a	CAD	1, 2, 5 g	Physically compatible. No loss in 1 hr at room temperature	2841, 2844	C
Sodium chloride 0.9%	a	CAD	1, 2, 5 g	Physically compatible. No loss in 1 hr at room temperature	2841, 2844	C

a Tested in glass containers.

Additive Compatibility

Acetaminophen

Test Drug	Mfr	Conc/L or %	Mfr	Conc/L or %	Test Solution	Remarks	Ref	C/I
Ketamine HCl a	PAN b	123 mg c	BMS	8.2 g		Physically compatible with less than 5% loss of either drug over 24 hr at 25°C	2842, 2843	C

a Test performed using the formulation containing chlorobutanol.

b Tested in polyolefin containers.

c Tested in sodium chloride 0.9%.

DOI: 10.37573/9781585286850.002

Y-Site Injection Compatibility (1:1 Mixture)

Acetaminophen

Test Drug	Mfr	Conc	Mfr	Conc	Remarks	Ref	C/I
Acyclovir sodium	APP	5 mg/mL[a]	CAD	10 mg/mL	Particle formation	2901	I
Blinatumomab	AMG	0.125 mcg/mL[a]	MAC	10 mg/mL	Thin flakes transiently appear when acetaminophen is added to blinatumomab; not observed when order of mixing was reversed	3405, 3417	?
Blinatumomab	AMG	0.375 mcg/mL[a]	MAC	10 mg/mL	Persistent particulate formation	3405, 3417	I
Buprenorphine HCl	HOS, BED	0.3 mg/mL	CAD	10 mg/mL	Physically compatible with less than 10% acetaminophen loss over 4 hr at room temperature	2841, 2844	C
Butorphanol tartrate	APO, BED	2 mg/mL	CAD	10 mg/mL	Physically compatible with less than 10% acetaminophen loss over 4 hr at room temperature	2841, 2844	C
Cefoxitin sodium	APO	100 mg/mL	CAD	10 mg/mL	Physically compatible for 4 hr at 23°C	2901, 2902	C
Ceftriaxone sodium	HOS	40 mg/mL	CAD	10 mg/mL	Physically compatible with no loss of either drug in 4 hr at 23°C	2901, 2902	C
Chlorpromazine HCl	BA	2 mg/mL[a]	CAD	10 mg/mL	Measured turbidity increased immediately	2840, 2844	I
Clindamycin phosphate	APP	10 mg/mL[a]	CAD	10 mg/mL	Physically compatible for 4 hr at 23°C	2901, 2902	C
Defibrotide sodium	JAZ	8 mg/mL[a]	BRN	10 mg/mL	Visually compatible for 4 hr at room temperature	3149	C
Dexamethasone sodium phosphate	APP	4 mg/mL	CAD	10 mg/mL	Physically compatible for 4 hr at 23°C	2901, 2902	C
Dexamethasone sodium phosphate	BA, SIC	10 mg/mL	CAD	10 mg/mL	Physically compatible with less than 10% acetaminophen loss over 4 hr at room temperature	2841, 2844	C
Diazepam	HOS	5 mg/mL	CAD	10 mg/mL	Yellowish-white precipitate forms immediately	2840, 2844	I
Diphenhydramine HCl	BA	50 mg/mL	CAD	10 mg/mL	Physically compatible with less than 10% acetaminophen loss over 4 hr at room temperature	2841, 2844	C
Diphenhydramine HCl	WW	50 mg/mL	CAD	10 mg/mL	Physically compatible with no loss of either drug in 4 hr at 23°C	2901, 2902	C
Dolasetron mesylate	SAA	20 mg/mL	CAD	10 mg/mL	Physically compatible with less than 10% acetaminophen loss over 4 hr at room temperature	2841, 2844	C
Droperidol	HOS	2.5 mg/mL	CAD	10 mg/mL	Physically compatible with less than 10% acetaminophen loss over 4 hr at room temperature	2841, 2844	C
Esmolol HCl	MYL	10 mg/mL	CAD	10 mg/mL	Physically compatible for 1 hr at 23°C	3533	C
Fentanyl citrate	TAY, HOS	50 mcg/mL	CAD	10 mg/mL	Physically compatible with less than 10% acetaminophen loss over 4 hr at room temperature	2841, 2844	C
Granisetron HCl	APO, TE	0.1 mg/mL	CAD	10 mg/mL	Physically compatible with less than 10% acetaminophen loss over 4 hr at room temperature	2841, 2844	C
Granisetron HCl	WOC	1 mg/mL	CAD	10 mg/mL	Physically compatible with little loss of either drug in 4 hr at 23°C	2901, 2902	C
Heparin sodium	HOS	100 units/mL	CAD	10 mg/mL	Physically compatible with less than 10% acetaminophen loss over 4 hr at room temperature	2841, 2844	C
Hydrocortisone sodium succinate	PF	50 mg/mL	CAD	10 mg/mL	Physically compatible with less than 10% acetaminophen loss over 4 hr at room temperature	2841, 2844	C
Hydrocortisone sodium succinate	PF	125 mg/mL	CAD	10 mg/mL	Physically compatible for 4 hr at 23°C	2901, 2902	C
Hydromorphone HCl	WW	2 mg/mL	CAD	10 mg/mL	Physically compatible for 4 hr at 23°C	2901, 2902	C

Y-Site Injection Compatibility (1:1 Mixture) (Cont.)

Test Drug	Mfr	Conc	Mfr	Conc	Remarks	Ref	C/I
Hydromorphone HCl	HOS	4 mg/mL	CAD	10 mg/mL	Physically compatible with less than 10% acetaminophen loss over 4 hr at room temperature	2841, 2844	C
Hydroxyzine HCl	ABX	2 mg/mL[a]	CAD	10 mg/mL	Physically compatible with less than 10% acetaminophen loss over 4 hr at room temperature	2841, 2844	C
Ketorolac tromethamine	WOC	15 mg/mL	CAD	10 mg/mL	Physically compatible with less than 10% acetaminophen loss over 4 hr at room temperature	2841, 2844	C
Ketorolac tromethamine	HOS	30 mg/mL	CAD	10 mg/mL	Physically compatible with no loss of either drug in 4 hr at 23°C	2901, 2902	C
Labetalol HCl	HOS	5 mg/mL	CAD	10 mg/mL	Physically compatible for 1 hr at 23°C	3533	C
Lidocaine HCl	HOS	20 mg/mL[b]	CAD	10 mg/mL	Physically compatible with less than 10% acetaminophen loss over 4 hr at room temperature	2841, 2844	C
Lorazepam	HOS	0.5 mg/mL[a]	CAD	10 mg/mL	Physically compatible with less than 10% acetaminophen loss over 4 hr at room temperature	2841, 2844	C
Mannitol	HOS	150 mg/mL	CAD	10 mg/mL	Physically compatible with less than 10% acetaminophen loss over 4 hr at room temperature	2841, 2844	C
Meperidine HCl	HOS	50 mg/mL	CAD	10 mg/mL	Physically compatible for 4 hr at 23°C	2901, 2902	C
Meperidine HCl	HOS	100 mg/mL	CAD	10 mg/mL	Physically compatible with less than 10% acetaminophen loss over 4 hr at room temperature	2841, 2844	C
Methylprednisolone sodium succinate	PF	62.5 mg/mL	CAD	10 mg/mL	Physically compatible for 4 hr at 23°C	2901, 2902	C
Methylprednisolone sodium succinate	PF	125 mg/mL	CAD	10 mg/mL	Physically compatible with less than 10% acetaminophen loss over 4 hr at room temperature	2841, 2844	C
Metoclopramide HCl	HOS	5 mg/mL	CAD	10 mg/mL	Physically compatible with less than 10% acetaminophen loss over 4 hr at room temperature	2841, 2844	C
Metoprolol tartrate	HOS	0.4 mg/mL[a]	CAD	10 mg/mL	Physically compatible for 1 hr at 23°C	3533	C
Midazolam HCl	ABX, BED	5 mg/mL	CAD	10 mg/mL	Physically compatible with less than 10% acetaminophen loss over 4 hr at room temperature	2841, 2844	C
Midazolam HCl	HOS	5 mg/mL	CAD	10 mg/mL	Physically compatible for 4 hr at 23°C	2901, 2902	C
Morphine sulfate	BA	15 mg/mL	CAD	10 mg/mL	Physically compatible with less than 10% acetaminophen loss over 4 hr at room temperature	2841, 2844	C
Morphine sulfate	WW	15 mg/mL	CAD	10 mg/mL	Physically compatible for 4 hr at 23°C	2901, 2902	C
Nalbuphine HCl	HOS	10 mg/mL	CAD	10 mg/mL	Physically compatible with little or no loss of either drug in 4 hr at 23°C	2901, 2902	C
Nalbuphine HCl	HOS	20 mg/mL	CAD	10 mg/mL	Physically compatible with less than 10% acetaminophen loss over 4 hr at room temperature	2841, 2844	C
Ondansetron HCl	WOC	2 mg/mL	CAD	10 mg/mL	Physically compatible with little or no loss of either drug in 4 hr at 23°C	2901, 2902	C
Ondansetron HCl	WW	2 mg/mL	CAD	10 mg/mL	Physically compatible with less than 10% acetaminophen loss over 4 hr at room temperature	2841, 2844	C
Piperacillin sodium–tazobactam sodium	WY	89 mg/mL[b]	CAD	10 mg/mL	Physically compatible with less than 2% loss of either drug in 4 hr at 23°C	2901, 2902	C
Potassium chloride	HOS, BED	0.1 mEq/mL[a]	CAD	10 mg/mL	Physically compatible with less than 10% acetaminophen loss over 4 hr at room temperature	2841, 2844	C
Prochlorperazine edisylate	BED	5 mg/mL	CAD	10 mg/mL	Physically compatible with less than 10% acetaminophen loss over 4 hr at room temperature	2841, 2844	C

Y-Site Injection Compatibility (1:1 Mixture) (Cont.)

Test Drug	Mfr	Conc	Mfr	Conc	Remarks	Ref	C/I
Ranitidine HCl	BED	1 mg/mL[c]	CAD	10 mg/mL	Physically compatible for 4 hr at 23°C	2901, 2902	C
Sufentanil citrate	BA, HOS	50 mcg/mL	CAD	10 mg/mL	Physically compatible with less than 10% acetamino-phen loss over 4 hr at room temperature	2841, 2844	C
Vancomycin HCl	HOS	5 mg/mL[a]	CAD	10 mg/mL	Physically compatible with little or no loss of either drug in 4 hr at 23°C	2901, 2902	C

[a] Tested in sodium chloride 0.9%.

[b] Piperacillin component. Piperacillin in an 8:1 fixed-ratio concentration with tazobactam.

[c] Tested in sodium chloride 0.45%.

Additional Compatibility Information
Infusion Solutions

Acetaminophen injection was found to be compatible with the following additional infusion solutions via simulated Y-site co-administration: Dextrose 5% in Ringer's injection, lactated; dextrose 5% in sodium chloride 0.9%; dextrose 10%; and Ringer's injection, lactated.[2841 2844]

Selected Revisions May 1, 2020. © Copyright, March 2017. American Society of Health-System Pharmacists, Inc.

Acetazolamide Sodium
AHFS 52:40.12

Products

Acetazolamide as the sodium salt is available in 500-mg (unpreserved) vials with sodium hydroxide and, if necessary, hydrochloric acid to adjust the pH.[3011] [3030] Each 500-mg vial should be reconstituted with at least 5 mL of sterile water for injection.[3011] [3030]

pH

Approximately 9.6.[3011] [3030]

Osmolality

The osmolality of acetazolamide sodium 500 mg was calculated for the following dilutions:[1054]

Diluent	Osmolality (mOsm/kg)	
	50 mL	100 mL
Dextrose 5%	321	291
Sodium chloride 0.9%	348	317

Sodium Content

2.049 mEq/500 mg (calculated).[846]

Administration

Administration by direct intravenous injection is preferred; intramuscular injection is not recommended.[3011] [3030]

Stability

Intact vials should be stored at controlled room temperature.[3011] [3030] Acetazolamide is a white to faintly yellowish white powder.[3011] [3030] The manufacturers state that the reconstituted solution is physically and chemically stable for 3 days at 2 to 8°C or for 12 hours at 20 to 25°C; however, storage of the reconstituted solution at 2 to 8°C and use of the solution within 12 hours after reconstitution is recommended.[3011] [3030] Any unused portion should be discarded.[3011] [3030]

pH Effects

The stability of acetazolamide sodium in aqueous solution appears to decrease as the pH increases above 9. At pH 8.8, a 0.25-mg/mL solution retained 96% of the initial amount after 3 days at 25°C; at pH 10.8 and 12.7, 88 and 83% of the concentration, respectively, remained after 4 days.[1230] Acetazolamide exhibits maximum stability at pH 4.[1424]

Sorption

Acetazolamide sodium was shown not to exhibit sorption to PVC bags and tubing, polyethylene tubing, Silastic tubing, and polypropylene syringes.[536] [606]

Compatibility Information

Solution Compatibility

Acetazolamide sodium

Test Soln Name	Mfr	Mfr	Conc/L or %	Remarks	Ref	C/I
Dextrose 2.5% in half-strength Ringer's injection	AB	LE	375 mg	Physically compatible	3	C
Dextrose 5% in Ringer's injection	AB	LE	375 mg	Physically compatible	3	C
Dextrose 2.5% in Ringer's injection, lactated	AB	LE	375 mg	Physically compatible	3	C
Dextrose 5% in half-strength Ringer's injection, lactated	AB	LE	375 mg	Physically compatible	3	C
Dextrose 5% in Ringer's injection, lactated	AB	LE	375 mg	Physically compatible	3	C
Dextrose 10% in Ringer's injection, lactated	AB	LE	375 mg	Physically compatible	3	C
Dextrose 2.5% in sodium chloride 0.45%	AB	LE	375 mg	Physically compatible	3	C
Dextrose 2.5% in sodium chloride 0.9%	AB	LE	375 mg	Physically compatible	3	C
Dextrose 5% in sodium chloride 0.225%	AB	LE	375 mg	Physically compatible	3	C
Dextrose 5% in sodium chloride 0.45%	AB	LE	375 mg	Physically compatible	3	C
Dextrose 5% in sodium chloride 0.9%	AB	LE	375 mg	Physically compatible	3	C
Dextrose 10% in sodium chloride 0.9%	AB	LE	375 mg	Physically compatible	3	C

DOI: 10.37573/9781585286850.003

Solution Compatibility (Cont.)

Test Soln Name	Mfr	Mfr	Conc/L or %	Remarks	Ref	C/I
Dextrose 2.5%	AB	LE	375 mg	Physically compatible	3	C
Dextrose 5%	AB	LE	375 mg	Physically compatible	3	C
Dextrose 5%	TR[a]	LE	375 mg	Physically compatible. Losses of 7% in 5 days at 25°C, 5% in 44 days at 5°C, and 3% in 44 days at −10°C	1085	C
Dextrose 10%	AB	LE	375 mg	Physically compatible	3	C
Ionosol B in dextrose 5%	AB	LE	375 mg	Physically compatible	3	C
Ionosol MB in dextrose 5%	AB	LE	375 mg	Physically compatible	3	C
Ringer's injection	AB	LE	375 mg	Physically compatible	3	C
Ringer's injection, lactated	AB	LE	375 mg	Physically compatible	3	C
Sodium chloride 0.45%	AB	LE	375 mg	Physically compatible	3	C
Sodium chloride 0.9%	AB	LE	375 mg	Physically compatible	3	C
Sodium chloride 0.9%	TR[a]	LE	375 mg	Physically compatible. Losses of 7% in 5 days at 25°C, 5% in 44 days at 5°C, and 3% in 44 days at −10°C	1085	C
Sodium lactate ⅙ M	AB	LE	375 mg	Physically compatible	3	C

[a] Tested in PVC containers.

Additive Compatibility

Acetazolamide sodium

Test Drug	Mfr	Conc/L or %	Mfr	Conc/L or %	Test Solution	Remarks	Ref	C/I
Ranitidine HCl	GL	50 mg and 2 g		5 g	D5W	Physically compatible. Ranitidine stable for 24 hr at 25°C. Acetazolamide not tested	1515	C

Drugs in Syringe Compatibility

Acetazolamide sodium

Test Drug	Mfr	Amt	Mfr	Amt	Remarks	Ref	C/I
Pantoprazole sodium	a	4 mg/1 mL		100 mg/1 mL	Clear solution	2574	C

[a] Test performed using the formulation WITHOUT edetate disodium.

Y-Site Injection Compatibility (1:1 Mixture)

Acetazolamide sodium

Test Drug	Mfr	Conc	Mfr	Conc	Remarks	Ref	C/I
Diltiazem HCl	MMD	5 mg/mL	LE	100 mg/mL	Precipitate forms	1807	I
Diltiazem HCl	MMD	1 mg/mL[b]	LE	100 mg/mL	Visually compatible	1807	C
TPN #203, #204[a]			LE	100 mg/mL	White precipitate forms immediately	1974	I

[a] Refer to Appendix for the composition of parenteral nutrition solutions. TPN indicates a 2-in-1 admixture.

[b] Tested in sodium chloride 0.9%.

Selected Revisions January 26, 2016. © Copyright, October 1982. American Society of Health-System Pharmacists, Inc.

Acetylcysteine
AHFS 92:12

Products

Acetylcysteine injection is available in 30-mL single-dose vials as a preservative-free concentrated solution containing 200 mg/mL of drug.[2861] The solution also contains sodium hydroxide to adjust the pH.[2861] This concentrate must be diluted for use.[2861]

pH

6 to 7.5.[2861]

Osmolarity

Acetylcysteine injection has an osmolarity of 2600 mOsm/L.[2861]

Trade Name(s)

Acetadote

Administration

Acetylcysteine injection is a concentrate that must be diluted in a compatible infusion solution (e.g., dextrose 5%, sodium chloride 0.45%) for intravenous infusion.[2861]

For patients weighing 41 kg or more, the manufacturer recommends a loading dose be added to 200 mL for infusion over 60 minutes.[2861] Subsequently, a first maintenance dose should be mixed in 500 mL and delivered over 4 hours.[2861] The second maintenance dose should be mixed in 1 L and delivered over 16 hours.[2861]

The total volume must be adjusted for patients weighing 40 kg or less and fluid-restricted patients.[2861] For patients weighing

21 to 40 kg, the manufacturer recommends a loading dose be added to 100 mL for infusion over 60 minutes.[2861] Subsequently, a first maintenance dose should be mixed in 250 mL and delivered over 4 hours.[2861] The second maintenance dose should be mixed in 500 mL and delivered over 16 hours.[2861]

For patients weighing 5 to 20 kg, the manufacturer recommends a loading dose be diluted in 3 mL/kg of body weight for infusion over 60 minutes.[2861] Subsequently, a first maintenance dose should be mixed in 7 mL/kg of body weight and delivered over 4 hours.[2861] The second maintenance dose should be mixed in 14 mL/kg of body weight and delivered over 16 hours.[2861]

Acetylcysteine is a reducing agent and is not compatible with oxidizing agents. The drug is incompatible with rubber, and some metals such as iron and copper, liberating hydrogen sulfide gas. Consequently, the use of preparation and administration equipment composed of plastic, glass, and stainless steel or other unreactive metal is recommended.[4]

Stability

Store intact vials of acetylcysteine injection at room temperature.[2861] The vials are for single use, and previously opened vials should be discarded and not used.[2861] The manufacturer states that the color of acetylcysteine injection may vary from colorless to slight pink or purple after stopper penetration, but this color change does not indicate an adverse effect on drug quality.[2861]

Compatibility Information

Solution Compatibility

Acetylcysteine

Test Soln Name	Mfr	Mfr	Conc/L or %	Remarks	Ref	C/I
Dextrose 5%				Compatible for 24 hr at room temperature	2861	C
Sodium chloride 0.45%				Compatible for 24 hr at room temperature	2861	C

Y-Site Injection Compatibility (1:1 Mixture)

Acetylcysteine

Test Drug	Mfr	Conc	Mfr	Conc	Remarks	Ref	C/I
Cefepime HCl	BMS	120 mg/mL		100 mg/mL	Over 10% cefepime loss occurs in 1 hr	2513	I
Ceftazidime	GSK	120 mg/mL		100 mg/mL	Over 10% ceftazidime loss occurs in 1 hr	2513	I
Cloxacillin sodium	SMX	100 mg/mL	ALV	200 mg/mL	Physically compatible for up to 4 hr at room temperature	3245	C
Meropenem		50 mg/mL	ALV	200 mg/mL	Physically compatible for 4 hr at room temperature	3538	C

Selected Revisions May 1, 2020. © Copyright, October 2006. American Society of Health-System Pharmacists, Inc.

DOI: 10.37573/9781585286850.004

Acyclovir Sodium
AHFS 8:18.32

Products

Acyclovir sodium is available in vials containing 500 mg or 1 g of acyclovir as the sodium salt. Reconstitute the 500-mg vial with 10 mL and the 1-g vial with 20 mL of sterile water for injection; shake well to ensure complete dissolution. Do not use bacteriostatic water for injection containing parabens or benzyl alcohol for reconstitution. The acyclovir concentration in the reconstituted solution is 50 mg/mL; the reconstituted solution must be diluted to a concentration of 7 mg/mL or less for use.[1(6/05)]

pH

The reconstituted solution has a pH of approximately 11.[1(6/05)] [4]

Osmolality

The osmolality of acyclovir sodium 500 mg was calculated for the following dilutions:[1054]

Diluent	Osmolality (mOsm/kg)	
	50 mL	100 mL
Dextrose 5%	316	289
Sodium chloride 0.9%	342	316

The osmolality of acyclovir sodium 7 mg/mL was determined to be 278 mOsm/kg in dextrose 5% and 299 mOsm/kg in sodium chloride 0.9%.[1375]

Sodium Content

Acyclovir sodium (Glaxo Wellcome) contains 4.2 mEq of sodium per gram of drug.[4]

Administration

Acyclovir sodium is administered by slow intravenous infusion at concentrations of 7 mg/mL or less over a period of 1 hour. Rapid intravenous administration and administration by other routes must be avoided.[1(6/05)] [4]

Stability

Intact vials of acyclovir sodium should be stored at controlled room temperature. The reconstituted solution should be used within 12 hours. Refrigeration of the reconstituted solution may cause a precipitate, but this precipitate will dissolve at room temperature, apparently without affecting potency. After dilution for administration, the dose may be stored at room temperature; it should be used within 24 hours.[1(6/05)] [4] However, storage of acyclovir admixtures at room temperature does not guarantee that no precipitate will form. Precipitation also has been observed in acyclovir sodium infusions in polyvinyl chloride (PVC) containers after a few days' storage at room temperature.[2190]

If acyclovir sodium is diluted in solutions with dextrose concentrations greater than 10%, a yellow discoloration may appear. This discoloration does not affect the drug's potency.[4]

Acyclovir sodium reconstituted with bacteriostatic water for injection containing benzyl alcohol is as stable as when reconstituted with unpreserved sterile water for injection. However, the manufacturer recommends not using the benzyl alcohol-containing diluent because of concerns about the risks to neonates. The paraben-containing form of bacteriostatic water for injection must not be used for reconstitution because of the potential for precipitate formation.[4]

Precipitation

Short-term refrigerated storage of acyclovir sodium admixtures with concentrations exceeding 1 mg/mL may result in formation of a precipitate that redissolves upon warming to room temperature. However, such solutions should be used immediately after warming to room temperature because of the subsequent appearance of persistent microprecipitates.[2098]

Physical instability is the principal limitation to long-term storage of acyclovir sodium admixtures. Persistent subvisual microprecipitate formation as well as frank persistent precipitation may occur in variable time periods. Such precipitation has been reported to occur after as little as 7 days and in varying time periods throughout a 35-day observation period; the appearance of a precipitate is not precisely predictable.[2098]

The formation of large amounts of subvisual particulates has been attributed to an interaction of the highly alkaline acyclovir sodium solution with PVC containers. Some increase in the number of particulates was observed in as little as 1 day, with substantial increases in 7 days. When packaged in ethylene vinyl acetate (EVA) containers, no significant increase in subvisual particulates occurs, even after 28 days of storage.[2190]

Freezing Solutions

Acyclovir (GlaxoSmithKline; Hospira) 5 mg/mL in sodium chloride 0.9% in polyolefin bags was found to be physically stable with less than 10% loss reported when frozen at −20°C for 90 days followed by thawing in a microwave oven and subsequent storage at 2 to 8°C for 15 days.[3300]

Syringes

Acyclovir sodium (American Pharmaceutical Partners) 10 mg/mL in sodium chloride 0.9% and packaged in polypropylene syringes (Becton Dickinson) was found to be stable for 30 days at room temperature but precipitated in 5 days under refrigeration.[2558]

Sorption

Acyclovir sodium was shown not to exhibit sorption to PVC, polyethylene, and glass containers as well as elastomeric reservoirs.[2014] [2289]

Central Venous Catheter

Acyclovir sodium (GlaxoWellcome) 1 mg/mL in dextrose 5% was found to be compatible with the ARROWg+ard Blue Plus (Arrow International) chlorhexidine-bearing triple-lumen central catheter. Essentially complete delivery of the drug was found with

DOI: 10.37573/9781585286850.005

little or no drug loss occurring. Furthermore, chlorhexidine delivered from the catheter remained at trace amounts with no substantial increase due to the delivery of the drug through the catheter.[2335]

Compatibility Information

Solution Compatibility

Acyclovir sodium

Test Soln Name	Mfr	Mfr	Conc/L or %	Remarks	Ref	C/I
Dextrose 5%	TR[a]	BW	5 g	Visually compatible with no loss in 37 days at 25 and 5°C	1343	C
Dextrose 5%	BA[a]	BW	1 g	Physically compatible with no loss after 35 days at 23°C and after 35 days at 4°C followed by 2 days at 23°C protected from light	2098	C
Dextrose 5%	BA[a]	BW	7 g	Physically compatible with 3% or less loss after 28 days at 23°C protected from light. Subvisible microprecipitate forms by 35 days	2098	C
Dextrose 5%	BA[a]	BW	7 g	Precipitate forms on refrigeration that redissolves on warming. No loss after 35 days at 4°C protected from light, but subvisible precipitate forms after 2 more days at 23°C	2098	C
Dextrose 5%	BA[a]	BW	10 g	Physically compatible with no loss after 21 days at 23°C protected from light. Subvisible microprecipitate forms in 28 days, and visible precipitate forms in 35 days	2098	C
Dextrose 5%	BA[a]	BW	10 g	Precipitate forms on refrigeration that redissolves on warming. No loss after 35 days at 4°C protected from light, but subvisible precipitate forms after 2 more days at 23°C	2098	C
Dextrose 5%	BA[a], BRN[c]	GW	5 g	Visually compatible with little or no loss in 24 hr at 4 and 22°C	2289	C
Sodium chloride 0.9%	TR[a]	BW	5 g	No loss in 37 days at 25 and 5°C. Storage at 5°C resulted in white precipitate that dissolved on warming to 25°C	1343	C
Sodium chloride 0.9%	BA[a]	BW	1, 7, 10 g	Physically compatible with no loss after 7 days at 23°C protected from light. Visible precipitate formed within 14 days	2098	C
Sodium chloride 0.9%	BA[a]	BW	1, 7, 10 g	Physically compatible with no loss after 35 days at 4°C followed by 2 days at 23°C protected from light	2098	C
Sodium chloride 0.9%	BA[a]	WEL	2.5 and 5 g	No loss in 28 days at 25°C, but subvisible particulates increase significantly after 7 days due to interaction with PVC containers	2190	C
Sodium chloride 0.9%	BA[b]	WEL	2.5 and 5 g	No loss and little change in subvisible particulates in 28 days at 25°C	2190	C
Sodium chloride 0.9%	BA[a], BRN[c]	GW	5 g	Visually compatible with little or no loss in 24 hr at 4 and 22°C	2289	C
Sodium chloride 0.9%	[d]	HOS	5 g	Physically stable with less than 10% loss reported in 21 days at 2 to 8°C	3300	C
Sodium chloride 0.9%	[d]	GSK	5 g	Physically stable with less than 10% loss reported in 15 days at 2 to 8°C	3300	C

[a] Tested in PVC containers.

[b] Tested in ethylene vinyl acetate (EVA) containers.

[c] Tested in polyethylene and glass containers.

[d] Tested in polyolefin containers.

Additive Compatibility

Acyclovir sodium

Test Drug	Mfr	Conc/L or %	Mfr	Conc/L or %	Test Solution	Remarks	Ref	C/I
Dobutamine HCl	LI	0.5 g	BW	2.5 g	D5W	Discoloration in 25 min. Cloudiness and brown color in 2 hr due to dobutamine oxidation. No acyclovir loss	1343	I
Dopamine HCl	SO	800 mg	BW	2.5 g	D5W	Yellow color developed in 1.5 hr due to dopamine oxidation. No acyclovir loss	1343	I

Additive Compatibility (Cont.)

Test Drug	Mfr	Conc/L or %	Mfr	Conc/L or %	Test Solution	Remarks	Ref	C/I
Fluconazole	PF	1 g	BW	5 g	D5W	Visually compatible with no fluconazole loss in 72 hr at 25°C under fluorescent light. Acyclovir not tested	1677	C
Meropenem	ZEN	1 g	BW	5 g	NS	Visually compatible for 4 hr at room temperature	1994	C
Meropenem	ZEN	20 g	BW	5 g	NS	Precipitates immediately	1994	I
Tramadol HCl	GRU	400 mg	WEL	5 g	NS	Precipitation and 20% tramadol loss in 1 hr	2652	I

Drugs in Syringe Compatibility

Acyclovir sodium

Test Drug	Mfr	Amt	Mfr	Amt	Remarks	Ref	C/I
Caffeine citrate		20 mg/1 mL	BW	50 mg/1 mL	Precipitates immediately	2440	I
Pantoprazole sodium	[a]	4 mg/1 mL		50 mg/1 mL	Precipitates within 4 hr	2574	I

[a] Test performed using the formulation WITHOUT edetate disodium.

Y-Site Injection Compatibility (1:1 Mixture)

Acyclovir sodium

Test Drug	Mfr	Conc	Mfr	Conc	Remarks	Ref	C/I
Acetaminophen	CAD	10 mg/mL	APP	5 mg/mL[b]	Particle formation	2901	I
Allopurinol sodium	BW	3 mg/mL[b]	BW	7 mg/mL[b]	Physically compatible for 4 hr at 22°C	1686	C
Amifostine	USB	10 mg/mL[a]	BW	7 mg/mL[a]	Subvisible needles form in 1 hr. Visible particles form in 4 hr	1845	I
Amikacin sulfate	BR	5 mg/mL[a]	BW	5 mg/mL[a]	Physically compatible for 4 hr at 25°C	1157	C
Ampicillin sodium	WY	20 mg/mL[b]	BW	5 mg/mL[a]	Physically compatible for 4 hr at 25°C	1157	C
Amsacrine	NCI	1 mg/mL[a]	BW	7 mg/mL[a]	Immediate dark orange turbidity, becoming brownish orange in 1 hr	1381	I
Anidulafungin	VIC	0.5 mg/mL[a]	APP	7 mg/mL[a]	Physically compatible for 4 hr at 23°C	2617	C
Aztreonam	SQ	40 mg/mL[a]	BW	7 mg/mL[a]	White needles form immediately and become dense precipitate in 4 hr	1758	I
Caspofungin acetate	ME	0.7 mg/mL[b]	BV	7 mg/mL[b]	Physically compatible for 4 hr at room temperature	2758	C
Caspofungin acetate	ME	0.5 mg/mL[b]	BED	5 mg/mL[b]	Fine clear crystals reported	2766	I
Cefazolin sodium	SKF	20 mg/mL[a]	BW	5 mg/mL[a]	Physically compatible for 4 hr at 25°C	1157	C
Cefotaxime sodium	HO	20 mg/mL[a]	BW	5 mg/mL[a]	Physically compatible for 4 hr at 25°C	1157	C
Cefoxitin sodium	MSD	20 mg/mL[a]	BW	5 mg/mL[a]	Physically compatible for 4 hr at 25°C	1157	C
Ceftaroline fosamil	FOR	2.22 mg/mL[a b g]	BV	7 mg/mL[a b g]	Physically compatible for 4 hr at 23°C	2826	C
Ceftazidime	SKF	20 mg/mL[a]	BW	5 mg/mL[a]	Physically compatible for 4 hr at 25°C	1157	C
Ceftriaxone sodium	RC	20 mg/mL[a]	BW	5 mg/mL[a]	Physically compatible for 4 hr at 25°C	1157	C
Cefuroxime sodium	GL	15 mg/mL[a]	BW	5 mg/mL[a]	Physically compatible for 4 hr at 25°C	1157	C
Chloramphenicol sodium succinate	ES	20 mg/mL[a]	BW	5 mg/mL[a]	Physically compatible for 4 hr at 25°C	1157	C
Cisatracurium besylate	GW	0.1 and 2 mg/mL[a]	BW	7 mg/mL[a]	Physically compatible for 4 hr at 23°C	2074	C
Cisatracurium besylate	GW	5 mg/mL[a]	BW	7 mg/mL[a]	White cloudiness forms immediately	2074	I

Y-Site Injection Compatibility (1:1 Mixture) (Cont.)

Test Drug	Mfr	Conc	Mfr	Conc	Remarks	Ref	C/I
Clindamycin phosphate	UP	12 mg/mL[a]	BW	5 mg/mL[a]	Physically compatible for 4 hr at 25°C	1157	C
Cloxacillin sodium	SMX	100 mg/mL	PPC	50 mg/mL	Physically compatible for up to 4 hr at room temperature	3245	C
Cyclosporine	BED	1 mg/mL[a]	BV	5 mg/mL[b]	Crystals form	2794	I
Defibrotide sodium	JAZ	8 mg/mL[b]	MYL	10 mg/mL[b]	Visually compatible for 4 hr at room temperature	3149	C
Dexamethasone sodium phosphate	ES	0.2 mg/mL[a]	BW	5 mg/mL[a]	Physically compatible for 4 hr at 25°C	1157	C
Dexamethasone sodium phosphate	APP	4 mg/mL	BV	5 mg/mL[b]	Physically compatible	2794	C
Diltiazem HCl	MMD	5 mg/mL	BW	5[a] and 7[b] mg/mL	Cloudiness and precipitate form	1807	I
Diltiazem HCl	MMD	1 mg/mL[b]	BW	5[a] and 7[b] mg/mL	Visually compatible	1807	C
Dimenhydrinate	SE	1 mg/mL[a]	BW	5 mg/mL[a]	Physically compatible for 4 hr at 25°C	1157	C
Diphenhydramine HCl	ES	1 mg/mL[a]	BW	5 mg/mL[a]	Physically compatible for 4 hr at 25°C	1157	C
Diphenhydramine HCl	BA	50 mg/mL	BV	5 mg/mL[b]	Cloudy upon mixing	2794	I
Dobutamine HCl	LI	1 mg/mL[a]	BW	5 mg/mL[a]	Cloudy and brown in 1 hr at 25°C	1157	I
Docetaxel	RPR	0.9 mg/mL[a]	GW	7 mg/mL[a]	Physically compatible for 4 hr at 23°C	2224	C
Dopamine HCl	AB	1.6 mg/mL[a]	BW	5 mg/mL[a]	Solution turns dark brown in 2 hr at 25°C	1157	I
Doripenem	JJ	5 mg/mL[a b]	BED	7 mg/mL[a b]	Physically compatible for 4 hr at 23°C	2743	C
Doxorubicin HCl liposomal	SEQ	0.4 mg/mL[a]	GW	7 mg/mL[a]	Physically compatible for 4 hr at 23°C	2087	C
Doxycycline hyclate	PF	1 mg/mL[a]	BW	5 mg/mL[a]	Physically compatible for 4 hr at 25°C	1157	C
Droperidol	MDX	2.5 mg/mL	BV	5 mg/mL[b]	Physically compatible	2794	C
Erythromycin lactobionate	AB	4 mg/mL[a]	BW	5 mg/mL[a]	Physically compatible for 4 hr at 25°C	1157	C
Etoposide phosphate	BR	5 mg/mL[a]	GW	7 mg/mL[a]	Physically compatible for 4 hr at 23°C	2218	C/I
Famotidine	ME	2 mg/mL[b]		7 mg/mL[a]	Visually compatible for 4 hr at 22°C	1936	C
Fentanyl citrate	HOS	50 mcg/mL	BV	5 mg/mL[b]	Physically compatible	2794	C
Filgrastim	AMG	30 mcg/mL[a]	BW	7 mg/mL[a]	Physically compatible for 4 hr at 22°C	1687	C
Fluconazole	RR	2 mg/mL	BW	10 mg/mL	Physically compatible for 24 hr at 25°C	1407	C
Fludarabine phosphate	BX	1 mg/mL[a]	BW	7 mg/mL[a]	Color darkens within 4 hr	1439	I
Foscarnet sodium	AST	24 mg/mL	BW	10 mg/mL	Precipitates immediately	1335	I
Foscarnet sodium	AST	24 mg/mL	BW	7 mg/mL[c]	Acyclovir crystals form immediately	1393	I
Gallium nitrate	FUJ	1 mg/mL[b]	BW	7 mg/mL[b]	Visually compatible for 24 hr at 25°C	1673	C
Gemcitabine HCl	LI	10 mg/mL[b]	GW	7 mg/mL[b]	Gross precipitation occurs immediately	2226	I
Gentamicin sulfate	TR	1.6 mg/mL[a]	BW	5 mg/mL[a]	Physically compatible for 4 hr at 25°C	1157	C
Gentamicin sulfate	AMS	30 mg/mL[i]	BV	5 mg/mL[b]	White paste-like precipitate	2794	I
Granisetron HCl	SKB	0.05 mg/mL[a]	BW	7 mg/mL[a]	Physically compatible for 4 hr at 23°C	2000	C
Granisetron HCl	RC	1 mg/mL	BV	5 mg/mL[b]	Crystals form	2794	I

Y-Site Injection Compatibility (1:1 Mixture) (Cont.)

Test Drug	Mfr	Conc	Mfr	Conc	Remarks	Ref	C/I
Heparin sodium	ES	50 units/mL[a]	BW	5 mg/mL[a]	Physically compatible for 4 hr at 25°C	1157	C
Heparin sodium	BD	100 units/mL	BV	5 mg/mL[b]	Physically compatible	2794	C
Hydrocortisone sodium succinate	LY	1 mg/mL[a]	BW	5 mg/mL[a]	Physically compatible for 4 hr at 25°C	1157	C
Hydromorphone HCl	WB	0.04 mg/mL[a]	BW	5 mg/mL[a]	Physically compatible for 4 hr at 25°C	1157	C
Idarubicin HCl	AD	1 mg/mL[b]	BW	5 mg/mL[b]	Haze forms and color changes immediately. Precipitate forms in 12 min	1525	I
Imipenem–cilastatin sodium	MSD	5 mg/mL[b i]	BW	5 mg/mL[a]	Physically compatible for 4 hr at 25°C	1157	C
Levofloxacin	OMN	5 mg/mL[a]	BW	50 mg/mL	Cloudy precipitate forms	2233	I
Linezolid	PHU	2 mg/mL[a]	APP	7 mg/mL[a]	Physically compatible for 4 hr at 23°C	2264	C
Lorazepam	WY	0.04 mg/mL[a]	BW	5 mg/mL[a]	Physically compatible for 4 hr at 25°C	1157	C
Magnesium sulfate	LY	20 mg/mL[a]	BW	5 mg/mL[a]	Physically compatible for 4 hr at 25°C	1157	C
Melphalan HCl	BW	0.1 mg/mL[b]	BW	7 mg/mL[b]	Physically compatible for 3 hr at 22°C	1557	C
Meperidine HCl	WB	1 mg/mL[a]	BW	5 mg/mL[a]	Physically compatible for 4 hr at 25°C	1157	C
Meperidine HCl	AB	10 mg/mL	BW	5 mg/mL[a]	White crystalline precipitate forms within 1 hr at 25°C	1397	I
Meperidine HCl	WY	100 mg/mL	BW	5 mg/mL[c]	Visually compatible for 24 hr at room temperature in test tubes. No precipitate found on filter from Y-site delivery	2063	C
Meropenem	ZEN	1 mg/mL[b]	BW	5 mg/mL[d]	Visually compatible for 4 hr at room temperature	1994	C
Meropenem	ZEN	50 mg/mL[b]	BW	5 mg/mL[d]	Precipitate forms	2068	I
Methylprednisolone sodium succinate	LY	0.8 mg/mL[a]	BW	5 mg/mL[a]	Physically compatible for 4 hr at 25°C	1157	C
Metoclopramide HCl	ES	0.2 mg/mL[a]	BW	5 mg/mL[a]	Physically compatible for 4 hr at 25°C	1157	C
Metoclopramide HCl	SIC	5 mg/mL	BV	5 mg/mL[b]	Crystals form	2794	I
Metronidazole	SE	5 mg/mL	BW	5 mg/mL[a]	Physically compatible for 4 hr at 25°C	1157	C
Milrinone lactate	SS	0.2 mg/mL[a]	APP	7 mg/mL[a]	Visually compatible for 4 hr at 25°C	2381	C
Morphine sulfate	WB	0.08 mg/mL[a]	BW	5 mg/mL[a]	Physically compatible for 4 hr at 25°C	1157	C
Morphine sulfate	AB	1 mg/mL	BW	5 mg/mL[a]	Precipitate forms in 2 hr at 25°C	1397	I
Multivitamins	LY	0.01 mL/mL[a]	BW	5 mg/mL[a]	Physically compatible for 4 hr at 25°C	1157	C
Nafcillin sodium	WY	20 mg/mL[a]	BW	5 mg/mL[a]	Physically compatible for 4 hr at 25°C	1157	C
Nalbuphine HCl	HOS	10 mg/mL	BV	5 mg/mL[b]	Physically compatible	2794	C
Ondansetron HCl	GL	1 mg/mL[b]	BW	7 mg/mL[a]	Precipitates immediately	1365	I
Oxacillin sodium	BE	20 mg/mL[a]	BW	5 mg/mL[a]	Physically compatible for 4 hr at 25°C	1157	C
Paclitaxel	NCI	1.2 mg/mL[a]	BW	7 mg/mL[a]	Physically compatible for 4 hr at 22°C	1556	C
Pemetrexed disodium	LI	20 mg/mL[b]	APP	7 mg/mL[a]	Physically compatible for 4 hr at 23°C	2564	C
Penicillin G potassium	PF	40,000 units/mL[a]	BW	5 mg/mL[a]	Physically compatible for 4 hr at 25°C	1157	C
Pentobarbital sodium	WY	2 mg/mL[a]	BW	5 mg/mL[a]	Physically compatible for 4 hr at 25°C	1157	C
Piperacillin sodium–tazobactam sodium	LE[h]	40 mg/mL[a j]	BW	7 mg/mL[a]	Particles form in 1 hr	1688	I

Y-Site Injection Compatibility (1:1 Mixture) (Cont.)

Test Drug	Mfr	Conc	Mfr	Conc	Remarks	Ref	C/I
Potassium chloride	IX	0.04 mEq/mL[a]	BW	5 mg/mL[a]	Physically compatible for 4 hr at 25°C	1157	C
Propofol	ZEN[o]	10 mg/mL	BW	7 mg/mL[a]	Physically compatible for 1 hr at 23°C	2066	C
Quinupristin–dalfopristin		2 mg/mL[a m]	[n]	5 mg/mL	Reported to be incompatible	3230	I
Ranitidine HCl	GL	1 mg/mL[a]	BW	5 mg/mL[a]	Physically compatible for 4 hr at 25°C	1157	C
Remifentanil HCl	GW	0.025 and 0.25 mg/mL[b]	BW	7 mg/mL[a]	Physically compatible for 4 hr at 23°C	2075	C
Sargramostim	IMM	10 mcg/mL[b]	BW	7 mg/mL[b]	Few small white particles form in 4 hr	1436	I
Sodium bicarbonate	IX	0.5 mEq/mL[a]	BW	5 mg/mL[a]	Physically compatible for 4 hr at 25°C	1157	C
Tacrolimus	FUJ				Significant tacrolimus loss within 15 min	191	I
Teniposide	BR	0.1 mg/mL[a]	BW	7 mg/mL[a]	Physically compatible for 4 hr at 23°C	1725	C
Theophylline	TR	1.6 mg/mL[a]	BW	5 mg/mL[a]	Physically compatible for 4 hr at 25°C	1157	C
Thiotepa	IMM[e]	1 mg/mL[a]	BW	7 mg/mL[a]	Physically compatible for 4 hr at 23°C	1861	C
TNA #218 to #226[f]			GW	7 mg/mL[a]	White precipitate forms immediately	2215	I
Tobramycin sulfate	DI	1.6 mg/mL[a]	BW	5 mg/mL[a]	Physically compatible for 4 hr at 25°C	1157	C
TPN #203, #204[f]			BW	7 mg/mL	White precipitate forms immediately	1974	I
TPN #212 to #215[f]			BW	7 mg/mL[a]	Crystalline needles form immediately, becoming a gross precipitate in 1 hr	2109	I
Trimethoprim–sulfame-thoxazole	RC	0.8 mg/mL[a k]	BW	5 mg/mL[a]	Physically compatible for 4 hr at 25°C	1157	C
Vancomycin HCl	LI	5 mg/mL[a]	BW	5 mg/mL[a]	Physically compatible for 4 hr at 25°C	1157	C
Vinorelbine tartrate	BW	1 mg/mL[b]	BW	7 mg/mL[b]	Immediate white precipitate	1558	I
Zidovudine	BW	4 mg/mL[a]	BW	7 mg/mL[a]	Physically compatible for 4 hr at 25°C	1193	C

[a] Tested in dextrose 5%.

[b] Tested in sodium chloride 0.9%.

[c] Tested in both dextrose 5% and sodium chloride 0.9%.

[d] Tested in sterile water for injection.

[e] Lyophilized formulation tested.

[f] Refer to Appendix for the composition of parenteral nutrition solutions. TNA indicates a 3-in-1 admixture, and TPN indicates a 2-in-1 admixture.

[g] Tested in Ringer's injection, lactated.

[h] Test performed using the formulation WITHOUT edetate disodium.

[i] Tested in sodium chloride 0.45%.

[j] Piperacillin component. Piperacillin in an 8:1 fixed-ratio concentration with tazobactam.

[k] Trimethoprim component. Trimethoprim in a 1:5 fixed-ratio concentration with sulfamethoxazole.

[l] Imipenem component. Imipenem in a 1:1 fixed-ratio concentration with cilastatin.

[m] Quinupristin and dalfopristin components combined.

[n] Salt not specified.

[o] Test performed using the formulation WITH edetate disodium.

Adenosine
AHFS 24:04.04.24

Products

Adenosine is available as a 3-mg/mL solution with sodium chloride 9 mg/mL in 2- and 4-mL disposable syringes and single-use vials for rapid intravenous bolus injection only.[2991 2993] Adenosine is also available as a 3-mg/mL solution in single-use vials with sodium chloride 9 mg/mL in 20- and 30-mL vials for intravenous infusion only.[2992]

pH

From 4.5 to 7.5.[2991 2992 2993]

Trade Name(s)

Adenocard IV, Adenoscan

Administration

Adenosine injections are administered intravenously.[2991 2992 2993] Adenosine for rapid intravenous bolus injection only is administered by the peripheral intravenous route directly into a vein or into an intravenous line close to the patient and is followed by a rapid sodium chloride 0.9% flush.[2991 2993] Adenosine for intravenous infusion only is administered by continuous peripheral intravenous infusion over 6 minutes.[2992]

Stability

Intact containers of adenosine injection should be stored at controlled room temperature.[2991 2992 2993] The drug should not be refrigerated due to the possibility of crystallization.[2991 2992 2993] If crystallization occurs, let the solution warm to room temperature to dissolve the crystals.[2991 2992 2993] The solution must be clear prior to administration.[2991 2992 2993]

Adenosine 6 mcg/mL in sodium chloride 0.9% was packaged in 5-mL glass ampuls. Based on analysis of high-temperature-accelerated decomposition, it was projected that the drug solution would be stable for at least 5 years at 4 and 25°C.[2115]

Adenosine 2 mg/mL in sodium chloride 0.9% was packaged in glass vials and stored for 6 months at temperatures ranging from 4 to 72°C. Analysis found no loss of adenosine in samples stored at 4, 22, and 37°C.[2277]

Adenosine 80 mg/L and 330 mg/L in cardioplegia solutions having high (100 mmol/L) and low (30 mmol/L) concentrations of potassium was stored at 4 and 23°C. The solutions also contained tromethamine (THAM) 12 mmol/L, magnesium sulfate 9 mmol/L, dextrose 250 mmol/L, and citrate-phosphate-dextrose-adenine solution 20 mL/L. No adenosine loss occurred after 14 days of storage in either solution.[2402]

Syringes

Undiluted adenosine (Fujisawa) 3 mg/mL was packaged as 25 mL in 60-mL polypropylene syringes (Becton Dickinson) and sealed with polyolefin tip caps (Sherwood Medical). The syringes were stored at 25, 5, and –15°C. The solutions remained visually clear, and analysis showed no loss of adenosine in 7 days at 25°C, 14 days at 5°C, and 28 days at –15°C. The drug's stability in glass vials was essentially identical under the same conditions.[2114]

Adenosine (Fujisawa) diluted to 0.75 mg/mL with several infusion solutions was packaged as 25 mL in 60-mL polypropylene syringes (Becton Dickinson) and sealed with polyolefin tip caps (Sherwood Medical). The syringes were stored at 25, 5, and –15°C. The solutions remained visually clear, and analysis showed no loss of adenosine in 14 days for dextrose 5% in Ringer's injection, lactated and Ringer's injection, lactated and 16 days for dextrose 5% and sodium chloride 0.9%.[2114]

Compatibility Information

Solution Compatibility

Adenosine

Test Soln Name	Mfr	Mfr	Conc/L or %	Remarks	Ref	C/I
Dextrose 5% in Ringer's injection, lactated	BA[a]	FUJ	750 mg	Visually compatible with no loss in 14 days at 25, 5, and –15°C	2114	C
Dextrose 5%	BA[a]	FUJ	750 mg	Visually compatible with no loss in 16 days at 25, 5, and –15°C	2114	C
Dextrose 5%	BRN[b]	APP	10 and 50 mg	Physically compatible with little to no loss in 14 days at 20 to 25°C and 2 to 8°C	2971	C
Dextrose 5%	HOS[a]	BV	50, 100, and 220 mg	Visually compatible with little to no loss in 14 days at 23 to 25°C and 2 to 8°C	2989, 2990	C
Ringer's injection, lactated	BA[a]	FUJ	750 mg	Visually compatible with no loss in 14 days at 25, 5, and –15°C	2114	C
Sodium chloride 0.9%	BA[a]	FUJ	750 mg	Visually compatible with no loss in 16 days at 25, 5, and –15°C	2114	C

DOI: 10.37573/9781585286850.006

Solution Compatibility (Cont.)

Test Soln Name	Mfr	Mfr	Conc/L or %	Remarks	Ref	C/I
Sodium chloride 0.9%	BRN[b]	APP	10 and 50 mg	Physically compatible with no loss in 14 days at 20 to 25°C and 2 to 8°C	2971	C
Sodium chloride 0.9%	HOS[a]	BV	50, 100, and 220 mg	Visually compatible with little to no loss in 14 days at 23 to 25°C and 2 to 8°C	2989, 2990	C
Sodium chloride 0.9%	BA[a]	TE	2 g	Physically compatible with little to no loss in 14 days at 20 to 25°C and 2 to 8°C	3561, 3562	C
Sodium chloride 0.9%	BA[c]	TE	2 g	Physically compatible with little to no loss in 14 days at 20 to 25°C and 2 to 8°C	3561, 3562	C

[a] Tested in PVC containers.

[b] Tested in polypropylene-polyethylene copolymer PAB bags.

[c] Tested in polyolefin containers.

Y-Site Injection Compatibility (1:1 Mixture)

Adenosine

Test Drug	Mfr	Conc	Mfr	Conc	Remarks	Ref	C/I
Abciximab	LI	36 mcg/mL[a]	FUJ	3 mg/mL	Visually compatible for 12 hr at 23°C	2374	C

[a] Tested in PVC containers.

Selected Revisions July 1, 2020. © Copyright, October 2000.
American Society of Health-System Pharmacists, Inc.

Albumin Human
AHFS 16:00

Products

Albumin human is available in 20-, 50-, and 100-mL vials as a 25% aqueous solution. Each 100 mL of solution contains 25 g of serum albumin. Albumin human is also available as a 5% aqueous solution in 50-, 250-, 500-, and 1000-mL sizes. The products also contain sodium carbonate, sodium bicarbonate, sodium hydroxide, and/or acetic acid to adjust the pH.[1(1/05) 4] The products are heat-treated for inactivation of hepatitis viruses. Sodium caprylate and sodium N-acetyltryptophanate are added to the products as stabilizers to prevent denaturation during the heat treatment. Low aluminum-containing albumin human products contain less than 200 mcg/L of aluminum.[1(1/05)]

pH
From 6.4 to 7.4.[1(1/05) 4]

Sodium Content
From 130 to 160 mEq/L.[1(1/05) 4]

Trade Name(s)
Albuminar, Albutein, Albumarc, Buminate, Plasbumin

Administration

Albumin human is administered intravenously either undiluted or diluted in an intravenous infusion solution having sufficient osmolality to be safely administered.[1(1/05) 4]

CAUTION—Substantial reduction in tonicity, creating the potential for fatal hemolysis and acute renal failure, may result from the use of sterile water as a diluent. The hemolysis and acute renal failure that result from the use of a sufficient volume of sterile water as a diluent may be life-threatening.[4 1942 2072 2073]

Stability

Albumin human has been variously described as clear amber to deep orange-brown and as a transparent or slightly opalescent pale straw to dark brown solution. The solution should not be used if it is turbid or contains a deposit. Since it contains no preservative, the manufacturer recommends use within 4 hours after opening the vial. The expiration date is 5 years after issue from the manufacturer if the labeling recommends storage between 2 and 8 or 10°C, or not more than 3 years after issue from the manufacturer if the labeling recommends storage at temperatures not greater than 30 or 37°C.[4]

The addition of albumin human to parenteral nutrition solutions has resulted in occlusion of filters at concentrations ranging from over 25 g/L to 10.8 g/L.[854 1634]

Freezing Solutions
Freezing the albumin human solutions may damage the container and result in contamination.[4]

Compatibility Information
Solution Compatibility

Albumin human

Test Soln Name	Mfr	Mfr	Conc/L or %	Remarks	Ref	C/I
Dextrose 2.5% in half-strength Ringer's injection	AB		5 g	Physically compatible	3	C
Dextrose 5% in Ringer's injection	AB		5 g	Physically compatible	3	C
Dextrose 2.5% in Ringer's injection, lactated	AB		5 g	Physically compatible	3	C
Dextrose 5% in half-strength Ringer's Injection, lactated	AB		5 g	Physically compatible	3	C
Dextrose 5% in Ringer's injection, lactated	AB		5 g	Physically compatible	3	C
Dextrose 10% in Ringer's injection, lactated	AB		5 g	Physically compatible	3	C
Dextrose 2.5% in sodium chloride 0.45%	AB		5 g	Physically compatible	3	C
Dextrose 2.5% in sodium chloride 0.9%	AB		5 g	Physically compatible	3	C
Dextrose 5% in sodium chloride 0.225%	AB		5 g	Physically compatible	3	C
Dextrose 5% in sodium chloride 0.45%	AB		5 g	Physically compatible	3	C
Dextrose 5% in sodium chloride 0.9%	AB		5 g	Physically compatible	3	C
Dextrose 10% in sodium chloride 0.9%	AB		5 g	Physically compatible	3	C

DOI: 10.37573/9781585286850.007

Solution Compatibility (Cont.)

Test Soln Name	Mfr	Mfr	Conc/L or %	Remarks	Ref	C/I
Dextrose 2.5%	AB		5 g	Physically compatible	3	C
Dextrose 5%	AB		5 g	Physically compatible	3	C
Dextrose 10%	AB		5 g	Physically compatible	3	C
Ionosol B in dextrose 5%	AB		5 g	Physically compatible	3	C
Ionosol MB in dextrose 5%	AB		5 g	Physically compatible	3	C
Ringer's injection	AB		5 g	Physically compatible	3	C
Ringer's injection, lactated	AB		5 g	Physically compatible	3	C
Sodium chloride 0.45%	AB		5 g	Physically compatible	3	C
Sodium chloride 0.9%	AB		5 g	Physically compatible	3	C
Sodium lactate ⅙ M	AB		5 g	Physically compatible	3	C
TNA #232[a]			9.5 g	Microscopically observed emulsion disruption found with increased fat globule size in 48 hr at room temperature	2267	?
TNA #233[a]			9.5 g	Visually apparent emulsion disruption with creaming in 4 hr at room temperature. Increased disruption attributed to the added effect of calcium and magnesium ions	2267	I
TNA #234[a]			18.2 g	Creaming and free oil formation visually observed in 24 hr at room temperature	2267	I
TNA #235[a]			18.2 g	Visually apparent emulsion disruption with creaming and free oil formation in 4 hr at room temperature. Increased disruption attributed to the added effect of calcium and magnesium ions	2267	I

[a] Refer to Appendix for the composition of parenteral nutrition solutions. TNA indicates a 3-in-1 admixture.

Additive Compatibility

Albumin human

Test Drug	Mfr	Conc/L or %	Mfr	Conc/L or %	Test Solution	Remarks	Ref	C/I
Verapamil HCl	KN	80 mg	ARC	25 g	D5W, NS	Cloudiness develops within 8 hr	764	I

Y-Site Injection Compatibility (1:1 Mixture)

Albumin human

Test Drug	Mfr	Conc	Mfr	Conc	Remarks	Ref	C/I
Blinatumomab	AMG	0.125 mcg/mL[b]	LFB	100 mg/mL	Persistent particulate formation when blinatumomab is added to albumin; haze transiently appeared when order of mixing was reversed	3405, 3417	I
Blinatumomab	AMG	0.375 mcg/mL[b]	LFB	100 mg/mL	Persistent particulate formation when blinatumomab is added to albumin; not observed when order of mixing was reversed	3405, 3417	?
Ceftolozane sulfate–tazobactam sodium	CUB	10 mg/mL[c] [d]	KED	250 mg/mL	Measured turbidity increases immediately	3262	I

Y-Site Injection Compatibility (1:1 Mixture) (Cont.)

Test Drug	Mfr	Conc	Mfr	Conc	Remarks	Ref	C/I
Cloxacillin sodium	SMX	100 mg/mL	BEH	250 mg/mL	Physically compatible for up to 4 hr at room temperature	3245	C
Defibrotide sodium	JAZ	8 mg/mL[b]	LFB	200 mg/mL	Visually compatible for 4 hr at room temperature	3149	C
Diltiazem HCl	MMD	5 mg/mL	AR, AT	5 and 25%	Visually compatible	1807	C
Eravacycline dihydrochloride	TET	0.6 mg/mL[b]	BXT	250 mg/mL	Measured turbidity increased immediately	3532	I
Esmolol HCl	MYL	10 mg/mL	OCT	250 mg/mL	Physically compatible for 1 hr at 23°C	3533	C
Fat emulsion, intravenous		20%		20%	Immediate emulsion destabilization	2267	I
Isavuconazo-nium sulfate	ASP	1.5 mg/mL[c]	CBH	250 mg/mL	Measured turbidity increases immediately	3263	I
Labetalol HCl	HOS	5 mg/mL	OCT	250 mg/mL	Measured turbidity increased	3533	I
Lorazepam	WY	0.33 mg/mL[b]		200 mg/mL	Visually compatible for 24 hr at 22°C	1855	C
Meropenem		50 mg/mL	CBH	250 mg/mL	Physically compatible for 4 hr at room temperature	3538	C
Meropenem–vaborbactam	TMC	8 mg/mL[b e]	BXT	250 mg/mL	Measured turbidity increases immediately	3380	I
Metoprolol tartrate	HOS	0.4 mg/mL[b]	OCT	250 mg/mL	Physically compatible for 1 hr at 23°C	3533	C
Micafungin sodium	ASP	1.5 mg/mL[b]	ZLB	25%	Immediate increase in measured haze	2683	I
Midazolam HCl	RC	5 mg/mL		200 mg/mL	White precipitate forms immediately	1855	I
Plazomicin sulfate	ACH	24 mg/mL[c]	BXT	250 mg/mL	Measured turbidity increases immediately	3432	I
Tedizolid phosphate	CUB	0.8 mg/mL[b]	CBH	250 mg/mL	Measured turbidity increases immediately	3244	I
Vancomycin HCl		20 mg/mL[a]		0.1 and 1%[b]	Heavy turbidity forms immediately and precipitate develops subsequently	1701	I
Verapamil HCl	LY	0.2 mg/mL[a]	HY	250 mg/mL[a]	Slight haze in 1 hr	1316	I
Verapamil HCl	LY	0.2 mg/mL[b]	HY	250 mg/mL[b]	Slight haze in 3 hr	1316	I

[a] Tested in dextrose 5%.

[b] Tested in sodium chloride 0.9%.

[c] Tested in both dextrose 5% and sodium chloride 0.9%.

[d] Ceftolozane component. Ceftolozane in a 2:1 fixed ratio concentration with tazobactam.

[e] Meropenem component. Meropenem in a 1:1 fixed-ratio concentration with vaborbactam.

Selected Revisions May 1, 2020. © Copyright, October 1982.
American Society of Health-System Pharmacists, Inc.

Aldesleukin
AHFS 10:00
Interleukin-2

Products

Aldesleukin is available in single-use vials containing 22 million international units (1.3 mg of protein). When reconstituted with 1.2 mL of sterile water for injection, each mL contains aldesleukin 18 million international units (1.1 mg) along with mannitol 50 mg, sodium dodecyl sulfate 0.18 mg, monobasic sodium phosphate 0.17 mg, and dibasic sodium phosphate 0.89 mg. During reconstitution, the sterile water for injection should be directed at the vial's sides. Swirl the contents gently to cause dissolution and avoid excess foaming. Do not shake the vial. Do not use bacteriostatic water for injection.[1(10/08)]

Units

The biological potency of aldesleukin is determined by the lymphocyte proliferation bioassay and is expressed in international units ("I.U."). Aldesleukin 18 million international units equals 1.1 mg of protein.[1(10/08)] During the development of aldesleukin, various unit systems were employed. However, the international unit is now the standard measure of its activity.

pH

The reconstituted product has a pH of 7.2 to 7.8.[1(10/08)]

Trade Name(s)

Proleukin

Administration

Aldesleukin is administered intravenously; the reconstituted solution should be diluted in 50 mL of dextrose 5% and infused over 15 minutes. Inline filters should not be used.[1(10/08) 4] The drug should be diluted within the concentration range of 30 to 70 mcg/mL for administration. Concentrations of aldesleukin below 30 mcg/mL and above 70 mcg/mL have shown increased variability in drug delivery. Dilution and drug delivery outside this concentration range should be avoided.[1(10/08)]

If aldesleukin concentrations less than 30 mcg/mL are necessary for short-term intravenous infusion of 15 minutes, the manufacturer recommends diluting the dose in dextrose 5% that contains albumin human 0.1% to prevent variability in the stability and bioactivity of the drug.[4 1890]

Stability

Aldesleukin is a white to off-white powder; it becomes a colorless to slightly yellow liquid when reconstituted.[1(10/08)]

Intact vials should be stored under refrigeration and protected from light.[1(10/08)] However, aldesleukin in intact vials is stable for at least 2 months at controlled room temperature.[1890] The reconstituted solution, as well as dilutions in infusion solutions for intravenous administration, should also be stored under refrigeration and protected from freezing. Intravenous infusions should be brought to room temperature before administration.[1(10/08)]

The manufacturer indicates that reconstituted and diluted aldesleukin is stable for 48 hours when stored at room temperature or under refrigeration. Refrigeration is recommended because the product contains no antibacterial preservative.[1(10/08)]

Syringes

Aldesleukin (Cetus), reconstituted according to label directions, was evaluated for stability when stored in 1-mL plastic syringes (Becton Dickinson). One- and 0.5-mL aliquots were drawn into these syringes and refrigerated for 5 days. The product was physically stable and retained activity by biological analysis (cell proliferation assay) throughout the study period.[1821]

Reconstituted aldesleukin diluted to a concentration of 220 mcg/mL with dextrose 5% was repackaged aseptically as 1 mL drawn into tuberculin syringes and stored under refrigeration at 2 to 8°C. The drug was found to be stable for the 14-day study period.[1890]

Ambulatory Pumps

For continuous intravenous infusion of aldesleukin in concentrations of 70 mcg/mL or less via an ambulatory pump at the accompanying higher temperature of near 32°C, the dose should be diluted in dextrose 5% to which albumin human at a concentration of 0.1% has been added to maintain aldesleukin stability.[1890] The albumin human helps keep aldesleukin in its microaggregate state and helps decrease sorption to surfaces, especially at concentrations below 10 mcg/mL.[4] In the absence of albumin human, visually observed precipitation and loss of aldesleukin activity has been found. At concentrations greater than 70 and less than 100 mcg/mL at 32°C, aldesleukin is unstable whether albumin human is present or not.[1890]

Aldesleukin (Cetus) 5 to 500 mcg/mL in dextrose 5% was evaluated for stability in polyvinyl chloride (PVC) containers during simulated administration from pumps (CADD-1, Pharmacia Deltec). At 100 to 500 mcg/mL, aldesleukin was stable for 6 days at 32°C and remained visually clear throughout the study period. At concentrations of 5 and 40 mcg/mL, however, albumin human 0.1% was necessary to maintain physical stability. The aldesleukin solutions with albumin human remained clear and remained active for 6 days at 32°C. Without albumin human, precipitation occurred within a few hours.[1821]

Sorption

Aldesleukin in low concentrations, particularly less than 10 mcg/mL, undergoes sorption to surfaces such as plastic bags, tubing, and administration devices. Addition of 0.1% albumin human to the solution decreases the extent of sorption.[4] Both glass and PVC containers have been used to infuse aldesleukin with comparable clinical results. However, drug delivery may be more consistent with PVC containers.[1(10/08) 4]

Filtration

Inline filters should not be used for aldesleukin.[1(10/08) 4]

DOI: 10.37573/9781585286850.008

Compatibility Information

Solution Compatibility

Aldesleukin

Test Soln Name	Mfr	Mfr	Conc/L or %	Remarks	Ref	C/I
Dextrose 5%				Recommended for dilution of aldesleukin	1(10/08)	C
Sodium chloride 0.9%				Increased aggregation occurs	1(10/08)	I

Y-Site Injection Compatibility (1:1 Mixture)

Aldesleukin

Test Drug	Mfr	Conc	Mfr	Conc	Remarks	Ref	C/I
Amphotericin B	SQ	1.6 mg/mL[a]	CHI	33,800 I.U./mL[a]	Visually compatible for 2 hr	1857	C
Calcium gluconate	LY	100 mg/mL	CHI	33,800 I.U./mL[a]	Visually compatible with little or no loss of aldesleukin activity	1857	C
Diphenhydramine HCl	SCN	50 mg/mL	CHI	33,800 I.U./mL[a]	Visually compatible for 2 hr	1857	C
Dopamine HCl	ES	1.6 mg/mL[a]	CHI	33,800 I.U./mL[a]	Visually compatible with little or no loss of aldesleukin activity	1857	C
Dopamine HCl			CHI	[c]	Unacceptable loss of aldesleukin activity	1890	I
Fluconazole	RR	2 mg/mL[a]	CHI	33,800 I.U./mL[a]	Visually compatible with little or no loss of aldesleukin activity	1857	C
Fluorouracil			CHI	[c]	Unacceptable loss of aldesleukin activity	1890	I
Foscarnet sodium	AST	24 mg/mL	CHI	33,800 I.U./mL[a]	Visually compatible with little or no loss of aldesleukin activity	1857	C
Ganciclovir sodium	SY	10 mg/mL[a]	CHI	33,800 I.U./mL[a]	Aldesleukin bioactivity inhibited	1857	I
Heparin sodium	BA	100 units/mL	CHI	33,800 I.U./mL[a]	Visually compatible with little or no loss of aldesleukin activity	1857	C
Heparin sodium			CHI	[c]	Visually compatible but aldesleukin activity was variable depending on rate of delivery. Heparin not tested	1890	?
Lorazepam	WY	2 mg/mL	CHI	33,800 I.U./mL[a]	Globules form immediately	1857	I
Magnesium sulfate	LY	20 mg/mL[a]	CHI	33,800 I.U./mL[a]	Visually compatible with little or no loss of aldesleukin activity	1857	C
Metoclopramide HCl	DU	5 mg/mL	CHI	33,800 I.U./mL[a]	Visually compatible with little or no loss of aldesleukin activity	1857	C
Ondansetron HCl	GL	0.7 mg/mL[a]	CHI	33,800 I.U./mL[a]	Visually compatible with little or no loss of aldesleukin activity	1857	C
Ondansetron HCl	GL		CHI	5 to 40 mcg/mL[c]	Visually compatible. Aldesleukin activity retained if each drug infused at a similar rate. Ondansetron not tested	1890	C
Pentamidine isethionate	FUJ	6 mg/mL[a]	CHI	33,800 I.U./mL[a]	Aldesleukin bioactivity inhibited	1857	I
Potassium chloride	AB	0.2 mEq/mL	CHI	33,800 I.U./mL[a]	Visually compatible with little or no loss of aldesleukin activity	1857	C
Potassium chloride			CHI	[c]	Loss of aldesleukin activity	1890	I

Y-Site Injection Compatibility (1:1 Mixture) (Cont.)

Test Drug	Mfr	Conc	Mfr	Conc	Remarks	Ref	C/I
Prochlorperazine edisylate	SKB	5 mg/mL	CHI	33,800 I.U./mL[a]	Aldesleukin bioactivity inhibited	1857	I
Promethazine HCl	ES	25 mg/mL	CHI	33,800 I.U./mL[a]	Aldesleukin bioactivity inhibited	1857	I
Ranitidine HCl	AB	1 mg/mL[b]	CHI	33,800 I.U./mL[a]	Visually compatible with little or no loss of aldesleukin activity	1857	C
Trimethoprim–sulfamethoxazole	BW	1.6 mg/mL[a] [d]	CHI	33,800 I.U./mL[a]	Visually compatible with little or no loss of aldesleukin activity	1857	C
Vancomycin HCl			CHI	[c]	Visually compatible. Aldesleukin activity retained. Vancomycin not tested	1890	C

[a] Tested in dextrose 5%.

[b] Tested in sodium chloride 0.45%.

[c] Tested in D5W with 0.1% human serum albumin.

[d] Trimethoprim component. Trimethoprim in a 1:5 fixed-ratio concentration with sulfamethoxazole.

Selected Revisions June 1, 2019. © Copyright, October 1994.
American Society of Health-System Pharmacists, Inc.

Alfentanil Hydrochloride
AHFS 28:08.08

Products

Alfentanil hydrochloride is available at a concentration equivalent to alfentanil base 500 mcg/mL with sodium chloride for isotonicity in 2-, 5-, 10-, and 20-mL ampuls.[1(10/06)]

pH

From 4 to 6.[1(10/06)]

Osmolality

Alfentanil hydrochloride injection is isotonic.[1(10/06)]

Trade Name(s)

Alfenta

Administration

Alfentanil hydrochloride is administered by intravenous injection or infusion. For infusion, dilution to 25 to 80 mcg/mL in a compatible solution has been utilized.[1(10/06)]

Stability

Alfentanil hydrochloride injection is stable at controlled room temperature when protected from light.[1(10/06)]

Syringes

Alfentanil hydrochloride (Janssen) 0.5 mg/mL in dextrose 5% was packaged in 20-mL polypropylene syringes (Becton Dickinson) and stored at 20°C exposed to light and at 8°C for 16 weeks. The solutions were visually clear and colorless throughout the study. No loss of alfentanil hydrochloride occurred and no leached substances from the plastic syringes appeared.[2191]

Alfentanil hydrochloride (Janssen) 0.167 mg/mL in sodium chloride 0.9% in polypropylene syringes (Sherwood) was physically stable and exhibited little loss in 24 hours stored at 4 and 23°C.[2191]

Sorption

Alfentanil hydrochloride (Janssen) (concentration unspecified) was found to be compatible with polyethylene, polypropylene, and polyvinyl chloride (PVC).[2468]

Compatibility Information

Solution Compatibility

Alfentanil HCl

Test Soln Name	Mfr	Mfr	Conc/L or %	Remarks	Ref	C/I
Dextrose 5% in sodium chloride 0.9%			25 to 80 mg	Physically and chemically stable	1(10/06)	C
Dextrose 5%			25 to 80 mg	Physically and chemically stable	1(10/06)	C
Ringer's injection, lactated			25 to 80 mg	Physically and chemically stable	1(10/06)	C
Sodium chloride 0.9%			25 to 80 mg	Physically and chemically stable	1(10/06)	C

Drugs in Syringe Compatibility

Alfentanil HCl

Test Drug	Mfr	Amt	Mfr	Amt	Remarks	Ref	C/I
Atracurium besylate	BW	10 mg/mL		0.5 mg/mL	Physically compatible and atracurium stable for 24 hr at 5 and 30°C	1694	C
Midazolam HCl	RC	0.2 mg/mL[a]	JN	0.5 mg/mL	Visually compatible. 8% midazolam and 2% alfentanil loss in 3 weeks at 20°C in light. No alfentanil loss and 7% midazolam loss in 4 weeks at 6°C in dark	2133	C
Morphine sulfate	DB	0.8 mg/mL[a]	ASZ	55 mcg/mL[a]	No loss of either drug in 182 days at room temperature or refrigerated	2527	C
Ondansetron HCl	GW	1.33 mg/mL[a]	JN	0.167 mg/mL[a]	Physically compatible. Little loss of either drug in 24 hr at 4 or 23°C	2199	C

[a] Diluted with sodium chloride 0.9%.

DOI: 10.37573/9781585286850.009

Y-Site Injection Compatibility (1:1 Mixture)

Alfentanil HCl

Test Drug	Mfr	Conc	Mfr	Conc	Remarks	Ref	C/I
Bivalirudin	TMC	5 mg/mL[a]	TAY	0.125 mg/mL[a]	Physically compatible for 4 hr at 23°C	2373	C
Cangrelor tetrasodium	TMC	1 mg/mL[b]		0.5 mg/mL	Physically compatible for 4 hr	3243	C
Cisatracurium besylate	GW	0.1, 2, 5 mg/mL[a]	JN	0.125 mg/mL[a]	Physically compatible for 4 hr at 23°C	2074	C
Dexmedetomidine HCl	AB	4 mcg/mL[b]	TAY	0.5 mg/mL	Physically compatible for 4 hr at 23°C	2383	C
Etomidate	AB	2 mg/mL	JN	0.5 mg/mL	Visually compatible for 7 days at 25°C	1801	C
Fenoldopam mesylate	AB	80 mcg/mL[b]	TAY	0.5 mg/mL	Physically compatible for 4 hr at 23°C	2467	C
Hetastarch in lactated electrolyte	AB	6%	TAY	0.125 mg/mL[a]	Physically compatible for 4 hr at 23°C	2339	C
Linezolid	PHU	2 mg/mL	TAY	0.5 mg/mL	Physically compatible for 4 hr at 23°C	2264	C
Propofol	ZEN[c]	10 mg/mL	JN	0.5 mg/mL	Physically compatible for 1 hr at 23°C	2066	C
Remifentanil HCl	GW	0.025 and 0.25 mg/mL[b]	JN	0.125 mg/mL[a]	Physically compatible for 4 hr at 23°C	2075	C

[a] Tested in dextrose 5%.

[b] Tested in sodium chloride 0.9%.

[c] Test performed using the formulation WITH edetate disodium.

Selected Revisions January 31, 2020. © Copyright, October 1996.
American Society of Health-System Pharmacists, Inc.

Allopurinol Sodium
AHFS 92:16

Products

Allopurinol sodium is available in single-use vials containing the equivalent of 500 mg of allopurinol in lyophilized form. Reconstitute with 25 mL of sterile water for injection to yield an almost colorless concentrated solution that is clear to slightly opalescent.[1(8/05)]

pH

From 11.1 to 11.8.[4]

Trade Name(s)

Aloprim

Administration

The reconstituted solution must be diluted for use in sodium chloride 0.9% or dextrose 5% to a final concentration of no greater than 6 mg/mL. The diluted infusion is given as a single infusion daily or in equally divided infusions at 6-, 8-, or 12-hour intervals. The rate of infusion depends on the volume to be infused.[1(8/05)]

Stability

Allopurinol sodium is supplied as a white lyophilized powder. The intact vials should be stored at controlled room temperature. Administration should begin within 10 hours of reconstitution. The reconstituted solution and diluted infusion solution should not be refrigerated.[1(8/05)]

Compatibility Information

Y-Site Injection Compatibility (1:1 Mixture)

Allopurinol sodium

Test Drug	Mfr	Conc	Mfr	Conc	Remarks	Ref	C/I
Acyclovir sodium	BW	7 mg/mL[b]	BW	3 mg/mL[b]	Physically compatible for 4 hr at 22°C	1686	C
Amikacin sulfate	BR	5 mg/mL[b]	BW	3 mg/mL[b]	Crystals and flakes form within 1 hr	1686	I
Aminophylline	AB	2.5 mg/mL[b]	BW	3 mg/mL[b]	Physically compatible for 4 hr at 22°C	1686	C
Amphotericin B	SQ	0.6 mg/mL[a b]	BW	3 mg/mL[b]	Amphotericin B haze lost immediately	1686	I
Aztreonam	SQ	40 mg/mL[b]	BW	3 mg/mL[b]	Physically compatible for 4 hr at 22°C	1686	C
Bleomycin sulfate	BR	1 unit/mL[b]	BW	3 mg/mL[b]	Physically compatible for 4 hr at 22°C	1686	C
Bumetanide	RC	0.04 mg/mL[b]	BW	3 mg/mL[b]	Physically compatible for 4 hr at 22°C	1686	C
Buprenorphine HCl	RKC	0.04 mg/mL[b]	BW	3 mg/mL[b]	Physically compatible for 4 hr at 22°C	1686	C
Butorphanol tartrate	BR	0.04 mg/mL[b]	BW	3 mg/mL[b]	Physically compatible for 4 hr at 22°C	1686	C
Calcium gluconate	AMR	40 mg/mL[b]	BW	3 mg/mL[b]	Physically compatible for 4 hr at 22°C	1686	C
Carboplatin	BR	5 mg/mL[b]	BW	3 mg/mL[b]	Physically compatible for 4 hr at 22°C	1686	C
Carmustine	BR	1.5 mg/mL[b]	BW	3 mg/mL[b]	Gas evolves immediately	1686	I
Cefazolin sodium	GEM	20 mg/mL[b]	BW	3 mg/mL[b]	Physically compatible for 4 hr at 22°C	1686	C
Cefotaxime sodium	HO	20 mg/mL[b]	BW	3 mg/mL[b]	Tiny particles form immediately	1686	I
Cefotetan disodium	STU	20 mg/mL[b]	BW	3 mg/mL[b]	Physically compatible for 4 hr at 22°C	1686	C
Ceftazidime	LI	40 mg/mL[b]	BW	3 mg/mL[b]	Physically compatible for 4 hr at 22°C	1686	C
Ceftriaxone sodium	RC	20 mg/mL[b]	BW	3 mg/mL[b]	Physically compatible for 4 hr at 22°C	1686	C
Cefuroxime sodium	GL	20 mg/mL[b]	BW	3 mg/mL[b]	Physically compatible for 4 hr at 22°C	1686	C
Chlorpromazine HCl	RU	2 mg/mL[b]	BW	3 mg/mL[b]	White precipitate forms immediately	1686	I

DOI: 10.37573/9781585286850.010

Y-Site Injection Compatibility (1:1 Mixture) (Cont.)

Test Drug	Mfr	Conc	Mfr	Conc	Remarks	Ref	C/I
Cisplatin	BR	1 mg/mL	BW	3 mg/mL[b]	Physically compatible for 4 hr at 22°C	1686	C
Clindamycin phosphate	AB	10 mg/mL[b]	BW	3 mg/mL[b]	Tiny particles form immediately and become more numerous over 4 hr	1686	I
Cyclophosphamide	MJ	10 mg/mL[b]	BW	3 mg/mL[b]	Physically compatible for 4 hr at 22°C	1686	C
Cytarabine	SCN	50 mg/mL	BW	3 mg/mL[b]	Tiny particles form within 4 hr	1686	I
Dacarbazine	MI	4 mg/mL[b]	BW	3 mg/mL[b]	Small particles form within 1 hr and become large pink pellets in 24 hr	1686	I
Dactinomycin	MSD	0.01 mg/mL[b]	BW	3 mg/mL[b]	Physically compatible for 4 hr at 22°C	1686	C
Daunorubicin HCl	WY	1 mg/mL[b]	BW	3 mg/mL[b]	Reddish-purple color and haze form immediately. Reddish-brown particles form within 1 hr	1686	I
Dexamethasone sodium phosphate	LY	1 mg/mL[b]	BW	3 mg/mL[b]	Physically compatible for 4 hr at 22°C	1686	C
Diphenhydramine HCl	PD	2 mg/mL[b]	BW	3 mg/mL[b]	White precipitate forms immediately	1686	I
Doxorubicin HCl	CET	2 mg/mL	BW	3 mg/mL[b]	Immediate dark red color and haze. Reddish-brown particles within 1 hr	1686	I
Doxorubicin HCl liposomal	SEQ	0.4 mg/mL[a]	BW	3 mg/mL	Physically compatible for 4 hr at 23°C	2087	C
Doxycycline hyclate	ES	1 mg/mL[b]	BW	3 mg/mL[b]	Immediate brown particles. Hazy brown solution with precipitate in 4 hr	1686	I
Droperidol	JN	0.4 mg/mL[b]	BW	3 mg/mL[b]	Immediate turbidity with particles	1686	I
Enalaprilat	MSD	0.1 mg/mL[b]	BW	3 mg/mL[b]	Physically compatible for 4 hr at 22°C	1686	C
Etoposide	BR	0.4 mg/mL[b]	BW	3 mg/mL[b]	Physically compatible for 4 hr at 22°C	1686	C
Famotidine	MSD	2 mg/mL[b]	BW	3 mg/mL[b]	Physically compatible for 4 hr at 22°C	1686	C
Filgrastim	AMG	30 mcg/mL[a]	BW	3 mg/mL[a]	Physically compatible for 4 hr at 22°C	1687	C
Floxuridine	RC	3 mg/mL[b]	BW	3 mg/mL[b]	Tiny particles form in 1 to 4 hr	1686	I
Fluconazole	RR	2 mg/mL	BW	3 mg/mL[b]	Physically compatible for 4 hr at 22°C	1686	C
Fludarabine phosphate	BX	1 mg/mL[b]	BW	3 mg/mL[b]	Physically compatible for 4 hr at 22°C	1686	C
Fluorouracil	RC	16 mg/mL[b]	BW	3 mg/mL[b]	Physically compatible for 4 hr at 22°C	1686	C
Furosemide	ES	3 mg/mL[b]	BW	3 mg/mL[b]	Physically compatible for 4 hr at 22°C	1686	C
Gallium nitrate	FUJ	0.4 mg/mL[b]	BW	3 mg/mL[b]	Physically compatible for 4 hr at 22°C	1686	C
Ganciclovir sodium	SY	20 mg/mL[b]	BW	3 mg/mL[b]	Physically compatible for 4 hr at 22°C	1686	C
Gentamicin sulfate	ES	5 mg/mL[b]	BW	3 mg/mL[b]	Hazy solution with crystals forms in 1 hr	1686	I
Granisetron HCl	SKB	0.05 mg/mL[a]	BW	3 mg/mL[a]	Physically compatible for 4 hr at 23°C	2000	C
Haloperidol lactate	MN	0.2 mg/mL[b]	BW	3 mg/mL[b]	Immediate turbidity. Crystals in 1 hr	1686	I
Heparin sodium	ES	100 units/mL[b]	BW	3 mg/mL[b]	Physically compatible for 4 hr at 22°C	1686	C
Hydrocortisone sodium succinate	UP	1 mg/mL[b]	BW	3 mg/mL[b]	Physically compatible for 4 hr at 22°C	1686	C
Hydromorphone HCl	KN	0.5 mg/mL[b]	BW	3 mg/mL[b]	Physically compatible for 4 hr at 22°C	1686	C
Hydroxyzine HCl	ES	4 mg/mL[b]	BW	3 mg/mL[b]	Immediate turbidity and precipitate	1686	I
Idarubicin HCl	AD	0.5 mg/mL[b]	BW	3 mg/mL[b]	Immediate reddish-purple color. Particles in 1 hr. Total color loss in 24 hr	1686	I
Ifosfamide	MJ	25 mg/mL[b]	BW	3 mg/mL[b]	Physically compatible for 4 hr at 22°C	1686	C
Imipenem–cilastatin sodium	MSD	10 mg/mL[b e]	BW	3 mg/mL[b]	Haze and particles form in 1 hr	1686	I

Y-Site Injection Compatibility (1:1 Mixture) (Cont.)

Test Drug	Mfr	Conc	Mfr	Conc	Remarks	Ref	C/I
Lorazepam	WY	0.1 mg/mL[b]	BW	3 mg/mL[b]	Physically compatible for 4 hr at 22°C	1686	C
Mannitol	BA	15%	BW	3 mg/mL[b]	Physically compatible for 4 hr at 22°C	1686	C
Mechlorethamine HCl	MSD	1 mg/mL	BW	3 mg/mL[b]	Haze and small particles form immediately. Numerous large particles in 4 hr	1686	I
Meperidine HCl	WY	4 mg/mL[b]	BW	3 mg/mL[b]	Tiny particles form immediately and increase in number over 4 hr	1686	I
Mesna	MJ	10 mg/mL[b]	BW	3 mg/mL[b]	Physically compatible for 4 hr at 22°C	1686	C
Methotrexate sodium	LE	15 mg/mL[b]	BW	3 mg/mL[b]	Physically compatible for 4 hr at 22°C	1686	C
Methylprednisolone sodium succinate	AB	5 mg/mL[b]	BW	3 mg/mL[b]	Haze forms in 1 hr with white precipitate in 24 hr	1686	I
Metoclopramide HCl	DU	5 mg/mL	BW	3 mg/mL[b]	Heavy white precipitate forms immediately	1686	I
Metronidazole	BA	5 mg/mL	BW	3 mg/mL[b]	Physically compatible for 4 hr at 22°C	1686	C
Mitoxantrone HCl	LE	0.5 mg/mL[b]	BW	3 mg/mL[b]	Physically compatible for 4 hr at 22°C	1686	C
Morphine sulfate	WI	1 mg/mL[b]	BW	3 mg/mL[b]	Physically compatible for 4 hr at 22°C	1686	C
Nalbuphine HCl	DU	10 mg/mL	BW	3 mg/mL[b]	Particles in 1 hr. Crystals in 4 hr	1686	I
Ondansetron HCl	GL	1 mg/mL[b]	BW	3 mg/mL[b]	Immediate turbidity becoming precipitate	1686	I
Potassium chloride	AB	0.1 mEq/mL[b]	BW	3 mg/mL[b]	Physically compatible for 4 hr at 22°C	1686	C
Prochlorperazine edisylate	SKB	0.5 mg/mL[b]	BW	3 mg/mL[b]	Heavy turbidity forms immediately	1686	I
Promethazine HCl	WY	2 mg/mL[b]	BW	3 mg/mL[b]	Immediate turbidity. Particles in 4 hr	1686	I
Ranitidine HCl	GL	2 mg/mL[b]	BW	3 mg/mL[b]	Physically compatible for 4 hr at 22°C	1686	C
Sodium bicarbonate	AB	1 mEq/mL	BW	3 mg/mL[b]	Small and large crystals form in 1 hr	1686	I
Streptozocin	UP	40 mg/mL[b]	BW	3 mg/mL[b]	Haze and small particles in 1 hr	1686	I
Teniposide	BR	0.1 mg/mL[a]	BW	3 mg/mL[a]	Physically compatible for 4 hr at 23°C	1725	C
Thiotepa	LE[c]	1 mg/mL[b]	BW	3 mg/mL[b]	Physically compatible for 4 hr at 22°C	1686	C
Tobramycin sulfate	LI	5 mg/mL[b]	BW	3 mg/mL[b]	Haze and crystals form in 1 hr	1686	I
Trimethoprim–sulfamethoxazole	ES	0.8 mg/mL[b] [d]	BW	3 mg/mL[b]	Physically compatible for 4 hr at 22°C	1686	C
Vancomycin HCl	LY	10 mg/mL[b]	BW	3 mg/mL[b]	Physically compatible for 4 hr at 22°C	1686	C
Vinblastine sulfate	LI	0.12 mg/mL[b]	BW	3 mg/mL[b]	Physically compatible for 4 hr at 22°C	1686	C
Vincristine sulfate	LI	0.05 mg/mL[b]	BW	3 mg/mL[b]	Physically compatible for 4 hr at 22°C	1686	C
Vinorelbine tartrate	BW	1 mg/mL[b]	BW	3 mg/mL[b]	Immediate white precipitate	1686	I
Zidovudine	BW	4 mg/mL[b]	BW	3 mg/mL[b]	Physically compatible for 4 hr at 22°C	1686	C

[a] Tested in dextrose 5%.

[b] Tested in sodium chloride 0.9%.

[c] Powder fill formulation tested.

[d] Trimethoprim component. Trimethoprim in a 1:5 fixed-ratio concentration with sulfamethoxazole.

[e] Not specified whether concentration refers to single component or combined components.

Alprostadil
AHFS 24:12.92

Products

Alprostadil for intravenous use is available as a 500-mcg/mL concentrate in dehydrated alcohol packaged in ampuls and vials. The concentrate must be diluted in a compatible infusion solution for use.[1(1/05)]

Administration

For continuous intravenous or intra-arterial infusion in neonates, alprostadil concentrate is diluted by adding 500 mcg (one vial of concentrate) to 25, 50, 100, or 250 mL of dextrose 5% or sodium chloride 0.9% to yield 20, 10, 5, or 2 mcg/mL, respectively. The diluted solution is administered using a controlled infusion device.[1(1/05)]

Stability

Intact containers of alprostadil concentrate should be stored under refrigeration. Alprostadil concentrate diluted for infusion is stable for up to 24 hours in the infusion solution.[1(1/05)]

Alprostadil is reported not to be subjected to increased degradation due to ambient light exposure.[2639]

Undiluted alprostadil concentrate may interact with plastic volumetric infusion chambers changing their appearance and resulting in a hazy solution. Consequently, the infusion solution should be added to the volumetric chamber first with the alprostadil concentrate added into the solution avoiding contact with the chamber walls.[1(1/05)]

pH Effects

Alprostadil is more stable at acidic pH values compared to neutral and especially alkaline pH. The pH of maximum stability has been reported to be pH 3.[2639]

Syringes

Alprostadil 500 mcg/mL undiluted and also diluted with sodium chloride 0.9% to concentrations near 250 and 125 mcg/mL was packaged in 1-mL polypropylene syringes (Becton Dickinson). After 30 days stored at 4°C, 5% or less alprostadil loss occurred.[2602]

Compatibility Information

Drugs in Syringe Compatibility

Alprostadil

Test Drug	Mfr	Amt	Mfr	Amt	Remarks	Ref	C/I
Caffeine citrate		20 mg/1 mL	UP	0.5 mg/1 mL	Visually compatible for 4 hr at 25°C	2440	C
Pantoprazole sodium	a	4 mg/1 mL		0.5 mg/1 mL	Clear solution	2574	C

[a] Test performed using the formulation WITHOUT edetate disodium.

Y-Site Injection Compatibility (1:1 Mixture)

Alprostadil

Test Drug	Mfr	Conc	Mfr	Conc	Remarks	Ref	C/I
Ampicillin sodium	SQ	100 mg/mL[b]	BED	7.5 mcg/mL[d]	Visually compatible for 1 hr	2746	C
Cefazolin sodium	LI	100 mg/mL[b]	BED	7.5 mcg/mL[d e]	Visually compatible for 1 hr	2746	C
Cefotaxime sodium	HO	100 mg/mL[b]	BED	7.5 mcg/mL[d e]	Visually compatible for 1 hr	2746	C
Chlorothiazide sodium	ME	25 mg/mL[b]	BED	7.5 mcg/mL[d]	Visually compatible for 1 hr	2746	C
Dobutamine HCl	AB	3 mg/mL[b]	BED	7.5 mcg/mL[d e]	Visually compatible for 1 hr	2746	C
Dopamine HCl	AB	3 mg/mL[b]	BED	7.5 mcg/mL[d e]	Visually compatible for 1 hr	2746	C
Fentanyl citrate	JN	10 mcg/mL[b]	BED	7.5 mcg/mL[d e]	Visually compatible for 1 hr	2746	C
Gentamicin sulfate	ES	1 mg/mL[b]	BED	7.5 mcg/mL[d e]	Visually compatible for 1 hr	2746	C
Levofloxacin	OMN	5 mg/mL[a]	UP	0.5 mg/mL	Precipitate forms	2233	I
Methylprednisolone sodium succinate	PH	40 mg/mL[b]	BED	7.5 mcg/mL[d e]	Visually compatible for 1 hr	2746	C

DOI: 10.37573/9781585286850.011

Y-Site Injection Compatibility (1:1 Mixture) (Cont.)

Test Drug	Mfr	Conc	Mfr	Conc	Remarks	Ref	C/I
Sodium nitroprusside	RC	0.3, 1.2, 3 mg/mL[a]	UP	2 mcg/mL[a]	Visually compatible for 48 hr at 24°C protected from light	2357	C
Sodium nitroprusside	RC	0.3, 1.2, 3 mg/mL[a]	UP	10 mcg/mL[a]	Visually compatible for 48 hr at 24°C protected from light	2357	C
Tobramycin sulfate	LI	1 mg/mL[b]	BED	7.5 mcg/mL[d e]	Visually compatible for 1 hr	2746	C
TPN #274[c]			BED	15 mcg/mL[a]	Visually compatible for 1 hr	2746	C
Vancomycin HCl	LI	5 mg/mL[b]	BED	7.5 mcg/mL[d e]	Visually compatible for 1 hr	2746	C
Vecuronium bromide	OR	1 mg/mL[b]	BED	7.5 mcg/mL[d e]	Visually compatible for 1 hr	2746	C

[a] Tested in dextrose 5%.

[b] Tested in either dextrose 5% or in sodium chloride 0.9%, but the report did not specify which solution.

[c] Refer to Appendix for the composition of parenteral nutrition solutions. TPN indicates a 2-in-1 admixture.

[d] Tested in a 1:1 mixture of (1) dextrose 5% and dextrose 5% in sodium chloride 0.45% with and without potassium chloride 20 mEq/L and also in (2) dextrose 10% in sodium chloride 0.45% with and without potassium chloride 20 mEq/L.

[e] Tested in a 1:1 mixture of dextrose 5% and TPN #274 (see Appendix).

Selected Revisions October 1, 2012. © Copyright, October 2004.
American Society of Health-System Pharmacists, Inc.

Alteplase
AHFS 20:12.20
t-PA

Products

Alteplase is available as a sterile lyophilized powder in 50- and 100-mg vials. The products also contain L-arginine, phosphoric acid, and polysorbate 80.[1(12/05)]

The pH may have been adjusted with phosphoric acid and/or sodium hydroxide. Intact 50-mg vials contain a vacuum, but the 100-mg vials do not.[1(12/05)]

The alteplase vials are accompanied by 50- and 100-mL vials of sterile water for injection for the 50- and 100-mg sizes, respectively. Alteplase should be reconstituted with sterile water for injection only; do not use solutions containing preservatives. Use of the accompanying diluent results in a 1-mg/mL concentration. The manufacturer recommends use of a large bore needle to direct the stream into the lyophilized cake of the 50-mg vials. For the 100-mg vials, the special transfer device should be used. The vials should be swirled gently—not shaken—to dissolve the drug. Excessive agitation should be avoided. Although slight foaming may occur, the bubbles will dissipate after standing for several minutes.[1(12/05)]

Cathflo Activase is available in alteplase 2.2-mg vials with L-arginine 77 mg, polysorbate 80 0.2 mg, and phosphoric acid to adjust pH. Reconstitute with 2.2 mL of sterile water for injection and gently swirl to yield a 1-mg/mL solution; do not shake. If slight foaming occurs, allow the solution to stand for a few minutes until the bubbles dissipate. Do not use bacteriostatic water for injection with a preservative as a diluent.[1(12/05)]

Specific Activity

Alteplase is a purified glycoprotein with a specific activity of 580,000 international units/mg. The 50-mg vial contains 29 million international units, and the 100-mg vial contains 58 million international units.[1(12/05)]

pH

Approximately 7.3.[1(12/05)]

Osmolality

The product has an osmolality of 215 mOsm/kg.[1(12/05)]

Trade Name(s)

Activase

Administration

Alteplase is administered by intravenous infusion, directly after reconstitution to a 1-mg/mL concentration or diluted with an equal volume of sodium chloride 0.9% or dextrose 5% to a 0.5-mg/mL concentration.[1(12/05) 4] Dilution to a lower concentration may result in precipitation.[4 1425]

Alteplase has been effective and well tolerated in catheter clearance.[1(12/05) 2328 2329 2330 2446 2635]

Stability

Alteplase, an off-white lyophilized powder, becomes a colorless to pale yellow solution on reconstitution. Intact vials should be refrigerated or stored at room temperature with protection from extended exposure to light. The 50-mg vials should not be used unless a vacuum is present. Cathflo Activase should be stored under refrigeration.[1(12/05)]

Because alteplase has no bacteriostat, the manufacturer recommends reconstitution immediately before use. However, the solution may be administered within 8 hours when stored at room temperature or under refrigeration.[1(12/05)] Exposure to light does not affect the potency of either reconstituted solutions of alteplase or dilutions in compatible infusion solutions.[1(12/05) 4]

Alteplase is stated to be incompatible with the preservatives used in bacteriostatic water for injection because preservatives can interact with the alteplase molecule.[4] Even so, alteplase was reconstituted with sterile water for injection and also bacteriostatic water for injection (benzyl alcohol 0.9%) to yield a 1-mg/mL solution. The test solutions were stored at 37°C and remained clear and colorless. In vitro clot lysis testing found activity was retained for at least 7 days. The USP antimicrobial effectiveness test was performed as well. The samples reconstituted with sterile water failed the test while the samples reconstituted with bacteriostatic water for injection passed.[2668]

pH Effects

Alteplase in solution is stable at pH 5 to 7.5.[4]

Freezing Solutions

A 50-mg vial of alteplase (Genentech), reconstituted with sterile water for injection to a concentration of 1 mg/mL, was diluted with balanced saline solution to a final concentration of 250 mcg/mL. Then 0.3-mL (75 mcg) portions of the diluted solution were drawn into 1-mL tuberculin syringes and frozen at –70°C. Alteplase activity was retained for at least 1 year.[2157]

However, others have objected to frozen storage of diluted alteplase solution. It was noted that the alteplase formulation has been designed for optimal stability, and dilution to a concentration lower than 500 mcg/mL might adversely affect the drug's solubility by diluting the formulation's solubilizing components. Furthermore, it was noted that the calcium or magnesium salts contained in some diluents might interact with the phosphates present in the alteplase formulation to form a precipitate. Indeed, precipitated protein has been found in diluted alteplase after room temperature storage for 24 hours. Frozen storage at –20°C with subsequent thawing has resulted in changed patterns of light scattering as well. It was recommended that dilution with balanced saline solution and storage of dilutions for any length of time at room temperature or frozen should be avoided.[2158]

DOI: 10.37573/9781585286850.012

Use of a diluent containing polysorbate 80, L-arginine, and phosphoric acid to reconstitute and dilute alteplase to 50 mcg/mL is reported to permit frozen storage. Although the report did not specify the exact concentrations of the diluent components, it may have duplicated the alteplase vehicle after reconstitution. Use of this diluent for dilution prevented precipitation of the protein upon frozen storage at –20°C. In addition, the activity in ophthalmic use was found to be unchanged after storage for 6 months in the frozen state.[2159]

Alteplase (Genentech) concentrations of 0.5, 1, and 2 mg/mL in sterile water for injection were packaged as 1 mL of solution in 5-mL polypropylene syringes and sealed with rubber tip caps. Sample syringes were stored frozen at –70 and –25°C for up to 14 days as well as refrigerated at 2°C. Frozen samples were thawed at room temperature and stored under refrigeration for determination of fibrinolytic activity. Fibrinolytic activity after frozen storage at both –70 and –25°C remained near nominal initial concentrations for at least 14 days. Furthermore, the activity remained greater than 90% for up to 48 hours in all thawed samples subsequently stored at 2°C and was comparable to the activity of refrigerated solutions that had never been frozen. However, substantial and unacceptable losses of activity occurred after 72 hours under refrigeration whether previously frozen or not.[2327]

Genentech evaluated the activity of alteplase 1 mg/mL when reconstituted with sterile water for injection, packaged in glass vials, and stored frozen at –20°C for 32 days, followed by thawing at room temperature. The frozen alteplase solution remained physically and chemically comparable to newly reconstituted alteplase for at least 8 hours at room temperature after thawing.[2328]

Alteplase (Genentech) 1 mg/mL in sterile water for injection packaged in polypropylene syringes was frozen at –20°C for 6 months. Similar solutions in glass vials were frozen at –70°C for 2 weeks, thawed and kept at 23°C for 24 hours, and then refrozen at –70°C for 19 days. Little or no loss of alteplase bioactivity was found.[2400]

Compatibility Information
Solution Compatibility

Alteplase

Test Soln Name	Mfr	Mfr	Conc/L or %	Remarks	Ref	C/I
Dextrose 5%	a	GEN	0.5 g	Stable for up to 8 hr at room temperature	1(12/05)	C
Dextrose 5%	MG	GEN	160 mg	Precipitates immediately	1425	I
Dextrose 5%	MG	GEN	90 mg	Precipitate forms in 4 hr	1425	I
Sodium chloride 0.9%	a	GEN	0.5 g	Stable for up to 8 hr at room temperature	1(12/05)	C
Sodium chloride 0.9%	BA	GEN	10 mg	Physically compatible. Alteplase stable for 24 hr at room temperature	2501	C

a Tested in glass and PVC containers.

Additive Compatibility

Alteplase

Test Drug	Mfr	Conc/L or %	Mfr	Conc/L or %	Test Solution	Remarks	Ref	C/I
Dobutamine HCl	LI	5 g	GEN	0.5 g	D5W, NS	Yellow discoloration and precipitate form	1856	I
Dopamine HCl	ACC	5 g	GEN	0.5 g	D5W, NS	About 30% alteplase clot-lysis activity loss in 24 hr at 25°C	1856	I
Eptifibatide	ME	750 mg		1 g		Physically compatible and chemically stable for up to 24 hr at 25°C	3049	C
Heparin sodium	ES	40,000 units	GEN	0.5 g	NS	Heparin interacts with alteplase. Opalescence forms within 5 min with peak intensity at 4 hr at 25°C. Alteplase clot-lysis activity reduced slightly	1856	I

Additive Compatibility (Cont.)

Test Drug	Mfr	Conc/L or %	Mfr	Conc/L or %	Test Solution	Remarks	Ref	C/I
Lidocaine HCl	AST	4 g	GEN	0.5 g	D5W	Visually compatible with no alteplase clot-lysis activity loss in 24 hr at 25°C	1856	C
Lidocaine HCl	AST	4 g	GEN	0.5 g	NS	Visually compatible with 7% alteplase clot-lysis activity loss in 24 hr at 25°C	1856	C
Morphine sulfate	WY	1 g	GEN	0.5 g	NS	Visually compatible with 5 to 8% alteplase clot-lysis activity loss in 24 hr at 25°C	1856	C
Nitroglycerin	ACC	400 mg	GEN	0.5 g	D5W, NS	Visually compatible with 2% or less clot-lysis activity loss in 24 hr at 25°C	1856	C

Y-Site Injection Compatibility (1:1 Mixture)

Alteplase

Test Drug	Mfr	Conc	Mfr	Conc	Remarks	Ref	C/I
Bivalirudin	TMC	5 mg/mL[a]	GEN	1 mg/mL	Small aggregates form immediately	2373	I
Cangrelor tetrasodium	TMC	1 mg/mL[b]		1 mg/mL	Measured haze increases immediately and microparticulates form	3243	I
Dobutamine HCl	LI	2 mg/mL[a]	GEN	1 mg/mL	Haze in 20 min spectrophotometrically and in 2 hr visually	1340	I
Dopamine HCl	DU	8 mg/mL[a]	GEN	1 mg/mL	Haze noted in 4 hr	1340	I
Heparin sodium	ES	100 units/mL[a]	GEN	1 mg/mL	Haze noted in 24 hr	1340	I
Lidocaine HCl	AB	8 mg/mL[a]	GEN	1 mg/mL	Physically compatible for 6 days	1340	C
Metoprolol tartrate	CI	1 mg/mL	GEN	1 mg/mL	Visually compatible with no alteplase clot-lysis activity loss in 24 hr at 25°C	1856	C
Nitroglycerin	DU	0.2 mg/mL[a]	GEN	1 mg/mL	Haze noted in 24 hr	1340	I
Propranolol HCl	AY	1 mg/mL	GEN	1 mg/mL	Visually compatible. 2% clot-lysis activity loss in 24 hr at 25°C	1856	C

[a] Tested in dextrose 5%.

[b] Tested in sodium chloride 0.9%.

Amifostine
AHFS 92:56

Products

Amifostine is available in vials containing, in lyophilized form, 500 mg of amifostine on the anhydrous basis. The vial contents are reconstituted with 9.7 mL of sodium chloride 0.9% to yield a solution containing amifostine 50 mg/mL.[1(4/08)]

pH

Approximately 7.[234]

Trade Name(s)

Ethyol

Administration

When used as a chemoprotectant in adults, amifostine is administered once daily as a 15-minute intravenous infusion. The infusion is started 30 minutes before chemotherapy. When used as a radioprotectant in adults, amifostine is administered once daily as a 3-minute intravenous infusion started 15 to 30 minutes prior to radiation therapy. Patients should be well hydrated prior to intravenous infusion of amifostine and should maintain a supine position during the infusion. Only limited experience in administration to children or elderly patients is available.[1(4/08)] [4]

Stability

The intact vials may be stored at controlled room temperatures of 20 to 25°C. The manufacturer states that the reconstituted solution is chemically stable for 24 hours under refrigeration but only 5 hours at 25°C. The product should not be used if cloudiness or a precipitate is observed.[1(4/08)]

Compatibility Information

Solution Compatibility

Amifostine

Test Soln Name	Mfr	Mfr	Conc/L or %	Remarks	Ref	C/I
Sodium chloride 0.9%	a		5 and 40 g	Stable for 24 hr at 4°C and 5 hr at 25°C	1(4/08)	C

[a] Tested in PVC containers.

Y-Site Injection Compatibility (1:1 Mixture)

Amifostine

Test Drug	Mfr	Conc	Mfr	Conc	Remarks	Ref	C/I
Acyclovir sodium	BW	7 mg/mL[a]	USB	10 mg/mL[a]	Subvisible needles form in 1 hr. Visible particles form in 4 hr	1845	I
Amikacin sulfate	DU	5 mg/mL[a]	USB	10 mg/mL[a]	Physically compatible for 4 hr at 23°C	1845	C
Aminophylline	AMR	2.5 mg/mL[a]	USB	10 mg/mL[a]	Physically compatible for 4 hr at 23°C	1845	C
Amphotericin B	AD	0.6 mg/mL[a]	USB	10 mg/mL[a]	Turbidity forms immediately	1845	I
Ampicillin sodium	WY	20 mg/mL[b]	USB	10 mg/mL[a]	Physically compatible for 4 hr at 23°C	1845	C
Ampicillin sodium–sulbactam sodium	RR	20 mg/mL[b d]	USB	10 mg/mL[a]	Physically compatible for 4 hr at 23°C	1845	C
Aztreonam	SQ	40 mg/mL[a]	USB	10 mg/mL[a]	Physically compatible for 4 hr at 23°C	1845	C
Bleomycin sulfate	MJ	1 unit/mL[b]	USB	10 mg/mL[a]	Physically compatible for 4 hr at 23°C	1845	C
Bumetanide	RC	0.04 mg/mL[a]	USB	10 mg/mL[a]	Physically compatible for 4 hr at 23°C	1845	C
Buprenorphine HCl	RKC	0.04 mg/mL[a]	USB	10 mg/mL[a]	Physically compatible for 4 hr at 23°C	1845	C
Butorphanol tartrate	BR	0.04 mg/mL[a]	USB	10 mg/mL[a]	Physically compatible for 4 hr at 23°C	1845	C
Calcium gluconate	AMR	40 mg/mL[a]	USB	10 mg/mL[a]	Physically compatible for 4 hr at 23°C	1845	C

DOI: 10.37573/9781585286850.013

Y-Site Injection Compatibility (1:1 Mixture) (Cont.)

Test Drug	Mfr	Conc	Mfr	Conc	Remarks	Ref	C/I
Carboplatin	BR	5 mg/mL[a]	USB	10 mg/mL[a]	Physically compatible for 4 hr at 23°C	1845	C
Carmustine	BR	1.5 mg/mL[a]	USB	10 mg/mL[a]	Physically compatible for 4 hr at 23°C	1845	C
Cefazolin sodium	MAR	20 mg/mL[a]	USB	10 mg/mL[a]	Physically compatible for 4 hr at 23°C	1845	C
Cefotaxime sodium	HO	20 mg/mL[a]	USB	10 mg/mL[a]	Physically compatible for 4 hr at 23°C	1845	C
Cefotetan disodium	STU	20 mg/mL[a]	USB	10 mg/mL[a]	Physically compatible for 4 hr at 23°C	1845	C
Cefoxitin sodium	MSD	20 mg/mL[a]	USB	10 mg/mL[a]	Physically compatible for 4 hr at 23°C	1845	C
Ceftazidime	LI	40 mg/mL[a]	USB	10 mg/mL[a]	Physically compatible for 4 hr at 23°C	1845	C
Ceftriaxone sodium	RC	20 mg/mL[a]	USB	10 mg/mL[a]	Physically compatible for 4 hr at 23°C	1845	C
Cefuroxime sodium	GL	30 mg/mL[a]	USB	10 mg/mL[a]	Physically compatible for 4 hr at 23°C	1845	C
Chlorpromazine HCl	SCN	2 mg/mL[a]	USB	10 mg/mL[a]	Subvisible haze forms immediately	1845	I
Ciprofloxacin	MI	1 mg/mL[a]	USB	10 mg/mL[a]	Physically compatible for 4 hr at 23°C	1845	C
Cisplatin	BR	1 mg/mL	USB	10 mg/mL[a]	Subvisible haze forms in 4 hr	1845	I
Clindamycin phosphate	AST	10 mg/mL[a]	USB	10 mg/mL[a]	Physically compatible for 4 hr at 23°C	1845	C
Cyclophosphamide	MJ	10 mg/mL[a]	USB	10 mg/mL[a]	Physically compatible for 4 hr at 23°C	1845	C
Cytarabine	CET	50 mg/mL	USB	10 mg/mL[a]	Physically compatible for 4 hr at 23°C	1845	C
Dacarbazine	MI	4 mg/mL[a]	USB	10 mg/mL[a]	Physically compatible for 4 hr at 23°C	1845	C
Dactinomycin	ME	0.01 mg/mL[a]	USB	10 mg/mL[a]	Physically compatible for 4 hr at 23°C	1845	C
Daunorubicin HCl	WY	1 mg/mL[a]	USB	10 mg/mL[a]	Physically compatible for 4 hr at 23°C	1845	C
Dexamethasone sodium phosphate	AMR	1 mg/mL[a]	USB	10 mg/mL[a]	Physically compatible for 4 hr at 23°C	1845	C
Diphenhydramine HCl	PD	2 mg/mL[a]	USB	10 mg/mL[a]	Physically compatible for 4 hr at 23°C	1845	C
Dobutamine HCl	LI	4 mg/mL[a]	USB	10 mg/mL[a]	Physically compatible for 4 hr at 23°C	1845	C
Docetaxel	RPR	0.9 mg/mL[a]	ALZ	10 mg/mL[b]	Physically compatible for 4 hr at 23°C	2224	C
Dopamine HCl	AST	3.2 mg/mL[a]	USB	10 mg/mL[a]	Physically compatible for 4 hr at 23°C	1845	C
Doxorubicin HCl	CET	2 mg/mL	USB	10 mg/mL[a]	Physically compatible for 4 hr at 23°C	1845	C
Doxycycline hyclate	LY	1 mg/mL[a]	USB	10 mg/mL[a]	Physically compatible for 4 hr at 23°C	1845	C
Droperidol	JN	0.4 mg/mL[a]	USB	10 mg/mL[a]	Physically compatible for 4 hr at 23°C	1845	C
Enalaprilat	MSD	0.1 mg/mL[a]	USB	10 mg/mL[a]	Physically compatible for 4 hr at 23°C	1845	C
Etoposide	BR	0.4 mg/mL[a]	USB	10 mg/mL[a]	Physically compatible for 4 hr at 23°C	1845	C
Famotidine	ME	2 mg/mL[a]	USB	10 mg/mL[a]	Physically compatible for 4 hr at 23°C	1845	C
Floxuridine	RC	3 mg/mL[a]	USB	10 mg/mL[a]	Physically compatible for 4 hr at 23°C	1845	C
Fluconazole	RR	2 mg/mL	USB	10 mg/mL[a]	Physically compatible for 4 hr at 23°C	1845	C
Fludarabine phosphate	BX	1 mg/mL[a]	USB	10 mg/mL[a]	Physically compatible for 4 hr at 23°C	1845	C
Fluorouracil	AD	16 mg/mL[a]	USB	10 mg/mL[a]	Physically compatible for 4 hr at 23°C	1845	C
Furosemide	AB	3 mg/mL[a]	USB	10 mg/mL[a]	Physically compatible for 4 hr at 23°C	1845	C
Gallium nitrate	FUJ	0.4 mg/mL[a]	USB	10 mg/mL[a]	Physically compatible for 4 hr at 23°C	1845	C
Ganciclovir sodium	SY	20 mg/mL[a]	USB	10 mg/mL[a]	Crystalline needles form immediately. Dense precipitate in 1 hr	1845	I

Y-Site Injection Compatibility (1:1 Mixture) (Cont.)

Test Drug	Mfr	Conc	Mfr	Conc	Remarks	Ref	C/I
Gemcitabine HCl	LI	10 mg/mL[b]	USB	10 mg/mL[b]	Physically compatible for 4 hr at 23°C	2226	C
Gentamicin sulfate	ES	5 mg/mL[a]	USB	10 mg/mL[a]	Physically compatible for 4 hr at 23°C	1845	C
Granisetron HCl	SKB	0.05 mg/mL[a]	USB	10 mg/mL[a]	Physically compatible for 4 hr at 23°C	2000	C
Haloperidol lactate	MN	0.2 mg/mL[a]	USB	10 mg/mL[a]	Physically compatible for 4 hr at 23°C	1845	C
Heparin sodium	ES	100 units/mL[a]	USB	10 mg/mL[a]	Physically compatible for 4 hr at 23°C	1845	C
Hydrocortisone sodium succinate	UP	1 mg/mL[a]	USB	10 mg/mL[a]	Physically compatible for 4 hr at 23°C	1845	C
Hydromorphone HCl	AST	0.5 mg/mL[a]	USB	10 mg/mL[a]	Physically compatible for 4 hr at 23°C	1845	C
Hydroxyzine HCl	WI	4 mg/mL[a]	USB	10 mg/mL[a]	Subvisible haze forms immediately	1845	I
Idarubicin HCl	AD	0.5 mg/mL[a]	USB	10 mg/mL[a]	Physically compatible for 4 hr at 23°C	1845	C
Ifosfamide	MJ	25 mg/mL[a]	USB	10 mg/mL[a]	Physically compatible for 4 hr at 23°C	1845	C
Imipenem–cilastatin sodium	MSD	10 mg/mL[a f]	USB	10 mg/mL[a]	Physically compatible for 4 hr at 23°C	1845	C
Leucovorin calcium	LE	2 mg/mL[a]	USB	10 mg/mL[a]	Physically compatible for 4 hr at 23°C	1845	C
Lorazepam	WY	0.1 mg/mL[a]	USB	10 mg/mL[a]	Physically compatible for 4 hr at 23°C	1845	C
Magnesium sulfate	AST	100 mg/mL[a]	USB	10 mg/mL[a]	Physically compatible for 4 hr at 23°C	1845	C
Mannitol	BA	15%	USB	10 mg/mL[a]	Physically compatible for 4 hr at 23°C	1845	C
Mechlorethamine HCl	MSD	1 mg/mL	USB	10 mg/mL[a]	Physically compatible for 4 hr at 23°C	1845	C
Meperidine HCl	WY	4 mg/mL[a]	USB	10 mg/mL[a]	Physically compatible for 4 hr at 23°C	1845	C
Mesna	MJ	10 mg/mL[a]	USB	10 mg/mL[a]	Physically compatible for 4 hr at 23°C	1845	C
Methotrexate sodium	LE	15 mg/mL[a]	USB	10 mg/mL[a]	Physically compatible for 4 hr at 23°C	1845	C
Methylprednisolone sodium succinate	AB	5 mg/mL[a]	USB	10 mg/mL[a]	Physically compatible for 4 hr at 23°C	1845	C
Metoclopramide HCl	ES	5 mg/mL	USB	10 mg/mL[a]	Physically compatible for 4 hr at 23°C	1845	C
Metronidazole	BA	5 mg/mL	USB	10 mg/mL[a]	Physically compatible for 4 hr at 23°C	1845	C
Mitomycin	BR	0.5 mg/mL	USB	10 mg/mL[a]	Physically compatible for 4 hr at 23°C	1845	C
Mitoxantrone HCl	LE	0.5 mg/mL[a]	USB	10 mg/mL[a]	Physically compatible for 4 hr at 23°C	1845	C
Morphine sulfate	AST	1 mg/mL[a]	USB	10 mg/mL[a]	Physically compatible for 4 hr at 23°C	1845	C
Nalbuphine HCl	AST	10 mg/mL	USB	10 mg/mL[a]	Physically compatible for 4 hr at 23°C	1845	C
Ondansetron HCl	GL	1 mg/mL[a]	USB	10 mg/mL[a]	Physically compatible for 4 hr at 23°C	1845	C
Pemetrexed disodium	LI	20 mg/mL[b]	MDI	10 mg/mL[b]	Physically compatible for 4 hr at 23°C	2564	C
Potassium chloride	AB	0.1 mEq/mL[a]	USB	10 mg/mL[a]	Physically compatible for 4 hr at 23°C	1845	C
Prochlorperazine edisylate	SN	0.5 mg/mL[a]	USB	10 mg/mL[a]	Immediate increase in measured haze	1845	I
Promethazine HCl	ES	2 mg/mL[a]	USB	10 mg/mL[a]	Physically compatible for 4 hr at 23°C	1845	C
Ranitidine HCl	GL	2 mg/mL[a]	USB	10 mg/mL[a]	Physically compatible for 4 hr at 23°C	1845	C
Sodium bicarbonate	AST	1 mEq/mL	USB	10 mg/mL[a]	Physically compatible for 4 hr at 23°C	1845	C
Streptozocin	UP	40 mg/mL[a]	USB	10 mg/mL[a]	Physically compatible for 4 hr at 23°C	1845	C
Teniposide	BR	0.1 mg/mL[a]	USB	10 mg/mL[a]	Physically compatible for 4 hr at 23°C	1845	C
Thiotepa	LE[c]	1 mg/mL[a]	USB	10 mg/mL[a]	Physically compatible for 4 hr at 23°C	1845	C

Y-Site Injection Compatibility (1:1 Mixture) (Cont.)

Test Drug	Mfr	Conc	Mfr	Conc	Remarks	Ref	C/I
Tobramycin sulfate	LI	5 mg/mL[a]	USB	10 mg/mL[a]	Physically compatible for 4 hr at 23°C	1845	C
Trimethoprim–sulfamethoxazole	ES	0.8 mg/mL[a][e]	USB	10 mg/mL[a]	Physically compatible for 4 hr at 23°C	1845	C
Vancomycin HCl	AB	10 mg/mL[a]	USB	10 mg/mL[a]	Physically compatible for 4 hr at 23°C	1845	C
Vinblastine sulfate	LI	0.12 mg/mL[a]	USB	10 mg/mL[a]	Physically compatible for 4 hr at 23°C	1845	C
Vincristine sulfate	LI	0.05 mg/mL[a]	USB	10 mg/mL[a]	Physically compatible for 4 hr at 23°C	1845	C
Zidovudine	BW	4 mg/mL[a]	USB	10 mg/mL[a]	Physically compatible for 4 hr at 23°C	1845	C

[a] Tested in dextrose 5%.

[b] Tested in sodium chloride 0.9%.

[c] Powder fill formulation tested.

[d] Ampicillin component. Ampicillin in a 2:1 fixed-ratio concentration with sulbactam.

[e] Trimethoprim component. Trimethoprim in a 1:5 fixed-ratio concentration with sulfamethoxazole.

[f] Not specified whether concentration refers to single component or combined components.

Selected Revisions December 13, 2018. © Copyright, October 1998. American Society of Health-System Pharmacists, Inc.

Amikacin Sulfate
AHFS 8:12.02

Products

Amikacin sulfate is available in a concentration of 250 mg/mL. Also present are sodium metabisulfite, sodium citrate, and sulfuric acid to adjust pH.[1(12/07)]

pH

4.5.[291] The range is 3.5 to 5.5.[4]

Osmolality

The osmolality of amikacin sulfate 500 mg was calculated for the following dilutions:[1054]

Diluent	Osmolality (mOsm/kg)	
	50 mL	100 mL
Dextrose 5%	353	319
Sodium chloride 0.9%	383	349

Sodium Content

The sodium content of amikacin sulfate 50 mg/mL is 0.064 mEq/mL; for the 250-mg/mL concentration, the sodium content is 0.319 mEq/mL.[291]

Administration

Amikacin sulfate may be administered by intramuscular injection and intravenous infusion; for intravenous infusion, 500 mg may be diluted in 100 to 200 mL of compatible infusion solution and administered to adults over 30 to 60 minutes. The diluent volume should be sufficient for drug infusion over 1 to 2 hours in infants and over 30 to 60 minutes in older children.[1(12/07) 4]

Stability

Amikacin sulfate is supplied as a colorless to pale yellow or light straw-colored solution.[4] It was reported that aqueous solutions of amikacin sulfate in concentrations of 37.5 to 250 mg/mL retained greater than 90% for up to 36 months at 25°C, 12 months at 37°C, and 3 months at 56°C.[291] Aqueous solutions of amikacin sulfate are subject to color darkening because of air oxidation. However, this change in color has no effect on potency.[291]

Syringes

Amikacin sulfate (Bristol) 750 mg diluted with 1 mL of sodium chloride 0.9% to a final volume of 4 mL was stable, showing about a 2% loss when stored in polypropylene syringes (Becton Dickinson) for 48 hours at 23°C under fluorescent light.[1159]

Sorption

Amikacin sulfate was shown not to exhibit sorption to polyvinyl chloride (PVC) bags or sets and multilayer bags composed of polyethylene, polyamide, and polypropylene.[2269]

Central Venous Catheter

Amikacin sulfate (Apothecon) 1 mg/mL in dextrose 5% was found to be compatible with the ARROWg+ard Blue Plus (Arrow International) chlorhexidine-bearing triple-lumen central catheter. Delivery of the amikacin sulfate ranged from 92 to 98% of the initial concentration among the 3 lumens. Furthermore, chlorhexidine delivered from the catheter remained at trace amounts with no substantial increase due to the delivery of the drug through the catheter.[2335]

Compatibility Information

Solution Compatibility

Amikacin sulfate

Test Soln Name	Mfr	Mfr	Conc/L or %	Remarks	Ref	C/I
Dextrose 5% in Ringer's injection	BA	BR	250 mg and 5 g	Compatible and stable for 24 hr at 25°C, 60 days at 4°C, 30 days at −15°C	292	C
Dextrose 5% in Ringer's injection, lactated	BA	BR	250 mg and 5 g	Compatible and stable for 24 hr at 25°C, 60 days at 4°C, 30 days at −15°C	292	C
Dextrose 2.5% in sodium chloride 0.45%	BA	BR	250 mg and 5 g	Compatible and stable for 24 hr at 25°C, 60 days at 4°C, 30 days at −15°C	292	C
Dextrose 2.5% in sodium chloride 0.9%	BA	BR	250 mg and 5 g	Compatible and stable for 24 hr at 25°C, 60 days at 4°C, 30 days at −15°C	292	C
Dextrose 5% in sodium chloride 0.225%	BA	BR	250 mg and 5 g	Compatible and stable for 24 hr at 25°C, 60 days at 4°C, 30 days at −15°C	292	C
Dextrose 5% in sodium chloride 0.45%	BA	BR	250 mg and 5 g	Compatible and stable for 24 hr at 25°C, 60 days at 4°C, 30 days at −15°C	292	C

DOI: 10.37573/9781585286850.014

Solution Compatibility (Cont.)

Test Soln Name	Mfr	Mfr	Conc/L or %	Remarks	Ref	C/I
Dextrose 5% in sodium chloride 0.9%	BA	BR	250 mg and 5 g	Compatible and stable for 24 hr at 25°C, 60 days at 4°C, 30 days at −15°C	292	C
Dextrose 10% in sodium chloride 0.9%	BA	BR	250 mg and 5 g	Compatible and stable for 24 hr at 25°C, 60 days at 4°C, 30 days at −15°C	292	C
Dextrose 5%	BA	BR	250 mg and 5 g	Compatible and stable for 24 hr at 25°C, 60 days at 4°C, 30 days at −15°C	292	C
Dextrose 5%	TR[a]	BR	5 g	Physically compatible and potency retained for 24 hr at room temperature	518	C
Dextrose 5%	TR[a]	BR	20 g	Physically compatible. 4% loss in 24 hr at room temperature and 6% loss frozen for 30 days at −20°C	555	C
Dextrose 5%	MG[b]	BR	4 g	Stable for 48 hr at 25°C in light	981	C
Dextrose 5%	AB[a]	BR	5 g	Visually compatible. Stable for 48 hr at 25°C in light and 4°C in dark	1541	C
Dextrose 10%	BA	BR	250 mg and 5 g	Compatible and stable for 24 hr at 25°C, 60 days at 4°C, 30 days at −15°C	292	C
Dextrose 10%	SO	BR	11.9 g[c]	Visually compatible with no loss in 30 days at 5°C	1731	C
Dextrose 10%	SO	BR	22.7 g[c]	Visually compatible with no loss in 30 days at 5°C	1731	C
Dextrose 20%	BA	BR	250 mg and 5 g	Compatible and stable for 24 hr at 25°C, 60 days at 4°C, 30 days at −15°C	292	C
Normosol M in dextrose 5%	AB	BR	250 mg and 5 g	Compatible and stable for 24 hr at 25°C, 60 days at 4°C, 30 days at −15°C	292	C
Normosol R	AB	BR	250 mg and 5 g	Compatible and stable for 24 hr at 25°C, 60 days at 4°C, 30 days at −15°C	292	C
Normosol R in dextrose 5%	AB	BR	250 mg and 5 g	Compatible and stable for 24 hr at 25°C, 60 days at 4°C, 30 days at −15°C	292	C
Ringer's injection	BA	BR	250 mg and 5 g	Compatible and stable for 24 hr at 25°C, 60 days at 4°C, 30 days at −15°C	292	C
Ringer's injection, lactated	BA	BR	250 mg and 5 g	Compatible and stable for 24 hr at 25°C, 60 days at 4°C, 30 days at −15°C	292	C
Sodium chloride 0.225%	BA	BR	250 mg and 5 g	Compatible and stable for 24 hr at 25°C, 60 days at 4°C, 30 days at −15°C	292	C
Sodium chloride 0.45%	BA	BR	250 mg and 5 g	Compatible and stable for 24 hr at 25°C, 60 days at 4°C, 30 days at −15°C	292	C
Sodium chloride 0.9%	BA	BR	250 mg and 5 g	Compatible and stable for 24 hr at 25°C, 60 days at 4°C, 30 days at −15°C	292	C
Sodium chloride 0.9%	TR[a]	BR	5 g	Physically compatible. Stable for 24 hr at room temperature	518	C
Sodium chloride 0.9%	MG[b]	BR	4 g	Stable for 48 hr at 25°C in light	981	C
Sodium chloride 0.9%	AB[a]	BR	5 g	Visually compatible. Stable for 48 hr at 25°C in light and 4°C in dark	1541	C
Sodium lactate ⅙ M	BA	BR	250 mg and 5 g	Compatible and stable for 24 hr at 25°C, 60 days at 4°C, 30 days at −15°C	292	C
TPN #107[d]			150 mg	Activity retained for 24 hr at 21°C	1326	C

[a] Tested in PVC containers.

[b] Tested in glass containers.

[c] Tested as a concentrate in glass vials.

[d] Refer to Appendix for the composition of parenteral nutrition solutions. TPN indicates a 2-in-1 admixture.

Additive Compatibility

Amikacin sulfate

Test Drug	Mfr	Conc/L or %	Mfr	Conc/L or %	Test Solution	Remarks	Ref	C/I
Aminophylline	SE	5 g	BR	5 g	LR, NS, R, SL	Physically compatible and amikacin stable for 24 hr at 25°C. Amino-phylline not analyzed	294	C
Aminophylline	SE	5 g	BR	5 g	D5LR, D5R, D5S, D5W, D10W	Over 10% amikacin loss after 8 hr but within 24 hr at 25°C. Amino-phylline not analyzed	294	I
Amphotericin B	SQ	100 mg	BR	5 g	D5LR, D5R, D5S, D5W, D10W, LR, NS, R, SL	Precipitates immediately	293	I
Ampicillin sodium	BR	30 g	BR	5 g	D5LR, D5R, D5S, D5W, D10W, LR, NS, R, SL	Over 10% ampicillin loss in 4 hr at 25°C	293	I
Ascorbic acid	CO[a]	5 g	BR	5 g	D5LR, D5R, D5S, D5W, D10W, LR, NS, R, SL	Physically compatible and both stable for 24 hr at 25°C	294	C
Bleomycin sulfate	BR	20 and 30 units	BR	1.25 g	NS	Physically compatible. Bleomycin stable for 1 week at 4°C. Amikacin not tested	763	C
Calcium chloride	UP	1 g	BR	5 g	D5LR, D5R, D5S, D5W, D10W, LR, NS, R, SL	Physically compatible and both stable for 24 hr at 25°C	294	C
Calcium gluconate	UP	500 mg	BR	5 g	D5LR, D5R, D5S, D5W, D10W, LR, NS, R, SL	Physically compatible and both stable for 24 hr at 25°C	294	C
Cefazolin sodium	LI	20 g	BR	5 g	D5LR, D5R, D5S, D5W, D10W, LR, NS, R, SL	Both drugs stable for 8 hr at 25°C. Turbidity observed at 24 hr	293	I
Cefepime HCl	BR	40 g	BR	6 g	D5W, NS	Visually compatible with 6% cefepime loss in 24 hr at room temperature and 4% loss in 7 days at 5°C. No amikacin loss	1681	C
Cefotaxime sodium	RS	50 mg	BR	25 mg	D5W	33% loss of amikacin in 2 hr at 22°C	504	I
Cefotaxime sodium	RS	50 mg	BR	15 mg	D5W	Under 8% loss of amikacin in 24 hr at 22°C	504	C
Cefoxitin sodium	MSD	5 g	BR	5 g	D5S	9% cefoxitin loss at 25°C and none at 5°C in 48 hr. No amikacin loss at 25°C and 1% at 5°C in 48 hr	308	C
Ceftazidime	GL	50 mg	BR	25 mg	D5W	28% loss of amikacin in 2 hr at 22°C	504	I
Ceftazidime	GL	50 mg	BR	15 mg	D5W	17% loss of amikacin in 24 hr at 22°C	504	I
Ceftriaxone sodium	RC	100 mg	BR	15 and 25 mg	D5W	6% loss of amikacin in 24 hr at 22°C	504	C
Chloramphenicol sodium succinate	PD	10 g	BR	5 g	D5LR, D5R, D5S, D5W, D10W, LR, NS, R, SL	Physically compatible and both stable for 24 hr at 25°C	293	C
Chlorothiazide sodium	MSD	10 mg	BR	5 g	D5LR, D5R, D5S, D5W, D10W, LR, NS, R, SL	Precipitate forms within 4 hr at 25°C	294	I
Ciprofloxacin	MI	1.6 g	BR	4.1 g	D5W, NS	Visually compatible and both stable for 48 hr at 25°C under fluo-rescent light	1541	C
Ciprofloxacin	BAY	2 g	APC	4.9 g	D5W	Visually compatible with no loss of ciprofloxacin in 24 hr at 22°C under fluorescent light. Amikacin not tested	2413	C
Clindamycin phos-phate	UP	6 g	BR	5 g	D5LR, D5R, D5S, D5W, D10W, LR, NS, R, SL	Physically compatible and amikacin stable for 24 hr at 25°C. Clinda-mycin not analyzed	293	C

Additive Compatibility (Cont.)

Test Drug	Mfr	Conc/L or %	Mfr	Conc/L or %	Test Solution	Remarks	Ref	C/I
Clindamycin phosphate	UP	9 g	BR	4 g	D5W, NS[b]	Both stable for 48 hr at 25°C under fluorescent light	981	C
Cloxacillin sodium	BR	10 g	BR	5 g	D5LR, D5R, D5S, D5W, D10W, LR, NS, R, SL	Physically compatible and both stable for 24 hr at 25°C	293	C
Colistimethate sodium	WC	500 mg	BR	5 g	D5LR, D5R, D5S, D5W, D10W, LR, NS, R, SL	Physically compatible and amikacin stable for 24 hr at 25°C. Colistimethate not analyzed	293	C
Dexamethasone sodium phosphate	MSD	40 mg	BR	5 g	D5LR, D5R, D5S, D5W, D10W, LR, NS, R, SL	Physically compatible and both stable for 24 hr at 25°C	294	C
Dexamethasone sodium phosphate	MSD	40 mg	BR	5 g	D2.5S	16% dexamethasone loss in 4 hr at 25°C	294	I
Dimenhydrinate	SE	100 mg	BR	5 g	D5LR, D5R, D5S, D5W, D10W, LR, NS, R, SL	Physically compatible and both stable for 24 hr at 25°C	294	C
Diphenhydramine HCl	PD	100 mg	BR	5 g	D5LR, D5R, D5S, D5W, D10W, LR, NS, R, SL	Physically compatible and both stable for 24 hr at 25°C	294	C
Epinephrine HCl	PD	2.5 mg	BR	5 g	D5LR, D5R, D5S, D5W, D10W, LR, NS, R, SL	Physically compatible and both stable for 24 hr at 25°C	294	C
Fluconazole	PF	1 g	BR	2.5 g	D5W	Visually compatible with no fluconazole loss in 72 hr at 25°C under fluorescent light. Amikacin not tested	1677	C
Furosemide	HO	160 mg	BR	2 g	D5W, NS	Transient cloudiness, then visually compatible for 24 hr at 21°C	876	?
Heparin sodium	AB	30,000 units	BR	5 g	D5LR, D5R, D5S, D5W, D10W, LR, NS, R, SL	Precipitates immediately	294	I
Hyaluronidase	SE	150 units	BR	5 g	D5LR, D5R, D5S, D5W, D10W, LR, NS, R, SL	Physically compatible and amikacin stable for 24 hr at 25°C. Hyaluronidase not analyzed	294	C
Hydrocortisone sodium succinate	UP	200 mg	BR	5 g	D5LR, D5R, D5S, D5W, D10W, LR, NS, R, SL	Physically compatible and both stable for 24 hr at 25°C	294	C
Lincomycin HCl	UP	10 g	BR	5 g	D5LR, D5R, D5S, D5W, D10W, LR, NS, R, SL	Physically compatible and both stable for 24 hr at 25°C	293	C
Mannitol	BA	20%	BR	250 mg and 5 g		Compatible and stable for 24 hr at 25°C, 60 days at 4°C, 30 days at –15°C	292	C
Norepinephrine bitartrate	WI	8 mg	BR	5 g	D5LR, D5R, D5S, D5W, D10W, LR, NS, R, SL	Physically compatible and both stable for 24 hr at 25°C	294	C
Oxacillin sodium	BR	2 g	BR	5 g	D5LR, D5R, D5S, D5W, D10W, LR, NS, R	Physically compatible and both stable for 24 hr at 25°C	293	C
Oxacillin sodium	BR	2 g	BR	5 g	NR, SL	Oxacillin stable for 8 hr at 25°C. Over 10% loss in 24 hr	293	I
Penicillin G potassium	LI	20 million units	BR	5 g	D5LR, D5R, D5S, D5W, D10W, LR, NS, R, SL	Physically compatible and both stable for 24 hr at 25°C	293	C
Pentobarbital sodium	AB	100 mg	BR	5 g	D5LR, D5R, D5S, D5W, D10W, LR, NS, R, SL	Physically compatible and both stable for 24 hr at 25°C	294	C
Phenobarbital sodium	LI	300 mg	BR	5 g	D5LR, D5R, D5S, D5W, D10W, LR, NS, R, SL	Physically compatible and both stable for 24 hr at 25°C	294	C
Phenytoin sodium	PD	250 mg	BR	5 g	D5LR, D5R, D5S, D5W, D10W, LR, NS, R, SL	Precipitates immediately	294	I

Additive Compatibility (Cont.)

Test Drug	Mfr	Conc/L or %	Mfr	Conc/L or %	Test Solution	Remarks	Ref	C/I
Phytonadione	MSD	200 mg	BR	5 g	D5LR, D5R, D5S, D5W, D10W, LR, NS, R, SL	Physically compatible and amikacin stable for 24 hr at 25°C. Phytonadione not analyzed	294	C
Polymyxin B sulfate	BW	200 mg	BR	5 g	D5LR, D5R, D5S, D5W, D10W, LR, NS, R, SL	Physically compatible and amikacin stable for 24 hr at 25°C. Polymyxin not analyzed	293	C
Potassium chloride	LI	3 g	BR	5 g	D5LR, D5R, D5S, D5W, D10W, LR, NS, R, SL	Physically compatible and both stable for 24 hr at 25°C	294	C
Prochlorperazine edisylate	SKF	20 mg	BR	5 g	D5LR, D5R, D5S, D5W, D10W, LR, NS, R, SL	Physically compatible and both stable for 24 hr at 25°C	294	C
Promethazine HCl	WY	100 mg	BR	5 g	D5LR, D5R, D5S, D5W, D10W, LR, NS, R, SL	Physically compatible and both stable for 24 hr at 25°C	294	C
Ranitidine HCl	GL	100 mg	BR	1 g	D5W	Physically compatible for 24 hr at ambient temperature in light	1151	C
Ranitidine HCl	GL	50 mg and 2 g		2.5 g	D5W	Physically compatible. Ranitidine stable for 24 hr at 25°C. Amikacin not tested	1515	C
Sodium bicarbonate	BR	15 g	BR	5 g	D5LR, D5R, D5S, D5W, D10W, LR, NS, R, SL	Physically compatible and both stable for 24 hr at 25°C	294	C
Succinylcholine chloride	SQ	2 g	BR	5 g	D5LR, D5R, D5S, D5W, D10W, LR, NS, R, SL	Physically compatible and both stable for 24 hr at 25°C	294	C
Vancomycin HCl	LI	2 g	BR	5 g	D5LR, D5R, D5S, D5W, D10W, LR, NS, R, SL	Physically compatible and amikacin stable for 24 hr at 25°C. Vancomycin not tested	293	C
Verapamil HCl	KN	80 mg	BR	2 g	D5W, NS	Physically compatible for 24 hr	764	C

[a] Present as calcium ascorbate.

[b] Tested in glass containers.

Drugs in Syringe Compatibility

Amikacin sulfate

Test Drug	Mfr	Amt	Mfr	Amt	Remarks	Ref	C/I
Caffeine citrate		20 mg/1 mL	BED	250 mg/1 mL	Visually compatible for 4 hr at 25°C	2440	C
Clindamycin phosphate	UP	900 mg/6 mL	BR	750 mg/4 mL[a]	Physically compatible with little loss of either drug in 48 hr at 25°C	1159	C
Doxapram HCl	RB	400 mg/20 mL		100 mg/2 mL	Physically compatible with no doxapram loss in 24 hr	1177	C
Heparin sodium		2500 units/1 mL		100 mg	Turbidity or precipitate forms within 5 min	1053	I
Pantoprazole sodium	[b]	4 mg/1 mL		250 mg/1 mL	Precipitates	2574	I

[a] Diluted to 4 mL with 1 mL of sodium chloride 0.9%.

[b] Test performed using the formulation WITHOUT edetate disodium.

Y-Site Injection Compatibility (1:1 Mixture)

Amikacin sulfate

Test Drug	Mfr	Conc	Mfr	Conc	Remarks	Ref	C/I
Acyclovir sodium	BW	5 mg/mL[a]	BR	5 mg/mL[a]	Physically compatible for 4 hr at 25°C	1157	C
Allopurinol sodium	BW	3 mg/mL[b]	BR	5 mg/mL[b]	Crystals and flakes form within 1 hr	1686	I
Amifostine	USB	10 mg/mL[a]	DU	5 mg/mL[a]	Physically compatible for 4 hr at 23°C	1845	C
Amiodarone HCl	LZ	4 mg/mL[c]	BR	5 mg/mL[c]	Physically compatible for 4 hr at room temperature	1444	C
Amsacrine	NCI	1 mg/mL[a]	BR	5 mg/mL[a]	Visually compatible for 4 hr at 22°C	1381	C
Anidulafungin	VIC	0.5 mg/mL[a]	APC	5 mg/mL[a]	Physically compatible for 4 hr at 23°C	2617	C
Azithromycin	PF	2 mg/mL[e]	VHA	100 mg/mL[e o]	Whitish-yellow microcrystals found	2368	I
Aztreonam	SQ	40 mg/mL[a]	BMS	5 mg/mL[a]	Physically compatible for 4 hr at 23°C	1758	C
Bivalirudin	TMC	5 mg/mL[a]	APO	5 mg/mL[a]	Physically compatible for 4 hr at 23°C	2373	C
Cangrelor tetrasodium	TMC	1 mg/mL[b]		5 mg/mL[b]	Physically compatible for 4 hr	3243	C
Caspofungin acetate	ME	0.7 mg/mL[b]	HOS	5 mg/mL[b]	Physically compatible for 4 hr at room temperature	2758	C
Cefepime HCl	BMS	120 mg/mL[n]		15 mg/mL	Physically compatible with less than 10% cefepime loss. Amikacin not tested	2513	C
Ceftaroline fosamil	FOR	2.22 mg/mL[a b d]	HOS	5 mg/mL[a b d]	Physically compatible for 4 hr at 23°C	2826	C
Ceftazidime	SKB	125 mg/mL		1.5 mg/mL	Visually compatible with less than 10% loss of both drugs in 1 hr	2434	C
Ceftazidime	GSK	120 mg/mL[n]		15 mg/mL	Physically compatible with less than 10% ceftazidime loss. Amikacin not tested	2513	C
Ceftazidime–avibactam sodium	ALL	20 mg/mL[u v]			Physically compatible for up to 4 hr at room temperature	3004	C
Ceftolozane sulfate–tazobactam sodium	CUB	10 mg/mL[c s]	HER	5 mg/mL[c]	Physically compatible for 2 hr	3262	C
Cisatracurium besylate	GW	0.1, 2, 5 mg/mL[a]	AB	5 mg/mL[a]	Physically compatible for 4 hr at 23°C	2074	C
Cloxacillin sodium	SMX	100 mg/mL	SZ	250 mg/mL	Large particles form immediately	3245	I
Cyclophosphamide	MJ	20 mg/mL[a]	BR	5 mg/mL[a]	Physically compatible for 4 hr at 25°C	1194	C
Defibrotide sodium	JAZ	8 mg/mL[b]	MYL	5 mg/mL[b]	Solution became milky white, opaque or opalescent	3149	I
Dexamethasone sodium phosphate	AMR	4 mg/mL	SQ	50 mg/mL[e]	Visually compatible for 24 hr at room temperature in test tubes. No precipitate found on filter from Y-site delivery	2063	C
Dexmedetomidine HCl	AB	4 mcg/mL[b]	APO	5 mg/mL[b]	Physically compatible for 4 hr at 23°C	2383	C
Diltiazem HCl	MMD	5 mg/mL	BR	5[b] and 250 mg/mL	Visually compatible	1807	C
Docetaxel	RPR	0.9 mg/mL[a]	AB	5 mg/mL[a]	Physically compatible for 4 hr at 23°C	2224	C
Doripenem	JJ	5 mg/mL[a b]	BED	5 mg/mL[a b]	Physically compatible for 4 hr at 23°C	2743	C
Enalaprilat	MSD	0.05 mg/mL[b]	BR	2 mg/mL[a]	Physically compatible for 24 hr at room temperature under fluorescent light	1355	C
Esmolol HCl	DCC	10 mg/mL[a]	BR	5 mg/mL[a]	Physically compatible for 24 hr at 22°C	1169	C
Etoposide phosphate	BR	5 mg/mL[a]	APC	5 mg/mL[a]	Physically compatible for 4 hr at 23°C	2218	C

Y-Site Injection Compatibility (1:1 Mixture) (Cont.)

Test Drug	Mfr	Conc	Mfr	Conc	Remarks	Ref	C/I
Fenoldopam mesylate	AB	80 mcg/mL[b]	APO	5 mg/mL[b]	Physically compatible for 4 hr at 23°C	2467	C
Filgrastim	AMG	30 mcg/mL[a]	ES	5 mg/mL[a]	Physically compatible for 4 hr at 22°C	1687	C
Filgrastim	AMG	10[f] and 40[a] mcg/mL	BMS	5 mg/mL[a]	Visually compatible. Little loss of filgrastim and fluconazole in 4 hr at 25°C	2060	C
Fluconazole	RR	2 mg/mL	BR	20 mg/mL	Physically compatible for 24 hr at 25°C	1407	C
Fludarabine phosphate	BX	1 mg/mL[a]	BR	5 mg/mL[a]	Visually compatible for 4 hr at 22°C	1439	C
Foscarnet sodium	AST	24 mg/mL	BR	20 mg/mL	Physically compatible for 24 hr at room temperature under fluorescent light	1335	C
Furosemide	HO	10 mg/mL	BR	2 mg/mL[c]	Physically compatible for 24 hr at 21°C	876	C
Gemcitabine HCl	LI	10 mg/mL[b]	APC	5 mg/mL[b]	Physically compatible for 4 hr at 23°C	2226	C
Granisetron HCl	SKB	0.05 mg/mL[a]	AB	5 mg/mL[a]	Physically compatible for 4 hr at 23°C	2000	C
Hetastarch in lactated electrolyte	AB	6%	APC	5 mg/mL[a]	Physically compatible for 4 hr at 23°C	2339	C
Hetastarch in sodium chloride 0.9%	DCC	6%	BR	5 mg/mL[a]	Small crystals form immediately after mixing and persist for 4 hr	1313	I
Hydromorphone HCl	WY	0.2 mg/mL[a]	BR	5 mg/mL[a]	Physically compatible for 4 hr at 25°C	987	C
Ibuprofen lysinate	OVA	10 mg/mL	HOS	50 mg/mL[a]	Measured turbidity increased immediately and solution became milky white and opaque	3541	I
Ibuprofen lysinate	OVA	10 mg/mL	HOS	50 mg/mL[b]	Measured turbidity increased immediately and solution became milky white and opaque with particulate matter present	3541	I
Ibuprofen lysinate	OVA	10 mg/mL	HOS	250 mg/mL	Measured turbidity increased immediately and solution became milky white and opaque with particulate matter present	3541	I
Idarubicin HCl	AD	1 mg/mL[b]	BR	5 mg/mL[a]	Visually compatible for 24 hr at 25°C	1525	C
Isavuconazonium sulfate	ASP	1.5 mg/mL[c]	HER	5 mg/mL[c]	Physically compatible for 2 hr	3263	C
Labetalol HCl	SC	1 mg/mL[a]	BR	5 mg/mL[a]	Physically compatible for 24 hr at 18°C	1171	C
Levofloxacin	OMN	5 mg/mL	BED	50 mg/mL	Visually compatible for 4 hr at 24°C	2233	C
Linezolid	PHU	2 mg/mL	AB	5 mg/mL[a]	Physically compatible for 4 hr at 23°C	2264	C
Lorazepam	WY	0.33 mg/mL[b]	BMS	5 mg/mL	Visually compatible for 24 hr at 22°C	1855	C
Magnesium sulfate	IX	16.7, 33.3, 66.7, 100 mg/mL[a]	BR	5 mg/mL[a]	Physically compatible for at least 4 hr at 32°C	813	C
Melphalan HCl	BW	0.1 mg/mL[b]	BR	5 mg/mL[b]	Physically compatible for 3 hr at 22°C	1557	C
Meperidine HCl	WY	10 mg/mL[a]	BR	5 mg/mL[a]	Physically compatible for 4 hr at 25°C	987	C
Meropenem		50 mg/mL	SZ	250 mg/mL	Physically compatible for 4 hr at room temperature	3538	C
Meropenem–vaborbactam	TMC	8 mg/mL[b t]	FRK	5 mg/mL[b]	Physically compatible for 3 hr at 20 to 25°C	3380	C
Midazolam HCl	RC	5 mg/mL	BMS	5 mg/mL	Visually compatible for 24 hr at 22°C	1855	C
Milrinone lactate	SS	0.2 mg/mL[a]	AB	5 mg/mL[a]	Visually compatible for 4 hr at 25°C	2381	C
Morphine sulfate	WI	1 mg/mL[a]	BR	5 mg/mL[a]	Physically compatible for 4 hr at 25°C	987	C
Nicardipine HCl	DCC	0.1 mg/mL[a]	BR	2 mg/mL[a]	Visually compatible for 24 hr at room temperature	235	C

Y-Site Injection Compatibility (1:1 Mixture) (Cont.)

Test Drug	Mfr	Conc	Mfr	Conc	Remarks	Ref	C/I
Ondansetron HCl	GL	1 mg/mL[b]	BR	5 mg/mL[a]	Visually compatible for 4 hr at 22°C	1365	C
Paclitaxel	NCI	1.2 mg/mL[a]	BR	5 mg/mL[a]	Physically compatible for 4 hr at 22°C	1556	C
Pemetrexed disodium	LI	20 mg/mL[b]	APC	5 mg/mL[a]	Physically compatible for 4 hr at 23°C	2564	C
Piperacillin sodium–tazo-bactam sodium	WY[q]	26.7 to 40 mg/mL[a b p]		1.75 to 7.5 mg/mL	Compatible	2918, 2922	C
Piperacillin sodium–tazo-bactam sodium	[r]			1.75 to 7.5 mg/mL	Stated to be compatible	2919, 2920, 2921, 2985	C
Posaconazole	ME	18 mg/mL		5 mg/mL[c]	Physically compatible	2911, 2912	C
Propofol	ZEN[q]	10 mg/mL	DU	5 mg/mL[a]	Immediate precipitate and yellow color	2066	I
Remifentanil HCl	GW	0.025 and 0.25 mg/mL[b]	AB	5 mg/mL[a]	Physically compatible for 4 hr at 23°C	2075	C
Sargramostim	IMM	10 mcg/mL[b]	BR	5 mg/mL[b]	Visually compatible for 4 hr at 22°C	1436	C
Tedizolid phosphate	CUB	0.8 mg/mL[b]	HER	5 mg/mL[b]	Physically compatible for 2 hr	3244	C
Teniposide	BR	0.1 mg/mL[a]	BR	5 mg/mL[a]	Physically compatible for 4 hr at 23°C	1725	C
Thiotepa	IMM[g]	1 mg/mL[a]	DU	5 mg/mL[a]	Physically compatible for 4 hr at 23°C	1861	C
Tigecycline	WY	1 mg/mL[b]		5 mg/mL[b]	Physically compatible for 4 hr	2714	C
Tigecycline	ACD, FRK, WY	[c]	[w]		Stated to be compatible	2915, 3459, 3460	C
TNA #97 to #104[h]			BR	250 mg/mL	Broken fat emulsion with floating oil	1324	I
TNA #218 to #226[h]			AB	5 mg/mL[a]	Visually compatible for 4 hr at 23°C	2215	C
TPN #54[h]				250 mg/mL	Physically compatible and activity retained over 6 hr at 22°C	1045	C
TPN #61[h]		[i]	BR	37.5 mg/0.15 mL[j]	Physically compatible	1012	C
TPN #61[h]		[k]	BR	225 mg/0.9 mL[j]	Physically compatible	1012	C
TPN #91[h]		[l]		15 mg[m]	Physically compatible	1170	C
TPN #203, #204[h]			APC	5 mg/mL	Visually compatible for 2 hr at 23°C	1974	C
TPN #212 to #215[h]			AB	5 mg/mL[a]	Physically compatible for 4 hr at 23°C	2109	C
Vinorelbine tartrate	BW	1 mg/mL[b]	BR	5 mg/mL[b]	Physically compatible for 4 hr at 22°C	1558	C
Zidovudine	BW	4 mg/mL[a]	BR	4 mg/mL[a]	Physically compatible for 4 hr at 25°C	1193	C

[a] Tested in dextrose 5%.

[b] Tested in sodium chloride 0.9%.

[c] Tested in both dextrose 5% and sodium chloride 0.9%.

[d] Tested in Ringer's injection, lactated.

[e] Tested in sodium chloride 0.45%.

[f] Tested in dextrose 5% with albumin human 2 mg/mL.

[g] Lyophilized formulation tested.

[h] Refer to Appendix for the composition of parenteral nutrition solutions. TNA indicates a 3-in-1 admixture, and TPN indicates a 2-in-1 admixture.

[i] Run at 21 mL/hr.

Y-Site Injection Compatibility (1:1 Mixture) (Cont.)

[j] Given over 30 minutes by syringe pump.

[k] Run at 94 mL/hr.

[l] Run at 10 mL/hr.

[m] Given over one hour by syringe pump.

[n] Tested in sterile water for injection.

[o] Injected via Y-site into an administration set running azithromycin.

[p] Piperacillin component. Piperacillin in an 8:1 fixed-ratio concentration with tazobactam.

[q] Test performed using the formulation WITH edetate disodium.

[r] Test performed using the formulation WITHOUT edetate disodium.

[s] Ceftolozane component. Ceftolozane in a 2:1 fixed-ratio concentration with tazobactam.

[t] Meropenem component. Meropenem in a 1:1 fixed-ratio concentration with vaborbactam.

[u] Ceftazidime component. Ceftazidime in a 4:1 fixed-ratio concentration with avibactam.

[v] Tested in dextrose 5%, sodium chloride 0.9%, and Ringer's injection, lactated.

[w] Salt not specified.

Additional Compatibility Information

β-Lactam Antibiotics

In common with other aminoglycoside antibiotics, amikacin activity may be impaired by β-lactam antibiotics. This inactivation is dependent on concentration, temperature, and time of exposure. However, amikacin appears to be less affected by the β-lactam antibiotics than other aminoglycosides such as gentamicin and tobramycin.[68 574 575 654 740 816 824 973 1052]

The clinical significance of these interactions appears to be primarily confined to patients with renal failure.[218 334 361 364 616 816 847] Literature reports of greatly reduced aminoglycoside levels in such patients have appeared frequently.[363 365 366 367 614 615 962] In addition, the interaction may be clinically important if assays for aminoglycoside levels in serum are sufficiently delayed.[576 618 814 824 847 1052]

Selected Revisions May 1, 2020. © Copyright, October 1982. American Society of Health-System Pharmacists, Inc.

Most authors believe that in vitro mixing of penicillins with aminoglycoside antibiotics should be avoided but that clinical use of the drugs in combination can be of great value. It is generally recommended that the drugs be given separately in such combined therapy.[157 218 222 224 361 364 368 369 370]

Peritoneal Dialysis Solutions

Amikacin base (Bristol) 10 and 50 mg/L in peritoneal dialysis concentrate with 50% dextrose (McGaw) retained about 70% of initial activity in 7 hours and about 40 to 50% in 24 hours at room temperature.[1044]

Amikacin sulfate (Bristol) 25 mcg/mL combined separately with the cephalosporins cefazolin sodium (Lilly) and cefoxitin (MSD) at a concentration of 125 mcg/mL in peritoneal dialysis solution (Dianeal 1.5%) exhibited enhanced rates of lethality to *Staphylococcus aureus, Escherichia coli,* and *Pseudomonas aeruginosa* compared to any of the drugs alone.[1623]

Amino Acids
AHFS 40:20

Products

Amino acids are supplied in a variety of concentrations and sizes, both alone and in kits with dextrose 50% injection. For components, concentrations, and characteristics, see the labeling for the individual products.

Administration

Parenteral nutrition solutions composed of amino acids and high-concentration dextrose, which are strongly hypertonic, may be safely administered only through an indwelling intravenous catheter with the tip in the superior vena cava; they are used for severely depleted patients or those requiring long-term therapy.[3267 3268] For moderately depleted patients in whom the central venous route is not indicated, parenteral nutrition solutions with dextrose concentrations of 5 to 10%, which are substantially less hypertonic, may be administered peripherally.[3267 3268]

It has been recommended that administration sets used to administer lipid emulsions be changed within 24 hours of initiating infusion because of the potential for bacterial and fungal contamination.[2342]

For non-lipid-containing (TPN, 2-in-1) parenteral nutrition, 0.22-μm filters, preferably endotoxin retaining, are recommended; for lipid-containing (TNA, 3-in-1, AIO) parenteral nutrition, 1.2-μm filters are recommended.[2346 3259]

Stability

Solution containers should be visually inspected for cloudiness, haze, discoloration, precipitates, and bottle cracks and checked for the presence of vacuum before mixing and prior to administration. Only clear solutions should be administered. It is also recommended that the containers be protected from light until ready for use and from extremes of temperature such as freezing or over 40°C. Because of the risk of microbiological contamination, manufacturers recommend storing mixed parenteral nutrition solutions for as little time as possible after preparation. Administration of a single bottle should not exceed 24 hours.

A study of the original FreAmine showed that the mixed solution was stable at 4°C for 12 weeks. Increased temperature enhanced degradation. Decomposition due to the Maillard reaction is visible as a color change from the clear, light, pale yellow of the freshly prepared solution to yellow to red to dark brown. It was noted that the possibility of microbiological contamination limits the desirable storage time. It was recommended that solutions be stored under refrigeration and used as soon as possible after mixing.[186]

The previous study did not report on the stability of tryptophan because of variable and nonreproducible results.[186] In another study, it was shown that the tryptophan content of the original FreAmine was reduced approximately 20% by the presence of the sodium bisulfite 0.1% antioxidant.[187]

An evaluation of amino acid 4.25% injection with dextrose 25% (prepared from FreAmine II 8.5%), without additional additives, stored at 4°C for 2 weeks showed little or no change in the concentrations of amino acids, including tryptophan, as well as pH. Particle counts were also normal over the period. When stored at 25°C, approximately 6% tryptophan loss occurred, but no other changes were observed.[581]

In contrast, parenteral nutrition solutions composed of amino acids solution with ethanol and vitamins (Aminofusin, Pfrimmer) along with dextrose and a variety of electrolytes exhibited a darkening of color on storage at 37, 25, and 5°C for 60 days. The rate of color change was less at the lowest temperature. A loss of ascorbic acid in the mixture was also demonstrated and was shown to be associated with the color changes. The rate of ascorbic acid decomposition was dependent on air space in the container and storage temperature. In addition, fine white crystals of calcium phosphate precipitated on day 12 at 25 and 37°C and on day 25 at 5°C.[580]

A photoreaction of the L-tryptophan in Nephramine essential amino acid injection was reported. The L-tryptophan in combination with bisulfite stabilizer, oxygen, and light yielded an indigo blue color. Although no toxicity was associated with the L-tryptophan degradation and blue color formation, it was recommended that Nephramine remain in its original carton until ready to be mixed with dextrose and that Nephramine mixtures be covered with amber, UV-light-resistant bags to retard the formation of the blue color. It was further noted that a slightly blue solution need not be changed for a colorless one, nor is it necessary to change a slightly blue filter for a white one.[579] However, it has been emphasized that the clinical importance of this reaction is largely undetermined and may not be entirely benign.[1055]

The effects of photoirradiation on a FreAmine II–dextrose 10% parenteral nutrition solution containing 1 mL/500 mL of multivitamins (USV) were evaluated. During simulated continuous administration to an infant at 0.156 mL/min, the amino acids did not change when the bottle, infusion tubing, and collection bottle were shielded with foil. Only 20 cm of tubing in the incubator was exposed to light. However, if the flow was stopped, a marked reduction in methionine (40%), tryptophan (44%), and histidine (22%) occurred in the solution exposed to light for 24 hours. In a similar solution without vitamins, only the tryptophan concentration decreased. The difference was attributed to the presence of riboflavin, a photosensitizer. The authors recommended administering the multivitamin separately and shielding from light.[833]

The stability of amino acids in a parenteral nutrition solution composed of amino acids 3.5%, dextrose 25%, and electrolytes in polyvinyl chloride (PVC) bags was assessed at 4 and 25°C over 30 days. No significant decreases of the amino acids occurred in the refrigerated samples. However, the sample stored at room temperature showed significant losses of methionine (10.2%) and arginine (8.2%) in 30 days.[1057]

DOI: 10.37573/9781585286850.015

The long-term stability of the components of a parenteral nutrition solution composed of amino acids, dextrose, electrolytes, and trace metals in PVC bags was determined over a 6-month period of storage at 4°C. None of the amino acids decomposed more than 10% during the first 2 months. However, at 6 months, all of the amino acids except tyrosine, lysine, and histidine had degraded by more than 10%; some losses exceeded 25%. The dextrose, electrolytes, and trace elements remained constant for the 6-month period. Water loss through the PVC bag was only 0.2%. Visually the color remained unchanged.[1058]

The long-term stability of the components of 6 parenteral nutrition solutions containing variable amounts of amino acids, dextrose, electrolytes, trace elements, and vitamins, stored in PVC bags at 4 and 25°C, was evaluated. No significant changes to the amino acids, dextrose, electrolytes, or trace elements were noted during 28 days.[1063]

Peroxide Formation

Potentially toxic peroxide is generated in parenteral nutrition admixtures as a reaction between oxygen and various components catalyzed by riboflavin in the presence of light. This is particularly true in neonatal formulations.[1650] [1653] [1947] [2306] [2309] [2316] Exposure of a neonatal parenteral nutrition admixture to ambient light resulted in the formation of peroxide concentrations up to 300 μM. Light protection from compounding through administration has been recommended as a more achievable approach to reduce the formation of peroxide than avoiding contact with oxygen.[2316]

Exposure of parenteral nutrition admixtures to light during phototherapy has been shown to generate substantially larger amounts of hydrogen peroxide.[2310] In a study of the rate of hydrogen peroxide formation in a TrophAmine 1%-based parenteral nutrition admixture exposed to light, levels of peroxide increased linearly for about 8 hours and then reached a plateau at about 940 μM. A similar solution kept in the dark did not generate any detectable peroxide. A hydrogen peroxide concentration of as little as 25 μM has been shown to be lethal to 90% of human cells in culture. The authors speculated that additive hepatic oxidant injury over time might increase hepatic dysfunction as the duration of exposure to parenteral nutrition increases. The presence of sulfite antioxidants in the amino acids helps to reduce the formation of hydrogen peroxide, but the antioxidants are present in insufficient quantities to offer adequate protection. Shielding parenteral nutrition admixtures from light was recommended for neonatal administration.[2309]

The formation of toxic peroxides due to exposure of parenteral nutrition admixtures to light was reduced substantially by using colored administration sets. Both 2-in-1 and 3-in-1 parenteral nutrition admixtures exhibited little protection from peroxide formation when only the bag was shielded from light. Peroxide formation was 2 to 3 times higher using light-protected bags with clear tubing when compared to colored tubing. Shielding the parenteral nutrition bags from light and using black, yellow, or orange tubing would reduce peroxide loads down to about 100 μM.[2306]

Freezing Solutions

The acceptability of frozen storage of some parenteral nutrition solutions has been determined. Parenteral nutrition solutions composed of equal parts of Travasol 8.5% with electrolytes and dextrose 70% injection (final concentrations of amino acids and dextrose were 4.25 and 35%, respectively), in PVC containers were stored frozen at –20°C for 60 days. Both overnight room temperature thawing and 30-minute microwave thawing were utilized. The results indicated that, with either thawing technique, the amino acids, electrolytes, and dextrose were unchanged after 60 days of frozen storage and subsequent thawing.[578]

Plasticizer Leaching

A parenteral nutrition solution containing an amino acid solution, dextrose, and electrolytes in a PVC bag did not leach measurable quantities of diethylhexyl phthalate (DEHP) plasticizer during 21 days of storage at 4 and 25°C. However, addition of fat emulsion 10 or 20% to the formula caused detectable leaching of DEHP from the PVC containers stored for 48 hours. Higher DEHP levels were found in the 25°C samples than in the 4°C samples. The authors recommended limiting the use of lipid-containing parenteral nutrition admixtures to 24 to 36 hours. Use of non-PVC containers and tubing is another option to eliminate the problem of plasticizer leaching.[1430]

Compatibility Information

Solution Compatibility

Amino acids

Test Soln Name	Mfr	Mfr	Conc/L or %	Remarks	Ref	C/I
Fat emulsion 10%, intravenous	VT	MG	AA 8.5%	Mixed in equal parts. Physically compatible for 48 hr at 4°C and room temperature	32	C
Fat emulsion 10%, intravenous	CU	AB	AA 7%	Mixed in equal parts. Physically compatible for 72 hr at room temperature	656	C
Fat emulsion 10%, intravenous	CU	MG	AA 8.5%	Mixed in equal parts. Physically compatible for 72 hr at room temperature	656	C
Fat emulsion 10%, intravenous	CU	TR	AA 8.5%	Mixed in equal parts. Physically compatible for 72 hr at room temperature	656	C
Fat emulsion 10%, intravenous	VT		AA 10%	Mixed in equal parts. Changes in 20 min. Coalescence and creaming in 8 hr at 8 and 25°C	825	I

Additive Compatibility

Amino acids

Test Drug	Mfr	Conc/L or %	Mfr	Conc/L or %	Test Solution	Remarks	Ref	C/I
Albumin human		9.5 g			TNA #232[a i]	Microscopically observed emulsion disruption found with increased fat globule size in 48 hr at room temperature	2267	?
Albumin human		9.5 g			TNA #233[a i]	Visually apparent emulsion disruption with creaming in 4 hr at room temperature. Increased disruption attributed to the added effect of calcium and magnesium ions	2267	I
Albumin human		18.2 g			TNA #234[a i]	Creaming and free oil formation visually observed in 24 hours at room temperature	2267	I
Albumin human		18.2 g			TNA #235[a i]	Visually apparent emulsion disruption with creaming and free oil formation in 4 hr at room temperature. Increased disruption attributed to the added effect of calcium and magnesium ions	2267	I
Amikacin sulfate		150 mg			TPN #107[a]	Activity retained for 24 hr at 21°C	1326	C
Aminophylline	SE	500 mg	MG		AA 4.25%, D 25%	No increase in particulate matter in 24 hr at 4°C	349	C
Aminophylline	SE	250 mg to 1.5 g			TPN #25 to #27[a]	Physically compatible and aminophylline stable for at least 24 hr at 25°C	755	C
Aminophylline	SE	1 g			TPN #25 to #27[a]	Physically compatible and aminophylline stable for at least 24 hr at 4°C	755	C
Aminophylline	SE	1 g			TPN #28 to #30[a]	Physically compatible and aminophylline stable for at least 24 hr at 25°C	755	C
Aminophylline		29.3 mg			[b]	No significant change in aminophylline content over 24 hr at 24 to 26°C	852	C
Aminophylline		284 and 638 mg			TNA #180[a]	No theophylline loss and no increase in fat particle size in 24 hr at room temperature	1617	C
Amphotericin B	SQ	100 mg	MG		AA 4.25%, D 25%	Turbidity and fine yellow particles form	349	I
Ampicillin sodium	BR	1 g	MG		TPN #21[a]	Activity retained for 24 hr at 4°C	87	C
Ampicillin sodium	BR	1 g	MG		TPN #21[a]	12 to 25% ampicillin loss in 24 hr at 25°C	87	I
Ampicillin sodium	BR	1 g	MG		AA 4.25%, D 25%	Increase in microscopic particles noted over 24 hr at 5°C	349	I
Ampicillin sodium	AST	1.5 g			TPN #52[a]	69% ampicillin loss in 24 hr at 29°C	440	I
Ampicillin sodium	AST	1.5 g			TPN #53[a]	22% ampicillin loss in 24 hr at 29°C	440	I
Ampicillin sodium		1 and 3 g			TPN #107[a]	Activity retained for 24 hr at 21°C	1326	C
Aztreonam		2 g			TPN #107[a]	Activity retained for 24 hr at 21°C	1326	C
Cefazolin sodium	LI	1 g	MG		AA 4.25%, D 25%	No increase in particulate matter in 24 hr at 4°C	349	C
Cefazolin sodium	SKF	10 g	TR		TPN #22[a]	Physically compatible with no loss of activity in 24 hr at 22°C in the dark	837	C
Cefazolin sodium		1 g			TPN #107[a]	9% cefazolin loss in 24 hr at 21°C	1326	C
Cefepime HCl	BR	1 and 4 g	AB		AA 4.25%, D 25%, electrolytes	5 to 6% cefepime loss in 8 hr at room temperature and 3 days at 5°C	1682	C
Cefotaxime sodium		1 g			TPN #107[a]	Activity retained for 24 hr at 21°C	1326	C
Cefoxitin sodium		1 g			TPN #107[a]	Activity retained for 24 hr at 21°C	1326	C
Ceftazidime		1 g			TPN #107[a]	Activity retained for 24 hr at 21°C	1326	C

Additive Compatibility (Cont.)

Test Drug	Mfr	Conc/L or %	Mfr	Conc/L or %	Test Solution	Remarks	Ref	C/I
Ceftazidime	GL	6 g	AB		AA 5%, D 25%	No substantial amino acid degradation in 48 hr at 22°C and 10 days at 4°C. Ceftazidime stability the determining factor	1535	C
Ceftazidime	GL	1 g			TPN #141 to #143[a]	Visually compatible with 8% ceftazidime loss in 6 hr and 10% loss in 24 hr at 22°C. 8% ceftazidime loss in 3 days at 4°C	1535	C
Ceftazidime	GL	6 g			TPN #141 to #143[a]	Visually compatible with 6% ceftazidime loss in 12 hr and 11 to 13% loss in 24 hr at 22°C. 7 to 9% ceftazidime loss in 3 days at 4°C	1535	C
Cefuroxime sodium		1 g			TPN #107[a]	Activity retained for 24 hr at 21°C	1326	C
Clindamycin phosphate	UP	250 mg	MG		TPN #21[a]	Stable for 24 hr at 4 and 25°C	87	C
Clindamycin phosphate	UP	600 mg	MG		AA 4.25%, D 25%	No increase in particulate matter in 24 hr at 4°C	349	C
Clindamycin phosphate	UP	3 g	TR		TPN #22[a]	Physically compatible with no loss in 24 hr at 22°C in the dark	837	C
Clindamycin phosphate		400 mg[c]			TPN #107[a]	Stable for 24 hr at 21°C	1326	C
Cyclophospha- mide	MJ	500 mg	MG		AA 4.25%, D 25%	No increase in particulate matter in 24 hr at 4°C	349	C
Cyclosporine	SZ	150 mg	MG		AA 5%, D 25%	Visually compatible with no cyclosporine loss in 72 hr at 21°C	1616	C
Cytarabine	UP	100 mg	MG		AA 4.25%, D 25%	No increase in particulate matter in 24 hr at 4°C	349	C
Cytarabine	UP	50 mg			TPN #57[a]	Physically compatible with no cytarabine loss in 48 hr at 25 or 8°C	996	C
Dopamine HCl	AS	400 mg	MG		AA 4.25%, D 25%	No increase in particulate matter in 24 hr at 4°C	349	C
Epoetin alfa	ORT	100 units			[d]	96% of the epoetin alfa delivered[e] over 24 hr	1878	C
Famotidine	MSD	20 and 40 mg			TPN #109, #110[a]	Physically compatible with no famotidine loss and little change in amino acids in 48 hr at 21°C and in 7 days at 4°C	1331	C
Famotidine	MSD	20 and 50 mg			TNA #111, #112[a]	Physically compatible. Little loss and no change in fat particle size in 48 hr at 4 and 21°C	1332	C
Famotidine	MSD	20 mg			TPN #113[a]	Physically compatible. Little loss in 35 days at 4°C in light	1334	C
Famotidine	MSD	20 and 40 mg			TNA #114[a]	Physically compatible. No loss and no change in fat particle size in 72 hr at 21°C in light	1333	C
Famotidine	MSD	20 mg			[f]	0 to 5% loss in 48 hr at 25°C in light or dark and at 5°C	1344	C
Famotidine	MSD	16.7 and 33.3 mg			TPN #115, #116[a]	No famotidine loss in 7 days at 23 and 4°C	1352	C
Famotidine	MSD	20 mg			TNA #182[a]	Visually compatible. No loss in 24 hr at 24°C in light	1576	C
Famotidine	MSD	20 mg			TNA #197 to #200[a]	Physically compatible. No loss in 48 hr at 22°C in light	1921	C
Famotidine	MSD	20 mg			TPN #196[a]	Physically compatible. No loss in 48 hr at 22°C in light	1921	C
Fluorouracil	RC	500 mg	MG		AA 4.25%, D 25%	No increase in particulate matter in 24 hr at 4°C	349	C

Additive Compatibility (Cont.)

Test Drug	Mfr	Conc/L or %	Mfr	Conc/L or %	Test Solution	Remarks	Ref	C/I
Fluorouracil	RC	1 and 4 g			TPN #23[a]	Physically compatible for 42 hr at room temperature in light. Erratic assay results	562	?
Fluorouracil	RC	1 g			TPN #23[a]	Physically compatible and fluorouracil stable for 48 hr at room temperature in ambient light	826	C
Folic acid		1 mg			TPN #74[a]	Folic acid stable over 8 hr at room temperature in fluorescent or sunlight	842	C
Folic acid	USP	0.2 and 10 mg	MG		AA 4.25%, D 25%	Physically compatible. Stable for 7 days at 4°C and room temperature in dark	895	C
Folic acid	USP	0.4 mg			TPN #69[a]	Physically compatible and folic acid stable for at least 7 days at 4 and 25°C protected from light	895	C
Folic acid	LE	0.25 to 1 mg			TPN #70[a]	Folic acid stable for at least 48 hr at 6 and 21°C in light or dark conditions	896	C
Furosemide	HO	40 mg	MG		AA 4.25%, D 25%	No increase in particulate matter in 24 hr at 4°C	349	C
Ganciclovir sodium	SY	3 and 5 g			TPN #183 to #185[a]	Precipitate forms	1744	I
Ganciclovir sodium	SY	2 g			TPN #183[a]	Precipitate forms	1744	I
Gentamicin sulfate	SC	80 mg	MG		AA 4.25%, D 25%	No increase in particulate matter in 24 hr at 4°C	349	C
Gentamicin sulfate	SC	800 mg	TR		TPN #22[a]	Physically compatible. No loss in 24 hr at 22°C in the dark	837	C
Gentamicin sulfate	SC	50 mg			TPN #52 and TPN #53[a]	Physically compatible. No loss in 24 hr at 29°C	440	C
Gentamicin sulfate		75 mg			TPN #107[a]	Physically compatible and stable for 24 hr at 21°C	1326	C
Heparin sodium	RI	20,000 units	MG		AA 4.25%, D 25%	No increase in particulate matter in 24 hr at 4°C	349	C
Heparin sodium		35,000 units			TPN #48 to #51[a]	Heparin activity retained for 24 hr at 25°C but fell significantly after 24 hr	900	C
Heparin sodium	LY	3000 to 20,000 units			TPN #205[a]	Heparin activity retained for 28 days at 4°C	2025	C
Hydrochloric acid		40, 60, 100 mEq	MG		TPN #24[a]	Physically compatible and changes in amino acid concentrations considered negligible over 24 hr at 25°C. Hydrochloric acid available from solution	582	C
Imipenem–cilastatin sodium		500[m][n] mg			TPN #107[a]	57% imipenem loss in 24 hr at 21°C	1326	I
Imipenem–cilastatin sodium	MSD	5[m] g			TPN #241, #242[a]	8 to 10% imipenem loss within 30 min at 25°C under fluorescent light	493	I
Insulin, regular	NOV	10 units	[a][i]		TNA #267[a][i]	40 to 60% loss likely due to sorption	2599	I
Iron dextran	FI	100 mg	TR		TPN #31 to #33[a]	Physically compatible with minimal changes to iron dextran and amino acids for 18 hr at room temperature	692	C
Iron dextran	FI	50 mg			TNA #122[a]	Lipid oiling out in 18 to 19 hr with formation of yellow-brown layer	1383	I
Iron dextran	FI				TNA #159 to #166[a]	Physically compatible with no change in particle size distribution in 48 hr at 4 and 25°C	1648	C
Iron dextran	SCN	10 mg			TPN #207, #208[a]	Rust-colored precipitate forms in 12 hr at 19°C protected from sunlight	2103	I

Additive Compatibility (Cont.)

Test Drug	Mfr	Conc/L or %	Mfr	Conc/L or %	Test Solution	Remarks	Ref	C/I
Iron dextran	SCN	10 mg			TPN #209[a]	Rust-colored precipitate forms in some samples in 18 to 24 hr at 19°C protected from sunlight	2103	I
Iron dextran	SCN	10 mg			TPN #210[a]	Visually compatible for 48 hr at 19°C protected from sunlight. Trace iron precipitation found after 48 hr	2103	?
Iron dextran	SCN	10 mg			TPN #211[a]	Visually compatible for 48 hr at 19°C protected from sunlight. No iron precipitation found after 48 hr	2103	C
Isoproterenol HCl	WI	2 mg	MG		AA 4.25%, D 25%	No increase in particulate matter in 24 hr at 4°C	349	C
Lidocaine HCl	AST	1 g	MG		AA 4.25%, D 25%	No increase in particulate matter in 24 hr at 4°C	349	C
Meperidine HCl	WI	100 mg			TPN #71[a g]	Physically compatible with no meperidine loss in 36 hr at 22°C	1000	C
Methotrexate sodium	LE	50 mg	MG		AA 4.25%, D 25%	No increase in particulate matter in 24 hr at 4°C	349	C
Methyldopate HCl	MSD	500 mg	MG		AA 4.25%, D 25%	No increase in particulate matter in 24 hr at 4°C	349	C
Methylprednisolone sodium succinate	UP	250 mg	MG		AA 4.25%, D 25%	No increase in particulate matter in 24 hr at 4°C	349	C
Methylprednisolone sodium succinate	PHU	25, 63, 125 mg			TNA #237[a i]	Physically compatible with no substantial change in lipid particle size. Variable assay results, but <10% change in drug concentration and <8% change in TNA components after 7 days at 4°C, followed by 24 hr at ambient temperature and light	2347	C
Methylprednisolone sodium succinate	PHU	25, 63, 125 mg			TPN #236[a i]	Variable assay results, but less than 10% change in drug concentration and less than 12% change in TPN components after 7 days at 4°C, followed by 24 hr at ambient temperature and light	2347	C
Metoclopramide HCl	RB	5 and 20 mg	TR		AA 2.75%, D 25%, electrolytes	Metoclopramide chemically stable for 72 hr at room temperature	854	C
Metoclopramide HCl	RB	5 mg			TPN #89[a]	Physically compatible with no metoclopramide loss in 24 hr and 10% loss in 48 hr at 25°C	1167	C
Metoclopramide HCl	RB	20 mg			TPN #89[a]	Physically compatible with no metoclopramide loss in 72 hr at 25°C	1167	C
Metoclopramide HCl	RB	5 mg			TPN #90[a]	Physically compatible with no metoclopramide loss in 72 hr at 25°C	1167	C
Metoclopramide HCl	RB	20 mg			TPN #90[a]	Physically compatible with 3% metoclopramide loss in 72 hr at 25°C	1167	C
Midazolam HCl	RC	600 mg to 1 g			TPN #174 to #176[a]	Precipitates immediately	1624	I
Midazolam HCl	RC	100 and 500 mg			TPN #174 to #176[a]	Visually compatible with no midazolam loss and less than 10% loss of any amino acid in 5 hr at 22°C	1624	C
Morphine sulfate	LI	100 mg			TPN #71[a g]	Physically compatible with no morphine loss in 36 hr at 22°C	1000	C
Multivitamins	USV	1 vial	TR		AA 4.25%, D 25%	No loss of thiamine HCl in 22 hr at 30°C	843	C
Multivitamins (M.V.I. Pediatric)	ROR	5 mL			AA 2%, D 12.5%, electrolytes	7% phytonadione loss in 4 hr and 27% loss in 24 hr under ambient temperature and light	1815	I
Multivitamins	LY	10 mL	AB[g h l]		AA 2.5%, D 25%	All vitamins stable for 24 hr at 4°C	926	C

Additive Compatibility (Cont.)

Test Drug	Mfr	Conc/L or %	Mfr	Conc/L or %	Test Solution	Remarks	Ref	C/I
Multivitamins	LY	10 mL	MG[g h l]		AA 4.25%, D 25%	All vitamins stable for 24 hr at 4°C	926	C
Nafcillin sodium		1 and 2 g			TPN #107[a]	Nafcillin activity retained for 24 hr at 21°C	1326	C
Norepinephrine bitartrate	WI	4 mg	MG		AA 4.25%, D 25%	No increase in particulate matter in 24 hr at 4°C	349	C
Octreotide acetate	SZ	1.5 mg			TPN #119, #120[a h]	Little octreotide loss over 48 hr at room temperature in ambient room light	1373	C
Octreotide acetate	SZ	450 mcg			TNA #139[a g i]	Physically compatible with no change in lipid particle size in 48 hr at 22°C under fluorescent light and 7 days at 4°C. Octreotide activity highly variable	1540	?
Ondansetron HCl	GL	0.03 and 0.3 g			TNA #190[a]	Physically compatible with no ondansetron loss in 48 hr at 24°C in light	1766	C
Oxacillin sodium	BR	500 mg	MG		AA 4.25%, D 25%	No increase in particulate matter in 24 hr at 4°C	349	C
Pantoprazole sodium	ALT[k]	13.3 mg			TPN #265[a]	Yellow discoloration and drug losses of 12% in 3 hr at room temperature in dark	2789	I
Penicillin G potassium	SQ	5 million units	MG		TPN #21[a]	Activity retained for 24 hr at 4 and 25°C	87	C
Penicillin G potassium	LI	1 million units	MG		AA 4.25%, D 25%	No increase in particulate matter in 24 hr at 4°C	349	C
Penicillin G potassium	AY	25 million units	TR		TPN #22[a]	Physically compatible with no loss of activity in 24 hr at 22°C in dark	837	C
Penicillin G potassium		2 g			TPN #107[a]	Activity retained for 24 hr at 21°C	1326	C
Penicillin G sodium		2 g			TPN #107[a]	Activity retained for 24 hr at 21°C	1326	C
Phytonadione	MSD	10 mg	MG		AA 4.25%, D 25%	No increase in particulate matter in 24 hr at 4°C	349	C
Polymyxin B sulfate	NOV	40 mg			TPN #52, #53[a]	Physically compatible with no polymyxin loss in 24 hr at 29°C	440	C
Ranitidine HCl	GL	83, 167, 250 mg			TPN #58[a]	10% ranitidine loss in 48 hr at 23°C	997	C
Ranitidine HCl	GL	50 and 100 mg			TPN #59, #60[a h]	No color change and 7 to 9% ranitidine loss in 24 hr at 24°C in light. Amino acids unaffected. Darkened color and 10 to 12% ranitidine loss in 48 hr	1010	C
Ranitidine HCl	GL	50 and 100 mg			TNA #92[a i]	7 to 10% ranitidine loss in 12 hr and 20 to 28% loss in 24 hr at 23°C in light	1183	I
Ranitidine HCl	GL	50 and 100 mg			TPN #117[a]	Physically compatible and 5% ranitidine loss in 48 hr refrigerated and at 25°C	1360	C
Ranitidine HCl	GL	50 and 100 mg			TNA #118[a]	Physically compatible. 6 to 10% ranitidine loss in 36 hr under refrigeration and at 25°C	1360	C
Ranitidine HCl	GL	75 mg			TNA #197 to #200[a]	Physically compatible with 7% or less ranitidine loss in 24 hr at 22°C in light. About 15% loss in 48 hr	1921	C
Ranitidine HCl	GL	75 mg			TPN #196[a]	Physically compatible with 7% or less ranitidine loss in 24 hr at 22°C in light. About 12% loss in 48 hr	1921	C
Ranitidine HCl		200 mg			TNA #245[a]	No ranitidine loss and no lipid change in 24 hr at room temperature	486	C
Ranitidine HCl	GL	72 mg			TNA #246[a]	Less than 7% ranitidine loss and no change in emulsion integrity in 14 days at 4°C	501	C

Additive Compatibility (Cont.)

Test Drug	Mfr	Conc/L or %	Mfr	Conc/L or %	Test Solution	Remarks	Ref	C/I
Ranitidine HCl	GL	72 mg			TPN #247[a]	2% ranitidine loss in 14 days at 4°C	501	C
Sodium bicar-bonate		50 and 150 mEq			TPN #62 to #65	Physically compatible with 10% or less carbon dioxide loss and unchanged pH in 7 days at 25°C protected from light	1011	C
Sodium bicar-bonate		100 mEq			TPN #66 to #68[a]	Physically compatible with 10% or less carbon dioxide loss and unchanged pH in 7 days at 25°C protected from light	1011	C
Tacrolimus	FUJ	100 mg			TPN #201[a g]	Visually compatible with no loss in 24 hr at 24°C	1922	C
Tobramycin sulfate	LI	80 mg	MG		AA 4.25%, D 25%	No increase in particulate matter in 24 hr at 4°C	349	C
Vancomycin HCl		400 mg			TPN #95, #96[a]	Physically compatible and no vancomycin loss for 8 days at room temperature and refrigerated	1321	C
Vancomycin HCl		1 and 6 g			TPN #105, #106[a]	Physically compatible with little or no vancomycin loss in 4 hr at 22°C	1325	C
Vancomycin HCl		200 mg			TPN #107[a]	Activity retained for 24 hr at 21°C	1326	C
Vancomycin HCl	LI	500 mg and 1 g			TPN #202[a h]	Visually compatible and activity retained for 35 days at 4°C plus 24 hr at 22°C	1933	C

[a] Refer to Appendix for the composition of parenteral nutrition solutions. TNA indicates a 3-in-1 admixture, and TPN indicates a 2-in-1 admixture.

[b] Tested in a pediatric parenteral nutrition solution containing 150 mL of dextrose 5% and 30 mL of Vamin glucose with electrolytes and vitamins.

[c] Expressed as clindamycin base.

[d] TPN composed of amino acids (TrophAmine) 0.5 or 2.25% with dextrose 12.5%, vitamins, trace elements, magnesium sulfate, calcium gluconate, sodium chloride, potassium acetate, and heparin sodium.

[e] Delivered from a syringe through microbore tubing, T-connector, and a Teflon neonatal 24-gauge intravenous catheter.

[f] Tested in Vamin 14, Vamin 18, Vamin glucose, and Vamin N.

[g] Tested in glass containers.

[h] Tested in PVC containers.

[i] Tested in ethylene vinyl acetate containers.

[j] Concentration of fosphenytoin expressed in milligrams of phenytoin sodium equivalents (PE) per mL.

[k] Test performed using the formulation WITH edetate disodium.

[l] Tested in polyolefin bags.

[m] Imipenem component. Imipenem in a 1:1 fixed-ratio concentration with cilastatin.

[n] Not specified whether concentration refers to single component or combined components.

Y-Site Injection Compatibility (1:1 Mixture)

Amino acids

Test Drug	Mfr	Conc	Mfr	Conc	Remarks	Ref	C/I
Acetazolamide sodium	LE	100 mg/mL		TPN #203, #204[g]	White precipitate forms immediately	1974	I
Acyclovir sodium	BW	7 mg/mL		TPN #203, #204[g]	White precipitate forms immediately	1974	I
Acyclovir sodium	BW	7 mg/mL[a]		TPN #212 to #215[g]	Crystalline needles form immediately, becoming a gross precipitate in 1 hr	2109	I
Acyclovir sodium	GW	7 mg/mL[a]		TNA #218 to #226[g]	White precipitate forms immediately	2215	I
Alprostadil	BED	15 mcg/mL[a]		TPN #274[g]	Visually compatible for 1 hr	2746	C
Amikacin sulfate		250 mg/mL		TPN #54[g]	Physically compatible and activity retained over 6 hr at 22°C	1045	C

Y-Site Injection Compatibility (1:1 Mixture) (Cont.)

Test Drug	Mfr	Conc	Mfr	Conc	Remarks	Ref	C/I
Amikacin sulfate	BR	37.5 mg/0.15 mL[j]		TPN #61[c g]	Physically compatible	1012	C
Amikacin sulfate	BR	225 mg/0.9 mL[j]		TPN #61[d g]	Physically compatible	1012	C
Amikacin sulfate	BR	15 mg[e]		TPN #91[f g]	Physically compatible	1170	C
Amikacin sulfate	BR	250 mg/mL		TNA #97 to #104[g]	Broken fat emulsion with floating oil	1324	I
Amikacin sulfate	APC	5 mg/mL		TPN #203, #204[g]	Visually compatible for 2 hr at 23°C	1974	C
Amikacin sulfate	AB	5 mg/mL[a]		TPN #212 to #215[g]	Physically compatible for 4 hr at 23°C	2109	C
Amikacin sulfate	AB	5 mg/mL[a]		TNA #218 to #226[g]	Visually compatible for 4 hr at 23°C	2215	C
Aminophylline	DB	1 mg/mL[b]		TPN #189[g]	Visually compatible for 24 hr at 22°C	1767	C
Aminophylline	AMR	5 and 25 mg/mL		TPN #203, #204[g]	White precipitate forms immediately	1974	I
Aminophylline	AB	2.5 mg/mL[a]		TPN #212 to #215[g]	Physically compatible for 4 hr at 23°C	2109	C
Aminophylline	AB	2.5 mg/mL[a]		TNA #218 to #226[g]	Visually compatible for 4 hr at 23°C	2215	C
Amoxicillin sodium		50 mg/mL[b]		TPN #189[g]	Visually compatible for 24 hr at 22°C	1767	C
Amphotericin B	PH	0.6 mg/mL[a]		TPN #212 to #215[g]	Precipitate forms immediately	2109	I
Amphotericin B	PH	0.6 mg/mL[a]		TNA #218 to #226[g]	Yellow precipitate forms immediately	2215	I
Ampicillin sodium	BR	40 mg/mL[b]		TNA #73[g h]	Visually compatible for 4 hr at 25°C	1008	C
Ampicillin sodium	WY	250 mg/1.3 mL[i]		TPN #61[c g]	Heavy precipitate of calcium phosphate	1012	I
Ampicillin sodium	WY	1.5 g/7.5 mL[i]		TPN #61[d g]	Heavy precipitate of calcium phosphate	1012	I
Ampicillin sodium				TPN #54[g]	Precipitate forms in 30 min at 22°C	1045	I
Ampicillin sodium	APC	100 and 250 mg/mL		TPN #203, #204[g]	White precipitate forms immediately	1974	I
Ampicillin sodium	SKB	20 mg/mL[b]		TPN #212 to #215[g]	Physically compatible for 4 hr at 23°C	2109	C
Ampicillin sodium	SKB	20 mg/mL[b]		TNA #218 to #226[g]	Visually compatible for 4 hr at 23°C	2215	C
Ampicillin sodium–sulbactam sodium	RR	20 mg/mL[b aa]		TPN #212 to #215[g]	Physically compatible for 4 hr at 23°C	2109	C
Ampicillin sodium–sulbactam sodium	PF	20 mg/mL[b aa]		TNA #218 to #226[g]	Visually compatible for 4 hr at 23°C	2215	C
Argatroban	SKB	1 mg/mL[a]		TPN #263[g]	Physically compatible for 24 hr at 23°C	2572	C
Ascorbic acid	DB	20 mg/mL[b]		TPN #189[g]	Visually compatible for 24 hr at 22°C	1767	C
Atracurium besylate	WEL	10 mg/mL		TPN #189[g]	Visually compatible for 24 hr at 22°C	1767	C
Aztreonam	SQ	40 mg/mL[a]		TPN #212 to #215[g]	Physically compatible for 4 hr at 23°C	2109	C
Aztreonam	SQ	40 mg/mL[a]		TNA #218 to #226[g]	Visually compatible for 4 hr at 23°C	2215	C
Bumetanide	RC	0.04 mg/mL[a]		TPN #212 to #215[g]	Physically compatible for 4 hr at 23°C	2109	C
Bumetanide	RC, BV	0.04 mg/mL[a]		TNA #218 to #226[g]	Visually compatible for 4 hr at 23°C	2215	C
Buprenorphine HCl	RKC	0.04 mg/mL[a]		TPN #212 to #215[g]	Physically compatible for 4 hr at 23°C	2109	C
Buprenorphine HCl	RKC	0.04 mg/mL[a]		TNA #218 to #226[g]	Visually compatible for 4 hr at 23°C	2215	C
Butorphanol tartrate	APC	0.04 mg/mL[a]		TPN #212 to #215[g]	Physically compatible for 4 hr at 23°C	2109	C
Butorphanol tartrate	APC	0.04 mg/mL[a]		TNA #218 to #226[g]	Visually compatible for 4 hr at 23°C	2215	C
Calcium gluconate	DB	10 mg/mL[b]		TPN #189[g]	Visually compatible for 24 hr at 22°C	1767	C

Y-Site Injection Compatibility (1:1 Mixture) (Cont.)

Test Drug	Mfr	Conc	Mfr	Conc	Remarks	Ref	C/I
Calcium gluconate	AB	40 mg/mL[a]		TPN #212 to #215[g]	Physically compatible for 4 hr at 23°C	2109	C
Calcium gluconate	AB	40 mg/mL[a]		TNA #218 to #226[g]	Visually compatible for 4 hr at 23°C	2215	C
Carboplatin	BMS	5 mg/mL[a]		TPN #212 to #215[g]	Physically compatible for 4 hr at 23°C	2109	C
Carboplatin	BMS	5 mg/mL[a]		TNA #218 to #226[g]	Visually compatible for 4 hr at 23°C	2215	C
Caspofungin acetate	ME	0.7 mg/mL[b]		TPN[w]	Immediate white turbid precipitate forms	2758	I
Cefazolin sodium	SKF	20 mg/mL[a]		TNA #73[g h]	Visually compatible for 4 hr at 25°C	1008	C
Cefazolin sodium	SKF	200 mg/0.9 mL[i]		TPN #61[c g]	Physically compatible	1012	C
Cefazolin sodium	SKF	1.2 g/5.3 mL[i]		TPN #61[d g]	Physically compatible	1012	C
Cefazolin sodium	SKB	20 mg/mL[a]		TPN #212, #213[g]	Physically compatible for 4 hr at 23°C	2109	C
Cefazolin sodium	SKB	20 mg/mL[a]		TPN #214, #215[g]	Microprecipitate forms immediately	2109	I
Cefazolin sodium	SKB	20 mg/mL[a]		TNA #218 to #226[g]	Visually compatible for 4 hr at 23°C	2215	C
Cefotaxime sodium	HO	200 mg/0.7 mL[i]		TPN #61[c g]	Physically compatible	1012	C
Cefotaxime sodium	HO	1.2 g/4 mL[i]		TPN #61[d g]	Physically compatible	1012	C
Cefotaxime sodium	RS	200 mg/mL[k]		TPN #189[g]	Visually compatible for 24 hr at 22°C	1767	C
Cefotaxime sodium	HO	60 mg/mL		TPN #203, #204[g]	Visually compatible for 2 hr at 23°C	1974	C
Cefotaxime sodium	HO	20 mg/mL[a]		TPN #212 to #215[g]	Physically compatible for 4 hr at 23°C	2109	C
Cefotaxime sodium	HO	20 mg/mL[a]		TNA #218 to #226[g]	Visually compatible for 4 hr at 23°C	2215	C
Cefotetan disodium	STU	20 mg/mL[a]		TPN #212 to #215[g]	Physically compatible for 4 hr at 23°C	2109	C
Cefotetan disodium	ZEN	20 mg/mL[a]		TNA #218 to #226[g]	Visually compatible for 4 hr at 23°C	2215	C
Cefoxitin sodium	MSD	20 mg/mL[a]		TNA #73[g h]	Visually compatible for 4 hr at 25°C	1008	C
Cefoxitin sodium	MSD	200 mg/2.1 mL[i]		TPN #61[c g]	Physically compatible	1012	C
Cefoxitin sodium	MSD	1.2 g/12.6 mL[i]		TPN #61[d g]	Physically compatible	1012	C
Cefoxitin sodium	MSD	200 mg/mL[k]		TPN #189[g]	Visually compatible for 24 hr at 22°C	1767	C
Cefoxitin sodium	ME	20 mg/mL[a]		TPN #212 to #215[d]	Physically compatible for 4 hr at 23°C	2109	C
Cefoxitin sodium	ME	20 mg/mL[a]		TNA #218 to #226[g]	Visually compatible for 4 hr at 23°C	2215	C
Ceftaroline fosamil	FOR	2.22 mg/mL[a b v]		TPN #296[g]	Physically compatible for 4 hr at 23°C	2826	C
Ceftazidime	GL	40 mg/mL[l]		TPN #141 to #143[g]	Visually compatible with 4% or less ceftazidime loss in 2 hr at 22°C in 1:1 and 1:3 ratios	1535	C
Ceftazidime	GL	200 mg/mL[k]		TPN #189[g]	Visually compatible for 24 hr at 22°C	1767	C
Ceftazidime	LI	60 mg/mL		TPN #203, #204[g]	Visually compatible for 2 hr at 23°C	1974	C
Ceftazidime	SKB	40 mg/mL[a]		TPN #212 to #215[g]	Physically compatible for 4 hr at 23°C	2109	C
Ceftazidime	SKB[cc]	40 mg/mL[a]		TNA #218 to #226[g]	Visually compatible for 4 hr at 23°C	2215	C
Ceftriaxone sodium	RC	20 mg/mL[a]		TNA #218 to #226[g]	Visually compatible for 4 hr at 23°C	2215	C
Cefuroxime sodium	LI	30 mg/mL[a]		TPN #212 to #215[g]	Physically compatible for 4 hr at 23°C	2109	C
Cefuroxime sodium	GL	30 mg/mL[a]		TNA #218 to #226[g]	Visually compatible for 4 hr at 23°C	2215	C
Chloramphenicol sodium succinate	PD	125 mg/1.25 mL[i]		TPN #61[c g]	Physically compatible	1012	C

Y-Site Injection Compatibility (1:1 Mixture) (Cont.)

Test Drug	Mfr	Conc	Mfr	Conc	Remarks	Ref	C/I
Chloramphenicol sodium succinate	PD	750 mg/7.5 mL[i]		TPN #61[d g]	Physically compatible	1012	C
Chlorothiazide sodium	ME	28 mg/mL		TPN #203, #204[g]	White precipitate forms immediately	1974	I
Chlorpromazine HCl	SCN	2 mg/mL[a]		TPN #212 to #215[g]	Physically compatible for 4 hr at 23°C	2109	C
Chlorpromazine HCl	SCN	2 mg/mL[a]		TNA #218 to #226[g]	Visually compatible for 4 hr at 23°C	2215	C
Ciprofloxacin	MI	2 mg/mL[a]	AB	AA 5%, D 25%	Visually compatible for 2 hr at 25°C under fluorescent light	1628	C
Ciprofloxacin	MI	1 mg/mL[a]		TPN #212 to #215[g]	Amber discoloration forms in 1 to 4 hr	2109	I
Ciprofloxacin	BAY	1 mg/mL[a]		TNA #218 to #226[g]	Visually compatible for 4 hr at 23°C	2215	C
Cisplatin	BMS	1 mg/mL		TPN #212 to #215[g]	Amber discoloration forms in 1 to 4 hr	2109	I
Cisplatin	BMS	1 mg/mL		TNA #218 to #226[g]	Visually compatible for 4 hr at 23°C	2215	C
Clevidipine butyrate	CHS	0.5 mg/mL		10%	Physically compatible for 24 hr at 23°C	3334	C
Clindamycin phosphate	UP	12 mg/mL[a]		TNA #73[g h]	Visually compatible for 4 hr at 25°C	1008	C
Clindamycin phosphate	UP	50 mg/0.33 mL[m]		TPN #61[c g]	Physically compatible	1012	C
Clindamycin phosphate	UP	300 mg/2 mL[m]		TPN #61[d g]	Physically compatible	1012	C
Clindamycin phosphate	AB	10 mg/mL[a]		TPN #212 to #215[g]	Physically compatible for 4 hr at 23°C	2109	C
Clindamycin phosphate	AST	10 mg/mL[a]		TNA #218 to #226[g]	Visually compatible for 4 hr at 23°C	2215	C
Clonazepam	RC	1 mg/mL[k]		TPN #189[g]	Visually compatible for 24 hr at 22°C	1767	C
Cyclophosphamide	MJ	10 mg/mL[a]		TPN #212 to #215[g]	Physically compatible for 4 hr at 23°C	2109	C
Cyclophosphamide	MJ	10 mg/mL[a]		TNA #218 to #226[g]	Visually compatible for 4 hr at 23°C	2215	C
Cyclosporine	SZ	5 mg/mL[a]		TPN #212, #213[g]	Physically compatible for 4 hr at 23°C	2109	C
Cyclosporine	SZ	5 mg/mL[a]		TPN #214, #215[g]	Small amount of subvisible precipitate forms in 4 hr	2109	I
Cyclosporine	SZ	5 mg/mL[a]		TNA #220, #223[g]	Small amount of precipitate forms immediately	2215	I
Cyclosporine	SZ	5 mg/mL[a]		TNA #218, #219, #221, #222, #224 to #226[g]	Visually compatible for 4 hr at 23°C	2215	C
Cytarabine	CHI	50 mg/mL		TPN #212 to #215[g]	Substantial loss of natural subvisible turbidity occurs immediately	2109	I
Cytarabine	BED	50 mg/mL		TNA #218 to #226[g]	Visually compatible for 4 hr at 23°C	2215	C
Dexamethasone sodium phosphate	AMR	4 mg/mL		TPN #203, #204[g]	Visually compatible for 2 hr at 23°C	1974	C
Dexamethasone sodium phosphate	AMR	1 mg/mL[a]		TPN #212 to #215[g]	Physically compatible for 4 hr at 23°C	2109	C
Dexamethasone sodium phosphate	FUJ, ES	1 mg/mL[a]		TNA #218 to #226[g]	Visually compatible for 4 hr at 23°C	2215	C
Digoxin	BW	12.5 mcg/mL[i]		TNA #73[g]	Visually compatible for 4 hr	1009	C
Digoxin	BW	0.25 mg/mL		TPN #212 to #215[g]	Physically compatible for 4 hr at 23°C	2109	C
Digoxin	ES, WY	0.25 mg/mL		TNA #218 to #226[g]	Visually compatible for 4 hr at 23°C	2215	C
Diphenhydramine HCl	SCN	2[a] and 50 mg/mL		TPN #212 to #215[g]	Physically compatible for 4 hr at 23°C	2109	C
Diphenhydramine HCl	PD	2 mg/mL[a]		TNA #218 to #226[g]	Visually compatible for 4 hr at 23°C	2215	C

Y-Site Injection Compatibility (1:1 Mixture) (Cont.)

Test Drug	Mfr	Conc	Mfr	Conc	Remarks	Ref	C/I
Diphenhydramine HCl	SCN	50 mg/mL		TNA #218 to #226[g]	Visually compatible for 4 hr at 23°C	2215	C
Dobutamine HCl	LI	1 mg/mL[n]		TPN #91[f g]	Physically compatible	1170	C
Dobutamine HCl	LI	50 mg/mL[b]		TPN #189[g]	Visually compatible for 24 hr at 22°C	1767	C
Dobutamine HCl	LI	5 mg/mL		TPN #203, #204[g]	Visually compatible for 4 hr at 23°C	1974	C
Dobutamine HCl	LI	4 mg/mL[a]		TPN #212 to #215[g]	Physically compatible for 4 hr at 23°C	2109	C
Dobutamine HCl	AST	4 mg/mL[a]		TNA #218 to #226[g]	Visually compatible for 4 hr at 23°C	2215	C
Dopamine HCl	AB	1.6 mg/mL[i]		TNA #73[g]	Visually compatible for 4 hr	1009	C
Dopamine HCl	DB	1.6 mg/mL[b]		TPN #189[g]	Visually compatible for 24 hr at 22°C	1767	C
Dopamine HCl	AMR	3.2 mg/mL		TPN #203, #204[g]	Visually compatible for 4 hr at 23°C	1974	C
Dopamine HCl	AB	3.2 mg/mL[a]		TPN #212 to #215[g]	Physically compatible for 4 hr at 23°C	2109	C
Dopamine HCl	AB	3.2 mg/mL[a]		TNA #222, #223[g]	Precipitate forms immediately	2215	I
Dopamine HCl	AB	3.2 mg/mL[a]		TNA #218 to #221, #224 to #226[g]	Visually compatible for 4 hr at 23°C	2215	C
Doxorubicin HCl	PH	2 mg/mL		TPN #212 to #215[g]	Substantial loss of natural subvisible haze occurs immediately	2109	I
Doxorubicin HCl	PH, GEN	2 mg/mL		TNA #218 to #226[g]	Damage to emulsion occurs immediately with free oil formation possible	2215	I
Doxycycline hyclate	PF	10 mg/1 mL[j]		TPN #61[c g]	Physically compatible	1012	C
Doxycycline hyclate	PF	60 mg/6 mL[j]		TPN #61[d g]	Physically compatible	1012	C
Doxycycline hyclate	LY	1 mg/mL[a]		TPN #212 to #215[g]	Physically compatible for 4 hr at 23°C	2109	C
Doxycycline hyclate	FUJ	1 mg/mL[a]		TNA #218 to #226[g]	Damage to emulsion occurs immediately with free oil formation possible	2215	I
Droperidol	AB	0.4 mg/mL[a]		TPN #212 to #215[g]	Physically compatible for 4 hr at 23°C	2109	C
Droperidol	AB	0.4 mg/mL[a]		TNA #218 to #226[g]	Damage to emulsion occurs in 1 to 4 hr with free oil formation possible	2215	I
Enalaprilat	MSD	0.1 mg/mL[a]		TPN #212 to #215[g]	Physically compatible for 4 hr at 23°C	2109	C/I
Enalaprilat	ME	0.1 mg/mL[a]		TNA #218 to #226[g]	Visually compatible for 4 hr at 23°C	2215	C
Epinephrine HCl	AST	0.2 mg/mL[b]		TPN #189[g]	Visually compatible for 24 hr at 22°C	1767	C
Erythromycin lactobionate	AB	20 mg/mL[b]		TNA #73[g h]	Visually compatible for 4 hr at 25°C	1008	C
Erythromycin lactobionate	AB	50 mg/1 mL[j]		TPN #61[c g]	Physically compatible	1012	C
Erythromycin lactobionate	AB	300 mg/6 mL[j]		TPN #61[d g]	Physically compatible	1012	C
Erythromycin lactobionate	DB	10 mg/mL[b]		TPN #189[g]	Visually compatible for 24 hr at 22°C	1767	C
Famotidine	ME	2 mg/mL[a]		TPN #212 to #215[g]	Physically compatible for 4 hr at 23°C	2109	C
Famotidine	ME	2 mg/mL[a]		TNA #218 to #226[g]	Visually compatible for 4 hr at 23°C	2215	C
Fentanyl citrate	ES	0.05 mg/mL		TPN #203, #204[g]	Visually compatible for 4 hr at 23°C	1974	C
Fentanyl citrate	ES	0.01 mg/mL[k]		TPN #216[g]	Mixed 1 mL of fentanyl with 9 mL of TPN. Visually compatible for 24 hr	2104	C

Y-Site Injection Compatibility (1:1 Mixture) (Cont.)

Test Drug	Mfr	Conc	Mfr	Conc	Remarks	Ref	C/I
Fentanyl citrate	AB, JN	0.0125[a] and 0.05 mg/mL		TPN #212 to #215[g]	Physically compatible for 4 hr at 23°C	2109	C
Fentanyl citrate	AB	0.0125[a] and 0.05 mg/mL		TNA #218 to #226[g]	Visually compatible for 4 hr at 23°C	2215	C
Floxacillin sodium	BE	50 mg/mL[b]		TPN #189[g]	Visually compatible for 24 hr at 22°C	1767	C
Fluconazole	PF	0.5 and 1.75 mg/mL[o]		TPN #146[g o]	Visually compatible with no fluconazole loss in 2 hr at 24°C in fluorescent light. Amino acids greater than 93%	1554	C
Fluconazole	PF	0.5 and 1.75 mg/mL[o]		TPN #147, #148[g o]	Visually compatible with no fluconazole loss in 2 hr at 24°C in fluorescent light. Amino acids not analyzed	1554	C
Fluconazole	RR	2 mg/mL		TPN #212 to #215[g]	Physically compatible for 4 hr at 23°C	2109	C
Fluconazole	PF	2 mg/mL		TNA #218 to #226[g]	Visually compatible for 4 hr at 23°C	2215	C
Fluorouracil	PH	16 mg/mL[a]		TPN #212, #213[g]	Slight subvisible haze, crystals, and amber discoloration form in 1 to 4 hr	2109	I
Fluorouracil	PH	16 mg/mL[a]		TPN #214, #215[g]	Turbidity forms immediately	2109	I
Fluorouracil	PH	16 mg/mL[a]		TNA #220, #223[g]	Small amount of white precipitate forms immediately	2215	I
Fluorouracil	PH	16 mg/mL[a]		TNA #218, #219, #221, #222, #224 to #226[g]	Visually compatible for 4 hr at 23°C	2215	C
Folic acid	AB	15 mg/mL		TPN #189[g]	Visually compatible for 24 hr at 22°C	1767	C
Foscarnet sodium	AST	24 mg/mL		TPN #121[g]	Physically compatible for 24 hr at 25°C	1393	C
Furosemide	ES	3.3 mg/mL[i]		TNA #73[g]	Visually compatible for 4 hr	1009	C
Furosemide		10 mg/mL[b]		TPN #189[g]	Visually compatible for 24 hr at 22°C	1767	C
Furosemide	AMR	10 mg/mL		TPN #203, #204[g]	Visually compatible for 2 hr at 23°C	1974	C
Furosemide	AB	3 mg/mL[a]		TPN #212 to #215[g]	Small amount of subvisible precipitate forms immediately	2109	I
Furosemide	AB	3 mg/mL[a]		TNA #218 to #226[g]	Visually compatible for 4 hr at 23°C	2215	C
Ganciclovir sodium	SY	1 and 5 mg/mL[a]		TPN #144[g]	Visually compatible for 2 hr at 20°C	1522	C
Ganciclovir sodium	SY	10 mg/mL[a]		TPN #144[g]	Heavy precipitate forms within 30 min	1522	I
Ganciclovir sodium	SY	3 and 5 mg/mL		TPN #183 to #185[g]	Precipitate forms	1744	I
Ganciclovir sodium	SY	2 mg/mL		TPN #183[g]	Precipitate forms	1744	I
Ganciclovir sodium	SY	1 mg/mL[p]		TPN #183[g]	Visually compatible with no ganciclovir loss in 3 hr at 24°C. Less than 10% amino acids loss in 2 hr	1744	C
Ganciclovir sodium	SY	2 mg/mL[q]		TPN #184, #185[g]	Visually compatible with no ganciclovir loss in 3 hr at 24°C. Less than 10% amino acid loss in 3 hr	1744	C
Ganciclovir sodium	SY	20 mg/mL[a]		TPN #212 to #215[g]	Gross white precipitate forms immediately	2109	I
Ganciclovir sodium	RC	20 mg/mL[a]		TNA #218 to #226[g]	White precipitate forms immediately	2215	I
Gentamicin sulfate	SC	1.6 mg/mL[a]		TNA #73[g h]	Visually compatible for 4 hr at 25°C	1008	C
Gentamicin sulfate	IX	12.5 mg/1.25 mL[j]		TPN #61[c g]	Physically compatible	1012	C
Gentamicin sulfate	IX	75 mg/1.9 mL[j]		TPN #61[d g]	Physically compatible	1012	C
Gentamicin sulfate		13 and 20 mg/mL		TPN #54[g]	Physically compatible and gentamicin activity retained over 6 hr at 22°C	1045	C

Y-Site Injection Compatibility (1:1 Mixture) (Cont.)

Test Drug	Mfr	Conc	Mfr	Conc	Remarks	Ref	C/I
Gentamicin sulfate	IX	5 mg[e]		TPN #91[f][g]	Physically compatible	1170	C
Gentamicin sulfate	ES	40 mg/mL		TNA #97 to #104[g]	Physically compatible and gentamicin content retained for 6 hr at 21°C	1324	C
Gentamicin sulfate	DB	1 mg/mL[b]		TPN #189[g]	Visually compatible for 24 hr at 22°C	1767	C
Gentamicin sulfate	ES	10 mg/mL		TPN #203, #204[g]	Visually compatible for 2 hr at 23°C	1974	C
Gentamicin sulfate	AB	5 mg/mL[a]		TPN #212 to #215[g]	Physically compatible for 4 hr at 23°C	2109	C
Gentamicin sulfate	AB, FUJ	5 mg/mL[a]		TNA #218 to #226[g]	Visually compatible for 4 hr at 23°C	2215	C
Granisetron HCl	SKB	0.05 mg/mL[a]		TPN #212 to #215[g]	Physically compatible for 4 hr at 23°C	2109	C
Granisetron HCl	SKB	0.05 mg/mL[a]		TNA #218 to #226[g]	Visually compatible for 4 hr at 23°C	2215	C
Haloperidol lactate	SE	10 mg/mL		TPN #189[g]	Visually compatible for 24 hr at 22°C	1767	C
Haloperidol lactate	MN	0.2 mg/mL[a]		TPN #212 to #215[g]	Physically compatible for 4 hr at 23°C	2109	C
Haloperidol lactate	MN	0.2 mg/mL[a]		TNA #218 to #226[g]	Damage to emulsion occurs immediately with free oil formation possible	2215	I
Heparin sodium	DB	500 units/mL[b]		TPN #189[g]	Visually compatible for 24 hr at 22°C	1767	C
Heparin sodium	AB	100 units/mL		TPN #212 to #215[g]	Physically compatible for 4 hr at 23°C	2109	C
Heparin sodium	AB	100 units/mL		TNA #218 to #226[g]	Damage to emulsion occurs immediately with free oil formation possible	2215	I
Hydrocortisone sodium succinate	UP	50 mg/mL[b]		TPN #189[g]	Visually compatible for 24 hr at 22°C	1767	C
Hydrocortisone sodium succinate	AB	1 mg/mL[a]		TPN #212 to #215[g]	Physically compatible for 4 hr at 23°C	2109	C
Hydrocortisone sodium succinate	AB	1 mg/mL[a]		TNA #218 to #226[g]	Visually compatible for 4 hr at 23°C	2215	C
Hydromorphone HCl	ES	0.5 mg/mL[a]		TPN #212 to #215[g]	Physically compatible for 4 hr at 23°C	2109	C
Hydromorphone HCl	ES	0.5 mg/mL[a]		TNA #219, #222, #224 to #226[g]	Damage to emulsion occurs immediately with free oil formation possible	2215	I
Hydromorphone HCl	ES	0.5 mg/mL[a]		TNA #218, #220, #221, #223[g]	Visually compatible for 4 hr at 23°C	2215	C
Hydroxyzine HCl	ES	2 mg/mL[a]		TPN #212 to #215[g]	Physically compatible for 4 hr at 23°C	2109	C
Hydroxyzine HCl	ES	2 mg/mL[a]		TNA #218 to #226[g]	Visually compatible for 4 hr at 23°C	2215	C
Ibuprofen lysinate	OVA	10 mg/mL	RRN	10%	Measured turbidity increased immediately and solution developed a cloudy haze	3541	I
Ibuprofen lysinate		1.25 mg/mL[b]		TPN #281, #282, #283[g]	Physically compatible for 4 hr at room temperature	3546	C
Ibuprofen lysinate		2.5 mg/mL[b]		TPN #281[g]	Slightly cloudy, opaque solution formed	3546	I
Ibuprofen lysinate		2.5 mg/mL[b]		TPN #282, #283[g]	Physically compatible for 4 hr at room temperature	3546	C
Ibuprofen lysinate		5 mg/mL[b]		TPN #281, #282, #283[g]	Cloudy, opaque solution formed with sediment detected after 24 hr	3546	I
Idarubicin HCl	AD	1 mg/mL[b]		TPN #140[g]	Visually compatible for 24 hr at 25°C	1525	C
Ifosfamide	MJ	25 mg/mL[a]		TPN #212 to #215[g]	Physically compatible for 4 hr at 23°C	2109	C
Ifosfamide	MJ	25 mg/mL[a]		TNA #218 to #226[g]	Visually compatible for 4 hr at 23°C	2215	C

Y-Site Injection Compatibility (1:1 Mixture) (Cont.)

Test Drug	Mfr	Conc	Mfr	Conc	Remarks	Ref	C/I
Imipenem–cilastatin sodium	ME	10 mg/mL[b y]		TPN #212 to #215[g]	Physically compatible for 4 hr at 23°C	2109	C
Imipenem–cilastatin sodium	ME	10 mg/mL[b y]		TNA #218 to #226[g]	Visually compatible for 4 hr at 23°C	2215	C
Indomethacin sodium trihydrate	MSD	1 mg/mL[b]	MG[r]	AA 1 and 2%, D 10%	Haze forms in 2 hr and white precipitate forms in 4 hr	1527	I
Indomethacin sodium trihydrate	MSD	1 mg/mL[b]	MG[r]	AA 1 and 2%, W	Haze forms in 30 min and white precipitate forms in 1 hr	1527	I
Insulin, regular	NOV	2 units/mL[s]		TPN #189[g]	Visually compatible for 24 hr at 22°C	1767	C
Insulin, regular	NOV	1 unit/mL[a]		TPN #212 to #215[g]	Physically compatible for 4 hr at 23°C	2109	C
Insulin, regular	NOV	1 unit/mL[a]		TNA #218 to #226[g]	Visually compatible for 4 hr at 23°C	2215	C
Isoproterenol HCl	BR	4 mcg/mL[l]		TNA #73[g]	Visually compatible for 4 hr	1009	C
Leucovorin calcium	IMM	2 mg/mL[a]		TPN #212 to #215[g]	Physically compatible for 4 hr at 23°C	2109	C
Leucovorin calcium	IMM	2 mg/mL[a]		TNA #218 to #226[g]	Visually compatible for 4 hr at 23°C	2215	C
Lidocaine HCl	ES	4 mg/mL[l]		TNA #73[g]	Visually compatible for 4 hr	1009	C
Lorazepam	WY	0.1 mg/mL[a]		TPN #212 to #215[g]	Physically compatible for 4 hr at 23°C	2109	C
Lorazepam	WY	0.1 mg/mL[a]		TNA #218 to #226[g]	Damage to emulsion occurs in 1 hr	2215	I
Magnesium sulfate	AB	100 mg/mL[a]		TPN #212 to #215[g]	Physically compatible for 4 hr at 23°C	2109	C
Magnesium sulfate	AB	100 mg/mL[a]		TNA #218 to #226[g]	Visually compatible for 4 hr at 23°C	2215	C
Mannitol	BA	15%		TPN #212 to #215[g]	Physically compatible for 4 hr at 23°C	2109	C
Mannitol	BA	15%		TNA #218 to #226[g]	Visually compatible for 4 hr at 23°C	2215	C
Meperidine HCl	AB	10 mg/mL		TPN #131, #132[g]	Physically compatible for 4 hr at 25°C under fluorescent light	1397	C
Meperidine HCl	DB	50 mg/mL		TPN #189[g]	Visually compatible for 24 hr at 22°C	1767	C
Meperidine HCl	AST	4 mg/mL[a]		TPN #212 to #215[g]	Physically compatible for 4 hr at 23°C	2109	C
Meperidine HCl	AST	4 mg/mL[a]		TNA #218 to #226[g]	Visually compatible for 4 hr at 23°C	2215	C
Meropenem	ZEN	20 mg/mL[a]		TNA #218 to #226[g]	Visually compatible for 4 hr at 23°C	2215	C
Mesna	MJ	10 mg/mL[a]		TPN #212 to #215[g]	Physically compatible for 4 hr at 23°C	2109	C
Mesna	MJ	10 mg/mL[a]		TNA #218 to #226[g]	Visually compatible for 4 hr at 23°C	2215	C
Methotrexate sodium	LE	15 mg/mL[a]		TPN #212 to #215[g]	Substantial loss of natural haze with a microprecipitate	2109	I
Methotrexate sodium	IMM	15 mg/mL[a]		TNA #218 to #226[g]	Visually compatible for 4 hr at 23°C	2215	C
Methyldopate HCl	MSD	5 mg/mL[a]		TNA #73[g]	Cracked the lipid emulsion	1009	I
Methyldopate HCl	MSD	5 mg/mL[b]		TNA #73[g]	Visually compatible for 4 hr	1009	C
Methylprednisolone sodium succinate	AB	5 mg/mL[a]		TPN #212 to #215[g]	Physically compatible for 4 hr at 23°C	2109	C
Methylprednisolone sodium succinate	AB	5 mg/mL[a]		TNA #218 to #226[g]	Visually compatible for 4 hr at 23°C	2215	C
Metoclopramide HCl	AB	5 mg/mL		TPN #212 to #215[g]	Substantial loss of natural haze occurs immediately	2109	I
Metoclopramide HCl	AB	5 mg/mL		TNA #218 to #226[g]	Visually compatible for 4 hr at 23°C	2215	C

Y-Site Injection Compatibility (1:1 Mixture) (Cont.)

Test Drug	Mfr	Conc	Mfr	Conc	Remarks	Ref	C/I
Metronidazole	DB	5 mg/mL		TPN #189[g]	Visually compatible for 24 hr at 22°C	1767	C
Metronidazole	AB	5 mg/mL		TPN #203, #204[g]	Visually compatible for 2 hr at 23°C	1974	C
Metronidazole	SCS	5 mg/mL		TPN #212 to #215[g]	Physically compatible for 4 hr at 23°C	2109	C
Metronidazole	AB	5 mg/mL		TNA #218 to #226[g]	Visually compatible for 4 hr at 23°C	2215	C
Micafungin sodium	ASP	1.5 mg/mL[b]		TPN #268[g]	Physically compatible for 4 hr at 23°C	2683	C
Midazolam HCl	RC	5 mg/mL		TPN #189[g]	White haze and precipitate form immediately. Crystals form in 24 hr	1767	I
Midazolam HCl	RC	2 mg/mL[a]		TPN #212 to #215[g]	White cloudiness forms rapidly	2109	I
Midazolam HCl	RC	2 mg/mL[a]		TNA #218 to #226[g]	Damage to emulsion occurs immediately with free oil formation possible	2215	I
Milrinone lactate	SW	0.4 mg/mL[a]		TPN #217[g]	Visually compatible with no loss of milrinone in 4 hr at 23°C	2214	C
Milrinone lactate	SS	0.2 mg/mL[a]		TPN #243, #244[g]	Visually compatible for 4 hr at 24°C	2381	C
Mitoxantrone HCl	IMM	0.5 mg/mL[a]		TPN #212 to #215[g]	Substantial loss of natural haze occurs immediately	2109	I
Mitoxantrone HCl	IMM	0.5 mg/mL[a]		TNA #218 to #226[g]	Visually compatible for 4 hr at 23°C	2215	C
Morphine sulfate	AB	1 mg/mL		TPN #131, #132[g]	Physically compatible for 4 hr at 25°C	1397	C
Morphine sulfate	DB	30 mg/mL		TPN #189[g]	Visually compatible for 24 hr at 22°C	1767	C
Morphine sulfate	ES	1 mg/mL		TPN #203, #204[g]	Visually compatible for 2 hr at 23°C	1974	C
Morphine sulfate	AST	1 mg/mL[a]		TPN #212 to #215[g]	Physically compatible for 4 hr at 23°C	2109	C
Morphine sulfate	ES	1 mg/mL[a]		TNA #218 to #226[g]	Visually compatible for 4 hr at 23°C	2215	C
Morphine sulfate	ES	15 mg/mL		TNA #218 to #226[g]	Damage to emulsion occurs immediately with free oil formation possible	2215	I
Multivitamins (M.V.I.-12)	ROR			TPN #189[g]	Visually compatible for 24 hr at 22°C	1767	C
Nafcillin sodium	WY	250 mg/1 mL[i]		TPN #61[c g]	Physically compatible	1012	C
Nafcillin sodium	WY	1.5 g/6 mL[i]		TPN #61[d g]	Physically compatible	1012	C
Nafcillin sodium		250 mg/mL		TPN #54[g]	Physically compatible and nafcillin activity retained over 6 hr at 22°C	1045	C
Nafcillin sodium	BE	20 mg/mL[a]		TPN #212 to #215[g]	Physically compatible for 4 hr at 23°C	2109	C
Nafcillin sodium	BE, APC	20 mg/mL[a]		TNA #218 to #226[g]	Visually compatible for 4 hr at 23°C	2215	C
Nalbuphine HCl	AB	10 mg/mL		TPN #212 to #215[g]	Physically compatible for 4 hr at 23°C	2109	C
Nalbuphine HCl	AB, AST	10 mg/mL		TNA #218 to #226[g]	Damage to emulsion occurs immediately with free oil formation possible	2215	I
Nitroglycerin	DU	0.4 mg/mL[a]		TPN #212 to #215[g]	Physically compatible for 4 hr at 23°C	2109	C
Nitroglycerin	DU	0.4 mg/mL[a]		TNA #218 to #226[g]	Visually compatible for 4 hr at 23°C	2215	C
Norepinephrine bitartrate	BN	8 mcg/mL[i]		TNA #73[g]	Visually compatible for 4 hr	1009	C
Norepinephrine bitartrate	AB	16 mcg/mL[a]		TPN #212 to #215[g]	Physically compatible for 4 hr at 23°C	2109	C
Octreotide acetate	SZ	0.01 mg/mL[a]		TPN #212 to #215[g]	Physically compatible for 4 hr at 23°C	2109	C
Octreotide acetate	SZ	0.01 mg/mL[a]		TNA #218 to #226[g]	Visually compatible for 4 hr at 23°C	2215	C

Y-Site Injection Compatibility (1:1 Mixture) (Cont.)

Test Drug	Mfr	Conc	Mfr	Conc	Remarks	Ref	C/I
Ondansetron HCl	GL	1 mg/mL[a]		TPN #212 to #215[g]	Physically compatible for 4 hr at 23°C	2109	C
Ondansetron HCl	CER	1 mg/mL[a]		TNA #218 to #226[g]	Damage to emulsion occurs immediately with free oil formation possible	2215	I
Oxacillin sodium	BE	20 mg/mL[a]		TNA #73[g h]	Visually compatible for 4 hr at 25°C	1008	C
Oxacillin sodium	BE	250 mg/1.5 mL[i]		TPN #61[c g]	Physically compatible	1012	C
Oxacillin sodium	BE	1.5 g/9 mL[i]		TPN #61[d g]	Physically compatible	1012	C
Oxacillin sodium		100 and 150 mg/mL		TPN #54[g]	Physically compatible and 88 to 94% oxacillin activity retained over 6 hr at 22°C	1045	C
Paclitaxel	MJ	1.2 mg/mL[a]		TPN #212 to #215[g]	Physically compatible for 4 hr at 23°C	2109	C
Paclitaxel	MJ	1.2 mg/mL[a]		TNA #218 to #226[g]	Visually compatible for 4 hr at 23°C	2215	C
Penicillin G	PF	200,000 units/2 mL[i]		TPN #61[c g]	Physically compatible	1012	C
Penicillin G	PF	1.2 million units/12 mL[i]		TPN #61[d g]	Physically compatible	1012	C
Penicillin G		320,000 and 500,000 units/mL		TPN #54[g]	Physically compatible and 88% penicillin activity retained over 6 hr at 22°C	1045	C
Penicillin G		300 mg/mL[b]		TPN #189[g]	Visually compatible for 24 hr at 22°C	1767	C
Penicillin G potassium	SQ	40,000 units/mL[a]		TNA #73[g h]	Visually compatible for 4 hr at 25°C	1008	C
Penicillin G potassium	MAR	500,000 units/mL		TPN #203, #204[g]	Visually compatible for 2 hr at 23°C	1974	C
Pentobarbital sodium	AB	5 mg/mL[a]		TPN #212 to #215[g]	Physically compatible for 4 hr at 23°C	2109	C
Pentobarbital sodium	AB	5 mg/mL[a]		TNA #218 to #226[g]	Damage to emulsion occurs immediately with free oil formation possible	2215	I
Phenobarbital sodium	WY	5 mg/mL[a]		TPN #212 to #215[g]	Physically compatible for 4 hr at 23°C	2109	C
Phenobarbital sodium	WY	5 mg/mL[a]		TNA #218 to #226[g]	Damage to emulsion occurs immediately with free oil formation possible	2215	I
Phenytoin sodium	PD	50 mg/mL		TPN #189[g]	Heavy white precipitate forms immediately	1767	I
Piperacillin sodium–tazobactam sodium	CY[x]	40 mg/mL[a z]		TPN #212 to #215[g]	Physically compatible for 4 hr at 23°C	2109	C
Piperacillin sodium–tazobactam sodium	LE[x]	40 mg/mL[a z]		TNA #218 to #226[g]	Visually compatible for 4 hr at 23°C	2215	C
Potassium chloride	AST	30 mg/mL[b]		TPN #189[g]	Visually compatible for 24 hr at 22°C	1767	C
Potassium chloride	AB	0.1 mEq/mL[a]		TPN #212 to #215[g]	Physically compatible for 4 hr at 23°C	2109	C
Potassium chloride	AB	0.1 mEq/mL[a]		TNA #218 to #226[g]	Visually compatible for 4 hr at 23°C	2215	C
Potassium phosphates	AB	3 mmol/mL		TPN #212 to #215[g]	Increased turbidity forms immediately	2109	I
Potassium phosphates	AB	3 mmol/mL		TNA #218 to #226[g]	Damage to emulsion occurs immediately with free oil formation possible	2215	I
Prochlorperazine edisylate	SCN	0.5 mg/mL[a]		TPN #212 to #215[g]	Physically compatible for 4 hr at 23°C	2109	C
Prochlorperazine edisylate	SCN, SO	0.5 mg/mL[a]		TNA #218 to #226[g]	Visually compatible for 4 hr at 23°C	2215	C
Promethazine HCl	SCN	2 mg/mL[a]		TPN #212, #214[g]	Physically compatible for 4 hr at 23°C	2109	C
Promethazine HCl	SCN	2 mg/mL[a]		TPN #213, #215[g]	Amber discoloration forms in 4 hr	2109	I

Y-Site Injection Compatibility (1:1 Mixture) (Cont.)

Test Drug	Mfr	Conc	Mfr	Conc	Remarks	Ref	C/I
Promethazine HCl	SCN	2 mg/mL[a]		TNA #218 to #226[g]	Visually compatible for 4 hr at 23°C	2215	C
Propofol	STU	2 and 3 g		TPN #186 to #188[g]	Physically compatible and 6% or less propofol loss in 5 hr at 22°C	1805	C
Propofol	STU	500 mg		TPN #186[g]	Physically compatible but 28% propofol loss in 5 hr at 22°C	1805	I
Propofol	STU	500 mg		TPN #187, #188[g]	Physically compatible and 6% or less propofol loss in 5 hr at 22°C	1805	C
Ranitidine HCl	GL	2.5 mg/mL[b]		TPN #189[g]	Visually compatible for 24 hr at 22°C	1767	C
Ranitidine HCl	GL	25 mg/mL		TPN #203, #204[g]	Visually compatible for 2 hr at 23°C	1974	C
Ranitidine HCl	GL	2 mg/mL[a]		TPN #212 to #215[g]	Physically compatible for 4 hr at 23°C	2109	C
Ranitidine HCl	GL	2 mg/mL[a]		TNA #218 to #226[g]	Visually compatible for 4 hr at 23°C	2215	C
Sargramostim	IMM	10 mcg/mL[b]		TPN #133[g]	Visually compatible for 4 hr at 22°C	1436	C
Sargramostim	IMM	6[t] and 15 mcg/mL[b]		TPN #181[g]	Visually compatible for 2 hr	1618	C
Sodium bicarbonate	AB	1 mEq/mL		TPN #212, #214[g]	Microprecipitate in 1 hr	2109	I
Sodium bicarbonate	AB	1 mEq/mL		TPN #213, #215[g]	Physically compatible for 4 hr at 23°C	2109	C
Sodium bicarbonate	AB	1 mEq/mL		TNA #218 to #226[g]	Visually compatible for 4 hr at 23°C	2215	C
Sodium nitroprusside	AB	0.4 mg/mL[a]		TPN #212 to #215[g]	Physically compatible for 4 hr at 23°C protected from light	2109	C
Sodium nitroprusside	AB	0.4 mg/mL[a]		TNA #218 to #226[g]	Visually compatible for 4 hr at 23°C protected from light	2215	C
Sodium phosphates	AB	3 mmol/mL		TPN #212 to #215[g]	Increased turbidity forms immediately	2109	I
Sodium phosphates	AB	3 mmol/mL		TNA #218 to #226[g]	Damage to emulsion occurs immediately with free oil formation possible	2215	I
Tacrolimus	FUJ	1 mg/mL[a]		TPN #212 to #215[g]	Physically compatible for 4 hr at 23°C	2109	C
Tacrolimus	FUJ	1 mg/mL[a]		TNA #218 to #226[g]	Visually compatible for 4 hr at 23°C	2215	C
Thiotepa	IMM[u]	1 mg/mL[a]		TPN #193[g]	Physically compatible for 4 hr at 23°C	1861	C
Tobramycin sulfate	LI	1.6 mg/mL[a]		TNA #73[g h]	Visually compatible for 4 hr at 25°C	1008	C
Tobramycin sulfate	DI	12.5 mg/1.25 mL[j]		TPN #61[c g]	Physically compatible	1012	C
Tobramycin sulfate	DI	75 mg/1.9 mL[j]		TPN #61[d g]	Physically compatible	1012	C
Tobramycin sulfate		20 mg/mL		TPN #54[g]	Physically compatible and tobramycin activity retained over 6 hr at 22°C	1045	C
Tobramycin sulfate	LI	5 mg[e]		TPN #91[f g]	Physically compatible	1170	C
Tobramycin sulfate	LI	40 mg/mL		TNA #97 to #104[g]	Physically compatible and tobramycin content retained for 6 hr at 21°C	1324	C
Tobramycin sulfate	AB	5 mg/mL[a]		TPN #212 to #215[g]	Physically compatible for 4 hr at 23°C	2109	C
Tobramycin sulfate	AB	5 mg/mL[a]		TNA #218 to #226[g]	Visually compatible for 4 hr at 23°C	2215	C
Trimethoprim–sulfamethoxazole	ES	0.8 mg/mL[a bb]		TNA #212 to #215[g]	Physically compatible for 4 hr at 23°C	2109	C
Trimethoprim–sulfamethoxazole	ES	0.8 mg/mL[a bb]		TNA #218 to #226[g]	Visually compatible for 4 hr at 23°C	2215	C

Y-Site Injection Compatibility (1:1 Mixture) (Cont.)

Test Drug	Mfr	Conc	Mfr	Conc	Remarks	Ref	C/I
Vancomycin HCl	LI	50 mg/1 mL[j]		TPN #61[c,g]	Physically compatible	1012	C
Vancomycin HCl	LI	300 mg/6 mL[j]		TPN #61[d,g]	Physically compatible	1012	C
Vancomycin HCl	LI	30 mg[e]		TPN #91[f,g]	Physically compatible	1170	C
Vancomycin HCl	DB	10 mg/mL[b]		TPN #189[g]	Visually compatible for 24 hr at 22°C	1767	C
Vancomycin HCl	AB	10 mg/mL[a]		TPN #212 to #215[g]	Physically compatible for 4 hr at 23°C	2109	C
Vancomycin HCl	AB	10 mg/mL[a]		TNA #218 to #226[g]	Visually compatible for 4 hr at 23°C	2215	C
Vecuronium bromide	OR	2 mg/mL[k]		TPN #189[g]	Visually compatible for 24 hr at 22°C	1767	C
Zidovudine	BW	4 mg/mL[a]		TPN #212 to #215[g]	Physically compatible for 4 hr at 23°C	2109	C
Zidovudine	GW	4 mg/mL[a]		TNA #218 to #226[g]	Visually compatible for 4 hr at 23°C	2215	C

[a] Tested in dextrose 5%.

[b] Tested in sodium chloride 0.9%.

[c] Run at 21 mL/hr.

[d] Run at 94 mL/hr.

[e] Given over one hour by syringe pump.

[f] Run at 10 mL/hr.

[g] Refer to Appendix for the composition of parenteral nutrition solutions. TNA indicates a 3-in-1 admixture, and TPN indicates a 2-in-1 admixture.

[h] A 32.5-mL sample of parenteral nutrition solution and 50 mL of antibiotic in a minibottle.

[i] Given over five minutes by syringe pump.

[j] Given over 30 minutes by syringe pump.

[k] Tested in sterile water for injection.

[l] Tested in both dextrose 5% and sodium chloride 0.9%.

[m] Given over 10 minutes by syringe pump.

[n] Tested in dextrose 5% infused at 1.2 mL/hr.

[o] Varying volumes to simulate varying administration rates.

[p] Ganciclovir sodium concentration after mixing was 0.83 mg/mL.

[q] Ganciclovir sodium concentration after mixing was 1.4 mg/mL.

[r] TrophAmine.

[s] Tested in Haemaccel (Behring).

[t] With albumin human 0.1%.

[u] Lyophilized formulation tested.

[v] Tested in Ringer's injection, lactated.

[w] Specific composition of the parenteral nutrition admixture not reported. TPN indicates a 2-in-1 admixture.

[x] Test performed using the formulation WITHOUT edetate disodium.

[y] Not specified whether concentration refers to single component or combined components.

[z] Piperacillin component. Piperacillin in an 8:1 fixed-ratio concentration with tazobactam.

[aa] Ampicillin component. Ampicillin in a 2:1 fixed-ratio concentration with sulbactam.

[bb] Trimethoprim component. Trimethoprim in a 1:5 fixed-ratio concentration with sulfamethoxazole.

[cc] Sodium carbonate-containing formulation tested.

Additional Compatibility Information
Multicomponent (3-in-1; TNA) Admixtures

Because of the potential benefits in terms of simplicity, efficiency, time, and cost savings, the concept of mixing amino acids, carbohydrates, electrolytes, fat emulsion, and other nutritional components together in the same container has been explored. Within limits, the feasibility of preparing such 3-in-1 parenteral nutrition admixtures has been demonstrated as long as a careful examination of the emulsion mixtures for signs of instability is performed prior to administration.

However, these 3-in-1 mixtures are very complex and inherently unstable. Emulsion stability is dependent on both zeta potential and van der Waals forces, influenced by the presence of dextrose.[2029] The ultimate stability of each unique mixture depends on numerous complicated factors, making definitive stability predictions impossible. Injury and death have resulted from administration of unrecognized precipitates in 3-in-1 parenteral nutrition admixtures.[1769][1782][1783] See the section on Calcium and Phosphate. In addition, the use of 3-in-1 admixtures is associated with a higher rate of catheter occlusion and reduced catheter life compared with giving the fat emulsion separately from the parenteral nutrition solution.[705][1518][2194]

The use of a 5-μm inline filter for a 3-in-1 admixture (containing Travasol 8.5%, dextrose, Intralipid 10%, various electrolytes, vitamins, and trace elements) showed that fat, in the form of large globules or aggregates, comprised 99.4% of the filter contents. These authors recommend the use of an appropriate filter for preventing catheter occlusion with 3-in-1 admixtures.[742]

Using light microscopy, the presence of glass particles, talc, and plastic has been observed in administration line samples drawn from 20 adults receiving 3-in-1 parenteral nutrition admixtures and in 20 children receiving 2-in-1 admixtures with separate fat emulsion infusions. Particles ranged from 3 to 5 μm to greater than 40 μm and were more consistently seen in the pediatric admixtures. The authors suggested the use of inline filters given that particulate contamination is present, has no therapeutic value, and can be harmful.[2458]

Combining an amino acids–glucose parenteral nutrition solution containing various electrolytes with fat emulsion 20%, intravenous (Intralipid, Vitrum), resulted in a mixture which, although apparently stable for a limited time, ultimately exhibited a creaming phenomenon. Within 12 hours, a distinct 2-cm layer separated on the upper surface. Microscopic examination revealed aggregates believed to be clumps of fat droplets. Fewer and smaller aggregates were noted in the lower layer.[560][561]

Amino acids were reported to have no adverse effect on the emulsion stability of Intralipid 10%. In addition, the amino acids appeared to prevent the adverse impact of dextrose and to slow the flocculation and coalescence resulting from mono- and divalent cations. However, significant coalescence did result after a longer time. Therefore, it was recommended that such cations not be mixed with fat emulsion, intravenous.[656]

Three-in-one TNA admixtures prepared with Intralipid 20% and containing mono- and divalent ions as well as heparin sodium 5 units/mL were found to undergo changes consistent with instability including fat particle shape and diameter changes as well as creaming and layering. The changes were evident within 48 hours at room temperature but were delayed to between 1 and 2 months when refrigerated.[58]

Travenol stated that 1:1:1 mixtures of amino acids 5.5, 8.5, or 10% (Travenol), fat emulsion 10 to 20% (Travenol), and dextrose 10 to 70% are physically stable but recommends administration within 24 hours. M.V.I.-12 3.3 mL/L and electrolytes may also be added to the admixtures up to the maximum amounts listed in Table 1.[850]

Table 1. Maximum electrolyte amounts for Travenol 3-in-1 admixtures[850]

Calcium	8.3 mEq/L
Magnesium	3.3 mEq/L
Sodium	23.3 mEq/L
Potassium	20 mEq/L
Chloride	23.3 mEq/L
Phosphate	20 mEq/L
Zinc	3.33 mg/L
Copper	1.33 mg/L
Manganese	0.33 mg/L
Chromium	13.33 mcg/L

The stability of mixtures of 1 L of Intralipid 20%, 1.5 L of Vamin glucose (amino acids with dextrose 10%), and 0.5 L of dextrose 10% with various electrolytes and vitamins was evaluated. Initial emulsion particle size was around 1 μm. The mixture containing only monovalent cations was stable for at least 9 days at 4°C, with little change in particle size. The mixtures containing the divalent cations, such as calcium and magnesium, demonstrated much greater particle size increases, with mean diameters of around 3.3 to 3.5 μm after 9 days at 4°C. After 48 hours of storage, however, these increases were more modest, around 1.5 to 1.85 μm. After storage at 4°C for 48 hours followed by 24 hours at room temperature, few particles exceeded 5 μm. It was found that the effect of particle aggregation caused by electrolytes demonstrates a critical concentration before the effect begins. For calcium and magnesium chlorides, the critical concentrations were 2.4 and 2.6 mmol/L, respectively. Sodium and potassium chloride had critical concentrations of 110 and 150 mmol/L, respectively. The rate of particle aggregation increased linearly with increasing electrolyte concentration. The quantity of emulsion in the mixture had a relatively small influence on stability, but higher concentrations exhibited a somewhat greater coalescence.[892]

Instability of the emulsion systems is manifested by (1) flocculation of oil droplets to form aggregates, producing a cream-like layer on top; or (2) coalescence of oil droplets, leading to an increase in the average droplet size and eventually a separation of free oil. The lowering of pH and the adding of electrolytes can adversely affect the mechanical and electrical properties at the oil–water interface, eventually leading to flocculation and coalescence. Amino acids act as buffering agents and provide a protective effect on emulsion stability. Adding electrolytes, especially the divalent ions Mg++ and Ca++ in excess of 2.5 mmol/L, to simple fat emulsions will cause flocculation. But in mixed parenteral nutrition solutions, the stability of the emulsion will be enhanced, depending on the quantity and nature of the amino acids present. The authors recommended a careful examination of emulsion mixtures for signs of instability prior to administration.[849]

Good stability was reported for an amino acid 4% (Travenol), dextrose 14%, and fat emulsion 4% (Pharmacia) parenteral nutrition solution. The solution also contained electrolytes, vitamins, and heparin sodium 4000 units/L. The aqueous solution was prepared first, with the fat emulsion added subsequently. This procedure allowed visual inspection of the aqueous phase and reduced the risk of emulsion breakdown by the divalent cations. Sample mixtures were stored at 18 to 25 and 3 to 8°C for up to 5 days. They were evaluated visually and with a Coulter counter for particle size measurements. Both room temperature and refrigerated mixtures were stable for 48 hours. A marked increase in particle size was noted in the room temperature sample after 72 hours, but refrigeration delayed the changes. The authors' experience with over 1400 mixtures for administration to patients resulted in one emulsion creaming and another cracking, but the authors had no explanation for the failure of these particular emulsions.[848]

Six parenteral nutrition solutions having various concentrations of amino acids, dextrose, soybean oil emulsion (Kabi-Vitrum), electrolytes, and multivitamins were evaluated. All of the admixtures were stable for 1 week under refrigeration followed by 24 hours at room temperature, with no visible changes, changes in pH, or significant changes in particle size.[1013] However, other researchers questioned this interpretation of the results.[1014 1015]

The stability of 3-in-1 parenteral nutrition solutions prepared with 500 mL of Intralipid 20%, compared to Soyacal 20%, along with 500 or 1000 mL of FreAmine III 8.5% and 500 mL of dextrose 70% was reported. Also present were relatively large amounts of electrolytes and other additives. All mixtures were similarly stable for 28 days at 4°C followed by 5 days at 21 to 25°C, with little change in the emulsion. A slight white cream layer appeared after 5 days at 4°C but was easily redispersed with gentle agitation. The appearance of this cream layer did not statistically affect particle size distribution. The authors concluded that the emulsion mixture remained suitable for clinical use throughout the study period. The stability of other components was not evaluated.[1019]

The stability of 3-in-1 parenteral nutrition admixtures prepared with Liposyn II 10 and 20%, Aminosyn pH 6, and dextrose along with electrolytes, trace metals, and vitamins was reported. Thirty-one different combinations were evaluated. Samples were stored at: (1) 25°C for 1 day, (2) 5°C for 2 days followed by 30°C for 1 day, and (3) 5°C for 9 days followed by 25°C for 1 day. In all cases, there was no visual evidence of creaming, free oil droplets, and other signs of emulsion instability. Furthermore, little

or no change in the particle size or zeta potential (electrostatic surface charge of lipid particles) was found, indicating emulsion stability. The dextrose and amino acids remained stable over the 10-day storage period. The greatest change of an amino acid occurred with tryptophan, which lost 6% in 10 days. Vitamin stability was not tested.[1025]

The stability of 4 parenteral nutrition admixtures, ranging from 1 L each of amino acids 5.5% (Travenol), dextrose 10%, and fat emulsion 10% (Travenol) up to a "worst case" of 1 L each of amino acids 10% with electrolytes (Travenol), dextrose 70%, and fat emulsion 10% (Travenol) was reported. The admixtures were stored for 48 hours at 5 to 9°C followed by 24 hours at room temperature. There were no visible signs of creaming, flocculation, and free oil. The mean emulsion particle size remained within acceptable limits for all admixtures, and there were no significant changes in glucose, soybean oil, and amino acid concentrations. The authors noted that 2 factors were predominant in determining the stability of such admixtures: electrolyte concentrations and pH.[1065]

Several parenteral nutrition solutions containing amino acids (Travenol), glucose, and lipid, with and without electrolytes and trace elements, produced no visible flocculation or any significant change in mean emulsion particle size during 24 hours at room temperature.[1066]

The compatibility of 10 parenteral nutrition admixtures, evaluated over 96 hours while stored at 20 to 25°C in both glass bottles and ethylene vinyl acetate bags was reported. A slight creaming occurred in all admixtures, but the cream layer was easily redispersed with gentle shaking. No fat globules were visually apparent. The mean drop size was larger in the cream layer, but no globules were larger than 5 μm. Analyses of the concentrations of amino acids, dextrose, and electrolytes showed no changes over the study period. The authors concluded that such parenteral nutrition admixtures could be safely prepared as long as the component concentrations are within the ranges found in Table 2.[1067]

Table 2. Range of component amounts for compatibility testing of 3-in-1 admixtures[1067]

Vamin glucose or Vamin N (amino acids 7%)	1000 to 2000 mL
Dextrose 10 to 30%	100 to 550 mL
Intralipid 10 or 20%	500 to 1000 mL
Electrolyte (mmol/L)	
Sodium	20 to 70
Potassium	20 to 55
Calcium	2.3 to 2.9
Magnesium	1.1 to 3.1
Phosphorus	0 to 9.2
Chloride	27 to 71
Zinc	0.005 to 0.03

The stability of 8 parenteral nutrition admixtures with various ratios of amino acids, carbohydrates, and fat was reported. FreAmine III 8.5%, dextrose 70%, and Soyacal 10 and 20% (mixed in ratios of 2:1:1, 1:1:1, 1:1:½, and 1:1:¼, where 1 = 500 mL) were evaluated. Additive concentrations were high to stress the admixtures and represent maximum doses likely to be encountered clinically. (See Table 3.)

Table 3. Range of component amounts for compatibility testing of 3-in-1 admixtures[1068]

Sodium acetate	150 mEq
Sodium chloride	210 mEq
Potassium acetate	45 mEq
Potassium chloride	90 mEq
Potassium phosphate	15 mM
Calcium gluconate	20 mEq
Magnesium sulfate	36 mEq
Trace elements	present
Folic acid	5 mg
M.V.I.-12	10 mL

The admixtures were stored at 4°C for 14 days followed by 4 days at 22 to 25°C. After 24 hours, all admixtures developed a thin white cream layer, which readily redispersed on gentle agitation. No free oil droplets were observed. The mean particle diameter remained near the original size of the Soyacal throughout the study. Few particles were larger than 3 μm. Osmolality and pH also remained relatively unchanged.[1068]

Parenteral nutrition 3-in-1 admixtures with Aminosyn and Liposyn have been a problem. Standard admixtures were prepared using Aminosyn 7% 1000 mL, dextrose 50% 1000 mL, and Liposyn 10% 500 mL. Concentrated admixtures were prepared using Aminosyn 10% 500 mL, dextrose 70% 500 mL, and Liposyn 20% 500 mL. Vitamins and trace elements were added to the admixtures along with the following electrolytes (see Table 4).

Table 4. Electrolyte amounts for compatibility testing of 3-in-1 admixtures[1069]

Electrolyte	Standard Admixture	Concentrated Admixture
Sodium	125 mEq	75 mEq
Potassium	95 mEq	74 mEq
Magnesium	25 mEq	25 mEq
Calcium	28 mEq	28 mEq
Phosphate	37 mM	36 mM
Chloride	83 mEq	50 mEq

Samples of each admixture were: (1) stored at 4°C, (2) adjusted to pH 6.6 with sodium bicarbonate and stored at 4°C,

or (3) adjusted to pH 6.6 and stored at room temperature. The compatibility was evaluated for 3 weeks.

Visible signs of emulsion deterioration were evident by 96 hours in the standard admixture and by 48 hours in the concentrated admixture. Clear rings formed at the meniscus, becoming thicker, yellow, and oily over time. Free-floating oil was obvious in 3 weeks in the standard admixture and 1 week in the concentrated admixture. The samples adjusted to pH 6.6 developed visible deterioration later than the others. The authors indicated that pH may play a greater role than temperature in emulsion stability. However, precipitation (probably calcium phosphate and possibly carbonate) occurred in 36 hours in the pH 6.6 concentrated admixture but not the unadjusted (pH 5.5) samples. Mean particle counts increased for all samples over time but were greatest in the concentrated admixtures. The authors concluded that the concentrated admixtures were unsatisfactory for clinical use because of the early increase in particles and precipitation. Furthermore, they recommended that the standard admixtures be prepared immediately prior to use.[1069]

The physical stability of 10 parenteral nutrition admixtures with different amino acid sources was studied. The admixtures contained 500 mL each of dextrose 70%, fat emulsion 20% (Alpha Therapeutic), and amino acids in various concentrations from each manufacturer. Also present were standard electrolytes, trace elements, and vitamins. The admixtures were stored for 14 days at 4°C, followed by 4 days at 22 to 25°C. Slight creaming was evident in all admixtures but redispersed easily with agitation. Emulsion particles were uniform in size, showing no tendency to aggregate. No cracked emulsions occurred.[1217]

The stability of parenteral nutrition solutions containing amino acids, dextrose, and fat emulsion along with electrolytes, trace elements, and vitamins has been described. In one study the admixtures were stable for 24 hours at room temperature and for 8 days at 4°C. The visual appearance and particle size of the fat emulsion showed little change over the observation periods.[1218] In another study variable stability periods were found, depending on electrolyte concentrations. Stability ranged from 4 to 25 days at room temperature.[1219]

The effects of dilution, dextrose concentration, amino acids, and electrolytes on the physical stability of 3-in-1 parenteral nutrition admixtures prepared with Intralipid 10% or Travamulsion 10% was studied. Travamulsion was affected by dilution up to 1:14, exhibiting an increase in mean particle size, while Intralipid remained virtually unchanged for 24 hours at 25°C and for 72 hours at 4°C. At dextrose concentrations above 15%, fat droplets larger than 5 μm formed during storage for 24 hours at either 4°C or room temperature. The presence of amino acids increased the stability of the fat emulsions in the presence of dextrose. Fat droplets larger than 5 μm formed at a total electrolyte concentration above approximately 240 mmol/L (monovalent cation equivalent) for Travamulsion 10% and 156 mmol/L for Intralipid 10% in 24 hours at room temperature, although creaming or breaking of the emulsion was not observed visually.[1221]

The stability of 43 parenteral nutrition admixtures composed of various ratios of amino acid products, dextrose 10 to 70%, and 4 lipid emulsions 10 and 20% with electrolytes, trace elements, and vitamins was studied. One group of admixtures included Travasol 5.5, 8.5, and 10%, FreAmine III 8.5 and 10%, Novamine 8.5 and 11.4%, Nephramine 5.4%, and RenAmine 6.5% with Liposyn II 10 and 20%. In another group, Aminosyn II 7, 8.5, and 10% was combined with Intralipid, Travamulsion, and Soyacal 10 and 20%. A third group consisted of Aminosyn II 7, 8.5, and 10% with electrolytes combined with the latter 3 lipid emulsions. The admixtures were stored for 24 hours at 25°C and for 9 days at 5°C followed by 24 hours at 25°C. A few admixtures containing FreAmine III and Novamine with Liposyn II developed faint yellow streaks after 10 days of storage. The streaks readily dispersed with gentle shaking, as did the creaming present in most admixtures. Other properties such as pH, zeta-potential, and osmolality underwent little change in all of the admixtures. Particle size increased fourfold in 1 admixture (Novamine 8.5%, dextrose 50%, and Liposyn II in a 1:1:1 ratio), which the authors noted signaled the onset of particle coalescence. Nevertheless, the authors concluded that all of the admixtures were stable for the storage conditions and time periods tested.[1222]

The stability of 24 parenteral nutrition admixtures composed of various ratios of Aminosyn II 7, 8.5, or 10%, dextrose, and Liposyn II 10 and 20% with electrolytes, trace elements, and vitamins was also studied. Four admixtures were stored for 24 hours at 25°C, 6 admixtures were stored for 2 days at 5°C followed by 1 day at 30°C, and 14 admixtures were stored for 9 days at 5°C followed by 1 day at 25°C. No visible instability was evident. Creaming was present in most admixtures but disappeared with gentle shaking. Other properties such as pH, zeta-potential, particle size, and potency of the amino acids and dextrose showed little or no change during storage.[1223]

The emulsion stability of 5 parenteral nutrition formulas (TNA #126 through #130 in Appendix) containing Liposyn II in concentrations ranging from 1.2 to 7.1% were reported. The parenteral nutrition solutions were prepared using simultaneous pumping of the components into empty containers (as with the Nutrimix compounder) and sequential pumping of the components (as with Automix compounders). The solutions were stored for 2 days at 5°C followed by 24 hours at 25°C. Similar results were obtained for both methods of preparation using visual assessment and oil globule size distribution.[1426]

The stability of 24 parenteral nutrition admixtures containing various concentrations of Aminosyn II, dextrose, and Liposyn II with a variety of electrolytes, trace elements, and multivitamins in dual-chamber, flexible, Nutrimix containers was studied as well. No instability was visible in the admixtures stored at 25°C for 24 hours or in those stored for 9 days at 5°C followed by 24 hours at 25°C. Creaming was observed, but neither particle coalescence nor free oil was noted. The pH, particle size distribution, and amino acid and dextrose concentrations remained acceptable during the observation period.[1432]

The physical stability of 10 parenteral nutrition formulas (TNA #149 through #158 in Appendix) containing TrophAmine and Intralipid 20%, Liposyn II 20%, and Nutrilipid 20% in varying concentrations with low and high electrolyte concentrations was studied. All test formulas were prepared with an automatic compounder and protected from light. TNA #149 through #156 were stored for 48 hours at 4°C followed by 24 hours at 21°C;

TNA #157 and #158 were stored for 24 hours at 4°C followed by 24 hours at 21°C. Although some minor creaming occurred in all formulas, it was completely reversible with agitation. No other changes were visible, and particle size analysis indicated little variation during the study period. The addition of cysteine hydrochloride 1 g/25 g of amino acids, alone or with L-carnitine 16 mg/g fat, to TNA #157 and #158 did not adversely affect the physical stability of 3-in-1 admixtures within the study period.[1620]

The physical stability of five 3-in-1 parenteral nutrition admixtures (TNA #167 through #171 in Appendix) was evaluated by visual observation, pH and osmolality determinations, and particle size distribution analysis. All 5 admixtures were physically stable for 90 days at 4°C. However, some irreversible flocculation occurred in all combinations after 180 days.[1651]

The stability of several parenteral nutrition formulas (TNA #159 through #166 in Appendix) with and without iron dextran 2 mg/L was studied. All formulas were physically compatible both visually and microscopically for 48 hours at 4 and 25°C, and particle size distribution remained unchanged. The order of mixing and deliberate agitation had no effect on physical compatibility.[1648]

The influence of 6 factors on the stability of fat emulsion in 45 different 3-in-1 parenteral nutrition mixtures was evaluated. The factors were amino acid concentration (2.5 to 7%); dextrose (5 to 20%); fat emulsion, intravenous (2 to 5%); monovalent cations (0 to 150 mEq/L); divalent cations (4 to 20 mEq/L); and trivalent cations from iron dextran (0 to 10 mg elemental iron/L). Although many formulations were unstable, visual examination could identify instability in only 65% of the samples. Electronic evaluation of particle size identified the remaining unstable mixtures. Furthermore, only the concentration of trivalent ferric ions significantly and consistently affected the emulsion stability during the 30-hour test period. Of the parenteral nutrition mixtures containing iron dextran, 16% were unstable, exhibiting emulsion cracking. The authors suggested that iron dextran should not be incorporated into 3-in-1 mixtures.[1814]

The compatibility of 8 parenteral nutrition admixtures, 4 with and 4 without electrolytes, comparing Liposyn II and Intralipid (TNA #250 through #257 in Appendix) was reported. The 3-in-1 admixtures were evaluated over 2 to 9 days at 4°C and then 24 hours at 25°C in ethylene vinyl acetate (EVA) bags. No substantial changes were noted in the fat particle sizes and no visual changes of emulsion breakage were observed. All admixtures tested had particle sizes in the 2- to 40-μm range.[2465]

The stability of 3-in-1 parenteral nutrition admixtures prepared with Vamin 14 with electrolytes and containing either Lipofundin MCT/LCT 20% or Intralipid 20% was evaluated. The admixtures contained 66.7 mmol/L of monovalent and 6.7 mmol/L of divalent cations. Stability of the fat emulsion was evaluated after 2, 7, and 21 days at 4°C in EVA bags followed by 24 hours of room temperature to simulate infusion. Microscopy, Coulter counter, photon correlation spectroscopy, and laser diffractometry techniques were used to determine stability. Droplet size by microscopy was noted to increase to 18 to 20 μm after 21 days in both of the admixtures with the Intralipid-containing admixture showing particles this large as early as day

2 and with Lipofundin MCT/LCT at day 7. The Coulter counter assessed particles greater than 2 μm to be approximately 1300 to 1500 with Lipofundin MCT/LCT and 37,000 in the Intralipid-containing admixtures immediately after their preparation. Heavy creaming with a thick firm layer was noted after 2 days with the Intralipid-containing admixture, making particle assessment difficult. The authors concluded that storage limitation of 2 days for the Intralipid-containing admixture and not more than 7 days for the Lipofundin-containing admixture appeared justified. They also noted that calcium and magnesium behaved identically in destabilizing fat emulsion with greater concentrations of divalent cations.[867]

The drop size of 3-in-1 parenteral nutrition solutions in drip chambers is variable, being altered by the constituents of the mixture. In one study, multivitamins (Multibionta, E. Merck) caused the greatest reductions in drop size, up to 37%. This change may affect the rate of delivery if the flow is estimated from drops per minute.[1016] Similarly, flow rates delivered by infusion controllers dependent on predictable drop size may be inaccurate. Flow rates up to 29% less than expected have been reported. Therefore, variable pressure volumetric pumps, which are independent of drop size, should be used rather than infusion controllers.[1215]

The physical instability of 3-in-1 total nutrient admixtures stored for 24 hours at room temperature was reported. The admixtures intended for use in neonates and infants were compounded with TrophAmine 2 to 3%, dextrose 18 to 24%, Liposyn II (Abbott) 2 to 3%, L-cysteine hydrochloride, and the following electrolytes in Table 5.

Table 5. Incompatible electrolyte ranges in neonatal 3-in-1 admixtures[2619]

Sodium	20 to 50 mEq/L
Potassium	13.3 to 40 mEq/L
Calcium chloride	20 to 26.6 mEq/L
Magnesium	3.4 to 5 mEq/L
Phosphates	6.7 to 15 mmol/L

The emulsion in the admixtures cracked and developed visible free oil within 24 hours after compounding. The incompatibility was considered to create a clinically significant risk of complications if administered. The authors determined that these 3-in-1 total nutrient admixtures containing these concentrations of electrolytes were unacceptable and should not be used.[2619]

Another evaluation of 3-in-1 total nutrient admixtures reported physical instabilities of several formulations evaluated over 7 days. The parenteral nutrition admixtures were prepared with dextrose 15% and Intralipos 4% (Fresenius Kabi) along with FreAmine 4.3%, NephrAmine 2.1%, TrophAmine 2.7%, Topanusol 5%, or HepatAmine 4%. Various electrolytes and other components were also present including sodium, potassium, calcium (salt form unspecified), magnesium, trace elements, vitamin K, and heparin. The admixtures were stored at 4°C and evaluated at 0, 3, and 7 days. After removal from refrigeration, the samples were subjected to additional exposure to room temperature and temperatures exceeding 28°C for 24 to 48 hours. Flocculation was found in the admixtures prepared with FreAmine and with TrophAmine after 24 hours storage at room temperature, and after 3 days under refrigeration followed by 24 hours at room temperature. All of the admixtures developed coalescence after 7 days under refrigeration followed by 24 hours at greater than 28°C.[2621]

The case of a 26-year-old female with Crohn's disease and enterocutaneous fistulae receiving a 3-in-1 parenteral nutrition admixture composed of Travasol 3.6%, dextrose 13.6%, Intralipid 1.5%, sodium chloride 52.3 mEq/L, sodium acetate 27.4 mEq/L, potassium chloride 27.4 mEq/L, potassium acetate 13.7 mEq/L, magnesium sulfate 4.5 mEq/L, calcium gluconate 3.2 mEq/L, MVI-12, and trace elements but no inorganic phosphates was presented. The patient became febrile, short of breath, and developed a dry cough with diffuse crackles in both lungs. After failing to respond to conventional medical therapy, an open lung biopsy was performed and showed widespread vascular pulmonary thromboses from irregularly shaped crystals leading to the lung perfusion defects. High levels of calcium, potassium, and carbon were detected in the crystals. Subsequent repeat testing in vitro failed to find crystallization. The patient's fever was postulated to contribute to the in vivo crystallization.[2621]

The physical stability of 5 highly concentrated 3-in-1 parenteral nutrition admixtures for fluid-restricted adults was evaluated. The admixtures were composed of Aminoplasmal (B. Braun) at concentrations over 7% as the amino acids source, dextrose concentrations of about 20%, and a 50:50 mixture of medium-chain triglycerides and long-chain triglycerides (Lipofundin MCT, B. Braun) at concentrations of about 2.5 to 2.7% as the lipid component with electrolytes and vitamins (TNA #269 through #273 in Appendix). The parenteral nutrition admixtures were prepared in EVA bags and stored at room temperature for 30 hours. Electronic evaluation of mean fat particle sizes and globule size distribution found little change over the 30-hour test period.[2721]

Considerations and Recommendations

When multicomponent, 3-in-1, parenteral nutrition admixtures are used, the following points should be considered:[490 703 892 893 1025 1064 1070 1214 1406 1951 2029 2030 2215 2282 2308 3251 3252 3253 3254 3255]

1. The order of mixing is important. The amino acid solution should be added to the dextrose prior to addition of the fat emulsion. This practice ensures that the protective effect of the amino acids to emulsion disruption by changes in pH and the presence of electrolytes is realized. Alternatively, some manufacturers of lipid emulsion state that all 3 components may be transferred to the admixture containers simultaneously, admixing with gentle agitation.

2. Electrolytes should not be added directly to the fat emulsions. Instead, they should be added to the amino acids or dextrose before the final mixing.

3. Such 3-in-1 admixtures containing electrolytes (especially divalent cations) are unstable and will eventually aggregate. The mixed systems should be carefully examined visually before use to ensure that a uniform emulsion still

exists and that separation of the emulsion (i.e., "breaking" or "oiling out"), indicated by yellowish streaking or accumulation of yellowish droplets in the admixed emulsion, has not occurred.

4. Avoid contact of 3-in-1 parenteral nutrition admixtures with heparin, which destabilizes and damages the fat emulsion upon contact. See Heparin section below.

5. The admixtures should be stored under refrigeration if not used immediately.

6. The ultimate stability of the admixtures will be the result of a complex interaction of pH, component concentrations, electrolyte concentrations, and, probably, storage temperature.

Furthermore, a 1.2-μm filter should be used in the administration of fat emulsion, intravenous, whether used alone or administered as a component of a TNA (3-in-1); filtration is necessary to remove large lipid particles, electrolyte precipitates, and other solid particulates and aggregates.[1106] [1657] [1769] [2061] [2135] [2346] [3251] [3252] [3253] [3254] [3255] [3259] [3260]

Blood Products

Amino acids injection should not be administered simultaneously with blood through the same infusion set because of possible pseudoagglutination.[341]

Calcium and Phosphate

UNRECOGNIZED CALCIUM PHOSPHATE PRECIPITATION IN A 3-IN-1 PARENTERAL NUTRITION MIXTURE RESULTED IN PATIENT DEATH.

The potential for the formation of a calcium phosphate precipitate in parenteral nutrition solutions is well studied and documented,[1771] [1777] but the information is complex and difficult to apply to the clinical situation.[1770] [1772] [1777] The incorporation of fat emulsion in 3-in-1 parenteral nutrition solutions obscures any precipitate that may be present, which has led to substantial debate about the dangers associated with 3-in-1 parenteral nutrition mixtures and when or if the danger to the patient is warranted therapeutically.[1770] [1771] [1772] [2031] [2032] [2033] [2034] [2035] [2036] Because such precipitation may be life threatening to patients,[2037] [2291] FDA issued a Safety Alert containing the following recommendations:[1769]

1. "The amounts of phosphorus and of calcium added to the admixture are critical. The solubility of the added calcium should be calculated from the volume at the time the calcium is added. It should not be based upon the final volume.

    Some amino acid injections for TPN admixtures contain phosphate ions (as a phosphoric acid buffer). These phosphate ions and the volume at the time the phosphate is added should be considered when calculating the concentration of phosphate additives. Also, when adding calcium and phosphate to an admixture, the phosphate should be added first.

    The line should be flushed between the addition of any potentially incompatible components.

2. A lipid emulsion in a 3-in-1 admixture obscures the presence of a precipitate. Therefore, if a lipid emulsion is needed, either (1) use a 2-in-1 admixture with the lipid infused separately, or (2) if a 3-in-1 admixture is medically necessary, then add the

calcium before the lipid emulsion and according to the recommendations in number 1 above.

    If the amount of calcium or phosphate which must be added is likely to cause a precipitate, some or all of the calcium should be administered separately. Such separate infusions must be properly diluted and slowly infused to avoid serious adverse events related to the calcium.

3. When using an automated compounding device, the above steps should be considered when programming the device. In addition, automated compounders should be maintained and operated according to the manufacturer's recommendations.

    Any printout should be checked against the programmed admixture and weight of components.

4. During the mixing process, pharmacists who mix parenteral nutrition admixtures should periodically agitate the admixture and check for precipitates. Medical or home care personnel who start and monitor these infusions should carefully inspect for the presence of precipitates both before and during infusion. Patients and care givers should be trained to visually inspect for signs of precipitation. They also should be advised to stop the infusion and seek medical assistance if precipitates are noted.

5. A filter should be used when infusing either central or peripheral parenteral nutrition admixtures. At this time, data have not been submitted to document which size filter is most effective in trapping precipitates.

    Standards of practice vary, but the following is suggested: a 1.2-μm air-eliminating filter for lipid-containing admixtures and a 0.22-μm air-eliminating filter for non-lipid-containing admixtures.

6. Parenteral nutrition admixtures should be administered within the following time frames: if stored at room temperature, the infusion should be started within 24 hours after mixing; if stored at refrigerated temperatures, the infusion should be started within 24 hours of rewarming. Because warming parenteral nutrition admixtures may contribute to the formation of precipitates, once administration begins, care should be taken to avoid excessive warming of the admixture.

    Persons administering home care parenteral nutrition admixtures may need to deviate from these time frames. Pharmacists who initially prepare these admixtures should check a reserve sample for precipitates over the duration and under the conditions of storage.

7. If symptoms of acute respiratory distress, pulmonary emboli, or interstitial pneumonitis develop, the infusion should be stopped immediately and thoroughly checked for precipitates. Appropriate medical interventions should be instituted. Home care personnel and patients should immediately seek medical assistance."

Calcium Phosphate Precipitation Fatalities

Fatal cases of paroxysmal respiratory failure in 2 previously healthy women receiving peripheral vein parenteral nutrition were reported. The patients experienced sudden cardiopulmonary arrest consistent with pulmonary emboli. The authors used in vitro simulations and an animal model to conclude that unrecognized calcium phosphate precipitation in a 3-in-1 total nutrition admixture caused the fatalities. The precipitation resulted during compounding by introducing calcium and phosphate near to one another in the compounding sequence and prior to complete fluid addition. This resulted in a temporarily high concentration of the drugs and precipitation of calcium phosphate. Observation of the precipitate was obscured by the incorporation of 20% fat emulsion, intravenous, into the nutrition mixture. No filter was used during infusion of the fatal nutrition admixtures.[2037]

In a follow-up retrospective review, 5 patients were identified who had respiratory distress associated with the infusion of the 3-in-1 admixtures at around the same time. Four of these 5 patients died, although the cause of death could be definitively determined for only 2.[2291]

Calcium and Phosphate Conditional Compatibility

Calcium salts are conditionally compatible with phosphate in parenteral nutrition solutions. The incompatibility is dependent on a solubility and concentration phenomenon and is not entirely predictable. Precipitation may occur during compounding or at some time after compounding is completed.

NOTE: Some amino acids solutions inherently contain calcium and phosphate, which must be considered in any projection of compatibility.

A study determined the maximum concentrations of calcium (as chloride and gluconate) and phosphate that can be maintained without precipitation in a parenteral nutrition solution consisting of FreAmine II 4.25% and dextrose 25% for 24 hours at 30°C. It was noted that the amino acids in parenteral nutrition solutions form soluble complexes with calcium and phosphate, reducing the available free calcium and phosphate that can form insoluble precipitates. The concentration of calcium available for precipitation is greater with the chloride salt compared to the gluconate salt, at least in part because of differences in dissociation characteristics. Consequently, a greater concentration of calcium gluconate than calcium chloride can be mixed with sodium phosphate.[608]

In addition to the concentrations of phosphate and calcium and the salt form of the calcium, the concentration of amino acids and the time and temperature of storage altered the formation of calcium phosphate in parenteral nutrition solutions. As the temperature was increased, the incidence of precipitate formation also increased. This finding was attributed, at least in part, to a greater degree of dissociation of the calcium and phosphate complexes and the decreased solubility of calcium phosphate. Therefore, a solution possibly may be stored at 4°C with no precipitation, but on warming to room temperature a precipitate will form over time.[608]

The compatibility of calcium and phosphate in several parenteral nutrition formulas for newborn infants was evaluated. Calcium gluconate 10% (Cutter) and potassium phosphate (Abbott) were used to achieve concentrations of 2.5 to 100 mEq/L of calcium and 2.5 to 100 mmol/L of phosphorus added. The parenteral nutrition solutions evaluated were as shown in Table 6. The results were reported as graphic depictions.

Table 6. Parenteral nutrition solutions evaluated[609]

| Component | Solution Number | | | |
	#1	#2	#3	#4
FreAmine III	4%	2%	1%	1%
Dextrose	25%	20%	10%	10%
pH	6.3	6.4	6.6	7.0[a]

[a] Adjusted with sodium hydroxide.

The pH dependence of the phosphate–calcium precipitation has been noted. Dibasic calcium phosphate is very insoluble, while monobasic calcium phosphate is relatively soluble. At low pH, the soluble monobasic form predominates; but as the pH increases, more dibasic phosphate becomes available to bind with calcium and precipitate. Therefore, the lower the pH of the parenteral nutrition solution, the more calcium and phosphate can be solubilized. Once again, the effects of temperature were observed. As the temperature is increased, more calcium ion becomes available and more dibasic calcium phosphate is formed. Therefore, temperature increases will increase the amount of precipitate.[609]

Similar calcium and phosphate solubility curves were reported for neonatal parenteral nutrition solutions using TrophAmine (McGaw) 2, 1.5, and 0.8% as the sources of amino acids. The solutions also contained dextrose 10%, with cysteine and pH adjustment being used in some admixtures. Calcium and phosphate solubility followed the patterns reported previously.[609] A slightly greater concentration of phosphate could be used in some mixtures, but this finding was not consistent.[1024]

Using a similar study design, 6 neonatal parenteral nutrition solutions based on Aminosyn-PF (Abbott) 2, 1.5, and 0.8%, with and without added cysteine hydrochloride and dextrose 10% were studied. Calcium concentrations ranged from 2.5 to 50 mEq/L, and phosphate concentrations ranged from 2.5 to 50 mmol/L. Solutions sat for 18 hours at 25°C and then were warmed to 37°C in a water bath to simulate the clinical situation of warming prior to infusion into a child. Solubility curves were markedly different than those for TrophAmine in the previous study.[1024] Solubilities were reported to decrease by 15 mEq/L for calcium and 15 mmol/L for phosphate. The solutions remained clear during room temperature storage, but crystals often formed on warming to 37°C.[1211]

However, these data were questioned by Mikrut, who noted the similarities between the Aminosyn-PF and TrophAmine products and found little difference in calcium and phosphate solubilities in a preliminary report.[1212] In the full report,[1213] parenteral nutrition solutions containing Aminosyn-PF or TrophAmine 1 or 2.5% with dextrose 10 or 25%, respectively, plus electrolytes and trace metals, with or without cysteine hydrochloride, were evaluated under the same conditions. Calcium concentrations ranged from 2.5 to 50 mEq/L, and phosphate concentrations ranged from 5 to 50 mmol/L. In contrast to the previous results,[1024] the solubility curves were very similar for the Aminosyn-PF and TrophAmine parenteral nutrition solutions but very different from those of the previous Aminosyn-PF study.[1211] The authors again showed that the solubility of calcium and phosphate is greater in solutions containing higher concentrations of amino acids and dextrose.[1213]

Calcium and phosphate solubility curves for TrophAmine 1 and 2% with dextrose 10% and electrolytes, vitamins, heparin, and trace elements were reported. Calcium concentrations ranged from 10 to 60 mEq/L, and phosphorus concentrations ranged from 10 to 40 mmol/L. Calcium and phosphate solubilities were assessed by analysis of the calcium concentrations and followed patterns similar to those reported previously.[608 609] The higher percentage of amino acids (TrophAmine 2%) permitted a slightly greater solubility of calcium and phosphate, especially in the 10 to 50-mEq/L and 10 to 35-mmol/L ranges, respectively.[1614]

The maximal product of the amount of calcium (as gluconate) times phosphate (as potassium) that can be added to a parenteral nutrition solution, composed of amino acids 1% (Travenol) and dextrose 10%, for preterm infants was reported. Turbidity was observed on initial mixing when the solubility product was around 115 to 130 $mmol^2$ (mmol squared) or greater. After storage at 7°C for 20 hours, visible precipitates formed at solubility products of 130 $mmol^2$ (mmol squared) or greater. If the solution was administered through a barium-impregnated silicone rubber catheter, crystalline precipitates obstructed the catheters in 12 hours at a solubility product of 100 $mmol^2$ (mmol squared) and in 10 days at 79 $mmol^2$ (mmol squared), much lower than the in vitro results.[1041]

The solubility characteristics of calcium and phosphate in pediatric parenteral nutrition solutions composed of Aminosyn 0.5, 2, and 4% with dextrose 10 to 25% were reported. Also present were electrolytes and vitamins. Sodium phosphate was added sequentially in phosphorus concentrations from 10 to 30 mmol/L. Calcium gluconate was added last in amounts ranging from 1 to 10 g/L. The solutions were stored at 25°C for 30 hours and examined visually and microscopically for precipitation. The authors found that higher concentrations of Aminosyn increased the solubility of calcium and phosphate. Precipitation occurred at lower calcium and phosphate concentrations in the 0.5% solution compared to the 2 and 4% solutions. For example, at a phosphorus concentration of 30 mmol/L, precipitation occurred at calcium gluconate concentrations of about 1, 2, and 4 g/L in the 0.5, 2, and 4% Aminosyn mixtures, respectively. Similarly, at a calcium gluconate concentration of 8 g/L and above, precipitation occurred at phosphorus concentrations of about 13, 17, and 22 mmol/L in the 0.5, 2, and 4% solutions, respectively. The dextrose concentration did not appear to affect the calcium and phosphate solubility significantly.[1042]

The solubility of calcium and phosphorus in neonatal parenteral nutrition solutions composed of amino acids (Abbott) 1.25 and 2.5% with dextrose 5 and 10%, respectively, was evaluated. Also present were multivitamins and trace elements. The solutions contained calcium (as gluconate) in amounts ranging from 25 to 200 mg/100 mL. The phosphorus (as potassium phosphate) concentrations evaluated ranged from 25 to 150 mg/100 mL. If calcium gluconate was added first, cloudiness occurred immediately. If potassium phosphate was added first, substantial quantities could be added with no precipitate formation in 48 hours at 4°C (Table 7). However, if stored at 22°C, the solutions were stable for only 24 hours, and all contained precipitates after 48 hours.[1210]

Table 7. Maximum calcium and phosphorus concentrations physically compatible for 48 hours at 4°C[1210]

Calcium (mg/100 mL)	Phosphorus (mg/100 mL)	
	Amino Acids 1.25% + Dextrose 5%[a]	Amino Acids 2.5% + Dextrose 10%[a]
200[b]	50	75
150	50	100
100	75	100
50	100	125
25	150[b]	150[b]

[a] Plus multivitamins and trace elements.

[b] Maximum concentration tested.

The physical compatibility of calcium gluconate 10 to 40 mEq/L and potassium phosphates 10 to 40 mmol/L in 3 neonatal parenteral nutrition solutions (TPN #123 to #125 in Appendix), alone and with retrograde administration of aminophylline 7.5 mg diluted with 1.5 mL of sterile water for injection was reported. Contact of the alkaline aminophylline solution with the parenteral nutrition solutions resulted in the precipitation of calcium phosphate at much lower concentrations than were compatible in the parenteral nutrition solutions alone.[1404]

Additional calcium and phosphate solubility curves were reported for specialty parenteral nutrition solutions based on NephrAmine and also HepatAmine at concentrations of 0.8, 1.5, and 2% as the sources of amino acids. The solutions also contained dextrose 10%, with cysteine and pH adjustment to simulate addition of fat emulsion used in some admixtures. Calcium and phosphate solubility followed the hyperbolic patterns previously reported.[609] Temperature, time, and pH affected calcium and phosphate solubility, with pH having the greatest effect.[2038]

The maximum sodium phosphate concentrations were reported for given amounts of calcium gluconate that could be admixed in parenteral nutrition solutions containing TrophAmine in varying quantities (with cysteine hydrochloride 40 mg/g of amino acid) and dextrose 10%. The solutions also contained magnesium sulfate 4 mEq/L, potassium acetate 24 mEq/L, sodium chloride 32 mEq/L, pediatric multivitamins, and trace elements. The presence of cysteine hydrochloride reduces the solution pH and increases the amount of calcium and phosphate that can be incorporated before precipitation occurs. The results of this study cannot be safely extrapolated to TPN solutions with compositions other than the ones tested. The admixtures were compounded with the sodium phosphate added last after thorough mixing of all other components. The authors noted that this is not the preferred order of mixing (usually phosphate is added first and thoroughly mixed before adding calcium last); however, they believed this reversed order of mixing would provide a margin of error in cases in which the proper order is not followed. After compounding, the solutions were stored for 24 hours at 40°C. The maximum calcium and phosphate amounts that could be mixed in the various solutions were reported tabularly and are shown in Table 8.[2039] However, these results are not entirely consistent with another study. See Table 9.

Table 8. Maximum amount of phosphate (as sodium) (mmol/L) not resulting in precipitation.[2039] See caution below.[a]

Calcium (as Gluconate)	Amino Acid (as TrophAmine) plus Cysteine HCl 40 mg/g Amino Acid				
	0%	0.4%	1%	2%	3%
9.8 mEq/L	0	27	42	60	66
14.7 mEq/L	0	15	18	30	36
19.6 mEq/L	0	6	15	27	30
29.4 mEq/L	0	3	6	21	24

[a] CAUTION: The results cannot be safely extrapolated to solutions with formulas other than the ones tested. See text.

The temperature dependence of the calcium–phosphate precipitation has resulted in the occlusion of a subclavian catheter by a solution apparently free of precipitation. The parenteral nutrition solution consisted of FreAmine III 500 mL, dextrose 70% 500 mL, sodium chloride 50 mEq, sodium phosphate 40 mmol, potassium acetate 10 mEq, potassium phosphate 40 mmol, calcium gluconate 10 mEq, magnesium sulfate 10 mEq, and Shil's trace metals solution 1 mL. Although there was no evidence of precipitation in the bottle, tubing and pump cassette, and filter (all at approximately 26°C) during administration, the occluded catheter and Vicra Loop Lock (next to the patient's body at 37°C) had numerous crystals identified as calcium phosphate. In vitro, this parenteral nutrition solution had a precipitate in 12 hours at 37°C but was clear for 24 hours at 26°C.[610]

Similarly, a parenteral nutrition solution that was clear and free of particulates after 2 weeks under refrigeration developed a precipitate in 4 to 6 hours when stored at room temperature. When the solution was warmed in a 37°C water bath, precipitation occurred in 1 hour. Administration of the solution before the precipitate was noticed led to interstitial pneumonitis due to deposition of calcium phosphate crystals.[1427]

The maximum allowable concentrations of calcium and phosphate in a 3-in-1 parenteral nutrition mixture for children (TNA #192 in Appendix) were reported. Added calcium was varied from 1.5 to 150 mmol/L, and added phosphate was varied from 21 to 300 mmol/L. These mixtures were stable for 48 hours at 22 and 37°C as long as the pH was not greater than 5.7, the calcium concentration was below 16 mmol/L, the phosphate concentration was below 52 mmol/L, and the product of the calcium and phosphate concentrations was below 250 $mmol^2/L^2$ (mmol squared per liter squared).[1773]

Calcium phosphate precipitation phenomena was evaluated in a series of parenteral nutrition admixtures composed of dextrose 22%, amino acids (FreAmine III) 2.7%, and fat emulsion (Abbott) 0, 1, and 3.2%. Incorporation of calcium gluconate 19 to 24 mEq/L and phosphate (as sodium) 22 to 28 mmol/L resulted in visible precipitation in the fat-free admixtures. New precipitate continued to form over 14 days, even after repeated filtrations of the solutions through 0.2-µm filters. The presence of the amino acids increased calcium and phosphate solubility, compared with simple aqueous solutions. However, the incorporation of the fat emulsion did not result in a statistically significant increase in calcium and phosphate solubility. The authors noted that the kinetics of calcium phosphate precipitate formation do not appear to be entirely predictable; both transient and permanent precipitation can occur either during the compounding process or at some time afterward. Because calcium phosphate precipitation can be very dangerous clinically, the use of inline filters was recommended. The authors suggested that the filters should have a porosity appropriate to the parenteral nutrition admixture—1.2 µm for fat-containing and 0.2 or 0.45 µm for fat-free nutrition mixtures.[2061]

Laser particle analysis was used to evaluate the formation of calcium phosphate precipitation in pediatric TPN solutions containing TrophAmine in concentrations ranging from 0.5 to 3% with dextrose 10% and also containing L-cysteine hydrochloride 1 g/L. The solutions also contained in each liter sodium chloride 20 mEq, sodium acetate 20 mEq, magnesium sulfate 3 mEq, trace elements 3 mL, and heparin sodium 500 units. The presence of L-cysteine hydrochloride reduces the solution pH and increases the amount of calcium and phosphate that can be incorporated before precipitation occurs. The results of this study cannot be safely extrapolated to TPN solutions with compositions other than the ones tested. The maximum amount of phosphate that was incorporated without the appearance of a measurable increase in particulates in 24 hours at 37°C for each of the amino acids concentrations is shown in Table 9.[2196] These results are not entirely consistent with previous results.[2039] See above. The use of more sensitive electronic particle measurement for the formation of subvisible particulates in this study may contribute to the differences in the results.

Table 9. Maximum amount of phosphate (as potassium) (mmol/L) not resulting in precipitation.[2196] See caution below.[a]

Calcium (as Gluconate) (mEq/L)	Amino Acid (as TrophAmine) plus Cysteine HCl 1 g/L					
	0.5%	1%	1.5%	2%	2.5%	3%
10	22	28	38	38	38	43
14	18	18	18	38	38	43
19	18	18	18	33	33	38
24	12	18	18	22	28	28
28	12	18	18	18	18	18
33	12	12	12	12	12	12
37	12	12	12	12	12	12
41	9	9	9	12	12	12
45	0	9	9	12	12	12
49	0	9	9	9	12	12
53	0	9	9	9	9	9

[a] CAUTION: The results cannot be safely extrapolated to solutions with formulas other than the ones tested. See text.

Calcium and phosphate compatibility was evaluated in a series of parenteral nutrition admixtures composed of Aminosyn II in concentrations ranging from 2% up to 5% (TPN #227 to #231 in Appendix). The solutions also contained dextrose ranging from 10% up to 25%. Also present were sodium chloride, potassium chloride, and magnesium sulfate in common amounts. Phosphates as the potassium salt and calcium as the acetate salt were added in variable quantities to determine the maximum amounts of calcium and phosphates that could be added to the representative TPN admixtures. The samples were evaluated at 23 and 37°C over 48 hours by visual inspection in ambient light and using a Tyndall beam and electronically measured for turbidity and microparticulates. The boundaries between the compatible and incompatible concentrations were presented graphically as hyperbolic curves.[2265]

The solubility of calcium acetate versus calcium gluconate with sodium phosphates was evaluated in pediatric parenteral nutrition solutions following storage for 30 hours at 25°C followed by 30 minutes at 37°C. Concentrations of Aminosyn PF studied varied from 1 to 3%, dextrose from 10 to 25%, calcium from 5 to 60 mEq/L, and phosphate from 1 to 60 mmol/L. L-cysteine hydrochloride at a dose of 40 mg/g of Aminosyn PF, magnesium 3.2 mEq/L, and pediatric trace elements-4 at 2.4 mL/L of pediatric parenteral nutrition solution were also added. Calcium acetate was found to be less soluble than calcium gluconate when prepared under these concentrations. The maximum concentrations of the calcium salts and sodium phosphates are shown in Table 10. Polarized light microscopy was used to identify the calcium acetate and sodium phosphate crystals adherent to the container walls because simple visual observation was not able to identify the precipitates. The authors recommended the use of calcium acetate to reduce the iatrogenic aluminum exposure often seen with calcium gluconate in the neonatal population receiving parenteral nutrition.[2466] However, care must be taken to avoid inadvertent calcium phosphate precipitation at the lower concentrations found with calcium acetate if it is substituted for the gluconate salt to reduce aluminum exposure.

Table 10. Maximum concentrations of sodium phosphates and calcium as acetate and as gluconate not resulting in precipitation[2466]

Aminosyn PF (%)	Sodium Phosphates (mmol/L)	Calcium Acetate (mEq/L)	Calcium Gluconate (mEq/L)
1	10	25	50
1	15	15	25
2	10	30	45
2	25	10	12.5
3	20	10	15
3	25	15	17.5

Calcium and phosphate compatibility was evaluated in a series of adult formula parenteral nutrition admixtures composed of FreAmine III, in concentrations ranging from 1 to 5% (TPN #258

through #262). The solutions also contained dextrose ranging from 15% up to 25%. Also present were sodium chloride, potassium chloride, and magnesium sulfate in common amounts. Cysteine hydrochloride was added in an amount of 25 mg/g of amino acids from FreAmine III to reduce the pH by about 0.5 pH unit and thereby increase the amount of calcium and phosphates that can be added to the TPN admixtures as has been done with pediatric parenteral nutrition admixtures. Phosphates as the potassium salts and calcium as the gluconate salt were added in variable quantities to determine the maximum amounts of calcium and phosphates that could be added to the test admixtures. The samples were evaluated at 23 and 37°C over 48 hours by visual inspection in ambient light and using a Tyndall beam and electronic measurement of turbidity and microparticulates. The addition of the cysteine hydrochloride resulted in an increase of calcium and phosphates solubility of about 30% by lowering the solution pH 0.5 pH unit. The boundaries between the compatible and incompatible concentrations were presented graphically as hyperbolic curves.[2469]

A 2-in-1 parenteral nutrition admixture with final concentrations of TrophAmine 0.5%, dextrose 5%, L-cysteine hydrochloride 40 mg/g of amino acids, calcium gluconate 60 mg/100 mL, and sodium phosphates 46.5 mg/mL was found to result in visible precipitation of calcium phosphate within 30 hours stored at 23 to 27°C. Despite the presence of the acidifying L-cysteine hydrochloride, precipitation occurred at clinically utilized amounts of calcium and phosphates.[2622]

The presence of magnesium in solutions may also influence the reaction between calcium and phosphate, including the nature and extent of precipitation.[158 159]

The interaction of calcium and phosphate in parenteral nutrition solutions is a complex phenomenon. Various factors play a role in the solubility or precipitation of a given combination, including:[608 609 1042 1063 1427 2038 2039 2061]

1. Concentration of calcium
2. Salt form of calcium
3. Concentration of phosphate
4. Concentration of amino acids
5. Amino acids composition
6. Concentration of dextrose
7. Temperature of solution
8. pH of solution
9. Presence of other additives
10. Order of mixing

Enhanced precipitate formation would be expected from such factors as high concentrations of calcium and phosphate, increases in solution pH, decreased amino acid concentrations, increases in temperature, addition of calcium prior to the phosphate, lengthy standing times or slow infusion rates, and use of calcium as the chloride salt.[854]

Even if precipitation does not occur in the bottle, it has been reported that crystallization of calcium phosphate may occur in a Silastic infusion pump chamber or tubing if the rate of administration is slow, as for premature infants. Water vapor may be transmitted outward and be replaced by air rapidly enough to produce supersaturation.[202] Several other cases of catheter occlusion also have been reported.[610 1427 1428 1429]

Vitamins

As might be expected, vitamin stability has been found to be better during nighttime when compared to daytime because of the influence of photodecomposition.[2307]

A patient receiving 3000 international units of retinol daily in a parenteral nutrition solution, nevertheless, experienced 2 episodes of night blindness. The pharmacy prepared the parenteral nutrition solution in 1-L PVC bags in weekly batches and stored them at 4°C in the dark until use. A subsequent in vitro study showed losses of vitamin A of 23 and 77% in 3- and 14-day periods, respectively, under these conditions. About 30% of the lost vitamin A could be extracted from the PVC bag.[1038]

Losses of vitamin A from multivitamins (USV) in a neonatal parenteral nutrition solution was reported. The solution was prepared in colorless glass bottles and run through an administration set with a burette (Travenol). The total loss of vitamin A was 75% in 24 hours, with about 16% as decomposition in the glass bottle. The decomposition was not noticeable during the first 12 hours, but then vitamin A levels fell rather precipitously to about one-third of the initial amount. The balance of the loss, averaging about 59%, occurred during transit through the administration set. Removal of the inline filter and treatment of the set with albumin human had no effect on vitamin A delivery. The authors recommended a threefold to fourfold increase in the amount of vitamin A to compensate for the losses.[1039]

A parenteral nutrition solution in glass bottles exposed to sunlight was reported. Vitamin A decomposed rapidly, losing more than 50% in 3 hours. The decomposition could be slowed by covering the bottle with a light-resistant vinyl bag, resulting in about a 25% loss in 3 hours.[1040]

Vitamin E was stable in the parenteral nutrition solution in glass bottles exposed to sunlight, with no loss occurring during 6 hours of exposure.[1040]

It was reported that 40% retinol losses occurred in 2 hours and 60% in 5 hours from parenteral nutrition solutions pumped at 10 mL/hr through standard infusion sets at room temperature. The retinol concentration in the bottle remained constant while the retinol in the effluent decreased. Antioxidants had no effect. Much of the vitamin A was recoverable from hexane washings of the tubing.[1050]

The delivery of vitamins A, D, and E from a parenteral nutrition solution composed of amino acids 3% solution (Pharmacia) in dextrose 10% with electrolytes, trace elements, vitamin K, folate, and vitamin B12 was evaluated. To this solution was added 6 mL of multivitamin infusion (USV). The solution was prepared in PVC bags (Travenol), and administration was simulated through a fluid chamber (Buretrol) and infusion tubing with a 0.5-μm filter at 10 mL/hr. During the first 60 to 90 minutes, minimal delivery of the vitamins occurred. This was followed by a rise and plateau in the delivered vitamins, which were attributed to an increasing saturation of adsorptive binding sites in the tubing. Total amounts delivered over 24 hours were 31% for vitamin A, 68% for vitamin D, and 64% for vitamin E. Sorption of the vitamins was found in the PVC bag, fluid chamber, and tubing. Decomposition was not a factor.[836]

Vitamin A was found to rapidly and significantly decompose when exposed to daylight. The extent and rate of loss were dependent on the degree of exposure to daylight which, in turn, depended on various factors such as the direction of the radiation, time of day, and climatic conditions. Delivery of less than 10% of the expected amount was reported.[1047] In controlled light experiments, the decomposition initially progressed exponentially. Subsequently, the rate of decomposition slowed. This result was attributed to a protective effect of the degradation products on the remaining vitamin A. The presence of amino acids provided greater protection. Compared to degradation rates in dextrose 5%, decomposition was reduced by up to 50% in some amino acid mixtures.[1048]

In a parenteral nutrition solution composed of amino acids, dextrose, electrolytes, trace elements, and multivitamins in PVC bags stored at 4 and 25°C, vitamin A rapidly deteriorated to 10% of the initial concentration in 8 hours at 25°C while exposed to light. The decomposition was slowed by light protection and refrigeration, with a loss of about 25% in 4 days. Folic acid concentration dropped 40% initially on admixture and then remained relatively constant for 28 days of storage. About 35% of the ascorbic acid was lost in 39 hours at 25°C with exposure to light. The loss was reduced to a negligible amount in 4 days by refrigeration and light protection. Thiamine content dropped by about 50% initially but then remained unchanged over 120 hours of storage.[1063]

A 50% loss of vitamin A from a bottle of parenteral nutrition solution prepared with multivitamin infusion (USV) after 5.5 hours of infusion was noted. The amount delivered through an Ivex-2 filter set was only 6.3% of the added amount. Similar quantities were found after 20 hours of infusion. A reduced light exposure and use of ³H-labeled vitamin A confirmed binding to the infusion bottles and tubing.[704]

Subsequently, solutions containing multivitamins (USV) spiked with ³H-labeled retinol were incubated in intravenous tubing protected from light and agitated to simulate flow for 5 hours. About half of the vitamin A was lost in 30 minutes, and 88 to 96% was lost in 5 hours. Spectrophotometric assays correlated closely with the radioisotope assays. Hexane rinses and radioactivity determinations on the tubing accounted for the decrease in radioactivity.[1049]

In another experiment, neonatal parenteral nutrition solutions containing multivitamins prepared in bags were delivered at 10 mL/hr through Buretrol sets (Travenol). The bags and sets were protected from light. Spectrophotometric and radioisotope assays showed that about 26% of the vitamin A was lost before the flow was started. At 10 mL/hr, about 67% was lost from the effluent. More rapid flow reduced the extent of loss. Analysis of clinical samples of parenteral nutrition solutions showed losses of 21 to 57% after 20 hours. Because losses after 5 hours were of the same magnitude, the authors concluded that the loss occurs fairly rapidly and is not due to gradual decomposition.[1049]

The quantity of retinol delivered from an M.V.I.-containing 2-in-1 parenteral nutrition solution and when M.V.I. was added to Intralipid 10% was evaluated during simulated administration through a PVC administration set. The parenteral nutrition solution was composed of amino acids 2.8%, dextrose 10%, and standard electrolytes; M.V.I. was added to yield a nominal retinol concentration of 455 mcg/150 mL. Retinol losses were about 80% of the admixed amount after being delivered through the PVC set. When M.V.I. was added to Intralipid 10% in a retinol concentration of 455 mcg/20 mL, retinol losses were reduced to about 10% of the admixed amount. The fat emulsion provides retinol protection from sorption to the PVC administration set.[2027]

Substantially higher amounts of retinol were found to be delivered using polyolefin administration set tubing when compared with PVC tubing during simulated neonatal intensive care administration. Retinol was added to a 2-in-1 parenteral nutrition solution (TPN #206) in concentrations of 25 and 50 international units/mL and run at 4 and 10 mL/hr through 3 meter lengths of polyolefin (MiniMed) and PVC (Baxter) intravenous extension set tubing protected from light and passed through a 37°C water bath. Delivered quantities of retinol varied from 19 to 74% through the PVC tubing and 47 to 87% through the polyolefin tubing. The authors noted that the loss of retinol to the PVC tubing appeared to be saturable. Even so, the use of polyolefin tubing increases the amount of retinol delivered during simulated neonatal administration.[2028]

Substantial loss of retinol all-*trans* palmitate and phytonadione from both TPN and TNA admixtures due to exposure to sunlight was reported. In 3 hours of exposure to sunlight, essentially total loss of retinol and 50% loss of phytonadione had occurred. The presence or absence of lipids did not affect stability. In contrast, tocopherol concentrations remained essentially unchanged by exposure to sunlight through 12 hours. The container material used to store the nutrition admixtures affected the concentration of the vitamins as well. Losses were greatest (10 to 25%) in PVC containers and were slightly better in EVA and glass containers.[2049]

The photodegradation of vitamins A and E in a 2-in-1 (Synthamin 9, dextrose 20%) admixture and a 3-in-1 (Synthamin 9, dextrose 20%, Intralipid 20%, electrolytes, vitamins, trace elements) admixture after exposure to 6 hours of indirect daylight was reported. The compounded admixtures were prepared in multilayer bags protected from light and stored at 5°C for a minimum of 5 days. The same admixtures were prepared in EVA bags 24 hours prior to use with vitamins added prior to study. Vitamin A decreased to 60 to 80% of the initial concentrations in 2 to 6 hours of exposure to indirect daylight. The type of bag had no influence on the photodegradation of vitamin A. Despite fat emulsion, no significant light protection was noted with the 3-in-1 admixture. Vitamin E losses were 15% in 6 hours with multilayer bags of both admixtures; however, 100% loss was noted with EVA bags within 1 hour for the 2-in-1 admixture. The presence of the opaque fat emulsion provided some protection; however, losses greater than 50% were noted by 6 hours in the EVA bags. The authors concluded that the use of multilayer bags prevents vitamin E losses during daylight exposure as compared to EVA bags but only light protection can minimize vitamin A losses.[2459]

The stability of retinol palmitate and tocopherols (δ, γ, and α) in 3-in-1 admixtures of amino acids 4%, dextrose 10%, fat emulsion 3% (Intralipid, Liposyn, and ClinOleic), various

electrolytes, vitamins, and trace elements in EVA bags over 3 days at 4, 25, and 37°C was evaluated. Retinol palmitate was found to be unstable at room temperature with 33 and 50% degradation at 24 and 72 hours after compounding, respectively. Refrigeration of the admixture reduced the degradation to 29% at 72 hours. The tocopherols displayed varying stability over the temperature range with 16 to 25% degradation after 72 hours. The variation in the tocopherols was theorized to be from the free conversion between the oxidized and reduced forms over the temperatures tested.[2460]

The stability of vitamin E (alpha-tocopherol acetate from M.V.I.-1000 or Soluzyme) and selenium (from Selepen) in amino acids (Abbott) and dextrose in PVC bags was evaluated. Exposure to fluorescent light and room temperature (23°C) for 24 hours and simulated infusion at 50 mL/hr for 8 hours through a Medlon TPN administration set with a 0.22-μm filter did not affect the concentrations of vitamin E and selenium.[1224]

The stability of numerous vitamins in parenteral nutrition solutions composed of amino acids (Kabi-Vitrum), dextrose 30%, and fat emulsion 20% (Kabi-Vitrum) in a 2:1:1 ratio with electrolytes, trace elements, and both fat- and water-soluble vitamins was reported. The admixtures were stored in darkness at 2 to 8°C for 96 hours with no significant loss of retinyl palmitate, alpha-tocopherol, thiamine mononitrate, sodium riboflavin-5′-phosphate, pyridoxine hydrochloride, nicotinamide, folic acid, biotin, sodium pantothenate, and cyanocobalamin. Sodium ascorbate and its biologically active degradation product, dehydroascorbic acid, totaled 59 and 42% of the nominal starting concentration at 24 and 96 hours, respectively. However, the actual initial concentration was only 66% of the nominal concentration.[1225]

When the admixture was subjected to simulated infusion over 24 hours at 20°C, either exposed to room light or light protected, or stored for 6 days in the dark under refrigeration and then subjected to the same simulated infusion, once again the retinyl palmitate, alpha-tocopherol, and sodium riboflavin-5′-phosphate did not undergo significant loss. However, sodium ascorbate and its degradation product, dehydroascorbic acid, had initial combined concentrations of 51 to 65% of the nominal initial concentration, with further declines during infusion. Light protection did not significantly alter the loss of total ascorbic acid.[1225]

The stability of several vitamins from M.V.I.-12 (Armour) admixed in parenteral nutrition solutions composed of different amino acid products, with or without Intralipid 10%, when stored in glass bottles and PVC bags at 25 and 5°C for 48 hours was reported. Riboflavin, folic acid, and vitamin E were stable in all samples. No vitamin A was lost in any formula in glass bottles, but samples in PVC containers lost as much as 35 and 60% at 5 and 25°C, respectively, in 48 hours. Thiamine hydrochloride was stable in the parenteral nutrition solutions prepared with amino acid products without sulfites. However, amino acid products containing sulfites (Travasol and FreAmine III) had a 25% thiamine loss in 12 hours and a 50% loss in 24 hours when the solutions were stored at 25°C; no loss occurred when the solutions were stored at 5°C. Ascorbic acid was lost from all samples stored at 25°C, with the greatest losses occurring in solutions stored in plastic bags. No losses occurring in any sample stored at 5°C.[1431]

In another study, the stability of vitamins A, E, C, riboflavin, thiamine, and folic acid following admixture (as M.V.I.-12) with 4 different amino acid products (Novamine, Neopham, FreAmine III, Travasol) with or without Intralipid when stored in glass bottles or PVC bags at 25°C for 48 hours was reported. They found that high-intensity phototherapy light did not affect folic acid, thiamine, or vitamin E; however, ascorbic acid and riboflavin losses were significant with all amino acid products tested. Furthermore, it was noted that vitamin A losses were reduced with the addition of Intralipid to the admixture. When bisulfite was added to the Neopham admixture, riboflavin, folic acid, and ascorbic acid were not affected; however, at a bisulfite concentration of 3 mEq/L, there was substantial losses of vitamin A and thiamine. The authors also noted that ascorbic acid losses were increased with a more alkaline pH and that bisulfite addition offered some protection presumably by bisulfite being preferentially oxidized. The authors concluded that intravenous multivitamins should be added to parenteral nutrition admixtures immediately prior to administration to reduce losses since commercially available amino acid products may contain bisulfites and have varying pH values.[487]

The stability of 5 B vitamins was studied over an 8-hour period in representative parenteral nutrition solutions exposed to fluorescent light, indirect sunlight, and direct sunlight. One 5-mL vial of multivitamin concentrate (Lyphomed) and 1 mg of folic acid (Lederle) were added to a liter of parenteral nutrition solution composed of amino acids 4.25%–dextrose 25% (Travenol) with standard electrolytes and trace elements. All 5 B vitamins tested were stable for 8 hours at room temperature when exposed to fluorescent light. In addition, folic acid and niacinamide were stable over 8 hours in direct or indirect sunlight. Exposure to indirect sunlight appeared to have little or no effect on thiamine hydrochloride and pyridoxine hydrochloride in 8 hours, but 47% of riboflavin-5'-phosphate was lost in that period. Direct sunlight caused a 26% loss of thiamine hydrochloride and an 86% loss of pyridoxine hydrochloride in 8 hours. Four-hour exposures of riboflavin-5'-phosphate to direct sunlight resulted in a 98% loss.[842]

The effects of photoirradiation on a FreAmine II–dextrose 10% parenteral nutrition solution containing 1 mL/500 mL of multivitamins (USV) were evaluated. During simulated continuous administration to an infant at 0.156 mL/min, no changes to the amino acids occurred when the bottle, infusion tubing, and collection bottle were shielded with foil. Only 20 cm of tubing in the incubator was exposed to light. However, if the flow was stopped, a marked reduction in methionine (40%), tryptophan (44%), and histidine (22%) occurred in the solution exposed to light for 24 hours. In a similar solution without vitamins, only the tryptophan concentration decreased. The difference was attributed to the presence of riboflavin, a photosensitizer. The authors recommended administering the multivitamins separately and shielding from light.[833]

In further work, the authors simulated more closely conditions occurring during phototherapy in neonatal intensive care units. Riboflavin 1 mg/100 mL was added to a solution of amino acids 2% (Abbott) with dextrose 10%. Infusion was simulated from glass bottles through PVC tubing with a Buretrol at a rate of 4 mL/hr. In addition to the fluorescent room lights, 8 daylight bulbs delivered phototherapy. After a simulated 24-hour infusion, riboflavin decreased to about 50% of its initial level. Also, a 7% reduction in total amino acids was noted, including individual losses of glycine (10%), leucine (14%), methionine (24%), proline (10%), serine (9%), tryptophan (35%), and tyrosine (16%). Although the authors did not believe that these losses of amino acids were nutritionally important, they were concerned about the possibility of toxicity from photo-oxidation products. In the same solution without riboflavin, the individual amino acids decreased only slightly.[974]

The extent and rapidity of ascorbic acid decomposition in parenteral nutrition solutions composed of amino acids, dextrose, electrolytes, multivitamins, and trace elements in 3-L PVC bags stored at 3 to 7°C was reported. About 30 to 40% was lost in 24 hours. The degradation then slowed as the oxygen supply was reduced to the diffusion through the bag. About a 55 to 65% loss occurred after 7 days of storage. The oxidation was catalyzed by metal ions, especially copper. In the absence of copper from the trace elements additive, less than 10% degradation of ascorbic acid occurred in 24 hours. The author estimated that 150 to 200 mg is degraded in 2 to 4 hours at ambient temperature in the presence of copper but that only 20 to 30 mg is broken down in 24 hours without copper. To minimize ascorbic acid loss, copper must be excluded. Alternatively, inclusion of excess ascorbic acid was suggested.[1056]

Extensive decomposition of ascorbic acid and folic acid was reported in a parenteral nutrition solution composed of amino acids 3.3%, dextrose 12.5%, electrolytes, trace elements, and M.V.I.-12 (USV) in PVC bags. Half-lives were 1.1, 2.9, and 8.9 hours for ascorbic acid and 2.7, 5.4, and 24 hours for folic acid stored at 24°C in daylight, 24°C protected from light, and 4°C protected from light, respectively. The decomposition was much greater than for solutions not containing catalyzing metal ions. Also, it was greater than for the vitamins singly because of interactions with the other vitamins present.[1059]

The stability of ascorbic acid in parenteral nutrition solutions, with and without fat emulsion, was studied. Both with and without fat emulsion, the total vitamin C content (ascorbic acid plus dehydroascorbic acid) remained above 90% for 12 hours when the solutions were exposed to fluorescent light and for 24 hours when they were protected from light. When stored in a cool dark place, the solutions were stable for 7 days.[1227]

The stability of several vitamins from M.V.I.-12 (Armour) admixed in parenteral nutrition solutions composed of different amino acid products, with or without Intralipid 10%, when stored in glass bottles and PVC bags at 25 and 5°C for 48 hours was reported. Ascorbic acid was lost from all samples stored at 25°C, with the greatest losses occurring in solutions stored in plastic bags. No losses occurred in any sample stored at 5°C.[1431]

The stability of ascorbic acid and dehydroascorbic acid in a 3-in-1 admixture containing Vamin 14, dextrose 30%, Intralipid 20%, potassium phosphate, Cernevit, and trace elements in EVA bags over a temperature range of 2 to 22°C was examined. They observed an 89% loss of ascorbic acid and a 37% loss of dehydroascorbic acid over 7 days. The authors concluded that oxygen, trace elements, temperature, and an underfilled bag were the greatest determinants of ascorbic acid loss.[2462]

The long-term stability of ascorbic acid in 3-in-1 admixtures containing amino acids (Eloamin) 10%, dextrose 20%, dextrose 5%, fat emulsion (Elolipid) 20%, calcium gluconate, M.V.C. 9 + 3, and trace elements mixed in EVA and multilayer (Ultrastab) bags at 5°C was compared. Ascorbic acid losses were greater than 75% in the first 24 hours and 100% after 48 to 72 hours in the EVA bags. In the multilayer bags, ascorbic acid showed a 20 and 40% loss over the first 24 hours with and without fat emulsion, respectively. The initial rapid fall in ascorbic acid was presumably due to the initial oxygen content of the admixtures despite the use of the less oxygen-permeable multilayer bags. The authors noted the ascorbic acid concentration remained stable for up to 28 days in the multilayer bags after the initial fall and recommended adding additional ascorbic acid to compensate for the losses to facilitate extended shelf-life.[2463]

The influence of several factors on the rate of ascorbic acid oxidation in parenteral nutrition solutions was evaluted. Ascorbic acid is regarded as the least stable component in TPN admixtures. The type of amino acid used in the TPN was important. Some, such as FreAmine III and Vamin 14, contain antioxidant compounds (e.g., sodium metabisulfite or cysteine). Ascorbic acid stability was better in such solutions compared with those amino acid solutions having no antioxidant present. Furthermore, the pH of the solution may play a small role, with greater degradation as the pH rises from about 5 to about 7. Adding air to a compounded TPN container can also accelerate ascorbic acid decomposition. The most important factor was the type of plastic container used for the TPN. EVA containers (Mixieva, Miramed) allow more oxygen permeation, which results in substantial losses of ascorbic acid in relatively short time periods. In multilayer TPN bags (Ultrastab, Miramed) designed to reduce gas permeability, the rate of ascorbic acid degradation was greatly reduced. TPNs without antioxidants packaged in EVA bags were found to have an almost total loss of ascorbic acid activity occurring in 1 or 2 days at 5°C. In contrast, in TPNs containing FreAmine III or Vamin 14 packaged in the multilayer bags, most of the ascorbic acid content was retained for 28 days at 5°C. The authors concluded that TPNs made with antioxidant-containing amino acids and packaged in multilayer bags that reduce gas permeability can safely be given extended expiration dates and still retain most of the ascorbic acid activity.[2163]

The initial degradation product of ascorbic acid (dehydroascorbic acid) in a 2-in-1 admixture containing Synthamin 14, glucose 20%, and trace elements over a temperature range of 5 to 35°C was evaluated. The presence of trace elements, including copper, had no influence on the degradation of dehydroascorbic acid. At room temperature and 5°C, there was a greater than 50% loss of dehydroascorbic acid noted within 2 and 24 hours, respectively. The authors concluded this degradation was temperature dependent.[2461]

The degradation of vitamins A, B1, C, and E from Cernevit (Roche) multivitamins in NuTRIflex Lipid Plus (B. Braun) admixtures prepared in ethylene vinyl acetate (EVA) bags and in multilayer bags was evaluated. After storage for up to 72 hours at

4, 21, and 40°C, greater vitamin losses occurred in the EVA bags: vitamin A (retinyl palmitate) losses were 20%, thiamine hydrochloride losses were 25%, alpha-tocopherol losses were 20%, and ascorbic acid losses were approximately 80 to 100%. In the multilayer bags (presumably a better barrier to oxygen transfer), losses were less: vitamin A (retinyl palmitate) losses were 5%, thiamine hydrochloride losses were 10%, alpha-tocopherol losses were 0%, and ascorbic acid losses were approximately 25 to 70%.[2618]

Phytonadione stability in a TPN solution containing amino acids 2%, dextrose 12.5%, "standard" electrolytes, and multivitamins (M.V.I. Pediatric) was evaluated over 24 hours while exposed to light. Vitamin loss, about 7% in 4 hours and 27% in 24 hours, was attributed partly to the light sensitivity of phytonadione.[1815]

Trace Elements

Because of interactions, recommendations to separate the administration of vitamins and trace elements have been made.[1056][1060][1061] Others have termed such recommendations premature based on differing reports[895][896] and the apparent absence of epidemic vitamin deficiency in parenteral nutrition patients.[1062]

The addition of trace elements to a 3-in-1 parenteral nutrition solution with electrolytes had no adverse effect on the particle size of the fat emulsion after 8 days of storage at 4°C.[1017]

The stability of a 3-in-1 parenteral nutrition mixture (TNA #191 in Appendix) was compared with trace elements added as gluconate salts or chloride salts. TNA #191 with copper 0.24 mg/L, iron 0.5 mg/L, and zinc 2 mg/L in either salt form was physically stable for 7 days at 4 and 25°C.[1787]

Trace elements additives, especially those containing copper ions, have the potential to be incompatible in TPN solutions, resulting in precipitation. In a TPN admixture containing 5% Synthamin 17, 25% dextrose, 1 g of ascorbic acid injection, 14 mmol of calcium chloride, and trace elements solution (David Bull), storage at 20 to 25°C and 2 to 8°C, protected from light, resulted in the formation of a discolored solution in 3 to 7 days and an off-white to yellow precipitate in 8 to 12 days, respectively. Electron microscopy revealed the presence of numerous bipyramidal, 8-sided crystals in sizes from 3 to 30 μm. The authors proposed that the crystals were calcium oxalate. They suggested that the ascorbic acid decomposed to oxalic acid; the oxalic acid then interacted with calcium ions to form calcium oxalate. The authors did not verify their supposition. They noted that the crystals were conformationally different from calcium phosphate crystals and that no phosphate had been added to the admixture. In addition, mixing ascorbic acid injection 500 mg/5 mL with trace elements solution 5 mL results in the formation of a transparent gel that becomes an opaque flocculent precipitate after 5 minutes. The authors recommended adding trace elements well away from injections that can act as ligands and with thorough mixing after each addition. Introduction of air and prolonged storage should be avoided. Incorporating trace elements and ascorbic acid on alternate days was also suggested.[2197]

The chromium and zinc contamination of various components of parenteral nutrition solutions by atomic absorption spectrophotometry was evaluated. They analyzed FreAmine III, Aminosyn, TrophAmine, and dextrose 70% and found chromium concentrations were below the limit of detection but zinc ranged from 0.11 to 4.97 mg/L. Additionally, detectable chromium and zinc concentrations were seen with various lots of L-cysteine, potassium and sodium salts (chloride, acetate, and phosphate), calcium gluconate, and magnesium sulfate. The zinc contamination was thought to be a product of manufacturing procedures as it is present in many rubber stoppers and in the materials to produce glass. The authors suggested that the amount of contamination of chromium and zinc present in most pediatric parenteral nutrition solutions may exceed current recommendations, especially for infants less than 10 kg.[2464]

Heparin

Flocculation of fat emulsion (Kabi-Vitrum) was reported during Y-site administration into a line used to infuse a parenteral nutrition admixture containing both calcium gluconate and heparin sodium. Subsequent evaluation indicated that the combination of calcium gluconate (0.46 and 1.8 mmol/125 mL) and heparin sodium (25 and 100 units/125 mL) in amino acids plus dextrose induced flocculation of the fat emulsion within 2 to 4 minutes at concentrations that resulted in no visually apparent flocculation in 30 minutes with either agent alone.[1214]

Calcium chloride quantities of 1 and 20 mmol normally result in slow flocculation of fat emulsion 20% over several hours. When heparin sodium 5 units/mL was added, the flocculation rate was accelerated greatly and a cream layer was observed visually in a few minutes. This effect was not observed when sodium ion was substituted for the divalent calcium.[1406]

Similar results were observed during simulated Y-site administration of heparin sodium into nine 3-in-1 nutrient admixtures having different compositions. Damage to the fat emulsion component was found to occur immediately, with the possible formation of free oil over time.[2215]

The destabilization of fat emulsion (Intralipid 20%) was also observed when administered simultaneously with a TPN admixture and heparin. The damage, detected by viscosity measurement, occurred immediately upon contact at the Y-site. The extent of the destabilization was dependent on the concentration of heparin and the presence of MVI Pediatric with its surfactant content. Additionally, phase separation was observed in 2 hours. The authors noted that TPN admixtures containing heparin should never be premixed with fat emulsion as a 3-in-1 total nutrient admixture because of this emulsion destabilization. The authors indicated their belief that the damage could be minimized during Y-site co-administration as long as the heparin was kept at a sufficiently low concentration (no visible separation occurred at a heparin concentration of 0.5 unit/mL) and the length of tubing between the Y-site and the patient was minimized.[2282]

However, because the damage to emulsion integrity has been found to occur immediately upon mixing with heparin in the presence of the calcium ions in TPN admixtures[1214] [2215] [2282] and no evaluation and documentation of the clinical safety of

using such destabilized emulsions has been performed, use of such damaged emulsions is suspect.

Ranitidine

The stability of ranitidine hydrochloride has been evaluated in a number of TPN solutions with variable results. See Additive Compatibility table. The major mechanism of ranitidine hydrochloride decomposition is oxidation. A number of factors have been found to contribute to ranitidine hydrochloride instability in TPN solutions, including the presence or absence of antioxidants (such as sodium metabisulfite) in the amino acids, the addition of trace elements (which can catalyze ranitidine oxidation), solution pH, and type of plastic container used. In a study of ranitidine hydrochloride stability in several TPN solutions stored at 5°C, the drug was most stable in FreAmine III–based (contains sodium metabisulfite) admixtures with additives when packaged in multilayer gas impermeable plastic containers (Ultrastab) with about 8% loss in 28 days. In contrast, in ethylene vinyl acetate (EVA) bags, which are permeable to oxygen, losses of approximately 50% occurred in this time period. If Vamin 14 with no antioxidant present was used as the amino acid source, and the solution was packaged in EVA bags, ranitidine hydrochloride losses of approximately 65% occurred in 28 days. Similarly, the addition of air to the bags during compounding increases the extent of ranitidine hydrochloride oxidation substantially.[2195]

Other Information

Titratable Acidity

The acidity of parenteral nutrition solutions can be a factor in the development of metabolic acidosis by a patient.[577] [851] Titratable acidity is a measure of the hydrogen ion content that must be neutralized to raise the pH to a given endpoint and is often expressed as milliequivalents of titrant per liter of reactant. In a study[577] of 5 amino acid injections and mixtures, the titratable acidities were determined for pH 7.4 by titrating with 0.1220 N sodium hydroxide and 7.54% (0.898 M) sodium bicarbonate. The results are noted in Table 11.

Table 11. Titratable acidity of several amino acids products[577]

	Titratable Acidity	
	NaOH (mEq/L)	NaHCO$_3$ (mEq/L)
Aminosyn 7%	37	314
FreAmine II 8.5%	16.8	176
Travasol 8.5%	34.7	354
Travasol 8.5% with electrolytes	45.2	420

Corresponding (although somewhat lower) values were also obtained for 1:1 mixtures with dextrose 50%. It was concluded that use of sodium bicarbonate to adjust to pH 7.4 was not usually feasible given the large volumes of fluid and increased sodium ion required. However, smaller amounts could be used for smaller pH adjustments.[577]

Aminocaproic Acid
AHFS 20:28.16

Products

Aminocaproic acid is available as a 250-mg/mL concentration in 20-mL vials containing 5 g of drug with hydrochloric acid for pH adjustment. Aminocaproic acid injection is available with benzyl alcohol 0.9% as a preservative and also in preservative-free form.[1(6/07)] [4]

pH

The pH is adjusted to approximately 6.8 with a range of 6 to 7.6.[1(6/07)]

Administration

Aminocaproic acid is administered by continuous intravenous infusion after dilution in a suitable infusion solution. Rapid intravenous injection of the undiluted drug should be avoided.[1(6/07)] [4]

Stability

Intact containers of aminocaproic acid injection should be stored at controlled room temperature. Freezing should be avoided.[1(6/07)] [4]

Compatibility Information

Solution Compatibility

Aminocaproic acid

Test Soln Name	Mfr	Mfr	Conc/L or %	Remarks	Ref	C/I
Dextrose 5%	BA[a]	IMM	10 and 100 g	Physically compatible with little or no loss in 7 days at 4 and 23°C. Yellow discoloration forms after 24 hr at 23°C but is not associated with drug loss	2096	C
Sodium chloride 0.9%	BA[a]	IMM	10 and 100 g	Physically compatible with little or no loss in 7 days at 4 and 23°C	2096	C

[a] Tested in PVC containers.

Y-Site Injection Compatibility (1:1 Mixture)

Aminocaproic acid

Test Drug	Mfr	Conc	Mfr	Conc	Remarks	Ref	C/I
Fenoldopam mesylate	AB	80 mcg/mL[a]	AMR	50 mg/mL[a]	Physically compatible for 4 hr at 23°C	2467	C

[a] Tested in sodium chloride 0.9%.

Selected Revisions October 1, 2012. © Copyright, October 1982.
American Society of Health-System Pharmacists, Inc.

DOI: 10.37573/9781585286850.016

Aminophylline
AHFS 86:16

Products

Aminophylline is available as a 25-mg/mL solution in 10-mL (250-mg) and 20-mL (500-mg) ampuls and vials for intravenous injection. Aminophylline is a 2:1 complex of theophylline and ethylenediamine. It contains excess ethylenediamine to ensure stability[6] and is approximately 79% theophylline by weight. Aminophylline 25 mg is equivalent to 19.7 mg of theophylline.[1(11/06)]

pH

From 8.6 to 9.[1(11/06)]

Osmolarity

The calculated osmolarity of the injection is 170 mOsm/L.[1(11/06)]

Osmolality

The osmolality was determined to be 114 mOsm/kg by freezing-point depression.[1071]

The osmolality of aminophylline 250 mg was calculated for the following dilutions:[1054]

Diluent	Osmolality (mOsm/kg)	
	50 mL	100 mL
Dextrose 5%	300	291
Sodium chloride 0.9%	327	318

Administration

Aminophylline may be administered by intravenous infusion or slow direct intravenous injection.[1(11/06) 4]

Stability

The containers should be stored at controlled room temperature and protected from freezing and light.[1(11/06) 4] Containers of aminophylline should be inspected for particulate matter and discoloration prior to use. Do not use if crystals are present.[1(11/06) 4]

pH Effects

Reports in the literature of aminophylline precipitating in acidic media do not apply to the dilute solutions found in intravenous infusions. Aminophylline should not be mixed in a syringe with other components of an admixture but should be added separately.[6]

Because of the alkalinity of aminophylline-containing solutions, drugs known to be alkali labile should be avoided in admixtures.[6]

Temperature Effects

Aminophylline under simulated summer conditions in paramedic vehicles was exposed to temperatures ranging from 26 to 38°C over 4 weeks. Analysis found no loss of the drug under these conditions.[2562]

Light Effects

A study of aminophylline (Squibb) 50 mg/mL found no change in theophylline after 8 weeks of storage with exposure to fluorescent light.[1231]

Syringes

Aminophylline (Abbott) 5 mg/mL in bacteriostatic water for injection containing benzyl alcohol 0.9% in plastic syringes (Becton Dickinson) exhibited 2 and 3% losses at 4 and 22°C, respectively, after 91 days of storage.[1586]

Sorption

Aminophylline was shown not to exhibit sorption to polyvinyl chloride (PVC) bags and tubing, polyethylene tubing, Silastic tubing, and polypropylene syringes.[536 606]

Filtration

Aminophylline 500 mg/L in dextrose 5% was passed through an Ivex-2 inline filter at a rate of 2 mL/min. No decrease in the aminophylline concentration occurred over the 8-hour study period.[556]

Central Venous Catheter

Aminophylline (Abbott) 2.5 mg/mL in dextrose 5% was found to be compatible with the ARROWg+ard Blue Plus (Arrow International) chlorhexidine-bearing triple-lumen central catheter. Essentially complete delivery of the drug was found with little or no drug loss occurring. Furthermore, chlorhexidine delivered from the catheter remained at trace amounts with no substantial increase due to the delivery of the drug through the catheter.[2335]

Compatibility Information
Solution Compatibility

Aminophylline

Test Soln Name	Mfr	Mfr	Conc/L or %	Remarks	Ref	C/I
Amino acids 4.25%, dextrose 25%	MG	SE	500 mg	No increase in particulate matter in 24 hr at 5°C	349	C
Dextrose 2.5% in half-strength Ringer's injection	AB	SE	500 mg	Physically compatible	3	C

DOI: 10.37573/9781585286850.017

Solution Compatibility (Cont.)

Test Soln Name	Mfr	Mfr	Conc/L or %	Remarks	Ref	C/I
Dextrose 5% in Ringer's injection	AB	SE	500 mg	Physically compatible	3	C
Dextrose 5% in half-strength Ringer's injection, lactated	AB	SE	500 mg	Physically compatible	3	C
Dextrose 2.5% in Ringer's injection, lactated	AB	SE	500 mg	Physically compatible	3	C
Dextrose 5% in Ringer's injection, lactated	AB	SE	500 mg	Physically compatible	3	C
Dextrose 5% in Ringer's injection, lactated	BA	SE	10 mg	Physically compatible for 24 hr	315	C
Dextrose 10% in Ringer's injection, lactated	AB	SE	500 mg	Physically compatible	3	C
Dextrose 2.5% in sodium chloride 0.45%	AB	SE	500 mg	Physically compatible	3	C
Dextrose 2.5% in sodium chloride 0.9%	AB	SE	500 mg	Physically compatible	3	C
Dextrose 5% in sodium chloride 0.225%	AB	SE	500 mg	Physically compatible	3	C
Dextrose 5% in sodium chloride 0.225%	MG	AQ	750 mg	Physically compatible with no aminophylline decomposition in 48 hr at 25°C. Yellow tinge at 48 hr due to slight dextrose decomposition	556	C
Dextrose 5% in sodium chloride 0.45%	AB	SE	500 mg	Physically compatible	3	C
Dextrose 5% in sodium chloride 0.9%	AB	SE	500 mg	Physically compatible	3	C
Dextrose 5% in sodium chloride 0.9%			250 mg	Physically compatible	74	C
Dextrose 5% in sodium chloride 0.9%	BA	SE	10 g	Physically compatible for 24 hr	315	C
Dextrose 5% in sodium chloride 0.9%	TRa	AQ	750 mg	Physically compatible with no aminophylline decomposition in 48 hr at 25°C. Yellow tinge at 48 hr due to slight dextrose decomposition	556	C
Dextrose 10% in sodium chloride 0.9%	AB	SE	500 mg	Physically compatible	3	C
Dextrose 2.5%	AB	SE	500 mg	Physically compatible	3	C
Dextrose 5%			500 mg to 2.5 g	Stable for 24 hr at room temperature	56	C
Dextrose 5%			250 mg	Physically compatible	74	C
Dextrose 5%	AB	SE	500 mg	Physically compatible	3	C
Dextrose 5%	AB	SE	450 mg	Stable for at least 24 hr at room temperature	6	C
Dextrose 5%	BA	SE	10 g	Physically compatible for 24 hr	315	C
Dextrose 5%	AB	ES	5 and 10 g	Physically compatible with little or no decomposition in 96 hr under refrigeration	537	C
Dextrose 5%	TRa	AQ	750 mg	Physically compatible with no aminophylline decomposition in 48 hr at 25°C and 7 days at 5°C. Yellow tinge in the 25°C admixture at 48 hr due to slight dextrose decomposition	556	C
Dextrose 5%	TRa	AQ	250 and 500 mg	Physically compatible with no aminophylline decomposition in 48 hr at 25°C. Yellow tinge in the admixture at 48 hr due to slight dextrose decomposition	556	C
Dextrose 5%			250 mg	Stable for at least 24 hr at 24 to 26°C	852	C
Dextrose 5%	TRa	IX	500 mg	Physically compatible with little or no loss in 48 hr at room temperature	1186	C
Dextrose 5%	AB	SE	1 g	Physically compatible with no loss in 24 hr at 24°C under fluorescent light	1198	C
Dextrose 5%	TRa	LY	1 g	Physically compatible with no loss in 24 hr at room temperature under fluorescent light	1358	C

Solution Compatibility (Cont.)

Test Soln Name	Mfr	Mfr	Conc/L or %	Remarks	Ref	C/I
Dextrose 5%	TR[a]		1 g	Yellow discoloration in 2 hr but theophylline content retained for at least 24 hr	1571	C
Dextrose 5%	TR[a]	ES	0.5 and 2 g	Visually compatible with little or no aminophylline loss in 48 hr at room temperature	1802	C
Dextrose 10%	AB	SE	500 mg	Physically compatible	3	C
Dextrose 10%	BA	SE	10 g	Physically compatible for 24 hr	315	C
Dextrose 10%			250 mg	Stable for at least 24 hr at 24 to 26°C. Yellow discoloration at 2 hr and increased with time	852	C
Dextrose 20%	BA	SE	10 g	Physically compatible for 24 hr	315	C
Dextrose 20%			250 mg	Stable for at least 24 hr at 24 to 26°C. Yellow discoloration at 2 hr and increased with time	852	C
Ionosol B in dextrose 5%	AB	SE	500 mg	Physically compatible	3	C
Ionosol MB in dextrose 5%	AB	SE	500 mg	Physically compatible	3	C
Ringer's injection	AB	SE	500 mg	Physically compatible	3	C
Ringer's injection, lactated			250 mg	Physically compatible	74	C
Ringer's injection, lactated	AB		500 mg	Physically compatible	3	C
Ringer's injection, lactated	BA	SE	10 g	Physically compatible for 24 hr	315	C
Sodium chloride 0.45%	AB	SE	500 mg	Physically compatible	3	C
Sodium chloride 0.9%	AB	SE	500 mg	Physically compatible	3	C
Sodium chloride 0.9%			250 mg	Physically compatible	74	C
Sodium chloride 0.9%	TR[a]	SE	500 mg	Stable for 24 hr	45	C
Sodium chloride 0.9%	BA[d]	SE	500 mg	Stable for 24 hr	45	C
Sodium chloride 0.9%	BA	SE	10 g	Physically compatible for 24 hr	315	C
Sodium chloride 0.9%	TR[a]	AQ	750 mg	Physically compatible with no decomposition in 48 hr at 25°C	556	C
Sodium chloride 0.9%	TR[a]		1 g	Theophylline content retained for 24 hr	1571	C/I
Sodium chloride 0.9%	TR[a]	ES	0.5 and 2 g	Visually compatible with no aminophylline loss in 48 hr at room temperature	1802	C
Sodium lactate ⅙ M	AB	SE	500 mg	Physically compatible	3	C
Sodium lactate ⅙ M	BA	SE	10 g	Physically compatible for 24 hr	315	C
TNA #180[b]			234 and 638 mg	No theophylline loss and no increase in fat particle size in 24 hr at room temperature	1617	C
TPN #25[b]		SE	250 mg to 1.5 g	Physically compatible and aminophylline stable for at least 24 hr at 25°C	755	C
TPN #25[b]		SE	1 g	Physically compatible and aminophylline stable for at least 24 hr at 4°C	755	C
TPN #26[b]		SE	250 mg to 1.5 g	Physically compatible and aminophylline stable for at least 24 hr at 25°C	755	C
TPN #26[b]		SE	1 g	Physically compatible and aminophylline stable for at least 24 hr at 4°C	755	C
TPN #27[b]		SE	250 mg to 1.5 g	Physically compatible and aminophylline stable for at least 24 hr at 25°C	755	C

Solution Compatibility (Cont.)

Test Soln Name	Mfr	Mfr	Conc/L or %	Remarks	Ref	C/I
TPN #27[b]		SE	1 g	Physically compatible and aminophylline stable for at least 24 hr at 4°C	755	C
TPN #28[b]		SE	1 g	Physically compatible and aminophylline stable for at least 24 hr at 25°C	755	C
TPN #29[b]		SE	1 g	Physically compatible and aminophylline stable for at least 24 hr at 25°C	755	C
TPN #30[b]		SE	1 g	Physically compatible and aminophylline stable for at least 24 hr at 25°C	755	C
TPN[c]			29.3 mg	No significant change in aminophylline content over 24 hr at 24 to 26°C	852	C

[a] Tested in PVC containers.

[b] Refer to Appendix for the composition of parenteral nutrition solutions. TNA indicates a 3-in-1 admixture, and TPN indicates a 2-in-1 admixture.

[c] Tested in a pediatric parenteral nutrition solution containing 150 mL of dextrose 5% and 30 mL of Vamin glucose with electrolytes and vitamins.

[d] Tested in glass containers.

Additive Compatibility

Aminophylline

Test Drug	Mfr	Conc/L or %	Mfr	Conc/L or %	Test Solution	Remarks	Ref	C/I
Amikacin sulfate	BR	5 g	SE	5 g	LR, NS, R, SL	Physically compatible and amikacin stable for 24 hr at 25°C. Aminophylline not analyzed	294	C
Amikacin sulfate	BR	5 g	SE	5 g	D5LR, D5R, D5S, D5W, D10W	Over 10% amikacin loss after 8 hr but within 24 hr at 25°C. Aminophylline not analyzed	294	I
Ascorbic acid	AB	500 mg	SE	500 mg		Physically compatible	6	C
Ascorbic acid	UP	500 mg	SE	1 g	D5W	Physically incompatible	15	I
Atracurium besylate	BW	500 mg		1 g	D5W	Atracurium unstable due to high pH	1694	I
Bleomycin sulfate	BR	20 and 30 units	ES	250 mg	NS	50% loss of bleomycin in 1 week at 4°C	763	I
Calcium gluconate		1 g		250 mg	D5W	Physically compatible	74	C
Cefepime HCl	BR	4 g	LY	1 g	NS	37% cefepime loss in 18 hr at room temperature and 32% loss in 3 days at 5°C. No aminophylline loss	1681	I
Ceftazidime	GL	2 g	ES	1 g	D5W, NS	20 to 23% ceftazidime loss in 6 hr at room temperature	1937	I
Ceftazidime	GL	6 g	ES	1 g	D5W, NS	8 to 10% ceftazidime loss in 6 hr at room temperature	1937	I
Ceftazidime	GL	2 g	ES	2 g	D5W, NS	35 to 40% ceftazidime loss in 6 hr at room temperature	1937	I
Ceftazidime	GL	6 g	ES	2 g	D5W, NS	22% ceftazidime loss in 6 hr at room temperature	1937	I
Ceftriaxone sodium	RC	20 g	AMR	1 g	D5W, NS[a]	Yellow color forms immediately. 3 to 6% ceftriaxone loss and 8 to 12% aminophylline loss in 24 hr	1727	I
Ceftriaxone sodium	RC	20 g	AMR	4 g	D5W, NS[a]	Yellow color forms immediately. 15 to 20% ceftriaxone loss and 7 to 9% aminophylline loss in 24 hr	1727	I
Ceftriaxone sodium	RC	40 g	AMR	1 g	D5W, NS[a]	Yellow color forms immediately. 15 to 18% ceftriaxone loss and 1 to 3% aminophylline loss in 24 hr	1727	I

Additive Compatibility (Cont.)

Test Drug	Mfr	Conc/L or %	Mfr	Conc/L or %	Test Solution	Remarks	Ref	C/I
Chloramphenicol sodium succinate	PD	500 mg		250 mg	D5W	Physically compatible	74	C
Chloramphenicol sodium succinate	PD	10 g	SE	1 g	D5W	Physically compatible	15	C
Chlorpromazine HCl	BP	200 mg	BP	1 g	D5W, NS	Precipitates immediately	26	I
Ciprofloxacin	MI	1.6 g	LY	2 g	D5W, NS	Precipitate forms in 4 hr at 4 and 25°C	1541	I
Ciprofloxacin						Physically incompatible with loss of ciprofloxacin reported due to pH over 6.0	1924	I
Clindamycin phosphate	UP	600 mg	SE	600 mg		Physically incompatible	101	I
Dexamethasone sodium phosphate		30 mg		625 mg	D5W	Physically compatible and chemically stable for 24 hr at 4 and 30°C	521	C
Dimenhydrinate	SE	50 mg		250 mg	D5W	Physically compatible	74	C
Dimenhydrinate	SE	500 mg	SE	1 g	D5W	Physically incompatible	15	I
Diphenhydramine HCl	PD	50 mg	SE	500 mg		Physically compatible	6	C
Dobutamine HCl	LI	1 g	SE	1 g	D5W, NS	Cloudy in 6 hr at 25°C	789	I
Dobutamine HCl	LI	1 g	ES	2.5 g	D5W, NS	White precipitate in 12 hr at 21°C	812	I
Dopamine HCl	ACC	800 mg	SE	500 mg	D5W	Physically compatible. At 25°C, 10% dopamine decomposition occurs in 111 hr	527	C
Doxapram HCl	WW					Precipitation or gas formation	3220	I
Doxorubicin HCl	AD					Discolors from red to purple	524	I
Epinephrine HCl	PD	4 mg	SE	500 mg	D5W	At 25°C, 10% epinephrine decomposition in 1.2 hr in light and 3 hr in dark	527	I
Epinephrine HCl		4 mg		500 mg	D5W	Pink to brown discoloration in 8 to 24 hr at room temperature	845	I
Erythromycin lactobionate	AB	1 g	SE	500 mg		Physically compatible. Erythromycin stable for 24 hr at 25°C	20	C
Esmolol HCl	DU	6 g	LY	1 g	D5W	Physically compatible with no loss of either drug in 24 hr at room temperature under fluorescent light	1358	C
Fat emulsion, intravenous	VT	10%	ES	1 g		Physically compatible for 48 hr at 4°C and room temperature	32	C
Fat emulsion, intravenous	VT	10%	DB	500 mg		Lipid coalescence in 24 hr at 25 and 8°C	825	I
Floxacillin sodium	BE	20 g	ANT	1 g	NS	Physically compatible for 72 hr at 15 and 30°C	1479	C
Flumazenil	RC	20 mg	AMR	2 g	D5Wb	Visually compatible. No flumazenil loss in 24 hr at 23°C in fluorescent light. Aminophylline not tested	1710	C
Furosemide	HO	1 g	ANT	1 g	NS	Physically compatible for 72 hr at 15 and 30°C	1479	C
Heparin sodium		12,000 units		250 mg	D5W	Physically compatible	74	C
Heparin sodium	UP	4000 units	SE	1 g	D5W	Physically compatible	15	C
Hydralazine HCl	BP	80 mg	BP	1 g	D5W	Yellow color produced	26	I
Hydrocortisone sodium succinate	UP	100 mg		250 mg	D5W	Physically compatible	74	C

Additive Compatibility (Cont.)

Test Drug	Mfr	Conc/L or %	Mfr	Conc/L or %	Test Solution	Remarks	Ref	C/I
Hydrocortisone sodium succinate	UP	500 mg	SE	1 g	D5W	Physically compatible	15	C
Hydrocortisone sodium succinate	UP	100 mg	SE	500 mg		Physically compatible	6	C
Hydrocortisone sodium succinate		250 mg		625 mg	D5W	Physically compatible and aminophylline stable for 24 hr at 4 and 30°C. Total hydrocortisone content changed little but substantial ester hydrolysis	521	C
Hydroxyzine HCl	RR	250 mg	SE	1 g	D5W	Physically incompatible	15	I
Isoproterenol HCl	BN	2 mg	SE	500 mg	D5W	At 25°C, 10% isoproterenol decomposition in 2.2 to 2.5 hr in light and dark	527	I
Lidocaine HCl	AST	2 g	SE	500 mg		Physically compatible	24	C
Lidocaine HCl	AST	2 g	AQ	1 g	D5W, LR, NS	Physically compatible for 24 hr at 25°C	775	C
Meropenem	ZEN	1 and 20 g	AMR	1 g	NS	Visually compatible for 4 hr at room temperature	1994	C
Methyldopate HCl	MSD	1 g	SE	500 mg	D5W, D10W, D2.5½S, D2.5S, D5¼S, D5½S, D5S, D10S, NS, ½S	Physically compatible	23	C
Methyldopate HCl	MSD	1 g	SE	500 mg	D5W	Physically compatible. At 25°C, 10% methyldopate decomposition in 90 hr	527	C
Methylprednisolone sodium succinate	UP	40 to 250 mg		500 mg	D5W, NS	Clear solution for 24 hr	329	C
Methylprednisolone sodium succinate	UP	80 mg		1 g	D5W	Clear solution for 24 hr	329	C
Methylprednisolone sodium succinate	UP	125 mg	SE	500 mg		Precipitate forms after 6 hr but within 24 hr	6	I
Methylprednisolone sodium succinate	UP	250 mg to 1 g		1 g	D5W	Precipitate forms	329	I
Methylprednisolone sodium succinate	UP	10 to 20 g		~400 mg	D5S, D5W, LR	Yellow color forms	329	I
Methylprednisolone sodium succinate	UP	500 mg and 2 g	SE	1 g	D5W	Physically compatible. No aminophylline or methylprednisolone alcohol loss in 3 hr at room temperature, but 7 to 10% ester hydrolysis	1022	C
Methylprednisolone sodium succinate	UP	500 mg and 2 g	SE	1 g	NS	Physically compatible. No aminophylline or methylprednisolone alcohol loss in 3 hr at room temperature, but 12 to 18% ester hydrolysis	1022	C
Midazolam HCl	RC	50 mg		720 mg	NS	Visually compatible for 4 hr	355	C
Midazolam HCl	RC	250 mg		720 mg	NS	Transient precipitate that dissipates	355	?
Midazolam HCl	RC	400 mg		720 mg	NS	Precipitate forms immediately	355	I
Nafcillin sodium	WY	30 g	SE	500 mg	D5W	Nafcillin retained for 24 hr at 25°C	27	C
Nafcillin sodium	WY	2 g	SE	500 mg	D5W	14% nafcillin loss in 24 hr at 25°C	27	I
Nitroglycerin	ACC	400 mg	IX	1 g	D5W^c	Physically compatible with 4% nitroglycerin loss in 24 hr and 6% loss in 48 hr at 23°C. Aminophylline not tested	929	C
Nitroglycerin	ACC	400 mg	IX	1 g	NS^c	Physically compatible with no nitroglycerin loss in 24 hr and 5% loss in 48 hr at 23°C. Aminophylline not tested	929	C

Additive Compatibility (Cont.)

Test Drug	Mfr	Conc/L or %	Mfr	Conc/L or %	Test Solution	Remarks	Ref	C/I
Norepinephrine bitartrate	WI	8 mg	SE	500 mg	D5W	10% norepinephrine loss in 3.6 hr at 25°C	527	I
Penicillin G potassium	SQ	1 million units	SE	500 mg	D5W	44% penicillin loss in 24 hr at 25°C	47	I
Penicillin G potassium	d	900,000 units	SE	500 mg	D5W	22% penicillin loss in 6 hr at 25°C	48	I
Pentazocine lactate	WI	300 mg	SE	1 g	D5W	Physically incompatible	15	I
Pentobarbital sodium	AB	500 mg		500 mg		Physically compatible	3	C
Pentobarbital sodium	AB	1 g	SE	1 g	D5W	Physically compatible	15	C
Pentobarbital sodium	AB	500 mg	SE	500 mg		Physically compatible	6	C
Phenobarbital sodium	WI	200 mg	SE	1 g	D5W	Physically compatible	15	C
Phenobarbital sodium	AB	100 mg	SE	500 mg		Physically compatible	6	C
Potassium chloride	AB	3 g		250 mg	D5W	Physically compatible	74	C
Potassium chloride	AB	40 mEq	SE	500 mg		Physically compatible	6	C
Prochlorperazine edisylate	SKF	100 mg	SE	1 g	D5W	Physically incompatible	15	I
Prochlorperazine mesylate	BP	100 mg	BP	1 g	D5W, NS	Precipitates immediately	26	I
Promethazine HCl	BP	100 mg	BP	1 g	D5W, NS	Precipitates immediately	26	I
Promethazine HCl	WY	250 mg	SE	1 g	D5W	Physically incompatible	15	I
Ranitidine HCl	GL	50 mg and 2 g	ES	500 mg and 2 g	D5W, NSb	Physically compatible. 4% or less ranitidine loss in 24 hr at room temperature in light. Aminophylline not tested	1361	C
Ranitidine HCl	GL	50 mg and 2 g	ES	0.5 and 2 g	D5W, NSb	Visually compatible. Little loss of either drug in 48 hr at room temperature	1802	C
Sodium bicarbonate	AB	80 mEq	SE	1 g	D5W	Physically compatible	15	C
Sodium bicarbonate	AB	40 mEq	SE	500 mg		Physically compatible	6	C
Terbutaline sulfate	CI	4 mg	SE	500 mg	D5W	Physically compatible. At 25°C, 10% terbutaline loss in 44 hr in light	527	C
Vancomycin HCl	LI	1 g		250 mg	D5W	Physically compatible	74	C
Vancomycin HCl	LI	5 g	SE	1 g	D5W	Physically incompatible	15	I
Verapamil HCl	KN	80 mg	SE	1 g	D5W, NS	Transient precipitate clears rapidly, then clear for 48 hr	739	?
Verapamil HCl	KN	400 mg	SE	1 g	D5W	Visible turbidity forms immediately. Filtration removes all verapamil	1198	I
Verapamil HCl	KN	100 mg	SE	1 g	D5W	Visually clear, but precipitate found by microscopic examination. Filtration removes all verapamil	1198	I

a Tested in polyolefin containers.

b Tested in PVC containers.

c Tested in glass containers.

d A buffered preparation was specified.

Drugs in Syringe Compatibility

Aminophylline

Test Drug	Mfr	Amt	Mfr	Amt	Remarks	Ref	C/I
Caffeine citrate		20 mg/1 mL	AB	25 mg/1 mL	Visually compatible for 4 hr at 25°C	2440	C
Dimenhydrinate		10 mg/1 mL		50 mg/1 mL	Light cloudiness forms immediately	2569	I
Doxapram HCl	RB	400 mg/20 mL		250 mg/10 mL	Immediate turbidity and precipitation	1177	I
Heparin sodium		2500 units/1 mL		240 mg/10 mL	Physically compatible for at least 5 min	1053	C
Metoclopramide HCl	RB	10 mg/2 mL	ES	80 mg/3.2 mL	Physically compatible for 24 hr at 25°C	1167	C
Metoclopramide HCl	RB	10 mg/2 mL	ES	500 mg/20 mL	Physically compatible for 24 hr at 25°C	1167	C
Metoclopramide HCl	RB	160 mg/32 mL	ES	500 mg/20 mL	Physically compatible for 24 hr at 25°C	1167	C
Pantoprazole sodium	a	4 mg/1 mL		50 mg/1 mL	Clear solution	2574	C
Pentobarbital sodium	AB	500 mg/10 mL[b]		500 mg/2 mL	Physically compatible	55	C

[a] Test performed using the formulation WITHOUT edetate disodium.

Y-Site Injection Compatibility (1:1 Mixture)

Aminophylline

Test Drug	Mfr	Conc	Mfr	Conc	Remarks	Ref	C/I
Allopurinol sodium	BW	3 mg/mL[b]	AB	2.5 mg/mL[b]	Physically compatible for 4 hr at 22°C	1686	C
Amifostine	USB	10 mg/mL[a]	AMR	2.5 mg/mL[a]	Physically compatible for 4 hr at 23°C	1845	C
Amiodarone HCl	LZ	4 mg/mL[c]	ES	5 mg/mL[c]	Haze forms within 15 min and white precipitate forms within 6 hr at 21°C	1032	I
Anidulafungin	VIC	0.5 mg/mL[a]	AB	2.5 mg/mL[a]	Physically compatible for 4 hr at 23°C	2617	C
Aztreonam	SQ	40 mg/mL[a]	AMR	2.5 mg/mL[a]	Physically compatible for 4 hr at 23°C	1758	C
Bivalirudin	TMC	5 mg/mL[a]	AB	2.5 mg/mL[a]	Physically compatible for 4 hr at 23°C	2373	C
Ceftaroline fosamil	FOR	2.22 mg/mL[d]	AMR	2.5 mg/mL[d]	Physically compatible for 4 hr at 23°C	2826	C
Ceftazidime	GL	40 mg/mL[a]	ES	2 mg/mL[a]	Visually compatible with 4% ceftazidime loss and 9% theophylline loss in 2 hr at room temperature	1937	C
Ceftazidime	GL	40 mg/mL[b]	ES	2 mg/mL[a]	Visually compatible with 5% ceftazidime loss and 4% theophylline loss in 2 hr at room temperature	1937	C
Ciprofloxacin	MI	2 mg/mL[c]	AB	2 mg/mL[c]	Fine white crystals form in 20 min in D5W and 2 min in NS	1655	I
Cisatracurium besylate	GW	0.1 and 2 mg/mL[a]	AB	2.5 mg/mL[a]	Physically compatible for 4 hr at 23°C	2074	C
Cisatracurium besylate	GW	5 mg/mL[a]	AB	2.5 mg/mL[a]	Gray subvisible haze forms in 1 hr	2074	I
Cladribine	ORT	0.015[b] and 0.5[e] mg/mL	AMR	2.5 mg/mL[b]	Physically compatible for 4 hr at 23°C	1969	C
Clarithromycin	AB	4 mg/mL[a]	EV	2 mg/mL[a]	Needle-like crystals form in 2 hr at 30°C and 4 hr at 17°C	2174	I
Clonidine HCl	BI	18 mcg/mL[b]	NYC	0.9 mg/mL[b]	Visually compatible	2642	C
Dexmedetomidine HCl	AB	4 mcg/mL[b]	AB	2.5 mg/mL[b]	Physically compatible for 4 hr at 23°C	2383	C
Diltiazem HCl	MMD	5 mg/mL	AMR	25 mg/mL[b]	Cloudiness forms	1807	I

Y-Site Injection Compatibility (1:1 Mixture) (Cont.)

Test Drug	Mfr	Conc	Mfr	Conc	Remarks	Ref	C/I
Diltiazem HCl	MMD	1 mg/mL[b]	AMR	25 mg/mL[b]	Visually compatible	1807	C
Diltiazem HCl	MMD	5 mg/mL	AMR	2 mg/mL[c]	Visually compatible	1807	C
Dobutamine HCl	LI	4 mg/mL[c]	ES	4 mg/mL[c]	Slight precipitate and color change in 1 hr	1316	I
Docetaxel	RPR	0.9 mg/mL[a]	AB	2.5 mg/mL[a]	Physically compatible for 4 hr at 23°C	2224	C
Doripenem	JJ	5 mg/mL[a b]	AMR	2.5 mg/mL[a b]	Physically compatible for 4 hr at 23°C	2743	C
Doxorubicin HCl liposomal	SEQ	0.4 mg/mL[a]	AB	2.5 mg/mL[a]	Physically compatible for 4 hr at 23°C	2087	C
Enalaprilat	MSD	0.05 mg/mL[b]	ES	1 mg/mL[a]	Physically compatible for 24 hr at room temperature under fluorescent light	1355	C
Esmolol HCl	DCC	10 mg/mL[a]	ES	1 mg/mL[a]	Physically compatible for 24 hr at 22°C	1169	C
Etoposide phosphate	BR	5 mg/mL[a]	AB	2.5 mg/mL[a]	Physically compatible for 4 hr at 23°C	2218	C
Famotidine	MSD	0.2 mg/mL[a]	LY	2.5 mg/mL[b]	Physically compatible for 14 hr	1196	C
Famotidine	ME	2 mg/mL[a]		2.5 mg/mL[a]	Visually compatible for 4 hr at 22°C	1936	C
Fenoldopam mesylate	AB	80 mcg/mL[b]	AB	2.5 mg/mL[b]	Haze and microparticulates form immediately. Yellow turbidity in 4 hr	2467	I
Filgrastim	AMG	30 mcg/mL[a]	AB	2.5 mg/mL[a]	Physically compatible for 4 hr at 22°C	1687	C
Fluconazole	RR	2 mg/mL	ES	25 mg/mL	Physically compatible for 24 hr at 25°C	1407	C
Fluconazole	PF	0.5 and 1.5 mg/mL[c]	AMR	0.8 and 1.5 mg/mL[c]	Visually compatible with no loss of either drug in 3 hr at 24°C	1626	C
Fludarabine phosphate	BX	1 mg/mL[a]	ES	2.5 mg/mL[a]	Visually compatible for 4 hr at 22°C	1439	C
Foscarnet sodium	AST	24 mg/mL	LY	25 mg/mL	Physically compatible for 24 hr at room temperature under fluorescent light	1335	C
Gallium nitrate	FUJ	1 mg/mL[b]	AMR	25 mg/mL	Visually compatible for 24 hr at 25°C	1673	C
Gemcitabine HCl	LI	10 mg/mL[b]	AB	2.5 mg/mL[b]	Physically compatible for 4 hr at 23°C	2226	C
Granisetron HCl	SKB	0.05 mg/mL[a]	AB	2.5 mg/mL[a]	Physically compatible for 4 hr at 23°C	2000	C
Heparin sodium[f]	RI	1000 units/L[d]	SE	25 mg/mL	Physically compatible for 4 hr at room temperature	322	C
Hetastarch in lactated electrolyte	AB	6%	AMR	2.5 mg/mL[a]	Physically compatible for 4 hr at 23°C	2339	C
Hydralazine HCl	SO	1 mg/mL[a]	ES	4 mg/mL[a]	Gross color change in 1 hr	1316	I
Hydralazine HCl	SO	1 mg/mL[b]	ES	4 mg/mL[b]	Color change in 1 hr and haze in 3 hr	1316	I
Hydrocortisone sodium succinate[g]	UP	100 mg/L[d]	SE	25 mg/mL	Physically compatible for 4 hr at room temperature	322	C
Labetalol HCl	SC	1 mg/mL[a]	ES	1 mg/mL[a]	Physically compatible for 24 hr at 18°C	1171	C
Levofloxacin	OMN	5 mg/mL[a]	AMR	25 mg/mL	Visually compatible for 4 hr at 24°C	2233	C
Linezolid	PHU	2 mg/mL	AB	2.5 mg/mL[a]	Physically compatible for 4 hr at 23°C	2264	C
Melphalan HCl	BW	0.1 mg/mL[b]	AB	2.5 mg/mL[b]	Physically compatible for 3 hr at 22°C	1557	C
Meropenem	ZEN	1 and 50 mg/mL[b]	AMR	25 mg/mL	Visually compatible for 4 hr at room temperature	1994	C
Micafungin sodium	ASP	1.5 mg/mL[b]	AMR	2.5 mg/mL[b]	Physically compatible for 4 hr at 23°C	2683	C
Morphine sulfate	WY	0.2 mg/mL[c]	ES	4 mg/mL[c]	Physically compatible for 3 hr	1316	C

Y-Site Injection Compatibility (1:1 Mixture) (Cont.)

Test Drug	Mfr	Conc	Mfr	Conc	Remarks	Ref	C/I
Nicardipine HCl	DCC	0.1 mg/mL[a]	ES	1 mg/mL[a]	Visually compatible for 24 hr at room temperature	235	C
Ondansetron HCl	GL	1 mg/mL[b]	AMR	2.5 mg/mL[a]	Immediate turbidity and precipitation	1365	I
Oritavancin diphosphate	TAR	0.8, 1.2, and 2 mg/mL[a]	AMR	1 mg/mL[a]	Haze or precipitate forms immediately	2928	I
Paclitaxel	NCI	1.2 mg/mL[a]	AB	2.5 mg/mL[a]	Physically compatible for 4 hr at 22°C	1556	C
Pancuronium bromide	ES	0.05 mg/mL[a]	AB	1 mg/mL[a]	Physically compatible for 24 hr at 28°C	1337	C
Pemetrexed disodium	LI	20 mg/mL[b]	AB	2.5 mg/mL[a]	Physically compatible for 4 hr at 23°C	2564	C
Piperacillin sodium-tazo-bactam sodium	LE[k]	40 mg/mL[a j]	AB	2.5 mg/mL[a]	Physically compatible for 4 hr at 22°C	1688	C
Potassium chloride		40 mEq/L[e]	SE	25 mg/mL	Physically compatible for 4 hr at room temperature	322	C
Propofol	ZEN[m]	10 mg/mL	AMR	2.5 mg/mL[a]	Physically compatible for 1 hr at 23°C	2066	C
Quinupristin–dalfopristin		2 mg/mL[a l]		2.5 mg/mL	Reported to be incompatible	3230	I
Ranitidine HCl	GL	0.5 mg/mL	LY	4 mg/mL[a]	Physically compatible for 24 hr	1323	C
Remifentanil HCl	GW	0.025 and 0.25 mg/mL[b]	AB	2.5 mg/mL[a]	Physically compatible for 4 hr at 23°C	2075	C
Sargramostim	IMM	10 mcg/mL[b]	ES	2.5 mg/mL[b]	Visually compatible for 4 hr at 22°C	1436	C
Tacrolimus	FUJ	1 mg/mL[b]	ES	2 mg/mL[a]	Visually compatible for 24 hr at 25°C	1630	C
Teniposide	BR	0.1 mg/mL[a]	AB	2.5 mg/mL[a]	Physically compatible for 4 hr at 23°C	1725	C
Thiotepa	IMM[h]	1 mg/mL[b]	AMR	2.5 mg/mL[b]	Physically compatible for 4 hr at 23°C	1861	C
TNA #218[i]			AB	2.5 mg/mL[a]	Visually compatible for 4 hr at 23°C	2215	C
TNA #219[i]			AB	2.5 mg/mL[a]	Visually compatible for 4 hr at 23°C	2215	C
TNA #220[i]			AB	2.5 mg/mL[a]	Visually compatible for 4 hr at 23°C	2215	C
TNA #221[i]			AB	2.5 mg/mL[a]	Visually compatible for 4 hr at 23°C	2215	C
TNA #222[i]			AB	2.5 mg/mL[a]	Visually compatible for 4 hr at 23°C	2215	C
TNA #223[i]			AB	2.5 mg/mL[a]	Visually compatible for 4 hr at 23°C	2215	C
TNA #224[i]			AB	2.5 mg/mL[a]	Visually compatible for 4 hr at 23°C	2215	C
TNA #225[i]			AB	2.5 mg/mL[a]	Visually compatible for 4 hr at 23°C	2215	C
TNA #226[i]			AB	2.5 mg/mL[a]	Visually compatible for 4 hr at 23°C	2215	C
TPN #189[i]			DB	1 mg/mL[b]	Visually compatible for 24 hr at 22°C	1767	C
TPN #203[i]			AMR	5 and 25 mg/mL	White precipitate forms immediately	1974	I
TPN #204[i]			AMR	5 and 25 mg/mL	White precipitate forms immediately	1974	I
TPN #212[i]			AB	2.5 mg/mL[a]	Physically compatible for 4 hr at 23°C	2109	C
TPN #213[i]			AB	2.5 mg/mL[a]	Physically compatible for 4 hr at 23°C	2109	C
TPN #214[i]			AB	2.5 mg/mL[a]	Physically compatible for 4 hr at 23°C	2109	C
TPN #215[i]			AB	2.5 mg/mL[a]	Physically compatible for 4 hr at 23°C	2109	C

Y-Site Injection Compatibility (1:1 Mixture) (Cont.)

Test Drug	Mfr	Conc	Mfr	Conc	Remarks	Ref	C/I
Vecuronium bromide	OR	0.1 mg/mL[a]	AB	1 mg/mL[a]	Physically compatible for 24 hr at 28°C	1337	C
Vinorelbine tartrate	BW	1 mg/mL[b]	AB	2.5 mg/mL[b]	Visible haze with large particles in 1 hr	1558	I

[a] Tested in dextrose 5%.

[b] Tested in sodium chloride 0.9%.

[c] Tested in both dextrose 5% and sodium chloride 0.9%.

[d] Tested in dextrose 5%, sodium chloride 0.9%, and Ringer's injection, lactated.

[e] Tested in bacteriostatic sodium chloride 0.9% preserved with benzyl alcohol 0.9%.

[f] Tested in combination with hydrocortisone sodium succinate (Upjohn) 100 mg/L.

[g] Tested in combination with heparin sodium (Riker) 1000 units/L.

[h] Lyophilized formulation tested.

[i] Refer to Appendix for the composition of parenteral nutrition solutions. TNA indicates a 3-in-1 admixture, and TPN indicates a 2-in-1 admixture.

[j] Piperacillin component. Piperacillin in an 8:1 fixed-ratio concentration with tazobactam.

[k] Test performed using the formulation WITHOUT edetate disodium.

[l] Quinupristin and dalfopristin components combined.

[m] Test performed using the formulation WITH edetate disodium.

Selected Revisions January 31, 2020. © Copyright, October 1982.
American Society of Health-System Pharmacists, Inc.

Amiodarone Hydrochloride
AHFS 24:04.04.20

Products

Amiodarone hydrochloride 50 mg/mL is available in 3-, 9-, and 18-mL vials. Each mL also contains polysorbate 80 100 mg, and benzyl alcohol 20.2 mg in water for injection.[1(5/08)]

pH

The pH is reported to be 4.08.[1053]

Administration

Amiodarone hydrochloride is a concentrate that is administered by intravenous infusion after dilution in a compatible diluent.[3279] Intravenous infusion at concentrations of 1 to 6 mg/mL is performed using a volumetric pump and a dedicated central venous catheter, when possible, with an inline filter; concentrations greater than 2 mg/mL require a central venous catheter.[3279] The injection contains polysorbate 80, a surface active agent that alters drop size. The drop size reduction may lead to substantial underdosage if a drop counter infusion set is used. Consequently, the drug must be delivered with a volumetric infusion pump.[1(5/08) 1445]

Stability

Amiodarone hydrochloride should be stored at room temperature and protected from light and excessive heat. Light protection is not necessary during administration,[1(5/08)] but exposure to direct sunlight should be avoided.[2258] It is recommended that amiodarone hydrochloride be added only to dextrose 5%.[1(5/08)] Information on the drug's compatibility in sodium chloride 0.9% has been conflicting.[1443 1031] Solutions containing less than 0.6 mg/mL of amiodarone hydrochloride in dextrose 5% are unstable and should not be used.[1442]

Precipitation

Amiodarone hydrochloride may precipitate when diluted. Studies found little or no precipitation when the formulation was diluted to very small or very large concentrations. In the middle range, however, at concentrations between 45 mg/mL (90% amiodarone hydrochloride formulation) and about 0.0025 mg/mL in phosphate buffer (pH 7.4), the drug concentration exceeds the solubility of amiodarone hydrochloride in the mixture. Precipitation may occur immediately or on standing. Such precipitation may occur when the drug enters the bloodstream, contributing to the phlebitis associated with amiodarone hydrochloride.[1818 1819]

The aqueous solubility of amiodarone hydrochloride is not substantially altered over the pH range of 1.5 to 7.5,[925] but precipitation may occur in alkaline media.[791 1032]

Amiodarone hydrochloride (Wyeth-Ayerst) 1.2 mg/mL in 250 mL of dextrose 5% has been reported to develop cloudiness upon standing when prepared in glass evacuated bottles (Abbott). The precipitation was attributed to the acetate buffers present in the small amount of residual fluid left in evacuated bottles from steam sterilization.[1982]

Syringes

Amiodarone hydrochloride (Sanofi) 600 mg/24 mL in dextrose 5% in a 50-mL polypropylene syringe (BD) was physically stable for 48 hours at room temperature.[3545]

Sorption

At concentrations of 1 to 6 mg/mL in dextrose 5% in polyolefin or glass containers, amiodarone hydrochloride is physically compatible, with no loss in 24 hours. In PVC containers, however, the amiodarone hydrochloride loss due to sorption occurs; acceptable potency (less than 10% loss) exists for 2 hours. Consequently, the manufacturer recommends that all infusions longer than 2 hours be made in glass or polyolefin containers only.[1(5/08)]

Similarly, amiodarone hydrochloride is lost due to sorption to PVC infusion sets.[1(5/08) 1443] However, the manufacturer states that these losses are accounted for by the recommended dosage schedule. Consequently, PVC sets should be used with this drug, but the recommended infusion regimen must be followed.[1(5/08)]

Amiodarone hydrochloride 1 mg/mL in dextrose 5% in VISIV polyolefin bags was tested for 24 hours at room temperature near 23°C. Little or no loss due to sorption was found within the 24-hour study period.[2660]

Plasticizer Leaching

Amiodarone hydrochloride leaches diethylhexyl phthalate (DEHP) plasticizer from PVC tubing. The degree of plasticizer leaching depends on the concentration and rate of administration. Higher concentrations and slower administration rates leach more plasticizer.[1(5/08)]

Filtration

Amiodarone hydrochloride (Labaz) 0.6 mg/mL in dextrose 5% and sodium chloride 0.9% was filtered through a 0.22-μm cellulose ester membrane filter (Ivex-HP, Millipore) over 6 hours. No significant drug loss due to binding to the filter was noted.[1034]

DOI: 10.37573/9781585286850.018

Compatibility Information

Solution Compatibility

Amiodarone HCl

Test Soln Name	Mfr	Mfr	Conc/L or %	Remarks	Ref	C/I
Dextrose 5%	MG[a]	LZ	1.8 g	Physically compatible. Little loss in 24 hr at 24°C in light	1031	C
Dextrose 5%	TR[b]	LZ	0.6 g	25% loss in 24 hr at room temperature	1443	I
Dextrose 5%	TR[c]	LZ	0.6 g	Physically compatible with little drug loss in 5 days at room temperature	1443	C
Dextrose 5%	BA[d]	WY	2 g	Visually compatible with no loss at 5°C and 3% loss at 25°C in 32 days	2110	C
Dextrose 5%	HOS[e]	BED	1 g	Less than 3% loss in 24 hr	2660	C
Sodium chloride 0.9%	MG[a]	LZ	1.8 g	Physically compatible. Little loss in 24 hr at 24°C in light	1031	C
Sodium chloride 0.9%	TR[c]	LZ	0.6 g	Incompatible in 24 hr at room temperature	1443	I
Sodium chloride 0.9%	BA[d]	WY	2 g	Visually compatible with no loss at 5°C and 3% loss at 25°C in 32 days	2110	C
Sodium chloride 0.9%	MYR[c]	EBE	0.84 g	5% loss in 6 hr at room temperature	2258	?

[a] Tested in polyolefin containers.

[b] Tested in PVC containers.

[c] Tested in glass containers.

[d] Tested in amber glass containers.

[e] Tested in VISIV polyolefin containers.

Additive Compatibility

Amiodarone HCl

Test Drug	Mfr	Conc/L or %	Mfr	Conc/L or %	Test Solution	Remarks	Ref	C/I
Dobutamine HCl	LI	1 g	LZ	2.5 g	D5W, NS	Physically compatible for 24 hr at 21°C	812	C
Floxacillin sodium	BE	20 g	LZ	4 g	D5W	Precipitates immediately	1479	I
Furosemide	ES	200 mg	LZ	1.8 g	D5W, NS[a]	Physically compatible. 8% or less amiodarone loss in 24 hr at 24°C in light	1031	C
Furosemide	HO	1 g	LZ	4 g	D5W	Haze in 5 hr and precipitate in 24 to 72 hr at 30°C. No changes at 15°C	1479	I
Lidocaine HCl	AB	4 g	LZ	1.8 g	D5W, NS[a]	Physically compatible. 9% or less amiodarone loss in 24 hr at 24°C in light	1031	C
Potassium chloride	AB	40 mEq	LZ	1.8 g	D5W, NS[a]	Physically compatible. No amiodarone loss in 24 hr at 24°C in light	1031	C
Procainamide HCl	SQ	4 g	LZ	1.8 g	D5W, NS[a]	Physically compatible. 5% or less amiodarone loss in 24 hr at 24°C in light	1031	C
Quinidine gluconate	LI	1 g	LZ	1.8 g	D5W[b]	Milky precipitation. 13% amiodarone loss in 6 hr and 23% in 24 hr at 24°C in light	1031	I
Quinidine gluconate	LI	1 g	LZ	1.8 g	D5W[c]	Milky precipitation. No amiodarone loss in 24 hr at 24°C in light	1031	I
Quinidine gluconate	LI	1 g	LZ	1.8 g	NS[b]	Physically compatible. 13% amiodarone loss in 24 hr at 24°C in light	1031	I

Additive Compatibility (Cont.)

Test Drug	Mfr	Conc/L or %	Mfr	Conc/L or %	Test Solution	Remarks	Ref	C/I
Quinidine gluconate	LI	1 g	LZ	1.8 g	NS[c]	Physically compatible. No amiodarone loss in 24 hr at 24°C in light	1031	C
Verapamil HCl	KN	50 mg	LZ	1.8 g	D5W, NS[a]	Physically compatible. 8% or less amiodarone loss in 24 hr at 24°C in light	1031	C

[a] Tested in both polyolefin and PVC containers.

[b] Tested in PVC containers.

[c] Tested in polyolefin containers.

Drugs in Syringe Compatibility

Amiodarone HCl

Test Drug	Mfr	Amt	Mfr	Amt	Remarks	Ref	C/I
Heparin sodium		2500 units/1 mL	LZ	150 mg/3 mL	Turbidity or precipitate forms within 5 min	1053	I
Pantoprazole sodium	[a]	4 mg/1 mL		50 mg/1 mL	Precipitates	2574	I

[a] Test performed using the formulation WITHOUT edetate disodium.

Y-Site Injection Compatibility (1:1 Mixture)

Amiodarone HCl

Test Drug	Mfr	Conc	Mfr	Conc	Remarks	Ref	C/I
Amikacin sulfate	BR	5 mg/mL[c]	LZ	4 mg/mL[c]	Physically compatible for 4 hr at room temperature	1444	C
Aminophylline	ES	5 mg/mL[c]	LZ	4 mg/mL[c]	Haze forms within 15 min and white precipitate forms within 6 hr at 21°C	1032	I
Amoxicillin sodium–clavulanic acid	GSK	10 mg/mL[g]	SAN	12.5 mg/mL	Turbidity appeared immediately	2727	I
Amphotericin B	BMS	0.5 mg/mL[a]	WY	6 mg/mL[a]	Visually compatible for 24 hr at 22°C	2352	C
Ampicillin sodium–sulbactam sodium	PF	20 mg/mL[b][h]	WY	6 mg/mL[a]	Immediate opaque white turbidity	2352	I
Argatroban	SKB	1 mg/mL[a]	NVP	1.8 mg/mL[a]	Trace precipitate forms immediately	2572	I
Atracurium besylate	BA	5 mg/mL[a]	WY	6 mg/mL[a]	Visually compatible for 24 hr at 22°C	2352	C
Atropine sulfate	AB	0.4 mg/mL	WY	6 mg/mL[a]	Visually compatible for 24 hr at 22°C	2352	C
Bivalirudin	TMC	5 mg/mL[a]	WAY	4 mg/mL[a]	Measured haze increases immediately	2373	I
Calcium chloride	APP	10 mg/mL[a]	WY	6 mg/mL[a]	Visually compatible for 24 hr at 22°C	2352	C
Calcium chloride	APP	100 mg/mL	WY	6 mg/mL[a]	Visually compatible for 24 hr at 22°C	2352	C
Calcium gluconate	AMR	10 mg/mL[a]	WY	6 mg/mL[a]	Visually compatible for 24 hr at 22°C	2352	C
Cangrelor tetrasodium	TMC	1 mg/mL[b]		4 mg/mL[b]	Physically compatible for 4 hr	3243	C
Caspofungin acetate	ME	0.7 mg/mL[b]	SIC	4 mg/mL[b]	Physically compatible for 4 hr at room temperature	2758	C
Cefazolin sodium	LI	20 mg/mL[a]	LZ	4 mg/mL[a]	Precipitate forms	1444	I
Cefazolin sodium	LI	20 mg/mL[b]	LZ	4 mg/mL[b]	Physically compatible for 4 hr at room temperature	1444	C

Y-Site Injection Compatibility (1:1 Mixture) (Cont.)

Test Drug	Mfr	Conc	Mfr	Conc	Remarks	Ref	C/I
Ceftaroline fosamil	FOR	2.22 mg/mL[a b f]	SIC	4 mg/mL[a b f]	Physically compatible for 4 hr at 23°C	2826	C
Ceftazidime	GW	40 mg/mL[a]	WY	6 mg/mL[a]	Immediate opaque white turbidity	2352	I
Ceftolozane sulfate–tazobactam sodium	CUB	10 mg/mL[c l]	APP	2 mg/mL[c]	Physically compatible for 2 hr	3262	C
Ceftriaxone sodium	RC	20 mg/mL[a]	WY	6 mg/mL[a]	Turned yellow in 24 hr at 22°C, but considered normal for cephalosporins	2352	C
Cefuroxime sodium	BA	30 mg/mL[a]	WY	6 mg/mL[a]	Turned yellow in 24 hr at 22°C, but considered normal for cephalosporins	2352	C
Ciprofloxacin	BAY	2 mg/mL[a]	WY	6 mg/mL[a]	Visually compatible for 24 hr at 22°C	2352	C
Clarithromycin	AB	4 mg/mL[a]	SW	3 mg/mL[a]	Visually compatible for 72 hr at both 30 and 17°C	2174	C
Clevidipine butyrate	CHS	0.5 mg/mL		4 mg/mL[m]	Physically incompatible	3334	I
Clindamycin phosphate	UP	6 mg/mL[c]	LZ	4 mg/mL[c]	Physically compatible for 4 hr at room temperature	1444	C
Cloxacillin sodium	SMX	100 mg/mL	SZ	50 mg/mL	Physically compatible for up to 4 hr at room temperature	3245	C
Dexmedetomidine HCl	AB	4 mcg/mL[b]	WAY	4 mg/mL[b]	Physically compatible for 4 hr at 23°C	2383	C
Digoxin	ES	0.25 mg/mL	WY	6 mg/mL[a]	Immediate opaque white turbidity	2352	I
Dobutamine HCl	LI	2 mg/mL[c]	LZ	4 mg/mL[c]	Physically compatible for 24 hr at 21°C	1032	C
Dopamine HCl	ES	1.6 mg/mL[c]	LZ	4 mg/mL[c]	Physically compatible for 24 hr at 21°C	1032	C
Doripenem	JJ	5 mg/mL[a b]	BED	4 mg/mL[a b]	Physically compatible for 4 hr at 23°C	2743	C
Doxycycline hyclate	ACC	0.25 mg/mL[c]	LZ	4 mg/mL[c]	Physically compatible for 4 hr at room temperature	1444	C
Epinephrine HCl	AMR	1 mg/mL	WY	6 mg/mL[a]	Visually compatible for 24 hr at 22°C	2352	C
Eptifibatide	KEY	0.75 mg/mL	WY	6 mg/mL[a]	Visually compatible for 24 hr at 22°C	2352	C
Eptifibatide	KEY	2 mg/mL	WY	6 mg/mL[a]	Visually compatible for 24 hr at 22°C	2352	C
Eravacycline dihydrochloride	TET	0.6 mg/mL[b]	MYL	2 mg/mL[b]	Measured turbidity increased immediately	3532	I
Erythromycin lactobionate	AB	2 mg/mL[c]	LZ	4 mg/mL[c]	Physically compatible for 4 hr at room temperature	1444	C
Esmolol HCl	DU	40 mg/mL[a]	WY	4.8 mg/mL[a]	Visually compatible for 24 hr at 23°C	1877	C
Famotidine	ME	10 mg/mL	WY	6 mg/mL[a]	Visually compatible for 24 hr at 22°C	2352	C
Fenoldopam mesylate	AB	80 mcg/mL[b]	WAY	4 mg/mL[b]	Physically compatible for 4 hr at 23°C	2467	C
Fentanyl citrate	BA	50 mcg/mL	WY	6 mg/mL[a]	Visually compatible for 24 hr at 22°C	2352	C
Fluconazole	PF	2 mg/mL[b]	WY	6 mg/mL[a]	Visually compatible for 24 hr at 22°C	2352	C
Furosemide	AMR	1 mg/mL[a]	WY	6 mg/mL[a]	Visually compatible for 24 hr at 22°C	2352	C
Furosemide	AMR	10 mg/mL	WY	6 mg/mL[a]	Immediate opaque white turbidity	2352	I
Gentamicin sulfate	LY	0.8 mg/mL[c]	LZ	4 mg/mL[c]	Physically compatible for 4 hr at room temperature	1444	C

Y-Site Injection Compatibility (1:1 Mixture) (Cont.)

Test Drug	Mfr	Conc	Mfr	Conc	Remarks	Ref	C/I
Gentamicin sulfate	APP	5 mg/mL[a]	WY	6 mg/mL[a]	Visually compatible for 24 hr at 22°C	2352	C
Heparin sodium		300 units/mL[b]			White precipitate forms upon sequential administration	791	I
Hetastarch in lactated electrolyte	AB	6%	WAY	4 mg/mL[a]	Physically compatible for 4 hr at 23°C	2339	C
Imipenem–cilastatin sodium	ME	5 mg/mL[a j]	WY	6 mg/mL[a]	Immediate haze. Becomes yellow in 24 hr	2352	I
Insulin, regular	LI	1 unit/mL[a]	WY	4.8 mg/mL[a]	Visually compatible for 24 hr at 23°C	1877	C
Isavuconazonium sulfate	ASP	1.5 mg/mL[c]	APP	2 mg/mL[c]	Physically compatible for 2 hr	3263	C
Isoproterenol HCl	ES	4 mcg/mL[c]	LZ	4 mg/mL[c]	Physically compatible for 24 hr at 21°C	1032	C
Labetalol HCl	GL	5 mg/mL	WY	4.8 mg/mL[a]	Visually compatible for 24 hr at 23°C	1877	C
Labetalol HCl	BED	5 mg/mL	WY	6 mg/mL[a]	Visually compatible for 24 hr at 22°C	2352	C
Letermovir	ME				Physically incompatible	3398	I
Lidocaine HCl	AST	8 mg/mL[c]	LZ	4 mg/mL[c]	Physically compatible for 24 hr at 21°C	1032	C
Lorazepam	WY	1 mg/mL[a]	WY	6 mg/mL[a]	Visually compatible for 24 hr at 22°C	2352	C
Magnesium sulfate	APP	500 mg/mL	WY	6 mg/mL[a]	Immediate opaque white turbidity becoming thick precipitate in 24 hr at 22°C	2352	I
Magnesium sulfate	APP	20 mg/mL[a]	WY	6 mg/mL[a]	Visually compatible for 24 hr at 22°C	2352	C
Meropenem		50 mg/mL	SZ	50 mg/mL	Solution became opaque within 1 hr	3538	I
Meropenem–vaborbactam	TMC	8 mg/mL[b n]	APP	2 mg/mL[b]	Measured turbidity increases immediately. pH increased by >3 units within 3 hr	3380	I
Methylprednisolone sodium succinate	PHU	125 mg/mL	WY	6 mg/mL[a]	Visually compatible for 24 hr at 22°C	2352	C
Metoprolol tartrate	BED	1 mg/mL	BIO	1.8 mg/mL[a]	Visually compatible for 24 hr at 19°C	2795	C
Micafungin sodium	ASP	1.5 mg/mL[b]	BA	4 mg/mL[b]	Gross milky white precipitate forms	2683	I
Midazolam HCl	RC	1 mg/mL[a]	WY	4.8 mg/mL[a]	Visually compatible for 24 hr at 23°C	1877	C
Midazolam HCl	RC	1 mg/mL[a]	WY	6 mg/mL[a]	Visually compatible for 24 hr at 22°C	2352	C
Milrinone lactate	SAN	0.4 mg/mL[a]	WY	6 mg/mL[a]	Visually compatible for 24 hr at 22°C	2352	C
Morphine sulfate	SX	1 mg/mL[a]	WY	4.8 mg/mL[a]	Visually compatible for 24 hr at 23°C	1877	C
Morphine sulfate	WY	1 mg/mL[a]	WY	6 mg/mL[a]	Visually compatible for 24 hr at 22°C	2352	C
Morphine sulfate	WY	10 mg/mL	WY	6 mg/mL[a]	Visually compatible for 24 hr at 22°C	2352	C
Nesiritide	SCI	50 mcg/mL[a b]		50 mg/mL	Physically compatible for 4 hr	2625	C
Nitroglycerin	AB	0.24 mg/mL[c]	LZ	4 mg/mL[c]	Physically compatible for 24 hr at 21°C	1032	C
Norepinephrine bitartrate	BN	64 mcg/mL[c]	LZ	4 mg/mL[c]	Physically compatible for 24 hr at 21°C	1032	C
Penicillin G potassium	PF	100,000 units/mL[c]	LZ	4 mg/mL[c]	Physically compatible for 4 hr at room temperature	1444	C

Y-Site Injection Compatibility (1:1 Mixture) (Cont.)

Test Drug	Mfr	Conc	Mfr	Conc	Remarks	Ref	C/I
Phentolamine mesylate	CI	0.04 mg/mL[c]	LZ	4 mg/mL[c]	Physically compatible for 24 hr at 21°C under fluorescent light	1032	C
Phenylephrine HCl	WI	0.04 mg/mL[c]	LZ	4 mg/mL[c]	Physically compatible for 24 hr at 21°C	1032	C
Piperacillin sodium–tazo-bactam sodium	LE[e]	60 mg/mL[a i]	WY	6 mg/mL[a]	White haze in 24 hr at 22°C	2352	I
Plazomicin sulfate	ACH	24 mg/mL[c]	MYL	2 mg/mL[c]	Measured turbidity increases immediately; pH increased by >1 unit within 30 min	3432	I
Potassium chloride	AB	0.04 mEq/mL[c]	LZ	4 mg/mL[c]	Physically compatible for 24 hr at 21°C	1032	C
Potassium phosphates	APP	0.12 mmol/mL[a]	WY	6 mg/mL[a]	Immediate white cloudiness	2352	I
Procainamide HCl	AHP	8 mg/mL[c]	LZ	4 mg/mL[c]	Physically compatible for 24 hr at 21°C	1032	C
Sodium bicarbonate	AB	1 mEq/mL	WY	3 mg/mL[a]	Precipitate forms immediately	1851	I
Sodium bicarbonate	AB	1 mEq/mL	WY	6 mg/mL[a]	Translucent haze in 1 hr	2352	I
Sodium nitroprusside	BA	0.4 mg/mL[a]	WY	6 mg/mL[a]	Visually compatible for 24 hr at 22°C	2352	C
Sodium nitroprusside	RC	0.3 mg/mL[a]	WAY	1.5 mg/mL[a]	Cloudy precipitate forms within 4 hr at 24°C protected from light	2357	I
Sodium nitroprusside	RC	1.2 and 3 mg/mL[a]	WAY	1.5 mg/mL[a]	Cloudy precipitate forms immediately	2357	I
Sodium nitroprusside	RC	0.3 mg/mL[a]	WAY	6 and 15 mg/mL[a]	Visually compatible for 48 hr at 24°C protected from light	2357	C
Sodium nitroprusside	RC	1.2 and 3 mg/mL[a]	WAY	6 and 15 mg/mL[a]	Cloudy precipitate forms immediately	2357	I
Sodium phosphates	APP	0.12 mmol/mL[a]	WY	6 mg/mL[a]	Immediate white cloudiness	2352	I
Sugammadex sodium		100 mg/mL	[k]	50 mg/mL	Precipitates immediately	3112	I
Tedizolid phosphate	CUB	0.8 mg/mL[b]	APP	2 mg/mL[b]	Physically compatible for 2 hr	3244	C
Tirofiban HCl	ME	0.25 mg/mL[a]	WY	6 mg/mL[a]	Visually compatible for 24 hr at 22°C	2352	C
Tobramycin sulfate	LI	0.8 mg/mL[c]	LZ	4 mg/mL[c]	Physically compatible for 4 hr at room temperature	1444	C
Tobramycin sulfate	LI	5 mg/mL[a]	WY	6 mg/mL[a]	Visually compatible for 24 hr at 22°C	2352	C
Vancomycin HCl	LI	5 mg/mL[c]	LZ	4 mg/mL[c]	Physically compatible for 4 hr at room temperature	1444	C
Vancomycin HCl	APP	4 mg/mL[a]	WY	6 mg/mL[a]	Visually compatible for 24 hr at 22°C	2352	C
Vancomycin HCl	APP	10 mg/mL[a]	WY	6 mg/mL[a]	Visually compatible for 24 hr at 22°C	2352	C
Vasopressin	AMR	0.2 unit/mL[b]	WY	6 mg/mL[a]	Visually compatible for 24 hr at 22°C	2352	C

Y-Site Injection Compatibility (1:1 Mixture) (Cont.)

Test Drug	Mfr	Conc	Mfr	Conc	Remarks	Ref	C/I
Vasopressin	AMR	2 and 4 units/mL[b]	WY	1.5 mg/mL[a]	Physically compatible with vasopressin pushed through a Y-site over 5 sec	2478	C
Vecuronium bromide	OR	1 mg/mL[a]	WY	6 mg/mL[a]	Visually compatible for 24 hr at 22°C	2352	C

[a] Tested in dextrose 5%.

[b] Tested in sodium chloride 0.9%.

[c] Tested in both dextrose 5% and sodium chloride 0.9%.

[d] Given over three minutes via a Y-site into a running infusion solution of heparin sodium in sodium chloride 0.9%.

[e] Test performed using the formulation WITHOUT edetate disodium.

[f] Tested in Ringer's injection, lactated.

[g] Amoxicillin sodium component. Amoxicillin sodium in a 5:1 fixed-ratio concentration with clavulanic acid.

[h] Ampicillin component. Ampicillin in a 2:1 fixed-ratio concentration with sulbactam.

[i] Piperacillin component. Piperacillin in an 8:1 fixed-ratio concentration with tazobactam.

[j] Not specified whether concentration refers to single component or combined components.

[k] Salt not specified.

[l] Ceftolozane component. Ceftolozane in a 2:1 fixed-ratio concentration with tazobactam.

[m] Tested in sterile water for injection.

[n] Meropenem component. Meropenem in a 1:1 fixed-ratio concentration with vaborbactam.

Selected Revisions May 1, 2020. © Copyright, October 1992.
American Society of Health-System Pharmacists, Inc.

Amisulpride
AHFS 56:22.92

Products

Amisulpride is available in single-dose vials containing 5 mg of the drug.[3548] Each mL of solution contains amisulpride 2.5 mg, citric acid monohydrate 9.35 mg, sodium chloride 1.8 mg, and trisodium citrate dihydrate 16.32 mg in water for injection.[3548] Hydrochloric acid and sodium hydroxide also may have been added to adjust the pH.[3548]

pH

The pH of amisulpride 2.5-mg/mL injection solution ranges from 4.75 to 5.25.[3548]

Osmolality

The osmolality of amisulpride 2.5-mg/mL injection solution ranges from 250 to 330 mOsmol/kg.[3548]

Trade Name(s)

Barhemsys

Administration

Amisulpride is administered as an intravenous injection over 1 to 2 minutes.[3548] Dilution of the injection solution prior to administration is not required.[3548] The intravenous line used to administer amisulpride may be flushed with either dextrose 5% or sodium chloride 0.9% prior to and following administration of the drug.[3548]

Stability

Amisulpride injection is a clear, colorless solution.[3548] Intact vials should be stored at controlled room temperature in the original carton to protect from light.[3548] Amisulpride should be administered within 12 hours after removal from the original carton since the drug is subject to photodegradation.[3548]

Compatibility Information

Solution Compatibility

Amisulpride

Test Soln Name	Mfr	Mfr	Conc/L or %	Remarks	Ref	C/I
Dextrose 5%		ACA		Stated to be physically and chemically compatible	3548	C
Sodium chloride 0.9%		ACA		Stated to be physically and chemically compatible	3548	C

DOI: 10.37573/9781585286850.019

Ammonium Chloride
AHFS 40:04

Products

Ammonium chloride additive solution is available in 20-mL vials containing 5.35 g of ammonium chloride, which provides 100 mEq (5 mEq/mL) of NH_4^+ and Cl^- ions. The solution also contains 2 mg/mL of disodium edetate as a stabilizer and hydrochloric acid to adjust the pH. The additive solution is intended to be used only after further dilution in a larger volume of sodium chloride 0.9% injection.[1(8/06)]

One gram of ammonium chloride contains 18.7 mEq each of ammonium and chloride ions.[4]

pH
About 4.4 with a range of 4 to 6.[1(8/06)]

Osmolarity
10 mOsm/mL (calculated).[1(8/06)]

Administration

Ammonium chloride injection is a concentrate that is generally administered by slow intravenous infusion after dilution of one or two vials (100 to 200 mEq) in 500 to 1000 mL of sodium chloride 0.9% injection. The infusion rate in adults of the diluted solution should not exceed 5 mL/min.[1(8/06)]

Stability

Store at controlled room temperature and protect from freezing. Highly concentrated solutions of ammonium chloride may crystallize when exposed to low temperatures. If such crystallization does occur, warming to room temperature in a water bath is recommended.[1(8/06) 4]

Ammonium chloride is stated to be incompatible with alkalies and their carbonates.[4]

Compatibility Information

Solution Compatibility

Ammonium chloride

Test Soln Name	Mfr	Mfr	Conc/L or %	Remarks	Ref	C/I
Dextrose 2.5% in half-strength Ringer's injection	AB	AB	400 mEq	Physically compatible	3	C
Dextrose 5% in Ringer's injection	AB	AB	400 mEq	Physically compatible	3	C
Dextrose 2.5% in Ringer's injection, lactated	AB	AB	400 mEq	Physically compatible	3	C
Dextrose 5% in half-strength Ringer's injection, lactated	AB	AB	400 mEq	Physically compatible	3	C
Dextrose 5% in Ringer's injection, lactated	AB	AB	400 mEq	Physically compatible	3	C
Dextrose 10% in Ringer's injection, lactated	AB	AB	400 mEq	Physically compatible	3	C
Dextrose 2.5% in sodium chloride 0.45%	AB	AB	400 mEq	Physically compatible	3	C
Dextrose 2.5% in sodium chloride 0.9%	AB	AB	400 mEq	Physically compatible	3	C
Dextrose 5% in sodium chloride 0.225%	AB	AB	400 mEq	Physically compatible	3	C
Dextrose 5% in sodium chloride 0.45%	AB	AB	400 mEq	Physically compatible	3	C
Dextrose 5% in sodium chloride 0.9%	AB	AB	400 mEq	Physically compatible	3	C
Dextrose 10% in sodium chloride 0.9%	AB	AB	400 mEq	Physically compatible	3	C
Dextrose 2.5%	AB	AB	400 mEq	Physically compatible	3	C
Dextrose 5%	AB	AB	400 mEq	Physically compatible	3	C
Dextrose 10%	AB	AB	400 mEq	Physically compatible	3	C
Ionosol B in dextrose 5%	AB	AB	400 mEq	Physically compatible	3	C
Ionosol MB in dextrose 5%	AB	AB	400 mEq	Physically compatible	3	C
Ringer's injection	AB	AB	400 mEq	Physically compatible	3	C

DOI: 10.37573/9781585286850.020

Solution Compatibility (Cont.)

Test Soln Name	Mfr	Mfr	Conc/L or %	Remarks	Ref	C/I
Ringer's injection, lactated	AB	AB	400 mEq	Physically compatible	3	C
Sodium chloride 0.45%	AB	AB	400 mEq	Physically compatible	3	C
Sodium chloride 0.9%	AB	AB	400 mEq	Physically compatible	3	C
Sodium lactate ⅙ M	AB	AB	400 mEq	Physically compatible	3	C

Additive Compatibility

Ammonium chloride

Test Drug	Mfr	Conc/L or %	Mfr	Conc/L or %	Test Solution	Remarks	Ref	C/I
Dimenhydrinate	SE	500 mg	AB	20 g	D5W	Physically compatible	15	C

Selected Revisions January 8, 2015. © Copyright, October 1982.
American Society of Health-System Pharmacists, Inc.

Amoxicillin Sodium
AHFS 8:12.16.08

Products

Amoxicillin sodium is available as a powder in vials containing the equivalent of amoxicillin 250 mg, 500 mg, and 1 g.[3553 3554 3555]

For intravenous injection, the 250-mg, 500-mg, and 1-g vials may be reconstituted with 5, 10, and 20 mL, respectively, of sterile water for injection when the dose reflects the entire contents of a vial and the entire vial contents are subsequently withdrawn.[3553 3554 3555] One manufacturer states that 500-mg and 1-g vials also may be reconstituted with 5 mL of sterile water for injection when the dose reflects the entire contents of the vial and the entire vial contents are subsequently withdrawn.[3555]

Alternatively, the 250-mg vials may be reconstituted with 4.8 mL of sterile water for injection to yield a 50-mg/mL solution, the 500-mg vials may be reconstituted with 4.6 mL of sterile water for injection to yield a 100-mg/mL solution, and the 1-g vials may be reconstituted with 4.2 mL of sterile water for injection to yield a 200-mg/mL solution.[3555] This allows for calculation of the volume required for a dose when only the partial contents of the vial are intended.[3555]

For intravenous infusion, the reconstituted drug should be added to a compatible intravenous infusion solution (e.g., using a minibag or an in-line burette).[3553 3554 3555] (See Solution Compatibility.)

For intramuscular injection, 250-mg vials should be reconstituted with 2 mL of sterile water for injection [3555] and 500-mg vials should be reconstituted with 2[3555] or 2.5 mL of sterile water for injection.[3553] Lidocaine hydrochloride (e.g., 1%) or procaine hydrochloride 0.5% injection solution (no longer commercially available in the US) may be used in place of sterile water for injection for reconstitution of the drug for intramuscular administration.[3553 3555] Vials containing 1 g of amoxicillin should be reconstituted with 4 mL of sterile water for injection[3555] or 2.5 mL of lidocaine hydrochloride injection solution for administration by intramuscular injection.[3554]

Final volumes of reconstituted amoxicillin sodium for intramuscular injection

Vial Size	Volume of Diluent	Final Volume
250 mg	2 mL	2.2 mL
500 mg	2 mL	2.4 mL
500 mg	2.5 mL	2.9 mL
1 g	2.5 mL	3.3 mL
1 g	4 mL	4.8 mL

Sodium Content

Sodium content in amoxicillin sodium vials varies;[3553 3554 3555] specific product labeling should be consulted for additional formulation details.

Trade Name(s)

Amoxil, Clamoxyl, Ibiamox

Administration

Amoxicillin sodium may be administered by slow direct intravenous injection over 3 to 4 minutes, intermittent intravenous infusion over 20 to 30 or 30 to 60 minutes, or intramuscular injection.[3553 3554 3555] Intramuscular administration should be considered only when the intravenous route is not possible or is less appropriate for the patient.[3553 3554]

Stability

Intact vials of amoxicillin sodium should be stored at or below 25°C;[3553 3554 3555] at least one manufacturer states the vials should be protected from light.[3555] After reconstitution with sterile water for injection, a transient pink color or slight opalescence may appear.[3553 3554 3555] Reconstituted solutions are normally colorless or a pale straw color.[3553 3554 3555] The reconstituted solution for intramuscular administration should be administered immediately[3553 3554] or within 1 hour[3555] after reconstitution. The reconstituted solution for direct intravenous injection should be administered within 20 minutes[3553 3554] or 1 hour[3555] after reconstitution. For intravenous infusion, the reconstituted solution should be added to the infusion solution without delay[3553 3554] and should be used immediately[3553 3554] (e.g., within 1 hour[3555]), though manufacturers provide stability data for the drug in various infusion solutions.[3553 3554 3555] (See Solution Compatibility.)

Concentration Effects

Degradation of amoxicillin is concentration dependent; the higher the concentration, the less stable the drug.[3556]

Amoxicillin sodium prepared at an amoxicillin concentration of 50 mg/mL is substantially less stable in all infusion solutions than at lower concentrations of 10 or 20 mg/mL.[1469]

Amoxicillin sodium prepared at an amoxicillin concentration of 125 mg/mL in sterile water for injection in Infusor elastomeric pumps (Baxter) demonstrated greater than 10% loss within about 1 hour at 24 to 26°C.[3556] Amoxicillin sodium prepared at an amoxicillin concentration of 50 mg/mL in sterile water for injection in FOLfusor elastomeric pumps (Baxter) demonstrated greater than 10% loss within about 5 hours at 24 to 26°C.[3556]

Temperature Effects

Degradation of amoxicillin also is temperature dependent; the higher the temperature, the less stable the drug.[3556] The rate of degradation of amoxicillin sodium prepared at an amoxicillin concentration of 125 mg/mL in sterile water for injection in Infusor elastomeric pumps (Baxter) was 1.92 and 3.29% per hour at 5 and 37°C, respectively.[3556]

DOI: 10.37573/9781585286850.021

Freezing Solutions

Amoxicillin sodium prepared at an amoxicillin concentration of 10 mg/mL in sterile water for injection was unstable when stored frozen at 0 and −20°C but was stable for 13 days when stored below −30°C. Amoxicillin sodium prepared at an amoxicillin concentration of 10 mg/mL in sterile water for injection was stable for only 2 days at 0°C in the unfrozen state.[1470]

Amoxicillin sodium prepared at an amoxicillin concentration of 10 mg/mL in sodium chloride 0.9% was stable for 10.5 days at 0°C (unfrozen) and for 14 hours when frozen at −19°C; in dextrose 5%, the comparative times were 12.5 and 8.4 hours, respectively.[1471]

The processes of freezing and thawing increase the degradation rate of amoxicillin sodium prepared at an amoxicillin concentration of 10 mg/mL in sodium chloride 0.9% in polyvinyl chloride (PVC) bags (Travenol). Freezing and thawing (natural or microwave) could account for a 5 to 10% loss of amoxicillin; the losses will be affected by the time to reach the equilibrium frozen temperature.[1472]

Elastomeric Reservoir Pumps

Amoxicillin sodium (Panpharma) prepared at an amoxicillin concentration of 25 mg/mL in equal volumes of sterile water for injection and sodium chloride 0.9% (Braun) in Accufuser elastomeric pumps (Wym) was stable for 12 hours at 18 to 26°C and 24 hours at 4 to 8°C.[3556]

Sorption

Amoxicillin sodium was shown not to exhibit sorption to PVC bags and tubing, polyethylene tubing, Silastic tubing, polypropylene syringes, and trilayer bags of polyethylene, polyamide, and polypropylene.[536 606 1918]

Filtration

Amoxicillin sodium prepared at an amoxicillin concentration of 1.98 mg/mL in sodium chloride 0.9% did not exhibit significant drug loss due to sorption to a 0.22-μm cellulose ester membrane filter (Ivex-HP, Millipore).[1034]

Compatibility Information

Solution Compatibility

Amoxicillin sodium

Test Soln Name	Mfr	Mfr	Conc/L or %	Remarks	Ref	C/I
Dextrose 5%		GSK	10 g	Unstable after 20 min at 20°C	3553, 3554	I
Dextrose 5%		DGL		Unstable after 1 hr at room temperature	3555	I
Dextrose 5%			1 g	9% loss in 4 hr and 34% loss in 24 hr at room temperature	768	I
Dextrose 5%			10, 20, 50 g	14 and 18% losses in 3 hr at 10 and 20 g/L, respectively, and 14% loss in 1.5 hr at 50 g/L at 25°C	1469	I
Sodium chloride 0.9%		GSK	10 g	Complete administration within 4 hr at 20°C	3553, 3554	C
Sodium chloride 0.9%		DGL		Stable for 6 hr at room temperature	3555	C
Sodium chloride 0.9%			1 g	10% loss in 24 hr at room temperature	768	C
Sodium chloride 0.9%			10, 20, 50 g	3 and 7% losses in 6 hr at 10 and 20 g/L, respectively, and 12% loss in 4 hr at 50 g/L at 25°C	1469	I
Sodium chloride 0.9%	TR		10 g	Less than 3% loss in 24 hr at 0°C	1472	C
Sodium chloride 0.9% with potassium chloride 0.3%			10, 20, 50 g	4 and 9% losses in 8 hr at 10 and 20 g/L, respectively, and 9% loss in 3 hr at 50 g/L at 25°C	1469	I
Sodium lactate ⅙ M			10, 20, 50 g	10% loss in 6 hr at 10 and 20 g/L and 14% loss in 4 hr at 50 g/L at 25°C	1469	I

[a] Tested in PVC containers.

Additive Compatibility

Amoxicillin sodium

Test Drug	Mfr	Conc/L or %	Mfr	Conc/L or %	Test Solution	Remarks	Ref	C/I
Ciprofloxacin		2 g		10 g	[a]	Precipitates immediately	1473	I
Dextran 40		10%		10, 20, 50 g	D5W	9, 12, and 12% amoxicillin loss at 10, 20, and 50 g/L, respectively, in 1 hr at 25°C	1469	I

Additive Compatibility (Cont.)

Test Drug	Mfr	Conc/L or %	Mfr	Conc/L or %	Test Solution	Remarks	Ref	C/I
Dextran 40		10%		10, 20, 50 g	NS	12, 14, and 20% amoxicillin loss at 10, 20, and 50 g/L, respectively, in 3 hr at 25°C	1469	I
Imipenem–cilastatin sodium	GSK	4[b] g	MSD	8 g	NS	Blue discoloration formed in 2 hr. Amoxicillin and imipenem losses of 40 and 72%, respectively, in 12 hr	2800	I
Midazolam HCl	RC	50 and 250 mg	BE	10 g	NS	Transient precipitate	355	?
Midazolam HCl	RC	400 mg	BE	10 g	NS	Precipitate forms immediately	355	I
Sodium bicarbonate		2.74%		10, 20, 50 g		9% amoxicillin loss in 6 and 4 hr at 10 and 20 g/L, respectively, and 15% loss in 4 hr at 50 g/L at 25°C	1469	I
Sodium bicarbonate		8.4%		10, 20, 50 g		10 and 13% amoxicillin loss in 4 hr at 10 and 20 g/L, respectively, and 17% loss in 3 hr at 50 g/L at 25°C	1469	I

[a] Amoxicillin sodium added to ciprofloxacin solution.

[b] Imipenem component. Imipenem in a 1:1 fixed-ratio concentration with cilastatin.

Y-Site Injection Compatibility (1:1 Mixture)

Amoxicillin sodium

Test Drug	Mfr	Conc	Mfr	Conc	Remarks	Ref	C/I
Defibrotide sodium	JAZ	8 mg/mL[a]	PAN	40 mg/mL[a]	Visually compatible for 4 hr at room temperature	3149	C
Lorazepam	WY	0.33 mg/mL[a]	SKB	50 mg/mL	Visually compatible for 24 hr at 22°C	1855	C
Midazolam HCl	RC	5 mg/mL	SKB	50 mg/mL	White precipitate forms immediately	1855	I
TPN #189[b]				50 mg/mL[a]	Visually compatible for 24 hr at 22°C	1767	C

[a] Tested in sodium chloride 0.9%.

[b] Refer to Appendix for the composition of parenteral nutrition solutions. TPN indicates a 2-in-1 admixture.

Additional Compatibility Information

Infusion Solutions

One manufacturer states that satisfactory concentrations of the drug are retained when administration of amoxicillin sodium (Amoxil, GlaxoSmithKline) prepared at an amoxicillin concentration of 10 g/L in sterile water for injection and compound sodium chloride (Ringer's solution) is completed within 6 and 2 hours, respectively, at 20°C.[3553][3554] Dilutions of the drug in compound sodium lactate (Hartmann's solution) and in dextrose 4% in sodium chloride 0.18% are unstable after 30 minutes at 20°C.[3553][3554]

One manufacturer states that a satisfactory degree of amoxicillin activity is retained when amoxicillin sodium (Ibiamox, Douglas) is diluted in compound sodium chloride (Ringer's solution), sodium lactate (concentration not specified), compound sodium lactate (Hartmann's solution), and dextrose 4% in sodium chloride (concentration not specified) for 6, 3, 3, and 1 hour, respectively, at room temperature.[3555]

Peritoneal Dialysis Solutions

The stability of amoxicillin (Aspen Pharmacare) 125 mg/L in pH-neutral Balance (Fresenius), icodextrin-based Extraneal (Baxter), and dextrose-based Dianeal PD-4 (Baxter) peritoneal dialysis solutions was evaluated.[2984] At 4, 25, and 37°C, amoxicillin was stable in Balance for 336, 12, and 12 hours, respectively; in Extraneal for 336, 48, and 24 hours, respectively; and in Dianeal PD-4 for 336, 72, and 24 hours, respectively.[2984]

Amoxicillin (Fisamox, Aspen Pharmacare) 1 g in 2 L of Dianeal PD-4 with dextrose 2.5% (Baxter) exhibited 10% drug loss over 6 hours at 37°C.[3108]

Selected Revisions July 1, 2020. © Copyright, October 1992. American Society of Health-System Pharmacists, Inc.

Amoxicillin Sodium–Clavulanate Potassium
AHFS 8:12.16.08
Co–amoxiclav

Products

The fixed combination of amoxicillin sodium–clavulanate potassium is available as a powder for injection in single-use vials or bottles containing 600 mg (amoxicillin 500 mg as the sodium salt plus clavulanate potassium equivalent to clavulanic acid 100 mg), 1.2 g (amoxicillin 1 g as the sodium salt plus clavulanate potassium equivalent to clavulanic acid 200 mg), and 2.2 g (amoxicillin 2 g as the sodium salt plus clavulanate potassium equivalent to clavulanic acid 200 mg).[3558] [3559] [3560] The 600-mg and 1.2-g vials should be reconstituted with 10 and 20 mL, respectively, of sterile water for injection, resulting in an amoxicillin to clavulanic acid ratio of 5:1.[3558] [3559] [3560] The 2.2-g vials should be reconstituted with 20 mL of sterile water for injection, resulting in an amoxicillin to clavulanic acid ratio of 10:1.[3558]

For administration by intravenous infusion, the reconstituted solution containing 500 mg of amoxicillin plus 100 mg of clavulanic acid should be diluted in 50 mL of, or to 50 mL with, a compatible diluent and the reconstituted solution containing 1 or 2 g of amoxicillin plus 200 mg of clavulanic acid should be diluted in 100 mL of, or to 100 mL with, a compatible diluent.[3558] [3559] [3560] (See Solution Compatibility.)

Sodium and Potassium Content

Sodium and potassium content of amoxicillin sodium–clavulanate potassium vials is variable.[3558] [3559] [3560] Several manufacturers state that 600-mg vials contain 1.4 mmol of sodium and 0.5 mmol of potassium.[3558] [3560] Manufacturers state that 1.2-g vials contain either 2.7[3558] [3560] or 3.1 mmol of sodium[3359] and 1 mmol of potassium. One manufacturer states that 2.2-g vials contain 5.5 mmol of sodium and 1 mmol of potassium.[3558] Specific product labeling should be consulted for additional formulation details.

Trade Name(s)

Augmentin, Clavulin, Flanamox

Administration

Amoxicillin sodium–clavulanate potassium is administered intravenously, either by slow injection over 3 to 4 minutes directly into a vein or via intravenous tubing or by intermittent infusion over 30 to 40 minutes following dilution.[3558] [3559] [3560] Some patients (e.g., pediatric patients younger than 3 months of age) should receive the drug only by intravenous infusion.[3558] Reconstituted solutions prepared from 2.2-g vials and resulting in an amoxicillin to clavulanic acid ratio of 10:1 should be administered only by intravenous infusion following dilution.[3558] Amoxicillin sodium–clavulanate potassium is not suitable for intramuscular administration.[3558] [3559] [3560]

Stability

Intact vials of the fixed combination of amoxicillin sodium–clavulanate potassium should be stored at 15 to 30°C[3558] or at a temperature not exceeding 25°C.[3559] [3560] After reconstitution with sterile water for injection, a transient pink color may appear,[3558] [3559] [3560] with solutions quickly becoming clear again thereafter.[3558] Reconstituted solutions are normally colorless or a yellow color.[3559] [3560] The injection should be administered by slow intravenous injection, if appropriate, or further diluted for intravenous infusion within 15[3558] or 20 minutes[3559] [3560] after reconstitution.

Amoxicillin–clavulanic acid is less stable in dextrose, dextran, or bicarbonate-containing infusion solutions and should not be mixed with such solutions.[3559] [3560] Manufacturers state that amoxicillin–clavulanic acid also should not be added to proteinaceous fluids (e.g., protein hydrolysates) or intravenous fat emulsions.[3559] [3560]

The stability of amoxicillin–clavulanic acid is governed by the more rapid degradation of clavulanic acid compared with amoxicillin.[1474]

Stability of amoxicillin–clavulanic acid also is concentration dependent;[3559] [3560] amoxicillin–clavulanic acid is less stable in high concentrations. Therefore, it is suggested that reconstituted solutions be used immediately or diluted without delay.[1474] [3558] [3559] [3560] If a more concentrated solution of amoxicillin–clavulanic acid is required, one manufacturer states that the stability period should be adjusted accordingly.[3559] [3560]

Freezing Solutions

The fixed combination of amoxicillin sodium–clavulanate potassium 1.2 g (amoxicillin 1 g as the sodium salt plus clavulanate potassium equivalent to clavulanic acid 200 mg) reconstituted with 20 mL and diluted in 100 mL of sterile water for injection was frozen at −20°C for 4 hours, followed by microwave thawing. Solutions retained only 65% of the initial clavulanic acid content.[1474]

Sorption

Amoxicillin–clavulanic acid did not undergo sorption to polyvinyl chloride (PVC) containers or administration tubing.[1474]

DOI: 10.37573/9781585286850.022

Compatibility Information

Solution Compatibility

Amoxicillin sodium–clavulanate potassium

Test Soln Name	Mfr .	Mfr	Conc/L or %	Remarks	Ref	C/I
Dextrose 5%	BT[a]	BE	8.33[c] g	Physically compatible with 10% loss within 30 min at 25°C and 1.2 hr at 5°C	1474	I
Ringer's injection	BT[a]	BE	8.33[c] g	Physically compatible with 10% loss in 4.1 hr at 25°C	1474	I[b]
Ringer's injection, lactated	BT[a]	BE	8.33[c] g	Physically compatible with 10% loss in 4.1 hr	1474	I[b]
Ringer's injection		SZ	10[c] g	Complete administration within 1 hr if stored at 25°C	3558	C
Ringer's injection		GSK	10[c] g	Complete administration within 3 hr if stored at 25°C	3559	C
Ringer's injection		GSK	10[c] g	Complete administration within 2 hr if stored at 25°C	3560	C
Ringer's injection		SZ	20[d] g	Complete administration within 1 hr if stored at 25°C	3558	C
Ringer's injection, lactated		SZ	10[c] g	Complete administration within 1 hr if stored at 25°C	3558	C
Ringer's injection, lactated		SZ	20[d] g	Complete administration within 1 hr if stored at 25°C	3558	C
Sodium chloride 0.9%	BT[a]	BE	8.33[c] g	Physically compatible with 10% loss in 4.4 hr at 25°C and 12.5 hr at 5°C	1474	I[b]
Sodium chloride 0.9%		SZ	10[c] g	Complete administration within 1 hr if stored at 25°C; also stable for 4 hr if added to pre-refrigerated bags and stored at 5°C	3558	C
Sodium chloride 0.9%		GSK	10[c] g	Complete administration within 4 hr if stored at 25°C; also stable for 8 hr if added to pre-refrigerated bags and stored at 5°C	3559	C
Sodium chloride 0.9%		GSK	10[c] g	Complete administration within 3 hr if stored at 25°C; also stable for 8 hr if added to pre-refrigerated bags and stored at 5°C	3560	C
Sodium chloride 0.9%		SZ	20[d] g	Complete administration within 1 hr if stored at 25°C; also stable for 4 hr if added to pre-refrigerated bags and stored at 5°C	3558	C
Sodium chloride 0.9% with potassium chloride 0.3%	BT[a]	BE	8.33[c] g	Physically compatible with 10% loss in 3.9 hr at 25°C	1474	I[b]
Sodium chloride 0.9% with potassium chloride 0.3%		GSK	10 g[c]	Complete administration within 2 hr if stored at 25°C	3560	C
Sodium lactate ⅙ M	BT[a]	BE	8.33[c] g	Physically compatible with 10% loss in 4.3 hr at 25°C	1474	I[b]
Sodium lactate ⅙ M		GSK	10 g[c]	Complete administration with 4 hr if stored at 25°C	3559	C

[a] Tested in polyethylene containers.

[b] Incompatible by conventional standards; may be used in shorter time periods.

[c] Amoxicillin component. Amoxicillin in a 5:1 fixed-ratio concentration with clavulanic acid.

[d] Amoxicillin component. Amoxicillin in a 10:1 fixed-ratio concentration with clavulanic acid.

Additive Compatibility

Amoxicillin sodium–clavulanate potassium

Test Drug	Mfr	Conc/L or %	Mfr	Conc/L or %	Test Solution	Remarks	Ref	C/I
Ciprofloxacin		2 g		10[b] g	[a]	Precipitates immediately	1473	I
Metronidazole	BAY	5 g	BE	20[c] g		Physically compatible with 8% clavulanate loss in 2 hr and 25% loss in 6 hr at 21°C. 7 to 8% amoxicillin and no metronidazole loss in 6 hr at 21°C	1920	I

[a] Amoxicillin sodium–clavulanate potassium added to ciprofloxacin solution.

[b] Amoxicillin component. Amoxicillin in a 5:1 fixed-ratio concentration with clavulanic acid.

[c] Amoxicillin component. Amoxicillin in a 10:1 fixed-ratio concentration with clavulanic acid.

Y-Site Injection Compatibility (1:1 Mixture)

Amoxicillin sodium–clavulanate potassium

Test Drug	Mfr	Conc	Mfr	Conc	Remarks	Ref	C/I
Amiodarone HCl	SAN	12.5 mg/mL	GSK	10 mg/mL[c]	Turbidity appeared immediately	2727	I
Clarithromycin	AB	4 mg/mL[a]	BE	20 mg/mL[a c]	Visually compatible for 72 hr at both 30 and 17°C	2174	C
Lorazepam	WY	0.33 mg/mL[b]	SKB	20 mg/mL[d]	Visually compatible for 24 hr at 22°C	1855	C
Midazolam HCl	RC	5 mg/mL	SKB	20 mg/mL[d]	White precipitate forms immediately	1855	I

[a] Tested in dextrose 5%.

[b] Tested in sodium chloride 0.9%.

[c] Amoxicillin component. Amoxicillin in a 5:1 fixed-ratio concentration with clavulanic acid.

[d] Amoxicillin component. Amoxicillin in a 10:1 fixed-ratio concentration with clavulanic acid.

Additional Compatibility Information

Infusion Solutions

One manufacturer (Sandoz Canada) states that satisfactory concentrations of the drug are retained for 1 hour at 25°C when prepared as directed in sterile water for injection, compound sodium lactate (Hartmann's solution), and sodium chloride with potassium chloride (concentrations unspecified).[3558]

One manufacturer (GlaxoSmithKline New Zealand) states that satisfactory concentrations of the drug are retained for 3 hours at 25°C when prepared as directed in compound sodium lactate (Hartmann's solution) and sodium chloride with potassium chloride (concentrations unspecified) and for 4 hours at 25°C and 8 hours at 5°C when prepared as directed in sterile water for injection.[3559]

One manufacturer (GlaxoSmithKline UK) states that satisfactory concentrations of the drug are retained for 2 hours at 25°C when prepared as directed in compound sodium lactate (Hartmann's solution) and for 3 hours at 25°C and 8 hours at 5°C when prepared as directed in sterile water for injection.[3560]

Selected Revisions July 1, 2020. © Copyright, October 1992. American Society of Health-System Pharmacists, Inc.

Amphotericin B
AHFS 8:14.28

Products

Amphotericin B is available in vials containing 50 mg of drug with sodium desoxycholate 41 mg and sodium phosphates 20.2 mg. Reconstitute with 10 mL of sterile water for injection without preservatives and shake until a clear colloidal dispersion is obtained. The resultant concentration is 5 mg/mL of amphotericin B. Use only sterile water for injection without preservatives for reconstitution because other diluents, such as sodium chloride 0.9% or solutions containing a bacteriostatic agent such as benzyl alcohol, may result in the precipitation of the antibiotic. For infusion, amphotericin B must be further diluted with dextrose 5% with a pH above 4.2.[1(4/07)] [4]

Although various lipid complex and liposomal products of amphotericin B exist, they are sufficiently different from conventional amphotericin B formulations that extrapolating information to or from the other forms would be inappropriate.

pH

The pH of amphotericin B (Squibb) 100 mg/L in dextrose 5% has been reported as 5.7.[149]

Osmolality

The osmolality of amphotericin B (Squibb) 0.1 mg/mL in dextrose 5% was determined to be 256 mOsm/kg.[1375]

Trade Name(s)

Fungizone

Administration

Amphotericin B is administered by slow intravenous infusion over approximately 2 to 6 hours. The recommended concentration of the infusion is 0.1 mg/mL.[1(4/07)] [4] The drug has also been given intra-articularly, intrathecally, intrapleurally, and by irrigation.[4]

CAUTION: Care should be taken to ensure that the correct drug product, dose, and administration procedure are used and that no confusion with other products occurs.

Stability

Store intact vials at 2 to 8°C and protect from light.[1(4/07)] [4] The manufacturer indicates that a 5 to 10% potency loss occurs in 1 month at room temperature.[1433]

Amphotericin B reconstituted with sterile water for injection without preservatives and stored in the dark is stable for 24 hours at room temperature and for 1 week under refrigeration at 2 to 8°C.[1(4/07)] [4] [108] One report indicates that aqueous solutions may be stable for over a week at both 5 and 28°C.[352]

Reconstituted amphotericin B may be added to dextrose 5% with a pH above 4.2. Buffers present in the formulation raise the pH of the admixture. If the dextrose 5% has a pH less than 4.2, additional buffer must be added.[1(4/07)] [4] One or 2 mL of a buffer solution composed of dibasic sodium phosphate anhydrous 1.59 g

and monobasic sodium phosphate anhydrous 0.96 g in water for injection is brought to 100 mL. The buffer solution should be sterilized either by filtration or by autoclaving for 30 minutes at 121°C at 15 pounds pressure.[1(4/07)] Failure to sterilize this buffer solution coupled with prolonged storage at room temperature has resulted in severe infection.[328]

Amphotericin B was reported to precipitate when added to some evacuated containers due to a small residual amount of fluid that may have acetic acid and sodium acetate buffer or sodium chloride 0.9% solution. Only evacuated containers with residual sterile water should be used for preparing amphotericin B admixtures.[1232]

In an effort to reduce toxicity, amphotericin B has been admixed in Intralipid instead of the more usual dextrose 5%.[1809] [1810] [1811] [2178] However, amphotericin B 0.75 mg/kg/day administered using this approach in 250 mL of Intralipid 20% has been associated with acute pulmonary toxicities, including sudden onset of coughing, tachypnea, cyanosis, and deterioration of oxygen saturation following administration. The temporal relationship between the drug administration and respiratory symptoms suggested a causal relationship. Furthermore, no reduction in renal toxicity or other side effects was observed. It was concluded amphotericin B should not be administered in Intralipid.[2177]

At a concentration of 0.6 mg/mL in Intralipid 10 or 20%, amphotericin B precipitates immediately or almost immediately. The precipitate is not visible to the unaided eye because of the emulsion's dense opacity. Particle size evaluation found thousands of particles larger than 10 μm per mL. In dextrose 5%, very few particles were larger than 10 μm. Centrifuging the Intralipid admixtures resulted in rapid visualization of the precipitate as a mass at the bottom of the test tubes.[1808]

However, amphotericin B precipitation is observed in fat emulsion within 2 to 4 hours without centrifuging. In concentrations ranging from 90 mg to 2 g/L in Intralipid 20%, amphotericin B precipitate is easily seen as yellow particulate matter on the bottom of the lipid emulsion containers.[1872] [1988] Damage to the emulsion integrity with creaming has also been reported.[1987]

In other reports, the appearance of problems was observed in as little as 15 minutes, and actual amphotericin B precipitate formed within 20 minutes of mixing. Analysis of the precipitate confirmed its identity as amphotericin B. The authors hypothesized that amphotericin B precipitates as a consequence of the excipient desoxycholic acid, which is an anion, attracting oppositely charged choline groups from the egg yolk components of the fat emulsion. As a consequence, desoxycholic acid and phosphatidylcholine form a precipitate and insufficient surfactant remains to keep the amphotericin B dispersed.[2204] [2205]

pH Effects

The pH range for optimum clarity and stability is 6 to 7.[148] At a pH of less than approximately 6, the colloidal dispersion may

DOI: 10.37573/9781585286850.023

become turbid.[40] [148] Colloidal particles tend to coagulate rapidly at a pH of less than 5.[4]

Light Effects

Although the manufacturer recommends light protection for aqueous solutions of amphotericin B,[1(4/07)] several reports indicate that for short-term exposure of 8 to 24 hours, little difference in potency is observed between light-protected and light-exposed solutions.[150] [335] [353] Longer exposure periods[150] or higher intensity light exposure[2414] may result in unacceptable potency losses, however.

Elastomeric Reservoir Pumps

Amphotericin B (Lyphomed) 0.25 mg/mL in dextrose 5% was evaluated for binding potential to natural rubber elastomeric reservoirs (Baxter). No binding was found after storage for 2 weeks at 35°C with gentle agitation.[2014]

Filtration

Various studies have assessed the effects of filtration on the amphotericin B colloidal dispersion with differing results. The use of a 0.22-μm membrane filter was reported to be unacceptable with colloidal solutions adjusted to pH 4.7, 5.6, and 6.5. The concentration of amphotericin B in the filtrate decreased substantially after several hours. A 0.45-μm filter was satisfactory for infusions with a pH of 6.5, but the results at pH 5.6 were inconclusive. At pH 5.6 and 6.5, 1- and 5-μm filters both proved satisfactory in that they did not reduce the concentration of amphotericin B. For the turbid mixtures resulting at pH 4.7, however, all filters sharply reduced the concentration.[148] A report tended to support this finding for the 0.22-μm filter. At pH 5.7, fine particles of amphotericin B formed and were retained by the 0.22-μm filter.[149] No appreciable reduction in concentration with a 0.45-μm filter was found; but with a 0.22-μm filter, after 1 hour the concentration of amphotericin B delivered was about 30% of the initial concentration.[152] When amphotericin B 50 mg/500 mL in dextrose 5% was filtered through a 0.22-μm circular cellulose ester membrane (Swinnex) or a 0.22-μm cylindrical cellulose ester filter (Ivex-2), the flow rate decreased dramatically after passage of as little as 30 mL. Flow ceased altogether after 100 to 200 mL. The last sample filtered contained no drug. With a 0.45-μm circular cellulose ester membrane (Swinnex), no loss of activity was determined after filtration of 200 mL. However, the flow rate had decreased.[598] On the other hand, no significant difference in the amount or concentration of amphotericin B in dextrose 5% with phosphate buffer was found after filtration with 0.22-, 0.45-, and 5-μm filters.[151]

For amphotericin B infusions, only filters with a pore size not less than 1 μm should be used for filtration.[1(4/07)] [4] [148] This would allow a margin for error that would compensate for possible variations in particle size.[148] Also, limiting the use of filtration to situations where it is believed to be necessary has been recommended.[598] [599]

Compatibility Information

Solution Compatibility

Amphotericin B

Test Soln Name	Mfr	Mfr	Conc/L or %	Remarks	Ref	C/I
Amino acids 4.25%, dextrose 25%	MG	SQ	100 mg	Turbidity and fine yellow particles form	349	I
Dextrose 5% in Ringer's injection, lactated	MG[a]	SQ	100 mg	Precipitate forms in 30 min. About 50% remains in 30 min	539	I
Dextrose 5% in sodium chloride 0.9%	MG[a]	SQ	100 mg	Precipitate forms within 2 hr. 30 to 70% remains in 2 hr	539	I
Dextrose 5%		SQ	70 and 140 mg	Bioactivity not affected over 24 hr at 25°C in light or dark	335	C
Dextrose 5%	MG[a]	SQ	100 mg	Physically compatible. Concentration unchanged in 48 hr	539	C
Dextrose 5%		SQ	50 and 100 mg	No loss of bioactivity in normal light at 25°C for 24 hr	540	C
Dextrose 5%	MG[b]	SQ	0.9, 1.2, 1.4 g	Physically compatible with little loss in 36 hr at 6 and 25°C	1434	C
Dextrose 5%	MG[b]	SQ	470, 660, 750 mg	Visually compatible with no loss in 24 hr at 25°C	1537	C
Dextrose 5%	BA[c]	SQ	100 mg	Visually compatible with no loss in 24 hr at 15 to 25°C	1544	C
Dextrose 5%	BA[c]	SQ	100 and 250 mg	Visually compatible with 4% loss in 35 days at 4°C in dark	1546	C
Dextrose 5%	BA[c]	SQ	0.2, 0.5, 1 g	Visually compatible. Little loss in 5 days at 4 and 25°C. Normal turbidity observed at 1 g/L	1728	C

Solution Compatibility (Cont.)

Test Soln Name	Mfr	Mfr	Conc/L or %	Remarks	Ref	C/I
Dextrose 5%	AB[c]	BMS	50 mg	Visually compatible. No loss protected from light and 5% loss exposed to fluorescent light in 24 hr at 24°C	2093	C
Dextrose 5%	AB[c]	BMS	500 mg	Visually compatible. No loss protected from or exposed to fluorescent light in 24 hr at 24°C	2093	C
Dextrose 5%			50, 100, 150 mg	Visually compatible with less than 5% loss in 24 hr at 4 and 25°C when protected from light	2414	C
Dextrose 10%	BA[c]	SQ	100 mg	Visually compatible with no loss in 24 hr at 15 to 25°C	1544	C
Dextrose 20%	BA[c]	SQ	100 mg	Visually compatible with no loss in 24 hr at 15 to 25°C	1544	C
Ringer's injection, lactated	MG[a]	SQ	100 mg	Precipitate forms within 2 hr. 80% remains in 2 hr	539	I
Sodium chloride 0.9%	AB	SQ	100 mg	Physically incompatible	15	I
Sodium chloride 0.9%	MG[a]	SQ	100 mg	Precipitate forms within 2 hr. 43% remains in 2 hr	539	I

[a] Tested in both glass and polyolefin containers.

[b] Tested in polyolefin containers.

[c] Tested in PVC containers.

Additive Compatibility

Amphotericin B

Test Drug	Mfr	Conc/L or %	Mfr	Conc/L or %	Test Solution	Remarks	Ref	C/I
Amikacin sulfate	BR	5 g	SQ	100 mg	D5LR, D5R, D5S, D5W, D10W, LR, NS, R, SL	Precipitates immediately	293	I
Calcium chloride	BP	4 g		200 mg	D5W	Haze develops over 3 hr	26	I
Calcium gluconate	BP	4 g		200 mg	D5W	Haze develops over 3 hr	26	I
Chlorpromazine HCl	BP	200 mg		200 mg	D5W	Precipitates immediately	26	I
Ciprofloxacin	MI	2 g		100 mg	D5W	Physically incompatible	888	I
Ciprofloxacin	BAY	2 g	APC	100 mg	D5W	Precipitates immediately	2413	I
Diphenhydramine HCl	PD	80 mg	SQ	100 mg	D5W	Physically incompatible	15	I
Dopamine HCl	AS	800 mg	SQ	200 mg	D5W	Precipitates immediately	78	I
Edetate calcium disodium	RI	4 g		200 mg	D5W	Haze develops over 3 hr	26	I
Fat emulsion, intravenous	CL	10 and 20%	APC, PHT	0.6 g		Precipitate forms immediately but is concealed by opaque emulsion	1808	I
Fat emulsion, intravenous		20%		90 mg		Yellow precipitate forms in 2 hr. Cumulative delivery of only 56% of total amphotericin B dose	1872	I
Fat emulsion, intravenous	CL	20%	APC	10, 50, 100, 500 mg, 1 and 5 g		Emulsion separation occurred rapidly with visible creaming within 4 hr at 27 and 8°C	1987	I
Fat emulsion, intravenous	KA	20%	SQ	500 mg, 1 and 2 g		Precipitated amphotericin noted on bottom of containers within 4 hr	1988	I

Additive Compatibility (Cont.)

Test Drug	Mfr	Conc/L or %	Mfr	Conc/L or %	Test Solution	Remarks	Ref	C/I
Fat emulsion, intravenous	CL[b]	20%	BMS	50 and 500 mg		Fat emulsion separates into two phases within 8 hr. Little loss protected from or exposed to fluorescent light in 24 hr at 24°C	2093	I
Fat emulsion, intravenous	KP	20%	BMS	1 and 3 g		Precipitate forms immediately	2518	I
Fat emulsion, intravenous	KP	20%	BMS	150 mg, 300 mg, 1.5 g	D5W[c]	Precipitate forms immediately	2518	I
Fluconazole	PF	1 g	LY	50 mg	D5W	Visually compatible with no fluconazole loss in 72 hr at 25°C. Amphotericin B not tested	1677	C
Gentamicin sulfate		320 mg		200 mg	D5W	Haze develops over 3 hr	26	I
Heparin sodium	UP	4000 units	SQ	100 mg	D5W	Physically compatible	15	C
Heparin sodium	AB	4000 units	SQ	100 mg	D	Physically compatible	21	C
Heparin sodium		2000 units	SQ	70 and 140 mg	D5W	Bioactivity not affected over 24 hr at 25°C	335	C
Hydrocortisone sodium succinate	UP	500 mg	SQ	100 mg	D5W	Physically compatible	15	C
Hydrocortisone sodium succinate		50 mg	SQ	70 and 140 mg	D5W	Bioactivity not significantly affected over 24 hr at 25°C	335	C
Magnesium sulfate	IMS	2 and 4 g	SQ	40 and 80 mg	D5W	Physically incompatible in 3 hr at 24°C with decreased clarity and development of supernatant	1578	I
Meropenem	ZEN	1 and 20 g	SQ	200 mg	NS	Precipitate forms	2068	I
Methyldopate HCl		1 g		200 mg	D5W	Haze develops over 3 hr	26	I
Penicillin G potassium	SQ	20 million units	SQ	100 mg	D5W	Physically incompatible	15	I
Penicillin G potassium	SQ	5 million units	SQ	50 mg		Precipitate forms within 1 hr	47	I
Penicillin G potassium	BP	10 million units		200 mg	D5W	Haze develops over 3 hr	26	I
Penicillin G sodium	UP	20 million units	SQ	100 mg	D5W	Physically incompatible	15	I
Penicillin G sodium	BP	10 million units		200 mg	D5W	Haze develops over 3 hr	26	I
Polymyxin B sulfate	BP	20 mg		200 mg	D5W	Haze develops over 3 hr	26	I
Potassium chloride	AB	100 mEq	SQ	100 mg	D5W	Physically incompatible	15	I
Potassium chloride	BP	4 g		200 mg	D5W	Haze develops over 3 hr	26	I
Prochlorperazine mesylate	BP	100 mg		200 mg	D5W	Haze develops over 3 hr	26	I
Ranitidine HCl	GL	100 mg	SQ	200 mg	D5W	Color change and particle formation	1151	I
Sodium bicarbonate	AB	2.4 mEq[a]	SQ	50 mg	D5W	Physically compatible for 24 hr	772	C
Streptomycin sulfate	BP	4 g		200 mg	D5W	Haze develops over 3 hr	26	I

Additive Compatibility (Cont.)

Test Drug	Mfr	Conc/L or %	Mfr	Conc/L or %	Test Solution	Remarks	Ref	C/I
Verapamil HCl	KN	80 mg	SQ	100 mg	D5W	Physically incompatible after 8 hr	764	I
Verapamil HCl	KN	80 mg	SQ	100 mg	NS	Immediate physical incompatibility	764	I

a One vial of Neut added to a liter of admixture.

b Tested in glass containers.

c Diluted in dextrose 5% before adding to the fat emulsion.

Drugs in Syringe Compatibility

Amphotericin B

Test Drug	Mfr	Amt	Mfr	Amt	Remarks	Ref	C/I
Heparin sodium		2500 units/1 mL		50 mg	Physically compatible for at least 5 min	1053	C
Pantoprazole sodium	a	4 mg/1 mL		5 mg/1 mL	Opacity within 1 hr	2574	I

a Test performed using the formulation WITHOUT edetate disodium.

Y-Site Injection Compatibility (1:1 Mixture)

Amphotericin B

Test Drug	Mfr	Conc	Mfr	Conc	Remarks	Ref	C/I
Aldesleukin	CHI	33,800 I.U./mL[a]	SQ	1.6 mg/mL[a]	Visually compatible for 2 hr	1857	C
Allopurinol sodium	BW	3 mg/mL[a]	SQ	0.6 mg/mL[a]	Amphotericin B haze lost immediately	1686	I
Amifostine	USB	10 mg/mL[a]	AD	0.6 mg/mL[a]	Turbidity forms immediately	1845	I
Amiodarone HCl	WY	6 mg/mL[a]	BMS	0.5 mg/mL[a]	Visually compatible for 24 hr at 22°C	2352	C
Amsacrine	NCI	1 mg/mL[a]	SQ	0.6 mg/mL[a]	Immediate yellow turbidity, becoming yellow flocculent precipitate in 15 min	1381	I
Anidulafungin	VIC	0.5 mg/mL[a]	PHT	0.6 mg/mL[a]	Measured haze went up immediately	2617	I
Aztreonam	SQ	40 mg/mL[a]	PHT	0.6 mg/mL[a]	Yellow turbidity forms immediately and becomes flocculent precipitate in 4 hr	1758	I
Bivalirudin	TMC	5 mg/mL[a]	APO	0.6 mg/mL[a]	Yellow precipitate forms immediately	2373	I
Caspofungin acetate	ME	0.7 mg/mL[b]	XGN	0.6 mg/mL[a]	Immediate yellow turbid precipitate forms	2758	I
Ceftaroline fosamil	FOR	2.22 mg/mL[a b c]	XGN	0.6 mg/mL[a]	Increased haze and microparticulates	2826	I
Ceftolozane sulfate–tazobactam sodium	CUB	10 mg/mL[a k]	XGN	0.1 mg/mL[a]	Measured turbidity increases immediately	3262	I
Cisatracurium besylate	GW	0.1 mg/mL[a]	PH	0.6 mg/mL[a]	Physically compatible for 4 hr at 23°C	2074	C
Cisatracurium besylate	GW	2 mg/mL[a]	PH	0.6 mg/mL[a]	Cloudiness forms immediately; gel-like precipitate forms in 1 hr	2074	I
Cisatracurium besylate	GW	5 mg/mL[a]	PH	0.6 mg/mL[a]	Turbidity forms immediately	2074	I
Dexmedetomidine HCl	AB	4 mcg/mL[b]	APO	0.6 mg/mL[a]	Yellow precipitate forms immediately	2383	I
Dexmedetomidine HCl	HOS, HQS	4 mcg/mL[b]			Stated to be incompatible	2848, 3179	I

Y-Site Injection Compatibility (1:1 Mixture) (Cont.)

Test Drug	Mfr	Conc	Mfr	Conc	Remarks	Ref	C/I
Diltiazem HCl	MMD	5 mg/mL	SQ	0.1 mg/mL[a]	Visually compatible	1807	C
Docetaxel	RPR	0.9 mg/mL[a]	PH	0.6 mg/mL[a]	Visible turbidity forms immediately	2224	I
Doripenem	JJ	5 mg/mL[a]	XGN	0.6 mg/mL[a]	Physically compatible for 4 hr at 23°C	2743	C
Doripenem	JJ	5 mg/mL[b]	XGN	0.6 mg/mL[a]	Yellow precipitate forms immediately	2743	I
Doxorubicin HCl liposomal	SEQ	0.4 mg/mL[a]	APC	0.6 mg/mL[a]	Fivefold increase in measured particulates in 4 hr	2087	I
Enalaprilat	MSD	1.25 mg/mL	SQ	0.1 mg/mL[a]	Layered haze develops in 4 hr at 21°C	1409	I
Etoposide phosphate	BR	5 mg/mL[a]	GNS	0.6 mg/mL[a]	Yellow-orange precipitate forms immediately	2218	I
Fenoldopam mesylate	AB	80 mcg/mL[b]	APO	0.6 mg/mL[b]	Yellow precipitate forms immediately	2467	I
Filgrastim	AMG	30 mcg/mL[a]	SQ	0.6 mg/mL[a]	Yellow turbidity and precipitate form	1687	I
Fluconazole	RR	2 mg/mL	SQ	5 mg/mL	Cloudiness and yellow precipitate	1407	I
Fludarabine phosphate	BX	1 mg/mL[a]	SQ	0.6 mg/mL[a]	Precipitate forms in 4 hr at 22°C	1439	I
Foscarnet sodium	AST	24 mg/mL	SQ	5 mg/mL	Cloudy yellow precipitate forms	1335	I
Foscarnet sodium	AST	24 mg/mL	SQ	0.6 mg/mL[a]	Dense haze forms immediately	1393	I
Gemcitabine HCl	LI	10 mg/mL[b]	PH	0.6 mg/mL[a]	Gross precipitation occurs immediately	2226	I
Granisetron HCl	SKB	0.05 mg/mL[a]	PH	0.6 mg/mL[a]	Large increase in measured turbidity occurs immediately	2000	I
Heparin sodium	SO	100 units/mL[b]	SQ	0.1 mg/mL[a]	Turbidity forms in 45 min	1435	I
Hetastarch in lactated electrolyte	AB	6%	APC	0.6 mg/mL[a]	Immediate gross precipitation	2339	I
Isavuconazonium sulfate	ASP	1.5 mg/mL[a]	XGN	0.1 mg/mL[a]	Measured turbidity increases immediately	3263	I
Linezolid	PHU	2 mg/mL	AB	0.6 mg/mL[a]	Yellow precipitate forms within 5 min	2264	I
Linezolid	PHU, HOS	2 mg/mL			Stated to be physically incompatible	3183, 3184	I
Melphalan HCl	BW	0.1 mg/mL[b]	SQ	0.6 mg/mL[a]	Immediate increase in measured turbidity	1557	I
Melphalan HCl	BW	0.1 mg/mL[a]	SQ	0.6 mg/mL[a]	Physically compatible but rapid melphalan loss in D5W precludes use	1557	I
Meropenem	ZEN	1 and 50 mg/mL[b]	SQ	5 mg/mL	Precipitate forms	2068	I
Ondansetron HCl	GL	1 mg/mL[a]	SQ	0.6 mg/mL[a]	Immediate yellow turbid precipitation	1365	I
Oritavancin diphosphate	TAR	0.8, 1.2, and 2 mg/mL[a]	XGN	0.1 mg/mL[a]	Slight haze forms immediately	2928	I
Paclitaxel	NCI	1.2 mg/mL[a]	SQ	0.6 mg/mL[a]	Immediate increase in measured turbidity followed by separation into two layers in 24 hr at 22°C	1556	I
Pemetrexed disodium	LI	20 mg/mL[b]	PHT	0.6 mg/mL[a]	Yellow precipitate forms immediately	2564	I
Piperacillin sodium–tazobactam sodium	LE[h]	40 mg/mL[a i]	SQ	0.6 mg/mL[a]	Yellow precipitate forms immediately	1688	I
Plazomicin sulfate	ACH	24 mg/mL[a]	XGN	0.1 mg/mL[a]	Measured turbidity increases immediately	3432	I
Propofol	ZEN[l]	10 mg/mL	APC	0.6 mg/mL[a]	Gel-like precipitate forms immediately	2066	I
Quinupristin–dalfopristin		2 mg/mL[a j]		0.6 mg/mL	Reported to be incompatible	3230	I
Remifentanil HCl	GW	0.025 mg/mL[a]	PHT	0.6 mg/mL[a]	Physically compatible for 4 hr at 23°C	2075	C

Y-Site Injection Compatibility (1:1 Mixture) (Cont.)

Test Drug	Mfr	Conc	Mfr	Conc	Remarks	Ref	C/I
Remifentanil HCl	GW	0.25 mg/mL[a]	PHT	0.6 mg/mL[a]	Yellow precipitate forms immediately	2075	I
Sargramostim	IMM	10 mcg/mL[a]	SQ	0.6 mg/mL[a]	Visually compatible for 4 hr at 22°C	1436	C
Sargramostim	IMM	10 mcg/mL[b]	SQ	0.6 mg/mL[b]	Yellow precipitate forms immediately	1436	I
Tacrolimus	FUJ	1 mg/mL[d]	LY	5 mg/mL[a]	Visually compatible for 24 hr at 25°C	1630	C
Telavancin HCl	ASP	7.5 mg/mL[a]	XGN	0.1 mg/mL[a]	Increase in measured turbidity	2830	I
Teniposide	BR	0.1 mg/mL[a]	SQ	0.6 mg/mL[a]	Physically compatible for 4 hr at 23°C	1725	C
Thiotepa	IMM[e]	1 mg/mL[a]	APC	0.6 mg/mL[a]	Physically compatible for 4 hr at 23°C	1861	C
Tigecycline	WY	1 mg/mL[b]		2 mg/mL[a]	Immediate cloudiness with particulates in 1 hr	2714	I
Tigecycline	ACD, FRK, WY				Stated to be incompatible	2915, 3459, 3460	I
TNA #218 to #226[g]			PH	0.6 mg/mL[a]	Yellow precipitate forms immediately	2215	I
TPN #212 to #215[g]			PH	0.6 mg/mL[a]	Precipitate forms immediately	2109	I
Vinorelbine tartrate	BW	1 mg/mL[b]	SQ	0.6 mg/mL[f]	Yellow precipitate forms immediately	1558	I
Zidovudine	BW	4 mg/mL[a]	SQ	600 mcg/mL[a]	Physically compatible for 4 hr at 25°C	1193	C

[a] Tested in dextrose 5%.

[b] Tested in sodium chloride 0.9%.

[c] Tested in Ringer's injection, lactated.

[d] Tested in sterile water.

[e] Lyophilized formulation tested.

[f] Tested in both dextrose 5% and sodium chloride 0.9%.

[g] Refer to Appendix for the composition of parenteral nutrition solutions. TNA indicates a 3-in-1 admixture, and TPN indicates a 2-in-1 admixture.

[h] Test performed using the formulation WITHOUT edetate disodium.

[i] Piperacillin component. Piperacillin in an 8:1 fixed-ratio concentration with tazobactam.

[j] Quinupristin and dalfopristin components combined.

[k] Ceftolozane component. Ceftolozane in a 2:1 fixed-ratio concentration with tazobactam.

[l] Test performed using the formulation WITH edetate disodium.

Selected Revisions January 31, 2020. © Copyright, October 1982.
American Society of Health-System Pharmacists, Inc.

Amphotericin B Lipid Complex
AHFS 8:14.28

Products

Amphotericin B lipid complex is available in single-use 20-mL vials containing amphotericin B complexed with 2 phospholipids in a 1:1 drug to lipid molar ratio; the injection is an opaque, yellow suspension.[3072] Each mL of the suspension contains amphotericin B 5 mg, L-α-dimyristoylphosphatidylcholine (DMPC) 3.4 mg, L-α-dimyristoylphosphatidylglycerol (DMPG) 1.5 mg, and sodium chloride 9 mg in water for injection.[3072]

To prepare the infusion, each vial should first be gently shaken until no yellow sediment is visible on the bottom of the vial.[3072] The appropriate dose should be withdrawn from the necessary number of vials using 1 or more syringes equipped with 18-gauge needles.[3072] The 18-gauge needle should then be removed from the syringe and replaced with the 5-μm filter needle that is supplied with each vial of the drug, and the drug suspension should be transferred into an infusion bag of dextrose 5%.[3072] One filter needle may be used to filter up to 4 vials of the drug.[3072] The final concentration of the drug diluted for infusion should be 1 mg/mL, although more concentrated infusions of 2 mg/mL may be used in some cases (e.g., pediatric patients, patients with cardiovascular disease).[3072]

Although other amphotericin B products exist, they are sufficiently different from amphotericin B lipid complex that extrapolating information to or from other forms is inappropriate.[3072]

pH

5 to 7.[3072]

Trade Name(s)

Abelcet

Administration

Amphotericin B lipid complex diluted to a concentration of 1 or 2 mg/mL in dextrose 5% is administered by intravenous infusion at a rate of 2.5 mg/kg/hr.[3072] The infusion bag should be shaken just prior to administration until the contents are thoroughly mixed.[3072] The admixture should not be used if evidence of foreign matter is present.[3072] If the infusion time exceeds 2 hours, the infusion bag should be shaken every 2 hours to mix the remaining contents.[3072] If an existing line is used to administer amphotericin B lipid complex, the line should be flushed with dextrose 5% prior to administration, otherwise a separate line should be used.[3072] **CAUTION: Care should be taken to ensure that the correct drug product, dose, and administration procedure are used and that no confusion with other products occurs.**

Stability

Intact vials of amphotericin B lipid complex are stored at 2 to 8°C.[3072] Vials should be kept in the original carton until time of use to protect from light and should not be frozen.[3072]

The manufacturer states that amphotericin B lipid complex diluted in dextrose 5% for administration may be stored for up to 48 hours at 2 to 8°C with an additional 6 hours at room temperature.[3072] The manufacturer also has confirmed that limited stability studies indicate that amphotericin B lipid complex 1 mg/mL in dextrose 5% is stable for up to 10 days stored at room temperature.[3074]

Amphotericin B lipid complex should not be mixed with saline or other electrolyte solutions.[3072]

Freezing Solutions

Admixtures of amphotericin B lipid complex in dextrose 5% should not be frozen.[3072]

Filtration

The manufacturer states that amphotericin B lipid complex is to be prepared using the 5-μm filter needle provided with the drug; however, the admixture should not be administered using an inline filter.[3072] Each 5-μm filter needle provided with the drug may be used to filter up to 4 vials of the drug.[3072]

Compatibility Information
Solution Compatibility

Amphotericin B lipid complex

Test Soln Name	Mfr	Mfr	Conc/L or %	Remarks	Ref	C/I
Dextrose 5%	MAC	ZNS	400 mg, 800 mg, 2 g	Physically compatible. Analytical results were variable but did not indicate substantial loss	2732	C
Dextrose 5%		SIG	1 and 2 g	Stable for 48 hr at 2 to 8°C and an additional 6 hr at room temperature	3072	C

DOI: 10.37573/9781585286850.024

Y-Site Injection Compatibility (1:1 Mixture)

Amphotericin B lipid complex

Test Drug	Mfr	Conc	Mfr	Conc	Remarks	Ref	C/I
Anidulafungin	VIC	0.5 mg/mL[a]	ELN	1 mg/mL[a]	Physically compatible for 4 hr at 23°C	2617	C
Caspofungin acetate	ME	0.7 mg/mL[b]	ENZ	1 mg/mL[a]	Immediate yellow turbid precipitate	2758	I
Ceftolozane sulfate–tazobactam sodium	CUB	10 mg/mL[a c]	SIG	1 mg/mL[a]	Immediate change in measured turbidity	3262	I
Doripenem	JJ	5 mg/mL[a]	ENZ	1 mg/mL[a]	Physically compatible for 4 hr at 23°C	2743	C
Doripenem	JJ	5 mg/mL[b]	ENZ	1 mg/mL[a]	Measured haze increases immediately	2743	I
Isavuconazonium sulfate	ASP	1.5 mg/mL[a]	SIG	1 mg/mL[a]	Immediate change in measured turbidity	3263	I
Letermovir	ME	[a]		[a]	Physically compatible	3398	C
Telavancin HCl	ASP	7.5 mg/mL[a]	ENZ	1 mg/mL[a]	Physically compatible for 2 hr	2830	C
Tigecycline	WY	1 mg/mL[b]	ENZ	2 mg/mL[a]	Incompatible with sodium chloride diluent	2714	I
Tigecycline	ACD, FRK, WY				Stated to be incompatible	2915, 3459, 3460	I

[a] Tested in dextrose 5%.

[b] Tested in sodium chloride 0.9%.

[c] Ceftolozane component. Ceftolozane in a 2:1 fixed-ratio concentration with tazobactam.

Additional Compatibility Information

Peritoneal Dialysis Solutions

Amphotericin B lipid complex (Abelcet, The Liposome Company) was evaluated for stability in Dianeal PD-1 with dextrose 1.5% (Baxter) and Dianeal PD-1 with dextrose 4.25% (Baxter) at concentrations of 0.5 mg/L, 2 mg/L, and 10 mg/L, with bags of each concentration stored at 4, 25, and 37°C.[3073] Although no visual changes were observed throughout the study period, results of the nuclear magnetic resonance (NMR) spectroscopy analysis demonstrated important changes in the resonances associated with the lipid component of the formulation, suggesting decomposition of the lipid component of the drug and/or bag adherence.[3073]

Selected Revisions January 31, 2020. © Copyright, October 2006. American Society of Health-System Pharmacists, Inc.

Amphotericin B Liposomal
AHFS 8:14.28

Products

Amphotericin B liposomal for injection is available as a lyophilized powder in vials containing the equivalent of amphotericin B 50 mg; the vial also contains hydrogenated soy phosphatidylcholine 213 mg, cholesterol 52 mg, distearoylphosphatidylglycerol 84 mg, and alpha tocopherol 0.64 mg, which form the liposomal membrane.[3068] Amphotericin B is intercalated into the liposomal membrane to form liposomes that are less than 100 nm in diameter.[3068] The vial also contains sucrose 900 mg and disodium succinate hexahydrate 27 mg.[3068]

Vials should be reconstituted only with 12 mL of sterile water for injection.[3068] No other diluent should be used because of potential drug precipitation.[3068] After addition of the sterile water for injection, vials should be shaken vigorously for 30 seconds to yield a liposomal suspension concentrate of amphotericin B 4 mg/mL.[3068] The vial should be visually inspected for particulate matter and shaken until completely dispersed.[3068]

To prepare for administration, the volume of reconstituted concentrate used to prepare the dose should be passed through the provided disposable 5-μm filters into an appropriate volume of dextrose 5%, using 1 filter per vial.[3068] The final concentration of the drug diluted for infusion generally should be 1 to 2 mg/mL, although lower concentrations of 0.2 to 0.5 mg/mL may be used for infants and small children.[3068]

Although other amphotericin B products exist, they are sufficiently different from amphotericin B liposomal that extrapolating information to or from other forms is inappropriate.[3068]

pH

From 5 to 6.[3068]

Trade Name(s)

AmBisome

Administration

Amphotericin B liposomal is administered by intravenous infusion following dilution in dextrose 5% using a controlled infusion device over approximately 120 minutes.[3068] The administration time may be reduced to 60 minutes for patients who tolerate the infusion well.[3068] If an existing line is used to administer amphotericin B liposomal, the line should be flushed with dextrose 5% prior to administration, otherwise a separate line must be used.[3068] **CAUTION: Care should be taken to ensure that the correct drug product, dose, and administration procedure are used and that no confusion with other products occurs.**

Stability

Intact vials of amphotericin B liposomal for injection are stored at room temperatures up to 25°C.[3068] The reconstituted concentrate is a yellow, translucent suspension.[3068]

The manufacturer states that the reconstituted concentrate may be stored at 2 to 8°C for up to 24 hours.[3068] The reconstituted concentrate should be protected from freezing.[3068] Vials contain no preservative; partially used vials should be discarded.[3068] The manufacturer also has confirmed that amphotericin B liposomal at a concentration of 4 mg/mL in sterile water for injection in the original glass vial is stable for 14 days at 2 to 8°C and protected from light.[3069]

The manufacturer states that administration of amphotericin B liposomal should begin within 6 hours of dilution in dextrose 5%.[3068] However, the manufacturer also has indicated that the drug diluted in dextrose 5% for administration is stable for longer time periods.[3069] (See Solution Compatibility.)

The manufacturer states that amphotericin B liposomal should not be mixed with saline or solutions containing bacteriostatic agents.[3068]

Syringes

The manufacturer states that amphotericin B liposomal 4 mg/mL packaged in syringes is stable for 14 days stored at 2 to 8°C and protected from light.[3069]

Filtration

The volume of reconstituted concentrate of amphotericin B liposomal used to prepare the dose should be passed through the disposable 5-μm filter (provided with each vial of drug) into an appropriate volume of dextrose 5% for dilution, using 1 filter per vial.[3068]

The manufacturer states that amphotericin B liposomal diluted for infusion may be administered through an inline filter as long as the mean pore diameter of the filter is not smaller than 1 μm.[3068]

Compatibility Information

Solution Compatibility

Amphotericin B liposomal

Test Soln Name	Mfr	Mfr	Conc/L or %	Remarks	Ref	C/I
Dextrose 5%	a	ASP	0.5 and 2 g	Stable for 14 days at 2 to 8°C protected from light	3069	C
Dextrose 5%	b	ASP	200 mg	Stable for 11 days at 2 to 8°C protected from light	3069	C

DOI: 10.37573/9781585286850.025

Solution Compatibility (Cont.)

Test Soln Name	Mfr	Mfr	Conc/L or %	Remarks	Ref	C/I
Dextrose 5%	b	ASP	2 g	Stable for 14 days at 2 to 8°C protected from light	3069	C
Dextrose 5%	c	ASP	200 mg	Stable for 7 days at 2 to 8°C protected from light	3069	C
Dextrose 5%	c	ASP	2 g	Stable for 14 days at 2 to 8°C protected from light	3069	C
Dextrose 5%	b	ASP	0.2 and 2 g	Stable for 24 hr at 23 to 27°C exposed to fluorescent light	3069	C
Dextrose 10%	b	ASP	0.2 and 2 g	Stable for 48 hr at 2 to 8°C protected from light	3069	C
Dextrose 20%	b	ASP	2 g	Stable for 48 hr at 2 to 8°C protected from light	3069	C
Dextrose 25%	b	ASP	2 g	Stable for 48 hr at 2 to 8°C protected from light	3069	C

[a] Tested in PVC containers.

[b] Tested in polyolefin containers.

[c] Tested in Homepump Eclipse elastomeric pump reservoirs.

Y-Site Injection Compatibility (1:1 Mixture)

Amphotericin B liposomal

Test Drug	Mfr	Conc	Mfr	Conc	Remarks	Ref	C/I
Anidulafungin	VIC	0.5 mg/mL[a]	FUJ	1 mg/mL[a]	Physically compatible for 4 hr at 23°C	2617	C
Blinatumomab	AMG	0.125 and 0.375 mcg/mL[b]	GIL	1 mg/mL[a]	Visually compatible for 12 hr at room temperature	3405, 3417	C
Caspofungin acetate	ME	0.7 mg/mL[b]	AST	1 mg/mL[a]	Immediate yellow turbid precipitate	2758	I
Ceftolozane sulfate–tazobactam sodium	CUB	10 mg/mL[a][c]	ASP	2 mg/mL[a]	Immediate change in measured turbidity	3262	I
Cloxacillin sodium	SMX	100 mg/mL	ASP	4 mg/mL	Physically compatible for up to 4 hr at room temperature	3245	C
Defibrotide sodium	JAZ	8 mg/mL[b]	GIL	2 mg/mL[a]	Visually compatible for 4 hr at room temperature	3149	C
Doripenem	JJ	5 mg/mL[a]	ASP	1 mg/mL[a]	Physically compatible for 4 hr at 23°C	2743	C
Doripenem	JJ	5 mg/mL[b]	ASP	1 mg/mL[a]	Measured haze increases immediately	2743	I
Isavuconazonium sulfate	ASP	1.5 mg/mL[a]	ASP	2 mg/mL[a]	Measured turbidity increases immediately	3263	I
Letermovir	ME				Physically incompatible	3398	I
Meropenem		50 mg/mL	ASP	2 mg/mL[a]	Physically compatible for 4 hr at room temperature	3538, 3547	C
Telavancin HCl	ASP	7.5 mg/mL[a]	ASP	1 mg/mL[a]	Increase in measured turbidity	2830	I

[a] Tested in dextrose 5%.

[b] Tested in sodium chloride 0.9%.

[c] Ceftolozane component. Ceftolozane in a 2:1 fixed-ratio concentration with tazobactam.

Selected Revisions May 1, 2020. © Copyright, October 2006.
American Society of Health-System Pharmacists, Inc.

Ampicillin Sodium
AHFS 8:12.16.08

Products

Ampicillin sodium is available in vials containing the equivalent of ampicillin 125 mg, 250 mg, 500 mg, 1 g, or 2 g as a powder.[3291]

For intramuscular injection, the vials should be reconstituted with sterile water for injection or bacteriostatic water for injection in the following amounts:[3291]

Vial Size	Volume of Diluent	Withdrawable Volume	Concentration
125 mg	1.2 mL	1 mL	125 mg/mL
250 mg	1 mL	1 mL	250 mg/mL
500 mg	1.8 mL	2 mL	250 mg/mL
1 g	3.5 mL	4 mL	250 mg/mL
2 g	6.8 mL	8 mL	250 mg/mL

For administration by direct intravenous injection, the 125-, 250-, and 500-mg vials should be reconstituted with 5 mL of sterile water for injection or bacteriostatic water for injection; the 1- or 2-g vials should be reconstituted with 7.4 or 14.8 mL, respectively, of sterile water for injection or bacteriostatic water for injection.[3291] For administration by intravenous infusion, the reconstituted solution as prepared for direct intravenous injection should be further diluted in a compatible infusion solution prior to administration.[3291]

Ampicillin sodium also is available in ADD-Vantage vials containing the equivalent of ampicillin 1 or 2 g as a powder.[3292] ADD-Vantage vials should be prepared with 50 or 100 mL of sodium chloride 0.9% or dextrose 5% in ADD-Vantage diluent bags.[3292]

Ampicillin sodium also is available in a pharmacy bulk package.[3293] The 10-g pharmacy bulk package should be reconstituted with 94 mL of sterile water for injection; the resulting solution contains ampicillin 100 mg/mL.[3293] The reconstituted pharmacy bulk package solution must be diluted further in a compatible infusion solution to achieve a solution with a final ampicillin concentration of 5 or 10 mg/mL.[3293]

pH

The reconstituted solution of ampicillin has a pH ranging from 8 to 10.[3293][3294] The pH values of various ampicillin solutions are shown below:[213]

Ampicillin Concentration	Diluent	Initial pH
20 mg/mL	Sterile water	8.8
50 mg/mL	Sterile water	8.92
100 mg/mL	Sterile water	9.15
20 mg/mL	Sodium chloride 0.9%	8.7
50 mg/mL	Sodium chloride 0.9%	8.9
100 mg/mL	Sodium chloride 0.9%	9.2
20 mg/mL	Dextrose 5%	8.9
50 mg/mL	Dextrose 5%	9.3
100 mg/mL	Dextrose 5%	9.3

Osmolality

Reconstituted with sterile water for injection, ampicillin (Wyeth) 100 mg/mL has an osmolality of 602 mOsm/kg.[50] At a concentration of 125 mg/mL, Wyeth's product was 702 mOsm/kg and Bristol's product was 675 mOsm/kg.[1071]

In another study, the osmolality of ampicillin sodium (Bristol) diluted in sodium chloride 0.9% was determined to be 493 mOsm/kg for ampicillin 50 mg/mL and 664 mOsm/kg for ampicillin 100 mg/mL.[1375]

The osmolality of ampicillin sodium 1 and 2 g was calculated for the following dilutions:[1054]

Diluent	Osmolality (mOsm/kg)	
	50 mL	100 mL
1 g		
Dextrose 5%	341	302
Sodium chloride 0.9%	368	328
2 g		
Dextrose 5%	418	346
Sodium chloride 0.9%	444	372

The following maximum ampicillin concentrations were recommended to achieve osmolalities suitable for peripheral infusion in fluid-restricted patients:[1180]

Diluent	Maximum Concentration (mg/mL)	Osmolality (mOsm/kg)
Dextrose 5%	62	583
Sodium chloride 0.9%	56	576
Sterile water for injection	112	588

Sodium Content

Ampicillin sodium contains approximately 2.9 mEq of sodium per gram of drug.[3291][3292][3293]

Administration

Ampicillin sodium is administered by intramuscular or direct intravenous injection[3291] or by intravenous infusion.[3291][3292][3293]

DOI: 10.37573/9781585286850.026

For direct intravenous injection, the reconstituted solutions of ampicillin prepared with 125-, 250-, and 500-mg vials should be administered slowly over 3 to 5 minutes; the reconstituted solutions of ampicillin prepared with 1- and 2-g vials should be administered slowly over at least 10 to 15 minutes.[3291] Solutions should not be administered more rapidly.[3291]

Stability

Intact vials of ampicillin sodium should be stored at controlled room temperature.[3291] [3292] [3293]

Reconstituted ampicillin solutions should be protected from freezing.[3291]

Manufacturers recommended the use of only freshly prepared solutions.[3291] [3292] [3293] Reconstituted solutions of ampicillin for intramuscular or direct intravenous injection should be administered within 1 hour after preparation.[3291] Reconstituted solutions of ampicillin prepared from the pharmacy bulk package should be further diluted for intravenous infusion within 1 hour after preparation.[3293]

The stability of ampicillin in solution under various conditions has been the subject of much work and numerous articles. Several characteristics of the stability of ampicillin have emerged from these studies:

. The stability is concentration dependent and decreases as the concentration increases.
. Sodium chloride 0.9% appears to be a suitable diluent for the intravenous infusion of ampicillin.
. The stability is greatly decreased in dextrose solutions.
. Storage temperature and the pH of solution affect the stability.

Storage and Usage Times

Savello and Shangraw offered the recommendations in Table 1 regarding storage conditions for ampicillin solutions.[210]

Table 1. Suggested storage conditions for ampicillin solutions[210]

Solution	Temperature (°C)	Maximum Storage
Reconstituted vial	−20	48 hr
	5	4 hr
	27	1 hr
Ampicillin 10 mg/mL in sodium chloride 0.9%	5	5 days
	27	24 hr
Ampicillin 10 mg/mL in dextrose 5%	5	4 hr
	27	2 hr

Concentration Effects

The effect of concentration on ampicillin stability has been attributed to a self-catalyzing effect.[210] As the concentration increases, so does the rate of decomposition.[170] [210] Savello and Shangraw reported that even though the initial pH values of various concentrations were 9.2 to 9.3, the higher concentrations of the drug maintained their pH longer because of their greater buffer capacity.[210] (See Table 2.)

Table 2. Percent degradation of ampicillin solutions after reconstitution with water for injection at 5°C after 8 hours[210]

Concentration	Percent Degradation
10 mg/mL	0.8
50 mg/mL	3.6
100 mg/mL	5.8
150 mg/mL	10.4
200 mg/mL	12.3
250 mg/mL	13.3

This concentration dependence of the stability of ampicillin has been related to the polymerization of penicillins in concentrated solutions.[601] [602] Dimerization is the predominant form of degradation with high ampicillin concentrations. The extent of this effect declines as the concentration drops but still remains significant in a 20-mg/mL solution. At lower concentrations, hydrolysis becomes the determining factor.[603]

At a concentration of 500 mg/mL, ampicillin formed dimers, trimers, tetramers, and pentamers during 24 hours of storage at 24°C in the dark. The polymer formed through a chain process by linkage of the amino group on the side chain to another molecule with a cleaved β-lactam ring.[1400]

In a 200-mg/mL solution of ampicillin adjusted to pH 8.5 and stored at 22°C, 90% of all decomposition products formed within 72 hours were dimers and polymers. In a 50-mg/mL solution, 70% of the decomposition products were dimers and polymers. However, a 10-mg/mL solution formed α-aminobenzylpenicilloic acid as the predominant decomposition product and a dimer concentration of 1 to 2%. The rate of dimerization was almost independent of pH in the range of 7 to 10, but increased strongly with increases in the initial ampicillin concentration.[858]

However, one study showed that if the pH of the solution was held constant at 8 or 9.15, there was little dependence of the rate of decomposition on concentration in the range of 20 to 100 mg/mL.[213]

Infusion Diluents

Infusion diluents also affect the stability of ampicillin. Sodium chloride 0.9% appears to be a suitable diluent for the intravenous infusion of ampicillin sodium.

Dextrose is thought to exhibit an immense catalytic effect on the hydrolysis of ampicillin sodium,[210] decreasing the stability about one-half when compared to sterile water or sodium chloride 0.9%.[213] This has been well documented and has been regarded as an incompatibility.[210] [213] (See Table 3.) This accelerated decomposition associated with dextrose extends to fructose as well, although it is not as extensive. It occurs in the alkaline pH range. Below pH 6 or 7, the decomposition rate with both dextrose and fructose appears to coincide with simple aqueous solutions.[604]

Table 3. Percent degradation of ampicillin 10 mg/ml in dextrose 5% in water according to temperature and time[210]

Temperature (°C)	4 hr	8 hr	24 hr
–20	13.6	22.3	45.6
0	6.2	11.6	26.3
5	10.1	15.2	29.7
27	21.3	31.1	46.5

Savello and Shangraw further showed that increasing the concentration of dextrose decreased the stability of ampicillin. (See Table 4.)

Table 4. Percent degradation of ampicillin 10 mg/ml at 5°C according to dextrose concentration and time[210]

Percent Dextrose	3 hr	7 hr
5	7.4	13.9
10	10.3	19.4
20	14.2	27.8

pH Effects

The pH of the solution also plays a role in its stability. Hydrolysis has been shown to be catalyzed by hydroxide ions. An increase of 1 pH unit in an ampicillin solution has been shown to increase the rate of decomposition 10-fold.[213]

The optimum pH for ampicillin stability has been variously reported as 5.8,[1072] 5.85 at 35°C,[215] approximately 5.2 at 25°C,[604] and 7.5 at room temperature.[209] The pH of ampicillin solutions, however, is in the alkaline range, with higher pH values having been reported at higher concentrations.[213] (See pH under Products.)

Ampicillin (Bristol) 10 g/L was tested for stability at pH 3.4 to 9.2 in various buffer additives. A 7.6% potency loss was reported in 12 hours at room temperature at pH 7.5. Significantly higher degradation rates occurred as the pH varied from 7.5, with about 70% degradation occurring in 12 hours at room temperature at pH 3.4 and 9.2.[209]

In another evaluation, rate constants for ampicillin degradation at various pH values were calculated for an aqueous solution at 25°C. The pH providing maximum stability was 5.2. When tested in dextrose 10%, a minimum rate of decomposition was observed at approximately pH 5 to 5.5. The amount of ampicillin degradation was 10% or less in 24 hours at 25°C within a pH range of about 2.75 to 6.75. At pH 8, the time to 10% decomposition was only about 2 hours.[604]

The stability of ampicillin (Beecham) 250 mg/50 mL and 1 g/100 mL in sodium chloride 0.9% in polyvinyl chloride (PVC) bags was compared with the stability of the same solutions buffered with potassium acid phosphate 13.6% injection. The 50- and 100-mL containers were buffered with 1 and 2 mL,

respectively, lowering the pH by nearly 2 pH units. Larger quantities of buffer caused precipitation. When stored at 5°C, the 250-mg/50 mL solution had a shelf life (t_{90}) of 12 days while the 1-g/100-mL solution had a shelf life of 6 days. This finding compares favorably to the shelf life of 1 to 2 days for the unbuffered solutions.[1820]

The stability of ampicillin 12 g/L prepared from ampicillin (AAP) 2 g/16 mL and ampicillin (Auromedics) 10 g/100 mL in sodium chloride 0.9% in 1-L bags was compared with the stability of the same solution buffered with sodium phosphate injection (American Regent) 10 mmol.[3418] Addition of the buffer lowered the average initial pH from 9.25 to 8.15.[3418] At a room temperature of 25°C, the buffered solution was stable for at least 48 hours (calculated time to 10% loss of 57.6 hours) as compared with at least 24 hours (calculated time to 10% loss ranging from 32 to 41.7 hours) for the unbuffered solution.[3418] The buffered solution also was stable for up to 48 hours at 2 to 8°C followed by up to 24 hours at a room temperature of 25°C.[3418]

Temperature Effects

The storage temperature of ampicillin solutions also may affect stability. It has been stated that freezing ampicillin solutions at –20°C increases the rate of decomposition over that at 5°C. For this reason, it has been recommended that ampicillin solutions not be stored in the frozen state.[123 213]

Apparent increased ampicillin decomposition was found at –20°C over that at 5°C in 2 of the 10-mg/mL solutions tested (Tables 3 and 5). In a study of ampicillin 20 mg/mL, about 4 to 6% greater loss was found at –20°C than at 5°C in 24 hours in both dextrose 5% and sodium chloride 0.9%.[208]

Table 5. Percent degradation of ampicillin 10 mg/ml in water according to temperature and time[210]

Temperature (°C)	4 hr	8 hr	24 hr
–20	1.3	1.9	5.2
5	0.4	0.8	2.0

An explanation of this phenomenon was proposed by Pincock and Kiovsky. Below the freezing point but above the eutectic temperature, there exists a liquid and solid phase in equilibrium. If it is assumed that –20°C is above the eutectic temperature, then liquid regions of a saturated solution of ampicillin exist, which result in increased decomposition.[214] Solutions of ampicillin stored at –78°C showed no decomposition within 24 hours.[210]

In a study of long-term storage, ampicillin (Ayerst) 1 g/50 mL in dextrose 5% and also sodium chloride 0.9% was tested in PVC containers frozen at –20°C for 30 days. In sodium chloride 0.9%, they reported approximately 10% decomposition in 1 day and approximately 70% decomposition in 30 days. In dextrose 5%, even greater decomposition occurred. They reported about 50% decomposition in 1 day and virtually total decomposition in 30 days.[299]

Ampicillin (Wyeth) 1 g/50 mL of dextrose 5% was tested in PVC bags frozen at –20°C for 30 days and then thawed by exposure to ambient temperature or microwave radiation. The admixtures showed essentially total loss of ampicillin activity determined microbiologically.[554] At −30°C, only 18% of the ampicillin remained in 30 days. A storage temperature of −70°C was required to retain at least 90% of the original activity for 30 days.[555]

The same concentration in sodium chloride 0.9% showed a 29% loss of ampicillin activity at −20°C but only about a 4% loss at −30 and −70°C after 30 days. Subsequent thawing of the −30 and −70°C samples by exposure to microwave radiation and storage at room temperature for 8 hours resulted in additional losses of activity, with the final concentration totaling about 90% of the initial amount. The authors concluded that ampicillin in sodium chloride 0.9% could be stored for 30 days at −30°C, which was presumably below the eutectic point for this admixture. However, −30°C was believed to be above the eutectic point for the dextrose 5% admixture because decomposition continued to occur.[555]

Even within acceptable limits for room temperature, significant differences in the rate of ampicillin decomposition can occur. In one solution at 20°C, a 10% ampicillin loss resulted in 44 hours. This same solution at 30°C exhibited a 10% loss in 12 hours. Over the range of 20 to 35°C, each 5°C rise approximately doubled the rate of decomposition.[604]

Sorption

Ampicillin was shown not to exhibit sorption to PVC bags and tubing, polyethylene tubing, Silastic tubing, polypropylene syringes, and trilayer solution bags composed of polyethylene, polyamide, and polypropylene.[536 606 1035 1918]

Filtration

Filtration of ampicillin sodium (Wyeth) is stated to result in no adsorption, yielding solutions that maintain their potency.[829]

Ampicillin (Bristol) 1.97 mg/mL in sodium chloride 0.9% was filtered through a 0.22-μm cellulose ester membrane filter (Ivex-HP, Millipore) over 5 hours. No significant drug loss due to binding to the filter was noted.[1034]

Central Venous Catheter

Ampicillin (Apothecon) 5 mg/mL in sodium chloride 0.9% was found to be compatible with the ARROWg+ard Blue Plus (Arrow International) chlorhexidine-bearing triple-lumen central catheter. Essentially complete delivery of the drug was found with little or no drug loss occurring. Furthermore, chlorhexidine delivered from the catheter remained at trace amounts with no substantial increase due to the delivery of the drug through the catheter.[2335]

Compatibility Information

Solution Compatibility

Ampicillin sodium

Test Soln Name	Mfr	Mfr	Conc/L or %	Remarks	Ref	C/I
Amino acids 4.25%, dextrose 25%	MG	BR	1 g	Increased microscopic particles in 24 hr at 5°C	349	I
Dextrose 5% in sodium chloride 0.45%		SZ	0 to 2 g	Less than 10% loss in 2 hr at 25°C	3291, 3293	C
Dextrose 5% in sodium chloride 0.45%		SZ	0 to 10 g	Less than 10% loss in 1 hr at 4°C	3291, 3293	C
Dextrose 5% in sodium chloride 0.9%	MG	BR	1 g	19% loss in 4 hr at 4°C and 17% in 2 hr at 25°C	105	I
Dextrose 5%		SZ	0 to 2 g	Less than 10% loss in 2 hr at 25°C	3291, 3293	C
Dextrose 5%		SZ	10 to 20 g	Less than 10% loss in 1 hr at 25°C	3291, 3293	C
Dextrose 5%		SZ	0 to 20 g	Less than 10% loss in 1 hr at 4°C	3291, 3293	C
Dextrose 5%		SZ	10 g	Stable for 2 hr at 25°C	3292	C
Dextrose 5%		SZ	20 g	Stable for 1 hr at 25°C	3292	C
Dextrose 5%		BE	1 g	24% loss in 8 hr at 25°C	211	I
Dextrose 5%		AY	2 and 4 g	10% loss in 4 hr at room temperature	99	I
Dextrose 5%	MG	BR	1 g	11% loss in 24 hr at 4°C and 21% in 24 hr at 25°C	105	I
Dextrose 5%	AB	AY	2 g	10% loss in 24 hr at 5°C and 20% in 24 hr at 25°C	88	I
Dextrose 5%		BR	20 g	19% loss in 4 hr at 25°C. 40% loss in 24 hr at 25°C	208	I
Dextrose 5%		BR	10 g	46% loss in 24 hr at −20°C. 30% loss in 24 hr at 5°C. 47% loss in 24 hr at 27°C	210	I

Solution Compatibility (Cont.)

Test Soln Name	Mfr	Mfr	Conc/L or %	Remarks	Ref	C/I
Dextrose 5%	BA[a], TR	AY	20 g	40% loss in 24 hr at 22°C and 30% in 24 hr at 5°C	298	I
Dextrose 5%			2 g	5% loss in 2 hr and 38% in 24 hr at 20 to 25°C	307	I
Dextrose 5%			4 g	10% loss in 2 hr and 45% in 24 hr at 25°C	307	I
Dextrose 5%			10 g	12% loss in 2 hr and 50% in 24 hr at 25°C	307	I
Dextrose 5%	TR[b]	WY	20 g	35% loss in 8 hr and 52% in 24 hr at room temperature	554	I
Dextrose 5%	PH	BAY	2 g	10% loss in 3.5 hr at 25°C	604	I
Dextrose 5%	PH	BAY	5 g	10% loss in 2.5 hr at 25°C	604	I
Dextrose 5%	PH	BAY	15 g	10% loss in 2 hr at 25°C	604	I
Dextrose 5%			4 g	10% loss in 4 hr and 28% in 24 hr at room temperature	768	I
Dextrose 5%			5 g	7% loss in 2 hr and 15% loss in 4 hr at 29°C. 8% loss in 8 hr at 4°C	773	I
Dextrose 5%	TR[b]	WY	10 and 20 g	60% loss in 48 hr at 25°C and in 7 days at 4°C	1001	I
Dextrose 5%	TR[b]	WY	20 g	50% loss at 24°C and 28% at 4°C in 1 day	1035	I
Dextrose 5%	[b]	BR	20 g	No loss during 2 hr storage and 1-hr simulated infusion	1774	C
Dextrose 10%	MG	BR	1 g	17% loss in 6 hr at 4°C and 18% in 4 hr at 25°C	105	I
Isolyte M in dextrose 5%	MG	BR	1 g	Stable for 24 hr at 4 and 25°C	105	C
Isolyte P in dextrose 5%	MG	BR	1 g	Stable for 24 hr at 4 and 25°C	105	C
Ringer's injection		AY	2 and 4 g	10% loss in 24 hr at room temperature	99	C
Ringer's injection		BAY	2 g	10% loss in 40 hr at 25°C	604	C
Ringer's injection		BAY	5 g	10% loss in 25 hr at 25°C	604	C
Ringer's injection		BAY	15 g	10% loss in 20 hr at 25°C	604	I
Ringer's injection			5 g	9% loss in 8 hr and 18% loss in 24 hr at 29°C. 3% loss in 24 hr at 4°C	773	I
Ringer's injection, lactated		SZ	0 to 30 g	Less than 10% loss in 8 hr at 25°C and 24 hr at 4°C	3291, 3293	C
Ringer's injection, lactated		BE	1 g	17% loss in 4 hr at 25°C	211	I
Ringer's injection, lactated		BR	1 g	11% loss in 12 hr at 25°C	87	I
Ringer's injection, lactated	MG	BR	1 g	17% loss in 6 hr at 4°C and 25% in 6 hr at 25°C	105	I
Ringer's injection, lactated			5 g	20% loss in 2 hr at 29°C and 11% in 4 hr at 4°C	773	I
Sodium chloride 0.9%		SZ	0 to 20 g	Less than 10% loss in 48 hr at 4°C	3291, 3293	C
Sodium chloride 0.9%		SZ	0 to 30 g	Less than 10% loss in 8 hr at 25°C	3291, 3293	C
Sodium chloride 0.9%		SZ	30 g	Less than 10% loss in 24 hr at 4°C	3291, 3293	C
Sodium chloride 0.9%		SZ	10 g	Stable for 8 hr at 25°C	3292	C
Sodium chloride 0.9%		SZ	40 g	Stable for 6 hr at 25°C	3292	C
Sodium chloride 0.9%		BAY	2 g	10% loss in over 48 hr at 25°C	604	C
Sodium chloride 0.9%		BAY	5 g	10% loss in 38 hr at 25°C	604	C
Sodium chloride 0.9%		BAY	15 g	10% loss in 33 hr at 25°C	604	C
Sodium chloride 0.9%		BE	10 g	Less than 10% decomposition in 24 hr at 25°C	113	C

Solution Compatibility (Cont.)

Test Soln Name	Mfr	Mfr	Conc/L or %	Remarks	Ref	C/I
Sodium chloride 0.9%		BR	6 g	9% loss in 24 hr at room temperature. 1% loss in 24 hr under refrigeration	127	C
Sodium chloride 0.9%	MG	BR	1 g	Activity retained for 24 hr at 4 and 25°C	105	C
Sodium chloride 0.9%		AY	2 to 30 g	10% loss in 24 hr at room temperature	99	C
Sodium chloride 0.9%		BR	20 g	4% loss in 24 hr at 5°C. 12 to 16% loss in 24 hr at 25°C	208	C
Sodium chloride 0.9%		BR	10 g	4% loss in 24 hr at −20°C. 3% loss in 24 hr at 5°C. 8% loss in 24 hr at 27°C	210	C
Sodium chloride 0.9%		BR	5, 10, 15, 20 g	6 to 12% loss in 24 hr at 25°C	212	C
Sodium chloride 0.9%		BR	5, 10, 15, 20, 30, 40 g	1 to 6% loss in 24 hr at 5°C	212	C
Sodium chloride 0.9%	BA[a], TR	AY	20 g	Activity retained for 24 hr at 5 and 22°C	298	C
Sodium chloride 0.9%			2, 4, 10 g	10% loss in 24 hr at 20 to 25°C	307	C
Sodium chloride 0.9%		BE	1 g	12% loss in 12 hr at 25°C and 28% in 24 hr at 25°C	211	I
Sodium chloride 0.9%		BR	30 and 40 g	15% loss in 24 hr at 25°C	212	I
Sodium chloride 0.9%			4 g	10% loss in 8 hr and 19% loss in 24 hr at room temperature	768	I
Sodium chloride 0.9%			5 g	10% loss in 8 hr at 29°C and 3% loss in 24 hr at 4°C	773	I
Sodium chloride 0.9%	TR[b]	WY	20 g	15% loss in 1 day and 30% in 4 days at 24°C. 6% loss in 1 day and 10% in 4 days at 4°C. 13% loss in 4 days at −7°C	1035	I
Sodium chloride 0.9%	[b]	BR	20 g	No loss during 2 hr storage and 1-hr simulated infusion	1774	C
Sodium chloride 0.9%	AB[c]	WY	60 g	Stable for 24 hr at 5°C. 10% loss in 6 hr and 20% loss in 24 hr during administration at 30°C via portable pump	1779	C
Sodium chloride 0.9%	BA[b]	BE	10 g	Visually compatible with 10% loss in 2 days at 5°C	1820	C
Sodium chloride 0.9%	BA[b]	BE	5 g	Visually compatible with 10% loss in 1 day at 5°C	1820	C
Sodium lactate ⅙ M		BR	1 g	37% loss in 4 hr at 25°C	211	I
Sodium lactate ⅙ M		AY	up to 30 g	10% loss in 6 hr at room temperature	99	I
TPN #21[d]		BR	1 g	Activity retained for 24 hr at 4°C	87	C
TPN #21[d]		BR	1 g	12 to 25% ampicillin loss in 24 hr at 25°C	87	I
TPN #52[d]		AST	1.5 g	69% ampicillin loss in 24 hr at 29°C	440	I
TPN #53[d]		AST	1.5 g	22% ampicillin loss in 24 hr at 29°C	440	I
TPN #107[d]			1 and 3 g	Activity retained for 24 hr at 21°C	1326	C

[a] Tested in both PVC and glass containers.

[b] Tested in PVC containers.

[c] Tested in portable pump reservoirs (Pharmacia Deltec).

[d] Refer to Appendix for the composition of parenteral nutrition solutions. TPN indicates a 2-in-1 admixture.

Additive Compatibility

Ampicillin sodium

Test Drug	Mfr	Conc/L or %	Mfr	Conc/L or %	Test Solution	Remarks	Ref	C/I
Amikacin sulfate	BR	5 g	BR	30 g	D5LR, D5R, D5S, D5W, D10W, LR, NS, R, SL	Over 10% ampicillin loss in 4 hr at 25°C	293	I
Aztreonam	SQ	10 g	WY	20 g	D5W[a]	10% ampicillin loss in 2 hr and 10% aztreonam loss in 3 hr at 25°C. 10% ampicillin loss in 24 hr and 10% aztreonam loss in 8 hr at 4°C	1001	I
Aztreonam	SQ	10 g	WY	5 g	D5W[a]	10% ampicillin loss in 3 hr and 10% aztreonam loss in 7 hr at 25°C. 10% loss of both drugs in 48 hr at 4°C	1001	I
Aztreonam	SQ	20 g	WY	20 g	D5W[a]	10% ampicillin loss in 4 hr and 10% aztreonam loss in 5 hr at 25°C. 10% loss of both drugs in 24 hr at 4°C	1001	I
Aztreonam	SQ	20 g	WY	5 g	D5W[a]	10% ampicillin loss in 5 hr and 10% aztreonam loss in 8 hr at 25°C. 10% ampicillin loss in 48 hr and 10% aztreonam loss in 72 hr at 4°C	1001	I
Aztreonam	SQ	10 g	WY	20 g	NS[a]	10% ampicillin loss in 24 hr and 2% aztreonam loss in 48 hr at 25°C. 10% ampicillin loss in 2 days and 9% aztreonam loss in 7 days at 4°C	1001	C
Aztreonam	SQ	10 g	WY	5 g	NS[a]	10% ampicillin loss and no aztreonam loss in 48 hr at 25°C. 10% ampicillin loss in 3 days and 8% aztreonam loss in 7 days at 4°C	1001	C
Aztreonam	SQ	20 g	WY	20 g	NS[a]	10% ampicillin loss in 24 hr and 5% aztreonam loss in 48 hr at 25°C. 10% ampicillin loss in 2 days and 7% aztreonam loss in 7 days at 4°C	1001	C
Aztreonam	SQ	20 g	WY	5 g	NS[a]	10% ampicillin loss and no aztreonam loss in 48 hr at 25°C. 10% ampicillin loss and 5% aztreonam loss in 7 days at 4°C	1001	C
Cefepime HCl	BR	40 g	BR	1 g	D5W	4% ampicillin loss in 8 hr at room temperature and 5°C. 7% cefepime loss in 8 hr at room temperature and no loss in 8 hr at 5°C	1682	?
Cefepime HCl	BR	40 g	BR	1 g	NS	No ampicillin loss in 24 hr at room temperature and 9% loss in 48 hr at 5°C. 5% cefepime loss in 24 hr at room temperature and 2% loss in 72 hr at 5°C	1682	C
Cefepime HCl	BR	40 g	BR	10 g	D5W	6% ampicillin loss in 2 hr at room temperature and 2% loss in 8 hr at 5°C. 7% cefepime loss in 2 hr at room temperature and 8 hr at 5°C	1682	I
Cefepime HCl	BR	40 g	BR	10 g	NS	6% ampicillin loss in 8 hr at room temperature and 9% loss in 48 hr at 5°C. 8% cefepime loss in 8 hr at room temperature and 10% loss in 48 hr at 5°C	1682	I
Cefepime HCl	BR	4 g	BR	40 g	D5W	10% ampicillin loss in 1 hr at room temperature and 9% loss in 2 hr at 5°C. 25% cefepime loss in 1 hr at room temperature and 9% loss in 2 hr at 5°C	1682	I
Cefepime HCl	BR	4 g	BR	40 g	NS	5% ampicillin loss in 8 hr at room temperature and 4% loss in 8 hr at 5°C. 4% cefepime loss in 8 hr at room temperature and 6% loss in 8 hr at 5°C	1682	?
Chlorpromazine HCl	BP	200 mg	BP	2 g	D5W, NS	Precipitates immediately	26	I
Clindamycin phosphate	UP	24 g	WY	10 and 20 g	NS	Physically compatible	1035	C
Clindamycin phosphate	UP	3 g	WY	3.7 g	NS	Physically compatible with 4% ampicillin loss in 1 day at 24°C	1035	C

Additive Compatibility (Cont.)

Test Drug	Mfr	Conc/L or %	Mfr	Conc/L or %	Test Solution	Remarks	Ref	C/I
Dextran 40		10%		4 g	D5W	46% ampicillin loss in 24 hr at 20°C	834	I
Dextran 40	PH	10%	AY	8 g	D5W	50% loss in 24 hr at room temperature	99	I
Dextran 40	PH	10%	BAY	15 g	D5W	10% ampicillin loss in 1.5 hr at 25°C	604	I
Dextran 40	PH	10%	BAY	2 g	D5W	10% ampicillin loss in 3.5 hr at 25°C	604	I
Dextran 40	PH	10%	BAY	5 g	D5W	10% ampicillin loss in 2.3 hr at 25°C	604	I
Dextran 40	PH	10%	AY	8 g	NS	25% loss in 24 hr at room temperature	99	I
Dextran 40	PH	10%	BAY	15 g	NS	10% ampicillin loss in 2.3 hr at 25°C	604	I
Dextran 40	PH	10%	BAY	2 g	NS	10% ampicillin loss in 2.8 hr at 25°C	604	I
Dextran 40	PH	10%	BAY	5 g	NS	10% ampicillin loss in 2.5 hr at 25°C	604	I
Dopamine HCl	AS	800 mg	BR	4 g	D5W	Color change. 36% ampicillin loss in 6 hr at 23 to 25°C. Dopamine loss in 6 hr	78	I
Erythromycin lactobionate	AB	3 g	WY	3.7 g	NS	Physically compatible with 6% ampicillin loss in 1 day at 24°C	1035	C
Fat emulsion, intravenous		10%		20 g		15% ampicillin loss in 24 hr at 23°C	37	I
Fat emulsion, intravenous	VT	10%	BE	2 g		Lipid coalescence in 24 hr at 25 and 8°C	825	I
Floxacillin sodium	BE	20 g	BE	20 g	NS	Physically compatible for 72 hr at 15 and 30°C	1479	C
Furosemide	HO	1 g	BE	20 g	NS	Physically compatible for 72 hr at 15 and 30°C	1479	C
Gentamicin sulfate	RS	160 mg	BE	8 g	D5¼S, D5W, NS	50% gentamicin loss in 2 hr at room temperature	157	I
Gentamicin sulfate		100 mg		1 g	TPN #107[b]	42% gentamicin loss and 25% ampicillin loss in 24 hr at 21°C	1326	I
Heparin sodium		32,000 units		2 g	NS	Physically compatible and heparin activity retained for 24 hr	57	C
Heparin sodium		12,000 units	BR	1 g	D10W, LR, NS	Ampicillin stable for 24 hr at 4°C	87	C
Heparin sodium	OR	20,000 units	BE	10 g	NS	Both stable for 24 hr at 25°C	113	C
Heparin sodium		12,000 units	BR	1 g	D5S	15% ampicillin decomposition in 24 hr at 4°C	87	I
Heparin sodium		12,000 units	BR	1 g	D5S, D10W, LR	20 to 25% ampicillin decomposition in 24 hr at 25°C	87	I
Hetastarch in sodium chloride 0.9%		6%		4 g	NS	18% loss in 6 hr and 35% in 24 hr at 20°C	834	I
Hydralazine HCl	BP	80 mg	BP	2 g	D5W	Yellow color produced	26	I
Hydrocortisone sodium succinate		200 and 400 mg	BR	1 g	LR	Ampicillin stable for 24 hr at 25°C	87	C
Hydrocortisone sodium succinate		50 and 100 mg	BR	1 g	LR	14% ampicillin loss in 12 hr at 25°C	87	I
Hydrocortisone sodium succinate		200 mg	BE	20 g	D2.5½S, D2.5S, D5¼S, D5½S, D5S, D10S	32% ampicillin loss in 6 hr at 25°C	89	I

Additive Compatibility (Cont.)

Test Drug	Mfr	Conc/L or %	Mfr	Conc/L or %	Test Solution	Remarks	Ref	C/I
Hydrocortisone sodium succinate		200 mg	BE	20 g	D5W	23% ampicillin loss in 6 hr at 25°C	89	I
Hydrocortisone sodium succinate		200 mg	BE	20 g	NS	18% ampicillin loss in 6 hr at 25°C	89	I
Hydrocortisone sodium succinate		1.8 g	BR	1 g	D5S, D10W, IM, IP, LR	11 to 28% ampicillin loss in 24 hr at 25°C	87	I
Hydrocortisone sodium succinate		1.8 g	BR	1 g	D5S, D5W, D10W, IM, IP, LR, NS	Ampicillin stable for 24 hr at 4°C	87	C
Lincomycin HCl	PHU, XGN					Physically compatible for 24 hr at room temperature	3164, 3165	C
Metronidazole	SE	5 g	BR	20 g		9% ampicillin loss in 22 hr at 25°C and in 12 days at 5°C. No metronidazole loss	993	C
Prochlorperazine mesylate	BP	100 mg	BP	2 g	D5W, NS	Precipitates immediately	26	I
Ranitidine HCl	GL	100 mg		2 g	D5W	Physically compatible for 24 hr at ambient temperature under fluorescent light. Ampicillin instability is determining factor	1151	?
Ranitidine HCl	GL	50 mg and 2 g		1 g	NS	Physically compatible. Ranitidine stable for 24 hr at 25°C. Ampicillin not tested	1515	C
Sodium bicarbonate		1.4%	AY	2 and 4 g		10% ampicillin loss in 6 hr at room temperature	99	I
Sodium bicarbonate		1.4%	BAY	15 g		10% ampicillin loss in 10 hr at 25°C	604	I
Sodium bicarbonate		1.4%	BAY	2 g		10% ampicillin loss in 17 hr at 25°C	604	I
Sodium bicarbonate		1.4%	BAY	5 g		10% ampicillin loss in 14 hr at 25°C	604	I
Verapamil HCl	KN	80 mg	BR	4 g	D5W, NS	Physically compatible for 24 hr	764	C
Verapamil HCl	SE	c	WY	40 g	D5W, NS	Cloudy solution clears with agitation	1166	?

a Tested in PVC containers.

b Refer to Appendix for the composition of parenteral nutrition solutions. TPN indicates a 2-in-1 admixture.

c Final concentration unspecified.

Drugs in Syringe Compatibility

Ampicillin sodium

Test Drug	Mfr	Amt	Mfr	Amt	Remarks	Ref	C/I
Chloramphenicol sodium succinate	PD	250 and 400 mg/mL in 1.5 to 2 mL	AY	500 mg	No precipitate or color change within 1 hr at room temperature	99	C
Chloramphenicol sodium succinate	PD	250 and 400 mg/1 mL	AY	500 mg	Physically compatible for 1 hr at room temperature	300	C
Colistimethate sodium	PX	40 mg/2 mL	AY	500 mg	No precipitate or color change within 1 hr at room temperature	99	C
Colistimethate sodium	PX	500 mg/2 mL	AY	500 mg	Physically compatible for 1 hr at room temperature	300	C

Drugs in Syringe Compatibility (Cont.)

Test Drug	Mfr	Amt	Mfr	Amt	Remarks	Ref	C/I
Dimenhydrinate		10 mg/1 mL		50 mg/1 mL	Clear solution	2569	C
Erythromycin lactobionate	AB	300 mg/6 mL	AY	500 mg	Precipitate forms in 1 hr at room temperature	300	I
Gentamicin sulfate		80 mg/2 mL	AY	500 mg	Physically incompatible within 1 hr at room temperature	99	I
Heparin sodium		2500 units/1 mL		2 g	Physically compatible for at least 5 min	1053	C
Hydromorphone HCl	KN	2, 10, 40 mg/1 mL	AY	250 mg/1 mL	Visually compatible but 10% loss of ampicillin in 5 hr at room temperature	2082	I
Iohexol	WI	64.7%, 5 mL	BR	30 mg/1 mL	Physically compatible for at least 2 hr	1438	C
Iopamidol	SQ	61%, 5 mL	BR	30 mg/1 mL	Physically compatible for at least 2 hr	1438	C
Iothalamate meglumine	MA	60%, 5 mL	BR	30 mg/1 mL	Physically compatible for at least 2 hr	1438	C
Ioxaglate meglumine–ioxaglate sodium	MA	5 mL	BR	30 mg/1 mL	Physically compatible for at least 2 hr	1438	C
Lidocaine HCl		0.5 and 2.5%/1.5 mL	BE	500 mg	Physically compatible	89	C
Lidocaine HCl		0.5 and 2.5%/1.5 mL	BE	250 mg	Occasional turbidity	89	I
Lincomycin HCl	UP	600 mg/2 mL	AY	500 mg	Physically incompatible within 1 hr at room temperature	99	I
Lincomycin HCl	UP	600 mg/2 mL	AY	500 mg	Precipitate forms within 1 hr at room temperature	300	I
Metoclopramide HCl	RB	10 mg/2 mL	BR	250 mg/2.5 mL	Incompatible. If mixed, use immediately	1167	I
Metoclopramide HCl	RB	10 mg/2 mL	BR	1 g/10 mL	Incompatible. If mixed, use immediately	1167	I
Metoclopramide HCl	RB	160 mg/32 mL	BR	1 g/10 mL	Incompatible. If mixed, use immediately	1167	I
Pantoprazole sodium	a	4 mg/1 mL		250 mg/1 mL	Clear solution	2574	C
Polymyxin B sulfate	BW	25 mg/1.5 mL	AY	500 mg	Physically compatible for 1 hr at room temperature	300	C
Polymyxin B sulfate	BW	25 mg/1.5 mL	AY	250 mg	Precipitate forms within 1 hr at room temperature	300	I
Streptomycin sulfate		1 g/2 mL	AY	500 mg	No precipitate or color change within 1 hr at room temperature	99	C
Streptomycin sulfate	BP	1 g/2 mL	AY	500 mg	Physically compatible for 1 hr at room temperature	300	C
Streptomycin sulfate	BP	1 g/1.5 mL	AY	500 mg	Syrupy solution forms	300	I

[a] Test performed using the formulation WITHOUT edetate disodium.

Y-Site Injection Compatibility (1:1 Mixture)

Ampicillin sodium

Test Drug	Mfr	Conc	Mfr	Conc	Remarks	Ref	C/I
Acyclovir sodium	BW	5 mg/mL[a]	WY	20 mg/mL[b]	Physically compatible for 4 hr at 25°C	1157	C
Alprostadil	BED	7.5 mcg/mL[m]	SQ	100 mg/mL[n]	Visually compatible for 1 hr	2746	C
Amifostine	USB	10 mg/mL[a]	WY	20 mg/mL[b]	Physically compatible for 4 hr at 23°C	1845	C
Anidulafungin	VIC	0.5 mg/mL[a]	APC	20 mg/mL[b]	Physically compatible for 4 hr at 23°C	2617	C
Aztreonam	SQ	40 mg/mL[a]	WY	20 mg/mL[b]	Physically compatible for 4 hr at 23°C	1758	C
Bivalirudin	TMC	5 mg/mL[a]	APO	20 mg/mL[b]	Physically compatible for 4 hr at 23°C	2373	C
Calcium gluconate	AST	4 mg/mL[b]	WY	40 mg/mL[b]	Physically compatible for 3 hr	1316	C

Y-Site Injection Compatibility (1:1 Mixture) (Cont.)

Test Drug	Mfr	Conc	Mfr	Conc	Remarks	Ref	C/I
Calcium gluconate	AST	4 mg/mL[a]	WY	40 mg/mL[b]	Slight color change in 1 hr	1316	I
Cangrelor tetrasodium	TMC	1 mg/mL[b]		20[b] and 40[b] mg/mL	Physically compatible for 4 hr	3243	C
Caspofungin acetate	ME	0.7 mg/mL[b]	APP	20 mg/mL[b]	Immediate white turbid precipitate forms	2758	I
Cisatracurium besylate	GW	0.1 and 2 mg/mL[a]	SKB	20 mg/mL[b]	Physically compatible for 4 hr at 23°C	2074	C
Cisatracurium besylate	GW	5 mg/mL[a]	SKB	20 mg/mL[b]	Gray subvisible haze forms in 1 hr	2074	I
Clarithromycin	AB	4 mg/mL[a]	BE	40 mg/mL[a]	Visually compatible for 72 hr at both 30 and 17°C	2174	C
Cloxacillin sodium	SMX	100 mg/mL	NOP	250 mg/mL	Physically compatible for up to 4 hr at room temperature	3245	C
Cyclophosphamide	MJ	20 mg/mL[a]	BR	20 mg/mL[b]	Physically compatible for 4 hr at 25°C	1194	C
Dexmedetomi-dine HCl	AB	4 mcg/mL[b]	APO	20 mg/mL[b]	Physically compatible for 4 hr at 23°C	2383	C
Diltiazem HCl	MMD	5 mg/mL	WY	100 mg/mL[b]	Cloudiness forms	1807	I
Diltiazem HCl	MMD	1 mg/mL[b]	WY	100 mg/mL[b]	Visually compatible	1807	C
Diltiazem HCl	MMD	5 mg/mL	WY	10 and 20 mg/mL[b]	Visually compatible	1807	C
Docetaxel	RPR	0.9 mg/mL[a]	SKB	20 mg/mL[b]	Physically compatible for 4 hr at 23°C	2224	C
Doxapram HCl	RB	2 mg/mL[a]	APO	50 mg/mL[b]	Visually compatible for 4 hr at 23°C	2470	C
Doxorubicin HCl liposomal	SEQ	0.4 mg/mL[a]	SKB	20 mg/mL[b]	Physically compatible for 4 hr at 23°C	2087	C
Enalaprilat	MSD	0.05 mg/mL[b]	BR	10 mg/mL[b]	Physically compatible for 24 hr at room temperature under fluorescent light	1355	C
Epinephrine HCl	ES	32 mcg/mL[c]	WY	40 mg/mL[b]	Slight color change in 3 hr	1316	I
Esmolol HCl	DCC	10 mg/mL[a]	WY	20 mg/mL[b]	Physically compatible for 24 hr at 22°C	1169	C
Etoposide phosphate	BR	5 mg/mL[a]	APC	20 mg/mL[b]	Physically compatible for 4 hr at 23°C	2218	C
Famotidine	MSD	0.2 mg/mL[a]	ES	20 mg/mL[b]	Physically compatible for 14 hr	1196	C
Famotidine	ME	2 mg/mL[b]		20 mg/mL[b]	Visually compatible for 4 hr at 22°C	1936	C
Fenoldopam mesylate	AB	80 mcg/mL[b]	APO	20 mg/mL[b]	Yellow color forms in 4 hr	2467	I
Filgrastim	AMG	30 mcg/mL[a]	WY	20 mg/mL[a]	Physically compatible for 4 hr at 22°C	1687	C
Fluconazole	RR	2 mg/mL	WY	20 mg/mL	Cloudiness develops	1407	I
Fludarabine phosphate	BX	1 mg/mL[a]	BR	20 mg/mL[b]	Visually compatible for 4 hr at 22°C	1439	C
Foscarnet sodium	AST	24 mg/mL	WY	20 mg/mL	Physically compatible for 24 hr at room temperature under fluorescent light	1335	C
Gemcitabine HCl	LI	10 mg/mL[b]	SKB	20 mg/mL[b]	Physically compatible for 4 hr at 23°C	2226	C
Granisetron HCl	SKB	0.05 mg/mL[a]	MAR	20 mg/mL[b]	Physically compatible for 4 hr at 23°C	2000	C
Heparin sodium	TR	50 units/mL	WY	20 mg/mL[b]	Visually compatible for 4 hr at 25°C	1793	C
Heparin sodium	LEO	10 and 5000 units/mL[b]	NOP	10 mg/mL[b]	Physically compatible with little change in heparin activity in 14 days at 4 and 37°C. Antibiotic not tested	2684	C

Y-Site Injection Compatibility (1:1 Mixture) (Cont.)

Test Drug	Mfr	Conc	Mfr	Conc	Remarks	Ref	C/I
Heparin sodium[o]	RI	1000 units/L[d]	BR	25, 50, 100, 125 mg/mL	Physically compatible for 4 hr at room temperature	322	C
Hetastarch in lactated electrolyte	AB	6%	APC	20 mg/mL[b]	Physically compatible for 4 hr at 23°C	2339	C
Hetastarch in sodium chloride 0.9%	DCC	6%	BR	20 mg/mL[a]	Visually compatible for 4 hr at room temperature	1313	C
Hetastarch in sodium chloride 0.9%	DCC	6%	BR	20 mg/mL[a]	One or two particles in one of five vials. Fine white strands appeared immediately during Y-site infusion	1315	I
Hydralazine HCl	SO	1 mg/mL[b]	WY	40 mg/mL[b]	Moderate color change in 3 hr	1316	I
Hydralazine HCl	SO	1 mg/mL[a]	WY	40 mg/mL[b]	Moderate color change in 1 hr	1316	I
Hydrocortisone sodium succinate[p]	UP	100 mg/L[d]	BR	25, 50, 100, 125 mg/mL	Physically compatible for 4 hr at room temperature	322	C
Hydromorphone HCl	WY	0.2 mg/mL[a]	BR	20 mg/mL[b]	Physically compatible for 4 hr at 25°C	987	C
Hydromorphone HCl	KN	2, 10, 40 mg/mL	AY	20[a] and 250 mg/mL	Visually compatible. Hydromorphone stable for 24 hr. 10% ampicillin loss in 5 hr	1532	I
Hydroxyethyl starch 130/0.4 in sodium chloride 0.9%	FRK	6%	NOP	10, 25, 40 mg/mL[a]	Visually compatible for 24 hr at room temperature	2770	C
Insulin, regular	LI	0.2 unit/mL[b]	WY	20 mg/mL[b]	Physically compatible for 2 hr at 25°C	1395	C
Labetalol HCl	SC	1 mg/mL[a]	WY	10 mg/mL[b]	Physically compatible for 24 hr at 18°C	1171	C
Letermovir	ME	[b]		[b]	Physically compatible	3398	C
Levofloxacin	OMN	5 mg/mL[a]	MAR	50 mg/mL	Visually compatible for 4 hr at 24°C	2233	C
Linezolid	PHU	2 mg/mL	APC	20 mg/mL[b]	Physically compatible for 4 hr at 23°C	2264	C
Magnesium sulfate	IX	16.7, 33.3, 66.7, 100 mg/mL[a]	WY	20 mg/mL[b]	Physically compatible for at least 4 hr at 32°C	813	C
Melphalan HCl	BW	0.1 mg/mL[b]	WY	20 mg/mL[b]	Physically compatible for 3 hr at 22°C	1557	C
Meperidine HCl	WY	10 mg/mL[a]	BR	20 mg/mL[b]	Physically compatible for 4 hr at 25°C	987	C
Meropenem		50 mg/mL	NOP	250 mg/mL	Physically compatible for 4 hr at room temperature	3538	C
Midazolam HCl	RC	1 mg/mL[a]	WY	20 mg/mL[b]	Haze forms immediately	1847	I
Milrinone lactate	SS	0.2 mg/mL[a]	APO	100 mg/mL[b]	Visually compatible for 4 hr at 25°C	2381	C
Morphine sulfate	WI	1 mg/mL[a]	BR	20 mg/mL[b]	Physically compatible for 4 hr at 25°C	987	C
Multivitamins	USV	5 mL/L[a]	AY	1 g/50 mL[c]	Physically compatible for 24 hr at room temperature	323	C
Nicardipine HCl	DCC	0.1 mg/mL[a b]	BR	10 mg/mL[a b]	Turbidity forms immediately	235	I
Ondansetron HCl	GL	1 mg/mL[b]	BR	20 mg/mL[b]	Immediate turbidity and precipitation	1365	I
Pantoprazole sodium	ALT[l]	0.16 to 0.8 mg/mL[b]	NVP	10 to 40 mg/mL[a]	Visually compatible for 12 hr at 23°C	2603	C
Pemetrexed disodium	LI	20 mg/mL[b]	APC	20 mg/mL[b]	Physically compatible for 4 hr at 23°C	2564	C
Phytonadione	MSD	0.4 mg/mL[c]	WY	40 mg/mL[b]	Physically compatible for 3 hr	1316	C
Potassium chloride		40 mEq/L[d]	BR	25, 50, 100, 125 mg/mL	Physically compatible for 4 hr at room temperature	322	C

Y-Site Injection Compatibility (1:1 Mixture) (Cont.)

Test Drug	Mfr	Conc	Mfr	Conc	Remarks	Ref	C/I
Propofol	ZEN[q]	10 mg/mL	WY	20 mg/mL[b]	Physically compatible for 1 hr at 23°C	2066	C
Remifentanil HCl	GW	0.025 and 0.25 mg/mL[b]	SKB	20 mg/mL[b]	Physically compatible for 4 hr at 23°C	2075	C
Sargramostim	IMM	10 mcg/mL[b]	BR	20 mg/mL[b]	Few small particles form in 4 hr	1436	I
Tacrolimus	FUJ	1 mg/mL[b]	WY	20 mg/mL[a]	Visually compatible for 24 hr at 25°C	1630	C
Teniposide	BR	0.1 mg/mL[a]	WY	20 mg/mL[b]	Physically compatible for 4 hr at 23°C	1725	C
Theophylline	TR	4 mg/mL	WY	20 mg/mL[b]	Visually compatible for 6 hr at 25°C	1793	C
Thiotepa	IMM[e]	1 mg/mL[a]	WY	20 mg/mL[b]	Physically compatible for 4 hr at 23°C	1861	C
TNA #73[f]		32.5 mL[g]	BR	40 mg/mL[b]	Visually compatible for 4 hr at 25°C	1008	C
TNA #218 to #226[f]			SKB	20 mg/mL[b]	Visually compatible for 4 hr at 23°C	2215	C
TPN #54[f]					Precipitate forms within 30 min at 22°C	1045	I
TPN #61[f]		[h]	WY	250 mg/1.3 mL[i]	Heavy precipitate of calcium phosphate	1012	I
TPN #61[f]		[j]	WY	1.5 g/7.5 mL[i]	Heavy precipitate of calcium phosphate	1012	I
TPN #203, #204[f]			APC	100 and 250 mg/mL	White precipitate forms immediately	1974	I
TPN #212 to #215[f]			SKB	20 mg/mL[b]	Visually compatible for 4 hr at 23°C	2109	C
Vancomycin HCl	AB	20 mg/mL[a]	SKB	250 mg/mL[k]	Transient precipitate forms	2189	?
Vancomycin HCl	AB	20 mg/mL[a]	SKB	1, 10, 50 mg/mL[b]	Physically compatible for 4 hr at 23°C	2189	C
Vancomycin HCl	AB	2 mg/mL[a]	SKB	1[b], 10[b], 50[b], 250[k] mg/mL	Physically compatible for 4 hr at 23°C	2189	C
Verapamil HCl	SE	2.5 mg/mL	WY	40 mg/mL[c]	White precipitate forms immediately. 91% of verapamil precipitated	1166	I
Vinorelbine tartrate	BW	1 mg/mL[b]	WY	20 mg/mL[b]	Tiny particles form immediately. White particles in turbidity in 1 hr	1558	I

[a] Tested in dextrose 5%.

[b] Tested in sodium chloride 0.9%.

[c] Tested in both dextrose 5% and sodium chloride 0.9%.

[d] Tested in dextrose 5%, sodium chloride 0.9%, and Ringer's injection, lactated.

[e] Lyophilized formulation tested.

[f] Refer to Appendix for the composition of parenteral nutrition solutions. TNA indicates a 3-in-1 admixture, and TPN indicates a 2-in-1 admixture.

[g] A 32.5-mL sample of parenteral nutrition solution mixed with 50 mL of antibiotic solution.

[h] Run at 21 mL/hr.

[i] Given over five minutes by syringe pump.

[j] Run at 94 mL/hr.

[k] Tested in sterile water for injection.

[l] Test performed using the formulation WITHOUT edetate disodium.

[m] Tested in either dextrose 5% or in sodium chloride 0.9%, but the report did not specify which solution.

[n] Tested in a 1:1 mixture of (1) dextrose 5% and dextrose 5% in sodium chloride 0.45% with and without potassium chloride 20 mEq/L and also in (2) dextrose 10% in sodium chloride 0.45% with and without potassium chloride 20 mEq/L.

[o] Tested in combination with hydrocortisone sodium succinate (Upjohn) 100 mg/L

[p] Tested in combination with heparin sodium (Rikers) 1000 units/L

[q] Test performed using the formulation WITH edetate disodium.

Additional Compatibility Information

Peritoneal Dialysis Solutions

The stability of ampicillin (Bristol) 50 mg/L in peritoneal dialysis solutions (Dianeal 137 and PD-2) with heparin sodium 500 units/L was evaluated at 25°C. Approximately 93 ± 10% activity remained after 24 hours.[1228] However, ampicillin (Bristol) 2.5 g/L in peritoneal dialysis concentrate (Travenol) containing dextrose 30% with and without heparin sodium 2500 units/L underwent substantial reduction in activity within as little as 10 minutes.[273]

The stability of ampicillin (Aspen Pharmacare) 125 mg/L in pH-neutral Balance (Fresenius), icodextrin-based Extraneal (Baxter), and dextrose-based Dianeal PD-4 (Baxter) peritoneal dialysis solutions was evaluated.[2984] At 4, 25, and 37°C, ampicillin was stable in Balance for 336, 12, and 12 hours, respectively; in Extraneal for 336, 48, and 24 hours, respectively; and in Dianeal PD-4 for 336, 72, and 24 hours, respectively.[2984]

Selected Revisions May 1, 2020. © Copyright, October 1982. American Society of Health-System Pharmacists, Inc.

Ampicillin Sodium–Sulbactam Sodium
AHFS 8:12.16.08

Products

Ampicillin sodium–sulbactam sodium is available in vials and piggyback bottles containing 1.5 g (ampicillin 1 g plus sulbactam 0.5 g) or 3 g (ampicillin 2 g plus sulbactam 1 g) as the sodium salts.[1(6/06)]

For intramuscular injection, reconstitute vials with sterile water for injection or lidocaine hydrochloride 0.5 or 2% in the following amounts:[1(6/06)]

Vial Size	Volume of Diluent	Withdrawable Volume	Concentration
1.5 g	3.2 mL	4 mL[a]	375 mg/mL[b]
3 g	6.4 mL	8 mL[a]	375 mg/mL[b]

[a] Sufficient excess is present to permit withdrawal of the volume noted.

[b] Ampicillin 250 mg plus sulbactam 125 mg per mL.

For intravenous use, reconstitute piggyback bottles directly with a compatible diluent to the desired concentration between 3 and 45 mg/mL (ampicillin 2 to 30 mg plus sulbactam 1 to 15 mg per mL). Standard vials of 1.5 and 3 g may be reconstituted with 3.2 and 6.4 mL of sterile water for injection, respectively, to yield 375-mg/mL solutions (ampicillin 250 mg plus sulbactam 125 mg per mL). The reconstituted solution should be diluted immediately in a compatible infusion solution to yield the desired concentration between 3 and 45 mg/mL.[1(6/06)]

Allow reconstituted solutions to stand so that any foaming may dissipate before inspecting them visually to ensure complete dissolution.[1(6/06)]

pH

From 8 to 10.[1(6/06)]

Sodium Content

Each 1.5 g (ampicillin 1 g plus sulbactam 0.5 g as the sodium salts) contains 5 mEq (115 mg) of sodium.[1(6/06)]

Trade Name(s)

Unasyn

Administration

Ampicillin sodium–sulbactam sodium may be administered by deep intramuscular injection or intravenous injection or infusion.[3285] For direct intravenous injection, the drug should be given slowly over at least 10 to 15 minutes.[3285] For intravenous infusion, the drug may be diluted in 50 to 100 mL of compatible diluent and infused over 15 to 30 minutes.[3285]

Stability

Intact vials of the white to off-white powder should be stored at or below 30°C.[3285] Aqueous solutions are pale yellow to yellow.[3285] Dilute solutions are colorless to pale yellow.[3285] The manufacturer recommends that intramuscular solutions be used within 1 hour after preparation.[3285]

Central Venous Catheter

Ampicillin sodium–sulbactam sodium (Pfizer-Roerig) 5 plus 2.5 mg/mL in sodium chloride 0.9% was found to be compatible with the ARROWg+ard Blue Plus (Arrow International) chlorhexidine-bearing triple-lumen central catheter. Essentially complete delivery of the drug was found with little or no drug loss occurring. Furthermore, chlorhexidine delivered from the catheter remained at trace amounts with no substantial increase due to the delivery of the drug through the catheter.[2335]

Compatibility Information

Solution Compatibility

Ampicillin sodium–sulbactam sodium

Test Soln Name	Mfr	Mfr	Conc/L or %	Remarks	Ref	C/I
Dextrose 5% in sodium chloride 0.45%			20[b], 10[b] g	Stable for only 4 hr at 4 and 25°C	1(6/06)	I
Dextrose 5%			2[b] g	Stable for only 4 hr at 25°C	1(6/06)	I
Dextrose 5%			20[b] g	Stable for only 4 hr at 4°C and 2 hr at 25°C	1(6/06)	I
Ringer's injection, lactated			30[b] g	Stable for 24 hr at 4°C but only 8 hr at 25°C	1(6/06)	I
Sodium chloride 0.9%			30[b] g	Stable for 48 hr at 4°C and 8 hr at 25°C	1(6/06)	C

DOI: 10.37573/9781585286850.027

Solution Compatibility (Cont.)

Test Soln Name	Mfr	Mfr	Conc/L or %	Remarks	Ref	C/I
Sodium chloride 0.9%	a	PF	20[b] g	Visually compatible with 10% loss in 32 hr at 24°C and 68 hr at 5°C	1691	C
Sodium lactate ⅙ M			30[b] g	Stable for only 8 hr at 4 and 25°C	1(6/06)	I

[a] Tested in PVC containers.

[b] Ampicillin component. Ampicillin in a 2:1 fixed-ratio concentration with sulbactam.

Additive Compatibility

Ampicillin sodium–sulbactam sodium

Test Drug	Mfr	Conc/L or %	Mfr	Conc/L or %	Test Solution	Remarks	Ref	C/I
Aztreonam	SQ	10 g	PF	20[b] g	NS[a]	Visually compatible with 10% ampicillin loss in 30 hr at 24°C and 94 hr at 5°C. Ampicillin loss is determining factor	1691	C
Ciprofloxacin	MI	2 g		20[b] g	D5W	Physically incompatible	888	I
Ciprofloxacin	BAY	2 g	RR	20[b] g	D5W	Precipitates immediately	2413	I
Tramadol HCl	GRU	400 mg	PF	20[b] g	NS	Visually compatible with up to 9% tramadol loss in 24 hr at room temperature	2652	C

[a] Tested in PVC containers.

[b] Ampicillin component. Ampicillin in a 2:1 fixed-ratio concentration with sulbactam.

Y-Site Injection Compatibility (1:1 Mixture)

Ampicillin sodium–sulbactam sodium

Test Drug	Mfr	Conc	Mfr	Conc	Remarks	Ref	C/I
Amifostine	USB	10 mg/mL[a]	RR	20 mg/mL[b h]	Physically compatible for 4 hr at 23°C	1845	C
Amiodarone HCl	WY	6 mg/mL[a]	PF	20 mg/mL[b h]	Immediate opaque white turbidity	2352	I
Anidulafungin	VIC	0.5 mg/mL[a]	LE	20 mg/mL[b h]	Physically compatible for 4 hr at 23°C	2617	C
Aztreonam	SQ	40 mg/mL[a]	RR	20 mg/mL[b h]	Physically compatible for 4 hr at 23°C	1758	C
Bivalirudin	TMC	5 mg/mL[a]	PF	20 mg/mL[b h]	Physically compatible for 4 hr at 23°C	2373	C
Cangrelor tetrasodium	TMC	1 mg/mL[b]		20[b h] and 30[b h] mg/mL	Physically compatible for 4 hr	3243	C
Ceftolozane sulfate–tazobactam sodium	CUB	10 mg/mL[i j]	APP	20 mg/mL[i h]	Physically compatible for 2 hr	3262	C
Ciprofloxacin		400 mg[c]		3 g[c h]	White crystals form immediately when administered sequentially through a Y-site into running D5S	1887	I
Cisatracurium besylate	GW	0.1 and 2 mg/mL[a]	RR	20 mg/mL[b h]	Physically compatible for 4 hr at 23°C	2074	C
Cisatracurium besylate	GW	5 mg/mL[a]	RR	20 mg/mL[b h]	Subvisible haze develops in 15 min	2074	I
Dexmedetomidine HCl	AB	4 mcg/mL[b]	PF	20 mg/mL[b h]	Physically compatible for 4 hr at 23°C	2383	C
Diltiazem HCl	MMD	5 mg/mL	RR	45 mg/mL[b h]	Cloudiness forms	1807	I
Diltiazem HCl	MMD	1 mg/mL[b]	RR	45 mg/mL[b h]	Visually compatible	1807	C
Diltiazem HCl	MMD	5 mg/mL	RR	2[b h] and 15[b h] mg/mL	Visually compatible	1807	C
Docetaxel	RPR	0.9 mg/mL[a]	RR	20 mg/mL[b h]	Physically compatible for 4 hr at 23°C	2224	C
Enalaprilat	MSD	0.05 mg/mL[b]	PF	10 mg/mL[b h]	Physically compatible for 24 hr at room temperature under fluorescent light	1355	C

Y-Site Injection Compatibility (1:1 Mixture) (Cont.)

Test Drug	Mfr	Conc	Mfr	Conc	Remarks	Ref	C/I
Etoposide phosphate	BR	5 mg/mL[a]	RR	20 mg/mL[b h]	Physically compatible for 4 hr at 23°C	2218	C
Famotidine	MSD	0.2 mg/mL[a]	RR	20 mg/mL[b h]	Physically compatible for 14 hr	1196	C
Fat emulsion, intravenous	OTS	20%[l]	PF	15 mg/mL[a m n]	No change in particle size ≥1.3 µm observed in 24 hr at 25°C in the dark	3452	C
Fenoldopam mesylate	AB	80 mcg/mL[b]	PF	20 mg/mL[b h]	Physically compatible for 4 hr at 23°C	2467	C
Filgrastim	AMG	30 mcg/mL[a]	RR	20 mg/mL[a h]	Physically compatible for 4 hr at 22°C	1687	C
Fluconazole	RR	2 mg/mL	PF	40 mg/mL[h]	Physically compatible for 24 hr at 25°C	1407	C
Fludarabine phosphate	BX	1 mg/mL[a]	RR	20 mg/mL[b h]	Visually compatible for 4 hr at 22°C	1439	C
Gallium nitrate	FUJ	1 mg/mL[b]	RR	45 mg/mL[b h]	Visually compatible for 24 hr at 25°C	1673	C
Gemcitabine HCl	LI	10 mg/mL[b]	RR	20 mg/mL[b h]	Physically compatible for 4 hr at 23°C	2226	C
Granisetron HCl	SKB	0.05 mg/mL[a]	RR	20 mg/mL[b h]	Physically compatible for 4 hr at 23°C	2000	C
Heparin sodium	TR	50 units/mL	PF	20 mg/mL[b h]	Visually compatible for 4 hr at 25°C	1793	C
Hetastarch in lactated electrolyte	AB	6%	PF	20 mg/mL[b h]	Physically compatible for 4 hr at 23°C	2339	C
Idarubicin HCl	AD	1 mg/mL[b]	RR	20 mg/mL[b h]	Haze forms and color changes immediately. Precipitate forms in 20 min	1525	I
Insulin, regular	LI	0.2 unit/mL[b]	RR	20 mg/mL[b h]	Physically compatible for 2 hr at 25°C	1395	C
Isavuconazonium sulfate	ASP	1.5 mg/mL[i]	FRK	20 mg/mL[h i]	Measured turbidity increases immediately with precipitation within 2 hr	3263	I
Letermovir	ME	[b]		[b]	Physically compatible	3398	C
Linezolid	PHU	2 mg/mL	PF	20 mg/mL[b h]	Physically compatible for 4 hr at 23°C	2264	C
Meperidine HCl	WY	10 mg/mL[b]	RR	20 mg/mL[b h]	Physically compatible for 1 hr at 25°C	1338	C
Meropenem–vaborbactam	TMC	8 mg/mL[b k]	PF	20 mg/mL[b h]	Physically compatible for 3 hr at 20 to 25°C	3380	C
Morphine sulfate	ES	1 mg/mL[b]	RR	20 mg/mL[b h]	Physically compatible for 1 hr at 25°C	1338	C
Nicardipine HCl	DCC	0.1 mg/mL[a b]	PF	10 mg/mL[a b h]	Turbidity forms immediately	235	I
Ondansetron HCl	GL	1 mg/mL[b]	RR	20 mg/mL[b h]	Immediate turbidity and precipitation	1365	I
Paclitaxel	NCI	1.2 mg/mL[a]	RR	20 mg/mL[b h]	Physically compatible for 4 hr at 22°C	1556	C
Palonosetron HCl	MGI	50 mcg/mL	RR	20 mg/mL[b h]	Physically compatible and no loss of either drug in 4 hr at room temperature	2749	C
Pemetrexed disodium	LI	20 mg/mL[b]	LE	20 mg/mL[b h]	Physically compatible for 4 hr at 23°C	2564	C
Plazomicin sulfate	ACH	24 mg/mL[i]	AUR	20 mg/mL[h i]	Physically compatible for 1 hr at 20 to 25°C	3432	C
Remifentanil HCl	GW	0.025 and 0.25 mg/mL[b]	RR	20 mg/mL[b h]	Physically compatible for 4 hr at 23°C	2075	C
Sargramostim	IMM	10 mcg/mL[b]	RR	20 mg/mL[b h]	Few small particles form in 4 hr	1436	I
Tacrolimus	FUJ	1 mg/mL[b]	RR	33.3 mg/mL[a h]	Visually compatible for 24 hr at 25°C	1630	C
Tedizolid phosphate	CUB	0.8 mg/mL[b]	FRK	20 mg/mL[b h]	Physically compatible for 2 hr	3244	C
Telavancin HCl	ASP	7.5 mg/mL[a b g]	BA	20 mg/mL[a b g h]	Physically compatible for 2 hr	2830	C
Teniposide	BR	0.1 mg/mL[a]	RR	20 mg/mL[b h]	Physically compatible for 4 hr at 23°C	1725	C
Theophylline	TR	4 mg/mL	PF	20 mg/mL[b h]	Visually compatible for 6 hr at 25°C	1793	C
Thiotepa	IMM[d]	1 mg/mL[a]	RR	20 mg/mL[b h]	Physically compatible for 4 hr at 23°C	1861	C

Y-Site Injection Compatibility (1:1 Mixture) (Cont.)

Test Drug	Mfr	Conc	Mfr	Conc	Remarks	Ref	C/I
TNA #218 to #226[e]			PF	20 mg/mL[b][h]	Visually compatible for 4 hr at 23°C	2215	C
TPN #212 to #215[e]			RR	20 mg/mL[b][h]	Physically compatible for 4 hr at 23°C	2109	C
Vancomycin HCl	AB	20 mg/mL[a]	PF	250 mg/mL[f][h]	Transient precipitate forms	2189	?
Vancomycin HCl	AB	20 mg/mL[a]	PF	1, 10, 50 mg/mL[b][h]	Physically compatible for 4 hr at 23°C	2189	C
Vancomycin HCl	AB	2 mg/mL[a]	PF	1[b][h], 10[b][h], 50[b][h], 250[f][h] mg/mL	Physically compatible for 4 hr at 23°C	2189	C

[a] Tested in dextrose 5%.

[b] Tested in sodium chloride 0.9%.

[c] Concentration and volume not specified.

[d] Lyophilized formulation tested.

[e] Refer to Appendix for the composition of parenteral nutrition solutions. TNA indicates a 3-in-1 admixture, and TPN indicates a 2-in-1 admixture.

[f] Tested in sterile water for injection.

[g] Tested in Ringer's injection, lactated.

[h] Ampicillin component. Ampicillin in a 2:1 fixed-ratio concentration with sulbactam.

[i] Tested in both dextrose 5% and sodium chloride 0.9%.

[j] Ceftolozane component. Ceftolozane in a 2:1 fixed-ratio concentration with tazobactam.

[k] Meropenem component. Meropenem in a 1:1 fixed-ratio concentration with vaborbactam.

[l] Run at 25 mL/hr with dextrose 5% run at 83 mL/hr.

[m] Run at 100 mL/hr.

[n] Not specified whether concentration refers to single component or combined components.

Selected Revisions September 30, 2019. © Copyright, October 1990. American Society of Health-System Pharmacists, Inc.

Amsacrine
AHFS 10:00

Products

Amsacrine is available in ampuls containing 1.5 mL of a 50-mg/mL solution (75 mg total) in anhydrous *N,N*-dimethylacetamide (DMA). It is packaged with a vial containing 13.5 mL of 0.0353 M L-lactic acid diluent.[1]

To prepare the drug for use, aseptically add 1.5 mL of the amsacrine solution to the vial of L-lactic acid diluent. The resulting orange-red solution contains amsacrine 5 mg/mL in 10% (v/v) *N,N*-dimethylacetamide and 0.0318 M L-lactic acid. This concentrated solution must be diluted in dextrose 5% for infusion; do not use chloride-containing solutions.[1]

Direct contact of amsacrine solutions with skin or mucous membranes may result in skin sensitization and should be avoided.[234]

Trade Name(s)

Amsidine, Amsidyl

Administration

Amsacrine is administered by central vein infusion over 60 to 90 minutes after the dose is diluted in 500 mL of dextrose 5%.[1]

Stability

Amsacrine in intact ampuls should be stored at room temperature.[1] When mixed with the L-lactic acid diluent, the amsacrine solution is physically and chemically stable for at least 48 hours at room temperature under ambient light.[234]

Light Effects

The effect of diffuse daylight and fluorescent light on amsacrine 150 mcg/mL in dextrose 5% was studied for 48 hours at 19 to 21°C; no loss due to light exposure occurred.[1308]

Syringes

Glass syringes are recommended for the transfer of amsacrine concentrate to the L-lactic acid diluent.[115] The DMA solvent may extract UV-absorbing species from plastics and rubber.[967]

The compatibility of amsacrine (Gödecke) concentrated solution in DMA with rubber-free plastic syringes (Injekt, B. Braun) was evaluated at 37°C and ambient temperature. Storage of the DMA diluent in the plastic syringes resulted in no visible changes to the drug or syringes and did not adversely affect the performance of the syringes. Analysis found a trace amount of oleic acid amide lubricant, about 50 mcg in the 2-mL syringe content, after storage for 24 hours at 37°C. Storage at ambient temperature resulted in substantially lower amounts of oleic acid amide. The authors concluded the rubber-free Injekt plastic syringes were acceptable alternatives to glass syringes to transfer the amsacrine concentrate. Other plastic syringes incorporating rubber components are not recommended because of the extraction of materials into the drug solution.[2284]

Sorption

Amsacrine 150 mcg/mL in dextrose 5% did not undergo sorption to cellulose propionate and methacrylate butadiene styrene burette chambers and PVC and polybutadiene tubing.[1308]

Compatibility Information
Solution Compatibility

Amsacrine

Test Soln Name	Mfr	Mfr	Conc/L or %	Remarks	Ref	C/I
Dextrose 5%		PD	150 mg[a]	Physically compatible with little or no loss in 48 hr at 20°C exposed to light	1308	C
Dextrose 5%		NCI	150 mg	Physically and chemically stable for 48 hours at room temperature in light	234	C
Sodium chloride 0.9%				Amsacrine is incompatible with chloride-containing solutions	1	I

[a] Tested in burette chambers composed of cellulose propionate or methacrylate butadiene styrene.

Additive Compatibility

Amsacrine

Test Drug	Mfr	Conc/L or %	Mfr	Conc/L or %	Test Solution	Remarks	Ref	C/I
Sodium bicarbonate		2 mEq	NCI	[a]	D5W	Amsacrine chemically stable for 96 hr at room temperature	234	C

[a] Concentration unspecified.

DOI: 10.37573/9781585286850.028

Y-Site Injection Compatibility (1:1 Mixture)

Amsacrine

Test Drug	Mfr	Conc	Mfr	Conc	Remarks	Ref	C/I
Acyclovir sodium	BW	7 mg/mL[a]	NCI	1 mg/mL[a]	Immediate dark orange turbidity, becoming brownish orange in 1 hr	1381	I
Amikacin sulfate	BR	5 mg/mL[a]	NCI	1 mg/mL[a]	Visually compatible for 4 hr at 22°C	1381	C
Amphotericin B	SQ	0.6 mg/mL[a]	NCI	1 mg/mL[a]	Immediate yellow turbidity, becoming yellow flocculent precipitate in 15 min	1381	I
Aztreonam	SQ	40 mg/mL[a]	NCI	1 mg/mL[a]	Immediate yellow-orange turbidity, becoming a precipitate in 4 hr	1381	I
Ceftazidime	GL	40 mg/mL[a]	NCI	1 mg/mL[a]	Immediate orange precipitate	1381	I
Ceftriaxone sodium	RC	40 mg/mL[a]	NCI	1 mg/mL[a]	Immediate orange turbidity, developing into flocculent precipitate in 4 hr	1381	I
Chlorpromazine HCl	ES	2 mg/mL[a]	NCI	1 mg/mL[a]	Visually compatible for 4 hr at 22°C	1381	C
Clindamycin phosphate	UP	10 mg/mL[a]	NCI	1 mg/mL[a]	Visually compatible for 4 hr at 22°C	1381	C
Cytarabine	QU	50 mg/mL	NCI	1 mg/mL[a]	Visually compatible for 4 hr at 22°C	1381	C
Dexamethasone sodium phosphate	QU	1 mg/mL[a]	NCI	1 mg/mL[a]	Visually compatible for 4 hr at 22°C	1381	C
Diphenhydramine HCl	PD	2 mg/mL[a]	NCI	1 mg/mL[a]	Visually compatible for 4 hr at 22°C	1381	C
Famotidine	MSD	2 mg/mL[a]	NCI	1 mg/mL[a]	Visually compatible for 4 hr at 22°C	1381	C
Fludarabine phosphate	BX	1 mg/mL[a]	NCI	1 mg/mL[a]	Visually compatible for 4 hr at 22°C	1439	C
Furosemide	ES	3 mg/mL[a]	NCI	1 mg/mL[a]	Yellow turbidity becoming colorless liquid with yellow precipitate	1381	I
Ganciclovir sodium	SY	20 mg/mL[a]	NCI	1 mg/mL[a]	Immediate dark orange turbidity	1381	I
Gentamicin sulfate	SO	5 mg/mL[a]	NCI	1 mg/mL[a]	Visually compatible for 4 hr at 22°C	1381	C
Granisetron HCl	SKB	0.05 mg/mL[a]	NCI	1 mg/mL[a]	Physically compatible for 4 hr at 23°C. Precipitate forms in 24 hr	2000	C
Haloperidol lactate	MN	0.2 mg/mL[a]	NCI	1 mg/mL[a]	Visually compatible for 4 hr at 22°C	1381	C
Heparin sodium	SO	40 units/mL[a]	NCI	1 mg/mL[a]	Orange precipitate forms immediately	1381	I
Hydrocortisone sodium succinate	UP	1 mg/mL[a]	NCI	1 mg/mL[a]	Visually compatible for 4 hr at 22°C	1381	C
Hydromorphone HCl	AST	0.5 mg/mL[a]	NCI	1 mg/mL[a]	Visually compatible for 4 hr at 22°C	1381	C
Lorazepam	WY	0.1 mg/mL[a]	NCI	1 mg/mL[a]	Visually compatible for 4 hr at 22°C	1381	C
Methylprednisolone sodium succinate	UP	5 mg/mL[a]	NCI	1 mg/mL[a]	Immediate orange turbidity and precipitate in 4 hr	1381	I
Metoclopramide HCl	RB	2.5 mg/mL[a]	NCI	1 mg/mL[a]	Orange turbidity becomes orange precipitate in 1 hr	1381	I
Morphine sulfate	ES	1 mg/mL[a]	NCI	1 mg/mL[a]	Visually compatible for 4 hr at 22°C	1381	C
Ondansetron HCl	GL	1 mg/mL[a]	NCI	1 mg/mL[a]	Orange precipitate forms within 30 min	1365	I
Prochlorperazine edisylate	SKF	0.5 mg/mL[a]	NCI	1 mg/mL[a]	Visually compatible for 4 hr at 22°C	1381	C
Promethazine HCl	ES	2 mg/mL[a]	NCI	1 mg/mL[a]	Visually compatible for 4 hr at 22°C	1381	C
Ranitidine HCl	GL	2 mg/mL[a]	NCI	1 mg/mL[a]	Visually compatible for 4 hr at 22°C	1381	C

Y-Site Injection Compatibility (1:1 Mixture) (Cont.)

Test Drug	Mfr	Conc	Mfr	Conc	Remarks	Ref	C/I
Sargramostim	IMM	10 mcg/mL[a]	NCI	1 mg/mL[a]	Visually compatible for 4 hr at 22°C	1436	C
Sargramostim	IMM	10 mcg/mL[b]	NCI	1 mg/mL[a]	Haze and yellow precipitate form	1436	I
Tobramycin sulfate	LI	5 mg/mL[a]	NCI	1 mg/mL[a]	Visually compatible for 4 hr at 22°C	1381	C
Vancomycin HCl	LI	10 mg/mL[a]	NCI	1 mg/mL[a]	Visually compatible for 4 hr at 22°C	1381	C

[a] Tested in dextrose 5%.

[b] Tested in sodium chloride 0.9%.

Anakinra
AHFS 92:36

Products

Anakinra is available in prefilled glass syringes containing 100 mg of drug in 0.67 mL of solution.[2859] The prefilled syringes have 27-gauge needles protected with latex rubber covers.[2859] Each syringe containing 0.67 mL of solution also contains anhydrous citric acid 1.29 mg, sodium chloride 5.48 mg, disodium EDTA 0.12 mg, and 0.7 mg of polysorbate 80 in water for injection.[2859]

pH

6.5.[2859]

Trade Name(s)

Kineret

Administration

Anakinra is administered subcutaneously.[2859]

Stability

Anakinra should be stored under refrigeration.[2859] Do not shake; protect from freezing and light. The injection contains no preservative and is for single use.[2859] Discard any unused portions.[2859]

Visually inspect the syringes prior to use.[2859] The solution may contain trace amounts of small, translucent to white, amorphous protein particles.[2859] If the number of these particles appears excessive or the solution is discolored, cloudy, or particulate matter is present, the syringe should be discarded.[2859]

Compatibility Information

Y-Site Injection Compatibility (1:1 Mixture)

Anakinra

Test Drug	Mfr	Conc	Mfr	Conc	Remarks	Ref	C/I
Aztreonam	BMS	20 mg/mL[b]	SYN	4 and 36 mg/mL[b]	Physically compatible. No aztreonam loss in 4 hr at 25°C. Anakinra uncertain	2508	?
Cefazolin sodium	GVA	15 mg/mL[b]	SYN	4 and 36 mg/mL[b]	Physically compatible. No cefazolin loss in 4 hr at 25°C. Anakinra uncertain	2508	?
Cefotaxime sodium	HO	10 mg/mL[b]	SYN	4 and 36 mg/mL[b]	Physically compatible. No cefotaxime loss in 4 hr at 25°C. Anakinra uncertain	2508	?
Cefoxitin sodium	ME	20 mg/mL[b]	SYN	4 and 36 mg/mL[b]	Physically compatible. No cefoxitin loss in 4 hr at 25°C. Anakinra uncertain	2508	?
Ceftriaxone sodium	RC	20 mg/mL[a]	SYN	4 and 36 mg/mL[a]	Ceftriaxone stable. 10% anakinra loss in 30 min and 20% in 4 hr at 22°C	2509	I
Ceftriaxone sodium	RC	20 mg/mL[b]	SYN	4 and 36 mg/mL[b]	Physically compatible with no loss of either drug in 4 hr at 22°C	2509	C
Clindamycin phosphate	AST	12 mg/mL[b]	SYN	4 and 36 mg/mL[b]	Physically compatible with little or no loss of either drug in 4 hr at 22°C	2510	C
Famotidine		1 mg/mL[b]	SYN	4 and 36 mg/mL[b]	Physically compatible with little or no loss of either drug in 4 hr at 22°C	2511	C
Fluconazole	PF	2 mg/mL[b]	SYN	4 and 36 mg/mL[b]	Physically compatible. No fluconazole loss in 4 hr at 25°C. Anakinra uncertain	2508	?
Lorazepam	WY	0.1 mg/mL[b]	SYN	4 and 36 mg/mL[b]	Physically compatible with no loss of either drug in 4 hr at 22°C	2512	C

[a] Tested in dextrose 5%.

[b] Tested in sodium chloride 0.9%.

Selected Revisions March 27, 2014. © Copyright, October 2006.
American Society of Health-System Pharmacists, Inc.

DOI: 10.37573/9781585286850.029

Angiotensin II Acetate
AHFS 68:44

Products

Angiotensin II acetate concentrate for injection is available as a solution in 1-mL single-dose vials with each mL containing the equivalent of 2.5 mg angiotensin II.[3397] Each mL of solution also contains mannitol 25 mg and sodium hydroxide and/or hydrochloric acid for pH adjustment in water for injection.[3397]

Angiotensin II acetate concentrate for injection must be diluted in sodium chloride 0.9% prior to administration.[3397] For fluid-restricted patients, 1 mL (2.5 mg) or 2 mL (5 mg) of the concentrate for injection should be diluted in a 250- or 500-mL infusion bag, respectively, of sodium chloride 0.9% for a resulting concentration of 10,000 ng/mL.[3397] For patients who are not fluid restricted, 1 mL (2.5 mg) of the concentrate for injection should be diluted in a 500-mL infusion bag of sodium chloride 0.9% for a resulting concentration of 5000 ng/mL.[3397]

pH
Adjusted to 5.5.[3397]

Osmolality
When diluted as directed in sodium chloride 0.9%, the diluted solution of angiotensin II will assume the same osmolality as the sodium chloride 0.9% solution.[3430]

Equivalency
Angiotensin II 2.5 mg is equivalent to an average of 2.9 mg of angiotensin II acetate.[3397]

Trade Name(s)
Giapreza

Administration

Angiotensin II acetate is administered as a continuous intravenous infusion following dilution in sodium chloride 0.9%.[3397] The manufacturer recommends administration of the infusion through a central venous line,[3397] preferably through a dedicated port.[3430]

Infusion of the diluted angiotensin II solution should be initiated at a rate of 20 ng/kg/min with an upward titration as frequently as every 5 minutes by increments of up to 15 ng/kg/min as needed to achieve or maintain target blood pressure.[3397] The infusion rate should not exceed 80 ng/kg/min during the first 3 hours of treatment; the maintenance infusion rate should not exceed 40 ng/kg/min.[3397]

Stability

Angiotensin II acetate concentrate for injection is a clear solution.[3397] Intact vials of the concentrate for injection should be stored under refrigeration at 2 to 8°C.[3397] Angiotensin II acetate solutions should be visually inspected for particulate matter and discoloration prior to administration.[3397]

Diluted solutions of angiotensin II for infusion may be stored at room temperature or under refrigeration for up to 24 hours; after this period, the diluted solutions should be discarded.[3397]

Sorption
Both polyvinyl chloride (PVC) and non-PVC infusion bags containing sodium chloride 0.9% may be used in the preparation of angiotensin II for infusion.[3430] Adherence of the peptide to the infusion bag has not been observed in compatibility studies.[3430]

Compatibility Information
Solution Compatibility

Angiotensin II acetate

Test Soln Name	Mfr	Mfr	Conc/L or %	Remarks	Ref	C/I
Sodium chloride 0.9%		LJ	5000 and 10,000 mcg	Discard after 24 hr at room temperature or under refrigeration	3397	C

Y-Site Injection Compatibility (1:1 Mixture)

Angiotensin II acetate

Test Drug	Mfr	Conc	Mfr	Conc	Remarks	Ref	C/I
Dopamine HCl			LJ	5 and 10 mcg/mL[a]	Stated to be compatible	3430	C
Epinephrine[b]			LJ	5 and 10 mcg/mL[a]	Stated to be compatible	3430	C
Norepinephrine bitartrate			LJ	5 and 10 mcg/mL[a]	Stated to be compatible	3430	C

DOI: 10.37573/9781585286850.030

Y-Site Injection Compatibility (1:1 Mixture) (Cont.)

Test Drug	Mfr	Conc	Mfr	Conc	Remarks	Ref	C/I
Phenylephrine HCl			LJ	5 and 10 mcg/mL[a]	Stated to be compatible	3430	C
Vasopressin			LJ	5 and 10 mcg/mL[a]	Stated to be compatible	3430	C

[a] Tested in sodium chloride 0.9%.

[b] Salt not specified.

Selected Revisions September 30, 2019. © Copyright, May 2018.
American Society of Health-System Pharmacists, Inc.

Anidulafungin
AHFS 8:14.16

Products

Anidulafungin is available in 50-mg vials with 50 mg of fructose, 250 mg of mannitol, 125 mg of polysorbate 80, 5.6 mg of tartaric acid, and sodium hydroxide and/or hydrochloric acid to adjust pH.[2862] Anidulafungin also is available in 100-mg vials with 100 mg of fructose, 500 mg of mannitol, 250 mg of polysorbate 80, 11.2 mg of tartaric acid, and sodium hydroxide and/or hydrochloric acid to adjust pH.[2862]

Reconstitute the 50- and 100-mg vials with 15 and 30 mL, respectively, of sterile water for injection to yield a concentrated solution containing anidulafungin 3.33 mg/mL.[2862] This concentrate must be diluted in dextrose 5% or sodium chloride 0.9% for administration.[2862] The manufacturer recommends diluting 50-, 100-, and 200-mg quantities of anidulafungin in 50, 100, and 200 mL, respectively.[2862]

Trade Name(s)

Eraxis

Administration

Anidulafungin is administered by intravenous infusion at a rate not exceeding 1.1 mg/min after dilution in dextrose 5% or sodium chloride 0.9%.[2862] No other solution should be used.[2862]

Stability

Intact vials of anidulafungin should be stored refrigerated and protected from freezing.[2862]

The reconstituted anidulafungin solution is stable at controlled room temperature for up to 24 hours prior to dilution.[2862] Anidulafungin diluted in dextrose 5% or sodium chloride 0.9% for infusion is stable at controlled room temperature for up to 48 hours or frozen for up to 72 hours from preparation.[2862]

Compatibility Information

Y-Site Injection Compatibility (1:1 Mixture)

Anidulafungin

Test Drug	Mfr	Conc	Mfr	Conc	Remarks	Ref	C/I
Acyclovir sodium	APP	7 mg/mL[a]	VIC	0.5 mg/mL[a]	Physically compatible for 4 hr at 23°C	2617	C
Amikacin sulfate	APC	5 mg/mL[a]	VIC	0.5 mg/mL[a]	Physically compatible for 4 hr at 23°C	2617	C
Aminophylline	AB	2.5 mg/mL[a]	VIC	0.5 mg/mL[a]	Physically compatible for 4 hr at 23°C	2617	C
Amphotericin B	PHT	0.6 mg/mL[a]	VIC	0.5 mg/mL[a]	Measured haze went up immediately	2617	I
Amphotericin B lipid complex	ELN	1 mg/mL[a]	VIC	0.5 mg/mL[a]	Physically compatible for 4 hr at 23°C	2617	C
Amphotericin B liposomal	FUJ	1 mg/mL[a]	VIC	0.5 mg/mL[a]	Physically compatible for 4 hr at 23°C	2617	C
Ampicillin sodium	APC	20 mg/mL[b]	VIC	0.5 mg/mL[a]	Physically compatible for 4 hr at 23°C	2617	C
Ampicillin sodium–sulbactam sodium	LE	20 mg/mL[b d]	VIC	0.5 mg/mL[a]	Physically compatible for 4 hr at 23°C	2617	C
Cangrelor tetrasodium	TMC	1 mg/mL[b]		0.5 mg/mL[b]	Physically compatible for 4 hr	3243	C
Carboplatin	BMS	5 mg/mL[a]	VIC	0.5 mg/mL[a]	Physically compatible for 4 hr at 23°C	2617	C
Cefazolin sodium	APC	20 mg/mL[a]	VIC	0.5 mg/mL[a]	Physically compatible for 4 hr at 23°C	2617	C
Cefepime HCl	DUR	20 mg/mL[a]	VIC	0.5 mg/mL[a]	Physically compatible for 4 hr at 23°C	2617	C
Cefoxitin sodium	APP	20 mg/mL[a]	VIC	0.5 mg/mL[a]	Physically compatible for 4 hr at 23°C	2617	C
Ceftazidime	GSK	40 mg/mL[a]	VIC	0.5 mg/mL[a]	Physically compatible for 4 hr at 23°C	2617	C
Ceftolozane sulfate–tazobactam sodium	CUB	10 mg/mL[j k]	PF	0.77 mg/mL[j]	Physically compatible for 2 hr	3262	C
Ceftriaxone sodium	RC	20 mg/mL[a]	VIC	0.5 mg/mL[a]	Physically compatible for 4 hr at 23°C	2617	C
Cefuroxime sodium	GSK	30 mg/mL[a]	VIC	0.5 mg/mL[a]	Physically compatible for 4 hr at 23°C	2617	C

DOI: 10.37573/9781585286850.031

Y-Site Injection Compatibility (1:1 Mixture) (Cont.)

Test Drug	Mfr	Conc	Mfr	Conc	Remarks	Ref	C/I
Ciprofloxacin	AB	2 mg/mL[a]	VIC	0.5 mg/mL[a]	Physically compatible for 4 hr at 23°C	2617	C
Cisplatin	SIC	1 mg/mL[b]	VIC	0.5 mg/mL[a]	Physically compatible for 4 hr at 23°C	2617	C
Clindamycin phosphate	AB	10 mg/mL[a]	VIC	0.5 mg/mL[a]	Physically compatible for 4 hr at 23°C	2617	C
Cyclophosphamide	MJ	10 mg/mL[a]	VIC	0.5 mg/mL[a]	Physically compatible for 4 hr at 23°C	2617	C
Cyclosporine	NOV	5 mg/mL[a]	VIC	0.5 mg/mL[a]	Physically compatible for 4 hr at 23°C	2617	C
Cytarabine	BED	50 mg/mL	VIC	0.5 mg/mL[a]	Physically compatible for 4 hr at 23°C	2617	C
Daunorubicin HCl	BED	1 mg/mL[a]	VIC	0.5 mg/mL[a]	Physically compatible for 4 hr at 23°C	2617	C
Dexamethasone sodium phosphate	AMR	1 mg/mL[a]	VIC	0.5 mg/mL[a]	Physically compatible for 4 hr at 23°C	2617	C
Digoxin	GW	0.25 mg/mL	VIC	0.5 mg/mL[a]	Physically compatible for 4 hr at 23°C	2617	C
Dobutamine HCl	AB	4 mg/mL[a]	VIC	0.5 mg/mL[a]	Physically compatible for 4 hr at 23°C	2617	C
Docetaxel	AVE	2 mg/mL[a]	VIC	0.5 mg/mL[a]	Physically compatible for 4 hr at 23°C	2617	C
Dopamine HCl	AMR	3.2 mg/mL[a]	VIC	0.5 mg/mL[a]	Physically compatible for 4 hr at 23°C	2617	C
Doripenem	JJ	5 mg/mL[a b]	PF	0.5 mg/mL[a b]	Physically compatible for 4 hr at 23°C	2743	C
Doxorubicin HCl	GNS	2 mg/mL[a]	VIC	0.5 mg/mL[a]	Physically compatible for 4 hr at 23°C	2617	C
Epinephrine HCl	AMR	50 mcg/mL	VIC	0.5 mg/mL[a]	Physically compatible for 4 hr at 23°C	2617	C
Ertapenem sodium	ME	20 mg/mL[b]	VIC	0.5 mg/mL[a]	Microparticulates form immediately	2617	I
Erythromycin lactobionate	AB	5 mg/mL[b]	VIC	0.5 mg/mL[a]	Physically compatible for 4 hr at 23°C	2617	C
Etoposide phosphate	BMS	5 mg/mL[a]	VIC	0.5 mg/mL[a]	Physically compatible for 4 hr at 23°C	2617	C
Famotidine	BV	2 mg/mL[a]	VIC	0.5 mg/mL[a]	Physically compatible for 4 hr at 23°C	2617	C
Fentanyl citrate	AB	50 mcg/mL	VIC	0.5 mg/mL[a]	Physically compatible for 4 hr at 23°C	2617	C
Fluconazole	PF	2 mg/mL	VIC	0.5 mg/mL[a]	Physically compatible for 4 hr at 23°C	2617	C
Fluorouracil	APP	16 mg/mL[a]	VIC	0.5 mg/mL[a]	Physically compatible for 4 hr at 23°C	2617	C
Furosemide	AB	3 mg/mL[a]	VIC	0.5 mg/mL[a]	Physically compatible for 4 hr at 23°C	2617	C
Ganciclovir sodium	RC	20 mg/mL[a]	VIC	0.5 mg/mL[a]	Physically compatible for 4 hr at 23°C	2617	C
Gemcitabine HCl	LI	10 mg/mL[a]	VIC	0.5 mg/mL[a]	Physically compatible for 4 hr at 23°C	2617	C
Gentamicin sulfate	AB	5 mg/mL[a]	VIC	0.5 mg/mL[a]	Physically compatible for 4 hr at 23°C	2617	C
Heparin sodium	AB	100 units/mL	VIC	0.5 mg/mL[a]	Physically compatible for 4 hr at 23°C	2617	C
Hydrocortisone sodium succinate	PHU	1 mg/mL[a]	VIC	0.5 mg/mL[a]	Physically compatible for 4 hr at 23°C	2617	C
Ifosfamide	BMS	25 mg/mL[a]	VIC	0.5 mg/mL[a]	Physically compatible for 4 hr at 23°C	2617	C
Imipenem–cilastatin sodium	ME	5 mg/mL[b h]	VIC	0.5 mg/mL[a]	Physically compatible for 4 hr at 23°C	2617	C
Isavuconazonium sulfate	ASP	1.5 mg/mL[j]	PF	0.77 mg/mL[j]	Physically compatible for 2 hr	3263	C
Letermovir	ME	[a]		[a]	Physically compatible	3398	C
Leucovorin calcium	BED	2 mg/mL[a]	VIC	0.5 mg/mL[a]	Physically compatible for 4 hr at 23°C	2617	C
Levofloxacin	OMN	5 mg/mL[a]	VIC	0.5 mg/mL[a]	Physically compatible for 4 hr at 23°C	2617	C
Linezolid	PH	2 mg/mL	VIC	0.5 mg/mL[a]	Physically compatible for 4 hr at 23°C	2617	C
Meperidine HCl	AB	10 mg/mL[a]	VIC	0.5 mg/mL[a]	Physically compatible for 4 hr at 23°C	2617	C
Meropenem	ASZ	2.5 mg/mL[b]	VIC	0.5 mg/mL[a]	Physically compatible for 4 hr at 23°C	2617	C

Y-Site Injection Compatibility (1:1 Mixture) (Cont.)

Test Drug	Mfr	Conc	Mfr	Conc	Remarks	Ref	C/I
Meropenem–vaborbactam	TMC	8 mg/mL[b i]	PF	0.77 mg/mL[b]	Immediate change in measured turbidity. pH increased by >3 units within 3 hr	3380	I
Methylprednisolone sodium succinate	PH	5 mg/mL[a]	VIC	0.5 mg/mL[a]	Physically compatible for 4 hr at 23°C	2617	C
Metronidazole	BA	5 mg/mL	VIC	0.5 mg/mL[a]	Physically compatible for 4 hr at 23°C	2617	C
Midazolam HCl	BA	1 mg/mL[a]	VIC	0.5 mg/mL[a]	Physically compatible for 4 hr at 23°C	2617	C
Morphine sulfate	ES	15 mg/mL	VIC	0.5 mg/mL[a]	Physically compatible for 4 hr at 23°C	2617	C
Mycophenolate mofetil HCl	RC	6 mg/mL[a]	VIC	0.5 mg/mL[a]	Physically compatible for 4 hr at 23°C	2617	C
Norepinephrine bitartrate	BED	0.12 mg/mL[a]	VIC	0.5 mg/mL[a]	Physically compatible for 4 hr at 23°C	2617	C
Paclitaxel	MJ	0.6 mg/mL[a]	VIC	0.5 mg/mL[a]	Physically compatible for 4 hr at 23°C	2617	C
Pantoprazole sodium	WAY[c]	0.4 mg/mL[a]	VIC	0.5 mg/mL[a]	Physically compatible for 4 hr at 23°C	2617	C
Phenylephrine HCl	BA	1 mg/mL[a]	VIC	0.5 mg/mL[a]	Physically compatible for 4 hr at 23°C	2617	C
Piperacillin sodium–tazobactam sodium	LE[c]	40 mg/mL[a e]	VIC	0.5 mg/mL[a]	Physically compatible for 4 hr at 23°C	2617	C
Plazomicin sulfate	ACH	24 mg/mL[j]	PF	0.77 mg/mL[j]	Measured turbidity increases within 15 min; pH increased by >1 unit within 30 min	3432	I
Potassium chloride	APP	0.1 mEq/mL[a]	VIC	0.5 mg/mL[a]	Physically compatible for 4 hr at 23°C	2617	C
Quinupristin–dalfopristin	AVE	5 mg/mL[a f]	VIC	0.5 mg/mL[a]	Physically compatible for 4 hr at 23°C	2617	C
Ranitidine HCl	GSK	2 mg/mL[a]	VIC	0.5 mg/mL[a]	Physically compatible for 4 hr at 23°C	2617	C
Sodium bicarbonate	APP	1 mEq/mL	VIC	0.5 mg/mL[a]	Haze increases immediately and microparticulates occur in 4 hr	2617	I
Tacrolimus	FUJ	20 mcg/mL[a]	VIC	0.5 mg/mL[a]	Physically compatible for 4 hr at 23°C	2617	C
Tedizolid phosphate	CUB	0.8 mg/mL[b]	PF	0.77 mg/mL[b]	Physically compatible for 2 hr	3244	C
Tobramycin sulfate	AB	5 mg/mL[a]	VIC	0.5 mg/mL[a]	Physically compatible for 4 hr at 23°C	2617	C
Trimethoprim–sulfamethoxazole	ES	0.8 mg/mL[a g]	VIC	0.5 mg/mL[a]	Physically compatible for 4 hr at 23°C	2617	C
Vancomycin HCl	APP	10 mg/mL[a]	VIC	0.5 mg/mL[a]	Physically compatible for 4 hr at 23°C	2617	C
Vincristine sulfate	FAU	50 mcg/mL[a]	VIC	0.5 mg/mL[a]	Physically compatible for 4 hr at 23°C	2617	C
Voriconazole	PF	4 mg/mL[a]	VIC	0.5 mg/mL[a]	Physically compatible for 4 hr at 23°C	2617	C
Zidovudine	GSK	4 mg/mL[a]	VIC	0.5 mg/mL[a]	Physically compatible for 4 hr at 23°C	2617	C

[a] Tested in dextrose 5%.

[b] Tested in sodium chloride 0.9%.

[c] Test performed using the formulation WITHOUT edetate disodium.

[d] Ampicillin component. Ampicillin in a 2:1 fixed-ratio concentration with sulbactam.

[e] Piperacillin component. Piperacillin in an 8:1 fixed-ratio concentration with tazobactam.

[f] Quinupristin and dalfopristin components combined.

[g] Trimethoprim component. Trimethoprim in a 1:5 fixed-ratio concentration with sulfamethoxazole.

[h] Not specified whether concentration refers to single component or combined components.

[i] Meropenem component. Meropenem in a 1:1 fixed-ratio concentration with vaborbactam.

[j] Tested in both dextrose 5% and sodium chloride 0.9%.

[k] Ceftolozane component. Ceftolozane sulfate in a fixed-ratio concentration with tazobactam sodium.

Additional Compatibility Information

Peritoneal Dialysis Solutions

Anidulafungin (Ecalta, Pfizer) 100 mg/L was visually compatible in both Dianeal PD-4 with dextrose 1.36% (Baxter) and Extraneal with icodextrin 7.5% (Baxter) peritoneal dialysis solutions at 4 and 25°C for up to 14 days in polyvinyl chloride (PVC) containers; however, cloudiness developed after 24 hours in the same solutions stored at 36°C.[3419]

Selected Revisions June 1, 2019. © Copyright, October 2008. American Society of Health-System Pharmacists, Inc.

Antihemophilic Factor (Recombinant)
AHFS 20:28.16

Products

Antihemophilic factor (recombinant) is available in forms prepared by differing processes. Helixate FS, Kogenate, and Kogenate FS are prepared using human factor VIII genes in baby hamster kidney cells while Advate, Recombinate, and ReFacto are prepared from human factor VIII genes in Chinese hamster ovary cells. The products are available in sizes of 250, 500, 1000, 2000, and 3000 international units with sterile water for injection diluent. The vials of drug are sealed under vacuum.[1(12/08) 4]

After reconstitution, Kogenate contains excipients of glycine 10 to 30 mg/mL, up to 500 mcg/1000 international units of imidazole, up to 600 mcg/1000 international units of polysorbate 80, calcium chloride 2 to 5 mM, human albumin 1 to 4 mg/mL, and sodium chloride.[1(12/08)]

Helixate FS and Kogenate FS are formulated with sucrose. After reconstitution, the products contain excipients of sucrose 0.9 to 1.3%, L-histidine 18 to 23 mM, glycine 21 to 25 mg/mL, calcium chloride 2 to 3 mM, up to 35 mcg/mL of polysorbate 80, up to 20 mcg/1000 international units of imidazole, up to 5 mcg/1000 international units of tri-n-butyl phosphate.[1(12/08)]

After reconstitution, Recombinate contains excipients of human albumin 12.5 mg/mL, calcium 0.2 mg/mL, polyethylene glycol 3350 1.5 mg/mL, histidine 55 mM, polysorbate 80 1.5 mcg/international unit, and sodium 0.18 mEq/mL.[1(12/08)]

Reconstituted ReFacto contains excipients of sodium chloride, sucrose, L-histidine, calcium chloride, and polysorbate 80.[1(12/08)]

To reconstitute, allow the vials to come to room temperature, and use the transfer needle provided or syringe and needle to transfer the diluent into the vial of drug. The vacuum will draw in the diluent. Direct the stream against the vial wall and avoid excessive foaming. Incomplete diluent transfer warrants discarding the vial. Remove the transfer needle and swirl the vial with gentle agitation to dissolve the powder. It should not be vigorously shaken. Do not refrigerate after reconstitution.[1(12/08)]

Trade Name(s)

Advate, Helixate FS, Kogenate, Kogenate FS, ReFacto

Selected Revisions June 1, 2019. © Copyright, October 2004. American Society of Health-System Pharmacists, Inc.

Administration

Antihemophilic factor (recombinant) is administered intravenously. The drug should be withdrawn from the vial into a syringe using the sterile filter needle provided. The use of plastic syringes has been suggested because proteins tend to adhere more to glass syringes than to plastic ones.[1(12/08)]

Stability

The products should be stored under refrigeration protected from light; freezing should be avoided because of possible damage to the diluent container. Intact vials of drug may be stored up to 3 months at room temperature up to 25°C (Kogenate, ReFacto) or 30°C (Recombinate). The products do not contain an antimicrobial preservative; use within 3 hours after reconstitution is recommended.[1(12/08) 4]

Antihemophilic factor VIII (ADVATE, Baxter) when reconstituted as directed was found to exhibit about 8% loss of activity within 24 hours when stored at controlled room temperature.[2748]

Sorption

Antihemophilic factor (recombinant) (Bayer) 1 international unit/mL in sodium chloride 0.9% was delivered at a rate of 1 mL/min through administration tubing composed of polyvinyl chloride (PVC) (Terumo) and polybutadiene (Terumo). No loss of antihemophilic factor (recombinant) occurred with the polybutadiene administration tubing. However, losses of 10 to 16% occurred through the PVC sets.[2448]

Filtration

Antihemophilic factor (recombinant) (Bayer) 1 international unit/mL in sodium chloride 0.9% was delivered at a rate of 1 mL/min through administration tubing composed of PVC with 0.2-μm inline filters composed of degenerated polysulfone (Terumo), polyethersulfone (JMS), and degenerated polyethersulfone (Nipro). No added loss of antihemophilic factor (recombinant) due to sorption to the filter occurred with the polysulfone filter. However, only 50 to 60% of the antihemophilic factor (recombinant) was delivered with the polyethersulfone filters. About 15% of the loss was attributable to the PVC tubing (see Sorption), but the balance resulted from the filters.[2448]

DOI: 10.37573/9781585286850.032

Antithymocyte Globulin (Rabbit)
AHFS 92:44

Products

Antithymocyte globulin (rabbit) is available as a lyophilized powder in 25-mg vials with glycine 50 mg, mannitol 50 mg, and sodium chloride 10 mg. The vial of drug is accompanied by a 5-mL vial of sterile water for injection for use as a diluent.[1(9/07)]

Allow the vials of antithymocyte globulin (rabbit) and diluent to warm to room temperature before reconstitution. Reconstitute the vial of drug with the diluent provided immediately before use. Direct the flow of diluent to the side of the vial. Rotate the vial gently to dissolve the drug, resulting in a 5-mg/mL solution. Inspect for particulate matter before use; the solution should be clear and not opaque. Should some particulate matter remain, continue rotating gently until all particulate matter is dissolved.[1(9/07) 4]

pH

From 6.6 to 7.4.[1(9/07)]

Trade Name(s)

Thymoglobulin

Administration

Antithymocyte globulin (rabbit) is administered intravenously into a high-flow vein after dilution in dextrose 5% or sodium chloride 0.9% to an approximate concentration of 0.5 mg/mL. The manufacturer recommends that each vial to be administered be diluted in 50 mL of infusion solution. The total volume usually ranges between 50 and 500 mL. Invert the bag gently once or twice to mix the solution before administration.[1(9/07) 4]

Antithymocyte globulin (rabbit) diluted for administration is infused through a 0.22-µm filter over a minimum of six hours for the first infusion and over at least four hours subsequently.

Stability

Intact vials of antithymocyte globulin (rabbit) should be stored under refrigeration and protected from light and freezing. After reconstitution, the drug is stable for 24 hours but should be used within four hours because of the absence of preservatives.[1(9/07) 4] Mixed in an infusion solution, immediate use is recommended.[1(9/07)]

Antithymocyte globulin (rabbit) is for single use and contains no preservative. Any unused drug remaining should be discarded.[1(9/07)]

Sorption

The manufacturer states that no interaction of antithymocyte globulin (rabbit) with glass bottles or PVC bags or administration sets has been found.[4]

Compatibility Information

Additive Compatibility

Antithymocyte globulin (rabbit)

Test Drug	Mfr	Conc/L or %	Mfr	Conc/L or %	Test Solution	Remarks	Ref	C/I
Heparin sodium	ES[a]	2000 units	SGS	200 and 300 mg	D5W	Immediate haze and precipitation	2488	I
Heparin sodium	ES[a]	2000 units	SGS	200 and 300 mg	NS	Physically compatible for 24 hr at 23°C	2488	C
Hydrocortisone sodium succinate	PHU[b]	50 mg	SGS	200 and 300 mg	D5W	Immediate haze and precipitation	2488	I
Hydrocortisone sodium succinate	PHU[b]	50 mg	SGS	200 and 300 mg	NS	Physically compatible for 24 hr at 23°C	2488	C

[a] Hydrocortisone sodium succinate (Pharmacia Upjohn) 50 mg/L was also present.

[b] Heparin sodium (Elkins-Sinn) 2000 units/L was also present.

Y-Site Injection Compatibility (1:1 Mixture)

Antithymocyte globulin (rabbit)

Test Drug	Mfr	Conc	Mfr	Conc	Remarks	Ref	C/I
Heparin sodium	ES	2 units/mL[a]	SGS	0.2 mg/mL[a]	Haze and precipitate form immediately	2488	I
Heparin sodium	ES	2 units/mL[a]	SGS	0.3 mg/mL[a]	Haze and precipitate form immediately	2488	I
Heparin sodium	ES	2 units/mL[b]	SGS	0.2 mg/mL[b]	Physically compatible for 4 hr at 23°C	2488	C
Heparin sodium	ES	2 units/mL[b]	SGS	0.3 mg/mL[b]	Physically compatible for 4 hr at 23°C	2488	C

DOI: 10.37573/9781585286850.033

Y-Site Injection Compatibility (1:1 Mixture) (Cont.)

Test Drug	Mfr	Conc	Mfr	Conc	Remarks	Ref	C/I
Heparin sodium	ES	100 units/mL[a][b]	SGS	0.2 mg/mL[a][b]	Physically compatible for 4 hr at 23°C	2488	C
Heparin sodium	ES	100 units/mL[a][b]	SGS	0.3 mg/mL[a][b]	Physically compatible for 4 hr at 23°C	2488	C
Hydrocortisone sodium succinate	PHU	0.5 mg/mL[a][b]	SGS	0.2 and 0.3 mg/mL[a][b]	Physically compatible for 4 hr at 23°C	2488	C
Hydrocortisone sodium succinate	PHU	1 mg/mL[a][b]	SGS	0.2 and 0.3 mg/mL[a][b]	Physically compatible for 4 hr at 23°C	2488	C

[a] Tested in dextrose 5%.

[b] Tested in sodium chloride 0.9%.

Selected Revisions October 1, 2012. © Copyright, October 2006.
American Society of Health-System Pharmacists, Inc.

Apomorphine Hydrochloride
AHFS 28:36.20.08

Products

Apomorphine hydrochloride is available as 10-mg/mL injections with sodium metabisulfite 1 mg in 1-, 2-, and 5-mL ampuls and may also contain sodium hydroxide and/or hydrochloric acid to adjust pH during manufacturing.[38] [115]

pH

From 3 to 4.[115]

Trade Name(s)

APO-go, Apokinon, Apomine

Administration

Apomorphine hydrochloride is administered subcutaneously by intermittent injection or continuous infusion using a controlled infusion device.[38] [115]

Stability

Containers should be stored under refrigeration[115] or at controlled room temperature[38] and protected from freezing and exposure to light.[38] [115] Apomorphine hydrochloride injection should be clear and colorless and should not be used if it has turned green.[38]

Light Effects

Apomorphine hydrochloride is very sensitive to exposure to light. In sodium chloride 0.9%, apomorphine hydrochloride (Teclapharm) 0.01 mg/mL and 0.1 mg/mL lost 44 and 24%, respectively, in one day when stored at room temperature without light protection.[2403]

Compatibility Information

Solution Compatibility

Apomorphine HCl

Test Soln Name	Mfr	Mfr	Conc/L or %	Remarks	Ref	C/I
Sodium chloride 0.9%	FRE[a]	TEC	100 mg	Physically compatible with about 8% loss in 14 days at room temperature and about 7% loss in 28 days at 4°C plus 7 days at room temperature when protected from light	2403	C
Sodium chloride 0.9%	FRE[a]	TEC	10 mg	Physically compatible with about 7% loss in 24 days at room temperature and about 9% loss in 7 days at 4°C plus 24 hr at room temperature when protected from light	2403	C

[a] Tested in PVC containers.

Selected Revisions October 1, 2012. © Copyright, October 2004.
American Society of Health-System Pharmacists, Inc.

DOI: 10.37573/9781585286850.034

Aprepitant
AHFS 56:22.32

Products

Aprepitant is available as an oil-in-water emulsion in single-dose vials containing 130 mg of aprepitant in 18 mL of emulsion.[3436] [3437] Also present in each 130-mg vial are egg lecithin 2.6 g, ethanol 0.5 g, sodium oleate 0.1 g, soybean oil 1.7 g, sucrose 1 g, and water for injection.[3436]

To prepare a 130-mg infusion, 18 mL of the emulsion should be withdrawn from the vial and transferred to a non-polyvinyl chloride (non-PVC) infusion bag containing 130 mL of sodium chloride 0.9% or dextrose 5%.[3436] To prepare a 100-mg infusion, 14 mL of the emulsion should be withdrawn from the vial and transferred to a non-PVC infusion bag containing 100 mL of sodium chloride 0.9% or dextrose 5%.[3436] After addition of the emulsion to the infusion bag, the bag should be inverted gently 4 to 5 times; shaking should be avoided.[3436] Infusion bags should be inspected for particulate matter and discoloration; if particulate matter is present or discoloration has occurred, the infusion bag should be discarded.[3436]

Trade Name(s)

Cinvanti

Administration

Aprepitant is administered by intravenous infusion over 30 minutes.[3436] Aprepitant should be administered using only non-diethylhexyl phthalate (non-DEHP) tubing after dilution of the emulsion in a non-PVC infusion bag containing the appropriate volume of sodium chloride 0.9% or dextrose 5%.[3436]

Stability

Aprepitant is an opaque, off-white to amber oil-in-water emulsion.[3436] [3437] Intact vials should be stored at 2 to 8°C and should not be frozen.[3436] Intact vials can be stored at room temperature for up to 60 days.[3436] The manufacturer states that the emulsion when diluted as recommended is stable for 6 hours at ambient room temperature in sodium chloride 0.9% or 12 hours at ambient room temperature in dextrose 5%.[3436]

Aprepitant is incompatible with any solutions containing divalent cations (e.g., calcium, magnesium), including Ringer's injection, lactated and Hartmann's solution.[3436]

Sorption

The diluted emulsion should be prepared using only non-PVC infusion bags and administered using only non-DEHP tubing.[3436]

Compatibility Information

Solution Compatibility

Aprepitant

Test Soln Name	Mfr	Mfr	Conc/L or %	Remarks	Ref	C/I
Dextrose 5% in Ringer's injection		HRN		Stated to be incompatible with calcium-containing solutions	3436	I
Dextrose 5% in Ringer's injection lactated		HRN		Stated to be incompatible with calcium-containing solutions	3436	I
Dextrose 5%		HRN	878 mg	Stated to be stable for 12 hours at ambient room temperature	3436	C
Dextrose 5%		HRN	887 mg	Stated to be stable for 12 hours at ambient room temperature	3436	C
Ringer's injection		HRN		Stated to be incompatible with calcium-containing solutions	3436	I
Ringer's injection, lactated		HRN		Stated to be incompatible with calcium-containing solutions	3436	I
Sodium chloride 0.9%		HRN	878 mg	Stated to be stable for 6 hours at ambient room temperature	3436	C
Sodium chloride 0.9%		HRN	887 mg	Stated to be stable for 6 hours at ambient room temperature	3436	C

© Copyright, June 2019. American Society of Health-System Pharmacists, Inc.

DOI: 10.37573/9781585286850.035

Argatroban
AHFS 20:12.04.12

Products

Argatroban concentrate for injection is available in 2.5-mL single-use vials containing 250 mg of the drug.[3186] Several different formulations of the concentrate for injection are available and excipients vary among them.[3186 3190 3191] Each mL of the concentrate for injection (GlaxoSmithKline) also contains D-sorbitol 300 mg and dehydrated alcohol 400 mg in water for injection.[3186] Each mL of the concentrate for injection (Fresenius Kabi) also contains propylene glycol 954 mg.[3190] Each mL of the concentrate for injection (West-Ward) also contains propylene glycol 1300 mg and dehydrated alcohol 760 mg.[3191] The concentrate for injection must be diluted 100-fold in sodium chloride 0.9%, dextrose 5%, or Ringer's injection, lactated to yield a final concentration of 1 mg/mL.[3186] The solution should be mixed thoroughly after dilution by repeated inversion of the infusion bag for 1 minute.[3186] Slight haziness may form due to transient microprecipitation, however, the microprecipitates should dissolve rapidly with mixing.[3186] Use of room temperature diluent is recommended for dilution as colder temperatures can slow down the dissolution rate of precipitates.[3186] The diluted solution for infusion must be clear for administration.[3186]

Argatroban also is available as a ready-to-use solution of 1 mg/mL of argatroban in 50- and 125-mL single-use vials and 250-mL single-use polyolefin bags.[3187 3188 3189] Each mL of solution in the 50-mL (50-mg) vial also contains lactobionic acid 2 mg, L-methionine 2 mg, sodium chloride 8 mg, and sodium hydroxide to adjust the pH in water for injection.[3187] Each mL of solution in the 125-mL (125-mg) vial and 250-mL (250-mg) bag also contains sodium chloride 9 mg and sorbitol 3 mg in water for injection.[3188 3189] The ready-to-use solution should not be diluted prior to administration.[3187 3188 3189]

pH

The pH of the concentrate for injection diluted to a concentration of 1 mg/mL for infusion and the 1-mg/mL ready-to-use solution in 125-mL vials and 250-mL bags ranges from 3.2 to 7.5.[3186 3188 3189] The pH of the 1-mg/mL ready-to-use solution in 50-mL vials is approximately 8.8.[3187]

Tonicity

The 1-mg/mL ready-to-use solution of argatroban in 125-mL vials and 250-mL bags is isotonic.[3188 3189]

Administration

Argatroban solutions of 1 mg/mL are administered by continuous intravenous infusion.[3186 3187 3188 3189] For certain indications, an initial bolus injection of the 1-mg/mL solution should be administered over 3 to 5 minutes through a large bore intravenous line; subsequent additional bolus injections of the 1-mg/mL solution may be warranted for dosage adjustment.[3186 3187 3188 3189] Specific labeling should be consulted for further dosage and administration details.

Vials of the ready-to-use solution of argatroban may be inverted and connected to an infusion set for administration.[3187 3188]

Stability

Argatroban concentrate for injection and ready-to-use solutions are clear and colorless to pale yellow in appearance.[3186 3187 3188 3189] The concentrate for injection is slightly viscous.[3186] Intact vials of the concentrate for injection and intact vials and bags of the ready-to-use solutions should be stored at controlled room temperature and retained in the original carton to protect from light.[3186 3187 3188 3189] At least one manufacturer states that its vials of the ready-to-use solution should not be refrigerated;[3187] all manufacturers of argatroban state that freezing should be avoided.[3186 3187 3188 3189]

The solution for infusion should be visually inspected for particulate matter and discoloration prior to administration; if precipitation is present or if cloudiness occurs, the solution should not be used and should be discarded.[3186 3187 3188 3189]

Several manufacturers of the concentrate for injection state that solutions of argatroban diluted for infusion as recommended are stable for 24 hours at 20 to 25°C in ambient indoor light, and therefore, light-resistant measures (e.g., foil protection of the intravenous line) are unnecessary.[3186 3191] Solutions diluted for infusion should not be exposed to direct sunlight.[3186]

Sorption

No substantial potency losses have been reported following simulated delivery of the diluted solution for infusion through intravenous tubing.[3186]

Compatibility Information

Solution Compatibility

Argatroban

Test Soln Name	Mfr	Mfr	Conc/L or %	Remarks	Ref	C/I
Dextrose 5%		GSK, WW	1 g	Stable for 24 hr at 20 to 25°C in normal room light	3186, 3191	C
Dextrose 5%		GSK, WW	1 g	Physically compatible and chemically stable for 96 hr at 20 to 25°C or 5°C protected from light	3186, 3191	C

DOI: 10.37573/9781585286850.036

Solution Compatibility (Cont.)

Test Soln Name	Mfr	Mfr	Conc/L or %	Remarks	Ref	C/I
Dextrose 5%		FRK	1 g	Physically compatible and chemically stable for 4 hr at 20 to 25°C or 2 to 8°C protected from light	3190	C
Ringer's injection, lactated		GSK, WW	1 g	Stable for 24 hr at 20 to 25°C in normal room light	3186, 3191	C
Ringer's injection, lactated		GSK, WW	1 g	Physically compatible and chemically stable for 96 hr at 20 to 25°C or 5°C protected from light	3186, 3191	C
Ringer's injection, lactated		FRK	1 g	Physically compatible and chemically stable for 4 hr at 20 to 25°C or 2 to 8°C protected from light	3190	C
Sodium chloride 0.9%		GSK, WW	1 g	Stable for 24 hr at 20 to 25°C in normal room light	3186, 3191	C
Sodium chloride 0.9%		GSK, WW	1 g	Physically compatible and chemically stable for 96 hr at 20 to 25°C or 5°C protected from light	3186, 3191	C
Sodium chloride 0.9%		FRK	1 g	Physically compatible and chemically stable for 96 hr at 20 to 25°C or 2 to 8°C protected from light	3190	C

Y-Site Injection Compatibility (1:1 Mixture)

Argatroban

Test Drug	Mfr	Conc	Mfr	Conc	Remarks	Ref	C/I
Abciximab	LI	36 mcg/mL[a b d]	GSK	1 mg/mL[a b d]	Physically compatible with no loss of argatroban in 4 hr at 23°C. Abciximab not tested	2630	C
Amiodarone HCl	NVP	1.8 mg/mL[a]	SKB	1 mg/mL[a]	Trace precipitate forms immediately	2572	I
Atropine sulfate	AMR	0.4 mg/mL	GSK	1 mg/mL[b]	Visually compatible for 24 hr at 23°C	2391	C
Diltiazem HCl	BV	5 mg/mL	GSK	1 mg/mL[b]	Visually compatible for 24 hr at 23°C	2391	C
Diltiazem HCl	AKN	1 mg/mL[a]	SZ	1 mg/mL	Physically compatible for up to 5 hr at 19 to 24°C in ambient light and 28 to 40% relative humidity	3192	C
Diphenhydramine HCl	ES	50 mg/mL	GSK	1 mg/mL[b]	Visually compatible for 24 hr at 23°C	2391	C
Dobutamine HCl	LI	12.5 mg/mL	GSK	1 mg/mL[b]	Visually compatible for 24 hr at 23°C	2391	C
Dopamine HCl	AMR	80 mg/mL	GSK	1 mg/mL[b]	Visually compatible for 24 hr at 23°C	2391	C
Eptifibatide	COR	2 mg/mL[e]	GSK	1 mg/mL[a b e]	Physically compatible with no loss of either drug in 4 hr at 23°C	2630	C
Esmolol HCl	BA	10 mg/mL	SZ	1 mg/mL	Physically compatible for up to 24 hr at 19 to 24°C in ambient light and 28 to 40% relative humidity	3192	C
Fenoldopam mesylate	AB	0.1 mg/mL[a]	SKB	1 mg/mL[a]	Physically compatible for 24 hr at 23°C	2572	C
Fentanyl citrate	ES	50 mcg/mL	GSK	1 mg/mL[b]	Visually compatible for 24 hr at 23°C	2391	C
Furosemide	AB	10 mg/mL	SKB	1 mg/mL[a]	Physically compatible for 24 hr at 23°C	2572	C
Hydrocortisone sodium succinate	PHU	50 mg/mL	GSK	1 mg/mL[b]	Visually compatible for 24 hr at 23°C	2391	C
Ibutilide fumarate	PF	0.017 mg/mL[a]	SZ	1 mg/mL	Increased turbidity and pH changes occur within 8 and 5 hr, respectively	3192, 3266	I
Lidocaine HCl	BA	8 mg/mL[a]	SKB	1 mg/mL[a]	Physically compatible for 24 hr at 23°C	2572	C
Metoprolol tartrate	AB	1 mg/mL	GSK	1 mg/mL[b]	Visually compatible for 24 hr at 23°C	2391	C
Midazolam HCl	AB	2 mg/mL	GSK	1 mg/mL[b]	Visually compatible for 24 hr at 23°C	2391	C
Milrinone lactate	NVP	0.4 mg/mL[a]	SKB	1 mg/mL[a]	Physically compatible for 24 hr at 23°C	2572	C

Y-Site Injection Compatibility (1:1 Mixture) (Cont.)

Test Drug	Mfr	Conc	Mfr	Conc	Remarks	Ref	C/I
Morphine sulfate	ES	10 mg/mL	GSK	1 mg/mL[b]	Visually compatible for 24 hr at 23°C	2391	C
Nesiritide	SCI	6 mcg/mL[a]	SKB	1 mg/mL[a]	Physically compatible for 24 hr at 23°C	2572	C
Nitroglycerin	BA	0.2 mg/mL[a]	SKB	1 mg/mL[a]	Physically compatible for 24 hr at 23°C	2572	C
Norepinephrine bitartrate	AB	1 mg/mL	GSK	1 mg/mL[b]	Visually compatible for 24 hr at 23°C	2391	C
Phenylephrine HCl	AMR	10 mg/mL	GSK	1 mg/mL[b]	Visually compatible for 24 hr at 23°C	2391	C
Procainamide HCl	HOS	4 mg/mL[a]	SZ	1 mg/mL	Physically compatible for up to 5 hr at 19 to 24°C in ambient light and 28 to 40% relative humidity	3192	C
Sodium nitroprusside	AB	0.2 mg/mL[a]	SKB	1 mg/mL[a]	Physically compatible for 24 hr at 23°C	2572	C
Tirofiban HCl	ME	0.05 mg/mL[f]	GSK	1 mg/mL[a b f]	Physically compatible with no loss of either drug in 4 hr at 23°C	2630	C
TPN #263[c]			SKB	1 mg/mL[a]	Physically compatible for 24 hr at 23°C	2572	C
Vasopressin	AMR	0.4 unit/mL[a]	SKB	1 mg/mL[a]	Physically compatible for 24 hr at 23°C	2572	C
Verapamil HCl	AMR	2.5 mg/mL	GSK	1 mg/mL[b]	Visually compatible for 24 hr at 23°C	2391	C

[a] Tested in dextrose 5%.

[b] Tested in sodium chloride 0.9%.

[c] Refer to Appendix for the composition of parenteral nutrition solutions. TPN indicates a 2-in-1 admixture.

[d] Mixed argatroban:abciximab 1:1 and 4:1.

[e] Mixed argatroban:eptifibatide 1:1 and 16:1.

[f] Mixed argatroban:tirofiban hydrochloride 1:1 and 8:1.

Selected Revisions June 16, 2017. © Copyright, October 2004.
American Society of Health-System Pharmacists, Inc.

Aripiprazole
AHFS 28:16.08.04

Products

Aripiprazole is available in 1.3-mL vials containing 9.75 mg (7.5 mg/mL) of drug with sulfobutylether β-cyclodextrin 150 mg/mL, tartaric acid, and sodium hydroxide in water for injection.[1(8/08)]

Trade Name(s)

Abilify

Administration

Aripiprazole injection is administered by deep intramuscular injection only. Other routes should not be used.[1(8/08)]

Stability

Intact vials of aripiprazole should be stored in the original cartons at controlled room temperature.[1(8/08)]

Compatibility Information

Drugs in Syringe Compatibility

Aripiprazole

Test Drug	Mfr	Amt	Mfr	Amt	Remarks	Ref	C/I
Lorazepam	HOS	0.2 mg/0.1 mL	BMS	6.75 mg/0.9 mL	Visually compatible for 30 min	2719	C
Lorazepam	HOS	0.6 mg/0.3 mL	BMS	5.25 mg/0.7 mL	Visually compatible for 30 min	2719	C
Lorazepam	HOS	1 mg/0.5 mL	BMS	3.75 mg/0.5 mL	Visually compatible for 30 min	2719	C
Lorazepam	HOS	1.4 mg/0.7 mL	BMS	2.25 mg/0.3 mL	Visually compatible for 30 min	2719	C
Lorazepam	HOS	1.8 mg/0.9 mL	BMS	0.75 mg/0.1 mL	Visually compatible for 30 min	2719	C

Selected Revisions October 1, 2012. © Copyright, October 2008.
American Society of Health-System Pharmacists, Inc.

DOI: 10.37573/9781585286850.037

Arsenic Trioxide
AHFS 10:00

Products

Arsenic trioxide is available as a 1-mg/mL solution in 10-mL ampuls.[2860] Sodium hydroxide and hydrochloric acid are used during manufacturing to adjust the pH.[2860]

pH

From 7.5 to 8.5.[2860]

Trade Name(s)

Trisenox

Administration

Arsenic trioxide must be diluted with 100 to 250 mL of dextrose 5% or sodium chloride 0.9% for use.[2860] After dilution, the drug is administered by intravenous infusion over 1 to 2 hours; the duration of infusion may be extended up to 4 hours in certain patients.[2860] A central venous catheter is *not* required for administration.[2860]

Stability

Arsenic trioxide injection is a clear and colorless solution.[2860] Intact ampuls should be stored at room temperature and protected from freezing.[2860] Discard unused portions of the drug properly.[2860]

Compatibility Information

Solution Compatibility

Arsenic trioxide

Test Soln Name	Mfr	Mfr	Conc/L or %	Remarks	Ref	C/I
Dextrose 5%		TE		Stated to be chemically and physically stable for 24 hr at room temperature and 48 hr under refrigeration	2860	C
Sodium chloride 0.9%		TE		Stated to be chemically and physically stable for 24 hr at room temperature and 48 hr under refrigeration	2860	C

Selected Revisions September 29, 2017. © Copyright, October 2004. American Society of Health-System Pharmacists, Inc.

DOI: 10.37573/9781585286850.038

Ascorbic Acid
AHFS 88:12

Products

Ascorbic acid is provided as a sodium ascorbate solution equivalent to 500 mg/mL of ascorbic acid in 1- and 2-mL containers. The pH may be adjusted with sodium bicarbonate or sodium hydroxide. Edetate disodium and sodium hydrosulfite 0.5% antioxidant may also be present.[1(6/07)]

Pressure may build up during storage of containers of ascorbic acid. At room temperature, the pressure may become excessive. When opening ascorbic acid, ampuls should be wrapped in a protective covering.[1(6/07)]

pH

From 5.5 to 7.[1(6/07)]

Administration

Intramuscular injection of ascorbic acid is preferred, but it may also be given subcutaneously or intravenously.[1(6/07)] [4] Intravenously, it should be added to a large volume of a compatible diluent and infused slowly.[1(6/07)]

Stability

To avoid excessive pressure inside the ampuls, they should be stored in the refrigerator and not allowed to stand at room temperature before use.[1(6/07)]

Although refrigeration is recommended, Lilly has stated that its ascorbic acid had a maximum room temperature stability of 96 hours.[853] Intact ampuls of commercial ascorbic acid (Vitarine) have been reported to be stable for 4 years at room temperatures not exceeding 25°C.[60]

Ascorbic acid in solution is rapidly oxidized in air and alkaline media.[4 2292]

The stability of ascorbic acid from a multiple vitamin product in dextrose 5% and sodium chloride 0.9%, in both PVC and ClearFlex containers, was evaluated. Analysis showed that ascorbic acid was stable at 23°C when protected from light, exhibiting less than a 10% loss in 24 hours. When exposed to light, however, ascorbic acid had losses of approximately 50 to 65% in 24 hours.[1509]

Ascorbic acid (Abbott) develops a grayish-brown color if left exposed to a stainless steel 5-μm filter needle (Monoject) for as little as 1 hour.[1645]

In one study, ascorbic acid (McGuff) was diluted to 30 mg/mL in sodium chloride 0.9% and 50 mg/mL in dextrose 5%.[3525] Spectrophotometric evaluation showed that the concentration of ascorbic acid remained greater than 90% for up to 96 hours in solutions stored at 4°C in the dark and in those stored at ambient temperature and light.[3525]

pH Effects

Literature reports of incompatibilities between various acid-labile drugs such as penicillin G potassium[47 165] and erythromycin lactobionate[20] with pure ascorbic acid do not pertain to ascorbic acid injection, USP. The official product has a pH of 5.5 to 7[4 17] and exists as a mixture of sodium ascorbate and ascorbic acid, with the sodium salt predominating. Pure ascorbic acid is quite acidic. A solution of ascorbic acid 500 mg in 2 mL of diluent had a pH of 2. The incompatibilities between pure ascorbic acid and penicillin G potassium have been attributed to the pH rather than being a characteristic of the ascorbate ion.[166]

Light Effects

Ascorbic acid gradually darkens on exposure to light. A slight color developed during storage does not impair the therapeutic activity.[4] Protect the intact containers from light by keeping them in the carton until ready for use.[1(6/07)]

Sorption

Pure ascorbic acid (Merck) did not display significant sorption to a PVC plastic test strip in 24 hours.[12]

Compatibility Information

Solution Compatibility

Ascorbic acid

Test Soln Name	Mfr	Mfr	Conc/L or %	Remarks	Ref	C/I
Dextrose 2.5% in half-strength Ringer's injection	AB	AB	1 g	Physically compatible	3	C
Dextrose 5% in Ringer's injection	AB	AB	1 g	Physically compatible	3	C
Dextrose 5% in half-strength Ringer's injection, lactated	AB	AB	1 g	Physically compatible	3	C

DOI: 10.37573/9781585286850.039

Solution Compatibility (Cont.)

Test Soln Name	Mfr	Mfr	Conc/L or %	Remarks	Ref	C/I
Dextrose 2.5% in Ringer's injection, lactated	AB	AB	1 g	Physically compatible	3	C
Dextrose 5% in Ringer's injection, lactated	AB	AB	1 g	Physically compatible	3	C
Dextrose 10% in Ringer's injection, lactated	AB	AB	1 g	Physically compatible	3	C
Dextrose 2.5% in sodium chloride 0.45%	AB	AB	1 g	Physically compatible	3	C
Dextrose 2.5% in sodium chloride 0.9%	AB	AB	1 g	Physically compatible	3	C
Dextrose 5% in sodium chloride 0.225%	AB	AB	1 g	Physically compatible	3	C
Dextrose 5% in sodium chloride 0.45%	AB	AB	1 g	Physically compatible	3	C
Dextrose 5% in sodium chloride 0.45%		BTK	1.25 g	5% loss in 24 hr at room temperature	1775	C
Dextrose 5% in sodium chloride 0.9%	AB	AB	1 g	Physically compatible	3	C
Dextrose 10% in sodium chloride 0.9%	AB	AB	1 g	Physically compatible	3	C
Dextrose 2.5%	AB	AB	1 g	Physically compatible	3	C
Dextrose 5%	AB	AB	1 g	Physically compatible	3	C
Dextrose 5%		BTK	1.25 g	5% loss in 24 hr at room temperature	1775	C
Dextrose 5%	BRN	AMR	10 g	Physically compatible with no loss in 24 hr at 24°C in the dark	2629	C
Dextrose 10%	AB	AB	1 g	Physically compatible	3	C
Dextrose 10%		BTK	1.25 g	4% loss in 24 hr at room temperature	1775	C
Ionosol B in dextrose 5%	AB	AB	1 g	Physically compatible	3	C
Ionosol MB in dextrose 5%	AB	AB	1 g	Physically compatible	3	C
Ringer's injection	AB	AB	1 g	Physically compatible	3	C
Ringer's injection		BTK	1.25 g	6% loss in 24 hr at room temperature	1775	C
Ringer's injection, lactated	AB	AB	1 g	Physically compatible	3	C
Ringer's injection, lactated		BTK	1.25 g	6% loss in 24 hr at room temperature	1775	C
Sodium chloride 0.45%	AB	AB	1 g	Physically compatible	3	C
Sodium chloride 0.9%	AB	AB	1 g	Physically compatible	3	C
Sodium chloride 0.9%		BTK	1.25 g	4% loss in 24 hr at room temperature	1775	C
Sodium chloride 0.9%	BRN	AMR	10 g	Physically compatible with 3% loss in 24 hr at 24°C in the dark	2629	C
Sodium lactate ⅙ M	AB	AB	1 g	Physically compatible	3	C

Additive Compatibility

Ascorbic acid

Test Drug	Mfr	Conc/L or %	Mfr	Conc/L or %	Test Solution	Remarks	Ref	C/I
Amikacin sulfate	BR	5 g	CO[a]	5 g	D5LR, D5R, D5S, D5W, D10W, LR, NS, R, SL	Physically compatible and both stable for 24 hr at 25°C	294	C
Aminophylline	SE	500 mg	AB	500 mg		Physically compatible	6	C
Aminophylline	SE	1 g	UP	500 mg	D5W	Physically incompatible	15	I
Bleomycin sulfate	BR	20 and 30 units	PD	2.5 and 5 g	NS	Loss of all bleomycin in 1 week at 4°C	763	I
Calcium chloride	UP	1 g	UP	500 mg	D5W	Physically compatible	15	C
Calcium gluconate	UP	1 g	UP	500 mg	D5W	Physically compatible	15	C
Chloramphenicol sodium succinate	PD	1 g	AB	1 g		Physically compatible	6	C
Chloramphenicol sodium succinate	PD		UP			Concentration-dependent incompatibility	15	I
Chlorpromazine HCl	SKF	250 mg	UP	500 mg	D5W	Physically compatible	15	C
Colistimethate sodium	WC	500 mg	UP	500 mg	D5W	Physically compatible	15	C
Cyanocobalamin	AB	1 mg	AB	1 g		Physically compatible	3	C
Cyanocobalamin						Stated to be incompatible	1729, 1736	I
Diphenhydramine HCl	PD	80 mg	UP	500 mg	D5W	Physically compatible	15	C
Erythromycin lactobionate	AB	1 g	AB	1 g		Physically compatible	3	C
Erythromycin lactobionate	AB	5 g	UP	500 mg	D5W	Physically incompatible	15	I
Fat emulsion, intravenous	VT	10%	VI	1 g		Physically compatible for 48 hr at 4°C and room temperature	32	C
Fat emulsion, intravenous	VT	10%	DB	500 mg		Lipid coalescence in 24 hr at 25 and 8°C	825	I
Heparin sodium	UP	4000 units	UP	500 mg	D5W	Physically compatible	15	C
Hydrocortisone sodium succinate	UP		UP			Concentration-dependent incompatibility	15	I
Methyldopate HCl	MSD	1 g	AB	1 g	D5W, D10W, D2.5½S, D2.5S, D5¼S, D5½S, D5S, D10S, NS, ½S	Physically compatible	23	C
Nafcillin sodium	WY	5 g	UP	500 mg	D5W	Physically incompatible	15	I
Penicillin G potassium		1 million units	AB	1 g		Physically compatible	3	C
Penicillin G potassium	SQ	10 million units	PD	500 mg	D5W	1% penicillin loss in 8 hr	166	C
Polymyxin B sulfate	BW	200 mg	UP	500 mg	D5W	Physically compatible	15	C
Prochlorperazine edisylate	SKF	100 mg	UP	500 mg	D5W	Physically compatible	15	C
Promethazine HCl	WY	250 mg	UP	500 mg	D5W	Physically compatible	15	C

Additive Compatibility (Cont.)

Test Drug	Mfr	Conc/L or %	Mfr	Conc/L or %	Test Solution	Remarks	Ref	C/I
Sodium bicarbonate	AB	80 mEq	UP	500 mg	D5W	Physically incompatible	15	I
Theophylline		2 g		1.9 g	D5W	Yellow discoloration. 8% ascorbic acid loss in 6 hr and 15% in 24 hr. No theophylline loss	1909	I
Verapamil HCl	KN	80 mg	LI	1 g	D5W, NS	Physically compatible for 24 hr	764	C

ª As calcium ascorbate.

Drugs in Syringe Compatibility

Ascorbic acid

Test Drug	Mfr	Amt	Mfr	Amt	Remarks	Ref	C/I
Cefazolin sodium	LI	1 g/3 mL	LI	1 mL	Precipitate forms within 3 min at 32°C	766	I
Doxapram HCl	RB	400 mg/20 mL		500 mg/2 mL	Immediate turbidity changing to precipitation in 24 hr	1177	I
Metoclopramide HCl	RB	10 mg/2 mL	AB	250 mg/0.5 mL	Physically compatible for 48 hr at 25°C	1167	C
Metoclopramide HCl	RB	160 mg/32 mL	AB	250 mg/0.5 mL	Physically compatible for 48 hr at 25°C	1167	C

Y-Site Injection Compatibility (1:1 Mixture)

Ascorbic acid

Test Drug	Mfr	Conc	Mfr	Conc	Remarks	Ref	C/I
Etomidate	AB	2 mg/mL	AB	500 mg/mL	Yellow color and precipitate form in 24 hr	1801	I
Propofol	STU	2 mg/mL	AB	500 mg/mL	No visible change in 24 hr at 25°C. Yellow color forms within 7 days	1801	?
TPN #189ª			DB	20 mg/mLᵇ	Visually compatible for 24 hr at 22°C	1767	C

ª Refer to Appendix for the composition of parenteral nutrition solutions. TPN indicates a 2-in-1 admixture.

ᵇ Tested in sodium chloride 0.9%.

Additional Compatibility Information

Parenteral Nutrition Solutions

A 35% ascorbic acid loss was reported from a parenteral nutrition solution, composed of amino acids, dextrose, electrolytes, trace elements, and multivitamins, in 39 hours at 25°C with exposure to light. The loss was reduced to a negligible amount in 4 days by refrigeration and light protection.[1063]

The extent and rapidity of ascorbic acid decomposition in parenteral nutrition solutions composed of amino acids, dextrose, electrolytes, multivitamins, and trace elements in 3-L PVC bags stored at 3 to 7°C was reported. About 30 to 40% was lost in 24 hours. The degradation then slowed as the oxygen supply was reduced to the diffusion through the bag. About a 55 to 65% loss occurred after 7 days of storage. The oxidation was catalyzed by metal ions, especially copper. In the absence of copper from the trace elements additive, less than 10% degradation of ascorbic acid occurred in 24 hours. The author estimated that 150 to 200 mg is degraded in 2 to 4 hours at ambient temperature in the presence of copper, but that only 20 to 30 mg is broken down in 24 hours without copper. To minimize ascorbic acid loss, copper must be excluded. Alternatively, inclusion of excess ascorbic acid was suggested.[1056]

Extensive decomposition of ascorbic acid and folic acid was reported in a parenteral nutrition solution composed of amino acids 3.3%, dextrose 12.5%, electrolytes, trace elements, and M.V.I.-12 (USV) in PVC bags. Half-lives were 1.1, 2.9, and 8.9 hours for ascorbic acid and 2.7, 5.4, and 24 hours for folic acid stored at 24°C in daylight, 24°C protected from light, and 4°C protected from light, respectively. The decomposition was much greater than for solutions not containing catalyzing metal ions. Also, it was greater than for the vitamins singly because of interactions with the other vitamins present.[1059]

Ascorbic acid decomposition in TPN admixtures has been reported to result in the formation of precipitated calcium oxalate. Oxalic acid forms as one of the decomposition products of ascorbic acid. The oxalic acid reacts with calcium in the TPN admixture to form the precipitate.[1060]

The stability of numerous vitamins in parenteral nutrition solutions composed of amino acids (Kabi-Vitrum), dextrose 30%, and fat emulsion 20% (Kabi-Vitrum) in a 2:1:1 ratio with electrolytes, trace elements, and both fat- and water-soluble vitamins was reported. The admixtures were stored in darkness at 2 to 8°C for 96 hours. Sodium ascorbate and its biologically active degradation product, dehydroascorbic acid, totaled 59 and 42% of the nominal starting concentration at 24 and 96 hours, respectively. However, the actual initial concentration was only 66% of the nominal concentration.[1225]

When the admixture was subjected to simulated infusion over 24 hours at 20°C, either exposed to room light or light protected, or stored for 6 days in the dark under refrigeration and then subjected to the same simulated infusion, once again the retinyl palmitate, alpha-tocopherol, and sodium riboflavin-5'-phosphate did not undergo significant loss. However, sodium ascorbate and its degradation product, dehydroascorbic acid, had initial combined concentrations of 51 to 65% of the nominal initial concentration, with further declines during infusion. Light protection did not significantly alter the loss of total ascorbic acid.[1225]

The stability of ascorbic acid in parenteral nutrition solutions, with and without fat emulsion, was studied. Both with and without fat emulsion, the total vitamin C content (ascorbic acid plus dehydroascorbic acid) remained above 90% for 12 hours when the solutions were exposed to fluorescent light and for 24 hours when they were protected from light. When stored in a cool dark place, the solutions were stable for 7 days.[1227]

The stability of several vitamins from M.V.I.-12 (Armour) was reported when admixed in parenteral nutrition solutions composed of different amino acid products, with or without Intralipid 10%, when stored in glass bottles and PVC bags at 25 and 5°C for 48 hours. Ascorbic acid was lost from all samples stored at 25°C, with the greatest losses occurring in solutions stored in plastic bags. No losses occurred in any sample stored at 5°C.[1431]

In another study, the stability of several vitamins (as M.V.I.-12) following admixture with 4 different amino acid products (Novamine, Neopham, FreAmine III, Travasol) with or without Intralipid was reported when stored in glass bottles or PVC bags at 25°C for 48 hours. Under high-intensity phototherapy light, ascorbic acid losses were significant with all amino acid products tested. When bisulfite was added to the Neopham admixture, ascorbic acid was unaffected. Ascorbic acid losses were increased with a more alkaline pH and that bisulfite addition offered some protection presumably by bisulfite being preferentially oxidized. The authors concluded that intravenous multivitamins should be added to parenteral nutrition admixtures immediately prior to administration to reduce losses since commercially available amino acid products may contain bisulfites and have varying pH values.[487]

The stability of ascorbic acid and dehydroascorbic acid was evaluated in a 3-in-1 admixture containing Vamin 14, dextrose 30%, Intralipid 20%, potassium phosphate, Cernevit, and trace elements in ethylene vinyl acetate (EVA) bags over a temperature range of 2 to 22°C. They observed an 89% loss of ascorbic acid and 37% loss of dehydroascorbic acid over 7 days. Oxygen, trace elements, temperature, and an underfilled bag were the greatest determinants of ascorbic acid loss.[2462]

The long-term stability of ascorbic acid in 3-in-1 admixtures containing amino acids (Eloamin) 10%, dextrose 20%, fat emulsion (Elolipid) 20%, calcium gluconate, M.V.C. 9 + 3, and trace elements mixed in EVA and multilayer (Ultrastab) bags at 5°C was evaluated. Ascorbic acid losses were greater than 75% in the first 24 hours and 100% after 48 to 72 hours in the EVA bags. In the multilayer bags, ascorbic acid showed a 20 and 40% loss over the first 24 hours with and without fat emulsion, respectively. The initial rapid fall in ascorbic acid was presumably due to the initial oxygen content of the admixtures despite the use of the less oxygen-permeable multilayer bags. The ascorbic acid concentration remained stable for up to 28 days in the multilayer bags after the initial fall. Adding additional ascorbic acid to compensate for the losses was recommended to facilitate extended shelf-life.[2463]

Because of these interactions, recommendations to separate the administration of vitamins and trace elements have been made.[1056] [1060] [1061] Other researchers have termed such recommendations premature based on differing reports[895] [896] and the apparent absence of epidemic vitamin deficiency in parenteral nutrition patients.[1062]

The influence of several factors on the rate of ascorbic acid oxidation in parenteral nutrition solutions was evaluated. Ascorbic acid is regarded as the least stable component in TPN admixtures. The type of amino acid used in the TPN was important. Some, such as FreAmine III and Vamin 14, contain antioxidant compounds (e.g., sodium metabisulfite or cysteine). Ascorbic acid stability was better in such solutions compared with those amino acid solutions having no antioxidant present. Furthermore, the pH of the solution may play a small role, with greater degradation as the pH rises from about 5 to about 7. Adding air to a compounded TPN container can also accelerate ascorbic acid decomposition. The most important factor was the type of plastic container used for the TPN. EVA containers (Mixieva, Miramed) allow more oxygen permeation, which results in substantial losses of ascorbic acid in relatively short time periods. In multilayer TPN bags (Ultrastab, Miramed) designed to reduce gas permeability, the rate of ascorbic acid degradation was greatly reduced. TPNs without antioxidants packaged in EVA bags had an almost total loss of ascorbic acid activity in 1 or 2 days at 5°C. In contrast, in TPNs containing FreAmine III or Vamin 14 and packaged in the multilayer bags, most of the ascorbic acid content was retained for 28 days at 5°C. The TPNs made with antioxidant-containing amino acids and packaged in multilayer bags that reduce gas permeability can safely be given extended expiration dates and still retain most of the ascorbic acid activity.[2163]

The initial degradation product of ascorbic acid (dehydroascorbic acid) was evaluated in a 2-in-1 admixture containing Synthamin 14, glucose 20%, and trace elements over a temperature range of 5 to 35°C. The presence of trace elements, including copper, had no influence on the degradation of dehydroascorbic acid. At room temperature and 5°C, there was a greater than 50% loss of dehydroascorbic acid noted within 2 and 24 hours, respectively. The authors concluded this degradation was temperature dependent.[2461]

The degradation of vitamins A, B1, C, and E from Cernevit (Roche) multivitamins was evaluated in NuTRIflex Lipid Plus (B. Braun) admixtures prepared in ethylene vinyl acetate (EVA) bags and in multilayer bags. After storage for up to 72 hours at 4, 21, and 40°C, greater vitamin losses occurred in the EVA bags: vitamin A (retinyl palmitate) losses were 20%, thiamine hydrochloride losses were 25%, alpha-tocopherol losses were 20%, and ascorbic acid losses were approximately 80 to 100%. In the multilayer bags (presumably a better barrier to oxygen transfer), losses were less: vitamin A (retinyl palmitate) losses were 5%, thiamine hydrochloride losses were 10%, alpha-tocopherol losses were 0%, and ascorbic acid losses were approximately 25 to 70%.[2618]

The vitamins in Cernevit (Baxter) diluted in three 2-in-1 parenteral nutrition admixtures were tested for stability over 48 hours. While all of the vitamins retained their initial concentrations, ascorbic acid exhibited losses of about 5%, 13%, and 17% in TPNs with dextrose concentrations of 10, 15, and 25%, respectively.[2796]

Asparaginase *Erwinia chrysanthemi*
AHFS 10:00

Products

Asparaginase *Erwinia chrysanthemi* is available as a lyophilized powder in vials containing 10,000 international units of the drug.[2896] Each vial also contains glucose monohydrate 5 mg and sodium chloride 0.5 mg.[2896]

Reconstitute each vial with 1 or 2 mL of preservative-free sodium chloride 0.9% to yield solutions of 10,000 or 5000 international units/mL, respectively.[2896] Direct the stream of diluent at the vial wall and not directly into the powder.[2896] Swirl or gently mix to dissolve the powder; do not shake or invert the vial.[2896]

Trade Name(s)

Erwinaze

Administration

Asparaginase *Erwinia chrysanthemi* is administered intramuscularly using a volume no greater than 2 mL; larger volumes require 2 injection sites.[2896]

Selected Revisions June 1, 2019. © Copyright, September 2014. American Society of Health-System Pharmacists, Inc.

Stability

Intact vials and cartons of asparaginase *Erwinia chrysanthemi* should be stored under refrigeration and protected from light.[2896]

Asparaginase *Erwinia chrysanthemi*, a white lyophilized powder, becomes a clear, colorless solution on reconstitution.[2896] If any visible particles or protein aggregates are present, the reconstituted solution should be discarded.[2896]

The volume of the reconstituted solution containing the calculated dose should be withdrawn from the vial into a polypropylene syringe within 15 minutes of reconstitution and administered within 4 hours.[2896] The manufacturer indicates that the reconstituted solution should not be stored under refrigeration or frozen.[2896] Any unused portions should be discarded.[2896]

DOI: 10.37573/9781585286850.040

Atracurium Besylate
AHFS 12:20.20

Products

Atracurium besylate is available as a 10-mg/mL aqueous solution in 5-mL single-use vials and 10-mL multiple-dose vials with benzyl alcohol 0.9% as a preservative. The pH is adjusted with benzenesulfonic acid.[1(1/04)]

pH

Adjusted to 3.25 to 3.65.[1(1/04)]

Administration

Atracurium besylate is administered by rapid intravenous injection or by intravenous infusion in concentrations of 0.2 and 0.5 mg/mL. It must not be given by intramuscular injection. Do not administer in the same syringe or through the same needle as an alkaline solution.[1(1/04)] [4]

Stability

Atracurium besylate injection is a clear, colorless solution; it should be stored under refrigeration and protected from freezing. Nevertheless, the drug undergoes slow decomposition of about 6% per year.[1(1/04)] [4] The estimated t_{90} at 5°C is approximately 18 months.[859] At 25°C, the rate of decomposition is stated to increase to about 5% per month.[1(1/04)] [4] The manufacturers have indicated that intact vials of atracurium besylate may be used for 14 days when stored at room temperature.[1(1/04)] [1181]

Other research indicates that atracurium besylate injection in intact containers may be stable even longer at room temperature. Intact containers were found to retain 92% of the concentration after 3 months at 20°C.[777]

pH Effects

Atracurium besylate is unstable in the presence of both acids and bases.[4] Maximum stability in aqueous solution was observed at about pH 2.5.[859]

Atracurium besylate, which has an acid pH, should not be mixed with alkaline solutions such as barbiturates. The atracurium besylate may be inactivated and precipitation of a free acid of the admixed drug may occur, depending on the resultant pH.[4]

Syringes

Atracurium besylate (Burroughs Wellcome) 10 mg/mL was repackaged as 10 mL of solution in 12-mL plastic syringes (Monoject) and stored at 5, 25, and 40°C. The samples remained visually clear throughout the study. No loss occurred in the refrigerated samples and about 4% loss occurred in the room temperature samples after 42 days of storage. At 40°C, 15% was lost in 21 days. Exposure of atracurium to elevated temperatures should be avoided.[2141]

Atracurium 10 mg/mL repackaged in polypropylene syringes exhibited little change in concentration after 4 weeks of storage at room temperature when not exposed to direct light.[2164]

Compatibility Information

Solution Compatibility

Atracurium besylate

Test Soln Name	Mfr	Mfr	Conc/L or %	Remarks	Ref	C/I
Dextrose 5% in sodium chloride 0.9%		BW	200 and 500 mg	Physically compatible and chemically stable for 24 hr at 5 and 25°C	1694	C
Dextrose 5%		BW	200 and 500 mg	Physically compatible and chemically stable for 24 hr at 5 and 30°C	1694	C
Dextrose 5%		BW	1 and 5 g	Chemically stable for 48 hr	1693	C
Dextrose 5%	BA[a]	BW	0.5 g	About 50% loss in 14 days stored at 5 and 25°C	2141	I
Ringer's injection, lactated		BW	200 and 500 mg	Increased rate of atracurium degradation limits utility time to 8 hr at 25°C	1694	I
Ringer's injection, lactated	TR	BW	500 mg	About 6% loss in 12 hr at 22°C	1692	I
Ringer's injection, lactated			1 and 5 g	About 10 to 12% loss in 24 hr at 30°C	1693	I
Sodium chloride 0.9%		BW	200 and 500 mg	Physically compatible and chemically stable for 24 hr at 5 and 25°C	1694	C
Sodium chloride 0.9%		BW	1 and 5 g	Chemically stable for 24 hr	1693	C
Sodium chloride 0.9%	BA[a]	BW	0.5 g	About 60% loss in 14 days at 5 and 25°C	2141	I
Sodium chloride 0.9%	TR	BW	500 mg	About 1% loss in 12 hr at 22°C	1692	C

[a] Tested in glass containers.

DOI: 10.37573/9781585286850.041

Additive Compatibility

Atracurium besylate

Test Drug	Mfr	Conc/L or %	Mfr	Conc/L or %	Test Solution	Remarks	Ref	C/I
Aminophylline		1 g	BW	500 mg	D5W	Atracurium unstable due to high pH	1694	I
Cefazolin sodium		10 g	BW	500 mg	D5W	Atracurium unstable and particles form	1694	I
Ciprofloxacin	BAY	1.6 g	GW	2 g	D5W	Visually compatible with no loss of ciprofloxacin in 24 hr at 22°C under fluorescent light. Atracurium not tested	2413	C
Dobutamine HCl		1 g	BW	500 mg	D5W	Physically compatible and atracurium stable for 24 hr at 5 and 30°C	1694	C
Dopamine HCl		1.6 g	BW	500 mg	D5W	Physically compatible and atracurium stable for 24 hr at 5 and 30°C	1694	C
Esmolol HCl		10 g	BW	500 mg	D5W	Physically compatible and atracurium stable for 24 hr at 5 and 30°C	1694	C
Gentamicin sulfate		2 g	BW	500 mg	D5W	Physically compatible and atracurium stable for 24 hr at 5 and 30°C	1694	C
Heparin sodium		40,000 units	BW	500 mg	D5W	Particles form at 5 and 30°C	1694	I
Isoproterenol HCl		4 mg	BW	500 mg	D5W	Physically compatible and atracurium stable for 24 hr at 5 and 30°C	1694	C
Lidocaine HCl		2 g	BW	500 mg	D5W	Physically compatible and atracurium stable for 24 hr at 5 and 30°C	1694	C
Morphine sulfate		1 g	BW	500 mg	D5W	Physically compatible and atracurium stable for 24 hr at 5 and 30°C	1694	C
Potassium chloride		80 mEq	BW	500 mg	D5W	Physically compatible and atracurium stable for 24 hr at 5 and 30°C	1694	C
Procainamide HCl		4 g	BW	500 mg	D5W	Physically compatible and atracurium stable for 24 hr at 5 and 30°C	1694	C
Quinidine gluconate		8.3 g	BW	500 mg	D5W	Particles form and atracurium unstable at 5 and 30°C	1694	I
Ranitidine HCl		500 mg	BW	500 mg	D5W	Atracurium unstable due to high pH	1694	I
Sodium nitroprusside		2 g	BW	500 mg	D5W	Physically incompatible. Haze, particles, and yellow color form	1694	I
Vancomycin HCl		5 g	BW	500 mg	D5W	Physically compatible and atracurium stable for 24 hr at 5 and 30°C	1694	C

Drugs in Syringe Compatibility

Atracurium besylate

Test Drug	Mfr	Amt	Mfr	Amt	Remarks	Ref	C/I
Alfentanil HCl		0.5 mg/mL	BW	10 mg/mL	Physically compatible and atracurium stable for 24 hr at 5 and 30°C	1694	C
Fentanyl citrate		50 mcg/mL	BW	10 mg/mL	Physically compatible and atracurium stable for 24 hr at 5 and 30°C	1694	C
Midazolam HCl		5 mg/mL	BW	10 mg/mL	Physically compatible and atracurium stable for 24 hr at 5 and 30°C	1694	C
Sufentanil citrate		50 mcg/mL	BW	10 mg/mL	Physically compatible and atracurium stable for 24 hr at 5 and 30°C	1694	C

Y-Site Injection Compatibility (1:1 Mixture)

Atracurium besylate

Test Drug	Mfr	Conc	Mfr	Conc	Remarks	Ref	C/I
Amiodarone HCl	WY	6 mg/mL[a]	BA	5 mg/mL[a]	Visually compatible for 24 hr at 22°C	2352	C
Cefazolin sodium	LY	10 mg/mL[a]	BW	0.5 mg/mL[a]	Physically compatible for 24 hr at 28°C	1337	C
Cefuroxime sodium	GL	7.5 mg/mL[a]	BW	0.5 mg/mL[a]	Physically compatible for 24 hr at 28°C	1337	C
Clarithromycin	AB	4 mg/mL[a]	GW	1 mg/mL[a]	Visually compatible for 72 hr at both 30 and 17°C	2174	C
Dexmedetomidine HCl	HOS	4 mcg/mL[d]			Stated to be compatible	3181	C
Diazepam	ES	5 mg/mL	BW	0.5 mg/mL[a]	Cloudy solution forms immediately	1337	I
Dobutamine HCl	LI	1 mg/mL[a]	BW	0.5 mg/mL[a]	Physically compatible for 24 hr at 28°C	1337	C
Dopamine HCl	SO	1.6 mg/mL[a]	BW	0.5 mg/mL[a]	Physically compatible for 24 hr at 28°C	1337	C
Epinephrine HCl	AB	4 mcg/mL[a]	BW	0.5 mg/mL[a]	Physically compatible for 24 hr at 28°C	1337	C
Esmolol HCl	DCC	10 mg/mL[a]	BW	0.5 mg/mL[a]	Physically compatible for 24 hr at 28°C	1337	C
Etomidate	AB	2 mg/mL	BW	10 mg/mL	Visually compatible for 7 days at 25°C	1801	C
Fenoldopam mesylate	AB	80 mcg/mL[b]	BA	0.5 mg/mL[b]	Physically compatible for 4 hr at 23°C	2467	C
Fentanyl citrate	ES	10 mcg/mL[a]	BW	0.5 mg/mL[a]	Physically compatible for 24 hr at 28°C	1337	C
Gentamicin sulfate	ES	2 mg/mL[a]	BW	0.5 mg/mL[a]	Physically compatible for 24 hr at 28°C	1337	C
Heparin sodium	SO	40 units/mL[a]	BW	0.5 mg/mL[a]	Physically compatible for 24 hr at 28°C	1337	C
Hetastarch in lactated electrolyte	AB	6%	GW	0.5 mg/mL[a]	Physically compatible for 4 hr at 23°C	2339	C
Hydrocortisone sodium succinate	AB	1 mg/mL[a]	BW	0.5 mg/mL[a]	Physically compatible for 24 hr at 28°C	1337	C
Isoproterenol HCl	ES	4 mcg/mL[a]	BW	0.5 mg/mL[a]	Physically compatible for 24 hr at 28°C	1337	C
Lorazepam	WY	0.5 mg/mL[a]	BW	0.5 mg/mL[a]	Physically compatible for 24 hr at 28°C	1337	C
Midazolam HCl	RC	0.05 mg/mL[a]	BW	0.5 mg/mL[a]	Physically compatible for 24 hr at 28°C	1337	C
Midazolam HCl	RC	0.1 mg/mL[a]	GW	1 and 5 mg/mL[a]	Visually compatible with no loss of either drug in 3 hr at 25°C	2112	C
Midazolam HCl	RC	0.5 mg/mL[a]	GW	5 mg/mL[a]	Visually compatible with no loss of either drug in 3 hr at 25°C	2112	C
Midazolam HCl	RC	0.5 mg/mL[a]	GW	1 mg/mL[a]	Visually compatible with no loss of midazolam and 4% loss of atracurium in 3 hr at 25°C	2112	C
Milrinone lactate	SW	0.4 mg/mL[a]	BW	1 mg/mL[a]	Visually compatible with little or no loss of either drug in 4 hr at 23°C	2214	C
Morphine sulfate	WY	1 mg/mL[a]	BW	0.5 mg/mL[a]	Physically compatible for 24 hr at 28°C	1337	C
Nitroglycerin	SO	0.4 mg/mL[a]	BW	0.5 mg/mL[a]	Physically compatible for 24 hr at 28°C	1337	C
Propofol	STU	2 mg/mL	BW	10 mg/mL	Oil droplets form within 24 hr, followed by phase separation at 25°C	1801	I
Propofol	ZEN[e]	10 mg/mL	BW	10 mg/mL	Emulsion broke and oiled out	2066	I
Propofol	ASZ[e]	10 mg/mL		10 mg/mL	Emulsion disruption upon mixing	2336	I
Propofol	BA[f]	10 mg/mL		10 mg/mL	Emulsion disruption upon mixing	2336	I

Y-Site Injection Compatibility (1:1 Mixture) (Cont.)

Test Drug	Mfr	Conc	Mfr	Conc	Remarks	Ref	C/I
Propofol	ASZ[e]	10 mg/mL		5 mg/mL	Emulsion disruption upon mixing	2336	I
Propofol	BA[f]	10 mg/mL		5 mg/mL	Emulsion disruption upon mixing	2336	I
Propofol	BA[f]	10 mg/mL		0.5 mg/mL[a]	Emulsion disruption upon mixing	2336	I
Propofol	ASZ[e]	10 mg/mL		0.5 mg/mL[a]	Physically compatible	2336	C
Ranitidine HCl	GL	0.5 mg/mL[a]	BW	0.5 mg/mL[a]	Physically compatible for 24 hr at 28°C	1337	C
Sodium nitroprusside	ES	0.2 mg/mL[a]	BW	0.5 mg/mL[a]	Physically compatible for 24 hr at 28°C	1337	C
TPN #189[b]			WEL	10 mg/mL	Visually compatible for 24 hr at 22°C	1767	C
Trimethoprim–sulfamethoxazole	ES	0.64 mg/mL[a][c]	BW	0.5 mg/mL[a]	Physically compatible for 24 hr at 28°C	1337	C
Vancomycin HCl	ES	5 mg/mL[a]	BW	0.5 mg/mL[a]	Physically compatible for 24 hr at 28°C	1337	C

[a] Tested in dextrose 5%.

[b] Refer to Appendix for the composition of parenteral nutrition solutions. TPN indicates a 2-in-1 admixture.

[c] Trimethoprim component. Trimethoprim in a 1:5 fixed-ratio concentration with sulfamethoxazole.

[d] Tested in sodium chloride 0.9%.

[e] Test performed using the formulation WITH edetate disodium.

[f] Test performed using the formulation WITHOUT edetate disodium.

Selected Revisions January 31, 2020. © Copyright, October 1986.
American Society of Health-System Pharmacists, Inc.

Atropine Sulfate
AHFS 12:08.08

Products

Atropine sulfate injection is available at concentrations of 0.4 mg/mL and 1 mg/mL in 1-mL single-dose (preservative-free) vials[3448] and at a concentration of 0.4 mg/mL in 20-mL multiple-dose vials.[3447 3450] Sodium chloride is present for isotonicity, and sulfuric acid may have been used to adjust the pH.[3447 3448 3450] Multiple-dose vials also contain benzyl alcohol as a preservative.[3447 3450]

Atropine sulfate also is available in a concentration of 0.05 mg/mL in 5-mL single-dose prefilled syringes and 0.1 mg/mL in 5- and 10-mL single-dose prefilled syringes.[3445 3446 3449] Sodium chloride is present for isotonicity.[3445 3446 3449] Some syringes may contain sodium hydroxide and/or sulfuric acid to adjust the pH.[3445 3446] Some syringes contain citric acid and sodium citrate as buffers and may contain additional amounts of citric acid and/or sodium citrate to adjust the pH.[3449]

Atropine sulfate also is available in 0.25-, 0.5-, 1-, and 2-mg auto-injector syringes for self or caregiver intramuscular administration in the treatment of nerve agent and insecticide poisoning only.[3451]

pH

Single-dose vials: From 3 to 6.5.[3448]

Multiple-dose vials: From 3 to 3.8 (Fresenius Kabi)[3447] or from 3 to 6.5 (West-Ward).[3450]

Prefilled syringes: From 3 to 6.5.[3445 3446 3449]

Auto-injector syringes: From 4 to 5.[3451]

Osmolarity

Atropine sulfate injection has a calculated osmolarity of 308 mOsm/L.[3445 3446]

Administration

Atropine sulfate injection may be administered by the intravenous, subcutaneous, intramuscular, or intraosseous routes.[3445 3446 3447 3448 3449 3450] Specific product labeling should be consulted for details on the routes of administration that are recommended for each individual product.

Stability

Atropine sulfate injection should be stored at controlled room temperature.[3445 3446 3447 3448 3449 3450] One manufacturer states that multiple-dose vials should be stored at 20 to 25°C after initial use and should be discarded within 24 hours.[3447]

pH Effects

Minimum hydrolysis occurs at pH 3.5.[1072]

Temperature Effects

Atropine sulfate 0.1 mg/mL in auto-injector syringes (Abbott) was evaluated for stability over 45 days under use conditions in paramedic vehicles. Temperatures fluctuated with locations and conditions and ranged from 6.5°C (43.7 °F) to 52°C (125.6 °F) in high desert conditions. No visually apparent changes occurred, and little or no loss of atropine sulfate was found.[2548]

In another study, atropine sulfate injection under simulated summer conditions in paramedic vehicles was exposed to temperatures ranging from 26 to 38°C over 4 weeks. Analysis found no loss of the drug under these conditions.[2562]

Syringes

In 2015, reports of decreased potency of certain drugs (e.g., atropine sulfate) stored in Becton Dickinson syringes for extended periods (i.e., exceeding 24 hours) were confirmed by the manufacturer of these syringes; the cause of this change was later identified to be the inclusion of an alternate rubber stopper in the plunger of certain product lots of syringes.[3029 3036 3037 3039 3041 3042] Decreased potency was not observed when the syringes were filled and used promptly.[3037] Use of the alternate stopper was later discontinued and use of the primary stopper in such syringes was resumed; however, Becton Dickinson states that its general-use syringes are cleared by FDA for immediate use in fluid aspiration and injection and that such syringes, regardless of the stopper material, have not been cleared by FDA for use as a closed-container system.[3391]

Atropine 1 mg/mL repackaged in polypropylene syringes exhibited little change in concentration after 4 weeks of storage at room temperature not exposed to direct light.[2164]

Extemporaneously compounded atropine sulfate 2-mg/mL injection in sodium chloride 0.9% for use in the event of a terrorist nerve gas attack was packaged in polypropylene syringes (Becton Dickinson) with sealed tips. The injection was adjusted to pH 3.5 with sulfuric acid during compounding. No visible changes were reported, and analysis found no loss of the drug over 364 days at 5°C protected from light, 364 days at 23°C exposed to light, and 28 days at 35°C exposed to light.[2781]

DOI: 10.37573/9781585286850.042

Compatibility Information

Solution Compatibility

Atropine sulfate

Test Soln Name	Mfr	Mfr	Conc/L or %	Remarks	Ref	C/I
Sodium chloride 0.9%	BA[a]		1 g	Physically compatible with little or no atropine loss in 72 hr at 6, 23, and 34°C	2522	C

[a] Tested in PVC containers.

Additive Compatibility

Atropine sulfate

Test Drug	Mfr	Conc/L or %	Mfr	Conc/L or %	Test Solution	Remarks	Ref	C/I
Dobutamine HCl	LI	167 mg	AB	16.7 mg	NS	Physically compatible for 24 hr	552	C
Dobutamine HCl	LI	1 g	ES	50 mg	D5W, NS	Physically compatible for 24 hr at 21°C	812	C
Eptifibatide	ME	750 mg		400 mg		Physically compatible and chemically stable for up to 24 hr at 25°C	3049	C
Floxacillin sodium	BE	20 g	ANT	60 mg	W	Haze forms in 24 hr and precipitate forms in 48 hr at 30°C. No change at 15°C	1479	I
Furosemide	HO	1 g	ANT	60 mg	W	Physically compatible for 72 hr at 15 and 30°C	1479	C
Meropenem	ZEN	1 and 20 g	ES	40 mg	NS	Visually compatible for 4 hr at room temperature	1994	C
Sodium bicarbonate	AB	2.4 mEq[a]		0.4 mg	D5W	Physically compatible for 24 hr	772	C
Verapamil HCl	KN	80 mg	IX	0.8 mg	D5W, NS	Physically compatible for 24 hr	764	C

[a] One vial of Neut added to a liter of admixture.

Drugs in Syringe Compatibility

Atropine sulfate

Test Drug	Mfr	Amt	Mfr	Amt	Remarks	Ref	C/I
Buprenorphine HCl					Physically and chemically compatible	4	C
Butorphanol tartrate	BR	4 mg/2 mL	ST	0.4 mg/1 mL	Physically compatible for 30 min at room temperature	566	C
Chlorpromazine HCl	SKF	50 mg/2 mL		0.6 mg/1.5 mL	Physically compatible for at least 15 min	14	C
Chlorpromazine HCl	PO	50 mg/2 mL	ST	0.4 mg/1 mL	Physically compatible for at least 15 min	326	C
Dimenhydrinate	HR	50 mg/1 mL	ST	0.4 mg/1 mL	Physically compatible for at least 15 min	326	C
Diphenhydramine HCl	PD	50 mg/1 mL	ST	0.4 mg/1 mL	Physically compatible for at least 15 min	326	C
Droperidol	MN	2.5 mg/1 mL	ST	0.4 mg/1 mL	Physically compatible for at least 15 min	326	C
Fentanyl citrate	MN	100 mcg/1 mL		0.6 mg/1.5 mL	Physically compatible for at least 15 min	14	C
Fentanyl citrate	MN	0.05 mg/1 mL	ST	0.4 mg/1 mL	Physically compatible for at least 15 min	326	C
Glycopyrrolate	RB	0.2 mg/1 mL	ES	0.4 mg/1 mL	Physically compatible. pH in glycopyrrolate stability range for 48 hr at 25°C	331	C
Glycopyrrolate	RB	0.2 mg/1 mL	ES	0.8 mg/2 mL	Physically compatible. pH in glycopyrrolate stability range for 48 hr at 25°C	331	C
Glycopyrrolate	RB	0.4 mg/2 mL	ES	0.4 mg/1 mL	Physically compatible. pH in glycopyrrolate stability range for 48 hr at 25°C	331	C

Drugs in Syringe Compatibility (Cont.)

Test Drug	Mfr	Amt	Mfr	Amt	Remarks	Ref	C/I
Heparin sodium		2500 units/1 mL		0.5 mg/1 mL	Physically compatible for at least 5 min	1053	C
Hydromorphone HCl	KN	4 mg/2 mL	ES	0.4 mg/0.5 mL	Physically compatible for 30 min	517	C
Hydroxyzine HCl	PF	100 mg/4 mL		0.6 mg/1.5 mL	Physically compatible for at least 15 min	14	C
Hydroxyzine HCl	NF	50 mg/1 mL	USP	0.4 mg/0.4 mL	Hydroxyzine stable for at least 10 days at 3 and 25°C	49	C
Hydroxyzine HCl	PF	50 mg/1 mL	ST	0.4 mg/1 mL	Physically compatible for at least 15 min	326	C
Hydroxyzine HCl	PF	100 mg/2 mL		0.4 mg/1 mL	Physically compatible	771	C
Hydroxyzine HCl	PF	50 mg/1 mL		0.4 mg/1 mL	Physically compatible	771	C
Meperidine HCl	WY	100 mg/1 mL		0.6 mg/1.5 mL	Physically compatible for at least 15 min	14	C
Meperidine HCl	WI	50 mg/1 mL	ST	0.4 mg/1 mL	Physically compatible for at least 15 min	326	C
Metoclopramide HCl	NO	10 mg/2 mL	GL	0.4 mg/1 mL	Physically compatible for 15 min at room temperature	565	C
Midazolam HCl	RC	5 mg/1 mL	IX	0.4 mg/1 mL	Physically compatible for 4 hr at 25°C	1145	C
Milrinone lactate	STR	5.25 mg/5.25 mL	IX	2 mg/2 mL	Physically compatible. No loss of either drug in 20 min at 23°C	1410	C
Morphine sulfate	WY	15 mg/1 mL		0.6 mg/1.5 mL	Physically compatible for at least 15 min	14	C
Morphine sulfate	ST	15 mg/1 mL	ST	0.4 mg/1 mL	Physically compatible for at least 15 min	326	C
Nalbuphine HCl	EN	10 mg/1 mL	WY	0.2 mg	Physically compatible for 36 hr at 27°C	762	C
Nalbuphine HCl	EN	5 mg/0.5 mL	WY	0.2 mg	Physically compatible for 36 hr at 27°C	762	C
Nalbuphine HCl	EN	10 mg/1 mL	WY	0.5 mg	Physically compatible for 36 hr at 27°C	762	C
Nalbuphine HCl	EN	5 mg/0.5 mL	WY	0.5 mg	Physically compatible for 36 hr at 27°C	762	C
Nalbuphine HCl	DU	10 mg/1 mL		0.4 and 1 mg	Physically compatible for 48 hr	128	C
Nalbuphine HCl	DU	20 mg/1 mL		0.4 and 1 mg	Physically compatible for 48 hr	128	C
Ondansetron HCl	GW	1.33 mg/mL[b]	GNS	0.133 mg/mL[b]	Physically compatible. Under 6% ondansetron and under 7% atropine losses in 24 hr at 4 or 23°C	2199	C
Pantoprazole sodium	[a]	4 mg/1 mL		0.4 mg/1 mL	Incompatible after 4 hr	2574	I
Pentazocine lactate	WI	30 mg/1 mL		0.6 mg/1.5 mL	Physically compatible for at least 15 min	14	C
Pentazocine lactate	WI	30 mg/1 mL	ST	0.4 mg/1 mL	Physically compatible for at least 15 min	326	C
Pentobarbital sodium	WY	100 mg/2 mL		0.6 mg/1.5 mL	Physically compatible for at least 15 min	14	C
Pentobarbital sodium	AB	50 mg/1 mL	ST	0.4 mg/1 mL	Physically compatible for at least 15 min	326	C
Pentobarbital sodium	AB	100 mg/2 mL	LI	0.6 mg/1.5 mL	Precipitate forms in 24 hr at room temperature	542	I
Prochlorperazine edisylate	SKF			0.6 mg/1.5 mL	Physically compatible for at least 15 min	14	C
Prochlorperazine edisylate	PO	5 mg/1 mL	ST	0.4 mg/1 mL	Physically compatible for at least 15 min	326	C
Promethazine HCl	WY	50 mg/2 mL		0.6 mg/1.5 mL	Physically compatible for at least 15 min	14	C
Promethazine HCl	PO	50 mg/2 mL	ST	0.4 mg/1 mL	Physically compatible for at least 15 min	326	C
Ranitidine HCl	GL	50 mg/2 mL	GL	0.4 mg/1 mL	Physically compatible for 1 hr at 25°C	978	C
Scopolamine HBr	ST	0.4 mg/1 mL	ST	0.4 mg/1 mL	Physically compatible for at least 15 min	326	C

[a] Test performed using the formulation WITHOUT edetate disodium.

[b] Tested in sodium chloride 0.9%.

Y-Site Injection Compatibility (1:1 Mixture)

Atropine sulfate

Test Drug	Mfr	Conc	Mfr	Conc	Remarks	Ref	C/I
Abciximab	LI	36 mcg/mL[a]	AMR	0.4 mg/mL	Visually compatible for 12 hr at 23°C	2374	C
Amiodarone HCl	WY	6 mg/mL[a]	AB	0.4 mg/mL	Visually compatible for 24 hr at 22°C	2352	C
Argatroban	GSK	1 mg/mL[b]	AMR	0.4 mg/mL	Visually compatible for 24 hr at 23°C	2391	C
Bivalirudin	TMC	5 mg/mL[a b]	AMR	0.4 mg/mL	Visually compatible for 6 hr at 23°C	2680	C
Cangrelor tetrasodium	TMC	1 mg/mL[b]		0.4 and 1 mg/mL	Physically compatible for 4 hr	3243	C
Cloxacillin sodium	SMX	100 mg/mL	SZ	0.4 mg/mL	Physically compatible for up to 4 hr at room temperature	3245	C
Dexmedetomidine HCl	HOS	4 mcg/mL[b]			Stated to be compatible	3181	C
Doripenem	JJ	5 mg/mL[a b]	BA	0.4 mg/mL	Physically compatible for 4 hr at 23°C	2743	C
Etomidate	AB	2 mg/mL	GNS	0.4 mg/mL	Visually compatible for 7 days at 25°C	1801	C
Famotidine	MSD	0.2 mg/mL[a]	AST	0.1 mg/mL[a]	Physically compatible for 4 hr at 25°C	1188	C
Fenoldopam mesylate	AB	80 mcg/mL[b]	APP	0.1 mg/mL[b]	Physically compatible for 4 hr at 23°C	2467	C
Fentanyl citrate	JN	25 mcg/mL[a]	LY	0.4 mg/mL	Physically compatible for 48 hr at 22°C	1706	C
Heparin sodium	UP	1000 units/L[c]	BW	0.5 mg/mL	Physically compatible for 4 hr at room temperature	534	C
Hydrocortisone sodium succinate	UP	10 mg/L[c]	BW	0.5 mg/mL	Physically compatible for 4 hr at room temperature	534	C
Hydromorphone HCl	AST	0.5 mg/mL[a]	LY	0.4 mg/mL	Physically compatible for 48 hr at 22°C	1706	C
Meropenem	ZEN	1 and 50 mg/mL[b]	ES	0.4 mg/mL	Visually compatible for 4 hr at room temperature	1994	C
Meropenem		50 mg/mL	ALV	0.4 mg/mL	Physically compatible for 4 hr at room temperature	3538	C
Methadone HCl	LI	1 mg/mL[a]	LY	0.4 mg/mL	Physically compatible for 48 hr at 22°C	1706	C
Morphine sulfate	AST	1 mg/mL[a]	LY	0.4 mg/mL	Physically compatible for 48 hr at 22°C	1706	C
Nafcillin sodium	WY	33 mg/mL[b]		0.4 mg/mL	No precipitation	547	C
Palonosetron HCl	MGI	50 mcg/mL	AMR	0.4 mg/mL	Physically compatible and no loss of either drug in 4 hr at room temperature	2771	C
Potassium chloride	AB	40 mEq/L[c]	BW	0.5 mg/mL	Physically compatible for 4 hr at room temperature	534	C
Propofol	STU	2 mg/mL	GNS	0.4 mg/mL	Oil droplets form within 7 days at 25°C. No visible change in 24 hr	1801	?
Propofol	ZEN[d]	10 mg/mL	AST	0.1 mg/mL[a]	Physically compatible for 1 hr at 23°C	2066	C
Tirofiban HCl	ME	50 mcg/mL[a b]	APP	0.4 mg/mL	Physically compatible with no loss of either drug in 4 hr at 23°C	2356	C
Tirofiban HCl	ME	50 mcg/mL[a b]	AMR	1 mg/mL	Physically compatible with no loss of either drug in 4 hr at 23°C	2356	C

[a] Tested in dextrose 5%.

[b] Tested in sodium chloride 0.9%.

[c] Tested in dextrose 5%, dextrose 5% in Ringer's injection, dextrose 5% in Ringer's injection, lactated, Ringer's injection, lactated, and sodium chloride 0.9%.

[d] Test performed using the formulation WITH edetate disodium.

Selected Revisions May 1, 2020. © Copyright, October 1982.
American Society of Health-System Pharmacists, Inc.

Azacitidine
AHFS 10:00

Products

Azacitidine is available as a lyophilized powder in single-use (preservative-free) vials in a formulation containing 100 mg of azacitidine and 100 mg of mannitol.[3325] Azacitidine (Actavis) also is available as a lyophilized powder in single-use (preservative-free) vials in a formulation containing 100 mg of azacitidine with sucrose 170 mg, monosodium phosphate monohydrate, and disodium hydrogen phosphate dihydrate.[3326]

To prepare a suspension of azacitidine for subcutaneous administration from either formulation, the powder contents of one vial should be reconstituted by slowly injecting 4 mL of sterile water for injection into the vial.[3325] [3326] The vial should be shaken vigorously or rolled until a uniform, cloudy suspension results.[3325] [3326] The suspension will have a final azacitidine concentration of 25 mg/mL.[3325] [3326]

To prepare a solution of azacitidine for intravenous administration from either formulation, each 100-mg vial of azacitidine should be reconstituted with 10 mL of sterile water for injection.[3325] [3326] Vials should be vigorously shaken or rolled until all solids are dissolved and a clear solution results.[3325] [3326] The solution will have a final azacitidine concentration of 10 mg/mL.[3325] [3326] The appropriate dose of the reconstituted solution should be withdrawn from the vial and diluted in 50 to 100 mL of sodium chloride 0.9% or Ringer's injection, lactated.[3325] [3326]

Trade Name(s)

Vidaza

Administration

Azacitidine may be administered subcutaneously as a suspension or intravenously as a solution.[3325] [3326]

Prior to subcutaneous administration, the reconstituted suspension may be allowed to come to room temperature for up to 30 minutes if it has been refrigerated.[3325] [3326] The suspension should be resuspended immediately prior to subcutaneous administration by vigorously rolling the container between the palms until a uniform, cloudy suspension is achieved.[3325] [3326] For doses exceeding a volume of 4 mL of the reconstituted suspension, the total dose should be divided equally into 2 syringes and injected into 2 separate sites.[3325] [3326] Injection sites should be rotated.[3325] [3326]

For intravenous infusion, the final diluted solution should be administered over 10 to 40 minutes.[3325] [3326]

As with other toxic drugs, applicable special handling and disposal procedures for azacitidine should be followed.[3325] [3326]

Stability

Azacitidine is a white to off-white powder.[3325] [3326] Intact vials should be stored at controlled room temperature.[3325] [3326]

The reconstituted suspension of azacitidine intended for immediate subcutaneous administration may be held at 25°C for up to 1 hour, but must be administered within 1 hour after reconstitution.[3325] [3326] One manufacturer recommends administration of the reconstituted suspension within 45 minutes of preparation when intended for immediate use.[3327]

Stability of the reconstituted suspension intended for delayed subcutaneous administration differs between the two formulations of azacitidine;[3325] [3326] the sucrose-containing formulation (Actavis) has demonstrated improved stability of the reconstituted suspension compared with the original mannitol-containing formulation.[3328] If either formulation of the reconstituted suspension is intended for delayed subcutaneous administration, the suspension must be stored in the refrigerator immediately following reconstitution, either in the vial or drawn into a syringe.[3325] [3326] For the mannitol-containing formulation, when cold sterile water for injection (stored at 2 to 8°C) is used for reconstitution, the resulting suspension may be stored at 2 to 8°C for up to 22 hours; when sterile water for injection that has not been refrigerated is used for reconstitution, the resulting suspension may be stored at 2 to 8°C for only up to 8 hours.[3325] For the sucrose-containing formulation, when cold sterile water for injection (stored at 2 to 8°C) is used for reconstitution, the resulting suspension may be stored at 2 to 8°C for up to 30 hours; when sterile water for injection that has not been refrigerated is used for reconstitution, the resulting suspension may be stored at 2 to 8°C for only up to 12 hours.[3326]

When cold sterile water for injection is used for reconstitution, some authors have noted that sterile water for injection in glass bottles and ampuls of various sizes stored at 2 to 8°C quickly increased in temperature within 15 minutes after removal from refrigeration, which could potentially impact the subsequent stability of the drug.[3329] To combat this problem, these authors have suggested freezing 20-mL ampuls of sterile water for injection and thawing them for 30 minutes prior to use.[3329] After thawing, ampuls should be agitated for 30 seconds prior to removing the volume needed for reconstitution.[3329]

If either formulation is reconstituted to a solution and further diluted for intravenous infusion, administration of the diluted solution for infusion must be completed within 1 hour of reconstitution.[3325] [3326]

Azacitidine (Celgene) 10-mg/mL solution and 25-mg/mL suspension prepared with room temperature sterile water for injection and stored in glass vials at 23°C demonstrated less than 10% loss in 2.4 hours;[3330] when prepared with cold (4°C) sterile water for injection and stored in glass vials at 4°C, this formulation demonstrated less than 10% loss in 1 day.[3330]

pH Effects

Maximum stability of azacitidine has been reported at a pH ranging from 6.5 to 7.[741] [969]

DOI: 10.37573/9781585286850.043

Temperature Effects

Azacitidine is very sensitive to temperature,[3329] [3330] degrading quickly at room temperature.[3325] [3326]

Freezing Solutions

Azacitidine (National Cancer Institute) 0.5- and 2-mg/mL solutions prepared with ice-cold (specific temperature not defined) Ringer's injection, lactated and stored in 50-mL polypropylene syringes (Becton Dickinson) were stable for 2 weeks at −20°C followed by 1 hour at room temperature after thawing over 30 to 45 minutes.[1519]

Azacitidine (Celgene) 10-mg/mL solution prepared with cold (4°C) sterile water for injection and stored in glass vials and polypropylene syringes (Becton Dickinson) at −20°C demonstrated little to no loss in 23 days.[3330]

Freezing Suspensions

Azacitidine (Celgene) 25-mg/mL suspension prepared with cold (4°C) sterile water for injection and stored in glass vials and polypropylene syringes (Becton Dickinson) at −20°C demonstrated little to no loss in 23 days.[3330]

Azacitidine (Celgene) 25-mg/mL suspension prepared with ice-cold water (specific temperature not defined) and stored in polypropylene syringes for 8 days at −20°C followed by thawing at room temperature (i.e., 23 to 25°C) for 30 minutes with or without subsequent storage for 8 hours at 2 to 8°C demonstrated a loss of less than 5%.[3331] Neither changes in color of the suspension nor partial dissolution of the suspension was noted throughout the study.[3331]

Syringes

Azacitidine (Celgene) 10-mg/mL solution and 25-mg/mL suspension prepared with cold (4°C) sterile water for injection and stored in polypropylene syringes (Becton Dickinson) at 4°C demonstrated less than 10% loss in 1 day.[3330]

Filtration

Filtration of azacitidine suspension could result in removal of the drug; the suspension should *not* be filtered.[3325] [3326]

Compatibility Information

Solution Compatibility

Azacitidine

Test Soln Name	Mfr	Mfr	Conc/L or %	Remarks	Ref	C/I
Dextrose 5%	AB[b]	NCI	200 mg	Initial reconstitution with ice-cold water prior to dilution in 25°C infusion solution. About 37% loss in 6 hr at 25°C; calculated time to 10% loss was 0.7 hr	969	I
Dextrose 5%	AB[a]	NCI	200 mg	Initial reconstitution with ice-cold water prior to dilution in 25°C infusion solution. About 26% loss in 6 hr at 25°C; calculated time to 10% loss was 0.8 hr	969	I
Dextrose 5%	AB[a]	NCI	2 g	Initial reconstitution with ice-cold water prior to dilution in 25°C infusion solution. About 16% loss in 6 hr at 25°C; calculated time to 10% loss was 3 hr	969	I
Dextrose 5%		CEL, ACT		Stated to be incompatible	3325, 3326	I
Normosol R	AB[a]	NCI	200 mg	Initial reconstitution with ice-cold water prior to dilution in 25°C infusion solution. About 24% loss in 6 hr at 25°C; calculated time to 10% loss was 1.9 hr	969	I
Normosol R	AB[a]	NCI	2 g	Initial reconstitution with ice-cold water prior to dilution in 25°C infusion solution. About 18% loss in 6 hr at 25°C; calculated time to 10% loss was 3 hr	969	I
Ringer's injection, lactated	AB[b]	NCI	200 mg	Initial reconstitution with ice-cold water prior to dilution in 25°C infusion solution. About 20% loss in 6 hr at 25°C; calculated time to 10% loss was 2 hr	969	I
Ringer's injection, lactated	AB[a]	NCI	200 mg	Initial reconstitution with ice-cold water prior to dilution in 25°C infusion solution. About 21% loss in 6 hr at 25°; calculated time to 10% loss was 1.9 hr	969	I
Ringer's injection, lactated	AB[a]	NCI	2 g	Initial reconstitution with ice-cold water prior to dilution in 25°C infusion solution. About 18% loss in 6 hr at 25°C; calculated time to 10% loss was 2.9 hr	969	I
Ringer's injection, lactated		CEL, ACT		Complete administration within 1 hr of reconstitution	3325, 3326	C

Solution Compatibility (Cont.)

Test Soln Name	Mfr	Mfr	Conc/L or %	Remarks	Ref	C/I
Sodium chloride 0.9%	AB[b]	NCl	200 mg	Initial reconstitution with ice-cold water prior to dilution in 25°C infusion solution. About 23% loss in 6 hr at 25°C; calculated time to 10% loss was 1.6 hr	969	I
Sodium chloride 0.9%	AB[a]	NCl	200 mg	Initial reconstitution with ice-cold water prior to dilution in 25°C infusion solution. About 21% loss in 6 hr at 25°C; calculated time to 10% loss was 1.9 hr	969	I
Sodium chloride 0.9%	AB[a]	NCl	2 g	Initial reconstitution with ice-cold water prior to dilution in 25°C infusion solution. About 18% loss in 6 hr at 25°C; calculated time to 10% loss was 2.4 hr	969	I
Sodium chloride 0.9%		CEL, ACT		Complete administration with 1 hr of reconstitution	3325, 3326	C

[a] Tested in glass containers.

[b] Tested in PVC containers.

Additive Compatibility

Azacitidine

Test Drug	Mfr	Conc/L or %	Mfr	Conc/L or %	Test Solution	Remarks	Ref	C/I
Hetastarch in sodium chloride 0.9%						Stated to be incompatible	3325, 3326	I
Sodium bicarbonate						Stated to be incompatible	3325, 3326	I

Azathioprine Sodium
AHFS 92:44

Products

Azathioprine sodium is available in 20-mL vials containing the equivalent of 100 mg of azathioprine with sodium hydroxide to adjust the pH. Reconstitute by adding 10 mL of sterile water for injection and swirling until a clear solution results.[1(5/08)]

pH

Approximately 9.6.[1(5/08)]

Trade Name(s)

Imuran

Administration

Azathioprine sodium is administered intravenously. Infusions are usually administered over 30 to 60 minutes but have been given over five minutes to eight hours.[1(5/08) 4]

In the event of spills or leaks, the manufacturer recommends sodium hypochlorite 5% (household bleach) and sodium hydroxide (concentration unspecified) to inactivate azathioprine.[1200]

Stability

Azathioprine sodium, a yellow powder, should be stored at controlled room temperature and protected from light. It is stated to be stable in neutral or acid solutions but is hydrolyzed to mercaptopurine in alkaline solutions,[1(5/08) 4] especially on warming.[1(5/08)] Maximum stability occurs at pH 5.5 to 6.5.[1633] Hydrolysis to mercaptopurine also occurs in the presence of sulfhydryl compounds such as cysteine.[1(5/08) 4]

Use of azathioprine sodium within 24 hours after reconstitution is recommended because the product contains no preservatives.[1(5/08) 4] Azathioprine sodium is stated to be incompatible with methylparaben, propylparaben, and phenol.[108] Chemically, azathioprine sodium 10 mg/mL in aqueous solution is stable for about two weeks at room temperature.[4] After this time, hydrolysis of azathioprine to mercaptopurine increases.

Storage of the reconstituted solution in the original vial and in plastic syringes (Jelco) at 20 to 25°C under fluorescent light resulted in no decomposition or precipitation in 16 days. At 4°C in the dark, a visible precipitate formed after four days.[605]

Azathioprine sodium (Burroughs Wellcome) 100 mg/50 mL diluted in dextrose 5%, sodium chloride 0.9%, or sodium chloride 0.45% in PVC bags (Travenol) was stored at 20 to 25°C under fluorescent light and at 4°C in the dark. No decomposition occurred in the solutions over 16 days of storage. However, a precipitate formed in the dextrose 5% admixtures by the 16th day. No precipitate was observed after eight days of storage.[605]

Compatibility Information

Solution Compatibility

Azathioprine sodium

Test Soln Name	Mfr	Mfr	Conc/L or %	Remarks	Ref	C/I
Dextrose 5%	TR[a]	BW	2 g	Physically compatible and chemically stable for 8 days at 23 and 4°C. Precipitate forms in 16 days	605	C
Sodium chloride 0.45%	TR[a]	BW	2 g	Physically compatible and chemically stable for 16 days at 23 and 4°C	605	C
Sodium chloride 0.9%	TR[a]	BW	2 g	Physically compatible and chemically stable for 16 days at 23 and 4°C	605	C

[a] Tested in PVC containers.

Selected Revisions October 1, 2012. © Copyright, October 1982.
American Society of Health-System Pharmacists, Inc.

DOI: 10.37573/9781585286850.044

Azithromycin
AHFS 8:12.12.92

Products

Azithromycin is available as a powder in vials containing the equivalent of 500 mg of azithromycin (as the dihydrate[2863] or monohydrate[3286]) along with citric acid and sodium hydroxide.[2863 3286] The drug is packaged under vacuum.[2863 3286] Each 500-mg vial should be reconstituted with 4.8 mL of sterile water for injection and shaken until the drug is dissolved yielding a 100-mg/mL solution.[2863 3286] Because of the vacuum, a non-automated syringe is recommended to ensure that the correct amount of diluent is added.[2863 3286]

Trade Name(s)

Zithromax

Administration

Azithromycin is administered only by intravenous infusion after dilution to a concentration of 1 or 2 mg/mL in a compatible infusion solution.[2863 3286] Diluted solutions with a final concentration of 1 mg/mL should be infused over 3 hours; diluted solutions with a final concentration of 2 mg/mL should be infused over 1 hour.[2863 3286] Azithromycin should not be given by direct intravenous or intramuscular injection.[2863 3286]

Stability

Intact vials should be stored at or below 30°C[2863] or at controlled room temperature.[3286] The reconstituted solution is stable for 24 hours below 30°C.[2863 3286]

Compatibility Information

Solution Compatibility

Azithromycin

Test Soln Name	Mfr	Mfr	Conc/L or %	Remarks	Ref	C/I
Dextrose 5% in Ringer's injection, lactated		PF, HOS	1 to 2 g	Stable for 24 hr at or below 30°C or 7 days at 5°C	2863, 3286	C
Dextrose 5% in sodium chloride 0.3%		PF, HOS	1 to 2 g	Stable for 24 hr at or below 30°C or 7 days at 5°C	2863, 3286	C
Dextrose 5% in sodium chloride 0.45%[a]		PF, HOS	1 to 2 g	Stable for 24 hr at or below 30°C or 7 days at 5°C	2863, 3286	C
Dextrose 5%		PF, HOS	1 to 2 g	Stable for 24 hr at or below 30°C or 7 days at 5°C	2863, 3286	C
Normosol M in dextrose 5%		PF, HOS	1 to 2 g	Stable for 24 hr at or below 30°C or 7 days at 5°C	2863, 3286	C
Normosol R in dextrose 5%		PF, HOS	1 to 2 g	Stable for 24 hr at or below 30°C or 7 days at 5°C	2863, 3286	C
Ringer's injection, lactated		PF, HOS	1 to 2 g	Stable for 24 hr at or below 30°C or 7 days at 5°C	2863, 3286	C
Sodium chloride 0.45%		PF, HOS	1 to 2 g	Stable for 24 hr at or below 30°C or 7 days at 5°C	2863, 3286	C
Sodium chloride 0.9%		PF, HOS	1 to 2 g	Stable for 24 hr at or below 30°C or 7 days at 5°C	2863, 3286	C

[a] Tested with and without potassium chloride 20 mEq present.

Additive Compatibility

Azithromycin

Test Drug	Mfr	Conc/L or %	Mfr	Conc/L or %	Test Solution	Remarks	Ref	C/I
Ciprofloxacin						Physically incompatible with loss of ciprofloxacin reported due to pH over 6.0	1924	I

DOI: 10.37573/9781585286850.045

Y-Site Injection Compatibility (1:1 Mixture)

Azithromycin

Test Drug	Mfr	Conc	Mfr	Conc	Remarks	Ref	C/I
Amikacin sulfate	VHA	100 mg/mL[c d]	PF	2 mg/mL[b]	Whitish-yellow microcrystals found	2368	I
Aztreonam	BMS	200 mg/mL[c d]	PF	2 mg/mL[b]	White microcrystals found	2368	I
Bivalirudin	TMC	5 mg/mL[a]	PF	2 mg/mL[a]	Physically compatible for 4 hr at 23°C	2373	C
Cangrelor tetrasodium	TMC	1 mg/mL[b]		2 mg/mL[b]	Physically compatible for 4 hr	3243	C
Caspofungin acetate	ME	0.5 mg/mL[b]	NVP	2 mg/mL[b]	Physically compatible over 60 min	2766	C
Cefotaxime sodium	HMR	200 mg/mL[c d]	PF	2 mg/mL[b]	White microcrystals found	2368	I
Ceftaroline fosamil	FOR	2.22 mg/mL[a b g]	BA	2 mg/mL[a b g]	Physically compatible for 4 hr at 23°C	2826	C
Ceftazidime	GW	80 mg/mL[c d]	PF	2 mg/mL[b]	Amber and white microcrystals found	2368	I
Ceftazidime–avibactam sodium	ALL	20 mg/mL[n o]			Physically compatible for up to 4 hr at room temperature	3004	C
Ceftolozane sulfate–tazobactam sodium	CUB	10 mg/mL[l m]	FRK	2 mg/mL[l]	Physically compatible for 2 hr	3262	C
Ceftriaxone sodium	RC	66.7 mg/mL[c d]	PF	2 mg/mL[b]	White and yellow microcrystals found	2368	I
Cefuroxime sodium	VHA	100 mg/mL[c d]	PF	2 mg/mL[b]	White and yellow microcrystals	2368	I
Ciprofloxacin	BAY	2 mg/mL[a d]	PF	2 mg/mL[b]	Amber microcrystals found	2368	I
Clindamycin phosphate	PHU	30 mg/mL[c d]	PF	2 mg/mL[b]	Amber and white microcrystals found	2368	I
Cloxacillin sodium	SMX	100 mg/mL	SMX[k]	100 mg/mL	Precipitates immediately	3245	I
Dexmedetomidine HCl	AB	4 mcg/mL[b]	PF	2 mg/mL[b]	Physically compatible for 4 hr at 23°C	2383	C
Diphenhydramine HCl	ES	50 mg/mL[d]	PF	2 mg/mL[b]	Visually compatible	2368	C
Dolasetron mesylate	HMR	20 mg/mL[d]	PF	2 mg/mL[b]	Visually compatible	2368	C
Doripenem	JJ	5 mg/mL[a b]	BA	2 mg/mL[a b]	Physically compatible for 4 hr at 23°C	2743	C
Droperidol	AMR	2.5 mg/mL[d]	PF	2 mg/mL[b]	Visually compatible	2368	C
Famotidine	ME	2 mg/mL[d]	PF	2 mg/mL[b]	Grayish-white microcrystals found	2368	I
Fentanyl citrate	AB	50 mcg/mL[d]	PF	2 mg/mL[b]	Whitish-yellow microcrystals found	2368	I
Furosemide	AMR	10 mg/mL[d]	PF	2 mg/mL[b]	White microcrystals found	2368	I
Gentamicin sulfate	AMR	21 mg/mL[c d]	PF	2 mg/mL[b]	Whitish-yellow microcrystals found	2368	I
Hetastarch in lactated electrolyte	AB	6%	PF	2 mg/mL[a]	Physically compatible for 4 hr at 23°C	2339	C
Imipenem–cilastatin sodium	ME	5 mg/mL[b d i]	PF	2 mg/mL[b]	Whitish-yellow microcrystals found	2368	I
Isavuconazonium sulfate	ASP	1.5 mg/mL[a]	APP	2 mg/mL[a]	Measured turbidity increases within 2 hr	3263	I
Isavuconazonium sulfate	ASP	1.5 mg/mL[b]	APP	2 mg/mL[b]	Physically compatible for 2 hr	3263	C
Ketorolac tromethamine	AB	15 mg/mL[d]	PF	2 mg/mL[b]	Amber microcrystals found	2368	I
Levofloxacin	ORT	5 mg/mL[d]	PF	2 mg/mL[b]	White and amber microcrystals found	2368	I
Meropenem		50 mg/mL	SMX	100 mg/mL	Physically compatible for 4 hr at room temperature	3538	C
Meropenem–vaborbactam	TMC	8 mg/mL[b j]	FRK	2 mg/mL[b]	Physically compatible for 3 hr at 20 to 25°C	3380	C

Y-Site Injection Compatibility (1:1 Mixture) (Cont.)

Test Drug	Mfr	Conc	Mfr	Conc	Remarks	Ref	C/I
Morphine sulfate	WY	1 mg/mL[d]	PF	2 mg/mL[b]	White microcrystals found	2368	I
Ondansetron HCl	GW	2 mg/mL[d]	PF	2 mg/mL[b]	Visually compatible	2368	C
Piperacillin sodium–tazobactam sodium	LE[e]	100 mg/mL[b d h]	PF	2 mg/mL[b]	White microcrystals found	2368	I
Plazomicin sulfate	ACH	24 mg/mL[l]	PF	2 mg/mL[l]	Physically compatible for 1 hr at 20 to 25°C	3432	C
Potassium chloride	BA	20 mEq/L[f]	PF	2 mg/mL[b]	White microcrystals found	2368	I
Tedizolid phosphate	CUB	0.8 mg/mL[b]	APP	2 mg/mL[b]	Physically compatible for 2 hr	3244	C
Telavancin HCl	ASP	7.5 mg/mL[a b g]	APP	2 mg/mL[a b g]	Physically compatible for 2 hr	2830	C
Tigecycline	WY	1 mg/mL[b]		2 mg/mL[b]	Physically compatible for 4 hr	2714	C
Tobramycin sulfate		21 mg/mL[d]	PF	2 mg/mL[b]	White microcrystals found	2368	I

[a] Tested in dextrose 5%.

[b] Tested in sodium chloride 0.9%.

[c] Tested in sodium chloride 0.45%.

[d] Injected via Y-site into an administration set running azithromycin.

[e] Test performed using the formulation WITHOUT edetate disodium.

[f] Tested in dextrose 5% in sodium chloride 0.45%.

[g] Tested in Ringer's injection, lactated.

[h] Piperacillin component. Piperacillin in an 8:1 fixed-ratio concentration with tazobactam.

[i] Imipenem component. Imipenem in a 1:1 fixed-ratio concentration with cilastatin.

[j] Meropenem component. Meropenem in a 1:1 fixed-ratio concentration with vaborbactam.

[k] Test performed using the monohydrate formulation.

[l] Tested in both dextrose 5% and sodium chloride 0.9%.

[m] Ceftolozane component. Ceftolozane in a 2:1 fixed-ratio concentration with tazobactam.

[n] Ceftazidime component. Ceftazidime in a 4:1 fixed-ratio concentration with avibactam.

[o] Tested in dextrose 5%, sodium chloride 0.9%, and Ringer's injection, lactated.

Selected Revisions May 1, 2020. © Copyright, October 2004.
American Society of Health-System Pharmacists, Inc.

Aztreonam
AHFS 8:12.07.16

Products

Aztreonam is available in vials containing 1 or 2 g of the drug.[2864] [2866] Aztreonam also is available in 1- and 2-g sizes as frozen premixed injection solutions in dextrose 3.4 and 1.4%, respectively, in single-dose Galaxy containers for intravenous infusion.[2865] Both preparations contain approximately 780 mg of arginine per gram of aztreonam.[2864] [2865] [2866]

For intramuscular injection, each gram of aztreonam in vials should be reconstituted with at least 3 mL of one of the following diluents:[2864] [2866]

- Sterile water for injection
- Bacteriostatic water for injection (benzyl alcohol or parabens)
- Sodium chloride 0.9%
- Bacteriostatic sodium chloride 0.9% (benzyl alcohol)

For intravenous bolus injection, vials should be used.[2864] [2866] A vial should be reconstituted with 6 to 10 mL of sterile water for injection.[2864] [2866]

For intravenous infusion, a vial of aztreonam should be reconstituted with at least 3 mL of sterile water for injection per gram of aztreonam and further diluted with a compatible infusion solution.[2864] [2866]

On adding the diluent to the vial or bottle, the contents should be shaken immediately and vigorously.[2864] [2866] Any unused portion of the reconstituted solution should be discarded.[2864] [2866]

The frozen premixed injection solutions also may be used for intravenous infusion after thawing at room temperature (25°C) or at 2 to 8°C.[2865]

pH

Aqueous solutions of aztreonam have pH values ranging from 4.5 to 7.5.[2864] [2865] [2866]

Sodium Content

Aztreonam is sodium free.[2864] [2865] [2866]

Trade Name(s)

Azactam

Administration

Aztreonam may be administered by intravenous injection or infusion[2864] [2865] [2866] or by deep intramuscular injection into a large muscle mass.[2864] [2866] By intravenous injection, the dose should be administered slowly, over 3 to 5 minutes, directly into a vein or into the tubing of a compatible infusion solution.[2864] [2866] Intermittent infusion of aztreonam should be completed within 20 to 60 minutes.[2864] [2865] [2866] If Y-site administration of aztreonam is employed, careful attention should be paid to ensure administration of the full intended dose.[2864] [2866] A volume-control administration set may be used to dilute aztreonam in a compatible infusion solution during administration; however, the final concentration of aztreonam administered in such a way should not exceed 2% (w/v).[2864] [2866]

Stability

Intact vials should be stored at controlled room temperature; excessive heat should be avoided.[2864] [2866] Exposure to strong light may cause yellowing of the powder.[3310]

Aztreonam solutions range from colorless to light straw to yellow.[2864] [2865] [2866] They may develop a slight pink tint on standing without potency being affected.[2864] [2866]

Aztreonam solutions at concentrations of 2% (w/v) or less must be used within 48 hours if stored at controlled room temperature (15 to 30°C) or within 7 days at 2 to 8°C.[2864] [2866] Solutions with concentrations exceeding 2% (w/v) should be used immediately after preparation unless sterile water for injection or sodium chloride 0.9% is used.[2864] [2866] In these 2 excepted solutions, aztreonam at concentrations exceeding 2% (w/v) must be used within 48 hours if stored at controlled room temperature or within 7 days under refrigeration.[2864] [2866]

Concentration Effects

In one study, aztreonam dissolved in sterile water for injection to concentrations greater than 100 g/L resulted in unacceptably viscous solutions that impeded flow from elastomeric pumps to less than 75% of the nominal flow rate.[3105]

pH Effects

In aqueous solutions, aztreonam undergoes hydrolysis of the β-lactam ring. Specific base catalysis occurs at pH greater than 6. At pH 2 to 5, isomerization of the side chain predominates. The lowest rates of decomposition occur at pH 5 to 7, with maximum stability occurring at pH 6.[1072]

Freezing Solutions

The commercially available frozen premixed injection solution should be stored in a freezer capable of maintaining the temperature at or below −20°C and should be thawed at room temperature (25°C) or at 2 to 8°C; solutions should not be refrozen.[2865] After thawing, the container should be inverted to ensure that the solution is well mixed.[2865] Solutions should not be subject to force thawing by immersion in water baths or microwaving.[2865] The manufacturer indicates that thawed solutions are stable for 48 hours at room temperature (25°C) or for 14 days at 2 to 8°C.[2865]

Central Venous Catheter

Aztreonam (Squibb) 10 mg/mL in dextrose 5% was found to be compatible with the ARROWg+ard Blue Plus (Arrow International) chlorhexidine-bearing triple-lumen central catheter. Essentially complete delivery of the drug was found with little or no drug loss occurring. Furthermore, chlorhexidine delivered from the catheter remained at trace amounts with no substantial increase due to the delivery of the drug through the catheter.[2335]

DOI: 10.37573/9781585286850.046

Compatibility Information

Solution Compatibility

Aztreonam

Test Soln Name	Mfr	Mfr	Conc/L or %	Remarks	Ref	C/I
Dextrose 5% in Ringer's injection, lactated		BMS, FRK		Manufacturer-recommended solution	2864, 2866	C
Dextrose 5% in sodium chloride 0.2%		BMS, FRK		Manufacturer-recommended solution	2864, 2866	C
Dextrose 5% in sodium chloride 0.45%		BMS, FRK		Manufacturer-recommended solution	2864, 2866	C
Dextrose 5% in sodium chloride 0.9%		BMS, FRK		Manufacturer-recommended solution	2864, 2866	C
Dextrose 5%	TR[a]	SQ	10 g	Physically compatible with 6% loss in 48 hr at 25°C and 3% in 7 days at 4°C	1001	C
Dextrose 5%	TR[a]	SQ	20 g	Physically compatible with 2% loss in 48 hr at 25°C and 3% in 7 days at 4°C	1001	C
Dextrose 5%	MG[b]	SQ	20 g	Physically compatible with no loss in 48 hr at 25°C under fluorescent light	1026	C
Dextrose 5%		BMS, FRK		Manufacturer-recommended solution	2864, 2866	C
Dextrose 10%		BMS, FRK		Manufacturer-recommended solution	2864, 2866	C
Ionosol B in dextrose 5%		BMS, FRK		Manufacturer-recommended solution	2864, 2866	C
Isolyte E		BMS, FRK		Manufacturer-recommended solution	2864, 2866	C
Isolyte E in dextrose 5%		BMS, FRK		Manufacturer-recommended solution	2864, 2866	C
Isolyte M in dextrose 5%		BMS, FRK		Manufacturer-recommended solution	2864, 2866	C
Normosol M in dextrose 5%		BMS, FRK		Manufacturer-recommended solution	2864, 2866	C
Normosol R		BMS, FRK		Manufacturer-recommended solution	2864, 2866	C
Normosol R in dextrose 5%		BMS, FRK		Manufacturer-recommended solution	2864, 2866	C
Plasma-Lyte M in dextrose 5%		BMS, FRK		Manufacturer-recommended solution	2864, 2866	C
Ringer's injection		BMS, FRK		Manufacturer-recommended solution	2864, 2866	C
Ringer's injection, lactated		BMS, FRK		Manufacturer-recommended solution	2864, 2866	C
Sodium chloride 0.9%	TR[a]	SQ	10 and 20 g	Physically compatible with little or no loss in 48 hr at 25°C and 7 days at 4°C	1001	C
Sodium chloride 0.9%	MG[b]	SQ	20 g	Physically compatible with no loss in 48 hr at 25°C under fluorescent light	1026	C
Sodium chloride 0.9%	BA	SQ	20 g	10% loss in 37 days at 25°C and more than 120 days at 4°C. No loss in 120 days at −20°C	1600	C
Sodium chloride 0.9%	[a]	SQ	10 g	Visually compatible with no loss in 96 hr at 5 and 24°C	1691	C
Sodium chloride 0.9%		BMS, FRK		Manufacturer-recommended solution	2864, 2866	C
Sodium chloride 0.9%	[d]		40 and 120 g	Less than 10% loss in theoretical concentration in 12 hr at ambient temperature when administered as a continuous infusion	3535	C
Sodium lactate ⅙ M		BMS, FRK		Manufacturer-recommended solution	2864, 2866	C
TPN #107[c]			2 g	Activity retained for 24 hr at 21°C	1326	C

[a] Tested in PVC containers.

[b] Tested in glass containers.

[c] Refer to Appendix for the composition of parenteral nutrition solutions. TPN indicates a 2-in-1 admixture.

[d] Tested in polypropylene syringes.

Additive Compatibility

Aztreonam

Test Drug	Mfr	Conc/L or %	Mfr	Conc/L or %	Test Solution	Remarks	Ref	C/I
Ampicillin sodium	WY	20 g	SQ	10 g	D5W[a]	10% ampicillin loss in 2 hr and 10% aztreonam loss in 3 hr at 25°C. 10% ampicillin loss in 24 hr and 10% aztreonam loss in 8 hr at 4°C	1001	I
Ampicillin sodium	WY	5 g	SQ	10 g	D5W[a]	10% ampicillin loss in 3 hr and 10% aztreonam loss in 7 hr at 25°C. 10% loss of both drugs in 48 hr at 4°C	1001	I
Ampicillin sodium	WY	20 g	SQ	20 g	D5W[a]	10% ampicillin loss in 4 hr and 10% aztreonam loss in 5 hr at 25°C. 10% loss of both drugs in 24 hr at 4°C	1001	I
Ampicillin sodium	WY	5 g	SQ	20 g	D5W[a]	10% ampicillin loss in 5 hr and 10% aztreonam loss in 8 hr at 25°C. 10% ampicillin loss in 48 hr and 10% aztreonam loss in 72 hr at 4°C	1001	I
Ampicillin sodium	WY	20 g	SQ	10 g	NS[a]	10% ampicillin loss in 24 hr and 2% aztreonam loss in 48 hr at 25°C. 10% ampicillin loss in 2 days and 9% aztreonam loss in 7 days at 4°C	1001	C
Ampicillin sodium	WY	5 g	SQ	10 g	NS[a]	10% ampicillin loss and no aztreonam loss in 48 hr at 25°C. 10% ampicillin loss in 3 days and 8% aztreonam loss in 7 days at 4°C	1001	C
Ampicillin sodium	WY	20 g	SQ	20 g	NS[a]	10% ampicillin loss in 24 hr and 5% aztreonam loss in 48 hr at 25°C. 10% ampicillin loss in 2 days and 7% aztreonam loss in 7 days at 4°C	1001	C
Ampicillin sodium	WY	5 g	SQ	20 g	NS[a]	10% ampicillin loss and no aztreonam loss in 48 hr at 25°C. 10% ampicillin loss and 5% aztreonam loss in 7 days at 4°C	1001	C
Ampicillin sodium–sulbactam sodium	PF	20 g[d]	SQ	10 g	NS[a]	Visually compatible with 10% ampicillin loss in 30 hr at 24°C and 94 hr at 5°C. Ampicillin loss is determining factor	1691	C
Cefazolin sodium	LI	5 and 20 g	SQ	10 and 20 g	D5W, NS[a]	Physically compatible. Little loss of either drug in 48 hr at 25°C and 7 days at 4°C in the dark	1020	C
Cefoxitin sodium	MSD	10 and 20 g	SQ	10 and 20 g	NS[a]	3 to 5% aztreonam loss and no cefoxitin loss in 7 days at 4°C	1023	C
Cefoxitin sodium	MSD	10 and 20 g	SQ	10 and 20 g	D5W[a]	3 to 6% cefoxitin loss and no aztreonam loss in 7 days at 4°C	1023	C
Cefoxitin sodium	MSD	10 and 20 g	SQ	10 and 20 g	D5W, NS[a]	Both drugs stable for 12 hr at 25°C. Yellow color and 6 to 12% aztreonam and 9 to 15% cefoxitin loss in 48 hr at 25°C	1023	I
Ciprofloxacin	BAY	1.6 g	SQ	39.7 g	D5W	Visually compatible with no loss of ciprofloxacin in 24 hr at 22°C under fluorescent light. Aztreonam not tested	2413	C
Clindamycin phosphate	UP	3 and 6 g	SQ	10 and 20 g	D5W, NS[a]	Physically compatible with little or no loss of either drug in 48 hr at 25°C and 7 days at 4°C	1002	C
Clindamycin phosphate	UP	9 g	SQ	20 g	D5W[b]	Physically compatible with 3% clindamycin loss and 5% aztreonam loss in 48 hr at 25°C under fluorescent light	1026	C
Clindamycin phosphate	UP	9 g	SQ	20 g	NS[b]	Physically compatible with 2% clindamycin loss and no aztreonam loss in 48 hr at 25°C under fluorescent light	1026	C
Gentamicin sulfate	SC	200 and 800 mg	SQ	10 and 20 g	D5W, NS[a]	Little aztreonam loss in 48 hr at 25°C and 7 days at 4°C. Gentamicin stable for 12 hr at 25°C and 24 hr at 4°C. Up to 10% loss in 48 hr at 25°C and 7 days at 4°C	1023	C
Linezolid	PHU	2 g	SQ	20 g	[c]	Physically compatible with no linezolid loss in 7 days at 4 and 23°C protected from light. About 9% aztreonam loss at 23°C and less than 4% loss at 4°C in 7 days	2263	C
Mannitol		50 and 100 g				Manufacturer-recommended solution	2864, 2866	C

Additive Compatibility (Cont.)

Test Drug	Mfr	Conc/L or %	Mfr	Conc/L or %	Test Solution	Remarks	Ref	C/I
Metronidazole	MG	5 g	SQ	10 and 20 g		Pink color develops in 12 hr, becoming cherry red in 48 hr at 25°C. Pink color develops in 3 days at 4°C. No loss of either drug detected	1023	I
Nafcillin sodium	BR	20 g	SQ	20 g	D5W, NSª	Cloudiness and precipitate form. 7% aztreonam and 11% nafcillin loss in 24 hr at room temperature	1028	I
Tobramycin sulfate	LI	200 and 800 mg	SQ	10 and 20 g	D5W, NSª	Little or no loss of either drug in 48 hr at 25°C and 7 days at 4°C	1023	C
Vancomycin HCl	AB	10 g	SQ	40 g	D5W, NS	Immediate microcrystalline precipitate. Turbidity and precipitate over 24 hr	1848	I
Vancomycin HCl	AB	1 g	SQ	4 g	D5W	Physically compatible. Little loss of either drug in 31 days at 4°C. 10% aztreonam loss in 14 days at 23°C and 7 days at 32°C	1848	C
Vancomycin HCl	AB	1 g	SQ	4 g	NS	Physically compatible. Little loss of either drug in 31 days at 4°C. 8% aztreonam loss in 31 days at 23°C and 7 days at 32°C	1848	C

ª Tested in PVC containers.

ᵇ Tested in glass containers.

ᶜ Admixed in the linezolid infusion container.

ᵈ Ampicillin component. Ampicillin in a 2:1 fixed-ratio concentration with sulbactam.

Drugs in Syringe Compatibility

Aztreonam

Test Drug	Mfr	Amt	Mfr	Amt	Remarks	Ref	C/I
Clindamycin phosphate	UP	600 mg/4 mL	SQ	2 g	Physically compatible with 2% clindamycin loss and 8% aztreonam loss in 48 hr at 25°C under fluorescent light	1164	C

Y-Site Injection Compatibility (1:1 Mixture)

Aztreonam

Test Drug	Mfr	Conc	Mfr	Conc	Remarks	Ref	C/I
Acyclovir sodium	BW	7 mg/mLª	SQ	40 mg/mLª	White needles form immediately and become dense precipitate in 4 hr	1758	I
Allopurinol sodium	BW	3 mg/mLᵇ	SQ	40 mg/mLᵇ	Physically compatible for 4 hr at 22°C	1686	C
Amifostine	USB	10 mg/mLª	SQ	40 mg/mLª	Physically compatible for 4 hr at 23°C	1845	C
Amikacin sulfate	BMS	5 mg/mLª	SQ	40 mg/mLª	Physically compatible for 4 hr at 23°C	1758	C
Aminophylline	AMR	2.5 mg/mLª	SQ	40 mg/mLª	Physically compatible for 4 hr at 23°C	1758	C
Amphotericin B	PHT	0.6 mg/mLª	SQ	40 mg/mLª	Yellow turbidity forms immediately and becomes flocculent precipitate in 4 hr	1758	I
Ampicillin sodium	WY	20 mg/mLᵇ	SQ	40 mg/mLª	Physically compatible for 4 hr at 23°C	1758	C
Ampicillin sodium–sulbactam sodium	RR	20 mg/mLᵇ ʲ	SQ	40 mg/mLª	Physically compatible for 4 hr at 23°C	1758	C
Amsacrine	NCI	1 mg/mLª	SQ	40 mg/mLª	Immediate yellow-orange turbidity, becoming a precipitate in 4 hr	1381	I
Anakinra	SYN	4 and 36 mg/mLᵇ	BMS	20 mg/mLᵇ	Physically compatible. No aztreonam loss in 4 hr at 25°C. Anakinra uncertain	2508	?
Azithromycin	PF	2 mg/mLᵇ	BMS	200 mg/mLᵍ ʰ	White microcrystals found	2368	I

Y-Site Injection Compatibility (1:1 Mixture) (Cont.)

Test Drug	Mfr	Conc	Mfr	Conc	Remarks	Ref	C/I
Bivalirudin	TMC	5 mg/mL[a]	DUR	40 mg/mL[a]	Physically compatible for 4 hr at 23°C	2373	C
Bleomycin sulfate	MJ	1 unit/mL[b]	SQ	40 mg/mL[a]	Physically compatible for 4 hr at 23°C	1758	C
Bumetanide	RC	0.04 mg/mL[a]	SQ	40 mg/mL[a]	Physically compatible for 4 hr at 23°C	1758	C
Buprenorphine HCl	RKC	0.04 mg/mL[a]	SQ	40 mg/mL[a]	Physically compatible for 4 hr at 23°C	1758	C
Butorphanol tartrate	BMS	0.04 mg/mL[a]	SQ	40 mg/mL[a]	Physically compatible for 4 hr at 23°C	1758	C
Calcium gluconate	AMR	40 mg/mL[a]	SQ	40 mg/mL[a]	Physically compatible for 4 hr at 23°C	1758	C
Cangrelor tetrasodium	TMC	1 mg/mL[b]		40 mg/mL[b]	Physically compatible for 4 hr	3243	C
Carboplatin	BMS	5 mg/mL[a]	SQ	40 mg/mL[a]	Physically compatible for 4 hr at 23°C	1758	C
Carmustine	BMS	1.5 mg/mL[a]	SQ	40 mg/mL[a]	Physically compatible for 4 hr at 23°C	1758	C
Caspofungin acetate	ME	0.7 mg/mL[b]	BMS	40 mg/mL[b]	Physically compatible for 4 hr at room temperature	2758	C
Caspofungin acetate	ME	0.5 mg/mL[b]	BMS	20 mg/mL[b]	Physically compatible over 60 min	2766	C
Cefazolin sodium	MAR	20 mg/mL[a]	SQ	40 mg/mL[a]	Physically compatible for 4 hr at 23°C	1758	C
Cefotaxime sodium	HO	20 mg/mL[a]	SQ	40 mg/mL[a]	Physically compatible for 4 hr at 23°C	1758	C
Cefotetan disodium	STU	20 mg/mL[a]	SQ	40 mg/mL[a]	Physically compatible for 4 hr at 23°C	1758	C
Cefoxitin sodium	MSD	20 mg/mL[a]	SQ	40 mg/mL[a]	Physically compatible for 4 hr at 23°C	1758	C
Ceftazidime	LI	40 mg/mL[a]	SQ	40 mg/mL[a]	Physically compatible for 4 hr at 23°C	1758	C
Ceftazidime–avibactam sodium	ALL	20 mg/mL[r s]			Physically compatible for up to 4 hr at room temperature	3004	C
Ceftolozane sulfate–tazobactam sodium	CUB	10 mg/mL[c q]	FRK	20 mg/mL[c]	Physically compatible for 2 hr	3262	C
Ceftriaxone sodium	RC	20 mg/mL[a]	SQ	40 mg/mL[a]	Physically compatible for 4 hr at 23°C	1758	C
Cefuroxime sodium	LI	30 mg/mL[a]	SQ	40 mg/mL[a]	Physically compatible for 4 hr at 23°C	1758	C
Chlorpromazine HCl	SCN	2 mg/mL[a]	SQ	40 mg/mL[a]	Dense white turbidity forms immediately	1758	I
Ciprofloxacin	MI	1 mg/mL[a]	SQ	20 mg/mL[c]	Physically compatible for 24 hr at 22°C	1189	C
Ciprofloxacin	MI	1 mg/mL[a]	SQ	40 mg/mL[a]	Physically compatible for 4 hr at 23°C	1758	C
Cisatracurium besylate	GW	0.1, 2, 5 mg/mL[a]	SQ	40 mg/mL[a]	Physically compatible for 4 hr at 23°C	2074	C
Cisplatin	BMS	1 mg/mL	SQ	40 mg/mL[a]	Physically compatible for 4 hr at 23°C	1758	C
Clindamycin phosphate	AST	10 mg/mL[a]	SQ	40 mg/mL[a]	Physically compatible for 4 hr at 23°C	1758	C
Cyclophosphamide	MJ	10 mg/mL[a]	SQ	40 mg/mL[a]	Physically compatible for 4 hr at 23°C	1758	C
Cytarabine	CET	50 mg/mL	SQ	40 mg/mL[a]	Physically compatible for 4 hr at 23°C	1758	C
Dacarbazine	MI	4 mg/mL[a]	SQ	40 mg/mL[a]	Physically compatible for 4 hr at 23°C	1758	C
Dactinomycin	ME	0.01 mg/mL[a]	SQ	40 mg/mL[a]	Physically compatible for 4 hr at 23°C	1758	C
Daptomycin	CUB[p]	16.7 mg/mL[b i]	BMS	16.7 mg/mL[b i]	Physically compatible with little loss of either drug in 2 hr at 25°C	2553	C
Daunorubicin HCl	WY	1 mg/mL[a]	SQ	40 mg/mL[a]	Haze forms immediately	1758	I
Dexamethasone sodium phosphate	AMR	1 mg/mL[a]	SQ	40 mg/mL[a]	Physically compatible for 4 hr at 23°C	1758	C
Dexmedetomidine HCl	AB	4 mcg/mL[b]	BMS	40 mg/mL[b]	Physically compatible for 4 hr at 23°C	2383	C
Diltiazem HCl	MMD	5 mg/mL	SQ	20 and 333 mg/mL[b]	Visually compatible	1807	C

Y-Site Injection Compatibility (1:1 Mixture) (Cont.)

Test Drug	Mfr	Conc	Mfr	Conc	Remarks	Ref	C/I
Diltiazem HCl	MMD	1 mg/mL[b]	SQ	333 mg/mL[b]	Visually compatible	1807	C
Diphenhydramine HCl	PD	2 mg/mL[a]	SQ	40 mg/mL[a]	Physically compatible for 4 hr at 23°C	1758	C
Dobutamine HCl	LI	4 mg/mL[a]	SQ	40 mg/mL[a]	Physically compatible for 4 hr at 23°C	1758	C
Docetaxel	RPR	0.9 mg/mL[a]	BMS	40 mg/mL[a]	Physically compatible for 4 hr at 23°C	2224	C
Dopamine HCl	AST	3.2 mg/mL[a]	SQ	40 mg/mL[a]	Physically compatible for 4 hr at 23°C	1758	C
Doxorubicin HCl	CET	2 mg/mL	SQ	40 mg/mL[a]	Physically compatible for 4 hr at 23°C	1758	C
Doxorubicin HCl liposomal	SEQ	0.4 mg/mL[a]	SQ	40 mg/mL[a]	Physically compatible for 4 hr at 23°C	2087	C
Doxycycline hyclate	ES	1 mg/mL[a]	SQ	40 mg/mL[a]	Physically compatible for 4 hr at 23°C	1758	C
Droperidol	JN	0.4 mg/mL[a]	SQ	40 mg/mL[a]	Physically compatible for 4 hr at 23°C	1758	C
Enalaprilat	MSD	0.05 mg/mL[b]	SQ	10 mg/mL[a]	Physically compatible for 24 hr at room temperature under fluorescent light	1355	C
Enalaprilat	MSD	0.1 mg/mL[a]	SQ	40 mg/mL[a]	Physically compatible for 4 hr at 23°C	1758	C
Eravacycline dihydro-chloride	TET	0.6 mg/mL[b]	BMS	20 mg/mL[b]	Physically compatible for 2 hr at room temperature	3532	C
Etoposide	BMS	0.4 mg/mL[a]	SQ	40 mg/mL[a]	Physically compatible for 4 hr at 23°C	1758	C
Etoposide phosphate	BR	5 mg/mL[a]	SQ	40 mg/mL[a]	Physically compatible for 4 hr at 23°C	2218	C
Famotidine	ME	2 mg/mL[a]	SQ	40 mg/mL[a]	Physically compatible for 4 hr at 23°C	1758	C
Fenoldopam mesylate	AB	80 mcg/mL[b]	BMS	40 mg/mL[b]	Physically compatible for 4 hr at 23°C	2467	C
Filgrastim	AMG	30 mcg/mL[a]	SQ	40 mg/mL[a]	Physically compatible for 4 hr at 22°C	1687	C
Filgrastim	AMG	30 mcg/mL[a]	SQ	40 mg/mL[a]	Physically compatible for 4 hr at 23°C	1758	C
Floxuridine	RC	3 mg/mL[a]	SQ	40 mg/mL[a]	Physically compatible for 4 hr at 23°C	1758	C
Fluconazole	RR	2 mg/mL	SQ	40 mg/mL	Visually compatible for 24 hr at 25°C	1407	C
Fluconazole	RR	2 mg/mL	SQ	40 mg/mL[a]	Physically compatible for 4 hr at 23°C	1758	C
Fludarabine phosphate	BX	1 mg/mL[a]	SQ	40 mg/mL[a]	Visually compatible for 4 hr at 22°C	1439	C
Fludarabine phosphate	BX	1 mg/mL[a]	SQ	40 mg/mL[a]	Physically compatible for 4 hr at 23°C	1758	C
Fluorouracil	AD	16 mg/mL[a]	SQ	40 mg/mL[a]	Physically compatible for 4 hr at 23°C	1758	C
Foscarnet sodium	AST	24 mg/mL	SQ	40 mg/mL	Physically compatible for 24 hr at room temperature under fluorescent light	1335	C
Foscarnet sodium	AST	24 mg/mL	SQ	40 mg/mL[c]	Physically compatible for 24 hr at 25°C under fluorescent light	1393	C
Furosemide	AB	3 mg/mL[a]	SQ	40 mg/mL[a]	Physically compatible for 4 hr at 23°C	1758	C
Gallium nitrate	FUJ	0.4 mg/mL[a]	SQ	40 mg/mL[a]	Physically compatible for 4 hr at 23°C	1758	C
Ganciclovir sodium	SY	20 mg/mL[a]	SQ	40 mg/mL[a]	White needles form immediately. Dense precipitate in 1 hr	1758	I
Gemcitabine HCl	LI	10 mg/mL[b]	SQ	40 mg/mL[b]	Physically compatible for 4 hr at 23°C	2226	C
Gentamicin sulfate	ES	5 mg/mL[a]	SQ	40 mg/mL[a]	Physically compatible for 4 hr at 23°C	1758	C
Granisetron HCl	SKB	0.05 mg/mL[a]	SQ	40 mg/mL[a]	Physically compatible for 4 hr at 23°C	2000	C
Haloperidol lactate	MN	0.2 mg/mL[a]	SQ	40 mg/mL[a]	Physically compatible for 4 hr at 23°C	1758	C
Heparin sodium	ES	100 units/mL[a]	SQ	40 mg/mL[a]	Physically compatible for 4 hr at 23°C	1758	C

Y-Site Injection Compatibility (1:1 Mixture) (Cont.)

Test Drug	Mfr	Conc	Mfr	Conc	Remarks	Ref	C/I
Heparin sodium	TR	50 units/mL	BV	20 mg/mL[a]	Visually compatible for 4 hr at 25°C	1793	C
Hetastarch in lactated electrolyte	AB	6%	BMS	40 mg/mL[a]	Physically compatible for 4 hr at 23°C	2339	C
Hydrocortisone sodium succinate	UP	1 mg/mL[a]	SQ	40 mg/mL[a]	Physically compatible for 4 hr at 23°C	1758	C
Hydromorphone HCl	KN	0.5 mg/mL[a]	SQ	40 mg/mL[a]	Physically compatible for 4 hr at 23°C	1758	C
Hydroxyzine HCl	WI	4 mg/mL[a]	SQ	40 mg/mL[a]	Physically compatible for 4 hr at 23°C	1758	C
Idarubicin HCl	AD	0.5 mg/mL[a]	SQ	40 mg/mL[a]	Physically compatible for 4 hr at 23°C	1758	C
Ifosfamide	MJ	25 mg/mL[a]	SQ	40 mg/mL[a]	Physically compatible for 4 hr at 23°C	1758	C
Imipenem–cilastatin sodium	MSD	10 mg/mL[a] [n]	SQ	40 mg/mL[a]	Physically compatible for 4 hr at 23°C	1758	C
Insulin, regular	LI	0.2 unit/mL[b]	SQ	20 mg/mL	Physically compatible for 2 hr at 25°C	1395	C
Isavuconazonium sulfate	ASP	1.5 mg/mL[c]	APP	20 mg/mL[c]	Physically compatible for 2 hr	3263	C
Letermovir	ME				Physically incompatible	3398	I
Leucovorin calcium	LE	2 mg/mL[a]	SQ	40 mg/mL[a]	Physically compatible for 4 hr at 23°C	1758	C
Linezolid	PHU	2 mg/mL	SQ	40 mg/mL[a]	Physically compatible for 4 hr at 23°C	2264	C
Lorazepam	WY	0.1 mg/mL[a]	SQ	40 mg/mL[a]	Haze forms within 1 hr	1758	I
Magnesium sulfate	AST	100 mg/mL[a]	SQ	40 mg/mL[a]	Physically compatible for 4 hr at 23°C	1758	C
Mannitol	BA	15%	SQ	40 mg/mL[a]	Physically compatible for 4 hr at 23°C	1758	C
Mechlorethamine HCl	MSD	1 mg/mL	SQ	40 mg/mL[a]	Physically compatible for 4 hr at 23°C	1758	C
Melphalan HCl	BW	0.1 mg/mL[b]	SQ	40 mg/mL[b]	Physically compatible for 3 at 22°C	1557	C
Meperidine HCl	AB	10 mg/mL	SQ	20 mg/mL[a]	Physically compatible for 4 hr at 25°C	1397	C
Meperidine HCl	WY	4 mg/mL[a]	SQ	40 mg/mL[a]	Physically compatible for 4 hr at 23°C	1758	C
Meropenem		50 mg/mL	SQ	100 mg/mL	Physically compatible for 4 hr at room temperature	3538	C
Meropenem–vabor-bactam	TMC	8 mg/mL[b] [o]	FRK	20 mg/mL[b]	Physically compatible for 3 hr at 20 to 25°C	3380	C
Mesna	MJ	10 mg/mL[a]	SQ	40 mg/mL[a]	Physically compatible for 4 hr at 23°C	1758	C
Methotrexate sodium	LE	15 mg/mL[a]	SQ	40 mg/mL[a]	Physically compatible for 4 hr at 23°C	1758	C
Methylprednisolone sodium succinate	AB	5 mg/mL[a]	SQ	40 mg/mL[a]	Physically compatible for 4 hr at 23°C	1758	C
Metoclopramide HCl	ES	5 mg/mL	SQ	40 mg/mL[a]	Physically compatible for 4 hr at 23°C	1758	C
Metronidazole	BA	5 mg/mL	SQ	40 mg/mL[a]	Orange color forms in 4 hr	1758	I
Mitomycin	BMS	0.5 mg/mL	SQ	40 mg/mL[a]	Reddish-purple color forms in 4 hr	1758	I
Mitoxantrone HCl	LE	0.5 mg/mL[a]	SQ	40 mg/mL[a]	Heavy precipitate forms in 1 hr	1758	I
Morphine sulfate	AB	1 mg/mL	SQ	20 mg/mL[a]	Physically compatible for 4 hr at 25°C	1397	C
Morphine sulfate	AST	1 mg/mL[a]	SQ	40 mg/mL[a]	Physically compatible for 4 hr at 23°C	1758	C
Nalbuphine HCl	AST	10 mg/mL	SQ	40 mg/mL[a]	Physically compatible for 4 hr at 23°C	1758	C
Nicardipine HCl	DCC	0.1 mg/mL[a]	SQ	10 mg/mL[a]	Visually compatible for 24 hr at room temperature	235	C

Y-Site Injection Compatibility (1:1 Mixture) (Cont.)

Test Drug	Mfr	Conc	Mfr	Conc	Remarks	Ref	C/I
Ondansetron HCl	GL	1 mg/mL[b]	SQ	40 mg/mL[a]	Visually compatible for 4 hr at 22°C	1365	C
Ondansetron HCl	GL	0.03 and 0.3 mg/mL[a]	SQ	40 mg/mL[a]	Visually compatible with little loss of either drug in 4 hr at 25°C	1732	C
Ondansetron HCl	GL	1 mg/mL[a]	SQ	40 mg/mL[a]	Physically compatible for 4 hr at 23°C	1758	C
Oritavancin diphosphate	TAR	0.8, 1.2, and 2 mg/mL[a]	BMS	20 mg/mL[a]	Precipitate forms immediately	2928	I
Pemetrexed disodium	LI	20 mg/mL[b]	BMS	40 mg/mL[a]	Physically compatible for 4 hr at 23°C	2564	C
Piperacillin sodium–tazobactam sodium	LE[f]	40 mg/mL[a k]	SQ	40 mg/mL[a]	Physically compatible for 4 hr at 22°C	1688	C
Plazomicin sulfate	ACH	24 mg/mL[c]	FRK	20 mg/mL[c]	Physically compatible for 1 hr at 20 to 25°C	3432	C
Potassium chloride	AB	0.1 mEq/mL[a]	SQ	40 mg/mL[a]	Physically compatible for 4 hr at 23°C	1758	C
Prochlorperazine edisylate	ES	0.5 mg/mL[a]	SQ	40 mg/mL[a]	Haze and tiny particles form within 4 hr	1758	I
Promethazine HCl	SCN	2 mg/mL[a]	SQ	40 mg/mL[a]	Physically compatible for 4 hr at 23°C	1758	C
Propofol	ZEN[t]	10 mg/mL	SQ	40 mg/mL[a]	Physically compatible for 1 hr at 23°C	2066	C
Quinupristin–dalfopristin	PF	2 mg/mL[a l]		20 mg/mL[a]	Physically compatible	3229	C
Ranitidine HCl	GL	1 mg/mL[b]	SQ	16.7 mg/mL[b]	No loss of either drug in 4 hr at 22°C	1632	C
Ranitidine HCl	GL	2 mg/mL[a]	SQ	40 mg/mL[a]	Physically compatible for 4 hr at 23°C	1758	C
Remifentanil HCl	GW	0.025 and 0.25 mg/mL[b]	SQ	40 mg/mL[a]	Physically compatible for 4 hr at 23°C	2075	C
Sargramostim	IMM	10 mcg/mL[b]	SQ	40 mg/mL[b]	Visually compatible for 4 hr at 22°C	1436	C
Sargramostim	IMM	10 mcg/mL[b]	SQ	40 mg/mL[b]	Physically compatible for 4 hr at 23°C	1758	C
Sodium bicarbonate	AB	1 mEq/mL	SQ	40 mg/mL[a]	Physically compatible for 4 hr at 23°C	1758	C
Streptozocin	UP	40 mg/mL[a]	SQ	40 mg/mL[a]	Red color forms in 1 hr	1758	I
Tedizolid phosphate	CUB	0.8 mg/mL[b]	APP	20 mg/mL[b]	Physically compatible for 2 hr	3244	C
Teniposide	BR	0.1 mg/mL[a]	SQ	40 mg/mL[a]	Physically compatible for 4 hr at 23°C	1725, 1758	C
Theophylline	TR	4 mg/mL	BV	20 mg/mL[a]	Visually compatible for 6 hr at 25°C	1793	C
Thiotepa	LE	1 mg/mL[a]	SQ	40 mg/mL[a]	Physically compatible for 4 hr at 23°C	1758	C
Thiotepa	IMM[d]	1 mg/mL[a]	SQ	40 mg/mL[a]	Physically compatible for 4 hr at 23°C	1861	C
Tigecycline	WY	1 mg/mL[b]		20 mg/mL[b]	Physically compatible for 4 hr	2714	C
TNA #218 to #226[e]			SQ	40 mg/mL[a]	Visually compatible for 4 hr at 23°C	2215	C
Tobramycin sulfate	LI	5 mg/mL[a]	SQ	40 mg/mL[a]	Physically compatible for 4 hr at 23°C	1758	C
TPN #212 to #215[e]			SQ	40 mg/mL[a]	Physically compatible for 4 hr at 23°C	2109	C
Trimethoprim–sulfamethoxazole	ES	0.8 mg/mL[a m]	SQ	40 mg/mL[a]	Physically compatible for 4 hr at 23°C	1758	C
Vancomycin HCl	LI	67 mg/mL[b]	SQ	200 mg/mL[b]	White granular precipitate forms immediately in tubing when given sequentially	1364	I
Vancomycin HCl	AB	10 mg/mL[a]	SQ	40 mg/mL[a]	Physically compatible for 4 hr at 23°C	1758	C
Vinblastine sulfate	LI	0.12 mg/mL[a]	SQ	40 mg/mL[a]	Physically compatible for 4 hr at 23°C	1758	C

Y-Site Injection Compatibility (1:1 Mixture) (Cont.)

Test Drug	Mfr	Conc	Mfr	Conc	Remarks	Ref	C/I
Vincristine sulfate	LI	0.05 mg/mL[a]	SQ	40 mg/mL[a]	Physically compatible for 4 hr at 23°C	1758	C
Vinorelbine tartrate	BW	1 mg/mL[b]	SQ	40 mg/mL[b]	Physically compatible for 4 hr at 23°C	1558	C
Zidovudine	BW	4 mg/mL[a]	SQ	40 mg/mL[a]	Physically compatible for 4 hr at 25°C	1193	C
Zidovudine	BW	4 mg/mL[a]	SQ	40 mg/mL[a]	Physically compatible for 4 hr at 23°C	1758	C

[a] Tested in dextrose 5%.

[b] Tested in sodium chloride 0.9%.

[c] Tested in both dextrose 5% and sodium chloride 0.9%.

[d] Lyophilized formulation tested.

[e] Refer to Appendix for the composition of parenteral nutrition solutions. TNA indicates a 3-in-1 admixture, and TPN indicates a 2-in-1 admixture.

[f] Test performed using the formulation WITHOUT edetate disodium.

[g] Tested in sodium chloride 0.45%.

[h] Injected via Y-site into an administration set running azithromycin.

[i] Final concentration after mixing.

[j] Ampicillin component. Ampicillin in a 2:1 fixed-ratio concentration with sulbactam.

[k] Piperacillin component. Piperacillin in an 8:1 fixed-ratio concentration with tazobactam.

[l] Quinupristin and dalfopristin components combined.

[m] Trimethoprim component. Trimethoprim in a 1:5 fixed-ratio concentration with sulfamethoxazole.

[n] Not specified whether concentration refers to single component or combined components.

[o] Meropenem component. Meropenem in a 1:1 fixed-ratio concentration with vaborbactam.

[p] Test performed using the Cubicin formulation.

[q] Ceftolozane component. Ceftolozane in a 2:1 fixed-ratio concentration with tazobactam.

[r] Ceftazidime component. Ceftazidime in a 4:1 fixed-ratio concentration with avibactam.

[s] Tested in dextrose 5%, sodium chloride 0.9%, and Ringer's injection, lactated.

[t] Test performed using the formulation WITH edetate disodium.

Additional Compatibility Information

Peritoneal Dialysis Solutions

Aztreonam (Bristol-Myers Squibb) was evaluated for stability at a concentration of 500 mg/L in Extraneal with icodextrin 7.5% (Baxter) and 400 mg/L in Nutrineal PD-4 with amino acids 1.1% (Baxter) at 6, 25, and 37°C protected from light.[3563] The drug also was evaluated for stability in 2-compartment Physioneal with dextrose 1.36% (Baxter) and Physioneal with dextrose 2.27% (Baxter).[3563] Bags of 2-compartment Physioneal with dextrose 1.36% and Physioneal with dextrose 2.27% contained aztreonam 1 g/L in one compartment (compartment composition unspecified) for storage at 6 and 25°C.[3563] For bags of Physioneal with dextrose intended for storage at 37°C, the initial concentration of aztreonam in one compartment also was 1 g/L; however, the 2 compartments were combined immediately prior to storage at 37°C for a final aztreonam concentration of 500 mg/L.[3563] Throughout the study, no color change or precipitation was noted on visual assessment.[3563] In Extraneal with icodextrin 7.5%, aztreonam underwent little loss in 14 days at 6°C, less than 7% loss in 14 days at 25°C, and less than 4% loss in 24 hours at 37°C.[3563] In Nutrineal PD-4 with amino acids 1.1%, aztreonam underwent about 7% loss in 14 days at 6°C, about 6% loss in 3 days at 25°C, and about 5% loss in 24 hours at 37°C.[3563] In Physioneal with dextrose 1.36%, aztreonam in one compartment underwent about 3% loss in 14 days at 6°C and about 7% loss in 3 days at 25°C; with the compartments combined, aztreonam loss was about 6% in 2 hours at 37°C.[3563] In Physioneal with dextrose 2.27%, aztreonam loss in one compartment was less than 6% in 14 days at 6°C and about 8% in 3 days at 25°C; with the compartments combined, aztreonam loss was about 7% in 1 hour at 37°C.[3563]

Aztreonam with cloxacillin sodium and aztreonam with vancomycin hydrochloride admixtures are stable in Dianeal 137 with dextrose 4.25% for 24 hours at room temperature.[2864] [2866]

Selected Revisions July 1, 2020. © Copyright, October 1988.
American Society of Health-System Pharmacists, Inc.

Bacitracin
AHFS 8:12.28.08

Products

Bacitracin for injection is available as a lyophilized powder in vials containing 50,000 units of bacitracin.[3317] Vial contents should be dissolved in sodium chloride with procaine hydrochloride 2%.[3317] Diluents containing parabens should not be used for reconstitution; cloudy solutions have resulted and precipitate formation has occurred with the use of such diluents.[3317] Bacitracin for injection should be reconstituted to form a solution with a bacitracin concentration of 5000 to 10,000 units/mL.[3317] Reconstitution of a 50,000-unit vial with 9.8 mL of diluent results in a solution with a bacitracin concentration of 5000 units/mL.[3317]

Administration

Bacitracin is administered by intramuscular injection only.[3317] Intramuscular injections of bacitracin should be administered into the upper outer quadrant of the buttocks, alternating between the right and left sides to avoid multiple injections into the same region.[3317] For infants, the daily dosage should be divided into 2 or 3 injections.[3317]

Stability

Intact vials of bacitracin for injection should be stored under refrigeration at 2 to 8°C.[3317] Reconstituted solutions of bacitracin are stable for 1 week under refrigeration at 2 to 8°C.[3317]

DOI: 10.37573/9781585286850.047

Baclofen
AHFS 12:20.12

Products

Baclofen injection is available as a preservative-free injection for intrathecal use only at a concentration of 0.5 mg/mL in 20-mL ampuls, vials, and prefilled syringes; at a concentration of 1 mg/mL in 20-mL vials and prefilled syringes; and at a concentration of 2 mg/mL in 5-mL ampuls and 20-mL ampuls, vials, and prefilled syringes.[2899] [2900] Each mL of solution contains baclofen 0.5, 1, or 2 mg (500, 1000, or 2000 mcg, respectively) with sodium chloride 9 mg in water for injection.[2899] [2900]

Baclofen injection is also available as a preservative-free injection for intrathecal use only at a concentration of 0.05 mg/mL in 1-mL ampuls and prefilled syringes for use in screening.[2899] [2900] Each mL of solution contains baclofen 0.05 mg (50 mcg) with sodium chloride 9 mg in water for injection.[2899] [2900]

pH

Gablofen: from 5.5 to 7.5.[2900] Lioresal Intrathecal: from 5 to 7.[2899]

Tonicity

Baclofen injection is an isotonic solution.[2899] [2900]

Trade Name(s)

Gablofen, Lioresal Intrathecal

Administration

For screening, 1-mL ampuls or prefilled syringes containing 50 mcg/mL of baclofen are used in the delivery of the drug by direct intrathecal injection via lumbar puncture or spinal catheter over at least one minute using barbotage.[2899] [2900]

For maintenance treatment, baclofen injection is administered intrathecally by chronic, continuous infusion through an implantable infusion pump.[2899] [2900] Baclofen injection (Gablofen) is intended for use only with the Medtronic SynchroMed II Programmable pump or other pumps labeled for intrathecal administration of Gablofen;[2900] baclofen injection (Lioresal Intrathecal) is intended for use only in implantable pumps specifically labeled for the administration of Lioresal Intrathecal.[2899] The concentration of the solution to be infused is dependent upon the rate of infusion and the total daily dosage, which is titrated according to the patient's response.[2899] [2900] For concentrations other than those that are commercially available, the drug must be diluted only with sterile, preservative-free sodium chloride.[2899] [2900] The drug may also require dilution in sterile, preservative-free sodium chloride when used with certain implantable infusion pumps;[2899] the pump manufacturer's manual should be consulted for specific details.[2899]

The pump manufacturer's instructions for programming of the pump and filling and refilling of the pump reservoir should be followed.[2899] [2900]

Stability

Baclofen injection should be stored at temperatures not exceeding 30°C and protected from freezing.[2899] [2900] The product is intended for use in implantable infusion pumps and is stable at a temperature of 37°C.[2899] [2900] It should not be heat sterilized.[2899] [2900] Each ampul, vial, or prefilled syringe contains no preservatives and is intended for single-use only; unused portions must be discarded.[2899] [2900]

If necessary, baclofen injection must be diluted only with sterile, preservative-free sodium chloride.[2899] [2900] The drug is also compatible with cerebrospinal fluid.[2899] [2900]

Implantable Pumps

Baclofen 0.5 mg/mL was filled into an implantable pump (Fresenius model VIP 30) and associated capillary tubing and stored at 37°C. No baclofen loss and no contamination from components of pump materials occurred during eight weeks of storage.[1903]

Compatibility Information
Solution Compatibility

Baclofen

Test Soln Name	Mfr	Mfr	Conc/L or %	Remarks	Ref	C/I
Sodium chloride 0.9%	BA		1 g	Visually compatible with no loss in 10 weeks at 37°C protected from light	2359	C

DOI: 10.37573/9781585286850.048

Additive Compatibility

Baclofen

Test Drug	Mfr	Conc/L or %	Mfr	Conc/L or %	Test Solution	Remarks	Ref	C/I
Clonidine HCl		0.2 g		1 g	NS	Visually compatible with no loss of either drug in 10 weeks at 37°C in dark	2359	C
Morphine sulfate	DB	1 and 1.5 g	CI	200 mg	NS[a]	Physically compatible. Little loss of either drug in 30 days at 37°C	1911	C
Morphine sulfate	DB	1 g	CI	800 mg	NS[a]	Physically compatible. Little baclofen loss and less than 7% morphine loss in 29 days at 37°C	1911	C
Morphine sulfate	DB	1.5 g	CI	800 mg	NS[a]	Physically compatible. Little loss of either drug in 30 days at 37°C	1911	C
Morphine sulfate	DB	7.5 g	CI	1.5 g	NS[a]	Physically compatible. Little loss of either drug in 30 days at 37°C	2170	C
Morphine sulfate	DB	15 g	CI	1 g	NS[a]	Physically compatible. Little loss of either drug in 30 days at 37°C	2170	C
Morphine sulfate	DB	21 g	CI	200 mg	NS[a]	Physically compatible. 7% baclofen loss and little morphine loss in 30 days at 37°C	2170	C

[a] Tested in glass containers.

Selected Revisions May 12, 2016. © Copyright, October 1998.
American Society of Health-System Pharmacists, Inc.

Bendamustine Hydrochloride
AHFS 10:00

Products

Bendamustine hydrochloride is available in several formulations that may differ in stability, incompatibilities, and directions for dilution and administration.[2994][3098][3456]

Bendamustine hydrochloride (Treanda) is available as a lyophilized powder in single-dose vials containing 25 or 100 mg of bendamustine hydrochloride and 42.5 or 170 mg of mannitol, respectively.[2994] The vials should be reconstituted only with sterile water for injection (5 or 20 mL, respectively) and shaken well to dissolve.[2994] The powder should completely dissolve within 5 minutes to yield a reconstituted solution with a bendamustine hydrochloride concentration of 5 mg/mL.[2994] If particulate matter is present, the reconstituted solution should be discarded.[2994] The reconstituted solution must be further diluted prior to administration.[2994] Within 30 minutes of reconstitution, the appropriate volume of the reconstituted solution should be withdrawn from the vial and immediately diluted in an infusion bag containing 500 mL of sodium chloride 0.9% or dextrose 2.5% in sodium chloride 0.45% prior to administration.[2994] The contents of the infusion bag should be thoroughly mixed following transfer of the reconstituted solution.[2994] The resulting concentration of bendamustine hydrochloride diluted in the infusion bag should be within the range of 0.2 to 0.6 mg/mL.[2994]

Bendamustine hydrochloride (Bendeka) is available as a 25 mg/mL ready-to-dilute concentrate for injection in 4-mL multidose vials containing 100 mg of bendamustine hydrochloride.[3098] Each mL of solution also contains propylene glycol 0.1 mL and monothioglycerol 5 mg in polyethylene glycol 400.[3098] Sodium hydroxide also may have been added to adjust the pH.[3098] Although the multidose vials do not contain any antimicrobial preservative, the drug is bacteriostatic.[3098] Bendamustine hydrochloride concentrate for injection must be diluted prior to infusion.[3098] Vials should be stored under refrigeration at 2 to 8°C; however, under such storage conditions, the contents of the vials may partially freeze.[3098] Vials should be allowed to reach room temperature prior to preparation of the infusion.[3098] If particulate matter is observed once the vial has warmed to room temperature, the vial should not be used.[3098] The appropriate volume of the solution should be withdrawn from the vial and immediately diluted in an infusion bag containing 50 mL of sodium chloride 0.9%, dextrose 2.5% in sodium chloride 0.45%, or dextrose 5%, and the contents of the infusion bag should be thoroughly mixed.[3098] The resulting concentration of bendamustine hydrochloride in the infusion bag should be within the range of 1.85 to 5.6 mg/mL.[3098]

Bendamustine hydrochloride (Eagle) is available as a 25-mg/mL ready-to-dilute concentrate for injection in 4-mL multidose vials containing 100 mg of bendamustine hydrochloride.[3456] Each mL of solution also contains propylene glycol 0.1 mL and monothioglycerol 5 mg in polyethylene glycol 400.[3456] Although the multidose vials do not contain any antimicrobial preservative, the drug is bacteriostatic.[3456] Bendamustine hydrochloride concentrate for injection must be diluted prior to infusion.[3456] Vials should be stored under refrigeration at 2 to 8°C; however, under such storage conditions, the contents of the vials may partially freeze.[3456] Vials should be allowed to reach room temperature prior to preparation of the infusion.[3456] If particulate matter is observed once the vial has warmed to room temperature, the vial should not be used.[3456] The appropriate volume of the solution should be withdrawn from the vial and immediately diluted in an infusion bag containing 500 mL of sodium chloride 0.9% or dextrose 2.5% in sodium chloride 0.45%, and the contents of the infusion bag should be thoroughly mixed.[3456] The resulting concentration of bendamustine hydrochloride in the infusion bag should be within the range of 0.2 to 0.7 mg/mL.[3456]

pH

The solution reconstituted from the lyophilized powder has a pH of 2.5 to 3.5.[2994]

Trade Name(s)

Bendeka, Treanda

Administration

Bendamustine hydrochloride is administered by intravenous infusion after dilution of the appropriate volume of the reconstituted solution or concentrate for injection in a compatible diluent;[2994][3098][3456] specific product labeling should be consulted for additional administration details.

Care should be taken to ensure good venous access prior to starting the infusion, and the infusion site should be monitored during and after the infusion;[2994][3098][3456] extravasation should be avoided.[2994][3098][3456]

As with other cytotoxic drugs, bendamustine hydrochloride should be prepared and administered using protective measures to avoid inadvertent contact with the drug in the case of breakage of the vial or other accidental spillage.[2994][2996][3098][3456] Hands should be washed both before and after handling the drug.[2996] Gloves and protective clothing (e.g., laboratory coat, eye protection) are recommended in the preparation of the drug.[2994][2996][3456] Gloves that come in contact with bendamustine hydrochloride concentrate prior to dilution should be removed and properly disposed of.[2994][3456] If skin contact with the drug occurs, the exposed area should be washed thoroughly with soap and water.[2994][3098][3456] For mucous membrane contact, the exposed area should be flushed thoroughly with water.[2994][3098][3456] Applicable disposal procedures for the drug should be followed.[2994][3098][3456]

DOI: 10.37573/9781585286850.049

Stability

Bendamustine hydrochloride lyophilized powder for injection (Treanda) is a white to off-white powder that forms a clear, colorless to pale yellow solution when reconstituted as directed with sterile water for injection.[2994] Intact vials of the lyophilized powder should be stored at controlled room temperature in the original package to protect from light.[2994] Short excursions not exceeding 2 days at −20 to 40°C are permitted for the intact 100-mg vials of lyophilized powder when stored in the original unopened carton.[2996] The reconstituted solution must be diluted within 30 minutes of reconstitution.[2994] Syringes containing the reconstituted solution and subsequently prepared infusions bags should be visually inspected to ensure the absence of particulate matter prior to administration.[2994] After dilution in sodium chloride 0.9% or dextrose 2.5% in sodium chloride 0.45%, the solution should be clear and colorless to slightly yellow in color.[2994]

Bendamustine hydrochloride concentrates for injection are clear, colorless to yellow solutions.[3098 3456] Intact vials of the concentrates for injection should be stored at 2 to 8°C in the original carton to protect from light.[3098 3456] When refrigerated, the contents of the vials may partially freeze.[3098 3456] Vials should be allowed to come to room temperature (15 to 30°C) prior to use.[3098 3456] Multidose vials do not contain any antimicrobial preservative, but the drug is bacteriostatic.[3098 3456] Partially used multidose vials may be stored for up to 28 days at 2 to 8°C in their original carton following initial puncture.[3098 3456] Vials should be discarded 28 days after initial entry and should not be used for more than a total of 6 withdrawals.[3098 3456] Vials and subsequently prepared infusion bags should be visually inspected to ensure the absence of particulate matter prior to administration.[3098 3456] After dilution in a compatible diluent, the solution should remain clear and colorless to yellow or slightly yellow.[3098 3456]

The manufacturers state that admixtures of bendamustine hydrochloride should be prepared (from any of the formulations) as close to the time of administration as possible.[2994 3098 3456]

Incompatibilities with Devices Containing Polycarbonate or Acrylonitrile-butadiene-styrene

Some previous formulations of bendamustine hydrochloride contained *N,N*-dimethylacetamide (DMA), which is incompatible with polycarbonate or acrylonitrile-butadiene-styrene (ABS) and devices containing these compounds (e.g., many closed-system transfer devices [CSTDs], adapters, syringes).[2994 2995 2997 3044 3045] Such devices had been shown to dissolve upon contact with DMA, leading to device failure (e.g., leaking, breaking or operational failure of CSTD components), potential contamination of the drug, and potential serious adverse effects in the patient (e.g., risk of small vessel blockage) or for the practitioner who prepared and/or administered the drug (e.g., skin reactions).[2994 2995 2997 3044 3045] Current commercially available formulations of bendamustine hydrochloride no longer contain DMA.[2994 3098 3456]

Compatibility Information

Solution Compatibility

Bendamustine HCl

Test Soln Name	Mfr	Mfr	Conc/L or %	Remarks	Ref	C/I
Dextrose 2.5% in sodium chloride 0.45%		TE[a]	200 to 600 mg	Complete administration within 3 hr after reconstitution and dilution if stored at 15 to 30°C or 24 hr if stored at 2 to 8°C	2994	C
Dextrose 2.5% in sodium chloride 0.45%		EGL[b]	200 to 700 mg	Complete administration within 3 hr after dilution if stored at 15 to 30°C or 24 hr if stored at 2 to 8°C	3456	C
Dextrose 2.5% in sodium chloride 0.45%		TE[c]	1.85 to 5.6 g	Complete administration within 6 hr after dilution if stored at 15 to 30°C or 24 hr if stored at 2 to 8°C	3098	C
Dextrose 5%		TE[c]	1.85 to 5.6 g	Complete administration within 3 hr after dilution if stored at 15 to 30°C or 24 hr if stored at 2 to 8°C	3098	C
Sodium chloride 0.9%		TE[a]	200 to 600 mg	Complete administration within 3 hr after reconstitution and dilution if stored at 15 to 30°C or 24 hr if stored at 2 to 8°C	2994	C
Sodium chloride 0.9%		TE[c]	1.85 to 5.6 g	Complete administration within 6 hr after dilution if stored at 15 to 30°C or 24 hr if stored at 2 to 8°C	3098	C
Sodium chloride 0.9%		EGL[b]	200 to 700 mg	Complete administration within 3 hr after dilution if stored at 15 to 30°C or 24 hr if stored at 2 to 8°C	3456	C

[a] Test performed using Treanda lyophilized formulation.

[b] Test performed using bendamustine HCl (Eagle) concentrate formulation.

[c] Test performed using Bendeka concentrate formulation.

Selected Revisions September 30, 2019. © Copyright, April 2016.
American Society of Health-System Pharmacists, Inc.

Benztropine Mesylate
AHFS 28:36.08

Products

Benztropine mesylate is available in 2-mL ampuls containing 2 mg of drug with sodium chloride in water for injection.[1(9/05)]

pH

From 5 to 8.[4]

Trade Name(s)

Cogentin

Administration

Benztropine mesylate may be administered by intramuscular or, rarely, intravenous injection.[1(9/05)] [4]

Stability

Store the ampuls at controlled room temperature. Avoid freezing and storing at temperatures over 40°C.[4]

Compatibility Information

Drugs in Syringe Compatibility

Benztropine mesylate

Test Drug	Mfr	Amt	Mfr	Amt	Remarks	Ref	C/I
Chlorpromazine HCl	STS	50 mg/2 mL	MSD	2 mg/2 mL	Visually compatible for 60 min	1784	C
Fluphenazine HCl	LY	5 mg/2 mL	MSD	2 mg/2 mL	Visually compatible for 60 min	1784	C
Haloperidol lactate	MN	0.25, 0.5, 1 mg	MSD	2 mg	Visually compatible for 24 hr at 21°C	1781	C
Haloperidol lactate	MN	2 mg	MSD	2 mg	Precipitate forms within 4 hr at 21°C	1781	I
Haloperidol lactate	MN	3, 4, 5 mg	MSD	2 mg	Precipitate forms within 15 min at 21°C	1781	I
Haloperidol lactate	MN	0.25 and 0.5 mg	MSD	1 mg	Visually compatible for 24 hr at 21°C	1781	C
Haloperidol lactate	MN	1 to 5 mg	MSD	1 mg	Precipitate forms within 15 min at 21°C	1781	I
Haloperidol lactate	MN	0.25 to 5 mg	MSD	0.5 mg	Precipitate forms within 15 min at 21°C	1781	I
Haloperidol lactate	MN	10 mg/2 mL	MSD	2 mg/2 mL	White precipitate forms within 5 min	1784	I
Metoclopramide HCl	RB	10 mg/2 mL	MSD	2 mg/2 mL	Physically compatible for 48 hr at 25°C	1167	C
Metoclopramide HCl	RB	160 mg/32 mL	MSD	2 mg/2 mL	Physically compatible for 48 hr at 25°C	1167	C

Y-Site Injection Compatibility (1:1 Mixture)

Benztropine mesylate

Test Drug	Mfr	Conc	Mfr	Conc	Remarks	Ref	C/I
Cloxacillin sodium	SMX	100 mg/mL	OM	1 mg/mL	Physically compatible for up to 4 hr at room temperature	3245	C
Fluconazole	RR	2 mg/mL	MSD	1 mg/mL	Physically compatible for 24 hr at 25°C	1407	C
Meropenem		50 mg/mL	OM	1 mg/mL	Physically compatible for 4 hr at room temperature	3538	C
Tacrolimus	FUJ	1 mg/mL[a]	MSD	1 mg/mL	Visually compatible for 24 hr at 25°C	1630	C

[a] Tested in sodium chloride 0.9%.

Selected Revisions May 1, 2020. © Copyright, October 1988.
American Society of Health-System Pharmacists, Inc.

DOI: 10.37573/9781585286850.050

Bevacizumab
AHFS 10:00

Products

Bevacizumab is available as a 25-mg/mL injection solution in 4- and 16-mL single-dose (preservative-free) vials.[1370] Each mL also contains α,α-trehalose dihydrate 60 mg, sodium phosphate monobasic monohydrate 5.8 mg, sodium phosphate dibasic anhydrous 1.2 mg, and polysorbate 20 0.4 mg in water for injection.[1370]

Bevacizumab injection solution should be visually inspected for particulate matter and discoloration prior to administration; if the solution is discolored or cloudy or if particulate matter is present, the vial should be discarded.[1370] The appropriate volume of the drug should be withdrawn from the vial and diluted in 100 mL of sodium chloride 0.9%.[1370]

pH

Bevacizumab injection has a pH of 6.2.[1370]

Trade Name(s)

Avastin

Administration

Bevacizumab is administered by intravenous infusion following dilution of the appropriate dose in 100 mL of sodium chloride 0.9%.[1370] The manufacturer recommends that the first infusion be administered over 90 minutes.[1370] Administration time of the second infusion may be reduced to 60 minutes if the 90-minute infusion was tolerated; administration time of subsequent infusions may be further reduced to 30 minutes if the 60-minute infusion was tolerated.[1370]

Bevacizumab must *not* be diluted in or administered with dextrose-containing solutions.[1370]

Bevacizumab also has been administered by intravitreal injection;[1372 1797 2117 2167 2237 2456 2457] this method of administration is not included in the manufacturer's prescribing information.[1370]

Stability

Bevacizumab injection is a clear to slightly opalescent, colorless to pale brown solution.[1370] Intact vials should be stored at 2 to 8°C in the original carton until time of use to protect from light.[1370] Vials or cartons of the drug should not be frozen or shaken.[1370] The manufacturer states that any unused portions should be discarded.[1370]

The diluted solution in sodium chloride 0.9% may be stored for up to 8 hours at 2 to 8°C.[1370] Bevacizumab must *not* be diluted in or administered with dextrose-containing solutions.[1370]

When bevacizumab has been administered by intravitreal injection, only small amounts of the injection have been withdrawn from a vial; stability and sterility of the remaining drug has been assessed.[1372 1797 2117]

Bevacizumab (Genentech) injection solution remaining in previously punctured vials was stored at 4°C for up to 6 months.[1372] An immunoassay was used to determine the drug's ability to bind vascular endothelial growth factor (VEGF)-165, and the concentration of bevacizumab was calculated by correlating the amount of bound bevacizumab to a standard curve.[1372] In 3 months, 9.6% degradation occurred; maximum degradation of 12.7% occurred in 6 months.[1372]

Bevacizumab injection solution remaining in vials that were previously punctured for clinical use (i.e., punctured 4 to 5 times during the first month) was stored at 4°C and sampled thereafter at 1, 3, and 6 months.[1797] Stability of bevacizumab was assessed by matrix-assisted laser desorption ionization/time-of-flight (MALDI-TOF) mass spectrometry (MS), and the authors concluded from these results that most of the molecular structure of bevacizumab did not degrade within 6 months.[1797] Activity of bevacizumab was assessed by the amount of residual active VEGF measured in the in vitro mixture of bevacizumab and VEGF-165 and was expressed as the percentage of VEGF-165 consumed; activity of bevacizumab was noted to be 94.5, 94, and 91.6% at 1, 3, and 6 months, respectively, relative to that of bevacizumab at 0 months.[1797] No bacterial or fungal growth was detected in any sample at any time throughout the study.[1797]

Bevacizumab (Hoffmann-La Roche) injection solution remaining in vials following the withdrawal of multiple 1.25-mg doses for multiple patients (average of 11 punctures for a single vial on a single day within 4 hours' time) was stored at 4°C for up to 6 months.[2117] Based on the results of reverse-phase high-performance liquid chromatography (RP-HPLC), the authors suggested that bevacizumab did not undergo degradation over the 6-month study period.[2117] Similarly, the authors suggested that bevacizumab is stable in structure and conformation over the 6-month period based on the results of circular dichroism spectroscopy and fluorescence measurements.[2117] While all samples tested negative for bacterial and fungal growth at 7 days, sterility was not evaluated over the entire 6-month period.[2117]

Freezing Solutions

The manufacturer states that bevacizumab injection solution should not be frozen.[1370]

Bevacizumab (Genentech) injection solution was packaged in 1-mL tuberculin syringes (Becton Dickinson) capped with a 30-gauge needle (Becton Dickinson) and stored at −10°C for 6 months.[1372] An immunoassay was used to determine the drug's ability to bind VEGF-165, and the concentration of bevacizumab was calculated by correlating the amount of bound bevacizumab to a standard curve.[1372] In 6 months, 12% degradation occurred.[1372]

DOI: 10.37573/9781585286850.051

Packaging of bevacizumab into syringes causes increases in particle concentrations, mostly due to the presence of silicone oil microdroplets.[2167] Freezing of bevacizumab injection solution and placebo (a solution closely resembling the vehicle of bevacizumab injection)[1370] in syringes at −20°C caused immediate increases in particle concentrations to greater than 1.2 million particles per mL; by comparison, the mean particle concentration in bevacizumab withdrawn directly from the original glass vials was about 64,000 particles per mL.[2167] While particle concentrations in bevacizumab syringes incubated at −20°C subsequently remained constant, particle concentrations in placebo syringes increased up to 6 million particles per mL over the 12-week study period.[2167] Repeated freeze-thaw cycles (e.g., 5 or 10 cycles) caused increased particle concentrations and greater than 10% bevacizumab monomer loss.[2167] Bevacizumab packaged as 0.05 mL in 1-mL tuberculin syringes (Becton Dickinson) and stored at −20°C demonstrated substantially lower particle counts (particularly for particles in the larger size range of 2 to 10 μm) than bevacizumab packaged as 0.05 mL in 0.3-mL plastic insulin syringes (Becton Dickinson).[2167]

Syringes

Bevacizumab (Genentech) injection solution was packaged in 1-mL tuberculin syringes (Becton Dickinson) capped with a 30-gauge needle (Becton Dickinson) and stored at 4°C for up to 6 months.[1372] An immunoassay was used to determine the drug's ability to bind VEGF-165, and the concentration of bevacizumab was calculated by correlating the amount of bound bevacizumab to a standard curve.[1372] In 3 months, 8.8% degradation occurred; maximum degradation of 15.9% occurred in 6 months.[1372]

Packaging of bevacizumab into syringes causes increases in particle concentrations, mostly due to the presence of silicone oil microdroplets.[2167] Bevacizumab injection solution was packaged as 0.05 mL in 0.3-mL plastic insulin syringes (Becton Dickinson) and stored at room temperature with or without exposure to fluorescent light and at 4°C.[2167] Mean baseline particle concentration in bevacizumab syringes was 283,675 particles per mL compared with a mean particle concentration in the range of 20,000 to 60,000 particles per mL in bevacizumab withdrawn directly from the original glass vial.[2167] Particle concentrations and particle size distribution remained relatively unchanged during 12 weeks of storage at 4°C.[2167] During the 12-week period, particle concentrations generally were slightly greater in syringes stored at room temperature than those stored at 4°C.[2167] Within 1 week, syringes stored at room temperature with light exposure developed clogged needles.[2167] Particle concentrations generally increased more in syringes stored at room temperature *with* light exposure compared with those stored at room temperature *without* light exposure over the 12-week period.[2167]

Bevacizumab (Roche) 25-mg/mL injection solution was packaged as 0.15 mL in 1-mL polypropylene tuberculin syringes (Becton Dickinson) with a 22-gauge capped needle attached and stored at 4°C for 3 months.[2237] A variety of techniques were used to assess the primary, secondary, and tertiary structure of bevacizumab, including cation exchange chromatography, size-exclusion chromatography, peptide mapping, second derivative ultraviolet (UV) and infrared (IR) spectroscopy, turbidimetry, diffraction laser spectroscopy, thermal denaturation curves, and microscopic examination and subsequent image analysis.[2237] The authors concluded that bevacizumab could be repackaged into polypropylene syringes and stored for up to 3 months at 4°C without changes to the primary, secondary, or tertiary structure of the drug.[2237] Silicone oil microdroplets were noted immediately upon repackaging of the drug into syringes and remained relatively constant in both number and size throughout the storage period.[2237]

Bevacizumab (Roche) 25-mg/mL injection solution was packaged as 1 mL in 1-mL tuberculin syringes (Henke-Sass Wolf) with syringe caps (Braun) and stored at 4°C for up to 54 days.[2456] Bevacizumab concentration (measured using only an HPLC method) and pH remained stable over 32 days.[2456] Another HPLC method used to screen for the presence of leachables did not show any additional peaks as compared with baseline.[2456] The number of particles increased during storage and exceeded USP limits by 7 days.[2456] The authors suggested that the particles could be silicone oil microdroplets from the syringes or bevacizumab protein aggregates.[2456] While the presence of subvisible particles in intravitreal injections is not tolerated by USP standards, the clinical relevance of such particles in intravitreal injections has not been extensively studied and remains unknown.[2456] Based on the results of the particle analysis, the authors concluded that storage of bevacizumab in such syringes should not exceed 3 days.[2456]

Bevacizumab (Genentech) 25-mg/mL injection solution was packaged as 0.13 mL in 1-mL polycarbonate (Braun) and polypropylene (Becton Dickinson) syringes and stored at 2 to 8°C.[2457] Physical stability of bevacizumab was assessed using a variety of techniques, including gel electrophoresis, size-exclusion chromatography, dynamic light scattering, and surface plasmon resonance.[2457] The authors concluded that no discernible changes in the physical stability of bevacizumab or its ability to bind VEGF were noted for up to 6 months as compared with bevacizumab injection solution from a freshly opened vial.[2457]

Sorption

Incompatibilities between bevacizumab injection solution and polyvinyl chloride (PVC) or polyolefin bags have not been observed.[1370]

Compatibility Information

Solution Compatibility

Bevacizumab

Test Soln Name	Mfr	Mfr	Conc/L or %	Remarks	Ref	C/I
Dextrose 5% in Ringer's injection		GEN		Must not be mixed with dextrose-containing solutions	1370	I
Dextrose 5% in Ringer's injection, lactated		GEN		Must not be mixed with dextrose-containing solutions	1370	I
Dextrose 5% in sodium chloride 0.45%		GEN		Must not be mixed with dextrose-containing solutions	1370	I
Dextrose 5% in sodium chloride 0.9%		GEN		Must not be mixed with dextrose-containing solutions	1370	I
Dextrose 5%		GEN		Must not be mixed with dextrose-containing solutions	1370	I
Sodium chloride 0.9%	a	GEN		May be stored for up to 8 hr at 2 to 8°C	1370	C

ᵃ Tested in PVC and polyolefin containers.

Additional Compatibility Information

Infusion Solutions

Bevacizumab must *not* be administered with any dextrose-containing solutions.[1370]

Bivalirudin
AHFS 20:12.04.12

Products

Bivalirudin is available as a white lyophilized powder or cake.[3287] Each single-dose vial contains bivalirudin 250 mg with mannitol 125 mg and sodium hydroxide to adjust the pH.[3287] Vials should be reconstituted with 5 mL of sterile water for injection and swirled to dissolve, yielding a 50-mg/mL solution.[3287] The reconstituted solution should be further diluted to a concentration of 0.5 or 5 mg/mL prior to administration.[3287]

Bivalirudin also is available as a lyophilized powder or cake in 250-mg single-use ADD-Vantage vials.[3308] Each ADD-Vantage vial also contains mannitol 125 mg and sodium hydroxide to adjust the pH.[3308] ADD-Vantage vials of bivalirudin should be prepared with 50 mL of dextrose 5% or sodium chloride 0.9% in ADD-Vantage diluent bags to yield a solution with a final concentration of 5 mg/mL.[3308]

pH

From 5 to 6.[3287 3308]

Sodium Content

Approximately 12.5 mg per vial.[3287 3308]

Trade Name(s)

Angiomax

Administration

Bivalirudin is administered by direct intravenous injection[3287] and continuous infusion.[3287 3308]

Stability

Bivalirudin vials should be stored at controlled room temperature.[3287 3308] The drug is a white lyophilized powder that forms a clear to slightly opalescent, colorless to slightly yellow solution upon reconstitution.[3287 3308] The reconstituted solution prepared from single-dose vials is stable for 24 hours at 2 to 8°C;[3287] freezing of reconstituted and diluted solutions should be avoided.[3287 3308] Unused portions should be discarded.[3287]

Compatibility Information
Solution Compatibility

Bivalirudin

Test Soln Name	Mfr	Mfr	Conc/L or %	Remarks	Ref	C/I
Dextrose 5%		TMC	0.5 to 5 g	Stable for 24 hr at room temperature	3287	C
Dextrose 5%		HOS	5 g	Stable for 24 hr at room temperature	3308	C
Sodium chloride 0.9%		TMC	0.5 to 5 g	Stable for 24 hr at room temperature	3287	C
Sodium chloride 0.9%		HOS	5 g	Stable for 24 hr at room temperature	3308	C

Y-Site Injection Compatibility (1:1 Mixture)

Bivalirudin

Test Drug	Mfr	Conc	Mfr	Conc	Remarks	Ref	C/I
Abciximab	CEN	10 mcg/mL[a]	TMC	5 mg/mL[a]	Physically compatible for 4 hr at 23°C	2373	C
Alfentanil HCl	TAY	0.125 mg/mL[a]	TMC	5 mg/mL[a]	Physically compatible for 4 hr at 23°C	2373	C
Alteplase	GEN	1 mg/mL	TMC	5 mg/mL[a]	Small aggregates form immediately	2373	I
Amikacin sulfate	APO	5 mg/mL[a]	TMC	5 mg/mL[a]	Physically compatible for 4 hr at 23°C	2373	C
Aminophylline	AB	2.5 mg/mL[a]	TMC	5 mg/mL[a]	Physically compatible for 4 hr at 23°C	2373	C
Amiodarone HCl	WAY	4 mg/mL[a]	TMC	5 mg/mL[a]	Measured haze increases immediately	2373	I
Amphotericin B	APO	0.6 mg/mL[a]	TMC	5 mg/mL[a]	Yellow precipitate forms immediately	2373	I
Ampicillin sodium	APO	20 mg/mL[b]	TMC	5 mg/mL[a]	Physically compatible for 4 hr at 23°C	2373	C

DOI: 10.37573/9781585286850.052

Y-Site Injection Compatibility (1:1 Mixture) (Cont.)

Test Drug	Mfr	Conc	Mfr	Conc	Remarks	Ref	C/I
Ampicillin sodium-sulbactam sodium	PF	20 mg/mL[b] [e]	TMC	5 mg/mL[a]	Physically compatible for 4 hr at 23°C	2373	C
Atropine sulfate	AMR	0.4 mg/mL	TMC	5 mg/mL[a] [b]	Visually compatible for 6 hr at 23°C	2680	C
Azithromycin	PF	2 mg/mL[a]	TMC	5 mg/mL[a]	Physically compatible for 4 hr at 23°C	2373	C
Aztreonam	DUR	40 mg/mL[a]	TMC	5 mg/mL[a]	Physically compatible for 4 hr at 23°C	2373	C
Bumetanide	OHM	40 mcg/mL[a]	TMC	5 mg/mL[a]	Physically compatible for 4 hr at 23°C	2373	C
Butorphanol tartrate	APO	40 mcg/mL[a]	TMC	5 mg/mL[a]	Physically compatible for 4 hr at 23°C	2373	C
Calcium gluconate	APP	40 mg/mL[a]	TMC	5 mg/mL[a]	Physically compatible for 4 hr at 23°C	2373	C
Cangrelor tetrasodium	TMC	1 mg/mL[b]	TMC	5 mg/mL[b]	Physically compatible for 4 hr	3243	C
Cefazolin sodium	APO	20 mg/mL[a]	TMC	5 mg/mL[a]	Physically compatible for 4 hr at 23°C	2373	C
Cefepime HCl	BMS	20 mg/mL[a]	TMC	5 mg/mL[a]	Physically compatible for 4 hr at 23°C	2373	C
Cefotaxime sodium	HO	20 mg/mL[a]	TMC	5 mg/mL[a]	Physically compatible for 4 hr at 23°C	2373	C
Cefotetan disodium	ZEN	20 mg/mL[a]	TMC	5 mg/mL[a]	Physically compatible for 4 hr at 23°C	2373	C
Cefoxitin sodium	ME	20 mg/mL[a]	TMC	5 mg/mL[a]	Physically compatible for 4 hr at 23°C	2373	C
Ceftazidime	GW	40 mg/mL[a]	TMC	5 mg/mL[a]	Physically compatible for 4 hr at 23°C	2373	C
Ceftriaxone sodium	RC	20 mg/mL[a]	TMC	5 mg/mL[a]	Physically compatible for 4 hr at 23°C	2373	C
Cefuroxime sodium	GW	30 mg/mL[a]	TMC	5 mg/mL[a]	Physically compatible for 4 hr at 23°C	2373	C
Chlorpromazine HCl	ES	2 mg/mL[a]	TMC	5 mg/mL[a]	Gross white precipitate forms immediately	2373	I
Ciprofloxacin	BAY	2 mg/mL[a]	TMC	5 mg/mL[a]	Physically compatible for 4 hr at 23°C	2373	C
Clevidipine butyrate	CHS	0.5 mg/mL		5 mg/mL[a]	pH shifted outside of specified pH range for clevidipine within 24 hr	3334	?
Clindamycin phosphate	AB	10 mg/mL[a]	TMC	5 mg/mL[a]	Physically compatible for 4 hr at 23°C	2373	C
Dexamethasone sodium phosphate	APP	1 mg/mL[a]	TMC	5 mg/mL[a]	Physically compatible for 4 hr at 23°C	2373	C
Diazepam	AB	5 mg/mL	TMC	5 mg/mL[a]	Yellowish precipitate forms immediately	2373	I
Digoxin	GW	0.25 mg/mL	TMC	5 mg/mL[a]	Physically compatible for 4 hr at 23°C	2373	C
Diltiazem HCl	BA	5 mg/mL	TMC	5 mg/mL[a]	Physically compatible for 4 hr at 23°C	2373	C
Diltiazem HCl	BV	5 mg/mL	TMC	5 mg/mL[a] [b]	Visually compatible for 6 hr at 23°C	2680	C
Diphenhydramine HCl	ES	2 mg/mL[a]	TMC	5 mg/mL[a]	Physically compatible for 4 hr at 23°C	2373	C
Dobutamine HCl	AB	4 mg/mL[a]	TMC	5 mg/mL[a]	Physically compatible for 4 hr at 23°C	2373	C
Dobutamine HCl	BV	12.5 mg/mL[d]	TMC	5 mg/mL[a] [b]	Cloudiness forms immediately	2680	I
Dopamine HCl	AB	3.2 mg/mL[a]	TMC	5 mg/mL[a]	Physically compatible for 4 hr at 23°C	2373	C
Dopamine HCl	AMR	80 mg/mL	TMC	5 mg/mL[a] [b]	Visually compatible for 6 hr at 23°C	2680	C
Doxycycline hyclate	APP	1 mg/mL[a]	TMC	5 mg/mL[a]	Physically compatible for 4 hr at 23°C	2373	C
Droperidol	AMR	2.5 mg/mL	TMC	5 mg/mL[a]	Physically compatible for 4 hr at 23°C	2373	C
Enalaprilat	BED	0.1 mg/mL[a]	TMC	5 mg/mL[a]	Physically compatible for 4 hr at 23°C	2373	C

Y-Site Injection Compatibility (1:1 Mixture) (Cont.)

Test Drug	Mfr	Conc	Mfr	Conc	Remarks	Ref	C/I
Ephedrine sulfate	TAY	5 mg/mL[a]	TMC	5 mg/mL[a]	Physically compatible for 4 hr at 23°C	2373	C
Epinephrine HCl	AMR	50 mcg/mL[a]	TMC	5 mg/mL[a]	Physically compatible for 4 hr at 23°C	2373	C
Epoprostenol sodium	GW[h]	10 mcg/mL[a]	TMC	5 mg/mL[a]	Physically compatible for 4 hr at 23°C	2373	C
Eptifibatide	KEY	2 mg/mL	TMC	5 mg/mL[a]	Physically compatible for 4 hr at 23°C	2373	C
Erythromycin lacto-bionate	AB	5 mg/mL[b]	TMC	5 mg/mL[a]	Physically compatible for 4 hr at 23°C	2373	C
Esmolol HCl	BA	10 mg/mL[a]	TMC	5 mg/mL[a]	Physically compatible for 4 hr at 23°C	2373	C
Famotidine	ME	2 mg/mL[a]	TMC	5 mg/mL[a]	Physically compatible for 4 hr at 23°C	2373	C
Fentanyl citrate	AB	50 mcg/mL	TMC	5 mg/mL[a]	Physically compatible for 4 hr at 23°C	2373	C
Fentanyl citrate	TAY	50 mcg/mL	TMC	5 mg/mL[a b]	Visually compatible for 6 hr at 23°C	2680	C
Fluconazole	PF	2 mg/mL	TMC	5 mg/mL[a]	Physically compatible for 4 hr at 23°C	2373	C
Furosemide	AMR	3 mg/mL[a]	TMC	5 mg/mL[a]	Physically compatible for 4 hr at 23°C	2373	C
Gentamicin sulfate	AB	5 mg/mL[a]	TMC	5 mg/mL[a]	Physically compatible for 4 hr at 23°C	2373	C
Haloperidol lactate	MN	0.2 mg/mL[a]	TMC	5 mg/mL[a]	Physically compatible for 4 hr at 23°C	2373	C
Heparin sodium	AB	100 units/mL	TMC	5 mg/mL[a]	Physically compatible for 4 hr at 23°C	2373	C
Hydrocortisone sodium succinate	PHU	1 mg/mL[a]	TMC	5 mg/mL[a]	Physically compatible for 4 hr at 23°C	2373	C
Hydrocortisone sodium succinate	PHU	50 mg/mL	TMC	5 mg/mL[a b]	Visually compatible for 6 hr at 23°C	2680	C
Hydromorphone HCl	AST	0.5 mg/mL[a]	TMC	5 mg/mL[a]	Physically compatible for 4 hr at 23°C	2373	C
Isoproterenol HCl	AB	20 mcg/mL[a]	TMC	5 mg/mL[a]	Physically compatible for 4 hr at 23°C	2373	C
Labetalol HCl	FP	2 mg/mL[a]	TMC	5 mg/mL[a]	Physically compatible for 4 hr at 23°C	2373	C
Levofloxacin	ORT	5 mg/mL[a]	TMC	5 mg/mL[a]	Physically compatible for 4 hr at 23°C	2373	C
Lidocaine HCl	AST	10 mg/mL[a]	TMC	5 mg/mL[a]	Physically compatible for 4 hr at 23°C	2373	C
Lorazepam	ESL	0.5 mg/mL[a]	TMC	5 mg/mL[a]	Physically compatible for 4 hr at 23°C	2373	C
Magnesium sulfate	APP	100 mg/mL[a]	TMC	5 mg/mL[a]	Physically compatible for 4 hr at 23°C	2373	C
Mannitol	BA	15%	TMC	5 mg/mL[a]	Physically compatible for 4 hr at 23°C	2373	C
Meperidine HCl	AST	10 mg/mL[a]	TMC	5 mg/mL[a]	Physically compatible for 4 hr at 23°C	2373	C
Methylprednisolone sodium succinate	PHU	5 mg/mL[a]	TMC	5 mg/mL[a]	Physically compatible for 4 hr at 23°C	2373	C
Metoclopramide HCl	FAU	5 mg/mL	TMC	5 mg/mL[a]	Physically compatible for 4 hr at 23°C	2373	C
Metoprolol tartrate	AB	1 mg/mL	TMC	5 mg/mL[a b]	Visually compatible for 6 hr at 23°C	2680	C
Metronidazole	BA	5 mg/mL	TMC	5 mg/mL[a]	Physically compatible for 4 hr at 23°C	2373	C
Midazolam HCl	BA	1 mg/mL[a]	TMC	5 mg/mL[a]	Physically compatible for 4 hr at 23°C	2373	C
Midazolam HCl	AB	2 mg/mL	TMC	5 mg/mL[a b]	Visually compatible for 6 hr at 23°C	2680	C
Milrinone lactate	SAN	0.2 mg/mL[a]	TMC	5 mg/mL[a]	Physically compatible for 4 hr at 23°C	2373	C
Morphine sulfate	AST	1 mg/mL[a]	TMC	5 mg/mL[a]	Physically compatible for 4 hr at 23°C	2373	C
Morphine sulfate	ES	10 mg/mL	TMC	5 mg/mL[a b]	Visually compatible for 6 hr at 23°C	2680	C

Y-Site Injection Compatibility (1:1 Mixture) (Cont.)

Test Drug	Mfr	Conc	Mfr	Conc	Remarks	Ref	C/I
Nalbuphine HCl	AST	10 mg/mL	TMC	5 mg/mL[a]	Physically compatible for 4 hr at 23°C	2373	C
Nitroglycerin	AMR	0.4 mg/mL[a]	TMC	5 mg/mL[a]	Physically compatible for 4 hr at 23°C	2373	C
Norepinephrine bitartrate	AB	0.12 mg/mL[a]	TMC	5 mg/mL[a]	Physically compatible for 4 hr at 23°C	2373	C
Phenylephrine HCl	AMR	1 mg/mL[a]	TMC	5 mg/mL[a]	Physically compatible for 4 hr at 23°C	2373	C
Phenylephrine HCl	AMR	10 mg/mL	TMC	5 mg/mL[a b]	Visually compatible for 6 hr at 23°C	2680	C
Piperacillin sodium-tazobactam sodium	LE[c]	40 mg/mL[a f]	TMC	5 mg/mL[a]	Physically compatible for 4 hr at 23°C	2373	C
Potassium chloride	APP	0.1 mEq/mL[a]	TMC	5 mg/mL[a]	Physically compatible for 4 hr at 23°C	2373	C
Procainamide HCl	ES	10 mg/mL[a]	TMC	5 mg/mL[a]	Physically compatible for 4 hr at 23°C	2373	C
Prochlorperazine edisylate	SKB	0.5 mg/mL[a]	TMC	5 mg/mL[a]	Gross white precipitate forms immediately	2373	I
Promethazine HCl	ES	2 mg/mL[a]	TMC	5 mg/mL[a]	Physically compatible for 4 hr at 23°C	2373	C
Ranitidine HCl	GW	2 mg/mL[a]	TMC	5 mg/mL[a]	Physically compatible for 4 hr at 23°C	2373	C
Reteplase	CEN	1 unit/mL[a]	TMC	5 mg/mL[a]	Small aggregates form immediately	2373	I
Sodium bicarbonate	AMR	1 mEq/mL	TMC	5 mg/mL[a]	Physically compatible for 4 hr at 23°C	2373	C
Sodium nitroprusside	BA	2 mg/mL[a]	TMC	5 mg/mL[a]	Physically compatible for 4 hr at 23°C protected from light	2373	C
Sufentanil citrate	ES	50 mcg/mL	TMC	5 mg/mL[a]	Physically compatible for 4 hr at 23°C	2373	C
Theophylline	BA	4 mg/mL[a]	TMC	5 mg/mL[a]	Physically compatible for 4 hr at 23°C	2373	C
Tirofiban HCl	ME	50 mcg/mL[a]	TMC	5 mg/mL[a]	Physically compatible for 4 hr at 23°C	2373	C
Tobramycin sulfate	GNS	5 mg/mL[a]	TMC	5 mg/mL[a]	Physically compatible for 4 hr at 23°C	2373	C
Trimethoprim-sulfamethoxazole	GNS	0.8 mg/mL[a g]	TMC	5 mg/mL[a]	Physically compatible for 4 hr at 23°C	2373	C
Vancomycin HCl	AB	10 mg/mL[a]	TMC	5 mg/mL[a]	Gross white precipitate forms immediately	2373	I
Verapamil HCl	AB	1.25 mg/mL[a]	TMC	5 mg/mL[a]	Physically compatible for 4 hr at 23°C	2373	C
Verapamil HCl	AMR	2.5 mg/mL	TMC	5 mg/mL[a b]	Visually compatible for 6 hr at 23°C	2680	C

[a] Tested in dextrose 5%.

[b] Tested in sodium chloride 0.9%.

[c] Test performed using the formulation WITHOUT edetate disodium.

[d] NOTE: Undiluted dobutamine hydrochloride concentrate must be diluted for administration. This concentration is not acceptable for intravenous administration.

[e] Ampicillin component. Ampicillin in a 2:1 fixed-ratio concentration with sulbactam.

[f] Piperacillin component. Piperacillin in an 8:1 fixed-ratio concentration with tazobactam.

[g] Trimethoprim component. Trimethoprim in a 1:5 fixed-ratio concentration with sulfamethoxazole.

[h] Test performed using the Flolan formulation.

Selected Revisions December 12, 2018. © Copyright, October 2004. American Society of Health-System Pharmacists, Inc.

Bleomycin Sulfate
AHFS 10:00

Products

Bleomycin sulfate is available in vials containing 15 and 30 units of bleomycin as the sulfate.[2936] [2937] Sulfuric acid or sodium hydroxide may have been added to some products to adjust the pH.[2937]

For intramuscular or subcutaneous administration, reconstitute the 15-unit vial with 1 to 5 mL and the 30-unit vial with 2 to 10 mL of sterile water for injection, sodium chloride 0.9%, or bacteriostatic water for injection.[2936] [2937] For intravenous injection, reconstitute the 15-unit or 30-unit vial with 5 or 10 mL, respectively, of sodium chloride 0.9%.[2936] [2937] For intrapleural administration, dissolve 60 units in 50 to 100 mL of sodium chloride 0.9%.[2936] [2937] The manufacturers state that dextrose-containing diluents should not be used for the reconstitution or dilution of bleomycin sulfate; analysis has revealed a loss in drug potency that occurs with the use of dextrose 5% that does not occur with the use of sodium chloride 0.9%.[2936] [2937]

Units

Bleomycin sulfate is a mixture of cytotoxic glycopeptide antibiotics.[2936] [2937] In the United States, a unit of bleomycin is equal to the term milligram activity, which was formerly used.[2936] [2937] One unit of bleomycin is equivalent in activity to 1 mg of bleomycin A_2 reference standard.[4]

Administration

Bleomycin sulfate may be administered by intramuscular, subcutaneous, or intravenous injection, or by intrapleural instillation through a thoracostomy tube.[2936] [2937] Intravenous injections should be given slowly over a 10-minute period.[2936] [2937]

Stability

Intact vials are stable under refrigeration.[2936] [2937] They also have been stated to be stable for 28 days at room temperature.[1181] [1433]

The manufacturers state that bleomycin in sodium chloride is stable for 24 hours at room temperature.[2936] [2937] Bleomycin sulfate solutions reconstituted with sodium chloride 0.9% also have been reported to be stable for 4 weeks when stored at 2 to 8°C,[4] [1369] for 2 weeks[4] to 4 weeks (protected from light)[1369] at room temperature, and for 10 days at 37°C.[1073]

Ogawa et al. reported that immersion of a needle with an aluminum component in bleomycin sulfate (Bristol) 3 units/mL resulted in no visually apparent reaction after 7 days at 24°C.[988]

In the event of spills or leaks, the use of sodium hypochlorite 5% (household bleach) or potassium permanganate 1% has been recommended to inactivate bleomycin sulfate.[1200]

pH Effects

Bleomycin sulfate (Bristol) is stable in solution over a pH range of 4 to 10.[763]

Filtration

Bleomycin sulfate was shown not to exhibit substantial sorption to cellulose ester (Ivex-2), cellulose nitrate/cellulose acetate (Millex OR), nylon, or Teflon (Millex FG) filters.[533] [1415] [1416] [1577]

Compatibility Information

Solution Compatibility

Bleomycin sulfate

Test Soln Name	Mfr	Mfr	Conc/L or %	Remarks	Ref	C/I
Dextrose 5%	a			About 54% loss in 28 days at room temperature in the dark	1369	I
Dextrose 5%	BA[b]	BR	300 and 3000 units	About 10% loss in 8 to 10 hr and 11 to 16% loss in 24 hr at 23°C in glass and PVC	1441	I
Dextrose 5%	c	BEL	15 units	No loss in 24 hr at room temperature in light	1577	C
Sodium chloride 0.9%				Stable for 24 hr at room temperature	2936, 2937	C
Sodium chloride 0.9%	a			About 4% loss in 28 days at room temperature in the dark	1369	C
Sodium chloride 0.9%	BA[b]	BR	300 and 3000 units	Little or no loss in 24 hr at 23°C in glass and PVC	1441	C
Sodium chloride 0.9%	c	BEL	15 units	No loss in 48 hr at room temperature in light	1577	C

[a] Tested in PVC containers.

[b] Tested in both glass and PVC containers.

[c] Tested in glass, PVC, and high-density polyethylene containers.

DOI: 10.37573/9781585286850.053

Additive Compatibility

Bleomycin sulfate

Test Drug	Mfr	Conc/L or %	Mfr	Conc/L or %	Test Solution	Remarks	Ref	C/I
Amikacin sulfate	BR	1.25 g	BR	20 and 30 units	NS	Physically compatible. Bleomycin stable for 1 week at 4°C. Amikacin not tested	763	C
Aminophylline	ES	250 mg	BR	20 and 30 units	NS	50% loss of bleomycin in 1 week at 4°C	763	I
Ascorbic acid	PD	2.5 and 5 g	BR	20 and 30 units	NS	Loss of all bleomycin in 1 week at 4°C	763	I
Cefazolin sodium	LI	1 g	BR	20 and 30 units	NS	43% loss of bleomycin activity in 1 week at 4°C	763	I
Dexamethasone sodium phosphate	MSD	50 mg	BR	20 and 30 units	NS	Physically compatible and bleomycin activity retained for 1 week at 4°C. Dexamethasone not tested	763	C
Diazepam	RC	50 and 100 mg	BR	20 and 30 units	NS	Physically incompatible	763	I
Diphenhydramine HCl	PD	100 mg	BR	20 and 30 units	NS	Physically compatible and bleomycin activity retained for 1 week at 4°C. Diphenhydramine not tested	763	C
Fluorouracil	RC	1 g	BR	20 and 30 units	NS	Physically compatible and bleomycin activity retained for 1 week at 4°C. Fluorouracil not tested	763	C
Gentamicin sulfate	SC	50, 100, 300, 600 mg	BR	20 and 30 units	NS	Physically compatible and bleomycin activity retained for 1 week at 4°C. Gentamicin not tested	763	C
Heparin sodium	RI	10,000 to 200,000 units	BR	20 and 30 units	NS	Physically compatible and bleomycin activity retained for 1 week at 4°C. Heparin not tested	763	C
Hydrocortisone sodium succinate	AB	300 mg, 750 mg, 1 g, 2.5 g	BR	20 and 30 units	NS	60 to 100% loss of bleomycin activity in 1 week at 4°C	763	I
Methotrexate sodium	LE	250 and 500 mg	BR	20 and 30 units	NS	About 60% loss of bleomycin activity in 1 week at 4°C	763	I
Mitomycin	BR	10 mg	BR	20 and 30 units	NS	20% loss of bleomycin activity in 1 week at 4°C	763	I
Mitomycin	BR	50 mg	BR	20 and 30 units	NS	52% loss of bleomycin activity in 1 week at 4°C	763	I
Nafcillin sodium	BR	2.5 g	BR	20 and 30 units	NS	Substantial loss of bleomycin activity in 1 week at 4°C	763	I
Penicillin G sodium	SQ	2 million units	BR	20 and 30 units	NS	77% loss of bleomycin activity in 1 week at 4°C	763	I
Penicillin G sodium	SQ	5 million units	BR	20 and 30 units	NS	41% loss of bleomycin activity in 1 week at 4°C	763	I
Streptomycin sulfate	PF	4 g	BR	20 and 30 units	NS	Physically compatible and bleomycin activity retained for 1 week at 4°C. Streptomycin not tested	763	C
Terbutaline sulfate	GG	7.5 mg	BR	20 and 30 units	NS	36% loss of bleomycin activity in 1 week at 4°C	763	I
Tobramycin sulfate	LI	500 mg	BR	20 and 30 units	NS	Physically compatible and bleomycin activity retained for 1 week at 4°C. Tobramycin not tested	763	C
Vinblastine sulfate	LI	10 and 100 mg	BR	20 and 30 units	NS	Physically compatible and bleomycin activity retained for 1 week at 4°C. Vinblastine not tested	763	C
Vincristine sulfate	LI	50 and 100 mg	BR	20 and 30 units	NS	Physically compatible and bleomycin activity retained for 1 week at 4°C. Vincristine not tested	763	C

Drugs in Syringe Compatibility

Bleomycin sulfate

Test Drug	Mfr	Amt	Mfr	Amt	Remarks	Ref	C/I
Cisplatin		0.5 mg/0.5 mL		1.5 units/0.5 mL	Physically compatible for 5 min at room temperature followed by 8 min of centrifugation	980	C
Cyclophosphamide		10 mg/0.5 mL		1.5 units/0.5 mL	Physically compatible for 5 min at room temperature followed by 8 min of centrifugation	980	C
Doxorubicin HCl		1 mg/0.5 mL		1.5 units/0.5 mL	Physically compatible for 5 min at room temperature followed by 8 min of centrifugation	980	C
Droperidol		1.25 mg/0.5 mL		1.5 units/0.5 mL	Physically compatible for 5 min at room temperature followed by 8 min of centrifugation	980	C
Fluorouracil		25 mg/0.5 mL		1.5 units/0.5 mL	Physically compatible for 5 min at room temperature followed by 8 min of centrifugation	980	C
Furosemide		5 mg/0.5 mL		1.5 units/0.5 mL	Physically compatible for 5 min at room temperature followed by 8 min of centrifugation	980	C
Heparin sodium		500 units/0.5 mL		1.5 units/0.5 mL	Physically compatible for 5 min at room temperature followed by 8 min of centrifugation	980	C
Leucovorin calcium		5 mg/0.5 mL		1.5 units/0.5 mL	Physically compatible for 5 min at room temperature followed by 8 min of centrifugation	980	C
Methotrexate sodium		12.5 mg/0.5 mL		1.5 units/0.5 mL	Physically compatible for 5 min at room temperature followed by 8 min of centrifugation	980	C
Metoclopramide HCl		2.5 mg/0.5 mL		1.5 units/0.5 mL	Physically compatible for 5 min at room temperature followed by 8 min of centrifugation	980	C
Mitomycin		0.25 mg/0.5 mL		1.5 units/0.5 mL	Physically compatible for 5 min at room temperature followed by 8 min of centrifugation	980	C
Vinblastine sulfate		0.5 mg/0.5 mL		1.5 units/0.5 mL	Physically compatible for 5 min at room temperature followed by 8 min of centrifugation	980	C
Vincristine sulfate		0.5 mg/0.5 mL		1.5 units/0.5 mL	Physically compatible for 5 min at room temperature followed by 8 min of centrifugation	980	C

Y-Site Injection Compatibility (1:1 Mixture)

Bleomycin sulfate

Test Drug	Mfr	Conc	Mfr	Conc	Remarks	Ref	C/I
Allopurinol sodium	BW	3 mg/mL[b]	BR	1 unit/mL[b]	Physically compatible for 4 hr at 22°C	1686	C
Amifostine	USB	10 mg/mL[a]	MJ	1 unit/mL[b]	Physically compatible for 4 hr at 23°C	1845	C
Aztreonam	SQ	40 mg/mL[a]	MJ	1 unit/mL[b]	Physically compatible for 4 hr at 23°C	1758	C
Cisplatin		1 mg/mL		3 units/mL	Drugs injected sequentially in Y-site with no flush. No precipitate seen	980	C
Cyclophosphamide		20 mg/mL		3 units/mL	Drugs injected sequentially in Y-site with no flush. No precipitate seen	980	C
Doxorubicin HCl		2 mg/mL		3 units/mL	Drugs injected sequentially in Y-site with no flush. No precipitate seen	980	C
Doxorubicin HCl liposomal	SEQ	0.4 mg/mL[a]	MJ	1 unit/mL[b]	Physically compatible for 4 hr at 23°C	2087	C

Y-Site Injection Compatibility (1:1 Mixture) (Cont.)

Test Drug	Mfr	Conc	Mfr	Conc	Remarks	Ref	C/I
Droperidol		2.5 mg/mL		3 units/mL	Drugs injected sequentially in Y-site with no flush. No precipitate seen	980	C
Etoposide phosphate	BR	5 mg/mL[a]	MJ	1 unit/mL[b]	Physically compatible for 4 hr at 23°C	2218	C
Filgrastim	AMG	30 mcg/mL[a]	BR	1 unit/mL[a]	Physically compatible for 4 hr at 22°C	1687	C
Fludarabine phosphate	BX	1 mg/mL[a]	BR	1 unit/mL[b]	Visually compatible for 4 hr at 22°C	1439	C
Fluorouracil		50 mg/mL		3 units/mL	Drugs injected sequentially in Y-site with no flush. No precipitate seen	980	C
Furosemide		10 mg/mL		3 units/mL	Drugs injected sequentially in Y-site with no flush. No precipitate seen	980	C
Gemcitabine HCl	LI	10 mg/mL[b]	MJ	1 unit/mL[b]	Physically compatible for 4 hr at 23°C	2226	C
Granisetron HCl	SKB	0.05 mg/mL[a]	MJ	1 unit/mL[b]	Physically compatible for 4 hr at 23°C	2000	C
Heparin sodium		1000 units/mL		3 units/mL	Drugs injected sequentially in Y-site with no flush. No precipitate seen	980	C
Leucovorin calcium		10 mg/mL		3 units/mL	Drugs injected sequentially in Y-site with no flush. No precipitate seen	980	C
Melphalan HCl	BW	0.1 mg/mL[b]	BR	1 unit/mL[b]	Physically compatible for 3 hr at 22°C	1557	C
Methotrexate sodium		25 mg/mL		3 units/mL	Drugs injected sequentially in Y-site with no flush. No precipitate seen	980	C
Metoclopramide HCl		5 mg/mL		3 units/mL	Drugs injected sequentially in Y-site with no flush. No precipitate seen	980	C
Mitomycin		0.5 mg/mL		3 units/mL	Drugs injected sequentially in Y-site with no flush. No precipitate seen	980	C
Ondansetron HCl	GL	1 mg/mL[b]	BR	1 unit/mL[b]	Visually compatible for 4 hr at 22°C	1365	C
Paclitaxel	NCI	1.2 mg/mL[a]	MJ	1 unit/mL[a]	Physically compatible for 4 hr at 22°C	1556	C
Piperacillin sodium–tazobactam sodium	LE[d]	40 mg/mL[a e]	BR	1 unit/mL[b]	Physically compatible for 4 hr at 22°C	1688	C
Sargramostim	IMM	10 mcg/mL[b]	MJ	1 unit/mL[b]	Visually compatible for 4 hr at 22°C	1436	C
Teniposide	BR	0.1 mg/mL[a]	BR	1 unit/mL[b]	Physically compatible for 4 hr at 23°C	1725	C
Thiotepa	IMM[c]	1 mg/mL[a]	MJ	1 unit/mL[b]	Physically compatible for 4 hr at 23°C	1861	C
Vinblastine sulfate		1 mg/mL		3 units/mL	Drugs injected sequentially in Y-site with no flush. No precipitate seen	980	C
Vincristine sulfate		1 mg/mL		3 units/mL	Drugs injected sequentially in Y-site with no flush. No precipitate seen	980	C
Vinorelbine tartrate	BW	1 mg/mL[b]	BR	1 unit/mL[b]	Physically compatible for 4 hr at 22°C	1558	C

[a] Tested in dextrose 5%.

[b] Tested in sodium chloride 0.9%.

[c] Lyophilized formulation tested.

[d] Test performed using the formulation WITHOUT edetate disodium.

[e] Piperacillin component. Piperacillin in an 8:1 fixed-ratio concentration with tazobactam.

Selected Revisions June 18, 2015. © Copyright, October 1982.
American Society of Health-System Pharmacists, Inc.

Blinatumomab

AHFS 10:00

Products

Blinatumomab is available as a lyophilized powder in preservative-free single-dose vials containing 35 mcg of the drug.[3095] Each vial also contains citric acid monohydrate 3.35 mg, lysine hydrochloride 23.23 mg, polysorbate 80 0.64 mg, trehalose dihydrate 95.5 mg, and sodium hydroxide to adjust the pH.[3095]

Each vial of blinatumomab is packaged with a 10-mL single-dose vial of preservative-free intravenous solution stabilizer.[3095] Each vial of intravenous solution stabilizer contains citric acid monohydrate 52.5 mg, lysine hydrochloride 2283.8 mg, polysorbate 80 10 mg, sodium hydroxide (to adjust the pH), and water for injection.[3095] The intravenous solution stabilizer is added to the infusion bag to coat the bag prior to the addition of the reconstituted blinatumomab solution, thereby preventing adhesion of the drug to the bag and administration tubing; *the solution stabilizer should not be used to reconstitute the drug.*[3095]

The manufacturer states that protective clothing and gloves should be worn in the preparation of blinatumomab.[3095] Gloves and surfaces that may have come in contact with the drug during preparation should be disinfected.[3095]

Because errors have occurred in the preparation of blinatumomab, the manufacturer's instructions for preparation of the drug should be strictly followed to minimize the risk of such errors.[3095]

To reconstitute a vial of blinatumomab, 3 mL of preservative-free sterile water for injection should be added to the vial containing 35 mcg of the drug.[3095] The stream of diluent should be directed along the walls of the vial (not directly into the lyophilized powder), and the vial should be gently swirled to avoid excess foaming.[3095] The vial should not be shaken.[3095] The concentration of blinatumomab in the reconstituted solution is 12.5 mcg/mL; this solution must be further diluted prior to administration.[3095] The reconstituted solution should be clear to slightly opalescent, colorless to slightly yellow.[3095] Reconstituted blinatumomab solution should be visually inspected for particulate matter and discoloration; the solution should not be used if it is cloudy or has precipitated.[3095]

To prepare a blinatumomab solution for infusion for administration over 24 or 48 hours at a rate of 10 or 5 mL/hr, respectively, 270 mL of sodium chloride 0.9% injection should be transferred to an empty polyolefin, diethylhexyl phthalate (DEHP)-free polyvinyl chloride (PVC), or ethyl vinyl acetate (EVA) infusion bag followed by 5.5 mL of intravenous solution stabilizer.[3095] The contents of the infusion bag should be mixed gently to avoid foaming.[3095] The remaining unused portion of intravenous solution stabilizer should be discarded.[3095] The appropriate amount of reconstituted blinatumomab solution should then be transferred to the infusion bag containing the sodium chloride 0.9% and intravenous solution stabilizer, and the contents of the infusion bag again should be mixed gently to avoid foaming.[3095]

Alternatively, diluted blinatumomab solution for infusion may be administered over 7 days in patients weighing at least 22 kg; this option is not recommended for use in patients weighing less than 22 kg.[3095] To prepare a blinatumomab solution for infusion for administration over 7 days at a rate of 0.6 mL/hr, 90 mL of bacteriostatic sodium chloride 0.9% preserved with benzyl alcohol should be transferred to an empty polyolefin, DEHP-free PVC, or EVA infusion bag followed by 2.2 mL of intravenous solution stabilizer.[3095] The contents of the infusion bag should be mixed gently to avoid foaming.[3095] The remaining unused portion of intravenous solution stabilizer should be discarded.[3095] The appropriate amount of reconstituted blinatumomab solution should then be transferred to the infusion bag containing bacteriostatic sodium chloride 0.9% and intravenous solution stabilizer, and the contents of the infusion bag again should be mixed gently to avoid foaming.[3095] A sufficient amount of sodium chloride 0.9% should be added to the infusion bag to yield a total volume of 110 mL resulting in a final benzyl alcohol concentration of 0.74%.[3095] The contents of the infusion bag again should be mixed gently to avoid foaming.[3095]

When prepared according to the manufacturer's directions for administration over 24 hours, 48 hours, or 7 days, the blinatumomab infusion solution will have a greater volume than will be administered to the patient to allow for priming of the line and to ensure that the patient receives the full dose of the drug.[3095] Intravenous tubing that is composed of polyolefin, DEHP-free PVC, or EVA and is compatible with the infusion pump used should be attached to the bag containing the diluted blinatumomab solution for infusion.[3095] Intravenous tubing used for the administration of a 24- or 48-hour infusion of blinatumomab must contain a low protein-binding 0.2-μm inline filter; intravenous tubing used for the administration of a 7-day infusion does not require an inline filter.[3095] Air should be removed from the infusion bag; removal of air from the bag is especially important for use with ambulatory infusion pumps.[3095] The attached intravenous tubing should be primed *only* with the prepared blinatumomab solution for infusion; the tubing should *not* be primed with sodium chloride 0.9%.[3095]

Trade Name(s)

Blincyto

Administration

Blinatumomab diluted for infusion is administered by continuous infusion, either over 24 or 48 hours at a rate of 10 or 5 mL/hr, respectively, or over 7 days at a rate of 0.6 mL/hr in patients weighing at least 22 kg.[3095] The diluted solution for infusion should be administered at a constant rate using a programmable, lockable, non-elastomeric infusion pump equipped with an alarm.[3095] Patients should receive appropriate premedication administered prior to blinatumomab infusion when indicated.[3095]

DOI: 10.37573/9781585286850.054

Because errors have occurred during administration of blinatumomab, the manufacturer's instructions for administration of the drug should be strictly followed to minimize the risk of such errors.[3095] The intravenous tubing should be primed *only* with the prepared blinatumomab solution for infusion; the tubing should *not* be primed with sodium chloride 0.9%.[3095] If a multi-lumen venous catheter is used for administration, the diluted solution of blinatumomab for infusion should be infused through a dedicated lumen.[3095] The infusion line or intravenous catheter through which blinatumomab is administered *must not be* flushed, especially when changing infusion bags.[3095] Flushing the line can result in the administration of an excess dose with resulting potential complications.[3095] Instead, any unused solution for infusion remaining in the infusion bag or line should be disposed of properly.[3095]

Stability

Blinatumomab is a white to off-white lyophilized powder that forms a clear to slightly opalescent, colorless to slightly yellow solution upon reconstitution.[3095] Intact vials of blinatumomab and intravenous solution stabilizer should be stored at 2 to 8°C in the original package to protect from light until the time of use.[3095] Vials of both blinatumomab lyophilized powder and intravenous solution stabilizer may be stored for a maximum of 8 hours at room temperature in the original carton to protect from light.[3095] Vials should not be frozen.[3095]

After reconstitution, a vial of blinatumomab may be stored for a maximum of 24 hours at 2 to 8°C or 4 hours at 23 to 27°C.[3095]

If not used immediately, final diluted solutions of blinatumomab for infusion should be stored at 2 to 8°C.[3095] The diluted solution intended for infusion over 24 or 48 hours and prepared with sodium chloride 0.9% may be stored for a maximum of 8 days at 2 to 8°C; if stored at 23 to 27°C, administration of these diluted solutions of blinatumomab must be completed within 48 hours.[3095] The diluted solution of blinatumomab intended for infusion over 7 days and prepared with bacteriostatic sodium chloride 0.9% (preserved with benzyl alcohol) may be stored for a maximum of 14 days at 2 to 8°C; if stored at 23 to 27°C, administration of this diluted solution of blinatumomab must be completed within 7 days.[3095]

Sorption

Intravenous solution stabilizer packaged with blinatumomab is added to the infusion bag to coat the bag prior to the addition of the reconstituted blinatumomab solution, thereby preventing adhesion of the drug to the bag and administration tubing.[3095] Only polyolefin, DEHP-free PVC, and EVA infusion bags, pump cassettes, and intravenous tubing should be used in the preparation and administration of blinatumomab.[3095]

Filtration

Blinatumomab solution for infusion must be administered through polyolefin, DEHP-free PVC, or EVA intravenous tubing.[3095] The final diluted solution of blinatumomab intended for infusion over 24 or 48 hours and prepared with sodium chloride 0.9% must be administered through intravenous tubing containing a low protein-binding 0.2-μm inline filter.[3095] An inline filter is *not* required for the administration of a 7-day infusion bag prepared with bacteriostatic sodium chloride 0.9% (preserved with benzyl alcohol).[3095]

Compatibility Information
Solution Compatibility

Blinatumomab

Test Soln Name	Mfr	Mfr	Conc/L or %	Remarks	Ref	C/I
Sodium chloride 0.9%	a	AMG		Stable for up to 8 days at 2 to 8°C	3095	C
Sodium chloride 0.9%	a	AMG		Complete administration within 48 hr if stored at 23 to 27°C	3095	C
Sodium chloride 0.9%	a b	AMG		Stable for up to 14 days at 2 to 8°C	3095	C
Sodium chloride 0.9%	a b	AMG		Complete administration within 7 days if stored at 23 to 27°C	3095	C

[a] Tested in polyolefin, non-DEHP PVC, and EVA containers.

[b] Diluted as directed in bacteriostatic sodium chloride 0.9% solutions preserved with benzyl alcohol.

Y-Site Injection Compatibility (1:1 Mixture)

Blinatumomab

Test Drug	Mfr	Conc	Mfr	Conc	Remarks	Ref	C/I
Acetaminophen	MAC	10 mg/mL	AMG	0.125 mcg/mL[b]	Thin flakes transiently appear when acetaminophen is added to blinatumomab; not observed when order of mixing was reversed	3405, 3417	?
Acetaminophen	MAC	10 mg/mL	AMG	0.375 mcg/mL[b]	Persistent particulate formation	3405, 3417	I

Y-Site Injection Compatibility (1:1 Mixture) (Cont.)

Test Drug	Mfr	Conc	Mfr	Conc	Remarks	Ref	C/I
Albumin human	LFB	100 mg/mL	AMG	0.125 mcg/mL[b]	Persistent particulate formation when blinatumomab is added to albumin; haze transiently appeared when order of mixing was reversed	3405, 3417	I
Albumin human	LFB	100 mg/mL	AMG	0.375 mcg/mL[b]	Persistent particulate formation when blinatumomab is added to albumin; not observed when order of mixing was reversed	3405, 3417	?
Amphotericin B liposomal	GIL	1 mg/mL[a]	AMG	0.125 and 0.375 mcg/mL[b]	Visually compatible for 12 hr at room temperature	3405, 3417	C
Caffeine citrate	CPR	25 mg/mL	AMG	0.125 and 0.375 mcg/mL[b]	Visually compatible for 12 hr at room temperature	3405, 3417	C
Caspofungin acetate	MCD	0.2 mg/mL[b]	AMG	0.125 and 0.375 mcg/mL[b]	Particles, flakes, thin needles, or haze transiently appears	3405, 3417	?
Ceftazidime	PAN	34.5 mg/mL[b]	AMG	0.125 and 0.375 mcg/mL[b]	Particles, flakes, thin needles, or haze transiently appears	3405, 3417	?
Ceftriaxone sodium	PAN	50 mg/mL[b]	AMG	0.125 and 0.375 mcg/mL[b]	Particles, flakes, thin needles, or haze transiently appears	3405, 3417	?
Ciprofloxacin	FRK	2 mg/mL	AMG	0.125 and 0.375 mcg/mL[b]	Persistent particulate formation	3405, 3417	I
Clonazepam	RC	0.02 mg/mL[b]	AMG	0.125 and 0.375 mcg/mL[b]	Particles, flakes, thin needles, or haze transiently appears	3405, 3417	?
Cloxacillin sodium	ASP	8.6 mg/mL[b]	AMG	0.125 mcg/mL[b]	Persistent particulate formation when blinatumomab is added to cloxacillin; not observed when order of mixing was reversed	3405, 3417	?
Cloxacillin sodium	ASP	8.6 mg/mL[b]	AMG	0.375 mcg/mL[b]	Visually compatible for 12 hr at room temperature	3405, 3417	C
Daptomycin	MSD	6.1 mg/mL[b]	AMG	0.125 and 0.375 mcg/mL[b]	Particles, flakes, thin needles, or haze transiently appears	3405, 3417	?
Dexamethasone sodium phosphate	MYL	0.19 mg/mL[b]	AMG	0.125 mcg/mL[b]	Persistent particulate formation	3405, 3417	I
Dexamethasone sodium phosphate	MYL	0.19 mg/mL[b]	AMG	0.375 mcg/mL[b]	Visually compatible for 12 hr at room temperature	3405, 3417	C
Furosemide	SAA	2.9 mg/mL	AMG	0.125 mcg/mL[b]	Visually compatible for 12 hr at room temperature	3405, 3417	C
Furosemide	SAA	2.9 mg/mL	AMG	0.375 mcg/mL[b]	Persistent particulate formation when furosemide is added to blinatumomab; small flakes transiently appeared when order of mixing was reversed	3405, 3417	I
Heparin sodium	PAN	192.3 units/mL[b]	AMG	0.125 mcg/mL[b]	Persistent particulate formation when blinatumomab is added to heparin; not observed when order of mixing was reversed	3405, 3417	?
Heparin sodium	PAN	192.3 units/mL[b]	AMG	0.375 mcg/mL[b]	Persistent particulate formation	3405, 3417	I
Hydrocortisone sodium succinate	SRB	0.98 mg/mL[b]	AMG	0.125 and 0.375 mcg/mL[b]	Visually compatible for 12 hr at room temperature	3405, 3417	C
Hydroxyzine HCl	REN	0.4 mg/mL[b]	AMG	0.125 mcg/mL[b]	Visually compatible for 12 hr at room temperature	3405, 3417	C
Hydroxyzine HCl	REN	0.4 mg/mL[b]	AMG	0.375 mcg/mL[b]	Persistent particulate formation when hydroxyzine is added to blinatumomab; not observed when order of mixing was reversed	3405, 3417	?
Imipenem–cilastatin sodium	PAN	5 mg/mL[b][c]	AMG	0.125 and 0.375 mcg/mL[b]	Particles, flakes, thin needles, or haze transiently appears when blinatumomab is added to imipenem–cilastatin; not observed when order of mixing was reversed	3405, 3417	?

Y-Site Injection Compatibility (1:1 Mixture) (Cont.)

Test Drug	Mfr	Conc	Mfr	Conc	Remarks	Ref	C/I
Meropenem	ARR	8.3 mg/mL[b]	AMG	0.125 mcg/mL[b]	Persistent particulate formation	3405, 3417	I
Meropenem	ARR	8.3 mg/mL[b]	AMG	0.375 mcg/mL[b]	Visually compatible for 12 hr at room temperature	3405, 3417	C
Methylprednisolone sodium succinate	MYL	5 mg/mL[b]	AMG	0.125 and 0.375 mcg/mL[b]	Persistent particulate formation when blinatumomab is added to methylprednisolone; not observed when order of mixing was reversed	3405, 3417	?
Metronidazole	BRN	2.5 mg/mL	AMG	0.125 mcg/mL[b]	Persistent particulate formation when blinatumomab is added to metronidazole; not observed when order of mixing was reversed	3405, 3417	?
Metronidazole	BRN	2.5 mg/mL	AMG	0.375 mcg/mL[b]	Flakes transiently appear when metronidazole is added to blinatumomab; not observed when order of mixing was reversed	3405, 3417	?
Nalbuphine HCl	MYL	1 mg/mL[b]	AMG	0.125 mcg/mL[b]	Persistent particulate formation	3405, 3417	I
Nalbuphine HCl	MYL	1 mg/mL[b]	AMG	0.375 mcg/mL[b]	Flakes transiently appear when blinatumomab is added to nalbuphine; not observed when order of mixing was reversed	3405, 3417	?
Naloxone HCl	MYL	0.2 mg/mL[b]	AMG	0.125 mcg/mL[b]	Particles, flakes, thin needles, or haze transiently appears when naloxone is added to blinatumomab; not observed when order of mixing was reversed	3405, 3417	?
Naloxone HCl	MYL	0.2 mg/mL[b]	AMG	0.375 mcg/mL[b]	Visually compatible for 12 hr at room temperature	3405, 3417	C
Pantoprazole sodium	ARR[d]	0.8 mg/mL[b]	AMG	0.125 mg/mL[b]	Visually compatible for 12 hr at room temperature	3405, 3417	C
Pantoprazole sodium	ARR[d]	0.8 mg/mL[b]	AMG	0.375 mcg/mL[b]	Particles, flakes, thin needles, or haze transiently appears when pantoprazole is added to blinatumomab; not observed when order of mixing was reversed	3405, 3417	?
Potassium chloride	AGT	0.0249 mg/mL[b]	AMG	0.125 mcg/mL[b]	Flakes transiently appear when blinatumomab is added to potassium chloride; not observed when order of mixing was reversed	3405, 3417	?
Potassium chloride	AGT	0.0249 mg/mL[b]	AMG	0.375 mcg/mL[b]	Persistent particulate formation when blinatumomab is added to potassium chloride; not observed when order of mixing was reversed	3405, 3417	?
Rasburicase	SAA	0.15 mg/mL[b]	AMG	0.125 mcg/mL[b]	Persistent particulate formation when blinatumomab is added to rasburicase; not observed when order of mixing was reversed	3405, 3417	?
Rasburicase	SAA	0.15 mg/mL[b]	AMG	0.375 mcg/mL[b]	Flakes transiently appear when rasburicase is added to blinatumomab; not observed when order of mixing was reversed	3405, 3417	?
Teicoplanin	SAA	4 mg/mL[a]	AMG	0.125 mcg/mL[b]	Persistent particulate formation when blinatumomab is added to teicoplanin; flakes transiently appeared when order of mixing was reversed	3405, 3417	I
Teicoplanin	SAA	4 mg/mL[a]	AMG	0.375 mcg/mL[b]	Persistent particulate formation when blinatumomab is added to teicoplanin; not observed when order of mixing was reversed	3405, 3417	?
Tranexamic acid	SAA	100 mg/mL	AMG	0.125 mcg/mL[b]	Haze or flakes transiently appear	3405, 3417	?
Tranexamic acid	SAA	100 mg/mL	AMG	0.375 mcg/mL[b]	Persistent particulate formation when blinatumomab is added to tranexamic acid; not observed when order of mixing was reversed	3405, 3417	?

Y-Site Injection Compatibility (1:1 Mixture) (Cont.)

Test Drug	Mfr	Conc	Mfr	Conc	Remarks	Ref	C/I
Trimethoprim–sulfamethoxazole	RC	3.2 mg/mL[b][c]	AMG	0.125 mcg/mL[b]	Visually compatible for 12 hr at room temperature	3405, 3417	C
Trimethoprim–sulfamethoxazole	RC	3.2 mg/mL[b][c]	AMG	0.375 mcg/mL[b]	Persistent particulate formation when trimethoprim–sulfamethoxazole is added to blinatumomab; flakes transiently appeared when order of mixing was reversed	3405, 3417	I

[a] Tested in dextrose 5%.

[b] Tested in sodium chloride 0.9%.

[c] Not specified whether concentration refers to single component or combined components.

[d] Presence or absence of edetate disodium not specified.

Selected Revisions June 6, 2018. © Copyright, June 2016. American Society of Health-System Pharmacists, Inc.

Bortezomib
AHFS 10:00

Products

Bortezomib is available as a lyophilized powder in single-use (unpreserved) vials containing 3.5 mg of drug with mannitol 35 mg.[2897]

For intravenous bolus injection, reconstitute vials with 3.5 mL of sodium chloride 0.9% to yield a solution containing 1 mg/mL.[2897] For subcutaneous administration, reconstitute vials with 1.4 mL of sodium chloride 0.9% to yield a solution containing 2.5 mg/mL.[2897] If subcutaneous injection results in local injection site reactions, the 1-mg/mL solution also may be administered subcutaneously.[2897]

Trade Name(s)

Velcade

Administration

Bortezomib is administered by intravenous bolus injection over 3 to 5 seconds or by subcutaneous injection only.[2897] It should not be given by any other route.[2897] Because the inadvertent intrathecal administration of bortezomib has resulted in fatalities and administration by this route is contraindicated, the manufacturer has provided stickers with each vial of the drug to be affixed to the prepared syringe of bortezomib to indicate the intended correct route of administration.[2897] [2898]

Stability

Intact vials should be stored at controlled room temperature and left in the original box to protect from light during storage.[2897] Bortezomib is a white to off-white lyophilized powder or cake that forms a clear, colorless solution when reconstituted with sodium chloride 0.9%.[2897]

The manufacturer states that bortezomib reconstituted as directed with sodium chloride 0.9% and stored at 25°C in the original vial or in a syringe should be used within 8 hours of preparation.[2897] However, bortezomib (Janssen-Cilag) reconstituted with sodium chloride 0.9% to a concentration of 1 mg/mL in the original vials was reported to be stable for at least 5 days under refrigeration protected from light.[2663]

Bortezomib reconstituted with sodium chloride 0.9% to a concentration of 1 mg/mL was found to undergo little or no loss for 42 days stored at 23°C or refrigerated at 4°C.[2768]

Bortezomib (Janssen) reconstituted with sodium chloride 0.9% to a concentration of 2.5 mg/mL was found to undergo less than 5% loss in 21 days when stored in the original vial at 23°C in fluorescent light or under refrigeration at 4°C in the dark.[2972]

Bortezomib (Janssen-Cilag) 1 mg/mL in sodium chloride 0.9% did not result in the loss of viability of *Staphylococcus aureus* within 120 hours at room temperature. Diluted solutions should be stored under refrigeration whenever possible, and the potential for microbiological growth should be considered when assigning expiration periods.[2740]

Syringes

Bortezomib (Janssen-Cilag) 1 mg/mL in sodium chloride 0.9% was packaged in 5-mL polypropylene plastic syringes (Becton-Dickinson) and stored at room temperature exposed to neon light and under refrigeration in the dark. The drug solutions remained clear and colorless throughout the study at both temperatures. About 8 to 9% loss occurred in 5 days at room temperature and in 7 days refrigerated and protected from light.[2663]

Bortezomib (Janssen) 2.5 mg/mL in sodium chloride 0.9% was packaged in 3-mL polypropylene syringes and stored at 23°C in fluorescent light or under refrigeration at 4°C in the dark.[2972] Less than 5% loss occurred in 21 days in syringes stored at either temperature.[2972]

Selected Revisions August 5, 2015. © Copyright, October 2008. American Society of Health-System Pharmacists, Inc.

DOI: 10.37573/9781585286850.055

Brexanolone
AHFS 28:16.04.92

Products

Brexanolone is available as a 5-mg/mL concentrate for injection in 20-mL single-dose (preservative-free) vials.[3461] The concentrate must be diluted prior to administration.[3461] Each mL of solution also contains betadex sulfobutyl ether sodium 250 mg, citric acid monohydrate 0.265 mg, sodium citrate dihydrate 2.57 mg, and water for injection.[3461] Hydrochloric acid or sodium hydroxide may have been added during manufacturing to adjust the pH.[3461]

Brexanolone concentrate for injection must be diluted prior to administration.[3461] Administration of the 60-hour infusion generally requires the preparation and administration of at least 5 infusion bags; additional bags will be necessary when the drug is administered to patients weighing at least 90 kg.[3461] Vials of brexanolone should be visually inspected for particulate matter and discoloration prior to administration; vials should not be used if the solution is discolored or if particulate matter is present.[3461] To prepare each infusion bag, 20 mL of brexanolone concentrate for injection should be withdrawn from the vial and transferred to a non-diethylhexyl phthalate (non-DEHP) and non-latex polyolefin infusion bag.[3461] The concentrate should then be diluted by adding 40 mL of sterile water for injection to the infusion bag followed by 40 mL of sodium chloride 0.9% for a total volume of 100 mL and a target brexanolone concentration of 1 mg/mL.[3461]

pH

The pH of admixtures with brexanolone (Sage) concentrations of 0.5 and 1.67 mg/mL ranges from 5.7 to 6.4.[3462]

Tonicity

Brexanolone 5-mg/mL concentrate for injection is hypertonic.[3461]

Osmolality

The measured osmolality of admixtures with brexanolone (Sage) concentrations of 0.5 and 1.67 mg/mL ranges from 243 to 286 mOsmol/kg.[3462]

Trade Name(s)

Zulresso

Administration

Brexanolone is administered as a continuous intravenous infusion over 60 hours following dilution as directed with sterile water for injection followed by sodium chloride 0.9%.[3461]

The diluted solution for infusion should be administered through a dedicated line using a programmable peristaltic infusion pump.[3461] The drug should be administered through a non-DEHP and non-latex polyvinyl chloride (PVC) infusion set; infusion sets with inline filters should *not* be used.[3461] Infusion sets should be fully primed with the diluted solution before inserting the set into the pump and connecting it to the venous catheter.[3461] The manufacturer states that other drugs should not be injected into the infusion bag or mixed with brexanolone.[3461]

The infusion should be initiated at a rate of 30 mcg/kg/hr for the first 4 hours.[3461] After the initial 4 hours, the infusion rate should be increased to 60 mcg/kg/hr for the next 20 hours and then increased further to 90 mcg/kg/hr for the following 28 hours.[3461] Alternatively, a reduction in the infusion rate back to 60 mcg/kg/hr may be considered during hours 24 to 52 for those who do not tolerate the recommended higher infusion rate.[3461] The infusion rate should be decreased to (or remain at) 60 mcg/kg/hr for hours 52 to 56, with a final reduction back to 30 mcg/kg/hr for the remaining 4 hours of the 60-hour infusion.[3461]

Stability

Brexanolone concentrate for injection is a clear, colorless solution.[3461] Intact vials should be stored at 2 to 8°C and protected from light; vials should not be frozen.[3461]

Administration of diluted solutions of brexanolone for infusion prepared as directed using both sterile water for injection and sodium chloride 0.9% should be completed within 12 hours after dilution; if not used immediately after dilution, the diluted solution may be stored under refrigeration for up to 96 hours.[3461]

Plasticizer Leaching

A non-DEHP and non-latex polyolefin infusion bag should be used to prepare diluted solutions of brexanolone for infusion.[3461]

A non-DEHP and non-latex PVC administration set should be used for administration of the diluted solution for infusion.[3461]

Filtration

Infusion sets with inline filters should *not* be used in the administration of the diluted solution.[3461]

DOI: 10.37573/9781585286850.056

Brivaracetam
AHFS 28:12.92

Products

Brivaracetam is available as a 10-mg/mL solution in 5-mL single-dose (unpreserved) vials.[3146] Each vial also contains sodium acetate trihydrate, sodium chloride, water for injection, and glacial acetic acid to adjust the pH.[3146]

pH

5.5.[3146]

Trade Name(s)

Briviact

Administration

Brivaracetam is administered intravenously over 2 to 15 minutes either undiluted or diluted in a compatible infusion solution.[3146] (See Solution Compatibility.)

Stability

Brivaracetam is a clear and colorless solution.[3146] Intact vials should be stored at room temperature and should not be frozen.[3146] Any unused portion of the contents from a single-dose vial should be discarded.[3146] Solutions should be visually inspected for particulate matter prior to administration; if particulate matter is present or if discoloration occurs, the solution should not be used.[3146]

Compatibility Information

Solution Compatibility

Brivaracetam

Test Soln Name	Mfr	Mfr	Conc/L or %	Remarks	Ref	C/I
Dextrose 5%	a	UCB		Stated to be stable for up to 4 hr at room temperature	3146	C
Ringer's injection, lactated	a	UCB		Stated to be stable for up to 4 hr at room temperature	3146	C
Sodium chloride 0.9%	a	UCB		Stated to be stable for up to 4 hr at room temperature	3146	C

a Tested in PVC containers.

DOI: 10.37573/9781585286850.057

Bumetanide
AHFS 40:28.08

Products

Bumetanide is available as a 0.25-mg/mL solution in 4-mL single-dose vials and 10-mL multidose vials.[3288] [3309] The solution also contains sodium chloride 0.85%, ammonium acetate 0.4%, disodium edetate 0.01%, and benzyl alcohol 1% with sodium hydroxide to adjust the pH.[3288] [3309]

pH

Adjusted to approximately 7[3288] or 6.8 to 7.8.[3309]

Administration

Bumetanide is administered by intramuscular injection,[3288] [3309] direct intravenous injection over 1 to 2 minutes,[3288] [3309] and by intravenous infusion.[4]

Stability

Bumetanide discolors when exposed to light. The injection should be stored at controlled room temperature and protected from light.[3288] [3309] Bumetanide is reported to be stable at pH 4 to 10.[4] Precipitation may occur at pH values less than 4.[1644]

Sorption

Substantial sorption to glass and PVC containers does not occur.[3288] [3309]

Central Venous Catheter

Bumetanide (Ohmeda) 0.04 mg/mL in dextrose 5% was found to be compatible with the ARROWg+ard Blue Plus (Arrow International) chlorhexidine-bearing triple-lumen central catheter. Essentially complete delivery of the drug was found with little or no drug loss occurring. Furthermore, chlorhexidine delivered from the catheter remained at trace amounts with no substantial increase due to the delivery of the drug through the catheter.[2335]

Compatibility Information
Solution Compatibility

Bumetanide

Test Soln Name	Mfr	Mfr	Conc/L or %	Remarks	Ref	C/I
Dextrose 5%				Compatible and stable for 24 hr	1(6/05)	C
Dextrose 5%	AB[a]	RC	20 mg	4 to 5% loss occurs within 3 hr with no further loss throughout 72 hr at 24°C under fluorescent light	2090	C
Dextrose 5%	AB[a]	RC	200 mg	Little or no loss occurs within 72 hr at 24°C under fluorescent light	2090	C
Ringer's injection, lactated				Compatible and stable for 24 hr	1(6/05)	C
Sodium chloride 0.9%				Compatible and stable for 24 hr	1(6/05)	C

[a] Tested in PVC containers.

Additive Compatibility

Bumetanide

Test Drug	Mfr	Conc/L or %	Mfr	Conc/L or %	Test Solution	Remarks	Ref	C/I
Dobutamine HCl	LI	1 g	RC	125 mg	D5W, NS	Immediate yellow discoloration with yellow precipitate within 6 hr at 21°C	812	I
Floxacillin sodium	BE	20 g	LEO	6 mg	NS	Physically compatible for 72 hr at 15 and 30°C	1479	C
Furosemide	HO	1 g	LEO	6 mg	NS	Physically compatible for 72 hr at 15 and 30°C	1479	C

DOI: 10.37573/9781585286850.058

Drugs in Syringe Compatibility

Bumetanide

Test Drug	Mfr	Amt	Mfr	Amt	Remarks	Ref	C/I
Doxapram HCl	RB	400 mg/20 mL		0.5 mg/1 mL	Physically compatible with 3% doxapram loss in 24 hr	1177	C

Y-Site Injection Compatibility (1:1 Mixture)

Bumetanide

Test Drug	Mfr	Conc	Mfr	Conc	Remarks	Ref	C/I
Allopurinol sodium	BW	3 mg/mL[b]	RC	0.04 mg/mL[b]	Physically compatible for 4 hr at 22°C	1686	C
Amifostine	USB	10 mg/mL[a]	RC	0.04 mg/mL[a]	Physically compatible for 4 hr at 23°C	1845	C
Aztreonam	SQ	40 mg/mL[a]	RC	0.04 mg/mL[a]	Physically compatible for 4 hr at 23°C	1758	C
Bivalirudin	TMC	5 mg/mL[a]	OHM	40 mcg/mL[a]	Physically compatible for 4 hr at 23°C	2373	C
Cangrelor tetrasodium	TMC	1 mg/mL[b]		0.25 mg/mL	Physically compatible for 4 hr	3243	C
Caspofungin acetate	ME	0.7 mg/mL[b]	BED	0.04 mg/mL[b]	Physically compatible for 4 hr at room temperature	2758	C
Ceftaroline fosamil	FOR	2.22 mg/mL[a b g]	HOS	40 mcg/mL[a b g]	Physically compatible for 4 hr at 23°C	2826	C
Ceftolozane sulfate–tazobactam sodium	CUB	10 mg/mL[i j]	HOS	0.25 mg/mL	Physically compatible for 2 hr	3262	C
Cisatracurium besylate	GW	0.1, 2, 5 mg/mL[a]	BV	0.04 mg/mL[a]	Physically compatible for 4 hr at 23°C	2074	C
Cladribine	ORT	0.015[b] and 0.5[c] mg/mL	RC	0.04 mg/mL[b]	Physically compatible for 4 hr at 23°C	1969	C
Clarithromycin	AB	4 mg/mL[a]	LEO	0.5 mg/mL	Visually compatible for 72 hr at both 30 and 17°C	2174	C
Dexmedetomidine HCl	AB	4 mcg/mL[b]	BED	40 mcg/mL[b]	Physically compatible for 4 hr at 23°C	2383	C
Diltiazem HCl	MMD	1[b] and 5 mg/mL	RC	0.25 mg/mL	Visually compatible	1807	C
Docetaxel	RPR	0.9 mg/mL[a]	RC	0.04 mg/mL[a]	Physically compatible for 4 hr at 23°C	2224	C
Doripenem	JJ	5 mg/mL[a b]	BED	0.04 mg/mL[a b]	Physically compatible for 4 hr at 23°C	2743	C
Eravacycline dihydrochloride	TET	0.6 mg/mL[b]	HOS	0.25 mg/mL	Physically compatible for 2 hr at room temperature	3532	C
Etoposide phosphate	BR	5 mg/mL[a]	RC	0.04 mg/mL[a]	Physically compatible for 4 hr at 23°C	2218	C
Fenoldopam mesylate	AB	80 mcg/mL[b]	BA	40 mcg/mL[b]	Trace haze forms immediately	2467	I
Filgrastim	AMG	30 mcg/mL[a]	RC	0.04 mg/mL[a]	Physically compatible for 4 hr at 22°C	1687	C
Gemcitabine HCl	LI	10 mg/mL[b]	RC	0.04 mg/mL[b]	Physically compatible for 4 hr at 23°C	2226	C
Granisetron HCl	SKB	0.05 mg/mL[a]	RC	0.04 mg/mL[a]	Physically compatible for 4 hr at 23°C	2000	C
Hetastarch in lactated electrolyte	AB	6%	OHM	0.04 mg/mL[a]	Physically compatible for 4 hr at 23°C	2339	C
Isavuconazonium sulfate	ASP	1.5 mg/mL[a]	HOS	0.25 mg/mL	Measured turbidity increases within 15 min	3263	I
Isavuconazonium sulfate	ASP	1.5 mg/mL[b]	HOS	0.25 mg/mL	Physically compatible for 2 hr	3263	C
Lorazepam	WY	0.33 mg/mL[b]	LEO	0.5 mg/mL	Visually compatible for 24 hr at 22°C	1855	C
Melphalan HCl	BW	0.1 mg/mL[b]	RC	0.04 mg/mL[b]	Physically compatible for 3 hr at 22°C	1557	C
Meperidine HCl	AB	10 mg/mL	RC	0.25 mg/mL	Physically compatible for 4 hr at 25°C	1397	C

Y-Site Injection Compatibility (1:1 Mixture) (Cont.)

Test Drug	Mfr	Conc	Mfr	Conc	Remarks	Ref	C/I
Meropenem–vaborbactam	TMC	8 mg/mL[b][k]	HOS	0.25 mg/mL	Physically compatible for 3 hr at 20 to 25°C	3380	C
Micafungin sodium	ASP	1.5 mg/mL[b]	BED	40 mcg/mL[b]	Physically compatible for 4 hr at 23°C	2683	C
Midazolam HCl	RC	5 mg/mL	LEO	0.5 mg/mL	White precipitate forms immediately	1855	I
Milrinone lactate	SW	0.4 mg/mL[a]	RC	0.25 mg/mL	Visually compatible with little or no loss of either drug in 4 hr at 23°C	2214	C
Morphine sulfate	AB	1 mg/mL	RC	0.25 mg/mL	Physically compatible for 4 hr at 25°C	1397	C
Nesiritide	SCI	50 mcg/mL[a][b]		0.25 mg/mL	Physically incompatible	2625	I
Oritavancin diphosphate	TAR	0.8, 1.2, and 2 mg/mL[a]	HOS	0.1 mg/mL[a]	Haze forms immediately with precipitate after 30 min	2928	I
Oxaliplatin	SS	0.5 mg/mL[a]	BA	0.04 mg/mL[a]	Physically compatible for 4 hr at 23°C	2566	C
Pemetrexed disodium	LI	20 mg/mL[b]	BA	0.04 mg/mL[a]	Physically compatible for 4 hr at 23°C	2564	C
Piperacillin sodium–tazobactam sodium	LE[f]	40 mg/mL[a][h]	RC	0.04 mg/mL[a]	Physically compatible for 4 hr at 22°C	1688	C
Plazomicin sulfate	ACH	24 mg/mL[i]	HOS	0.25 mg/mL	Physically compatible for 1 hr at 20 to 25°C	3432	C
Propofol	ZEN[j]	10 mg/mL	RC	0.04 mg/mL[a]	Physically compatible for 1 hr at 23°C	2066	C
Remifentanil HCl	GW	0.025 and 0.25 mg/mL[b]	RC	0.04 mg/mL[a]	Physically compatible for 4 hr at 23°C	2075	C
Tedizolid phosphate	CUB	0.8 mg/mL[b]	HOS	0.25 mg/mL	Physically compatible for 2 hr	3244	C
Teniposide	BR	0.1 mg/mL[a]	RC	0.04 mg/mL[a]	Physically compatible for 4 hr at 23°C	1725	C
Thiotepa	IMM[d]	1 mg/mL[a]	RC	0.04 mg/mL[a]	Physically compatible for 4 hr at 23°C	1861	C
TNA #218 to #226[e]			RC, BV	0.04 mg/mL[a]	Visually compatible for 4 hr at 23°C	2215	C
TPN #212 to #215[e]			RC	0.04 mg/mL[a]	Physically compatible for 4 hr at 23°C	2109	C
Vinorelbine tartrate	BW	1 mg/mL[b]	RC	0.04 mg/mL[b]	Physically compatible for 4 hr at 22°C	1558	C

[a] Tested in dextrose 5%.

[b] Tested in sodium chloride 0.9%.

[c] Tested in bacteriostatic sodium chloride 0.9% preserved with benzyl alcohol 0.9%.

[d] Lyophilized formulation tested.

[e] Refer to Appendix for the composition of parenteral nutrition solutions. TNA indicates a 3-in-1 admixture, and TPN indicates a 2-in-1 admixture.

[f] Test performed using the formulation WITHOUT edetate disodium.

[g] Tested in Ringer's injection, lactated.

[h] Piperacillin component. Piperacillin in an 8:1 fixed-ratio concentration with tazobactam.

[i] Tested in both dextrose 5% and sodium chloride 0.9%.

[j] Ceftolozane component. Ceftolozane in a 2:1 fixed-ratio concentration with tazobactam.

[k] Meropenem component. Meropenem in a 1:1 fixed-ratio concentration with vaborbactam.

[l] Test performed using the formulation WITH edetate disodium.

Selected Revisions May 1, 2020. © Copyright, October 1986.
American Society of Health-System Pharmacists, Inc.

Bupivacaine Hydrochloride
AHFS 72:00

Products

Bupivacaine hydrochloride is available in concentrations of 0.25, 0.5, and 0.75% (2.5, 5, and 7.5 mg/mL, respectively) in single-dose containers. The 0.25 and 0.5% concentrations also come in 50-mL multiple-dose vials with methylparaben 1 mg/mL as a preservative. Sodium hydroxide or hydrochloric acid is used to adjust the pH.[1](11/06) [4]

Bupivacaine hydrochloride is also available in concentrations of 0.25, 0.5, and 0.75% with epinephrine 1:200,000 as the bitartrate. In addition to bupivacaine hydrochloride, each mL contains epinephrine bitartrate 0.005 mg, sodium metabisulfite 0.5 mg, and disodium edetate 0.1 mg. Multiple-dose vials contain methylparaben 1 mg/mL as a preservative while single-dose containers are preservative free. Sodium hydroxide or hydrochloric acid is used to adjust the pH.[1](11/06) [4]

A hyperbaric solution of bupivacaine hydrochloride is available in 2-mL ampuls. Each mL contains bupivacaine hydrochloride 7.5 mg and dextrose 82.5 mg (8.25%) with sodium hydroxide or hydrochloric acid to adjust the pH.[1](11/06) [4]

pH

Bupivacaine hydrochloride injection and the hyperbaric solution have a pH of 4 to 6.5. Bupivacaine hydrochloride with epinephrine 1:200,000 has a pH of 3.3 to 5.5.[4]

Specific Gravity

The hyperbaric solution has a specific gravity of 1.030 to 1.035 at 25°C and 1.03 at 37°C.[4]

Trade Name(s)

Marcaine, Sensorcaine, Sensorcaine-MPF

Administration

Bupivacaine hydrochloride may be administered by infiltration or by epidural, spinal, or peripheral or sympathetic nerve block as a single injection or repeat injections. Injections should be made slowly, with frequent aspirations, to guard against intravascular injection. Products containing preservatives should not be used for epidural or caudal block.[1](11/06) [4]

Stability

Bupivacaine hydrochloride injections should be stored at controlled room temperature; freezing should be avoided.[1](11/06) [4]

Products containing epinephrine should be protected from light during storage. Partially used containers that do not contain antibacterial preservatives should be discarded after entry.[4]

Bupivacaine hydrochloride without epinephrine and the hyperbaric solution may be autoclaved at 121°C and 15 psi for 15 minutes. Products containing epinephrine should not be autoclaved.[1](11/06) [4]

Bupivacaine hydrochloride with epinephrine should not be used if a pinkish color, a color darker than "slightly" yellow, or a precipitate develops.[1](11/06) [4]

Syringes

The stability of bupivacaine (salt form unspecified) 5 mg/mL repackaged in polypropylene syringes was evaluated. Little or no change in concentration was found after four weeks of storage at room temperature not exposed to direct light.[2164]

Bupivacaine hydrochloride (Astra) 1 mg/mL in sodium chloride 0.9% was packaged in two types in polypropylene syringes. The Omnifix (B. Braun) syringes had polyisoprene piston tips while the Terumo syringes had no natural or synthetic rubber in the product. Stored at 4, 21, and 35°C for 30 days, the test solutions exhibited no visible or pH changes. Although the pH remained within the stability range for the drug, this does not demonstrate stability.[2387]

Ambulatory Pumps

Bupivacaine hydrochloride (Astra) 7.5 mg/mL was filled into 50-mL ambulatory pump cassette reservoirs (Pharmacia Deltec) and stored at room temperature protected from light for 90 days. The drug concentration increased 12% during the observation period, possibly because of loss of water from the solutions.[1850]

Implantable Pumps

Bupivacaine hydrochloride 7.5 mg/mL in dextrose 8.25% (Marcaine spinal) stability was evaluated in SynchroMed implantable pumps over 12 weeks at 37°C. Little or no loss of bupivacaine hydrochloride and no adverse effects on the pumps occurred.[2583]

An admixture of bupivacaine hydrochloride 25 mg/mL, clonidine hydrochloride 2 mg/mL, and morphine sulfate 50 mg/mL in sterile water for injection was reported to be physically and chemically stable for 90 days at 37°C in SynchroMed implantable pumps. Little or no loss of any of the drugs occurred.[2585]

DOI: 10.37573/9781585286850.059

Compatibility Information

Solution Compatibility

Bupivacaine HCl

Test Soln Name	Mfr	Mfr	Conc/L or %	Remarks	Ref	C/I
Sodium chloride 0.9%	AB[b]	AST	1.25 g	Visually compatible with no loss in 32 days at 3°C in the dark and 23°C exposed to light	1718	C
Sodium chloride 0.9%	AB[a]	AB	625 mg and 1.25 g	Visually compatible with no loss in 72 hr at 24°C under fluorescent light	1870, 2058	C
Sodium chloride 0.9%	GRI[a]		850 mg	No change in concentration in 28 days at 4°C and room temperature	1910	C

[a] Tested in PVC containers.

[b] Tested in polypropylene syringes.

Additive Compatibility

Bupivacaine HCl

Test Drug	Mfr	Conc/L or %	Mfr	Conc/L or %	Test Solution	Remarks	Ref	C/I
Buprenorphine HCl	RC	180 mg	AST	3 g	[a]	No loss of either drug in 30 days at 18°C	1932	C
Clonidine HCl	BI[i]	9 mg	AST	1 g	NS[a]	Visually compatible with less than 10% change of any drug in 28 days at 4°C and 24 days at 25°C in the dark	2437	C
Diamorphine HCl		0.125 g	GL	1.25 g	NS	Visually compatible with 8% diamorphine loss and no bupivacaine loss in 28 days at room temperature	1791	C
Diamorphine HCl	NAP	20 mg	AST	150 mg	NS[c]	5% diamorphine and no bupivacaine loss in 14 days at 7°C. Both drugs were stable for 6 months at −20°C	2070	C
Epinephrine bitartrate	PHX[h]	2 mg	IVX	1 g		Visually compatible with less than 10% loss of epinephrine and no loss of other drugs in 182 days at 4 and 22°C	2613	C
Epinephrine HCl	AB[g]	0.69 mg	WI	440 mg	[d]	No bupivacaine and fentanyl loss and 10% epinephrine loss in 30 days at 3 and 23°C then 48 hr at 30°C	1627	C
Fentanyl citrate	JN	20 mg	WI	1.25 g	NS[a]	Physically compatible with little or no loss of either drug in 30 days at 3 and 23°C	1396	C
Fentanyl citrate		2 mg		1.25 g	NS[a]	Physically compatible with no bupivacaine loss and about 6 to 7% fentanyl loss in 30 days at 4 and 23°C	2305	C
Fentanyl citrate		2 mg		600 mg	NS[a]	Physically compatible with no bupivacaine loss and about 2 to 4% fentanyl loss in 30 days at 4 and 23°C	2305	C
Fentanyl citrate	JN[j]	35 mg	AST	1 g	NS[a]	Visually compatible with less than 10% change of any drug in 28 days at 4°C and 24 days at 25°C in the dark	2437	C
Fentanyl citrate	JN[k]	1.25 mg	WI	440 mg	[d]	No bupivacaine and fentanyl loss and 10% epinephrine loss in 30 days at 3 and 23°C then 48 hr at 30°C	1627	C
Fentanyl citrate	IVX[l]	2 mg	IVX	1 g		Visually compatible with less than 10% loss of epinephrine and no loss of other drugs in 182 days at 4 and 22°C	2613	C

Additive Compatibility (Cont.)

Test Drug	Mfr	Conc/L or %	Mfr	Conc/L or %	Test Solution	Remarks	Ref	C/I
Hydromorphone HCl	KN	20 mg	AB	625 mg and 1.25 g	NS[a]	Visually compatible with little or no loss of either drug in 72 hr at 24°C under fluorescent light	1870	C
Hydromorphone HCl	KN	100 mg	AB	625 mg and 1.25 g	NS[a]	Visually compatible with little or no loss of either drug in 72 hr at 24°C under fluorescent light	1870	C
Morphine sulfate		1 g	AST	3 g	[a]	Little loss of either drug in 30 days at 18°C	1932	C
Morphine sulfate	SCN	100 mg	AB	625 mg and 1.25 g	NS[a]	Visually compatible. No loss of either drug in 72 hr at 24°C in light	2058	C
Morphine sulfate	SCN	500 mg	AB	625 mg and 1.25 g	NS[a]	Visually compatible. No loss of either drug in 72 hr at 24°C in light	2058	C
Sufentanil citrate	JN	5 mg	AST	2 g	NS[b]	9% sufentanil loss and 5% bupivacaine loss in 30 days at 32°C. No loss of either drug in 30 days at 4°C	1756	C
Sufentanil citrate	JN	20 mg		3 g	NS[b]	5% sufentanil loss and no bupivacaine loss in 10 days at 5, 26, and 37°C	1751	C
Sufentanil citrate	JN	5 mg	AST	2 g	NS[a]	Buffered with pH 4.6 citrate buffer. Visually compatible with no loss of either drug in 48 hr at 32°C	2042	C
Sufentanil citrate	JN	12 mg	AST	40 mg	NS[a]	Visually compatible with no loss of either drug in 43 days at 4 and 25°C	2455	C
Ziconotide acetate	ELN	25 mg[f]	BB	5 g[e]		90% ziconotide retained for 22 days at 37°C. No bupivacaine loss in 30 days	2751	C

[a] Tested in PVC containers.

[b] Tested in PVC/Kalex 3000 (phthalate ester) CADD pump reservoirs.

[c] Tested in PVC containers.

[d] Tested in portable infusion pump reservoirs (Pharmacia Deltec).

[e] Drug powder dissolved in ziconotide acetate injection.

[f] Tested in SynchroMed II implantable pumps.

[g] Tested with fentanyl citrate (JN) 1.25 mg.

[h] Tested with fentanyl citrate (IVX) 2 mg.

[i] Tested with fentanyl citrate (JN) 35 mg.

[j] Tested with clonidine HCl (BI) 9 mg.

[k] Tested with epinephrine HCl (AB) 0.69 mg.

[l] Tested with epinephrine bitartrate 2 mg.

Drugs in Syringe Compatibility

Bupivacaine HCl

Test Drug	Mfr	Amt	Mfr	Amt	Remarks	Ref	C/I
Clonidine HCl	FUJ	100 mcg/1 mL	SAN	3.75 mg/1 mL	Physically and chemically stable for 14 days at room temperature	2069	C
Clonidine HCl	FUJ	100 mcg/1 mL	SAN	60 mg/8 mL	Physically and chemically stable for 14 days at room temperature	2069	C
Clonidine HCl with fentanyl citrate	BI JN	0.45 mg 1.75 mg	AST	50 mg	Diluted to 50 mL with NS. Visually compatible with less than 10% loss of any drug in 25 days at 4 and 25°C in the dark	2437	C

Drugs in Syringe Compatibility (Cont.)

Test Drug	Mfr	Amt	Mfr	Amt	Remarks	Ref	C/I
Clonidine HCl with morphine sulfate	BI ES	0.03 mg/mL 0.2 mg/mL	SW	1.5 mg/mL	Diluted to 5 mL with NS. Visually compatible with no new GC/MS peaks in 1 hr at room temperature	1956	C
Diamorphine HCl	EV	1 and 10 mg/mL	AST	0.5%	10 to 11% diamorphine loss in 5 weeks at 20°C and 3 to 7% loss in 8 weeks at 6°C. No bupivacaine loss at 6 or 20°C in 8 weeks	1952	C
Fentanyl citrate with clonidine HCl	JN BI	1.75 mg 0.45 mg	AST	50 mg	Diluted to 50 mL with NS. Visually compatible with less than 10% loss of any drug in 25 days at 4 and 25°C in the dark	2437	C
Fentanyl citrate with ketamine HCl	JN PD	0.01 mg/mL 2 mg/mL	SW	1.5 mg/mL	Diluted to 5 mL with NS. Visually compatible with no new GC/MS peaks in 1 hr at room temperature	1956	C
Hydromorphone HCl	KN	65 mg/mL	AST	7.5 mg/mL	Visually compatible for 30 days at 25°C	1660	C
Iohexol		64.7%, 1 mL	AST	0.25 and 0.125%[a], 4 mL	Visually compatible with no bupivacaine loss in 24 hr at room temperature. Iohexol not tested	1611	C
Ketamine HCl with fentanyl citrate	PD JN	2 mg/mL 0.01 mg/mL	SW	1.5 mg/mL	Diluted to 5 mL with NS. Visually compatible with no new GC/MS peaks in 1 hr at room temperature	1956	C
Morphine sulfate		1 mg/mL	AST	3 mg/mL	Little loss of either drug in 30 days at 18°C	1932	C
Morphine sulfate	[d]	5 mg/mL[e]	[d]	2.5 mg/mL[e]	Physically compatible. Little morphine or bupivacaine loss in 60 days at 23°C in fluorescent light and at 4°C	2378	C
Morphine sulfate	[d]	5 mg/mL[e]	[d]	2.5 mg/mL[e]	Little or no loss of either drug in 2 days at 37°C	2378	C
Morphine sulfate	[d]	5 mg/mL[e]	[d]	2.5 mg/mL[e]	Formation of large amounts of microparticulates upon thawing following little or no loss of either drug in 2 days at –20°C		I
Morphine sulfate	[d]	50 mg/mL[f]	[d]	25 mg/mL[f]	Physically compatible. Little morphine or bupivacaine loss in 60 days at 23°C in fluorescent light and at 4°C in dark. Slight yellow discoloration at 23°C not indicative of decomposition	2378	C
Morphine sulfate	[d]	50 mg/mL[f]	[d]	25 mg/mL[f]	Little or no loss of either drug in 2 days at 37°C	2378	C
Morphine sulfate	[d]	50 mg/mL[f]	[d]	25 mg/mL[f]	Formation of large amounts of microparticulates upon thawing following little or no loss of either drug in 2 days at –20°C	2378	I
Morphine sulfate with clonidine HCl	ES BI	0.2 mg/mL 0.03 mg/mL	SW	1.5 mg/mL	Diluted to 5 mL with NS. Visually compatible with no new GC/MS peaks in 1 hr at room temperature	1956	C
Sodium bicarbonate	AB	4%, 0.05 to 0.6 mL	AST, WI	0.25, 0.5[b], 0.75%[b], 20 mL	Precipitate forms in 1 to 2 min up to 2 hr at lowest amount of bicarbonate	1724	I

Drugs in Syringe Compatibility (Cont.)

Test Drug	Mfr	Amt	Mfr	Amt	Remarks	Ref	C/I
Sodium bicarbonate		1.4%, 1.5 mL	BEL	0.5%[c], 20 mL	No epinephrine loss in 7 days at room temperature. Bupivacaine not tested	1743	C
Sodium bicarbonate		4.2 and 8.4%, 1.5 mL	BEL	0.5%[c], 20 mL	5 to 7% epinephrine loss in 7 days at room temperature. Bupivacaine not tested	1743	C

[a] Diluted 1:1 in sodium chloride 0.9%.

[b] Tested with and without epinephrine hydrochloride 1:200,000 added.

[c] Tested with epinephrine hydrochloride 1:200,000 added.

[d] Extemporaneously compounded from bulk drug powders.

[e] Tested in sodium chloride 0.9%.

[f] Tested in sterile water for injection.

Y-Site Injection Compatibility (1:1 Mixture)

Bupivacaine HCl

Test Drug	Mfr	Conc	Mfr	Conc	Remarks	Ref	C/I
Meropenem		50 mg/mL	HOS	5 mg/mL	Solution became opaque immediately	3538	I

Selected Revisions May 1, 2020. © Copyright, October 1994.
American Society of Health-System Pharmacists, Inc.

Buprenorphine Hydrochloride
AHFS 28:08.12

Products

Buprenorphine hydrochloride is available in 1-mL ampuls. Each mL contains buprenorphine 0.3 mg (as the hydrochloride) with anhydrous dextrose 50 mg in water for injection. The pH is adjusted with hydrochloric acid.[1(4/05)]

Osmolality

The osmolality was 297 mOsm/kg.[1233]

Trade Name(s)

Buprenex

Administration

Buprenorphine hydrochloride is administered by deep intramuscular injection or by intravenous injection slowly over at least 2 minutes.[1(4/05)] [4] It also has been given by continuous intravenous infusion at a concentration of 15 mcg/mL in sodium chloride 0.9% and by epidural injection at a concentration of 6 to 30 mcg/mL.[4]

Stability

The clear solution should be stored at 15 to 30°C and protected from prolonged exposure to light and exposure to temperatures in excess of 40°C and freezing.[1(4/05)] [4] Buprenorphine hydrochloride may undergo substantial decomposition when autoclaved.[4]

Central Venous Catheter

Buprenorphine hydrochloride (Reckitt & Colman) 0.04 mg/mL in dextrose 5% was found to be compatible with the ARROW-g+ard Blue Plus (Arrow International) chlorhexidine-bearing triple-lumen central catheter. Essentially complete delivery of the drug was found with little or no drug loss occurring. Furthermore, chlorhexidine delivered from the catheter remained at trace amounts with no substantial increase due to the delivery of the drug through the catheter.[2335]

Compatibility Information

Solution Compatibility

Buprenorphine HCl

Test Soln Name	Mfr	Mfr	Conc/L or %	Remarks	Ref	C/I
Dextrose 5%			150 mg	Stated to be compatible	4	C
Ringer's injection, lactated			150 mg	Stated to be compatible	4	C
Sodium chloride 0.9%			150 mg	Stated to be compatible	4	C

Additive Compatibility

Buprenorphine HCl

Test Drug	Mfr	Conc/L or %	Mfr	Conc/L or %	Test Solution	Remarks	Ref	C/I
Bupivacaine HCl	AST	3 g	RC	180 mg	a	No loss of either drug in 30 days at 18°C	1932	C
Floxacillin sodium	BE	20 g		75 mg	W	Thick haze forms in 24 hr and precipitate forms in 47 hr at 30°C. No change at 15°C	1479	I
Furosemide	HO	1 g		75 mg	W	Haze for 6 hr at 30°C. No change at 15°C	1479	I
Glycopyrrolate with haloperidol lactate	ON	25 mg 104 mg	RKC	84 mg	NS[a]	Visually compatible with less than 10% loss of any drug in 30 days at 4 and 25°C in the dark	2436	C
Haloperidol lactate with glycopyrrolate	ON	104 mg 25 mg	RKC	84 mg	NS[a]	Visually compatible with less than 10% loss of any drug in 30 days at 4 and 25°C in the dark	2436	C

[a] Tested in PVC containers.

DOI: 10.37573/9781585286850.060

Drugs in Syringe Compatibility

Buprenorphine HCl

Test Drug	Mfr	Amt	Mfr	Amt	Remarks	Ref	C/I
Atropine sulfate					Physically and chemically compatible	4	C
Diazepam					Incompatible	4	I
Diphenhydramine HCl					Physically and chemically compatible	4	C
Droperidol					Physically and chemically compatible	4	C
Glycopyrrolate with haloperidol lactate	ON	1.2 mg 5 mg	RKC	4 mg	Diluted to 48 mL with NS. Visually compatible with less than 10% loss of any drug in 30 days at 4 and 25°C in the dark	2436	C
Haloperidol lactate with glycopyrrolate	ON	5 mg 1.2 mg	RKC	4 mg	Diluted to 48 mL with NS. Visually compatible with less than 10% loss of any drug in 30 days at 4 and 25°C in the dark	2436	C
Heparin sodium		2500 units/1 mL	BM	300 mg/1 mL	Visually compatible for at least 5 min	1053	C
Hydroxyzine HCl					Physically and chemically compatible	4	C
Lorazepam					Incompatible	4	I
Midazolam HCl	RC	5 mg/1 mL	NE	0.3 mg/1 mL	Physically compatible for 4 hr at 25°C	1145	C
Promethazine HCl					Physically and chemically compatible	4	C
Scopolamine HBr					Physically and chemically compatible	4	C

Y-Site Injection Compatibility (1:1 Mixture)

Buprenorphine HCl

Test Drug	Mfr	Conc	Mfr	Conc	Remarks	Ref	C/I
Acetaminophen	CAD	10 mg/mL	HOS, BED	0.3 mg/mL	Physically compatible with less than 10% acetaminophen loss over 4 hr at room temperature	2841, 2844	C
Allopurinol sodium	BW	3 mg/mL[b]	RKC	0.04 mg/mL[b]	Physically compatible for 4 hr at 22°C	1686	C
Amifostine	USB	10 mg/mL[a]	RKC	0.04 mg/mL[a]	Physically compatible for 4 hr at 23°C	1845	C
Aztreonam	SQ	40 mg/mL[a]	RKC	0.04 mg/mL[a]	Physically compatible for 4 hr at 23°C	1758	C
Cisatracurium besylate	GW	0.1, 2, 5 mg/mL[a]	RKC	0.04 mg/mL[a]	Physically compatible for 4 hr at 23°C	2074	C
Cladribine	ORT	0.015[b] and 0.5[c] mg/mL	RKC	0.04 mg/mL[b]	Physically compatible for 4 hr at 23°C	1969	C
Docetaxel	RPR	0.9 mg/mL[a]	RKC	0.04 mg/mL[a]	Physically compatible for 4 hr at 23°C	2224	C
Doxorubicin HCl liposomal	SEQ	0.4 mg/mL[a]	RKC	0.04 mg/mL[a]	Partial loss of measured natural turbidity	2087	I
Etoposide phosphate	BR	5 mg/mL[a]	RKC	0.04 mg/mL[a]	Physically compatible for 4 hr at 23°C	2218	C
Filgrastim	AMG	30 mcg/mL[a]	RKC	0.04 mg/mL[a]	Physically compatible for 4 hr at 22°C	1687	C
Gemcitabine HCl	LI	10 mg/mL[b]	RKC	0.04 mg/mL[b]	Physically compatible for 4 hr at 23°C	2226	C
Granisetron HCl	SKB	0.05 mg/mL[a]	RKC	0.04 mg/mL[a]	Physically compatible for 4 hr at 23°C	2000	C
Linezolid	PHU	2 mg/mL	RKC	0.04 mg/mL[a]	Physically compatible for 4 hr at 23°C	2264	C
Melphalan HCl	BW	0.1 mg/mL[b]	RKC	0.04 mg/mL[b]	Physically compatible for 3 hr at 22°C	1557	C
Oxaliplatin	SS	0.5 mg/mL[a]	RKC	0.04 mg/mL[a]	Physically compatible for 4 hr at 23°C	2566	C
Pemetrexed disodium	LI	20 mg/mL[b]	RKB	0.04 mg/mL[a]	Physically compatible for 4 hr at 23°C	2564	C

Y-Site Injection Compatibility (1:1 Mixture) (Cont.)

Test Drug	Mfr	Conc	Mfr	Conc	Remarks	Ref	C/I
Piperacillin sodium–tazobactam sodium	LE[f]	40 mg/mL[a g]	RKC	0.04 mg/mL[a]	Physically compatible for 4 hr at 22°C	1688	C
Propofol	ZEN[h]	10 mg/mL	RKC	0.04 mg/mL[a]	Physically compatible for 1 hr at 23°C	2066	C
Remifentanil HCl	GW	0.025 and 0.25 mg/mL[b]	RKC	0.04 mg/mL[a]	Physically compatible for 4 hr at 23°C	2075	C
Teniposide	BR	0.1 mg/mL[a]	RKC	0.04 mg/mL[a]	Physically compatible for 4 hr at 23°C	1725	C
Thiotepa	IMM[d]	1 mg/mL[a]	RKC	0.04 mg/mL[a]	Physically compatible for 4 hr at 23°C	1861	C
TNA #218 to #226[e]			RKC	0.04 mg/mL[a]	Visually compatible for 4 hr at 23°C	2215	C
TPN #212 to #215[e]			RKC	0.04 mg/mL[a]	Physically compatible for 4 hr at 23°C	2109	C
Vinorelbine tartrate	BW	1 mg/mL[b]	RKC	0.04 mg/mL[b]	Physically compatible for 4 hr at 22°C	1558	C

[a] Tested in dextrose 5%.

[b] Tested in sodium chloride 0.9%.

[c] Tested in bacteriostatic sodium chloride 0.9% preserved with benzyl alcohol 0.9%.

[d] Lyophilized formulation tested.

[e] Refer to Appendix for the composition of parenteral nutrition solutions. TNA indicates a 3-in-1 admixture, and TPN indicates a 2-in-1 admixture.

[f] Test performed using the formulation WITHOUT edetate disodium.

[g] Piperacillin component. Piperacillin in an 8:1 fixed-ratio concentration with tazobactam.

[h] Test performed using the formulation WITH edetate disodium.

Selected Revisions January 31, 2020. © Copyright, October 1990.
American Society of Health-System Pharmacists, Inc.

Busulfan
AHFS 10:00

Products

Busulfan is available as a 6-mg/mL concentrate for injection; busulfan is dissolved in a vehicle composed of 33% (v/v) *N, N*-dimethylacetamide (DMA) (approximately 309 mg DMA per mL of busulfan solution) and 67% (v/v) polyethylene glycol 400.[2982][3047] The concentrate for injection is packaged in 10-mL single-dose vials and must be diluted for administration.[2982]

pH

Busulfan diluted for infusion to a concentration of approximately 0.5 mg/mL with sodium chloride 0.9% or dextrose 5% has a pH of 3.4 to 3.9, depending on which solution is used.[2982]

Trade Name(s)

Busulfex

Administration

Busulfan concentrate for injection must be diluted prior to administration.[2982] Sodium chloride 0.9% and dextrose 5% are both recommended diluents for dilution of busulfan concentrate for injection.[2982] The volume of infusion solution used for dilution should be 10 times the volume of the busulfan concentrate for injection dose to ensure that the final concentration is approximately 0.5 mg/mL.[2982]

Busulfan admixtures should be administered intravenously through a central venous catheter as a 2-hour infusion.[2982] More rapid infusion has not been tested and is not recommended.[2982] An infusion pump should be used to control the flow rate.[2982] The central venous catheter should be flushed before and after busulfan administration with approximately 5 mL of sodium chloride 0.9% or dextrose 5%.[2982] The manufacturer states that an administration set with a minimal residual volume (2 to 5 mL) should be used for busulfan administration.[2982]

As with other toxic drugs, caution should be exercised in the handling and preparation of busulfan, and applicable special handling and disposal procedures should be followed.[2982] Appropriate gloves should be worn during preparation; accidental skin exposure may result in skin reactions.[2982] The busulfan is added into an intravenous solution bag that already contains the appropriate amount of sodium chloride 0.9% or dextrose 5%.[2982] The drug should always be added to the diluent, not the diluent to the drug.[2982] The solution should be mixed thoroughly by inverting the bag several times.[2982] Other diluents should not be used.[2982]

Busulfan (Pierre Fabre) 6 mg/mL was found to be incompatible with the silicone SmartSite needle-free valve of the MFX 2301E tubing set (CareFusion).[2983] Slight turbidity was noted immediately on injection of the busulfan into the valve and persisted throughout the 5-hour study period.[2983]

Polycarbonate syringes and filter needles should not be used with busulfan;[2982] the manufacturer notes that a precipitate has been known to form when syringes composed of or containing polycarbonate are used to withdraw busulfan from the vial.[3046]

Stability

Busulfan concentrate for injection is a clear, colorless solution.[2982] Intact vials must be stored under refrigeration at 2 to 8°C.[2982] Solutions should be visually inspected for particulate matter and discoloration prior to administration; if particulate matter is observed in the vial, the concentrate for injection should not be used.[2982]

Administration of busulfan diluted for infusion in sodium chloride 0.9% or dextrose 5% should be completed within 8 hours when stored at 25°C.[2982] Administration of busulfan diluted for infusion in sodium chloride 0.9% should be completed within 12 hours when stored under refrigeration at 2 to 8°C.[2982]

Busulfan (Pierre Fabre) 6 mg/mL did not support the growth of *Staphylococcus aureus* and *Candida albicans* within 2 hours at room temperature.[2740] Busulfan 0.5 mg/mL in sodium chloride 0.9% did not support the growth of *Staphylococcus aureus*, *Enterococcus faecium*, or *Pseudomonas aeruginosa* with loss of viability over 24 to 48 hours at room temperature but had no effect on the growth of *Candida albicans*.[2740] Diluted solutions should be stored under refrigeration whenever possible, and the potential for microbiological growth should be considered when assigning expiration periods.[2740]

Syringes

Busulfan (Pierre Fabre) 0.54 mg/mL in 0.9% sodium chloride stored in 50-mL polypropylene syringes (Becton Dickinson) fitted with tip caps (Braun) and protected from light at 2 to 8°C or 23 to 27°C was visually compatible and demonstrated less than 10% loss in 30 or 12 hours, respectively.[3399] White crystals were detected on the surface of the syringes after 33 hours at 2 to 8°C.[3399]

DOI: 10.37573/9781585286850.061

Compatibility Information

Solution Compatibility

Busulfan

Test Soln Name	Mfr	Mfr	Conc/L or %	Remarks	Ref	C/I
Dextrose 5%	BA[a], MG[b]		0.5 g	Physically compatible. Under 10% loss in 8 hr at 23°C but over 20% loss in 24 hr	2183	I[c]
Dextrose 5%	BA[a], MG[b]		0.1 g	Physically compatible. Under 10% loss in 4 hr at 23°C but 19% loss in 8 hr	2183	I[c]
Dextrose 5%		OTS	500 mg	Complete administration within 8 hr after dilution if stored at 25°C	2982	C
Sodium chloride 0.9%	BA[a], MG[b]		0.5 g	Physically compatible. Under 10% loss in 8 hr at 23°C but over 20% loss in 24 hr	2183	I[c]
Sodium chloride 0.9%	BA[a], MG[b]		0.1 g	Physically compatible. Under 10% loss in 4 hr at 23°C but 13% loss in 8 hr	2183	I[c]
Sodium chloride 0.9%	[d]	ORP	0.5 g	Precipitation in about 19 hr at 4°C. Substantial busulfan loss from precipitation	2739	I
Sodium chloride 0.9%	[e]	ORP	0.5 g	Precipitation appears when frozen. Precipitation in about 19 hr at 4°C. Substantial busulfan loss from precipitation	2739	I
Sodium chloride 0.9%	[d] [e]	ORP	0.5 g	Physically stable for 19 to 36 hr at 13 to 15°C. Under 10% loss until precipitation	2739	?
Sodium chloride 0.9%	[b]	PRF	0.24 g	10% loss in 8 hr at 25°C. 12% loss in 24 hr at 4°C	2785	I[c]
Sodium chloride 0.9%	[b]	PRF	0.12 g	10% loss in 12 hr at 25°C and 4°C	2785	I[c]
Sodium chloride 0.9%		OTS	500 mg	Complete administration within 8 hr after dilution if stored at 25°C or 12 hr if stored at 2 to 8°C	2982	C
Sodium chloride 0.9%	SB[f]	PRF	540 mg	Visually compatible with less than 10% loss in 3 hr at 23 to 27°C or 9 hr at 2 to 8°C; however, variability observed among 3 lots and between different container sizes	3399	?

[a] Tested in PVC containers.

[b] Tested in polyolefin containers.

[c] Incompatible by conventional standards but may be used in shorter periods of time.

[d] Tested in Freeflex polypropylene bags.

[e] Tested in glass containers.

[f] Tested in polypropylene containers.

Butorphanol Tartrate
AHFS 28:08.12

Products

Butorphanol tartrate is available in concentrations of 1 mg/mL (in 1-mL vials) and 2 mg/mL (in 1- and 2-mL single-use vials and 10-mL multidose [preserved] vials).[2904] [2905]

Each mL of solution also contains citric acid 3.3 mg, sodium citrate 7.29 mg (equivalent to sodium citrate anhydrous 6.4 mg),[2904] and sodium chloride 6.4 mg.[2904] [2905] Also present in the multidose vials is 0.1 mg/mL of benzethonium chloride as a preservative.[2904]

pH

From 3 to 5.5.[2904]

Administration

Butorphanol tartrate may be administered by intramuscular or intravenous injection.[2904] [2905]

Stability

Butorphanol tartrate injection should be stored at controlled room temperature and retained in the original carton to protect from light.[2904] [2905]

Central Venous Catheter

Butorphanol tartrate (Apothecon) 0.04 mg/mL in dextrose 5% was found to be compatible with the ARROWg+ard Blue Plus (Arrow International) chlorhexidine-bearing triple-lumen central catheter. Essentially complete delivery of the drug was found with little or no drug loss occurring. Furthermore, chlorhexidine delivered from the catheter remained at trace amounts with no substantial increase due to the delivery of the drug through the catheter.[2335]

Compatibility Information

Additive Compatibility

Butorphanol tartrate

Test Drug	Mfr	Conc/L or %	Mfr	Conc/L or %	Test Solution	Remarks	Ref	C/I
Droperidol	XU	50 mg	HE	80 mg	NS[a]	Physically compatible with less than 2% loss of either drug in 15 days at 4 and 25°C protected from light	2908	C
Granisetron HCl	NIN	30 and 60 mg	HE	80 mg	NS[b]	Physically compatible with little to no loss of either drug in 14 days at 4°C protected from light or 48 hr at 25°C in room light	3120	C
Granisetron HCl	NIN	30 and 60 mg	HE	80 mg	NS[c]	Physically compatible with little to no loss of either drug in 14 days at 4°C protected from light or 48 hr at 25°C in room light	3120	C
Ketamine HCl	QI	1, 2, 4 g	HE	50 mg	NS[b]	Physically compatible with little to no loss of either drug in 15 days at 4, 25, and 37°C in the dark	3119	C
Ketamine HCl	QI	1, 2, 4 g	HE	100 mg	NS[b]	Physically compatible with little to no loss of either drug in 15 days at 4, 25, and 37°C in the dark	3119	C
Ketamine HCl	QI	1, 2, 4 g	HE	150 mg	NS[b]	Physically compatible with little to no loss of either drug in 15 days at 4, 25, and 37°C in the dark	3119	C
Tropisetron HCl	COM	50 mg	HE	80 mg	NS[b]	Physically compatible with little to no loss of either drug in 14 days at 4 and 25°C in the dark	3121	C
Tropisetron HCl	COM	50 mg	HE	80 mg	NS[c]	Physically compatible with little to no loss of either drug in 14 days at 4 and 25°C in the dark	3121	C

[a] Tested in PVC and glass containers.

[b] Tested in polyolefin containers.

[c] Tested in glass containers.

DOI: 10.37573/9781585286850.062

Drugs in Syringe Compatibility

Butorphanol tartrate

Test Drug	Mfr	Amt	Mfr	Amt	Remarks	Ref	C/I
Atropine sulfate	ST	0.4 mg/1 mL	BR	4 mg/2 mL	Physically compatible for 30 min at room temperature	566	C
Chlorpromazine HCl	MB	25 mg/1 mL	BR	4 mg/2 mL	Physically compatible for 30 min at room temperature	566	C
Dimenhydrinate	HR	50 mg/1 mL	BR	4 mg/2 mL	Gas evolves	761	I
Diphenhydramine HCl	PD	50 mg/1 mL	BR	4 mg/2 mL	Physically compatible for 30 min at room temperature	566	C
Droperidol	MN	5 mg/2 mL	BR	4 mg/2 mL	Physically compatible for 30 min at room temperature	566	C
Fentanyl citrate	MN	0.1 mg/2 mL	BR	4 mg/2 mL	Physically compatible for 30 min at room temperature	566	C
Hydroxyzine HCl	PF	50 mg/1 mL	BR	2 mg/1 mL	Physically compatible	771	C
Hydroxyzine HCl	PF	100 mg/2 mL	BR	1 mg/1 mL	Physically compatible	771	C
Meperidine HCl	WI	50 mg/1 mL	BR	4 mg/2 mL	Physically compatible for 30 min at room temperature	566	C
Methotrimeprazine HCl		25 mg/1 mL	BR	4 mg/2 mL	Physically compatible for 30 min at room temperature	566	C
Metoclopramide HCl	NO	10 mg/2 mL	BR	4 mg/2 mL	Physically compatible for 30 min at room temperature	566	C
Midazolam HCl	RC	5 mg/1 mL	BR	2 mg/1 mL	Physically compatible for 4 hr at 25°C	1145	C
Morphine sulfate	AH	15 mg/1 mL	BR	4 mg/2 mL	Physically compatible for 30 min at room temperature	566	C
Pentazocine lactate	WI	30 mg/1 mL	BR	4 mg/2 mL	Physically compatible for 30 min at room temperature	566	C
Pentobarbital sodium	AB	50 mg/1 mL	BR	4 mg/2 mL	Precipitates immediately	761	I
Prochlorperazine edisylate	MB	5 mg/1 mL	BR	4 mg/2 mL	Physically compatible for 30 min at room temperature	566	C
Promethazine HCl	WY	25 mg/1 mL	BR	4 mg/2 mL	Physically compatible for 30 min at room temperature	566	C
Scopolamine HBr	ST	0.4 mg/1 mL	BR	4 mg/2 mL	Physically compatible for 30 min at room temperature	566	C

Y-Site Injection Compatibility (1:1 Mixture)

Butorphanol tartrate

Test Drug	Mfr	Conc	Mfr	Conc	Remarks	Ref	C/I
Acetaminophen	CAD	10 mg/mL	APO, BED	2 mg/mL	Physically compatible with less than 10% acetaminophen loss over 4 hr at room temperature	2841, 2844	C
Allopurinol sodium	BW	3 mg/mL[b]	BR	0.04 mg/mL[b]	Physically compatible for 4 hr at 22°C	1686	C
Amifostine	USB	10 mg/mL[a]	BR	0.04 mg/mL[a]	Physically compatible for 4 hr at 23°C	1845	C
Aztreonam	SQ	40 mg/mL[a]	BMS	0.04 mg/mL[a]	Physically compatible for 4 hr at 23°C	1758	C

Y-Site Injection Compatibility (1:1 Mixture) (Cont.)

Test Drug	Mfr	Conc	Mfr	Conc	Remarks	Ref	C/I
Bivalirudin	TMC	5 mg/mL[a]	APO	40 mcg/mL[a]	Physically compatible for 4 hr at 23°C	2373	C
Cangrelor tetrasodium	TMC	1 mg/mL[b]		40 mcg/mL[b]	Physically compatible for 4 hr	3243	C
Cangrelor tetrasodium	TMC	1 mg/mL[b]		2 mg/mL	Gross white turbid precipitate forms immediately	3243	I
Cisatracurium besylate	GW	0.1, 2, 5 mg/mL[a]	APC	0.04 mg/mL[a]	Physically compatible for 4 hr at 23°C	2074	C
Cladribine	ORT	0.015[b] and 0.5[c] mg/mL	APC	0.04 mg/mL[b]	Physically compatible for 4 hr at 23°C	1969	C
Dexmedetomidine HCl	AB	4 mcg/mL[b]	APO	40 mcg/mL[b]	Physically compatible for 4 hr at 23°C	2383	C
Docetaxel	RPR	0.9 mg/mL[a]	APC	0.04 mg/mL[a]	Physically compatible for 4 hr at 23°C	2224	C
Doxorubicin HCl liposomal	SEQ	0.4 mg/mL[a]	APC	0.04 mg/mL[a]	Physically compatible for 4 hr at 23°C	2087	C
Enalaprilat	MSD	0.05 mg/mL[b]	BR	0.4 mg/mL[a]	Physically compatible for 24 hr at room temperature under fluorescent light	1355	C
Esmolol HCl	DCC	10 mg/mL[a]	BR	0.04 mg/mL[a]	Physically compatible for 24 hr at 22°C	1169	C
Etoposide phosphate	BR	5 mg/mL[a]	APC	0.04 mg/mL[a]	Physically compatible for 4 hr at 23°C	2218	C
Fenoldopam mesylate	AB	80 mcg/mL[b]	APO	40 mcg/mL[b]	Physically compatible for 4 hr at 23°C	2467	C
Filgrastim	AMG	30 mcg/mL[a]	BR	0.04 mg/mL[a]	Physically compatible for 4 hr at 22°C	1687	C
Fludarabine phosphate	BX	1 mg/mL[a]	BR	0.04 mg/mL[a]	Visually compatible for 4 hr at 22°C	1439	C
Gemcitabine HCl	LI	10 mg/mL[b]	APC	0.04 mg/mL[b]	Physically compatible for 4 hr at 23°C	2226	C
Granisetron HCl	SKB	0.05 mg/mL[a]	APC	0.04 mg/mL[a]	Physically compatible for 4 hr at 23°C	2000	C
Hetastarch in lactated electrolyte	AB	6%	APC	0.04 mg/mL[a]	Physically compatible for 4 hr at 23°C	2339	C
Labetalol HCl	SC	1 mg/mL[a]	BR	0.04 mg/mL[a]	Physically compatible for 24 hr at 18°C	1171	C
Linezolid	PHU	2 mg/mL	APC	0.04 mg/mL[a]	Physically compatible for 4 hr at 23°C	2264	C
Melphalan HCl	BW	0.1 mg/mL[b]	BR	0.04 mg/mL[b]	Physically compatible for 3 hr at 22°C	1557	C
Midazolam HCl	RC	[f]	BR	[f]	Crystalline midazolam precipitate forms	2144	I
Nicardipine HCl	DCC	0.1 mg/mL[a]	BR	0.4 mg/mL[a]	Visually compatible for 24 hr at room temperature	235	C
Oxaliplatin	SS	0.5 mg/mL[a]	APO	0.04 mg/mL[a]	Physically compatible for 4 hr at 23°C	2566	C
Paclitaxel	NCI	1.2 mg/mL[a]	BR	0.04 mg/mL[a]	Physically compatible for 4 hr at 22°C	1556	C
Pemetrexed disodium	LI	20 mg/mL[b]	BMS	0.04 mg/mL[a]	Physically compatible for 4 hr at 23°C	2564	C
Piperacillin sodium–tazobactam sodium	LE[g]	40 mg/mL[a] [h]	BR	0.04 mg/mL[a]	Physically compatible for 4 hr at 23°C	1688	C
Propofol	ZEN[i]	10 mg/mL	APC	0.04 mg/mL[a]	Physically compatible for 1 hr at 23°C	2066	C
Remifentanil HCl	GW	0.025 and 0.25 mg/mL[b]	APC	0.04 mg/mL[a]	Physically compatible for 4 hr at 23°C	2075	C
Sargramostim	IMM	10 mcg/mL[b]	BR	0.04 mg/mL[b]	Visually compatible for 4 hr at 22°C	1436	C
Teniposide	BR	0.1 mg/mL[a]	BR	0.04 mg/mL[a]	Physically compatible for 4 hr at 23°C	1725	C

Y-Site Injection Compatibility (1:1 Mixture) (Cont.)

Test Drug	Mfr	Conc	Mfr	Conc	Remarks	Ref	C/I
Thiotepa	IMM[d]	1 mg/mL[a]	APC	0.04 mg/mL[a]	Physically compatible for 4 hr at 23°C	1861	C
TNA #218 to #226[e]			APC	0.04 mg/mL[a]	Visually compatible for 4 hr at 23°C	2215	C
TPN #212 to #215[e]			APC	0.04 mg/mL[a]	Physically compatible for 4 hr at 23°C	2109	C
Vinorelbine tartrate	BW	1 mg/mL[b]	BR	0.04 mg/mL[b]	Physically compatible for 4 hr at 22°C	1558	C

[a] Tested in dextrose 5%.

[b] Tested in sodium chloride 0.9%.

[c] Tested in bacteriostatic sodium chloride 0.9% preserved with benzyl alcohol 0.9%.

[d] Lyophilized formulation tested.

[e] Refer to Appendix for the composition of parenteral nutrition solutions. TNA indicates a 3-in-1 admixture, and TPN indicates a 2-in-1 admixture.

[f] Concentration unspecified.

[g] Test performed using the formulation WITHOUT edetate disodium.

[h] Piperacillin component. Piperacillin in an 8:1 fixed-ratio concentration with tazobactam.

[i] Test performed using the formulation WITH edetate disodium.

Selected Revisions January 31, 2020. © Copyright, October 1982.
American Society of Health-System Pharmacists, Inc.

Caffeine Citrate
AHFS 28:20.32

Products

Caffeine citrate is available as a 20-mg/mL solution in 3-mL (60-mg) vials. Each mL provides caffeine base 10 mg/mL with citric acid monohydrate 5 mg and sodium citrate dihydrate 8.3 mg/mL in water for injection.[1(5/08)]

pH

The pH is adjusted to 4.7.[1(5/08)]

Trade Name(s)

Cafcit

Administration

Caffeine citrate injection is administered slowly intravenously using a syringe pump over 30 minutes as a loading dose and over 10 minutes as a maintenance dose.[1(5/08)] [4]

Stability

Intact vials of the clear, colorless injection should be stored at room temperature. The injection contains no antibacterial preservative and unused portions should be discarded.[1(5/08)]

Syringes

Caffeine (salt form unspecified) 10 mg/mL was repackaged in glass and plastic syringes (Becton Dickinson) and stored at room temperature and 4°C. Less than 4% loss occurred over 60 days.[139]

Compatibility Information

Solution Compatibility

Caffeine citrate

Test Soln Name	Mfr	Mfr	Conc/L or %	Remarks	Ref	C/I
Dextrose 5%			10 g	Physically compatible and chemically stable for 24 hr at room temperature	1(5/08)	C
Dextrose 5% in sodium chloride 0.225%			5 g	Physically compatible and chemically stable for 24 hr at room temperature	193, 483	C
Dextrose 5% in sodium chloride 0.225%	a		5 g	Physically compatible and chemically stable for 24 hr at room temperature	193, 483	C

a Tested with potassium chloride 20 mEq/L.

Drugs in Syringe Compatibility

Caffeine citrate

Test Drug	Mfr	Amt	Mfr	Amt	Remarks	Ref	C/I
Acyclovir sodium	BW	50 mg/1 mL		20 mg/1 mL	Precipitates immediately	2440	I
Alprostadil	UP	0.5 mg/1 mL		20 mg/1 mL	Visually compatible for 4 hr at 25°C	2440	C
Amikacin sulfate	BED	250 mg/1 mL		20 mg/1 mL	Visually compatible for 4 hr at 25°C	2440	C
Aminophylline	AB	25 mg/1 mL		20 mg/1 mL	Visually compatible for 4 hr at 25°C	2440	C
Calcium gluconate		100 mg/1 mL		20 mg/1 mL	Physically compatible and chemically stable for 24 hr at room temperature	1(5/08)	C
Cefotaxime sodium	HO	200 mg/1 mL		20 mg/1 mL	Visually compatible for 4 hr at 25°C	2440	C
Clindamycin phosphate	UP	150 mg/1 mL		20 mg/1 mL	Visually compatible for 4 hr at 25°C	2440	C

DOI: 10.37573/9781585286850.063

Drugs in Syringe Compatibility (Cont.)

Test Drug	Mfr	Amt	Mfr	Amt	Remarks	Ref	C/I
Dexamethasone sodium phosphate	ES	4 mg/1 mL		20 mg/1 mL	Visually compatible for 4 hr at 25°C	2440	C
Dimenhydrinate		10 mg/1 mL		10 mg/1 mL	Clear solution	2569	C
Dobutamine HCl	GNS	12.5 mg/1 mL		20 mg/1 mL	Visually compatible for 4 hr at 25°C	2440	C
Dopamine HCl	SO	80 mg/1 mL		20 mg/1 mL	Visually compatible for 4 hr at 25°C	2440	C
Epinephrine HCl	IMS	0.1 mg/1 mL		20 mg/1 mL	Visually compatible for 4 hr at 25°C	2440	C
Fentanyl citrate	ES	50 mcg/1 mL		20 mg/1 mL	Visually compatible for 4 hr at 25°C	2440	C
Furosemide	AST	10 mg/1 mL		20 mg/1 mL	Precipitates immediately	2440	I
Gentamicin sulfate	ES	10 mg/1 mL		20 mg/1 mL	Visually compatible for 4 hr at 25°C	2440	C
Heparin sodium	AB	10 units/1 mL		20 mg/1 mL	Visually compatible for 4 hr at 25°C	2440	C
Isoproterenol HCl	SW	0.2 mg/1 mL		20 mg/1 mL	Visually compatible for 4 hr at 25°C	2440	C
Lidocaine HCl	AB	1%, 1 mL		20 mg/1 mL	Visually compatible for 4 hr at 25°C	2440	C
Lorazepam	SW	2 mg/1 mL		20 mg/1 mL	Haze forms immediately becoming two layers over time	2440	I
Metoclopramide HCl	ES	5 mg/1 mL		20 mg/1 mL	Visually compatible for 4 hr at 25°C	2440	C
Morphine sulfate	SW	4 mg/1 mL		20 mg/1 mL	Visually compatible for 4 hr at 25°C	2440	C
Nitroglycerin	SO	5 mg/1 mL		20 mg/1 mL	White precipitate forms immediately becoming two layers over time	2440	I
Oxacillin sodium	APC	50 mg/1 mL		20 mg/1 mL	White precipitate forms immediately becoming two layers over time	2440	I
Pancuronium bromide	GNS	1 mg/1 mL		20 mg/1 mL	Visually compatible for 4 hr at 25°C	2440	C
Pantoprazole sodium	[a]	4 mg/1 mL		10 mg/1 mL	Precipitates	2574	I
Phenobarbital sodium	ES	130 mg/1 mL		20 mg/1 mL	Visually compatible for 4 hr at 25°C	2440	C
Phenylephrine HCl	ES	10 mg/1 mL		20 mg/1 mL	Visually compatible for 4 hr at 25°C	2440	C
Sodium bicarbonate	AST	4.2%, 1 mL		20 mg/1 mL	Visually compatible for 4 hr at 25°C	2440	C
Sodium nitroprusside	ES	25 mg/1 mL		20 mg/1 mL	Visually compatible for 4 hr at 25°C	2440	C
Vancomycin HCl	LI	50 mg/1 mL		20 mg/1 mL	Visually compatible for 4 hr at 25°C	2440	C

[a] Test performed using the formulation WITHOUT edetate disodium.

Y-Site Injection Compatibility (1:1 Mixture)

Caffeine citrate

Test Drug	Mfr	Conc	Mfr	Conc	Remarks	Ref	C/I
Blinatumomab	AMG	0.125 and 0.375 mcg/mL[b]	CPR	25 mg/mL	Visually compatible for 12 hr at room temperature	3405, 3417	C
Dopamine HCl		0.6 mg/mL[a]		20 mg/mL	Compatible and stable for 24 hr at room temperature	1(5/08)	C
Doxapram HCl	RB	2 mg/mL[a]	BI	20 mg/mL	Visually compatible for 4 hr at 23°C	2470	C
Fentanyl citrate		10 mcg/mL[a]		20 mg/mL	Compatible and stable for 24 hr at room temperature	1(5/08)	C
Heparin sodium		1 unit/mL[a]		20 mg/mL	Compatible and stable for 24 hr at room temperature	1(5/08)	C

Y-Site Injection Compatibility (1:1 Mixture) (Cont.)

Test Drug	Mfr	Conc	Mfr	Conc	Remarks	Ref	C/I
Ibuprofen lysinate	OVA	10 mg/mL	MJ	20 mg/mL	Measured turbidity increased immediately and solution became milky white and opaque with a white precipitate	3541	I
Levofloxacin	OMN	5 mg/mL[a]		5 mg/mL	Visually compatible for 4 hr at 24°C	2233	C
Meropenem		50 mg/mL	SGT	20 mg/mL	Physically compatible for 4 hr at room temperature	3538	C

[a] Tested in dextrose 5%.

[b] Tested in sodium chloride 0.9%.

Selected Revisions September 10, 2020. © Copyright, October 2004. American Society of Health-System Pharmacists, Inc.

Calcitriol
AHFS 88:16

Products

Calcitriol is available as 1 mL of solution in ampuls. Each mL of the Calcijex (Abbott) aqueous solution contains calcitriol 1 mcg, polysorbate 20 4 mg, sodium ascorbate 2.5 mg, and hydrochloric acid and/or sodium hydroxide to adjust pH.[1(11/07)]

Calcitriol injection (American Regent) utilizes a different formulation. Each mL of solution contains calcitriol 1 mcg, polysorbate 20 4 mg, sodium ascorbate 10 mg, sodium chloride 1.5 mg, dibasic sodium phosphate anhydrous 7.6 mg, monobasic sodium phosphate monohydrate 1.8 mg, and edetate disodium dihydrate.[1(11/07)]

pH

The Calcijex (Abbott) injection has a target pH of 6.5 with a range of 5.9 to 7.0. Calcitriol injection (American Regent) has a pH in the range of 6.7 to 7.7.[1(11/07)]

Tonicity

The injection is an isotonic solution.[1(11/07)]

Trade Name(s)

Calcijex

Administration

Calcitriol is given by intravenous injection. For patients undergoing hemodialysis, it may be administered by rapid intravenous injection through the catheter after a period of hemodialysis.[4]

Stability

Calcitriol injection is a clear, colorless to yellow solution. It should be stored at controlled room temperature and protected from light.[1(11/07)] [4] Freezing and excessive heat should be avoided, although brief exposure to temperatures up to 40°C does not adversely affect the injection.[4]

The product does not contain a preservative, and the manufacturers recommend discarding any unused solution.[1(11/07)] [4]

Syringes

Calcitriol (Abbott) 1 and 2 mcg/mL undiluted and 0.5 mcg/mL diluted in dextrose 5%, sodium chloride 0.9%, and water for injection was evaluated for stability. It was stored in 1-mL polypropylene tuberculin syringes (Becton Dickinson) for eight hours at room temperature while exposed to normal room light. Little or no loss occurred during the study period.[1662]

Sorption

The sorption potential of calcitriol (Abbott) to PVC bags and administration sets and to polypropylene syringes was evaluated by determining the apparent calcitriol polymer–water partition coefficients. The mean apparent partition coefficient was 66 times greater for PVC than polypropylene. In this test, 50% of the calcitriol was lost to PVC within two hours while approximately 4% was lost to polypropylene in 20 days.[1662]

Similar results were reported for calcitriol 1.5 mcg in 2000 mL of Dianeal PD-2, Midpeliq 250, and Peritoliq 250 in polyvinyl chloride peritoneal dialysis solution bags. Losses of up to 75% occurred in 72 hours due to sorption to the container material. However, the same combinations in polypropylene and glass containers exhibited only about 10 to 20% loss in 72 hours.[2695]

Peritoneal Dialysis Solutions

Calcitriol (Abbott) in concentrations of 0.5 to 2 mcg/L in Dianeal (Baxter) with dextrose 1.5 and 4.5% and in Inpersol (Abbott) with dextrose 1.5% lost about 50% in two hours and about 75% in 20 hours due to sorption to the plastic bag.[502]

Selected Revisions October 1, 2012. © Copyright, October 1994. American Society of Health-System Pharmacists, Inc.

DOI: 10.37573/9781585286850.064

Calcium Chloride
AHFS 40:12

Products

Calcium chloride is available in 10-mL single-dose vials and prefilled syringes containing 1 g of calcium chloride (dihydrate), providing 13.6 mEq (270 mg) of calcium and 13.6 mEq of chloride in water for injection. The pH may have been adjusted with hydrochloric acid and/or calcium hydroxide.[1(5/06) 4]

pH

From 5.5 to 7.5 diluted in water to a 5% concentration.[1(5/06) 4]

Osmolarity

The 10% injection is labeled as having an osmolarity of 2.04 mOsm/mL.[1(5/06)]

Osmolality

The osmolality of a calcium chloride 10% solution was determined by osmometer to be 1765 mOsm/kg.[1233]

Administration

Calcium chloride is administered by direct intravenous injection or by continuous or intermittent intravenous infusion. Intravenous administration should be performed slowly at a rate not exceeding 0.7 to 1.8 mEq/min. The drug may also be injected into the ventricular cavity in cardiac resuscitation. It must not be injected into the myocardium. Severe necrosis and sloughing may result if calcium chloride is injected intramuscularly or subcutaneously or leaks into the perivascular tissue.[1(5/06) 4]

Stability

The injection is clear and colorless. Intact vials should be stored at controlled room temperature. The single-use vials do not contain a preservative; the manufacturer recommends discarding any unused solution.[1(5/06)]

Calcium chloride injection under simulated summer conditions in paramedic vehicles was exposed to temperatures ranging from 26 to 38°C over 4 weeks. Analysis found no loss of the drug under these conditions.[2562]

Compatibility Information

Additive Compatibility

Calcium chloride

Test Drug	Test	Conc/L or %	Mfr	Conc/L or %	Test Solution	Remarks	Ref	C/I
Amikacin sulfate	BR	5 g	UP	1 g	D5LR, D5R, D5S, D5W, D10W, LR, NS, R, SL	Physically compatible and both stable for 24 hr at 25°C	294	C
Amphotericin B		200 mg	BP	4 g	D5W	Haze develops over 3 hr	26	I
Ascorbic acid	UP	500 mg	UP	1 g	D5W	Physically compatible	15	C
Ceftriaxone sodium						Incompatible. Precipitate may form in calcium-containing solutions	2222, 2731, 2784	I
Chloramphenicol sodium succinate	PD	10 g	UP	1 g	D5W	Physically compatible	15	C
Dobutamine HCl	LI	182 mg	UP	9 g	NS	Physically compatible for 20 hr. Haze forms at 24 hr	552	I
Dobutamine HCl	LI	1 g	ES	2 g	D5W, NS	Deeply pink in 24 hr at 25°C	789	I
Dobutamine HCl	LI	1 g	ES	50 g	D5W, NS	Physically compatible for 24 hr at 21°C	812	C
Dopamine HCl	AS	800 mg	UP		D5W	No dopamine loss in 24 hr at 25°C	312	C
Fat emulsion, intravenous	CU	10%		1 g		Immediate flocculation with visually apparent layer in 2 hr at room temperature	656	I

DOI: 10.37573/9781585286850.065

Additive Compatibility (Cont.)

Test Drug	Test	Conc/L or %	Mfr	Conc/L or %	Test Solution	Remarks	Ref	C/I
Fat emulsion, intravenous	CU	10%		500 mg		Flocculation within 4 hr at room temperature	656	I
Fat emulsion, intravenous	VT	10%	DB	1 g		Coalescence and creaming in 8 hr at 8 and 25°C	825	I
Fat emulsion, intravenous	KV	10%		10 and 20 mEq		Immediate flocculation, aggregation, and creaming	1018	I
Hydrocortisone sodium succinate	UP	500 mg	UP	1 g	D5W	Physically compatible	15	C
Isoproterenol HCl	WI	4 mg	UP	1 g		Physically compatible	59	C
Lidocaine HCl	AST	2 g	UP	1 g		Physically compatible	24	C
Magnesium sulfate	DB	10 to 50 g	DB	4 to 20 g	D5W, NS	Visible precipitate or microprecipitate forms at room temperature	2597	I
Magnesium sulfate	DB	4 g	DB	2 g	D5W, NS	No visible precipitate. Microscopic examination was inconclusive	2597	?
Magnesium sulfate	DB	2.5 g	DB	2 g	TPN #266[a]	No visible precipitate or microprecipitate in 24 hr at room temperature	2597	C
Norepinephrine bitartrate	WI	8 mg	UP	1 g	D5W, D10W, D2.5½S, D2.5S, D5¼S, D5½S, D5S, D10S, NS, ½S	Physically compatible	77	C
Penicillin G potassium	SQ	20 million units	UP	1 g	D5W	Physically compatible	15	C
Penicillin G sodium	UP	20 million units	UP	1 g	D5W	Physically compatible	15	C
Pentobarbital sodium	AB	1 g	UP	1 g	D5W	Physically compatible	15	C
Phenobarbital sodium	WI	200 mg	UP	1 g	D5W	Physically compatible	15	C
Potassium phosphates						Compatibility dependent on solubility and concentration and is not entirely predictable. See the monograph discussion under Additional Compatibility Information	1777, 2803	?
Sodium bicarbonate	AB		UP		D5W	Conditionally compatible depending on concentrations	15	?
Sodium bicarbonate	AB	2.4 mEq[b]		1 g	D5W	Physically compatible for 24 hr	772	C
Sodium phosphates						Compatibility dependent on solubility and concentration and is not entirely predictable. See the monograph discussion under Additional Compatibility Information	1777, 2803	?
Verapamil HCl	KN	80 mg	ES	2 g	D5W, NS	Physically compatible for 24 hr	764	C

[a] Refer to Appendix for the composition of parenteral nutrition solutions. TPN indicates a 2-in-1 admixture.

[b] One vial of Neut added to a liter of admixture.

Drugs in Syringe Compatibility

Calcium chloride

Test Drug	Mfr	Amt	Mfr	Amt	Remarks	Ref	C/I
Milrinone lactate	STR	5.25 mg/5.25 mL	AB	3 g/30 mL	Physically compatible. No milrinone loss in 20 min at 23°C	1410	C
Pantoprazole sodium	a	4 mg/1 mL		100 mg/1 mL	Precipitates	2574	I

[a] Test performed using the formulation WITHOUT edetate disodium.

Y-Site Injection Compatibility (1:1 Mixture)

Calcium chloride

Test Drug	Mfr	Conc	Mfr	Conc	Remarks	Ref	C/I
Amiodarone HCl	WY	6 mg/mL[a]	APP	10 mg/mL[a]	Visually compatible for 24 hr at 22°C	2352	C
Amiodarone HCl	WY	6 mg/mL[a]	APP	100 mg/mL	Visually compatible for 24 hr at 22°C	2352	C
Ceftaroline fosamil	FOR	2.22 mg/mL[a b e]	AMR	40 mg/mL[a b e]	Physically compatible for 4 hr at 23°C	2826	C
Ceftolozane sulfate–tazobactam sodium	CUB	10 mg/mL[c f]	HOS	20 mg/mL[c]	Physically compatible for 2 hr	3262	C
Cloxacillin sodium	SMX	100 mg/mL	HOS	100 mg/mL	Physically compatible for up to 4 hr at room temperature	3245	C
Dobutamine HCl	LI	4 mg/mL[c]	AB	4 mg/mL[c]	Physically compatible for 3 hr	1316	C
Doxapram HCl	RB	2 mg/mL[a]	APP	100 mg/mL	Visually compatible for 4 hr at 23°C	2470	C
Epinephrine HCl	ES	0.032 mg/mL[c]	AB	4 mg/mL[c]	Physically compatible for 3 hr	1316	C
Eravacycline dihydro-chloride	TET	0.6 mg/mL[b]	HOS	20 mg/mL[b]	Physically compatible for 2 hr at room temperature	3532	C
Esmolol HCl	DCC	10 mg/mL[a]	AB	20 mg/mL[a]	Physically compatible for 24 hr at 22°C	1169	C
Hydroxyethyl starch 130/0.4 in sodium chloride 0.9%	FRK	6%	HOS	20, 40, 80 mg/mL[a]	Visually compatible for 24 hr at room temperature	2770	C
Isavuconazonium sulfate	ASP	1.5 mg/mL[c]	HOS, AMP	20 mg/mL[c]	Physically compatible for 2 hr	3263	C
Meropenem		50 mg/mL	LIF	100 mg/mL	Physically compatible for 4 hr at room temperature	3538	C
Meropenem–vabor-bactam	TMC	8 mg/mL[b g]	HOS	20 mg/mL[b]	Precipitation and increase in measured turbidity within 30 min. pH increased by >3 units within 3 hr	3380	I
Micafungin sodium	ASP	1.5 mg/mL[b]	AB	40 mg/mL[b]	Physically compatible for 4 hr at 23°C	2683	C
Milrinone lactate	SS	0.2 mg/mL[a]	AMR	20 mg/mL[a]	Visually compatible for 4 hr at 25°C	2381	C
Morphine sulfate	WY	0.2 mg/mL[c]	AB	4 mg/mL[c]	Physically compatible for 3 hr	1316	C
Paclitaxel	NCI	1.2 mg/mL[a]	AST	20 mg/mL[a]	Physically compatible for 4 hr at 22°C	1556	C
Plazomicin sulfate	ACH	24 mg/mL[c]	HOS	20 mg/mL[c]	White particulates form within 1 hr; pH increased by >1 unit within 30 min	3432	I
Propofol	ZEN[h]	10 mg/mL	AST	40 mg/mL[a]	White precipitate forms in 1 hr	2066	I
Sodium bicarbonate	AB	1 mEq/mL	AB	4 mg/mL[c]	Slight haze or precipitate in 1 hr	1316	I

Y-Site Injection Compatibility (1:1 Mixture) (Cont.)

Test Drug	Mfr	Conc	Mfr	Conc	Remarks	Ref	C/I
Sodium nitroprusside	RC	0.3, 1.2, 3 mg/mL[a]	AST	0.4 and 1.36 mEq/mL[d]	Visually compatible for 48 hr at 24°C protected from light	2357	C
Sodium nitroprusside	RC	1.2 and 3 mg/mL[a]	AST	0.8 mEq/mL[d]	Visually compatible for 48 hr at 24°C protected from light	2357	C
Tedizolid phosphate	CUB	0.8 mg/mL[b]	HOS	20 mg/mL[b]	Immediate precipitation and increase in measured turbidity	3244	I

[a] Tested in dextrose 5%.

[b] Tested in sodium chloride 0.9%.

[c] Tested in both dextrose 5% and sodium chloride 0.9%.

[d] Tested in dextrose 5% in sodium chloride 0.225%.

[e] Tested in Ringer's injection, lactated.

[f] Ceftolozane component. Ceftolozane in a 2:1 fixed-ratio concentration with tazobactam.

[g] Meropenem component. Meropenem in a 1:1 fixed-ratio concentration with vaborbactam.

[h] Test performed using the formulation WITH edetate disodium.

Additional Compatibility Information

Calcium and Phosphate

UNRECOGNIZED CALCIUM PHOSPHATE PRECIPITATION IN A 3-IN-1 PARENTERAL NUTRITION MIXTURE RESULTED IN PATIENT DEATH.

The potential for the formation of a calcium phosphate precipitate in parenteral nutrition solutions is well studied and documented,[1771 1777] but the information is complex and difficult to apply to the clinical situation.[1770 1772 1777] The incorporation of fat emulsion in 3-in-1 parenteral nutrition solutions obscures any precipitate that is present, which has led to substantial debate on the dangers associated with 3-in-1 parenteral nutrition mixtures and when or if the danger to the patient is warranted therapeutically.[1770 1771 1772 2031 2032 2033 2034 2035 2036] Because such precipitation may be life-threatening to patients,[2037 2291] FDA issued a Safety Alert containing the following recommendations:[1769]

1. "The amounts of phosphorus and of calcium added to the admixture are critical. The solubility of the added calcium should be calculated from the volume at the time the calcium is added. It should not be based upon the final volume.

   Some amino acid injections for TPN admixtures contain phosphate ions (as a phosphoric acid buffer). These phosphate ions and the volume at the time the phosphate is added should be considered when calculating the concentration of phosphate additives. Also, when adding calcium and phosphate to an admixture, the phosphate should be added first.

   The line should be flushed between the addition of any potentially incompatible components.

2. A lipid emulsion in a 3-in-1 admixture obscures the presence of a precipitate. Therefore, if a lipid emulsion is needed, either (1) use a 2-in-1 admixture with the lipid infused separately, or (2) if a 3-in-1 admixture is medically necessary, then add the calcium before the lipid emulsion and according to the recommendations in number 1 above.

   If the amount of calcium or phosphate which must be added is likely to cause a precipitate, some or all of the calcium should be administered separately. Such separate infusions must be properly diluted and slowly infused to avoid serious adverse events related to the calcium.

3. When using an automated compounding device, the above steps should be considered when programming the device. In addition, automated compounders should be maintained and operated according to the manufacturer's recommendations.

   Any printout should be checked against the programmed admixture and weight of components.

4. During the mixing process, pharmacists who mix parenteral nutrition admixtures should periodically agitate the admixture and check for precipitates. Medical or home care personnel who start and monitor these infusions should carefully inspect for the presence of precipitates both before and during infusion. Patients and care givers should be trained to visually inspect for signs of precipitation. They also should be advised to stop the infusion and seek medical assistance if precipitates are noted.

5. A filter should be used when infusing either central or peripheral parenteral nutrition admixtures. At this time, data have not been submitted to document which size filter is most effective in trapping precipitates.

   Standards of practice vary, but the following is suggested: a 1.2-μm air-eliminating filter for lipid-containing admixtures and a 0.22-μm air-eliminating filter for non-lipid-containing admixtures.

6. Parenteral nutrition admixtures should be administered within the following time frames: if stored at room temperature, the infusion should be started within 24 hours after mixing; if stored at refrigerated temperatures, the infusion should be started within 24 hours of rewarming. Because warming parenteral nutrition admixtures may contribute to the formation of precipitates, once administration begins, care should be taken to avoid excessive warming of the admixture.

Persons administering home care parenteral nutrition admixtures may need to deviate from these time frames. Pharmacists who initially prepare these admixtures should check a reserve sample for precipitates over the duration and under the conditions of storage.

7. If symptoms of acute respiratory distress, pulmonary emboli, or interstitial pneumonitis develop, the infusion should be stopped immediately and thoroughly checked for precipitates. Appropriate medical interventions should be instituted. Home care personnel and patients should immediately seek medical assistance."[1769]

Calcium Phosphate Precipitation Fatalities

Fatal cases of paroxysmal respiratory failure in 2 previously healthy women receiving peripheral vein parenteral nutrition were reported. The patients experienced sudden cardiopulmonary arrest consistent with pulmonary emboli. The authors used in vitro simulations and an animal model to conclude that unrecognized calcium phosphate precipitation in a 3-in-1 total nutrition admixture caused the fatalities. The precipitation resulted during compounding by introducing calcium and phosphate near to one another in the compounding sequence and prior to complete fluid addition. This resulted in a temporarily high concentration of the drugs and precipitation of calcium phosphate. Observation of the precipitate was obscured by the incorporation of 20% fat emulsion, intravenous, into the nutrition mixture. No filter was used during infusion of the fatal nutrition admixtures.[2037]

In a follow-up retrospective review, 5 patients were identified who had respiratory distress associated with the infusion of the 3-in-1 admixtures at around the same time. Four of these 5 patients died, although the cause of death could be definitively determined for only 2.[2291]

Calcium and Phosphate Conditional Compatibility

Calcium salts are conditionally compatible with phosphate in parenteral nutrition solutions. The incompatibility is dependent on a solubility and concentration phenomenon and is not entirely predictable. Precipitation may occur during compounding or at some time after compounding is completed.

NOTE: Some amino acid solutions inherently contain calcium and phosphate, which must be considered in any projection of compatibility.

A study determined the maximum concentrations of calcium (as chloride and gluconate) and phosphate (as sodium phosphates) that can be maintained without precipitation in a parenteral nutrition solution consisting of FreAmine II 4.25% and dextrose 25% for 24 hours at 30°C. It was noted that the amino acids in parenteral nutrition solutions form soluble complexes with calcium and phosphate, reducing the available free calcium and phosphate that can form insoluble precipitates. The concentration of calcium available for precipitation is greater with the chloride salt compared to the gluconate salt, at least in part

because of differences in dissociation characteristics. Consequently, a greater concentration of calcium gluconate than calcium chloride can be mixed with sodium phosphate.[608]

In addition to the concentrations of phosphate and calcium and the salt form of the calcium, the concentration of amino acids and the time and temperature of storage altered the formation of calcium phosphate in parenteral nutrition solutions. As the temperature was increased, the incidence of precipitate formation also increased. This finding was attributed, at least in part, to a greater degree of dissociation of the calcium and phosphate complexes and the decreased solubility of calcium phosphate. Therefore, a solution possibly may be stored at 4°C with no precipitation, but on warming to room temperature a precipitate will form over time.[608]

The maximum allowable concentrations of calcium and phosphate in a 3-in-1 parenteral nutrition mixture for children (TNA #192 in Appendix) were reported. Added calcium was varied from 1.5 to 150 mmol/L, and added phosphate was varied from 21 to 300 mmol/L. These mixtures were stable for 48 hours at 22 and 37°C as long as the pH was not greater than 5.7, the calcium concentration was below 16 mmol/L, the phosphate concentration was below 52 mmol/L, and the product of the calcium and phosphate concentrations was below 250 $mmol^2/L^2$ (mmol squared per liter squared).[1773]

The presence of magnesium in solutions may also influence the reaction between calcium and phosphate, including the nature and extent of precipitation.[158][159]

The interaction of calcium and phosphate in parenteral nutrition solutions is a complex phenomenon. Various factors play a role in the solubility or precipitation of a given combination, including:[608][609][1042][1063][1210][1234][1427][2778]

1. Concentration of calcium
2. Salt form of calcium
3. Concentration of phosphate
4. Concentration of amino acids
5. Amino acids composition
6. Concentration of dextrose
7. Temperature of solution
8. pH of solution
9. Presence of other additives
10. Order of mixing

Enhanced precipitate formation would be expected from such factors as high concentrations of calcium and phosphate, increases in solution pH, decreases in amino acid concentrations, increases in temperature, addition of calcium before phosphate, lengthy standing times or slow infusion rates, and use of calcium as the chloride salt.[854]

Even if precipitation does not occur in the container, it has been reported that crystallization of calcium phosphate may occur in a Silastic infusion pump chamber or tubing if the rate of administration is slow, as for premature infants. Water vapor may be transmitted outward and be replaced by air rapidly enough to produce supersaturation.[202] Several other cases of catheter occlusion have been reported.[610][1427][1428][1429]

Calcium Gluconate
AHFS 40:12

Products

Calcium gluconate is available in 10- and 50-mL single-dose (preservative-free) vials and 100-mL pharmacy bulk packages as a 10% solution.[3289] Each mL contains 100 mg of calcium gluconate (equivalent to 94 mg of calcium gluconate with 4.5 mg of calcium saccharate tetrahydrate) and hydrochloric acid and/or sodium hydroxide for pH adjustment in water for injection, providing 9.3 mg (0.465 mEq) of elemental calcium.[3289] Aluminum also is present.[3289]

For direct intravenous injection, the calcium gluconate dose should be diluted in dextrose 5% or sodium chloride 0.9% to a concentration of 10 to 50 mg/mL.[3289] For continuous intravenous infusion, the calcium gluconate dose should be diluted in dextrose 5% or sodium chloride 0.9% to a concentration of 5.8 to 10 mg/mL.[3289]

pH

From 6 to 8.2.[3289]

Osmolarity

The osmolarity is stated to be 680 mOsm/L.[3313]

Osmolality

The osmolality of a calcium gluconate 10% solution was determined by osmometer to be 276 mOsm/kg.[1233]

Administration

Calcium gluconate usually is administered intravenously, slowly by direct intravenous injection, or by continuous or intermittent intravenous infusion, following appropriate dilution in dextrose 5% or sodium chloride 0.9%.[3289] The drug diluted for infusion should be administered through a secure intravenous line.[3289] When calcium gluconate diluted in a compatible infusion solution is administered slowly by direct intravenous injection or by continuous or intermittent intravenous infusion, the infusion rate should not exceed 200 mg of calcium gluconate per minute in adults or 100 mg of calcium gluconate per minute in pediatric patients, including neonates.[3289]

Intramuscular or subcutaneous injection of the drug is *not* recommended because of possible severe necrosis and sloughing.[183][184][185][359][3313] If extravasation occurs or if clinical manifestations of calcinosis cutis are present, administration at that site should be discontinued and appropriate treatment should be instituted.[3289]

Stability

Calcium gluconate injection is a supersaturated solution that has been stabilized by the addition of calcium saccharate.[3313] Intact vials should be stored at controlled room temperature.[3289] Freezing should be avoided.[3289] The solution should appear clear and colorless to slightly yellow; the solution should not be used if particulate matter or a precipitate is present or if discoloration has occurred.[3289]

The manufacturer states that doses dispensed from the pharmacy bulk package and diluted solutions must be used immediately.[3289] Unused portions of single-dose vials should be discarded immediately, and pharmacy bulk packages should be discarded after 4 hours of initial puncture.[3289]

Precipitation

Calcium gluconate injection is a supersaturated solution, and such solutions are susceptible to precipitation.[3289] If precipitates have formed, they may be dissolved by warming affected vials to 60 to 80°C with occasional agitation until a clear solution results, followed by vigorous shaking of the vials.[3289] Warmed vials should be allowed to cool to room temperature prior to dispensing.[3289] Contents of such vials should only be used if they are clear immediately prior to use.[3289]

Compatibility Information

Solution Compatibility

Calcium gluconate

Test Soln Name	Mfr	Mfr	Conc/L or %	Remarks	Ref	C/I
Dextrose 5% in Ringer's injection, lactated	BA	PD	2 g	Physically compatible for 24 hr	315	C
Dextrose 5% in sodium chloride 0.9%			1 g	Physically compatible	74	C
Dextrose 5% in sodium chloride 0.9%	BA	PD	2 g	Physically compatible for 24 hr	315	C
Dextrose 5%			1 g	Physically compatible	74	C
Dextrose 5%	BA	PD	2 g	Physically compatible for 24 hr	315	C

DOI: 10.37573/9781585286850.066

Solution Compatibility (Cont.)

Test Soln Name	Mfr	Mfr	Conc/L or %	Remarks	Ref	C/I
Dextrose 10%	BA	PD	2 g	Physically compatible for 24 hr	315	C
Dextrose 10%		BP	18 g	Physically compatible for 30 hr at room temperature under fluorescent light	1347	C
Dextrose 20%	BA	PD	2 g	Physically compatible for 24 hr	315	C
Ringer's injection, lactated			1 g	Physically compatible	74	C
Ringer's injection, lactated	BA	PD	2 g	Physically compatible for 24 hr	315	C
Sodium chloride 0.9%			1 g	Physically compatible	74	C
Sodium chloride 0.9%	BA	PD	2 g	Physically compatible for 24 hr	315	C
Sodium lactate ⅙ M	BA	PD	2 g	Physically compatible for 24 hr	315	C

Additive Compatibility

Calcium gluconate

Test Drug	Mfr	Conc/L or %	Mfr	Conc/L or %	Test Solution	Remarks	Ref	C/I
Amikacin sulfate	BR	5 g	UP	500 mg	D5LR, D5R, D5S, D5W, D10W, LR, NS, R, SL	Physically compatible and both stable for 24 hr at 25°C	294	C
Aminophylline		250 mg		1 g	D5W	Physically compatible	74	C
Amphotericin B		200 mg	BP	4 g	D5W	Haze develops over 3 hr	26	I
Ascorbic acid	UP	500 mg	UP	1 g	D5W	Physically compatible	15	C
Ceftriaxone sodium						Incompatible. Precipitate may form in calcium-containing solutions	2222, 2731, 2784	I
Chloramphenicol sodium succinate	PD	500 mg		1 g	D5W	Physically compatible	74	C
Chloramphenicol sodium succinate	PD	10 g	UP	1 g	D5W	Physically compatible	15	C
Chloramphenicol sodium succinate	PD	10 g	UP	1 g		Physically compatible	6	C
Dobutamine HCl	LI	182 mg	VI	9 g	NS	Small particles form within 4 hr. White precipitate and haze after 15 hr	552	I
Dobutamine HCl	LI	1 g	ES	2 g	D5W, NS	Deeply pink in 24 hr at 25°C	789	I
Dobutamine HCl	LI	1 g	IX	50 g	D5W, NS	Small white particles in 24 hr at 21°C	812	I
Fat emulsion, intravenous	VT	10%	PR	2 g		Produced cracked emulsion	32	I
Fat emulsion, intravenous	KV	10%		7.2 and 9.6 mEq		Immediate flocculation, aggregation, and creaming	1018	I
Floxacillin sodium	BE	20 g	ANT	2 g	NS	White precipitate forms immediately	1479	I
Furosemide	HO	1 g	ANT	2 g	NS	Physically compatible for 72 hr at 15 and 30°C	1479	C
Heparin sodium		12,000 units		1 g	D5W	Physically compatible	74	C
Heparin sodium	UP	4000 units	UP	1 g	D5W	Physically compatible	15	C

Additive Compatibility (Cont.)

Test Drug	Mfr	Conc/L or %	Mfr	Conc/L or %	Test Solution	Remarks	Ref	C/I
Heparin sodium	AB	20,000 units	UP	1 g		Physically compatible	21	C
Hydrocortisone sodium succinate	UP	100 mg		1 g	D5W	Physically compatible	74	C
Hydrocortisone sodium succinate	UP	500 mg	UP	1 g	D5W	Physically compatible	15	C
Lidocaine HCl	AST	2 g	ES	2 g	D5W, LR, NS	Physically compatible for 24 hr at 25°C	775	C
Magnesium sulfate	DB	10 to 50 g	DB	12 to 60 g	D5W, NS	Visible precipitate or microprecipitate forms at room temperature	2597	I
Magnesium sulfate	DB	5 g	DB	6 g	D5W, NS	No visible precipitate or microprecipitate in 24 hr at room temperature	2597	C
Magnesium sulfate	SZ	4 g	PP	4 g	D5W, NS	Physically compatible for 7 days at 5 and 25°C protected from light	2909	C
Magnesium sulfate	SZ	10 g	PP	10 g	D5W, NS	Physically compatible for 7 days at 5 and 25°C protected from light	2909	C
Methylprednisolone sodium succinate	UP	40 mg		1 g	D5S	Physically incompatible	329	I
Norepinephrine bitartrate	WI	8 mg		1 g	D5W	Physically compatible	74	C
Penicillin G potassium		1 million units		1 g	D5W	Physically compatible	74	C
Penicillin G potassium	SQ	20 million units	UP	1 g	D5W	Physically compatible	15	C
Penicillin G sodium	UP	20 million units	UP	1 g	D5W	Physically compatible	15	C
Phenobarbital sodium	WI	200 mg	UP	1 g	D5W	Physically compatible	15	C
Potassium chloride		3 g		1 g	D5W	Physically compatible	74	C
Potassium phosphates						Compatibility dependent on solubility and concentration and is not entirely predictable. See the monograph discussion under Additional Compatibility Information	1777, 2803	?
Prochlorperazine edisylate	SKF	100 mg	UP	1 g	D5W	Physically compatible	15	C
Sodium bicarbonate	AB		UP		D5W	Conditionally compatible depending on concentrations	15	?
Sodium phosphates						Compatibility dependent on solubility and concentration and is not entirely predictable. See the monograph discussion under Additional Compatibility Information	1777, 2803	?
Tobramycin sulfate	LI	5 g		16 g	D5W	Physically compatible. No tobramycin loss in 60 min at room temperature	984	C
Tobramycin sulfate	LI	1 g		33 g	D5W	Physically compatible. No tobramycin loss in 60 min at room temperature	984	C
Vancomycin HCl	LI	1 g		1 g	D5W	Physically compatible	74	C
Verapamil HCl	KN	80 mg	IX	2 g	D5W, NS	Physically compatible for 48 hr	739	C

Drugs in Syringe Compatibility

Calcium gluconate

Test Drug	Mfr	Amt	Mfr	Amt	Remarks	Ref	C/I
Caffeine citrate		20 mg/1 mL		100 mg/1 mL	Physically compatible and chemically stable for 24 hr at room temperature	1(12/07)	C
Dimenhydrinate		10 mg/1 mL		100 mg/1 mL	Clear solution	2569	C
Metoclopramide HCl	RB	10 mg/2 mL	ES	1 g/10 mL	Possible precipitate formation	924	I
Metoclopramide HCl	RB	160 mg/32 mL	ES	1 g/10 mL	Incompatible. If mixed, use immediately	1167	I
Pantoprazole sodium	a	4 mg/1 mL		100 mg/1 mL	Precipitates	2574	I

[a] Test performed using the formulation WITHOUT edetate disodium.

Y-Site Injection Compatibility (1:1 Mixture)

Calcium gluconate

Test Drug	Mfr	Conc	Mfr	Conc	Remarks	Ref	C/I
Aldesleukin	CHI	33800 I.U./mL[a]	LY	100 mg/mL	Visually compatible with little or no loss of aldesleukin activity	1857	C
Allopurinol sodium	BW	3 mg/mL[b]	AMR	40 mg/mL[b]	Physically compatible for 4 hr at 22°C	1686	C
Amifostine	USB	10 mg/mL[a]	AMR	40 mg/mL[a]	Physically compatible for 4 hr at 23°C	1845	C
Amiodarone HCl	WY	6 mg/mL[a]	AMR	10 mg/mL[a]	Visually compatible for 24 hr at 22°C	2352	C
Ampicillin sodium	WY	40 mg/mL[b]	AST	4 mg/mL[b]	Physically compatible for 3 hr	1316	C
Ampicillin sodium	WY	40 mg/mL[b]	AST	4 mg/mL[a]	Slight color change in 1 hr	1316	I
Aztreonam	SQ	40 mg/mL[a]	AMR	40 mg/mL[a]	Physically compatible for 4 hr at 23°C	1758	C
Bivalirudin	TMC	5 mg/mL[a]	APP	40 mg/mL[a]	Physically compatible for 4 hr at 23°C	2373	C
Cangrelor tetrasodium	TMC	1 mg/mL[b]		40 mg/mL[b]	Cloudy white precipitate with particulates appears immediately	3243	I
Cefazolin sodium	LI	40 mg/mL[c]	AST	4 mg/mL[c]	Physically compatible for 3 hr	1316	C
Ceftaroline fosamil	FOR	2.22 mg/mL[e]	ABX	40 mg/mL[e]	Physically compatible for 4 hr at 23°C	2826	C
Ceftolozane sulfate–tazobactam sodium	CUB	10 mg/mL[c n]	FRK	20 mg/mL[c]	Physically compatible for 2 hr	3262	C
Ciprofloxacin	MI	2 mg/mL[a]	LY	10%	Visually compatible for 2 hr at 25°C	1628	C
Cisatracurium besylate	GW	0.1, 2, 5 mg/mL[a]	AB	40 mg/mL[a]	Physically compatible for 4 hr at 23°C	2074	C
Cisatracurium besylate	AB	1 mg/mL[b]	APP	20 mg/mL[b]	Physically compatible for 1 hr at 23°C	3157	C
Cladribine	ORT	0.015[b] and 0.5[d] mg/mL	AMR	40 mg/mL[b]	Physically compatible for 4 hr at 23°C	1969	C
Clevidipine butyrate	CHS	0.5 mg/mL		40 mg/mL[f]	Physically compatible for 24 hr at 23°C	3334	C
Cloxacillin sodium	SMX	100 mg/mL	PPC	100 mg/mL	Physically compatible for up to 4 hr at room temperature	3245	C
Dexmedetomidine HCl	AB	4 mcg/mL[b]	APP	40 mg/mL[b]	Physically compatible for 4 hr at 23°C	2383	C
Dobutamine HCl	LI	4 mg/mL[c]	AST	4 mg/mL[c]	Physically compatible for 3 hr	1316	C
Docetaxel	RPR	0.9 mg/mL[a]	FUJ	40 mg/mL[a]	Physically compatible for 4 hr at 23°C	2224	C

Y-Site Injection Compatibility (1:1 Mixture) (Cont.)

Test Drug	Mfr	Conc	Mfr	Conc	Remarks	Ref	C/I
Doripenem	JJ	5 mg/mL[a] [b]	AMR	40 mg/mL[a] [b]	Physically compatible for 4 hr at 23°C	2743	C
Doxapram HCl	RB	2 mg/mL[a]	APP	100 mg/mL	Visually compatible for 4 hr at 23°C	2470	C
Doxorubicin HCl liposomal	SEQ	0.4 mg/mL[a]	AB	40 mg/mL[a]	Physically compatible for 4 hr at 23°C	2087	C
Enalaprilat	MSD	0.05 mg/mL[b]	ES	0.092 mEq/mL[a]	Physically compatible for 24 hr at room temperature	1355	C
Epinephrine HCl	ES	0.032 mg/mL[c]	AST	4 mg/mL[c]	Physically compatible for 3 hr	1316	C
Eravacycline dihydrochloride	TET	0.6 mg/mL[b]	FRK	20 mg/mL[b]	Physically compatible for 2 hr at room temperature	3532	C
Etoposide phosphate	BR	5 mg/mL[a]	FUJ	40 mg/mL[a]	Physically compatible for 4 hr at 23°C	2218	C
Famotidine	MSD	0.2 mg/mL[a]	LY	0.00465 mEq/mL[b]	Physically compatible for 14 hr	1196	C
Fenoldopam mesylate	AB	80 mcg/mL[b]	APP	40 mg/mL[b]	Physically compatible for 4 hr at 23°C	2467	C
Filgrastim	AMG	30 mcg/mL[a]	AST	40 mg/mL[a]	Physically compatible for 4 hr at 22°C	1687	C
Fluconazole	RR	2 mg/mL	ES	100 mg/mL	Cloudiness develops	1407	I
Gemcitabine HCl	LI	10 mg/mL[b]	FUJ	40 mg/mL[b]	Physically compatible for 4 hr at 23°C	2226	C
Granisetron HCl	SKB	0.05 mg/mL[a]	AB	40 mg/mL[a]	Physically compatible for 4 hr at 23°C	2000	C
Heparin sodium[k]	RI	1000 units/L[e]	ES	100 mg/mL	Physically compatible for 4 hr at room temperature	322	C
Hetastarch in lactated electrolyte	AB	6%	FUJ	40 mg/mL[a]	Physically compatible for 4 hr at 23°C	2339	C
Hydrocortisone sodium succinate[l]	UP	100 mg/L[e]	ES	100 mg/mL	Physically compatible for 4 hr at room temperature	322	C
Hydroxyethyl starch 130/0.4 in sodium chloride 0.9%	FRK	6%	PP	20, 30, 40 mg/mL[a]	Visually compatible for 24 hr at room temperature	2770	C
Indomethacin sodium trihydrate	MSD	1 mg/mL[b]	AMR	100 mg/mL	Fine yellow precipitate forms within 1 hr	1527	I
Isavuconazonium sulfate	ASP	1.5 mg/mL[c]	APP	20 mg/mL[c]	Physically compatible for 2 hr	3263	C
Labetalol HCl	SC	1 mg/mL[a]	AMR	0.23 mEq/mL[a]	Physically compatible for 24 hr at 18°C	1171	C
Linezolid	PHU	2 mg/mL	AMR	40 mg/mL[a]	Physically compatible for 4 hr at 23°C	2264	C
Melphalan HCl	BW	0.1 mg/mL[b]	AST	40 mg/mL[b]	Physically compatible for 3 hr at 22°C	1557	C
Meropenem	ZEN	1 mg/mL[b]	AMR	4 mg/mL[f]	Visually compatible for 4 hr at room temperature	1994	C
Meropenem	ZEN	50 mg/mL[b]	AMR	4 mg/mL[f]	Yellow discoloration forms in 4 hr at room temperature	1994	I
Meropenem		50 mg/mL	FRK	100 mg/mL	Yellow color change occurred within 4 hr	3538	I
Meropenem–vaborbactam	TMC	8 mg/mL[b] [o]	FRK	20 mg/mL[b]	Physically compatible for 3 hr at 20 to 25°C	3380	C
Micafungin sodium	ASP	1.5 mg/mL[b]	AMR	40 mg/mL[b]	Physically compatible for 4 hr at 23°C	2683	C

Y-Site Injection Compatibility (1:1 Mixture) (Cont.)

Test Drug	Mfr	Conc	Mfr	Conc	Remarks	Ref	C/I
Midazolam HCl	RC	1 mg/mL[a]	FUJ	100 mg/mL	Visually compatible for 24 hr at 23°C	1847	C
Milrinone lactate	SW	0.4 mg/mL[a]	LY	0.465 mEq/mL	Visually compatible with no loss of milrinone in 4 hr at 23°C	2214	C
Milrinone lactate	SS	0.2 mg/mL[a]	AMR	50 mg/mL[a]	Visually compatible for 4 hr at 25°C	2381	C
Nicardipine HCl	DCC	0.1 mg/mL[a]	ES	0.092 mEq/mL[a]	Visually compatible for 24 hr at room temperature	235	C
Oritavancin diphosphate	TAR	0.8, 1.2, and 2 mg/mL[a]	AMR	40 mg/mL[a]	Visually compatible for 4 hr at 20 to 24°C	2928	C
Oxaliplatin	SS	0.5 mg/mL[a]	APP	40 mg/mL[a]	Physically compatible for 4 hr at 23°C	2566	C
Pemetrexed disodium	LI	20 mg/mL[b]	APP	40 mg/mL[a]	White microparticulates form within 4 hr	2564	I
Piperacillin sodium-tazobactam sodium	LE[j]	40 mg/mL[a m]	AMR	40 mg/mL[a]	Physically compatible for 4 hr at 22°C	1688	C
Plazomicin sulfate	ACH	24 mg/mL[c]	FRK	20 mg/mL[c]	Physically compatible for 1 hr at 20 to 25°C	3432	C
Potassium chloride		40 mEq/L[e]	ES	100 mg/mL	Physically compatible for 4 hr at room temperature	322	C
Prochlorperazine edisylate	SCN	5 mg/mL	AMR	10 mg/mL[b]	Visually compatible for 24 hr at room temperature	2063	C
Propofol	ZEN[p]	10 mg/mL	AMR	40 mg/mL[a]	Physically compatible for 1 hr at 23°C	2066	C
Remifentanil HCl	GW	0.025 and 0.25 mg/mL[b]	AB	40 mg/mL[a]	Physically compatible for 4 hr at 23°C	2075	C
Sargramostim	IMM	10 mcg/mL[b]	AMR	40 mg/mL[b]	Visually compatible for 4 hr at 22°C	1436	C
Tacrolimus	FUJ	1 mg/mL[b]	ES	100 mg/mL	Visually compatible for 24 hr at 25°C	1630	C
Tedizolid phosphate	CUB	0.8 mg/mL[b]	APP	20 mg/mL[b]	Immediate precipitation and increase in measured turbidity	3244	I
Telavancin HCl	ASP	7.5 mg/mL[e]	APP	40 mg/mL[e]	Physically compatible for 2 hr	2830	C
Teniposide	BR	0.1 mg/mL[a]	AMR	40 mg/mL[a]	Physically compatible for 4 hr at 23°C	1725	C
Thiotepa	IMM[h]	1 mg/mL[a]	AMR	40 mg/mL[a]	Physically compatible for 4 hr at 23°C	1861	C
TNA #218[i]			AB	40 mg/mL[a]	Visually compatible for 4 hr at 23°C	2215	C
TNA #219[i]			AB	40 mg/mL[a]	Visually compatible for 4 hr at 23°C	2215	C
TNA #220[i]			AB	40 mg/mL[a]	Visually compatible for 4 hr at 23°C	2215	C
TNA #221[i]			AB	40 mg/mL[a]	Visually compatible for 4 hr at 23°C	2215	C
TNA #222[i]			AB	40 mg/mL[a]	Visually compatible for 4 hr at 23°C	2215	C
TNA #223[i]			AB	40 mg/mL[a]	Visually compatible for 4 hr at 23°C	2215	C
TNA #224[i]			AB	40 mg/mL[a]	Visually compatible for 4 hr at 23°C	2215	C
TNA #225[i]			AB	40 mg/mL[a]	Visually compatible for 4 hr at 23°C	2215	C
TNA #226[i]			AB	40 mg/mL[a]	Visually compatible for 4 hr at 23°C	2215	C
TPN #189[i]			DB	10 mg/mL[b]	Visually compatible for 24 hr at 22°C	1767	C
TPN #212[i]			AB	40 mg/mL[a]	Physically compatible for 4 hr at 23°C	2109	C

Y-Site Injection Compatibility (1:1 Mixture) (Cont.)

Test Drug	Mfr	Conc	Mfr	Conc	Remarks	Ref	C/I
TPN #213[i]			AB	40 mg/mL[a]	Physically compatible for 4 hr at 23°C	2109	C
TPN #214			AB	40 mg/mL[a]	Physically compatible for 4 hr at 23°C	2109	C
TPN #215[i]			AB	40 mg/mL[a]	Physically compatible for 4 hr at 23°C	2109	C
Vinorelbine tartrate	BW	1 mg/mL[b]	AMR	40 mg/mL[b]	Physically compatible for 4 hr at 22°C	1558	C

[a] Tested in dextrose 5%.

[b] Tested in sodium chloride 0.9%.

[c] Tested in both dextrose 5% and sodium chloride 0.9%.

[d] Tested in bacteriostatic sodium chloride 0.9% preserved with benzyl alcohol 0.9%.

[e] Tested in dextrose 5%, Ringer's injection, lactated, and sodium chloride 0.9%.

[f] Tested in sterile water for injection.

[g] Tested in dextrose 5% in sodium chloride 0.9%.

[h] Lyophilized formulation tested.

[i] Refer to Appendix for the composition of parenteral nutrition solutions. TNA indicates a 3-in-1 admixture, and TPN indicates a 2-in-1 admixture.

[j] Test performed using the formulation WITHOUT edetate disodium.

[k] Tested in combination with hydrocortisone sodium succinate (Upjohn) 100 mg/L.

[l] Tested in combination with heparin sodium (Riker) 1000 units/L.

[m] Piperacillin component. Piperacillin in an 8:1 fixed-ratio concentration with tazobactam.

[n] Ceftolozane component. Ceftolozane in a 2:1 fixed-ratio concentration with tazobactam.

[o] Meropenem component. Meropenem in a 1:1 fixed-ratio concentration with vaborbactam.

[p] Test performed using the formulation WITH edetate disodium.

Additional Compatibility Information

Calcium and Phosphate

UNRECOGNIZED CALCIUM PHOSPHATE PRECIPITATION IN A 3-IN-1 PARENTERAL NUTRITION MIXTURE RESULTED IN PATIENT DEATH.

The potential for the formation of a calcium phosphate precipitate in parenteral nutrition solutions is well studied and documented,[1771 1777] but the information is complex and difficult to apply to the clinical situation.[1770 1772 1777] The incorporation of fat emulsion in 3-in-1 parenteral nutrition solutions obscures any precipitate that is present, which has led to substantial debate on the dangers associated with 3-in-1 parenteral nutrition mixtures and when or if the danger to the patient is warranted therapeutically.[1770 1771 1772 2031 2032 2033 2034 2035 2036] Because such precipitation may be life-threatening to patients,[2037 2291] FDA issued a Safety Alert containing the following recommendations:[1769]

1. "The amounts of phosphorus and of calcium added to the admixture are critical. The solubility of the added calcium should be calculated from the volume at the time the calcium is added. It should not be based upon the final volume.

   Some amino acid injections for TPN admixtures contain phosphate ions (as a phosphoric acid buffer). These phosphate ions and the volume at the time the phosphate is added should be considered when calculating the concentration of phosphate additives. Also, when adding calcium and phosphate to an admixture, the phosphate should be added first.

   The line should be flushed between the addition of any potentially incompatible components.

2. A lipid emulsion in a 3-in-1 admixture obscures the presence of a precipitate. Therefore, if a lipid emulsion is needed, either (1) use a 2-in-1 admixture with the lipid infused separately, or (2) if a 3-in-1 admixture is medically necessary, then add the calcium before the lipid emulsion and according to the recommendations in number 1 above.

   If the amount of calcium or phosphate which must be added is likely to cause a precipitate, some or all of the calcium should be administered separately. Such separate infusions must be properly diluted and slowly infused to avoid serious adverse events related to the calcium.

3. When using an automated compounding device, the above steps should be considered when programming the device. In addition, automated compounders should be maintained and operated according to the manufacturer's recommendations.

   Any printout should be checked against the programmed admixture and weight of components.

4. During the mixing process, pharmacists who mix parenteral nutrition admixtures should periodically agitate the admixture and check for precipitates. Medical or home care personnel who start and monitor these infusions should carefully inspect for the presence of precipitates both before and during infusion. Patients and care givers should be trained to visually inspect for signs of precipitation. They also should be advised to stop the infusion and seek medical assistance if precipitates are noted.

5. A filter should be used when infusing either central or peripheral parenteral nutrition admixtures. At this time, data have not been submitted to document which size filter is most effective in trapping precipitates.

Standards of practice vary, but the following is suggested: a 1.2-μm air-eliminating filter for lipid-containing admixtures and a 0.22-μm air-eliminating filter for non-lipid-containing admixtures.

6. Parenteral nutrition admixtures should be administered within the following time frames: if stored at room temperature, the infusion should be started within 24 hours after mixing; if stored at refrigerated temperatures, the infusion should be started within 24 hours of rewarming. Because warming parenteral nutrition admixtures may contribute to the formation of precipitates, once administration begins, care should be taken to avoid excessive warming of the admixture.

Persons administering home care parenteral nutrition admixtures may need to deviate from these time frames. Pharmacists who initially prepare these admixtures should check a reserve sample for precipitates over the duration and under the conditions of storage.

7. If symptoms of acute respiratory distress, pulmonary emboli, or interstitial pneumonitis develop, the infusion should be stopped immediately and thoroughly checked for precipitates. Appropriate medical interventions should be instituted. Home care personnel and patients should immediately seek medical assistance."[1769]

Calcium Phosphate Precipitation Fatalities

Fatal cases of paroxysmal respiratory failure in 2 previously healthy women receiving peripheral vein parenteral nutrition were reported. The patients experienced sudden cardiopulmonary arrest consistent with pulmonary emboli. The authors used in vitro simulations and an animal model to conclude that unrecognized calcium phosphate precipitation in a 3-in-1 total nutrition admixture caused the fatalities. The precipitation resulted during compounding by introducing calcium and phosphate near to one another in the compounding sequence and prior to complete fluid addition. This resulted in a temporarily high concentration of the drugs and precipitation of calcium phosphate. Observation of the precipitate was obscured by the incorporation of 20% fat emulsion, intravenous, into the nutrition mixture. No filter was used during infusion of the fatal nutrition admixtures.[2037]

In a follow-up retrospective review, 5 patients were identified who had respiratory distress associated with the infusion of the 3-in-1 admixtures at around the same time. Four of these 5 patients died, although the cause of death could be definitively determined for only 2.[2291]

Calcium and Phosphate Conditional Compatibility

Calcium salts are conditionally compatible with phosphate in parenteral nutrition solutions. The incompatibility is dependent on a solubility and concentration phenomenon and is not entirely predictable. Precipitation may occur during compounding or at some time after compounding is completed.

NOTE: Some amino acid solutions inherently contain both calcium and phosphate, which must be considered in any projection of compatibility.

A study determined the maximum concentrations of calcium (as chloride and gluconate) and phosphate (as sodium phosphates) that can be maintained without precipitation in a parenteral nutrition solution consisting of FreAmine II 4.25% and dextrose 25% for 24 hours at 30°C. It was noted that the amino acids in parenteral nutrition solutions form soluble complexes with calcium and phosphate, reducing the available free calcium and phosphate that can form insoluble precipitates. The concentration of calcium available for precipitation is greater with the chloride salt compared to the gluconate salt, at least in part because of differences in dissociation characteristics. Consequently, a greater concentration of calcium gluconate than calcium chloride can be mixed with sodium phosphate.[608]

In addition to the concentrations of phosphate and calcium and the salt form of the calcium, the concentration of amino acids and the time and temperature of storage altered the formation of calcium phosphate in parenteral nutrition solutions. As the temperature was increased, the incidence of precipitate formation also increased. This finding was attributed, at least in part, to a greater degree of dissociation of the calcium and phosphate complexes and the decreased solubility of calcium phosphate. Therefore, a solution possibly may be stored at 4°C with no precipitation, but on warming to room temperature a precipitate will form over time.[608]

The compatibility of calcium and phosphate in several parenteral nutrition formulas for newborn infants was evaluated. Calcium gluconate 10% (Cutter) and potassium phosphate (Abbott) were used to achieve concentrations of 2.5 to 100 mEq/L of calcium and 2.5 to 100 mmol/L of phosphorus added. The parenteral nutrition solutions evaluated were as shown in Table 1. The results were reported as graphic depictions.

Table 1. Parenteral nutrition solutions[609]

| Component | Solution Number | | | |
	#1	#2	#3	#4
FreAmine III	4%	2%	1%	1%
Dextrose	25%	20%	10%	10%
pH	6.3	6.4	6.6	7[a]

[a] Adjusted with sodium hydroxide.

The pH dependence of the phosphate–calcium precipitation has been noted. Dibasic calcium phosphate is very insoluble, while monobasic calcium phosphate is relatively soluble. At low pH, the soluble monobasic form predominates; but as the pH increases, more dibasic phosphate becomes available to bind with calcium and precipitate. Therefore, the lower the pH of the parenteral nutrition solution, the more calcium and phosphate can be solubilized. Once again, the effects of temperature were observed. As the temperature is increased, more calcium ion becomes available and more dibasic calcium phosphate is formed. Therefore, temperature increases will increase the amount of precipitate.[609]

Similar calcium and phosphate solubility curves were reported for neonatal parenteral nutrition solutions using TrophAmine (McGaw) 2, 1.5, and 0.8% as the sources of amino acids. The solutions also contained dextrose 10%, with cysteine and pH adjustment being used in some admixtures. Calcium and phosphate solubility followed the patterns reported previously.[609] A slightly greater concentration of phosphate could be used in some mixtures, but this finding was not consistent.[1024]

Using a similar study design, 6 neonatal parenteral nutrition solutions based on Aminosyn-PF (Abbott) 2, 1.5, and 0.8%, with and without added cysteine hydrochloride and dextrose 10% were studied. Calcium concentrations ranged from 2.5 to 50 mEq/L, and phosphate concentrations ranged from 2.5 to 50 mmol/L. Solutions sat for 18 hours at 25°C and then were warmed to 37°C in a water bath to simulate the clinical situation of warming prior to infusion into a child. Solubility curves were markedly different than those for TrophAmine in the previous study.[1024] Solubilities were reported to decrease by 15 mEq/L for calcium and 15 mmol/L for phosphate. The solutions remained clear during room temperature storage, but crystals often formed on warming to 37°C.[1211]

However, these data were questioned by Mikrut, who noted the similarities between the Aminosyn-PF and TrophAmine products and found little difference in calcium and phosphate solubilities in a preliminary report.[1212] In the full report,[1213] parenteral nutrition solutions containing Aminosyn-PF or TrophAmine 1 or 2.5% with dextrose 10 or 25%, respectively, plus electrolytes and trace metals, with or without cysteine hydrochloride, were evaluated under the same conditions. Calcium concentrations ranged from 2.5 to 50 mEq/L, and phosphate concentrations ranged from 5 to 50 mmol/L. In contrast to the previous results,[1024] the solubility curves were very similar for the Aminosyn-PF and TrophAmine parenteral nutrition solutions but very different from those of the previous Aminosyn-PF study.[1211] The authors again showed that the solubility of calcium and phosphate is greater in solutions containing higher concentrations of amino acids and dextrose.[1213]

Calcium and phosphate solubility curves for TrophAmine 1 and 2% with dextrose 10% and electrolytes, vitamins, heparin, and trace elements were reported. Calcium concentrations ranged from 10 to 60 mEq/L, and phosphorus concentrations ranged from 10 to 40 mmol/L. Calcium and phosphate solubilities were assessed by analysis of the calcium concentrations and followed patterns similar to those reported previously.[608 609] The higher percentage of amino acids (TrophAmine 2%) permitted a slightly greater solubility of calcium and phosphate, especially in the 10 to 50-mEq/L and 10 to 35-mmol/L ranges, respectively.[1614]

The maximal product of the amount of calcium (as gluconate) times phosphate (as potassium) that can be added to a parenteral nutrition solution, composed of amino acids 1% (Travenol) and dextrose 10%, for preterm infants was reported. Turbidity was observed on initial mixing when the solubility product was around 115 to 130 mmol² (mmol squared) or greater. After storage at 7°C for 20 hours, visible precipitates formed at solubility products of 130 mmol² (mmol squared) or greater. If the solution was administered through a barium-impregnated silicone rubber catheter, crystalline precipitates obstructed the catheters in 12 hours at a solubility product of 100 mmol² (mmol squared) and in 10 days at 79 mmol² (mmol squared), much lower than the in vitro results.[1041]

The solubility characteristics of calcium and phosphate in pediatric parenteral nutrition solutions composed of Aminosyn 0.5, 2, and 4% with dextrose 10 to 25% were reported. Also present were electrolytes and vitamins. Sodium phosphate was added sequentially in phosphorus concentrations from 10 to 30 mmol/L. Calcium gluconate was added last in amounts ranging from 1 to 10 g/L. The solutions were stored at 25°C for 30 hours and examined visually and microscopically for precipitation. The authors found that higher concentrations of Aminosyn increased the solubility of calcium and phosphate. Precipitation occurred at lower calcium and phosphate concentrations in the 0.5% solution compared to the 2 and 4% solutions. For example, at a phosphorus concentration of 30 mmol/L, precipitation occurred at calcium gluconate concentrations of about 1, 2, and 4 g/L in the 0.5, 2, and 4% Aminosyn mixtures, respectively. Similarly, at a calcium gluconate concentration of 8 g/L and above, precipitation occurred at phosphorus concentrations of about 13, 17, and 22 mmol/L in the 0.5, 2, and 4% solutions, respectively. The dextrose concentration did not appear to affect the calcium and phosphate solubility significantly.[1042]

The solubility of calcium and phosphorus in neonatal parenteral nutrition solutions composed of amino acids (Abbott) 1.25 and 2.5% with dextrose 5 and 10%, respectively, was evaluated. Also present were multivitamins and trace elements. The solutions contained calcium (as gluconate) in amounts ranging from 25 to 200 mg/100 mL. The phosphorus (as potassium phosphate) concentrations evaluated ranged from 25 to 150 mg/100 mL. If calcium gluconate was added first, cloudiness occurred immediately. If potassium phosphate was added first, substantial quantities could be added with no precipitate formation in 48 hours at 4°C (Table 2). However, if stored at 22°C, the solutions were stable for only 24 hours, and all contained precipitates after 48 hours.[1210]

Table 2. Maximum calcium and phosphorus concentrations physically compatible for 48 hours at 4°C[1210]

Calcium (mg/100 mL)	Phosphorus (mg/100 mL)	
	Amino Acids 1.25% + Dextrose 5%[a]	Amino Acids 2.5% + Dextrose 10%[a]
200[b]	50	75
150	50	100
100	75	100
50	100	125
25	150[b]	150[b]

[a] Plus multivitamins and trace elements.

[b] Maximum concentration tested.

The physical compatibility of calcium gluconate 10 to 40 mEq/L and potassium phosphates 10 to 40 mmol/L in 3 neonatal parenteral nutrition solutions (TPN #123 to #125 in Appendix), alone and with retrograde administration of aminophylline 7.5 mg diluted with 1.5 mL of sterile water for injection was reported. Contact of the alkaline aminophylline solution with the parenteral nutrition solutions resulted in the precipitation of calcium phosphate at much lower concentrations than were compatible in the parenteral nutrition solutions alone.[1404]

The maximum allowable concentrations of calcium and phosphate in a 3-in-1 parenteral nutrition mixture for children (TNA #192 in Appendix) were reported. Added calcium was varied from 1.5 to 150 mmol/L, while added phosphate was varied from 21 to 300 mmol/L. The mixtures were stable for 48 hours at 22 and 37°C as long as the pH was not greater than 5.7, the calcium concentration was below 16 mmol/L, the phosphate concentration was below 52 mmol/L, and the product of the calcium and phosphate concentrations was below 250 $mmol^2/L^2$ (mmol squared per liter squared).[1773]

Additional calcium and phosphate solubility curves were reported for specialty parenteral nutrition solutions based on NephrAmine and also HepatAmine at concentrations of 0.8, 1.5, and 2% as the sources of amino acids. The solutions also contained dextrose 10%, with cysteine and pH adjustment to simulate addition of fat emulsion used in some admixtures. Calcium and phosphate solubility followed the hyperbolic patterns previously reported.[609] Temperature, time, and pH affected calcium and phosphate solubility, with pH having the greatest effect.[2038]

The maximum sodium phosphate concentrations were reported for given amounts of calcium gluconate that could be admixed in parenteral nutrition solutions containing TrophAmine in varying quantities (with cysteine hydrochloride 40 mg/g of amino acid) and dextrose 10%. The solutions also contained magnesium sulfate 4 mEq/L, potassium acetate 24 mEq/L, sodium chloride 32 mEq/L, pediatric multivitamins, and trace elements. The presence of cysteine hydrochloride reduces the solution pH and increases the amount of calcium and phosphate that can be incorporated before precipitation occurs. The results of this study cannot be safely extrapolated to TPN solutions with compositions other than the ones tested. The admixtures were compounded with the sodium phosphate added last after thorough mixing of all other components. The authors noted that this is not the preferred order of mixing (usually phosphate is added first and thoroughly mixed before adding calcium last); however, they believed this reversed order of mixing would provide a margin of error in cases in which the proper order is not followed. After compounding, the solutions were stored for 24 hours at 40°C. The maximum calcium and phosphate amounts that could be mixed in the various solutions were reported tabularly and are shown in Table 3.[2039] However, these results are not entirely consistent with another study.[2196] See below.

Table 3. Maximum amount of phosphate (as sodium) (mmol/L) not resulting in precipitation.[2039] See CAUTION below.[a]

Calcium (as Gluconate)	Amino Acid (as TrophAmine) with Cysteine HCl 40 mg/g of Amino Acid				
	0%	0.4%	1%	2%	3%
9.8 mEq/L	0	27	42	60	66
14.7 mEq/L	0	15	18	30	36
19.6 mEq/L	0	6	15	27	30
29.4 mEq/L	0	3	6	21	24

[a] CAUTION: The results cannot be safely extrapolated to solutions with formulas other than the ones tested. See text.

The temperature dependence of the calcium–phosphate precipitation has resulted in the occlusion of a subclavian catheter by a solution apparently free of precipitation. The parenteral nutrition solution consisted of FreAmine III 500 mL, dextrose 70% 500 mL, sodium chloride 50 mEq, sodium phosphate 40 mmol, potassium acetate 10 mEq, potassium phosphate 40 mmol, calcium gluconate 10 mEq, magnesium sulfate 10 mEq, and Shil's trace metals solution 1 mL. Although there was no evidence of precipitation in the bottle, tubing and pump cassette, and filter (all at approximately 26°C) during administration, the occluded catheter and Vicra Loop Lock (next to the patient's body at 37°C) had numerous crystals identified as calcium phosphate. In vitro, this parenteral nutrition solution had a precipitate in 12 hours at 37°C but was clear for 24 hours at 26°C.[610]

Similarly, a parenteral nutrition solution that was clear and free of particulates after 2 weeks under refrigeration developed a precipitate in 4 to 6 hours when stored at room temperature. When the solution was warmed in a 37°C water bath, precipitation occurred in 1 hour. Administration of the solution before the precipitate was noticed led to interstitial pneumonitis due to deposition of calcium phosphate crystals.[1427]

A 2-mL fluid barrier of dextrose 5% in a microbore retrograde infusion set failed to prevent precipitation when used between calcium gluconate 200 mg/2 mL and sodium phosphate 0.3 mmol/0.1 mL.[1385]

Calcium phosphate precipitation phenomena was evaluated in a series of parenteral nutrition admixtures composed of dextrose 22%, amino acids (FreAmine III) 2.7%, and fat emulsion (Abbott) 0, 1, and 3.2%. Incorporation of calcium gluconate 19 to 24 mEq/L and phosphate (as sodium) 22 to 28 mmol/L resulted in visible precipitation in the fat-free admixtures. New precipitate continued to form over 14 days, even after repeated filtrations of the solutions through 0.2-μm filters. The presence of the amino acids increased calcium and phosphate solubility, compared with simple aqueous solutions. However, the incorporation of the fat emulsion did not result in a statistically significant increase in calcium and phosphate solubility. The authors noted that the kinetics of calcium phosphate precipitate formation do not appear to be entirely predictable; both transient and permanent precipitation can occur either during the compounding process or at some time afterward. Because calcium phosphate precipitation can be very dangerous clinically, the use of inline filters was recommended. The authors suggested that the filters should have a porosity appropriate to the parenteral nutrition admixture—1.2 μm for fat-containing and 0.2 or 0.45 μm for fat-free nutrition mixtures.[2061]

Laser particle analysis was used to evaluate the formation of calcium phosphate precipitation in pediatric TPN solutions containing TrophAmine in concentrations ranging from 0.5 to 3% with dextrose 10% and also containing L-cysteine hydrochloride 1 g/L. The solutions also contained in each liter sodium chloride 20 mEq, sodium acetate 20 mEq, magnesium sulfate 3 mEq, trace elements 3 mL, and heparin sodium 500 units. The presence of L-cysteine hydrochloride reduces the solution pH and increases the amount of calcium and phosphate that can be incorporated before precipitation occurs. The results of this study cannot be safely extrapolated to TPN solutions with compositions other than the ones tested. The maximum amount of phosphate that was incorporated without the appearance of a measurable increase in particulates in 24 hours at 37°C for each of the amino acids concentrations is shown in Table 4.[2196] These results are not entirely consistent with previous results.[2039] See Table 3. The use of more sensitive electronic particle measurement for the formation of subvisual particulates in this study may contribute to the differences in the results.

Table 4. Maximum amount of phosphate (as potassium) (mmol/L) not resulting in precipitation.[2196] See CAUTION below.[a]

Calcium (as Gluconate) (mEq/L)	Amino Acid (as TrophAmine) plus Cysteine HCl 1 g/L					
	0.5%	1%	1.5%	2%	2.5%	3%
10	22	28	38	38	38	43
14	18	18	18	38	38	43
19	18	18	18	33	33	38
24	12	18	18	22	28	28
28	12	18	18	18	18	18
33	12	12	12	12	12	12
37	12	12	12	12	12	12
41	9	9	9	12	12	12
45	0	9	9	12	12	12
49	0	9	9	9	12	12
53	0	9	9	9	9	9

[a] CAUTION: The results cannot be safely extrapolated to solutions with formulas other than the ones tested. See text.

The solubility of calcium acetate versus calcium gluconate with sodium phosphates was evaluated in pediatric parenteral nutrition solutions following storage for 30 hours at 25°C followed by 30 minutes at 37°C. Concentrations of Aminosyn PF studied varied from 1 to 3%, dextrose from 10 to 25%, calcium from 5 to 60 mEq/L, and phosphate from 1 to 60 mmol/L. L-Cysteine hydrochloride at a dose of 40 mg/g of Aminosyn PF, magnesium 3.2 mEq/L, and pediatric trace elements-4 at 2.4 mL/L of pediatric parenteral nutrition solution were also added. Calcium acetate was found to be less soluble than calcium gluconate when prepared under these concentrations. The maximum concentrations of the calcium salts and sodium phosphates are shown in Table 5. Polarized light microscopy was used to identify the calcium acetate and sodium phosphate crystals adherent to the container walls because simple visual observation was not able to identify the precipitates. The authors recommended the use of calcium acetate to reduce the iatrogenic aluminum exposure often seen with calcium gluconate in the neonatal population receiving parenteral nutrition.[2466] However, care must be taken to avoid inadvertent calcium phosphate precipitation at the lower concentrations found with calcium acetate if it is substituted for the gluconate salt to reduce aluminum exposure.

Table 5. Maximum concentrations of sodium phosphates and calcium as acetate and as gluconate not resulting in precipitation[2466]

Aminosyn PF (%)	Sodium Phosphates (mmol/L)	Calcium Acetate (mEq/L)	Calcium Gluconate (mEq/L)
1	10	25	50
1	15	15	25
2	10	30	45
2	25	10	12.5
3	20	10	15
3	25	15	17.5

Calcium and phosphate compatibility was evaluated in a series of adult formula parenteral nutrition admixtures composed of FreAmine III, in concentrations ranging from 1 to 5% (TPN #258 through #262). The solutions also contained dextrose ranging from 15% up to 25%. Also present were sodium chloride, potassium chloride, and magnesium sulfate in common amounts. Cysteine hydrochloride was added in an amount of 25 mg/g of amino acids from FreAmine III to reduce the pH by about 0.5 pH unit and thereby increase the amount of calcium and phosphates that can be added to the TPN admixtures as has been done with pediatric parenteral nutrition admixtures. Phosphates as the potassium salts and calcium as the gluconate salt were added in variable quantities to determine the maximum amounts of calcium and phosphates that could be added to the test admixtures. The samples were evaluated at 23 and 37°C over 48 hours by visual inspection in ambient light and using a Tyndall beam and electronic measurement of turbidity and microparticulates. The addition of the cysteine hydrochloride resulted in an increase of calcium and phosphates solubility of about 30% by lowering the solution pH 0.5 pH unit. The boundaries between the compatible and incompatible concentrations were presented graphically as hyperbolic curves.[2469]

A 2-in-1 parenteral nutrition admixture with final concentrations of TrophAmine 0.5%, dextrose 5%, L-cysteine hydrochloride 40 mg/g of amino acids, calcium gluconate 60 mg/100 mL, and sodium phosphates 46.5 mg/mL was found to result in visible precipitation of calcium phosphate within 30 hours stored at 23 to 27°C. Despite the presence of the acidifying L-cysteine hydrochloride, precipitation occurred at clinically utilized amounts of calcium and phosphates.[2622]

The presence of magnesium in solutions may also influence the reaction between calcium and phosphate, including the nature and extent of precipitation.[158 159]

The interaction of calcium and phosphate in parenteral nutrition solutions is a complex phenomenon. Various factors play a role in the solubility or precipitation of a given combination, including:[608 609 1042 1063 1210 1234 1427 2778]

1. Concentration of calcium
2. Salt form of calcium
3. Concentration of phosphate
4. Concentration of amino acids
5. Amino acids composition
6. Concentration of dextrose
7. Temperature of solution
8. pH of solution
9. Presence of other additives
10. Order of mixing

Enhanced precipitate formation would be expected from such factors as high concentrations of calcium and phosphate, increases in solution pH, decreases in amino acid concentrations, increases in temperature, addition of calcium before phosphate, lengthy standing times or slow infusion rates, and use of calcium as the chloride salt.[854]

Even if precipitation does not occur in the container, it has been reported that crystallization of calcium phosphate may occur in a Silastic infusion pump chamber or tubing if the rate of administration is slow, as for premature infants. Water vapor may be transmitted outward and be replaced by air rapidly enough to produce supersaturation.[202] Several other cases of catheter occlusion also have been reported.[610 1427 1428 1429]

Aluminum

Calcium gluconate injection in glass vials is a significant source of aluminum, which has been associated with neurological impairment in premature neonates. Aluminum is leached from the glass vial during the autoclaving of the vials for sterilization. The use of calcium gluconate injection in polyethylene plastic vials in countries where it is available has been recommended to reduce the aluminum burden for neonates.[2322]

Cangrelor Tetrasodium
AHFS 20:12.18

Products

Cangrelor is available as a lyophilized powder in single-use vials containing 50 mg of cangrelor as the tetrasodium salt.[3023] Each vial also contains mannitol, sorbitol, and sodium hydroxide to adjust the pH.[3023]

Each 50-mg vial of cangrelor should be reconstituted with 5 mL of sterile water for injection.[3023] The vial should be gently swirled until all of the powder has fully dissolved; vigorous mixing should be avoided.[3023] Any foam that forms should be allowed to settle.[3023] The reconstituted solution should be visually inspected for particulate matter.[3023]

The reconstituted solution must be diluted prior to administration.[3023] The entire contents of the vial should be withdrawn and diluted in an infusion bag containing 250 mL of sodium chloride 0.9% or dextrose 5% to yield a solution containing cangrelor 200 mcg/mL.[3023] The solution should be thoroughly mixed.[3023]

Trade Name(s)

Kengreal

Administration

Cangrelor tetrasodium is administered by rapid intravenous injection of a bolus dose followed by continuous intravenous infusion via a dedicated line.[3023] The bolus dose should be withdrawn from the bag containing the diluted drug and administered (by manual intravenous push or by pump) over less than 1 minute.[3023] The continuous intravenous infusion should immediately follow administration of the bolus.[3023]

Stability

Intact vials of cangrelor tetrasodium should be stored at controlled room temperature.[3023] Cangrelor tetrasodium is a white to off-white lyophilized powder that forms a clear, colorless to pale yellow solution when reconstituted with sterile water for injection.[3023]

The manufacturer states that the reconstituted solution should be diluted immediately.[3023] The drug is noted to be stable for up to 12 hours at room temperature when diluted in dextrose 5% or up to 24 hours at room temperature if diluted in sodium chloride 0.9%.[3023] Any unused portion should be discarded.[3023]

Compatibility Information

Solution Compatibility

Cangrelor tetrasodium

Test Soln Name	Mfr	Mfr	Conc/L or %	Remarks	Ref	C/I
Dextrose 5%		TMC	200 mg	Stated to be stable for up to 12 hr at room temperature	3023	C
Sodium chloride 0.9%		TMC	200 mg	Stated to be stable for up to 24 hr at room temperature	3023	C

Y-Site Injection Compatibility (1:1 Mixture)

Cangrelor tetrasodium

Test Drug	Mfr	Conc	Mfr	Conc	Remarks	Ref	C/I
Abciximab		10 mcg/mL[b]	TMC	1 mg/mL[b]	Physically compatible for 4 hr	3243	C
Alfentanil HCl		0.5 mg/mL	TMC	1 mg/mL[b]	Physically compatible for 4 hr	3243	C
Alteplase		1 mg/mL	TMC	1 mg/mL[b]	Measured haze increases immediately and microparticulates form	3243	I
Amikacin sulfate		5 mg/mL[b]	TMC	1 mg/mL[b]	Physically compatible for 4 hr	3243	C
Amiodarone HCl		4 mg/mL[b]	TMC	1 mg/mL[b]	Physically compatible for 4 hr	3243	C
Ampicillin sodium		20[b] and 40[b] mg/mL	TMC	1 mg/mL[b]	Physically compatible for 4 hr	3243	C
Ampicillin sodium–sulbactam sodium		20[b d] and 30[b d] mg/mL	TMC	1 mg/mL[b]	Physically compatible for 4 hr	3243	C
Anidulafungin		0.5 mg/mL[b]	TMC	1 mg/mL[b]	Physically compatible for 4 hr	3243	C

DOI: 10.37573/9781585286850.067

Y-Site Injection Compatibility (1:1 Mixture) (Cont.)

Test Drug	Mfr	Conc	Mfr	Conc	Remarks	Ref	C/I
Atropine sulfate		0.4 and 1 mg/mL	TMC	1 mg/mL[b]	Physically compatible for 4 hr	3243	C
Azithromycin		2 mg/mL[b]	TMC	1 mg/mL[b]	Physically compatible for 4 hr	3243	C
Aztreonam		40 mg/mL[b]	TMC	1 mg/mL[b]	Physically compatible for 4 hr	3243	C
Bivalirudin	TMC	5 mg/mL[b]	TMC	1 mg/mL[b]	Physically compatible for 4 hr	3243	C
Bumetanide		0.25 mg/mL	TMC	1 mg/mL[b]	Physically compatible for 4 hr	3243	C
Butorphanol tartrate		40 mcg/mL[b]	TMC	1 mg/mL[b]	Physically compatible for 4 hr	3243	C
Butorphanol tartrate		2 mg/mL	TMC	1 mg/mL[b]	Gross white turbid precipitate forms immediately	3243	I
Calcium gluconate		40 mg/mL[b]	TMC	1 mg/mL[b]	Cloudy white precipitate with particulates appears immediately	3243	I
Cefotaxime sodium		20 mg/mL[b]	TMC	1 mg/mL[b]	Physically compatible for 4 hr	3243	C
Cefoxitin sodium		20[b] and 95 mg/mL	TMC	1 mg/mL[b]	Physically compatible for 4 hr	3243	C
Ceftazidime		40[b] and 100 mg/mL	TMC	1 mg/mL[b]	Physically compatible for 4 hr	3243	C
Ceftriaxone sodium		20[b] and 30[b] mg/mL	TMC	1 mg/mL[b]	Physically compatible for 4 hr	3243	C
Chlorpromazine HCl		2 mg/mL[b]	TMC	1 mg/mL[b]	Gross white turbid precipitate forms immediately	3243	I
Ciprofloxacin		1 mg/mL[b]	TMC	1 mg/mL[b]	Measured haze increases immediately	3243	I
Clevidipine butyrate	TMC	0.5 mg/mL	TMC	1 mg/mL[b]	Physically compatible for 4 hr	3243	C
Clindamycin phosphate		10 mg/mL[b]	TMC	1 mg/mL[b]	Physically compatible for 4 hr	3243	C
Daptomycin	[g]	10 mg/mL[b]	TMC	1 mg/mL[b]	Physically compatible for 4 hr	3243	C
Dexamethasone sodium phosphate		1[b] and 4 mg/mL	TMC	1 mg/mL[b]	Physically compatible for 4 hr	3243	C
Diazepam		5 mg/mL	TMC	1 mg/mL[b]	Gross white turbid precipitate forms immediately	3243	I
Digoxin		0.25 mg/mL	TMC	1 mg/mL[b]	Physically compatible for 4 hr	3243	C
Diltiazem HCl		5 mg/mL	TMC	1 mg/mL[b]	Physically compatible for 4 hr	3243	C
Diphenhydramine HCl		2 mg/mL[b]	TMC	1 mg/mL[b]	Physically compatible for 4 hr	3243	C
Diphenhydramine HCl		25 mg/mL[b]	TMC	1 mg/mL[b]	Gross white turbid precipitate forms immediately	3243	I
Dobutamine HCl		4 mg/mL[b]	TMC	1 mg/mL[b]	Physically compatible for 4 hr	3243	C
Dopamine HCl		4 mg/mL[b]	TMC	1 mg/mL[b]	Physically compatible for 4 hr	3243	C
Doxycycline hyclate		1 mg/mL[b]	TMC	1 mg/mL[b]	Physically compatible for 4 hr	3243	C
Droperidol		2.5 mg/mL	TMC	1 mg/mL[b]	Gross white turbid precipitate forms immediately	3243	I
Enalaprilat		0.1 mg/mL[b]	TMC	1 mg/mL[b]	Physically compatible for 4 hr	3243	C
Ephedrine sulfate		5 mg/mL[b]	TMC	1 mg/mL[b]	Physically compatible for 4 hr	3243	C
Epinephrine HCl		50 mcg/mL[b]	TMC	1 mg/mL[b]	Physically compatible for 4 hr	3243	C
Eptifibatide		2 mg/mL	TMC	1 mg/mL[b]	Physically compatible for 4 hr	3243	C
Ertapenem[i]		20 mg/mL[b]	TMC	1 mg/mL[b]	Physically compatible for 4 hr	3243	C
Erythromycin lactobionate		5 mg/mL[b]	TMC	1 mg/mL[b]	Physically compatible for 4 hr	3243	C
Esmolol[i]		10 mg/mL	TMC	1 mg/mL[b]	Physically compatible for 4 hr	3243	C
Famotidine		2 mg/mL[b]	TMC	1 mg/mL[b]	Physically compatible for 4 hr	3243	C

Y-Site Injection Compatibility (1:1 Mixture) (Cont.)

Test Drug	Mfr	Conc	Mfr	Conc	Remarks	Ref	C/I
Fentanyl citrate		12.5 mcg/mL[b]	TMC	1 mg/mL[b]	Physically compatible for 4 hr	3243	C
Fluconazole		2 mg/mL	TMC	1 mg/mL[b]	Physically compatible for 4 hr	3243	C
Furosemide		3[b] and 10 mg/mL	TMC	1 mg/mL[b]	Physically compatible for 4 hr	3243	C
Gentamicin sulfate		5 mg/mL[b]	TMC	1 mg/mL[b]	Gross white turbid precipitate forms immediately	3243	I
Haloperidol lactate		0.2 mg/mL[b]	TMC	1 mg/mL[b]	Physically compatible for 4 hr	3243	C
Heparin sodium		100 units/mL	TMC	1 mg/mL[b]	Physically compatible for 4 hr	3243	C
Hydrocortisone sodium succinate		1 mg/mL[b]	TMC	1 mg/mL[b]	Physically compatible for 4 hr	3243	C
Hydromorphone HCl		0.5[b] and 1[b] mg/mL	TMC	1 mg/mL[b]	Physically compatible for 4 hr	3243	C
Isoproterenol HCl		20 mcg/mL[b]	TMC	1 mg/mL[b]	Physically compatible for 4 hr	3243	C
Labetalol HCl		2[b] and 5 mg/mL	TMC	1 mg/mL[b]	Gross white turbid precipitate forms immediately	3243	I
Levofloxacin		5 mg/mL[b]	TMC	1 mg/mL[b]	Physically compatible for 4 hr	3243	C
Lidocaine HCl		8 mg/mL[b]	TMC	1 mg/mL[b]	Physically compatible for 4 hr	3243	C
Linezolid		2 mg/mL	TMC	1 mg/mL[b]	Physically compatible for 4 hr	3243	C
Lorazepam		0.5 mg/mL[b]	TMC	1 mg/mL[b]	Physically compatible for 4 hr	3243	C
Magnesium sulfate		100 mg/mL[b]	TMC	1 mg/mL[b]	Physically compatible for 4 hr	3243	C
Mannitol		15%	TMC	1 mg/mL[b]	Physically compatible for 4 hr	3243	C
Meperidine HCl		4 mg/mL[b]	TMC	1 mg/mL[b]	Physically compatible for 4 hr	3243	C
Meropenem		2.5 mg/mL[b]	TMC	1 mg/mL[b]	Physically compatible for 4 hr	3243	C
Methylprednisolone sodium succinate		5 mg/mL[b]	TMC	1 mg/mL[b]	Physically compatible for 4 hr	3243	C
Metoclopramide HCl		5 mg/mL	TMC	1 mg/mL[b]	Physically compatible for 4 hr	3243	C
Metoprolol tartrate		1 mg/mL	TMC	1 mg/mL[b]	Physically compatible for 4 hr	3243	C
Metronidazole		5 mg/mL	TMC	1 mg/mL[b]	Physically compatible for 4 hr	3243	C
Micafungin sodium		1.5 mg/mL[b]	TMC	1 mg/mL[b]	Physically compatible for 4 hr	3243	C
Midazolam HCl		1 mg/mL[b]	TMC	1 mg/mL[b]	Physically compatible for 4 hr	3243	C
Midazolam HCl		5 mg/mL	TMC	1 mg/mL[b]	Cloudy white precipitate with particulates appears immediately	3243	I
Milrinone lactate		0.2 mg/mL[b]	TMC	1 mg/mL[b]	Physically compatible for 4 hr	3243	C
Morphine sulfate		1 mg/mL[b]	TMC	1 mg/mL[b]	Physically compatible for 4 hr	3243	C
Moxifloxacin HCl		1.6 mg/mL	TMC	1 mg/mL[b]	Physically compatible for 4 hr	3243	C
Mycophenolate mofetil HCl		6 mg/mL[a]	TMC	1 mg/mL[b]	Gross white turbid precipitate forms immediately	3243	I
Nalbuphine HCl		10 mg/mL	TMC	1 mg/mL[b]	Physically compatible for 4 hr	3243	C
Nitroglycerin		0.4 mg/mL[b]	TMC	1 mg/mL[b]	Physically compatible for 4 hr	3243	C
Norepinephrine bitartrate		120 mcg/mL[b]	TMC	1 mg/mL[b]	Physically compatible for 4 hr	3243	C
Pantoprazole sodium		0.4 mg/mL[b]	TMC	1 mg/mL[b]	Physically compatible for 4 hr	3243	C
Phenylephrine HCl		1 mg/mL[b]	TMC	1 mg/mL[b]	Physically compatible for 4 hr	3243	C

Y-Site Injection Compatibility (1:1 Mixture) (Cont.)

Test Drug	Mfr	Conc	Mfr	Conc	Remarks	Ref	C/I
Piperacillin sodium–tazobactam sodium		40 mg/mL[b][e]	TMC	1 mg/mL[b]	Physically compatible for 4 hr	3243	C
Potassium chloride		0.1 mEq/mL[b]	TMC	1 mg/mL[b]	Physically compatible for 4 hr	3243	C
Procainamide HCl		10 mg/mL[b]	TMC	1 mg/mL[b]	Physically compatible for 4 hr	3243	C
Prochlorperazine edisylate		0.5 mg/mL[b]	TMC	1 mg/mL[b]	Gross white turbid precipitate forms immediately	3243	I
Promethazine HCl		2 mg/mL[b]	TMC	1 mg/mL[b]	Gross white turbid precipitate forms immediately	3243	I
Propofol		10 mg/mL[b]	TMC	1 mg/mL[b]	Physically compatible for 4 hr	3243	C
Quinupristin–dalfopristin		5 mg/mL[b][f]	TMC	1 mg/mL[b]	Gross white turbid precipitate with fluffy particulates forms immediately	3243	I
Ranitidine HCl		2[b] and 5[b] mg/mL	TMC	1 mg/mL[b]	Physically compatible for 4 hr	3243	C
Reteplase		1 unit/mL	TMC	1 mg/mL[b]	Cloudy white precipitate with fluffy particulates forms immediately	3243	I
Sodium bicarbonate		1 mEq/mL	TMC	1 mg/mL[b]	Physically compatible for 4 hr	3243	C
Sodium nitroprusside		2 mg/mL[b]	TMC	1 mg/mL[b]	Physically compatible for 4 hr	3243	C
Sufentanil citrate		12.5 mcg/mL[b]	TMC	1 mg/mL[b]	Physically compatible for 4 hr	3243	C
Theophylline		1.6 mg/mL	TMC	1 mg/mL[b]	Physically compatible for 4 hr	3243	C
Tigecycline		1 mg/mL[b]	TMC	1 mg/mL[b]	Physically compatible for 4 hr	3243	C
Tirofiban HCl		50 mcg/mL	TMC	1 mg/mL[b]	Physically compatible for 4 hr	3243	C
Tobramycin sulfate		5 mg/mL[b]	TMC	1 mg/mL[b]	Gross white turbid precipitate forms immediately	3243	I
Trimethoprim–sulfamethoxazole		0.8[c][h] and 1.6[c][h] mg/mL	TMC	1 mg/mL[b]	Physically compatible for 4 hr	3243	C
Vancomycin HCl		10 mg/mL[b]	TMC	1 mg/mL[b]	Physically compatible for 4 hr	3243	C
Verapamil HCl		1.25[b] and 2.5 mg/mL	TMC	1 mg/mL[b]	Physically compatible for 4 hr	3243	C
Voriconazole		4 mg/mL[b]	TMC	1 mg/mL[b]	Physically compatible for 4 hr	3243	C

[a] Tested in dextrose 5%.

[b] Tested in sodium chloride 0.9%.

[c] Tested in both dextrose 5% and sodium chloride 0.9%.

[d] Ampicillin component. Ampicillin in a 2:1 fixed-ratio concentration with sulbactam.

[e] Piperacillin component. Piperacillin in an 8:1 fixed-ratio concentration with tazobactam.

[f] Quinupristin and dalfopristin components combined.

[g] Formulation not specified.

[h] Trimethoprim component. Trimethoprim in a 1:5 fixed-ratio concentration with sulfamethoxazole.

[i] Salt not specified.

Selected Revisions December 12, 2018. © Copyright, May 2016.
American Society of Health-System Pharmacists, Inc.

Carbamazepine
AHFS 28:12.92

Products

Carbamazepine is available as a 10-mg/mL concentrate for injection in 20-mL single-dose vials.[3318] Each mL of the concentrate also contains betadex sulfobutyl ether sodium 250 mg and sodium phosphate monobasic dihydrate 0.78 mg in water for injection and may contain sodium hydroxide and/or hydrochloric acid for pH adjustment.[3318] The concentrate must be diluted prior to administration.[3318]

pH

Carbamazepine 10-mg/mL concentrate for injection has an adjusted pH of 6.2.[3318]

Trade Name(s)

Carnexiv

Administration

Carbamazepine concentrate for injection is administered by intravenous infusion over 30 minutes following dilution of the appropriate dose in 100 mL of a compatible infusion solution.[3318]

Stability

Carbamazepine concentrate for injection is a clear, colorless solution.[3318] Intact vials should be stored at controlled room temperature.[3318] Vials are for single-dose only; any unused portion should be discarded.[3318]

Carbamazepine concentrate for injection diluted in a compatible infusion solution may be stored for 4 hours at 20 to 25°C or 24 hours at 2 to 8°C.[3318] Carbamazepine solution should be visually inspected prior to administration; if particulate matter is present or if cloudiness or discoloration occurs, the solution should be discarded.[3318]

Compatibility Information

Solution Compatibility

Carbamazepine

Test Soln Name	Mfr	Mfr	Conc/L or %	Remarks	Ref	C/I
Dextrose 5%		LUN		Stable for 4 hr at 20 to 25°C or 24 hr at 2 to 8°C	3318	C
Ringer's injection, lactated		LUN		Stable for 4 hr at 20 to 25°C or 24 hr at 2 to 8°C	3318	C
Sodium chloride 0.9%		LUN		Stable for 4 hr at 20 to 25°C or 24 hr at 2 to 8°C	3318	C

DOI: 10.37573/9781585286850.068

Carboplatin
AHFS 10:00

Products

Carboplatin is available as a 10-mg/mL aqueous solution in 5-mL (50-mg), 15-mL (150-mg), 45-mL (450-mg), 60-mL (600-mg), and 100-mL (1-g) multidose vials.[2939] [2940] In addition to water for injection, some products also contain mannitol 10 mg in each mL of solution.[2939]

pH

A 1% (10-mg/mL) solution has a pH of 5 to 7.[2939] [2940]

Administration

Carboplatin usually is administered by intravenous infusion over a period of 15 minutes or longer.[2939] [2940] The drug also has been administered as a continuous intravenous infusion over 24 hours.[2939] [2940] Manufacturers state that carboplatin solution may be diluted in dextrose 5% or sodium chloride 0.9% to a concentration as low as 0.5 mg/mL for administration.[2939] [2940]

Because of an interaction occurring between carboplatin and aluminum (resulting in precipitate formation and loss of drug potency), only administration equipment (e.g., needles, intravenous sets) that does *not* contain aluminum should be used for the preparation or administration of this drug.[2939] [2940]

Stability

Intact vials should be stored at controlled room temperature and protected from light.[2939] [2940]

Manufacturers state that reconstituted solutions are stable for 8 hours at room temperature (25°C).[2939] [2940] Because no antibacterial preservative is present, the manufacturers recommend that carboplatin solutions for infusion be discarded 8 hours after dilution.[2939] [2940] However, other information indicates that the drug may be stable for a much longer time. At a concentration of 15 mg/mL in sterile water for injection or at concentrations of 0.5 and 2 mg/mL in dextrose 5%, no decomposition occurred in 24 hours at 22 to 25°C.[234]

Formation of cisplatin in solutions of carboplatin 1 mg/mL in sodium chloride 0.9% at 25°C with exposure to fluorescent light was evaluated. Less than 0.1% of the carboplatin had converted to cisplatin in 2 hours, and 0.7% had converted in 24 hours.[1695]

Carboplatin 1 mg/mL in sterile water for injection was reported to exhibit less than 10% loss in 14 days at room temperature.[1379]

Carboplatin (Bristol-Myers Oncology) 1 mg/mL in sterile water for injection was stable in polyvinyl chloride (PVC) reservoirs (Parker Micropump) for 14 days at 4 and 37°C, exhibiting no loss.[1696]

Manufacturers state that carboplatin 10 mg/mL aqueous injection in multidose vials is stable for up to 14 days at 25°C, even with multiple needle entries.[2939] [2940]

pH Effects

The pH range of maximum stability has been reported to be pH 4 to 6[1919] or 6.5.[1369] The degradation rate increases above pH 6.5.[1369]

Syringes

Carboplatin 10-mg/mL aqueous solution prefilled into plastic syringes exhibited no decomposition in 5 days at 4°C and only 3% loss in 24 hours at 37°C.[1238]

Carboplatin 10 mg/mL (Bristol-Myers Squibb) was repackaged into 30-mL polypropylene syringes for use in the Intelliject portable syringe pump. The carboplatin solution exhibited no visual changes, and no loss of carboplatin content was found when stored at 25°C for 8 days. No evidence of interaction between carboplatin and the syringe plastic was identified, and no impact on the functioning of the syringe pump was observed.[2147]

Sorption

Carboplatin (Ribosepharm) 0.72 mg/mL in dextrose 5% exhibited little or no loss due to sorption in polyethylene and PVC containers compared to glass containers over 72 hours at room and refrigeration temperatures.[2420] [2430] Simulated infusion of carboplatin 10 mg/mL through a Silastic catheter over 24 hours at 37°C did not affect the delivered drug concentration.[1238]

Compatibility Information

Solution Compatibility

Carboplatin

Test Soln Name	Mfr	Mfr	Conc/L or %	Remarks	Ref	C/I
Dextrose 5% in sodium chloride 0.225%	AB[a]	NCI	1 g	Physically compatible. 2% loss in 24 hr at 25°C	1087	C
Dextrose 5% in sodium chloride 0.45%	AB[b]	NCI	1 g	Physically compatible. 2% loss in 24 hr at 25°C	1087	C

DOI: 10.37573/9781585286850.069

Solution Compatibility (Cont.)

Test Soln Name	Mfr	Mfr	Conc/L or %	Remarks	Ref	C/I
Dextrose 5% in sodium chloride 0.9%	AB[a]	NCI	1 g	Physically compatible. 4% loss in 24 hr at 25°C	1087	C
Dextrose 5%	[a]	NCI	500 mg and 2 g	Physically compatible. No loss for 24 hr at 25°C	234	C
Dextrose 5%	AB[a]	NCI	100 mg and 1 g	Physically compatible. 1.5% loss in 6 hr at 25°C	1087	C
Dextrose 5%	[c]	BR	2.4 g	No loss in 9 days at 23°C in the dark	1757	C
Dextrose 5%	[c]	BR	1 g	Visually compatible. Little loss in 28 days at 4, 22, and 35°C	1823	C
Dextrose 5%	[a]	BR	1 g	Visually compatible. 6% loss in 28 days at 4, 22, and 35°C	1823	C
Dextrose 5%	[d]	BR	1 g	Visually compatible. No loss in 28 days at 4, 22, and 35°C	1823	C
Dextrose 5%	[e]	BR	1 g	Visually compatible. Little loss in 28 days at 4 and 22°C. Concentration increased by 14% in 28 days at 35°C due to moisture transfer through container	1823	C
Dextrose 5%	BA[a]	BMS	500 mg and 4 g	Visually compatible. 5% loss at 25°C and no loss at 4°C in the dark in 21 days	2099	C
Dextrose 5%	BA[a]	BMS	750 mg and 2 g	Visually compatible with no loss at 25 and 4°C in the dark in 7 days	2099	C
Dextrose 5%	[f]	BR	6 g	Little loss in 14 days at 37°C in the dark	2321	C
Dextrose 5%	FRE,[c] MAC[g]	TE	0.7 and 2.15 g	Physically compatible. Stable for 84 days at 4°C and 24 hr at 25°C	2777	C
Dextrose 5%		TE		Use within 8 hr	2939, 2940	C
Dextrose 5%	FRK[h]	TE	20 mg	Alteration of UV spectra; concentration increased to >105% of initial within 3 hr at room temperature protected from light	3557	I
Dextrose 5%	FRK[h]	TE	200 mg	Physically stable with little to no loss in 24 hr at room temperature protected from light	3557	C
Sodium chloride 0.9%		TE		Use within 8 hr	2939, 2940	C
Sodium chloride 0.9%	AB[a]	NCI	1 g	Physically compatible. 5% loss in 24 hr at 25°C	1087	C
Sodium chloride 0.9%			7 g	8% loss in 24 hr at 27°C	1379	C
Sodium chloride 0.9%	BA[c]	TE	0.5 g	Physically compatible. 5% loss in 7 days at 4°C in the dark and 9% loss in 3 days at 23°C	3350	C
Sodium chloride 0.9%	BA[c]	TE	2 g	Physically compatible. 5% loss in 7 days at 4°C in the dark and 9% loss in 5 days at 23°C	3350	C
Sodium chloride 0.9%	BA[c]	TE	4 g	Physically compatible. 4% loss in 7 days at 4°C in the dark and 8% loss in 7 days at 23°C	3350	C

[a] Tested in glass containers.

[b] Tested in both glass and PVC containers.

[c] Tested in PVC containers.

[d] Tested in ethylene vinyl acetate containers.

[e] Tested in elastomeric balloon reservoirs (Baxter Infusor).

[f] Tested in Pharmacia Deltec medication cassette reservoirs.

[g] Tested in polyolefin containers.

[h] Tested in polypropylene containers.

Additive Compatibility

Carboplatin

Test Drug	Mfr	Conc/L or %	Mfr	Conc/L or %	Test Solution	Remarks	Ref	C/I
Cisplatin		200 mg		1 g	NS	Under 10% drug loss in 7 days at 23°C	1954	C
Etoposide		200 mg		1 g	W	Under 10% drug loss in 7 days at 23°C	1954	C
Floxuridine		10 g		1 g	W	Under 10% drug loss in 7 days at 23°C	1954	C
Fluorouracil		10 g		1 g	W	Greater than 20% carboplatin loss in 24 hr at room temperature	1379	I
Fluorouracil	DB	1 g	BR	100 mg	D5W	9% carboplatin loss in 5 hr at 25°C	2415	I
Ifosfamide		1 g		1 g	W	Both drugs stable for 5 days at room temperature	1379	C
Mesna		1 g		1 g	W	More than 10% carboplatin loss in 24 hr at room temperature	1379	I
Paclitaxel	BMS	300 mg and 1.2 g	BMS	2 g	NS	No paclitaxel loss but carboplatin losses of less than 2, 5, and 6 to 7% at 4, 24, and 32°C, respectively, in 24 hr. Physically compatible for 24 hr but microparticles of paclitaxel form after 3 to 5 days	2094	C
Paclitaxel	BMS	300 mg and 1.2 g	BMS	2 g	D5W	No paclitaxel and carboplatin loss at 4, 24, and 32°C in 24 hr. Physically compatible for 24 hr but microparticles of paclitaxel form after 3 to 5 days	2094	C
Sodium bicarbonate		200 mmol		1 g		13% carboplatin loss in 24 hr at 27°C	1379	I

Y-Site Injection Compatibility (1:1 Mixture)

Carboplatin

Test Drug	Mfr	Conc	Mfr	Conc	Remarks	Ref	C/I
Allopurinol sodium	BW	3 mg/mL[b]	BR	5 mg/mL[b]	Physically compatible for 4 hr at 22°C	1686	C
Amifostine	USB	10 mg/mL[a]	BR	5 mg/mL[a]	Physically compatible for 4 hr at 23°C	1845	C
Anidulafungin	VIC	0.5 mg/mL[a]	BMS	5 mg/mL[a]	Physically compatible for 4 hr at 23°C	2617	C
Aztreonam	SQ	40 mg/mL[a]	BMS	5 mg/mL[a]	Physically compatible for 4 hr at 23°C	1758	C
Caspofungin acetate	ME	0.7 mg/mL[b]	MAY	5 mg/mL[b]	Physically compatible for 4 hr at room temperature	2758	C
Cladribine	ORT	0.015[b] and 0.5[c] mg/mL	BR	5 mg/mL[b]	Physically compatible for 4 hr at 23°C	1969	C
Doripenem	JJ	5 mg/mL[a b]	SIC	5 mg/mL[a b]	Physically compatible for 4 hr at 23°C	2743	C
Doxorubicin HCl liposomal	SEQ	0.4 mg/mL[a]	BR	5 mg/mL[a]	Physically compatible for 4 hr at 23°C	2087	C
Etoposide phosphate	BR	5 mg/mL[a]	BR	5 mg/mL[a]	Physically compatible for 4 hr at 23°C	2218	C
Filgrastim	AMG	30 mcg/mL[a]	BR	5 mg/mL[a]	Physically compatible for 4 hr at 22°C	1687	C
Fludarabine phosphate	BX	1 mg/mL[a]	BR	5 mg/mL[a]	Visually compatible for 4 hr at 22°C	1439	C
Gemcitabine HCl	LI	10 mg/mL[b]	BR	5 mg/mL[b]	Physically compatible for 4 hr at 23°C	2226	C
Granisetron HCl	SKB	1 mg/mL	BR	1 mg/mL[b]	Physically compatible with little or no loss of either drug in 4 hr at 22°C	1883	C

Y-Site Injection Compatibility (1:1 Mixture) (Cont.)

Test Drug	Mfr	Conc	Mfr	Conc	Remarks	Ref	C/I
Linezolid	PHU	2 mg/mL	BR	5 mg/mL[a]	Physically compatible for 4 hr at 23°C	2264	C
Melphalan HCl	BW	0.1 mg/mL[b]	BR	5 mg/mL[b]	Physically compatible for 3 hr at 22°C	1557	C
Micafungin sodium	ASP	1.5 mg/mL[b]	BA	5 mg/mL[b]	Physically compatible for 4 hr at 23°C	2683	C
Ondansetron HCl	GL	1 mg/mL[b]	BR	5 mg/mL[a]	Visually compatible for 4 hr at 22°C	1365	C
Ondansetron HCl	GL	16 to 160 mcg/mL		0.18 to 9.9 mg/mL	Physically compatible when carboplatin given over 10 to 60 min via Y-site	1366	C
Oxaliplatin	SS	0.5 mg/mL[a]	BR	5 mg/mL[a]	Physically compatible for 4 hr at 23°C	2566	C
Paclitaxel	NCI	1.2 mg/mL[a]		5 mg/mL[a]	Physically compatible for 4 hr at 22°C	1528	C
Palonosetron HCl	MGI	50 mcg/mL	BMS	5 mg/mL[a]	Physically compatible. No palonosetron and 2% carboplatin loss in 4 hr	2579	C
Pemetrexed disodium	LI	20 mg/mL[b]	BMS	5 mg/mL[a]	Physically compatible for 4 hr at 23°C	2564	C
Piperacillin sodium–tazobactam sodium	LE[f]	40 mg/mL[a] [g]	BR	5 mg/mL[a]	Physically compatible for 4 hr at 22°C	1688	C
Propofol	ZEN[h]	10 mg/mL	BR	5 mg/mL[a]	Physically compatible for 1 hr at 23°C	2066	C
Sargramostim	IMM	10 mcg/mL[b]	BR	5 mg/mL[b]	Visually compatible for 4 hr at 22°C	1436	C
Teniposide	BR	0.1 mg/mL[a]	BR	5 mg/mL[a]	Physically compatible for 4 hr at 23°C	1725	C
Thiotepa	IMM[d]	1 mg/mL[a]	BMS	5 mg/mL[a]	Physically compatible for 4 hr at 23°C	1861	C
TNA #218 to #226[e]			BMS	5 mg/mL[a]	Visually compatible for 4 hr at 23°C	2215	C
Topotecan HCl	SKB	56 mcg/mL[a] [b]	BR	0.9 mg/mL[a] [b]	Visually compatible. Little loss of either drug in 4 hr at 22°C	2245	C
TPN #212 to #215[e]			BMS	5 mg/mL[a]	Physically compatible for 4 hr at 23°C	2109	C
Vinorelbine tartrate	BW	1 mg/mL[b]	BR	5 mg/mL[b]	Physically compatible for 4 hr at 22°C	1558	C

[a] Tested in dextrose 5%.

[b] Tested in sodium chloride 0.9%.

[c] Tested in bacteriostatic sodium chloride 0.9% preserved with benzyl alcohol 0.9%.

[d] Lyophilized formulation tested.

[e] Refer to Appendix for the composition of parenteral nutrition solutions. TNA indicates a 3-in-1 admixture, and TPN indicates a 2-in-1 admixture.

[f] Test performed using the formulation WITHOUT edetate disodium.

[g] Piperacillin component. Piperacillin in an 8:1 fixed-ratio concentration with tazobactam.

[h] Test performed using the formulation WITH edetate disodium.

Selected Revisions July 1, 2020. © Copyright, October 1990.
American Society of Health-System Pharmacists, Inc.

Carmustine (BCNU)
AHFS 10:00

Products

Carmustine is available in vials containing 100 mg of drug, packaged with a vial containing 3 mL of dehydrated alcohol injection, USP, for use as a diluent.[1(8/07)]

Dissolve the contents of the vial of carmustine with 3 mL of dehydrated alcohol injection, USP. Further dilute with 27 mL of sterile water for injection. The resultant solution will contain 3.3 mg/mL of carmustine in 10% ethanol.[1(8/07)]

Avoid accidental contact of the reconstituted solution with the skin. Transient hyperpigmentation in the affected areas has occurred.[1(8/07) 4]

Trade Name(s)

BiCNU

Administration

Carmustine is administered as an intravenous infusion over one to two hours. Shorter durations may result in pain and burning at the injection site and flushing.[1(8/07) 4]

Stability

The product consists of vacuum-dried pale yellow flakes or is a congealed mass. Intact vials are stored under refrigeration and are stable for at least three years.[1(8/07)] Intact vials are stable for seven days at room temperatures not exceeding 25°C.[1181 1236 1433] Room temperature storage of intact vials results in slow decomposition, with approximately 3% degradation occurring in 36 days.[285]

Reconstitution as directed results in a colorless to pale yellow solution. This solution is stable for eight hours at room temperature protected from light.[4] About a 6% loss occurs in three hours and about an 8% loss occurs in six hours.[285] A loss of 20% in 21 hours was also reported.[484]

Refrigeration of the solution significantly increases its stability. In 24 hours at 2 to 8°C with protection from light, approximately 4% decomposition occurs.[1(8/07) 285]

Carmustine has a melting point of approximately 30.5 to 32°C. At this temperature, the drug liquifies, becoming an oily film on the bottom of the vial. Should this occur, the manufacturer recommends that the vials be discarded, because the melting is a sign of decomposition.[1(8/07)] However, one study showed that storage of the vials at 37°C for 15 minutes followed by storage at 22 to 25°C resulted in no decomposition in eight days and about an 8% loss in 37 days. Storage of the vials at 37°C for seven days resulted in about 10% decomposition.[862]

In 95% ethanol, carmustine 2 mg/mL is reported to be stable for at least 24 hours at 22 to 25 and 37°C.[862] Under refrigeration, carmustine 0.5 to 0.6 mg/mL in 95% ethanol or absolute ethanol is stable at 0 to 5°C for up to three months.[863]

pH Effects

The degradation rate for carmustine in aqueous solution was reported to be at a minimum between pH 5.2 and 5.5[619] and 3.3 and 4.8.[1237] Above pH 6, the degradation rate increases greatly.[619] Decomposition of 10% occurred in less than two hours at pH 6.5 but in 5.5 hours at optimum pH.[1237]

Light Effects

Increased decomposition rates were reported when carmustine, in solution, was exposed to increasing intensities of light.[1237] However, in another study, no clear effect on rate of carmustine loss from exposure to light was demonstrated. Some samples seemed to demonstrate increased rate of loss due to light exposure while others did not.[2337]

Sorption

The manufacturer recommends the use of glass containers for carmustine administration.[1(8/07) 4] The rate of loss of carmustine from infusion admixtures in dextrose 5% in PVC containers is substantially greater than the rate of loss in glass[519 1237 1658 2430] or polyolefin[1237 1658] containers.

Substantial loss to PVC, ethylene vinyl acetate, and polyurethane infusion sets was also noted. Only a set lined with polyethylene proved resistant to carmustine sorption, resulting in little loss in two hours.[1237]

Carmustine (Bristol-Myers Squibb) 0.2 mg/mL in dextrose 5% was evaluated for loss of drug content in glass, polyethylene, and PVC containers. At room temperature, about 40% loss of drug occurred in glass containers in 72 hours. In polyethylene containers, a slightly larger loss occurred, about 50% loss in 72 hours. The greatest loss occurred in PVC containers with about 65% loss in 72 hours. Carmustine losses of 5% occurred in 5.5 hours, 2.5 hours, and 45 minutes in glass, polyethylene, and PVC containers, respectively. The increased losses in polyethylene and PVC containers were attributed to sorption. Under refrigeration, glass and polyethylene containers were similar with less than 10% loss in 72 hours. However, in PVC containers about 20% loss due to sorption occurred in that time frame.[2420 2430]

DOI: 10.37573/9781585286850.070

Compatibility Information

Solution Compatibility

Carmustine

Test Soln Name	Mfr	Mfr	Conc/L or %	Remarks	Ref	C/I
Dextrose 5%	a	BMS	200 mg	Stable for 8 hr at room temperature	1(8/07)	C
Dextrose 5%	TR[a]	BR	1.25 g	10% loss in 7.7 hr at room temperature	519	I
Dextrose 5%	TR[b]	BR	1.25 g	18.5% loss in 1 hr at room temperature	519	I
Dextrose 5%	CU	BR	100 mg	No decomposition over 90-min study period	523	C
Dextrose 5%	MG, TR[a]		1.25 g	10% loss in 7.7 to 8.3 hr at room temperature exposed to light	1658	I
Dextrose 5%	MG[c]		1.25 g	10% loss in 7 hr at room temperature exposed to light	1658	I
Dextrose 5%	TR[b]		1.25 g	10% loss in 0.6 hr at room temperature exposed to light	1658	I
Dextrose 5%	FAN[a]	BMS	100 mg	7% loss in 2 hr and 12% loss in 4 hr at 25°C in light or dark. 7% loss in 48 hr at 4°C	2337	I[e]
Dextrose 5%	MAC[b]	BMS	100 mg	10% loss in 1 hr at 25°C in light or dark. 5% loss in 12 hr and 12% loss in 24 hr at 4°C	2337	I
Dextrose 5%	BFM[d]	BMS	100 mg	5 to 8% loss in 4 hr and 11 to 14% loss in 6 hr at 25°C in light or dark. 5% loss in 48 hr and 15% loss in 7 days at 4°C	2337	I[e]
Dextrose 5%	FAN[a]	BMS	500 mg	9% loss in 4 hr and 17% loss in 6 hr at 25°C in light or dark. 9% loss in 48 hr at 4°C	2337	I[e]
Dextrose 5%	MAC[b]	BMS	500 mg	7% loss in 1 hr and 10 to 13% loss in 2 hr at 25°C in light or dark. 7% loss in 12 hr and 18% loss in 24 hr at 4°C	2337	I
Dextrose 5%	BFM[d]	BMS	500 mg	9% loss in 6 hr and 13 to 15% loss in 8 hr at 25°C in light or dark. 5% loss in 48 hr and 15% loss in 7 days at 4°C	2337	I[e]
Dextrose 5%	FAN[a]	BMS	1 g	4% loss in 4 hr and 9% loss in 6 hr in dark and 9% loss in 4 hr in light at 25°C. 4% loss in 48 hr and 13% loss in 7 days at 4°C	2337	I[e]
Dextrose 5%	MAC[b]	BMS	1 g	4 to 7% loss in 1 hr and 10% loss in 2 hr at 25°C in light or dark. 7% loss in 6 hr and 12% loss in 24 hr at 4°C	2337	I
Dextrose 5%	BFM[d]	BMS	1 g	7 to 10% loss in 6 hr and 10 to 14% loss in 8 hr at 25°C in light or dark. 9% loss in 48 hr and 14% loss in 7 days at 4°C	2337	I[e]
Dextrose 5%	HOS[f]	BMS	1 g	About 7% loss in 6 hr	2660, 2792	I[e]
Sodium chloride 0.9%	CU	BR	100 mg	No decomposition over 90-min study period	523	C

[a] Tested in glass containers.

[b] Tested in PVC containers.

[c] Tested in polyolefin containers.

[d] Polyethylene-lined trilayer containers.

[e] Incompatible by conventional standards but may be used in lesser time periods.

[f] Tested in VISIV polyolefin containers.

Additive Compatibility

Carmustine

Test Drug	Mfr	Conc/L or %	Mfr	Conc/L or %	Test Solution	Remarks	Ref	C/I
Sodium bicarbonate	AB	100 mEq	BR	100 mg	D5W, NS	10% carmustine loss in 15 min and 27% in 90 min	523	I

Y-Site Injection Compatibility (1:1 Mixture)

Carmustine

Test Drug	Mfr	Conc	Mfr	Conc	Remarks	Ref	C/I
Allopurinol sodium	BW	3 mg/mL[b]	BR	1.5 mg/mL[b]	Gas evolves immediately	1686	I
Amifostine	USB	10 mg/mL[a]	BR	1.5 mg/mL[a]	Physically compatible for 4 hr at 23°C	1845	C
Aztreonam	SQ	40 mg/mL[a]	BMS	1.5 mg/mL[a]	Physically compatible for 4 hr at 23°C	1758	C
Etoposide phosphate	BR	5 mg/mL[a]	BR	1.5 mg/mL[a]	Physically compatible for 4 hr at 23°C	2218	C
Filgrastim	AMG	30 mcg/mL[a]	BR	1.5 mg/mL[a]	Physically compatible for 4 hr at 22°C	1687	C
Fludarabine phosphate	BX	1 mg/mL[a]	BR	1.5 mg/mL[a]	Visually compatible for 4 hr at 22°C	1439	C
Gemcitabine HCl	LI	10 mg/mL[b]	BR	1.5 mg/mL[b]	Physically compatible for 4 hr at 23°C	2226	C
Granisetron HCl	SKB	0.05 mg/mL[a]	BMS	1.5 mg/mL[a]	Physically compatible for 4 hr at 23°C	2000	C
Melphalan HCl	BW	0.1 mg/mL[b]	BR	1.5 mg/mL[b]	Physically compatible for 3 hr at 22°C	1557	C
Ondansetron HCl	GL	1 mg/mL[b]	BR	1.5 mg/mL[a]	Visually compatible for 4 hr at 22°C	1365	C
Piperacillin sodium–tazobactam sodium	LE[d]	40 mg/mL[a] [e]	BR	1.5 mg/mL[a]	Physically compatible for 4 hr at 22°C	1688	C
Sargramostim	IMM	10 mcg/mL[b]	BR	1.5 mg/mL[b]	Visually compatible for 4 hr at 22°C	1436	C
Teniposide	BR	0.1 mg/mL[a]	BR	1.5 mg/mL[a]	Physically compatible for 4 hr at 23°C	1725	C
Thiotepa	IMM[c]	1 mg/mL[a]	BMS	1.5 mg/mL[a]	Physically compatible for 4 hr at 23°C	1861	C
Vinorelbine tartrate	BW	1 mg/mL[b]	BR	1.5 mg/mL[b]	Physically compatible for 4 hr at 22°C	1558	C

[a] Tested in dextrose 5%.

[b] Tested in sodium chloride 0.9%.

[c] Lyophilized formulation tested.

[d] Test performed using the formulation WITHOUT edetate disodium.

[e] Piperacillin component. Piperacillin in an 8:1 fixed-ratio concentration with tazobactam.

Selected Revisions May 28, 2014. © Copyright, October 1982.
American Society of Health-System Pharmacists, Inc.

Caspofungin Acetate
AHFS 8:14.16

Products

Caspofungin acetate is available in 2 different formulations.[3344] [3345] [3346] In addition to varying inactive ingredients, the formulations differ in their storage requirements.[3344] [3345] [3346]

Caspofungin acetate (Cancidas, Merck; generic) is available as a lyophilized powder or cake in single-dose vials containing 50 or 70 mg of caspofungin.[3344] [3346] The 50-mg vial also contains sucrose 39 mg and mannitol 26 mg.[3344] [3346] The 70-mg vial also contains sucrose 54 mg and mannitol 36 mg.[3344] [3346] Both vial sizes contain glacial acetic acid and sodium hydroxide to adjust the pH.[3344] [3346] The 50- and 70-mg vials contain an overfill of caspofungin (4.6 and 5.6 mg, respectively) to permit withdrawal of a full 50- or 70-mg dose of the reconstituted product.[3344] [3346]

Caspofungin acetate (Fresenius Kabi) is available as a lyophilized powder or cake in single-dose vials containing 50 or 70 mg of caspofungin.[3345] The 50- and 70-mg vials also contain arginine 100 and 140 mg, respectively.[3345] Both vial sizes contain hydrochloric acid and/or sodium hydroxide to adjust the pH.[3345] The 50- and 70-mg vials contain an overfill of caspofungin (4.6 and 7.2 mg, respectively) to permit withdrawal of a full 50- or 70-mg dose of the reconstituted product.[3345]

To prepare a solution of caspofungin for intravenous infusion, vials of caspofungin acetate that have been stored under refrigeration should be allowed to come to room temperature prior to reconstitution.[3344] [3346] Both the 50- and 70-mg vials should be reconstituted with 10.8 mL of sterile water for injection, sodium chloride 0.9%, or bacteriostatic water for injection (containing methyl- or propylparabens or benzyl alcohol 0.9%) and should be mixed gently until the powder or cake has completely dissolved and a clear solution forms.[3344] [3345] [3346] The resulting caspofungin concentrations of the reconstituted solutions prepared from the 50- and 70-mg vials are 5 and 7 mg/mL, respectively.[3344] [3345] [3346] To prepare doses intended for pediatric patients, manufacturers recommend use of the 50-mg vial for doses less than or equal to 50 mg; the 70-mg vial should be reserved for pediatric doses exceeding 50 mg.[3344] [3345] [3346]

The reconstituted caspofungin solution should be diluted for infusion within 1 hour after reconstitution.[3344] [3345] [3346] The appropriate volume of the reconstituted solution should be withdrawn from the vial and transferred to a 250-mL bag or bottle of sodium chloride 0.9%, sodium chloride 0.45%, sodium chloride 0.225%, or Ringer's injection, lactated.[3344] [3345] [3346]

Alternatively, the appropriate volume of the reconstituted solution may be added to a smaller volume of these infusion solutions for a final caspofungin concentration not exceeding 0.5 mg/mL.[3344] [3345] [3346] Reconstituted and diluted solutions should be visually inspected for particulate matter and discoloration; if the solution has precipitated or if cloudiness occurs, the solution should not be used.[3344] [3345] [3346]

pH
The pH of a saturated aqueous solution of caspofungin is approximately 6.6.[3344] [3345] [3346]

Osmolality
Caspofungin acetate diluted as directed for infusion is near isotonicity.[2722]

Trade Name(s)
Cancidas

Administration
Caspofungin acetate is administered by slow intravenous infusion over approximately 1 hour.[3344] [3345] [3346] Caspofungin acetate should *not* be administered by intravenous bolus.[3344] [3345] [3346]

Stability
Caspofungin acetate is available as a lyophilized white to off-white cake or powder that forms a clear solution upon reconstitution.[3344] [3345] [3346] Intact vials of caspofungin acetate (Cancidas, Merck; generic) should be stored at 2 to 8°C.[3344] [3346] Intact vials of caspofungin acetate (Fresenius Kabi) should be stored at controlled room temperature.[3345] Vials are for single use only; unused portions should be discarded.[3344] [3345] [3346]

The reconstituted solution may be stored for up to 1 hour after reconstitution at room temperature up to 25°C, but should be withdrawn within 1 hour after reconstitution to prepare the intravenous infusion solution.[3344] [3345] [3346]

The diluted solution for infusion in the intravenous bag or bottle must be used within 24 hours if stored at room temperature up to 25°C or within 48 hours if stored at 2 to 8°C.[3344] [3345] [3346]

Caspofungin acetate is unstable in dextrose-containing solutions; such solutions should not be used for reconstitution or dilution of the drug.[3344] [3345] [3346] The manufacturers recommend that caspofungin acetate not be mixed with or co-infused with other drugs.[3344] [3345] [3346]

DOI: 10.37573/9781585286850.071

Compatibility Information

Solution Compatibility

Caspofungin acetate

Test Soln Name	Mfr	Mfr	Conc/L or %	Remarks	Ref	C/I
Dextrose 5%		ME, MYL		Unstable in dextrose-containing solutions	3344, 3346	I
Dextrose 5%		FRK		Unstable in dextrose-containing solutions	3345	I
Ringer's injection, lactated		ME, MYL		Stable for 24 hr at ≤25°C and 48 hr at 2 to 8°C	3344, 3346	C
Ringer's injection, lactated		FRK		Stable for 24 hr at ≤25°C and 48 hr at 2 to 8°C	3345	C
Sodium chloride 0.225%		ME, MYL		Stable for 24 hr at ≤25°C and 48 hr at 2 to 8°C	3344, 3346	C
Sodium chloride 0.225%		FRK		Stable for 24 hr at ≤25°C and 48 hr at 2 to 8°C	3345	C
Sodium chloride 0.45%		ME, MYL		Stable for 24 hr at ≤25°C and 48 hr at 2 to 8°C	3344, 3346	C
Sodium chloride 0.45%		FRK		Stable for 24 hr at ≤25°C and 48 hr at 2 to 8°C	3345	C
Sodium chloride 0.9%		ME, MYL		Stable for 24 hr at ≤25°C and 48 hr at 2 to 8°C	3344, 3346	C
Sodium chloride 0.9%		FRK		Stable for 24 hr at ≤25°C and 48 hr at 2 to 8°C	3345	C
Sodium chloride 0.9%	[a]	ME	0.2, 0.28, 0.5 g	Physically compatible with less than 10% drug loss in 60 hr at 25°C and 14 days at 5°C	2828	C

[a] Tested in Intermate and Homepump Eclipse elastomeric pump reservoirs.

Y-Site Injection Compatibility (1:1 Mixture)

Caspofungin acetate

Test Drug	Mfr	Conc	Mfr	Conc	Remarks	Ref	C/I
Acyclovir sodium	BV	7 mg/mL[b]	ME	0.7 mg/mL[b]	Physically compatible for 4 hr at room temperature	2758	C
Acyclovir sodium	BED	5 mg/mL[b]	ME	0.5 mg/mL[b]	Fine clear crystals reported	2766	I
Amikacin sulfate	HOS	5 mg/mL[b]	ME	0.7 mg/mL[b]	Physically compatible for 4 hr at room temperature	2758	C
Amiodarone HCl	SIC	4 mg/mL[b]	ME	0.7 mg/mL[b]	Physically compatible for 4 hr at room temperature	2758	C
Amphotericin B	XGN	0.6 mg/mL[a]	ME	0.7 mg/mL[b]	Immediate yellow turbid precipitate forms	2758	I
Amphotericin B lipid complex	ENZ	1 mg/mL[a]	ME	0.7 mg/mL[b]	Immediate yellow turbid precipitate	2758	I
Amphotericin B liposomal	AST	1 mg/mL[a]	ME	0.7 mg/mL[b]	Immediate yellow turbid precipitate	2758	I
Ampicillin sodium	APP	20 mg/mL[b]	ME	0.7 mg/mL[b]	Immediate white turbid precipitate forms	2758	I
Azithromycin	NVP	2 mg/mL[b]	ME	0.5 mg/mL[b]	Physically compatible over 60 min	2766	C
Aztreonam	BMS	40 mg/mL[b]	ME	0.7 mg/mL[b]	Physically compatible for 4 hr at room temperature	2758	C
Aztreonam	BMS	20 mg/mL[b]	ME	0.5 mg/mL[b]	Physically compatible over 60 min	2766	C
Blinatumomab	AMG	0.125 and 0.375 mcg/mL[b]	MCD	0.2 mg/mL[b]	Particles, flakes, thin needles, or haze transiently appears	3405, 3417	?
Bumetanide	BED	0.04 mg/mL[b]	ME	0.7 mg/mL[b]	Physically compatible for 4 hr at room temperature	2758	C
Carboplatin	MAY	5 mg/mL[b]	ME	0.7 mg/mL[b]	Physically compatible for 4 hr at room temperature	2758	C
Cefazolin sodium	CUR	20 mg/mL[b]	ME	0.7 mg/mL[b]	Immediate white turbid precipitate forms	2758	I

Y-Site Injection Compatibility (1:1 Mixture) (Cont.)

Test Drug	Mfr	Conc	Mfr	Conc	Remarks	Ref	C/I
Cefazolin sodium	SZ	100 mg/mL[b]	ME	0.5 mg/mL[b]	Fine white crystals reported	2766	I
Cefepime HCl	BMS	20 mg/mL[b]	ME	0.7 mg/mL[b]	Immediate white turbid precipitate forms	2758	I
Ceftaroline fosamil	FOR	2.22 mg/mL[a b h]	ME	0.5 mg/mL[b h]	Increased haze and particulates	2826	I
Ceftazidime	GSK	40 mg/mL[b]	ME	0.7 mg/mL[b]	Immediate white turbid precipitate forms	2758	I
Ceftolozane sulfate–tazobactam sodium	CUB	10 mg/mL[b p]	ME	0.5 mg/mL[b]	Measured turbidity increases immediately	3262	I
Ceftriaxone sodium	ORC	20 mg/mL[b]	ME	0.7 mg/mL[b]	Immediate white turbid precipitate forms	2758	I
Ceftriaxone sodium	NVP	20 mg/mL[b]	ME	0.5 mg/mL[b]	Amber crystals and white paste form	2766	I
Ciprofloxacin	HOS	2 mg/mL[b]	ME	0.7 mg/mL[b]	Physically compatible for 4 hr at room temperature	2758	C
Ciprofloxacin	BAY	2 mg/mL	ME	0.5 mg/mL[b]	Physically compatible over 60 min	2766	C
Cisplatin	APP	0.5 mg/mL[b]	ME	0.7 mg/mL[b]	Physically compatible for 4 hr at room temperature	2758	C
Clindamycin phosphate	BED	10 mg/mL[b]	ME	0.7 mg/mL[b]	Immediate white turbid precipitate forms	2758	I
Clindamycin phosphate	HOS	60 mg/mL[d]	ME	0.5 mg/mL[b]	Fine white crystals reported	2766	I
Cloxacillin sodium	SMX	100 mg/mL	ME	5 mg/mL	Physically compatible for up to 4 hr at room temperature	3245	C
Cyclosporine	BED	5 mg/mL[b]	ME	0.7 mg/mL[b]	Physically compatible for 4 hr at room temperature	2758	C
Cytarabine	MAY	50 mg/mL	ME	0.7 mg/mL[b]	Microparticles form within 4 hr	2758	I
Daptomycin	CUB°	10 mg/mL[b]	ME	0.7 mg/mL[b]	Physically compatible for 4 hr at room temperature	2758	C
Daunorubicin HCl	BED	1 mg/mL[b]	ME	0.7 mg/mL[b]	Physically compatible for 4 hr at room temperature	2758	C
Defibrotide sodium	JAZ	8 mg/mL[b]	MCD	0.4 mg/mL[b]	Visually compatible for 4 hr at room temperature	3149	C
Diltiazem HCl	HOS	5 mg/mL	ME	0.7 mg/mL[b]	Physically compatible for 4 hr at room temperature	2758	C
Diphenhydramine HCl	BA	50 mg/mL	ME	0.5 mg/mL[b]	Physically compatible with diphenhydramine HCl given i.v. push over 2 to 5 min	2766	C
Dobutamine HCl	HOS	4 mg/mL[b]	ME	0.7 mg/mL[b]	Physically compatible for 4 hr at room temperature	2758	C
Dobutamine HCl	BA	1 mg/mL	ME	0.5 mg/mL[b]	Physically compatible over 60 min	2766	C
Dolasetron mesylate	SAA	20 mg/mL	ME	0.5 mg/mL[b]	Physically compatible with dolasetron mesylate given i.v. push over 2 to 5 min	2766	C
Dopamine HCl	AMR	3.2 mg/mL[b]	ME	0.7 mg/mL[b]	Physically compatible for 4 hr at room temperature	2758	C
Dopamine HCl	BA	3.2 mg/mL	ME	0.5 mg/mL[b]	Physically compatible over 60 min	2766	C
Doripenem	JJ	5 mg/mL[a b]	ME	0.5 mg/mL[b]	Physically compatible for 4 hr at 23°C	2743	C
Doxorubicin HCl	BED	1 mg/mL[b]	ME	0.7 mg/mL[b]	Physically compatible for 4 hr at room temperature	2758	C
Epinephrine HCl	AMP	0.05 mg/mL[b]	ME	0.7 mg/mL[b]	Physically compatible for 4 hr at room temperature	2758	C
Ertapenem sodium	ME	20 mg/mL[b]	ME	0.7 mg/mL[b]	Immediate white turbid precipitate forms	2758	I
Etoposide phosphate	SIC	5 mg/mL[b]	ME	0.7 mg/mL[b]	Physically compatible for 4 hr at room temperature	2758	C
Famotidine	BA	2 mg/mL[b]	ME	0.5 mg/mL[b]	Physically compatible with famotidine i.v. push over 2 to 5 min	2766	C
Fentanyl citrate	HOS	0.05 mg/mL	ME	0.7 mg/mL[b]	Physically compatible for 4 hr at room temperature	2758	C

Y-Site Injection Compatibility (1:1 Mixture) (Cont.)

Test Drug	Mfr	Conc	Mfr	Conc	Remarks	Ref	C/I
Fentanyl citrate	HOS	0.05 mg/mL	ME	0.5 mg/mL[b]	Physically compatible with fentanyl citrate i.v. push over 2 to 5 min	2766	C
Fluconazole	HOS	2 mg/mL	ME	0.5 mg/mL[b]	Physically compatible over 60 min	2766	C
Furosemide	AMR	3 mg/mL[b]	ME	0.7 mg/mL[b]	Immediate white turbid precipitate forms	2758	I
Furosemide	HOS	10 mg/mL	ME	0.5 mg/mL[b]	Gelatinous material reported	2766	I
Ganciclovir sodium	RC	20 mg/mL[b]	ME	0.7 mg/mL[b]	Physically compatible for 4 hr at room temperature	2758	C
Gentamicin sulfate	HOS	5 mg/mL[b]	ME	0.7 mg/mL[b]	Physically compatible for 4 hr at room temperature	2758	C
Heparin sodium	HOS	100 units/mL	ME	0.7 mg/mL[b]	Immediate white turbid precipitate forms	2758	I
Heparin sodium	BA	100 units/mL	ME	0.5 mg/mL[b]	Fine white crystalline material reported	2766	I
Hydralazine HCl	APP	20 mg/mL	ME	0.5 mg/mL[b]	Physically compatible with hydralazine HCl i.v. push over 2 to 5 min	2766	C
Hydrocortisone sodium succinate	HOS	1 mg/mL[b]	ME	0.7 mg/mL[b]	Physically compatible for 4 hr at room temperature	2758	C
Hydromorphone HCl	BA	1 mg/mL[b]	ME	0.7 mg/mL[b]	Physically compatible for 4 hr at room temperature	2758	C
Hydromorphone HCl	HOS	1 mg/mL	ME	0.5 mg/mL[b]	Physically compatible with hydromorphone HCl i.v. push over 2 to 5 min	2766	C
Ifosfamide	BA	20 mg/mL[b]	ME	0.7 mg/mL[b]	Physically compatible for 4 hr at room temperature	2758	C
Imipenem–cilastatin sodium	ME	5 mg/mL[b l]	ME	0.7 mg/mL[b]	Physically compatible for 4 hr at room temperature	2758	C
Insulin, regular	NOV	1 unit/mL[b]	ME	0.7 mg/mL[b]	Physically compatible for 4 hr at room temperature	2758	C
Insulin, regular	NOV	1 unit/mL[b]	ME	0.5 mg/mL[b]	Physically compatible over 60 min	2766	C
Isavuconazonium sulfate	ASP	1.5 mg/mL[b]	ME	0.5 mg/mL[b]	Physically compatible for 2 hr	3263	C
Levofloxacin	JN	5 mg/mL[b]	ME	0.7 mg/mL[b]	Physically compatible for 4 hr at room temperature	2758	C
Levofloxacin	HOS	5 mg/mL[a]	ME	0.5 mg/mL[b]	Physically compatible over 60 min	2766	C
Linezolid	PHU	2 mg/mL[b]	ME	0.7 mg/mL[b]	Physically compatible for 4 hr at room temperature	2758	C
Linezolid	PF	2 mg/mL	ME	0.5 mg/mL[b]	Physically compatible over 60 min	2766	C
Lorazepam	HOS	0.5 mg/mL[b]	ME	0.7 mg/mL[b]	Physically compatible for 4 hr at room temperature	2758	C
Magnesium sulfate	AMR	100 mg/mL[b]	ME	0.7 mg/mL[b]	Physically compatible for 4 hr at room temperature	2758	C
Magnesium sulfate	HOS	40 mg/mL	ME	0.5 mg/mL[b]	Physically compatible over 60 min	2766	C
Melphalan HCl	CAR	1 mg/mL[b]	ME	0.7 mg/mL[b]	Physically compatible for 4 hr at room temperature	2758	C
Meperidine HCl	HOS	10 mg/mL[b]	ME	0.7 mg/mL[b]	Physically compatible for 4 hr at room temperature	2758	C
Meropenem	ASZ	2.5 mg/mL[b]	ME	0.7 mg/mL[b]	Physically compatible for 4 hr at room temperature	2758	C
Meropenem	ASZ	10 mg/mL[b]	ME	0.5 mg/mL[b]	Physically compatible over 30 min	2766	C
Meropenem		50 mg/mL	ME	0.5 mg/mL	Physically compatible for 4 hr at room temperature	3538, 3547	C
Meropenem–vabor-bactam	TMC	8 mg/mL[b c]	ME	0.5 mg/mL[b]	Measured turbidity increases immediately. pH increased by >2 units within 3 hr	3380	I
Methylprednisolone sodium succinate	PHU	5 mg/mL[b]	ME	0.7 mg/mL[b]	Immediate white turbid precipitate forms	2758	I
Metronidazole	BA	5 mg/mL	ME	0.7 mg/mL[b]	Physically compatible for 4 hr at room temperature	2758	C

Y-Site Injection Compatibility (1:1 Mixture) (Cont.)

Test Drug	Mfr	Conc	Mfr	Conc	Remarks	Ref	C/I
Metronidazole	BA	5 mg/mL	ME	0.5 mg/mL[b]	Physically compatible over 60 min	2766	C
Midazolam HCl	APP	2 mg/mL[b]	ME	0.7 mg/mL[b]	Physically compatible for 4 hr at room temperature	2758	C
Milrinone lactate	BA	0.2 mg/mL[b]	ME	0.7 mg/mL[b]	Physically compatible for 4 hr at room temperature	2758	C
Mitomycin	BED	0.5 mg/mL[b]	ME	0.7 mg/mL[b]	Physically compatible for 4 hr at room temperature	2758	C
Morphine sulfate	BA	15 mg/mL	ME	0.7 mg/mL[b]	Physically compatible for 4 hr at room temperature	2758	C
Morphine sulfate	HOS	2 mg/mL	ME	0.5 mg/mL[b]	Physically compatible with morphine sulfate i.v. push over 2 to 5 min	2766	C
Mycophenolate mofetil HCl	RC	6 mg/mL[b]	ME	0.7 mg/mL[b]	Physically compatible for 4 hr at room temperature	2758	C
Nafcillin sodium	SZ	20 mg/mL[b]	ME	0.7 mg/mL[b]	Transient turbidity becomes white precipitate	2758	I
Norepinephrine bitartrate	BED	0.128 mg/mL[b]	ME	0.7 mg/mL[b]	Physically compatible for 4 hr at room temperature	2758	C
Ondansetron HCl	BED	2 mg/mL	ME	0.5 mg/mL[b]	Physically compatible with ondansetron HCl i.v. push over 2 to 5 min	2766	C
Pantoprazole sodium	WY[e]	0.4 mg/mL[b]	ME	0.7 mg/mL[b]	Physically compatible for 4 hr at room temperature	2758	C
Pantoprazole sodium	WY[e]	0.4 mg/mL[b]	ME	0.5 mg/mL[b]	White particles reported	2766	I
Phenylephrine HCl	BA	1 mg/mL[b]	ME	0.7 mg/mL[b]	Physically compatible for 4 hr at room temperature	2758	C
Piperacillin sodium–tazobactam sodium	WY[e]	40 mg/mL[b i]	ME	0.7 mg/mL[b]	Immediate white turbid precipitate forms	2758	I
Piperacillin sodium–tazobactam sodium	WY[m]	80 mg/mL[b i]	ME	0.5 mg/mL[b]	Black particles reported	2766	I
Plazomicin sulfate	ACH	24 mg/mL[b]	ME	0.5 mg/mL[b]	Physically compatible for 1 hr at 20 to 25°C	3432	C
Posaconazole	ME	18 mg/mL		0.28 mg/mL[n]	Physically compatible	2911, 2912	C
Potassium chloride	APP	0.1 mEq/mL[b]	ME	0.7 mg/mL[b]	Physically compatible for 4 hr at room temperature	2758	C
Potassium chloride	BA	0.04 mEq/mL[b]	ME	0.5 mg/mL[b]	Physically compatible over 60 min	2766	C
Potassium phosphates	APP	0.5 mmol/mL[b]	ME	0.7 mg/mL[b]	Immediate white turbid precipitate forms	2758	I
Quinupristin–dalfopristin	MON	5 mg/mL[b j]	ME	0.7 mg/mL[b]	Physically compatible for 4 hr at room temperature	2758	C
Tacrolimus	AST	0.02 mg/mL[b]	ME	0.7 mg/mL[b]	Physically compatible for 4 hr at room temperature	2758	C
Tedizolid phosphate	CUB	0.8 mg/mL[b]	ME	0.5 mg/mL[h]	Immediate precipitation and increase in measured turbidity	3244	I
Telavancin HCl	ASP	7.5 mg/mL[b]	ME	0.5 mg/mL[b]	Physically compatible for 2 hr	2830	C
Tobramycin sulfate	SIC	5 mg/mL[b]	ME	0.7 mg/mL[b]	Physically compatible for 4 hr at room temperature	2758	C
TPN[g]			ME	0.7 mg/mL[b]	Immediate white turbid precipitate forms	2758	I
Trimethoprim–sulfamethoxazole	SIC	0.8 mg/mL[b k]	ME	0.7 mg/mL[b]	Immediate white turbid precipitate forms	2758	I
Vancomycin HCl	HOS	10 mg/mL[b]	ME	0.7 mg/mL[b]	Physically compatible for 4 hr at room temperature	2758	C
Vancomycin HCl	HOS	4 mg/mL[b]	ME	0.5 mg/mL[b]	Physically compatible over 60 min	2766	C
Vasopressin	APP	0.2 unit/mL[b]	ME	0.5 mg/mL[b]	Physically compatible	2641	C
Vincristine sulfate	MAY	0.05 mg/mL[b]	ME	0.7 mg/mL[b]	Physically compatible for 4 hr at room temperature	2758	C

Y-Site Injection Compatibility (1:1 Mixture) (Cont.)

Test Drug	Mfr	Conc	Mfr	Conc	Remarks	Ref	C/I
Voriconazole	PF	4 mg/mL[b]	ME	0.7 mg/mL[b]	Physically compatible for 4 hr at room temperature	2758	C
Voriconazole	PF	2 mg/mL[b]	ME	0.5 mg/mL[b]	Physically compatible over 60 min	2766	C

[a] Tested in dextrose 5%.

[b] Tested in sodium chloride 0.9%.

[c] Meropenem component. Meropenem in a 1:1 fixed-ratio concentration with vaborbactam.

[d] Tested in sodium chloride 0.45%.

[e] Test performed using the formulation WITH edetate disodium.

[f] Test performed using the formulation WITHOUT edetate disodium.

[g] Specific composition of the parenteral nutrition admixture not reported. TPN indicates a 2-in-1 admixture.

[h] Tested in Ringer's injection, lactated.

[i] Piperacillin component. Piperacillin in an 8:1 fixed-ratio concentration with tazobactam.

[j] Quinupristin and dalfopristin components combined.

[k] Trimethoprim component. Trimethoprim in a 1:5 fixed-ratio concentration with sulfamethoxazole.

[l] Not specified whether concentration refers to single component or combined components.

[m] Presence or absence of edetate disodium not specified.

[n] Tested in both dextrose 5% and sodium chloride 0.9%.

[o] Test performed using the Cubicin formulation.

[p] Ceftolozane component. Ceftolozane in a 2:1 fixed-ratio concentration with tazobactam.

Selected Revisions June 1, 2019. © Copyright, October 2008.
American Society of Health-System Pharmacists, Inc.

Cefazolin Sodium
AHFS 8:12.06.04

Products

Cefazolin as the sodium salt is available in 500-mg and 1-, 10-, and 20-g vials. For intramuscular administration, reconstitute the 500-mg vial with 2 mL and the 1-g vial with 2.5 mL and shake well until dissolved, yielding 225 and 330 mg/mL, respectively. Sterile water for injection or bacteriostatic water for injection may be used for either the 500-mg or 1-g vials while sodium chloride 0.9% only may be used for the 500-mg vial.[1(4/08)] [4]

For direct intravenous injection, further dilute the reconstituted cefazolin sodium with approximately 5 mL of sterile water for injection.[1(4/08)] [4]

For intermittent intravenous infusion, reconstituted cefazolin sodium should be diluted further in 50 to 100 mL of compatible infusion solution.[1(4/08)] [4]

The 10-g bulk vials may be reconstituted with sterile water for injection, bacteriostatic water for injection, or sodium chloride 0.9%. The 10-g vial should be reconstituted with 45 or 96 mL to yield concentrations of 1 g/5 mL or 1 g/10 mL, respectively.[1(4/08)]

Cefazolin sodium (Braun) is available as 1 g in a dual-chamber flexible container. The diluent chamber contains dextrose solution.[1(4/08)]

Cefazolin sodium is also available frozen in polyvinyl chloride (PVC) bags in concentrations of 500 mg and 1 g in 50 mL of dextrose 5%.[4]

pH

From 4.5 to 6. The frozen premixed solutions have a pH of 4.5 to 7.[4]

Osmolality

The osmolality of a 225-mg/mL solution in sterile water for injection was determined to be 636 mOsm/kg by freezing-point depression.[1071]

The osmolality of cefazolin sodium 1 and 2 g was calculated for the following dilutions:[1054]

Diluent	Osmolality (mOsm/kg)	
	50 mL	100 mL
1 g		
Dextrose 5%	321	291
Sodium chloride 0.9%	344	317
2 g		
Dextrose 5%	379	324
Sodium chloride 0.9%	406	351

Cefazolin sodium (Braun) 1 g in dual-chamber flexible containers has an osmolality of 290 mOsm/kg when activated with the dextrose solution diluent.[1(4/08)]

The frozen premixed solutions have osmolalities of 260 to 320 mOsm/kg for the 500 mg/50-mL concentration and 310 to 380 mOsm/kg for the 1-g/50-mL concentration.[4]

The following maximum cefazolin sodium concentrations were recommended to achieve osmolalities suitable for peripheral infusion in fluid-restricted patients:[1180]

Diluent	Maximum Concentration (mg/mL)	Osmolality (mOsm/kg)
Dextrose 5%	77	507
Sodium chloride 0.9%	69	494
Sterile water for injection	138	404

Sodium Content

Each gram of cefazolin sodium contains 48 mg or approximately 2 mEq of sodium.[1(4/08)] [4]

Administration

Cefazolin sodium may be administered by deep intramuscular injection or by intravenous injection. By direct intravenous injection, it is given over 3 to 5 minutes directly into the vein or tubing of a running infusion solution. It may also be given by intermittent infusion in 50 to 100 mL of compatible diluent or by continuous infusion.[1(4/08)]

Stability

Intact containers of the sterile powder should be stored at controlled room temperature. Reconstituted solutions of cefazolin sodium are light yellow to yellow. Protection from light is recommended for both the powder and its solutions.[1(4/08)] [4]

The manufacturer recommends that solutions of cefazolin sodium be discarded after 24 hours at room temperature or 10 days under refrigeration.[1(4/08)] This recommendation is made to reduce the potential for the growth of microorganisms and to minimize an increase in color and a change in pH.[276] A test of cefazolin sodium 250 mg/mL in water for injection showed that the drug lost less than 3% in 14 days at 5°C. A loss of 8 to 10% was noted in 4 days at 25°C.[276]

Cefazolin sodium (Braun) 1 g in dual-chamber flexible plastic containers with dextrose solution diluent should be used within 24 hours after activation if stored at room temperature and in 7 days if stored under refrigeration.[1(4/08)]

DOI: 10.37573/9781585286850.072

Crystallization

Crystal formation has also been observed in reconstituted cefazolin sodium 330 mg/mL stored at room temperature after complete dissolution when sodium chloride 0.9% is the diluent. The crystals formed initially are fine and may be easily overlooked. At 330 mg/mL, cefazolin sodium is near its saturation point, and the room temperature and ionic content of the diluent are important for maintaining the drug in solution. In an evaluation of cefazolin sodium reconstituted with 2.5 mL of either sodium chloride 0.9% or sterile water for injection and stored at 24 or 26°C, none of the vials reconstituted with sterile water for injection formed crystals within 24 hours. However, when sodium chloride 0.9% was the diluent, all vials had crystals. Consequently, sterile water for injection was recommended as the diluent when possible.[875] The crystals of cefazolin sodium can be redissolved by hand-warming the vials or by immersion in a 35°C water bath for 2 minutes. The clear solution will then be suitable for use.[1075]

pH Effects

Cefazolin sodium solutions are relatively stable at pH 4.5 to 8.5. Above pH 8.5, rapid hydrolysis of the drug occurs. Below pH 4.5, precipitation of the insoluble free acid may occur.[4 284]

Cefazolin sodium in solutions containing dextrose, fructose, sucrose, dextran 40 or 70, mannitol, sorbitol, or glycerol in concentrations up to 15% was most stable at pH 5 to 6.5. At neutral and alkaline pH, the rate of degradation was accelerated by the carbohydrates and alcohols.[820]

Cefazolin sodium 3.33 mg/mL was evaluated in several aqueous buffer solutions. The drug was most stable in pH 4.5 acetate buffer, exhibiting 10% decomposition in 3 days at 35°C and in 5 days at 25°C. In pH 5.7 acetate buffer, a 13% loss occurred in 3 days at 35°C and a 10% loss occurred in 5 days at 25°C. No loss occurred in either acetate buffer in 7 days at 4°C.[1147]

In pH 7.5 phosphate buffer, a yellow color and particulate matter developed after 3 to 4 days at 35°C. This change was accompanied by a 6% cefazolin loss in 1 day and an 18% loss in 3 days. At 25 and 4°C, 10 and 5% cefazolin losses occurred, respectively, in 5 days.[1147]

Freezing Solutions

Solutions of cefazolin sodium 125, 225, and 330 mg/mL frozen in the original containers at −20°C immediately after reconstitution with sterile water for injection, bacteriostatic water for injection, or sodium chloride 0.9% are stated to be stable for 12 weeks. Thawed solutions are stable for 24 hours at room temperature or 10 days under refrigeration; they should not be refrozen.[4]

When reconstituted with water for injection, dextrose 5%, or sodium chloride 0.9% in concentrations of 1 g/2.5 mL, 500 mg/100 mL, and 10 g/45 mL, cefazolin sodium retained more than 90% potency for up to 26 weeks when frozen within 1 hour after reconstitution at −10 and −20°C. In a concentration of 500 mg/100 mL in dextrose 5% in Ringer's injection, lactated, Ionosol B in dextrose 5%, Normosol M in dextrose

5%, Plasma-Lyte in dextrose 5%, or Ringer's injection, lactated, cefazolin sodium was stable for up to 4 weeks when frozen within 1 hour after reconstitution at −10°C.[277]

In another study, cefazolin sodium (SKF) 1 g/50 mL of dextrose 5% and also sodium chloride 0.9% in PVC containers was frozen at −20°C for 30 days. The results indicate that potency was retained for the duration of the study.[299]

Cefazolin sodium (Lilly) 1 g/100 mL in dextrose 5% in PVC bags was frozen at −20°C for 30 days and then thawed by exposure to ambient temperature or microwave radiation. The solutions showed no evidence of precipitation or color change and showed no loss of potency as determined microbiologically. Subsequent storage of the admixture at room temperature for 24 hours also yielded a physically compatible solution which exhibited a 3 to 6% loss of potency.[554]

In an additional study, cefazolin sodium (Lilly and SKF) 10 mg/mL in 50, 100, and 250 mL of dextrose 5% and sodium chloride 0.9% in PVC bags was frozen at −20°C for 48 hours. Thawing was then performed by exposure to microwave radiation carefully applied so that the solution temperature did not exceed 20°C and so that a small amount of ice remained at the endpoint. This procedure avoids accelerated decomposition due to inadvertent excessive temperature increases. The solutions were stored for 4 hours at room temperature. Both brands of cefazolin sodium retained at least 90% of the initial activity as determined by microbiological assay. In addition, the solutions did not exhibit color changes or significant pH changes.[627]

An approximate fourfold increase in particles of 2 to 60 μm was produced by freezing and thawing cefazolin sodium (Lilly) 2 g/100 mL of dextrose 5% (Travenol). The reconstituted drug was filtered through a 0.45-μm filter into PVC bags of solution and frozen for 7 days at −20°C. Thawing was performed at room temperature (29°C) for 12 hours. Although the total number of particles increased significantly, no particles greater than 60 μm were observed; the solution complied with USP standards for particle sizes and numbers in large volume parenteral solutions.[822]

No loss of cefazolin sodium (SKF) was reported from a solution containing 73.2 mg/mL in sterile water for injection in PVC and glass containers after 30 days at −20°C. Subsequent thawing and storage for 4 days at 5°C, followed by 24 hours at 37°C to simulate the use of a portable infusion pump, also did not result in a cefazolin loss.[1391]

The manufacturer warns against continued heating of a completely thawed solution, which can result in accelerated drug decomposition and possibly dangerous pressure increases in the container.[627]

Cefazolin sodium (Braun) 1 g in dual-chamber flexible containers should not be frozen.[1(4/08)]

Syringes

Cefazolin sodium (SKF) 1 and 2 g/10 mL in sterile water for injection, packaged in plastic syringes (Monoject), exhibited a 10% cefazolin loss in 13 days at 24°C. At 4°C, the drug exhibited less than a 10% loss during the 28-day study period. Frozen at −15°C, less than 10% drug loss occurred in 3 months.[1178]

Cefazolin sodium (Apothecon) 50 mg/mL in sodium chloride 0.9% was packaged in 5-mL polypropylene syringes (Becton Dickinson) and stored at 23 and 5°C. About 10% loss was found after 12 days of storage at 23°C. About 3% loss was found after 22 days of refrigerated storage.[2474]

Cefazolin sodium (Apotex) 100 and 200 mg/mL in sterile water for injection was packaged in polypropylene syringes and stored at 5°C protected from light.[2986] A slight increase in yellow discoloration of the solution occurred with less than 10% loss in 30 days at 5°C with light protection followed by 72 hours at 21 to 25°C with light exposure.[2986]

Filtration

Cefazolin sodium (SKF) 10 g/L in dextrose 5% and also in sodium chloride 0.9% was filtered through 0.45- and 0.22-μm Millipore membrane filters at time zero and at 4, 8, and 24 hours after mixing. No significant difference in concentration occurred between any of the filtered samples compared to unfiltered solutions at these time intervals. It was concluded that filtra-tion of cefazolin sodium solutions through these membrane filters could be performed without adversely affecting the drug concentration.[375]

Central Venous Catheter

Cefazolin sodium (SmithKline Beecham) 5 mg/mL in dextrose 5% was found to be compatible with the ARROWg+ard Blue Plus (Arrow International) chlorhexidine-bearing triple-lumen central catheter. Essentially complete delivery of the drug was found with little or no drug loss occurring. Furthermore, chlorhexidine delivered from the catheter remained at trace amounts with no substantial increase due to the delivery of the drug through the catheter.[2335]

Cefazolin sodium 10 mg/mL with heparin sodium 5000 units/mL as an antibiotic lock in polyurethane central hemodi-alysis catheters lost about 50% of the antibiotic over 72 hours at 37°C. The loss was attributed to sorption to the catheters. Nevertheless, the reduced antibiotic concentration (about 5 mg/mL) remained effective against common microorganisms in catheter-related bacteremia in hemodialysis patients.[2515] [2516]

Compatibility Information

Solution Compatibility

Cefazolin sodium

Test Soln Name	Mfr	Mfr	Conc/L or %	Remarks	Ref	C/I
Amino acids 4.25%, dextrose 25%	MG	LI	1 g	No increase in particulate matter in 24 hr at 5°C	349	C
Dextrose 5% in Ringer's injection, lactated		SZ		Manufacturer-recommended solution	1(4/08)	C
Dextrose 5% in Ringer's injection, lactated		LI	5 g	Stable for 14 days at 5°C. 8% loss in 4 days at 25°C	276	C
Dextrose 2.5% in sodium chloride 0.45%	AB	SZ		Manufacturer-recommended solution	1(4/08)	C
Dextrose 2.5% in sodium chloride 0.9%	AB	SZ		Manufacturer-recommended solution	1(4/08)	C
Dextrose 5% in sodium chloride 0.225%	AB	SZ		Manufacturer-recommended solution	1(4/08)	C
Dextrose 5% in sodium chloride 0.45%	AB	SZ		Manufacturer-recommended solution	1(4/08)	C
Dextrose 5% in sodium chloride 0.9%	AB	SZ		Manufacturer-recommended solution	1(4/08)	C
Dextrose 10% in sodium chloride 0.9%	AB	SZ		Manufacturer-recommended solution	1(4/08)	C
Dextrose 5%		SZ		Manufacturer-recommended solution	1(4/08)	C
Dextrose 5%		LI	5 g	4% loss in 14 days at 5°C, 6% loss in 4 days at 25°C	276	C
Dextrose 5%	BA[a], TR	SKF	20 g	Stable for 24 hr at 5 and 22°C	298	C
Dextrose 5%	TR[b]	LI	10 g	Physically compatible with 3% loss in 24 hr at room temperature	554	C

Solution Compatibility (Cont.)

Test Soln Name	Mfr	Mfr	Conc/L or %	Remarks	Ref	C/I
Dextrose 5%	MG[c]	SKF	10 g	Physically compatible with no loss in 48 hr at room temperature under fluorescent light	983	C
Dextrose 5%	BA[a]	BR	10 g	Visually compatible with 7% loss in 30 days at 4°C	2142	C
Dextrose 5%	TR[a]	LI	20 g	7% loss in 5 days at 24°C and 5% loss in 24 days at 4°C	336	C
Dextrose 5%	BA[e]	NOP	5 and 40 g	Less than 10% loss in 7 days at 23°C and 28 days at 4°C	2819	C
Dextrose 5%	[b]	APO	20 and 40 g	Slight increase in yellow discoloration with less than 10% loss in 30 days at 5°C with light protection followed by 72 hr at 21 to 25°C with light exposure	2986	C
Dextrose 5%	BA[f]	AFT	12.5 and 25 g	Physically compatible with less than 6% loss in 3 days at 4°C followed by 12 hr at 35°C and an additional 12 hr at 25°C	3564	C
Dextrose 10%		SZ		Manufacturer-recommended solution	1(4/08)	C
Ionosol B in dextrose 5%		LI	5 g	2% loss in 14 days at 5°C, 1 to 4% loss in 4 days at 25°C	276	C
Normosol M in dextrose 5%		LI	5 g	3% loss in 14 days at 5°C, 1 to 4% loss in 4 days at 25°C	276	C
Ringer's injection		SZ		Manufacturer-recommended solution	1(4/08)	C
Ringer's injection, lactated		SZ		Manufacturer-recommended solution	1(4/08)	C
Ringer's injection, lactated		LI	5 g	Stable for 14 days at 5°C. 9% loss in 7 days at 25°C	276	C
Sodium chloride 0.9%		SZ		Manufacturer-recommended solution	1(4/08)	C
Sodium chloride 0.9%		LI	5 g	4% loss in 7 days at 5°C, 8% loss in 4 days at 25°C	276	C
Sodium chloride 0.9%	BA[a], TR	SKF	20 g	Stable for 24 hr at 5 and 22°C	298	C
Sodium chloride 0.9%	MG[c]	SKF	10 g	Physically compatible with no loss in 48 hr at room temperature under fluorescent light	983	C
Sodium chloride 0.9%		LI	3.33 g	Physically compatible with 5% loss at 25°C in 3 days. No loss in 7 days at 4°C	1147	C
Sodium chloride 0.9%	TR[b]	LI	20 g	9% loss in 7 days at 24°C and 5% loss in 15 days at 4°C	336	C
Sodium chloride 0.9%	HOS[e]	NOP	5 and 40 g	Less than 10% loss in 7 days at 23°C and 28 days at 4°C	2819	C
Sodium chloride 0.9%	[b]	APO	20 and 40 g	Slight increase in yellow discoloration with less than 10% loss in 30 days at 5°C with light protection followed by 72 hours at 21 to 25°C with light exposure	2986	C
Sodium chloride 0.9%	BA[f]	AFT	12.5 and 25 g	Physically compatible with less than 5% loss in 3 days at 4°C followed by 12 hr at 35°C and an additional 12 hr at 25°C	3564	C
TPN #22[d]		SKF	10 g	Physically compatible with no loss of activity in 24 hr at 22°C in the dark	837	C
TPN #107[d]			1 g	9% cefazolin loss in 24 hr at 21°C	1326	C

[a] Tested in both glass and PVC containers.

[b] Tested in PVC containers.

[c] Tested in glass containers.

[d] Refer to Appendix for the composition of parenteral nutrition solutions. TPN indicates a 2-in-1 admixture.

[e] Tested in Accufusor reservoirs.

[f] Tested in Infusor LV (Baxter) elastomeric reservoirs.

Additive Compatibility

Cefazolin sodium

Test Drug	Mfr	Conc/L or %	Mfr	Conc/L or %	Test Solution	Remarks	Ref	C/I
Amikacin sulfate	BR	5 g	LI	20 g	D5LR, D5R, D5S, D5W, D10W, LR, NS, R, SL	Both drugs stable for 8 hr at 25°C. Turbidity observed at 24 hr	293	I
Atracurium besylate	BW	500 mg		10 g	D5W	Atracurium unstable and particles form	1694	I
Aztreonam	SQ	10 and 20 g	LI	5 and 20 g	D5W, NS[a]	Physically compatible. Little loss of either drug in 48 hr at 25°C and 7 days at 4°C in the dark	1020	C
Bleomycin sulfate	BR	20 and 30 units	LI	1 g	NS	43% loss of bleomycin activity in 1 week at 4°C	763	I
Clindamycin phosphate	UP	9 g	SKF	10 g	D5W[b]	Physically compatible with no clindamycin loss and 8% cefazolin loss in 48 hr at room temperature under fluorescent light	983	C
Clindamycin phosphate	UP	9 g	SKF	10 g	NS[b]	Physically compatible with no clindamycin loss and 3% cefazolin loss in 48 hr at room temperature under fluorescent light	983	C
Clindamycin phosphate[d]	UP	9 g	SKF	10 g	D5W, NS[b]	10% cefazolin loss in 4 hr in D5W and 12 hr in NS at 25°C. No clindamycin and gentamicin loss in 24 hr	1328	I
Famotidine	YAM	200 mg	FUJ	10 g	D5W	Visually compatible with 10% cefazolin and 5% famotidine loss in 24 hr at 25°C. 9% cefazolin and 5% famotidine loss in 48 hr at 4°C	1763	C
Fluconazole	PF	1 g	SM	10 g	D5W	Visually compatible with no fluconazole loss in 72 hr at 25°C under fluorescent light. Cefazolin not tested	1677	C
Gentamicin sulfate[e]	ES	800 mg	SKF	10 g	D5W, NS[b]	10% cefazolin loss in 4 hr in D5W and 12 hr in NS at 25°C. No clindamycin and gentamicin loss in 24 hr	1328	I
Linezolid	PHU	2 g	APC	10 g	[c]	Physically compatible with 5% or less loss of each drug in 3 days at 23°C and 7 days at 4°C protected from light	2262	C
Meperidine HCl		0.5 g	FUJ	10 g	D5W	Visually compatible. 5% loss of each drug in 5 days at 25°C. 5% cefazolin and 7% meperidine loss in 20 days at 4°C	1966	C
Metronidazole	SE	5 g	LI	10 g		5% cefazolin loss and no metronidazole loss in 7 days at 25°C. No loss of either drug in 12 days at 5°C	993	C
Metronidazole	AB	5 g	LI	10 g		Visually compatible with no loss of either drug in 72 hr at 8°C	1649	C
Promethazine HCl	ES	250 mg	LI	10 g	D5W	Cloudiness forms then dissipates	1753	?
Ranitidine HCl	GL	100 mg		2 g	D5W	Color change within 24 hr	1151	?
Ranitidine HCl	GL	50 mg and 2 g		1 g	D5W	Ranitidine stable for only 6 hr at 25°C. Cefazolin not tested	1515	I

Additive Compatibility (Cont.)

Test Drug	Mfr	Conc/L or %	Mfr	Conc/L or %	Test Solution	Remarks	Ref	C/I
Tenoxicam	RC	200 mg	FUJ	5 g	D5W	Visually compatible with less than 10% loss of both drugs in 48 hr at 25°C and in 72 hr at 4°C in the dark	2441	C
Verapamil HCl	KN	80 mg	SKF	2 g	D5W, NS	Physically compatible for 24 hr	764	C

[a] Tested in PVC containers.

[b] Tested in glass containers.

[c] Admixed in the linezolid infusion container.

[d] Tested in combination with gentamicin sulfate 800 mg/L.

[e] Tested in combination with clindamycin phosphate 9 g/L.

Drugs in Syringe Compatibility

Cefazolin sodium

Test Drug	Mfr	Amt	Mfr	Amt	Remarks	Ref	C/I
Ascorbic acid	LI	1 mL	LI	1 g/3 mL	Precipitate forms within 3 min at 32°C	766	I
Dimenhydrinate		10 mg/1 mL		100 mg/1 mL	Clear solution	2569	C
Heparin sodium		2500 units/1 mL		2 g	Physically compatible for at least 5 min	1053	C
Hydromorphone HCl	KN	2, 10, 40 mg/1 mL	SKF	>200 mg/1 mL	Precipitate forms	2082	I
Hydromorphone HCl	KN	2, 10, 40 mg/1 mL	SKF	150 mg/1 mL	Visually compatible with less than 10% loss of each drug in 24 hr at room temperature	2082	C
Lidocaine HCl	AST	0.5%, 3 mL	SKF	1 g	Precipitate forms within 3 to 4 hr at 4°C	532	I
Pantoprazole sodium	[a]	4 mg/1 mL		100 mg/1 mL	Precipitates immediately	2574	I

[a] Test performed using the formulation WITHOUT edetate disodium.

Y-Site Injection Compatibility (1:1 Mixture)

Cefazolin sodium

Test Drug	Mfr	Conc	Mfr	Conc	Remarks	Ref	C/I
Acyclovir sodium	BW	5 mg/mL[a]	SKF	20 mg/mL[a]	Physically compatible for 4 hr at 25°C	1157	C
Allopurinol sodium	BW	3 mg/mL[b]	GEM	20 mg/mL[b]	Physically compatible for 4 hr at 22°C	1686	C
Alprostadil	BED	7.5 mcg/mL[o] [p]	LI	100 mg/mL[n]	Visually compatible for 1 hr	2746	C
Amifostine	USB	10 mg/mL[a]	MAR	20 mg/mL[a]	Physically compatible for 4 hr at 23°C	1845	C
Amiodarone HCl	LZ	4 mg/mL[a]	LI	20 mg/mL[a]	Precipitate forms	1444	I
Amiodarone HCl	LZ	4 mg/mL[b]	LI	20 mg/mL[b]	Physically compatible for 4 hr at room temperature	1444	C
Anakinra	SYN	4 and 36 mg/mL[b]	GVA	15 mg/mL[b]	Physically compatible. No cefazolin loss in 4 hr at 25°C. Anakinra uncertain	2508	?
Anidulafungin	VIC	0.5 mg/mL[a]	APC	20 mg/mL[a]	Physically compatible for 4 hr at 23°C	2617	C
Atracurium besylate	BW	0.5 mg/mL[a]	LY	10 mg/mL[a]	Physically compatible for 24 hr at 28°C	1337	C
Aztreonam	SQ	40 mg/mL[a]	MAR	20 mg/mL[a]	Physically compatible for 4 hr at 23°C	1758	C
Bivalirudin	TMC	5 mg/mL[a]	APO	20 mg/mL[a]	Physically compatible for 4 hr at 23°C	2373	C
Calcium gluconate	AST	4 mg/mL[c]	LI	40 mg/mL[c]	Physically compatible for 3 hr	1316	C

Y-Site Injection Compatibility (1:1 Mixture) (Cont.)

Test Drug	Mfr	Conc	Mfr	Conc	Remarks	Ref	C/I
Caspofungin acetate	ME	0.7 mg/mL[b]	CUR	20 mg/mL[b]	Immediate white turbid precipitate forms	2758	I
Caspofungin acetate	ME	0.5 mg/mL[b]	SZ	100 mg/mL[b]	Fine white crystals reported	2766	I
Ceftolozane sulfate–tazobactam sodium	CUB	10 mg/mL[c q]	HOS	20 mg/mL[c]	Physically compatible for 2 hr	3262	C
Cisatracurium besylate	GW	0.1 mg/mL[a]	SKB	20 mg/mL[a]	Physically compatible for 4 hr at 23°C	2074	C
Cisatracurium besylate	GW	2 mg/mL[a]	SKB	20 mg/mL[a]	Gray subvisible haze forms immediately	2074	I
Cisatracurium besylate	GW	5 mg/mL[a]	SKB	20 mg/mL[a]	Gray haze forms immediately	2074	I
Cloxacillin sodium	SMX	100 mg/mL	NOP	10 mg/mL	Physically compatible for up to 4 hr at room temperature	3245	C
Cyclophosphamide	MJ	20 mg/mL[a]	SKF	20 mg/mL[a]	Physically compatible for 4 hr at 25°C	1194	C
Dexmedetomidine HCl	AB	4 mcg/mL[b]	LI	20 mg/mL[b]	Physically compatible for 4 hr at 23°C	2383	C
Diltiazem HCl	MMD	5 mg/mL	LI	20 and 200 mg/mL[b]	Visually compatible	1807	C
Diltiazem HCl	MMD	1 mg/mL[b]	LI	200 mg/mL[b]	Visually compatible	1807	C
Docetaxel	RPR	0.9 mg/mL[a]	APC	20 mg/mL[a]	Physically compatible for 4 hr at 23°C	2224	C
Doxapram HCl	RB	2 mg/mL[a]	APO	100 mg/mL[a]	Visually compatible for 4 hr at 23°C	2470	C
Doxorubicin HCl liposomal	SEQ	0.4 mg/mL[a]	SKB	20 mg/mL[a]	Physically compatible for 4 hr at 23°C	2087	C
Enalaprilat	MSD	0.05 mg/mL[b]	SKF	20 mg/mL[e]	Physically compatible for 24 hr at room temperature under fluorescent light	1355	C
Esmolol HCl	DCC	10 mg/mL[a]	LI	10 mg/mL[a]	Physically compatible for 24 hr at 22°C	1169	C
Etoposide phosphate	BR	5 mg/mL[a]	APC	20 mg/mL[a]	Physically compatible for 4 hr at 23°C	2218	C
Famotidine	MSD	0.2 mg/mL[a]	LY	20 mg/mL[b]	Physically compatible for 14 hr	1196	C
Famotidine	ME	2 mg/mL[b]		20 mg/mL[a]	Visually compatible for 4 hr at 22°C	1936	C
Fenoldopam mesylate	AB	80 mcg/mL[b]	APO	20 mg/mL[b]	Physically compatible for 4 hr at 23°C	2467	C
Filgrastim	AMG	30 mcg/mL[a]	LI	20 mg/mL[a]	Physically compatible for 4 hr at 22°C	1687	C
Fluconazole	RR	2 mg/mL	LY	40 mg/mL	Physically compatible for 24 hr at 25°C	1407	C
Fludarabine phosphate	BX	1 mg/mL[a]	LEM	20 mg/mL[a]	Visually compatible for 4 hr at 22°C	1439	C
Foscarnet sodium	AST	24 mg/ml	SKF	40 mg/mL	Physically compatible for 24 hr at room temperature under fluorescent light	1335	C
Gallium nitrate	FUJ	1 mg/mL[b]	GEM	100 mg/mL[b]	Visually compatible for 24 hr at 25°C	1673	C
Gemcitabine HCl	LI	10 mg/mL[b]	APC	20 mg/mL[b]	Physically compatible for 4 hr at 23°C	2226	C
Granisetron HCl	SKB	0.05 mg/mL[a]	SKB	20 mg/mL[a]	Physically compatible for 4 hr at 23°C	2000	C
Heparin sodium	TR	50 units/mL	SKB	20 mg/mL[a]	Visually compatible for 4 hr at 25°C	1793	C
Heparin sodium	LEO	10 and 5000 units/mL[b]	NOP	10 mg/mL[b]	Physically compatible with little change in heparin activity in 14 days at 4 and 37°C. Antibiotic not tested	2684	C
Hetastarch in lactated electrolyte	AB	6%	LI	20 mg/mL[a]	Physically compatible for 4 hr at 23°C	2339	C
Hetastarch in sodium chloride 0.9%	DCC	6%	SKF	20 mg/mL[a]	Visually compatible for 4 hr at room temperature	1313	C

Y-Site Injection Compatibility (1:1 Mixture) (Cont.)

Test Drug	Mfr	Conc	Mfr	Conc	Remarks	Ref	C/I
Hetastarch in sodium chloride 0.9%	DCC	6%	SKF	20 mg/mL[a]	Simulation in vials showed no incompatibility, but white precipitate formed in Y-site during infusion	1315	I
Hydromorphone HCl	WY	0.2 mg/mL[a]	SKF	20 mg/mL[a]	Physically compatible for 4 hr at 25°C	987	C
Hydromorphone HCl	KN	2, 10, 40 mg/mL	SKF	20[a] and 150 mg/mL	Visually compatible and both drugs stable for 24 hr	1532	C
Hydromorphone HCl	KN	2, 10, 40 mg/mL	SKF	>200 mg/mL	Precipitate forms immediately	1532	I
Hydroxyethyl starch 130/0.4 in sodium chloride 0.9%	FRK	6%	NOP	20, 30, 40 mg/mL[a]	Visually compatible for 24 hr at room temperature	2770	C
Idarubicin HCl	AD	1 mg/mL[b]	LI	20 mg/mL[a]	Precipitate forms in 1 hr	1525	I
Insulin, regular	LI	0.2 unit/mL[b]	LI	20 mg/mL[a]	Physically compatible for 2 hr at 25°C	1395	C
Isavuconazonium sulfate	ASP	1.5 mg/mL[c]	APO	20 mg/mL[c]	Measured turbidity increases immediately	3263	I
Labetalol HCl	SC	1 mg/mL[a]	LI	10 mg/mL[a]	Physically compatible for 24 hr at 18°C	1171	C
Letermovir	ME	[a]		[a]	Physically compatible	3398	C
Lidocaine HCl	AB	8 mg/mL[c]	LI	40 mg/mL[c]	Physically compatible for 3 hr	1316	C
Linezolid	PHU	2 mg/mL	SKB	20 mg/mL[a]	Physically compatible for 4 hr at 23°C	2264	C
Magnesium sulfate	IX	16.7, 33.3, 66.7, 100 mg/mL[a]	LI	20 mg/mL[a]	Physically compatible for at least 4 hr at 32°C	813	C
Melphalan HCl	BW	0.1 mg/mL[b]	GEM	20 mg/mL[b]	Physically compatible for 3 hr at 22°C	1557	C
Meperidine HCl	WY	10 mg/mL[a]	SKF	20 mg/mL[a]	Physically compatible for 4 hr at 25°C	987	C
Meropenem		50 mg/mL	HOS	100 mg/mL	Physically compatible for 4 hr at room temperature	3538	C
Meropenem–vaborbactam	TMC	8 mg/mL[b r]	SGT	20 mg/mL[b]	Physically compatible for 3 hr at 20 to 25°C	3380	C
Midazolam HCl	RC	1 mg/mL[a]	MAR	20 mg/mL[a]	Visually compatible for 24 hr at 23°C	1847	C
Milrinone lactate	SS	0.2 mg/mL[a]	APO	100 mg/mL[a]	Visually compatible for 4 hr at 25°C	2381	C
Morphine sulfate	WI	1 mg/mL[a]	SKF	20 mg/mL[a]	Physically compatible for 4 hr at 25°C	987	C
Multivitamins	USV	5 mL/L[a]	SKF	1 g/50 mL[a]	Physically compatible for 24 hr at room temperature	323	C
Nicardipine HCl	DCC	0.1 mg/mL[a]	SKF	20 mg/mL[a]	Visually compatible for 24 hr at room temperature	235	C
Ondansetron HCl	GL	1 mg/mL[b]	LEM	20 mg/mL[a]	Visually compatible for 4 hr at 22°C	1365	C
Ondansetron HCl	GL	0.03 and 0.3 mg/mL[a]	LI	20 mg/mL[a]	Visually compatible with little loss of either drug in 4 hr at 25°C	1732	C
Palonosetron HCl	MGI	50 mcg/mL	WAT	20 mg/mL[a]	Physically compatible and no loss of either drug in 4 hr at room temperature	2749	C
Pancuronium bromide	ES	0.05 mg/mL[a]	LY	10 mg/mL[a]	Physically compatible for 24 hr at 28°C	1337	C
Pantoprazole sodium	ALT[m]	0.16 to 0.8 mg/mL[b]	NOP	20 to 40 mg/mL[a]	Visually compatible for 12 hr at 23°C	2603	C
Pemetrexed disodium	LI	20 mg/mL[b]	GVA	20 mg/mL[a]	Slight color darkening occurs over 4 hr	2564	I
Pentamidine isethionate	FUJ	3 mg/mL[a]	SKB	20 mg/mL[a]	Cloudy precipitation forms immediately	1880	I

Y-Site Injection Compatibility (1:1 Mixture) (Cont.)

Test Drug	Mfr	Conc	Mfr	Conc	Remarks	Ref	C/I
Plazomicin sulfate	ACH	24 mg/mL[c]	SGT	20 mg/mL[c]	Physically compatible for 1 hr at 20 to 25°C	3432	C
Promethazine HCl	ES	25 mg/mL	LI	10 mg/mL[a]	Cloudiness forms then dissipates	1753	?
Propofol	ZEN[s]	10 mg/mL	MAR	20 mg/mL[a]	Physically compatible for 1 hr at 23°C	2066	C
Ranitidine HCl	GL	1 mg/mL[b]	FUJ	20 mg/mL[b]	Visually compatible with little loss of either drug in 4 hr at 25°C	2259	C
Ranitidine HCl	GL	1 mg/mL[b]	FUJ	20 mg/mL[b]	Visually compatible with no cefazolin loss and 3% ranitidine loss in 4 hr	2362	C
Remifentanil HCl	GW	0.025 and 0.25 mg/mL[b]	SKB	20 mg/mL[a]	Physically compatible for 4 hr at 23°C	2075	C
Sargramostim	IMM	10 mcg/mL[b]	LEM	20 mg/mL[b]	Visually compatible for 4 hr at 22°C	1436	C
Tacrolimus	FUJ	1 mg/mL[b]	BR	40 mg/mL[a]	Visually compatible for 24 hr at 25°C	1630	C
Tedizolid phosphate	CUB	0.8 mg/mL[b]	APO	20 mg/mL[b]	Physically compatible for 2 hr	3244	C
Teniposide	BR	0.1 mg/mL[a]	MAR	20 mg/mL[a]	Physically compatible for 4 hr at 23°C	1725	C
Theophylline	TR	4 mg/mL	SKB	20 mg/mL	Visually compatible for 6 hr at 25°C	1793	C
Thiotepa	IMM[f]	1 mg/mL[a]	MAR	20 mg/mL[a]	Physically compatible for 4 hr at 23°C	1861	C
TNA #73[g]		32.5 mL[h]	SKF	20 mg/mL[a]	Visually compatible for 4 hr at 25°C	1008	C
TNA #218[g]			SKB	20 mg/mL[a]	Visually compatible for 4 hr at 23°C	2215	C
TNA #219[g]			SKB	20 mg/mL[a]	Visually compatible for 4 hr at 23°C	2215	C
TNA #220[g]			SKB	20 mg/mL[a]	Visually compatible for 4 hr at 23°C	2215	C
TNA #221[g]			SKB	20 mg/mL[a]	Visually compatible for 4 hr at 23°C	2215	C
TNA #222[g]			SKB	20 mg/mL[a]	Visually compatible for 4 hr at 23°C	2215	C
TNA #223[g]			SKB	20 mg/mL[a]	Visually compatible for 4 hr at 23°C	2215	C
TNA #224[g]			SKB	20 mg/mL[a]	Visually compatible for 4 hr at 23°C	2215	C
TNA #225[g]			SKB	20 mg/mL[a]	Visually compatible for 4 hr at 23°C	2215	C
TNA #226[g]			SKB	20 mg/mL[a]	Visually compatible for 4 hr at 23°C	2215	C
TPN #61[g]		[i]	SKF	200 mg/0.9 mL[j]	Physically compatible	1012	C
TPN #61[g]		[k]	SKF	1.2 g/5.3 mL[j]	Physically compatible	1012	C
TPN #212[g]			SKB	20 mg/mL[a]	Physically compatible for 4 hr at 23°C	2109	C
TPN #213[g]			SKB	20 mg/mL[a]	Physically compatible for 4 hr at 23°C	2109	C
TPN #214[g]			SKB	20 mg/mL[a]	Microprecipitate forms immediately	2109	I
TPN #215[g]			SKB	20 mg/mL[a]	Microprecipitate forms immediately	2109	I
Vancomycin HCl	AB	20 mg/mL[a]	SKB	200 mg/mL[l]	Transient precipitate forms	2189	?
Vancomycin HCl	AB	20 mg/mL[a]	SKB	10 and 50 mg/mL[a]	Gross white precipitate forms immediately	2189	I
Vancomycin HCl	AB	20 mg/mL[a]	SKB	1 mg/mL[a]	Physically compatible for 4 hr at 23°C	2189	C
Vancomycin HCl	AB	2 mg/mL[a]	SKB	200 mg/mL[l]	Physically compatible for 4 hr at 23°C	2189	C
Vancomycin HCl	AB	2 mg/mL[a]	SKB	50 mg/mL[a]	Subvisible haze forms immediately	2189	I

Y-Site Injection Compatibility (1:1 Mixture) (Cont.)

Test Drug	Mfr	Conc	Mfr	Conc	Remarks	Ref	C/I
Vancomycin HCl	AB	2 mg/mL[a]	SKB	1 and 10 mg/mL[a]	Physically compatible for 4 hr at 23°C	2189	C
Vecuronium bromide	OR	0.1 mg/mL[a]	LY	10 mg/mL[a]	Physically compatible for 24 hr at 28°C	1337	C
Vinorelbine tartrate	BW	1 mg/mL[b]	GEM	20 mg/mL[b]	Measured turbidity increases immediately	1558	I

[a] Tested in dextrose 5%.

[b] Tested in sodium chloride 0.9%.

[c] Tested in both dextrose 5% and sodium chloride 0.9%.

[d] Tested in dextrose 5%, Ringer's injection, lactated, sodium chloride 0.45%, and sodium chloride 0.9%.

[e] Tested as the premixed infusion solution.

[f] Lyophilized formulation tested.

[g] Refer to Appendix for the composition of parenteral nutrition solutions. TNA indicates a 3-in-1 admixture, and TPN indicates a 2-in-1 admixture.

[h] A 32.5-mL sample of parenteral nutrition solution combined with 50 mL of antibiotic solution.

[i] Run at 21 mL/hr.

[j] Given over five minutes by syringe pump.

[k] Run at 94 mL/hr.

[l] Tested in sterile water for injection.

[m] Test performed using the formulation WITHOUT edetate disodium.

[n] Tested in either dextrose 5% or in sodium chloride 0.9%, but the report did not specify which solution.

[o] Tested in a 1:1 mixture of (1) dextrose 5% and dextrose 5% in sodium chloride 0.45% with and without potassium chloride 20 mEq/L and also in (2) dextrose 10% in sodium chloride 0.45% with and without potassium chloride 20 mEq/L.

[p] Tested in a 1:1 mixture of dextrose 5% and TPN #274 (see Appendix).

[q] Ceftolozane component. Ceftolozane in a 2:1 fixed-ratio concentration with tazobactam.

[r] Meropenem component. Meropenem in a 1:1 fixed-ratio concentration with vaborbactam.

[s] Test performed using the formulation WITH edetate disodium.

Additional Compatibility Information

Peritoneal Dialysis Solutions

The stability of cefazolin sodium 75 and 150 mg/L, alone and with gentamicin sulfate 8 mg/L, was evaluated in a peritoneal dialysis solution of dextrose 1.5% with heparin sodium 1000 units/L. Cefazolin activity was retained for 48 hours at both 4 and 26°C at both concentrations, alone and with gentamicin. Gentamicin activity also was retained over the study period. At 37°C, however, cefazolin losses were greater, with about a 10 to 12% loss occurring in 48 hours. Gentamicin losses ranged from 4 to 8% in this time period.[1029]

Gentamicin 4 mcg/mL in Dianeal PDS with dextrose 1.5 and 4.25% (Travenol) was evaluated with cefazolin sodium 125 mcg/mL, heparin 500 units, and albumin 80 mg in 2-L bags. The gentamicin content was retained for 72 hours.[1413]

The stability of cefazolin sodium (Lilly) 0.5 mg/mL in Dianeal PD-1 with dextrose 1.5 and 4.25% (Travenol) was studied. The drug was stable, exhibiting losses of 10.5% or less in 14 days at 4°C, 8 days at 25°C, and 24 hours at 37°C. However, losses of 11.7 and 14.6% occurred in the solutions containing dextrose 1.5% and dextrose 4.25%, respectively, in 11 days at 25°C.[1480]

Cefazolin sodium (Lilly) 125 mcg/mL combined separately with the aminoglycosides amikacin sulfate (Bristol), gentamicin sulfate (Schering), and tobramycin sulfate (Lilly) at a concentration of 25 mcg/mL in peritoneal dialysis solution (Dianeal 1.5%) exhibited enhanced rates of lethality to *Staphylococcus aureus*, *Escherichia coli*, and *Pseudomonas aeruginosa* compared to any of the drugs alone.[1623]

Cefazolin sodium (Fujisawa) 0.333 mg/mL in PD-2 with dextrose 1.5% (Baxter) peritoneal dialysis solution with and without heparin sodium 1000 units/1.5 L was stored at 4, 25, and 37°C. No visible changes occurred, and less than 10% loss of cefazolin occurred in 20 days at 4°C, 11 days at 25°C, and 24 hours at 37°C.[2388]

Cefazolin sodium (Fujisawa) 0.5 mg/mL in Extraneal PD (Baxter) containing 7.5% icodextrin was physically compatible and chemically stable for 30 days at 4°C with about 7% cefazolin loss and for 7 days at room temperature with about 9% loss. At 37°C, 8% cefazolin loss occurred in 24 hours.[2480]

Cefazolin sodium 125 and 500 mg/mL (Apothecon) was evaluated for stability at 38°C in Dianeal PD-2 with dextrose 1.5, 2.5, and 4.25% and in Extraneal 7.5% with and without added heparin. Less than 10% loss occurred in 48 hours and 10 to 14% loss in 60 hours.[2655]

Cefazolin sodium (Hospira) 500 mg/L in Extraneal with icodextrin 7.5% (Baxter) peritoneal dialysis solution bags exhibited less than 10% loss in 14 days at 4°C, 7 days at 25°C, and 6 hours at 37°C.[3537] Cefazolin sodium (Hospira) 500 mg/L with gentamicin sulfate (Pfizer) 20 mg/L in Extraneal with icodextrin 7.5% (Baxter) peritoneal dialysis solution bags exhibited less than 10% loss of either drug in 14 days at 4°C, 7% loss of cefazolin and no loss of gentamicin in 4 days at 25°C, and 5% loss of cefazolin and 1% loss of gentamicin in 1 day at 37°C.[3537] Cefazolin sodium (Hospira) 500 mg/L with ceftazidime (Sandoz) 500 mg/L in Extraneal with icodextrin 7.5% (Baxter) peritoneal dialysis solution bags exhibited less than 10% loss of either drug in 14 days at 4°C, 2% loss of cefazolin and 6% loss of ceftazidime in 2 days at 25°C, and 2% loss of cefazolin and no loss of ceftazidime in 6 hours at 37°C.[3537]

Cefepime Hydrochloride
AHFS 8:12.06.16

Products

Cefepime hydrochloride is available as 1 and 2 g of cefepime in vials.[3295] The drug also may be available in a 500-mg vial.[3295] [3324] The products contain L-arginine in an approximate concentration of 707 mg/g of cefepime to control the pH of the reconstituted solution.[3295]

For intramuscular administration, reconstitute the 500-mg and 1-g vials with 1.3 and 2.4 mL, respectively, of sterile water for injection, sodium chloride 0.9%, dextrose 5%, lidocaine hydrochloride 0.5 or 1%, or bacteriostatic water for injection preserved with parabens or benzyl alcohol to yield a solution with a cefepime concentration of 280 mg/mL.[3295]

For intravenous injection, reconstitute the 500-mg and 1-g vials with 5 and 10 mL, respectively, of a compatible diluent to yield a solution with a cefepime concentration of 100 mg/mL; reconstitute the 2-g vial with 10 mL of a compatible diluent to yield a solution with a cefepime concentration of 160 mg/mL.[3295] The reconstituted solutions should be added to compatible intravenous solutions for intermittent intravenous infusion.[3295]

Cefepime hydrochloride also is available as 1 and 2 g of cefepime in ADD-Vantage vials.[3295] Each ADD-Vantage vial also contains L-arginine in an approximate concentration of 707 mg/g of cefepime.[3295] ADD-Vantage vials of cefepime hydrochloride should be prepared with 50 or 100 mL of dextrose 5% or sodium chloride 0.9% in ADD-Vantage diluent bags.[3295]

Cefepime hydrochloride is available as 1 and 2 g of cefepime in a dual-chamber flexible container.[3297] The drug chamber also contains L-arginine in an approximate concentration of 725 mg/g of cefepime.[3297] The diluent chamber contains approximately 50 mL of dextrose 5% for use as a diluent.[3297]

Cefepime is available in 1- and 2-g sizes as a frozen premixed solution in 50- and 100-mL bags, respectively.[3296] Approximately 1.03 or 2.06 g of dextrose hydrous has been added to the 50- or 100-mL bags, respectively, to adjust the osmolality.[3296] The frozen premixed solution also contains L-arginine in an approximate concentration of 725 mg/g of cefepime with or without hydrochloric acid in water for injection for intravenous infusion.[3296]

pH

The pH of the reconstituted solution and the frozen premixed solution ranges from 4 to 6.[3295] [3296] [3297]

Osmolality

Cefepime 1 and 2 g in dual-chamber flexible containers has an approximate osmolality of 431 and 577 mOsm/kg, respectively, when activated with the dextrose solution diluent.[3297]

Frozen premixed solutions of cefepime are iso-osmotic.[3296]

Trade Name(s)

Maxipime

Administration

Cefepime hydrochloride is administered by intermittent intravenous infusion over approximately 30 minutes;[3295] [3296] [3297] the manufacturer states that the drug also can be given by intramuscular injection for certain indications.[3295]

Stability

Intact vials of cefepime hydrochloride should be stored at controlled room temperature and protected from light.[3295] Reconstituted solutions may vary from pale yellow to amber.[3295] Both the powder and reconstituted solutions may darken during storage like other cephalosporins.[3295] [3297] In one study, solutions of cefepime in sterile water for injection at concentrations greater than 50 g/L underwent marked color changes (i.e., from light yellow to dark red) in 2 hours at 37°C.[3105] When stored as recommended, the drug is not adversely affected.[3295] [3279]

Reconstituted solutions of cefepime hydrochloride in compatible diluents are stable for 24 hours at room temperatures of 20 to 25°C and for 7 days under refrigeration at 2 to 8°C.[3295] Cefepime 1 and 2 g in dual-chamber flexible plastic containers with dextrose solution diluent should be used within 12 hours after activation if stored at room temperature and in 5 days if stored under refrigeration.[3297]

pH Effects

Cefepime hydrochloride is most stable at pH values in the range of 4 to 5. At higher pH values, cefepime hydrochloride is less stable. Cefepime hydrochloride decomposition results in alkaline degradation products, which may increase the rate of loss.[2513] [2514] [2515]

Freezing Solutions

The commercially available frozen injection should be thawed at room temperature of 25°C or under refrigeration at 5°C; solutions should not be subject to force thawing by immersion in water baths or microwaving.[3296] The manufacturer indicates that the thawed solution is stable for 24 hours at room temperature of 25°C or 7 days under refrigeration at 5°C.[3296] Thawed solutions should not be refrozen.[3296]

Syringes

Cefepime (Bristol-Myers Squibb) 100 and 200 mg/mL in dextrose 5%, sodium chloride 0.9%, and sterile water for injection was packaged as 10 mL of solution in 10-mL polypropylene syringes and capped (Becton Dickinson). The samples were stored frozen at −20°C for 90 days and were also tested without having been frozen. The solutions remained stable for up to 14

DOI: 10.37573/9781585286850.073

days refrigerated at 4°C, losing 10% or less of the cefepime. In samples stored at room temperature of about 23°C, less than 10% loss occurred in 1 day in most cases, but losses as high as 13% occurred in 2 days in some (but not all) samples that were evaluated.[2220][2221] Samples refrigerated up to 5 days followed by room temperature storage exhibited similar stability, exhibiting less than 10% loss in 1 day but higher losses after 2 days.[2220]

Cefepime (Bristol-Myers Squibb) 20 mg/mL in sodium chloride 0.9% was packaged in 10-mL polypropylene syringes (Becton Dickinson) and stored at 25 and 5°C. The drug solutions remained clear, but the color deepened to a darker yellow during storage at room temperature. About 5% loss occurred in 2 days and 11% loss in 4 days at 25°C. About 3% loss was found after 21 days at 5°C. The losses were comparable to the drug solution stored in a glass flask, indicating sorption to syringe components did not occur.[2341]

Central Venous Catheter

Cefepime (Bristol-Myers Squibb) 5 mg/mL in dextrose 5% was found to be compatible with the ARROWg+ard Blue Plus (Arrow International) chlorhexidine-bearing triple-lumen central catheter. Delivery of the cefepime hydrochloride ranged from 92 to 95% of the initial concentration among the 3 lumens. Furthermore, chlorhexidine delivered from the catheter remained at trace amounts with no substantial increase due to the delivery of the drug through the catheter.[2335]

Compatibility Information

Solution Compatibility

Cefepime HCl

Test Soln Name	Mfr	Mfr	Conc/L or %	Remarks	Ref	C/I
Amino acids 4.25%, dextrose 25% with electrolytes	AB	BR	1 and 4 g	5 to 6% loss in 8 hr at room temperature and 3 days at 5°C	1682	C
Dextrose 5% in Ringer's injection, lactated	a	BR	1 and 40 g	Visually compatible with 2 to 6% loss in 24 hr at room temperature exposed to light and about 2 to 3% loss in 7 days at 5°C	1680	C
Dextrose 5% in sodium chloride 0.9%	a	BR	1 and 40 g	Visually compatible with 3 to 5% loss in 24 hr at room temperature exposed to light and 1 to 3% loss in 7 days at 5°C	1680	C
Dextrose 5%	b	BR	1 g	Visually compatible with 2 to 4% loss in 24 hr at room temperature exposed to light and 1 to 2% loss in 7 days at 5°C	1680	C
Dextrose 5%	b	BR	40 g	Visually compatible with 4 to 7% loss in 24 hr at room temperature exposed to light and about 2% loss in 7 days at 5°C	1680	C
Dextrose 5%	BAa	BMS	20 g	6% loss in 2 days at 25°C and in 23 days at 5°C. Increase in yellow color	2102	C
Dextrose 5%	BFMc	BMS	8 g	8 to 9% loss in 48 hr at 24°C and in 15 days at 4°C. Amber discoloration	2150	C
Dextrose 5%	BAa	BMS	20 g	Visually compatible and stable for 30 days frozen at −20°C followed by 11 days at 4°C	2390	C
Dextrose 10%	a	BR	1 and 40 g	Visually compatible with 3 to 5% loss in 24 hr at room temperature exposed to light and 1 to 3% loss in 7 days at 5°C	1680	C
Normosol M in dextrose 5%	ABa	BR	1 and 40 g	Visually compatible with 2 to 5% loss in 24 hr at room temperature exposed to light and 2% loss in 7 days at 5°C	1680	C
Normosol R	ABa	BR	1 and 40 g	Visually compatible with 2 to 5% loss in 24 hr at room temperature exposed to light and 1 to 2% loss in 7 days at 5°C	1680	C
Normosol R in dextrose 5%	ABa	BR	1 g	Visually compatible with 2% loss in 24 hr at room temperature exposed to light	1680	C
Sodium chloride 0.9%	b	BR	1 and 40 g	Visually compatible with 2 to 5% loss in 24 hr at room temperature exposed to light and about 1 to 3% loss in 7 days at 5°C	1680	C
Sodium chloride 0.9%	BAa	BMS	20 g	6% loss in 2 days at 25°C and in 23 days at 5°C. Increase in yellow color	2102	C
Sodium chloride 0.9%	BFMc	BMS	8 g	8% loss in 72 hr at 24°C and in 15 days at 4°C. Amber discoloration	2150	C

Solution Compatibility (Cont.)

Test Soln Name	Mfr	Mfr	Conc/L or %	Remarks	Ref	C/I
Sodium chloride 0.9%	d	e	20 g	Less than 10% loss in theoretical concentration in 12 hr at ambient temperature when administered as a continuous infusion	3535	C
Sodium chloride 0.9%	d	e	40 g	Less than 10% loss in theoretical concentration in 10 hr at ambient temperature when administered as a continuous infusion	3535	C

[a] Tested in PVC containers.

[b] Tested in both glass and PVC containers.

[c] Tested in polyethylene-lined trilayer (Clear-Flex) containers.

[d] Tested in polypropylene syringes.

[e] Salt not specified.

Additive Compatibility

Cefepime HCl

Test Drug	Mfr	Conc/L or %	Mfr	Conc/L or %	Test Solution	Remarks	Ref	C/I
Amikacin sulfate	BR	6 g	BR	40 g	D5W, NS	Visually compatible with 6% cefepime loss in 24 hr at room temperature and 4% loss in 7 days at 5°C. No amikacin loss	1681	C
Aminophylline	LY	1 g	BR	4 g	NS	37% cefepime loss in 18 hr at room temperature and 32% loss in 3 days at 5°C. No aminophylline loss	1681	I
Ampicillin sodium	BR	1 g	BR	40 g	D5W	4% ampicillin loss in 8 hr at room temperature and 5°C. 7% cefepime loss in 8 hr at room temperature and no loss in 8 hr at 5°C	1682	?
Ampicillin sodium	BR	1 g	BR	40 g	NS	No ampicillin loss in 24 hr at room temperature and 9% loss in 48 hr at 5°C. 5% cefepime loss in 24 hr at room temperature and 2% loss in 72 hr at 5°C	1682	C
Ampicillin sodium	BR	10 g	BR	40 g	D5W	6% ampicillin loss in 2 hr at room temperature and 2% loss in 8 hr at 5°C. 7% cefepime loss in 2 hr at room temperature and 8 hr at 5°C	1682	I
Ampicillin sodium	BR	10 g	BR	40 g	NS	6% ampicillin loss in 8 hr at room temperature and 9% loss in 48 hr at 5°C. 8% cefepime loss in 8 hr at room temperature and 10% loss in 48 hr at 5°C	1682	I
Ampicillin sodium	BR	40 g	BR	4 g	D5W	10% ampicillin loss in 1 hr at room temperature and 9% loss in 2 hr at 5°C. 25% cefepime loss in 1 hr at room temperature and 9% loss in 2 hr at 5°C	1682	I
Ampicillin sodium	BR	40 g	BR	4 g	NS	5% ampicillin loss in 8 hr at room temperature and 4% loss in 8 hr at 5°C. 4% cefepime loss in 8 hr at room temperature and 6% loss in 8 hr at 5°C	1682	?
Clindamycin phosphate	UP	0.25 g	BR	40 g	D5W, NS	7% or less cefepime loss in 24 hr at room temperature and 10% or less loss in 7 days at 5°C. No clindamycin loss in 24 hr at room temperature and 8% or less loss in 7 days at 5°C	1682	C
Clindamycin phosphate	UP	6 g	BR	4 g	D5W, NS	7% or less cefepime loss in 24 hr at room temperature and 10% or less loss in 7 days at 5°C. No clindamycin loss in 24 hr at room temperature and 8% or less loss in 7 days at 5°C	1682	C
Gentamicin sulfate	ES	1.2 g	BR	40 g	D5W, NS	Cloudy in 18 hr at room temperature	1681	I

Additive Compatibility (Cont.)

Test Drug	Mfr	Conc/L or %	Mfr	Conc/L or %	Test Solution	Remarks	Ref	C/I
Heparin sodium	MG	10,000 and 50,000 units	BR	4 g	D5W, NS	Visually compatible with 4% cefepime loss in 24 hr at room temperature and 3% in 7 days at 5°C. No heparin loss	1681	C
Metronidazole	AB, ES, SE	5 g	BR	4 and 40 g		4 to 5% cefepime loss in 24 hr at room temperature exposed to light and up to 10% loss in 7 days at 5°C. No metronidazole loss. Orange color develops in 18 hr at room temperature and 24 hr at 5°C	1682	?
Metronidazole	SCS	5 g	BMS	2.5, 5, 10, and 20 g	a	Visually compatible. 7 to 9% cefepime loss in 48 hr at 23°C; 2 to 8% cefepime loss in 7 days at 4°C. 7% or less metronidazole loss in 7 days at 4 and 23°C	2324	C
Metronidazole	AB	5 g	ELN	3.3, 6.6, 10, 20 g	a	Physically compatible and less than 6% metronidazole loss at 4 and 23°C in 14 days. 2 to 5% cefepime loss in 14 days at 4°C. At 23°C, 10 to 12% cefepime loss in 72 hr	2726	C
Potassium chloride	AB	10 and 40 mEq	BR	4 g	D5W, NS	Visually compatible with 2% cefepime loss in 24 hr at room temperature or 7 days at 5°C	1681	C
Theophylline	BA	800 mg	BR	4 g	D5W	Visually compatible. 3% cefepime loss in 24 hr at room temperature and 7 days at 5°C. No theophylline loss	1681	C
Tobramycin sulfate	AB	0.4 g	BR	40 g	D5W, NS	Cloudiness forms immediately	1682	I
Tobramycin sulfate	AB	2 g	BR	2.5 g	D5W, NS	Cloudiness forms immediately	1682	I
Vancomycin HCl	LI	5 g	BR	4 g	D5W, NS	4% cefepime loss in 24 hr at room temperature in light and 2% loss in 7 days at 5°C. No vancomycin loss. Cloudiness in 5 days at 5°C	1682	C
Vancomycin HCl	LI	1 g	BR	40 g	D5W, NS	4% cefepime loss in 24 hr at room temperature in light and 2% loss in 7 days at 5°C. No vancomycin loss and no cloudiness	1682	C

[a] Tested in PVC containers.

Y-Site Injection Compatibility (1:1 Mixture)

Cefepime HCl

Test Drug	Mfr	Conc	Mfr	Conc	Remarks	Ref	C/I
Acetylcysteine		100 mg/mL	BMS	120 mg/mL[c]	Over 10% cefepime loss occurs in 1 hr	2513	I
Amikacin sulfate		15 mg/mL	BMS	120 mg/mL[c]	Physically compatible with less than 10% cefepime loss. Amikacin not tested	2513	C
Anidulafungin	VIC	0.5 mg/mL[a]	DUR	20 mg/mL[a]	Physically compatible for 4 hr at 23°C	2617	C
Bivalirudin	TMC	5 mg/mL[a]	BMS	20 mg/mL[a]	Physically compatible for 4 hr at 23°C	2373	C
Caspofungin acetate	ME	0.7 mg/mL[b]	BMS	20 mg/mL[b]	Immediate white turbid precipitate forms	2758	I
Ceftolozane sulfate–tazobactam sodium	CUB	10 mg/mL[e f]	SGT	40 mg/mL[e]	Physically compatible for 2 hr	3262	C
Clarithromycin		50 mg/mL	BMS	120 mg/mL[c]	Physically compatible with less than 10% cefepime loss. Clarithromycin not tested	2513	C
Dexmedetomidine HCl	AB	4 mcg/mL[b]	BMS	20 mg/mL[b]	Physically compatible for 4 hr at 23°C	2383	C
Dobutamine HCl		1 mg/mL	BMS	120 mg/mL[c]	Physically compatible with less than 10% cefepime loss. Dobutamine not tested	2513	C

Y-Site Injection Compatibility (1:1 Mixture) (Cont.)

Test Drug	Mfr	Conc	Mfr	Conc	Remarks	Ref	C/I
Dobutamine HCl		250 mg/mL	BMS	120 mg/mL[c]	Precipitates	2513	I
Docetaxel	RPR	0.9 mg/mL[a]	BMS	20 mg/mL[a]	Physically compatible for 4 hr at 23°C	2224	C
Dopamine HCl		0.4 mg/mL	BMS	120 mg/mL[c]	Physically compatible with less than 10% cefepime loss. Dopamine not tested	2513	C
Doxorubicin HCl liposomal	SEQ	0.4 mg/mL[a]	BMS	20 mg/mL[a]	Physically compatible for 4 hr at 23°C	2087	C
Eravacycline dihydrochloride	TET	0.6 mg/mL[b]	WG	40 mg/mL[b]	Physically compatible for 2 hr at room temperature	3532	C
Erythromycin lactobionate		5 mg/mL	BMS	120 mg/mL[c]	Over 10% cefepime loss occurs in 1 hr	2513	I
Esmolol HCl	MYL	10 mg/mL	APP	40 mg/mL[b]	Physically compatible for 1 hr at 23°C	3533	C
Etoposide phosphate	BR	5 mg/mL[a]	BMS	20 mg/mL[a]	Increased haze and particulates form within 1 hr	2218	I
Fenoldopam mesylate	AB	80 mcg/mL[b]	BMS	20 mg/mL[b]	Physically compatible for 4 hr at 23°C	2467	C
Fluconazole		2 mg/mL	BMS	120 mg/mL[c]	Physically compatible with less than 10% cefepime loss. Fluconazole not tested	2513	C
Furosemide		10 mg/mL	BMS	120 mg/mL[c]	Physically compatible with less than 10% cefepime loss. Furosemide not tested	2513	C
Gentamicin sulfate		6 mg/mL	BMS	120 mg/mL[c]	Physically compatible with less than 10% cefepime loss. Gentamicin not tested	2513	C
Granisetron HCl	SKB	0.05 mg/mL[a]	BMS	20 mg/mL[a]	Physically compatible for 4 hr at 23°C	2000	C
Hetastarch in lactated electrolyte	AB	6%	BMS	20 mg/mL[a]	Physically compatible for 4 hr at 23°C	2339	C
Insulin, regular		100 units/mL	BMS	120 mg/mL[c]	Physically compatible with less than 10% cefepime loss. Insulin not tested	2513	C
Isavuconazonium sulfate	ASP	1.5 mg/mL[e]	SGT	40 mg/mL[e]	Measured turbidity increases immediately	3263	I
Isosorbide dinitrate		0.2 mg/mL	BMS	120 mg/mL[c]	Physically compatible with less than 10% cefepime loss. Isosorbide not tested	2513	C
Ketamine HCl		10 mg/mL	BMS	120 mg/mL[c]	Physically compatible with less than 10% cefepime loss. Ketamine not tested	2513	C
Labetalol HCl	HOS	5 mg/mL	APP	40 mg/mL[b]	Slight haze and particulate matter forms immediately	3533	I
Letermovir	ME				Physically incompatible	3398	I
Meropenem–vaborbactam	TMC	8 mg/mL[b g]	HOS	40 mg/mL[b]	Physically compatible for 3 hr at 20 to 25°C	3380	C
Methylprednisolone sodium succinate		50 mg/mL	BMS	120 mg/mL[c]	Physically compatible with less than 10% cefepime loss. Methylprednisolone not tested	2513	C
Metoprolol tartrate	HOS	0.4 mg/mL[b]	APP	40 mg/mL[b]	Physically compatible for 1 hr at 23°C	3533	C
Midazolam HCl		5 mg/mL	BMS	120 mg/mL[c]	Over 10% cefepime loss occurs in 1 hr	2513	I
Milrinone lactate	SS	0.2 mg/mL[a]	BMS	100 mg/mL[a]	Visually compatible for 4 hr at 25°C	2381	C
Morphine sulfate		1 mg/mL	BMS	120 mg/mL[c]	Physically compatible with less than 10% cefepime loss. Morphine not tested	2513	C
Mycophenolate mofetil HCl	RC	5.9 mg/mL[a]		20 mg/mL[a]	Physically compatible with no mycophenolate mofetil loss in 4 hr	2738	C

Y-Site Injection Compatibility (1:1 Mixture) (Cont.)

Test Drug	Mfr	Conc	Mfr	Conc	Remarks	Ref	C/I
Nicardipine HCl		1 mg/mL	BMS	120 mg/mL[c]	Precipitates	2513	I
Phenytoin sodium		50 mg/mL	BMS	120 mg/mL[c]	Precipitates	2513	I
Plazomicin sulfate	ACH	24 mg/mL[e]	WG	40 mg/mL[e]	Physically compatible for 1 hr at 20 to 25°C	3432	C
Propofol		1 mg/mL	BMS	120 mg/mL[c]	Precipitates	2513	I
Remifentanil HCl		0.2 mg/mL	BMS	120 mg/mL[c]	Physically compatible with less than 10% cefepime loss. Remifentanil not tested	2513	C
Sufentanil citrate		5 mcg/mL	BMS	120 mg/mL[c]	Physically compatible with less than 10% cefepime loss. Sufentanil not tested	2513	C
Tedizolid phosphate	CUB	0.8 mg/mL[b]	SGT	40 mg/mL[b]	Physically compatible for 2 hr	3244	C
Telavancin HCl	ASP	7.5 mg/mL[a b d]	SAG	40 mg/mL[a b d]	Physically compatible for 2 hr	2830	C
Theophylline		20 mg/mL	BMS	120 mg/mL[c]	Over 25% cefepime loss in 1 hr	2513	I
Tigecycline	WY	1 mg/mL[b]	ELN	40 mg/mL[b]	Physically compatible for 4 hr	2714	C
Tobramycin sulfate		6 mg/mL	BMS	120 mg/mL[c]	Physically compatible with less than 10% cefepime loss. Tobramycin not tested	2513	C
Valproate sodium		100 mg/mL	BMS	120 mg/mL[c]	Physically compatible. Under 10% cefepime loss. Valproate not tested	2513	C
Vancomycin HCl		30 mg/mL	BMS	120 mg/mL[c]	Physically compatible with less than 10% cefepime loss. Vancomycin not tested	2513	C
Vancomycin HCl	NVP	4 mg/mL[b]	APO	20 mg/mL[b]	Samples from 4-hr cefepime and 1-hr vancomycin infusions physically compatible during infusion and after 24 hr at 22.5°C in dark. Cefepime chemically stable during infusion and after 12 hr at 22.5°C in dark; vancomycin not measured using an assay noted to be stability indicating	3475	C
Vancomycin HCl	NVP	5 mg/mL[a]	APO	20 mg/mL[a]	Samples from 4-hr cefepime and 1-hr vancomycin infusions physically compatible during infusion and after 24 hr at 22.5°C in dark. Cefepime chemically stable during infusion and after 12 hr at 22.5°C in dark; vancomycin not measured using an assay noted to be stability indicating	3475	C
Vancomycin HCl	NVP	4 mg/mL[b]	APO	20 mg/mL[a]	Samples from 4-hr cefepime and 1-hr vancomycin infusions physically compatible during infusion and after 24 hr at 22.5°C in dark. Cefepime chemically stable during infusion and after 12 hr at 22.5°C in dark; vancomycin not measured using an assay noted to be stability indicating	3475	C
Vancomycin HCl	NVP	5 mg/mL[a]	APO	20 mg/mL[b]	Samples from 4-hr cefepime and 1-hr vancomycin infusions physically compatible during infusion and after 24 hr at 22.5°C in dark. Cefepime chemically stable during infusion and after 12 hr at 22.5°C in dark; vancomycin not measured using an assay noted to be stability indicating	3475	C

[a] Tested in dextrose 5%.

[b] Tested in sodium chloride 0.9%.

[c] Tested in sterile water for injection.

[d] Tested in Ringer's injection, lactated.

[e] Tested in both dextrose 5% and sodium chloride 0.9%.

[f] Ceftolozane component. Ceftolozane in a 2:1 fixed-ratio concentration with tazobactam.

[g] Meropenem component. Meropenem in a 1:1 fixed-ratio concentration with vaborbactam.

Additional Compatibility Information

Peritoneal Dialysis Solutions

Cefepime (Bristol-Myers Squibb) 0.125 and 0.25 mg/mL in Inpersol peritoneal dialysis solution with dextrose 4.25% is stable, exhibiting 3% loss in 7 days at 5°C, 2% loss in 24 hours at room temperature, and 8% loss in 24 hours at 37°C.[1682]

Cefepime (Bristol-Myers Squibb) 0.1 mg/mL in Delflex solution with dextrose 1.5% stored at various temperatures was evaluated for physical and chemical stability. No visible particulates or changes in color or clarity were observed in any sample. Cefepime exhibited no loss in 14 days at 4°C, 7% loss in 7 days at 25°C, and 4% loss in 24 hours and 9% loss in 48 hours at body temperature.[2283]

Cefepime (Bristol-Myers Squibb) 0.48 mg/mL was found to exhibit less than 10% loss in icodextrin 7.5% peritoneal dialysis solution (Extraneal) after 7 days at refrigerator temperature, 2 days at room temperature, and 4 hours at 37°C.[2616]

Cefepime hydrochloride was evaluated for stability in pH-neutral Balance with dextrose 1.5% (Fresenius).[3270] Bags of 2-compartment pH-neutral Balance with 1.5% dextrose contained cefepime 250 mg/L in the non-dextrose (i.e., buffer solution) compartment for storage at 4 and 25°C; for bags intended for storage at 37°C, the initial concentration of cefepime in the non-dextrose compartment also was 250 mg/L; however, the 2 compartments were combined immediately prior to storage at 37°C for a final cefepime concentration of 125 mg/L.[3270] No color change or precipitation was noted on visual assessment and no meaningful pH changes occurred.[3270] Less than 10% loss of cefepime occurred in 7 days at 4°C, 3 days at 25°C, and 12 hours at 37°C.[3270]

Cefiderocol Sulfate Tosylate
AHFS 8:12.06.28

Products

Cefiderocol sulfate tosylate is available as a lyophilized powder in single-dose vials containing the equivalent of 1 g of cefiderocol.[3531] Each vial also contains sucrose 900 mg, sodium chloride 216 mg, and sodium hydroxide to adjust the pH.[3531]

The contents of each 1-g vial of cefiderocol should be reconstituted with 10 mL of sodium chloride 0.9% or dextrose 5% and the vial should be shaken gently to dissolve the powder.[3531] Vials should be allowed to stand until any foam that has been generated on the surface has disappeared (usually about 2 minutes).[3531] The reconstituted solution must be diluted prior to infusion.[3531]

The manufacturer's instructions for preparing various doses of cefiderocol from the reconstituted solution are as follows:[3531]

For a 2-g dose, withdraw the entire contents of 2 vials (i.e., approximately 11.2 mL per vial).

For a 1.5-g dose, withdraw the entire contents of 1 vial (i.e., approximately 11.2 mL) and 5.6 mL from a second vial.

For a 1-g dose, withdraw the entire contents of 1 vial (i.e., approximately 11.2 mL).

For a 0.75-g dose, withdraw 8.4 mL from 1 vial.

All doses should then be added to an infusion bag containing 100 mL of sodium chloride 0.9% or dextrose 5%.[3531][3544]

pH

The pH of the resulting solution that forms when 1 g of cefiderocol is dissolved in 10 mL of water is within the range of 5.2 to 5.8.[3531]

Equivalency

Cefiderocol sulfate tosylate 1.6 g is equivalent to 1 g of cefiderocol.[3531]

Sodium Content

Each 1-g vial of cefiderocol contains approximately 176 mg of sodium.[3531]

Trade Name(s)

Fetroja

Administration

Cefiderocol sulfate tosylate is administered by intravenous infusion over 3 hours following reconstitution and further dilution.[3531]

Stability

Cefiderocol sulfate tosylate is a white to off-white powder that forms a clear, colorless solution upon reconstitution and dilution.[3531] Intact vials of cefiderocol sulfate tosylate should be stored at 2 to 8°C in the original carton until time of use to protect from light.[3531]

After reconstitution with an appropriate diluent as instructed, the drug may be stored for up to 1 hour at room temperature.[3531] Following dilution, the drug is stable for 4 hours at room temperature.[3531]

Compatibility Information
Solution Compatibility

Cefiderocol sulfate tosylate

Test Soln Name	Mfr	Mfr	Conc/L or %	Remarks	Ref	C/I
Dextrose 5%		SHI		Stable for 4 hr at room temperature	3531	C
Sodium chloride 0.9%		SHI		Stable for 4 hr at room temperature	3531	C

DOI: 10.37573/9781585286850.074

Cefotaxime Sodium
AHFS 8:12.06.12

Products

Cefotaxime sodium is available in vials containing the equivalent of 500 mg and 1 and 2 g of cefotaxime (as sodium) and in infusion bottles containing the equivalent of 1 g of cefotaxime (as sodium). It is also available in 10- and 20-g pharmacy bulk packages.[1(9/08)]

For intravenous administration, the contents of any size vial may be reconstituted with 10 mL of sterile water for injection. (See Table 1.) The 1- and 2-g infusion bottles may be reconstituted with 50 or 100 mL of dextrose 5% or sodium chloride 0.9%. For intramuscular injection, reconstitute with sterile water for injection or bacteriostatic water for injection in the amounts shown in Table 1.[1(9/08)]

Table 1. Reconstitution of cefotaxime sodium[1(9/08)]

Vial Size	Volume of Diluent	Withdrawable Volume	Approximate Concentration
Intravenous			
500 mg	10 mL	10.2 mL	50 mg/mL
1 g	10 mL	10.4 mL	95 mg/mL
2 g	10 mL	11 mL	180 mg/mL
Intramuscular			
500 mg	2 mL	2.2 mL	230 mg/mL
1 g	3 mL	3.4 mL	300 mg/mL
2 g	5 mL	6 mL	330 mg/mL

The pharmacy bulk packages may be reconstituted according to the manufacturer's directions, and the dose should be diluted appropriately for administration.[1(9/08) 4]

After addition of the diluent, shake to dissolve the contents and inspect for particulate matter or discoloration.[1(9/08)]

For intravenous infusion, the primary solution may be diluted further to 50 to 1000 mL in a compatible diluent.[1(9/08)]

Cefotaxime sodium also is available as a frozen premixed iso-osmotic infusion solution of 1 or 2 g in dextrose 3.4 or 1.4%, respectively, buffered with sodium citrate. Hydrochloric acid and sodium hydroxide, if needed, are used to adjust the pH during manufacturing.[1(9/08) 4]

pH

Injectable solutions of the drug have pH values ranging from 5 to 7.5.[1(9/08)]

Tonicity

A solution of cefotaxime sodium 1 g/14 mL of sterile water for injection is isotonic.[1(9/08)]

Osmolality

The osmolality of cefotaxime sodium 1, 2, and 3 g was calculated for the following dilutions:[1054]

Diluent	Osmolality (mOsm/kg)	
	50 mL	100 mL
1 g		
Dextrose 5%	350	319
Sodium chloride 0.9%	375	344
2 g		
Dextrose 5%	343	327
Sodium chloride 0.9%	406	351
3 g		
Dextrose 5%	433	344
Sodium chloride 0.9%	458	382

The frozen premixed solutions have osmolalities of 340 to 420 mOsm/kg for the 1-g/50 mL concentration and 450 to 540 mOsm/kg for the 2-g/50 mL concentration.[4]

The osmolality of cefotaxime sodium (Hoechst) 50 mg/mL was determined to be 326 mOsm/kg in dextrose 5% and 333 mOsm/kg in sodium chloride 0.9%.[1375]

The following maximum cefotaxime sodium concentrations were recommended to achieve osmolalities suitable for peripheral infusion in fluid-restricted patients:[1180]

Diluent	Maximum Concentration (mg/mL)	Osmolality (mOsm/kg)
Dextrose 5%	86	577
Sodium chloride 0.9%	73	555
Sterile water for injection	147	525

Sodium Content

Cefotaxime sodium contains approximately 2.2 mEq (50.5 mg) of sodium per gram of cefotaxime activity.[1(9/08)]

Trade Name(s)

Claforan

Administration

Cefotaxime sodium may be administered by deep intramuscular injection; doses of 2 g should be divided between different injection sites. Cefotaxime also may be administered by direct intravenous injection over 3 to 5 minutes directly into the vein or into the tubing of a running compatible infusion solution. In addition, cefo-

DOI: 10.37573/9781585286850.075

taxime sodium may be administered in 50 to 100 mL of compatible diluent over 20 to 30 minutes by intermittent intravenous infusion or by continuous intravenous infusion.[1(9/08)] [4]

The manufacturer states that cefotaxime sodium should not be admixed with aminoglycosides; however, they may be administered separately to the same patient.[1(9/08)] [792]

Stability

Intact vials of cefotaxime sodium should be stored below 30°C. The dry powder is off-white to pale yellow in color. Solutions may range from light yellow to amber, depending on the diluent, concentration, and storage conditions. Both the dry material and solutions may darken and should be protected from elevated temperatures and excessive light. Discoloration of the powder or solution may indicate a loss of potency.[1(9/08)] [4]

Store the frozen premixed cefotaxime sodium infusions at –20°C or below. Thaw at room temperature or under refrigeration. Accelerated thawing using water bath immersion or microwave irradiation should not be used. Thawed solutions should not be refrozen.[1(9/08)] [4]

When reconstituted as described in the Products section, cefotaxime sodium is stable in the original containers as indicated in Table 2. Storage of reconstituted solutions in disposable glass or plastic syringes for 5 days under refrigeration is also recommended.[1(9/08)]

Table 2. Manufacturer's recommended storage times of reconstituted cefotaxime sodium[1(9/08)]

Vial Size	Concentration	Storage Temperature	
		22°C	5°C
500 mg	230 mg/mL	12 hr	7 days
	50 mg/mL	24 hr	7 days
1 g	300 mg/mL	12 hr	7 days
	95 mg/mL	24 hr	7 days
(Infusion bottle)	10 to 20 mg/mL	24 hr	10 days
2 g	330 mg/mL	12 hr	7 days
	180 mg/mL	12 hr	7 days
(Infusion bottle)	20 to 40 mg/ml	24 hr	10 days

Cefotaxime sodium (Hoechst-Roussel) 1 g/10 mL reconstituted with sterile water for injection or 1 g/50 mL in dextrose 5% in PVC bags exhibited no visible changes in 24 hours at 5 and 25°C. Although increased levels of particulate matter were observed in most solutions, the increases were significant only in solutions stored at 25°C.[986]

The stability of cefotaxime sodium (Hoechst-Roussel) 125 mg/L in peritoneal dialysis solutions (Dianeal 137 and PD2) with heparin sodium 500 units/L was evaluated at 25°C by microbiological assay. Approximately 95 ± 6% activity remained after 24 hours.[1228]

The stability of cefotaxime sodium (Hoechst-Roussel) 1 mg/mL in Dianeal PD-1 with dextrose 1.5 and 4.25% (Travenol) was reported. At 25°C, the drug exhibited an 8% loss in 24 hours and a 16% loss in 48 hours in both solutions. Storage at 37°C for 12 hours resulted in 11 and 14% losses in the solutions containing dextrose 1.5% and dextrose 4.25%, respectively.[1481]

pH Effects

The primary factor in the stability of cefotaxime sodium is solution pH.[792] Cefotaxime sodium in aqueous solutions is stable at pH 5 to 7[1(9/08)] or 4.3 to 6.2.[1077] The theoretical pH of minimum decomposition is 5.13.[793] However, between pH 3 and 7, the hydrolysis rate is virtually independent of pH.[1072] Determination of decomposition kinetics in various aqueous buffer systems at 25°C showed 10% decomposition occurring in 24 hours or longer over a pH range of 3.9 to 7.6. At pH 2.2 and 8.4, 10% decomposition occurred in about 13 hours.[793]

The manufacturer recommends that cefotaxime sodium not be diluted in solutions with a pH greater than 7.5.[1(9/08)] [4]

Freezing Solutions

When reconstituted as recommended, cefotaxime sodium may be stored frozen in the vial or in disposable glass or plastic syringes for 13 weeks. Similarly, dilutions of cefotaxime sodium in dextrose 5% or sodium chloride 0.9% in PVC bags may be stored frozen for 13 weeks. Thawing at room temperature is recommended; frozen solutions should not be heated. Once thawed, the solutions are stable for 24 hours at room temperature or 5 days at less than 5°C. Thawed solutions should not be refrozen.[1(9/08)] [4]

Syringes

Cefotaxime sodium (Aventis) 50 mg/mL in sodium chloride 0.9% packaged in 5-mL polypropylene plastic syringes is visually compatible and undergoes about 10% loss in 2 days at 25°C and about 3% loss in 18 days at 5°C.[2371]

Sorption

Cefotaxime sodium (Aventis) 50 mg/mL in sodium chloride 0.9% packaged in polypropylene plastic syringes exhibited no evidence of sorption when compared to glass containers.[2371]

Central Venous Catheter

Cefotaxime sodium (Hoechst-Roussel) 5 mg/mL in dextrose 5% was found to be compatible with the ARROWg+ard Blue Plus (Arrow International) chlorhexidine-bearing triple-lumen central catheter. Delivery of the cefotaxime sodium ranged from 93 to 95% of the initial concentration among the 3 lumens. Furthermore, chlorhexidine delivered from the catheter remained at trace amounts with no substantial increase due to the delivery of the drug through the catheter.[2335]

Compatibility Information

Solution Compatibility

Cefotaxime sodium

Test Soln Name	Mfr	Mfr	Conc/L or %	Remarks	Ref	C/I
Dextrose 5% in sodium chloride 0.225%		SAA		Stable for 24 hr at room temperature and 5 days refrigerated	1(9/08)	C
Dextrose 5% in sodium chloride 0.45%		SAA		Stable for 24 hr at room temperature and 5 days refrigerated	1(9/08)	C
Dextrose 5% in sodium chloride 0.9%		SAA		Stable for 24 hr at room temperature and 5 days refrigerated	1(9/08)	C
Dextrose 5%				Stable for 24 hr at room temperature and 5 days refrigerated	1(9/08)	C
Dextrose 5%	TR[a]	HO	10 g	Physically compatible. 3% loss in 24 hr at 24°C. No loss in 22 days at 4°C and 63 days at −10°C	751, 1077	C
Dextrose 5%	AB[b]	HO	20 g	Physically compatible. Little loss in 24 hr at 25°C	994	C
Dextrose 10%				Stable for 24 hr at room temperature and 5 days refrigerated	1(9/08)	C
Ringer's injection, lactated				Stable for 24 hr at room temperature and 5 days refrigerated	1(9/08)	C
Sodium chloride 0.9%				Stable for 24 hr at room temperature and 5 days refrigerated	1(9/08)	C
Sodium chloride 0.9%	TR[a]	HO	10 g	Physically compatible with 2% loss in 24 hr at 24°C. No loss in 22 days at 4°C and 63 days at −10°C	751, 1077	C
Sodium chloride 0.9%	AB[b]	HO	20 g	Physically compatible. Little loss in 24 hr at 25°C	994	C
Sodium lactate ⅙ M				Stable for 24 hr at room temperature and 5 days refrigerated	1(9/08)	C
TPN #107[c]			1 g	Activity retained for 24 hr at 21°C	1326	C

[a] Tested in PVC containers.

[b] Tested in both glass bottles and PVC bags.

[c] Refer to Appendix for the composition of parenteral nutrition solutions. TPN indicates a 2-in-1 admixture.

Additive Compatibility

Cefotaxime sodium

Test Drug	Mfr	Conc/L or %	Mfr	Conc/L or %	Test Solution	Remarks	Ref	C/I
Amikacin sulfate	BR	25 mg	RS	50 mg	D5W	33% loss of amikacin in 2 hr at 22°C	504	I
Amikacin sulfate	BR	15 mg	RS	50 mg	D5W	Under 8% loss of amikacin in 24 hr at 22°C	504	C
Clindamycin phosphate	UP	9 g	HO	20 g	D5W, NS[a]	Physically compatible with no clindamycin loss and 3% cefotaxime loss in 24 hr at 25°C	994	C
Fusidate sodium	LEO	500 mg		2.5 g	D2.5½S, D2.5S, D5¼S, D5½S, D5S, D10S	Physically compatible and chemically stable for 48 hr at room temperature	1800	C
Gentamicin sulfate	SC	9 mg	RS	50 mg	D5W	30% loss of gentamicin in 2 hr at 22°C	504	I
Gentamicin sulfate	SC	6 mg	RS	50 mg	D5W	4% loss of gentamicin in 24 hr at 22°C	504	C

Additive Compatibility (Cont.)

Test Drug	Mfr	Conc/L or %	Mfr	Conc/L or %	Test Solution	Remarks	Ref	C/I
Metronidazole	AB	5 g	HO	10 g		Both drugs stable for 72 hr at 8°C	1547	C
Metronidazole	AB	5 g	HO	10 g		Visually compatible with 10% cefotaxime loss in 19 hr at 28°C and 8% loss in 96 hr at 5°C. No metronidazole loss in 96 hr at 5 or 28°C	1754	C
Verapamil HCl	KN	80 mg	HO	4 g	D5W, NS	Physically compatible for 24 hr	764	C

[a] Tested in both glass and PVC containers.

Drugs in Syringe Compatibility

Cefotaxime sodium

Test Drug	Mfr	Amt	Mfr	Amt	Remarks	Ref	C/I
Caffeine citrate		20 mg/1 mL	HO	200 mg/1 mL	Visually compatible for 4 hr at 25°C	2440	C
Dimenhydrinate		10 mg/1 mL		100 mg/1 mL	Clear solution	2569	C
Doxapram HCl	RB	400 mg/20 mL		500 mg/4 mL	Precipitates immediately	1177	I
Heparin sodium		2500 units/1 mL	HO	2 g	Physically compatible for at least 5 min	1053	C
Heparin sodium	HOS	5000 units/mL	WW	10 mg/mL	Physically compatible. No cefotaxime loss in 3 days at 4°C. Losses of 7 and 14% in 1 and 2 days at 27°C	2820	C
Pantoprazole sodium	[a]	4 mg/1 mL		100 mg/1 mL	Precipitates immediately	2574	I

[a] Test performed using the formulation WITHOUT edetate disodium.

Y-Site Injection Compatibility (1:1 Mixture)

Cefotaxime sodium

Test Drug	Mfr	Conc	Mfr	Conc	Remarks	Ref	C/I
Acyclovir sodium	BW	5 mg/mL[a]	HO	20 mg/mL[a]	Physically compatible for 4 hr at 25°C	1157	C
Allopurinol sodium	BW	3 mg/mL[b]	HO	20 mg/mL[b]	Tiny particles form immediately	1686	I
Alprostadil	BED	7.5 mcg/mL[l m]	HO	100 mg/mL[k]	Visually compatible for 1 hr	2746	C
Amifostine	USB	10 mg/mL[a]	HO	20 mg/mL[a]	Physically compatible for 4 hr at 23°C	1845	C
Anakinra	SYN	4 and 36 mg/mL[b]	HO	10 mg/mL[b]	Physically compatible. No cefotaxime loss in 4 hr at 25°C. Anakinra uncertain	2508	?
Azithromycin	PF	2 mg/mL[b]	HMR	200 mg/mL[i j]	White microcrystals found	2368	I
Aztreonam	SQ	40 mg/mL[a]	HO	20 mg/mL[a]	Physically compatible for 4 hr at 23°C	1758	C
Bivalirudin	TMC	5 mg/mL[a]	HO	20 mg/mL[a]	Physically compatible for 4 hr at 23°C	2373	C
Cangrelor tetrasodium	TMC	1 mg/mL[b]		20 mg/mL[b]	Physically compatible for 4 hr	3243	C
Cisatracurium besylate	GW	0.1 mg/mL[a]	HO	20 mg/mL[a]	Physically compatible for 4 hr at 23°C	2074	C
Cisatracurium besylate	GW	2 mg/mL[a]	HO	20 mg/mL[a]	Subvisible haze forms in 4 hr	2074	I
Cisatracurium besylate	GW	5 mg/mL[a]	HO	20 mg/mL[a]	Subvisible haze forms immediately	2074	I
Cloxacillin sodium	SMX	100 mg/mL	SAN	95 mg/mL	Physically compatible for up to 4 hr at room temperature	3245	C
Cyclophosphamide	MJ	20 mg/mL[a]	HO	20 mg/mL[a]	Physically compatible for 4 hr at 25°C	1194	C

Y-Site Injection Compatibility (1:1 Mixture) (Cont.)

Test Drug	Mfr	Conc	Mfr	Conc	Remarks	Ref	C/I
Dexmedetomidine HCl	AB	4 mcg/mL[b]	HO	20 mg/mL[b]	Physically compatible for 4 hr at 23°C	2383	C
Diltiazem HCl	MMD	5 mg/mL	HO	10 and 180 mg/mL[b]	Visually compatible	1807	C
Diltiazem HCl	MMD	1 mg/mL[b]	HO	180 mg/mL[b]	Visually compatible	1807	C
Docetaxel	RPR	0.9 mg/mL[a]	HO	20 mg/mL[a]	Physically compatible for 4 hr at 23°C	2224	C
Etoposide phosphate	BR	5 mg/mL[a]	HO	20 mg/mL[a]	Physically compatible for 4 hr at 23°C	2218	C
Famotidine	MSD	0.2 mg/mL[a]	HO	20 mg/mL[b]	Physically compatible for 14 hr	1196	C
Famotidine	ME	2 mg/mL[b]		20 mg/mL[a]	Visually compatible for 4 hr at 22°C	1936	C
Fenoldopam mesylate	AB	80 mcg/mL[b]	HO	20 mg/mL[b]	Physically compatible for 4 hr at 23°C	2467	C
Filgrastim	AMG	30 mcg/mL[a]	HO	20 mg/mL[a]	Particles form in 4 hr	1687	I
Fluconazole	RR	2 mg/mL	HO	20 mg/mL	Cloudiness and amber color develop	1407	I
Fludarabine phosphate	BX	1 mg/mL[a]	HO	20 mg/mL[a]	Visually compatible for 4 hr at 22°C	1439	C
Gemcitabine HCl	LI	10 mg/mL[b]	HO	20 mg/mL[b]	Subvisible haze forms in 1 hr. Increased haze and a microprecipitate in 4 hr	2226	I
Granisetron HCl	SKB	0.05 mg/mL[a]	HO	20 mg/mL[a]	Physically compatible for 4 hr at 23°C	2000	C
Hetastarch in lactated electrolyte	AB	6%	HO	20 mg/mL[a]	Physically compatible for 4 hr at 23°C	2339	C
Hetastarch in sodium chloride 0.9%	DCC	6%	HO	20 mg/mL[a]	Small crystals form immediately after mixing and persist for 4 hr	1313	I
Hydromorphone HCl	WY	0.2 mg/mL[a]	HO	20 mg/mL[a]	Physically compatible for 4 hr at 25°C	987	C
Levofloxacin	OMN	5 mg/mL[a]	HO	200 mg/mL	Visually compatible for 4 hr at 24°C	2233	C
Lorazepam	WY	0.33 mg/mL[b]	RS	10 mg/mL	Visually compatible for 24 hr at 22°C	1855	C
Magnesium sulfate	IX	16.7, 33.3, 66.7, 100 mg/mL[a]	HO	20 mg/mL[a]	Physically compatible for at least 4 hr at 32°C	813	C
Melphalan HCl	BW	0.1 mg/mL[b]	HO	20 mg/mL[b]	Physically compatible for 3 hr at 22°C	1557	C
Meperidine HCl	WY	10 mg/mL[a]	HO	20 mg/mL[a]	Physically compatible for 4 hr at 25°C	987	C
Meropenem		50 mg/mL	SMX	100 mg/mL	Physically compatible for 4 hr at room temperature	3538, 3547	C
Midazolam HCl	RC	1 mg/mL[a]	HO	20 mg/mL[a]	Visually compatible for 24 hr at 23°C	1847	C
Midazolam HCl	RC	5 mg/mL	RS	10 mg/mL	Visually compatible for 24 hr at 22°C	1855	C
Milrinone lactate	SS	0.2 mg/mL[a]	HO	150 mg/mL[a]	Visually compatible for 4 hr at 25°C	2381	C
Morphine sulfate	WI	1 mg/mL[a]	HO	20 mg/mL[a]	Physically compatible for 4 hr at 25°C	987	C
Ondansetron HCl	GL	1 mg/mL[b]	HO	20 mg/mL[a]	Visually compatible for 4 hr at 22°C	1365	C
Pemetrexed disodium	LI	20 mg/mL[b]	APP	20 mg/mL[a]	Slight color darkening occurs over 4 hr	2564	I
Pentamidine isethionate	FUJ	3 mg/mL[a]	HO	20 mg/mL[a]	Fine precipitate forms immediately	1880	I
Propofol	ZEN°	10 mg/mL	HO	20 mg/mL[a]	Physically compatible for 1 hr at 23°C	2066	C
Quinupristin–dalfopristin		2 mg/mL[a] [n]		20 mg/mL	Reported to be incompatible	3230	I
Remifentanil HCl	GW	0.025 and 0.25 mg/mL[b]	HO	20 mg/mL[a]	Physically compatible for 4 hr at 23°C	2075	C
Sargramostim	IMM	10 mcg/mL[b]	HO	20 mg/mL[b]	Visually compatible for 4 hr at 22°C	1436	C

Y-Site Injection Compatibility (1:1 Mixture) (Cont.)

Test Drug	Mfr	Conc	Mfr	Conc	Remarks	Ref	C/I
Teniposide	BR	0.1 mg/mL[a]	HO	20 mg/mL[a]	Physically compatible for 1 hr at 23°C	1725	C
Thiotepa	IMM[c]	1 mg/mL[a]	HO	20 mg/mL[a]	Physically compatible for 1 hr at 23°C	1861	C
Tigecycline	WY	1 mg/mL[b]		40 mg/mL[b]	Physically compatible for 4 hr	2714	C
TNA #218 to #226[d]			HO	20 mg/mL[a]	Visually compatible for 4 hr at 23°C	2215	C
TPN #61[d]		[e]	HO	200 mg/0.7 mL[f]	Physically compatible	1012	C
TPN #61[d]		[g]	HO	1.2 g/4 mL[f]	Physically compatible	1012	C
TPN #189[d]			RS	200 mg/mL[e]	Visually compatible for 24 hr at 22°C	1767	C
TPN #203, #204[d]			HO	60 mg/mL	Visually compatible for 2 hr at 23°C	1974	C
TPN #212 to #215[d]			HO	20 mg/mL[a]	Physically compatible for 4 hr at 23°C	2109	C
Vancomycin HCl		12.5, 25, 30, 50 mg/mL[h]		100 mg/mL[h]	White precipitate forms immediately	1721	I
Vancomycin HCl		5 mg/mL[h]		100 mg/mL[h]	No precipitate visually observed over 7 days at room temperature, but nonvisible incompatibility cannot be ruled out	1721	?
Vancomycin HCl	AB	20 mg/mL[a]	HO	200 mg/mL[h]	Transient precipitate forms	2189	?
Vancomycin HCl	AB	20 mg/mL[a]	HO	50 mg/mL[a]	White cloudiness forms immediately	2189	I
Vancomycin HCl	AB	20 mg/mL[a]	HO	1 and 10 mg/mL[a]	Physically compatible for 4 hr at 23°C	2189	C
Vancomycin HCl	AB	2 mg/mL[a]	HO	1[a], 10[a], 50[a], 200[h] mg/mL	Physically compatible for 4 hr at 23°C	2189	C
Vinorelbine tartrate	BW	1 mg/mL[b]	HO	20 mg/mL[b]	Physically compatible for 4 hr at 22°C	1558	C

[a] Tested in dextrose 5%.

[b] Tested in sodium chloride 0.9%.

[c] Lyophilized formulation tested.

[d] Refer to Appendix for the composition of parenteral nutrition solutions. TNA indicates a 3-in-1 admixture, and TPN indicates a 2-in-1 admixture.

[e] Run at 21 mL/hr.

[f] Given over five minutes by syringe pump.

[g] Run at 94 mL/hr.

[h] Tested in sterile water for injection.

[i] Tested in sodium chloride 0.45%.

[j] Injected via Y site into an administration set running azithromycin.

[k] Tested in either dextrose 5% or in sodium chloride 0.9%, but the report did not specify which solution.

[l] Tested in a 1:1 mixture of (1) dextrose 5% and dextrose 5% in sodium chloride 0.45% with and without potassium chloride 20 mEq/L and also in (2) dextrose 10% in sodium chloride 0.45% with and without potassium chloride 20 mEq/L.

[m] Tested in a 1:1 mixture of dextrose 5% and TPN #274 (see Appendix).

[n] Quinupristin and dalfopristin components combined.

[o] Test performed using the formulation WITH edetate disodium.

Selected Revisions May 1, 2020. © Copyright, October 1984.
American Society of Health-System Pharmacists, Inc.

Cefotetan Disodium
AHFS 8:12.07.12

Products

Cefotetan disodium is available in 1- and 2-g vials and infusion bottles and 10-g pharmacy bulk packages.[1(8/07)]

For intramuscular injection, reconstitute the vials with sterile water for injection, bacteriostatic water for injection, sodium chloride 0.9%, or lidocaine hydrochloride 0.5 or 1%. Then shake well to dissolve and let stand until clear. Recommended volumes for reconstitution are shown in Table 1.[1(8/07)]

For intravenous use, reconstitute the vials with sterile water for injection in the amounts noted in Table 1, shake well to dissolve, and let stand until clear.[1(8/07)]

Reconstitute the 10-g pharmacy bulk package with sterile water for injection, dextrose 5%, or sodium chloride 0.9% according to the instructions on the package label. Then shake it well to dissolve and let stand until clear.[1(8/07)]

Table 1. Recommended dilutions of cefotetan disodium vials[1(8/07) 4]

Vial Size	Volume of Diluent	Withdrawable Volume	Approximate Concentration
Intramuscular			
1 g	2 mL	2.5 mL	400 mg/mL
2 g	3 mL	4.0 mL	500 mg/mL
Intravenous			
1 g	10 mL	10.5 mL	95 mg/mL
2 g	10 to 20 mL	11 to 21 mL	182 to 95 mg/mL

Cefotetan disodium (Braun) is available as 1 and 2 g in a dual chamber flexible container. The diluent chamber contains dextrose solution 3.58% for the 1-g container and 2.08% for the 2-g container for use as a diluent.[1(8/07)]

pH

Reconstituted solutions have a pH of 4.5 to 6.5.[1(8/07)]

Osmolarity

Concentrations of 100 to 200 mg/mL in sterile water for injection have osmolarities of 400 to 800 mOsm/L, respectively. Intramuscular concentrations of 375 to 471.5 mg/mL are extremely hypertonic, with osmolarities greater than 1500 mOsm/L.[4]

Osmolality

Cefotetan disodium (Braun) 1 and 2 g in dual chamber flexible containers has an osmolality of 290 mOsm/kg when activated with the dextrose solution diluent.[1(8/07)]

Sodium Content

Each gram of cefotetan disodium contains approximately 3.5 mEq (80 mg) of sodium.[1(8/07)]

Administration

Cefotetan disodium may be administered by deep intramuscular injection, direct intravenous injection over 3 to 5 minutes, and intermittent intravenous infusion in 50 to 100 mL of dextrose 5% or sodium chloride 0.9% infused over 20 to 60 minutes. The manufacturer recommends temporarily discontinuing other solutions being administered at the same site.[1(8/07) 4]

Stability

Intact vials should be stored at 22°C or less and protected from light. Cefotetan disodium powder is white to pale yellow. Solutions may vary from colorless to yellow, depending on the concentration.[1(8/07)]

When reconstituted as recommended, cefotetan disodium solutions are stable for 24 hours at room temperature (25°C) and 96 hours under refrigeration (5°C). In disposable glass or plastic syringes, the drug also is stable for 24 hours at room temperature and 96 hours under refrigeration.[1(8/07) 4]

Cefotetan disodium (Braun) 1 and 2 g in dual chamber flexible plastic containers with dextrose solution diluent should be used within 12 hours after activation if stored at room temperature and in 5 days if stored under refrigeration.[1(8/07)]

Freezing Solutions

The manufacturer states that solutions reconstituted as recommended are stable for at least 1 week when frozen at −20°C.[1(8/07)] The manufacturer also has stated that cefotetan disodium as the reconstituted solution in vials is stable for 1 year at −20°C; in a large volume parenteral solution, it is stable for 30 weeks at −20°C.[283] Thawing should be performed at room temperature, and thawed solutions should not be refrozen.[1(8/07) 4]

Cefotetan disodium (Braun) 1 and 2 g in dual chamber flexible containers should not be frozen.[1(8/07)]

Central Venous Catheter

Cefotetan disodium (Zeneca) 5 mg/mL in dextrose 5% was found to be compatible with the ARROWg+ard Blue Plus (Arrow International) chlorhexidine-bearing triple-lumen central catheter. Essentially complete delivery of the drug was found with little or no drug loss occurring. Furthermore, chlorhexidine delivered from the catheter remained at trace amounts with no substantial increase due to the delivery of the drug through the catheter.[2335]

DOI: 10.37573/9781585286850.076

Compatibility Information

Solution Compatibility

Cefotetan disodium

Test Soln Name	Mfr	Mfr	Conc/L or %	Remarks	Ref	C/I
Dextrose 5%	TR[a]	STU	2 g	4% loss at 20°C and 0 to 2% loss at 4 and −20°C in 14 days	966	C
Dextrose 5%	[a]	AY	20 and 40 g	Visually compatible with 10% loss in 3.5 days at 23°C and 13 days at 4°C	1591	C
Dextrose 5%	TR[a]	STU	20 g	8% loss in 2 days and 11% loss in 3 days at 25°C. 6% loss in 41 days at 5°C. No loss in 60 days at −10°C	1598	C
Sodium chloride 0.9%	[a]	AY	20 and 40 g	Visually compatible with 10% loss in 3.5 days at 23°C and 14 days at 4°C	1591	C
Sodium chloride 0.9%	TR[a]	STU	20 g	8% loss in 2 days and 11% loss in 3 days at 25°C. 5% loss in 41 days at 5°C. No loss in 60 days at −10°C	1598	C

[a] Tested in PVC containers.

Additive Compatibility

Cefotetan disodium

Test Drug	Mfr	Conc/L or %	Mfr	Conc/L or %	Test Solution	Remarks	Ref	C/I
Promethazine HCl	ES	250 mg	ZEN	10 g	D5W	Precipitates immediately	1753	I

Drugs in Syringe Compatibility

Cefotetan disodium

Test Drug	Mfr	Amt	Mfr	Amt	Remarks	Ref	C/I
Doxapram HCl	RB	400 mg/20 mL		1 g/10 mL	Immediate turbidity	1177	I
Promethazine HCl	ES	25 mg/1 mL	ZEN	50 mg/5 mL[a]	White precipitate, resembling cottage cheese, forms immediately	1753	I

[a] Tested in dextrose 5%.

Y-Site Injection Compatibility (1:1 Mixture)

Cefotetan disodium

Test Drug	Mfr	Conc	Mfr	Conc	Remarks	Ref	C/I
Allopurinol sodium	BW	3 mg/mL[h]	STU	20 mg/mL[b]	Physically compatible for 4 hr at 22°C	1686	C
Amifostine	USB	10 mg/mL[a]	STU	20 mg/mL[a]	Physically compatible for 4 hr at 23°C	1845	C
Aztreonam	SQ	40 mg/mL[b]	STU	20 mg/mL[b]	Physically compatible for 4 hr at 23°C	1758	C
Bivalirudin	TMC	5 mg/mL[a]	ZEN	20 mg/mL[a]	Physically compatible for 4 hr at 23°C	2373	C
Dexmedetomidine HCl	AB	4 mcg/mL[b]	ZEN	20 mg/mL[b]	Physically compatible for 4 hr at 23°C	2383	C
Diltiazem HCl	MMD	5 mg/mL	STU	10 and 200 mg/mL[b]	Visually compatible	1807	C
Diltiazem HCl	MMD	1 mg/mL[b]	STU	200 mg/mL[b]	Visually compatible	1807	C
Docetaxel	RPR	0.9 mg/mL[a]	ZEN	20 mg/mL[a]	Physically compatible for 4 hr at 23°C	2224	C

Y-Site Injection Compatibility (1:1 Mixture) (Cont.)

Test Drug	Mfr	Conc	Mfr	Conc	Remarks	Ref	C/I
Etoposide phosphate	BR	5 mg/mL[a]	ZEN	20 mg/mL[a]	Physically compatible for 4 hr at 23°C	2218	C
Famotidine	MSD	0.2 mg/mL[a]	STU	20 mg/mL[b]	Physically compatible for 14 hr	1196	C
Fenoldopam mesylate	AB	80 mcg/mL[b]	ZEN	20 mg/mL[b]	Physically compatible for 4 hr at 23°C	2467	C
Filgrastim	AMG	30 mcg/mL[a]	STU	20 mg/mL[a]	Physically compatible for 4 hr at 22°C	1687	C
Fluconazole	RR	2 mg/mL	STU	40 mg/mL	Physically compatible for 24 hr at 25°C	1407	C
Fludarabine phosphate	BX	1 mg/mL[a]	STU	20 mg/mL[a]	Visually compatible for 4 hr at 22°C	1439	C
Gemcitabine HCl	LI	10 mg/mL[b]	ZEN	20 mg/mL[b]	Physically compatible for 4 hr at 23°C	2226	C
Granisetron HCl	SKB	0.05 mg/mL[a]	STU	20 mg/mL[a]	Physically compatible for 4 hr at 23°C	2000	C
Heparin sodium	TR	50 units/mL	STU	40 mg/mL[a]	Visually compatible for 4 hr at 25°C	1793	C
Hetastarch in lactated electrolyte	AB	6%	ZEN	20 mg/mL[a]	Physically compatible for 4 hr at 23°C	2339	C
Insulin, regular	LI	0.2 unit/mL[b]	STU	20 and 40 mg/mL[a]	Physically compatible for 2 hr at 25°C	1395	C
Linezolid	PHU	2 mg/mL	ZEN	20 mg/mL[a]	Physically compatible for 4 hr at 23°C	2264	C
Melphalan HCl	BW	0.1 mg/mL[b]	STU	20 mg/mL[b]	Physically compatible for 3 hr at 22°C	1557	C
Meperidine HCl	WY	10 mg/mL[b]	STU	20 and 40 mg/mL[a]	Physically compatible for 1 hr at 25°C	1338	C
Morphine sulfate	ES	1 mg/mL[b]	STU	20 and 40 mg/mL[a]	Physically compatible for 1 hr at 25°C	1338	C
Paclitaxel	NCI	1.2 mg/mL[a]	STU	20 mg/mL[a]	Physically compatible for 4 hr at 22°C	1556	C
Palonosetron HCl	MGI	50 mcg/mL	ASZ	20 mg/mL[b]	Physically compatible and no loss of either drug in 4 hr at room temperature	2749	C
Pemetrexed disodium	LI	20 mg/mL[b]	ASZ	20 mg/mL[a]	Color darkening and brownish discoloration occur immediately	2564	I
Promethazine HCl	ES	25 mg/mL	ZEN	10 mg/mL[a]	White precipitate forms immediately despite flushing of line with NS	1753	I
Propofol	ZEN[f]	10 mg/mL	STU	20 mg/mL[a]	Physically compatible for 1 hr at 23°C	2066	C
Remifentanil HCl	GW	0.025 and 0.25 mg/mL[b]	ZEN	20 mg/mL[a]	Physically compatible for 4 hr at 23°C	2075	C
Sargramostim	IMM	10 mcg/mL[b]	STU	20 mg/mL[b]	Visually compatible for 4 hr at 22°C	1436	C
Tacrolimus	FUJ	1 mg/mL[b]	STU	40 mg/mL[a]	Visually compatible for 24 hr at 25°C	1630	C
Teniposide	BR	0.1 mg/mL[a]	STU	20 mg/mL[a]	Physically compatible for 4 hr at 23°C	1725	C
Theophylline	TR	4 mg/mL	STU	40 mg/mL[a]	Visually compatible for 6 hr at 25°C	1793	C
Thiotepa	IMM[c]	1 mg/mL[a]	STU	20 mg/mL[a]	Physically compatible for 4 hr at 23°C	1861	C
TNA #218 to #226[d]			ZEN	20 mg/mL[a]	Visually compatible for 4 hr at 23°C	2215	C
TPN #212 to #215[d]			STU	20 mg/mL[a]	Physically compatible for 4 hr at 23°C	2109	C
Vancomycin HCl	AB	20 mg/mL[a]	ZEN	200 mg/mL[e]	Transient precipitate forms followed by white precipitate in 4 hr	2189	I
Vancomycin HCl	AB	20 mg/mL[a]	ZEN	10 and 50 mg/mL[a]	Gross white precipitate forms immediately	2189	I
Vancomycin HCl	AB	20 mg/mL[a]	ZEN	1 mg/mL[a]	Subvisible haze forms immediately. White precipitate in 4 hr	2189	I

Y-Site Injection Compatibility (1:1 Mixture) (Cont.)

Test Drug	Mfr	Conc	Mfr	Conc	Remarks	Ref	C/I
Vancomycin HCl	AB	2 mg/mL[a]	ZEN	1[a], 10[a], 50[a], 200[e] mg/mL	Physically compatible for 4 hr at 23°C	2189	C
Vinorelbine tartrate	BW	1 mg/mL[b]	STU	20 mg/mL[b]	Tiny particles form immediately. Turbidity in 4 hr	1558	I

[a] Tested in dextrose 5%.

[b] Tested in sodium chloride 0.9%.

[c] Lyophilized formulation tested.

[d] Refer to Appendix for the composition of parenteral nutrition solutions. TNA indicates a 3-in-1 admixture, and TPN indicates a 2-in-1 admixture.

[e] Tested in sterile water for injection.

[f] Test performed using the formulation WITH edetate disodium.

Selected Revisions January 31, 2020. © Copyright, October 1990. American Society of Health-System Pharmacists, Inc.

Cefoxitin Sodium
AHFS 8:12.07.12

Products

Cefoxitin sodium is available in vials containing the equivalent of 1 and 2 g of cefoxitin (as sodium). It is also available in 10-g bulk bottles.[1(4/08)]

For intravenous administration, reconstitute the vial contents with sterile water for injection. The 1-g vials may be reconstituted with 10 mL resulting in a 95-mg/mL concentration. The 2-g vials may be reconstituted with 20 or 10 mL resulting in 95 or 180 mg/mL, respectively. The 10-g bulk bottles may be reconstituted with 93 or 43 mL resulting in 100 or 200 mg/mL, respectively. After addition of the diluent, shake the vial and allow the solution to stand until it becomes clear.[1(4/08) 4]

For intravenous infusion, the primary solution may be diluted further in 50 to 1000 mL of compatible diluent.[1(4/08)]

Cefoxitin sodium (Braun) is available as 1 and 2 g in a dual-chamber flexible container. The diluent chamber contains dextrose solution.[1(4/08)]

pH

Reconstituted solutions have a pH of 4.2 to 7. The frozen premixed infusion and reconstituted drug in dual-chamber containers have a pH of about 6.5.[1(4/08) 4]

Osmolality

The osmolality of cefoxitin sodium 1 and 2 g was calculated for the following dilutions:[1054]

Diluent	Osmolality (mOsm/kg)	
	50 mL	100 mL
1 g		
Dextrose 5%	326	293
Sodium chloride 0.9%	352	319
2 g		
Dextrose 5%	388	329
Sodium chloride 0.9%	415	355

The osmolality of cefoxitin sodium (MSD) 50 mg/mL was determined to be 348 mOsm/kg in dextrose 5% and 361 mOsm/kg in sodium chloride 0.9%.[1375]

Cefoxitin sodium (Braun) 1 and 2 g in dual-chamber flexible containers has an osmolality of 290 mOsm/kg when activated with the dextrose solution diluent.[1(4/08)]

The following maximum cefoxitin sodium concentrations were recommended to achieve osmolalities suitable for peripheral infusion in fluid-restricted patients:[1180]

Diluent	Maximum Concentration (mg/mL)	Osmolality (mOsm/kg)
Dextrose 5%	62	531
Sodium chloride 0.9%	56	508
Sterile water for injection	112	437

Sodium Content

Each gram of cefoxitin sodium contains 2.3 mEq (53.8 mg) of sodium.[1(4/08)]

Administration

Cefoxitin sodium may be administered by direct intravenous injection over 3 to 5 minutes directly into the vein or slowly into the tubing of a running compatible infusion solution, or by continuous or intermittent intravenous infusion. The manufacturer recommends temporarily discontinuing other solutions being administered at the site.[1(4/08) 4]

The manufacturer recommends that cefoxitin sodium not be mixed with aminoglycoside antibiotics such as amikacin sulfate, gentamicin sulfate, and tobramycin sulfate.[1(4/08)] However, compatibility studies show that such admixtures may indeed be sufficiently stable to allow combined mixture in the same solution.

Stability

Intact vials of cefoxitin sodium should be stored between 2 and 25°C. Exposure to temperatures above 50°C should be avoided. The powder is white to off-white in color. Solutions may range from colorless to light amber.[1(4/08)] Both the dry material and solutions may darken, depending on storage conditions. Although moisture plays a role in the rate and intensity of the darkening, exposure to oxygen is the most significant factor. However, this discoloration is stated not to affect potency or relate to any significant chemical change. The concern over color is purely aesthetic.[865]

Exposure of cefoxitin sodium (MSD) 40 mg/mL in sterile water for injection to 37°C for 24 hours, to simulate the use of a portable infusion pump, resulted in about a 3 to 4% cefoxitin loss.[1391]

DOI: 10.37573/9781585286850.077

Cefoxitin sodium solutions reconstituted as indicated in Table 1 are stable for 48 hours at 25°C and at least 7 days and, in some cases, up to 1 month at 5°C.[308]

Table 1. Stability of reconstituted cefoxitin sodium 1 g[308]

Diluent	Volume	Remarks
Bacteriostatic water for injection (benzyl alcohol)	2 mL	9% decomposition in 48 hr at 25°C. 4% in 7 days and 10% in 1 month at 5°C
Bacteriostatic water for injection (para-bens)	2 mL	9% decomposition in 48 hr at 25°C. 5% in 7 days and 12% in 1 month at 5°C
Dextrose 5%	10 mL	9% decomposition in 48 hr at 25°C, 2% in 7 days at 5°C
Lidocaine HCl 0.5% (with parabens)	2 mL	8% decomposition in 48 hr at 25°C. 5% in 7 days and 10% in 1 month at 5°C
Lidocaine HCl 1% (with parabens)	2 mL	7% decomposition in 48 hr at 25°C. 2% in 7 days and 10% in 1 month at 5°C
Sodium chloride 0.9%	10 mL	8% decomposition in 48 hr at 25°C
Water for injection	10 mL	10% decomposition in 48 hr at 25°C, 1% in 7 days at 5°C
Water for injection	4 mL	7% decomposition in 48 hr at 25°C, 2% in 7 days at 5°C
Water for injection	2 mL	8% decomposition in 48 hr at 25°C. 2% in 7 days and 10% in 1 month at 5°C
(In plastic syringe)	10 mL	6% decomposition in 24 hr and 11% in 48 hr at 25°C

Cefoxitin sodium (MSD) 1 and 2 g/10 mL in sterile water for injection, packaged in plastic syringes (Monoject), exhibited a 10% cefoxitin sodium loss in 2 days at 24°C and 23 days at 4°C. Less than 10% loss occurred in 3 months frozen at −15°C.[1178]

pH Effects

Cefoxitin sodium at 1 and 10 mg/mL in aqueous solution is stable over pH 4 to 8. The time to 10% decomposition when stored at 25°C was essentially independent of pH, ranging from 40 to 44 hours at pH 4 to 5 to 33 hours at pH 8. Under refrigeration, a pH 7 (unbuffered) aqueous solution showed 10% decomposition in 26 days. At pH less than 4, precipitation of the free acid may occur. Above pH 8, hydrolysis of the β-lactam group may result.[308]

In another study, cefoxitin sodium in aqueous solution at 25°C exhibited minimum rates of decomposition at pH 5 to 7. The solutions in this pH range showed 10% decomposition in about 2 days. At pH 3, about 40 hours elapsed before 10% decomposition occurred. However, at pH 9, only 14 hours was required to incur a 10% loss.[630]

Freezing Solutions

The stability of cefoxitin sodium reconstituted with the diluents as shown in Table 2 was evaluated in the frozen state at −20°C. The solutions retained adequate potency for at least 30 weeks.[308] Thawed solutions should not be refrozen.[1(4/08)] Frozen premixed cefoxitin solutions also should not be refrozen after thawing. The manufacturer states that the thawed solution may be stored for 24 hours at room temperature or 21 days under refrigeration.[1(4/08)]

An approximate twofold increase in particles of 2 to 60 μm produced by freezing and thawing cefoxitin sodium (MSD) 2 g/100 mL of dextrose 5% (Travenol) was reported. The reconstituted drug was filtered through a 0.45-μm filter into polyvinyl chloride (PVC) bags of solution and frozen for 7 days at −20°C. Thawing was performed at room temperature (29°C) for 12 hours. Although the total number of particles increased significantly, no particles greater than 60 μm were observed; the solutions complied with USP standards for particle sizes and numbers in large volume parenteral solutions.[822]

Table 2. Stability of reconstituted cefoxitin sodium 1 g frozen at −20°C[308]

Diluent	Volume	Remarks
Bacteriostatic water for injection (benzyl alcohol)	10 mL	2% decomposition in 30 weeks. Thawed solutions showed 6% decomposition in 24 hr at 25°C and 1% in 7 days at 5°C
Bacteriostatic water for injection (parabens)	10 mL	2% decomposition in 30 weeks. Thawed solutions showed no decomposition in 24 hr at 25°C and 1% in 7 days at 5°C
Dextrose 5%	10 mL	3% decomposition in 30 weeks. Thawed solutions showed 8% decomposition in 24 hr at 25°C and 6% in 7 days at 5°C
Lidocaine HCl 0.5%	2 mL	2% cefoxitin decomposition in 26 weeks. Thawed solutions showed 6% decomposition in 24 hr at 25°C. Lidocaine stable
Sodium chloride 0.9%	10 mL	5% decomposition in 30 weeks. Thawed solutions showed 3% decomposition in 24 hr at 25°C and 6% in 7 days at 5°C
Water for injection	10 mL	1% decomposition in 30 weeks. Thawed solutions showed 3% decomposition in 24 hr at 25°C and 5% in 7 days at 5°C
Water for injection	4 mL	No decomposition in 13 weeks

A 3% or less cefoxitin sodium (MSD) loss was reported from a solution containing 40 mg/mL in sterile water for injection in PVC and glass containers after 30 days at −20°C. Subsequent thawing and storage for 4 days at 5°C, followed by 24 hours at 37°C to simulate the use of a portable infusion pump, resulted in an additional 3 to 4% cefoxitin sodium loss.[1391]

Cefoxitin sodium in sodium chloride 0.9%, Ringer's injection, lactated, and dextrose 5% in PVC bags is stable for 26 weeks if kept frozen.[4]

Cefoxitin sodium (Braun) 1 and 2 g in dual-chamber flexible containers should not be frozen.[1(4/08)]

Sorption

Cefoxitin sodium was shown not to exhibit sorption to PVC bags and tubing, polyethylene tubing, Silastic tubing, and polypropylene syringes.[536 606]

Central Venous Catheter

Cefoxitin sodium (Merck) 5 mg/mL in dextrose 5% was found to be compatible with the ARROWg+ard Blue Plus (Arrow International) chlorhexidine-bearing triple-lumen central catheter.

Essentially complete delivery of the drug was found with little or no drug loss occurring. Furthermore, chlorhexidine delivered from the catheter remained at trace amounts with no substantial increase due to the delivery of the drug through the catheter.[2335]

Compatibility Information

Solution Compatibility

Cefoxitin sodium

Test Soln Name	Mfr	Mfr	Conc/L or %	Remarks	Ref	C/I
Dextrose 5% in Ringer's injection, lactated	a	MSD	1, 2, 10, 20 g	5 to 8% loss in 24 hr and 12 to 13% in 48 hr at 25°C. 3 to 5% in 7 days at 5°C	308	C
Dextrose 5% in sodium chloride 0.225%	a	MSD	1 g	5% loss in 24 hr and 11% in 48 hr at 25°C	308	C
Dextrose 5% in sodium chloride 0.45%	a	MSD	1 g	4% loss in 24 hr and 10% in 48 hr at 25°C	308	C
Dextrose 5% in sodium chloride 0.9%	a	MSD	1 g	4% loss in 24 hr and 10% in 48 hr at 25°C	308	C
Dextrose 5%	a	MSD	1, 2, 10 g	6 to 7% loss in 24 hr and 11 to 13% in 48 hr at 25°C. 3 to 6% in 7 days at 5°C	308	C
Dextrose 5%	a	MSD	20 g	7.5% loss in 24 hr and 13% in 48 hr at 25°C. 4% in 7 days at 5°C. No loss noted in 13 weeks at –20°C	308	C
Dextrose 5%	TR[b]	MSD	1 g	9% loss in 24 hr and 11% in 48 hr at 25°C	308	C
Dextrose 5%	TR[b]	MSD	20 g	No loss noted in 24 hr but 11% loss in 48 hr at 24°C. 3% loss in 13 days at 5°C	525	C
Dextrose 5%	TR[b]	MSD	20 g	Physically compatible with 5% loss in 24 hr at room temperature. No loss in 30 days at –20°C	554	C
Dextrose 5%	b		10 and 20 g	Visually compatible and 3% loss after storage at –20°C for 72 hr, thawed, and 6 hr at room temperature	629	C
Dextrose 5%	MG[a]	MSD	20 g	Physically compatible with no loss in 24 hr and 6% loss in 48 hr at room temperature	983	C
Dextrose 10%	a	MSD	1 g	6% loss in 24 hr and 11% in 48 hr at 25°C	308	C
Ionosol B in dextrose 5%	AB[a]	MSD	1, 2, 10 g	6 to 8% loss in 24 hr and 12 to 13% in 48 hr at 25°C. 3 to 6% in 7 days at 5°C	308	C
Normosol M in dextrose 5%	AB[a]	MSD	1, 2, 10, 20 g	4 to 6% loss in 24 hr and 11 to 12% in 48 hr at 25°C. 3 to 5% in 7 days at 5°C	308	C
Ringer's injection	a	MSD	1 g	2% loss in 24 hr and 12% in 48 hr at 25°C	308	C
Ringer's injection, lactated	a	MSD	1, 2, 10, 20 g	5 to 7% loss in 24 hr and 10 to 12% in 48 hr at 25°C. 3% in 7 days at 5°C	308	C
Ringer's injection, lactated	TR[b]	MSD	1 g	7% loss in 24 hr and 9% in 48 hr at 25°C	308	C
Sodium chloride 0.9%	a	MSD	1 g	5% loss in 24 hr and 11% in 48 hr at 25°C	308	C
Sodium chloride 0.9%	a	MSD	10 and 20 g	8 to 10% loss in 24 hr and 13 and 15% in 48 hr at 25°C. 4 to 5% in 48 hr at 5°C	308	C
Sodium chloride 0.9%	b	MSD	1 g	4 to 7% loss in 24 hr and 8 to 9% loss in 48 hr at 25°C	308	C
Sodium chloride 0.9%	TR[b]	MSD	20 g	No loss noted in 24 hr but 12% loss in 48 hr at 24°C. 3% loss in 13 days at 5°C	525	C
Sodium chloride 0.9%	b		10 and 20 g	Visually compatible and 3% loss after storage at –20°C for 72 hr, thawing, and 6 hr at room temperature	629	C

Solution Compatibility (Cont.)

Test Soln Name	Mfr	Mfr	Conc/L or %	Remarks	Ref	C/I
Sodium chloride 0.9%	MG[a]	MSD	20 g	Physically compatible with no loss in 24 hr and 6% loss in 48 hr at room temperature	983	C
Sodium lactate ⅙ M	[a]	MSD	1 g	5% loss in 24 hr and 8% in 48 hr at 25°C	308	C
TPN #107[c]			1 g	Activity retained for 24 hr at 21°C	1326	C

[a] Tested in glass containers.

[b] Tested in PVC containers.

[c] Refer to Appendix for the composition of parenteral nutrition solutions. TPN indicates a 2-in-1 admixture.

Additive Compatibility

Cefoxitin sodium

Test Drug	Mfr	Conc/L or %	Mfr	Conc/L or %	Test Solution	Remarks	Ref	C/I
Amikacin sulfate	BR	5 g	MSD	5 g	D5S	9% cefoxitin loss at 25°C and none at 5°C in 48 hr. No amikacin loss at 25°C and 1% at 5°C in 48 hr	308	C
Aztreonam	SQ	10 and 20 g	MSD	10 and 20 g	D5W, NS[a]	Both drugs stable for 12 hr at 25°C. Yellow color and 6 to 12% aztreonam and 9 to 15% cefoxitin loss in 48 hr at 25°C	1023	I
Aztreonam	SQ	10 and 20 g	MSD	10 and 20 g	D5W[a]	3 to 6% cefoxitin loss and no aztreonam loss in 7 days at 4°C	1023	C
Aztreonam	SQ	10 and 20 g	MSD	10 and 20 g	NS[a]	3 to 5% aztreonam loss and no cefoxitin loss in 7 days at 4°C	1023	C
Clindamycin phosphate	UP	9 g	MSD	20 g	D5W[b]	Physically compatible with no loss of either drug in 48 hr at room temperature	983	C
Clindamycin phosphate	UP	9 g	MSD	20 g	NS[b]	Physically compatible with no clindamycin loss and 7% cefoxitin loss in 48 hr at room temperature	983	C
Gentamicin sulfate	SC	400 mg	MSD	5 g	D5S	4% cefoxitin loss in 24 hr and 11% in 48 hr at 25°C. 2% in 48 hr at 5°C. 9% gentamicin loss in 24 hr and 23% in 48 hr at 25°C. 2% in 48 hr at 5°C	308	C
Mannitol		10%	MSD	1, 2, 10, 20 g		4 to 5% cefoxitin loss in 24 hr and 10 to 11% in 48 hr at 25°C. 2 to 5% cefoxitin loss in 7 days at 5°C	308	C
Metronidazole	SE	5 g	MSD	30 g		9% cefoxitin loss in 48 hr at 25°C and 3% in 12 days at 5°C. No metronidazole loss	993	C
Multivitamins	USV	50 mL	MSD	10 g	W	5% cefoxitin loss in 24 hr and 10% in 48 hr at 25°C; 3% in 48 hr at 5°C	308	C
Ranitidine HCl	GL	50 mg and 2 g		10 g	D5W	Ranitidine stable for only 4 hr at 25°C. Cefoxitin not tested	1515	I
Sodium bicarbonate	AB	200 mg	MSD	1 g	W	5 to 6% cefoxitin loss in 24 hr and 11 to 12% in 48 hr at 25°C. 2 to 3% loss in 7 days at 5°C	308	C
Tobramycin sulfate	LI	400 mg	MSD	5 g	D5S	5% cefoxitin loss in 24 hr and 11% in 48 hr at 25°C. 3% in 48 hr at 5°C. 8% tobramycin loss in 24 hr and 37% in 48 hr at 25°C. 3% in 48 hr at 5°C	308	C
Verapamil HCl	KN	80 mg	MSD	4 g	D5W, NS	Physically compatible for 24 hr	764	C

[a] Tested in PVC containers.

[b] Tested in glass containers.

Drugs in Syringe Compatibility

Cefoxitin sodium

Test Drug	Mfr	Amt	Mfr	Amt	Remarks	Ref	C/I
Heparin sodium		2500 units/1 mL	MSD	2 g	Physically compatible for at least 5 min	1053	C
Pantoprazole sodium	a	4 mg/1 mL		100 mg/1 mL	Precipitates immediately	2574	I

[a] Test performed using the formulation WITHOUT edetate disodium.

Y-Site Injection Compatibility (1:1 Mixture)

Cefoxitin sodium

Test Drug	Mfr	Conc	Mfr	Conc	Remarks	Ref	C/I
Acetaminophen	CAD	10 mg/mL	APO	100 mg/mL	Physically compatible for 4 hr at 23°C	2901, 2902	C
Acyclovir sodium	BW	5 mg/mL[a]	MSD	20 mg/mL[a]	Physically compatible for 4 hr at 25°C	1157	C
Amifostine	USB	10 mg/mL[a]	MSD	20 mg/mL[a]	Physically compatible for 4 hr at 23°C	1845	C
Anakinra	SYN	4 and 36 mg/mL[b]	ME	20 mg/mL[b]	Physically compatible. No cefoxitin loss in 4 hr at 25°C. Anakinra uncertain	2508	?
Anidulafungin	VIC	0.5 mg/mL[a]	APP	20 mg/mL[a]	Physically compatible for 4 hr at 23°C	2617	C
Aztreonam	SQ	40 mg/mL[a]	MSD	20 mg/mL[a]	Physically compatible for 4 hr at 23°C	1758	C
Bivalirudin	TMC	5 mg/mL[a]	ME	20 mg/mL[a]	Physically compatible for 4 hr at 23°C	2373	C
Cangrelor tetrasodium	TMC	1 mg/mL[b]		20[b] and 95 mg/mL	Physically compatible for 4 hr	3243	C
Cisatracurium besylate	GW	0.1 mg/mL[a]	ME	20 mg/mL[a]	Physically compatible for 4 hr at 23°C	2074	C
Cisatracurium besylate	GW	2 and 5 mg/mL[a]	ME	20 mg/mL[a]	Subvisible haze forms immediately	2074	I
Cloxacillin sodium	SMX	100 mg/mL	HOS	100 mg/mL	Physically compatible for up to 4 hr at room temperature	3245	C
Cyclophosphamide	MJ	20 mg/mL[a]	MSD	20 mg/mL[a]	Physically compatible for 4 hr at 25°C	1194	C
Dexmedetomidine HCl	AB	4 mcg/mL[b]	ME	20 mg/mL[b]	Physically compatible for 4 hr at 23°C	2383	C
Diltiazem HCl	MMD	5 mg/mL	MSD	10 and 200 mg/mL[b]	Visually compatible	1807	C
Diltiazem HCl	MMD	1 mg/mL[b]	MSD	200 mg/mL[b]	Visually compatible	1807	C
Docetaxel	RPR	0.9 mg/mL[a]	ME	20 mg/mL[a]	Physically compatible for 4 hr at 23°C	2224	C
Doxorubicin HCl liposomal	SEQ	0.4 mg/mL[a]	ME	20 mg/mL[a]	Physically compatible for 4 hr at 23°C	2087	C
Etoposide phosphate	BR	5 mg/mL[a]	ME	20 mg/mL[a]	Physically compatible for 4 hr at 23°C	2218	C
Famotidine	MSD	0.2 mg/mL[a]	MSD	20 mg/mL[b]	Physically compatible for 14 hr	1196	C
Famotidine	ME	2 mg/mL[b]		20 mg/mL[a]	Visually compatible for 4 hr at 22°C	1936	C

Y-Site Injection Compatibility (1:1 Mixture) (Cont.)

Test Drug	Mfr	Conc	Mfr	.Conc	Remarks	Ref	C/I
Fenoldopam mesylate	AB	80 mcg/mL[b]	ME	20 mg/mL[b]	Microparticulates form immediately	2467	I
Filgrastim	AMG	30 mcg/mL[a]	MSD	20 mg/mL[a]	Haze, particles, and filaments form immediately	1687	I
Fluconazole	RR	2 mg/mL	MSD	40 mg/mL	Physically compatible for 24 hr at 25°C	1407	C
Foscarnet sodium	AST	24 mg/mL	MSD	40 mg/mL	Physically compatible for 24 hr at room temperature under fluorescent light	1335	C
Gemcitabine HCl	LI	10 mg/mL[b]	ME	20 mg/mL[b]	Physically compatible for 4 hr at 23°C	2226	C
Granisetron HCl	SKB	0.05 mg/mL[a]	ME	20 mg/mL[a]	Physically compatible for 4 hr at 23°C	2000	C
Hetastarch in lactated electrolyte	AB	6%	ME	20 mg/mL[a]	Physically compatible for 4 hr at 23°C	2339	C
Hetastarch in sodium chloride 0.9%	DCC	6%	MSD	20 mg/mL[a]	Precipitate in 1 hr at room temperature	1313	I
Hydromorphone HCl	WY	0.2 mg/mL[a]	MSD	20 mg/mL[a]	Physically compatible for 4 hr at 25°C	987	C
Linezolid	PHU	2 mg/mL	ME	20 mg/mL[a]	Physically compatible for 4 hr at 23°C	2264	C
Magnesium sulfate	IX	16.7, 33.3, 66.7, 100 mg/mL[a]	MSD	20 mg/mL[a]	Physically compatible for at least 4 hr at 32°C	813	C
Meperidine HCl	WY	10 mg/mL[a]	MSD	20 mg/mL[a]	Physically compatible for 4 hr at 25°C	987	C
Meperidine HCl	WY	10 mg/mL[b]	MSD	40 mg/mL[a]	Physically compatible for 1 hr at 25°C	1338	C
Meropenem		50 mg/mL	NOP	100 mg/mL	Physically compatible for 4 hr at room temperature	3538	C
Morphine sulfate	WI	1 mg/mL[a]	MSD	20 mg/mL[a]	Physically compatible for 4 hr at 25°C	987	C
Morphine sulfate	ES	1 mg/mL[b]	MSD	40 mg/mL[a]	Physically compatible for 1 hr at 25°C	1338	C
Ondansetron HCl	GL	1 mg/mL[b]	MSD	20 mg/mL[a]	Visually compatible for 4 hr at 22°C	1365	C
Pemetrexed disodium	LI	20 mg/mL[b]	APP	20 mg/mL[a]	Immediate brown discoloration	2564	I
Pentamidine isethionate	FUJ	3 mg/mL[a]	ME	20 mg/mL[c]	Immediate cloudy precipitation	1880	I
Plazomicin sulfate	ACH	24 mg/mL[i]	FRK	20 mg/mL[i]	Physically compatible for 1 hr at 20 to 25°C	3432	C
Propofol	ZEN[d]	10 mg/mL	ME	20 mg/mL[a]	Physically compatible for 1 hr at 23°C	2066	C
Ranitidine HCl	GL	1 mg/mL[b]	BAN	20 mg/mL[h]	Visually compatible. No cefoxitin loss. Under 8% ranitidine loss in 4 hr at 25°C	2259	C
Ranitidine HCl	GL	1 mg/mL[b]	BAN	20 mg/mL[b]	Visually compatible with no cefoxitin loss and 7% ranitidine loss in 4 hr	2362	C
Remifentanil HCl	GW	0.025 and 0.25 mg/mL[b]	ME	20 mg/mL[a]	Physically compatible for 4 hr at 23°C	2075	C
Teniposide	BR	0.1 mg/mL[a]	MSD	20 mg/mL[a]	Physically compatible for 4 hr at 23°C	1725	C
Thiotepa	IMM[e]	1 mg/mL[a]	ME	20 mg/mL[a]	Physically compatible for 4 hr at 23°C	1861	C
TNA #73[f]		32.5 mL[g]	MSD	20 mg/mL[a]	Visually compatible for 4 hr at 25°C	1008	C
TNA #218 to #226[f]			ME	20 mg/mL[a]	Visually compatible for 4 hr at 23°C	2215	C
TPN #61[f]		[h]	MSD	200 mg/2.1 mL[i]	Physically compatible	1012	C

Y-Site Injection Compatibility (1:1 Mixture) (Cont.)

Test Drug	Mfr	Conc	Mfr	Conc	Remarks	Ref	C/I
TPN #61[f]		[j]	MSD	1.2 g/12.6 mL[i]	Physically compatible	1012	C
TPN #189[f]			MSD	200 mg/mL[k]	Visually compatible for 24 hr at 22°C	1767	C
TPN #212 to #215[f]			ME	20 mg/mL[a]	Physically compatible for 4 hr at 23°C	2109	C
Vancomycin HCl	AB	20 mg/mL[a]	ME	180 mg/mL[k]	Transient precipitate forms	2189	?
Vancomycin HCl	AB	20 mg/mL[a]	ME	50 mg/mL[a]	Immediate gross white precipitate	2189	I
Vancomycin HCl	AB	20 mg/mL[a]	ME	10 mg/mL[a]	Visible haze forms in 4 hr at 23°C	2189	I
Vancomycin HCl	AB	20 mg/mL[a]	ME	1 mg/mL[a]	Physically compatible for 4 hr at 23°C	2189	C
Vancomycin HCl	AB	2 mg/mL[a]	ME	1[a], 10[a], 50[a], 180[k] mg/mL	Physically compatible for 4 hr at 23°C	2189	C

[a] Tested in dextrose 5%.

[b] Tested in sodium chloride 0.9%.

[c] Tested in dextrose 4%.

[d] Test performed using the formulation WITH edetate disodium.

[e] Lyophilized formulation tested.

[f] Refer to Appendix for the composition of parenteral nutrition solutions. TNA indicates a 3-in-1 admixture, and TPN indicates a 2-in-1 admixture.

[g] A 32.5-mL sample of parenteral nutrition solution combined with 50 mL of antibiotic solution.

[h] Run at 21 mL/hr.

[i] Given over five minutes by syringe pump.

[j] Run at 94 mL/hr.

[k] Tested in sterile water for injection.

[l] Tested in both dextrose 5% and sodium chloride 0.9%.

Selected Revisions May 1, 2020. © Copyright, October 1982.
American Society of Health-System Pharmacists, Inc.

Ceftaroline Fosamil
AHFS 8:12.06.20

Products

Ceftaroline fosamil is available in vials containing 400 and 600 mg of anhydrous ceftaroline fosamil with L-arginine.[2832]

The 400- and 600-mg vials of ceftaroline fosamil should be reconstituted with 20 mL of sterile water for injection, sodium chloride 0.9%, dextrose 5%, or Ringer's injection, lactated and mixed gently, yielding concentrations of 20 and 30 mg/mL, respectively.[2832] The reconstituted solution must be further diluted in a suitable infusion solution prior to administration.[2832] The same diluent should be used for both reconstitution and further dilution unless the drug was reconstituted with sterile water, in which case any compatible infusion solution should be used for further dilution.[2832] (See Solution Compatibility.)

For adults and pediatric patients *at least 2 years of age weighing more than 33 kg* and requiring doses of 400 or 600 mg, the entire reconstituted contents of a 400- or 600-mg vial, respectively, must be diluted in 50 to 250 mL of a compatible infusion solution.[2832] For adults requiring doses less than 400 mg (e.g., those with renal impairment requiring dosage adjustment), the appropriate volume of the reconstituted solution must be withdrawn from the vial and diluted in 50 to 250 mL of a compatible infusion solution.[2832] For pediatric patients *weighing 33 kg or less*, the appropriate volume of the reconstituted solution must be withdrawn from the vial and diluted in a compatible infusion solution to yield an infusion solution with a ceftaroline fosamil concentration not exceeding 12 mg/mL.[2832]

The manufacturer recommends the following instructions specifically for the dilution of ceftaroline fosamil in 50-mL infusion bags: When ceftaroline fosamil is prepared for administration in a 50-mL infusion bag for adults, 20 mL of the diluent should be removed from the infusion bag prior to injecting the entire reconstituted contents of a 600-mg vial of the drug to yield an approximate concentration of 12 mg/mL.[2832] When the drug is prepared for administration in a 50-mL infusion bag for adults or pediatric patients *weighing more than 33 kg*, 20 mL of the diluent should be removed from the infusion bag prior to injecting the entire reconstituted contents of a 400-mg vial of the drug to yield an approximate concentration of 8 mg/mL.[2832] When the drug is prepared for administration in a 50-mL infusion bag for pediatric patients *weighing 33 kg or less*, the appropriate volume of the reconstituted solution should be withdrawn from the vial and transferred to an infusion bag to yield a concentration not exceeding 12 mg/mL.[2832]

pH

The reconstituted solution has a pH ranging from 4.8 to 6.5.[2832]

Trade Name(s)

Teflaro

Administration

Following dilution in a compatible infusion solution, ceftaroline fosamil is administered by intravenous infusion over 5 to 60 minutes in patients 2 months of age or older and over 30 to 60 minutes in patients less than 2 months of age.[2832]

Stability

Intact vials should be stored at controlled room temperature.[2832] The powder is pale yellowish-white to light yellow in color.[2832] After reconstitution, ceftaroline fosamil solution is clear and light to dark yellow in color.[2832]

Compatibility Information

Solution Compatibility

Ceftaroline fosamil

Test Soln Name	Mfr	Mfr	Conc/L or %	Remarks	Ref	C/I
Dextrose 2.5%		ALL		Use within 6 hr at room temperature or 24 hr at 2 to 8°C	2832	C
Dextrose 5%		ALL		Use within 6 hr at room temperature or 24 hr at 2 to 8°C	2832	C
Dextrose 5%	b	FOR	12 g	Physically compatible. Little or no loss in 24 hr at 2 to 8°C followed by 6 hr at room temperature	3138	C
Dextrose 5%	BA[d]	ASZ	6 g	Physically compatible with less than 10% loss in 6 days at 4°C, 24 hr at 25°C, 12 hr at 30°C, and 6 hr at 35°C	3494	C
Ringer's injection, lactated		ALL		Use within 6 hr at room temperature or 24 hr at 2 to 8°C	2832	C
Sodium chloride 0.45%		ALL		Use within 6 hr at room temperature or 24 hr at 2 to 8°C	2832	C
Sodium chloride 0.9%		ALL		Use within 6 hr at room temperature or 24 hr at 2 to 8°C	2832	C
Sodium chloride 0.9%	BA[a]	ALL	4 to 12 g	Stable for up to 6 hr at room temperature or 24 hr at 2 to 8°C	2832	C

DOI: 10.37573/9781585286850.078

Solution Compatibility (Cont.)

Test Soln Name	Mfr	Mfr	Conc/L or %	Remarks	Ref	C/I
Sodium chloride 0.9%	BA[a]	FOR	4, 6, 12 g	Physically compatible. Little or no loss in 24 hr at 2 to 8°C followed by 6 hr at room temperature	3138	C
Sodium chloride 0.9%	[c]	FOR	12 g	Physically compatible. Little or no loss in 24 hr at 2 to 8°C followed by 6 hr at room temperature	3138	C
Sodium chloride 0.9%	BA[d]	ASZ	6 g	Physically compatible with less than 10% loss in 6 days at 4°C, 24 hr at 25°C, and 12 hr at 30 and 35°C	3494	C

[a] Tested in 50- or 100-mL Mini-Bag Plus container systems.

[b] Tested in Intermate, Homepump Eclipse, and AccuRx elastomeric pump reservoirs.

[c] Tested in Intermate elastomeric pump reservoirs.

[d] Tested in Infusor LV 10 elastomeric pump reservoirs (Baxter).

Y-Site Injection Compatibility (1:1 Mixture)

Ceftaroline fosamil

Test Drug	Mfr	Conc	Mfr	Conc	Remarks	Ref	C/I
Acyclovir sodium	BV	7 mg/mL[a b c]	FOR	2.22 mg/mL[a b c]	Physically compatible for 4 hr at 23°C	2826	C
Amikacin sulfate	HOS	5 mg/mL[a b c]	FOR	2.22 mg/mL[a b c]	Physically compatible for 4 hr at 23°C	2826	C
Aminophylline	AMR	2.5 mg/mL[a b c]	FOR	2.22 mg/mL[a b c]	Physically compatible for 4 hr at 23°C	2826	C
Amiodarone HCl	SIC	4 mg/mL[a b c]	FOR	2.22 mg/mL[a b c]	Physically compatible for 4 hr at 23°C	2826	C
Amphotericin B	XGN	0.6 mg/mL[a]	FOR	2.22 mg/mL[a b c]	Increased haze and microparticulates	2826	I
Azithromycin	BA	2 mg/mL[a b c]	FOR	2.22 mg/mL[a b c]	Physically compatible for 4 hr at 23°C	2826	C
Bumetanide	HOS	40 mcg/mL[a b c]	FOR	2.22 mg/mL[a b c]	Physically compatible for 4 hr at 23°C	2826	C
Calcium chloride	AMR	40 mg/mL[a b c]	FOR	2.22 mg/mL[a b c]	Physically compatible for 4 hr at 23°C	2826	C
Calcium gluconate	ABX	40 mg/mL[a b c]	FOR	2.22 mg/mL[a b c]	Physically compatible for 4 hr at 23°C	2826	C
Caspofungin acetate	ME	0.5 mg/mL[b c]	FOR	2.22 mg/mL[a b c]	Increased haze and particulates	2826	I
Ceftazidime–avibactam sodium	ALL	20 mg/mL[i k]			Physically compatible for up to 4 hr at room temperature	3004	C
Ceftolozane sulfate–tazobactam sodium	CUB	10 mg/mL[g h]	FOR	12 mg/mL[g]	Physically compatible for 2 hr	3262	C
Ciprofloxacin	BED	2 mg/mL[a b c]	FOR	2.22 mg/mL[a b c]	Physically compatible for 4 hr at 23°C	2826	C
Cisatracurium besylate	HOS	0.5 mg/mL[a b c]	FOR	2.22 mg/mL[a b c]	Physically compatible for 4 hr at 23°C	2826	C
Clindamycin phosphate	BED	10 mg/mL[a b c]	FOR	2.22 mg/mL[a b c]	Physically compatible for 4 hr at 23°C	2826	C
Cyclosporine	BED	5 mg/mL[a b c]	FOR	2.22 mg/mL[a b c]	Physically compatible for 4 hr at 23°C	2826	C
Dexamethasone sodium phosphate	SIC	1 mg/mL[a b c]	FOR	2.22 mg/mL[a b c]	Physically compatible for 4 hr at 23°C	2826	C
Diazepam	HOS	5 mg/mL	FOR	2.22 mg/mL[a b c]	Turbid precipitation forms	2826	I
Digoxin	BA	0.25 mg/mL	FOR	2.22 mg/mL[a b c]	Physically compatible for 4 hr at 23°C	2826	C
Diltiazem HCl	HOS	5 mg/mL	FOR	2.22 mg/mL[a b c]	Physically compatible for 4 hr at 23°C	2826	C
Diphenhydramine HCl	BA	2 mg/mL[a b c]	FOR	2.22 mg/mL[a b c]	Physically compatible for 4 hr at 23°C	2826	C
Dobutamine HCl	HOS	4 mg/mL[a]	FOR	2.22 mg/mL[a]	Haze increases and particulates appear	2826	I
Dobutamine HCl	HOS	4 mg/mL[b c]	FOR	2.22 mg/mL[b c]	Physically compatible for 4 hr at 23°C	2826	C

Y-Site Injection Compatibility (1:1 Mixture) (Cont.)

Test Drug	Mfr	Conc	Mfr	Conc	Remarks	Ref	C/I
Dopamine HCl	HOS	3.2 mg/mL[a b c]	FOR	2.22 mg/mL[a b c]	Physically compatible for 4 hr at 23°C	2826	C
Doripenem	SHI	5 mg/mL[b]	FOR	2.22 mg/mL[a b c]	Physically compatible for 4 hr at 23°C	2826	C
Enalaprilat	SIC	0.1 mg/mL[a b c]	FOR	2.22 mg/mL[a b c]	Physically compatible for 4 hr at 23°C	2826	C
Eravacycline dihydro-chloride	TET	0.3 and 0.6 mg/mL[b]	FOR	12 mg/mL[b]	Measured turbidity increased within 2 hr	3532	I
Esomeprazole sodium	ASZ	0.4 mg/mL[a b c]	FOR	2.22 mg/mL[a b c]	Physically compatible for 4 hr at 23°C	2826	C
Famotidine	ABX	2 mg/mL[a b c]	FOR	2.22 mg/mL[a b c]	Physically compatible for 4 hr at 23°C	2826	C
Fentanyl citrate	HOS	50 mcg/mL	FOR	2.22 mg/mL[a b c]	Physically compatible for 4 hr at 23°C	2826	C
Filgrastim	AMG	30 mcg/mL[a]	FOR	2.22 mg/mL[a b c]	Microparticulates formed	2826	I
Fluconazole	BED	2 mg/mL	FOR	2.22 mg/mL[a b c]	Physically compatible for 4 hr at 23°C	2826	C
Furosemide	HOS	3 mg/mL[a b c]	FOR	2.22 mg/mL[a b c]	Physically compatible for 4 hr at 23°C	2826	C
Gentamicin sulfate	HOS	5 mg/mL[a b c]	FOR	2.22 mg/mL[a b c]	Physically compatible for 4 hr at 23°C	2826	C
Granisetron HCl	CUP	50 mcg/mL[a b c]	FOR	2.22 mg/mL[a b c]	Physically compatible for 4 hr at 23°C	2826	C
Haloperidol lactate	BED	0.2 mg/mL[a b c]	FOR	2.22 mg/mL[a b c]	Physically compatible for 4 hr at 23°C	2826	C
Heparin sodium	HOS	100 units/mL	FOR	2.22 mg/mL[a b c]	Physically compatible for 4 hr at 23°C	2826	C
Hydrocortisone sodium succinate	PF	1 mg/mL[a b c]	FOR	2.22 mg/mL[a b c]	Physically compatible for 4 hr at 23°C	2826	C
Hydromorphone HCl	HOS	0.5 mg/mL[a b c]	FOR	2.22 mg/mL[a b c]	Physically compatible for 4 hr at 23°C	2826	C
Hydroxyzine HCl	ABX	2 mg/mL[a b c]	FOR	2.22 mg/mL[a b c]	Physically compatible for 4 hr at 23°C	2826	C
Insulin, regular	NOV	1 unit/mL[a b c]	FOR	2.22 mg/mL[a b c]	Physically compatible for 4 hr at 23°C	2826	C
Isavuconazonium sulfate	ASP	1.5 mg/mL[g]	FOR	12 mg/mL[g]	Measured turbidity increases within 1 hr	3263	I
Labetalol HCl	HOS	5 mg/mL	FOR	2.22 mg/mL[a]	Increase in measured haze and microparticulates	2826	I
Labetalol HCl	HOS	5 mg/mL	FOR	2.22 mg/mL[b c]	Increase in measured haze	2826	I
Levofloxacin	OMN	5 mg/mL[a b c]	FOR	2.22 mg/mL[a b c]	Physically compatible for 4 hr at 23°C	2826	C
Lidocaine HCl	HOS	10 mg/mL	FOR	2.22 mg/mL[a b c]	Physically compatible for 4 hr at 23°C	2826	C
Lorazepam	HOS	0.5 mg/mL[a b c]	FOR	2.22 mg/mL[a b c]	Physically compatible for 4 hr at 23°C	2826	C
Magnesium sulfate	AMR	100 mg/mL[a b]	FOR	2.22 mg/mL[a b]	Physically compatible for 4 hr at 23°C	2826	C
Magnesium sulfate	AMR	100 mg/mL[c]	FOR	2.22 mg/mL[c]	Increase in measured haze	2826	I
Mannitol	HOS	15%	FOR	2.22 mg/mL[a b c]	Physically compatible for 4 hr at 23°C	2826	C
Meperidine HCl	HOS	10 mg/mL[a b c]	FOR	2.22 mg/mL[a b c]	Physically compatible for 4 hr at 23°C	2826	C
Meropenem–vaborbactam	TMC	8 mg/mL[b i]	FOR	12 mg/mL[b]	Measured turbidity increases within 30 min. pH increased by >2 units within 3 hr	3380	I
Methylprednisolone sodium succinate	PHU	5 mg/mL[a b c]	FOR	2.22 mg/mL[a b c]	Physically compatible for 4 hr at 23°C	2826	C
Metoclopramide HCl	HOS	5 mg/mL	FOR	2.22 mg/mL[a b c]	Physically compatible for 4 hr at 23°C	2826	C
Metoprolol tartrate	HOS	1 mg/mL	FOR	2.22 mg/mL[a b c]	Physically compatible for 4 hr at 23°C	2826	C
Metronidazole	BA	5 mg/mL	FOR	2.22 mg/mL[a b c]	Physically compatible for 4 hr at 23°C	2826	C
Midazolam HCl	BV	2 mg/mL[a b c]	FOR	2.22 mg/mL[a b c]	Physically compatible for 4 hr at 23°C	2826	C

Y-Site Injection Compatibility (1:1 Mixture) (Cont.)

Test Drug	Mfr	Conc	Mfr	Conc	Remarks	Ref	C/I
Milrinone lactate	BED	0.2 mg/mL[a b c]	FOR	2.22 mg/mL[a b c]	Physically compatible for 4 hr at 23°C	2826	C
Morphine sulfate	BA	15 mg/mL	FOR	2.22 mg/mL[a b c]	Physically compatible for 4 hr at 23°C	2826	C
Moxifloxacin HCl	BAY	1.6 mg/mL	FOR	2.22 mg/mL[a b c]	Physically compatible for 4 hr at 23°C	2826	C
Multivitamins	BA	5 mL/L[a b c]	FOR	2.22 mg/mL[a b c]	Physically compatible for 4 hr at 23°C	2826	C
Norepinephrine bitartrate	BED	0.128 mg/mL[a b c]	FOR	2.22 mg/mL[a b c]	Physically compatible for 4 hr at 23°C	2826	C
Ondansetron HCl	WOC	1 mg/mL[a b c]	FOR	2.22 mg/mL[a b c]	Physically compatible for 4 hr at 23°C	2826	C
Pantoprazole sodium	WY[d]	0.4 mg/mL[a b c]	FOR	2.22 mg/mL[a b c]	Physically compatible for 4 hr at 23°C	2826	C
Plazomicin sulfate	ACH	24 mg/mL[g]	FAC	12 mg/mL[g]	Physically compatible for 1 hr at 20 to 25°C	3432	C
Potassium chloride	HOS	0.1 mEq/mL[a b c]	FOR	2.22 mg/mL[a b c]	Physically compatible for 4 hr at 23°C	2826	C
Potassium phosphates	HOS	0.5 mmol/mL[a]	FOR	2.22 mg/mL[a]	Increase in measured haze and microparticulates	2826	I
Potassium phosphates	HOS	0.5 mmol/mL[b c]	FOR	2.22 mg/mL[b c]	Increase in measured haze	2826	I
Promethazine HCl	SIC	2 mg/mL[a b c]	FOR	2.22 mg/mL[a b c]	Physically compatible for 4 hr at 23°C	2826	C
Propofol	HOS[l]	10 mg/mL	FOR	2.22 mg/mL[a b c]	Physically compatible for 4 hr at 23°C	2826	C
Ranitidine HCl	BED	2 mg/mL[a b c]	FOR	2.22 mg/mL[a b c]	Physically compatible for 4 hr at 23°C	2826	C
Remifentanil HCl	HOS	0.25 mg/mL[a b c]	FOR	2.22 mg/mL[a b c]	Physically compatible for 4 hr at 23°C	2826	C
Sodium bicarbonate	HOS	1 mEq/mL	FOR	2.22 mg/mL[a b c]	Physically compatible for 4 hr at 23°C	2826	C
Sodium phosphates	HOS	0.5 mmol/mL[a b c]	FOR	2.22 mg/mL[a b c]	Increase in measured haze	2826	I
Tedizolid phosphate	CUB	0.8 mg/mL[b]	FOR	12 mg/mL[b]	Measured turbidity increases after 15 min	3244	I
Tobramycin sulfate	SIC	5 mg/mL[a b c]	FOR	2.22 mg/mL[a b c]	Physically compatible for 4 hr at 23°C	2826	C
Trimethoprim–sulfamethoxazole	SIC	0.8 mg/mL[a b c f]	FOR	2.22 mg/mL[a b c]	Physically compatible for 4 hr at 23°C	2826	C
TPN #276[e]			FOR	2.22 mg/mL[a b c]	Physically compatible for 4 hr at 23°C	2826	C
Vasopressin	APP	1 unit/mL[a b c]	FOR	2.22 mg/mL[a b c]	Physically compatible for 4 hr at 23°C	2826	C
Voriconazole	PF	4 mg/mL[a b c]	FOR	2.22 mg/mL[a b c]	Physically compatible for 4 hr at 23°C	2826	C

[a] Tested in dextrose 5%.

[b] Tested in sodium chloride 0.9%.

[c] Tested in Ringer's injection, lactated.

[d] Test performed using the formulation WITH edetate disodium.

[e] Refer to Appendix for the composition of parenteral nutrition solutions. TPN indicates a 2-in-1 admixture.

[f] Trimethoprim component. Trimethoprim in a 1:5 fixed-ratio concentration with sulfamethoxazole.

[g] Tested in both dextrose 5% and sodium chloride 0.9%.

[h] Ceftolozane component. Ceftolozane in a 2:1 fixed-ratio concentration with tazobactam.

[i] Meropenem component. Meropenem in 1:1 fixed-ratio concentration with vaborbactam.

[j] Ceftazidime component. Ceftazidime in a 4:1 fixed-ratio concentration with avibactam.

[k] Tested in dextrose 5%, sodium chloride 0.9%, and Ringer's injection, lactated.

[l] Test performed using the formulation WITHOUT edetate disodium.

Ceftazidime
AHFS 8:12.06.12

Products

Ceftazidime is supplied in vials containing 500 mg, 1 g, and 2 g of drug (under reduced pressure), infusion packs containing 1 and 2 g of drug, and 6-g pharmacy bulk packages. The dosage forms contain sodium carbonate 118 mg per gram of ceftazidime. The sodium salt of ceftazidime and carbon dioxide are formed during reconstitution.[1(2/07)] [4] The use of a venting needle has been suggested for ease of use.[1136] Spraying or leaking of the solution after needle withdrawal has been reported, especially with smaller vials.[1137] The use of larger vials reduces the occurrence of such leakage.[1137] [1138] Care must be taken if a multiple-additive set with a 2-way valve is used for reconstitution. The negative pressure in the product may cause inaccuracies in the volume of diluent added to the vial. In one test, almost 3 mL extra entered the vial during reconstitution.[1240] Vials have been vented prior to reconstitution but clamping the tubing from the supply bottle prior to adding the diluent to the vial when multiple-additive sets are used is recommended.[1241]

Ceftazidime is also supplied in frozen solutions containing 1 and 2 g/50 mL of dextrose 4.4 and 3.2%, respectively.[1(2/07)] [4]

For intramuscular injection, ceftazidime should be reconstituted with sterile water for injection, bacteriostatic water for injection, or lidocaine hydrochloride 0.5 or 1% using 1.5 mL for the 500-mg vial and 3 mL for the 1-g vial. Any carbon dioxide bubbles that are withdrawn into the syringe should be expelled prior to injection.[1(2/07)] [4]

For direct intravenous injection, ceftazidime should be reconstituted with sterile water for injection. Carbon dioxide will form during dissolution, but the solution will clear in about 1 to 2 minutes.[1(2/07)] [4]

Table 1. Reconstitution for intravenous injection[1(2/07)]

Product	Volume of Diluent	Withdrawable Volume	Concentration
500 mg	5.3 mL	5.7 mL	100 mg/mL
1 g	10 mL	10.6 mL	100 mg/mL
2 g	10 mL	11.5 ml	170 mq/mL

For intravenous infusion, the reconstituted solution can be added to a compatible infusion solution (after expelling any carbon dioxide bubbles that have entered the syringe). Alternatively, the 1- or 2-g infusion packs can be reconstituted with 100 mL of compatible infusion solution, yielding a 10- or 20-mg/mL solution, respectively.[1(2/07)] [4] To reconstitute the infusion packs, add the diluent in 2 increments. Initially, add 10 mL with shaking to dissolve the drug. To release the carbon dioxide pressure, insert a venting needle through the closure only after the drug has dissolved and become clear (about 1 to 2 minutes). Then add the remaining 90 mL and remove the venting needle. Additional pressure may develop, especially during storage, and should be released prior to use.[4]

The 6-g pharmacy bulk package should be reconstituted with 26 mL of a compatible diluent to yield 30 mL of solution containing 200 mg/mL of ceftazidime. The carbon dioxide pressure that develops should be released using a venting needle. The 200-mg/mL concentrated solution must be diluted further for intravenous use.[1(2/07)]

pH
From 5 to 8.[1(2/07)] [4]

Osmolality

The osmolality of ceftazidime (Fortaz, Glaxo) 50 mg/mL was determined to be 321 mOsm/kg in dextrose 5% and 330 mOsm/kg in sodium chloride 0.9%.[1375]

The following maximum ceftazidime concentrations were recommended to achieve osmolalities suitable for peripheral infusion in fluid-restricted patients:[1180]

Diluent	Maximum Concentration (mg/mL)	Osmolality (mOsm/kg)
Dextrose 5%	70	503
Sodium chloride 0.9%	63	486
Sterile water for injection	126	302

Sodium Content

Each gram of ceftazidime activity provides 2.3 mEq (54 mg) of sodium from the sodium carbonate present in the formulation.[1(2/07)] [4]

Trade Name(s)

Fortaz, Tazicef

Administration

Ceftazidime may be administered by deep intramuscular injection, by direct intravenous injection over 3 to 5 minutes directly into a vein or through the tubing of a running compatible infusion solution, or by intermittent intravenous infusion over 15 to 30 minutes. The manufacturer recommends temporarily discontinuing other solutions being administered at the same site during ceftazidime infusion. The drug may be instilled intraperitoneally in a concentration of 250 mg/2 L of compatible dialysis solution.[1(2/07)] [4]

Stability

Intact vials should be stored at controlled room temperature and protected from light.[1(2/07)] Approximately 2% decomposition has been reported after 12 months of storage at 37°C with protection from light.[1136]

Reconstituted ceftazidime solutions are light yellow to amber, depending on the diluent and concentration, and may darken on storage. Color changes do not necessarily indicate a potency loss.[1(2/07)] [4]

DOI: 10.37573/9781585286850.079

Solutions in sterile water for injection at 95 to 280 mg/mL, in lidocaine hydrochloride 0.5 or 1% or bacteriostatic water for injection at 280 mg/mL, and in sodium chloride 0.9% or dextrose 5% at 10 or 20 mg/mL in piggyback infusion packs are stable for 24 hours at room temperature and 7 days under refrigeration. Tazicef and Tazidime in sterile water for injection at 95 to 280 mg/mL or in sodium chloride 0.9% at 10 to 20 mg/mL are stable for 24 hours at room temperature and 7 days under refrigeration.[1(2/07)]

One report of ceftazidime in concentrations of 1, 40, and 333 mg/mL in water indicated no loss after 24 hours at 4°C and 6 hours at 25°C. About a 4 to 6% loss was reported after 24 hours at 25°C.[1136]

Ceftazidime vials reconstituted with sterile water for injection to a concentration of 270 mg/mL were evaluated for stability at 4 temperatures. About 8 to 9% ceftazidime loss occurred in 7 days under refrigeration at 4°C and in 4 days at 10°C. At 20°C about 7 to 8% loss occurred in 24 hours, but at a higher room temperature of 30°C about 5% loss occurred in 6 hours and 12% loss occurred in 18 hours.[2285]

Freezing Solutions

Ceftazidime products differ in their reported stabilities, both during frozen storage of their solutions and after thawing. Table 2 summarizes the reported stabilities.[4]

Table 2. Reported stabilities of frozen and thawed solutions of ceftazidime products[1(2/07) 4]

Concentration	Fortaz	Tazicef
280 mg/mL		
Frozen	3 months[a]	3 months[a]
Thawed/RT[b]	8 hr	8 hr
Thawed/4°C[c]	4 days	4 days
100 to 180 mg/mL		
Frozen	6 months[a d]	3 months[e]
Thawed/RT	24 hr	8 hr
Thawed/4°C	7 days	4 days
10 to 20 mg/mL[f]		
Frozen	9 months[a]	
Thawed/RT	24 hr	
Thawed/4°C	7 days	

[a] In sterile water for injection.

[b] Thawed and stored at room temperature.

[c] Thawed and stored at 4 to 5°C.

[d] In sodium chloride 0.9%.

[e] In sodium chloride 0.9% and dextrose 5%.

[f] In infusion packs.

The commercially available frozen ceftazidime solutions (Fortaz, Glaxo) of 1 and 2 g/50 mL of sodium chloride 0.9%, when thawed, are stable for 24 hours at room temperature or 7 days under refrigeration.[4]

Ceftazidime (Fortaz, Glaxo) 1 g/50 mL in sodium chloride 0.9% was stored frozen at −20°C. About 7% loss occurred in 97 days. After thawing at room temperature, subsequent storage refrigerated for 4 days and at room temperature for 24 hours resulted in additional loss with only about 90% of the ceftazidime remaining.[500]

Less than a 2% ceftazidime (Fortaz, Glaxo) loss was reported from a solution containing 36.6 mg/mL in sterile water for injection in polyvinyl choride (PVC) and glass containers after 30 days at −20°C. Subsequent thawing and storage for 4 days at 5°C, followed by 24 hours at 37°C to simulate the use of a portable infusion pump, resulted in little additional ceftazidime loss.[1391]

Ceftazidime (Fortaz, Glaxo) 100 and 200 mg/mL in sterile water for injection in glass vials and polypropylene syringes (Becton Dickinson) was stored frozen at −20°C for 91 days followed by 8 hours at 22°C. Losses of about 5 and 10% occurred in the 100- and 200-mg/mL concentrations, respectively. Freezing at −20°C for 91 days followed by refrigeration at 4°C for 4 days resulted in losses of about 10 and 6% in the 100- and 200-mg/mL concentrations, respectively. Particle counts remained within USP limits throughout the study.[1580]

Usually, frozen solutions should be thawed at room temperature or under refrigeration. Other techniques are not recommended. Thawed solutions should not be refrozen.[1(2/07) 4]

Light Effects

Ceftazidime reconstituted with sterile water for injection to a concentration of 270 mg/mL exhibited no substantial difference in stability when stored protected from light or exposed to daylight.[2285]

Syringes

Ceftazidime (Fortaz, Glaxo) 100 and 200 mg/mL in sterile water for injection in polypropylene syringes (Becton Dickinson) and glass vials exhibited a 5% or less loss in 8 hours at 22°C and 96 hours at 4°C.[1580]

Ceftazidime (Hospira) 1 mg/mL in sodium chloride 0.9% in plastic syringes was stored at room temperature, refrigerated, and frozen at −20°C. About 10% ceftazidime loss occurred in 3 days at room temperature and in 17 days refrigerated. No loss occurred in the frozen samples over 60 days.[2793]

Ambulatory Pumps

Ceftazidime (Fortaz, Glaxo) at a concentration of 60 mg/mL in water for injection was filled into PVC portable infusion pump reservoirs (Pharmacia Deltec). Storage at −20°C resulted in less than 3% loss in 14 days. The thawed reservoirs were then stored under refrigeration at 6°C. Losses totaled 10% after 5 days of refrigerated storage. Under simulated use conditions at 30°C, ceftazidime decomposes at a rate of about 10% in 18 hours. The authors concluded prefilling of reservoirs with ceftazidime solutions for home use was not advisable.[2008]

Central Venous Catheter

Ceftazidime (Fortaz, Glaxo Wellcome) 10 mg/mL in dextrose 5% was found to be compatible with the ARROWg+ard Blue Plus (Arrow International) chlorhexidine-bearing triple-lumen central catheter. Furthermore, chlorhexidine delivered from the catheter remained at trace amounts with no substantial increase due to the delivery of the drug through the catheter.[2335]

Ceftazidime 10 mg/mL with heparin sodium 5000 units/mL as an antibiotic lock in polyurethane central hemodialysis

catheters lost about 50% of the antibiotic over 72 hours at 37°C. The loss was attributed to sorption to the catheters. Nevertheless, the reduced antibiotic concentration (about 5 mg/mL) remained effective against common microorganisms in catheter-related bacteremia in hemodialysis patients.[2515] [2516]

Compatibility Information

Solution Compatibility

Ceftazidime

Test Soln Name	Mfr	Mfr	Conc/L or %	Remarks	Ref	C/I
Amino acids 5%, dextrose 25%	AB	GL	6 g	No substantial amino acid degradation in 48 hr at 22°C and 10 days at 4°C. Ceftazidime stability the determining factor	1535	C
Dextrose 5% in sodium chloride 0.225%		GSK	1 to 40 g	Physically and chemically stable for 24 hr at room temperature and 7 days refrigerated	1(2/07)	C
Dextrose 5% in sodium chloride 0.45%		GSK	1 to 40 g	Physically and chemically stable for 24 hr at room temperature and 7 days refrigerated	1(2/07)	C
Dextrose 5% in sodium chloride 0.9%		GSK	1 to 40 g	Physically and chemically stable for 24 hr at room temperature and 7 days refrigerated	1(2/07)	C
Dextrose 5% in sodium chloride 0.9%		GL	20 g	5% loss in 24 hr at 25°C and no loss in 48 hr at 4°C	1136	C
Dextrose 5%			1 to 40 g	Physically and chemically stable for 24 hr at room temperature and 7 days refrigerated	1(2/07)	C
Dextrose 5%	MG[a]	GL	20 g	Physically compatible with 5% drug loss in 24 hr and 9% in 48 hr at 25°C under fluorescent light	1026	C
Dextrose 5%		GL	20 g	6% loss in 24 hr at 25°C. No loss in 24 hr and 3% loss in 48 hr at 4°C	1136	C
Dextrose 5%	TR[a]		40 g	Physically compatible with 8% loss in 2 days at 25°C, 6% loss in 21 days at 5°C, and 6% loss in 90 days at −10°C	1341	C
Dextrose 5%	[b]	GL	40 g	Physically compatible with 7% loss in 1 day and 19% loss in 3 days at 23°C; 8% loss in 10 days at 4°C	1353	C
Dextrose 5%	BA[b]	GL	2 and 6 g	Visually compatible with 7 to 9% loss in 24 hr at room temperature	1937	C
Dextrose 5%	[b]		4 g	Visually compatible with little or no loss in 24 hr at room temperature and 4°C	1953	C
Dextrose 5%	BA[b], BRN[a c]	GW	10 g	Visually compatible with little or no loss in 24 hr at 4 and 22°C	2289	C
Dextrose 5%	BA[d]	GW	40 g	10% loss in about 12 hr at 37°C in the dark	2421	I
Dextrose 5%	[f]	GW	40 g	Losses of 5, 8, and 10% in 20 hr at 20°C, and losses of 9, 17, and 21% in 20 hr at 35°C in glass, polypropylene, and PVC containers, respectively	2539	C
Dextrose 10%			1 to 40 g	Physically and chemically stable for 24 hr at room temperature and 7 days refrigerated	1(2/07)	C
Ringer's injection			1 to 40 g	Physically and chemically stable for 24 hr at room temperature and 7 days refrigerated	1(2/07)	C
Ringer's injection, lactated			1 to 40 g	Physically and chemically stable for 24 hr at room temperature and 7 days refrigerated	1(2/07)	C
Ringer's injection, lactated		GL	20 g	6% loss in 24 hr at 25°C and 1% loss in 48 hr at 4°C	1136	C
Sodium chloride 0.9%			1 to 40 g	Physically and chemically stable for 24 hr at room temperature and 7 days refrigerated	1(2/07)	C

Solution Compatibility (Cont.)

Test Soln Name	Mfr	Mfr	Conc/L or %	Remarks	Ref	C/I
Sodium chloride 0.9%	MG[a]	GL	20 g	Physically compatible with 2% drug loss in 24 hr and 5% in 48 hr at 25°C under fluorescent light	1026	C
Sodium chloride 0.9%		GL	20 g	7% loss in 24 hr at 25°C and no loss in 48 hr at 4°C	1136	C
Sodium chloride 0.9%	TR[a]		40 g	Physically compatible with 5% loss in 2 days and 12% loss in 3 days at 25°C; 7% loss in 28 days at 5°C and 6% loss in 90 days at −10°C	1341	C
Sodium chloride 0.9%	[b]	GL	40 g	Physically compatible with 3% loss in 1 day and 14% loss in 3 days at 25°C; 10% loss in 14 days at 5°C	1353	C
Sodium chloride 0.9%	BA[b]	GL	2 and 6 g	Visually compatible with 4 to 6% loss in 24 hr at room temperature	1937	C
Sodium chloride 0.9%	[b]		4 g	Visually compatible with little or no loss in 24 hr at room temperature and 4°C	1953	C
Sodium chloride 0.9%	KA[h]	GL	60 g	Visually compatible with little or no loss of ceftazidime and little formation of pyridine in 14 days frozen at −20°C	2113	C
Sodium chloride 0.9%	KA[h]	GL	60 g	Visually compatible with 9% loss of ceftazidime but formation of potentially toxic pyridine 0.53 mg/mL in 14 days at 4°C	2113	?
Sodium chloride 0.9%	BA[b], BRN[a c]	GW	10 g	Visually compatible with little or no loss in 24 hr at 4 and 22°C	2289	C
Sodium chloride 0.9%	BA[d]	GW	40 g	10% loss occurred in about 12 to 16 hr at 37°C in the dark	2421	I
Sodium chloride 0.9%	[f]	GW	40 g	Losses of 1, 3, and 6% in 20 hr at 20°C, and losses of 6, 11, and 13% in 20 hr at 35°C in glass, polypropylene, and PVC containers, respectively	2539	C
Sodium chloride 0.9%	[i]		40 g	Less than 10% loss in theoretical concentration in 8 hr at ambient temperature when administered as a continuous infusion	3535	C
Sodium lactate ⅙ M			1 to 40 g	Physically and chemically stable for 24 hr at room temperature and 7 days refrigerated	1(2/07)	C
TPN #107[g]			1 g	Activity retained for 24 hr at 21°C	1326	C
TPN #141 to #143[g]		GL	1 g	Visually compatible with 8% ceftazidime loss in 6 hr and 10% loss in 24 hr at 22°C. 8% ceftazidime loss in 3 days at 4°C	1535	C
TPN #141 to #143[g]		GL	6 g	Visually compatible with 6% ceftazidime loss in 12 hr and 11 to 13% loss in 24 hr at 22°C. 7 to 9% ceftazidime loss in 3 days at 4°C	1535	C

[a] Tested in glass containers.

[b] Tested in PVC containers.

[c] Tested in polyethylene plastic containers.

[d] Tested in Infusor LV 10 (elastomeric), Easypump LT 125 (elastomeric), Ultra-Flow (PVC), and Outbound (polyethylene) infusion device reservoirs.

[e] Tested in Singleday Infusors (Baxter).

[f] Tested in glass, polypropylene, and PVC containers.

[g] Refer to Appendix for the composition of parenteral nutrition solutions. TPN indicates a 2-in-1 admixture.

[h] Tested in elastomeric ambulatory pumps (Homepump, Block Medical).

[i] Tested in polypropylene syringes.

Additive Compatibility

Ceftazidime

Test Drug	Mfr	Conc/L or %	Mfr	Conc/L or %	Test Solution	Remarks	Ref	C/I
Amikacin sulfate	BR	25 mg	GL	50 mg	D5W	28% loss of amikacin in 2 hr at 22°C	504	I
Amikacin sulfate	BR	15 mg	GL	50 mg	D5W	17% loss of amikacin in 24 hr at 22°C	504	I
Aminophylline	ES	1 g	GL	2 g	D5W, NS	20 to 23% ceftazidime loss in 6 hr at room temperature	1937	I
Aminophylline	ES	1 g	GL	6 g	D5W, NS	8 to 10% ceftazidime loss in 6 hr at room temperature	1937	I
Aminophylline	ES	2 g	GL	2 g	D5W, NS	35 to 40% ceftazidime loss in 6 hr at room temperature	1937	I
Aminophylline	ES	2 g	GL	6 g	D5W, NS	22% ceftazidime loss in 6 hr at room temperature	1937	I
Ciprofloxacin	MI	2 g		20 g	D5W	Physically incompatible	888	I
Ciprofloxacin	BAY	2 g	SKB	19.8 g	D5W	Visually compatible but pH changed by more than 1 unit	2413	?
Clindamycin phosphate	UP	9 g	GL	20 g	D5W[b]	Physically compatible with 9% clindamycin loss and 11% ceftazidime loss in 48 hr at 25°C under fluorescent light	1026	C
Clindamycin phosphate	UP	9 g	GL	20 g	NS[b]	Physically compatible with 5% clindamycin loss and 7% ceftazidime loss in 48 hr at 25°C under fluorescent light	1026	C
Floxacillin sodium	GSK	40 g	GSK	40 g	NS, W	Physically compatible. Under 10% loss in 24 hr at room temperature and 4°C	2658	C
Floxacillin sodium	GSK	120 g	GSK	60 g	NS, W	Physically compatible. Under 10% loss in 24 hr at room temperature and 4°C	2658	C
Floxacillin sodium	GSK	240 g	GSK	180 g	NS, W	Physically compatible. Under 10% loss in 24 hr at room temperature and 4°C	2658	C
Fluconazole	PF	1 g	GL	20 g	D5W	Visually compatible with no fluconazole loss in 72 hr at 25°C under fluorescent light. Ceftazidime not tested	1677	C
Gentamicin sulfate	SC	6 and 9 mg	GL	50 mg	D5W	10 to 20% gentamicin loss in 2 hr at 22°C	504	I
Heparin sodium		10,000 and 50,000 units		4 g	D5W, NS	Ceftazidime stable for 24 hr at room temperature and 7 days refrigerated	4	C
Linezolid	PHU	2 g	GW	20 g	[c]	Physically compatible with no linezolid loss in 7 days at 4 and 23°C protected from light. Ceftazidime losses of 5% in 24 hr and 12% in 3 days at 23°C and about 3% in 7 days at 4°C	2262	C
Metronidazole		5 g	GL	20 g		No loss of either drug in 4 hr	1345	C
Metronidazole	AB	5 g	LI	10 g		Visually compatible with little or no loss of either drug in 72 hr at 8°C	1849	C
Potassium chloride		10 and 40 mEq		4 g	D5W, NS	Ceftazidime stable for 24 hr at room temperature and 7 days refrigerated	4	C
Ranitidine HCl	GL	500 mg	GL	10 g	D2.5½S	8% ranitidine loss in 4 hr and 37% loss in 24 hr at 22°C	1632	I
Sodium bicarbonate		4.2%	GL	20 g		11% ceftazidime loss in 24 hr at 25°C. 3% loss in 48 hr at 4°C	1136	C
Tenoxicam	RC	200 mg	LI	5 g	D5W[a]	Visually compatible for up to 72 hr with yellow discoloration. 10% loss of ceftazidime in 96 hr and of tenoxicam in 168 hr at 4 and 25°C	2557	C
Tenoxicam	RC	200 mg	LI	5 g	D5W[b]	Visually compatible with about 10% loss of both drugs in 168 hr at 4 and 25°C	2557	C

[a] Tested in PVC containers.

[b] Tested in glass containers.

[c] Admixed in the linezolid infusion container.

Drugs in Syringe Compatibility

Ceftazidime

Test Drug	Mfr	Amt	Mfr	Amt	Remarks	Ref	C/I
Dimenhydrinate		10 mg/1 mL		100 mg/1 mL	Clear solution	2569	C
Hydromorphone HCl	KN	2, 10, 40 mg/1 mL	GL	180 mg/1 mL	Visually compatible with less than 10% loss of either drug in 24 hr at room temperature	2082	C
Pantoprazole sodium	a	4 mg/1 mL		100 mg/1 mL	Precipitates immediately	2574	I

[a] Test performed using the formulation WITHOUT edetate disodium.

Y-Site Injection Compatibility (1:1 Mixture)

Ceftazidime

Test Drug	Mfr	Conc	Mfr	Conc	Remarks	Ref	C/I
Acetylcysteine		100 mg/mL	GSK	120 mg/mL[k]	Over 10% ceftazidime loss occurs in 1 hr	2513	I
Acyclovir sodium	BW	5 mg/mL[a]	SKF	20 mg/mL[a]	Physically compatible for 4 hr at 25°C	1157	C
Allopurinol sodium	BW	3 mg/mL[b]	LI	40 mg/mL[a]	Physically compatible for 4 hr at 22°C	1686	C
Amifostine	USB	10 mg/mL[a]	LI	40 mg/mL[a]	Physically compatible for 4 hr at 23°C	1845	C
Amikacin sulfate		1.5 mg/mL	SKB	125 mg/mL	Visually compatible with less than 10% loss of both drugs in 1 hr	2434	C
Amikacin sulfate		15 mg/mL	GSK	120 mg/mL[k]	Physically compatible with less than 10% ceftazidime loss. Amikacin not tested	2513	C
Aminophylline	ES	2 mg/mL[a]	GL	40 mg/mL[a]	Visually compatible with 4% ceftazidime loss and 9% theophylline loss in 2 hr at room temperature	1937	C
Aminophylline	ES	2 mg/mL[a]	GL	40 mg/mL[b]	Visually compatible with 5% ceftazidime loss and 4% theophylline loss in 2 hr at room temperature	1937	C
Amiodarone HCl	WY	6 mg/mL[a]	GW	40 mg/mL[a]	Immediate opaque white turbidity	2352	I
Amsacrine	NCI	1 mg/mL[a]	GL	40 mg/mL[a]	Immediate orange precipitate	1381	I
Anidulafungin	VIC	0.5 mg/mL[a]	GSK	40 mg/mL[a]	Physically compatible for 4 hr at 23°C	2617	C
Azithromycin	PF	2 mg/mL[b]	GW	80 mg/mL[c d]	Amber and white microcrystals found	2368	I
Aztreonam	SQ	40 mg/mL[a]	LI	40 mg/mL[a]	Physically compatible for 4 hr at 23°C	1758	C
Bivalirudin	TMC	5 mg/mL[a]	GW	40 mg/mL[a]	Physically compatible for 4 hr at 23°C	2373	C
Blinatumomab	AMG	0.125 and 0.375 mcg/mL[b]	PAN	34.5 mg/mL[b]	Particles, flakes, thin needles, or haze transiently appears	3405, 3417	?
Cangrelor tetrasodium	TMC	1 mg/mL[b]		40[b] and 100 mg/mL	Physically compatible for 4 hr	3243	C
Caspofungin acetate	ME	0.7 mg/mL[b]	GSK	40 mg/mL[b]	Immediate white turbid precipitate forms	2758	I
Ceftolozane sulfate–tazobactam sodium	CUB	10 mg/mL[f o]	SZ	40 mg/mL[f]	Physically compatible for 2 hr	3262	C
Ciprofloxacin	MI	1 mg/mL[a]	SKF	20 mg/mL[f]	Physically compatible for 24 hr at 22°C	1189	C
Cisatracurium besylate	GW	0.1 and 2 mg/mL[a]	SKB	40 mg/mL[a]	Physically compatible for 4 hr at 23°C	2074	C
Cisatracurium besylate	GW	5 mg/mL[a]	SKB	40 mg/mL[a]	Subvisible haze forms immediately	2074	I
Clarithromycin		50 mg/mL	SKB	125 mg/mL	Precipitates immediately	2434	I
Clarithromycin		10 mg/mL	SKB	125 mg/mL	Trace precipitation	2434	I

Y-Site Injection Compatibility (1:1 Mixture) (Cont.)

Test Drug	Mfr	Conc	Mfr	Conc	Remarks	Ref	C/I
Clarithromycin		50 mg/mL	GSK	120 mg/mL[k]	Precipitates	2513	I
Cloxacillin sodium	SMX	100 mg/mL	PPC	95 mg/mL	Physically compatible for up to 4 hr at room temperature	3245	C
Colistimethate sodium	MIL	1.5 mg/mL[b]	GSK	5 mg/mL[b]	Visually compatible for 1 hr at 26°C	3335	C
Daptomycin	CUB[n]	16.7 mg/mL[b e]	GSK	16.7 mg/mL[b e]	Physically compatible with no loss of either drug in 2 hr at 25°C	2553	C
Defibrotide sodium	JAZ	8 mg/mL[b]	PAN	80 mg/mL[b]	Visually compatible for 4 hr at room temperature	3149	C
Dexmedetomidine HCl	AB	4 mcg/mL[b]	GW	40 mg/mL[b]	Physically compatible for 4 hr at 23°C	2383	C
Diltiazem HCl	MMD	5 mg/mL	GL	10 and 170 mg/mL[b]	Visually compatible	1807	C
Diltiazem HCl	MMD	1 mg/mL[b]	GL	170 mg/mL[b]	Visually compatible	1807	C
Dobutamine HCl		1 mg/mL	GSK	120 mg/mL[k]	Physically compatible with less than 10% ceftazidime loss. Dobutamine not tested	2513	C
Dobutamine HCl		250 mg/mL	GSK	120 mg/mL[k]	Precipitates	2513	I
Docetaxel	RPR	0.9 mg/mL[a]	SKB	40 mg/mL[a]	Physically compatible for 4 hr at 23°C	2224	C
Dopamine HCl		0.4 mg/mL	GSK	120 mg/mL[k]	Physically compatible with less than 10% ceftazidime loss. Dopamine not tested	2513	C
Doxapram HCl	RB	2 mg/mL[a]	GW	40 mg/mL[a]	Visually compatible for 4 hr at 23°C	2470	C
Doxorubicin HCl liposomal	SEQ	0.4 mg/mL[a]	SKB	40 mg/mL[a]	Partial loss of measured natural turbidity	2087	I
Enalaprilat	MSD	0.05 mg/mL[b]	GL	10 mg/mL[a]	Physically compatible for 24 hr at room temperature under fluorescent light	1355	C
Epinephrine HCl		50 mcg/mL	GSK	120 mg/mL[k]	Physically compatible with less than 10% ceftazidime loss. Epinephrine not tested	2513	C
Eravacycline dihydrochloride	TET	0.6 mg/mL[b]	PPR	40 mg/mL[b]	Physically compatible for 2 hr at room temperature	3532	C
Erythromycin lactobionate		50 mg/mL	SKB	125 mg/mL	Precipitates immediately	2434	I
Erythromycin lactobionate		10 mg/mL	SKB	125 mg/mL	Trace precipitation	2434	I
Erythromycin lactobionate		5 mg/mL	GSK	120 mg/mL[k]	Precipitates	2513	I
Esmolol HCl	DCC	10 mg/mL[a]	GL	10 mg/mL[a]	Physically compatible for 24 hr at 22°C	1169	C
Etoposide phosphate	BR	5 mg/mL[a]	SKB	40 mg/mL[a]	Physically compatible for 4 hr at 23°C	2218	C
Famotidine	MSD	0.2 mg/mL[a]	GL	20 mg/mL[b]	Physically compatible for 14 hr	1196	C
Famotidine	ME	2 mg/mL[b]		20 mg/mL[a]	Visually compatible for 4 hr at 22°C	1936	C
Fenoldopam mesylate	AB	80 mcg/mL[b]	GW	40 mg/mL[b]	Physically compatible for 4 hr at 23°C	2467	C
Filgrastim	AMG	30 mcg/mL[a]	LI	40 mg/mL[b]	Physically compatible for 4 hr at 22°C	1687	C
Filgrastim	AMG	10[g] and 40[a] mcg/mL	LI	10 mg/mL[a]	Visually compatible. Little loss of filgrastim and fluconazole in 4 hr at 25°C	2060	C
Fluconazole	RR	2 mg/mL	GL	20 mg/mL	Precipitates immediately	1407	I
Fluconazole		2 mg/mL	SKB	125 mg/mL	Visually compatible with less than 10% loss of ceftazidime in 30 min. Fluconazole not tested	2434	C
Fluconazole		2 mg/mL	GSK	120 mg/mL[k]	Physically compatible with less than 10% ceftazidime loss. Fluconazole not tested	2513	C
Fludarabine phosphate	BX	1 mg/mL[a]	GL	40 mg/mL[a]	Visually compatible for 4 hr at 22°C	1439	C
Foscarnet sodium	AST	24 mg/mL	GL	20 mg/mL	Physically compatible for 24 hr at room temperature under fluorescent light	1335	C

Y-Site Injection Compatibility (1:1 Mixture) (Cont.)

Test Drug	Mfr	Conc	Mfr	Conc	Remarks	Ref	C/I
Foscarnet sodium	AST	24 mg/mL	GL	20 mg/mL[f]	Physically compatible for 24 hr at 25°C under fluorescent light	1393	C
Furosemide		10 mg/mL	SKB	125 mg/mL	Visually compatible with less than 10% loss of ceftazidime in 30 min. Furosemide not tested	2434	C
Furosemide		10 mg/mL	GSK	120 mg/mL[k]	Physically compatible with less than 10% ceftazidime loss. Furosemide not tested	2513	C
Gallium nitrate	FUJ	1 mg/mL[b]	LI	100 mg/mL[b]	Visually compatible for 24 hr at 25°C	1673	C
Gemcitabine HCl	LI	10 mg/mL[b]	SKB	40 mg/mL[b]	Physically compatible for 4 hr at 23°C	2226	C
Gentamicin sulfate		0.6 mg/mL	SKB	125 mg/mL	Visually compatible with less than 10% loss of both drugs in 1 hr	2434	C
Gentamicin sulfate		6 mg/mL	GSK	120 mg/mL[k]	Physically compatible with less than 10% ceftazidime loss. Gentamicin not tested	2513	C
Granisetron HCl	SKB	1 mg/mL	SKB	16.7 mg/mL[b]	Physically compatible with little or no loss of either drug in 4 hr at 22°C	1883	C
Heparin sodium	TR	50 units/mL	LI	20 mg/mL	Visually compatible for 4 hr at 25°C	1793	C
Hetastarch in lactated electrolyte	AB	6%	GW	40 mg/mL[a]	Physically compatible for 4 hr at 23°C	2339	C
Hydromorphone HCl	KN	2, 10, 40 mg/mL	GL	40[a] and 180 mg/mL	Visually compatible and both drugs stable for 24 hr	1532	C
Ibuprofen lysinate	OVA	10 mg/mL	GSK	200 mg/mL[f]	Slight turbidity increase	3541	I
Idarubicin HCl	AD	1 mg/mL[b]	LI	20 mg/mL[a]	Haze forms in 1 hr	1525	I
Insulin, regular		100 units/mL	GSK	120 mg/mL[k]	Physically compatible with less than 10% ceftazidime loss. Insulin not tested	2513	C
Isavuconazonium sulfate	ASP	1.5 mg/mL[f]	HOS	40 mg/mL[f]	Measured turbidity increases immediately	3263	I
Isosorbide dinitrate		0.2 mg/mL	GSK	120 mg/mL[k]	Physically compatible with less than 10% ceftazidime loss. Isosorbide not tested	2513	C
Ketamine HCl		10 mg/mL	SKB	125 mg/mL	Visually compatible with less than 10% loss of ceftazidime in 24 hr. Ketamine not tested	2434	C
Ketamine HCl		10 mg/mL	GSK	120 mg/mL[k]	Physically compatible with less than 10% ceftazidime loss. Ketamine not tested	2513	C
Labetalol HCl	SC	1 mg/mL[a]	GL	10 mg/mL[a]	Physically compatible for 24 hr at 18°C	1171	C
Linezolid	PHU	2 mg/mL	SKB	40 mg/mL[a]	Physically compatible for 4 hr at 23°C	2264	C
Melphalan HCl	BW	0.1 mg/mL[b]	LI	40 mg/mL[b]	Physically compatible for 3 hr at 22°C	1557	C
Meperidine HCl	AB	10 mg/mL	LI	20 and 40 mg/mL[a]	Physically compatible for 4 hr at 25°C	1397	C
Meropenem		50 mg/mL	FRK	100 mg/mL	Physically compatible for 4 hr at room temperature	3538	C
Meropenem–vaborbactam	TMC	8 mg/mL[b p]	SGT	40 mg/mL[b]	Physically compatible for 3 hr at 20 to 25°C	3380	C
Methylprednisolone sodium succinate		50 mg/mL	GSK	120 mg/mL[k]	Physically compatible. Less than 10% ceftazidime loss. Methylprednisolone not tested	2513	C
Midazolam HCl	RC	1 mg/mL[a]	LI	20 mg/mL[a]	Haze forms in 1 hr	1847	I
Midazolam HCl		5 mg/mL	SKB	125 mg/mL	Precipitates immediately	2434	I
Midazolam HCl		5 mg/mL	GSK	120 mg/mL[k]	Precipitates	2513	I
Milrinone lactate	SS	0.2 mg/mL[a]	GW	100 mg/mL[a]	Visually compatible for 4 hr at 25°C	2381	C

Y-Site Injection Compatibility (1:1 Mixture) (Cont.)

Test Drug	Mfr	Conc	Mfr	Conc	Remarks	Ref	C/I
Morphine sulfate	AB	1 mg/mL	LI	20 and 40 mg/mL[a]	Physically compatible for 4 hr at 25°C	1397	C
Morphine sulfate		1 mg/mL	GSK	120 mg/mL[k]	Physically compatible with less than 10% ceftazidime loss. Morphine not tested	2513	C
Nicardipine HCl	DCC	0.1 mg/mL[a]	GL	10 mg/mL[a]	Visually compatible for 24 hr at room temperature	235	C
Nicardipine HCl		1 mg/mL	SKB	125 mg/mL	Precipitates immediately	2434	I
Nicardipine HCl		1 mg/mL	GSK	120 mg/mL[k]	Precipitates	2513	I
Ondansetron HCl	GL	1 mg/mL[b]	GL	40 mg/mL[a]	Visually compatible for 4 hr at 22°C	1365	C
Ondansetron HCl	GL	16 to 160 mcg/mL		100 to 200 mg/mL	Physically compatible when ceftazidime given as 5-min bolus via Y-site	1366	C
Ondansetron HCl	GL	0.03 and 0.3 mg/mL[a]	LI	40 mg/mL[a]	Visually compatible with less than 10% loss of either drug in 4 hr at 25°C	1732	C
Paclitaxel	NCI	1.2 mg/mL[a]	LI	40 mg/mL[a]	Physically compatible for 4 hr at 22°C	1556	C
Pemetrexed disodium	LI	20 mg/mL[b]	GW	40 mg/mL[a]	Color darkening and brownish discoloration occur over 4 hr	2564	I
Pentamidine isethionate	FUJ	3 mg/mL[a]	LI	20 mg/mL[a]	Fine precipitate forms immediately	1880	I
Phenytoin sodium		50 mg/mL	GSK	120 mg/mL[k]	Precipitates	2513	I
Plazomicin sulfate	ACH	24 mg/mL[f]	SGT	40 mg/mL[f]	Physically compatible for 1 hr at 20 to 25°C	3432	C
Propofol	ZEN[r]	10 mg/mL	SKB	40 mg/mL[a]	Physically compatible for 1 hr at 23°C	2066	C
Propofol		1 mg/mL	SKB	125 mg/mL	Physically incompatible	2434	I
Propofol		1 mg/mL	GSK	120 mg/mL[k]	Precipitates	2513	I
Quinupristin–dalfopristin		2 mg/mL[a m]		20 mg/mL	Reported to be incompatible	3230	I
Ranitidine HCl	GL	1 mg/mL[b]	GL	20 mg/mL[a]	8% ranitidine loss and no ceftazidime loss in 4 hr at 22°C	1632	C
Remifentanil HCl		0.2 mg/mL	GSK	120 mg/mL[k]	Physically compatible with less than 10% ceftazidime loss. Remifentanil not tested	2513	C
Sargramostim	IMM	10 mcg/mL[b]	GL	40 mg/mL[b]	Particles and filaments form in 4 hr	1436	I
Sargramostim	IMM	6[h] and 15 mcg/mL[b]	LI	40 mg/mL[f]	Visually compatible for 2 hr	1618	C
Sufentanil citrate		50 mcg/mL	SKB	125 mg/mL	Visually compatible with less than 10% loss of ceftazidime in 24 hr. Sufentanil not tested	2434	C
Sufentanil citrate		5 mcg/mL	GSK	120 mg/mL[k]	Physically compatible with less than 10% ceftazidime loss. Sufentanil not tested	2513	C
Tacrolimus	FUJ	1 mg/mL[b]	GL	20 mg/mL[a]	Visually compatible for 24 hr at 25°C	1630	C
Tacrolimus	FUJ	10 and 40 mcg/mL[a]	GW	40 and 200 mg/mL[a]	Visually compatible with no loss of either drug in 4 hr at 24°C	2216	C
Tedizolid phosphate	CUB	0.8 mg/mL[b]	SZ	40 mg/mL[b]	Physically compatible for 2 hr	3244	C
Telavancin HCl	ASP	7.5 mg/mL[a b l]	HOS	40 mg/mL	Physically compatible for 2 hr	2830	C
Teniposide	BR	0.1 mg/mL[a]	LI	40 mg/mL[a]	Physically compatible for 4 hr at 23°C	1725	C
Theophylline	TR	4 mg/mL	LI	20 mg/mL	Visually compatible for 6 hr at 25°C	1793	C
Theophylline		20 mg/mL	GSK	120 mg/mL[k]	Over 25% ceftazidime loss in 1 hr	2513	I
Thiotepa	IMM[i]	1 mg/mL[a]	LI	40 mg/mL[a]	Physically compatible for 4 hr at 23°C	1861	C

Y-Site Injection Compatibility (1:1 Mixture) (Cont.)

Test Drug	Mfr	Conc	Mfr	Conc	Remarks	Ref	C/I
Tigecycline	WY	1 mg/mL[b]		40 mg/mL[b]	Physically compatible for 4 hr	2714	C
TNA #218 to #226[j]			SKB[q]	40 mg/mL[a]	Visually compatible for 4 hr at 23°C	2215	C
Tobramycin sulfate		0.6 mg/mL	SKB	125 mg/mL	Visually compatible with less than 10% loss of both drugs in 1 hr	2434	C
Tobramycin sulfate		6 mg/mL	GSK	120 mg/mL[k]	Physically compatible with less than 10% ceftazidime loss. Tobramycin not tested	2513	C
TPN #141 to #143[j]			GL	40 mg/mL[f]	Visually compatible with 4% or less ceftazidime loss in 2 hr at 22°C in 1:1 and 1:3 ratios	1535	C
TPN #189[j]			GL	200 mg/mL[k]	Visually compatible for 24 hr at 22°C	1767	C
TPN #203, #204[j]			LI	60 mg/mL	Visually compatible for 2 hr at 23°C	1974	C
TPN #212 to #215[j]			SKB	40 mg/mL[a]	Physically compatible for 4 hr at 23°C	2109	C
Valproate sodium		100 mg/mL	SKB	125 mg/mL	Physically compatible. Under 10% ceftazidime loss. Valproate not tested	2434	C
Valproate sodium		100 mg/mL	GSK	120 mg/mL[k]	Physically compatible. Under 10% ceftazidime loss. Valproate not tested	2513	C
Vancomycin HCl		10 mg/mL[a]		50 mg/mL[k]	Precipitates immediately	873	I
Vancomycin HCl	AB	20 mg/mL[a]	SKB	10[a], 50[a], 200[k] mg/mL	Gross white precipitate forms immediately	2189	I
Vancomycin HCl	AB	20 mg/mL[a]	SKB	1 mg/mL[a]	Physically compatible for 4 hr at 23°C	2189	C
Vancomycin HCl	AB	2 mg/mL[a]	SKB	1[a], 10[a], 50[a], 200[k] mg/mL	Physically compatible for 4 hr at 23°C	2189	C
Vancomycin HCl		30 mg/mL	SKB	125 mg/mL	Precipitates immediately	2434	I
Vancomycin HCl		30 mg/mL	GSK	120 mg/mL[k]	Precipitates	2513	I
Vancomycin HCl	LI	10 mg/mL[a]		125 mg/mL	Physically incompatible	3536	I
Vinorelbine tartrate	BW	1 mg/mL[b]	LI	40 mg/mL[b]	Physically compatible for 4 hr at 22°C	1558	C
Zidovudine	BW	4 mg/mL[a]	GL	20 mg/mL[a]	Physically compatible for 4 hr at 25°C	1193	C

[a] Tested in dextrose 5%.

[b] Tested in sodium chloride 0.9%.

[c] Tested in sodium chloride 0.45%.

[d] Injected via Y-site into an administration set running azithromycin.

[e] Final concentration after mixing.

[f] Tested in both dextrose 5% and sodium chloride 0.9%.

[g] Tested in dextrose 5% with human albumin 2 mg/mL.

[h] With human albumin 0.1%.

[i] Lyophilized formulation tested.

[j] Refer to Appendix for the composition of parenteral nutrition solutions. TNA indicates a 3-in-1 admixture, and TPN indicates a 2-in-1 admixture.

[k] Tested in sterile water for injection.

[l] Tested in Ringer's injection, lactated.

[m] Quinupristin and dalfopristin components combined.

[n] Test performed using the Cubicin formulation.

[o] Ceftolozane component. Ceftolozane in a 2:1 fixed-ratio concentration with tazobactam.

[p] Meropenem component. Meropenem in a 1:1 fixed-ratio concentration with vaborbactam.

[q] Sodium carbonate-containing formulation tested.

[r] Test performed using the formulation WITH edetate disodium.

Additional Compatibility Information

Peritoneal Dialysis Solutions

Ceftazidime 2 mg/mL in Dianeal with dextrose 1.5% is stated to be stable for 10 days under refrigeration, 24 hours at room temperature, and at least 4 hours at 37°C.[4]

Ceftazidime (Glaxo) 125 mg/L and tobramycin sulfate (Lilly) 8 mg/L in Dianeal PD-2 with dextrose 2.5% (Baxter) were visually compatible and chemically stable. After 16 hours of storage at 25°C under fluorescent light, the loss of both drugs was less than 3%. Additional storage for 8 hours at 37°C, to simulate the maximum peritoneal dwell time, showed tobramycin sulfate concentrations of 96% and ceftazidime concentrations of 92 to 96%.[1652]

Ceftazidime (Glaxo) 0.1 mg/mL in Dianeal PD-2 with dextrose 1.5% in PVC containers was physically and chemically stable for 24 hours at 25°C exposed to light, exhibiting about 9% loss; additional storage for 8 hours at 37°C resulted in additional loss of about 6%. Under refrigeration at 4°C protected from light, no loss occurred in 7 days. Additional storage for 16 hours at 25°C followed by 8 hours at 37°C resulted in about 6% loss.[1989]

Ceftazidime (Glaxo) 0.1 mg/mL admixed with teicoplanin (Marion Merrell Dow) 0.025 mg/mL in Dianeal PD-2 with dextrose 1.5% in PVC containers did not result in a stable mixture. Large (but variable) teicoplanin losses generally in the 20% range were noted in as little as 2 hours at 25°C exposed to light. Ceftazidime losses of about 9% occurred in 16 hours. Refrigeration and protection from light of the peritoneal dialysis admixture reduced losses of both drugs to negligible levels. Even so, the authors did not recommend admixing these 2 drugs because of the high levels of teicoplanin loss at room temperature.[1989]

Ceftazidime (Glaxo) 0.1 mg/mL in Dianeal PD-2 with dextrose 1.5% with or without heparin sodium 1 unit/mL in PVC bags was chemically stable for up to 6 days at 4°C (about 3 to 4% loss), 4 days at 25°C (about 9 to 10% loss), and less than 12 hours at body temperature of 37°C.[866]

The addition of vancomycin hydrochloride (Lederle) 0.05 mg/mL to this peritoneal dialysis solution demonstrated similar stability with the ceftazidime being the defining component. Ceftazidime was chemically stable for up to 6 days at 4°C (about 3% loss), 3 days at 25°C (about 9 to 10% loss), and 12 hours at body temperature of 37°C with the vancomycin exhibiting less loss throughout.[866]

Vancomycin hydrochloride (Lilly) 1 mg/mL admixed with ceftazidime (Lilly) 0.5 mg/mL in Dianeal PD-2 (Baxter) with 1.5% and also 4.25% dextrose were evaluated for compatibility and stability. Samples were stored under fluorescent light at 4 and 24°C for 24 hours and at 37°C for 12 hours. No precipitation or other change was observed by visual inspection in any sample. No loss of either drug occurred in the samples stored at 4°C and no loss of vancomycin hydrochloride and about 4 to 5% ceftazidime loss occurred in the samples stored at 24°C in 24 hours. Vancomycin hydrochloride losses of 3% or less and ceftazidime loss of about 6% were found in the samples stored at 37°C for 12 hours. No difference in stability was found between samples at either dextrose concentration.[2217]

Ceftazidime (GlaxoWellcome) 0.125 mg/mL in Delflex peritoneal dialysis solution bags with 2.5% dextrose (Fresenius) was stable with 10% loss occurring in 7 days at refrigerator temperature and 3 days at room temperature.[2573]

Ceftazidime (Sandoz) 500 mg/L in Extraneal with icodextrin 7.5% (Baxter) peritoneal dialysis solution bags exhibited less than 10% loss in 14 days at 4°C and 2 days at 25°C; the drug was unstable at 37°C.[3537] Ceftazidime (Sandoz) 500 mg/L with cefazolin sodium (Hospira) 500 mg/L in Extraneal with icodextrin 7.5% (Baxter) peritoneal dialysis solution bags exhibited less than 10% loss of either drug in 14 days at 4°C, 6% loss of ceftazidime and 2% loss of cefazolin in 2 days at 25°C, and no loss of ceftazidime and 2% loss of cefazolin in 6 hours at 37°C.[3537]

Ceftazidime–Avibactam Sodium
AHFS 8:12.06.12

Products

The fixed combination of ceftazidime–avibactam sodium is available as a powder in single-use vials containing 2.5 g (ceftazidime 2 g as the pentahydrate plus avibactam 0.5 g as the sodium salt).[3004] Each vial also contains sodium carbonate 239.6 mg.[3004]

Each 2.5-g vial should be reconstituted with 10 mL of sterile water for injection, sodium chloride 0.9%, dextrose 5%, Ringer's injection, lactated, or solutions containing any combination of dextrose and sodium chloride with concentrations not exceeding 2.5 and 0.45%, respectively;[3004][3005] the vial contents should be mixed gently.[3004] Each mL of the resultant reconstituted solution contains approximately 167 mg of ceftazidime plus 42 mg of avibactam.[3004] The reconstituted solution is *not* suitable for direct injection and must be diluted prior to infusion.[3004]

For adult and pediatric patients *weighing 40 kg or more*, the manufacturer's instructions for preparing various dosages of ceftazidime–avibactam with final ceftazidime and avibactam concentrations of 8 to 40 and 2 to 10 mg/mL, respectively, from the reconstituted solution are as follows:[3004]

For 2.5 g (ceftazidime 2 g plus avibactam 0.5 g), withdraw the entire vial contents (i.e., 12 mL) and add to an infusion bag to achieve a total volume of 50 to 250 mL in a compatible diluent.

For 1.25 g (ceftazidime 1 g plus avibactam 0.25 g), withdraw 6 mL and add to an infusion bag to achieve a total volume of at least 50 mL (but less than 250 mL) in a compatible diluent.

For 940 mg (ceftazidime 750 mg plus avibactam 190 mg), withdraw 4.5 mL and add to an infusion bag to achieve a total volume of at least 50 mL (but less than 250 mL) in a compatible diluent.

For pediatric patients *weighing less than 40 kg*, the appropriate volume of the reconstituted solution to achieve the prescribed dose should be withdrawn from the vial and diluted in a compatible diluent to final ceftazidime and avibactam concentrations of 8 to 40 and 2 to 10 mg/mL, respectively.[3004]

The same diluent should be used for both reconstitution and further dilution unless the drug was reconstituted with sterile water, in which case any compatible diluent should be used for further dilution.[3004] The diluted solution for infusion should be mixed gently to ensure complete dissolution and visually inspected for particulate matter and discoloration.[3004]

Sodium Content

Each 2.5-g vial contains approximately 6.4 mEq (146 mg) of sodium.[3004]

Trade Name(s)

Avycaz

Administration

Ceftazidime–avibactam sodium is administered by intravenous infusion over 2 hours following dilution of the reconstituted solution in a suitable infusion solution.[3004]

Stability

Intact vials should be stored at controlled room temperature and protected from light by storing in the original carton.[3004] Ceftazidime-avibactam sodium is a white to yellow powder that ultimately forms a clear to light yellow solution upon reconstitution and subsequent dilution.[3004] After reconstitution with an appropriate diluent as instructed, the drug may be stored for no longer than 30 minutes prior to dilution.[3004] Following dilution, the drug should be used within 12 hours when stored at room temperature; alternatively, the diluted solution may be stored up to 24 hours at 2 to 8°C and then should be used within 12 hours of subsequent storage at room temperature.[3004]

Compatibility Information

Solution Compatibility

Ceftazidime–avibactam sodium

Test Soln Name	Mfr	Mfr	Conc/L or %	Remarks	Ref	C/I
Dextrose 2.5% in sodium chloride 0.45%		ALL	8 to 40 g[a]	Use within 12 hr if stored at room temperature or store up to 24 hr at 2 to 8°C and use within 12 hr of subsequent storage at room temperature	3004, 3005	C
Dextrose 5%		ALL	8 to 40 g[a]	Use within 12 hr if stored at room temperature or store up to 24 hr at 2 to 8°C and use within 12 hr of subsequent storage at room temperature	3004	C
Ringer's injection, lactated		ALL	8 to 40 g[a]	Use within 12 hr if stored at room temperature or store up to 24 hr at 2 to 8°C and use within 12 hr of subsequent storage at room temperature	3004	C
Sodium chloride 0.9%		ALL	8 to 40 g[a]	Use within 12 hr if stored at room temperature or store up to 24 hr at 2 to 8°C and use within 12 hr of subsequent storage at room temperature	3004	C

[a] Ceftazidime component. Ceftazidime in a 4:1 fixed-ratio concentration with avibactam.

DOI: 10.37573/9781585286850.080

Y-Site Injection Compatibility (1:1 Mixture)

Ceftazidime–avibactam sodium

Test Drug	Mfr	Conc	Mfr	Conc	Remarks	Ref	C/I
Amikacin sulfate			ALL	20 mg/mL[e h]	Physically compatible for up to 4 hr at room temperature	3004	C
Azithromycin			ALL	20 mg/mL[e h]	Physically compatible for up to 4 hr at room temperature	3004	C
Aztreonam			ALL	20 mg/mL[e h]	Physically compatible for up to 4 hr at room temperature	3004	C
Ceftaroline fosamil			ALL	20 mg/mL[e h]	Physically compatible for up to 4 hr at room temperature	3004	C
Colistimethate[i]			ALL	20 mg/mL[e h]	Physically compatible for up to 4 hr at room temperature	3004	C
Daptomycin[i]			ALL	20 mg/mL[e h]	Physically compatible for up to 4 hr at room temperature	3004	C
Dexmedetomidine[i]			ALL	20 mg/mL[e h]	Physically compatible for up to 4 hr at room temperature	3004	C
Dopamine HCl			ALL	20 mg/mL[e h]	Physically compatible for up to 4 hr at room temperature	3004	C
Eravacycline dihydrochloride	TET	0.6 mg/mL[b]	GSK	40 mg/mL[b e]	Physically compatible for 2 hr at room temperature	3532	C
Ertapenem sodium			ALL	20 mg/mL[e d]	Physically compatible for up to 4 hr at room temperature	3004	C
Furosemide			ALL	20 mg/mL[e h]	Physically compatible for up to 4 hr at room temperature	3004	C
Gentamicin[i]			ALL	20 mg/mL[e h]	Physically compatible for up to 4 hr at room temperature	3004	C
Heparin sodium			ALL	20 mg/mL[e g]	Physically compatible for up to 4 hr at room temperature	3004	C
Imipenem–cilastatin[i]			ALL	20 mg/mL[e h]	Physically compatible for up to 4 hr at room temperature	3004	C
Levofloxacin			ALL	20 mg/mL[e h]	Physically compatible for up to 4 hr at room temperature	3004	C
Linezolid			ALL	20 mg/mL[e g]	Physically compatible for up to 4 hr at room temperature	3004	C
Magnesium sulfate			ALL	20 mg/mL[e h]	Physically compatible for up to 4 hr at room temperature	3004	C
Meropenem			ALL	20 mg/mL[b e]	Physically compatible for up to 4 hr at room temperature	3004	C
Meropenem–vaborbactam	TMC	8 mg/mL[b c]	GSK	40 mg/mL[b e]	Physically compatible for 3 hr at 20 to 25°C	3380	C
Metronidazole			ALL	20 mg/mL[e h]	Physically compatible for up to 4 hr at room temperature	3004	C
Norepinephrine bitartrate			ALL	20 mg/mL[e h]	Physically compatible for up to 4 hr at room temperature	3004	C
Phenylephrine HCl			ALL	20 mg/mL[e h]	Physically compatible for up to 4 hr at room temperature	3004	C
Plazomicin sulfate	ACH	24 mg/mL[d]	GSK	40 mg/mL[d e]	Physically compatible for 1 hr at 20 to 25°C	3432	C
Potassium chloride		0.4 mEq/mL	ALL	20 mg/mL[e f]	Physically compatible for up to 4 hr at room temperature	3004	C
Potassium phosphates			ALL	20 mg/mL[d e]	Physically compatible for up to 4 hr at room temperature	3004	C
Sodium bicarbonate			ALL	20 mg/mL[a e]	Physically compatible for up to 4 hr at room temperature	3004	C
Tedizolid phosphate			ALL	20 mg/mL[a e]	Physically compatible for up to 4 hr at room temperature	3004	C
Tobramycin[i]			ALL	20 mg/mL[e g]	Physically compatible for up to 4 hr at room temperature	3004	C
Vancomycin HCl	HOS	5, 10, 15, 20 mg/mL[a]	FOR	8 mg/mL[a e]	Physically incompatible	3480	I
Vancomycin HCl	HOS	5 mg/mL[a]	FOR	20 mg/mL[a e]	Physically compatible for up to 24 hr at room temperature with no loss of antimicrobial activity	3480	C
Vancomycin HCl	HOS	10, 15, 20 mg/mL[a]	FOR	20 mg/mL[a e]	Physically incompatible	3480	I

Y-Site Injection Compatibility (1:1 Mixture) (Cont.)

Test Drug	Mfr	Conc	Mfr	Conc	Remarks	Ref	C/I
Vancomycin HCl	HOS	5, 10 mg/mL[a]	FOR	40 mg/mL[a] [e]	Physically compatible for up to 24 hr at room temperature with no loss of antimicrobial activity	3480	C
Vancomycin HCl	HOS	15, 20 mg/mL[a]	FOR	40 mg/mL[a] [e]	Physically incompatible	3480	I
Vasopressin			ALL	20 mg/mL[e] [h]	Physically compatible for up to 4 hr at room temperature	3004	C
Vecuronium bromide			ALL	20 mg/mL[e] [h]	Physically compatible for up to 4 hr at room temperature	3004	C

[a] Tested in dextrose 5%.

[b] Tested in sodium chloride 0.9%.

[c] Meropenem component. Meropenem in a 1:1 fixed-ratio concentration with vaborbactam.

[d] Tested in both dextrose 5% and sodium chloride 0.9%.

[e] Ceftazidime component. Ceftazidime in a 4:1 fixed-ratio concentration with avibactam.

[f] Tested in Ringer's injection, lactated.

[g] Tested in both dextrose 5% and Ringer's injection, lactated.

[h] Tested in dextrose 5%, sodium chloride 0.9%, and Ringer's injection, lactated.

[i] Salt not specified.

Selected Revisions May 1, 2020. © Copyright, February 2016.
American Society of Health-System Pharmacists, Inc.

Ceftolozane Sulfate-Tazobactam Sodium
AHFS 8:12.06.12

Products

The fixed combination of ceftolozane sulfate–tazobactam sodium is available as a lyophilized powder for injection in single-use (preservative-free) vials containing 1.5 g (ceftolozane 1 g as the sulfate plus tazobactam 0.5 g as the sodium salt).[2958] Each vial also contains sodium chloride 487 mg, citric acid 21 mg, and L-arginine approximately 600 mg.[2958]

Reconstitute each 1.5-g vial with 10 mL of sterile water for injection or sodium chloride 0.9% and gently shake to dissolve.[2958] The reconstituted solution is *not* suitable for direct injection.[2958]

The manufacturer's instructions for preparing various dosages of ceftolozane–tazobactam from the reconstituted solution are as follows:[2958]

For a 3-g dose (ceftolozane 2 g plus tazobactam 1 g), withdraw the entire contents of 2 vials (i.e., approximately 11.4 mL per vial).

For a 2.25-g dose (ceftolozane 1.5 g plus tazobactam 0.75 g), withdraw the entire contents of 1 vial (i.e., approximately 11.4 mL) and 5.7 mL from a second vial.

For a 1.5-g dose (ceftolozane 1 g plus tazobactam 0.5 g), withdraw the entire contents of 1 vial (i.e., approximately 11.4 mL).

For a 750-mg dose (ceftolozane 500 mg plus tazobactam 250 mg), withdraw 5.7 mL.

For a 450-mg dose (ceftolozane 300 mg plus tazobactam 150 mg), withdraw 3.5 mL.

For a 375-mg dose (ceftolozane 250 mg plus tazobactam 125 mg), withdraw 2.9 mL.

For a 150-mg dose (ceftolozane 100 mg plus tazobactam 50 mg), withdraw 1.2 mL.

All doses should be added to an infusion bag containing 100 mL of a compatible diluent.

Trade Name(s)

Zerbaxa

Administration

Ceftolozane sulfate–tazobactam sodium is administered by intravenous infusion over 1 hour after dilution in an infusion bag containing 100 mL of sodium chloride 0.9% or dextrose 5%.[2958]

Stability

Intact vials of ceftolozane sulfate–tazobactam sodium should be stored under refrigeration at 2 to 8°C and protected from light.[2958] Ceftolozane sulfate–tazobactam sodium is a white to yellow lyophilized powder that forms a clear, colorless to slightly yellow solution for infusion; variations in color within this range do not affect the potency of the product.[2958] The drug reconstituted as instructed with sterile water for injection or sodium chloride 0.9% may be stored for 1 hour prior to dilution.[2958] Following dilution in sodium chloride 0.9% or dextrose 5%, the drug is stable for 24 hours when stored at room temperature or 7 days when stored under refrigeration at 2 to 8°C.[2958] Neither the reconstituted nor the diluted solutions should be frozen.[2958]

Compatibility Information

Solution Compatibility

Ceftolozane sulfate–tazobactam sodium

Test Soln Name	Mfr	Mfr	Conc/L or %	Remarks	Ref	C/I
Dextrose 5%	b	ME	1 to 20ᵃ g	Stable for 24 hr at room temperature or 7 days at 2 to 8°C	2958	C
Sodium chloride 0.9%	b	ME	1 to 20ᵃ g	Stable for 24 hr at room temperature or 7 days at 2 to 8°C	2958	C

ᵃ Ceftolozane component. Ceftolozane in a 2:1 fixed-ratio concentration with tazobactam.

ᵇ Tested in PVC containers.

Y-Site Injection Compatibility (1:1 Mixture)

Ceftolozane sulfate–tazobactam sodium

Test Drug	Mfr	Conc	Mfr	Conc	Remarks	Ref	C/I
Albumin human	KED	250 mg/mL	CUB	10 mg/mLᵃ ᵈ	Measured turbidity increases immediately	3262	I
Amikacin sulfate	HER	5 mg/mLᵈ	CUB	10 mg/mLᵃ ᵈ	Physically compatible for 2 hr	3262	C
Amiodarone HCl	APP	2 mg/mLᵈ	CUB	10 mg/mLᵃ ᵈ	Physically compatible for 2 hr	3262	C
Amphotericin B	XGN	0.1 mg/mLᵇ	CUB	10 mg/mLᵃ ᵇ	Measured turbidity increases immediately	3262	I

DOI: 10.37573/9781585286850.081

Y-Site Injection Compatibility (1:1 Mixture) (Cont.)

Test Drug	Mfr	Conc	Mfr	Conc	Remarks	Ref	C/I
Amphotericin B lipid complex	SIG	1 mg/mL[b]	CUB	10 mg/mL[a b]	Immediate change in measured turbidity	3262	I
Amphotericin B liposomal	ASP	2 mg/mL[b]	CUB	10 mg/mL[a b]	Immediate change in measured turbidity	3262	I
Ampicillin sodium–sulbactam sodium	APP	20 mg/mL[d e]	CUB	10 mg/mL[a d]	Physically compatible for 2 hr	3262	C
Anidulafungin	PF	0.77 mg/mL[d]	CUB	10 mg/mL[a d]	Physically compatible for 2 hr	3262	C
Azithromycin	FRK	2 mg/mL[d]	CUB	10 mg/mL[a d]	Physically compatible for 2 hr	3262	C
Aztreonam	FRK	20 mg/mL[d]	CUB	10 mg/mL[a d]	Physically compatible for 2 hr	3262	C
Bumetanide	HOS	0.25 mg/mL	CUB	10 mg/mL[a d]	Physically compatible for 2 hr	3262	C
Calcium chloride	HOS	20 mg/mL[d]	CUB	10 mg/mL[a d]	Physically compatible for 2 hr	3262	C
Calcium gluconate	FRK	20 mg/mL[d]	CUB	10 mg/mL[a d]	Physically compatible for 2 hr	3262	C
Caspofungin acetate	ME	0.5 mg/mL[c]	CUB	10 mg/mL[a c]	Measured turbidity increases immediately	3262	I
Cefazolin sodium	HOS	20 mg/mL[d]	CUB	10 mg/mL[a d]	Physically compatible for 2 hr	3262	C
Cefepime HCl	SGT	40 mg/mL[d]	CUB	10 mg/mL[a d]	Physically compatible for 2 hr	3262	C
Ceftaroline fosamil	FOR	12 mg/mL[d]	CUB	10 mg/mL[a d]	Physically compatible for 2 hr	3262	C
Ceftazidime	SZ	40 mg/mL[d]	CUB	10 mg/mL[a d]	Physically compatible for 2 hr	3262	C
Ceftriaxone sodium	HOS	40 mg/mL[d]	CUB	10 mg/mL[a d]	Physically compatible for 2 hr	3262	C
Cefuroxime sodium	COV	30 mg/mL[d]	CUB	10 mg/mL[a d]	Physically compatible for 2 hr	3262	C
Ciprofloxacin	HOS	2 mg/mL[d]	CUB	10 mg/mL[a d]	Physically compatible for 2 hr	3262	C
Cisatracurium besylate	ABV	0.4 mg/mL[d]	CUB	10 mg/mL[a d]	Physically compatible for 2 hr	3262	C
Colistimethate sodium	APP	4.5 mg/mL[d]	CUB	10 mg/mL[a d]	Physically compatible for 2 hr	3262	C
Cyclosporine	PAD	5 mg/mL[d]	CUB	10 mg/mL[a d]	Immediate change in measured turbidity	3262	I
Daptomycin	CUB[j]	10 mg/mL[c]	CUB	10 mg/mL[a c]	Physically compatible for 2 hr	3247, 3262	C
Dexamethasone sodium phosphate	FRK	1 mg/mL[d]	CUB	10 mg/mL[a d]	Physically compatible for 2 hr	3262	C
Dexmedetomidine HCl	MYL	4 mcg/mL[d]	CUB	10 mg/mL[a d]	Physically compatible for 2 hr	3262	C
Digoxin	SZ	0.25 mg/mL	CUB	10 mg/mL[a d]	Physically compatible for 2 hr	3262	C
Diltiazem HCl	WW	5 mg/mL	CUB	10 mg/mL[a d]	Physically compatible for 2 hr	3262	C
Diphenhydramine HCl	APP	50 mg/mL	CUB	10 mg/mL[a d]	Physically compatible for 2 hr	3262	C
Dobutamine HCl	HOS	4 mg/mL[d]	CUB	10 mg/mL[a d]	Physically compatible for 2 hr	3262	C
Dopamine HCl		3.2 mg/mL	CUB	30 mg/mL[a d]	Physically compatible with no loss of either drug in 24 hr at 25°C	2959	C
Dopamine HCl	HOS	0.8 mg/mL[d]	CUB	10 mg/mL[a d]	Physically compatible for 2 hr	3262	C
Doripenem	SHI	4.5 mg/mL[d]	CUB	10 mg/mL[a d]	Physically compatible for 2 hr	3262	C
Doxycycline hyclate	FRK	1 mg/mL[d]	CUB	10 mg/mL[a d]	Physically compatible for 2 hr	3262	C
Epinephrine[k]	JHP	16 mcg/mL[d]	CUB	10 mg/mL[a d]	Physically compatible for 2 hr	3247, 3262	C
Eptifibatide	ME	2 mg/mL	CUB	10 mg/mL[a d]	Physically compatible for 2 hr	3262	C
Eravacycline dihydrochloride	TET	0.6 mg/mL[c]	ME	20 mg/mL[a c]	Physically compatible for 2 hr at room temperature	3532	C

Y-Site Injection Compatibility (1:1 Mixture) (Cont.)

Test Drug	Mfr	Conc	Mfr	Conc	Remarks	Ref	C/I
Ertapenem sodium	ME	20 mg/mL[c]	CUB	10 mg/mL[a c]	Physically compatible for 2 hr	3262	C
Esmolol HCl	MYL	10 mg/mL	CUB	10 mg/mL[a d]	Physically compatible for 2 hr	3262	C
Esomeprazole sodium	ASZ	0.8 mg/mL[d]	CUB	10 mg/mL[a d]	Physically compatible for 2 hr	3262	C
Famotidine	WW	4 mg/mL[d]	CUB	10 mg/mL[a d]	Physically compatible for 2 hr	3262	C
Fentanyl citrate	WW	50 mcg/mL	CUB	10 mg/mL[a d]	Physically compatible for 2 hr	3247, 3262	C
Filgrastim	AMG	15 mcg/mL[b]	CUB	10 mg/mL[a b]	Physically compatible for 2 hr	3262	C
Fosphenytoin sodium	WW	25 mg PE/mL[d i]	CUB	10 mg/mL[a d]	Physically compatible for 2 hr	3247, 3262	C
Furosemide	HOS	3 mg/mL[d]	CUB	10 mg/mL[a d]	Physically compatible for 2 hr	3262	C
Gentamicin sulfate	FRK	5 mg/mL[d]	CUB	10 mg/mL[a d]	Physically compatible for 2 hr	3262	C
Heparin sodium	SGT	1000 units/mL	CUB	10 mg/mL[a d]	Physically compatible for 2 hr	3262	C
Hydrocortisone sodium succinate	PF	1 mg/mL[d]	CUB	10 mg/mL[a d]	Physically compatible for 2 hr	3262	C
Hydromorphone HCl	AKN	1 mg/mL[d]	CUB	10 mg/mL[a d]	Physically compatible for 2 hr	3262	C
Imipenem–cilastatin sodium	FRK	5 mg/mL[d f]	CUB	10 mg/mL[a d]	Physically compatible for 2 hr	3247, 3262	C
Insulin, regular	NVN	1 unit/mL[d]	CUB	10 mg/mL[a d]	Physically compatible for 2 hr	3262	C
Isavuconazonium sulfate	ASP	1.5 mg/mL[d]	CUB	10 mg/mL[a d]	Physically compatible for 2 hr	3262, 3263	C
Labetalol HCl	HOS	2 mg/mL[d]	CUB	10 mg/mL[a d]	Physically compatible for 2 hr	3262	C
Levofloxacin	CLA	5 mg/mL[d]	CUB	10 mg/mL[a d]	Physically compatible for 2 hr	3262	C
Lidocaine HCl	APP	8 mg/mL[d]	CUB	10 mg/mL[a d]	Physically compatible for 2 hr	3262	C
Linezolid	PF	2 mg/mL[b]	CUB	10 mg/mL[a d]	Physically compatible for 2 hr	3247, 3262	C
Lorazepam		2 mg/mL	CUB	30 mg/mL[a b]	Physically compatible with no loss of either drug in 4 hr at 25°C	2959	C
Lorazepam		2 mg/mL	CUB	30 mg/mL[a c]	Physically compatible with no loss of either drug in 24 hr at 25°C	2959	C
Lorazepam	WW	1 mg/mL[d]	CUB	10 mg/mL[a d]	Physically compatible for 2 hr	3262	C
Magnesium sulfate	APP	100 mg/mL[d]	CUB	10 mg/mL[a d]	Physically compatible for 2 hr	3262	C
Mannitol	HOS	25%	CUB	10 mg/mL[a d]	Physically compatible for 2 hr	3262	C
Meperidine HCl	WW	10 mg/mL[d]	CUB	10 mg/mL[a d]	Physically compatible for 2 hr	3262	C
Meropenem	FRK	10 mg/mL[d]	CUB	10 mg/mL[a d]	Physically compatible for 2 hr	3262	C
Meropenem–vabor-bactam	TMC	8 mg/mL[c i]	ME	20 mg/mL[a c]	Physically compatible for 3 hr at 20 to 25°C	3380	C
Mesna	TE	20 mg/mL[d]	CUB	10 mg/mL[a d]	Physically compatible for 2 hr	3262	C
Methylprednisolone sodium succinate	PF	20 mg/mL[d]	CUB	10 mg/mL[a d]	Physically compatible for 2 hr	3247, 3262	C
Metoclopramide HCl	TE	0.2 mg/mL[d]	CUB	10 mg/mL[a d]	Physically compatible for 2 hr	3247, 3262	C
Metronidazole	BA	5 mg/mL[d]	CUB	10 mg/mL[a d]	Physically compatible for 2 hr	3262	C
Micafungin sodium	ASP	2 mg/mL[d]	CUB	10 mg/mL[a d]	Physically compatible for 2 hr	3262	C
Midazolam HCl	APP	1 mg/mL[d]	CUB	10 mg/mL[a d]	Physically compatible for 2 hr	3262	C

Y-Site Injection Compatibility (1:1 Mixture) (Cont.)

Test Drug	Mfr	Conc	Mfr	Conc	Remarks	Ref	C/I
Milrinone lactate	APP	0.2 mg/mL[d]	CUB	10 mg/mL[a d]	Physically compatible for 2 hr	3262	C
Morphine sulfate		1 mg/mL	CUB	30 mg/mL[a b]	Physically compatible with no loss of either drug in 4 hr at 25°C	2959	C
Morphine sulfate		1 mg/mL	CUB	30 mg/mL[a c]	Physically compatible with no loss of either drug in 24 hr at 25°C	2959	C
Morphine sulfate	WW	1 mg/mL[d]	CUB	10 mg/mL[a d]	Physically compatible for 2 hr	3262	C
Mycophenolate mofetil HCl	GEN	6 mg/mL[b]	CUB	10 mg/mL[a b]	Physically compatible for 2 hr	3262	C
Naloxone HCl	MYL	0.04 mg/mL[d]	CUB	10 mg/mL[a d]	Physically compatible for 2 hr	3262	C
Nicardipine HCl	EXL	0.1 mg/mL[d]	CUB	10 mg/mL[a d]	Immediate gross precipitation and increase in measured turbidity	3247, 3262	I
Nitroglycerin	BA	0.4 mg/mL[d]	CUB	10 mg/mL[a d]	Physically compatible for 2 hr	3262	C
Norepinephrine bitartrate		32 mcg/mL	CUB	30 mg/mL[a d]	Physically compatible with no loss of either drug in 4 hr at 25°C	2959	C
Norepinephrine bitartrate	HOS	32 mcg/mL[d]	CUB	10 mg/mL[a d]	Physically compatible for 2 hr	3262	C
Octreotide acetate	APP, FRK	4 mcg/mL[d]	CUB	10 mg/mL[a d]	Physically compatible for 2 hr	3262	C
Ondansetron HCl	HOS	0.16 mg/mL[d]	CUB	10 mg/mL[a d]	Physically compatible for 2 hr	3262	C
Pantoprazole sodium	PF[h]	0.4 mg/mL[d]	CUB	10 mg/mL[a d]	Physically compatible for 2 hr	3247, 3262	C
Penicillin G potassium	PF	100,000 units/mL[d]	CUB	10 mg/mL[a d]	Physically compatible for 2 hr	3262	C
Phenylephrine HCl	WW	1 mg/mL[d]	CUB	10 mg/mL[a d]	Physically compatible for 2 hr	3262	C
Phenytoin sodium	WW	10 mg/mL[c]	CUB	10 mg/mL[a c]	Immediate gross precipitation and increase in measured turbidity	3262	I
Piperacillin sodium–tazobactam sodium	WY[h]	40 mg/mL[d g]	CUB	10 mg/mL[a d]	Physically compatible for 2 hr	3247, 3262	C
Plazomicin sulfate	ACH	24 mg/mL[d]	ME	20 mg/mL[a d]	Physically compatible for 1 hr at 20 to 25°C	3432	C
Potassium chloride	HOS	0.1 mEq/mL[d]	CUB	10 mg/mL[a d]	Physically compatible for 2 hr	3262	C
Potassium phosphates	HOS	0.3 mmol/mL[d]	CUB	10 mg/mL[a d]	Physically compatible for 2 hr	3262	C
Propofol	FRK[h]	10 mg/mL	CUB	10 mg/mL[a b]	Immediate formation of free oil layer atop fat plug	3262	I
Ranitidine HCl	ZY	2.5 mg/mL[d]	CUB	10 mg/mL[a d]	Physically compatible for 2 hr	3262	C
Rocuronium bromide	HOS	5 mg/mL[d]	CUB	10 mg/mL[a d]	Physically compatible for 2 hr	3262	C
Sodium bicarbonate	HOS	1 mEq/mL	CUB	10 mg/mL[a d]	Physically compatible for 2 hr	3262	C
Sodium nitroprusside	MTN	0.4 mg/mL[d]	CUB	10 mg/mL[a d]	Physically compatible for 2 hr	3262	C
Sodium phosphates	HOS	0.5 mmol/mL[d]	CUB	10 mg/mL[a d]	Physically compatible for 2 hr	3262	C
Tacrolimus	ASP	0.02 mg/mL[d]	CUB	10 mg/mL[a d]	Physically compatible for 2 hr	3262	C
Tedizolid phosphate	CUB	0.8 mg/mL[c]	CUB	10 mg/mL[a c]	Physically compatible for 2 hr	3244, 3262	C
Tigecycline	PF	1 mg/mL[d]	CUB	10 mg/mL[a d]	Physically compatible for 2 hr	3262	C
Tobramycin sulfate	MYL	5 mg/mL[d]	CUB	10 mg/mL[a d]	Physically compatible for 2 hr	3262	C
Vancomycin HCl	APP	5 mg/mL[d]	CUB	10 mg/mL[a d]	Physically compatible for 2 hr	3262	C

Y-Site Injection Compatibility (1:1 Mixture) (Cont.)

Test Drug	Mfr	Conc	Mfr	Conc	Remarks	Ref	C/I
Vancomycin HCl	HOS	5, 10 mg/mL[b]	ME	15 mg/mL[a b]	Physically compatible for up to 24 hr at room temperature with no loss of antimicrobial activity	3480	C
Vancomycin HCl	HOS	15, 20 mg/mL[b]	ME	15 mg/mL[a b]	Physically incompatible	3480	I
Vasopressin	JHP	1 unit/mL[d]	CUB	10 mg/mL[a d]	Physically compatible for 2 hr	3262	C
Vecuronium bromide	SUN	1 mg/mL[d]	CUB	10 mg/mL[a d]	Physically compatible for 2 hr	3262	C

[a] Ceftolozane component. Ceftolozane in a 2:1 fixed-ratio concentration with tazobactam.

[b] Tested in dextrose 5%.

[c] Tested in sodium chloride 0.9%.

[d] Tested in both dextrose 5% and sodium chloride 0.9%.

[e] Ampicillin component. Ampicillin in a 2:1 fixed-ratio concentration with sulbactam.

[f] Imipenem component. Imipenem in a 1:1 fixed-ratio concentration with cilastatin.

[g] Piperacillin component. Piperacillin in an 8:1 fixed-ratio concentration with tazobactam.

[h] Test performed using the formulation WITH edetate disodium.

[i] Concentration of fosphenytoin expressed in milligrams of phenytoin sodium equivalents (PE) per mL.

[j] Test performed using the Cubicin formulation.

[k] As epinephrine base rather than the salt.

[l] Meropenem component. Meropenem in a 1:1 fixed-ratio concentration with vaborbactam.

Additional Compatibility Information

Peritoneal Dialysis Solutions

The fixed combination of ceftolozane sulfate–tazobactam sodium (Merck Sharpe & Dohme) was evaluated for stability in Dianeal with dextrose 1.5% (Baxter), Dianeal with dextrose 2.5% (Baxter), Dianeal with dextrose 4.25% (Baxter), and Extraneal with icodextrin 7.5% (Baxter) at ceftolozane and tazobactam concentrations of 20 and 10 mg/L, respectively, with bags stored at 25, 4, and 37°C.[3565] The fixed combination also was evaluated for stability in 2-compartment pH-neutral Balance with dextrose 1.3% (Fresenius), pH-neutral Balance with dextrose 2.3% (Fresenius), Physioneal with 1.36% dextrose (Baxter), Physioneal with 2.27% dextrose (Fresenius), and Physioneal with 3.86% dextrose (Fresenius).[3565] Bags of 2-compartment pH-neutral Balance contained ceftolozane and tazobactam at concentrations of 40 and 20 mg/L, respectively, in the non-dextrose compartment for storage at 25 and 4°C; for storage at 37°C, the 2 compartments were combined immediately prior to storage for final ceftolozane and tazobactam concentrations of 20 and 10 mg/L, respectively.[3565] Bags of 2-compartment Physioneal contained ceftolozane and tazobactam at concentrations of 55.1 and 27.5 mg/L, respectively, in the dextrose compartment for storage at 25 and 4°C; for storage at 37°C, the 2 compartments were combined immediately prior to storage for final ceftolozane and tazobactam concentrations of 20 and 10 mg/L, respectively.[3565] No color change or particle formation was noted on visual assessment and no meaningful pH changes occurred.[3565] In all solutions, losses of both drugs were less than 3% in 6 hours at 25°C followed by 7 days at 4°C and an additional 12 hours at 37°C.[3565]

Ceftriaxone Sodium
AHFS 8:12.06.12

Products

Ceftriaxone sodium is available in vials containing the equivalent of 250 mg, 500 mg, 1 g, and 2 g of ceftriaxone. It also is available in 1- and 2-g piggyback bottles and 10-g bulk pharmacy containers.[1(9/08)]

For intramuscular use, reconstitute the vials with a compatible diluent in the amounts indicated:[1(9/08)]

Vial Size	Volume of Diluent for 250 mg/mL	Volume of Diluent for 350 mg/mL
250 mg	0.9 mL	a
500 mg	1.8 mL	1 mL
1 g	3.6 mL	2.1 mL
2 g	7.2 mL	4.2 mL

a This vial size not recommended for 350-mg/mL concentration because withdrawal of the entire contents may not be possible.

More dilute solutions for intramuscular injection may be prepared if required.[1(9/08)]

For intermittent intravenous infusion, reconstitute the vials with a compatible diluent in the amounts indicated to yield a 100-mg/mL solution:[1(9/08)]

Vial Size	Volume of Diluent
250 mg	2.4 mL
500 mg	4.8 mL
1 g	9.6 mL
2 g	19.2 mL

After reconstitution, withdraw the entire vial contents and further dilute in a compatible infusion solution to the desired concentration. Concentrations between 10 and 40 mg/mL are recommended, but lower concentrations may be used.[1(9/08)]

The piggyback bottles should be reconstituted with 10 or 20 mL of compatible diluent for the 1- or 2-g size, respectively. After reconstitution, further dilution to 50 to 100 mL with a compatible infusion solution is recommended.[1(9/08)]

The bulk pharmacy container should be reconstituted with 95 mL of a compatible diluent. The solution is not for direct administration and must be diluted further before use.[4]

Ceftriaxone sodium (Braun) is available as 1 or 2 g in a dual-chamber flexible container. The diluent chamber contains dextrose solution.[1(9/08)]

Ceftriaxone sodium also is available as a frozen premixed infusion solution of 1 or 2 g in 50 mL of dextrose 3.8 or 2.4%, respectively, in water. It should be thawed at room temperature.[1(9/08) 4]

pH

The pH of the reconstituted drug in dual-chamber containers is approximately 6.7.[1(9/08)] The frozen premixed infusion solutions have a pH of approximately 6.6 (range 6 to 8).[4]

Osmolality

The frozen premixed infusion solutions have osmolalities of 276 to 324 mOsm/kg.[4]

The osmolality of ceftriaxone sodium (Roche) 50 mg/mL was determined to be 351 mOsm/kg in dextrose 5% and 364 mOsm/kg in sodium chloride 0.9%.[1375]

Ceftriaxone sodium (Braun) 1 or 2 g in dual-chamber flexible containers has an osmolality of 290 mOsm/kg when activated with the dextrose diluent.[1(9/08)]

Sodium Content

Ceftriaxone sodium contains approximately 3.6 mEq (83 mg) of sodium per gram of ceftriaxone activity.[1(9/08)]

Trade Name(s)

Rocephin

Administration

Ceftriaxone sodium is administered by deep intramuscular injection or intermittent intravenous infusion over 15 to 30 minutes in adults or over 10 to 30 minutes in pediatric patients.[1(9/08) 4]

Stability

Intact vials of ceftriaxone sodium should be stored at room temperature of 25°C or below and protected from light. After reconstitution, normal exposure to light is permitted. Solutions may vary from light yellow to amber, depending on length of storage, diluent, and concentration.[1(9/08)]

Reconstituted solutions of ceftriaxone sodium are stable, exhibiting less than a 10% potency loss for the time periods indicated:[1(9/08)]

Diluent	Ceftriaxone Concentration (mg/mL)	25°C	4°C
Sterile water for injection	100	2 days	10 days
Sterile water for injection	250, 350	24 hr	3 days
Sodium chloride 0.9%	100	2 days	10 days
Sodium chloride 0.9%	250, 350	24 hr	3 days
Dextrose 5%	100	2 days	10 days
Dextrose 5%	250, 350	24 hr	3 days
Bacteriostatic water for injection (benzyl alcohol 0.9%)	100	24 hr	10 days

DOI: 10.37573/9781585286850.082

Diluent	Ceftriaxone Concentration (mg/mL)	25°C	4°C
Bacteriostatic water for injection (benzyl alcohol 0.9%)	250, 350	24 hr	3 days
Lidocaine HCl 1% (without epinephrine)	100	24 hr	10 days
Lidocaine HCl 1% (without epinephrine)	250, 350	24 hr	3 days

Ceftriaxone sodium (Braun) 1 or 2 g in dual-chamber flexible plastic containers with dextrose solution diluent should be used within 24 hours after activation if stored at room temperature and in 7 days if stored under refrigeration.[1(9/08)]

Ceftriaxone sodium at concentrations of 10 to 40 mg/mL is incompatible with calcium-containing solutions, including Ringer's injection and Ringer's injection, lactated. Precipitation has been observed to form rapidly.[2222] Fatalities in neonates and infants have been reported to the FDA.

The FDA states that ceftriaxone sodium and calcium-containing solutions should not be given concomitantly to neonates less than 28 days of age; ceftriaxone sodium should not be used in these neonates if they are receiving or expected to receive calcium-containing intravenous solutions.[2731 2784]

For patients over 28 days of age, the FDA states that ceftriaxone sodium and calcium-containing intravenous solutions may be administered sequentially as long as the infusion lines are thoroughly flushed between the separate infusions. The FDA states that ceftriaxone sodium and calcium-containing intravenous solutions should not be given simultaneously via Y-site to any patient regardless of age.[2731 2784]

pH Effects

The pH of maximum stability for ceftriaxone sodium has been variously reported as 2.5 to 4.5[1080] and 7.2.[1244]

Freezing Solutions

The manufacturer indicates that ceftriaxone sodium 10 to 40 mg/mL in dextrose 5% or sodium chloride 0.9%, when frozen at −20°C in polyvinyl chloride (PVC) or polyolefin containers, is stable for 26 weeks. Thawing should be performed at room temperature; thawed solutions should not be refrozen.[1(9/08)]

The frozen premixed infusion solutions are stable for at least 90 days at −20°C. Thawed solutions are stable for 72 hours at room temperature or 21 days at 5°C.[4]

Ceftriaxone sodium (Roche) 250 and 450 mg/mL in dextrose 5%, 250 mg/mL in bacteriostatic water for injection, and 450 mg/mL in lidocaine hydrochloride 1% (Lyphomed) were evaluated for stability and pharmaceutical integrity during frozen storage at −15°C. The solutions were packaged in 10-mL polypropylene syringes with attached needles (Becton Dickinson) and frozen for 8 weeks. Some syringes were stored further at 4°C for 10 days for at 20°C for 3 days. Ceftriaxone sodium losses of 5% or less were found after 8 weeks of frozen storage. However, particulate matter levels were unacceptable in most samples. While additional storage at 4°C for 10 days did not cause unacceptable drug loss, storage at 20°C for 3 days resulted in 12% drug loss.[1824]

Ceftriaxone sodium (Roche) 2 g/100 mL of dextrose 5% in polyolefin containers was found to remain stable for 14 weeks frozen at −20°C with no loss of drug occurring. Subsequent thawing in a microwave oven and storage at about 4°C resulted in 10% drug loss in 44 to 56 days, depending on the power level used for thawing.[2724]

Ceftriaxone sodium (Braun) 1 or 2 g in dual-chamber flexible containers should not be frozen.[1(9/08)]

Syringes

Bailey et al. reported the stability of ceftriaxone sodium (Roche) 10 and 40 mg/mL in dextrose 5% and sodium chloride 0.9% packaged in polypropylene syringes. The solutions were visually compatible and lost 5% or less ceftriaxone in 48 hours at 4 and 20°C and 10 days stored frozen at −10°C.[1720]

Plumridge et al. reported on the stability of ceftriaxone sodium (Roche) 100 mg/mL in sterile water for injection packaged in polypropylene syringes (Terumo). About 9 to 10% loss of ceftriaxone occurred in 5 days at 20°C and 40 days at 4°C. However, the room temperature samples underwent color intensification that the authors found unacceptable after about 72 hours. Little or no loss occurred during 180 days of frozen storage at −20°C.[1990]

O'Connell et al. evaluated the stability of reconstituted ceftriaxone sodium 100 mg/mL packaged in 10-mL polypropylene syringes. Stored under refrigeration at 8°C, about 5% loss occurred in 10 days and 8% in 13 days.[1999]

Elastomeric Reservoir Pumps

Ceftriaxone sodium (Roche) 10 mg/mL in both dextrose 5% and sodium chloride 0.9% was evaluated for binding potential to natural rubber elastomeric reservoirs (Baxter). No binding was found after storage for 2 weeks at 35°C with gentle agitation.[2014]

Central Venous Catheter

Ceftriaxone sodium (Roche) 5 mg/mL in dextrose 5% was found to be compatible with the ARROWg+ard Blue Plus (Arrow International) chlorhexidine-bearing triple-lumen central catheter. Essentially complete delivery of the drug was found with little or no drug loss occurring. Furthermore, chlorhexidine delivered from the catheter remained at trace amounts with no substantial increase due to the delivery of the drug through the catheter.[2335]

Compatibility Information

Solution Compatibility

Ceftriaxone sodium

Test Soln Name	Mfr	Mfr	Conc/L or %	Remarks	Ref	C/I
Dextrose 5% in sodium chloride 0.45%		RC	10 to 40 g	Less than 10% loss in 2 days at 25°C. Incompatible if refrigerated	1(9/08)	C
Dextrose 5% in sodium chloride 0.45%		RC	10 g	3% loss in 48 hr at 20°C. 5% loss in 72 hr and 9% in 96 hr at 4°C	965	C
Dextrose 5% in sodium chloride 0.9%		RC	10 to 40 g	Less than 10% loss in 2 days at 25°C. Incompatible if refrigerated	1(9/08)	C
Dextrose 5%		RC	10 to 40 g	Less than 10% loss in 2 days at 25°C and 10 days at 4°C	1(9/08)	C
Dextrose 5%		RC	10 g	No loss in 48 hr and 8% in 72 hr at 20°C. 4% loss in 72 hr and 9% in 96 hr at 4°C	965	C
Dextrose 5%	TR[b]	RC	2 g	Little or no loss in 14 days at 20, 4, and −20°C	966	C
Dextrose 5%	MG[c]	RC	20 g	Physically compatible with 5% drug loss in 24 hr and 9% in 48 hr at 25°C	1026	C
Dextrose 5%	[b]	RC	40 g	Physically compatible with 12% loss in 3 days at 23°C and 10% loss in 14 days at 4°C	1243	C
Dextrose 5%	[a]	RC	1 g	10% loss calculated to occur in 48 hr at 20°C	1244	C
Dextrose 5%		RC	10 g	Physically compatible with 8% loss in 7 days at room temperature. 5 to 8% loss in 12 weeks at 5 and −20°C	1245	C
Dextrose 5%		RC	50 g	Physically compatible with no loss in 24 hr but 12 to 17% loss in 7 days at room temperature. 5 to 7% loss in 12 weeks at 5 and −20°C	1245	C
Dextrose 5%	BA[d]	RC	5 and 40 g	Less than 10% loss in 4 days at 23°C and 21 days at 4°C	2819	C
Dextrose 5%			5 and 40 g	Color darkening occurs but only about 3% ceftriaxone loss occurs in 20 days at 4°C	2598	C
Dextrose 10%		RC	10 to 40 g	Less than 10% loss in 2 days at 25°C and 10 days at 4°C	1(9/08)	C
Dextrose 10%		RC	10 g	No loss in 48 hr and 8% in 72 hr at 20°C. 2% loss in 72 hr and 8% in 96 hr at 4°C	965	C
Ionosol B in dextrose 5%		RC	10 to 40 g	Less than 10% loss in 24 hours at 25°C	1(9/08)	C
Normosol M in dextrose 5%	[a]	RC	1 to 40 g	Less than 10% loss in 24 hours at 25°C	1(9/08)	C
Ringer's injection, lactated		RC	10 and 13 g	Precipitate forms relatively rapidly	2222	I
Sodium chloride 0.9%		RC	10 to 40 g	Less than 10% loss in 2 days at 25°C and 10 days at 4°C	1(9/08)	C
Sodium chloride 0.9%		RC	10 g	4% loss in 48 hr and 14% in 72 hr at 20°C. 3% loss in 48 hr and 9% in 72 hr at 4°C	965	C
Sodium chloride 0.9%	MG[c]	RC	20 g	Physically compatible with 10% drug loss in 24 hr and 16% in 48 hr at 25°C under fluorescent light	1026	C
Sodium chloride 0.9%	[b]	RC	40 g	Physically compatible with 5% loss in 3 days at 23°C and 9% loss in 30 days at 4°C	1243	C
Sodium chloride 0.9%	[a]	RC	1 g	10% loss calculated to occur in 10 days at 20°C	1244	C
Sodium chloride 0.9%		RC	10 g	Physically compatible with 9% loss in 7 days at room temperature. 11 to 12% loss in 6 weeks at 5°C	1245	C
Sodium chloride 0.9%		RC	50 g	Physically compatible with 8 to 9% loss in 7 days at room temperature. 5% loss in 5 weeks and 15% in 8 weeks at 5°C	1245	C
Sodium chloride 0.9%			5 and 40 g	Color darkening occurs but only about 3% ceftriaxone loss occurs in 20 days at 4°C	2598	C

Solution Compatibility (Cont.)

Test Soln Name	Mfr	Mfr	Conc/L or %	Remarks	Ref	C/I
Sodium chloride 0.9%	HOS[d]	RC	40 g	Less than 10% loss in 4 days at 23°C and 14 days at 4°C	2819	C
Sodium chloride 0.9%	HOS[d]	RC	5 g	Less than 10% loss in 7 days at 23°C and 21 days at 4°C	2819	C
Sodium lactate ⅙ M		RC	10 to 40 g	Less than 10% loss in 24 hr at 25°C	1(9/08)	C

[a] Tested in glass, PVC, and polyethylene containers.

[b] Tested in PVC containers.

[c] Tested in glass containers.

[d] Tested in Accufusor reservoirs.

Additive Compatibility

Ceftriaxone sodium

Test Drug	Mfr	Conc/L or %	Mfr	Conc/L or %	Test Solution	Remarks	Ref	C/I
Amikacin sulfate	BR	15 and 25 mg	RC	100 mg	D5W	6% loss of amikacin in 24 hr at 22°C	504	C
Aminophylline	AMR	1 g	RC	20 g	D5W, NS[a]	Yellow color forms immediately. 3 to 6% ceftriaxone loss and 8 to 12% aminophylline loss in 24 hr	1727	I
Aminophylline	AMR	4 g	RC	20 g	D5W, NS[a]	Yellow color forms immediately. 15 to 20% ceftriaxone loss and 7 to 9% aminophylline loss in 24 hr	1727	I
Aminophylline	AMR	1 g	RC	40 g	D5W, NS[a]	Yellow color forms immediately. 15 to 18% ceftriaxone loss and 1 to 3% aminophylline loss in 24 hr	1727	I
Calcium chloride						Incompatible. Precipitate may form in calcium-containing solutions	2222, 2731, 2784	I
Calcium gluconate						Incompatible. Precipitate may form in calcium-containing solutions	2222, 2731, 2784	I
Clindamycin phosphate	UP	12 g	RC	20 g	D5W[b]	10% ceftriaxone loss in 4 hr and 17% in 24 hr at 25°C under fluorescent light. No clindamycin loss in 48 hr	1026	I
Clindamycin phosphate	UP	12 g	RC	20 g	NS[b]	10% ceftriaxone loss in 1 hr and 12% in 24 hr at 25°C under fluorescent light. 6% clindamycin loss in 48 hr	1026	I
Gentamicin sulfate	SC	9 mg	RC	100 mg	D5W	13% loss of gentamicin in 8 hr at 22°C	504	I
Gentamicin sulfate	SC	6 mg	RC	100 mg	D5W	5% loss of gentamicin in 24 hr at 22°C	504	C
Linezolid	PHU	2 g	RC	10 g	[d]	Physically compatible, but up to 37% ceftriaxone loss in 24 hr at 23°C and 10% loss in 3 days at 4°C	2262	I
Linezolid	PHU, HOS					Stated to be chemically incompatible	3183, 3184	I
Mannitol		5 and 10%	RC	10 to 40 g		Less than 10% loss in 24 hr at 25°C	1(9/08)	C
Metronidazole	AB	5 g	RC	10 g		Visually compatible with little or no loss of either drug in 72 hr at 8°C	1849	C
Metronidazole	BA	5 g	RC	10 g		Visually compatible with no metronidazole loss and with 6% ceftriaxone loss in 3 days and 8% in 4 days at 25°C	2101	C

Additive Compatibility (Cont.)

Test Drug	Mfr	Conc/L or %	Mfr	Conc/L or %	Test Solution	Remarks	Ref	C/I
Sodium bicarbonate		5%	RC	10 to 40 g		Less than 10% loss in 24 hr at 25°C	1(9/08)	C
Theophylline	BA^c	4 g	RC	40 g		Yellow color forms immediately. 14% ceftriaxone loss and no theophylline loss in 24 hr	1727	I

^a Tested in polyolefin containers.

^b Tested in glass containers.

^c Tested in PVC containers.

^d Admixed in the linezolid infusion container.

Drugs in Syringe Compatibility

Ceftriaxone sodium

Test Drug	Mfr	Amt	Mfr	Amt	Remarks	Ref	C/I
Lidocaine HCl	LY	1%	RC	450 mg/mL	5% ceftriaxone loss in 8 weeks at −15°C but solution failed the particulate matter test	1824	I
Lidocaine HCl	DW	1%	RC	250 and 450 mg/mL	10% ceftriaxone loss in 3 days at 20°C, 7 to 8% loss in 35 days at 4°C, and 4 to 6% loss in 168 days at −20°C. Lidocaine not tested	1991	C

Y-Site Injection Compatibility (1:1 Mixture)

Ceftriaxone sodium

Test Drug	Mfr	Conc	Mfr	Conc	Remarks	Ref	C/I
Acetaminophen	CAD	10 mg/mL	HOS	40 mg/mL	Physically compatible with no loss of either drug in 4 hr at 23°C	2901, 2902	C
Acyclovir sodium	BW	5 mg/mL^a	RC	20 mg/mL^a	Physically compatible for 4 hr at 25°C	1157	C
Allopurinol sodium	BW	3 mg/mL^b	RC	20 mg/mL^b	Physically compatible for 4 hr at 22°C	1686	C
Amifostine	USB	10 mg/mL^a	RC	20 mg/mL^a	Physically compatible for 4 hr at 23°C	1845	C
Amiodarone HCl	WY	6 mg/mL^a	RC	20 mg/mL^a	Turned yellow in 24 hr at 22°C, but considered normal for cephalosporins	2352	C
Amsacrine	NCI	1 mg/mL^a	RC	40 mg/mL^a	Immediate orange turbidity, developing into flocculent precipitate in 4 hr	1381	I
Anakinra	SYN	4 and 36 mg/mL^a	RC	20 mg/mL^a	Ceftriaxone stable. 10% anakinra loss in 30 min and 20% in 4 hr at 22°C	2509	I
Anakinra	SYN	4 and 36 mg/mL^b	RC	20 mg/mL^b	Physically compatible with no loss of either drug in 4 hr at 22°C	2509	C
Anidulafungin	VIC	0.5 mg/mL^a	RC	20 mg/mL^a	Physically compatible for 4 hr at 23°C	2617	C
Azithromycin	PF	2 mg/mL^b	RC	66.7 mg/mL^f g	White and yellow microcrystals found	2368	I
Aztreonam	SQ	40 mg/mL^a	RC	20 mg/mL^a	Physically compatible for 4 hr at 23°C	1758	C
Bivalirudin	TMC	5 mg/mL^a	RC	20 mg/mL^a	Physically compatible for 4 hr at 23°C	2373	C
Blinatumomab	AMG	0.125 and 0.375 mcg/mL^b	PAN	50 mg/mL^b	Particles, flakes, thin needles, or haze transiently appears	3405, 3417	?
Cangrelor tetrasodium	TMC	1 mg/mL^b		20^b and 30^b mg/mL	Physically compatible for 4 hr	3243	C

Y-Site Injection Compatibility (1:1 Mixture) (Cont.)

Test Drug	Mfr	Conc	Mfr	Conc	Remarks	Ref	C/I
Caspofungin acetate	ME	0.7 mg/mL[b]	ORC	20 mg/mL[b]	Immediate white turbid precipitate forms	2758	I
Caspofungin acetate	ME	0.5 mg/mL[b]	NVP	20 mg/mL[b]	Amber crystals and white paste form	2766	I
Ceftolozane sulfate–tazobactam sodium	CUB	10 mg/mL[c k]	HOS	40 mg/mL[c]	Physically compatible for 2 hr	3262	C
Cisatracurium besylate	GW	0.1, 2, 5 mg/mL[a]	RC	20 mg/mL[a]	Physically compatible for 4 hr at 23°C	2074	C
Cloxacillin sodium	SMX	100 mg/mL	SZ	100 mg/mL	Physically compatible for up to 4 hr at room temperature	3245	C
Daptomycin	CUB[j]	16.7 mg/mL[b h]	RC	16.7 mg/mL[b h]	Physically compatible with 4 to 5% loss of both drugs in 2 hr at 25°C	2553	C
Defibrotide sodium	JAZ	8 mg/mL[b]	PAN	100 mg/mL[b]	Visually compatible for 4 hr at room temperature	3149	C
Dexmedetomidine HCl	AB	4 mcg/mL[b]	RC	20 mg/mL[b]	Physically compatible for 4 hr at 23°C	2383	C
Diltiazem HCl	MMD	5 mg/mL	RC	40 mg/mL[b]	Visually compatible	1807	C
Docetaxel	RPR	0.9 mg/mL[a]	RC	20 mg/mL[a]	Physically compatible for 4 hr at 23°C	2224	C
Doxorubicin HCl liposomal	SEQ	0.4 mg/mL[a]	RC	20 mg/mL[a]	Physically compatible for 4 hr at 23°C	2087	C
Etoposide phosphate	BR	5 mg/mL[a]	RC	20 mg/mL[a]	Physically compatible for 4 hr at 23°C	2218	C
Famotidine	ME	2 mg/mL[b]		20 mg/mL[a]	Visually compatible for 4 hr at 22°C	1936	C
Fenoldopam mesylate	AB	80 mcg/mL[b]	RC	20 mg/mL[b]	Physically compatible for 4 hr at 23°C	2467	C
Filgrastim	AMG	30 mcg/mL[a]	RC	20 mg/mL[a]	Particles and filaments form in 1 hr	1687	I
Fluconazole	RR	2 mg/mL	RC	40 mg/mL	Precipitates immediately	1407	I
Fludarabine phosphate	BX	1 mg/mL[a]	RC	20 mg/mL[a]	Visually compatible for 4 hr at 22°C	1439	C
Foscarnet sodium	AST	24 mg/mL	RC	20 mg/mL[c]	Physically compatible for 24 hr at 25°C under fluorescent light	1393	C
Gallium nitrate	FUJ	1 mg/mL[b]	RC	40 mg/mL[b]	Visually compatible for 24 hr at 25°C	1673	C
Gemcitabine HCl	LI	10 mg/mL[b]	RC	20 mg/mL[b]	Physically compatible for 4 hr at 23°C	2226	C
Granisetron HCl	SKB	0.05 mg/mL[a]	RC	20 mg/mL[a]	Physically compatible for 4 hr at 23°C	2000	C
Heparin sodium	TR	50 units/mL	RC	20 mg/mL	Visually compatible for 4 hr at 25°C	1793	C
Hydroxyethyl starch 130/0.4 in sodium chloride 0.9%	FRK	6%	RC	20, 30, 40 mg/mL[a]	Visually compatible for 24 hr at room temperature	2770	C
Isavuconazonium sulfate	ASP	1.5 mg/mL[c]	WOC	20 mg/mL[c]	Measured turbidity increases immediately with precipitation within 1 hr	3263	I
Labetalol HCl	GL	2.5[d] and 5 mg/mL	RC	20[a b] and 100[d] mg/mL	Fluffy white precipitate forms immediately	1964	I
Letermovir	ME	[a]		[a]	Physically compatible	3398	C

Y-Site Injection Compatibility (1:1 Mixture) (Cont.)

Test Drug	Mfr	Conc	Mfr	Conc	Remarks	Ref	C/I
Linezolid	PHU	2 mg/mL	RC	20 mg/mL[a]	Physically compatible for 4 hr at 23°C	2264	C
Melphalan HCl	BW	0.1 mg/mL[b]	RC	20 mg/mL[b]	Physically compatible for 3 hr at 22°C	1557	C
Meperidine HCl	AB	10 mg/mL	RC	20 and 40 mg/mL[a]	Physically compatible for 4 hr at 25°C	1397	C
Meropenem		50 mg/mL	SMX	100 mg/mL	Physically compatible for 4 hr at room temperature	3538	C
Meropenem–vaborbactam	TMC	8 mg/mL[b l]	SGT	20 mg/mL[b]	Physically compatible for 3 hr at 20 to 25°C	3380	C
Methotrexate sodium		30 mg/mL	RC	100 mg/mL	Visually compatible for 4 hr at room temperature	1788	C
Morphine sulfate	AB	1 mg/mL	RC	20 and 40 mg/mL[a]	Physically compatible for 4 hr at 25°C	1397	C
Paclitaxel	NCI	1.2 mg/mL[a]	RC	20 mg/mL[a]	Physically compatible for 4 hr at 22°C	1556	C
Pantoprazole sodium	ALT[i]	0.16 to 0.8 mg/mL[b]	RC	20 to 40 mg/mL[a]	Visually compatible for 12 hr at 23°C	2603	C
Pemetrexed disodium	LI	20 mg/mL[b]	RC	20 mg/mL[a]	Physically compatible for 4 hr at 23°C	2564	C
Pentamidine isethionate	FUJ	3 mg/mL[a]	RC	20 mg/mL[a]	Heavy white precipitate forms immediately	1880	I
Plazomicin sulfate	ACH	24 mg/mL[c]	HOS	20 mg/mL[c]	Physically compatible for 1 hr at 20 to 25°C	3432	C
Propofol	ZEN[n]	10 mg/mL	RC	20 mg/mL[a]	Physically compatible for 1 hr at 23°C	2066	C
Remifentanil HCl	GW	0.025 and 0.25 mg/mL[b]	RC	20 mg/mL[a]	Physically compatible for 4 hr at 23°C	2075	C
Sargramostim	IMM	10 mcg/mL[b]	RC	20 mg/mL[b]	Visually compatible for 4 hr at 22°C	1436	C
Sodium bicarbonate		1.4%	RC	100 mg/mL	Visually compatible for 4 hr at room temperature	1788	C
Tacrolimus	FUJ	1 mg/mL[b]	RC	40 mg/mL[a]	Visually compatible for 24 hr at 25°C	1630	C
Tedizolid phosphate	CUB	0.8 mg/mL[b]	WOC	20 mg/mL[b]	Physically compatible for 2 hr	3244	C
Telavancin HCl	ASP	7.5 mg/mL[a b]	HOS	20 mg/mL[a b]	Physically compatible for 2 hr	2830	C
Teniposide	BR	0.1 mg/mL[a]	RC	20 mg/mL[a]	Physically compatible for 4 hr at 23°C	1725	C
Theophylline	TR	4 mg/mL	RC	20 mg/mL	Visually compatible for 6 hr at 25°C	1793	C
Thiotepa	IMM[e]	1 mg/mL[a]	RC	20 mg/mL[a]	Physically compatible for 4 hr at 23°C	1861	C
Tigecycline	WY	1 mg/mL[b]		40 mg/mL[b]	Physically compatible for 4 hr	2714	C
TNA #218 to #226[m]			RC	20 mg/mL[a]	Visually compatible for 4 hr at 23°C	2215	C
Vancomycin HCl	LI	20 mg/mL	RC	100 mg/mL	White precipitate forms immediately	1398	I
Vancomycin HCl	AB	20 mg/mL[a]	RC	250 mg/mL[d]	Transient precipitate forms	2189	?
Vancomycin HCl	AB	20 mg/mL[a]	RC	10 and 50 mg/mL[a]	Gross white precipitate forms immediately	2189	I
Vancomycin HCl	AB	20 mg/mL[a]	RC	1 mg/mL[a]	Subvisible haze forms immediately	2189	I
Vancomycin HCl	AB	2 mg/mL[a]	RC	1[a], 10[a], 50[a], 250[d] mg/mL	Physically compatible for 4 hr at 23°C	2189	C

Y-Site Injection Compatibility (1:1 Mixture) (Cont.)

Test Drug	Mfr	Conc	Mfr	Conc	Remarks	Ref	C/I
Vinorelbine tartrate	BW	1 mg/mL[b]	RC	20 mg/mL[b]	Tiny particles form immediately, becoming more numerous in 4 hr at 22°C	1558	I
Zidovudine	BW	4 mg/mL[a]	RC	20 mg/mL[a]	Physically compatible for 4 hr at 25°C	1193	C

[a] Tested in dextrose 5%.

[b] Tested in sodium chloride 0.9%.

[c] Tested in both dextrose 5% and sodium chloride 0.9%.

[d] Tested in sterile water for injection.

[e] Lyophilized formulation tested.

[f] Tested in sodium chloride 0.45%.

[g] Injected via Y-site into an administration set running azithromycin.

[h] Final concentration after mixing.

[i] Test performed using the formulation WITHOUT edetate disodium.

[j] Test performed using the Cubicin formulation.

[k] Ceftolozane component. Ceftolozane in a 2:1 fixed-ratio concentration with tazobactam.

[l] Meropenem component. Meropenem in a 1:1 fixed-ratio concentration with vaborbactam.

[m] Refer to Appendix for the composition of parenteral nutrition solutions. TNA indicates a 3-in-1 admixture, and TPN indicates a 2-in-1 admixture.

[n] Test performed using the formulation WITH edetate disodium.

Additional Compatibility Information
Peritoneal Dialysis Solutions

Ceftriaxone sodium (Roche) 1 mg/mL in Dianeal PD-1 with dextrose 1.5 and 4.25% was stable, retaining at least 90% for 14 days at 4°C, 24 hours at 23°C, or 6 hours at 37°C.[1592]

Selected Revisions May 1, 2020. © Copyright, October 1986. American Society of Health-System Pharmacists, Inc.

Cefuroxime Sodium
AHFS 8:12.06.08

Products

Cefuroxime sodium is available in vials containing 750 mg and 1.5 g of cefuroxime as the sodium salt.[3567]

For intravenous administration, the 750-mg and 1.5-g vials should be reconstituted with 8.3 and 16 mL, respectively, of sterile water for injection to yield a solution with an approximate cefuroxime concentration of 90 mg/mL.[3567]

For intramuscular administration, the 750-mg vial only should be reconstituted with 3 mL of sterile water for injection to yield a suspension with an approximate cefuroxime concentration of 225 mg/mL.[3567] The suspension should be dispersed with shaking before the dose is withdrawn.[3567]

pH

The pH of freshly reconstituted solutions ranges from 6 to 8.5.[3567]

Osmolality

The osmolality of cefuroxime sodium (Glaxo) diluted to a cefuroxime concentration of 30 mg/mL in dextrose 5% was determined to be 315 mOsm/kg and in sodium chloride 0.9% was determined to be 314 mOsm/kg. At a cefuroxime concentration of 50 mg/mL, the osmolality was determined to be 329 mOsm/kg in dextrose 5% and 335 mOsm/kg in sodium chloride 0.9%.[1375]

The following maximum cefuroxime concentrations were recommended to achieve osmolalities suitable for peripheral infusion in fluid-restricted patients:[1180]

Diluent	Maximum Concentration (mg/mL)	Osmolality (mOsm/kg)
Dextrose 5%	76	568
Sodium chloride 0.9%	68	541
Sterile water for injection	137	489

Sodium Content

Cefuroxime sodium (Teligent) vials contain approximately 2.4 mEq (54.2 mg) of sodium per gram of cefuroxime.[3567]

Trade Name(s)

Kefurox, Zinacef

Administration

Cefuroxime sodium is administered by deep intramuscular injection, by direct intravenous injection over 3 to 5 minutes directly into the vein or into the tubing of a running infusion solution, by intermittent intravenous infusion, or by continuous intravenous infusion.[3567] The manufacturer recommends temporarily discontinuing any other solutions infusing at the same site when administering the drug by Y-site infusion.[3567]

Stability

Intact vials of cefuroxime sodium should be stored at 15 to 30°C and protected from light.[3567] The drug is present as a white to off-white powder.[3567] Solutions may range in color from light yellow to amber, depending on the concentration and diluent used.[3567] Cefuroxime sodium powder and solutions and suspensions prepared from cefuroxime sodium tend to darken, depending on storage conditions, without affecting their potency.[3567]

The reconstituted suspension for intramuscular injection and solution for intravenous administration prepared as directed are stable for 24 hours at room temperature and 48 hours refrigerated at 5°C.[3567]

pH Effects

The pH of maximum stability is in the range of 4.5 to 7.3.[712]

Freezing Solutions

Solutions of cefuroxime prepared as directed by reconstituting 750-mg or 1.5-g vials and immediately adding the reconstituted solution to 50 or 100 mL of sodium chloride 0.9% or dextrose 5% in a compatible container are stable for 6 months at −20°C.[3567] The manufacturer states that frozen solutions should be thawed at room temperature; the use of water baths or microwaves for force thawing is not recommended.[3567] Following thawing at room temperature, the solutions are stable for 24 hours at room temperature or 7 days under refrigeration.[3567] Thawed solutions should not be refrozen.[3567]

Minibags of cefuroxime sodium in dextrose 5% or sodium chloride 0.9% were frozen at −20°C for up to 35 days and subsequently thawed at room temperature and in a microwave oven with care taken that the thawed solution temperature never exceeded 25°C. No significant differences in cefuroxime concentrations occurred between the thawing methods.[1192]

Cefuroxime sodium (Glaxo) diluted to cefuroxime concentrations of 30 and 60 mg/mL in sterile water for injection in polyvinyl chloride (PVC) portable infusion pump reservoirs (Pharmacia Deltec) and glass vials exhibited a 4% loss after 30 days at −20°C. Subsequent storage for 4 days at 3°C resulted in about a 10% loss in the PVC bags and a 4% loss in the glass vials.[1581]

Cefuroxime sodium diluted to a cefuroxime concentration of 15 mg/mL (i.e., 1.5 g/100 mL) in dextrose 5% in polyolefin bags was reported to be physically and chemically stable for 98 days stored at −20°C. Less than 10% drug loss occurred upon microwave thawing and subsequent refrigerated storage for 18 to 21 days.[2592]

Cefuroxime sodium (Panpharma) diluted to a cefuroxime concentration of 10 mg/mL in sodium chloride 0.9% and stored in polypropylene syringes (Becton Dickinson) protected from light at −20°C was stable for 365 days.[3271]

DOI: 10.37573/9781585286850.083

Syringes

Cefuroxime sodium (Panpharma) diluted to a cefuroxime concentration of 10 mg/mL in sodium chloride 0.9% and stored in polypropylene syringes (Becton Dickinson) protected from light at 5°C and 25°C with 60% relatively humidity was stable for 21 days and 9 hours, respectively.[3271]

Cefuroxime sodium (GlaxoSmithKline) diluted to a cefuroxime concentration of 90 mg/mL in sodium chloride 0.9% was stored as 50 mL in 50-mL polypropylene syringes.[3566] Syringes stored at 2 to 8°C protected from light demonstrated less than 4% loss in theoretical concentration in 14 days with no significant change in physical appearance.[3566] Syringes stored at 20 to 25°C both protected from and exposed to light demonstrated less than 10% loss in 2 days; syringes stored without light protection underwent a more intense yellowing in color than did those protected from light.[3566] Syringes stored at 38 to 42°C protected from light exhibited losses of more than 40% of theoretical concentra-

tion after as little as 1 day.[3566] pH of the solutions was not measured.[3566]

Ambulatory Pumps

Cefuroxime sodium (Glaxo) diluted to cefuroxime concentrations of 22.5 and 45 mg/mL in sterile water for injection in PVC portable infusion pump reservoirs (Pharmacia Deltec) exhibited a 4 to 6% loss in 8 hours and an 11 to 12% loss in 16 hours at 30°C. No loss occurred in 7 days at 3°C.[1581]

Central Venous Catheter

Cefuroxime sodium (Glaxo Wellcome) diluted to a cefuroxime concentration of 10 mg/mL in dextrose 5% was found to be compatible with the ARROWg+ard Blue Plus (Arrow International) chlorhexidine-bearing triple-lumen central catheter. Essentially complete delivery of the drug was found with little or no drug loss occurring. Furthermore, chlorhexidine delivered from the catheter remained at trace amounts with no substantial increase due to the delivery of the drug through the catheter.[2335]

Compatibility Information

Solution Compatibility

Cefuroxime sodium

Test Soln Name	Mfr	Mfr	Conc/L or %	Remarks	Ref	C/I
Dextrose 5% in sodium chloride 0.225%		TEL	1 to 30 g	Less than 10% loss in 24 hr at room temperature and 7 days refrigerated	3567	C
Dextrose 5% in sodium chloride 0.45%		TEL	1 to 30 g	Less than 10% loss in 24 hr at room temperature and 7 days refrigerated	3567	C
Dextrose 5% in sodium chloride 0.9%		TEL	1 to 30 g	Less than 10% loss in 24 hr at room temperature and 7 days refrigerated	3567	C
Dextrose 5%		TEL	1 to 30 g	Less than 10% loss in 24 hr at room temperature and 7 days refrigerated	3567	C
Dextrose 5%		TEL	7.5 and 15 g	Stable for 24 hr at room temperature and 7 days refrigerated	3567	C
Dextrose 5%	MG[a]	GL	15 g	5% loss in 48 hr at 25°C under fluorescent light	1164	C
Dextrose 5%	[b]		6 g	Visually compatible with little or no loss in 24 hr at room temperature and 4°C	1953	C
Dextrose 5%	BA[a]	GL	15 g	Visually compatible with 7% loss in 11 days at 4°C	2142	C
Dextrose 5%	BA[a b]	GL	5 and 10 g	Physically compatible with about 7% cefuroxime loss in 24 hr and 13% loss in 48 hr at 25°C. About 4% loss at 5°C and no loss at −10°C in 30 days	712	C
Dextrose 5%	[d]		15 g	Visually compatible with about 6% loss by in 31 days at 4°C	2661	C
Dextrose 10%		TEL	1 to 30 g	Less than 10% loss in 24 hr at room temperature and 7 days refrigerated	3567	C
Invert sugar 10%		TEL	1 to 30 g	Less than 10% loss in 24 hr at room temperature and 7 days refrigerated	3567	C
Ringer's injection		TEL	1 to 30 g	Less than 10% loss in 24 hr at room temperature and 7 days refrigerated	3567	C
Ringer's injection, lactated		TEL	1 to 30 g	Less than 10% loss in 24 hr at room temperature and 7 days refrigerated	3567	C
Sodium chloride 0.9%		TEL	1 to 30 g	Less than 10% loss in 24 hr at room temperature and 7 days refrigerated	3567	C
Sodium chloride 0.9%		TEL	7.5 and 15 g	Stable for 24 hr at room temperature and 7 days refrigerated	3567	C
Sodium chloride 0.9%	MG[a]	GL	15 g	5% loss in 48 hr at 25°C under fluorescent light	1164	C
Sodium chloride 0.9%	[b]		6 g	Visually compatible with little or no loss in 24 hr at room temperature and 4°C	1953	C

Solution Compatibility (Cont.)

Test Soln Name	Mfr	Mfr	Conc/L or %	Remarks	Ref	C/I
Sodium chloride 0.9%	BA[a][b]	GL	5 and 10 g	Physically compatible with about 7% cefuroxime loss in 24 hr and 13% loss in 48 hr at 25°C. About 4% loss at 5°C and no loss at −10°C in 30 days	712	C
Sodium chloride 0.9%	[e]	PAN	10 g	Less than 10% loss in 365 days, 21 days, and 16 hours protected from light at −20, 5, and 25°C with 60% relatively humidity, respectively	3271	C
Sodium lactate ⅙ M		TEL	1 to 30 g	Less than 10% loss in 24 hr at room temperature and 7 days refrigerated	3567	C
TPN #107[c]			1 g	Activity retained for 24 hr at 21°C	1326	C

[a] Tested in glass containers.

[b] Tested in PVC containers.

[c] Refer to Appendix for the composition of parenteral nutrition solutions. TPN indicates a 2-in-1 admixture.

[d] Tested in polyolefin containers.

[e] Tested in cyclic olefin copolymer (COC) Crystal vials filled using an automated primary packaging system.

Additive Compatibility

Cefuroxime sodium

Test Drug	Mfr	Conc/L or %	Mfr	Conc/L or %	Test Solution	Remarks	Ref	C/I
Ciprofloxacin	MI	2 g		30 g	D5W	Physically incompatible	888	I
Ciprofloxacin	BAY	2 g	GW	30 g	D5W	Visually compatible for 6 hr, but small particles appeared by 24 hr at about 22°C	2413	I
Clindamycin phosphate	UP	9 g	GL	15 g	D5W	Physically compatible with 4% clindamycin loss and 6 to 8% cefuroxime loss in 48 hr at 25°C under fluorescent light	1164	C
Clindamycin phosphate	UP	9 g	GL	15 g	NS	Physically compatible with 9% clindamycin and cefuroxime losses in 48 hr at 25°C under fluorescent light	1164	C
Floxacillin sodium	BE	20 g	GL	37.5 g	W	Physically compatible for 72 hr at 15 and 30°C	1479	C
Floxacillin sodium	BE	10 g	GL	7.5 g	D5W, NS	Physically compatible for 48 hr. Both drugs stable for 1 hr at room temperature	1036	C
Furosemide	HO	1 g	GL	37.5 g	W	Physically compatible for 72 hr at 15 and 30°C	1479	C
Gentamicin sulfate	EX	800 mg	GL	7.5 g	D5W, NS[b]	Physically compatible with no loss of either drug in 1 hr	1036	C
Gentamicin sulfate		100 mg		1 g	TPN #107[c]	32% gentamicin loss in 24 hr at 21°C	1326	I
Heparin sodium		10,000 and 50,000 units	TEL		NS	Stable for 24 hr at room temperature	3567	C
Metronidazole		5 g	GL	7.5 g	[b]	Physically compatible with no loss of either drug in 1 hr	1036	C
Metronidazole		5 g	GL	15 g		No loss of either drug in 4 hr at 24°C	1376	C
Metronidazole		5 g	GL	7.5 g		10% cefuroxime loss in 16 days at 4°C and 35 hr at 25°C. No metronidazole loss in 15 days at 4 and 25°C	1565	C
Metronidazole	IVX	5 g	GL	7.5 and 15 g		Physically compatible. No loss of metronidazole and about 6% cefuroxime loss in 49 days at 5°C	2192	C
Midazolam HCl	RC	50, 250, 400 mg	GL	7.5 g	NS	Visually compatible for 4 hr	355	C
Potassium chloride		10 and 40 mEq	TEL		NS	Stable for 24 hr at room temperature	3567	C

Additive Compatibility (Cont.)

Test Drug	Mfr	Conc/L or %	Mfr	Conc/L or %	Test Solution	Remarks	Ref	C/I
Ranitidine HCl	GL	100 mg	GL	1.5 g	D5W	Color change in 24 hr at ambient temperature in light	1151	?
Ranitidine HCl	GL	50 mg and 2 g		6 g	D5W	Ranitidine stable for only 6 hr at 25°C. Cefuroxime not tested	1515	I

ª Tested in both glass and PVC containers.

ᵇ Tested in PVC containers.

ᶜ Refer to Appendix for the composition of parenteral nutrition solutions. TPN indicates a 2-in-1 admixture.

ᵈ Tested in glass containers.

Drugs in Syringe Compatibility

Cefuroxime sodium

Test Drug	Mfr	Amt	Mfr	Amt	Remarks	Ref	C/I
Dimenhydrinate		10 mg/1 mL		100 mg/1 mL	Clear solution	2569	C
Doxapram HCl	RB	400 mg/20 mL	GL	750 mg/7 mL	Immediate turbidity	1177	I
Pantoprazole sodium	ª	4 mg/1 mL		100 mg/1 mL	Precipitates immediately	2574	I

ª Test performed using the formulation WITHOUT edetate disodium.

Y-Site Injection Compatibility (1:1 Mixture)

Cefuroxime sodium

Test Drug	Mfr	Conc	Mfr	Conc	Remarks	Ref	C/I
Acyclovir sodium	BW	5 mg/mLª	GL	15 mg/mLª	Physically compatible for 4 hr at 25°C	1157	C
Allopurinol sodium	BW	3 mg/mLᵇ	GL	20 mg/mLᵇ	Physically compatible for 4 hr at 22°C	1686	C
Amifostine	USB	10 mg/mLª	GL	30 mg/mLª	Physically compatible for 4 hr at 23°C	1845	C
Amiodarone HCl	WY	6 mg/mLª	BA	30 mg/mLª	Turned yellow in 24 hr at 22°C, but considered normal for cephalosporins	2352	C
Anidulafungin	VIC	0.5 mg/mLª	GSK	30 mg/mLª	Physically compatible for 4 hr at 23°C	2617	C
Atracurium besylate	BW	0.5 mg/mLª	GL	7.5 mg/mLª	Physically compatible for 24 hr at 28°C	1337	C
Azithromycin	PF	2 mg/mLᵇ	VHA	100 mg/mLᶠ ᵍ	White and yellow microcrystals	2368	I
Aztreonam	SQ	40 mg/mLª	LI	30 mg/mLª	Physically compatible for 4 hr at 23°C	1758	C
Bivalirudin	TMC	5 mg/mLª	GW	30 mg/mLª	Physically compatible for 4 hr at 23°C	2373	C
Ceftolozane sulfate–tazobactam sodium	CUB	10 mg/mLʰ ⁱ	COV	30 mg/mLʰ	Physically compatible for 2 hr	3262	C
Cisatracurium besylate	GW	0.1 mg/mLª	LI	30 mg/mLª	Physically compatible for 4 hr at 23°C	2074	C
Cisatracurium besylate	GW	2 mg/mLª	LI	30 mg/mLª	White cloudiness forms immediately	2074	I
Cisatracurium besylate	GW	5 mg/mLª	LI	30 mg/mLª	Turbidity forms immediately	2074	I
Clarithromycin	AB	4 mg/mLª	GW	60 mg/mLª	White precipitate forms in 3 hr at 30°C and 24 hr at 17°C	2174	I
Cloxacillin sodium	SMX	100 mg/mL	PPC	90 mg/mL	Physically compatible for up to 4 hr at room temperature	3245	C
Cyclophosphamide	MJ	20 mg/mLª	GL	30 mg/mLª	Physically compatible for 4 hr at 25°C	1194	C

Y-Site Injection Compatibility (1:1 Mixture) (Cont.)

Test Drug	Mfr	Conc	Mfr	Conc	Remarks	Ref	C/I
Dexmedetomidine HCl	AB	4 mcg/mL[b]	GW	30 mg/mL[b]	Physically compatible for 4 hr at 23°C	2383	C
Diltiazem HCl	MMD	5 mg/mL	LI	15 and 100 mg/mL[b]	Visually compatible	1807	C
Diltiazem HCl	MMD	1 mg/mL[b]	LI	100 mg/mL[b]	Visually compatible	1807	C
Docetaxel	RPR	0.9 mg/mL[a]	LI	30 mg/mL[a]	Physically compatible for 4 hr at 23°C	2224	C
Etoposide phosphate	BR	5 mg/mL[a]	GW	30 mg/mL[a]	Physically compatible for 4 hr at 23°C	2218	C
Famotidine	MSD	0.2 mg/mL[a]	GL	15 mg/mL[b]	Physically compatible for 14 hr	1196	C
Famotidine	ME	2 mg/mL[b]		20 mg/mL[a]	Visually compatible for 4 hr at 22°C	1936	C
Fenoldopam mesylate	AB	80 mcg/mL[b]	GW	30 mg/mL[b]	Physically compatible for 4 hr at 23°C	2467	C
Filgrastim	AMG	30 mcg/mL[a]	GL	20 mg/mL[a]	Haze, particles, and filaments form immediately	1687	I
Fluconazole	RR	2 mg/mL	GL	30 mg/mL	Precipitates immediately	1407	I
Fludarabine phosphate	BX	1 mg/mL[a]	GL	30 mg/mL[a]	Visually compatible for 4 hr at 22°C	1439	C
Foscarnet sodium	AST	24 mg/mL[b]	GL	30 mg/mL	Physically compatible for 24 hr at room temperature under fluorescent light	1335	C
Gemcitabine HCl	LI	10 mg/mL[b]	GW	30 mg/mL[b]	Physically compatible for 4 hr at 23°C	2226	C
Granisetron HCl	SKB	0.05 mg/mL[a]	LI	30 mg/mL[a]	Physically compatible for 4 hr at 23°C	2000	C
Hetastarch in lactated electrolyte	AB	6%	LI	30 mg/mL[a]	Physically compatible for 4 hr at 23°C	2339	C
Hydromorphone HCl	WY	0.2 mg/mL[a]	GL	30 mg/mL[a]	Physically compatible for 4 hr at 25°C	987	C
Isavuconazonium sulfate	ASP	1.5 mg/mL[h]	COV	30 mg/mL[h]	Measured turbidity increases immediately	3263	I
Linezolid	PHU	2 mg/mL	GL	30 mg/mL[a]	Physically compatible for 4 hr at 23°C	2264	C
Melphalan HCl	BW	0.1 mg/mL[b]	GL	20 mg/mL[b]	Physically compatible for 3 hr at 22°C	1557	C
Meperidine HCl	WY	10 mg/mL[a]	GL	30 mg/mL[a]	Physically compatible for 4 hr at 25°C	987	C
Meropenem		50 mg/mL	SMX	100 mg/mL	Physically compatible for 4 hr at room temperature	3538	C
Meropenem–vaborbactam	TMC	8 mg/mL[b j]	SGT	30 mg/mL[b]	Physically compatible for 3 hr at 20 to 25°C	3380	C
Midazolam HCl	RC	1 mg/mL[a]	LI	15 mg/mL[a]	Particles form in 8 hr	1847	I
Milrinone lactate	SS	0.2 mg/mL[a]	LI	100 mg/mL[a]	Visually compatible for 4 hr at 25°C	2381	C
Morphine sulfate	WI	1 mg/mL[a]	GL	30 mg/mL[a]	Physically compatible for 4 hr at 25°C	987	C
Ondansetron HCl	GL	1 mg/mL[b]	LI	30 mg/mL[a]	Visually compatible for 4 hr at 22°C	1365	C
Pancuronium bromide	ES	0.05 mg/mL[a]	GL	7.5 mg/mL[a]	Physically compatible for 24 hr at 28°C	1337	C
Pemetrexed disodium	LI	20 mg/mL[b]	GSK	30 mg/mL[a]	Physically compatible for 4 hr at 23°C	2564	C
Plazomicin sulfate	ACH	24 mg/mL[h]	HIK	30 mg/mL[h]	Physically compatible for 1 hr at 20 to 25°C	3432	C
Propofol	ZEN[k]	10 mg/mL	LI	30 mg/mL[a]	Physically compatible for 1 hr at 23°C	2066	C
Remifentanil HCl	GW	0.025 and 0.25 mg/mL[b]	LI	30 mg/mL[a]	Physically compatible for 4 hr at 23°C	2075	C
Sargramostim	IMM	10 mcg/mL[b]	GL	30 mg/mL[b]	Visually compatible for 4 hr at 22°C	1436	C
Tacrolimus	FUJ	1 mg/mL[b]	LI	30 mg/mL[a]	Visually compatible for 24 hr at 25°C	1630	C
Tedizolid phosphate	CUB	0.8 mg/mL[b]	COV	30 mg/mL[b]	Physically compatible for 2 hr	3244	C

Y-Site Injection Compatibility (1:1 Mixture) (Cont.)

Test Drug	Mfr	Conc	Mfr	Conc	Remarks	Ref	C/I
Teniposide	BR	0.1 mg/mL[a]	GL	20 mg/mL[a]	Physically compatible for 4 hr at 23°C	1725	C
Thiotepa	IMM[c]	1 mg/mL[a]	LI	30 mg/mL[a]	Physically compatible for 4 hr at 23°C	1861	C
TNA #218 to #226[d]			GL	30 mg/mL[a]	Visually compatible for 4 hr at 23°C	2215	C
TPN #212 to #215[d]			LI	30 mg/mL[a]	Physically compatible for 4 hr at 23°C	2109	C
Vancomycin HCl	AB	20 mg/mL[a]	GW	150 mg/mL[e]	Transient precipitate forms followed by a subvisible haze	2189	I
Vancomycin HCl	AB	20 mg/mL[a]	GW	50 mg/mL[a]	Gross white precipitate forms immediately	2189	I
Vancomycin HCl	AB	20 mg/mL[a]	GW	10 mg/mL[a]	Subvisible haze forms immediately	2189	I
Vancomycin HCl	AB	20 mg/mL[a]	GW	1 mg/mL[a]	Physically compatible for 4 hr at 23°C	2189	C
Vancomycin HCl	AB	2 mg/mL[a]	GW	1[a], 10[a], 50[a], 150[e] mg/mL	Physically compatible for 4 hr at 23°C	2189	C
Vecuronium bromide	OR	0.1 mg/mL[a]	GL	7.5 mg/mL[a]	Physically compatible for 24 hr at 28°C	1337	C
Vinorelbine tartrate	BW	1 mg/mL[b]	GL	20 mg/mL[b]	Large increase in measured turbidity occurs immediately	1558	I

[a] Tested in dextrose 5%.

[b] Tested in sodium chloride 0.9%.

[c] Lyophilized formulation tested.

[d] Refer to Appendix for the composition of parenteral nutrition solutions. TNA indicates a 3-in-1 admixture, and TPN indicates a 2-in-1 admixture.

[e] Tested in sterile water for injection.

[f] Tested in sodium chloride 0.45%.

[g] Injected via Y-site into an administration set running azithromycin.

[h] Tested in both dextrose 5% and sodium chloride 0.9%.

[i] Ceftolozane component. Ceftolozane in a 2:1 fixed-ratio concentration with tazobactam.

[j] Meropenem component. Meropenem in a 1:1 fixed-ratio concentration with vaborbactam.

[k] Test performed using the formulation WITH edetate disodium.

Selected Revisions July 1, 2020. © Copyright, October 1986.
American Society of Health-System Pharmacists, Inc.

Chloramphenicol Sodium Succinate
AHFS 8:12.08

Products

Chloramphenicol sodium succinate is available in vials containing the equivalent of chloramphenicol 1 g as the sodium succinate salt. The manufacturer recommends reconstitution with 10 mL of an aqueous diluent such as water for injection or dextrose 5% to yield a solution containing 100 mg/mL (10%) of chloramphenicol.[1(4/07)] [4]

pH

From 6.4 to 7.[4] [6]

Osmolality

Chloramphenicol sodium succinate 100 mg/mL in sterile water for injection has an osmolality of 533 mOsm/kg as determined by freezing-point depression.[1071]

The osmolality of chloramphenicol sodium succinate 1 g was calculated for the following dilutions:[1054]

Diluent	Osmolality (mOsm/kg)	
	50 mL	100 mL
Dextrose 5%	341	303
Sodium chloride 0.9%	368	330

The osmolality of chloramphenicol sodium succinate (Parke-Davis) 20 mg/mL was determined to be 330 mOsm/kg in dextrose 5% and 344 mOsm/kg in sodium chloride 0.9%. At 50 mg/mL, the osmolality was determined to be 417 and 422 mOsm/kg, respectively.[1375]

The following maximum chloramphenicol sodium succinate concentrations were recommended to achieve osmolalities suitable for peripheral infusion in fluid-restricted patients:[1180]

Diluent	Maximum Concentration (mg/mL)	Osmolality (mOsm/kg)
Dextrose 5%	71	554
Sodium chloride 0.9%	64	538
Sterile water for injection	128	473

Sodium Content

Chloramphenicol sodium succinate contains 2.25 mEq (52 mg) of sodium per gram of drug.[1(4/07)] [4]

Administration

Chloramphenicol sodium succinate injection at a concentration not exceeding 100 mg/mL may be administered by direct intravenous injection over at least 1 minute.[1(4/07)] [4]

Stability

Intact vials should be stored at controlled room temperature. The reconstituted solution is stable for 30 days at room temperature.[4] [6] Cloudy solutions should not be used.[4]

pH Effects

Chloramphenicol is stable over a pH range of 2 to 7, with maximum stability at pH 6.[1072] Chloramphenicol activity was retained for 24 hours at pH 3.6 to 7.5 in dextrose 5%.[6]

Sorption

Chloramphenicol sodium succinate was shown not to exhibit sorption to PVC bags and tubing, polyethylene tubing, Silastic tubing, and polypropylene syringes.[536] [606]

Compatibility Information

Solution Compatibility

Chloramphenicol sodium succinate

Test Soln Name	Mfr	Mfr	Conc/L or %	Remarks	Ref	C/I
Dextrose 2.5% in half-strength Ringer's injection	AB	PD	1 g	Physically compatible	3	C
Dextrose 5% in Ringer's injection	AB	PD	1 g	Physically compatible	3	C
Dextrose 5% in half-strength Ringer's injection, lactated	AB	PD	1 g	Physically compatible	3	C
Dextrose 2.5% in Ringer's injection, lactated	AB	PD	1 g	Physically compatible	3	C
Dextrose 5% in Ringer's injection, lactated	AB	PD	1 g	Physically compatible	3	C
Dextrose 5% in Ringer's injection, lactated	AB			Stable for 24 hr	6	C
Dextrose 10% in Ringer's injection, lactated	AB	PD	1 g	Physically compatible	3	C
Dextrose 2.5% in sodium chloride 0.45%	AB	PD	1 g	Physically compatible	3	C

DOI: 10.37573/9781585286850.084

Solution Compatibility (Cont.)

Test Soln Name	Mfr	Mfr	Conc/L or %	Remarks	Ref	C/I
Dextrose 2.5% in sodium chloride 0.9%	AB	PD	1 g	Physically compatible	3	C
Dextrose 5% in sodium chloride 0.225%	AB	PD	1 g	Physically compatible	3	C
Dextrose 5% in sodium chloride 0.45%	AB	PD	1 g	Physically compatible	3	C
Dextrose 5% in sodium chloride 0.9%	AB	PD	1 g	Physically compatible	3	C
Dextrose 5% in sodium chloride 0.9%		PD	500 mg	Physically compatible	74	C
Dextrose 5% in sodium chloride 0.9%	AB			Stable for 24 hr	6	C
Dextrose 5% in sodium chloride 0.9%		PD	2 g	Stable for 24 hr	109	C
Dextrose 10% in sodium chloride 0.9%	AB	PD	1 g	Physically compatible	3	C
Dextrose 2.5%	AB	PD	1 g	Physically compatible	3	C
Dextrose 5%	AB	PD	1 g	Physically compatible	3	C
Dextrose 5%		PD	500 mg	Physically compatible	74	C
Dextrose 5%	AB			Stable for 24 hr	6	C
Dextrose 5%		PD	2 g	Stable for 24 hr	109	C
Dextrose 5%			10 g	4% loss in 24 hr at room temperature	768	C
Dextrose 10%	AB	PD	1 g	Physically compatible	3	C
Dextrose 10%	AB			Stable for 24 hr	6	C
Dextrose 10%		PD	2 g	Stable for 24 hr	109	C
Ionosol B in dextrose 5%	AB	PD	1 g	Physically compatible	3	C
Ionosol MB in dextrose 5%	AB	PD	1 g	Physically compatible	3	C
Normosol M in dextrose 5%	AB			Stable for 24 hr	6	C
Normosol R	AB			Stable for 24 hr	6	C
Ringer's injection	AB	PD	1 g	Physically compatible	3	C
Ringer's injection	AB			Stable for 24 hr	6	C
Ringer's injection, lactated	AB	PD	1 g	Physically compatible	3	C
Ringer's injection, lactated		PD	500 mg	Physically compatible	74	C
Ringer's injection, lactated	AB			Stable for 24 hr	6	C
Sodium chloride 0.45%	AB	PD	1 g	Physically compatible	3	C
Sodium chloride 0.9%	AB	PD	1 g	Physically compatible	3	C
Sodium chloride 0.9%		PD	500 mg	Physically compatible	74	C
Sodium chloride 0.9%	AB			Stable for 24 hr	6	C
Sodium chloride 0.9%		PD	2 g	Stable for 24 hr	109	C
Sodium chloride 0.9%			10 g	4% loss in 24 hr at room temperature	768	C
Sodium lactate ⅙ M	AB	PD	1 g	Physically compatible	3	C

Additive Compatibility

Chloramphenicol sodium succinate

Test Drug	Mfr	Conc/L or %	Mfr	Conc/L or %	Test Solution	Remarks	Ref	C/I
Amikacin sulfate	BR	5 g	PD	10 g	D5LR, D5R, D5S, D5W, D10W, LR, NS, R, SL	Physically compatible and both stable for 24 hr at 25°C	293	C
Aminophylline	SE	1 g	PD	10 g	D5W	Physically compatible	15	C
Aminophylline		250 mg	PD	500 mg	D5W	Physically compatible	74	C
Ascorbic acid	AB	1 g	PD	1 g		Physically compatible	6	C
Ascorbic acid	UP		PD			Concentration-dependent incompatibility	15	I
Calcium chloride	UP	1 g	PD	10 g	D5W	Physically compatible	15	C
Calcium gluconate		1 g	PD	500 mg	D5W	Physically compatible	74	C
Calcium gluconate	UP	1 g	PD	10 g	D5W	Physically compatible	15	C
Calcium gluconate	UP	1 g	PD	10 g		Physically compatible	6	C
Chlorpromazine HCl	BP	200 mg	BP	4 g	D5W	Precipitates immediately	26	I
Chlorpromazine HCl	BP	200 mg	BP	4 g	NS	Haze develops over 3 hr	26	I
Colistimethate sodium	WC	500 mg	PD	10 g	D5W	Physically compatible	15	C
Colistimethate sodium	WC	500 mg	PD	10 g		Physically compatible	6	C
Cyanocobalamin	AB	1 mg	PD	1 g		Physically compatible	6	C
Dimenhydrinate	SE	50 mg	PD	500 mg	D5W	Physically compatible	74	C
Dopamine HCl	AS	800 mg	PD	4 g	D5W	Both drugs stable for 24 hr at 25°C	78	C
Ephedrine sulfate	AB	50 mg	PD	1 g		Physically compatible	6	C
Erythromycin lactobionate	AB		PD		D5W	May precipitate at some concentrations	15	I
Fat emulsion, intravenous	VT	10%	PD	2 g		Physically compatible for 48 hr at 4°C and room temperature	32	C
Fat emulsion, intravenous	VT	10%	PD	2 g		Physically compatible for 24 hr at 8 and 25°C	825	C
Heparin sodium	UP	4000 units	PD	10 g	D5W	Physically compatible	15	C
Heparin sodium	AB	20,000 units	PD	1 g		Physically compatible	6, 21	C
Heparin sodium		12,000 units	PD	500 mg	D5W	Physically compatible	74	C
Hydrocortisone sodium succinate	UP	500 mg	PD	10 g	D5W	Physically compatible	15	C
Hydrocortisone sodium succinate	UP	500 mg	PD	1 g		Physically compatible	6	C
Hydrocortisone sodium succinate	UP	100 mg	PD	500 mg	D5W	Physically compatible	74	C
Hydroxyzine HCl	RR	250 mg	PD	10 g	D5W	Physically incompatible	15	I
Lidocaine HCl	AST	2 g	PD	1 g		Physically compatible	24	C
Lincomycin HCl	PHU, XGN					Physically compatible for 24 hr at room temperature	3164, 3165	C
Magnesium sulfate	LI	16 mEq	PD	10 g	D5W	Physically compatible	15	C
Methyldopate HCl	MSD	1 g	PD	1 g	D5W, D10W, D2.5½S, D2.5S, D5¼S, D5½S, D5S, D10S, NS, ½S	Physically compatible	23	C

Additive Compatibility (Cont.)

Test Drug	Mfr	Conc/L or %	Mfr	Conc/L or %	Test Solution	Remarks	Ref	C/I
Methylprednisolone sodium succinate	UP	40 mg	PD	1 g	D5W	Clear solution for 20 hr	329	C
Methylprednisolone sodium succinate	UP	80 mg	PD	2 g	D5W	Clear solution for 20 hr	329	C
Nafcillin sodium	WY	500 mg	PD	1 g		Physically compatible	27	C
Oxacillin sodium	BR	2 g	PD	1 g		Physically compatible	6	C
Oxacillin sodium	BR	500 mg	PD	500 mg	D5S, D5W	Therapeutic availability maintained	110	C
Oxacillin sodium	BR	2 g	PD	1 g	D5S, D5W	Therapeutic availability maintained	110	C
Oxytocin	PD	5 units	PD	1 g		Physically compatible	6	C
Penicillin G potassium		1 million units	PD	1 g		Physically compatible	3	C
Penicillin G potassium	SQ	1 million units	PD	500 mg	D5S, D5W	Therapeutic availability maintained	110	C
Penicillin G potassium	SQ	5 million units	PD	1 g		Physically compatible	47	C
Penicillin G potassium	SQ	10 million units	PD	1 g		Physically compatible	6	C
Penicillin G potassium	SQ	5 and 10 million units	PD	1 g	D5S, D5W	Therapeutic availability maintained	110	C
Penicillin G potassium	SQ	20 million units	PD	10 g	D5W	Physically compatible	15	C
Penicillin G sodium	UP	20 million units	PD	10 g	D5W	Physically compatible	15	C
Pentobarbital sodium	AB	200 mg	PD	1 g		Physically compatible	6	C
Phenylephrine HCl[a]	WI	2.5 g	PD	500 mg	D5W, NS	Phenylephrine stable for 24 hr at 22°C	132	C
Phytonadione	MSD	50 mg	PD	1 g		Physically compatible	6	C
Polymyxin B sulfate	BW	200 mg	PD	10 g	D5W	Physically incompatible	15	I
Polymyxin B sulfate	BW	200 mg	PD	10 g		Precipitate forms within 1 hr	6	I
Potassium chloride		20 and 40 mEq	PD	500 mg and 1 g	D2.5½S, D5W	Therapeutic availability maintained	110	C
Potassium chloride	AB	40 mEq	PD	1 g		Physically compatible	6	C
Potassium chloride		3 g	PD	500 mg	D5W	Physically compatible	74	C
Prochlorperazine edisylate	SKF	100 mg	PD	10 g	D5W	Physically incompatible	15	I
Prochlorperazine mesylate	BP	100 mg	BP	4 g	NS	Haze develops over 3 hr	26	I
Promethazine HCl	WY	250 mg	PD	10 g	D5W	Physically incompatible	15	I
Ranitidine HCl	GL	100 mg		2 g	D5W	Physically compatible for 24 hr at ambient temperature	1151	C
Sodium bicarbonate	AB	80 mEq	PD	1 g		Physically compatible	6	C
Sodium bicarbonate	AB	80 mEq	PD	10 g	D5W	Physically compatible	15	C
Vancomycin HCl	LI	5 g	PD	10 g	D5W	Physically incompatible	15	I
Verapamil HCl	KN	80 mg	PD	2 g	D5W, NS	Physically compatible for 24 hr	764	C

[a] Tested both with and without sodium bicarbonate 7.5 g/L.

Drugs in Syringe Compatibility

Chloramphenicol sodium succinate

Test Drug	Mfr	Amt	Mfr	Amt	Remarks	Ref	C/I
Ampicillin sodium	AY	500 mg	PD	250 and 400 mg/mL in 1.5 to 2 mL	No precipitate or color change within 1 hr at room temperature	99	C
Ampicillin sodium	AY	500 mg	PD	250 and 400 mg/1 mL	Physically compatible for 1 hr at room temperature	300	C
Cloxacillin sodium	BE	250 mg	PD	250 and 400 mg/1.5 to 2 mL	No precipitate or color change within 1 hr at room temperature	99	C
Cloxacillin sodium	AY	250 mg	PD	250 and 400 mg/mL	Physically compatible for 1 hr at room temperature	300	C
Glycopyrrolate	RB	0.2 mg/1 mL	PD	100 mg/1 mL	Gas evolves	331	I
Glycopyrrolate	RB	0.2 mg/1 mL	PD	200 mg/2 mL	Gas evolves	331	I
Glycopyrrolate	RB	0.4 mg/2 mL	PD	100 mg/1 mL	Gas evolves	331	I
Heparin sodium	AB	20,000 units/1 mL	PD	1 g	Physically compatible for at least 30 min	21	C
Heparin sodium		2500 units/1 mL		1 g	Physically compatible for at least 5 min	1053	C
Iohexol	WI	64.7%, 5 mL	PD	33 mg/1 mL	Physically compatible for at least 2 hr	1438	C
Iopamidol	SQ	61%, 5 mL	PD	33 mg/1 mL	Physically compatible for at least 2 hr	1438	C
Iothalamate meglumine	MA	60%, 5 mL	PD	33 mg/1 mL	Physically compatible for at least 2 hr	1438	C
Ioxaglate meglumine–ioxaglate sodium	MA	5 mL	PD	33 mg/1 mL	Physically compatible for at least 2 hr	1438	C
Metoclopramide HCl	RB	10 mg/2 mL	PD	250 mg/2.5 mL	White precipitate forms immediately at 25°C	1167	I
Metoclopramide HCl	RB	10 mg/2 mL	PD	2 g/20 mL	White precipitate forms immediately at 25°C	1167	I
Metoclopramide HCl	RB	160 mg/32 mL	PD	2 g/20 mL	White precipitate forms immediately at 25°C	1167	I
Penicillin G sodium		1 million units	PD	250 and 400 mg/1.5 mL	No precipitate or color change within 1 hr at room temperature	99	C
Penicillin G sodium		1 million units	PD	250 and 400 mg/2 mL	No precipitate or color change within 1 hr at room temperature	99	C

Y-Site Injection Compatibility (1:1 Mixture)

Chloramphenicol sodium succinate

Test Drug	Mfr	Conc	Mfr	Conc	Remarks	Ref	C/I
Acyclovir sodium	BW	5 mg/mL[a]	ES	20 mg/mL[a]	Physically compatible for 4 hr at 25°C	1157	C
Cyclophosphamide	MJ	20 mg/mL[a]	ES	20 mg/mL[a]	Physically compatible for 4 hr at 25°C	1194	C
Enalaprilat	MSD	0.05 mg/mL[b]	PD	10 mg/mL[a]	Physically compatible for 24 hr at room temperature under fluorescent light	1355	C
Esmolol HCl	DCC	10 mg/mL[a]	PD	10 mg/mL[a]	Physically compatible for 24 hr at 22°C	1169	C
Fluconazole	RR	2 mg/mL	PD	20 mg/mL	Gas production	1407	I
Foscarnet sodium	AST	24 mg/mL	PD	20 mg/mL	Physically compatible for 24 hr at room temperature under fluorescent light	1335	C
Hydromorphone HCl	WY	0.2 mg/mL[a]	LY	20 mg/mL[a]	Physically compatible for 4 hr at 25°C	987	C
Labetalol HCl	SC	1 mg/mL[a]	PD	10 mg/mL[a]	Physically compatible for 24 hr at 18°C	1171	C

Y-Site Injection Compatibility (1:1 Mixture) (Cont.)

Test Drug	Mfr	Conc	Mfr	Conc	Remarks	Ref	C/I
Magnesium sulfate	IX	16.7, 33.3, 66.7, 100 mg/mL[a]	PD	20 mg/mL[a]	Physically compatible for at least 4 hr at 32°C	813	C
Meperidine HCl	WY	10 mg/mL[a]	LY	20 mg/mL[a]	Physically compatible for 4 hr at 25°C	987	C
Morphine sulfate	WI	1 mg/mL[a]	LY	20 mg/mL[a]	Physically compatible for 4 hr at 25°C	987	C
Nicardipine HCl	DCC	0.1 mg/mL[a]	PD	10 mg/mL[a]	Visually compatible for 24 hr at room temperature	235	C
Tacrolimus	FUJ	1 mg/mL[b]	PD	20 mg/mL[a]	Visually compatible for 24 hr at 25°C	1630	C
TPN #61[c]		[d]	PD	125 mg/1.25 mL[e]	Physically compatible	1012	C
TPN #61[c]		[f]	PD	750 mg/7.5 mL[e]	Physically compatible	1012	C

[a] Tested in dextrose 5%.

[b] Tested in sodium chloride 0.9%.

[c] Refer to Appendix for the composition of parenteral nutrition solutions. TPN indicates a 2-in-1 admixture.

[d] Run at 21 mL/hr.

[e] Given over five minutes by syringe pump.

[f] Run at 94 mL/hr.

Selected Revisions March 16, 2017. © Copyright, October 1982.
American Society of Health-System Pharmacists, Inc.

Chlorothiazide Sodium
AHFS 40:28.20

Products

Chlorothiazide sodium is supplied in vials containing lyophilized drug equivalent to 500 mg of chlorothiazide with mannitol 250 mg and sodium hydroxide to adjust the pH.[3132] [3133] Each vial should be reconstituted with 18 mL of sterile water for injection to obtain an isotonic solution yielding a concentration of 28 mg/mL of drug.[3132] [3133] No less than 18 mL of sterile water for injection should be used for reconstitution.[3132] [3133]

pH

From 9.2 to 10.[7]

Trade Name(s)

Sodium Diuril

Administration

Chlorothiazide sodium is administered intravenously by direct injection or infusion.[3132] [3133] It should not be administered intramuscularly or subcutaneously, and extravasation must be avoided.[3132] [3133]

Stability

Intact vials should be stored between 2 and 25°C[3133] or between 20 and 25°C at controlled room temperature;[3132] specific product labeling should be consulted for details. Vials are intended for single dose only and unused portions of the reconstituted solution should be discarded. The manufacturers state that the solution should be used immediately after reconstitution.[3132] [3133] However, the reconstituted solution has been stated to be stable for 24 hours.[7]

Chlorothiazide sodium (APP) reconstituted with bacteriostatic water for injection, diluted in dextrose 5% to a chlorothiazide concentration of 10 mg/mL, and packaged as 10 mL in 15-mL polypropylene tubes (BD Biosciences) was physically compatible with less than 6% loss of chlorothiazide in 48 hours at 25°C in the dark.[3568]

pH Effects

Chlorothiazide sodium appears to be stable at pH 7.5 to 9.5 in dextrose 5%.[7] No loss of potency was noted over a 24-hour study period.[7]

The solubility of chlorothiazide sodium is very pH sensitive.[7] Depending on concentration, precipitation occurs at approximately pH 7.4 and below.[7] Additives that result in a final pH in this range should not be mixed.[7] Chlorothiazide sodium is sufficiently alkaline to raise the pH of unbuffered solutions such as dextrose, saline, and their combinations;[7] however, if an acidic buffer is present, such as lactate or acetate buffers, the resultant pH may fall below pH 7.4, causing precipitation.[7]

Chlorothiazide sodium possesses some alkalizing power.[7] Therefore, it should not be combined with drugs known to be unstable in alkaline media.[7]

Syringes

Chlorothiazide (APP) 25 mg/mL (as the sodium salt) diluted in sterile water for injection was packaged as 0.5 mL in 1-mL polypropylene syringes (Monoject) sealed with luer-tip caps (Becton Dickinson) and stored at 2 to 8°C protected from light for 10 days.[3134] Neither changes in color or clarity nor appreciable changes in pH from baseline values occurred.[3134] Samples exhibited a loss of approximately 8% by 6 days.[3134]

Compatibility Information

Solution Compatibility

Chlorothiazide sodium

Test Soln Name	Mfr	Mfr	Conc/L or %	Remarks	Ref	C/I
Dextrose 2.5% in half-strength Ringer's injection	AB	MSD	2 g	Physically compatible	3	C
Dextrose 5% in Ringer's injection	AB	MSD	2 g	Physically compatible	3	C
Dextrose 5% in half-strength Ringer's injection, lactated	AB	MSD	2 g	Physically compatible	3	C
Dextrose 2.5% in Ringer's injection, lactated	AB	MSD	2 g	Physically compatible	3	C
Dextrose 5% in Ringer's injection, lactated	AB	MSD	2 g	Physically compatible	3	C
Dextrose 10% in Ringer's injection, lactated	AB	MSD	2 g	Physically compatible	3	C
Dextrose 2.5% in sodium chloride 0.45%	AB	MSD	2 g	Physically compatible	3	C
Dextrose 2.5% in sodium chloride 0.9%	AB	MSD	2 g	Physically compatible	3	C
Dextrose 5% in sodium chloride 0.225%	AB	MSD	2 g	Physically compatible	3	C

DOI: 10.37573/9781585286850.085

Solution Compatibility (Cont.)

Test Soln Name	Mfr	Mfr	Conc/L or %	Remarks	Ref	C/I
Dextrose 5% in sodium chloride 0.45%	AB	MSD	2 g	Physically compatible	3	C
Dextrose 5% in sodium chloride 0.9%	AB	MSD	2 g	Physically compatible	3	C
Dextrose 5% in sodium chloride 0.9%	AB	MSD	1 g	Stable for 24 hr	7	C
Dextrose 10% in sodium chloride 0.9%	AB	MSD	2 g	Physically compatible	3	C
Dextrose 2.5%	AB	MSD	2 g	Physically compatible	3	C
Dextrose 5%	AB	MSD	1 g	Stable for 24 hr	7	C
Dextrose 5%	AB	MSD	2 g	Physically compatible	3	C
Dextrose 10%	AB	MSD	2 g	Physically compatible	3	C
Ionosol B in dextrose 5%	AB	MSD	500 mg	Physically incompatible	15	I
Ionosol B in dextrose 5%	AB	MSD	2 g	Precipitate forms after 6 hr	7	I
Ionosol B in dextrose 5%	AB	MSD	2 g	Haze or precipitate forms within 24 hr	3	I
Ionosol MB in dextrose 5%	AB	MSD	2 g	Physically compatible	3	C
Ionosol T in dextrose 5%	AB	MSD	2 g	Physically compatible	3	C
Normosol M in dextrose 5%	AB	MSD	2 g	Precipitate forms after 6 hr	7	I
Normosol R in dextrose 5%	AB	MSD	2 g	Precipitate forms after 6 hr	7	I
Ringer's injection	AB	MSD	1 g	Stable for 24 hr	7	C
Ringer's injection	AB	MSD	2 g	Physically compatible	3	C
Ringer's injection, lactated	AB	MSD	1 g	Stable for 24 hr	7	C
Ringer's injection, lactated	AB	MSD	2 g	Physically compatible	3	C
Sodium chloride 0.45%	AB	MSD	2 g	Physically compatible	3	C
Sodium chloride 0.9%	AB	MSD	1 g	Stable for 24 hr	7	C
Sodium chloride 0.9%	AB	MSD	2 g	Physically compatible	3	C
Sodium lactate ⅙ M	AB	MSD	2 g	Physically compatible	3	C

Additive Compatibility

Chlorothiazide sodium

Test Drug	Mfr	Conc/L or %	Mfr	Conc/L or %	Test Solution	Remarks	Ref	C/I
Amikacin sulfate	BR	5 g	MSD	10 mg	D5LR, D5R, D5S, D5W, D10W, LR, NS, R, SL	Precipitate forms within 4 hr at 25°C	294	I
Chlorpromazine HCl	BP	200 mg	BP	2 g	D5W, NS	Precipitates immediately	26	I
Furosemide	HOS	1 g	APP	10 g	D5W[a]	Physically compatible with less than 10% loss of either drug for 96 hours at 25°C in the dark	3568	C
Hydralazine HCl	BP	80 mg	BP	2 g	D5W, NS	Yellow color with precipitate in 3 hr	26	I
Lidocaine HCl	AST	2 g	MSD	500 mg		Physically compatible	24	C
Nafcillin sodium	WY	500 mg	MSD	500 mg		Physically compatible	27	C
Polymyxin B sulfate	BP	20 mg	BP	2 g	D5W	Yellow color produced	26	I

Additive Compatibility (Cont.)

Test Drug	Mfr	Conc/L or %	Mfr	Conc/L or %	Test Solution	Remarks	Ref	C/I
Prochlorperazine mesylate	BP	100 mg	BP	2 g	D5W	Precipitates immediately	26	I
Prochlorperazine mesylate	BP	100 mg	BP	2 g	NS	Haze develops over 3 hr	26	I
Promethazine HCl	BP	100 mg	BP	2 g	D5W, NS	Precipitates immediately	26	I
Ranitidine HCl	GL	50 mg and 2 g		5 g	D5W	Physically compatible. Ranitidine stable for 24 hr at 25°C. Chlorothiazide not tested	1515	C

[a] Tested in polypropylene containers.

Y-Site Injection Compatibility (1:1 Mixture)

Chlorothiazide sodium

Test Drug	Mfr	Conc	Mfr	Conc	Remarks	Ref	C/I
Alprostadil	BED	7.5 mcg/mL[c]	ME	25 mg/mL[b]	Visually compatible for 1 hr	2746	C
TPN #203[a]			ME	28 mg/mL	White precipitate forms immediately	1974	I
TPN #204[a]			ME	28 mg/mL	White precipitate forms immediately	1974	I

[a] Refer to Appendix for the composition of the parenteral nutrition solutions. TPN indicates a 2-in-1 admixture.

[b] Tested in either dextrose 5% or in sodium chloride 0.9%, but the report did not specify which solution.

[c] Tested in a 1:1 mixture of (1) dextrose 5% and dextrose 5% in sodium chloride 0.45% with and without potassium chloride 20 mEq/L and also in (2) dextrose 10% in sodium chloride 0.45% with and without potassium chloride 20 mEq/L.

Selected Revisions July 1, 2020. © Copyright, October 1982.
American Society of Health-System Pharmacists, Inc.

Chlorpromazine Hydrochloride
AHFS 28:16.08.24

Products

Chlorpromazine hydrochloride 25 mg/mL is available in 1- and 2-mL ampuls and vials. Each mL of solution also contains ascorbic acid 2 mg, sodium metabisulfite 1 mg, sodium sulfite 1 mg, and sodium chloride 6 mg in water for injection.[1(10/06)]

pH

From 3.4 to 5.4.[1(10/06)] [17]

Administration

Chlorpromazine hydrochloride may be administered slowly by deep intramuscular injection into the upper outer quadrant of the buttock. Dilution with sodium chloride 0.9% or procaine hydrochloride 2% (no longer commercially available in the US) has been recommended for intramuscular injection if local irritation is a problem. Subcutaneous injection is not recommended. The drug may be diluted to 1 mg/mL with sodium chloride 0.9% and administered by direct intravenous injection at a rate of 1 mg/min to adults and 0.5 mg/min to children. For infusion, it may be diluted in 500 to 1000 mL of sodium chloride 0.9%.[1(10/06)] [4]

Stability

Intact containers should be stored at controlled room temperature. Freezing should be avoided. Protect the solution from light during storage or it may discolor. A slightly yellowed solution does not indicate potency loss. However, a markedly discolored solution should be discarded.[1(10/06)]

pH Effects

The pH of maximum stability is 6.[67] Oxidation of chlorpromazine hydrochloride occurs in alkaline media.[4] The titration of chlorpromazine hydrochloride in sodium chloride 0.9% with alkali resulted in precipitation of chlorpromazine base at pH 6.7 to 6.8.[138] Precipitation may occur if chlorpromazine hydrochloride is admixed with alkaline drugs or solutions.

Light Effects

Chlorpromazine hydrochloride ampuls and vials should be protected from light during storage.[1(10/06)] [4] However, chlorpromazine hydrochloride infusion solutions in polyvinyl chloride (PVC) bags exposed to light during administration lost less than 2% of the drug over a 6-hour administration period. Light protection of infusion sets during administration was found not to be necessary.[2280]

Sorption

Chlorpromazine hydrochloride (May & Baker) 9 mg/L in sodium chloride 0.9% (Travenol) in PVC bags exhibited only about 5% sorption to the plastic bag during 1 week of storage at room temperature (15 to 20°C). However, when the solution was buffered from its initial pH of 5 to pH 7.4, approximately 86% of the drug was lost in 1 week due to sorption.[536]

Chlorpromazine hydrochloride (May & Baker) 9 mg/L in sodium chloride 0.9% exhibited a cumulative 41% loss due to sorption during a 7-hour simulated infusion through an infusion set (Travenol) consisting of a cellulose propionate burette chamber and 170 cm of PVC tubing. Both the burette chamber and the tubing contributed to the loss. The extent of sorption was found to be independent of concentration.[606]

The drug also was tested as a simulated infusion over at least 1 hour by a syringe pump system. A glass syringe on a syringe pump was fitted with 20 cm of polyethylene tubing or 50 cm of Silastic tubing. A negligible amount of drug was lost with the polyethylene tubing, but a cumulative loss of 79% occurred during the 1-hour infusion through the Silastic tubing.[606]

A 25-mL aliquot of chlorpromazine hydrochloride 9 mg/L in sodium chloride 0.9% was stored in all-plastic syringes composed of polypropylene barrels and polyethylene plungers for 24 hours at room temperature in the dark. The solution did not exhibit any loss due to sorption.[606]

In a continuation of this work, chlorpromazine hydrochloride (May & Baker) 90 mg/L in sodium chloride 0.9% in a glass bottle was delivered through a polyethylene administration set (Tridilset) over 8 hours at 15 to 20°C. The flow rate was set at 1 mL/min. No appreciable loss due to sorption occurred.[769] This finding is in contrast to a 41% loss using a conventional administration set.[606]

Central Venous Catheter

Chlorpromazine hydrochloride (Elkins-Sinn) 2 mg/mL in dextrose 5% was found to be compatible with the ARROWg+ard Blue Plus (Arrow International) chlorhexidine-bearing triple-lumen central catheter. Essentially complete delivery of the drug was found with little or no drug loss occurring. Furthermore, chlorhexidine delivered from the catheter remained at trace amounts with no substantial increase due to the delivery of the drug through the catheter.[2335]

DOI: 10.37573/9781585286850.086

Compatibility Information

Solution Compatibility

Chlorpromazine HCl

Test Soln Name	Mfr	Mfr	Conc/L or %	Remarks	Ref	C/I
Dextrose 2.5% in half-strength Ringer's injection	AB	SKF	50 mg	Physically compatible	3	C
Dextrose 5% in Ringer's injection	AB	SKF	50 mg	Physically compatible	3	C
Dextrose 2.5% in Ringer's injection, lactated	AB	SKF	50 mg	Physically compatible	3	C
Dextrose 5% in half-strength Ringer's injection, lactated	AB	SKF	50 mg	Physically compatible	3	C
Dextrose 5% in Ringer's injection, lactated	AB	SKF	50 mg	Physically compatible	3	C
Dextrose 10% in Ringer's injection, lactated	AB	SKF	50 mg	Physically compatible	3	C
Dextrose 2.5% in sodium chloride 0.45%	AB	SKF	50 mg	Physically compatible	3	C
Dextrose 2.5% in sodium chloride 0.9%	AB	SKF	50 mg	Physically compatible	3	C
Dextrose 5% in sodium chloride 0.225%	AB	SKF	50 mg	Physically compatible	3	C
Dextrose 5% in sodium chloride 0.45%	AB	SKF	50 mg	Physically compatible	3	C
Dextrose 5% in sodium chloride 0.9%	AB	SKF	50 mg	Physically compatible	3	C
Dextrose 10% in sodium chloride 0.9%	AB	SKF	50 mg	Physically compatible	3	C
Dextrose 2.5%	AB	SKF	50 mg	Physically compatible	3	C
Dextrose 5%	AB	SKF	50 mg	Physically compatible	3	C
Dextrose 10%	AB	SKF	50 mg	Physically compatible	3	C
Ionosol B in dextrose 5%	AB	SKF	50 mg	Physically compatible	3	C
Ionosol MB in dextrose 5%	AB	SKF	50 mg	Physically compatible	3	C
Ringer's injection	AB	SKF	50 mg	Physically compatible	3	C
Ringer's injection, lactated	AB	SKF	50 mg	Physically compatible	3	C
Sodium chloride 0.45%	AB	SKF	50 mg	Physically compatible	3	C
Sodium chloride 0.9%	AB	SKF	50 mg	Physically compatible	3	C
Sodium chloride 0.9%		SKF	1 g	Variable assay results over 30 days at 23°C	1083	?
Sodium lactate ⅙ M	AB	SKF	50 mg	Physically compatible	3	C

Additive Compatibility

Chlorpromazine HCl

Test Drug	Mfr	Conc/L or %	Mfr	Conc/L or %	Test Solution	Remarks	Ref	C/I
Aminophylline	BP	1 g	BP	200 mg	D5W, NS	Precipitates immediately	26	I
Amphotericin B		200 mg	BP	200 mg	D5W	Precipitates immediately	26	I
Ampicillin sodium	BP	2 g	BP	200 mg	D5W, NS	Precipitates immediately	26	I
Ascorbic acid	UP	500 mg	SKF	250 mg	D5W	Physically compatible	15	C
Chloramphenicol sodium succinate	BP	4 g	BP	200 mg	D5W	Precipitates immediately	26	I
Chloramphenicol sodium succinate	BP	4 g	BP	200 mg	NS	Haze develops over 3 hr	26	I

Additive Compatibility (Cont.)

Test Drug	Mfr	Conc/L or %	Mfr	Conc/L or %	Test Solution	Remarks	Ref	C/I
Chlorothiazide sodium	BP	2 g	BP	200 mg	D5W, NS	Precipitates immediately	26	I
Cloxacillin sodium	BP	1 g	BP	200 mg	NS	Haze forms over 3 hr	26	I
Ethacrynate sodium	MSD	50 mg	SKF	50 mg	NS	Little alteration of UV spectra within 8 hr at room temperature	16	C
Floxacillin sodium	BE	20 g	ANT	5 g	W	Yellow precipitate forms immediately	1479	I
Furosemide	HO	1 g	ANT	5 g	W	Precipitates immediately	1479	I
Methohexital sodium	BP	2 g	BP	200 mg	D5W, NS	Precipitates immediately	26	I
Penicillin G potassium	BP	10 million units	BP	200 mg	NS	Haze develops over 3 hr	26	I
Penicillin G sodium	BP	10 million units	BP	200 mg	NS	Haze develops over 3 hr	26	I
Phenobarbital sodium	BP	800 mg	BP	200 mg	D5W, NS	Precipitates immediately	26	I
Theophylline		2 g		200 mg	D5W	Visually compatible. 7% chlorpromazine and no theophylline loss in 48 hr	1909	C

Drugs in Syringe Compatibility

Chlorpromazine HCl

Test Drug	Mfr	Amt	Mfr	Amt	Remarks	Ref	C/I
Atropine sulfate		0.6 mg/1.5 mL	SKF	50 mg/2 mL	Physically compatible for at least 15 min	14	C
Atropine sulfate	ST	0.4 mg/1 mL	PO	50 mg/2 mL	Physically compatible for at least 15 min	326	C
Benztropine mesylate	MSD	2 mg/2 mL	STS	50 mg/2 mL	Visually compatible for 60 min	1784	C
Butorphanol tartrate	BR	4 mg/2 mL	MB	25 mg/1 mL	Physically compatible for 30 min at room temperature	566	C
Dimenhydrinate	HR	50 mg/1 mL	PO	50 mg/2 mL	Physically incompatible within 15 min	326	I
Dimenhydrinate		10 mg/1 mL		25 mg/1 mL	Clear solution	2569	C
Diphenhydramine HCl	PD	50 mg/1 mL	PO	50 mg/2 mL	Physically compatible for at least 15 min	326	C
Diphenhydramine HCl	ES	100 mg/2 mL	STS	50 mg/2 mL	Visually compatible for 60 min	1784	C
Doxapram HCl	RB	400 mg/20 mL		250 mg/5 mL	Physically compatible with no doxapram loss in 24 hr	1177	C
Droperidol	MN	2.5 mg/1 mL	PO	50 mg/2 mL	Physically compatible for at least 15 min	326	C
Fentanyl citrate	MN	0.05 mg/1 mL	PO	50 mg/2 mL	Physically compatible for at least 15 min	326	C
Glycopyrrolate	RB	0.2 mg/1 mL	SKF	25 mg/1 mL	Physically compatible. pH in glycopyrrolate stability range for 48 hr at 25°C	331	C
Glycopyrrolate	RB	0.2 mg/1 mL	SKF	50 mg/2 mL	Physically compatible. pH in glycopyrrolate stability range for 48 hr at 25°C	331	C
Glycopyrrolate	RB	0.4 mg/2 mL	SKF	25 mg/1 mL	Physically compatible. pH in glycopyrrolate stability range for 48 hr at 25°C	331	C
Heparin sodium		2500 units/1 mL		50 mg/2 mL	Turbidity or precipitate forms within 5 min	1053	I
Hydromorphone HCl	KN	4 mg/2 mL	ES	25 mg/1 mL	Physically compatible for 30 min	517	C
Hydroxyzine HCl	PF	50 mg/1 mL	PO	50 mg/2 mL	Physically compatible for at least 15 min	326	C
Hydroxyzine HCl	ES	100 mg/2 mL	STS	50 mg/2 mL	Visually compatible for 60 min	1784	C
Meperidine HCl	WY	100 mg/1 mL	SKF	50 mg/2 mL	Physically compatible for at least 15 min	14	C
Meperidine HCl	WI	50 mg/1 mL	PO	50 mg/2 mL	Physically compatible for at least 15 min	326	C

Drugs in Syringe Compatibility (Cont.)

Test Drug	Mfr	Amt	Mfr	Amt	Remarks	Ref	C/I
Metoclopramide HCl	NO	10 mg/2 mL	MB	25 mg/1 mL	Physically compatible for 15 min at room temperature	565	C
Midazolam HCl	RC	5 mg/1 mL	SKF	50 mg/2 mL	Physically compatible for 4 hr at 25°C	1145	C
Morphine sulfate	WY	15 mg/1 mL	SKF	50 mg/2 mL	Physically compatible for at least 15 min	14	C
Morphine sulfate	ST	15 mg/1 mL	PO	50 mg/2 mL	Physically compatible for at least 15 min	326	C
Pantoprazole sodium	a	4 mg/1 mL		25 mg/1 mL	Precipitates immediately	2574	I
Pentazocine lactate	WI	30 mg/1 mL	SKF	50 mg/2 mL	Physically compatible for at least 15 min	14	C
Pentazocine lactate	WI	30 mg/1 mL	PO	50 mg/2 mL	Physically compatible for at least 15 min	326	C
Pentobarbital sodium	WY	100 mg/2 mL	SKF	50 mg/2 mL	Precipitate forms within 15 min	14	I
Pentobarbital sodium	AB	500 mg/10 mL	SKF	50 mg/2 mL	Physically incompatible	55	I
Pentobarbital sodium	AB	50 mg/1 mL	PO	50 mg/2 mL	Physically incompatible within 15 min	326	I
Prochlorperazine edisylate	SKF		SKF	50 mg/2 mL	Physically compatible for at least 15 min	14	C
Prochlorperazine edisylate	PO	5 mg/1 mL	PO	50 mg/2 mL	Physically compatible for at least 15 min	326	C
Promethazine HCl	PO	50 mg/2 mL	PO	50 mg/2 mL	Physically compatible for at least 15 min	326	C
Ranitidine HCl	GL	50 mg/2 mL	RP	25 mg/1 mL	Physically compatible for 1 hr at 25°C	978	C
Ranitidine HCl	GL	50 mg/5 mL	RP	25 mg	Gas formation	1151	I
Scopolamine HBr		0.6 mg/1.5 mL	SKF	50 mg/2 mL	Physically compatible for at least 15 min	14	C
Scopolamine HBr	ST	0.4 mg/1 mL	PO	50 mg/2 mL	Physically compatible for at least 15 min	326	C

[a] Test performed using the formulation WITHOUT edetate disodium.

Y-Site Injection Compatibility (1:1 Mixture)

Chlorpromazine HCl

Test Drug	Mfr	Conc	Mfr	Conc	Remarks	Ref	C/I
Acetaminophen	CAD	10 mg/mL	BA	2 mg/mL[b]	Measured turbidity increased immediately	2840, 2844	I
Allopurinol sodium	BW	3 mg/mL[b]	RU	2 mg/mL[b]	White precipitate forms immediately	1686	I
Amifostine	USB	10 mg/mL[a]	SCN	2 mg/mL[a]	Subvisible haze forms immediately	1845	I
Amsacrine	NCI	1 mg/mL[a]	ES	2 mg/mL[a]	Visually compatible for 4 hr at 22°C	1381	C
Aztreonam	SQ	40 mg/mL[a]	SCN	2 mg/mL[a]	Dense white turbidity forms immediately	1758	I
Bivalirudin	TMC	5 mg/mL[a]	ES	2 mg/mL[a]	Gross white precipitate forms immediately	2373	I
Cangrelor tetrasodium	TMC	1 mg/mL[b]		2 mg/mL[b]	Gross white turbid precipitation forms immediately	3243	I
Cisatracurium besylate	GW	0.1, 2, 5 mg/mL[a]	SCN	2 mg/mL[a]	Physically compatible for 4 hr at 23°C	2074	C
Cladribine	ORT	0.015[b] and 0.5[c] mg/mL	SCN	2 mg/mL[b]	Physically compatible for 4 hr at 23°C	1969	C
Cloxacillin sodium	SMX	100 mg/mL	SZ	25 mg/mL	Precipitates immediately	3245	I
Dexmedetomidine HCl	AB	4 mcg/mL[b]	ES	2 mg/mL[b]	Physically compatible for 4 hr at 23°C	2383	C
Docetaxel	RPR	0.9 mg/mL[a]	SCN	2 mg/mL[a]	Physically compatible for 4 hr at 23°C	2224	C

Y-Site Injection Compatibility (1:1 Mixture) (Cont.)

Test Drug	Mfr	Conc	Mfr	Conc	Remarks	Ref	C/I
Doxorubicin HCl liposomal	SEQ	0.4 mg/mL[a]	ES	2 mg/mL[a]	Physically compatible for 4 hr at 23°C	2087	C
Etoposide phosphate	BR	5 mg/mL[a]	ES	2 mg/mL[a]	Cloudy solution forms immediately with particulates in 4 hr	2218	I
Famotidine	ME	2 mg/mL[b]		2 mg/mL[a]	Visually compatible for 4 hr at 22°C	1936	C
Fenoldopam mesylate	AB	80 mcg/mL[b]	ES	2 mg/mL[b]	Physically compatible for 4 hr at 23°C	2467	C
Filgrastim	AMG	30 mcg/mL[a]	RU	2 mg/mL[a]	Physically compatible for 4 hr at 22°C	1687	C
Fluconazole	RR	2 mg/mL	ES	25 mg/mL	Physically compatible for 24 hr at 25°C	1407	C
Fludarabine phosphate	BX	1 mg/mL[a]	ES	2 mg/mL[a]	Initial light haze intensifies within 30 min	1439	I
Furosemide	HMR	2.6 mg/mL[a]	RPR	0.13 mg/mL[a]	Precipitate forms immediately	2244	I
Gemcitabine HCl	LI	10 mg/mL[b]	ES	2 mg/mL[b]	Physically compatible for 4 hr at 23°C	2226	C
Granisetron HCl	SKB	0.05 mg/mL[a]	SCN	2 mg/mL[a]	Physically compatible for 4 hr at 23°C	2000	C
Heparin sodium	UP	1000 units/L[d]	SKF	25 mg/mL	Physically compatible for 4 hr at room temperature	534	C
Heparin sodium	NOV	29.2 units/mL[a]	RPR	0.13 mg/mL[a]	Visually compatible for 150 min	2244	C
Hetastarch in lactated electrolyte	AB	6%	ES	2 mg/mL[a]	Physically compatible for 4 hr at 23°C	2339	C
Hydrocortisone sodium succinate	UP	10 mg/L[d]	SKF	25 mg/mL	Physically compatible for 4 hr at room temperature	534	C
Linezolid	PHU	2 mg/mL	ES	2 mg/mL[a]	Measured haze level increases immediately	2264	I
Linezolid	PHU, HOS	2 mg/mL			Stated to be physically incompatible	3183, 3184	I
Melphalan HCl	BW	0.1 mg/mL[b]	ES	2 mg/mL[b]	Large increase in measured turbidity occurs within 1 hr and grows over 3 hr	1557	I
Ondansetron HCl	GL	1 mg/mL[b]	ES	2 mg/mL[a]	Visually compatible for 4 hr at 22°C	1365	C
Oxaliplatin	SS	0.5 mg/mL[a]	ES	2 mg/mL[a]	Physically compatible for 4 hr at 23°C	2566	C
Paclitaxel	NCI	1.2 mg/mL[a]	ES	2 mg/mL[a]	Normal inherent haze from paclitaxel decreases immediately	1556	I
Pemetrexed disodium	LI	20 mg/mL[b]	ES	2 mg/mL[a]	Cloudy precipitate forms immediately	2564	I
Piperacillin sodium–tazobactam sodium	LE[e]	40 mg/mL[a h]	RU	2 mg/mL[a]	Heavy white turbidity forms immediately. White precipitate forms in 4 hr	1688	I
Potassium chloride	AB	40 mEq/L[d]	SKF	25 mg/mL	Physically compatible for 4 hr at room temperature	534	C
Potassium chloride	BRN	0.625 mEq/mL[a]	RPR	0.13 mg/mL[a]	Visually compatible for 150 min	2244	C
Propofol	ZEN[i]	10 mg/mL	SCN	2 mg/mL[a]	Physically compatible for 1 hr at 23°C	2066	C
Remifentanil HCl	GW	0.025 mg/mL[b]	SCN	2 mg/mL[a]	Slight haze forms in 1 hr	2075	I
Remifentanil HCl	GW	0.25 mg/mL[b]	SCN	2 mg/mL[a]	Physically compatible for 4 hr at 23°C	2075	C
Sargramostim	IMM	10 mcg/mL[b]	ES	2 mg/mL[b]	Slight haze forms immediately	1436	I
Teniposide	BR	0.1 mg/mL[a]	SCN	2 mg/mL[a]	Physically compatible for 4 hr at 23°C	1725	C
Thiotepa	IMM[f]	1 mg/mL[a]	SCN	2 mg/mL[a]	Physically compatible for 4 hr at 23°C	1861	C
Tigecycline	WY	1 mg/mL[b]		1 mg/mL[b]	Precipitates immediately	2714	I
TNA #218 to #226[g]			SCN	2 mg/mL[a]	Visually compatible for 4 hr at 23°C	2215	C

Y-Site Injection Compatibility (1:1 Mixture) (Cont.)

Test Drug	Mfr	Conc	Mfr	Conc	Remarks	Ref	C/I
TPN #212 to #215[g]			SCN	2 mg/mL[a]	Physically compatible for 4 hr at 23°C	2109	C
Vinorelbine tartrate	BW	1 mg/mL[b]	RU	2 mg/mL[b]	Physically compatible for 4 hr at 22°C	1558	C

[a] Tested in dextrose 5%.

[b] Tested in sodium chloride 0.9%.

[c] Tested in bacteriostatic sodium chloride 0.9% preserved with benzyl alcohol 0.9%.

[d] Tested in dextrose 5% in Ringer's injection, dextrose 5% in Ringer's injection, lactated, dextrose 5%, Ringer's injection, lactated, and sodium chloride 0.9%.

[e] Test performed using the formulation WITHOUT edetate disodium.

[f] Lyophilized formulation tested.

[g] Refer to Appendix for the composition of parenteral nutrition solutions. TNA indicates a 3-in-1 admixture, and TPN indicates a 2-in-1 admixture.

[h] Piperacillin component. Piperacillin in an 8:1 fixed-ratio concentration with tazobactam.

[i] Test performed using the formulation WITH edetate disodium.

Additional Compatibility Information

Hydroxyzine and Meperidine

Chlorpromazine hydrochloride (Elkins-Sinn) 6.25 mg/mL, hydroxyzine hydrochloride (Pfizer) 12.5 mg/mL, and meperidine hydrochloride (Winthrop) 25 mg/mL, in both glass and plastic syringes, have been reported to be physically compatible and chemically stable for at least 1 year at 4 and 25°C when protected from light.[989]

Meperidine and Promethazine

Chlorpromazine hydrochloride, meperidine hydrochloride, and promethazine hydrochloride combined as an extemporaneous mixture for preoperative sedation, developed a brownish-yellow color after 2 weeks of storage with protection from light. The discoloration was attributed to the metacresol preservative content of the meperidine hydrochloride product used. Use of meperidine hydrochloride which contains a different preservative resulted in a solution that remained clear and colorless for at least 3 months when protected from light.[1148]

Chlorocresol

Chlorpromazine hydrochloride is incompatible with chlorocresol preservative.[467] [468]

Selected Revisions January 31, 2020. © Copyright, October 1982. American Society of Health-System Pharmacists, Inc.

Cidofovir

AHFS 8:18.32

Products

Cidofovir is available in single-use (unpreserved) 5-mL vials.[2924][2925] Each mL contains cidofovir 75 mg with sodium hydroxide and/or hydrochloric acid to adjust pH.[2924][2925] The drug must be diluted in 100 mL of sodium chloride 0.9% prior to administration.[2924][2925]

Take appropriate safety precautions for handling mutagenic substances in accordance with current guidelines and manufacturers' safe handling guidance.[2924][2925] If cidofovir solution contacts skin or mucosa, wash the affected area immediately with soap and water.[2924][2925]

Partially used vials, diluted solutions, and materials used in admixture preparation and administration should be sealed in leak- and puncture-proof containers and incinerated at high temperature.[2924][2925]

pH

Cidofovir has a pH adjusted to 7.4[2924] or from 7.1 to 7.7.[2925]

The pH values of cidofovir admixtures in three infusion solutions were:[1963]

Solution	Concentration	pH
Dextrose 5% in sodium chloride 0.45%	0.085 and 3.51 mg/mL	6.7 to 7
Dextrose 5%	0.21 and 8.12 mg/mL	7.2 to 7.6
Sodium chloride 0.9%	0.21 and 8.12 mg/mL	7.1 to 7.5

Osmolality

Cidofovir is hypertonic and is diluted for administration.[2924] The osmolalities of cidofovir admixtures in three infusion solutions were:[1963]

Solution	Concentration	Osmolality (mOsm/kg)
Dextrose 5% in sodium chloride 0.45%	0.085 and 3.51 mg/mL	382 and 392
Dextrose 5%	0.21 and 8.12 mg/mL	241 and 286
Sodium chloride 0.9%	0.21 and 8.12 mg/mL	275 and 315

Trade Name(s)

Vistide

Administration

Cidofovir is administered by intravenous infusion in 100 mL of sodium chloride 0.9% at a constant rate over one hour.[2924][2925] Use of an infusion pump is recommended for administration.[2924][2925] Shorter periods must not be used.[2924][2925] Patients must be hydrated with at least 1 L of intravenous sodium chloride 0.9% infused over 1 to 2 hours immediately prior to each cidofovir infusion.[2924][2925] In patients who can tolerate additional hydration, a second liter of intravenous sodium chloride 0.9% should be infused over 1 to 3 hours, either at the start of the cidofovir infusion or immediately afterwards.[2924][2925] Patients must also be treated with oral probenecid with each infusion of cidofovir.[2924][2925]

Intraocular administration of cidofovir is contraindicated.[2924][2925]

Stability

Cidofovir should be stored at controlled room temperature.[2924][2925] If any particulate matter or discoloration is present, the vial should be discarded.[2924][2925] The manufacturer states that, diluted in 100 mL of sodium chloride 0.9% for administration, cidofovir should be used within 24 hours of preparation.[2924][2925] Admixtures not used immediately should be stored under refrigeration at 2 to 8°C but should still be used within 24 hours of preparation; refrigeration or freezing should not be used to extend beyond the 24-hour limit.[2924][2925] Refrigerated admixtures should be allowed to come to room temperature prior to use.[2924][2925]

Syringes

Cidofovir 6.25 mg/mL in sodium chloride 0.9% packaged in polypropylene syringes (Becton Dickinson) has been reported to be stable by HPLC analysis for 150 days at room and refrigeration temperatures.[2607]

Sorption

Cidofovir is stated to be compatible with glass, PVC, and ethylene/propylene copolymer infusion solution containers.[2924][2925]

DOI: 10.37573/9781585286850.087

Compatibility Information

Solution Compatibility

Cidofovir

Test Soln Name	Mfr	Mfr	Conc/L or %	Remarks	Ref	C/I
Dextrose 5% in sodium chloride 0.45%	AB[a], BA[a], MG[b]	GIL	85 mg and 3.51 g	Physically compatible with no increase in subvisual particulates in 24 hr at 4 and 30°C	1963	C
Dextrose 5%	AB[a], BA[a], MG[b]	GIL	210 mg and 8.12 g	Physically compatible with no increase in subvisual particulates and no loss by HPLC in 24 hr at 4 and 30°C	1963	C
Sodium chloride 0.9%	AB[a], BA[a], MG[b]	GIL	210 mg and 8.12 g	Physically compatible with no increase in subvisual particulates and no loss by HPLC in 24 hr at 4 and 30°C	1963	C
Sodium chloride 0.9%	AB[a], BA[a], MG[b]	GIL	200 mg and 8.1 g	Physically compatible with no increase in subvisual particulates and no loss by HPLC in 5 days at 4 and –20°C	2076	C

[a] Tested in PVC containers.

[b] Tested in polyolefin containers.

Selected Revisions April 20, 2015. © Copyright, October 1998.
American Society of Health-System Pharmacists, Inc.

Ciprofloxacin
AHFS 8:12.18

Products

Ciprofloxacin is available as a premixed, ready-to-use solution in 100- and 200-mL polyvinyl chloride (PVC) containers. Each mL contains 2 mg of ciprofloxacin with dextrose 5%, lactic acid as a solubilizer, and hydrochloric acid to adjust the pH.[1(10/08)]

pH

From 3.5 to 4.6.[1(10/08) 17]

Trade Name(s)

Cipro I.V.

Administration

Ciprofloxacin is administered at a concentration of 1 to 2 mg/mL by intravenous infusion into a large vein slowly over 60 minutes. When given intermittently through a Y-site, the primary solution should be discontinued temporarily.[1(10/08) 4]

Stability

Ciprofloxacin is a clear, colorless to slightly yellow solution. It should be stored between 5 and 25°C and protected from light and freezing.[1(10/08) 4]

pH Effects

Ciprofloxacin in aqueous solution is stated to be stable for up to 14 days at room temperature in the pH range of 1.5 to 7.5.[4] However, Teraoka et al. reported substantial loss of ciprofloxacin content in admixtures with a pH over 6.[1924]

Light Effects

Ciprofloxacin undergoes slow degradation when exposed to natural daylight. Exposure to mixed natural daylight and fluorescent light resulted in about 2% loss after 12 hours of exposure and about 9% loss after about 96 hours of exposure.[2399]

Central Venous Catheter

Ciprofloxacin (Bayer) 1 mg/mL in dextrose 5% was found to be compatible with the ARROWg+ard Blue Plus (Arrow International) chlorhexidine-bearing triple-lumen central catheter. Essentially complete delivery of the drug was found with little or no drug loss occurring. Furthermore, chlorhexidine delivered from the catheter remained at trace amounts with no substantial increase due to the delivery of the drug through the catheter.[2335]

Compatibility Information

Solution Compatibility

Ciprofloxacin

Test Soln Name	Mfr	Mfr	Conc/L or %	Remarks	Ref	C/I
Dextrose 5% in sodium chloride 0.225%		MI	0.5 to 2 g	Stable for 14 days at 5 and 25°C	888	C
Dextrose 5% in sodium chloride 0.45%		MI	0.5 to 2 g	Stable for 14 days at 5 and 25°C	888	C
Dextrose 5%	AB[a]	MI	1.5 g	Visually compatible with no loss in 48 hr at 25°C under fluorescent light	1541	C
Dextrose 5%	[a]	BAY	800 mg	Visually compatible with no significant loss in 6 hr at 22°C exposed to light	1698	C
Dextrose 5%		MI	0.5 to 2 g	Stable for 14 days at 5 and 25°C	888	C
Dextrose 5%	BA[a]	MI	2.86 g	Visually compatible with no loss in 90 days at room temperature and 5°C	1891	C
Dextrose 10%		MI	0.5 to 2 g	Stable for 14 days at 5 and 25°C	888	C
Ringer's injection		MI	0.5 to 1 g	Stable for 14 days at 5 and 25°C	888	C
Ringer's injection, lactated		MI	0.5 to 2 g	Stable for 14 days at 5 and 25°C	888	C
Sodium chloride 0.9%	AB[a]	MI	1.5 g	Visually compatible with no loss in 48 hr at 25°C under fluorescent light	1541	C
Sodium chloride 0.9%	[a]	BAY	800 mg	Visually compatible with no significant loss in 6 hr at 22°C exposed to light	1698	C
Sodium chloride 0.9%		MI	0.5 to 2 g	Stable for 14 days at 5 and 25°C	888	C
Sodium chloride 0.9%	BA[a]	MI	2.86 g	Visually compatible with no loss in 90 days at room temperature and 5°C	1891	C
Sodium chloride 0.9%	AB	BAY	2 g	Visually compatible with no loss in 24 hr at 25°C	1934	C

[a] Tested in PVC containers.

DOI: 10.37573/9781585286850.088

Additive Compatibility

Ciprofloxacin

Test Drug	Mfr	Conc/L or %	Mfr	Conc/L or %	Test Solution	Remarks	Ref	C/I
Amikacin sulfate	BR	4.1 g	MI	1.6 g	D5W, NS	Visually compatible and both stable for 48 hr at 25°C under fluorescent light	1541	C
Amikacin sulfate	APC	4.9 g	BAY	2 g	D5W	Visually compatible with no loss of ciprofloxacin in 24 hr at 22°C under fluorescent light. Amikacin not tested	2413	C
Aminophylline	LY	2 g	MI	1.6 g	D5W, NS	Precipitate forms in 4 hr at 4 and 25°C	1541	I
Aminophylline						Physically incompatible with loss of ciprofloxacin reported due to pH over 6.0	1924	I
Amoxicillin sodium		10 g		2 g	a	Precipitates immediately	1473	I
Amoxicillin sodium–clavulanate potassium		10d g		2 g	a	Precipitates immediately	1473	I
Amphotericin B		100 mg	MI	2 g	D5W	Physically incompatible	888	I
Amphotericin B	APC	100 mg	BAY	2 g	D5W	Precipitates immediately	2413	I
Ampicillin sodium–sulbactam sodium		20e g	MI	2 g	D5W	Physically incompatible	888	I
Ampicillin sodium–sulbactam sodium	RR	20e g	BAY	2 g	D5W	Precipitates immediately	2413	I
Atracurium besylate	GW	2 g	BAY	1.6 g	D5W	Visually compatible with no loss of ciprofloxacin in 24 hr at 22°C under fluorescent light. Atracurium not tested	2413	C
Azithromycin						Physically incompatible with loss of ciprofloxacin reported due to pH over 6.0	1924	I
Aztreonam	SQ	39.7 g	BAY	1.6 g	D5W	Visually compatible with no loss of ciprofloxacin in 24 hr at 22°C under fluorescent light. Aztreonam not tested	2413	C
Ceftazidime		20 g	MI	2 g	D5W	Physically incompatible	888	I
Ceftazidime	SKB	19.8 g	BAY	2 g	D5W	Visually compatible but pH changed by more than 1 unit	2413	?
Cefuroxime sodium		30 g	MI	2 g	D5W	Physically incompatible	888	I
Cefuroxime sodium	GW	30 g	BAY	2 g	D5W	Visually compatible for 6 hr, but small particles appeared by 24 hr at about 22°C	2413	I
Clindamycin phosphate	LY	7.1 g	MI	1.6 g	D5W, NS	Precipitate forms immediately	1541	I
Cyclosporine	SZ	500 mg	BAY	2 g	NS	Visually compatible with 8% ciprofloxacin loss in 24 hr at 25°C. Cyclosporine not tested	1934	C
Dobutamine HCl	LI	2 g	BAY	1.7 g	D5W	Visually compatible with no loss of ciprofloxacin in 24 hr at 22°C under fluorescent light. Dobutamine not tested	2413	C
Dopamine HCl		400 mg	MI	2 g	NS	Compatible for 24 hr at 25°C	888	C
Dopamine HCl		1.04 g	MI	2 g	NS	Compatible for 24 hr at 25°C	888	C
Floxacillin sodium		10 g		2 g	a	Precipitates immediately	1473	I
Fluconazole	RR	1 g	BAY	1 g		Visually compatible with no loss of ciprofloxacin in 24 hr at 22°C under fluorescent light. Fluconazole not tested	2413	C

Additive Compatibility (Cont.)

Test Drug	Mfr	Conc/L or %	Mfr	Conc/L or %	Test Solution	Remarks	Ref	C/I
Fluorouracil						Physically incompatible with loss of ciprofloxacin reported due to pH over 6.0	1924	I
Gentamicin sulfate	LY	1 g	MI	1.6 g	D5W, NS	Visually compatible and both drugs stable for 48 hr at 25°C under fluorescent light and 4°C in the dark	1541	C
Gentamicin sulfate	SC	10 g	BAY	2 g	NS	Visually compatible. Little ciprofloxacin loss in 24 hr at 25°C. Gentamicin not tested	1934	C
Gentamicin sulfate	SC	1.6 g	BAY	2 g	D5W	Visually compatible with no loss of ciprofloxacin in 24 hr at 22°C under fluorescent light. Gentamicin not tested	2413	C
Heparin sodium	CP	10,000, 100,000, 1 million units	BAY	2 g	NS	White precipitate forms immediately	1934	I
Heparin sodium		4100 units	MI	2 g	NS	Physically incompatible	888	I
Heparin sodium		8300 units	MI	2 g	NS	Physically incompatible	888	I
Lidocaine HCl		1 g	MI	2 g	NS	Compatible for 24 hr at 25°C	888	C
Lidocaine HCl		1.5 g	MI	2 g	NS	Compatible for 24 hr at 25°C	888	C
Linezolid	PHU	2 g	BAY	4 g	b	Physically compatible with little or no loss of either drug in 7 days at 23°C protected from light. Refrigeration results in precipitation after 1 day	2334	C
Meropenem	ASZ	10 g	SZ	1 g	f	White precipitate forms	3107	I
Metronidazole		5 g		2 g		No loss of either drug in 4 hr at 24°C	1346	C
Metronidazole	SE	4.2 g	MI	1.6 g		Visually compatible. Both drugs stable for 48 hr at 25°C in light and 4°C in dark	1541	C
Metronidazole	RPR	2.5 g		1 g		Under 3% metronidazole loss in 24 hr at 25°C in light or dark. Ciprofloxacin not tested	2361	C
Metronidazole	SCS	2.5 g	BAY	1 g		Visually compatible. No ciprofloxacin loss in 24 hr at 22°C in light. Metronidazole not tested	2413	C
Midazolam HCl	RC	200 mg	BAY	2 g	D5W	Visually compatible. No ciprofloxacin loss in 24 hr at 22°C in light. Midazolam not tested	2413	C
Norepinephrine bitartrate	SW	64 mg	BAY	2 g	D5W	Visually compatible. No ciprofloxacin loss in 24 hr at 22°C in light. Norepinephrine not tested	2413	C
Pancuronium bromide	OR	200 mg	BAY	1.6 g	D5W	Visually compatible with no loss of ciprofloxacin in 24 hr at 22°C under fluorescent light. Pancuronium not tested	2413	C
Potassium chloride	AB	40 mEq	BAY	2 g	NS	Visually compatible with little or no ciprofloxacin loss in 24 hr at 25°C	1934	C
Potassium chloride		40 mEq	MI	2 g	NS	Compatible for 24 hr at 25°C	888	C
Potassium chloride	LY	2.9 g	BAY	2 g	D5W	Visually compatible with no loss of ciprofloxacin in 24 hr at 22°C under fluorescent light. Potassium chloride not tested	2413	C
Potassium phosphates		60 mg		2 g	D5W	Precipitation occurs	671	I
Ranitidine HCl	GL	500 mg and 1 g	BAY	2 g	NS	Visually compatible. Little ciprofloxacin loss in 24 hr at 25°C. Ranitidine not tested	1934	C
Sodium bicarbonate		c	MI	2 g	D5W	Physically incompatible	888	I

Additive Compatibility (Cont.)

Test Drug	Mfr	Conc/L or %	Mfr	Conc/L or %	Test Solution	Remarks	Ref	C/I
Sodium bicarbonate	AST	4 g	BAY	2 g	D5W	Precipitates immediately	2413	I
Tobramycin sulfate	LI	1 g	MI	1.6 g	D5W, NS	Visually compatible and both drugs stable for 48 hr at 25°C under fluorescent light and 4°C in the dark	1541	C
Tobramycin sulfate	LI	1.6 g	BAY	2 g	D5W	Visually compatible with no loss of ciprofloxacin in 24 hr at 22°C under fluorescent light. Tobramycin not tested	2413	C
Vecuronium bromide	OR	200 mg	BAY	1.6 g	D5W	Visually compatible with no loss of ciprofloxacin in 24 hr at 22°C under fluorescent light. Vecuronium not tested	2413	C

[a] Drug added to ciprofloxacin solution.

[b] Admixed in the linezolid infusion container.

[c] Final sodium bicarbonate concentration not specified.

[d] Amoxicillin sodium component. Amoxicillin sodium in a 5:1 fixed-ratio concentration with clavulanic acid.

[e] Ampicillin component. Ampicillin in a 2:1 fixed-ratio concentration with sulbactam.

[f] Tested in glass containers.

Drugs in Syringe Compatibility

Ciprofloxacin

Test Drug	Mfr	Amt	Mfr	Amt	Remarks	Ref	C/I
Pantoprazole sodium	[a]	4 mg/1 mL		2 mg/1 mL	Precipitates immediately	2574	I

[a] Test performed using the formulation WITHOUT edetate disodium.

Y-Site Injection Compatibility (1:1 Mixture)

Ciprofloxacin

Test Drug	Mfr	Conc	Mfr	Conc	Remarks	Ref	C/I
Amifostine	USB	10 mg/mL[a]	MI	1 mg/mL[a]	Physically compatible for 4 hr at 23°C	1845	C
Amino acids, dextrose	AB	AA 5%, D 25%	MI	2 mg/mL[a]	Visually compatible for 2 hr at 25°C	1628	C
Aminophylline	AB	2 mg/mL[a] [b]	MI	2 mg/mL[a] [b]	Fine white crystals form in 20 min in D5W and 2 min in NS	1655	I
Amiodarone HCl	WY	6 mg/mL[a]	BAY	2 mg/mL[a]	Visually compatible for 24 hr at 22°C	2352	C
Ampicillin sodium–sulbactam sodium		3 g[c] [l]		400 mg[c]	White crystals form immediately when administered sequentially through a Y-site into running D5S	1887	I
Anidulafungin	VIC	0.5 mg/mL[a]	AB	2 mg/mL[a]	Physically compatible for 4 hr at 23°C	2617	C
Azithromycin	PF	2 mg/mL[b]	BAY	2 mg/mL[d] [e]	Amber microcrystals found	2368	I
Aztreonam	SQ	20 mg/mL[a] [b]	MI	1 mg/mL[a]	Physically compatible for 24 hr at 22°C	1189	C
Aztreonam	SQ	40 mg/mL[a]	MI	1 mg/mL[a]	Physically compatible for 4 hr at 23°C	1758	C
Bivalirudin	TMC	5 mg/mL[a]	BAY	2 mg/mL[a]	Physically compatible for 4 hr at 23°C	2373	C
Blinatumomab	AMG	0.125 and 0.375 mcg/mL[b]	FRK	2 mg/mL	Persistent particulate formation	3405, 3417	I
Calcium gluconate	LY	10%	MI	2 mg/mL[a]	Visually compatible for 2 hr at 25°C	1628	C
Cangrelor tetrasodium	TMC	1 mg/mL[b]		1 mg/mL[b]	Measured haze increases immediately	3243	I

Y-Site Injection Compatibility (1:1 Mixture) (Cont.)

Test Drug	Mfr	Conc	Mfr	Conc	Remarks	Ref	C/I
Caspofungin acetate	ME	0.7 mg/mL[b]	HOS	2 mg/mL[b]	Physically compatible for 4 hr at room temperature	2758	C
Caspofungin acetate	ME	0.5 mg/mL[b]	BAY	2 mg/mL	Physically compatible over 60 min	2766	C
Ceftaroline fosamil	FOR	2.22 mg/mL[a b k]	BED	2 mg/mL[a b k]	Physically compatible for 4 hr at 23°C	2826	C
Ceftazidime	SKF	20 mg/mL[a b]	MI	1 mg/mL[a]	Physically compatible for 24 hr at 22°C	1189	C
Ceftolozane sulfate–tazobactam sodium	CUB	10 mg/mL[n o]	HOS	2 mg/mL[n]	Physically compatible for 2 hr	3262	C
Cisatracurium besylate	GW	0.1, 2, 5 mg/mL[a]	BAY	1 mg/mL[a]	Physically compatible for 4 hr at 23°C	2074	C
Clarithromycin	AB	4 mg/mL[a]	BAY	2 mg/mL[a]	Visually compatible for 72 hr at both 30 and 17°C	2174	C
Cloxacillin sodium	SMX	100 mg/mL	OM[m]	2 mg/mL	Large particles form immediately	3245	I
Defibrotide sodium	JAZ	8 mg/mL[b]	FRK	2 mg/mL	Visually compatible for 4 hr at room temperature	3149	C
Dexamethasone sodium phosphate	LY	4 mg/mL	MI	2 mg/mL[a b]	Cloudiness rapidly dissipates. White crystals form in 1 hr at 24°C	1655	I
Dexmedetomidine HCl	AB	4 mcg/mL[b]	BAY	1 mg/mL[b]	Physically compatible for 4 hr at 23°C	2383	C
Digoxin	ES	0.25 mg/mL	MI	2 mg/mL[a b]	Visually compatible for 24 hr at 24°C	1655	C
Digoxin	BW	0.25 mg/mL	BAY	2 mg/mL[b]	Visually compatible with no ciprofloxacin loss in 15 min. Digoxin not tested	1934	C
Diltiazem HCl	MMD	5 mg/mL	MI	2 and 10 mg/mL[b]	Visually compatible	1807	C
Dimenhydrinate		10 mg/mL		2 mg/mL	Clear solution	2569	C
Diphenhydramine HCl	ES	50 mg/mL	MI	2 mg/mL[a b]	Visually compatible for 24 hr at 24°C	1655	C
Dobutamine HCl	LI	250 mcg/mL[a b]	MI	2 mg/mL[a b]	Visually compatible for 24 hr at 24°C	1655	C
Docetaxel	RPR	0.9 mg/mL[a]	BAY	1 mg/mL[a]	Physically compatible for 4 hr at 23°C	2224	C
Dopamine HCl	AB	1.6 mg/mL[a b]	MI	2 mg/mL[a b]	Visually compatible for 24 hr at 24°C	1655	C
Doripenem	JJ	5 mg/mL[a b]	BED	2 mg/mL[a b]	Physically compatible for 4 hr at 23°C	2743	C
Doxorubicin HCl liposomal	SEQ	0.4 mg/mL[a]	BAY	1 mg/mL[a]	Physically compatible for 4 hr at 23°C	2087	C
Eravacycline dihydrochloride	TET	0.6 mg/mL[b]	CLA	2 mg/mL[r]	Physically compatible for 2 hr at room temperature	3532	C
Esmolol HCl	MYL	10 mg/mL	SZ	2 mg/mL	Physically incompatible	3533	I
Etoposide phosphate	BR	5 mg/mL[a]	BAY	1 mg/mL[a]	Physically compatible for 4 hr at 23°C	2218	C
Fat emulsion, intravenous	OTS	20%[q]	BAY	2 mg/mL[j]	Coarsening of particle diameter observed immediately after preparation	3452	I
Fenoldopam mesylate	AB	80 mcg/mL[b]	BAY	2 mg/mL[b]	Physically compatible for 4 hr at 23°C	2467	C
Furosemide	AB	10 mg/mL	MI	2 mg/mL[a b]	Precipitates immediately	1655	I
Furosemide	DMX	5 mg/mL	BAY	2 mg/mL[b]	White precipitate forms immediately	1934	I
Gallium nitrate	FUJ	1 mg/mL[b]	MI	2 mg/mL[b]	Visually compatible for 24 hr at 25°C	1673	C
Gemcitabine HCl	LI	10 mg/mL[b]	BAY	1 mg/mL[b]	Physically compatible for 4 hr at 23°C	2226	C
Gentamicin sulfate	LY	1.6 mg/mL[a b]	MI	2 mg/mL[a b]	Visually compatible for 24 hr at 24°C	1655	C
Granisetron HCl	SKB	0.05 mg/mL[a]	MI	1 mg/mL[a]	Physically compatible for 4 hr at 23°C	2000	C

Y-Site Injection Compatibility (1:1 Mixture) (Cont.)

Test Drug	Mfr	Conc	Mfr	Conc	Remarks	Ref	C/I
Heparin sodium		10 units/mL		2 mg/mL	Turbidity forms rapidly with subsequent white precipitate	1483	I
Heparin sodium	LY	100 units/mL[a b]	MI	2 mg/mL[a b]	Crystals form immediately	1655	I
Heparin sodium	CP	10, 100, 1000 units/mL[b]	BAY	2 mg/mL[b]	White precipitate forms immediately	1934	I
Hetastarch in lactated electrolyte	AB	6%	BAY	2 mg/mL[a]	Physically compatible for 4 hr at 23°C	2339	C
Hydrocortisone sodium succinate	UP	50 mg/mL	MI	2 mg/mL[a b]	Transient cloudiness rapidly dissipates. Crystals form in 1 hr at 24°C	1655	I
Hydroxyethyl starch 130/0.4 in sodium chloride 0.9%	FRK	6%	AB	0.5, 1, 2 mg/mL[a]	Visually compatible for 24 hr at room temperature	2770	C
Hydroxyzine HCl	ES	50 mg/mL	MI	2 mg/mL[a b]	Visually compatible for 24 hr at 24°C	1655	C
Isavuconazonium sulfate	ASP	1.5 mg/mL[n]	HOS	2 mg/mL[n]	Physically compatible for 2 hr	3263	C
Labetalol HCl	HOS	5 mg/mL	SZ	2 mg/mL	Physically compatible for 1 hr at 23°C	3533	C
Letermovir	ME				Physically incompatible	3398	I
Lidocaine HCl	AB	4[a] and 20 mg/mL	MI	2 mg/mL[a b]	Visually compatible for 24 hr at 24°C	1655	C
Linezolid	PHU	2 mg/mL	BAY	1 mg/mL[a]	Physically compatible for 4 hr at 23°C	2264	C
Lorazepam	WY	0.33 mg/mL[b]	BAY	2 mg/mL	Visually compatible for 24 hr at 22°C	1855	C
Magnesium sulfate	AB	4 mEq/mL	MI	2 mg/mL[a b]	Precipitate forms in 4 hr in D5W and 1 hr in NS at 24°C	1655	I
Magnesium sulfate	LY	50%	MI	2 mg/mL[a]	Visually compatible for 2 hr at 25°C	1628	C
Meropenem		50 mg/mL	SZ[m]	2 mg/mL	Crystallization occurred within 4 hr	3538	I
Meropenem–vaborbactam	TMC	8 mg/mL[b p]	HOS	2 mg/mL[b]	Precipitation and increase in measured turbidity within 30 min. pH increased by >3 units within 3 hr	3380, 3382	I
Methylprednisolone sodium succinate	UP	62.5 mg/mL	MI	2 mg/mL[a b]	Transient cloudiness rapidly dissipates. Crystals form in 2 hr at 24°C	1655	I
Metoclopramide HCl	DU	5 mg/mL	MI	2 mg/mL[a b]	Visually compatible for 24 hr at 24°C	1655	C
Metoclopramide HCl		5 mg/mL	BAY	2 mg/mL[b]	Visually compatible. No ciprofloxacin loss in 15 min. Metoclopramide not tested	1934	C
Metoprolol tartrate	HOS	0.4 mg/mL[b]	SZ	2 mg/mL	Physically compatible for 1 hr at 23°C	3533	C
Midazolam HCl	RC	5 mg/mL	BAY	2 mg/mL	Visually compatible for 24 hr at 22°C	1855	C
Milrinone lactate	SS	0.2 mg/mL[a]	BAY	2 mg/mL	Visually compatible for 4 hr at 25°C	2381	C
Oritavancin diphosphate	TAR	0.8, 1.2, and 2 mg/mL[a]	HOS[m]	2 mg/mL[a]	Visually compatible for 4 hr at 20 to 24°C	2928	C
Pemetrexed disodium	LI	20 mg/mL[b]	BAY	2 mg/mL[a]	Slight color darkening occurs over 4 hr	2564	I
Phenytoin sodium	PD	50 mg/mL	MI	2 mg/mL[a b]	Immediate crystal formation	1655	I
Plazomicin sulfate	ACH	24 mg/mL[n]	CLA	2 mg/mL[n]	Physically compatible for 1 hr at 20 to 25°C	3432	C
Posaconazole	ME	18 mg/mL		2 mg/mL[n]	Physically compatible	2911, 2912	C
Potassium acetate	LY	2 mEq/mL	MI	2 mg/mL[a]	Visually compatible for 2 hr at 25°C	1628	C

Y-Site Injection Compatibility (1:1 Mixture) (Cont.)

Test Drug	Mfr	Conc	Mfr	Conc	Remarks	Ref	C/I
Potassium chloride	LY	0.04 mEq/mL	MI	2 mg/mL[a b]	Visually compatible for 24 hr at 24°C	1655	C
Potassium chloride	AMR	2 mEq/mL	MI	2 mg/mL[a]	Visually compatible for 2 hr at 25°C	1628	C
Promethazine HCl	ES	25 mg/mL	MI	2 mg/mL[a b]	Visually compatible for 24 hr at 24°C	1655	C
Quinupristin–dalfo-pristin	PF	2 mg/mL[a h]		1 mg/mL[a]	Physically compatible	3229	C
Ranitidine HCl	GL	0.5 mg/mL[a b]	MI	2 mg/mL[a b]	Visually compatible for 24 hr at 24°C	1655	C
Remifentanil HCl	GW	0.025 and 0.25 mg/mL[b]	BAY	1 mg/mL[a]	Physically compatible for 4 hr at 23°C	2075	C
Sodium bicarbonate	AB	1 mEq/mL	MI	2 mg/mL[a]	Visually compatible for 24 hr at 24°C	1655	C
Sodium bicarbonate	AB	1 mEq/mL	MI	2 mg/mL[b]	Very fine crystals form in 20 min in NS	1655	I
Sodium bicarbonate	AB	1 mEq/mL	MI	2 mg/mL[a]	Physically compatible for 4 hr at 23°C	1869	C
Sodium bicarbonate	AB	0.1 mEq/mL[a]	MI	2 mg/mL[a]	Subvisible haze forms immediately. Crystalline precipitate in 4 hr at 23°C	1869	I
Sodium bicarbonate	AB	1 and 0.75[a] mEq/mL	BAY	1 and 2 mg/mL[a]	Physically compatible for 4 hr at 23°C	2065	C
Sodium bicarbonate	AB	1 and 0.75[b] mEq/mL	BAY	1 mg/mL[b]	Physically compatible for 4 hr at 23°C	2065	C
Sodium bicarbonate	AB	1 and 0.75[b] mEq/mL	BAY	2 mg/mL[b]	Particles form immediately, becoming more numerous over 4 hr at 23°C	2065	I
Sodium bicarbonate	AB	0.5, 0.25, 0.1 mEq/mL[a]	BAY	1 and 2 mg/mL[a]	Particles form immediately, becoming more numerous over 4 hr at 23°C	2065	I
Sodium bicarbonate	AB	0.5, 0.25, 0.1 mEq/mL[b]	BAY	1 mg/mL[b]	Particles form immediately, becoming more numerous over 4 hr at 23°C	2065	I
Sodium bicarbonate	AB	0.5, 0.25, 0.1 mEq/mL[b]	BAY	2 mg/mL[b]	Precipitate forms immediately	2065	I
Sodium chloride	AMR	4 mEq/mL	MI	2 mg/mL[a]	Visually compatible for 2 hr at 25°C	1628	C
Sodium phosphates	AB	3 mmol/mL	BAY	2 mg/mL[a]	Microcrystals form in 1 hr at 23°C	1972	I
Sodium phosphates	AB	3 mmol/mL	BAY	2 mg/mL[f]	White crystalline precipitate forms immediately	1971, 1972	I
Tacrolimus	FUJ	1 mg/mL[b]	MI	1 mg/mL[a]	Visually compatible for 24 hr at 25°C	1630	C
Tedizolid phosphate	CUB	0.8 mg/mL[b]	HOS	2 mg/mL[b]	Physically compatible for 2 hr	3244	C
Teicoplanin	GRP	60 mg/mL	BAY	2 mg/mL[b]	White precipitate forms immediately but disappears with shaking	1934	?
Telavancin HCl	ASP	7.5 mg/mL[a]	HOS	2 mg/mL[a]	Physically compatible for 2 hr	2830	C
Teniposide	BR	0.1 mg/mL[a]	MI	2 mg/mL[a]	Physically compatible for 4 hr at 23°C	1725	C
Thiotepa	IMM[g]	1 mg/mL[a]	MI	1 mg/mL[a]	Physically compatible for 4 hr at 23°C	1861	C
Tigecycline	WY	1 mg/mL[b]		1 mg/mL[b]	Physically compatible for 4 hr	2714	C
TNA #218 to #226[i]			BAY	1 mg/mL[a]	Visually compatible for 4 hr at 23°C	2215	C
Tobramycin sulfate	LI	1.6 mg/mL[a b]	MI	1 mg/mL[a]	Physically compatible for 24 hr at 22°C	1189	C
TPN #212 to #215[i]			MI	1 mg/mL[a]	Amber discoloration forms in 1 to 4 hr	2109	I

Y-Site Injection Compatibility (1:1 Mixture) (Cont.)

Test Drug	Mfr	Conc	Mfr	Conc	Remarks	Ref	C/I
Vasopressin	APP	0.2 unit/mL[b]	BAY	2 mg/mL[a]	Physically compatible	2641	C
Verapamil HCl	KN	2.5 mg/mL	MI	2 mg/mL[a b]	Visually compatible for 24 hr at 24°C	1655	C

[a] Tested in dextrose 5%.

[b] Tested in sodium chloride 0.9%.

[c] Concentration and volume not specified.

[d] Tested in sodium chloride 0.45%.

[e] Injected via Y-site into an administration set running azithromycin.

[f] Tested in both sodium chloride 0.9% and 0.45%.

[g] Lyophilized formulation tested.

[h] Quinupristin and dalfopristin components combined.

[i] Refer to Appendix for the composition of parenteral nutrition solutions. TNA indicates a 3-in-1 admixture, and TPN indicates a 2-in-1 admixture.

[j] Run at 100 mL/hr.

[k] Tested in Ringer's injection, lactated.

[l] Ampicillin component. Ampicillin in a 2:1 fixed-ratio concentration with sulbactam.

[m] Test performed using the lactate salt formulation.

[n] Tested in both dextrose 5% and sodium chloride 0.9%.

[o] Ceftolozane component. Ceftolozane in a 2:1 fixed-ratio concentration with tazobactam.

[p] Meropenem component. Meropenem in a 1:1 fixed-ratio concentration with vaborbactam.

[q] Run at 25 mL/hr with dextrose 5% run at 83 mL/hr.

[r] Tested as the premixed infusion solution.

Additional Compatibility Information
Peritoneal Dialysis Solutions

Ciprofloxacin 25 mg/L in Dianeal 137 peritoneal dialysis solution exhibited little or no loss after 42 days at 4, 22, and 37°C when protected from light.[1585] At 37°C over 48 hours, losses of up to 10% occurred in Dianeal PD-1 with dextrose 1.5%; losses of up to 7% occurred in Dianeal PD-1 with dextrose 4.5%.[1826] Ciprofloxacin 25 and 50 mg/L in Dianeal PD-2 with dextrose 1.5, 2.5, and 4.25% and Extraneal, all solutions both with and without heparin, were found to be stable for 4 days at 38°C.[2686]

Selected Revisions May 1, 2020. © Copyright, October 1992. American Society of Health-System Pharmacists, Inc.

Cisatracurium Besylate
AHFS 12:20.20

Products

Cisatracurium besylate is available as a 2-mg/mL solution in 5- and 10-mL vials.[2868] The drug is also available as a 10-mg/mL solution in 20-mL vials intended for use in intensive care units only.[2868] The pH is adjusted with benzenesulfonic acid.[2868] The 2-mg/mL concentration in 10-mL vials also contains benzyl alcohol 0.9%.[2868] The other dosage forms have no preservative and are for single use only.[2868]

pH

From 3.25 to 3.65.[2868]

Trade Name(s)

Nimbex

Administration

Cisatracurium besylate is administered intravenously only.[2868] Both initial bolus doses and continuous intravenous infusion have been used.[2868] Rates of administration depend on the drug concentration in the solution, desired dose, and patient weight.[2868] Avoid contact with alkaline drugs during administration.[2868]

Stability

Cisatracurium besylate injection is a colorless to slightly yellow or greenish-yellow solution.[2868] Intact vials of cisatracurium besylate should be stored at 2 to 8°C protected from light and freezing.[2868] Potency losses of 5% per year occur under refrigeration.[2868] However, at 25°C, potency losses increase to about 5% per month.[2868] The manufacturer recommends that vials that have been warmed to room temperature be used within 21 days even if rerefrigerated.[2868]

In an independent study, cisatracurium besylate 2 mg/mL in 5- and 10-mL vials and the 10-mg/mL solution in 20-mL vials was stored at 4 and 23°C both protected from light and exposed to fluorescent light. All the samples remained physically stable throughout the 90-day study period. Samples stored under refrigeration exhibited little or no drug loss in 90 days whether exposed to or protected from light. At 23°C, samples were stable through 45 days of storage with losses near 5 to 7% in most samples. However, most samples became unacceptable after 90 days of storage at 23°C, exhibiting losses of 9 to 14%.[2116]

pH Effects

The manufacturer indicates that cisatracurium besylate may not be compatible with barbiturates and other alkaline solutions having a pH greater than 8.5.[2868]

Syringes

In 2015, reports of decreased potency of certain drugs (e.g., cisatracurium besylate) stored in Becton Dickinson syringes for extended periods (i.e., exceeding 24 hours) were confirmed by the manufacturer of these syringes; the cause of this change was later identified to be the inclusion of an alternate rubber stopper in the plunger of certain product lots of syringes.[3029 3036 3037 3039 3041 3042] Decreased potency was not observed when the syringes were filled and used promptly.[3037] Use of the alternate stopper was later discontinued and use of the primary stopper in such syringes was resumed; however, Becton Dickinson states that its general-use syringes are cleared by FDA for immediate use in fluid aspiration and injection and that such syringes, regardless of the stopper material, have not been cleared by FDA for use as a closed-container system.[3391]

Cisatracurium besylate 2 mg/mL was repackaged in 3-mL plastic syringes (Becton Dickinson) and sealed with tip caps (Red Cap, Burron). The syringes were stored at 4 and 23°C both protected from light and exposed to fluorescent light. All of the samples remained physically stable throughout the 30-day study period. Little or no loss occurred when stored under refrigeration, whereas samples stored at 23°C exhibited 4 to 7% loss in 30 days.[2116]

Compatibility Information

Solution Compatibility

Cisatracurium besylate

Test Soln Name	Mfr	Mfr	Conc/L or %	Remarks	Ref	C/I
Dextrose 5%			100 mg	Stable for 24 hr at 4 and 25°C	2868	C
Dextrose 5%	BA[a]	GW	100 mg	Physically compatible with 8% loss in 7 days and 15% loss in 14 days at 23°C under fluorescent light. Little loss in 30 days at 4°C	2116	C
Dextrose 5%	BA[a]	GW	2 g	Physically compatible with 10% loss in 14 days and 14% loss in 30 days at 23°C under fluorescent light. Little loss in 30 days at 4°C	2116	C
Dextrose 5%	BA[a]	GW	5 g	Physically compatible with 4% loss in 30 days at 23°C under fluorescent light. Little loss in 30 days at 4°C	2116	C

DOI: 10.37573/9781585286850.089

Solution Compatibility (Cont.)

Test Soln Name	Mfr	Mfr	Conc/L or %	Remarks	Ref	C/I
Dextrose 5% in Ringer's injection, lactated			100 to 200 mg	Stable for 24 hr at 4°C	2868	C
Dextrose 5% in sodium chloride 0.9%			100 mg	Stable for 24 hr at 4 and 25°C	2868	C
Ringer's injection, lactated				Cisatracurium unstable	2868	I
Sodium chloride 0.9%			100 mg	Stable for 24 hr at 4 and 25°C	2868	C
Sodium chloride 0.9%	BA[a]	GW	100 mg	Physically compatible with 8% loss in 14 days and 14% loss in 30 days at 23°C under fluorescent light. Little loss in 30 days at 4°C	2116	C
Sodium chloride 0.9%	BA[a]	GW	2 g	Physically compatible with 6% loss in 30 days at 23°C under fluorescent light. Little loss in 30 days at 4°C	2116	C
Sodium chloride 0.9%	BA[a]	GW	5 g	Physically compatible with 3% loss in 30 days at 23°C under fluorescent light. Little loss in 30 days at 4°C	2116	C

[a] Tested in PVC containers.

Y-Site Injection Compatibility (1:1 Mixture)

Cisatracurium besylate

Test Drug	Mfr	Conc	Mfr	Conc	Remarks	Ref	C/I
Acyclovir sodium	BW	7 mg/mL[a]	GW	0.1 and 2 mg/mL[a]	Physically compatible for 4 hr at 23°C	2074	C
Acyclovir sodium	BW	7 mg/mL[a]	GW	5 mg/mL[a]	White cloudiness forms immediately	2074	I
Alfentanil HCl	JN	0.125 mg/mL[a]	GW	0.1, 2, 5 mg/mL[a]	Physically compatible for 4 hr at 23°C	2074	C
Amikacin sulfate	AB	5 mg/mL[a]	GW	0.1, 2, 5 mg/mL[a]	Physically compatible for 4 hr at 23°C	2074	C
Aminophylline	AB	2.5 mg/mL[a]	GW	0.1 and 2 mg/mL[a]	Physically compatible for 4 hr at 23°C	2074	C
Aminophylline	AB	2.5 mg/mL[a]	GW	5 mg/mL[a]	Gray subvisible haze forms in 1 hr	2074	I
Amphotericin B	PH	0.6 mg/mL[a]	GW	0.1 mg/mL[a]	Physically compatible for 4 hr at 23°C	2074	C
Amphotericin B	PH	0.6 mg/mL[a]	GW	2 mg/mL[a]	Cloudiness forms immediately; gel-like precipitate forms in 1 hr	2074	I
Amphotericin B	PH	0.6 mg/mL[a]	GW	5 mg/mL[a]	Turbidity forms immediately	2074	I
Ampicillin sodium	SKB	20 mg/mL[b]	GW	0.1 and 2 mg/mL[a]	Physically compatible for 4 hr at 23°C	2074	C
Ampicillin sodium	SKB	20 mg/mL[b]	GW	5 mg/mL[a]	Gray subvisible haze forms in 1 hr	2074	I
Ampicillin sodium–sulbactam sodium	RR	20 mg/mL[b e]	GW	0.1 and 2 mg/mL[a]	Physically compatible for 4 hr at 23°C	2074	C
Ampicillin sodium–sulbactam sodium	RR	20 mg/mL[b e]	GW	5 mg/mL[a]	Subvisible haze develops in 15 min	2074	I
Aztreonam	SQ	40 mg/mL[a]	GW	0.1, 2, 5 mg/mL[a]	Physically compatible for 4 hr at 23°C	2074	C
Bumetanide	BV	0.04 mg/mL[a]	GW	0.1, 2, 5 mg/mL[a]	Physically compatible for 4 hr at 23°C	2074	C
Buprenorphine HCl	RKC	0.04 mg/mL[a]	GW	0.1, 2, 5 mg/mL[a]	Physically compatible for 4 hr at 23°C	2074	C
Butorphanol tartrate	APC	0.04 mg/mL[a]	GW	0.1, 2, 5 mg/mL[a]	Physically compatible for 4 hr at 23°C	2074	C
Calcium gluconate	AB	40 mg/mL[a]	GW	0.1, 2, 5 mg/mL[a]	Physically compatible for 4 hr at 23°C	2074	C
Calcium gluconate	APP	20 mg/mL[b]	AB	1 mg/mL[b]	Physically compatible for 1 hr at 23°C	3157	C
Cefazolin sodium	SKB	20 mg/mL[a]	GW	0.1 mg/mL[a]	Physically compatible for 4 hr at 23°C	2074	C
Cefazolin sodium	SKB	20 mg/mL[a]	GW	2 mg/mL[a]	Gray subvisible haze forms immediately	2074	I

Y-Site Injection Compatibility (1:1 Mixture) (Cont.)

Test Drug	Mfr	Conc	Mfr	Conc	Remarks	Ref	C/I
Cefazolin sodium	SKB	20 mg/mL[a]	GW	5 mg/mL[a]	Gray haze forms immediately	2074	I
Cefotaxime sodium	HO	20 mg/mL[a]	GW	0.1 mg/mL[a]	Physically compatible for 4 hr at 23°C	2074	C
Cefotaxime sodium	HO	20 mg/mL[a]	GW	2 mg/mL[a]	Subvisible haze forms in 4 hr	2074	I
Cefotaxime sodium	HO	20 mg/mL[a]	GW	5 mg/mL[a]	Subvisible haze forms immediately	2074	I
Cefoxitin sodium	ME	20 mg/mL[a]	GW	0.1 mg/mL[a]	Physically compatible for 4 hr at 23°C	2074	C
Cefoxitin sodium	ME	20 mg/mL[a]	GW	2 and 5 mg/mL[a]	Subvisible haze forms immediately	2074	I
Ceftaroline fosamil	FOR	2.22 mg/mL[a b c]	HOS	0.5 mg/mL[a b c]	Physically compatible for 4 hr at 23°C	2826	C
Ceftazidime	SKB	40 mg/mL[a]	GW	0.1 and 2 mg/mL[a]	Physically compatible for 4 hr at 23°C	2074	C
Ceftazidime	SKB	40 mg/mL[a]	GW	5 mg/mL[a]	Subvisible haze forms immediately	2074	I
Ceftolozane sulfate–tazobactam sodium	CUB	10 mg/mL[k l]	ABV	0.4 mg/mL[k]	Physically compatible for 2 hr	3262	C
Ceftriaxone sodium	RC	20 mg/mL[a]	GW	0.1, 2, 5 mg/mL[a]	Physically compatible for 4 hr at 23°C	2074	C
Cefuroxime sodium	LI	30 mg/mL[a]	GW	0.1 mg/mL[a]	Physically compatible for 4 hr at 23°C	2074	C
Cefuroxime sodium	LI	30 mg/mL[a]	GW	2 mg/mL[a]	White cloudiness forms immediately	2074	I
Cefuroxime sodium	LI	30 mg/mL[a]	GW	5 mg/mL[a]	Turbidity forms immediately	2074	I
Chlorpromazine HCl	SCN	2 mg/mL[a]	GW	0.1, 2, 5 mg/mL[a]	Physically compatible for 4 hr at 23°C	2074	C
Ciprofloxacin	BAY	1 mg/mL[a]	GW	0.1, 2, 5 mg/mL[a]	Physically compatible for 4 hr at 23°C	2074	C
Clindamycin phosphate	AST	10 mg/mL[a]	GW	0.1, 2, 5 mg/mL[a]	Physically compatible for 4 hr at 23°C	2074	C
Dexamethasone sodium phosphate	FUJ	2 mg/mL[a]	GW	0.1, 2, 5 mg/mL[a]	Physically compatible for 4 hr at 23°C	2074	C
Dexmedetomidine HCl	AB	4 mcg/mL[b]	GW	0.5 mg/mL[b]	Physically compatible for 4 hr at 23°C	2383	C
Diazepam	ES	5 mg/mL	GW	0.1, 2, 5 mg/mL[a]	White turbidity forms immediately	2074	I
Diazepam	ES	0.25 mg/mL[a]	GW	0.1, 2, 5 mg/mL[a]	Physically compatible for 4 hr at 23°C	2074	C
Digoxin	ES	0.25 mg/mL	GW	0.1, 2, 5 mg/mL[a]	Physically compatible for 4 hr at 23°C	2074	C
Diltiazem HCl	BA	1 mg/mL[b]	AB	1 mg/mL[b]	Physically compatible for 1 hr at 23°C	3157	C
Diphenhydramine HCl	SCN	2 mg/mL[a]	GW	0.1, 2, 5 mg/mL[a]	Physically compatible for 4 hr at 23°C	2074	C
Dobutamine HCl	LI	4 mg/mL[a]	GW	0.1, 2, 5 mg/mL[a]	Physically compatible for 4 hr at 23°C	2074	C
Dopamine HCl	AB	3.2 mg/mL[a]	GW	0.1, 2, 5 mg/mL[a]	Physically compatible for 4 hr at 23°C	2074	C
Doxycycline hyclate	FUJ	1 mg/mL[a]	GW	0.1, 2, 5 mg/mL[a]	Physically compatible for 4 hr at 23°C	2074	C
Droperidol	AB	2.5 mg/mL	GW	0.1, 2, 5 mg/mL[a]	Physically compatible for 4 hr at 23°C	2074	C
Enalaprilat	ME	0.1 mg/mL[a]	GW	0.1, 2, 5 mg/mL[a]	Physically compatible for 4 hr at 23°C	2074	C
Epinephrine HCl	AMR	0.05 mg/mL[a]	GW	0.1, 2, 5 mg/mL[a]	Physically compatible for 4 hr at 23°C	2074	C
Eravacycline dihydrochloride	TET	0.6 mg/mL[b]	ABV	0.4 mg/mL[b]	Physically compatible for 2 hr at room temperature	3532	C
Esmolol HCl	OHM	10 mg/mL[a]	GW	0.1, 2, 5 mg/mL[a]	Physically compatible for 4 hr at 23°C	2074	C
Esmolol HCl	MYL	10 mg/mL[a]	AB	2 mg/mL	Physically compatible for 1 hr at 23°C	3533	C
Esomeprazole sodium	ASZ	0.4 mg/mL[b]	AB	1 mg/mL[b]	Physically compatible for 1 hr at 23°C	3157	C

Y-Site Injection Compatibility (1:1 Mixture) (Cont.)

Test Drug	Mfr	Conc	Mfr	Conc	Remarks	Ref	C/I
Famotidine	ME	2 mg/mL[a]	GW	0.1, 2, 5 mg/mL[a]	Physically compatible for 4 hr at 23°C	2074	C
Fenoldopam mesylate	AB	80 mcg/mL[b]	AB	0.5 mg/mL[b]	Physically compatible for 4 hr at 23°C	2467	C
Fentanyl citrate	AB	12.5 mcg/mL[a]	GW	0.1, 2, 5 mg/mL[a]	Physically compatible for 4 hr at 23°C	2074	C
Fluconazole	RR	2 mg/mL	GW	0.1, 2, 5 mg/mL[a]	Physically compatible for 4 hr at 23°C	2074	C
Furosemide	AB	3 mg/mL[a]	GW	0.1 mg/mL[a]	Physically compatible for 4 hr at 23°C	2074	C
Furosemide	AB	3 mg/mL[a]	GW	2 and 5 mg/mL[a]	White cloudiness forms immediately	2074	I
Ganciclovir sodium	SY	20 mg/mL[a]	GW	0.1 and 2 mg/mL[a]	Physically compatible for 4 hr at 23°C	2074	C
Ganciclovir sodium	SY	20 mg/mL[a]	GW	5 mg/mL[a]	White cloudiness forms immediately	2074	I
Gentamicin sulfate	ES	5 mg/mL[a]	GW	0.1, 2, 5 mg/mL[a]	Physically compatible for 4 hr at 23°C	2074	C
Haloperidol lactate	MN	0.2 mg/mL[a]	GW	0.1, 2, 5 mg/mL[a]	Physically compatible for 4 hr at 23°C	2074	C
Heparin sodium	AB	100 units/mL	GW	0.1 and 2 mg/mL[a]	Physically compatible for 4 hr at 23°C	2074	C
Heparin sodium	AB	100 units/mL	GW	5 mg/mL[a]	White cloudiness forms immediately	2074	I
Hetastarch in lactated electrolyte	AB	6%	GW	0.5 mg/mL[a]	Physically compatible for 4 hr at 23°C	2339	C
Hydrocortisone sodium succinate	AB	1 mg/mL[a]	GW	0.1, 2, 5 mg/mL[a]	Physically compatible for 4 hr at 23°C	2074	C
Hydromorphone HCl	ES	0.5 mg/mL[a]	GW	0.1, 2, 5 mg/mL[a]	Physically compatible for 4 hr at 23°C	2074	C
Hydroxyzine HCl	ES	2 mg/mL[a]	GW	0.1, 2, 5 mg/mL[a]	Physically compatible for 4 hr at 23°C	2074	C
Imipenem–cilastatin sodium	ME	10 mg/mL[b h]	GW	0.1, 2, 5 mg/mL[a]	Physically compatible for 4 hr at 23°C	2074	C
Insulin, regular	LI	1 unit/mL[b]	AB	1 mg/mL[b]	Physically compatible for 1 hr at 23°C	3157	C
Isavuconazonium sulfate	ASP	1.5 mg/mL[k]	ABV	0.4 mg/mL[k]	Physically compatible for 2 hr	3263	C
Isoproterenol HCl	AB	0.02 mg/mL[a]	GW	0.1, 2, 5 mg/mL[a]	Physically compatible for 4 hr at 23°C	2074	C
Ketorolac tromethamine	RC	15 mg/mL[a]	GW	0.1, 2, 5 mg/mL[a]	Physically compatible for 4 hr at 23°C	2074	C
Ketorolac tromethamine			ABV		Manufacturer states incompatible	2868	I
Labetalol HCl	HOS	5 mg/mL	AB	2 mg/mL	Physically compatible for 1 hr at 23°C	3533	C
Lidocaine HCl	AST	8 mg/mL[a]	GW	0.1, 2, 5 mg/mL[a]	Physically compatible for 4 hr at 23°C	2074	C
Linezolid	PHU	2 mg/mL	GW	2 mg/mL	Physically compatible for 4 hr at 23°C	2264	C
Lorazepam	WY	0.5 mcg/mL[a]	GW	0.1, 2, 5 mg/mL[a]	Physically compatible for 4 hr at 23°C	2074	C
Magnesium sulfate	AB	100 mg/mL[a]	GW	0.1, 2, 5 mg/mL[a]	Physically compatible for 4 hr at 23°C	2074	C
Mannitol	BA	15%	GW	0.1, 2, 5 mg/mL[a]	Physically compatible for 4 hr at 23°C	2074	C
Meperidine HCl	AST	4 mg/mL[a]	GW	0.1, 2, 5 mg/mL[a]	Physically compatible for 4 hr at 23°C	2074	C
Meropenem–vaborbactam	TMC	8 mg/mL[b i]	ABV	0.4 mg/mL[b]	Physically compatible for 3 hr at 20 to 25°C	3380	C
Methylprednisolone sodium succinate	AB	5 mg/mL[a]	GW	0.1 mg/mL[a]	Physically compatible for 4 hr at 23°C	2074	C
Methylprednisolone sodium succinate	AB	5 mg/mL[a]	GW	2 mg/mL[a]	Subvisible haze forms immediately	2074	I
Methylprednisolone sodium succinate	AB	5 mg/mL[a]	GW	5 mg/mL[a]	Haze forms immediately	2074	I

Y-Site Injection Compatibility (1:1 Mixture) (Cont.)

Test Drug	Mfr	Conc	Mfr	Conc	Remarks	Ref	C/I
Metoclopramide HCl	AB	5 mg/mL	GW	0.1, 2, 5 mg/mL[a]	Physically compatible for 4 hr at 23°C	2074	C
Metoprolol tartrate	HOS	0.4 mg/mL[b]	AB	2 mg/mL	Physically compatible for 1 hr at 23°C	3533	C
Metronidazole	AB	5 mg/mL	GW	0.1, 2, 5 mg/mL[a]	Physically compatible for 4 hr at 23°C	2074	C
Micafungin sodium	ASP	1.5 mg/mL[b]	AB	0.5 mg/mL[b]	Gross precipitate forms immediately	2683	I
Midazolam HCl	RC	1 mg/mL[a]	GW	0.1, 2, 5 mg/mL[a]	Physically compatible for 4 hr at 23°C	2074	C
Morphine sulfate	AST	1 mg/mL[a]	GW	0.1, 2, 5 mg/mL[a]	Physically compatible for 4 hr at 23°C	2074	C
Nalbuphine HCl	AST	10 mg/mL	GW	0.1, 2, 5 mg/mL[a]	Physically compatible for 4 hr at 23°C	2074	C
Nicardipine HCl	CRC	0.5 mg/mL[b]	AB	1 mg/mL[b]	Physically compatible for 1 hr at 23°C	3157	C
Nitroglycerin	DU	0.4 mg/mL[a]	GW	0.1, 2, 5 mg/mL[a]	Physically compatible for 4 hr at 23°C	2074	C
Norepinephrine bitartrate	SW	0.12 mg/mL[a]	GW	0.1, 2, 5 mg/mL[a]	Physically compatible for 4 hr at 23°C	2074	C
Ondansetron HCl	CER	1 mg/mL[a]	GW	0.1, 2, 5 mg/mL[a]	Physically compatible for 4 hr at 23°C	2074	C
Palonosetron HCl	MGI	50 mcg/mL	AB	0.5 mg/mL[a]	Physically compatible with no loss of either drug in 4 hr at room temperature	2764	C
Pantoprazole sodium	PF	0.8 mg/mL[b j]	AB	1 mg/mL[b]	Increase in measured turbidity	3157	I
Phenylephrine HCl	GNS	1 mg/mL[a]	GW	0.1, 2, 5 mg/mL[a]	Physically compatible for 4 hr at 23°C	2074	C
Piperacillin sodium–tazobactam sodium	CY[d]	40 mg/mL[a f]	GW	0.1 and 2 mg/mL[a]	Physically compatible for 4 hr at 23°C	2074	C
Piperacillin sodium–tazobactam sodium	CY[d]	40 mg/mL[a f]	GW	5 mg/mL[a]	Particles and subvisible haze within 4 hr	2074	I
Plazomicin sulfate	ACH	24 mg/mL[k]	ABV	0.4 mg/mL[k]	Physically compatible for 1 hr at 20 to 25°C	3432	C
Potassium chloride	AB	0.1 mEq/mL[a]	GW	0.1, 2, 5 mg/mL[a]	Physically compatible for 4 hr at 23°C	2074	C
Procainamide HCl	ES	10 mg/mL[a]	GW	0.1, 2, 5 mg/mL[a]	Physically compatible for 4 hr at 23°C	2074	C
Prochlorperazine edisylate	SO	0.5 mg/mL[a]	GW	0.1, 2, 5 mg/mL[a]	Physically compatible for 4 hr at 23°C	2074	C
Promethazine HCl	ES	2 mg/mL[a]	GW	0.1, 2, 5 mg/mL[a]	Physically compatible for 4 hr at 23°C	2074	C
Propofol	ASZ[m]	10 mg/mL	GW	5 mg/mL	Emulsion disruption upon mixing	2336	I
Propofol	BA[d]	10 mg/mL	GW	5 mg/mL	Emulsion disruption upon mixing	2336	I
Propofol	BA[d]	10 mg/mL	GW	0.5 mg/mL[a]	Emulsion disruption upon mixing	2336	I
Propofol	ASZ[m]	10 mg/mL	GW	0.5 mg/mL[a]	Physically compatible	2336	C
Propofol	[m]		ABV		Manufacturer states incompatible	2868	I
Ranitidine HCl	GL	2 mg/mL[a]	GW	0.1, 2, 5 mg/mL[a]	Physically compatible for 4 hr at 23°C	2074	C
Remifentanil HCl	GW	0.025 and 0.25 mg/mL[b]	GW	2 mg/mL[a]	Physically compatible for 4 hr at 23°C	2075	C
Sodium bicarbonate	AB	1 mEq/mL	GW	0.1 mg/mL[a]	Physically compatible for 4 hr at 23°C	2074	C
Sodium bicarbonate	AB	1 mEq/mL	GW	2 mg/mL[a]	Subvisible brown color and haze in 1 hr	2074	I
Sodium bicarbonate	AB	1 mEq/mL	GW	5 mg/mL[a]	Subvisible haze forms immediately with brown color and turbidity in 4 hr	2074	I
Sodium nitroprusside	AB	2 mg/mL[a]	GW	0.1 mg/mL[a]	Physically compatible for 4 hr at 23°C protected from light	2074	C

Y-Site Injection Compatibility (1:1 Mixture) (Cont.)

Test Drug	Mfr	Conc	Mfr	Conc	Remarks	Ref	C/I
Sodium nitroprusside	AB	2 mg/mL[a]	GW	2 and 5 mg/mL[a]	White cloudiness forms immediately	2074	I
Sufentanil citrate	ES	0.0125 mg/mL[a]	GW	0.1, 2, 5 mg/mL[a]	Physically compatible for 4 hr at 23°C	2074	C
Tedizolid phosphate	CUB	0.8 mg/mL[b]	ABV	0.4 mg/mL[b]	Physically compatible for 2 hr	3244	C
Theophylline	AB	3.2 mg/mL	GW	0.1, 2, 5 mg/mL[a]	Physically compatible for 4 hr at 23°C	2074	C
Tobramycin sulfate	AB	5 mg/mL[a]	GW	0.1, 2, 5 mg/mL[a]	Physically compatible for 4 hr at 23°C	2074	C
Trimethoprim–sulfamethoxazole	ES	0.8 mg/mL[a g]	GW	0.1 mg/mL[a]	Physically compatible for 4 hr at 23°C	2074	C
Trimethoprim–sulfamethoxazole	ES	0.8 mg/mL[a g]	GW	2 mg/mL[a]	Subvisible haze forms in 1 hr	2074	I
Trimethoprim–sulfamethoxazole	ES	0.8 mg/mL[a g]	GW	5 mg/mL[a]	Subvisible haze forms immediately	2074	I
Vancomycin HCl	AB	10 mg/mL[a]	GW	0.1, 2, 5 mg/mL[a]	Physically compatible for 4 hr at 23°C	2074	C
Vasopressin	AMR	1 unit/mL[b]	AB	1 mg/mL[b]	Physically compatible for 1 hr at 23°C	3157	C
Zidovudine	BW	4 mg/mL[a]	GW	0.1, 2, 5 mg/mL[a]	Physically compatible for 4 hr at 23°C	2074	C

[a] Tested in dextrose 5%.

[b] Tested in sodium chloride 0.9%.

[c] Tested in Ringer's injection, lactated.

[d] Test performed using the formulation WITHOUT edetate disodium.

[e] Ampicillin component. Ampicillin in a 2:1 fixed-ratio concentration with sulbactam.

[f] Piperacillin component. Piperacillin in an 8:1 fixed-ratio concentration with tazobactam.

[g] Trimethoprim component. Trimethoprim in a 1:5 fixed-ratio concentration with sulfamethoxazole.

[h] Not specified whether concentration refers to single component or combined components.

[i] Meropenem component. Meropenem in a 1:1 fixed-ratio concentration with vaborbactam.

[j] Presence or absence of edetate disodium not specified.

[k] Tested in both dextrose 5% and sodium chloride 0.9%.

[l] Ceftolozane component. Ceftolozane in a 2:1 fixed-ratio concentration with tazobactam.

[m] Test performed using the formulation WITH edetate disodium.

Selected Revisions May 1, 2020. © Copyright, October 2000.
American Society of Health-System Pharmacists, Inc.

Cisplatin
AHFS 10:00

Products

Cisplatin is available as a sterile aqueous injection containing cisplatin 1 mg/mL and sodium chloride 9 mg/mL, with hydrochloric acid and/or sodium hydroxide to adjust the pH. This aqueous solution is available in 50-mL (50-mg), 100-mL (100-mg), and 200-mL (200-mg) vials.[1(1/08)] [4]

pH

From 3.5 to 4.5.[1(1/08)]

Osmolality

The aqueous injection has an osmolality of about 285 mOsm/kg.[4]

Sodium Content

Each 10 mg of cisplatin contains 1.54 mEq of sodium.[846] [869]

Administration

Cisplatin is administered by intravenous infusion with a regimen of hydration (with or without mannitol and/or furosemide) prior to therapy. One regimen consists of 1 to 2 L of fluid given over 8 to 12 hours prior to cisplatin administration. In addition, adequate hydration and urinary output must be maintained for 24 hours after therapy. The official labeling recommends diluting the cisplatin dose in 2 L of compatible infusion solution containing mannitol 37.5 g and infusing over 6 to 8 hours.[1(1/08)] [4] Other dilutions and rates of administration have been used, including intravenous infusions over periods from 15 to 120 minutes and continuous infusion over 1 to 5 days. Intra-arterial infusion and intraperitoneal instillation have been used.[4]

Because of an interaction occurring between cisplatin and the metal aluminum, only administration equipment such as needles, syringes, catheters, and sets that contain no aluminum should be used for this drug. Aluminum in contact with cisplatin solution will result in a replacement oxidation–reduction reaction, forcing platinum from the cisplatin molecule out of solution and appearing as a black or brown precipitate. Other metal components such as stainless steel needles and plated brass hubs do not elicit an observable reaction within 24 hours.[1(1/08)] [203] [204] [512] [988]

Stability

Intact vials of the clear, colorless aqueous injection should be stored between 20 and 25°C and protected from light; they should not be refrigerated.[1(1/08)] [4]

After initial vial entry, the aqueous cisplatin injection in amber vials is stable for 28 days if it is protected from light or for 7 days if it is exposed to fluorescent room light.[1(1/08)]

Concern has been expressed that storage of cisplatin solutions for several weeks might result in substantial amounts of the toxic mono- and di-aquo species.[1199] However, the solution's chloride content, rather than extended storage time periods, appears to determine the extent of aquated product formation. (See Effect of Chloride Ion below.)

Kristjansson et al. evaluated the long-term stability of cisplatin 1 mg/mL in an aqueous solution containing sodium chloride 9 mg/mL and mannitol 10 mg/mL in glass vials. After 22 months at 5°C, the 4% loss of cisplatin could be explained as the expected equilibrium between cisplatin and its aquated products. Furthermore, a precipitate formed and required sonication at 40°C for about 20 to 30 minutes to redissolve. Storage of the cisplatin solution at 40°C for 10 months resulted in no physical change. After an additional 1 year at 5°C, these samples exhibited an average 15% loss, which the authors concluded was not the result of the formation of aquated species or the toxic and inactive oligomeric species. These proposed degradation products were not present in the 40°C sample.[1246]

Theuer et al. reported little or no loss of cisplatin potency, after 27 days at room temperature with protection from light, from a solution of cisplatin 500 mcg/mL in sodium chloride 0.9% at pH 4.75 and 3.25.[1605]

Cisplatin may react with sodium thiosulfate, sodium metabisulfite, and sodium bisulfite in solution, rapidly and completely inactivating the cisplatin.[4] [1089] [1175]

Cisplatin 1 mg/mL did not support the growth of several microorganisms and may impart an antimicrobial effect at this concentration. Loss of viability was observed for *Staphylococcus aureus*, *Escherichia coli*, *Pseudomonas aeruginosa*, *Pseudomonas cepacia*, *Candida albicans*, and *Aspergillus niger*.[1187]

pH Effects

The pH of maximum stability is 3.5 to 5.5. Alkaline media should be avoided because of increased hydrolysis.[1379]

In the dark at pH 6.3, cisplatin (Bristol) 1 mg/mL in sodium chloride 0.9% reached the maximum amount of decomposition product permitted in the *USP* in 34 days. Half of that amount was formed in 96 days at pH 4.3.[1647]

Cisplatin degradation results in ammonia formation, which increases the solution pH. Thus, the initial cisplatin degradation rate may be slow but increases with time.[1647]

Temperature Effects

It is recommended that cisplatin not be refrigerated because of the formation of a crystalline precipitate.[1(1/08)] [4] [633] [636] [1246] In a study of cisplatin at concentrations of 0.4 to 1 mg/mL in sodium chloride 0.9%, it was found that at 0.6 mg/mL or greater a precipitate formed on refrigeration at 2 to 6°C. At 1 mg/mL the precipitation was noted in 1 hour. However, the 0.6-mg/mL solution did not have a precipitate until after 48 hours under refrigeration. The 0.5-mg/mL and lower solutions did not precipitate for up to 72 hours at 2 to 6°C. In solutions where precipitate did form, redissolution occurred very slowly with warming back to

DOI: 10.37573/9781585286850.090

room temperature.[317] Sonication at 40°C has been used to redissolve the precipitate in about 20 to 30 minutes.[1246] The warming of precipitated cisplatin solutions to effect redissolution is not recommended, however. Solutions containing a precipitate should not be used.[4 633]

Freezing Solutions

Cisplatin (Bristol) 50 and 200 mg/L in dextrose 5% in sodium chloride 0.45% in polyvinyl chloride (PVC) bags and admixed with either mannitol 18.75 g/L or magnesium sulfate 1 or 2 g/L is reportedly stable for 30 days when frozen at −15°C followed by an additional 48 hours at 25°C.[1088]

Light Effects

Although changes in the UV spectra of cisplatin solutions on exposure to intense light have long been recognized,[317] their significance was questioned. It was reported that exposure to normal laboratory light for 72 hours had no significant effect on cisplatin's stability.[635]

More recently, however, Zieske et al. reported substantial cisplatin decomposition after exposure to typical laboratory light, a mixture of incandescent and fluorescent illumination. As much as 12% degraded to trichloroammineplatinate (II) after 25 hours. Cisplatin was most sensitive to light in the UV to blue region and had little sensitivity to yellow or red light. It was protected from light-induced degradation by low-actinic amber glass flasks but not by PVC bags, clear glass vials, or polyethylene syringes. The authors concluded that exposure to moderately intense white light for more than 1 hour should be avoided.[1647]

The manufacturer recommends that a cisplatin solution removed from its amber vial be protected from light if it is not used within 6 hours. Even in the amber vial, the cisplatin solution should be discarded after 7 days if exposed to fluorescent room light.[1(1/08)]

Chloride Ion Effects

The stability of cisplatin in solution is dependent on the chloride ion concentration present. Cisplatin is stable in solutions containing an adequate amount of chloride ion but is incompatible in solutions having a low chloride content.[4 316 317 634 635 637]

In solutions with an inadequate chloride content, one or both chloride ions in the cisplatin molecule are displaced by water, forming mono- and di-aquo species. The minimum acceptable chloride ion concentration is about 0.040 mol/L, the equivalent of about 0.2% sodium chloride.[317 634 635]

At a cisplatin concentration of 200 mg/L in sodium chloride 0.9% with the pH adjusted to 4, about 3% decomposition occurs in less than 1 hour at room temperature. An equilibrium is then reached, with the cisplatin remaining stable thereafter. At lesser concentrations of chloride ion, greater decomposition of cisplatin occurs. In sodium chloride 0.45 and 0.2%, approximately 4 and 7% decomposition occurred at equilibrium, respectively. In very low chloride-containing solutions, most of the drug may be decomposed. The decomposition appears to be reversible, with cisplatin being reformed in the presence of high chloride concentrations.[317]

In another study, the stability of cisplatin 50 and 500 mg/L was evaluated in aqueous solutions containing sodium chloride 0.9, 0.45, and 0.1% and also in water over 24 hours at 25°C exposed to light. Approximately 2 and 4% of the cisplatin were lost in the sodium chloride 0.9 and 0.45% solutions, respectively. In the 0.1% solution, about 4 to 10% decomposition occurred in 4 to 6 hours, increasing to approximately 11 to 15% at both 12 and 24 hours. In aqueous solution with no chloride content, cisplatin decomposed rapidly, with about a 30 to 35% loss in 4 hours increasing to a 70 to 80% loss in 24 hours.[635]

Ambulatory Pumps

Cisplatin (David Bull) reconstituted to concentrations of 1 and 1.6 mg/mL with sterile water for injection was evaluated for stability for 14 days protected from light in Pharmacia Deltec medication cassettes at 24 and 37°C. The 1.6-mg/mL concentration developed a yellow crystalline precipitate rendering it unfit for use. For the 1-mg/mL concentration, little change in cisplatin concentration was found, but water loss due to evaporation was found to be about 1% at 24°C and 3% at 37°C in 14 days.[2319]

Filtration

Cisplatin 10 to 300 mcg/mL exhibited no loss due to sorption to cellulose nitrate/cellulose acetate ester (Millex OR) or Teflon (Millex FG) filters.[1415 1416]

Compatibility Information

Solution Compatibility

Cisplatin

Test Soln Name	Mfr	Mfr	Conc/L or %	Remarks	Ref	C/I
Dextrose 5% in sodium chloride 0.225%	AB[a]	NCI	300 mg	3% loss in 23 hr at 25°C under fluorescent light	1087	C
Dextrose 5% in sodium chloride 0.45%		BV	50 and 500 mg	Less than 10% loss in 24 hr at room temperature	234	C
Dextrose 5% in sodium chloride 0.45%	AB[b]	NCI	300 mg	2% loss in 23 hr at 25°C under fluorescent light	1087	C
Dextrose 5% in sodium chloride 0.9%		BV	50 and 500 mg	Less than 10% loss in 24 hr at room temperature	234	C
Dextrose 5% in sodium chloride 0.9%			500 mg	2% loss in 24 hr at 25°C	635	C

Solution Compatibility (Cont.)

Test Soln Name	Mfr	Mfr	Conc/L or %	Remarks	Ref	C/I
Dextrose 5% in sodium chloride 0.9%	AB[a]	NCI	300 mg	1% loss in 23 hr at 25°C under fluorescent light	1087	C
Dextrose 5% in sodium chloride 0.45%[f]		BR	50, 100, 200 mg	Physically compatible. Stable for 72 hr at 25 and 4°C plus 8-hr infusion with 2 to 10% loss	636	C
Dextrose 5% in sodium chloride 0.33%[f g]		BR	50, 100, 200 mg	Physically compatible. Stable for 72 hr at 25 and 4°C plus 8-hr infusion with 0 to 8% loss	636	C
Dextrose 5%	TR	BV	100 mg	Decomposition occurs in under 2 hr	316	I
Dextrose 5%	AB[a]	NCI	300 mg	4% loss in 2 hr and 6% in 23 hr at 25°C	1087	C
Dextrose 5%	AB[a]	NCI	75 mg	10% loss in 2 hr and 16% in 6 hr at 25°C	1087	I
Sodium chloride 0.9%			50 and 500 mg	2% loss in 24 hr at 25°C	635	C
Sodium chloride 0.9%	TR	BV	100 mg	No loss in 24 hr at room temperature	316	C
Sodium chloride 0.9%		BV	200 mg	2 to 3% loss in 1 hr and no further loss for 24 hr at room temperature and pH adjusted to 4	317	C
Sodium chloride 0.9%	AB[a]	NCI	300 mg	1% loss in 23 hr at 25°C under fluorescent light	1087	C
Sodium chloride 0.9%	[c]	BEL	600 mg	Little loss in 9 days at 23°C in dark	1757	C
Sodium chloride 0.9%	[d]	BEL	500 and 900 mg	Little loss in 28 days at 22 and 35°C in dark	1827	C
Sodium chloride 0.9%	[e]	WAS	167 mg	Little loss in 14 days at 30°C in dark	1828	C
Sodium chloride 0.9%		EBE	100 mg	9% loss in 5 days and 13% loss in 6 days at 22°C in dark. 3% loss in 7 days at 4°C in dark	2293	C
Sodium chloride 0.45%			50 and 500 mg	Approximately 4% loss in 24 hr at 25°C	635	C
Sodium chloride 0.45%		BV	200 mg	4 to 5% loss in 1 hr and no further loss for 24 hr at room temperature and pH adjusted to 4	317	C
Sodium chloride 0.3%		BR	50, 100, 200 mg	Physically compatible and 2 to 3% loss over 72 hr at 25 and 4°C	636	C
Sodium chloride 0.225%		BR	50, 100, 200 mg	Physically compatible and 2 to 5% loss over 72 hr at 25 and 4°C	636	C

[a] Tested in glass containers.

[b] Tested in both glass and PVC containers.

[c] Tested in PVC containers.

[d] Tested in ethylene vinyl acetate containers.

[e] Tested in glass, PVC, polyethylene, and polypropylene containers.

[f] Tested with mannitol 1.875% present.

[g] Tested with and without potassium chloride 20 mEq/L present.

Additive Compatibility

Cisplatin

Test Drug	Mfr	Conc/L or %	Mfr	Conc/L or %	Test Solution	Remarks	Ref	C/I
Carboplatin		1 g		200 mg	NS	Under 10% drug loss in 7 days at 23°C	1954	C
Cyclophosphamide with etoposide		2 g 200 mg		200 mg	NS	All drugs stable for 7 days at room temperature	1379	C
Etoposide	BR	200 and 400 mg	BR	200 mg	NS[a]	Physically compatible. Under 10% loss of both drugs in 24 hr at 22°C	1329	C

Additive Compatibility (Cont.)

Test Drug	Mfr	Conc/L or %	Mfr	Conc/L or %	Test Solution	Remarks	Ref	C/I
Etoposide	BR	200 and 400 mg	BR	200 mg	D5½S[a]	Physically compatible. Under 10% loss of both drugs in 24 hr at 22°C	1329	C
Etoposide		400 mg		200 mg	NS	10% etoposide loss and no cisplatin loss in 7 days at room temperature	1388	C
Etoposide		200 mg		200 mg	NS	Both drugs stable for 14 days at room temperature protected from light	1379	C
Etoposide[e]	BR	400 mg	BR	200 mg	D5½S, NS[a]	Physically compatible. Drugs stable for 8 hr at 22°C. Precipitate within 24 to 48 hr	1329	I
Etoposide with cyclo-phosphamide		200 mg 2 g		200 mg	NS	All drugs stable for 7 days at room temperature	1379	C
Etoposide with flox-uridine		300 mg 700 mg		200 mg	NS	All drugs stable for 7 days at room temperature	1379	C
Etoposide with ifos-famide		200 mg 2 g		200 mg	NS	All drugs stable for 5 days at room temperature	1379	C
Floxuridine	RC	10 g	BR	500 mg	NS	13% floxuridine loss in 7 days at room temperature in dark	1386	C
Floxuridine with etoposide		700 mg 300 mg		200 mg	NS	All drugs stable for 7 days at room temperature	1379	C
Floxuridine with leucovorin calcium		700 mg 140 mg		200 mg	NS	All drugs stable for 7 days at room temperature	1379	C
Fluorouracil	SO	1 g	BR	200 mg	NS[b]	10% cisplatin loss in 1.5 hr and 25% loss in 4 hr at 25°C	1339	I
Fluorouracil	SO	10 g	BR	500 mg	NS[b]	10% cisplatin loss in 1.2 hr and 25% loss in 3 hr at 25°C	1339	I
Fluorouracil	AD	10 g	BR	500 mg	NS	80% cisplatin loss in 24 hr at room temperature due to low pH	1386	I
Hydroxyzine HCl	LY	500 mg	BR	200 mg	NS[c]	Physically compatible for 48 hr	1190	C
Ifosfamide		2 g		200 mg	NS	Both drugs stable for 7 days at room temperature	1379	C
Ifosfamide with etoposide		2 g 200 mg		200 mg	NS	All drugs stable for 5 days at room temperature	1379	C
Leucovorin calcium		140 mg		200 mg	NS	Both drugs stable for 15 days at room temperature protected from light	1379	C
Leucovorin calcium with floxuridine		140 mg 700 mg		200 mg	NS	All drugs stable for 7 days at room temperature	1379	C
Magnesium sulfate		1 and 2 g	BR	50 and 200 mg	D5½S[b]	Compatible for 48 hr at 25°C and 96 hr at 4°C followed by 48 hr at 25°C	1088	C
Mannitol		18.75 g	BR	50 and 200 mg	D5½S[b]	Compatible for 48 hr at 25°C and 96 hr at 4°C followed by 48 hr at 25°C	1088	C
Mesna		3.33 g		67 mg	NS	Cisplatin not detectable after 1 hr	1291	I
Mesna		110 mg		67 mg	NS	Cisplatin weakly detected after 1 hr	1291	I
Ondansetron HCl	GL	1.031 g	BR	485 mg	NS[b]	Physically compatible. Little loss of drugs in 24 hr at 4°C then 7 days at 30°C	1846	C
Ondansetron HCl	GL	479 mg	BR	219 mg	NS[d]	Physically compatible. Little loss of drugs in 7 days at 4°C then 24 hr at 30°C	1846	C

Additive Compatibility (Cont.)

Test Drug	Mfr	Conc/L or %	Mfr	Conc/L or %	Test Solution	Remarks	Ref	C/I
Paclitaxel	BMS	300 mg	BMS	200 mg	NS	No paclitaxel loss and cisplatin losses of 1, 4, and 5% at 4, 24, and 32°C, respectively, in 24 hr. Physically compatible for 24 hr but microparticles of paclitaxel form after 3 to 5 days	2094	C
Paclitaxel	BMS	1.2 g	BMS	200 mg	NS	No paclitaxel loss but cisplatin losses of 10, 19, and 22% at 4, 24, and 32°C, respectively, in 24 hr. Physically compatible for 24 hr but microparticles of paclitaxel form after 3 to 5 days	2094	I
Sodium bicarbonate		5%		50 and 500 mg		Bright gold precipitate forms in 8 to 24 hr at 25°C	635	I
Thiotepa		1 g		200 mg	NS	Yellow precipitation	1379	I

[a] Tested in both glass and PVC containers.

[b] Tested in PVC containers.

[c] Tested in glass containers.

[d] Tested in polyisoprene reservoirs (Travenol Infusors).

[e] Tested with mannitol 1.875% and potassium chloride 20 mEq/L present.

Drugs in Syringe Compatibility

Cisplatin

Test Drug	Mfr	Amt	Mfr	Amt	Remarks	Ref	C/I
Bleomycin sulfate		1.5 units/0.5 mL		0.5 mg/0.5 mL	Physically compatible for 5 min at room temperature followed by 8 min of centrifugation	980	C
Cyclophosphamide		10 mg/0.5 mL		0.5 mg/0.5 mL	Physically compatible for 5 min at room temperature followed by 8 min of centrifugation	980	C
Doxapram HCl	RB	400 mg/20 mL		10 mg/20 mL	Physically compatible with no doxapram loss in 24 hr	1177	C
Doxorubicin HCl		1 mg/0.5 mL		0.5 mg/0.5 mL	Physically compatible for 5 min at room temperature followed by 8 min of centrifugation	980	C
Doxorubicin HCl with mitomycin	BED BMS	25 mg 5 mg	BMS	50 mg	Brought to a 5-mL final volume with NS. Visually compatible but more than 10% loss of mitomycin in 4 hr at 25°C. At 4°C, less than 10% loss of all three drugs in 12 hr, but about 16% mitomycin loss in 24 hr	2423	I
Droperidol		1.25 mg/0.5 mL		0.5 mg/0.5 mL	Physically compatible for 5 min at room temperature followed by 8 min of centrifugation	980	C
Fluorouracil		25 mg/0.5 mL		0.5 mg/0.5 mL	Physically compatible for 5 min at room temperature followed by 8 min of centrifugation	980	C
Furosemide		5 mg/0.5 mL		0.5 mg/0.5 mL	Physically compatible for 5 min at room temperature followed by 8 min of centrifugation	980	C
Heparin sodium		500 units/0.5 mL		0.5 mg/0.5 mL	Physically compatible for 5 min at room temperature followed by 8 min of centrifugation	980	C
Leucovorin calcium		5 mg/0.5 mL		0.5 mg/0.5 mL	Physically compatible for 5 min at room temperature followed by 8 min of centrifugation	980	C
Methotrexate sodium		12.5 mg/0.5 mL		0.5 mg/0.5 mL	Physically compatible for 5 min at room temperature followed by 8 min of centrifugation	980	C
Metoclopramide HCl		2.5 mg/0.5 mL		0.5 mg/0.5 mL	Physically compatible for 5 min at room temperature followed by 8 min of centrifugation	980	C

Drugs in Syringe Compatibility (Cont.)

Test Drug	Mfr	Amt	Mfr	Amt	Remarks	Ref	C/I
Mitomycin		0.25 mg/0.5 mL		0.5 mg/0.5 mL	Physically compatible for 5 min at room temperature followed by 8 min of centrifugation	980	C
Mitomycin with doxorubicin HCl	BMS BED	5 mg 25 mg	BMS	50 mg	Brought to a 5-mL final volume with NS. Visually compatible but more than 10% loss of mitomycin in 4 hr at 25°C. At 4°C, less than 10% loss of all three drugs in 12 hr, but about 16% mitomycin loss in 24 hr	2423	I
Vinblastine sulfate		0.5 mg/0.5 mL		0.5 mg/0.5 mL	Physically compatible for 5 min at room temperature followed by 8 min of centrifugation	980	C
Vincristine sulfate		0.5 mg/0.5 mL		0.5 mg/0.5 mL	Physically compatible for 5 min at room temperature followed by 8 min of centrifugation	980	C

Y-Site Injection Compatibility (1:1 Mixture)

Cisplatin

Test Drug	Mfr	Conc	Mfr	Conc	Remarks	Ref	C/I
Allopurinol sodium	BW	3 mg/mL[b]	BR	1 mg/mL	Physically compatible for 4 hr at 22°C	1686	C
Amifostine	USB	10 mg/mL[a]	BR	1 mg/mL	Subvisible haze forms in 4 hr	1845	I
Anidulafungin	VIC	0.5 mg/mL[a]	SIC	1 mg/mL[b]	Physically compatible for 4 hr at 23°C	2617	C
Aztreonam	SQ	40 mg/mL[a]	BMS	1 mg/mL	Physically compatible for 4 hr at 23°C	1758	C
Bleomycin sulfate		3 units/mL		1 mg/mL	Drugs injected sequentially in Y-site with no flush. No precipitate seen	980	C
Caspofungin acetate	ME	0.7 mg/mL[b]	APP	0.5 mg/mL[b]	Physically compatible for 4 hr at room temperature	2758	C
Cladribine	ORT	0.015[b] and 0.5[c] mg/mL	BR	1 mg/mL	Physically compatible for 4 hr at 23°C	1969	C
Cyclophosphamide		20 mg/mL		1 mg/mL	Drugs injected sequentially in Y-site with no flush. No precipitate seen	980	C
Doripenem	JJ	5 mg/mL[a b]	SIC	0.5 mg/mL[b]	Physically compatible for 4 hr at 23°C	2743	C
Doxorubicin HCl		2 mg/mL		1 mg/mL	Drugs injected sequentially in Y-site with no flush. No precipitate seen	980	C
Doxorubicin HCl liposomal	SEQ	0.4 mg/mL[a]	BR	1 mg/mL	Physically compatible for 4 hr at 23°C	2087	C
Droperidol		2.5 mg/mL		1 mg/mL	Drugs injected sequentially in Y-site with no flush. No precipitate seen	980	C
Etoposide phosphate	BR	5 mg/mL[a]	BR	1 mg/mL	Physically compatible for 4 hr at 23°C	2218	C
Filgrastim	AMG	30 mcg/mL[a]	BR	1 mg/mL	Physically compatible for 4 hr at 22°C	1687	C
Fludarabine phosphate	BX	1 mg/mL[a]	BR	1 mg/mL	Visually compatible for 4 hr at 22°C	1439	C
Fluorouracil		50 mg/mL		1 mg/mL	Drugs injected sequentially in Y-site with no flush. No precipitate seen	980	C

Y-Site Injection Compatibility (1:1 Mixture) (Cont.)

Test Drug	Mfr	Conc	Mfr	Conc	Remarks	Ref	C/I
Furosemide		10 mg/mL		1 mg/mL	Drugs injected sequentially in Y-site with no flush. No precipitate seen	980	C
Gallium nitrate	FUJ	1 mg/mL[b]	BR	1 mg/mL	Precipitates immediately	1673	I
Gemcitabine HCl	LI	10 mg/mL[b]	BR	1 mg/mL	Physically compatible for 4 hr at 23°C	2226	C
Granisetron HCl	SKB	1 mg/mL	BR	0.05 mg/mL[b]	Physically compatible with little or no granisetron loss in 4 hr at 22°C	1883	C
Granisetron HCl	SKB	1 mg/mL	BR	1 mg/mL	Physically compatible with little or no loss of either drug in 4 hr at 22°C	1883	C
Heparin sodium		1000 units/mL		1 mg/mL	Drugs injected sequentially in Y-site with no flush. No precipitate seen	980	C
Leucovorin calcium		10 mg/mL		1 mg/mL	Drugs injected sequentially in Y-site with no flush. No precipitate seen	980	C
Linezolid	PHU	2 mg/mL	BR	1 mg/mL	Physically compatible for 4 hr at 23°C	2264	C
Melphalan HCl	BW	0.1 mg/mL[b]	BR	1 mg/mL	Physically compatible for 3 hr at 22°C	1557	C
Methotrexate sodium		25 mg/mL		1 mg/mL	Drugs injected sequentially in Y-site with no flush. No precipitate seen	980	C
Metoclopramide HCl		5 mg/mL		1 mg/mL	Drugs injected sequentially in Y-site with no flush. No precipitate seen	980	C
Mitomycin		0.5 mg/mL		1 mg/mL	Drugs injected sequentially in Y-site with no flush. No precipitate seen	980	C
Ondansetron HCl	GL	1 mg/mL[b]	BR	1 mg/mL	Visually compatible for 4 hr at 22°C	1365	C
Ondansetron HCl	GL	16 to 160 mcg/mL		0.48 mg/mL	Physically compatible when cisplatin given over 1 to 8 hr via Y-site	1366	C
Paclitaxel	NCI	1.2 mg/mL[a]		1 mg/mL	Physically compatible for 4 hr at 22°C	1528	C
Palonosetron HCl	MGI	50 mcg/mL	BMS	0.5 mg/mL[b]	Physically compatible. No palonosetron and 5% cisplatin loss in 4 hr	2579	C
Pemetrexed disodium	LI	20 mg/mL[b]	BMS	0.5 mg/mL[b]	Physically compatible for 4 hr at 23°C	2564	C
Piperacillin sodium–tazobactam sodium	LE[f]	40 mg/mL[a g]	BR	1 mg/mL	Haze and particles form in 1 hr	1688	I
Propofol	ZEN[h]	10 mg/mL	BR	1 mg/mL	Physically compatible for 1 hr at 23°C	2066	C
Sargramostim	IMM	10 mcg/mL[b]	BR	1 mg/mL	Visually compatible for 4 hr at 22°C	1436	C
Teniposide	BR	0.1 mg/mL[a]	BR	1 mg/mL	Physically compatible for 4 hr at 23°C	1725	C
Thiotepa	IMM[d]	1 mg/mL[a]	BMS	1 mg/mL[b]	White cloudiness appears in 4 hr at 23°C	1861	I
TNA #218 to #226[e]			BMS	1 mg/mL	Visually compatible for 4 hr at 23°C	2215	C
Topotecan HCl	SKB	56 mcg/mL[b]	BR	0.168 mg/mL[b]	Visually compatible. Little loss of either drug in 4 hr at 22°C	2245	C
TPN #212 to #215[e]			BMS	1 mg/mL	Amber discoloration formed in 1 to 4 hr	2109	I
Vinblastine sulfate		1 mg/mL		1 mg/mL	Drugs injected sequentially in Y-site with no flush. No precipitate seen	980	C

Y-Site Injection Compatibility (1:1 Mixture) (Cont.)

Test Drug	Mfr	Conc	Mfr	Conc	Remarks	Ref	C/I
Vincristine sulfate		1 mg/mL		1 mg/mL	Drugs injected sequentially in Y-site with no flush. No precipitate seen	980	C
Vinorelbine tartrate	BW	1 mg/mL[b]	BR	1 mg/mL	Physically compatible for 4 hr at 22°C	1558	C

[a] Tested in dextrose 5%.

[b] Tested in sodium chloride 0.9%.

[c] Tested in bacteriostatic sodium chloride 0.9% preserved with benzyl alcohol 0.9%.

[d] Lyophilized formulation tested.

[e] Refer to Appendix for the composition of parenteral nutrition solutions. TNA indicates a 3-in-1 admixture, and TPN indicates a 2-in-1 admixture.

[f] Test performed using the formulation WITHOUT edetate disodium.

[g] Piperacillin component. Piperacillin in an 8:1 fixed-ratio concentration with tazobactam.

[h] Test performed using the formulation WITH edetate disodium.

Selected Revisions January 31, 2020. © Copyright, October 1982. American Society of Health-System Pharmacists, Inc.

Cladribine

AHFS 10:00

Products

Cladribine is available as a 1-mg/mL concentrate for injection in single-use preservative-free vials containing 10 mL of the concentrate.[2938] Each mL of the solution contains cladribine 1 mg, sodium chloride 9 mg, and phosphoric acid and/or dibasic sodium phosphate to adjust the pH.[2938] The injection is a concentrate that must be diluted for administration.[2938]

pH

From 5.5 to 8.[2938]

Tonicity

Cladribine injection is isotonic.[2938]

Sodium Content

Each mL of cladribine injection contains 0.15 mEq of sodium.[2938]

Administration

Cladribine is administered by continuous intravenous infusion over 24 hours after dilution in 500 mL of sodium chloride 0.9% for repeated single daily doses.[2938] Some manufacturers recommend that the injection be passed through a 0.22-μm filter prior to being introduced into the infusion bag in the preparation of single daily doses.[2938]

Alternatively, to prepare a solution for 7-day continuous infusion, cladribine should be diluted only in bacteriostatic sodium chloride 0.9% containing benzyl alcohol 0.9%.[2938] The 7-day solution should be prepared by sequentially transferring the volume of the total 7-day dose followed by the calculated volume of solution required to bring the final volume to 100 mL to the pump reservoir through a 0.22-μm hydrophilic syringe filter.[2938] Air in the reservoir should be removed by aspiration using a syringe and a new filter or a vent-filter assembly.[2938] The finished preserved solution is then administered continuously over 7 days.[2938]

The use of dextrose 5% as a diluent is not recommended because of an increased rate of cladribine degradation.[2938]

Stability

Intact cladribine vials should be stored under refrigeration and protected from light.[2938] The solution is clear and colorless.[2938]

Solutions prepared for a single daily dose are stated to be both physically and chemically stable at room temperature under normal lighting conditions for at least 24 hours in polyvinyl chloride (PVC) containers; however, the manufacturers recommend that diluted solutions of cladribine be administered promptly or stored under refrigeration for no more than 8 hours prior to administration.[2938]

A precipitate may develop upon low-temperature storage; the precipitate may be redissolved by allowing the solution to warm to room temperature with vigorous shaking.[2938] Heating the solution is not recommended.[2938] However, less than 5% loss of activity is reported to occur in 7 days when the solution is stored at 37°C.[1369]

Freezing does not adversely affect stability of the product.[2938] Thawing should be allowed to occur naturally by exposure to room temperature.[2938] The vials should not be heated or exposed to microwaves.[2938] After thawing, the vial contents are stable under refrigeration until expiration.[2938] Thawed vials should not be refrozen.[2938]

Cladribine (Ortho Biotech) 0.025 mg/mL in sodium chloride 0.9% did not exhibit an antimicrobial effect on *Enterococcus faecium*, *Staphylococcus aureus*, *Pseudomonas aeruginosa*, and *Candida albicans* inoculated into the solution. Admixtures should be stored under refrigeration whenever possible, and the potential for microbiological growth should be considered when assigning expiration periods.[2160]

Ambulatory Pumps

Prepared in bacteriostatic sodium chloride 0.9% preserved with benzyl alcohol 0.9%, cladribine exhibits both chemical and physical stability for at least 7 days in Sims Deltec ambulatory infusion pump reservoirs.[2938] Preservative effectiveness may be reduced in solutions prepared for patients weighing more than 85 kg due to greater benzyl alcohol dilution in such patients.[2938] In solutions of cladribine at concentrations of 0.15 to 0.3 mg/mL in bacteriostatic sodium chloride 0.9% containing benzyl alcohol, the drug is stated to be stable for at least 14 days.[1369]

Compatibility Information

Solution Compatibility

Cladribine

Test Soln Name	Mfr	Mfr	Conc/L or %	Remarks	Ref	C/I
Dextrose 5%				Increased cladribine decomposition	2938	I
Sodium chloride 0.9%	a			Stable for at least 24 hr at room temperature exposed to light, but refrigeration and use within 8 hr recommended	2938	C

DOI: 10.37573/9781585286850.091

Solution Compatibility (Cont.)

Test Soln Name	Mfr	Mfr	Conc/L or %	Remarks	Ref	C/I
Sodium chloride 0.9%	a b	JC	16 mg	Visually compatible and little or no loss in 30 days at 4 and 18°C	2154	C
Sodium chloride 0.9%	c		24 mg	No loss of drug in 2 weeks at 4°C	2398	C

[a] Tested in PVC containers.

[b] Tested in polyethylene-lined trilayer (Clearflex) containers.

[c] Tested in glass infusion bottles.

Y-Site Injection Compatibility (1:1 Mixture)

Cladribine

Test Drug	Mfr	Conc	Mfr	Conc	Remarks	Ref	C/I
Aminophylline	AMR	2.5 mg/mL[a]	ORT	0.015[a] and 0.5[b] mg/mL	Physically compatible for 4 hr at 23°C	1969	C
Bumetanide	RC	0.04 mg/mL[a]	ORT	0.015[a] and 0.5[b] mg/mL	Physically compatible for 4 hr at 23°C	1969	C
Buprenorphine HCl	RKC	0.04 mg/mL[a]	ORT	0.015[a] and 0.5[b] mg/mL	Physically compatible for 4 hr at 23°C	1969	C
Butorphanol tartrate	APC	0.04 mg/mL[a]	ORT	0.015[a] and 0.5[b] mg/mL	Physically compatible for 4 hr at 23°C	1969	C
Calcium gluconate	AMR	40 mg/mL[a]	ORT	0.015[a] and 0.5[b] mg/mL	Physically compatible for 4 hr at 23°C	1969	C
Carboplatin	BR	5 mg/mL[a]	ORT	0.015[a] and 0.5[b] mg/mL	Physically compatible for 4 hr at 23°C	1969	C
Chlorpromazine HCl	SCN	2 mg/mL[a]	ORT	0.015[a] and 0.5[b] mg/mL	Physically compatible for 4 hr at 23°C	1969	C
Cisplatin	BR	1 mg/mL	ORT	0.015[a] and 0.5[b] mg/mL	Physically compatible for 4 hr at 23°C	1969	C
Cyclophosphamide	MJ	10 mg/mL[a]	ORT	0.015[a] and 0.5[b] mg/mL	Physically compatible for 4 hr at 23°C	1969	C
Cytarabine	CHI	50 mg/mL	ORT	0.015[a] and 0.5[b] mg/mL	Physically compatible for 4 hr at 23°C	1969	C
Dexamethasone sodium phosphate	AMR	1 mg/mL[a]	ORT	0.015[a] and 0.5[b] mg/mL	Physically compatible for 4 hr at 23°C	1969	C
Diphenhydramine HCl	SCN	2 mg/mL[a]	ORT	0.015[a] and 0.5[b] mg/mL	Physically compatible for 4 hr at 23°C	1969	C
Dobutamine HCl	LI	4 mg/mL[a]	ORT	0.015[a] and 0.5[b] mg/mL	Physically compatible for 4 hr at 23°C	1969	C
Dopamine HCl	AST	3.2 mg/mL[a]	ORT	0.015[a] and 0.5[b] mg/mL	Physically compatible for 4 hr at 23°C	1969	C
Doxorubicin HCl	CHI	2 mg/mL	ORT	0.015[a] and 0.5[b] mg/mL	Physically compatible for 4 hr at 23°C	1969	C
Droperidol	JN	0.4 mg/mL[a]	ORT	0.015[a] and 0.5[b] mg/mL	Physically compatible for 4 hr at 23°C	1969	C
Enalaprilat	MSD	0.1 mg/mL[a]	ORT	0.015[a] and 0.5[b] mg/mL	Physically compatible for 4 hr at 23°C	1969	C
Etoposide	BR	0.4 mg/mL[a]	ORT	0.015[a] and 0.5[b] mg/mL	Physically compatible for 4 hr at 23°C	1969	C
Famotidine	ME	2 mg/mL[a]	ORT	0.015[a] and 0.5[b] mg/mL	Physically compatible for 4 hr at 23°C	1969	C
Furosemide	AB	3 mg/mL[a]	ORT	0.015[a] and 0.5[b] mg/mL	Physically compatible for 4 hr at 23°C	1969	C
Gallium nitrate	FUJ	0.4 mg/mL[b]	ORT	0.015[a] and 0.5[b] mg/mL	Physically compatible for 4 hr at 23°C	1969	C
Granisetron HCl	SKB	0.05 mg/mL[a]	ORT	0.015[a] and 0.5[b] mg/mL	Physically compatible for 4 hr at 23°C	1969	C
Haloperidol lactate	MN	0.2 mg/mL[a]	ORT	0.015[a] and 0.5[b] mg/mL	Physically compatible for 4 hr at 23°C	1969	C
Heparin sodium	WY	100 units/mL[a]	ORT	0.015[a] and 0.5[b] mg/mL	Physically compatible for 4 hr at 23°C	1969	C
Hydrocortisone sodium succinate	UP	1 mg/mL[a]	ORT	0.015[a] and 0.5[b] mg/mL	Physically compatible for 4 hr at 23°C	1969	C
Hydromorphone HCl	KN	0.5 mg/mL[a]	ORT	0.015[a] and 0.5[b] mg/mL	Physically compatible for 4 hr at 23°C	1969	C

Y-Site Injection Compatibility (1:1 Mixture) (Cont.)

Test Drug	Mfr	Conc	Mfr	Conc	Remarks	Ref	C/I
Hydroxyzine HCl	ES	4 mg/mL[a]	ORT	0.015[a] and 0.5[b] mg/mL	Physically compatible for 4 hr at 23°C	1969	C
Idarubicin HCl	AD	0.5 mg/mL[a]	ORT	0.015[a] and 0.5[b] mg/mL	Physically compatible for 4 hr at 23°C	1969	C
Leucovorin calcium	IMM	2 mg/mL[a]	ORT	0.015[a] and 0.5[b] mg/mL	Physically compatible for 4 hr at 23°C	1969	C
Lorazepam	WY	0.1 mg/mL[a]	ORT	0.015[a] and 0.5[b] mg/mL	Physically compatible for 4 hr at 23°C	1969	C
Mannitol	BA	15%	ORT	0.015[a] and 0.5[b] mg/mL	Physically compatible for 4 hr at 23°C	1969	C
Meperidine HCl	WY	4 mg/mL[a]	ORT	0.015[a] and 0.5[b] mg/mL	Physically compatible for 4 hr at 23°C	1969	C
Mesna	MJ	10 mg/mL[a]	ORT	0.015[a] and 0.5[b] mg/mL	Physically compatible for 4 hr at 23°C	1969	C
Methylprednisolone sodium succinate	AB	5 mg/mL[a]	ORT	0.015[a] and 0.5[b] mg/mL	Physically compatible for 4 hr at 23°C	1969	C
Metoclopramide HCl	RB	5 mg/mL	ORT	0.015[a] and 0.5[b] mg/mL	Physically compatible for 4 hr at 23°C	1969	C
Mitoxantrone HCl	LE	0.5 mg/mL[a]	ORT	0.015[a] and 0.5[b] mg/mL	Physically compatible for 4 hr at 23°C	1969	C
Morphine sulfate	AST	1 mg/mL[a]	ORT	0.015[a] and 0.5[b] mg/mL	Physically compatible for 4 hr at 23°C	1969	C
Nalbuphine HCl	AST	10 mg/mL	ORT	0.015[a] and 0.5[b] mg/mL	Physically compatible for 4 hr at 23°C	1969	C
Ondansetron HCl	CER	1 mg/mL[a]	ORT	0.015[a] and 0.5[b] mg/mL	Physically compatible for 4 hr at 23°C	1969	C
Paclitaxel	BR	0.6 mg/mL[a]	ORT	0.015[a] and 0.5[b] mg/mL	Physically compatible for 4 hr at 23°C	1969	C
Potassium chloride	AB	0.1 mEq/mL[a]	ORT	0.015[a] and 0.5[b] mg/mL	Physically compatible for 4 hr at 23°C	1969	C
Prochlorperazine edisylate	SCN	0.5 mg/mL[a]	ORT	0.015[a] and 0.5[b] mg/mL	Physically compatible for 4 hr at 23°C	1969	C
Promethazine HCl	SCN	2 mg/mL[a]	ORT	0.015[a] and 0.5[b] mg/mL	Physically compatible for 4 hr at 23°C	1969	C
Ranitidine HCl	GL	2 mg/mL[a]	ORT	0.015[a] and 0.5[b] mg/mL	Physically compatible for 4 hr at 23°C	1969	C
Sodium bicarbonate	AB	1 mEq/mL	ORT	0.015[a] and 0.5[b] mg/mL	Physically compatible for 4 hr at 23°C	1969	C
Teniposide	BR	0.1 mg/mL[a]	ORT	0.015[a] and 0.5[b] mg/mL	Physically compatible for 4 hr at 23°C	1969	C
Vincristine sulfate	LI	0.05 mg/mL[a]	ORT	0.015[a] and 0.5[b] mg/mL	Physically compatible for 4 hr at 23°C	1969	C

[a] Tested in sodium chloride 0.9%.

[b] Tested in bacteriostatic sodium chloride 0.9% preserved with benzyl alcohol 0.9%.

Selected Revisions June 18, 2015. © Copyright, October 1998.
American Society of Health-System Pharmacists, Inc.

Clarithromycin
AHFS 8:12.12.92

Products

Clarithromycin is available in 500-mg vials with lactobionic acid as a solubilizing agent and sodium hydroxide to adjust pH. Reconstitute with 10 mL of sterile water for injection, and shake to dissolve the powder. Do not use diluents containing preservatives or inorganic salts. Each mL of the resultant solution contains 50 mg of clarithromycin. This solution must be diluted before use. See Administration below.[38][115]

Trade Name(s)

Klacid, Klaricid, Zeclar

Administration

Clarithromycin is administered by intravenous infusion after dilution in an appropriate infusion solution. It should not be given by intravenous bolus or intramuscular injection. The reconstituted drug solution (500 mg) is added to 250 mL of compatible infusion solution yielding a 2-mg/mL final solution. The final diluted solution is administered by intravenous infusion over 60 minutes into one of the larger proximal veins.[38][115]

Stability

Intact containers of the white to off-white lyophilized powder should be stored at 30°C or below and protected from light. When reconstituted as directed, the 50-mg/mL solution should be used within 24 hours stored at room temperature of 25°C[38][115] and 48 hours stored under refrigeration at 5°C.[115]

Compatibility Information

Solution Compatibility

Clarithromycin

Test Soln Name	Mfr	Mfr	Conc/L or %	Remarks	Ref	C/I
Dextrose 5%			2 g	Use within 6 hr at 25°C or 48 hr at 5°C	115	C
Dextrose 5% in Ringer's injection, lactated			2 g	Use within 6 hr at 25°C or 48 hr at 5°C	115	C
Dextrose 5% in sodium chloride 0.45%			2 g	Use within 6 hr at 25°C or 48 hr at 5°C	115	C
Normosol M in dextrose 5%			2 g	Use within 6 hr at 25°C or 48 hr at 5°C	115	C
Normosol R in dextrose 5%			2 g	Use within 6 hr at 25°C or 48 hr at 5°C	115	C
Ringer's injection, lactated			2 g	Use within 6 hr at 25°C or 48 hr at 5°C	115	C
Sodium chloride 0.9%			2 g	Use within 6 hr at 25°C or 48 hr at 5°C	115	C

Y-Site Injection Compatibility (1:1 Mixture)

Clarithromycin

Test Drug	Mfr	Conc	Mfr	Conc	Remarks	Ref	C/I
Aminophylline	EV	2 mg/mL[a]	AB	4 mg/mL[a]	Needle-like crystals form in 2 hr at 30°C and 4 hr at 17°C	2174	I
Amiodarone HCl	SW	3 mg/mL[a]	AB	4 mg/mL[a]	Visually compatible for 72 hr at both 30 and 17°C	2174	C
Amoxicillin sodium–clavulanate potassium	BE	20 mg/mL[a][c]	AB	4 mg/mL[a]	Visually compatible for 72 hr at both 30 and 17°C	2174	C
Ampicillin sodium	BE	40 mg/mL[a]	AB	4 mg/mL[a]	Visually compatible for 72 hr at both 30 and 17°C	2174	C
Atracurium besylate	GW	1 mg/mL[a]	AB	4 mg/mL[a]	Visually compatible for 72 hr at both 30 and 17°C	2174	C
Bumetanide	LEO	0.5 mg/mL	AB	4 mg/mL[a]	Visually compatible for 72 hr at both 30 and 17°C	2174	C

DOI: 10.37573/9781585286850.092

Y-Site Injection Compatibility (1:1 Mixture) (Cont.)

Test Drug	Mfr	Conc	Mfr	Conc	Remarks	Ref	C/I
Cefepime HCl	BMS	120 mg/mL[b]		50 mg/mL	Physically compatible with less than 10% cefepime loss. Clarithromycin not tested	2513	C
Ceftazidime	SKB	125 mg/mL		50 mg/mL	Precipitates immediately	2434	I
Ceftazidime	SKB	125 mg/mL		10 mg/mL	Trace precipitation	2434	I
Ceftazidime	GSK	120 mg/mL[b]		50 mg/mL	Precipitates	2513	I
Cefuroxime sodium	GW	60 mg/mL[a]	AB	4 mg/mL[a]	White precipitate forms in 3 hr at 30°C and 24 hr at 17°C	2174	I
Ciprofloxacin	BAY	2 mg/mL[a]	AB	4 mg/mL[a]	Visually compatible for 72 hr at both 30 and 17°C	2174	C
Dobutamine HCl	BI	2 mg/mL[a]	AB	4 mg/mL[a]	Visually compatible for 72 hr at both 30 and 17°C	2174	C
Dopamine HCl	DB	3.2 mg/mL[a]	AB	4 mg/mL[a]	Visually compatible for 72 hr at both 30 and 17°C	2174	C
Floxacillin sodium	BE	40 mg/mL[a]	AB	4 mg/mL[a]	Translucent precipitate in 1 to 2 hr becoming a gel in 3 hr at 30 and 17°C	2174	I
Furosemide	ANT	10 mg/mL	AB	4 mg/mL[a]	White cloudiness forms immediately, becoming an obvious precipitate in 15 min	2174	I
Gentamicin sulfate	RS	40 mg/mL	AB	4 mg/mL[a]	Visually compatible for 72 hr at both 30 and 17°C	2174	C
Heparin sodium	CPP	1000 units/mL[a]	AB	4 mg/mL[a]	White cloudiness forms immediately	2174	I
Insulin, human	NOV	4 units/mL[a]	AB	4 mg/mL[a]	Visually compatible for 72 hr at both 30 and 17°C	2174	C
Lidocaine HCl	ANT	4 mg/mL[a]	AB	4 mg/mL[a]	Visually compatible for 72 hr at both 30 and 17°C	2174	C
Metoclopramide HCl	ANT	5 mg/mL	AB	4 mg/mL[a]	Visually compatible for 72 hr at both 30 and 17°C	2174	C
Metronidazole	PRK	5 mg/mL	AB	4 mg/mL[a]	Visually compatible for 72 hr at both 30 and 17°C	2174	C
Penicillin G sodium	BRT	24 mg/mL[a]	AB	4 mg/mL[a]	Visually compatible for 72 hr at both 30 and 17°C	2174	C
Phenytoin sodium	ANT	20 mg/mL[a]	AB	4 mg/mL[a]	White cloudy precipitate in 1 hr at both 30 and 17°C	2174	I
Prochlorperazine mesylate	ANT	12.5 mg/mL	AB	4 mg/mL[a]	Visually compatible for 72 hr at both 30 and 17°C	2174	C
Potassium chloride	ANT	0.08 mmol/mL[a]	AB	4 mg/mL[a]	Visually compatible for 72 hr at both 30 and 17°C	2174	C
Ranitidine HCl	GW	5 mg/mL[a]	AB	4 mg/mL[a]	Visually compatible for 72 hr at both 30 and 17°C	2174	C
Vancomycin HCl	DB	10 mg/mL[a]	AB	4 mg/mL[a]	Visually compatible for 72 hr at both 30 and 17°C	2174	C
Vecuronium bromide	OR	2 mg/mL[a]	AB	4 mg/mL[a]	Visually compatible for 72 hr at both 30 and 17°C	2174	C
Verapamil HCl	BKN	2.5 mg/mL	AB	4 mg/mL[a]	Visually compatible for 72 hr at both 30 and 17°C	2174	C

[a] Tested in dextrose 5%.

[b] Tested in sterile water for injection.

[c] Amoxicillin component. Amoxicillin in a 5:1 fixed-ratio concentration with clavulanic acid.

Selected Revisions July 1, 2020. © Copyright, October 2000.
American Society of Health-System Pharmacists, Inc.

Clevidipine Butyrate
AHFS 24:28.08

Products

Clevidipine is available as a ready-to-use oil-in-water emulsion in 50-, 100-, and 250-mL single-use vials.[3200] Each mL contains clevidipine butyrate 0.5 mg along with soybean oil 200 mg, glycerin 22.5 mg, purified egg yolk phospholipids 12 mg, oleic acid 0.3 mg, and disodium edetate 0.05 mg (0.005%) with sodium hydroxide to adjust the pH.[3200] [3236]

pH

From 6 to 8[3200] or 8.8.[3236]

Trade Name(s)

Cleviprex

Administration

Clevidipine butyrate is administered by intravenous infusion into either a central line or peripheral line using an infusion device that allows calibrated infusion rates.[3200]

Vials of clevidipine should be inverted gently several times prior to administration to ensure uniformity of the emulsion.[3200] Commercially available standard plastic cannulae may be used to administer the infusion.[3200]

Clevidipine ready-to-use emulsion should not be diluted.[3200]

Stability

Clevidipine butyrate is a milky white, oil-in-water emulsion.[3200] Intact vials should be stored at 2 to 8°C in the carton to protect from light and should not be frozen.[3200] Intact vials may be stored for up to 2 months at controlled room temperature; vials stored at room temperature should be marked with the date of removal from refrigeration and a "DISCARD BY" date of 2 months after transfer to room temperature storage or the expiration date, whichever comes first.[3200] Once moved to storage at room temperature, vials should not be returned to refrigerated storage.[3200]

The lipid base of the oil-in-water emulsion supports microbiological growth.[3200] The disodium edetate in the formulation retards the growth of microorganisms, but the product can still support growth and is not antimicrobially preserved.[3200] Aseptic technique should be maintained during handling.[3200]

Once the vial stopper is punctured, administration of clevidipine butyrate should be completed within 12 hours and any unused portion should be discarded.[3200] The emulsion should be visually inspected for particulate matter and discoloration prior to administration.[3200]

Temperature Effects

Clevidipine should be stored at 2 to 8°C;[3200] however, clevidipine butyrate (Chiesi) 0.5 mg/mL in intact vials has been reported to be physically and chemically stable after 5 cycles of alternating storage at 5°C for 24 hours followed by 25°C for 24 hours.[3334]

Freezing Solutions

Clevidipine should not be frozen;[3200] however, clevidipine butyrate (Chiesi) 0.5 mg/mL in intact vials has been reported to be physically and chemically stable for up to 12 hours at −15°C followed by storage for 24 hours at 5°C.[3334]

Compatibility Information

Y-Site Injection Compatibility (1:1 Mixture)

Clevidipine butyrate

Test Drug	Mfr	Conc	Mfr	Conc	Remarks	Ref	C/I
Amino acids		10%	CHS	0.5 mg/mL	Physically compatible for 24 hr at 23°C	3334	C
Amiodarone HCl		4 mg/mL[c]	CHS	0.5 mg/mL	Physically incompatible	3334	I
Bivalirudin		5 mg/mL[a]	CHS	0.5 mg/mL	pH shifted outside of specified pH range for clevidipine within 24 hr	3334	?
Calcium gluconate		40 mg/mL[c]	CHS	0.5 mg/mL	Physically compatible for 24 hr at 23°C	3334	C
Cangrelor tetrasodium	TMC	1 mg/mL[b]	TMC	0.5 mg/mL	Physically compatible for 4 hr	3243	C
Dobutamine HCl		4 mg/mL[c]	CHS	0.5 mg/mL	pH shifted outside of specified pH range for clevidipine within 24 hr	3334	?
Ephedrine sulfate		50 mg/mL	CHS	0.5 mg/mL	pH shifted outside of specified pH range for clevidipine within 24 hr	3334	?
Epinephrine HCl		1 mg/mL	CHS	0.5 mg/mL	Emulsion broke	3334	I

DOI: 10.37573/9781585286850.093

Y-Site Injection Compatibility (1:1 Mixture) (Cont.)

Test Drug	Mfr	Conc	Mfr	Conc	Remarks	Ref	C/I
Esmolol HCl		10 mg/mL	CHS	0.5 mg/mL	pH shifted outside of specified pH range for clevidipine within 24 hr	3334	?
Heparin sodium		100 units/mL[b]	CHS	0.5 mg/mL	Physically compatible for 24 hr at 23°C	3334	C
Hetastarch in sodium chloride 0.9%		6%	CHS	0.5 mg/mL	Emulsion broke	3334	I
Hydromorphone HCl		10 mg/mL	CHS	0.5 mg/mL	Physically incompatible	3334	I
Insulin, regular		100 units/mL	CHS	0.5 mg/mL	Physically compatible for 24 hr at 23°C	3334	C
Metoprolol tartrate		1 mg/mL	CHS	0.5 mg/mL	Physically compatible for 24 hr at 23°C	3334	C
Milrinone lactate		0.5 mg/mL[a]	CHS	0.5 mg/mL	Physically incompatible	3334	I
Nicardipine HCl		0.1 mg/mL[c]	CHS	0.5 mg/mL	pH shifted outside of specified pH range for clevidipine within 24 hr	3334	?
Nitroglycerin		0.4 mg/mL[a]	CHS	0.5 mg/mL	Physically compatible for 24 hr at 23°C	3334	C
Potassium chloride		[b]	CHS	0.5 mg/mL	Physically compatible for 24 hr at 23°C	3334	C
Propofol		10 mg/mL	CHS	0.5 mg/mL	Physically compatible for 24 hr at 23°C	3334	C
Propranolol HCl		1 mg/mL	CHS	0.5 mg/mL	Physically incompatible	3334	I
Sodium nitroprusside		2 mg/mL[a]	CHS	0.5 mg/mL	Physically compatible for 24 hr at 23°C	3334	C
Tranexamic acid		20 mg/mL[a]	CHS	0.5 mg/mL	Physically compatible for 24 hr at 23°C	3334	C

[a] Tested in dextrose 5%.

[b] Tested in sodium chloride 0.9%.

[c] Tested in sterile water for injection.

Additional Compatibility Information

Infusion Solutions

Clevidipine ready-to-use oil-in-water emulsion should not be diluted; however, the drug may be administered with dextrose 5% in Ringer's injection, lactated; dextrose 5% in sodium chloride 0.9%; dextrose 5%; Ringer's injection, lactated; sodium chloride 0.45%, and sodium chloride 0.9%.[3200][3334]

Selected Revisions February 21, 2018. © Copyright, september 2017. American Society of Health-System Pharmacists, Inc.

Clindamycin Phosphate
AHFS 8:12.28.20

Products

Clindamycin phosphate is available in 2-, 4-, and 6-mL single-dose and ADD-Vantage vials and a 60-mL pharmacy bulk package containing the equivalent of clindamycin base 150 mg/mL.[3384] Single-dose vials and the pharmacy bulk package are intended for intravenous or intramuscular use; ADD-Vantage vials are intended for intravenous use only.[3384] Each mL of solution also contains benzyl alcohol 9.45 mg and disodium edetate 0.5 mg.[3384] Sodium hydroxide and/or hydrochloric acid may have been added to adjust the pH.[3384] For intravenous administration, the injection solution should be diluted in a compatible diluent; clindamycin doses of 300 and 600 mg should be diluted in 50 mL, doses of 900 mg should be diluted in 50 to 100 mL, and doses of 1200 mg should be diluted in 100 mL.[3384] The injection solution should be used undiluted for intramuscular administration.[3384] ADD-Vantage vials of clindamycin should be prepared with 50 mL (for the 300- and 600-mg vials) or 100 mL (for the 900-mg vials) of dextrose 5% or sodium chloride 0.9% in ADD-Vantage diluent bags.[3384]

Clindamycin phosphate also is available in several ready-to-use formulations.[3384] [3385] [3386] [3387] Clindamycin phosphate is available as a premixed injection solution containing the equivalent of 300, 600, and 900 mg of clindamycin base in 50 mL of dextrose 5% in single-dose Galaxy[3384] and Cryovac[3387] plastic containers and glass bottles[3386] and in 50 mL of sodium chloride 0.9% in single-dose Galaxy containers.[3385] Premixed injection solutions also contain disodium edetate 0.04 mg/mL.[3384] [3385] [3386] [3387] Sodium hydroxide and/or hydrochloric acid have been added to adjust the pH.[3384] [3385] [3386] [3387]

pH

Clindamycin (Alvogen) 150-mg/mL injection solution has a pH ranging from 5.5 to 7.[3388]

Clindamycin (Akorn) 6-, 12-, and 18-mg/mL premixed infusion solutions in dextrose 5% have a pH ranging from 5.9 to 6.3.[3390]

Clindamycin (Baxter) 6-, 12-, and 18-mg/mL premixed infusion solutions in sodium chloride 0.9% have a pH ranging from 5.5 to 6.5.[3389]

Osmolality

Clindamycin (Upjohn) 150 mg/mL has been reported to have an osmolality of 795 mOsm/kg[50] or 835 mOsm/kg[1071] as determined by freezing-point depression. However, the manufacturer has stated that the osmolality is usually 825 to 880 mOsm/kg.[1705]

The osmolality of clindamycin (Upjohn) 12 mg/mL was determined to be 293 mOsm/kg in dextrose 5% and 309 mOsm/kg in sodium chloride 0.9%.[1375]

One manufacturer has stated that the osmolalities of clindamycin (Akorn) 300-, 600-, and 900-mg premixed infusion solutions in dextrose 5% are 260 to 340, 280 to 370, and 300 to 400 mOsm/kg, respectively.[3390] One manufacturer has stated that the osmolalities of clindamycin (Baxter) 300-, 600-, and 900-mg premixed infusions in sodium chloride 0.9% are 285 to 345, 305 to 370, and 335 to 395 mOsm/kg, respectively.[3389]

The osmolality of clindamycin 600 mg was calculated for the following dilutions:[1054]

Diluent	Osmolality (mOsm/kg)	
	50 mL	100 mL
Dextrose 5%	279	268
Sodium chloride 0.9%	306	294

Trade Name(s)

Cleocin Phosphate

Administration

Clindamycin phosphate is administered by intermittent intravenous infusion at concentrations not exceeding 18 mg/mL of clindamycin.[3384] [3384] [3385] [3386] [3387] Intermittent infusions should be administered over 10 to 60 minutes at a rate not exceeding 30 mg/min; clindamycin doses of 300, 600, 900, and 1200 mg should be infused over 10, 20, 30, and 40 minutes, respectively.[3384] [3385] [3386] Not more than 1200 mg of clindamycin should be administered in a single 1-hour infusion period.[3384] [3386] Alternatively, following an initial single rapid infusion over 30 minutes with an infusion rate ranging from 10 to 20 mg/min, the drug also can be administered by continuous intravenous infusion at maintenance infusion rates of 0.75 to 1.25 mg/min in adult patients, with infusion rates determined by the desired serum clindamycin concentration.[3384] [3385] [3386] The drug should not be administered undiluted as a bolus.[3384]

Clindamycin phosphate also can be administered by intramuscular injection as an undiluted solution in some patients.[3384] Single injections exceeding 600 mg are not recommended.[3384]

Stability

Intact containers of clindamycin phosphate should be stored at controlled room temperature; exposure to heat should be minimized and temperatures above 30°C should be avoided.[3384] [3385] [3386] [3387] Some manufacturers state that vials should not be refrigerated.[3388] Crystallization may occur if refrigerated; the crystals resolubilize when warmed to room temperature, but care should be exercised to ensure that all crystals have redissolved.[102] Solutions should be visually inspected for particulate matter and discoloration prior to administration; only clear solutions should be used.[3384] [3385] [3386] [3387] [3388]

Less than 10% decomposition occurs in 2 years at 25°C at pH 3.5 to 6.5.[102] [103]

DOI: 10.37573/9781585286850.094

pH Effects

Maximum stability occurs at pH 4, but an acceptable long-term shelf life is attained at pH 1 to 6.5.[1072]

Freezing Solutions

Manufacturers state that clindamycin 6, 9, and 12 mg/mL in dextrose 5%, sodium chloride 0.9%, or Ringer's injection, lactated is physically compatible and chemically stable for 56 days at −10°C.[3384][3388] Frozen solutions should be thawed at room temperature and should not be refrozen.[3384][3388]

Some manufacturers state that vials of clindamycin phosphate should not be refrigerated.[3384][3388] Crystallization may occur if refrigerated; the crystals resolubilize when warmed to room temperature, but care should be exercised to ensure that all crystals have redissolved. This would also apply if the product is frozen.[102]

Syringes

Clindamycin 900 mg/6 mL in polypropylene syringes (Becton Dickinson) retained more than 95% of the initial concentration over at least 48 hours at room temperature.[172] Diluted with sterile water for injection to concentrations of 20, 40, 60, and 120 mg/mL and stored in Monoject plastic syringes or glass vials, clindamycin exhibited little change in concentration and was free of particulate matter over 30 days at 25°C and 60 days at −15°C.[173]

Clindamycin (Upjohn) 900 mg/6 mL showed no more than a 4 to 5% loss when stored in polypropylene syringes (Becton Dickinson) for 48 hours at 25°C under fluorescent light.[1159]

Clindamycin (Upjohn) 600 mg stored in polypropylene syringes (3M) at 25°C under fluorescent light exhibited no loss in 48 hours.[1164]

Vials

Dilution of clindamycin 300 and 900 mg in glass vials containing 20 mL of dextrose 10% resulted in no visual changes and less than a 10% loss after 30 days of refrigeration at 10°C.[1604]

Clindamycin (Abbott) injection was diluted with sterile water for injection to a concentration of 15 mg/mL for use in minimizing measurement errors in pediatric dosing. The dilution was packaged in glass vials, and samples were stored at 22 and 4°C. The dilution remained visually free of particulate matter at both storage conditions throughout the study. No clindamycin loss occurred after 91 days at either 4 or 22°C.[1714]

Clindamycin phosphate is incompatible with natural rubber closures because of the extraction of crystalline particulate matter, primarily β-sitosterol and stigmasterol. Simple cleaning procedures for the closures do not effectively remove the source of contamination. It is recommended that if clindamycin phosphate is repackaged in vials or disposable syringes, storage at room temperature should be limited to a few days.[102]

Central Venous Catheter

Clindamycin (Upjohn) 2 mg/mL in dextrose 5% was found to be compatible with the ARROWg+ard Blue Plus (Arrow International) chlorhexidine-bearing triple-lumen central catheter. Essentially complete delivery of the drug was found with little or no drug loss occurring. Furthermore, chlorhexidine delivered from the catheter remained at trace amounts with no substantial increase due to the delivery of the drug through the catheter.[2335]

Compatibility Information

Solution Compatibility

Clindamycin phosphate

Test Soln Name	Mfr	Mfr	Conc/L or %	Remarks	Ref	C/I
Amino acids 4.25%, dextrose 25%	MG	UP	600 mg	No increase in particulate matter in 24 hr at 5°C	349	C
Dextrose 2.5% in Ringer's injection, lactated		UP	600 mg	Physically compatible and stable for 24 hr at room temperature	104	C
Dextrose 5% in Ringer's injection		UP	600 mg	Physically compatible and stable for 24 hr at room temperature	104	C
Dextrose 5% in sodium chloride 0.45%		UP	600 mg	Stable for 24 hr	101	C
Dextrose 5% in sodium chloride 0.9%	MG	UP	250 mg	Stable for 24 hr at 4 and 25°C	105	C
Dextrose 5% in sodium chloride 0.9%		UP	600 mg	Physically compatible and stable for 24 hr at room temperature	104	C
Dextrose 5%	MG	UP	250 mg	Stable for 24 hr at 4 and 25°C	105	C
Dextrose 5%		UP	600 mg	Physically compatible and stable for 24 hr at room temperature	104	C
Dextrose 5%		UP	6, 9, 12 g	Stable for 24 hr	101	C

Solution Compatibility (Cont.)

Test Soln Name	Mfr	Mfr	Conc/L or %	Remarks	Ref	C/I
Dextrose 5%			6 g	3% loss in 79 days frozen at −10°C	174	C
Dextrose 5%	TR[a]	UP	6 g	Physically compatible and 9% loss in 24 hr at room temperature. Little to no loss in 30 days at −20°C	555	C
Dextrose 5%	TR[g]	UP	6, 9, 12 g	Physically compatible and stable for 16 days at 25°C, 32 days at 4°C, and 56 days at −10°C	753	C
Dextrose 5%	AB[g]	UP	9 g	Physically compatible and no loss in 24 hr at 25°C	994	C
Dextrose 5%	AB[a]	UP	18 g	3% loss in 28 days frozen at −20°C	981	C
Dextrose 5%	TR[a]	QU	6 and 12 g	Physically compatible with no loss in 22 days at 25°C, 54 days at 5°C, and 68 days at −10°C	1351	C
Dextrose 5%	MG[c]	UP	7.6 g	Visually compatible with no loss in 30 days at −20°C then 14 days at 4°C	1539	C
Dextrose 5%	BA[a], BRN[b c]	GW	3 g	Visually compatible with little loss in 24 hr at 4 and 22°C	2289	C
Dextrose 5%	BA[f]	SZ	1 and 12 g	Little loss in 7 days at 23°C and 21 days at 4°C	2819	C
Dextrose 5%	[g]	PHU, AVG	6, 9, and 12 g	Physically compatible and chemically stable for 16 days at 25°C and 32 days at 4°C	3384, 3388	C
Dextrose 5%	[a]	PHU, AVG	6, 9, and 12 g	Physically compatible and chemically stable for 56 days at −10°C	3384, 3388	C
Dextrose 5%	[a]	PHU, AVG	18 g	Physically compatible and chemically stable for 16 days at 25°C	3384, 3388	C
Dextrose 10%	MG	UP	250 mg	Stable for 24 hr at 4 and 25°C	105	C
Isolyte M in dextrose 5%	MG	UP	250 mg	Stable for 24 hr at 4 and 25°C	105	C
Isolyte P in dextrose 5%	MG	UP	250 mg	Stable for 24 hr at 4 and 25°C	105	C
Normosol R	AB	UP	1.2 g	Stable for 24 hr	101	C
Ringer's injection, lactated	MG	UP	250 mg	Stable for 24 hr at 4 and 25°C	105	C
Ringer's injection, lactated	TR[g]	UP	6, 9, 12 g	Physically compatible with no loss in 16 days at 25°C, 32 days at 5°C, and 56 days at −10°C	753	C
Ringer's injection, lactated	[g]	PHU, AVG	6, 9, and 12 g	Physically compatible and chemically stable for 16 days at 25°C and 32 days at 4°C	3384, 3388	C
Ringer's injection, lactated	[a]	PHU, AVG	6, 9, and 12 g	Physically compatible and chemically stable for 56 days at −10°C	3384, 3388	C
Sodium chloride 0.9%		UP	600 mg	Physically compatible and stable for 24 hr at room temperature	104	C
Sodium chloride 0.9%		UP	6 g	Stable for 24 hr	101	C
Sodium chloride 0.9%	MG	UP	250 mg	Stable for 24 hr at 4 and 25°C	105	C
Sodium chloride 0.9%	TR[g]	UP	6, 9, 12 g	Physically compatible with no loss in 16 days at 25°C, 32 days at 4°C, and 56 days at −10°C	753	C
Sodium chloride 0.9%	AB[g]	UP	9 g	Physically compatible and no loss in 24 hr at 25°C	994	C
Sodium chloride 0.9%	AB[a]	UP	18 g	4% loss in 28 days frozen at −20°C	981	C
Sodium chloride 0.9%	TR[a]	QU	6 and 12 g	Physically compatible with no loss in 22 days at 25°C, 54 days at 5°C, and 68 days at −10°C	1351	C
Sodium chloride 0.9%	BR[a], BRN[b c]	GW	3 g	Visually compatible with little loss in 24 hr at 4 and 22°C	2289	C
Sodium chloride 0.9%	HOS[f]	SZ	1 and 12 g	Little loss in 7 days at 23°C and 21 days at 4°C	2819	C
Sodium chloride 0.9%	[g]	PHU, AVG	6, 9, and 12 g	Physically compatible and chemically stable for 16 days at 25°C and 32 days at 4°C	3384, 3388	C

Solution Compatibility (Cont.)

Test Soln Name	Mfr	Mfr	Conc/L or %	Remarks	Ref	C/I
Sodium chloride 0.9%	a	PHU, AVG	6, 9, and 12 g	Physically compatible and chemically stable for 56 days at –10°C	3384, 3388	C
TPN #21[d]		UP	250 mg	Stable for 24 hr at 4 and 25°C	87	C
TPN #22[d]		UP	3 g	Physically compatible with no loss in 24 hr at 22°C in the dark	837	C
TPN #107[d]			400 mg[e]	Stable for 24 hr at 21°C	1326	C

[a] Tested in PVC containers.

[b] Tested in glass containers.

[c] Tested in polyolefin containers.

[d] Refer to Appendix for the composition of parenteral nutrition solutions. TPN indicates a 2-in-1 admixture.

[e] As clindamycin base.

[f] Tested in Accufusor reservoirs.

[g] Tested in both PVC and glass containers.

Additive Compatibility

Clindamycin phosphate

Test Drug	Mfr	Conc/L or %	Mfr	Conc/L or %	Test Solution	Remarks	Ref	C/I
Amikacin sulfate	BR	5 g	UP	6 g	D5LR, D5R, D5S, D5W, D10W, LR, NS, R, SL	Physically compatible and amikacin stable for 24 hr at 25°C. Clindamycin not analyzed	293	C
Amikacin sulfate	BR	4 g	UP	9 g	D5W, NS[a]	Both stable for 48 hr at 25°C under fluorescent light	981	C
Aminophylline	SE	600 mg	UP	600 mg		Physically incompatible	101	I
Ampicillin sodium		10 and 20 g	UP,	24 g	NS	Physically compatible	1035	C
Ampicillin sodium	WY	3.7 g	UP	3 g	NS	Physically compatible with 4% ampicillin loss in 1 day at 24°C	1035	C
Aztreonam	SQ	10 and 20 g	UP	3 and 6 g	D5W, NS[b]	Physically compatible with little or no loss of either drug in 48 hr at 25°C and 7 days at 4°C	1002	C
Aztreonam	SQ	20 g	UP	9 g	D5W[a]	Physically compatible with 3% clindamycin loss and 5% aztreonam loss in 48 hr at 25°C under fluorescent light	1026	C
Aztreonam	SQ	20 g	UP	9 g	NS[a]	Physically compatible with 2% clindamycin loss and no aztreonam loss in 48 hr at 25°C under fluorescent light	1026	C
Cefazolin sodium	SKF	10 g	UP	9 g	D5W[a]	Physically compatible with no clindamycin loss and 8% cefazolin loss in 48 hr at room temperature under fluorescent light	983	C
Cefazolin sodium	SKF	10 g	UP	9 g	NS[a]	Physically compatible with no clindamycin loss and 3% cefazolin loss in 48 hr at room temperature under fluorescent light	983	C
Cefazolin sodium[f]	SKF	10 g	UP	9 g	D5W, NS[a]	10% cefazolin loss in 4 hr in D5W and 12 hr in NS at 25°C. No clindamycin and gentamicin loss in 24 hr	1328	I
Cefepime HCl	BR	40 g	UP	0.25 g	D5W, NS	7% or less cefepime loss in 24 hr at room temperature and 10% or less loss in 7 days at 5°C. No clindamycin loss in 24 hr at room temperature and 8% or less loss in 7 days at 5°C	1682	C

Additive Compatibility (Cont.)

Test Drug	Mfr	Conc/L or %	Mfr	Conc/L or %	Test Solution	Remarks	Ref	C/I
Cefepime HCl	BR	4 g	UP	6 g	D5W, NS	7% or less cefepime loss in 24 hr at room temperature and 10% or less loss in 7 days at 5°C. No clindamycin loss in 24 hr at room temperature and 8% or less loss in 7 days at 5°C	1682	C
Cefotaxime sodium	HO	20 g	UP	9 g	D5W, NSc	Physically compatible with no clindamycin loss and 3% cefotaxime loss in 24 hr at 25°C	994	C
Cefoxitin sodium	MSD	20 g	UP	9 g	D5Wa	Physically compatible with no loss of either drug in 48 hr at room temperature	983	C
Cefoxitin sodium	MSD	20 g	UP	9 g	NSa	Physically compatible with no clindamycin loss and 7% cefoxitin loss in 48 hr at room temperature	983	C
Ceftazidime	GL	20 g	UP	9 g	D5Wa	Physically compatible with 9% clindamycin loss and 11% ceftazidime loss in 48 hr at 25°C under fluorescent light	1026	C
Ceftazidime	GL	20 g	UP	9 g	NSa	Physically compatible with 5% clindamycin loss and 7% ceftazidime loss in 48 hr at 25°C under fluorescent light	1026	C
Ceftriaxone sodium	RC	20 g	UP	12 g	D5Wa	10% ceftriaxone loss in 4 hr and 17% in 24 hr at 25°C under fluorescent light. No clindamycin loss in 48 hr	1026	I
Ceftriaxone sodium	RC	20 g	UP	12 g	NSa	10% ceftriaxone loss in 1 hr and 12% in 24 hr at 25°C under fluorescent light. 6% clindamycin loss in 48 hr	1026	I
Cefuroxime sodium	GL	15 g	UP	9 g	D5W	Physically compatible with 4% clindamycin loss and 6 to 8% cefuroxime loss in 48 hr at 25°C under fluorescent light	1164	C
Cefuroxime sodium	GL	15 g	UP	9 g	NS	Physically compatible with 9% clindamycin and cefuroxime losses in 48 hr at 25°C under fluorescent light	1164	C
Ciprofloxacin	MI	1.6 g	LY	7.1 g	D5W, NS	Precipitate forms immediately	1541	I
Fluconazole	PF	1 g	AST	6 g	D5W	Visually compatible with no fluconazole loss in 72 hr at 25°C under fluorescent light. Clindamycin not tested	1677	C
Gentamicin sulfate		120 mg	UP	2.4 g	D5W	Physically compatible. Clindamycin stable for 24 hr at room temperature	104	C
Gentamicin sulfate		60 mg	UP	1.2 g	D5W	Physically compatible. Clindamycin stable for 24 hr at room temperature	104	C
Gentamicin sulfate		600 mg	UP	12 g	D5W	Physically compatible	101	C
Gentamicin sulfate		800 mg	UP	9 g	D5W	Clindamycin stable for 24 hr	101	C
Gentamicin sulfate	AB	1 g	UP	9 g	D5W, NSc	Physically compatible and both drugs stable for 48 hr at room temperature exposed to light and 1 week frozen	174	C
Gentamicin sulfate	LY	1.2 g	UP	9 g	D5Wa	Physically compatible and both drugs stable for 7 days at 4 and 25°C	174	C
Gentamicin sulfate	LY	1.2 g	UP	9 g	NSa	Physically compatible and both drugs stable for 14 days at 4 and 25°C	174	C
Gentamicin sulfate	LY	2.4 g	UP	18 g	D5W, NSc	Physically compatible and both drugs stable for 14 days at 4 and 25°C	174	C
Gentamicin sulfate	ES	1.2 g	UP	9 g	D5W, NSa	Physically compatible and both drugs stable for 28 days frozen at –20°C	174	C
Gentamicin sulfate	ES	2.4 g	UP	18 g	D5W, NSb	Both drugs stable for 28 days frozen at –20°C	981	C

Additive Compatibility (Cont.)

Test Drug	Mfr	Conc/L or %	Mfr	Conc/L or %	Test Solution	Remarks	Ref	C/I
Gentamicin sulfate	ES	667 mg	UP	6 g	D5W[b]	Physically compatible with no clindamycin loss and 9% gentamicin loss in 24 hr at room temperature	995	C
Gentamicin sulfate		75 mg		400 mg[d]	TPN #107[e]	19% gentamicin loss and 15% clindamycin loss in 24 hr at 21°C	1326	I
Gentamicin sulfate[g]	ES	800 mg	UP	9 g	D5W, NS[a]	10% cefazolin loss in 4 hr in D5W and 12 hr in NS at 25°C. No clindamycin and gentamicin loss in 24 hr	1328	I
Heparin sodium		100,000 units	UP	9 g	D5W	Clindamycin stable for 24 hr	101	C
Hydrocortisone sodium succinate	UP	1 g	UP	1.2 g	W	Clindamycin stable for 24 hr	101	C
Methylprednisolone sodium succinate	UP	500 mg	UP	1.2 g	D5W, W	Clindamycin stable for 24 hr	101	C
Metoclopramide HCl	RB	100 and 200 mg	UP	6 g		Physically compatible for 24 hr at 25°C	1167	C
Metoclopramide HCl	RB	1.9 g	UP	3.5 g		Physically compatible for 24 hr at 25°C	1167	C
Metoclopramide HCl	RB	1.2 g	UP	4.4 g		Physically compatible for 24 hr at 25°C	1167	C
Potassium chloride		40 mEq	UP	600 mg	D5½S	Physically compatible and clindamycin stable for 24 hr at room temperature	104	C
Potassium chloride		100 mEq	UP	600 mg	D5W, NS	Physically compatible	101	C
Potassium chloride		400 mEq	UP	6 g	D5½S	Clindamycin stable for 24 hr	101	C
Ranitidine HCl	GL	100 mg	UP	1.2 g	D5W	Color change and gas formation	1151	I
Ranitidine HCl	GL	50 mg and 2 g		1.2 g	D5W, NS	Physically compatible. Ranitidine stable for 24 hr at 25°C. Clindamycin not tested	1515	C
Sodium bicarbonate		44 mEq	UP	1.2 g	D5S, D5W	Clindamycin stable for 24 hr	101	C
Tobramycin sulfate	DI	1 g	UP	9 g	D5W, NS[c]	Physically compatible and both drugs stable for 48 hr at room temperature exposed to light and for 1 week frozen	174	C
Tobramycin sulfate	DI	1.2 g	UP	9 g	D5W[a]	Physically compatible and clindamycin stable for 28 days frozen. 8% tobramycin loss in 14 days and 17% in 28 days	174	C
Tobramycin sulfate	DI	1.2 g	UP	9 g	NS[a]	Physically compatible and both drugs stable for 28 days frozen	174	C
Tobramycin sulfate	DI	2.4 g	UP	18 g	D5W[b]	8% tobramycin lost in 14 days and 17% in 28 days at –20°C. Clindamycin stable	981	C
Tobramycin sulfate	DI	2.4 g	UP	18 g	NS[b]	Both drugs stable for 28 days frozen at –20°C	981	C
Tramadol HCl	GRU	400 mg	AB	6 g	NS	Tramadol losses of 20% in 4 hr at room temperature with precipitate	2652	I
Verapamil HCl	KN	80 mg	UP	1.2 g	D5W, NS	Physically compatible for 24 hr	764	C

[a] Tested in glass containers.

[b] Tested in PVC containers.

[c] Tested in both glass and PVC containers.

[d] Present as clindamycin base.

[e] Refer to Appendix for the composition of parenteral nutrition solutions. TPN indicates a 2-in-1 admixture.

[f] Tested in combination with gentamicin sulfate 800 mg/L.

[g] Tested in combination with cefazolin sodium 10 g/L.

Drugs in Syringe Compatibility

Clindamycin phosphate

Test Drug	Mfr	Amt	Mfr	Amt	Remarks	Ref	C/I
Amikacin sulfate	BR	750 mg/4 mL[a]	UP	900 mg/6 mL	Physically compatible with little loss of either drug in 48 hr at 25°C	1159	C
Aztreonam	SQ	2 g	UP	600 mg/4 mL	Physically compatible with 2% clindamycin loss and 8% aztreonam loss in 48 hr at 25°C under fluorescent light	1164	C
Caffeine citrate		20 mg/1 mL	UP	150 mg/1 mL	Visually compatible for 4 hr at 25°C	2440	C
Dimenhydrinate		10 mg/1 mL		150 mg/1 mL	Clear solution	2569	C
Gentamicin sulfate	ES	120 mg/4 mL[a]	UP	900 mg/6 mL	Physically compatible with little loss of either drug for 48 hr at 25°C	1159	C
Heparin sodium		2500 units/1 mL	UP	300 mg	Physically compatible for at least 5 min	1053	C
Pantoprazole sodium	[b]	4 mg/1 mL		150 mg/1 mL	Precipitates within 1 hr	2574	I
Tobramycin sulfate	DI	120 mg/4 mL[a]	UP	900 mg/6 mL	Cloudy white precipitate forms immediately and changes to gel-like precipitate	1159	I

[a] Diluted to 4 mL with 1 mL of sodium chloride 0.9%.

[b] Test performed using the formulation WITHOUT edetate disodium.

Y-Site Injection Compatibility (1:1 Mixture)

Clindamycin phosphate

Test Drug	Mfr	Conc	Mfr	Conc	Remarks	Ref	C/I
Acetaminophen	CAD	10 mg/mL	APP	10 mg/mL[b]	Physically compatible for 4 hr at 23°C	2901, 2902	C
Acyclovir sodium	BW	5 mg/mL[a]	UP	12 mg/mL[a]	Physically compatible for 4 hr at 25°C	1157	C
Allopurinol sodium	BW	3 mg/mL[b]	AB	10 mg/mL[b]	Tiny particles form immediately and become more numerous over 4 hr	1686	I
Amifostine	USB	10 mg/mL[a]	AST	10 mg/mL[a]	Physically compatible for 4 hr at 23°C	1845	C
Amiodarone HCl	LZ	4 mg/mL[c]	UP	6 mg/mL[c]	Physically compatible for 4 hr at room temperature	1444	C
Amsacrine	NCI	1 mg/mL[a]	UP	10 mg/mL[a]	Visually compatible for 4 hr at 22°C	1381	C
Anakinra	SYN	4 and 36 mg/mL[b]	AST	12 mg/mL[b]	Physically compatible with little or no loss of either drug in 4 hr at 22°C	2510	C
Anidulafungin	VIC	0.5 mg/mL[a]	AB	10 mg/mL[a]	Physically compatible for 4 hr at 23°C	2617	C
Azithromycin	PF	2 mg/mL[b]	PHU	30 mg/mL[k l]	Amber and white microcrystals found	2368	I
Aztreonam	SQ	40 mg/mL[a]	AST	10 mg/mL[a]	Physically compatible for 4 hr at 23°C	1758	C
Bivalirudin	TMC	5 mg/mL[a]	AB	10 mg/mL[a]	Physically compatible for 4 hr at 23°C	2373	C
Cangrelor tetrasodium	TMC	1 mg/mL[b]		10 mg/mL[b]	Physically compatible for 4 hr	3243	C
Caspofungin acetate	ME	0.7 mg/mL[b]	BED	10 mg/mL[b]	Immediate white turbid precipitate forms	2758	I
Caspofungin acetate	ME	0.5 mg/mL[b]	HOS	60 mg/mL[k]	Fine white crystals reported	2766	I
Ceftaroline fosamil	FOR	2.22 mg/mL[a b m]	BED	10 mg/mL[a b m]	Physically compatible for 4 hr at 23°C	2826	C
Cisatracurium besylate	GW	0.1, 2, 5 mg/mL[a]	AST	10 mg/mL[a]	Physically compatible for 4 hr at 23°C	2074	C
Cloxacillin sodium	SMX	100 mg/mL	SZ	150 mg/mL	Physically compatible for up to 4 hr at room temperature	3245	C

Y-Site Injection Compatibility (1:1 Mixture) (Cont.)

Test Drug	Mfr	Conc	Mfr	Conc	Remarks	Ref	C/I
Cyclophosphamide	MJ	20 mg/mL[a]	UP	12 mg/mL[a]	Physically compatible for 4 hr at 25°C	1194	C
Dexmedetomidine HCl	AB	4 mcg/mL[b]	AB	10 mg/mL[b]	Physically compatible for 4 hr at 23°C	2383	C
Diltiazem HCl	MMD	5 mg/mL	UP	12[b] and 150 mg/mL	Visually compatible	1807	C
Docetaxel	RPR	0.9 mg/mL[a]	AST	10 mg/mL[a]	Physically compatible for 4 hr at 23°C	2224	C
Doxapram HCl	RB	2 mg/mL[a]	PHU	10 mg/mL[a]	Gas bubbles evolve immediately	2470	I
Doxorubicin HCl liposomal	SEQ	0.4 mg/mL[a]	AST	10 mg/mL[a]	Physically compatible for 4 hr at 23°C	2087	C
Enalaprilat	MSD	0.05 mg/mL[b]	UP	9 mg/mL[a]	Physically compatible for 24 hr at room temperature under fluorescent light	1355	C
Esmolol HCl	DCC	10 mg/mL[a]	UP	9 mg/mL[a]	Physically compatible for 24 hr at 22°C	1169	C
Etoposide phosphate	BR	5 mg/mL[a]	AST	10 mg/mL[a]	Physically compatible for 4 hr at 23°C	2218	C
Fat emulsion, intravenous	OTS	20%[o]	PF	5.77 mg/mL[a p]	No change in particle size ≥1.3 μm observed in 24 hr at 25°C in the dark	3452	C
Fenoldopam mesylate	AB	80 mcg/mL[b]	AB	10 mg/mL[b]	Physically compatible for 4 hr at 23°C	2467	C
Filgrastim	AMG	30 mcg/mL[a]	AB	10 mg/mL[a]	Particles and filaments form immediately	1687	I
Fluconazole	RR	2 mg/mL	AB	24 mg/mL	Precipitates immediately	1407	I
Fludarabine phosphate	BX	1 mg/mL[a]	LY	10 mg/mL[a]	Visually compatible for 4 hr at 22°C	1439	C
Foscarnet sodium	AST	24 mg/mL	AB	24 mg/mL	Physically compatible for 24 hr at room temperature under fluorescent light	1335	C
Foscarnet sodium	AST	24 mg/mL	UP	12 mg/mL[c]	Physically compatible for 24 hr at 25°C under fluorescent light	1393	C
Gemcitabine HCl	LI	10 mg/mL[b]	AST	10 mg/mL[b]	Physically compatible for 4 hr at 23°C	2226	C
Granisetron HCl	SKB	0.05 mg/mL[a]	AB	10 mg/mL[a]	Physically compatible for 4 hr at 23°C	2000	C
Heparin sodium	TR	50 units/mL	UP	12 mg/mL[a]	Visually compatible for 4 hr at 25°C	1793	C
Hetastarch in lactated electrolyte	AB	6%	PHU	10 mg/mL[a]	Physically compatible for 4 hr at 23°C	2339	C
Hydromorphone HCl	WY	0.2 mg/mL[a]	UP	12 mg/mL[a]	Physically compatible for 4 hr at 25°C	987	C
Hydroxyethyl starch 130/0.4 in sodium chloride 0.9%	FRK	6%	SZ	6, 12, 24 mg/mL[a]	Visually compatible for 24 hr at room temperature	2770	C
Idarubicin HCl	AD	1 mg/mL[b]	AST	12 mg/mL[a]	Haze and precipitate form immediately	1525	I
Labetalol HCl	SC	1 mg/mL[a]	UP	9 mg/mL[a]	Physically compatible for 24 hr at 18°C	1171	C
Levofloxacin	OMN	5 mg/mL[a]	UP	150 mg/mL	Visually compatible for 4 hr at 24°C	2233	C
Linezolid	PHU	2 mg/mL	UP	10 mg/mL[a]	Physically compatible for 4 hr at 23°C	2264	C
Magnesium sulfate	IX	16.7, 33.3, 66.7, 100 mg/mL[a]	UP	12 mg/mL[a]	Physically compatible for at least 4 hr at 32°C	813	C
Melphalan HCl	BW	0.1 mg/mL[b]	AB	10 mg/mL[b]	Physically compatible for 3 hr at 22°C	1557	C
Meperidine HCl	WY	10 mg/mL[a]	UP	12 mg/mL[a]	Physically compatible for 4 hr at 25°C	987	C
Meropenem		50 mg/mL	SZ	150 mg/mL	Physically compatible for 4 hr at room temperature	3538	C
Midazolam HCl	RC	1 mg/mL[a]	UP	9 mg/mL[a]	Visually compatible for 24 hr at 23°C	1847	C
Milrinone lactate	SS	0.2 mg/mL[a]	PHU	18 mg/mL[a]	Visually compatible for 4 hr at 25°C	2381	C

Y-Site Injection Compatibility (1:1 Mixture) (Cont.)

Test Drug	Mfr	Conc	Mfr	Conc	Remarks	Ref	C/I
Morphine sulfate	WI	1 mg/mL[a]	UP	12 mg/mL[a]	Physically compatible for 4 hr at 25°C	987	C
Multivitamins	USV	5 mL/L[a]	UP	600 mg/100 mL[a]	Physically compatible for 24 hr at room temperature	323	C
Nicardipine HCl	DCC	0.1 mg/mL[a]	UP	9 mg/mL[a]	Visually compatible for 24 hr at room temperature	235	C
Ondansetron HCl	GL	1 mg/mL[b]	LY	10 mg/mL[a]	Visually compatible for 4 hr at 22°C	1365	C
Oritavancin diphosphate	TAR	0.8, 1.2, and 2 mg/mL[a]	HOS	12 mg/mL[a]	Haze forms immediately with precipitate after 30 to 60 min	2928	I
Pemetrexed disodium	LI	20 mg/mL[b]	PHU	10 mg/mL[a]	Physically compatible for 4 hr at 23°C	2564	C
Piperacillin sodium–tazobactam sodium	LE[d]	40 mg/mL[a][n]	AB	10 mg/mL[a]	Physically compatible for 4 hr at 22°C	1688	C
Propofol	ZEN[q]	10 mg/mL	AST	10 mg/mL[a]	Physically compatible for 1 hr at 23°C	2066	C
Remifentanil HCl	GW	0.025 and 0.25 mg/mL[b]	AST	10 mg/mL[a]	Physically compatible for 4 hr at 23°C	2075	C
Sargramostim	IMM	10 mcg/mL[b]	LY	10 mg/mL[b]	Visually compatible for 4 hr at 22°C	1436	C
Tacrolimus	FUJ	1 mg/mL[b]	ES	12 mg/mL[a]	Visually compatible for 24 hr at 25°C	1630	C
Teniposide	BR	0.1 mg/mL[a]	AST	10 mg/mL[a]	Physically compatible for 4 hr at 23°C	1725	C
Theophylline	TR	4 mg/mL	UP	12 mg/mL[a]	Visually compatible for 6 hr at 25°C	1793	C
Thiotepa	IMM[e]	1 mg/mL[a]	AST	10 mg/mL[a]	Physically compatible for 4 hr at 23°C	1861	C
TNA #73[f]		32.5 mL[g]	UP	12 mg/mL[a]	Visually compatible for 4 hr at 25°C	1008	C
TNA #218 to #226[f]			AST	10 mg/mL[a]	Visually compatible for 4 hr at 23°C	2215	C
TPN #61[f]		[h]	UP	50 mg/0.33 mL[i]	Physically compatible	1012	C
TPN #61[f]		[j]	UP	300 mg/2 mL[i]	Physically compatible	1012	C
TPN #212 to #215[f]			AB	10 mg/mL[a]	Physically compatible for 4 hr at 23°C	2109	C
Vinorelbine tartrate	BW	1 mg/mL[b]	AB	10 mg/mL[b]	Physically compatible for 4 hr at 22°C	1558	C
Zidovudine	BW	4 mg/mL[a]	UP	12 mg/mL[a]	Physically compatible for 4 hr at 25°C	1193	C

[a] Tested in dextrose 5%.

[b] Tested in sodium chloride 0.9%.

[c] Tested in both dextrose 5% and sodium chloride 0.9%.

[d] Test performed using the formulation WITHOUT edetate disodium.

[e] Lyophilized formulation tested.

[f] Refer to Appendix for the composition of parenteral nutrition solutions. TNA indicates a 3-in-1 admixture, and TPN indicates a 2-in-1 admixture.

[g] A 32.5-mL sample of parenteral nutrition solution mixed with 50 mL of antibiotic solution.

[h] Run at 21 mL/hr.

[i] Given over 10 minutes by syringe pump.

[j] Run at 94 mL/hr.

[k] Tested in sodium chloride 0.45%.

[l] Injected via Y-site into an administration set running azithromycin.

[m] Tested in Ringer's injection, lactated.

[n] Piperacillin component. Piperacillin in an 8:1 fixed-ratio concentration with tazobactam.

[o] Run at 25 mL/hr with dextrose 5% run at 83 mL/hr.

[p] Run at 100 mL/hr.

[q] Test performed using the formulation WITH edetate disodium.

Additional Compatibility Information

Infusion Solutions

Manufacturers state that clindamycin phosphate demonstrated no inactivation or incompatibility in intravenous solutions containing sodium chloride, dextrose, and calcium or potassium and in solutions containing vitamin B complex in concentrations used clinically.[3384] [3388]

Other Drugs

Manufacturers state that clindamycin phosphate is physically incompatible with aminophylline, ampicillin sodium, barbiturates, calcium gluconate, magnesium sulfate, and phenytoin sodium, but that no incompatibility has been demonstrated with cephalothin, kanamycin, gentamicin, penicillin, and carbenicillin.[3384] [3388]

Peritoneal Dialysis Solutions

Clindamycin (Upjohn) 10 mg/L stability in peritoneal dialysis solutions (Dianeal 137 and PD-2) with heparin sodium 500 units/L was evaluated. Approximately 102 ± 9% activity remained after 24 hours at 25°C.[1228]

Clindamycin (Dalacin C Phosphate, Pfizer) 300 mg in 2 L of Dianeal PD-4 with dextrose 2.5% (Baxter) exhibited little to no loss of drug over 6 hours at 37°C.[3108]

Selected Revisions January 31, 2020. © Copyright, October 1982. American Society of Health-System Pharmacists, Inc.

Clofarabine

AHFS 10:00

Products

Clofarabine is available as a 1-mg/mL solution in 20-mL single-use (preservative-free) vials.[3213] Each vial also contains water for injection and sodium chloride.[3213]

To prepare for administration, clofarabine injection should be passed through a 0.2-μm syringe filter and then diluted in an appropriate amount of dextrose 5% or sodium chloride 0.9% to yield a final clofarabine concentration between 0.15 and 0.4 mg/mL.[3213]

pH

The pH of the undiluted solution ranges from 4.5 to 7.5.[3213]

Osmolarity

The osmolarity of the undiluted solution (Evoltra) is from 270 to 310 mOsm/L.[3215]

Trade Name(s)

Clolar, Evoltra

Administration

Clofarabine is administered as an intravenous infusion over 2 hours following dilution of the drug with dextrose 5% or sodium chloride 0.9%.[3213]

As with other toxic drugs, applicable special handling and disposal procedures for clofarabine should be followed.[3213]

Stability

Clofarabine injection is a clear, practically colorless solution.[3213] Intact vials should be stored at controlled room temperature.[3213]

Diluted solutions of clofarabine should be stored at room temperature (15 to 30°C) and must be used within 24 hours of preparation.[3213]

The undiluted 1-mg/mL solution of clofarabine in the original glass vial was found to be physically and chemically stable for 4 weeks after first opening the vial at 2 to 8°C or 25°C both with and without light protection.[3216]

Filtration

Clofarabine injection should be filtered through a 0.2-μm syringe filter prior to dilution.[3213]

Compatibility Information

Solution Compatibility

Clofarabine

Test Soln Name	Mfr	Mfr	Conc/L or %	Remarks	Ref	C/I
Dextrose 5%		SAA	150 to 400 mg	Use within 24 hr	3213	C
Dextrose 5%	FRK[a]	GZ	200 and 600 mg	Physically and chemically stable for 4 weeks at 2 to 8°C or 25°C both with and without light protection	3216	C
Sodium chloride 0.9%			150 to 400 mg	Use within 24 hr	3213	C
Sodium chloride 0.9%		GZ		Physically and chemically stable for 3 days at 2 to 8°C and room temperature up to 25°C	3215	C
Sodium chloride 0.9%	FRK[a]	GZ	100, 200, 300, and 400 mg	Physically and chemically stable for 48 hours at 2 to 8°C protected from light	3216	C
Sodium chloride 0.9%	FRK[b]	GZ	200, 300, and 400 mg	Physically and chemically stable for 48 hours at 2 to 8°C protected from light	3216	C

DOI: 10.37573/9781585286850.095

Solution Compatibility (Cont.)

Test Soln Name	Mfr	Mfr	Conc/L or %	Remarks	Ref	C/I
Sodium chloride 0.9%	FRK[c]	GZ	100, 200, and 300 mg	Physically and chemically stable for 48 hours at 2 to 8°C protected from light	3216	C
Sodium chloride 0.9%	FRK[a]	GZ	200 and 600 mg	Physically and chemically stable for 4 weeks at 2 to 8°C or 25°C both with and without light protection	3216	C

[a] Tested in Freeflex polypropylene/polyethylene containers.

[b] Tested in glass containers.

[c] Tested in PVC containers.

Clonazepam
AHFS 28:12.08

Products

Clonazepam is available as a concentrate for injection in 1-mL ampuls containing 1 mg of the drug in a solvent composed of ethanol, benzyl alcohol, propylene glycol, and glacial acetic acid.[3406] [3407] Each ampul of the drug is packaged with an ampul containing 1 mL of sterile water for injection diluent.[3406] [3407]

For intravenous injection, the contents of the clonazepam ampul must be mixed thoroughly with the contents of the diluent ampul of sterile water for injection; to avoid local irritation of the veins, the mixture should be prepared immediately prior to administration.[3406] [3407]

For intravenous infusion, the contents of each clonazepam ampul (1 mg) should be diluted to at least 85 mL (e.g., 3 mg of clonazepam in 250 mL) with sodium chloride 0.9%, dextrose 2.5% in sodium chloride 0.45%, dextrose 5%, or dextrose 10% to avoid precipitation.[3406] [3407]

pH

Clonazepam (Roche) 0.125, 0.222, and 0.5 mg/mL in sodium chloride 0.9% for continuous subcutaneous infusion had pH values of 3.6, 3.5, and 3.6, respectively.[2161]

Trade Name(s)

Rivotril

Administration

Clonazepam is administered after dilution by slow intravenous injection or intravenous infusion.[3406] [3407] When administered by intravenous injection, the diluted drug must be administered very slowly into a sufficiently large vein at a rate not exceeding 0.25 to 0.5 mg/min.[3406] [3407] If the injection is administered rapidly or the vein into which the diluted drug is administered is not sufficiently large, there is a risk of thrombophlebitis and subsequent thrombosis.[3406] [3407]

Clonazepam has been administered intramuscularly after being mixed thoroughly with the contents of the diluent ampul of sterile water for injection, but this route should be used only in exceptional cases or if intravenous administration is not possible.[3407] Efficacy of clonazepam administered by the intramuscular route has not been demonstrated.[3406]

Stability

Clonazepam concentrate for injection is a colorless to slightly green-yellow solution.[3406] [3407] Intact ampuls should be stored below 25[3406] or 30°C[3407] in the outer carton to protect from light.[3406] [3407] If intended for administration by slow intravenous injection, the manufacturer recommends that the drug be used immediately after mixing with the supplied sterile water for injection diluent.[3406] [3407] After clonazepam is diluted in a compatible infusion solution as instructed, the infusion is stated to be stable for 24 hours at room temperature;[3406] [3407] however, if prepared in a polyvinyl chloride (PVC) container, the infusion should be infused immediately and usually within 4 hours, and the infusion time should not exceed 8 hours.[3407]

Clonazepam should not be mixed with sodium bicarbonate because of the potential for precipitation.[3406] [3407]

Syringes

Clonazepam (Roche) 5 and 10 mg, diluted to 48 mL with sodium chloride 0.9% and stored in polyethylene syringes, was physically compatible and exhibited no clonazepam loss in 10 hours at room temperature.[1708]

Reconstituted clonazepam (Roche) 0.5 mg/mL packaged in polypropylene syringes was evaluated. Less than 2% clonazepam loss occurred in 48 hours stored at room temperature exposed to normal room light.[2172]

Sorption

Clonazepam can adsorb to plastic infusion bags and infusion sets, especially those made of PVC.[3406] [3407] Clonazepam has demonstrated sorption losses of up to 50% when in contact with PVC, especially when prepared bags are stored for more than 24 hours and/or when bags are stored in warm ambient conditions or when long tubing sets or slow rates of infusion are used.[3406] [3407] It is recommended that PVC-containing bags and infusion sets be avoided if possible and that alternative materials be used.[3406] [3407] If PVC bags are used, the admixture should be infused immediately and usually within 4 hours, and the infusion time should not exceed 8 hours.[3407] Caution should be exercised when switching between PVC and non-PVC-containing bags and infusion sets.[3406] [3407]

Hooymans et al. compared losses of clonazepam to PVC and polyethylene-lined infusion tubing. Clonazepam (Roche) 5 and 10 mg, diluted in sodium chloride 0.9% to a final volume of 48 mL in polyethylene syringes, was delivered at room temperature through tubing at flow rates of 2 or 4 mL/hr (5 mg in 48 mL) and 2 mL/hr (10 mg in 48 mL). No losses were observed in the plastic syringes or to the polyethylene-lined tubing over 10 hours. Losses to the PVC tubing were dependent on the flow rate and concentration, being greater at 2 mL/hr and at 5 mg/48 mL, respectively. Potency decreased to approximately 40 and 55% of the original strength after 0.6 hour for the 5-mg/48 mL concentration at 2 and 4 mL/hr, respectively. After 0.6 hour, the 10-mg/48 mL concentration retained 55% of original potency when delivered at 2 mL/hr. Effluent concentrations gradually increased after the first hour, reaching approximately 80 to 90% of original concentrations after 10 hours.[1708]

Clonazepam (Roche) (concentration unspecified) in dextrose 5% in PVC containers was delivered over 4 hours through PVC administration sets. Losses due to sorption ranged from about 13 to 18% determined by UV spectroscopy.[2045]

DOI: 10.37573/9781585286850.096

Compatibility Information

Solution Compatibility

Clonazepam

Test Soln Name	Mfr	Mfr	Conc/L or %	Remarks	Ref	C/I
Dextrose 2.5% in sodium chloride 0.45%		RC		Physically and chemically stable for 24 hr at room temperature	3406, 3407	C
Dextrose 2.5% in sodium chloride 0.45%	b	RC		Use within 4 hr and complete administration within 8 hr	3407	C
Dextrose 5%	AB[a]	RC	6 mg	Physically compatible with no loss in 10 hr	1707	C
Dextrose 5%	TR[b]	RC	6 mg	7% loss in 7 hr, 17 to 20% loss in 24 hr, and 31 to 33% loss in 6 days at room temperature protected from light	1707	I
Dextrose 5%		RC		Physically and chemically stable for 24 hr at room temperature	3406, 3407	C
Dextrose 5%	b	RC		Use within 4 hr and complete administration within 8 hr	3407	C
Dextrose 10%		RC		Physically and chemically stable for 24 hr at room temperature	3406, 3407	C
Dextrose 10%	b	RC		Use within 4 hr and complete administration within 8 hr	3407	C
Sodium chloride 0.9%	AB[a]	RC	6 mg	Physically compatible with no loss in 10 hr	1707	C
Sodium chloride 0.9%	TR[b]	RC	6 mg	14% loss in 7 hr, 17 to 20% loss in 24 hr, and 31 to 33% loss in 6 days at room temperature protected from light	1707	I
Sodium chloride 0.9%		RC		Physically and chemically stable for 24 hr at room temperature	3406, 3407	C
Sodium chloride 0.9%	b	RC		Use within 4 hr and complete administration within 8 hr	3407	C

[a] Tested in glass containers.

[b] Tested in PVC containers.

Drugs in Syringe Compatibility

Clonazepam

Test Drug	Mfr	Amt	Mfr	Amt	Remarks	Ref	C/I
Heparin sodium		2500 units/1 mL	RC	1 mg/2 mL	Visually compatible for at least 5 min	1053	C

Y-Site Injection Compatibility (1:1 Mixture)

Clonazepam

Test Drug	Mfr	Conc	Mfr	Conc	Remarks	Ref	C/I
Blinatumomab	AMG	0.125 and 0.375 mcg/mL[c]	RC	0.02 mg/mL[c]	Particles, flakes, thin needles, or haze transiently appears	3405, 3417	?
Defibrotide sodium	JAZ	8 mg/mL[c]	RC	0.02 mg/mL[c]	Visually compatible for 4 hr at room temperature	3149	C
TPN #189[a]			RC	10 mg/mL[b]	Visually compatible for 24 hr at 22°C	1767[a]	C

[a] Refer to Appendix for the composition of parenteral nutrition solutions. TPN indicates a 2-in-1 admixture.

[b] Tested in sterile water for injection.

[c] Tested in sodium chloride 0.9%.

Clonidine Hydrochloride
AHFS 24:08.16

Products

Clonidine hydrochloride is available in concentrations of 0.1 mg/ mL (100 mcg/mL) and 0.5 mg/mL (500 mcg/mL) in 10-mL vials. Each mL of the preservative-free solution also contains sodium chloride 9 mg in water for injection. Hydrochloric acid and/or sodium hydroxide may have been added to adjust the pH.[1(2/06)]

pH

From 5 to 7.[1(2/06)]

Trade Name(s)

Duraclon

Administration

Clonidine hydrochloride injection is administered by continuous epidural infusion using an appropriate epidural infusion device. The 0.5-mg/mL concentration must be diluted with sodium chloride 0.9% to 0.1 mg/mL for use. Clonidine hydrochloride injection must not be used with a preservative.[1(2/06)]

Stability

Intact vials containing the clear, colorless solution should be stored at controlled room temperature.[1(2/06)] They are stable for 6 months stored at an elevated temperature of 40°C, remaining clear and colorless with no loss of clonidine hydrochloride.[2069]

Clonidine hydrochloride (Roxane) 100 mcg/mL was filled into plastic syringes (Becton Dickinson), pump reservoirs (Bard), and glass vials and stored at 22 to 27°C for 7 days. The solution was also filled into administration set tubing (Kendall McGaw) and stored under the same conditions. In all cases, the solution remained clear and colorless and no loss of potency was found.[2069]

Clonidine hydrochloride 100 mcg/mL was delivered at a rate of 0.1 mL/hr for 7 days through 2 epidural catheter sets, Epi-Cath (Abbott) and Port-A-Cath (Pharmacia Deltec). The temperature was maintained at 37°C to simulate internal use of the set. The delivered solution remained clear and colorless throughout the study. Furthermore, the solution delivered through the Epi-Cath resulted in little or no loss. With the Port-A-Cath, a concentrating effect due to a loss of water was countered by a small clonidine hydrochloride loss of drug (about 5%). The net effect was delivery of about 95% of the clonidine hydrochloride dose.[2069]

Syringes

Clonidine hydrochloride (Boehringer Ingelheim) 9 mcg/mL in sodium chloride 0.9% was packaged in 2 types of polypropylene syringes. The Omnifix (B. Braun) syringes had polyisoprene piston tips while the Terumo syringes had no natural or synthetic rubber in the product. Stored at 4, 21, and 35°C for 30 days, the test solutions in Terumo syringes exhibited no visual changes or changes in measured pH. Stored at 4, 21, and 35°C for 30 days, the test solutions in Omnifix syringes exhibited no visual changes but substantial changes in measured pH occurred in some samples. An acceptable pH was maintained for 30 days at 4°C, 5 days at 21°C, and less than 1 day at 35°C. Although the pH remained within the stability range for the drug in most of the samples, this does not definitively demonstrate stability.[2387]

Clonidine hydrochloride (Medicianz) 0.5 and 5 mcg/mL in dextrose 5%, dextrose 10%, and sodium chloride 0.9% was packaged in 20-mL plastic syringes (MicroAnalytix).[3506] Solutions were physically stable with little to no loss of drug in 24 hours at 35°C.[3506]

Implantable Pumps

An admixture of bupivacaine hydrochloride 25 mg/mL, clonidine hydrochloride 2 mg/mL, and morphine sulfate 50 mg/mL in sterile water for injection was reported to be physically and chemically stable for 90 days at 37°C in SynchroMed implantable pumps. Little or no loss of any drug occurred.[2585]

Clonidine hydrochloride and morphine sulfate powders were dissolved in ziconotide acetate (Elan) injection to yield concentrations of 2 and 35 mg/mL and 25 mcg/mL, respectively. Stored at 37°C, 11% ziconotide loss in 7 days, 4% clonidine loss in 20 days, and no morphine loss in 28 days occurred.[2752]

Morphine sulfate (Infumorph) 20 mg/mL with clonidine hydrochloride (Boehringer Ingelheim) 50 mcg/mL and morphine sulfate 2 mg/mL with clonidine hydrochloride 1.84 mg/mL were evaluated in SynchroMed EL (Medtronic) implantable pumps with silicone elastomer intrathecal catheters at 37°C for 3 months. No visible incompatibilities were observed, and delivered concentrations of both drugs were in the range of 94 to 99.6% of the theoretical concentrations throughout the study. Furthermore, no impairment of mechanical performance of the pump or any of its components was found.[2477]

Compatibility Information

Solution Compatibility

Clonidine HCl

Test Soln Name	Mfr	Mfr	Conc/L or %	Remarks	Ref	C/I
Dextrose 5%	BA[a]	MDZ	0.5 and 5 mg	Physically stable with little to no loss of drug in 7 days at 4°C	3506	C
Dextrose 10%	BA[a]	MDZ	0.5 and 5 mg	Physically stable with little to no loss of drug in 7 days at 4°C	3506	C

DOI: 10.37573/9781585286850.097

Solution Compatibility (Cont.)

Test Soln Name	Mfr	Mfr	Conc/L or %	Remarks	Ref	C/I
Sodium chloride 0.9%	BA		200 mg	Visually compatible with no loss of drug in 10 weeks at 37°C protected from light	2359	C
Sodium chloride 0.9%	BA[a]	MDZ	0.5 and 5 mg	Physically stable with little to no loss of drug in 7 days at 4°C	3506	C

[a] Tested in amber glass containers.

Additive Compatibility

Clonidine HCl

Test Drug	Mfr	Conc/L or %	Mfr	Conc/L or %	Test Solution	Remarks	Ref	C/I
Baclofen		1 g		0.2 g	NS	Visually compatible with no loss of either drug in 10 weeks at 37°C in dark	2359	C
Bupivacaine HCl with fentanyl citrate	AST JN	1 g 35 mg	BI	9 mg	NS[a]	Visually compatible with less than 10% change of any drug in 28 days at 4°C and 24 days at 25°C in the dark	2437	C
Fentanyl citrate with bupivacaine HCl	JN AST	35 mg 1 g	BI	9 mg	NS[a]	Visually compatible with less than 10% change of any drug in 28 days at 4°C and 24 days at 25°C in the dark	2437	C
Hydromorphone HCl		25 mg	BI	150 mg	[c]	No clonidine loss in 35 days at 37°C	2593	C
Meperidine HCl		8 g	BI	3 mg	NS[a]	Visually compatible with no loss of either drug in 21 days at room temperature	2710	C
Ropivacaine HCl	ASZ	1 g	BI	5 and 50 mg	NS[b]	Physically compatible. No loss of either drug in 30 days at 30°C in the dark	2433	C
Ropivacaine HCl	ASZ	2 g	BI	5 mg	[b]	Physically compatible. No loss of either drug in 30 days at 30°C in the dark	2433	C
Ziconotide acetate	ELN	25 mg[d]	BB	2 g[e]		No loss of either drug in 28 days at 37°C	2703	C

[a] Tested in PVC containers.

[b] Tested in polypropylene bags (Mark II Polybags).

[c] Tested in SynchroMed implantable pumps.

[d] Tested in SynchroMed II implantable pumps.

[e] Clonidine HCl powder dissolved in ziconotide acetate injection.

Drugs in Syringe Compatibility

Clonidine HCl

Test Drug	Mfr	Amt	Mfr	Amt	Remarks	Ref	C/I
Bupivacaine HCl	SAN	3.75 mg/1 mL	FUJ	100 mcg/1 mL	Physically and chemically stable for 14 days at room temperature	2069	C
Bupivacaine HCl	SAN	60 mg/8 mL	FUJ	100 mcg/1 mL	Physically and chemically stable for 14 days at room temperature	2069	C
Bupivacaine HCl with fentanyl citrate	AST JN	50 mg 1.75 mg	BI	0.45 mg	Diluted to 50 mL with NS. Visually compatible with less than 10% loss of any drug in 25 days at 4 and 25°C in the dark	2437	C
Bupivacaine HCl with morphine sulfate	SW ES	1.5 mg/mL 0.2 mg/mL	BI	0.03 mg/mL	Diluted to 5 mL with NS. Visually compatible with no new GC/MS peaks in 1 hr at room temperature	1956	C
Fentanyl citrate with bupivacaine HCl	JN AST	1.75 mg 50 mg	BI	0.45 mg	Diluted to 50 mL with NS. Visually compatible with less than 10% loss of any drug in 25 days at 4 and 25°C in the dark	2437	C

Drugs in Syringe Compatibility (Cont.)

Test Drug	Mfr	Amt	Mfr	Amt	Remarks	Ref	C/I
Fentanyl citrate with lidocaine HCl	JN AST	0.01 mg/mL 2 mg/mL	BI	0.03 mg/mL	Diluted to 5 mL with NS. Visually compatible with no new GC/MS peaks in 1 hr at room temperature	1956	C
Heparin sodium		2500 units/1 mL	BI	0.15 mg/1 mL	Visually compatible for at least 5 min	1053	C
Ketamine HCl with tetracaine HCl	PD SW	2 mg/mL 2 mg/mL	BI	0.03 mg/mL	Diluted to 5 mL with NS. Visually compatible with no new GC/MS peaks in 1 hr at room temperature	1956	C
Lidocaine HCl with fentanyl citrate	AST JN	2 mg/mL 0.01 mg/mL	BI	0.03 mg/mL	Diluted to 5 mL with NS. Visually compatible with no new GC/MS peaks in 1 hr at room temperature	1956	C
Morphine sulfate	ES	10 mg/1 mL	FUJ	100 mcg/1 mL	Physically and chemically stable for 14 days at room temperature	2069	C
Morphine sulfate	a	5 mg/mL[b]	a	0.25 mg/mL[b]	Physically compatible. Little morphine or clonidine loss in 60 days at 23°C in light and at 4°C in dark	2380	C
Morphine sulfate	a	50 mg/mL[c]	a	4 mg/mL[c]	Physically compatible. Little morphine or clonidine loss in 60 days at 23°C in light and at 4°C in dark. Slight yellow discoloration at 23°C not indicative of decomposition	2380	C
Morphine sulfate with bupivacaine HCl	ES SW	0.2 mg/mL 1.5 mg/mL	BI	0.03 mg/mL	Diluted to 5 mL with NS. Visually compatible with no new GC/MS peaks in 1 hr at room temperature	1956	C
Tetracaine HCl with ketamine HCl	SW PD	2 mg/mL 2 mg/mL	BI	0.03 mg/mL	Diluted to 5 mL with NS. Visually compatible with no new GC/MS peaks in 1 hr at room temperature	1956	C
Ziconotide acetate	ELN	25 mcg/mL	BB	2 mg/mL[d]	No loss of either drug in 28 days at 5°C	2703	C

[a] Extemporaneously compounded from bulk drug powders.

[b] Tested in sodium chloride 0.9%.

[c] Tested in sterile water for injection.

[d] Clonidine HCl powder dissolved in ziconotide acetate.

Y-Site Injection Compatibility (1:1 Mixture)

Clonidine HCl

Test Drug	Mfr	Conc	Mfr	Conc	Remarks	Ref	C/I
Aminophylline	NYC	0.9 mg/mL[b]	BI	18 mcg/mL[b]	Visually compatible	2642	C
Defibrotide sodium	JAZ	8 mg/mL[b]	BI	2.4 mcg/mL[a]	Visually compatible for 4 hr at room temperature	3149	C
Dobutamine HCl	LI	2 mg/mL[a]	BI	18 mcg/mL[b]	Visually compatible	2642	C
Dopamine HCl	NYC	2 mg/mL[a]	BI	18 mcg/mL[b]	Visually compatible	2642	C
Epinephrine HCl	NYC	20 mcg/mL[a]	BI	18 mcg/mL[b]	Visually compatible	2642	C
Fentanyl citrate	ALP	50 mcg/mL	BI	18 mcg/mL[b]	Visually compatible	2642	C
Labetalol HCl	GSK	1 mg/mL[a b]	BI	18 mcg/mL[b]	Visually compatible	2642	C
Lorazepam	WY	0.33 mg/mL[b]	BI	0.015 mg/mL	Visually compatible for 24 hr at 22°C	1855	C
Magnesium sulfate	BRN	9.6 mg/mL[a]	BI	18 mcg/mL[b]	Visually compatible	2642	C
Midazolam HCl	RC	5 mg/mL	BI	0.015 mg/mL	Orange color in 24 hr at 22°C	1855	I
Midazolam HCl	ALP	1 mg/mL	BI	18 mcg/mL[b]	Visually compatible	2642	C
Nitroglycerin	NYC	0.4 mg/mL[a]	BI	18 mcg/mL[b]	Visually compatible	2642	C
Norepinephrine bitartrate	APO	20 mcg/mL[a]	BI	18 mcg/mL[b]	Visually compatible	2642	C

Y-Site Injection Compatibility (1:1 Mixture) (Cont.)

Test Drug	Mfr	Conc	Mfr	Conc	Remarks	Ref	C/I
Potassium chloride	BRN	1 mEq/mL	BI	18 mcg/mL[b]	Visually compatible	2642	C
Theophylline	ASZ	1 mg/mL	BI	18 mcg/mL[b]	Visually compatible	2642	C
Verapamil HCl	AB	2.5 mg/mL	BI	18 mcg/mL[b]	Visually compatible	2642	C

[a] Tested in dextrose 5%.

[b] Tested in sodium chloride 0.9%.

Selected Revisions January 31, 2020. © Copyright, October 1998. American Society of Health-System Pharmacists, Inc.

Cloxacillin Sodium
AHFS 8:12.16.12

Products

Cloxacillin sodium is available as a dry powder in vials containing 500 mg, 1 g, and 2 g of cloxacillin as the sodium salt.[3248] The drug also is available in a pharmacy bulk package containing 10 g of cloxacillin as the sodium salt.[3248]

For intramuscular use, 1.7 mL of sterile water for injection should be added to the 500-mg vial, and the vial should be shaken well to yield a solution with a nominal concentration of 250 mg/mL.[3248]

For intravenous use, 4.8 or 9.6 mL of sterile water for injection should be added to a 500-mg or 1-g vial, respectively, and the vial should be shaken well to yield a solution with a nominal concentration of 100 mg/mL.[3248]

For intravenous infusion, 3.4 or 6.8 mL of sterile water for injection should be added to the 1- or 2-g vial, respectively, and the vial should be shaken well to yield a solution with a nominal concentration of 250 mg/mL, which is then added to an appropriate infusion solution for administration.[3248] The 10-g pharmacy bulk package should be reconstituted with 34 mL of sterile water for injection and shaken well to yield a solution with a nominal concentration of 250 mg/mL, which is then added to an appropriate infusion solution for administration.[3248]

Sodium Content

Each gram of cloxacillin sodium contains approximately 50 mg of sodium.[3248]

Administration

Cloxacillin sodium may be administered by intramuscular injection, direct intravenous injection slowly over 2 to 4 minutes, or by intravenous infusion (following dilution in an appropriate infusion solution) over 30 to 40 minutes.[3248]

Stability

Intact vials containing the drug in dry form should be stored at controlled room temperature.[3248] After reconstitution with sterile water for injection, cloxacillin solutions are stable for up to 24 hours at controlled room temperature not exceeding 25°C or 48 hours under refrigeration at 2 to 8°C.[3248]

Cloxacillin sodium (Beecham) 250 mg reconstituted with 1.5 mL and 500 mg reconstituted with 2 mL of sterile water for injection exhibited a 5% loss in 7 days at 5°C and a 15% loss in 4 days at 23°C.[99]

Cloxacillin sodium (Ayerst) 20 g/L in sodium chloride 0.9% or dextrose 5% was stored in polyvinyl chloride (PVC) minibags (Travenol) or glass bottles (Travenol) for 24 hours at 5 and 22°C. No significant decrease in antibiotic stability was observed at 24 hours in sodium chloride 0.9% in either container. With dextrose 5%, a decrease in cloxacillin was observed at 24 hours. The results indicated that cloxacillin sodium was stable for 24 hours in sodium chloride 0.9% and for 8 hours in dextrose 5%.[298]

pH Effects

Cloxacillin sodium is most stable at a pH of 5.5 to 7, with a minimum decomposition rate at pH 6.3.[1476][1477]

Freezing Solutions

Cloxacillin sodium (Beecham) at concentrations of 1 to 10%, buffered to pH 6.05, lost no more than 1% potency in 1 month when frozen at −20°C.[99]

Cloxacillin sodium (Beecham) 1 g in 50 mL of dextrose 5% or sodium chloride 0.9% in PVC containers (Travenol) was frozen at −20°C for 30 days, followed by natural thawing and storage at 5°C for 21 hours. The cloxacillin concentration was retained for the duration of the study.[299]

Cloxacillin sodium 2 g in 100 mL in dextrose 5% or sodium chloride 0.9% in PVC containers was frozen at −27°C for up to 9 months and then thawed by microwave. The results indicated that at least 90% of the concentration was retained. A distinct yellow discoloration was observed in solutions in dextrose 5% stored for 6 months. Consequently, the authors recommended that such frozen solutions not be stored for more than 3 months.[1176]

Cloxacillin sodium (Beecham) 500 mg in 50-mL PVC bags (Travenol) stored at −20°C and thawed under natural conditions was stable for at least 100 days. In addition, the drug was stable under refrigeration for 4 days followed by 24 hours at room temperature after thawing.[1478]

Sorption

Cloxacillin sodium was shown not to exhibit sorption to PVC bags and tubing, polyethylene tubing, Silastic tubing, and polypropylene syringes.[536][606]

Filtration

Cloxacillin sodium (Beecham) 1.97 mg/mL in sodium chloride 0.9% or dextrose 5% was filtered through a 0.22-μm cellulose acetate membrane filter (Ivex-HP, Millipore) over 6 hours. No significant loss due to binding was noted.[1034]

DOI: 10.37573/9781585286850.098

Compatibility Information

Solution Compatibility

Cloxacillin sodium

Test Soln Name	Mfr	Mfr	Conc/L or %	Remarks	Ref	C/I
Dextrose 5%		BE	10 g	Less than 5% loss in 24 hr at room temperature	99	C
Dextrose 5%	TR[a]	AY	20 g	Potency retained for 24 hr at 5°C	298	C
Dextrose 5%	TR[b]	AY	20 g	3% loss in 1 hr and 12% loss in 24 hr at 22°C	298	I
Dextrose 5%	BA[b]	AY	20 g	1 to 7% loss in 8 hr and 13 to 15% loss in 24 hr at 5 and 22°C	298	I
Dextrose 5%		AST	2.25 g	Less than 4% cloxacillin loss in 48 hr at 25°C	1476	C
Dextrose 5%	BA[a]	NVP	5 to 50 g	Physically compatible with less than 7% loss in 18 days at 4°C	2372	C
Dextrose 5%	BA[a]	NVP	5 g	Physically compatible with 10% loss calculated in 3.8 days at 23°C	2372	C
Dextrose 5%	BA[a]	NVP	10 g	Physically compatible with 10% loss calculated in 3 days at 23°C	2372	C
Dextrose 5%	BA[a]	NVP	20 g	Physically compatible with 10% loss calculated in 2.6 days at 23°C	2372	C
Dextrose 5%	BA[a]	NVP	40 g	Physically compatible with 10% loss calculated in 1.9 days at 23°C	2372	C
Dextrose 5%	BA[a]	NVP	50 g	Physically compatible with 10% loss calculated in 1.7 days at 23°C	2372	C
Dextrose 5%		SMX	1 and 2 g	Stable for up to 12 hr at controlled room temperature not exceeding 25°C	3248	C
Ringer's injection		BE	10 g	Less than 10% loss in 24 hr at room temperature	99	C
Sodium chloride 0.9%		BE	10 g	Less than 5% loss in 24 hr at room temperature	99	C
Sodium chloride 0.9%	TR[b], BA[a]	AY	20 g	Potency retained for 24 hr at 5 and 22°C	298	C
Sodium chloride 0.9%	BA[a]	NVP	5 to 50 g	Physically compatible with less than 7% loss in 18 days at 4°C	2372	C
Sodium chloride 0.9%	BA[a]	NVP	5 g	Physically compatible with 10% loss calculated in 2.1 days at 23°C	2372	C
Sodium chloride 0.9%	BA[a]	NVP	10 g	Physically compatible with 10% loss calculated in 1.9 days at 23°C	2372	C
Sodium chloride 0.9%	BA[a]	NVP	20 g	Physically compatible with 10% loss calculated in 1.9 days at 23°C	2372	C
Sodium chloride 0.9%	BA[a]	NVP	40 g	Physically compatible with 10% loss calculated in 1.5 days at 23°C	2372	C
Sodium chloride 0.9%	BA[a]	NVP	50 g	Physically compatible with 10% loss calculated in 1.5 days at 23°C	2372	C
Sodium lactate (⅙) M		BE	10 g	15% loss in 24 hr at room temperature	99	I
Sodium lactate (⅙) M		AST	2.25 g	10% cloxacillin loss in 7 hr at 25°C	1476	I
Sodium lactate (⅙) M		SMX	1 and 2 g	Stable for up to 12 hr at controlled room temperature not exceeding 25°C	3248	C
TPN #22[c]		AY	10 g	Physically compatible with no activity loss in 24 hr at 22°C in the dark	837	C

[a] Tested in PVC containers.

[b] Tested in glass containers.

[c] Refer to Appendix for the composition of parenteral nutrition solutions. TPN indicates a 2-in-1 admixture.

Additive Compatibility

Cloxacillin sodium

Test Drug	Mfr	Conc/L or %	Mfr	Conc/L or %	Test Solution	Remarks	Ref	C/I
Amikacin sulfate	BR	5 g	BR	10 g	D5LR, D5R, D5S, D5W, D10W, LR, NS, R, SL	Physically compatible and both stable for 24 hr at 25°C	293	C
Chlorpromazine HCl	BP	200 mg	BP	1 g	NS	Haze forms over 3 hr	26	I

Additive Compatibility (Cont.)

Test Drug	Mfr	Conc/L or %	Mfr	Conc/L or %	Test Solution	Remarks	Ref	C/I
Dextran 40	PH	10%	AST	2.25 g	D5W	Under 4% cloxacillin loss in 48 hr at 25°C	1476	C
Dextran 40	PH	10%	BE	4 g	D5W	2% cloxacillin loss in 24 hr at 20°C	834	C
Dextran 40	PH	10%	BE	8 g	D5W, NS	Under 5% loss in 24 hr at room temperature	99	C
Fat emulsion, intravenous		10%		10 g		Aggregation of oil droplets	37	I
Floxacillin sodium	BE	20 g	BE	20 g	NS	Physically compatible for 24 hr at 15 and 30°C. Haze forms in 48 hr at 30°C. No change at 15°C	1479	C
Furosemide	HO	1 g	BE	20 g	NS	Physically compatible for 72 hr at 15 and 30°C	1479	C
Gentamicin sulfate	RS	160 mg	BE	4 g	D5¼S, D5W, NS	Precipitate forms	157	I
Heparin sodium		32,000 units		2 g	NS	Physically compatible and heparin stable for 24 hr	57	C
Hydrocortisone sodium succinate	GL	200 mg	BE	20 g	D5S, D5W, NS	Physically compatible and cloxacillin stable for 24 hr at 25°C	89	C
Potassium chloride		60 mEq	AST	2.25 g	D5W	10% cloxacillin loss in 48 hr at 25°C	1476	C

Drugs in Syringe Compatibility

Cloxacillin sodium

Test Drug	Mfr	Amt	Mfr	Amt	Remarks	Ref	C/I
Chloramphenicol sodium succinate	PD	250 and 400 mg/1.5 to 2 mL	BE	250 mg	No precipitate or color change within 1 hr at room temperature	99	C
Chloramphenicol sodium succinate	PD	250 and 400 mg/mL	AY	250 mg	Physically compatible for 1 hr at room temperature	300	C
Colistimethate sodium	PX	40 mg/2 mL	BE	250 mg	No precipitate or color change within 1 hr at room temperature	99	C
Colistimethate sodium	PX	500 mg/2 mL	AY	250 mg	Physically compatible for 1 hr at room temperature	300	C
Dimenhydrinate		10 mg/1 mL		100 mg/1 mL	Clear solution	2569	C
Erythromycin lactobionate	AB	300 mg/6 mL	AY	250 mg	Precipitate forms within 1 hr at room temperature	300	I
Gentamicin sulfate		80 mg/2 mL	BE	250 mg	Physically incompatible within 1 hr at room temperature	99	I
Hydromorphone HCl	KN	2, 10, 40 mg/1 mL	AY	250 mg/1 mL	Precipitate forms but dissipates with shaking. Under 10% loss of both drugs in 24 hr at room temperature	2082	?
Lidocaine HCl			BE		Physically compatible	89	C
Lincomycin HCl	UP	600 mg/2 mL	BE	250 mg	No precipitate or color change within 1 hr at room temperature	99	C
Lincomycin HCl	UP	600 mg/2 mL	AY	250 mg	Physically compatible for 1 hr at room temperature	300	C
Pantoprazole sodium	a	4 mg/1 mL		100 mg/1 mL	Precipitates immediately	2574	I

Drugs in Syringe Compatibility (Cont.)

Test Drug	Mfr	Amt	Mfr	Amt	Remarks	Ref	C/I
Polymyxin B sulfate	BE	250,000 units/1.5 to 2 mL	BE	250 mg	Physically incompatible within 1 hr at room temperature	99	I
Streptomycin sulfate		1 g/2 mL	BE	250 mg	No precipitate or color change within 1 hr at room temperature	99	C
Streptomycin sulfate	BP	1 g/2 mL	AY	250 mg	Physically compatible for 1 hr at room temperature	300	C
Streptomycin sulfate	BP	1 g/1.5 mL	AY	250 mg	Syrupy solution forms	300	I
Streptomycin sulfate	BP	750 mg/1.5 mL	AY	250 mg	Precipitate forms within 1 hr at room temperature	300	I

[a] Test performed using the formulation WITHOUT edetate disodium.

Y-Site Injection Compatibility (1:1 Mixture)

Cloxacillin sodium

Test Drug	Mfr	Conc	Mfr	Conc	Remarks	Ref	C/I
Acetylcysteine	ALV	200 mg/mL	SMX	100 mg/mL	Physically compatible for up to 4 hr at room temperature	3245	C
Acyclovir sodium	PPC	50 mg/mL	SMX	100 mg/mL	Physically compatible for up to 4 hr at room temperature	3245	C
Albumin human	BEH	250 mg/mL	SMX	100 mg/mL	Physically compatible for up to 4 hr at room temperature	3245	C
Amikacin sulfate	SZ	250 mg/mL	SMX	100 mg/mL	Large particles form immediately	3245	I
Amiodarone HCl	SZ	50 mg/mL	SMX	100 mg/mL	Physically compatible for up to 4 hr at room temperature	3245	C
Amphotericin B liposomal	ASP	4 mg/mL	SMX	100 mg/mL	Physically compatible for up to 4 hr at room temperature	3245	C
Ampicillin sodium	NOP	250 mg/mL	SMX	100 mg/mL	Physically compatible for up to 4 hr at room temperature	3245	C
Atropine sulfate	SZ	0.4 mg/mL	SMX	100 mg/mL	Physically compatible for up to 4 hr at room temperature	3245	C
Azithromycin[h]	SMX	100 mg/mL	SMX	100 mg/mL	Precipitates immediately	3245	I
Benztropine mesylate	OM	1 mg/mL	SMX	100 mg/mL	Physically compatible for up to 4 hr at room temperature	3245	C
Blinatumomab	AMG	0.125 mcg/mL[b]	ASP	8.6 mg/mL[b]	Persistent particulate formation when blinatumomab is added to cloxacillin; not observed when order of mixing was reversed	3405, 3417	?
Blinatumomab	AMG	0.375 mcg/mL[b]	ASP	8.6 mg/mL[b]	Visually compatible for 12 hr at room temperature	3405, 3417	C
Calcium chloride	HOS	100 mg/mL	SMX	100 mg/mL	Physically compatible for up to 4 hr at room temperature	3245	C
Calcium gluconate	PPC	100 mg/mL	SMX	100 mg/mL	Physically compatible for up to 4 hr at room temperature	3245	C
Caspofungin acetate	ME	5 mg/mL	SMX	100 mg/mL	Physically compatible for up to 4 hr at room temperature	3245	C
Cefazolin sodium	NOP	10 mg/mL	SMX	100 mg/mL	Physically compatible for up to 4 hr at room temperature	3245	C
Cefotaxime sodium	SAN	95 mg/mL	SMX	100 mg/mL	Physically compatible for up to 4 hr at room temperature	3245	C
Cefoxitin sodium	HOS	100 mg/mL	SMX	100 mg/mL	Physically compatible for up to 4 hr at room temperature	3245	C
Ceftazidime	PPC	95 mg/mL	SMX	100 mg/mL	Physically compatible for up to 4 hr at room temperature	3245	C
Ceftriaxone sodium	SZ	100 mg/mL	SMX	100 mg/mL	Physically compatible for up to 4 hr at room temperature	3245	C
Cefuroxime sodium	PPC	90 mg/mL	SMX	100 mg/mL	Physically compatible for up to 4 hr at room temperature	3245	C

Y-Site Injection Compatibility (1:1 Mixture) (Cont.)

Test Drug	Mfr	Conc	Mfr	Conc	Remarks	Ref	C/I
Chlorpromazine HCl	SZ	25 mg/mL	SMX	100 mg/mL	Precipitates immediately	3245	I
Ciprofloxacin[c]	OM	2 mg/mL	SMX	100 mg/mL	Large particles form immediately	3245	I
Clindamycin phosphate	SZ	150 mg/mL	SMX	100 mg/mL	Physically compatible for up to 4 hr at room temperature	3245	C
Cyclosporine	NVA	5 mg/mL[d]	SMX	100 mg/mL	Physically compatible for up to 4 hr at room temperature	3245	C
Dexamethasone sodium phosphate	OM	4 mg/mL	SMX	100 mg/mL	Physically compatible for up to 4 hr at room temperature	3245	C
Diazepam	SZ	5 mg/mL	SMX	100 mg/mL	Large particles form immediately	3245	I
Digoxin	SZ	0.05 mg/mL	SMX	100 mg/mL	Physically compatible for up to 4 hr at room temperature	3245	C
Dimenhydrinate	SZ	10 mg/mL	SMX	100 mg/mL	Physically compatible for up to 4 hr at room temperature	3245	C
Diphenhydramine HCl	PPC	50 mg/mL	SMX	100 mg/mL	Precipitates immediately	3245	I
Dobutamine HCl	HOS	12.5 mg/mL	SMX	100 mg/mL	Precipitates immediately	3245	I
Dopamine HCl	BA	3.2 mg/mL	SMX	100 mg/mL	Physically compatible for up to 4 hr at room temperature	3245	C
Droperidol	SZ	2.5 mg/mL	SMX	100 mg/mL	Precipitates immediately	3245	I
Epinephrine[g]	HOS	0.1 mg/mL	SMX	100 mg/mL	Physically compatible for up to 4 hr at room temperature	3245	C
Epinephrine HCl	ERF	1 mg/mL	SMX	100 mg/mL	Physically compatible for up to 4 hr at room temperature	3245	C
Erythromycin lactobionate	AMD	50 mg/mL	SMX	100 mg/mL	Precipitates immediately	3245	I
Esmolol HCl	BA	10 mg/mL	SMX	100 mg/mL	Physically compatible for up to 4 hr at room temperature	3245	C
Fentanyl citrate	SZ	50 mcg/mL	SMX	100 mg/mL	Physically compatible for up to 4 hr at room temperature	3245	C
Fluconazole	SZ	2 mg/mL	SMX	100 mg/mL	Physically compatible for up to 4 hr at room temperature	3245	C
Furosemide	OM	10 mg/mL	SMX	100 mg/mL	Physically compatible for up to 4 hr at room temperature	3245	C
Gentamicin sulfate	SZ	40 mg/mL	SMX	100 mg/mL	Precipitates immediately	3245	I
Heparin sodium	PPC	100 units/mL	SMX	100 mg/mL	Physically compatible for up to 4 hr at room temperature	3245	C
Hydralazine HCl	SMX	20 mg/mL	SMX	100 mg/mL	Opaque yellow turbidity forms within 4 hr	3245	I
Hydrocortisone sodium succinate	NOP	125 mg/mL	SMX	100 mg/mL	Physically compatible for up to 4 hr at room temperature	3245	C
Hydromorphone HCl	KN	2, 10, 40 mg/mL	AY	250 mg/mL	Turbidity forms but dissipates with shaking and solution remains clear. Both drugs stable for 24 hr	1532	?
Hydromorphone HCl	KN	2, 10, 40 mg/mL	AY	40 mg/mL[a]	Turbidity forms immediately and cloxacillin precipitate develops	1532	I
Hydromorphone HCl	KN	2, 10, 40 mg/mL	AY	27 mg/mL[a]	Turbidity forms immediately	1532	I
Hydromorphone HCl	KN	2, 10, 40 mg/mL	AY	12 mg/mL[a]	Visually compatible for 24 hr; precipitate forms in 96 hr	1532	C
Hydromorphone HCl	SZ	10 mg/mL	SMX	100 mg/mL	Physically compatible for up to 4 hr at room temperature	3245	C
Insulin, regular	LI	100 units/mL	SMX	100 mg/mL	Physically compatible for up to 4 hr at room temperature	3245	C
Isoproterenol HCl	SZ	0.2 mg/mL	SMX	100 mg/mL	Physically compatible for up to 4 hr at room temperature	3245	C
Ketamine HCl	SZ	50 mg/mL	SMX	100 mg/mL	Physically compatible for up to 4 hr at room temperature	3245	C
Labetalol HCl	SZ	5 mg/mL	SMX	100 mg/mL	Precipitates immediately	3245	I
Levocarnitine	SIG	200 mg/mL	SMX	100 mg/mL	Physically compatible for up to 4 hr at room temperature	3245	C

Y-Site Injection Compatibility (1:1 Mixture) (Cont.)

Test Drug	Mfr	Conc	Mfr	Conc	Remarks	Ref	C/I
Levofloxacin	HOS	5 mg/mL	SMX	100 mg/mL	Physically compatible for up to 4 hr at room temperature	3245	C
Lidocaine HCl	ALV	1 mg/mL	SMX	100 mg/mL	Physically compatible for up to 4 hr at room temperature	3245	C
Lorazepam	SZ	4 mg/mL	SMX	100 mg/mL	Large particles form within 4 hr	3245	I
Magnesium sulfate	PPC	500 mg/mL	SMX	100 mg/mL	Physically compatible for up to 4 hr at room temperature	3245	C
Mannitol	HOS	250 mg/mL	SMX	100 mg/mL	Physically compatible for up to 4 hr at room temperature	3245	C
Meropenem	SZ	50 mg/mL	SMX	100 mg/mL	Physically compatible for up to 4 hr at room temperature	3245	C
Meropenem		50 mg/mL	SMX	250 mg/mL	Physically compatible for 4 hr at room temperature	3538	C
Methylprednisolone sodium succinate	NOP	62.5 mg/mL	SMX	100 mg/mL	Physically compatible for up to 4 hr at room temperature	3245	C
Metoclopramide HCl	SZ	5 mg/mL	SMX	100 mg/mL	Physically compatible for up to 4 hr at room temperature	3245	C
Metronidazole	HOS	5 mg/mL	SMX	100 mg/mL	Physically compatible for up to 4 hr at room temperature	3245	C
Midazolam HCl	PPC	5 mg/mL	SMX	100 mg/mL	Precipitates immediately	3245	I
Milrinone lactate	PPC	1 mg/mL	SMX	100 mg/mL	Physically compatible for up to 4 hr at room temperature	3245	C
Morphine sulfate	SZ	50 mg/mL	SMX	100 mg/mL	Precipitates immediately	3245	I
Multivitamins	SZ		SMX	100 mg/mL	Physically compatible for up to 4 hr at room temperature	3245	C
Naloxone HCl	SZ	0.4 mg/mL	SMX	100 mg/mL	Physically compatible for up to 4 hr at room temperature	3245	C
Nitroglycerin	OM	5 mg/mL	SMX	100 mg/mL	Large particles form within 4 hr	3245	I
Norepinephrine bitartrate	SZ	1 mg/mL	SMX	100 mg/mL	Physically compatible for up to 4 hr at room temperature	3245	C
Ondansetron HCl	SZ	2 mg/mL	SMX	100 mg/mL	Physically compatible for up to 4 hr at room temperature	3245	C
Oxytocin	PPC	10 units/mL	SMX	100 mg/mL	Physically compatible for up to 4 hr at room temperature	3245	C
Pantoprazole sodium	SZ[e]	4 mg/mL	SMX	100 mg/mL	Physically compatible for up to 4 hr at room temperature	3245	C
Penicillin G sodium	PPC	500,000 units/mL	SMX	100 mg/mL	Physically compatible for up to 4 hr at room temperature	3245	C
Phenytoin sodium	SZ	50 mg/mL	SMX	100 mg/mL	Precipitates within 1 hr	3245	I
Piperacillin sodium–tazobactam sodium	SZ[e]	200 mg/mL[f]	SMX	100 mg/mL	Physically compatible for up to 4 hr at room temperature	3245	C
Potassium chloride	HOS	2 mEq/mL	SMX	100 mg/mL	Physically compatible for up to 4 hr at room temperature	3245	C
Potassium phosphates	PPC	3 mmol/mL	SMX	100 mg/mL	Large particles form within 4 hr	3245	I
Promethazine HCl	SZ	25 mg/mL	SMX	100 mg/mL	Precipitates immediately	3245	I
Propranolol HCl	SZ	1 mg/mL	SMX	100 mg/mL	Physically compatible for up to 4 hr at room temperature	3245	C
Ranitidine HCl	GSK	25 mg/mL	SMX	100 mg/mL	Physically compatible for up to 4 hr at room temperature	3245	C
Rocuronium bromide	ME	10 mg/mL	SMX	100 mg/mL	Precipitates immediately	3245	I
Salbutamol sulfate	GSK	1 mg/mL	SMX	100 mg/mL	Physically compatible for up to 4 hr at room temperature	3245	C
Sodium bicarbonate	HOS	84 mg/mL	SMX	100 mg/mL	Physically compatible for up to 4 hr at room temperature	3245	C
Sodium nitroprusside	HOS	25 mg/mL	SMX	100 mg/mL	Physically compatible for up to 4 hr at room temperature	3245	C
Sufentanil citrate	SZ	50 mcg/mL	SMX	100 mg/mL	Physically compatible for up to 4 hr at room temperature	3245	C
Tobramycin sulfate	SZ	40 mg/mL	SMX	100 mg/mL	Precipitates immediately	3245	I

Y-Site Injection Compatibility (1:1 Mixture) (Cont.)

Test Drug	Mfr	Conc	Mfr	Conc	Remarks	Ref	C/I
Trimethoprim–sulfamethoxazole	APT	16 mg/mL^i	SMX	100 mg/mL	Large particles form immediately and within 4 hr	3245	I
Valproate sodium	AB	100 mg/mL	SMX	100 mg/mL	Physically compatible for up to 4 hr at room temperature	3245	C
Vancomycin HCl	PPC	50 mg/mL	SMX	100 mg/mL	Precipitates immediately	3245	I
Vancomycin HCl	PPC	0.3 mg/mL^b	SMX	0.8^b and 1.25^b mg/mL	Visually compatible for up to 1 hr at 25°C	3246	C
Vancomycin HCl	PPC	0.5 mg/mL^b	SMX	23.75 mg/mL^b	Visually compatible for up to 1 hr at 25°C	3246	C
Vancomycin HCl	PPC	0.6 mg/mL^b	SMX	1.25^b and 1.75^b mg/mL	Visually compatible for up to 1 hr at 25°C	3246	C
Vancomycin HCl	PPC	1.3 mg/mL^b	SMX	1.25^b and 3.4^b mg/mL	Visually compatible for up to 1 hr at 25°C	3246	C
Vancomycin HCl	PPC	2 mg/mL^b	SMX	0.8^b, 1.75^b, 3.4^b, and 6.8^b mg/mL	Visually compatible for up to 1 hr at 25°C	3246	C
Vancomycin HCl	PPC	2 mg/mL^b	SMX	12.5^b and 20^b mg/mL	White, gel-like precipitate forms immediately	3246	I
Vancomycin HCl	PPC	2.5 mg/mL^b	SMX	1.25 mg/mL^b	White, gel-like precipitate forms within 1 hr	3246	I
Vancomycin HCl	PPC	2.5 mg/mL^b	SMX	6.8 mg/mL^b	White, gel-like precipitate forms immediately	3246	I
Vancomycin HCl	PPC	5 mg/mL^b	SMX	1.25^b and 12.5^b mg/mL	White, gel-like precipitate forms immediately	3246	I
Vancomycin HCl	PPC	8 mg/mL^b	SMX	5 mg/mL^b	White, gel-like precipitate forms immediately	3246	I
Vancomycin HCl	PPC	9.5 mg/mL^b	SMX	1.25 mg/mL^b	White, gel-like precipitate forms immediately	3246	I
Voriconazole	PF	10 mg/mL	SMX	100 mg/mL	Physically compatible for up to 4 hr at room temperature	3245	C

^{a} Tested in dextrose 5%.

^{b} Tested in sodium chloride 0.9%.

^{c} Test performed using the lactate salt formulation.

^{d} Tested in sterile water for injection.

^{e} Presence or absence of edetate disodium not specified.

^{f} Piperacillin component. Piperacillin in an 8:1 fixed-ratio concentration with tazobactam.

^{g} As epinephrine base rather than the salt.

^{h} Test performed using the monohydrate formulation.

^{i} Trimethoprim component. Trimethoprim in a 1:5 fixed-ratio concentration with sulfamethoxazole.

Selected Revisions May 1, 2020. © Copyright, October 2004.
American Society of Health-System Pharmacists, Inc.

Colistimethate Sodium
AHFS 8:12.28.28

Products

Colistimethate sodium is a prodrug that undergoes hydrolysis in vivo to form primarily the active drug, colistin, which is a mixture of the 2 active components colistin A (polymyxin E1) and colistin B (polymyxin E2).[2734][3152][3153][3154] Colistimethate sodium is available as a lyophilized cake of a complex mixture, containing colistimethate sodium or pentasodium colistinmethanesulfonate, in vials containing the equivalent of 150 mg of colistin base activity.[3150][3151][3154]

Each 150-mg vial should be reconstituted with 2 mL of sterile water for injection to yield a solution containing 75 mg/mL of colistin base activity.[3150][3151] During reconstitution, the contents of the vials should be gently swirled to avoid frothing.[3150][3151] Reconstituted solutions should be visually inspected for particulate matter and discoloration prior to administration; if particulate matter is present or discoloration occurs, the solution should not be used.[3150][3151]

Units

The strength of colistimethate for injection products is expressed in terms of equivalent colistin base activity, *not* in terms of the prodrug.[3150][3151][3153] In the US, it has been recommended that all prescribing of the drug consistently be in terms of colistin base activity to avoid dosing errors that could result from confusion between the 2 forms.[3153] The manufacturers provide dosage recommendations in terms of colistin base activity.[3150][3151][3153] If the drug is ordered as colistimethate or colistimethate sodium, the dosage should be clarified in terms of colistin base activity.[3153]

Sodium Content

Colistimethate sodium (Perrigo) contains approximately 0.099 mg (0.0043 mEq) of sodium per mg of colistin.[3151]

Trade Name(s)

Coly-Mycin M Parenteral

Administration

Colistimethate sodium may be administered intravenously or intramuscularly.[3150][3151]

For intravenous administration, half of the total daily dose should be administered as an intermittent direct intravenous injection over 3 to 5 minutes every 12 hours.[3150][3151] Alternatively, half of the total daily dose should be administered as a direct intravenous injection over 3 to 5 minutes and the remaining half of the total daily dose should be diluted in a compatible infusion solution and administered by slow intravenous infusion over 22 to 23 hours beginning 1 to 2 hours after administration of the direct intravenous injection.[3150][3151] Slower rates of infusion may be warranted in specific populations (e.g., those with renal impairment).[3150][3151]

The reconstituted solution also may be administrated by deep intramuscular injection into a large muscle mass (e.g., gluteal muscles, lateral part of the thigh).[3150][3151]

Stability

Colistimethate sodium is a white to slightly yellow lyophilized cake.[3150][3151] Intact vials should be stored at controlled room temperature.[3150][3151]

In addition to undergoing hydrolysis in vivo, colistimethate sodium also may undergo spontaneous hydrolysis to colistin in aqueous solution prior to administration.[2734][3152][3154] In 2007, FDA warned healthcare professionals that prolonged storage (longer than 24 hours) of the reconstituted drug resulted in increased concentrations of colistin in solution.[2734] The FDA warning followed the death of a cystic fibrosis patient who received the injectable colistimethate sodium product prepared in advance and administered by inhalation via nebulization; the drug is not FDA-labeled for such use.[2734][3150][3151] It was not known how far in advance of administration the drug was prepared or whether it was prepared with saline or water;[3154] however, some studies have indicated that hydrolysis of colistimethate sodium to colistin is both temperature and concentration dependent[3152] and that the drug is substantially less stable when diluted in saline.[3154] The FDA recommends that colistimethate sodium be administered promptly after mixing.[2734]

The manufacturers state that the reconstituted solution may be stored at 2 to 8°C or between 20 and 25°C and used within 7 days.[3150][3151] Solutions diluted for intravenous infusion should be used after preparation or within 24 hours.[3150][3151]

One study found that the reconstituted solution of 75 mg/mL of colistin base activity (APP) prepared with sterile water for injection and stored at −70, −20, 4, and 21°C for 24 hours exhibited formation of less than 1% colistin A and B combined.[3154][3231] A single freeze-thaw cycle did not appear to substantially affect hydrolysis.[3154]

In another study, less than 0.1% of the initial colistimethate sodium concentration was present as colistin after storage of the reconstituted solution of 75 mg/mL of colistin base activity (Pfizer) prepared with sterile water for injection at 4 or 25°C for 7 days in the dark.[3155]

Diluted solutions of 0.333 mg/mL of colistin base activity (Foster) were prepared using sodium chloride 0.9% and stored at 4°C in an elastomeric pump (Braun Easypump).[3152] Degradation of colistimethate sodium to colistin was not detected within the first 3 days of storage at 4°C; however, after 7 days of storage at 4°C and a subsequent 24 hours of storage at 20 to 25°C, the drug was rapidly hydrolyzed to colistin (more than 30%).[3152]

In a diluted solution of 1.5 mg/mL of colistin base activity (Pfizer) prepared using sodium chloride 0.9% or dextrose 5% and stored at 4 or 25°C for 48 hours in the dark, colistin formation was 0.3% of the initial colistimethate sodium concentration at 4°C and 4% at 25°C in both diluents.[3155]

DOI: 10.37573/9781585286850.099

Filtration

Colistimethate sodium (R. Bellon) 0.16 mg/mL in dextrose 5% and sodium chloride 0.9% was filtered through a 0.22-μm cellulose ester member filter (Ivex-HP, Millipore) over 6 hours. No significant drug loss due to binding to the filter was noted.[1034]

Compatibility Information

Solution Compatibility

Colistimethate sodium

Test Soln Name	Mfr	Mfr	Conc/L or %	Remarks	Ref	C/I
Dextrose 5% in sodium chloride 0.225%		JHP		Use within 24 hr	3150	C
Dextrose 5% in sodium chloride 0.45%		JHP		Use within 24 hr	3150	C
Dextrose 5% in sodium chloride 0.9%		JHP		Use within 24 hr	3150	C
Dextrose 5%		JHP		Use within 24 hr	3150	C
Invert sugar 10%		JHP		Use within 24 hr	3150	C
Ringer's injection, lactated		JHP		Use within 24 hr	3150	C
Sodium chloride 0.9%		JHP		Use within 24 hr	3150	C

Additive Compatibility

Colistimethate sodium

Test Drug	Mfr	Conc/L or %	Mfr	Conc/L or %	Test Solution	Remarks	Ref	C/I
Amikacin sulfate	BR	5 g	WC	500 mg	D5LR, D5R, D5S, D5W, D10W, LR, NS, R, SL	Physically compatible and amikacin stable for 24 hr at 25°C. Colistimethate not analyzed	293	C
Ascorbic acid	UP	500 mg	WC	500 mg	D5W	Physically compatible	15	C
Chloramphenicol sodium succinate	PD	10 g	WC	500 mg	D5W	Physically compatible	15	C
Chloramphenicol sodium succinate	PD	10 g	WC	500 mg		Physically compatible	6	C
Diphenhydramine HCl	PD	80 mg	WC	500 mg	D5W	Physically compatible	15	C
Erythromycin lactobionate	AB	5 g	WC	500 mg	D5W	Physically incompatible	15	I
Erythromycin lactobionate	AB	1 g	WC	500 mg	D	Precipitate forms within 1 hr	20	I
Heparin sodium	UP	4000 units	WC	500 mg	D5W	Physically compatible	15	C
Heparin sodium	AB	20,000 units	WC	500 mg	D	Physically compatible	21	C
Hydrocortisone sodium succinate	UP	500 mg	WC	500 mg	D5W	Physically incompatible	15	I
Penicillin G potassium	SQ	20 million units	WC	500 mg	D5W	Physically compatible	15	C
Penicillin G potassium	SQ	5 million units	WC	500 mg	D	Physically compatible	47	C
Penicillin G sodium	UP	20 million units	WC	500 mg	D5W	Physically compatible	15	C
Phenobarbital sodium	WI	200 mg	WC	500 mg	D5W	Physically compatible	15	C

Additive Compatibility (Cont.)

Test Drug	Mfr	Conc/L or %	Mfr	Conc/L or %	Test Solution	Remarks	Ref	C/I
Polymyxin B sulfate	BW	200 mg	WC	500 mg	D5W	Physically compatible	15	C
Ranitidine HCl	GL	50 mg and 2 g		1.5 g	D5W	Physically compatible. Ranitidine stable for 24 hr at 25°C. Colistimethate not tested	1515	C

Drugs in Syringe Compatibility

Colistimethate sodium

Test Drug	Mfr	Amt	Mfr	Amt	Remarks	Ref	C/I
Ampicillin sodium	AY	500 mg	PX	40 mg/2 mL	No precipitate or color change within 1 hr at room temperature	99	C
Ampicillin sodium	AY	500 mg	PX	500 mg/2 mL	Physically compatible for 1 hr at room temperature	300	C
Cloxacillin sodium	BE	250 mg	PX	40 mg/2 mL	No precipitate or color change within 1 hr at room temperature	99	C
Cloxacillin sodium	AY	250 mg	PX	500 mg/2 mL	Physically compatible for 1 hr at room temperature	300	C
Penicillin G sodium		1 million units	PX	40 mg/2 mL	No precipitate or color change within 1 hr at room temperature	99	C

Y-Site Injection Compatibility (1:1 Mixture)

Colistimethate sodium

Test Drug	Mfr	Conc	Mfr	Conc	Remarks	Ref	C/I
Ceftazidime	GSK	5 mg/mL[b]	MIL	1.5 mg/mL[b]	Visually compatible for 1 hr at 26°C	3335	C
Ceftazidime–avibactam sodium	ALL	20 mg/mL[i][k]	[l]		Physically compatible for up to 4 hr at room temperature	3004	C
Ceftolozane sulfate–tazobactam sodium	CUB	10 mg/mL[d][e]	APP	4.5 mg/mL[d]	Physically compatible for 2 hr	3262	C
Eravacycline dihydrochloride	TET	0.3 and 0.6 mg/mL[b]	FRK	4.5 mg/mL[b]	Measured turbidity inreased within 30 min	3532	I
Ertapenem sodium	MSD	5 mg/mL[b]	MIL	1.5 mg/mL[b]	Visually compatible for 1 hr at 26°C	3335	C
Imipenem–cilastatin sodium	MSD	5 mg/mL[b][f]	MIL	1.5 mg/mL[b]	Visually compatible for 1 hr at 26°C	3335	C
Isavuconazonium sulfate	ASP	1.5 mg/mL[d]	APP	4.5 mg/mL[d]	Measured turbidity increases immediately	3263	I
Linezolid	PF	2 mg/mL	MIL	1.5 mg/mL[b]	Visually compatible for 1 hr at 26°C	3335	C
Meropenem	ASZ	10 mg/mL[b]	MIL	1.5 mg/mL[b]	Visually compatible for 1 hr at 26°C	3335	C
Meropenem		50 mg/mL	SMX	75 mg/mL	Physically compatible for 4 hr at room temperature	3538	C
Meropenem–vaborbactam	TMC	8 mg/mL[b][i]	APP	4.5 mg/mL[b]	Physically compatible for 3 hr at 20 to 25°C	3380	C
Piperacillin sodium–tazobactam sodium	ASZ[h]	40 mg/mL[b][g]	MIL	1.5 mg/mL[b]	Visually compatible for 1 hr at 26°C	3335	C
Plazomicin sulfate	ACH	24 mg/mL[d]	PAR	4.5 mg/mL[d]	Physically compatible for 1 hr at 20 to 25°C	3432	C
Tedizolid phosphate	CUB	0.8 mg/mL[b]	APP	4.5 mg/mL[b]	Physically compatible for 2 hr	3244	C
Telavancin HCl	ASP	7.5 mg/mL[a]	PAD	4.5 mg/mL[a]	Visible turbidity formed	2830	I

Y-Site Injection Compatibility (1:1 Mixture) (Cont.)

Test Drug	Mfr	Conc	Mfr	Conc	Remarks	Ref	C/I
Telavancin HCl	ASP	7.5 mg/mL[b][c]	PAD	4.5 mg/mL[b][c]	Physically compatible for 2 hr	2830	C
Vancomycin HCl	SIA	10 mg/mL[b]	MIL	1.5 mg/mL[b]	Visually compatible for 1 hr at 26°C	3335	C

[a] Tested in dextrose 5%.

[b] Tested in sodium chloride 0.9%.

[c] Tested in Ringer's injection, lactated.

[d] Tested in both dextrose 5% and sodium chloride 0.9%.

[e] Ceftolozane component. Ceftolozane in a 2:1 fixed-ratio concentration with tazobactam.

[f] Imipenem component. Imipenem in a 1:1 fixed-ratio concentration with cilastatin.

[g] Piperacillin component. Piperacillin in an 8:1 fixed-ratio concentration with tazobactam.

[h] Presence or absence of edetate disodium not specified.

[i] Meropenem component. Meropenem in a 1:1 fixed-ratio concentration with vaborbactam.

[j] Ceftazidime component. Ceftazidime in a 4:1 fixed-ratio concentration with avibactam.

[k] Tested in dextrose 5%, sodium chloride 0.9%, and Ringer's injection, lactated.

[l] Salt not specified.

Selected Revisions May 1, 2020. © Copyright, October 1982.
American Society of Health-System Pharmacists, Inc.

Conivaptan Hydrochloride
AHFS 40:28.28

Products

Conivaptan hydrochloride is available as a single-use ready-to-use solution of 20 mg conivaptan hydrochloride in 100 mL dextrose 5% in a flexible plastic container.[2838] The solution also contains lactic acid for pH adjustment.[2838]

pH

The pH is adjusted to the range of 3.4 to 3.8.[2838]

Osmolality

The osmolality of conivaptan hydrochloride ready-to-use solution is within the range of 250 to 330 mOsm/kg.[2839]

Trade Name(s)

Vaprisol

Administration

Conivaptan hydrochloride in dextrose ready-to-use solution is administered only by intravenous infusion.[2838] No further dilution is required.[2838] A loading dose of conivaptan hydrochloride is administered over 30 minutes, followed by a continuous infusion.[2838] The drug should be administered through large veins with the infusion site changed every 24 hours to minimize the risk of vascular irritation.[2838]

Stability

Conivaptan hydrochloride ready-to-use solution should be stored at 25°C and protected from light, freezing, and excessive heat; however, brief exposure to temperatures up to 40°C was not noted to adversely affect the product.[2838] The plastic container should remain in its overwrap until ready for use.[2838]

Little to no change in stability of the ready-to-use product was noted when stored in its foil overwrap for up to 6 months at 40°C and 20% relative humidity.[2839] Out of its overwrap, the product was stable at 25°C and 40% relative humidity for up to 31 days.[2839] Storage of the product at 5°C resulted in long-term stability of up to 38 months.[2839]

Following administration, any remaining product should be discarded.[2838]

Compatibility Information

Solution Compatibility

Conivaptan HCl

Test Soln Name	Mfr	Mfr	Conc/L or %	Remarks	Ref	C/I
Dextrose 5%		BA		Stated to be compatible	2838	C
Sodium chloride 0.9%		BA		Physically and chemically compatible with Y-site administration for up to 48 hr at flow rates of 2:1 and 3:2 conivaptan HCl:sodium chloride 0.9%	2838	C
Ringer's injection, lactated		BA		Stated to be incompatible	2838	I

Additive Compatibility

Conivaptan HCl

Test Drug	Mfr	Conc/L or %	Mfr	Conc/L or %	Test Solution	Remarks	Ref	C/I
Furosemide			BA			Stated to be incompatible	2838	I

DOI: 10.37573/9781585286850.100

Cyanocobalamin
AHFS 88:08

Products

Cyanocobalamin is available in a concentration of 1 mg/mL with sodium chloride 0.9%, benzyl alcohol 1.5%, and sodium hydroxide and/or hydrochloric acid to adjust pH during manufacturing.[1(6/05)] [4]

pH

From 4.5 to 7.[1(6/05)]

Administration

Cyanocobalamin is administered by intramuscular or deep subcutaneous injection. The intravenous route is not recommended because the drug is excreted more rapidly and almost all of the cyanocobalamin is lost in the urine.[1(6/05)] [4]

Stability

The clear pink to red solutions are stable at room temperature and may be autoclaved at 121°C for short periods such as 15 to 20 minutes. Cyanocobalamin is light sensitive, so protection from light is recommended.[1(6/05)] [4] Exposure to light results in the organometallic bond being cleaved, with the extent of degradation generally increasing with increasing light intensity.[1072]

The vitamins in Cernevit (Baxter) diluted in three 2-in-1 parenteral nutrition admixtures were tested for stability over 48 hours. Most of the vitamins, including cyanocobalamin, retained their initial concentrations.[2796]

pH Effects

Cyanocobalamin is stable at pH 3 to 7 but is most stable at pH 4.5 to 5.[1072] It is stated to be incompatible with alkaline and strongly acidic solutions.[4]

Sorption

Cyanocobalamin (Organon) 30 mg/L did not display significant sorption to a PVC plastic test strip in 24 hours.[12]

Filtration

Cyanocobalamin (Wyeth) 1 mg/L in dextrose 5% and in sodium chloride 0.9% was filtered at a rate of 120 mL/hr for 6 hours through a 0.22-μm cellulose ester membrane filter (Ivex-2). No significant reduction in potency due to binding to the filter was noted.[533]

Compatibility Information

Solution Compatibility

Cyanocobalamin

Test Soln Name	Mfr	Mfr	Conc/L or %	Remarks	Ref	C/I
Dextrose 2.5% in half-strength Ringer's injection	AB	AB	1 mg	Physically compatible	3	C
Dextrose 5% in Ringer's injection	AB	AB	1 mg	Physically compatible	3	C
Dextrose 2.5% in Ringer's injection, lactated	AB	AB	1 mg	Physically compatible	3	C
Dextrose 5% in half-strength Ringer's injection, lactated	AB	AB	1 mg	Physically compatible	3	C
Dextrose 5% in Ringer's injection, lactated	AB	AB	1 mg	Physically compatible	3	C
Dextrose 10% in Ringer's injection, lactated	AB	AB	1 mg	Physically compatible	3	C
Dextrose 2.5% in sodium chloride 0.45%	AB	AB	1 mg	Physically compatible	3	C
Dextrose 2.5% in sodium chloride 0.9%	AB	AB	1 mg	Physically compatible	3	C
Dextrose 5% in sodium chloride 0.225%	AB	AB	1 mg	Physically compatible	3	C
Dextrose 5% in sodium chloride 0.45%	AB	AB	1 mg	Physically compatible	3	C
Dextrose 5% in sodium chloride 0.9%	AB	AB	1 mg	Physically compatible	3	C
Dextrose 10% in sodium chloride 0.9%	AB	AB	1 mg	Physically compatible	3	C
Dextrose 2.5%	AB	AB	1 mg	Physically compatible	3	C
Dextrose 5%	AB	AB	1 mg	Physically compatible	3	C

DOI: 10.37573/9781585286850.101

Solution Compatibility (Cont.)

Test Soln Name	Mfr	Mfr	Conc/L or %	Remarks	Ref	C/I
Dextrose 10%	AB	AB	1 mg	Physically compatible	3	C
Ionosol B in dextrose 5%	AB	AB	1 mg	Physically compatible	3	C
Ionosol MB in dextrose 5%	AB	AB	1 mg	Physically compatible	3	C
Ringer's injection	AB	AB	1 mg	Physically compatible	3	C
Ringer's injection, lactated	AB	AB	1 mg	Physically compatible	3	C
Sodium chloride 0.45%	AB	AB	1 mg	Physically compatible	3	C
Sodium chloride 0.9%	AB	AB	1 mg	Physically compatible	3	C
Sodium lactate ⅙ M	AB	AB	1 mg	Physically compatible	3	C

Additive Compatibility

Cyanocobalamin

Test Drug	Mfr	Conc/L or %	Mfr	Conc/L or %	Test Solution	Remarks	Ref	C/I
Ascorbic acid	AB	1 g	AB	1 mg		Physically compatible	3	C
Ascorbic acid						Stated to be incompatible	1729, 1736	I
Chloramphenicol sodium succinate	PD	1 g	AB	1 mg		Physically compatible	6	C

Y-Site Injection Compatibility (1:1 Mixture)

Cyanocobalamin

Test Drug	Mfr	Conc	Mfr	Conc	Remarks	Ref	C/I
Heparin sodium	UP	1000 units/L[a]	PD	0.1 mg/mL	Physically compatible for 4 hr at room temperature	534	C
Hydrocortisone sodium succinate	UP	10 mg/L[a]	PD	0.1 mg/mL	Physically compatible for 4 hr at room temperature	534	C
Potassium chloride	AB	40 mEq/L[a]	PD	0.1 mg/mL	Physically compatible for 4 hr at room temperature	534	C

[a] Tested in dextrose 5% in Ringer's injection, dextrose 5% in Ringer's injection, lactated, dextrose 5%, Ringer's injection, lactated, and sodium chloride 0.9%.

Selected Revisions September 29, 2017. © Copyright, October 1982. American Society of Health-System Pharmacists, Inc.

Cyclizine Lactate
AHFS 56:22.08

Products

Cyclizine lactate is available in 1-mL ampuls containing 50 mg of drug in water for injection.[38] [115]

pH

From 3.3 to 3.7.[176]

Trade Name(s)

Valoid

Administration

Cyclizine lactate is administered by intramuscular or intravenous injection. When administered intravenously, it should be injected slowly, with minimal withdrawal of blood in the syringe.[38] [115]

Stability

Cyclizine lactate injection, a colorless solution, should be stored below 25°C and protected from light.[38] [115]

Crystallization

Cyclizine lactate has an aqueous solubility of 8 mg/mL. When the drug was diluted to concentrations of 7.5 and 3.75 mg/mL in water or dextrose 5%, it remained in solution for at least 24 hours at 23°C. However, when these dilutions were made with sodium chloride 0.9%, crystals formed within 24 hours at 23°C.[1761]

Compatibility Information

Additive Compatibility

Cyclizine lactate

Test Drug	Mfr	Conc/L or %	Mfr	Conc/L or %	Test Solution	Remarks	Ref	C/I
Oxycodone HCl	NAP	1 g	GW	1 g	NS	Crystals form in a few hours	2600	I
Oxycodone HCl	NAP	1 g	GW	1 g	W	Visually compatible. Under 4% concentration change in 24 hr at 25°C	2600	C
Oxycodone HCl	NAP	1 g	GW	500 mg	NS	Crystals form in a few hours	2600	I
Oxycodone HCl	NAP	1 g	GW	500 mg	W	Visually compatible. Under 4% concentration change in 24 hr at 25°C	2600	C

Drugs in Syringe Compatibility

Cyclizine lactate

Test Drug	Mfr	Amt	Mfr	Amt	Remarks	Ref	C/I
Diamorphine HCl	MB	20, 50, 100 mg/1 mL	CA	5 mg/1 mLa	Physically compatible and diamorphine stable for 24 hr at room temperature	1454	C
Diamorphine HCl	EV	15 mg/1 mL	CA	15 mg/1 mL	Physically compatible for 24 hr at room temperature	1455	C
Diamorphine HCl	EV	37.5 to 150 mg/1 mL	CA	12.5 to 50 mg/1 mL	Precipitate forms within 24 hr	1455	I
Diamorphine HCl	HC	25 to 100 mg/mL	CA	10 mg/mL	Visually incompatible	1672	I
Diamorphine HCl	HC	20 mg/mL	CA	10 mg/mL	Visually compatible for 48 hr at 5 and 20°C	1672	C
Diamorphine HCl	HC	100 mg/mL	CA	6.7 mg/mL	Visually compatible for 48 hr at 5 and 20°C	1672	C
Diamorphine HCl	HC	2 mg/mL	CA	6.7 mg/mL	5% diamorphine loss in 9.9 days at 20°C. Cyclizine stable for 45 days	1672	C
Diamorphine HCl	HC	20 mg/mL	CA	6.7 mg/mL	5% diamorphine loss in 13.6 days at 20°C. Cyclizine stable for 45 days	1672	C

DOI: 10.37573/9781585286850.102

Drugs in Syringe Compatibility (Cont.)

Test Drug	Mfr	Amt	Mfr	Amt	Remarks	Ref	C/I
Diamorphine HCl	BP	6 mg/mL	WEL	51 mg/mL	Physically compatible. 10% diamorphine loss in 1.7 days. Little cyclizine loss at 23°C	2071	C
Diamorphine HCl	BP	9 mg/mL	WEL	32 mg/mL	Physically compatible. Under 10% diamorphine loss and little cyclizine loss in 4 days at 23°C	2071	C
Diamorphine HCl	BP	10 mg/mL	WEL	39 mg/mL	Physically compatible. Under 10% diamorphine loss and little cyclizine loss in 4 days at 23°C	2071	C
Diamorphine HCl	BP	10 mg/mL	WEL	28 mg/mL	Physically compatible. 10% diamorphine loss in 3.1 days and little cyclizine loss at 23°C	2071	C
Diamorphine HCl	BP	12 mg/mL	WEL	51 mg/mL	Physically compatible. 10% diamorphine loss in 2.2 days and little cyclizine loss at 23°C	2071	C
Diamorphine HCl	BP	14 mg/mL	WEL	40 mg/mL	Crystals form	2071	I
Diamorphine HCl	BP	17 mg/mL	WEL	26 mg/mL	Physically compatible. 10% diamorphine loss in 1.1 days and 10% cyclizine loss in 2.5 days at 23°C	2071	C
Diamorphine HCl	BP	18 mg/mL	WEL	52 mg/mL	Crystals form	2071	I
Diamorphine HCl	BP	20 mg/mL	WEL	10 mg/mL	Physically compatible. Under 10% diamorphine loss and little cyclizine loss in 7 days at 23°C	2071	C
Diamorphine HCl	BP	20 mg/mL	WEL	15 mg/mL	Physically compatible. Little diamorphine loss and 10% cyclizine loss in 0.5 days at 23°C	2071	I
Diamorphine HCl	BP	21 mg/mL	WEL	26 mg/mL	Physically compatible. 10% diamorphine loss in 4.9 days. 10% cyclizine loss in 3.2 days at 23°C	2071	C
Diamorphine HCl	BP	23 mg/mL	WEL	18 mg/mL	Physically compatible. Little diamorphine loss and 10% cyclizine loss in 3.2 days at 23°C	2071	C
Diamorphine HCl	BP	26 mg/mL	WEL	23 mg/mL	Physically compatible. 10% diamorphine loss in 1.9 days. 10% cyclizine loss in 9 hr at 23°C	2071	I
Diamorphine HCl	BP	30 mg/mL	WEL	30 mg/mL	Physically compatible. 10% diamorphine loss in 21 hr and 10% cyclizine loss in 9 hr at 23°C	2071	I
Diamorphine HCl	BP	49 mg/mL	WEL	10 mg/mL	Physically compatible. Little diamorphine loss and 10% cyclizine loss in 5.5 days at 23°C	2071	C
Diamorphine HCl	BP	51 mg/mL	WEL	4 mg/mL	Physically compatible. Little diamorphine or cyclizine loss in 7 days at 23°C	2071	C
Diamorphine HCl	BP	61 mg/mL	WEL	8 mg/mL	Physically compatible. 10% diamorphine loss in 1.4 days. 10% cyclizine loss in 1.1 days at 23°C	2071	C
Diamorphine HCl	BP	65 mg/mL	WEL	13 mg/mL	Physically compatible. 10% diamorphine loss in 1.6 days. 10% cyclizine loss in 12 hr at 23°C	2071	I
Diamorphine HCl	BP	92 mg/mL	WEL	10 mg/mL	Physically compatible. Little diamorphine loss and 10% cyclizine loss in 2.4 days at 23°C	2071	C
Diamorphine HCl	BP	99 mg/mL	WEL	4 mg/mL	Physically compatible. Little diamorphine or cyclizine loss in 7 days at 23°C	2071	C
Diamorphine HCl with haloperidol lactate	BP JC	11 mg/mL 2.2 mg/mL	WEL	16 mg/mL	Physically compatible with less than 10% loss of any drug in 7 days at 23°C	2071	C
Diamorphine HCl with haloperidol lactate	BP JC	16 mg/mL 2.2 mg/mL	WEL	25 mg/mL	Physically compatible with less than 10% loss of any drug in 7 days at 23°C	2071	C
Diamorphine HCl with haloperidol lactate	BP JC	40 mg/mL 2.2 mg/mL	WEL	11 mg/mL	Physically compatible with less than 10% loss of any drug in 7 days at 23°C	2071	C

Drugs in Syringe Compatibility (Cont.)

Test Drug	Mfr	Amt	Mfr	Amt	Remarks	Ref	C/I
Diamorphine HCl with haloperidol lactate	BP JC	42 mg/mL 2.1 mg/mL	WEL	13 mg/mL	Physically compatible with less than 10% loss of any drug in 7 days at 23°C	2071	C
Diamorphine HCl with haloperidol lactate	BP JC	55 mg/mL 2.1 mg/mL	WEL	9 mg/mL	Physically compatible with less than 10% loss of any drug in 7 days at 23°C	2071	C
Diamorphine HCl with haloperidol lactate	BP JC	56 mg/mL 2.1 mg/mL	WEL	13 mg/mL	Physically compatible with less than 10% loss of any drug in 7 days at 23°C	2071	C
Haloperidol lactate	SE	1.5 mg/0.3 mL	WEL	150 mg/3 mL	Diluted with 17 mL of NS. Crystals of cyclizine form within 24 hr at 25°C	1761	I
Haloperidol lactate	SE	1.5 mg/0.3 mL	WEL	150 mg/3 mL	Diluted with 17 mL of D5W or W. Visually compatible for 24 hr at 25°C	1761	C
Haloperidol lactate with diamorphine HCl	JC BP	2.2 mg/mL 11 mg/mL	WEL	16 mg/mL	Physically compatible with less than 10% loss of any drug in 7 days at 23°C	2071	C
Haloperidol lactate with diamorphine HCl	JC BP	2.2 mg/mL 16 mg/mL	WEL	25 mg/mL	Physically compatible with less than 10% loss of any drug in 7 days at 23°C	2071	C
Haloperidol lactate with diamorphine HCl	JC BP	2.2 mg/mL 40 mg/mL	WEL	11 mg/mL	Physically compatible with less than 10% loss of any drug in 7 days at 23°C	2071	C
Haloperidol lactate with diamorphine HCl	JC BP	2.1 mg/mL 42 mg/mL	WEL	13 mg/mL	Physically compatible with less than 10% loss of any drug in 7 days at 23°C	2071	C
Haloperidol lactate with diamorphine HCl	JC BP	2.1 mg/mL 55 mg/mL	WEL	9 mg/mL	Physically compatible with less than 10% loss of any drug in 7 days at 23°C	2071	C
Haloperidol lactate with diamorphine HCl	JC BP	2.1 mg/mL 56 mg/mL	WEL	13 mg/mL	Physically compatible with less than 10% loss of any drug in 7 days at 23°C	2071	C
Ketorolac tromethamine	RC	30 mg/mL	WEL	50 mg/mL	White precipitate forms	2495	I
Oxycodone HCl	NAP	200 mg/20 mL	GW	150 mg/3 mL	Crystals form in 5 hr	2600	I
Oxycodone HCl	NAP	70 mg/7 mL	GW	50 mg/1 mL	Crystals form in 5 hr	2600	I
Oxycodone HCl	NAP	100 mg/10 mL	GW	50 mg/1 mL	Visually compatible. Under 4% concentration change in 24 hr at 25°C	2600	C
Oxycodone HCl	NAP	150 mg/15 mL	GW	50 mg/1 mL	Visually compatible. Under 4% concentration change in 24 hr at 25°C	2600	C
Oxycodone HCl	NAP	200 mg/20 mL	GW	50 mg/1 mL	Visually compatible. Under 4% concentration change in 24 hr at 25°C	2600	C
Oxycodone HCl	NAP	200 mg/20 mL	GW	100 mg/2 mL	Visually compatible. Under 4% concentration change in 24 hr at 25°C	2600	C
Ranitidine HCl	GL	50 mg/2 mL	CA	50 mg/1 mL	Physically compatible for 1 hr at 25°C	978	C

[a] Diluted with sterile water for injection.

Selected Revisions October 1, 2012. © Copyright, October 1988.
American Society of Health-System Pharmacists, Inc.

Cyclophosphamide
AHFS 10:00

Products

Cyclophosphamide is available as a dry powder in vials containing cyclophosphamide monohydrate equivalent to 500 mg, 1 g, or 2 g of cyclophosphamide.[2962] Reconstitute each vial with 25, 50, or 100 mL, respectively, of sodium chloride 0.9%.[2962] Sterile water for injection also may be used for reconstitution, but *only* if the dose is to be administered by intravenous infusion, in which case the reconstituted solution must be further diluted with a compatible intravenous infusion solution.[2962] Gently swirl the vials to dissolve the powder, yielding a solution containing cyclophosphamide 20 mg/mL.[2962]

pH

A 22-mg/mL solution was found to have a pH of 6.87.[126]

Administration

Cyclophosphamide reconstituted with sodium chloride 0.9% may be administered by direct intravenous injection or by intravenous infusion.[2962]

Cyclophosphamide reconstituted with sterile water for injection is very hypotonic and is *not* suitable for direct intravenous injection.[2962]

For intravenous infusion, the reconstituted solution must be further diluted in a compatible intravenous infusion solution.[2962]

Stability

Vials containing cyclophosphamide powder should be stored at or below 25°C.[2962] Vials contain no preservatives and are for single use.[2962]

Do not use vials that show signs of cyclophosphamide melting (e.g., clear or yellowish viscous liquid as a connected phase or in droplets).[2962]

Visually inspect the solution for particulate matter and discoloration prior to administration.[2962] If not used immediately, solutions formed by reconstituting the dry powder with sodium chloride 0.9% may be stored for up to 24 hours at room temperature or up to 6 days under refrigeration.[2962] Solutions formed by reconstituting the dry powder with sterile water for injection should be further diluted for intravenous infusion immediately; do not store.[2962]

Total time (from reconstitution through administration) for solutions that are further diluted with dextrose 5% or dextrose 5% in sodium chloride 0.9% should not exceed 24 hours if stored at room temperature or 36 hours if stored under refrigeration; total time for solutions further diluted with sodium chloride 0.45% should not exceed 24 hours at room temperature or 6 days under refrigeration.[2962]

When reconstituted with sterile water for injection or paraben-preserved bacteriostatic water for injection to a concentration of 21 mg/mL, less than 1.5% cyclophosphamide decomposition occurred within 8 hours at 24 to 27°C and within 6 days at 5°C. The rate constant for decomposition of cyclophosphamide when reconstituted with benzyl alcohol-preserved bacteriostatic water for injection was significantly higher than with sterile water for injection. It was suggested that benzyl alcohol may catalyze the decomposition of cyclophosphamide.[125]

The stability of cyclophosphamide 20 mg/mL, reconstituted with sterile water for injection and stored in various containers at several temperatures, was evaluated. In glass ampuls at 20 to 23°C, approximately 13 and 35% were lost in 1 and 4 weeks, respectively. Under refrigeration at 4°C or frozen at −20°C, the solution lost not more than 3% over 4 weeks.[1090]

Cyclophosphamide (Bristol-Myers Squibb) reconstituted with sterile water for injection to a concentration of 20 mg/mL was found to undergo about 10% degradation in 4 days at 25°C. When the solutions were stored under refrigeration at 5°C, approximately 6% loss occurred in 52 days and 10 to 12% loss occurred in 119 days.[2255]

Immersion of a needle with an aluminum component in cyclophosphamide (Adria) 20 mg/mL resulted in a slight darkening of the aluminum and gas production after a few days at 24°C with protection from light.[988]

pH Effects

Cyclophosphamide exhibits maximum solution stability over the range of 2 to 10; the rate of decomposition is essentially the same over this broad pH range.[1369] At pH values less than 2 and above 11, increased rates of decomposition have been observed.[1369] [2002]

Syringes

In polypropylene syringes (Plastipak, Becton Dickinson) sealed with blind Luer locking hubs, the 20-mg/mL cyclophosphamide solution lost about 3% in 4 weeks at 4°C and about 10% in 11 to 14 weeks. When frozen at −20°C (with microwave thawing), the solution lost about 4% in 19 weeks. However, the syringe plungers contracted markedly during freezing, resulting in drug solution seeping past the plunger onto the inner surface of the barrel. This seeping poses the risk of bacterial contamination. Furthermore, cyclophosphamide precipitated during microwave thawing and required vigorous shaking for 5 minutes to redissolve. This precipitation during thawing appears not to occur at concentrations less than 8 mg/mL.[1090]

Central Venous Catheter

Cyclophosphamide (Mead Johnson) 2 mg/mL in dextrose 5% was found to be compatible with the ARROWg+ard Blue Plus (Arrow International) chlorhexidine-bearing triple-lumen central catheter. Essentially complete delivery of the drug was found with little or no drug loss occurring. Furthermore, chlorhexidine delivered from the catheter remained at trace amounts with no substantial increase due to the delivery of the drug through the catheter.[2335]

DOI: 10.37573/9781585286850.103

Compatibility Information

Solution Compatibility

Cyclophosphamide

Test Soln Name	Mfr	Mfr	Conc/L or %	Remarks	Ref	C/I
Amino acids 4.25%, dextrose 25%	MG	MJ	500 mg	No increase in particulate matter in 24 hr at 5°C	349	C
Dextrose 5% in sodium chloride 0.9%				Stable up to 24 hr at room temperature or 36 hr under refrigeration	2962	C
Dextrose 5% in sodium chloride 0.9%	CU	MJ	100 mg	1.5% loss in 8 hr at 27°C and 6 days at 5°C	125	C
Dextrose 5% in sodium chloride 0.9%	CU	MJ	3.1 g	1.5% loss in 8 hr at 27°C and 6 days at 5°C	125	C
Dextrose 5%				Stable up to 24 hr at room temperature or 36 hr under refrigeration	2962	C
Dextrose 5%	CU	MJ	100 mg	1.5% loss in 8 hr at 27°C and 6 days at 5°C	125	C
Dextrose 5%	CU	MJ	3.1 g	1.5% loss in 8 hr at 27°C and 6 days at 5°C	125	C
Dextrose 5%	TR[a]	MJ	6.6 g	Less than 10% loss in 24 hr at room temperature	519	C
Dextrose 5%	MG, TR[b]		6.7 g	Less than 10% loss in 24 hr at room temperature exposed to light	1658	C
Sodium chloride 0.45%				Stable up to 24 hr at room temperature or 6 days under refrigeration	2962	C
Sodium chloride 0.9%		MJ	4 g	3.5% loss in 24 hr at room temperature	127	C
Sodium chloride 0.9%		MJ	4 g	1% loss in 4 weeks under refrigeration	127	C
Sodium chloride 0.9%	TR	CE	4 g[c]	Physically compatible with no loss in 4 weeks and 8% in 19 weeks at 4 and −20°C	1090	C
Sodium chloride 0.9%		BMS	400 mg	8% loss in 6 days at 23°C. Less than 2% loss in 14 days at 4°C	2255	C

[a] Tested in both glass and PVC containers.

[b] Tested in glass, PVC, and polyolefin containers.

[c] Tested in PVC containers.

Additive Compatibility

Cyclophosphamide

Test Drug	Mfr	Conc/L or %	Mfr	Conc/L or %	Test Solution	Remarks	Ref	C/I
Cisplatin with etoposide		200 mg 200 mg		2 g	NS	All drugs stable for 7 days at room temperature	1379	C
Etoposide with cisplatin		200 mg 200 mg		2 g	NS	All drugs stable for 7 days at room temperature	1379	C
Fluorouracil		8.3 g		1.67 g	NS	Both drugs stable for 14 days at room temperature	1389	C
Fluorouracil with methotrexate sodium		8.3 g 25 mg		1.67 g	NS	9.3% cyclophosphamide loss in 7 days at room temperature. No loss of other drugs observed	1389	C
Hydroxyzine HCl	LY	500 mg	AD	1 g	D5W[a]	Physically compatible for 48 hr	1190	C

Additive Compatibility (Cont.)

Test Drug	Mfr	Conc/L or %	Mfr	Conc/L or %	Test Solution	Remarks	Ref	C/I
Mesna	AM	3.2 g	AM	10.8 g	D5W	Physically compatible with about 5% loss of both drugs in 24 hr at 22°C. 7% cyclophosphamide loss and 10% mesna loss occurred in 72 hr at 4°C	2486	C
Mesna	AM	540 mg	AM	1.8 g	D5W	Physically compatible with about 10% loss of both drugs in 12 hr at 22°C	2486	I
Mesna	AM	540 mg	AM	1.8 g	D5W	Physically compatible with about 9% loss of both drugs in 72 hr at 4°C	2486	C
Methotrexate sodium		25 mg		1.67 g	NS	6.6% cyclophosphamide loss in 14 days at room temperature	1379, 1389	C
Methotrexate sodium with fluorouracil		25 mg 8.3 g		1.67 g	NS	9.3% cyclophosphamide loss in 7 days at room temperature. No loss of other drugs observed	1389	C
Mitoxantrone HCl	LE	500 mg	AD	10 g	D5W	Visually compatible. Mitoxantrone stable for 24 hr at room temperature. Cyclophosphamide not tested	1531	C
Ondansetron HCl	GL	50 mg	MJ	300 mg	D5W[b], NS[b]	Visually compatible with 9 to 10% cyclophosphamide loss and no ondansetron loss in 5 days at 24°C. No loss of either drug in 8 days at 4°C	1812	C
Ondansetron HCl	GL	400 mg	MJ	2 g	D5W[b], NS[b]	Visually compatible with 10% cyclophosphamide loss and no ondansetron loss in 5 days at 24°C. No loss of either drug in 8 days at 4°C	1812	C

[a] Tested in glass containers.

[b] Tested in PVC containers.

Drugs in Syringe Compatibility

Cyclophosphamide

Test Drug	Mfr	Amt	Mfr	Amt	Remarks	Ref	C/I
Bleomycin sulfate		1.5 units/0.5 mL		10 mg/0.5 mL	Physically compatible for 5 min at room temperature followed by 8 min of centrifugation	980	C
Cisplatin		0.5 mg/0.5 mL		10 mg/0.5 mL	Physically compatible for 5 min at room temperature followed by 8 min of centrifugation	980	C
Doxapram HCl	RB	400 mg/20 mL		100 mg/5 mL	Physically compatible with 2% doxapram loss in 24 hr	1177	C
Doxorubicin HCl		1 mg/0.5 mL		10 mg/0.5 mL	Physically compatible for 5 min at room temperature followed by 8 min of centrifugation	980	C
Droperidol		1.25 mg/0.5 mL		10 mg/0.5 mL	Physically compatible for 5 min at room temperature followed by 8 min of centrifugation	980	C
Fluorouracil		25 mg/0.5 mL		10 mg/0.5 mL	Physically compatible for 5 min at room temperature followed by 8 min of centrifugation	980	C
Furosemide		5 mg/0.5 mL		10 mg/0.5 mL	Physically compatible for 5 min at room temperature followed by 8 min of centrifugation	980	C
Heparin sodium		500 units/0.5 mL		10 mg/0.5 mL	Physically compatible for 5 min at room temperature followed by 8 min of centrifugation	980	C
Leucovorin calcium		5 mg/0.5 mL		10 mg/0.5 mL	Physically compatible for 5 min at room temperature followed by 8 min of centrifugation	980	C
Methotrexate sodium		12.5 mg/0.5 mL		10 mg/0.5 mL	Physically compatible for 5 min at room temperature followed by 8 min of centrifugation	980	C

Drugs in Syringe Compatibility (Cont.)

Test Drug	Mfr	Amt	Mfr	Amt	Remarks	Ref	C/I
Metoclopramide HCl		2.5 mg/0.5 mL		10 mg/0.5 mL	Physically compatible for 5 min at room temperature followed by 8 min of centrifugation	980	C
Metoclopramide HCl	RB	10 mg/2 mL	MJ	40 mg/2 mL	Physically compatible for 24 hr at 25°C	1167	C
Metoclopramide HCl	RB	10 mg/2 mL	MJ	1 g/50 mL	Physically compatible for 24 hr at 25°C	1167	C
Metoclopramide HCl	RB	160 mg/32 mL	MJ	1 g/50 mL	Physically compatible for 24 hr at 25°C	1167	C
Mitomycin		0.25 mg/0.5 mL		10 mg/0.5 mL	Physically compatible for 5 min at room temperature followed by 8 min of centrifugation	980	C
Vinblastine sulfate		0.5 mg/0.5 mL		10 mg/0.5 mL	Physically compatible for 5 min at room temperature followed by 8 min of centrifugation	980	C
Vincristine sulfate		0.5 mg/0.5 mL		10 mg/0.5 mL	Physically compatible for 5 min at room temperature followed by 8 min of centrifugation	980	C

Y-Site Injection Compatibility (1:1 Mixture)

Cyclophosphamide

Test Drug	Mfr	Conc	Mfr	Conc	Remarks	Ref	C/I
Allopurinol sodium	BW	3 mg/mL[b]	MJ	10 mg/mL[b]	Physically compatible for 4 hr at 22°C	1686	C
Amifostine	USB	10 mg/mL[a]	MJ	10 mg/mL[a]	Physically compatible for 4 hr at 23°C	1845	C
Amikacin sulfate	BR	5 mg/mL[a]	MJ	20 mg/mL[a]	Physically compatible for 4 hr at 25°C	1194	C
Ampicillin sodium	BR	20 mg/mL[b]	MJ	20 mg/mL[a]	Physically compatible for 4 hr at 25°C	1194	C
Anidulafungin	VIC	0.5 mg/mL[a]	MJ	10 mg/mL[a]	Physically compatible for 4 hr at 23°C	2617	C
Aztreonam	SQ	40 mg/mL[a]	MJ	10 mg/mL[a]	Physically compatible for 4 hr at 23°C	1758	C
Bleomycin sulfate		3 units/mL		20 mg/mL	Drugs injected sequentially in Y-site with no flush. No precipitate seen	980	C
Cefazolin sodium	SKF	20 mg/mL[a]	MJ	20 mg/mL[a]	Physically compatible for 4 hr at 25°C	1194	C
Cefotaxime sodium	HO	20 mg/mL[a]	MJ	20 mg/mL[a]	Physically compatible for 4 hr at 25°C	1194	C
Cefoxitin sodium	MSD	20 mg/mL[a]	MJ	20 mg/mL[a]	Physically compatible for 4 hr at 25°C	1194	C
Cefuroxime sodium	GL	30 mg/mL[a]	MJ	20 mg/mL[a]	Physically compatible for 4 hr at 25°C	1194	C
Chloramphenicol sodium succinate	ES	20 mg/mL[a]	MJ	20 mg/mL[a]	Physically compatible for 4 hr at 25°C	1194	C
Cisplatin		1 mg/mL		20 mg/mL	Drugs injected sequentially in Y-site with no flush. No precipitate seen	980	C
Cladribine	ORT	0.015[b] and 0.5[c] mg/mL	MJ	10 mg/mL[b]	Physically compatible for 4 hr at 23°C	1969	C
Clindamycin phosphate	UP	12 mg/mL[a]	MJ	20 mg/mL[a]	Physically compatible for 4 hr at 25°C	1194	C
Doripenem	JJ	5 mg/mL[a][b]	BMS	10 mg/mL[a][b]	Physically compatible for 4 hr at 23°C	2743	C
Doxorubicin HCl		2 mg/mL		20 mg/mL	Drugs injected sequentially in Y-site with no flush. No precipitate seen	980	C
Doxorubicin HCl liposomal	SEQ	0.4 mg/mL[a]	MJ	10 mg/mL[a]	Physically compatible for 4 hr at 23°C	2087	C

Y-Site Injection Compatibility (1:1 Mixture) (Cont.)

Test Drug	Mfr	Conc	Mfr	Conc	Remarks	Ref	C/I
Doxycycline hyclate	ES	1 mg/mL[a]	MJ	20 mg/mL[a]	Physically compatible for 4 hr at 25°C	1194	C
Droperidol		2.5 mg/mL		20 mg/mL	Drugs injected sequentially in Y-site with no flush. No precipitate seen	980	C
Erythromycin lactobionate	AB	5 mg/mL[a]	MJ	20 mg/mL[a]	Physically compatible for 4 hr at 25°C	1194	C
Etoposide phosphate	BR	5 mg/mL[a]	MJ	10 mg/mL[a]	Physically compatible for 4 hr at 23°C	2218	C
Filgrastim	AMG	30 mcg/mL[a]	MJ	10 mg/mL[a]	Physically compatible for 4 hr at 22°C	1687	C
Fludarabine phosphate	BX	1 mg/mL[a]	MJ	10 mg/mL[a]	Visually compatible for 4 hr at 22°C	1439	C
Fluorouracil		50 mg/mL		20 mg/mL	Drugs injected sequentially in Y-site with no flush. No precipitate seen	980	C
Furosemide		10 mg/mL		20 mg/mL	Drugs injected sequentially in Y-site with no flush. No precipitate seen	980	C
Gallium nitrate	FUJ	1 mg/mL[b]	MJ	20 mg/mL	Visually compatible for 24 hr at 25°C	1673	C
Gemcitabine HCl	LI	10 mg/mL[b]	BR	10 mg/mL[b]	Physically compatible for 4 hr at 23°C	2226	C
Gentamicin sulfate	TR	1.6 mg/mL[a]	MJ	20 mg/mL[a]	Physically compatible for 4 hr at 25°C	1194	C
Granisetron HCl	SKB	1 mg/mL	MJ	2 mg/mL[b]	Physically compatible with little loss of either drug in 4 hr at 22°C	1883	C
Heparin sodium		1000 units/mL		20 mg/mL	Drugs injected sequentially in Y-site with no flush. No precipitate seen	980	C
Idarubicin HCl	AD	1 mg/mL[b]	AD	4 mg/mL[a]	Visually compatible for 24 hr at 25°C	1525	C
Leucovorin calcium		10 mg/mL		20 mg/mL	Drugs injected sequentially in Y-site with no flush. No precipitate seen	980	C
Linezolid	PHU	2 mg/mL	MJ	10 mg/mL[a]	Physically compatible for 4 hr at 23°C	2264	C
Melphalan HCl	BW	0.1 mg/mL[b]	BR	10 mg/mL[b]	Physically compatible for 3 hr at 22°C	1557	C
Methotrexate sodium		25 mg/mL		20 mg/mL	Drugs injected sequentially in Y-site with no flush. No precipitate seen	980	C
Methotrexate sodium		30 mg/mL		20 mg/mL[a]	Visually compatible for 4 hr at room temperature	1788	C
Metoclopramide HCl		5 mg/mL		20 mg/mL	Drugs injected sequentially in Y-site with no flush. No precipitate seen	980	C
Metronidazole	SE	5 mg/mL	MJ	20 mg/mL[a]	Physically compatible for 4 hr at 25°C	1194	C
Mitomycin		0.5 mg/mL		20 mg/mL	Drugs injected sequentially in Y-site with no flush. No precipitate seen	980	C
Nafcillin sodium	WY	20 mg/mL[a]	MJ	20 mg/mL[a]	Physically compatible for 4 hr at 25°C	1194	C
Ondansetron HCl	GL	1 mg/mL[b]	MJ	10 mg/mL[a]	Visually compatible for 4 hr at 22°C	1365	C
Ondansetron HCl	GL	16 to 160 mcg/mL		20 mg/mL	Physically compatible when cyclophospha-mide given as 5-min bolus via Y-site	1366	C
Oxacillin sodium	BE	20 mg/mL[a]	MJ	20 mg/mL[a]	Physically compatible for 4 hr at 25°C	1194	C
Oxaliplatin	SS	0.5 mg/mL[a]	MJ	10 mg/mL[a]	Physically compatible for 4 hr at 23°C	2566	C
Paclitaxel	NCI	1.2 mg/mL[a]		10 mg/mL[a]	Physically compatible for 4 hr at 22°C	1528	C
Palonosetron HCl	MGI	50 mcg/mL	MJ	10 mg/mL[a]	Physically compatible and no loss of either drug in 4 hr	2640	C

Y-Site Injection Compatibility (1:1 Mixture) (Cont.)

Test Drug	Mfr	Conc	Mfr	Conc	Remarks	Ref	C/I
Pemetrexed disodium	LI	20 mg/mL[b]	MJ	10 mg/mL[a]	Physically compatible for 4 hr at 23°C	2564	C
Penicillin G potassium	PF	100,000 units/mL[a]	MJ	20 mg/mL[a]	Physically compatible for 4 hr at 25°C	1194	C
Piperacillin sodium–tazo-bactam sodium	LE[f]	40 mg/mL[a g]	MJ	10 mg/mL[a]	Physically compatible for 4 hr at 22°C	1688	C
Propofol	ZEN[i]	10 mg/mL	MJ	10 mg/mL[a]	Physically compatible for 1 hr at 23°C	2066	C
Sargramostim	IMM	10 mcg/mL[b]	MJ	10 mg/mL[b]	Visually compatible for 4 hr at 22°C	1436	C
Sodium bicarbonate		1.4%		20 mg/mL[a]	Visually compatible for 4 hr at room temperature	1788	C
Teniposide	BR	0.1 mg/mL[a]	MJ	10 mg/mL[a]	Physically compatible for 4 hr at 23°C	1725	C
Thiotepa	IMM[d]	1 mg/mL[a]	MJ	10 mg/mL[a]	Physically compatible for 4 hr at 23°C	1861	C
TNA #218 to #226[e]			MJ	10 mg/mL[a]	Visually compatible for 4 hr at 23°C	2215	C
Tobramycin sulfate	DI	0.8 mg/mL[a]	MJ	20 mg/mL[a]	Physically compatible for 4 hr at 25°C	1194	C
Topotecan HCl	SKB	56 mcg/mL[a b]	MJ	20 mg/mL	Visually compatible. Little loss of either drug in 4 hr at 22°C	2245	C
TPN #212 to #215[e]			MJ	10 mg/mL[a]	Physically compatible for 4 hr at 23°C	2109	C
Trimethoprim–sulfame-thoxazole	BW	0.8 mg/mL[a h]	MJ	20 mg/mL[a]	Physically compatible for 4 hr at 25°C	1194	C
Vancomycin HCl	LI	5 mg/mL[a]	MJ	20 mg/mL[a]	Physically compatible for 4 hr at 25°C	1194	C
Vinblastine sulfate		1 mg/mL		20 mg/mL	Drugs injected sequentially in Y-site with no flush. No precipitate seen	980	C
Vincristine sulfate		1 mg/mL		20 mg/mL	Drugs injected sequentially in Y-site with no flush. No precipitate seen	980	C
Vinorelbine tartrate	BW	1 mg/mL[b]	MJ	10 mg/mL[b]	Physically compatible for 4 hr at 22°C	1558	C

[a] Tested in dextrose 5%.

[b] Tested in sodium chloride 0.9%.

[c] Tested in bacteriostatic sodium chloride 0.9% preserved with benzyl alcohol 0.9%.

[d] Lyophilized formulation tested.

[e] Refer to Appendix for the composition of parenteral nutrition solutions. TNA indicates a 3-in-1 admixture, and TPN indicates a 2-in-1 admixture.

[f] Test performed using the formulation WITHOUT edetate disodium.

[g] Piperacillin component. Piperacillin in an 8:1 fixed-ratio concentration with tazobactam.

[h] Trimethoprim component. Trimethoprim in a 1:5 fixed-ratio concentration with sulfamethoxazole.

[i] Test performed using the formulation WITH edetate disodium.

Selected Revisions July 1, 2020. © Copyright, October 1982.
American Society of Health-System Pharmacists, Inc.

Cyclosporine

AHFS 92:44

Products

Cyclosporine is available as a concentrate in 5-mL ampuls.[2929] Each mL of the solution contains cyclosporine 50 mg, polyoxyethylated castor oil (Cremophor EL) 650 mg, and alcohol 278 mg (32.9%).[874 2929 2930]

Cyclosporine concentrate must be diluted prior to administration.[874 2929]

Trade Name(s)

Sandimmune

Administration

Cyclosporine concentrate for injection is administered over 2 to 6 hours by intravenous infusion only after dilution.[2929] Each mL of concentrate should be diluted in 20 to 100 mL of dextrose 5% or sodium chloride 0.9%.[2929]

Stability

Intact ampuls of cyclosporine concentrate should be stored below 30°C and protected from light.[874 2929] Light protection is not required for intravenous admixtures of cyclosporine.[4 1091] The manufacturer recommends that cyclosporine diluted for infusion be discarded after 24 hours.[2929]

Syringes

The stability of cyclosporine (Novartis) after dilution to a concentration of 0.2 or 2.5 mg/mL in dextrose 5% or sodium chloride 0.9% and packaged as 60 mL in 60-mL polypropylene syringes (Becton Dickinson) was evaluated at room temperature.[2930] Although no physical changes were detected by visual inspection and chemical stability of cyclosporine did not appear to be affected, HPLC analysis revealed the development of an impurity after 1 day that substantially increased until termination of the study after 7 days.[2930] This impurity was not detected in similar samples of cyclosporine that were stored in polypropylene-polyolefin bags.[2930] The authors suggested that the diluted cyclosporine solution could have leached an ingredient used in the manufacture of the black rubber component of the syringe plunger.[2930]

Because such syringes are commonly used to transfer cyclosporine during preparation of IV solutions, an additional shorter test was conducted using 0.4 or 1 mL of undiluted cyclosporine concentrate 50 mg/mL in 1- or 5-mL polypropylene syringes.[2930] The suspected leached component from the black rubber portion of the syringe plunger was not detected within the 10-minute study period.[2930] Therefore, such short-term use of these syringes was considered appropriate provided the period of contact with the drug was less than 10 minutes.[2930]

Sorption

Simulated infusion studies of cyclosporine (Sandoz) 2 mg/mL in dextrose 5% and sodium chloride 0.9% were performed at a rate of 0.67 mL/minute over 75 minutes through 70-inch microdrip administration sets (Abbott). Significant amounts of cyclosporine were lost, presumably as a result of sorption to the tubing. Approximately 7% of the dose was lost from the dextrose 5% admixture, and about 13% was lost from the sodium chloride 0.9% admixture. The authors noted that as much as 30% of a pediatric dose could be lost.[1091]

In contrast, no significant cyclosporine loss occurred when 2.38 and 0.495 mg/mL in dextrose 5% and sodium chloride 0.9%, in either glass or polyvinyl chloride (PVC) containers, were delivered over 6 hours by an electronic infusion pump.[1154]

Cyclosporine 0.495 mg/mL in sodium chloride 0.9%, dextrose 5%, maltose 10%, and an electrolyte maintenance solution exhibited loss of delivered cyclosporine due to sorption when run through PVC administration tubing. The delivered cyclosporine concentrations were reduced to about 70% during the first 2 to 4 hours but rose to over 90% after 8 to 24 hours. The extent of sorption was somewhat higher in the electrolyte solutions compared with the sugar solutions. No loss occurred when the cyclosporine solutions were run through polybutadiene administration tubing.[2443]

Stability of cyclosporine 0.2 or 2.5 mg/mL diluted in dextrose 5% or sodium chloride 0.9% in ethylene vinyl acetate (EVA) containers was evaluated at 25°C.[2931] The 2.5-mg/mL solution appeared to be stable for at least 2 weeks under the study conditions.[2931] However, drug concentrations in the 0.2-mg/mL solution decreased to less than 90% within the 2-week study period.[2931] The authors concluded that the absence of impurities detected within this study period combined with the drug loss suggest sorption to the EVA container as the cause for such decreases.[2931]

Plasticizer Leaching

Polyoxyethylated castor oil (Cremophor EL), a nonionic surfactant, may leach phthalate from PVC containers such as bags of infusion solutions.[4 2929] In 1996, an acceptability limit of no more than 5 parts per million (5 mcg/mL) for diethylhexyl phthalate (DEHP) plasticizer leached from PVC-containing devices (e.g., containers, administration sets, other equipment) was proposed based on a review of metabolic and toxicologic considerations.[2185] FDA later evaluated the safety of DEHP exposure by comparing doses of DEHP received by patients undergoing various medical procedures with a defined tolerable intake value of DEHP, a value that was based upon the results of selected critical toxicity studies in experimental animals.[3100] Based on the results of the safety assessment, FDA concluded that there is little risk posed by exposure to the amount of DEHP released from PVC bags used to store and administer drugs that require an excipient for solubilization *when label instructions for preparation and administration are followed*.[3100] However, such conclusions do not take into account increased risk for adverse effects from DEHP exposure in certain patients (e.g., critically ill male neonates or infants, male infants less than 1 year of age, male

DOI: 10.37573/9781585286850.104

offspring of pregnant or breast-feeding women undergoing certain medical treatments) or potential adverse effects related to aggregate exposure for patients exposed to multiple medical devices, procedures, or intravenous medications known to leach DEHP, for which there are varying levels of concern.[3100] [3101]

Cyclosporine (Sandoz) 3 mg/mL in dextrose 5% leached relatively large amounts of DEHP plasticizer from PVC bags. This leaching was due to the surfactant Cremophor EL in the formulation. After 4 hours at 24°C, the DEHP concentration in 50-mL bags of infusion solution was as much as 13 mcg/mL and it increased through 24 hours to 104 mcg/mL. This finding is consistent with the high surfactant concentration (3.9%) in the final admixture solution. The actual amount of DEHP leached from PVC containers and administration sets may vary in clinical situations, depending on surfactant concentration, bag size, and contact time. Non-PVC containers and administration sets should be used to administer cyclosporine solutions.[1683]

Storage of cyclosporine (Sandoz) 3 mg/mL in dextrose 5% in PVC bags at 24°C was shown to cause leaching of significant amounts of DEHP due to the vehicle containing Cremophor EL and alcohol. Use of glass containers and tubing that does not contain DEHP to administer cyclosporine was recommended.[1092]

Cyclosporine 0.495 mg/mL in sodium chloride 0.9%, dextrose 5%, maltose 10%, and an electrolyte maintenance solution leached relatively large amounts of DEHP plasticizer when run through PVC administration tubing. The bulk of the leaching occurred during the first 4 hours but reached a plateau after 8 hours. About 94 mcg/mL was delivered over 12 hours in the saline solution. The cyclosporine admixtures in electrolyte solutions leached a greater amount of DEHP than those prepared in sugar-containing solutions.[2443]

Filtration

Use of either a 0.22- or 0.45-μm filter reduced the delivered cyclosporine concentration from 2.38- and 0.495-mg/mL solutions in dextrose 5% and sodium chloride 0.9%. A significant (but unspecified) decrease was found in the first sample, taken at 1 minute. At the 6-hour time point, the concentration had returned to the original concentration. The total amount of drug delivered over 6 hours was not quantified.[1154]

Compatibility Information

Solution Compatibility

Cyclosporine

Test Soln Name	Mfr	Mfr	Conc/L or %	Remarks	Ref	C/I
Amino acids 5%, dextrose 25%	MG	SZ	150 mg	Visually compatible with no cyclosporine loss in 72 hr at 21°C	1616	C
Dextrose 5%	AB[a]	SZ	2 g	Physically compatible with no cyclosporine loss in 24 hr at 24°C in the dark or light	1091	C
Dextrose 5%	AB[b]	SZ	2 g	Physically compatible with 5% cyclosporine loss in 48 hr at 24°C under fluorescent light and refrigerated at 6°C	1330	C
Dextrose 5%	BA	SZ	1 g	Visually compatible with no cyclosporine loss in 72 hr at 21°C	1616	C
Dextrose 5%			2 g	Physically compatible with little or no loss in 24 hr at room temperature or refrigerated	2503	C
Dextrose 5%	BA[c]	NVA	200 mg	Physically compatible with little loss of drug in 14 days at 25°C	2930	C
Dextrose 5%	BA[c]	NVA	2.5 g	Physically compatible with little loss of drug in 14 days at 25°C	2930	C
Sodium chloride 0.9%	AB[a]	SZ	2 g	Physically compatible with 7 to 8% cyclosporine loss in 24 hr at 24°C in the dark or light	1091	C
Sodium chloride 0.9%			2 g	Physically compatible with little loss in 24 hr at room temperature or refrigerated	2503	C
Sodium chloride 0.9%	BA[c]	NVA	200 mg	Physically compatible with no loss of drug in 14 days at 25°C	2930	C
Sodium chloride 0.9%	BA[c]	NVA	2.5g	Physically compatible with little loss of drug in 14 days at 25°C	2930	C

[a] Tested in both glass and PVC containers.

[b] Tested in glass containers.

[c] Tested in Aviva polypropylene-polyolefin containers.

Additive Compatibility

Cyclosporine

Test Drug	Mfr	Conc/L or %	Mfr	Conc/L or %	Test Solution	Remarks	Ref	C/I
Ciprofloxacin	BAY	2 g	SZ	500 mg	NS	Visually compatible with 8% ciprofloxacin loss in 24 hr at 25°C. Cyclosporine not tested	1934	C
Fat emulsion, intravenous	AB	10%	SZ	400 mg		No cyclosporine loss in 72 hr at 21°C	1616	C
Fat emulsion, intravenous	KA	10 and 20%	SZ	500 mg and 2 g		Physically compatible with no cyclosporine loss in 48 hr at 24°C under fluorescent light	1625	C
Magnesium sulfate	LY	30 g	SZ	2 g	D5W	Transient turbidity upon preparation. 5% cyclosporine loss in 6 hr and 10% loss in 12 hr at 24°C under fluorescent light	1629	I

Drugs in Syringe Compatibility

Cyclosporine

Test Drug	Mfr	Amt	Mfr	Amt	Remarks	Ref	C/I
Dimenhydrinate		10 mg/1 mL		50 mg/1 mL	Clear solution	2569	C
Pantoprazole sodium	a	4 mg/1 mL		50 mg/1 mL	Precipitates	2574	I

a Test performed using the formulation WITHOUT edetate disodium.

Y-Site Injection Compatibility (1:1 Mixture)

Cyclosporine

Test Drug	Mfr	Conc	Mfr	Conc	Remarks	Ref	C/I
Acyclovir sodium	BV	5 mg/mL[b]	BED	1 mg/mL[a]	Crystals form	2794	I
Anidulafungin	VIC	0.5 mg/mL[a]	NOV	5 mg/mL[a]	Physically compatible for 4 hr at 23°C	2617	C
Caspofungin acetate	ME	0.7 mg/mL[b]	BED	5 mg/mL[b]	Physically compatible for 4 hr at room temperature	2758	C
Ceftaroline fosamil	FOR	2.22 mg/mL[a b e]	BED	5 mg/mL[a b e]	Physically compatible for 4 hr at 23°C	2826	C
Ceftolozane sulfate–tazobactam sodium	CUB	10 mg/mL[g h]	PAD	5 mg/mL[g]	Immediate change in measured turbidity	3262	I
Cloxacillin sodium	SMX	100 mg/mL	NVA	5 mg/mL[f]	Physically compatible for up to 4 hr at room temperature	3245	C
Defibrotide sodium	JAZ	8 mg/mL[b]	NVA	1.27 mg/mL[b]	Visually compatible for 4 hr at room temperature	3149	C
Doripenem	JJ	5 mg/mL[a b]	BED	5 mg/mL[a b]	Physically compatible for 4 hr at 23°C	2743	C
Isavuconazonium sulfate	ASP	1.5 mg/mL[g]	DRX	5 mg/mL[g]	Immediate change in measured turbidity	3263	I
Letermovir	ME				Physically incompatible	3398	I
Linezolid	PHU	2 mg/mL	SZ	5 mg/mL[a]	Physically compatible for 4 hr at 23°C	2264	C
Meropenem	ASZ	10 mg/mL[b]	BED	1 mg/mL[a]	Physically compatible	2794	C
Meropenem		50 mg/mL	NVA	5 mg/mL	Physically compatible for 4 hr at room temperature	3538	C

Y-Site Injection Compatibility (1:1 Mixture) (Cont.)

Test Drug	Mfr	Conc	Mfr	Conc	Remarks	Ref	C/I
Meropenem		50 mg/mL	NVA	50 mg/mL	Unacceptably viscous	3538	I
Micafungin sodium	ASP	1.5 mg/mL[b]	BED	5 mg/mL[b]	Physically compatible for 4 hr at 23°C	2683	C
Mycophenolate mofetil HCl	RC	5.9 mg/mL[a]	BED	1 mg/mL[a]	Effervescence reported. No mycophenolate mofetil loss in 4 hr	2738	?
Propofol	ZEN[i]	10 mg/mL	SZ	5 mg/mL[a]	Physically compatible for 1 hr at 23°C	2066	C
Sargramostim	IMM	6[c] and 15[b] mcg/mL	SZ	5 mg/mL[b]	Visually compatible for 2 hr	1618	C
Tedizolid phosphate	CUB	0.8 mg/mL[b]	DRX	5 mg/mL[b]	Immediate change in measured turbidity	3244	I
Telavancin HCl	ASP	7.5 mg/mL[a]	BED	5 mg/mL[a]	Physically compatible for 2 hr	2830	C
Telavancin HCl	ASP	7.5 mg/mL[b e]	BED	5 mg/mL[b e]	Increase in measured turbidity	2830	I
TNA #220, #223[d]			SZ	5 mg/mL[a]	Small amount of precipitate forms immediately	2215	I
TNA #218, #219, #221, #222, #224 to #226[d]			SZ	5 mg/mL[a]	Visually compatible for 4 hr at 23°C	2215	C
TPN #212, #213[d]			SZ	5 mg/mL[a]	Physically compatible for 4 hr at 23°C	2109	C
TPN #214, #215[d]			SZ	5 mg/mL[a]	Small amount of subvisible precipitate forms in 4 hr	2109	I

[a] Tested in dextrose 5%.

[b] Tested in sodium chloride 0.9%.

[c] Tested in sodium chloride 0.9% with albumin human 0.1%.

[d] Refer to Appendix for the composition of parenteral nutrition solutions. TNA indicates a 3-in-1 admixture, and TPN indicates a 2-in-1 admixture.

[e] Tested in Ringer's injection, lactated.

[f] Tested in sterile water for injection.

[g] Tested in both dextrose 5% and sodium chloride 0.9%.

[h] Ceftolozane component. Ceftolozane in a 2:1 fixed-ratio concentration with tazobactam.

[i] Test performed using the formulation WITH edetate disodium.

Selected Revisions May 1, 2020. © Copyright, October 1986.
American Society of Health-System Pharmacists, Inc.

Cytarabine
AHFS 10:00
Cytosine Arabinoside

Products

Cytarabine injection is available as a 20-mg/mL solution in 5-mL single-use vials,[2942] 25-mL multidose vials,[2944] and 50-mL pharmacy bulk vials.[2943] Preservative-free 5-mL vials and 50-mL pharmacy bulk vials contain sodium chloride 6.8 mg/mL in water for injection.[2942 2943] The 25-mL multidose vial contains benzyl alcohol 0.9% in water for injection.[2944] Hydrochloric acid and/or sodium hydroxide may have been added to any of these vials during manufacturing to adjust pH.[2942 2943 2944]

Cytarabine injection also is available as a 100-mg/mL solution in preservative-free, single-use 20-mL vials in water for injection.[2941 2942] Hydrochloric acid and/or sodium hydroxide may have been added during manufacturing to adjust pH.[2941 2942]

CAUTION: Care should be taken to ensure that the correct drug product, dose, and administration procedures are used and that no confusion with other products occurs.

pH

Preservative-free cytarabine 20-mg/mL injection solution has a pH of 7.4.[2942 2943] Cytarabine 20-mg/mL injection solution in multidose vials containing benzyl alcohol has a pH of 7.6.[2944] Preservative-free cytarabine 100-mg/mL injection solution has a pH of 7.7.[2941 2942]

Sodium Content

Preservative-free cytarabine 20-mg/mL injection contains 0.12 mEq of sodium per mL.[2942 2943]

Administration

Cytarabine may be administered by subcutaneous or intrathecal (preservative-free preparations *only*) routes, or intravenously by direct injection or continuous or intermittent infusion.[2941 2942 2943 2944] Some preparations contain preservatives and should *not* be used for intrathecal administration.[2944] Preservative-free pharmacy bulk vials are intended *only* for the preparation of solutions for intravenous infusion.[2943]

CAUTION: Care should be taken to ensure that the correct drug product, dose, and administration procedures are used and that no confusion with other products occurs.

Stability

Intact vials of cytarabine injection should be stored at controlled room temperature.[2941 2942 2943 2944]

A stability study of cytarabine in aqueous solution showed maximum stability in the neutral pH range. It was calculated to retain 90% for 6.5 months at pH 6.9 at 25°C. The rate of decomposition of cytarabine in alkaline solutions is about 10 times as great as in acid solutions.[82]

One manufacturer indicated that for concentrations of 20 and 250 mg/mL in bacteriostatic water for injection, greater than 99% was retained after 5 days of storage at room temperature.[174] However, cytarabine has an aqueous solubility of 100 mg/mL,[4 1369] and precipitation from more highly concentrated solutions has been observed in varying time frames. In another test, concentrations of 40 and 80 mg/mL in bacteriostatic water for injection were stored in plastic syringes (Becton Dickinson) at 37, 25, 4, and −20°C. Cytarabine remained stable for at least 15 days at 25 and 4°C and for 7 days at 37°C. However, storage at −20°C resulted in a precipitate.[174]

Immersion of a needle with an aluminum component in cytarabine (Upjohn) 20 mg/mL resulted in no visually apparent reaction after 7 days at 24°C.[988]

Cytarabine 12.5 mg/mL in sodium chloride 0.9% did not inhibit the growth of inoculated *Staphylococcus epidermidis* during 21 days at 35°C. At a concentration of 50 mg/mL in sodium chloride, the viability was reduced but not eliminated.[1659] The potential for microbiological growth should be considered when assigning expiration periods.

Syringes

Cytarabine (Upjohn) 50 mg/mL in polypropylene syringes containing 5, 10, and 20 mL was stable for 29 days at 8 and 21°C in the dark, exhibiting losses of 8.5% or less.[1566]

Cytarabine (Upjohn) 50 mg/2.5 mL was stored at 5 and 25°C in 5-mL plastic syringes (Becton Dickinson) with rubber tip caps and in glass flasks covered with parafilm. After 7 days, samples in the plastic syringes showed a 2 to 3% loss of cytarabine at both temperatures. The 25°C sample in glass also showed a 2% loss, but the 5°C sample in glass showed no loss after 7 days.[759]

Intrathecal Injections

Bacterially contaminated intrathecal solutions could pose very grave risks; consequently, solutions for intrathecal use should be administered as soon as possible after preparation.[328]

The stability and compatibility of cytarabine (Upjohn), methotrexate (NCI), and hydrocortisone (Upjohn), mixed together in intrathecal injections, were evaluated. Two combinations were tested: (1) cytarabine 50 mg, methotrexate 12 mg (as the sodium salt), and hydrocortisone 25 mg (as the sodium succinate salt); and (2) cytarabine 30 mg, methotrexate 12 mg (as the sodium salt), and hydrocortisone 15 mg (as the sodium succinate salt). Each drug combination was added to 12 mL of Elliott's B solution (NCI), sodium chloride 0.9% (Abbott), dextrose 5% (Abbott), and Ringer's injection, lactated (Abbott), and stored for 24 hours at 25°C. Cytarabine and methotrexate were both chemically stable, with no drug loss after the full 24 hours in all solutions. Hydrocortisone was also stable in sodium chloride

DOI: 10.37573/9781585286850.105

0.9%, dextrose 5%, and Ringer's injection, lactated, with about a 2% drug loss. However, in Elliott's B solution, hydrocortisone was significantly less stable, with a 6% loss in the solution containing 25 mg of hydrocortisone over 24 hours. The solution containing 15 mg of hydrocortisone was worse, with a 5% loss in 10 hours and a 13% loss in 24 hours. The higher pH of Elliott's B solution and the lower concentration of hydrocortisone may have been factors in this increased decomposition. All mixtures were physically compatible during this study, but a precipitate formed after several days of storage.[819]

Elliott's B solution has been recommended as a diluent for cytarabine for intrathecal administration because it is more nearly physiologic.[435] The patient's own spinal fluid also has been recommended.[830]

Cytarabine (Upjohn) 3 mg/mL diluted in Elliott's B solution (Orphan Medical) was packaged as 20 mL in 30-mL glass vials and 20-mL plastic syringes (Becton Dickinson) with Red Cap (Burron) Luer-Lok syringe tip caps. The solution was physically compatible and was chemically stable, exhibiting little or no loss during storage for 48 hours at 4 and 23°C.[1976]

Implantable Pumps

Cytarabine (Upjohn) 1 mg/mL in Elliott's B solution was evaluated for stability in an implantable infusion pump (Infusaid model 400). In this in vitro assessment, no cytarabine loss occurred in 15 days at 37°C with mild agitation.[767]

Sorption

Cytarabine (Mack) 0.144 mg/mL in dextrose 5% and in sodium chloride 0.9% exhibited little or no loss due to sorption in polyethylene and polyvinyl chloride (PVC) containers compared to glass containers over 72 hours at room and refrigeration temperatures.[2420,2430]

Filtration

Cytarabine 100 mg/15 mL was injected as a bolus through a 0.2-μm nylon, air-eliminating filter (Ultipor, Pall) to evaluate the effect of filtration on simulated intravenous push delivery. Spectrophotometric evaluation showed that about 96% of the drug was delivered through the filter after flushing with 10 mL of sodium chloride 0.9%.[809]

Cytarabine 10 to 100 mcg/mL exhibited no loss due to sorption to either cellulose nitrate/cellulose acetate ester (Millex OR) or polytetrafluoroethylene (Millex FG) filters.[1416]

Central Venous Catheter

Cytarabine (Fujisawa) 5 mg/mL in dextrose 5% was found to be compatible with the ARROWg+ard Blue Plus (Arrow International) chlorhexidine-bearing triple-lumen central catheter. Essentially complete delivery of the drug was found with little or no drug loss occurring. Furthermore, chlorhexidine delivered from the catheter remained at trace amounts with no substantial increase due to the delivery of the drug through the catheter.[2335]

Compatibility Information

Solution Compatibility

Cytarabine

Test Soln Name	Mfr	Mfr	Conc/L or %	Remarks	Ref	C/I
Amino acids 4.25%, dextrose 25%	MG	UP	100 mg	No increase in particulate matter in 24 hr at 5°C	349	C
Dextrose 5% in Ringer's injection, lactated	TR[a]	UP	500 mg	Stable for 24 hr at 5°C	282	C
Dextrose 5% in sodium chloride 0.225%	[a]	UP	8, 24, 32 g	No loss in 7 days at room temperature or 4 or –20°C	174	C
Dextrose 5% in sodium chloride 0.9%	TR[a]	UP	500 mg	Stable for 24 hr at 5°C	282	C
Dextrose 5% in sodium chloride 0.9%		UP	3.6 g	Physically compatible	174	C
Dextrose 10% in sodium chloride 0.9%		UP	3.6 g	Physically compatible	174	C
Dextrose 5%	[d]			Little to no loss over 8 days at room temperature	2943, 2944	C
Dextrose 5%	TR[a]	UP	500 mg	Stable for 24 hr at 5°C	282	C
Dextrose 5%	TR[a]	UP	1.87 g	Under 10% loss in 24 hr at room temperature	519	C
Dextrose 5%		UP	500 mg	Stable for 7 days at room temperature	174	C
Dextrose 5%	[a]	UP	8, 24, 32 g	No loss in 7 days at room temperature or 4 or –20°C	174	C

Solution Compatibility (Cont.)

Test Soln Name	Mfr	Mfr	Conc/L or %	Remarks	Ref	C/I
Dextrose 5%			0.5 to 5 g	Under 10% loss in 14 days at room temperature	1379	C
Dextrose 5%	b	UP	1.25 and 25 g	Visually compatible with less than 6% cytarabine loss in 28 days at 4 and 22°C and 7 days at 35°C protected from light. Excessive decomposition products in 14 days at 35°C	1548	C
Dextrose 5%	MG, TRa		1.83 g	Less than 10% cytarabine loss in 24 hr at room temperature exposed to light	1658	C
Dextrose 5%		UP	157 mg	Less than 2% loss in 48 hr at room temperature, exposed to light and in the dark, and at 4°C	1955	C
Ringer's injection		UP	3.6 g	Physically compatible	174	C
Ringer's injection			0.5 to 5 g	Under 10% loss in 14 days at room temperature	1379	C
Ringer's injection, lactated	TRa	UP	500 mg	Stable for 24 hr at 5°C	282	C
Sodium chloride 0.9%	d			Little to no loss over 8 days at room temperature	2943, 2944	C
Sodium chloride 0.9%	TRa	UP	500 mg	Stable for 24 hr at 5°C	282	C
Sodium chloride 0.9%		UP	500 mg	Stable for 7 days at room temperature	174	C
Sodium chloride 0.9%	a	UP	8, 24, 32 g	No loss in 7 days at room temperature or 4 or −20°C	174	C
Sodium chloride 0.9%		UP	3.6 g	Physically compatible	174	C
Sodium chloride 0.9%			0.5 to 5 g	Under 10% loss in 14 days at room temperature	1379	C
Sodium chloride 0.9%	b	UP	1.25 and 25 g	Visually compatible with less than 6% cytarabine loss in 28 days at 4 and 22°C and 7 days at 35°C protected from light. Excessive decomposition products in 14 days at 35°C	1548	C
Sodium lactate (⅙) M		UP	3.6 g	Physically compatible	174	C
TPN #57c		UP	50 mg	Physically compatible with no loss in 48 hr at 25 or 8°C	996	C

a Tested in both glass and PVC containers.

b Tested in ethylene vinyl acetate (EVA) containers.

c Refer to Appendix for the composition of parenteral nutrition solutions. TPN indicates a 2-in-1 admixture.

d Tested in both glass and plastic (not otherwise specified) containers.

Additive Compatibility

Cytarabine

Test Drug	Mfr	Conc/L or %	Mfr	Conc/L or %	Test Solution	Remarks	Ref	C/I
Daunorubicin HCl with etoposide	RP BR	33 mg 400 mg	UP	267 mg	D5½S	Physically compatible with about 6% cytarabine loss and no loss of other drugs in 72 hr at 20°C	1162	C
Daunorubicin HCl with etoposide	BEL SZ	15.7 mg 157 mg	UP	157 mg	D5W	Less than 10% loss of any drug in 48 hr at room temperature, exposed to light and in the dark, and at 4°C	1955	C
Etoposide with daunorubicin HCl	BR RP	400 mg 33 mg	UP	267 mg	D5½S	Physically compatible with about 6% cytarabine loss and no loss of other drugs in 72 hr at 20°C	1162	C

Additive Compatibility (Cont.)

Test Drug	Mfr	Conc/L or %	Mfr	Conc/L or %	Test Solution	Remarks	Ref	C/I
Etoposide with daunorubicin HCl	SZ BEL	157 mg 15.7 mg	UP	157 mg	D5W	Less than 10% loss of any drug in 48 hr at room temperature, exposed to light and in the dark, and at 4°C	1955	C
Fluorouracil	RC	250 mg	UP	400 mg	D5W	Altered UV spectra for cytarabine within 1 hr at room temperature	207	I
Gentamicin sulfate		80 mg	UP	100 mg	D5W	Physically compatible for 24 hr	174	C
Gentamicin sulfate		240 mg	UP	300 mg	D5W	Physically incompatible	174	I
Heparin sodium		10,000 units	UP	500 mg	NS	Haze formation	174	I
Heparin sodium		20,000 units	UP	100 mg	D5W	Haze formation	174	I
Hydrocortisone sodium succinate	UP	500 mg	UP	360 mg	D5S, D10S	Physically compatible for 40 hr	174	C
Hydrocortisone sodium succinate	UP	500 mg	UP	360 mg	R, SL	Physically incompatible	174	I
Hydroxyzine HCl	LY	500 mg	UP	1 g	D5W[a]	Physically compatible for 48 hr	1190	C
Insulin, regular		40 units	UP	100 and 500 mg	D5W	Fine precipitate forms	174	I
Lincomycin HCl		1, 1.5, 2, 2.4, 3 g	UP	500 mg		Physically compatible for 48 hr	174	C
Methotrexate sodium	LE	200 mg	UP	400 mg	D5W	Physically compatible. Very little change in UV spectra in 8 hr at room temperature	207	C
Methylprednisolone sodium succinate	UP	250 mg	UP	360 mg	D5S, D10S, NS	Clear solution for 24 hr	329	C
Methylprednisolone sodium succinate	UP	250 mg	UP	360 mg	R, SL	Physically incompatible	329	I
Mitoxantrone HCl	LE	500 mg	UP	500 mg	D5W	Visually compatible. Mitoxantrone stable for 24 hr at room temperature. Cytarabine not tested	1531	C
Nafcillin sodium		4 g	UP	100 mg	D5W	Heavy crystalline precipitation	174	I
Ondansetron HCl	GL	30 and 300 mg	UP	200 mg	D5W[b]	Physically compatible with little loss of either drug in 48 hr at 23°C	1876	C
Ondansetron HCl	GL	30 and 300 mg	UP	40 g	D5W[b]	Physically compatible with little loss of either drug in 48 hr at 23°C	1876	C
Oxacillin sodium		2 g	UP	100 mg	D5W	pH outside stability range for oxacillin	174	I
Penicillin G sodium		2 million units	UP	200 mg	D5W	pH outside stability range for penicillin G	174	I
Potassium chloride		80 mEq	UP	170 mg	D5S	Physically compatible for 24 hr	174	C
Potassium chloride		100 mEq	UP	2 g	D5S	Physically compatible. Stable for 8 days	174	C
Sodium bicarbonate	AB	50 mEq	UP	200 mg and 1 g	D5W[c]	Physically compatible with no cytarabine loss in 7 days at 8 and 22°C	748	C
Sodium bicarbonate	AB	50 mEq	UP	200 mg	D5¼S[c]	Physically compatible with no cytarabine loss in 7 days at 8 and 22°C	748	C

Additive Compatibility (Cont.)

Test Drug	Mfr	Conc/L or %	Mfr	Conc/L or %	Test Solution	Remarks	Ref	C/I
Vincristine sulfate	LI	4 mg	UP	16 mg	D5W	Physically compatible. No alteration in UV spectra in 8 hr at room temperature	207	C

[a] Tested in glass containers.

[b] Tested in PVC containers.

[c] Tested in both glass and PVC containers.

Drugs in Syringe Compatibility

Cytarabine

Test Drug	Mfr	Amt	Mfr	Amt	Remarks	Ref	C/I
Metoclopramide HCl	RB	10 mg/2 mL	UP	50 mg/1 mL	Physically compatible for 48 hr at 25°C	1167	C
Metoclopramide HCl	RB	160 mg/32 mL	UP	500 mg/10 mL	Physically compatible for 48 hr at 25°C	1167	C

Y-Site Injection Compatibility (1:1 Mixture)

Cytarabine

Test Drug	Mfr	Conc	Mfr	Conc	Remarks	Ref	C/I
Allopurinol sodium	BW	3 mg/mL[b]	SCN	50 mg/mL	Tiny particles form within 4 hr	1686	I
Amifostine	USB	10 mg/mL[a]	CET	50 mg/mL	Physically compatible for 4 hr at 23°C	1845	C
Amsacrine	NCI	1 mg/mL[a]	QU	50 mg/mL	Visually compatible for 4 hr at 22°C	1381	C
Anidulafungin	VIC	0.5 mg/mL[a]	BED	50 mg/mL	Physically compatible for 4 hr at 23°C	2617	C
Aztreonam	SQ	40 mg/mL[a]	CET	50 mg/mL	Physically compatible for 4 hr at 23°C	1758	C
Caspofungin acetate	ME	0.7 mg/mL[b]	MAY	50 mg/mL	Microparticles form within 4 hr	2758	I
Cladribine	ORT	0.015[b] and 0.5[c] mg/mL	CHI	50 mg/mL	Physically compatible for 4 hr at 23°C	1969	C
Doxorubicin HCl liposomal	SEQ	0.4 mg/mL[a]	CHI	50 mg/mL	Physically compatible for 4 hr at 23°C	2087	C
Etoposide phosphate	BR	5 mg/mL[a]	BED	50 mg/mL	Physically compatible for 4 hr at 23°C	2218	C
Filgrastim	AMG	30 mcg/mL[a]	CET	50 mg/mL	Physically compatible for 4 hr at 22°C	1687	C
Fludarabine phosphate	BX	1 mg/mL[a]	UP	50 mg/mL	Visually compatible for 4 hr at 22°C	1439	C
Gallium nitrate	FUJ	1 mg/mL[b]	CET	50 mg/mL	Precipitates immediately	1673	I
Gemcitabine HCl	LI	10 mg/mL[b]	BED	50 mg/mL	Physically compatible for 4 hr at 23°C	2226	C
Gentamicin sulfate	GNS	15 mg/mL[d]	UP	16 mg/mL[b]	Visually compatible for 24 hr at room temperature in test tubes. No precipitate found on filter from Y-site delivery	2063	C
Granisetron HCl	SKB	1 mg/mL	UP	2 mg/mL[b]	Physically compatible with little loss of either drug in 4 hr at 22°C	1883	C
Granisetron HCl	SKB	0.05 mg/mL[a]	UP	50 mg/mL	Physically compatible for 4 hr at 23°C	2000	C
Hydrocortisone sodium succinate	UP	125 mg/mL	UP	16 mg/mL[b]	Visually compatible for 24 hr at room temperature in test tubes. No precipitate found on filter from Y-site delivery	2063	C

Y-Site Injection Compatibility (1:1 Mixture) (Cont.)

Test Drug	Mfr	Conc	Mfr	Conc	Remarks	Ref	C/I
Idarubicin HCl	AD	1 mg/mL[b]	CET	6 mg/mL[a]	Visually compatible for 24 hr at 25°C	1525	C
Linezolid	PHU	2 mg/mL	BED	50 mg/mL	Physically compatible for 4 hr at 23°C	2264	C
Melphalan HCl	BW	0.1 mg/mL[b]	UP	50 mg/mL	Physically compatible for 3 hr at 22°C	1557	C
Methotrexate sodium		30 mg/mL	UP	0.6 mg/mL[a]	Visually compatible for 4 hr at room temperature	1788	C
Methylprednisolone sodium succinate	UP	5 mg/mL[a]	UP	16 mg/mL[b]	Visually compatible for 24 hr at room temperature in test tubes. No precipitate found on filter from Y-site delivery	2063	C
Ondansetron HCl	GL	1 mg/mL[b]	UP	50 mg/mL	Visually compatible for 4 hr at 22°C	1365	C
Paclitaxel	NCI	1.2 mg/mL[a]		50 mg/mL	Physically compatible for 4 hr at 22°C	1528	C
Pemetrexed disodium	LI	20 mg/mL[b]	PHU	50 mg/mL	Physically compatible for 4 hr at 23°C	2564	C
Piperacillin sodium–tazobactam sodium	LE[g]	40 mg/mL[a h]	SCN	50 mg/mL	Physically compatible for 4 hr at 22°C	1688	C
Propofol	ZEN[i]	10 mg/mL	CHI	50 mg/mL	Physically compatible for 1 hr at 23°C	2066	C
Sargramostim	IMM	10 mcg/mL[b]	SCN	50 mg/mL	Visually compatible for 4 hr at 22°C	1436	C
Sodium bicarbonate		1.4%	UP	0.6 mg/mL[a]	Visually compatible for 4 hr at room temperature	1788	C
Teniposide	BR	0.1 mg/mL[a]	CET	50 mg/mL	Physically compatible for 4 hr at 23°C	1725	C
Thiotepa	IMM[e]	1 mg/mL[a]	CET	50 mg/mL	Physically compatible for 4 hr at 23°C	1861	C
TNA #218 to #226[f]			BED	50 mg/mL	Visually compatible for 4 hr at 23°C	2215	C
TPN #212 to #215[f]			CHI	50 mg/mL	Substantial loss of natural subvisible turbidity occurs immediately	2109	I
Vinorelbine tartrate	BW	1 mg/mL[b]	CET	50 mg/mL	Physically compatible for 4 hr at 22°C	1558	C

[a] Tested in dextrose 5%.

[b] Tested in sodium chloride 0.9%.

[c] Tested in bacteriostatic sodium chloride 0.9% preserved with benzyl alcohol 0.9%.

[d] Tested in sodium chloride 0.45%.

[e] Lyophilized formulation tested.

[f] Refer to Appendix for the composition of parenteral nutrition solutions. TNA indicates a 3-in-1 admixture, and TPN indicates a 2-in-1 admixture.

[g] Test performed using the formulation WITHOUT edetate disodium.

[h] Piperacillin component. Piperacillin in an 8:1 fixed-ratio concentration with tazobactam.

[i] Test performed using the formulation WITH edetate disodium.

Dacarbazine
AHFS 10:00

Products

Dacarbazine is available in vials containing 100 and 200 mg of drug along with anhydrous citric acid and mannitol. Reconstitute the 100- and 200-mg vials with 9.9 and 19.7 mL of sterile water for injection, respectively, to yield solutions containing 10 mg/mL of dacarbazine.[1(1/08)]

pH

From 3 to 4.[1(1/08)]

Administration

Dacarbazine is administered as a direct intravenous injection over one minute and as an intravenous infusion in up to 250 mL of dextrose 5% or sodium chloride 0.9% over 15 to 30 minutes.[4] Extravasation may result in severe pain and tissue damage.[1(1/08) 4 377]

In the event of spills or leaks, the manufacturer recommends the use of sulfuric acid 10% in contact for 24 hours to inactivate dacarbazine.[1200]

Stability

Intact vials of dacarbazine should be stored at 2 to 8°C and protected from light.[1(1/08) 4] However, dacarbazine in intact vials stored at controlled room temperature has been stated to be stable for periods of four weeks[1239 1433] to three months.[1433 2745] The manufacturer also recommends storage of reconstituted solutions for up to eight hours at normal room temperatures and light or up to 72 hours at 4°C.[1(1/08)] However, it has been reported that solutions are stable for at least 24 hours at room temperature (1% decomposition) and at least 96 hours under refrigeration (less than 1% decomposition) when protected from light.[285] A change in color from pale yellow or ivory to pink or red is a sign of decomposition.[4 285 1093]

Immersion of a needle with an aluminum component in dacarbazine (Miles) 10 mg/mL resulted in no visually apparent unexpected reaction after seven days at 24°C.[988]

Light Effects

Administration of dacarbazine in a room illuminated only with a red photographic light apparently reduced the incidence of disagreeable side effects. The authors attributed this result to a reduced amount of photodegradation of dacarbazine.[469]

Multiple photodegradation products of dacarbazine have been identified and specific concentrations of each are crucially dependent on the pH of the solution.[496]

The effects of daylight and fluorescent light on dacarbazine (Bayer) 4 mg/mL in sodium chloride 0.9% were reported. Exposure to direct sunlight resulted in up to a 12% loss in 30 minutes, and a pink color formed in 35 to 40 minutes. Exposure to indirect daylight resulted in less than a 2% loss in 30 minutes. Solutions protected from light or exposed to fluorescent light lost about 4% of their dacarbazine in 24 hours.[1248]

The photostability of dacarbazine has been shown to increase with the addition of reduced glutathione at about 5 mg/100 mL.[1829]

Dacarbazine (Aventis) 11 mg/mL reconstituted with sterile water for injection in original amber glass vials stored at room temperature exposed to fluorescent light formed a visible precipitate and became yellow in 24 hours and turned pink after 96 hours. About 4% dacarbazine loss occurred in 96 hours, but precipitation limited the utility period to 24 hours. Formation of 2-azahypoxanthine, a potentially toxic decomposition product, was also noted. Under refrigeration protected from light, no precipitation was seen, but red discoloration appeared after 96 hours; little or no loss of dacarbazine occurred in seven days. Reconstituted dacarbazine was stated to be stable for 24 hours at room temperature under fluorescent light and 96 hours refrigerated in the dark.[2386]

Dacarbazine (Aventis) 1.4 mg/mL in dextrose 5% in PVC bags (Fresenius) was stored under a variety of temperature and light conditions. In PVC bags exposed to natural sunlight, the solution turned pink in six hours and red in 48 hours; it developed a precipitate in 96 hours. About 11% dacarbazine loss in three hours and 35% loss in 24 hours. Exposed to or protected from fluorescent light at room temperature and refrigerated, no visible changes occurred in seven days. At room temperature, dacarbazine losses were about 6% in 24 hours exposed to fluorescent light and 7% in 48 hours protected from light. Refrigerated samples protected from light exhibited little or no loss in seven days.[2386]

Simulated infusion of the dacarbazine 1.4-mg/mL solution through transparent (Baxter) and opaque (Codan) infusion tubing over about 110 minutes exposed to light resulted in the delivery of 94% (transparent tubing) and 98% (opaque tubing) of the dacarbazine.[2386]

Sorption

Dacarbazine (Medac) 0.64 mg/mL in sodium chloride 0.9% exhibited no loss due to sorption in polyethylene and PVC containers compared to glass containers over 48 hours at refrigeration temperature.[2420 2430]

DOI: 10.37573/9781585286850.106

Compatibility Information

Solution Compatibility

Dacarbazine

Test Soln Name	Mfr	Mfr	Conc/L or %	Remarks	Ref	C/I
Dextrose 5%	a		1.7 g	Less than 10% loss in 24 hr at room temperature	519	C
Dextrose 5%	MG, TR[b]		1.7 g	Less than 10% loss in 24 hr at room temperature exposed to light	1658	C
Dextrose 5%	BA[c]	MI	1 and 3 g	Physically compatible with 4% loss in 8 hr and 10 to 15% loss in 24 hr at 23°C	1876	I
Dextrose 5%	FRE[c]	AVE	1.4 g	Exposed to sunlight, pink color formed in 3 hr and red color in 6 hr with precipitation in 96 hr at 23°C. 11% loss in 3 hr	2386	I
Dextrose 5%	FRE[c]	AVE	1.4 g	Exposed to or protected from fluorescent light, visually compatible for 7 days. 6% loss in 24 hr exposed to fluorescent light and 7% loss in 48 hr in the dark. Little loss at 4°C in 7 days	2386	C

[a] Tested in both glass and PVC containers.

[b] Tested in glass, PVC, and polyolefin containers.

[c] Tested in PVC containers.

Additive Compatibility

Dacarbazine

Test Drug	Mfr	Conc/L or %	Mfr	Conc/L or %	Test Solution	Remarks	Ref	C/I
Doxorubicin HCl with ondansetron HCl	AD GL	800 mg 640 mg	LY	8 g	D5W[a]	Visually compatible. Under 10% ondansetron and doxorubicin loss in 24 hr at 30°C and 7 days at 4°C then 24 hr at 30°C. Dacarbazine stable for 8 hr but 13% loss in 24 hr	2092	I
Doxorubicin HCl with ondansetron HCl	AD GL	800 mg 640 mg	LY	8 g	D5W[b]	Visually compatible. Under 10% loss of all drugs in 24 hr at 30°C and 7 days at 4°C then 24 hr at 30°C	2092	C
Doxorubicin HCl with ondansetron HCl	AD GL	1.5 g 640 mg	LY	20 g	D5W[a b]	Visually compatible. Under 10% loss of all drugs in 24 hr at 30°C and 7 days at 4°C then 24 hr at 30°C	2092	C
Ondansetron HCl	GL	30 and 300 mg	MI	1 g	D5W[a]	Physically compatible with little loss of ondansetron in 48 hr at 23°C. 8 to 12% dacarbazine loss in 24 hr and 20% loss in 48 hr at 23°C	1876	C
Ondansetron HCl	GL	30 and 300 mg	MI	3 g	D5W[a]	Physically compatible with little loss of ondansetron in 48 hr at 23°C. 8% dacarbazine loss in 24 hr and 15% loss in 48 hr at 23°C	1876	C
Ondansetron HCl with doxorubicin HCl	GL AD	640 mg 800 mg	LY	8 g	D5W[a]	Visually compatible. Under 10% ondansetron and doxorubicin loss in 24 hr at 30°C and 7 days at 4°C then 24 hr at 30°C. Dacarbazine stable for 8 hr but 13% loss in 24 hr	2092	I
Ondansetron HCl with doxorubicin HCl	GL AD	640 mg 800 mg	LY	8 g	D5W[b]	Visually compatible. Under 10% loss of all drugs in 24 hr at 30°C and 7 days at 4°C then 24 hr at 30°C	2092	C
Ondansetron HCl with doxorubicin HCl	GL AD	640 mg 1.5 g	LY	20 g	D5W[a b]	Visually compatible. Under 10% loss of all drugs in 24 hr at 30°C and 7 days at 4°C then 24 hr at 30°C	2092	C

[a] Tested in PVC containers.

[b] Tested in polyisoprene infusion pump reservoirs.

Y-Site Injection Compatibility (1:1 Mixture)

Dacarbazine

Test Drug	Mfr	Conc	Mfr	Conc	Remarks	Ref	C/I
Allopurinol sodium	BW	3 mg/mL[b]	MI	4 mg/mL[b]	Small particles form within 1 hr and become large pink pellets in 24 hr	1686	I
Amifostine	USB	10 mg/mL[a]	MI	4 mg/mL[a]	Physically compatible for 4 hr at 23°C	1845	C
Aztreonam	SQ	40 mg/mL[a]	MI	4 mg/mL[a]	Physically compatible for 4 hr at 23°C	1758	C
Doxorubicin HCl liposomal	SEQ	0.4 mg/mL[a]	MI	4 mg/mL[a]	Physically compatible for 4 hr at 23°C	2087	C
Etoposide phosphate	BR	5 mg/mL[a]	MI	4 mg/mL[a]	Physically compatible for 4 hr at 23°C	2218	C
Filgrastim	AMG	30 mcg/mL[a]	MI	4 mg/mL[a]	Physically compatible for 4 hr at 22°C	1687	C
Fludarabine phosphate	BX	1 mg/mL[a]	MI	4 mg/mL[a]	Visually compatible for 4 hr at 22°C	1439	C
Granisetron HCl	SKB	1 mg/mL	MI	1.7 mg/mL[b]	Physically compatible with little loss of either drug in 4 hr at 22°C	1883	C
Heparin sodium	WY	100 units/mL	MI	25 mg/mL[b]	White precipitate forms immediately[c]	1158	I
Heparin sodium	WY	100 units/mL	MI	10 mg/mL[b]	No observable precipitation[c]	1158	C
Hydrocortisone sodium succinate					Pink precipitate forms immediately	524	I
Melphalan HCl	BW	0.1 mg/mL[b]	MI	4 mg/mL[b]	Physically compatible for 3 hr at 22°C	1557	C
Ondansetron HCl	GL	1 mg/mL[b]	MI	4 mg/mL[a]	Visually compatible for 4 hr at 22°C	1365	C
Paclitaxel	NCI	1.2 mg/mL[a]	MI	4 mg/mL[a]	Physically compatible for 4 hr at 22°C	1556	C
Palonosetron HCl	MGI	50 mcg/mL	BV	4 mg/mL[a]	Physically compatible and no loss of either drug in 4 hr	2681	C
Piperacillin sodium–tazobactam sodium	LE[e]	40 mg/mL[a] [f]	MI	4 mg/mL[a]	Turbidity and particles form immediately and increase over 4 hr	1688	I
Sargramostim	IMM	10 mcg/mL[b]	MI	4 mg/mL[b]	Visually compatible for 4 hr at 22°C	1436	C
Teniposide	BR	0.1 mg/mL[a]	MI	4 mg/mL[a]	Physically compatible for 4 hr at 23°C	1725	C
Thiotepa	IMM[d]	1 mg/mL[a]	MI	4 mg/mL[a]	Physically compatible for 4 hr at 23°C	1861	C
Vinorelbine tartrate	BW	1 mg/mL[b]	MI	4 mg/mL[b]	Physically compatible for 4 hr at 22°C	1558	C

[a] Tested in dextrose 5%.

[b] Tested in sodium chloride 0.9%.

[c] Dacarbazine in intravenous tubing flushed with heparin sodium.

[d] Lyophilized formulation tested.

[e] Test performed using the formulation WITHOUT edetate disodium.

[f] Piperacillin component. Piperacillin in an 8:1 fixed-ratio concentration with tazobactam.

Selected Revisions May 28, 2014. © Copyright, October 1982.
American Society of Health-System Pharmacists, Inc.

Dactinomycin

AHFS 10:00
Actinomycin D

Products

Dactinomycin is available in vials containing 0.5 mg of drug with mannitol 20 mg.[2945] Reconstitute with 1.1 mL of sterile water for injection *without* preservatives to yield a gold-colored solution containing approximately 0.5 mg/mL of dactinomycin.[2945] The use of water for injection containing preservatives (e.g., benzyl alcohol, parabens) causes precipitation.[2945]

pH

The pH of the reconstituted solution is 5.5 to 7.[1369]

Trade Name(s)

Cosmegen

Administration

Dactinomycin is administered intravenously or by regional perfusion techniques.[2945] The manufacturer states that only products diluted to concentrations greater than 10 mcg/mL are recommended for administration.[2945] Extravasation should be avoided because of possible corrosion of soft tissue.[377][2945] An inline cellulose ester membrane filter should *not* be used for administration of dactinomycin.[2945] (See Filtration.)

In the event of spills or leaks, the manufacturer recommends the use of trisodium phosphate 5% to inactivate dactinomycin.[1200]

Stability

Intact vials of dactinomycin should be stored at controlled room temperature and protected from light and humidity.[2945] The clear, gold-colored, reconstituted solution is stable at room temperature; however, this solution contains no preservative so it has been suggested that unused portions of the injection be discarded.[2945]

Solutions of dactinomycin diluted to concentrations of 10 mcg/mL or greater in water for injection, sodium chloride 0.9%, or dextrose 5% demonstrated chemical stability for up to 10 hours at room temperature in both glass and PVC containers.[2945] Solutions diluted to concentrations less than 10 mcg/mL, however, demonstrated significant losses.[2945] The manufacturer recommends that the reconstituted and diluted product be used within 4 hours of reconstitution when stored at room temperature.[2945]

The drug is reported to be most stable at pH 5 to 7.[1369] A 30-mcg/mL concentration at this pH range exhibits about a 2 to 3% loss in 6 hours at 25°C; at pH 9, an 80% loss occurs under these conditions.[51]

Dactinomycin, reconstituted according to the manufacturer's instructions, was cultured with human lymphoblasts to determine whether its cytotoxic activity was retained. The solution retained cytotoxicity for 24 hours at 4°C and room temperature.[1575]

Filtration

Dactinomycin may exhibit considerable binding to cellulose acetate/nitrate (Millex OR) and polytetrafluoroethylene (Millex GV) filters.[1249]

Dactinomycin (MSD) 0.5 mg/L in dextrose 5%, sodium chloride 0.9%, and Ringer's injection, lactated, was filtered over 12 hours through a 5-μm stainless steel depth filter (Argyle Filter Connector), a 0.22-μm cellulose ester membrane filter (Ivex-2 Filter Set), and a 0.22-μm polycarbonate membrane filter (In-Sure Filter Set). No significant reduction in potency due to binding was observed with the stainless steel filter. Approximately 25% of the drug delivered through the polycarbonate filter in the first 10 mL of solution was bound, but binding decreased rapidly thereafter, resulting in only 0.3% of the total delivered dose in 12 hours being bound.[320]

In contrast, filtration through the cellulose ester filter resulted in the binding of about 95 to 99% of the drug in the first 10 mL, with the total cumulative amount of drug bound in 12 hours being 13%. Approximately 50% of the bound drug was released by rinsing 3 times with 100 mL of the same intravenous solutions used in the admixtures.[320]

In another study, dactinomycin 0.5 mg/mL was injected as a bolus through a 0.2-μm nylon, air-eliminating filter (Ultipor, Pall) to evaluate the effect of filtration on simulated intravenous push delivery. Spectrophotometric evaluation showed that about 87% of the drug was delivered through the filter after flushing with 10 mL of sodium chloride 0.9%.[809]

Dactinomycin 4 to 50 mcg/mL exhibited a greater than 95% loss due to sorption to cellulose nitrate/cellulose acetate ester filters (Millex OR) and a 50 to 60% loss with polytetrafluoroethylene filters (Millex FG).[1415][1416]

DOI: 10.37573/9781585286850.107

Compatibility Information

Solution Compatibility

Dactinomycin

Test Soln Name	Mfr	Mfr	Conc/L or %	Remarks	Ref	C/I
Dextrose 5%				Manufacturer recommended solution	2945	C
Dextrose 5%	a	MSD	9.8 mg	Less than 10% loss in 24 hr at room temperature	519	C
Dextrose 5%	MG, TR[a]	MSD	9.8 mg	Less than 10% loss in 24 hr at room temperature exposed to light	1658	C
Dextrose 5%	MG, TR[b]	MSD	7.5 mg	Less than 10% loss in 24 hr at room temperature exposed to light	1658	C
Sodium chloride 0.9%				Manufacturer recommended solution	3003	C

[a] Tested in both glass and PVC containers.

[b] Tested in both glass and polyolefin containers.

Y-Site Injection Compatibility (1:1 Mixture)

Dactinomycin

Test Drug	Mfr	Conc	Mfr	Conc	Remarks	Ref	C/I
Allopurinol sodium	BW	3 mg/mL[b]	MSD	0.01 mg/mL[b]	Physically compatible for 4 hr at 22°C	1686	C
Amifostine	USB	10 mg/mL[a]	ME	0.01 mg/mL[a]	Physically compatible for 4 hr at 23°C	1845	C
Aztreonam	SQ	40 mg/mL[a]	ME	0.01 mg/mL[a]	Physically compatible for 4 hr at 23°C	1758	C
Etoposide phosphate	BR	5 mg/mL[a]	ME	0.01 mg/mL[a]	Physically compatible for 4 hr at 23°C	2218	C
Filgrastim	AMG	30 mcg/mL[a]	MSD	0.01 mg/mL[a]	Particles and filaments form immediately	1687	I
Fludarabine phosphate	BX	1 mg/mL[a]	MSD	0.01 mg/mL[a]	Visually compatible for 4 hr at 22°C	1439	C
Gemcitabine HCl	LI	10 mg/mL[b]	ME	0.01 mg/mL[b]	Physically compatible for 4 hr at 23°C	2226	C
Granisetron HCl	SKB	0.05 mg/mL[a]	ME	0.01 mg/mL[a]	Physically compatible for 4 hr at 23°C	2000	C
Melphalan HCl	BW	0.1 mg/mL[b]	MSD	0.01 mg/mL[b]	Physically compatible for 3 hr at 22°C	1557	C
Ondansetron HCl	GL	1 mg/mL[b]	MSD	0.01 mg/mL[a]	Visually compatible for 4 hr at 22°C	1365	C
Sargramostim	IMM	10 mcg/mL[b]	MSD	0.01 mg/mL[b]	Visually compatible for 4 hr at 22°C	1436	C
Teniposide	BR	0.1 mg/mL[a]	MSD	0.01 mg/mL[a]	Physically compatible for 4 hr at 23°C	1725	C
Thiotepa	IMM[c]	1 mg/mL[a]	ME	0.01 mg/mL[a]	Physically compatible for 4 hr at 23°C	1861	C
Vinorelbine tartrate	BW	1 mg/mL[b]	MSD	0.01 mg/mL[b]	Physically compatible for 4 hr at 22°C	1558	C

[a] Tested in dextrose 5%.

[b] Tested in sodium chloride 0.9%.

[c] Lyophilized formulation tested.

Selected Revisions July 28, 2015. © Copyright, October 1982.
American Society of Health-System Pharmacists, Inc.

Dalbavancin Hydrochloride
AHFS 8:12.28.16

Products

Dalbavancin is available as a lyophilized powder in single-use vials containing dalbavancin hydrochloride equivalent to anhydrous dalbavancin 500 mg as the free base.[2910] Also present in each vial are lactose monohydrate 129 mg and mannitol 129 mg as excipients.[2910] Sodium hydroxide or hydrochloric acid may have been added during manufacturing to adjust the pH.[2910]

Each 500-mg vial should be reconstituted with 25 mL sterile water for injection to yield a solution containing dalbavancin 20 mg/mL.[2910] Alternate between gently swirling and inverting the vial to avoid foaming until contents are completely dissolved; do not shake.[2910] The appropriate dose must be withdrawn and further diluted only in dextrose 5% to a final concentration of 1 to 5 mg/mL.[2910] Saline-based infusion solutions must not be used for dilution as precipitation may result.[2910] The diluted solution should be inspected for particulate matter prior to infusion; if present, the solution should not be used.[2910]

Trade Name(s)

Dalvance

Administration

Dalbavancin is administered by intravenous infusion over 30 minutes after dilution only in dextrose 5% to a concentration of 1 to 5 mg/mL.[2910] If a common infusion line is being used to administer other drugs in addition to dalbavancin, the line should be flushed with dextrose 5% prior to and following infusion of dalbavancin.[2910]

Stability

Intact vials of dalbavancin hydrochloride should be stored at controlled room temperature.[2910] Dalbavancin hydrochloride is a white to off-white to pale yellow powder that forms a clear, colorless to yellow solution when reconstituted with sterile water for injection.[2910]

The manufacturer states that the reconstituted drug and the diluted solution may be stored under refrigeration or at room temperature; do not freeze.[2910] The total time from reconstitution to dilution to administration should not exceed 48 hours.[2910] Any unused portion should be discarded.[2910]

Compatibility Information

Solution Compatibility

Dalbavancin HCl

Test Soln Name	Mfr	Mfr	Conc/L or %	Remarks	Ref	C/I
Dextrose 5%		DRT	1 to 5 g	Use within 48 hours at room temperature or refrigerated	2910	C
Sodium chloride 0.45%		DRT		Physically incompatible	2910	I
Sodium chloride 0.9%		DRT		Physically incompatible	2910	I

DOI: 10.37573/9781585286850.108

Dalteparin Sodium
AHFS 20:12.04.16

Products

Dalteparin sodium is available as an injection solution with each mL containing 10,000, 12,500, or 25,000 anti-factor Xa international units in water for injection.[3403] The 10,000-international unit/mL concentration is available in preservative-free, single-dose, graduated prefilled syringes containing 10,000 international units (1 mL); the 12,500-international unit/mL concentration is available in preservative-free, single-dose, prefilled syringes containing 2500 international units/0.2 mL.[3403] The 25,000-international unit/mL concentration is available in preservative-free, single-dose, prefilled syringes containing 5000 international units/0.2 mL, 7500 international units/0.3 mL, 12,500 international units/0.5 mL, 15,000 international units/0.6 mL, and 18,000 international units/0.72 mL.[3403] Sodium chloride also may be present.[3403]

Dalteparin sodium injection solution also is available in 3.8-mL multidose vials with each mL containing 25,000 anti-factor Xa international units in water for injection; the solution is preserved with benzyl alcohol 14 mg/mL.[3403]

pH

The pH of both the unpreserved and preserved injection solutions ranges from 5 to 7.5.[3403]

Units

Each milligram of dalteparin sodium is equivalent to 156.25 anti-factor Xa international units.[3403]

Trade Name(s)

Fragmin

Administration

Dalteparin sodium injection solution is administered by deep subcutaneous injection to patients who are seated or lying down; administration sites should be alternated among a U-shaped area around the navel, the upper outer side of the thigh, and the upper outer quadrangle of the buttock.[3403] Dalteparin sodium injection solution must *not* be administered by intramuscular injection.[3403]

To avoid loss of drug when administering the 12,500- and 25,000-international unit/mL single-dose, prefilled syringes, the air bubble from the syringe should *not* be expelled prior to injection of the drug.[3403]

The manufacturer states that dalteparin sodium should not be mixed with other injections or infusions unless specific compatibility data are available that support such mixing.[3403]

Stability

Intact containers of dalteparin sodium should be stored at controlled room temperature.[3403] Dalteparin sodium injection solution in prefilled syringes and vials should be visually inspected for particulate matter and discoloration prior to administration.[3403]

Multidose vials of dalteparin sodium are stable at room temperature for up to 2 weeks from initial vial puncture; any unused solution remaining after 2 weeks should be discarded.[3403]

Syringes

Dalteparin sodium (Pharmacia & Upjohn) 10,000 international units/mL was packaged in 1-mL polypropylene tuberculin syringes (Becton Dickinson), apparently with the needles left attached, and stored at 25°C exposed to fluorescent light and 2 to 5°C in the dark for 15 days.[2323] Chromogenic assays of the dalteparin activity were variable, but there was no indication of substantial loss of activity.[2323] Dalteparin activity remained at 95% or above of the initial level throughout.[2323] An 8% loss of the benzyl alcohol preservative occurred in 10 days and a 10% loss in 15 days in the samples stored at 25°C.[2323] Benzyl alcohol losses from samples stored at 2 to 5°C were minimal.[2323] Unfortunately, many syringes became nonfunctional during the study with the fluid unable to be expressed through the attached needles, thus necessitating removal of the needles.[2323] The cause of this needle blockage was not addressed.[2323]

Dalteparin sodium (Pharmacia & Upjohn) 10,000 international units/mL from preservative-free ampules and 25,000 international units/mL from multidose vials preserved with benzyl alcohol was packaged in 1-mL (Becton Dickinson) and 3-mL (Sherwood) plastic syringes and stored for 30 days at room temperature and 4°C.[2484] Dalteparin sodium (Pharmacia & Upjohn) 10,000 international units/mL from multidose vials preserved with benzyl alcohol was packaged as 0.75 mL and 1 mL in 1-mL (Becton Dickinson) and 3-mL (Sherwood) plastic syringes, respectively, and stored for 30 days at room temperature and 4°C.[2484] No loss of anti-factor Xa activity was found.[2484]

In another report, the stability of dalteparin sodium (manufacturer unspecified) 25,000 units/mL from multidose vials packaged in 1-mL polypropylene tuberculin syringes (manufacturer unspecified) was evaluated over 10 days stored at 22 and 4°C.[2546] Losses of 7 and 4%, respectively, were found at the two storage temperatures; however, 8 of 45 test syringes stored at 22°C could not be operated to eject the drug.[2546] None of the refrigerated samples exhibited this failure.[2546] The authors speculated that precipitation had resulted in blockage.[2546]

Dalteparin sodium (manufacturer unspecified) 25,000-units/mL injection solution from multidose vials diluted in sodium chloride 0.9% to 2500 units/mL was packaged in tuberculin syringes (manufacturer unspecified) and stored for 28 days under refrigeration at 4°C.[2774] Anti-Xa activity determined by chromogenic assay found no significant differences over the course of 28 days.[2774]

DOI: 10.37573/9781585286850.109

Dalteparin sodium (Pfizer) injection solution (as 10,000-units/mL prefilled syringe) diluted in sodium chloride 0.9% to 1000 units/mL and packaged as 0.5 mL in 1-mL polypropylene tuberculin syringes (Monoject) fitted with Luer-Lok tip caps (Becton Dickinson) was physically and chemically stable for 30 days under refrigeration at 2 to 8°C when exposed to ambient fluorescent light.[3404]

Selected Revisions June 1, 2019. © Copyright, October 2002. American Society of Health-System Pharmacists, Inc.

Dantrolene Sodium
AHFS 12:20.08

Products

Dantrolene sodium (Dantrium, Par; Revonto, US WorldMeds) is available as a lyophilized powder in vials containing 20 mg of dantrolene sodium.[3159] [3160] Each vial also contains mannitol 3000 mg and sodium hydroxide to adjust the pH.[3159] [3160] The powder should be reconstituted by adding 60 mL of sterile water for injection (without a bacteriostatic agent) to each vial; dextrose 5%, sodium chloride 0.9%, and other acidic solutions are incompatible with the drug and should not be used for reconstitution.[3159] [3160] Vials should be shaken for approximately 20 seconds[3160] or until the reconstituted solution is clear.[3159] [3160] For prophylactic infusion, the contents of the appropriate number of dantrolene vials should be transferred to a sterile intravenous plastic bag; large glass bottles should not be used because precipitate formation has been observed with the use of some glass bottles.[3159] [3160] Reconstituted solutions should be visually inspected for particulate matter, discoloration, cloudiness and/or precipitation prior to administration; such solutions should not be used.[3159] [3160]

Dantrolene sodium (Ryanodex, Eagle) also is available as a lyophilized powder in single-use vials containing 250 mg of dantrolene sodium.[3161] Each vial also contains mannitol 125 mg, polysorbate 80 25 mg, povidone 4 mg, and sodium hydroxide or hydrochloric acid to adjust the pH.[3161] The powder should be reconstituted by adding 5 mL of sterile water for injection (without a bacteriostatic agent) to each vial; other solutions (e.g., dextrose 5%, sodium chloride 0.9%) should not be used.[3161] Vials should be shaken until the contents form an orange-colored uniform suspension.[3161] The reconstituted suspension should be visually inspected for particulate matter and discoloration prior to administration.[3161] The reconstituted suspension should not be diluted or transferred to another container for infusion.[3161]

pH

The reconstituted solution of dantrolene sodium (Dantrium, Par; Revonto, US WorldMeds) has a pH of approximately 9.5.[3159] [3160]

The reconstituted suspension of dantrolene sodium (Ryanodex Eagle) has a pH of approximately 10.3.[3161]

Trade Name(s)

Dantrium, Revonto, Ryanodex

Administration

Dantrolene sodium (Dantrium, Revonto) solution is administered by continuous rapid intravenous push injection or, for prophylactic use, as an intravenous infusion over approximately 1 hour.[3159] [3160]

Dantrolene sodium (Ryanodex) suspension is administered by intravenous push (bolus) injection, or, for prophylactic use, intravenously over at least 1 minute.[3161] The drug should be administered into an intravenous catheter while an intravenous infusion solution of sodium chloride 0.9% or dextrose 5% is freely infusing or into a patent indwelling catheter without a freely running infusion solution, in which case the line should be flushed following administration of dantrolene sodium to remove residual drug from the catheter.[3161]

Care should be taken to prevent extravasation of the reconstituted dantrolene sodium solutions or suspension into the surrounding tissues due to the high pH of the formulations and the potential for tissue necrosis.[3159] [3160] [3161]

Stability

Intact vials should be stored at controlled room temperature; prolonged exposure to light should be avoided.[3159] [3160] [3161]

The reconstituted solution should be stored at 15 to 30°C[3159] or 20 to 25°C[3160] and protected from direct light;[3159] [3160] the reconstituted suspension should be stored at 20 to 25°C.[3161] The reconstituted solutions or suspension must be used within 6 hours after reconstitution.[3159] [3160] [3161] Solutions for prophylactic infusion should be prepared immediately prior to administration but are stated to be stable for 6 hours.[3159] [3160]

Additional Compatibility Information
Infusion Solutions

Dantrolene sodium (Ryanodex) suspension may be administered into an intravenous catheter while an intravenous infusion solution of sodium chloride 0.9% or dextrose 5% is freely infusing.[3161]

DOI: 10.37573/9781585286850.110

Daptomycin
AHFS 8:12.28.12

Products

Daptomycin is available in 2 different formulations: daptomycin (Cubicin, Merck; generic) and Cubicin RF (Merck).[2977] [3221] The formulations differ in storage requirements and directions for reconstitution; in addition, there are differences in stability of the products following reconstitution or dilution.[2977] [3221]

Daptomycin (Cubicin, Merck; generic) is available as a lyophilized powder or cake in 500-mg single-dose vials with sodium hydroxide to adjust the pH.[2977] [3222] Each vial should be reconstituted slowly with 10 mL of sodium chloride 0.9% using a beveled, 21-gauge or smaller transfer needle or a needleless device to direct the stream of diluent against the vial wall.[2977] [3222] The vial should be gently rotated to ensure that all of the daptomycin powder becomes wetted.[2977] [3222] The reconstituted vial should be allowed to stand undisturbed for 10 minutes, then gently rotated or swirled to ensure complete dissolution.[2977] [3222] Vigorous agitation or shaking of the vial should be avoided to minimize foaming.[2977] [3222] The reconstituted solution has a daptomycin concentration of 50 mg/mL.[2977] [3222]

Cubicin RF (Merck) is available as a lyophilized powder in 500-mg single-dose vials.[3221] Each vial also contains sucrose 713 mg and sodium hydroxide to adjust the pH.[3221] Each vial should be reconstituted *only* with 10 mL of sterile water for injection or bacteriostatic water for injection; a syringe with a beveled, 21-gauge or smaller transfer needle should be used to slowly direct the stream of diluent against the vial wall.[3221] Saline-based diluents must *not* be used to reconstitute Cubicin RF because the resulting solution is hyperosmotic and may lead to infusion-site reactions if administered as a direct injection (e.g., over 2 minutes).[3221] The vial should be rotated or swirled for a few minutes, as needed, to ensure complete dissolution of the powder.[3221] The reconstituted solution has a daptomycin concentration of 50 mg/mL.[3221]

pH

The pH of the 50-mg/mL reconstituted solution of Cubicin RF is 6.8.[3221]

Trade Name(s)

Cubicin, Cubicin RF

Administration

Daptomycin is administered by intravenous injection (*only* in adult patients) or by intravenous infusion (in adult and pediatric patients).[2977] [3221] [3222]

For intravenous injection in adult patients *only*, the appropriate volume of the reconstituted solution should be withdrawn from the vial using a syringe with a beveled, 21-gauge or smaller needle and may be administered without further dilution over 2 minutes.[2977] [3221] [3222] The drug should *not* be administered to pediatric patients by direct intravenous injection.[2977] [3221]

To prepare intravenous infusions of daptomycin, a syringe with a beveled, 21-gauge or smaller needle should be used to withdraw the appropriate volume of reconstituted solution from the vial and transfer the drug to a bag containing the appropriate volume of infusion solution.[2977] [3221] [3222]

For intravenous infusion in adult patients, the appropriate volume of the reconstituted solution should be withdrawn from the vial and transferred to an infusion bag containing 50 mL of sodium chloride 0.9% to be administered over 30 minutes.[2977] [3221] [3222]

For intravenous infusion in pediatric patients 1–6 years of age, the appropriate volume of the reconstituted solution should be withdrawn from the vial and transferred to an infusion bag containing 25 mL of sodium chloride 0.9%.[2977] [3221] The diluted solution should be administered over 60 minutes; the infusion rate should be maintained at 0.42 mL/min over the 60-minute period of infusion.[2977] [3221] The manufacturer states that the drug should be avoided in infants younger than 12 months of age based on adverse effects observed in animals.[2977] [3221]

For intravenous infusion in pediatric patients 7–17 years of age, the appropriate volume of the reconstituted solution should be withdrawn from the vial and transferred to an infusion bag containing 50 mL of sodium chloride 0.9%.[2977] [3221] The diluted solution should be administered over 30 minutes; the infusion rate should be maintained at 1.67 mL/min over the 30-minute period of infusion.[2977] [3221]

If a common infusion line is being used to administer other drugs, the line should be flushed with a compatible infusion solution prior to and following infusion of daptomycin.[2977] [3221] [3222]

Stability

Daptomycin is a pale yellow to light brown powder or cake that forms a pale yellow to light brown solution upon reconstitution.[2977] [3221] [3222] Vials of daptomycin are for single dose only; any unused portion should be discarded.[2977] [3221] [3222]

Intact vials of daptomycin (Cubicin, Merck; generic) should be stored under refrigeration at 2 to 8°C.[2977] [3222] Although refrigerated storage is required, one manufacturer has stated that the drug may be stored at room temperature for 12 months.[2745] Exposure to excessive heat should be avoided.[2977] [3222] When reconstituted as directed, this formulation of daptomycin is stable in the vial for 12 hours at room temperature and up to 48 hours under refrigeration at 2 to 8°C; once diluted for infusion, the drug also is stable in the infusion bag for 12 hours at room temperature and 48 hours under refrigeration at 2 to 8°C.[2977] [3222] However, the time after reconstitution in the vial and after dilution for infusion in the bag should not exceed a combined time of 12 hours at room temperature or 48 hours under refrigeration for this formulation.[2977] [3222]

Intact vials of the Cubicin RF (Merck) formulation of daptomycin should be stored at controlled room temperature.[3221] When reconstituted as directed with sterile water for injection, Cubicin RF is stable in the vial for 1 day at 20 to 25°C or

DOI: 10.37573/9781585286850.111

3 days at 2 to 8°C; if diluted in sodium chloride 0.9% immediately following reconstitution, the drug is stable in the infusion bag for 19 hours at 20 to 25°C or 3 days at 2 to 8°C.[3221] When reconstituted as directed with bacteriostatic water for injection, Cubicin RF is stable in the vial for 2 days at 20 to 25°C or 3 days at 2 to 8°C; if diluted in sodium chloride 0.9% immediately following reconstitution, the drug is stable in the infusion bag for 2 days at 20 to 25°C or 5 days at 2 to 8°C.[3221]

The manufacturer states that daptomycin is *not* compatible in dextrose-containing solutions.[2977 3221 3222] (See Additional Compatibility Information: Peritoneal Dialysis Solutions.)

Syringes

The Cubicin RF formulation of daptomycin reconstituted with sterile water for injection to yield a concentration of 50 mg/mL and packaged in polypropylene syringes with an elastomeric plunger stopper is stable for 1 day at 20 to 25°C or 3 days at 2 to 8°C; when similarly reconstituted with bacteriostatic water for injection, the drug is stable for 2 days at 20 to 25°C or 5 days at 2 to 8°C.[3221]

Ambulatory Pumps

During stability studies of daptomycin stored in ReadyMed elastomeric infusion pumps, an impurity (i.e., 2-mercaptobenzothiazole) was found to leach from the pump system into the daptomycin solution.[2977 3221 3222] Therefore, manufacturers state that the drug should not be used in conjunction with ReadyMed elastomeric infusion pumps.[2977 3221 3222]

Filtration

A study was performed on the compatibility of various syringe filters with the Cubicin (Cubist) formulation of daptomycin after reconstitution of each vial with 10 mL of sodium chloride 0.9%.[3198 3199] Visual assessment and potency of the filtered solution were compared with those of the unfiltered control.[3198 3199] No changes in color or clarity occurred.[3198 3199] Decreases in potency of the reconstituted and filtered solutions compared with the reconstituted and unfiltered solutions ranged from 0.39 to 2.23%.[3198 3199] The syringe filters noted in Table 1 were found to be compatible with the reconstituted drug.[3198 3199]

Table 1. Syringe filters compatible with reconstituted Cubicin[3198 3199]

Manufacturer	Syringe Filter
Covidien	Monoject 5-μm stainless steel (M305)
Becton Dickinson	Nokor 5-μm acrylic copolymer/nylon (305200)
Millipore	Millex-GS 0.22-μm mixed cellulose esters (SLGS025NB)
Millipore	Millex-GV 0.22-μm polyvinylidene difluoride (SLGV033NS)
Thermo	Scientific/Nalgene 0.2-μm nylon (195-2520)

Compatibility Information

Solution Compatibility

Daptomycin

Test Soln Name	Mfr	Mfr	Conc/L or %	Remarks	Ref	C/I
Dextrose 5%		ME[a]		Incompatible with dextrose-containing solutions	2977	I
Dextrose 5%		ME[b]		Incompatible with dextrose-containing solutions	3221	I
Dextrose 5%		FRK		Incompatible with dextrose-containing solutions	3222	I
Ringer's injection, lactated		ME[a]		Stated to be compatible	2977	C
Ringer's injection, lactated		FRK		Stated to be compatible	3222	C
Sodium chloride 0.9%		ME[a]		Stable for 12 hr at room temperature or 48 hr at 2 to 8°C	2977	C
Sodium chloride 0.9%		FRK		Stable for 12 hr at room temperature or 48 hr at 2 to 8°C	3222	C
Sodium chloride 0.9%		ME[b]	c	Stable for 19 hr at 20 to 25°C or 3 days at 2 to 8°C	3221	C
Sodium chloride 0.9%		ME[b]	d	Stable for 2 days at 20 to 25°C or 5 days at 2 to 8°C	3221	C

[a] Test performed using the Cubicin formulation.

[b] Test performed using the Cubicin RF formulation.

[c] Reconstituted with sterile water for injection.

[d] Reconstituted with bacteriostatic water for injection.

Y-Site Injection Compatibility (1:1 Mixture)

Daptomycin

Test Drug	Mfr	Conc	Mfr	Conc	Remarks	Ref	C/I
Aztreonam	BMS	16.7 mg/mL[a][b]	CUB[d]	16.7 mg/mL[a][b]	Physically compatible with little loss of either drug in 2 hr at 25°C	2553	C
Blinatumomab	AMG	0.125 and 0.375 mcg/mL[b]	MSD	6.1 mg/mL[b]	Particles, flakes, thin needles, or haze transiently appears	3405, 3417	?
Cangrelor tetrasodium	TMC	1 mg/mL[b]	e	10 mg/mL[b]	Physically compatible for 4 hr	3243	C
Caspofungin acetate	ME	0.7 mg/mL[b]	CUB[d]	10 mg/mL[b]	Physically compatible for 4 hr at room temperature	2758	C
Ceftazidime	GSK	16.7 mg/mL[a][b]	CUB[d]	16.7 mg/mL[a][b]	Physically compatible with no loss of either drug in 2 hr at 25°C	2553	C
Ceftazidime–avibactam sodium	ALL	20 mg/mL[h][i]			Physically compatible for up to 4 hr at room temperature	3004	C
Ceftolozane sulfate–tazobactam sodium	CUB	10 mg/mL[b][f]	CUB[d]	10 mg/mL[b]	Physically compatible for 2 hr	3247, 3262	C
Ceftriaxone sodium	RC	16.7 mg/mL[a][b]	CUB[d]	16.7 mg/mL[a][b]	Physically compatible with 4 to 5% loss of both drugs in 2 hr at 25°C	2553	C
Dopamine HCl	AMR	3.6 mg/mL[a]	CUB[d]	18.2 mg/mL[a][b]	Physically compatible with no loss of either drug in 2 hr at 25°C	2553	C
Doripenem	JJ	5 mg/mL[a][b]	CUB[d]	10 mg/mL[b]	Physically compatible for 4 hr at 23°C	2743	C
Fluconazole	PF	1.3 mg/mL[a]	CUB[d]	6.3 mg/mL[a][b]	Physically compatible. No daptomycin loss and 4% fluconazole loss in 2 hr at 25°C	2553	C
Gentamicin sulfate	AB	1.5 mg/mL[a]	CUB[d]	19.2 mg/mL[a][b]	Physically compatible with no loss of either drug in 2 hr at 25°C	2553	C
Heparin sodium	ES	98 units/mL[a][b]	CUB[d]	19.6 mg/mL[a][b]	Physically compatible with no loss of either drug in 2 hr at 25°C	2553	C
Isavuconazonium sulfate	ASP	1.5 mg/mL[b]	CUB[d]	10 mg/mL[b]	Physically compatible for 2 hr	3247, 3263	C
Letermovir	ME	[b]		[b]	Physically compatible	3398	C
Levofloxacin	OMN	7.1 mg/mL[a][b]	CUB[d]	14.3 mg/mL[a][b]	Physically compatible with no loss of either drug in 2 hr at 25°C	2553	C
Lidocaine HCl	ASZ	3.3 mg/mL[a][b]	CUB[d]	16.7 mg/mL[a][b]	Physically compatible with no loss of either drug in 2 hr at 25°C	2553	C
Meropenem–vaborbactam	TMC	8 mg/mL[b][g]	TE	20 mg/mL[b]	Immediate change in measured turbidity. pH increased by 2 units within 3 hr	3380	I
Plazomicin sulfate	ACH	24 mg/mL[b]	TE	20 mg/mL[b]	Measured turbidity increases immediately	3432	I
Posaconazole	ME	18 mg/mL		20 mg/mL[c]	Physically compatible	2911, 2912	C
Tedizolid phosphate	CUB	0.8 mg/mL[b]	CUB[d]	10 mg/mL[b]	Physically compatible for 2 hr	3244	C

[a] Final concentration after mixing.

[b] Tested in sodium chloride 0.9%.

[c] Tested in both dextrose 5% and sodium chloride 0.9%.

[d] Test performed using the Cubicin formulation.

[e] Formulation not specified.

[f] Ceftolozane component. Ceftolozane in a 2:1 fixed-ratio concentration with tazobactam.

[g] Meropenem component. Meropenem in a 1:1 fixed-ratio concentration with vaborbactam.

[h] Ceftazidime component. Ceftazidime in a 4:1 fixed-ratio concentration with avibactam.

[i] Tested in dextrose 5%, sodium chloride 0.9%, and Ringer's injection, lactated.

Additional Compatibility Information

Peritoneal Dialysis Solutions

Daptomycin (Cubicin, Novartis) 20 mg/L was physically compatible with both Physioneal 35 with dextrose 1.36% (Baxter) and Physioneal 35 with dextrose 2.27% (Baxter) peritoneal dialysis solutions at 25°C for up to 24 hours in polyvinyl chloride (PVC) containers.[2979] Daptomycin also was physically compatible with both of these solutions at 37°C for up to 6 hours in PVC containers.[2979]

Daptomycin (Cubicin, Cubist) 50 mg/L, 100 mg/L, and 200 mg/L was physically compatible with Physioneal 40 with 1.36% dextrose (Baxter) and Nutrineal (Baxter) at 4, 25, and 37°C in PVC and glass containers for at least 24 hours.[2980]

Heparin Locks

A combination of daptomycin (Cubicin, Cubist) 5 mg/mL and heparin sodium (Hospira) 100 units/mL in Ringer's injection, lactated was evaluated for stability as a lock solution stored in 5-mL aliquots in 5-mL polypropylene syringes (Becton Dickinson) at 4 and −20°C.[2978] The solution remained clear and colorless on visual inspection and little or no loss of either drug occurred throughout the 14-day study period.[2978]

Selected Revisions May 1, 2020. © Copyright, October 2006. American Society of Health-System Pharmacists, Inc.

Daunorubicin–Cytarabine Liposomal
AHFS 10:00

Products

The fixed combination of daunorubicin–cytarabine liposomal is available as a purple, lyophilized cake in single-dose (preservative-free) vials containing 44 mg of daunorubicin and 100 mg of cytarabine encapsulated in liposomes.[3369] Each vial also contains distearoyl phosphatidylcholine (DSPC) 454 mg, distearoyl phosphatidylglycerol (DSPG) 132 mg, and cholesterol HP 32 mg, which form the liposomal membrane, as well as copper gluconate 100 mg, triethanolamine 4 mg, and sucrose 2.054 g.[3369]

CAUTION: Care should be taken to ensure that the correct drug product, dose, and administration procedures are used and that no confusion with other products occurs. Although other daunorubicin and cytarabine products exist, they are sufficiently different from daunorubicin–cytarabine liposomal that extrapolating information to or from other formulations or substituting other products is inappropriate.[3369]

To prepare a diluted solution for infusion, the number of vials of the drug required to achieve the appropriate dose (based on the daunorubicin component) should be allowed to equilibrate to room temperature for 30 minutes.[3369] Each vial should then be reconstituted with 19 mL of sterile water for injection.[3369] Using a timer set for 5 minutes, each vial should be swirled, gently inverting the vial every 30 seconds.[3369] Vials should not be heated, vortexed, or shaken vigorously.[3369] Each mL of the resulting reconstituted product contains 2.2 mg of daunorubicin and 5 mg of cytarabine.[3369] The reconstituted product should be allowed to rest for 15 minutes.[3369] After resting, each vial should be gently inverted 5 times prior to withdrawing the total volume required of the reconstituted product and transferring this volume to an infusion bag containing 500 mL of sodium chloride 0.9% or dextrose 5%.[3369] The bag should be gently inverted to mix the solution.[3369]

Copper Content

The reconstituted daunorubicin–cytarabine product contains copper gluconate 5 mg/mL, 14% of which is elemental copper.[3369] Copper gluconate is required for stable daunorubicin encapsulation inside the liposome.[1711]

Trade Name(s)

Vyxeos

Administration

Daunorubicin–cytarabine liposomal should be administered only by the intravenous route; the drug should *not* be administered by the intramuscular or subcutaneous routes.[3369]

Diluted solutions of daunorubicin–cytarabine liposomal for infusion should be administered at a constant rate over 90 minutes through a central venous catheter or a peripherally inserted central catheter (PICC) using an infusion pump.[3369] The line used to administer the drug should be flushed with sodium chloride 0.9% or dextrose 5% following completion of the infusion.[3369] Interruption of the infusion, reduction in the rate of infusion, or discontinuance of the drug may be necessary if hypersensitivity reactions occur; the product labeling should be consulted for additional details on management of hypersensitivity reactions.[3369]

Severe local necrosis has occurred with extravasation of daunorubicin; care should be taken to avoid extravasation.[3369]

As with other toxic drugs, applicable special handling and disposal procedures for daunorubicin–cytarabine liposomal should be followed.[3369]

CAUTION: Care should be taken to ensure that the correct drug product, dose, and administration procedures are used and that no confusion with other products occurs.

Stability

Intact vials of daunorubicin–cytarabine liposomal for injection should be stored under refrigeration at 2 to 8°C.[3369] Vials should be stored upright and in the original carton to protect from light.[3369] The reconstituted product is a homogenous opaque purple dispersion essentially free of visible particulates; a homogenous translucent deep purple dispersion free from visible particulates forms upon dilution in sodium chloride 0.9% or dextrose 5%.[3369] The solution should be visually inspected for particulate matter and discoloration prior to administration; only solutions without visible particles should be administered.[3369]

The reconstituted product, if not diluted immediately, is stable for up to 4 hours at 2 to 8°C; the diluted solution for infusion, if not administered immediately following dilution of the reconstituted product, is stable for up to 4 hours at 2 to 8°C.[3369] Any unused portion should be discarded.[3369]

Filtration

Diluted solutions of daunorubicin–cytarabine liposomal for infusion should *not* be infused through an inline filter.[3369]

DOI: 10.37573/9781585286850.112

Compatibility Information

Solution Compatibility

Daunorubicin–cytarabine liposomal

Test Soln Name	Mfr	Mfr	Conc/L or %	Remarks	Ref	C/I
Dextrose 5%		JAZ		Stable for up to 4 hr at 2 to 8°C	3369	C
Sodium chloride 0.9%		JAZ		Stable for up to 4 hr at 2 to 8°C	3369	C

Daunorubicin Hydrochloride
AHFS 10:00

Products

Daunorubicin hydrochloride injection is available as a 5-mg/mL solution in single-dose vials containing daunorubicin base 20 mg.[2950] Each mL also contains sodium chloride 9 mg, hydrochloric acid to adjust the pH, and water for injection.[2950]

CAUTION: Care should be taken to ensure that the correct drug product, dose, and administration procedures are used and that no confusion with other products occurs.

pH

From 3 to 4.[2950]

Trade Name(s)

Cerubidine

Administration

Daunorubicin hydrochloride is administered intravenously *only*.[2950] The drug must never be given by the intramuscular or subcutaneous routes.[2950] Extravasation will result in severe local tissue necrosis.[2950]

The dose may be diluted by drawing the desired dose into a syringe containing 10 to 15 mL of sodium chloride 0.9% and injecting the contents into the sidearm or tubing of a rapidly flowing intravenous infusion of dextrose 5% or sodium chloride 0.9%.[2950]

In the event of spills or leaks, Wyeth-Ayerst recommends the use of sodium hypochlorite 5% (household bleach) to inactivate daunorubicin hydrochloride until a colorless liquid results.[1200]

CAUTION: Care should be taken to ensure that the correct drug product, dose, and administration procedures are used and that no confusion with other products occurs.

Stability

Intact vials of daunorubicin hydrochloride injection should be stored under refrigeration at 2 to 8°C in the original carton to protect from light.[2950] The manufacturer states that the solution prepared for administration is stable for 24 hours at 20 to 25°C.[2950]

Immersion of a needle with an aluminum component in daunorubicin hydrochloride (Ives) 5 mg/mL resulted in a darkening of the solution, with black patches forming on the aluminum in 12 to 24 hours at 24°C with protection from light.[988]

pH Effects

Daunorubicin hydrochloride appears to have pH-dependent stability in solution.[526][1250] Solutions of daunorubicin hydrochloride are less stable at pH values above 8. Decomposition occurs, as indicated by a color change from red to blue-purple. The drug becomes progressively more stable as the pH of drug–infusion solution admixtures becomes more acidic, from 7.4 down to 4.5.[526] The pH range of maximum stability was reported to be approximately 4.5 to 5.5. Below pH 4, decomposition increases substantially.[1207]

Light Effects

Protection of the injection from light is recommended.[2950] Photoinactivation of daunorubicin hydrochloride exposed to radiation of 366 nm and fluorescent light has been reported.[1094] One source indicates that significant losses due to light exposure for a sufficient time may occur at concentrations below 100 mcg/mL.[1369] However, in clinical concentrations at or above 500 mcg/mL, no special light protection appeared to be necessary.[1369]

Syringes

Daunorubicin hydrochloride (Rhone-Poulenc) 2 mg/mL in polypropylene syringes exhibited little loss in 43 days at 4°C.[1460]

Filtration

Daunorubicin hydrochloride binds only slightly to cellulose acetate/nitrate (Millex OR) and polytetrafluoroethylene (Millex FG) filters.[1249][1415][1416]

Compatibility Information

Solution Compatibility

Daunorubicin HCl

Test Soln Name	Mfr	Mfr	Conc/L or %	Remarks	Ref	C/I
Dextrose 3.3% in sodium chloride 0.3%		RP	100 mg	5% or less loss in 4 weeks at 25°C in the dark	1007	C
Dextrose 5%	AB	NCI	20 mg	Physically compatible with 2% loss in 24 hr at 21°C	526	C
Dextrose 5%		RP	100 mg	5% or less loss in 4 weeks at 25°C in the dark	1007	C
Dextrose 5%	a	BEL	16 mg	No loss in 7 days at 4°C protected from light	1700	C
Dextrose 5%	TR[a]	RP	100 mg	7% or less loss in 43 days at 4 and 25°C in the dark and at –20°C	1460	C

DOI: 10.37573/9781585286850.113

Solution Compatibility (Cont.)

Test Soln Name	Mfr	Mfr	Conc/L or %	Remarks	Ref	C/I
Dextrose 5%		BEL	15.7 mg	5 to 8% loss in 48 hr at room temperature, exposed to light and in the dark, and at 4°C	1955	C
Ringer's injection, lactated	AB	NCI	20 mg	Physically compatible. 5% loss in 24 hr at 21°C	526	C
Ringer's injection, lactated		RP	100 mg	5% or less loss in 4 weeks at 25°C in the dark	1007	C
Sodium chloride 0.9%	AB	NCI	20 mg	Physically compatible. 3% loss in 24 hr at 21°C	526	C
Sodium chloride 0.9%		RP	100 mg	5% or less loss in 4 weeks at 25°C in the dark	1007	C
Sodium chloride 0.9%	a	BEL	16 mg	No loss in 7 days at 4°C protected from light	1700	C
Sodium chloride 0.9%	TRa	RP	100 mg	10% or less loss in 43 days at 4 and 25°C in the dark and at −20°C	1460	C

a Tested in PVC containers.

Additive Compatibility

Daunorubicin HCl

Test Drug	Mfr	Conc/L or %	Mfr	Conc/L or %	Test Solution	Remarks	Ref	C/I
Cytarabine with etoposide	UP BR	267 mg 400 mg	RP	33 mg	D5½S	Physically compatible with about 6% cytarabine loss and no loss of other drugs in 72 hr at 20°C	1162	C
Cytarabine with etoposide	UP SZ	157 mg 157 mg	BEL	15.7 mg	D5W	Less than 10% loss of any drug in 48 hr at room temperature, exposed to light and in the dark, and at 4°C	1955	C
Dexamethasone sodium phosphate						Immediate milky precipitation	524	I
Etoposide with cytarabine	BR UP	400 mg 267 mg	RP	33 mg	D5½S	Physically compatible with about 6% cytarabine loss and no loss of other drugs in 72 hr at 20°C	1162	C
Etoposide with cytarabine	SZ UP	157 mg 157 mg	BEL	15.7 mg	D5W	Less than 10% loss of any drug in 48 hr at room temperature, exposed to light and in the dark, and at 4°C	1955	C
Heparin sodium	UP	4000 units	FA	200 mg	D5W	Physically incompatible	15	I
Hydrocortisone sodium succinate	UP	500 mg	FA	200 mg	D5W	Physically compatible	15	C

Y-Site Injection Compatibility (1:1 Mixture)

Daunorubicin HCl

Test Drug	Mfr	Conc	Mfr	Conc	Remarks	Ref	C/I
Allopurinol sodium	BW	3 mg/mLb	WY	1 mg/mLb	Reddish-purple color and haze form immediately. Reddish-brown particles form within 1 hr	1686	I
Amifostine	USB	10 mg/mLa	WY	1 mg/mLa	Physically compatible for 4 hr at 23°C	1845	C
Anidulafungin	VIC	0.5 mg/mLa	BED	1 mg/mLa	Physically compatible for 4 hr at 23°C	2617	C
Aztreonam	SQ	40 mg/mLa	WY	1 mg/mLa	Haze forms immediately	1758	I
Caspofungin acetate	ME	0.7 mg/mLb	BED	1 mg/mLb	Physically compatible for 4 hr at room temperature	2758	C
Etoposide phosphate	BR	5 mg/mLa	BED	1 mg/mLa	Physically compatible for 4 hr at 23°C	2218	C
Filgrastim	AMG	30 mcg/mLa	WY	1 mg/mLa	Physically compatible for 4 hr at 22°C	1687	C
Fludarabine phosphate	BX	1 mg/mLa	WY	2 mg/mLa	Slight haze forms in 4 hr at 22°C	1439	I

Y-Site Injection Compatibility (1:1 Mixture) (Cont.)

Test Drug	Mfr	Conc	Mfr	Conc	Remarks	Ref	C/I
Gemcitabine HCl	LI	10 mg/mL[b]	BED	1 mg/mL[b]	Physically compatible for 4 hr at 23°C	2226	C
Granisetron HCl	SKB	0.05 mg/mL[a]	CHI	1 mg/mL[a]	Physically compatible for 4 hr at 23°C	2000	C
Melphalan HCl	BW	0.1 mg/mL[b]	WY	1 mg/mL[b]	Physically compatible for 3 hr at 22°C	1557	C
Methotrexate sodium		30 mg/mL	BEL	0.52 mg/mL[a]	Visually compatible for 4 hr at room temperature	1788	C
Ondansetron HCl	GL	1 mg/mL[b]	WY	2 mg/mL[a]	Visually compatible for 4 hr at 22°C	1365	C
Piperacillin sodium–tazobactam sodium	LE[d]	40 mg/mL[a e]	WY	1 mg/mL[a]	Turbidity increases immediately	1688	I
Sodium bicarbonate		1.4%	BEL	0.52 mg/mL[a]	Visually compatible for 4 hr at room temperature	1788	C
Teniposide	BR	0.1 mg/mL[a]	WY	1 mg/mL[a]	Physically compatible for 4 hr at 23°C	1725	C
Thiotepa	IMM[c]	1 mg/mL[a]	WY	1 mg/mL[a]	Physically compatible for 4 hr at 23°C	1861	C
Vinorelbine tartrate	BW	1 mg/mL[b]	WY	1 mg/mL[b]	Physically compatible for 4 hr at 22°C	1558	C

[a] Tested in dextrose 5%.

[b] Tested in sodium chloride 0.9%.

[c] Lyophilized formulation tested.

[d] Test performed using the formulation WITHOUT edetate disodium.

[e] Piperacillin component. Piperacillin in an 8:1 fixed-ratio concentration with tazobactam.

Selected Revisions June 26, 2018. © Copyright, October 1982.
American Society of Health-System Pharmacists, Inc.

Deferoxamine Mesylate
AHFS 64:00

Products

Deferoxamine mesylate is available in vials containing 500 mg and 2 g of sterile drug in dry form. For intramuscular injection, reconstitute the 500-mg and 2-g vials with 2 and 8 mL, respectively, to yield solutions providing deferoxamine mesylate 213 mg/mL. For intravenous and subcutaneous infusion, reconstitute the 500-mg and 2-g vials with 5 and 20 mL, respectively, to yield solutions providing deferoxamine mesylate 95 mg/mL.[1(2/09)]

Tonicity

Reconstituted deferoxamine 95 mg/mL is isotonic.[1(2/09)]

Trade Name(s)

Desferal

Administration

Deferoxamine mesylate is administered by intramuscular injection, subcutaneous infusion using a portable infusion control device, and by slow intravenous infusion after dilution at an initial rate not exceeding 15 mg/kg/hr for the first 1000 mg. Subsequent dosing should be at a decreased rate not exceeding 125 mg/hr.[1(2/09)]

Stability

Store the intact vials at temperatures not exceeding 25°C. Deferoxamine mesylate is a white to off-white powder that forms a clear colorless to yellow solution when reconstituted with sterile water for injection. The manufacturer states that reconstitution with other diluents may result in precipitation. Turbid solutions should not be used. The reconstituted solution is stable for 24 hours at room temperature. The solution should not be refrigerated.[1(2/09)]

For intravenous infusion, sodium chloride 0.9%, dextrose 5%, or Ringer's injection, lactated are recommended for use as diluents.[1(2/09)]

Syringes

Deferoxamine mesylate (Ciba-Geigy) 250 mg/mL in sterile water for injection 3 mL in 10-mL polypropylene infusion pump syringes (Pharmacia Deltec) had little loss in 14 days of storage at 30°C.[1967]

Ambulatory Pumps

Deferoxamine mesylate stability was evaluated at concentrations of 210, 285, and 370 mg/mL in sterile water for injection in PVC infusion cassette reservoirs (Pharmacia Deltec) stored at 20 to 23°C. Analysis was inconclusive because of an inordinate degree of assay variation. However, a white precipitate formed in varying time periods, depending on the concentration. Higher concentrations precipitated more rapidly than lower concentrations. In the 370-mg/mL concentration, precipitation was observed in as little as 1 day while the 285- and 210-mg/mL concentrations developed precipitation in 9 and 17 days, respectively. This study's inordinate degree of assay variability coupled with the propensity for precipitation preclude a reasonable determination of stability for these high concentrations of deferoxamine mesylate.[672]

Elastomeric Reservoir Pumps

Deferoxamine mesylate (Ciba-Geigy) 5 mg/mL in both dextrose 5% and sodium chloride 0.9% was evaluated for binding potential to natural rubber elastomeric reservoirs (Baxter). No binding was found after storage for 2 weeks at 35°C with gentle agitation.[2014]

Compatibility Information

Y-Site Injection Compatibility (1:1 Mixture)

Deferoxamine mesylate

Test Drug	Mfr	Conc	Mfr	Conc	Remarks	Ref	C/I
Defibrotide sodium	JAZ	8 mg/mL[a]	NVA	6.7 mg/mL[a]	Visually compatible for 4 hr at room temperature	3149	C

[a] Tested in sodium chloride 0.9%.

Selected Revisions March 1, 2017. © Copyright, October 1998. American Society of Health-System Pharmacists, Inc.

DOI: 10.37573/9781585286850.114

Defibrotide Sodium
AHFS 20:12.92

Products

Defibrotide sodium is available as an 80-mg/mL concentrate for injection in vials containing 2.5 mL of solution; vials contain no preservative and are intended for single-patient use.[3148] Each mL of solution also contains sodium citrate 10 mg in water for injection.[3148] Hydrochloric acid and/or sodium hydroxide may have been added to adjust the pH.[3148]

Defibrotide sodium concentrate for injection must be diluted prior to administration.[3148] The appropriate volume of the concentrate should be withdrawn from the vial and transferred to an infusion bag containing dextrose 5% or sodium chloride 0.9%.[3148] The diluted solution for infusion should be gently mixed and should have a final concentration of 4 to 20 mg/mL.[3148]

pH

Defibrotide sodium concentrate for injection has a pH ranging from 6.8 to 7.8.[3148]

Trade Name(s)

Defitelio

Administration

Defibrotide sodium is administered intravenously as an infusion over 2 hours after dilution in dextrose 5% or sodium chloride 0.9%.[3148] The final diluted solution for infusion should be administered through an infusion set containing a 0.2-μm inline filter.[3148] The intravenous infusion line being used to administer defibrotide sodium should be flushed with dextrose 5% or sodium chloride 0.9% immediately prior to and following administration of the drug.[3148]

Stability

Intact vials of defibrotide sodium should be stored at controlled room temperature.[3148] Defibrotide sodium concentrate for injection is a clear, light yellow to brown solution; the diluted solution for infusion may vary from colorless to light yellow, depending upon the diluent and the final concentration of the drug in the solution.[3148] The diluted solution for infusion should be visually inspected for particulate matter and discoloration prior to administration; only clear solutions without visible particulates should be used.[3148]

The manufacturer states that diluted solutions for infusion should be used within 4 hours if stored at room temperature or 24 hours if stored under refrigeration.[3148]

Vials are intended for single-patient use only.[3148] The manufacturer states that up to 4 doses of the diluted solution for infusion may be prepared at one time if refrigerated.[3148] Partially used vials should be discarded.[3148]

Filtration

Defibrotide solution diluted for infusion should be administered through an infusion set containing a 0.2-μm inline filter.[3148]

Compatibility Information

Solution Compatibility

Defibrotide sodium

Test Soln Name	Mfr	Mfr	Conc/L or %	Remarks	Ref	C/I
Dextrose 5%		JAZ	4 to 20 g	Use within 4 hr at room temperature or 24 hr under refrigeration	3148	C
Sodium chloride 0.9%		JAZ	4 to 20 g	Use within 4 hr at room temperature or 24 hr under refrigeration	3148	C

Y-Site Injection Compatibility (1:1 Mixture)

Defibrotide sodium

Test Drug	Mfr	Conc	Mfr	Conc	Remarks	Ref	C/I
Acetaminophen	BRN	10 mg/mL	JAZ	8 mg/mL[b]	Visually compatible for 4 hr at room temperature	3149	C
Acyclovir sodium	MYL	10 mg/mL[b]	JAZ	8 mg/mL[b]	Visually compatible for 4 hr at room temperature	3149	C
Albumin human	LFB	200 mg/mL	JAZ	8 mg/mL[b]	Visually compatible for 4 hr at room temperature	3149	C
Amikacin sulfate	MYL	5 mg/mL[b]	JAZ	8 mg/mL[b]	Solution became milky white, opaque or opalescent	3149	I
Amoxicillin sodium	PAN	40 mg/mL[b]	JAZ	8 mg/mL[b]	Visually compatible for 4 hr at room temperature	3149	C
Amphotericin B liposomal	GIL	2 mg/mL[a]	JAZ	8 mg/mL[b]	Visually compatible for 4 hr at room temperature	3149	C

DOI: 10.37573/9781585286850.115

Y-Site Injection Compatibility (1:1 Mixture) (Cont.)

Test Drug	Mfr	Conc	Mfr	Conc	Remarks	Ref	C/I
Caspofungin acetate	MCD	0.4 mg/mL[b]	JAZ	8 mg/mL[b]	Visually compatible for 4 hr at room temperature	3149	C
Ceftazidime	PAN	80 mg/mL[b]	JAZ	8 mg/mL[b]	Visually compatible for 4 hr at room temperature	3149	C
Ceftriaxone sodium	PAN	100 mg/mL[b]	JAZ	8 mg/mL[b]	Visually compatible for 4 hr at room temperature	3149	C
Ciprofloxacin	FRK	2 mg/mL	JAZ	8 mg/mL[b]	Visually compatible for 4 hr at room temperature	3149	C
Clonazepam	RC	0.02 mg/mL[b]	JAZ	8 mg/mL[b]	Visually compatible for 4 hr at room temperature	3149	C
Clonidine HCl	BI	2.4 mcg/mL[a]	JAZ	8 mg/mL[b]	Visually compatible for 4 hr at room temperature	3149	C
Cyclosporine	NVA	1.27 mg/mL[b]	JAZ	8 mg/mL[b]	Visually compatible for 4 hr at room temperature	3149	C
Deferoxamine mesylate	NVA	6.7 mg/mL[b]	JAZ	8 mg/mL[b]	Visually compatible for 4 hr at room temperature	3149	C
Fluconazole	FRK	2 mg/mL	JAZ	8 mg/mL[b]	Visually compatible for 4 hr at room temperature	3149	C
Foscarnet sodium	NVX	24 mg/mL	JAZ	8 mg/mL[b]	Visually compatible for 4 hr at room temperature	3149	C
Furosemide	REN	10 mg/mL	JAZ	8 mg/mL[b]	Slight and transient bubbling occurs only when defibrotide added to furosemide; not observed when order of mixing was reversed	3149	?
Ganciclovir sodium	RC	10 mg/mL[b]	JAZ	8 mg/mL[b]	Visually compatible for 4 hr at room temperature	3149	C
Heparin sodium	SAA	373 units/mL[b]	JAZ	8 mg/mL[b]	Visually compatible for 4 hr at room temperature	3149	C
Hydrocortisone sodium succinate	UP	1.9 mg/mL[b]	JAZ	8 mg/mL[b]	Visually compatible for 4 hr at room temperature	3149	C
Hydroxyzine HCl	REN	0.79 mg/mL[b]	JAZ	8 mg/mL[b]	Visually compatible for 4 hr at room temperature	3149	C
Imipenem–cilastatin sodium	PAN	9.94 mg/mL[b c]	JAZ	8 mg/mL[b]	Visually compatible for 4 hr at room temperature	3149	C
Mesna	BA	4.76 mg/mL[b]	JAZ	8 mg/mL[b]	Visually compatible for 4 hr at room temperature	3149	C
Methylprednisolone sodium succinate	MYL	10 mg/mL[b]	JAZ	8 mg/mL[b]	Visually compatible for 4 hr at room temperature	3149	C
Metronidazole	BRN	5 mg/mL	JAZ	8 mg/mL[b]	Visually compatible for 4 hr at room temperature	3149	C
Midazolam HCl	PAN	5 mg/mL	JAZ	8 mg/mL[b]	A fine and transient suspension forms within 2.5 hr only when midazolam HCl added to defibrotide; not observed when order of mixing was reversed	3149	?
Mycophenolate mofetil HCl	RC	11.9 mg/mL[a]	JAZ	8 mg/mL[b]	Solution became milky white and opaque	3149	I
Nalbuphine HCl	MYL	2 mg/mL[b]	JAZ	8 mg/mL[b]	Visually compatible for 4 hr at room temperature	3149	C
Naloxone HCl	MYL	0.4 mg/mL	JAZ	8 mg/mL[b]	Visually compatible for 4 hr at room temperature	3149	C
Nicardipine HCl	AGT	0.5 mg/mL[b]	JAZ	8 mg/mL[b]	Small particles form in 4 hr	3149	I
Ondansetron HCl	ACD	0.16 mg/mL[b]	JAZ	8 mg/mL[b]	Visually compatible for 4 hr at room temperature	3149	C
Pantoprazole sodium	TAK	1.6 mg/mL[b]	JAZ	8 mg/mL[b]	Visually compatible for 4 hr at room temperature	3149	C
Teicoplanin	SAA	125 mg/mL	JAZ	8 mg/mL[b]	Visually compatible for 4 hr at room temperature	3149	C
Tobramycin sulfate	ERM	10 mg/mL	JAZ	8 mg/mL[b]	Solution immediately became milky white, opaque or opalescent; precipitate formed within 2.5 hr	3149	I
Tranexamic acid	SAA	100 mg/mL	JAZ	8 mg/mL[b]	Visually compatible for 4 hr at room temperature	3149	C
Trimethoprim–sulfamethoxazole	RC	0.64 mg/mL[b d]	JAZ	8 mg/mL[b]	Visually compatible for 4 hr at room temperature	3149	C

Y-Site Injection Compatibility (1:1 Mixture) (Cont.)

Test Drug	Mfr	Conc	Mfr	Conc	Remarks	Ref	C/I
Vancomycin HCl	MYL	10.4 mg/mL[b]	JAZ	8 mg/mL[b]	Solution became milky white and opalescent. Precipitate formed within 1 hr when defibrotide added to vancomycin HCl, but developed immediately when order of mixing was reversed	3149	I

[a] Tested in dextrose 5%.

[b] Tested in sodium chloride 0.9%.

[c] Imipenem component. Imipenem in a 1:1 fixed-ratio concentration with cilastatin.

[d] Trimethoprim component. Trimethoprim in a 1:5 fixed-ratio concentration with sulfamethoxazole.

Delafloxacin Meglumine
AHFS 8:12.18

Products

Delafloxacin meglumine is available as a lyophilized powder in single-dose vials containing 300 mg of delafloxacin.[3332] Each vial also contains edetate disodium 3.4 mg, meglumine 59 mg, and sulfobutylether β-cyclodextrin 2400 mg.[3332] The contents of each 300-mg vial should be reconstituted with 10.5 mL of dextrose 5% or sodium chloride 0.9%, and the vial should be shaken vigorously until all of the powder is dissolved to yield a 25-mg/mL solution.[3332]

The reconstituted solution must be further diluted with dextrose 5% or sodium chloride 0.9% to a total volume of 250 mL prior to intravenous administration.[3332] To prepare a 300-mg dose, 12 mL of the infusion solution should be removed from the bag prior to addition of 12 mL (300 mg) of the drug;[3332] to prepare a 200-mg dose, 8 mL of the infusion solution should be removed from the bag prior to addition of 8 mL (200 mg) of the drug.[3332] [3333]

Equivalency

Delafloxacin meglumine 433 mg is equivalent to 300 mg of delafloxacin as the free acid.[3332]

Trade Name(s)

Baxdela

Administration

Delafloxacin meglumine is administered intravenously over 60 minutes following dilution of the reconstituted solution in sodium chloride 0.9% or dextrose 5%.[3332] If a common infusion line is being used to administer other drugs in addition to delafloxacin meglumine, the line should be flushed with sodium chloride 0.9% or dextrose 5% prior to and following infusion of delafloxacin meglumine.[3332] Delafloxacin is incompatible with any solutions that contain multivalent cations (e.g., calcium, magnesium).[3332]

Stability

Delafloxacin meglumine lyophilized powder is a light yellow to tan cake that may have cracking, shrinkage, and slight variations in texture and color; upon reconstitution, a clear yellow to amber-colored solution forms.[3332] Intact vials of delafloxacin meglumine should be stored at controlled room temperature.[3332] The reconstituted solution and solutions diluted for infusion may be stored at 2 to 8°C or 20 to 25°C for up to 24 hours and should not be frozen.[3332] Any unused portions should be discarded.[3332] Solutions should be visually inspected for particulate matter and discoloration prior to administration.[3332]

Compatibility Information

Solution Compatibility

Delafloxacin meglumine

Test Soln Name	Mfr	Mfr	Conc/L or %	Remarks	Ref	C/I
Dextrose 5% in Ringer's injection		MEL		Must not be mixed with calcium-containing solutions	3332	I
Dextrose 5% in Ringer's injection, lactated		MEL		Must not be mixed with calcium-containing solutions	3332	I
Dextrose 5%		MEL	0.8, 1.2 g	Stable for up to 24 hr at 2 to 8°C or 20 to 25°C	3332, 3333	C
Dextrose 5%	BRN[b]	MEL	0.2, 3.2, and 3.75 g	Compatible and stable for up to 48 hr protected from light at 2 to 8°C or 25°C with 60% relative humidity	3333	C
Dextrose 5%	BA[b]	MEL	1.1 g	Compatible for up to 48 hr protected from light at 5°C or 25°C with 60% relative humidity	3333	C
Dextrose 5%	HOS[a]	MEL	1.1 g	Compatible for up to 48 hr protected from light at 5°C or 25°C with 60% relative humidity	3333	C
Dextrose 5%	BA[c]	MEL	1.1 g	Compatible for up to 48 hr protected from light at 5°C or 25°C with 60% relative humidity	3333	C
Ringer's injection		MEL		Must not be mixed with calcium-containing solutions	3332	I
Ringer's injection, lactated		MEL		Must not be mixed with calcium-containing solutions	3332	I
Sodium chloride 0.9%		MEL	0.8, 1.2 g	Stable for up to 24 hr at 2 to 8°C or 20 to 25°C	3332, 3333	C

[a] Tested in PVC containers.

[b] Tested in polyolefin containers.

[c] Tested in polyethylene containers.

DOI: 10.37573/9781585286850.116

Dexamethasone Sodium Phosphate
AHFS 68:04

Products

Dexamethasone sodium phosphate is available as dexamethasone phosphate 4 mg/mL with sodium sulfite 1 mg/mL, benzyl alcohol 10 mg/mL, sodium citrate for isotonicity, and citric acid and sodium hydroxide to adjust pH in water for injection. It is also available as dexamethasone phosphate 10 mg/mL with sodium metabisulfite 1 mg/mL, benzyl alcohol 10 mg/mL, sodium citrate 10 mg/mL, and citric acid and sodium hydroxide to adjust pH in water for injection.[1(6/06)]

pH

Dexamethasone sodium phosphate injections have a pH range from 7 to 8.5.[1(6/06)] [17] Dexamethasone sodium phosphate (David Bull) 0.5, 1, and 2 mg/mL in sodium chloride 0.9% for continuous subcutaneous infusion had pH values of 7.3, 7.3, and 7.5, respectively.[2161]

Osmolality

The osmolality of the 4-mg/mL concentration of dexamethasone sodium phosphate (Elkins-Sinn) was determined by freezing-point depression to be 356 mOsm/kg.[1071] Another study reported the osmolality of a dexamethasone injection (manufacturer unspecified) to be 255 mOsm/kg.[1233]

Dexamethasone sodium phosphate (David Bull) 0.5, 1, and 2 mg/mL in sodium chloride 0.9% for continuous subcutaneous infusion had osmolalities of 269, 260, and 238 mOsm/kg, respectively.[2161]

Administration

Dexamethasone sodium phosphate 4- and 10-mg/mL may be administered intravenously by direct injection slowly over 1 to several minutes or by continuous or intermittent intravenous infusion and by intramuscular, intra-articular, intrasynovial, intralesional, or soft-tissue injection.[1(6/06)] [4]

Stability

The injections should be protected from light and freezing. In addition, dexamethasone sodium phosphate is heat labile and should not be autoclaved to sterilize the vial's exterior.[1(6/06)] [4]

Dexamethasone sodium phosphate (Lyphomed) was diluted to a concentration of 1 mg/mL with bacteriostatic sodium chloride 0.9% and packaged in 10-mL sterile glass vials. The dilutions remained clear and colorless, and little or no loss of dexamethasone was found after 28 days of storage at 4 and 22°C.[1940]

Dexamethasone sodium phosphate under simulated summer conditions in paramedic vehicles was exposed to temperatures ranging from 26 to 38°C over 4 weeks. Analysis found no loss of the drug under these conditions.[2562]

Syringes

The stability of dexamethasone sodium phosphate (Organon Teknica) 10 mg/mL repackaged into 1- and 2.5-mL Glaspak (Becton Dickinson) and 1- and 3-mL plastic (Monoject, Sherwood) syringes was reported. Samples in the Glaspak syringes were stored at 4 and 23°C, exposed to light and both shaken and unshaken during storage. Samples in plastic syringes were stored only at 23°C. Not more than 5% loss occurred in the Glaspak syringes after 91 days at either temperature. Similarly, losses in the 3-mL plastic syringes were 7% or less after 55 days while losses in the 1-mL plastic syringes were 3% or less in 35 days; these time periods were the maximum that the plastic syringes were evaluated in this study. No contamination by the rubber components was found to leach into the drug solution.[1897]

Sorption

Dexamethasone sodium phosphate was shown not to exhibit sorption to polyvinyl chloride (PVC) bags and tubing, polyethylene tubing, Silastic tubing, and polypropylene syringes.[536 606]

Filtration

Dexamethasone sodium phosphate (MSD) 4 mg/L in dextrose 5%, sodium chloride 0.9%, and Ringer's injection, lactated filtered over 12 hours through a 5-μm stainless steel depth filter (Argyle Filter Connector), a 0.22-μm cellulose ester membrane filter (Ivex-2 Filter Set), and a 0.22-μm polycarbonate membrane filter (In-Sure Filter Set), showed no significant reduction due to binding to the filters.[320]

In another study, dexamethasone sodium phosphate (MSD) 4 mg/L in dextrose 5% and sodium chloride 0.9% did not display significant sorption to a 0.45-μm cellulose membrane filter (Abbott S-A-I-F) during an 8-hour simulated infusion.[567]

Central Venous Catheter

Dexamethasone sodium phosphate (American Regent) 0.5 mg/mL in dextrose 5% was found to be compatible with the ARROWg+ard Blue Plus (Arrow International) chlorhexidine-bearing triple-lumen central catheter. Essentially complete delivery of the drug was found with little or no drug loss occurring. Furthermore, chlorhexidine delivered from the catheter remained at trace amounts with no substantial increase due to the delivery of the drug through the catheter.[2335]

DOI: 10.37573/9781585286850.117

Compatibility Information

Solution Compatibility

Dexamethasone sodium phosphate

Test Soln Name	Mfr	Mfr	Conc/L or %	Remarks	Ref	C/I
Dextrose 5%	a	AMR	94 and 658 mg	Visually compatible with no loss in 14 days stored at 24°C protected from light	1875	C
Sodium chloride 0.9%	a	AMR	92 and 660 mg	Visually compatible with no loss in 14 days stored at 24°C protected from light	1875	C
Sodium chloride 0.9%	BAa	ES	200 and 400 mg	Visually compatible with no loss in 30 days at 4°C then 2 days at 23°C	1882	C
Sodium chloride 0.9%	BA	APP	0.1 and 1 gb	Visually compatible with less than 3% loss in 22 days at 25°C	2392	C
Sodium chloride 0.9%	BA	DB	250 and 500 mg	Visually compatible with 3% or less loss in 48 hr at room temperature	2531	C

a Tested in PVC containers.

b Tested in polypropylene syringes.

Additive Compatibility

Dexamethasone sodium phosphate

Test Drug	Mfr	Conc/L or %	Mfr	Conc/L or %	Test Solution	Remarks	Ref	C/I
Amikacin sulfate	BR	5 g	MSD	40 mg	D5LR, D5R, D5S, D5W, D10W, LR, NS, R, SL	Physically compatible and both stable for 24 hr at 25°C	294	C
Amikacin sulfate	BR	5 g	MSD	40 mg	D2.5S	16% dexamethasone loss in 4 hr at 25°C	294	I
Aminophylline		625 mg		30 mg	D5W	Physically compatible and chemically stable for 24 hr at 4 and 30°C	521	C
Bleomycin sulfate	BR	20 and 30 units	MSD	50 mg	NS	Physically compatible and bleomycin activity retained for 1 week at 4°C. Dexamethasone not tested	763	C
Daunorubicin HCl						Immediate milky precipitation	524	I
Diphenhydramine HCl with lorazepam and metoclopramide HCl	ES WY DU	2 g 40 mg 4 g	AMR	400 mg	NSa	Rapid lorazepam losses of 8, 10, and 15% at 3, 23, and 30°C, respectively, in 24 hr. Other drugs stable for 14 days at all three storage temperatures	1733	I
Floxacillin sodium	BE	20 g	MSD	4 g	NS	Physically compatible for 72 hr at 15 and 30°C	1479	C
Fosaprepitant dimeglumine	MSDg	1 g		100 mg	NS	Physically compatible for 24 hr at 25°C in light	2999	C
Fosaprepitant dimeglumine	MSDh	1 g		100 mg	NS	Physically compatible for 24 hr at 25°C in light	2999	C
Fosaprepitant dimeglumine	MSDi	1 g		100 mg	NS	Physically compatible for 24 hr at 25°C in light	2999	C
Furosemide	HO	1 g	MSD	4 g	NS	Physically compatible for 72 hr at 15 and 30°C	1479	C
Granisetron HCl	SKB	10 and 40 mg	AMR	92 mg	D5W, NSb	Visually compatible. Little loss of either drug in 14 days at 4 and 24°C in dark	1875	C
Granisetron HCl	SKB	10 and 40 mg	AMR	660 mg	D5W, NSb	Visually compatible. Little dexamethasone and 8% granisetron loss in 14 days at 4 and 24°C in dark	1875	C
Granisetron HCl	BE	55 and 51 mg	MSD	75 and 345 mg	D5W, NSb	Visually compatible. Little loss of either drug in 72 hr at room temperature	1884	C
Granisetron HCl	j	26 mg		100 mg	NS	Physically compatible for 24 hr at 25°C in light	2999	C
Lidocaine HCl	AST	2 g	MSD	4 mg		Physically compatible	24	C
Lorazepam with diphenhydramine HCl and metoclopramide HCl	WY ES DU	40 mg 2 g 4 g	AMR	400 mg	NSa	Rapid lorazepam losses of 8, 10, and 15% at 3, 23, and 30°C, respectively, in 24 hr. Other drugs stable for 14 days at all three storage temperatures	1733	I

Additive Compatibility (Cont.)

Test Drug	Mfr	Conc/L or %	Mfr	Conc/L or %	Test Solution	Remarks	Ref	C/I
Meropenem	ZEN	1 and 20 g	MSD	4 g	NS	Visually compatible for 4 hr at room temperature	1994	C
Metoclopramide HCl with diphenhydramine HCl and lorazepam	DU ES WY	4 g 2 g 40 mg	AMR	400 mg	NS[a]	Rapid lorazepam losses of 8, 10, and 15% at 3, 23, and 30°C, respectively, in 24 hr. Other drugs stable for 14 days at all three storage temperatures	1733	I
Mitomycin	BR	100 mg	LY	5 g	NS[c]	Visually compatible. 10% calculated loss of mitomycin in 68 hr and dexamethasone in 250 hr at 25°C	1866	C
Mitomycin	BR	100 mg	LY	5 g	NS[b]	Visually compatible. 10% calculated loss of mitomycin in 91 hr and dexamethasone in 154 hr at 25°C	1866	C
Mitomycin	BR	100 mg	LY	5 g	NS[c]	Visually compatible. 10% calculated loss of mitomycin in 211 hr and dexamethasone in 98 hr at 4°C	1866	C
Mitomycin	BR	100 mg	LY	5 g	NS[b]	Visually compatible. 10% calculated loss of mitomycin in 238 hr and dexamethasone in 355 hr at 4°C	1866	C
Nafcillin sodium	WY	500 mg	MSD	4 mg		Physically compatible	27	C
Ondansetron HCl	GL	48 mg		20 and 40 mg	D5W, NS	Visually compatible for 24 hr at 22°C	1608	C
Ondansetron HCl	GL	160 mg		200 and 400 mg	NS	Visually compatible for 24 hr at 22°C	1608	C
Ondansetron HCl	CER	100 mg	ES	200 mg	NS[b]	Visually compatible. No dexamethasone and 8% ondansetron loss in 30 days at 4°C then 2 days at 23°C	1882	C
Ondansetron HCl	CER	100 and 200 mg	ES	400 mg	NS[b]	Visually compatible. No dexamethasone and 7 to 10% ondansetron loss in 30 days at 4°C then 2 days at 23°C	1882	C
Ondansetron HCl	CER	200, 400, 640 mg	ES	200 mg	NS[b]	Visually compatible. No dexamethasone and 5% ondansetron loss in 30 days at 4°C then 2 days at 23°C	1882	C
Ondansetron HCl	CER	400 and 640 mg	ES	400 mg	NS[b]	Visually compatible. No dexamethasone and 3% ondansetron loss in 30 days at 4°C then 2 days at 23°C	1882	C
Ondansetron HCl	CER	640 mg	ES	200 and 400 mg	D5W[d]	Visually compatible. 7% dexamethasone and no ondansetron loss in 30 days at 4°C then 2 days at 23°C	1882	C
Ondansetron HCl	GL	150 mg	MSD	400 mg	NS[b]	Visually compatible. 4% or less loss of either drug in 28 days at 4 and 22°C	2084	C
Ondansetron HCl	GL	150 mg	MSD	400 mg	D5W[b]	Visually compatible. 4% or less loss of either drug in 28 days at 4°C. 10% ondansetron loss in 3 days at 22°C	2084	C
Ondansetron HCl	GL	750 mg	MSD	230 mg	NS[b]	Visually compatible. 4% or less loss of either drug in 28 days at 4°C. 10% ondansetron loss in 7 days at 22°C	2084	C
Ondansetron HCl	GL	750 mg	MSD	230 mg	D5W[b]	Visually compatible. Up to 13% ondansetron loss in 3 days at 4 and 22°C	2084	?
Ondansetron HCl	GSK	80 mg	OR	100 mg	D5W[f]	Visually compatible. Under 3% ondansetron and 8% dexamethasone loss when frozen for 3 months then stored refrigerated for 30 days	2822	C
Ondansetron HCl	j	70 mg		100 mg	NS	Physically compatible for 24 hr at 25°C in light	2999	C
Oxycodone HCl	NAP	0.8 g	FAU	0.8 g	NS, W	Visually compatible. Under 4% concentration change in 24 hr at 25°C	2600	C

Additive Compatibility (Cont.)

Test Drug	Mfr	Conc/L or %	Mfr	Conc/L or %	Test Solution	Remarks	Ref	C/I
Palonosetron HCl	MGI	5 mg	AMR	200 and 400 mg	D5W, NS[b]	Physically compatible. Little loss of either drug in 48 hr at 23°C in light and 14 days at 4°C	2552	C
Prochlorperazine edisylate	SKF	100 mg	MSD	20 mg	D5W	Physically compatible	15	C
Ranitidine HCl	GL	50 mg and 2 g		40 mg	D5W	Physically compatible. Ranitidine stable for 24 hr at 25°C. Dexamethasone not tested	1515	C
Rolapitant HCl	TES	1.8 g	APP	105.3 mg	[k]	Physically compatible. No loss of either drug in 6 hr at 20 to 25°C	3372	C
Rolapitant HCl	TES	1.7 g	APP	205.1 mg	[k]	Physically compatible. No loss of either drug in 6 hr at 20 to 25°C	3372	C
Tramadol HCl	AND	11.18 g	ME	440 mg	NS[e]	Visually compatible for 7 days at 25°C protected from light	2701	C
Tramadol HCl	AND	33.3 g	ME	1.33 g	NS[e]	Visually compatible for 7 days at 25°C protected from light	2701	C
Tropisetron HCl	[j]	43 mg		100 mg	NS	Physically compatible for 24 hr at 25°C in light	2999	C
Verapamil HCl	KN	80 mg	MSD	40 mg	D5W, NS	Physically compatible for 24 hr	764	C

[a] Tested in Pharmacia-Deltec PVC pump reservoirs.

[b] Tested in PVC containers.

[c] Tested in glass containers.

[d] Tested in ondansetron hydrochloride ready-to-use CR3 polyester bags.

[e] Tested in elastomeric pump reservoirs (Baxter).

[f] Tested in polyolefin containers.

[g] Tested with granisetron HCl 26 mg/L.

[h] Tested with ondansetron HCl 70 mg/L.

[i] Tested with tropisetron HCl 43 mg/L.

[j] Tested with fosaprepitant dimeglumine (MSD) 1 g/L.

[k] Tested in cyclic olefin copolymer (COC) and glass containers.

Drugs in Syringe Compatibility

Dexamethasone sodium phosphate

Test Drug	Mfr	Amt	Mfr	Amt	Remarks	Ref	C/I
Caffeine citrate		20 mg/1 mL	ES	4 mg/1 mL	Visually compatible for 4 hr at 25°C	2440	C
Dimenhydrinate		10 mg/1 mL		10 mg/1 mL	Clear solution	2569	C
Diphenhydramine HCl	PD	50 mg/mL[a]	DB, SX	4 and 10 mg/mL[a]	White turbidity and precipitate form immediately	1542	I
Diphenhydramine HCl	PD	4.54 mg/mL[b]	DB	9.52 mg/mL[b]	Visually compatible for 24 hr at 24°C	1542	C
Diphenhydramine HCl	PD	4.54 to 15 mg/mL[b]	DB	5 to 9.02 mg/mL[b]	Precipitate forms	1542	I
Diphenhydramine HCl	PD	34.8 to 40 mg/mL[b]	SX	2 mg/mL[b]	Visually compatible for 24 hr at 24°C	1542	C
Diphenhydramine HCl	PD	25 mg/mL[b]	SX	1 mg/mL[b]	Precipitate forms	1542	I
Doxapram HCl	RB	400 mg/20 mL	MSD	3.3 mg/1 mL	Immediate turbidity and precipitation	1177	I
Furosemide	HO	3.33 to 10 mg/mL	ME	0.33 to 3.33 mg/mL	Tested in NS. No visible precipitation with under 10% loss of either drug in 5 days at 4 and 25°C. Precipitation with over 10% drug loss in 15 days	2711	C

Drugs in Syringe Compatibility (Cont.)

Test Drug	Mfr	Amt	Mfr	Amt	Remarks	Ref	C/I
Glycopyrrolate	RB	0.2 mg/1 mL	MSD	4 mg/1 mL	Physically compatible for 48 hr at 25°C. pH >6.0. 5% glycopyrrolate loss may occur in 4 to 7 hr	331	I
Glycopyrrolate	RB	0.2 mg/1 mL	MSD	8 mg/2 mL	Physically compatible for 48 hr at 25°C. pH >6.0. 5% glycopyrrolate loss may occur in 4 to 7 hr	331	I
Glycopyrrolate	RB	0.4 mg/2 mL	MSD	4 mg/1 mL	Physically compatible for 48 hr at 25°C. pH >6.0. 5% glycopyrrolate loss may occur in 4 to 7 hr	331	I
Glycopyrrolate	RB	0.2 mg/1 mL	MSD	24 mg/1 mL	Physically compatible for 48 hr at 25°C. pH >6.0. 5% glycopyrrolate loss may occur in 4 to 7 hr	331	I
Glycopyrrolate	RB	0.2 mg/1 mL	MSD	48 mg/2 mL	Physically compatible for 48 hr at 25°C. pH >6.0. 5% glycopyrrolate loss may occur in 4 to 7 hr	331	I
Glycopyrrolate	RB	0.4 mg/2 mL	MSD	24 mg/1 mL	Physically compatible for 48 hr at 25°C. pH >6.0. 5% glycopyrrolate loss may occur in 4 to 7 hr	331	I
Granisetron HCl	BE	0.15 mg/mL[c]	MSD	0.2 and 1 mg/mL[c]	Visually compatible. Little loss of either drug in 72 hr at room temperature	1884	C
Hydromorphone HCl	KN	2, 10, 40 mg/mL[a]	SX	4 mg/mL[a]	Visually compatible and both drugs stable for 24 hr at 24°C	1542	C
Hydromorphone HCl	KN	2 and 10 mg/mL[a]	DB	10 mg/mL[a]	Visually compatible and both drugs stable for 24 hr at 24°C	1542	C
Hydromorphone HCl	KN	40 mg/mL[a]	DB	10 mg/mL[a]	White turbidity forms immediately	1542	I
Hydromorphone HCl	KN	11.6 mg/mL[b]	DB	7.1 mg/mL[b]	Visually compatible for 24 hr at 24°C	1542	C
Hydromorphone HCl	KN	13.3 to 17.5 mg/mL[b]	DB	5.5 to 6.6 mg/mL[b]	Precipitate forms	1542	I
Hydromorphone HCl	KN	10.5 mg/mL[b]	DB	4.75 mg/mL[b]	Visually compatible for 24 hr at 24°C	1542	C
Hydromorphone HCl	KN	14.75 to 25 mg/mL[b]	DB	3 to 4.1 mg/mL[b]	Precipitate forms	1542	I
Hydromorphone HCl	KN	26.66 mg/mL[b]	SX	3.34 mg/mL[b]	Visually compatible for 24 hr at 24°C	1542	C
Ketamine HCl	PF	1 mg	OR	50 and 600 mg	Diluted to 14 mL with NS. Physically compatible with no loss of either drug in 8 days at 4 and 23°C	2677	C
Metoclopramide HCl	RB	10 mg/2 mL	ES, MSD	8 mg/2 mL	Physically compatible for 48 hr at 25°C	1167	C
Metoclopramide HCl	RB	160 mg/32 mL	ES, MSD	8 mg/2 mL	Physically compatible for 48 hr at 25°C	1167	C
Midazolam HCl	RC	2.5 mg/8 mL	DB	2 mg/8 mL	Diluted in NS. Visually clear. No dexamethasone loss in 48 hr. Midazolam losses over 10% beyond 24 hr at room temperature	2531	C
Midazolam HCl	RC	5 mg/8 mL	DB	2 mg/8 mL	Diluted in NS. Visually clear. No dexamethasone loss in 48 hr. Midazolam losses were 7% in 48 hr at room temperature	2531	C
Midazolam HCl	RC	5 mg/8 mL	DB	4 mg/8 mL	Diluted in NS. Cloudiness forms immediately	2531	I
Midazolam HCl	RC	7.5 mg/8 mL	DB	4 mg/8 mL	Diluted in NS. Cloudiness forms immediately	2531	I
Midazolam HCl	RC	7.5 mg/8 mL	DB	2 mg/8 mL	Diluted in NS. Crystals form in some samples within 24 hr	2531	I
Ondansetron HCl	CER	0.17 mg/mL[d]	ES	0.33 and 0.67 mg/mL[d]	Visually compatible. No loss of either drug in 30 days at 4°C then 2 days at 23°C	1882	C
Ondansetron HCl	CER	0.25 mg/mL[d]	ES	0.5 mg/mL[d]	Visually compatible. No loss of either drug in 30 days at 4°C then 2 days at 23°C	1882	C

Drugs in Syringe Compatibility (Cont.)

Test Drug	Mfr	Amt	Mfr	Amt	Remarks	Ref	C/I
Ondansetron HCl	CER	0.25 mg/mL[d]	ES	1 mg/mL[d]	Visually compatible for 3 days at 4°C. Precipitation of ondansetron observed at 7 days as opaque white ring	1882	C
Ondansetron HCl	CER	0.33 mg/mL[d]	ES	0.33 and 0.67 mg/mL[d]	Visually compatible. No loss of either drug in 30 days at 4°C then 2 days at 23°C	1882	C
Ondansetron HCl	CER	0.5 mg/mL[d]	ES	0.5 mg/mL[d]	Visually compatible. No loss of either drug in 30 days at 4°C then 2 days at 23°C	1882	C
Ondansetron HCl	CER	0.5 mg/mL[d]	ES	1 mg/mL[d]	Visually compatible for 3 days at 4°C. Precipitation of ondansetron observed at 5 days as opaque white ring	1882	C
Ondansetron HCl	CER	0.67 mg/mL[d]	ES	0.33 and 0.67 mg/mL[d]	Visually compatible. No loss of either drug in 30 days at 4°C then 2 days at 23°C	1882	C
Ondansetron HCl	CER	1.07 mg/mL[d]	ES	0.33 mg/mL[d]	Visually compatible. No loss of either drug in 30 days at 4°C then 2 days at 23°C	1882	C
Ondansetron HCl	CER	1.07 mg/mL[d]	ES	0.67 mg/mL[d]	Heavy white precipitate in 72 hr at 4°C. 25 to 30% loss of both drugs	1882	I
Ondansetron HCl		4 mg/2 mL	OM[h]	4 mg/1 mL	Physically incompatible within 3 min	2767	I
Ondansetron HCl		4 mg/2 mL	[i]	4 mg/1 mL	Physically compatible	2767	C
Oxycodone HCl	NAP	200 mg/20 mL	FAU	40 mg/10 mL	Visually compatible. Under 4% concentration change in 24 hr at 25°C	2600	C
Palonosetron HCl	MGI	0.25 mg/5 mL	AMR	3.3 mg/5 mL[e f]	Physically compatible. Little loss of either drug in 48 hr at 23°C in light and 14 days at 4°C	2552	C
Pantoprazole sodium	[g]	4 mg/1 mL		10 mg/1 mL	Precipitates immediately	2574	I
Ranitidine HCl	GL	50 mg/5 mL	ME	4 mg	Physically compatible for 4 hr at ambient temperature under fluorescent light	1151	C
Tramadol HCl	GRU	33.33, 16.66, 8.33 mg/mL[f]	ME	3.33, 1.67, 1.33, 0.33 mg/mL[f]	Physically compatible and both drugs chemically stable for 5 days at 25°C protected from light	2747	C

[a] Mixed in equal quantities. Final concentration is one-half the indicated concentration.

[b] Mixed in varying quantities to yield the final concentrations noted.

[c] Diluted with water.

[d] Diluted with sodium chloride 0.9% drawn into a syringe prior to drugs to yield the concentrations cited.

[e] Tested in dextrose 5%.

[f] Tested in sodium chloride 0.9%.

[g] Test performed using the formulation WITHOUT edetate disodium.

[h] Contained benzyl alcohol as a preservative.

[i] Contained parabens as preservatives.

Y-Site Injection Compatibility (1:1 Mixture)

Dexamethasone sodium phosphate

Test Drug	Mfr	Conc	Mfr	Conc	Remarks	Ref	C/I
Acetaminophen	CAD	10 mg/mL	APP	4 mg/mL	Physically compatible for 4 hr at 23°C	2901, 2902	C
Acetaminophen	CAD	10 mg/mL	BA, SIC	10 mg/mL	Physically compatible with less than 10% acetaminophen loss over 4 hr at room temperature	2841, 2844	C
Acyclovir sodium	BW	5 mg/mL[a]	ES	0.2 mg/mL[a]	Physically compatible for 4 hr at 25°C	1157	C
Acyclovir sodium	BV	5 mg/mL[b]	APP	4 mg/mL	Physically compatible	2794	C

Y-Site Injection Compatibility (1:1 Mixture) (Cont.)

Test Drug	Mfr	Conc	Mfr	Conc	Remarks	Ref	C/I
Allopurinol sodium	BW	3 mg/mL[b]	LY	1 mg/mL[b]	Physically compatible for 4 hr at 22°C	1686	C
Amifostine	USB	10 mg/mL[a]	AMR	1 mg/mL[a]	Physically compatible for 4 hr at 23°C	1845	C
Amikacin sulfate	SQ	50 mg/mL[c]	AMR	4 mg/mL	Visually compatible for 24 hr at room temperature in test tubes. No precipitate found on filter from Y-site delivery	2063	C
Amsacrine	NCI	1 mg/mL[a]	QU	1 mg/mL[a]	Visually compatible for 4 hr at 22°C	1381	C
Anidulafungin	VIC	0.5 mg/mL[a]	AMR	1 mg/mL[a]	Physically compatible for 4 hr at 23°C	2617	C
Aztreonam	SQ	40 mg/mL[a]	AMR	1 mg/mL[a]	Physically compatible for 4 hr at 23°C	1758	C
Bivalirudin	TMC	5 mg/mL[a]	APP	1 mg/mL[a]	Physically compatible for 4 hr at 23°C	2373	C
Blinatumomab	AMG	0.125 mcg/mL[b]	MYL	0.19 mg/mL[b]	Persistent particulate formation	3405, 3417	I
Blinatumomab	AMG	0.375 mcg/mL[b]	MYL	0.19 mg/mL[b]	Visually compatible for 12 hr at room temperature	3405, 3417	C
Cangrelor tetrasodium	TMC	1 mg/mL[b]		1[b] and 4 mg/mL	Physically compatible for 4 hr	3243	C
Ceftaroline fosamil	FOR	2.22 mg/mL[g]	SIC	1 mg/mL[g]	Physically compatible for 4 hr at 23°C	2826	C
Ceftolozane sulfate–tazobactam sodium	CUB	10 mg/mL[e][p]	FRK	1 mg/mL[e]	Physically compatible for 2 hr	3262	C
Ciprofloxacin	MI	2 mg/mL[e]	LY	4 mg/mL	Cloudiness rapidly dissipates. White crystals form in 1 hr at 24°C	1655	I
Cisatracurium besylate	GW	0.1, 2, 5 mg/mL[a]	FUJ	2 mg/mL[a]	Physically compatible for 4 hr at 23°C	2074	C
Cladribine	ORT	0.015[b] and 0.5[f] mg/mL	AMR	1 mg/mL[b]	Physically compatible for 4 hr at 23°C	1969	C
Cloxacillin sodium	SMX	100 mg/mL	OM	4 mg/mL	Physically compatible for up to 4 hr at room temperature	3245	C
Dexmedetomidine HCl	AB	4 mcg/mL[b]	AMR	1 mg/mL[b]	Physically compatible for 4 hr at 23°C	2383	C
Docetaxel	RPR	0.9 mg/mL[a]	ES	2 mg/mL[a]	Physically compatible for 4 hr at 23°C	2224	C
Doripenem	JJ	5 mg/mL[a][b]	APP	1 mg/mL[a][b]	Physically compatible for 4 hr at 23°C	2743	C
Doxorubicin HCl liposomal	SEQ	0.4 mg/mL[a]	ES	2 mg/mL[a]	Physically compatible for 4 hr at 23°C	2087	C
Etoposide phosphate	BR	5 mg/mL[a]	ES	1 mg/mL[a]	Physically compatible for 4 hr at 23°C	2218	C
Famotidine	MSD	0.2 mg/mL[a]	ES	10 mg/mL	Physically compatible for 14 hr	1196	C
Famotidine	ME	2 mg/mL[b]		1 mg/mL[a]	Visually compatible for 4 hr at 22°C	1936	C
Fenoldopam mesylate	AB	80 mcg/mL[b]	AMR	1 mg/mL[b]	Trace haze forms immediately	2467	I
Fentanyl citrate	JN	0.025 mg/mL[a]	AMR	1 mg/mL[a]	Physically compatible for 48 hr at 22°C	1706	C
Filgrastim	AMG	30 mcg/mL[a]	LY	1 mg/mL[a]	Physically compatible for 4 hr at 22°C	1687	C
Fluconazole	RR	2 mg/mL	ES	4 mg/mL	Physically compatible for 24 hr at 25°C	1407	C
Fludarabine phosphate	BX	1 mg/mL[a]	MSD	1 mg/mL[a]	Visually compatible for 4 hr at 22°C	1439	C
Foscarnet sodium	AST	24 mg/mL	OR	10 mg/mL	Physically compatible for 24 hr at room temperature under fluorescent light	1335	C
Gallium nitrate	FUJ	1 mg/mL[b]	AMR	4 mg/mL	Visually compatible for 24 hr at 25°C	1673	C
Gemcitabine HCl	LI	10 mg/mL[b]	ES	1 mg/mL[b]	Physically compatible for 4 hr at 23°C	2226	C
Granisetron HCl	SKB	1 mg/mL	ME	0.24 mg/mL[b]	Physically compatible with little or no loss of either drug in 4 hr at 22°C	1883	C

Y-Site Injection Compatibility (1:1 Mixture) (Cont.)

Test Drug	Mfr	Conc	Mfr	Conc	Remarks	Ref	C/I
Heparin sodium	TR	50 units/mL	ES	0.08 mg/mL[a]	Visually compatible for 4 hr at 25°C	1793	C
Heparin sodium[m]	RI	1000 units/L[g]	MSD	4 mg/mL	Physically compatible for 4 hr at room temperature	322	C
Hetastarch in lactated electrolyte	AB	6%	APP	1 mg/mL[a]	Physically compatible for 4 hr at 23°C	2339	C
Hydrocortisone sodium succinate[n]	UP	100 mg/L[g]	MSD	4 mg/mL	Physically compatible for 4 hr at room temperature	322	C
Hydromorphone HCl	AST	0.5 mg/mL[a]	AMR	1 mg/mL[a]	Physically compatible for 48 hr at 22°C	1706	C
Idarubicin HCl	AD	1 mg/mL[b]	OR	10 mg/mL	Haze forms immediately and precipitate forms in 20 min	1525	I
Idarubicin HCl	AD	1 mg/mL[b]	AMR	0.2 mg/mL[b]	Haze forms in 20 min	1525	I
Isavuconazonium sulfate	ASP	1.5 mg/mL[e]	FRK	1 mg/mL[e]	Measured turbidity increases within 1 hr	3263	I
Levofloxacin	OMN	5 mg/mL[a]	ES	4 mg/mL	Visually compatible for 4 hr at 24°C	2233	C
Linezolid	PHU	2 mg/mL	FUJ	1 mg/mL[a]	Physically compatible for 4 hr at 23°C	2264	C
Lorazepam	WY	0.33 mg/mL[b]		4 mg/mL	Visually compatible for 24 hr at 22°C	1855	C
Melphalan HCl	BW	0.1 mg/mL[b]	LY	1 mg/mL[b]	Physically compatible for 3 hr at 22°C	1557	C
Meperidine HCl	AB	10 mg/mL	LY	0.2 mg/mL[a]	Physically compatible for 4 hr at 25°C	1397	C
Meropenem	ZEN	1 and 50 mg/mL[b]	MSD	10 mg/mL[h]	Visually compatible for 4 hr at room temperature	1994	C
Meropenem		50 mg/mL	SZ	4 mg/mL	Physically compatible for 4 hr at room temperature	3538	C
Meropenem–vaborbactam	TMC	8 mg/mL[b q]	FRK	1 mg/mL[b]	Physically compatible for 3 hr at 20 to 25°C	3380	C
Methadone HCl	LI	1 mg/mL[a]	AMR	1 mg/mL[a]	Physically compatible for 48 hr at 22°C	1706	C
Methotrexate sodium		30 mg/mL	MSD	4 mg/mL	Visually compatible for 2 hr at room temperature. Precipitate forms in 4 hr	1788	I
Midazolam HCl	RC	1 mg/mL[a]	ES	4 mg/mL	Immediate haze. Precipitate in 8 hr	1847	I
Midazolam HCl	RC	5 mg/mL		4 mg/mL	White precipitate forms immediately	1855	I
Milrinone lactate	SS	0.2 mg/mL[a]	ES	10 mg/mL[a]	Visually compatible for 4 hr at 25°C	2381	C
Morphine sulfate	AB	1 mg/mL	LY	0.2 mg/mL[a]	Physically compatible for 4 hr at 25°C	1397	C
Morphine sulfate	AST	1 mg/mL[a]	AMR	1 mg/mL[a]	Physically compatible for 48 hr at 22°C	1706	C
Ondansetron HCl	GL	1 mg/mL[b]	MSD	1 mg/mL[a]	Visually compatible for 4 hr at 22°C	1365	C
Oxaliplatin	SS	0.5 mg/mL[a]	AMR	1 mg/mL[a]	Physically compatible for 4 hr at 23°C	2566	C
Paclitaxel	NCI	1.2 mg/mL[a]		1 mg/mL[a]	Physically compatible for 4 hr at 22°C	1528	C
Pemetrexed disodium	LI	20 mg/mL[b]	AMR	1 mg/mL[a]	Physically compatible for 4 hr at 23°C	2564	C
Piperacillin sodium–tazobactam sodium	LE[l]	40 mg/mL[a o]	LY	1 mg/mL[a]	Physically compatible for 4 hr at 22°C	1688	C
Plazomicin sulfate	ACH	24 mg/mL[e]	FRK	1 mg/mL[e]	Physically compatible for 1 hr at 20 to 25°C	3432	C
Potassium chloride		40 mEq/L[g]	MSD	4 mg/mL	Physically compatible for 4 hr at room temperature	322	C
Propofol	ZEN[r]	10 mg/mL	AMR	1 mg/mL[a]	Physically compatible for 1 hr at 23°C	2066	C
Remifentanil HCl	GW	0.025 and 0.25 mg/mL[b]	FUJ	2 mg/mL[a]	Physically compatible for 4 hr at 23°C	2075	C
Sargramostim	IMM	10 mcg/mL[b]	ES	1 mg/mL[b]	Visually compatible for 4 hr at 22°C	1436	C

Y-Site Injection Compatibility (1:1 Mixture) (Cont.)

Test Drug	Mfr	Conc	Mfr	Conc	Remarks	Ref	C/I
Sodium bicarbonate		1.4%	MSD	4 mg/mL	Visually compatible for 4 hr at room temperature	1788	C
Tacrolimus	FUJ	1 mg/mL[b]	ES	4 mg/mL[a]	Visually compatible for 24 hr at 25°C	1630	C
Tedizolid phosphate	CUB	0.8 mg/mL[b]	FRK	1 mg/mL[b]	Physically compatible for 2 hr	3244	C
Telavancin HCl	ASP	7.5 mg/mL[g]	AMR	1 mg/mL[g]	Physically compatible for 2 hr	2830	C
Teniposide	BR	0.1 mg/mL[a]	LY	1 mg/mL[a]	Physically compatible for 4 hr at 23°C	1725	C
Theophylline	TR	4 mg/mL	ES	0.08 mg/mL[a]	Visually compatible for 6 hr at 25°C	1793	C
Thiotepa	IMM[j]	1 mg/mL[a]	AMR	1 mg/mL[a]	Physically compatible for 4 hr at 23°C	1861	C
TNA #218 to #226[k]			FUJ, ES	1 mg/mL[a]	Visually compatible for 4 hr at 23°C	2215	C
Topotecan HCl	SKB	56 mcg/mL[b]	RU	4 mg/mL	Haze and color change to intense yellow occur immediately	2245	I
TPN #203, #204[k]			AMR	4 mg/mL	Visually compatible for 2 hr at 23°C	1974	C
TPN #212 to #215[k]			AMR	1 mg/mL[a]	Physically compatible for 4 hr at 23°C	2109	C
Vinorelbine tartrate	BW	1 mg/mL[b]	LY	1 mg/mL[b]	Physically compatible for 4 hr at 22°C	1558	C
Zidovudine	BW	4 mg/mL[a]	ES	0.16 mg/mL[a]	Physically compatible for 4 hr at 25°C	1193	C

[a] Tested in dextrose 5%.

[b] Tested in sodium chloride 0.9%.

[c] Tested in sodium chloride 0.45%.

[d] Tested in dextrose 5%, Ringer's injection, lactated, sodium chloride 0.45%, and sodium chloride 0.9%.

[e] Tested in both dextrose 5% and sodium chloride 0.9%.

[f] Tested in bacteriostatic sodium chloride 0.9% preserved with benzyl alcohol 0.9%.

[g] Tested in dextrose 5%, Ringer's injection, lactated, and sodium chloride 0.9%.

[h] Tested in sterile water for injection.

[i] Tested in dextrose 5% with sodium bicarbonate 0.05 mEq/mL.

[j] Lyophilized formulation tested.

[k] Refer to Appendix for the composition of the parenteral nutrition solutions. TNA indicates a 3-in-1 admixture, and TPN indicates a 2-in-1 admixture.

[l] Test performed using the formulation WITHOUT edetate disodium.

[m] Tested in combination with hydrocortisone sodium succinate (Upjohn) 100 mg/L.

[n] Tested in combination with heparin sodium (Riker) 1000 units/L.

[o] Piperacillin component. Piperacillin in an 8:1 fixed-ratio concentration with tazobactam.

[p] Ceftolozane component. Ceftolozane in a 2:1 fixed-ratio concentration with tazobactam.

[q] Meropenem component. Meropenem in a 1:1 fixed-ratio concentration with vaborbactam.

[r] Test performed using the formulation WITH edetate disodium.

Selected Revisions May 1, 2020. © Copyright, October 1982.
American Society of Health-System Pharmacists, Inc.

Dexmedetomidine Hydrochloride
AHFS 28:24.92

Products

Dexmedetomidine hydrochloride (Precedex, Hospira) is available as a concentrate for injection providing 100 mcg/mL of dexmedetomidine as the hydrochloride in single-use (preservative-free) 2-mL (200-mcg) vials.[2848] Each mL of the concentrate also contains sodium chloride 9 mg in water for injection.[2848]

Dexmedetomidine hydrochloride (Fresenius Kabi) also is available as a concentrate for injection providing 100 mcg/mL of dexmedetomidine as the hydrochloride in single-use (preservative-free) 2-mL (200-mcg) vials.[3180] Each mL of the concentrate also contains sodium acetate trihydrate 597 mcg, glacial acetic acid 27 mcg, and sodium chloride 9 mg in water for injection.[3180]

The concentrates for injection must be diluted in sodium chloride 0.9% prior to administration.[2848] [3180] To prepare the required concentration solution for infusion (i.e., 4 mcg/mL), 2 mL of the concentrate should be added to 48 mL of sodium chloride 0.9% and shaken gently to mix.[2848]

Dexmedetomidine hydrochloride (Precedex, Hospira) also is available as a premixed, ready-to-use solution in sodium chloride 0.9% at a concentration of 4 mcg/mL in single-use 20-mL vials and 50- and 100-mL glass bottles for intravenous infusion.[2848] No further dilution of the ready-to-use solution is necessary.[2848]

Dexmedetomidine hydrochloride (HQ Specialty) also is available as a concentrate providing 100 mcg/mL of dexmedetomidine as the hydrochloride in multidose 4- and 10-mL vials.[3179] Each mL of the concentrate also contains methylparaben 1.6 mg, propylparaben 0.2 mg, and sodium chloride 9 mg in water for injection.[3179] The concentrate for injection must be diluted in sodium chloride 0.9% prior to administration.[3179] To prepare the required concentration solution for infusion (i.e., 4 mcg/mL), 2 or 4 mL of the concentrate should be added to 48 or 96 mL, respectively, of sodium chloride 0.9% and shaken gently to mix.[3179]

Tonicity

Dexmedetomidine hydrochloride concentrates for injection and premixed, ready-to-use solution in sodium chloride 0.9% are isotonic.[2848] [3179] [3180]

Equivalency

Dexmedetomidine hydrochloride 118 mcg is equivalent to 100 mcg of dexmedetomidine as the base.[2848] [3179] [3180]

pH

Dexmedetomidine hydrochloride concentrates for injection in both single-use and multidose vials have a pH ranging from 4.5 to 7.[2848] [3179] [3180]

Dexmedetomidine hydrochloride premixed, ready-to-use solution in sodium chloride 0.9% has a pH ranging from 4.5 to 8.[2848]

Trade Name(s)

Precedex

Administration

Dexmedetomidine hydrochloride is administered by intravenous infusion using a controlled infusion device over periods not exceeding 24 hours.[2848] [3179] [3180] The concentrates for injection must be diluted in sodium chloride 0.9% to a concentration of 4 mcg/mL prior to administration;[2848] [3179] [3180] the premixed, ready-to-use solution does not require any further dilution.[2848]

Stability

Dexmedetomidine hydrochloride concentrates for injection and premixed, ready-to-use solution should be clear and colorless.[2848] [3179] [3180] Intact single-use and multidose vials containing the concentrates for injection and single-use vials and glass bottles containing the drug diluted for intravenous infusion in sodium chloride 0.9% should be stored at controlled room temperature;[2848] [3179] [3180] consult specific labeling for additional storage details.

Dexmedetomidine hydrochloride solutions should be visually inspected for particulate matter and discoloration prior to administration.[2848] [3179] [3180]

Diluted solutions of dexmedetomidine hydrochloride (HQ Specialty) prepared from multidose vials of the concentrate for injection may be stored for up to 4 hours at room temperature or 24 hours at 2 to 8°C prior to administration.[3179] Any unused portion of the solution should be discarded.[3179]

Syringes

The stability of dexmedetomidine hydrochloride concentrate (Hospira) after dilution to a concentration of 4 mcg/mL in sodium chloride 0.9% and packaged as 25 mL in 60-mL natural rubber-free polypropylene syringes (Becton Dickinson) was evaluated at ambient room temperature with light exposure and under refrigeration in the dark.[2849] No changes in color or clarity occurred.[2849] Samples stored at 20 to 25°C in light exhibited a loss of less than 10% over 48 hours; those stored at 5°C in the dark exhibited a loss of less than 5% over 14 days.[2849]

Sorption

Dexmedetomidine hydrochloride is known to undergo sorption to some types of natural rubber.[2848] [3179] [3180] Although the drug is dosed to effect, the manufacturer recommends the use of administration equipment with synthetic rubber or coated natural rubber gaskets.[2848] [3179] [3180]

DOI: 10.37573/9781585286850.118

Compatibility Information

Solution Compatibility

Dexmedetomidine HCl

Test Soln Name	Mfr	Mfr	Conc/L or %	Remarks	Ref	C/I
Sodium chloride 0.9%		HOS, HQS, FRK	4 mg	Manufacturer-recommended solution	2848, 3179, 3180	C
Sodium chloride 0.9%	HOS[a]	HOS	4 mg	Little to no loss in 14 days at 3 to 4°C or 20 to 25°C	3383	C
Sodium chloride 0.9%	BRN[b]	HOS	4 mg	Little to no loss in 14 days at 3 to 4°C or 20 to 25°C	3383	C

[a] Tested in PVC containers.

[b] Tested in polyethylene-polypropylene copolymer PAB bags.

Y-Site Injection Compatibility (1:1 Mixture)

Dexmedetomidine HCl

Test Drug	Mfr	Conc	Mfr	Conc	Remarks	Ref	C/I
Alfentanil HCl	TAY	0.5 mg/mL	AB	4 mcg/mL[b]	Physically compatible for 4 hr at 23°C	2383	C
Amikacin sulfate	APO	5 mg/mL[b]	AB	4 mcg/mL[b]	Physically compatible for 4 hr at 23°C	2383	C
Aminophylline	AB	2.5 mg/mL[b]	AB	4 mcg/mL[b]	Physically compatible for 4 hr at 23°C	2383	C
Amiodarone HCl	WAY	4 mg/mL[b]	AB	4 mcg/mL[b]	Physically compatible for 4 hr at 23°C	2383	C
Amphotericin B	APO	0.6 mg/mL[a]	AB	4 mcg/mL[b]	Yellow precipitate forms immediately	2383	I
Amphotericin B			HOS, HQS	4 mcg/mL[b]	Stated to be incompatible	2848, 3179	I
Ampicillin sodium	APO	20 mg/mL[b]	AB	4 mcg/mL[b]	Physically compatible for 4 hr at 23°C	2383	C
Ampicillin sodium–sulbactam sodium	PF	20 mg/mL[b d]	AB	4 mcg/mL[b]	Physically compatible for 4 hr at 23°C	2383	C
Atracurium besylate			HOS	4 mcg/mL[b]	Stated to be compatible	3181	C
Atropine sulfate			HOS	4 mcg/mL[b]	Stated to be compatible	3181	C
Azithromycin	PF	2 mg/mL[b]	AB	4 mcg/mL[b]	Physically compatible for 4 hr at 23°C	2383	C
Aztreonam	BMS	40 mg/mL[b]	AB	4 mcg/mL[b]	Physically compatible for 4 hr at 23°C	2383	C
Bumetanide	BED	40 mcg/mL[b]	AB	4 mcg/mL[b]	Physically compatible for 4 hr at 23°C	2383	C
Butorphanol tartrate	APO	40 mcg/mL[b]	AB	4 mcg/mL[b]	Physically compatible for 4 hr at 23°C	2383	C
Calcium gluconate	APP	40 mg/mL[b]	AB	4 mcg/mL[b]	Physically compatible for 4 hr at 23°C	2383	C
Cefazolin sodium	LI	20 mg/mL[b]	AB	4 mcg/mL[b]	Physically compatible for 4 hr at 23°C	2383	C
Cefepime HCl	BMS	20 mg/mL[b]	AB	4 mcg/mL[b]	Physically compatible for 4 hr at 23°C	2383	C
Cefotaxime sodium	HO	20 mg/mL[b]	AB	4 mcg/mL[b]	Physically compatible for 4 hr at 23°C	2383	C
Cefotetan disodium	ZEN	20 mg/mL[b]	AB	4 mcg/mL[b]	Physically compatible for 4 hr at 23°C	2383	C
Cefoxitin sodium	ME	20 mg/mL[b]	AB	4 mcg/mL[b]	Physically compatible for 4 hr at 23°C	2383	C
Ceftazidime	GW	40 mg/mL[b]	AB	4 mcg/mL[b]	Physically compatible for 4 hr at 23°C	2383	C
Ceftazidime–avibactam sodium	ALL	20 mg/mL[j k]	l		Physically compatible for up to 4 hr at room temperature	3004	C

Y-Site Injection Compatibility (1:1 Mixture) (Cont.)

Test Drug	Mfr	Conc	Mfr	Conc	Remarks	Ref	C/I
Ceftolozane sulfate-tazobactam sodium	CUB	10 mg/mL[h i]	MYL	4 mcg/mL[h]	Physically compatible for 2 hr	3262	C
Ceftriaxone sodium	RC	20 mg/mL[b]	AB	4 mcg/mL[b]	Physically compatible for 4 hr at 23°C	2383	C
Cefuroxime sodium	GW	30 mg/mL[b]	AB	4 mcg/mL[b]	Physically compatible for 4 hr at 23°C	2383	C
Chlorpromazine HCl	ES	2 mg/mL[b]	AB	4 mcg/mL[b]	Physically compatible for 4 hr at 23°C	2383	C
Ciprofloxacin	BAY	1 mg/mL[b]	AB	4 mcg/mL[b]	Physically compatible for 4 hr at 23°C	2383	C
Cisatracurium besylate	GW	0.5 mg/mL[b]	AB	4 mcg/mL[b]	Physically compatible for 4 hr at 23°C	2383	C
Clindamycin phosphate	AB	10 mg/mL[b]	AB	4 mcg/mL[b]	Physically compatible for 4 hr at 23°C	2383	C
Dexamethasone sodium phosphate	AMR	1 mg/mL[b]	AB	4 mcg/mL[b]	Physically compatible for 4 hr at 23°C	2383	C
Diazepam	AB	5 mg/mL	AB	4 mcg/mL[b]	White turbid precipitate forms immediately	2383	I
Diazepam			HOS	4 mcg/mL[b]	Stated to be incompatible	2848, 3179	I
Digoxin	ES	0.25 mg/mL	AB	4 mcg/mL[b]	Physically compatible for 4 hr at 23°C	2383	C
Diltiazem HCl	BA	5 mg/mL	AB	4 mcg/mL[b]	Physically compatible for 4 hr at 23°C	2383	C
Diphenhydramine HCl	PD	2 mg/mL[b]	AB	4 mcg/mL[b]	Physically compatible for 4 hr at 23°C	2383	C
Dobutamine HCl	AST	4 mg/mL[b]	AB	4 mcg/mL[b]	Physically compatible for 4 hr at 23°C	2383	C
Dolasetron mesylate	HO	2 mg/mL[b]	AB	4 mcg/mL[b]	Physically compatible for 4 hr at 23°C	2383	C
Dopamine HCl	AB	3.2 mg/mL[b]	AB	4 mcg/mL[b]	Physically compatible for 4 hr at 23°C	2383	C
Doxycycline hyclate	APP	1 mg/mL[b]	AB	4 mcg/mL[b]	Physically compatible for 4 hr at 23°C	2383	C
Droperidol	AMR	2.5 mg/mL	AB	4 mcg/mL[b]	Physically compatible for 4 hr at 23°C	2383	C
Enalaprilat	BED	0.1 mg/mL[b]	AB	4 mcg/mL[b]	Physically compatible for 4 hr at 23°C	2383	C
Ephedrine sulfate	TAY	5 mg/mL[b]	AB	4 mcg/mL[b]	Physically compatible for 4 hr at 23°C	2383	C
Epinephrine HCl	AMR	50 mcg/mL[b]	AB	4 mcg/mL[b]	Physically compatible for 4 hr at 23°C	2383	C
Eravacycline dihydrochloride	TET	0.6 mg/mL[b]	HOS	4 mcg/mL	Physically compatible for 2 hr at room temperature	3532	C
Erythromycin lactobionate	AB	5 mg/mL[b]	AB	4 mcg/mL[b]	Physically compatible for 4 hr at 23°C	2383	C
Esmolol HCl	BA	10 mg/mL[b]	AB	4 mcg/mL[b]	Physically compatible for 4 hr at 23°C	2383	C
Etomidate			HOS	4 mcg/mL[b]	Stated to be compatible	3181	C
Famotidine	ME	2 mg/mL[b]	AB	4 mcg/mL[b]	Physically compatible for 4 hr at 23°C	2383	C
Fenoldopam mesylate	AB	80 mcg/mL[b]	AB	4 mcg/mL[b]	Physically compatible for 4 hr at 23°C	2383	C
Fentanyl citrate			HOS	4 mcg/mL[b]	Stated to be compatible	3181	C
Fluconazole	PF	2 mg/mL	AB	4 mcg/mL[b]	Physically compatible for 4 hr at 23°C	2383	C
Furosemide	AMR	3 mg/mL[b]	AB	4 mcg/mL[b]	Physically compatible for 4 hr at 23°C	2383	C
Gentamicin sulfate	APP	5 mg/mL[b]	AB	4 mcg/mL[b]	Physically compatible for 4 hr at 23°C	2383	C
Granisetron HCl	SKB	50 mcg/mL[b]	AB	4 mcg/mL[b]	Physically compatible for 4 hr at 23°C	2383	C
Haloperidol lactate	MN	0.2 mg/mL[b]	AB	4 mcg/mL[b]	Physically compatible for 4 hr at 23°C	2383	C

Y-Site Injection Compatibility (1:1 Mixture) (Cont.)

Test Drug	Mfr	Conc	Mfr	Conc	Remarks	Ref	C/I
Heparin sodium	AB	100 units/mL	AB	4 mcg/mL[b]	Physically compatible for 4 hr at 23°C	2383	C
Hydrocortisone sodium succinate			HOS	4 mcg/mL[b]	Stated to be compatible	3181	C
Hydromorphone HCl	AST	0.5 mg/mL[b]	AB	4 mcg/mL[b]	Physically compatible for 4 hr at 23°C	2383	C
Hydroxyzine HCl	ES	2 mg/mL[b]	AB	4 mcg/mL[b]	Physically compatible for 4 hr at 23°C	2383	C
Isavuconazonium sulfate	ASP	1.5 mg/mL[h]	HOS	4 mcg/mL[h]	Physically compatible for 2 hr	3263	C
Isoproterenol HCl	AB	20 mcg/mL[b]	AB	4 mcg/mL[b]	Physically compatible for 4 hr at 23°C	2383	C
Ketorolac tromethamine	AB	15 mg/mL	AB	4 mcg/mL[b]	Physically compatible for 4 hr at 23°C	2383	C
Labetalol HCl	AB	2 mg/mL[b]	AB	4 mcg/mL[b]	Physically compatible for 4 hr at 23°C	2383	C
Levofloxacin	ORT	5 mg/mL[b]	AB	4 mcg/mL[b]	Physically compatible for 4 hr at 23°C	2383	C
Lidocaine HCl	AST	10 mg/mL[b]	AB	4 mcg/mL[b]	Physically compatible for 4 hr at 23°C	2383	C
Linezolid	PHU	2 mg/mL	AB	4 mcg/mL[b]	Physically compatible for 4 hr at 23°C	2383	C
Lorazepam	ESL	0.5 mg/mL[b]	AB	4 mcg/mL[b]	Physically compatible for 4 hr at 23°C	2383	C
Magnesium sulfate	APP	100 mg/mL[b]	AB	4 mcg/mL[b]	Physically compatible for 4 hr at 23°C	2383	C
Magnesium sulfate		100 mg/mL	HOS, HQS	4 mcg/mL[b]	Stated to be compatible	2848, 3179	C
Mannitol		20%	HOS, HQS	4 mcg/mL[b]	Stated to be compatible	2848, 3179	C
Meperidine HCl	AST	10 mg/mL[b]	AB	4 mcg/mL[b]	Physically compatible for 4 hr at 23°C	2383	C
Meropenem		50 mg/mL	HOS	0.1 mg/mL	Physically compatible for 4 hr at room temperature	3538	C
Meropenem–vaborbactam	TMC	8 mg/mL[b g]	HOS	4 mcg/mL	Physically compatible for 3 hr at 20 to 25°C	3380	C
Methylprednisolone sodium succinate	PHU	5 mg/mL[b]	AB	4 mcg/mL[b]	Physically compatible for 4 hr at 23°C	2383	C
Metoclopramide HCl	FAU	5 mg/mL	AB	4 mcg/mL[b]	Physically compatible for 4 hr at 23°C	2383	C
Metronidazole	BA	5 mg/mL	AB	4 mcg/mL[b]	Physically compatible for 4 hr at 23°C	2383	C
Midazolam HCl			HOS	4 mcg/mL[b]	Stated to be compatible	3181	C
Milrinone lactate	SAN	0.2 mg/mL[b]	AB	4 mcg/mL[b]	Physically compatible for 4 hr at 23°C	2383	C
Morphine sulfate			HOS	4 mcg/mL[b]	Stated to be compatible	3181	C
Nalbuphine HCl	AST	10 mg/mL	AB	4 mcg/mL[b]	Physically compatible for 4 hr at 23°C	2383	C
Nitroglycerin	AMR	0.4 mg/mL[b]	AB	4 mcg/mL[b]	Physically compatible for 4 hr at 23°C	2383	C
Norepinephrine bitartrate	AB	0.12 mg/mL[b]	AB	4 mcg/mL[b]	Physically compatible for 4 hr at 23°C	2383	C
Ondansetron HCl	GW	1 mg/mL[b]	AB	4 mcg/mL[b]	Physically compatible for 4 hr at 23°C	2383	C
Oritavancin diphosphate	TAR	0.8, 1.2, and 2 mg/mL[a]	HOS	4 mcg/mL[a]	Visually compatible for 4 hr at 20 to 24°C	2928	C
Pancuronium bromide			HOS	4 mcg/mL[b]	Stated to be compatible	3181	C
Phenylephrine HCl			HOS	4 mcg/mL[b]	Stated to be compatible	3181	C

Y-Site Injection Compatibility (1:1 Mixture) (Cont.)

Test Drug	Mfr	Conc	Mfr	Conc	Remarks	Ref	C/I
Piperacillin sodium–tazobactam sodium	LE[c]	40 mg/mL[b e]	AB	4 mcg/mL[b]	Physically compatible for 4 hr at 23°C	2383	C
Plazomicin sulfate	ACH	24 mg/mL[h]	HOS	4 mcg/mL	Physically compatible for 1 hr at 20 to 25°C	3432	C
Potassium chloride	AB	0.1 mEq/mL[b]	AB	4 mcg/mL[b]	Physically compatible for 4 hr at 23°C	2383	C
Potassium chloride		0.04 mEq/mL	HOS, HQS	4 mcg/mL[b]	Stated to be compatible	2848, 3179	C
Procainamide HCl	ES	10 mg/mL[b]	AB	4 mcg/mL[b]	Physically compatible for 4 hr at 23°C	2383	C
Prochlorperazine edisylate	SKB	0.5 mg/mL[b]	AB	4 mcg/mL[b]	Physically compatible for 4 hr at 23°C	2383	C
Promethazine HCl	ES	2 mg/mL[b]	AB	4 mcg/mL[b]	Physically compatible for 4 hr at 23°C	2383	C
Propofol	ASZ[m]	10 mg/mL	AB	4 mcg/mL[b]	Physically compatible for 4 hr at 23°C	2383	C
Ranitidine HCl	GW	2 mg/mL[b]	AB	4 mcg/mL[b]	Physically compatible for 4 hr at 23°C	2383	C
Remifentanil HCl	AB	0.25 mg/mL[b]	AB	4 mcg/mL[b]	Physically compatible for 4 hr at 23°C	2383	C
Rocuronium bromide	OR	1 mg/mL[b]	AB	4 mcg/mL[b]	Physically compatible for 4 hr at 23°C	2383	C
Sodium bicarbonate	AMR	1 mEq/mL	AB	4 mcg/mL[b]	Physically compatible for 4 hr at 23°C	2383	C
Sodium nitroprusside	BA	2 mg/mL[b]	AB	4 mcg/mL[b]	Physically compatible for 4 hr at 23°C protected from light	2383	C
Succinylcholine chloride			HOS	4 mcg/mL[b]	Stated to be compatible	3181	C
Sufentanil citrate	AB	50 mcg/mL	AB	4 mcg/mL[b]	Physically compatible for 4 hr at 23°C	2383	C
Tedizolid phosphate	CUB	0.8 mg/mL[b]	HOS	4 mcg/mL[b]	Physically compatible for 2 hr	3244	C
Theophylline	AB	4 mg/mL[a]	AB	4 mcg/mL[b]	Physically compatible for 4 hr at 23°C	2383	C
Tobramycin sulfate	GNS	5 mg/mL[b]	AB	4 mcg/mL[b]	Physically compatible for 4 hr at 23°C	2383	C
Trimethoprim–sulfamethoxazole	GNS	0.8 mg/mL[b f]	AB	4 mcg/mL[b]	Physically compatible for 4 hr at 23°C	2383	C
Vancomycin HCl	AB	10 mg/mL[b]	AB	4 mcg/mL[b]	Physically compatible for 4 hr at 23°C	2383	C
Vecuronium bromide			HOS	4 mcg/mL[b]	Stated to be compatible	3181	C
Verapamil HCl	AB	1.25 mg/mL[b]	AB	4 mcg/mL[b]	Physically compatible for 4 hr at 23°C	2383	C

[a] Tested in dextrose 5%.

[b] Tested in sodium chloride 0.9%.

[c] Test performed using the formulation WITHOUT edetate disodium.

[d] Ampicillin component. Ampicillin in a 2:1 fixed ratio concentration with sulbactam.

[e] Piperacillin component. Piperacillin in an 8:1 fixed-ratio concentration with tazobactam.

[f] Trimethoprim component. Trimethoprim in a 1:5 fixed-ratio concentration with sulfamethoxazole.

[g] Meropenem component. Meropenem in a 1:1 fixed-ratio concentration with vaborbactam.

[h] Tested in both dextrose 5% and sodium chloride 0.9%.

[i] Ceftolozane component. Ceftolozane in a 2:1 fixed-ratio concentration with tazobactam.

[j] Ceftazidime component. Ceftazidime in a 4:1 fixed-ratio concentration with avibactam.

[k] Tested in dextrose 5%, sodium chloride 0.9%, and Ringer's injection, lactated.

[l] Salt not specified.

[m] Test performed using the formulation WITH edetate disodium.

Additional Compatibility Information

Infusion Solutions

Manufacturers state that dexmedetomidine hydrochloride is compatible when administered with dextrose 5% or Ringer's injection, lactated.[2848] [3179] [3180]

Selected Revisions May 1, 2020. © Copyright, October 2004. American Society of Health-System Pharmacists, Inc.

Dexrazoxane Hydrochloride
AHFS 92:56

Products

Dexrazoxane hydrochloride (Zinecard) is available as a lyophilized powder in single-dose vials containing the equivalent of 250 or 500 mg of dexrazoxane.[3392] Reconstitution of the contents of the 250- or 500-mg Zinecard vial with 25 or 50 mL, respectively, of sterile water for injection results in a solution with a dexrazoxane concentration of 10 mg/mL.[3392] The pH has been adjusted during manufacturing with hydrochloric acid.[3392] The reconstituted solution should be diluted in an infusion bag with Ringer's injection, lactated to a final dexrazoxane concentration of 1.3 to 3 mg/mL.[3392]

Dexrazoxane hydrochloride (generic; Mylan) also is available as a lyophilized powder in single-use vials containing the equivalent of 250 or 500 mg of dexrazoxane.[3393] Each vial is packaged with a 25- or 50-mL vial, respectively, of 0.167 M (i.e., ⅙ M) sodium lactate for use as a diluent for reconstituting the drug.[3393] Reconstitution of the contents of the 250- or 500-mg vials with 25 or 50 mL, respectively, of the provided diluent results in a solution with a dexrazoxane concentration of 10 mg/mL.[3393] The pH has been adjusted during manufacturing with hydrochloric acid.[3393] The reconstituted solution may be transferred to an empty infusion bag or may be diluted in an infusion bag with sodium chloride 0.9% or dextrose 5% to a final dexrazoxane concentration of 1.3 to 5 mg/mL.[3393]

Dexrazoxane hydrochloride (Totect) is available as a lyophilized powder in single-dose vials containing the equivalent of 500 mg of dexrazoxane.[3394] Reconstitution of the contents of the 500-mg Totect vial with 50 mL of 0.167 M sodium lactate results in a solution with a dexrazoxane concentration of 10 mg/mL.[3394] The resulting solution also contains hydrochloric acid, sodium hydroxide, and lactic acid in water for injection.[3394] The appropriate volume of the reconstituted solution should be diluted in 1 L of sodium chloride 0.9%.[3394]

pH

The pH of reconstituted Zinecard solutions ranges from 1 to 3 while the pH of Zinecard diluted for infusion ranges from 3.5 to 5.5.[3392]

The pH of reconstituted solutions of dexrazoxane (generic; Mylan) ranges from 3.5 to 5.5.[3393]

Trade Name(s)

Totect, Zinecard

Administration

Diluted solutions of Zinecard for infusion should be administered by rapid intravenous drip infusion over 15 minutes.[3392]

The reconstituted solution of dexrazoxane (generic; Mylan) is administered by slow intravenous push; alternatively, the reconstituted solution may be diluted and administered by rapid intravenous drip infusion.[3393]

Diluted solutions of Totect for infusion should be administered by intravenous infusion over 1 to 2 hours at room temperature and under normal light conditions into a large caliber vein in an extremity or area other than the one affected by the anthracycline extravasation.[3394] Any cooling methods (e.g., ice packs) used for the extravasation being treated should be removed from the area at least 15 minutes prior to Totect administration.[3394]

As with other toxic drugs, caution should be exercised in the handling and preparation of dexrazoxane and applicable special handling and disposal procedures should be followed.[3392] [3393] [3394] Manufacturers recommend the use of gloves.[3392] [3393] [3394] If skin contact with the drug occurs, the affected area(s) should be washed immediately and thoroughly with soap and water.[3392] [3393] [3394]

Stability

Intact vials of dexrazoxane should be stored at controlled room temperature.[3392] [3393] [3394] One manufacturer recommends that Totect vials remain in the original carton to protect from light.[3394]

Reconstituted solutions of Zinecard are stable for 30 minutes at room temperature or for up to 3 hours at 2 to 8°C.[3392] Diluted solutions of Zinecard for infusion are stable for 1 hour at room temperature or for up to 4 hours at 2 to 8°C.[3392]

The manufacturer states that reconstituted solutions of dexrazoxane (generic; Mylan) are stable for 6 hours from the time of reconstitution when stored in an empty infusion bag at controlled room temperature of 20 to 25°C or at 2 to 8°C; this preparation of dexrazoxane diluted for infusion in sodium chloride 0.9% or dextrose 5% is stable for 6 hours at 20 to 25°C or 2 to 8°C.[3393]

Reconstituted solutions of Totect should be diluted within 2 hours after reconstitution.[3394] Diluted solutions of Totect for infusion should be used immediately after preparation, but are stable for 4 hours from the time of preparation when stored below 25°C.[3394]

Solutions should be visually inspected for particulate matter and discoloration prior to administration; solutions containing a precipitate should be discarded.[3392] [3393] [3394] Any unused portions should be discarded.[3392] [3393] [3394]

In one study, reconstituted solutions of dexrazoxane (National Cancer Institute) 10 mg/mL were found to be stable for about 24 hours at 20 to 22°C exposed to or protected from fluorescent light; about 7% loss occurred when reconstituted with dextrose 5% and about 9% loss occurred when reconstituted with sodium chloride 0.9%.[2395] Refrigeration resulted in precipitation after 1 day.[2395]

In another study, reconstituted solutions of Zinecard 10 mg/mL prepared with sterile water for injection and dexrazoxane (generic; Mylan) prepared with 0.167 M sodium lactate were stable for

DOI: 10.37573/9781585286850.119

8 hours at room temperature; the reconstituted solutions exhibited a mean drug loss of 11 and 13%, respectively, at 24 hours.[3395]

pH Effects

Dexrazoxane is most stable at acidic pH and is highly unstable in alkaline solutions.[2395] Dexrazoxane degrades rapidly at pH values above 7;[3392][3393] more than 10% loss occurred in less than 2 hours at such pH values.[2395]

Light Effects

No adverse effect on drug stability was found in 1- and 10-mg/mL solutions when exposed to fluorescent light.[2395]

Compatibility Information
Solution Compatibility

Dexrazoxane HCl

Test Soln Name	Mfr	Mfr	Conc/L or %	Remarks	Ref	C/I
Dextrose 5%		MYL	1.3 to 5 g	Stable for 6 hr at room temperature or 2 to 8°C	3393	C
Dextrose 5%	a	NCI	1 g	Visually compatible with less than 10% loss in 24 hr at 21°C exposed to and protected from light and in 3 days at 4°C in the dark	2395	C
Dextrose 5%	BA[b]	MYL	1 g	Physically and chemically stable with 8.9% loss in 24 hr at room temperature	3395	C
Dextrose 5%	BA[b]	MYL	3 g	Physically and chemically stable with 4.9% loss in 8 hr at room temperature	3395	C
Ringer's injection, lactated		PF	1.3 to 3 g	Stable for 1 hr at room temperature or 4 hr at 2 to 8°C	3392	C
Ringer's injection, lactated	BA[b]	PF	1 and 3 g	Physically and chemically stable with less than 5% loss in 8 hr at room temperature	3395	C
Sodium chloride 0.9%		MYL	1.3 to 5 g	Stable for 6 hr at room temperature or 2 to 8°C	3393	C
Sodium chloride 0.9%	a	NCI	1 g	Visually compatible with less than 10% loss in 24 hr at 21°C exposed to and protected from light and in 3 days at 4°C in the dark	2395	C
Sodium chloride 0.9%	BA[b]	MYL	1 g	Physically and chemically stable with 9.2% loss in 24 hr at room temperature	3395	C
Sodium chloride 0.9%	BA[b]	MYL	3 g	Physically and chemically stable with 4.2% loss in 8 hr at room temperature	3395	C
Sodium chloride 0.9%		CMB		Stable for 4 hr at temperatures less than 25°C	3394	C

[a] Tested in both glass and PVC containers.

[b] Tested in PVC containers.

Y-Site Injection Compatibility (1:1 Mixture)

Dexrazoxane HCl

Test Drug	Mfr	Conc	Mfr	Conc	Remarks	Ref	C/I
Gemcitabine HCl	LI	10 mg/mL[b]	PH	5 mg/mL[b]	Physically compatible for 4 hr at 23°C	2226	C
Pemetrexed disodium	LI	20 mg/mL[b]	PHU	5 mg/mL[a]	Physically compatible for 4 hr at 23°C	2564	C

[a] Tested in dextrose 5%.

[b] Tested in sodium chloride 0.9%.

Selected Revisions April 16, 2018. © Copyright, October 2004.
American Society of Health-System Pharmacists, Inc.

Dextran 40

AHFS 40:12

Products

Dextran 40 products are available as 10% injections in dextrose 5% or sodium chloride 0.9% in 500-mL containers. The colloidal products contain low molecular weight dextran (average molecular weight of 40,000) with either dextrose, hydrous, 5 g/100 mL or sodium chloride 0.9 g/100 mL in water for injection.[1(10/05)] [4]

pH

The pH of dextran 40 10% in dextrose 5% ranges from 3 to 7. The pH of dextran 40 10% in sodium chloride 0.9% ranges from 3.5 to 7.[1(10/05)] [4]

Osmolarity

Dextran 40 10% in dextrose 5% has a calculated osmolarity of 255 mOsm/L. Dextran 40 10% in sodium chloride 0.9% has a calculated osmolarity of 310 mOsm/L.[1(10/05)]

Sodium Content

Dextran 40 10% in sodium chloride 0.9% provides 77 mEq of sodium per 500-mL bottle.[1(10/05)] [4]

Trade Name(s)

LMD

Administration

Dextran 40 10% injection is administered by intravenous infusion.[1(10/05)] [4]

Stability

Dextran 40 products should not be administered unless they are clear. Long periods of storage or exposure to temperature fluctuations may cause the formation of dextran flakes or crystals. Therefore, solutions should be stored at a constant temperature, preferably 25°C, and protected from freezing and extreme heat. Do not use dextran solutions that contain crystals.[1(10/05)] However, if flakes or crystals do appear, they can be dissolved by heating in a water bath at 100°C or autoclaving at 110°C for 15 minutes.[4] [1484] [1485] Because no antibacterial preservative is present, partially used containers should be discarded.[4]

Compatibility Information

Additive Compatibility

Dextran 40

Test Drug	Mfr	Conc/L or %	Mfr	Conc/L or %	Test Solution	Remarks	Ref	C/I
Amoxicillin sodium		10, 20, 50 g		10%	D5W	9, 12, and 12% amoxicillin loss at 10, 20, and 50 g/L, respectively, in 1 hr at 25°C	1469	I
Amoxicillin sodium		10, 20, 50 g		10%	NS	12, 14, and 20% amoxicillin loss at 10, 20, and 50 g/L, respectively, in 3 hr at 25°C	1469	I
Ampicillin sodium		4 g		10%	D5W	46% ampicillin loss in 24 hr at 20°C	834	I
Ampicillin sodium	AY	8 g	PH	10%	D5W	50% loss in 24 hr at room temperature	99	I
Ampicillin sodium	BAY	15 g	PH	10%	D5W	10% ampicillin loss in 1.5 hr at 25°C	604	I
Ampicillin sodium	BAY	2 g	PH	10%	D5W	10% ampicillin loss in 3.5 hr at 25°C	604	I
Ampicillin sodium	BAY	5 g	PH	10%	D5W	10% ampicillin loss in 2.3 hr at 25°C	604	I
Ampicillin sodium	AY	8 g	PH	10%	NS	25% loss in 24 hr at room temperature	99	I
Ampicillin sodium	BAY	15 g	PH	10%	NS	10% ampicillin loss in 2.3 hr at 25°C	604	I
Ampicillin sodium	BAY	2 g	PH	10%	NS	10% ampicillin loss in 2.8 hr at 25°C	604	I
Ampicillin sodium	BAY	5 g	PH	10%	NS	10% ampicillin loss in 2.5 hr at 25°C	604	I
Cloxacillin sodium	AST	2.25 g	PH	10%	D5W	Under 4% cloxacillin loss in 48 hr at 25°C	1476	C
Cloxacillin sodium	BE	4 g	PH	10%	D5W	2% cloxacillin loss in 24 hr at 20°C	834	C
Cloxacillin sodium	BE	8 g	PH	10%	D5W, NS	Under 5% loss in 24 hr at room temperature	99	C

DOI: 10.37573/9781585286850.120

Additive Compatibility (Cont.)

Test Drug	Mfr	Conc/L or %	Mfr	Conc/L or %	Test Solution	Remarks	Ref	C/I
Enalaprilat	MSD	25 mg	TR	10%	D5W	Physically compatible for 24 hr at room temperature under fluorescent light	1355	C
Floxacillin sodium				10%	D5W, NS	Under 10% loss in 24 hr at room temperature	1475	C
Gentamicin sulfate				10%	D5W	Gentamicin stable for 24 hr at room temperature	227	C
Nafcillin sodium	WY	2 and 30 g	PH	10%	D5W	Physically compatible and stable for 24 hr at 25°C	27	C
Oxacillin sodium		4 g		10%	D5W	3% loss in 24 hr at 20°C	834	C
Penicillin G potassium		6 million units		10%	D5W	34% loss in 24 hr at 20°C	834	I
Penicillin G sodium	KA	6 million units	PH	10%		Stable for 24 hr at 25°C	131	C
Tobramycin sulfate	LI	200 mg and 1 g	TR	10%	D5W	Physically compatible and stable for 24 hr at 25°C. Not more than 9% loss	147	C
Tranexamic acid	PF					Manufacturer-recommended solution	2887	C
Verapamil HCl	KN	80 mg	TR	10%	NS	Physically compatible for 24 hr	764	C

Y-Site Injection Compatibility (1:1 Mixture)

Dextran 40

Test Drug	Mfr	Conc	Mfr	Conc	Remarks	Ref	C/I
Enalaprilat	MSD	0.05 mg/mL[b]	TR	100 mg/mL[a]	Physically compatible for 24 hr at room temperature under fluorescent light	1355	C
Famotidine	MSD	0.2 mg/mL[a]	PH	100 mg/mL[a]	Physically compatible for 4 hr at 25°C	1188	C
Nicardipine HCl	DCC	0.1 mg/mL[a]	TR	10%	Visually compatible for 24 hr at room temperature	235	C

[a] Tested in dextrose 5%.

[b] Tested in sodium chloride 0.9%.

Selected Revisions September 1, 2014. © Copyright, October 1990. American Society of Health-System Pharmacists, Inc.

Diamorphine Hydrochloride
AHFS 28:08.08
Diacetylmorphine HCl

Products

Diamorphine hydrochloride is available as a lyophilized product in 10-, 30-, 100-, and 500-mg ampuls.[38]

Diamorphine hydrochloride is very soluble in water. Up to 100 mg can be reconstituted in 1 mL of diluent; a minimum of 2 mL of diluent is recommended for the 500-mg size. The preferred diluent is dextrose 5%, but sodium chloride 0.9% also may be used.[1442]

Administration

Diamorphine hydrochloride is given by intramuscular, intravenous, or subcutaneous injection. Administration can also be by slow continuous subcutaneous or intravenous injection with an infusion control device.[38]

Stability

Ampuls of lyophilized diamorphine hydrochloride should be stored at or below 25°C and protected from light.[38]

Diamorphine hydrochloride 1 mg/mL as an aqueous solution in flint glass ampuls stored at 25°C exhibited 10% loss in 50 days.[1958]

In another study, diamorphine hydrochloride up to 25 mg/mL in sterile water for injection was stable for up to 24 hours at ambient temperature when protected from light.[1454]

pH Effects

The stability of the reconstituted injection depends on its pH; it is most stable at acidic pH, around 3.8 to 4.4[1442] to pH 4.5.[1958] Degradation increases greatly at neutral or basic pH.[1448]

Diamorphine hydrochloride exhibits a pH-dependent incompatibility in sodium chloride injection. To remain in solution, the pH must be below 6.[1458] Solutions containing up to 250 mg/mL of diamorphine hydrochloride have been shown to be compatible in sodium chloride 0.9%.[1457 1458 1459]

Temperature Effects

Solutions of diamorphine hydrochloride in sterile water for injection at concentrations greater than 15 mg/mL exhibited precipitation when stored at 21 and 37°C for longer than two weeks. At concentrations of 1 to 250 mg/mL in sterile water for injection in glass containers, diamorphine hydrochloride was stable for eight weeks at –20°C, exhibiting less than 10% degradation. At 4°C, degradation was inversely related to concentration. Diamorphine hydrochloride 31 and 250 mg/mL was stable, but solutions containing 1 and 7.81 mg/mL showed 15 and 12% losses, respectively, after eight weeks of storage.[1452]

Syringes

The stability of diamorphine hydrochloride solutions containing 1 and 20 mg/mL in sodium chloride 0.9% in glass syringes was determined. At ambient temperature, diamorphine hydrochloride in glass syringes was stable for seven days at 1 mg/mL and for 12 days at 20 mg/mL. This was somewhat less than the drug's stability at these concentrations in PVC containers; adequate stability was maintained for at least 15 days in PVC containers.[1449]

Diamorphine hydrochloride stability in plastic syringes was reported to be 14 days at room temperature and greater than 40 days at 4°C.[982]

Diamorphine hydrochloride (Hillcross) 2 and 20 mg/mL in water for injection was stored in plastic syringes (Becton Dickinson) sealed with blind hubs. A 5% loss occurred in 18 days at 20°C.[1672]

Infusion Pumps

Solutions containing diamorphine hydrochloride 250 mg/mL in an Act-a-Pump (Pharmacia) reservoir were stable for at least 14 days during simulated patient use.[1450] Degradation was both temperature and concentration dependent. Solutions of diamorphine hydrochloride 1 mg/mL in water stored at 21°C for 42 days showed 10.6% degradation. At 37°C, 32.6% degradation occurred.[1451]

However, at a concentration of 250 mg/mL, diamorphine hydrochloride losses of 11 and 85.8% at 21 and 37°C, respectively,[1451] were partially attributed to precipitation.[1452]

Diamorphine hydrochloride (Evans Medical) 5 mg/mL in sterile water for injection was stable in Parker Micropump PVC reservoirs for 14 days at 4°C, exhibiting no loss. At 37°C, about a 2% loss occurred in seven days and a 7% loss occurred in 14 days.[1696]

Elastomeric Reservoir Pumps

Diamorphine hydrochloride 1 and 20 mg/mL in sodium chloride 0.9% was evaluated for stability in two elastomeric disposable infusion devices, Infusor (Travenol) and Intermate 200 (I.S.C.). The drug was stable for 15 days in most cases. However, solutions containing diamorphine hydrochloride 1 mg/mL in the Intermate reservoir stored at 31°C were only stable for two days.[1449]

DOI: 10.37573/9781585286850.121

Compatibility Information
Solution Compatibility

Diamorphine HCl

Test Soln Name	Mfr	Mfr	Conc/L or %	Remarks	Ref	C/I
Sodium chloride 0.9%	TR[a]	EV	1 and 20 g	Little or no loss in 15 days at 4 and 24°C	1449	C

[a] Tested in PVC containers.

Additive Compatibility

Diamorphine HCl

Test Drug	Mfr	Conc/L or %	Mfr	Conc/L or %	Test Solution	Remarks	Ref	C/I
Bupivacaine HCl	GL	1.25 g		0.125 g	NS	Visually compatible with 8% diamorphine loss and no bupivacaine loss in 28 days at room temperature	1791	C
Bupivacaine HCl	AST	150 mg	NAP	20 mg	NS[a]	5% diamorphine and no bupivacaine loss in 14 days at 7°C. Both drugs were stable for 6 months at −20°C	2070	C
Floxacillin sodium	BE	20 g	EV	500 mg	W	Physically compatible for 24 hr at 15 and 30°C. Haze forms in 48 hr at 30°C. No change at 15°C	1479	C
Furosemide	HO	1 g	EV	500 mg	W	Physically compatible for 72 hr at 15 and 30°C	1479	C
Ropivacaine HCl	ASZ	2 g		25 mg	[a]	No ropivacaine and 10% diamorphine loss in 70 days at 4°C and 28 days at 21°C	2517	C

[a] Tested in PVC containers.

Drugs in Syringe Compatibility

Diamorphine HCl

Test Drug	Mfr	Amt	Mfr	Amt	Remarks	Ref	C/I
Bupivacaine HCl	AST	0.5%	EV	1 and 10 mg/mL	10 to 11% diamorphine loss in 5 weeks at 20°C and 3 to 7% loss in 8 weeks at 6°C. No bupivacaine loss at 6 or 20°C in 8 weeks	1952	C
Cyclizine lactate	CA	5 mg/1 mL[a]	MB	20, 50, 100 mg/1 mL	Physically compatible and diamorphine stable for 24 hr at room temperature	1454	C
Cyclizine lactate	CA	15 mg/1 mL	EV	15 mg/1 mL	Physically compatible for 24 hr at room temperature	1455	C
Cyclizine lactate	CA	12.5 to 50 mg/1 mL	EV	37.5 to 150 mg/1 mL	Precipitate forms within 24 hr	1455	I
Cyclizine lactate	CA	10 mg/mL	HC	25 to 100 mg/mL	Visually incompatible	1672	I
Cyclizine lactate	CA	10 mg/mL	HC	20 mg/mL	Visually compatible for 48 hr at 5 and 20°C	1672	C
Cyclizine lactate	CA	6.7 mg/mL	HC	100 mg/mL	Visually compatible for 48 hr at 5 and 20°C	1672	C
Cyclizine lactate	CA	6.7 mg/mL	HC	2 mg/mL	5% diamorphine loss in 9.9 days at 20°C. Cyclizine stable for 45 days	1672	C
Cyclizine lactate	CA	6.7 mg/mL	HC	20 mg/mL	5% diamorphine loss in 13.6 days at 20°C. Cyclizine stable for 45 days	1672	C
Cyclizine lactate	WEL	51 mg/mL	BP	6 mg/mL	Physically compatible. 10% diamorphine loss in 1.7 days. Little cyclizine loss at 23°C	2071	C

Drugs in Syringe Compatibility (Cont.)

Test Drug	Mfr	Amt	Mfr	Amt	Remarks	Ref	C/I
Cyclizine lactate	WEL	32 mg/mL	BP	9 mg/mL	Physically compatible. Under 10% diamorphine loss and little cyclizine loss in 4 days at 23°C	2071	C
Cyclizine lactate	WEL	39 mg/mL	BP	10 mg/mL	Physically compatible. Under 10% diamorphine loss and little cyclizine loss in 4 days at 23°C	2071	C
Cyclizine lactate	WEL	28 mg/mL	BP	10 mg/mL	Physically compatible. 10% diamorphine loss in 3.1 days and little cyclizine loss at 23°C	2071	C
Cyclizine lactate	WEL	51 mg/mL	BP	12 mg/mL	Physically compatible. 10% diamorphine loss in 2.2 days and little cyclizine loss at 23°C	2071	C
Cyclizine lactate	WEL	40 mg/mL	BP	14 mg/mL	Crystals form	2071	I
Cyclizine lactate	WEL	26 mg/mL	BP	17 mg/mL	Physically compatible. 10% diamorphine loss in 1.1 days and 10% cyclizine loss in 2.5 days at 23°C	2071	C
Cyclizine lactate	WEL	52 mg/mL	BP	18 mg/mL	Crystals form	2071	I
Cyclizine lactate	WEL	10 mg/mL	BP	20 mg/mL	Physically compatible. Under 10% diamorphine loss and little cyclizine loss in 7 days at 23°C	2071	C
Cyclizine lactate	WEL	15 mg/mL	BP	20 mg/mL	Physically compatible. Little diamorphine loss and 10% cyclizine loss in 0.5 days at 23°C	2071	I
Cyclizine lactate	WEL	26 mg/mL	BP	21 mg/mL	Physically compatible. 10% diamorphine loss in 4.9 days. 10% cyclizine loss in 3.2 days at 23°C	2071	C
Cyclizine lactate	WEL	18 mg/mL	BP	23 mg/mL	Physically compatible. Little diamorphine loss and 10% cyclizine loss in 3.2 days at 23°C	2071	C
Cyclizine lactate	WEL	23 mg/mL	BP	26 mg/mL	Physically compatible. 10% diamorphine loss in 1.9 days. 10% cyclizine loss in 9 hr at 23°C	2071	I
Cyclizine lactate	WEL	30 mg/mL	BP	30 mg/mL	Physically compatible. 10% diamorphine loss in 21 hr and 10% cyclizine loss in 9 hr at 23°C	2071	I
Cyclizine lactate	WEL	10 mg/mL	BP	49 mg/mL	Physically compatible. Little diamorphine loss and 10% cyclizine loss in 5.5 days at 23°C	2071	C
Cyclizine lactate	WEL	4 mg/mL	BP	51 mg/mL	Physically compatible. Little diamorphine or cyclizine loss in 7 days at 23°C	2071	C
Cyclizine lactate	WEL	8 mg/mL	BP	61 mg/mL	Physically compatible. 10% diamorphine loss in 1.4 days. 10% cyclizine loss in 1.1 days at 23°C	2071	C
Cyclizine lactate	WEL	13 mg/mL	BP	65 mg/mL	Physically compatible. 10% diamorphine loss in 1.6 days. 10% cyclizine loss in 12 hr at 23°C	2071	I
Cyclizine lactate	WEL	10 mg/mL	BP	92 mg/mL	Physically compatible. Little diamorphine loss and 10% cyclizine loss in 2.4 days at 23°C	2071	C
Cyclizine lactate	WEL	4 mg/mL	BP	99 mg/mL	Physically compatible. Little diamorphine or cyclizine loss in 7 days at 23°C	2071	C
Cyclizine lactate with haloperidol lactate	WEL JC	16 mg/mL 2.2 mg/mL	BP	11 mg/mL	Physically compatible with less than 10% loss of any drug in 7 days at 23°C	2071	C
Cyclizine lactate with haloperidol lactate	WEL JC	25 mg/mL 2.2 mg/mL	BP	16 mg/mL	Physically compatible with less than 10% loss of any drug in 7 days at 23°C	2071	C
Cyclizine lactate with haloperidol lactate	WEL JC	11 mg/mL 2.2 mg/mL	BP	40 mg/mL	Physically compatible with less than 10% loss of any drug in 7 days at 23°C	2071	C

Drugs in Syringe Compatibility (Cont.)

Test Drug	Mfr	Amt	Mfr	Amt	Remarks	Ref	C/I
Cyclizine lactate with haloperidol lactate	WEL JC	13 mg/mL 2.1 mg/mL	BP	42 mg/mL	Physically compatible with less than 10% loss of any drug in 7 days at 23°C	2071	C
Cyclizine lactate with haloperidol lactate	WEL JC	9 mg/mL 2.1 mg/mL	BP	55 mg/mL	Physically compatible with less than 10% loss of any drug in 7 days at 23°C	2071	C
Cyclizine lactate with haloperidol lactate	WEL JC	13 mg/mL 2.1 mg/mL	BP	56 mg/mL	Physically compatible with less than 10% loss of any drug in 7 days at 23°C	2071	C
Haloperidol lactate	SE	1.5 mg/1 mL[a]	MB	10, 25, 50 mg/1 mL	Physically compatible and diamorphine content retained for 24 hr at room temperature	1454	C
Haloperidol lactate	SE	2 mg/1 mL	EV	20 mg/1 mL	Crystallization with 58% haloperidol loss in 7 days at room temperature	1455	I
Haloperidol lactate	SE	5 mg/1 mL	EV	50 and 150 mg/1 mL	Precipitates immediately	1455	I
Haloperidol lactate	SE	2.5 mg/8 mL	EV	100 mg/8 mL	Physically compatible for 24 hr at room temperature and 7 days at 6°C	1456	C
Haloperidol lactate	SE	0.75 mg/mL	HC	20 to 100 mg/mL	Visually compatible for 48 hr at 5 and 20°C	1672	C
Haloperidol lactate	SE	0.75 mg/mL	HC	2 mg/mL	5% diamorphine loss in 14.8 days at 20°C. Haloperidol stable for 45 days	1672	C
Haloperidol lactate	SE	0.75 mg/mL	HC	20 mg/mL	5% diamorphine loss in 20.7 days at 20°C. Haloperidol stable for 45 days	1672	C
Haloperidol lactate	JC	2 and 3 mg/mL	BP	20, 50, 100 mg/mL	Physically compatible with less than 10% loss of either drug in 7 days at 23°C	2071	C
Haloperidol lactate	JC	4 mg/mL	BP	20 and 50 mg/mL	Physically compatible with less than 10% loss of either drug in 7 days at 23°C	2071	C
Haloperidol lactate with cyclizine lactate	JC WEL	2.2 mg/mL 16 mg/mL	BP	11 mg/mL	Physically compatible with less than 10% loss of any drug in 7 days at 23°C	2071	C
Haloperidol lactate with cyclizine lactate	JC WEL	2.2 mg/mL 25 mg/mL	BP	16 mg/mL	Physically compatible with less than 10% loss of any drug in 7 days at 23°C	2071	C
Haloperidol lactate with cyclizine lactate	JC WEL	2.2 mg/mL 11 mg/mL	BP	40 mg/mL	Physically compatible with less than 10% loss of any drug in 7 days at 23°C	2071	C
Haloperidol lactate with cyclizine lactate	JC WEL	2.1 mg/mL 13 mg/mL	BP	42 mg/mL	Physically compatible with less than 10% loss of any drug in 7 days at 23°C	2071	C
Haloperidol lactate with cyclizine lactate	JC WEL	2.1 mg/mL 9 mg/mL	BP	55 mg/mL	Physically compatible with less than 10% loss of any drug in 7 days at 23°C	2071	C
Haloperidol lactate with cyclizine lactate	JC WEL	2.1 mg/mL 13 mg/mL	BP	56 mg/mL	Physically compatible with less than 10% loss of any drug in 7 days at 23°C	2071	C
Methotrimeprazine HCl	MB	1.25 and 2.5 mg/1 mL[a]	MB	50 mg/1 mL	Physically compatible and diamorphine stable for 24 hr at room temperature	1454	C
Metoclopramide HCl	BK	5 mg/1 mL	MB	10, 25, 50 mg/1 mL	Physically compatible and diamorphine stable for 24 hr at room temperature	1454	C
Metoclopramide HCl	LA	5 mg/1 mL	EV	50 and 150 mg/1 mL	Slight discoloration with 8% metoclopramide loss and 9% diamorphine loss in 7 days at room temperature	1455	C
Midazolam HCl	RC	10[b] and 75[c] mg	EV	10 mg	Visually compatible. 10% diamorphine and no midazolam loss in 15.9 days at 22°C	1792	C
Midazolam HCl	RC	10[b] and 75[c] mg	EV	500 mg	Visually compatible. 10% diamorphine and no midazolam loss in 22.2 days at 22°C	1792	C

Drugs in Syringe Compatibility (Cont.)

Test Drug	Mfr	Amt	Mfr	Amt	Remarks	Ref	C/I
Octreotide acetate	NVA	300 mcg/8 mL[a]	EV	50 mg/8 mL[a]	Visually compatible with no octreotide loss in 48 hr. Diamorphine not tested	2709	C
Octreotide acetate	NVA	600 mcg/8 mL[a]	EV	50 mg/8 mL[a]	Visually compatible with no octreotide loss in 48 hr. Diamorphine not tested	2709	C
Octreotide acetate	NVA	900 mcg/8 mL[a]	EV	50 mg/8 mL[a]	Visually compatible with 1% octreotide loss in 48 hr. Diamorphine not tested	2709	C
Octreotide acetate	NVA	300 mcg/8 mL[a]	EV	100 mg/8 mL[a]	Visually compatible with 4% octreotide loss in 48 hr. Diamorphine not tested	2709	C
Octreotide acetate	NVA	600 mcg/8 mL[a]	EV	100 mg/8 mL[a]	Visually compatible with 6% octreotide loss in 48 hr. Diamorphine not tested	2709	C
Octreotide acetate	NVA	900 mcg/8 mL[a]	EV	100 mg/8 mL[a]	Visually compatible with 5% octreotide loss in 48 hr. Diamorphine not tested	2709	C
Octreotide acetate	NVA	600 mcg/8 mL[a]	EV	200 mg/8 mL[a]	Visually compatible with 6% octreotide loss in 48 hr. Diamorphine not tested	2709	C
Prochlorperazine edisylate	MB	1.25 mg/1 mL[a]	MB	10, 25, 50 mg/1 mL	Physically compatible and diamorphine content retained for 24 hr at room temperature	1454	C
Ropivacaine HCl	ASZ	10 g		45 mg	No ropivacaine loss and 10% diamorphine loss in 30 days at 4°C and 16 days at 21°C	2517	C
Scopolamine butylbromide	BI	20 mg/1 mL	EV	50 and 150 mg/1 mL	Physically compatible with no scopolamine loss and 4% diamorphine loss in 7 days at room temperature	1455	C
Scopolamine HBr	EV	60 mcg/1 mL[a]	MB	10, 25, 50 mg/1 mL	Physically compatible and diamorphine stable for 24 hr at room temperature	1454	C
Scopolamine HBr	EV	0.4 mg/1 mL	EV	50 and 150 mg/1 mL	Physically compatible with 7% diamorphine loss in 7 days at room temperature	1455	C

[a] Diluted with sterile water for injection.

[b] Diluted with sterile water to 15 mL.

[c] Diamorphine hydrochloride reconstituted with midazolam injection.

Selected Revisions October 1, 2012. © Copyright, October 1992.
American Society of Health-System Pharmacists, Inc.

Diazepam
AHFS 28:24.08

Products

Diazepam 5 mg/mL is available in 2-mL ampuls and vials, 10-mL vials, and 2-mL syringe cartridges. Each mL of solution also contains propylene glycol 40%, ethanol 10%, sodium benzoate and benzoic acid 5%, and benzyl alcohol 1.5%.[1(1/08)]

pH

From 6.2 to 6.9.[17]

Osmolality

The osmolality of diazepam (Roche) was determined to be 7775 mOsm/kg. Diazemuls (Kabi) has an osmolality of 349 mOsm/kg.[1233]

Administration

Diazepam is administered by direct intravenous injection into a large vein[1(1/08)] [4] or, if necessary, into the tubing of a running infusion solution.[4] Extravasation should be avoided. It is recommended that the rate of administration in adults not exceed 5 mg/min; for children, it is recommended that the dose be administered over not less than 3 minutes. Diazepam can be given by deep intramuscular injection,[1(1/08)] [4] but this route may yield low or erratic plasma levels.[4 121 638] Intravenous infusion of diazepam diluted in infusion solutions has been performed but is not recommended.[1(1/08) 4]

Stability

The commercial product should be stored at controlled room temperature and protected from light.[1(1/08)]

The drug is most stable at pH 4 to 8 and is subject to acid-catalyzed hydrolysis below pH 3.[643]

In tropical climates, diazepam injection is subject to discoloration from degradation by an oxidative hydrolytic mechanism. The rate of degradation leading to discoloration is dependent on various factors including the polarity/dielectric constant of the vehicle, pH, oxygen and electrolyte content, access to light, and storage temperature.[1749]

Diazepam injection under simulated summer conditions in paramedic vehicles was exposed to temperatures ranging from 26 to 38°C over 4 weeks. Analysis found no loss of the drug under these conditions.[2562]

Syringes

Diazepam 5 mg/mL was filled into 3-mL plastic syringes (Becton Dickinson, Sherwood Monoject, and Terumo) and stored at –20, 4, and 25°C in the dark. Losses, presumably due to sorption to surfaces and/or the elastomeric plunger seal, ranged from 6% at 25°C to 2 or 3% at 4°C to 1% or less at –20°C in 1 day. Storage for 7 days at 4°C and 30 days at –20°C resulted in losses of 4 to 8% and 5 to 13%, respectively.[1562]

Diazepam (Roche) 10 mg/2 mL stored in plastic syringes composed of polypropylene and polyethylene exhibited no loss of diazepam in 4 hours.[351]

Diazepam (Roche) 5 mg/mL was stored in 1.5-mL disposable glass syringes with slit rubber plunger-stoppers (Hy-Pod) for 90 days at 30 and 4°C in light-resistant bags. Diazepam was gradually lost from the solution, with the disappearance being essentially complete in 60 days. At 4°C, about 5% was lost at the 60- and 90-day intervals; about 9 to 10% was lost at 30°C in this period. The loss was attributed to sorption to the rubber plunger-stoppers.[794]

Sorption

The stability of diazepam in several infusion fluids in glass containers[321] does not extend to the solutions in polyvinyl chloride (PVC) bags, in which substantial sorption occurs. At 10 mg in 100 and 200 mL, over 24% loss occurred in 30 minutes and 80 to 90% loss occurred in 24 hours.[330]

Diazepam 8 mg/L in sodium chloride 0.9% in PVC bags exhibited 20% loss in 24 hours and 32% loss in 1 week at 15 to 20°C due to sorption.[536]

The sorption of diazepam to PVC infusion bags was evaluated at concentrations of 5 and 20 mg/100 mL in dextrose 5% and sodium chloride 0.9%. Diazepam concentration was under 45% in 2 hours and 20 to 25% in 8 hours.[647]

Diazepam sorption that results from plastic infusion sets was evaluated. Dilutions of 7.5 and 30 mg in 150 mL of dextrose 5% and sodium chloride 0.9% were prepared in the burette chamber of a Buretrol. The solutions flowed through the tubing at 30 mL/hr for 2 hours. Less than 10% decrease in diazepam occurred in the burette chamber. However, running the solution through the tubing resulted in steep declines to 43% of the initial amount. When diazepam 25 and 100 mg/500 mL of dextrose 5% and sodium chloride 0.9% prepared in glass bottles and 100-mL aliquots were run through the Buretrol over 1 hour, only about 60 to 70% of the diazepam was delivered. The presence of a 0.5-μm inline filter did not affect the concentration delivered.[647]

Over 90% loss due to sorption to the administration set (Abbott) and the extension tubing (Extracorporeal) both with and without a 0.22-μm inline filter (Abbott) was reported. Diazepam 0.02 to 0.04 mg/mL in dextrose 5% had no precipitation, and solutions in glass bottles were stable over 24 hours. However, the amount delivered through the tubing was only 40 to 55% at time zero, and this amount dropped to 2 to 7% at 24 hours. No difference was noted from the inline filter.[645]

The sorption of diazepam to administration sets from solutions of diazepam 25 and 50 mg/500 mL in glass bottles of dextrose 5% and Ringer's injection, lactated or 12.5 and 25 mg/250 mL of these same solutions in Soluset burette chambers

DOI: 10.37573/9781585286850.122

was tested. The admixtures showed no evidence of physical incompatibility over 4 hours at room temperature. The solutions in glass bottles were run through Venosets composed of PVC drip chambers and tubing at 2.5 and 5 mg/hr. The solutions stored in the cellulose propionate burette chambers of the Solusets were also run through their PVC tubing at the same rates. The solution delivered through the Venosets contained about 91 to 97% of the initial concentration, with the more dilute solution having slightly more drug remaining. However, the Soluset delivered only about 50 to 60% in 2 hours and about 35 to 45% of the initial concentration after 4 hours. Most of the loss was due to sorption to the cellulose propionate burette chamber. This result was attributed to the larger surface area of the burette compared with the tubing and/or the difference in plastic composition. Almost all of the lost diazepam could be recovered through desorption from the burettes. The use of 0.45-μm inline filters had no effect on the drug concentration.[646]

Diazepam 50-mg/500 mL solution in dextrose 5% prepared in glass bottles and run through an administration set (Travenol) at 100 mL/hr was assessed. Only 63% of the diazepam was initially delivered but gradually climbed to 81% at the end of 5 hours.[649]

A 27 to 33% diazepam loss was noted from admixtures in both dextrose 5% and sodium chloride 0.9% in PVC bags. Diazepam concentrations ranged from 0.05 to 0.2 mg/mL. No drug decomposition could be detected. Diazepam solutions in dextrose 5% were also run through a 70-inch Travenol set. A steep decline to under 70% was delivered during the first 15 minutes, after which the delivered amount increased to between 80 and 90% over the next 85 minutes as saturation of the tubing occurred. A quantitatively smaller, but qualitatively similar, effect was observed when diazepam was administered by intravenous push through an intravenous catheter (Abbott Venocath-18) of 11.5-inch total length. The decline in delivered diazepam reached a nadir of 95% in about 8 minutes before returning to 100% at 10 minutes. The smaller effect of the intravenous catheter relates to its relatively shorter length.[650]

Diazepam 8 mg/L in sodium chloride 0.9% in glass bottles exhibited a cumulative 7% loss due to sorption during a 7-hour simulated infusion through an infusion set (Travenol). The set consisted of a cellulose propionate burette chamber and 170 cm of PVC tubing. Diazepam sorption was attributed mainly to the tubing. The extent of sorption was found to be independent of concentration.[606]

Diazepam was also tested as a simulated infusion over at least 1 hour by a syringe pump system. A glass syringe on a syringe pump was fitted with 20 cm of polyethylene tubing or 50 cm of Silastic tubing. A negligible amount of drug was lost with the polyethylene tubing, but a cumulative loss of 21% occurred during the 1-hour infusion through the Silastic tubing.[606]

Storage of a 25-mL aliquot of the 8-mg/L diazepam solution in all-plastic syringes composed of polypropylene barrels and polyethylene plungers for 24 hours at room temperature in the dark did not result in any drug loss due to sorption.[606]

Diazepam 20 mg/500 mL in dextrose 5% was delivered at 4 mL/hr through PVC tubing by means of an infusion pump. Under 20% of the diazepam was delivered at any time point over 24 hours. Increasing the concentration to 50 mg/500 mL in dextrose 5% and increasing the infusion rate to 20 mL/hr decreased the amount of diazepam lost from the solution. After 30 minutes of solution delivery, the diazepam in the tubing effluent was about 30% of the initial concentration. Subsequently, the delivered diazepam concentration climbed to about 60% over 24 hours.[351]

The partition coefficients of diazepam with various plastics from intravenous containers and administration sets were determined. PVC bags and tubings from a variety of suppliers were all similar in partitioning and hundreds of times greater than polyolefin containers. Volume-control chambers made from cellulose propionate had partition coefficients smaller than those of PVC but still sufficient to cause serious depletion of diazepam from the chambers.[644]

The uptake of diazepam into PVC is absorption into the plastic matrix rather than adsorption to the surface. The absorption is independent of concentration but related to contact time with the plastic. Decreasing the flow rate or increasing the tubing length increases the amount of diazepam absorbed.

Increasing the flow rate from 10 to 264 mL/hr through 198 cm of PVC tubing decreased the amount of diazepam absorbed from 88 down to 28%. Increasing the tubing length from 100 to 350 cm increased the amount absorbed from 17 to 59%. However, it was noted that absorption is not markedly affected by tubing length within the range of lengths commercially available.[644]

Diazepam 50 mg/L in sodium chloride 0.9% in a glass bottle was delivered through a polyethylene administration set (Tridilset) over 8 hours at 15 to 20°C. The flow rate was 1 mL/min. No appreciable loss due to sorption occurred. This finding is in contrast to a 20% loss using a conventional administration set.[769]

The sorption of diazepam 40 and 120 mg/L in sodium chloride 0.9% was evaluated in 100- and 500-mL PVC infusion bags. After 8 hours at 20 to 24°C, 58 to 60% of the diazepam was lost in the 100-mL bag and 31% was lost in the 500-mL bag. The extent of sorption was independent of concentration but was influenced by the size of the PVC container. This difference results from the ratio of the surface area of plastic to the volume of solution. As the volume of solution in the bag decreases, the extent of sorption increases.[770]

Diazepam showed negligible (<3%) loss when aqueous solutions were stored in polypropylene bags.[770]

Extensive sorption of diazepam in dextrose 5% and sodium chloride 0.9% to PVC containers was found. Solutions of 10 to 80 mg/L showed a 12 to 20% diazepam loss in 1 hour. In 6 hours, the loss was 30% at 5°C and 40% at room temperature. Over 30% of the missing diazepam could be recovered by washing the PVC with methanol. Sorption did not occur to glass or polyethylene containers, which showed losses of about 6 to 8% in 24 hours.[796]

No loss of diazepam occurred to glass or polyethylene containers in 200-mg/L concentrations in dextrose 5% or sodium chloride 0.9%. In PVC containers, drug losses of 37 to 43% occurred in 24 hours at 25°C.[797]

Testing the administration of diazepam with a glass syringe on an infusion pump connected with high-density polyethylene tubing resulted in negligible drug loss.[795]

Plastic syringes having polypropylene barrels and polyethylene plungers (Pharma-Plast, AHS Australia) and all-glass containers were compared for the possible sorption of diazepam. After 24 hours of storage, no drug loss was found in either container. The authors indicated that these plastic syringes could be used with syringe pumps.[782]

The effect of several factors on the rate and extent of sorption of diazepam by PVC was evaluated. Sorption proved to be independent of changes in ethanol–propylene glycol concentrations in the vehicle, pH changes in the admixtures over 4.2 to 7.5, and the diazepam concentration. The rate and extent of sorption could be minimized by decreasing the storage temperature, minimizing the storage time, and increasing the surface area to volume ratio by storing the largest possible fluid volume in a given PVC bag and using short lengths of small diameter infusion tubing. Use of glass or polyolefin solution bottles and polyolefin infusion tubing avoids the loss of diazepam.[880]

The sorption of diazepam 20 mg/500 mL in sodium chloride 0.9%, run at 1 mL/min through PVC and polybutadiene (PBD) administration sets (Avon Medicals, U.K.), was reported. The delivered concentration through the PVC set was 80% initially and then climbed to 90% after 4 hours. For a concentration of 10 mg/120 mL prepared in a cellulose propionate burette, 10 to 15% sorption occurred in the burette. Use of the PBD set, with or without a methacrylate butadiene styrene burette chamber, resulted in no loss of diazepam.[1027]

The delivery of diazepam 50 and 100 mg/500 mL in dextrose 5% and sodium chloride 0.9% through a PVC administration set (Accuset 9210, IMED) and a set composed of ethylene vinyl acetate with a polyethylene inner wall (Accuset 9630, IMED) was evaluated. The solutions were run through the sets at 50 and 100 mL/hr. The delivered diazepam concentration varied between 44 and 71% at 50 mL/hr and between 62 and 89% at 100 mL/hr, increasing from the lower to the higher percentage over the 5-hour study period. The non-PVC set exhibited no sorption of diazepam, delivering 100% of the diazepam.[1096]

The percentage of diazepam delivered through PVC administration sets varied with the length of the tubing; the longer the tubing, the smaller was the percentage delivered. For a 25-mg/500 mL admixture in sodium chloride 0.9%, delivery through PVC tubing in lengths from 23 to 185 cm varied from 88% of the theoretical amount for the shortest length to 53% for the 185-cm length.[1097]

The effect of container type and flow rate on the sorption of diazepam was evaluated. Glass and polyethylene containers showed 0 and 5% sorption, respectively, of the diazepam content of a 25-mg/500 mL admixture in sodium chloride 0.9% in 7 days at 25°C. PVC containers showed a 75% loss in this time period. Simulated infusion of this solution from glass bottles through PVC sets at flow rates of 30 to 120 mL/hr showed that a greater percentage of diazepam was lost at the slower infusion rates. At 30 mL/hr, 63% was lost after 4 hours, while only 23% was lost after 4 hours at 120 mL/hr.[1098]

A rapid diazepam loss from a 40-mcg/mL solution in sodium chloride 0.9% in a PVC container at 21°C was reported. A 15% loss occurred in 2 hours, and a 55% loss occurred in 24 hours. Little or no diazepam loss occurred in 24 hours in glass bottles or polyethylene-lined laminated bags.[1392]

Diazepam 100 mcg/mL in sodium chloride 0.9% exhibited no loss due to sorption in 24 hours at 21°C in glass bottles and polypropylene trilayer bags (Softbag, Orion). However, about a 70% loss occurred due to sorption in PVC bags.[1796]

Diazepam 40 mcg/mL in 0.9% sodium chloride and in pH 7 buffer also underwent sorption to ethylene vinyl acetate (EVA) plastic bags. Losses exceeding 25% occurred within 24 hours stored at 30°C. The solutions appeared to reach equilibrium after 96 hours of storage.[1917]

Diazepam 0.04 mg/mL in dextrose 5% and sodium chloride 0.9% in PVC, polyethylene, and glass containers exhibited only 4 to 5% loss in glass and polyethylene containers but 66% loss due to sorption in PVC containers stored at 4 and 22°C for 24 hours.[2289]

To minimize the sorption of diazepam, glass or polyolefin containers should be used. If PVC bags are used, the lowest possible surface-to-volume ratio should be selected and storage time should be minimized. The use of non-PVC administration sets will reduce loss. If PVC tubing is used, it should be the shortest possible length with a small diameter, and the set should not contain a burette chamber. More rapid flow rates (consistent with safe clinical use) will also reduce the loss of diazepam.

Filtration

Diazepam (Roche) 50 mcg/mL in dextrose 5% and sodium chloride 0.9% was delivered over 7 hours through 4 kinds of 0.2-μm membrane filters varying in size and composition. Diazepam concentration losses of 7 to 17% were found during the first 60 minutes; subsequent diazepam levels returned to the original concentration when the binding sites became saturated.[1399]

Compatibility Information

Solution Compatibility

Diazepam

Test Soln Name	Mfr	Mfr	Conc/L or %	Remarks	Ref	C/I
Dextrose 5%	BA[a]	RC	>250 mg	Immediate white precipitation	321	I
Dextrose 5%	BA[a]	RC	250 mg	No precipitate in 24 hr. 6% loss in 4 hr	321	I

Solution Compatibility (Cont.)

Test Soln Name	Mfr	Mfr	Conc/L or %	Remarks	Ref	C/I
Dextrose 5%	BAª	RC	100 and 125 mg	No precipitate and 8 to 10% loss in 24 hr	321	C
Dextrose 5%	BAª	RC	50 and 67 mg	No precipitate and 0 to 1% loss in 24 hr	321	C
Dextrose 5%	BAᵇ	RC	100 mg	35% loss in 30 min. 90% loss in 24 hr at room temperature	330	I
Dextrose 5%	BAᵇ	RC	50 mg	35% loss in 30 min. 77% loss in 24 hr at room temperature	330	I
Dextrose 5%		RC	370 mg	Precipitate formed	640	I
Dextrose 5%	TRᵇ	RC	50 and 200 mg	Solution initially cloudy but clears. 55 to 60% loss within 2 hr	647	I
Dextrose 5%	BTᵇ	RC	40 mg	No precipitate but 12 to 14% loss in 1 hr at room temperature and 5°C	796	I
Dextrose 5%	BTᶜ	RC	40 mg	No precipitate and about 10% loss in 24 hr at room temperature	796	C
Dextrose 5%	ONª ᶜ	ON	200 mg	No precipitate and negligible loss in 24 hr at 25°C	797	C
Dextrose 5%	ᵇ	ON	200 mg	No precipitate but about 10% loss in 3.5 hr and about 37% in 24 hr at 25°C	797	I
Dextrose 5%	BAᵇ	BRN	40 mg	Visually compatible but 66% loss due to sorption to the PVC container in 24 hr at 4 and 22°C	2289	I
Dextrose 5%	BRNª ᶜ	BRN	40 mg	Visually compatible with 4 to 5% loss in 24 hr at 4 and 22°C	2289	C
Ringer's injection	BAª	RC	250 mg	Immediate white precipitation in all concentrations >250 mg/L	321	I
Ringer's injection	BAª	RC	250 mg	White precipitate in 6 to 8 hr. 8% loss in 4 hr	321	I
Ringer's injection	BAª	RC	100 and 125 mg	No precipitate and 7 to 12% loss in 24 hr	321	C
Ringer's injection	BAª	RC	50 and 67 mg	No precipitate and 0 to 3% loss in 24 hr	321	C
Ringer's injection	BAᵇ	RC	100 mg	38% loss in 30 min. 89% loss in 24 hr at room temperature	330	I
Ringer's injection	BAᵇ	RC	50 mg	29% loss in 30 min. 78% loss in 24 hr at room temperature	330	I
Ringer's injection, lactated	BAª	RC	250 mg	Immediate white precipitation in all concentrations >250 mg/L	321	I
Ringer's injection, lactated	BAª	RC	250 mg	White precipitate in 8 to 12 hr. 5% loss in 4 hr	321	I
Ringer's injection, lactated		RC	200 mg	Transient cloudiness followed by clear solution	392	?
Ringer's injection, lactated	BAª	RC	100 and 125 mg	No precipitate and 8 to 10% loss in 24 hr	321	C
Ringer's injection, lactated	BAª	RC	50 and 67 mg	No precipitate and 6% loss in 24 hr	321	C
Ringer's injection, lactated	BAᵇ	RC	100 mg	35% loss in 30 min. 89% loss in 24 hr at room temperature	330	I
Ringer's injection, lactated	BAᵇ	RC	50 mg	40% loss in 30 min. 78% loss in 24 hr at room temperature	330	I
Sodium chloride 0.9%	BAª	RC	>250 mg	Immediate white precipitation	321	I
Sodium chloride 0.9%	BAª	RC	250 mg	No precipitate in 24 hr. 6% loss in 4 hr	321	I
Sodium chloride 0.9%	BAª	RC	125 mg	No precipitate and 6% loss in 24 hr	321	C
Sodium chloride 0.9%	BAª	RC	100 mg	No precipitate and 4 to 5% loss in 24 hr	321, 330	C
Sodium chloride 0.9%	BAª	RC	67 mg	No precipitate and 6% loss in 24 hr	321	C

Solution Compatibility (Cont.)

Test Soln Name	Mfr	Mfr	Conc/L or %	Remarks	Ref	C/I
Sodium chloride 0.9%	BA[a]	RC	50 mg	No precipitate and 1 to 3% loss in 24 hr	321, 330	C
Sodium chloride 0.9%	BA[b]	RC	100 mg	29% loss in 30 min. 89% loss in 24 hr at room temperature	330	I
Sodium chloride 0.9%	BA[b]	RC	50 mg	24% loss in 30 min. 80% loss in 24 hr at room temperature	330	I
Sodium chloride 0.9%	TR[b]	RC	50 and 200 mg	Solution initially cloudy but clears. 55 to 60% loss within 2 hr	647	I
Sodium chloride 0.9%	[a]	RC	40 mg	No precipitate and 6% loss in 24 hr at room temperature	796	C
Sodium chloride 0.9%	BT, TR[b]	RC	10 to 80 mg	No precipitate but 12 to 20% loss in 1 hr at room temperature and 5°C	796	I
Sodium chloride 0.9%	BT[c]	RC	10 to 80 mg	No precipitate and 2 to 8% loss in 24 hr at room temperature and 5°C	796	C
Sodium chloride 0.9%	ON[a c]	ON	200 mg	No precipitate and negligible loss in 24 hr at 25°C	797	C
Sodium chloride 0.9%	[b]	ON	200 mg	No precipitate but 10% loss in 1 hr and 43% in 24 hr at 25°C	797	I
Sodium chloride 0.9%	[a]		400 mg	Precipitate forms immediately or within 1 min	1095	I
Sodium chloride 0.9%	[a]		333 mg	Precipitate forms after 30 min	1095	I
Sodium chloride 0.9%	[a]		100 and 200 mg	Remained clear for 10 days	1095	C
Sodium chloride 0.9%	[a]		50 mg	No diazepam loss in 7 days at 25°C	1098	C
Sodium chloride 0.9%	[b]		50 mg	Over 40% loss in 1 day and 75% in 7 days at 25°C	1098	I
Sodium chloride 0.9%	[c]		50 mg	5% loss in 7 days at 25°C	1098	C
Sodium chloride 0.9%	[b]		40 mg	15% diazepam loss in 2 hr and 55% loss in 24 hr at 21°C in dark	1392	I
Sodium chloride 0.9%	[a c]		40 mg	Little diazepam loss in 24 hr at 21°C in dark	1392	C
Sodium chloride 0.9%	ON[d]	ON	100 mg	Visually compatible with no loss in 24 hr at 21°C	1796	C
Sodium chloride 0.9%	ON[b]	ON	100 mg	Visually compatible but 70% loss due to sorption in 24 hr at 21°C	1796	I
Sodium chloride 0.9%	BA[b]	BRN	40 mg	Visually compatible but 66% loss due to sorption to the PVC container in 24 hr at 4 and 22°C	2289	I
Sodium chloride 0.9%	BRN[a c]	BRN	40 mg	Visually compatible with 4 to 5% loss in 24 hr at 4 and 22°C	2289	C

[a] Tested in glass containers.

[b] Tested in PVC containers.

[c] Tested in polyethylene containers.

[d] Tested in glass containers and polypropylene trilayer containers.

Additive Compatibility

Diazepam

Test Drug	Mfr	Conc/L or %	Mfr	Conc/L or %	Test Solution	Remarks	Ref	C/I
Bleomycin sulfate	BR	20 and 30 units	RC	50 and 100 mg	NS	Physically incompatible	763	I
Dobutamine HCl	LI	1 g	RC	2.5 g	D5W, NS	Rapid clouding of solution with yellow precipitate within 24 hr at 21°C	812	I
Doxorubicin HCl	AD		RC			Precipitates immediately	524	I
Floxacillin sodium	BE	20 g	PHX	1 g	D5W	Haze forms in 7 hr at 30°C and 48 hr at 15°C	1479	I
Fluorouracil			RC			Precipitates immediately	524	I
Furosemide	HO	1 g	PHX	1 g	D5W	Precipitates immediately	1479	I
Levetiracetam	UCB				D5W, LR, NSa	Stable for 4 hr at 15 to 30°C	2833	C
Verapamil HCl	KN	80 mg	RC	20 mg	D5W, NS	Physically compatible for 24 hr	764	C

a Tested in PVC containers.

Drugs in Syringe Compatibility

Diazepam

Test Drug	Mfr	Amt	Mfr	Amt	Remarks	Ref	C/I
Buprenorphine HCl					Incompatible	4	I
Dimenhydrinate		10 mg/1 mL		5 mg/1 mL	Loss of clarity	2569	I
Doxapram HCl	RB	400 mg/20 mL		10 mg/2 mL	Immediate turbidity and precipitation	1177	I
Glycopyrrolate	RB	0.2 mg/1 mL	RC	5 mg/1 mL	Precipitates immediately	331	I
Glycopyrrolate	RB	0.2 mg/1 mL	RC	10 mg/2 mL	Precipitates immediately	331	I
Glycopyrrolate	RB	0.4 mg/2 mL	RC	5 mg/1 mL	Precipitates immediately	331	I
Heparin sodium		2500 units/1 mL		10 mg/2 mL	Turbidity or precipitate forms within 5 min	1053	I
Hydromorphone HCl	KN	2, 10, 40 mg/1 mL	SX	5 mg/1 mL	Diazepam precipitate forms immediately due to aqueous dilution	2082	I
Ketorolac tromethamine	SY	180 mg/6 mL	ES	15 mg/3 mL	Visually compatible for 4 hr at 24°C. Increase in absorbance occurs immediately, persists for 30 min, and dissipates by 1 hr	1703	?
Nalbuphine HCl	EN	10 mg/1 mL	RC	5 mg/1 mL	Immediate milky precipitate that persists for 36 hr at 27°C	762	I
Nalbuphine HCl	EN	5 mg/0.5 mL	RC	5 mg/1 mL	Immediate milky precipitate that clears upon shaking. Clear for 36 hr at 27°C	762	?
Nalbuphine HCl	EN	2.5 mg/0.25 mL	RC	5 mg/1 mL	Immediate milky precipitate that clears upon shaking. Clear for 36 hr at 27°C	762	?
Nalbuphine HCl	DU	10 mg/1 mL	RC	10 mg/2 mL	Physically incompatible	128	I
Nalbuphine HCl	DU	20 mg/1 mL	RC	10 mg/2 mL	Physically incompatible	128	I
Pantoprazole sodium	a	4 mg/1 mL		5 mg/1 mL	Red precipitate forms immediately	2574	I
Ranitidine HCl	GL	50 mg/2 mL	RC	10 mg/2 mL	Immediate white haze that disappears following vortex mixing	978	?
Ranitidine HCl	GL	50 mg/5 mL		10 mg	Physically compatible for 4 hr at ambient temperature under fluorescent light	1151	C

a Test performed using the formulation WITHOUT edetate disodium.

Y-Site Injection Compatibility (1:1 Mixture)

Diazepam

Test Drug	Mfr	Conc	Mfr	Conc	Remarks	Ref	C/I
Acetaminophen	CAD	10 mg/mL	HOS	5 mg/mL	Yellowish-white precipitate forms immediately	2840, 2844	I
Atracurium besylate	BW	0.5 mg/mL[a]	ES	5 mg/mL	Cloudy solution forms immediately	1337	I
Bivalirudin	TMC	5 mg/mL[a]	AB	5 mg/mL	Yellowish precipitate forms immediately	2373	I
Cangrelor tetrasodium	TMC	1 mg/mL[b]		5 mg/mL	Gross white turbid precipitate forms immediately	3243	I
Ceftaroline fosamil	FOR	2.22 mg/mL[a b d]	HOS	5 mg/mL	Turbid precipitation forms	2826	I
Cisatracurium besylate	GW	0.1, 2, 5 mg/mL[a]	ES	5 mg/mL	White turbidity forms immediately	2074	I
Cisatracurium besylate	GW	0.1, 2, 5 mg/mL[a]	ES	0.25 mg/mL[a]	Physically compatible for 4 hr at 23°C	2074	C
Cloxacillin sodium	SMX	100 mg/mL	SZ	5 mg/mL	Large particles form immediately	3245	I
Dexmedetomidine HCl	AB	4 mcg/mL[b]	AB	5 mg/mL	White turbid precipitate forms immediately	2383	I
Dexmedetomidine HCl	HOS, HQS	4 mcg/mL[b]			Stated to be incompatible	2848, 3179	I
Diltiazem HCl	MMD	1[b] and 5 mg/mL	ES	5 mg/mL	Cloudiness and precipitate form	1807	I
Dobutamine HCl	LI	4 mg/mL[a b]	ES	0.2 mg/mL[a b]	Physically compatible for 3 hr	1316	C
Doripenem	JJ	5 mg/mL[a b]	HOS	5 mg/mL	Gross white turbid precipitate forms	2743	I
Fenoldopam mesylate	AB	80 mcg/mL[b]	AB	5 mg/mL	Gross white turbidity forms immediately	2467	I
Fentanyl citrate	JN	0.025 mg/mL[a]	ES	0.5 mg/mL[a]	Physically compatible for 48 hr at 22°C	1706	C
Fluconazole	RR	2 mg/mL	ES	5 mg/mL	Precipitates immediately	1407	I
Foscarnet sodium	AST	24 mg/mL	ES	5 mg/mL	Gas production	1335	I
Heparin sodium[f]	RI	1000 units/L[a b d]	RC	5 mg/mL	Immediate haziness and globule formation	322	I
Hetastarch in lactated electrolyte	AB	6%	AB	5 mg/mL	White turbidity forms immediately	2339	I
Hydrocortisone sodium succinate[g]	UP	100 mg/L[a b d]	RC	5 mg/mL	Immediate haziness and globule formation	322	I
Hydromorphone HCl	KN	2, 10, 40 mg/mL	SX	5 mg/mL	Turbidity forms immediately and diazepam precipitate develops	1532	I
Hydromorphone HCl	AST	0.5 mg/mL[a]	ES	0.5 mg/mL[a]	Physically compatible for 48 hr at 22°C	1706	C
Linezolid	PHU	2 mg/mL	AB	5 mg/mL	Turbid precipitate forms immediately	2264	I
Linezolid	PHU, HOS	2 mg/mL			Stated to be physically incompatible	3183, 3184	I
Meropenem	ZEN	1 and 50 mg/mL[b]	RC	5 mg/mL	White precipitate forms immediately	1994	I
Meropenem		50 mg/mL	SZ	5 mg/mL	Precipitates immediately	3538	I
Methadone HCl	LI	1 mg/mL[a]	ES	0.5 mg/mL[a]	Physically compatible for 48 hr at 22°C	1706	C
Morphine sulfate	AST	1 mg/mL[a]	ES	0.5 mg/mL[a]	Physically compatible for 48 hr at 22°C	1706	C
Nafcillin sodium	WY	33 mg/mL[b]		5 mg/mL	No precipitation	547	C
Oxaliplatin	SS	0.5 mg/mL[a]	AB	5 mg/mL	Gross white turbidity forms immediately	2566	I
Pancuronium bromide	ES	0.05 mg/mL[a]	ES	5 mg/mL	Cloudy solution forms immediately	1337	I
Potassium chloride		40 mEq/L[a b d]	RC	5 mg/mL	Immediate haziness and globule formation	322	I
Propofol	ZEN[h]	10 mg/mL	ES	5 mg/mL	Emulsion broke and oiled out	2066	I
Quinidine gluconate	LI	6 mg/mL[a b]	ES	0.2 mg/mL[a b]	Physically compatible for 3 hr	1316	C

Y-Site Injection Compatibility (1:1 Mixture) (Cont.)

Test Drug	Mfr	Conc	Mfr	Conc	Remarks	Ref	C/I
Remifentanil HCl	GW	0.025 and 0.25 mg/mL[b]	ES	5 mg/mL	White turbidity forms immediately	2075	I
Remifentanil HCl	GW	0.025 and 0.25 mg/mL[b]	ES	0.25 mg/mL[a]	Physically compatible for 4 hr at 23°C	2075	C
Tigecycline	ACD, FRK, WY				Stated to be incompatible	2915, 3459, 3460	I
Tirofiban HCl	ME	50 mcg/mL[a b]	ES	5 mg/mL	Precipitate forms immediately	2356	I
Vecuronium bromide	OR	0.1 mg/mL[a]	ES	5 mg/mL	Cloudy solution forms immediately	1337	I

[a] Tested in dextrose 5%.

[b] Tested in sodium chloride 0.9%.

[c] Given over three minutes via a Y-site into the running heparin admixture.

[d] Tested in Ringer's injection, lactated.

[e] Refer to Appendix for the composition of parenteral nutrition solutions. TPN indicates a 2-in-1 admixture.

[f] Tested in combination with hydrocortisone sodium succinate (Upjohn) 100 mg/L.

[g] Tested in combination with heparin sodium (Riker) 1000 units/L.

[h] Test performed using the formulation WITH edetate disodium.

Additional Compatibility Information

Infusion Solutions

Although the package insert for diazepam contains a caveat against dilution of the product before intravenous administration,[1(1/08)] interest in the intravenous administration of diluted diazepam has been expressed repeatedly in the literature.

Roche indicated that an ampul of diazepam should be diluted in no more than 5 mL or, alternatively, all the way to 20 mL to avoid precipitation. Between these concentrations, a fine white precipitate may occur.[379]

Dilution of diazepam in a volume of 25% or more of the diazepam volume is stated to result in the immediate precipitation of diazepam. No precipitation was observed if aqueous dilution was made with a volume of less than 25% of the diazepam volume.[2082]

Diazepam injection added to sodium chloride 0.9% caused the immediate formation of a light yellow to white precipitate. The maximum dilution that produced such a precipitate was 15-fold, representing a mixture of about 0.3 to 0.4 mg/mL. Analysis of the diazepam injection–sodium chloride 0.9% precipitate showed that it was almost entirely diazepam. A precipitate also formed in human plasma. A solution composed of all ingredients of diazepam injection except diazepam was tried, but dilution yielded no precipitate. It was estimated that injection of 5 mg/min into the tubing of an intravenous infusion of sodium chloride 0.9% would result in a precipitate unless the solution rate exceeded 17 mL/min.[381]

It was determined that the precipitate induced by adding 2 mL of sterile water for injection to 1 mL of diazepam injection

is only diazepam. The precipitate appeared to be oily and adhered to the walls of the container, leaving a clear solution. This may explain the reports of the clearing of cloudy solutions with time.[641 642]

As little as 10 mg of diazepam in 100 mL of dextrose 5% resulted in a precipitate. It was also found that an infusion rate of over 15 to 20 mL/min was required to prevent precipitation of diazepam being injected at a rate of 5 mg/min in running infusions of dextrose 5% and sodium chloride 0.9%.[382]

Nevertheless, interest in infusing diazepam has persisted because of bioavailability problems associated with intramuscular injection[121 383 384 638] and a belief in the utility of diazepam infusions.[386 387 388 389 390 391 392 1099]

Diazepam 10 mg in 250 mL and 5 mg in 50 mL of sodium chloride 0.9% resulted in no observable precipitate.[385]

A transient cloudiness occurred when 100 mg of diazepam was added to 500 mL of Ringer's injection, lactated. The solution thereafter remained clear, and the clinical response to the diazepam infusion was good.[392]

A study was conducted on the compatibility and stability of diazepam in a variety of intravenous infusion solutions. Results indicate that a visible precipitate is produced in dilutions of 1:1 to 1:10. Haziness was reported at 1:15, and delayed precipitates forming after 6 to 8 hours were seen in some solutions at 1:20. Dilutions of 1:40 to 1:100 remained clear for 24 hours. Further, the concentration of the 1:40 to 1:100 dilutions was retained for 24 hours.[321]

The equilibrium solubilities of diazepam in water for injection, sodium chloride 0.9%, dextrose 5%, and Ringer's injection, lactated were determined. The equilibrium solubilities were found to be about 0.04 to 0.05 mg/mL in all of the solutions at 25°C. This finding corroborated the work of others which indicated the solubility to be about 0.05 to 0.06 mg/mL. It was concluded that a more conservative 1:100 dilution should be used for diazepam infusion to guarantee solubility for 24 hours.[643]

The aqueous solubility of diazepam over a pH range of approximately 3 to 8 in phosphate buffer adjusted with hydrochloric acid or sodium hydroxide as well as dextrose 5%, sodium chloride 0.9%, and Ringer's injection, lactated was determined. In the pH range of 4 to 8, which included all 3 infusion solutions, the solubility was approximately 0.05 to 0.06 mg/mL at 25°C. Dilution to at least 0.04 mg/mL was recommended to ensure rapid and complete re-solution upon addition to the infusion solution.[644]

Various dilutions of diazepam in water for injection and sodium chloride 0.9% were tested. The observations are tabulated here:[1095]

Diazepam Concentration	Diluent	Observation
10 mg/5 mL	W, NS	Clear for 1 min but then precipitate forms
10 mg/10 mL	W, NS	Precipitates immediately

Diazepam Concentration	Diluent	Observation
10 mg/20 mL	NS	Precipitates immediately
10 mg/25 mL	NS	Precipitates immediately
10 mg/30 mL	NS	Clear for 30 min but then precipitate forms
10 mg/50 mL	NS	Clear for 10 days
10 mg/100 mL	NS	Clear for 10 days

Order of Mixing

It has been reported that addition of diazepam to dextrose 5% and sodium chloride 0.9% to form concentrations of 50 and 200 mg/L results in an immediate and persistent yellow precipitate. However, addition of the diluent to the diazepam injection to these same concentrations results initially in a cloudy solution which clears before the completion of admixture. It was recommended that admixtures of diazepam be prepared by adding the infusion solution to the diazepam injection.[647] [648]

Diclofenac Sodium
AHFS 28:08.04.92

Products

Diclofenac is available as 37.5-mg/mL solution of diclofenac as the sodium salt in single-use vials.[2821] Each mL of solution also contains hydroxypropyl-beta-cyclodextrin 333 mg and monothioglycerol 5 mg in water for injection with sodium hydroxide and/or hydrochloric acid for pH adjustment.[2821]

Trade Name(s)

Dyloject

Administration

Diclofenac sodium is administered by intravenous bolus injection over 15 seconds.[2821]

Stability

Diclofenac sodium is a clear, colorless solution.[2821] Intact vials should be stored at controlled room temperature and protected from freezing and light.[2821]

DOI: 10.37573/9781585286850.123

Digoxin
AHFS 24:04.08

Products

Digoxin is available in 1- and 2-mL ampuls and vials containing 0.25 mg/mL in propylene glycol 40% and alcohol 10%, along with sodium phosphate 0.17% and citric acid 0.08%.[1(6/06)]

Digoxin pediatric injection is available in 1-mL ampuls containing 0.1 mg/mL in propylene glycol 40% and alcohol 10%, along with sodium phosphate 0.17% and citric acid 0.08%.[1(6/06)]

pH

From 6.8 to 7.2.[1(6/06)]

Osmolality

The osmolality of digoxin pediatric injection (Burroughs Wellcome) was determined to be 9105 mOsm/kg by freezing-point depression and 5885 mOsm/kg by vapor pressure.[1071]

Trade Name(s)

Lanoxin

Administration

Digoxin is administered by direct intravenous injection slowly over a minimum of 5 minutes or longer given undiluted or diluted with a fourfold or greater volume of sterile water for injection, dextrose 5%, or sodium chloride 0.9%. If a tuberculin syringe is used for very small doses, the possibility of inadvertent overdosage exists. Following intravenous administration, the syringe should not be flushed with parenteral solution.[1(6/06) 4] Deep intramuscular injection of not more than 2 mL at a single site followed by massage has been performed. However, it is painful and causes severe local irritation.[4]

Stability

Intact containers of digoxin should be stored at controlled room temperature and protected from light.[1(6/06)]

pH Effects

Digoxin is hydrolyzed in acidic solutions with a pH less than 3. At pH 5 to 8, however, digoxin is not hydrolyzed in aqueous solutions.[798 799 800 801]

Plasticizer Leaching

Digoxin (Elkins-Sinn) 0.04 mg/mL in dextrose 5% did not leach diethylhexyl phthalate (DEHP) plasticizer from 50-mL polyvinyl chloride (PVC) bags in 24 hours at 24°C.[1683]

Filtration

Digoxin (Burroughs Wellcome) 1 mg/L in dextrose 5%, sodium chloride 0.9%, and Ringer's injection, lactated filtered over 12 hours through a 5-µm stainless steel depth filter (Argyle Filter Connector), a 0.22-µm cellulose ester membrane filter (Ivex-2 Filter Set), and a 0.22-µm polycarbonate membrane filter (In-Sure Filter Set), showed no significant reduction due to binding to the filters.[320]

In another evaluation, digoxin (Burroughs Wellcome) 3 mg/L in dextrose 5% and sodium chloride 0.9% did not display significant sorption to a 0.45-µm cellulose membrane filter (Abbott S-A-I-F) during an 8-hour simulated infusion.[567]

Digoxin (Wellcome) 1 mcg/mL in dextrose 5% and sodium chloride 0.9% was delivered over 8 hours through 4 kinds of 0.2-µm membrane filters varying in size and composition. In the first 20 minutes, digoxin concentration losses were 10 to 23% through the Sterifix filter and 24 to 32% through the Pall ELD-96LL filter. However, losses of 63 to 73% occurred in the first 20 minutes with the Ivex-HP and Pall FAE-020LL filters. Subsequent digoxin levels returned to the original concentration when the binding sites became saturated.[1399]

Compatibility Information

Solution Compatibility

Digoxin

Test Soln Name	Mfr	Mfr	Conc/L or %	Remarks	Ref	C/I
Dextrose 5%	AB	BW	2.5 mg	Physically compatible with no loss of digoxin in 48 hr at 4 and 23°C	778	C
Dextrose 5% in sodium chloride 0.45%[a]	AB	BW	2.5 mg	Physically compatible with no loss of digoxin in 6-hr study period at 23°C	778	C
Ringer's injection, lactated	AB	BW	2.5 mg	Physically compatible with no loss of digoxin in 6-hr study period at 23°C	778	C
Sodium chloride 0.45%		ES	125 mg	Physically compatible with no loss of digoxin in 4 hr at 22°C	1419	C
Sodium chloride 0.9%	AB	BW	2.5 mg	Physically compatible with no loss of digoxin in 48 hr at 4 and 23°C	778	C

[a] Tested in combination with potassium chloride 20 mEq/L.

DOI: 10.37573/9781585286850.124

Additive Compatibility

Digoxin

Test Drug	Mfr	Conc/L or %	Mfr	Conc/L or %	Test Solution	Remarks	Ref	C/I
Dobutamine HCl	LI	1 g	BW	4 mg	D5W, NS	Slightly pink in 24 hr at 25°C	789	I
Floxacillin sodium	BE	20 g	BW	25 mg	NS	Physically compatible for 72 hr at 15 and 30°C	1479	C
Furosemide	HO	1 g	BW	25 mg	NS	Physically compatible for 72 hr at 15 and 30°C	1479	C
Lidocaine HCl	AST	2 g	ES	1 mg	D5W, LR, NS	Physically compatible for 24 hr at 25°C	775	C
Ranitidine HCl	GL	50 mg and 2 g		2.5 mg	D5W	Physically compatible. Ranitidine stable for 24 hr at 25°C. Digoxin not tested	1515	C
Verapamil HCl	KN	80 mg	BW	2 mg	D5W, NS	Physically compatible for 48 hr	739	C

Drugs in Syringe Compatibility

Digoxin

Test Drug	Mfr	Amt	Mfr	Amt	Remarks	Ref	C/I
Dimenhydrinate		10 mg/1 mL		0.05 mg/1 mL	Clear solution	2569	C
Doxapram HCl	RB	400 mg/20 mL		0.25 mg/1 mL	10% doxapram loss in 9 hr and 17% in 24 hr	1177	I
Heparin sodium		2500 units/1 mL		0.25 mg/1 mL	Physically compatible for at least 5 min	1053	C
Milrinone lactate	WI	3.5 mg/3.5 mL	BW	0.5 mg/2 mL	Brought to 10-mL total volume with D5W. Physically compatible with no loss of either drug in 4 hr at 23°C	1191	C
Pantoprazole sodium	a	4 mg/1 mL		0.05 mg/1 mL	Precipitates within 4 hr	2574	I

a Test performed using the formulation without edetate disodium.

Y-Site Injection Compatibility (1:1 Mixture)

Digoxin

Test Drug	Mfr	Conc	Mfr	Conc	Remarks	Ref	C/I
Amiodarone HCl	WY	6 mg/mL[a]	ES	0.25 mg/mL	Immediate opaque white turbidity	2352	I
Anidulafungin	VIC	0.5 mg/mL[a]	GW	0.25 mg/mL	Physically compatible for 4 hr at 23°C	2617	C
Bivalirudin	TMC	5 mg/mL[a]	GW	0.25 mg/mL	Physically compatible for 4 hr at 23°C	2373	C
Cangrelor tetrasodium	TMC	1 mg/mL[b]		0.25 mg/mL	Physically compatible for 4 hr	3243	C
Ceftaroline fosamil	FOR	2.22 mg/mL[d]	BA	0.25 mg/mL	Physically compatible for 4 hr at 23°C	2826	C
Ceftolozane sulfate–tazobactam sodium	CUB	10 mg/mL[c i]	SZ	0.25 mg/mL	Physically compatible for 2 hr	3262	C
Ciprofloxacin	MI	2 mg/mL[c]	ES	0.25 mg/mL	Visually compatible for 24 hr at 24°C	1655	C
Ciprofloxacin	BAY	2 mg/mL[b]	BW	0.25 mg/mL	Visually compatible with no ciprofloxacin loss in 15 min. Digoxin not tested	1934	C
Cisatracurium besylate	GW	0.1, 2, 5 mg/mL[a]	ES	0.25 mg/mL	Physically compatible for 4 hr at 23°C	2074	C
Cloxacillin sodium	SMX	100 mg/mL	SZ	0.05 mg/mL	Physically compatible for up to 4 hr at room temperature	3245	C
Dexmedetomidine HCl	AB	4 mcg/mL[b]	ES	0.25 mg/mL	Physically compatible for 4 hr at 23°C	2383	C

Y-Site Injection Compatibility (1:1 Mixture) (Cont.)

Test Drug	Mfr	Conc	Mfr	Conc	Remarks	Ref	C/I
Diltiazem HCl	MMD	1[b] and 5 mg/mL	ES	0.5 mg/mL	Visually compatible	1807	C
Doripenem	JJ	5 mg/mL[a b]	BA	0.25 mg/mL	Physically compatible for 4 hr at 23°C	2743	C
Famotidine	MSD	0.2 mg/mL[a]	ES	0.25 mg/mL	Physically compatible for 14 hr	1196	C
Fenoldopam mesylate	AB	80 mcg/mL[b]	ES	0.25 mg/mL	Physically compatible for 4 hr at 23°C	2467	C
Fluconazole	RR	2 mg/mL	BW	0.25 mg/mL	Gas production	1407	I
Foscarnet sodium	AST	24 mg/mL	WY	0.25 mg/mL	Gas production	1335	I
Heparin sodium[f]	RI	1000 units/L[d]	BW	0.25 mg/mL	Physically compatible for 4 hr at room temperature	322	C
Hetastarch in lactated electrolyte	AB	6%	ES	0.25 mg/mL	Physically compatible for 4 hr at 23°C	2339	C
Hydrocortisone sodium succinate[g]	UP	100 mg/L[d]	BW	0.25 mg/mL	Physically compatible for 4 hr at room temperature	322	C
Insulin, regular	LI	1 unit/mL[b]	ES	0.005 mg/mL[b]	Physically compatible for 3 hr	1316	C
Insulin, regular	LI	1 unit/mL[a]	ES	0.005 mg/mL[a]	Slight haze in 1 hr	1316	I
Isavuconazonium sulfate	ASP	1.5 mg/mL[c]	SZ	0.25 mg/mL	Physically compatible for 2 hr	3263	C
Linezolid	PHU	2 mg/mL	ES	0.25 mg/mL	Physically compatible for 4 hr at 23°C	2264	C
Meperidine HCl	AB	10 mg/mL	BW	0.25 mg/mL	Physically compatible for 4 hr at 25°C	1397	C
Meropenem	ZEN	1 and 50 mg/mL[b]	BW	0.25 mg/mL	Visually compatible for 4 hr at room temperature	1994	C
Meropenem		50 mg/mL	SZ	0.25 mg/mL	Physically compatible for 4 hr at room temperature	3538	C
Meropenem–vaborbactam	TMC	8 mg/mL[b j]	SZ	0.25 mg/mL	Physically compatible for 3 hr at 20 to 25°C	3380	C
Midazolam HCl	RC	1 mg/mL[a]	BW	0.1 mg/mL	Visually compatible for 24 hr at 23°C	1847	C
Milrinone lactate	WI	200 mcg/mL[a]	BW	0.25 mg/mL	Physically compatible with no loss of either drug in 4 hr at 23°C	1191	C
Morphine sulfate	AB	1 mg/mL	BW	0.25 mg/mL	Physically compatible for 4 hr at 25°C	1397	C
Nesiritide	SCI	50 mcg/mL[a b]		0.25 mg/mL	Physically compatible for 4 hr	2625	C
Plazomicin sulfate	ACH	24 mg/mL[c]	WW	0.25 mg/mL	Physically compatible for 1 hr at 20 to 25°C	3432	C
Potassium chloride		40 mEq/L[d]	BW	0.25 mg/mL	Physically compatible for 4 hr at room temperature	322	C
Quinupristin–dalfopristin		2 mg/mL[a h]		0.25 mg/mL	Reported to be incompatible	3230	I
Remifentanil HCl	GW	0.025 and 0.25 mg/mL[b]	ES	0.25 mg/mL	Physically compatible for 4 hr at 23°C	2075	C
Tacrolimus	FUJ	1 mg/mL[b]	WY	0.25 mg/mL	Visually compatible for 24 hr at 25°C	1630	C
Tedizolid phosphate	CUB	0.8 mg/mL[b]	SZ	0.25 mg/mL	Physically compatible for 2 hr	3244	C
Telavancin HCl	ASP	7.5 mg/mL[d]	BA	0.25 mg/mL	Visible turbidity formed	2830	I
TNA #73[e]			BW	12.5 mcg/mL[c]	Visually compatible for 4 hr	1009	C

Y-Site Injection Compatibility (1:1 Mixture) (Cont.)

Test Drug	Mfr	Conc	Mfr	Conc	Remarks	Ref	C/I
TNA #218 to #226[e]			ES, WY	0.25 mg/mL	Visually compatible for 4 hr at 23°C	2215	C
TPN #212 to #215[e]			BW	0.25 mg/mL	Physically compatible for 4 hr at 23°C	2109	C

[a] Tested in dextrose 5%.

[b] Tested in sodium chloride 0.9%.

[c] Tested in both dextrose 5% and sodium chloride 0.9%.

[d] Tested in dextrose 5%, Ringer's injection, lactated, and sodium chloride 0.9%.

[e] Refer to Appendix for the composition of parenteral nutrition solutions. TNA indicates a 3-in-1 admixture, and TPN indicates a 2-in-1 admixture.

[f] Tested in combination with hydrocortisone sodium succinate (Upjohn) 100 mg/L.

[g] Tested in combination with heparin sodium (Riker) 1000 units/L.

[h] Quinupristin and dalfopristin components combined.

[i] Ceftolozane component. Ceftolozane in a 2:1 fixed-ratio concentration with tazobactam.

[j] Meropenem component. Meropenem in a 1:1 fixed-ratio concentration with vaborbactam.

Selected Revisions June 1, 2019. © Copyright, October 1982.
American Society of Health-System Pharmacists, Inc.

Diltiazem Hydrochloride
AHFS 24:28.92

Products

Diltiazem hydrochloride is available as a 5-mg/mL solution in 5-mL (25-mg), 10-mL (50-mg), and 25-mL (125-mg) single-use vials.[2875] Also present in each mL of solution are citric acid hydrous 0.75 mg, sodium citrate dihydrate 0.65 mg, sorbitol solution 71.4 mg, and water for injection.[2875] Sodium hydroxide or hydrochloric acid is used to adjust the pH.[2875]

Diltiazem hydrochloride also is available as a lyophilized powder in 100-mg single-use ADD-Vantage vials.[2876] Each ADD-Vantage vial also contains mannitol base 75 mg.[2876] ADD-Vantage vials of diltiazem hydrochloride should be prepared with 100 mL of dextrose 5% or sodium chloride 0.9% in ADD-Vantage diluent bags.[2876]

pH

From 3.7 to 4.1.[2875]

Administration

Diltiazem hydrochloride in single-use vials is administered by direct intravenous injection over 2 minutes and by continuous intravenous infusion after dilution.[2875]

Following reconstitution using ADD-Vantage diluent bags, ADD-Vantage vials are intended for continuous intravenous infusion and should *not* be used for direct intravenous injection.[2876]

Stability

Intact vials of the liquid injection should be stored under refrigeration and protected from freezing.[2875] Diltiazem hydrochloride may be stored for up to 1 month at room temperature but should then be destroyed.[2875]

Intact ADD-Vantage vials of diltiazem hydrochloride should be stored at controlled room temperature and protected from freezing.[2876] Reconstituted ADD-Vantage diltiazem hydrochloride injection is stable for 24 hours at controlled room temperature or under refrigeration.[2876]

pH Effects

An increased rate of diltiazem hydrochloride hydrolysis occurs with increasing pH. Hydrolysis was lowest at pH 5 and 6 but increased substantially at pH 7 and 8. Diltiazem hydrochloride 100 mcg/mL in sodium chloride 0.9% with a pH between 5 and 6 exhibited no loss in 24 hours. Buffered to pH 7, losses of 3 to 4% in 24 hours were found.[1915]

Light Effects

Diltiazem hydrochloride reconstituted with distilled water to a concentration of 10 mg/mL was exposed to UVA-UVB radiation with a solar simulator for 28 hours. Only 5.6% degradation occurred under this intense light exposure. The drug maintained adequate stability and light protection was not required.[2432]

Freezing Solutions

Diltiazem hydrochloride (Baxter) 1 mg/mL in dextrose 5% was stored in polyolefin bags and frozen at −20°C.[2874] The solution was physically stable and demonstrated less than 3% loss after 30 days of storage followed by warming to room temperature.[2874]

Sorption

A pH-dependent loss of diltiazem hydrochloride occurs due to sorption to polyvinyl chloride (PVC) containers and administration sets. Diltiazem hydrochloride 100 mcg/mL in sodium chloride 0.9% buffered to neutrality exhibits a loss of 11% in 24 hours in PVC containers but only 3 to 4% in glass and polypropylene containers. Similar results were found with PVC administration sets. Buffered to pH 8, diltiazem hydrochloride concentration was initially reduced to about 83% when delivered at 0.52 mL/min through a 100-cm PVC administration set. At pH 6 and 7, initial losses were much less, about 1 and 5%, respectively. Delivered diltiazem hydrochloride returned to full concentration in less than 1 hour at pH 6 and 7 but at pH 8 was only about 93% in 2 hours.[1915]

Diltiazem hydrochloride 0.05 mg/mL in dextrose 5% and sodium chloride 0.9% packaged in PVC, polyethylene, and glass containers exhibited little or no loss due to sorption to any of the container types when stored at 4 and 22°C for 24 hours protected from light.[2289]

Diltiazem hydrochloride (Synthelabo) 1 g/L in dextrose 5% and in sodium chloride 0.9% was evaluated for loss due to sorption to a variety of polymer container types compared to glass containers. No significant loss due to sorption was found at 21°C after 48 hours of contact time to PVC and polyethylene containers and 24 hours of contact time to polyamide containers.[274]

Similarly, no significant loss of diltiazem hydrochloride occurred from 1-g/L solutions in dextrose 5% and in sodium chloride 0.9% in cellulose propionate (Abbott), butadiene styrene (B. Braun), and metacrylate butadiene styrene (Avon) burettes for 24 hours at 21°C and when delivered over 5 hours through PVC (Abbott and Baxter), PVC/polyethylene double polymer (Abbott), and polybutadiene (Avon) administration tubing.[274]

Filtration

Cellulose ester filters (B. Braun and Millipore) were found to result in a temporary reduction in the concentration of delivered diltiazem hydrochloride from a 1-g/L solution in sodium chloride 0.9%. The concentration of delivered diltiazem hydrochloride returned to near 100% after about 1 to 2 hours of infusion through the filter. No reduction in delivered concentration was found if dextrose 5% was used as the vehicle. No loss occurred in either infusion solution with polyamide (Pall) filters.[274]

DOI: 10.37573/9781585286850.125

Compatibility Information

Solution Compatibility

Diltiazem HCl

Test Soln Name	Mfr	Mfr	Conc/L or %	Remarks	Ref	C/I
Dextrose 5%	d		1 g	Compatible and stable for 24 hr at room and refrigeration temperatures	2875	C
Dextrose 5%	e	HOS	1 g	Compatible and stable for 24 hr at room and refrigeration temperatures	2876	C
Dextrose 5%	BA[a]	GO	50 mg	Visually compatible. 4% loss in 24 hr at 22°C and little loss at 4°C	2289	C
Dextrose 5%	BRN[b]	GO	50 mg	Visually compatible. Little loss in 24 hr at 4 and 22°C	2289	C
Dextrose 5%		SYO	1 g	No loss occurred in 48 hr at 21°C	274	C
Dextrose 5%	GRI[a]	BED	1 g	Physically compatible. No loss in 90 days at 25 and 5°C	2750	C
Dextrose 5%	BRN[c]	BA	1 g	Physically compatible with <1% loss in 30 days under refrigeration and at room temperature	2874	C
Dextrose 5% in sodium chloride 0.45%	d		1 g	Compatible and stable for 24 hr at room and refrigeration temperatures	2875	C
Sodium chloride 0.9%	d		1 g	Compatible and stable for 24 hr at room and refrigeration temperatures	2875	C
Sodium chloride 0.9%	e	HOS	1 g	Compatible and stable for 24 hr at room and refrigeration temperatures	2876	C
Sodium chloride 0.9%	BA[a]	GO	50 mg	Visually compatible. 4% loss in 24 hr at 22°C and little or no loss at 4°C	2289	C
Sodium chloride 0.9%	BRN[b]	GO	50 mg	Visually compatible. Little loss in 24 hr at 4 and 22°C	2289	C
Sodium chloride 0.9%		SYO	1 g	No loss occurred in 48 hr at 21°C	274	C
Sodium chloride 0.9%	GRI[a]	BED	1 g	Physically compatible. No loss in 90 days at 25 and 5°C	2750	C

[a] Tested in PVC containers.

[b] Tested in polyethylene and glass containers.

[c] Tested in polyolefin containers.

[d] Tested in glass and PVC containers.

[e] Tested in the ADD-Vantage system.

Y-Site Injection Compatibility (1:1 Mixture)

Diltiazem HCl

Test Drug	Mfr	Conc	Mfr	Conc	Remarks	Ref	C/I
Acetazolamide sodium	LE	100 mg/mL	MMD	5 mg/mL	Precipitate forms	1807	I
Acetazolamide sodium	LE	100 mg/mL	MMD	1 mg/mL[b]	Visually compatible	1807	C
Acyclovir sodium	BW	5[a] and 7[b] mg/mL	MMD	5 mg/mL	Cloudiness and precipitate form	1807	I
Acyclovir sodium	BW	5[a] and 7[b] mg/mL	MMD	1 mg/mL[b]	Visually compatible	1807	C
Albumin human	AR, AT	5 and 25%	MMD	5 mg/mL	Visually compatible	1807	C
Amikacin sulfate	BR	5[b] and 250 mg/mL	MMD	5 mg/mL	Visually compatible	1807	C
Aminophylline	AMR	25 mg/mL[b]	MMD	5 mg/mL	Cloudiness forms	1807	I
Aminophylline	AMR	25 mg/mL[b]	MMD	1 mg/mL[b]	Visually compatible	1807	C

Y-Site Injection Compatibility (1:1 Mixture) (Cont.)

Test Drug	Mfr	Conc	Mfr	Conc	Remarks	Ref	C/I
Aminophylline	AMR	2 mg/mL[a] [b]	MMD	5 mg/mL	Visually compatible	1807	C
Amphotericin B	SQ	0.1 mg/mL[a]	MMD	5 mg/mL[b]	Visually compatible	1807	C
Ampicillin sodium	WY	100 mg/mL[b]	MMD	5 mg/mL	Cloudiness forms	1807	I
Ampicillin sodium	WY	100 mg/mL[b]	MMD	1 mg/mL[b]	Visually compatible	1807	C
Ampicillin sodium	WY	10 and 20 mg/mL[b]	MMD	5 mg/mL	Visually compatible	1807	C
Ampicillin sodium–sulbactam sodium	RR	45 mg/mL[b] [g]	MMD	5 mg/mL	Cloudiness forms	1807	I
Ampicillin sodium–sulbactam sodium	RR	45 mg/mL[b] [g]	MMD	1 mg/mL[b]	Visually compatible	1807	C
Ampicillin sodium–sulbactam sodium	RR	2 and 15 mg/mL[b] [g]	MMD	5 mg/mL	Visually compatible	1807	C
Argatroban	GSK	1 mg/mL[b]	BV	5 mg/mL	Visually compatible for 24 hr at 23°C	2391	C
Argatroban	SZ	1 mg/mL	AKN	1 mg/mL[a]	Physically compatible for up to 5 hr at 19 to 24°C in ambient light and 28 to 40% relative humidity	3192	C
Aztreonam	SQ	20 and 333 mg/mL[b]	MMD	5 mg/mL	Visually compatible	1807	C
Aztreonam	SQ	333 mg/mL[b]	MMD	1 mg/mL[b]	Visually compatible	1807	C
Bivalirudin	TMC	5 mg/mL[a]	BA	5 mg/mL	Physically compatible for 4 hr at 23°C	2373	C
Bivalirudin	TMC	5 mg/mL[a] [b]	BV	5 mg/mL	Visually compatible for 6 hr at 23°C	2680	C
Bumetanide	RC	0.25 mg/mL	MMD	1[b] and 5 mg/mL	Visually compatible	1807	C
Cangrelor tetrasodium	TMC	1 mg/mL[b]		5 mg/mL	Physically compatible for 4 hr	3243	C
Caspofungin acetate	ME	0.7 mg/mL[b]	HOS	5 mg/mL	Physically compatible for 4 hr at room temperature	2758	C
Cefazolin sodium	LI	20 and 200 mg/mL[b]	MMD	5 mg/mL	Visually compatible	1807	C
Cefazolin sodium	LI	200 mg/mL[b]	MMD	1 mg/mL[b]	Visually compatible	1807	C
Cefotaxime sodium	HO	10 and 180 mg/mL[b]	MMD	5 mg/mL	Visually compatible	1807	C
Cefotaxime sodium	HO	180 mg/mL[b]	MMD	1 mg/mL[b]	Visually compatible	1807	C
Cefotetan disodium	STU	10 and 200 mg/mL[b]	MMD	5 mg/mL	Visually compatible	1807	C
Cefotetan disodium	STU	200 mg/mL[b]	MMD	1 mg/mL[b]	Visually compatible	1807	C
Cefoxitin sodium	MSD	10 and 200 mg/mL[b]	MMD	5 mg/mL	Visually compatible	1807	C
Cefoxitin sodium	MSD	200 mg/mL[b]	MMD	1 mg/mL[b]	Visually compatible	1807	C
Ceftaroline fosamil	FOR	2.22 mg/mL[a] [b] [f]	HOS	5 mg/mL	Physically compatible for 4 hr at 23°C	2826	C
Ceftazidime	GL	10 and 170 mg/mL[b]	MMD	5 mg/mL	Visually compatible	1807	C
Ceftazidime	GL	170 mg/mL[b]	MMD	1 mg/mL[b]	Visually compatible	1807	C
Ceftolozane sulfate–tazobactam sodium	CUB	10 mg/mL[c] [k]	WW	5 mg/mL	Physically compatible for 2 hr	3262	C

Y-Site Injection Compatibility (1:1 Mixture) (Cont.)

Test Drug	Mfr	Conc	Mfr	Conc	Remarks	Ref	C/I
Ceftriaxone sodium	RC	40 mg/mL[b]	MMD	5 mg/mL	Visually compatible	1807	C
Cefuroxime sodium	LI	15 and 100 mg/mL[b]	MMD	5 mg/mL	Visually compatible	1807	C
Cefuroxime sodium	LI	100 mg/mL[b]	MMD	1 mg/mL[b]	Visually compatible	1807	C
Ciprofloxacin	MI	2 and 10 mg/mL[b]	MMD	5 mg/mL	Visually compatible	1807	C
Cisatracurium besylate	AB	1 mg/mL[b]	BA	1 mg/mL[b]	Physically compatible for 1 hr at 23°C	3157	C
Clindamycin phosphate	UP	12[b] and 150 mg/mL	MMD	5 mg/mL	Visually compatible	1807	C
Dexmedetomidine HCl	AB	4 mcg/mL[b]	BA	5 mg/mL	Physically compatible for 4 hr at 23°C	2383	C
Diazepam	ES	5 mg/mL	MMD	1[b] and 5 mg/mL	Cloudiness and precipitate form	1807	I
Digoxin	ES	0.5 mg/mL	MMD	1[b] and 5 mg/mL	Visually compatible	1807	C
Dobutamine HCl	LI	2 mg/mL[a]	MMD	1 mg/mL[a]	Visually compatible for 24 hr at 25°C	1530	C
Dobutamine HCl	LI	1 mg/mL[c]	MMD	5 mg/mL	Visually compatible	1807	C
Dobutamine HCl	LI	4 mg/mL[a]	MMD	1 mg/mL[a]	Visually compatible for 4 hr at 27°C	2062	C
Dopamine HCl	AB	1.6 mg/mL[a]	MMD	1 mg/mL[a]	Visually compatible for 24 hr at 25°C	1530	C
Dopamine HCl	AB, SO	0.8 mg/mL[c]	MMD	5 mg/mL	Visually compatible	1807	C
Dopamine HCl	AB	3.2 mg/mL[a]	MMD	1 mg/mL[a]	Visually compatible for 4 hr at 27°C	2062	C
Doripenem	JJ	5 mg/mL[a b]	BED	5 mg/mL	Physically compatible for 4 hr at 23°C	2743	C
Doxycycline hyclate	RR	1 and 10 mg/mL[b]	MMD	5 mg/mL	Visually compatible	1807	C
Epinephrine HCl	PD	0.004 and 0.05 mg/mL[b]	MMD	5 mg/mL	Visually compatible	1807	C
Epinephrine HCl	PD	0.05 mg/mL[b]	MMD	1 mg/mL[b]	Visually compatible	1807	C
Epinephrine HCl	AB	0.02 mg/mL[a]	MMD	1 mg/mL[a]	Visually compatible for 4 hr at 27°C	2062	C
Eravacycline dihydrochloride	TET	0.6 mg/mL[b]	AKN	5 mg/mL	Physically compatible for 2 hr at room temperature	3532	C
Erythromycin lactobionate	ES	5 and 50 mg/mL[b]	MMD	5 mg/mL	Visually compatible	1807	C
Esmolol HCl	DU	10 mg/mL[a]	MMD	1 mg/mL[a]	Visually compatible for 24 hr at 25°C	1530	C
Fenoldopam mesylate	AB	80 mcg/mL[b]	BA	5 mg/mL	Physically compatible for 4 hr at 23°C	2467	C
Fentanyl citrate	ES	0.05 mg/mL	MMD	1 mg/mL[a]	Visually compatible for 4 hr at 27°C	2062	C
Fluconazole	RR	2 mg/mL	MMD	5 mg/mL	Visually compatible	1807	C
Furosemide	AMR	10 mg/mL	MMD	1[b] and 5 mg/mL	Heavy precipitate forms	1807	I
Furosemide	AMR	10 mg/mL	MMD	1 mg/mL[a]	Precipitate forms immediately	2062	I
Gentamicin sulfate	SC	2.4[b] and 40 mg/mL	MMD	1[b] and 5 mg/mL	Visually compatible	1807	C
Heparin sodium	LY	20,000 units/mL	MMD	5 mg/mL	Precipitate forms	1807	I
Heparin sodium	LY	20,000 units/mL	MMD	1 mg/mL[b]	Visually compatible	1807	C

Y-Site Injection Compatibility (1:1 Mixture) (Cont.)

Test Drug	Mfr	Conc	Mfr	Conc	Remarks	Ref	C/I
Heparin sodium	SCN	5000 and 10,000 units/mL	MMD	1[b] and 5 mg/mL	Visually compatible	1807	C
Heparin sodium	LY, SCN	80 units/mL[c]	MMD	5 mg/mL	Visually compatible	1807	C
Heparin sodium	ES	100 units/mL[a]	MMD	1 mg/mL[a]	Visually compatible for 4 hr at 27°C	2062	C
Hetastarch in lactated electrolyte	AB	6%	BA	5 mg/mL	Physically compatible for 4 hr at 23°C	2339	C
Hetastarch in sodium chloride 0.9%	DU	6%	MMD	5 mg/mL	Visually compatible	1807	C
Hydrocortisone sodium succinate	UP	50 and 125 mg/mL	MMD	5 mg/mL	Precipitate forms but clears with swirling	1807	?
Hydrocortisone sodium succinate	UP	50 and 125 mg/mL	MMD	1 mg/mL[b]	Visually compatible	1807	C
Hydrocortisone sodium succinate	UP	1[b] and 2[a] mg/mL	MMD	5 mg/mL	Visually compatible	1807	C
Hydromorphone HCl	KN	1 mg/mL	MMD	1 mg/mL[a]	Visually compatible for 4 hr at 27°C	2062	C
Imipenem–cilastatin sodium	MSD	5 mg/mL[c i]	MMD	5 mg/mL	Visually compatible	1807	C
Insulin, regular		100 units/mL	BED		Physically incompatible	2875	I
Isavuconazonium sulfate	ASP	1.5 mg/mL[c]	AKN	5 mg/mL	Physically compatible for 2 hr	3263	C
Labetalol HCl	AH	2 mg/mL[a]	MMD	1 mg/mL[a]	Visually compatible for 4 hr at 27°C	2062	C
Letermovir	ME				Physically incompatible	3398	I
Lidocaine HCl	AST	8 mg/mL[a]	MMD	1 mg/mL[a]	Visually compatible for 24 hr at 25°C	1530	C
Lidocaine HCl	AB	10 mg/mL[b]	MMD	1[b] and 5 mg/mL	Visually compatible	1807	C
Lidocaine HCl	AB, SCN	4 and 8 mg/mL[a]	MMD	5 mg/mL	Visually compatible	1807	C
Lorazepam	WY	4 mg/mL	MMD	5 mg/mL	Visually compatible	1807	C
Lorazepam	WY	2 mg/mL[b]	MMD	1 mg/mL[b]	Visually compatible	1807	C
Lorazepam	WY	0.5 mg/mL[a]	MMD	1 mg/mL[a]	Visually compatible for 4 hr at 27°C	2062	C
Meperidine HCl	WY	100 mg/mL	MMD	1[b] and 5 mg/mL	Visually compatible	1807	C
Meperidine HCl	WY	10 mg/mL[b]	MMD	5 mg/mL	Visually compatible	1807	C
Meropenem–vaborbactam	TMC	8 mg/mL[b j]	AKN	5 mg/mL	Physically compatible for 3 hr at 20 to 25°C	3380	C
Methylprednisolone sodium succinate	UP	2.5[a], 20[b], 62.5 mg/mL	MMD	1 mg/mL[b]	Visually compatible	1807	C
Methylprednisolone sodium succinate	UP	2.5 mg/mL[a]	MMD	5 mg/mL	Cloudiness forms	1807	I
Methylprednisolone sodium succinate	UP	20 mg/mL[b]	MMD	5 mg/mL	Precipitate forms	1807	I
Methylprednisolone sodium succinate	UP	62.5 mg/mL	MMD	5 mg/mL	Cloudiness forms but clears with swirling	1807	?
Metoclopramide HCl	RB	5 mg/mL	MMD	1[b] and 5 mg/mL	Visually compatible	1807	C
Metoclopramide HCl	RB	0.2 mg/mL[b]	MMD	5 mg/mL	Visually compatible	1807	C

Y-Site Injection Compatibility (1:1 Mixture) (Cont.)

Test Drug	Mfr	Conc	Mfr	Conc	Remarks	Ref	C/I
Metoprolol tartrate	BED	1 mg/mL	NVP	1 mg/mL[a]	Visually compatible for 24 hr at 19°C	2795	C
Metronidazole	SE	5 mg/mL	MMD	5 mg/mL	Visually compatible	1807	C
Micafungin sodium	ASP	1.5 mg/mL[b]	BA	5 mg/mL	Gross precipitate forms immediately	2683	I
Midazolam HCl	RC	2 mg/mL[a]	MMD	1 mg/mL[a]	Visually compatible for 4 hr at 27°C	2062	C
Milrinone lactate	SW	0.2 mg/mL[a]	MMD	1 mg/mL[a]	Visually compatible for 4 hr at 27°C	2062	C
Milrinone lactate	SW	0.4 mg/mL[a]	MMD	1 mg/mL[a]	Visually compatible with little loss of either drug in 4 hr at 23°C	2214	C
Morphine sulfate	SCN	15 mg/mL	MMD	1[b] and 5 mg/mL	Visually compatible	1807	C
Morphine sulfate	SCN	0.4 mg/mL[b]	MMD	5 mg/mL	Visually compatible	1807	C
Morphine sulfate	SCN	2 mg/mL[a]	MMD	1 mg/mL[a]	Visually compatible for 4 hr at 27°C	2062	C
Multivitamins		[d]	MMD	5 mg/mL	Visually compatible	1807	C
Nafcillin sodium	WY	10 mg/mL[b]	MMD	5 mg/mL	Cloudiness forms and persists	1807	I
Nafcillin sodium	WY	200 mg/mL[b]	MMD	5 mg/mL	Cloudiness forms but clears with swirling	1807	?
Nafcillin sodium	WY	10 and 200 mg/mL[b]	MMD	1 mg/mL[b]	Visually compatible	1807	C
Nesiritide	SCI	50 mcg/mL[a b]		5 mg/mL	Physically compatible for 4 hr	2625	C
Nicardipine HCl	WY	1 mg/mL[a]	MMD	1 mg/mL[a]	Visually compatible for 4 hr at 27°C	2062	C
Nitroglycerin	DU	0.032 mg/mL[a]	MMD	1 mg/mL[a]	Visually compatible for 24 hr at 25°C	1530	C
Nitroglycerin	DU	400 mcg/mL[b]	MMD	1[b] and 5 mg/mL	Visually compatible	1807	C
Nitroglycerin	DU	400 mcg/mL[a]	MMD	5 mg/mL	Visually compatible	1807	C
Nitroglycerin	AB	0.4 mg/mL[a]	MMD	1 mg/mL[a]	Visually compatible for 4 hr at 27°C	2062	C
Norepinephrine bitartrate	WI	0.12 mg/mL[a]	MMD	1 mg/mL[a]	Visually compatible for 24 hr at 25°C	1530	C
Norepinephrine bitartrate	AB	0.128 mg/mL[a]	MMD	1 mg/mL[a]	Visually compatible for 4 hr at 27°C	2062	C
Oxacillin sodium		100 mg/mL[b]	MMD	1[b] and 5 mg/mL	Visually compatible	1807	C
Oxacillin sodium		10 mg/mL[b]	MMD	5 mg/mL	Visually compatible	1807	C
Penicillin G potassium	RR	1 million units/mL	MMD	1[b] and 5 mg/mL	Visually compatible	1807	C
Penicillin G potassium	RR	100,000 units/mL[b]	MMD	5 mg/mL	Visually compatible	1807	C
Pentamidine isethionate	LY	6 and 30 mg/mL[a]	MMD	5 mg/mL	Visually compatible	1807	C
Phenytoin sodium	PD	50 mg/mL	MMD	1 mg/mL[b]	Precipitate forms	1807	I
Plazomicin sulfate	ACH	24 mg/mL[c]	AKN	5 mg/mL	Physically compatible for 1 hr at 20 to 25°C	3432	C
Potassium chloride	LY	0.08[a] and 2 mEq/mL	MMD	5 mg/mL	Visually compatible	1807	C
Potassium phosphates	AMR	0.015 mmol/mL	MMD	5 mg/mL	Visually compatible	1807	C
Procainamide HCl	ES	500 mg/mL	MMD	5 mg/mL	Cloudiness forms but clears within 2 min	1807	?

Y-Site Injection Compatibility (1:1 Mixture) (Cont.)

Test Drug	Mfr	Conc	Mfr	Conc	Remarks	Ref	C/I
Procainamide HCl	ES	50 mg/mL[a]	MMD	1 mg/mL[b]	Visually compatible	1807	C
Procainamide HCl	ES	2 mg/mL[a]	MMD	5 mg/mL	Visually compatible	1807	C
Ranitidine HCl	GL	25 mg/mL	MMD	1[b] and 5 mg/mL	Visually compatible	1807	C
Ranitidine HCl	GL	0.5[e] and 1[b] mg/mL	MMD	5 mg/mL	Visually compatible	1807	C
Ranitidine HCl	GL	1 mg/mL[a]	MMD	1 mg/mL[a]	Visually compatible for 4 hr at 27°C	2062	C
Rifampin	MMD	6 mg/mL[b]	MMD	1[b] and 5 mg/mL	Precipitate forms	1807	I
Sodium bicarbonate	LY	1 mEq/mL	MMD	5 mg/mL	Precipitate forms	1807	I
Sodium bicarbonate	LY	1 mEq/mL	MMD	1 mg/mL[b]	Visually compatible	1807	C
Sodium bicarbonate	AMR	0.05 mEq/mL[a]	MMD	5 mg/mL	Visually compatible	1807	C
Sodium nitroprusside	AB	0.2 mg/mL[a]	MMD	5 mg/mL	Visually compatible	1807	C
Tedizolid phosphate	CUB	0.8 mg/mL[b]	AKN	5 mg/mL	Physically compatible for 2 hr	3244	C
Telavancin HCl	ASP	7.5 mg/mL[a b f]	BED	5 mg/mL	Physically compatible for 2 hr	2830	C
Theophylline	AB	0.8 mg/mL[a]	MMD	5 mg/mL	Visually compatible	1807	C
Tobramycin sulfate	LI	2.4[b] and 40 mg/mL	MMD	5 mg/mL	Visually compatible	1807	C
Trimethoprim–sulfa-methoxazole	BW, RC	0.21 and 0.63 mg/mL[a h]	MMD	5 mg/mL	Visually compatible	1807	C
Vancomycin HCl	LI	5 and 50 mg/mL[b]	MMD	5 mg/mL	Visually compatible	1807	C
Vasopressin	AMR	2 and 4 units/mL[b]	NVP	1 mg/mL[b]	Physically compatible with vaso-pressin pushed through a Y-site over 5 sec	2478	C
Vecuronium bromide	OR	1 mg/mL	MMD	1 mg/mL[a]	Visually compatible for 4 hr at 27°C	2062	C

[a] Tested in dextrose 5%.

[b] Tested in sodium chloride 0.9%.

[c] Tested in both dextrose 5% and sodium chloride 0.9%.

[d] Concentration not specified.

[e] Tested in sodium chloride 0.45%.

[f] Tested in Ringer's injection, lactated.

[g] Ampicillin component. Ampicillin in a 2:1 fixed-ratio concentration with sulbactam.

[h] Trimethoprim component. Trimethoprim in a 1:5 fixed-ratio concentration with sulfamethoxazole.

[i] Not specified whether concentration refers to single component or combined components.

[j] Meropenem component. Meropenem in a 1:1 fixed-ratio concentration with vaborbactam.

[k] Ceftolozane component. Ceftolozane in a 2:1 fixed-ratio concentration with tazobactam.

Selected Revisions May 1, 2020. © Copyright, October 1994.
American Society of Health-System Pharmacists, Inc.

Dimenhydrinate
AHFS 56:22.08

Products

Dimenhydrinate is available in 1-mL and 10-mL vials containing dimenhydrinate 50 mg/mL in propylene glycol 50% and water. Sodium hydroxide and/or hydrochloric acid may be used to adjust the pH and benzyl alcohol is present in multiple-dose vials as a preservative. Dimenhydrinate contains 53 to 55.5% of diphenhydramine and 44 to 47% of 8-chlorotheophylline.[1(6/06) 4]

pH

From 6.4 to 7.2.[1(6/06) 4]

Administration

Dimenhydrinate is administered by intramuscular injection or by intravenous injection over 2 minutes after dilution with 10 mL of sodium chloride 0.9%.[1(6/06) 4]

Stability

Intact containers should be stored at controlled room temperature and protected from freezing.[1(6/06) 4]

pH Effects

A test of dimenhydrinate solutions at pH 2 to 10 showed no separation or precipitation at pH 5.4 to 8.6 on extended room temperature storage. Below pH 5.4, a white powdery precipitate of 8-chlorotheophylline formed within 24 hours. Above pH 8.6, an oily liquid separated within 30 minutes.[279]

Compatibility Information

Solution Compatibility

Dimenhydrinate

Test Soln Name	Mfr	Mfr	Conc/L or %	Remarks	Ref	C/I
Dextrose 2.5% in half-strength Ringer's injection	AB	SE	50 mg	Physically compatible	3	C
Dextrose 5% in Ringer's injection	AB	SE	50 mg	Physically compatible	3	C
Dextrose 5% in half-strength Ringer's injection, lactated	AB	SE	50 mg	Physically compatible	3	C
Dextrose 2.5% in Ringer's injection, lactated	AB	SE	50 mg	Physically compatible	3	C
Dextrose 5% in Ringer's injection, lactated	AB	SE	50 mg	Physically compatible	3	C
Dextrose 10% in Ringer's injection, lactated	AB	SE	50 mg	Physically compatible	3	C
Dextrose 2.5% in sodium chloride 0.45%	AB	SE	50 mg	Physically compatible	3	C
Dextrose 2.5% in sodium chloride 0.9%	AB	SE	50 mg	Physically compatible	3	C
Dextrose 5% in sodium chloride 0.225%	AB	SE	50 mg	Physically compatible	3	C
Dextrose 5% in sodium chloride 0.45%	AB	SE	50 mg	Physically compatible	3	C
Dextrose 5% in sodium chloride 0.9%	AB	SE	50 mg	Physically compatible	3	C
Dextrose 5% in sodium chloride 0.9%		SE	50 mg	Physically compatible	74	C
Dextrose 10% in sodium chloride 0.9%	AB	SE	50 mg	Physically compatible	3	C
Dextrose 2.5%	AB	SE	50 mg	Physically compatible	3	C
Dextrose 5%	AB	SE	50 mg	Physically compatible	3	C
Dextrose 5%		SE	50 mg	Physically compatible	74	C
Dextrose 5%				Stable for 10 days at room temperature	279	C

DOI: 10.37573/9781585286850.126

Solution Compatibility (Cont.)

Test Soln Name	Mfr	Mfr	Conc/L or %	Remarks	Ref	C/I
Dextrose 10%	AB	SE	50 mg	Physically compatible	3	C
Ionosol B in dextrose 5%	AB	SE	50 mg	Physically compatible	3	C
Ionosol MB in dextrose 5%	AB	SE	50 mg	Physically compatible	3	C
Ringer's injection	AB	SE	50 mg	Physically compatible	3	C
Ringer's injection, lactated	AB	SE	50 mg	Physically compatible	3	C
Ringer's injection, lactated		SE	50 mg	Physically compatible	74	C
Sodium chloride 0.45%	AB	SE	50 mg	Physically compatible	3	C
Sodium chloride 0.9%	AB	SE	50 mg	Physically compatible	3	C
Sodium chloride 0.9%		SE	50 mg	Physically compatible	74	C
Sodium chloride 0.9%				Stable for 10 days at room temperature	279	C
Sodium lactate ⅙ M	AB	SE	50 mg	Physically compatible	3	C

Additive Compatibility

Dimenhydrinate

Test Drug	Mfr	Conc/L or %	Mfr	Conc/L or %	Test Solution	Remarks	Ref	C/I
Amikacin sulfate	BR	5 g	SE	100 mg	D5LR, D5R, D5S, D5W, D10W, LR, NS, R, SL	Physically compatible and both stable for 24 hr at 25°C	294	C
Aminophylline		250 mg	SE	50 mg	D5W	Physically compatible	74	C
Aminophylline	SE	1 g	SE	500 mg	D5W	Physically incompatible	15	I
Ammonium chloride	AB	20 g	SE	500 mg	D5W	Physically compatible	15	C
Chloramphenicol sodium succinate	PD	500 mg	SE	50 mg	D5W	Physically compatible	74	C
Heparin sodium		12,000 units	SE	50 mg	D5W	Physically compatible	74	C
Heparin sodium	UP	4000 units	SE	500 mg	D5W	Physically compatible	15	C
Heparin sodium	AB	20,000 units	SE	50 mg	D	Physically compatible	21	C
Hydrocortisone sodium succinate	UP	100 mg	SE	50 mg	D5W	Physically compatible	74	C
Hydrocortisone sodium succinate	UP	500 mg	SE	500 mg	D5W	Physically incompatible	15	I
Hydroxyzine HCl	RR	250 mg	SE	500 mg	D5W	Physically compatible	15	C
Norepinephrine bitartrate	WI	8 mg	SE	50 mg	D5W	Physically compatible	74	C
Penicillin G potassium		1 million units	SE	50 mg	D5W	Physically compatible	74	C
Pentobarbital sodium	AB	1 g	SE	500 mg	D5W	Physically compatible	15	C
Phenobarbital sodium	WI	200 mg	SE	500 mg	D5W	Physically compatible	15	C
Potassium chloride		3 g	SE	50 mg	D5W	Physically compatible	74	C
Prochlorperazine edisylate	SKF	100 mg	SE	500 mg	D5W	Physically compatible	15	C
Vancomycin HCl	LI	1 g	SE	50 mg	D5W	Physically compatible	74	C

Drugs in Syringe Compatibility

Dimenhydrinate

Test Drug	Mfr	Amt	Mfr	Amt	Remarks	Ref	C/I
Aminophylline		50 mg/1 mL		10 mg/1 mL	Light cloudiness forms immediately	2569	I
Ampicillin sodium		50 mg/1 mL		10 mg/1 mL	Clear solution	2569	C
Atropine sulfate	ST	0.4 mg/1 mL	HR	50 mg/1 mL	Physically compatible for at least 15 min	326	C
Butorphanol tartrate	BR	4 mg/2 mL	HR	50 mg/1 mL	Gas evolves	761	I
Caffeine citrate		10 mg/1 mL		10 mg/1 mL	Clear solution	2569	C
Calcium gluconate		100 mg/1 mL		10 mg/1 mL	Clear solution	2569	C
Cefazolin sodium		100 mg/1 mL		10 mg/1 mL	Clear solution	2569	C
Cefotaxime sodium		100 mg/1 mL		10 mg/1 mL	Clear solution	2569	C
Ceftazidime		100 mg/1 mL		10 mg/1 mL	Clear solution	2569	C
Cefuroxime sodium		100 mg/1 mL		10 mg/1 mL	Clear solution	2569	C
Chlorpromazine HCl	PO	50 mg/2 mL	HR	50 mg/1 mL	Physically incompatible within 15 min	326	I
Chlorpromazine HCl		25 mg/1 mL		10 mg/1 mL	Clear solution	2569	C
Clindamycin phosphate		150 mg/1 mL		10 mg/1 mL	Clear solution	2569	C
Cloxacillin sodium		100 mg/1 mL		10 mg/1 mL	Clear solution	2569	C
Cyclosporine		50 mg/1 mL		10 mg/1 mL	Clear solution	2569	C
Dexamethasone sodium phosphate		10 mg/1 mL		10 mg/1 mL	Clear solution	2569	C
Diazepam		5 mg/1 mL		10 mg/1 mL	Loss of clarity	2569	I
Digoxin		0.05 mg/1 mL		10 mg/1 mL	Clear solution	2569	C
Diphenhydramine HCl	PD	50 mg/1 mL	HR	50 mg/1 mL	Physically compatible for at least 15 min	326	C
Dobutamine HCl		12.5 mg/1 mL		10 mg/1 mL	Clear solution	2569	C
Droperidol	MN	2.5 mg/1 mL	HR	50 mg/1 mL	Physically compatible for at least 15 min	326	C
Fentanyl citrate	MN	0.05 mg/1 mL	HR	50 mg/1 mL	Physically compatible for at least 15 min	326	C
Furosemide		10 mg/1 mL		10 mg/1 mL	Precipitate forms	2569	I
Gentamicin sulfate		10 mg/1 mL		10 mg/1 mL	Clear solution	2569	C
Gentamicin sulfate		40 mg/1 mL		10 mg/1 mL	Clear solution	2569	C
Glycopyrrolate	RB	0.2 mg/1 mL	SE	50 mg/1 mL	Precipitates immediately	331	I
Glycopyrrolate	RB	0.2 mg/1 mL	SE	100 mg/2 mL	Precipitates immediately	331	I
Glycopyrrolate	RB	0.4 mg/2 mL	SE	50 mg/1 mL	Precipitates immediately	331	I
Heparin sodium		2500 units/1 mL		65 mg/10 mL	Physically compatible for at least 5 min	1053	C
Heparin sodium		25,000 units/1 mL		10 mg/1 mL	Precipitate forms	2569	I
Hydrocortisone sodium succinate		125 mg/1 mL		10 mg/1 mL	Clear solution	2569	C
Hydromorphone HCl	KN	2, 10, 40 mg/1 mL	SQ	50 mg/1 mL	Visually compatible with both drugs stable for 24 hr at 4, 23, and 37°C. Precipitate forms after 24 hr	1776	C

Drugs in Syringe Compatibility (Cont.)

Test Drug	Mfr	Amt	Mfr	Amt	Remarks	Ref	C/I
Hydromorphone HCl		50 mg/1 mL		10 mg/1 mL	Precipitate forms in about 2 hr	2569	I
Hydroxyzine HCl	PF	50 mg/1 mL	HR	50 mg/1 mL	Physically incompatible within 15 min	326	I
Iodipamide meglumine		52%, 40 mL		1 mL[d]	Forms a precipitate initially but clears within 1 hr and remains clear for 48 hr	530	?
Iodipamide meglumine		52%, 2 to 20 mL		1 mL[d]	Forms a precipitate initially but clears within 1 hr. Precipitate reforms on standing	530	I
Iodipamide meglumine		52%, 1 mL		1 mL[d]	Precipitates immediately	530	I
Iothalamate meglumine		60%, 1 to 40 mL		1 mL[d]	Physically compatible for 48 hr	530	C
Lorazepam		4 mg/1 mL		10 mg/1 mL	Clear solution	2569	C
Magnesium sulfate		500 mg/1 mL		10 mg/1 mL	Clear solution	2569	C
Meperidine HCl	WI	50 mg/1 mL	HR	50 mg/1 mL	Physically compatible for at least 15 min	326	C
Metoclopramide HCl	NO	10 mg/2 mL	HR	50 mg/1 mL	Physically compatible for 15 min at room temperature	565	C
Midazolam HCl	RC	5 mg/1 mL	SE	50 mg/1 mL	White precipitate forms immediately	1145	I
Morphine sulfate	ST	15 mg/1 mL	HR	50 mg/1 mL	Physically compatible for at least 15 min	326	C
Naloxone HCl		0.4 mg/1 mL		10 mg/1 mL	Clear solution	2569	C
Octreotide acetate		0.5 mg/1 mL		10 mg/1 mL	Precipitate forms in about 1 hr	2569	I
Oxytocin		10 units/1 mL		10 mg/1 mL	Precipitate forms	2569	I
Pantoprazole sodium	[a]	4 mg/1 mL		50 mg/1 mL	White precipitate	2574	I
Penicillin G sodium		500,000 units/1 mL		10 mg/1 mL	Clear solution	2569	C
Pentazocine lactate	WI	30 mg/1 mL	HR	50 mg/1 mL	Physically compatible for at least 15 min	326	C
Pentobarbital sodium	AB	500 mg/10 mL	SE	50 mg/1 mL	Physically incompatible	55	I
Pentobarbital sodium	AB	50 mg/1 mL	HR	50 mg/1 mL	Physically incompatible within 15 min	326	I
Piperacillin sodium–tazobactam sodium	[a]	200 mg/1 mL[b]		10 mg/1 mL	Clear solution	2569	C
Potassium chloride		2 mEq/1 mL		10 mg/1 mL	Precipitate forms in about 1 hr	2569	I
Prochlorperazine edisylate	PO	5 mg/1 mL	HR	50 mg/1 mL	Physically incompatible within 15 min	326	I
Promethazine HCl	PO	50 mg/2 mL	HR	50 mg/1 mL	Physically incompatible within 15 min	326	I
Promethazine HCl		25 mg/1 mL		10 mg/1 mL	Solution discolors	2569	I
Ranitidine HCl	GL	50 mg/2 mL	HR	50 mg/1 mL	Physically compatible for 1 hr at 25°C	978	C
Salbutamol[e]		1 mg/1 mL		10 mg/1 mL	Precipitate forms	2569	I
Scopolamine HBr	ST	0.4 mg/1 mL	HR	50 mg/1 mL	Physically compatible for at least 15 min	326	C
Sodium bicarbonate		1 mEq/1 mL		10 mg/1 mL	Precipitates immediately	2569	I
Tobramycin sulfate		40 mg/1 mL		10 mg/1 mL	Clear solution	2569	C
Trimethoprim–sulfamethoxazole		16 mg/1 mL[c]		10 mg/1 mL	Clear solution	2569	C

Drugs in Syringe Compatibility (Cont.)

Test Drug	Mfr	Amt	Mfr	Amt	Remarks	Ref	C/I
Vancomycin HCl		50 mg/1 mL		10 mg/1 mL	Precipitate forms	2569	I
Verapamil HCl		2.5 mg/1 mL		10 mg/1 mL	Clear solution	2569	C

[a] Test performed using the formulation WITHOUT edetate disodium.

[b] Piperacillin component. Piperacillin in an 8:1 fixed-ratio concentration with tazobactam.

[c] Trimethoprim component. Trimethoprim in a 1:5 fixed-ratio concentration with sulfamethoxazole.

[d] Concentration unspecified.

[e] Salt not specified.

Y-Site Injection Compatibility (1:1 Mixture)

Dimenhydrinate

Test Drug	Mfr	Conc	Mfr	Conc	Remarks	Ref	C/I
Acyclovir sodium	BW	5 mg/mL[a]	SE	1 mg/mL[a]	Physically compatible for 4 hr at 25°C	1157	C
Ciprofloxacin		2 mg/mL		10 mg/mL	Clear solution	2569	C
Cloxacillin sodium	SMX	100 mg/mL	SZ	10 mg/mL	Physically compatible for up to 4 hr at room temperature	3245	C
Fluconazole		2 mg/mL		10 mg/mL	Clear solution	2569	C
Hydroxyethyl starch 130/0.4 in sodium chloride 0.9%	FRK	6%	SZ	0.5, 0.75, 1 mg/mL[a]	Visually compatible for 24 hr at room temperature	2770	C
Meropenem		50 mg/mL	SZ	10 mg/mL	Physically compatible for 4 hr at room temperature	3538	C
Metronidazole		5 mg/mL		10 mg/mL	Clear solution	2569	C
Pantoprazole sodium	ALT[c]	0.16 to 0.8 mg/mL[b]	AST	0.5 to 1 mg/mL[a]	Visually compatible for 12 hr at 23°C	2603	C

[a] Tested in dextrose 5%.

[b] Tested in sodium chloride 0.9%.

[c] Test performed using the formulation WITHOUT edetate disodium.

Selected Revisions July 1, 2020. © Copyright, October 1982.
American Society of Health-System Pharmacists, Inc.

Diphenhydramine Hydrochloride
AHFS 4:04

Products

Diphenhydramine hydrochloride is available as a 50-mg/mL solution in 1-mL vials and disposable syringes. Also present in the vials is 0.1 mg/mL of benzethonium chloride. The pH may have been adjusted with sodium hydroxide or hydrochloric acid.[1(1/08)]

pH

From 4 to 6.5.[17]

Trade Name(s)

Benadryl

Administration

Diphenhydramine hydrochloride is administered by deep intramuscular injection, slow direct intravenous injection, or continuous or intermittent intravenous infusion.[1(1/08)] [4] Subcutaneous or perivascular injection should be avoided due to irritation.[4]

Stability

Diphenhydramine hydrochloride in intact containers should be stored in light-resistant containers at controlled room temperature. Freezing should be avoided.[1(1/08)] [4]

Diphenhydramine hydrochloride under simulated summer conditions in paramedic vehicles was exposed to temperatures ranging from 26 to 38°C over 4 weeks. Analysis found no loss of the drug under these conditions.[2562]

Central Venous Catheter

Diphenhydramine hydrochloride (Schein) 2 mg/mL in dextrose 5% was found to be compatible with the ARROWg+ard Blue Plus (Arrow International) chlorhexidine-bearing triple-lumen central catheter. Essentially complete delivery of the drug was found with little or no drug loss occurring. Furthermore, chlorhexidine delivered from the catheter remained at trace amounts with no substantial increase due to the delivery of the drug through the catheter.[2335]

Compatibility Information

Solution Compatibility

Diphenhydramine HCl

Test Soln Name	Mfr	Mfr	Conc/L or %	Remarks	Ref	C/I
Dextrose 2.5% in half-strength Ringer's injection	AB	PD	100 mg	Physically compatible	3	C
Dextrose 5% in Ringer's injection	AB	PD	100 mg	Physically compatible	3	C
Dextrose 2.5% in Ringer's injection, lactated	AB	PD	100 mg	Physically compatible	3	C
Dextrose 5% in half-strength Ringer's injection, lactated	AB	PD	100 mg	Physically compatible	3	C
Dextrose 5% in Ringer's injection, lactated	AB	PD	100 mg	Physically compatible	3	C
Dextrose 10% in Ringer's injection, lactated	AB	PD	100 mg	Physically compatible	3	C
Dextrose 2.5% in sodium chloride 0.45%	AB	PD	100 mg	Physically compatible	3	C
Dextrose 2.5% in sodium chloride 0.9%	AB	PD	100 mg	Physically compatible	3	C
Dextrose 5% in sodium chloride 0.225%	AB	PD	100 mg	Physically compatible	3	C
Dextrose 5% in sodium chloride 0.45%	AB	PD	100 mg	Physically compatible	3	C
Dextrose 5% in sodium chloride 0.9%	AB	PD	100 mg	Physically compatible	3	C
Dextrose 10% in sodium chloride 0.9%	AB	PD	100 mg	Physically compatible	3	C
Dextrose 2.5%	AB	PD	100 mg	Physically compatible	3	C
Dextrose 5%	AB	PD	100 mg	Physically compatible	3	C
Dextrose 5%	BA[a]	FRK	0.2 and 1 g	Physically compatible with little to no loss in 14 days at 2 to 8°C	3539	C
Dextrose 10%	AB	PD	100 mg	Physically compatible	3	C

DOI: 10.37573/9781585286850.127

Solution Compatibility (Cont.)

Test Soln Name	Mfr	Mfr	Conc/L or %	Remarks	Ref	C/I
Ionosol B in dextrose 5%	AB	PD	100 mg	Physically compatible	3	C
Ionosol MB in dextrose 5%	AB	PD	100 mg	Physically compatible	3	C
Ringer's injection	AB	PD	100 mg	Physically compatible	3	C
Ringer's injection, lactated	AB	PD	100 mg	Physically compatible	3	C
Sodium chloride 0.45%	AB	PD	100 mg	Physically compatible	3	C
Sodium chloride 0.9%	AB	PD	100 mg	Physically compatible	3	C
Sodium chloride 0.9%	BA[a]	FRK	0.2 and 1 g	Physically compatible with no loss in 14 days at 2 to 8°C	3539	C
Sodium lactate ⅙ M	AB	PD	100 mg	Physically compatible	3	C

[a] Tested in PVC containers.

Additive Compatibility

Diphenhydramine HCl

Test Drug	Mfr	Conc/L or %	Mfr	Conc/L or %	Test Solution	Remarks	Ref	C/I
Amikacin sulfate	BR	5 g	PD	100 mg	D5LR, D5R, D5S, D5W, D10W, LR, NS, R, SL	Physically compatible and both stable for 24 hr at 25°C	294	C
Aminophylline	SE	500 mg	PD	50 mg		Physically compatible	6	C
Amphotericin B	SQ	100 mg	PD	80 mg	D5W	Physically incompatible	15	I
Ascorbic acid	UP	500 mg	PD	80 mg	D5W	Physically compatible	15	C
Bleomycin sulfate	BR	20 and 30 units	PD	100 mg	NS	Physically compatible and bleomycin activity retained for 1 week at 4°C. Diphenhydramine not tested	763	C
Colistimethate sodium	WC	500 mg	PD	80 mg	D5W	Physically compatible	15	C
Dexamethasone sodium phosphate with lorazepam and metoclopramide HCl	AMR WY DU	400 mg 40 mg 4 g	ES	2 g	NS[a]	Rapid lorazepam losses of 8, 10, and 15% at 3, 23, and 30°C, respectively, in 24 hr. Other drugs stable for 14 days at all three storage temperatures	1733	I
Erythromycin lactobionate	AB	1 g	PD	50 mg		Physically compatible. Erythromycin stable for 24 hr at 25°C	20	C
Erythromycin lactobionate	AB	1 g	PD	50 mg	D5W	Erythromycin stable for 24 hr at 25°C	48	C
Fat emulsion, intravenous	VT	10%	PD	100 mg		Physically compatible for 48 hr at 4°C and room temperature	32	C
Iodipamide meglumine	SQ	52%	PD	20 to 200 mg	NS	Dense putty-like white precipitate forms immediately	309	I
Lidocaine HCl	AST	2 g	PD	50 mg		Physically compatible	24	C
Lorazepam with dexamethasone sodium phosphate and metoclopramide HCl	WY AMR DU	40 mg 400 mg 4 g	ES	2 g	NS[a]	Rapid lorazepam losses of 8, 10, and 15% at 3, 23, and 30°C, respectively, in 24 hr. Other drugs stable for 14 days at all three storage temperatures	1733	I

Additive Compatibility (Cont.)

Test Drug	Mfr	Conc/L or %	Mfr	Conc/L or %	Test Solution	Remarks	Ref	C/I
Methyldopate HCl	MSD	1 g	PD	50 mg	D5W, D10W, D2.5½S, D2.5S, D5¼S, D5½S, D5S, D10S, NS, ½S	Physically compatible	23	C
Metoclopramide HCl with dexamethasone sodium phosphate and lorazepam	DU, AMR, WY	4 g, 400 mg, 40 mg	ES	2 g	NS[a]	Rapid lorazepam losses of 8, 10, and 15% at 3, 23, and 30°C, respectively, in 24 hr. Other drugs stable for 14 days at all three storage temperatures	1733	I
Nafcillin sodium	WY	500 mg	PD	50 mg		Physically compatible	27	C
Penicillin G potassium	SQ	20 million units	PD	80 mg	D5W	Physically compatible	15	C
Penicillin G potassium	SQ	1 million units	PD	50 mg	D5W	Physically compatible. Penicillin stable for 24 hr at 25°C	47	C
Penicillin G sodium	UP	20 million units	PD	80 mg	D5W	Physically compatible	15	C
Polymyxin B sulfate	BW	200 mg	PD	80 mg	D5W	Physically compatible	15	C

[a] Tested in Pharmacia-Deltec PVC pump reservoirs.

Drugs in Syringe Compatibility

Diphenhydramine HCl

Test Drug	Mfr	Amt	Mfr	Amt	Remarks	Ref	C/I
Atropine sulfate	ST	0.4 mg/1 mL	PD	50 mg/1 mL	Physically compatible for at least 15 min	326	C
Buprenorphine HCl					Physically and chemically compatible	4	C
Butorphanol tartrate	BR	4 mg/2 mL	PD	50 mg/1 mL	Physically compatible for 30 min at room temperature	566	C
Chlorpromazine HCl	PO	50 mg/2 mL	PD	50 mg/1 mL	Physically compatible for at least 15 min	326	C
Chlorpromazine HCl	STS	50 mg/2 mL	ES	100 mg/2 mL	Visually compatible for 60 min	1784	C
Dexamethasone sodium phosphate	DB, SX	4 and 10 mg/mL[a]	PD	50 mg/mL[a]	White turbidity and precipitate form immediately	1542	I
Dexamethasone sodium phosphate	DB	9.52 mg/mL[b]	PD	4.54 mg/mL[b]	Visually compatible for 24 hr at 24°C	1542	C
Dexamethasone sodium phosphate	DB	5 to 9.02 mg/mL[b]	PD	4.54 to 15 mg/mL[b]	Precipitate forms	1542	I
Dexamethasone sodium phosphate	SX	2 mg/mL[b]	PD	34.8 to 40 mg/mL[b]	Visually compatible for 24 hr at 24°C	1542	C
Dexamethasone sodium phosphate	SX	1 mg/mL[b]	PD	25 mg/mL[b]	Precipitate forms	1542	I
Dimenhydrinate	HR	50 mg/1 mL	PD	50 mg/1 mL	Physically compatible for at least 15 min	326	C
Droperidol	MN	2.5 mg/1 mL	PD	50 mg/1 mL	Physically compatible for at least 15 min	326	C
Fentanyl citrate	MN	0.05 mg/1 mL	PD	50 mg/1 mL	Physically compatible for at least 15 min	326	C
Fluphenazine HCl	LY	5 mg/2 mL	ES	100 mg/2 mL	Visually compatible for 60 min	1784	C
Glycopyrrolate	RB	0.2 mg/1 mL	PD	10 mg/1 mL	Physically compatible. pH in glycopyrrolate stability range for 48 hr at 25°C	331	C

Drugs in Syringe Compatibility (Cont.)

Test Drug	Mfr	Amt	Mfr	Amt	Remarks	Ref	C/I
Glycopyrrolate	RB	0.2 mg/1 mL	PD	20 mg/2 mL	Physically compatible. pH in glycopyrrolate stability range for 48 hr at 25°C	331	C
Glycopyrrolate	RB	0.4 mg/2 mL	PD	10 mg/1 mL	Physically compatible. pH in glycopyrrolate stability range for 48 hr at 25°C	331	C
Glycopyrrolate	RB	0.2 mg/1 mL	PD	50 mg/1 mL	Physically compatible. pH in glycopyrrolate stability range for 48 hr at 25°C	331	C
Glycopyrrolate	RB	0.2 mg/1 mL	PD	100 mg/2 mL	Physically compatible. pH in glycopyrrolate stability range for 48 hr at 25°C	331	C
Glycopyrrolate	RB	0.4 mg/2 mL	PD	50 mg/1 mL	Physically compatible. pH in glycopyrrolate stability range for 48 hr at 25°C	331	C
Haloperidol lactate	MN	10 mg/2 mL	ES	100 mg/2 mL	White precipitate forms within 5 min	1784	I
Haloperidol lactate	MN	5 mg/1 mL	ES	50 mg/1 mL	White cloudy precipitate forms in 2 hr at room temperature	1886	I
Hydromorphone HCl	KN	4 mg/2 mL	PD	50 mg/1 mL	Physically compatible for 30 min	517	C
Hydroxyzine HCl	PF	50 mg/1 mL	PD	50 mg/1 mL	Physically compatible for at least 15 min	326	C
Iodipamide meglumine	SQ		PD	5 mg/0.1 mL to 50 mg/1 mL	Dense putty-like white precipitate forms immediately	309	I
Iodipamide meglumine		52%, 1 to 40 mL		1 mL[c]	Forms a precipitate initially but clears within 1 hr and remains clear for 48 hr	530	?
Iohexol	WI	64.7%, 5 mL	PD	12.5 mg/0.25 mL	Physically compatible for at least 2 hr	1438	C
Iopamidol	SQ	61%, 5 mL	PD	12.5 mg/0.25 mL	Physically compatible for at least 2 hr	1438	C
Iothalamate meglumine	MA	5 mL	PD	50 mg/1 mL	No precipitate observed	309	C
Iothalamate meglumine		60%, 1 to 40 mL		1 mL[c]	Physically compatible for 48 hr	530	C
Iothalamate meglumine	MA	60%, 5 mL	PD	12.5 mg/0.25 mL	Physically compatible for at least 2 hr	1438	C
Ioxaglate meglumine–ioxaglate sodium	MA	5 mL	PD	12.5 mg/0.25 mL	Precipitate forms immediately and persists for at least 2 hr	1438	I
Meperidine HCl	WY	100 mg/1 mL	PD	50 mg/1 mL	Physically compatible for at least 15 min	14	C
Meperidine HCl	WI	50 mg/1 mL	PD	50 mg/1 mL	Physically compatible for at least 15 min	326	C
Metoclopramide HCl	NO	10 mg/2 mL	PD	50 mg/1 mL	Physically compatible for 15 min at room temperature	565	C
Metoclopramide HCl	RB	10 mg/2 mL	PD	50 mg/5 mL	Physically compatible for 48 hr at 25°C	1167	C
Metoclopramide HCl	RB	10 mg/2 mL	PD	250 mg/25 mL	Physically compatible for 48 hr at 25°C	1167	C
Metoclopramide HCl	RB	160 mg/32 mL	PD	40 mg/4 mL	Physically compatible for 48 hr at 25°C	1167	C
Metoclopramide HCl	RB	160 mg/32 mL	PD	200 mg/20 mL	Physically compatible for 48 hr at 25°C	1167	C
Midazolam HCl	RC	5 mg/1 mL	ES	50 mg/1 mL	Physically compatible for 4 hr at 25°C	1145	C
Morphine sulfate	WY	15 mg/1 mL	PD	50 mg/1 mL	Physically compatible for at least 15 min	14	C
Morphine sulfate	ST	15 mg/1 mL	PD	50 mg/1 mL	Physically compatible for at least 15 min	326	C
Nalbuphine HCl	DU	10 mg/1 mL	PD	50 mg/1 mL	Physically compatible for 48 hr	128	C
Nalbuphine HCl	DU	20 mg/1 mL	PD	50 mg/1 mL	Physically compatible for 48 hr	128	C
Pantoprazole sodium	[d]	4 mg/1 mL		50 mg/1 mL	Precipitates immediately	2574	I

Drugs in Syringe Compatibility (Cont.)

Test Drug	Mfr	Amt	Mfr	Amt	Remarks	Ref	C/I
Pentazocine lactate	WI	30 mg/1 mL	PD	50 mg/1 mL	Physically compatible for at least 15 min	326	C
Pentobarbital sodium	WY	100 mg/2 mL	PD	50 mg/1 mL	Precipitate observed within 15 min	14	I
Pentobarbital sodium	AB	500 mg/10 mL	PD	50 mg/1 mL	Physically incompatible	55	I
Pentobarbital sodium	AB	50 mg/1 mL	PD	50 mg/1 mL	Physically incompatible within 15 min	326	I
Prochlorperazine edisylate	PO	5 mg/1 mL	PD	50 mg/1 mL	Physically compatible for at least 15 min	326	C
Promethazine HCl	WY	50 mg/2 mL	PD	50 mg/1 mL	Physically compatible for at least 15 min	14	C
Promethazine HCl	PO	50 mg/2 mL	PD	50 mg/1 mL	Physically compatible for at least 15 min	326	C
Ranitidine HCl	GL	50 mg/2 mL	PD	50 mg/1 mL	Physically compatible for 1 hr at 25°C	978	C
Scopolamine HBr	ST	0.4 mg/1 mL	PD	50 mg/1 mL	Physically compatible for at least 15 min	326	C

[a] Mixed in equal quantities. Final concentration is one-half the indicated concentration.

[b] Mixed in varying quantities to yield the final concentrations noted.

[c] Concentration unspecified.

[d] Test performed using the formulation WITHOUT edetate disodium.

Y-Site Injection Compatibility (1:1 Mixture)

Diphenhydramine HCl

Test Drug	Mfr	Conc	Mfr	Conc	Remarks	Ref	C/I
Abciximab	LI	36 mcg/mL[a]	ES	25 mg/mL	Visually compatible for 12 hr at 23°C	2374	C
Acetaminophen	CAD	10 mg/mL	BA	50 mg/mL	Physically compatible with less than 10% acetaminophen loss over 4 hr at room temperature	2841, 2844	C
Acetaminophen	CAD	10 mg/mL	WW	50 mg/mL	Physically compatible with no loss of either drug in 4 hr at 23°C	2901, 2902	C
Acyclovir sodium	BW	5 mg/mL[a]	ES	1 mg/mL[a]	Physically compatible for 4 hr at 25°C	1157	C
Acyclovir sodium	BV	5 mg/mL[b]	BA	50 mg/mL	Cloudy upon mixing	2794	I
Aldesleukin	CHI	33,800 I.U./mL[a]	SCN	50 mg/mL	Visually compatible for 2 hr	1857	C
Allopurinol sodium	BW	3 mg/mL[b]	PD	2 mg/mL[b]	White precipitate forms immediately	1686	I
Amifostine	USB	10 mg/mL[a]	PD	2 mg/mL[a]	Physically compatible for 4 hr at 23°C	1845	C
Amsacrine	NCI	1 mg/mL[a]	PD	2 mg/mL[a]	Visually compatible for 4 hr at 22°C	1381	C
Argatroban	GSK	1 mg/mL[b]	ES	50 mg/mL	Visually compatible for 24 hr at 23°C	2391	C
Azithromycin	PF	2 mg/mL[b]	ES	50 mg/mL[i]	Visually compatible	2368	C
Aztreonam	SQ	40 mg/mL[a]	PD	2 mg/mL[a]	Physically compatible for 4 hr at 23°C	1758	C
Bivalirudin	TMC	5 mg/mL[a]	ES	2 mg/mL[a]	Physically compatible for 4 hr at 23°C	2373	C
Cangrelor tetrasodium	TMC	1 mg/mL[b]		2 mg/mL[b]	Physically compatible for 4 hr	3243	C
Cangrelor tetrasodium	TMC	1 mg/mL[b]		25 mg/mL[b]	Gross white turbid precipitate forms immediately	3243	I

Y-Site Injection Compatibility (1:1 Mixture) (Cont.)

Test Drug	Mfr	Conc	Mfr	Conc	Remarks	Ref	C/I
Caspofungin acetate	ME	0.5 mg/mL[b]	BA	50 mg/mL	Physically compatible with diphenhydramine HCl given i.v. push over 2 to 5 min	2766	C
Ceftaroline fosamil	FOR	2.22 mg/mL[a b k]	BA	2 mg/mL[a b k]	Physically compatible for 4 hr at 23°C	2826	C
Ceftolozane sulfate–tazobactam sodium	CUB	10 mg/mL[c m]	APP	50 mg/mL	Physically compatible for 2 hr	3262	C
Ciprofloxacin	MI	2 mg/mL[c]	ES	50 mg/mL	Visually compatible for 24 hr at 24°C	1655	C
Cisatracurium besylate	GW	0.1, 2, 5 mg/mL[a]	SCN	2 mg/mL[a]	Physically compatible for 4 hr at 23°C	2074	C
Cladribine	ORT	0.015[b] and 0.5[d] mg/mL	SCN	2 mg/mL[b]	Physically compatible for 4 hr at 23°C	1969	C
Cloxacillin sodium	SMX	100 mg/mL	PPC	50 mg/mL	Precipitates immediately	3245	I
Dexmedetomidine HCl	AB	4 mcg/mL[b]	PD	2 mg/mL[b]	Physically compatible for 4 hr at 23°C	2383	C
Docetaxel	RPR	0.9 mg/mL[a]	ES	2 mg/mL[a]	Physically compatible for 4 hr at 23°C	2224	C
Doripenem	JJ	5 mg/mL[a b]	BA	2 mg/mL[a b]	Physically compatible for 4 hr at 23°C	2743	C
Doxorubicin HCl liposomal	SEQ	0.4 mg/mL[a]	SCN	2 mg/mL[a]	Physically compatible for 4 hr at 23°C	2087	C
Etoposide phosphate	BR	5 mg/mL[a]	ES	2 mg/mL[a]	Physically compatible for 4 hr at 23°C	2218	C
Famotidine	ME	2 mg/mL[b]		2 mg/mL[a]	Visually compatible for 4 hr at 22°C	1936	C
Fenoldopam mesylate	AB	80 mcg/mL[b]	ES	2 mg/mL[b]	Physically compatible for 4 hr at 23°C	2467	C
Fentanyl citrate	JN	0.025 mg/mL[a]	SCN	2 mg/mL[a]	Physically compatible for 48 hr at 22°C	1706	C
Filgrastim	AMG	30 mcg/mL[a]	ES	2 mg/mL[a]	Physically compatible for 4 hr at 22°C	1687	C
Fluconazole	RR	2 mg/mL	ES	50 mg/mL	Physically compatible for 24 hr at 25°C	1407	C
Fludarabine phosphate	BX	1 mg/mL[a]	WY	2 mg/mL[a]	Visually compatible for 4 hr at 22°C	1439	C
Foscarnet sodium	AST	24 mg/mL	PD	50 mg/mL	Cloudy solution	1335	I
Gallium nitrate	FUJ	1 mg/mL[b]	ES	50 mg/mL	Visually compatible for 24 hr at 25°C	1673	C
Gemcitabine HCl	LI	10 mg/mL[b]	SCN	2 mg/mL[b]	Physically compatible for 4 hr at 23°C	2226	C
Granisetron HCl	SKB	1 mg/mL	PD	1 mg/mL[b]	Physically compatible with little loss of either drug in 4 hr at 22°C	1883	C
Granisetron HCl	SKB	0.05 mg/mL[a]	SCN	2 mg/mL[a]	Physically compatible for 4 hr at 23°C	2000	C
Heparin sodium	UP	1000 units/L[e]	PD	50 mg/mL	Physically compatible for 4 hr at room temperature	534	C
Hetastarch in lactated electrolyte	AB	6%	SCN	2 mg/mL[a]	Physically compatible for 4 hr at 23°C	2339	C
Hydrocortisone sodium succinate	UP	10 mg/L[e]	PD	50 mg/mL	Physically compatible for 4 hr at room temperature	534	C
Hydromorphone HCl	AST	0.5 mg/mL[a]	SCN	2 mg/mL[a]	Physically compatible for 48 hr at 22°C	1706	C

Y-Site Injection Compatibility (1:1 Mixture) (Cont.)

Test Drug	Mfr	Conc	Mfr	Conc	Remarks	Ref	C/I
Idarubicin HCl	AD	1 mg/mL[b]	ES	1[a] and 50 mg/mL	Visually compatible for 24 hr at 25°C	1525	C
Isavuconazonium sulfate	ASP	1.5 mg/mL[c]	APP	50 mg/mL	Physically compatible for 2 hr	3263	C
Linezolid	PHU	2 mg/mL	ES	2 mg/mL[a]	Physically compatible for 4 hr at 23°C	2264	C
Melphalan HCl	BW	0.1 mg/mL[b]	WY	2 mg/mL[b]	Physically compatible for 3 hr at 22°C	1557	C
Meperidine HCl	AB	10 mg/mL	ES	1[a] and 50 mg/mL	Physically compatible for 4 hr at 25°C	1397	C
Meropenem	ZEN	1 and 50 mg/mL[b]	PD	50 mg/mL	Visually compatible for 4 hr at room temperature	1994	C
Meropenem		50 mg/mL	FRK	50 mg/mL	Physically compatible for 4 hr at room temperature	3538	C
Meropenem–vabor-bactam	TMC	8 mg/mL[b n]	FRK	50 mg/mL	Immediate change in measured turbidity with precipitation within 3 hr. pH increased by >2 units within 3 hr	3380	I
Methadone HCl	LI	1 mg/mL[a]	SCN	2 mg/mL[a]	Physically compatible for 48 hr at 22°C	1706	C
Morphine sulfate	AST	1 mg/mL[a]	SCN	2 mg/mL[a]	Physically compatible for 48 hr at 22°C	1706	C
Ondansetron HCl	GL	1 mg/mL[b]	PD	2 mg/mL[a]	Visually compatible for 4 hr at 22°C	1365	C
Oxaliplatin	SS	0.5 mg/mL[a]	ES	2 mg/mL[a]	Physically compatible for 4 hr at 23°C	2566	C
Paclitaxel	NCI	1.2 mg/mL[a]		2 mg/mL[a]	Physically compatible for 4 hr at 22°C	1528	C
Pemetrexed disodium	LI	20 mg/mL[b]	ES	2 mg/mL[a]	Physically compatible for 4 hr at 23°C	2564	C
Piperacillin sodium–tazobactam sodium	LE[j]	40 mg/mL[a l]	WY	2 mg/mL[a]	Physically compatible for 4 hr at 22°C	1688	C
Plazomicin sulfate	ACH	24 mg/mL[c]	FRK	50 mg/mL	Physically compatible for 1 hr at 20 to 25°C	3432	C
Potassium chloride	AB	40 mEq/L[e]	PD	50 mg/mL	Physically compatible for 4 hr at room temperature	534	C
Propofol	ZEN[o]	10 mg/mL	SCN	2 mg/mL[a]	Physically compatible for 1 hr at 23°C	2066	C
Remifentanil HCl	GW	0.025 and 0.25 mg/mL[b]	SCN	2 mg/mL[a]	Physically compatible for 4 hr at 23°C	2075	C
Sargramostim	IMM	10 mcg/mL[b]	RU	1 mg/mL[b]	Visually compatible for 4 hr at 22°C	1436	C
Tacrolimus	FUJ	1 mg/mL[b]	ES	1 mg/mL[a]	Visually compatible for 24 hr at 25°C	1630	C
Tedizolid phosphate	CUB	0.8 mg/mL[b]	APP	50 mg/mL	Measured turbidity increases within 2 hr	3244	I
Teniposide	BR	0.1 mg/mL[a]	ES	2 mg/mL[a]	Physically compatible for 4 hr at 23°C	1725	C
Thiotepa	IMM[g]	1 mg/mL[a]	WY	2 mg/mL[a]	Physically compatible for 4 hr at 23°C	1861	C
TNA #218 to #226[h]			PD	2 mg/mL[a]	Visually compatible for 4 hr at 23°C	2215	C
TNA #218 to #226[h]			SCN	50 mg/mL	Visually compatible for 4 hr at 23°C	2215	C
TPN #212 to #215[h]			SCN	2[a] and 50 mg/mL	Physically compatible for 4 hr at 23°C	2109	C

Y-Site Injection Compatibility (1:1 Mixture) (Cont.)

Test Drug	Mfr	Conc	Mfr	Conc	Remarks	Ref	C/I
Vinorelbine tartrate	BW	1 mg/mL[b]	ES	2 mg/mL[b]	Physically compatible for 4 hr at 22°C	1558	C

[a] Tested in dextrose 5%.

[b] Tested in sodium chloride 0.9%.

[c] Tested in both dextrose 5% and sodium chloride 0.9%.

[d] Tested in bacteriostatic sodium chloride 0.9% preserved with benzyl alcohol 0.9%.

[e] Tested in dextrose 5% in Ringer's injection, dextrose 5% in Ringer's injection, lactated, dextrose 5%, Ringer's injection, lactated, and sodium chloride 0.9%.

[f] Tested in dextrose 5% with sodium bicarbonate 0.05 mEq/mL.

[g] Lyophilized formulation tested.

[h] Refer to Appendix for the composition of parenteral nutrition solutions. TNA indicates a 3-in-1 admixture, and TPN indicates a 2-in-1 admixture.

[i] Injected via Y-site into an administration set running azithromycin.

[j] Test performed using the formulation WITHOUT edetate disodium.

[k] Tested in Ringer's injection, lactated.

[l] Piperacillin component. Piperacillin in an 8:1 fixed-ratio concentration with tazobactam.

[m] Ceftolozane component. Ceftolozane in a 2:1 fixed-ratio concentration with tazobactam.

[n] Meropenem component. Meropenem in a 1:1 fixed-ratio concentration with vaborbactam.

[o] Test performed using the formulation WITH edetate disodium.

Selected Revisions May 1, 2020. © Copyright, October 1982.
American Society of Health-System Pharmacists, Inc.

Dobutamine Hydrochloride
AHFS 12:12.08.08

Products

Dobutamine hydrochloride is available in 20-, 40-, and 100-mL single-dose vials as a concentrate for injection. Each mL contains 12.5 mg of dobutamine (as the hydrochloride), sodium bisulfite 0.24 mg, and hydrochloric acid and/or sodium hydroxide to adjust the pH. Dobutamine hydrochloride concentrate for injection must be diluted further to a concentration not greater than 5 mg/mL before administration.[1(1/07)] [4]

Dobutamine hydrochloride also is available in plastic bags as premixed solutions in concentrations of 1, 2, and 4 mg/mL in dextrose 5%. Sodium metabisulfite and edetate disodium dihydrate also may be present.[4]

pH

From 2.5 to 5.5.[1(1/07)] [4] [17] The premixed infusion solutions in dextrose 5% have a pH ranging from 2.5 to 5.5.[4]

Osmolality

The osmolality of dobutamine hydrochloride injection (Lilly) was determined to be 273 mOsm/kg by freezing-point depression and vapor pressure.[1071] At a concentration of 5 mg/mL (manufacturer and diluent unspecified), the osmolality was determined to be 361 mOsm/kg by freezing-point depression.[1233]

The premixed infusion solutions in dextrose 5% have osmolalities ranging from 260 to 284 mOsm/kg for the 4 concentrations available.[4]

Administration

Dobutamine hydrochloride is administered by intravenous infusion after dilution to a concentration no greater than 5 mg/mL. The concentration used is dependent on the patient's dosage and fluid requirements. An infusion pump or other infusion control device should be used to control the flow rate.[1(1/07)] [4]

Stability

Intact containers should be stored at controlled room temperature and protected from excessive heat and freezing. Solutions that are further diluted for intravenous infusion should be used within 24 hours.[1(1/07)] [4]

Dobutamine hydrochloride concentrate for injection is a clear, colorless to pale straw-colored solution. Solutions of dobutamine hydrochloride may have a pink discoloration. This discoloration, which will increase with time, results from a slight oxidation of the drug. However, there is no significant loss of drug within the recommended storage times for solutions of the drug.[4]

Dobutamine hydrochloride has been stated to be incompatible with alkaline solutions.[1(1/07)] [4]

Syringes

Dobutamine hydrochloride (Lilly) 250 mg/50 mL in dextrose 5% exhibited no change in appearance and no drug loss when stored in 60-mL plastic syringes (Becton Dickinson) for 24 hours at 25°C.[1579]

Dobutamine hydrochloride (Lilly) 5 mg/mL in dextrose 5% was packaged in 50-mL polypropylene syringes (Becton Dickinson) and stored at 4 and 24°C in the dark and exposed to room light for 48 hours. Dobutamine losses were less than 10% throughout the study.[1961]

To assess the stability of dobutamine 500 mg in 50-mL syringes, dobutamine hydrochloride (Phoenix) 12.5-mg/mL concentrate for injection was mixed with dextrose 5% for final dobutamine and dextrose concentrations of 10 mg/mL and 1%, respectively, and packaged as 3 mL in 50-mL syringes (Becton Dickinson).[3511] Syringes were stored at 4 and 40°C protected from light and at room temperature, both protected from and exposed to light.[3511] Calculated times to 5% loss from initial concentrations were approximately 111, 74, 56, and 45 days for samples stored at 4°C protected from light, room temperature protected from light, room temperature exposed to light, and 40°C protected from light, respectively.[3511] However, syringes stored at room temperature protected from light, 40°C protected from light, and room temperature exposed to light demonstrated discoloration at 42, 35, and 28 days, respectively; syringes stored at 4°C protected from light did not demonstrate any such discoloration.[3511] While all samples demonstrated less than 10% loss from initial concentrations in 42 days, the authors concluded that syringes stored at 4°C protected from light and room temperature protected from light have a shelf life of 42 and 35 days, respectively.[3511]

Sorption

Delivering dobutamine hydrochloride (Lilly) 5 mg/mL in dextrose 5% by syringe pump over 12 hours at 24°C through polyvinyl chloride (PVC) and polyethylene tubing did not result in substantial dobutamine losses.[1961]

Filtration

Dobutamine hydrochloride (Lilly) 0.5 mg/mL in dextrose 5% and sodium chloride 0.9% was filtered through a 0.22-μm cellulose ester membrane filter (Ivex-HP, Millipore) over 6 hours. No significant drug loss due to binding to the filter was noted.[1034]

Central Venous Catheter

Dobutamine hydrochloride (Astra) 4 mg/mL in dextrose 5% was found to be compatible with the ARROWg+ard Blue Plus (Arrow International) chlorhexidine-bearing triple-lumen central catheter. Essentially complete delivery of the drug was found with little or no drug loss occurring. Furthermore, chlorhexidine delivered from the catheter remained at trace amounts with no substantial increase due to the delivery of the drug through the catheter.[2335]

DOI: 10.37573/9781585286850.128

Compatibility Information

Solution Compatibility

Dobutamine HCl

Test Soln Name	Mfr	Mfr	Conc/L or %	Remarks	Ref	C/I
Dextrose 2.5% in half-strength Ringer's injection, lactated	MG[a]	LI	1 g	No loss in 48 hr at 25°C. Slight pink color at 8 hr becoming slightly brown at 24 hr	789	C
Dextrose 5% in Ringer's injection, lactated				Use within 24 hr	1(1/07)	C
Dextrose 5% in Ringer's injection, lactated	MG[a]	LI	1 g	No loss in 48 hr at 25°C. Slight pink color at 8 hr becoming slightly brown at 48 hr	789	C
Dextrose 2.5% in sodium chloride 0.45%	MG[a]	LI	1 g	No loss in 48 hr at 25°C. Slight pink color at 24 hr becoming slightly brown at 48 hr	789	C
Dextrose 5% in sodium chloride 0.45%				Use within 24 hr	1(1/07)	C
Dextrose 5% in sodium chloride 0.45%	AB[b], CU[a]	LI	1 g	No loss in 48 hr at 25°C. Slight pink color at 24 hr becoming slightly brown at 48 hr	749	C
Dextrose 5% in sodium chloride 0.9%				Use within 24 hr	1(1/07)	C
Dextrose 5% in sodium chloride 0.9%	MG[b]	LI	1 g	No loss in 48 hr at 25°C. Slight pink color at 24 hr becoming slightly brown at 48 hr	789	C
Dextrose 5%				Use within 24 hr	1(1/07)	C
Dextrose 5%	CU[a], TR[b]	LI	1 g	No loss in 48 hr at 25°C. Slight pink color at 24 hr becoming slightly brown at 48 hr	749	C
Dextrose 5%	TR[b]	LI	250 mg	Physically compatible with no loss in 48 hr at 24°C. Transient light pink color. No loss after 7 days at 5°C	811	C
Dextrose 5%	[a]		2 to 8 g	Pale pink discoloration with 4% or less dobutamine loss in 24 hr exposed to light	1412	C
Dextrose 5%	BA[b]	LI	5 g	5% loss in 100 days at 5°C protected from light	1610	C
Dextrose 5%	BA[b]	LI	1 g	5% loss in 234.7 days at 5°C protected from light	1610	C
Dextrose 5%	TR[b]	LI	0.25 and 1 g	Visually compatible with no dobutamine loss in 48 hr at room temperature	1802	C
Dextrose 5%	AB[b]	AB	4 g	Visually compatible with no loss in 30 days at 4 and 23°C protected from light	2241	C
Dextrose 5%	BA[b], BRN[a c]	GIU	0.5 g	Visually compatible with little loss in 24 hr at 4 and 22°C	2289	C
Dextrose 5%	BA[d]	HOS	10 g	Physically stable with little to no loss of drug in 7 days at 4°C followed by 12 hr at 35°C and an additional 12 hr at 25°C	3507	C
Dextrose 10%				Use within 24 hr	1(1/07)	C
Normosol M in dextrose 5%				Use within 24 hr	1(1/07)	C
Ringer's injection, lactated				Use within 24 hr	1(1/07)	C
Ringer's injection, lactated	CU[a], TR[b]	LI	1 g	No loss in 48 hr at 25°C. Slight pink color at 3 hr becoming slightly brown at 48 hr	749	C
Sodium chloride 0.45%	MG[a]	LI	1 g	No loss in 48 hr at 25°C. Slight pink color at 24 hr becoming slightly brown at 48 hr	789	C

Solution Compatibility (Cont.)

Test Soln Name	Mfr	Mfr	Conc/L or %	Remarks	Ref	C/I
Sodium chloride 0.9%				Use within 24 hr	1(1/07)	C
Sodium chloride 0.9%		LI	200 mg	Physically compatible for 24 hr	552	C
Sodium chloride 0.9%	CU[a], TR[b]	LI	1 g	No loss in 48 hr at 25°C. Slight pink color at 24 hr becoming slightly brown at 48 hr	749	C
Sodium chloride 0.9%	TR[b]	LI	250 mg	About 3% dobutamine loss in 48 hr at 24°C. Initially colorless solution becomes pink with time. No decomposition after 7 days at 5°C	811	C
Sodium chloride 0.9%	[a]		2 to 8 g	Pale pink discoloration with 3% or less dobutamine loss in 24 hr exposed to light	1412	C
Sodium chloride 0.9%	TR[a]	LI	0.25 and 1 g	Visually compatible with no loss in 48 hr at room temperature	1802	C
Sodium chloride 0.9%	BA[b], BRN[a c]	GIU	0.5 g	Visually compatible with little loss in 24 hr at 4 and 22°C	2289	C
Sodium chloride 0.9%	BA[d]	HOS	10 g	Physically stable with little to no loss of drug in 7 days at 4°C followed by 12 hr at 35°C and an additional 12 hr at 25°C	3507	C
Sodium lactate ⅙ M				Use within 24 hr	1(1/07)	C

[a] Tested in glass containers.

[b] Tested in PVC containers.

[c] Tested in polyethylene containers.

[d] Tested in medication cassette reservoirs.

Additive Compatibility

Dobutamine HCl

Test Drug	Mfr	Conc/L or %	Mfr	Conc/L or %	Test Solution	Remarks	Ref	C/I
Acyclovir sodium	BW	2.5 g	LI	0.5 g	D5W	Discoloration in 25 min. Cloudiness and brown color in 2 hr due to dobutamine oxidation. No acyclovir loss	1343	I
Alteplase	GEN	0.5 g	LI	5 g	D5W, NS	Yellow discoloration and precipitate form	1856	I
Aminophylline	SE	1 g	LI	1 g	D5W, NS	Cloudy in 6 hr at 25°C	789	I
Aminophylline	ES	2.5 g	LI	1 g	D5W, NS	White precipitate in 12 hr at 21°C	812	I
Amiodarone HCl	LZ	2.5 g	LI	1 g	D5W, NS	Physically compatible for 24 hr at 21°C	812	C
Atracurium besylate	BW	500 mg		1 g	D5W	Physically compatible and atracurium stable for 24 hr at 5 and 30°C	1694	C
Atropine sulfate	AB	16.7 mg	LI	167 mg	NS	Physically compatible for 24 hr	552	C
Atropine sulfate	ES	50 mg	LI	1 g	D5W, NS	Physically compatible for 24 hr at 21°C	812	C
Bumetanide	RC	125 mg	LI	1 g	D5W, NS	Immediate yellow discoloration with yellow precipitate within 6 hr at 21°C	812	I
Calcium chloride	UP	9 g	LI	182 mg	NS	Physically compatible for 20 hr. Haze forms at 24 hr	552	I
Calcium chloride	ES	2 g	LI	1 g	D5W, NS	Deeply pink in 24 hr at 25°C	789	I
Calcium chloride	ES	50 g	LI	1 g	D5W, NS	Physically compatible for 24 hr at 21°C	812	C

Additive Compatibility (Cont.)

Test Drug	Mfr	Conc/L or %	Mfr	Conc/L or %	Test Solution	Remarks	Ref	C/I
Calcium gluconate	VI	9 g	LI	182 mg	NS	Small particles form within 4 hr. White precipitate and haze after 15 hr	552	I
Calcium gluconate	ES	2 g	LI	1 g	D5W, NS	Deeply pink in 24 hr at 25°C	789	I
Calcium gluconate	IX	50 g	LI	1 g	D5W, NS	Small white particles in 24 hr at 21°C	812	I
Ciprofloxacin	BAY	1.7 g	LI	2 g	D5W	Visually compatible with no loss of ciprofloxacin in 24 hr at 22°C under fluorescent light. Dobutamine not tested	2413	C
Diazepam	RC	2.5 g	LI	1 g	D5W, NS	Rapid clouding of solution with yellow precipitate within 24 hr at 21°C	812	I
Digoxin	BW	4 mg	LI	1 g	D5W, NS	Slightly pink in 24 hr at 25°C	789	I
Dopamine HCl	AS	5.5 g	LI	172 mg	NS	Physically compatible for 24 hr	552	C
Dopamine HCl	ACC	1.6 g	LI	1 g	D5W, NS	Physically compatible with no color change in 24 hr at 25°C	789	C
Dopamine HCl	ES	800 mg	LI	1 g	D5W, NS	Physically compatible for 24 hr at 21°C	812	C
Enalaprilat	MSD	12 mg	LI	1 g	D5W[a]	Visually compatible. Little enalaprilat loss in 24 hr at room temperature under fluorescent light. Dobutamine not tested	1572	C
Epinephrine HCl	BR	50 mg	LI	1 g	D5W, NS	Physically compatible for 24 hr at 21°C	812	C
Eptifibatide	ME	750 mg		5 g		Physically compatible and chemically stable for up to 24 hr at 25°C	3049	C
Floxacillin sodium	BE	20 g	LI	500 mg	NS	Haze forms immediately and precipitate forms in 24 to 48 hr at 15 and 30°C	1479	I
Flumazenil	RC	20 mg	LI	2 g	D5W[a]	Visually compatible. No flumazenil loss in 24 hr at 23°C in fluorescent light. Dobutamine not tested	1710	C
Furosemide	HO	1 g	LI	1 g	D5W, NS	Cloudy in 1 hr at 25°C	789	I
Furosemide	WY	5 g	LI	1 g	D5W, NS	Immediate white precipitate	812	I
Furosemide	HO	1 g	LI	500 mg	NS	Haze forms immediately	1479	I
Heparin sodium	ES	40,000 units	LI	1 g	D5W, NS	Physically compatible with no color change in 24 hr at 25°C	789	C
Heparin sodium	LY	50,000 units	LI	1 g	D5W, NS	Physically compatible for 24 hr at 21°C	812	C
Heparin sodium	ES	5 million units	LI	1 g	D5W, NS	Pink discoloration within 6 hr at 21°C	812	I
Heparin sodium	ES	50,000 units	LI	1 g	D5W	Precipitate forms within 3 min	841	I
Heparin sodium	LY	50,000 units	LI	1.5 g	D5W, NS	Obvious precipitation	1318	I
Heparin sodium	LY	50,000 units	LI	900 mg	D5W, W	Physically compatible for 4 hr, but heat of reaction detected by microcalorimetry	1318	I
Heparin sodium	LY	50,000 units	LI	900 mg	NS	Physically compatible for 4 hr with no heat of reaction detected by microcalorimetry	1318	C
Hydralazine HCl	CI	200 mg	LI	200 mg	NS	Physically compatible for 24 hr	552	C
Isoproterenol HCl	ES	2 mg	LI	1 g	D5W, NS	Physically compatible for 24 hr at 21°C	812	C
Lidocaine HCl	ES	4 g	LI	1 g	D5W, NS	Visually compatible for 24 hr at 25°C	789	C
Lidocaine HCl	AST	4 and 10 g	LI	1 g	D5W, NS	Physically compatible for 24 hr at 21°C	812	C
Magnesium sulfate	TO	2 g	LI	1 g	D5W, NS	Slightly pink in 24 hr at 25°C	789	I

Additive Compatibility (Cont.)

Test Drug	Mfr	Conc/L or %	Mfr	Conc/L or %	Test Solution	Remarks	Ref	C/I
Magnesium sulfate	ES	83 g[b]	LI	167 mg	NS	Haze forms between 20 and 24 hr	552	I
Meperidine HCl	ES	50 g	LI	1 g	D5W, NS	Physically compatible for 24 hr at 21°C	812	C
Meropenem	ZEN	1 and 20 g	LI	1 g	NS	Visually compatible for 4 hr at room temperature	1994	C
Morphine sulfate	ES	5 g	LI	1 g	D5W, NS	Physically compatible for 24 hr at 21°C	812	C
Nitroglycerin	AB	120 mg	LI	1 g	D5W, NS	Physically compatible for 24 hr at 21°C	812	C
Nitroglycerin	ACC	100 mg	LI	500 mg	D5S	Stable with no loss of either drug after 24 hr at 25°C. Pink color after 4 hr	990	C
Nitroglycerin with sodium nitroprusside		200 to 800 mg 200 to 800 mg		2 to 8 g	D5W[c]	Pink color with small amount of dark brown precipitate and 11 to 19% nitroglycerin loss in 24 hr exposed to light	1412	I
Nitroglycerin with sodium nitroprusside		200 to 800 mg 200 to 800 mg		2 to 8 g	NS[c]	Pink color with 8% or less loss for any drug for 24 hr exposed to light	1412	C
Norepinephrine bitartrate	BN	32 mg	LI	1 g	D5W, NS	Physically compatible for 24 hr at 21°C	812	C
Phentolamine mesylate	CI	20 mg	LI	1 g	D5W, NS	Physically compatible for 24 hr at 21°C	812	C
Phenylephrine HCl	WI	20 mg	LI	1 g	D5W, NS	Physically compatible for 24 hr at 21°C	812	C
Phenytoin sodium	AHP	25 g	LI	1 g	D5W, NS	White precipitate forms rapidly, with brown solution in 6 hr at 21°C	812	I
Phenytoin sodium	ES	1 g	LI	1 g	D5W, NS	White precipitate forms within 5 to 10 min	789	I
Potassium chloride	ES	160 mEq	LI	1 g	D5W, NS	Slightly pink in 24 hr at 25°C	789	I
Potassium chloride	AB	20 mEq	LI	1 g	D5W, NS	Physically compatible for 24 hr at 21°C	812	C
Potassium phosphates	AB	100 mmol	LI	200 mg	NS	Small particles form after 1 hr. White precipitate noted after 15 hr	552	I
Procainamide HCl	SQ	1 g	LI	1 g	D5W, NS	Physically compatible with no color change in 24 hr at 25°C	789	C
Procainamide HCl	AHP	4 and 50 g	LI	1 g	D5W, NS	Physically compatible for 24 hr at 21°C	812	C
Propranolol HCl	AY	50 mg	LI	1 g	D5W, NS	Physically compatible for 24 hr at 21°C	812	C
Ranitidine HCl	GL	2 g	LI	250 mg and 1 g	D5W, NS[a]	Physically compatible. No ranitidine loss in 48 hr at room temperature in light. Dobutamine not tested	1361	C
Ranitidine HCl	GL	50 mg	LI	250 mg and 1 g	D5W[a]	Physically compatible. 7% ranitidine loss in 48 hr at room temperature in light. Dobutamine not tested	1361	C
Ranitidine HCl	GL	50 mg	LI	250 mg and 1 g	NS[a]	Physically compatible. No ranitidine loss in 48 hr at room temperature in light. Dobutamine not tested	1361	C
Ranitidine HCl	GL	50 mg and 2 g	LI	0.25 and 1 g	D5W, NS[a]	Visually compatible. Little loss of either drug in 48 hr at room temperature	1802	C
Sodium bicarbonate	MG	5%	LI	1 g		Cloudy brown with precipitate in 3 hr at 25°C. 18% dobutamine loss in 24 hr	789	I
Sodium bicarbonate	IX	500 mEq	LI	1 g	D5W, NS	White precipitate in 6 hr at 21°C	812	I

Additive Compatibility (Cont.)

Test Drug	Mfr	Conc/L or %	Mfr	Conc/L or %	Test Solution	Remarks	Ref	C/I
Sodium nitroprusside with nitroglycerin		200 to 800 mg 200 to 800 mg		2 to 8 g	D5W[c]	Pink color with small amount of dark brown precipitate and 11 to 19% nitroglycerin loss in 24 hr exposed to light	1412	I
Sodium nitroprusside with nitroglycerin		200 to 800 mg 200 to 800 mg		2 to 8 g	NS[c]	Pink color with 8% or less loss for any drug for 24 hr exposed to light	1412	C
Valproate sodium	WW	4.5 g	BA	1 g	[a]	Physically compatible for 24 hr at 22 to 25°C in ambient light and 34 to 38% relative humidity	3424	C
Verapamil HCl	KN	80 mg	LI	500 mg	D5W, NS	Slight pink color develops after 24 hr because of dobutamine oxidation	764	I
Verapamil HCl	KN	160 mg	LI	250 mg	D5W	No loss of either drug in 48 hr at 24°C or 7 days at 5°C. Transient pink color	811	C
Verapamil HCl	KN	160 mg	LI	250 mg	NS	Pink color and no verapamil and 3% dobutamine loss in 48 hr at 24°C. At 5°C, no loss of either drug in 7 days	811	C
Verapamil HCl	KN	1.25 g	LI	1 g	D5W, NS	Physically compatible for 24 hr at 21°C	812	C
Zidovudine	GW	2 g	AB	1 g	D5W	No more than 5% loss for either drug at 23°C and 2% loss at 4°C in 24 hr	2489	C
Zidovudine	GW	2 g	AB	1 g	NS	No more than 4% loss for either drug at 23°C and 2% loss at 4°C in 24 hr	2489	C

[a] Tested in PVC containers.

[b] Tested as 1 g/12 mL final concentration.

[c] Tested in glass containers.

Drugs in Syringe Compatibility

Dobutamine HCl

Test Drug	Mfr	Amt	Mfr	Amt	Remarks	Ref	C/I
Caffeine citrate		20 mg/1 mL	GNS	12.5 mg/1 mL	Visually compatible for 4 hr at 25°C	2440	C
Dimenhydrinate		10 mg/1 mL		12.5 mg/1 mL	Clear solution	2569	C
Doxapram HCl	RB	400 mg/20 mL	LI	100 mg/10 mL	5% doxapram loss in 3 hr and 11% in 24 hr	1177	I
Heparin sodium		2500 units/1 mL	LI	250 mg/10 mL	Physically compatible for at least 5 min	1053	C
Pantoprazole sodium	[a]	4 mg/1 mL		12.5 mg/1 mL	White precipitate forms within 1 hr	2574	I
Ranitidine HCl	GL	50 mg/5 mL	LI	25 mg	Physically compatible for 4 hr at ambient temperature under fluorescent light	1151	C

[a] Test performed using the formulation WITHOUT edetate disodium.

Y-Site Injection Compatibility (1:1 Mixture)

Dobutamine HCl

Test Drug	Mfr	Conc	Mfr	Conc	Remarks	Ref	C/I
Acyclovir sodium	BW	5 mg/mL[a]	LI	1 mg/mL[a]	Cloudy and brown in 1 hr at 25°C	1157	I
Alprostadil	BED	7.5 mcg/mL[p] [q]	AB	3 mg/mL[o]	Visually compatible for 1 hr	2746	C

Y-Site Injection Compatibility (1:1 Mixture) (Cont.)

Test Drug	Mfr	Conc	Mfr	Conc	Remarks	Ref	C/I
Alteplase	GEN	1 mg/mL	LI	2 mg/mL[a]	Haze in 20 min spectrophotometrically and in 2 hr visually	1340	I
Amifostine	USB	10 mg/mL[a]	LI	4 mg/mL[a]	Physically compatible for 4 hr at 23°C	1845	C
Aminophylline	ES	4 mg/mL[c]	LI	4 mg/mL[c]	Slight precipitate and color change in 1 hr	1316	I
Amiodarone HCl	LZ	4 mg/mL[c]	LI	2 mg/mL[c]	Physically compatible for 24 hr at 21°C	1032	C
Anidulafungin	VIC	0.5 mg/mL[a]	AB	4 mg/mL[a]	Physically compatible for 4 hr at 23°C	2617	C
Argatroban	GSK	1 mg/mL[b]	LI	12.5 mg/mL	Visually compatible for 24 hr at 23°C	2391	C
Atracurium besylate	BW	0.5 mg/mL[a]	LI	1 mg/mL[a]	Physically compatible for 24 hr at 28°C	1337	C
Aztreonam	SQ	40 mg/mL[a]	LI	4 mg/mL[a]	Physically compatible for 4 hr at 23°C	1758	C
Bivalirudin	TMC	5 mg/mL[a]	AB	4 mg/mL[a]	Physically compatible for 4 hr at 23°C	2373	C
Bivalirudin	TMC	5 mg/mL[a b]	BV	12.5 mg/mL	Cloudiness forms immediately	2680	I
Calcium chloride	AB	4 mg/mL[c]	LI	4 mg/mL[c]	Physically compatible for 3 hr	1316	C
Calcium gluconate	AST	4 mg/mL[c]	LI	4 mg/mL[c]	Physically compatible for 3 hr	1316	C
Cangrelor tetrasodium	TMC	1 mg/mL[b]		4 mg/mL[b]	Physically compatible for 4 hr	3243	C
Caspofungin acetate	ME	0.7 mg/mL[b]	HOS	4 mg/mL[b]	Physically compatible for 4 hr at room temperature	2758	C
Caspofungin acetate	ME	0.5 mg/mL[b]	BA	1 mg/mL	Physically compatible over 60 min	2766	C
Cefepime HCl	BMS	120 mg/mL[c]		1 mg/mL	Physically compatible with less than 10% cefepime loss. Dobutamine not tested	2513	C
Cefepime HCl	BMS	120 mg/mL[c]		250 mg/mL	Precipitates	2513	I
Ceftaroline fosamil	FOR	2.22 mg/mL[a]	HOS	4 mg/mL[a]	Haze increases and particulates appear	2826	I
Ceftaroline fosamil	FOR	2.22 mg/mL[b i]	HOS	4 mg/mL[b i]	Physically compatible for 4 hr at 23°C	2826	C
Ceftazidime	GSK	120 mg/mL[d]		1 mg/mL	Physically compatible with less than 10% ceftazidime loss. Dobutamine not tested	2513	C
Ceftazidime	GSK	120 mg/mL[d]		250 mg/mL	Precipitates	2513	I
Ceftolozane sulfate–tazobactam sodium	CUB	10 mg/mL[c u]	HOS	4 mg/mL[c]	Physically compatible for 2 hr	3262	C
Ciprofloxacin	MI	2 mg/mL[c]	LI	250 mcg/mL[c]	Visually compatible for 24 hr at 24°C	1655	C
Cisatracurium besylate	GW	0.1, 2, 5 mg/mL[a]	LI	4 mg/mL[a]	Physically compatible for 4 hr at 23°C	2074	C
Cladribine	ORT	0.015[b] and 0.5[e] mg/mL	LI	4 mg/mL[b]	Physically compatible for 4 hr at 23°C	1969	C
Clarithromycin	AB	4 mg/mL[a]	BI	2 mg/mL[a]	Visually compatible for 72 hr at both 30 and 17°C	2174	C
Clevidipine butyrate	CHS	0.5 mg/mL		4 mg/mL[d]	pH shifted outside of specified pH range for clevidipine within 24 hr	3334	?
Clonidine HCl	BI	18 mcg/mL[b]	LI	2 mg/mL[a]	Visually compatible	2642	C
Cloxacillin sodium	SMX	100 mg/mL	HOS	12.5 mg/mL	Precipitates immediately	3245	I
Dexmedetomidine HCl	AB	4 mcg/mL[b]	AST	4 mg/mL[b]	Physically compatible for 4 hr at 23°C	2383	C

Y-Site Injection Compatibility (1:1 Mixture) (Cont.)

Test Drug	Mfr	Conc	Mfr	Conc	Remarks	Ref	C/I
Diazepam	ES	0.2 mg/mL[c]	LI	4 mg/mL[c]	Physically compatible for 3 hr	1316	C
Diltiazem HCl	MMD	1 mg/mL[a]	LI	2 mg/mL[a]	Visually compatible for 24 hr at 25°C	1530	C
Diltiazem HCl	MMD	5 mg/mL	LI	1 mg/mL[c]	Visually compatible	1807	C
Diltiazem HCl	MMD	1 mg/mL[a]	LI	4 mg/mL[a]	Visually compatible for 4 hr at 27°C	2062	C
Docetaxel	RPR	0.9 mg/mL[a]	AST	4 mg/mL[a]	Physically compatible for 4 hr at 23°C	2224	C
Dopamine HCl	DCC	3.2 mg/mL[c]	LI	4 mg/mL[c]	Physically compatible for 3 hr	1316	C
Dopamine HCl	AB	3.2 mg/mL[a]	LI	4 mg/mL[a]	Visually compatible for 4 hr at 27°C	2062	C
Dopamine HCl with lidocaine HCl	DCC AB	3.2 mg/mL[c] 8 mg/mL[c]	LI	4 mg/mL[c]	Physically compatible for 3 hr	1316	C
Dopamine HCl with nitroglycerin	DCC LY	3.2 mg/mL[c] 0.4 mg/mL[c]	LI	4 mg/mL[c]	Physically compatible for 3 hr	1316	C
Dopamine HCl with sodium nitroprusside	DCC ES	3.2 mg/mL[c] 0.4 mg/mL[c]	LI	4 mg/mL[c]	Physically compatible for 3 hr	1316	C
Doripenem	JJ	5 mg/mL[a b]	HOS	4 mg/mL[a b]	Physically compatible for 4 hr at 23°C	2743	C
Doxorubicin HCl liposomal	SEQ	0.4 mg/mL[a]	BA	4 mg/mL[a]	Physically compatible for 4 hr at 23°C	2087	C
Enalaprilat	MSD	0.05 mg/mL[b]	LI	1 mg/mL[a]	Physically compatible for 24 hr at room temperature under fluorescent light	1355	C
Epinephrine HCl	AB	0.02 mg/mL[a]	LI	4 mg/mL[a]	Visually compatible for 4 hr at 27°C	2062	C
Eravacycline dihydrochloride	TET	0.6 mg/mL[b]	HOS	4.1 mg/mL[b]	Physically compatible for 2 hr at room temperature	3532	C
Etoposide phosphate	BR	5 mg/mL[a]	AST	4 mg/mL[a]	Physically compatible for 4 hr at 23°C	2218	C
Famotidine	MSD	0.2 mg/mL[a]	LI	1 mg/mL[a]	Physically compatible for 4 hr at 25°C	1188	C
Famotidine	ME	2 mg/mL[b]		4 mg/mL[a]	Visually compatible for 4 hr at 22°C	1936	C
Fenoldopam mesylate	AB	80 mcg/mL[b]	BED	4 mg/mL[b]	Physically compatible for 4 hr at 23°C	2467	C
Fentanyl citrate	ES	0.05 mg/mL	LI	4 mg/mL[a]	Visually compatible for 4 hr at 27°C	2062	C
Fluconazole	RR	2 mg/mL	LI	2 mg/mL[a]	Visually compatible for 24 hr at 28°C under fluorescent light	1760	C
Foscarnet sodium	AST	24 mg/mL	LI	12.5 mg/mL	Delayed formation of muddy precipitate	1335	I
Furosemide	ES	1 mg/mL[b]	LI	4 mg/mL[b]	Physically compatible for 3 hr	1316	C
Furosemide	ES	1 mg/mL[a]	LI	4 mg/mL[a]	Slight precipitate in 1 hr	1316	I
Furosemide	AMR	10 mg/mL	LI	4 mg/mL[a]	Precipitate forms immediately	2062	I
Gemcitabine HCl	LI	10 mg/mL[b]	AST	4 mg/mL[b]	Physically compatible for 4 hr at 23°C	2226	C
Granisetron HCl	SKB	0.05 mg/mL[a]	BA	4 mg/mL[a]	Physically compatible for 4 hr at 23°C	2000	C
Haloperidol lactate	MN	0.5[a] and 5 mg/mL	LI	4 mg/mL[a]	Visually compatible for 24 hr at 21°C	1523	C
Heparin sodium	ES	50 units/mL[b]	LI	4 mg/mL[b]	Physically compatible for 3 hr	1316	C
Heparin sodium	ES	50 units/mL[a]	LI	4 mg/mL[a]	Immediate gross precipitation	1316	I
Heparin sodium	TR	50 units/mL	LI	1 mg/mL[a]	Visually compatible for 4 hr at 25°C	1793	C

Y-Site Injection Compatibility (1:1 Mixture) (Cont.)

Test Drug	Mfr	Conc	Mfr	Conc	Remarks	Ref	C/I
Heparin sodium	OR	100 units/mL[a]	LI	4 mg/mL[a]	Haze and white precipitate form	1877	I
Heparin sodium	ES	100 units/mL[a]	LI	4 mg/mL[a]	Precipitate forms in 4 hr at 27°C	2062	I
Hetastarch in lactated electrolyte	AB	6%	AST	4 mg/mL[a]	Physically compatible for 4 hr at 23°C	2339	C
Hydromorphone HCl	KN	1 mg/mL	LI	4 mg/mL[a]	Visually compatible for 4 hr at 27°C	2062	C
Hydroxyethyl starch 130/0.4 in sodium chloride 0.9%	FRK	6%	SZ	1, 2, 4 mg/mL[a]	Visually compatible for 24 hr at room temperature	2770	C
Ibuprofen lysinate	OVA	10 mg/mL	HOS	1 mg/mL[f]	Measured turbidity increased immediately and solution became hazy white with a white precipitate	3541	I
Indomethacin sodium trihydrate	MSD	1 mg/mL[b]	LI	1.2 mg/mL[a]	Hazy precipitate forms immediately	1527	I
Insulin, regular	LI	1 unit/mL[c]	LI	4 mg/mL[c]	Physically compatible for 3 hr	1316	C
Isavuconazonium sulfate	ASP	1.5 mg/mL[c]	HOS	4.1 mg/mL[c]	Physically compatible for 2 hr	3263	C
Labetalol HCl	GL	1 mg/mL[a]	LI	2.5 mg/mL[a]	Visually compatible. Little loss of either drug in 4 hr at room temperature	1762	C
Labetalol HCl	GL	5 mg/mL	LI	4 mg/mL[a]	Visually compatible for 24 hr at 23°C	1877	C
Labetalol HCl	AH	2 mg/mL[a]	LI	4 mg/mL[a]	Visually compatible for 4 hr at 27°C	2062	C
Levofloxacin	OMN	5 mg/mL[a]	AB	12.5 mg/mL	Visually compatible for 4 hr at 24°C	2233	C
Lidocaine HCl	AB	8 mg/mL[c]	LI	4 mg/mL[c]	Physically compatible for 3 hr	1316	C
Lidocaine HCl with dopamine HCl	AB DCC	8 mg/mL[c] 3.2 mg/mL[c]	LI	4 mg/mL[c]	Physically compatible for 3 hr	1316	C
Lidocaine HCl with nitroglycerin	AB LY	8 mg/mL[c] 0.4 mg/mL[c]	LI	4 mg/mL[c]	Physically compatible for 3 hr	1316	C
Lidocaine HCl with sodium nitroprusside	AB ES	8 mg/mL[c] 0.4 mg/mL[c]	LI	4 mg/mL[c]	Physically compatible for 3 hr	1316	C
Linezolid	PHU	2 mg/mL	AST	4 mg/mL[a]	Physically compatible for 4 hr at 23°C	2264	C
Lorazepam	WY	0.5 mg/mL[a]	LI	4 mg/mL[a]	Visually compatible for 4 hr at 27°C	2062	C
Magnesium sulfate	LY	40 mg/mL[c]	LI	4 mg/mL[c]	Physically compatible for 3 hr	1316	C
Meperidine HCl	AB	10 mg/mL	LI	1 mg/mL[a]	Physically compatible for 4 hr at 25°C	1397	C
Meropenem		50 mg/mL	HOS	12.5 mg/mL	Precipitation occurred within 4 hr	3538	I
Meropenem–vaborbactam	TMC	8 mg/mL[b, v]	HOS	4.1 mg/mL[b]	Measured turbidity increases within 1 hr. pH increased by >3 units within 3 hr	3380	I
Micafungin sodium	ASP	1.5 mg/mL[b]	AB	4 mg/mL[b]	Gross precipitate forms immediately	2683	I
Midazolam HCl	RC	1 mg/mL[a]	GNS	2 mg/mL[a]	Particles form in 8 hr	1847	I
Midazolam HCl	RC	1 mg/mL[a]	LI	4 mg/mL[a]	Visually compatible for 24 hr at 23°C	1877	C
Midazolam HCl	RC	2 mg/mL[a]	LI	4 mg/mL[a]	Visually compatible for 4 hr at 27°C	2062	C
Milrinone lactate	SW	0.2 mg/mL[a]	LI	4 mg/mL[a]	Visually compatible for 4 hr at 27°C	2062	C

Y-Site Injection Compatibility (1:1 Mixture) (Cont.)

Test Drug	Mfr	Conc	Mfr	Conc	Remarks	Ref	C/I
Milrinone lactate	SW	0.4 mg/mL[a]	GEN	8 mg/mL[a]	Visually compatible. Little loss of either drug in 4 hr at 23°C	2214	C
Morphine sulfate	SCN	2 mg/mL[a]	LI	4 mg/mL[a]	Visually compatible for 4 hr at 27°C	2062	C
Nesiritide	SCI	50 mcg/mL[a][b]		12.5 mg/mL	Physically compatible for 4 hr. May be chemically incompatible with nesiritide[m]	2625	?
Nicardipine HCl	WY	1 mg/mL[a]	LI	4 mg/mL[a]	Visually compatible for 4 hr at 27°C	2062	C
Nicardipine HCl	DCC	0.1 mg/mL[a]	LI	1 mg/mL[a]	Visually compatible for 24 hr at room temperature	235	C
Nitroglycerin	LY	0.4 mg/mL[c]	LI	4 mg/mL[c]	Physically compatible for 3 hr	1316	C
Nitroglycerin	AB	0.4 mg/mL[a]	LI	4 mg/mL[a]	Visually compatible for 4 hr at 27°C	2062	C
Nitroglycerin with dopamine HCl	LY DCC	0.4 mg/mL[c] 3.2 mg/mL[c]	LI	4 mg/mL[c]	Physically compatible for 3 hr	1316	C
Nitroglycerin with lidocaine HCl	LY AB	0.4 mg/mL[c] 8 mg/mL[c]	LI	4 mg/mL[c]	Physically compatible for 3 hr	1316	C
Nitroglycerin with sodium nitroprusside	LY ES	0.4 mg/mL[c] 0.4 mg/mL[c]	LI	4 mg/mL[c]	Physically compatible for 3 hr	1316	C
Norepinephrine bitartrate	AB	0.128 mg/mL[a]	LI	4 mg/mL[a]	Visually compatible for 4 hr at 27°C	2062	C
Oritavancin diphosphate	TAR	0.8, 1.2, and 2 mg/mL[a]	HOS	4 mg/mL[a]	Visually compatible for 4 hr at 20 to 24°C	2928	C
Oxaliplatin	SS	0.5 mg/mL[a]	BED	4 mg/mL[a]	Physically compatible for 4 hr at 23°C	2566	C
Pancuronium bromide	ES	0.05 mg/mL[a]	LI	1 mg/mL[a]	Physically compatible for 24 hr at 28°C	1337	C
Pantoprazole sodium	ALT[n]	0.16 to 0.8 mg/mL[b]	LI	1 to 4 mg/mL[a]	Cloudiness forms over time	2603	I
Pemetrexed disodium	LI	20 mg/mL[b]	AB	4 mg/mL[a]	White cloudy precipitate with microparticulates forms immediately	2564	I
Phytonadione	MSD	0.4 mg/mL[c]	LI	4 mg/mL[c]	Slight haze in 3 hr	1316	I
Piperacillin sodium–tazobactam sodium	LE[n]	40 mg/mL[a][r]	LI	4 mg/mL[a]	Heavy white turbidity forms immediately	1688	I
Plazomicin sulfate	ACH	24 mg/mL[c]	HOS	4.1 mg/mL[c]	Physically compatible for 1 hr at 20 to 25°C	3432	C
Posaconazole	ME	18 mg/mL		5 mg/mL[c]	Physically compatible	2911, 2912	C
Potassium chloride	AB	0.06 mEq/mL[c]	LI	4 mg/mL[c]	Physically compatible for 3 hr	1316	C
Propofol	ZEN[w]	10 mg/mL	LI	4 mg/mL[a]	Physically compatible for 1 hr at 23°C	2066	C
Quinupristin–dalfopristin		2 mg/mL[a][t]	[s]	4 mg/mL	Reported to be incompatible	3230	I
Ranitidine HCl	GL	0.5 mg/mL[f]	LI	1 mg/mL[a]	Physically compatible for 24 hr	1323	C
Ranitidine HCl	GL	1 mg/mL[a]	LI	4 mg/mL[a]	Visually compatible for 4 hr at 27°C	2062	C
Remifentanil HCl	GW	0.025 and 0.25 mg/mL[b]	LI	4 mg/mL[a]	Physically compatible for 4 hr at 23°C	2075	C
Sodium nitroprusside	ES	0.4 mg/mL[c]	LI	4 mg/mL[c]	Physically compatible for 3 hr	1316	C

Y-Site Injection Compatibility (1:1 Mixture) (Cont.)

Test Drug	Mfr	Conc	Mfr	Conc	Remarks	Ref	C/I
Sodium nitroprusside	RC	0.3, 1.2, 3 mg/mL[a]	LI	1.5 mg/mL[k]	Visually compatible for 48 hr at 24°C protected from light	2357	C
Sodium nitroprusside	RC	1.2 and 3 mg/mL[a]	LI	6 mg/mL[k]	Color darkening occurs over 48 hr at 24°C protected from light	2357	?
Sodium nitroprusside	RC	0.3 and 1.2 mg/mL[a]	LI	12.5 mg/mL[k]	Visually compatible for 48 hr at 24°C protected from light	2357	C
Sodium nitroprusside	RC	3 mg/mL[a]	LI	12.5 mg/mL[k]	Color darkening occurs over 48 hr at 24°C protected from light	2357	?
Sodium nitroprusside with dopamine HCl	ES DCC	0.4 mg/mL[c] 3.2 mg/mL[c]	LI	4 mg/mL[c]	Physically compatible for 3 hr	1316	C
Sodium nitroprusside with lidocaine HCl	ES AB	0.4 mg/mL[c] 8 mg/mL[c]	LI	4 mg/mL[c]	Physically compatible for 3 hr	1316	C
Sodium nitroprusside with nitroglycerin	ES LY	0.4 mg/mL[c] 0.4 mg/mL[c]	LI	4 mg/mL[c]	Physically compatible for 3 hr	1316	C
Sugammadex sodium		100 mg/mL	s	12.5 mg/mL	Precipitates immediately	3112	I
Tacrolimus	FUJ	1 mg/mL[b]	LI	1 mg/mL[a]	Visually compatible for 24 hr at 25°C	1630	C
Tedizolid phosphate	CUB	0.8 mg/mL[b]	HOS	4.1 mg/mL[b]	Immediate precipitation and increase in measured turbidity	3244	I
Telavancin HCl	ASP	7.5 mg/mL[a b l]	HOS	4 mg/mL[a b l]	Physically compatible for 2 hr	2830	C
Theophylline	TR	4 mg/mL	LI	1 mg/mL[a]	Visually compatible for 6 hr at 25°C	1793	C
Thiotepa	IMM[g]	1 mg/mL[a]	LI	4 mg/mL[a]	Physically compatible for 4 hr at 23°C	1861	C
Tigecycline	WY	1 mg/mL[b]		0.2 and 1 mg/mL[b]	Physically compatible for 4 hr	2714	C
Tigecycline	ACD, FRK, WY	c	s		Stated to be compatible	2915, 3459, 3460	C
Tirofiban HCl	ME	50 mcg/mL[a b]	AB	0.25 and 5 mg/mL[a b]	Physically compatible with no loss of either drug in 4 hr at 23°C	2356	C
TNA #218 to #226[h]			AST	4 mg/mL[a]	Visually compatible for 4 hr at 23°C	2215	C
TPN #91[h]		i	LI	1 mg/mL[j]	Physically compatible	1170	C
TPN #189[h]			LI	50 mg/mL[b]	Visually compatible for 24 hr at 22°C	1767	C
TPN #203, #204[h]			LI	5 mg/mL	Visually compatible for 4 hr at 23°C	1974	C
TPN #212 to #215[h]			LI	4 mg/mL[a]	Physically compatible for 4 hr at 23°C	2109	C
Vasopressin	AMR	2 and 4 units/mL[b]	AB	4.2 mg/mL[a]	Physically compatible with vasopressin pushed through a Y-site over 5 sec	2478	C
Vecuronium bromide	OR	0.1 mg/mL[a]	LI	1 mg/mL[a]	Physically compatible for 24 hr at 28°C	1337	C
Vecuronium bromide	OR	1 mg/mL	LI	4 mg/mL[a]	Visually compatible for 4 hr at 27°C	2062	C
Verapamil HCl	LY	0.2 mg/mL[c]	LI	4 mg/mL[c]	Physically compatible for 3 hr	1316	C

Y-Site Injection Compatibility (1:1 Mixture) (Cont.)

Test Drug	Mfr	Conc	Mfr	Conc	Remarks	Ref	C/I
Zidovudine	BW	4 mg/mL[a]	LI	5 mg/mL[a]	Physically compatible for 4 hr at 25°C	1193	C

[a] Tested in dextrose 5%.

[b] Tested in sodium chloride 0.9%.

[c] Tested in both dextrose 5% and sodium chloride 0.9%.

[d] Tested in sterile water for injection.

[e] Tested in bacteriostatic sodium chloride 0.9% preserved with benzyl alcohol 0.9%.

[f] Tested as the premixed infusion solution.

[g] Lyophilized formulation tested.

[h] Refer to Appendix for the composition of parenteral nutrition solutions. TNA indicates a 3-in-1 admixture, and TPN indicates a 2-in-1 admixture.

[i] Run at 10 mL/hr.

[j] In dextrose 5% infused at 1.2 mL/hr.

[k] Tested in dextrose 5% in sodium chloride 0.45%.

[l] Tested in Ringer's injection, lactated.

[m] Nesiritide is incompatible with bisulfite antioxidants used in some drug formulations. The specific formulation of the product to be used should be checked to assure that no sulfite antioxidants are present.

[n] Test performed using the formulation WITHOUT edetate disodium.

[o] Tested in either dextrose 5% or in sodium chloride 0.9%, but the report did not specify which solution.

[p] Tested in a 1:1 mixture of (1) dextrose 5% and dextrose 5% in sodium chloride 0.45% with and without potassium chloride 20 mEq/L and also in (2) dextrose 10% in sodium chloride 0.45% with and without potassium chloride 20 mEq/L.

[q] Tested in a 1:1 mixture of dextrose 5% and TPN #274 (see Appendix).

[r] Piperacillin component. Piperacillin in an 8:1 fixed-ratio concentration with tazobactam.

[s] Salt not specified.

[t] Quinupristin and dalfopristin components combined.

[u] Ceftolozane component. Ceftolozane in a 2:1 fixed-ratio concentration with tazobactam.

[v] Meropenem component. Meropenem in a 1:1 fixed-ratio concentration with vaborbactam.

[w] Test performed using the formulation WITH edetate disodium.

Additional Compatibility Information

Peritoneal Dialysis Solutions

Dobutamine hydrochloride (Lilly) 2.5, 5, and 7.5 mcg/mL in Dianeal PD-1 (Baxter) with dextrose 1.5 and 4.25% retained at least 90% when stored for 24 hours at 4, 26, and 37°C.[1417] [1702]

Selected Revisions May 1, 2020. © Copyright, October 1982. American Society of Health-System Pharmacists, Inc.

Docetaxel
AHFS 10:00

Products

Several different formulations of docetaxel injection products are available.[3012] [3013] [3014] [3015] [3099] **CAUTION: Care should be taken to ensure that the correct drug product, dose, and preparation procedure are used and that no confusion among differing products and concentrations occurs.**

The use of gloves during preparation of docetaxel doses is recommended.[3012] [3013] [3014] [3015] [3099] If docetaxel concentrate, powder, or any reconstituted or diluted solution comes in contact with skin, the affected area should be washed thoroughly with soap and water.[3012] [3013] [3014] [3015] [3099] If contact with mucosa occurs, thorough flushing with water is required.[3012] [3013] [3014] [3015] [3099]

Docetaxel concentrate with diluent (2-vial package). Docetaxel concentrate is available in a 2-vial package: the first vial contains docetaxel concentrate 0.5 mL (20 mg) or 2 mL (80 mg), while the second vial contains 1.95 or 7.2 mL, respectively, of the special diluent.[3014] Each mL of docetaxel concentrate in the first vial contains docetaxel (anhydrous) 40 mg, polysorbate 80 1040 mg, and dehydrated alcohol 60 mg.[3014] Citric acid anhydrous also may have been added to adjust the pH.[3014] The diluent vial contains the special diluent, which is composed of polyethylene glycol 400 13% (w/v) in water for injection.[3014] Both the docetaxel vials and the accompanying diluent vials contain an overfill.[3014]

Preparation of the final diluted solution for infusion from this 2-vial formulation requires a 2-step dilution procedure prior to administration.[3014] Step 1 is the preparation of the *initial* diluted solution, which is then further diluted to the *final* diluted solution for infusion in step 2.[3014]

To prepare the initial diluted solution (step 1), the vial of accompanying diluent should be partially inverted to withdraw the entire contents (approximately 1.95 mL for docetaxel 20 mg and approximately 7.2 mL for docetaxel 80 mg) and the contents should be added to the appropriate corresponding vial of docetaxel concentrate.[3014] Using repeated inversions, each vial of diluted docetaxel concentrate should then be thoroughly mixed for about 45 seconds; vials should not be shaken.[3014] This initial diluted solution is a clear solution having a docetaxel concentration of 10 mg/mL.[3014] If foam appears on the surface of the solution from the surfactant (i.e., polysorbate 80) in the formulation, the vials should be allowed to stand until any foam has dissipated; however, it is not necessary for all of the foam to have dissipated before proceeding with the rest of the preparation steps.[3014]

To prepare the final diluted solution (step 2), the appropriate dose of the docetaxel 10-mg/mL initial diluted solution should be withdrawn from the vial and added to 250 mL of sodium chloride 0.9% or dextrose 5% in a glass or plastic (e.g., polypropylene, polyolefin) infusion container to produce a final diluted solution for infusion with a concentration of 0.3 to 0.74 mg/mL.[3014] For docetaxel doses exceeding 200 mg, a larger volume of infusion solution should be used so that the concentration of the final diluted solution for infusion does not exceed 0.74 mg/mL.[3014] The final diluted solution for infusion should be thoroughly mixed by rotation.[3014]

The manufacturer cautions that the 2-vial and 1-vial formulations of docetaxel concentrate should not be used together.[3014]

Docetaxel concentrate (1-vial package). Docetaxel also is available in single-use and multidose 1-vial formulations as concentrates of either 10[3013] or 20 mg/mL[3012] [3014] in polysorbate 80 and dehydrated alcohol.[3012] [3013] [3014] Anhydrous citric acid,[3013] [3014] polyethylene glycol,[3013] propylene glycol,[3016] edetate disodium,[3016] and povidone[3018] also may be present in some products; specific product labeling should be consulted for additional formulation details.[3012] [3013] [3014] [3016] [3018] These concentrates do not require a 2-step dilution process; instead, these concentrates may be added directly to an infusion solution as a single step.[3012] [3013] [3014]

Manufacturer recommendations differ on storage of the various 1-vial formulations;[3012] [3013] [3014] if stored under refrigeration, the appropriate number of vials should be allowed to stand at room temperature for approximately 5 minutes prior to use.[3012] The appropriate dose of the docetaxel concentrate should be withdrawn from the vials using *only* a 21-gauge needle;[3012] [3013] [3014] larger bore needles (e.g., 18- or 19-gauge) may result in coring of the stopper and the presence of rubber particulates.[3012] [3014] The dose should be added to 250 mL of sodium chloride 0.9% or dextrose 5% in a glass or plastic (e.g., polypropylene, polyolefin) infusion container to produce a diluted solution for infusion with a docetaxel concentration of 0.3 to 0.74 mg/mL.[3012] [3013] [3014] For docetaxel doses exceeding 200 mg, a larger volume of infusion solution should be used so that the concentration of the diluted solution for infusion does not exceed 0.74 mg/mL.[3012] [3013] [3014] The diluted solution for infusion should be thoroughly mixed by gentle manual rotation.[3012] [3013] [3014]

Docetaxel alcohol-free concentrate (1-vial package). An alcohol-free 1-vial formulation of docetaxel 20 mg/mL concentrate also is available for dilution as a single step.[3099] This formulation is available in 1-mL (20 mg) single-dose vials and 4-mL (80 mg) and 8-mL (160 mg) multidose vials.[3099] Each mL contains docetaxel (anhydrous) 20 mg, soybean oil 27.5 mg, polysorbate 80 585 mg, citric acid 10 mg, and polyethylene glycol 300 442.2 mg.[3099] The appropriate dose of the docetaxel injection should be withdrawn from the vials using a 20-gauge needle and transferred to 250 mL of sodium chloride 0.9% or dextrose 5% in a glass or plastic (e.g., polypropylene, polyolefin) infusion container in a single injection to produce a diluted solution for infusion with a concentration of 0.3 to 0.74 mg/mL.[3099] For docetaxel doses exceeding 200 mg, a larger volume of infusion solution should be used so that the concentration of the diluted solution for infusion does not exceed 0.74 mg/mL.[3099] The diluted solution for infusion should be thoroughly mixed by gentle manual rotation.[3099]

DOI: 10.37573/9781585286850.129

Docetaxel lyophilized powder with diluent (2-vial package). Docetaxel also is available as a lyophilized powder in a single-use vial containing 20 or 80 mg of docetaxel (anhydrous) packaged with a diluent vial containing approximately 1 or 4 mL of diluent (ethanol 35.4% [w/w] in polysorbate 80).[3015] Both the docetaxel vials and the accompanying diluent vials contain a slight overfill.[3015]

To prepare the solution for infusion, the appropriate number of vials of powder and accompanying diluent should be allowed to stand at room temperature for approximately 5 minutes prior to use.[3015] The diluent vials should be partially inverted to withdraw the diluent using an 18- to 21-gauge, 1½-inch needle.[3015] The diluent should be transferred to the powder vial, and the vial should be shaken well to completely dissolve the powder.[3015] The 20-mg vial should be reconstituted with 1 mL of the accompanying diluent to yield a solution containing 20 mg/0.8 mL (equivalent to 25 mg/mL); the 80-mg vial should be reconstituted with 4 mL of the accompanying diluent to yield a solution with a concentration of 24 mg/mL.[3015] If bubbles appear in the solution from the surfactant (i.e., polysorbate 80) in the formulation, the vials should be allowed to stand until any bubbles have dissipated.[3015]

The appropriate dose of the docetaxel reconstituted solution should be withdrawn from the vial and added to 250 mL of sodium chloride 0.9% or dextrose 5% in a glass or plastic (e.g., polypropylene, polyolefin) infusion container to produce a final diluted solution for infusion with a concentration of 0.3 to 0.74 mg/mL.[3015] For docetaxel doses exceeding 200 mg, a larger volume of infusion solution should be used so that the concentration of the final diluted solution for infusion does not exceed 0.74 mg/mL.[3015] The final diluted solution for infusion should be thoroughly mixed by manual rotation.[3015]

Alcohol Content

Docetaxel injection products differ in the amount of alcohol (ethanol) present in the formulation:[3012 3013 3014 3015 3019 3025 3099]

Manufacturer	Formulation	Alcohol (ethanol) Content (g/m^2) per Docetaxel 100 mg/m^2 dose	Ref
Accord	1-vial concentrate	1.975	3014
Accord	2-vial concentrate	0.15	3014
Actavis	1-vial concentrate	2	3018
Eagle	Alcohol-free concentrate	0	3099
Hospira	1-vial concentrate	1.8	3013
Pfizer	1-vial concentrate	3.2	3016
Sandoz	1-vial concentrate	2.6	3017
Sanofi-Aventis	1-vial concentrate	2	3012
Sun Pharma Global	Lyophilized powder	1.425	3015

The manufacturers and FDA state that consideration should be given to the alcohol content of docetaxel injection products when prescribing or administering the drug, especially in patients in whom alcohol intake should be avoided or minimized[3012 3013 3014 3015 3019] or when used in conjunction with other medications.[3019]

Trade Name(s)

Docefrez, Taxotere

Administration

Docetaxel is administered as a 1-hour intravenous infusion at ambient temperature and light to patients who have been adequately premedicated to control adverse effects.[3012 3013 3014 3015] To minimize patient exposure to the diethylhexyl phthalate (DEHP) plasticizer, the infusion solution should be infused using polyethylene-lined administration sets.[3012 3013 3014 3015 3099]

Stability

All diluted docetaxel solutions for infusion should be visually inspected for particulate matter and discoloration prior to administration; any solution that is not clear or that appears to contain a precipitate should be discarded.[3012 3013 3014 3015]

Docetaxel concentrate with diluent (2-vial package) is a viscous clear yellow to brownish-yellow solution.[3014] Intact vials of docetaxel with the accompanying special diluent should be stored at controlled room temperature and protected from light.[3014]

The manufacturer states that the *initial* diluted solution is stable for up to 8 hours after preparation when stored under refrigeration or at room temperature.[3014] Thiesen and Kramer evaluated the stability of docetaxel 10-mg/mL initial diluted solution over 28 days at 25 and 4°C.[2242] The initial diluted solution remained visually clear with no color change and no docetaxel loss at either temperature.[2242]

The manufacturer states that the *final* diluted solution for infusion is stable for 4 hours, including the 1-hour infusion time, if stored between 2 and 25°C.[3014]

Docetaxel concentrate (1-vial package) formulations vary in color from clear, colorless to pale yellow to brownish-yellow.[3012 3013 3014 3016 3017 3018] Recommended storage conditions of intact vials also vary; however, most products should be stored between 2 and 25°C in the original container to protect from light.[3012 3013 3014 3016 3017 3018] Freezing of the docetaxel concentrate vials does not adversely affect most 1-vial concentrate products.[3012 3013 3014 3016 3017] Multidose vials are stable for up to 28 days from initial vial puncture; however, temperature storage requirements and light protection recommendations during that time vary among products.[3013 3014 3016 3017] Specific product labeling should be consulted for additional storage and stability details.

The diluted solution prepared from docetaxel concentrate (Taxotere, Sanofi-Aventis) is stable for up to 6 hours, including the 1-hour infusion time, if stored between 2 and 25°C;[3012] diluted solutions prepared from some generic 1-vial concentrate products have been described as stable for up to 4 hours under the same conditions.[3013 3014 3016 3017 3018] In addition, the physical and chemical stability of the diluted solution for infusion in non-polyvinyl chloride (non-PVC) bags has been demonstrated for up to 48 hours for solutions prepared as recommended and stored at 2 to 8°C for certain products.[3012] Specific product labeling should be consulted for additional stability details.

Docetaxel alcohol-free concentrate (1-vial package) is a clear, colorless to yellow viscous solution.[3099] Intact vials of the drug should be stored at 20 to 25°C in the original package to protect from light.[3099] Following dilution of the alcohol-free formulation in sodium chloride 0.9% or dextrose 5% for infusion, the solution is stable for 24 hours if stored between 2 and 25°C.[3099] Multidose vials are stable for up to 28 days from initial vial puncture with multiple needle entries and withdrawals when stored at 2 to 8°C and protected from light.[3099]

Docetaxel lyophilized powder with diluent (2-vial package) is a white powder that forms a clear solution when reconstituted.[3015] Intact vials of the drug and accompanying diluent should be stored at 2 to 8°C in the original package to protect against bright light.[3015] The manufacturer states that the reconstituted solution is stable for up to 8 hours after preparation when stored under refrigeration or at room temperature.[3015] The final diluted solution for infusion is stable for 6 hours, including the 1-hour infusion time, if stored between 2 and 25°C.[3015] Physical and chemical stability of the final diluted solution for infusion in non-PVC bags also has been demonstrated for up to 48 hours for solutions prepared as recommended and stored at 2 to 8°C.[3015]

Docetaxel 0.8 mg/mL in sodium chloride 0.9% did not exhibit an antimicrobial effect on *Enterococcus faecium*, *Staphylococcus aureus*, *Pseudomonas aeruginosa*, and *Candida albicans* inoculated into the solution. Diluted solutions should be stored under refrigeration whenever possible, and the potential for microbiological growth should be considered when assigning expiration periods.[2160]

Freezing Solutions

Although freezing is not noted to adversely affect most 1-vial docetaxel concentrate products,[3012] [3013] [3014] [3016] one manufacturer states that the diluted docetaxel solution for infusion should not be frozen.[3017]

Crystallization

Some docetaxel products are supersaturated and may crystallize over time.[3012] [3015] [3016] If crystallization is noted, the drug must no longer be used and should be discarded.[3012] [3015] [3016]

Plasticizer Leaching

The surfactant (polysorbate 80) contained in docetaxel formulations can leach plasticizer from DEHP-plasticized PVC containers and administration sets.[1683] The amount of DEHP plasticizer leached is time and concentration dependent;[1683] it is also a function of the lipophilicity of the fluid that comes into contact with the DEHP-plasticized PVC container or device.[3100] The manufacturers recommend that docetaxel not be allowed to contact such containers and equipment.[3012] [3013] [3014] [3015] [3099] To minimize patient exposure to the plasticizer, the infusion solution should be stored in glass or plastic (e.g., polyolefin, polypropylene) containers and infused using polyethylene-lined administration sets.[3012] [3013] [3014] [3015] [3099]

In 1996, an acceptability limit of no more than 5 parts per million (5 mcg/mL) for DEHP plasticizer leached from PVC-containing devices (e.g., containers) was proposed based on a

review of metabolic and toxicologic considerations.[2185] FDA later evaluated the safety of DEHP exposure by comparing doses of DEHP received by patients undergoing various medical procedures with a defined tolerable intake value of DEHP, a value that was based upon the results of selected critical toxicity studies in experimental animals.[3100] Based on the results of the safety assessment, FDA concluded that there is little risk posed by exposure to the amount of DEHP released from PVC bags used to store and administer drugs that require an excipient for solubilization *when label instructions for preparation and administration are followed*.[3100] However, such conclusions do not take into account increased risk for adverse effects from DEHP exposure in certain patients (e.g., critically ill male neonates or infants, male infants less than 1 year of age, male offspring of pregnant or breast-feeding women undergoing certain medical treatments) or potential adverse effects related to aggregate exposure for patients exposed to multiple medical devices, procedures, or intravenous medications known to leach DEHP, for which there are varying levels of concern.[3100] [3101]

Mazzo et al. evaluated the leaching of DEHP plasticizer by docetaxel 0.56 and 0.96 mg/mL in dextrose 5% and in sodium chloride 0.9%. PVC bags of the solutions were used to prepare the admixtures. The leaching of the plasticizer was found to be time and concentration dependent; however, there was little difference between the 2 infusion solutions. After storage for 8 hours at 21°C, leached DEHP was found in the range of 30 to 51 mcg/mL for the 0.96-mg/mL concentration and 25 to 36 mcg/mL for the 0.56-mg/mL concentration. During a simulated 1-hour infusion, the amount of leached DEHP did not exceed 14 mcg/mL.[1825]

A study was performed on the compatibility of docetaxel 0.31 and 0.88 mg/mL in dextrose 5% or sodium chloride 0.9% with various infusion sets. The docetaxel solutions were run through the administration sets and the effluent was analyzed for DEHP plasticizer. At the higher concentration of docetaxel tested (0.88 mg/mL), unacceptable amounts of DEHP were leached from the Baxter vented nitroglycerin set (2C7552S), the Baxter vented volumetric pump nitroglycerin set (2C1042), and the IMED standard PVC set (9210). At both the low and high concentrations tested (0.31 and 0.88 mg/mL), unacceptable amounts of DEHP were leached from the IVAC MiniMed Uni-Set microbore (28026) and MiniMed Uni-Set macrobore full set (28034). The sets cited in Table 1 and Table 2 leached little or no DEHP.[2451]

In another study, 20 mg of docetaxel (Taxotere, Sanofi-Aventis) was first dissolved in 1 mL of dehydrated alcohol and then diluted in 100 mL of sodium chloride 0.9%.[3110] The solution was circulated through an 85-cm length of commercial PVC intravenous infusion tubing (Becton Dickinson) containing 25% DEHP by weight at a rate of 1.2 to 3 mL/min over a period of 1 hour.[3110] A decrease in light transmittance was first detected at 30 minutes and precipitation of the drug was noted by 1 hour.[3110] Precipitation was thought to be the result of leached DEHP interacting with surfactant (polysorbate 80) molecules in the docetaxel formulation, thereby decreasing the solubility of the drug.[3110] This phenomenon was not observed with the use of low-DEHP content (10% by weight) PVC and non-PVC intravenous infusion tubings (Polysciencetech).[3110]

With use of infusion bags and tubing that are free of DEHP plasticizer and the elimination of PVC precision flow regulators, a reduction in leached DEHP of up to 99% has been reported.[2679]

Docetaxel vehicle equivalent to docetaxel 0.74 mg/mL in dextrose 5% was tested in VISIV polyolefin bags at room temperature near 23°C for 24 hours. No leached plastic components were found within the 24-hour study period.[2660] [2792]

Docetaxel in PVC containers leached 200 to 500 mcg/mL of DEHP in 48 hours when stored under refrigeration and at room temperature, respectively. The use of nonplasticized containers such as polyethylene plastic containers was recommended.[2718]

Table 1. Administration sets compatible with docetaxel infusions at concentrations of 0.88 mg/mL or less[2451]

Manufacturer	Administration Set
Abbott	LifeCare 5000 Plum non-PVC specialty set (11594)
	LifeCare model 4P specialty set, non-PVC (11434)
	Life Shield anesthesia pump set OL with cartridge (13503)
	Nitroglycerin primary i.v. pump set OL, vented (1772)
	Omni-Flow universal primary i.v. pump short minibore (40527)
Block Medical	Verifuse nonvented administration set with 0.22-μm filter, check valve, and non-DEHP PVC tubing (V021015)
I-Flow	Vivus-400 polyethylene-lined infusion set (5000-784)
IMED	Closed system non-PVC fluid path nonvented quick spike set (9630)
	Non-PVC set with inline filter (9986)
	Gemini 20 nonvented primary administration set for nitroglycerin and emulsions (2260)
IVAC	Universal set with low-sorbing tubing (52053, 59953, S75053)
	Reduced-PVC full set MiniMed Uni-Set macrobore (28190)
Ivion/Medex	WalkMed spike set (SP-06) with pump set (PS-401, PS-360, PS-560)
McGaw	Horizon pump vented nitroglycerin i.v. set (V7450)
	Intelligent pump vented nitroglycerin i.v. set (V7150)
SoloPak	Primary solution set with universal spike, 0.22-μm filter, and injection site (73600)

Table 2. Extension sets compatible with docetaxel infusions at concentrations of 0.88 mg/mL or less[2451]

Manufacturer	Administration Set
Abbott	IVEX-HP filter set (4524)
	IVEX-2 filter set (2679)
Baxter	Polyethylene-lined extension set with 0.22-μm air-eliminating filter (1C8363)
Becton Dickinson	E-Z infusion set (38-53121)
	E-Z infusion set shorty (38-53741)
	Intima i.v. catheter placement set (38-6918-1)
	J-loop connector (38-1252-2)
Braun	0.2-μm filter extension set (FE-2012L)
	Small-bore 0.2-μm filter extension set (PFE-2007)
	Small-bore extension set with T-fitting (ET-04T)
	Small-bore extension set with reflux valve (ET-116L)
	Whin-winged extension set 90° Huber needle (HW-2276)
	Whin extension set with Y-site and Huber needle (HW-2276 YHRF)
	Y-extension set with valve (ET-08-YL)
Gish Biomedical	VasTack noncoring portal-access needle system (VT 2022)
IMED	0.2-μm add-on filter set (9400XL)
IVAC	Spec-Sets extension set with 0.2-μm inline filter (C20028, C20350)
Pall	SetSaver extended-life disposable set with 0.2-μm filter (ELD-96P)
	SetSaver extended-life disposable set with 0.2-μm filter (ELD-96LL)
	SetSaver extended-life disposable microbore extension tubing with 0.2-μm Posidyne filter (ELD-96LYL)
	SetSaver extended-life disposable intravenous filter 0.2-μm with standard bore extension tubing with injection site (ELD-96LYLS)
Pfizer/Strato Medical	Lifeport vascular-access system infusion set with Y-site (LPS 3009)

Compatibility Information

Solution Compatibility

Docetaxel

Test Soln Name	Mfr	Mfr	Conc/L or %	Remarks	Ref	C/I
Dextrose 5%	BRN[a]	RPR	0.3 and 0.9 g	Visually compatible with little or no loss in 28 days at 25°C protected from light	2242	C
Dextrose 5%	BRN[b]	RPR	0.3 and 0.9 g	Visually compatible with little or no loss in 28 days at 25°C protected from light	2242	C
Dextrose 5%	BR[c]	RPR	0.3 and 0.9 g	Visually compatible with little or no loss in 5 days at 25°C protected from light. Precipitation and accompanying loss of drug occurred after 5 days in some samples	2242	C

Solution Compatibility (Cont.)

Test Soln Name	Mfr	Mfr	Conc/L or %	Remarks	Ref	C/I
Sodium chloride 0.9%	BRN[a]	RPR	0.3 and 0.9 g	Visually compatible with little or no loss in 28 days at 25°C protected from light	2242	C
Sodium chloride 0.9%	BRN[d]	RPR	0.3 and 0.9 g	Visually compatible with little or no loss in 28 days at 25°C protected from light	2242	C
Sodium chloride 0.9%	BR[c]	RPR	0.3 and 0.9 g	Visually compatible with little or no loss in 3 days at 25°C protected from light. Precipitation and accompanying loss of drug occurred after 3 days in some samples	2242	C
Sodium chloride 0.9%	BRN[d], FRE[c]	SAA	740 mg	Precipitation when stored at 23°C. No precipitation or loss of docetaxel in 48 hr when stored at 4°C followed by 4 hr at 23°C	2718	?
Sodium chloride 0.9%	BRN[e]	AVE	0.4 and 0.8 g	Visually compatible. No docetaxel loss in 35 days at 23°C exposed to fluorescent light	2761	C
Sodium chloride 0.9%	BA[b], GRI[a]	RP	0.3 and 0.9 g	Physically and chemically stable for 24 hr at 20°C. Precipitation after that time	2804	C
Sodium chloride 0.9%	[d]	SAA	0.77 g	Physically and chemically stable for 7 days at 5°C followed by 24 hr at approximately 20°C	3242	C

[a] Tested in glass containers.

[b] Tested in polypropylene containers.

[c] Tested in PVC containers.

[d] Tested in polyethylene containers.

[e] Tested in polypropylene-polyethylene copolymer PAB bags.

Y-Site Injection Compatibility (1:1 Mixture)

Docetaxel

Test Drug	Mfr	Conc	Mfr	Conc	Remarks	Ref	C/I
Acyclovir sodium	GW	7 mg/mL[a]	RPR	0.9 mg/mL[a]	Physically compatible for 4 hr at 23°C	2224	C
Amifostine	ALZ	10 mg/mL[b]	RPR	0.9 mg/mL[a]	Physically compatible for 4 hr at 23°C	2224	C
Amikacin sulfate	AB	5 mg/mL[a]	RPR	0.9 mg/mL[a]	Physically compatible for 4 hr at 23°C	2224	C
Aminophylline	AB	2.5 mg/mL[a]	RPR	0.9 mg/mL[a]	Physically compatible for 4 hr at 23°C	2224	C
Amphotericin B	PH	0.6 mg/mL[a]	RPR	0.9 mg/mL[a]	Visible turbidity forms immediately	2224	I
Ampicillin sodium	SKB	20 mg/mL[b]	RPR	0.9 mg/mL[a]	Physically compatible for 4 hr at 23°C	2224	C
Ampicillin sodium–sulbactam sodium	RR	20 mg/mL[b][d]	RPR	0.9 mg/mL[a]	Physically compatible for 4 hr at 23°C	2224	C
Anidulafungin	VIC	0.5 mg/mL[a]	AVE	2 mg/mL[a]	Physically compatible for 4 hr at 23°C	2617	C
Aztreonam	BMS	40 mg/mL[a]	RPR	0.9 mg/mL[a]	Physically compatible for 4 hr at 23°C	2224	C
Bumetanide	RC	0.04 mg/mL[a]	RPR	0.9 mg/mL[a]	Physically compatible for 4 hr at 23°C	2224	C
Buprenorphine HCl	RKC	0.04 mg/mL[a]	RPR	0.9 mg/mL[a]	Physically compatible for 4 hr at 23°C	2224	C
Butorphanol tartrate	APC	0.04 mg/mL[a]	RPR	0.9 mg/mL[a]	Physically compatible for 4 hr at 23°C	2224	C
Calcium gluconate	FUJ	40 mg/mL[a]	RPR	0.9 mg/mL[a]	Physically compatible for 4 hr at 23°C	2224	C
Cefazolin sodium	APC	20 mg/mL[a]	RPR	0.9 mg/mL[a]	Physically compatible for 4 hr at 23°C	2224	C
Cefepime HCl	BMS	20 mg/mL[a]	RPR	0.9 mg/mL[a]	Physically compatible for 4 hr at 23°C	2224	C
Cefotaxime sodium	HO	20 mg/mL[a]	RPR	0.9 mg/mL[a]	Physically compatible for 4 hr at 23°C	2224	C

Y-Site Injection Compatibility (1:1 Mixture) (Cont.)

Test Drug	Mfr	Conc	Mfr	Conc	Remarks	Ref	C/I
Cefotetan disodium	ZEN	20 mg/mL[a]	RPR	0.9 mg/mL[a]	Physically compatible for 4 hr at 23°C	2224	C
Cefoxitin sodium	ME	20 mg/mL[a]	RPR	0.9 mg/mL[a]	Physically compatible for 4 hr at 23°C	2224	C
Ceftazidime	SKB	40 mg/mL[a]	RPR	0.9 mg/mL[a]	Physically compatible for 4 hr at 23°C	2224	C
Ceftriaxone sodium	RC	20 mg/mL[a]	RPR	0.9 mg/mL[a]	Physically compatible for 4 hr at 23°C	2224	C
Cefuroxime sodium	LI	30 mg/mL[a]	RPR	0.9 mg/mL[a]	Physically compatible for 4 hr at 23°C	2224	C
Chlorpromazine HCl	SCN	2 mg/mL[a]	RPR	0.9 mg/mL[a]	Physically compatible for 4 hr at 23°C	2224	C
Ciprofloxacin	BAY	1 mg/mL[a]	RPR	0.9 mg/mL[a]	Physically compatible for 4 hr at 23°C	2224	C
Clindamycin phosphate	AST	10 mg/mL[a]	RPR	0.9 mg/mL[a]	Physically compatible for 4 hr at 23°C	2224	C
Dexamethasone sodium phosphate	ES	2 mg/mL[a]	RPR	0.9 mg/mL[a]	Physically compatible for 4 hr at 23°C	2224	C
Diphenhydramine HCl	ES	2 mg/mL[a]	RPR	0.9 mg/mL[a]	Physically compatible for 4 hr at 23°C	2224	C
Dobutamine HCl	AST	4 mg/mL[a]	RPR	0.9 mg/mL[a]	Physically compatible for 4 hr at 23°C	2224	C
Dopamine HCl	AB	3.2 mg/mL[a]	RPR	0.9 mg/mL[a]	Physically compatible for 4 hr at 23°C	2224	C
Doripenem	JJ	5 mg/mL[a b]	SAA	0.8 mg/mL[a b]	Physically compatible for 4 hr at 23°C	2743	C
Doxorubicin HCl liposomal	SEQ	0.4 mg/mL[a]	RPR	2 mg/mL[a]	Partial loss of measured natural turbidity	2087	I
Doxycycline hyclate	FUJ	1 mg/mL[a]	RPR	0.9 mg/mL[a]	Physically compatible for 4 hr at 23°C	2224	C
Droperidol	AST	0.4 mg/mL[a]	RPR	0.9 mg/mL[a]	Physically compatible for 4 hr at 23°C	2224	C
Enalaprilat	ME	0.1 mg/mL[a]	RPR	0.9 mg/mL[a]	Physically compatible for 4 hr at 23°C	2224	C
Famotidine	ME	2 mg/mL[a]	RPR	0.9 mg/mL[a]	Physically compatible for 4 hr at 23°C	2224	C
Fluconazole	RR	2 mg/mL	RPR	0.9 mg/mL[a]	Physically compatible for 4 hr at 23°C	2224	C
Furosemide	AMR	3 mg/mL[a]	RPR	0.9 mg/mL[a]	Physically compatible for 4 hr at 23°C	2224	C
Ganciclovir sodium	RC	20 mg/mL[a]	RPR	0.9 mg/mL[a]	Physically compatible for 4 hr at 23°C	2224	C
Gemcitabine HCl	LI	10 mg/mL[b]	RPR	2 mg/mL[a]	Physically compatible for 4 hr at 23°C	2226	C
Gentamicin sulfate	AB	5 mg/mL[a]	RPR	0.9 mg/mL[a]	Physically compatible for 4 hr at 23°C	2224	C
Granisetron HCl	SKB	0.05 mg/mL[a]	RPR	0.9 mg/mL[a]	Physically compatible for 4 hr at 23°C	2224	C
Haloperidol lactate	MN	0.2 mg/mL[a]	RPR	0.9 mg/mL[a]	Physically compatible for 4 hr at 23°C	2224	C
Heparin sodium	ES	100 units/mL	RPR	0.9 mg/mL[a]	Physically compatible for 4 hr at 23°C	2224	C
Hydrocortisone sodium succinate	AB	1 mg/mL[a]	RPR	0.9 mg/mL[a]	Physically compatible for 4 hr at 23°C	2224	C
Hydromorphone HCl	AST	0.5 mg/mL[a]	RPR	0.9 mg/mL[a]	Physically compatible for 4 hr at 23°C	2224	C
Hydroxyzine HCl	ES	2 mg/mL[a]	RPR	0.9 mg/mL[a]	Physically compatible for 4 hr at 23°C	2224	C
Imipenem–cilastatin sodium	ME	10 mg/mL[b g]	RPR	0.9 mg/mL[a]	Physically compatible for 4 hr at 23°C	2224	C
Leucovorin calcium	ES	2 mg/mL[a]	RPR	0.9 mg/mL[a]	Physically compatible for 4 hr at 23°C	2224	C
Lorazepam	WY	0.5 mg/mL[a]	RPR	0.9 mg/mL[a]	Physically compatible for 4 hr at 23°C	2224	C
Magnesium sulfate	AST	100 mg/mL[a]	RPR	0.9 mg/mL[a]	Physically compatible for 4 hr at 23°C	2224	C

Y-Site Injection Compatibility (1:1 Mixture) (Cont.)

Test Drug	Mfr	Conc	Mfr	Conc	Remarks	Ref	C/I
Mannitol	BA	15%	RPR	0.9 mg/mL[a]	Physically compatible for 4 hr at 23°C	2224	C
Meperidine HCl	AST	4 mg/mL[a]	RPR	0.9 mg/mL[a]	Physically compatible for 4 hr at 23°C	2224	C
Meropenem	ZEN	20 mg/mL[b]	RPR	0.9 mg/mL[a]	Physically compatible for 4 hr at 23°C	2224	C
Mesna	MJ	10 mg/mL[a]	RPR	0.9 mg/mL[a]	Physically compatible for 4 hr at 23°C	2224	C
Methylprednisolone sodium succinate	PHU	5 mg/mL[a]	RPR	0.9 mg/mL[a]	Partial loss of measured natural turbidity occurs immediately	2224	I
Metoclopramide HCl	AB	5 mg/mL	RPR	0.9 mg/mL[a]	Physically compatible for 4 hr at 23°C	2224	C
Metronidazole	BA	5 mg/mL	RPR	0.9 mg/mL[a]	Physically compatible for 4 hr at 23°C	2224	C
Morphine sulfate	ES	1 mg/mL[a]	RPR	0.9 mg/mL[a]	Physically compatible for 4 hr at 23°C	2224	C
Nalbuphine HCl	AST	10 mg/mL	RPR	0.9 mg/mL[a]	Increase in measured subvisible turbidity occurs immediately	2224	I
Ondansetron HCl	GW	1 mg/mL[a]	RPR	0.9 mg/mL[a]	Physically compatible for 4 hr at 23°C	2224	C
Oxaliplatin	SS	0.5 mg/mL[a]	AVE	2 mg/mL[a]	Physically compatible for 4 hr at 23°C	2566	C
Palonosetron HCl	MGI	50 mcg/mL	AVE	0.8 mg/mL[a]	Physically compatible and no loss of either drug in 4 hr	2533	C
Pemetrexed disodium	LI	20 mg/mL[b]	AVE	0.8 mg/mL[a]	Physically compatible for 4 hr at 23°C	2564	C
Piperacillin sodium–tazo-bactam sodium	CY[c]	40 mg/mL[a e]	RPR	0.9 mg/mL[a]	Physically compatible for 4 hr at 23°C	2224	C
Potassium chloride	AB	0.1 mEq/mL[a]	RPR	0.9 mg/mL[a]	Physically compatible for 4 hr at 23°C	2224	C
Prochlorperazine edisylate	SO	0.5 mg/mL[a]	RPR	0.9 mg/mL[a]	Physically compatible for 4 hr at 23°C	2224	C
Promethazine HCl	SCN	2 mg/mL[a]	RPR	0.9 mg/mL[a]	Physically compatible for 4 hr at 23°C	2224	C
Ranitidine HCl	GL	2 mg/mL[a]	RPR	0.9 mg/mL[a]	Physically compatible for 4 hr at 23°C	2224	C
Sodium bicarbonate	AB	1 mEq/mL	RPR	0.9 mg/mL[a]	Physically compatible for 4 hr at 23°C	2224	C
Tobramycin sulfate	LI	5 mg/mL[a]	RPR	0.9 mg/mL[a]	Physically compatible for 4 hr at 23°C	2224	C
Trimethoprim–sulfame-thoxazole	ES	0.8 mg/mL[a f]	RPR	0.9 mg/mL[a]	Physically compatible for 4 hr at 23°C	2224	C
Vancomycin HCl	LI	10 mg/mL[a]	RPR	0.9 mg/mL[a]	Physically compatible for 4 hr at 23°C	2224	C
Zidovudine	GW	4 mg/mL[a]	RPR	0.9 mg/mL[a]	Physically compatible for 4 hr at 23°C	2224	C

[a] Tested in dextrose 5%.

[b] Tested in sodium chloride 0.9%.

[c] Test performed using the formulation WITHOUT edetate disodium.

[d] Ampicillin component. Ampicillin in a 2:1 fixed-ratio concentration with sulbactam.

[e] Piperacillin component. Piperacillin in an 8:1 fixed-ratio concentration with tazobactam.

[f] Trimethoprim component. Trimethoprim in a 1:5 fixed-ratio concentration with sulfamethoxazole.

[g] Not specified whether concentration refers to single component or combined components.

Selected Revisions December 12, 2018. © Copyright, October 2000. American Society of Health-System Pharmacists, Inc.

Dolasetron Mesylate

AHFS 56:22.20

Products

Dolasetron mesylate is available in 0.625-mL (12.5-mg) single-use ampuls and 5-mL (100-mg) single-use vials. Each mL of solution contains 20 mg of dolasetron mesylate and 38.2 mg of mannitol with acetate buffer in water for injection.[1(8/08)]

Dolasetron mesylate is also available in 25-mL (500-mg) multidose vials. Each mL of solution contains 20 mg of dolasetron mesylate, 29 mg of mannitol, and 5 mg of phenol with acetate buffer in water for injection.[1(8/08)]

pH

From 3.2 to 3.8.[1(8/08)]

Trade Name(s)

Anzemet

Administration

Dolasetron mesylate is administered intravenously undiluted up to a rate of 100 mg/30 seconds or diluted in a compatible infusion solution to a volume of 50 mL for infusion over 15 minutes. The administration line should be flushed both before and after dolasetron mesylate administration.[1(8/08)]

Stability

Dolasetron mesylate injection is a clear, colorless solution. Intact containers should be stored at controlled room temperature and protected from light.[1(8/08)]

Syringes

Dolasetron mesylate (Aventis) 12.5 mg/0.63 mL was packaged in 1-mL syringes sealed with tip caps. No loss of dolasetron mesylate occurred after 240 days of storage at 22°C.[2626]

Compatibility Information

Solution Compatibility

Dolasetron mesylate

Test Soln Name	Mfr	Mfr	Conc/L or %	Remarks	Ref	C/I
Dextrose 5% in Ringer's injection, lactated				Stable for 24 hr at room temperature and 48 hr refrigerated	1(8/08)	C
Dextrose 5% in sodium chloride 0.45%				Stable for 24 hr at room temperature and 48 hr refrigerated	1(8/08)	C
Dextrose 5%				Stable for 24 hr at room temperature and 48 hr refrigerated	1(8/08)	C
Dextrose 5%		HMR	10 g	Physically compatible with no loss in 31 days at 4 and 23°C	2675	C
Ringer's injection, lactated				Stable for 24 hr at room temperature and 48 hr refrigerated	1(8/08)	C
Sodium chloride 0.9%				Stable for 24 hr at room temperature and 48 hr refrigerated	1(8/08)	C
Sodium chloride 0.9%		HMR	10 g	Physically compatible with no loss in 31 days at 4 and 23°C	2675	C
Sodium chloride 0.9%			12.5 g[a]	Visually compatible and no loss in 31 days at room temperature	2736	C

[a] Tested in polypropylene syringes.

Y-Site Injection Compatibility (1:1 Mixture)

Dolasetron mesylate

Test Drug	Mfr	Conc	Mfr	Conc	Remarks	Ref	C/I
Acetaminophen	CAD	10 mg/mL	SAA	20 mg/mL	Physically compatible with less than 10% acetaminophen loss over 4 hr at room temperature	2841, 2844	C
Azithromycin	PF	2 mg/mL[b]	HMR	20 mg/mL[c]	Visually compatible	2368	C
Caspofungin acetate	ME	0.5 mg/mL[b]	SAA	20 mg/mL	Physically compatible with dolasetron mesylate given i.v. push over 2 to 5 min	2766	C

DOI: 10.37573/9781585286850.130

Y-Site Injection Compatibility (1:1 Mixture) (Cont.)

Test Drug	Mfr	Conc	Mfr	Conc	Remarks	Ref	C/I
Dexmedetomidine HCl	AB	4 mcg/mL[b]	HO	2 mg/mL[b]	Physically compatible for 4 hr at 23°C	2383	C
Fenoldopam mesylate	AB	80 mcg/mL[b]	AVE	2 mg/mL[b]	Physically compatible for 4 hr at 23°C	2467	C
Hetastarch in lactated electrolyte	AB	6%	HO	2 mg/mL[a]	Physically compatible for 4 hr at 23°C	2339	C
Oxaliplatin	SS	0.5 mg/mL[a]	AVE	2 mg/mL[a]	Physically compatible for 4 hr at 23°C	2566	C

[a] Tested in dextrose 5%.

[b] Tested in sodium chloride 0.9%.

[c] Injected via Y-site into an administration set running azithromycin.

Selected Revisions January 17, 2014. © Copyright, October 2002. American Society of Health-System Pharmacists, Inc.

Dopamine Hydrochloride
AHFS 12:12.08.08

Products

Dopamine hydrochloride is available in 200-mg (40 mg/mL), 400-mg (40 mg/mL), 400-mg (80 mg/mL), 800-mg (80 mg/mL), and 800-mg (160 mg/mL) vials and prefilled syringes. The solutions also contain sodium metabisulfite 0.9% as an antioxidant, citric acid and sodium citrate buffer, and hydrochloric acid or sodium hydroxide to adjust the pH in water for injection.[1(4/07)] [4]

Dopamine hydrochloride is available premixed for infusion in concentrations of 0.8, 1.6, and 3.2 mg/mL in dextrose 5%. Also present are sodium metabisulfite 0.5 mg/mL and hydrochloric acid and/or sodium hydroxide for pH adjustment.[1(4/07)]

pH

Dopamine hydrochloride injection has a pH of about 3.3 (range 2.5 to 5). The premixed dopamine hydrochloride infusions have a pH of about 3.3 to 3.8 (range 2.5 to 4.5).[1(4/07)] [4]

Osmolality

The osmolality of dopamine hydrochloride 40 mg/mL was 619 mOsm/kg by freezing-point depression and 581 mOsm/kg by vapor pressure.[1071] At a concentration of 10 mg/mL (diluent unspecified), the osmolality was determined to be 277 mOsm/kg.[1233]

Osmolarity

The osmolarity of premixed dopamine hydrochloride in dextrose 5% (Hospira) is 261, 269, and 286 mOsm/L for the 0.8-, 1.6-, and 3.2-mg/mL concentrations, respectively.[1(4/07)] [4]

Administration

Dopamine hydrochloride is administered by intravenous infusion into a large vein using an infusion pump or other infusion control device. The premixed infusion solutions are suitable for administration without dilution, but the concentrated injection must be diluted for use. Often the dose of concentrate is added to 250 or 500 mL of compatible solution. The concentration used depends on the patient's requirements. Concentrations as high as 3200 mcg/mL have been used.[1(4/07)] [4]

Stability

Intact containers of dopamine hydrochloride should be stored at controlled room temperature. The injections should be protected from excessive heat and from freezing.[1(4/07)] [4] Do not use the injection if it is darker than slightly yellow or discolored in any other way.[1(4/07)]

Dopamine hydrochloride under simulated summer conditions in paramedic vehicles was exposed to temperatures ranging from 26 to 38°C over 4 weeks. Analysis found no loss of the drug under these conditions.[2562]

pH Effects

The pH of the solution is one of the most critical factors determining dopamine hydrochloride stability. Dopamine hydrochlo-ride is stable over a pH range of 4 to 6.4 when mixed with other drugs in dextrose 5%,[312] but it is most stable at pH 5 or below.[79] In alkaline solutions, the catechol moieties are oxidized, cyclized, and polymerized to colored materials,[312] forming a pink to violet color.[78] Decomposition is also indicated by the formation of a yellow or brown discoloration of the solution.[4] Discolored solutions should not be used.[1(4/07)] [4] [312]

Freezing Solutions

Dopamine hydrochloride 0.5 mg/mL in dextrose 5% was frozen at –20°C in polypropylene syringes (Codan Medical and B. Braun) for 6 months. No visible precipitation or color change was observed. However, layering or stratification occurred in the frozen samples. Repeated inversion of the syringes was required to yield a clear and uniform solution. Less than 2% dopamine loss occurred in 6 months to samples in the Codan syringes. However, samples frozen in the Braun syringes were less stable, with dopamine losses up to 14%. The Braun syringes when frozen allowed air to enter into the product, which could compromise sterility as well as stability.[2530]

Light Effects

Exposure of dopamine hydrochloride 100 mg/100 mL in dextrose 5% to fluorescent and blue phototherapy light for 36 hours at 25°C, while static or flowing through tubing at 2 mL/hr, resulted in no significant difference in drug concentration compared to controls stored in the dark. Because no unacceptable loss occurs, protection of dopamine hydrochloride infusions from blue phototherapy lights is not necessary.[1100]

Syringes

Dopamine hydrochloride (Abbott) 200 mg/50 mL in dextrose 5% exhibited no change in appearance and no drug loss when stored in 60-mL plastic syringes (Becton Dickinson) for 24 hours at 25°C.[1579]

Dopamine hydrochloride (Therabel Lucien Pharma) 4 mg/mL in dextrose 5% was packaged in 50-mL polypropylene syringes (Becton Dickinson) and stored at 4 and 24°C in the dark and exposed to room light for 48 hours. Dopamine losses were less than 10% throughout the study.[1961]

Sorption

Dopamine hydrochloride has been shown not to exhibit sorption to polyvinyl chloride (PVC) bags and tubing, polyethylene tubing, polypropylene syringes, and polypropylene-polystyrene syringes.[536] [784] [1961]

Filtration

Dopamine hydrochloride 100 mcg/mL in dextrose 5% or sodium chloride 0.9% was delivered over 5 hours through 4 kinds of 0.2-μm membrane filters varying in size and composition. Dopamine concentration losses of 3 to 5% were found during the first 60 minutes; subsequent dopamine levels returned to the original concentration when the binding sites became saturated.[1399]

DOI: 10.37573/9781585286850.131

Central Venous Catheter

Dopamine hydrochloride (Abbott) 3.2 mg/mL in dextrose 5% was found to be compatible with the ARROWg+ard Blue Plus (Arrow International) chlorhexidine-bearing triple-lumen central catheter. Essentially complete delivery of the drug was found with little or no drug loss occurring. Furthermore, chlorhexidine delivered from the catheter remained at trace amounts with no substantial increase due to the delivery of the drug through the catheter.[2335]

Compatibility Information

Solution Compatibility

Dopamine HCl

Test Soln Name	Mfr	Mfr	Conc/L or %	Remarks	Ref	C/I
Amino acids 4.25%, dextrose 25%	MG	AS	400 mg	No increase in particulate matter in 24 hr at 4°C	349	C
Dextrose 5% in Ringer's injection, lactated	MG	AS	800 mg	Less than 5% loss in 48 hr at 25°C	79	C
Dextrose 5% in sodium chloride 0.45%	MG	AS	800 mg	Less than 5% loss in 48 hr at 25°C	79	C
Dextrose 5% in sodium chloride 0.9%	MG	AS	800 mg	Less than 5% loss in 48 hr at 25°C	79	C
Dextrose 10% in sodium chloride 0.18%	TRa		300 mg	Visually compatible with no loss in 96 hr at room temperature under fluorescent light	1569	C
Dextrose 5%	MG	AS	800 mg	Less than 5% loss in 48 hr at 25°C	79	C
Dextrose 5%	TRa	AS	800 mg	Stable for 24 hr at 25°C	79	C
Dextrose 5%		AS	800 mg	Stable for 7 days at 5°C	79	C
Dextrose 5%	AB	ACC	800 mg	Physically compatible. 10% loss calculated to occur after 142 hr at 25°C	527	C
Dextrose 5%	BAa	DB	3.2 g	5% loss in 14.75 days at 5°C protected from light	1610	C
Dextrose 5%	TRa	ES	0.4 and 3.2 g	Visually compatible with no loss in 48 hr at room temperature	1802	C
Dextrose 5%	BAa	SO	6.1 g	3% loss in 24 hr at 23°C	2085	C
Dextrose 5%	FRE	NYC	500 mg	Visually compatible. Losses of 4% in 7 days at room temperature and 2% in 3 months refrigerated	2530	C
Dextrose 10%	TRa		300 mg	Visually compatible with no loss in 96 hr at room temperature under fluorescent light	1569	C
Ringer's injection, lactated	MG	AS	800 mg	Less than 5% loss in 48 hr at 25°C	79	C
Sodium chloride 0.9%	MG	AS	800 mg	Less than 5% loss in 48 hr at 25°C	79	C
Sodium chloride 0.9%	TRa	ES	0.4 and 3.2 g	Visually compatible. 5% loss in 48 hr at room temperature	1802	C
Sodium lactate ⅙ M	MG	AS	800 mg	Less than 5% loss in 48 hr at 25°C	79	C

a Tested in PVC containers.

Additive Compatibility

Dopamine HCl

Test Drug	Mfr	Conc/L or %	Mfr	Conc/L or %	Test Solution	Remarks	Ref	C/I
Acyclovir sodium	BW	2.5 g	SO	800 mg	D5W	Yellow color developed in 1.5 hr due to dopamine oxidation. No acyclovir loss	1343	I
Alteplase	GEN	0.5 g	ACC	5 g	D5W, NS	About 30% alteplase clot-lysis activity loss in 24 hr at 25°C	1856	I

Additive Compatibility (Cont.)

Test Drug	Mfr	Conc/L or %	Mfr	Conc/L or %	Test Solution	Remarks	Ref	C/I
Aminophylline	SE	500 mg	ACC	800 mg	D5W	Physically compatible. At 25°C, 10% dopamine decomposition occurs in 111 hr	527	C
Amphotericin B	SQ	200 mg	AS	800 mg	D5W	Precipitates immediately	78	I
Ampicillin sodium	BR	4 g	AS	800 mg	D5W	Color change. 36% ampicillin loss in 6 hr at 23 to 25°C. Dopamine loss in 6 hr	78	I
Atracurium besylate	BW	500 mg		1.6 g	D5W	Physically compatible and atracurium stable for 24 hr at 5 and 30°C	1694	C
Calcium chloride	UP		AS	800 mg	D5W	No dopamine loss in 24 hr at 25°C	312	C
Chloramphenicol sodium succinate	PD	4 g	AS	800 mg	D5W	Both drugs stable for 24 hr at 25°C	78	C
Ciprofloxacin	MI	2 g		400 mg	NS	Compatible for 24 hr at 25°C	888	C
Ciprofloxacin	MI	2 g		1.04 g	NS	Compatible for 24 hr at 25°C	888	C
Dobutamine HCl	LI	172 mg	AS	5.5 g	NS	Physically compatible for 24 hr	552	C
Dobutamine HCl	LI	1 g	ACC	1.6 g	D5W, NS	Physically compatible with no color change in 24 hr at 25°C	789	C
Dobutamine HCl	LI	1 g	ES	800 mg	D5W, NS	Physically compatible for 24 hr at 21°C	812	C
Enalaprilat	MSD	12 mg	AMR	1.6 g	D5W[b]	Visually compatible. 5% enalaprilat loss in 24 hr at room temperature under fluorescent light. Dopamine not tested	1572	C
Flumazenil	RC	20 mg	AB	3.2 g	D5W[b]	Visually compatible. 7% flumazenil loss in 24 hr at 23°C in fluorescent light. Dopamine not tested	1710	C
Gentamicin sulfate	SC	2 g	AS	800 mg	D5W	No dopamine and 7% gentamicin loss in 24 hr at 25°C	312	C
Gentamicin sulfate	SC	320 mg	AS	800 mg	D5W	Gentamicin stable through 6 hr. 80% gentamicin loss in 24 hr at 25°C. Dopamine stable for 24 hr	78	I
Heparin sodium	AB	200,000 units	AS	800 mg	D5W	No dopamine or heparin loss in 24 hr at 25°C	312	C
Hydrocortisone sodium succinate	UP	1 g	AS	800 mg	D5W	No dopamine loss in 18 hr at 25°C	312	C
Lidocaine HCl	AST	4 g	AS	800 mg	D5W[b]	No dopamine or lidocaine loss in 24 hr at 25°C	312	C
Lidocaine HCl	AST	2 g	ACC	800 mg	D5W, LR, NS	Physically compatible for 24 hr at 25°C	775	C
Mannitol	MG	20%	AS	800 mg		Under 5% dopamine loss in 48 hr at 25°C	79	C
Meropenem	ZEN	1 and 20 g	DU	800 mg	NS	Visually compatible for 4 hr at room temperature	1994	C
Methylprednisolone sodium succinate	UP	500 mg	AS	800 mg	D5W	No dopamine loss in 18 hr at 25°C	312	C
Methylprednisolone sodium succinate	UP	500 mg	AS	800 mg	D5W	Clear solution for 24 hr	329	C
Nitroglycerin	ACC	400 mg	ACC	800 mg	D5W, NS[c]	Physically compatible with little or no nitroglycerin loss in 48 hr at 23°C. Dopamine not tested	929	C
Oxacillin sodium	BR	2 g	AS	800 mg	D5W	No dopamine and 2% oxacillin loss in 24 hr at 25°C	312	C
Penicillin G potassium	LI	20 million units	AS	800 mg	D5W	14% penicillin loss in 24 hr at 25°C. Dopamine stable for 24 hr	78	I
Potassium chloride	MG		AS	800 mg	D5W	No dopamine loss in 24 hr at 25°C	312	C
Ranitidine HCl	GL	50 mg and 2 g	ES	400 mg and 3.2 g	D5W, NS[b]	Physically compatible. 6% ranitidine loss in 48 hr at room temperature in light. Dopamine not tested	1361	C

Additive Compatibility (Cont.)

Test Drug	Mfr	Conc/L or %	Mfr	Conc/L or %	Test Solution	Remarks	Ref	C/I
Ranitidine HCl	GL	50 mg and 2 g	ES	0.4 and 3.2 g	D5W, NS[a]	Visually compatible. No dopamine and 7% ranitidine loss in 48 hr at room temperature	1802	C
Sodium bicarbonate	MG	5%	AS	800 mg		Color change 5 min after mixing	79	I
Valproate sodium	WW	4.5 g	BA	800 mg	[b]	Physically compatible for 24 hr at 22 to 25°C in ambient light and 34 to 38% relative humidity	3424	C
Verapamil HCl	KN	80 mg	ES	400 mg	D5W, NS	Physically compatible for 24 hr	764	C

[a] Tested in both glass and PVC containers.

[b] Tested in PVC containers.

[c] Tested in glass containers.

Drugs in Syringe Compatibility

Dopamine HCl

Test Drug	Mfr	Amt	Mfr	Amt	Remarks	Ref	C/I
Caffeine citrate		20 mg/1 mL	SO	80 mg/1 mL	Visually compatible for 4 hr at 25°C	2440	C
Doxapram HCl	RB	400 mg/20 mL		100 mg/5 mL	Physically compatible with 3% doxapram loss in 24 hr	1177	C
Heparin sodium		2500 units/1 mL		50 mg/5 mL	Physically compatible for at least 5 min	1053	C
Pantoprazole sodium	[a]	4 mg/1 mL		40 mg/1 mL	Whitish precipitate forms within 1 hr	2574	I
Ranitidine HCl	GL	50 mg/5 mL		40 mg	Physically compatible for 4 hr at ambient temperature under fluorescent light	1151	C

[a] Test performed using the formulation WITHOUT edetate disodium.

Y-Site Injection Compatibility (1:1 Mixture)

Dopamine HCl

Test Drug	Mfr	Conc	Mfr	Conc	Remarks	Ref	C/I
Acyclovir sodium	BW	5 mg/mL[a]	AB	1.6 mg/mL[a]	Solution turns dark brown in 2 hr at 25°C	1157	I
Aldesleukin	CHI	33,800 I.U./mL[a]	ES	1.6 mg/mL[a]	Visually compatible with little or no loss of aldesleukin activity	1857	C
Aldesleukin	CHI[i]	[a]			Unacceptable loss of aldesleukin activity	1890	I
Alprostadil	BED	7.5 mcg/mL[t u]	AB	3 mg/mL[s]	Visually compatible for 1 hr	2746	C
Alteplase	GEN	1 mg/mL	DU	8 mg/mL[a]	Haze noted in 4 hr	1340	I
Amifostine	USB	10 mg/mL[a]	AST	3.2 mg/mL[a]	Physically compatible for 4 hr at 23°C	1845	C
Amiodarone HCl	LZ	4 mg/mL[c]	ES	1.6 mg/mL[c]	Physically compatible for 24 hr at 21°C	1032	C
Angiotensin II acetate	LJ	5 and 10 mcg/mL[b]			Stated to be compatible	3430	C
Anidulafungin	VIC	0.5 mg/mL[a]	AMR	3.2 mg/mL[a]	Physically compatible for 4 hr at 23°C	2617	C
Argatroban	GSK	1 mg/mL[b]	AMR	80 mg/mL	Visually compatible for 24 hr at 23°C	2391	C

Y-Site Injection Compatibility (1:1 Mixture) (Cont.)

Test Drug	Mfr	Conc	Mfr	Conc	Remarks	Ref	C/I
Atracurium besylate	BW	0.5 mg/mL[a]	SO	1.6 mg/mL[a]	Physically compatible for 24 hr at 28°C	1337	C
Aztreonam	SQ	40 mg/mL[a]	AST	3.2 mg/mL[a]	Physically compatible for 4 hr at 23°C	1758	C
Bivalirudin	TMC	5 mg/mL[a]	AB	3.2 mg/mL[a]	Physically compatible for 4 hr at 23°C	2373	C
Bivalirudin	TMC	5 mg/mL[a b]	AMR	80 mg/mL	Visually compatible for 6 hr at 23°C	2680	C
Caffeine citrate		20 mg/mL		0.6 mg/mL[a]	Compatible and stable for 24 hr at room temperature	1(4/07)	C
Cangrelor tetrasodium	TMC	1 mg/mL[b]		4 mg/mL[b]	Physically compatible for 4 hr	3243	C
Caspofungin acetate	ME	0.7 mg/mL[b]	AMR	3.2 mg/mL[b]	Physically compatible for 4 hr at room temperature	2758	C
Caspofungin acetate	ME	0.5 mg/mL[b]	BA	3.2 mg/mL	Physically compatible over 60 min	2766	C
Cefepime HCl	BMS	120 mg/mL[d]		0.4 mg/mL	Physically compatible with less than 10% cefepime loss. Dopamine not tested	2513	C
Ceftaroline fosamil	FOR	2.22 mg/mL[a b n]	HOS	3.2 mg/mL[a b n]	Physically compatible for 4 hr at 23°C	2826	C
Ceftazidime	GSK	120 mg/mL[d]		0.4 mg/mL	Physically compatible with less than 10% ceftazidime loss. Dopamine not tested	2513	C
Ceftazidime–avibactam sodium	ALL	20 mg/mL[bb cc]			Physically compatible for up to 4 hr at room temperature	3004	C
Ceftolozane sulfate–tazobactam sodium	CUB[w]	30 mg/mL[a b]		3.2 mg/mL	Physically compatible with no loss of either drug in 24 hr at 25°C	2959	C
Ceftolozane sulfate–tazobactam sodium	CUB	10 mg/mL[c w]	HOS	0.8 mg/mL[c]	Physically compatible for 2 hr	3262	C
Ciprofloxacin	MI	2 mg/mL[c]	AB	1.6 mg/mL[c]	Visually compatible for 24 hr at 24°C	1655	C
Cisatracurium besylate	GW	0.1, 2, 5 mg/mL[a]	AB	3.2 mg/mL[a]	Physically compatible for 4 hr at 23°C	2074	C
Cladribine	ORT	0.015[b] and 0.5[f] mg/mL	AST	3.2 mg/mL[b]	Physically compatible for 4 hr at 23°C	1969	C
Clarithromycin	AB	4 mg/mL[a]	DB	3.2 mg/mL[a]	Visually compatible for 72 hr at both 30 and 17°C	2174	C
Clonidine HCl	BI	18 mcg/mL[b]	NYC	2 mg/mL[a]	Visually compatible	2642	C
Cloxacillin sodium	SMX	100 mg/mL	BA	3.2 mg/mL	Physically compatible for up to 4 hr at room temperature	3245	C
Daptomycin	CUB[z]	18.2 mg/mL[b o]	AMR	3.6 mg/mL[o]	Physically compatible with no loss of either drug in 2 hr at 25°C	2553	C
Dexmedetomidine HCl	AB	4 mcg/mL[b]	AB	3.2 mg/mL[b]	Physically compatible for 4 hr at 23°C	2383	C
Diltiazem HCl	MMD	1 mg/mL[a]	AB	1.6 mg/mL[a]	Visually compatible for 24 hr at 25°C	1530	C
Diltiazem HCl	MMD	5 mg/mL	AB, SO	0.8 mg/mL[c]	Visually compatible	1807	C
Diltiazem HCl	MMD	1 mg/mL[a]	AB	3.2 mg/mL[a]	Visually compatible for 4 hr at 27°C	2062	C
Dobutamine HCl	LI	4 mg/mL[b]	DCC	3.2 mg/mL[c]	Physically compatible for 3 hr	1316	C
Dobutamine HCl	LI	4 mg/mL[a]	AB	3.2 mg/mL[a]	Visually compatible for 4 hr at 27°C	2062	C
Dobutamine HCl with lidocaine HCl	LI AB	4 mg/mL[c] 8 mg/mL[c]	DCC	3.2 mg/mL[c]	Physically compatible for 3 hr	1316	C

Y-Site Injection Compatibility (1:1 Mixture) (Cont.)

Test Drug	Mfr	Conc	Mfr	Conc	Remarks	Ref	C/I
Dobutamine HCl with nitroglycerin	LI LY	4 mg/mL[c] 0.4 mg/mL[c]	DCC	3.2 mg/mL[c]	Physically compatible for 3 hr	1316	C
Dobutamine HCl with sodium nitroprusside	LI ES	4 mg/mL[c] 0.4 mg/mL[c]	DCC	3.2 mg/mL[c]	Physically compatible for 3 hr	1316	C
Docetaxel	RPR	0.9 mg/mL[a]	AB	3.2 mg/mL[a]	Physically compatible for 4 hr at 23°C	2224	C
Doripenem	JJ	5 mg/mL[a b]	AMR	3.2 mg/mL[a b]	Physically compatible for 4 hr at 23°C	2743	C
Doxorubicin HCl liposomal	SEQ	0.4 mg/mL[a]	AB	3.2 mg/mL[a]	Physically compatible for 4 hr at 23°C	2087	C
Enalaprilat	MSD	0.05 mg/mL[b]	IMS	1.6 mg/mL[a]	Physically compatible for 24 hr at room temperature under fluorescent light	1355	C
Epinephrine HCl	AB	0.02 mg/mL[a]	AB	3.2 mg/mL[a]	Visually compatible for 4 hr at 27°C	2062	C
Eravacycline dihydrochloride	TET	0.6 mg/mL[b]	BA	0.8 mg/mL[h]	Physically compatible for 2 hr at room temperature	3532	C
Esmolol HCl	DCC	10 mg/mL[a]	IMS	1.6 mg/mL[a]	Physically compatible for 24 hr at 22°C	1169	C
Etoposide phosphate	BR	5 mg/mL[a]	AST	3.2 mg/mL[a]	Physically compatible for 4 hr at 23°C	2218	C
Famotidine	MSD	0.2 mg/mL[a]	TR	1.6 mg/mL[a]	Physically compatible for 4 hr at 25°C	1188	C
Famotidine	ME	2 mg/mL[b]		1.6 mg/mL[a]	Visually compatible for 4 hr at 22°C	1936	C
Fenoldopam mesylate	AB	80 mcg/mL[b]	AB	3.2 mg/mL[b]	Physically compatible for 4 hr at 23°C	2467	C
Fentanyl citrate	ES	0.05 mg/mL	AB	3.2 mg/mL[a]	Visually compatible for 4 hr at 27°C	2062	C
Fluconazole	RR	2 mg/mL	AMR	1.6 mg/mL[a]	Visually compatible for 24 hr at 28°C under fluorescent light	1760	C
Foscarnet sodium	AST	24 mg/mL	DU	80 mg/mL	Physically compatible for 24 hr at room temperature under fluorescent light	1335	C
Furosemide	AB, AMR	5 mg/mL	AST, DU	12.8 mg/mL	Physically compatible for 3 hr at room temperature	1978	C
Furosemide	AB, AMR	5 mg/mL	AB, AMR	12.8 mg/mL	White precipitate forms immediately	1978	I
Furosemide	AMR	10 mg/mL	AB	3.2 mg/mL[a]	Precipitate forms in 4 hr at 27°C	2062	I
Gemcitabine HCl	LI	10 mg/mL[b]	AB	3.2 mg/mL[b]	Physically compatible for 4 hr at 23°C	2226	C
Granisetron HCl	SKB	0.05 mg/mL[a]	AB	3.2 mg/mL[a]	Physically compatible for 4 hr at 23°C	2000	C
Haloperidol lactate	MN	0.5[a] and 5 mg/mL	DU	1.6 mg/mL[a]	Visually compatible for 24 hr at 21°C	1523	C
Heparin sodium	UP	1000 units/L[g]	ACC	40 mg/mL	Physically compatible for 4 hr at room temperature	534	C
Heparin sodium	ES	100 units/mL[a]	AB	3.2 mg/mL[a]	Visually compatible for 4 hr at 27°C	2062	C
Heparin sodium	TR	50 units/mL	BA	1.6 mg/mL	Visually compatible for 4 hr at 25°C	1793	C
Hetastarch in lactated electrolyte	AB	6%	AB	3.2 mg/mL[a]	Physically compatible for 4 hr at 23°C	2339	C
Hydrocortisone sodium succinate	UP	10 mg/L[g]	ACC	40 mg/mL	Physically compatible for 4 hr at room temperature	534	C
Hydromorphone HCl	KN	1 mg/mL	AB	3.2 mg/mL[a]	Visually compatible for 4 hr at 27°C	2062	C

Y-Site Injection Compatibility (1:1 Mixture) (Cont.)

Test Drug	Mfr	Conc	Mfr	Conc	Remarks	Ref	C/I
Hydroxyethyl starch 130/0.4 in sodium chloride 0.9%	FRK	6%	BMS	0.8, 3.2, 6.4 mg/mL[a]	Visually compatible for 24 hr at room temperature	2770	C
Ibuprofen lysinate	OVA	10 mg/mL	HOS	3.2 mg/mL[h]	Precipitate formed within 4 hr	3541	I
Indomethacin sodium trihydrate	MSD	1 mg/mL[b]	AB	1.2 mg/mL[a]	Hazy precipitate forms immediately	1527	I
Insulin, regular	LI	1 unit/mL[a]	DU	3.2 mg/mL[a]	White precipitate forms immediately, dissolves quickly, and reforms in 24 hr at 23°C	1877	I
Isavuconazonium sulfate	ASP	1.5 mg/mL[c]	HOS	0.8 mg/mL[c]	Physically compatible for 2 hr	3263	C
Labetalol HCl	SC	1 mg/mL[a]	IMS	1.6 mg/mL[a]	Physically compatible for 24 hr at 18°C	1171	C
Labetalol HCl	GL	1 mg/mL[a]	ES	1.6 mg/mL[a]	Visually compatible. Little loss of either drug in 4 hr at room temperature	1762	C
Labetalol HCl	AH	2 mg/mL[a]	AB	3.2 mg/mL[a]	Visually compatible for 4 hr at 27°C	2062	C
Levofloxacin	OMN	5 mg/mL[a]	AMR	80 mg/mL	Visually compatible for 4 hr at 24°C	2233	C
Lidocaine HCl	AB	8 mg/mL[c]	DCC	3.2 mg/mL[c]	Physically compatible for 3 hr	1316	C
Lidocaine HCl with dobutamine HCl	AB LI	8 mg/mL[c] 4 mg/mL[c]	DCC	3.2 mg/mL[c]	Physically compatible for 3 hr	1316	C
Lidocaine HCl with nitroglycerin	AB LY	8 mg/mL[c] 0.4 mg/mL[c]	DCC	3.2 mg/mL[c]	Physically compatible for 3 hr	1316	C
Lidocaine HCl with sodium nitroprusside	AB ES	8 mg/mL[c] 0.4 mg/mL[c]	DCC	3.2 mg/mL[c]	Physically compatible for 3 hr	1316	C
Linezolid	PHU	2 mg/mL	AB	3.2 mg/mL[a]	Physically compatible for 4 hr at 23°C	2264	C
Lorazepam	WY	0.5 mg/mL[a]	AB	3.2 mg/mL[a]	Visually compatible for 4 hr at 27°C	2062	C
Meperidine HCl	AB	10 mg/mL	AB	1.6 mg/mL[a]	Physically compatible for 4 hr at 25°C	1397	C
Meropenem		50 mg/mL	HOS	32 mg/mL[h]	Physically compatible for 4 hr at room temperature	3538	C
Meropenem–vaborbactam	TMC	8 mg/mL[b aa]	HOS	0.8 mg/mL[b]	Physically compatible for 3 hr at 20 to 25°C	3380	C
Methylprednisolone sodium succinate	UP	5 mg/mL[a]	AB	0.8 mg/mL[a]	Visually compatible for 24 hr at room temperature in test tubes. No precipitate found on filter from Y-site delivery	2063	C
Metronidazole	MG	5 mg/mL	AB	0.8 mg/mL[a]	Visually compatible for 24 hr at room temperature in test tubes. No precipitate found on filter from Y-site delivery	2063	C
Micafungin sodium	ASP	1.5 mg/mL[b]	AMR	3.2 mg/mL[b]	Physically compatible for 4 hr at 23°C	2683	C
Midazolam HCl	RC	1 mg/mL[a]	AB	1.6 mg/mL[a]	Visually compatible for 24 hr at 23°C	1847	C
Midazolam HCl	RC	1 mg/mL[a]	DU	3.2 mg/mL[a]	Visually compatible for 24 hr at 23°C	1877	C
Midazolam HCl	RC	2 mg/mL[a]	AB	3.2 mg/mL[a]	Visually compatible for 4 hr at 27°C	2062	C
Milrinone lactate	SW	0.2 mg/mL[a]	AB	3.2 mg/mL[a]	Visually compatible for 4 hr at 27°C	2062	C

Y-Site Injection Compatibility (1:1 Mixture) (Cont.)

Test Drug	Mfr	Conc	Mfr	Conc	Remarks	Ref	C/I
Milrinone lactate	SW	0.4 mg/mL[a]	SO	6.4 mg/mL[a]	Visually compatible. Little loss of either drug in 4 hr at 23°C	2214	C
Morphine sulfate	AB	1 mg/mL	AB	1.6 mg/mL[a]	Physically compatible for 4 hr at 25°C	1397	C
Morphine sulfate	SCN	2 mg/mL[a]	AB	3.2 mg/mL[a]	Visually compatible for 4 hr at 27°C	2062	C
Mycophenolate mofetil HCl	RC	5.9 mg/mL[a]	AMR	4 mg/mL[a]	Physically compatible and 4% mycophenolate mofetil loss in 4 hr	2738	C
Nesiritide	SCI	50 mcg/mL[a b]		80 mg/mL	Physically compatible for 4 hr. May be chemically incompatible with nesiritide[p]	2625	?
Nicardipine HCl	WY	1 mg/mL[a]	AB	3.2 mg/mL[a]	Visually compatible for 4 hr at 27°C	2062	C
Nicardipine HCl	DCC	0.1 mg/mL[a]	IMS	1.6 mg/mL[a]	Visually compatible for 24 hr at room temperature	235	C
Nitroglycerin	LY	0.4 mg/mL[c]	DCC	3.2 mg/mL[c]	Physically compatible for 3 hr	1316	C
Nitroglycerin	AB	0.4 mg/mL[a]	AB	3.2 mg/mL[a]	Visually compatible for 4 hr at 27°C	2062	C
Nitroglycerin with dobutamine HCl	LY LI	0.4 mg/mL[c] 4 mg/mL[c]	DCC	3.2 mg/mL[c]	Physically compatible for 3 hr	1316	C
Nitroglycerin with lidocaine HCl	LY AB	0.4 mg/mL[c] 8 mg/mL[c]	DCC	3.2 mg/mL[c]	Physically compatible for 3 hr	1316	C
Nitroglycerin with sodium nitroprusside	LY ES	0.4 mg/mL[c] 0.4 mg/mL[c]	DCC	3.2 mg/mL[c]	Physically compatible for 3 hr	1316	C
Norepinephrine bitartrate	STR	0.064 mg/mL[a]	DU	3.2 mg/mL[a]	Visually compatible for 24 hr at 23°C	1877	C
Norepinephrine bitartrate	AB	0.128 mg/mL[a]	AB	3.2 mg/mL[a]	Visually compatible for 4 hr at 27°C	2062	C
Ondansetron HCl	GL	0.32 mg/mL[b]	AB	0.8 mg/mL[a]	Visually compatible for 24 hr at room temperature in test tubes. No precipitate found on filter from Y-site delivery	2063	C
Oritavancin diphosphate	TAR	0.8, 1.2, and 2 mg/mL[a]	HOS	3.2 mg/mL[a]	Visually compatible for 4 hr at 20 to 24°C	2928	C
Oxaliplatin	SS	0.5 mg/mL[a]	AB	3.2 mg/mL[a]	Physically compatible for 4 hr at 23°C	2566	C
Pancuronium bromide	ES	0.05 mg/mL[a]	SO	1.6 mg/mL[a]	Physically compatible for 24 hr at 28°C	1337	C
Pantoprazole sodium	ALT[q]	0.16 to 0.8 mg/mL[b]	DU	0.8 to 3.2 mg/mL[a]	Visually compatible for 12 hr at 23°C	2603	C
Pemetrexed disodium	LI	20 mg/mL[b]	AB	3.2 mg/mL[a]	Physically compatible for 4 hr at 23°C	2564	C
Piperacillin sodium–tazobactam sodium	LE[q]	40 mg/mL[a v]	AST	3.2 mg/mL[a]	Physically compatible for 4 hr at 22°C	1688	C
Plazomicin sulfate	ACH	24 mg/mL[c]	HOS	0.8 mg/mL[c]	Physically compatible for 1 hr at 20 to 25°C	3432	C
Potassium chloride	AB	40 mEq/L[g]	ACC	40 mg/mL	Physically compatible for 4 hr at room temperature	534	C
Propofol	ZEN[r]	10 mg/mL	AST	3.2 mg/mL[a]	Physically compatible for 1 hr at 23°C	2066	C
Quinupristin–dalfopristin		2 mg/mL[a x]	[y]	2.2 mg/mL	Reported to be incompatible	3230	I
Ranitidine HCl	GL	0.5 mg/mL[h]	ES	1.6 mg/mL[a]	Physically compatible for 24 hr	1323	C
Ranitidine HCl	GL	1 mg/mL[a]	AB	3.2 mg/mL[a]	Visually compatible for 4 hr at 27°C	2062	C

Y-Site Injection Compatibility (1:1 Mixture) (Cont.)

Test Drug	Mfr	Conc	Mfr	Conc	Remarks	Ref	C/I
Remifentanil HCl	GW	0.025 and 0.25 mg/mL[b]	AB	3.2 mg/mL[a]	Physically compatible for 4 hr at 23°C	2075	C
Sargramostim	IMM	6[b i] and 15[b] mcg/mL	DU	1.6 mg/mL[c]	Visually compatible for 2 hr	1618	C
Sodium nitroprusside	ES	0.4 mg/mL[c]	DCC	3.2 mg/mL[c]	Physically compatible for 3 hr	1316	C
Sodium nitroprusside	RC	0.3, 1.2, 3 mg/mL[a]	DU	1.5, 6, 15 mg/mL[m]	Visually compatible for 48 hr at 24°C protected from light	2357	C
Sodium nitroprusside with dobutamine HCl	ES LI	0.4 mg/mL[c] 4 mg/mL[c]	DCC	3.2 mg/mL[c]	Physically compatible for 3 hr	1316	C
Sodium nitroprusside with lidocaine HCl	ES AB	0.4 mg/mL[c] 8 mg/mL[c]	DCC	3.2 mg/mL[c]	Physically compatible for 3 hr	1316	C
Sodium nitroprusside with nitroglycerin	ES LY	0.4 mg/mL[c] 0.4 mg/mL[c]	DCC	3.2 mg/mL[c]	Physically compatible for 3 hr	1316	C
Tacrolimus	FUJ	1 mg/mL[b]	ES	1.6 mg/mL[a]	Visually compatible for 24 hr at 25°C	1630	C
Tedizolid phosphate	CUB	0.8 mg/mL[b]	HOS	0.8 mg/mL[b]	Physically compatible for 2 hr	3244	C
Telavancin HCl	ASP	7.5 mg/mL[a b n]	HOS	3.2 mg/mL[a b n]	Physically compatible for 2 hr	2830	C
Theophylline	TR	4 mg/mL	BA	1.6 mg/mL	Visually compatible for 6 hr at 25°C	1793	C
Thiotepa	IMM[j]	1 mg/mL[a]	AST	3.2 mg/mL[a]	Physically compatible for 4 hr at 23°C	1861	C
Tigecycline	WY	1 mg/mL[b]		1.6 mg/mL[b]	Physically compatible for 4 hr	2714	C
Tigecycline	ACD, FRK, WY	[c]			Stated to be compatible	2915, 3459, 3460	C
Tirofiban HCl	ME	0.05 mg/mL[a b]	AMR	0.2 and 3.2 mg/mL[a b]	Physically compatible. Little loss of either drug in 4 hr at room temperature	2250	C
TNA #73[k]			AB	1.6 mg/mL[c]	Visually compatible for 4 hr	1009	C
TNA #222, #223[k]			AB	3.2 mg/mL[a]	Precipitate forms immediately	2215	I
TNA #218 to #221, #224 to #226[k]			AB	3.2 mg/mL[a]	Visually compatible for 4 hr at 23°C	2215	C
TPN #189[k]			DB	1.6 mg/mL[b]	Visually compatible for 24 hr at 22°C	1767	C
TPN #203, #204[k]			AMR	3.2 mg/mL	Visually compatible for 4 hr at 23°C	1974	C
TPN #212 to #215[k]			AB	3.2 mg/mL[a]	Physically compatible for 4 hr at 23°C	2109	C
Vasopressin	AMR	2 and 4 units/mL[b]	AMR	4.2 mg/mL[a]	Physically compatible with vasopressin pushed through a Y-site over 5 sec	2478	C
Vasopressin	APP	0.2 unit/mL[b]	BA	3.2 mg/mL[a]	Physically compatible	2641	C
Vecuronium bromide	OR	0.1 mg/mL[a]	SO	1.6 mg/mL[a]	Physically compatible for 24 hr at 28°C	1337	C
Vecuronium bromide	OR	1 mg/mL	AB	3.2 mg/mL[a]	Visually compatible for 4 hr at 27°C	2062	C
Verapamil HCl				[l]	Physically compatible	840	C

Y-Site Injection Compatibility (1:1 Mixture) (Cont.)

Test Drug	Mfr	Conc	Mfr	Conc	Remarks	Ref	C/I
Zidovudine	BW	4 mg/mL[a]	AB	1.6 mg/mL[a]	Physically compatible for 4 hr at 25°C	1193	C

[a] Tested in dextrose 5%.

[b] Tested in sodium chloride 0.9%.

[c] Tested in both dextrose 5% and sodium chloride 0.9%.

[d] Tested in sterile water for injection.

[e] Tested in dextrose 5%, Ringer's injection, lactated, sodium chloride 0.45%, and sodium chloride 0.9%.

[f] Tested in bacteriostatic sodium chloride 0.9% preserved with benzyl alcohol 0.9%.

[g] Tested in dextrose 5% in Ringer's injection, dextrose 5% in Ringer's injection, lactated, dextrose 5%, Ringer's injection, lactated, and sodium chloride 0.9%.

[h] Tested as the premixed infusion solution.

[i] Tested with albumin human 0.1%.

[j] Lyophilized formulation tested.

[k] Refer to Appendix for the composition of parenteral nutrition solutions. TNA indicates a 3-in-1 admixture, and TPN indicates a 2-in-1 admixture.

[l] Injected into a line being used to infuse dopamine hydrochloride in dextrose 5% in sodium chloride 0.3% with potassium chloride 20 mEq.

[m] Tested in dextrose 5% in sodium chloride 0.45%.

[n] Tested in Ringer's injection, lactated.

[o] Final concentration after mixing.

[p] Nesiritide is incompatible with bisulfite antioxidants used in some drug formulations. The specific formulation of the product to be used should be checked to assure that no sulfite antioxidants are present.

[q] Test performed using the formulation WITHOUT edetate disodium.

[r] Test performed using the formulation WITH edetate disodium.

[s] Tested in either dextrose 5% or in sodium chloride 0.9%, but the report did not specify which solution.

[t] Tested in a 1:1 mixture of (1) dextrose 5% and dextrose 5% in sodium chloride 0.45% with and without potassium chloride 20 mEq/L and also in (2) dextrose 10% in sodium chloride 0.45% with and without potassium chloride 20 mEq/L.

[u] Tested in a 1:1 mixture of dextrose 5% and TPN #274 (see Appendix).

[v] Piperacillin component. Piperacillin in an 8:1 fixed-ratio concentration with tazobactam.

[w] Ceftolozane component. Ceftolozane in a 2:1 fixed-ratio concentration with tazobactam.

[x] Quinupristin and dalfopristin components combined.

[y] Salt not specified.

[z] Test performed using the Cubicin formulation.

[aa] Meropenem component. Meropenem in a 1:1 fixed-ratio concentration with vaborbactam.

[bb] Ceftazidime component. Ceftazidime in a 4:1 fixed-ratio concentration with avibactam.

[cc] Tested in dextrose 5%, sodium chloride 0.9%, and Ringer's injection, lactated.

Selected Revisions May 1, 2020. © Copyright, October 1982.
American Society of Health-System Pharmacists, Inc.

Doripenem
AHFS 8:12.07.08

Products

Doripenem is available in single-use vials containing doripenem 250 or 500 mg on the anhydrous basis.[2916] Reconstitute each vial with 10 mL of sterile water for injection or sodium chloride 0.9% and gently shake to form a 25- or 50-mg/mL suspension, respectively.[2916] These suspensions are not suitable for administration.[2916]

To prepare as a solution suitable for intravenous infusion, withdraw the vial contents using a syringe with a 21-gauge needle and transfer to an appropriately-sized infusion bag of dextrose 5% or sodium chloride 0.9%, shaking gently after addition until the solution is clear.[2916] For a 250-mg dose prepared using the 250-mg vial, the vial contents should be transferred to a 50- or 100-mL infusion bag to yield a doripenem concentration of approximately 4.2 or 2.3 mg/mL, respectively.[2916] For a 500-mg dose prepared using the 500-mg vial, the vial contents should be transferred to a 100-mL infusion bag to yield a doripenem concentration of approximately 4.5 mg/mL.[2916]

Alternatively, for a 250-mg dose prepared using the 500-mg vial, the vial contents should be withdrawn from the vial using a syringe with a 21-gauge needle and added to a 100-mL infusion bag of dextrose 5% or sodium chloride 0.9%.[2916] The bag should be gently shaken until the solution is clear.[2916] Then 55 mL of this solution should be removed and discarded;[2916] the remaining solution delivers 250 mg of doripenem at a concentration of approximately 4.5 mg/mL.[2916]

pH

From 4.5 to 5.5.[2916]

Trade Name(s)

Doribax

Administration

Doripenem is administered by intravenous infusion over 1 hour after dilution in dextrose 5% or sodium chloride 0.9%.[2916]

Stability

Intact vials of doripenem should be stored at controlled room temperature.[2916] After initial reconstitution, the suspension may be stored for up to 1 hour prior to adding to the intravenous solution.[2916]

After dilution in dextrose 5% or sodium chloride 0.9%, the solution may range from colorless to slightly yellow in appearance; variations in color within this range are not indications of differences in drug stability.[2916] The manufacturer states that doripenem is stable for 4 hours in dextrose 5% and 12 hours in sodium chloride 0.9% at room temperature.[2916] If stored under refrigeration, doripenem is stated to be stable for 24 hours in dextrose 5% and 72 hours in sodium chloride 0.9%.[2916] These time frames include both storage and administration.[2916]

Freezing Solutions

The manufacturer states that the initial reconstituted doripenem suspension or diluted solutions for infusion should not be frozen.[2916]

Solutions of doripenem 5 and 10 mg/mL in sodium chloride 0.9% were frozen at −20°C. Upon thawing a visible white precipitate was found. Vigorous shaking for 3 to 12 minutes resulted in the precipitate no longer being visible. Not more than 5% doripenem loss occurred upon 14 days of frozen storage followed by 24 hours of thawing under refrigeration and then 2 hours at room temperature; a similar amount of loss occurred upon 28 days of frozen storage followed by 4 to 6 hours of thawing at room temperature.[2809]

Compatibility Information

Solution Compatibility

Doripenem

Test Soln Name	Mfr	Mfr	Conc/L or %	Remarks	Ref	C/I
Dextrose 5%		JJ	5 g	Physically compatible and less than 5% loss in 4 hr at 25°C and 48 hr at 4°C	2757	C
Dextrose 5%	a b	OMN	1 and 10 g	Visually compatible. Up to 3.6% loss in 8 hr at 25°C under fluorescent light and 48 hr at 4°C	2801	C
Dextrose 5%	a	OMN	5 and 10 g	Visually compatible. 8 to 10% loss in 18 hr at 23°C in dark	2808	C
Dextrose 5%	c	OMN	5 and 10 g	Visually compatible. 6 to 8% loss in 18 hr and 10 to 12% loss in 24 hr at 23°C in dark	2808	C
Dextrose 5%	a c	OMN	5 g	Visually compatible. Up to 10% loss in 16 hours at 25°C and 10 days at 4°C	2809	C

DOI: 10.37573/9781585286850.132

Solution Compatibility (Cont.)

Test Soln Name	Mfr	Mfr	Conc/L or %	Remarks	Ref	C/I
Dextrose 5%	a c	OMN	10 g	Visually compatible. Up to 10% loss in 16 hours at 25°C and 7 days at 4°C	2809	C
Sodium chloride 0.9%		JJ	5 g	Physically compatible and less than 8% loss in 12 hr at 25°C and 72 hr at 4°C	2757	C
Sodium chloride 0.9%	a b	OMN	1 and 10 g	Visually compatible. Up to 6.8% loss in 12 hr at 25°C under fluorescent light and 72 hr at 4°C	2801	C
Sodium chloride 0.9%	a c	OMN	5 and 10 g	Visually compatible. 8 to 10% loss in 24 hr at 23°C in dark	2809	C
Sodium chloride 0.9%	a c	OMN	5 g	Visually compatible. Up to 10% loss in 24 hours at 25°C and 10 days at 4°C	2809	C
Sodium chloride 0.9%	a c	OMN	10 g	Visually compatible. Up to 10% loss in 24 hours at 25°C and 7 days at 4°C	2809	C
Sodium chloride 0.9%		OMJ	5 g	More than 10% loss by 16, 12, and 8 hr at temperatures of 30, 35, and 40°C, respectively	3109	I

a Tested in PVC bags.

b Tested in polyethylene bags.

c Tested in Eclipse elastomeric containers.

Y-Site Injection Compatibility (1:1 Mixture)

Doripenem

Test Drug	Mfr	Conc	Mfr	Conc	Remarks	Ref	C/I
Acyclovir sodium	BED	7 mg/mL[a b]	JJ	5 mg/mL[a b]	Physically compatible for 4 hr at 23°C	2743	C
Amikacin sulfate	BED	5 mg/mL[a b]	JJ	5 mg/mL[a b]	Physically compatible for 4 hr at 23°C	2743	C
Aminophylline	AMR	2.5 mg/mL[a b]	JJ	5 mg/mL[a b]	Physically compatible for 4 hr at 23°C	2743	C
Amiodarone HCl	BED	4 mg/mL[a b]	JJ	5 mg/mL[a b]	Physically compatible for 4 hr at 23°C	2743	C
Amphotericin B	XGN	0.6 mg/mL[a]	JJ	5 mg/mL[a]	Physically compatible for 4 hr at 23°C	2743	C
Amphotericin B	XGN	0.6 mg/mL[a]	JJ	5 mg/mL[b]	Yellow precipitate forms immediately	2743	I
Amphotericin B lipid complex	ENZ	1 mg/mL[a]	JJ	5 mg/mL[a]	Physically compatible for 4 hr at 23°C	2743	C
Amphotericin B lipid complex	ENZ	1 mg/mL[a]	JJ	5 mg/mL[b]	Measured haze increases immediately	2743	I
Amphotericin B liposomal	ASP	1 mg/mL[a]	JJ	5 mg/mL[a]	Physically compatible for 4 hr at 23°C	2743	C
Amphotericin B liposomal	ASP	1 mg/mL[a]	JJ	5 mg/mL[b]	Measured haze increases immediately	2743	I
Anidulafungin	PF	0.5 mg/mL[a b]	JJ	5 mg/mL[a b]	Physically compatible for 4 hr at 23°C	2743	C
Atropine sulfate	BA	0.4 mg/mL	JJ	5 mg/mL[a b]	Physically compatible for 4 hr at 23°C	2743	C
Azithromycin	BA	2 mg/mL[a b]	JJ	5 mg/mL[a b]	Physically compatible for 4 hr at 23°C	2743	C
Bumetanide	BED	0.04 mg/mL[a b]	JJ	5 mg/mL[a b]	Physically compatible for 4 hr at 23°C	2743	C
Calcium gluconate	AMR	40 mg/mL[a b]	JJ	5 mg/mL[a b]	Physically compatible for 4 hr at 23°C	2743	C
Carboplatin	SIC	5 mg/mL[a b]	JJ	5 mg/mL[a b]	Physically compatible for 4 hr at 23°C	2743	C
Caspofungin acetate	ME	0.5 mg/mL[b]	JJ	5 mg/mL[a b]	Physically compatible for 4 hr at 23°C	2743	C
Ceftaroline fosamil	FOR	2.22 mg/mL[a b d]	SHI	5 mg/mL[b]	Physically compatible for 4 hr at 23°C	2826	C
Ceftolozane sulfate–tazobactam sodium	CUB	10 mg/mL[f g]	SHI	4.5 mg/mL[f]	Physically compatible for 2 hr	3262	C

Y-Site Injection Compatibility (1:1 Mixture) (Cont.)

Test Drug	Mfr	Conc	Mfr	Conc	Remarks	Ref	C/I
Ciprofloxacin	BED	2 mg/mL[a b]	JJ	5 mg/mL[a b]	Physically compatible for 4 hr at 23°C	2743	C
Cisplatin	SIC	0.5 mg/mL[b]	JJ	5 mg/mL[a b]	Physically compatible for 4 hr at 23°C	2743	C
Cyclophosphamide	BMS	10 mg/mL[a b]	JJ	5 mg/mL[a b]	Physically compatible for 4 hr at 23°C	2743	C
Cyclosporine	BED	5 mg/mL[a b]	JJ	5 mg/mL[a b]	Physically compatible for 4 hr at 23°C	2743	C
Daptomycin	CUB[e]	10 mg/mL[b]	JJ	5 mg/mL[a b]	Physically compatible for 4 hr at 23°C	2743	C
Dexamethasone sodium phosphate	APP	1 mg/mL[a b]	JJ	5 mg/mL[a b]	Physically compatible for 4 hr at 23°C	2743	C
Diazepam	HOS	5 mg/mL	JJ	5 mg/mL[a b]	Gross white turbid precipitate forms	2743	I
Digoxin	BA	0.25 mg/mL	JJ	5 mg/mL[a b]	Physically compatible for 4 hr at 23°C	2743	C
Diltiazem HCl	BED	5 mg/mL	JJ	5 mg/mL[a b]	Physically compatible for 4 hr at 23°C	2743	C
Diphenhydramine HCl	BA	2 mg/mL[a b]	JJ	5 mg/mL[a b]	Physically compatible for 4 hr at 23°C	2743	C
Dobutamine HCl	HOS	4 mg/mL[a b]	JJ	5 mg/mL[a b]	Physically compatible for 4 hr at 23°C	2743	C
Docetaxel	SAA	0.8 mg/mL[a b]	JJ	5 mg/mL[a b]	Physically compatible for 4 hr at 23°C	2743	C
Dopamine HCl	AMR	3.2 mg/mL[a b]	JJ	5 mg/mL[a b]	Physically compatible for 4 hr at 23°C	2743	C
Doxorubicin HCl	BED	1 mg/mL[a b]	JJ	5 mg/mL[a b]	Physically compatible for 4 hr at 23°C	2743	C
Enalaprilat	SIC	0.1 mg/mL[a b]	JJ	5 mg/mL[a b]	Physically compatible for 4 hr at 23°C	2743	C
Esmolol HCl	BED	10 mg/mL[a b]	JJ	5 mg/mL[a b]	Physically compatible for 4 hr at 23°C	2743	C
Esmolol HCl	MYL	10 mg/mL	SHI	4.5 mg/mL[b]	Physically compatible for 1 hr at 23°C	3533	C
Esomeprazole sodium	ASZ	0.4 mg/mL[b]	JJ	5 mg/mL[a b]	Physically compatible for 4 hr at 23°C	2743	C
Etoposide phosphate	SIC	5 mg/mL[a b]	JJ	5 mg/mL[a b]	Physically compatible for 4 hr at 23°C	2743	C
Famotidine	BED	2 mg/mL[a b]	JJ	5 mg/mL[a b]	Physically compatible for 4 hr at 23°C	2743	C
Fentanyl citrate	HOS	0.05 mg/mL	JJ	5 mg/mL[a b]	Physically compatible for 4 hr at 23°C	2743	C
Fluconazole	HAE	2 mg/mL	JJ	5 mg/mL[a b]	Physically compatible for 4 hr at 23°C	2743	C
Fluorouracil	ABX	16 mg/mL[a b]	JJ	5 mg/mL[a b]	Physically compatible for 4 hr at 23°C	2743	C
Foscarnet sodium	HOS	24 mg/mL	JJ	5 mg/mL[a b]	Physically compatible for 4 hr at 23°C	2743	C
Furosemide	AMR	3 mg/mL[a b]	JJ	5 mg/mL[a b]	Physically compatible for 4 hr at 23°C	2743	C
Gemcitabine HCl	LI	10 mg/mL[b]	JJ	5 mg/mL[a b]	Physically compatible for 4 hr at 23°C	2743	C
Gentamicin sulfate	HOS	5 mg/mL[a b]	JJ	5 mg/mL[a b]	Physically compatible for 4 hr at 23°C	2743	C
Granisetron HCl	RC	0.05 mg/mL[a b]	JJ	5 mg/mL[a b]	Physically compatible for 4 hr at 23°C	2743	C
Heparin sodium	HOS	100 units/mL	JJ	5 mg/mL[a b]	Physically compatible for 4 hr at 23°C	2743	C
Hydrocortisone sodium succinate	PHU	1 mg/mL[a b]	JJ	5 mg/mL[a b]	Physically compatible for 4 hr at 23°C	2743	C
Hydromorphone HCl	BA	1 mg/mL[a b]	JJ	5 mg/mL[a b]	Physically compatible for 4 hr at 23°C	2743	C
Ifosfamide	BMS	20 mg/mL[a b]	JJ	5 mg/mL[a b]	Physically compatible for 4 hr at 23°C	2743	C
Insulin, regular	NOV	1 unit/mL[a b]	JJ	5 mg/mL[a b]	Physically compatible for 4 hr at 23°C	2743	C
Isavuconazonium sulfate	ASP	1.5 mg/mL[f]	SHI	4.5 mg/mL[f]	Physically compatible for 2 hr	3263	C
Labetalol HCl	HOS	2 mg/mL[a b]	JJ	5 mg/mL[a b]	Physically compatible for 4 hr at 23°C	2743	C
Labetalol HCl	HOS	5 mg/mL	SHI	4.5 mg/mL[b]	Physically compatible for 1 hr at 23°C	3533	C

Y-Site Injection Compatibility (1:1 Mixture) (Cont.)

Test Drug	Mfr	Conc	Mfr	Conc	Remarks	Ref	C/I
Letermovir	ME	a		a	Physically compatible	3398	C
Levofloxacin	OMN	5 mg/mL[a][b]	JJ	5 mg/mL[a][b]	Physically compatible for 4 hr at 23°C	2743	C
Linezolid	PHU	2 mg/mL	JJ	5 mg/mL[a][b]	Physically compatible for 4 hr at 23°C	2743	C
Lorazepam	BED	0.5 mg/mL[a][b]	JJ	5 mg/mL[a][b]	Physically compatible for 4 hr at 23°C	2743	C
Magnesium sulfate	AMR	100 mg/mL[a][b]	JJ	5 mg/mL[a][b]	Physically compatible for 4 hr at 23°C	2743	C
Mannitol	HOS	15%	JJ	5 mg/mL[a][b]	Physically compatible for 4 hr at 23°C	2743	C
Meperidine HCl	HOS	10 mg/mL[a][b]	JJ	5 mg/mL[a][b]	Physically compatible for 4 hr at 23°C	2743	C
Meropenem–vaborbactam	TMC	8 mg/mL[b][h]	APO	10 mg/mL[b]	Physically compatible for 3 hr at 20 to 25°C	3380	C
Methotrexate sodium	BED	12.5 mg/mL[a][b]	JJ	5 mg/mL[a][b]	Physically compatible for 4 hr at 23°C	2743	C
Methylprednisolone sodium succinate	PHU	5 mg/mL[a][b]	JJ	5 mg/mL[a][b]	Physically compatible for 4 hr at 23°C	2743	C
Metoclopramide HCl	HOS	5 mg/mL	JJ	5 mg/mL[a][b]	Physically compatible for 4 hr at 23°C	2743	C
Metoprolol tartrate	HOS	0.4 mg/mL[b]	SHI	4.5 mg/mL[b]	Physically compatible for 1 hr at 23°C	3533	C
Metronidazole	BA	5 mg/mL	JJ	5 mg/mL[a][b]	Physically compatible for 4 hr at 23°C	2743	C
Micafungin sodium	ASP	1.5 mg/mL[a][b]	JJ	5 mg/mL[a][b]	Physically compatible for 4 hr at 23°C	2743	C
Midazolam HCl	BED	2 mg/mL[a][b]	JJ	5 mg/mL[a][b]	Physically compatible for 4 hr at 23°C	2743	C
Milrinone lactate	BA	0.2 mg/mL[a][b]	JJ	5 mg/mL[a][b]	Physically compatible for 4 hr at 23°C	2743	C
Morphine sulfate	BA	15 mg/mL	JJ	5 mg/mL[a][b]	Physically compatible for 4 hr at 23°C	2743	C
Moxifloxacin HCl	BAY	1.6 mg/mL	JJ	5 mg/mL[a][b]	Physically compatible for 4 hr at 23°C	2743	C
Norepinephrine bitartrate	BED	0.128 mg/mL[a][b]	JJ	5 mg/mL[a][b]	Physically compatible for 4 hr at 23°C	2743	C
Ondansetron HCl	WOC	1 mg/mL[a][b]	JJ	5 mg/mL[a][b]	Physically compatible for 4 hr at 23°C	2743	C
Paclitaxel	MAY	0.6 mg/mL[a][b]	JJ	5 mg/mL[a][b]	Physically compatible for 4 hr at 23°C	2743	C
Pantoprazole sodium	WY[c]	0.4 mg/mL[a][b]	JJ	5 mg/mL[a][b]	Physically compatible for 4 hr at 23°C	2743	C
Phenobarbital sodium	BA	5 mg/mL[a][b]	JJ	5 mg/mL[a][b]	Physically compatible for 4 hr at 23°C	2743	C
Phenylephrine HCl	GNS	1 mg/mL[a][b]	JJ	5 mg/mL[a][b]	Physically compatible for 4 hr at 23°C	2743	C
Plazomicin sulfate	ACH	24 mg/mL[f]	SHI	10 mg/mL[f]	Physically compatible for 1 hr at 20 to 25°C	3432	C
Potassium chloride	APP	0.1 mEq/mL[a][b]	JJ	5 mg/mL[a][b]	Physically compatible for 4 hr at 23°C	2743	C
Potassium phosphates	APP	0.5 mmol/mL[a][b]	JJ	5 mg/mL[a][b]	Measured haze increases after 1 hr	2743	I
Propofol	BED	10 mg/mL	JJ	5 mg/mL[a][b]	Precipitation forms immediately	2743	I
Ranitidine HCl	BED	2 mg/mL[a][b]	JJ	5 mg/mL[a][b]	Physically compatible for 4 hr at 23°C	2743	C
Sodium bicarbonate	HOS	1 mEq/mL	JJ	5 mg/mL[a][b]	Physically compatible for 4 hr at 23°C	2743	C
Sodium phosphates	AMR	0.5 mmol/mL[a][b]	JJ	5 mg/mL[a][b]	Physically compatible for 4 hr at 23°C	2743	C
Tacrolimus	ASP	0.02 mg/mL[a][b]	JJ	5 mg/mL[a][b]	Physically compatible for 4 hr at 23°C	2743	C
Tedizolid phosphate	CUB	0.8 mg/mL[b]	SHI	5 mg/mL[b]	Physically compatible for 2 hr	3244	C

Y-Site Injection Compatibility (1:1 Mixture) (Cont.)

Test Drug	Mfr	Conc	Mfr	Conc	Remarks	Ref	C/I
Telavancin HCl	ASP	7.5 mg/mL[a b]	OMN	10 mg/mL[a b]	Physically compatible for 2 hr	2830	C
Tigecycline	WY	1 mg/mL[a b]	JJ	5 mg/mL[a b]	Physically compatible for 4 hr at 23°C	2743	C
Tobramycin sulfate	SIC	5 mg/mL[a b]	JJ	5 mg/mL[a b]	Physically compatible for 4 hr at 23°C	2743	C
Vancomycin HCl	HOS	10 mg/mL[a b]	JJ	5 mg/mL[a b]	Physically compatible for 4 hr at 23°C	2743	C
Voriconazole	PF	4 mg/mL[a b]	JJ	5 mg/mL[a b]	Physically compatible for 4 hr at 23°C	2743	C
Zidovudine	GSK	4 mg/mL[a b]	JJ	5 mg/mL[a b]	Physically compatible for 4 hr at 23°C	2743	C

[a] Tested in dextrose 5%.

[b] Tested in sodium chloride 0.9%.

[c] Test performed using the formulation WITH edetate disodium.

[d] Tested in Ringer's injection, lactated.

[e] Test performed using the Cubicin formulation.

[f] Tested in both dextrose 5% and sodium chloride 0.9%.

[g] Ceftolozane component. Ceftolozane in a 2:1 fixed-ratio concentration with tazobactam.

[h] Meropenem component. Meropenem in a 1:1 fixed-ratio concentration with vaborbactam.

Selected Revisions May 1, 2020. © Copyright, October 2010.
American Society of Health-System Pharmacists, Inc.

Doxapram Hydrochloride
AHFS 28:20.32

Products

Doxapram hydrochloride is available in 20-mL multiple-dose vials.[3220] Each mL of solution contains doxapram hydrochloride 20 mg and benzyl alcohol 0.9% in water for injection.[3220]

Infusions of doxapram may be prepared by transferring 12.5 mL (250 mg) of doxapram hydrochloride to an infusion bag containing 250 mL of dextrose 5%, dextrose 10%, or sodium chloride 0.9% or adding 20 mL (400 mg) of doxapram hydrochloride to 180 mL of dextrose 5%, dextrose 10%, or sodium chloride 0.9%; the concentration to be prepared is dependent upon the indication.[3220]

pH

The pH of the undiluted injection ranges from 3.5 to 5.[3220]

Trade Name(s)

Dopram

Administration

Doxapram hydrochloride is administered by intravenous injection or by intravenous infusion following dilution in a compatible infusion solution.[3220]

Stability

Doxapram hydrochloride is a clear, colorless solution.[3220] Intact vials of doxapram hydrochloride injection should be stored at controlled room temperature.[3220]

pH Effects

Doxapram hydrochloride in solution became turbid when the pH was adjusted from 3.8 to 5.7 with 0.1 N sodium hydroxide.[1177] When the pH was adjusted down to 1.9 with 0.1 N hydrochloric acid, no visible change occurred to the clear solution.[1177] The drug is stated to be incompatible with alkaline drugs.[3220]

At pH 2.5 to 6.5, doxapram hydrochloride remained chemically stable for 24 hours.[1177] At pH 7.5 and above, a 10 to 15% doxapram hydrochloride loss occurred in about 6 hours.[1177]

Compatibility Information

Solution Compatibility

Doxapram HCl

Test Soln Name	Mfr	Mfr	Conc/L or %	Remarks	Ref	C/I
Dextrose 5%		WW	1 and 2 g	Stated to be stable	3220	C
Dextrose 10%		WW	1 and 2 g	Stated to be stable	3220	C
Sodium chloride 0.9%		WW	1 and 2 g	Stated to be stable	3220	C

Additive Compatibility

Doxapram HCl

Test Drug	Mfr	Conc/L or %	Mfr	Conc/L or %	Test Solution	Remarks	Ref	C/I
Aminophylline			WW			Precipitation or gas formation	3220	I
Furosemide			WW			Precipitation or gas formation	3220	I
Minocycline HCl			WW			8% doxapram loss in 3 hr and 13% loss in 6 hr	3220	I
Sodium bicarbonate			WW			Precipitation or gas formation	3220	I

DOI: 10.37573/9781585286850.133

Drugs in Syringe Compatibility

Doxapram HCl

Test Drug	Mfr	Amt	Mfr	Amt	Remarks	Ref	C/I
Amikacin sulfate		100 mg/2 mL	RB	400 mg/20 mL	Physically compatible with no doxapram loss in 24 hr	1177	C
Aminophylline		250 mg/10 mL	RB	400 mg/20 mL	Immediate turbidity and precipitation	1177	I
Ascorbic acid		500 mg/2 mL	RB	400 mg/20 mL	Immediate turbidity changing to precipitation in 24 hr	1177	I
Bumetanide		0.5 mg/1 mL	RB	400 mg/20 mL	Physically compatible with 3% doxapram loss in 24 hr	1177	C
Cefotaxime sodium		500 mg/4 mL	RB	400 mg/20 mL	Precipitates immediately	1177	I
Cefotetan disodium		1 g/10 mL	RB	400 mg/20 mL	Immediate turbidity	1177	I
Cefuroxime sodium	GL	750 mg/7 mL	RB	400 mg/20 mL	Immediate turbidity	1177	I
Chlorpromazine HCl		250 mg/5 mL	RB	400 mg/20 mL	Physically compatible with no doxapram loss in 24 hr	1177	C
Cisplatin		10 mg/20 mL	RB	400 mg/20 mL	Physically compatible with no doxapram loss in 24 hr	1177	C
Cyclophosphamide		100 mg/5 mL	RB	400 mg/20 mL	Physically compatible with 2% doxapram loss in 24 hr	1177	C
Dexamethasone sodium phosphate	MSD	3.3 mg/1 mL	RB	400 mg/20 mL	Immediate turbidity and precipitation	1177	I
Diazepam		10 mg/2 mL	RB	400 mg/20 mL	Immediate turbidity and precipitation	1177	I
Digoxin		0.25 mg/1 mL	RB	400 mg/20 mL	10% doxapram loss in 9 hr and 17% in 24 hr	1177	I
Dobutamine HCl	LI	100 mg/10 mL	RB	400 mg/20 mL	5% doxapram loss in 3 hr and 11% in 24 hr	1177	I
Dopamine HCl		100 mg/5 mL	RB	400 mg/20 mL	Physically compatible with 3% doxapram loss in 24 hr	1177	C
Doxycycline hyclate		100 mg/5 mL	RB	400 mg/20 mL	Physically compatible with 3% doxapram loss in 24 hr	1177	C
Epinephrine HCl		1 mg/1 mL	RB	400 mg/20 mL	Physically compatible with no doxapram loss in 24 hr	1177	C
Folic acid		15 mg/1 mL	RB	400 mg/20 mL	Immediate turbidity	1177	I
Furosemide	HO	100 mg/10 mL	RB	400 mg/20 mL	Immediate turbidity	1177	I
Hydrocortisone sodium succinate	UP	500 mg/2 mL	RB	400 mg/20 mL	Immediate turbidity and precipitation	1177	I
Hydroxyzine HCl		25 mg/1 mL	RB	400 mg/20 mL	Physically compatible with no doxapram loss in 24 hr	1177	C
Isoniazid		100 mg/2 mL	RB	400 mg/20 mL	Physically compatible with 2% doxapram loss in 24 hr	1177	C
Ketamine HCl	PD	200 mg/20 mL	RB	400 mg/20 mL	Physically compatible with no doxapram loss in 9 hr but 12% loss in 24 hr	1177	I
Lincomycin HCl		300 mg/1 mL	RB	400 mg/20 mL	Physically compatible with no doxapram loss in 24 hr	1177	C
Methotrexate sodium		50 mg/20 mL	RB	400 mg/20 mL	Physically compatible with 4% doxapram loss in 24 hr	1177	C
Methylprednisolone sodium succinate	UP	40 mg/2 mL	RB	400 mg/20 mL	Immediate turbidity and precipitation	1177	I
Phytonadione		10 mg/1 mL	RB	400 mg/20 mL	Physically compatible with no doxapram loss in 24 hr	1177	C
Pyridoxine HCl		10 mg/1 mL	RB	400 mg/20 mL	Physically compatible with 6% doxapram loss in 24 hr	1177	C
Terbutaline sulfate		0.2 mg/1 mL	RB	400 mg/20 mL	Physically compatible with 6% doxapram loss in 24 hr	1177	C
Thiamine HCl		10 mg/2 mL	RB	400 mg/20 mL	Physically compatible with 6% doxapram loss in 24 hr	1177	C
Tobramycin sulfate		60 mg/1.5 mL	RB	400 mg/20 mL	Physically compatible with no doxapram loss in 24 hr	1177	C
Tranexamic acid		250 mg/5 mL	RB	400 mg/20 mL	5% doxapram loss in 9 hr and 12% in 24 hr	1177	I
Vincristine sulfate		1 mg/10 mL	RB	400 mg/20 mL	Physically compatible with 7% doxapram loss in 24 hr	1177	C

Y-Site Injection Compatibility (1:1 Mixture)

Doxapram HCl

Test Drug	Mfr	Conc	Mfr	Conc	Remarks	Ref	C/I
Ampicillin sodium	APO	50 mg/mL[b]	RB	2 mg/mL[a]	Visually compatible for 4 hr at 23°C	2470	C
Caffeine citrate	BI	20 mg/mL	RB	2 mg/mL[a]	Visually compatible for 4 hr at 23°C	2470	C
Calcium chloride	APP	100 mg/mL	RB	2 mg/mL[a]	Visually compatible for 4 hr at 23°C	2470	C
Calcium gluconate	APP	100 mg/mL	RB	2 mg/mL[a]	Visually compatible for 4 hr at 23°C	2470	C
Cefazolin sodium	APO	100 mg/mL[a]	RB	2 mg/mL[a]	Visually compatible for 4 hr at 23°C	2470	C
Ceftazidime	GW	40 mg/mL[a]	RB	2 mg/mL[a]	Visually compatible for 4 hr at 23°C	2470	C
Clindamycin phosphate	PHU	10 mg/mL[a]	RB	2 mg/mL[a]	Gas bubbles evolve immediately	2470	I
Erythromycin lactobionate	AB	5 mg/mL[a]	RB	2 mg/mL[a]	Visually compatible for 4 hr at 23°C	2470	C
Fentanyl citrate	ESL	25 mcg/mL[a]	RB	2 mg/mL[a]	Visually compatible for 4 hr at 23°C	2470	C
Gentamicin sulfate	APP	10 mg/mL[a]	RB	2 mg/mL[a]	Visually compatible for 4 hr at 23°C	2470	C
Heparin sodium	APP	1 unit/mL[c]	RB	2 mg/mL[a]	Visually compatible for 4 hr at 23°C	2470	C
Insulin, regular	NOV	1 unit/mL[c]	RB	2 mg/mL[a]	Visually compatible for 4 hr at 23°C	2470	C
Metoclopramide HCl	AB	1 mg/mL	RB	2 mg/mL[a]	Visually compatible for 4 hr at 23°C	2470	C
Metronidazole	AB	5 mg/mL	RB	2 mg/mL[a]	Visually compatible for 4 hr at 23°C	2470	C
Oxacillin sodium	APO	20 mg/mL[a]	RB	2 mg/mL[a]	Visually compatible for 4 hr at 23°C	2470	C
Phenobarbital sodium	ES	10 mg/mL[b]	RB	2 mg/mL[a]	Visually compatible for 4 hr at 23°C	2470	C
Ranitidine HCl	GSK	5 mg/mL[a]	RB	2 mg/mL[a]	Visually compatible for 4 hr at 23°C	2470	C
Vancomycin HCl	APP	5 mg/mL[a]	RB	2 mg/mL[a]	Visually compatible for 4 hr at 23°C	2470	C

[a] Tested in dextrose 5%.

[b] Tested in sodium chloride 0.9%.

[c] Tested in sodium chloride 0.45%.

Selected Revisions June 16, 2017. © Copyright, October 1990.
American Society of Health-System Pharmacists, Inc.

Doxorubicin Hydrochloride
AHFS 10:00

Products

Doxorubicin hydrochloride is available as a lyophilized product in 10-, 20-, and 50-mg single-dose glass vials with 50 mg of lactose for each 10 mg of doxorubicin hydrochloride.[1(10/06)]

Reconstitution of the lyophilized products should be performed with sodium chloride 0.9%. Bacteriostatic diluents are not recommended. Add 5, 10, or 25 mL sodium chloride 0.9% to the 10-, 20-, or 50-mg vial, respectively. After the diluent is added, the vial should be shaken and the drug allowed to dissolve, forming a 2-mg/mL solution.[1(10/06)]

Additionally, doxorubicin hydrochloride is available in 5-, 10-, 25-, and 100-mL vials as a 2-mg/mL solution without preservatives. The solution also contains sodium chloride 0.9% and hydrochloric acid to adjust the pH in water for injection.[1(10/06)]

pH

The pH of lyophilized doxorubicin hydrochloride reconstituted with sodium chloride 0.9% is 3.8 to 6.5.[4] The pH of the solution products is adjusted to 3.[1(10/06)]

Trade Name(s)

Adriamycin

Administration

Doxorubicin hydrochloride is administered intravenously, preferably into the tubing of a running intravenous infusion of sodium chloride 0.9% or dextrose 5% over not less than 3 to 5 minutes.[1(10/06)] [4] The drug should not be administered intramuscularly or subcutaneously, and extravasation should be avoided because of local tissue necrosis.[1(10/06)]

In the event of spills or leaks, a doxorubicin hydrochloride manufacturer recommends the use of sodium hypochlorite 5% (household bleach) for inactivation.[1200]

Stability

Doxorubicin hydrochloride liquid injections should be stored under refrigeration and protected from light. Intact vials should be kept in their cartons until use.[1(10/06)] [4]

The lyophilized products in intact vials should be stored at room temperature and protected from light. The manufacturer states that its reconstituted lyophilized products are stable for 7 days at room temperature and 15 days under refrigeration.[1(10/06)]

For 50-mcg/mL and 0.5-mg/mL doxorubicin hydrochloride solutions, Janssen et al. reported that a greater rate of decomposition occurred in the more concentrated solution.[1206] However, most other studies found no concentration dependence for the degradation rate.[489 526 1208 1255]

A darkening of doxorubicin hydrochloride color has been noted when solutions of the drug contact aluminum metal. This change was initially noticed in the first small amount of drug to be injected through a needle with an aluminum hub. When solutions of doxorubicin hydrochloride containing aluminum are allowed to stand, the color becomes much darker than the control. Precipitation may also occur. As a precautionary measure, the author recommended not using any aluminum-containing apparatus for preparing or administering doxorubicin hydrochloride.[653]

In another evaluation, stainless steel needles with steel or plastic hubs and pieces of aluminum were immersed in doxorubicin hydrochloride 2 mg/mL in sterile water for injection or sodium chloride 0.9%. After 24 hours, the solutions containing the needles were unchanged in appearance and pH. The solution containing the aluminum was darker in color, and the pH had changed from 4.8 to 5.2. The concentrations of all solutions remained the same after 6 hours, but after 3 days, the solution containing aluminum was down to 91.9% while the others were only down to 94.4%. The authors concluded that doxorubicin hydrochloride does react with aluminum but at a slow rate and without major loss. They recommended not storing the drug in syringes capped with aluminum-hubbed needles but thought that doxorubicin could be injected safely through aluminum-hubbed needles.[887]

Immersion of a needle with an aluminum component in doxorubicin hydrochloride (Adria) 2 mg/mL resulted in a darkening of the solution, with black patches forming on the aluminum in 12 to 24 hours at 24°C with protection from light.[988]

Doxorubicin hydrochloride 0.5 mg/mL in sodium chloride 0.9% supported the growth of *Escherichia coli*, *Klebsiella pneumoniae*, *Pseudomonas aeruginosa*, and *Candida albicans*, which are implicated in nosocomial infections. The arbitrary extension of expiration dates to doxorubicin hydrochloride solutions is highly questionable.[827]

Doxorubicin hydrochloride, etoposide phosphate, and vincristine sulfate admixtures at a variety of concentrations were unable to pass the USP test for antimicrobial effectiveness. Mixtures of these drugs are not "self-preserving" and permit microbial growth.[2343] The potential for microbiological growth should be considered when assigning expiration periods.

pH Effects

Doxorubicin hydrochloride appears to have pH-dependent stability in solution.[526 1007 1037] It becomes progressively more stable as the pH of drug–infusion solution admixtures becomes more acidic at 7.4 to 4.5.[526] The pH range of maximum stability has been variously stated to be about 4 to 5,[1007 1460] 3 to 4,[1037] and about 4.[1208] At a concentration of 0.1 mg/mL in buffer solutions stored at 4°C, no significant doxorubicin loss occurred in 60 days at pH 4, but substantial decomposition occurred at pH 7.4.[1206] Doxorubicin hydrochloride is unstable at pH values less than 3 or greater than 7.[4] In acidic media, splitting of the glycosidic bond results in a red-colored, water-insoluble aglycone and

DOI: 10.37573/9781585286850.134

a water-soluble amino sugar.[4] In alkaline media, a color change to deep purple is indicative of decomposition. This color change also occurs with other anthracyclines.[394] It is thought to reflect cleavage of the amino sugar, resulting in an ineffective moiety.[524]

Freezing Solutions

Hoffman et al. found that doxorubicin hydrochloride, reconstituted to 2 mg/mL with sterile water for injection and kept at 4°C, exhibited a 1.5% loss in 1 month and a 10.5% loss in 6 months. Freezing the solutions at −20°C resulted in no loss over 30 days. It was indicated that filtration of stored solutions through a 0.22-μm filter was appropriate to ensure sterility.[652]

Doxorubicin hydrochloride (Farmitalia) 70 mg/50 mL in polyvinyl chloride (PVC) bags of sodium chloride 0.9% (Travenol) could be frozen at −20°C for at least 30 days and thawed by exposure to microwave radiation for 2 minutes with no significant change in concentration. However, the doxorubicin hydrochloride concentration apparently began declining after the fourth repetition of the freeze-thaw treatment with a loss of about 5%.[818]

The stability of doxorubicin hydrochloride 1 mg/mL in sodium chloride 0.9% in PVC containers at −20°C was evaluated. No drug loss occurred after 2 weeks of storage and thawing for 150 minutes at room temperature or 180 seconds in a microwave oven. Refreezing the solutions and rethawing at room temperature or in a microwave oven 3 weeks later (total of 5 weeks of frozen storage) resulted in 3% drug loss.[1256]

Although the thawing of frozen doxorubicin hydrochloride solutions in microwave ovens has been suggested,[818 1256] Williamson recommended only room temperature thawing because of the risks of drug decomposition from overheating and exposure if the bags burst.[1257]

Light Effects

Doxorubicin hydrochloride is sensitive to light, especially in very dilute solutions.[489 1073 1094] However, the photolability of dilute solutions is not observed with more concentrated solutions. A 10-fold difference in photolability half-life was found between concentrations of 0.01 and 0.1 mg/mL.[1594] The manufacturers recommend protecting the solutions from exposure to sunlight and that any unused solution be discarded.[1(10/06) 4]

An evaluation of etoposide phosphate (Bristol-Myers Squibb) 2 mg/mL, doxorubicin hydrochloride 0.4 mg/mL, and vincristine sulfate 0.016 mg/mL (16 mcg/mL) in sodium chloride 0.9% in polyolefin plastic bags (McGaw) found little or no effect of constant exposure to normal fluorescent room light for 124 hours. The admixtures were physically compatible, and all 3 drugs in the admixture remained stable throughout the time period stored at an elevated temperature of 35 to 40°C.[2343]

Syringes

Doxorubicin hydrochloride (Farmitalia) 2 mg/mL repackaged in polypropylene syringes exhibited little loss after storage for 43 days at 4°C.[1460]

Doxorubicin hydrochloride (Adria) 2 mg/mL in sodium chloride 0.9% in glass vials and plastic syringes (Monoject and Terumo) and also 1 mg/mL in sodium chloride 0.9% in plastic

syringes (Monoject) exhibited no visual changes and little or no loss when stored at 4 and 23°C while exposed to light for 124 days. Potential extractable materials from the syringes were not detected during the study period.[1594]

Implantable Pumps

Vogelzang et al. reported the stability of 3- and 5-mg/mL concentrations in sodium chloride 0.9% in the reservoir of a Medtronic DAD implantable pump at 37°C. Losses of about 5 to 6% in 1 week and 9 to 11% in 2 weeks occurred. Analyses after longer periods continued to show about a 5 to 6% loss per week at 37°C.[1255]

Sorption

Doxorubicin hydrochloride 16 mcg/mL in dextrose 5% and sodium chloride 0.9% in PVC containers was infused through PVC infusion sets at 21 mL/hr over 24 hours at 22°C while exposed to light. No evidence of sorption was found.[1700]

Doxorubicin hydrochloride (Farmitalia) 1 mg/mL in sodium chloride 0.9% exhibited no loss due to sorption to PVC and polyethylene administration lines during simulated infusions at 0.875 mL/hr for 2.5 hours via a syringe pump.[1795]

Filtration

Although doxorubicin hydrochloride was reported to undergo considerable binding to cellulose ester and polytetrafluoroethylene filters,[1249 1415 1416] other studies did not confirm unacceptable losses at clinical concentrations. Doxorubicin hydrochloride 2 mg/mL in sterile water for injection showed no loss due to filtration when filtered through a 0.22-μm Millex filter.[652]

In another study, doxorubicin hydrochloride (Adria) 30 mg/15 mL was injected as a bolus through a 0.2-μm nylon, air-eliminating filter (Ultipor, Pall) to evaluate the effect of filtration on simulated intravenous push delivery. About 92% of the drug was delivered through the filter after flushing with 10 mL of sodium chloride 0.9%.[809]

Doxorubicin hydrochloride 1 mg/mL in sodium chloride 0.9% exhibited little loss due to sorption to cellulose acetate (Minisart 45, Sartorius), polysulfone (Acrodisc 45, Gelman), and nylon (Nylaflo, Gelman) filters. However, a 20 to 25% loss due to sorption occurred during the first 60 minutes of infusion through nylon filters (Utipore, Pall). A 35% loss was found during the first 15 min using a nylon filter (Posidyne ELD96, Pall). Return to the full concentrations occurred gradually within 1.5 to 2.5 hours.[1795]

Central Venous Catheter

Doxorubicin hydrochloride (Pharmacia) 0.25 mg/mL in dextrose 5% was found to be compatible with the ARROWg+ard Blue Plus (Arrow International) chlorhexidine-bearing triple-lumen central catheter. Essentially complete delivery of the drug was found with little or no drug loss occurring. Furthermore, chlorhexidine delivered from the catheter remained at trace amounts with no substantial increase due to the delivery of the drug through the catheter.[2335]

Compatibility Information

Solution Compatibility

Doxorubicin HCl

Test Soln Name	Mfr	Mfr	Conc/L or %	Remarks	Ref	C/I
Dextrose 3.3% in sodium chloride 0.3%			100 mg	5% loss in 4 weeks at 25°C in the dark	1007	C
Dextrose 5%	TR[a]	AD	180 mg	10% loss in 40 hr at room temperature along with a color change and an increase in pH	519	C
Dextrose 5%	TR[b]	AD	180 mg	No decrease in 48 hr at room temperature	519	C
Dextrose 5%	AB[a]	AD	10 and 20 mg	Physically compatible. 2% loss in 24 hr at 21°C in fluorescent light	526	C
Dextrose 5%			100 mg	5% loss in 4 weeks at 25°C in the dark	1007	C
Dextrose 5%	[c]	BEL	0.5 g	Visually compatible. 5% loss in 28 days at 4°C and 14 days at 22 and 35°C in the dark	1548	C
Dextrose 5%	[c]	BEL	1.25 g	Visually compatible. 5% loss in 28 days at 4 and 22°C and 7 days at 35°C in the dark	1548	C
Dextrose 5%	MG[d], TR[b]		180 mg	Less than 10% loss in 48 hr at room temperature in light	1658	C
Dextrose 5%	[b]		40 mg	10% loss in 7 days at 4°C in the dark	1700	C
Dextrose 5%	TR[b]	FA	100 mg	10% or less loss in 43 days at −20, 4, and 25°C in the dark	1460	C
Ringer's injection, lactated	AB[a]	AD	10 and 20 mg	Physically compatible. 8% loss in 24 hr at 21°C in fluorescent light	526	C
Ringer's injection, lactated			100 mg	10% loss in 1.7 days at 25°C in the dark	1007	C
Sodium chloride 0.9%	AB[a]	AD	10 and 20 mg	Physically compatible. 5% in 24 hr at 21°C in fluorescent light	526	C
Sodium chloride 0.9%			100 mg	10% loss in 6 days at 25°C in the dark	1007	C
Sodium chloride 0.9%	TR[b]	FA	100 mg	10% or less loss in 43 days at −20, 4, and 25°C in the dark	1460	C
Sodium chloride 0.9%	BA[e]	CET	2 g	Stable for 14 days at 3 and 23°C plus 28 days at 30°C	1538	C
Sodium chloride 0.9%	[c]	BEL	0.5 g	Visually compatible. 5% or less loss in 14 days at 4 and 22°C and 7 days at 35°C in the dark	1548	C
Sodium chloride 0.9%	[c]	BEL	1.25 g	Visually compatible. 5% or less loss in 28 days at 4 and 22°C and 7 days at 35°C in the dark	1548	C
Sodium chloride 0.9%	[b]		40 mg	6% loss in 7 days at 4°C in the dark	1700	C

[a] Tested in glass containers.

[b] Tested in PVC containers.

[c] Tested in ethylene vinyl acetate (EVA) containers.

[d] Tested in both glass and polyolefin containers.

[e] Tested in Pharmacia Deltec reservoirs.

Additive Compatibility

Doxorubicin HCl

Test Drug	Mfr	Conc/L or %	Mfr	Conc/L or %	Test Solution	Remarks	Ref	C/I
Aminophylline			AD			Discolors from red to purple	524	I
Dacarbazine with ondansetron HCl	LY GL	8 g 640 mg	AD	800 mg	D5W[a]	Visually compatible. Under 10% ondansetron and doxorubicin loss in 24 hr at 30°C and 7 days at 4°C then 24 hr at 30°C. Dacarbazine stable for 8 hr but 13% loss in 24 hr	2092	I

Additive Compatibility (Cont.)

Test Drug	Mfr	Conc/L or %	Mfr	Conc/L or %	Test Solution	Remarks	Ref	C/I
Dacarbazine with ondansetron HCl	LY GL	8 g 640 mg	AD	800 mg	D5W[b]	Visually compatible. Under 10% loss of all drugs in 24 hr at 30°C and 7 days at 4°C then 24 hr at 30°C	2092	C
Dacarbazine with ondansetron HCl	LY GL	20 g 640 mg	AD	1.5 g	D5W[a b]	Visually compatible. Under 10% loss of all drugs in 24 hr at 30°C and 7 days at 4°C then 24 hr at 30°C	2092	C
Diazepam	RC		AD			Precipitates immediately	524	I
Etoposide with vincristine sulfate	BMS LI	200 mg 1.6 mg	PHU	40 mg	NS[c]	Visually compatible. All drugs stable for 72 hr at 30°C in the dark	2239	C
Etoposide with vincristine sulfate	BMS LI	125 mg 1 mg	PHU	25 mg	NS[c]	Visually compatible. All drugs stable for 96 hr at 24°C in light or dark	2239	C
Etoposide with vincristine sulfate	BMS LI	175 mg 1.4 mg	PHU	35 mg	NS[c]	Visually compatible. All drugs stable for 96 hr at 24°C in light or dark	2239	C
Etoposide with vincristine sulfate	BMS LI	250 mg 2 mg	PHU	50 mg	NS[c]	Visually compatible. All drugs stable for 48 hr at 24°C in light or dark. Etoposide precipitate in 72 hr	2239	C
Etoposide with vincristine sulfate	BMS LI	350 mg 2.8 mg	PHU	70 mg	NS[c]	Visually compatible. All drugs stable for 24 hr at 24°C in light or dark. Etoposide precipitate in 36 hr	2239	C
Etoposide with vincristine sulfate	BMS LI	500 mg 4 mg	PHU	100 mg	NS[c]	Etoposide precipitate formed in 12 hr at 24°C in light or dark	2239	I
Etoposide phosphate with vincristine sulfate	BMS LI	600 mg 5 mg	PHU	120 mg	NS[c]	Physically compatible. Little loss of any drug in 124 hr at 4 and 40°C	2343	C
Etoposide phosphate with vincristine sulfate	BMS LI	1.2 g 10 mg	PHU	240 mg	NS[c]	Physically compatible. Little loss of any drug in 124 hr at 4 and 40°C	2343	C
Etoposide phosphate with vincristine sulfate	BMS LI	2 g 16 mg	PHU	400 mg	NS[c]	Physically compatible. Under 4% loss of any drug in 124 hr at 4 and 40°C	2343	C
Fluorouracil			AD			Discolors from red to blue-purple	524	I
Fluorouracil	RC	250 mg	AD	10 mg	D5W	Color changes to deep purple	296	I
Ondansetron HCl	GL	30 and 300 mg	MJ	100 mg and 2 g	D5W[a]	Physically compatible with little loss of either drug in 48 hr at 23°C	1876	C
Ondansetron HCl with dacarbazine	GL LY	640 mg 8 g	AD	800 mg	D5W[a]	Visually compatible. Under 10% ondansetron and doxorubicin loss in 24 hr at 30°C and 7 days at 4°C then 24 hr at 30°C. Dacarbazine stable for 8 hr but 13% loss in 24 hr	2092	I
Ondansetron HCl with dacarbazine	GL LY	640 mg 8 g	AD	800 mg	D5W[b]	Visually compatible. Under 10% loss of all drugs in 24 hr at 30°C and 7 days at 4°C then 24 hr at 30°C	2092	C
Ondansetron HCl with dacarbazine	GL LY	640 mg 20 g	AD	1.5 g	D5W[a b]	Visually compatible. Under 10% loss of all drugs in 24 hr at 30°C and 7 days at 4°C then 24 hr at 30°C	2092	C
Ondansetron HCl with vincristine sulfate	GL LI	480 mg 14 mg	AD	400 mg	D5W[b]	Visually compatible. Under 10% loss of all drugs in 5 days at 4°C then 24 hr at 30°C	2092	C
Ondansetron HCl with vincristine sulfate	GL LI	960 mg 28 mg	AD	800 mg	D5W[a]	Visually compatible. Under 10% loss of all drugs after 120 hr at 30°C	2092	C
Paclitaxel	BMS	300 mg	PH	200 mg	D5W, NS	Visually compatible for 1 day with microprecipitation in 3 to 5 days and gross precipitation in 7 days at 4, 23, and 32°C in the dark. No paclitaxel and under 8% doxorubicin loss in 7 days	2247	C

Additive Compatibility (Cont.)

Test Drug	Mfr	Conc/L or %	Mfr	Conc/L or %	Test Solution	Remarks	Ref	C/I
Paclitaxel	BMS	1.2 g	PH	200 mg	D5W, NS	Visually compatible for 1 day with microprecipitation in 3 to 5 days and gross precipitation in 7 days at 4, 23, and 32°C in the dark. No paclitaxel and less than 7% doxorubicin loss in 7 days	2247	C
Vinblastine sulfate	LI	75 mg	AD	500 mg	NSa	Physically compatible for 10 days at 8, 25, and 32°C. Assays highly erratic	838	?
Vinblastine sulfate	LI	150 mg	AD	1.5 g	NSa	Physically compatible for 10 days at 8, 25, and 32°C. Assays highly erratic	838	?
Vincristine sulfate	LI	33 mg	FA	1.4 g	D5½S, NS	Visually compatible. Less than 10% loss of both drugs for 14 days at 25, 30, and 37°C	1030	C
Vincristine sulfate	LI	50 mg	FA	1.88 and 2.37 g	D5½S, NS	Visually compatible. Less than 10% loss of both drugs for 14 days at 25 and 30°C. Up to 16% doxorubicin loss at 37°C in 14 days	1030	C
Vincristine sulfate	LI	36 mg	NYC	1.67 g	NSa b	Visually compatible and both drugs stable for 7 days at 4°C then 4 days at 37°C	1874	C
Vincristine sulfate	FAU	200 mg	PHU	2 g	Wd	Physically compatible. No loss of either drug in 7 days at 37°C. 4% loss of both drugs in 14 days at 4°C	2288	C
Vincristine sulfate	PHC	33 mg	PHC	1.4 g	D5½S	Physically compatible. Little loss of either drug in 14 days at 4 and 25°C. 12% loss of both drugs at 37°C	2674	C
Vincristine sulfate	PHC	33 mg	PHC	1.4 g	NS	Physically compatible. Little loss of either drug in 14 days at 4 and 25°C. 4% loss of both drugs at 37°C	2674	C
Vincristine sulfate	PHC	53 mg	PHC	1.4 g	D5½S	Physically compatible. Little loss of either drug in 14 days at 4 and 25°C. 8% loss of both drugs at 37°C	2674	C
Vincristine sulfate	PHC	53 mg	PHC	1.4 g	NS	Physically compatible. Little loss of either drug in 14 days at 4 and 25°C. 9% loss of both drugs at 37°C	2674	C
Vincristine sulfate with etoposide	LI BMS	1.6 mg 200 mg	PHU	40 mg	NSc	Visually compatible. All drugs stable for 72 hr at 30°C in the dark	2239	C
Vincristine sulfate with etoposide	LI BMS	1 mg 125 mg	PHU	25 mg	NSc	Visually compatible. All drugs stable for 96 hr at 24°C in light or dark	2239	C
Vincristine sulfate with etoposide	LI BMS	1.4 mg 175 mg	PHU	35 mg	NSc	Visually compatible. All drugs stable for 96 hr at 24°C in light or dark	2239	C
Vincristine sulfate with etoposide	LI BMS	2 mg 250 mg	PHU	50 mg	NSc	Visually compatible. All drugs stable for 48 hr at 24°C in light or dark. Etoposide precipitate in 72 hr	2239	C
Vincristine sulfate with etoposide	LI BMS	2.8 mg 350 mg	PHU	70 mg	NSc	Visually compatible. All drugs stable for 24 hr at 24°C in light or dark. Etoposide precipitate in 36 hr	2239	C
Vincristine sulfate with etoposide	LI BMS	4 mg 500 mg	PHU	100 mg	NSc	Etoposide precipitate formed in 12 hr at 24°C in light or dark	2239	I
Vincristine sulfate with etoposide phosphate	LI BMS	5 mg 600 mg	PHU	120 mg	NSc	Physically compatible. Little loss of any drug in 124 hr at 4 and 40°C	2343	C
Vincristine sulfate with etoposide phosphate	LI BMS	10 mg 1.2 g	PHU	240 mg	NSc	Physically compatible. Little loss of any drug in 124 hr at 4 and 40°C	2343	C
Vincristine sulfate with etoposide phosphate	LI BMS	16 mg 2 g	PHU	400 mg	NSc	Physically compatible. Under 4% loss of any drug in 124 hr at 4 and 40°C	2343	C

Additive Compatibility (Cont.)

Test Drug	Mfr	Conc/L or %	Mfr	Conc/L or %	Test Solution	Remarks	Ref	C/I
Vincristine sulfate with ondansetron HCl	LI GL	14 mg 480 mg	AD	400 mg	D5W[b]	Visually compatible. Under 10% loss of all drugs in 5 days at 4°C then 24 hr at 30°C	2092	C
Vincristine sulfate with ondansetron HCl	LI GL	28 mg 960 mg	AD	800 mg	D5W[a]	Visually compatible. Under 10% loss of all drugs after 120 hr at 30°C	2092	C

[a] Tested in PVC containers.

[b] Tested in polyisoprene infusion pump reservoirs.

[c] Tested in polyolefin-lined plastic bags.

[d] Tested in PVC reservoirs for the Graseby 9000 ambulatory pumps.

Drugs in Syringe Compatibility

Doxorubicin HCl

Test Drug	Mfr	Amt	Mfr	Amt	Remarks	Ref	C/I
Bleomycin sulfate		1.5 units/0.5 mL		1 mg/0.5 mL	Physically compatible for 5 min at room temperature followed by 8 min of centrifugation	980	C
Cisplatin		0.5 mg/0.5 mL		1 mg/0.5 mL	Physically compatible for 5 min at room temperature followed by 8 min of centrifugation	980	C
Cisplatin with mitomycin	BMS BMS	50 mg 5 mg	BED	25 mg	Brought to a 5-mL final volume with NS. Visually compatible but more than 10% loss of mitomycin in 4 hr at 25°C. At 4°C, less than 10% loss of all three drugs in 12 hr, but about 16% mitomycin loss in 24 hr	2423	I
Cyclophosphamide		10 mg/0.5 mL		1 mg/0.5 mL	Physically compatible for 5 min at room temperature followed by 8 min of centrifugation	980	C
Droperidol		1.25 mg/0.5 mL		1 mg/0.5 mL	Physically compatible for 5 min at room temperature followed by 8 min of centrifugation	980	C
Fluorouracil		25 mg/0.5 mL		1 mg/0.5 mL	Physically compatible for 5 min at room temperature followed by 8 min of centrifugation	980	C
Fluorouracil		500 mg/10 mL		5 and 10 mg/10 mL[a]	Precipitate forms within several hours of mixing	1564	I
Furosemide		5 mg/0.5 mL		1 mg/0.5 mL	Precipitates immediately	980	I
Heparin sodium		500 units/0.5 mL		1 mg/0.5 mL	Precipitates immediately	980	I
Leucovorin calcium		5 mg/0.5 mL		1 mg/0.5 mL	Physically compatible for 5 min at room temperature followed by 8 min of centrifugation	980	C
Methotrexate sodium		12.5 mg/0.5 mL		1 mg/0.5 mL	Physically compatible for 5 min at room temperature followed by 8 min of centrifugation	980	C
Metoclopramide HCl		2.5 mg/0.5 mL		1 mg/0.5 mL	Physically compatible for 5 min at room temperature followed by 8 min of centrifugation	980	C
Metoclopramide HCl	RB	10 mg/2 mL	AD	40 mg/20 mL	Physically compatible for 48 hr at 25°C	1167	C
Metoclopramide HCl	RB	160 mg/32 mL	AD	90 mg/45 mL	Physically compatible for 48 hr at 25°C	1167	C
Mitomycin		0.25 mg/0.5 mL		1 mg/0.5 mL	Physically compatible for 5 min at room temperature followed by 8 min of centrifugation	980	C
Mitomycin with cisplatin	BMS BMS	5 mg 50 mg	BED	25 mg	Brought to a 5-mL final volume with NS. Visually compatible but more than 10% loss of mitomycin in 4 hr at 25°C. At 4°C, less than 10% loss of all three drugs in 12 hr, but about 16% mitomycin loss in 24 hr	2423	I

Drugs in Syringe Compatibility (Cont.)

Test Drug	Mfr	Amt	Mfr	Amt	Remarks	Ref	C/I
Vinblastine sulfate	LI	4.5 mg/4.5 mL	AD	45 mg/22.5 mL	Brought to 30-mL total volume with NS. Physically compatible for 10 days at 8, 25, and 32°C. Assays highly erratic	838	?
Vinblastine sulfate	LI	2.25 mg/2.25 mL	AD	15 mg/7.5 mL	Brought to 30-mL total volume with NS. Physically compatible for 10 days at 8, 25, and 32°C. Assays highly erratic	838	?
Vinblastine sulfate		0.5 mg/0.5 mL		1 mg/0.5 mL	Physically compatible for 5 min at room temperature followed by 8 min of centrifugation	980	C
Vincristine sulfate		0.5 mg/0.5 mL		1 mg/0.5 mL	Physically compatible for 5 min at room temperature followed by 8 min of centrifugation	980	C

^a Diluted in sodium chloride 0.9%.

Y-Site Injection Compatibility (1:1 Mixture)

Doxorubicin HCl

Test Drug	Mfr	Conc	Mfr	Conc	Remarks	Ref	C/I
Allopurinol sodium	BW	3 mg/mL[b]	CET	2 mg/mL	Immediate dark red color and haze. Reddish-brown particles within 1 hr	1686	I
Amifostine	USB	10 mg/mL[a]	CET	2 mg/mL	Physically compatible for 4 hr at 23°C	1845	C
Anidulafungin	VIC	0.5 mg/mL[a]	GNS	2 mg/mL[a]	Physically compatible for 4 hr at 23°C	2617	C
Aztreonam	SQ	40 mg/mL[a]	CET	2 mg/mL	Physically compatible for 4 hr at 23°C	1758	C
Bleomycin sulfate		3 units/mL		2 mg/mL	Drugs injected sequentially in Y-site with no flush. No precipitate seen	980	C
Caspofungin acetate	ME	0.7 mg/mL[b]	BED	1 mg/mL[b]	Physically compatible for 4 hr at room temperature	2758	C
Cisplatin		1 mg/mL		2 mg/mL	Drugs injected sequentially in Y-site with no flush. No precipitate seen	980	C
Cladribine	ORT	0.015[b] and 0.5[c] mg/mL	CHI	2 mg/mL	Physically compatible for 4 hr at 23°C	1969	C
Cyclophosphamide		20 mg/mL		2 mg/mL	Drugs injected sequentially in Y-site with no flush. No precipitate seen	980	C
Doripenem	JJ	5 mg/mL[a][b]	BED	1 mg/mL[a][b]	Physically compatible for 4 hr at 23°C	2743	C
Droperidol		2.5 mg/mL		2 mg/mL	Drugs injected sequentially in Y-site with no flush. No precipitate seen	980	C
Etoposide phosphate	BR	5 mg/mL[a]	GEN	2 mg/mL	Physically compatible for 4 hr at 23°C	2218	C
Filgrastim	AMG	30 mcg/mL[a]	CET	2 mg/mL	Physically compatible for 4 hr at 22°C	1687	C
Fludarabine phosphate	BX	1 mg/mL[a]	CET	2 mg/mL	Visually compatible for 4 hr at 22°C	1439	C
Fluorouracil		50 mg/mL		2 mg/mL	Drugs injected sequentially in Y-site with no flush. No precipitate seen	980	C
Furosemide		10 mg/mL		2 mg/mL	Drugs injected sequentially in Y-site with no flush. Precipitates immediately	980	I
Gallium nitrate	FUJ	1 mg/mL[b]	CET	2 mg/mL	Precipitates immediately	1673	I

Y-Site Injection Compatibility (1:1 Mixture) (Cont.)

Test Drug	Mfr	Conc	Mfr	Conc	Remarks	Ref	C/I
Gemcitabine HCl	LI	10 mg/mL[b]	PH	2 mg/mL	Physically compatible for 4 hr at 23°C	2226	C
Granisetron HCl	SKB	1 mg/mL	AD	0.2 mg/mL[b]	Physically compatible with little loss of either drug in 4 hr at 22°C	1883	C
Heparin sodium		1000 units/mL		2 mg/mL	Drugs injected sequentially in Y-site with no flush. Precipitates immediately	980	I
Leucovorin calcium		10 mg/mL		2 mg/mL	Drugs injected sequentially in Y-site with no flush. No precipitate seen	980	C
Linezolid	PHU	2 mg/mL	FUJ	2 mg/mL	Physically compatible for 4 hr at 23°C	2264	C
Melphalan HCl	BW	0.1 mg/mL[b]	AD	2 mg/mL	Physically compatible for 3 hr at 22°C	1557	C
Methotrexate sodium		25 mg/mL		2 mg/mL	Drugs injected sequentially in Y-site with no flush. No precipitate seen	980	C
Methotrexate sodium		30 mg/mL	FA	0.4 mg/mL[a]	Visually compatible for 4 hr at room temperature	1788	C
Metoclopramide HCl		5 mg/mL		2 mg/mL	Drugs injected sequentially in Y-site with no flush. No precipitate seen	980	C
Mitomycin		0.5 mg/mL		2 mg/mL	Drugs injected sequentially in Y-site with no flush. No precipitate seen	980	C
Ondansetron HCl	GL	1 mg/mL[b]	CET	2 mg/mL	Visually compatible for 4 hr at 22°C	1365	C
Ondansetron HCl	GL	16 to 160 mcg/mL		2 mg/mL	Physically compatible when doxorubicin given as 5-min bolus via Y-site	1366	C
Oxaliplatin	SS	0.5 mg/mL[a]	APP	1 mg/mL[a]	Physically compatible for 4 hr at 23°C	2566	C
Paclitaxel	NCI	1.2 mg/mL[a]		2 mg/mL	Physically compatible for 4 hr at 22°C	1528	C
Pemetrexed disodium	LI	20 mg/mL[b]	BED	1 mg/mL[a]	Dark-red discoloration forms immediately	2564	I
Piperacillin sodium–tazobactam sodium	LE[f]	40 mg/mL[a g]	CET	2 mg/mL	Turbidity forms immediately	1688	I
Sargramostim	IMM	10 mcg/mL[b]	CET	2 mg/mL	Visually compatible for 4 hr at 22°C	1436	C
Sodium bicarbonate		1.4%	FA	0.4 mg/mL[a]	Visually compatible for 2 hr at room temperature	1788	C
Teniposide	BR	0.1 mg/mL[a]	CET	2 mg/mL	Physically compatible for 4 hr at 23°C	1725	C
Thiotepa	IMM[d]	1 mg/mL[a]	CHI	2 mg/mL	Physically compatible for 4 hr at 23°C	1861	C
TNA #218 to #226[e]			PH, GEN	2 mg/mL	Damage to emulsion occurs immediately with free oil formation possible	2215	I
Topotecan HCl	SKB	56 mcg/mL[a b]	PH	2 mg/mL	Visually compatible. Little loss of either drug in 4 hr at 22°C	2245	C
TPN #212 to #215[e]			PH	2 mg/mL	Substantial loss of natural subvisible haze occurs immediately	2109	I
Vinblastine sulfate		1 mg/mL		2 mg/mL	Drugs injected sequentially in Y-site with no flush. No precipitate seen	980	C
Vincristine sulfate		1 mg/mL		2 mg/mL	Drugs injected sequentially in Y-site with no flush. No precipitate seen	980	C

Y-Site Injection Compatibility (1:1 Mixture) (Cont.)

Test Drug	Mfr	Conc	Mfr	Conc	Remarks	Ref	C/I
Vinorelbine tartrate	BW	1 mg/mL[b]	CET	2 mg/mL	Physically compatible for 4 hr at 22°C	1558	C

[a] Tested in dextrose 5%.

[b] Tested in sodium chloride 0.9%.

[c] Tested in bacteriostatic sodium chloride 0.9% preserved with benzyl alcohol 0.9%.

[d] Lyophilized formulation tested.

[e] Refer to Appendix for the composition of parenteral nutrition solutions. TNA indicates a 3-in-1 admixture, and TPN indicates a 2-in-1 admixture.

[f] Test performed using the formulation WITHOUT edetate disodium.

[g] Piperacillin component. Piperacillin in an 8:1 fixed-ratio concentration with tazobactam.

Selected Revisions December 13, 2018. © Copyright, October 1982. American Society of Health-System Pharmacists, Inc.

Doxorubicin Hydrochloride Liposomal
AHFS 10:00

Products

Doxorubicin hydrochloride liposomal is available as a red translucent liposomal dispersion providing 2 mg/mL of doxorubicin hydrochloride packaged in vials containing 20 and 50 mg of drug.[1(1/08)]

Over 90% of the doxorubicin hydrochloride is provided inside liposome carriers composed of N-(carbonyl-methoxypolyethylene glycol 2000)-1,2-distearoyl-sn-glycero-3-phosphoethanolamine sodium, 3.19 mg/mL; fully hydrogenated soy phosphatidylcholine, 9.58 mg/mL; and cholesterol, 3.19 mg/mL. The product also contains about 2 mg/mL of ammonium sulfate, histidine as a buffer, hydrochloric acid and/or sodium hydroxide to adjust pH, and sucrose to adjust tonicity.[1(1/08)]

CAUTION: Care should be taken to ensure that the correct drug product, dose, and administration procedures are used and that no confusion with other products occurs.

Trade Name(s)

Doxil

Administration

Doxorubicin hydrochloride liposomal is administered intravenously after dilution in dextrose 5%. Doses of 90 mg or less should be diluted in 250 mL, while doses exceeding 90 mg should be diluted in 500 mL of dextrose 5%. The product should not be administered as a bolus injection, as the undiluted dispersion, as a rapid infusion, or by other routes. Extravasation should be avoided; the drug is extremely irritating to tissues. The use of protective gloves during dose preparation is recommended.[1(1/08)]

The functional properties of a drug incorporated into a liposomal dispersion like this one may differ substantially from the functional properties of the conventional aqueous formulation.[1(1/08)]

CAUTION: Care should be taken to ensure that the correct drug product, dose, and administration procedures are used and that no confusion with other products occurs.

Stability

Intact vials of doxorubicin hydrochloride liposomal should be stored under refrigeration at 2 to 8°C. After dilution in dextrose 5% for administration, the drug should be stored under refrigeration and administered within 24 hours after preparation. Freezing should be avoided because prolonged freezing may adversely affect liposomal products. However, short-term freezing (less than 1 month) did not adversely affect this product.[1(1/08)]

Doxorubicin hydrochloride liposomal 0.15 mg/mL in dextrose 5% did not result in the loss of viability of *Staphylococcus aureus*, *Enterococcus faecium*, *Pseudomonas aeruginosa*, and *Candida albicans* within 120 hours at 22°C. Diluted solutions should be stored under refrigeration whenever possible, and the potential for microbiological growth should be considered when assigning expiration periods.[2740]

Filtration

Doxorubicin hydrochloride liposomal is a liposomal dispersion; filtration, including inline filtration, should not be performed.[1(1/08)]

Compatibility Information

Solution Compatibility

Doxorubicin HCl liposomal

Test Soln Name	Mfr	Mfr	Conc/L or %	Remarks	Ref	C/I
Dextrose 5%				Store at 4°C and use within 24 hr	1(1/08)	C

Y-Site Injection Compatibility (1:1 Mixture)

Doxorubicin HCl liposomal

Test Drug	Mfr	Conc	Mfr	Conc	Remarks	Ref	C/I
Acyclovir sodium	GW	7 mg/mL[a]	SEQ	0.4 mg/mL[a]	Physically compatible for 4 hr at 23°C	2087	C
Allopurinol sodium	BW	3 mg/mL[a]	SEQ	0.4 mg/mL[a]	Physically compatible for 4 hr at 23°C	2087	C
Aminophylline	AB	2.5 mg/mL[a]	SEQ	0.4 mg/mL[a]	Physically compatible for 4 hr at 23°C	2087	C
Amphotericin B	APC	0.6 mg/mL[a]	SEQ	0.4 mg/mL[a]	Fivefold increase in measured particulates in 4 hr	2087	I

DOI: 10.37573/9781585286850.135

Y-Site Injection Compatibility (1:1 Mixture) (Cont.)

Test Drug	Mfr	Conc	Mfr	Conc	Remarks	Ref	C/I
Ampicillin sodium	SKB	20 mg/mL[b]	SEQ	0.4 mg/mL[a]	Physically compatible for 4 hr at 23°C	2087	C
Aztreonam	SQ	40 mg/mL[a]	SEQ	0.4 mg/mL[a]	Physically compatible for 4 hr at 23°C	2087	C
Bleomycin sulfate	MJ	1 unit/mL[b]	SEQ	0.4 mg/mL[a]	Physically compatible for 4 hr at 23°C	2087	C
Buprenorphine HCl	RKC	0.04 mg/mL[a]	SEQ	0.4 mg/mL[a]	Partial loss of measured natural turbidity	2087	I
Butorphanol tartrate	APC	0.04 mg/mL[a]	SEQ	0.4 mg/mL[a]	Physically compatible for 4 hr at 23°C	2087	C
Calcium gluconate	AB	40 mg/mL[a]	SEQ	0.4 mg/mL[a]	Physically compatible for 4 hr at 23°C	2087	C
Carboplatin	BR	5 mg/mL[a]	SEQ	0.4 mg/mL[a]	Physically compatible for 4 hr at 23°C	2087	C
Cefazolin sodium	SKB	20 mg/mL[a]	SEQ	0.4 mg/mL[a]	Physically compatible for 4 hr at 23°C	2087	C
Cefepime HCl	BMS	20 mg/mL[a]	SEQ	0.4 mg/mL[a]	Physically compatible for 4 hr at 23°C	2087	C
Cefoxitin sodium	ME	20 mg/mL[a]	SEQ	0.4 mg/mL[a]	Physically compatible for 4 hr at 23°C	2087	C
Ceftazidime	SKB	40 mg/mL[a]	SEQ	0.4 mg/mL[a]	Partial loss of measured natural turbidity	2087	I
Ceftriaxone sodium	RC	20 mg/mL[a]	SEQ	0.4 mg/mL[a]	Physically compatible for 4 hr at 23°C	2087	C
Chlorpromazine HCl	ES	2 mg/mL[a]	SEQ	0.4 mg/mL[a]	Physically compatible for 4 hr at 23°C	2087	C
Ciprofloxacin	BAY	1 mg/mL[a]	SEQ	0.4 mg/mL[a]	Physically compatible for 4 hr at 23°C	2087	C
Cisplatin	BR	1 mg/mL	SEQ	0.4 mg/mL[a]	Physically compatible for 4 hr at 23°C	2087	C
Clindamycin phosphate	AST	10 mg/mL[a]	SEQ	0.4 mg/mL[a]	Physically compatible for 4 hr at 23°C	2087	C
Cyclophosphamide	MJ	10 mg/mL[a]	SEQ	0.4 mg/mL[a]	Physically compatible for 4 hr at 23°C	2087	C
Cytarabine	CHI	50 mg/mL	SEQ	0.4 mg/mL[a]	Physically compatible for 4 hr at 23°C	2087	C
Dacarbazine	MI	4 mg/mL[a]	SEQ	0.4 mg/mL[a]	Physically compatible for 4 hr at 23°C	2087	C
Dexamethasone sodium phosphate	ES	2 mg/mL[a]	SEQ	0.4 mg/mL[a]	Physically compatible for 4 hr at 23°C	2087	C
Diphenhydramine HCl	SCN	2 mg/mL[a]	SEQ	0.4 mg/mL[a]	Physically compatible for 4 hr at 23°C	2087	C
Dobutamine HCl	BA	4 mg/mL[a]	SEQ	0.4 mg/mL[a]	Physically compatible for 4 hr at 23°C	2087	C
Docetaxel	RPR	2 mg/mL[a]	SEQ	0.4 mg/mL[a]	Partial loss of measured natural turbidity	2087	I
Dopamine HCl	AB	3.2 mg/mL[a]	SEQ	0.4 mg/mL[a]	Physically compatible for 4 hr at 23°C	2087	C
Droperidol	AST	0.4 mg/mL[a]	SEQ	0.4 mg/mL[a]	Physically compatible for 4 hr at 23°C	2087	C
Enalaprilat	MSD	0.1 mg/mL[a]	SEQ	0.4 mg/mL[a]	Physically compatible for 4 hr at 23°C	2087	C
Etoposide	BR	0.4 mg/mL[a]	SEQ	0.4 mg/mL[a]	Physically compatible for 4 hr at 23°C	2087	C
Famotidine	ME	2 mg/mL[a]	SEQ	0.4 mg/mL[a]	Physically compatible for 4 hr at 23°C	2087	C
Fluconazole	RR	2 mg/mL	SEQ	0.4 mg/mL[a]	Physically compatible for 4 hr at 23°C	2087	C
Fluorouracil	PH	16 mg/mL[a]	SEQ	0.4 mg/mL[a]	Physically compatible for 4 hr at 23°C	2087	C
Furosemide	AMR	3 mg/mL[a]	SEQ	0.4 mg/mL[a]	Physically compatible for 4 hr at 23°C	2087	C
Ganciclovir sodium	RC	20 mg/mL[a]	SEQ	0.4 mg/mL[a]	Physically compatible for 4 hr at 23°C	2087	C
Gentamicin sulfate	ES	5 mg/mL[a]	SEQ	0.4 mg/mL[a]	Physically compatible for 4 hr at 23°C	2087	C
Granisetron HCl	SKB	0.05 mg/mL[a]	SEQ	0.4 mg/mL[a]	Physically compatible for 4 hr at 23°C	2087	C

Y-Site Injection Compatibility (1:1 Mixture) (Cont.)

Test Drug	Mfr	Conc	Mfr	Conc	Remarks	Ref	C/I
Haloperidol lactate	MN	0.2 mg/mL[a]	SEQ	0.4 mg/mL[a]	Physically compatible for 4 hr at 23°C	2087	C
Heparin sodium	ES	1000 units/mL[a]	SEQ	0.4 mg/mL[a]	Physically compatible for 4 hr at 23°C	2087	C
Hydrocortisone sodium succinate	AB	1 mg/mL[a]	SEQ	0.4 mg/mL[a]	Physically compatible for 4 hr at 23°C	2087	C
Hydromorphone HCl	ES	0.5 mg/mL[a]	SEQ	0.4 mg/mL[a]	Physically compatible for 4 hr at 23°C	2087	C
Hydroxyzine HCl	ES	2 mg/mL[a]	SEQ	0.4 mg/mL[a]	10-fold increase in particles ≥10 μm in 4 hr	2087	I
Ifosfamide	MJ	25 mg/mL[a]	SEQ	0.4 mg/mL[a]	Physically compatible for 4 hr at 23°C	2087	C
Leucovorin calcium	IMM	2 mg/mL[a]	SEQ	0.4 mg/mL[a]	Physically compatible for 4 hr at 23°C	2087	C
Lorazepam	WY	0.1 mg/mL[a]	SEQ	0.4 mg/mL[a]	Physically compatible for 4 hr at 23°C	2087	C
Magnesium sulfate	AST	100 mg/mL[a]	SEQ	0.4 mg/mL[a]	Physically compatible for 4 hr at 23°C	2087	C
Mannitol	BA	15%	SEQ	0.4 mg/mL[a]	Partial loss of measured natural turbidity	2087	I
Meperidine HCl	AST	4 mg/mL[a]	SEQ	0.4 mg/mL[a]	Increase in measured turbidity	2087	I
Mesna	MJ	10 mg/mL[a]	SEQ	0.4 mg/mL[a]	Physically compatible for 4 hr at 23°C	2087	C
Methotrexate sodium	IMM	15 mg/mL[a]	SEQ	0.4 mg/mL[a]	Physically compatible for 4 hr at 23°C	2087	C
Methylprednisolone sodium succinate	UP	5 mg/mL[a]	SEQ	0.4 mg/mL[a]	Physically compatible for 4 hr at 23°C	2087	C
Metoclopramide HCl	GNS	5 mg/mL	SEQ	0.4 mg/mL[a]	Increase in measured turbidity	2087	I
Metronidazole	AB	5 mg/mL	SEQ	0.4 mg/mL[a]	Physically compatible for 4 hr at 23°C	2087	C
Mitoxantrone HCl	IMM	0.5 mg/mL[a]	SEQ	0.4 mg/mL[a]	Partial loss of measured natural turbidity	2087	I
Morphine sulfate	ES	1 mg/mL[a]	SEQ	0.4 mg/mL[a]	Partial loss of measured natural turbidity	2087	I
Ondansetron HCl	CER	1 mg/mL[a]	SEQ	0.4 mg/mL[a]	Physically compatible for 4 hr at 23°C	2087	C
Paclitaxel	MJ	0.6 mg/mL[a]	SEQ	0.4 mg/mL[a]	Partial loss of measured natural turbidity	2087	I
Piperacillin sodium–tazobactam sodium	CY[c]	40 mg/mL[a d]	SEQ	0.4 mg/mL[a]	Partial loss of measured natural turbidity	2087	I
Potassium chloride	AB	0.1 mEq/mL[a]	SEQ	0.4 mg/mL[a]	Physically compatible for 4 hr at 23°C	2087	C
Prochlorperazine edisylate	SO	0.5 mg/mL[a]	SEQ	0.4 mg/mL[a]	Physically compatible for 4 hr at 23°C	2087	C
Promethazine HCl	ES	2 mg/mL[a]	SEQ	0.4 mg/mL[a]	Increase in measured turbidity	2087	I
Ranitidine HCl	GL	2 mg/mL[a]	SEQ	0.4 mg/mL[a]	Physically compatible for 4 hr at 23°C	2087	C
Sodium bicarbonate	AB	1 mEq/mL	SEQ	0.4 mg/mL[a]	Partial loss of measured natural turbidity	2087	I
Tobramycin sulfate	AB	5 mg/mL[a]	SEQ	0.4 mg/mL[a]	Physically compatible for 4 hr at 23°C	2087	C
Trimethoprim–sulfamethoxazole	ES	0.8 mg/mL[a e]	SEQ	0.4 mg/mL[a]	Physically compatible for 4 hr at 23°C	2087	C
Vancomycin HCl	AB	10 mg/mL[a]	SEQ	0.4 mg/mL[a]	Physically compatible for 4 hr at 23°C	2087	C
Vinblastine sulfate	FAU	0.12 mg/mL[a]	SEQ	0.4 mg/mL[a]	Physically compatible for 4 hr at 23°C	2087	C
Vincristine sulfate	FAU	0.05 mg/mL[a]	SEQ	0.4 mg/mL[a]	Physically compatible for 4 hr at 23°C	2087	C

Y-Site Injection Compatibility (1:1 Mixture) (Cont.)

Test Drug	Mfr	Conc	Mfr	Conc	Remarks	Ref	C/I
Vinorelbine tartrate	BW	1 mg/mL[a]	SEQ	0.4 mg/mL[a]	Physically compatible for 4 hr at 23°C	2087	C
Zidovudine	BW	4 mg/mL[a]	SEQ	0.4 mg/mL[a]	Physically compatible for 4 hr at 23°C	2087	C

[a] Tested in dextrose 5%.

[b] Tested in sodium chloride 0.9%.

[c] Test performed using the formulation WITHOUT edetate disodium.

[d] Piperacillin component. Piperacillin in an 8:1 fixed-ratio concentration with tazobactam.

[e] Trimethoprim component. Trimethoprim in a 1:5 fixed-ratio concentration with sulfamethoxazole.

Selected Revisions December 12, 2018. © Copyright, October 2000. American Society of Health-System Pharmacists, Inc.

Doxycycline Hyclate
AHFS 8:12.24

Products

Doxycycline hyclate is available as a lyophilized powder in vials containing the equivalent of 100 mg of doxycycline with ascorbic acid 480 mg and mannitol 300 mg or the equivalent of 200 mg of doxycycline with ascorbic acid 960 mg and mannitol 600 mg.[3071]

The 100- or 200-mg vials should be reconstituted with 10 mL or 20 mL, respectively, of sterile water for injection; sodium chloride; dextrose 5%; Ringer's injection; invert sugar 10%; Ringer's injection, lactated; dextrose 5% in Ringer's injection, lactated; Normosol M or R in dextrose 5%; or Plasma-Lyte 56 or 148 in dextrose 5%.[3071] The resultant solution contains the equivalent of 10 mg/mL of doxycycline.[3071] This reconstituted solution must be further diluted to a concentration of 0.1 to 1 mg/mL with a compatible infusion solution prior to use.[3071] (See Solution Compatibility.)

pH

The pH range for reconstituted solutions of 10 mg/mL is 1.8 to 3.3.[3071]

Osmolality

The osmolality of doxycycline (Elkins-Sinn) 1 mg/mL was determined to be 292 mOsm/kg in dextrose 5% and 310 mOsm/kg in sodium chloride 0.9%.[1375]

Administration

Doxycycline hyclate is administered by intravenous infusion, usually over 1 to 4 hours.[3071] Rapid administration should be avoided.[3071] The reconstituted solution should be diluted further with a compatible infusion solution to a concentration of 0.1 to 1 mg/mL.[3071] Other parenteral routes (e.g., intramuscular, subcutaneous) are not recommended, and extravasation should be avoided.[3071]

Stability

Intact vials should be stored at 20 to 25°C and should remain in the carton until time of use to protect from light.[3071]

Solutions of doxycycline at concentrations of 0.1 to 1 mg/mL prepared with sodium chloride, dextrose 5%, Ringer's injection, or invert sugar 10% may be stored for up to 72 hours prior to starting the infusion when kept in the refrigerator and protected from both direct sunlight and artificial light.[3071] Infusions must then be completed within 12 hours.[3071]

Doxycycline prepared in sodium chloride or dextrose 5% is noted to be stable under fluorescent light for 48 hours, but must be protected from direct sunlight during storage and infusion.[3071] Doxycycline prepared in Ringer's injection, invert sugar 10%, Ringer's injection, lactated, or dextrose 5% in Ringer's injection, lactated also must be protected from direct sunlight during infusion.[3071]

Because of the acidity of the solution, doxycycline hyclate may precipitate the free acids of barbiturate salts and sulfonamide derivatives. It may also adversely affect the stability of acid-labile drugs.[6 20 22 27]

Freezing Solutions

The manufacturer states that at a concentration of 10 mg/mL in sterile water for injection, doxycycline is stable for 8 weeks when frozen at −20°C immediately following reconstitution.[3071] Frozen solutions that have been completely thawed should not be heated.[3071] Thawed solutions should not be refrozen.[3071]

Doxycycline (Pfizer) 10 mg/mL in sterile water for injection was stable for 8 weeks when frozen at −20°C. At a concentration of 1 mg/mL in dextrose 5%, doxycycline also showed no significant decomposition over 8 weeks at −20°C.[310]

Sorption

Doxycycline was shown not to exhibit sorption to PVC bags and tubing, polyethylene tubing, Silastic tubing, and polypropylene syringes.[536 606]

Central Venous Catheter

Doxycycline (Fujisawa) 0.5 mg/mL in dextrose 5% was found to be compatible with the ARROWg+ard Blue Plus (Arrow International) chlorhexidine-bearing triple-lumen central catheter. Essentially complete delivery of the drug was found with little or no drug loss occurring. Furthermore, chlorhexidine delivered from the catheter remained at trace amounts with no substantial increase due to the delivery of the drug through the catheter.[2335]

Compatibility Information

Solution Compatibility

Doxycycline hyclate

Test Soln Name	Mfr	Mfr	Conc/L or %	Remarks	Ref	C/I
Dextrose 5%			0.1 to 1 g	Stable for 48 hr at 25°C	3071	C
Dextrose 5%	BAᵃ	PF	800 mg and 1 g	Visually compatible with 5 to 8% loss in 96 hr at 23°C. 2% loss in 7 days at 4°C	1928	C

DOI: 10.37573/9781585286850.136

Solution Compatibility (Cont.)

Test Soln Name	Mfr	Mfr	Conc/L or %	Remarks	Ref	C/I
Dextrose 5% in Ringer's injection, lactated		APP	0.1 and 1 g	Complete administration within 6 hr after reconstitution	3071	C
Invert sugar 10%		APP	0.1 to 1 g	Complete administration within 12 hr after reconstitution	3071	C
Normosol M in dextrose 5%	AB		0.1 to 1 g	Complete administration within 12 hr if refrigerated and protected from sunlight and artificial light	3071	C
Normosol R in dextrose 5%	AB		0.1 to 1 g	Complete administration within 12 hr if refrigerated and protected from sunlight and artificial light	3071	C
Plasma-Lyte 56 in dextrose 5%	BA		0.1 to 1 g	Complete administration within 12 hr if refrigerated and protected from sunlight and artificial light	3071	C
Plasma-Lyte 148 in dextrose 5%	BA		0.1 to 1 g	Complete administration within 12 hr if refrigerated and protected from sunlight and artificial light	3071	C
Ringer's injection			0.1 to 1 g	Complete administration within 12 hr after reconstitution	3071	C
Ringer's injection, lactated		APP	0.1 and 1 g	Complete administration within 6 hr after reconstitution	3071	C
Sodium chloride			0.1 to 1 g	Stable for 48 hr at 25°C	3071	C
Sodium chloride 0.9%	AB[b]	ES	2 g	5% loss for freshly prepared solutions during 24-hr simulated administration at 30°C. Stored at 5°C for 24 hr, then at 30°C, >5% loss in 6 hr	1779	C
Sodium chloride 0.9%	BA[a]	PF	800 mg and 1 g	Visually compatible with 8% loss in 96 hr at 23°C. 4% or less loss in 7 days at 4°C	1928	C

[a] Tested in PVC containers.

[b] Tested in portable pump reservoirs (Pharmacia Deltec).

Additive Compatibility

Doxycycline hyclate

Test Drug	Mfr	Conc/L or %	Mfr	Conc/L or %	Test Solution	Remarks	Ref	C/I
Meropenem	ZEN	1 g	RR	200 mg	NS	Visually compatible for 4 hr at room temperature	1994	C
Meropenem	ZEN	20 g	RR	200 mg	NS	Brown discoloration forms in 1 hr at room temperature	1994	I
Ranitidine HCl	GL	100 mg	PF	200 mg	D5W	Physically compatible for 24 hr at ambient temperature in light	1151	C

Drugs in Syringe Compatibility

Doxycycline hyclate

Test Drug	Mfr	Amt	Mfr	Amt	Remarks	Ref	C/I
Doxapram HCl	RB	400 mg/20 mL		100 mg/5 mL	Physically compatible with 3% doxapram loss in 24 hr	1177	C

Y-Site Injection Compatibility (1:1 Mixture)

Doxycycline hyclate

Test Drug	Mfr	Conc	Mfr	Conc	Remarks	Ref	C/I
Acyclovir sodium	BW	5 mg/mL[a]	PF	1 mg/mL[a]	Physically compatible for 4 hr at 25°C	1157	C
Allopurinol sodium	BW	3 mg/mL[b]	ES	1 mg/mL[b]	Immediate brown particles. Hazy brown solution with precipitate in 4 hr	1686	I

Y-Site Injection Compatibility (1:1 Mixture) (Cont.)

Test Drug	Mfr	Conc	Mfr	Conc	Remarks	Ref	C/I
Amifostine	USB	10 mg/mL[a]	LY	1 mg/mL[a]	Physically compatible for 4 hr at 23°C	1845	C
Amiodarone HCl	LZ	4 mg/mL[c]	ACC	0.25 mg/mL[c]	Physically compatible for 4 hr at room temperature	1444	C
Aztreonam	SQ	40 mg/mL[a]	ES	1 mg/mL[a]	Physically compatible for 4 hr at 23°C	1758	C
Bivalirudin	TMC	5 mg/mL[a]	APP	1 mg/mL[a]	Physically compatible for 4 hr at 23°C	2373	C
Cangrelor tetra-sodium	TMC	1 mg/mL[b]		1 mg/mL[b]	Physically compatible for 4 hr	3243	C
Ceftolozane sulfate–tazo-bactam sodium	CUB	10 mg/mL[c m]	FRK	1 mg/mL[c]	Physically compatible for 2 hr	3262	C
Cisatracurium besylate	GW	0.1, 2, 5 mg/mL[a]	FUJ	1 mg/mL[a]	Physically compatible for 4 hr at 23°C	2074	C
Cyclophospha-mide	MJ	20 mg/mL[a]	ES	1 mg/mL[a]	Physically compatible for 4 hr at 25°C	1194	C
Dexmedetomi-dine HCl	AB	4 mcg/mL[b]	APP	1 mg/mL[b]	Physically compatible for 4 hr at 23°C	2383	C
Diltiazem HCl	MMD	5 mg/mL	RR	1 and 10 mg/mL[b]	Visually compatible	1807	C
Docetaxel	RPR	0.9 mg/mL[a]	FUJ	1 mg/mL[a]	Physically compatible for 4 hr at 23°C	2224	C
Etoposide phos-phate	BR	5 mg/mL[a]	FUJ	1 mg/mL[a]	Physically compatible for 4 hr at 23°C	2218	C
Fenoldopam mesylate	AB	80 mcg/mL[b]	APP	1 mg/mL[b]	Physically compatible for 4 hr at 23°C	2467	C
Filgrastim	AMG	30 mcg/mL[a]	ES	1 mg/mL[a]	Physically compatible for 4 hr at 22°C	1687	C
Fludarabine phosphate	BX	1 mg/mL[a]	ES	1 mg/mL[a]	Visually compatible for 4 hr at 22°C	1439	C
Gemcitabine HCl	LI	10 mg/mL[b]	FUJ	1 mg/mL[b]	Physically compatible for 4 hr at 23°C	2226	C
Granisetron HCl	SKB	0.05 mg/mL[a]	LY	1 mg/mL[a]	Physically compatible for 4 hr at 23°C	2000	C
Heparin sodium	TR	50 units/mL	ES	1 mg/mL[a]	Visually incompatible within 4 hr at 25°C	1793	I
Hetastarch in lactated electro-lyte	AB	6%	APP	1 mg/mL[a]	Physically compatible for 4 hr at 23°C	2339	C
Hetastarch in sodium chloride 0.9%	DCC	6%	LY	1 mg/mL[a]	Visually compatible for 4 hr at room temperature	1313	C
Hetastarch in sodium chloride 0.9%	DCC	6%	LY	1 mg/mL[a]	White particle in one of five tests. No incompatibility during Y-site infusion	1315	?
Hydromorphone HCl	WY	0.2 mg/mL[a]	ES	1 mg/mL[c]	Physically compatible for 4 hr at 25°C	987	C
Isavuconazonium sulfate	ASP	1.5 mg/mL[c]	PRP	1 mg/mL[c]	Physically compatible for 2 hr	3263	C
Linezolid	PHU	2 mg/mL	FUJ	1 mg/mL[a]	Physically compatible for 4 hr at 23°C	2264	C
Magnesium sulfate	IX	16.7, 33.3, 66.7, 100 mg/mL[a]	PF	1 mg/mL[a]	Physically compatible for at least 4 hr at 32°C	813	C
Melphalan HCl	BW	0.1 mg/mL[b]	LY	1 mg/mL[b]	Physically compatible for 3 hr at 22°C	1557	C

Y-Site Injection Compatibility (1:1 Mixture) (Cont.)

Test Drug	Mfr	Conc	Mfr	Conc	Remarks	Ref	C/I
Meperidine HCl	WY	10 mg/mL[a]	ES	1 mg/mL[a]	Physically compatible for 4 hr at 25°C	987	C
Meropenem	ZEN	1 mg/mL[b]	RR	1 mg/mL[d]	Visually compatible for 4 hr at room temperature	1994	C
Meropenem	ZEN	50 mg/mL[b]	RR	1 mg/mL[d]	Amber discoloration forms within 30 min	1994	I
Meropenem–vaborbactam	TMC	8 mg/mL[b n]	FRK	1 mg/mL[b]	Physically compatible for 3 hr at 20 to 25°C	3380	C
Morphine sulfate	WI	1 mg/mL[a]	ES	1 mg/mL[a]	Physically compatible for 4 hr at 25°C	987	C
Ondansetron HCl	GL	1 mg/mL[b]	ES	1 mg/mL[a]	Visually compatible for 4 hr at 22°C	1365	C
Pemetrexed disodium	LI	20 mg/mL[b]	APP	1 mg/mL[a]	Cloudy precipitate forms immediately	2564	I
Piperacillin sodium–tazobactam sodium	LE[j]	40 mg/mL[a l]	ES	1 mg/mL[a]	Heavy white turbidity forms immediately	1688	I
Plazomicin sulfate	ACH	24 mg/mL[c]	FRK	1 mg/mL[c]	Physically compatible for 1 hr at 20 to 25°C	3432	C
Propofol	ZEN[o]	10 mg/mL	LY	1 mg/mL[a]	Physically compatible for 1 hr at 23°C	2066	C
Remifentanil HCl	GW	0.025 and 0.25 mg/mL[b]	FUJ	1 mg/mL[a]	Physically compatible for 4 hr at 23°C	2075	C
Sargramostim	IMM	10 mcg/mL[b]	LY	1 mg/mL[b]	Visually compatible for 4 hr at 22°C	1436	C
Tacrolimus	FUJ	1 mg/mL[b]	RR	5 mg/mL[a]	Visually compatible for 24 hr at 25°C	1630	C
Tedizolid phosphate	CUB	0.8 mg/mL[b]	PRP	1 mg/mL[b]	Measured turbidity increases immediately	3244	I
Telavancin HCl	ASP	7.5 mg/mL[a b k]	APP	1 mg/mL[a b k]	Physically compatible for 2 hr	2830	C
Teniposide	BR	0.1 mg/mL[a]	LY	1 mg/mL[a]	Physically compatible for 4 hr at 23°C	1725	C
Theophylline	TR	4 mg/mL	ES	1 mg/mL[a]	Visually compatible for 6 hr at 25°C	1793	C
Thiotepa	IMM[e]	1 mg/mL[a]	LY	1 mg/mL[a]	Physically compatible for 4 hr at 23°C	1861	C
TNA #218 to #226[f]			FUJ	1 mg/mL[a]	Damage to emulsion occurs immediately with free oil formation possible	2215	I
TPN #61[f]		[g]	PF	10 mg/mL[h]	Physically compatible	987	C
TPN #61[f]		[i]	PF	60 mg/6 mL[h]	Physically compatible	987	C
TPN #212 to #215[f]			LY	1 mg/mL[a]	Physically compatible for 4 hr at 23°C	2109	C
Vinorelbine tartrate	BW	1 mg/mL[b]	ES	1 mg/mL[b]	Physically compatible for 4 hr at 22°C	1558	C

[a] Tested in dextrose 5%.

[b] Tested in sodium chloride 0.9%.

[c] Tested in both dextrose 5% and sodium chloride 0.9%.

[d] Tested in sterile water for injection.

[e] Lyophilized formulation tested.

[f] Refer to Appendix for the composition of parenteral nutrition solutions. TNA indicates a 3-in-1 admixture, and TPN indicates a 2-in-1 admixture.

[g] Run at 21 mL/hr.

[h] Given over 30 minutes by syringe pump.

[i] Run at 94 mL/hr.

Y-Site Injection Compatibility (1:1 Mixture) (Cont.)

[j] Test performed using the formulation WITHOUT edetate disodium.

[k] Tested in Ringer's injection, lactated.

[l] Piperacillin component. Piperacillin in an 8:1 fixed-ratio concentration with tazobactam.

[m] Ceftolozane component. Ceftolozane in a 2:1 fixed-ratio concentration with tazobactam.

[n] Meropenem component. Meropenem in a 1:1 fixed-ratio concentration with vaborbactam.

[o] Test performed using the formulation WITH edetate disodium.

Selected Revisions January 31, 2020. © Copyright, October 1982. American Society of Health-System Pharmacists, Inc.

Droperidol
AHFS 28:24.92

Products

Droperidol is available in 1- and 2-mL ampuls and vials.[2906] [2907] Each mL of solution contains droperidol 2.5 mg with lactic acid and, if necessary, sodium hydroxide[2907] to adjust the pH.[2906] [2907]

pH

From 3 to 3.8.[2906] [2907]

Osmolality

The osmolality of droperidol 2.5 mg/mL was determined to be 16 mOsm/kg.[1233]

Administration

Droperidol may be administered intramuscularly or slowly intravenously.[2906] [2907]

Stability

Intact ampuls and vials of droperidol should be stored at controlled room temperature and retained in the original container to protect from light.[2906] [2907]

Precipitation may occur if droperidol is mixed with barbiturates.[4]

Syringes

The stability of droperidol 2.5 mg/mL repackaged in polypropylene syringes was evaluated. Little change in concentration was found after 4 weeks at room temperature out of direct light.[2164]

Central Venous Catheter

Droperidol (Abbott) 0.4 mg/mL in dextrose 5% was found to be compatible with the ARROWg+ard Blue Plus (Arrow International) chlorhexidine-bearing triple-lumen central catheter. Essentially complete delivery of the drug was found with little or no drug loss occurring. Furthermore, chlorhexidine delivered from the catheter remained at trace amounts with no substantial increase due to the delivery of the drug through the catheter.[2335]

Compatibility Information

Solution Compatibility

Droperidol

Test Soln Name	Mfr	Mfr	Conc/L or %	Remarks	Ref	C/I
Dextrose 5%	AB[a], TR[b]	JN	20 mg	Physically compatible and stable for 7 days at 27°C	750	C
Ringer's injection, lactated	TR[a]	JN	20 mg	Physically compatible and stable for 7 days at 27°C	750	C
Ringer's injection, lactated	TR[b]	JN	20 mg	Physically compatible. Stable with no loss for 24 hr at 27°C. 15% loss in 48 hr attributed to sorption	750	C
Sodium chloride 0.9%	AB[a]	JN	20 mg	Physically compatible with about 5% drug loss in 7 days at 27°C	750	C
Sodium chloride 0.9%	TR[b]	JN	20 mg	Physically compatible and stable for 7 days at 27°C	750	C
Sodium chloride 0.9%	[c]	AMR	1.25 g	Compatible and stable for 24 hr at 23°C. Droperidol precipitates if refrigerated	2199	C

[a] Tested in glass containers.

[b] Tested in PVC containers.

[c] Tested in polypropylene syringes.

DOI: 10.37573/9781585286850.137

Additive Compatibility

Droperidol

Test Drug	Mfr	Conc/L or %	Mfr	Conc/L or %	Test Solution	Remarks	Ref	C/I
Butorphanol tartrate	HE	80 mg	XU	50 mg	NS[c]	Physically compatible with less than 2% loss of either drug in 15 days at 4 and 25°C protected from light	2908	C
Fentanyl citrate with ketamine HCl	DB JN	10 mg 1 g	JN	50 mg	NS[a]	Visually compatible. 5% increase in all drugs in 30 days at 4 and 25°C due to water loss	2653	C
Fentanyl citrate with ketamine HCl	DB JN	10 mg 1 g	JN	50 mg	NS[b]	Visually compatible with little loss of the drugs in 30 days at 25°C	2653	C
Ketamine HCl with fentanyl citrate	JN DB	1 g 10 mg	JN	50 mg	NS[a]	Visually compatible. 5% increase in all drugs in 30 days at 4 and 25°C due to water loss	2653	C
Ketamine HCl with fentanyl citrate	JN DB	1 g 10 mg	JN	50 mg	NS[b]	Visually compatible with little loss of the drugs in 30 days at 25°C	2653	C

[a] Tested in PVC containers.

[b] Tested in glass containers.

[c] Tested in PVC and glass containers.

Drugs in Syringe Compatibility

Droperidol

Test Drug	Mfr	Amt	Mfr	Amt	Remarks	Ref	C/I
Atropine sulfate	ST	0.4 mg/1 mL	MN	2.5 mg/1 mL	Physically compatible for at least 15 min	326	C
Bleomycin sulfate		1.5 units/0.5 mL		1.25 mg/0.5 mL	Physically compatible for 5 min at room temperature followed by 8 min of centrifugation	980	C
Buprenorphine HCl					Physically and chemically compatible	4	C
Butorphanol tartrate	BR	4 mg/2 mL	MN	5 mg/2 mL	Physically compatible for 30 min at room temperature	566	C
Chlorpromazine HCl	PO	50 mg/2 mL	MN	2.5 mg/1 mL	Physically compatible for at least 15 min	326	C
Cisplatin		0.5 mg/0.5 mL		1.25 mg/0.5 mL	Physically compatible for 5 min at room temperature followed by 8 min of centrifugation	980	C
Cyclophosphamide		10 mg/0.5 mL		1.25 mg/0.5 mL	Physically compatible for 5 min at room temperature followed by 8 min of centrifugation	980	C
Dimenhydrinate	HR	50 mg/1 mL	MN	2.5 mg/1 mL	Physically compatible for at least 15 min	326	C
Diphenhydramine HCl	PD	50 mg/1 mL	MN	2.5 mg/1 mL	Physically compatible for at least 15 min	326	C
Doxorubicin HCl		1 mg/0.5 mL		1.25 mg/0.5 mL	Physically compatible for 5 min at room temperature followed by 8 min of centrifugation	980	C
Fentanyl citrate	MN	0.05 mg/1 mL	MN	2.5 mg/1 mL	Physically compatible for at least 15 min	326	C
Fluorouracil		25 mg/0.5 mL		1.25 mg/0.5 mL	Precipitates immediately	980	I
Furosemide		5 mg/0.5 mL		1.25 mg/0.5 mL	Precipitates immediately	980	I
Glycopyrrolate	RB	0.2 mg/1 mL	MN	2.5 mg/1 mL	Physically compatible. pH in glycopyrrolate stability range for 48 hr at 25°C	331	C

Drugs in Syringe Compatibility (Cont.)

Test Drug	Mfr	Amt	Mfr	Amt	Remarks	Ref	C/I
Glycopyrrolate	RB	0.2 mg/1 mL	MN	5 mg/2 mL	Physically compatible. pH in glycopyrrolate stability range for 48 hr at 25°C	331	C
Glycopyrrolate	RB	0.4 mg/2 mL	MN	2.5 mg/1 mL	Physically compatible. pH in glycopyrrolate stability range for 48 hr at 25°C	331	C
Heparin sodium		500 units/0.5 mL		1.25 mg/0.5 mL	Precipitates immediately	980	I
Heparin sodium		2500 units/1 mL	JN	5 mg/2 mL	Turbidity or precipitate forms within 5 min	1053	I
Hydroxyzine HCl	PF	50 mg/1 mL	MN	2.5 mg/1 mL	Physically compatible for at least 15 min	326	C
Leucovorin calcium		5 mg/0.5 mL		1.25 mg/0.5 mL	Precipitates immediately	980	I
Meperidine HCl	WI	50 mg/1 mL	MN	2.5 mg/1 mL	Physically compatible for at least 15 min	326	C
Methotrexate sodium		12.5 mg/0.5 mL		1.25 mg/0.5 mL	Precipitates immediately	980	I
Metoclopramide HCl	NO	10 mg/2 mL	MN	2.5 mg/1 mL	Physically compatible for 15 min at room temperature	565	C
Metoclopramide HCl		2.5 mg/0.5 mL		1.25 mg/0.5 mL	Physically compatible for 5 min at room temperature followed by 8 min of centrifugation	980	C
Midazolam HCl	RC	5 mg/1 mL	JN	2.5 mg/1 mL	Physically compatible for 4 hr at 25°C	1145	C
Mitomycin		0.25 mg/0.5 mL		1.25 mg/0.5 mL	Physically compatible for 5 min at room temperature followed by 8 min of centrifugation	980	C
Morphine sulfate	ST	15 mg/1 mL	MN	2.5 mg/1 mL	Physically compatible for at least 15 min	326	C
Nalbuphine HCl	EN	5 mg/0.5 mL	JN	5 mg/2 mL	Physically compatible for 36 hr at 27°C	762	C
Nalbuphine HCl	EN	10 mg/1 mL	JN	2.5 mg/1 mL	Physically compatible for 36 hr at 27°C	762	C
Nalbuphine HCl	EN	5 mg/0.5 mL	JN	2.5 mg/1 mL	Physically compatible for 36 hr at 27°C	762	C
Nalbuphine HCl	DU	10 mg/1 mL	JN	5 mg/2 mL	Physically compatible for 48 hr	128	C
Nalbuphine HCl	DU	20 mg/1 mL	JN	5 mg/2 mL	Physically compatible for 48 hr	128	C
Ondansetron HCl	GW	1 mg/mL[a]	AMR	1.25 mg/mL[a]	Droperidol precipitates at 4°C. At 23°C, little or no loss of either drug in 8 hr, but droperidol precipitates after that time	2199	I
Pentazocine lactate	WI	30 mg/1 mL	MN	2.5 mg/1 mL	Physically compatible for at least 15 min	326	C
Pentobarbital sodium	AB	50 mg/1 mL	MN	2.5 mg/1 mL	Physically incompatible within 15 min	326	I
Prochlorperazine edisylate	PO	5 mg/1 mL	MN	2.5 mg/1 mL	Physically compatible for at least 15 min	326	C
Promethazine HCl	PO	50 mg/2 mL	MN	2.5 mg/1 mL	Physically compatible for at least 15 min	326	C
Scopolamine HBr	ST	0.4 mg/1 mL	MN	2.5 mg/1 mL	Physically compatible for at least 15 min	326	C
Vinblastine sulfate		0.5 mg/0.5 mL		1.25 mg/0.5 mL	Physically compatible for 5 min at room temperature followed by 8 min of centrifugation	980	C
Vincristine sulfate		0.5 mg/0.5 mL		1.25 mg/0.5 mL	Physically compatible for 5 min at room temperature followed by 8 min of centrifugation	980	C

[a] Tested in sodium chloride 0.9%.

Y-Site Injection Compatibility (1:1 Mixture)

Droperidol

Test Drug	Mfr	Conc	Mfr	Conc	Remarks	Ref	C/I
Acetaminophen	CAD	10 mg/mL	HOS	2.5 mg/mL	Physically compatible with less than 10% acetaminophen loss over 4 hr at room temperature	2841, 2844	C
Acyclovir sodium	BV	5 mg/mL[b]	MDX	2.5 mg/mL	Physically compatible	2794	C
Allopurinol sodium	BW	3 mg/mL[b]	JN	0.4 mg/mL[b]	Immediate turbidity with particles	1686	I
Amifostine	USB	10 mg/mL[a]	JN	0.4 mg/mL[a]	Physically compatible for 4 hr at 23°C	1845	C
Azithromycin	PF	2 mg/mL[b]	AMR	2.5 mg/mL[i]	Visually compatible	2368	C
Aztreonam	SQ	40 mg/mL[a]	JN	0.4 mg/mL[a]	Physically compatible for 4 hr at 23°C	1758	C
Bivalirudin	TMC	5 mg/mL[a]	AMR	2.5 mg/mL	Physically compatible for 4 hr at 23°C	2373	C
Bleomycin sulfate		3 units/mL		2.5 mg/mL	Drugs injected sequentially in Y-site with no flush. No precipitate seen	980	C
Cangrelor tetrasodium	TMC	1 mg/mL[b]		2.5 mg/mL	Gross white turbid precipitate forms immediately	3243	I
Cisatracurium besylate	GW	0.1, 2, 5 mg/mL[a]	AB	2.5 mg/mL	Physically compatible for 4 hr at 23°C	2074	C
Cisplatin		1 mg/mL		2.5 mg/mL	Drugs injected sequentially in Y-site with no flush. No precipitate seen	980	C
Cladribine	ORT	0.015[b] and 0.5[c] mg/mL	JN	0.4 mg/mL[b]	Physically compatible for 4 hr at 23°C	1969	C
Cloxacillin sodium	SMX	100 mg/mL	SZ	2.5 mg/mL	Precipitates immediately	3245	I
Cyclophosphamide		20 mg/mL		2.5 mg/mL	Drugs injected sequentially in Y-site with no flush. No precipitate seen	980	C
Dexmedetomidine HCl	AB	4 mcg/mL[b]	AMR	2.5 mg/mL	Physically compatible for 4 hr at 23°C	2383	C
Docetaxel	RPR	0.9 mg/mL[a]	AST	0.4 mg/mL[a]	Physically compatible for 4 hr at 23°C	2224	C
Doxorubicin HCl		2 mg/mL		2.5 mg/mL	Drugs injected sequentially in Y-site with no flush. No precipitate seen	980	C
Doxorubicin HCl liposomal	SEQ	0.4 mg/mL[a]	AST	0.4 mg/mL[a]	Physically compatible for 4 hr at 23°C	2087	C
Etoposide phosphate	BR	5 mg/mL[a]	AST	0.4 mg/mL[a]	Physically compatible for 4 hr at 23°C	2218	C
Famotidine	ME	2 mg/mL[b]		0.4 mg/mL[a]	Visually compatible for 4 hr at 22°C	1936	C
Fenoldopam mesylate	AB	80 mcg/mL[b]	AB	2.5 mg/mL	Physically compatible for 4 hr at 23°C	2467	C
Filgrastim	AMG	30 mcg/mL[a]	JN	0.4 mg/mL[a]	Physically compatible for 4 hr at 22°C	1687	C
Fluconazole	RR	2 mg/mL	DU	2.5 mg/mL	Physically compatible for 24 hr at 25°C	1407	C
Fludarabine phosphate	BX	1 mg/mL[a]	JN	0.4 mg/mL[a]	Visually compatible for 4 hr at 22°C	1439	C
Fluorouracil		50 mg/mL		2.5 mg/mL	Drugs injected sequentially in Y-site with no flush. Precipitates immediately	980	I
Foscarnet sodium	AST	24 mg/mL	QU	2.5 mg/mL	Delayed formation of yellow precipitate	1335	I
Furosemide		10 mg/mL		2.5 mg/mL	Drugs injected sequentially in Y-site with no flush. Precipitates immediately	980	I
Furosemide		10 mg/mL		2.5 mg/mL	Precipitate forms	977	I

Y-Site Injection Compatibility (1:1 Mixture) (Cont.)

Test Drug	Mfr	Conc	Mfr	Conc	Remarks	Ref	C/I
Gemcitabine HCl	LI	10 mg/mL[b]	AST	0.4 mg/mL[b]	Physically compatible for 4 hr at 23°C	2226	C
Granisetron HCl	SKB	0.05 mg/mL[a]	AB	0.4 mg/mL[a]	Physically compatible for 4 hr at 23°C	2000	C
Heparin sodium		1000 units/mL		2.5 mg/mL	Drugs injected sequentially in Y-site with no flush. Precipitates immediately	980	I
Heparin sodium	UP	1000 units/L[e]	CR	1.25 mg/mL	Physically compatible for 4 hr at room temperature	534	C
Hetastarch in lactated electrolyte	AB	6%	AMR	2.5 mg/mL	Physically compatible for 4 hr at 23°C	2339	C
Hydrocortisone sodium succinate	UP	10 mg/L[e]	CR	1.25 mg/mL	Physically compatible for 4 hr at room temperature	534	C
Idarubicin HCl	AD	1 mg/mL[b]	AMR	0.04[a] and 2.5 mg/mL	Visually compatible for 24 hr at 25°C	1525	C
Leucovorin calcium		10 mg/mL		2.5 mg/mL	Drugs injected sequentially in Y-site with no flush. Precipitates immediately	980	I
Linezolid	PHU	2 mg/mL	AMR	0.4 mg/mL[a]	Physically compatible for 4 hr at 23°C	2264	C
Melphalan HCl	BW	0.1 mg/mL[b]	JN	0.4 mg/mL[b]	Physically compatible for 3 hr at 22°C	1557	C
Meperidine HCl	AB	10 mg/mL	AMR	2.5 mg/mL	Physically compatible for 4 hr at 25°C	1397	C
Methotrexate sodium		25 mg/mL		2.5 mg/mL	Precipitate forms	977	I
Methotrexate sodium		25 mg/mL		2.5 mg/mL	Drugs injected sequentially in Y-site with no flush. Precipitates immediately	980	I
Metoclopramide HCl		5 mg/mL		2.5 mg/mL	Drugs injected sequentially in Y-site with no flush. No precipitate seen	980	C
Mitomycin		0.5 mg/mL		2.5 mg/mL	Drugs injected sequentially in Y-site with no flush. No precipitate seen	980	C
Nafcillin sodium	WY	33 mg/mL[b]		2.5 mg/mL	Precipitate forms, probably free nafcillin	547	I
Ondansetron HCl	GL	1 mg/mL[b]	JN	0.4 mg/mL[a]	Visually compatible for 4 hr at 22°C	1365	C
Oxaliplatin	SS	0.5 mg/mL[a]	AB	2.5 mg/mL	Physically compatible for 4 hr at 23°C	2566	C
Paclitaxel	NCI	1.2 mg/mL[a]	JN	0.4 mg/mL[a]	Physically compatible for 4 hr at 22°C	1556	C
Pemetrexed disodium	LI	20 mg/mL[b]	AB	2.5 mg/mL	Gross white precipitate forms immediately	2564	I
Piperacillin sodium–tazobactam sodium	LE[f]	40 mg/mL[a j]	JN	0.4 mg/mL[a]	Heavy white turbidity with white precipitate forms immediately	1688	I
Potassium chloride	AB	40 mEq/L[e]	CR	1.25 mg/mL	Physically compatible for 4 hr at room temperature	534	C
Propofol	ZEN[k]	10 mg/mL	JN	0.4 mg/mL[a]	Physically compatible for 1 hr at 23°C	2066	C
Remifentanil HCl	GW	0.025 and 0.25 mg/mL[b]	AST	2.5 mg/mL	Physically compatible for 4 hr at 23°C	2075	C
Sargramostim	IMM	10 mcg/mL[b]	DU	0.4 mg/mL[b]	Visually compatible for 4 hr at 22°C	1436	C
Teniposide	BR	0.1 mg/mL[a]	JN	0.4 mg/mL[a]	Physically compatible for 4 hr at 23°C	1725	C
Thiotepa	IMM[g]	1 mg/mL[a]	JN	0.4 mg/mL[a]	Physically compatible for 4 hr at 23°C	1861	C
TNA #218 to #226[h]			AB	0.4 mg/mL[a]	Damage to emulsion occurs in 1 to 4 hr with free oil formation possible	2215	I
TPN #212 to #215[h]			AB	0.4 mg/mL[a]	Physically compatible for 4 hr at 23°C	2109	C
Vinblastine sulfate		1 mg/mL		2.5 mg/mL	Drugs injected sequentially in Y-site with no flush. No precipitate seen	980	C

Y-Site Injection Compatibility (1:1 Mixture) (Cont.)

Test Drug	Mfr	Conc	Mfr	Conc	Remarks	Ref	C/I
Vincristine sulfate		1 mg/mL		2.5 mg/mL	Drugs injected sequentially in Y-site with no flush. No precipitate seen	980	C
Vinorelbine tartrate	BW	1 mg/mL[b]	JN	0.4 mg/mL[b]	Physically compatible for 4 hr at 22°C	1558	C

[a] Tested in dextrose 5%.

[b] Tested in sodium chloride 0.9%.

[c] Tested in bacteriostatic sodium chloride 0.9% preserved with benzyl alcohol 0.9%.

[d] Given over three minutes via a Y-site into a running infusion solution of heparin sodium in sodium chloride 0.9%.

[e] Tested in dextrose 5% in Ringer's injection, dextrose 5% in Ringer's injection, lactated, dextrose 5%, Ringer's injection, lactated, and sodium chloride 0.9%.

[f] Test performed using the formulation WITHOUT edetate disodium.

[g] Lyophilized formulation tested.

[h] Refer to Appendix for the composition of parenteral nutrition solutions. TNA indicates a 3-in-1 admixture, and TPN indicates a 2-in-1 admixture.

[i] Injected via Y-site into an administration set running azithromycin.

[j] Piperacillin component. Piperacillin in an 8:1 fixed-ratio concentration with tazobactam.

[k] Test performed using the formulation WITH edetate disodium.

Selected Revisions January 31, 2020. © Copyright, October 1982. American Society of Health-System Pharmacists, Inc.

Edetate Calcium Disodium
AHFS 64:00

Products

Edetate calcium disodium is available in 5-mL ampuls containing 200 mg/mL of the drug in water for injection.[3237] For intravenous infusion, the appropriate dose of edetate calcium disodium should be added to 250 to 500 mL of dextrose 5% or sodium chloride 0.9%, or the drug should be diluted to a concentration of approximately 0.5% (5 mg/mL) or less in one of these solutions.[3237] [3238]

Trade Name(s)

Calcium Disodium Versenate

Administration

After establishment of adequate urine flow with intravenous fluid administration prior to the first dose, edetate calcium disodium may be administered intravenously or intramuscularly.[3237] [3238] The manufacturer states that intravenous and intramuscular routes of administration have been found to be equally effective.[3237] Because of the pain associated with intramuscular injection, continuous intravenous infusion generally is preferred; however, the intramuscular route is used in all patients with overt lead encephalopathy and is preferred in patients with lead encephalopathy and cerebral edema.[3237] [3238] The intramuscular route also is preferred by some for use in young pediatric patients[3237] or may be considered when fluid restriction is required.[3238]

For intravenous infusion, the appropriate dose of the drug should be added to 250 to 500 mL of dextrose 5% or sodium chloride 0.9% and infused over 8 to 12 hours.[3237] The drug also has been diluted to a concentration of approximately 0.5% (5 mg/mL) or less in dextrose 5% or sodium chloride 0.9% and administered as a continuous infusion over 24 hours.[3238] When the intravenous route of administration is used, rapid infusion should be avoided.[3237]

The total daily dose may be given by intramuscular injection in equally divided doses at 8- to 12-hour intervals.[3237] To minimize pain at the injection site, the drug should be mixed in equal volumes with lidocaine hydrochloride 1% or procaine hydrochloride 1% injection (no longer commercially available in the US) (e.g., 1 mL of local anesthetic for each mL of edetate calcium disodium injection) or 0.25 mL of lidocaine hydrochloride 10% injection can be added to 5 mL of edetate calcium disodium injection to yield a final local anesthetic concentration of 0.5%.[3237] [3238]

Stability

Edetate calcium disodium in intact ampuls should be stored at controlled room temperature.[3237]

Compatibility Information

Solution Compatibility

Edetate calcium disodium

Test Soln Name	Mfr	Mfr	Conc/L or %	Remarks	Ref	C/I
Dextrose 5%				Manufacturer-recommended solution	3237	C
Dextrose 10%				Stated to be incompatible	3237	I
Ringer's injection				Stated to be incompatible	3237	I
Ringer's injection, lactated				Stated to be incompatible	3237	I
Sodium chloride 0.9%				Manufacturer-recommended solution	3237	C
Sodium lactate ⅙ M				Stated to be incompatible	3237	I

Additive Compatibility

Edetate calcium disodium

Test Drug	Mfr	Conc/L or %	Mfr	Conc/L or %	Test Solution	Remarks	Ref	C/I
Amphotericin B		200 mg	RI	4 g	D5W	Haze develops over 3 hr	26	I
Hydralazine HCl	BP	80 mg	RI	4 g	D5W	Yellow color produced	26	I

Selected Revisions June 16, 2017. © Copyright, October 1982.
American Society of Health-System Pharmacists, Inc.

DOI: 10.37573/9781585286850.138

Edrophonium Chloride
AHFS 36:56

Products

Edrophonium chloride is available in 15-mL multiple-dose vials.[3227] Each mL of solution contains edrophonium chloride 10 mg with phenol 0.45% and sodium sulfite 0.2%; the solution also contains sodium citrate and citric acid as buffers.[3227]

pH

Approximately 5.4.[3227]

Trade Name(s)

Enlon

Administration

Edrophonium chloride is administered intravenously.[3227] The drug also may be administered intramuscularly in adults with inaccessible veins or in pediatric patients, owing to the difficulty of intravenous injection in pediatric patients.[3227] The drug also has been administered subcutaneously in infants.[3228]

Stability

Intact vials should be stored at controlled room temperature.[3227]

Compatibility Information

Y-Site Injection Compatibility (1:1 Mixture)

Edrophonium chloride

Test Drug	Mfr	Conc	Mfr	Conc	Remarks	Ref	C/I
Heparin sodium	UP	1000 units/L[a]	RC	10 mg/mL	Physically compatible for 4 hr at room temperature	534	C
Hydrocortisone sodium succinate	UP	10 mg/L[a]	RC	10 mg/mL	Physically compatible for 4 hr at room temperature	534	C
Potassium chloride	AB	40 mEq/L[a]	RC	10 mg/mL	Physically compatible for 4 hr at room temperature	534	C

[a] Tested in dextrose 5% in Ringer's injection, dextrose 5% in Ringer's injection, lactated, dextrose 5%, Ringer's injection, lactated, and sodium chloride 0.9%.

Selected Revisions June 16, 2017. © Copyright, October 1982.
American Society of Health-System Pharmacists, Inc.

DOI: 10.37573/9781585286850.139

Enalaprilat
AHFS 24:32.04

Products

Enalaprilat is available in 1- and 2-mL vials.[3249] Each mL of solution contains enalaprilat 1.25 mg with sodium chloride to adjust tonicity and benzyl alcohol 9 mg in water for injection.[3249] The solution also may contain sodium hydroxide to adjust the pH.[3249]

Administration

Enalaprilat is administered intravenously slowly over at least 5 minutes either undiluted or diluted with up to 50 mL of a compatible intravenous infusion solution.[3249]

Stability

Enalaprilat is a clear, colorless solution.[3249] Intact vials should be stored at controlled room temperature.[3249]

Enalaprilat solution should be visually inspected for particulate matter and discoloration prior to administration.[3249]

Central Venous Catheter

Enalaprilat (Merck) 0.1 mg/mL in dextrose 5% was found to be compatible with the ARROWg+ard Blue Plus (Arrow International) chlorhexidine-bearing triple-lumen central catheter. Essentially complete delivery of the drug was found with little or no drug loss occurring. Furthermore, chlorhexidine delivered from the catheter remained at trace amounts with no substantial increase due to the delivery of the drug through the catheter.[2335]

Compatibility Information

Solution Compatibility

Enalaprilat

Test Soln Name	Mfr	Mfr	Conc/L or %	Remarks	Ref	C/I
Dextrose 5%		HOS		Stable for 24 hr at room temperature	3249	C
Dextrose 5%	TR[a]	MSD	12 mg	Visually compatible with no loss in 24 hr at room temperature under fluorescent light	1572	C
Dextrose 5% in Ringer's injection, lactated		HOS		Stable for 24 hr at room temperature	3249	C
Dextrose 5% in sodium chloride 0.9%		HOS		Stable for 24 hr at room temperature	3249	C
Isolyte E	BRN	HOS		Stable for 24 hr at room temperature	3249	C
Normosol R	AB	MSD	25 mg	Physically compatible for 24 hr at room temperature under fluorescent light	1355	C
Sodium chloride 0.9%		HOS		Stable for 24 hr at room temperature	3249	C

[a] Tested in PVC containers.

Additive Compatibility

Enalaprilat

Test Drug	Mfr	Conc/L or %	Mfr	Conc/L or %	Test Solution	Remarks	Ref	C/I
Dextran 40	TR	10%	MSD	25 mg	D5W	Physically compatible for 24 hr at room temperature under fluorescent light	1355	C
Dobutamine HCl	LI	1 g	MSD	12 mg	D5W[a]	Visually compatible. Little enalaprilat loss in 24 hr at room temperature under fluorescent light. Dobutamine not tested	1572	C

DOI: 10.37573/9781585286850.140

Additive Compatibility (Cont.)

Test Drug	Mfr	Conc/L or %	Mfr	Conc/L or %	Test Solution	Remarks	Ref	C/I
Dopamine HCl	AMR	1.6 g	MSD	12 mg	D5W[a]	Visually compatible. 5% enalaprilat loss in 24 hr at room temperature under fluorescent light. Dopamine not tested	1572	C
Heparin sodium	ES	50,000 units	MSD	12 mg	D5W[a]	Visually compatible. Little enalaprilat loss in 24 hr at room temperature under fluorescent light. Heparin not tested	1572	C
Hetastarch in sodium chloride 0.9%	DU	6%	MSD	25 mg		Physically compatible for 24 hr at room temperature under fluorescent light	1355	C
Meropenem	ZEN	1 and 20 g	MSD	50 mg	NS	Visually compatible for 4 hr at room temperature	1994	C
Nitroglycerin	DU	200 mg	MSD	12 mg	D5W[b]	Visually compatible. 4% enalaprilat loss in 24 hr at room temperature in light. Nitroglycerin not tested	1572	C
Potassium chloride	AB	3 g	MSD	12 mg	D5W[a]	Visually compatible. Little enalaprilat loss in 24 hr at room temperature in light	1572	C
Sodium nitroprusside	ES	1 g	MSD	12 mg	D5W[a]	Visually compatible. Little enalaprilat loss in 24 hr at room temperature under fluorescent light. Sodium nitroprusside not tested	1572	C

[a] Tested in PVC containers.

[b] Tested in glass containers.

Drugs in Syringe Compatibility

Enalaprilat

Test Drug	Mfr	Amt	Mfr	Amt	Remarks	Ref	C/I
Pantoprazole sodium	a	4 mg/1 mL		1.25 mg/1 mL	Precipitate forms within 1 hr	2574	I

[a] Test performed using the formulation WITHOUT edetate disodium.

Y-Site Injection Compatibility (1:1 Mixture)

Enalaprilat

Test Drug	Mfr	Conc	Mfr	Conc	Remarks	Ref	C/I
Allopurinol sodium	BW	3 mg/mL[b]	MSD	0.1 mg/mL[b]	Physically compatible for 4 hr at 22°C	1686	C
Amifostine	USB	10 mg/mL[a]	MSD	0.1 mg/mL[a]	Physically compatible for 4 hr at 23°C	1845	C
Amikacin sulfate	BR	2 mg/mL[a]	MSD	0.05 mg/mL[b]	Physically compatible for 24 hr at room temperature under fluorescent light	1355	C
Aminophylline	ES	1 mg/mL[a]	MSD	0.05 mg/mL[b]	Physically compatible for 24 hr at room temperature under fluorescent light	1355	C
Amphotericin B	SQ	0.1 mg/mL[a]	MSD	1.25 mg/mL	Layered haze develops in 4 hr at 21°C	1409	I
Ampicillin sodium	BR	10 mg/mL[b]	MSD	0.05 mg/mL[b]	Physically compatible for 24 hr at room temperature under fluorescent light	1355	C
Ampicillin sodium–sulbactam sodium	PF	10 mg/mL[b k]	MSD	0.05 mg/mL[b]	Physically compatible for 24 hr at room temperature under fluorescent light	1355	C
Aztreonam	SQ	10 mg/mL[a]	MSD	0.05 mg/mL[b]	Physically compatible for 24 hr at room temperature under fluorescent light	1355	C

Y-Site Injection Compatibility (1:1 Mixture) (Cont.)

Test Drug	Mfr	Conc	Mfr	Conc	Remarks	Ref	C/I
Aztreonam	SQ	40 mg/mL[a]	MSD	0.1 mg/mL[a]	Physically compatible for 4 hr at 23°C	1758	C
Bivalirudin	TMC	5 mg/mL[a]	BED	0.1 mg/mL[a]	Physically compatible for 4 hr at 23°C	2373	C
Butorphanol tartrate	BR	0.4 mg/mL[a]	MSD	0.05 mg/mL[b]	Physically compatible for 24 hr at room temperature under fluorescent light	1355	C
Calcium gluconate	ES	0.092 mEq/mL[a]	MSD	0.05 mg/mL[b]	Physically compatible for 24 hr at room temperature	1355	C
Cangrelor tetrasodium	TMC	1 mg/mL[b]		0.1 mg/mL[b]	Physically compatible for 4 hr	3243	C
Cefazolin sodium	SKF	20 mg/mL[c]	MSD	0.05 mg/mL[b]	Physically compatible for 24 hr at room temperature under fluorescent light	1355	C
Ceftaroline fosamil	FOR	2.22 mg/mL[a b i]	SIC	0.1 mg/mL[a b i]	Physically compatible for 4 hr at 23°C	2826	C
Ceftazidime	GL	10 mg/mL[a]	MSD	0.05 mg/mL[b]	Physically compatible for 24 hr at room temperature under fluorescent light	1355	C
Chloramphenicol sodium succinate	PD	10 mg/mL[a]	MSD	0.05 mg/mL[b]	Physically compatible for 24 hr at room temperature under fluorescent light	1355	C
Cisatracurium besylate	GW	0.1, 2, 5 mg/mL[a]	ME	0.1 mg/mL[a]	Physically compatible for 4 hr at 23°C	2074	C
Cladribine	ORT	0.015[b] and 0.5[d] mg/mL	MSD	0.1 mg/mL[b]	Physically compatible for 4 hr at 23°C	1969	C
Clindamycin phosphate	UP	9 mg/mL[a]	MSD	0.05 mg/mL[b]	Physically compatible for 24 hr at room temperature under fluorescent light	1355	C
Dexmedetomidine HCl	AB	4 mcg/mL[b]	BED	0.1 mg/mL[b]	Physically compatible for 4 hr at 23°C	2383	C
Dextran 40	TR	100 mg/mL[a]	MSD	0.05 mg/mL[b]	Physically compatible for 24 hr at room temperature under fluorescent light	1355	C
Dobutamine HCl	LI	1 mg/mL[a]	MSD	0.05 mg/mL[b]	Physically compatible for 24 hr at room temperature under fluorescent light	1355	C
Docetaxel	RPR	0.9 mg/mL[a]	ME	0.1 mg/mL[a]	Physically compatible for 4 hr at 23°C	2224	C
Dopamine HCl	IMS	1.6 mg/mL[a]	MSD	0.05 mg/mL[b]	Physically compatible for 24 hr at room temperature under fluorescent light	1355	C
Doripenem	JJ	5 mg/mL[a b]	SIC	0.1 mg/mL[a b]	Physically compatible for 4 hr at 23°C	2743	C
Doxorubicin HCl liposomal	SEQ	0.4 mg/mL[a]	MSD	0.1 mg/mL[a]	Physically compatible for 4 hr at 23°C	2087	C
Erythromycin lactobionate	AB	5 mg/mL[a]	MSD	0.05 mg/mL[b]	Physically compatible for 24 hr at room temperature under fluorescent light	1355	C
Esmolol HCl	DU	10 mg/mL[a]	MSD	0.05 mg/mL[b]	Physically compatible for 24 hr at room temperature under fluorescent light	1355	C
Etoposide phosphate	BR	5 mg/mL[a]	ME	0.1 mg/mL[a]	Physically compatible for 4 hr at 23°C	2218	C
Famotidine	MSD	0.2 mg/mL[a]	MSD	0.05 mg/mL[b]	Physically compatible for 24 hr at room temperature under fluorescent light	1355	C
Fenoldopam mesylate	AB	80 mcg/mL[b]	BA	0.1 mg/mL[b]	Physically compatible for 4 hr at 23°C	2467	C
Fentanyl citrate	ES	2 mcg/mL[a]	MSD	0.05 mg/mL[b]	Physically compatible for 24 hr at room temperature under fluorescent light	1355	C
Filgrastim	AMG	30 mcg/mL[a]	MSD	0.1 mg/mL[a]	Physically compatible for 4 hr at 22°C	1687	C
Ganciclovir sodium	SY	5 mg/mL[e]	MSD	1.25 mg/mL	Physically compatible for 4 hr at 21°C	1409	C

Y-Site Injection Compatibility (1:1 Mixture) (Cont.)

Y-Site Injection Compatibility (1:1 Mixture) (Cont.)

Test Drug	Mfr	Conc	Mfr	Conc	Remarks	Ref	C/I
Gemcitabine HCl	LI	10 mg/mL[b]	ME	0.1 mg/mL[b]	Physically compatible for 4 hr at 23°C	2226	C
Gentamicin sulfate	ES	0.8 mg/mL[a]	MSD	0.05 mg/mL[b]	Physically compatible for 24 hr at room temperature under fluorescent light	1355	C
Granisetron HCl	SKB	0.05 mg/mL[a]	MSD	0.1 mg/mL[a]	Physically compatible for 4 hr at 23°C	2000	C
Heparin sodium	IX	40 units/mL[a]	MSD	0.05 mg/mL[b]	Physically compatible for 24 hr at room temperature under fluorescent light	1355	C
Hetastarch in lactated electrolyte	AB	6%	ME	0.1 mg/mL[a]	Physically compatible for 4 hr at 23°C	2339	C
Hetastarch in sodium chloride 0.9%	DCC	6%	MSD	0.05 mg/mL[b]	Physically compatible for 24 hr at room temperature under fluorescent light	1355	C
Hydrocortisone sodium succinate	UP	2 mg/mL[a]	MSD	0.05 mg/mL[b]	Physically compatible for 24 hr at room temperature under fluorescent light	1355	C
Labetalol HCl	GL	1 mg/mL[a]	MSD	0.05 mg/mL[b]	Physically compatible for 24 hr at room temperature under fluorescent light	1355	C
Lidocaine HCl	AST	4 mg/mL[a]	MSD	0.05 mg/mL[b]	Physically compatible for 24 hr at room temperature under fluorescent light	1355	C
Linezolid	PHU	2 mg/mL	ME	0.1 mg/mL[a]	Physically compatible for 4 hr at 23°C	2264	C
Magnesium sulfate	LY	10 mEq/mL[a]	MSD	0.05 mg/mL[b]	Physically compatible for 24 hr at room temperature under fluorescent light	1355	C
Melphalan HCl	BW	0.1 mg/mL[b]	MSD	0.1 mg/mL[b]	Physically compatible for 3 hr at 22°C	1557	C
Meropenem	ZEN	1 and 50 mg/mL[b]	MSD	0.05 mg/mL[f]	Visually compatible for 4 hr at room temperature	1994	C
Methylprednisolone sodium succinate	UP	0.8 mg/mL[a]	MSD	0.05 mg/mL[b]	Physically compatible for 24 hr at room temperature under fluorescent light	1355	C
Metronidazole	SE	5 mg/mL	MSD	0.05 mg/mL[b]	Physically compatible for 24 hr at room temperature under fluorescent light	1355	C
Morphine sulfate	WY	0.2 mg/mL[a]	MSD	0.05 mg/mL[b]	Physically compatible for 24 hr at room temperature under fluorescent light	1355	C
Nafcillin sodium	BR	10 mg/mL[a]	MSD	0.05 mg/mL[b]	Physically compatible for 24 hr at room temperature under fluorescent light	1355	C
Nesiritide	SCI	50 mcg/mL[a b]		1.25 mg/mL	Physically incompatible	2625	I
Nicardipine HCl	DU	0.1 mg/mL[a]	MSD	0.05 mg/mL[b]	Physically compatible for 24 hr at room temperature under fluorescent light	1355	C
Nicardipine HCl	DCC	0.1 mg/mL[a]	MSD	0.5 mg/mL[a]	Visually compatible for 24 hr at room temperature	235	C
Oxaliplatin	SS	0.5 mg/mL[a]	BA	0.1 mg/mL[a]	Physically compatible for 4 hr at 23°C	2566	C
Pemetrexed disodium	LI	20 mg/mL[b]	BED	0.1 mg/mL[a]	Physically compatible for 4 hr at 23°C	2564	C
Penicillin G potassium	PF	50,000 units/mL[a]	MSD	0.05 mg/mL[b]	Physically compatible for 24 hr at room temperature under fluorescent light	1355	C
Phenobarbital sodium	WY	0.32 mg/mL[e]	MSD	1.25 mg/mL	Physically compatible for 4 hr at 21°C	1409	C
Phenytoin sodium	PD	1 mg/mL[b]	MSD	1.25 mg/mL	Crystalline precipitate forms immediately	1409	I
Piperacillin sodium–tazobactam sodium	LE[j]	40 mg/mL[a l]	MSD	0.1 mg/mL[a]	Physically compatible for 4 hr at 22°C	1688	C

Y-Site Injection Compatibility (1:1 Mixture) (Cont.)

Test Drug	Mfr	Conc	Mfr	Conc	Remarks	Ref	C/I
Potassium chloride	LY	0.4 mEq/mL[a]	MSD	0.05 mg/mL[b]	Physically compatible for 24 hr at room temperature under fluorescent light	1355	C
Potassium phosphates	LY	0.44 mEq/mL[a]	MSD	0.05 mg/mL[b]	Physically compatible for 24 hr at room temperature under fluorescent light	1355	C
Propofol	ZEN[n]	10 mg/mL	MSD	0.1 mg/mL[a]	Physically compatible for 1 hr at 23°C	2066	C
Ranitidine HCl	GL	0.5 mg/mL[a]	MSD	0.05 mg/mL[b]	Physically compatible for 24 hr at room temperature under fluorescent light	1355	C
Remifentanil HCl	GW	0.025 and 0.25 mg/mL[b]	ME	0.1 mg/mL[a]	Physically compatible for 4 hr at 23°C	2075	C
Sodium acetate	LY	0.4 mEq/mL[a]	MSD	0.05 mg/mL[b]	Physically compatible for 24 hr at room temperature under fluorescent light	1355	C
Sodium nitroprusside	LY	0.2 mg/mL[a]	MSD	0.05 mg/mL[b]	Physically compatible for 24 hr at room temperature protected from light	1355	C
Teniposide	BR	0.1 mg/mL[a]	MSD	0.1 mg/mL[a]	Physically compatible for 4 hr at 23°C	1725	C
Thiotepa	IMM[g]	1 mg/mL[a]	ME	0.1 mg/mL[a]	Physically compatible for 4 hr at 23°C	1861	C
TNA #218 to #226[h]			ME	0.1 mg/mL[a]	Visually compatible for 4 hr at 23°C	2215	C
Tobramycin sulfate	LI	0.8 mg/mL[a]	MSD	0.05 mg/mL[b]	Physically compatible for 24 hr at room temperature under fluorescent light	1355	C
TPN #212 to #215[h]			MSD	0.1 mg/mL[a]	Physically compatible for 4 hr at 23°C	2109	C
Trimethoprim–sulfamethoxazole	QU	0.16 mg/mL[a] [m]	MSD	0.05 mg/mL[b]	Physically compatible for 24 hr at room temperature under fluorescent light	1355	C
Vancomycin HCl	LE	5 mg/mL[a]	MSD	0.05 mg/mL[b]	Physically compatible for 24 hr at room temperature under fluorescent light	1355	C
Vinorelbine tartrate	BW	1 mg/mL[b]	MSD	0.1 mg/mL[b]	Physically compatible for 4 hr at 22°C	1558	C

[a] Tested in dextrose 5%.

[b] Tested in sodium chloride 0.9%.

[c] Tested as the premixed infusion solution.

[d] Tested in bacteriostatic sodium chloride 0.9% preserved with benzyl alcohol 0.9%.

[e] Tested in both dextrose 5% and sodium chloride 0.9%.

[f] Tested in sterile water for injection.

[g] Lyophilized formulation tested.

[h] Refer to Appendix for the composition of parenteral nutrition solutions. TNA indicates a 3-in-1 admixture, and TPN indicates a 2-in-1 admixture.

[i] Tested in Ringer's injection, lactated.

[j] Test performed using the formulation WITHOUT edetate disodium.

[k] Ampicillin component. Ampicillin in a 2:1 fixed-ratio concentration with sulbactam.

[l] Piperacillin component. Piperacillin in an 8:1 fixed-ratio concentration with tazobactam.

[m] Trimethoprim component. Trimethoprim in a 1:5 fixed-ratio concentration with sulfamethoxazole.

[n] Test performed using the formulation WITH edetate disodium.

Selected Revisions June 1, 2020. © Copyright, October 1992.
American Society of Health-System Pharmacists, Inc.

Enoxaparin Sodium
AHFS 20:12.04.16

Products

Enoxaparin sodium is available as a solution with each mL containing 100 or 150 mg of the drug in water for injection.[3351] The 100-mg/mL concentration is available in both preservative-free, single-dose, prefilled syringes, containing 30 mg/0.3 mL and 40 mg/0.4 mL, and preservative-free, single-dose, graduated prefilled syringes, containing 60 mg/0.6 mL, 80 mg/0.8 mL, and 100 mg/1 mL.[3351] The 100-mg/mL concentration also is available in 3-mL multidose vials preserved with benzyl alcohol 15 mg/mL.[3351] The 150-mg/mL concentration is available in preservative-free, single-dose, graduated prefilled syringes, containing 120 mg/0.8 mL and 150 mg/1 mL.[3351]

pH

From 5.5 to 7.5.[3351]

Units

The approximate anti-factor Xa activity is 1000 international units for every 10 mg of enoxaparin sodium.[3351]

Trade Name(s)

Lovenox

Administration

Enoxaparin sodium is administered by deep subcutaneous injection, without dilution, alternating administration sites between the left and right anterolateral and left and right posterolateral abdominal wall.[3351] To avoid loss of drug when administering the 30- and 40-mg prefilled syringes, the air bubble from the syringe should *not* be expelled prior to injection of the drug.[3351] To minimize bruising, the injection site should not be rubbed after completion of the injection.[3351]

Enoxaparin sodium solution in multidose vials is administered by intravenous bolus injection into an intravenous line.[3351] The drug may be mixed with sodium chloride 0.9% or dextrose 5%.[3351] The line used to administer enoxaparin sodium should be flushed with a sufficient volume of dextrose or sodium chloride prior to and following intravenous bolus injection of enoxaparin sodium.[3351] The manufacturer states that enoxaparin sodium should not be mixed or co-administered with other drugs.[3351]

Enoxaparin sodium is not intended for intramuscular administration and must not be administered by this route.[3351]

Stability

Enoxaparin sodium injection is a clear, colorless to pale yellow solution.[3351] Intact containers should be stored at controlled room temperature.[3351] Enoxaparin sodium solutions should be visually inspected for particulate matter and discoloration prior to administration.[3351] One manufacturer has noted that degradation in the color of enoxaparin is a known phenomenon

and that such color changes outside of product specifications have been observed at increased temperatures (e.g., 40°C) over periods of 3 to greater than 6 months; however, the manufacturer states that this color degradation does not affect the potency of the drug.[3356]

One manufacturer of enoxaparin sodium (Sanofi) has stated that prefilled graduated syringes containing 60 mg/0.6 mL and 100 mg/1 mL were stable for 12 months at 4°C, 25°C with 60% relative humidity, and 30°C with 60% relative humidity and that such syringes containing 30 mg/0.3 mL were stable for 36 months at 4°C.[3356] Enoxaparin sodium 100-mg/mL solution in 3-mL multidose vials was stable for 3 months at 25°C with 60% relative humidity, 30°C with 60% relative humidity, and 40°C with 75% relative humidity and for 24 months at 25°C with 60% relative humidity.[3356] The stability of the solution in the multidose vial was similar to that of the 100-mg/mL solution in prefilled syringes, and the presence of benzyl alcohol in the multidose vial did not affect stability.[3356]

Multidose vials should not be stored for more than 28 days after first use.[3351]

Enoxaparin sodium (Aventis) 100-mg/mL solution (as 60-mg/0.6 mL prefilled syringes) diluted to 20 mg/mL in sterile water for injection has been reported to undergo little or no change in anti-factor Xa activity for 29 days at 22 to 26°C when the dilution was packaged in glass vials.[2499]

Enoxaparin sodium (Aventis) 100-mg/mL solution diluted to 20 mg/mL with dextrose 4% and stored in glass vials had 0.7 and 2.8% losses of baseline anti-factor Xa activity when stored for 31 days at 4 and −12°C, respectively; solutions stored at −80°C had a 6.6% loss in 14 days.[3352]

Temperature Effects

Solutions of enoxaparin sodium heated to 70°C exhibited a rapid decline in anti-factor Xa activity within 8 hours, with a maximum loss of 27%.[3365] Anti-factor Xa activity returned to 94% of initial activity after 12 hours, with a subsequent decline to 84% of initial anti-factor Xa activity after 48 hours and 80% after 22 days.[3365]

Freezing Solutions

Freezing solutions of enoxaparin sodium at or below temperatures of −26°C resulted in substantial losses of anti-factor Xa activity, with greater losses associated with lower temperatures.[3364] Samples frozen at −12°C exhibited no loss, whereas samples frozen at −26 and −196°C exhibited losses of 14 and 67%, respectively.[3364] Losses of anti-factor Xa activity appeared to be independent of the duration of freezing time.[3364] Anti-factor Xa activity also decreased with increasing freeze-thaw cycles; only 13% of anti-factor Xa activity remained after 50 such cycles of freezing at −196°C and subsequent thawing at room temperature.[3364] Rapid freezing with subsequent slow thawing or slow

DOI: 10.37573/9781585286850.141

freezing with subsequent rapid thawing resulted in negligible losses in anti-factor Xa activity as compared with rapid freezing with subsequent rapid thawing.[3364]

Syringes

Enoxaparin sodium (Rhone-Poulenc Rorer) 100-mg/mL solution (as 30-mg/0.3 mL prefilled syringes) was packaged in 1-mL tuberculin syringes (Monoject, Sherwood) fitted with 27-gauge, ½-inch needles.[2272] The syringes were stored at 22 and 3°C for 10 days.[2272] A 7 to 8% loss in anti-factor Xa activity occurred in 10 days under refrigeration at 3°C, but 15 to 25% losses occurred in as little as 2 days at 22°C.[2272]

One manufacturer of enoxaparin sodium (Sanofi) has indicated that the 100-mg/mL undiluted solution containing benzyl alcohol 15 mg/mL repackaged in 3 types of plastic syringes (tuberculin, Terumo; Safety-Lok, Becton Dickinson; Monoject, Sherwood) is stable for 5 days at room temperature.[3355] Because benzyl alcohol was not found to influence the stability of enoxaparin sodium 100-mg/mL solution,[3355] [3356] it has been proposed that a preservative-free solution of the same strength also would be stable in such plastic syringes.[3355]

Enoxaparin sodium (Aventis) 100-mg/mL solution (as 60-mg/0.6 mL prefilled syringes) diluted to 20 mg/mL in sterile water for injection packaged as 0.3 mL in 1-mL plastic tuberculin syringes has been reported to undergo little or no change in anti-factor Xa activity for about 14 days at 22 to 26°C and at 2 to 6°C.[2499]

The stability of enoxaparin sodium 100-mg/mL solution packaged in 1-mL polypropylene tuberculin syringes was evaluated over 10 days stored at 22 and 4°C. Enoxaparin losses did not exceed 10% at either storage temperature; however, 7 of 45 test syringes stored at room temperature could not be operated to eject the enoxaparin. None of the refrigerated samples exhibited this failure. The authors speculated that precipitation had resulted in blockage.[2546]

Enoxaparin sodium (Clexane, Sanofi Aventis) preservative-free 150-mg/mL solution diluted to 20 mg/mL with sodium chloride 0.9% and stored in polypropylene syringes retained at least 90% of baseline anti-factor Xa and anti-factor IIa activity when stored for up to 43 days at 22 to 26°C exposed to natural light and at 2 to 8°C in the dark; the anti-factor Xa activity of solutions stored at 22 to 26°C in the dark decreased to 89% by day 8, but exhibited anti-factor Xa activity greater than 90% at the next test (i.e., day 15) and throughout the remainder of the study (i.e., up to 43 days).[3353] Authors noted that some solutions exhibited a trend towards an increase in anti-factor Xa activity during this time period due to an unknown mechanism.[3353]

Enoxaparin sodium (Aventis) 100-mg/mL solution diluted with either dextrose 4% or sterile water for injection or undiluted was stored in 1-mL plastic tuberculin syringes at 4, –12, and –80°C for 31 days.[3352] Enoxaparin sodium diluted to 20 mg/mL with dextrose 4% had 0.6 and 2.2% losses of baseline anti-factor Xa activity when stored for 31 days at 4 and –12°C, respectively; solutions stored at –80°C had a 6.6% loss in 14 days.[3352] Enoxaparin sodium diluted to 20 mg/mL with sterile water for injection had a 6.3% loss in 14 days at 4°C and a 3% loss in 7 days at –12°C; solutions stored at –80°C had a loss of more than 10% in 7 days.[3352] Undiluted enoxaparin sodium 100-mg/mL solution had no loss at 4°C in 31 days, 4.9% loss at –12°C in 7 days, and more than 10% loss at –80°C in 7 days.[3352]

Enoxaparin sodium (Aventis) 100-mg/mL solution (as 40-mg/0.4 mL prefilled syringes) was diluted to 8 mg/mL with sterile water for injection and stored in polypropylene syringes (Becton Dickinson) at 2 to 6°C for 30 days.[3354] Solutions retained greater than 90% anti-factor Xa activity for 14 days; however, authors noted that there was a substantial amount of variability in anti-factor Xa activity due to an unknown mechanism.[3354]

Compatibility Information

Solution Compatibility

Enoxaparin sodium

Test Soln Name	Mfr	Mfr	Conc/L or %	Remarks	Ref	C/I
Sodium chloride 0.9%	AB[a]	RP	1.2 g	No loss of activity in 48 hr at 21°C under fluorescent light	1871	C

[a] Tested in PVC containers.

Selected Revisions June 1, 2019. © Copyright, October 1998. American Society of Health-System Pharmacists, Inc.

Ephedrine Sulfate
AHFS 12:12.12

Products

Ephedrine sulfate is available as a concentrate for injection in single-dose 1-mL vials and ampuls.[2754] [3336] [3337] Each mL of the concentrate for injection contains ephedrine sulfate 50 mg in water for injection.[2754] [3336] [3337] The pH may have been adjusted with sodium hydroxide and/or glacial acetic acid, if necessary.[2754] [3337]

The concentrate for injection must be diluted prior to intravenous administration.[2754] [3336] [3337] For bolus administration, 1 mL (50 mg) of ephedrine sulfate should be diluted in 9 mL of sodium chloride 0.9% or dextrose 5% to a final concentration of 5 mg/mL.[2754] [3336] [3337] An appropriate dose of the diluted solution of ephedrine sulfate should be withdrawn for administration.[2754] [3336] [3337]

Equivalency

Ephedrine sulfate 50 mg is equivalent to 38 mg of ephedrine base.[2754] [3336] [3337]

pH

From 4.5 to 7.[2754] [3336] [3337]

Trade Name(s)

Akovaz, Corphedra

Administration

Ephedrine sulfate concentrate for injection must be diluted prior to intravenous administration.[2754] [3336] [3337] The drug is administered as an intravenous bolus[2754] [3336] [3337] or infusion.[3336]

The drug also has been administered by subcutaneous or intramuscular injection;[2314] however, FDA-approved labeling does not include these routes.[2754] [3336] [3337]

Stability

Intact ampuls and vials of ephedrine sulfate should be stored at controlled room temperature in their original cartons to protect from light.[2754] [3336] [3337] The drug should be visually inspected for particulate matter and discoloration prior to administration;[2754] [3336] [3337] if particulate matter is present or if discoloration or cloudiness occurs, the solution should not be used.[3336] [3337] Ampuls and vials of ephedrine sulfate are intended for single use only, and any remaining drug should be discarded.[2754] [3336] [3337]

Syringes

The stability of ephedrine (salt form unspecified) 10 mg/mL repackaged in polypropylene syringes was evaluated. Little or no change in concentration was found after 4 weeks of storage at room temperature not exposed to direct light.[2164]

Ephedrine sulfate (Ben Venue) 5 mg/mL in sodium chloride 0.9% was packaged in 10-mL polypropylene syringes (Becton Dickinson) and stored at 25°C in fluorescent light and at 4°C. Ephedrine sulfate losses were less than 3% after 60 days under both conditions.[2365]

Ephedrine sulfate 50 mg/mL packaged in polypropylene syringes (Becton Dickinson) was stable for 4 days at room temperature. Analysis found little or no loss of ephedrine sulfate, and no change in solution appearance occurred.[2649]

Compatibility Information

Solution Compatibility

Ephedrine sulfate

Test Soln Name	Mfr	Mfr	Conc/L or %	Remarks	Ref	C/I
Dextrose 2.5% in half-strength Ringer's injection	AB		50 mg	Physically compatible	3	C
Dextrose 5% in Ringer's injection	AB		50 mg	Physically compatible	3	C
Dextrose 2.5% in Ringer's injection, lactated	AB		50 mg	Physically compatible	3	C
Dextrose 5% in half-strength Ringer's injection, lactated	AB		50 mg	Physically compatible	3	C
Dextrose 5% in Ringer's injection, lactated	AB		50 mg	Physically compatible	3	C
Dextrose 10% in Ringer's injection, lactated	AB		50 mg	Physically compatible	3	C
Dextrose 2.5% in sodium chloride 0.45%	AB		50 mg	Physically compatible	3	C
Dextrose 2.5% in sodium chloride 0.9%	AB		50 mg	Physically compatible	3	C
Dextrose 5% in sodium chloride 0.225%	AB		50 mg	Physically compatible	3	C

DOI: 10.37573/9781585286850.142

Solution Compatibility (Cont.)

Test Soln Name	Mfr	Mfr	Conc/L or %	Remarks	Ref	C/I
Dextrose 5% in sodium chloride 0.45%	AB		50 mg	Physically compatible	3	C
Dextrose 5% in sodium chloride 0.9%	AB		50 mg	Physically compatible	3	C
Dextrose 10% in sodium chloride 0.9%	AB		50 mg	Physically compatible	3	C
Dextrose 2.5%	AB		50 mg	Physically compatible	3	C
Dextrose 5%	AB		50 mg	Physically compatible	3	C
Dextrose 5%		AKN, AVD, PAR	5 g	Manufacturer-recommended solution	2754, 3336, 3337	C
Dextrose 10%	AB		50 mg	Physically compatible	3	C
Ionosol B in dextrose 5%	AB		50 mg	Physically compatible	3	C
Ionosol MB in dextrose 5%	AB		50 mg	Physically compatible	3	C
Ringer's injection	AB		50 mg	Physically compatible	3	C
Ringer's injection, lactated	AB		50 mg	Physically compatible	3	C
Sodium chloride 0.45%	AB		50 mg	Physically compatible	3	C
Sodium chloride 0.9%	AB		50 mg	Physically compatible	3	C
Sodium chloride 0.9%		AKN, AVD, PAR	5 g	Manufacturer-recommended solution	2754, 3336, 3337	C
Sodium lactate ⅙ M	AB		50 mg	Physically compatible	3	C

Additive Compatibility

Ephedrine sulfate

Test Drug	Mfr	Conc/L or %	Mfr	Conc/L or %	Test Solution	Remarks	Ref	C/I
Chloramphenicol sodium succinate	PD	1 g	AB	50 mg		Physically compatible	6	C
Lidocaine HCl	AST	2 g		50 mg		Physically compatible	24	C
Nafcillin sodium	WY	500 mg		50 mg		Physically compatible	27	C
Penicillin G potassium		1 million units		50 mg		Physically compatible	3	C
Penicillin G potassium	SQ	5 million units	AB	50 mg		Physically compatible	47	C
Pentobarbital sodium	AB	1 g	LI	250 mg	D5W	Physically incompatible	15	I
Phenobarbital sodium	WI	200 mg	LI	250 mg	D5W	Physically incompatible	15	I

Drugs in Syringe Compatibility

Ephedrine sulfate

Test Drug	Mfr	Amt	Mfr	Amt	Remarks	Ref	C/I
Pentobarbital sodium	AB	500 mg/10 mL		50 mg/1 mL	Physically compatible	55	C

Y-Site Injection Compatibility (1:1 Mixture)

Ephedrine sulfate

Test Drug	Mfr	Conc	Mfr	Conc	Remarks	Ref	C/I
Bivalirudin	TMC	5 mg/mL[a]	TAY	5 mg/mL[a]	Physically compatible for 4 hr at 23°C	2373	C
Cangrelor tetrasodium	TMC	1 mg/mL[b]		5 mg/mL[b]	Physically compatible for 4 hr	3243	C
Clevidipine butyrate	CHS	0.5 mg/mL		50 mg/mL	pH shifted outside of specified pH range for clevidipine within 24 hr	3334	?
Dexmedetomidine HCl	AB	4 mcg/mL[b]	TAY	5 mg/mL[b]	Physically compatible for 4 hr at 23°C	2383	C
Etomidate	AB	2 mg/mL	AB	50 mg/mL	Visually compatible for 7 days at 25°C	1801	C
Fenoldopam mesylate	AB	80 mcg/mL[b]	BED	5 mg/mL[b]	Physically compatible for 4 hr at 23°C	2467	C
Hetastarch in lactated electrolyte	AB	6%	TAY	5 mg/mL[a]	Physically compatible for 4 hr at 23°C	2339	C
Propofol	ZEN[c]	10 mg/mL	AB	5 mg/mL[a]	Physically compatible for 1 hr at 23°C	2066	C

[a] Tested in dextrose 5%.

[b] Tested in sodium chloride 0.9%.

[c] Test performed using the formulation WITH edetate disodium.

Selected Revisions January 31, 2020. © Copyright, October 1982. American Society of Health-System Pharmacists, Inc.

Epinephrine Hydrochloride
AHFS 12:12.12

Products

Epinephrine hydrochloride 1 mg/mL is available in 1-mL ampuls, 30-mL vials, and 0.3-mL auto-injector syringes. Epinephrine hydrochloride is also available at a concentration of 0.1 mg/mL (1:10,000) in vials and prefilled syringes. Some products also contain sodium chloride, a bisulfite antioxidant, and an antibacterial preservative such as chlorobutanol.[1(11/05)] [4]

pH

From 2.2 to 5.[4] [17]

Osmolality

The osmolality of epinephrine hydrochloride (Abbott) 0.1 mg/mL was determined to be 273 mOsm/kg by freezing-point depression.[1071] A 1-mg/mL solution was determined to have an osmolality of 348 mOsm/kg.[1233]

Trade Name(s)

Adrenalin Chloride, Epipen

Administration

Epinephrine hydrochloride may be administered by subcutaneous, intramuscular, intravenous, or intracardiac injection. Intramuscular injection into the buttocks should be avoided.[1(11/05)] [4] Intravenous infusion at a rate of 1 to 10 mcg/min has also been described.[4]

Stability

Epinephrine hydrochloride is sensitive to light and air.[4] [1259] Protection from light is recommended. Withdrawal of doses from multiple-dose vials introduces air, which results in oxidation. As epinephrine oxidizes, it changes from colorless to pink, as adrenochrome forms, to brown, as melanin forms.[4] [1072] Discolored solutions or solutions containing a precipitate should not be used.[4] The various epinephrine preparations have varying stabilities, depending on the form and the preservatives present. The manufacturer's recommendations should be followed with regard to storage.[4]

The stability of epinephrine hydrochloride in intact ampuls subjected to resterilization to provide a sterile outer surface was evaluated. Epinephrine hydrochloride (adrenalin injection, BP) ampuls were resterilized by the following methods:

1. Autoclaved at 121°C for 15 minutes.
2. Autoclaved at 115°C for 30 minutes.
3. Exposed to ethylene oxide–freon (12:88) at 55°C for 4 hours followed by aeration at 50°C for 12 hours.

No loss of epinephrine hydrochloride concentration was found in samples from any of these methods. However, if ampuls were resterilized by autoclaving 2 times at 121°C for 15 minutes, 8% of the drug was lost.[803]

Epinephrine hydrochloride is rapidly destroyed by alkalies or oxidizing agents including sodium bicarbonate, halogens, permanganates, chromates, nitrates, nitrites, and salts of easily reducible metals such as iron, copper, and zinc.[4]

Visual inspection for color changes may be inadequate to assess compatibility of epinephrine hydrochloride admixtures. In one evaluation with aminophylline stored at 25°C, a color change was not noted until 8 hours had elapsed. However, only 40% of the initial epinephrine hydrochloride was still present in the admixture at 24 hours.[527]

pH Effects

The primary determinant of catecholamine stability in intravenous admixtures is the pH of the solution.[527] Epinephrine hydrochloride is unstable in dextrose 5% at a pH above 5.5.[48] The pH of optimum stability is 3 to 4.[1072] In one study, the decomposition rate increased twofold (from 5 to 10% in 200 days at 30°C) when the pH was increased from 2.5 to 4.5.[1259]

When lidocaine hydrochloride is mixed with epinephrine hydrochloride, the buffering capacity of the lidocaine hydrochloride may raise the pH of intravenous admixtures above 5.5, the maximum necessary for stability of epinephrine hydrochloride. The final pH is usually about 6. Epinephrine hydrochloride will begin to deteriorate within several hours. Therefore, admixtures should be used promptly after preparation or the separate administration of the epinephrine hydrochloride should be considered. This restriction does not apply to commercial lidocaine–epinephrine combinations that have had the pH adjusted for epinephrine stability.[24]

Syringes

Epinephrine hydrochloride was diluted to 1 and 7 mg/10 mL with sterile water for injection and repackaged into 10-mL glass vials and plastic syringes with 18-gauge needles (Becton Dickinson). The diluted injections were stored at room temperature protected from light. Epinephrine stability was evaluated over 56 days of storage. The 1-mg/10-mL samples had an epinephrine loss of 4 to 6% in 7 days and 13% in 14 days. The 7-mg/10-mL samples lost 2% in the glass vials and 5% in the syringes in 56 days.[1902]

Epinephrine hydrochloride 1:10,000 in autoinjector syringes was evaluated for stability over 45 days under use conditions in paramedic vehicles. Temperatures fluctuated with locations and conditions and ranged from 6.5°C (43.7 °F) to 52°C (125.6 °F) in high desert conditions. No visually apparent changes occurred, and not more than 6% loss of epinephrine hydrochloride was found. Most samples exhibited no loss.[2548]

Epinephrine hydrochloride under simulated summer conditions in paramedic vehicles was exposed to temperatures ranging from 26 to 38°C over 4 weeks. Analysis found no loss of the drug under these conditions. However, the buffer in the injection was altered, resulting in an increase in pH.[2562]

DOI: 10.37573/9781585286850.143

Central Venous Catheter

Epinephrine hydrochloride (American Regent) 0.1 mg/mL in dextrose 5% was found to be compatible with the ARROW-g+ard Blue Plus (Arrow International) chlorhexidine-bearing triple-lumen central catheter. Essentially complete delivery of the drug was found with little or no drug loss occurring. Furthermore, chlorhexidine delivered from the catheter remained at trace amounts with no substantial increase due to the delivery of the drug through the catheter.[2335]

Compatibility Information

Solution Compatibility

Epinephrine HCl

Test Soln Name	Mfr	Mfr	Conc/L or %	Remarks	Ref	C/I
Dextrose 2.5% in half-strength Ringer's injection	AB	PD	4 mg	Physically compatible	3	C
Dextrose 5% in Ringer's injection	AB	PD	4 mg	Physically compatible	3	C
Dextrose 5% in half-strength Ringer's injection, lactated	AB	PD	4 mg	Physically compatible	3	C
Dextrose 2.5% in Ringer's injection, lactated	AB	PD	4 mg	Physically compatible	3	C
Dextrose 5% in Ringer's injection, lactated	AB	PD	4 mg	Physically compatible	3	C
Dextrose 5% in Ringer's injection, lactated	TR[a]	PD	1 mg	Stable for 24 hr at 5°C	282	C
Dextrose 10% in Ringer's injection, lactated	AB	PD	4 mg	Physically compatible	3	C
Dextrose 2.5% in sodium chloride 0.45%	AB	PD	4 mg	Physically compatible	3	C
Dextrose 2.5% in sodium chloride 0.9%	AB	PD	4 mg	Physically compatible	3	C
Dextrose 5% in sodium chloride 0.225%	AB	PD	4 mg	Physically compatible	3	C
Dextrose 5% in sodium chloride 0.45%	AB	PD	4 mg	Physically compatible	3	C
Dextrose 5% in sodium chloride 0.9%	AB	PD	4 mg	Physically compatible	3	C
Dextrose 5% in sodium chloride 0.9%	TR[a]	PD	1 mg	Stable for 24 hr at 5°C	282	C
Dextrose 10% in sodium chloride 0.9%	AB	PD	4 mg	Physically compatible	3	C
Dextrose 2.5%	AB	PD	4 mg	Physically compatible	3	C
Dextrose 5%	AB	PD	4 mg	Physically compatible	3	C
Dextrose 5%	TR[a]	PD	1 mg	Stable for 24 hr at 5°C	282	C
Dextrose 5%	AB	PD	4 mg	Physically compatible and stable. At 25°C, 10% loss is calculated to occur in 50 hr in light and in 1000 hr in the dark	527	C
Dextrose 5%	BA[b]	ANT	16 mg	5% loss in 20.75 days at 5°C protected from light	1610	C
Dextrose 5%	BA[a]	AMR	87 mg	No epinephrine loss in 24 hr at 23°C protected from light	2085	C
Dextrose 10%	AB	PD	4 mg	Physically compatible	3	C
Ionosol B in dextrose 5%	AB	PD	4 mg	Physically compatible	3	C
Ionosol MB in dextrose 5%	AB	PD	4 mg	Physically compatible	3	C
Ionosol T in dextrose 5%	AB	PD	4 mg	Haze or precipitate within 6 to 24 hr	3	I
Ringer's injection	AB	PD	4 mg	Physically compatible	3	C

Solution Compatibility (Cont.)

Test Soln Name	Mfr	Mfr	Conc/L or %	Remarks	Ref	C/I
Ringer's injection, lactated	AB	PD	4 mg	Physically compatible	3	C
Ringer's injection, lactated	TR[a]	PD	1 mg	Stable for 24 hr at 5°C	282	C
Sodium chloride 0.9%	TR[a]	PD	1 mg	Stable for 24 hr at 5°C	282	C
Sodium lactate ⅙ M	AB	PD	4 mg	Physically compatible	3	C

[a] Tested in both glass and PVC containers.

[b] Tested in PVC containers.

Additive Compatibility

Epinephrine HCl

Test Drug	Mfr	Conc/L or %	Mfr	Conc/L or %	Test Solution	Remarks	Ref	C/I
Amikacin sulfate	BR	5 g	PD	2.5 mg	D5LR, D5R, D5S, D5W, D10W, LR, NS, R, SL	Physically compatible and both stable for 24 hr at 25°C	294	C
Aminophylline	SE	500 mg	PD	4 mg	D5W	At 25°C, 10% epinephrine decomposition in 1.2 hr in light and 3 hr in dark	527	I
Aminophylline		500 mg		4 mg	D5W	Pink to brown discoloration in 8 to 24 hr at room temperature	845	I
Bupivacaine HCl	WI[c]	440 mg	AB	0.69 mg	[b]	No bupivacaine and fentanyl loss and 10% epinephrine loss in 30 days at 3 and 23°C then 48 hr at 30°C	1627	C
Bupivacaine HCl	IVX[d]	1 g	PHX	2 mg		Visually compatible with less than 10% loss of epinephrine and no loss of other drugs in 182 days at 4 and 22°C. Bitartrate salt of epinephrine tested	2613	C
Dobutamine HCl	LI	1 g	BR	50 mg	D5W, NS	Physically compatible for 24 hr at 21°C	812	C
Fentanyl citrate	JN[e]	1.25 mg	AB	0.69 mg	[b]	No bupivacaine and fentanyl loss and 10% epinephrine loss in 30 days at 3 and 23°C then 48 hr at 30°C	1627	C
Fentanyl citrate	IVX[f]	2 mg	PHX	2 mg		Visually compatible with less than 10% loss of epinephrine and no loss of other drugs in 182 days at 4 and 22°C. Bitartrate salt of epinephrine tested	2613	C
Floxacillin sodium	BE	20 g	ANT	8 mg	W	Physically compatible for 72 hr at 15 and 30°C	1479	C
Furosemide	HO	1 g	ANT	8 mg	W	Physically compatible for 72 hr at 15 and 30°C	1479	C
Ranitidine HCl	GL	50 mg and 2 g		50 mg	D5W	Physically compatible. Ranitidine stable for 24 hr at 25°C. Epinephrine not tested	1515	C
Sodium bicarbonate	AB	2.4 mEq[a]		4 mg	D5W	Epinephrine inactivated	772	I

Additive Compatibility (Cont.)

Test Drug	Mfr	Conc/L or %	Mfr	Conc/L or %	Test Solution	Remarks	Ref	C/I
Sodium bicarbonate		5%		4 mg		Epinephrine rapidly decomposes. 58% loss immediately after mixing	48	I
Verapamil HCl	KN	80 mg	PD	2 mg	D5W, NS	Physically compatible for 24 hr	764	C

[a] One vial of Neut added to a liter of admixture.

[b] Tested in portable infusion pump reservoirs (Pharmacia Deltec).

[c] Tested with fentanyl citrate (JN) 1.25 mg.

[d] Tested with fentanyl citrate (IVX) 2 mg.

[e] Tested with bupivacaine HCl (WI) 440 mg.

[f] Tested with bupivacaine HCl (IVX) 1 g.

Drugs in Syringe Compatibility

Epinephrine HCl

Test Drug	Mfr	Amt	Mfr	Amt	Remarks	Ref	C/I
Caffeine citrate		20 mg/1 mL	IMS	0.1 mg/1 mL	Visually compatible for 4 hr at 25°C	2440	C
Doxapram HCl	RB	400 mg/20 mL		1 mg/1 mL	Physically compatible with no doxapram loss in 24 hr	1177	C
Heparin sodium		2500 units/1 mL		1 mg/1 mL	Physically compatible for at least 5 min	1053	C
Iohexol	WI	64.7%, 5 mL	PD	1 mg/1 mL	Physically compatible for at least 2 hr	1438	C
Iopamidol	SQ	61%, 5 mL	PD	1 mg/1 mL	Physically compatible for at least 2 hr	1438	C
Iothalamate meglumine	MA	60%, 5 mL	PD	1 mg/1 mL	Physically compatible for at least 2 hr	1438	C
Ioxaglate meglumine–ioxaglate sodium	MA	5 mL	PD	1 mg/1 mL	Physically compatible for at least 2 hr	1438	C
Milrinone lactate	STR	5.25 mg/5.25 mL	AB	0.5 mg/0.5 mL	Physically compatible. No loss of either drug in 20 min at 23°C	1410	C
Pantoprazole sodium	[a]	4 mg/1 mL		1 mg/1 mL	Precipitates	2574	I

[a] Test performed using the formulation WITHOUT edetate disodium.

Y-Site Injection Compatibility (1:1 Mixture)

Epinephrine HCl

Test Drug	Mfr	Conc	Mfr	Conc	Remarks	Ref	C/I
Amiodarone HCl	WY	6 mg/mL[a]	AMR	1 mg/mL	Visually compatible for 24 hr at 22°C	2352	C
Ampicillin sodium	WY	40 mg/mL[b]	ES	32 mcg/mL[c]	Slight color change in 3 hr	1316	I
Angiotensin II acetate	LJ	5 and 10 mcg/mL[b]	[n]		Stated to be compatible	3430	C
Anidulafungin	VIC	0.5 mg/mL[a]	AMR	50 mcg/mL	Physically compatible for 4 hr at 23°C	2617	C
Atracurium besylate	BW	0.5 mg/mL[a]	AB	4 mcg/mL[a]	Physically compatible for 24 hr at 28°C	1337	C
Bivalirudin	TMC	5 mg/mL[a]	AMR	50 mcg/mL[a]	Physically compatible for 4 hr at 23°C	2373	C
Calcium chloride	AB	4 mg/mL[c]	ES	0.032 mg/mL[c]	Physically compatible for 3 hr	1316	C
Calcium gluconate	AST	4 mg/mL[c]	ES	0.032 mg/mL[c]	Physically compatible for 3 hr	1316	C
Cangrelor tetrasodium	TMC	1 mg/mL[b]		50 mcg/mL[b]	Physically compatible for 4 hr	3243	C

Y-Site Injection Compatibility (1:1 Mixture) (Cont.)

Test Drug	Mfr	Conc	Mfr	Conc	Remarks	Ref	C/I
Caspofungin acetate	ME	0.7 mg/mL[b]	AMP	0.05 mg/mL[b]	Physically compatible for 4 hr at room temperature	2758	C
Ceftazidime	GSK	120 mg/mL[e]		50 mcg/mL	Physically compatible with less than 10% ceftazidime loss. Epinephrine not tested	2513	C
Ceftolozane sulfate–tazobactam sodium	CUB	10 mg/mL[c i]	JHP[k]	16 mcg/mL[c]	Physically compatible for 2 hr	3247, 3262	C
Cisatracurium besylate	GW	0.1, 2, 5 mg/mL[a]	AMR	0.05 mg/mL[a]	Physically compatible for 4 hr at 23°C	2074	C
Clevidipine butyrate	CHS	0.5 mg/mL		1 mg/mL	Emulsion broke	3334	I
Clonidine HCl	BI	18 mcg/mL[b]	NYC	20 mcg/mL[a]	Visually compatible	2642	C
Cloxacillin sodium	SMX	100 mg/mL	HOS[k]	0.1 mg/mL	Physically compatible for up to 4 hr at room temperature	3245	C
Cloxacillin sodium	SMX	100 mg/mL	ERF	1 mg/mL	Physically compatible for up to 4 hr at room temperature	3245	C
Dexmedetomidine HCl	AB	4 mcg/mL[b]	AMR	50 mcg/mL[b]	Physically compatible for 4 hr at 23°C	2383	C
Diltiazem HCl	MMD	5 mg/mL	PD	0.004 and 0.05 mg/mL[b]	Visually compatible	1807	C
Diltiazem HCl	MMD	1 mg/mL[b]	PD	0.05 mg/mL[b]	Visually compatible	1807	C
Diltiazem HCl	MMD	1 mg/mL[a]	AB	0.02 mg/mL[a]	Visually compatible for 4 hr at 27°C	2062	C
Dobutamine HCl	LI	4 mg/mL[a]	AB	0.02 mg/mL[a]	Visually compatible for 4 hr at 27°C	2062	C
Dopamine HCl	AB	3.2 mg/mL[a]	AB	0.02 mg/mL[a]	Visually compatible for 4 hr at 27°C	2062	C
Eravacycline dihydro-chloride	TET	0.6 mg/mL[b]	BPI[k]	16 mcg/mL[b]	Physically compatible for 2 hr at room temperature	3532	C
Esmolol HCl	MYL	10 mg/mL	AMP[n]	0.128 mg/mL[b]	Physically compatible for 1 hr at 23°C	3533	C
Famotidine	MSD	0.2 mg/mL[a]	ES	4 mcg/mL[a]	Physically compatible for 4 hr at 25°C	1188	C
Fenoldopam mesylate	AB	80 mcg/mL[b]	AMR	50 mcg/mL[b]	Physically compatible for 4 hr at 23°C	2467	C
Fentanyl citrate	ES	0.05 mg/mL	AB	0.02 mg/mL[a]	Visually compatible for 4 hr at 27°C	2062	C
Furosemide	AMR	10 mg/mL	AB	0.02 mg/mL[a]	Visually compatible for 4 hr at 27°C	2062	C
Heparin sodium	UP	1000 units/L[d]	AB	0.1 mg/mL	Physically compatible for 4 hr at room temperature	534	C
Heparin sodium	ES	100 units/mL[a]	AB	0.02 mg/mL[a]	Visually compatible for 4 hr at 27°C	2062	C
Hetastarch in lactated electrolyte	AB	6%	AB	0.05 mg/mL[a]	Physically compatible for 4 hr at 23°C	2339	C
Hydrocortisone sodium succinate	UP	10 mg/L[d]	AB	0.1 mg/mL	Physically compatible for 4 hr at room temperature	534	C
Hydromorphone HCl	KN	1 mg/mL	AB	0.02 mg/mL[a]	Visually compatible for 4 hr at 27°C	2062	C
Hydroxyethyl starch 130/0.4 in sodium chloride 0.9%	FRK	6%	BIO	16, 24, 32 mcg/mL[a]	Color change within 4 hr	2770	I
Ibuprofen lysinate	OVA	10 mg/mL	AMR[n]	8, 64, and 100 mcg/mL[a]	Physically compatible for 4 hr at room temperature	3541	C
Isavuconazonium sulfate	ASP	1.5 mg/mL[c]	JHP[k]	16 mcg/mL[c]	Physically compatible for 2 hr	3247, 3263	C
Labetalol HCl	AH	2 mg/mL[a]	AB	0.02 mg/mL[a]	Visually compatible for 4 hr at 27°C	2062	C

Y-Site Injection Compatibility (1:1 Mixture) (Cont.)

Test Drug	Mfr	Conc	Mfr	Conc	Remarks	Ref	C/I
Labetalol HCl	HOS	5 mg/mL	AMP[n]	0.128 mg/mL[b]	Physically compatible for 1 hr at 23°C	3533	C
Levofloxacin	OMN	5 mg/mL[a]	AB	1 mg/mL	Visually compatible for 4 hr at 24°C	2233	C
Lorazepam	WY	0.5 mg/mL[a]	AB	0.02 mg/mL[a]	Visually compatible for 4 hr at 27°C	2062	C
Meropenem		50 mg/mL	ERF	1 mg/mL	Physically compatible for 4 hr at room temperature	3538	C
Meropenem–vaborbactam	TMC	8 mg/mL[b m]	HOS[k]	16 mcg/mL[b]	Physically compatible for 3 hr at 20 to 25°C	3380	C
Metoprolol tartrate	HOS	0.4 mg/mL[b]	AMP[n]	0.128 mg/mL[b]	Physically compatible for 1 hr at 23°C	3533	C
Micafungin sodium	ASP	1.5 mg/mL[b]	AB	50 mcg/mL[b]	Microparticulates form in 4 hr	2683	I
Midazolam HCl	RC	2 mg/mL[a]	AB	0.02 mg/mL[a]	Visually compatible for 4 hr at 27°C	2062	C
Milrinone lactate	SW	0.2 mg/mL[a]	AB	0.02 mg/mL[a]	Visually compatible for 4 hr at 27°C	2062	C
Milrinone lactate	SW	0.4 mg/mL[a]	AB	0.064 mg/mL[a]	Visually compatible. Little loss of either drug in 4 hr at 23°C	2214	C
Morphine sulfate	SCN	2 mg/mL[a]	AB	0.02 mg/mL[a]	Visually compatible for 4 hr at 27°C	2062	C
Nesiritide	SCI	50 mcg/mL[a b]		1 mg/mL	Physically compatible for 4 hr. May be chemically incompatible with nesiritide[j]	2625	?
Nicardipine HCl	WY	1 mg/mL[a]	AB	0.02 mg/mL[a]	Visually compatible for 4 hr at 27°C	2062	C
Nitroglycerin	AB	0.4 mg/mL[a]	AB	0.02 mg/mL[a]	Visually compatible for 4 hr at 27°C	2062	C
Norepinephrine bitartrate	AB	0.128 mg/mL[a]	AB	0.02 mg/mL[a]	Visually compatible for 4 hr at 27°C	2062	C
Oritavancin diphosphate	TAR	0.8, 1.2, and 2 mg/mL[a]	HOS	40 mcg/mL[a]	Visually compatible for 4 hr at 20 to 24°C	2928	C
Pancuronium bromide	ES	0.05 mg/mL[a]	AB	4 mcg/mL[a]	Physically compatible for 24 hr at 28°C	1337	C
Pantoprazole sodium	ALT[i]	0.16 to 0.8 mg/mL[b]	AB	16 to 32 mcg/mL[a]	Visually compatible for 12 hr at 23°C	2603	C
Phytonadione	MSD	0.4 mg/mL[c]	ES	0.032 mg/mL[c]	Physically compatible for 3 hr	1316	C
Plazomicin sulfate	ACH	24 mg/mL[c]	HOS[k]	16 mcg/mL[c]	Physically compatible for 1 hr at 20 to 25°C	3432	C
Potassium chloride	AB	40 mEq/L[d]	AB	0.1 mg/mL	Physically compatible for 4 hr at room temperature	534	C
Propofol	ZEN[o]	10 mg/mL	AMR	0.1 mg/mL	Physically compatible for 1 hr at 23°C	2066	C
Ranitidine HCl	GL	1 mg/mL[a]	AB	0.02 mg/mL[a]	Visually compatible for 4 hr at 27°C	2062	C
Remifentanil HCl	GW	0.025 and 0.25 mg/mL[b]	AMR	0.05 mg/mL[a]	Physically compatible for 4 hr at 23°C	2075	C
Sodium nitroprusside	RC	1.2 and 3 mg/mL[a]	AB	0.03, 0.12, 0.3 mg/mL[h]	Visually compatible for 48 hr at 24°C protected from light	2357	C
Tedizolid phosphate	CUB	0.8 mg/mL[b]	JHP[k]	16 mcg/mL[b]	Physically compatible for 2 hr; however, mean pH change >1 unit within 2 hr	3244, 3247	?
Tigecycline	WY	1 mg/mL[b]		4 mcg/mL[b]	Physically compatible for 4 hr	2714	C
Tirofiban HCl	ME	50 mcg/mL[a b]	AMR	2 and 100 mcg/mL[a b]	Physically compatible. No loss of either drug in 4 hr at 23°C	2356	C
TPN #189[f]			AST	0.2 mg/mL[b]	Visually compatible for 24 hr at 22°C	1767	C

Y-Site Injection Compatibility (1:1 Mixture) (Cont.)

Test Drug	Mfr	Conc	Mfr	Conc	Remarks	Ref	C/I
Vasopressin	AMR	2 and 4 units/mL[b]	AMR	4 mcg/mL[b]	Physically compatible with vasopressin pushed through a Y-site over 5 sec	2478	C
Vecuronium bromide	OR	0.1 mg/mL[a]	AB	4 mcg/mL[a]	Physically compatible for 24 hr at 28°C	1337	C
Vecuronium bromide	OR	1 mg/mL	AB	0.02 mg/mL[a]	Visually compatible for 4 hr at 27°C	2062	C

[a] Tested in dextrose 5%.

[b] Tested in sodium chloride 0.9%.

[c] Tested in both dextrose 5% and sodium chloride 0.9%.

[d] Tested in dextrose 5% in Ringer's injection, dextrose 5% in Ringer's injection, lactated, dextrose 5%, Ringer's injection, lactated, and sodium chloride 0.9%.

[e] Tested in sterile water for injection.

[f] Refer to Appendix for the composition of parenteral nutrition solutions. TPN indicates a 2-in-1 admixture.

[g] Tested in dextrose 5%, Ringer's injection, lactated, sodium chloride 0.45%, and sodium chloride 0.9%.

[h] Tested in dextrose 5% in sodium chloride 0.45%.

[i] Test performed using the formulation WITHOUT edetate disodium.

[j] Nesiritide is incompatible with bisulfite antioxidants used in some drug formulations. The specific formulation of the product to be used should be checked to assure that no sulfite antioxidants are present.

[k] As epinephrine base rather than the salt.

[l] Ceftolozane component. Ceftolozane in a 2:1 fixed-ratio concentration with tazobactam.

[m] Meropenem component. Meropenem in a 1:1 fixed-ratio concentration with vaborbactam.

[n] Salt not specified.

[o] Test performed using the formulation WITH edetate disodium.

Selected Revisions May 1, 2020. © Copyright, October 1982.
American Society of Health-System Pharmacists, Inc.

Epirubicin Hydrochloride
AHFS 10:00

Products

Epirubicin hydrochloride is available as a clear, red, preservative-free, ready-to-use 2-mg/mL solution in single-use 25- and 100-mL vials containing 50 and 200 mg of drug, respectively.[3377] The solution also contains sodium chloride and water for injection.[3377] The pH has been adjusted with hydrochloric acid.[3377]

pH

Adjusted to 3.[3377]

Trade Name(s)

Ellence

Administration

Epirubicin hydrochloride is administered slowly by intravenous infusion into the tubing of a freely running intravenous infusion of sodium chloride 0.9% or dextrose 5%.[3377] The manufacturer states that initial therapy at the recommended starting dosage generally should be infused over 15 to 20 minutes.[3377] For patients receiving reduced dosages (e.g., due to organ dysfunction and/or dosage modification for toxicity), the infusion time may be proportionally decreased; however, the drug should not be infused over less than 3 minutes.[3377] Administration by direct push injection is not recommended because of the risk of extravasation.[3377]

Extravasation may occur even in the presence of adequate blood return upon needle aspiration.[3377] Extravasation may cause local pain, severe tissue lesions (e.g., vesication, severe cellulitis), and necrosis and should be avoided.[3377] Burning or stinging may indicate perivenous infiltration, which requires immediately terminating the infusion and restarting it in another vein.[3377] Perivenous infiltration also may occur without pain.[3377] Venous sclerosis may result from injection of the drug into a small vessel or from repeated injection into the same vein.[3377] Facial flushing and erythematous streaking along the vein may result from excessively rapid administration and may precede local phlebitis or thrombophlebitis.[3377] Decreasing the duration of infusion of the drug proportionally with an indicated dosage reduction is intended to reduce the risk of thrombosis or perivenous extravasation, which could in turn reduce the risk of severe cellulitis, vesication, or tissue necrosis.[3377] Infusion of the drug into veins occurring over joints or in extremities with compromised venous or lymphatic drainage should be avoided if possible.[3377] Epirubicin hydrochloride must *not* be administered by intramuscular or subcutaneous injection.[3377]

As with other toxic drugs, caution should be exercised in the handling and preparation of epirubicin hydrochloride.[3377] Personnel preparing and administering the drug should take protective measures to avoid contact with the solution, including use of disposable gloves, gowns, masks, and goggles.[3377] Dose preparation preferably should be performed in a suitable laminar airflow device on a work surface protected by disposable, plastic-backed, absorbent paper.[3377] Procedures for the proper disposal of epirubicin hydrochloride should be considered; all equipment and materials used in the preparation and administration of doses and for cleaning should be disposed of safely in high-risk waste disposal bags intended for high-temperature incineration.[3377] In the event of spills or leaks, the manufacturer recommends preferably soaking first with a dilute sodium hypochlorite (1% available chlorine) solution, followed by water.[3377] Hands always should be washed after removing gloves.[3377] If accidental skin or eye contact with the drug occurs, the affected area(s) should be flushed immediately with a large amount of water, soap and water, or a sodium bicarbonate solution; the skin should not be abraded by using a scrub brush.[3377] Medical attention should be sought.[3377]

Stability

Intact vials should be stored at 2 to 8°C and protected from freezing and exposure to light.[3377] Although vials should be stored under refrigeration, manufacturers note that refrigeration of epirubicin hydrochloride injection can result in the formation of a gelled product; however, the gelled product will return to a slightly viscous to mobile solution after 2 to 4 hours (maximum) at a controlled room temperature of 15 to 25°C.[3377] Epirubicin hydrochloride solution should be visually inspected for particulate matter and discoloration prior to administration.[3377] Vials are for single use only and any unused portion should be discarded.[3377] Manufacturers recommend that any unused solution from the single-dose vials be discarded within 24 hours after initial puncture of the vial stopper.[3377]

The manufacturer states that the drug should not be mixed with other drugs in the same syringe.[3377]

pH Effects

Epirubicin hydrochloride stability is pH dependent. The drug becomes progressively more stable at acid pH, with maximum stability at pH 4 to 5.[1007][1460] Prolonged contact of epirubicin hydrochloride with any solution having an alkaline pH should be avoided because of the resulting hydrolysis of the drug.[3377]

Light Effects

Although epirubicin hydrochloride is photosensitive, no special precautions are necessary to protect solutions containing epirubicin hydrochloride 500 mcg/mL or greater during intravenous administration,[1463] even over periods extending to 14 days in room light.[2081]

Syringes

Epirubicin hydrochloride 2 mg/mL in sterile water for injection was stable for at least 43 days at 4°C in Plastipak (Becton Dickinson) plastic syringes.[1460]

DOI: 10.37573/9781585286850.144

Epirubicin hydrochloride 0.5 mg/mL in sodium chloride 0.9% was reported to be stable for at least 28 days at 4 and 20°C when stored in plastic syringes.[1564]

Epirubicin hydrochloride 2 mg/mL in sodium chloride 0.9% in 50-mL polypropylene syringes with blind luer hubs was stored at 25°C both in light and dark and at 4°C in dark. About 2 to 4% loss occurred in 14 days at 25°C whether in light or dark. No loss was found after 180 days of refrigerated storage.[2081]

Epirubicin hydrochloride (Farmorubicine, Pfizer) lyophilized powder formulation containing methylparaben and lactose was reconstituted with sodium chloride 0.9% to a final concentration of 8.33 mg/mL and stored as 6 mL in 50-mL brown polypropylene syringes (Becton Dickinson) with polypropylene caps protected from light.[3378] The solution was reported to be physically and chemically stable, retaining at least 95% of the initial concentration for 72 hours at 4°C with or without additional storage for 4 hours at 22°C.[3378]

Sorption

Although epirubicin hydrochloride was initially reported to undergo sorptive losses to PVC containers, subsequent studies have shown no loss to glass, PVC, and high-density polyethylene containers, PVC, polyethylene, and polybutadiene infusion sets, and polypropylene syringes.[1460][1577][1700]

Filtration

Epirubicin hydrochloride 50 mg/1000 mL in dextrose 5% and sodium chloride 0.9% was infused over 24 hours and exhibited a drug loss during the initial period of filtration through cellulose ester and nylon filters; however, the concentrations returned to expected levels within minutes, and the total amount of drug lost was deemed negligible.[1577]

Compatibility Information

Solution Compatibility

Epirubicin HCl

Test Soln Name	Mfr	Mfr	Conc/L or %	Remarks	Ref	C/I
Dextrose 3.3% in sodium chloride 0.3%		FA	100 mg	5% or less loss in 4 weeks at 25°C in the dark	1007	C
Dextrose 5%		FA	100 mg	5% or less loss in 4 weeks at 25°C in the dark	1007	C
Dextrose 5%	TR[a]	FA	100 mg	10% or less loss in 43 days at –20, 4, and 25°C in the dark	1460	C
Dextrose 5%	[b]	FA	50 mg	9% loss in 30 days at 4°C in the dark	1577	C
Dextrose 5%	[a]	FA	40 mg	Stable for 7 days at 4°C in the dark	1700	C
Ringer's injection, lactated		FA	100 mg	10% loss in 3 days at 25°C in the dark	1007	C
Sodium chloride 0.9%		FA	100 mg	10% loss in 8 days at 25°C in the dark	1007	C
Sodium chloride 0.9%	TR[a]	FA	100 mg	10% or less loss in 43 days at –20, 4, and 25°C in the dark	1460	C
Sodium chloride 0.9%	RS[a]		1 g	Under 5% loss in 4 weeks at –20°C	1462	C
Sodium chloride 0.9%	[b]	FA	50 mg	6% or less loss in 25 days at 4°C in the dark	1577	C
Sodium chloride 0.9%	[a]	FA	40 mg	Stable for 7 days at 4°C in the dark	1700	C
Sodium chloride 0.9%		PH	1 g	Physically stable. No loss in 84 days at 8°C	2534	C

[a] Tested in PVC containers.

[b] Tested in glass, PVC, and high density polyethylene containers.

Additive Compatibility

Epirubicin HCl

Test Drug	Mfr	Conc/L or %	Mfr	Conc/L or %	Test Solution	Remarks	Ref	C/I
Fluorouracil		10 g		0.5 to 1 g	NS	Greater than 10% epirubicin loss in 1 day	1379	I
Fluorouracil			PHU			Potential precipitation	3377	I
Heparin sodium			PHU			Potential precipitation	3377	I

Additive Compatibility (Cont.)

Test Drug	Mfr	Conc/L or %	Mfr	Conc/L or %	Test Solution	Remarks	Ref	C/I
Ifosfamide		2.5 g		1 g	NS	Under 10% loss of either drug in 14 days	1379	C
Irinotecan HCl	RPR	640 mg	CE	560 mg	NS	UV spectrum changes immediately upon mixing	2670	I

Drugs in Syringe Compatibility

Epirubicin HCl

Test Drug	Mfr	Amt	Mfr	Amt	Remarks	Ref	C/I
Fluorouracil		500 mg/10 mL		5 and 10 mg/10 mL[a]	Precipitate forms within several hours of mixing	1564	I
Ifosfamide		50 mg/mL[a]		1 mg/mL[a]	Little or no loss of either drug in 28 days at 4 and 20°C	1564	C
Ifosfamide with mesna		50 mg/mL[a] 40 mg/mL[a]		1 mg/mL[a]	50% epirubicin loss in 7 days at 4 and 20°C. No loss of other drugs in 7 days	1564	I
Mesna with ifosfamide		40 mg/mL[a] 50 mg/mL[a]		1 mg/mL[a]	50% epirubicin loss in 7 days at 4 and 20°C. No loss of other drugs in 7 days	1564	I

[a] Tested in sodium chloride 0.9%.

Y-Site Injection Compatibility (1:1 Mixture)

Epirubicin HCl

Test Drug	Mfr	Conc	Mfr	Conc	Remarks	Ref	C/I
Oxaliplatin	SS	0.5 mg/mL[a]	PHU	0.5 mg/mL[a]	Physically compatible for 4 hr at 23°C	2566	C

[a] Tested in dextrose 5%.

Selected Revisions April 16, 2018. © Copyright, October 1992.
American Society of Health-System Pharmacists, Inc.

Epoetin Alfa
AHFS 20:16

Products

Epoetin alfa is available in 1-mL single-use (unpreserved) vials containing 2000, 3000, 4000, and 10,000 units/mL. The solution also contains in each mL albumin human 2.5 mg, sodium citrate 5.8 mg, sodium chloride 5.8 mg, and citric acid 0.06 mg in water for injection.[1(8/08)]

Preservative-free single-dose epoetin alfa is also available in 1-mL vials containing 40,000 units along with albumin human 2.5 mg, sodium phosphate monobasic monohydrate 1.2 mg, sodium phosphate dibasic anhydrate 1.8 mg, sodium citrate 0.7 mg, sodium chloride 5.8 mg, and citric acid 6.8 mg in water for injection.[1(8/08)]

Epoetin alfa is also available in 2-mL multidose (preserved) vials containing 10,000 units/mL and 1-mL multidose (preserved) vials containing 20,000 units/mL. The solution also contains in each mL albumin human 2.5 mg, sodium citrate 1.3 mg, sodium chloride 8.2 mg, citric acid 0.11 mg, and benzyl alcohol 1% in water for injection.[1(8/08)]

pH

Single-use vials: from 6.6 to 7.2. Multidose vials: from 5.8 to 6.4.[1(8/08)]

Tonicity

The injection is isotonic.[1(8/08)]

Trade Name(s)

Epogen, Procrit

Administration

Epoetin alfa is administered by intravenous or subcutaneous injection. For subcutaneous injection, epoetin alfa (single-dose) may be diluted at the time of administration with an equal quantity of bacteriostatic sodium chloride 0.9% containing benzyl alcohol 0.9% to help ameliorate local discomfort at the subcutaneous injection site.[1(8/08)] [4]

Stability

Epoetin alfa is a colorless solution. It should not be used if it contains particulate matter or is discolored. Intact vials should be stored under refrigeration and protected from freezing.[1(8/08)] Although refrigerated storage is required, the manufacturer has stated the single-dose form may be stored at room temperature for 14 days while the multidose form may be stored at room temperature for seven days.[2745] To prevent foaming and inactivation, the product should not be shaken; vigorous prolonged shaking may denature the protein, inactivating it.[1(8/08)] [4] However, a small amount of flocculated protein in the solution does not affect potency. In addition, exposure to light for less than 24 hours does not adversely affect the product.[4]

The single-dose vials have no preservative. After a single dose has been removed from this product, the vial should not be re-entered and should be discarded.[1(8/08)] Drawn into plastic tuberculin syringes, the preservative-free products at 2000 or 10,000 units/mL are reported to be stable for two weeks at room temperature or under refrigeration. However, use shortly after drawing up in syringes is recommended because of the absence of preservative.[4]

Usually, epoetin alfa should not be diluted and transferred to new containers or admixed with other drugs and solutions because of possible protein loss from adsorption to PVC containers and tubing. However, when 10,000-unit/mL single-use product is diluted in the original vial with benzyl alcohol-preserved sodium chloride 0.9% injection to a concentration of 4000 units/mL for subcutaneous use, it is stated to be stable for at least 12 weeks stored at 5 and 30°C. Furthermore, the final benzyl alcohol concentration of 0.54% enabled the dilution to pass the USP preservative effectiveness test.[1905] Restriction of this dilution to 28 days used as a multiple-dose vial has been recommended.[1906] Higher concentrations of epoetin alfa (e.g., 5000 units/mL), which would have lower benzyl alcohol concentrations, were found to fail the preservative effectiveness test.[1905]

Epoetin alfa (Amgen) 20,000 units/1 mL was packaged in 1-mL hubless Medsaver (Becton Dickinson) plastic syringes and stored under refrigeration for six weeks. No loss of epoetin alfa biological activity was found.[2472]

The multidose vials contain a preservative and may be stored under refrigeration after initial dose removal. The vials should be discarded 21 days after initial entry.[1(8/08)]

DOI: 10.37573/9781585286850.145

Compatibility Information

Solution Compatibility

Epoetin alfa

Test Soln Name	Mfr	Mfr	Conc/L or %	Remarks	Ref	C/I
Dextrose 10%[b]	a	ORT	100 units	40 to 50% of epoetin alfa lost over 24-hr delivery	1878	I
Dextrose 10%[c]	a	ORT	100 units	96% of the epoetin alfa delivered over 24 hr	1878	C
Sodium chloride 0.9%	a	ORT	100 units	15% of epoetin alfa lost over 24-hr delivery	1878	I
TPN[d]	a	ORT	100 units	96% of the epoetin alfa delivered over 24 hr	1878	C

[a] Delivered from a syringe through microbore tubing, T-connector, and a Teflon neonatal 24-gauge intravenous catheter.

[b] Tested with and without albumin human 0.01%.

[c] Tested with albumin human 0.05 and 0.1%.

[d] TPN composed of amino acids (TrophAmine) 0.5% or 2.25% with dextrose 12.5%, vitamins, trace elements, magnesium sulfate, calcium gluconate, sodium chloride, potassium acetate, and heparin sodium.

Selected Revisions October 1, 2012. © Copyright, October 1998.
American Society of Health-System Pharmacists, Inc.

Epoprostenol Sodium
AHFS 48:48

Products

Epoprostenol sodium is available as a lyophilized powder in vials containing 0.5 mg (500,000 ng) and 1.5 mg (1,500,000 ng) of epoprostenol.[2879][2880][2881] Several different formulations of epoprostenol sodium products are available; instructions for reconstitution and administration may differ, and epoprostenol stability may vary depending on formulation-specific factors.[2879][2880][2881]

Epoprostenol sodium (Flolan, Glaxo; generic, Teva) vials also contain glycine 3.76 mg, sodium chloride 2.93 mg, and mannitol 50 mg.[2879][2881] Sodium hydroxide may have been added during manufacturing to adjust the pH.[2879][2881] These epoprostenol sodium vials must be reconstituted and further diluted using only a special diluent that is recommended by the manufacturer.[2879][2881] Flolan must be reconstituted only with one of 2 special diluents, which are labeled as either "sterile diluent for Flolan" (in a 50-mL glass vial) or "pH 12 sterile diluent for Flolan" (in a 50-mL plastic vial).[2879] The choice of which of these 2 special diluents is used in the reconstitution and dilution of Flolan affects the drug's stability.[2879] (See Stability.) Epoprostenol sodium (Teva) must be reconstituted only with the sterile diluent that is labeled as "sterile diluent for epoprostenol sodium for injection" (in a 50-mL glass vial).[2881] Regardless of the formulation, these vials of special diluent contain glycine 94 mg, sodium chloride 73.3 mg, and sodium hydroxide to adjust the pH in water for injection.[2879][2881]

Epoprostenol sodium (Veletri, Actelion) has a differing formulation.[2880] In addition to epoprostenol sodium, vials of Veletri contain sucrose 100 mg, arginine 50 mg, and sodium hydroxide to adjust the pH.[2880] Vials of this formulation may be reconstituted with either sterile water for injection or sodium chloride 0.9% and further diluted with the same diluent used for reconstitution.[2880]

Each 0.5-mg (500,000-ng) or 1.5-mg (1,500,000-ng) vial of any formulation of epoprostenol sodium should be reconstituted with 5 mL of an appropriate diluent.[2879][2880][2881] The reconstituted solutions must be diluted prior to administration to provide a final concentration that is compatible with the maximum and minimum flow rates of the infusion pump, the reservoir capacity, and other infusion pump-specific criteria as stated by the manufacturers.[2879][2880][2881] In general, a 3000- to 10,000-ng/mL concentration of epoprostenol is sufficient to accommodate infusion rates of 2 to 16 ng/kg/min in adults, although higher concentrations may be required for some patients.[2879][2880][2881]

The manufacturers' instructions for preparing various concentrations of epoprostenol from the reconstituted solution using the identical diluent that was used for reconstitution are as follows:[2879][2880][2881]

For 3000 ng/mL, withdraw 3 mL from one 0.5-mg (500,000-ng) vial and add a sufficient amount of diluent to make a total of 100 mL.

For 5000 ng/mL, withdraw the entire contents of one 0.5-mg (500,000-ng) vial and add a sufficient amount of diluent to make a total of 100 mL.

For 10,000 ng/mL, withdraw the entire contents of two 0.5-mg (500,000-ng) vials and add a sufficient amount of diluent to make a total of 100 mL.

For 15,000 ng/mL, withdraw the entire contents of one 1.5-mg (1,500,000-ng) vial and add a sufficient amount of diluent to make a total of 100 mL.

For 30,000 ng/mL, withdraw the entire contents of two 1.5-mg (1,500,000-ng) vials and add a sufficient amount of diluent to make a total of 100 mL.[2880]

The manufacturers state that higher concentrations of the drug may be prepared for those receiving long-term therapy.[2879][2880][2881]

pH

Sterile diluent for Flolan has a pH ranging from 10.2 to 10.8; pH 12 sterile diluent for Flolan has a pH ranging from 11.7 to 12.3.[2879]

Reconstituted solutions of epoprostenol (Teva) prepared with the provided sterile diluent for epoprostenol sodium for injection have a pH ranging from 11 to 11.8.[2881]

Reconstituted solutions of Veletri have a pH ranging from 11 to 13.[2880]

Trade Name(s)

Flolan, Veletri

Administration

Following reconstitution and dilution to the selected final concentration, epoprostenol solution is administered by continuous intravenous infusion through a central venous catheter using an ambulatory infusion pump.[2879][2880][2881] The drug may be given temporarily by peripheral infusion until a central line can be established.[2879][2880][2881] The pump reservoirs used should be made of polyvinyl chloride (PVC), polypropylene, or glass.[2879][2880][2881]

Epoprostenol solutions prepared with sterile diluent for Flolan or sterile diluent for epoprostenol sodium for injection must be used with a cold pouch if not administered within 8 hours of reconstitution or removal from refrigeration.[2879][2881] (See Stability.)

Stability

Epoprostenol Sodium (Flolan, Glaxo)

Intact vials of the Flolan formulation of epoprostenol sodium should be stored at 15 to 25°C in the carton to protect from light.[2879] Intact vials of sterile diluent for Flolan and pH 12 sterile diluent for Flolan also should be stored at 15 to 25°C and should not be frozen.[2879] Flolan must be reconstituted and diluted

DOI: 10.37573/9781585286850.146

only with one of these 2 diluents; the reconstituted epoprostenol solutions should not be diluted or administered with other parenteral solutions or medications.[2879] If not used immediately following preparation, these solutions of epoprostenol should be refrigerated at 2 to 8°C and protected from light.[2879] The solutions should *not* be frozen; any solution that has been frozen should be discarded.[2879] Solutions should be visually inspected for particulate matter and discoloration and should not be used if either is noted.[2879] Vials are for single dose only; any unused solution or diluent should be discarded.[2879]

Epoprostenol solutions prepared with sterile diluent for Flolan are stable for up to 8 hours when used at 15 to 25°C following reconstitution.[2879] These solutions may be stored for up to 40 hours at 2 to 8°C prior to use and are stable for up to 8 hours when used at 15 to 25°C following removal from refrigeration; solutions should be discarded after more than 40 hours of refrigerated storage.[2879] Solutions prepared with sterile diluent for Flolan must be used with a cold pouch if not administered within 8 hours.[2879] These solutions may be stored for up to 24 hours at 2 to 8°C prior to use and are stable for up to 24 hours when used with a cold pouch that is changed every 12 hours.[2879] Solutions may be stored at 2 to 8°C prior to use as long as the total combined time of refrigerated storage and infusion does not exceed 48 hours; solutions should be discarded after more than 48 hours of refrigerated storage.[2879]

Epoprostenol solutions prepared with *pH 12* sterile diluent for Flolan may be administered for up to 72 hours at up to 25°C, 48 hours at up to 30°C, 24 hours at up to 35°C, or 12 hours at up to 40°C, either immediately following preparation or following refrigerated storage at 2 to 8°C for up to 8 days; these solutions do *not* require the use of a cold pouch during administration.[2879] Solutions prepared with *pH 12* sterile diluent for Flolan should be discarded after 8 days of refrigerated storage.[2879]

Epoprostenol Sodium (Teva)

Intact vials of this formulation of epoprostenol sodium should be stored at 20 to 25°C in the carton to protect from light.[2881] Intact vials of sterile diluent for epoprostenol sodium for injection also should be stored at 20 to 25°C and should *not* be frozen.[2881] This epoprostenol sodium formulation must be reconstituted and diluted only with sterile diluent for epoprostenol sodium for injection; the reconstituted epoprostenol solutions should not be diluted or administered with other parenteral medications or solutions.[2881] If not used immediately following preparation, these solutions of epoprostenol should be refrigerated at 2 to 8°C and protected from light.[2881] The solutions should *not* be frozen; any solution that has been frozen should be discarded.[2881] Solutions should be visually inspected for particulate matter and discoloration and should not be used if either is noted.[2881] Vials are for single dose only; any unused solution or diluent should be discarded.[2881]

Epoprostenol solutions prepared with sterile diluent for epoprostenol sodium for injection are stable for up to 8 hours when used at 15 to 25°C following reconstitution.[2881] These solutions may be stored for up to 40 hours at 2 to 8°C prior to use and are stable for up to 8 hours when used at 15 to 25°C following removal from refrigeration; solutions should be discarded after more than 40 hours of refrigerated storage.[2881] Solutions prepared with sterile diluent for epoprostenol sodium for injection must be used with a cold pouch if not administered within 8 hours.[2881] These solutions may be stored for up to 24 hours at 2 to 8°C prior to use and are stable for up to 24 hours when used with a cold pouch that is changed every 12 hours.[2881] Solutions may be stored at 2 to 8°C prior to use as long as the total combined time of refrigerated storage and infusion does not exceed 48 hours; solutions should be discarded after more than 48 hours of refrigerated storage.[2881]

Epoprostenol Sodium (Veletri, Actelion)

Intact vials of the Veletri formulation of epoprostenol sodium should be stored at 20 to 25°C in the carton and protected from direct sunlight.[2880] The manufacturer states that this formulation of epoprostenol sodium is stable only when reconstituted and diluted as directed with sterile water for injection or sodium chloride 0.9%; the drug should not be mixed with any other drugs or solutions prior to or during administration.[2880] Solutions should be visually inspected for particulate matter and discoloration and should not be used if either is noted.[2880] Vials are for single use only; any unused solution should be discarded.[2880]

For administration at 25°C, reconstituted and diluted epoprostenol solutions of 3000 to less than 15,000 ng/mL (prepared as directed using 0.5-mg [500,000-ng] vials) may be administered for a maximum duration of 48 hours beginning immediately after reconstitution and dilution or a maximum duration of 24 hours after storage under refrigeration at 2 to 8°C for up to 8 days.[2880] Solutions of 15,000 to less than 60,000 ng/mL (prepared as directed using 1.5-mg [1,500,000-ng] vials) may be administered at 25°C for a maximum duration of 48 hours beginning either immediately after reconstitution and dilution or after storage under refrigeration at 2 to 8°C for up to 8 days.[2880] Solutions of 60,000 ng/mL or more (prepared using 1.5-mg [1,500,000-ng] vials) may be administered at 25°C for a maximum duration of 72 hours beginning immediately after reconstitution and dilution or a maximum duration of 48 hours after storage under refrigeration at 2 to 8°C for up to 8 days.[2880] Short excursions at 40°C are permitted for up to 2, 4, or 8 hours for solutions of less than 15,000 ng/mL, 15,000 to 60,000 ng/mL, or greater than 60,000 ng/mL, respectively.[2880]

Epoprostenol solutions of 60,000 ng/mL or more (prepared using 1.5-mg [1,500,000-ng] vials) may be administered at temperatures greater than 25°C up to 30°C for a maximum duration of 48 hours, either beginning immediately after reconstitution and dilution or after refrigeration at 2 to 8°C for up to 8 days.[2880] Such solutions also may be administered at temperatures up to 40°C for a maximum duration of 24 hours immediately after reconstitution and dilution.[2880] For solutions with a concentration less than 60,000 ng/mL, the pump reservoir should be changed every 24 hours.[2880]

pH Effects

Epoprostenol is best stabilized in basic solutions,[2882] and the reconstituted solution becomes increasingly unstable at pH values below the respective normal ranges of each formulation.[2880] [2881] Veletri uses arginine as a buffer, which provides a higher pH than that provided by the glycine buffer in other epoprostenol sodium products (Glaxo, Teva) and likely contributes to the relative improvement in stability.[2879] [2880] [2881] [2882] Flolan prepared with the provided *pH 12* sterile diluent for Flolan results in a reconstituted solution with a higher pH than if prepared with the alternative provided sterile diluent for Flolan and demonstrates increased stability as a result.[2879]

Light Effects

Epoprostenol sodium (Flolan, Glaxo; generic, Teva) as unopened vials and reconstituted solutions should be protected from light during storage.[2879] [2881] The manufacturer of Veletri notes that this formulation of epoprostenol sodium should not be exposed to direct sunlight either in the unopened vial during storage or in solution.[2880]

Filtration

A 60-inch microbore non-diethylhexyl phthalate (non-DEHP) extension set with proximal antisyphon valve, low priming volume (0.9 mL), and inline 0.22-μm filter was used during trials with epoprostenol[2880] [2881] and is recommended for Flolan administration.[2879] Infusion sets with an inline 0.22-μm filter should be used for the administration of Veletri.[2880]

Compatibility Information

Y-Site Injection Compatibility (1:1 Mixture)

Epoprostenol sodium

Test Drug	Mfr	Conc	Mfr	Conc	Remarks	Ref	C/I
Bivalirudin	TMC	5 mg/mL[a]	GW[b]	10 mcg/mL[a]	Physically compatible for 4 hr at 23°C	2373	C

[a] Tested in dextrose 5%.

[b] Test performed using the Flolan formulation.

Eptifibatide
AHFS 20:12.18

Products

Eptifibatide is available at a concentration of 2 mg/mL in 10- and 100-mL vials and at a concentration of 0.75 mg/mL in 100-mL vials.[3048] Each mL of injection also contains citric acid 5.25 mg and sodium hydroxide to adjust the pH.[3048]

pH

The pH is adjusted to near 5.35 during manufacturing.[3048]

Trade Name(s)

Integrilin

Administration

Eptifibatide is administered by intravenous bolus (push) injection; the appropriate dose should be withdrawn from the 10-mL vial.[3048] The bolus dose should be followed immediately by a continuous intravenous infusion; using an infusion pump, the appropriate concentration of eptifibatide in a 100-mL vial should be spiked with a vented infusion set and administered directly (undiluted) at a rate that is appropriate for the specific patient.[3048] For some indications, a second bolus injection of eptifibatide is administered 10 minutes after the initial bolus.[3048]

Stability

Intact vials of eptifibatide should be stored under refrigeration and protected from light until the time of administration.[3048] The drug may be stored for up to 2 months at room temperature; the cartons of the vials stored at room temperature should be marked with a "DISCARD BY" date of 2 months after transfer to room temperature storage or the expiration date, whichever comes first.[3048]

pH Effects

The minimum rate of decomposition occurs in the pH range of 5 to 6.[2417]

Compatibility Information

Solution Compatibility

Eptifibatide

Test Soln Name	Mfr	Mfr	Conc/L or %	Remarks	Ref	C/I
Normosol R in dextrose 5%	HOS	ME	50 and 250 mg	Physically compatible and chemically stable for up to 24 hr at 25°C	3049	C
Normosol R in dextrose 5%	HOS	ME	75 and 375 mg	Physically compatible and chemically stable for up to 24 hr at 25°C	3049	C
Sodium chloride 0.9%		ME	50 and 250 mg	Physically compatible and chemically stable for up to 24 hr at 25°C	3049	C
Sodium chloride 0.9%		ME	75 and 375 mg	Physically compatible and chemically stable for up to 24 hr at 25°C	3049	C

Additive Compatibility

Eptifibatide

Test Drug	Mfr	Conc/L or %	Mfr	Conc/L or %	Test Solution	Remarks	Ref	C/I
Alteplase		1 g	ME	750 mg		Physically compatible and chemically stable for up to 24 hr at 25°C	3049	C
Atropine sulfate		400 mg	ME	750 mg		Physically compatible and chemically stable for up to 24 hr at 25°C	3049	C
Dobutamine HCl		5 g	ME	750 mg		Physically compatible and chemically stable for up to 24 hr at 25°C	3049	C
Furosemide		10 g	ME	750 mg		Precipitation and crystallization occurred after 1 hr	3049	I

DOI: 10.37573/9781585286850.147

Additive Compatibility (Cont.)

Test Drug	Mfr	Conc/L or %	Mfr	Conc/L or %	Test Solution	Remarks	Ref	C/I
Heparin sodium		24,000 units	ME	750 mg		Physically compatible and chemically stable for up to 24 hr at 25°C	3049	C
Lidocaine HCl		2 g	ME	750 mg		Physically compatible and chemically stable for up to 24 hr at 25°C	3049	C
Meperidine HCl		10 g	ME	750 mg		Physically compatible and chemically stable for up to 24 hr at 25°C	3049	C
Metoprolol tartrate		1 g	ME	750 mg		Physically compatible and chemically stable for up to 24 hr at 25°C	3049	C
Midazolam HCl		1 g	ME	750 mg		Physically compatible and chemically stable for up to 24 hr at 25°C	3049	C
Morphine sulfate		1 g	ME	750 mg		Physically compatible and chemically stable for up to 24 hr at 25°C	3049	C
Nitroglycerin		400 mg	ME	750 mg		Physically compatible and chemically stable for up to 24 hr at 25°C	3049	C
Potassium chloride		40 mEq	ME	50 and 250 mg	NRD5W	Physically compatible and chemically stable for up to 24 hr at 25°C	3049	C
Potassium chloride		40 mEq	ME	75 and 375 mg	NRD5W	Physically compatible and chemically stable for up to 24 hr at 25°C	3049	C
Potassium chloride		40 mEq	ME	50 and 250 mg	NS	Physically compatible and chemically stable for up to 24 hr at 25°C	3049	C
Potassium chloride		40 mEq	ME	75 and 375 mg	NS	Physically compatible and chemically stable for up to 24 hr at 25°C	3049	C
Potassium chloride		60 mEq	ME	50 and 250 mg	NRD5W	Physically compatible and chemically stable for up to 24 hr at 25°C	3049	C
Potassium chloride		60 mEq	ME	75 and 375 mg	NRD5W	Physically compatible and chemically stable for up to 24 hr at 25°C	3049	C
Potassium chloride		60 mEq	ME	50 and 250 mg	NS	Physically compatible and chemically stable for up to 24 hr at 25°C	3049	C
Potassium chloride		60 mEq	ME	75 and 375 mg	NS	Physically compatible and chemically stable for up to 24 hr at 25°C	3049	C
Verapamil HCl		2.5 g	ME	750 mg		Physically compatible and chemically stable for up to 24 hr at 25°C	3049	C

Y-Site Injection Compatibility (1:1 Mixture)

Eptifibatide

Test Drug	Mfr	Conc	Mfr	Conc	Remarks	Ref	C/I
Amiodarone HCl	WY	6 mg/mL[a]	KEY	0.75 mg/mL	Visually compatible for 24 hr at 22°C	2352	C
Amiodarone HCl	WY	6 mg/mL[a]	KEY	2 mg/mL	Visually compatible for 24 hr at 22°C	2352	C
Argatroban	GSK	1 mg/mL[a b c]	COR	2 mg/mL[c]	Physically compatible with no loss of either drug in 4 hr at 23°C	2630	C
Bivalirudin	TMC	5 mg/mL[a]	KEY	2 mg/mL	Physically compatible for 4 hr at 23°C	2373	C
Cangrelor tetrasodium	TMC	1 mg/mL[b]		2 mg/mL	Physically compatible for 4 hr	3243	C

Y-Site Injection Compatibility (1:1 Mixture) (Cont.)

Test Drug	Mfr	Conc	Mfr	Conc	Remarks	Ref	C/I
Ceftolozane sulfate–tazobactam sodium	CUB	10 mg/mL[d e]	ME	2 mg/mL	Physically compatible for 2 hr	3262	C
Isavuconazonium sulfate	ASP	1.5 mg/mL[b]	ME	0.75 mg/mL	Physically compatible for 2 hr	3263	C
Meropenem–vaborbactam	TMC	8 mg/mL[b f]	AMB	2 mg/mL	Physically compatible for 3 hr at 20 to 25°C	3380	C
Metoprolol tartrate	BED	1 mg/mL	SC	0.75 mg/mL	Visually compatible for 24 hr at 19°C	2795	C
Micafungin sodium	ASP	1.5 mg/mL[b]	SC	0.75 mg/mL	Physically compatible for 4 hr at 23°C	2683	C
Plazomicin sulfate	ACH	24 mg/mL[b]	ME	2 mg/mL	Physically compatible for 1 hr at 20 to 25°C	3432	C
Tedizolid phosphate	CUB	0.8 mg/mL[b]	ME	0.75 mg/mL	Physically compatible for 2 hr	3244	C

[a] Tested in dextrose 5%.

[b] Tested in sodium chloride 0.9%.

[c] Mixed argatroban:eptifibatide 1:1 and 16:1.

[d] Tested in both dextrose 5% and sodium chloride 0.9%.

[e] Ceftolozane component. Ceftolozane in a 2:1 fixed-ratio concentration with tazobactam.

[f] Meropenem component. Meropenem in a 1:1 fixed-ratio concentration with vaborbactam.

Additional Compatibility Information

Other Drugs

The manufacturer states that eptifibatide may be administered in the same intravenous administration line as alteplase, atropine, dobutamine, heparin, lidocaine, meperidine, metoprolol, midazolam, morphine, nitroglycerin, and verapamil.[3048]

Furosemide

Eptifibatide must not be administered in the same intravenous administration line as furosemide.[3048] Admixtures of eptifibatide and furosemide demonstrated precipitation and crystal formation 1 hour after mixing.[3049]

Selected Revisions June 1, 2019. © Copyright, October 2004. American Society of Health-System Pharmacists, Inc.

Eravacycline Dihydrochloride
AHFS 8:12.24.08

Products

Eravacycline dihydrochloride is available as a lyophilized powder in single-dose (preservative-free) vials containing the equivalent of 50 mg of eravacycline and 150 mg of mannitol in each vial.[3434] Each vial also may contain sodium hydroxide and hydrochloric acid for pH adjustment.[3434]

Each 50-mg vial should be reconstituted with 5 mL of sterile water for injection or sodium chloride 0.9% to yield a reconstituted solution with an eravacycline concentration of 10 mg/mL.[3434] During reconstitution, vials should be swirled gently to completely dissolve the vial contents; shaking or rapid movement should be avoided as it may cause foaming.[3434] If any particles are present or if cloudiness is observed, the reconstituted solution should not be used.[3434] The reconstituted solution must be further diluted prior to administration.[3434] The appropriate volume of the reconstituted solution should be withdrawn from the vial(s) and diluted in an infusion bag containing sodium chloride 0.9% for a target eravacycline concentration of 0.3 mg/mL (within the range of 0.2 to 0.6 mg/mL).[3434] The infusion bag should not be shaken.[3434] The diluted solution for infusion also should be visually inspected for particulate matter and discoloration prior to administration.[3434] Unused portions of reconstituted or diluted solutions should be discarded.[3434]

pH

The pH is adjusted to the range of 5.5 to 7.[3434]

Equivalency

Eravacycline dihydrochloride 63.5 mg is equivalent to 50 mg of eravacycline.[3434]

Trade Name(s)

Xerava

Administration

Eravacycline dihydrochloride is administered by intravenous infusion over 60 minutes after reconstitution and further dilution.[3434] The reconstituted solution is *not* for direct injection.[3434]

Eravacycline dihydrochloride may be administered intravenously through a dedicated line or through a Y-site.[3434] If the intravenous line is used to administer other drugs, it should be flushed with sodium chloride injection 0.9% prior to and following eravacycline dihydrochloride administration.[3434]

Stability

Eravacycline dihydrochloride lyophilized powder is a yellow to orange powder that forms a clear, pale yellow to orange solution upon reconstitution and a clear, light yellow to orange solution upon dilution.[3434] Intact vials of eravacycline dihydrochloride should be stored at 2 to 8°C in the original carton until time of use.[3434]

The manufacturer states that the drug should not be mixed with any other drugs or solutions.[3434]

The reconstituted solution may be stored for up to 1 hour after reconstitution at room temperature up to 25°C, but should be diluted in an infusion bag within 1 hour after reconstitution.[3434] Admixtures prepared as directed from the lyophilized powder should be infused within 7 days if stored at 2 to 8°C or 24 hours if stored at room temperature up to 25°C.[3434]

Freezing Solutions

The manufacturer states that neither the reconstituted nor diluted solutions should be frozen.[3434]

Compatibility Information

Solution Compatibility

Eravacycline dihydrochloride

Test Soln Name	Mfr	Mfr	Conc/L or %	Remarks	Ref	C/I
Sodium chloride 0.9%		TET	200 to 600 mg	Infuse within 24 hr if stored at room temperature up to 25°C or 7 days if stored at 2 to 8°C	3434	C

Y-Site Injection Compatibility (1:1 Mixture)

Eravacycline dihydrochloride

Test Drug	Mfr	Conc	Mfr	Conc	Remarks	Ref	C/I
Albumin human	BXT	250 mg/mL	TET	0.6 mg/mL[a]	Measured turbidity increased immediately	3532	I
Amiodarone HCl	MYL	2 mg/mL[a]	TET	0.6 mg/mL[a]	Measured turbidity increased immediately	3532	I

DOI: 10.37573/9781585286850.148

Y-Site Injection Compatibility (1:1 Mixture) (Cont.)

Test Drug	Mfr	Conc	Mfr	Conc	Remarks	Ref	C/I
Aztreonam	BMS	20 mg/mL[a]	TET	0.6 mg/mL[a]	Physically compatible for 2 hr at room temperature	3532	C
Bumetanide	HOS	0.25 mg/mL	TET	0.6 mg/mL[a]	Physically compatible for 2 hr at room temperature	3532	C
Calcium chloride	HOS	20 mg/mL[a]	TET	0.6 mg/mL[a]	Physically compatible for 2 hr at room temperature	3532	C
Calcium gluconate	FRK	20 mg/mL[a]	TET	0.6 mg/mL[a]	Physically compatible for 2 hr at room temperature	3532	C
Cefepime HCl	WG	40 mg/mL[a]	TET	0.6 mg/mL[a]	Physically compatible for 2 hr at room temperature	3532	C
Ceftaroline fosamil	FOR	12 mg/mL[a]	TET	0.3 and 0.6 mg/mL[a]	Measured turbidity increased within 2 hr	3532	I
Ceftazidime	PPR	40 mg/mL[a]	TET	0.6 mg/mL[a]	Physically compatible for 2 hr at room temperature	3532	C
Ceftazidime–avibactam sodium	GSK	40 mg/mL[a] [d]	TET	0.6 mg/mL[a]	Physically compatible for 2 hr at room temperature	3532	C
Ceftolozane sulfate–tazobactam sodium	ME	20 mg/mL[a] [e]	TET	0.6 mg/mL[a]	Physically compatible for 2 hr at room temperature	3532	C
Ciprofloxacin	CLA	2 mg/mL[b]	TET	0.6 mg/mL[a]	Physically compatible for 2 hr at room temperature	3532	C
Cisatracurium besylate	ABV	0.4 mg/mL[a]	TET	0.6 mg/mL[a]	Physically compatible for 2 hr at room temperature	3532	C
Colistimethate sodium	FRK	4.5 mg/mL[a]	TET	0.3 and 0.6 mg/mL[a]	Measured turbidity increased within 30 min	3532	I
Dexmedetomidine HCl	HOS	4 mcg/mL	TET	0.6 mg/mL[a]	Physically compatible for 2 hr at room temperature	3532	C
Diltiazem HCl	AKN	5 mg/mL	TET	0.6 mg/mL[a]	Physically compatible for 2 hr at room temperature	3532	C
Dobutamine HCl	HOS	4.1 mg/mL[a]	TET	0.6 mg/mL[a]	Physically compatible for 2 hr at room temperature	3532	C
Dopamine HCl	BA	0.8 mg/mL[b]	TET	0.6 mg/mL[a]	Physically compatible for 2 hr at room temperature	3532	C
Epinephrine[c]	BPI	16 mcg/mL[a]	TET	0.6 mg/mL[a]	Physically compatible for 2 hr at room temperature	3532	C
Esmolol HCl	FRK	10 mg/mL	TET	0.6 mg/mL[a]	Physically compatible for 2 hr at room temperature	3532	C
Fentanyl citrate	WW	50 mcg/mL	TET	0.6 mg/mL[a]	Physically compatible for 2 hr at room temperature	3532	C
Fluconazole	SGT	2 mg/mL[b]	TET	0.6 mg/mL[a]	Physically compatible for 2 hr at room temperature	3532	C
Furosemide	FRK	3 mg/mL[a]	TET	0.3 and 0.6 mg/mL[a]	Measured turbidity increased immediately; pH decreased by >1 unit within 60 min	3532	I
Gentamicin sulfate	FRK	5 mg/mL[a]	TET	0.6 mg/mL[a]	Physically compatible for 2 hr at room temperature	3532	C
Heparin sodium	SGT	1000 units/mL[a]	TET	0.6 mg/mL[a]	Physically compatible for 2 hr at room temperature	3532	C
Hydromorphone HCl	AKN	1 mg/mL[a]	TET	0.6 mg/mL[a]	Physically compatible for 2 hr at room temperature	3532	C
Imipenem–cilastatin sodium	FRK	5 mg/mL[a] [f]	TET	0.6 mg/mL[a]	Physically compatible for 2 hr at room temperature	3532	C
Insulin, regular	LI	1 unit/mL[a]	TET	0.6 mg/mL[a]	Physically compatible for 2 hr at room temperature	3532	C
Levofloxacin	AUR	5 mg/mL[a]	TET	0.6 mg/mL[a]	Physically compatible for 2 hr at room temperature	3532	C
Linezolid	PF	2 mg/mL[b]	TET	0.6 mg/mL[a]	Physically compatible for 2 hr at room temperature	3532	C
Magnesium sulfate	FRK	100 mg/mL[a]	TET	0.6 mg/mL[a]	Physically compatible for 2 hr at room temperature	3532	C
Meropenem	FRK	20 mg/mL[a]	TET	0.3 and 0.6 mg/mL[a]	Measured turbidity increased immediately	3532	I
Meropenem–vaborbactam	FAC	8 mg/mL[a] [g]	TET	0.6 mg/mL[a]	Measured turbidity increased immediately	3532	I

Y-Site Injection Compatibility (1:1 Mixture) (Cont.)

Test Drug	Mfr	Conc	Mfr	Conc	Remarks	Ref	C/I
Metronidazole	BA	5 mg/mL[b]	TET	0.6 mg/mL[a]	Physically compatible for 2 hr at room temperature	3532	C
Micafungin sodium	ASP	4 mg/mL[a]	TET	0.6 mg/mL[a]	Measured turbidity increased immediately; pH increased by >2 units within 60 min	3532	I
Midazolam HCl	HOS	1 mg/mL[a]	TET	0.6 mg/mL[a]	Physically compatible for 2 hr at room temperature	3532	C
Morphine sulfate	WW	1 mg/mL[a]	TET	0.6 mg/mL[a]	Physically compatible for 2 hr at room temperature	3532	C
Nicardipine HCl	EXL	0.1 mg/mL[a]	TET	0.6 mg/mL[a]	Physically compatible for 2 hr at room temperature	3532	C
Norepinephrine bitartrate	CLA	32 mcg/mL[a]	TET	0.6 mg/mL[a]	Physically compatible for 2 hr at room temperature	3532	C
Octreotide acetate	FRK	4 mcg/mL[a]	TET	0.6 mg/mL[a]	Physically compatible for 2 hr at room temperature	3532	C
Pantoprazole sodium	PF	0.4 mg/mL[a]	TET	0.6 mg/mL[a]	Physically compatible for 2 hr at room temperature	3532	C
Phenylephrine HCl	AVD	1 mg/mL[a]	TET	0.6 mg/mL[a]	Physically compatible for 2 hr at room temperature	3532	C
Piperacillin sodium–tazobactam sodium	FRK[i]	40 mg/mL[a] [h]	TET	0.6 mg/mL[a]	Physically compatible for 2 hr at room temperature	3532	C
Propofol	FRK[j]	10 mg/mL	TET	0.3 and 0.6 mg/mL[a]	Physically incompatible; pH decreased by >1 unit within 60 min	3532	I
Sodium bicarbonate	FRK	1 mEq/mL	TET	0.3 and 0.6 mg/mL[a]	Measured turbidity increased immediately	3532	I
Tobramycin sulfate	FRK	5 mg/mL[a]	TET	0.6 mg/mL[a]	Physically compatible for 2 hr at room temperature	3532	C
Vancomycin HCl	AVG	5 mg/mL[a]	TET	0.6 mg/mL[a]	Physically compatible for 2 hr at room temperature	3532	C
Vasopressin	PAR	1 unit/mL[a]	TET	0.6 mg/mL[a]	Physically compatible for 2 hr at room temperature	3532	C
Vecuronium bromide	TE	1 mg/mL	TET	0.6 mg/mL[a]	Physically compatible for 2 hr at room temperature	3532	C

[a] Tested in sodium chloride 0.9%.

[b] Tested as the premixed infusion solution.

[c] As epinephrine base rather than the salt.

[d] Ceftazidime component. Ceftazidime in a 4:1 fixed-ratio concentration with avibactam.

[e] Ceftolozane component. Ceftolozane in a 2:1 fixed-ratio concentration with tazobactam.

[f] Imipenem component. Imipenem in a 1:1 fixed-ratio concentration with cilastatin.

[g] Meropenem component. Meropenem in a 1:1 fixed-ratio concentration with vaborbactam.

[h] Piperacillin component. Piperacillin in an 8:1 fixed-ratio concentration with tazobactam.

[i] Test performed using the formulation WITHOUT edetate disodium.

[j] Test performed using the formulation WITH edetate disodium.

Selected Revisions May 1, 2020. © Copyright, June 2019. American Society of Health-System Pharmacists, Inc.

Eribulin Mesylate
AHFS 10:00

Products

Eribulin mesylate is available as a 0.5-mg/mL solution in 2-mL single-use vials containing a total of eribulin mesylate 1 mg (equivalent to eribulin 0.88 mg), dehydrated alcohol 5% (v/v), and water for injection 95% (v/v).[3027] [3028] Sodium hydroxide and/or hydrochloric acid may have been added during manufacturing to adjust the pH.[2805] [3028]

pH

From 6.5 to 8.5.[2805]

Trade Name(s)

Halaven

Administration

Eribulin mesylate is administered intravenously over 2 to 5 minutes.[3027] The drug may be administered undiluted or diluted in 100 mL of sodium chloride 0.9%.[3027]

Eribulin mesylate should not be diluted in dextrose-containing solutions nor administered through an intravenous line that is infusing dextrose-containing solutions.[3027]

Stability

Intact vials should be stored at controlled room temperature in the original carton; vials should not be refrigerated nor frozen.[3027] Eribulin mesylate is a clear, colorless solution.[3027]

The manufacturer states that undiluted eribulin mesylate may be stored in a syringe for up to 4 hours at room temperature or up to 24 hours at 4°C.[3027] Similarly, diluted solutions of eribulin mesylate may be stored for up to 4 hours at room temperature or 24 hours under refrigeration.[3027] Unused portions remaining in the vials should be discarded.[3027]

Stability of the undiluted product (Eisai) was tested in the original glass vial with light protection at 25°C and at 2 to 8°C.[3028] The solution was found to be physically compatible and chemically stable with little to no loss in 28 days.[3028]

pH Effects

Eribulin mesylate stability is pH dependent.[3028] The drug has been noted to be stable over a pH range of 5 to 9.[3028] Mixing eribulin mesylate with dextrose-containing solutions is not recommended given the acid sensitivity of the drug.[3027] [3028]

Syringes

Eribulin mesylate (Eisai) 205 mcg/mL in sodium chloride 0.9% packaged in 10-mL polypropylene syringes (Becton Dickinson) was physically compatible and chemically stable with little to no loss in 28 days stored with light protection at 25 and 2 to 8°C.[3028]

Compatibility Information

Solution Compatibility

Eribulin mesylate

Test Soln Name	Mfr	Mfr	Conc/L or %	Remarks	Ref	C/I
Dextrose 5% in Ringer's injection		EI		Must not be mixed with dextrose-containing solutions	3027	I
Dextrose 5% in Ringer's injection, lactated		EI		Must not be mixed with dextrose-containing solutions	3027	I
Dextrose 5% in sodium chloride 0.45%		EI		Must not be mixed with dextrose-containing solutions	3027	I
Dextrose 5% in sodium chloride 0.9%		EI		Must not be mixed with dextrose-containing solutions	3027	I
Dextrose 5%		EI		Must not be mixed with dextrose-containing solutions	3027	I
Sodium chloride 0.9%		EI		Manufacturer-recommended solution	3027	C
Sodium chloride 0.9%	FRK[a]	EI	20 mg	Physically compatible and chemically stable with little to no loss for up to 28 days with light protection at 25 and 2 to 8°C	3028	C

[a] Tested in Freeflex polyolefin containers.

DOI: 10.37573/9781585286850.149

Ertapenem Sodium
AHFS 8:12.07.08

Products

Ertapenem is available as a lyophilized powder in 1-g single-use vials as the sodium salt with sodium bicarbonate 175 mg and sodium hydroxide to adjust the pH.[2973] For intravenous administration, reconstitute the contents of a 1-g vial with 10 mL of sterile water for injection, bacteriostatic water for injection, or sodium chloride 0.9% and shake well,[2973] yielding a concentration of 100 mg/mL.[2975] For adult patients, immediately transfer the appropriate dose of the reconstituted solution to 50 mL of sodium chloride 0.9%.[2973] For pediatric patients, transfer the appropriate dose of reconstituted solution to a volume of sodium chloride 0.9% that is sufficient to yield a final concentration of 20 mg/mL or less.[2973]

Ertapenem also is available as a lyophilized powder in 1-g single-use ADD-Vantage vials as the sodium salt.[2973] Each ADD-Vantage vial also contains sodium bicarbonate 175 mg and sodium hydroxide to adjust the pH.[2973] Prepare ADD-Vantage vials of ertapenem sodium with 50 or 100 mL of sodium chloride 0.9% in ADD-Vantage diluent containers.[2973]

For intramuscular injection, reconstitute the contents of a 1-g vial with 3.2 mL of lidocaine hydrochloride 1% (without epinephrine) and shake well,[2973] yielding a final volume of approximately 3.6 mL and a concentration of approximately 280 mg/mL.[2975] Upon dissolution, administer within 1 hour.[2973] Do *not* administer the reconstituted intramuscular injection intravenously.[2973]

pH

7.5.[2973]

Sodium Content

Each 1-g vial contains approximately 137 mg or 6 mEq of sodium.[2973]

Trade Name(s)

Invanz

Administration

Ertapenem sodium diluted in sodium chloride 0.9% may be administered by intravenous infusion over 30 minutes.[2973] Ertapenem sodium prepared with lidocaine hydrochloride 1% for intramuscular administration may be administered by deep intramuscular injection into a large muscle mass (e.g., gluteal muscle, lateral part of the thigh).[2973]

Stability

Intact vials of ertapenem sodium should be stored at a temperature not exceeding 25°C.[2973] The reconstituted drug solution for intravenous administration should be diluted immediately in sodium chloride 0.9%,[2973] but has been noted to remain stable in the vial for 2 hours at 25°C or 6 hours at 5°C when reconstituted with sterile water for injection, sodium chloride 0.9%, bacteriostatic water with benzyl alcohol 0.9%, or Ringer's injection, lactated.[2975] The manufacturer recommends that solutions of ertapenem not be frozen.[2973]

Dextrose-containing solutions should *not* be used to dilute ertapenem[2973] as an unacceptable loss due to degradation has been observed with their use; however, limited contact over a short period of time (e.g., ertapenem run as a piggyback into the same line as dextrose) should not adversely affect ertapenem stability.[2975]

Ertapenem diluted for infusion from both single-use vials and ADD-Vantage single-use vials may be stored and used within 6 hours at room temperature or may be stored for 24 hours under refrigeration and used within 4 hours after removal from refrigeration.[2973]

Ertapenem prepared for intramuscular administration should be used within 1 hour.[2973]

Freezing Solutions

The manufacturer recommends that solutions of ertapenem not be frozen due to degradation of the drug.[2973][2975]

Ertapenem (Merck) 100 mg/mL in sodium chloride 0.9% in polypropylene syringes was frozen at −20°C for 14 or 28 days immediately after preparation, followed by thawing at room temperature for 1 hour.[2974] Upon thawing for 1 hour, the solution frozen for 28 days was found to have undergone about 5% loss.[2974] The solution frozen for 14 days was found to have undergone about 7% loss after 5 hours at room temperature (including the 1 hour of thawing time).[2974]

Syringes

Ertapenem (Merck) 100 mg/mL in sodium chloride 0.9% was packaged as 10 mL in 20-mL polypropylene syringes (Monoject).[2974] The drug was found to be stable for approximately 30 minutes at room temperature or 24 hours under refrigeration followed by up to 4 hours at room temperature after removal from refrigeration.[2974]

DOI: 10.37573/9781585286850.150

Compatibility Information

Solution Compatibility

Ertapenem sodium

Test Soln Name	Mfr	Mfr	Conc/L or %	Remarks	Ref	C/I
Dextrose 5% in sodium chloride 0.225%	AB	ME	10 and 20 g	Visually compatible. 10% loss in 6 hr at 25°C. 8% loss in 32 hr and 11% loss in 48 hr at 4°C	2487	I
Dextrose 5% in sodium chloride 0.9%	AB	ME	10 and 20 g	Visually compatible. 11% loss in 6 hr at 25°C and 10% loss in 32 hr at 4°C	2487	I
Dextrose 5%	AB	ME	10 and 20 g	Visually compatible. 10% loss in 6 hr at 25°C and 5 to 8% loss in 24 hr at 4°C	2487	I
Ringer's injection	AB	ME	10 and 20 g	Visually compatible. 10 to 12% ertapenem loss in 20 hr at 25°C and 11% loss in 5 days at 4°C	2487	I[a]
Ringer's injection, lactated	AB	ME	10 and 20 g	Visually compatible. 18% loss in 20 hr at 25°C and 9% loss in 3 days at 4°C	2487	I
Sodium chloride 0.225%	AB	ME	10 and 20 g	Visually compatible. 9 to 12% loss in 20 hr at 25°C and 8 to 11% loss in 5 days at 4°C	2487	I[a]
Sodium chloride 0.9%	AB	ME	10 and 20 g	Visually compatible. 9 to 11% loss in 20 hr at 25°C and 8 to 11% loss in 5 days at 4°C	2487	I[a]
Sodium chloride 0.9%	[b]	ME	10 g	Physically compatible with less than 10% drug loss in 24 hr at 25°C and 7 days at 5°C	2723	C
Sodium chloride 0.9%	[c]	ME	10 g	Physically compatible with less than 10% drug loss in 30 hr at 25°C and 8 days at 5°C	2723	C
Sodium chloride 0.9%	[b]	ME	20 g	Physically compatible with less than 10% drug loss in 18 hr at 25°C and 5 days at 5°C	2723	C
Sodium chloride 0.9%	[c]	ME	20 g	Physically compatible with less than 10% drug loss in 24 hr at 25°C and 7 days at 5°C	2723	C
Sodium lactate ⅙ M	AB	ME	10 and 20 g	Visually compatible. 7 to 9% loss in 6 hr at 25°C and 8 to 11% loss in 2 days at 4°C	2487	I

[a] Incompatible by conventional standards but recommended for dilution of ertapenem with use in shorter periods of time.

[b] Tested in the Homepump Eclipse elastomeric pump reservoirs.

[c] Tested in Intermate elastomeric pump reservoirs.

Additive Compatibility

Ertapenem sodium

Test Drug	Mfr	Conc/L or %	Mfr	Conc/L or %	Test Solution	Remarks	Ref	C/I
Mannitol	AB	5%	ME	10 and 20 g		Precipitate in <1 hr. 15% loss in 20 hr at 25°C. 7% loss in 2 days at 4°C	2487	I
Mannitol	AB	20%	ME	10 and 20 g		Precipitate in <1 hr. 13% loss in 6 hr at 25°C. 8% loss in 1 day at 4°C	2487	I
Sodium bicarbonate	AB	5%	ME	10 and 20 g		Visually compatible. 11% loss in 3 hr at 25°C. 16 to 19% loss in 1 day at 4°C	2487	I

Y-Site Injection Compatibility (1:1 Mixture)

Ertapenem sodium

Test Drug	Mfr	Conc	Mfr	Conc	Remarks	Ref	C/I
Anidulafungin	VIC	0.5 mg/mL[a]	ME	20 mg/mL[b]	Microparticulates form immediately	2617	I
Cangrelor tetrasodium	TMC	1 mg/mL[b]	[d]	20 mg/mL[b]	Physically compatible for 4 hr	3243	C
Caspofungin acetate	ME	0.7 mg/mL[b]	ME	20 mg/mL[b]	Immediate white turbid precipitate forms	2758	I
Ceftazidime–avibactam sodium	ALL	20 mg/mL[g][h]			Physically compatible for up to 4 hr at room temperature	3004	C
Ceftolozane sulfate–tazobactam sodium	CUB	10 mg/mL[b][e]	ME	20 mg/mL[b]	Physically compatible for 2 hr	3262	C
Colistimethate sodium	MIL	1.5 mg/mL[b]	MSD	5 mg/mL[b]	Visually compatible for 1 hr at 26°C	3335	C
Heparin sodium	APP	40 and 100 units/mL[a]	ME	10 mg/mL[b]	Visually compatible with about 4% ertapenem loss in 4 hr	2487	C
Heparin sodium	APP	50 and 100 units/mL[b]	ME	10 mg/mL[b]	Visually compatible with about 3% ertapenem loss in 4 hr	2487	C
Hetastarch in sodium chloride 0.9%	AB	6%	ME	10 mg/mL[b]	Visually compatible with about 3% ertapenem loss in 8 hr	2487	C
Isavuconazonium sulfate	ASP	1.5 mg/mL[b]	ME	20 mg/mL[b]	Measured turbidity increases within 1 hr	3263	I
Meropenem		50 mg/mL	ME	100 mg/mL	Physically compatible for 4 hr at room temperature	3538	C
Meropenem–vaborbactam	TMC	8 mg/mL[b][f]	ME	20 mg/mL[b]	Physically compatible for 3 hr at 20 to 25°C	3380	C
Plazomicin sulfate	ACH	24 mg/mL[b]	ME	20 mg/mL[b]	Physically compatible for 1 hr at 20 to 25°C	3432	C
Potassium chloride	AB	0.01 and 0.04 mEq/mL[c]	ME	10 mg/mL[b]	Visually compatible with about 2% ertapenem loss in 4 hr	2487	C
Tedizolid phosphate	CUB	0.8 mg/mL[b]	ME	20 mg/mL[b]	Physically compatible for 2 hr	3244	C
Telavancin HCl	ASP	7.5 mg/mL[b]	ME	20 mg/mL[b]	Physically compatible for 2 hr	2830	C
Tigecycline	WY	1 mg/mL[b]		20 mg/mL[b]	Physically compatible for 4 hr	2714	C

[a] Tested in dextrose 5%.

[b] Tested in sodium chloride 0.9%.

[c] Tested in sterile water for injection.

[d] Salt not specified.

[e] Ceftolozane component. Ceftolozane in a 2:1 fixed-ratio concentration with tazobactam.

[f] Meropenem component. Meropenem in a 1:1 fixed-ratio concentration with vaborbactam.

[g] Ceftazidime component. Ceftazidime in a 4:1 fixed-ratio concentration with avibactam.

[h] Tested in both dextrose 5% and sodium chloride 0.9%.

Selected Revisions May 1, 2020. © Copyright, October 2006.
American Society of Health-System Pharmacists, Inc.

Erythromycin Lactobionate
AHFS 8:12.12.04

Products

Erythromycin lactobionate is available in vials containing the equivalent of 1 g of erythromycin and in vials containing the equivalent of 500 mg of erythromycin. Reconstitute the 1-g vials with at least 20 mL and the 500-mg vials with 10 mL of sterile water for injection without preservatives. The resultant concentration is 5% (50 mg/mL). The drug is also available in 500-mg and 1-g ADD-Vantage vials without preservative.[1(11/06)] [4]

pH

Reconstitution with sterile water for injection to a 50-mg/mL concentration results in a solution with a pH of 6.5 to 7.5.[20]

Osmolality

Erythromycin lactobionate 50 mg/mL in sterile water for injection has an osmolality of 223 mOsm/kg.[50]

The osmolality of erythromycin lactobionate was calculated for the following dilutions:[1054]

Diluent	Osmolality (mOsm/kg)	
	50 mL	100 mL
500 mg		
Dextrose 5%	273	265
Sodium chloride 0.9%	299	291
1 g		
Dextrose 5%	287	273
Sodium chloride 0.9%	313	300

Trade Name(s)

Erythrocin Lactobionate-I.V.

Administration

Erythromycin lactobionate may be administered by continuous or intermittent intravenous infusion; it must not be given by direct intravenous injection. To minimize venous irritation, slow continuous infusion of a 1-mg/mL concentration is recommended. By intermittent infusion, one-fourth of the daily dose at a concentration of 1 to 5 mg/mL in at least 100 mL of infusion solution may be given over 20 to 60 minutes every 6 hours.[1(11/06)] [4]

Stability

Do not use sodium chloride 0.9% or other solutions containing inorganic ions in the initial reconstitution of the regular vials. Such solutions result in the formation of a precipitate.[4] [20] (Note: This restriction does not apply to the drug in ADD-Vantage containers.)

The commercial vials are stable at room temperature.[20] Reconstituted (5%) solutions are stable for 14 days when stored under refrigeration[20] or for 24 hours when kept at room temperature.[1(11/06)]

pH Effects

The stability of erythromycin lactobionate is extremely pH dependent. It is most stable at pH 6 to 8[20] [1935] or 9.[1101] [2596] Erythromycin lactobionate is unstable in acidic solutions. Decomposition occurs at an increasingly more rapid rate as the pH approaches 4.[20] A pH over 5.5 is recommended for the final diluted solution. At pH 5.5 or below and at pH 10 or above, erythromycin lactobionate is particularly unstable, with 10% decomposition occurring in about eight or nine hours. The following pH profile was determined for erythromycin in solution:[1101]

Solution pH	Approximate Time for 10% Decomposition (t_{90})
5	2.5 hr
5.5	8.8 hr
6	1 day
7	4.6 days
8	7.3 days
9	2.6 days
10	8.8 hr
11	53 min

Erythromycin lactobionate can alter the pH of solutions and give itself some protection against decomposition for varying periods. The length of time is dependent on the initial pH and the buffer capacity of the solution.[48] The pH of unbuffered dextrose 5% is raised 1 pH unit by the addition of erythromycin lactobionate.[20] The use of admixtures with a pH of less than 5 is not recommended. If the admixture pH is 5 to 6, it should be used immediately.[48]

The effect of buffering erythromycin lactobionate (Abbott) solutions was evaluated. Erythromycin lactobionate 2 mg/mL in sodium chloride 0.9% (pH 7.15 to 7.25) exhibited 5% losses in about 20 days at 5°C. However, buffering with sodium bicarbonate to pH 7.5 to 8 extended stability, with 5% losses occurring in about 85 days at 5°C.[1587]

Freezing Solutions

Erythromycin lactobionate (Abbott) 500 mg/110 mL in sodium chloride 0.9% in PVC bags was frozen at −20°C; no loss occurred after 12 months of storage followed by microwave thawing. Furthermore, the solution was physically compatible, with no increase in subvisible particles. In addition, no erythromycin loss was found after 6 months at −20°C followed by 3 freeze–thaw cycles.[1612]

DOI: 10.37573/9781585286850.151

Compatibility Information

Solution Compatibility

Erythromycin lactobionate

Test Soln Name	Mfr	Mfr	Conc/L or %	Remarks	Ref	C/I
Dextrose 5% in Ringer's injection, lactated	AB	AB	1 g	10% loss in 3 hr at 25°C	20	I
Dextrose 5% in Ringer's injection, lactated	TRa	AB	1 g	10 to 24% loss in 24 hr at 5°C	282	I
Dextrose 5% in sodium chloride 0.9%	TRa	AB	1 g	Stable for 24 hr at 5°C	282	C
Dextrose 5% in sodium chloride 0.9%	AB	AB	1 g	33% loss in 24 hr	46	I
Dextrose 5% in sodium chloride 0.9%		AB	1 g	12% loss in 6 hr at 25°C	48	I
Dextrose 5% in sodium chloride 0.9%		AB	2 g	15% loss in 6 hr	109	I
Dextrose 5%	TRa	AB	1 g	Stable for 24 hr at 5°C	282	C
Dextrose 5%	AB	AB	1 g	15% loss in 24 hr	46	I
Dextrose 5%	AB	AB	1 g	10% loss in 10 hr at 25°C	20	I
Dextrose 5%		AB	1 g	15% loss in 24 hr at 25°C	48	I
Dextrose 5%		AB	2 g	14% loss in 6 hr	109	I
Dextrose 5%	TRb	AB	4 g	21% loss in activity in 24 hr at room temperature	518	I
Dextrose 5%	TRb c	AB	4 g	Physically compatible and stable for 24 hr at room temperature	518	C
Dextrose 10%		AB	2 g	14% loss in 6 hr	109	I
Normosol M in dextrose 5%	AB	AB	1 g	10% loss in 6 hr at 25°C	20	I
Normosol R		AB	1 g	14% loss in 24 hr at 25°C	48	I
Ringer's injection	AB	AB	1 g	10% loss in 11 hr at 25°C	20	I
Ringer's injection, lactated	TRa	AB	1 g	Stable for 24 hr at 5°C	282	C
Ringer's injection, lactated	AB	AB	1 g	10% loss in 18 hr at 25°C	20	I
Sodium chloride 0.9%		AB	1 g	Stable for 24 hr at 25°C	48	C
Sodium chloride 0.9%		AB	2 g	Stable for 24 hr	109	C
Sodium chloride 0.9%	AB	AB	1 g	Stable for 24 hr	46	C
Sodium chloride 0.9%	AB	AB	1 g	10% loss in 22 hr at 25°C	20	C
Sodium chloride 0.9%	TRa	AB	1 g	Stable for 24 hr at 5°C	282	C
Sodium chloride 0.9%	TRb	AB	4 g	Physically compatible and stable for 24 hr at room temperature	518	C
Sodium chloride 0.9%	TRb c	AB	4 g	Physically compatible and stable for 24 hr at room temperature	518	C
Sodium chloride 0.9%		AB	2 g	5% loss in about 20 days at 5°C	1587	C

Solution Compatibility (Cont.)

Test Soln Name	Mfr	Mfr	Conc/L or %	Remarks	Ref	C/I
Sodium chloride 0.9%	BA[b]	AB	8.3 g	No more than 5% loss after 60 days at 5°C	1597	C
Sodium chloride 0.9%	AB[d]	ES	20 g	Little or no loss with 24-hr storage at 5°C followed by 24-hr simulated administration at 30°C via portable pump	1779	C

[a] Tested in both glass and PVC containers.

[b] Tested in PVC containers.

[c] Buffered with sodium bicarbonate 4% (Neut, Abbott).

[d] Tested in portable pump reservoirs (Pharmacia Deltec).

Additive Compatibility

Erythromycin lactobionate

Test Drug	Mfr	Conc/L or %	Mfr	Conc/L or %	Test Solution	Remarks	Ref	C/I
Aminophylline	SE	500 mg	AB	1 g		Physically compatible. Erythromycin stable for 24 hr at 25°C	20	C
Ampicillin sodium	WY	3.7 g	AB	3 g	NS	Physically compatible with 6% ampicillin loss in 1 day at 24°C	1035	C
Ascorbic acid	AB	1 g	AB	1 g		Physically compatible	3	C
Ascorbic acid	UP	500 mg	AB	5 g	D5W	Physically incompatible	15	I
Chloramphenicol sodium succinate	PD		AB		D5W	May precipitate at some concentrations	15	I
Colistimethate sodium	WC	500 mg	AB	5 g	D5W	Physically incompatible	15	I
Colistimethate sodium	WC	500 mg	AB	1 g	D	Precipitate forms within 1 hr	20	I
Diphenhydramine HCl	PD	50 mg	AB	1 g		Physically compatible. Erythromycin stable for 24 hr at 25°C	20	C
Diphenhydramine HCl	PD	50 mg	AB	1 g	D5W	Erythromycin stable for 24 hr at 25°C	48	C
Floxacillin sodium	BE	20 g	AB	5 g	NS	Precipitates immediately. Crystals form in 5 hr at 15°C	1479	I
Furosemide	HO	1 g	AB	5 g	NS	Precipitates immediately. Crystals form in 12 to 24 hr at 15 and 30°C	1479	I
Fusidate sodium	LEO	1 g		5 g	D2.5½S, D2.5S, D5¼S, D5½S, D5S, D10S	Physically compatible and chemically stable for 48 hr at room temperature	1800	C
Heparin sodium	UP	4000 units	AB	5 g	D5W	Physically incompatible	15	I
Heparin sodium	AB	1500 units	AB	1 g		Precipitate forms within 1 hr	20	I
Heparin sodium	AB	20,000 units	AB	1 g		Precipitate forms within 1 hr	21	I
Heparin sodium	OR	20,000 units	AB	1.5 g	D5W, NS	Precipitate forms	113	I
Hydrocortisone sodium succinate	UP	500 mg	AB	5 g	D5W	Physically compatible	15	C
Hydrocortisone sodium succinate	UP	250 mg	AB	1 g		Physically compatible	20	C
Lidocaine HCl	AST	2 g	AB	1 g		Physically compatible	24	C

Additive Compatibility (Cont.)

Test Drug	Mfr	Conc/L or %	Mfr	Conc/L or %	Test Solution	Remarks	Ref	C/I
Linezolid	PHU	2 g	AB	5 g	b	Erythromycin loss of 15% in 1 hr and 30% in 4 hr at 23°C. Loss of 45% in 1 day at 4°C	2333	I
Metoclopramide HCl	RB	400 mg	AB	4 g	NS	Incompatible. If mixed, use immediately	924	I
Metoclopramide HCl	RB	100 mg	AB	5 g	NS	Incompatible. If mixed, use immediately	924	I
Metoclopramide HCl	RB	416 mg	AB	4.1 g		Incompatible. If mixed, use immediately	1167	I
Metoclopramide HCl	RB	1.1 g	AB	3.5 g		Incompatible. If mixed, use immediately	1167	I
Penicillin G potassium		1 million units	AB	1 g		Physically compatible	3	C
Penicillin G potassium	SQ	20 million units	AB	5 g	D5W	Physically compatible	15	C
Penicillin G potassium	SQ	5 million units	AB	1 g		Physically compatible	20, 47	C
Penicillin G sodium	UP	20 million units	AB	5 g	D5W	Physically compatible	15	C
Pentobarbital sodium	AB	500 mg	AB	1 g		Physically compatible. Erythromycin stable for 24 hr at 25°C	20	C
Polymyxin B sulfate	BW	200 mg	AB	5 g	D5W	Physically compatible	15	C
Potassium chloride	AB	40 mEq	AB	1 g		Physically compatible	20	C
Prochlorperazine edisylate	SKF	10 mg	AB	1 g		Physically compatible. Erythromycin stable for 24 hr at 25°C	20	C
Ranitidine HCl	GL	50 mg and 2 g		5 g	NS	Physically compatible. Ranitidine stable for 24 hr at 25°C. Erythromycin not tested	1515	C
Sodium bicarbonate	AB	3.75 g	AB	1 g		Physically compatible. Erythromycin stable for 24 hr at 25°C	20	C
Sodium bicarbonate	AB	2.4 mEq[a]	AB	1 g	D5W	Physically compatible for 24 hr	772	C
Verapamil HCl	KN	80 mg	AB	2 g	D5W, NS	Physically compatible for 24 hr	764	C

[a] One vial of Neut added to a liter of admixture.

[b] Admixed in the linezolid infusion container.

Drugs in Syringe Compatibility

Erythromycin lactobionate

Test Drug	Mfr	Amt	Mfr	Amt	Remarks	Ref	C/I
Ampicillin sodium	AY	500 mg	AB	300 mg/6 mL	Precipitate forms in 1 hr at room temperature	300	I
Cloxacillin sodium	AY	250 mg	AB	300 mg/6 mL	Precipitate forms within 1 hr at room temperature	300	I
Heparin sodium	AB	20,000 units/1 mL	AB	1 g	Physically incompatible	21	I

Y-Site Injection Compatibility (1:1 Mixture)

Erythromycin lactobionate

Test Drug	Mfr	Conc	Mfr	Conc	Remarks	Ref	C/I
Acyclovir sodium	BW	5 mg/mL[a]	AB	4 mg/mL[a]	Physically compatible for 4 hr at 25°C	1157	C
Amiodarone HCl	LZ	4 mg/mL[c]	AB	2 mg/mL[c]	Physically compatible for 4 hr at room temperature	1444	C
Anidulafungin	VIC	0.5 mg/mL[a]	AB	5 mg/mL[b]	Physically compatible for 4 hr at 23°C	2617	C
Bivalirudin	TMC	5 mg/mL[a]	AB	5 mg/mL[b]	Physically compatible for 4 hr at 23°C	2373	C
Cangrelor tetrasodium	TMC	1 mg/mL[b]		5 mg/mL[b]	Physically compatible for 4 hr	3243	C
Cefepime HCl	BMS	120 mg/mL[j]		5 mg/mL	Over 10% cefepime loss occurs in 1 hr	2513	I
Ceftazidime	SKB	125 mg/mL		50 mg/mL	Precipitates immediately	2434	I
Ceftazidime	SKB	125 mg/mL		10 mg/mL	Trace precipitation	2434	I
Ceftazidime	GSK	120 mg/mL[j]		5 mg/mL	Precipitates	2513	I
Cloxacillin sodium	SMX	100 mg/mL	AMD	50 mg/mL	Precipitates immediately	3245	I
Cyclophosphamide	MJ	20 mg/mL[a]	AB	5 mg/mL[a]	Physically compatible for 4 hr at 25°C	1194	C
Dexmedetomidine HCl	AB	4 mcg/mL[b]	AB	5 mg/mL[b]	Physically compatible for 4 hr at 23°C	2383	C
Diltiazem HCl	MMD	5 mg/mL	ES	5 and 50 mg/mL[b]	Visually compatible	1807	C
Doxapram HCl	RB	2 mg/mL[a]	AB	5 mg/mL[a]	Visually compatible for 4 hr at 23°C	2470	C
Enalaprilat	MSD	0.05 mg/mL[b]	AB	5 mg/mL[a]	Physically compatible for 24 hr at room temperature under fluorescent light	1355	C
Esmolol HCl	DCC	10 mg/mL[a]	AB	5 mg/mL[a]	Physically compatible for 24 hr at 22°C	1169	C
Famotidine	MSD	0.2 mg/mL[a]	ES	2 mg/mL[b]	Physically compatible for 14 hr	1196	C
Fenoldopam mesylate	AB	80 mcg/mL[b]	AB	5 mg/mL[b]	Physically compatible for 4 hr at 23°C	2467	C
Foscarnet sodium	AST	24 mg/mL	AB	20 mg/mL	Physically compatible for 24 hr at room temperature under fluorescent light	1335	C
Foscarnet sodium	AST	24 mg/mL	ES	20 mg/mL[c]	Physically compatible for 24 hr at 25°C under fluorescent light	1393	C
Heparin sodium	TR	50 units/mL	AB	3.3 mg/mL[b]	Visually compatible for 4 hr at 25°C	1793	C
Hetastarch in lactated electrolyte	AB	6%	AB	5 mg/mL[b]	Physically compatible for 4 hr at 23°C	2339	C
Hydromorphone HCl	WY	0.2 mg/mL[a]	AB	5 mg/mL[a]	Physically compatible for 4 hr at 25°C	987	C
Idarubicin HCl	AD	1 mg/mL[b]	ES	2 mg/mL[b]	Visually compatible for 24 hr at 25°C	1525	C
Labetalol HCl	SC	1 mg/mL[a]	AB	5 mg/mL[a]	Physically compatible for 24 hr at 18°C	1171	C
Linezolid	PHU, HOS	2 mg/mL			Stated to be physically incompatible	3183, 3184	I
Lorazepam	WY	0.33 mg/mL[b]	AB	5 mg/mL	Visually compatible for 24 hr at 22°C	1855	C
Magnesium sulfate	IX	16.7, 33.3, 66.7, 100 mg/mL[a]	AB	5 mg/mL[a]	Physically compatible for at least 4 hr at 32°C	813	C
Meperidine HCl	WY	10 mg/mL[a]	AB	5 mg/mL[a]	Physically compatible for 4 hr at 25°C	987	C
Meropenem		50 mg/mL	AMD	50 mg/mL	Physically compatible for 4 hr at room temperature	3538	C

Y-Site Injection Compatibility (1:1 Mixture) (Cont.)

Test Drug	Mfr	Conc	Mfr	Conc	Remarks	Ref	C/I
Midazolam HCl	RC	5 mg/mL	AB	5 mg/mL	Visually compatible for 24 hr at 22°C	1855	C
Morphine sulfate	WI	1 mg/mL[a]	AB	5 mg/mL[a]	Physically compatible for 4 hr at 25°C	987	C
Multivitamins	USV	5 mL/L[a]	AB	500 mg/250 mL[b]	Physically compatible for 24 hr at room temperature	323	C
Nicardipine HCl	DCC	0.1 mg/mL[a]	AB	5 mg/mL[a]	Visually compatible for 24 hr at room temperature	235	C
Quinupristin–dalfopristin		2 mg/mL[a k]		5 mg/mL	Reported to be incompatible	3230	I
Tacrolimus	FUJ	1 mg/mL[b]	AB	20 mg/mL[a]	Visually compatible for 24 hr at 25°C	1630	C
Theophylline	TR	4 mg/mL	AB	3.3 mg/mL[b]	Visually compatible for 6 hr at 25°C	1793	C
TNA #73[d]		32.5 mL[e]	AB	20 mg/mL[b]	Visually compatible for 4 hr at 25°C	1008	C
TPN #61[d]		[f]	AB	50 mg/1 mL[g]	Physically compatible	1012	C
TPN #61[d]		[h]	AB	300 mg/6 mL[g]	Physically compatible	1012	C
TPN #189[d]			DB	10 mg/mL[a]	Visually compatible for 24 hr at 22°C	1767	C
Zidovudine	BW	4 mg/mL[a]	AB	20 mg/mL[a i]	Physically compatible for 4 hr at 25°C	1193	C

[a] Tested in dextrose 5%.

[b] Tested in sodium chloride 0.9%.

[c] Tested in both dextrose 5% and sodium chloride 0.9%.

[d] Refer to Appendix for the composition of parenteral nutrition solutions. TNA indicates a 3-in-1 admixture, and TPN indicates a 2-in-1 admixture.

[e] A 32.5-mL sample of parenteral nutrition solution mixed with 50 mL of antibiotic solution.

[f] Run at 21 mL/hr.

[g] Given over 30 minutes by syringe pump.

[h] Run at 94 mL/hr.

[i] Sodium bicarbonate 2.5 mEq added to adjust pH.

[j] Tested in sterile water for injection.

[k] Quinupristin and dalfopristin components combined.

Selected Revisions May 1, 2020. © Copyright, October 1982.
American Society of Health-System Pharmacists, Inc.

Esmolol Hydrochloride
AHFS 24:24

Products

Esmolol hydrochloride is available as a 10-mg/mL premixed, ready-to-use solution in 10-mL single-dose (preservative-free) vials and 250-mL bags.[2869][3234] Each mL of the ready-to-use solution also contains sodium acetate trihydrate 2.8 mg and glacial acetic acid 0.546 mg in water for injection with or without sodium chloride 5.9 mg, and may contain sodium hydroxide and/or hydrochloric acid for pH adjustment during manufacturing.[2869][3234] Vials may be used to prepare loading doses for administration by hand-held syringe while the maintenance infusion is being readied.[2869][3234]

Esmolol hydrochloride also is available as a double-strength 20-mg/mL premixed, ready-to-use solution in 100-mL bags.[2869] Each mL of the double-strength ready-to-use solution also contains sodium chloride 4.1 mg, sodium acetate trihydrate 2.8 mg, and glacial acetic acid 0.546 mg, and also may contain sodium hydroxide and/or hydrochloric acid for pH adjustment during manufacturing.[2869]

Esmolol hydrochloride (WG Critical Care) is available as a premixed, ready-to-use, preservative-free solution at a concentration of 10 mg/mL in 250-mL bags and 20 mg/mL (double strength) in 100-mL bags intended for single-patient use.[3235] Each mL of the ready-to-use solution also contains ethanol 1.23% (v/v), propylene glycol 10 mg, sodium acetate trihydrate 0.68 mg, and glacial acetic acid 0.27 mg in water for injection, and may contain sodium hydroxide for pH adjustment during manufacturing.[3235]

pH

Esmolol hydrochloride 10- and 20-mg/mL solutions (Brevibloc, Baxter; generic) have a pH ranging from 4.5 to 5.5.[2869][3234]

Esmolol hydrochloride 10- and 20-mg/mL solutions (WG Critical Care) have a pH ranging from 4.5 to 6.5.[3235]

Osmolarity

Esmolol hydrochloride 10- and 20-mg/mL solutions (Brevibloc, Baxter) are iso-osmotic having an osmolarity of 312 mOsm/L.[2869]

Esmolol hydrochloride 10- and 20-mg/mL solutions (WG Critical Care) have an osmolarity of 320 to 450 mOsmol/L and 440 to 500 mOsm/L, respectively.[3235]

Trade Name(s)

Brevibloc

Administration

Esmolol hydrochloride may be administered as a continuous infusion at a concentration of 10 or 20 mg/mL with or without a loading dose administered by intravenous bolus injection over 30 to 60 seconds.[2869][3234][3235]

Esmolol hydrochloride may cause serious venous irritation, including thrombophlebitis, and more serious local reactions, including skin necrosis and blistering, especially when associated with extravasation.[2869][3234][3235] The manufacturer recommends avoiding infusions into a small vein or through a butterfly catheter.[2869][3234][3235] If a local infusion site reaction develops, an alternative infusion site should be used; extravasation should be avoided.[2869][3234][3235]

Stability

Esmolol hydrochloride is a clear, colorless to light yellow solution.[2869][3234][3235] Intact vials and bags should be stored at controlled room temperature and protected from elevated temperatures and freezing.[2869][3234][3235] Bags should remain in their overwrap until ready for use.[2869][3235]

Esmolol hydrochloride solutions should be visually inspected for particulate matter and discoloration prior to administration.[2869][3234][3235] Following withdrawal of solution from the bag (e.g., a bolus dose), infusion of the remaining solution should begin immediately and any unused portion not infused by 24 hours after withdrawal from the bag should be discarded.[2869][3235]

pH Effects

Esmolol hydrochloride is relatively stable at neutral pH; the optimal pH is 4.5 to 5.5. However, ester hydrolysis occurs rapidly in strongly acidic or basic solutions.[1358][1359]

Compatibility Information

Solution Compatibility

Esmolol HCl

Test Soln Name	Mfr	Mfr	Conc/L or %	Remarks	Ref	C/I
Dextrose 5% in Ringer's injection		BA, FRK	10 g	Compatible and stable for 24 hr under refrigeration and at controlled room temperature	2869, 3234	C
Dextrose 5% in Ringer's injection		WG	10 g	Compatible and stable for 24 hr under refrigeration and at controlled room temperature	3235	C

DOI: 10.37573/9781585286850.152

Solution Compatibility (Cont.)

Test Soln Name	Mfr	Mfr	Conc/L or %	Remarks	Ref	C/I
Dextrose 5% in Ringer's injection, lactated		BA, FRK	10 g	Compatible and stable for 24 hr under refrigeration and at controlled room temperature	2869, 3234	C
Dextrose 5% in Ringer's injection, lactated		WG	10 g	Compatible and stable for 24 hr under refrigeration and at controlled room temperature	3235	C
Dextrose 5% in Ringer's injection, lactated	BA[a], MG[b]	ACC	10 g	Visually compatible with little or no drug loss in 7 days at 5 or 27°C, 48 hr at 40°C, and 24 hr under intense light	1831	C
Dextrose 5% in sodium chloride 0.45%		BA, FRK	10 g	Compatible and stable for 24 hr under refrigeration and at controlled room temperature	2869, 3234	C
Dextrose 5% in sodium chloride 0.45%		WG	10 g	Compatible and stable for 24 hr under refrigeration and at controlled room temperature	3235	C
Dextrose 5% in sodium chloride 0.45%	BA[a], MG[b]	ACC	10 g	Visually compatible with little or no drug loss in 7 days at 5 or 27°C, 48 hr at 40°C, and 24 hr under intense light	1831	C
Dextrose 5% in sodium chloride 0.9%		BA, FRK	10 g	Compatible and stable for 24 hr under refrigeration and at controlled room temperature	2869, 3234	C
Dextrose 5% in sodium chloride 0.9%		WG	10 g	Compatible and stable for 24 hr under refrigeration and at controlled room temperature	3235	C
Dextrose 5% in sodium chloride 0.9%	BA[a], MG[b]	ACC	10 g	Visually compatible with little or no drug loss in 7 days at 5 or 27°C, 48 hr at 40°C, and 24 hr under intense light	1831	C
Dextrose 5%	TR[a]	DU	6 g	Physically compatible with no loss in 24 hr at room temperature under fluorescent light	1358	C
Dextrose 5%	BA[a]	DU	10, 20, 30 g	Visually compatible with little or no drug loss in 48 hr at 23°C	1830	C
Dextrose 5%[c]	BA[a], MG[b]	ACC	10 g	Visually compatible with little or no drug loss in 7 days at 5 or 27°C, 48 hr at 40°C, and 24 hr under intense light	1831	C
Dextrose 5%[c]		BA, FRK	10 g	Compatible and stable for 24 hr under refrigeration and at controlled room temperature	2869, 3234	C
Dextrose 5%[c]		WG	10 g	Compatible and stable for 24 hr under refrigeration and at controlled room temperature	3235	C
Ringer's injection, lactated		BA, FRK	10 g	Compatible and stable for 24 hr under refrigeration and at controlled room temperature	2869, 3234	C
Ringer's injection, lactated		WG	10 g	Compatible and stable for 24 hr under refrigeration and at controlled room temperature	3235	C
Ringer's injection, lactated	BA[a], MG[b]	ACC	10 g	Visually compatible with little or no drug loss in 7 days at 5 or 27°C, 48 hr at 40°C, and 24 hr under intense light	1831	C
Sodium chloride 0.45%		BA, FRK	10 g	Compatible and stable for 24 hr under refrigeration and at controlled room temperature	2869, 3234	C
Sodium chloride 0.45%		WG	10 g	Compatible and stable for 24 hr under refrigeration and at controlled room temperature	3235	C
Sodium chloride 0.45%	BA[a], MG[b]	ACC	10 g	Visually compatible with little or no drug loss in 7 days at 5 or 27°C, 48 hr at 40°C, and 24 hr under intense light	1831	C
Sodium chloride 0.9%		BA, FRK	10 g	Compatible and stable for 24 hr under refrigeration and at controlled room temperature	2869, 3234	C

Solution Compatibility (Cont.)

Test Soln Name	Mfr	Mfr	Conc/L or %	Remarks	Ref	C/I
Sodium chloride 0.9%		WG	10 g	Compatible and stable for 24 hr under refrigeration and at controlled room temperature	3235	C
Sodium chloride 0.9%	BA[a], MG[b]	ACC	10 g	Visually compatible with little or no drug loss in 7 days at 5 or 27°C, 48 hr at 40°C, and 24 hr under intense light	1831	C

[a] Tested in PVC containers.

[b] Tested in glass containers.

[c] Tested with and without potassium chloride 40 mEq/L.

Additive Compatibility

Esmolol HCl

Test Drug	Mfr	Conc/L or %	Mfr	Conc/L or %	Test Solution	Remarks	Ref	C/I
Aminophylline	LY	1 g	DU	6 g	D5W	Physically compatible with no loss of either drug in 24 hr at room temperature under fluorescent light	1358	C
Atracurium besylate	BW	500 mg		10 g	D5W	Physically compatible and atracurium stable for 24 hr at 5 and 30°C	1694	C
Heparin sodium	LY	50,000 units	DU	6 g	D5W	Physically compatible with no esmolol loss in 24 hr at room temperature under fluorescent light. Heparin not tested	1358	C
Procainamide HCl	ES	4 g	DU	6 g	D5W	43% procainamide loss in 24 hr at room temperature under fluorescent light	1358	I
Sodium bicarbonate	MG[a]	5%	ACC	10 g		Visually compatible. 5 and 8% esmolol losses in 7 days at 4 and 27°C, respectively	1831	C

[a] Tested in glass containers.

Y-Site Injection Compatibility (1:1 Mixture)

Esmolol HCl

Test Drug	Mfr	Conc	Mfr	Conc	Remarks	Ref	C/I
Acetaminophen	CAD	10 mg/mL	MYL	10 mg/mL	Physically compatible for 1 hr at 23°C	3533	C
Albumin human	OCT	250 mg/mL	MYL	10 mg/mL	Physically compatible for 1 hr at 23°C	3533	C
Amikacin sulfate	BR	5 mg/mL[a]	DCC	10 mg/mL[a]	Physically compatible for 24 hr at 22°C	1169	C
Aminophylline	ES	1 mg/mL[a]	DCC	10 mg/mL[a]	Physically compatible for 24 hr at 22°C	1169	C
Amiodarone HCl	WY	4.8 mg/mL[a]	DU	40 mg/mL[a]	Visually compatible for 24 hr at 23°C	1877	C
Ampicillin sodium	WY	20 mg/mL[b]	DCC	10 mg/mL[a]	Physically compatible for 24 hr at 22°C	1169	C
Argatroban	SZ	1 mg/mL	BA	10 mg/mL	Physically compatible for up to 24 hr at 19 to 24°C in ambient light and 28 to 40% relative humidity	3192	C
Atracurium besylate	BW	0.5 mg/mL[a]	DCC	10 mg/mL[a]	Physically compatible for 24 hr at 28°C	1337	C
Bivalirudin	TMC	5 mg/mL[a]	BA	10 mg/mL[a]	Physically compatible for 4 hr at 23°C	2373	C
Butorphanol tartrate	BR	0.04 mg/mL[a]	DCC	10 mg/mL[a]	Physically compatible for 24 hr at 22°C	1169	C
Calcium chloride	AB	20 mg/mL[a]	DCC	10 mg/mL[a]	Physically compatible for 24 hr at 22°C	1169	C

Y-Site Injection Compatibility (1:1 Mixture) (Cont.)

Test Drug	Mfr	Conc	Mfr	Conc	Remarks	Ref	C/I
Cangrelor tetrasodium	TMC	1 mg/mL[b]	[h]	10 mg/mL	Physically compatible for 4 hr	3243	C
Cefazolin sodium	LI	10 mg/mL[a]	DCC	10 mg/mL[a]	Physically compatible for 24 hr at 22°C	1169	C
Cefepime HCl	APP	40 mg/mL[b]	MYL	10 mg/mL	Physically compatible for 1 hr at 23°C	3533	C
Ceftazidime	GL	10 mg/mL[a]	DCC	10 mg/mL[a]	Physically compatible for 24 hr at 22°C	1169	C
Ceftolozane sulfate–tazobactam sodium	CUB	10 mg/mL[f i]	MYL	10 mg/mL	Physically compatible for 2 hr	3262	C
Chloramphenicol sodium succinate	PD	10 mg/mL[a]	DCC	10 mg/mL[a]	Physically compatible for 24 hr at 22°C	1169	C
Ciprofloxacin	SZ	2 mg/mL	MYL	10 mg/mL	Physically incompatible	3533	I
Cisatracurium besylate	GW	0.1, 2, 5 mg/mL[a]	OHM	10 mg/mL[a]	Physically compatible for 4 hr at 23°C	2074	C
Cisatracurium besylate	AB	2 mg/mL	MYL	10 mg/mL	Physically compatible for 1 hr at 23°C	3533	C
Clevidipine butyrate	CHS	0.5 mg/mL		10 mg/mL	pH shifted outside of specified pH range for clevidipine within 24 hr	3334	?
Clindamycin phosphate	UP	9 mg/mL[a]	DCC	10 mg/mL[a]	Physically compatible for 24 hr at 22°C	1169	C
Cloxacillin sodium	SMX	100 mg/mL	BA	10 mg/mL	Physically compatible for up to 4 hr at room temperature	3245	C
Dexmedetomidine HCl	AB	4 mcg/mL[b]	BA	10 mg/mL[b]	Physically compatible for 4 hr at 23°C	2383	C
Diltiazem HCl	MMD	1 mg/mL[a]	DU	10 mg/mL[a]	Visually compatible for 24 hr at 25°C	1530	C
Dopamine HCl	IMS	1.6 mg/mL[a]	DCC	10 mg/mL[a]	Physically compatible for 24 hr at 22°C	1169	C
Doripenem	JJ	5 mg/mL[a b]	BED	10 mg/mL[a b]	Physically compatible for 4 hr at 23°C	2743	C
Doripenem	SHI	4.5 mg/mL[b]	MYL	10 mg/mL	Physically compatible for 1 hr at 23°C	3533	C
Enalaprilat	MSD	0.05 mg/mL[b]	DU	10 mg/mL[a]	Physically compatible for 24 hr at room temperature under fluorescent light	1355	C
Epinephrine[h]	AMP	0.128 mg/mL[b]	MYL	10 mg/mL	Physically compatible for 1 hr at 23°C	3533	C
Eravacycline dihydrochloride	TET	0.6 mg/mL[b]	FRK	10 mg/mL	Physically compatible for 2 hr at room temperature	3532	C
Erythromycin lactobionate	AB	5 mg/mL[a]	DCC	10 mg/mL[a]	Physically compatible for 24 hr at 22°C	1169	C
Esomeprazole sodium	ASZ	0.8 mg/mL[b]	MYL	10 mg/mL	Initial light champagne color that intensifies over 1 hr	3533	I
Famotidine	MSD	0.2 mg/mL[a]	DU	10 mg/mL[b]	Physically compatible for 4 hr at 25°C	1188	C
Fenoldopam mesylate	AB	80 mcg/mL[b]	BA	10 mg/mL[b]	Physically compatible for 4 hr at 23°C	2467	C
Fentanyl citrate	JN	0.05 mg/1 mL	DCC	1 g/100 mL[d]	Physically compatible when fentanyl is injected into Y-site of flowing admixture[e]	1168	C
Fentanyl citrate	JN	0.05 mg/mL	DCC	10 mg/mL[d]	Physically compatible. No drug loss in 8 hr at room temperature in light	1168	C
Furosemide	HO	10 mg/mL	ACC	10 mg/mL[f]	Cloudy precipitate forms immediately	1146	I
Gentamicin sulfate	ES	0.8 mg/mL[a]	DCC	10 mg/mL[a]	Physically compatible for 24 hr at 22°C	1169	C
Heparin sodium	IX	40 units/mL[a]	DCC	10 mg/mL[a]	Physically compatible for 24 hr at 22°C	1169	C
Hetastarch in lactated electrolyte	AB	6%	OHM	10 mg/mL	Physically compatible for 4 hr at 23°C	2339	C

Y-Site Injection Compatibility (1:1 Mixture) (Cont.)

Test Drug	Mfr	Conc	Mfr	Conc	Remarks	Ref	C/I
Hydrocortisone sodium succinate	LY	1 mg/mL[a]	DCC	10 mg/mL[a]	Physically compatible for 24 hr at 22°C	1169	C
Hydrocortisone sodium succinate	PF	1 mg/mL[b]	MYL	10 mg/mL	Physically compatible for 1 hr at 23°C	3533	C
Hydroxyethyl starch 130/0.4 in sodium chloride 0.9%	FRK	6%	BA	10 mg/mL[a]	Visually compatible for 24 hr at room temperature	2770	C
Ibuprofen	CMB	4 mg/mL	MYL	10 mg/mL	White cloudy solution forms upon mixing	3533	I
Insulin, regular	LI	1 unit/mL[a]	DU	40 mg/mL[a]	Visually compatible for 24 hr at 23°C	1877	C
Isavuconazonium sulfate	ASP	1.5 mg/mL[f]	MYL, FRK	10 mg/mL	Physically compatible for 2 hr	3263	C
Labetalol HCl	GL	5 mg/mL	DU	40 mg/mL[a]	Visually compatible for 24 hr at 23°C	1877	C
Levofloxacin	SGT	5 mg/mL	MYL	10 mg/mL	Physically compatible for 1 hr at 23°C	3533	C
Levothyroxine sodium	PRP	0.4 mcg/mL[b]	MYL	10 mg/mL	Physically compatible for 1 hr at 23°C	3533	C
Linezolid	PHU	2 mg/mL	OHM	10 mg/mL	Physically compatible for 4 hr at 23°C	2264	C
Magnesium sulfate	LY	10 mg/mL[a]	DCC	10 mg/mL[a]	Physically compatible for 24 hr at 22°C	1169	C
Meropenem	NVP	20 mg/mL[b]	MYL	10 mg/mL	Physically compatible for 1 hr at 23°C	3533	C
Meropenem		50 mg/mL	BA	10 mg/mL	Physically compatible for 4 hr at room temperature	3538	C
Meropenem–vaborbactam	TMC	8 mg/mL[b j]	MYL	10 mg/mL	Physically compatible for 3 hr at 20 to 25°C	3380	C
Methyldopate HCl	MSD	5 mg/mL[a]	DCC	10 mg/mL[a]	Physically compatible for 24 hr at 22°C	1169	C
Metronidazole	SE	5 mg/mL	DCC	10 mg/mL[a]	Physically compatible for 24 hr at 22°C	1169	C
Micafungin sodium	ASP	1.5 mg/mL[b]	BA	10 mg/mL[b]	Physically compatible for 4 hr at 23°C	2683	C
Midazolam HCl	RC	1 mg/mL[a]	DU	40 mg/mL[a]	Visually compatible for 24 hr at 23°C	1877	C
Morphine sulfate	ES	15 mg/1 mL	DCC	1 g/100 mL[d]	Physically compatible when morphine is injected in Y-site[d]	1168	C
Morphine sulfate	ES	15 mg/mL	DCC	10 mg/mL[d]	Physically compatible. No drug loss in 8 hr at room temperature in light	1168	C
Nafcillin sodium	BR	10 mg/mL[a]	DCC	10 mg/mL[a]	Physically compatible for 24 hr at 22°C	1169	C
Nicardipine HCl	DCC	0.1 mg/mL[a]	DU	10 mg/mL[a]	Visually compatible for 24 hr at room temperature	235	C
Nitroglycerin	OM	0.2 mg/mL[a]	DU	40 mg/mL[a]	Visually compatible for 24 hr at 23°C	1877	C
Norepinephrine bitartrate	STR	0.064 mg/mL[a]	DU	40 mg/mL[a]	Visually compatible for 24 hr at 23°C	1877	C
Norepinephrine bitartrate	HOS	0.128 mg/mL[b]	MYL	10 mg/mL	Physically compatible for 1 hr at 23°C	3533	C
Pancuronium bromide	ES	0.05 mg/mL[a]	DCC	10 mg/mL[a]	Physically compatible for 24 hr at 28°C	1337	C
Pantoprazole sodium	ALT[g]	0.16 to 0.8 mg/mL[b]	BA	10 to 20 mg/mL[a]	Discoloration and reddish-brown precipitate form	2603	I
Penicillin G potassium	PF	50,000 units/mL[a]	DCC	10 mg/mL[a]	Physically compatible for 24 hr at 22°C	1169	C
Phenytoin sodium	IX	1 mg/mL[a]	DCC	10 mg/mL[a]	Physically compatible for 24 hr at 22°C	1169	C

Y-Site Injection Compatibility (1:1 Mixture) (Cont.)

Test Drug	Mfr	Conc	Mfr	Conc	Remarks	Ref	C/I
Plazomicin sulfate	ACH	24 mg/mL[f]	MYL	10 mg/mL	Physically compatible for 1 hr at 20 to 25°C	3432	C
Polymyxin B sulfate	PF	0.005 unit/mL[a]	DCC	10 mg/mL[a]	Physically compatible for 24 hr at 22°C	1169	C
Potassium chloride	IX	0.4 mEq/mL[a]	DCC	10 mg/mL[a]	Physically compatible for 24 hr at 22°C	1169	C
Potassium phosphates	LY	0.44 mEq/mL[a]	DCC	10 mg/mL[a]	Physically compatible for 24 hr at 22°C	1169	C
Propofol	ZEN[k]	10 mg/mL	OHM	10 mg/mL	Physically compatible for 1 hr at 23°C	2066	C
Ranitidine HCl	GL	0.5 mg/mL[a]	DCC	10 mg/mL[a]	Physically compatible for 24 hr at 22°C	1169	C
Remifentanil HCl	GW	0.025 and 0.25 mg/mL[b]	OHM	10 mg/mL[a]	Physically compatible for 4 hr at 23°C	2075	C
Sodium acetate	LY	0.4 mEq/mL[a]	DCC	10 mg/mL[a]	Physically compatible for 24 hr at 22°C	1169	C
Sodium nitroprusside	RC	0.2 mg/mL[a]	DU	40 mg/mL[a]	Visually compatible for 24 hr at 23°C	1877	C
Streptomycin sulfate	PF	10 mg/mL[a]	DCC	10 mg/mL[a]	Physically compatible for 24 hr at 22°C	1169	C
Tacrolimus	FUJ	1 mg/mL[b]	DU	10 mg/mL[a]	Visually compatible for 24 hr at 25°C	1630	C
Tedizolid phosphate	CUB	0.8 mg/mL[b]	BA	10 mg/mL	Measured turbidity increases immediately	3244	I
Tobramycin sulfate	LI	0.8 mg/mL[a]	DCC	10 mg/mL[a]	Physically compatible for 24 hr at 22°C	1169	C
Trimethoprim–sulfamethoxazole	BW	0.64 mg/mL[a] [c]	DCC	10 mg/mL[a]	Physically compatible for 24 hr at 22°C	1169	C
Vancomycin HCl	LE	5 mg/mL[a]	DCC	10 mg/mL[a]	Physically compatible for 24 hr at 22°C	1169	C
Vecuronium bromide	OR	0.1 mg/mL[a]	DCC	10 mg/mL[a]	Physically compatible for 24 hr at 28°C	1337	C

[a] Tested in dextrose 5%.

[b] Tested in sodium chloride 0.9%.

[c] Trimethoprim component. Trimethoprim in a 1:5 fixed-ratio concentration with sulfamethoxazole.

[d] Tested in dextrose 5% in sodium chloride 0.9%.

[e] Flowing at 1.6 mL/min.

[f] Tested in both dextrose 5% and sodium chloride 0.9%.

[g] Test performed using the formulation WITHOUT edetate disodium.

[h] Salt not specified.

[i] Ceftolozane component. Ceftolozane in a 2:1 fixed-ratio concentration with tazobactam.

[j] Meropenem component. Meropenem in a 1:1 fixed-ratio concentration with vaborbactam.

[k] Test performed using the formulation WITH edetate disodium.

Selected Revisions May 1, 2020. © Copyright, October 1990.
American Society of Health-System Pharmacists, Inc.

Esomeprazole Sodium
AHFS 56:28.36

Products

Esomeprazole is available as a lyophilized powder in 20- and 40-mg vials as the sodium salt with edetate disodium 1.5 mg and sodium hydroxide to adjust pH during manufacturing. For direct intravenous injection, reconstitute either size vial with 5 mL of sodium chloride 0.9%.[1(3/05)]

For intravenous infusion, reconstitute either size vial with 5 mL of sodium chloride 0.9%; Ringer's injection, lactated; or dextrose 5%, and then dilute the reconstituted solution to 50 mL with additional infusion solution.[1(3/05)]

pH

From 9 to 11.[1(3/05)]

Trade Name(s)

Nexium I.V.

Administration

Esomeprazole sodium is administered by direct intravenous injection over at least 3 minutes or by intravenous infusion over 10 to 30 minutes.[1(3/05)]

Stability

Intact vials of esomeprazole sodium should be stored at controlled room temperature and protected from light. The drug reconstituted with sodium chloride 0.9% for direct intravenous injection should be administered within 12 hours after reconstitution when stored at room temperature. Esomeprazole sodium reconstituted and diluted for intravenous infusion should be administered within 12 hours at room temperature after reconstitution and dilution if sodium chloride 0.9% or Ringer's injection, lactated, is the reconstitution and dilution solution. If dextrose 5% is used for reconstitution and dilution, the drug should be used within 6 hours at room temperature. The manufacturer states that refrigeration is not required for esomeprazole solutions.[1(3/05)]

The manufacturer states that esomeprazole sodium administration requires flushing the administration line with sodium chloride 0.9%; Ringer's injection, lactated; or dextrose 5% both before and after administering the drug, and that esomeprazole sodium should not be administered concomitantly with other drugs.[1(3/05)]

pH Effects

The stability of esomeprazole sodium in solution is strongly dependent on pH. The stability of the drug decreases with decreasing pH.[1(3/05)]

Compatibility Information

Solution Compatibility

Esomeprazole sodium

Test Soln Name	Mfr	Mfr	Conc/L or %	Remarks	Ref	C/I
Dextrose 5%	BA[a]	ASZ	400 and 800 mg	Physically compatible with less than 7% loss in 48 hr at room temperature and no loss in 120 hr at 4°C	2760	C
Dextrose 5%	[b]	ASZ	400 mg	Less than 10% loss after −20°C storage for 30 days, microwave thawing, and storage at 5°C for 20 days	3272	C
Dextrose 5%	[b]	ASZ	800 mg	Less than 10% loss after −20°C storage for 30 days, microwave thawing, and storage at 5°C for 29 days	3272	C
Ringer's injection, lactated	BA[a]	ASZ	400 and 800 mg	Physically compatible with less than 4% loss in 48 hr at room temperature and little or no loss in 120 hr at 4°C	2760	C
Sodium chloride 0.9%	BA[a]	ASZ	400 and 800 mg	Physically compatible with less than 3% loss in 48 hr at room temperature and about 1% loss in 120 hr at 4°C	2760	C

[a] Tested in PVC containers.

[b] Tested in polyolefin containers.

DOI: 10.37573/9781585286850.153

Y-Site Injection Compatibility (1:1 Mixture)

Esomeprazole sodium

Test Drug	Mfr	Conc	Mfr	Conc	Remarks	Ref	C/I
Ceftaroline fosamil	FOR	2.22 mg/mL[a b c]	ASZ	0.4 mg/mL[a b c]	Physically compatible for 4 hr at 23°C	2826	C
Ceftolozane sulfate–tazobactam sodium	CUB	10 mg/mL[d e]	ASZ	0.8 mg/mL[d]	Physically compatible for 2 hr	3262	C
Cisatracurium besylate	AB	1 mg/mL[b]	ASZ	0.4 mg/mL[b]	Physically compatible for 1 hr at 23°C	3157	C
Doripenem	JJ	5 mg/mL[a b]	ASZ	0.4 mg/mL[b]	Physically compatible for 4 hr at 23°C	2743	C
Esmolol HCl	MYL	10 mg/mL	ASZ	0.8 mg/mL[b]	Initial light champagne color that intensifies over 1 hr	3533	I
Isavuconazonium sulfate	ASP	1.5 mg/mL[d]	ASZ	0.8 mg/mL[d]	Measured turbidity increases immediately with color changes within 15 to 60 min	3263	I
Labetalol HCl	HOS	5 mg/mL	ASZ	0.8 mg/mL[b]	Light pink solution forms immediately	3533	I
Meropenem–vaborbactam	TMC	8 mg/mL[b f]	ASZ	0.8 mg/mL[b]	Physically compatible for 3 hr at 20 to 25°C	3380	C
Metoprolol tartrate	HOS	0.4 mg/mL[b]	ASZ	0.8 mg/mL[b]	Physically compatible for 1 hr at 23°C	3533	C
Plazomicin sulfate	ACH	24 mg/mL[d]	ASZ	0.8 mg/mL[d]	Measured turbidity increases within 1 hr; pH decreased by nearly 3 units within 30 min	3432	I
Tedizolid phosphate	CUB	0.8 mg/mL[b]	ASZ	0.8 mg/mL[b]	Physically compatible for 2 hr	3244	C
Telavancin HCl	ASP	7.5 mg/mL[a b c]	ASZ	0.4 mg/mL[a b c]	Discoloration and increase in measured turbidity	2830	I
Tigecycline	ACD, FRK, WY		[g]		Stated to be incompatible	2915, 3459, 3460	I

[a] Tested in dextrose 5%.

[b] Tested in sodium chloride 0.9%.

[c] Tested in Ringer's injection, lactated.

[d] Tested in both dextrose 5% and sodium chloride 0.9%.

[e] Ceftolozane component. Ceftolozane in a 2:1 fixed-ratio concentration with tazobactam.

[f] Meropenem component. Meropenem in a 1:1 fixed-ratio concentration with vaborbactam.

[g] Salt not specified.

Selected Revisions May 1, 2020. © Copyright, October 2010.
American Society of Health-System Pharmacists, Inc.

Estrogens, Conjugated
AHFS 68:16.04

Products

Estrogens, conjugated is available in packages containing a vial with lyophilized estrogens, conjugated, 25 mg; lactose 200 mg; sodium citrate 12.2 mg; simethicone 0.2 mg; and sodium hydroxide or hydrochloric acid for pH adjustment. Reconstitute the vial with 5 mL of sterile water for injection flowing along the side of the vial and agitate gently – not violently.[1(3/08)]

Trade Name(s)

Premarin Intravenous

Administration

Estrogens, conjugated may be administered by deep intramuscular injection or slow direct intravenous injection. Intravenous infusion is not recommended, but injection into the tubing of a running infusion may be performed.[1(3/08)] [4]

Stability

The manufacturer recommends refrigeration of the intact containers at 2 to 8°C.[1(3/08)] Such storage provides a shelflife of up to 60 months. Although refrigerated storage is required, the manufacturer has stated the drug may be stored at room temperature for seven days.[2745] The manufacturer recommends use immediately after reconstitution.[1(3/08)]

pH Effects

Estrogens, conjugated, has been stated to be incompatible with any solution with an acid pH.[1(3/08)] [4]

Compatibility Information

Solution Compatibility

Estrogens, conjugated

Test Soln Name	Mfr	Mfr	Conc/L or %	Remarks	Ref	C/I
Dextrose 5%				Compatible	1(3/08)	C
Sodium chloride 0.9%				Compatible	1(3/08)	C

Drugs in Syringe Compatibility

Estrogens, conjugated

Test Drug	Mfr	Amt	Mfr	Amt	Remarks	Ref	C/I
Pantoprazole sodium	a	4 mg/1 mL		5 mg/1 mL	Possible precipitate within 1 hr	2574	I

[a] Test performed using the formulation WITHOUT edetate disodium.

Y-Site Injection Compatibility (1:1 Mixture)

Estrogens, conjugated

Test Drug	Mfr	Conc	Mfr	Conc	Remarks	Ref	C/I
Heparin sodium[b]	RI	1000 units/L[a]	AY	5 mg/mL	Physically compatible for 4 hr at room temperature	322	C
Hydrocortisone sodium succinate[c]	UP	100 mg/L[a]	AY	5 mg/mL	Physically compatible for 4 hr at room temperature	322	C
Potassium chloride		40 mEq/L[a]	AY	5 mg/mL	Physically compatible for 4 hr at room temperature	322	C

[a] Tested in dextrose 5%, sodium chloride 0.9%, and Ringer's injection, lactated.

[b] Tested in combination with hydrocortisone sodium succinate (Upjohn) 100 mg/L.

[c] Tested in combination with heparin sodium (Riker) 1000 units/L.

DOI: 10.37573/9781585286850.154

Ethacrynate Sodium

AHFS 40:28.08

Products

Each vial has ethacrynate sodium equivalent to ethacrynic acid 50 mg and mannitol 62.5 mg. Reconstitute with 50 mL of dextrose 5% or sodium chloride 0.9% to yield a 1-mg/mL solution. Some dextrose 5% has a pH below 5 and results in a hazy or opalescent solution, which is not recommended for use.[1(2/05)] [4]

pH

Reconstitution with dextrose 5% or sodium chloride 0.9% results in a solution having a pH of 6.3 to 7.7.[4]

Sodium Content

Ethacrynate sodium contains 0.165 mEq of sodium per 50 mg of ethacrynic acid equivalent.[846]

Trade Name(s)

Sodium Edecrin

Administration

Ethacrynate sodium may be given slowly through the tubing of a running intravenous solution or directly into a vein over several minutes.[1(2/05)] [4] Subcutaneous or intramuscular injection should not be used because of local pain and irritation.[1(2/05)] [4]

Stability

Solutions of ethacrynate sodium are relatively stable for short periods at pH 7 at room temperature; but as the pH or temperature or both increase, the solutions are less stable. Ethacrynate sodium is incompatible with solutions or drugs with a final pH below 5. The reconstituted solution should be discarded after 24 hours.[1(2/05)] [4]

Compatibility Information

Solution Compatibility

Ethacrynate sodium

Test Soln Name	Mfr	Mfr	Conc/L or %	Remarks	Ref	C/I
Dextrose 5%				Compatible	4	C
Dextrose 5% in sodium chloride 0.9%				Compatible	4	C
Ringer's injection				Compatible	4	C
Ringer's injection, lactated				Compatible	4	C
Sodium chloride 0.9%				Compatible	4	C

Additive Compatibility

Ethacrynate sodium

Test Drug	Mfr	Conc/L or %	Mfr	Conc/L or %	Test Solution	Remarks	Ref	C/I
Chlorpromazine HCl	SKF	50 mg	MSD	50 mg	NS	Little alteration of UV spectra within 8 hr at room temperature	16	C
Hydralazine HCl	CI	20 mg	MSD	50 mg	NS	Altered UV spectra at room temperature	16	I
Procainamide HCl	SQ	1 g	MSD	50 mg	NS	Altered UV spectra at room temperature	16	I
Prochlorperazine edisylate	SKF	20 mg	MSD	80 mg	NS	Little alteration of UV spectra within 8 hr at room temperature	16	C
Ranitidine HCl	GL	50 mg and 2 g		500 mg	D5W	Ranitidine stable for only 6 hr at 25°C. Ethacrynate not tested	1515	I
Triflupromazine HCl	SQ		MSD		NS	Occasional gas bubble formation	16	I

DOI: 10.37573/9781585286850.155

Y-Site Injection Compatibility (1:1 Mixture)

Ethacrynate sodium

Test Drug	Mfr	Conc	Mfr	Conc	Remarks	Ref	C/I
Heparin sodium[d]	RI	1000 units/L[a b c]	MSD	1 mg/mL	Physically compatible for 4 hr at room temperature	322	C
Hydrocortisone sodium succinate[e]	UP	100 mg/L[a b c]	MSD	1 mg/mL	Physically compatible for 4 hr at room temperature	322	C
Nesiritide	SCI	50 mcg/mL[a b]		1 mg/mL	Physically incompatible	2625	I
Potassium chloride		40 mEq/L[a b c]	MSD	1 mg/mL	Physically compatible for 4 hr at room temperature	322	C

[a] Tested in dextrose 5%.

[b] Tested in sodium chloride 0.9%.

[c] Tested in Ringer's injection, lactated.

[d] Tested in combination with hydrocortisone sodium succinate (Upjohn) 100 mg/L.

[e] Tested in combination with heparin sodium (Riker) 1000 units/L.

Selected Revisions October 1, 2012. © Copyright, October 1982.
American Society of Health-System Pharmacists, Inc.

Etomidate
AHFS 28:04.92

Products

Etomidate injection is available as a 2-mg/mL solution in 10- and 20-mL single-dose vials and ampuls and 20-mL syringes.[3319] Each mL of etomidate injection also contains propylene glycol 35% (v/v).[3319]

pH
From 4 to 7.[3319]

Trade Name(s)
Amidate

Administration

Etomidate is administered only by the intravenous route as an injection over 30 to 60 seconds.[3319] Manufacturers state that the drug should *not* be administered by prolonged infusion.[3319]

Stability

Intact containers of etomidate should be stored at controlled room temperature.[3319]

Etomidate injection should be visually inspected for particulate matter and discoloration prior to administration; the solution should not be used unless it is clear and the container is undamaged.[3319] Unused portions should be discarded.[3319]

Compatibility Information

Drugs in Syringe Compatibility

Etomidate

Test Drug	Mfr	Amt	Mfr	Amt	Remarks	Ref	C/I
Heparin sodium		2500 units/1 mL	JN	20 mg/10 mL	Visually compatible for at least 5 min	1053	C

Y-Site Injection Compatibility (1:1 Mixture)

Etomidate

Test Drug	Mfr	Conc	Mfr	Conc	Remarks	Ref	C/I
Alfentanil HCl	JN	0.5 mg/mL	AB	2 mg/mL	Visually compatible for 7 days at 25°C	1801	C
Ascorbic acid	AB	500 mg/mL	AB	2 mg/mL	Yellow color and precipitate form in 24 hr	1801	I
Atracurium besylate	BW	10 mg/mL	AB	2 mg/mL	Visually compatible for 7 days at 25°C	1801	C
Atropine sulfate	GNS	0.4 mg/mL	AB	2 mg/mL	Visually compatible for 7 days at 25°C	1801	C
Dexmedetomidine HCl	HOS	4 mcg/mL[a]			Stated to be compatible	3181	C
Ephedrine sulfate	AB	50 mg/mL	AB	2 mg/mL	Visually compatible for 7 days at 25°C	1801	C
Fentanyl citrate	ES	0.05 mg/mL	AB	2 mg/mL	Visually compatible for 7 days at 25°C	1801	C
Lidocaine HCl	AST	20 mg/mL	AB	2 mg/mL	Visually compatible for 7 days at 25°C	1801	C
Lorazepam	WY	2 mg/mL	AB	2 mg/mL	Visually compatible for 7 days at 25°C	1801	C
Midazolam HCl	RC	5 mg/mL	AB	2 mg/mL	Visually compatible for 7 days at 25°C	1801	C
Morphine sulfate	ES	10 mg/mL	AB	2 mg/mL	Visually compatible for 7 days at 25°C	1801	C
Pancuronium bromide	GNS	2 mg/mL	AB	2 mg/mL	Visually compatible for 7 days at 25°C	1801	C
Phenylephrine HCl	ES	10 mg/mL	AB	2 mg/mL	Visually compatible for 7 days at 25°C	1801	C

DOI: 10.37573/9781585286850.156

Y-Site Injection Compatibility (1:1 Mixture) (Cont.)

Test Drug	Mfr	Conc	Mfr	Conc	Remarks	Ref	C/I
Succinylcholine chloride	AB	20 mg/mL	AB	2 mg/mL	Visually compatible for 7 days at 25°C	1801	C
Sufentanil citrate	JN	0.05 mg/mL	AB	2 mg/mL	Visually compatible for 7 days at 25°C	1801	C
Vecuronium bromide	OR	1 mg/mL	AB	2 mg/mL	Slight turbidity and white particles form	1801	I

ᵃ Tested in sodium chloride 0.9%.

Selected Revisions February 21, 2018. © Copyright, October 1996. American Society of Health-System Pharmacists, Inc.

Etoposide

AHFS 10:00

Products

Etoposide 20 mg/mL concentrate for injection is available in 5-, 25-, and 50-mL multiple-dose vials.[2951] Each mL also contains polyethylene glycol 300 650 mg, ethanol 30.5% (v/v), polysorbate 80 80 mg, benzyl alcohol 30 mg, and citric acid 2 mg.[2951]

pH

From 3 to 4.[2951]

Administration

Etoposide concentrate for injection must be diluted to a final concentration of 0.2 to 0.4 mg/mL prior to administration.[2951] The drug is recommended to be given by slow intravenous infusion over at least 30 to 60 minutes; however, a longer duration of administration may be considered if the volume of the infusion solution is a concern.[2951]

Continuous intravenous infusion also has been used.[4] The drug should *not* be given by rapid intravenous injection.[2951]

The surfactant content of the etoposide formulation decreases surface tension and has been found to produce a 30% reduction in drop size compared to simple aqueous solutions. The altered drop size may interfere with accurate infusion rates if infusion devices that rely on drop counting are used. The use of infusion devices that operate independently of drop size has been recommended.[181]

The manufacturer notes that accidental exposure to this potentially toxic agent may cause skin reactions.[2951] Therefore, protective gloves should be used during preparation of solutions.[2951] A soap and water wash should be employed after accidental contact with the skin and accidentally exposed mucosa should be flushed with water.[2951]

In the event of spills or leaks, the use of sodium hypochlorite 5% (household bleach) or potassium permanganate 1% to inactivate etoposide has been recommended.[1200]

Stability

Etoposide concentrate for injection is a clear yellow solution.[2951] Intact vials should be stored at controlled room temperature.[2951] Stability is not affected by exposure to normal room fluorescent light.[1374]

Plastic devices composed of acrylic or a polymer of acrylonitrile, butadiene, and styrene (ABS) may crack and leak when used with undiluted etoposide.[2951] In one study, a multiport disposable infusion cassette (Omni-Flow) developed cracks within 5 minutes after infusion was started and leakage was evident within 15 minutes. This phenomenon did not occur when etoposide was diluted to concentrations up to 1 mg/mL. In addition, a venting pin and a connector on an extension set reportedly cracked. Exposure to the polyethylene glycol 300 content of the etoposide formulation can cause cracks in minutes. However, dehydrated alcohol did not cause any cracks within 1 hour.[1261]

Immersion of a needle with an aluminum component in etoposide (Bristol) 20 mg/mL resulted in no visually apparent reaction after 7 days at 24°C.[988]

Precipitation

Dextrose 5% and sodium chloride 0.9% have been recommended as diluents for the infusion of etoposide.[2951] Unlike etoposide phosphate, the aqueous solubility of etoposide is poor (0.03 mg/mL), but the formulation temporarily increases its miscibility in an aqueous medium. Nevertheless, the drug will eventually crystallize in varying time periods, and the crystallization is reported to be exacerbated by peristaltic pumps.[1949] At concentrations of 0.2 and 0.4 mg/mL in dextrose 5% or sodium chloride 0.9%, the solutions are stable for 96 and 24 hours, respectively, at 25°C under normal fluorescent light in either glass or plastic containers.[2951] However, precipitation in shorter time periods has been observed. At concentrations of 0.2 and 0.4 mg/mL in Ringer's injection, lactated, or mannitol 10% in glass containers under the same conditions, the solutions are stable for 8 hours. No precipitate formed in 72 hours at 20°C in solutions of etoposide 0.4 mg/mL in dextrose 5% in sodium chloride 0.45%.[1162] However, at 1 mg/mL, crystallization may occur in 30 minutes in a standing solution or 5 minutes if the solution is stirred. Occasionally, 1-mg/mL concentrations may remain in solution for extended periods.[1374] Nevertheless, concentrations greater than 0.4 mg/mL are not recommended by the manufacturer.[2951] Because of the poor solubility of etoposide in aqueous media, monitor closely for precipitation before and during administration.[915] [916]

The rate of precipitation of a supersaturated etoposide solution depends on the presence of crystalline nuclei, agitation, contact with incompatible surfaces, and possibly other factors.[1374]

Etoposide 1 mg/mL in sodium chloride 0.9% in polypropylene syringes (Braun Omnifix) developed a pure etoposide precipitate in about 10% of the prefilled syringes. It also precipitated at various locations in subclavian lines.[1564]

Precipitation of etoposide from infusion solutions is reportedly exacerbated by the use of peristaltic pumps, especially at concentrations of 0.4 mg/mL or above. Use of volumetric pumps has been recommended to reduce this problem.[1832] [1949]

pH Effects

Etoposide is most stable at a pH of about 3.5 to 6, with a calculated minimum degradation rate occurring at pH 4.8.[1262] Epimerization to the less active *cis*-etoposide may occur at pH values above 6. Hydrolysis may occur in alkaline solutions.[1379]

DOI: 10.37573/9781585286850.157

Syringes

When etoposide 1 mg/mL in sodium chloride 0.9% was stored in plastic syringes (Gillette), seizing of the syringes occurred.[1564]

Ambulatory Pumps

Etoposide (Bristol-Myers Squibb) 0.5 mg/mL in sterile water for injection was evaluated for stability and compatibility in polyvinyl chloride (PVC) reservoirs of Graseby 9000 ambulatory pumps. Etoposide was chemically stable at 37°C for 7 days with no loss of drug. However, refrigerated storage at 4°C resulted in precipitation of the etoposide in some samples. In addition, substantial amounts of diethylhexyl phthalate (DEHP) plasticizer (up to 90 mcg/mL) were leached from the PVC reservoirs. The authors concluded that etoposide was unsuitable for use in this pump reservoir and recommended consideration of etoposide phosphate, which should not be subject to precipitation and leaching of plasticizer.[2288]

Sorption

No loss of etoposide because of sorption to PVC containers has been observed.[1374]

In an admixture composed of cytarabine (Upjohn) 0.157 mg/mL, daunorubicin hydrochloride (Bellon) 15.7 mcg/mL, and etoposide (Sandoz) 0.157 mg/mL in dextrose 5%, little or no loss of the drugs due to sorption occurred when delivered through PVC, PVC with polyethylene-lined sets, and silicone central catheter.[1955]

Plasticizer Leaching

The surfactant in the etoposide formulation leaches DEHP plasticizer from PVC containers and tubing. The amount of DEHP leached is variable, depending on surfactant concentration, container size, tubing diameter and length, ambient temperature, DEHP concentration in the plastic, and contact time. The use of non-PVC containers and tubing has been recommended to reduce patient exposure to DEHP. If there is sufficient concern, the use of the water-soluble ester form, etoposide phosphate, which does not leach DEHP plasticizer, could be used.

Etoposide 0.4 mg/mL in PVC bags of dextrose 5% leached relatively minor amounts of DEHP plasticizer from PVC bags. This leaching was due to the surfactant polysorbate 80 (Tween 80) in the formulation. After 24 hours at 24°C, the DEHP concentration in 50-mL bags of infusion solution was 2.6 mcg/mL. This finding is consistent with the low surfactant concentration

(0.16%) in the final admixture solution. The actual amount of DEHP leached from PVC containers and administration sets may vary in clinical situations, depending on surfactant concentration, bag size, and contact time.[1683]

Etoposide (Sandoz) 0.4 mg/mL in sodium chloride 0.9% in PVC containers leached DEHP plasticizer from the container material. This leaching increased with storage time from about 12 mcg/mL in 8 hours to over 50 mcg/mL in 96 hours at 24°C. Refrigeration reduced, but did not eliminate, DEHP leaching.[1833]

Etoposide (Novartis) 0.4 mg/mL in dextrose 5% and sodium chloride 0.9% was evaluated for the leaching of DEHP plasticizer from PVC bags of the infusion solution from 4 manufacturers (Aguettant, Baxter, Biosedra-Fresenius, and Macopharma) over 24 hours stored at 24°C. Both solutions from all manufacturers leached DEHP in amounts near 20 mcg/mL.[2447]

The low-density polyethylene inner linings of trilayer Vygon tubing and bilayer Cair tubing have been reported not to act as effective barriers to DEHP leaching from the outer PVC layers. Leached DEHP was nearly identical to plain PVC tubing.[2587] [2605]

Filtration

Etoposide 0.1 to 0.4 mg/mL in dextrose 5% or sodium chloride 0.9% has been filtered through several commercially available filters (such as the 0.22-µm Millex-GS or Millex GV) without filter decomposition.[4]

Etoposide (Sandoz) 0.2 mg/mL in dextrose 5% and sodium chloride 0.9% was filtered through a 0.22-µm cellulose ester membrane filter (Ivex-HP, Millipore) over 6 hours. No significant drug loss due to binding to the filter was noted.[1034]

Central Venous Catheter

Etoposide infused undiluted at a rate of 30 mL/hr for 24 hours through a polyurethane central catheter caused substantial damage to the catheter. In addition to cracking the catheter, a 36% decrease in elasticity, a 3.7% increase in catheter length, and damage similar to melting on the internal catheter wall were found. The damage also occurred with the etoposide vehicle and ethanol alone. Consequently, the damage was attributed to the ethanol component of the formulation.[2286]

The damage to polyurethane catheters caused by the etoposide formulation did not extend to silicone central catheters. Administration of undiluted etoposide could be performed using silicone catheters.[2286]

Compatibility Information

Solution Compatibility

Etoposide

Test Soln Name	Mfr	Mfr	Conc/L or %	Remarks	Ref	C/I
Dextrose 5%	a	BR	400 mg	Physically compatible. 4% loss in 4 days at 21°C in dark or fluorescent light	1374	C
Dextrose 5%		SZ	157 mg	2% or less loss in 48 hr at room temperature, in light and dark, and at 4°C	1955	C
Ringer's injection, lactated	a	BR	400 mg	Physically compatible. 5% loss in 4 days at 21°C in fluorescent light	1374	C

Solution Compatibility (Cont.)

Test Soln Name	Mfr	Mfr	Conc/L or %	Remarks	Ref	C/I
Sodium chloride 0.9%	b	BR	400 mg	Physically compatible. 1 to 5% loss in 4 days at 21°C in dark or in fluorescent light	1374	C
Sodium chloride 0.9%	a	BR	50 to 400 mg	Physically compatible for at least 4 days	1374	C
Sodium chloride 0.9%	a	BR	500 mg	Precipitate forms after 48 hr at 21°C exposed to fluorescent light	1374	C
Sodium chloride 0.9%	a	BR	600 and 700 mg	Precipitate forms within 24 hr at 21°C exposed to fluorescent light	1374	I
Sodium chloride 0.9%	c		400 mg	Stable for 24 hr at 4 and 24°C. Precipitation at varying times after 24 hr	1833	C
Sodium chloride 0.9%	BA		0.2 g	Compatible and stable for 22 days at 24 and 4°C	2541	C
Sodium chloride 0.9%	BA		0.3 g	Compatible and stable for 2 days at 24°C and 7 days at 4°C. Precipitate forms after these times	2541	C
Sodium chloride 0.9%	BA		0.4 g	Compatible and stable for 1 day at 24°C and 2 days at 4°C. Precipitate forms after these times	2541	C
Sodium chloride 0.9%	BA		0.5 g	Compatible and stable for 1 day at 24 and 4°C. Precipitate forms after this time	2541	C
Sodium chloride 0.9%	BA		1 to 8 g	Precipitate forms within a few hours	2541	I
Sodium chloride 0.9%	BA		9.5 g	Compatible and stable for 1 day at 24°C and 2 days at 4°C. Precipitate forms after these times	2541	C
Sodium chloride 0.9%	BA		10 g	Compatible and stable for 5 days at 24°C and 7 days at 4°C. Precipitate forms after these times	2541	C
Sodium chloride 0.9%	BA		11 g	Compatible and stable for 7 days at 24°C and 22 days at 4°C	2541	C
Sodium chloride 0.9%	BA		12 g	Compatible and stable for 7 days at 24°C and 14 days at 4°C	2541	C

[a] Tested in glass containers.

[b] Tested in both glass and PVC containers.

[c] Tested in glass, PVC, and polyethylene containers.

Additive Compatibility

Etoposide

Test Drug	Mfr	Conc/L or %	Mfr	Conc/L or %	Test Solution	Remarks	Ref	C/I
Carboplatin		1 g		200 mg	W	Under 10% drug loss in 7 days at 23°C	1954	C
Cisplatin	BR	200 mg	BR	200 and 400 mg	NS[a]	Physically compatible. Under 10% loss of both drugs in 24 hr at 22°C	1329	C
Cisplatin	BR	200 mg	BR	200 and 400 mg	D5½S[a]	Physically compatible. Under 10% loss of both drugs in 24 hr at 22°C	1329	C
Cisplatin		200 mg		200 mg	NS	Both drugs stable for 14 days at room temperature protected from light	1379	C
Cisplatin		200 mg		400 mg	NS	10% etoposide loss and no cisplatin loss in 7 days at room temperature	1388	C
Cisplatin[d]	BR	200 mg	BR	400 mg	D5½S, NS[a]	Physically compatible. Drugs stable for 8 hr at 22°C. Precipitate within 24 to 48 hr	1329	I
Cisplatin with cyclophosphamide		200 mg 2 g		200 mg	NS	All drugs stable for 7 days at room temperature	1379	C
Cisplatin with floxuridine		200 mg 700 mg		300 mg	NS	All drugs stable for 7 days at room temperature	1379	C

Additive Compatibility (Cont.)

Test Drug	Mfr	Conc/L or %	Mfr	Conc/L or %	Test Solution	Remarks	Ref	C/I
Cisplatin with ifosfamide		200 mg 2 g		200 mg	NS	All drugs stable for 5 days at room temperature	1379	C
Cyclophosphamide with cisplatin		2 g 200 mg		200 mg	NS	All drugs stable for 7 days at room temperature	1379	C
Cytarabine with daunorubicin HCl	UP RP	267 mg 33 mg	BR	400 mg	D5½S	Physically compatible with about 6% cytarabine loss and no loss of other drugs in 72 hr at 20°C	1162	C
Cytarabine with daunorubicin HCl	UP BEL	157 mg 15.7 mg	SZ	157 mg	D5W[b]	Less than 10% loss of any drug in 48 hr at room temperature, exposed to light and in the dark, and at 4°C	1955	C
Daunorubicin HCl with cytarabine	RP UP	33 mg 267 mg	BR	400 mg	D5½S	Physically compatible with about 6% cytarabine loss and no loss of other drugs in 72 hr at 20°C	1162	C
Daunorubicin HCl with cytarabine	BEL UP	15.7 mg 157 mg	SZ	157 mg	D5W[b]	Less than 10% loss of any drug in 48 hr at room temperature, exposed to light and in the dark, and at 4°C	1955	C
Doxorubicin HCl with vincristine sulfate	PHU LI	40 mg 1.6 mg	BMS	200 mg	NS	Visually compatible. All drugs stable for 72 hr at 30°C in the dark	2239	C
Doxorubicin HCl with vincristine sulfate	PHU LI	25 mg 1 mg	BMS	125 mg	NS	Visually compatible. All drugs stable for 96 hr at 24°C in light or dark	2239	C
Doxorubicin HCl with vincristine sulfate	PHU LI	35 mg 1.4 mg	BMS	175 mg	NS	Visually compatible. All drugs stable for 96 hr at 24°C in light or dark	2239	C
Doxorubicin HCl with vincristine sulfate	PHU LI	50 mg 2 mg	BMS	250 mg	NS	Visually compatible. All drugs stable for 48 hr at 24°C in light or dark. Etoposide precipitate in 72 hr	2239	C
Doxorubicin HCl with vincristine sulfate	PHU LI	70 mg 2.8 mg	BMS	350 mg	NS	Visually compatible. All drugs stable for 24 hr at 24°C in light or dark. Etoposide precipitate in 36 hr	2239	C
Doxorubicin HCl with vincristine sulfate	PHU LI	100 mg 4 mg	BMS	500 mg	NS	Etoposide precipitate formed in 12 hr at 24°C in light or dark	2239	I
Floxuridine		10 g		200 mg	NS	Both drugs stable for 15 days at room temperature	1379	C
Floxuridine with cisplatin		700 mg 200 mg		300 mg	NS	All drugs stable for 7 days at room temperature	1379	C
Fluorouracil		10 g		200 mg	NS	Both drugs stable for 7 days at room temperature and 1 day at 35°C	1379	C
Hydroxyzine HCl	LY	500 mg	BR	1 g	D5W[c]	Physically compatible for 48 hr	1190	C
Ifosfamide		2 g		200 mg	NS	Both drugs stable for 5 days at room temperature	1379	C
Ifosfamide with cisplatin		2 g 200 mg		200 mg	NS	All drugs stable for 5 days at room temperature	1379	C
Mitoxantrone HCl	LE	50 mg	BR	500 mg	NS	Visually compatible with no loss of either drug in 22 hr at room temperature	2271	C
Ondansetron HCl	GL	30 and 300 mg	BR	100 mg	D5W[b]	Physically compatible. Little or no loss of ondansetron in 48 hr at 23°C. 4% etoposide loss in 24 hr and 6% loss in 48 hr at 23°C	1876	C
Ondansetron HCl	GL	30 and 300 mg	BR	400 mg	D5W[b]	Physically compatible with little or no loss of either drug in 48 hr at 23°C	1876	C

Additive Compatibility (Cont.)

Test Drug	Mfr	Conc/L or %	Mfr	Conc/L or %	Test Solution	Remarks	Ref	C/I
Vincristine sulfate with doxorubicin HCl	LI PHU	1.6 mg 40 mg	BMS	200 mg	NS	Visually compatible. All drugs stable for 72 hr at 30°C in the dark	2239	C
Vincristine sulfate with doxorubicin HCl	LI PHU	1 mg 25 mg	BMS	125 mg	NS	Visually compatible. All drugs stable for 96 hr at 24°C in light or dark	2239	C
Vincristine sulfate with doxorubicin HCl	LI PHU	1.4 mg 35 mg	BMS	175 mg	NS	Visually compatible. All drugs stable for 96 hr at 24°C in light or dark	2239	C
Vincristine sulfate with doxorubicin HCl	LI PHU	2 mg 50 mg	BMS	250 mg	NS	Visually compatible. All drugs stable for 48 hr at 24°C in light or dark. Etoposide precipitate in 72 hr	2239	C
Vincristine sulfate with doxorubicin HCl	LI PHU	2.8 mg 70 mg	BMS	350 mg	NS	Visually compatible. All drugs stable for 24 hr at 24°C in light or dark. Etoposide precipitate in 36 hr	2239	C
Vincristine sulfate with doxorubicin HCl	LI PHU	4 mg 100 mg	BMS	500 mg	NS	Etoposide precipitate formed in 12 hr at 24°C in light or dark	2239	I

[a] Tested in both glass and PVC containers.

[b] Tested in PVC containers.

[c] Tested in glass containers.

[d] Tested with mannitol 1.875% and potassium chloride 20 mEq/L present.

Y-Site Injection Compatibility (1:1 Mixture)

Etoposide

Test Drug	Mfr	Conc	Mfr	Conc	Remarks	Ref	C/I
Allopurinol sodium	BW	3 mg/mL[b]	BR	0.4 mg/mL[b]	Physically compatible for 4 hr at 22°C	1686	C
Amifostine	USB	10 mg/mL[a]	BR	0.4 mg/mL[a]	Physically compatible for 4 hr at 23°C	1845	C
Aztreonam	SQ	40 mg/mL[a]	BMS	0.4 mg/mL[a]	Physically compatible for 4 hr at 23°C	1758	C
Cladribine	ORT	0.015[b] and 0.5[c] mg/mL	BR	0.4 mg/mL[b]	Physically compatible for 4 hr at 23°C	1969	C
Doxorubicin HCl liposomal	SEQ	0.4 mg/mL[a]	BR	0.4 mg/mL[a]	Physically compatible for 4 hr at 23°C	2087	C
Filgrastim	AMG	30 mcg/mL[a]	BR	0.4 mg/mL[a]	Particles form immediately. Filaments form in 1 hr	1687	I
Fludarabine phosphate	BX	1 mg/mL[a]	BR	0.4 mg/mL[a]	Visually compatible for 4 hr at 22°C	1439	C
Gallium nitrate	FUJ	1 mg/mL[b]	RR	0.4 mg/mL[b]	Precipitate forms after 60 min	1673	I
Gemcitabine HCl	LI	10 mg/mL[b]	BR	0.4 mg/mL[b]	Physically compatible for 4 hr at 23°C	2226	C
Granisetron HCl	SKB	1 mg/mL	BMS	0.4 mg/mL[b]	Physically compatible with little or no loss of either drug in 4 hr at 22°C	1883	C
Granisetron HCl	SKB	0.05 mg/mL[a]	BR	0.4 mg/mL[a]	Physically compatible for 4 hr at 23°C	2000	C
Idarubicin HCl	AD	1 mg/mL[b]	BR	0.4 mg/mL[a]	Gas forms immediately	1525	I
Melphalan HCl	BW	0.1 mg/mL[b]	BR	0.4 mg/mL[b]	Physically compatible for 3 hr at 22°C	1557	C
Methotrexate sodium		30 mg/mL	BR	0.6 mg/mL[b]	Visually compatible for 4 hr at room temperature	1788	C
Micafungin sodium	ASP	1.5 mg/mL[b]	SIC	0.4 mg/mL[b]	Physically compatible for 4 hr at 23°C	2683	C
Mitoxantrone HCl	LE	2 mg/mL	BR	20 mg/mL	Visually compatible with no loss of either drug in 22 hr at room temperature	2271	C

Y-Site Injection Compatibility (1:1 Mixture) (Cont.)

Test Drug	Mfr	Conc	Mfr	Conc	Remarks	Ref	C/I
Ondansetron HCl	GL	1 mg/mL[b]	BR	0.4 mg/mL[a]	Visually compatible for 4 hr at 22°C	1365	C
Ondansetron HCl	GL	16 to 160 mcg/mL		0.144 to 0.25 mg/mL	Physically compatible when etoposide given over 30 to 60 min via Y-site	1366	C
Paclitaxel	NCI	1.2 mg/mL[a]		0.4 mg/mL[a]	Physically compatible for 4 hr at 22°C	1528	C
Piperacillin sodium–tazobactam sodium	LE[e]	40 mg/mL[a f]	BR	0.4 mg/mL[a]	Physically compatible for 4 hr at 22°C	1688	C
Sargramostim	IMM	10 mcg/mL[b]	BR	0.4 mg/mL[b]	Visually compatible for 4 hr at 22°C	1436	C
Sodium bicarbonate		1.4%	BR	0.6 mg/mL[b]	Visually compatible for 4 hr at room temperature	1788	C
Teniposide	BR	0.1 mg/mL[a]	BR	0.4 mg/mL[a]	Physically compatible for 4 hr at 23°C	1725	C
Thiotepa	IMM[d]	1 mg/mL[a]	BR	0.4 mg/mL[a]	Physically compatible for 4 hr at 23°C	1861	C
Topotecan HCl	SKB	56 mcg/mL[a b]	BR	0.4 mg/mL[a b]	Visually compatible. Little loss of either drug in 4 hr at 22°C	2245	C
Vinorelbine tartrate	BW	1 mg/mL[b]	BR	0.4 mg/mL[b]	Physically compatible for 4 hr at 22°C	1558	C

[a] Tested in dextrose 5%.

[b] Tested in sodium chloride 0.9%.

[c] Tested in bacteriostatic sodium chloride 0.9% preserved with benzyl alcohol 0.9%.

[d] Lyophilized formulation tested.

[e] Test performed using the formulation WITHOUT edetate disodium.

[f] Piperacillin component. Piperacillin in an 8:1 fixed-ratio concentration with tazobactam.

Selected Revisions June 18, 2015. © Copyright, October 1986.
American Society of Health-System Pharmacists, Inc.

Etoposide Phosphate
AHFS 10:00

Products

Etoposide phosphate is available in single-dose vials containing the equivalent of 100 mg of etoposide as the phosphate along with sodium citrate 32.7 mg and 300 mg of dextran 40. Reconstitute with 5 or 10 mL of compatible diluent to yield solutions of 20 or 10 mg/mL, respectively. Sterile water for injection, dextrose 5%, sodium chloride 0.9%, bacteriostatic water for injection preserved with benzyl alcohol, or bacteriostatic sodium chloride 0.9% preserved with benzyl alcohol may be used for reconstitution.[1(6/07)]

pH

Reconstitution with sterile water for injection to a concentration of 1 mg/mL results in a pH of approximately 2.9.[4]

Trade Name(s)

Etopophos

Administration

Etoposide phosphate is administered by intravenous infusion from 5 to 210 minutes. The reconstituted drug may be given without further dilution or may be diluted to a concentration as low as 0.1 mg/mL with dextrose 5% or sodium chloride 0.9%.[1(6/07) 4]

Stability

Etoposide phosphate is a white to off-white powder.[4] Intact vials should be stored under refrigeration at 2 to 8°C and protected from light.[1(6/07)]

The manufacturer states that etoposide phosphate reconstituted with an unpreserved diluent (such as sterile water for injection, dextrose 5%, or sodium chloride 0.9%) is stable for 24 hours at room temperatures of 20 to 25°C and 7 days under refrigeration at 2 to 8°C. If a diluent containing benzyl alcohol as a preservative (such as bacteriostatic water for injection or bacteriostatic sodium chloride 0.9%) is used to reconstitute etoposide phosphate, the solution is stable for 48 hours at room temperatures of 20 to 25°C and for 7 days under refrigeration at 2 to 8°C.[1(6/07) 4]

Unlike etoposide, the phosphate ester is highly water soluble, having a solubility over 100 mg/mL.[4] Consequently, the potential for precipitation in aqueous media is reduced greatly compared with the older surfactant- and organic solvent-based formulation.[2219]

Etoposide production by hydrolysis from infusion admixtures of etoposide phosphate (Bristol-Myers Squibb) was measured. The admixtures, equivalent to etoposide 1.5 mg/mL in 66.7 mL and 15 mg/mL in 20 mL of sodium chloride 0.9%, were filled into polyvinyl chloride (PVC) ambulatory infusion pump reservoirs (Pharmacia Deltec) and stored at 20 and 37°C protected from light. Etoposide levels in the etoposide phosphate admixtures increased at both temperatures; in 7 days the increase in concentration was about 2% at 20°C and about 7% at 37°C. The authors concluded that etoposide phosphate is suitable for multiple-day ambulatory infusion.[2024]

Doxorubicin hydrochloride, etoposide phosphate, and vincristine sulfate admixtures at a variety of concentrations were unable to pass the USP test for antimicrobial effectiveness. Mixtures of these drugs are not "self-preserving" and permit microbial growth.[2343]

Etoposide phosphate (Bristol Myers Squibb) 0.09 mg/mL in sodium chloride 0.9% did not result in the loss of viability of *Staphylococcus aureus*, *Enterococcus faecium*, *Pseudomonas aeruginosa*, and *Candida albicans* within 120 hours at 22°C. Diluted solutions should be stored under refrigeration whenever possible, and the potential for microbiological growth should be considered when assigning expiration periods.[2740]

Light Effects

An evaluation of etoposide phosphate (Bristol-Myers Squibb) 2 mg/mL, doxorubicin hydrochloride 0.4 mg/mL, and vincristine sulfate 0.016 mg/mL (16 mcg/mL) in sodium chloride 0.9% in polyolefin plastic bags (McGaw) found little or no effect of constant exposure to normal fluorescent room light for 124 hours. The admixtures were physically compatible, and all 3 drugs in the admixture remained stable throughout the time stored at an elevated temperature of 35 to 40°C.[2343]

Syringes

Etoposide phosphate (Bristol Laboratories Oncology Products) 10 and 20 mg/mL was prepared with bacteriostatic water for injection preserved with benzyl alcohol 0.9% (Abbott). The solutions were packaged as 4 mL of solution in 5 mL polypropylene syringes (Becton Dickinson) and sealed with tip caps (Red Cap, Burron Medical). The syringes were stored at 32°C for 7 days, 23°C for 31 days, and 4°C for 31 days. All samples were physically stable, with no visual change and no increase in measured haze or particle content, and little drug loss occurred. At 32°C, 2 to 4% loss occurred in 7 days. At 23°C, about 6 to 7% loss occurred in 31 days. Losses under refrigeration were 4% or less in 31 days.[2219]

DOI: 10.37573/9781585286850.158

Compatibility Information

Solution Compatibility

Etoposide phosphate

Test Soln Name	Mfr	Mfr°	Conc/L or %	Remarks	Ref	C/I
Dextrose 5%	a b	BMS	100 mg	Compatible and stable for 24 hr at 4 and 25°C	1(6/07)	C
Dextrose 5%	BAª	BR	0.1 and 10 g	Physically compatible and little loss in 7 days at 32°C and in 31 days at 23 and 4°C	2219	C
Sodium chloride 0.9%	a b	BMS	100 mg	Compatible and stable for 24 hr at 4 and 25°C	1(6/07)	C
Sodium chloride 0.9%	BAª	BR	0.1 and 10 g	Physically compatible and little loss in 7 days at 32°C and in 31 days at 23 and 4°C	2219	C

ª Tested in PVC containers.

ᵇ Tested in glass containers.

Additive Compatibility

Etoposide phosphate

Test Drug	Mfr	Conc/L or %	Mfr	Conc/L or %	Test Solution	Remarks	Ref	C/I
Doxorubicin HCl with vincristine sulfate	PHU LI	120 mg 5 mg	BMS	600 mg	NSª	Physically compatible. Little loss of any drug in 124 hr at 4 and 40°C	2343	C
Doxorubicin HCl with vincristine sulfate	PHU LI	240 mg 10 mg	BMS	1.2 g	NSª	Physically compatible. Little loss of any drug in 124 hr at 4 and 40°C	2343	C
Doxorubicin HCl with vincristine sulfate	PHU LI	400 mg 16 mg	BMS	2 g	NSª	Physically compatible. Under 4% loss of any drug in 124 hr at 4 and 40°C	2343	C
Vincristine sulfate with doxorubicin HCl	LI PHU	5 mg 120 mg	BMS	600 mg	NSª	Physically compatible. Little loss of any drug in 124 hr at 4 and 40°C	2343	C
Vincristine sulfate with doxorubicin HCl	LI PHU	10 mg 240 mg	BMS	1.2 g	NSª	Physically compatible. Little loss of any drug in 124 hr at 4 and 40°C	2343	C
Vincristine sulfate with doxorubicin HCl	LI PHU	16 mg 400 mg	BMS	2 g	NSª	Physically compatible. Under 4% loss of any drug in 124 hr at 4 and 40°C	2343	C

ª Tested in polyolefin-lined plastic bags.

Y-Site Injection Compatibility (1:1 Mixture)

Etoposide phosphate

Test Drug	Mfr	Conc	Mfr	Conc	Remarks	Ref	C/I
Acyclovir sodium	GW	7 mg/mLª	BR	5 mg/mLª	Physically compatible for 4 hr at 23°C	2218	C
Amikacin sulfate	APC	5 mg/mLª	BR	5 mg/mLª	Physically compatible for 4 hr at 23°C	2218	C
Aminophylline	AB	2.5 mg/mLª	BR	5 mg/mLª	Physically compatible for 4 hr at 23°C	2218	C
Amphotericin B	GNS	0.6 mg/mLª	BR	5 mg/mLª	Yellow-orange precipitate forms immediately	2218	I
Ampicillin sodium	APC	20 mg/mLᵇ	BR	5 mg/mLª	Physically compatible for 4 hr at 23°C	2218	C
Ampicillin sodium–sulbactam sodium	RR	20 mg/mLᵇ ᵈ	BR	5 mg/mLª	Physically compatible for 4 hr at 23°C	2218	C
Anidulafungin	VIC	0.5 mg/mLª	BMS	5 mg/mLª	Physically compatible for 4 hr at 23°C	2617	C
Aztreonam	SQ	40 mg/mLª	BR	5 mg/mLª	Physically compatible for 4 hr at 23°C	2218	C

Y-Site Injection Compatibility (1:1 Mixture) (Cont.)

Test Drug	Mfr	Conc	Mfr	Conc	Remarks	Ref	C/I
Bleomycin sulfate	MJ	1 unit/mL[b]	BR	5 mg/mL[a]	Physically compatible for 4 hr at 23°C	2218	C
Bumetanide	RC	0.04 mg/mL[a]	BR	5 mg/mL[a]	Physically compatible for 4 hr at 23°C	2218	C
Buprenorphine HCl	RKC	0.04 mg/mL[a]	BR	5 mg/mL[a]	Physically compatible for 4 hr at 23°C	2218	C
Butorphanol tartrate	APC	0.04 mg/mL[a]	BR	5 mg/mL[a]	Physically compatible for 4 hr at 23°C	2218	C
Calcium gluconate	FUJ	40 mg/mL[a]	BR	5 mg/mL[a]	Physically compatible for 4 hr at 23°C	2218	C
Carboplatin	BR	5 mg/mL[a]	BR	5 mg/mL[a]	Physically compatible for 4 hr at 23°C	2218	C
Carmustine	BR	1.5 mg/mL[a]	BR	5 mg/mL[a]	Physically compatible for 4 hr at 23°C	2218	C
Caspofungin acetate	ME	0.7 mg/mL[b]	SIC	5 mg/mL[b]	Physically compatible for 4 hr at room temperature	2758	C
Cefazolin sodium	APC	20 mg/mL[a]	BR	5 mg/mL[a]	Physically compatible for 4 hr at 23°C	2218	C
Cefepime HCl	BMS	20 mg/mL[a]	BR	5 mg/mL[a]	Increased haze and particulates form within 1 hr	2218	I
Cefotaxime sodium	HO	20 mg/mL[a]	BR	5 mg/mL[a]	Physically compatible for 4 hr at 23°C	2218	C
Cefotetan disodium	ZEN	20 mg/mL[a]	BR	5 mg/mL[a]	Physically compatible for 4 hr at 23°C	2218	C
Cefoxitin sodium	ME	20 mg/mL[a]	BR	5 mg/mL[a]	Physically compatible for 4 hr at 23°C	2218	C
Ceftazidime	SKB	40 mg/mL[a]	BR	5 mg/mL[a]	Physically compatible for 4 hr at 23°C	2218	C
Ceftriaxone sodium	RC	20 mg/mL[a]	BR	5 mg/mL[a]	Physically compatible for 4 hr at 23°C	2218	C
Cefuroxime sodium	GW	30 mg/mL[a]	BR	5 mg/mL[a]	Physically compatible for 4 hr at 23°C	2218	C
Chlorpromazine HCl	ES	2 mg/mL[a]	BR	5 mg/mL[a]	Cloudy solution forms immediately with particulates in 4 hr	2218	I
Ciprofloxacin	BAY	1 mg/mL[a]	BR	5 mg/mL[a]	Physically compatible for 4 hr at 23°C	2218	C
Cisplatin	BR	1 mg/mL	BR	5 mg/mL[a]	Physically compatible for 4 hr at 23°C	2218	C
Clindamycin phosphate	AST	10 mg/mL[a]	BR	5 mg/mL[a]	Physically compatible for 4 hr at 23°C	2218	C
Cyclophosphamide	MJ	10 mg/mL[a]	BR	5 mg/mL[a]	Physically compatible for 4 hr at 23°C	2218	C
Cytarabine	BED	50 mg/mL	BR	5 mg/mL[a]	Physically compatible for 4 hr at 23°C	2218	C
Dacarbazine	MI	4 mg/mL[a]	BR	5 mg/mL[a]	Physically compatible for 4 hr at 23°C	2218	C
Dactinomycin	ME	0.01 mg/mL[a]	BR	5 mg/mL[a]	Physically compatible for 4 hr at 23°C	2218	C
Daunorubicin HCl	BED	1 mg/mL[a]	BR	5 mg/mL[a]	Physically compatible for 4 hr at 23°C	2218	C
Dexamethasone sodium phosphate	ES	1 mg/mL[a]	BR	5 mg/mL[a]	Physically compatible for 4 hr at 23°C	2218	C
Diphenhydramine HCl	ES	2 mg/mL[a]	BR	5 mg/mL[a]	Physically compatible for 4 hr at 23°C	2218	C
Dobutamine HCl	AST	4 mg/mL[a]	BR	5 mg/mL[a]	Physically compatible for 4 hr at 23°C	2218	C
Dopamine HCl	AST	3.2 mg/mL[a]	BR	5 mg/mL[a]	Physically compatible for 4 hr at 23°C	2218	C
Doripenem	JJ	5 mg/mL[a b]	SIC	5 mg/mL[a b]	Physically compatible for 4 hr at 23°C	2743	C
Doxorubicin HCl	GEN	2 mg/mL	BR	5 mg/mL[b]	Physically compatible for 4 hr at 23°C	2218	C
Doxycycline hyclate	FUJ	1 mg/mL[a]	BR	5 mg/mL[a]	Physically compatible for 4 hr at 23°C	2218	C
Droperidol	AST	0.4 mg/mL[a]	BR	5 mg/mL[a]	Physically compatible for 4 hr at 23°C	2218	C
Enalaprilat	ME	0.1 mg/mL[a]	BR	5 mg/mL[a]	Physically compatible for 4 hr at 23°C	2218	C
Famotidine	ME	2 mg/mL[a]	BR	5 mg/mL[a]	Physically compatible for 4 hr at 23°C	2218	C

Y-Site Injection Compatibility (1:1 Mixture) (Cont.)

Test Drug	Mfr	Conc	Mfr	Conc	Remarks	Ref	C/I
Floxuridine	RC	3 mg/mL[a]	BR	5 mg/mL[a]	Physically compatible for 4 hr at 23°C	2218	C
Fluconazole	RR	2 mg/mL	BR	5 mg/mL[a]	Physically compatible for 4 hr at 23°C	2218	C
Fludarabine phosphate	BX	1 mg/mL[a]	BR	5 mg/mL[a]	Physically compatible for 4 hr at 23°C	2218	C
Fluorouracil	PH	16 mg/mL[a]	BR	5 mg/mL[a]	Physically compatible for 4 hr at 23°C	2218	C
Furosemide	AMR	3 mg/mL[a]	BR	5 mg/mL[a]	Physically compatible for 4 hr at 23°C	2218	C
Ganciclovir sodium	RC	20 mg/mL[a]	BR	5 mg/mL[a]	Physically compatible for 4 hr at 23°C	2218	C
Gemcitabine HCl	LI	10 mg/mL[b]	BR	5 mg/mL[b]	Physically compatible for 4 hr at 23°C	2226	C
Gentamicin sulfate	AB	5 mg/mL[a]	BR	5 mg/mL[a]	Physically compatible for 4 hr at 23°C	2218	C
Granisetron HCl	SKB	0.05 mg/mL[a]	BR	5 mg/mL[a]	Physically compatible for 4 hr at 23°C	2218	C
Haloperidol lactate	MN	0.2 mg/mL[a]	BR	5 mg/mL[a]	Physically compatible for 4 hr at 23°C	2218	C
Heparin sodium	ES	100 units/mL[a]	BR	5 mg/mL[a]	Physically compatible for 4 hr at 23°C	2218	C
Hydrocortisone sodium succinate	UP	1 mg/mL[a]	BR	5 mg/mL[a]	Physically compatible for 4 hr at 23°C	2218	C
Hydromorphone HCl	ES	0.5 mg/mL[a]	BR	5 mg/mL[a]	Physically compatible for 4 hr at 23°C	2218	C
Hydroxyzine HCl	ES	4 mg/mL[a]	BR	5 mg/mL[a]	Physically compatible for 4 hr at 23°C	2218	C
Idarubicin HCl	AD	0.5 mg/mL[a]	BR	5 mg/mL[a]	Physically compatible for 4 hr at 23°C	2218	C
Ifosfamide	MJ	25 mg/mL[a]	BR	5 mg/mL[a]	Physically compatible for 4 hr at 23°C	2218	C
Imipenem–cilastatin sodium	ME	10 mg/mL[b g]	BR	5 mg/mL[a]	Yellow color forms in 4 hr at 23°C	2218	I
Leucovorin calcium	IMM	2 mg/mL[a]	BR	5 mg/mL[a]	Physically compatible for 4 hr at 23°C	2218	C
Linezolid	PHU	2 mg/mL	BR	5 mg/mL[a]	Physically compatible for 4 hr at 23°C	2264	C
Lorazepam	WY	0.5 mg/mL[a]	BR	5 mg/mL[a]	Physically compatible for 4 hr at 23°C	2218	C
Magnesium sulfate	AST	100 mg/mL[a]	BR	5 mg/mL[a]	Physically compatible for 4 hr at 23°C	2218	C
Mannitol	BA	15%	BR	5 mg/mL[a]	Physically compatible for 4 hr at 23°C	2218	C
Meperidine HCl	AST	4 mg/mL[a]	BR	5 mg/mL[a]	Physically compatible for 4 hr at 23°C	2218	C
Mesna	MJ	10 mg/mL[a]	BR	5 mg/mL[a]	Physically compatible for 4 hr at 23°C	2218	C
Methotrexate sodium	IMM	15 mg/mL[a]	BR	5 mg/mL[a]	Physically compatible for 4 hr at 23°C	2218	C
Methylprednisolone sodium succinate	AB	5 mg/mL[a]	BR	5 mg/mL[a]	Haze with subvisible microparticles forms immediately. Particle content increases fivefold over 4 hr at 23°C	2218	I
Metoclopramide HCl	FAU	5 mg/mL	BR	5 mg/mL[a]	Physically compatible for 4 hr at 23°C	2218	C
Metronidazole	AB	5 mg/mL	BR	5 mg/mL[a]	Physically compatible for 4 hr at 23°C	2218	C
Mitomycin	BR	0.5 mg/mL	BR	5 mg/mL[a]	Color changed from light blue to reddish purple in 4 hr at 23°C	2218	I
Mitoxantrone HCl	IMM	0.5 mg/mL[a]	BR	5 mg/mL[a]	Physically compatible for 4 hr at 23°C	2218	C
Morphine sulfate	ES	1 mg/mL[a]	BR	5 mg/mL[a]	Physically compatible for 4 hr at 23°C	2218	C
Nalbuphine HCl	AST	10 mg/mL	BR	5 mg/mL[a]	Physically compatible for 4 hr at 23°C	2218	C
Ondansetron HCl	GW	1 mg/mL[a]	BR	5 mg/mL[a]	Physically compatible for 4 hr at 23°C	2218	C

Y-Site Injection Compatibility (1:1 Mixture) (Cont.)

Test Drug	Mfr	Conc	Mfr	Conc	Remarks	Ref	C/I
Oxaliplatin	SS	0.5 mg/mL[a]	BR	5 mg/mL[a]	Physically compatible for 4 hr at 23°C	2566	C
Paclitaxel	MJ	1.2 mg/mL[a]	BR	5 mg/mL[a]	Physically compatible for 4 hr at 23°C	2218	C
Piperacillin sodium–tazobactam sodium	LE[c]	40 mg/mL[b e]	BR	5 mg/mL[a]	Physically compatible for 4 hr at 23°C	2218	C
Potassium chloride	AB	0.1 mEq/mL[a]	BR	5 mg/mL[a]	Physically compatible for 4 hr at 23°C	2218	C
Prochlorperazine edisylate	ES	0.5 mg/mL[a]	BR	5 mg/mL[a]	White cloudy solution forms immediately with precipitate in 4 hr	2218	I
Promethazine HCl	SCN	2 mg/mL[a]	BR	5 mg/mL[a]	Physically compatible for 4 hr at 23°C	2218	C
Ranitidine HCl	GL	2 mg/mL[a]	BR	5 mg/mL[a]	Physically compatible for 4 hr at 23°C	2218	C
Sodium bicarbonate	AB	1 mEq/mL	BR	5 mg/mL[a]	Physically compatible for 4 hr at 23°C	2218	C
Streptozocin	UP	40 mg/mL[a]	BR	5 mg/mL[a]	Physically compatible for 4 hr at 23°C	2218	C
Teniposide	BR	0.1 mg/mL[a]	BR	5 mg/mL[a]	Physically compatible for 4 hr at 23°C	2218	C
Thiotepa	IMM	1 mg/mL[a]	BR	5 mg/mL[a]	Physically compatible for 4 hr at 23°C	2218	C
Tobramycin sulfate	LI	5 mg/mL[a]	BR	5 mg/mL[a]	Physically compatible for 4 hr at 23°C	2218	C
Trimethoprim–sulfamethoxazole	ES	0.8 mg/mL[a f]	BR	5 mg/mL[a]	Physically compatible for 4 hr at 23°C	2218	C
Vancomycin HCl	LI	10 mg/mL[a]	BR	5 mg/mL[a]	Physically compatible for 4 hr at 23°C	2218	C
Vinblastine sulfate	FAU	0.12 mg/mL[a]	BR	5 mg/mL[a]	Physically compatible for 4 hr at 23°C	2218	C
Vincristine sulfate	FAU	0.05 mg/mL[a]	BR	5 mg/mL[a]	Physically compatible for 4 hr at 23°C	2218	C
Zidovudine	BW	4 mg/mL[a]	BR	5 mg/mL[a]	Physically compatible for 4 hr at 23°C	2218	C

[a] Tested in dextrose 5%.

[b] Tested in sodium chloride 0.9%.

[c] Test performed using the formulation WITHOUT edetate disodium.

[d] Ampicillin component. Ampicillin in a 2:1 fixed-ratio concentration with sulbactam.

[e] Piperacillin component. Piperacillin in an 8:1 fixed-ratio concentration with tazobactam.

[f] Trimethoprim component. Trimethoprim in a 1:5 fixed-ratio concentration with sulfamethoxazole.

[g] Not specified whether concentration refers to single component or combined components.

Selected Revisions December 12, 2018. © Copyright, October 1998. American Society of Health-System Pharmacists, Inc.

Factor Xa (Recombinant), Inactivated-zhzo
AHFS 20:28.92
Andexanet alfa

Products

Factor Xa (recombinant), inactivated-zhzo is available in single-use (preservative-free) vials as a lyophilized cake or powder containing 100 or 200 mg of the drug.[3429] Each 100-mg vial also contains tromethamine (TRIS), L-arginine hydrochloride, sucrose 2% (w/v), mannitol 5% (w/v), and polysorbate 80 0.01% (w/v).[3429] Each 200-mg vial also contains tromethamine (TRIS), tromethamine hydrochloride, L-arginine hydrochloride, sucrose 1% (w/v), mannitol 2.5% (w/v), and polysorbate 80 0.01% (w/v).[3429]

Factor Xa (recombinant), inactivated-zhzo is administered as an intravenous bolus infusion, followed by a continuous intravenous infusion.[3429] (See Administration.)

To prepare the bolus dose for intravenous infusion, the total number of vials required should be determined and all vials necessary to achieve the required dose should be reconstituted in succession in order to reduce the total reconstitution time.[3429] Each 100- or 200-mg vial should be reconstituted with 10 or 20 mL, respectively, of sterile water for injection using a 20-mL or larger syringe with a 20-gauge or larger needle to slowly inject the diluent onto the inside wall of the vial to minimize foaming.[3429] Vials should be swirled gently until the contents are completely dissolved, typically for about 3 to 5 minutes each, to yield a 10-mg/mL solution.[3429] Vials should *not* be shaken, because foaming may occur.[3429] The reconstituted solution should be visually inspected for particulate matter and discoloration.[3429] Vials exhibiting incomplete dissolution should be discarded and should not be used.[3429] To prepare the initial intravenous bolus dose for infusion, a 60-mL or larger syringe with a 20-gauge or larger needle should be used to withdraw the appropriate volume of the reconstituted solution from the vials to achieve the dose.[3429] The reconstituted solution should be transferred to an appropriately sized empty 250-mL or smaller polyolefin or polyvinyl chloride (PVC) bag.[3429] Any unused portion of the reconstituted solution should be discarded.[3429]

To prepare the continuous intravenous infusion, the same procedure should be followed as that used to prepare the bolus infusion dose; however, multiple 40- to 60-mL syringes or an equivalent 100-mL syringe may be used to withdraw the appropriate volume of the reconstituted solution from the vials to achieve the dose.[3429]

Trade Name(s)

Andexxa

Administration

Factor Xa (recombinant), inactivated-zhzo is administered intravenously only.[3429] The reconstituted solution should be infused through a 0.2- or 0.22-μm polyethersulfone or equivalent low protein-binding inline filter.[3429]

An initial intravenous bolus dose should be infused, beginning at a target rate of approximately 30 mg/min.[3429]

Within 2 minutes of completing infusion of the bolus dose, a continuous intravenous infusion should be started and administered at a rate of 4 or 8 mg/min, depending on the dosing regimen used, for up to 120 minutes.[3429]

Stability

Factor Xa (recombinant), inactivated-zhzo is a white to off-white cake or powder that forms a clear, colorless to slightly yellow solution upon reconstitution.[3429] Intact vials should be stored under refrigeration at 2 to 8°C; vials should *not* be frozen.[3429]

The reconstituted solution is stable *in vials* for up to 8 hours at room temperature or may be stored for up to 24 hours at 2 to 8°C.[3429] The reconstituted solution *in the listed plastic intravenous infusion bags* is stable for up to 8 hours at room temperature.[3429]

Sorption

The manufacturer recommends the use of polyolefin or PVC intravenous infusion bags in the preparation of the drug for bolus and continuous intravenous infusions.[3429]

Filtration

The reconstituted solution for infusion should be administered through a 0.2- or 0.22-μm polyethersulfone or equivalent low protein-binding inline filter.[3429]

DOI: 10.37573/9781585286850.159

Famotidine
AHFS 56:28.12

Products

Famotidine is available as a 10-mg/mL concentrated injection in 2-mL single-dose vials and 4- and 20-mL multiple-dose vials. Each mL of the solution also contains L-aspartic acid 4 mg and mannitol 20 mg. Benzyl alcohol 0.9% is present as a preservative in the multiple-dose product.[1(10/06)]

Famotidine is also available premixed at a concentration of 20 mg/50 mL. Each 50 mL of solution also contains L-aspartic acid 6.8 mg and sodium chloride 450 mg in water for injection. Additional L-aspartic acid or sodium hydroxide may be added to adjust the pH.[1(10/06)]

pH

The injection has a pH from 5 to 5.6.[4] The premixed solution has a pH from 5.7 to 6.4.[1(10/06)]

Osmolarity

The osmolarities of the single- and multiple-dose products are 217 and 290 mOsm/L, respectively.[4]

Sodium Content

Famotidine premixed infusion solution has 7.8 mEq of sodium per 50 mL.[4]

Trade Name(s)

Pepcid

Administration

Famotidine is administered by slow intravenous injection or infusion. For injection, 20 mg should be diluted to 5 to 10 mL with a compatible diluent and injected no faster than 10 mg/min. For infusion, 20 mg should be diluted in 100 mL of dextrose 5% or another compatible diluent and infused over 15 to 30 minutes. Alternatively, famotidine premixed solution may be administered by intravenous infusion over 15 to 30 minutes.[1(10/06)] [4]

Stability

Famotidine injection is a clear, colorless solution. The vials should be stored under refrigeration and protected from freezing. If freezing occurs, thaw at room temperature; make sure that all components have resolubilized.[1(10/06)] [4] Use of a microwave oven for thawing is not recommended because of the potential hazard of vapor pressure increases in the vials.[4]

Although refrigeration is recommended, the manufacturer has indicated that the drug may be stored at room temperature for 26 weeks[1239] and for 3 months[2745] at controlled room temperature in differing statements.

Famotidine premixed infusion solution should be stored at controlled room temperature (25°C) and protected from excessive heat. Brief exposure to temperatures up to 35°C does not affect the stability of the product adversely.[1(10/06)]

Freezing Solutions

Famotidine (MSD) 200 mcg/mL in dextrose 5% or sodium chloride 0.9% in polyvinyl chloride (PVC) bags showed no loss when frozen at −20°C for 28 days followed by storage at 4°C for 14 days.[1271]

Famotidine (MSD) 2 mg/mL in dextrose 5%, sodium chloride 0.9%, or sterile water for injection stored in polypropylene syringes (Becton Dickinson) exhibited a 5 to 8% loss in 8 weeks when frozen at −20°C.[1486]

Syringes

Famotidine (MSD) 2 mg/mL in dextrose 5%, sodium chloride 0.9%, or sterile water for injection stored in plastic syringes (Becton Dickinson) exhibited no loss in 14 days at 4°C.[1487]

Central Venous Catheter

Famotidine (Merck) 2 mg/mL in dextrose 5% was found to be compatible with the ARROWg+ard Blue Plus (Arrow International) chlorhexidine-bearing triple-lumen central catheter. Essentially complete delivery of the drug was found with little or no drug loss occurring. Furthermore, chlorhexidine delivered from the catheter remained at trace amounts with no substantial increase due to the delivery of the drug through the catheter.[2335]

Compatibility Information

Solution Compatibility

Famotidine

Test Soln Name	Mfr	Mfr	Conc/L or %	Remarks	Ref	C/I
Dextrose 5%				Under 10% loss in 7 days at room temperature	1(10/06)	C
Dextrose 5%	TR[a]		200 mg	Physically compatible with 6% loss in 15 days at 25°C and no loss in 63 days at 5°C	1342	C

DOI: 10.37573/9781585286850.160

Solution Compatibility (Cont.)

Test Soln Name	Mfr	Mfr	Conc/L or %	Remarks	Ref	C/I
Dextrose 5%		MSD	20 mg	No loss in 48 hr at 25°C in light or dark and at 5°C	1344	C
Dextrose 5%	AB[a][b]	ME	200 mg	Visually compatible with less than 5% loss in 15 days at 22°C both in dark and light	1936	C
Dextrose 10%				Under 10% loss in 7 days at room temperature	1(10/06)	C
Ringer's injection, lactated				Under 10% loss in 7 days at room temperature	1(10/06)	C
Sodium chloride 0.9%				Under 10% loss in 7 days at room temperature	1(10/06)	C
Sodium chloride 0.9%	TR[a]		200 mg	Physically compatible with little or no loss in 15 days at 25°C and in 63 days at 5°C	1342	C
Sodium chloride 0.9%		MSD	20 mg	No loss in 48 hr at 25°C in light or dark and at 5°C	1344	C
Sodium chloride 0.9%	AB[a][b]	ME	200 mg	Visually compatible with less than 5% loss in 15 days at 22°C both in dark and light	1936	C
TNA #111, #112[c]		MSD	20 and 50 mg	Physically compatible. Little loss and no change in fat particle size in 48 hr at 4 and 21°C	1332	C
TNA #114[c]		MSD	20 and 40 mg	Physically compatible. No loss and no change in fat particle size in 72 hr at 21°C in light	1333	C
TNA #182[c]		MSD	20 mg	Visually compatible. No loss in 24 hr at 24°C in light	1576	C
TNA #197 to #200[c]		MSD	20 mg	Physically compatible. No loss in 48 hr at 22°C in light	1921	C
TPN #109, #110[c]		MSD	20 and 40 mg	Physically compatible with no famotidine loss and little change in amino acids in 48 hr at 21°C and in 7 days at 4°C	1331	C
TPN #113[c]		MSD	20 mg	Physically compatible. Little loss in 35 days at 4°C in light	1334	C
TPN #115, #116[c]		MSD	16.7 and 33.3 mg	No famotidine loss in 7 days at 23 and 4°C	1352	C
TPN #196[c]		MSD	20 mg	Physically compatible. No loss in 48 hr at 22°C in light	1921	C

[a] Tested in PVC containers.

[b] Tested in polypropylene syringes.

[c] Refer to Appendix for the composition of parenteral nutrition solutions. TNA indicates a 3-in-1 admixture, and TPN indicates a 2-in-1 admixture.

Additive Compatibility

Famotidine

Test Drug	Mfr	Conc/L or %	Mfr	Conc/L or %	Test Solution	Remarks	Ref	C/I
Cefazolin sodium	FUJ	10 g	YAM	200 mg	D5W	Visually compatible with 10% cefazolin and 5% famotidine loss in 24 hr at 25°C. 9% cefazolin and 5% famotidine loss in 48 hr at 4°C	1763	C
Fat emulsion, intravenous		10%	MSD	200 mg		Little loss in 48 hr at 25°C in light or dark and at 5°C	1344	C
Flumazenil	RC	20 mg	MSD	80 mg	D5W[a]	Visually compatible. 3% flumazenil loss in 24 hr at 23°C in fluorescent light. Famotidine not tested	1710	C
Vancomycin HCl	AB	5 g	YAM	200 mg	D5W[b]	Visually compatible. 9% vancomycin and 6% famotidine loss in 14 days at 25°C. At 4°C, 4% loss of both drugs in 14 days	2111	C

[a] Tested in PVC containers.

[b] Tested in methyl-methacrylate-butadiene-styrene plastic containers.

Y-Site Injection Compatibility (1:1 Mixture)

Famotidine

Test Drug	Mfr	Conc	Mfr	Conc	Remarks	Ref	C/I
Acyclovir sodium		7 mg/mL[a]	ME	2 mg/mL[b]	Visually compatible for 4 hr at 22°C	1936	C
Allopurinol sodium	BW	3 mg/mL[b]	MSD	2 mg/mL[b]	Physically compatible for 4 hr at 22°C	1686	C
Amifostine	USB	10 mg/mL[a]	ME	2 mg/mL[a]	Physically compatible for 4 hr at 23°C	1845	C
Aminophylline	LY	2.5 mg/mL[b]	MSD	0.2 mg/mL[a]	Physically compatible for 14 hr	1196	C
Aminophylline		2.5 mg/mL[a]	ME	2 mg/mL	Visually compatible for 4 hr at 22°C	1936	C
Amiodarone HCl	WY	6 mg/mL[a]	ME	10 mg/mL	Visually compatible for 24 hr at 22°C	2352	C
Ampicillin sodium	ES	20 mg/mL[b]	MSD	0.2 mg/mL[a]	Physically compatible for 14 hr	1196	C
Ampicillin sodium		20 mg/mL[b]	ME	2 mg/mL[b]	Visually compatible for 4 hr at 22°C	1936	C
Ampicillin sodium–sulbactam sodium	RR	20 mg/mL[b l]	MSD	0.2 mg/mL[a]	Physically compatible for 14 hr	1196	C
Amsacrine	NCI	1 mg/mL[a]	MSD	2 mg/mL[a]	Visually compatible for 4 hr at 22°C	1381	C
Anakinra	SYN	4 and 36 mg/mL[b]		1 mg/mL[b]	Physically compatible with little or no loss of either drug in 4 hr at 22°C	2511	C
Anidulafungin	VIC	0.5 mg/mL[a]	BV	2 mg/mL[a]	Physically compatible for 4 hr at 23°C	2617	C
Atropine sulfate	AST	0.1 mg/mL[a]	MSD	0.2 mg/mL[a]	Physically compatible for 4 hr at 25°C	1188	C
Azithromycin	PF	2 mg/mL[b]	ME	2 mg/mL[j]	Grayish-white microcrystals found	2368	I
Aztreonam	SQ	40 mg/mL[a]	ME	2 mg/mL[a]	Physically compatible for 4 hr at 23°C	1758	C
Bivalirudin	TMC	5 mg/mL[a]	ME	2 mg/mL[a]	Physically compatible for 4 hr at 23°C	2373	C
Calcium gluconate	LY	0.00465 mEq/mL[b]	MSD	0.2 mg/mL[a]	Physically compatible for 14 hr	1196	C
Cangrelor tetrasodium	TMC	1 mg/mL[b]		2 mg/mL[b]	Physically compatible for 4 hr	3243	C
Caspofungin acetate	ME	0.5 mg/mL[b]	BA	2 mg/mL[b]	Physically compatible with famotidine i.v. push over 2 to 5 min	2766	C
Cefazolin sodium	LY	20 mg/mL[b]	MSD	0.2 mg/mL[a]	Physically compatible for 14 hr	1196	C
Cefazolin sodium		20 mg/mL[a]	ME	2 mg/mL[b]	Visually compatible for 4 hr at 22°C	1936	C
Cefotaxime sodium	HO	20 mg/mL[b]	MSD	0.2 mg/mL[a]	Physically compatible for 14 hr	1196	C
Cefotaxime sodium		20 mg/mL[a]	ME	2 mg/mL[b]	Visually compatible for 4 hr at 22°C	1936	C
Cefotetan disodium	STU	20 mg/mL[b]	MSD	0.2 mg/mL[a]	Physically compatible for 14 hr	1196	C
Cefoxitin sodium	MSD	20 mg/mL[h]	MSD	0.2 mg/mL[a]	Physically compatible for 14 hr	1196	C
Cefoxitin sodium		20 mg/mL[a]	ME	2 mg/mL[b]	Visually compatible for 4 hr at 22°C	1936	C
Ceftaroline fosamil	FOR	2.22 mg/mL[a b c]	ABX	2 mg/mL[a b c]	Physically compatible for 4 hr at 23°C	2826	C
Ceftazidime	GL	20 mg/mL[b]	MSD	0.2 mg/mL[a]	Physically compatible for 14 hr	1196	C
Ceftazidime		20 mg/mL[a]	ME	2 mg/mL[b]	Visually compatible for 4 hr at 22°C	1936	C
Ceftolozane sulfate–tazobactam sodium	CUB	10 mg/mL[p q]	WW	4 mg/mL[p]	Physically compatible for 2 hr	3262	C
Ceftriaxone sodium		20 mg/mL[a]	ME	2 mg/mL[b]	Visually compatible for 4 hr at 22°C	1936	C
Cefuroxime sodium	GL	15 mg/mL[b]	MSD	0.2 mg/mL[a]	Physically compatible for 14 hr	1196	C

Y-Site Injection Compatibility (1:1 Mixture) (Cont.)

Test Drug	Mfr	Conc	Mfr	Conc	Remarks	Ref	C/I
Cefuroxime sodium		20 mg/mL[a]	ME	2 mg/mL[b]	Visually compatible for 4 hr at 22°C	1936	C
Chlorpromazine HCl		2 mg/mL[a]	ME	2 mg/mL[b]	Visually compatible for 4 hr at 22°C	1936	C
Cisatracurium besylate	GW	0.1, 2, 5 mg/mL[a]	ME	2 mg/mL[a]	Physically compatible for 4 hr at 23°C	2074	C
Cladribine	ORT	0.015[b] and 0.5[d] mg/mL	ME	2 mg/mL[b]	Physically compatible for 4 hr at 23°C	1969	C
Dexamethasone sodium phosphate	ES	10 mg/mL	MSD	0.2 mg/mL[a]	Physically compatible for 14 hr	1196	C
Dexamethasone sodium phosphate		1 mg/mL[a]	ME	2 mg/mL[b]	Visually compatible for 4 hr at 22°C	1936	C
Dexmedetomidine HCl	AB	4 mcg/mL[b]	ME	2 mg/mL[b]	Physically compatible for 4 hr at 23°C	2383	C
Dextran 40	PH	100 mg/mL[a]	MSD	0.2 mg/mL[a]	Physically compatible for 4 hr at 25°C	1188	C
Digoxin	ES	0.25 mg/mL	MSD	0.2 mg/mL[a]	Physically compatible for 14 hr	1196	C
Diphenhydramine HCl		2 mg/mL[a]	ME	2 mg/mL[b]	Visually compatible for 4 hr at 22°C	1936	C
Dobutamine HCl	LI	1 mg/mL[a]	MSD	0.2 mg/mL[a]	Physically compatible for 4 hr at 25°C	1188	C
Dobutamine HCl		4 mg/mL[a]	ME	2 mg/mL[b]	Visually compatible for 4 hr at 22°C	1936	C
Docetaxel	RPR	0.9 mg/mL[a]	ME	2 mg/mL[a]	Physically compatible for 4 hr at 23°C	2224	C
Dopamine HCl	TR	1.6 mg/mL[a]	MSD	0.2 mg/mL[a]	Physically compatible for 4 hr at 25°C	1188	C
Dopamine HCl		1.6 mg/mL[a]	ME	2 mg/mL[b]	Visually compatible for 4 hr at 22°C	1936	C
Doripenem	JJ	5 mg/mL[a b]	BED	2 mg/mL[a b]	Physically compatible for 4 hr at 23°C	2743	C
Doxorubicin HCl liposomal	SEQ	0.4 mg/mL[a]	ME	2 mg/mL[a]	Physically compatible for 4 hr at 23°C	2087	C
Droperidol		0.4 mg/mL[a]	ME	2 mg/mL[b]	Visually compatible for 4 hr at 22°C	1936	C
Enalaprilat	MSD	0.05 mg/mL[b]	MSD	0.2 mg/mL[a]	Physically compatible for 24 hr at room temperature under fluorescent light	1355	C
Epinephrine HCl	ES	4 mcg/mL[a]	MSD	0.2 mg/mL[a]	Physically compatible for 4 hr at 25°C	1188	C
Erythromycin lactobionate	ES	2 mg/mL[b]	MSD	0.2 mg/mL[a]	Physically compatible for 14 hr	1196	C
Esmolol HCl	DU	10 mg/mL[b]	MSD	0.2 mg/mL[a]	Physically compatible for 4 hr at 25°C	1188	C
Etoposide phosphate	BR	5 mg/mL[a]	ME	2 mg/mL[a]	Physically compatible for 4 hr at 23°C	2218	C
Fenoldopam mesylate	AB	80 mcg/mL[b]	ME	2 mg/mL[b]	Physically compatible for 4 hr at 23°C	2467	C
Filgrastim	AMG	30 mcg/mL[a]	MSD	2 mg/mL[a]	Physically compatible for 4 hr at 22°C	1687	C
Fluconazole	RR	2 mg/mL	MSD	10 mg/mL	Physically compatible for 24 hr at 25°C	1407	C
Fluconazole		2 mg/mL[a]	ME	2 mg/mL[b]	Visually compatible for 4 hr at 22°C	1936	C
Fludarabine phosphate	BX	1 mg/mL[a]	MSD	2 mg/mL[a]	Visually compatible for 4 hr at 22°C	1439	C
Folic acid	LE	5 mg/mL	MSD	0.2 mg/mL[a]	Physically compatible for 14 hr	1196	C
Furosemide	ES	10 mg/mL	MSD	0.2 mg/mL[a]	Physically compatible for 14 hr	1196	C
Furosemide	IMS	0.8 mg/mL[a]	MSD	0.2 mg/mL[a]	Physically compatible for 4 hr at 25°C	1188	C
Furosemide		3 mg/mL[a]	ME	2 mg/mL[b]	White precipitate forms immediately	1936	I
Gemcitabine HCl	LI	10 mg/mL[b]	ME	2 mg/mL[b]	Physically compatible for 4 hr at 23°C	2226	C

Y-Site Injection Compatibility (1:1 Mixture) (Cont.)

Test Drug	Mfr	Conc	Mfr	Conc	Remarks	Ref	C/I
Gentamicin sulfate	ES	0.8 mg/mL[b]	MSD	0.2 mg/mL[a]	Physically compatible for 14 hr	1196	C
Gentamicin sulfate		5 mg/mL[a]	ME	2 mg/mL[b]	Visually compatible for 4 hr at 22°C	1936	C
Granisetron HCl	SKB	0.05 mg/mL[a]	ME	2 mg/mL[a]	Physically compatible for 4 hr at 23°C	2000	C
Haloperidol lactate	MN	0.5[a] and 5 mg/mL	MSD	0.267 mg/mL[a]	Visually compatible for 24 hr at 21°C	1523	C
Haloperidol lactate		0.2 mg/mL[a]	ME	2 mg/mL[b]	Visually compatible for 4 hr at 22°C	1936	C
Heparin sodium	ES	40 units/mL[b]	MSD	0.2 mg/mL[a]	Physically compatible for 14 hr	1196	C
Heparin sodium	TR	50 units/mL[a]	MSD	0.2 mg/mL[a]	Physically compatible for 4 hr at 25°C	1188	C
Heparin sodium		40 units/mL[a]	ME	2 mg/mL[b]	Visually compatible for 4 hr at 22°C	1936	C
Hetastarch in lactated electrolyte	AB	6%	ME	2 mg/mL[a]	Physically compatible for 4 hr at 23°C	2339	C
Hydrocortisone sodium succinate	AB	1 mg/mL[a]	MSD	0.2 mg/mL[a]	Physically compatible for 4 hr at 25°C	1188	C
Hydrocortisone sodium succinate	AB	125 mg/mL	MSD	0.2 mg/mL[a]	Physically compatible for 14 hr	1196	C
Hydromorphone HCl		0.5 mg/mL[a]	ME	2 mg/mL[b]	Visually compatible for 4 hr at 22°C	1936	C
Hydroxyzine HCl		4 mg/mL[a]	ME	2 mg/mL[b]	Visually compatible for 4 hr at 22°C	1936	C
Imipenem–cilastatin sodium	MSD	10 mg/mL[b n]	MSD	0.2 mg/mL[a]	Physically compatible for 14 hr	1196	C
Imipenem–cilastatin sodium		5 mg/mL[b n]	ME	2 mg/mL[b]	Visually compatible for 4 hr at 22°C	1936	C
Insulin, regular	LI	0.03 unit/mL[a]	MSD	0.2 mg/mL[a]	Physically compatible for 4 hr at 25°C	1188	C
Isavuconazonium sulfate	ASP	1.5 mg/mL[p]	WW	4 mg/mL[p]	Physically compatible for 2 hr	3263	C
Isoproterenol HCl	ES	0.004 mg/mL[a]	MSD	0.2 mg/mL[a]	Physically compatible for 4 hr at 25°C	1188	C
Labetalol HCl	SC	1 mg/mL[a]	MSD	0.2 mg/mL[a]	Physically compatible for 4 hr at 25°C	1188	C
Letermovir	ME	[a]		[a]	Physically compatible	3398	C
Lidocaine HCl	LY	1 mg/mL[a]	MSD	0.2 mg/mL[a]	Physically compatible for 14 hr	1196	C
Lidocaine HCl	TR	4 mg/mL[a]	MSD	0.2 mg/mL[a]	Physically compatible for 4 hr at 25°C	1188	C
Linezolid	PHU	2 mg/mL	ME	2 mg/mL[a]	Physically compatible for 4 hr at 23°C	2264	C
Lorazepam		0.1 mg/mL[a]	ME	2 mg/mL[b]	Visually compatible for 4 hr at 22°C	1936	C
Magnesium sulfate	SO	100 mg/mL[h]	MSD	0.2 mg/mL[a]	Physically compatible for 14 hr	1196	C
Magnesium sulfate		100 mg/mL[a]	ME	2 mg/mL[b]	Visually compatible for 4 hr at 22°C	1936	C
Melphalan HCl	BW	0.1 mg/mL[b]	MSD	2 mg/mL[b]	Physically compatible for 3 hr at 22°C	1557	C
Meperidine HCl	AB	10 mg/mL	MSD	0.2 mg/mL[a]	Physically compatible for 4 hr at 25°C	1397	C
Meperidine HCl		4 mg/mL[a]	ME	2 mg/mL[b]	Visually compatible for 4 hr at 22°C	1936	C
Meropenem–vabor-bactam	TMC	8 mg/mL[b o]	FRK	4 mg/mL[b]	Physically compatible for 3 hr at 20 to 25°C	3380	C
Methylprednisolone sodium succinate	QU	40 mg/mL	MSD	0.2 mg/mL[a]	Physically compatible for 14 hr	1196	C
Methylprednisolone sodium succinate	AB	1 mg/mL[a]	MSD	0.2 mg/mL[a]	Physically compatible for 4 hr at 25°C	1188	C

Y-Site Injection Compatibility (1:1 Mixture) (Cont.)

Test Drug	Mfr	Conc	Mfr	Conc	Remarks	Ref	C/I
Methylprednisolone sodium succinate		5 mg/mL[a]	ME	2 mg/mL[b]	Visually compatible for 4 hr at 22°C	1936	C
Metoclopramide HCl	RB	5 mg/mL	MSD	0.2 mg/mL[a]	Physically compatible for 14 hr	1196	C
Metoclopramide HCl		5 mg/mL	ME	2 mg/mL[b]	Visually compatible for 4 hr at 22°C	1936	C
Midazolam HCl	RC	0.15 mg/mL[a]	MSD	0.2 mg/mL[a]	Physically compatible for 4 hr at 25°C	1188	C
Midazolam HCl		1.5 mg/mL[a]	ME	2 mg/mL[b]	Visually compatible for 4 hr at 22°C	1936	C
Morphine sulfate	ES	0.2 mg/mL[a]	MSD	0.2 mg/mL[a]	Physically compatible for 4 hr at 25°C	1188	C
Morphine sulfate	AB	1 mg/mL	MSD	0.2 mg/mL[a]	Physically compatible for 4 hr at 25°C	1397	C
Morphine sulfate		1 mg/mL[a]	ME	2 mg/mL[b]	Visually compatible for 4 hr at 22°C	1936	C
Nafcillin sodium	WY	15 mg/mL[b]	MSD	0.2 mg/mL[a]	Physically compatible for 14 hr	1196	C
Nicardipine HCl	DCC	0.1 mg/mL[a]	MSD	0.2 mg/mL[a]	Visually compatible for 24 hr at room temperature	235	C
Nitroglycerin	PD	85 mcg/mL[b]	MSD	0.2 mg/mL[a]	Physically compatible for 14 hr	1196	C
Nitroglycerin	IMS	0.8 mg/mL[a]	MSD	0.2 mg/mL[a]	Physically compatible for 4 hr at 25°C	1188	C
Norepinephrine bitartrate	WI	0.004 mg/mL[a]	MSD	0.2 mg/mL[a]	Physically compatible for 4 hr at 25°C	1188	C
Ondansetron HCl	GL	1 mg/mL[b]	MSD	2 mg/mL[a]	Visually compatible for 4 hr at 22°C	1365	C
Oritavancin diphosphate	TAR	0.8, 1.2, and 2 mg/mL[a]	BED	0.2 mg/mL[a]	Visually compatible for 4 hr at 20 to 24°C	2928	C
Oxacillin sodium	BE	20 mg/mL[b]	MSD	0.2 mg/mL[a]	Physically compatible for 14 hr	1196	C
Oxaliplatin	SS	0.5 mg/mL[a]	ESL	2 mg/mL[a]	Physically compatible for 4 hr at 23°C	2566	C
Paclitaxel	NCI	1.2 mg/mL[a]	MSD	2 mg/mL[a]	Physically compatible for 4 hr at 22°C	1556	C
Palonosetron HCl	MGI	50 mcg/mL	BED	2 mg/mL[a]	Physically compatible and no loss of either drug in 4 hr at room temperature	2771	C
Pemetrexed disodium	LI	20 mg/mL[b]	ESL	2 mg/mL[a]	Physically compatible for 4 hr at 23°C	2564	C
Phenylephrine HCl	WI	0.02 mg/mL[a]	MSD	0.2 mg/mL[a]	Physically compatible for 4 hr at 25°C	1188	C
Phenytoin sodium	PD	50 mg/mL	MSD	0.2 mg/mL[a]	Physically compatible for 14 hr	1196	C
Phytonadione	MSD	2 mg/mL	MSD	0.2 mg/mL[a]	Physically compatible for 14 hr	1196	C
Piperacillin sodium–tazobactam sodium	LE[k]	40 mg/mL[a] [m]	MSD	2 mg/mL[a]	Particles form immediately	1688	I
Plazomicin sulfate	ACH	24 mg/mL[p]	FRK	4 mg/mL[p]	Physically compatible for 1 hr at 20 to 25°C	3432	C
Posaconazole	ME	18 mg/mL		4 mg/mL[p]	Physically compatible	2911, 2912	C
Potassium chloride	AB	0.04 mEq/mL[a]	MSD	0.2 mg/mL[a]	Physically compatible for 4 hr at 25°C	1188	C
Potassium chloride		0.1 mEq/mL[a]	ME	2 mg/mL[b]	Visually compatible for 4 hr at 22°C	1936	C
Potassium phosphates	LY	0.03 mmol/mL[b]	MSD	0.2 mg/mL[a]	Physically compatible for 14 hr	1196	C
Procainamide HCl	ASC	5 mg/mL[a]	MSD	0.2 mg/mL[a]	Physically compatible for 4 hr at 25°C	1188	C
Propofol	ZEN[r]	10 mg/mL	ME	2 mg/mL[a]	Physically compatible for 1 hr at 23°C	2066	C
Remifentanil HCl	GW	0.025 and 0.25 mg/mL[b]	MSD	2 mg/mL[a]	Physically compatible for 4 hr at 23°C	2075	C
Sargramostim	IMM	10 mcg/mL[b]	MSD	2 mg/mL[b]	Visually compatible for 4 hr at 22°C	1436	C

Y-Site Injection Compatibility (1:1 Mixture) (Cont.)

Test Drug	Mfr	Conc	Mfr	Conc	Remarks	Ref	C/I
Sodium bicarbonate	AB	1 mEq/mL	MSD	0.2 mg/mL[a]	Physically compatible for 4 hr at 25°C	1188	C
Sodium nitroprusside	ES	0.2 mg/mL[a]	MSD	0.2 mg/mL[a]	Physically compatible for 4 hr at 25°C protected from light	1188	C
Tedizolid phosphate	CUB	0.8 mg/mL[b]	WW	4 mg/mL[b]	Physically compatible for 2 hr	3244	C
Telavancin HCl	ASP	7.5 mg/mL[a b c]	BED	2 mg/mL[a b c]	Physically compatible for 2 hr	2830	C
Teniposide	BR	0.1 mg/mL[a]	MSD	2 mg/mL[a]	Physically compatible for 4 hr at 23°C	1725	C
Theophylline	TR	1.6 mg/mL[a]	MSD	0.2 mg/mL[a]	Physically compatible for 4 hr at 25°C	1188	C
Thiamine HCl	ES	100 mg/mL	MSD	0.2 mg/mL[a]	Physically compatible for 14 hr	1196	C
Thiotepa	IMM[g]	1 mg/mL[a]	ME	2 mg/mL[a]	Physically compatible for 4 hr at 23°C	1861	C
Tirofiban HCl	ME	0.05 mg/mL[b]	ME	2 and 4 mg/mL[a]	Physically compatible. Little loss of either drug in 4 hr at room temperature	2250	C
Tirofiban HCl	ME	0.05 mg/mL[a]	ME	2 and 4 mg/mL[b]	Physically compatible. Little loss of either drug in 4 hr at room temperature	2250	C
TNA #218 to #226[h]			ME	2 mg/mL[a]	Visually compatible for 4 hr at 23°C	2215	C
TPN #212 to #215[h]			ME	2 mg/mL[a]	Physically compatible for 4 hr at 23°C	2109	C
Verapamil HCl	KN	0.1 mg/mL[a]	MSD	0.2 mg/mL[a]	Physically compatible for 4 hr at 25°C	1188	C
Vinorelbine tartrate	BW	1 mg/mL[b]	MSD	2 mg/mL[b]	Physically compatible for 4 hr at 22°C	1558	C

[a] Tested in dextrose 5%.

[b] Tested in sodium chloride 0.9%.

[c] Tested in Ringer's injection, lactated.

[d] Tested in bacteriostatic sodium chloride 0.9% preserved with benzyl alcohol 0.9%.

[e] Form not specified.

[f] Tested in dextrose 5% with sodium bicarbonate 0.05 mEq/mL.

[g] Lyophilized formulation tested.

[h] Refer to Appendix for the composition of parenteral nutrition solutions. TNA indicates a 3-in-1 admixture, and TPN indicates a 2-in-1 admixture.

[i] Diluent not specified.

[j] Injected via Y-site into an administration set running azithromycin.

[k] Test performed using the formulation WITHOUT edetate disodium.

[l] Ampicillin component. Ampicillin in a 2:1 fixed-ratio concentration with sulbactam.

[m] Piperacillin component. Piperacillin in an 8:1 fixed-ratio concentration with tazobactam.

[n] Not specified whether concentration refers to single component or combined components.

[o] Meropenem component. Meropenem in a 1:1 fixed-ratio concentration with vaborbactam.

[p] Tested in both dextrose 5% and sodium chloride 0.9%.

[q] Ceftolozane component. Ceftolozane in a 2:1 fixed-ratio concentration with tazobactam.

[r] Test performed using the formulation WITH edetate disodium.

Selected Revisions June 1, 2019. © Copyright, October 1990.
American Society of Health-System Pharmacists, Inc.

Fat Emulsion, Intravenous
AHFS 40:20

Products

The compositions and characteristics of fat emulsion, intravenous, products are listed in Table 1.

In addition, fat emulsion, intravenous (as Intralipid 20%), is available as one component of 3-chamber bag products that also contain amino acids with electrolytes and dextrose in a fixed volume and concentration (i.e., Kabiven and Perikabiven, both by Fresenius Kabi).[3264][3265] The specific product labeling should be consulted for additional details on the formulation, administration, and stability of these products.[3264][3265]

pH

The pH of fat emulsion, intravenous, products is adjusted with sodium hydroxide to a pH ranging from 6 to 8.9[3251][3252][3253][3254] or 9.[3255][3444]

Osmolality

The osmolality of Intralipid 30% is approximately 310 mOsm/kg.[3253]

The osmolality of Omegaven 10% is approximately 342 mOsm/kg.[3444]

The osmolality of Intralipid 20% is approximately 350 mOsm/kg.[3251][3252]

The osmolality of Smoflipid 20% is approximately 380 mOsm/kg.[3255]

The osmolality of Nutrilipid 20% is 390 mOsm/kg.[3254]

Osmolarity

The osmolarity of Intralipid 30% is 200 mOsm/L.[3253]

The osmolarity of Intralipid 20% is 260 mOsm/L.[3251][3252]

The osmolarity of Smoflipid 20% is 270 mOsm/L.[3255]

The osmolarity of Omegaven 10% is 273 mOsm/L.[3444]

The osmolarity of Nutrilipid 20% is 290 mOsm/L.[3257]

Phosphate Content

The phosphate content of Smoflipid 20% and Omegaven 10% is 15 mmol/L.[3255][3444]

Aluminum Content

Fat emulsion, intravenous, products contain no more than 25 mcg of aluminum per L.[3251][3252][3253][3254][3255][3444]

Trade Name(s)

Intralipid, Nutrilipid, Omegaven, Smoflipid

Administration

Fat emulsion, intravenous 10 and 20%, may be administered alone by intravenous infusion via a peripheral or central vein.[3251][3254][3255][3444] Fat emulsion, intravenous, also may be administered by intravenous infusion in total nutrient admixtures (TNA, "3-in-1") in combination with amino acids, dextrose, and other nutrients; however, selection of the peripheral or central venous route depends upon the osmolarity of the final infusate.[3251][3252][3253][3254][3255][3444] Some manufacturers state that solutions with an osmolarity of 900 mOsm/L or more must be infused through a central vein.[3255][3444]

Fat emulsion, intravenous, in pharmacy bulk packages is used as a component in parenteral nutrition admixtures; fat emulsion, intravenous, in pharmacy bulk packages is *not* intended for direct intravenous administration.[3252][3253][3254]

The specific product labeling should be consulted for additional details on initial infusion rates, titration, and maximum infusion rates in various populations.[3251][3252][3253][3254][3255][3444]

Stability

Fat emulsion, intravenous, products may be stored in the intact containers at controlled room temperature[3255] or at temperatures of 25°C or less; the specific manufacturer's instructions should be consulted.[3251][3252][3253][3254][3444] The emulsions should be protected from freezing; any product that has been frozen should be discarded.[3251][3252][3253][3254][3255][3444] Excessive heat also should be avoided.[3255][3444]

In general, admixtures containing fat emulsion, intravenous, should be used immediately after preparation, but may be stored for up to 24 hours under refrigeration at 2 to 8°C; admixtures should be infused within 24 hours after removal from such storage at 2 to 8°C.[3251][3252][3253][3254][3255][3444] The specific product labeling should be consulted for additional details on stability of admixtures. If pharmacy bulk packages of fat emulsion, intravenous, are used to prepare such admixtures, the contents of the pharmacy bulk package should be transferred to a suitable admixture container as soon as possible within 4 hours after the bulk package closure has been penetrated.[3252][3253][3254]

Excessive acidity (e.g., pH less than 5) and inappropriate electrolyte content are the primary destabilizers of emulsions.[3251][3252][3253][3254][3255][3444] A 2-year study of Intralipid 10% found an increase in free fatty acids and a decrease in pH on storage. Gross particles formed and toxicity to rabbits increased with time. These changes were greatest during storage at 40°C but were measurable at 20 and even 4°C. The toxicity of the emulsions to rabbits could be correlated to the extent of free fatty acid formation in the emulsions. The formation of free fatty acids, with a consequent lowering of pH, is the major route of degradation of fat emulsions. The rate of degradation is minimized at pH 6 to 7.[889]

The container-closure system is important for long-term stability. Plastic containers are generally permeable to oxygen, which can readily oxidize the lipid emulsions, so glass bottles

DOI: 10.37573/9781585286850.161

Table 1. Composition and characteristics of several fat emulsion, intravenous, products

Component or Characteristic	Intralipid 20% (Baxter)[3251 3252]	Intralipid 30% (Baxter)[3253]	Nutrilipid 20% (B. Braun)[3254]	Smoflipid 20% (Fresenius Kabi)[3255 3258]	Omegaven 10% (Fresenius Kabi)[3444]
Soybean oil	20%	30%	20%	6%	-
Medium chain triglycerides	-	-	-	6%	-
Olive oil	-	-	-	5%	-
Fish oil	-	-	-	3%	10%
Linoleic acid	44–62%	44–62%	48–58%	14–25%	1.5%
Oleic acid	19–30%	19–30%	17–30%	23–35%	4–11%
Palmitic acid	7–14%	7–14%	9–13%	7–12%	4–12%
Linolenic acid	4–11%	4–11%	4–11%	1.5–3.5%	1.1%
Palmitoleic acid	-	-	-	-	4–10%
Stearic acid	1.4–5.5%	1.4–5.5%	2.5–5%	1.5–4%	-
Caprylic acid	-	-	-	13–24%	-
Capric acid	-	-	-	5–15%	-
Eicosapentaenoic acid (EPA)	-	-	-	1–3.5%	13–26%
Docosahexaenoic acid (DHA)	-	-	-	1–3.5%	14–27%
Myristic acid	-	-	-	-	2–7%
Arachidonic acid	-	-	-	-	0.2–2%
Egg yolk phospholipids	1.2%	1.2%	1.2%	1.2%	1.2%
Glycerin	2.25%	1.7%	2.5%	2.5%	2.5%
Sodium oleate	-	-	0.03%	0.3%	0.03%
dl-α-Tocopherol	-	-	-	0.0163–0.0225%	0.015–0.03%
Water for injection	qs	qs	qs	qs	qs
Fat particle diameter (μm)	0.5	0.5	0.26	≤0.5	-
Caloric value (kcal/mL)	2	3	2	2	1.12
Available as	100-, 250-, and 500-mL and 1000-mL (pharmacy bulk package[a]) bags	500-mL (pharmacy bulk package[a b]) bags	250-, 350-, and 500-mL and 1000-mL (pharmacy bulk package[a]) bags	100-, 250-, and 500-mL bags	50- and 100-mL bottles

[a] Not for direct infusion.
[b] Must be combined with dextrose and amino acid solutions such that the final concentration of fat in the total nutrient admixture (TNA) does not exceed 20%.

have been used. Furthermore, the stoppers must not be permeable to oxygen and must not soften on contact with the emulsions. Teflon-coated stoppers have been recommended. Finally, the emulsions are packed under an atmosphere of nitrogen.[889 3420 3421 3422] More recently, specifically designed lipid-compatible plastic (e.g., polypropylene) containers made of multilayered film have been used.[3251 3252 3253]

The long-term room temperature stability of the emulsions is lost when the intact containers are entered. The integrity of the nitrogen layer in the sealed container is essential for room temperature stability. Exposure of Intralipid 10% to the atmosphere has resulted in gradual changes in the emulsion system. No changes in the particle size distribution occurred during the first 36 hours of room temperature storage. After 48 hours at room temperature, globule coalescence was noticeable. By 72 hours, the changes had become significant; however, the visual appearance after 72 hours was unchanged. Long-term storage for 15 months at room temperature resulted in formation of a nonhomogeneous cream layer with oil globules on top.[656] [657] If the pH of the emulsion is optimal and the emulsion is stored under nitrogen and not exposed to direct sunlight, oxidative degradation is not likely to be significant.[889]

The manufacturers state that partially used containers should be discarded[3254] [3255] [3444] and that no container should be used if the emulsion appears to be oiling out.[3251] [3252] [3253] [3255] [3444]

Fat emulsion, intravenous, has been shown to support the growth of various microbes, including both bacterial and fungal species. No visual changes occurred in the emulsions to suggest contamination.[1102] [1103] [1104] [1216] The potential for microbiological growth should be considered when assigning expiration periods.

The 3-in-1 parenteral nutrition solutions that have a lower pH and higher osmolality due to the presence of amino acids and dextrose reportedly do not support microbial growth as well as fat emulsion alone;[1216] however, this risk still exists and the use of strict aseptic technique in the preparation of such admixtures is essential.[3251] [3252] [3253] [3254] [3255] [3444]

See Additional Compatibility Information for other information on stability of fat emulsion, intravenous, including stability of multicomponent (3-in-1) admixtures.

Freezing Emulsions

Freezing may cause physical damage. The emulsions may become coarse and coalesce, and they can undergo irreversible phase separation.[559]

The emulsions should *not* be frozen.[3251] [3252] [3253] [3254] [3255] [3444] If accidental freezing occurs, the products should be discarded.[3251] [3252] [3253] [3254] [3255] [3444]

Syringes

The physical stability of fat emulsion, intravenous (ClinOleic 20%, Baxter; Intralipid 20%, Fresenius Kabi; Lipofundin MCT/LCT, Braun; Omegaven 10%, Fresenius Kabi; Smoflipid, Fresenius Kabi) packaged as 20 mL in 20-mL polypropylene syringe (Becton Dickinson) was evaluated at 4°C, 25°C with 60% relative humidity, and 40°C with 75% relatively humidity.[3457] [3458] Visual and microscopic observations, pH analysis, measurement of oil droplet size (via laser diffraction and photon correlation spectroscopy methods), and zeta potential analysis were performed.[3457] The author concluded that the emulsions were physically stable for 30 days at 4 and 25°C and for 21 days at 40°C.[3457]

Plasticizer Leaching

Diethylhexyl phthalate (DEHP)-containing devices (e.g., containers, administration sets, lines) should *not* be used for the administration of fat emulsion, intravenous.[3251] [3252] [3253] [3254] [3255] [3259] [3444] Fat emulsion extracts DEHP plasticizer from polyvinyl chloride (PVC) equipment.[3251] [3252] [3253] The amount of plasticizer leached from PVC sets by fat emulsion is directly related to the length of administration time and inversely related to the flow rate; these two factors influence the amount of contact time between the fat emulsion and the PVC tubing. Longer administration times and slower administration rates increase the amount of leached plasticizer. Non-PVC plastic containers, such as an ethylene vinyl acetate (EVA) bag, may be used to avoid plasticizer exposure.[658] [661] [673] [893] [1105]

Storage of Intralipid 10 and 20% for 24 hours in PVC sets resulted in phthalate contents of 64 to 70 mcg/mL at 5°C and 144 to 160 mcg/mL at ambient temperature. When the fat emulsions were simply infused through PVC sets, phthalate content dropped to 3.6 to 8.5 mcg/mL. A patient being administered 500 mL of fat emulsion per day would receive about 1.5 to 2.75 mg of phthalate per day. Negligible levels of phthalate were delivered from a parenteral nutrition admixture containing fat emulsion.[1264]

A parenteral nutrition solution containing an amino acid solution, dextrose, and electrolytes in a PVC bag did not leach measurable quantities of DEHP plasticizer during 21 days of storage at 4 and 25°C. However, addition of fat emulsion 10 or 20% to the formula caused detectable leaching of DEHP from the PVC containers stored for 48 hours. Higher DEHP levels were found in the 25°C samples than in the 4°C samples. The authors recommended limiting the use of lipid-containing parenteral nutrition admixtures to 24 to 36 hours. Use of non-PVC containers and tubing is another option.[1430]

Total nutrient admixtures with fat emulsion concentrations ranging from 1 to 3.85% were found to leach DEHP plasticizer even though they were packaged in EVA bags. The bags had PVC sites in their composition, which contributed the DEHP. Use of PVC administration sets added additional DEHP. Leached DEHP ranged from about 200 mcg to 2 mg during simulated infusions conducted immediately after preparation. The authors concluded that children who are treated regularly with TNA are exposed to significant amounts of DEHP.[2588]

Filtration

A 1.2-μm inline filter should be used in the administration of fat emulsion, intravenous, when used alone and when administered as a component of a 3-in-1 admixture (TNA), to reduce the potential for patient harm due to particulates, microprecipitates, and air emboli.[3251] [3252] [3253] [3254] [3255] [3259] [3260] [3444]

Only a 1.2-μm filter should be used; filters with a pore size smaller than 1.2-μm must not be used with lipid emulsions.[3251] [3252] [3253] The particle size of the fat emulsion products may exceed the porosity of some inline filters, and such small porosity filters should not be used with fat emulsion products.[658] [1106]

Compatibility Information

Solution Compatibility

Fat emulsion, intravenous

Test Soln Name	Mfr	Mfr	Conc/L or %	Remarks	Ref	C/I
Amino acids 8.5%	MG	VT	10%	Mixed in equal parts. Physically compatible for 48 hr at 4°C and room temperature	32	C
Amino acids 8.5%	MG	CU	10%	Mixed in equal parts. Physically compatible for 72 hr at room temperature	656	C
Amino acids 8.5%	TR	CU	10%	Mixed in equal parts. Physically compatible for 72 hr at room temperature	656	C
Amino acids 7%	AB	CU	10%	Mixed in equal parts. Physically compatible for 72 hr at room temperature	656	C
Amino acids 10%		VT	10%	Mixed in equal parts. Changes in 20 min. Coalescence and creaming in 8 hr at 8 and 25°C	825	I
Dextrose 5% in Ringer's injection, lactated	CU	VT	10%	Mixed in equal parts. Physically compatible for 48 hr at 4°C and room temperature	32	C
Dextrose 10%	MG	CU		Mixed in equal parts. Increased globule association in 8 hr at room temperature, considered significant at 48 hr. Formation of a top cream layer by 72 hr	656	I
Dextrose 25%	MG	CU	10%	Mixed in equal parts. Increased globule association in 8 hr, progressing to globule coalescence at 48 hr at room temperature. Formation of a top cream layer by 72 hr	656	I
Dextrose 50%		VT	10%	Mixed in equal parts. Physically compatible for 48 hr at 4°C and room temperature	32	C
Dextrose 50%	AB	VT	10%	Mixed in equal parts. Physically compatible for 24 hr at 8 and 25°C	825	C
Ringer's injection, lactated	CU	VT	10%	Mixed in equal parts. Physically compatible for 48 hr at 4°C and room temperature	32	C
Sodium chloride 0.9%	CU	VT	10%	Mixed in equal parts. Physically compatible for 48 hr at 4°C and room temperature	32	C

Additive Compatibility

Fat emulsion, intravenous

Test Drug	Mfr	Conc/L or %	Mfr	Conc/L or %	Test Solution	Remarks	Ref	C/I
Aminophylline	ES	1 g	VT	10%		Physically compatible for 48 hr at 4°C and room temperature	32	C
Aminophylline	DB	500 mg	VT	10%		Lipid coalescence in 24 hr at 25 and 8°C	825	I
Amphotericin B	APC, PHT	0.6 g	CL	10 and 20%		Precipitate forms immediately but is concealed by opaque emulsion	1808	I
Amphotericin B		90 mg		20%		Yellow precipitate forms in 2 hr. Cumulative delivery of only 56% of total amphotericin B dose	1872	I
Amphotericin B	APC	10, 50, 100, and 500 mg, 1 and 5 g	CL	20%		Emulsion separation occurred rapidly, with visible creaming within 4 hr at 27 and 8°C	1987	I
Amphotericin B	SQ	500 mg, 1 and 2 g	KA	20%		Precipitated amphotericin noted on bottom of containers within 4 hr	1988	I
Amphotericin B	BMS	50 and 500 mg	CL[a]	20%		Fat emulsion separates into two phases within 8 hr. Little loss protected from or exposed to fluorescent light in 24 hr at 24°C	2093	I
Amphotericin B	KP	1 and 3 g	BMS	20%		Precipitate forms immediately	2518	I
Amphotericin B	KP	150 mg, 300 mg, 1.5 g	BMS	20%	D5W[b]	Precipitate forms immediately	2518	I
Ampicillin sodium		20 g		10%		15% ampicillin loss in 24 hr at 23°C	37	I

Additive Compatibility (Cont.)

Test Drug	Mfr	Conc/L or %	Mfr	Conc/L or %	Test Solution	Remarks	Ref	C/I
Ampicillin sodium	BE	2 g	VT	10%		Lipid coalescence in 24 hr at 25 and 8°C	825	I
Ascorbic acid	VI	1 g	VT	10%		Physically compatible for 48 hr at 4°C and room temperature	32	C
Ascorbic acid	DB	500 mg	VT	10%		Lipid coalescence in 24 hr at 25 and 8°C	825	I
Calcium chloride		1 g	CU	10%		Immediate flocculation with visually apparent layer in 2 hr at room temperature	656	I
Calcium chloride		500 mg	CU	10%		Flocculation within 4 hr at room temperature	656	I
Calcium chloride	DB	1 g	VT	10%		Coalescence and creaming in 8 hr at 8 and 25°C	825	I
Calcium chloride		10 and 20 mEq	KV	10%		Immediate flocculation, aggregation, and creaming	1018	I
Calcium gluconate	PR	2 g	CU	10%		Produced cracked emulsion	32	I
Calcium gluconate		7.2 and 9.6 mEq	KV	10%		Immediate flocculation, aggregation, and creaming	1018	I
Chloramphenicol sodium succinate	PD	2 g	VT	10%		Physically compatible for 48 hr at 4°C and room temperature	32	C
Chloramphenicol sodium succinate	PD	2 g	VT	10%		Physically compatible for 24 hr at 8 and 25°C	825	C
Cloxacillin sodium		10 g		10%		Aggregation of oil droplets	37	I
Cyclosporine	SZ	400 mg	AB	10%		No cyclosporine loss in 72 hr at 21°C	1616	C
Cyclosporine	SZ	500 mg and 2 g	KA	10 and 20%		Physically compatible with no cyclosporine loss in 48 hr at 24°C under fluorescent light	1625	C
Diphenhydramine HCl	PD	200 mg	VT	10%		Physically compatible for 48 hr at 4°C and room temperature	32	C
Famotidine	MSD	20 mg		10%		Little or no famotidine loss in 48 hr at 25°C in light or dark and at 5°C	1344	C
Folic acid	USP	20 and 0.2 mg	KV	10%		Physically compatible for 2 weeks at 4°C and room temperature in the dark but erratic assays	895	?
Fusidate sodium	LEO	1 g		10%		Physically incompatible	1800	I
Gentamicin sulfate	RS	160 mg	VT	10%		Lipid coalescence in 24 hr at 8 and 25°C	825	I
Hydrocortisone sodium succinate	GL	200 mg	VT	10%		Physically compatible for 24 hr at 8 and 25°C	825	C
Multivitamins	USV	4 mL	VT	10%		Physically compatible for 48 hr at 4°C and room temperature	32	C
Multivitamins	KA		KA	10%		Physically compatible for 24 hr at 26°C. Little loss of most vitamins; up to 52% ascorbate loss	2050	C
Octreotide acetate	SZ	1.5 mg	KV	10%		Octreotide content unstable	1373	I
Phenytoin sodium	PD	1 g	VT	10%		Phenytoin crystal precipitation	32	I
Potassium chloride		100 mEq	VT	10%		Physically compatible for 48 hr at 4°C and room temperature	32	C
Potassium chloride		100 mEq	CU	10%		No change in 24 hr at room temperature, but lipid coalescence in 48 hr	656	C

Additive Compatibility (Cont.)

Test Drug	Mfr	Conc/L or %	Mfr	Conc/L or %	Test Solution	Remarks	Ref	C/I
Potassium chloride		200 mEq	CU	10%		Coalescence with surface creaming in 4 hr at room temperature. Oil globules on surface at 48 hr	656	I
Potassium chloride	DB	4 g	VT	10%		Lipid coalescence in 24 hr at 8 and 25°C	825	I
Ranitidine HCl	GL	50 and 100 mg	KV	10%		Physically compatible. 4% or less ranitidine loss in 48 hr at 25°C in light or dark	1360	C
Sodium bicarbonate	BR	7.5 g	VT	10%		Physically compatible for 48 hr at 4°C and room temperature	32	C
Sodium bicarbonate		3.4 g	VT	10%		Lipid coalescence in 24 hr at 8 and 25°C	825	I
Sodium chloride		100 mEq	CU	10%		No change for 24 hr at room temperature, but lipid coalescence in 48 hr	656	C
Sodium chloride		200 mEq	CU	10%		Lipid coalescence with surface creaming in 4 hr at room temperature. Oil globules on surface at 48 hr	656	I

[a] Tested in glass containers.

[b] Diluted in dextrose 5% before adding to the fat emulsion.

Y-Site Injection Compatibility (1:1 Mixture)

Fat emulsion, intravenous

Test Drug	Mfr	Conc	Mfr	Conc	Remarks	Ref	C/I
Acyclovir sodium	GW	7 mg/mL[a]		TNA #218 to #226[c]	White precipitate forms immediately	2215	I
Albumin human		20%		20%	Immediate emulsion destabilization	2267	I
Amikacin sulfate	BR	250 mg/mL		TNA #97 to #104[c]	Broken fat emulsion with floating oil	1324	I
Amikacin sulfate	AB	5 mg/mL[a]		TNA #218 to #226[c]	Visually compatible for 4 hr at 23°C	2215	C
Aminophylline	AB	2.5 mg/mL[a]		TNA #218 to #226[c]	Visually compatible for 4 hr at 23°C	2215	C
Amphotericin B	PH	0.6 mg/mL[a]		TNA #218 to #226[c]	Yellow precipitate forms immediately	2215	I
Ampicillin sodium	BR	40 mg/mL[b]		TNA #73[c l]	Visually compatible for 4 hr at 25°C	1008	C
Ampicillin sodium	SKB	20 mg/mL[b]		TNA #218 to #226[c]	Visually compatible for 4 hr at 23°C	2215	C
Ampicillin sodium–sulbactam sodium	PF	20 mg/mL[b h]		TNA #218 to #226[c]	Visually compatible for 4 hr at 23°C	2215	C
Ampicillin sodium–sulbactam sodium	PF	15 mg/mL[a g i]	OTS	20%[f]	No change in particle size >1.3 μm observed in 24 hr at 25°C in the dark	3452	C
Aztreonam	SQ	40 mg/mL[a]		TNA #218 to #226[c]	Visually compatible for 4 hr at 23°C	2215	C
Bumetanide	RC, BV	0.04 mg/mL[a]		TNA #218 to #226[c]	Visually compatible for 4 hr at 23°C	2215	C
Buprenorphine HCl	RKC	0.04 mg/mL[a]		TNA #218 to #226[c]	Visually compatible for 4 hr at 23°C	2215	C
Butorphanol tartrate	APC	0.04 mg/mL[a]		TNA #218 to #226[c]	Visually compatible for 4 hr at 23°C	2215	C
Calcium gluconate	AB	40 mg/mL[a]		TNA #218 to #226[c]	Visually compatible for 4 hr at 23°C	2215	C
Carboplatin	BMS	5 mg/mL[a]		TNA #218 to #226[c]	Visually compatible for 4 hr at 23°C	2215	C
Cefazolin sodium	SKF	20 mg/mL[a]		TNA #73[c l]	Visually compatible for 4 hr at 25°C	1008	C
Cefazolin sodium	SKB	20 mg/mL[a]		TNA #218 to #226[c]	Visually compatible for 4 hr at 23°C	2215	C

Y-Site Injection Compatibility (1:1 Mixture) (Cont.)

Test Drug	Mfr	Conc	Mfr	Conc	Remarks	Ref	C/I
Cefotaxime sodium	HO	20 mg/mL[a]		TNA #218 to #226[c]	Visually compatible for 4 hr at 23°C	2215	C
Cefotetan disodium	ZEN	20 mg/mL[a]		TNA #218 to #226[c]	Visually compatible for 4 hr at 23°C	2215	C
Cefoxitin sodium	MSD	20 mg/mL[a]		TNA #73[c l]	Visually compatible for 4 hr at 25°C	1008	C
Cefoxitin sodium	ME	20 mg/mL[a]		TNA #218 to #226[c]	Visually compatible for 4 hr at 23°C	2215	C
Ceftazidime	SKB[d]	40 mg/mL[a]		TNA #218 to #226[c]	Visually compatible for 4 hr at 23°C	2215	C
Ceftriaxone sodium	RC	20 mg/mL[a]		TNA #218 to #226[c]	Visually compatible for 4 hr at 23°C	2215	C
Cefuroxime sodium	GL	30 mg/mL[a]		TNA #218 to #226[c]	Visually compatible for 4 hr at 23°C	2215	C
Chlorpromazine HCl	SCN	2 mg/mL[a]		TNA #218 to #226[c]	Visually compatible for 4 hr at 23°C	2215	C
Ciprofloxacin	BAY	1 mg/mL[a]		TNA #218 to #226[c]	Visually compatible for 4 hr at 23°C	2215	C
Ciprofloxacin	BAY	2 mg/mL[g]	OTS	20%[f]	Coarsening of particle diameter observed immediately after preparation	3452	I
Cisplatin	BMS	1 mg/mL		TNA #218 to #226[c]	Visually compatible for 4 hr at 23°C	2215	C
Clindamycin phosphate	UP	12 mg/mL[a]		TNA #73[c l]	Visually compatible for 4 hr at 25°C	1008	C
Clindamycin phosphate	AST	10 mg/mL[a]		TNA #218 to #226[c]	Visually compatible for 4 hr at 2°C	2215	C
Clindamycin phosphate	PF	5.77 mg/mL[a g]	OTS	20%[f]	No change in particle size ≥1.3 µm observed in 24 hr at 25°C in the dark	3452	C
Cyclophosphamide	MJ	10 mg/mL[a]		TNA #218 to #226[c]	Visually compatible for 4 hr at 23°C	2215	C
Cyclosporine	SZ	5 mg/mL[a]		TNA #220, #223[c]	Small amount of precipitate forms immediately	2215	I
Cyclosporine	SZ	5 mg/mL[a]		TNA #218, #219, #221, #222, #224 to #226[c]	Visually compatible for 4 hr at 23°C	2215	C
Cytarabine	BED	50 mg/mL		TNA #218 to #226[c]	Visually compatible for 4 hr at 23°C	2215	C
Dexamethasone sodium phosphate	FUJ, ES	1 mg/mL[a]		TNA #218 to #226[c]	Visually compatible for 4 hr at 23°C	2215	C
Digoxin	BW	12.5 mcg/mL[m]		TNA #73[c]	Visually compatible for 4 hr	1009	C
Digoxin	ES, WY	0.25 mg/mL		TNA #218 to #226[c]	Visually compatible for 4 hr at 23°C	2215	C
Diphenhydramine HCl	PD	2 mg/mL[a]		TNA #218 to #226[c]	Visually compatible for 4 hr at 23°C	2215	C
Diphenhydramine HCl	SCN	50 mg/mL		TNA #218 to #226[c]	Visually compatible for 4 hr at 23°C	2215	C
Dobutamine HCl	AST	4 mg/mL[a]		TNA #218 to #226[c]	Visually compatible for 4 hr at 23°C	2215	C
Dopamine HCl	AB	1.6 mg/mL[m]		TNA #73[c]	Visually compatible for 4 hr	1009	C
Dopamine HCl	AB	3.2 mg/mL[a]		TNA #222, #223[c]	Precipitate forms immediately	2215	I
Dopamine HCl	AB	3.2 mg/mL[a]		TNA #218 to #221, #224 to #226[c]	Visually compatible for 4 hr at 23°C	2215	C
Doxorubicin HCl	PH, GEN	2 mg/mL		TNA #218 to #226[c]	Damage to emulsion occurs immediately with free oil formation possible	2215	I
Doxycycline hyclate	FUJ	1 mg/mL[a]		TNA #218 to #226[c]	Damage to emulsion occurs immediately with free oil formation possible	2215	I
Droperidol	AB	0.4 mg/mL[a]		TNA #218 to #226[c]	Damage to emulsion occurs in 1 to 4 hr with free oil formation possible	2215	I
Enalaprilat	ME	0.1 mg/mL[a]		TNA #218 to #226[c]	Visually compatible for 4 hr at 23°C	2215	C

Y-Site Injection Compatibility (1:1 Mixture) (Cont.)

Test Drug	Mfr	Conc	Mfr	Conc	Remarks	Ref	C/I
Erythromycin lactobionate	AB	20 mg/mL[b]		TNA #73[c i]	Visually compatible for 4 hr at 25°C	1008	C
Famotidine	ME	2 mg/mL[a]		TNA #218 to #226[c]	Visually compatible for 4 hr at 23°C	2215	C
Fentanyl citrate	AB	0.0125[a] and 0.05 mg/mL		TNA #218 to #226[c]	Visually compatible for 4 hr at 23°C	2215	C
Fluconazole	PF	2 mg/mL		TNA #218 to #226[c]	Visually compatible for 4 hr at 23°C	2215	C
Fluconazole	PF	1 mg/mL[g]	OTS	20%[f]	Fine particles increased after preparation and continued to increase over time	3452	I
Fluorouracil	PH	16 mg/mL[a]		TNA #220, #223[c]	Small amount of white precipitate forms immediately	2215	I
Fluorouracil	PH	16 mg/mL[a]		TNA #218, #219, #221, #222, #224 to #226[c]	Visually compatible for 4 hr at 23°C	2215	C
Furosemide	ES	3.3 mg/mL[m]		TNA #73[c]	Visually compatible for 4 hr	1009	C
Furosemide	AB	3 mg/mL[a]		TNA #218 to #226[c]	Visually compatible for 4 hr at 23°C	2215	C
Ganciclovir sodium	RC	20 mg/mL[a]		TNA #218 to #226[c]	White precipitate forms immediately	2215	I
Gentamicin sulfate	SC	1.6 mg/mL[a]		TNA #73[c i]	Visually compatible for 4 hr at 25°C	1008	C
Gentamicin sulfate	ES	40 mg/mL		TNA #97 to #104[c]	Physically compatible and gentamicin content retained for 6 hr at 21°C	1324	C
Gentamicin sulfate	AB, FUJ	5 mg/mL[a]		TNA #218 to #226[c]	Visually compatible for 4 hr at 23°C	2215	C
Gentamicin sulfate	MSD	0.4 mg/mL[a g]	OTS	20%[f]	Coarsening of particle diameter observed immediately after preparation	3452	I
Granisetron HCl	SKB	0.05 mg/mL[a]		TNA #218 to #226[c]	Visually compatible for 4 hr at 23°C	2215	C
Haloperidol lactate	MN	0.2 mg/mL[a]		TNA #218 to #226[c]	Damage to emulsion occurs immediately with free oil formation possible	2215	I
Heparin sodium	AB	100 units/mL		TNA #218 to #226[c]	Damage to emulsion occurs immediately with free oil formation possible	2215	I
Hydrocortisone sodium succinate	AB	1 mg/mL[a]		TNA #218 to #226[c]	Visually compatible for 4 hr at 23°C	2215	C
Hydromorphone HCl	ES	0.5 mg/mL[a]		TNA #219, #222, #224 to #226[c]	Damage to emulsion occurs immediately with free oil formation possible	2215	I
Hydromorphone HCl	ES	0.5 mg/mL[a]		TNA #218, #220, #221, #223[c]	Visually compatible for 4 hr at 23°C	2215	C
Hydroxyzine HCl	ES	2 mg/mL[a]		TNA #218 to #226[c]	Visually compatible for 4 hr at 23°C	2215	C
Ibuprofen lysinate	OVA	10 mg/mL	BA	10%	Could not be evaluated because of initial milky white opaque appearance and high turbidity	3541	?
Ibuprofen lysinate		1.25, 2.5, and 5 mg/mL[b]		20%	Physically compatible	3546	C
Ifosfamide	MJ	25 mg/mL[a]		TNA #218 to #226[c]	Visually compatible for 4 hr at 23°C	2215	C
Imipenem–cilastatin sodium	ME	10 mg/mL[b i]		TNA #218 to #226[c]	Visually compatible for 4 hr at 23°C	2215	C
Imipenem–cilastatin sodium	MSD	5 mg/mL[a g i]	OTS	20%[f]	No change in particle size ≥1.3 μm observed in 24 hr at 25°C in the dark	3452	C
Insulin, regular	NOV	1 unit/mL[a]		TNA #218 to #226[c]	Visually compatible for 4 hr at 23°C	2215	C
Isoproterenol HCl	BR	4 mcg/mL[m]		TNA #73[c]	Visually compatible for 4 hr	1009	C

Y-Site Injection Compatibility (1:1 Mixture) (Cont.)

Test Drug	Mfr	Conc	Mfr	Conc	Remarks	Ref	C/I
Leucovorin calcium	IMM	2 mg/mL[a]		TNA #218 to #226[c]	Visually compatible for 4 hr at 23°C	2215	C
Lidocaine HCl	ES	4 mg/mL[m]		TNA #73[c]	Visually compatible for 4 hr	1009	C
Lorazepam	WY	0.1 mg/mL[a]		TNA #218 to #226	Damage to emulsion occurs in 1 hr	2215	I
Magnesium sulfate	AB	100 mg/mL[a]		TNA #218 to #226[c]	Visually compatible for 4 hr at 23°C	2215	C
Mannitol	BA	15%		TNA #218 to #226[c]	Visually compatible for 4 hr at 23°C	2215	C
Meperidine HCl	AST	4 mg/mL[a]		TNA #218 to #226[c]	Visually compatible for 4 hr at 23°C	2215	C
Meropenem	ZEN	20 mg/mL[a]		TNA #218 to #226[c]	Visually compatible for 4 hr at 23°C	2215	C
Mesna	MJ	10 mg/mL[a]		TNA #218 to #226[c]	Visually compatible for 4 hr at 23°C	2215	C
Methotrexate sodium	IMM	15 mg/mL[a]		TNA #218 to #226[c]	Visually compatible for 4 hr at 23°C	2215	C
Methyldopate HCl	MSD	5 mg/mL[a]		TNA #73[c]	Cracked the lipid emulsion	1009	I
Methyldopate HCl	MSD	5 mg/mL[b]		TNA #73[c]	Visually compatible for 4 hr	1009	C
Methylprednisolone sodium succinate	AB	5 mg/mL[a]		TNA #218 to #226[c]	Visually compatible for 4 hr at 23°C	2215	C
Metoclopramide HCl	AB	5 mg/mL		TNA #218 to #226[c]	Visually compatible for 4 hr at 23°C	2215	C
Metronidazole	AB	5 mg/mL		TNA #218 to #226[c]	Visually compatible for 4 hr at 23°C	2215	C
Metronidazole	PF	5 mg/mL[g]	OTS	20%[f]	Fine particles increased after preparation and continued to increase over time	3452	I
Micafungin sodium	ASP	0.25 mg/mL[a g]	OTS	20%[f]	No change in particle size ≥1.3 µm observed in 24 hr at 25°C in the dark	3452	C
Midazolam HCl	RC	2 mg/mL[a]		TNA #218 to #226[c]	Damage to emulsion occurs immediately with free oil formation possible	2215	I
Minocycline HCl	PF	1 mg/mL[a g]	OTS	20%[f]	Coarsening of particle diameter observed immediately after preparation	3452	I
Mitoxantrone HCl	IMM	0.5 mg/mL[a]		TNA #218 to #226[c]	Visually compatible for 4 hr at 23°C	2215	C
Morphine sulfate	ES	1 mg/mL[a]		TNA #218 to #226[c]	Visually compatible for 4 hr at 23°C	2215	C
Morphine sulfate	ES	15 mg/mL		TNA #218 to #226[c]	Damage to emulsion occurs immediately with free oil formation possible	2215	I
Nafcillin sodium	BE, APC	20 mg/mL[a]		TNA #218 to #226[c]	Visually compatible for 4 hr at 23°C	2215	C
Nalbuphine HCl	AB, AST	10 mg/mL		TNA #218 to #226[c]	Damage to emulsion occurs immediately with free oil formation possible	2215	I
Nitroglycerin	DU	0.4 mg/mL[a]		TNA #218 to #226[c]	Visually compatible for 4 hr at 23°C	2215	C
Norepinephrine bitartrate	BN	8 mcg/mL[m]		TNA #73[c]	Visually compatible for 4 hr	1009	C
Octreotide acetate	SZ	0.01 mg/mL[a]		TNA #218 to #226[c]	Visually compatible for 4 hr at 23°C	2215	C
Ondansetron HCl	CER	1 mg/mL[a]		TNA #218 to #226[c]	Damage to emulsion occurs immediately with free oil formation possible	2215	I
Oxacillin sodium	BE	20 mg/mL[a]		TNA #73[c l]	Visually compatible for 4 hr at 25°C	1008	C
Paclitaxel	MJ	1.2 mg/mL[a]		TNA #218 to #226[c]	Visually compatible for 4 hr at 23°C	2215	C
Penicillin G potassium	SQ	40,000 units/mL[a]		TNA #73[c l]	Visually compatible for 4 hr at 25°C	1008	C
Pentobarbital sodium	AB	5 mg/mL[a]		TNA #218 to #226[c]	Damage to emulsion occurs immediately with free oil formation possible	2215	I

Y-Site Injection Compatibility (1:1 Mixture) (Cont.)

Test Drug	Mfr	Conc	Mfr	Conc	Remarks	Ref	C/I
Phenobarbital sodium	WY	5 mg/mL[a]		TNA #218 to #226[c]	Damage to emulsion occurs immediately with free oil formation possible	2215	I
Piperacillin sodium–tazobactam sodium	LE[e]	40 mg/mL[a k]		TNA #218 to #226[c]	Visually compatible for 4 hr at 23°C	2215	C
Potassium chloride	AB	0.1 mEq/mL[a]		TNA #218 to #226[c]	Visually compatible for 4 hr at 23°C	2215	C
Potassium phosphates	AB	3 mmol/mL		TNA #218 to #226[c]	Damage to emulsion occurs immediately with free oil formation possible	2215	I
Prochlorperazine edisylate	SCN, SO	0.5 mg/mL[a]		TNA #218 to #226[c]	Visually compatible for 4 hr at 23°C	2215	C
Promethazine HCl	SCN	2 mg/mL[a]		TNA #218 to #226[c]	Visually compatible for 4 hr at 23°C	2215	C
Ranitidine HCl	GL	2 mg/mL[a]		TNA #218 to #226[c]	Visually compatible for 4 hr at 23°C	2215	C
Sodium bicarbonate	AB	1 mEq/mL		TNA #218 to #226[c]	Visually compatible for 4 hr at 23°C	2215	C
Sodium nitroprusside	AB	0.4 mg/mL[a]		TNA #218 to #226[c]	Visually compatible for 4 hr at 23°C protected from light	2215	C
Sodium phosphates	AB	3 mmol/mL		TNA #218 to #226[c]	Damage to emulsion occurs immediately with free oil formation possible	2215	I
Tacrolimus	FUJ	1 mg/mL[a]		TNA #218 to #226[c]	Visually compatible for 4 hr at 23°C	2215	C
Teicoplanin	SAN	2 mg/mL[a g]	OTS	20%[f]	No change in particle size ≥1.3 µm observed in 24 hr at 25°C in the dark	3452	C
Tobramycin sulfate	LI	1.6 mg/mL[a]		TNA #73[c l]	Visually compatible for 4 hr at 25°C	1008	C
Tobramycin sulfate	LI	40 mg/mL		TNA #97 to #104[c]	Physically compatible and tobramycin content retained for 6 hr at 21°C	1324	C
Tobramycin sulfate	AB	5 mg/mL[a]		TNA #218 to #226[c]	Visually compatible for 4 hr at 23°C	2215	C
Trimethoprim–sulfamethoxazole	ES	0.8 mg/mL[a j]		TNA #218 to #226[c]	Visually compatible for 4 hr at 23°C	2215	C
Trimethoprim–sulfamethoxazole	CHU	0.76 mg/mL[a g j]	OTS	20%[f]	No change in particle size ≥1.3 µm observed in 24 hr at 25°C in the dark	3452	C
Vancomycin HCl	AB	10 mg/mL[a]		TNA #218 to #226[c]	Visually compatible for 4 hr at 23°C	2215	C
Vancomycin HCl	SHI	5 mg/mL[a g]	OTS	20%[f]	Fine particles increased after preparation and continued to increase over time	3452	I
Zidovudine	GW	4 mg/mL[a]		TNA #218 to #226[c]	Visually compatible for 4 hr at 23°C	2215	C

[a] Tested in dextrose 5%.

[b] Tested in sodium chloride 0.9%.

[c] Refer to Appendix for the composition of parenteral nutrition solutions. TNA indicates a 3-in-1 admixture.

[d] Sodium carbonate-containing formulation tested.

[e] Test performed using the formulation WITHOUT edetate disodium.

[f] Run at 25 mL/hr with dextrose 5% run at 83 mL/hr.

[g] Run at 100 mL/hr.

[h] Ampicillin component. Ampicillin in a 2:1 fixed-ratio concentration with sulbactam.

[i] Not specified whether concentration refers to single component or combined components.

[j] Trimethoprim component. Trimethoprim in a 1:5 fixed-ratio concentration with sulfamethoxazole.

[k] Piperacillin component. Piperacillin in an 8:1 fixed-ratio concentration with tazobactam.

[l] A 32.5-mL sample of parenteral nutrition solution and 50 mL of antibiotic in a minibottle.

[m] Tested in both dextrose 5% and sodium chloride 0.9%.

Additional Compatibility Information

Calcium and Phosphate

UNRECOGNIZED CALCIUM PHOSPHATE PRECIPITATION IN A 3-IN-1 PARENTERAL NUTRITION MIXTURE RESULTED IN PATIENT DEATH.

The potential for the formation of a calcium phosphate precipitate in parenteral nutrition solutions is well studied and documented,[1771] [1777] but the information is complex and difficult to apply to the clinical situation.[1770] [1772] [1777] The incorporation of fat emulsion in 3-in-1 parenteral nutrition solutions obscures any precipitate that is present, which has led to substantial debate on the dangers associated with 3-in-1 parenteral nutrition mixtures and when or if the danger to the patient is warranted therapeutically.[1770] [1771] [1772] [2031] [2032] [2033] [2034] [2035] [2036] Because such precipitation may be life-threatening to patients,[2037] [2291] FDA issued a Safety Alert containing the following recommendations:[1769]

1. "The amounts of phosphorus and of calcium added to the admixture are critical. The solubility of the added calcium should be calculated from the volume at the time the calcium is added. It should not be based upon the final volume.

   Some amino acid injections for TPN admixtures contain phosphate ions (as a phosphoric acid buffer). These phosphate ions and the volume at the time the phosphate is added should be considered when calculating the concentration of phosphate additives. Also, when adding calcium and phosphate to an admixture, the phosphate should be added first.

   The line should be flushed between the addition of any potentially incompatible components.
2. A lipid emulsion in a 3-in-1 admixture obscures the presence of a precipitate. Therefore, if a lipid emulsion is needed, either (1) use a 2-in-1 admixture with the lipid infused separately, or (2) if a 3-in-1 admixture is medically necessary, then add the calcium before the lipid emulsion and according to the recommendations in number 1 above.

   If the amount of calcium or phosphate which must be added is likely to cause a precipitate, some or all of the calcium should be administered separately. Such separate infusions must be properly diluted and slowly infused to avoid serious adverse events related to the calcium.
3. When using an automated compounding device, the above steps should be considered when programming the device. In addition, automated compounders should be maintained and operated according to the manufacturer's recommendations.

   Any printout should be checked against the programmed admixture and weight of components.
4. During the mixing process, pharmacists who mix parenteral nutrition admixtures should periodically agitate the admixture and check for precipitates. Medical or home care personnel who start and monitor these infusions should carefully inspect for the presence of precipitates both before and during infusion. Patients and care givers should be trained to visually inspect for signs of precipitation. They also should be advised to stop the infusion and seek medical assistance if precipitates are noted.
5. A filter should be used when infusing either central or peripheral parenteral nutrition admixtures. At this time, data have

not been submitted to document which size filter is most effective in trapping precipitates.

   Standards of practice vary, but the following is suggested: a 1.2-μm air-eliminating filter for lipid-containing admixtures and a 0.22-μm air-eliminating filter for non-lipid-containing admixtures.
6. Parenteral nutrition admixtures should be administered within the following time frames: if stored at room temperature, the infusion should be started within 24 hours after mixing; if stored at refrigerated temperatures, the infusion should be started within 24 hours of rewarming. Because warming parenteral nutrition admixtures may contribute to the formation of precipitates, once administration begins, care should be taken to avoid excessive warming of the admixture.

   Persons administering home care parenteral nutrition admixtures may need to deviate from these time frames. Pharmacists who initially prepare these admixtures should check a reserve sample for precipitates over the duration and under the conditions of storage.
7. If symptoms of acute respiratory distress, pulmonary emboli, or interstitial pneumonitis develop, the infusion should be stopped immediately and thoroughly checked for precipitates. Appropriate medical interventions should be instituted. Home care personnel and patients should immediately seek medical assistance."

Calcium Phosphate Precipitation Fatalities

Fatal cases of paroxysmal respiratory failure in 2 previously healthy women receiving peripheral vein parenteral nutrition were reported. The patients experienced sudden cardiopulmonary arrest consistent with pulmonary emboli. The authors used in vitro simulations and an animal model to conclude that unrecognized calcium phosphate precipitation in a 3-in-1 TNA caused the fatalities. The precipitation resulted during compounding by introducing calcium and phosphate near to one another in the compounding sequence and prior to complete fluid addition. This resulted in a temporarily high concentration of the drugs and precipitation of calcium phosphate. Observation of the precipitate was obscured by the incorporation of 20% fat emulsion, intravenous, into the nutrition mixture. No filter was used during infusion of the fatal nutrition admixtures.[2037]

In a follow-up retrospective review, 5 patients were identified who had respiratory distress associated with the infusion of the 3-in-1 admixtures at around the same time. Four of these 5 patients died, although the cause of death could be definitively determined for only 2.[2291]

Calcium and Phosphate Conditional Compatibility

Calcium salts are conditionally compatible with phosphates in parenteral nutrition mixtures. The incompatibility is dependent on a solubility and concentration phenomenon and is not entirely predictable. Precipitation may occur during compounding or at some time after compounding is completed.

NOTE: Some amino acid solutions inherently contain calcium and phosphate, which must be considered in any projection of compatibility.

Dextrose

Dextrose in final concentrations of 5 to 12.5% has been shown to cause a progressive coalescence of the globules in Intralipid 10% due to its alteration of pH from about 7 down to about 3.5 in 48 hours.[656]

Monovalent Cations

Monovalent cations such as potassium and sodium also cause progressive globule coalescence in Intralipid 10 and 20%, leading to surface creaming.[480 490 656 890] The degree and rate of this effect are dependent on the concentration of the ions. A decreasing degree and rate of coalescence were noted as concentrations of sodium chloride or potassium chloride decreased. At 200 mEq/L, the rate is rapid and the effect is severe. In the range of 100 mEq/L or less, significant effects may not occur for over 24 hours.[490 656]

Divalent Cations

Divalent cations such as calcium and magnesium cause immediate flocculation, with a nonhomogeneous white granular layer forming at the surface of the Intralipid 10%. This is followed by a substantial, visibly distinct layer, which does not redisperse on shaking.[480 490 656]

The creaming of Intralipid 20% when calcium chloride was admixed in concentrations from 0.25 to 5% was found to be concentration dependent, with maximum creaming occurring with the 5% additive in 30 minutes.[890]

Multicomponent (3-in-1) Admixtures

Because of the potential benefits in terms of simplicity, efficiency, time, and cost savings, the concept of mixing amino acids, carbohydrates, electrolytes, fat emulsion, and other nutritional components together in the same container has been explored. Within limits, the feasibility of preparing such 3-in-1 parenteral nutrition admixtures has been demonstrated as long as a careful examination of the emulsion mixtures for signs of instability is performed prior to administration.[1813]

However, these 3-in-1 mixtures are very complex and inherently unstable. Emulsion stability is dependent on both zeta potential and van der Waals forces, influenced by the presence of dextrose.[2029] Because the ultimate stability of each mixture is the result of various complicated factors, a definitive prediction of stability is impossible. Death and injury have resulted from administration of unrecognized precipitates in 3-in-1 parenteral nutrition admixtures. In addition, the use of 3-in-1 admixtures is associated with a higher rate of catheter occlusion and reduced catheter life compared with giving the fat emulsion separately from the parenteral nutrition solution.[705 1518 2194]

Intravenous administration of unstable fat emulsion with a large amount of large fat globules greater than 5 μm is potentially embolic and has been demonstrated to result in liver toxicity.[2690]

The use of a 5-μm inline filter for a 3-in-1 admixture (containing Travasol 8.5%, dextrose, Intralipid 10%, various electrolytes, vitamins, and trace elements) showed that fat, in the form of large globules or aggregates, comprised 99.4% of the filter contents. These authors recommended the use of an appropriate filter for preventing catheter occlusion with 3-in-1 admixtures.[742]

The presence of glass particles, talc, and plastic has been observed in administration line samples drawn from 20 adults receiving 3-in-1 parenteral nutrition admixtures and in 20 children receiving 2-in-1 admixtures with separate fat emulsion infusions. Particles ranged from 3 to 5 μm to greater than 40 μm and were more consistently seen in the pediatric admixtures. The authors suggested the use of inline filters given that particulate contamination is present, has no therapeutic value, and can be harmful.[2458]

Combining an amino acids–dextrose parenteral nutrition solution containing various electrolytes with fat emulsion 20%, intravenous (Intralipid, Vitrum), resulted in a mixture that was apparently stable for a limited time. However, it ultimately exhibited a creaming phenomenon. Within 12 hours, a distinct 2-cm layer separated on the upper surface. Aggregates believed to be clumps of fat droplets were found. Fewer and smaller aggregates were noted in the lower layer.[560 561]

Amino acids have been reported to have no adverse effect on the emulsion stability of Intralipid 10%. In addition, the amino acids appeared to prevent the adverse impact of dextrose and to slow the coalescence and flocculation resulting from mono- and divalent cations. However, significant coalescence did result after a somewhat longer time. Therefore, it was recommended that such cations not be mixed with fat emulsion, intravenous.[656]

Three-in-one TNA admixtures prepared with Intralipid 20% and containing mono- and divalent ions as well as heparin sodium 5 units/mL were found to undergo changes consistent with instability, including fat particle shape and diameter changes as well as creaming and layering. The changes were evident within 48 hours at room temperature but were delayed to between 1 and 2 months when refrigerated.[58]

Travenol stated that 1:1:1 mixtures of amino acids 5.5, 8.5, or 10% (Travenol), fat emulsion 10 or 20% (Travenol), and dextrose 10 to 70% are physically stable but recommended administration within 24 hours. M.V.I.-12 3.3 mL/L and electrolytes may also be added to the admixtures up to the maximum amounts listed below:[850]

Calcium	8.3 mEq/L
Magnesium	3.3 mEq/L
Sodium	23.3 mEq/L
Potassium	20 mEq/L
Chloride	23.3 mEq/L
Phosphate	20 mEq/L
Zinc	3.33 mg/L
Copper	1.33 mg/L
Manganese	0.33 mg/L
Chromium	13.33 mcg/L

The stability of mixtures of Intralipid 20% 1 L, Vamin glucose (amino acids with dextrose 10%) 1.5 L, and dextrose 10% 0.5 L with various electrolytes and vitamins was evaluated. Initial emulsion particle size was around 1 μm. The mixture containing only monovalent cations was stable for at least 9 days at 4°C, with little change in particle size. The mixtures containing the divalent cations, such as calcium and magnesium, demonstrated much greater particle size increases, with mean diameters of around 3.3 to 3.5 μm after 9 days at 4°C. After 48 hours of storage, however, these increases were more modest, around 1.5 to 1.85 μm. After storage at 4°C for 48 hours followed by 24 hours at room temperature, very few particles exceeded 5 μm. It was found that the effect of particle aggregation caused by electrolytes demonstrates a critical concentration before the effect begins. For calcium and magnesium chlorides, the critical concentrations were 2.4 and 2.6 mmol/L, respectively. Sodium and potassium chloride had critical concentrations of 110 and 150 mmol/L, respectively. The rate of particle aggregation increased linearly with increasing electrolyte concentration. Heparin 667 units/L had no effect on emulsion stability. The quantity of emulsion in the mixture had a relatively small influence on stability, but higher concentrations exhibited a somewhat greater coalescence.[892]

Instability of the emulsion systems is manifested by (1) flocculation of oil droplets to form aggregates that produce a cream-like layer on top or (2) coalescence of oil droplets leading to an increase in the average droplet size and eventually to a separation of free oil. The lowering of pH and addition of electrolytes can adversely affect the mechanical and electrical properties at the oil–water interface, eventually leading to flocculation and coalescence. Amino acids act as buffering agents and provide a protective effect on emulsion stability. Addition of electrolytes, especially the divalent ions Mg^{++} and Ca^{++} in excess of 2.5 mmol/L, to simple fat emulsions causes flocculation. But in mixed parenteral nutrition solutions, the stability of the emulsion is enhanced, depending on the quantity and nature of the amino acids present. The authors recommended a careful examination of emulsion mixtures for instability prior to administration.[849]

The stability of an amino acid 4% (Travenol), dextrose 14%, and fat emulsion 4% (Pharmacia) parenteral nutrition solution was reported to be quite good. The solution also contained electrolytes, vitamins, and heparin sodium 4000 units/L. The aqueous solution was prepared first, with the fat emulsion added subsequently. This procedure allowed visual inspection of the aqueous phase and reduced the risk of emulsion breakdown by the divalent cations. Sample mixtures were stored at 18 to 25 and 3 to 8°C for up to 5 days. They were evaluated visually and with a Coulter counter for particle size measurements. Both room temperature and refrigerated mixtures were stable for 48 hours. A marked increase in particle size was noted in the room temperature sample after 72 hours, but refrigeration delayed the changes. The authors' experience with over 1400 mixtures for administration to patients resulted in one emulsion creaming and another cracking. The authors had no explanation for the failure of these particular emulsions.[848]

Six parenteral nutrition solutions having various concentrations of amino acids, dextrose, soybean oil emulsion (Kabi-Vitrum), electrolytes, and multivitamins were reported.

All of the admixtures were stable for 1 week under refrigeration followed by 24 hours at room temperature, with no visible changes, pH changes, or significant particle size changes.[1013] However, other researchers questioned this interpretation of the results.[1014 1015]

The stability of 3-in-1 parenteral nutrition solutions prepared with 500 mL of Intralipid 20%, compared to Soyacal 20%, along with 500 or 1000 mL of FreAmine III 8.5% and 500 mL of dextrose 70% was reported. Also present were relatively large amounts of electrolytes and other additives. All mixtures were similarly stable for 28 days at 4°C followed by 5 days at 21 to 25°C, with little change in the emulsion. A slight white cream layer appeared after 5 days at 4°C, but it was easily dispersed with gentle agitation. The appearance of this cream layer did not statistically affect particle size distribution. The authors concluded that the emulsion mixture remained suitable for clinical use throughout the study period. The stability of other components was not evaluated.[1019]

The stability of 3-in-1 parenteral nutrition admixtures prepared with Liposyn II 10 and 20%, Aminosyn pH 6, and dextrose along with electrolytes, trace metals, and vitamins was reported. Thirty-one different combinations were evaluated. Samples were stored under the following conditions: (1) 25°C for 1 day, (2) 5°C for 2 days followed by 30°C for 1 day, or (3) 5°C for 9 days followed by 25°C for 1 day. In all cases, there was no visual evidence of creaming, free oil droplets, and other signs of emulsion instability. Furthermore, little or no change in the particle size or zeta potential (electrostatic surface charge of lipid particles) was found, indicating emulsion stability. The dextrose and amino acids remained stable over the 10-day storage period. The greatest change of an amino acid occurred with tryptophan, which lost 6% in 10 days. Vitamin stability was not tested.[1025]

The stability of 4 parenteral nutrition admixtures, ranging from 1 L each of amino acids 5.5% (Travenol), dextrose 10%, and fat emulsion 10% (Travenol) up to a "worst case" of 1 L each of amino acids 10% with electrolytes (Travenol), dextrose 70%, and fat emulsion 10% (Travenol) was reported. The admixtures were stored for 48 hours at 5 to 9°C followed by 24 hours at room temperature. There were no visible signs of creaming, flocculation, or free oil. The mean emulsion particle size remained within acceptable limits for all admixtures, and there were no significant changes in glucose, soybean oil, and amino acid concentrations. The authors noted that 2 factors were predominant in determining the stability of such admixtures: electrolyte concentrations and pH.[1065]

Several parenteral nutrition solutions containing amino acids (Travenol), glucose, and lipid, with and without electrolytes and trace elements, produced no visible flocculation or any significant change in mean emulsion particle size during 24 hours at room temperature.[1066]

The compatibility of 10 parenteral nutrition admixtures, evaluated over 96 hours while stored at 20 to 25°C in both glass bottles and EVA bags, was reported. A slight creaming occurred in all admixtures, but this cream layer was easily dispersed by gentle shaking. No fat globules were visually apparent. The mean drop size was larger in the cream layer, but no globules were larger than 5 μm. Analyses of the concentrations of amino acids, dextrose, and electrolytes showed no changes over the study period. The authors concluded that such parenteral nutrition admixtures can be prepared safely as long as the component concentrations are within the following ranges:[1067]

Vamin glucose or Vamin N (amino acids 7%)	1000 to 2000 mL
Dextrose 10 to 30%	100 to 550 mL
Intralipid 10 or 20%	500 to 1000 mL
Electrolytes (mmol/L)	
Sodium	20 to 70
Potassium	20 to 55
Calcium	2.3 to 2.9
Magnesium	1.1 to 3.1
Phosphorus	0 to 9.2
Chloride	27 to 71
Zinc	0.005 to 0.03

The stability of 8 parenteral nutrition admixtures with various ratios of amino acids, carbohydrates, and fat, consisting of FreAmine III 8.5%, dextrose 70%, and Soyacal 10 and 20% (mixed in ratios of 2:1:1, 1:1:1, 1:1:½, and 1:1:¼, where 1 = 500 mL), was evaluated. Additive concentrations were high to stress the admixtures and represent maximum doses likely to be encountered clinically:

Sodium acetate	150 mEq
Sodium chloride	210 mEq
Potassium acetate	45 mEq
Potassium chloride	90 mEq
Potassium phosphate	15 mM
Calcium gluconate	20 mEq
Magnesium sulfate	36 mEq
Trace elements	present
Folic acid	5 mg
M.V.I.-12	10 mL

The admixtures were stored at 4°C for 14 days followed by 4 days at 22 to 25°C. After 24 hours, all admixtures developed a thin white cream layer, which was readily dispersed by gentle agitation. No free oil droplets were observed. The mean particle diameter remained near the original size of the Soyacal throughout the study. Few particles were larger than 3 μm. Osmolality and pH also remained relatively unchanged.[1068]

Parenteral nutrition 3-in-1 admixtures with Aminosyn and Liposyn have been a problem. Standard admixtures were prepared using Aminosyn 7% 1000 mL, dextrose 50% 1000 mL, and Liposyn 10% 500 mL. Concentrated admixtures were prepared using Aminosyn 10% 500 mL, dextrose 70% 500 mL, and Liposyn 20% 500 mL. Vitamins and trace elements were added to the admixtures along with the following electrolytes:

Electrolyte	Standard Admixture	Concentrated Admixture
Sodium	125 mEq	75 mEq
Potassium	95 mEq	74 mEq
Magnesium	25 mEq	25 mEq
Calcium	28 mEq	28 mEq
Phosphate	37 mmol	36 mmol
Chloride	83 mEq	50 mEq

Samples of each admixture were (1) stored at 4°C, (2) adjusted to pH 6.6 with sodium bicarbonate and stored at 4°C, or (3) adjusted to pH 6.6 and stored at room temperature. Compatibility was evaluated for 3 weeks.

Signs of emulsion deterioration were visible by 96 hours in the standard admixture and by 48 hours in the concentrated admixture. Clear rings formed at the meniscus, becoming thicker, yellow, and oily over time. Free-floating oil was obvious in 3 weeks in the standard admixture and in 1 week in the concentrated admixture. The samples adjusted to pH 6.6 developed visible deterioration later than the others. The authors indicated that pH may play a greater role than temperature in emulsion stability. However, precipitation (probably calcium phosphate and possibly carbonate) occurred in 36 hours in the pH 6.6 concentrated admixture but not the unadjusted (pH 5.5) samples. Mean particle counts increased for all samples over time but were greatest in the concentrated admixtures. The concentrated admixtures were unsatisfactory for clinical use because of the early increase in particles and precipitation. Furthermore, the standard admixtures should be prepared immediately prior to use.[1069]

The physical stability of 10 parenteral nutrition admixtures with different amino acid sources was studied. The admixtures contained 500 mL each of dextrose 70%, fat emulsion 20% (Alpha Therapeutics), and amino acids in various concentrations from each manufacturer. Also present were standard electrolytes, trace elements, and vitamins. The admixtures were stored for 14 days at 4°C, followed by 4 days at 22 to 25°C. Slight creaming was evident in all admixtures but redispersed easily with agitation. Emulsion particles were uniform in size, showing no tendency to aggregate. No cracked emulsions occurred.[1217]

The stability of parenteral nutrition solutions containing amino acids, dextrose, and fat emulsion along with electrolytes, trace elements, and vitamins has been described. In one study the admixtures were stable for 24 hours at room temperature and for 8 days at 4°C. The visual appearance and particle size of the fat emulsion showed little change over the observation periods.[1218] In another study variable stability periods were found, depending on electrolyte concentrations. Stability ranged from 4 to 25 days at room temperature.[1219]

The effects of dilution, dextrose concentration, amino acids, and electrolytes on the physical stability of 3-in-1 parenteral nutrition admixtures prepared with Intralipid 10% or Travamulsion 10% was studied. Travamulsion was affected by dilution up to 1:14, exhibiting an increase in mean particle size, while Intralipid remained virtually unchanged for 24 hours at 25°C and for 72 hours at 4°C. At dextrose concentrations above 15%, fat droplets larger than 5 μm formed during storage for 24 hours at either 4°C or room temperature. The presence of amino acids increased the stability of the fat emulsions in the presence of dextrose. Fat droplets larger than 5 μm formed at a total electrolyte concentration above approximately 240 mmol/L (monovalent cation equivalent) for Travamulsion 10% and 156 mmol/L for Intralipid 10% in 24 hours at room temperature, although creaming or breaking of the emulsion was not observed visually.[1221]

The stability of 43 parenteral nutrition admixtures composed of various ratios of amino acid products, dextrose 10 to 70%, and 4 lipid emulsions 10 and 20% with electrolytes, trace elements, and vitamins was studied. One group of admixtures included Travasol 5.5, 8.5, and 10%, FreAmine III 8.5 and 10%, Novamine 8.5 and 11.4%, Nephramine 5.4%, and RenAmine 6.5% with Liposyn II 10 and 20%. In another group, Aminosyn II 7, 8.5, and 10% was combined with Intralipid, Travamulsion, and Soyacal 10 and 20%. A third group consisted of Aminosyn II 7, 8.5, and 10% with electrolytes combined with the latter 3 lipid emulsions. The admixtures were stored for 24 hours at 25°C and for 9 days at 5°C followed by 24 hours at 25°C. A few admixtures containing FreAmine III and Novamine with Liposyn II developed faint yellow streaks after 10 days of storage. The streaks readily dispersed with gentle shaking, as did the creaming present in most admixtures. Other properties such as pH, zeta potential, and osmolality underwent little change in all of the admixtures. Particle size increased fourfold in one admixture (Novamine 8.5%, dextrose 50%, and Liposyn II in a 1:1:1 ratio), which the authors noted signaled the onset of particle coalescence. Nevertheless, the authors concluded that all of the admixtures were stable for the storage conditions and time periods tested.[1222]

The stability of 24 parenteral nutrition admixtures composed of various ratios of Aminosyn II 7, 8.5, or 10%, dextrose, and Liposyn II 10 and 20% with electrolytes, trace elements, and vitamins was studied. Four admixtures were stored for 24 hours at 25°C, 6 admixtures were stored for 2 days at 5°C followed by 1 day at 30°C, and 14 admixtures were stored for 9 days at 5°C followed by 1 day at 25°C. No visible instability was evident. Creaming was present in most admixtures but disappeared with gentle shaking. Other properties such as pH, zeta potential, particle size, and concentrations of the amino acids and dextrose showed little or no change during storage.[1223]

The emulsion stability of 5 parenteral nutrition formulas (TNA #126 through #130 in Appendix) containing Liposyn II in concentrations ranging from 1.2 to 7.1% were reported. The parenteral nutrition solutions were prepared using simultaneous pumping of the components into empty containers (as with the Nutrimix compounder) and sequential pumping of the

components (as with Automix compounders). The solutions were stored for 2 days at 5°C followed by 24 hours at 25°C. Similar results were obtained for both methods of preparation using visual assessment and oil globule size distribution.[1426]

The stability of 24 parenteral nutrition admixtures containing various concentrations of Aminosyn II, dextrose, and Liposyn II with a variety of electrolytes, trace elements, and multivitamins in dual-chamber, flexible, Nutrimix containers was studied as well. No instability was visible in the admixtures stored at 25°C for 24 hours or in those stored for 9 days at 5°C followed by 24 hours at 25°C. Creaming was observed, but neither particle coalescence nor free oil was noted. The pH, particle size distribution, and amino acid and dextrose concentrations remained acceptable during the observation period.[1432]

The physical stability of 10 parenteral nutrition formulas (TNA #149 through #158 in Appendix) containing TrophAmine and Intralipid 20%, Liposyn II 20%, and Nutrilipid 20% in varying concentrations with low and high electrolyte concentrations was studied. All test formulas were prepared with an automatic compounder and protected from light. TNA #149 through #156 were stored for 48 hours at 4°C followed by 24 hours at 21°C; TNA #157 and #158 were stored for 24 hours at 4°C followed by 24 hours at 21°C. Although some minor creaming occurred in all formulas, it was completely reversible with agitation. No other changes were visible, and particle size analysis indicated little variation during the study period. The addition of cysteine hydrochloride 1 g/25 g of amino acids, alone or with L-carnitine 16 mg/g fat, to TNA #157 and #158 did not adversely affect the physical stability of 3-in-1 admixtures within the study period.[1620]

The physical stability of five 3-in-1 parenteral nutrition admixtures (TNA #167 through #171 in Appendix) was evaluated by visual observation, pH and osmolality determinations, and particle size distribution analysis. All 5 admixtures were physically stable for 90 days at 4°C. However, some irreversible flocculation occurred in all combinations after 180 days.[1651]

The stability of several parenteral nutrition formulas (TNA #159 through #166 in Appendix) with and without iron dextran 2 mg/L was studied. All formulas were physically compatible both visually and microscopically for 48 hours at 4 and 25°C, and particle size distribution remained unchanged. The order of mixing and deliberate agitation had no effect on physical compatibility.[1648]

The maximum allowable concentrations of calcium and phosphate in a 3-in-1 parenteral nutrition mixture for children (TNA #192 in Appendix) were reported. Added calcium varied from 1.5 to 150 mmol/L, while added phosphate varied from 21 to 300 mmol/L. The mixtures were stable for 48 hours at 22 and 37°C as long as the pH was not greater than 5.7, the calcium concentration was below 16 mmol/L, the phosphate concentration was below 52 mM/L, and the product of the calcium and phosphate concentrations was below 250 $mmol^2/L^2$ (mmol squared/liter squared).[1773]

The influence of 6 factors on the stability of fat emulsion in 45 different 3-in-1 parenteral nutrition mixtures was evaluated. The factors were amino acid concentration (2.5 to 7%); dextrose (5 to 20%); fat emulsion, intravenous (2 to 5%);

monovalent cations (0 to 150 mEq/L); divalent cations (4 to 20 mEq/L); and trivalent cations from iron dextran (0 to 10 mg elemental iron/L). Although many formulations were unstable, visual examination could identify instability in only 65% of the samples. Electronic evaluation of particle size identified the remaining unstable mixtures. Furthermore, only the concentration of trivalent ferric ions significantly and consistently affected the emulsion stability during the 30-hour test period. Of the parenteral nutrition mixtures containing iron dextran, 16% were unstable, exhibiting emulsion cracking. The authors suggested that iron dextran should not be incorporated into 3-in-1 mixtures.[1814]

The compatibility of 8 parenteral nutrition admixtures, 4 with and 4 without electrolytes, comparing Liposyn II and Intralipid (TNA #250 through #257 in Appendix) was reported. The 3-in-1 admixtures were evaluated over 2 to 9 days at 4°C and then 24 hours at 25°C in EVA bags. No substantial changes were noted in the fat particle sizes and no visual changes of emulsion breakage were observed. All admixtures tested had particle sizes in the 2- to 40-μm range.[2465]

The stability of 3-in-1 parenteral nutrition admixtures prepared with Vamin 14 with electrolytes and containing either Lipofundin MCT/LCT 20% or Intralipid 20% was evaluated. The admixtures contained 66.7 mmol/L of monovalent and 6.7 mmol/L of divalent cations. Stability of the fat emulsion was evaluated after 2, 7, and 21 days at 4°C in EVA bags followed by 24 hours at room temperature to simulate infusion. Microscopy, Coulter counter, photon correlation spectroscopy, and laser diffractometry techniques were used to determine stability. Droplet size by microscopy was noted to increase to 18 to 20 μm after 21 days in both of the admixtures with the Intralipid-containing admixture showing particles this large as early as day 2 and with Lipofundin MCT/LCT at day 7. The Coulter counter assessed particles greater than 2 μm to be approximately 1300 to 1500 with Lipofundin MCT/LCT and 37,000 in the Intralipid-containing admixtures immediately after their preparation. Heavy creaming with a thick firm layer was noted after 2 days with the Intralipid-containing admixture, making particle assessment difficult. The authors concluded that storage limitation of 2 days for the Intralipid-containing admixture and not more than 7 days for the Lipofundin-containing admixture appeared justified. They also noted that calcium and magnesium behaved identically in destabilizing fat emulsion with greater concentrations of divalent cations.[867]

The physical instability of 3-in-1 TNA stored for 24 hours at room temperature was reported. The admixtures intended for use in neonates and infants were compounded with TrophAmine 2 to 3%, dextrose 18 to 24%, Liposyn II (Abbott) 2 to 3%, L-cysteine hydrochloride, and the following electrolytes:

Sodium	20 to 50 mEq/L
Potassium	13.3 to 40 mEq/L
Calcium chloride	20 to 26.6 mEq/L
Magnesium	3.4 to 5 mEq/L
Phosphates	6.7 to 15 mmol/L

The emulsion in the admixtures cracked and developed visible free oil within 24 hours after compounding. The incompatibility was considered to create a clinically significant risk of complications if the admixture was administered. The authors determined that these 3-in-1 TNA containing these concentrations of electrolytes were unacceptable and should not be used.[2619]

Another evaluation of 3-in-1 TNA reported physical instabilities of several formulations evaluated over 7 days. The parenteral nutrition admixtures were prepared with dextrose 15%, and Intralipos 4% (Fresenius Kabi) along with FreAmine 4.3%, NephrAmine 2.1%, TrophAmine 2.7%, Topanusol 5%, or Hepat-Amine 4%. Various electrolytes and other components were also present including sodium, potassium, calcium (salt form unspecified), magnesium, trace elements, vitamin K, and heparin. The admixtures were stored at 4°C and evaluated at 0, 3, and 7 days. After removal from refrigeration, the samples were subjected to additional exposure to room temperature and temperatures exceeding 28°C for 24 to 48 hours. Flocculation was found in the admixtures prepared with FreAmine and with TrophAmine after 24 hours of storage at room temperature and after 3 days under refrigeration followed by 24 hours at room temperature. All of the admixtures developed coalescence after 7 days under refrigeration followed by 24 hours at greater than 28°C.[2621]

The physical stability of 5 highly concentrated 3-in-1 parenteral nutrition admixtures for fluid-restricted adults was evaluated. The admixtures were composed of Aminoplasmal (B. Braun) at concentrations over 7% as the amino acids source, dextrose concentrations of about 20%, and a 50:50 mixture of medium-chain triglycerides and long-chain triglycerides (Lipofundin MCT, B. Braun) at concentrations of about 2.5 to 2.7% as the lipid component with electrolytes and vitamins (TNA #269 through #273 in Appendix). The parenteral nutrition admixtures were prepared in EVA bags and stored at room temperature for 30 hours. Electronic evaluation of mean fat particle sizes and globule size distribution found little change over the 30-hour test period.[2721]

The physical stability of 64 formulations of 3-in-1 parenteral nutrition admixtures containing Smoflipid 20% (TNA #277 in Appendix) and 16 formulations of 3-in-1 parenteral nutrition admixtures containing Lipoplus 20% (TNA #278 in Appendix), both in combination with fixed amounts of dextrose 40% and amino acids (Neonutrin 15%) and variable amounts of electrolytes, was evaluated.[3261] Admixtures were stored in EVA bags for up to 29 days at 2 to 8°C followed by 24 hours at 23 to 25°C.[3261] Particle counts were assessed by optical microscopy.[3261] Although particle counts increased over time in admixtures containing either fat emulsion product, all admixtures remained stable throughout the study period and particle counts remained within limits.[3261] Formulations with Lipoplus 20% contained fewer large fat particles than those with Smoflipid 20%.[3261]

The drop size of 3-in-1 parenteral nutrition solutions in drip chambers is variable, being altered by the constituents of the mixture. In one study, multivitamins (Multibionta, E. Merck) caused the greatest reductions in drop size, up to 37%. This change may affect the rate of delivery if flow is estimated from drops per minute.[1016] Similarly, flow rates delivered by infusion controllers dependent on predictable drop size may be inaccurate. Flow rates up to 29% less than expected have been reported. Therefore, variable-pressure volumetric pumps, which are independent of drop size, should be used rather than infusion controllers.[1215]

When using multicomponent, 3-in-1, parenteral nutrition admixtures, the following points should be considered:[490 703 892 893 1025 1064 1070 1214 1324 1406 1670 2215 2282 2308 3251 3252 3253 3254 3255 3444]

1. The order of mixing is important. The amino acid solution should be added to the dextrose prior to addition of the fat emulsion. This practice ensures that the protective effect of the amino acids to emulsion disruption by changes in pH and the presence of electrolytes is realized. Alternatively, some manufacturers of lipid emulsion state that all 3 components may be transferred to the admixture containers simultaneously, admixing with gentle agitation.
2. Electrolytes should not be added directly to the fat emulsion. Instead, they should be added to the amino acids or dextrose before the final mixing.
3. Such 3-in-1 admixtures containing electrolytes (especially divalent cations) are unstable and will eventually aggregate. The mixed systems should be carefully examined visually before use to ensure that a uniform emulsion still exists and that separation of the emulsion (i.e., "breaking" or "oiling out"), indicated by yellowish streaking or accumulation of yellowish droplets in the admixed emulsion, has not occurred.
4. Avoid contact of 3-in-1 parenteral nutrition admixtures with heparin, which destabilizes and damages the fat emulsion upon contact.
5. The admixtures should be stored under refrigeration if not used immediately.
6. The ultimate stability of the admixtures will be the result of a complex interaction of pH, component concentrations, electrolyte concentrations, and, probably, storage temperature.

Furthermore, a 1.2-μm filter should be used in the administration of fat emulsion, intravenous, whether used alone or administered as a component of a TNA (3-in-1); filtration is necessary to remove large lipid particles, electrolyte precipitates, other solid particulates and aggregates.[1106 1657 1769 2061 2135 2346 3251 3252 3253 3254 3255 3259 3260 3444]

Heparin

Heparin sodium has been stated to be compatible in fat emulsion.[480 660] The addition of heparin sodium (Abbott) 1 and 2 units/mL to Liposyn 10% and Intralipid 10% did not break the emulsion and effectively reversed the blood hypercoagulability associated with intravenous fat emulsion administration.[568]

Flocculation of fat emulsion (Kabi-Vitrum), however, has been reported during Y-site administration into a line used to infuse a parenteral nutrition solution containing both calcium gluconate and heparin sodium. Subsequent evaluation indicated that the combination of calcium gluconate (0.46 and 1.8 mmol/125 mL) and heparin sodium (25 and 100 units/125 mL) in amino acids plus dextrose induced flocculation of the fat emulsion within 2 to 4 minutes at concentrations that resulted in no visually apparent flocculation in 30 minutes with either agent alone.[1214]

Calcium chloride quantities of 1 to 20 mmol normally result in slow flocculation of fat emulsion 20% over several hours. When heparin sodium 5 units/mL was added, the flocculation rate was accelerated greatly and a cream layer was observed visually in a few minutes. This effect was not observed when sodium ion was substituted for the divalent calcium.[1406]

Similar results were observed during simulated Y-site administration of heparin sodium into nine 3-in-1 nutrient admixtures having different compositions. Damage to the fat emulsion component was found to occur immediately, with the possible formation of free oil over time.[2215]

The destabilization of fat emulsion (Intralipid 20%) when administered simultaneously with a TPN admixture and heparin was observed. The damage, detected by viscosity measurement, occurred immediately upon contact at the Y-site. The extent of the destabilization was dependent on the concentration of heparin and the presence of MVI Pediatric with its surfactant content. Additionally, phase separation was observed in 2 hours. The authors noted that TPN admixtures containing heparin should never be premixed with fat emulsion as a 3-in-1 TNA because of this emulsion destabilization. The authors indicated their belief that the damage could be minimized during Y-site co-administration as long as the heparin was kept at a sufficiently low concentration (no visible separation occurred at a heparin concentration of 0.5 unit/mL) and the length of tubing between the Y-site and the patient was minimized.[2282]

However, because the damage to emulsion integrity has been found to occur immediately upon mixing with heparin in the presence of the calcium ions in TPN admixtures[1214 2215 2282] and no evaluation and documentation of the clinical safety of using such destabilized emulsions has been performed, use of such damaged emulsions in patients is suspect.

Amphotericin B

In an effort to reduce toxicity, amphotericin B has been admixed in Intralipid instead of the more usual dextrose 5%.[1809 1810 1811 2178] However, amphotericin B 0.75 mg/kg/day administered using this approach in 250 mL of Intralipid 20% has been associated with acute pulmonary toxicities, including sudden onset of coughing, tachypnea, agitation, cyanosis, and deterioration of oxygen saturation. The temporal relationship between the drug administration and respiratory symptoms suggested a causal relationship. Furthermore, no reduction in renal toxicity or other side effects associated with amphotericin B was observed. The authors concluded amphotericin B should not be administered to patients in Intralipid.[2177]

At a concentration of 0.6 mg/mL in Intralipid 10 or 20%, amphotericin B precipitated immediately or almost immediately. The precipitate was not visible to the unaided eye because of the emulsion's dense opacity. Particle size evaluation found thousands of particles larger than 10 μm per mL. In dextrose 5%, very few particles were larger than 10 μm. Centrifuging the Intralipid admixtures resulted in rapid visualization of the precipitate as a mass at the bottom of the test tubes.[1808]

Amphotericin B precipitation is observed in fat emulsion within 2 to 4 hours without centrifuging. In concentrations ranging from 90 mg/L to 2 g/L in Intralipid 20%, amphotericin precipitate is easily seen as yellow particulate matter on the bottom of the lipid emulsion containers.[1872] [1988] Damage to the emulsion integrity with creaming also has been reported.[1987]

In other reports, the appearance of problems was observed in as little as 15 minutes, and actual amphotericin B precipitate formed within 20 minutes of mixing. Analysis of the precipitate confirmed its identity as amphotericin B. The authors hypothesized that amphotericin B precipitates because the excipient deoxycholic acid, an anion, attracts oppositely charged choline groups from the egg yolk components of the fat emulsion and forms a precipitate with phosphatidylcholine, leaving insufficient surfactant to keep the amphotericin B dispersed.[2204] [2205]

Plasma Expanders

Fat emulsion (Abbott) 10 and 20% were combined with the plasma expanders Macrodex 6% in sodium chloride 0.9% (Schiwa), Gelafundin (Braun), Haes Steril 10% (Fresenius), and Expafusin Sine (Pfrimmer); fat particles exceeding 5 µm resulted, as observed by microscopic examination. These combinations were incompatible.[1668]

Selected Revisions May 1, 2020. © Copyright, October 1982. American Society of Health-System Pharmacists, Inc.

Fenoldopam Mesylate
AHFS 24:08.20

Products

Fenoldopam mesylate is available as a concentrate for injection in 1- and 2-mL single-use ampuls.[3241] Each mL of the concentrate for injection contains fenoldopam 10 mg (as the mesylate salt), propylene glycol 518 mg, citric acid 3.44 mg, sodium citrate dihydrate 0.61 mg, and sodium metabisulfite 1 mg.[3241] The concentrate must be diluted for use.[3241]

To prepare a diluted solution of fenoldopam for continuous intravenous infusion in adult patients, 1, 2, or 4 mL of the concentrate for injection should be added to 250, 500, or 1000 mL, respectively, of sodium chloride 0.9% or dextrose 5% to yield a solution with a fenoldopam concentration of 40 mcg/mL.[3241]

To prepare a diluted solution for continuous intravenous infusion in pediatric patients, 0.6, 1.5, or 3 mL of the concentrate for injection should be added to 100, 250, or 500 mL, respectively, of sodium chloride 0.9% or dextrose 5% to yield a solution with a fenoldopam concentration of 60 mcg/mL.[3241]

Trade Name(s)

Corlopam

Administration

Fenoldopam mesylate is administered by continuous intravenous infusion only after dilution in dextrose 5% or sodium chloride 0.9%.[3241]

Stability

Intact ampuls should be stored at 2 to 30°C.[3241] After dilution in dextrose 5% or sodium chloride 0.9%, fenoldopam mesylate is stable for 4 hours at room temperature or 24 hours when refrigerated prior to administration.[3241]

Solutions should be visually inspected for particulate matter and discoloration prior to administration; if particulate matter is present or cloudiness occurs, the solution should be discarded.[3241]

Compatibility Information

Solution Compatibility

Fenoldopam mesylate

Test Soln Name	Mfr	Mfr	Conc/L or %	Remarks	Ref	C/I
Dextrose 5%	AB[a]	AB	4, 8, 40, 80, 200, 300 mg	Physically compatible. Little loss in 72 hr at 4°C in dark and at 23°C in light	2369	C
Dextrose 5%		HOS	40 and 60 mg	Stable for 4 hr at room temperature or 24 hr under refrigeration	3241	C
Sodium chloride 0.9%	AB[a]	AB	4, 8, 40, 80, 200, 300 mg	Physically compatible. Little loss in 72 hr at 4°C in dark and at 23°C in light	2369	C
Sodium chloride 0.9%		HOS	40 and 60 mg	Stable for 4 hr at room temperature or 24 hr under refrigeration	3241	C

[a] Tested in PVC containers.

Y-Site Injection Compatibility (1:1 Mixture)

Fenoldopam mesylate

Test Drug	Mfr	Conc	Mfr	Conc	Remarks	Ref	C/I
Alfentanil HCl	TAY	0.5 mg/mL	AB	80 mcg/mL[b]	Physically compatible for 4 hr at 23°C	2467	C
Amikacin sulfate	APO	5 mg/mL[b]	AB	80 mcg/mL[b]	Physically compatible for 4 hr at 23°C	2467	C
Aminocaproic acid	AMR	50 mg/mL[b]	AB	80 mcg/mL[b]	Physically compatible for 4 hr at 23°C	2467	C
Aminophylline	AB	2.5 mg/mL[b]	AB	80 mcg/mL[b]	Haze and microparticulates form immediately. Yellow turbidity in 4 hr	2467	I
Amiodarone HCl	WAY	4 mg/mL[b]	AB	80 mcg/mL[b]	Physically compatible for 4 hr at 23°C	2467	C

DOI: 10.37573/9781585286850.162

Y-Site Injection Compatibility (1:1 Mixture) (Cont.)

Test Drug	Mfr	Conc	Mfr	Conc	Remarks	Ref	C/I
Amphotericin B	APO	0.6 mg/mL[b]	AB	80 mcg/mL[b]	Yellow precipitate forms immediately	2467	I
Ampicillin sodium	APO	20 mg/mL[b]	AB	80 mcg/mL[b]	Yellow color forms in 4 hr	2467	I
Ampicillin sodium–sulbactam sodium	PF	20 mg/mL[b e]	AB	80 mcg/mL[b]	Physically compatible for 4 hr at 23°C	2467	C
Argatroban	SKB	1 mg/mL[a]	AB	0.1 mg/mL[a]	Physically compatible for 24 hr at 23°C	2572	C
Atracurium besylate	BA	0.5 mg/mL[b]	AB	80 mcg/mL[b]	Physically compatible for 4 hr at 23°C	2467	C
Atropine sulfate	APP	0.1 mg/mL[b]	AB	80 mcg/mL[b]	Physically compatible for 4 hr at 23°C	2467	C
Aztreonam	BMS	40 mg/mL[b]	AB	80 mcg/mL[b]	Physically compatible for 4 hr at 23°C	2467	C
Bumetanide	BA	40 mcg/mL[b]	AB	80 mcg/mL[b]	Trace haze forms immediately	2467	I
Butorphanol tartrate	APO	40 mcg/mL[b]	AB	80 mcg/mL[b]	Physically compatible for 4 hr at 23°C	2467	C
Calcium gluconate	APP	40 mg/mL[b]	AB	80 mcg/mL[b]	Physically compatible for 4 hr at 23°C	2467	C
Cefazolin sodium	APO	20 mg/mL[b]	AB	80 mcg/mL[b]	Physically compatible for 4 hr at 23°C	2467	C
Cefepime HCl	BMS	20 mg/mL[b]	AB	80 mcg/mL[b]	Physically compatible for 4 hr at 23°C	2467	C
Cefotaxime sodium	HO	20 mg/mL[b]	AB	80 mcg/mL[b]	Physically compatible for 4 hr at 23°C	2467	C
Cefotetan disodium	ZEN	20 mg/mL[b]	AB	80 mcg/mL[b]	Physically compatible for 4 hr at 23°C	2467	C
Cefoxitin sodium	ME	20 mg/mL[b]	AB	80 mcg/mL[b]	Microparticulates form immediately	2467	I
Ceftazidime	GW	40 mg/mL[b]	AB	80 mcg/mL[b]	Physically compatible for 4 hr at 23°C	2467	C
Ceftriaxone sodium	RC	20 mg/mL[b]	AB	80 mcg/mL[b]	Physically compatible for 4 hr at 23°C	2467	C
Cefuroxime sodium	GW	30 mg/mL[b]	AB	80 mcg/mL[b]	Physically compatible for 4 hr at 23°C	2467	C
Chlorpromazine HCl	ES	2 mg/mL[b]	AB	80 mcg/mL[b]	Physically compatible for 4 hr at 23°C	2467	C
Ciprofloxacin	BAY	2 mg/mL[b]	AB	80 mcg/mL[b]	Physically compatible for 4 hr at 23°C	2467	C
Cisatracurium besylate	AB	0.5 mg/mL[b]	AB	80 mcg/mL[b]	Physically compatible for 4 hr at 23°C	2467	C
Clindamycin phosphate	AB	10 mg/mL[b]	AB	80 mcg/mL[b]	Physically compatible for 4 hr at 23°C	2467	C
Dexamethasone sodium phosphate	AMR	1 mg/mL[b]	AB	80 mcg/mL[b]	Trace haze forms immediately	2467	I
Dexmedetomidine HCl	AB	4 mcg/mL[b]	AB	80 mcg/mL[b]	Physically compatible for 4 hr at 23°C	2383	C
Diazepam	AB	5 mg/mL	AB	80 mcg/mL[b]	Gross white turbidity forms immediately	2467	I
Digoxin	ES	0.25 mg/mL	AB	80 mcg/mL[b]	Physically compatible for 4 hr at 23°C	2467	C
Diltiazem HCl	BA	5 mg/mL	AB	80 mcg/mL[b]	Physically compatible for 4 hr at 23°C	2467	C
Diphenhydramine HCl	ES	2 mg/mL[b]	AB	80 mcg/mL[b]	Physically compatible for 4 hr at 23°C	2467	C
Dobutamine HCl	BED	4 mg/mL[b]	AB	80 mcg/mL[b]	Physically compatible for 4 hr at 23°C	2467	C
Dolasetron mesylate	AVE	2 mg/mL[b]	AB	80 mcg/mL[b]	Physically compatible for 4 hr at 23°C	2467	C
Dopamine HCl	AB	3.2 mg/mL[b]	AB	80 mcg/mL[b]	Physically compatible for 4 hr at 23°C	2467	C
Doxycycline hyclate	APP	1 mg/mL[b]	AB	80 mcg/mL[b]	Physically compatible for 4 hr at 23°C	2467	C
Droperidol	AB	2.5 mg/mL	AB	80 mcg/mL[b]	Physically compatible for 4 hr at 23°C	2467	C
Enalaprilat	BA	0.1 mg/mL[b]	AB	80 mcg/mL[b]	Physically compatible for 4 hr at 23°C	2467	C
Ephedrine sulfate	BED	5 mg/mL[b]	AB	80 mcg/mL[b]	Physically compatible for 4 hr at 23°C	2467	C

Y-Site Injection Compatibility (1:1 Mixture) (Cont.)

Test Drug	Mfr	Conc	Mfr	Conc	Remarks	Ref	C/I
Epinephrine HCl	AMR	50 mcg/mL[b]	AB	80 mcg/mL[b]	Physically compatible for 4 hr at 23°C	2467	C
Erythromycin lactobionate	AB	5 mg/mL[b]	AB	80 mcg/mL[b]	Physically compatible for 4 hr at 23°C	2467	C
Esmolol HCl	BA	10 mg/mL[b]	AB	80 mcg/mL[b]	Physically compatible for 4 hr at 23°C	2467	C
Famotidine	ME	2 mg/mL[b]	AB	80 mcg/mL[b]	Physically compatible for 4 hr at 23°C	2467	C
Fentanyl citrate	AB	12.5 mcg/mL[b]	AB	80 mcg/mL[b]	Physically compatible for 4 hr at 23°C	2467	C
Fluconazole	PF	2 mg/mL	AB	80 mcg/mL[b]	Physically compatible for 4 hr at 23°C	2467	C
Fosphenytoin sodium	PD[c]	20 mg PE/mL[b]	AB	80 mcg/mL[b]	Trace haze and microparticulates form in 4 hr	2467	I
Furosemide	AMR	3 mg/mL[b]	AB	80 mcg/mL[b]	Trace haze forms immediately	2467	I
Gentamicin sulfate	APP	5 mg/mL[b]	AB	80 mcg/mL[b]	Physically compatible for 4 hr at 23°C	2467	C
Granisetron HCl	SKB	50 mcg/mL[b]	AB	80 mcg/mL[b]	Physically compatible for 4 hr at 23°C	2467	C
Haloperidol lactate	APP	0.2 mg/mL[b]	AB	80 mcg/mL[b]	Physically compatible for 4 hr at 23°C	2467	C
Heparin sodium	AB	100 units/mL	AB	80 mcg/mL[b]	Physically compatible for 4 hr at 23°C	2467	C
Hetastarch in lactated electrolyte	AB	6%	AB	80 mcg/mL[b]	Physically compatible for 4 hr at 23°C	2467	C
Hydrocortisone sodium succinate	PHU	1 mg/mL[b]	AB	80 mcg/mL[b]	Physically compatible for 4 hr at 23°C	2467	C
Hydromorphone HCl	ES	0.5 mg/mL[b]	AB	80 mcg/mL[b]	Physically compatible for 4 hr at 23°C	2467	C
Hydroxyzine HCl	ES	2 mg/mL[b]	AB	80 mcg/mL[b]	Physically compatible for 4 hr at 23°C	2467	C
Iodixanol	NYC	55%	AB	80 mcg/mL[b]	Physically compatible for 4 hr at 23 and 37°C	2467	C
Iohexol	NYC	51.8%	AB	80 mcg/mL[b]	Physically compatible for 4 hr at 23 and 37°C	2467	C
Iopamidol	BRD	51%	AB	80 mcg/mL[b]	Physically compatible for 4 hr at 23 and 37°C	2467	C
Ioxaglate meglumine–ioxaglate sodium	MA	39.3%	AB	80 mcg/mL[b]	Physically compatible for 4 hr at 23 and 37°C	2467	C
Isoproterenol HCl	AB	20 mcg/mL[b]	AB	80 mcg/mL[b]	Physically compatible for 4 hr at 23°C	2467	C
Ketorolac tromethamine	AB	15 mg/mL[b]	AB	80 mcg/mL[b]	Trace haze forms immediately	2467	I
Labetalol HCl	AB	2 mg/mL[b]	AB	80 mcg/mL[b]	Physically compatible for 4 hr at 23°C	2467	C
Levofloxacin	OMN	5 mg/mL[b]	AB	80 mcg/mL[b]	Physically compatible for 4 hr at 23°C	2467	C
Lidocaine HCl	AST	10 mg/mL[b]	AB	80 mcg/mL[b]	Physically compatible for 4 hr at 23°C	2467	C
Linezolid	PHU	2 mg/mL	AB	80 mcg/mL[b]	Physically compatible for 4 hr at 23°C	2467	C
Lorazepam	ES	0.5 mg/mL[b]	AB	80 mcg/mL[b]	Physically compatible for 4 hr at 23°C	2467	C
Magnesium sulfate	APP	100 mg/mL[b]	AB	80 mcg/mL[b]	Physically compatible for 4 hr at 23°C	2467	C
Mannitol	BA	15%	AB	80 mcg/mL[b]	Physically compatible for 4 hr at 23°C	2467	C
Meperidine HCl	AB	4 mg/mL[b]	AB	80 mcg/mL[b]	Physically compatible for 4 hr at 23°C	2467	C
Methohexital sodium	JP	10 mg/mL[b]	AB	80 mcg/mL[b]	Microparticulates and yellow color form immediately	2467	I
Methylprednisolone sodium succinate	PHU	5 mg/mL[b]	AB	80 mcg/mL[b]	Microparticulates form immediately	2467	I
Metoclopramide HCl	RB	5 mg/mL	AB	80 mcg/mL[b]	Physically compatible for 4 hr at 23°C	2467	C

Y-Site Injection Compatibility (1:1 Mixture) (Cont.)

Test Drug	Mfr	Conc	Mfr	Conc	Remarks	Ref	C/I
Metronidazole	BA	5 mg/mL	AB	80 mcg/mL[b]	Physically compatible for 4 hr at 23°C	2467	C
Micafungin sodium	ASP	1.5 mg/mL[b]	BA	80 mcg/mL[b]	Physically compatible for 4 hr at 23°C	2683	C
Midazolam HCl	APP	1 mg/mL[b]	AB	80 mcg/mL[b]	Physically compatible for 4 hr at 23°C	2467	C
Milrinone lactate	SAN	0.2 mg/mL[b]	AB	80 mcg/mL[b]	Physically compatible for 4 hr at 23°C	2467	C
Morphine sulfate	ES	1 mg/mL[b]	AB	80 mcg/mL[b]	Physically compatible for 4 hr at 23°C	2467	C
Nalbuphine HCl	EN	10 mg/mL	AB	80 mcg/mL[b]	Physically compatible for 4 hr at 23°C	2467	C
Naloxone HCl	AB	0.4 mg/mL[b]	AB	80 mcg/mL[b]	Physically compatible for 4 hr at 23°C	2467	C
Nicardipine HCl	WAY	1 mg/mL[b]	AB	80 mcg/mL[b]	Physically compatible for 4 hr at 23°C	2467	C
Nitroglycerin	AMR	0.4 mg/mL[b]	AB	80 mcg/mL[b]	Physically compatible for 4 hr at 23°C	2467	C
Norepinephrine bitartrate	AB	0.12 mg/mL[b]	AB	80 mcg/mL[b]	Physically compatible for 4 hr at 23°C	2467	C
Ondansetron HCl	GW	1 mg/mL[b]	AB	80 mcg/mL[b]	Physically compatible for 4 hr at 23°C	2467	C
Pancuronium bromide	BA	0.1 mg/mL[b]	AB	80 mcg/mL[b]	Physically compatible for 4 hr at 23°C	2467	C
Pentobarbital sodium	AB	5 mg/mL[b]	AB	80 mcg/mL[b]	Trace haze and microparticulates form immediately	2467	I
Phenylephrine HCl	AMR	1 mg/mL[b]	AB	80 mcg/mL[b]	Physically compatible for 4 hr at 23°C	2467	C
Phenytoin sodium	ES	50 mg/mL	AB	80 mcg/mL[b]	Microcrystals and yellowish darkening form immediately	2467	I
Piperacillin sodium–tazobactam sodium	LE[d]	40 mg/mL[b f]	AB	80 mcg/mL[b]	Physically compatible for 4 hr at 23°C	2467	C
Potassium chloride	APP	0.1 mEq/mL[b]	AB	80 mcg/mL[b]	Physically compatible for 4 hr at 23°C	2467	C
Procainamide HCl	ES	10 mg/mL[b]	AB	80 mcg/mL[b]	Physically compatible for 4 hr at 23°C	2467	C
Prochlorperazine edisylate	SKB	0.5 mg/mL[b]	AB	80 mcg/mL[b]	Trace haze forms in 4 hr	2467	I
Promethazine HCl	ES	2 mg/mL[b]	AB	80 mcg/mL[b]	Physically compatible for 4 hr at 23°C	2467	C
Propofol	ASZ[i]	10 mg/mL	AB	80 mcg/mL[b]	Physically compatible for 4 hr at 23°C	2467	C/I
Propranolol HCl	WAY	1 mg/mL	AB	80 mcg/mL[b]	Physically compatible for 4 hr at 23°C	2467	C
Quinupristin–dalfopristin	AVE	5 mg/mL[b g]	AB	80 mcg/mL[b]	Physically compatible for 4 hr at 23°C	2467	C
Ranitidine HCl	GW	2 mg/mL[b]	AB	80 mcg/mL[b]	Physically compatible for 4 hr at 23°C	2467	C
Remifentanil HCl	AB	0.2 mg/mL[b]	AB	80 mcg/mL[b]	Physically compatible for 4 hr at 23°C	2467	C
Rocuronium bromide	OR	1 mg/mL[b]	AB	80 mcg/mL[b]	Physically compatible for 4 hr at 23°C	2467	C
Sodium bicarbonate	APP	1 mEq/mL	AB	80 mcg/mL[b]	Trace haze and microparticulates form immediately with turbidity in 4 hr	2467	I
Sufentanil citrate	BA	12.5 mcg/mL[b]	AB	80 mcg/mL[b]	Physically compatible for 4 hr at 23°C	2467	C
Theophylline	BA	4 mg/mL[a]	AB	80 mcg/mL[b]	Physically compatible for 4 hr at 23°C	2467	C
Tobramycin sulfate	LI	5 mg/mL[b]	AB	80 mcg/mL[b]	Physically compatible for 4 hr at 23°C	2467	C
Trimethoprim–sulfamethoxazole	ES	0.8 mg/mL[b h]	AB	80 mcg/mL[b]	Physically compatible for 4 hr at 23°C	2467	C
Vancomycin HCl	APP	10 mg/mL[b]	AB	80 mcg/mL[b]	Physically compatible for 4 hr at 23°C	2467	C

Y-Site Injection Compatibility (1:1 Mixture) (Cont.)

Test Drug	Mfr	Conc	Mfr	Conc	Remarks	Ref	C/I
Vecuronium bromide	ES	0.2 mg/mL[b]	AB	80 mcg/mL[b]	Physically compatible for 4 hr at 23°C	2467	C
Verapamil HCl	AB	1.25 mg/mL[b]	AB	80 mcg/mL[b]	Physically compatible for 4 hr at 23°C	2467	C

[a] Tested in dextrose 5%.

[b] Tested in sodium chloride 0.9%.

[c] Concentration expressed in milligrams of phenytoin sodium equivalents (PE) per mL.

[d] Test performed using the formulation WITHOUT edetate disodium.

[e] Ampicillin component. Ampicillin in a 2:1 fixed-ratio concentration with sulbactam.

[f] Piperacillin component. Piperacillin in an 8:1 fixed-ratio concentration with tazobactam.

[g] Quinupristin and dalfopristin components combined.

[h] Trimethoprim component. Trimethoprim in a 1:5 fixed-ratio concentration with sulfamethoxazole.

[i] Test performed using the formulation WITH edetate disodium.

Selected Revisions January 31, 2020. © Copyright, October 2004. American Society of Health-System Pharmacists, Inc.

Fentanyl Citrate
AHFS 28:08.08

Products

Fentanyl citrate is available in 2-, 5-, 10-, and 20-mL ampuls, 2- and 5-mL syringe cartridges, and 30- and 50-mL vials. Each mL contains fentanyl (as the citrate) 50 mcg (0.05 mg) with hydrochloric acid and/or sodium hydroxide for pH adjustment.[1(1/08) 4]

pH

From 4 to 7.5.[1(1/08) 4]

Osmolality

The product osmolality was determined to be essentially 0 mOsm/kg.[1233]

Trade Name(s)

Sublimaze

Administration

Fentanyl citrate is administered by intramuscular or intravenous injection.[1(1/08)]

Stability

Intact containers should be stored at controlled room temperature and protected from light. Brief exposure to temperatures up to 40°C does not affect concentration.[1(1/08) 4]

pH Effects

Fentanyl citrate is most stable at pH 3.5 to 7.5.[1638] Fentanyl is hydrolyzed in acidic solutions.[4]

Syringes

In 2015, reports of decreased potency of certain drugs (e.g., fentanyl citrate) stored in Becton Dickinson syringes for extended periods (i.e., exceeding 24 hours) were confirmed by the manufacturer of these syringes; the cause of this change was later identified to be the inclusion of an alternate rubber stopper in the plunger of certain product lots of syringes.[3029 3036 3037 3039 3041 3042] Decreased potency was not observed when the syringes were filled and used promptly.[3037] Use of the alternate stopper was later discontinued and use of the primary stopper in such syringes was resumed; however, Becton Dickinson states that its general-use syringes are cleared by FDA for immediate use in fluid aspiration and injection and that such syringes, regardless of the stopper material, have not been cleared by FDA for use as a closed-container system.[3391]

Undiluted fentanyl citrate 50 mcg/mL was tested for stability in polypropylene syringes. The fentanyl citrate injection was filled into polypropylene syringes that were then capped off. The samples were stored for 28 days under refrigeration at 5°C and at room temperature of 22°C exposed to light. No change in color or clarity occurred. No loss of fentanyl citrate at either set of storage conditions occurred.[2648]

Fentanyl citrate (Elkins Sinn) 0.0167 mg/mL in sodium chloride 0.9% packaged in polypropylene syringes (Sherwood) was physically stable and exhibited little or no loss in 24 hours stored at 4 or 23°C in the dark.[2199]

Fentanyl citrate (David Bull) 12.5 mcg/mL in sodium chloride 0.9% was packaged as 8 mL in 10-mL polypropylene syringes (Terumo) with attached needles. Fentanyl citrate (David Bull) 33.3 mcg/mL in sodium chloride 0.9% was packaged as 18 mL in 20-mL polypropylene syringes (Terumo) with attached needles. The syringes were stored at 5, 22, and 38°C for 7 days. The solutions were visually unchanged with no loss of drug at 5 and 22°C. At 38°C, the 12.5-mcg/mL solution had under 7% loss and the 33.3-mcg/mL solution had no loss.[2202]

Fentanyl citrate (Janssen) 35 mcg/mL in sodium chloride 0.9% was packaged in 2 types of polypropylene syringes. The Omnifix (B. Braun) syringes had polyisoprene piston tips while the Terumo syringes had no natural or synthetic rubber in the product. Stored at 4, 21, and 35°C for 30 days, the test solutions exhibited no visible or pH changes. Although the pH remained within the stability range for the drug, this does not demonstrate stability.[2387]

Fentanyl citrate (Hospira) was diluted to a concentration of 5 mcg/mL in sodium chloride 0.9% and packaged as 1.1 mL in 12-mL polypropylene syringes (Terumo).[2791] The syringes were stored for 90 days at a controlled temperature of 23 to 27°C and relative humidity of 55 to 65% while being protected from light.[2791] Neither changes in color or clarity nor appreciable changes in pH from baseline values occurred.[2791] Samples exhibited a loss of less than 1% at 90 days.[2791]

Ambulatory Pumps

Fentanyl citrate (Merck) 50 and 30 mcg/mL in sodium chloride 0.9% was evaluated in CADD-1 and CADD-PRIZM medication cassettes. About 4% drug loss occurred in 14 days at room and refrigeration temperatures.[2717]

Sorption

Fentanyl citrate 2 mcg/mL in various buffer solutions ranging from pH 5.5 to pH 6.7 packaged in polyvinyl chloride (PVC) containers (Baxter) was shown to undergo slow sorption to the PVC in amounts dependent on the pH of the solution. The lower pH solutions exhibited less loss with increasing loss as the pH increased. At the highest pH tested of 6.7, 17% fentanyl loss occurred in 1 day. Refrigeration decreased the extent of loss but did not eliminate it. See Table 1. Little or no fentanyl loss was found in identical fentanyl citrate 2-mcg/mL solutions packaged in glass containers.[2305]

Undiluted fentanyl citrate 50 mcg/mL was tested for stability in PVC bags. The fentanyl citrate injection was filled into PVC bags that were stored for 28 days under refrigeration at 5°C and

DOI: 10.37573/9781585286850.163

at room temperature of 22°C exposed to light. No change in color or clarity occurred. No loss of fentanyl citrate at either set of storage conditions occurred.[2648]

Table 1. Percentage of fentanyl citrate 2 mcg/mL remaining after storage for 30 days at 23°C in PVC containers[2305]

Buffer pH	Fentanyl Remaining (%)
5.5	85
5.8	77
6.3	56
6.7	27

Filtration

Fentanyl citrate (Janssen) 2.5 mcg/mL in dextrose 5% or sodium chloride 0.9% was delivered over 4 hours through 3 kinds of 0.2-μm membrane filters varying in size and composition. No fentanyl loss occurred due to sorption to the filter.[1399]

Central Venous Catheter

Fentanyl citrate (Abbott) 10 mcg/mL in dextrose 5% was found to be compatible with the ARROWg+ard Blue Plus (Arrow International) chlorhexidine-bearing triple-lumen central catheter. Essentially complete delivery of the drug was found with little or no drug loss occurring. Furthermore, chlorhexidine delivered from the catheter remained at trace amounts with no substantial increase due to the delivery of the drug through the catheter.[2335]

Compatibility Information

Solution Compatibility

Fentanyl citrate

Test Soln Name	Mfr	Mfr	Conc/L or %	Remarks	Ref	C/I
Dextrose 5%	DB,[a] TR[b]	JN	5 mg	Physically compatible. No loss in 48 hr at 22°C in light	1357	C
Dextrose 5%	AB	JN	20 and 40 mg	Visually compatible. 3% or less loss in 3 hr at 24°C	1852	C
Sodium chloride 0.9%	TR[b]	JN	20 mg	Physically compatible. Little loss in 30 days at 3 and 23°C	1356	C
Sodium chloride 0.9%	DB,[a] TR[b]	JN	5 mg	Physically compatible. No loss in 48 hr at 22°C in light	1357	C

[a] Tested in glass containers.

[b] Tested in PVC containers.

Additive Compatibility

Fentanyl citrate

Test Drug	Mfr	Conc/L or %	Mfr	Conc/L or %	Test Solution	Remarks	Ref	C/I
Bupivacaine HCl	WI	1.25 g	JN	20 mg	NS[a]	Physically compatible with little or no loss of either drug in 30 days at 3 and 23°C	1396	C
Bupivacaine HCl		1.25 g		2 mg	NS[a]	Physically compatible with no bupivacaine loss and about 6 to 7% fentanyl loss in 30 days at 4 and 23°C	2305	C
Bupivacaine HCl		600 mg		2 mg	NS[a]	Physically compatible with no bupivacaine loss and about 2 to 4% fentanyl loss in 30 days at 4 and 23°C	2305	C
Bupivacaine HCl	AST[g]	1 g	JN	35 mg	NS[a]	Visually compatible with less than 10% change of any drug in 28 days at 4°C and 24 days at 25°C in the dark	2437	C
Bupivacaine HCl	WI[h]	440 mg	JN	1.25 mg	[e]	No bupivacaine and fentanyl loss and 10% epinephrine loss in 30 days at 3 and 23°C then 48 hr at 30°C	1627	C
Bupivacaine HCl	IVX[i]	1 g	IVX	2 mg		Visually compatible with less than 10% loss of epinephrine and no loss of other drugs in 182 days at 4 and 22°C	2613	C

Additive Compatibility (Cont.)

Test Drug	Mfr	Conc/L or %	Mfr	Conc/L or %	Test Solution	Remarks	Ref	C/I
Clonidine HCl	BI[j]	9 mg	JN	35 mg	NS[a]	Visually compatible with less than 10% change of any drug in 28 days at 4°C and 24 days at 25°C in the dark	2437	C
Droperidol with ketamine HCl	JN JN	50 mg 1 g	DB	10 mg	NS[a]	Visually compatible. 5% increase in all drugs in 30 days at 4 and 25°C due to water loss	2653	C
Droperidol with ketamine HCl	JN JN	50 mg 1 g	DB	10 mg	NS[d]	Visually compatible with little loss of the drugs in 30 days at 25°C	2653	C
Epinephrine bitartrate	PHX[i]	2 mg	IVX	2 mg		Visually compatible with less than 10% loss of epinephrine and no loss of other drugs in 182 days at 4 and 22°C	2613	C
Epinephrine HCl	AB[k]	0.69 mg	JN	1.25 mg	[e]	No bupivacaine and fentanyl loss and 10% epinephrine loss in 30 days at 3 and 23°C then 48 hr at 30°C	1627	C
Fluorouracil	AB	1 and 16 g	AB	12.5 mg	D5W, NS[a]	25% fentanyl loss in 15 min due to sorption to PVC	2064	I
Ketamine HCl with droperidol	JN JN	1 g 50 mg	DB	10 mg	NS[a]	Visually compatible. 5% increase in all drugs in 30 days at 4 and 25°C due to water loss	2653	C
Ketamine HCl with droperidol	JN JN	1 g 50 mg	DB	10 mg	NS[d]	Visually compatible with little loss of the drugs in 30 days at 25°C	2653	C
Lidocaine HCl	AST	2.5 g		2 mg	NS[a]	Physically compatible with no loss of lidocaine or fentanyl at pH 5.8 in 30 days at 4 and 23°C	2305	C
Lidocaine HCl	BRN	2.5 g		2 mg	NS[a]	Physically compatible with little lidocaine loss but 18% fentanyl loss at 23°C and 10% loss at 4°C in 2 days due to sorption at pH 6.7 from higher pH lidocaine product	2305	I
Ropivacaine HCl	ASZ	1 g	JN	1 mg	NS[b]	Physically compatible. No loss of either drug in 30 days at 30°C in the dark	2433	C
Ropivacaine HCl	ASZ	2 g	JN	1 and 10 mg	[b]	Physically compatible. No loss of either drug in 30 days at 30°C in the dark	2433	C
Ropivacaine HCl	ASZ	1.5 g	CUR	3 mg	NS[c]	Physically compatible. No loss of either drug in 51 days at 20 and 4°C	2498	C
Ropivacaine HCl	ASZ	1.5 g	CUR	3 mg	NS[a]	Physically compatible. No loss of either drug in 7 days at 20 and 4°C	2498	C
Ziconotide acetate	ELN	25 mg[b]	BB	1 g[f]		10% ziconotide loss in 26 days. No fentanyl loss in 40 days at 37°C	2772	C

[a] Tested in PVC containers.

[b] Tested in polypropylene bags (Mark II Polybags).

[c] Tested in glass and ethylene vinyl acetate containers.

[d] Tested in glass containers.

[e] Tested in portable infusion pump reservoirs (Pharmacia Deltec).

[f] Fentanyl citrate powder dissolved in ziconotide acetate injection.

[g] Tested with clonidine HCl (BI) 9 mg.

[h] Tested with epinephrine HCl (AB) 0.69 mg.

[i] Tested with epinephrine bitartrate (PHX) 2 mg.

[j] Tested with bupivacaine HCl (AST) 1 g.

[k] Tested with bupivacaine HCl (WI) 440 mg.

[l] Tested with bupivacaine HCl (IVX) 1 g.

Drugs in Syringe Compatibility

Fentanyl citrate

Test Drug	Mfr	Amt	Mfr	Amt	Remarks	Ref	C/I
Atracurium besylate	BW	10 mg/mL		50 mcg/mL	Physically compatible and atracurium stable for 24 hr at 5 and 30°C	1694	C
Atropine sulfate		0.6 mg/1.5 mL	MN	100 mcg/1 mL	Physically compatible for at least 15 min	14	C
Atropine sulfate	ST	0.4 mg/1 mL	MN	0.05 mg/1 mL	Physically compatible for at least 15 min	326	C
Bupivacaine HCl with clonidine HCl	AST BI	50 mg 0.45 mg	JN	1.75 mg	Diluted to 50 mL with NS. Visually compatible with less than 10% loss of any drug in 25 days at 4 and 25°C in the dark	2437	C
Bupivacaine HCl with ketamine HCl	SW PD	1.5 mg/mL 2 mg/mL	JN	0.01 mg/mL	Diluted to 5 mL with NS. Visually compatible with no new GC/MS peaks in 1 hr at room temperature	1956	C
Butorphanol tartrate	BR	4 mg/2 mL	MN	0.1 mg/2 mL	Physically compatible for 30 min at room temperature	566	C
Caffeine citrate		20 mg/1 mL	ES	50 mcg/1 mL	Visually compatible for 4 hr at 25°C	2440	C
Chlorpromazine HCl	PO	50 mg/2 mL	MN	0.05 mg/1 mL	Physically compatible for at least 15 min	326	C
Clonidine HCl with bupivacaine HCl	BI AST	0.45 mg 50 mg	JN	1.75 mg	Diluted to 50 mL with NS. Visually compatible with less than 10% loss of any drug in 25 days at 4 and 25°C in the dark	2437	C
Clonidine HCl with lidocaine HCl	BI AST	0.03 mg/mL 2 mg/mL	JN	0.01 mg/mL	Diluted to 5 mL with NS. Visually compatible with no new GC/MS peaks in 1 hr at room temperature	1956	C
Dimenhydrinate	HR	50 mg/1 mL	MN	0.05 mg/1 mL	Physically compatible for at least 15 min	326	C
Diphenhydramine HCl	PD	50 mg/1 mL	MN	0.05 mg/1 mL	Physically compatible for at least 15 min	326	C
Droperidol	MN	2.5 mg/1 mL	MN	0.05 mg/1 mL	Physically compatible for at least 15 min	326	C
Heparin sodium		2500 units/1 mL	JN	0.1 mg/2 mL	Physically compatible for at least 5 min	1053	C
Hydromorphone HCl	KN	4 mg/2 mL	MN	0.05 mg/1 mL	Physically compatible for 30 min	517	C
Hydroxyzine HCl	PF	50 mg/1 mL	MN	0.05 mg/1 mL	Physically compatible for at least 15 min	326	C
Hydroxyzine HCl	PF	50 mg/1 mL	CR	0.05 mg/1 mL	Physically compatible	771	C
Hydroxyzine HCl	PF	100 mg/2 mL	CR	0.05 mg/1 mL	Physically compatible	771	C
Ketamine HCl	PF	1 mg/mL		40 mcg/mL	Diluted in sodium chloride 0.9%. Physically compatible for 96 hr at 25°C	2563	C
Ketamine HCl with bupivacaine HCl	PD SW	2 mg/mL 1.5 mg/mL	JN	0.01 mg/mL	Diluted to 5 mL with NS. Visually compatible with no new GC/MS peaks in 1 hr at room temperature	1956	C
Lidocaine HCl with clonidine HCl	AST BI	2 mg/mL 0.03 mg/mL	JN	0.01 mg/mL	Diluted to 5 mL with NS. Visually compatible with no new GC/MS peaks in 1 hr at room temperature	1956	C
Meperidine HCl	WI	50 mg/1 mL	MN	0.05 mg/1 mL	Physically compatible for at least 15 min	326	C
Metoclopramide HCl	NO	10 mg/2 mL	MN	0.05 mg/1 mL	Physically compatible for 15 min at room temperature	565	C
Metoclopramide HCl with midazolam HCl	AST RC	20 mg/4 mL 15 mg/3 mL	DB	1 mg/20 mL	Visually compatible with 7% or less loss of each drug in 10 days at 32°C	2268	C
Midazolam HCl	RC	5 mg/1 mL	ES	0.1 mg/2 mL	Physically compatible for 4 hr at 25°C	1145	C

Drugs in Syringe Compatibility (Cont.)

Test Drug	Mfr	Amt	Mfr	Amt	Remarks	Ref	C/I
Midazolam HCl	RC	0.625 and 0.938 mg/mL[a]	DB	12.5 mcg/mL[a]	Visually compatible. Little fentanyl loss. 7 and 9% midazolam loss in 7 days at 5 and 22°C, respectively	2202	C
Midazolam HCl	RC	0.625 mg/mL[a]	DB	37.5 mcg/mL[a]	Visually compatible. No fentanyl loss. 5 and 8% midazolam loss in 7 days at 5 and 22°C, respectively	2202	C
Midazolam HCl	RC	0.938 mg/mL[a]	DB	37.5 mcg/mL[a]	Visually compatible. Little fentanyl loss. 7 and 9% midazolam loss in 7 days at 5 and 22°C, respectively	2202	C
Midazolam HCl	RC	0.278 and 0.833 mg/mL[a]	DB	33.3 mcg/mL[a]	Visually compatible. No fentanyl loss. 5 and 7% midazolam loss in 7 days at 5 and 22°C, respectively	2202	C
Midazolam HCl with metoclopramide HCl	RC AST	15 mg/3 mL 20 mg/4 mL	DB	1 mg/20 mL	Visually compatible with 7% or less loss of each drug in 10 days at 32°C	2268	C
Morphine sulfate	ST	15 mg/1 mL	MN	0.05 mg/1 mL	Physically compatible for at least 15 min	326	C
Ondansetron HCl	GW	1.33 mg/mL[a]	ES	16.7 mcg/mL[a]	Physically compatible. Little loss of either drug in 24 hr at 4 or 23°C	2199	C
Pantoprazole sodium	[b]	4 mg/1 mL		50 mcg/1 mL	Possible precipitate within 15 min	2574	I
Pentazocine lactate	WI	30 mg/1 mL	MN	0.05 mg/1 mL	Physically compatible for at least 15 min	326	C
Pentobarbital sodium	AB	50 mg/1 mL	MN	0.05 mg/1 mL	Physically incompatible within 15 min	326	I
Prochlorperazine edisylate	PO	5 mg/1 mL	MN	0.05 mg/1 mL	Physically compatible for at least 15 min	326	C
Promethazine HCl	PO	50 mg/2 mL	MN	0.05 mg/1 mL	Physically compatible for at least 15 min	326	C
Ranitidine HCl	GL	50 mg/2 mL	JN	0.1 mg/2 mL	Physically compatible for 1 hr at 25°C	978	C
Scopolamine HBr		0.6 mg/1.5 mL	MN	100 mcg/1 mL	Physically compatible for at least 15 min	14	C
Scopolamine HBr	ST	0.4 mg/1 mL	MN	0.05 mg/1 mL	Physically compatible for at least 15 min	326	C

[a] Tested in sodium chloride 0.9%.

[b] Test performed using the formulation WITHOUT edetate disodium.

Y-Site Injection Compatibility (1:1 Mixture)

Fentanyl citrate

Test Drug	Mfr	Conc	Mfr	Conc	Remarks	Ref	C/I
Abciximab	LI	36 mcg/mL[a]	AB	50 mcg/mL	Visually compatible for 12 hr at 23°C	2374	C
Acetaminophen	CAD	10 mg/mL	TAY, HOS	50 mcg/mL	Physically compatible with less than 10% acetaminophen loss over 4 hr at room temperature	2841, 2844	C
Acyclovir sodium	BV	5 mg/mL[b]	HOS	50 mcg/mL	Physically compatible	2794	C
Alprostadil	BED	7.5 mcg/mL[k l]	JN	10 mcg/mL[j]	Visually compatible for 1 hr	2746	C
Amiodarone HCl	WY	6 mg/mL[a]	BA	50 mcg/mL	Visually compatible for 24 hr at 22°C	2352	C
Anidulafungin	VIC	0.5 mg/mL[a]	AB	50 mcg/mL	Physically compatible for 4 hr at 23°C	2617	C
Argatroban	GSK	1 mg/mL[b]	ES	50 mcg/mL	Visually compatible for 24 hr at 23°C	2391	C

Y-Site Injection Compatibility (1:1 Mixture) (Cont.)

Test Drug	Mfr	Conc	Mfr	Conc	Remarks	Ref	C/I
Atracurium besylate	BW	0.5 mg/mL[a]	ES	10 mcg/mL[a]	Physically compatible for 24 hr at 28°C	1337	C
Atropine sulfate	LY	0.4 mg/mL	JN	25 mcg/mL[a]	Physically compatible for 48 hr at 22°C	1706	C
Azithromycin	PF	2 mg/mL[b]	AB	50 mcg/mL[i]	Whitish-yellow microcrystals found	2368	I
Bivalirudin	TMC	5 mg/mL[a]	AB	50 mcg/mL	Physically compatible for 4 hr at 23°C	2373	C
Bivalirudin	TMC	5 mg/mL[a b]	TAY	50 mcg/mL	Visually compatible for 6 hr at 23°C	2680	C
Caffeine citrate		20 mg/mL		10 mcg/mL[a]	Compatible and stable for 24 hr at room temperature	1(1/08)	C
Cangrelor tetrasodium	TMC	1 mg/mL[b]		12.5 mcg/mL[b]	Physically compatible for 4 hr	3243	C
Caspofungin acetate	ME	0.7 mg/mL[b]	HOS	0.05 mg/mL	Physically compatible for 4 hr at room temperature	2758	C
Caspofungin acetate	ME	0.5 mg/mL[b]	HOS	0.05 mg/mL	Physically compatible with fentanyl citrate i.v. push over 2 to 5 min	2766	C
Ceftaroline fosamil	FOR	2.22 mg/mL[a b m]	HOS	50 mcg/mL	Physically compatible for 4 hr at 23°C	2826	C
Ceftolozane sulfate–tazobactam sodium	CUB	10 mg/mL[o p]	WW	50 mcg/mL	Physically compatible for 2 hr	3247, 3262	C
Cisatracurium besylate	GW	0.1, 2, 5 mg/mL[a]	AB	12.5 mcg/mL[a]	Physically compatible for 4 hr at 23°C	2074	C
Clonidine HCl	BI	18 mcg/mL[b]	ALP	50 mcg/mL	Visually compatible	2642	C
Cloxacillin sodium	SMX	100 mg/mL	SZ	50 mcg/mL	Physically compatible for up to 4 hr at room temperature	3245	C
Dexamethasone sodium phosphate	AMR	1 mg/mL[a]	JN	0.025 mg/mL[a]	Physically compatible for 48 hr at 22°C	1706	C
Dexmedetomidine HCl	HOS	4 mcg/mL[b]			Stated to be compatible	3181	C
Diazepam	ES	0.5 mg/mL[a]	JN	0.025 mg/mL[a]	Physically compatible for 48 hr at 22°C	1706	C
Diltiazem HCl	MMD	1 mg/mL[a]	ES	0.05 mg/mL	Visually compatible for 4 hr at 27°C	2062	C
Diphenhydramine HCl	SCN	2 mg/mL[a]	JN	0.025 mg/mL[a]	Physically compatible for 48 hr at 22°C	1706	C
Dobutamine HCl	LI	4 mg/mL[a]	ES	0.05 mg/mL	Visually compatible for 4 hr at 27°C	2062	C
Dopamine HCl	AB	3.2 mg/mL[a]	ES	0.05 mg/mL	Visually compatible for 4 hr at 27°C	2062	C
Doripenem	JJ	5 mg/mL[a b]	HOS	0.05 mg/mL	Physically compatible for 4 hr at 23°C	2743	C
Doxapram HCl	RB	2 mg/mL[a]	ESL	25 mcg/mL[a]	Visually compatible for 4 hr at 23°C	2470	C
Enalaprilat	MSD	0.05 mg/mL[b]	ES	2 mcg/mL[a]	Physically compatible for 24 hr at room temperature under fluorescent light	1355	C
Epinephrine HCl	AB	0.02 mg/mL[a]	ES	0.05 mg/mL	Visually compatible for 4 hr at 27°C	2062	C
Eravacycline dihydrochloride	TET	0.6 mg/mL[b]	WW	50 mcg/mL	Physically compatible for 2 hr at room temperature	3532	C
Esmolol HCl	DCC	1 g/100 mL[c]	JN	0.05 mg/1 mL	Physically compatible when fentanyl is injected into Y-site of flowing admixture[d]	1168	C
Esmolol HCl	DCC	10 mg/mL[c]	JN	0.05 mg/mL	Physically compatible. No drug loss in 8 hr at room temperature in light	1168	C
Etomidate	AB	2 mg/mL	ES	0.05 mg/mL	Visually compatible for 7 days at 25°C	1801	C
Fenoldopam mesylate	AB	80 mcg/mL[b]	AB	12.5 mcg/mL[b]	Physically compatible for 4 hr at 23°C	2467	C
Furosemide	AMR	10 mg/mL	ES	0.05 mg/mL	Visually compatible for 4 hr at 27°C	2062	C
Haloperidol lactate	MN	0.2 mg/mL[a]	JN	0.025 mg/mL[a]	Physically compatible for 48 hr at 22°C	1706	C

Y-Site Injection Compatibility (1:1 Mixture) (Cont.)

Test Drug	Mfr	Conc	Mfr	Conc	Remarks	Ref	C/I
Heparin sodium	UP	1000 units/L[e]	MN	0.05 mg/mL	Physically compatible for 4 hr at room temperature	534	C
Heparin sodium	ES	100 units/mL[a]	ES	0.05 mg/mL	Visually compatible for 4 hr at 27°C	2062	C
Hetastarch in lactated electrolyte	AB	6%	ES	12.5 mcg/mL[a]	Physically compatible for 4 hr at 23°C	2339	C
Hydrocortisone sodium succinate	UP	10 mg/L[e]	MN	0.05 mg/mL	Physically compatible for 4 hr at room temperature	534	C
Hydromorphone HCl	KN	1 mg/mL	ES	0.05 mg/mL	Visually compatible for 4 hr at 27°C	2062	C
Hydroxyethyl starch 130/0.4 in sodium chloride 0.9%	FRK	6%	SZ	20[a], 35[a], 50 mcg/mL	Visually compatible for 24 hr at room temperature	2770	C
Hydroxyzine HCl	WI	4 mg/mL[a]	JN	0.025 mg/mL[a]	Physically compatible for 48 hr at 22°C	1706	C
Isavuconazonium sulfate	ASP	1.5 mg/mL[o]	WW	50 mcg/mL	Physically compatible for 2 hr	3263	C
Ketorolac tromethamine	WY	1 mg/mL[a]	JN	0.025 mg/mL[a]	Physically compatible for 48 hr at 22°C	1706	C
Labetalol HCl	SC	1 mg/mL[a]	JN	10 mcg/mL[a]	Physically compatible for 24 hr at 18°C	1171	C
Labetalol HCl	AH	2 mg/mL[a]	ES	0.05 mg/mL	Visually compatible for 4 hr at 27°C	2062	C
Letermovir	ME	[b]		[b]	Physically compatible	3398	C
Levofloxacin	OMN	5 mg/mL[a]	AB	0.05 mg/mL	Visually compatible for 4 hr at 24°C	2233	C
Linezolid	PHU	2 mg/mL	AB	0.05 mg/mL	Physically compatible for 4 hr at 23°C	2264	C
Lorazepam	WY	0.33 mg/mL[b]		0.05 mg/mL	Visually compatible for 24 hr at 22°C	1855	C
Lorazepam	WY	0.5 mg/mL[a]	ES	0.05 mg/mL	Visually compatible for 4 hr at 27°C	2062	C
Lorazepam	WY	0.1 mg/mL[a]	JN	0.025 mg/mL[a]	Physically compatible for 48 hr at 22°C	1706	C
Meropenem		50 mg/mL	SZ	50 mcg/mL	Physically compatible for 4 hr at room temperature	3538	C
Meropenem–vaborbactam	TMC	8 mg/mL[b q]	HOS	50 mcg/mL	Physically compatible for 3 hr at 20 to 25°C	3380	C
Methotrimeprazine HCl	LE	0.2 mg/mL[a]	JN	0.025 mg/mL[a]	Physically compatible for 48 hr at 22°C	1706	C
Metoclopramide HCl	DU	5 mg/mL	JN	0.025 mg/mL[a]	Physically compatible for 48 hr at 22°C	1706	C
Midazolam HCl	RC	1 mg/mL[a]	ES	0.05 mg/mL	Visually compatible for 24 hr at 23°C	1847	C
Midazolam HCl	RC	0.1 and 0.5 mg/mL[a]	JN	0.02 mg/mL[a]	Visually compatible. No midazolam and 4% fentanyl loss in 3 hr at 24°C	1852	C
Midazolam HCl	RC	0.1 and 0.5 mg/mL[a]	JN	0.04 mg/mL[a]	Visually compatible with no loss of either drug in 3 hr at 24°C	1852	C
Midazolam HCl	RC	5 mg/mL		0.05 mg/mL[a]	Visually compatible for 24 hr at 22°C	1855	C
Midazolam HCl	RC	2 mg/mL[a]	ES	0.05 mg/mL	Visually compatible for 4 hr at 27°C	2062	C
Midazolam HCl	RC	0.2 mg/mL[a]	JN	0.025 mg/mL[a]	Physically compatible for 48 hr at 22°C	1706	C
Milrinone lactate	SW	0.2 mg/mL[a]	ES	0.05 mg/mL	Visually compatible for 4 hr at 27°C	2062	C
Milrinone lactate	SW	0.4 mg/mL[a]	ES	50 mcg/mL	Visually compatible. Little loss of either drug in 4 hr at 23°C	2214	C

Y-Site Injection Compatibility (1:1 Mixture) (Cont.)

Test Drug	Mfr	Conc	Mfr	Conc	Remarks	Ref	C/I
Morphine sulfate	SCN	2 mg/mL[a]	ES	0.05 mg/mL	Visually compatible for 4 hr at 27°C	2062	C
Nafcillin sodium	WY	33 mg/mL[b]		0.05 mg/mL	No precipitation	547	C
Nesiritide	SCI	50 mcg/mL[a b]		0.05 mg/mL	Physically compatible for 4 hr	2625	C
Nicardipine HCl	WY	1 mg/mL[a]	ES	0.05 mg/mL	Visually compatible for 4 hr at 27°C	2062	C
Nicardipine HCl	DCC	0.1 mg/mL[a]	ES	2 mcg/mL[a]	Visually compatible for 24 hr at room temperature	235	C
Nitroglycerin	AB	0.4 mg/mL[a]	ES	0.05 mg/mL	Visually compatible for 4 hr at 27°C	2062	C
Norepinephrine bitartrate	AB	0.128 mg/mL[a]	ES	0.05 mg/mL	Visually compatible for 4 hr at 27°C	2062	C
Oritavancin diphosphate	TAR	0.8, 1.2, and 2 mg/mL[a]	HOS	50 mcg/mL[n]	Visually compatible for 4 hr at 20 to 24°C	2928	C
Oxaliplatin	SS	0.5 mg/mL[a]	AB	0.05 mg/mL[a]	Physically compatible for 4 hr at 23°C	2566	C
Palonosetron HCl	MGI	50 mcg/mL	AB	50 mcg/mL	Physically compatible and no loss of either drug in 4 hr	2720	C
Pancuronium bromide	ES	0.05 mg/mL[a]	ES	10 mcg/mL[a]	Physically compatible for 24 hr at 28°C	1337	C
Phenobarbital sodium	WY	2 mg/mL[a]	JN	0.025 mg/mL[a]	Physically compatible for 48 hr at 22°C	1706	C
Phenytoin sodium	ES	2 mg/mL[a b]	JN	0.025 mg/mL[a]	Precipitate forms within 1 hr	1706	I
Plazomicin sulfate	ACH	24 mg/mL[o]	WW	50 mcg/mL	Physically compatible for 1 hr at 20 to 25°C	3432	C
Posaconazole	ME	18 mg/mL		0.05 mg/mL[o]	Physically compatible	2912	C
Potassium chloride	AB	40 mEq/L[e]	MN	0.05 mg/mL	Physically compatible for 4 hr at room temperature	534	C
Propofol	ZEN[r]	10 mg/mL	AB	0.05 mg/mL	Physically compatible for 1 hr at 23°C	2066	C
Ranitidine HCl	GL	1 mg/mL[a]	ES	0.05 mg/mL	Visually compatible for 4 hr at 27°C	2062	C
Remifentanil HCl	GW	0.025 and 0.25 mg/mL[b]	ES	12.5 mcg/mL[a]	Physically compatible for 4 hr at 23°C	2075	C
Sargramostim	IMM	6[f] and 15 mcg/mL[b]	ES	50 mcg/mL	Visually compatible for 2 hr	1618	C
Scopolamine HBr	LY	0.05 mg/mL[a]	JN	0.025 mg/mL[a]	Physically compatible for 48 hr at 22°C	1706	C
Tedizolid phosphate	CUB	0.8 mg/mL[b]	WW	50 mcg/mL	Physically compatible for 2 hr	3244	C
TNA #218[h]			AB	12.5[a] and 50 mcg/mL	Visually compatible for 4 hr at 23°C	2215	C
TNA #219[h]			AB	12.5[a] and 50 mcg/mL	Visually compatible for 4 hr at 23°C	2215	C
TNA #220[h]			AB	12.5[a] and 50 mcg/mL	Visually compatible for 4 hr at 23°C	2215	C
TNA #221[h]			AB	12.5[a] and 50 mcg/mL	Visually compatible for 4 hr at 23°C	2215	C
TNA #222[h]			AB	12.5[a] and 50 mcg/mL	Visually compatible for 4 hr at 23°C	2215	C
TNA #223[h]			AB	12.5[a] and 50 mcg/mL	Visually compatible for 4 hr at 23°C	2215	C
TNA #224[h]			AB	12.5[a] and 50 mcg/mL	Visually compatible for 4 hr at 23°C	2215	C

Y-Site Injection Compatibility (1:1 Mixture) (Cont.)

Test Drug	Mfr	Conc	Mfr	Conc	Remarks	Ref	C/I
TNA #225[h]			AB	12.5[a] and 50 mcg/mL	Visually compatible for 4 hr at 23°C	2215	C
TNA #226[h]			AB	12.5[a] and 50 mcg/mL	Visually compatible for 4 hr at 23°C	2215	C
TPN #203[h]			ES	0.05 mg/mL	Visually compatible for 4 hr at 23°C	1974	C
TPN #204[h]			ES	0.05 mg/mL	Visually compatible for 4 hr at 23°C	1974	C
TPN #212[h]			AB	0.0125 and 0.05 mg/mL[a]	Physically compatible for 4 hr at 23°C	2109	C
TPN #213[h]			AB	0.0125 and 0.05 mg/mL[a]	Physically compatible for 4 hr at 23°C	2109	C
TPN #214[h]			AB	0.0125 and 0.05 mg/mL[a]	Physically compatible for 4 hr at 23°C	2109	C
TPN #215[h]			AB	0.0125 and 0.05 mg/mL[a]	Physically compatible for 4 hr at 23°C	2109	C
TPN #216[h]			ES	0.01 mg/mL[g]	Mixed 1 mL of fentanyl with 9 mL of TPN. Visually compatible for 24 hr	2104	C
Vecuronium bromide	OR	0.1 mg/mL[a]	ES	10 mcg/mL[a]	Physically compatible for 24 hr at 28°C	1337	C
Vecuronium bromide	OR	1 mg/mL	ES	0.05 mg/mL	Visually compatible for 4 hr at 27°C	2062	C

[a] Tested in dextrose 5%.

[b] Tested in sodium chloride 0.9%.

[c] Tested in dextrose 5% in sodium chloride 0.9%.

[d] Flowing at 1.6 mL/min.

[e] Tested in dextrose 5% in Ringer's injection, dextrose 5% in Ringer's injection, lactated, dextrose 5%, Ringer's injection, lactated, and sodium chloride 0.9%.

[f] Tested with albumin human 0.1%.

[g] Tested in sterile water for injection.

[h] Refer to Appendix for the composition of parenteral nutrition solutions. TNA indicates a 3-in-1 admixture, and TPN indicates a 2-in-1 admixture.

[i] Injected via Y-site into an administration set running azithromycin.

[j] Tested in either dextrose 5% or in sodium chloride 0.9%, but the report did not specify which solution.

[k] Tested in a 1:1 mixture of (1) dextrose 5% and dextrose 5% in sodium chloride 0.45% with and without potassium chloride 20 mEq/L and also in (2) dextrose 10% in sodium chloride 0.45% with and without potassium chloride 20 mEq/L.

[l] Tested in a 1:1 mixture of dextrose 5% and TPN #274 (see Appendix).

[m] Tested in Ringer's injection, lactated.

[n] Tested undiluted.

[o] Tested in both dextrose 5% and sodium chloride 0.9%.

[p] Ceftolozane component. Ceftolozane in a 2:1 fixed-ratio concentration with tazobactam.

[q] Meropenem component. Meropenem in a 1:1 fixed-ratio concentration with vaborbactam.

[r] Test performed using the formulation WITH edetate disodium.

Selected Revisions May 1, 2020. © Copyright, October 1982.
American Society of Health-System Pharmacists, Inc.

Ferric Carboxymaltose
AHFS 20:04.04

Products

Ferric carboxymaltose injection is available as a dark brown colloidal solution in 15-mL single-use vials containing 750 mg of elemental iron.[3374] Each mL of the solution contains 50 mg of elemental iron in water for injection.[3374] Vials also may contain sodium hydroxide and/or hydrochloric acid to adjust the pH.[3374]

pH

From 5 to 7.[3374]

Tonicity

The undiluted solution of ferric carboxymaltose injection containing 50 mg of elemental iron per mL is isotonic.[3374]

Trade Name(s)

Injectafer

Administration

Ferric carboxymaltose injection is administered intravenously, either injected undiluted as a slow intravenous push or diluted in a compatible infusion solution for intravenous infusion.[3374]

For slow intravenous push administration, the drug should be administered undiluted at a rate of approximately 100 mg (2 mL)/min.[3374]

For intravenous infusion, doses of up to 750 mg of elemental iron should be diluted in up to 250 mL of sodium chloride 0.9% to yield a diluted solution for infusion with a concentration of elemental iron that is at least 2 mg/mL.[3374] Such diluted solutions for infusion should be administered over at least 15 minutes.[3374]

Extravasation of ferric carboxymaltose injection should be avoided as it may cause a persistent brown discoloration at the extravasation site.[3374] Patients should be monitored for extravasation of the drug during administration; if extravasation occurs, administration at that site should be discontinued.[3374]

Stability

Intact vials should be stored at controlled room temperature; freezing should be avoided.[3374]

In colloidal solutions such as ferric carboxymaltose colloidal solution, the complex may be destabilized if diluted too much;[3375] in order to maintain stability, ferric carboxymaltose injection should not be diluted to a concentration of elemental iron that is less than 2 mg/mL.[3374]

Ferric carboxymaltose injection should be visually inspected for particulate matter and discoloration prior to administration.[3374] Vials are for single use; any unused portion should be discarded.[3374]

Evaluating the stability of non-biological complex drugs, like ferric carboxymaltose, which are large, synthetic, and complex products, requires the use of a variety of assessments.[3375] In one study, ferric carboxymaltose (Vifor Pharma) injection was diluted in sodium chloride 0.9% to elemental iron concentrations of 1, 2, and 5 mg/mL in polypropylene bottles and bags.[3375] Stability tests showed that the total iron content in solutions (as assessed by complexometric titration with ethylenediaminetetraacetic acid [EDTA]) was within 10% of the theoretical iron content for up to 72 hours at room temperature (30°C) and 70 to 80% relative humidity.[3375] Additionally, the molecular weight distribution of ferric carboxymaltose was essentially unchanged.[3375] Diluted solutions of ferric carboxymaltose injection also were found to be free from sediment on visual inspection and had pH values and particle counts that were within the limits of acceptability during this study period.[3375]

Sorption

In one study, ferric carboxymaltose (Vifor Pharma) injection diluted in sodium chloride 0.9% to elemental iron concentrations of 1, 2, and 5 mg/mL and stored for up to 72 h at 30°C and 70 to 80% relative humidity in polypropylene bottles and bags showed no measurable sorption of iron to the surface of the containers.[3375]

Compatibility Information

Solution Compatibility

Ferric carboxymaltose

Test Soln Name	Mfr	Mfr	Conc/L or %	Remarks	Ref	C/I
Sodium chloride 0.9%		AMR	2 to 4 g	Physically and chemically stable for 72 hr at room temperature	3374	C

DOI: 10.37573/9781585286850.164

Ferric Derisomaltose
AHFS 20:04.04

Products

Ferric derisomaltose injection is available as a dark brown, nontransparent solution in 1-, 5-, and 10-mL single-dose (preservative-free) vials containing 100, 500, and 1000 mg of elemental iron, respectively.[3549] Each mL of the solution contains 100 mg of elemental iron in water for injection.[3549]

pH

Ferric derisomaltose injection has a pH ranging from 5 to 7.[3549]

Trade Name(s)

Monoferric

Administration

Ferric derisomaltose is administered as an intravenous infusion over at least 20 minutes after dilution of the drug in 100 to 500 mL of sodium chloride 0.9% to a final concentration exceeding 1 mg of elemental iron per mL.[3549]

Extravasation of ferric derisomaltose injection should be avoided as it may cause a persistent brown discoloration at the extravasation site.[3549] Patients should be monitored for extravasation of the drug during administration; if extravasation occurs, administration at that site should be discontinued.[3549]

Stability

Intact vials of ferric derisomaltose should be stored at controlled room temperature; freezing should be avoided.[3549]

Ferric derisomaltose injection should be visually inspected for particulate matter and discoloration prior to administration.[3549] The manufacturer states that the drug should not be mixed with or added to solutions containing other drugs.[3549]

Compatibility Information

Solution Compatibility

Ferric derisomaltose

Test Soln Name	Mfr	Mfr	Conc/L or %	Remarks	Ref	C/I
Sodium chloride 0.9%		PHM		May be stored for up to 8 hr at room temperature	3549	C

© Copyright, July 2020. American Society of Health-System Pharmacists, Inc.

DOI: 10.37573/9781585286850.165

Ferumoxytol
AHFS 20:04.04

Products

Ferumoxytol injection is available as a black to reddish brown colloidal solution in single-use (preservative-free) vials containing 510 mg of elemental iron.[3550] Each mL of the solution contains 30 mg of elemental iron, as well as polyglucose sorbitol carboxymethylether 30 mg and mannitol 44 mg.[3550]

pH

Ferumoxytol injection has a pH ranging from 6 to 8.[3550]

Tonicity

Ferumoxytol injection is isotonic.[3550]

Osmolality

Ferumoxytol injection has an osmolality of 270 to 330 mOsmol/kg.[3550]

Trade Name(s)

Feraheme

Administration

Ferumoxytol is administered only as an intravenous infusion over at least 15 minutes after dilution of the drug in 50 to 200 mL of sodium chloride 0.9% or dextrose 5%.[3550]

Stability

Intact vials of ferumoxytol should be stored at controlled room temperature.[3550]

Ferumoxytol injection should be visually inspected for particulate matter and discoloration prior to administration.[3550]

Compatibility Information

Solution Compatibility

Ferumoxytol

Test Soln Name	Mfr	Mfr	Conc/L or %	Remarks	Ref	C/I
Dextrose 5%		AMA	2 to 8 g	May be stored at room temperature of 23 to 27°C for up to 4 hr or refrigerated at 2 to 8°C for up to 48 hr	3550	C
Sodium chloride 0.9%		AMAG	2 to 8 g	May be stored at room temperature of 23 to 27°C for up to 4 hr or refrigerated at 2 to 8°C for up to 48 hr	3550	C

DOI: 10.37573/9781585286850.166

Filgrastim

AHFS 20:16

Products

Filgrastim is available in 300- and 480-mcg vials and syringes with the product compositions and package configurations shown in Table 1.[2873]

Table 1. Filgrastim products and compositions[2873]

	300 mcg/ 1-mL Vial	480 mcg/ 1.6-mL Vial	300 mcg/ 0.5-mL Syringe	480 mcg/ 0.8-mL Syringe
Filgrastim	300 mcg	480 mcg	300 mcg	480 mcg
Acetate	0.59 mg	0.94 mg	0.295 mg	0.472 mg
Sorbitol	50 mg	80 mg	25 mg	40 mg
Polysorbate 80	0.004%	0.004%	0.004%	0.004%
Sodium	0.035 mg	0.056 mg	0.0175 mg	0.028 mg
Water for injection qs	1 mL	1.6 mL	0.5 mL	0.8 mL

Trade Name(s)

Neupogen

Administration

Filgrastim is administered by subcutaneous injection undiluted or by intravenous or subcutaneous infusion.[4][2873] For intravenous infusion, it is diluted in 50 to 100 mL of dextrose 5% and given over 15 to 30 minutes, 60 minutes, or 4 hours or over 24 hours by continuous infusion.[4][2873] It may also be given over 24 hours by continuous subcutaneous infusion[2873] after diluting the dose in 10 to 50 mL of dextrose 5% and infusing at a rate not exceeding 10 mL/24 hours.[4] For extended infusions by either route, a controlled-infusion device is used.[4] For filgrastim concentrations of 5 to 15 mcg/mL, albumin human should be added to the infusion solution at a final concentration of 0.2% (2 mg/mL).[2873] The drug should not be diluted to concentrations less than 5 mcg/mL.[2873]

Stability

Filgrastim injection is a clear, colorless solution.[2873] Intact containers should be refrigerated at 2 to 8°C and protected from direct sunlight.[2873] The product also should be protected from freezing[2873] and temperatures above 30°C to avoid aggregation.[4] The solution should not be shaken since this may damage the drug.[2873] If vigorous shaking and subsequent foaming has occurred, the solution should not be used.[2873]

Although refrigerated storage is required, the manufacturer has stated that filgrastim may be stored at room temperature for up to 24 hours,[2873] while others have stated that the drug is stable for 7 days at room temperature.[2745] The product is packaged in single-use containers with no antibacterial preservative.[2873] The manufacturer recommends that vials not be reentered and that unused portions be discarded.[2873]

Filgrastim dilutions in dextrose 5% prepared for infusion should be stored under refrigeration and used within 24 hours of preparation because of concern about possible bacterial contamination.[4]

pH Effects

Filgrastim is stable at pH 3.8 to 4.2, but stability is limited at neutral pH.[4]

Syringes

Undiluted filgrastim is stable for 24 hours at 15 to 30°C and for 7 days refrigerated at 2 to 8°C repackaged in tuberculin syringes (Becton Dickinson). However, refrigeration and use within 24 hours are recommended because of concern about bacterial contamination.[4]

Although studies have found filgrastim in syringes remained sterile stored under refrigeration,[1764][2186] the sterility of repackaged injections is a function of the quality of the specific aseptic process of packaging, the quality of the environment in which the sterile product is packaged, and the capability of the personnel involved rather than a property of this unpreserved injection. Consequently, sterility is only valid for the specific facilities and operators for that specific test. The adequacy and safety of repackaging in another location or with other individuals or on another occasion should be verified independently for each institution and batch of repackaged filgrastim injection. Each institution needs to establish specific validation testing results for its own aseptic processing facilities, equipment, procedures, and personnel.[1765][2187] The potential for microbiological growth should be considered when assigning expiration periods.

The sterility of filgrastim 0.2 mL (60 mcg) extemporaneously drawn aseptically into tuberculin syringes and kept under "patient use" storage conditions was evaluated. The syringes were sent home with patients to be stored in their home refrigerators for 7 days and then were returned for sterility testing. A contamination rate as high as 1.25% was reported. The authors expressed the opinion and hope that the high rate of contamination was an artifact of the sterility testing itself. However, contamination during storage in the patients' refrigerators may have occurred.[2294]

Sorption

Filgrastim in dextrose 5% at concentrations above 15 mcg/mL and between 2 and 15 mcg/mL with added albumin human 0.2% is compatible with common plastics used in syringes, administration sets, solution containers, and pump cassettes including polyvinyl chloride (PVC), polyolefin, and polypropylene.[4]

Filgrastim sorption occurs to a greater extent with lower concentrations and with longer infusion tubing.[2601] For filgrastim

DOI: 10.37573/9781585286850.167

concentrations between 5 and 15 mcg/mL, albumin human should be added to the infusion solution to make a final albumin human concentration of 0.2% (2 mg/mL) to minimize filgrastim adsorption to infusion containers and equipment.[4] At filgrastim concentrations above 15 mcg/mL, albumin human is unnecessary.[4] The product should not be diluted to a final concentration of less than 5 mcg/mL.[2873]

The amount of loss of filgrastim (Amgen) from the undiluted injection at a concentration of 300 mcg/mL when delivered through 6.6-French, single-lumen, silicone rubber, Broviac catheters (Bard) was evaluated. The catheters were filled with dextrose 5% (about 0.45 mL) and flushed before and after introduction of the filgrastim. Injected amounts of filgrastim 300 mcg/mL ranged from 0.17 to 1 mL. The delivered flush solution was collected and analyzed for filgrastim content and activity. The lowest volume (0.17 mL) incurred about 32% loss of filgrastim upon delivery. The other volumes incurred lower losses, ranging from 12% to none. A second repeat filgrastim injection incurred similar losses. The filgrastim that was delivered through the catheters remained active.[2017]

Compatibility Information

Solution Compatibility

Filgrastim

Test Soln Name	Mfr	Mfr	Conc/L or %	Remarks	Ref	C/I
Dextrose 5%		AMG	a	Manufacturer-recommended solution	2873	C
Dextrose 5%		AMG	2 mg[a]	Stable for 7 days at 2 to 8°C	4	C
Sodium chloride 0.45%		AMG		Physically incompatible	2873, 2892	I
Sodium chloride 0.9%		AMG		Physically incompatible	2873, 2892	I

[a] Concentrations between 5 and 15 mcg/mL require human albumin 2 mg/mL.

Y-Site Injection Compatibility (1:1 Mixture)

Filgrastim

Test Drug	Mfr	Conc	Mfr	Conc	Remarks	Ref	C/I
Acyclovir sodium	BW	7 mg/mL[a]	AMG	30 mcg/mL[a]	Physically compatible for 4 hr at 22°C	1687	C
Allopurinol sodium	BW	3 mg/mL[a]	AMG	30 mcg/mL[a]	Physically compatible for 4 hr at 22°C	1687	C
Amikacin sulfate	ES	5 mg/mL[a]	AMG	30 mcg/mL[a]	Physically compatible for 4 hr at 22°C	1687	C
Amikacin sulfate	BMS	5 mg/mL[a]	AMG	10[d] and 40[a] mcg/mL	Visually compatible. Little loss of filgrastim and fluconazole in 4 hr at 25°C	2060	C
Aminophylline	AB	2.5 mg/mL[a]	AMG	30 mcg/mL[a]	Physically compatible for 4 hr at 22°C	1687	C
Amphotericin B	SQ	0.6 mg/mL[a]	AMG	30 mcg/mL[a]	Yellow turbidity and precipitate form	1687	I
Ampicillin sodium	WY	20 mg/mL[a]	AMG	30 mcg/mL[a]	Physically compatible for 4 hr at 22°C	1687	C
Ampicillin sodium–sulbactam sodium	RR	20 mg/mL[a, e]	AMG	30 mcg/mL[a]	Physically compatible for 4 hr at 22°C	1687	C
Aztreonam	SQ	40 mg/mL[a]	AMG	30 mcg/mL[a]	Physically compatible for 4 hr at 22°C	1687	C
Aztreonam	SQ	40 mg/mL[a]	AMG	30 mcg/mL[a]	Physically compatible for 4 hr at 23°C	1758	C
Bleomycin sulfate	BR	1 unit/mL[a]	AMG	30 mcg/mL[a]	Physically compatible for 4 hr at 22°C	1687	C
Bumetanide	RC	0.04 mg/mL[a]	AMG	30 mcg/mL[a]	Physically compatible for 4 hr at 22°C	1687	C
Buprenorphine HCl	RKC	0.04 mg/mL[a]	AMG	30 mcg/mL[a]	Physically compatible for 4 hr at 22°C	1687	C
Butorphanol tartrate	BR	0.04 mg/mL[a]	AMG	30 mcg/mL[a]	Physically compatible for 4 hr at 22°C	1687	C
Calcium gluconate	AST	40 mg/mL[a]	AMG	30 mcg/mL[a]	Physically compatible for 4 hr at 22°C	1687	C

Y-Site Injection Compatibility (1:1 Mixture) (Cont.)

Test Drug	Mfr	Conc	Mfr	Conc	Remarks	Ref	C/I
Carboplatin	BR	5 mg/mL[a]	AMG	30 mcg/mL[a]	Physically compatible for 4 hr at 22°C	1687	C
Carmustine	BR	1.5 mg/mL[a]	AMG	30 mcg/mL[a]	Physically compatible for 4 hr at 22°C	1687	C
Cefazolin sodium	LI	20 mg/mL[a]	AMG	30 mcg/mL[a]	Physically compatible for 4 hr at 22°C	1687	C
Cefotaxime sodium	HO	20 mg/mL[a]	AMG	30 mcg/mL[a]	Particles form in 4 hr	1687	I
Cefotetan disodium	STU	20 mg/mL[a]	AMG	30 mcg/mL[a]	Physically compatible for 4 hr at 22°C	1687	C
Cefoxitin sodium	MSD	20 mg/mL[a]	AMG	30 mcg/mL[a]	Haze, particles, and filaments form immediately	1687	I
Ceftaroline fosamil	FOR	2.22 mg/mL[a b c]	AMG	30 mcg/mL[a]	Microparticulates formed	2826	I
Ceftazidime	LI	40 mg/mL[a]	AMG	30 mcg/mL[a]	Physically compatible for 4 hr at 22°C	1687	C
Ceftazidime	LI	10 mg/mL[a]	AMG	10[d] and 40[a] mcg/mL	Visually compatible. Little loss of filgrastim and fluconazole in 4 hr at 25°C	2060	C
Ceftolozane sulfate–tazobactam sodium	CUB	10 mg/mL[a i]	AMG	15 mcg/mL[a]	Physically compatible for 2 hr	3262	C
Ceftriaxone sodium	RC	20 mg/mL[a]	AMG	30 mcg/mL[a]	Particles and filaments form in 1 hr	1687	I
Cefuroxime sodium	GL	20 mg/mL[a]	AMG	30 mcg/mL[a]	Haze, particles, and filaments form immediately	1687	I
Chlorpromazine HCl	RU	2 mg/mL[a]	AMG	30 mcg/mL[a]	Physically compatible for 4 hr at 22°C	1687	C
Cisplatin	BR	1 mg/mL	AMG	30 mcg/mL[a]	Physically compatible for 4 hr at 22°C	1687	C
Clindamycin phosphate	AB	10 mg/mL[a]	AMG	30 mcg/mL[a]	Particles and filaments form immediately	1687	I
Cyclophosphamide	MJ	10 mg/mL[a]	AMG	30 mcg/mL[a]	Physically compatible for 4 hr at 22°C	1687	C
Cytarabine	CET	50 mg/mL	AMG	30 mcg/mL[a]	Physically compatible for 4 hr at 22°C	1687	C
Dacarbazine	MI	4 mg/mL[a]	AMG	30 mcg/mL[a]	Physically compatible for 4 hr at 22°C	1687	C
Dactinomycin	MSD	0.01 mg/mL[a]	AMG	30 mcg/mL[a]	Particles and filaments form immediately	1687	I
Daunorubicin HCl	WY	1 mg/mL[a]	AMG	30 mcg/mL[a]	Physically compatible for 4 hr at 22°C	1687	C
Dexamethasone sodium phosphate	LY	1 mg/mL[a]	AMG	30 mcg/mL[a]	Physically compatible for 4 hr at 22°C	1687	C
Diphenhydramine HCl	ES	2 mg/mL[a]	AMG	30 mcg/mL[a]	Physically compatible for 4 hr at 22°C	1687	C
Doxorubicin HCl	CET	2 mg/mL	AMG	30 mcg/mL[a]	Physically compatible for 4 hr at 22°C	1687	C
Doxycycline hyclate	ES	1 mg/mL[a]	AMG	30 mcg/mL[a]	Physically compatible for 4 hr at 22°C	1687	C
Droperidol	JN	0.4 mg/mL[a]	AMG	30 mcg/mL[a]	Physically compatible for 4 hr at 22°C	1687	C
Enalaprilat	MSD	0.1 mg/mL[a]	AMG	30 mcg/mL[a]	Physically compatible for 4 hr at 22°C	1687	C
Etoposide	BR	0.4 mg/mL[a]	AMG	30 mcg/mL[a]	Particles form immediately. Filaments form in 1 hr	1687	I
Famotidine	MSD	2 mg/mL[a]	AMG	30 mcg/mL[a]	Physically compatible for 4 hr at 22°C	1687	C
Floxuridine	RC	3 mg/mL[a]	AMG	30 mcg/mL[a]	Physically compatible for 4 hr at 22°C	1687	C
Fluconazole	RR	2 mg/mL	AMG	30 mcg/mL[a]	Physically compatible for 4 hr at 22°C	1687	C
Fluconazole	RR	2 mg/mL[a]	AMG	10[d] and 40[a] mcg/mL	Visually compatible. Little loss of filgrastim and fluconazole in 4 hr at 25°C	2060	C
Fludarabine phosphate	BX	1 mg/mL[a]	AMG	30 mcg/mL[a]	Physically compatible for 4 hr at 22°C	1687	C

Y-Site Injection Compatibility (1:1 Mixture) (Cont.)

Test Drug	Mfr	Conc	Mfr	Conc	Remarks	Ref	C/I
Fluorouracil	RC	16 mg/mL[a]	AMG	30 mcg/mL[a]	Particles and long filaments form in 1 hr	1687	I
Furosemide	AB	3 mg/mL[a]	AMG	30 mcg/mL[a]	Turbidity forms immediately. Filaments and particles form in 1 hr	1687	I
Gallium nitrate	FUJ	0.4 mg/mL[a]	AMG	30 mcg/mL[a]	Physically compatible for 4 hr at 22°C	1687	C
Ganciclovir sodium	SY	20 mg/mL[a]	AMG	30 mcg/mL[a]	Physically compatible for 4 hr at 22°C	1687	C
Gentamicin sulfate	LY	5 mg/mL[a]	AMG	30 mcg/mL[a]	Physically compatible for 4 hr at 22°C	1687	C
Gentamicin sulfate	GNS	1.6 mg/mL[a]	AMG	40 mcg/mL[a]	Visually compatible. Little loss of filgrastim and gentamicin in 4 hr at 25°C	2060	C
Gentamicin sulfate	GNS	1.6 mg/mL[a]	AMG	10 mcg/mL[d]	23% loss of filgrastim in 4 hr at 25°C. Little gentamicin loss	2060	I
Granisetron HCl	SKB	0.05 mg/mL[a]	AMG	30 mcg/mL[a]	Physically compatible for 4 hr at 23°C	2000	C
Haloperidol lactate	MN	0.2 mg/mL[a]	AMG	30 mcg/mL[a]	Physically compatible for 4 hr at 22°C	1687	C
Heparin sodium	ES	100 units/mL[a]	AMG	30 mcg/mL[a]	Particles and filaments form immediately	1687	I
Hydrocortisone sodium succinate	UP	1 mg/mL[a]	AMG	30 mcg/mL[a]	Physically compatible for 4 hr at 22°C	1687	C
Hydromorphone HCl	KN	0.5 mg/mL[a]	AMG	30 mcg/mL[a]	Physically compatible for 4 hr at 22°C	1687	C
Hydroxyzine HCl	ES	4 mg/mL[a]	AMG	30 mcg/mL[a]	Physically compatible for 4 hr at 22°C	1687	C
Idarubicin HCl	AD	0.5 mg/mL[a]	AMG	30 mcg/mL[a]	Physically compatible for 4 hr at 22°C	1687	C
Ifosfamide	MJ	25 mg/mL[a]	AMG	30 mcg/mL[a]	Physically compatible for 4 hr at 22°C	1687	C
Imipenem–cilastatin sodium	MSD	10 mg/mL[a,h]	AMG	30 mcg/mL[a]	Physically compatible for 4 hr at 22°C	1687	C
Imipenem–cilastatin sodium	ME	5 mg/mL[a,g]	AMG	40 mcg/mL[a]	16% loss of filgrastim in 4 hr at 25°C. Little imipenem–cilastatin loss	2060	I
Imipenem–cilastatin sodium	ME	5 mg/mL[a,g]	AMG	10 mcg/mL[d]	Visually compatible. Little loss of filgrastim and imipenem–cilastatin in 4 hr at 25°C	2060	C
Isavuconazonium sulfate	ASP	1.5 mg/mL[a]	AMG	15 mcg/mL[a]	Measured turbidity increases within 15 min	3263	I
Letermovir	ME				Physically incompatible	3398	I
Leucovorin calcium	LE	2 mg/mL[a]	AMG	30 mcg/mL[a]	Physically compatible for 4 hr at 22°C	1687	C
Lorazepam	WY	0.1 mg/mL[a]	AMG	30 mcg/mL[a]	Physically compatible for 4 hr at 22°C	1687	C
Mannitol	BA	15%	AMG	30 mcg/mL[a]	Filaments form immediately	1687	I
Mechlorethamine HCl	MSD	1 mg/mL	AMG	30 mcg/mL[a]	Physically compatible for 4 hr at 22°C	1687	C
Melphalan HCl	BW	0.1 mg/mL[a]	AMG	30 mcg/mL[a]	Physically compatible for 4 hr at 22°C	1687	C
Meperidine HCl	WY	4 mg/mL[a]	AMG	30 mcg/mL[a]	Physically compatible for 4 hr at 22°C	1687	C
Mesna	MJ	10 mg/mL[a]	AMG	30 mcg/mL[a]	Physically compatible for 4 hr at 22°C	1687	C
Methotrexate sodium	LE	15 mg/mL[a]	AMG	30 mcg/mL[a]	Physically compatible for 4 hr at 22°C	1687	C
Methylprednisolone sodium succinate	AB	5 mg/mL[a]	AMG	30 mcg/mL[a]	Haze, particles, and filaments form immediately	1687	I
Metoclopramide HCl	ES	5 mg/mL	AMG	30 mcg/mL[a]	Physically compatible for 4 hr at 22°C	1687	C
Metronidazole	BA	5 mg/mL	AMG	30 mcg/mL[a]	Particles form immediately. Filaments form in 1 hr	1687	I

Y-Site Injection Compatibility (1:1 Mixture) (Cont.)

Test Drug	Mfr	Conc	Mfr	Conc	Remarks	Ref	C/I
Mitomycin	BR	0.5 mg/mL	AMG	30 mcg/mL[a]	Color changes to reddish purple in 1 hr	1687	I
Mitoxantrone HCl	LE	0.5 mg/mL[a]	AMG	30 mcg/mL[a]	Physically compatible for 4 hr at 22°C	1687	C
Morphine sulfate	WY	1 mg/mL[a]	AMG	30 mcg/mL[a]	Physically compatible for 4 hr at 22°C	1687	C
Nalbuphine HCl	DU	10 mg/mL	AMG	30 mcg/mL[a]	Physically compatible for 4 hr at 22°C	1687	C
Ondansetron HCl	GL	1 mg/mL[a]	AMG	30 mcg/mL[a]	Physically compatible for 4 hr at 22°C	1687	C
Posaconazole	ME	18 mg/mL		6 mcg/mL[j]	Physically compatible	2911, 2912	C
Potassium chloride	AB	0.1 mEq/mL[a]	AMG	30 mcg/mL[a]	Physically compatible for 4 hr at 22°C	1687	C
Prochlorperazine edisylate	SCN	0.5 mg/mL[a]	AMG	30 mcg/mL[a]	Particles form immediately. Filaments form in 1 hr	1687	I
Promethazine HCl	SCN	2 mg/mL[a]	AMG	30 mcg/mL[a]	Physically compatible for 4 hr at 22°C	1687	C
Ranitidine HCl	GL	2 mg/mL[a]	AMG	30 mcg/mL[a]	Physically compatible for 4 hr at 22°C	1687	C
Sodium bicarbonate	AB	1 mEq/mL	AMG	30 mcg/mL[a]	Physically compatible for 4 hr at 22°C	1687	C
Streptozocin	UP	40 mg/mL[a]	AMG	30 mcg/mL[a]	Physically compatible for 4 hr at 22°C	1687	C
Thiotepa	LE	1 mg/mL[a]	AMG	30 mcg/mL[a]	Particles and filaments form immediately	1687	I
Tobramycin sulfate	LI	5 mg/mL[a]	AMG	30 mcg/mL[a]	Physically compatible for 4 hr at 22°C	1687	C
Tobramycin sulfate	LI	1.6 mg/mL[a]	AMG	10[d] and 40[a] mcg/mL	Visually compatible. Little loss of filgrastim and tobramycin in 4 hr at 25°C	2060	C
Trimethoprim–sulfamethoxazole	ES	0.8 mg/mL[a f]	AMG	30 mcg/mL[a]	Physically compatible for 4 hr at 22°C	1687	C
Vancomycin HCl	AB	10 mg/mL[a]	AMG	30 mcg/mL[a]	Physically compatible for 4 hr at 22°C	1687	C
Vinblastine sulfate	LI	0.12 mg/mL[a]	AMG	30 mcg/mL[a]	Physically compatible for 4 hr at 22°C	1687	C
Vincristine sulfate	LI	0.05 mg/mL[a]	AMG	30 mcg/mL[a]	Physically compatible for 4 hr at 22°C	1687	C
Vinorelbine tartrate	BW	1 mg/mL[a]	AMG	30 mcg/mL[a]	Physically compatible for 4 hr at 22°C	1687	C
Zidovudine	BW	4 mg/mL[a]	AMG	30 mcg/mL[a]	Physically compatible for 4 hr at 22°C	1687	C

[a] Tested in dextrose 5%.

[b] Tested in sodium chloride 0.9%.

[c] Tested in Ringer's injection, lactated.

[d] Tested in dextrose 5% with albumin human 2 mg/mL.

[e] Ampicillin component. Ampicillin in a 2:1 fixed-ratio concentration with sulbactam.

[f] Trimethoprim component. Trimethoprim in a 1:5 fixed-ratio concentration with sulfamethoxazole.

[g] Imipenem component. Imipenem in a 1:1 fixed-ratio concentration with cilastatin.

[h] Not specified whether concentration refers to single component or combined components.

[i] Ceftolozane component. Ceftolozane in a 2:1 fixed-ratio concentration with tazobactam.

[j] Tested in both dextrose 5% and sodium chloride 0.9%.

Floxacillin Sodium
AHFS 8:12.16.12
Flucloxacillin Sodium

Products

Floxacillin sodium is available in vials containing 250 mg, 500 mg, and 1 g of floxacillin as the sodium salt. To reconstitute for intramuscular use, add 1.5 mL of sterile water for injection to the 250-mg vial, 2 mL to the 500-mg vial, or 2.5 mL to the 1-g vial.[38] [115]

For intravenous use, reconstitute the 250- or 500-mg vial with 5 to 10 mL and the 1-g vial with 15 to 20 mL of sterile water for injection. For intravenous infusion, the solution may be diluted further in a compatible infusion fluid.[38] [115]

For intrapleural use, reconstitute the 250-mg vial with 5 to 10 mL of sterile water for injection. For intra-articular use, reconstitute the 250- or 500-mg vial with up to 5 mL of sterile water for injection or lidocaine hydrochloride 0.5% injection.[38] [115]

For smaller doses, the reconstitution volumes in Table 1 will yield the indicated concentrations.

Table 1. Floxacillin reconstitution volumes for smaller doses[38] [115]

Vial Size	Concentration (mg/1 mL)					
	50	100	125	200	250	500
250 mg	4.8 mL	2.3 mL	1.8 mL	1.05 mL		
500 mg		4.7 mL	3.7 mL	2.2 mL	1.7 mL	
1 g		9.3 mL			3.3 mL	1.3 mL

Sodium and Magnesium Content

Each gram of drug contains 2.2 mmol (51 mg) of sodium and 1 mmol of magnesium.[38] [89] [115]

Trade Name(s)

Floxapen, Ladropen

Administration

Floxacillin sodium may be administered by intramuscular injection, direct intravenous injection slowly over three to four minutes, continuous intravenous infusion, and intrapleural and intra-articular injection.[38]

Stability

Floxacillin sodium in intact vials should be stored below 25°C. The injection reconstituted for intramuscular or direct intravenous injection should be freshly prepared and administered within 30 minutes. However, reconstituted floxacillin sodium injection is stated to be stable for 24 hours when stored under refrigeration.[38] [115]

Losses of 8% in three days were reported for reconstituted solutions containing floxacillin sodium (Beecham) 100 mg/mL stored at 20 to 25°C.[89]

Freezing Solutions

Floxacillin sodium (Beecham) 20 mg/mL in sodium chloride 0.9% or dextrose 5% in PVC bags (Travenol) retained greater than 90% after being frozen and stored at −27°C for up to 270 days. Thawing by microwave radiation and subsequent storage for 24 hours at 4°C did not cause drug loss below 90% of the stated concentration. However, a distinct yellow discoloration was produced after 90 days of storage, rendering the solutions unacceptable.[1176]

Floxacillin sodium (Beecham) 1 g in 50 mL of sodium chloride 0.9% or dextrose 5% in PVC bags (Travenol) was stored at −20°C for 30 days, followed by natural thawing and storage at 5°C for 21 hours. The drug was stable under these conditions for the duration of the study.[299]

Sorption

Floxacillin sodium was shown not to exhibit sorption to PVC bags and tubing, polyethylene tubing, Silastic tubing, and polypropylene syringes.[536] [606]

Compatibility Information
Solution Compatibility

Floxacillin sodium

Test Soln Name	Mfr	Mfr	Conc/L or %	Remarks	Ref	C/I
Dextrose 2.5% in sodium chloride 0.45%		BE	1 g	6% loss in 24 hr at 20 to 25°C	89	C
Dextrose 5%				Under 10% loss in 24 hr at room temperature	1475	C
Dextrose 5%		BE	1 g	1% loss in 24 hr at 20 to 25°C	89	C

DOI: 10.37573/9781585286850.168

Solution Compatibility (Cont.)

Test Soln Name	Mfr	Mfr	Conc/L or %	Remarks	Ref	C/I
Ringer's injection, lactated				Under 10% loss in 24 hr at room temperature	1475	C
Sodium chloride 0.9%				Under 10% loss in 24 hr at room temperature	1475	C
Sodium chloride 0.9%		BE	1 g	3% loss in 24 hr at 20 to 25°C	89	C
Sodium chloride 0.9%	BA	BE	5, 10, 20 g	Visually compatible. 2 to 3% loss in 14 days and 7 to 9% loss in 28 days at 5°C	1844	C
Sodium chloride 0.9%	BA[a]		120 g	Stable for 6 days at 4°C. 28% loss in 24 hr at 37°C	2206	C
Sodium chloride 0.9%	[b]		50 g	2% loss in 6 days at 4°C, 6% loss in 24 hr at 31°C, and 13% in 7 hr at 37°C	2715	C
Sodium lactate ⅙ M				Under 10% loss in 24 hr at room temperature	1475	C
Sodium lactate ⅙ M		BE	1 g	4% loss in 24 hr at 20 to 25°C	89	C

[a] Tested in PVC containers.

[b] Tested in Infusor LV reservoirs.

Additive Compatibility

Floxacillin sodium

Test Drug	Mfr	Conc/L or %	Mfr	Conc/L or %	Test Solution	Remarks	Ref	C/I
Aminophylline	ANT	1 g	BE	20 g	NS	Physically compatible for 72 hr at 15 and 30°C	1479	C
Amiodarone HCl	LZ	4 g	BE	20 g	D5W	Precipitates immediately	1479	I
Ampicillin sodium	BE	20 g	BE	20 g	NS	Physically compatible for 72 hr at 15 and 30°C	1479	C
Atropine sulfate	ANT	60 mg	BE	20 g	W	Haze forms in 24 hr and precipitate forms in 48 hr at 30°C. No change at 15°C	1479	I
Bumetanide	LEO	6 mg	BE	20 g	NS	Physically compatible for 72 hr at 15 and 30°C	1479	C
Buprenorphine HCl		75 mg	BE	20 g	W	Thick haze forms in 24 hr and precipitate forms in 47 hr at 30°C. No change at 15°C	1479	I
Calcium gluconate	ANT	2 g	BE	20 g	NS	White precipitate forms immediately	1479	I
Ceftazidime	GSK	40 g	GSK	40 g	NS, W	Physically compatible. Under 10% loss in 24 hr at room temperature and 4°C	2658	C
Ceftazidime	GSK	60 g	GSK	120 g	NS, W	Physically compatible. Under 10% loss in 24 hr at room temperature and 4°C	2658	C
Ceftazidime	GSK	180 g	GSK	240 g	NS, W	Physically compatible. Under 10% loss in 24 hr at room temperature and 4°C	2658	C
Cefuroxime sodium	GL	37.5 g	BE	20 g	W	Physically compatible for 72 hr at 15 and 30°C	1479	C
Cefuroxime sodium	GL	7.5 g	BE	10 g	D5W, NS	Physically compatible for 48 hr. Both drugs stable for 1 hr at room temperature	1036	C
Chlorpromazine HCl	ANT	5 g	BE	20 g	W	Yellow precipitate forms immediately	1479	I
Ciprofloxacin		2 g		10 g	[a]	Precipitates immediately	1473	I
Cloxacillin sodium	BE	20 g	BE	20 g	NS	Physically compatible for 24 hr at 15 and 30°C. Haze forms in 48 hr at 30°C. No change at 15°C	1479	C
Dexamethasone sodium phosphate	MSD	4 g	BE	20 g	NS	Physically compatible for 72 hr at 15 and 30°C	1479	C
Dextran 40		10%			D5W, NS	Under 10% loss in 24 hr at room temperature	1475	C
Diamorphine HCl	EV	500 mg	BE	20 g	W	Physically compatible for 24 hr at 15 and 30°C. Haze forms in 48 hr at 30°C. No change at 15°C	1479	C

Additive Compatibility (Cont.)

Test Drug	Mfr	Conc/L or %	Mfr	Conc/L or %	Test Solution	Remarks	Ref	C/I
Diazepam	PHX	1 g	BE	20 g	D5W	Haze forms in 7 hr at 30°C and 48 hr at 15°C	1479	I
Digoxin	BW	25 mg	BE	20 g	NS	Physically compatible for 72 hr at 15 and 30°C	1479	C
Dobutamine HCl	LI	500 mg	BE	20 g	NS	Haze forms immediately and precipitate forms in 24 to 48 hr at 15 and 30°C	1479	I
Epinephrine HCl	ANT	8 mg	BE	20 g	W	Physically compatible for 72 hr at 15 and 30°C	1479	C
Erythromycin lactobionate	AB	5 g	BE	20 g	NS	Precipitates immediately. Crystals form in 5 hr at 15°C	1479	I
Fusidate sodium	LEO	500 mg		2.5 g	D2.5½S, D2.5S, D5¼S, D5½S, D5S, D10S	Physically compatible and chemically stable for 48 hr at room temperature	1800	C
Gentamicin sulfate	RS	8 g	BE	20 g	NS	Haze forms immediately and precipitate forms in 2 hr	1479	I
Gentamicin sulfate	EX	8 g	BE	10 g	NS	Physically compatible for 48 hr. Both drugs stable for 1 hr at room temperature	1036	C
Gentamicin sulfate	EX	8 g	BE	10 g	D5W	Precipitates immediately	1036	I
Heparin sodium	WED	20,000 units	BE	20 g	NS	Physically compatible for 24 hr at 15 and 30°C. Haze forms in 48 hr at 30°C. No change at 15°C	1479	C
Hydrocortisone sodium succinate	UP	50 g	BE	20 g	NS	Physically compatible for 72 hr at 15 and 30°C	1479	C
Isoproterenol HCl	PX	4 mg	BE	20 g	D5W	Physically compatible for 24 hr at 15 and 30°C. Haze forms in 48 hr and precipitate forms in 72 hr	1479	C
Isosorbide dinitrate		1 g	BE	20 g		Physically compatible for 24 hr at 15 and 30°C. Haze forms in 48 hr and precipitate forms in 72 hr at 30°C. No change at 15°C	1479	C
Lidocaine HCl	ANT	2 g	BE	20 g	NS	Physically compatible for 72 hr at 15 and 30°C	1479	C
Meperidine HCl	RC	5 g	BE	20 g	W	Haze forms immediately and precipitate forms in 5 to 24 hr	1479	I
Metoclopramide HCl	ANT	1 g	BE	20 g	NS	White precipitate forms immediately	1479	I
Metronidazole		5 g	BE	10 g		Physically compatible for 48 hr. Both drugs stable for 1 hr at room temperature	1036	C
Morphine sulfate	EV	1 g	BE	20 g	W	Haze forms in 24 hr and precipitate forms in 48 hr at 30°C. No change at 15°C	1479	I
Potassium chloride	ANT	40 mmol	BE	20 g	W	Physically compatible for 72 hr at 15 and 30°C	1479	C
Prochlorperazine edisylate	MB	1.25 g	BE	20 g	W	Precipitates immediately	1479	I
Promethazine HCl	MB	5 g	BE	20 g	W	White precipitate forms immediately	1479	I
Ranitidine HCl	GL	500 mg	BE	20 g	NS	Physically compatible for 72 hr at 15 and 30°C	1479	C
Scopolamine butylbromide	BI	2 g	BE	20 g	W	Physically compatible for 24 hr at 15 and 30°C. Precipitate forms in 48 hr at 30°C. No change in 48 hr at 15°C	1479	C
Tobramycin sulfate	LI	8 g	BE	20 g	NS	White precipitate forms in 7 hr	1479	I
Verapamil HCl	AB	500 mg	BE	20 g	NS	Haze and precipitate form in 24 hr at 30°C. No change at 15°C	1479	I

ᵃ Floxacillin sodium added to ciprofloxacin solvent.

Drugs in Syringe Compatibility

Floxacillin sodium

Test Drug	Mfr	Amt	Mfr	Amt	Remarks	Ref	C/I
Heparin sodium		2500 units/1 mL	BE	1 g	Visually compatible for at least 5 min	1053	C

Y-Site Injection Compatibility (1:1 Mixture)

Floxacillin sodium

Test Drug	Mfr	Conc	Mfr	Conc	Remarks	Ref	C/I
Clarithromycin	AB	4 mg/mL[a]	BE	40 mg/mL[a]	Translucent precipitate in 1 to 2 hr becoming a gel in 3 hr at 30 and 17°C	2174	I
Lorazepam	WY	0.33 mg/mL[b]	SKB	50 mg/mL	White opalescence forms in 4 hr	1855	I
Midazolam HCl	RC	5 mg/mL	SKB	50 mg/mL	White precipitate forms immediately	1855	I
TPN #189[c]			BE	50 mg/mL[b]	Visually compatible for 24 hr at 22°C	1767	C
Vancomycin HCl	LI	10 mg/mL[a]	[d]	250 mg/mL	Physically incompatible	3536	I

[a] Tested in dextrose 5%.

[b] Tested in sodium chloride 0.9%.

[c] Refer to Appendix for the composition of parenteral nutrition solutions. TPN indicates a 2-in-1 admixture.

[d] Salt not specified.

Selected Revisions May 1, 2020. © Copyright, October 1992.
American Society of Health-System Pharmacists, Inc.

Floxuridine

AHFS 10:00

Products

Floxuridine is supplied in 5-mL vials containing 500 mg of drug.[3070] Each vial should be reconstituted with 5 mL of sterile water for injection to yield a solution with a concentration of approximately 100 mg/mL.[3070]

pH

A 2% aqueous solution has a pH of 4 to 5.5.[3070]

Administration

Floxuridine is administered only by continuous regional intra-arterial infusion using an infusion pump after dilution in dextrose 5% or sodium chloride 0.9% to a volume appropriate for the device to be used.[3070]

Stability

Intact vials of floxuridine should be stored at 20 to 25°C.[3070] The reconstituted solution in vials should be stored under refrigeration at 2 to 8°C for no longer than 2 weeks.[3070]

The pH of optimum stability is 4 to 7. Extreme acidity or alkalinity may result in hydrolysis.[1379]

At a concentration of 5 mg/mL in sodium chloride 0.9%, floxuridine supported the growth of several microorganisms commonly implicated in nosocomial infections, including

Escherichia coli, *Pseudomonas aeruginosa*, and *Candida albicans*. The arbitrary application of an extended expiration date to floxuridine solutions is, therefore, highly questionable.[827]

Syringes

Floxuridine (Roche) 50 mg/mL and 1 mg/mL in sodium chloride 0.9% was packaged as 3 mL in 10-mL polypropylene infusion pump syringes (Pharmacia Deltec). Little or no loss occurred during 21 days of storage at 30°C.[1967]

Implantable Pumps

Floxuridine 10 mg/mL was filled into an implantable infusion pump (Fresenius VIP 30) and associated capillary tubing and stored at 37°C. No floxuridine loss and no contamination from components of pump materials occurred during 6 weeks of storage. However, an unidentified substance appeared in 7 weeks, and 22% loss of floxuridine occurred by 8 weeks.[1903]

Floxuridine (Roche) at concentrations ranging from about 2.5 to 12 mg/mL with heparin sodium 200 units/mL in bacteriostatic sodium chloride 0.9% was evaluated for stability in an implantable infusion pump (Infusaid model 400). In this in vivo assessment, the floxuridine concentrations were determined prior to implantation in patients and again at the time of pump refills. No appreciable floxuridine loss occurred during 8 courses of therapy, from 4 to 12 days in duration, in 5 patients.[767]

Compatibility Information

Solution Compatibility

Floxuridine

Test Soln Name	Mfr	Mfr	Conc/L or %	Remarks	Ref	C/I
Dextrose 5%			5 to 10 g	Under 10% loss in 14 days at room temperature	1379	C
Dextrose 5%		APP		Manufacturer-recommended solution	3070	C
Sodium chloride 0.9%			5 to 10 g	Under 10% loss in 14 days at room temperature	1379	C
Sodium chloride 0.9%		APP		Manufacturer-recommended solution	3070	C

Additive Compatibility

Floxuridine

Test Drug	Mfr	Conc/L or %	Mfr	Conc/L or %	Test Solution	Remarks	Ref	C/I
Carboplatin		1 g		10 g	W	Under 10% drug loss in 7 days at 23°C	1954	C
Cisplatin	BR	500 mg	RC	10 g	NS	13% floxuridine loss in 7 days at room temperature in dark	1386	C
Cisplatin with etoposide		200 mg 300 mg		700 mg	NS	All drugs stable for 7 days at room temperature	1379	C

DOI: 10.37573/9781585286850.169

Additive Compatibility (Cont.)

Test Drug	Mfr	Conc/L or %	Mfr	Conc/L or %	Test Solution	Remarks	Ref	C/I
Cisplatin with leucovorin calcium		200 mg 140 mg		700 mg	NS	All drugs stable for 7 days at room temperature	1379	C
Etoposide		200 mg		10 g	NS	Both drugs stable for 15 days at room temperature	1379	C
Etoposide with cisplatin		300 mg 200 mg		700 mg	NS	All drugs stable for 7 days at room temperature	1379	C
Fluorouracil		10 g		10 g	NS	Both drugs stable for 15 days at room temperature	1390	C
Leucovorin calcium	QU	30 mg	QU	1 g	NS	Physically compatible. Stable for 48 hr at 4 and 20°C. No floxuridine and 10% leucovorin loss in 48 hr at 40°C	1317	C
Leucovorin calcium	QU	240 mg	QU	2 g	NS	Physically compatible. Stable for 48 hr at 4 and 20°C. No floxuridine and 7% leucovorin loss in 48 hr at 40°C	1317	C
Leucovorin calcium	QU	960 mg	QU	4 g	NS	Physically compatible. Stable for 48 hr at 4, 20, and 40°C	1317	C
Leucovorin calcium		200 mg		10 g	NS	Both drugs stable for 15 days at room temperature protected from light	1387	C
Leucovorin calcium with cisplatin		140 mg 200 mg		700 mg	NS	All drugs stable for 7 days at room temperature	1379	C

Y-Site Injection Compatibility (1:1 Mixture)

Floxuridine

Test Drug	Mfr	Conc	Mfr	Conc	Remarks	Ref	C/I
Allopurinol sodium	BW	3 mg/mL[b]	RC	3 mg/mL[b]	Tiny particles form in 1 to 4 hr	1686	I
Amifostine	USB	10 mg/mL[a]	RC	3 mg/mL[a]	Physically compatible for 4 hr at 23°C	1845	C
Aztreonam	SQ	40 mg/mL[a]	RC	3 mg/mL[a]	Physically compatible for 4 hr at 23°C	1758	C
Etoposide phosphate	BR	5 mg/mL[a]	RC	3 mg/mL[a]	Physically compatible for 4 hr at 23°C	2218	C
Filgrastim	AMG	30 mcg/mL[a]	RC	3 mg/mL[a]	Physically compatible for 4 hr at 22°C	1687	C
Fludarabine phosphate	BX	1 mg/mL[a]	RC	3 mg/mL[a]	Visually compatible for 4 hr at 22°C	1439	C
Gemcitabine HCl	LI	10 mg/mL[b]	RC	3 mg/mL[b]	Physically compatible for 4 hr at 23°C	2226	C
Granisetron HCl	SKB	0.05 mg/mL[a]	RC	3 mg/mL[a]	Physically compatible for 4 hr at 23°C	2000	C
Melphalan HCl	BW	0.1 mg/mL[b]	RC	3 mg/mL[b]	Physically compatible for 3 hr at 22°C	1557	C
Ondansetron HCl	GL	1 mg/mL[b]	RC	3 mg/mL[a]	Visually compatible for 4 hr at 22°C	1365	C
Paclitaxel	NCI	1.2 mg/mL[a]	RC	3 mg/mL[a]	Physically compatible for 4 hr at 22°C	1556	C
Piperacillin sodium–tazobactam sodium	LE[d]	40 mg/mL[a e]	RC	3 mg/mL[a]	Physically compatible for 4 hr at 22°C	1688	C
Sargramostim	IMM	10 mcg/mL[b]	RC	3 mg/mL[b]	Visually compatible for 4 hr at 22°C	1436	C
Teniposide	BR	0.1 mg/mL[a]	RC	3 mg/mL[a]	Physically compatible for 4 hr at 23°C	1725	C

Y-Site Injection Compatibility (1:1 Mixture) (Cont.)

Test Drug	Mfr	Conc	Mfr	Conc	Remarks	Ref	C/I
Thiotepa	IMM[c]	1 mg/mL[a]	RC	3 mg/mL[a]	Physically compatible for 4 hr at 23°C	1861	C
Vinorelbine tartrate	BW	1 mg/mL[b]	RC	3 mg/mL[b]	Physically compatible for 4 hr at 22°C	1558	C

[a] Tested in dextrose 5%.

[b] Tested in sodium chloride 0.9%.

[c] Lyophilized formulation tested.

[d] Test performed using the formulation WITHOUT edetate disodium.

[e] Piperacillin component. Piperacillin in an 8:1 fixed-ratio concentration with tazobactam.

Selected Revisions May 10, 2016. © Copyright, October 1984.
American Society of Health-System Pharmacists, Inc.

Fluconazole
AHFS 8:14.08

Products

Fluconazole is available for intravenous infusion in 100- and 200-mL glass bottles and polyvinyl chloride (PVC) bags in sodium chloride or dextrose diluents. Each mL of solution contains fluconazole 2 mg and either sodium chloride 9 mg or dextrose 56 mg.[1(6/06)]

pH

From 4 to 8 in the sodium chloride diluent and from 3.5 to 6.5 in the dextrose diluent.[1(6/06)]

Osmolarity

The infusion solution is iso-osmotic,[1(6/06)] having an osmolarity of 300 to 315 mOsm/L.[4]

Trade Name(s)

Diflucan

Administration

Fluconazole is administered by intravenous infusion at a rate not exceeding 200 mg/hr.[1(6/06) 4]

Stability

Fluconazole injection in glass bottles or PVC bags should be stored between 5 and 30°C or between 5 and 25°C, respectively, and protected from freezing. Brief exposure to temperatures up to 40°C does not adversely affect the product in PVC bags. The overwrap moisture barrier should not be removed from the PVC bags until ready for use. The solution should not be used if it is cloudy or precipitated.[1(6/06) 4]

Elastomeric Reservoir Pumps

Fluconazole (Pfizer) 2 mg/mL in sodium chloride 0.9% was evaluated for binding to natural rubber elastomeric reservoirs (Baxter). Less than 2% binding was found after storage for 2 weeks at 35°C with gentle agitation.[2014]

Central Venous Catheter

Fluconazole (Roerig) 2 mg/mL in dextrose 5% was found to be compatible with the ARROWg+ard Blue Plus (Arrow International) chlorhexidine-bearing triple-lumen central catheter. Essentially complete delivery of the drug was found with little or no drug loss occurring. Furthermore, chlorhexidine delivered from the catheter remained at trace amounts with no substantial increase due to the delivery of the drug through the catheter.[2335]

Compatibility Information

Solution Compatibility

Fluconazole

Test Soln Name	Mfr	Mfr	Conc/L or %	Remarks	Ref	C/I
Dextrose 5%	BA[a]	PF	1 g	Stable for 24 hr at 25°C in fluorescent light	1676	C
Ringer's injection, lactated	BA[a]	PF	1 g	Stable for 24 hr at 25°C in fluorescent light	1676	C

[a] Tested in PVC containers.

Additive Compatibility

Fluconazole

Test Drug	Mfr	Conc/L or %	Mfr	Conc/L or %	Test Solution	Remarks	Ref	C/I
Acyclovir sodium	BW	5 g	PF	1 g	D5W	Visually compatible with no fluconazole loss in 72 hr at 25°C under fluorescent light. Acyclovir not tested	1677	C
Amikacin sulfate	BR	2.5 g	PF	1 g	D5W	Visually compatible with no fluconazole loss in 72 hr at 25°C under fluorescent light. Amikacin not tested	1677	C
Amphotericin B	LY	50 mg	PF	1 g	D5W	Visually compatible with no fluconazole loss in 72 hr at 25°C. Amphotericin B not tested	1677	C

DOI: 10.37573/9781585286850.170

Additive Compatibility (Cont.)

Test Drug	Mfr	Conc/L or %	Mfr	Conc/L or %	Test Solution	Remarks	Ref	C/I
Cefazolin sodium	SM	10 g	PF	1 g	D5W	Visually compatible with no fluconazole loss in 72 hr at 25°C under fluorescent light. Cefazolin not tested	1677	C
Ceftazidime	GL	20 g	PF	1 g	D5W	Visually compatible with no fluconazole loss in 72 hr at 25°C under fluorescent light. Ceftazidime not tested	1677	C
Ciprofloxacin	BAY	1 g	RR	1 g		Visually compatible with no loss of ciprofloxacin in 24 hr at 22°C under fluorescent light. Fluconazole not tested	2413	C
Clindamycin phosphate	AST	6 g	PF	1 g	D5W	Visually compatible with no fluconazole loss in 72 hr at 25°C under fluorescent light. Clindamycin not tested	1677	C
Gentamicin sulfate	SO	0.5 g	PF	1 g	D5W	Visually compatible with no fluconazole loss in 72 hr at 25°C under fluorescent light. Gentamicin not tested	1677	C
Heparin sodium	BA	50,000 units	PF	1 g	D5W[a]	Fluconazole stable for 24 hr at 25°C in fluorescent light. Heparin not tested	1676	C
Meropenem	ZEN	1 and 20 g	RR	2 g	NS	Visually compatible for 4 hr at room temperature	1994	C
Metronidazole	AB	2.5 g	PF	1 g		Visually compatible with no fluconazole loss in 72 hr at 25°C under fluorescent light. Metronidazole not tested	1677	C
Morphine sulfate	ES	0.25 g	PF	1 g	D5W[a]	Fluconazole stable for 24 hr at 25°C in fluorescent light. Morphine not tested	1676	C
Ondansetron HCl with ranitidine HCl	GL GL	100 mg 500 mg	RR	2 g	[a]	Visually compatible with no loss of any drug in 4 hr	1730	C
Potassium chloride	AB	10 mEq	PF	1 g	D5W[a]	Fluconazole stable for 24 hr at 25°C in fluorescent light	1676	C
Ranitidine HCl with ondansetron HCl	GL GL	500 mg 100 mg	RR	2 g	[a]	Visually compatible with no loss of any drug in 4 hr	1730	C
Theophylline	BA	0.4 g	PF	1 g	D5W[a]	Fluconazole stable for 72 hr at 25°C in fluorescent light. Theophylline not tested	1676	C
Trimethoprim–sulfamethoxazole	ES	0.4[b] g	PF	1 g	D5W	Delayed cloudiness and precipitation. No fluconazole loss in 72 hr at 25°C under fluorescent light	1677	I

[a] Tested in PVC containers.

[b] Trimethoprim component. Trimethoprim in a 1:5 fixed-ratio concentration with sulfamethoxazole.

Drugs in Syringe Compatibility

Fluconazole

Test Drug	Mfr	Amt	Mfr	Amt	Remarks	Ref	C/I
Pantoprazole sodium	[a]	4 mg/1 mL		2 mg/1 mL	Possible precipitate within 4 hr	2574	I

[a] Test performed using the formulation WITHOUT edetate disodium.

Y-Site Injection Compatibility (1:1 Mixture)

Fluconazole

Test Drug	Mfr	Conc	Mfr	Conc	Remarks	Ref	C/I
Acyclovir sodium	BW	10 mg/mL	RR	2 mg/mL	Physically compatible for 24 hr at 25°C	1407	C
Aldesleukin	CHI	33,800 I.U./mL[a]	RR	2 mg/mL[a]	Visually compatible with little or no loss of aldesleukin activity	1857	C

Y-Site Injection Compatibility (1:1 Mixture) (Cont.)

Test Drug	Mfr °	Conc	Mfr	Conc	Remarks	Ref	C/I
Allopurinol sodium	BW	3 mg/mL[b]	RR	2 mg/mL	Physically compatible for 4 hr at 22°C	1686	C
Amifostine	USB	10 mg/mL[a]	RR	2 mg/mL	Physically compatible for 4 hr at 23°C	1845	C
Amikacin sulfate	BR	20 mg/mL	RR	2 mg/mL	Physically compatible for 24 hr at 25°C	1407	C
Aminophylline	ES	25 mg/mL	RR	2 mg/mL	Physically compatible for 24 hr at 25°C	1407	C
Aminophylline	AMR	0.8 and 1.5 mg/mL[a b]	PF	0.5 and 1.5 mg/mL[a b]	Visually compatible with no loss of either drug in 3 hr at 24°C	1626	C
Amiodarone HCl	WY	6 mg/mL[a]	PF	2 mg/mL[b]	Visually compatible for 24 hr at 22°C	2352	C
Amphotericin B	SQ	5 mg/mL	RR	2 mg/mL	Cloudiness and yellow precipitate	1407	I
Ampicillin sodium	WY	20 mg/mL	RR	2 mg/mL	Cloudiness develops	1407	I
Ampicillin sodium–sulbactam sodium	PF	40 mg/mL[m]	RR	2 mg/mL	Physically compatible for 24 hr at 25°C	1407	C
Anakinra	SYN	4 and 36 mg/mL[b]	PF	2 mg/mL[b]	Physically compatible. No fluconazole loss in 4 hr at 25°C. Anakinra uncertain	2508	?
Anidulafungin	VIC	0.5 mg/mL[a]	PF	2 mg/mL	Physically compatible for 4 hr at 23°C	2617	C
Aztreonam	SQ	40 mg/mL	RR	2 mg/mL	Visually compatible for 24 hr at 25°C	1407	C
Aztreonam	SQ	40 mg/mL[a]	RR	2 mg/mL	Physically compatible for 4 hr at 23°C	1758	C
Benztropine mesylate	MSD	1 mg/mL	RR	2 mg/mL	Physically compatible for 24 hr at 25°C	1407	C
Bivalirudin	TMC	5 mg/mL[a]	PF	2 mg/mL	Physically compatible for 4 hr at 23°C	2373	C
Calcium gluconate	ES	100 mg/mL	RR	2 mg/mL	Cloudiness develops	1407	I
Cangrelor tetrasodium	TMC	1 mg/mL[b]		2 mg/mL	Physically compatible for 4 hr	3243	C
Caspofungin acetate	ME	0.5 mg/mL[b]	HOS	2 mg/mL	Physically compatible over 60 min	2766	C
Cefazolin sodium	LY	40 mg/mL	RR	2 mg/mL	Physically compatible for 24 hr at 25°C	1407	C
Cefepime HCl	BMS	120 mg/mL[k]		2 mg/mL	Physically compatible with less than 10% cefepime loss. Fluconazole not tested	2513	C
Cefotaxime sodium	HO	20 mg/mL	RR	2 mg/mL	Cloudiness and amber color develop	1407	I
Cefotetan disodium	STU	40 mg/mL	RR	2 mg/mL	Physically compatible for 24 hr at 25°C	1407	C
Cefoxitin sodium	MSD	40 mg/mL	RR	2 mg/mL	Physically compatible for 24 hr at 25°C	1407	C
Ceftaroline fosamil	FOR	2.22 mg/mL[a b j]	BED	2 mg/mL	Physically compatible for 4 hr at 23°C	2826	C
Ceftazidime	GL	20 mg/mL	RR	2 mg/mL	Precipitates immediately	1407	I
Ceftazidime	SKB	125 mg/mL		2 mg/mL	Visually compatible with less than 10% loss of ceftazidime in 30 min. Fluconazole not tested	2434	C
Ceftazidime	GSK	120 mg/mL[k]		2 mg/mL	Physically compatible with less than 10% ceftazidime loss. Fluconazole not tested	2513	C
Ceftriaxone sodium	RC	40 mg/mL	RR	2 mg/mL	Precipitates immediately	1407	I
Cefuroxime sodium	GL	30 mg/mL	RR	2 mg/mL	Precipitates immediately	1407	I
Chloramphenicol sodium succinate	PD	20 mg/mL	RR	2 mg/mL	Gas production	1407	I
Chlorpromazine HCl	ES	25 mg/mL	RR	2 mg/mL	Physically compatible for 24 hr at 25°C	1407	C

Y-Site Injection Compatibility (1:1 Mixture) (Cont.)

Test Drug	Mfr	Conc	Mfr	Conc	Remarks	Ref	C/I
Cisatracurium besylate	GW	0.1, 2, 5 mg/mL[a]	RR	2 mg/mL	Physically compatible for 4 hr at 23°C	2074	C
Clindamycin phosphate	AB	24 mg/mL	RR	2 mg/mL	Precipitates immediately	1407	I
Cloxacillin sodium	SMX	100 mg/mL	SZ	2 mg/mL	Physically compatible for up to 4 hr at room temperature	3245	C
Daptomycin	CUB[r]	6.3 mg/mL[b c]	PF	1.3 mg/mL[c]	Physically compatible. No daptomycin loss and 4% fluconazole loss in 2 hr at 25°C	2553	C
Defibrotide sodium	JAZ	8 mg/mL[b]	FRK	2 mg/mL	Visually compatible for 4 hr at room temperature	3149	C
Dexamethasone sodium phosphate	ES	4 mg/mL	RR	2 mg/mL	Physically compatible for 24 hr at 25°C	1407	C
Dexmedetomidine HCl	AB	4 mcg/mL[b]	PF	2 mg/mL	Physically compatible for 4 hr at 23°C	2383	C
Diazepam	ES	5 mg/mL	RR	2 mg/mL	Precipitates immediately	1407	I
Digoxin	BW	0.25 mg/mL	RR	2 mg/mL	Gas production	1407	I
Diltiazem HCl	MMD	5 mg/mL	RR	2 mg/mL	Visually compatible	1807	C
Dimenhydrinate		10 mg/mL		2 mg/mL	Clear solution	2569	C
Diphenhydramine HCl	ES	50 mg/mL	RR	2 mg/mL	Physically compatible for 24 hr at 25°C	1407	C
Dobutamine HCl	LI	2 mg/mL[a]	RR	2 mg/mL	Visually compatible for 24 hr at 28°C under fluorescent light	1760	C
Docetaxel	RPR	0.9 mg/mL[a]	RR	2 mg/mL	Physically compatible for 4 hr at 23°C	2224	C
Dopamine HCl	AMR	1.6 mg/mL[a]	RR	2 mg/mL	Visually compatible for 24 hr at 28°C under fluorescent light	1760	C
Doripenem	JJ	5 mg/mL[a b]	HAE	2 mg/mL	Physically compatible for 4 hr at 23°C	2743	C
Doxorubicin HCl liposomal	SEQ	0.4 mg/mL[a]	RR	2 mg/mL	Physically compatible for 4 hr at 23°C	2087	C
Droperidol	DU	2.5 mg/mL	RR	2 mg/mL	Physically compatible for 24 hr at 25°C	1407	C
Eravacycline dihydrochloride	TET	0.6 mg/mL[b]	SGT	2 mg/mL[w]	Physically compatible for 2 hr at room temperature	3532	C
Etoposide phosphate	BR	5 mg/mL[a]	RR	2 mg/mL	Physically compatible for 4 hr at 23°C	2218	C
Famotidine	MSD	10 mg/mL	RR	2 mg/mL	Physically compatible for 24 hr at 25°C	1407	C
Famotidine	ME	2 mg/mL[b]		2 mg/mL[a]	Visually compatible for 4 hr at 22°C	1936	C
Fat emulsion, intravenous	OTS	20%[t]	PF	1 mg/mL[u]	Fine particles increased after preparation and continued to increase over time	3452	I
Fenoldopam mesylate	AB	80 mcg/mL[b]	PF	2 mg/mL	Physically compatible for 4 hr at 23°C	2467	C
Filgrastim	AMG	30 mcg/mL[a]	RR	2 mg/mL	Physically compatible for 4 hr at 22°C	1687	C
Filgrastim	AMG	10[e] and 40[a] mcg/mL	RR	2 mg/mL[a]	Visually compatible. Little loss of filgrastim and fluconazole in 4 hr at 25°C	2060	C
Fludarabine phosphate	BX	1 mg/mL[a]	RR	2 mg/mL	Visually compatible for 4 hr at 22°C	1439	C
Foscarnet sodium	AST	24 mg/mL	RR	2 mg/mL	Physically compatible for 24 hr at 25°C	1407	C
Furosemide	ES	10 mg/mL	RR	2 mg/mL	Precipitate forms	1407	I
Gallium nitrate	FUJ	1 mg/mL[b]	PF	2 mg/mL	Visually compatible for 24 hr at 25°C	1673	C
Ganciclovir sodium	SY	50 mg/mL	RR	2 mg/mL	Physically compatible for 24 hr at 25°C	1407	C

Y-Site Injection Compatibility (1:1 Mixture) (Cont.)

Test Drug	Mfr	Conc	Mfr	Conc	Remarks	Ref	C/I
Gemcitabine HCl	LI	10 mg/mL[b]	RR	2 mg/mL	Physically compatible for 4 hr at 23°C	2226	C
Gentamicin sulfate	ES	4 mg/mL	RR	2 mg/mL	Physically compatible for 24 hr at 25°C	1407	C
Granisetron HCl	SKB	0.05 mg/mL[a]	PF	2 mg/mL	Physically compatible for 4 hr at 23°C	2000	C
Haloperidol lactate	MN	5 mg/mL	RR	2 mg/mL	Precipitate forms	1407	I
Heparin sodium	LY	1000 units/mL	RR	2 mg/mL	Physically compatible for 24 hr at 25°C	1407	C
Heparin sodium	TR	50 units/mL	PF	2 mg/mL	Visually compatible for 4 hr at 25°C	1793	C
Hetastarch in lactated electrolyte	AB	6%	PF	2 mg/mL[b]	Physically compatible for 4 hr at 23°C	2339	C
Hydroxyzine HCl	ES	50 mg/mL	RR	2 mg/mL	Cloudiness develops	1407	I
Imipenem–cilastatin sodium	MSD	10 mg/mL[q]	RR	2 mg/mL	Precipitates immediately	1407	I
Immune globulin human	CU	50 mg/mL	RR	2 mg/mL	Physically compatible for 24 hr at 25°C	1407	C
Letermovir	ME	[b]		[b]	Physically compatible	3398	C
Leucovorin calcium	LE	10 mg/mL	RR	2 mg/mL	Physically compatible for 24 hr at 25°C	1407	C
Linezolid	PHU	2 mg/mL	RR	2 mg/mL	Physically compatible for 4 hr at 23°C	2264	C
Lorazepam	WY	0.33 mg/mL[b]	PF	2 mg/mL	Visually compatible for 24 hr at 22°C	1855	C
Melphalan HCl	BW	0.1 mg/mL[b]	RR	2 mg/mL	Physically compatible for 3 hr at 22°C	1557	C
Meperidine HCl	AB	10 mg/mL	RR	2 mg/mL	Physically compatible for 4 hr at 25°C	1397	C
Meropenem	ZEN	1 and 50 mg/mL[b]	RR	2 mg/mL	Visually compatible for 4 hr at room temperature	1994	C
Meropenem		50 mg/mL	SZ	2 mg/mL	Physically compatible for 4 hr at room temperature	3538	C
Metoclopramide HCl	RB	5 mg/mL	RR	2 mg/mL	Physically compatible for 24 hr at 25°C	1407	C
Metronidazole	AB	5 mg/mL	RR	2 mg/mL	Physically compatible for 24 hr at 25°C	1407	C
Midazolam HCl	RC	5 mg/mL	RR	2 mg/mL	Physically compatible for 24 hr at 25°C	1407	C
Midazolam HCl	RC	5 mg/mL	PF	2 mg/mL	Visually compatible for 24 hr at 22°C	1855	C
Morphine sulfate	IMS	25 mg/mL	RR	2 mg/mL	Physically compatible for 24 hr at 25°C	1407	C
Morphine sulfate	AB	1 mg/mL	RR	2 mg/mL	Physically compatible for 4 hr at 25°C	1397	C
Nafcillin sodium	BR	20 mg/mL	RR	2 mg/ml	Physically compatible for 24 hr at 25°C	1407	C
Nitroglycerin	AMR	0.2 mg/mL[a]	RR	2 mg/mL	Visually compatible for 24 hr at 28°C under fluorescent light	1760	C
Ondansetron HCl	GL	1 mg/mL[b]	PF	2 mg/mL	Visually compatible for 4 hr at 22°C	1365	C
Ondansetron HCl	GL	0.03 and 0.3 mg/mL[a]	RR	2 mg/mL[b]	Visually compatible. Little loss of either drug in 4 hr at 25°C in light	1732	C
Ondansetron HCl	GL	0.03, 0.1, 0.3 mg/mL[a b]	RR	2 mg/mL	Visually compatible. Little loss of both drugs in 4 hr. 5% or less loss of both in 12 hr at room temperature	2168	C
Oritavancin diphosphate	TAR	0.8, 1.2, and 2 mg/mL[a]	BED	2 mg/mL[a]	Visually compatible for 4 hr at 20 to 24°C	2928	C
Oxacillin sodium	BE	40 mg/mL	RR	2 mg/mL	Physically compatible for 24 hr at 25°C	1407	C

Y-Site Injection Compatibility (1:1 Mixture) (Cont.)

Test Drug	Mfr	Conc	Mfr	Conc	Remarks	Ref	C/I
Paclitaxel	NCI	1.2 mg/mL[a]	RR	2 mg/mL	Physically compatible for 4 hr at 22°C	1556	C
Paclitaxel	BR	0.3 and 1.2 mg/mL[a]	PF	2 mg/mL	Visually compatible. No loss of either drug in 4 hr at 23°C	1790	C
Pancuronium bromide	GNS	0.5 mg/mL[b]	RR	2 mg/mL	Visually compatible for 24 hr at 28°C under fluorescent light	1760	C
Pemetrexed disodium	LI	20 mg/mL[b]	PF	2 mg/mL	Physically compatible for 4 hr at 23°C	2564	C
Penicillin G potassium	RR	100,000 units/mL	RR	2 mg/mL	Physically compatible for 24 hr at 25°C	1407	C
Pentamidine isethionate	LY	6 mg/mL	RR	2 mg/mL	Cloudiness develops	1407	I
Phenytoin sodium	PD	50 mg/mL	RR	2 mg/mL	Physically compatible for 24 hr at 25°C	1407	C
Piperacillin sodium–tazobactam sodium	LE[i]	40 mg/mL[a n]	RR	2 mg/mL	Physically compatible for 4 hr at 22°C	1688	C
Plazomicin sulfate	ACH	24 mg/mL[s]	SGT	2 mg/mL[s]	Physically compatible for 1 hr at 20 to 25°C	3432	C
Prochlorperazine edisylate	SKF	5 mg/mL	RR	2 mg/mL	Physically compatible for 24 hr at 25°C	1407	C
Promethazine HCl	ES	50 mg/mL	RR	2 mg/mL	Physically compatible for 24 hr at 25°C	1407	C
Propofol	ZEN[v]	10 mg/mL	PF	2 mg/mL[a]	Physically compatible for 1 hr at 23°C	2066	C
Quinupristin–dalfopristin	PF	2 mg/mL[a o]		2 mg/mL	Physically compatible	3229	C
Ranitidine HCl	GL	0.5 and 2 mg/mL[a]	RR	2 mg/mL[b]	Visually compatible. No loss of either drug in 4 hr	1730	C
Remifentanil HCl	GW	0.025 and 0.25 mg/mL[b]	RR	2 mg/mL	Physically compatible for 4 hr at 23°C	2075	C
Sargramostim	IMM	10 mcg/mL[b]	RR	2 mg/mL	Visually compatible for 4 hr at 22°C	1436	C
Tacrolimus	FUJ	1 mg/mL[b]	RR	2 mg/mL[a]	Visually compatible for 24 hr at 25°C	1630	C
Tacrolimus	FUJ	5 and 20 mcg/mL[b]	PF	0.5 and 1.5 mg/mL[b]	Visually compatible. No loss of either drug in 3 hr at 24°C	2236	C
Telavancin HCl	ASP	7.5 mg/mL[b]	SAG	2 mg/mL[b]	Physically compatible for 2 hr	2830	C
Teniposide	BR	0.1 mg/mL[a]	RR	2 mg/mL	Physically compatible for 4 hr at 23°C	1725	C
Theophylline	AMR	1.6 mg/mL[a]	RR	2 mg/mL	Visually compatible for 24 hr at 28°C under fluorescent light	1760	C
Theophylline	TR	4 mg/mL	PF	2 mg/mL	Visually compatible for 6 hr at 25°C	1793	C
Thiotepa	IMM[f]	1 mg/mL[a]	RR	2 mg/mL	Physically compatible for 4 hr at 23°C	1861	C
Tigecycline	WY	1 mg/mL[b]		2 mg/mL	Physically compatible for 4 hr	2714	C
Tobramycin sulfate	LI	40 mg/mL	RR	2 mg/mL	Physically compatible for 24 hr at 25°C	1407	C
TNA #218 to #226[g]			PF	2 mg/mL	Visually compatible for 4 hr at 23°C	2215	C
TPN #146[g]		[h]	PF	0.5 and 1.75 mg/mL[h]	Visually compatible with no fluconazole loss in 2 hr at 24°C in fluorescent light. Amino acids greater than 93%	1554	C
TPN #147, #148[g]		[h]	PF	0.5 and 1.75 mg/mL[h]	Visually compatible with no fluconazole loss in 2 hr at 24°C in fluorescent light. Amino acids not analyzed	1554	C
TPN #212 to #215[g]			RR	2 mg/mL	Physically compatible for 4 hr at 23°C	2109	C

Y-Site Injection Compatibility (1:1 Mixture) (Cont.)

Test Drug	Mfr	Conc	Mfr	Conc °	Remarks	Ref	C/I
Trimethoprim–sulfame-thoxazole	BW	16 mg/mL[p]	RR	2 mg/mL	Viscous gel-like substance forms	1407	I
Vancomycin HCl	LY	20 mg/mL	RR	2 mg/mL	Physically compatible for 24 hr at 25°C	1407	C
Vasopressin	APP	0.2 unit/mL[b]	PF	2 mg/mL	Physically compatible	2641	C
Vecuronium bromide	OR	1 mg/mL[a]	RR	2 mg/mL	Visually compatible for 24 hr at 28°C under fluorescent light	1760	C
Vinorelbine tartrate	BW	1 mg/mL[b]	RR	2 mg/mL	Physically compatible for 4 hr at 22°C	1558	C
Zidovudine	BW	10 mg/mL	RR	2 mg/mL	Physically compatible for 24 hr at 25°C	1407	C

[a] Tested in dextrose 5%.

[b] Tested in sodium chloride 0.9%.

[c] Final concentration after mixing.

[d] Tested in dextrose 5%, Ringer's injection, lactated, sodium chloride 0.45%, and sodium chloride 0.9%.

[e] Tested in dextrose 5% with albumin human 2 mg/mL.

[f] Lyophilized formulation tested.

[g] Refer to Appendix for the composition of parenteral nutrition solutions. TNA indicates a 3-in-1 admixture, and TPN indicates a 2-in-1 admixture.

[h] Varying volumes to simulate varying administration rates.

[i] Final concentrations were 1.5 mg/mL of fluconazole and 5 and 20 mcg/mL of tacrolimus.

[j] Tested in Ringer's injection, lactated.

[k] Tested in sterile water for injection.

[l] Test performed using the formulation WITHOUT edetate disodium.

[m] Ampicillin component. Ampicillin in a 2:1 fixed-ratio concentration with sulbactam.

[n] Piperacillin component. Piperacillin in an 8:1 fixed-ratio concentration with tazobactam.

[o] Quinupristin and dalfopristin components combined.

[p] Trimethoprim component. Trimethoprim in a 1:5 fixed-ratio concentration with sulfamethoxazole.

[q] Not specified whether concentration refers to single component or combined components.

[r] Test performed using the Cubicin formulation.

[s] Tested in both dextrose 5% and sodium chloride 0.9%.

[t] Run at 25 mL/hr with dextrose 5% run at 83 mL/hr.

[u] Run at 100 mL/hr.

[v] Test performed using the formulation WITH edetate disodium.

[w] Tested as the premixed infusion solution.

Selected Revisions May 1, 2020. © Copyright, October 1992.
American Society of Health-System Pharmacists, Inc.

Fludarabine Phosphate
AHFS 10:00

Products

Fludarabine phosphate is supplied as a lyophilized product in 6-mL vials containing 50 mg of drug with mannitol 50 mg and sodium hydroxide for pH adjustment. Reconstitute with 2 mL of sterile water for injection to yield a 25-mg/mL concentration.[1(9/06)]

Fludarabine phosphate is also available as a 50-mg/2 mL solution with disodium phosphate dihydrate and sodium hydroxide for pH adjustment.[1(9/06)]

pH

From pH 7.2 to 8.2 for the reconstituted powder. From pH 7.3 to 7.7 for the liquid.[1(9/06)]

Trade Name(s)

Fludara

Administration

Fludarabine phosphate is administered by intravenous infusion over 30 minutes in 100 or 125 mL of dextrose 5% or sodium chloride 0.9%.[1(9/06)] [4] The drug also has been administered by rapid intravenous injection and continuous infusion, although the risk of toxicity may be increased.[4]

Stability

Intact vials should be stored under refrigeration. The manufacturer recommends use of the reconstituted solution within 8 hours because it does not contain an antibacterial preservative.[1(9/06)] Nevertheless, the drug is chemically stable in solution, exhibiting less than 2% decomposition in 16 days when stored at room temperature and exposed to normal laboratory light.[234]

Fludarabine phosphate (Berlex) 0.2 mg/mL diluted in sodium chloride 0.9% and stored at 22°C did not exhibit an antimicrobial effect on the growth of *Enterococcus faecium*, *Staphylococcus aureus*, *Pseudomonas aeruginosa*, and *Candida albicans* inoculated into the solution. Diluted solutions should be stored under refrigeration whenever possible, and the potential for microbiological growth should be considered when assigning expiration dates.[2160]

pH Effects

Fludarabine phosphate is stable in aqueous solution at pH 4.5 to 8. The pH of optimum stability is approximately 7.6.[234]

Sorption

Fludarabine phosphate 0.04 mg/mL in dextrose 5% or sodium chloride 0.9% was equally stable in either glass or polyvinyl chloride (PVC) containers, exhibiting no loss due to sorption during 48 hours at room temperature or under refrigeration.[234]

Compatibility Information

Solution Compatibility

Fludarabine phosphate

Test Soln Name	Mfr	Mfr	Conc/L or %	Remarks	Ref	C/I
Dextrose 5%			1 g	Under 3% loss in 16 days at room temperature in light	234	C
Dextrose 5%			40 mg	No loss in 48 hr at room temperature or refrigerated	234	C
Sodium chloride 0.9%			1 g	Under 3% loss in 16 days at room temperature in light	234	C

Y-Site Injection Compatibility (1:1 Mixture)

Fludarabine phosphate

Test Drug	Mfr	Conc	Mfr	Conc	Remarks	Ref	C/I
Acyclovir sodium	BW	7 mg/mL[a]	BX	1 mg/mL[a]	Color darkens within 4 hr	1439	I
Allopurinol sodium	BW	3 mg/mL[b]	BX	1 mg/mL[b]	Physically compatible for 4 hr at 22°C	1686	C
Amifostine	USB	10 mg/mL[a]	BX	1 mg/mL[a]	Physically compatible for 4 hr at 23°C	1845	C

DOI: 10.37573/9781585286850.171

Y-Site Injection Compatibility (1:1 Mixture) (Cont.)

Test Drug	Mfr	Conc	Mfr	Conc	Remarks	Ref	C/I
Amikacin sulfate	BR	5 mg/mL[a]	BX	1 mg/mL[a]	Visually compatible for 4 hr at 22°C	1439	C
Aminophylline	ES	2.5 mg/mL[a]	BX	1 mg/mL[a]	Visually compatible for 4 hr at 22°C	1439	C
Amphotericin B	SQ	0.6 mg/mL[a]	BX	1 mg/mL[a]	Precipitate forms in 4 hr at 22°C	1439	I
Ampicillin sodium	BR	20 mg/mL[b]	BX	1 mg/mL[a]	Visually compatible for 4 hr at 22°C	1439	C
Ampicillin sodium–sulbactam sodium	RR	20 mg/mL[b e]	BX	1 mg/mL[a]	Visually compatible for 4 hr at 22°C	1439	C
Amsacrine	NCI	1 mg/mL[a]	BX	1 mg/mL[a]	Visually compatible for 4 hr at 22°C	1439	C
Aztreonam	SQ	40 mg/mL[a]	BX	1 mg/mL[a]	Visually compatible for 4 hr at 22°C	1439	C
Aztreonam	SQ	40 mg/mL[a]	BX	1 mg/mL[a]	Physically compatible for 4 hr at 23°C	1758	C
Bleomycin sulfate	BR	1 unit/mL[b]	BX	1 mg/mL[a]	Visually compatible for 4 hr at 22°C	1439	C
Butorphanol tartrate	BR	0.04 mg/mL[a]	BX	1 mg/mL[a]	Visually compatible for 4 hr at 22°C	1439	C
Carboplatin	BR	5 mg/mL[a]	BX	1 mg/mL[a]	Visually compatible for 4 hr at 22°C	1439	C
Carmustine	BR	1.5 mg/mL[a]	BX	1 mg/mL[a]	Visually compatible for 4 hr at 22°C	1439	C
Cefazolin sodium	LEM	20 mg/mL[a]	BX	1 mg/mL[a]	Visually compatible for 4 hr at 22°C	1439	C
Cefotaxime sodium	HO	20 mg/mL[a]	BX	1 mg/mL[a]	Visually compatible for 4 hr at 22°C	1439	C
Cefotetan disodium	STU	20 mg/mL[a]	BX	1 mg/mL[a]	Visually compatible for 4 hr at 22°C	1439	C
Ceftazidime	GL	40 mg/mL[a]	BX	1 mg/mL[a]	Visually compatible for 4 hr at 22°C	1439	C
Ceftriaxone sodium	RC	20 mg/mL[a]	BX	1 mg/mL[a]	Visually compatible for 4 hr at 22°C	1439	C
Cefuroxime sodium	GL	30 mg/mL[a]	BX	1 mg/mL[a]	Visually compatible for 4 hr at 22°C	1439	C
Chlorpromazine HCl	ES	2 mg/mL[a]	BX	1 mg/mL[a]	Initial light haze intensifies within 30 min	1439	I
Cisplatin	BR	1 mg/mL	BX	1 mg/mL[a]	Visually compatible for 4 hr at 22°C	1439	C
Clindamycin phosphate	LY	10 mg/mL[a]	BX	1 mg/mL[a]	Visually compatible for 4 hr at 22°C	1439	C
Cyclophosphamide	MJ	10 mg/mL[a]	BX	1 mg/mL[a]	Visually compatible for 4 hr at 22°C	1439	C
Cytarabine	UP	50 mg/mL	BX	1 mg/mL[a]	Visually compatible for 4 hr at 22°C	1439	C
Dacarbazine	MI	4 mg/mL[a]	BX	1 mg/mL[a]	Visually compatible for 4 hr at 22°C	1439	C
Dactinomycin	MSD	0.01 mg/mL[a]	BX	1 mg/mL[a]	Visually compatible for 4 hr at 22°C	1439	C
Daunorubicin HCl	WY	2 mg/mL[a]	BX	1 mg/mL[a]	Slight haze forms in 4 hr at 22°C	1439	I
Dexamethasone sodium phosphate	MSD	1 mg/mL[a]	BX	1 mg/mL[a]	Visually compatible for 4 hr at 22°C	1439	C
Diphenhydramine HCl	WY	2 mg/mL[a]	BX	1 mg/mL[a]	Visually compatible for 4 hr at 22°C	1439	C
Doxorubicin HCl	CET	2 mg/mL	BX	1 mg/mL[a]	Visually compatible for 4 hr at 22°C	1439	C
Doxycycline hyclate	ES	1 mg/mL[a]	BX	1 mg/mL[a]	Visually compatible for 4 hr at 22°C	1439	C
Droperidol	JN	0.4 mg/mL[a]	BX	1 mg/mL[a]	Visually compatible for 4 hr at 22°C	1439	C
Etoposide	BR	0.4 mg/mL[a]	BX	1 mg/mL[a]	Visually compatible for 4 hr at 22°C	1439	C
Etoposide phosphate	BR	5 mg/mL[a]	BX	1 mg/mL[a]	Physically compatible for 4 hr at 23°C	2218	C
Famotidine	MSD	2 mg/mL[a]	BX	1 mg/mL[a]	Visually compatible for 4 hr at 22°C	1439	C
Filgrastim	AMG	30 mcg/mL[a]	BX	1 mg/mL[a]	Physically compatible for 4 hr at 22°C	1687	C

Y-Site Injection Compatibility (1:1 Mixture) (Cont.)

Test Drug	Mfr	Conc	Mfr	Conc	Remarks	Ref	C/I
Floxuridine	RC	3 mg/mL[a]	BX	1 mg/mL[a]	Visually compatible for 4 hr at 22°C	1439	C
Fluconazole	RR	2 mg/mL	BX	1 mg/mL[a]	Visually compatible for 4 hr at 22°C	1439	C
Fluorouracil	LY	16 mg/mL[a]	BX	1 mg/mL[a]	Visually compatible for 4 hr at 22°C	1439	C
Furosemide	AB	3 mg/mL[a]	BX	1 mg/mL[a]	Visually compatible for 4 hr at 22°C	1439	C
Ganciclovir sodium	SY	20 mg/mL[a]	BX	1 mg/mL[a]	Darker color forms within 4 hr	1439	I
Gemcitabine HCl	LI	10 mg/mL[b]	BX	1 mg/mL[b]	Physically compatible for 4 hr at 23°C	2226	C
Gentamicin sulfate	ES	5 mg/mL[a]	BX	1 mg/mL[a]	Visually compatible for 4 hr at 22°C	1439	C
Granisetron HCl	SKB	0.05 mg/mL[a]	BX	1 mg/mL[a]	Physically compatible for 4 hr at 23°C	2000	C
Haloperidol lactate	MN	0.2 mg/mL[a]	BX	1 mg/mL[a]	Visually compatible for 4 hr at 22°C	1439	C
Heparin sodium	SO, WY	40[a] , 100, 1000 units/mL	BX	1 mg/mL[a]	Visually compatible for 4 hr at 22°C	1439	C
Hydrocortisone sodium succinate	UP	1 mg/mL[a]	BX	1 mg/mL[a]	Visually compatible for 4 hr at 22°C	1439	C
Hydromorphone HCl	KN	0.5 mg/mL[a]	BX	1 mg/mL[a]	Visually compatible for 4 hr at 22°C	1439	C
Hydroxyzine HCl	WI	4 mg/mL[a]	BX	1 mg/mL[a]	Slight haze forms immediately	1439	I
Ifosfamide	MJ	25 mg/mL[a]	BX	1 mg/mL[a]	Visually compatible for 4 hr at 22°C	1439	C
Imipenem–cilastatin sodium	MSD	5 mg/mL[b h]	BX	1 mg/mL[a]	Visually compatible for 4 hr at 22°C	1439	C
Lorazepam	WY	0.1 mg/mL[a]	BX	1 mg/mL[a]	Visually compatible for 4 hr at 22°C	1439	C
Magnesium sulfate	SO	100 mg/mL[a]	BX	1 mg/mL[a]	Visually compatible for 4 hr at 22°C	1439	C
Mannitol	BA	15%	BX	1 mg/mL[a]	Visually compatible for 4 hr at 22°C	1439	C
Mechlorethamine HCl	MSD	1 mg/mL	BX	1 mg/mL[a]	Visually compatible for 4 hr at 22°C	1439	C
Melphalan HCl	BW	0.1 mg/mL[b]	BX	1 mg/mL[b]	Physically compatible for 3 hr at 22°C	1557	C
Meperidine HCl	WI	4 mg/mL[a]	BX	1 mg/mL[a]	Visually compatible for 4 hr at 22°C	1439	C
Mesna	BR	10 mg/mL[a]	BX	1 mg/mL[a]	Visually compatible for 4 hr at 22°C	1439	C
Methotrexate sodium	CET	15 mg/mL[a]	BX	1 mg/mL[a]	Visually compatible for 4 hr at 22°C	1439	C
Methylprednisolone sodium succinate	UP	5 mg/mL[a]	BX	1 mg/mL[a]	Visually compatible for 4 hr at 22°C	1439	C
Metoclopramide HCl	DU	5 mg/mL	BX	1 mg/mL[a]	Visually compatible for 4 hr at 22°C	1439	C
Mitoxantrone HCl	LE	0.5 mg/mL[a]	BX	1 mg/mL[a]	Visually compatible for 4 hr at 22°C	1439	C
Morphine sulfate	WI	1 mg/mL[a]	BX	1 mg/mL[a]	Visually compatible for 4 hr at 22°C	1439	C
Multivitamins	ROR	0.01 mL/mL[a]	BX	1 mg/mL[a]	Visually compatible for 4 hr at 22°C	1439	C
Nalbuphine HCl	DU	10 mg/mL	BX	1 mg/mL[a]	Visually compatible for 4 hr at 22°C	1439	C
Ondansetron HCl	GL	0.5 mg/mL[a]	BX	1 mg/mL[a]	Visually compatible for 4 hr at 22°C	1439	C
Pentostatin	NCI	0.4 mg/mL[b]	BX	1 mg/mL[a]	Visually compatible for 4 hr at 22°C	1439	C
Piperacillin sodium–tazobactam sodium	LE[d]	40 mg/mL[a f]	BX	1 mg/mL[a]	Physically compatible for 4 hr at 22°C	1688	C
Potassium chloride	AB	0.1 mEq/mL[a]	BX	1 mg/mL[a]	Visually compatible for 4 hr at 22°C	1439	C
Prochlorperazine edisylate	WY	0.5 mg/mL[a]	BX	1 mg/mL[a]	Slight haze forms within 30 min	1439	I

Y-Site Injection Compatibility (1:1 Mixture) (Cont.)

Test Drug	Mfr	Conc	Mfr	Conc	Remarks	Ref	C/I
Promethazine HCl	WY	2 mg/mL[a]	BX	1 mg/mL[a]	Visually compatible for 4 hr at 22°C	1439	C
Ranitidine HCl	GL	2 mg/mL[a]	BX	1 mg/mL[a]	Visually compatible for 4 hr at 22°C	1439	C
Sodium bicarbonate	AB	1 mEq/mL	BX	1 mg/mL[a]	Visually compatible for 4 hr at 22°C	1439	C
Teniposide	BR	0.1 mg/mL[a]	BX	1 mg/mL[a]	Physically compatible for 4 hr at 23°C	1725	C
Thiotepa	IMM[c]	1 mg/mL[a]	BX	1 mg/mL[a]	Physically compatible for 4 hr at 23°C	1861	C
Tobramycin sulfate	LI	5 mg/mL[a]	BX	1 mg/mL[a]	Visually compatible for 4 hr at 22°C	1439	C
Trimethoprim–sulfamethox-azole	ES	0.8 mg/mL[a] [g]	BX	1 mg/mL[a]	Visually compatible for 4 hr at 22°C	1439	C
Vancomycin HCl	LI	10 mg/mL[a]	BX	1 mg/mL[a]	Visually compatible for 4 hr at 22°C	1439	C
Vinblastine sulfate	LY	0.12 mg/mL[a]	BX	1 mg/mL[a]	Visually compatible for 4 hr at 22°C	1439	C
Vincristine sulfate	LY	1 mg/mL	BX	1 mg/mL[a]	Visually compatible for 4 hr at 22°C	1439	C
Vinorelbine tartrate	BW	1 mg/mL[b]	BX	1 mg/mL[b]	Physically compatible for 4 hr at 22°C	1558	C
Zidovudine	BW	4 mg/mL[a]	BX	1 mg/mL[a]	Visually compatible for 4 hr at 22°C	1439	C

[a] Tested in dextrose 5%.

[b] Tested in sodium chloride 0.9%.

[c] Lyophilized formulation tested.

[d] Test performed using the formulation WITHOUT edetate disodium.

[e] Ampicillin component. Ampicillin in a 2:1 fixed-ratio concentration with sulbactam.

[f] Piperacillin component. Piperacillin in an 8:1 fixed-ratio concentration with tazobactam.

[g] Trimethoprim component. Trimethoprim in a 1:5 fixed-ratio concentration with sulfamethoxazole.

[h] Not specified whether concentration refers to single component or combined components.

Selected Revisions December 12, 2018. © Copyright, October 1992. American Society of Health-System Pharmacists, Inc.

Flumazenil
AHFS 28:92

Products

Flumazenil is available as a 0.1-mg/mL solution in 5- and 10-mL multiple-dose vials. In addition to flumazenil, each mL also contains methylparaben 1.8 mg, propylparaben 0.2 mg, sodium chloride 0.9%, edetate disodium 0.01%, and acetic acid 0.01%. The pH is adjusted with hydrochloric acid and, if necessary, sodium hydroxide.[1(12/07)]

pH

The injection has a pH of approximately 4.[1(12/07)]

Trade Name(s)

Romazicon

Administration

Flumazenil is administered intravenously over 15 to 30 seconds. To minimize pain at the injection site, flumazenil should be administered through a freely running intravenous infusion line into a large vein. Extravasation should be avoided.[1(12/07)] [4]

Stability

Flumazenil injection is a stable aqueous solution; it should be stored at controlled room temperature. Discard the product 24 hours after removal from its original vial, whether admixed in an infusion solution or simply drawn into a syringe.[1(12/07)]

Compatibility Information

Solution Compatibility

Flumazenil

Test Soln Name	Mfr	Mfr	Conc/L or %	Remarks	Ref	C/I
Dextrose 5%				Compatible	1(12/07)	C
Dextrose 5%	BA[a]	RC	20 mg	Visually compatible. No loss in 24 hr at 23°C in fluorescent light	1710	C
Ringer's injection, lactated				Compatible	1(12/07)	C
Sodium chloride 0.9%				Compatible	1(12/07)	C

[a] Tested in PVC containers.

Additive Compatibility

Flumazenil

Test Drug	Mfr	Conc/L or %	Mfr	Conc/L or %	Test Solution	Remarks	Ref	C/I
Aminophylline	AMR	2 g	RC	20 mg	D5W[a]	Visually compatible. No flumazenil loss in 24 hr at 23°C in fluorescent light. Aminophylline not tested	1710	C
Dobutamine HCl	LI	2 g	RC	20 mg	D5W[a]	Visually compatible. No flumazenil loss in 24 hr at 23°C in fluorescent light. Dobutamine not tested	1710	C
Dopamine HCl	AB	3.2 g	RC	20 mg	D5W[a]	Visually compatible. 7% flumazenil loss in 24 hr at 23°C in fluorescent light. Dopamine not tested	1710	C
Famotidine	MSD	80 mg	RC	20 mg	D5W[a]	Visually compatible. 3% flumazenil loss in 24 hr at 23°C in fluorescent light. Famotidine not tested	1710	C
Heparin sodium	ES	50,000 units	RC	20 mg	D5W[a]	Visually compatible. 4% flumazenil loss in 24 hr at 23°C in fluorescent light. Heparin not tested	1710	C
Lidocaine HCl	AB	4 g	RC	20 mg	D5W[a]	Visually compatible. 4% flumazenil loss in 24 hr at 23°C in fluorescent light. Lidocaine not tested	1710	C

DOI: 10.37573/9781585286850.172

Additive Compatibility (Cont.)

Test Drug	Mfr	Conc/L or %	Mfr	Conc/L or %	Test Solution	Remarks	Ref	C/I
Procainamide HCl	ES	4 g	RC	20 mg	D5W[a]	Visually compatible. No flumazenil loss in 24 hr at 23°C in fluorescent light. Procainamide not tested	1710	C
Ranitidine HCl	GL	300 mg	RC	20 mg	D5W[a]	Visually compatible. 3% flumazenil loss in 24 hr at 23°C in light. Ranitidine not tested	1710	C

[a] Tested in PVC containers.

Selected Revisions October 1, 2012. © Copyright, October 1996.
American Society of Health-System Pharmacists, Inc.

Fluorouracil

AHFS 10:00

5-Fluorouracil

Products

Fluorouracil injection is available in 10- and 20-mL single-use vials[2955] [2957] and in 50- and 100-mL pharmacy bulk packages for preparation of individual doses.[2954] [2956] Each mL contains fluorouracil 50 mg with sodium hydroxide for pH adjustment.[2954] [2955] [2956] [2957]

pH

The pH is adjusted to approximately 9.2[2954] [2955] [2957] with a range of 8.6 to 9.4.[2956]

Administration

Fluorouracil is administered intravenously.[2954] [2955] [2956] [2957] Care should be taken to avoid extravasation.[2954] [2955] [2956] [2957] Dilution of the injection is not required for administration.[2954] [2955] [2956] [2957] Fluorouracil also has been given by portal vein or hepatic artery infusion.[4]

In the event of spills or leaks, the use of sodium hypochlorite 5% (household bleach) to inactivate fluorouracil is recommended.[1200]

Stability

Fluorouracil is normally colorless to faint yellow[2956] or yellow.[2954] [2955] Its stability and safety are not affected by slight discoloration that may occur during storage.[2954] [2955] [2956] [2957] It should be stored at controlled room temperature and protected from light[2954] [2955] [2956] [2957] and freezing.[2954] [2955] Some manufacturers recommend storing the vials in the original cartons until the time of use.[2956] [2957] The color of the solution results from the presence of free fluorine. A dark yellow indicates greater decomposition. Such decomposition may result from storage for several months at temperatures above room temperature. It is suggested that solutions having a darker yellow color be discarded.[398] Exposure to sunlight or intense incandescent light also has caused degradation. The solutions changed to dark amber to brown.[760] A precipitate may form from exposure to low temperatures and may be resolubilized by heating to 60°C with vigorous shaking.[2954] [2955] [2956] [2957] The solution should then be allowed to cool to body temperature before administration.[2954] [2955] [2956] [2957]

Microwave radiation also has been used to resolubilize the precipitate. Ampuls of fluorouracil (no longer commercially available in the US) containing a precipitate were exposed to microwave radiation and shaken until clear. These ampuls were then compared to ampuls that were heated to 60°C and shaken until clear and also to unheated controls. The precipitate was redissolved by microwave radiation without significantly affecting the drug. No significant decrease in concentration was observed. There was a slight change in pH. The authors concluded that microwave radiation was a suitable method for solubilizing the precipitate that may form in fluorouracil ampuls. However, they warned that extreme care should be taken to avoid overheating and the resulting explosions from excessive pressure in the ampuls.[662]

Fluorouracil (Roche) 1 mg/mL in dextrose 5% was evaluated for stability in translucent containers (Perfupack Y, Baxter) and 5 opaque containers (green polyvinyl chloride [PVC] Opafuseur [Bruneau], white ethylene vinyl acetate [EVA] Perfu-opaque [Baxter], orange PVC PF170 [Cair], white PVC V86 [Codan], and white EVA Perfecran [Fandre]) when exposed to sunlight for 28 days. No photodegradation or sorption was found. However, an increase in concentration due to moisture permeation was detected after 2 weeks.[1750]

Immersion of a needle with an aluminum component in fluorouracil (Adria) 50 mg/mL resulted in no visually apparent reaction after 7 days at 24°C.[988]

Fluorouracil (Adria) 500 mg/10 mL did not support the growth of several microorganisms commonly implicated in nosocomial infections. The bacteriostatic properties were observed against *Escherichia coli*, *Klebsiella pneumoniae*, *Staphylococcus epidermidis*, *Pseudomonas aeruginosa*, *Candida albicans*, and *Clostridium perfringens*.[828]

In another study, fluorouracil (Adria) 1 g/20 mL transferred to PVC containers did not support the growth of several microorganisms and may have imparted an antimicrobial effect at this concentration. Loss of viability was observed for *Staphylococcus aureus*, *Escherichia coli*, *Pseudomonas aeruginosa*, *Pseudomonas cepacia*, *Candida albicans*, and *Aspergillus niger*.[1187]

Fluorouracil eliminated the viability of *Staphylococcus epidermidis* (10^6 to 10^7 CFU/mL) in varying time periods, depending on concentration and diluent, when stored at near-body temperature (35°C). At 50 mg/mL, no viability was found after 5 days of incubation. At 10 mg/mL in sodium chloride 0.9% and dextrose 5%, no viability was found after 7 and 5 days, respectively. Following dilution to 10 mg/mL with bacteriostatic sodium chloride 0.9%, no viability was found after 2 days.[1659]

pH Effects

At a pH greater than 11, slow hydrolysis of fluorouracil occurs. At a pH less than 8, solubility is reduced and precipitation may or may not occur, depending on the concentration.[1369] [1379]

Fluorouracil 50 mg/mL (Lyphomed, Roche, and SoloPak) exhibited precipitation in 2 to 4 hours at pH 8.6 to 8.68; precipitation occurred immediately at pH 8.52 or less. The precipitate consisted of needle-shaped crystals at pH 8.26 to 8.68. Cluster-shaped crystals formed at pH 8.18 and below.[1489]

Admixture with acidic drugs or drugs that decompose in an alkaline environment should be avoided.[524]

DOI: 10.37573/9781585286850.173

A color change to deep purple was reported for the mixtures of doxorubicin hydrochloride (Adria) 10 mg/L with fluorouracil (Roche) 250 mg/L in dextrose 5%.[296] This color change is indicative of decomposition occurring in solutions with an alkaline pH. It also occurs with other anthracyclines.[394]

Freezing Solutions

Fluorouracil (Abic) 5 mg/0.5 mL in sodium chloride 0.9% in polypropylene syringes (Plastipak, Becton Dickinson) was stored frozen at –20°C. No fluorouracil loss occurred in 8 weeks. Refreezing and further storage at –20°C for another 2 weeks also did not result in a fluorouracil loss.[1666]

Fluorouracil (Teva) near 6.8 mg/mL in sodium chloride 0.9% in PVC bags was stored frozen at –20°C for 79 days, thawed in a microwave oven, and stored for an additional 28 days under refrigeration. No precipitation or crystallization occurred. No fluorouracil loss occurred after frozen storage and about 6% loss occurred after the subsequent refrigerated storage.[2807]

Syringes

Fluorouracil 25 mg/mL in polypropylene syringes (Braun Omnifix) was stable for 28 days at 4 and 20°C.[1564]

Fluorouracil (Roche) 50 mg/mL was packaged as 3 mL in 10-mL polypropylene infusion pump syringes (Pharmacia Deltec). Little or no loss occurred during 21 days of storage at 30°C.[1967]

Fluorouracil (Roche) 12 and 40 mg/mL diluted with sodium chloride 0.9% and dextrose 5% was packaged in 60-mL polypropylene syringes and stored at 25°C protected from light. Losses of 5% or less occurred in the solutions after storage for 72 hours. Furthermore, the solutions had no visually apparent precipitate or discoloration.[1983]

Ambulatory Pumps

The stability of undiluted fluorouracil 50 mg/mL from 3 manufacturers (Lyphomed, Roche, and SoloPak) in the reservoirs of 4 portable infusion pumps (Pharmacia Deltec CADD-1, Model 5100; Cormed II, Model 10500; Medfusion Infumed 200; and Pancretec Provider I.V., Model 2000) was evaluated. The fluorouracil was delivered by the pumps at a rate of 10 mL/day over a 7-day cycle at 25 and 37°C. All fluorouracil samples in all pump reservoirs were stable over the 7-day study period, exhibiting little or no drug loss and only minimal leached plasticizer, diethylhexyl phthalate (DEHP), at either temperature.[1489]

However, precipitation of the Roche fluorouracil was observed with all pumps; a fine white precipitate originated close to the connection junction and migrated in both directions until it occupied most of the tubing and was in the drug reservoir. In some cases, the pumps stopped due to the extent of precipitation. The authors noted that various factors, including solution pH, temperature, drug concentration and solubility, and the manipulative techniques used could contribute to precipitate formation.[1489]

Undiluted fluorouracil (Roche) 50 mg/mL in EVA bags for use with portable infusion pumps remained stable, with little or no loss after 28 days at 4, 22, and 35°C. The containers at 35°C did sustain approximately a 3% water loss due to evaporation during storage, increasing the fluorouracil concentration slightly.[1548]

Fluorouracil (David Bull Laboratories) 25 mg/mL was stable in PVC reservoirs (Parker Micropump) for 14 days at 4 and 37°C, exhibiting no loss.[1696]

The stability of undiluted fluorouracil injection (Roche) 50 mg/mL in EVA reservoirs (Celsa) and PVC reservoirs (Pharmacia) for use with ambulatory infusion pumps was evaluated. The filled reservoirs were stored for 14 days at 4°C and at 33°C to simulate the conditions of prolonged infusion from the reservoirs kept under patients' clothing. No loss of fluorouracil due to decomposition was found. However, the refrigerated samples exhibited substantial (up to 15%) loss of drug content from solution due to gross precipitation. Flocculent precipitation was observed in as little as 3 days, though subvisible precipitation may occur earlier. At the elevated temperature, substantial increases in concentration of fluorouracil occurred in the EVA reservoirs due to water loss from permeation through the plastic reservoir. Approximately 5% increase in drug concentration occurred in 14 days. No change in concentration occurred in the PVC reservoirs during this time frame.[2004]

Implantable Pumps

Fluorouracil 50 mg/mL was filled into an implantable infusion pump (Fresenius VIP 30) and associated capillary tubing and stored at 37°C. No fluorouracil loss and no contamination from components of pump materials occurred during 8 weeks of storage.[1903]

Fluorouracil combined with leucovorin calcium for repeated administration using a Fresenius implanted port resulted in blockage of the pump catheter and necessitated surgical removal of the port. The blockage was caused by precipitation of calcium carbonate in the catheter.[2504]

Sorption

Fluorouracil was shown not to exhibit sorption to PVC bags and tubing, polyethylene bags or tubing, Silastic tubing, and polypropylene and polyethylene syringes.[536 606 760 2420 2430]

Fluorouracil may be more extensively adsorbed to glass surfaces than to plastic. In one report, significant loss occurred from solutions in glass vials, but almost quantitative recovery was obtained from polyethylene and polypropylene plastic vials. The loss was attributed to adsorption to the glass surface.[663] This difference was also observed in dextrose 5% in glass and PVC infusion containers. A 10% loss of fluorouracil occurred in 43 hours in the PVC containers but in only 7 hours in the glass containers.[519]

Filtration

Fluorouracil 10 to 75 mcg/mL exhibited little or no loss due to sorption to either cellulose nitrate/cellulose acetate ester (Millex OR) or Teflon (Millex FG) filters.[1415 1416]

Central Venous Catheter

Fluorouracil (Roche) 5 mg/mL in dextrose 5% was found to be compatible with the ARROWg+ard Blue Plus (Arrow International) chlorhexidine-bearing triple-lumen central catheter. Essentially complete delivery of the drug was found with little or no drug loss occurring. Furthermore, chlorhexidine delivered from the catheter remained at trace amounts with no substantial increase due to the delivery of the drug through the catheter.[2335]

Compatibility Information

Solution Compatibility

Fluorouracil

Test Soln Name	Mfr	Mfr	Conc/L or %	Remarks	Ref	C/I
Amino acids 4.25%, dextrose 25%	MG	RC	500 mg	No increase in particulate matter in 24 hr at 5°C	349	C
Dextrose 5% in Ringer's injection, lactated	MG[a]		500 mg	No decomposition in 24 hr	399	C
Dextrose 5%	[d]	RC	10 g	No loss in 16 weeks at 5°C. Little change in 7 days at 25°C	894	C
Dextrose 5%	[h]	RC	10 g	No loss in 16 weeks at 5°C	894	C
Dextrose 5%	TR[b]	RC	1.5 g	Physically compatible. Stable for 8 weeks at ambient temperature both in dark and light	1153	C
Dextrose 5%			1 and 2 g	Physically compatible and no loss in 48 hr at room temperature and 7°C	1152	C
Dextrose 5%	[c]	RC	10 g	Visually compatible with little loss in 28 days at 4, 22, and 35°C in dark. At 35°C, concentration increased due to water evaporation	1548	C
Dextrose 5%	MG[a]		8.3 g	Less than 10% loss in 48 hr at room temperature exposed to light	1658	C
Dextrose 5%	BA[d]	RC	1 and 10 g	Visually compatible with less than 3% loss in 14 days at 4 and 21°C	2004	C
Dextrose 5%	BA[d]	RC[e]	0.5 and 5 g	Little or no loss in 13 days at 4 and 25°C	2175	C
Dextrose 5%	BA[g]	ICN	25 g	Physically compatible. Little loss in 14 days at 4°C, 21 days at 25 and 31°C	2483	C
Sodium chloride 0.9%	TR[b]	RC	1.5 g	Physically compatible and chemically stable for 8 weeks at ambient temperature both in the dark and exposed to fluorescent light	1153	C
Sodium chloride 0.9%			1 and 2 g	Physically compatible and no loss in 48 hr at room temperature and 7°C	1152	C
Sodium chloride 0.9%	[c]	RC	10 g	Visually compatible with little loss in 28 days at 4, 22, and 35°C in dark. At 35°C, concentration increased due to water evaporation	1548	C
Sodium chloride 0.9%	[b]	FA, RC	5 and 50 g	Visually compatible. Little loss in 91 days at 4°C followed by 7 days at 25°C in the dark	1567	C
Sodium chloride 0.9%	[c]	RC	15 and 45 g	Visually compatible with little or no loss in 72 hr at 25°C protected from light	1983	C
Sodium chloride 0.9%	BA[d]	RC	1 and 10 g	Visually compatible with less than 3% loss in 14 days at 4 and 21°C	2004	C
Sodium chloride 0.9%	BA[d]	RC[e]	0.5 and 5 g	Little or no loss in 13 days at 4 and 25°C	2175	C
Sodium chloride 0.9%	BA[g]	ICN	25 g	Physically compatible. Little loss in 14 days at 4°C, 21 days at 25 and 31°C	2483	C
TPN #23[f]		RC	1 and 4 g	Physically compatible for 42 hr at room temperature in light. Erratic assay results	562	?

Solution Compatibility (Cont.)

Test Soln Name	Mfr	Mfr	Conc/L or %	Remarks	Ref	C/I
TPN #23[f]		RC	1 g	Physically compatible and fluorouracil stable for 48 hr at room temperature in ambient light	826	C

[a] Tested in both glass and polyolefin containers.

[b] Tested in both glass and PVC containers.

[c] Tested in ethylene vinyl acetate (EVA) containers.

[d] Tested in PVC containers.

[e] A modified fluorouracil formulation containing tromethamine (TRIS, THAM, trometamol) instead of sodium hydroxide.

[f] Refer to Appendix for the composition of parenteral nutrition solutions. TPN indicates a 2-in-1 admixture.

[g] Tested in Easypump (Braun) elastomeric reservoir pumps.

[h] Tested in Infusor (Travenol) elastomeric reservoir pumps.

Additive Compatibility

Fluorouracil

Test Drug	Mfr	Conc/L or %	Mfr	Conc/L or %	Test Solution	Remarks	Ref	C/I
Bleomycin sulfate	BR	20 and 30 units	RC	1 g	NS	Physically compatible and bleomycin activity retained for 1 week at 4°C. Fluorouracil not tested	763	C
Carboplatin		1 g		10 g	W	Greater than 20% carboplatin loss in 24 hr at room temperature	1379	I
Carboplatin	BR	100 mg	DB	1 g	D5W	9% carboplatin loss in 5 hr at 25°C	2415	I
Ciprofloxacin						Physically incompatible with loss of ciprofloxacin reported due to pH over 6.0	1924	I
Cisplatin	BR	200 mg	SO	1 g	NS[a]	10% cisplatin loss in 1.5 hr and 25% loss in 4 hr at 25°C	1339	I
Cisplatin	BR	500 mg	SO	10 g	NS[a]	10% cisplatin loss in 1.2 hr and 25% loss in 3 hr at 25°C	1339	I
Cisplatin	BR	500 mg	AD	10 g	NS	80% cisplatin loss in 24 hr at room temperature due to low pH	1386	I
Cyclophosphamide		1.67 g		8.3 g	NS	Both drugs stable for 14 days at room temperature	1389	C
Cyclophosphamide with methotrexate sodium		1.67 g 25 mg		8.3 g	NS	9.3% cyclophosphamide loss in 7 days at room temperature. No loss of other drugs observed	1389	C
Cytarabine	UP	400 mg	RC	250 mg	D5W	Altered UV spectra for cytarabine within 1 hr at room temperature	207	I
Diazepam	RC					Precipitates immediately	524	I
Doxorubicin HCl	AD					Discolors from red to blue-purple	524	I
Doxorubicin HCl	AD	10 mg	RC	250 mg	D5W	Color changes to deep purple	296	I
Epirubicin HCl		0.5 to 1 g		10 g	NS	Greater than 10% epirubicin loss in 1 day	1379	I
Epirubicin HCl	PHU					Potential precipitation	3377	I
Etoposide		200 mg		10 g	NS	Both drugs stable for 7 days at room temperature and 1 day at 35°C	1379	C

Additive Compatibility (Cont.)

Test Drug	Mfr	Conc/L or %	Mfr	Conc/L or %	Test Solution	Remarks	Ref	C/I
Fentanyl citrate	AB	12.5 mg	AB	1 and 16 g	D5W, NS[a]	25% fentanyl loss in 15 min due to sorption to PVC	2064	I
Floxuridine		10 g		10 g	NS	Both drugs stable for 15 days at room temperature	1390	C
Hydromorphone HCl	AST	500 mg	AB	1 g	D5W, NS[a]	Physically compatible. Little loss of either drug in 7 days at 32°C and 35 days at 23, 4, and –20°C	1977	C
Hydromorphone HCl	AST	500 mg	AB	16 g	D5W, NS[a]	Physically compatible. Little loss of either drug in 3 days at 32°C, 7 days at 23°C, and 35 days at 4 and –20°C	1977	C
Ifosfamide		2 g		10 g	NS	Both drugs stable for 5 days at room temperature	1379	C
Leucovorin calcium	LE	1.5 to 13.3 g	AD	16.7 to 46.2 g	[b]	Subvisible particulates form in all combinations in variable periods from 1 to 4 days at 4, 23, and 32°C	1816	I
Levoleucovorin calcium	CY	1.5 to 13.3 g	AD	16.7 to 46.2 g	[b]	Subvisible particulates form in all combinations in variable periods from 1 to 4 days at 4, 23, and 32°C	1816	I
Methotrexate sodium		30 mg		10 g	NS	Both drugs stable for 15 days at room temperature	1379	C
Methotrexate sodium with cyclophosphamide		25 mg 1.67 g		8.3 g	NS	9.3% cyclophosphamide loss in 7 days at room temperature. No loss of other drugs observed	1389	C
Metoclopramide HCl	FUJ	100 mg	RC	2.5 g	D5W	10% metoclopramide loss in 6 hr and 27% loss in 24 hr at 25°C. 5% metoclopramide loss in 120 hr at 4°C. 5 and 7% fluorouracil losses in 120 hr at 4 and 25°C, respectively	1780	I
Mitoxantrone HCl	LE	500 mg		25 g	D5W	Visually compatible. Mitoxantrone stable for 24 hr at room temperature. Fluorouracil not tested	1531	C
Morphine sulfate	AST	1 g	AB	1 and 16 g	D5W, NS[a]	Subvisible morphine precipitate forms immediately, becoming grossly visible within 24 hr. Morphine losses of 60 to 80% occur within 1 day	1977	I
Vincristine sulfate	LI	4 mg	RC	10 mg	D5W	Physically compatible. No alteration in UV spectra in 8 hr at room temperature	207	C

[a] Tested in PVC containers.

[b] Tested with both drugs undiluted and diluted by 25% with dextrose 5%.

Drugs in Syringe Compatibility

Fluorouracil

Test Drug	Mfr	Amt	Mfr	Amt	Remarks	Ref	C/I
Bleomycin sulfate		1.5 units/0.5 mL		25 mg/0.5 mL	Physically compatible for 5 min at room temperature followed by 8 min of centrifugation	980	C
Cisplatin		0.5 mg/0.5 mL		25 mg/0.5 mL	Physically compatible for 5 min at room temperature followed by 8 min of centrifugation	980	C
Cyclophosphamide		10 mg/0.5 mL		25 mg/0.5 mL	Physically compatible for 5 min at room temperature followed by 8 min of centrifugation	980	C
Doxorubicin HCl		1 mg/0.5 mL		25 mg/0.5 mL	Physically compatible for 5 min at room temperature followed by 8 min of centrifugation	980	C

Drugs in Syringe Compatibility (Cont.)

Test Drug	Mfr	Amt	Mfr	Amt	Remarks	Ref	C/I
Doxorubicin HCl		5 and 10 mg/10 mL[a]		500 mg/10 mL	Precipitate forms within several hours of mixing	1564	I
Droperidol		1.25 mg/0.5 mL		25 mg/0.5 mL	Precipitates immediately	980	I
Epirubicin HCl		5 and 10 mg/10 mL[a]		500 mg/10 mL	Precipitate forms within several hours of mixing	1564	I
Furosemide		5 mg/0.5 mL		25 mg/0.5 mL	Physically compatible for 5 min at room temperature followed by 8 min of centrifugation	980	C
Heparin sodium		500 units/0.5 mL		25 mg/0.5 mL	Physically compatible for 5 min at room temperature followed by 8 min of centrifugation	980	C
Heparin sodium	LEO	20,000 units/0.8 mL	DB	500 mg/20 mL	Visually compatible with no loss of either drug in 7 days at 25°C and 14 days at 4°C in the dark	2415	C
Leucovorin calcium		5 mg/0.5 mL		25 mg/0.5 mL	Physically compatible for 5 min at room temperature followed by 8 min of centrifugation	980	C
Methotrexate sodium		12.5 mg/0.5 mL		25 mg/0.5 mL	Physically compatible for 5 min at room temperature followed by 8 min of centrifugation	980	C
Metoclopramide HCl		2.5 mg/0.5 mL		25 mg/0.5 mL	Physically compatible for 5 min at room temperature followed by 8 min of centrifugation	980	C
Mitomycin		0.25 mg/0.5 mL		25 mg/0.5 mL	Physically compatible for 5 min at room temperature followed by 8 min of centrifugation	980	C
Vinblastine sulfate		0.5 mg/0.5 mL		25 mg/0.5 mL	Physically compatible for 5 min at room temperature followed by 8 min of centrifugation	980	C
Vincristine sulfate		0.5 mg/0.5 mL		25 mg/0.5 mL	Physically compatible for 5 min at room temperature followed by 8 min of centrifugation	980	C

[a] Diluted in sodium chloride 0.9%.

Y-Site Injection Compatibility (1:1 Mixture)

Fluorouracil

Test Drug	Mfr	Conc	Mfr	Conc	Remarks	Ref	C/I
Aldesleukin	CHI[g]	[a]			Unacceptable loss of aldesleukin activity	1890	I
Allopurinol sodium	BW	3 mg/mL[b]	RC	16 mg/mL[b]	Physically compatible for 4 hr at 22°C	1686	C
Amifostine	USB	10 mg/mL[a]	AD	16 mg/mL[b]	Physically compatible for 4 hr at 23°C	1845	C
Anidulafungin	VIC	0.5 mg/mL[a]	APP	16 mg/mL[a]	Physically compatible for 4 hr at 23°C	2617	C
Aztreonam	SQ	40 mg/ml[a]	AD	16 mg/mL[a]	Physically compatible for 4 hr at 23°C	1758	C
Bleomycin sulfate		3 units/mL		50 mg/mL	Drugs injected sequentially in Y-site with no flush. No precipitate seen	980	C
Cisplatin		1 mg/mL		50 mg/mL	Drugs injected sequentially in Y-site with no flush. No precipitate seen	980	C
Cyclophosphamide		20 mg/mL		50 mg/mL	Drugs injected sequentially in Y-site with no flush. No precipitate seen	980	C
Doripenem	JJ	5 mg/mL[a b]	ABX	16 mg/mL[a b]	Physically compatible for 4 hr at 23°C	2743	C
Doxorubicin HCl		2 mg/mL		50 mg/mL	Drugs injected sequentially in Y-site with no flush. No precipitate seen	980	C
Doxorubicin HCl liposomal	SEQ	0.4 mg/mL[a]	PH	16 mg/mL[a]	Physically compatible for 4 hr at 23°C	2087	C

Y-Site Injection Compatibility (1:1 Mixture) (Cont.)

Test Drug	Mfr	Conc	Mfr	Conc	Remarks	Ref	C/I
Droperidol		2.5 mg/mL		50 mg/mL	Drugs injected sequentially in Y-site with no flush. Precipitates immediately	980	I
Etoposide phosphate	BR	5 mg/mL[a]	PH	16 mg/mL[a]	Physically compatible for 4 hr at 23°C	2218	C
Filgrastim	AMG	30 mcg/mL[a]	RC	16 mg/mL[a]	Particles and long filaments form in 1 hr	1687	I
Fludarabine phosphate	BX	1 mg/mL[a]	LY	16 mg/mL[a]	Visually compatible for 4 hr at 22°C	1439	C
Furosemide		10 mg/mL		50 mg/mL	Drugs injected sequentially in Y-site with no flush. No precipitate seen	980	C
Gallium nitrate	FUJ	1 mg/mL[b]	RC	50 mg/mL	Precipitate forms immediately but clears after 60 min	1673	I
Gemcitabine HCl	LI	10 mg/mL[b]	PH	16 mg/mL[b]	Physically compatible for 4 hr at 23°C	2226	C
Granisetron HCl	SKB	0.05 mg/mL[b]	AD	16 mg/mL[b]	Physically compatible for 4 hr at 23°C	1804	C
Granisetron HCl	SKB	1 mg/mL	RC	2 mg/mL[b]	Physically compatible with little or no loss of either drug in 4 hr at 22°C	1883	C
Granisetron HCl	SKB	0.05 mg/mL[a]	AD	16 mg/mL[a]	Physically compatible for 4 hr at 23°C	2000	C
Heparin sodium		1000 units/mL		50 mg/mL	Drugs injected sequentially in Y-site with no flush. No precipitate seen	980	C
Heparin sodium	UP	1000 units/L[c]	RC	50 mg/mL	Physically compatible for 4 hr at room temperature	534	C
Hydrocortisone sodium succinate	UP	10 mg/L[c]	RC	50 mg/mL	Physically compatible for 4 hr at room temperature	534	C
Leucovorin calcium		10 mg/mL		50 mg/mL	Drugs injected sequentially in Y-site with no flush. No precipitate seen	980	C
Linezolid	PHU	2 mg/mL	PH	16 mg/mL[a]	Physically compatible for 4 hr at 23°C	2264	C
Mannitol		20%	SO	1 and 2 mg/mL[d]	Physically compatible and fluorouracil stable for 24 hr. Mannitol not tested	1526	C
Melphalan HCl	BW	0.1 mg/mL[b]	LY	16 mg/mL[b]	Physically compatible for 3 hr at 22°C	1557	C
Methotrexate sodium		25 mg/mL		50 mg/mL	Drugs injected sequentially in Y-site with no flush. No precipitate seen	980	C
Metoclopramide HCl		5 mg/mL		50 mg/mL	Drugs injected sequentially in Y-site with no flush. No precipitate seen	980	C
Mitomycin		0.5 mg/mL		50 mg/mL	Drugs injected sequentially in Y-site with no flush. No precipitate seen	980	C
Ondansetron HCl	GL	1 mg/mL[b]	SO	16 mg/mL[a]	Precipitates immediately	1365	I
Ondansetron HCl	GL	16 to 160 mcg/mL		≤0.8 mg/mL	Physically compatible when fluorouracil given at 20 mL/hr via Y-site	1366	C
Paclitaxel	NCI	1.2 mg/mL[a]		16 mg/mL[a]	Physically compatible for 4 hr at 22°C	1528	C
Palonosetron HCl	MGI	50 mcg/mL	APP	16 mg/mL[a]	Physically compatible and no loss of either drug in 4 hr	2627	C
Pemetrexed disodium	LI	20 mg/mL[b]	APP	16 mg/mL[a]	Physically compatible for 4 hr at 23°C	2564	C
Piperacillin sodium–tazobactam sodium	LE[h]	40 mg/mL[a i]	LY	16 mg/mL[a]	Physically compatible for 4 hr at 22°C	1688	C
Potassium chloride	AB	40 mEq/L[c]	RC	50 mg/mL	Physically compatible for 4 hr at room temperature	534	C

Y-Site Injection Compatibility (1:1 Mixture) (Cont.)

Test Drug	Mfr	Conc	Mfr	Conc	Remarks	Ref	C/I
Propofol	ZEN[j]	10 mg/mL	AD	16 mg/mL[a]	Physically compatible for 1 hr at 23°C	2066	C
Sargramostim	IMM	10 mcg/mL[b]	SO	16 mg/mL[b]	Visually compatible for 4 hr at 22°C	1436	C
Teniposide	BR	0.1 mg/mL[a]	AD	16 mg/mL[a]	Physically compatible for 4 hr at 23°C	1725	C
Thiotepa	IMM[e]	1 mg/mL[a]	AD	16 mg/mL[a]	Physically compatible for 4 hr at 23°C	1861	C
TNA #218, #219, #221, #222, #224 to #226[f]			PH	16 mg/mL[a]	Visually compatible for 4 hr at 23°C	2215	C
TNA #220, #223[f]			PH	16 mg/mL[a]	Small amount of white precipitate forms immediately	2215	I
Topotecan HCl	SKB	56 mcg/mL[b]	RC	50 mg/mL	Immediate haze and yellow color	2245	I
TPN #212, #213[f]			PH	16 mg/mL[a]	Slight subvisible haze, crystals, and amber discoloration form in 1 to 4 hr	2109	I
TPN #214, #215[f]			PH	16 mg/mL[a]	Turbidity forms immediately	2109	I
Vinblastine sulfate		1 mg/mL		50 mg/mL	Drugs injected sequentially in Y-site with no flush. No precipitate seen	980	C
Vincristine sulfate		1 mg/mL		50 mg/mL	Drugs injected sequentially in Y-site with no flush. No precipitate seen	980	C
Vinorelbine tartrate	BW	1 mg/mL[b]	RC	16 mg/mL[b]	Heavy white precipitate forms immediately	1558	I

[a] Tested in dextrose 5%.

[b] Tested in sodium chloride 0.9%.

[c] Tested in dextrose 5% in Ringer's injection, dextrose 5% in Ringer's injection, lactated, dextrose 5%, Ringer's injection, lactated, and sodium chloride 0.9%.

[d] Tested in dextrose 5% in sodium chloride 0.45%, dextrose 5%, and sodium chloride 0.9%.

[e] Lyophilized formulation tested.

[f] Refer to Appendix for the composition of parenteral nutrition solutions. TNA indicates a 3-in-1 admixture, and TPN indicates a 2-in-1 admixture.

[g] Tested with albumin human 0.1%.

[h] Test performed using the formulation WITHOUT edetate disodium.

[i] Piperacillin component. Piperacillin in an 8:1 fixed-ratio concentration with tazobactam.

[j] Test performed using the formulation WITH edetate disodium.

Selected Revisions January 31, 2020. © Copyright, October 1982. American Society of Health-System Pharmacists, Inc.

Fluphenazine Hydrochloride
AHFS 28:16.08.24

Products

Fluphenazine hydrochloride is available in 10-mL multiple-dose vials. Each mL contains fluphenazine hydrochloride 2.5 mg with sodium chloride for isotonicity, sodium hydroxide or hydrochloric acid to adjust the pH, and methylparaben 0.1% and propylparaben 0.01% as preservatives.[1(9/08)]

pH

From 4.8 to 5.2.[1(9/08) 4]

Administration

Fluphenazine hydrochloride is administered by intramuscular injection.[1(9/08) 4]

Stability

Intact vials should be stored at controlled room temperature and protected from freezing and light. Parenteral solutions of fluphenazine hydrochloride vary from colorless to light amber. Solutions that are darker than light amber, are discolored in some other way, or contain a precipitate should not be used.[1(9/08) 4]

Compatibility Information

Drugs in Syringe Compatibility

Fluphenazine HCl

Test Drug	Mfr	Amt	Mfr	Amt	Remarks	Ref	C/I
Benztropine mesylate	MSD	2 mg/2 mL	LY	5 mg/2 mL	Visually compatible for 60 min	1784	C
Diphenhydramine HCl	ES	100 mg/2 mL	LY	5 mg/2 mL	Visually compatible for 60 min	1784	C
Hydroxyzine HCl	ES	100 mg/2 mL	LY	5 mg/2 mL	Visually compatible for 60 min	1784	C

Selected Revisions October 1, 2012. © Copyright, October 1996.
American Society of Health-System Pharmacists, Inc.

DOI: 10.37573/9781585286850.174

Folic Acid
AHFS 88:08

Products

Folic acid 5 mg/mL injection is available in 10-mL vials. Each mL of solution also contains edetate sodium 5 mg, benzyl alcohol 2 mg, and hydrochloric acid and/or sodium hydroxide to adjust pH in water for injection.[1(1/08)]

pH

From 8 to 11.[1(1/08) 4]

Administration

Folic acid injection is administered by deep intramuscular, intravenous, or subcutaneous injection.[1(1/08) 4]

Stability

Intact vials should be stored at controlled room temperature and protected from light.[1(1/08)] The yellow to orange-yellow solutions are heat sensitive and should be protected from light[4] for long-term storage. However, exposure of folic acid in parenteral nutrition solutions to fluorescent light for 48 hours did not cause any significant loss of folic acid.[896]

pH Effects

Folic acid is soluble in solutions of pH 5.6 or above at room temperature to a concentration of 1 g/L. However, below about pH 4.5 to 5, folic acid may precipitate in varying time periods, depending on the acidity of the solution. In the small concentrations used for parenteral nutrition, a pH of above 5 ensures that folic acid will remain in solution. Most parenteral nutrition solutions are buffered by the amino acids to pH 5 to 6.[895]

The rate of folic acid photodegradation is higher in an acidic medium compared to the rate in an alkaline medium.[2496]

Sorption

A parenteral nutrition solution containing 13 mcg/L of folic acid injection in a 3-L polyvinyl chloride (PVC) bag and run through an administration set delivered the full amount of folic acid, with no loss.[895]

Filtration

Folic acid (Lederle) 0.5 mg/L in dextrose 5% and sodium chloride 0.9% was filtered at 120 mL/hr for 6 hours through a 0.22-μm cellulose ester membrane filter (Ivex-2). No significant reduction due to binding to the filter was noted.[533]

Compatibility Information

Solution Compatibility

Folic acid

Test Soln Name	Mfr	Mfr	Conc/L or %	Remarks	Ref	C/I
Amino acids 4.25%, dextrose 25%	MG	USP	0.2 and 10 mg	Physically compatible. Stable for 7 days at 4°C and room temperature in dark	895	C
Dextrose 20%		USP	0.2 and 20 mg	Physically compatible. Stable for 7 days at 4°C and room temperature in dark	895	C
Dextrose 40%		USP	0.2 and 20 mg	17 to 25% loss in 24 hr at 4°C and room temperature in dark, with precipitation at the higher concentration after 48 hr	895	I
Dextrose 50%		USP	20 mg	Precipitate forms within 24 hr at 4°C and room temperature protected from light	895	I
TPN #69[a]		USP	0.4 mg	Physically compatible and folic acid stable for at least 7 days at 4 and 25°C protected from light	895	C
TPN #70[a]		LE	0.25 to 1 mg	Folic acid stable for at least 48 hr at 6 and 21°C in the light or dark	896	C
TPN #74[a]			1 mg	Folic acid stable over 8 hr at room temperature in fluorescent or sunlight	842	C
TPN #189[a]		AB	15 mg/mL	Visually compatible for 24 hr at 22°C	1767	C

[a] Refer to Appendix for the composition of parenteral nutrition solutions. TPN indicates a 2-in-1 admixture.

DOI: 10.37573/9781585286850.175

Additive Compatibility

Folic acid

Test Drug	Mfr	Conc/L or %	Mfr	Conc/L or %	Test Solution	Remarks	Ref	C/I
Fat emulsion, intravenous	KV	10%	USP	0.2 and 20 mg		Physically compatible for 2 weeks at 4°C and room temperature in the dark but erratic assays	895	?

Drugs in Syringe Compatibility

Folic acid

Test Drug	Mfr	Amt	Mfr	Amt	Remarks	Ref	C/I
Doxapram HCl	RB	400 mg/20 mL		15 mg/1 mL	Immediate turbidity	1177	I

Y-Site Injection Compatibility (1:1 Mixture)

Folic acid

Test Drug	Mfr	Conc	Mfr	Conc	Remarks	Ref	C/I
Famotidine	MSD	0.2 mg/mL[a]	LE	5 mg/mL	Physically compatible for 14 hr	1196	C
Letermovir	ME	[a]		[a]	Physically compatible	3398	C

[a] Tested in dextrose 5%.

Additional Compatibility Information

Parenteral Nutrition Solutions

A 40% drop in folic acid concentration occurred immediately after admixture in a parenteral nutrition solution composed of amino acids, dextrose, electrolytes, trace elements, and multivitamins in PVC bags. The folic acid concentration then remained relatively constant for 28 days when stored at both 4 and 25°C.[1063]

Extensive decomposition of ascorbic acid and folic acid was reported in a parenteral nutrition solution composed of amino acids 3.3%, dextrose 12.5%, electrolytes, trace elements, and M.V.I.-12 (USV) in PVC bags. Half-lives were 1.1, 2.9, and 8.9 hours for ascorbic acid and 2.7, 5.4, and 24 hours for folic acid stored at 24°C in daylight, 24°C protected from light, and 4°C protected from light, respectively. The decomposition was much greater than for solutions not containing catalyzing metal ions. Also, it was greater than for the vitamins singly because of interactions with the other vitamins present.[1059]

Because of these interactions, recommendations to separate the administration of vitamins and trace elements have been made.[1056] [1060] [1061] Other researchers have termed such recommendations premature based on differing reports[895] [896] and the apparent absence of epidemic vitamin deficiency in parenteral nutrition patients.[1062]

The stability of several vitamins from M.V.I.-12 (Armour) admixed in parenteral nutrition solutions composed of different amino acid products, with or without Intralipid 10%, in glass bottles and PVC bags at 25 and 5°C for 48 hours was reported. Folic acid was stable in all samples.[1431]

In another study, the stability of several vitamins (from M.V.I.-12) following admixture with 4 different amino acid products (FreAmine III, Neopham, Novamine, Travasol) with or without Intralipid when stored in glass bottles or PVC bags at 25°C for 48 hours was reported. High-intensity phototherapy light did not affect folic acid. When bisulfite was added to the Neopham admixture, folic acid was unaffected. The authors concluded that intravenous multivitamins should be added to parenteral nutrition admixtures immediately prior to administration to reduce losses of vitamins other than folic acid since commercially available amino acid products may contain bisulfites and have varying pH values.[487]

The vitamins in Cernevit (Baxter) diluted in three 2-in-1 parenteral nutrition admixtures were tested for stability over 48 hours. Most of the other vitamins, including folic acid, retained their initial concentrations.[2796]

Selected Revisions June 19, 2018. © Copyright, October 1982. American Society of Health-System Pharmacists, Inc.

Fomepizole
AHFS 92:12

Products

Fomepizole concentrate for injection is available in single-use (unpreserved) vials containing 1.5 g of fomepizole.[3130] [3131] The concentrate must be diluted prior to administration.[3130] [3131] The appropriate dose of the concentrate should be withdrawn from the vial with a syringe and diluted in at least 100 mL of sodium chloride 0.9% or dextrose 5%; the solution should be mixed well.[3130] [3131]

Trade Name(s)

Antizol

Administration

Fomepizole concentrate for injection is administered intravenously as a slow infusion over 30 minutes following dilution of the drug in at least 100 mL of sodium chloride 0.9% or dextrose 5%.[3130] [3131] Fomepizole should *not* be administered undiluted or by bolus injection.[3130] [3131]

Stability

Fomepizole concentrate for injection is a clear to yellow solution at room temperature.[3130] [3131] Intact vials should be stored at controlled room temperature.[3130] [3131]

Solutions diluted for infusion in sodium chloride 0.9% or dextrose 5% are stated to be stable for 24 hours when stored under refrigeration or at room temperature; solutions should not be used beyond 24 hours.[3130] [3131]

Solutions diluted for infusion should be visually inspected for particulate matter prior to administration.[3130] [3131] If haziness, particulate matter, discoloration, or precipitation is present or if leakage occurs, the solution should not be used.[3130] [3131]

Fomepizole concentrate solidifies at temperatures less than 25°C.[3130] [3131] If the fomepizole concentrate becomes solid in the vial, the vial should be passed under warm water or held in the hand to liquify the drug.[3130] [3131] Solidification does not affect the efficacy, safety, or stability of fomepizole.[3130] [3131]

Compatibility Information

Solution Compatibility

Fomepizole

Test Soln Name	Mfr	Mfr	Conc/L or %	Remarks	Ref	C/I
Dextrose 5%		PAL		Stated to be stable for 24 hr if stored under refrigeration or at room temperature	3131	C
Sodium chloride 0.9%		PAL		Stated to be stable for 24 hr if stored under refrigeration or at room temperature	3131	C

DOI: 10.37573/9781585286850.176

Fosaprepitant Dimeglumine
AHFS 56:22.32

Products

Fosaprepitant is available as a lyophilized powder in single-use vials containing fosaprepitant dimeglumine equivalent to 150 mg of fosaprepitant as the free acid.[2998] Also present in each vial are edetate disodium 18.8 mg, polysorbate 80 75 mg, lactose anhydrous 375 mg, and sodium hydroxide and/or hydrochloric acid to adjust the pH.[2998]

Each 150-mg vial should be reconstituted with 5 mL of sodium chloride 0.9%, directing the stream of diluent along the vial wall to prevent foaming.[2998] The vial should be gently swirled to dissolve the powder; shaking should be avoided.[2998] After reconstitution, the solution should be further diluted to a concentration of 1 mg/mL by transferring the entire vial contents to an infusion bag containing 145 mL of sodium chloride 0.9% and gently inverting the bag 2 to 3 times.[2998] The diluted solution should be inspected for particulate matter and discoloration prior to infusion.[2998]

Trade Name(s)

Emend

Administration

Fosaprepitant dimeglumine is administered by intravenous infusion over 15 minutes or 20 to 30 minutes (depending on the indicated use) after dilution in sodium chloride 0.9% to a concentration of 1 mg/mL.[2998]

Stability

Intact vials should be stored under refrigeration at 2 to 8°C.[2998] The manufacturer states that the diluted solution is stable for 24 hours at or below 25°C.[2998]

Fosaprepitant is incompatible with any solutions containing divalent cations (e.g., calcium, magnesium), including Ringer's injection, lactated and Hartmann's solution.[2998]

Compatibility Information

Solution Compatibility

Fosaprepitant dimeglumine

Test Soln Name	Mfr	Mfr	Conc/L or %	Remarks	Ref	C/I
Dextrose 5% in Ringer's injection		MSD		Stated to be incompatible	2998	I
Dextrose 5% in Ringer's injection, lactated		MSD		Stated to be incompatible	2998	I
Sodium chloride 0.9%		MSD	1 g	Stable for 24 hr at or below 25°C	2998	C
Ringer's injection		MSD		Stated to be incompatible	2998	I
Ringer's injection, lactated		MSD		Stated to be incompatible	2998	I

Additive Compatibility

Fosaprepitant dimeglumine

Test Drug	Mfr	Conc/L or %	Mfr	Conc/L or %	Test Solution	Remarks	Ref	C/I
Dexamethasone sodium phosphate	b	100 mg	MSD	1 g	NS	Physically compatible for 24 hr at 25°C in light	2999	C
Dexamethasone sodium phosphate	d	100 mg	MSD	1 g	NS	Physically compatible for 24 hr at 25°C in light	2999	C
Dexamethasone sodium phosphate	e	100 mg	MSD	1 g	NS	Physically compatible for 24 hr at 25°C in light	2999	C
Granisetron HCl		26 mg	MSD	1 g	NS	Physically compatible for 24 hr at 25°C in light	2999	C
Granisetron HCl	a	26 mg	MSD	1 g	NS	Physically compatible for 24 hr at 25°C in light	2999	C
Granisetron HCl	c	26 mg	MSD	1 g	NS	Physically compatible for 24 hr at 25°C in light	2999	C
Methylprednisolone sodium succinate	b	700 mg	MSD	1 g	NS	Physically compatible for 24 hr at 25°C in light	2999	C

DOI: 10.37573/9781585286850.177

Additive Compatibility (Cont.)

Test Drug	Mfr	Conc/L or %	Mfr	Conc/L or %	Test Solution	Remarks	Ref	C/I
Methylprednisolone sodium succinate	d	700 mg	MSD	1 g	NS	Physically compatible for 24 hr at 25°C in light	2999	C
Methylprednisolone sodium succinate	e	700 mg	MSD	1 g	NS	Physically compatible for 24 hr at 25°C in light	2999	C
Ondansetron HCl		70 mg	MSD	1 g	NS	Physically compatible for 24 hr at 25°C in light	2999	C
Ondansetron HCl	a	70 mg	MSD	1 g	NS	Physically compatible for 24 hr at 25°C in light	2999	C
Ondansetron HCl	c	70 mg	MSD	1 g	NS	Physically compatible for 24 hr at 25°C in light	2999	C
Tropisetron HCl	a	43 mg	MSD	1 g	NS	Physically compatible for 24 hr at 25°C in light	2999	C
Tropisetron HCl	c	43 mg	MSD	1 g	NS	Physically compatible for 24 hr at 25°C in light	2999	C

[a] Tested with dexamethasone sodium phosphate 100 mg/L.

[b] Tested with granisetron HCl 26 mg/L.

[c] Tested with methylprednisolone sodium succinate 700 mg/L.

[d] Tested with ondansetron HCl 70 mg/L.

[e] Tested with tropisetron HCl 43 mg/L.

Foscarnet Sodium
AHFS 8:18.92

Products

Foscarnet sodium is available as a 24-mg/mL solution of the drug (as the hexahydrate) in water for injection in 250-mL (6 g of foscarnet sodium hexahydrate) glass bottles.[3022] Hydrochloric acid may have been added to adjust the pH.[3022]

pH

Adjusted to pH 7.4.[3022]

Sodium Content

Foscarnet sodium contains 5.5 mg of sodium per mL of solution.[3022]

Tonicity

Foscarnet sodium injection is isotonic.[3022]

Trade Name(s)

Foscavir

Administration

Foscarnet sodium is administered by intravenous infusion.[3022] An infusion pump *must* be used for administration to prevent rapid infusion; the drug should *not* be administered by rapid or bolus intravenous injection.[3022]

Foscarnet sodium should only be infused into veins with adequate blood flow to allow for rapid dilution and distribution.[3022] For peripheral administration, foscarnet sodium solution must be diluted to a concentration of 12 mg/mL with dextrose 5% or sodium chloride 0.9% to avoid local irritation of peripheral veins.[3022] For administration through a central venous catheter, the 24-mg/mL solution may be infused undiluted.[3022]

Adequate hydration to establish diuresis is recommended in patients receiving foscarnet sodium provided there are no clinical contraindications.[3022] It is recommended that patients receive hydration with 750 to 1000 mL of sodium chloride 0.9% or dextrose 5% prior to the first infusion of foscarnet sodium.[3022] With subsequent infusions, hydration should be administered concurrently with each infusion of foscarnet sodium.[3022] For foscarnet sodium doses of 90 to 120 mg/kg, 750 to 1000 mL of hydration fluid should be administered; for doses of 40 to 60 mg/kg, 500 mL of hydration fluid should be administered, although hydration may be decreased if clinically warranted.[3022]

Foscarnet sodium should be infused over at least 1 to 2 hours, depending upon the indication, dosage, and regimen (e.g., induction, maintenance).[3022] The rate of infusion must not exceed 1 mg/kg/min.[3022] Recommended dosage, frequency, and administration rates should not be exceeded.[3022]

Stability

Foscarnet sodium injection is a clear, colorless solution.[3022] Intact bottles should be stored at controlled room temperature and protected from temperatures above 40°C and from freezing.[3022] Refrigerated products or products exposed to temperatures below freezing may exhibit precipitation; however, the precipitate can be dissolved by bringing the bottle to room temperature and with repeated shaking.[3022] The product should be used only if the bottle and seal are intact and a vacuum is present.[3022]

The manufacturer states that foscarnet sodium solutions diluted for infusion should be used within 24 hours of initial entry into a sealed bottle.[3022]

Foscarnet sodium may chelate divalent metal ions (e.g., calcium, magnesium) and is chemically incompatible with solutions containing calcium, such as Ringer's injection, lactated, and parenteral nutrition solutions.[3022]

Foscarnet sodium (Astra) diluted to a concentration of 13 mg/mL in sodium chloride 0.9% and stored at 22°C did not exhibit an antibacterial effect on the growth of 3 organisms (*Enterococcus faecium*, *Staphylococcus aureus*, and *Pseudomonas aeruginosa*) that were inoculated into the solution. Foscarnet sodium exhibited moderate antifungal activity against *Candida albicans*. The authors recommended that ready-to-use solutions be stored under refrigeration whenever possible and that the potential for microbiological growth be considered when assigning expiration periods.[2160]

Autoclaving

The concentration of foscarnet sodium (Astra), diluted in sodium chloride 0.9% to a concentration of 12 mg/mL and packaged in glass infusion bottles with rubber bungs, was compared before and after autoclaving at 30 psi for 15 minutes at 121°C. The foscarnet sodium concentration did not change after autoclaving. Therefore, the dilution may be autoclaved to avoid limiting its shelf life due to sterility concerns.[1835]

Elastomeric Reservoir Pumps

Foscarnet sodium (Astra) 24 mg/mL was evaluated for binding potential to natural rubber elastomeric reservoirs (Baxter). No binding was found after storage for 2 weeks at 35°C with gentle agitation.[2014]

DOI: 10.37573/9781585286850.178

Compatibility Information

Solution Compatibility

Foscarnet sodium

Test Soln Name	Mfr	Mfr	Conc/L or %	Remarks	Ref	C/I
Dextrose 5% in Ringer's injection		HOS		Chemically incompatible with calcium-containing solutions	3022	I
Dextrose 5% in Ringer's injection, lactated		HOS		Chemically incompatible with calcium-containing solutions	3022	I
Dextrose 5%	BAª	AST	12 g	Visually compatible and chemically stable for 35 days at 5 and 25°C	1834	C
Dextrose 5%		HOS	12 g	Manufacturer-recommended solution	3022	C
Ringer's injection		HOS		Chemically incompatible with calcium-containing solutions	3022	I
Ringer's injection, lactated		HOS		Chemically incompatible with calcium-containing solutions	3022	I
Sodium chloride 0.9%	MGª	AST	12 g	Visually compatible. Stable for 30 days at 25°C in light or dark and at 5°C in dark	1726	C
Sodium chloride 0.9%	BAª	AST	12 g	Visually compatible and chemically stable for 35 days at 5 and 25°C	1834	C
Sodium chloride 0.9%		HOS	12 g	Manufacturer-recommended solution	3022	C

ª Tested in PVC containers.

Additive Compatibility

Foscarnet sodium

Test Drug	Mfr	Conc/L or %	Mfr	Conc/L or %	Test Solution	Remarks	Ref	C/I
Potassium chloride		20 to 120 mmol	AST	12 g	NS	Foscarnet concentrations of 93 to 99% were maintained for at least 65 hr	2156	C

Y-Site Injection Compatibility (1:1 Mixture)

Foscarnet sodium

Test Drug	Mfr	Conc	Mfr	Conc	Remarks	Ref	C/I
Acyclovir sodium	BW	10 mg/mL	AST	24 mg/mL	Precipitates immediately	1335	I
Acyclovir sodium	BW	7 mg/mLª ᵇ	AST	24 mg/mL	Acyclovir crystals form immediately	1393	I
Aldesleukin	CHI	33,800 I.U./mLª	AST	24 mg/mL	Visually compatible with little or no loss of aldesleukin activity	1857	C
Amikacin sulfate	BR	20 mg/mL	AST	24 mg/mL	Physically compatible for 24 hr at room temperature under fluorescent light	1335	C
Aminophylline	LY	25 mg/mL	AST	24 mg/mL	Physically compatible for 24 hr at room temperature under fluorescent light	1335	C
Amphotericin B	SQ	5 mg/mL	AST	24 mg/mL	Cloudy yellow precipitate forms	1335	I
Amphotericin B	SQ	0.6 mg/mLª	AST	24 mg/mL	Dense haze forms immediately	1393	I
Ampicillin sodium	WY	20 mg/mL	AST	24 mg/mL	Physically compatible for 24 hr at room temperature under fluorescent light	1335	C
Aztreonam	SQ	40 mg/mL	AST	24 mg/mL	Physically compatible for 24 hr at room temperature under fluorescent light	1335	C
Aztreonam	SQ	40 mg/mLª ᵇ	AST	24 mg/mL	Physically compatible for 24 hr at 25°C under fluorescent light	1393	C

Y-Site Injection Compatibility (1:1 Mixture) (Cont.)

Test Drug	Mfr	Conc	Mfr	Conc	Remarks	Ref	C/I
Cefazolin sodium	SKF	40 mg/mL	AST	24 mg/mL	Physically compatible for 24 hr at room temperature under fluorescent light	1335	C
Cefoxitin sodium	MSD	40 mg/mL	AST	24 mg/mL	Physically compatible for 24 hr at room temperature under fluorescent light	1335	C
Ceftazidime	GL	20 mg/mL	AST	24 mg/mL	Physically compatible for 24 hr at room temperature under fluorescent light	1335	C
Ceftazidime	GL	20 mg/mL[a b]	AST	24 mg/mL	Physically compatible for 24 hr at 25°C under fluorescent light	1393	C
Ceftriaxone sodium	RC	20 mg/mL[a b]	AST	24 mg/mL	Physically compatible for 24 hr at 25°C under fluorescent light	1393	C
Cefuroxime sodium	GL	30 mg/mL	AST	24 mg/mL	Physically compatible for 24 hr at room temperature under fluorescent light	1335	C
Chloramphenicol sodium succinate	PD	20 mg/mL	AST	24 mg/mL	Physically compatible for 24 hr at room temperature under fluorescent light	1335	C
Clindamycin phosphate	AB	24 mg/mL	AST	24 mg/mL	Physically compatible for 24 hr at room temperature under fluorescent light	1335	C
Clindamycin phosphate	UP	12 mg/mL[a b]	AST	24 mg/mL	Physically compatible for 24 hr at 25°C under fluorescent light	1393	C
Defibrotide sodium	JAZ	8 mg/mL[b]	NVX	24 mg/mL	Visually compatible for 4 hr at room temperature	3149	C
Dexamethasone sodium phosphate	OR	10 mg/mL	AST	24 mg/mL	Physically compatible for 24 hr at room temperature under fluorescent light	1335	C
Diazepam	ES	5 mg/mL	AST	24 mg/mL	Gas production	1335	I
Digoxin	WY	0.25 mg/mL	AST	24 mg/mL	Gas production	1335	I
Diphenhydramine HCl	PD	50 mg/mL	AST	24 mg/mL	Cloudy solution	1335	I
Dobutamine HCl	LI	12.5 mg/mL	AST	24 mg/mL	Delayed formation of muddy precipitate	1335	I
Dopamine HCl	DU	80 mg/mL	AST	24 mg/mL	Physically compatible for 24 hr at room temperature under fluorescent light	1335	C
Doripenem	JJ	5 mg/mL[a b]	HOS	24 mg/mL	Physically compatible for 4 hr at 23°C	2743	C
Droperidol	QU	2.5 mg/mL	AST	24 mg/mL	Delayed formation of yellow precipitate	1335	I
Erythromycin lactobionate	AB	20 mg/mL	AST	24 mg/mL	Physically compatible for 24 hr at room temperature under fluorescent light	1335	C
Erythromycin lactobionate	ES	20 mg/mL[a b]	AST	24 mg/mL	Physically compatible for 24 hr at 25°C under fluorescent light	1393	C
Fluconazole	RR	2 mg/mL	AST	24 mg/mL	Physically compatible for 24 hr at 25°C	1407	C
Furosemide	AB	10 mg/mL	AST	24 mg/mL	Physically compatible for 24 hr at room temperature under fluorescent light	1335	C
Ganciclovir sodium		50 mg/mL	AST	24 mg/mL	Precipitates immediately	1335	I
Gentamicin sulfate	ES	4 mg/mL	AST	24 mg/mL	Physically compatible for 24 hr at room temperature under fluorescent light	1335	C
Gentamicin sulfate	ES	2 mg/mL[a b]	AST	24 mg/mL	Physically compatible for 24 hr at 25°C under fluorescent light	1393	C
Haloperidol lactate	LY	5 mg/mL	AST	24 mg/mL	Delayed formation of fine white precipitate	1335	I

Y-Site Injection Compatibility (1:1 Mixture) (Cont.)

Test Drug	Mfr	Conc	Mfr	Conc	Remarks	Ref	C/I
Heparin sodium	ES	1000 units/mL	AST	24 mg/mL	Physically compatible for 24 hr at room temperature under fluorescent light	1335	C
Heparin sodium	LY	100 units/mL^{a b}	AST	24 mg/mL	Physically compatible for 24 hr at 25°C under fluorescent light	1393	C
Hydrocortisone sodium succinate	UP	50 mg/mL	AST	24 mg/mL	Physically compatible for 24 hr at room temperature under fluorescent light	1335	C
Hydromorphone HCl	KN	10 mg/mL	AST	24 mg/mL	Physically compatible for 24 hr at room temperature under fluorescent light	1335	C
Hydroxyzine HCl	LY	50 mg/mL	AST	24 mg/mL	Physically compatible for 24 hr at room temperature under fluorescent light	1335	C
Imipenem–cilastatin sodium	MSD	10 mg/mL^f	AST	24 mg/mL	Physically compatible for 24 hr at room temperature under fluorescent light	1335	C
Imipenem–cilastatin sodium	MSD	5 mg/mL^{a f}	AST	24 mg/mL	Physically compatible for 24 hr at 25°C under fluorescent light	1393	C
Leucovorin calcium	QU	10 mg/mL	AST	24 mg/mL	Cloudy yellow solution	1335	I
Lorazepam	WY	4 mg/mL	AST	24 mg/mL	Gas production	1335	I
Lorazepam	WY	0.08 mg/mL^{a b}	AST	24 mg/mL	Physically compatible for 24 hr at 25°C under fluorescent light	1393	C
Meropenem		50 mg/mL	CLN	24 mg/mL	Physically compatible for 4 hr at room temperature	3538	C
Metoclopramide HCl	RB	4 mg/mL	AST	24 mg/mL	Physically compatible for 24 hr at room temperature under fluorescent light	1335	C
Metoclopramide HCl	RB	2 mg/mL^{a b}	AST	24 mg/mL	Physically compatible for 24 hr at 25°C under fluorescent light	1393	C
Metronidazole	AB	5 mg/mL	AST	24 mg/mL	Physically compatible for 24 hr at room temperature under fluorescent light	1335	C
Metronidazole	SE	5 mg/mL	AST	24 mg/mL	Physically compatible for 24 hr at 25°C under fluorescent light	1393	C
Midazolam HCl	RC	5 mg/mL	AST	24 mg/mL	Gas production	1335	I
Morphine sulfate	IMS	1 mg/mL	AST	24 mg/mL	Physically compatible for 24 hr at room temperature under fluorescent light	1335	C
Morphine sulfate	ES	1 mg/mL^{a b}	AST	24 mg/mL	Physically compatible for 24 hr at 25°C under fluorescent light	1393	C
Morphine sulfate	ES	5^b and 15 mg/mL	AST	24 mg/mL	Visually compatible for 24 hr at 23°C under fluorescent light	1529	C
Nafcillin sodium	BR	20 mg/mL^{a b}	AST	24 mg/mL	Physically compatible for 24 hr at 25°C under fluorescent light	1393	C
Oxacillin sodium	BR	40 mg/mL	AST	24 mg/mL	Physically compatible for 24 hr at room temperature under fluorescent light	1335	C
Oxacillin sodium	BE	20 mg/mL^{a b}	AST	24 mg/mL	Physically compatible for 24 hr at 25°C under fluorescent light	1393	C
Penicillin G potassium	SQ	100,000 units/mL	AST	24 mg/mL	Physically compatible for 24 hr at room temperature under fluorescent light	1335	C
Pentamidine isethionate	LY	6 mg/mL	AST	24 mg/mL	Precipitates immediately	1335	I
Pentamidine isethionate	LY	6 mg/mL^{a b}	AST	24 mg/mL	Pentamidine crystals form immediately	1393	I
Prochlorperazine edisylate	SKF	5 mg/mL	AST	24 mg/mL	Cloudy brown solution	1335	I
Promethazine HCl	ES	50 mg/mL	AST	24 mg/mL	Gas production	1335	I

Y-Site Injection Compatibility (1:1 Mixture) (Cont.)

Test Drug	Mfr	Conc	Mfr	Conc	Remarks	Ref	C/I
Ranitidine HCl	GL	2 mg/mL[a][b]	AST	24 mg/mL	Physically compatible for 24 hr at 25°C under fluorescent light	1393	C
Tobramycin sulfate	LI	40 mg/mL	AST	24 mg/mL	Physically compatible for 24 hr at room temperature under fluorescent light	1335	C
TPN #121[d]		[c]	AST	24 mg/mL	Physically compatible for 24 hr at 25°C	1393	C
Trimethoprim–sulfamethoxazole	RC	16 mg/mL[e]	AST	24 mg/mL	Precipitates immediately and gas production	1335	I
Trimethoprim–sulfamethoxazole	BW	0.53 mg/mL[a][e]	AST	24 mg/mL	Physically compatible for 24 hr at 25°C under fluorescent light	1393	C
Vancomycin HCl	LE	20 mg/mL	AST	24 mg/mL	Precipitates immediately	1335	I
Vancomycin HCl	LE	15 mg/mL[a][b]	AST	24 mg/mL	Physically compatible for 24 hr at 25°C under fluorescent light	1393	C
Vancomycin HCl	LE	10 mg/mL[b]	AST	24 mg/mL	Visually compatible for 24 hr at room temperature. No precipitate found	2063	C

[a] Tested in dextrose 5%.

[b] Tested in sodium chloride 0.9%.

[c] Tested in equal quantities.

[d] Refer to Appendix for the composition of parenteral nutrition solutions. TPN indicates a 2-in-1 admixture.

[e] Trimethoprim component. Trimethoprim in a 1:5 fixed-ratio concentration with sulfamethoxazole.

[f] Not specified whether concentration refers to single component or combined components.

Selected Revisions May 1, 2020. © Copyright, October 1992.
American Society of Health-System Pharmacists, Inc.

Fosnetupitant Chloride Hydrochloride–Palonosetron Hydrochloride
AHFS 56:22.32

Products

Fosnetupitant is a prodrug that is converted in vivo to netupitant via metabolic hydrolysis.[3428] Fosnetupitant–palonosetron is available as a lyophilized powder in single-dose (preservative-free) vials containing fosnetupitant chloride hydrochloride equivalent to 235 mg of fosnetupitant and palonosetron hydrochloride equivalent to 0.25 mg of palonosetron.[3428] Also present in each vial are edetate disodium 6.4 mg, mannitol 760 mg, and sodium hydroxide and/or hydrochloric acid to adjust the pH.[3428]

Each vial of fosnetupitant chloride hydrochloride–palonosetron hydrochloride should be reconstituted with 20 mL of dextrose 5% or sodium chloride 0.9%, directing the stream of diluent along the vial wall and swirling the vial gently to prevent foaming.[3428] The entire volume of the reconstituted solution should then be withdrawn from the vial and transferred to an infusion vial or bag containing 30 mL of dextrose 5% or sodium chloride 0.9% to yield a final total volume of 50 mL.[3428] The vial or bag should be gently inverted until dissolution is complete.[3428]

Equivalency

Fosnetupitant chloride hydrochloride 260 mg is equivalent to fosnetupitant 235 mg.[3428]

Palonosetron hydrochloride 0.28 mg is equivalent to palonosetron 0.25 mg.[3428]

Trade Name(s)

Akynzeo

Administration

Fosnetupitant chloride hydrochloride–palonosetron hydrochloride should be administered as an intravenous infusion over 30 minutes after reconstitution and dilution.[3428] The infusion line should be flushed at the end of the infusion with the same solution used for reconstitution and dilution of the drug.[3428] In addition, if a common infusion line is being used to administer other drugs, the line should be flushed with sodium chloride 0.9% prior to and following infusion of fosnetupitant chloride hydrochloride–palonosetron hydrochloride.[3428]

Stability

Fosnetupitant chloride hydrochloride–palonosetron hydrochloride is a white to off-white lyophilized powder.[3428] Intact vials should be stored at 2 to 8°C in the original carton to protect from light.[3428] The reconstituted solution and the final diluted solution for infusion should be stored at room temperature.[3428] The final diluted solution for infusion should be inspected for particulate matter and discoloration; if either is observed, the vial or bag should be discarded.[3428] Administration of the infusion should begin within 3 hours after reconstitution.[3428]

Because of limited compatibility data, the manufacturer states that other drugs should not be mixed or infused simultaneously with fosnetupitant chloride hydrochloride–palonosetron hydrochloride.[3428] Fosnetupitant chloride hydrochloride–palonosetron hydrochloride is incompatible with any solutions that contain divalent cations (e.g., calcium, magnesium), including Hartmann's solution and Ringer's injection, lactated.[3428]

Compatibility Information
Solution Compatibility

Fosnetupitant chloride HCl–palonosetron HCl

Test Soln Name	Mfr	Mfr	Conc/L or %	Remarks	Ref	C/I
Dextrose 5% in Ringer's injection		HEL		Stated to be incompatible with calcium-containing solutions	3428	I
Dextrose 5% in Ringer's injection, lactated		HEL		Stated to be incompatible with calcium-containing solutions	3428	I
Dextrose 5%		HEL	4.7 g[a]	Begin administration within 3 hr after reconstitution	3428	C
Ringer's injection		HEL		Stated to be incompatible with calcium-containing solutions	3428	I
Ringer's injection, lactated		HEL		Stated to be incompatible with calcium-containing solutions	3428	I
Sodium chloride 0.9%		HEL	4.7 g[a]	Begin administration within 3 hr after reconstitution	3428	C

[a] Fosnetupitant component. Fosnetupitant in a 940:1 fixed-ratio concentration with palonosetron.

DOI: 10.37573/9781585286850.179

Fosphenytoin Sodium
AHFS 28:12.12

Products

Fosphenytoin is the prodrug for its active metabolite, phenytoin.[3280] Fosphenytoin sodium is available as a solution containing 50 mg phenytoin sodium equivalents (PE)/mL in single-dose 2-mL (100-mg) and 10-mL (500-mg) vials.[3280] Each mL of solution also contains tromethamine (TRIS) buffer along with hydrochloric acid or sodium hydroxide to adjust the pH in water for injection.[3280]

CAUTION: Care should be taken to avoid confusion between the two different forms (i.e., fosphenytoin sodium and phenytoin sodium) to prevent dosing errors.[3280]

Units

Each 1.5 mg of fosphenytoin sodium is equivalent to phenytoin sodium 1 mg and is referred to as 1 mg of phenytoin sodium equivalents (PE).[3280] The amount and concentration of fosphenytoin sodium are expressed in terms of the equivalent mass of phenytoin sodium.[3280] Manufacturers indicate that this avoids the need to perform conversions between the two forms based on molecular weight; however, it necessitates that all prescribing, preparation, and dosing be consistently expressed in terms of PE to avoid dosing errors that could result from confusion between the two forms.[3280]

pH

From 8.6 to 9[3280] or 8.3 to 9.3.[3281]

Phosphate Content

Each 1 mg PE contains 0.0037 mmol phosphate.[3280]

Trade Name(s)

Cerebyx

Administration

Fosphenytoin sodium is dosed in terms of phenytoin sodium equivalents (PE).[3280]

CAUTION: Care should be taken to ensure that all prescribing, preparation, and dosing is performed using the correct units and that any confusion between the two forms (i.e., fosphenytoin sodium and phenytoin sodium) is avoided.[3280]

Fosphenytoin sodium is administered intravenously.[3280] For intravenous infusion, fosphenytoin sodium must be diluted in dextrose 5% or sodium chloride 0.9% to a concentration ranging from 1.5 mg PE/mL to a maximum of 25 mg PE/mL.[3280] The drug also has been administered intramuscularly in certain situations when intravenous access is not possible.[3280]

For the treatment of status epilepticus in adult patients, a loading dose of fosphenytoin sodium should be administered by intravenous infusion at a rate of 100 to 150 mg PE/min; the rate of administration must not exceed 150 mg PE/min.[3280] The intramuscular route of administration generally should not be used in the treatment of status epilepticus.[3280] For non-emergent situations in adult patients in which fosphenytoin sodium is indicated, the loading dose may be administered intravenously or intramuscularly.[3280] For non-emergent indications, intravenous fosphenytoin sodium infusion should be administered more slowly.[3280] The rate of administration of maintenance doses in adults also should not exceed 150 mg PE/min.[3280]

For the treatment of status epilepticus in pediatric patients, a loading dose of fosphenytoin sodium should be administered by intravenous infusion at a rate of 2 mg PE/kg/min (or 150 mg PE/min, whichever is slower); the rate of administration must not exceed 2 mg PE/kg/min (or 150 mg PE/min, whichever is slower).[3280] For non-emergent indications, intravenous fosphenytoin sodium infusion should be administered more slowly.[3280] For non-emergent situations in pediatric patients in which fosphenytoin sodium is indicated, the loading dose should be administered intravenously at a rate of 1 to 2 mg PE/kg/min (or 150 mg PE/min, whichever is slower).[3280] Following administration of a loading dose, maintenance doses in pediatric patients should be administered at a rate of 1 to 2 mg PE/kg/min (or 100 mg PE/min, whichever is slower).[3280] The intramuscular route of administration generally should not be used in pediatric patients.[3280]

Purple glove syndrome, characterized by edema, discoloration, and pain distal to the site of infusion, has been reported following intravenous administration of fosphenytoin sodium through a peripheral vein and may or may not be associated with extravasation.[3280]

Stability

Fosphenytoin sodium injection is a clear, colorless to pale yellow solution.[3280] Intact vials should be stored under refrigeration at 2 to 8°C.[3280] Storage at room temperature should not exceed 48 hours.[3280]

Fosphenytoin sodium injection solution should be visually inspected for particulate matter and discoloration prior to administration.[3280] Any unused portions should be discarded.[3280]

Freezing Solutions

Fosphenytoin sodium (Parke-Davis) 1, 8, and 20 mg PE/mL in dextrose 5% (Baxter) and sodium chloride 0.9% (Baxter) in PVC containers and undiluted fosphenytoin sodium 50 mg PE/mL were packaged in 3-mL polypropylene syringes sealed with tip caps (Becton Dickinson). The samples were frozen at −20°C. Little or no loss occurred after 30 days of frozen storage followed by 7 days at 4 or 25°C. Stability also was maintained if the thawed samples that had been stored at 25°C were returned to the freezer for an additional 7 days.[2083]

Syringes

Fosphenytoin sodium (Parke-Davis) 50 mg PE/mL was packaged in 3-mL polypropylene syringes with syringe caps (Becton Dickinson) and stored at −20, 4, and 25°C. The samples stored at 4

DOI: 10.37573/9781585286850.180

and 25°C exhibited little or no loss of fosphenytoin sodium in 30 days. The samples stored at −20°C also showed little or no loss of fosphenytoin sodium after 30 days of storage followed by 7 days at 4°C or at 25°C. Stability was maintained if the thawed samples that had been stored at 25°C were returned to the freezer for an additional 7 days.[2083]

Compatibility Information

Solution Compatibility

Fosphenytoin sodium

Test Soln Name	Mfr	Mfr	Conc/L or %	Remarks	Ref	C/I
Dextrose 5% in Ringer's injection, lactated	BA[a]	PD[c]	1, 8, 20 mg PE/mL	Visually compatible with little or no loss in 7 days at 25°C under fluorescent light	2083	C
Dextrose 5% in sodium chloride 0.45%	BA[a]	PD[c]	1, 8, 20 mg PE/mL	Visually compatible with little or no loss in 7 days at 25°C under fluorescent light	2083	C
Dextrose 5%	BA[a b]	PD[c]	1, 8, 20 mg PE/mL	Visually compatible with little or no loss in 7 days at 25°C under fluorescent light	2083	C
Dextrose 10%	BA[a]	PD[c]	1, 8, 20 mg PE/mL	Visually compatible with little or no loss in 7 days at 25°C under fluorescent light	2083	C
Plasma-Lyte A, pH 7.4	BA[a]	PD[c]	1, 8, 20 mg PE/mL	Visually compatible with little or no loss in 7 days at 25°C under fluorescent light	2083	C
Ringer's injection, lactated	BA[a]	PD[c]	1, 8, 20 mg PE/mL	Visually compatible with little or no loss in 7 days at 25°C under fluorescent light	2083	C
Sodium chloride 0.9%	BA[a b]	PD[c]	1, 8, 20 mg PE/mL	Visually compatible with little or no loss in 7 days at 25°C under fluorescent light	2083	C

[a] Tested in PVC containers.

[b] Tested in glass containers.

[c] Concentration of fosphenytoin expressed in milligrams of phenytoin sodium equivalents (PE) per mL.

Additive Compatibility

Fosphenytoin sodium

Test Drug	Mfr	Conc/L or %	Mfr	Conc/L or %	Test Solution	Remarks	Ref	C/I
Hetastarch in sodium chloride 0.9%	MG	6%	PD[b]	1, 8, 20 mg PE/mL	NS	Visually compatible with little or no loss in 7 days at 25°C under fluorescent light	2083	C
Mannitol	BA[a]	20%	PD[b]	2, 8, 20 mg PE/mL		Visually compatible with little or no loss in 7 days at 25°C under fluorescent light	2083	C
Potassium chloride	BA	20 and 40 mEq	PD[b]	1, 8, 20 mg PE/mL	D5½S[a]	Visually compatible with little or no loss in 7 days at 25°C under fluorescent light	2083	C

[a] Tested in PVC containers.

[b] Concentration of fosphenytoin expressed in milligrams of phenytoin sodium equivalents (PE) per mL.

Y-Site Injection Compatibility (1:1 Mixture)

Fosphenytoin sodium

Test Drug	Mfr	Conc	Mfr	Conc	Remarks	Ref	C/I
Ceftolozane sulfate–tazobactam sodium	CUB	10 mg/mL[c d]	WW[b]	25 mg PE/mL[c]	Physically compatible for 2 hr	3247, 3262	C
Fenoldopam mesylate	AB	80 mcg/mL[a]	PD[b]	20 mg PE/mL[a]	Trace haze and microparticulates form in 4 hr	2467	I
Isavuconazonium sulfate	ASP	1.5 mg/mL[c]	WW[b]	25 mg PE/mL[c]	Measured turbidity increases immediately	3247, 3263	I

Y-Site Injection Compatibility (1:1 Mixture) (Cont.)

Test Drug	Mfr	Conc	Mfr	Conc	Remarks	Ref	C/I
Lorazepam	WY	2 mg/mL	PD[b]	1 mg PE/mL[a]	Samples remained clear with no loss of either drug in 8 hr	2223	C
Midazolam HCl	RC	2 mg/mL[a]	PD[b]	1 mg PE/mL[a]	Midazolam base precipitates immediately	2223	I
Meropenem–vaborbactam	TMC	8 mg/mL[a e]	AMB[b]	25 mg PE/mL[a]	Physically compatible for 3 hr at 20 to 25°C	3380, 3382	C
Phenobarbital sodium		130 mg/mL	PD[b]	10 mg PE/mL[a]	Visually compatible with no loss of either drug in 8 hr at room temperature	2212	C
Plazomicin sulfate	ACH	24 mg/mL[c]	AMB	25 mg/mL[b c]	Physically compatible for 1 hr at 20 to 25°C	3432	C
Tedizolid phosphate	CUB	0.8 mg/mL[a]	WW[b]	25 mg PE/mL[a]	Physically compatible for 2 hr	3244, 3247	C

[a] Tested in sodium chloride 0.9%.

[b] Concentration of fosphenytoin expressed in milligrams of phenytoin sodium equivalents (PE) per mL.

[c] Tested in both dextrose 5% and sodium chloride 0.9%.

[d] Ceftolozane component. Ceftolozane in a 2:1 fixed-ratio concentration with tazobactam.

[e] Meropenem component. Meropenem in a 1:1 fixed-ratio concentration with vaborbactam.

Selected Revisions June 1, 2019. © Copyright, October 2000.
American Society of Health-System Pharmacists, Inc.

Furosemide
AHFS 40:28.08
Frusemide

Products

Furosemide is available in 2-, 4-, and 10-mL amber ampuls, single-use vials, prefilled syringes, and syringe cartridges. Each mL of solution contains furosemide 10 mg, water for injection, with sodium chloride for isotonicity, sodium hydroxide, and, if necessary, hydrochloric acid to adjust pH.[1(9/06)] [4]

pH

From 8 to 9.3.[1(9/06)] [4]

Osmolality

Furosemide (Hoechst-Roussel) 10 mg/mL has an osmolality of 287 mOsm/kg.[50] The osmolality of the Elkins-Sinn product has been determined to be 289 mOsm/kg by freezing-point depression.[1071]

In another study, the osmolality of furosemide injection (manufacturer unspecified) was determined to be 291 mOsm/kg.[1233]

Sodium Content

The injection contains 0.162 mEq of sodium per mL.[4]

Trade Name(s)

Lasix

Administration

Furosemide may be administered by intramuscular injection, by direct intravenous injection over 1 to 2 minutes, and by intravenous infusion at a rate not exceeding 4 mg/min.[1(9/06)] [4]

Stability

Exposure to light may cause discoloration; protection from light for the syringes once they are removed from the package is recommended. Do not use furosemide solutions if they have a yellow color. Furosemide products should be stored at controlled room temperature.[1(9/06)] [4] Refrigeration may result in precipitation or crystallization. However, resolubilization at room temperature or on warming may be performed without affecting the drug's stability.[593]

Furosemide under simulated summer conditions in paramedic vehicles was exposed to temperatures from 26 to 38°C over 4 weeks. Analysis found no loss of drug under these conditions.[2562]

Furosemide (Hospira) 1 mg/mL diluted in dextrose 5% and packaged as 10 mL in 15-mL polypropylene tubes (BD Biosciences) was physically compatible with less than 4% loss of furosemide in 96 hours at 25°C in the dark.[3568]

pH Effects

Furosemide is soluble in alkaline solutions and is prepared as a mildly buffered alkaline product.[1(9/06)] [4] It can usually be mixed with infusion solutions that are neutral or weakly basic (pH 7 to 10) and with some weakly acidic solutions that have a low buffer capacity.[4] It should not be mixed with acidic solutions having a pH below 5.5. Solutions such as sodium chloride 0.9%, Ringer's injection, lactated, and dextrose 5% have been recommended. If the solution pH is below 5.5, pH adjustment has been recommended.[1(9/06)] [4] In addition, furosemide has been found to be unstable in acidic media,[96] [664] but very stable in basic media.[664]

A 2-mL fluid barrier of dextrose 5% in a microbore retrograde infusion set failed to prevent precipitation when used between gentamicin sulfate 5 mg/0.5 mL and furosemide 2 mg/0.2 mL.[1385]

Autoclaving

Autoclaving of furosemide 1 mg/mL in sodium chloride 0.9% in glass bottles at 115°C for 34 minutes resulted in no loss of furosemide. Storage of the solution for 70 days at room temperature with protection from light also showed no detectable change in furosemide content. However, storage at room temperature with exposure to light for 70 days resulted in about a 60% loss of furosemide and the formation of a yellow-orange precipitate.[1108]

Light Effects

Furosemide is subject to photodegradation by several mechanisms.[358] [400] [2067] Photodegradation is minimized at pH 7; rates of decomposition increase as the pH becomes more acidic or basic.[400] [2067] Photodegradation is unaffected by ionic strength and initial concentration (in the range of 10 mcg/mL to 1 mg/mL), but the rate of loss may decrease at the higher concentration due to a light-filtering effect of the yellow discoloration. In pH 7 phosphate buffer, more than 60% furosemide loss occurred in transparent glass vials exposed to fluorescent light for 90 hours; little or no loss occurred if the transparent vials were covered with aluminum foil or if amber glass containers were used.[2067]

Syringes

Furosemide (Hoechst) 10 mg/mL was filled into 25-mL polypropylene syringes (Becton Dickinson) and stored at 25°C while exposed to normal room light or in the dark for 24 hours. There was no detectable change in furosemide content in either light-exposed or light-protected syringes.[1108]

Furosemide (Abbott) 1, 2, 4, and 8 mg/mL diluted in sodium chloride 0.9% was packaged in polypropylene syringes. Samples were stored for 84 days at 22°C and also at 4°C protected from light for 84 days. This was followed by an additional 7 days of storage at 22°C exposed to fluorescent light. No visible changes occurred and little or no loss of furosemide occurred in any of the samples.[2389]

Furosemide 5 mg/mL packaged as 8 mL in 12-mL transparent polypropylene syringes (Terumo) and 50 mL in 60-mL transparent polypropylene syringes (Becton Dickinson) was

DOI: 10.37573/9781585286850.181

physically stable and exhibited little to no loss in 35 days stored at 4°C protected from light followed by 24 hours at 20°C exposed to light.[3569]

Filtration

Furosemide (Hoechst) 0.04 mg/mL in dextrose 5% and sodium chloride 0.9% was filtered through a 0.22-μm cellulose ester membrane filter (Ivex-HP, Millipore) over 6 hours. No significant drug loss due to binding to the filter was noted.[1034]

Central Venous Catheter

Furosemide (American Regent) 1 mg/mL in dextrose 5% was found to be compatible with the ARROWg+ard Blue Plus (Arrow International) chlorhexidine-bearing triple-lumen central catheter. Essentially complete delivery of the drug was found with little or no drug loss occurring. Furthermore, chlorhexidine delivered from the catheter remained at trace amounts with no substantial increase due to the delivery of the drug through the catheter.[2335]

Compatibility Information

Solution Compatibility

Furosemide

Test Soln Name	Mfr	Mfr	Conc/L or %	Remarks	Ref	C/I
Amino acids 4.25%, dextrose 25%	MG	HO	40 mg	No increase in particulate matter in 24 hr at 25°C	349	C
Dextrose 5% in Ringer's injection, lactated	BA	HO	600 mg	Physically compatible for 24 hr	315	C
Dextrose 5% in sodium chloride 0.9%	BA	HO	600 mg	Physically compatible for 24 hr	315	C
Dextrose 5%	BA	HO	600 mg	Physically compatible for 24 hr	315	C
Dextrose 5%			200 and 400 mg	4 to 5% loss in 24 hr at 25°C	1348	C
Dextrose 10%	BA	HO	600 mg	Physically compatible for 24 hr	315	C
Dextrose 20%	BA	HO	600 mg	Physically compatible for 24 hr	315	C
Ringer's injection, lactated	BA	HO	600 mg	Physically compatible for 24 hr	315	C
Ringer's injection, lactated	TR[a]	HO	1 g	No furosemide loss in 24 hr at 25°C exposed to light or in the dark	1108	C
Sodium chloride 0.9%	BA	HO	600 mg	Physically compatible for 24 hr	315	C
Sodium chloride 0.9%	TR[a]	HO	1 g	No furosemide loss in 24 hr at 25°C exposed to light or in the dark. 10% loss in 26 days at 6°C	1108	C
Sodium chloride 0.9%			200 and 400 mg	5 to 7% loss in 24 hr at 25°C	1348	C
Sodium chloride 0.9%	BA[a]	AB	1.2, 2.4, 3.2 g	Visually compatible. Little loss in 84 days at 4 and 22°C in dark then 7 days at 22°C in fluorescent light	2389	C
Sodium lactate ⅙ M	BA	HO	600 mg	Physically compatible for 24 hr	315	C

[a] Tested in PVC containers.

Additive Compatibility

Furosemide

Test Drug	Mfr	Conc/L or %	Mfr	Conc/L or %	Test Solution	Remarks	Ref	C/I
Amikacin sulfate	BR	2 g	HO	160 mg	D5W, NS	Transient cloudiness, then visually compatible for 24 hr at 21°C	876	?
Aminophylline	ANT	1 g	HO	1 g	NS	Physically compatible for 72 hr at 15 and 30°C	1479	C
Amiodarone HCl	LZ	1.8 g	ES	200 mg	D5W, NS[a]	Physically compatible. 8% or less amiodarone loss in 24 hr at 24°C in light	1031	C
Amiodarone HCl	LZ	4 g	HO	1 g	D5W	Haze in 5 hr and precipitate in 24 to 72 hr at 30°C. No changes at 15°C	1479	I

Additive Compatibility (Cont.)

Test Drug	Mfr	Conc/L or %	Mfr	Conc/L or %	Test Solution	Remarks	Ref	C/I
Ampicillin sodium	BE	20 g	HO	1 g	NS	Physically compatible for 72 hr at 15 and 30°C	1479	C
Atropine sulfate	ANT	60 mg	HO	1 g	W	Physically compatible for 72 hr at 15 and 30°C	1479	C
Bumetanide	LEO	6 mg	HO	1 g	NS	Physically compatible for 72 hr at 15 and 30°C	1479	C
Buprenorphine HCl		75 mg	HO	1 g	W	Haze for 6 hr at 30°C. No change at 15°C	1479	I
Calcium gluconate	ANT	2 g	HO	1 g	NS	Physically compatible for 72 hr at 15 and 30°C	1479	C
Cefuroxime sodium	GL	37.5 g	HO	1 g	W	Physically compatible for 72 hr at 15 and 30°C	1479	C
Chlorothiazide sodium	APP	10 g	HOS	1 g	D5W[d]	Physically compatible with less than 10% loss of either drug for 96 hours at 25°C in the dark	3568	C
Chlorpromazine HCl	ANT	5 g	HO	1 g	W	Precipitates immediately	1479	I
Cloxacillin sodium	BE	20 g	HO	1 g	NS	Physically compatible for 72 hr at 15 and 30°C	1479	C
Conivaptan HCl	BA					Stated to be incompatible	2838	I
Dexamethasone sodium phosphate	MSD	4 g	HO	1 g	NS	Physically compatible for 72 hr at 15 and 30°C	1479	C
Diamorphine HCl	EV	500 mg	HO	1 g	W	Physically compatible for 72 hr at 15 and 30°C	1479	C
Diazepam	PHX	1 g	HO	1 g	D5W	Precipitates immediately	1479	I
Digoxin	BW	25 mg	HO	1 g	NS	Physically compatible for 72 hr at 15 and 30°C	1479	C
Dobutamine HCl	LI	1 g	HO	1 g	D5W, NS	Cloudy in 1 hr at 25°C	789	I
Dobutamine HCl	LI	1 g	WY	5 g	D5W, NS	Immediate white precipitate	812	I
Dobutamine HCl	LI	500 mg	HO	1 g	NS	Haze forms immediately	1479	I
Doxapram HCl	WW					Precipitation or gas formation	3220	I
Epinephrine HCl	ANT	8 mg	HO	1 g	W	Physically compatible for 72 hr at 15 and 30°C	1479	C
Eptifibatide	ME	750 mg		10 g		Precipitation and crystallization occurred after 1 hr	3049	I
Erythromycin lactobionate	AB	5 g	HO	1 g	NS	Precipitates immediately. Crystals form in 12 to 24 hr at 15 and 30°C	1479	I
Gentamicin sulfate	SC	1.6 g	HO	800 mg	D5W, NS	Furosemide precipitates immediately	876	I
Gentamicin sulfate	RS	8 g	HO	1 g	NS	Physically compatible for 24 hr at 15 and 30°C. Precipitate forms in 48 to 72 hr	1479	C
Heparin sodium	WED	20,000 units	HO	1 g	NS	Physically compatible for 72 hr at 15 and 30°C	1479	C
Hydrocortisone sodium succinate		1 g		200 and 400 mg	D5W, NS	6 to 8% hydrocortisone loss and 5 to 6% furosemide loss in 24 hr at 25°C	1348	C
Hydrocortisone sodium succinate		300 mg		200 and 400 mg	D5W, NS	6 to 8% hydrocortisone loss in 6 hr and 10 to 14% loss in 24 hr at 25°C. 5 to 6% furosemide loss in 24 hr	1348	I
Hydrocortisone sodium succinate	UP	50 g	HO	1 g	NS	Physically compatible for 72 hr at 15 and 30°C	1479	C
Isoproterenol HCl	PX	4 mg	HO	1 g	D5W	Precipitates immediately	1479	I
Isosorbide dinitrate		1 g	HO	1 g		Physically compatible for 72 hr at 15 and 30°C	1479	C
Lidocaine HCl	ANT	2 g	HO	1 g	NS	Physically compatible for 72 hr at 15 and 30°C	1479	C
Mannitol	BA[c]	20%	AB	200, 400, 800 mg		Visually compatible for 72 hr at 22°C	1803	C

Additive Compatibility (Cont.)

Test Drug	Mfr	Conc/L or %	Mfr	Conc/L or %	Test Solution	Remarks	Ref	C/I
Meperidine HCl	RC	5 g	HO	1 g	W	Fine precipitate forms immediately	1479	I
Meropenem	ZEN	1 and 20 g	HO	1 g	NS	Visually compatible for 4 hr at room temperature	1994	C
Metoclopramide HCl	ANT	1 g	HO	1 g	NS	Precipitates immediately	1479	I
Midazolam HCl	RC	50 and 250 mg		80 mg	NS	Visually compatible for 4 hr	355	C
Morphine sulfate	EV	1 g	HO	1 g	W	Physically compatible for 72 hr at 15 and 30°C	1479	C
Nitroglycerin	ACC	400 mg	HO	1 g	D5W[b]	Physically compatible with no nitroglycerin loss in 48 hr at 23°C. Furosemide not tested	929	C
Nitroglycerin	ACC	400 mg	HO	1 g	NS[b]	Physically compatible with 3% nitroglycerin loss in 48 hr at 23°C. Furosemide not tested	929	C
Potassium chloride	ANT	40 mmol	HO	1 g	W	Physically compatible for 72 hr at 15 and 30°C	1479	C
Prochlorperazine edisylate	MB	1.25 g	HO	1 g	W	Yellow precipitate forms immediately	1479	I
Promethazine HCl	MB	5 g	HO	1 g	W	White precipitate forms immediately	1479	I
Ranitidine HCl	GL	500 mg	HO	1 g	NS	Physically compatible for 72 hr at 15 and 30°C	1479	C
Ranitidine HCl	GL	50 mg and 2 g		400 mg	D5W	Physically compatible. Ranitidine stable for 24 hr at 25°C. Furosemide not tested	1515	C
Scopolamine butylbromide	BI	2 g	HO	1 g	W	Physically compatible for 72 hr at 15 and 30°C	1479	C
Sodium bicarbonate	IMS	8.4%	HO	1 g		Physically compatible for 72 hr at 15 and 30°C	1479	C
Theophylline		2 g		330 mg	D5W	Visually compatible. Little theophylline and 10% furosemide loss in 48 hr	1909	C
Tobramycin sulfate	DI	1.6 g	HO	800 mg	D5W, NS	Transient cloudiness then physically compatible for 24 hr at 21°C	876	?
Tobramycin sulfate	LI	8 g	HO	1 g	NS	Physically compatible for 72 hr at 15 and 30°C	1479	C
Verapamil HCl	KN	80 mg	HO	200 mg	D5W, NS	Physically compatible for 24 hr	764	C
Verapamil HCl	AB	500 mg	HO	1 g	NS	Slight precipitate forms but dissipates	1479	?

[a] Tested in both polyolefin and PVC containers.

[b] Tested in glass containers.

[c] Tested in PVC containers.

[d] Tested in polypropylene containers.

Drugs in Syringe Compatibility

Furosemide

Test Drug	Mfr	Amt	Mfr	Amt	Remarks	Ref	C/I
Bleomycin sulfate		1.5 units/0.5 mL		5 mg/0.5 mL	Physically compatible for 5 min at room temperature followed by 8 min of centrifugation	980	C
Caffeine citrate		20 mg/1 mL	AST	10 mg/1 mL	Precipitates immediately	2440	I
Cisplatin		0.5 mg/0.5 mL		5 mg/0.5 mL	Physically compatible for 5 min at room temperature followed by 8 min of centrifugation	980	C

Drugs in Syringe Compatibility (Cont.)

Test Drug	Mfr	Amt	Mfr	Amt	Remarks	Ref	C/I
Cyclophosphamide		10 mg/0.5 mL		5 mg/0.5 mL	Physically compatible for 5 min at room temperature followed by 8 min of centrifugation	980	C
Dexamethasone sodium phosphate	ME	0.33 to 3.33 mg/mL	HO	3.33 to 10 mg/mL	Tested in NS. No visible precipitation with under 10% loss of either drug in 5 days at 4 and 25°C. Precipitation with over 10% drug loss in 15 days	2711	C
Dimenhydrinate		10 mg/1 mL		10 mg/1 mL	Precipitate forms	2569	I
Doxapram HCl	RB	400 mg/20 mL	HO	100 mg/10 mL	Immediate turbidity	1177	I
Doxorubicin HCl		1 mg/0.5 mL		5 mg/0.5 mL	Precipitates immediately	980	I
Droperidol		1.25 mg/0.5 mL		5 mg/0.5 mL	Precipitates immediately	980	I
Fluorouracil		25 mg/0.5 mL		5 mg/0.5 mL	Physically compatible for 5 min at room temperature followed by 8 min of centrifugation	980	C
Heparin sodium		500 units/0.5 mL		5 mg/0.5 mL	Physically compatible for 5 min at room temperature followed by 8 min of centrifugation	980	C
Heparin sodium		2500 units/1 mL		20 mg/2 mL	Physically compatible for at least 5 min	1053	C
Leucovorin calcium		5 mg/0.5 mL		5 mg/0.5 mL	Physically compatible for 5 min at room temperature followed by 8 min of centrifugation	980	C
Methotrexate sodium		12.5 mg/0.5 mL		5 mg/0.5 mL	Physically compatible for 5 min at room temperature followed by 8 min of centrifugation	980	C
Metoclopramide HCl		2.5 mg/0.5 mL		5 mg/0.5 mL	Precipitates immediately	980	I
Milrinone lactate	WI	3.5 mg/3.5 mL	LY	40 mg/4 mL	Brought to 10-mL total volume with D5W. Precipitates immediately	1191	I
Mitomycin		0.25 mg/0.5 mL		5 mg/0.5 mL	Physically compatible for 5 min at room temperature followed by 8 min of centrifugation	980	C
Pantoprazole sodium	[a]	4 mg/1 mL		10 mg/1 mL	Possible precipitate within 15 min	2574	I
Vinblastine sulfate		0.5 mg/0.5 mL		5 mg/0.5 mL	Precipitates immediately	980	I
Vincristine sulfate		0.5 mg/0.5 mL		5 mg/0.5 mL	Precipitates immediately	980	I

[a] Test performed using the formulation WITHOUT edetate disodium.

Y-Site Injection Compatibility (1:1 Mixture)

Furosemide

Test Drug	Mfr	Conc	Mfr	Conc	Remarks	Ref	C/I
Allopurinol sodium	BW	3 mg/mL[b]	ES	3 mg/mL[b]	Physically compatible for 4 hr at 22°C	1686	C
Amifostine	USB	10 mg/mL[a]	AB	3 mg/mL[a]	Physically compatible for 4 hr at 23°C	1845	C
Amikacin sulfate	BR	2 mg/mL[c]	HO	10 mg/mL	Physically compatible for 24 hr at 21°C	876	C
Amiodarone HCl	WY	6 mg/mL[a]	AMR	1 mg/mL[a]	Visually compatible for 24 hr at 22°C	2352	C
Amiodarone HCl	WY	6 mg/mL[a]	AMR	10 mg/mL	Immediate opaque white turbidity	2352	I
Amsacrine	NCI	1 mg/mL[a]	ES	3 mg/mL[a]	Yellow turbidity becoming colorless liquid with yellow precipitate	1381	I
Anidulafungin	VIC	0.5 mg/mL[a]	AB	3 mg/mL[a]	Physically compatible for 4 hr at 23°C	2617	C

Y-Site Injection Compatibility (1:1 Mixture) (Cont.)

Test Drug	Mfr	Conc	Mfr	Conc	Remarks	Ref	C/I
Argatroban	SKB	1 mg/mLª	AB	10 mg/mL	Physically compatible for 24 hr at 23°C	2572	C
Azithromycin	PF	2 mg/mLᵇ	AMR	10 mg/mLˡ	White microcrystals found	2368	I
Aztreonam	SQ	40 mg/mLª	AB	3 mg/mLª	Physically compatible for 4 hr at 23°C	1758	C
Bivalirudin	TMC	5 mg/mLª	AMR	3 mg/mLª	Physically compatible for 4 hr at 23°C	2373	C
Bleomycin sulfate		3 units/mL		10 mg/mL	Drugs injected sequentially in Y-site with no flush. No precipitate seen	980	C
Blinatumomab	AMG	0.125 mcg/mLᵇ	SAA	2.9 mg/mL	Visually compatible for 12 hr at room temperature	3405, 3417	C
Blinatumomab	AMG	0.375 mcg/mLᵇ	SAA	2.9 mg/mL	Persistent particulate formation when furosemide is added to blinatumomab; small flakes transiently appeared when order of mixing was reversed	3405, 3417	I
Cangrelor tetrasodium	TMC	1 mg/mLᵇ		3ᵇ and 10 mg/mL	Physically compatible for 4 hr	3243	C
Caspofungin acetate	ME	0.7 mg/mLᵇ	AMR	3 mg/mLᵇ	Immediate white turbid precipitate forms	2758	I
Caspofungin acetate	ME	0.5 mg/mLᵇ	HOS	10 mg/mL	Gelatinous material reported	2766	I
Cefepime HCl	BMS	120 mg/mLᶜ		10 mg/mLª	Physically compatible with less than 10% cefepime loss. Furosemide not tested	2513	C
Ceftaroline fosamil	FOR	2.22 mg/mLª ᵇ ᵐ	HOS	3 mg/mLª ᵇ ᵐ	Physically compatible for 4 hr at 23°C	2826	C
Ceftazidime	SKB	125 mg/mL		10 mg/mL	Visually compatible with less than 10% loss of ceftazidime in 30 min. Furosemide not tested	2434	C
Ceftazidime	GSK	120 mg/mLᵈ		10 mg/mL	Physically compatible with less than 10% ceftazidime loss. Furosemide not tested	2513	C
Ceftazidime–avibactam sodium	ALL	20 mg/mLᵗ ᵘ			Physically compatible for up to 4 hr at room temperature	3004	C
Ceftolozane sulfate–tazobactam sodium	CUB	10 mg/mLᶜ ʳ	HOS	3 mg/mLᶜ	Physically compatible for 2 hr	3262	C
Chlorpromazine HCl	RPR	0.13 mg/mLª	HMR	2.6 mg/mLª	Precipitate forms immediately	2244	I
Ciprofloxacin	MI	2 mg/mLᶜ	AB	10 mg/mL	Precipitates immediately	1655	I
Ciprofloxacin	BAY	2 mg/mLᵇ	DMX	5 mg/mL	White precipitate forms immediately	1934	I
Cisatracurium besylate	GW	0.1 mg/mLª	AB	3 mg/mLª	Physically compatible for 4 hr at 23°C	2074	C
Cisatracurium besylate	GW	2 and 5 mg/mLª	AB	3 mg/mLª	White cloudiness forms immediately	2074	I
Cisplatin		1 mg/mL		10 mg/mL	Drugs injected sequentially in Y-site with no flush. No precipitate seen	980	C
Cladribine	ORT	0.015ᵇ and 0.5ᵉ mg/mL	AB	3 mg/mLᵇ	Physically compatible for 4 hr at 23°C	1969	C
Clarithromycin	AB	4 mg/mLª	ANT	10 mg/mL	White cloudiness forms immediately, becoming an obvious precipitate in 15 min	2174	I
Cloxacillin sodium	SMX	100 mg/mL	OM	10 mg/mL	Physically compatible for up to 4 hr at room temperature	3245	C
Cyclophosphamide		20 mg/mL		10 mg/mL	Drugs injected sequentially in Y-site with no flush. No precipitate seen	980	C

Y-Site Injection Compatibility (1:1 Mixture) (Cont.)

Test Drug	Mfr	Conc	Mfr	Conc	Remarks	Ref	C/I
Defibrotide sodium	JAZ	8 mg/mL[b]	REN	10 mg/mL	Slight and transient bubbling occurs only when defibrotide added to furosemide; not observed when order of mixing was reversed	3149	?
Dexmedetomidine HCl	AB	4 mcg/mL[b]	AMR	3 mg/mL[b]	Physically compatible for 4 hr at 23°C	2383	C
Diltiazem HCl	MMD	1[b] and 5 mg/mL	AMR	10 mg/mL	Heavy precipitate forms	1807	I
Diltiazem HCl	MMD	1 mg/mL[a]	AMR	10 mg/mL	Precipitate forms immediately	2062	I
Dobutamine HCl	LI	4 mg/mL[b]	ES	1 mg/mL[b]	Physically compatible for 3 hr	1316	C
Dobutamine HCl	LI	4 mg/mL[a]	ES	1 mg/mL[a]	Slight precipitate in 1 hr	1316	I
Dobutamine HCl	LI	4 mg/mL[a]	AMR	10 mg/mL	Precipitate forms immediately	2062	I
Docetaxel	RPR	0.9 mg/mL[a]	AMR	3 mg/mL[a]	Physically compatible for 4 hr at 23°C	2224	C
Dopamine HCl	AST, DU	12.8 mg/mL	AB, AMR	5 mg/mL	Physically compatible for 3 hr at room temperature	1978	C
Dopamine HCl	AB, AMR	12.8 mg/mL	AB, AMR	5 mg/mL	White precipitate forms immediately	1978	I
Dopamine HCl	AB	3.2 mg/mL[a]	AMR	10 mg/mL	Precipitate forms in 4 hr at 27°C	2062	I
Doripenem	JJ	5 mg/mL[a b]	AMR	3 mg/mL[a b]	Physically compatible for 4 hr at 23°C	2743	C
Doxorubicin HCl		2 mg/mL		10 mg/mL	Drugs injected sequentially in Y-site with no flush. Precipitates immediately	980	I
Doxorubicin HCl liposomal	SEQ	0.4 mg/mL[a]	AMR	3 mg/mL[a]	Physically compatible for 4 hr at 23°C	2087	C
Droperidol		2.5 mg/mL		10 mg/mL	Drugs injected sequentially in Y-site with no flush. Precipitates immediately	980	I
Droperidol		2.5 mg/mL		10 mg/mL	Precipitate forms	977	I
Epinephrine HCl	AB	0.02 mg/mL[a]	AMR	10 mg/mL	Visually compatible for 4 hr at 27°C	2062	C
Eravacycline dihydrochloride	TET	0.3 and 0.6 mg/mL[b]	FRK	3 mg/mL[b]	Measured turbidity increased immediately; pH decreased by >1 unit within 60 min	3532	I
Esmolol HCl	ACC	10 mg/mL[c]	HO	10 mg/mL	Cloudy precipitate forms immediately	1146	I
Etoposide phosphate	BR	5 mg/mL[a]	AMR	3 mg/mL[a]	Physically compatible for 4 hr at 23°C	2218	C
Famotidine	MSD	0.2 mg/mL[a]	IMS	0.8 mg/mL[a]	Physically compatible for 4 hr at 25°C	1188	C
Famotidine	MSD	0.2 mg/mL[a]	ES	10 mg/mL	Physically compatible for 14 hr	1196	C
Famotidine	ME	2 mg/mL[b]		3 mg/mL[a]	White precipitate forms immediately	1936	I
Fenoldopam mesylate	AB	80 mcg/mL[b]	AMR	3 mg/mL[b]	Trace haze forms immediately	2467	I
Fentanyl citrate	ES	0.05 mg/mL	AMR	10 mg/mL	Visually compatible for 4 hr at 27°C	2062	C
Filgrastim	AMG	30 mcg/mL[a]	AB	3 mg/mL[a]	Turbidity forms immediately. Filaments and particles form in 1 hr	1687	I
Fluconazole	RR	2 mg/mL	ES	10 mg/mL	Precipitate forms	1407	I
Fludarabine phosphate	BX	1 mg/mL[a]	AB	3 mg/mL[a]	Visually compatible for 4 hr at 22°C	1439	C
Fluorouracil		50 mg/mL		10 mg/mL	Drugs injected sequentially in Y-site with no flush. No precipitate seen	980	C

Y-Site Injection Compatibility (1:1 Mixture) (Cont.)

Test Drug	Mfr	Conc	Mfr	Conc	Remarks	Ref	C/I
Foscarnet sodium	AST	24 mg/mL	AB	10 mg/mL	Physically compatible for 24 hr at room temperature under fluorescent light	1335	C
Gallium nitrate	FUJ	1 mg/mL[b]	AB	10 mg/mL	Visually compatible for 24 hr at 25°C	1673	C
Gemcitabine HCl	LI	10 mg/mL[b]	AMR	3 mg/mL[b]	Gross precipitation occurs immediately	2226	I
Gentamicin sulfate	SC	1.6 mg/mL[c]	HO	10 mg/mL	Furosemide precipitates immediately	876	I
Granisetron HCl	SKB	0.05 mg/mL[a]	AB	3 mg/mL[a]	Physically compatible for 4 hr at 23°C	1804	C
Granisetron HCl	SKB	1 mg/mL	HO	0.4 mg/mL[b]	Physically compatible with little or no loss of either drug in 4 hr at 22°C	1883	C
Heparin sodium		1000 units/mL		10 mg/mL	Drugs injected sequentially in Y-site with no flush. No precipitate seen	980	C
Heparin sodium	UP	1000 units/L[f]	HO	10 mg/mL	Physically compatible for 4 hr at room temperature	534	C
Heparin sodium	ES	100 units/mL[a]	AMR	10 mg/mL	Visually compatible for 4 hr at 27°C	2062	C
Heparin sodium	NOV	29.2 units/mL[a]	HMR	2.6 mg/mL[a]	Visually compatible for 150 min	2244	C
Hetastarch in lactated electrolyte	AB	6%	AMR	3 mg/mL[a]	Physically compatible for 4 hr at 23°C	2339	C
Hydralazine HCl	SO	1 mg/mL[c]	ES	1 mg/mL[c]	Slight color change in 3 hr	1316	I
Hydrocortisone sodium succinate	UP	10 mg/L[f]	HO	10 mg/mL	Physically compatible for 4 hr at room temperature	534	C
Hydromorphone HCl	KN	1 mg/mL	AMR	10 mg/mL	Visually compatible for 4 hr at 27°C	2062	C
Hydroxyethyl starch 130/0.4 in sodium chloride 0.9%	FRK	6%	SZ	1, 1.5, 2 mg/mL[a]	Visually compatible for 24 hr at room temperature	2770	C
Ibuprofen lysinate	OVA	10 mg/mL	HOS	10 mg/mL	Physically compatible for 4 hr at room temperature	3541	C
Idarubicin HCl	AD	1 mg/mL[b]	AB	10 mg/mL	Precipitate forms immediately	1525	I
Idarubicin HCl	AD	1 mg/mL[b]	AB	0.8 mg/mL[b]	Haze forms immediately	1525	I
Indomethacin sodium trihydrate	MSD	1 mg/mL[b]	AB	10 mg/mL	Visually compatible for 24 hr at 28°C	1527	C
Isavuconazonium sulfate	ASP	1.5 mg/mL[c]	HOS	3 mg/mL[c]	Immediate precipitation and increase in measured turbidity	3263	I
Labetalol HCl	SC	1.6 mg/mL[g]	ES	10 mg/mL[g]	White precipitate forms immediately	1715	I
Labetalol HCl	AH	2 mg/mL[a]	AMR	10 mg/mL	Precipitate forms immediately	2062	I
Letermovir	ME	[b]		[b]	Physically compatible	3398	C
Leucovorin calcium		10 mg/mL		10 mg/mL	Drugs injected sequentially in Y-site with no flush. No precipitate seen	980	C
Levofloxacin	OMN	5 mg/mL[a]	AST	10 mg/mL	Cloudy precipitate forms	2233	I
Linezolid	PHU	2 mg/mL	AMR	3 mg/mL[a]	Physically compatible for 4 hr at 23°C	2264	C
Lorazepam	WY	0.33 mg/mL[b]	CNF	10 mg/mL	Visually compatible for 24 hr at 22°C	1855	C
Lorazepam	WY	0.5 mg/mL[a]	AMR	10 mg/mL	Visually compatible for 4 hr at 27°C	2062	C
Melphalan HCl	BW	0.1 mg/mL[b]	AB	3 mg/mL[b]	Physically compatible for 3 hr at 22°C	1557	C
Meperidine HCl	AB	10 mg/mL	ES	0.8 mg/mL[a]	Physically compatible for 4 hr at 25°C	1397	C

Y-Site Injection Compatibility (1:1 Mixture) (Cont.)

Test Drug	Mfr	Conc	Mfr	Conc	Remarks	Ref	C/I
Meperidine HCl	AB	10 mg/mL	ES	2.4 mg/mL[a]	White cloudiness forms immediately	1397	I
Meperidine HCl	AB	10 mg/mL	ES	10 mg/mL	White precipitate forms immediately	1397	I
Meropenem	ZEN	1 and 50 mg/mL[b]	HO	10 mg/mL	Visually compatible for 4 hr at room temperature	1994	C
Meropenem		50 mg/mL	OM	10 mg/mL	Physically compatible for 4 hr at room temperature	3538	C
Meropenem–vaborbactam	TMC	8 mg/mL[b s]	CLA	3 mg/mL[b]	Physically compatible for 3 hr at 20 to 25°C	3380	C
Methotrexate sodium		25 mg/mL		10 mg/mL	Drugs injected sequentially in Y-site with no flush. No precipitate seen	980	C
Metoclopramide HCl		5 mg/mL		10 mg/mL	Drugs injected sequentially in Y-site with no flush. Precipitates immediately	980	I
Metoprolol tartrate	BED	1 mg/mL	HOS	10 mg/mL	Visually compatible for 24 hr at 19°C	2795	C
Micafungin sodium	ASP	1.5 mg/mL[b]	AMR	3 mg/mL[b]	Physically compatible for 4 hr at 23°C	2683	C
Midazolam HCl	RC	1 mg/mL[a]	AST	10 mg/mL	Immediate haze. Precipitate in 2 hr	1847	I
Midazolam HCl	RC	5 mg/mL	CNF	10 mg/mL	White precipitate forms immediately	1855	I
Midazolam HCl	RC	2 mg/mL[a]	AMR	10 mg/mL	Precipitate forms immediately	2062	I
Milrinone lactate	WI	200 mcg/mL[a]	LY	10 mg/mL	Precipitates immediately	1191	I
Milrinone lactate	SW	0.2 mg/mL[a]	AMR	10 mg/mL	Precipitate forms in 4 hr at 27°C	2062	I
Mitomycin		0.5 mg/mL		10 mg/mL	Drugs injected sequentially in Y-site with no flush. No precipitate seen	980	C
Morphine sulfate	AB	1 mg/mL	ES	0.8[a], 2.4[a], 10 mg/mL	White precipitate in 1 hr at 25°C	1397	I
Morphine sulfate	SCN	2 mg/mL[a]	AMR	10 mg/mL	Visually compatible for 4 hr at 27°C	2062	C
Nesiritide	SCI	50 mcg/mL[a b]		10 mg/mL	Physically incompatible	2625	I
Nicardipine HCl	WY	1 mg/mL[a]	AMR	10 mg/mL	Precipitate forms immediately	2062	I
Nitroglycerin	AB	0.4 mg/mL[a]	AMR	10 mg/mL	Visually compatible for 4 hr at 27°C	2062	C
Nitroglycerin	BA	0.1 mg/mL[o]	AMR	10 mg/mL	Precipitation occurs immediately	2725	I
Nitroglycerin	AMR	0.1 mg/mL[a]	AMR	10 mg/mL	Physically compatible for 48 hr at room temperature	2725	C
Norepinephrine bitartrate	AB	0.128 mg/mL[a]	AMR	10 mg/mL	Visually compatible for 4 hr at 27°C	2062	C
Ondansetron HCl	GL	1 mg/mL[b]	AB	3 mg/mL[a]	Immediate turbidity and precipitation	1365	I
Oritavancin diphosphate	TAR	0.8, 1.2, and 2 mg/mL[a]	AMR	5 mg/mL[a]	Haze forms immediately with precipitate after 30 min	2928	I
Oxaliplatin	SS	0.5 mg/mL[a]	AMR	3 mg/mL[a]	Physically compatible for 4 hr at 23°C	2566	C
Paclitaxel	NCI	1.2 mg/mL[a]	AST	3 mg/mL[a]	Physically compatible for 4 hr at 22°C	1556	C
Pantoprazole sodium	ALT[n]	0.16 to 0.8 mg/mL[b]	SX	1 to 2 mg/mL[a]	Visually compatible for 12 hr at 23°C	2603	C
Phenylephrine HCl	BA	0.64 mg/mL[a b]	AB	4 mg/mL[a b]	Precipitates in 5 to 15 min	2687	I
Piperacillin sodium–tazobactam sodium	LE[n]	40 mg/mL[a p]	AB	3 mg/mL[a]	Physically compatible for 4 hr at 22°C	1688	C

Y-Site Injection Compatibility (1:1 Mixture) (Cont.)

Test Drug	Mfr	Conc	Mfr	Conc	Remarks	Ref	C/I
Plazomicin sulfate	ACH	24 mg/mL^c	CLA	3 mg/mL^c	Physically compatible for 1 hr at 20 to 25°C	3432	C
Potassium chloride	AB	40 mEq/L^f	HO	10 mg/mL	Physically compatible for 4 hr at room temperature	534	C
Potassium chloride	BRN	0.625 mEq/mL^a	HMR	2.6 mg/mL^a	Visually compatible for 150 min	2244	C
Propofol	ZEN^v	10 mg/mL	AB	3 mg/mL^a	Physically compatible for 1 hr at 23°C	2066	C
Quinidine gluconate	LI	6 mg/mL^c	ES	4 mg/mL^c	Immediate gross precipitation	1316	I
Quinupristin–dalfopristin		2 mg/mL$^{a\ q}$		3 mg/mL	Reported to be incompatible	3230	I
Ranitidine HCl	GL	1 mg/mL^a	AMR	10 mg/mL	Visually compatible for 4 hr at 27°C	2062	C
Remifentanil HCl	GW	0.025 and 0.25 mg/mL^b	AMR	3 mg/mL^a	Physically compatible for 4 hr at 23°C	2075	C
Sargramostim	IMM	10 mcg/mL^b	AB	3 mg/mL^b	Visually compatible for 4 hr at 22°C	1436	C
Sodium nitroprusside	RC	0.3, 1.2, 3 mg/mL^a	SX	1.2^k and 10 mg/mL	Visually compatible for 48 hr at 24°C protected from light	2357	C
Sodium nitroprusside	RC	1.2 and 3 mg/mL^a	SX	5 mg/mL^a	Visually compatible for 48 hr at 24°C protected from light	2357	C
Tacrolimus	FUJ	1 mg/mL^b	ES	10 mg/mL	Visually compatible for 24 hr at 25°C	1630	C
Tedizolid phosphate	CUB	0.8 mg/mL^b	HOS	3 mg/mL^b	Physically compatible for 2 hr	3244	C
Telavancin HCl	ASP	7.5 mg/mL$^{a\ b\ m}$	HOS	3 mg/mL$^{a\ b\ m}$	Immediate precipitation	2830	I
Teniposide	BR	0.1 mg/mL^a	AB	3 mg/mL^a	Physically compatible for 4 hr at 23°C	1725	C
Thiotepa	IMM^i	1 mg/mL^a	AMR	3 mg/mL^a	Physically compatible for 4 hr at 23°C	1861	C
Tirofiban HCl	ME	50 mcg/mL$^{a\ b}$	AB	0.5$^{a\ b}$ and 10 mg/mL	Physically compatible with no loss of either drug in 4 hr at 23°C	2356	C
TNA #73^j			ES	3.3 mg/mL^c	Visually compatible for 4 hr	1009	C
TNA #218 to #226^j			AB	3 mg/mL^a	Visually compatible for 4 hr at 23°C	2215	C
Tobramycin sulfate	DI	1.6 mg/mL^c	HO	10 mg/mL	Physically compatible for 24 hr at 21°C	876	C
TPN #189^j				10 mg/mL^b	Visually compatible for 24 hr at 22°C	1767	C
TPN #203, #204^j			AMR	10 mg/mL	Visually compatible for 2 hr at 23°C	1974	C
TPN #212 to #215^j			AB	3 mg/mL^a	Small amount of subvisible precipitate forms immediately	2109	I
Vancomycin HCl	LI	10 mg/mL		10 mg/mL	Physically incompatible	3536	I
Vasopressin	APP	0.4 unit/mL$^{a\ b}$	AB	4 mg/mL$^{a\ b}$	Precipitates in 5 to 15 min	2687	I
Vecuronium bromide	OR	1 mg/mL	AMR	10 mg/mL	Precipitate forms immediately	2062	I
Vinblastine sulfate		1 mg/mL		10 mg/mL	Drugs injected sequentially in Y-site with no flush. Precipitates immediately	980	I

Y-Site Injection Compatibility (1:1 Mixture) (Cont.)

Test Drug	Mfr	Conc	Mfr	Conc	Remarks	Ref	C/I
Vincristine sulfate		1 mg/mL		10 mg/mL	Drugs injected sequentially in Y-site with no flush. Precipitates immediately	980	I
Vinorelbine tartrate	BW	1 mg/mL[b]	ES	3 mg/mL[b]	Heavy white precipitate forms immediately	1558	I

[a] Tested in dextrose 5%.

[b] Tested in sodium chloride 0.9%.

[c] Tested in both dextrose 5% and sodium chloride 0.9%.

[d] Tested in sterile water for injection.

[e] Tested in bacteriostatic sodium chloride 0.9% preserved with benzyl alcohol 0.9%.

[f] Tested in dextrose 5% in Ringer's injection, dextrose 5% in Ringer's injection, lactated, dextrose 5%, Ringer's injection, lactated, and sodium chloride 0.9%.

[g] Furosemide 0.5 mL injected in the Y-site port of a running infusion of labetalol hydrochloride in dextrose 5%.

[h] Tested in dextrose 5% with sodium bicarbonate 0.05 mEq/mL.

[i] Lyophilized formulation tested.

[j] Refer to Appendix for the composition of parenteral nutrition solutions. TNA indicates a 3-in-1 admixture, and TPN indicates a 2-in-1 admixture.

[k] Tested in dextrose 5% in sodium chloride 0.225%.

[l] Injected via Y-site into an administration set running azithromycin.

[m] Tested in Ringer's injection, lactated.

[n] Test performed using the formulation WITHOUT edetate disodium.

[o] Tested using premixed nitroglycerin infusion in dextrose 5% with citrate buffer (Baxter Healthcare).

[p] Piperacillin component. Piperacillin in an 8:1 fixed-ratio concentration with tazobactam.

[q] Quinupristin and dalfopristin components combined.

[r] Ceftolozane component. Ceftolozane in a 2:1 fixed-ratio concentration with tazobactam.

[s] Meropenem component. Meropenem in a 1:1 fixed-ratio concentration with vaborbactam.

[t] Ceftazidime component. Ceftazidime in a 4:1 fixed-ratio concentration with avibactam.

[u] Tested in dextrose 5%, sodium chloride 0.9%, and Ringer's injection, lactated.

[v] Test performed using the formulation WITH edetate disodium.

Selected Revisions July 1, 2020. © Copyright, October 1982.
American Society of Health-System Pharmacists, Inc.

Fusidate Sodium
AHFS 8:12.28.92

Products

Fusidate sodium is available as a dry powder in vials containing 500 mg (equivalent to 480 mg of fusidic acid). It is packaged with a diluent vial containing 10 mL of phosphate–citrate buffer (pH 7.4 to 7.6). The drug should be reconstituted with the diluent and diluted further with sodium chloride 0.9% or other compatible diluent for administration.[38]

Sodium and Phosphate Content

Each vial of fusidate sodium contains 3.1 mmol of sodium and 1.1 mmol of phosphate.[38]

Trade Name(s)

Fucidin

Administration

Fusidate sodium is administered by slow intravenous infusion over not less than six hours if a superficial vein is employed. If a central venous line is used, the infusion should be given over two to four hours. The reconstituted fusidate sodium in 10 mL of buffer solution is diluted in 500 mL of sodium chloride 0.9% or other compatible infusion solution for administration. The drug must not be given by other routes.[38]

Stability

Fusidate sodium should be stored below 25°C and protected from light. Reconstituted solutions that are added to 500 mL of compatible infusion solutions are stable for 24 hours at room temperature. Unused portions of the reconstituted solution should be discarded.[38]

Fusidate sodium reconstituted with the buffer solution to 50 mg/mL is physically incompatible with infusion solutions containing amino acids solutions, dextrose 20% or greater, and lipid infusions.[38]

Fusidate sodium (Leo) at a concentration of 0.125 mg/mL is stated to be physically incompatible with the following peritoneal dialysis solutions[1800]:

Dianeal PD2 with dextrose 1.36%
Dianeal PD3 with dextrose 1.36%
Dianeal with dextrose 3.86%
Peritoneal Dialysis Solution 6.36%
Peritoneal Dialysis Solution 6.36% + acetate
Peritoneal Dialysis Solution with dextrose 2.27%

pH Effects

Precipitation may occur upon dilution if the resulting pH is less than 7.4.[38]

Freezing Solutions

Fusidate sodium (Leo) 1 mg/mL in sodium chloride 0.9% and dextrose 5% is stated to be stable frozen at –20°C for 24 hours followed by thawing in a microwave oven.[1800]

Fusidic acid (Leo) 500 mg, reconstituted in buffer and diluted to 550 mL in sodium chloride 0.9% in PVC bags, was stored frozen at –20°C. No loss was found after 12 months of storage followed by microwave thawing. Furthermore, the solution was physically compatible, with no increase in subvisible particles. In addition, there was no loss of fusidate sodium after six months of storage at –20°C followed by three freeze–thaw cycles.[1612]

Compatibility Information
Solution Compatibility

Fusidate sodium

Test Soln Name	Mfr	Mfr	Conc/L or %	Remarks	Ref	C/I
Dextrose 5%	BA[a]	LEO	1.16 and 2.32 g	Physically compatible. Under 10% loss in 162 days at 4°C. 10% loss in 10.4 days at 25°C or 2.1 days at 37°C	1709	C
Dextrose 5%[b]	BP	LEO	1 and 2 g	Physically compatible and chemically stable for 48 hr at room temperature	1800	C
Sodium chloride 0.9%[b]	BP	LEO	1 and 2 g	Physically compatible and chemically stable for 48 hr at room temperature	1800	C
Sodium chloride 0.18% and dextrose 4%	BP	LEO	1 g	Physically compatible and chemically stable for 48 hr at room temperature	1800	C
Sodium lactate ⅙ M	BP	LEO	1 g	Physically compatible and chemically stable for 48 hr at room temperature	1800	C

[a] Tested in PVC containers.

[b] Tested both with and without potassium chloride 0.3%.

DOI: 10.37573/9781585286850.182

Additive Compatibility

Fusidate sodium

Test Drug	Mfr	Conc/L or %	Mfr	Conc/L or %	Test Solution	Remarks	Ref	C/I
Cefotaxime sodium		2.5 g	LEO	500 mg	D2.5½S, D2.5S, D5¼S, D5½S, D5S, D10S	Physically compatible and chemically stable for 48 hr at room temperature	1800	C
Erythromycin lactobionate		5 g	LEO	1 g	D2.5½S, D2.5S, D5¼S, D5½S, D5S, D10S	Physically compatible and chemically stable for 48 hr at room temperature	1800	C
Fat emulsion, intravenous		10%	LEO	1 g		Physically incompatible	1800	I
Floxacillin sodium		2.5 g	LEO	500 mg	D2.5½S, D2.5S, D5¼S, D5½S, D5S, D10S	Physically compatible and chemically stable for 48 hr at room temperature	1800	C
Gentamicin sulfate		160 mg	LEO	1 g	D2.5½S, D2.5S, D5¼S, D5½S, D5S, D10S	Physically compatible and chemically stable for 48 hr at room temperature	1800	C
Gentamicin sulfate		1.5 g	LEO	1 g	D2.5½S, D2.5S, D5¼S, D5½S, D5S, D10S	Physically incompatible	1800	I
Vancomycin HCl		25 g	LEO	500 mg	D2.5½S, D2.5S, D5¼S, D5½S, D5S, D10S	Physically incompatible	1800	I

Selected Revisions March 13, 2017. © Copyright, October 1994.
American Society of Health-System Pharmacists, Inc.

Gallium Nitrate
AHFS 92:24

Products

Gallium nitrate is available in 20-mL vials. Each mL of solution contains gallium nitrate 25 mg, sodium citrate dihydrate 28.75 mg, and sodium hydroxide or hydrochloric acid for pH adjustment during manufacturing in water for injection.[1(2/08)]

pH
From 6 to 7.[1(2/08)]

Trade Name(s)
Ganite

Administration

Gallium nitrate is administered by intravenous infusion over 24 hours after dilution in 1000 mL of dextrose 5% or sodium chloride 0.9%.[1(2/08)]

Stability

Gallium nitrate in intact vials should be stored at controlled room temperature. The manufacturer states that unused portions of the vials should be discarded because no preservative is present.[1(2/08)]

Gallium nitrate diluted in 1000 mL of dextrose 5% or sodium chloride 0.9% is stable for 48 hours at room temperature and for 7 days stored under refrigeration.[1(2/08)]

Compatibility Information

Y-Site Injection Compatibility (1:1 Mixture)

Gallium nitrate

Test Drug	Mfr	Conc	Mfr	Conc	Remarks	Ref	C/I
Acyclovir sodium	BW	7 mg/mL[b]	FUJ	1 mg/mL[b]	Visually compatible for 24 hr at 25°C	1673	C
Allopurinol sodium	BW	3 mg/mL[b]	FUJ	0.4 mg/mL[b]	Physically compatible for 4 hr at 22°C	1686	C
Amifostine	USB	10 mg/mL[a]	FUJ	0.4 mg/mL[a]	Physically compatible for 4 hr at 23°C	1845	C
Aminophylline	AMR	25 mg/mL	FUJ	1 mg/mL[b]	Visually compatible for 24 hr at 25°C	1673	C
Ampicillin sodium–sulbactam sodium	RR	45 mg/mL[b f]	FUJ	1 mg/mL[b]	Visually compatible for 24 hr at 25°C	1673	C
Aztreonam	SQ	40 mg/mL[a]	FUJ	0.4 mg/mL[a]	Physically compatible for 4 hr at 23°C	1758	C
Cefazolin sodium	GEM	100 mg/mL[b]	FUJ	1 mg/mL[b]	Visually compatible for 24 hr at 25°C	1673	C
Ceftazidime	LI	100 mg/mL[b]	FUJ	1 mg/mL[b]	Visually compatible for 24 hr at 25°C	1673	C
Ceftriaxone sodium	RC	40 mg/mL[b]	FUJ	1 mg/mL[b]	Visually compatible for 24 hr at 25°C	1673	C
Ciprofloxacin	MI	2 mg/mL[b]	FUJ	1 mg/mL[b]	Visually compatible for 24 hr at 25°C	1673	C
Cisplatin	BR	1 mg/mL	FUJ	1 mg/mL[b]	Precipitates immediately	1673	I
Cladribine	ORT	0.015[b] and 0.5[c] mg/mL	FUJ	0.4 mg/mL[b]	Physically compatible for 4 hr at 23°C	1969	C
Cyclophosphamide	MJ	20 mg/mL	FUJ	1 mg/mL[b]	Visually compatible for 24 hr at 25°C	1673	C
Cytarabine	CET	50 mg/mL	FUJ	1 mg/mL[b]	Precipitates immediately	1673	I
Dexamethasone sodium phosphate	AMR	4 mg/mL	FUJ	1 mg/mL[b]	Visually compatible for 24 hr at 25°C	1673	C
Diphenhydramine HCl	ES	50 mg/mL	FUJ	1 mg/mL[b]	Visually compatible for 24 hr at 25°C	1673	C
Doxorubicin HCl	CET	2 mg/mL	FUJ	1 mg/mL[b]	Precipitates immediately	1673	I

DOI: 10.37573/9781585286850.183

Y-Site Injection Compatibility (1:1 Mixture) (Cont.)

Test Drug	Mfr	Conc	Mfr	Conc	Remarks	Ref	C/I
Etoposide	BR	0.4 mg/mL[b]	FUJ	1 mg/mL[b]	Precipitate forms after 60 min	1673	I
Filgrastim	AMG	30 mcg/mL[a]	FUJ	0.4 mg/mL[a]	Physically compatible for 4 hr at 22°C	1687	C
Fluconazole	PF	2 mg/mL	FUJ	1 mg/mL[b]	Visually compatible for 24 hr at 25°C	1673	C
Fluorouracil	RC	50 mg/mL	FUJ	1 mg/mL[b]	Precipitate forms immediately but clears after 60 min	1673	I
Furosemide	AB	10 mg/mL	FUJ	1 mg/mL[b]	Visually compatible for 24 hr at 25°C	1673	C
Granisetron HCl	SKB	0.05 mg/mL[a]	FUJ	0.4 mg/mL[a]	Physically compatible for 4 hr at 23°C	2000	C
Haloperidol lactate	MN	5 mg/mL	FUJ	1 mg/mL[b]	Immediate white cloudiness	1673	I
Heparin sodium	ES	40 units/mL[b]	FUJ	1 mg/mL[b]	Visually compatible for 24 hr at 25°C	1673	C
Hydrocortisone sodium succinate	AB	50 mg/mL	FUJ	1 mg/mL[b]	Visually compatible for 24 hr at 25°C	1673	C
Hydromorphone HCl	WY	4 mg/mL	FUJ	1 mg/mL[b]	Precipitate forms in 24 hr at 25°C	1673	I
Ifosfamide	MJ	20 mg/mL[b]	FUJ	1 mg/mL[b]	Visually compatible for 24 hr at 25°C	1673	C
Imipenem–cilastatin sodium	MSD	5 mg/mL[b i]	FUJ	1 mg/mL[b]	Precipitates immediately	1673	I
Lorazepam	WY	1 mg/mL[b]	FUJ	1 mg/mL[b]	White haze and precipitate form immediately but clear in 30 min	1673	I
Magnesium sulfate	AMR	200 mg/mL[b]	FUJ	1 mg/mL[b]	Visually compatible for 24 hr at 25°C	1673	C
Mannitol	AB	250 mg/mL	FUJ	1 mg/mL[b]	Visually compatible for 24 hr at 25°C	1673	C
Melphalan HCl	BW	0.1 mg/mL[b]	FUJ	0.4 mg/mL[b]	Physically compatible for 3 hr at 22°C	1557	C
Meperidine HCl	WY	50 mg/mL	FUJ	1 mg/mL[b]	Visually compatible for 24 hr at 25°C	1673	C
Mesna	MJ	20 mg/mL	FUJ	1 mg/mL[b]	Visually compatible for 24 hr at 25°C	1673	C
Methotrexate sodium	LE	25 mg/mL[b]	FUJ	1 mg/mL[b]	Visually compatible for 24 hr at 25°C	1673	C
Metoclopramide HCl	SO	5 mg/mL	FUJ	1 mg/mL[b]	Visually compatible for 24 hr at 25°C	1673	C
Morphine sulfate	SCN	1 mg/mL[b]	FUJ	1 mg/mL[b]	Precipitate forms in 24 hr at 25°C	1673	I
Ondansetron HCl	GL	0.3 mg/mL[b]	FUJ	1 mg/mL[b]	Visually compatible for 24 hr at 25°C	1673	C
Piperacillin sodium–tazobactam sodium	LE[e]	40 mg/mL[a g]	FUJ	0.4 mg/mL[a]	Physically compatible for 4 hr at 22°C	1688	C
Potassium chloride	AB	0.3 mEq/mL[b]	FUJ	1 mg/mL[b]	Visually compatible for 24 hr at 25°C	1673	C
Prochlorperazine edisylate	SCN	5 mg/ml	FUJ	1 mg/mL[b]	Precipitates immediately	1673	I
Ranitidine HCl	GL	2.5 mg/mL[b]	FUJ	1 mg/mL[b]	Visually compatible for 24 hr at 25°C	1673	C
Sodium bicarbonate	AB	1 mEq/mL	FUJ	1 mg/mL[b]	Visually compatible for 24 hr at 25°C	1673	C
Teniposide	BR	0.1 mg/mL[a]	FUJ	0.4 mg/mL[a]	Physically compatible for 4 hr at 23°C	1725	C
Thiotepa	IMM[d]	1 mg/mL[a]	FUJ	0.4 mg/mL[a]	Physically compatible for 4 hr at 23°C	1861	C
Trimethoprim–sulfamethoxazole	ES	0.8 mg/mL[b h]	FUJ	1 mg/mL[b]	Visually compatible for 24 hr at 25°C	1673	C

Y-Site Injection Compatibility (1:1 Mixture) (Cont.)

Test Drug	Mfr	Conc	Mfr	Conc	Remarks	Ref	C/I
Vancomycin HCl	AB	5 mg/mL[b]	FUJ	1 mg/mL[b]	Visually compatible for 24 hr at 25°C	1673	C
Vinorelbine tartrate	BW	1 mg/mL[b]	FUJ	0.4 mg/mL[b]	Physically compatible for 4 hr at 22°C	1558	C

[a] Tested in dextrose 5%.

[b] Tested in sodium chloride 0.9%.

[c] Tested in bacteriostatic water for injection preserved with benzyl alcohol 0.9%.

[d] Lyophilized formulation tested.

[e] Test performed using the formulation WITHOUT edetate disodium.

[f] Ampicillin component. Ampicillin in a 2:1 fixed-ratio concentration with sulbactam.

[g] Piperacillin component. Piperacillin in an 8:1 fixed-ratio concentration with tazobactam.

[h] Trimethoprim component. Trimethoprim in a 1:5 fixed-ratio concentration with sulfamethoxazole.

[i] Imipenem component. Imipenem in a 1:1 fixed-ratio concentration with cilastatin.

Selected Revisions December 13, 2018. © Copyright, October 2006. American Society of Health-System Pharmacists, Inc.

Ganciclovir Sodium
AHFS 8:18.32

Products

Ganciclovir sodium is available as a lyophilized powder in single-dose vials containing the equivalent of 500 mg of ganciclovir.[3361 3366] Vials also may include hydrochloric acid and sodium hydroxide to adjust the pH.[3361] Each vial should be reconstituted with 10 mL of sterile water for injection and swirled gently or shaken to fully wet the product and dissolve the drug to yield a 50-mg/mL solution of ganciclovir.[3361 3366] Paraben-containing diluents (e.g., bacteriostatic water for injection containing parabens) should not be used to reconstitute ganciclovir sodium because precipitation may result.[3361 3366] Reconstituted solutions should be visually inspected for particulate matter and discoloration prior to dilution; if particulate matter is present or discoloration occurs, the vial should be discarded.[3361 3366] The appropriate volume of the reconstituted solution should be withdrawn from the vial and diluted in an appropriate volume (usually 100 mL) of sodium chloride 0.9%, dextrose 5%, Ringer's injection, or Ringer's injection, lactated to obtain a ganciclovir concentration of 10 mg/mL or less prior to administration; concentrations greater than 10 mg/mL are not recommended.[3361 3366]

Ganciclovir also is available as a 2-mg/mL premixed, ready-to-use solution in 250-mL single-dose (preservative-free) bags containing 500 mg of ganciclovir; this product does not contain the sodium salt of ganciclovir.[3362] Each mL also contains sodium chloride 8 mg in water for injection and may contain sodium hydroxide and/or hydrochloric acid to adjust the pH.[3362] Solutions should be visually inspected for particulate matter and discoloration prior to administration.[3362]

pH

Ganciclovir 50-mg/mL solution (reconstituted from ganciclovir sodium) has a pH of 11.[3361 3366]

Ganciclovir 2-mg/mL premixed, ready-to-use solution has a pH of 7.5.[3362]

Sodium Content

Each 500-mg vial of ganciclovir sodium (Par) contains 46 mg of sodium.[3366]

Trade Name(s)

Cytovene-IV

Administration

Solutions of ganciclovir must be administered only by intravenous infusion at a constant rate over 1 hour.[3361 3362 3366] The recommended infusion rate should not be exceeded.[3361 3362 3366] The drug should *not* be administered by intramuscular, subcutaneous, or rapid or bolus intravenous injection.[3361 3362 3366] Intramuscular or subcutaneous administration can result in severe tissue irritation due to the high pH of the drug; rapid or bolus intravenous injection can increase the risk of toxicity.[3361 3366]

Administration of ganciclovir should be accompanied by adequate hydration.[3361 3362 3366] The drug must only be infused into a vein with adequate blood flow, preferably through a plastic cannula, to permit rapid dilution and distribution of the drug in an attempt to avoid phlebitis and/or pain at the infusion site.[3361 3362 3366] Phlebitis and/or pain at the site of intravenous infusion still may occur despite further dilution of the reconstituted solution of the drug in intravenous infusion solutions.[3366]

As with other toxic drugs, caution should be exercised in the handling and preparation of ganciclovir.[3361 3362 3366] Direct contact of the drug with the skin or mucous membrane should be avoided, and the use of disposable gloves during handling has been recommended.[3361 3366] If skin or mucosal membrane contact with the solution occurs, the exposed area should be washed thoroughly with soap and water; for eye contact, the eyes should be flushed thoroughly with water.[3361 3366] Procedures and guidelines for the proper disposal of ganciclovir should be considered.[3361 3362 3366]

Stability

Ganciclovir sodium is a white to off-white powder that forms a clear solution upon reconstitution.[3361 3366] Intact vials should be stored at controlled room temperature.[3361 3366] The reconstituted solution is stable in the vial for 12 hours at room temperature (25°C).[3361 3366] Manufacturers do not recommend refrigeration of the reconstituted solution;[3361 3366] however, ganciclovir 500 mg/10 mL in sterile water for injection had no significant loss in 60 days when stored at 4°C.[1637] One manufacturer states that diluted solutions of ganciclovir may be stored at 2 to 8°C for up to 24 hours.[3361] Neither reconstituted nor diluted solutions of ganciclovir should be frozen.[3361 3362]

Ganciclovir premixed, ready-to-use solution is clear and colorless.[3362] Intact containers should be stored at controlled room temperature.[3362] Crystals may form during transportation or storage at temperatures that are lower than those recommended for storage.[3362] Bags should be gently shaken to redissolve such crystals.[3362] The solution must be clear at the time of use.[3362] Any unused portion should be discarded.[3362]

Ganciclovir sodium (Syntex) 0.35 mg/mL diluted in sodium chloride 0.9% and stored at 22°C did not exhibit a substantial antimicrobial effect on the growth of 4 organisms (*Enterococcus faecium*, *Staphylococcus aureus*, *Pseudomonas aeruginosa*, and *Candida albicans*) inoculated into the solution. *S. aureus* and *C. albicans* remained viable for 24 hours, and the others remained viable to the end of the study at 120 hours. The author recommended that diluted solutions of ganciclovir be stored under refrigeration whenever possible and that the potential for microbiological growth should be considered when assigning expiration periods.[2160]

Freezing Solutions

The manufacturers do not recommend freezing reconstituted and/or diluted solutions of ganciclovir;[3361 3362] however, ganciclovir sodium (Syntex), prepared at a ganciclovir concentration of 1.4, 4, and 7 mg/mL in sodium chloride 0.9% packaged in polypropylene syringes and 0.28 and 1.4 mg/mL in sodium chloride 0.9%

DOI: 10.37573/9781585286850.184

packaged in polyvinyl chloride (PVC) containers was evaluated. All samples exhibited 4% or less drug loss after 364 days at –20°C.[1836]

No ganciclovir loss occurred in a 10-mg/mL solution in sodium chloride 0.9% in 48 weeks when stored frozen at –8°C.[2595]

Syringes

Ganciclovir sodium (Syntex), prepared at a ganciclovir concentration of 5.8 mg/mL in sodium chloride 0.9%, packaged in polypropylene infusion-pump syringes (Healthtek), exhibited 3% or less drug loss in 10 days at 4°C and no loss in 12 hours at 25°C.[1742]

Ganciclovir sodium (Syntex), prepared at a ganciclovir concentration of 1.4, 4, and 7 mg/mL in sodium chloride 0.9% was packaged in polypropylene syringes and stored at 20, 4, and –20°C. Drug loss of 4% or less occurred in 7 days at 20°C, in 80 days at 4°C, and in 364 days at –20°C.[1836]

Ganciclovir sodium (Roche), prepared at a ganciclovir concentration of 5 mg/mL in sodium chloride 0.9% packaged as 20 mL in 50-mL polypropylene syringes (Becton Dickinson) and protected from light remained stable and clear for up to 185 days at 23 to 27°C and 2 to 8°C.[3363]

Central Venous Catheter

Ganciclovir sodium (Roche), prepared at a ganciclovir concentration of 5 mg/mL in dextrose 5% was found to be compatible with the ARROWg+ard Blue Plus (Arrow International) chlorhexidine-bearing triple-lumen central catheter. Essentially complete delivery of the drug was found with little or no drug loss occurring. Furthermore, chlorhexidine delivered from the catheter remained at trace amounts with no substantial increase due to the delivery of the drug through the catheter.[2335]

Compatibility Information

Solution Compatibility

Ganciclovir sodium

Test Soln Name	Mfr	Mfr	Conc/L or %	Remarks	Ref	C/I
Dextrose 5%		GEN		Stable for up to 24 hr at 2 to 8°C	3361	C
Dextrose 5%	TR[a]	SY	2.44 g	Physically compatible with no loss in 5 days at 25°C in light or dark and at 4°C	1288	C
Dextrose 5%	BA[a]	SY	1, 5, 10 g	Visually compatible with 3 to 7% loss in 35 days at 4 to 8°C in the dark	1545	C
Dextrose 5%	AB[a]	SY	1 and 5 g	Visually compatible with 1% or less loss in 35 days at 5 and 25°C	1643	C
Ringer's injection		GEN		Stable for up to 24 hr at 2 to 8°C	3361	C
Ringer's injection, lactated		GEN		Stable for up to 24 hr at 2 to 8°C	3361	C
Sodium chloride 0.9%		GEN		Stable for up to 24 hr at 2 to 8°C	3361	C
Sodium chloride 0.9%	SB[d]	RC	0.25 and 5 g	Visually compatible. Less than 10% loss in 185 days at 23 to 27°C and 2 to 8°C protected from light	3363	C
Sodium chloride 0.9%	[a]	PAR		Physically compatible and stable for 14 days at 5°C but use within 24 hr recommended	3366	C
Sodium chloride 0.9%	TR[a]	SY	2.59 g	Physically compatible with no loss in 5 days at 25°C in light or dark and at 4°C	1288	C
Sodium chloride 0.9%	AB[a]	SY	1 and 5 g	Visually compatible with 1% or less loss in 35 days at 5 and 25°C	1643	C
Sodium chloride 0.9%		SY	2.2 g	Little or no loss in 14 days at 4°C	1637	C
Sodium chloride 0.9%	[a]	SY	0.28 and 1.4 g	4% or less loss in 7 days at 20°C, 80 days at 4°C, and 364 days at –20°C	1836	C
Sodium chloride 0.9%	BA[a]	RC	1 and 5 g	No ganciclovir loss in 35 days at 4°C in the dark. No visible particles but an increase in microparticulates under 10 μm in size	2251	C
Sodium chloride 0.9%	BA[b]	RC	1 and 5 g	Physically compatible with no loss in 35 days at 4°C protected from light	2251	C
TPN #183[c]		SY	2 g	Precipitate forms	1744	I
TPN #183 to #185[c]		SY	3 and 5 g	Precipitate forms	1744	I

[a] Tested in PVC containers.

[b] Tested in latex elastomeric pump reservoirs (Baxter Intermate).

[c] Refer to Appendix for the composition of parenteral nutrition solutions. TPN indicates a 2-in-1 admixture.

[d] Tested in polypropylene containers.

Y-Site Injection Compatibility (1:1 Mixture)

Ganciclovir sodium

Test Drug	Mfr	Conc	Mfr	Conc	Remarks	Ref	C/I
Aldesleukin	CHI	33,800 I.U./mL[a]	SY	10 mg/mL[a]	Aldesleukin bioactivity inhibited	1857	I
Allopurinol sodium	BW	3 mg/mL[b]	SY	20 mg/mL[b]	Physically compatible for 4 hr at 22°C	1686	C
Amifostine	USB	10 mg/mL[a]	SY	20 mg/mL[a]	Crystalline needles form immediately. Dense precipitate in 1 hr	1845	I
Amsacrine	NCI	1 mg/mL[a]	SY	20 mg/mL[a]	Immediate dark orange turbidity	1381	I
Anidulafungin	VIC	0.5 mg/mL[a]	RC	20 mg/mL[a]	Physically compatible for 4 hr at 23°C	2617	C
Aztreonam	SQ	40 mg/mL[a]	SY	20 mg/mL[a]	White needles form immediately. Dense precipitate in 1 hr	1758	I
Caspofungin acetate	ME	0.7 mg/mL[b]	RC	20 mg/mL[b]	Physically compatible for 4 hr at room temperature	2758	C
Cisatracurium besylate	GW	0.1 and 2 mg/mL[a]	SY	20 mg/mL[a]	Physically compatible for 4 hr at 23°C	2074	C
Cisatracurium besylate	GW	5 mg/mL[a]	SY	20 mg/mL[a]	White cloudiness forms immediately	2074	I
Defibrotide sodium	JAZ	8 mg/mL[b]	RC	10 mg/mL[b]	Visually compatible for 4 hr at room temperature	3149	C
Docetaxel	RPR	0.9 mg/mL[a]	RC	20 mg/mL[a]	Physically compatible for 4 hr at 23°C	2224	C
Doxorubicin HCl liposomal	SEQ	0.4 mg/mL[a]	RC	20 mg/mL[a]	Physically compatible for 4 hr at 23°C	2087	C
Enalaprilat	MSD	1.25 mg/mL	SY	5 mg/mL[c]	Physically compatible for 4 hr at 21°C	1409	C
Etoposide phosphate	BR	5 mg/mL[a]	RC	20 mg/mL[a]	Physically compatible for 4 hr at 23°C	2218	C
Filgrastim	AMG	30 mcg/mL[a]	SY	20 mg/mL[a]	Physically compatible for 4 hr at 22°C	1687	C
Fluconazole	RR	2 mg/mL	SY	50 mg/mL	Physically compatible for 24 hr at 25°C	1407	C
Fludarabine phosphate	BX	1 mg/mL[a]	SY	20 mg/mL[a]	Darker color forms within 4 hr	1439	I
Foscarnet sodium	AST	24 mg/mL		50 mg/mL	Precipitates immediately	1335	I
Gemcitabine HCl	LI	10 mg/mL[b]	RC	20 mg/mL[b]	Subvisible crystals form immediately. Gross precipitate in 1 hr	2226	I
Granisetron HCl	SKB	0.05 mg/mL[a]	SY	20 mg/mL[a]	Physically compatible for 4 hr at 23°C	2000	C
Letermovir	ME	[a]		[a]	Physically compatible	3398	C
Linezolid	PHU	2 mg/mL	RC	20 mg/mL[a]	Physically compatible for 4 hr at 23°C	2264	C
Melphalan HCl	BW	0.1 mg/mL[b]	SY	20 mg/mL[b]	Physically compatible for 3 hr at 22°C	1557	C
Ondansetron HCl	GL	1 mg/mL[b]	SY	20 mg/mL[a]	Immediate turbidity and precipitation	1365	I
Paclitaxel	NCI	1.2 mg/mL[a]	SY	20 mg/mL[a]	Physically compatible for 4 hr at 22°C	1556	C
Pemetrexed disodium	LI	20 mg/mL[b]	RC	20 mg/mL[a]	Physically compatible for 4 hr at 23°C	2564	C
Piperacillin sodium–tazobactam sodium	LE[d]	40 mg/mL[a][i]	SY	20 mg/mL[a]	Large crystals form in 1 hr and become heavy white precipitate in 4 hr	1688	I
Propofol	ZEN[j]	10 mg/mL	SY	20 mg/mL[a]	Physically compatible for 1 hr at 23°C	2066	C
Remifentanil HCl	GW	0.025 and 0.25 mg/mL[b]	SY	20 mg/mL[a]	Physically compatible for 4 hr at 23°C	2075	C
Sargramostim	IMM	10 mcg/mL[b]	SY	20 mg/mL[b]	Small particles form in 4 hr	1436	I
Tacrolimus	FUJ				Significant tacrolimus loss within 15 min	191	I
Teniposide	BR	0.1 mg/mL[a]	SY	20 mg/mL[a]	Physically compatible for 4 hr at 23°C	1725	C

Y-Site Injection Compatibility (1:1 Mixture) (Cont.)

Test Drug	Mfr	Conc	Mfr	Conc	Remarks	Ref	C/I
Thiotepa	IMM[e]	1 mg/mL[a]	SY	20 mg/mL[a]	Physically compatible for 4 hr at 23°C	1861	C
TNA #218 to #226[f]			RC	20 mg/mL[a]	White precipitate forms immediately	2215	I
TPN #144[f]			SY	1 and 5 mg/mL[a]	Visually compatible for 2 hr at 20°C	1522	C
TPN #144[f]			SY	10 mg/mL[a]	Heavy precipitate forms within 30 min	1522	I
TPN #183[f]			SY	2 mg/mL	Precipitate forms	1744	I
TPN #183[f]			SY	1 mg/mL[g]	Visually compatible with no ganciclovir loss in 3 hr at 24°C. Less than 10% amino acids loss in 2 hr	1744	C
TPN #183 to #185[f]			SY	3 and 5 mg/mL	Precipitate forms	1744	I
TPN #184, #185[f]			SY	2 mg/mL[h]	Visually compatible with no ganciclovir loss in 3 hr at 24°C. Less than 10% amino acid loss in 3 hr	1744	C
TPN #212 to #215[f]			SY	20 mg/mL[a]	Gross white precipitate forms immediately	2109	I
Vinorelbine tartrate	BW	1 mg/mL[b]	SY	20 mg/mL[b]	Turbid precipitate forms immediately	1558	I

[a] Tested in dextrose 5%.

[b] Tested in sodium chloride 0.9%.

[c] Tested in both dextrose 5% and sodium chloride 0.9%.

[d] Test performed using the formulation WITHOUT edetate disodium.

[e] Lyophilized formulation tested.

[f] Refer to Appendix for the composition of parenteral nutrition solutions. TNA indicates a 3-in-1 admixture, and TPN indicates a 2-in-1 admixture.

[g] Ganciclovir sodium concentration after mixing was 0.83 mg/mL.

[h] Ganciclovir sodium concentration after mixing was 1.4 mg/mL.

[i] Piperacillin component. Piperacillin in an 8:1 fixed-ratio concentration with tazobactam.

[j] Test performed using the formulation WITH edetate disodium.

Selected Revisions January 31, 2020. © Copyright, October 1990.
American Society of Health-System Pharmacists, Inc.

Gemcitabine Hydrochloride
AHFS 10:00

Products

Gemcitabine hydrochloride is available as a lyophilized powder in single-dose (preservative-free) vials containing 200 mg, 1 g, or 2 g of drug (as the base).[3526][3527] For each 200 mg of gemcitabine lyophilized powder contained in each vial, mannitol 200 mg and sodium acetate 12.5 mg also are present.[3526][3527] The contents of the 200-mg, 1-g, and 2-g vials should be reconstituted with 5, 25, and 50 mL, respectively, of sodium chloride 0.9% and shaken to dissolve the powder to yield a solution with a gemcitabine concentration of 38 mg/mL.[3526][3527] Prior to administration, the appropriate dose of the reconstituted solution should be diluted with sodium chloride 0.9% to a final gemcitabine concentration of not less than 0.1 mg/mL.[3526][3527]

Gemcitabine hydrochloride also is available as a concentrate for injection.[3528][3529] In 200-mg, 1-g, and 2-g single-dose vials, each mL of the concentrate contains 38 mg of gemcitabine in water for injection.[3529] In 200-mg and 1-, 1.5-, and 2-g multidose vials, each mL of the concentrate for injection contains 100 mg of gemcitabine, 250 mg of polyethylene glycol (PEG) 300, 150 mg of propylene glycol, and 16 mg of sodium hydroxide in dehydrated alcohol.[3528] Prior to administration, the appropriate dose of the concentrate for injection must be diluted with sodium chloride 0.9% to a final gemcitabine concentration of not less than 0.1 mg/mL.[3528][3529] The diluted solution should be mixed by gentle inversion and should not be shaken.[3528]

Gemcitabine hydrochloride also is available as a premixed, ready-to-use solution for infusion in single-dose bags containing 120, 130, 140, 150, 160, 170, 180, 190, 200, and 220 mL.[3530] Each 100 mL of the ready-to-use solution for infusion contains 1 g of gemcitabine and 900 mg of sodium chloride in water for injection.[3530] The ready-to-use solution for infusion should not be further diluted and should *not* be used in patients requiring less than the entire dose of a single-dose bag.[3530]

The pH of all of the gemcitabine products may have been adjusted by the manufacturers with sodium hydroxide and/or hydrochloric acid.[3526][3527][3528][3529][3530]

Solutions of gemcitabine (e.g., reconstituted solutions, commercially available solutions, solutions diluted for infusion, commercially available solutions for infusion) should be inspected for particulate matter and discoloration prior to administration; if particulate matter is present or discoloration has occurred, solutions should be discarded.[3526][3527][3528][3529][3530]

Equivalency

Gemcitabine hydrochloride 113.85 mg is equivalent to 100 mg of gemcitabine base.[3527][3528][3529][3530]

Trade Name(s)

Gemzar, Infugem

Administration

Gemcitabine hydrochloride is administered by intravenous infusion over 30 minutes.[3526][3527][3528][3529][3530] When 2 bags of the premixed, ready-to-use solution for infusion are required to achieve the appropriate dose, the combined volume of both infusion bags should be infused over 30 minutes.[3530] Prolongation of the infusion time of gemcitabine hydrochloride beyond 60 minutes has resulted in an increased incidence of adverse effects.[3526][3527][3528][3529][3530]

As with other toxic drugs, caution should be exercised in the handling and preparation of gemcitabine hydrochloride and applicable special handling and disposal procedures should be followed.[3526][3527][3528][3529][3530] Gloves are recommended to be worn in the preparation of the drug.[3526][3527][3528][3529][3530] If skin or mucosal contact with the drug occurs, the affected area(s) should be washed immediately and thoroughly with copious amounts of water.[3526][3527][3528][3529][3530]

Stability

Gemcitabine hydrochloride is a white to off-white lyophilized powder that forms a clear, colorless to light straw-colored solution upon reconstitution.[3526][3527] Intact vials of gemcitabine hydrochloride should be stored at controlled room temperature.[3526][3527] Manufacturers state that reconstituted and diluted solutions for infusion prepared from the lyophilized powder may be stored at controlled room temperature for up to 24 hours; solutions not used within 24 hours after reconstitution should be discarded.[3526][3527] However, other information indicates the reconstituted solution may be stable for longer periods.[2227] (See Reconstituted Solutions). Manufacturers state that reconstituted and diluted solutions of gemcitabine hydrochloride should not be refrigerated because crystallization may occur.[3526][3527]

Gemcitabine hydrochloride concentrate for injection is a clear, colorless to pale yellow[3528] or light straw-colored[3529] solution. Intact multidose vials of gemcitabine hydrochloride concentrate for injection should be stored at controlled room temperature.[3528] Multidose vials are stable for up to 28 days from initial vial puncture when stored at room temperature.[3528] Intact single-dose vials of gemcitabine hydrochloride concentrate for injection should be stored at 2 to 8°C and should not be frozen.[3529] Manufacturers state that diluted solutions for infusion prepared from the concentrate for injection may be stored at controlled room temperature for up to 24 hours; solutions not used within 24 hours after dilution should be discarded.[3528][3529]

Gemcitabine hydrochloride premixed, ready-to-use solution for infusion is a clear, colorless solution.[3530] Intact containers should be stored at controlled room temperature.[3530] The solution should not be frozen because crystallization may occur.[3530]

DOI: 10.37573/9781585286850.185

Gemcitabine hydrochloride (Lilly) 2.4 mg/mL diluted in sodium chloride 0.9% and stored at 22°C did not exhibit a substantial antimicrobial effect on the growth of 4 organisms (*Enterococcus faecium, Staphylococcus aureus, Pseudomonas aeruginosa,* and *Candida albicans*) inoculated into the solution. *C. albicans* maintained viability for 120 hours, and the others were viable for 24 hours. The author recommended that diluted solutions of gemcitabine hydrochloride be stored under refrigeration whenever possible and that the potential for microbiological growth should be considered when assigning expiration periods.[2160]

Reconstituted Solutions

The contents of gemcitabine hydrochloride (Lilly) 200-mg and 1-g vials were reconstituted to a gemcitabine concentration of 38 mg/mL with sterile water for injection and also sodium chloride 0.9% in the original vials and evaluated over periods of 35 days at 23°C exposed to and protected from fluorescent light and at 4°C protected from light.[2227] The samples stored at 23°C were physically stable throughout the study period.[2227] Under 4% loss occurred in 35 days at 23°C.[2227] When refrigerated, the solutions remained physically and chemically stable for at least 7 days, but large colorless crystals formed in some samples after that time.[2227] The crystals did not redissolve on warming to room temperature.[2227] No loss occurred in the refrigerated solutions unless crystals formed; gemcitabine losses of 20 to 35%

were determined in samples containing crystals.[2227] Exposure to or protection from fluorescent light did not affect gemcitabine stability.[2227]

Syringes

Gemcitabine hydrochloride (Lilly) 38 mg/mL in sodium chloride 0.9% was repackaged as 10 mL of solution in 20-mL plastic syringes (Becton Dickinson) and sealed with tip caps (Red Cap, Burron).[2227] Sample syringes were stored at 23°C both exposed to and protected from fluorescent light and at 4°C protected from light for 35 days.[2227] All samples were physically stable throughout the study period.[2227] Although not observed in the solutions packaged in plastic syringes in this study,[2227] crystallization can occur in reconstituted solutions stored under refrigeration.[3526 3527] Little to no loss occurred in 35 days under any of the conditions.[2227]

Sorption

Gemcitabine hydrochloride has not exhibited any incompatibilities with bottles or polyvinyl chloride (PVC) bags and administration sets.[3526 3527 3528 3529]

Gemcitabine hydrochloride (Lilly) 5.12 mg/mL in sodium chloride 0.9% exhibited no loss due to sorption in polyethylene and PVC containers compared to glass containers over 48 hours at room temperature.[2420 2430]

Compatibility Information

Solution Compatibility

Gemcitabine HCl

Test Soln Name	Mfr	Mfr	Conc/L or %	Remarks	Ref	C/I
Dextrose 5%	BA[a]	LI	0.1 and 10 g	Physically compatible and chemically stable with little to no loss in 35 days at 23°C in light and dark and at 4°C in dark	2227	C
Dextrose 5%	BA[a]	LI	0.1, 10, and 38 g	Physically compatible and chemically stable with no loss in 7 days at 32°C in dark	2227	C
Sodium chloride 0.9%	BA[a]	LI	0.1 and 10 g	Physically compatible and chemically stable with little to no loss in 35 days at 23°C in light and dark and at 4°C in dark	2227	C
Sodium chloride 0.9%	BA[a]	LI	0.1, 10, and 38 g	Physically compatible and chemically stable with little to no loss in 7 days at 32°C in dark	2227	C
Sodium chloride 0.9%	GRI[a b]	LI	7.5 and 25 g	Visually compatible. Under 4% loss in 27 days at 25°C in light and dark	2741	C

[a] Tested in PVC containers.

[b] Tested in glass containers.

Y-Site Injection Compatibility (1:1 Mixture)

Gemcitabine HCl

Test Drug	Mfr	Conc	Mfr	Conc	Remarks	Ref	C/I
Acyclovir sodium	GW	7 mg/mL[b]	LI	10 mg/mL[b]	Gross precipitation occurs immediately	2226	I
Amifostine	USB	10 mg/mL[b]	LI	10 mg/mL[b]	Physically compatible for 4 hr at 23°C	2226	C
Amikacin sulfate	APC	5 mg/mL[b]	LI	10 mg/mL[b]	Physically compatible for 4 hr at 23°C	2226	C
Aminophylline	AB	2.5 mg/mL[b]	LI	10 mg/mL[b]	Physically compatible for 4 hr at 23°C	2226	C

Y-Site Injection Compatibility (1:1 Mixture) (Cont.)

Test Drug	Mfr	Conc	Mfr	Conc	Remarks	Ref	C/I
Amphotericin B	PH	0.6 mg/mL[a]	LI	10 mg/mL[b]	Gross precipitation occurs immediately	2226	I
Ampicillin sodium	SKB	20 mg/mL[b]	LI	10 mg/mL[b]	Physically compatible for 4 hr at 23°C	2226	C
Ampicillin sodium–sulbactam sodium	RR	20 mg/mL[b d]	LI	10 mg/mL[b]	Physically compatible for 4 hr at 23°C	2226	C
Anidulafungin	VIC	0.5 mg/mL[a]	LI	10 mg/mL[a]	Physically compatible for 4 hr at 23°C	2617	C
Aztreonam	SQ	40 mg/mL[b]	LI	10 mg/mL[b]	Physically compatible for 4 hr at 23°C	2226	C
Bleomycin sulfate	MJ	1 unit/mL[b]	LI	10 mg/mL[b]	Physically compatible for 4 hr at 23°C	2226	C
Bumetanide	RC	0.04 mg/mL[b]	LI	10 mg/mL[b]	Physically compatible for 4 hr at 23°C	2226	C
Buprenorphine HCl	RKC	0.04 mg/mL[b]	LI	10 mg/mL[b]	Physically compatible for 4 hr at 23°C	2226	C
Butorphanol tartrate	APC	0.04 mg/mL[b]	LI	10 mg/mL[b]	Physically compatible for 4 hr at 23°C	2226	C
Calcium gluconate	FUJ	40 mg/mL[b]	LI	10 mg/mL[b]	Physically compatible for 4 hr at 23°C	2226	C
Carboplatin	BR	5 mg/mL[b]	LI	10 mg/mL[b]	Physically compatible for 4 hr at 23°C	2226	C
Carmustine	BR	1.5 mg/mL[b]	LI	10 mg/mL[b]	Physically compatible for 4 hr at 23°C	2226	C
Cefazolin sodium	APC	20 mg/mL[b]	LI	10 mg/mL[b]	Physically compatible for 4 hr at 23°C	2226	C
Cefotaxime sodium	HO	20 mg/mL[b]	LI	10 mg/mL[b]	Subvisible haze forms in 1 hr. Increased haze and a microprecipitate in 4 hr	2226	I
Cefotetan disodium	ZEN	20 mg/mL[b]	LI	10 mg/mL[b]	Physically compatible for 4 hr at 23°C	2226	C
Cefoxitin sodium	ME	20 mg/mL[b]	LI	10 mg/mL[b]	Physically compatible for 4 hr at 23°C	2226	C
Ceftazidime	SKB	40 mg/mL[b]	LI	10 mg/mL[b]	Physically compatible for 4 hr at 23°C	2226	C
Ceftriaxone sodium	RC	20 mg/mL[b]	LI	10 mg/mL[b]	Physically compatible for 4 hr at 23°C	2226	C
Cefuroxime sodium	GW	30 mg/mL[b]	LI	10 mg/mL[b]	Physically compatible for 4 hr at 23°C	2226	C
Chlorpromazine HCl	ES	2 mg/mL[b]	LI	10 mg/mL[b]	Physically compatible for 4 hr at 23°C	2226	C
Ciprofloxacin	BAY	1 mg/mL[b]	LI	10 mg/mL[b]	Physically compatible for 4 hr at 23°C	2226	C
Cisplatin	BR	1 mg/mL	LI	10 mg/mL[b]	Physically compatible for 4 hr at 23°C	2226	C
Clindamycin phosphate	AST	10 mg/mL[b]	LI	10 mg/mL[b]	Physically compatible for 4 hr at 23°C	2226	C
Cyclophosphamide	BR	10 mg/mL[b]	LI	10 mg/mL[b]	Physically compatible for 4 hr at 23°C	2226	C
Cytarabine	BED	50 mg/mL	LI	10 mg/mL[b]	Physically compatible for 4 hr at 23°C	2226	C
Dactinomycin	ME	0.01 mg/mL[b]	LI	10 mg/mL[b]	Physically compatible for 4 hr at 23°C	2226	C
Daunorubicin HCl	BED	1 mg/mL[b]	LI	10 mg/mL[b]	Physically compatible for 4 hr at 23°C	2226	C
Dexamethasone sodium phosphate	ES	1 mg/mL[b]	LI	10 mg/mL[b]	Physically compatible for 4 hr at 23°C	2226	C
Dexrazoxane HCl	PH	5 mg/mL[b]	LI	10 mg/mL[b]	Physically compatible for 4 hr at 23°C	2226	C
Diphenhydramine HCl	SCN	2 mg/mL[b]	LI	10 mg/mL[b]	Physically compatible for 4 hr at 23°C	2226	C
Dobutamine HCl	AST	4 mg/mL[b]	LI	10 mg/mL[b]	Physically compatible for 4 hr at 23°C	2226	C
Docetaxel	RPR	2 mg/mL[a]	LI	10 mg/mL[b]	Physically compatible for 4 hr at 23°C	2226	C
Dopamine HCl	AB	3.2 mg/mL[b]	LI	10 mg/mL[b]	Physically compatible for 4 hr at 23°C	2226	C
Doripenem	JJ	5 mg/mL[a b]	LI	10 mg/mL[b]	Physically compatible for 4 hr at 23°C	2743	C
Doxorubicin HCl	PH	2 mg/mL	LI	10 mg/mL[b]	Physically compatible for 4 hr at 23°C	2226	C
Doxycycline hyclate	FUJ	1 mg/mL[b]	LI	10 mg/mL[b]	Physically compatible for 4 hr at 23°C	2226	C

Y-Site Injection Compatibility (1:1 Mixture) (Cont.)

Test Drug	Mfr	Conc	Mfr	Conc	Remarks	Ref	C/I
Droperidol	AST	0.4 mg/mL[b]	LI	10 mg/mL[b]	Physically compatible for 4 hr at 23°C	2226	C
Enalaprilat	ME	0.1 mg/mL[b]	LI	10 mg/mL[b]	Physically compatible for 4 hr at 23°C	2226	C
Etoposide	BR	0.4 mg/mL[b]	LI	10 mg/mL[b]	Physically compatible for 4 hr at 23°C	2226	C
Etoposide phosphate	BR	5 mg/mL[b]	LI	10 mg/mL[b]	Physically compatible for 4 hr at 23°C	2226	C
Famotidine	ME	2 mg/mL[b]	LI	10 mg/mL[b]	Physically compatible for 4 hr at 23°C	2226	C
Floxuridine	RC	3 mg/mL[b]	LI	10 mg/mL[b]	Physically compatible for 4 hr at 23°C	2226	C
Fluconazole	RR	2 mg/mL	LI	10 mg/mL[b]	Physically compatible for 4 hr at 23°C	2226	C
Fludarabine phosphate	BX	1 mg/mL[b]	LI	10 mg/mL[b]	Physically compatible for 4 hr at 23°C	2226	C
Fluorouracil	PH	16 mg/mL[b]	LI	10 mg/mL[b]	Physically compatible for 4 hr at 23°C	2226	C
Furosemide	AMR	3 mg/mL[b]	LI	10 mg/mL[b]	Gross precipitation occurs immediately	2226	I
Ganciclovir sodium	RC	20 mg/mL[b]	LI	10 mg/mL[b]	Subvisible crystals form immediately. Gross precipitate in 1 hr	2226	I
Gentamicin sulfate	AB	5 mg/mL[b]	LI	10 mg/mL[b]	Physically compatible for 4 hr at 23°C	2226	C
Granisetron HCl	SKB	0.05 mg/mL[b]	LI	10 mg/mL[b]	Physically compatible for 4 hr at 23°C	2226	C
Haloperidol lactate	MN	0.2 mg/mL[b]	LI	10 mg/mL[b]	Physically compatible for 4 hr at 23°C	2226	C
Heparin sodium	ES	100 units/mL[b]	LI	10 mg/mL[b]	Physically compatible for 4 hr at 23°C	2226	C
Hydrocortisone sodium succinate	UP	1 mg/mL[b]	LI	10 mg/mL[b]	Physically compatible for 4 hr at 23°C	2226	C
Hydromorphone HCl	AST	0.5 mg/mL[b]	LI	10 mg/mL[b]	Physically compatible for 4 hr at 23°C	2226	C
Hydroxyzine HCl	ES	2 mg/mL[b]	LI	10 mg/mL[b]	Physically compatible for 4 hr at 23°C	2226	C
Idarubicin HCl	AD	0.5 mg/mL[b]	LI	10 mg/mL[b]	Physically compatible for 4 hr at 23°C	2226	C
Ifosfamide	MJ	25 mg/mL[b]	LI	10 mg/mL[b]	Physically compatible for 4 hr at 23°C	2226	C
Imipenem–cilastatin sodium	ME	10 mg/mL[b] [g]	LI	10 mg/mL[b]	Yellow-green discoloration forms in 1 hr	2226	I
Irinotecan HCl	PHU	5 mg/mL[b]	LI	10 mg/mL[b]	Subvisible haze with green discoloration forms immediately	2226	I
Leucovorin calcium	IMM	2 mg/mL[b]	LI	10 mg/mL[b]	Physically compatible for 4 hr at 23°C	2226	C
Linezolid	PHU	2 mg/mL	LI	10 mg/mL[a]	Physically compatible for 4 hr at 23°C	2264	C
Lorazepam	WY	0.5 mg/mL[a]	LI	10 mg/mL[b]	Physically compatible for 4 hr at 23°C	2226	C
Mannitol	BA	15%	LI	10 mg/mL[b]	Physically compatible for 4 hr at 23°C	2226	C
Meperidine HCl	AST	4 mg/mL[b]	LI	10 mg/mL[b]	Physically compatible for 4 hr at 23°C	2226	C
Mesna	MJ	10 mg/mL[b]	LI	10 mg/mL[b]	Physically compatible for 4 hr at 23°C	2226	C
Methotrexate sodium	IMM	15 mg/mL[b]	LI	10 mg/mL[b]	Precipitate forms immediately, redissolves, but reprecipitates in 15 to 20 min	2226	I
Methylprednisolone sodium succinate	AB	5 mg/mL[b]	LI	10 mg/mL[b]	Gross precipitation occurs immediately	2226	I
Metoclopramide HCl	FAU	5 mg/mL	LI	10 mg/mL[b]	Physically compatible for 4 hr at 23°C	2226	C
Metronidazole	AB	5 mg/mL	LI	10 mg/mL[b]	Physically compatible for 4 hr at 23°C	2226	C
Mitomycin	BR	0.5 mg/mL	LI	10 mg/mL[b]	Reddish-purple color forms in 1 hr	2226	I
Mitoxantrone HCl	IMM	0.5 mg/mL[b]	LI	10 mg/mL[b]	Physically compatible for 4 hr at 23°C	2226	C

Y-Site Injection Compatibility (1:1 Mixture) (Cont.)

Test Drug	Mfr	Conc	Mfr	Conc	Remarks	Ref	C/I
Morphine sulfate	ES	1 mg/mL[b]	LI	10 mg/mL[b]	Physically compatible for 4 hr at 23°C	2226	C
Nalbuphine HCl	AST	10 mg/mL	LI	10 mg/mL[b]	Physically compatible for 4 hr at 23°C	2226	C
Ondansetron HCl	GW	1 mg/mL[b]	LI	10 mg/mL[b]	Physically compatible for 4 hr at 23°C	2226	C
Oxaliplatin	SS	0.5 mg/mL[a]	LI	10 mg/mL[a]	Physically compatible for 4 hr at 23°C	2566	C
Paclitaxel	MJ	1.2 mg/mL[a]	LI	10 mg/mL[b]	Physically compatible for 4 hr at 23°C	2226	C
Palonosetron HCl	MGI	50 mcg/mL	LI	10 mg/mL[a]	Physically compatible and no loss of either drug in 4 hr	2627	C
Pemetrexed disodium	LI	20 mg/mL[b]	LI	10 mg/mL[a]	Cloudy precipitate forms immediately	2564	I
Piperacillin sodium–tazobactam sodium	LE[c]	40 mg/mL[b e]	LI	10 mg/mL[b]	Cloudiness forms immediately, becoming flocculent precipitate in 1 hr	2226	I
Potassium chloride	AB	0.1 mEq/mL[b]	LI	10 mg/mL[b]	Physically compatible for 4 hr at 23°C	2226	C
Prochlorperazine edisylate	SCN	0.5 mg/mL[b]	LI	10 mg/mL[b]	Subvisible haze forms immediately	2226	I
Promethazine HCl	SCN	2 mg/mL[b]	LI	10 mg/mL[b]	Physically compatible for 4 hr at 23°C	2226	C
Ranitidine HCl	GL	2 mg/mL[b]	LI	10 mg/mL[b]	Physically compatible for 4 hr at 23°C	2226	C
Sodium bicarbonate	AB	1 mEq/mL	LI	10 mg/mL[b]	Physically compatible for 4 hr at 23°C	2226	C
Streptozocin	UP	40 mg/mL[b]	LI	10 mg/mL[b]	Physically compatible for 4 hr at 23°C	2226	C
Teniposide	BR	0.1 mg/mL[a]	LI	10 mg/mL[b]	Physically compatible for 4 hr at 23°C	2226	C
Thiotepa	IMM	1 mg/mL[b]	LI	10 mg/mL[b]	Physically compatible for 4 hr at 23°C	2226	C
Tobramycin sulfate	LI	5 mg/mL[b]	LI	10 mg/mL[b]	Physically compatible for 4 hr at 23°C	2226	C
Topotecan HCl	SKB	0.1 mg/mL[b]	LI	10 mg/mL[b]	Physically compatible for 4 hr at 23°C	2226	C
Trimethoprim–sulfamethoxazole	ES	0.8 mg/mL[b f]	LI	10 mg/mL[b]	Physically compatible for 4 hr at 23°C	2226	C
Vancomycin HCl	LI	10 mg/mL[b]	LI	10 mg/mL[b]	Physically compatible for 4 hr at 23°C	2226	C
Vinblastine sulfate	FAU	0.12 mg/mL[b]	LI	10 mg/mL[b]	Physically compatible for 4 hr at 23°C	2226	C
Vincristine sulfate	FAU	0.05 mg/mL[b]	LI	10 mg/mL[b]	Physically compatible for 4 hr at 23°C	2226	C
Vinorelbine tartrate	GW	1 mg/mL[b]	LI	10 mg/mL[b]	Physically compatible for 4 hr at 23°C	2226	C
Zidovudine	GW	4 mg/mL[b]	LI	10 mg/mL[b]	Physically compatible for 4 hr at 23°C	2226	C

[a] Tested in dextrose 5%.

[b] Tested in sodium chloride 0.9%.

[c] Test performed using the formulation WITHOUT edetate disodium.

[d] Ampicillin component. Ampicillin in a 2:1 fixed-ratio concentration with sulbactam.

[e] Piperacillin component. Piperacillin in an 8:1 fixed-ratio concentration with tazobactam.

[f] Trimethoprim component. Trimethoprim in a 1:5 fixed-ratio concentration with sulfamethoxazole.

[g] Not specified whether concentration refers to single component or combined components.

Selected Revisions January 31, 2020. © Copyright, October 2000. American Society of Health-System Pharmacists, Inc.

Gentamicin Sulfate
AHFS 8:12.02

Products

Gentamicin (as the sulfate) is available at a concentration of 40 mg/mL in 2- and 20-mL vials. The drug is also available at a concentration of 10 mg/mL for pediatric use. The products also may contain edetate disodium, sodium bisulfite, and parabens.[1(10/04)] [4]

Gentamicin sulfate also is available from several manufacturers premixed in various concentrations in sodium chloride 0.9%.[4]

pH

The injection for intravenous or intramuscular administration has a pH of 3 to 5.5. Premixed infusions of gentamicin sulfate in sodium chloride 0.9% have a pH of around 4 to 4.5.[4]

Osmolality

Gentamicin sulfate (Wyeth) 40 mg/mL has an osmolality of 160 mOsm/kg.[50] Gentamicin sulfate pediatric injection (Elkins-Sinn) 10 mg/mL has an osmolality of 116 mOsm/kg by freezing-point depression or 212 mOsm/kg by vapor pressure.[1071]

The osmolality of gentamicin sulfate 1 mg/mL was 262 mOsm/kg in dextrose 5% and 278 mOsm/kg in sodium chloride 0.9%. At a 2.5-mg/mL concentration, the osmolality was 278 mOsm/kg in dextrose 5% and 293 mOsm/kg in sodium chloride 0.9%.[1375]

The osmolality of gentamicin sulfate 80 mg was calculated for the following dilutions:[1054]

Diluent	Osmolality (mOsm/kg)	
	50 mL	100 mL
Dextrose 5%	293	285
Sodium chloride 0.9%	320	315

Osmolarity

The osmolarity of the premixed infusions in sodium chloride 0.9% is approximately 284 to 308 mOsm/L.[4]

Administration

Gentamicin sulfate is administered by intramuscular injection or intermittent intravenous infusion over 0.5 to 2 hours. For adults, intravenous administration in 50 to 200 mL of sodium chloride 0.9% or dextrose 5% is recommended, while the volume for pediatric patients should be reduced to meet patients' needs.[1(10/04)] [4]

Stability

Gentamicin sulfate injection is colorless to slightly yellow.[4] Intact containers should be stored at controlled room temperature and protected from freezing.[1(10/04)] [4] Drug concentration is unrelated to color intensity of gentamicin sulfate solutions.[2139]

Freezing Solutions

Gentamicin sulfate (Schering) 50 mg in 50 mL of dextrose 5% and also sodium chloride 0.9% in polyvinyl chloride (PVC) containers frozen at –20°C was stable for 30 days.[299]

Gentamicin sulfate (Schering) 80 mg/100 mL of dextrose 5% in PVC bags was frozen at –20°C for 30 days and then thawed by exposure to ambient temperature or microwave radiation. No precipitation or color change was observed, and no drug loss occurred. Subsequent storage of the admixture at room temperature for 24 hours also yielded a physically compatible solution, exhibiting little or no drug loss.[554]

Gentamicin sulfate (Elkins-Sinn) 120 mg/50 mL lost 6% in dextrose 5% and 2% in sodium chloride 0.9% in 28 days when frozen at –20°C.[981]

The stability of gentamicin sulfate (Schering) 5.45 mg/mL in dextrose 5% frozen in an ambulatory pump reservoir was studied. The drug-filled reservoirs were stored at –20°C for 30 days and then thawed at 5°C for 4 days. This thawing was then followed by 2 days of drug delivery through the pump at 37°C. No visible changes and no loss occurred during storage and delivery. Furthermore, plasticizer diethylhexyl phthalate (DEHP) levels were insignificant.[1490]

Syringes

The stability of gentamicin sulfate (Schering) repackaged in plastic syringes (Monoject) was significantly less than in glass syringes (Glaspak, Becton Dickinson) at both 4 and 25°C. The commercial concentrations were tested in the following amounts: 40 mg/mL—1, 0.75, 0.5, and 0.25 mL; and 10 mg/mL—1.5, 1, and 0.5 mL. Storage in plastic syringes resulted in an average loss of 16% in 30 days and in the formation of a brown precipitate. In glass syringes, the average loss was 7% at 30 days. The brown precipitate did not appear after 30 days but was present at 60 days. It appeared in the cannula of the needle in both glass and plastic syringes. For the 40-mg/mL concentration, the volume of the sample also affected stability. Significantly less loss was noted in the smaller volumes (0.25 and 0.5 mL) than in the larger volumes (0.5 and 1 mL). This volume-related phenomenon was not demonstrated in the 10-mg/mL pediatric concentration. Storage temperature had no effect on stability over 90 days.[297]

The manufacturer also expressed concern about plastic packaging of gentamicin, noting a possibly inadequate oxygen and moisture barrier both through the tip and the walls of the syringe. It was indicated that gentamicin is oxygen sensitive and that depletion of the antioxidant present could result in instability. Further, loss of moisture at the tip could result in occlusion by the dried product.[403]

DOI: 10.37573/9781585286850.186

Gentamicin sulfate 40 mg/1 mL was packaged in polypropylene syringes (Plastipak, Becton Dickinson). No significant change in concentration occurred over 30 days at 4 or 25°C.[401]

Gentamicin sulfate (Elkins-Sinn) 120 mg, diluted with 1 mL of sodium chloride 0.9% to a final volume of 4 mL, was stable (less than 10% loss) when stored in polypropylene syringes (Becton Dickinson) for 48 hours at 23°C under fluorescent light.[1159]

The stability of gentamicin sulfate (Elkins-Sinn) diluted to 10 mg/mL with sodium chloride 0.9% and stored in glass syringes (Becton Dickinson) at 4°C was studied. No loss of gentamicin sulfate was found during 12 weeks of storage.[1265]

Sorption

Gentamicin sulfate was shown not to exhibit sorption to PVC bags and tubing, polyethylene bags and tubing, multilayer bags of polyethylene, polyamide, and polypropylene, Silastic tubing, polypropylene syringes, and elastomeric reservoirs.[536 606 2014 2269]

Filtration

The effect of several filters on the delivered concentration of gentamicin sulfate (Roussel) from simulated pediatric infusions was studied. A syringe containing dextrose 10% on a syringe pump set at 8.26 mL/hr was connected by intravenous tubing to a 0.5-μm air-blocking filter set (Travenol), a 0.22-μm air-eliminating filter set (Travenol), and a 0.2-μm air-eliminating filter set (Pall). Gentamicin doses of 2.5 and 7.5 mg were injected antegrade to the filter. The effluents were sampled at 1, 1.5, 2, and 4 hours. No significant drug sorption to the plastic tubing or inline filters occurred. However, because of the difference in specific gravity of the drug (1.010) and intravenous solution (1.032), variations in delivered gentamicin did occur due to filter design and position. With the Travenol filters, gentamicin delivery was more rapid with ascending flow in both horizontal and vertical positions. Drug delivery was significantly delayed with descending flow in both positions. The Pall filter delivered gentamicin more rapidly in the horizontal position with either ascending or descending flow. The vertical filter position significantly delayed drug delivery in both flow directions.[804]

However, in another study, gentamicin sulfate 60 mg/15 mL was injected as a bolus through a 0.2-μm nylon air-eliminating filter (Ultipor, Pall) to evaluate the effect of filtration on simulated intravenous push delivery. About 38% of the drug was delivered through the filter after flushing with 10 mL of sodium chloride 0.9%.[809]

Gentamicin sulfate 5 and 10 mg/55 mL of dextrose 5% and sodium chloride 0.9% was filtered over 20 minutes through a 0.22-μm cellulose ester filter set (Ivex-2, Millipore). Virtually all of the drug was delivered through the filter.[1003]

The binding of gentamicin sulfate to the filter of a set used for continuous ambulatory peritoneal dialysis (CAPD) was studied. Gentamicin sulfate 60 mg/2 L in Dianeal 137 with dextrose 4.25 and 1.5% was filtered through a Peridex CAPD filter set (Millipore); this set has a surface area 27 times larger than an inline intravenous filter. About 25% binding occurred from the solution containing dextrose 4.25%, but only 7.5% was bound with the 1.5% solution.[1112]

Gentamicin sulfate (Unicet-Unilabo) 0.32 mg/mL in dextrose 5% and sodium chloride 0.9% was filtered through a 0.22-μm cellulose ester membrane filter (Ivex-HP, Millipore) over 6 hours. No significant drug loss due to binding to the filter was noted.[1034]

Central Venous Catheter

Gentamicin sulfate (Fujisawa) 1 mg/mL in dextrose 5% was found to be compatible with the ARROWg+ard Blue Plus (Arrow International) chlorhexidine-bearing triple-lumen central catheter. Essentially complete delivery of the drug was found with little or no drug loss occurring. Furthermore, chlorhexidine delivered from the catheter remained at trace amounts with no substantial increase due to the delivery of the drug through the catheter.[2335]

Compatibility Information

Solution Compatibility

Gentamicin sulfate

Test Soln Name	Mfr	Mfr	Conc/L or %	Remarks	Ref	C/I
Amino acids 4.25%, dextrose 25%	MG	SC	80 mg	No increase in particulate matter in 24 hr at 5°C	349	C
Dextrose 5%		RS	160 mg	Stable for 48 hr at room temperature	157	C
Dextrose 5%	AB	SC	160 mg	Stable for 24 hr at 5 and 25°C	88	C
Dextrose 5%	BA[a], TR	SC	1 g	Stable for 24 hr at 5 and 22°C	298	C
Dextrose 5%	TR[b]	SC	800 mg	Physically compatible with little loss in 24 hr at room temperature	554	C
Dextrose 5%			120 mg	Physically compatible. Stable for 24 hr at 25°C	897	C
Dextrose 5%	AB[b]	LY	1.2 g	Visually compatible. Stable for 48 hr at 25°C in light and 4°C	1541	C
Dextrose 5%			600 mg	Decomposition products in 48 hr at room temperature. Gentamicin not quantified	2139	?

Solution Compatibility (Cont.)

Test Soln Name	Mfr	Mfr	Conc/L or %	Remarks	Ref	C/I
Dextrose 10%	SO	SC	60 mg/21.5 mL[c]	Visually compatible with no loss in 30 days at 5°C in the dark	1731	C
Dextrose 10%	SO	SC	120 mg/23 mL[c]	Visually compatible with no loss in 30 days at 5°C in the dark	1731	C
Isolyte M in dextrose 5%	BRN			Stable for 24 hr at room temperature	227	C
Isolyte P in dextrose 5%	BRN			Stable for 24 hr at room temperature	227	C
Normosol M in dextrose 5%	HOS			Stable for 24 hr at room temperature	227	C
Normosol R	HOS			Stable for 24 hr at room temperature	227	C
Normosol R in dextrose 5%	HOS			Stable for 24 hr at room temperature	227	C
Ringer's injection			120 mg	Physically compatible and stable for 24 hr at 25°C	897	C
Ringer's injection, lactated				Stable for 24 hr at room temperature	227	C
Sodium chloride 0.9%			120 mg	Physically compatible and stable for 24 hr at 25°C	897	C
Sodium chloride 0.9%		RS	160 mg	Stable for 48 hr at room temperature	157	C
Sodium chloride 0.9%	BA[a], TR	SC	1 g	Stable for 24 hr at 5 and 22°C	298	C
Sodium chloride 0.9%	AB[b]	LY	1.2 g	Visually compatible and stable for 48 hr at 25°C in light and 4°C	1541	C
TPN #22[d]		SC	800 mg	Physically compatible. No loss in 24 hr at 22°C in the dark	837	C
TPN #52[d]		SC	50 mg	Physically compatible. No loss in 24 hr at 29°C	440	C
TPN #53[d]		SC	50 mg	Physically compatible. No loss in 24 hr at 29°C	440	C
TPN #107[d]			75 mg	Physically compatible and stable for 24 hr at 21°C	1326	C

[a] Tested in both glass and PVC containers.

[b] Tested in PVC containers.

[c] Tested in glass vials as a concentrate.

[d] Refer to Appendix for the composition of parenteral nutrition solutions. TPN indicates a 2-in-1 admixture.

Additive Compatibility

Gentamicin sulfate

Test Drug	Mfr	Conc/L or %	Mfr	Conc/L or %	Test Solution	Remarks	Ref	C/I
Amphotericin B		200 mg		320 mg	D5W	Haze develops over 3 hr	26	I
Ampicillin sodium	BE	8 g	RS	160 mg	D5¼S, D5W, NS	50% gentamicin loss in 2 hr at room temperature	157	I
Ampicillin sodium		1 g		100 mg	TPN #107[a]	42% gentamicin loss and 25% ampicillin loss in 24 hr at 21°C	1326	I
Atracurium besylate	BW	500 mg		2 g	D5W	Physically compatible and atracurium stable for 24 hr at 5 and 30°C	1694	C
Aztreonam	SQ	10 and 20 g	SC	200 and 800 mg	D5W, NS[b]	Little aztreonam loss in 48 hr at 25°C and 7 days at 4°C. Gentamicin stable for 12 hr at 25°C and 24 hr at 4°C. Up to 10% loss in 48 hr at 25°C and 7 days at 4°C	1023	C
Bleomycin sulfate	BR	20 and 30 units	SC	50, 100, 300, 600 mg	NS	Physically compatible and bleomycin activity retained for 1 week at 4°C. Gentamicin not tested	763	C
Cefazolin sodium[f]	SKF	10 g	ES	800 mg	D5W, NS[c]	10% cefazolin loss in 4 hr in D5W and 12 hr in NS at 25°C. No clindamycin and gentamicin loss in 24 hr	1328	I

Additive Compatibility (Cont.)

Test Drug	Mfr	Conc/L or %	Mfr	Conc/L or %	Test Solution	Remarks	Ref	C/I
Cefepime HCl	BR	40 g	ES	1.2 g	D5W, NS	Cloudy in 18 hr at room temperature	1681	I
Cefotaxime sodium	RS	50 mg	SC	9 mg	D5W	30% loss of gentamicin in 2 hr at 22°C	504	I
Cefotaxime sodium	RS	50 mg	SC	6 mg	D5W	4% loss of gentamicin in 24 hr at 22°C	504	C
Cefoxitin sodium	MSD	5 g	SC	400 mg	D5S	4% cefoxitin loss in 24 hr and 11% in 48 hr at 25°C. 2% in 48 hr at 5°C. 9% gentamicin loss in 24 hr and 23% in 48 hr at 25°C. 2% in 48 hr at 5°C	308	C
Ceftazidime	GL	50 mg	SC	6 and 9 mg	D5W	10 to 20% gentamicin loss in 2 hr at 22°C	504	I
Ceftriaxone sodium	RC	100 mg	SC	9 mg	D5W	13% loss of gentamicin in 8 hr at 22°C	504	I
Ceftriaxone sodium	RC	100 mg	SC	6 mg	D5W	5% loss of gentamicin in 24 hr at 22°C	504	C
Cefuroxime sodium	GL	7.5 g	EX	800 mg	D5W, NS[b]	Physically compatible with no loss of either drug in 1 hr	1036	C
Cefuroxime sodium		1 g		100 mg	TPN #107[a]	32% gentamicin loss in 24 hr at 21°C	1326	I
Ciprofloxacin	MI	1.6 g	LY	1 g	D5W, NS	Visually compatible and both drugs stable for 48 hr at 25°C under fluorescent light and 4°C in the dark	1541	C
Ciprofloxacin	BAY	2 g	SC	10 g	NS	Visually compatible. Little ciprofloxacin loss in 24 hr at 25°C. Gentamicin not tested	1934	C
Ciprofloxacin	BAY	2 g	SC	1.6 g	D5W	Visually compatible with no loss of ciprofloxacin in 24 hr at 22°C under fluorescent light. Gentamicin not tested	2413	C
Clindamycin phosphate	UP	2.4 g		120 mg	D5W	Physically compatible. Clindamycin stable for 24 hr at room temperature	104	C
Clindamycin phosphate	UP	1.2 g		60 mg	D5W	Physically compatible. Clindamycin stable for 24 hr at room temperature	104	C
Clindamycin phosphate	UP	12 g		600 mg	D5W	Physically compatible	101	C
Clindamycin phosphate	UP	9 g		800 mg	D5W	Clindamycin stable for 24 hr	101	C
Clindamycin phosphate	UP	9 g	AB	1 g	D5W, NS[d]	Physically compatible and both drugs stable for 48 hr at room temperature exposed to light and 1 week frozen	174	C
Clindamycin phosphate	UP	9 g	LY	1.2 g	D5W[c]	Physically compatible and both drugs stable for 7 days at 4 and 25°C	174	C
Clindamycin phosphate	UP	9 g	LY	1.2 g	NS[c]	Physically compatible and both drugs stable for 14 days at 4 and 25°C	174	C
Clindamycin phosphate	UP	18 g	LY	2.4 g	D5W, NS[b]	Physically compatible and both drugs stable for 14 days at 4 and 25°C	174	C
Clindamycin phosphate	UP	9 g	ES	1.2 g	D5W, NS[c]	Physically compatible and both drugs stable for 28 days frozen at –20°C	174	C
Clindamycin phosphate	UP	18 g	ES	2.4 g	D5W, NS[b]	Both drugs stable for 28 days frozen at –20°C	981	C
Clindamycin phosphate	UP	6 g	ES	667 mg	D5W[b]	Physically compatible with no clindamycin loss and 9% gentamicin loss in 24 hr at room temperature	995	C
Clindamycin phosphate		400 mg		75 mg	TPN #107[a]	19% gentamicin loss and 15% clindamycin loss in 24 hr at 21°C	1326	I
Clindamycin phosphate[g]	UP	9 g	ES	800 mg	D5W, NS[c]	10% cefazolin loss in 4 hr in D5W and 12 hr in NS at 25°C. No clindamycin and gentamicin loss in 24 hr	1328	I

Additive Compatibility (Cont.)

Test Drug	Mfr	Conc/L or %	Mfr	Conc/L or %	Test Solution	Remarks	Ref	C/I
Cloxacillin sodium	BE	4 g	RS	160 mg	D5¼S, D5W, NS	Precipitate forms	157	I
Cytarabine	UP	100 mg		80 mg	D5W	Physically compatible for 24 hr	174	C
Cytarabine	UP	300 mg		240 mg	D5W	Physically incompatible	174	I
Dextran 40		10%			D5W	Gentamicin stable for 24 hr at room temperature	227	C
Dopamine HCl	AS	800 mg	SC	2 g	D5W	No dopamine and 7% gentamicin loss in 24 hr at 25°C	312	C
Dopamine HCl	AS	800 mg	SC	320 mg	D5W	Gentamicin stable through 6 hr. 80% gentamicin loss in 24 hr at 25°C. Dopamine stable for 24 hr	78	I
Fat emulsion, intra-venous	OTS	20%	MSD	0.4 mg/mL[a]		Coarsening of particle diameter observed immediately after preparation	3452	I
Floxacillin sodium	BE	20 g	RS	8 g	NS	Haze forms immediately and precipitate forms in 2 hr	1479	I
Floxacillin sodium	BE	10 g	EX	8 g	NS	Physically compatible for 48 hr. Both drugs stable for 1 hr at room temperature	1036	C
Floxacillin sodium	BE	10 g	EX	8 g	D5W	Precipitates immediately	1036	I
Fluconazole	PF	1 g	SO	0.5 g	D5W	Visually compatible with no fluconazole loss in 72 hr at 25°C under fluorescent light. Gentamicin not tested	1677	C
Furosemide	HO	800 mg	SC	1.6 g	D5W, NS	Furosemide precipitates immediately	876	I
Furosemide	HO	1 g	RS	8 g	NS	Physically compatible for 24 hr at 15 and 30°C. Precipitate forms in 48 to 72 hr	1479	C
Fusidate sodium	LEO	1 g		160 mg	D2.5½S, D2.5S, D5¼S, D5½S, D5S, D10S	Physically compatible and chemically stable for 48 hr at room temperature	1800	C
Fusidate sodium	LEO	1 g		1.5 g	D2.5½S, D2.5S, D5¼S, D5½S, D5S, D10S	Physically incompatible	1800	I
Heparin sodium	BP	20,000 units		320 mg	D5W, NS	Precipitates immediately	26	I
Heparin sodium	OR	20,000 units	SC	1 g	D5W, NS	Opalescence	113	I
Heparin sodium	BRN	1000 to 6000 units	ME	88 mg	D10W, NS	Activity of both drugs greatly reduced	1570	I
Linezolid	PHU	2 g	AB	800 mg	e	Physically compatible. Little linezolid loss in 7 days at 4 and 23°C in dark. Gentamicin losses of 5 to 7% in 7 days at 4°C and 8% in 5 days at 23°C	2332	C
Mannitol		20%		120 mg		Physically compatible and gentamicin stable for 24 hr at 25°C	897	C
Meropenem	ZEN	1 and 20 g	SC	800 mg	NS	Visually compatible for 4 hr at room temperature	1994	C
Metronidazole	SE	5 g	SC	800 mg and 1.2 g		Physically compatible with no loss of either drug in 2 days at 18°C. At 4°C, no metronidazole loss but up to 10% gentamicin loss in 7 days	1242	C
Metronidazole	RP	5 g		800 mg		Visually compatible with no loss of metronidazole in 15 days at 5 and 25°C. 10% gentamicin loss in 63 hr at 25°C and 10.6 days at 5°C	1931	C
Midazolam HCl	RC	50, 250, 400 mg	EX	800 mg	NS	Visually compatible for 4 hr	355	C
Nafcillin sodium		1 g		75 mg	TPN #107[a]	10% gentamicin loss in 24 hr at 21°C	1326	I

Additive Compatibility (Cont.)

Test Drug	Mfr	Conc/L or %	Mfr	Conc/L or %	Test Solution	Remarks	Ref	C/I
Penicillin G sodium	GL	13 and 40 million units	RS	160 mg	D5¼S, D5W, NS	Gentamicin stable for 24 hr at room temperature	157	C
Ranitidine HCl	GL	100 mg		160 mg	D5W	Physically compatible for 24 hr at ambient temperature in light	1151	C
Ranitidine HCl	GL	50 mg and 2 g		80 mg	D5W, NS	Physically compatible. Ranitidine stable for 24 hr at 25°C. Gentamicin not tested	1515	C
Verapamil HCl	KN	80 mg	SC	160 mg	D5W, NS	Physically compatible for 24 hr	764	C

[a] Refer to Appendix for the composition of parenteral nutrition solutions. TPN indicates a 2-in-1 admixture.

[b] Tested in PVC containers.

[c] Tested in glass containers.

[d] Tested in both glass and PVC containers.

[e] Admixed in the linezolid infusion container.

[f] Tested in combination with clindamycin phosphate 9 g/L.

[g] Tested in combination with cefazolin sodium 10 g/L.

Drugs in Syringe Compatibility

Gentamicin sulfate

Test Drug	Mfr	Amt	Mfr	Amt	Remarks	Ref	C/I
Ampicillin sodium	AY	500 mg		80 mg/2 mL	Physically incompatible within 1 hr at room temperature	99	I
Caffeine citrate		20 mg/1 mL	ES	10 mg/1 mL	Visually compatible for 4 hr at 25°C	2440	C
Clindamycin phosphate	UP	900 mg/6 mL	ES	120 mg/4 mL[a]	Physically compatible with little loss of either drug for 48 hr at 25°C	1159	C
Cloxacillin sodium	BE	250 mg		80 mg/2 mL	Physically incompatible within 1 hr at room temperature	99	I
Dimenhydrinate		10 mg/1 mL		10 mg/1 mL	Clear solution	2569	C
Dimenhydrinate		10 mg/1 mL		40 mg/1 mL	Clear solution	2569	C
Heparin sodium		2500 units/1 mL		40 mg	Turbidity or precipitate forms within 5 min	1053	I
Iohexol	WI	64.7%, 5 mL	SC	0.8 mg/1 mL	Physically compatible for at least 2 hr	1438	C
Iopamidol	SQ	61%, 5 mL	SC	0.8 mg/1 mL	Physically compatible for at least 2 hr	1438	C
Iothalamate meglumine	MA	60%, 5 mL	SC	0.8 mg/1 mL	Physically compatible for at least 2 hr	1438	C
Ioxaglate meglumine–ioxaglate sodium	MA	5 mL	SC	0.8 mg/1 mL	Transient precipitate clears within 5 min	1438	?
Pantoprazole sodium	[b]	4 mg/1 mL		40 mg/1 mL	Whitish precipitate	2574	I
Penicillin G sodium		1 million units		80 mg/2 mL	No precipitate or color change within 1 hr at room temperature	99	C

[a] Diluted to 4 mL with 1 mL of sodium chloride 0.9%.

[b] Test performed using the formulation WITHOUT edetate disodium.

Y-Site Injection Compatibility (1:1 Mixture)

Gentamicin sulfate

Test Drug	Mfr	Conc	Mfr	Conc	Remarks	Ref	C/I
Acyclovir sodium	BW	5 mg/mL[a]	TR	1.6 mg/mL[a]	Physically compatible for 4 hr at 25°C	1157	C
Acyclovir sodium	BV	5 mg/mL[b]	AMS	30 mg/mL[e]	White paste-like precipitate	2794	I
Allopurinol sodium	BW	3 mg/mL[b]	ES	5 mg/mL[b]	Hazy solution with crystals forms in 1 hr	1686	I
Alprostadil	BED	7.5 mcg/mL[t u]	ES	1 mg/mL[s]	Visually compatible for 1 hr	2746	C
Amifostine	USB	10 mg/mL[a]	ES	5 mg/mL[a]	Physically compatible for 4 hr at 23°C	1845	C
Amiodarone HCl	LZ	4 mg/mL[c]	LY	0.8 mg/mL[c]	Physically compatible for 4 hr at room temperature	1444	C
Amiodarone HCl	WY	6 mg/mL[a]	APP	5 mg/mL[a]	Visually compatible for 24 hr at 22°C	2352	C
Amsacrine	NCI	1 mg/mL[a]	SO	5 mg/mL[a]	Visually compatible for 4 hr at 22°C	1381	C
Anidulafungin	VIC	0.5 mg/mL[a]	AB	5 mg/mL[a]	Physically compatible for 4 hr at 23°C	2617	C
Atracurium besylate	BW	0.5 mg/mL[a]	ES	2 mg/mL[a]	Physically compatible for 24 hr at 28°C	1337	C
Azithromycin	PF	2 mg/mL[b]	AMR	21 mg/mL[e p]	Whitish-yellow microcrystals found	2368	I
Aztreonam	SQ	40 mg/mL[a]	ES	5 mg/mL[a]	Physically compatible for 4 hr at 23°C	1758	C
Bivalirudin	TMC	5 mg/mL[a]	AB	5 mg/mL[a]	Physically compatible for 4 hr at 23°C	2373	C
Cangrelor tetrasodium	TMC	1 mg/mL[b]		5 mg/mL[b]	Gross white turbid precipitate forms immediately	3243	I
Caspofungin acetate	ME	0.7 mg/mL[b]	HOS	5 mg/mL[b]	Physically compatible for 4 hr at room temperature	2758	C
Cefepime HCl	BMS	120 mg/mL[c]		6 mg/mL	Physically compatible with less than 10% cefepime loss. Gentamicin not tested	2513	C
Ceftaroline fosamil	FOR	2.22 mg/mL[a b q]	HOS	5 mg/mL[a b q]	Physically compatible for 4 hr at 23°C	2826	C
Ceftazidime	SKB	125 mg/mL		0.6 mg/mL	Visually compatible with less than 10% loss of both drugs in 1 hr	2434	C
Ceftazidime	GSK	120 mg/mL[g]		6 mg/mL	Physically compatible with less than 10% ceftazidime loss. Gentamicin not tested	2513	C
Ceftazidime–avibactam sodium	ALL	20 mg/mL[ff gg]	[aa]		Physically compatible for up to 4 hr at room temperature	3004	C
Ceftolozane sulfate–tazobactam sodium	CUB	10 mg/mL[c dd]	FRK	5 mg/mL[c]	Physically compatible for 2 hr	3262	C
Ciprofloxacin	MI	2 mg/mL[c]	LY	1.6 mg/mL[c]	Visually compatible for 24 hr at 24°C	1655	C
Cisatracurium besylate	GW	0.1, 2, 5 mg/mL[a]	ES	5 mg/mL[a]	Physically compatible for 4 hr at 23°C	2074	C
Clarithromycin	AB	4 mg/mL[a]	RS	40 mg/mL	Visually compatible for 72 hr at both 30 and 17°C	2174	C
Cloxacillin sodium	SMX	100 mg/mL	SZ	40 mg/mL	Precipitates immediately	3245	I
Cyclophosphamide	MJ	20 mg/mL[a]	TR	1.6 mg/mL[a]	Physically compatible for 4 hr at 25°C	1194	C
Cytarabine	UP	16 mg/mL[b]	GNS	15 mg/mL[e]	Visually compatible for 24 hr at room temperature in test tubes. No precipitate found on filter from Y-site delivery	2063	C

Y-Site Injection Compatibility (1:1 Mixture) (Cont.)

Test Drug	Mfr	Conc	Mfr	Conc	Remarks	Ref	C/I
Daptomycin	CUB[cc]	19.2 mg/mL[b r]	AB	1.5 mg/mL[r]	Physically compatible with no loss of either drug in 2 hr at 25°C	2553	C
Dexmedetomidine HCl	AB	4 mcg/mL[b]	APP	5 mg/mL[b]	Physically compatible for 4 hr at 23°C	2383	C
Diltiazem HCl	MMD	1[b] and 5 mg/mL	SC	2.4[b] and 40 mg/mL	Visually compatible	1807	C
Docetaxel	RPR	0.9 mg/mL[a]	AB	5 mg/mL[a]	Physically compatible for 4 hr at 23°C	2224	C
Doripenem	JJ	5 mg/mL[a b]	HOS	5 mg/mL[a b]	Physically compatible for 4 hr at 23°C	2743	C
Doxapram HCl	RB	2 mg/mL[a]	APP	10 mg/mL[a]	Visually compatible for 4 hr at 23°C	2470	C
Doxorubicin HCl liposomal	SEQ	0.4 mg/mL[a]	ES	5 mg/mL[a]	Physically compatible for 4 hr at 23°C	2087	C
Enalaprilat	MSD	0.05 mg/mL[b]	ES	0.8 mg/mL[a]	Physically compatible for 24 hr at room temperature under fluorescent light	1355	C
Eravacycline dihydro-chloride	TET	0.6 mg/mL[b]	FRK	5 mg/mL[b]	Physically compatible for 2 hr at room temperature	3532	C
Esmolol HCl	DCC	10 mg/mL[a]	ES	0.8 mg/mL[a]	Physically compatible for 24 hr at 22°C	1169	C
Etoposide phosphate	BR	5 mg/mL[a]	AB	5 mg/mL[a]	Physically compatible for 4 hr at 23°C	2218	C
Famotidine	MSD	0.2 mg/mL[a]	ES	0.8 mg/mL[b]	Physically compatible for 14 hr	1196	C
Famotidine	ME	2 mg/mL[b]		5 mg/mL[a]	Visually compatible for 4 hr at 22°C	1936	C
Fat emulsion, intravenous	OTS	20%[hh]	MSD	0.4 mg/mL[a ii]	Coarsening of particle diameter observed immediately after preparation	3452	I
Fenoldopam mesylate	AB	80 mcg/mL[b]	APP	5 mg/mL[b]	Physically compatible for 4 hr at 23°C	2467	C
Filgrastim	AMG	30 mcg/mL[a]	LY	5 mg/mL[a]	Physically compatible for 4 hr at 22°C	1687	C
Filgrastim	AMG	40 mcg/mL[a]	GNS	1.6 mg/mL[a]	Visually compatible. Little loss of filgrastim and gentamicin in 4 hr at 25°C	2060	C
Filgrastim	AMG	10 mcg/mL[f]	GNS	1.6 mg/mL[a]	23% loss of filgrastim in 4 hr at 25°C. Little gentamicin loss	2060	I
Fluconazole	RR	2 mg/mL	ES	4 mg/mL	Physically compatible for 24 hr at 25°C	1407	C
Fludarabine phosphate	BX	1 mg/mL[a]	ES	5 mg/mL[a]	Visually compatible for 4 hr at 22°C	1439	C
Foscarnet sodium	AST	24 mg/mL	ES	4 mg/mL	Physically compatible for 24 hr at room temperature under fluorescent light	1335	C
Foscarnet sodium	AST	24 mg/mL	ES	2 mg/mL[c]	Physically compatible for 24 hr at 25°C under fluorescent light	1393	C
Furosemide	HO	10 mg/mL	SC	1.6 mg/mL[c]	Furosemide precipitates immediately	876	I
Gemcitabine HCl	LI	10 mg/mL[b]	AB	5 mg/mL[b]	Physically compatible for 4 hr at 23°C	2226	C
Granisetron HCl	SKB	1 mg/mL	ES	1.5 mg/mL[b]	Physically compatible with little loss of either drug in 4 hr at 22°C	1883	C
Heparin sodium		[b]	RS	80 mg	Precipitates immediately	528	I
Heparin sodium	ES	50 units/mL[c]	ES	3.2 mg/mL[c]	Immediate gross haze	1316	I
Heparin sodium	TR	50 units/mL	TR	2 mg/mL	Visually incompatible within 4 hr at 25°C	1793	I
Hetastarch in lactated electrolyte	AB	6%	SC	5 mg/mL[a]	Physically compatible for 4 hr at 23°C	2339	C

Y-Site Injection Compatibility (1:1 Mixture) (Cont.)

Test Drug	Mfr	Conc	Mfr	Conc	Remarks	Ref	C/I
Hetastarch in sodium chloride 0.9%	DCC	6%	TR	0.8 mg/mLᶻ	Precipitates immediately but disappears after 1 hr at room temperature	1313	I
Hydromorphone HCl	WY	0.2 mg/mLᵃ	TR	0.8 mg/mLᵃ	Physically compatible for 4 hr at 25°C	987	C
Hydroxyethyl starch 130/0.4 in sodium chloride 0.9%	FRK	6%	SX	1, 3, 5 mg/mLᵃ	Visually compatible for 24 hr at room temperature	2770	C
Indomethacin sodium trihydrate	MSD	0.5 and 1 mg/mLᵃ		1 mg/mLᵃ	White turbidity forms immediately and becomes white flakes in 1 hr	1550	I
Insulin	LI	0.2 unit/mLᵇ	TR	1.2 mg/mLᵇ	Physically compatible for 2 hr at 25°C	1395	C
Iodipamide meglumine	SQ	52%			White precipitate forms immediately downstream to Y-site when given into a set through which gentamicin was administered previously	324	I
Isavuconazonium sulfate	ASP	1.5 mg/mLᶜ	PPR	5 mg/mLᶜ	Physically compatible for 2 hr	3263	C
Labetalol HCl	SC	1 mg/mLᵃ	ES	0.8 mg/mLᵃ	Physically compatible for 24 hr at 18°C	1171	C
Letermovir	ME				Physically incompatible	3398	I
Levofloxacin	OMN	5 mg/mLᵃ	ES	10 mg/mL	Visually compatible for 4 hr at 24°C	2233	C
Linezolid	PHU	2 mg/mL	FUJ	5 mg/mLᵃ	Physically compatible for 4 hr at 23°C	2264	C
Lorazepam	WY	0.33 mg/mLᵇ	CNF	3 mg/mL	Visually compatible for 24 hr at 22°C	1855	C
Magnesium sulfate	IX	16.7, 33.3, 66.7, 100 mg/mLᵃ	SC	0.8 mg/mLᵃ	Physically compatible for at least 4 hr at 32°C	813	C
Melphalan HCl	BW	0.1 mg/mLᵇ	LY	5 mg/mLᵇ	Physically compatible for 3 hr at 22°C	1557	C
Meperidine HCl	WY	10 mg/mLᵃ	TR	0.8 mg/mLᵃ	Physically compatible for 4 hr at 25°C	987	C
Meperidine HCl	WY	10 mg/mLᵇ	ES	1.2 and 2 mg/mLᵇ	Physically compatible for 1 hr at 25°C	1338	C
Meropenem	ZEN	1 and 50 mg/mLᵇ	SC	4 mg/mLᵍ	Visually compatible for 4 hr at room temperature	1994	C
Meropenem	ASZ	10 mg/mLᵇ	AMS	30 mg/mLᵉ	Physically compatible	2794	C
Meropenem		50 mg/mL	SZ	40 mg/mL	Physically compatible for 4 hr at room temperature	3538	C
Meropenem–vaborbactam	TMC	8 mg/mLᵇ ᵉᵉ	FRK	5 mg/mLᵇ	Physically compatible for 3 hr at 20 to 25°C	3380	C
Midazolam HCl	RC	1 mg/mLᵃ	ES	10 mg/mL	Visually compatible for 24 hr at 23°C	1847	C
Midazolam HCl	RC	5 mg/mL	CNF	3 mg/mL	Visually compatible for 24 hr at 22°C	1855	C
Milrinone lactate	SS	0.2 mg/mLᵃ	APP	10 mg/mLᵃ	Visually compatible for 4 hr at 25°C	2381	C
Morphine sulfate	WI	1 mg/mLᵃ	TR	0.8 mg/mLᵃ	Physically compatible for 4 hr at 25°C	987	C
Morphine sulfate	ES	1 mg/mLᵇ	ES	1.2 and 2 mg/mLᵇ	Physically compatible for 1 hr at 25°C	1338	C
Multivitamins	USV	5 mL/Lᵃ	SC	80 mg/100 mLᵃ	Physically compatible for 24 hr at room temperature	323	C
Nicardipine HCl	DCC	0.1 mg/mLᵃ	ES	0.8 mg/mLᵃ	Visually compatible for 24 hr at room temperature	235	C
Ondansetron HCl	GL	1 mg/mLᵇ	ES	5 mg/mLᵃ	Visually compatible for 4 hr at 22°C	1365	C

Y-Site Injection Compatibility (1:1 Mixture) (Cont.)

Test Drug	Mfr	Conc	Mfr	Conc	Remarks	Ref	C/I
Oritavancin diphosphate	TAR	0.8, 1.2, and 2 mg/mL[a]	ABX	5 mg/mL[a]	Visually compatible for 4 hr at 20 to 24°C	2928	C
Paclitaxel	NCI	1.2 mg/mL[a]	ES	5 mg/mL[a]	Physically compatible for 4 hr at 22°C	1556	C
Palonosetron HCl	MGI	50 mcg/mL	APP	5 mg/mL[a]	Physically compatible. No loss of either drug in 4 hr at room temperature	2765	C
Pancuronium bromide	ES	0.05 mg/mL[a]	ES	2 mg/mL[a]	Physically compatible for 24 hr at 28°C	1337	C
Pemetrexed disodium	LI	20 mg/mL[b]	AB	5 mg/mL[a]	Gross white precipitate forms immediately	2564	I
Piperacillin sodium–tazobactam sodium	WY[x]	26.7 to 40 mg/mL[a b y]		0.7 to 3.32 mg/mL	Compatible	2918, 2922	C
Piperacillin sodium–tazobactam sodium	WY[x]	40 mg/mL[y z]		0.7 to 3.32 mg/mL	Compatible	2918, 2922	C
Piperacillin sodium–tazobactam sodium	WY[x]	60 mg/mL[y z]		0.7 to 3.32 mg/mL	Incompatible	2918, 2922	I
Piperacillin sodium–tazobactam sodium	[w]			0.7 to 3.32 mg/mL	Stated to be compatible	2919, 2920, 2921, 2985	C
Posaconazole	ME	18 mg/mL		1.6 mg/mL[c]	Physically compatible	2911, 2912	C
Potassium chloride	BA	0.02 mEq/mL[v]	AMS	30 mg/mL[e]	Physically compatible	2794	C
Propofol	ZEN[x]	10 mg/mL	ES	5 mg/mL[a]	White precipitate forms immediately	2066	I
Quinupristin–dalfopristin		2 mg/mL[a bb]	[aa]	3 mg/mL	Reported to be incompatible	3230	I
Remifentanil HCl	GW	0.025 and 0.25 mg/mL[b]	ES	5 mg/mL[a]	Physically compatible for 4 hr at 23°C	2075	C
Sargramostim	IMM	10 mcg/mL[b]	SO	5 mg/mL[a]	Visually compatible for 4 hr at 22°C	1436	C
Tacrolimus	FUJ	1 mg/mL[b]	SCN	4 mg/mL[a]	Visually compatible for 24 hr at 25°C	1630	C
Tedizolid phosphate	CUB	0.8 mg/mL[b]	PRP	5 mg/mL[b]	Measured turbidity increases immediately	3244	I
Telavancin HCl	ASP	7.5 mg/mL[a b q]	HOS	5 mg/mL[a b q]	Physically compatible for 2 hr	2830	C
Teniposide	BR	0.1 mg/mL[a]	LY	5 mg/mL[a]	Physically compatible for 4 hr at 23°C	1725	C
Theophylline	TR	4 mg/mL	TR	2 mg/mL	Visually compatible for 6 hr at 25°C	1793	C
Thiotepa	IMM[h]	1 mg/mL[a]	ES	5 mg/mL[a]	Physically compatible for 4 hr at 23°C	1861	C
Tigecycline	WY	1 mg/mL[b]		1.4 mg/mL[b]	Physically compatible for 4 hr	2714	C
Tigecycline	ACD, FRK, WY	[c]	[aa]		Stated to be compatible	2915, 3459, 3460	C
TNA #73[i]		32.5 mL[j]	SC	1.6 mg/mL[a]	Visually compatible for 4 hr at 25°C	1008	C
TNA #97[i]			ES	40 mg/mL	Physically compatible and gentamicin content retained for 6 hr at 21°C	1324	C
TNA #98[i]			ES	40 mg/mL	Physically compatible and gentamicin content retained for 6 hr at 21°C	1324	C

Y-Site Injection Compatibility (1:1 Mixture) (Cont.)

Test Drug	Mfr	Conc	Mfr	Conc	Remarks	Ref	C/I
TNA #99[i]			ES	40 mg/mL	Physically compatible and gentamicin content retained for 6 hr at 21°C	1324	C
TNA #100[i]			ES	40 mg/mL	Physically compatible and gentamicin content retained for 6 hr at 21°C	1324	C
TNA #101[i]			ES	40 mg/mL	Physically compatible and gentamicin content retained for 6 hr at 21°C	1324	C
TNA #102[i]			ES	40 mg/mL	Physically compatible and gentamicin content retained for 6 hr at 21°C	1324	C
TNA #103[i]			ES	40 mg/mL	Physically compatible and gentamicin content retained for 6 hr at 21°C	1324	C
TNA #104[i]			ES	40 mg/mL	Physically compatible and gentamicin content retained for 6 hr at 21°C	1324	C
TNA #218[i]			AB, FUJ	5 mg/mL[a]	Visually compatible for 4 hr at 23°C	2215	C
TNA #219[i]			AB, FUJ	5 mg/mL[a]	Visually compatible for 4 hr at 23°C	2215	C
TNA #220[i]			AB, FUJ	5 mg/mL[a]	Visually compatible for 4 hr at 23°C	2215	C
TNA #221[i]			AB, FUJ	5 mg/mL[a]	Visually compatible for 4 hr at 23°C	2215	C
TNA #222[i]			AB, FUJ	5 mg/mL[a]	Visually compatible for 4 hr at 23°C	2215	C
TNA #223[i]			AB, FUJ	5 mg/mL[a]	Visually compatible for 4 hr at 23°C	2215	C
TNA #224[i]			AB, FUJ	5 mg/mL[a]	Visually compatible for 4 hr at 23°C	2215	C
TNA #225[i]			AB, FUJ	5 mg/mL[a]	Visually compatible for 4 hr at 23°C	2215	C
TNA #226[i]			AB, FUJ	5 mg/mL[a]	Visually compatible for 4 hr at 23°C	2215	C
TPN #54[i]				13 and 20 mg/mL	Physically compatible and gentamicin activity retained over 6 hr at 22°C	1045	C
TPN #61[i]		[k]	IX	12.5 mg/1.25 mL[l]	Physically compatible	1012	C
TPN #61[i]		[m]	IX	75 mg/1.9 mL[l]	Physically compatible	1012	C
TPN #91[i]		[n]	IX	5 mg[o]	Physically compatible	1170	C
TPN #189[i]			DB	1 mg/mL[b]	Visually compatible for 24 hr at 22°C	1767	C
TPN #203[i]			ES	10 mg/mL	Visually compatible for 2 hr at 23°C	1974	C
TPN #204[i]			ES	10 mg/mL	Visually compatible for 2 hr at 23°C	1974	C
TPN #212[i]			AB	5 mg/mL[a]	Physically compatible for 4 hr at 23°C	2109	C
TPN #213[i]			AB	5 mg/mL[a]	Physically compatible for 4 hr at 23°C	2109	C
TPN #214[i]			AB	5 mg/mL[a]	Physically compatible for 4 hr at 23°C	2109	C
TPN #215[i]			AB	5 mg/mL[a]	Physically compatible for 4 hr at 23°C	2109	C
Vasopressin	APP	0.2 unit/mL[b]	APP	1.2 mg/mL[e]	Physically compatible	2641	C
Vecuronium bromide	OR	0.1 mg/mL[a]	ES	2 mg/mL[a]	Physically compatible for 24 hr at 28°C	1337	C
Vinorelbine tartrate	BW	1 mg/mL[b]	ES	5 mg/mL[b]	Physically compatible for 4 hr at 22°C	1558	C
Zidovudine	BW	4 mg/mL[a]	IMS	2 mg/mL[a]	Physically compatible for 4 hr at 25°C	1193	C

Y-Site Injection Compatibility (1:1 Mixture) (Cont.)

[a] Tested in dextrose 5%.

[b] Tested in sodium chloride 0.9%.

[c] Tested in both dextrose 5% and sodium chloride 0.9%.

[d] Tested in dextrose 5%, Ringer's injection, lactated, sodium chloride 0.45%, and sodium chloride 0.9%.

[e] Tested in sodium chloride 0.45%.

[f] Tested in dextrose 5% with albumin human 2 mg/mL.

[g] Tested in sterile water for injection.

[h] Lyophilized formulation tested.

[i] Refer to Appendix for the composition of parenteral nutrition solutions. TNA indicates a 3-in-1 admixture, and TPN indicates a 2-in-1 admixture.

[j] A 32.5-mL sample of parenteral nutrition solution mixed with 50 mL of antibiotic solution.

[k] Run at 21 mL/hr.

[l] Given over 30 minutes by syringe pump.

[m] Run at 94 mL/hr.

[n] Run at 10 mL/hr.

[o] Given over one hour by syringe pump.

[p] Injected via Y-site into an administration set running azithromycin.

[q] Tested in Ringer's injection, lactated.

[r] Final concentration after mixing.

[s] Tested in either dextrose 5% or in sodium chloride 0.9%, but the report did not specify which solution.

[t] Tested in a 1:1 mixture of (1) dextrose 5% and dextrose 5% in sodium chloride 0.45% with and without potassium chloride 20 mEq/L and also in (2) dextrose 10% in sodium chloride 0.45% with and without potassium chloride 20 mEq/L.

[u] Tested in a 1:1 mixture of dextrose 5% and TPN #274 (see Appendix).

[v] Tested in dextrose 5% in sodium chloride 0.45%.

[w] Test performed using the formulation WITHOUT edetate disodium.

[x] Test performed using the formulation WITH edetate disodium.

[y] Piperacillin component. Piperacillin in an 8:1 fixed-ratio concentration with tazobactam.

[z] Tested as the premixed infusion solution.

[aa] Salt not specified.

[bb] Quinupristin and dalfopristin components combined.

[cc] Test performed using the Cubicin formulation.

[dd] Ceftolozane component. Ceftolozane in a 2:1 fixed-ratio concentration with tazobactam.

[ee] Meropenem component. Meropenem in a 1:1 fixed-ratio concentration with vaborbactam.

[ff] Ceftazidime component. Ceftazidime in a 4:1 fixed-ratio concentration with avibactam.

[gg] Tested in dextrose 5%, sodium chloride 0.9%, and Ringer's injection, lactated.

[hh] Run at 25 mL/hr with dextrose 5% run at 83 mL/hr.

[ii] Run at 100 mL/hr.

Additional Compatibility Information

Peritoneal Dialysis Solutions

The activity of gentamicin 10 mg/L was evaluated in peritoneal dialysis fluids containing 1.5 or 4.25% dextrose (Dianeal 137, Travenol). Storage at 25°C resulted in no loss of antimicrobial activity in 24 hours.[515]

Gentamicin sulfate (Schering) 3 and 10 mg/L in peritoneal dialysis concentrate with 50% dextrose retained about 90% of initial activity in 7 hours and about 50 to 70% in 24 hours at room temperature.[1044]

The stability of gentamicin sulfate 8 mg/L, alone and with cefazolin sodium 75 and 150 mg/L, was evaluated in a peritoneal dialysis solution of dextrose 1.5% with heparin sodium 1000 units/L. Gentamicin activity was retained for 48 hours at both 4 and 26°C, alone and with both concentrations of cefazolin. Cefazolin activity was also retained over the study period. At 37°C, gentamicin losses ranged from 4 to 8% and cefazolin losses ranged from 10 to 12% in 48 hours.[1029]

In another study, the stability of gentamicin sulfate (Schering) was evaluated in peritoneal dialysate concentrates containing dextrose 30 and 50% (Dianeal) as well as in a diluted solution containing dextrose 2.5%. The gentamicin sulfate concentrations were 100 and 160 mg/L in the peritoneal dialysate concentrates and 5 and 8 mg/L in the diluted solutions. Gentamicin sulfate was found to be stable in all of these solutions for at least 24 hours at 23°C.[1229]

Gentamicin 4 mcg/mL was evaluated in Dianeal PDS with dextrose 1.5 and 4.25% (Travenol) with cefazolin 125 mcg/mL, heparin 500 units, and albumin human 80 mg in 2-L bags. The gentamicin content was retained for 72 hours.[1413]

The retention of antimicrobial activity of gentamicin sulfate (SoloPak) 120 mg/L alone and with vancomycin hydrochloride (Lilly) 1 g/L was evaluated in Dianeal PD-2 (Travenol) with dextrose 1.5%. Little or no loss of either antibiotic occurred in 8 hours at 37°C. Gentamicin sulfate alone retained activity for at least 48 hours at 4 and 25°C. In combination with vancomycin hydrochloride, antimicrobial activity of both antibiotics was retained for up to 48 hours. However, the authors recommended refrigeration at 4°C for storage periods greater than 24 hours.[1414]

Gentamicin sulfate (Schering) 25 mcg/mL combined separately with the cephalosporins cefazolin sodium (Lilly) and cefoxitin (MSD) at a concentration of 125 mcg/mL in peritoneal dialysis solution (Dianeal 1.5%) exhibited enhanced rates of lethality to *Staphylococcus aureus*, *Escherichia coli*, and *Pseudomonas aeruginosa* compared to any of the drugs alone.[1623]

Gentamicin sulfate (American Pharmaceutical Partners) 8 mcg/mL in Delflex peritoneal dialysis solution bags with 2.5% dextrose (Fresenius) is stable with little or no loss occurring in 14 days refrigerated and at room temperature.[2573]

Gentamicin sulfate (American Pharmaceutical Partners) 8 mcg/mL with vancomycin hydrochloride (Lederle) 25 mcg/mL in Delflex peritoneal dialysis solution bags with 2.5% dextrose (Fresenius) is stable with little or no loss of either drug occurring in 14 days refrigerated and at room temperature.[2573]

Gentamicin sulfate (Pfizer) 20 mg/L in Extraneal with icodextrin 7.5% (Baxter) peritoneal dialysis solution bags exhibited less than 10% loss in 14 days at 37, 25, and 4°C.[3537] Gentamicin sulfate (Pfizer) 20 mg/L with vancomycin hydrochloride (Hospira) 1 g/L in Extraneal with icodextrin 7.5% (Baxter) peritoneal dialysis solution bags exhibited less than 10% loss of either drug in 14 days at 25 and 4°C and 3% loss of gentamicin and 7% loss of vancomycin in 4 days at 37°C.[3537] Gentamicin sulfate (Pfizer) 20 mg/L and cefazolin sodium (Hospira) 500 mg/L in Extraneal with icodextrin 7.5% (Baxter) peritoneal dialysis solution bags exhibited less than 10% loss of either drug in 14 days at 4°C, no loss of gentamicin and 7% loss of cefazolin in 4 days at 25°C, and 1% loss of gentamicin and 5% loss of cefazolin in 1 day at 37°C.[3537]

β-Lactam Antibiotics

In common with other aminoglycoside antibiotics, gentamicin activity may be impaired by β-lactam antibiotics. The inactivation is dependent on concentration, temperature, and time of exposure.[68 219 504 574 575 654 667 740 792 816 824 973 1052 1382]

The clinical significance of these interactions in patients appears to be primarily confined to those with renal failure.[218 334 361 364 616 737 816 847] Literature reports of greatly reduced aminoglycoside levels in such patients have appeared frequently.[363 365 366 367 614 666 962] In addition, the interaction may be clinically important if assays for aminoglycoside levels in serum are sufficiently delayed.[576 618 735 832 847 1052 1382]

Most authors believe that in vitro mixing of penicillins with aminoglycoside antibiotics should be avoided but that clinical use of the drugs in combination can be of great value. It is generally recommended that the drugs be given separately in such combined therapy.[157 218 222 224 361 364 368 369 370]

Local Anesthetics

Gentamicin sulfate 80 mg (2 mL) was physically compatible with 1 mL of each of the following local anesthetics and did not show significant loss in 24 hours at room temperature or under refrigeration:[227]

Lidocaine hydrochloride 1 and 2% (Astra)
Lidocaine hydrochloride 1 and 2% with epinephrine 1:100,000 (Astra)
Mepivacaine hydrochloride 1 and 2% (Winthrop)

Heparin

Addition of gentamicin sulfate (Roussel) 80 mg to the tubing of an infusion solution of sodium chloride 0.9% containing heparin resulted in immediate precipitation.[528]

Gentamicin sulfate 10 mg/L with heparin sodium 1000 units/L in Dianeal with dextrose 5% peritoneal dialysis solution was reported to be conditionally compatible. No significant reduction in gentamicin sulfate concentration occurred in 4 to 6 hours.[228] However, a marked reduction in the anticoagulant activity of heparin sodium occurred if opalescence or a precipitate formed (which results if the undiluted drugs are combined), even if the precipitate redissolved. Heparin activity was retained if one drug was added to a dilute solution of the other and no precipitate formed.[295]

The incompatibility of heparin sodium with gentamicin sulfate is said to result from coprecipitation.[230]

A white precipitate may result from the administration of gentamicin sulfate through a heparinized intravenous cannula.[976] Flushing heparin locks with sodium chloride 0.9% before and after administering drugs incompatible with heparin has been recommended.[4]

Sodium Citrate

The physical stability of gentamicin sulfate (Schering) 1, 2, and 5 mg/mL in sodium citrate 4% anticoagulant solution (Baxter) was evaluated. The combination has been used in preventing hemodialysis catheter-related infections. The gentamicin dilutions were packaged in 3-mL syringes and were stored at 4 and 23°C. The solutions remained clear and colorless for 35 days at both temperatures. The pH was found to be near 5.1 initially and did not change throughout the study. Although the gentamicin content was not measured, the authors pointed out that other studies had reported that the drug in solutions within the pH range of 4 to 7 was stable for up to 90 days. Furthermore, in another study, sodium citrate also had been documented to be stable for 28 days at room temperature.[2631]

Gentamicin sulfate (Sandoz) 2.5 mg/mL in sodium citrate 4% (Cytasol) was found to be physically and chemically stable for 112 days at 24°C packaged in polyethylene plastic syringes sealed with tip caps.[2824]

Selected Revisions May 1, 2020. © Copyright, October 1982. American Society of Health-System Pharmacists, Inc.

Glycopyrrolate
AHFS 12:08.08

Products

Glycopyrrolate is available in 1- and 2-mL single-dose vials and 5- and 20-mL multiple-dose vials. Each mL contains glycopyrrolate 0.2 mg, sodium hydroxide and/or hydrochloric acid to adjust the pH, and benzyl alcohol 0.9% in water for injection.[1(8/06)]

pH

From 2 to 3.[1(8/06)]

Trade Name(s)

Robinul

Administration

Glycopyrrolate may be administered by intravenous or intramuscular injection without dilution. The drug may also be given via the tubing of a running intravenous infusion.[1(8/06) 4]

Stability

Glycopyrrolate is a clear, colorless solution; intact vials should be stored at controlled room temperature.[1(8/06)]

pH Effects

The stability of glycopyrrolate in solution is pH dependent. At pH 2 to 3, the drug is very stable. Above pH 6, the stability becomes questionable because of ester hydrolysis. The speed of this hydrolysis is increased with increasing pH. A significant decline in glycopyrrolate stability as the pH is increased above 6 can be seen in Table 1.[331]

Table 1. Stability of glycopyrrolate 0.8 mg/L in dextrose 5% adjusted to various pH values (25°C)

Admixture pH	Approximate Time for 5% Decomposition (hr)
4	>48
5	>48
6	30
6.5	7
7	4
8	2

Glycopyrrolate 0.8 mg/L in Ringer's injection, lactated, is physically compatible for 48 hours at 25°C. The pH of the solution (6.1) is slightly higher than the pH range yielding acceptable glycopyrrolate stability (2 to 6). However, the drug can be administered via the tubing of a running intravenous infusion of Ringer's injection, lactated.[1(8/06) 4]

Because of the low pH of glycopyrrolate, mixtures with alkaline drugs such as barbiturates result in precipitation of the free acid. If the pH of the admixture is increased above 6 by an alkaline additive or solution, rapid ester hydrolysis of the glycopyrrolate results.[331]

Syringes

Glycopyrrolate (American Regent) 0.1 mg/mL in sodium chloride 0.9% in polypropylene syringes (Sherwood) was physically stable and exhibited little loss in 24 hours stored at 4 and 23°C.[2199]

Glycopyrrolate (Robins) 0.2 mg/mL packaged as 4 mL of undiluted injection in 6-mL polypropylene syringes (Becton Dickinson) was stored at 4 and 25°C exposed to fluorescent light. The injection remained visually clear, and little loss of glycopyrrolate occurred in 90 days at both storage conditions.[2439]

Compatibility Information

Solution Compatibility

Glycopyrrolate

Test Soln Name	Mfr	Mfr	Conc/L or %	Remarks	Ref	C/I
Dextrose 5% in sodium chloride 0.45%	MG	RB	0.8 mg	Physically compatible. pH in glycopyrrolate stability range for 48 hr at 25°C	331	C
Dextrose 5%	AB	RB	0.8 mg	Physically compatible. pH in glycopyrrolate stability range for 48 hr at 25°C	331	C
Dextrose 10%			0.8 mg	Physically compatible	1(8/06)	C
Ringer's injection	AB	RB	0.8 mg	Physically compatible. pH in glycopyrrolate stability range for 48 hr at 25°C	331	C

DOI: 10.37573/9781585286850.187

Solution Compatibility (Cont.)

Test Soln Name	Mfr	Mfr	Conc/L or %	Remarks	Ref	C/I
Ringer's injection, lactated			0.8 mg	Physically compatible for 48 hr at 25°C but pH outside stability range	1(8/06)	I
Sodium chloride 0.9%	CU	RB	0.8 mg	Physically compatible. pH in glycopyrrolate stability range for 48 hr at 25°C	331	C

Additive Compatibility

Glycopyrrolate

Test Drug	Mfr	Conc/L or %	Mfr	Conc/L or %	Test Solution	Remarks	Ref	C/I
Buprenorphine HCl with haloperidol lactate	RKC ON	84 mg 104 mg		25 mg	NS[a]	Visually compatible with less than 10% loss of any drug in 30 days at 4 and 25°C in the dark	2436	C
Haloperidol lactate with buprenorphine HCl	ON RKC	104 mg 84 mg		25 mg	NS[a]	Visually compatible with less than 10% loss of any drug in 30 days at 4 and 25°C in the dark	2436	C
Methylprednisolone sodium succinate	UP	250 mg	RB	1.33 mg	D5½S	Physically incompatible	329	I

[a] Tested in PVC containers.

Drugs in Syringe Compatibility

Glycopyrrolate

Test Drug	Mfr	Amt	Mfr	Amt	Remarks	Ref	C/I
Atropine sulfate	ES	0.4 mg/1 mL	RB	0.2 mg/1 mL	Physically compatible. pH in glycopyrrolate stability range for 48 hr at 25°C	331	C
Atropine sulfate	ES	0.8 mg/2 mL	RB	0.2 mg/1 mL	Physically compatible. pH in glycopyrrolate stability range for 48 hr at 25°C	331	C
Atropine sulfate	ES	0.4 mg/1 mL	RB	0.4 mg/2 mL	Physically compatible. pH in glycopyrrolate stability range for 48 hr at 25°C	331	C
Buprenorphine HCl with haloperidol lactate	RKC ON	4 mg 5 mg		1.2 mg	Diluted to 48 mL with NS. Visually compatible with less than 10% loss of any drug in 30 days at 4 and 25°C in the dark	2436	C
Chloramphenicol sodium succinate	PD	100 mg/1 mL	RB	0.2 mg/1 mL	Gas evolves	331	I
Chloramphenicol sodium succinate	PD	200 mg/2 mL	RB	0.2 mg/1 mL	Gas evolves	331	I
Chloramphenicol sodium succinate	PD	100 mg/1 mL	RB	0.4 mg/2 mL	Gas evolves	331	I
Chlorpromazine HCl	SKF	25 mg/1 mL	RB	0.2 mg/1 mL	Physically compatible. pH in glycopyrrolate stability range for 48 hr at 25°C	331	C
Chlorpromazine HCl	SKF	50 mg/2 mL	RB	0.2 mg/1 mL	Physically compatible. pH in glycopyrrolate stability range for 48 hr at 25°C	331	C
Chlorpromazine HCl	SKF	25 mg/1 mL	RB	0.4 mg/2 mL	Physically compatible. pH in glycopyrrolate stability range for 48 hr at 25°C	331	C
Dexamethasone sodium phosphate	MSD	4 mg/1 mL	RB	0.2 mg/1 mL	Physically compatible for 48 hr at 25°C. pH >6.0. 5% glycopyrrolate loss may occur in 4 to 7 hr	331	I
Dexamethasone sodium phosphate	MSD	8 mg/2 mL	RB	0.2 mg/1 mL	Physically compatible for 48 hr at 25°C. pH >6.0. 5% glycopyrrolate loss may occur in 4 to 7 hr	331	I
Dexamethasone sodium phosphate	MSD	4 mg/1 mL	RB	0.4 mg/2 mL	Physically compatible for 48 hr at 25°C. pH >6.0. 5% glycopyrrolate loss may occur in 4 to 7 hr	331	I

Drugs in Syringe Compatibility (Cont.)

Test Drug	Mfr	Amt	Mfr	Amt	Remarks	Ref	C/I
Dexamethasone sodium phosphate	MSD	24 mg/1 mL	RB	0.2 mg/1 mL	Physically compatible for 48 hr at 25°C. pH >6.0. 5% glycopyrrolate loss may occur in 4 to 7 hr	331	I
Dexamethasone sodium phosphate	MSD	48 mg/2 mL	RB	0.2 mg/1 mL	Physically compatible for 48 hr at 25°C. pH >6.0. 5% glycopyrrolate loss may occur in 4 to 7 hr	331	I
Dexamethasone sodium phosphate	MSD	24 mg/1 mL	RB	0.4 mg/2 mL	Physically compatible for 48 hr at 25°C. pH >6.0. 5% glycopyrrolate loss may occur in 4 to 7 hr	331	I
Diazepam	RC	5 mg/1 mL	RB	0.2 mg/1 mL	Precipitates immediately	331	I
Diazepam	RC	10 mg/2 mL	RB	0.2 mg/1 mL	Precipitates immediately	331	I
Diazepam	RC	5 mg/1 mL	RB	0.4 mg/2 mL	Precipitates immediately	331	I
Dimenhydrinate	SE	50 mg/1 mL	RB	0.2 mg/1 mL	Precipitates immediately	331	I
Dimenhydrinate	SE	100 mg/2 mL	RB	0.2 mg/1 mL	Precipitates immediately	331	I
Dimenhydrinate	SE	50 mg/1 mL	RB	0.4 mg/2 mL	Precipitates immediately	331	I
Diphenhydramine HCl	PD	10 mg/1 mL	RB	0.2 mg/1 mL	Physically compatible. pH in glycopyrrolate stability range for 48 hr at 25°C	331	C
Diphenhydramine HCl	PD	20 mg/2 mL	RB	0.2 mg/1 mL	Physically compatible. pH in glycopyrrolate stability range for 48 hr at 25°C	331	C
Diphenhydramine HCl	PD	10 mg/1 mL	RB	0.4 mg/2 mL	Physically compatible. pH in glycopyrrolate stability range for 48 hr at 25°C	331	C
Diphenhydramine HCl	PD	50 mg/1 mL	RB	0.2 mg/1 mL	Physically compatible. pH in glycopyrrolate stability range for 48 hr at 25°C	331	C
Diphenhydramine HCl	PD	100 mg/2 mL	RB	0.2 mg/1 mL	Physically compatible. pH in glycopyrrolate stability range for 48 hr at 25°C	331	C
Diphenhydramine HCl	PD	50 mg/1 mL	RB	0.4 mg/2 mL	Physically compatible. pH in glycopyrrolate stability range for 48 hr at 25°C	331	C
Droperidol	MN	2.5 mg/1 mL	RB	0.2 mg/1 mL	Physically compatible. pH in glycopyrrolate stability range for 48 hr at 25°C	331	C
Droperidol	MN	5 mg/2 mL	RB	0.2 mg/1 mL	Physically compatible. pH in glycopyrrolate stability range for 48 hr at 25°C	331	C
Droperidol	MN	2.5 mg/1 mL	RB	0.4 mg/2 mL	Physically compatible. pH in glycopyrrolate stability range for 48 hr at 25°C	331	C
Haloperidol lactate with buprenorphine HCl	ON RKC	5 mg 4 mg		1.2 mg	Diluted to 48 mL with NS. Visually compatible with less than 10% loss of any drug in 30 days at 4 and 25°C in the dark	2436	C
Hydromorphone HCl	KN	2 mg/1 mL	RB	0.2 mg/1 mL	Physically compatible. pH in glycopyrrolate stability range for 48 hr at 25°C	331	C
Hydromorphone HCl	KN	4 mg/2 mL	RB	0.2 mg/1 mL	Physically compatible. pH in glycopyrrolate stability range for 48 hr at 25°C	331	C
Hydromorphone HCl	KN	2 mg/1 mL	RB	0.4 mg/2 mL	Physically compatible. pH in glycopyrrolate stability range for 48 hr at 25°C	331	C
Hydroxyzine HCl	PF	25 mg/1 mL	RB	0.2 mg/1 mL	Physically compatible. pH in glycopyrrolate stability range for 48 hr at 25°C	331	C
Hydroxyzine HCl	PF	50 mg/2 mL	RB	0.2 mg/1 mL	Physically compatible. pH in glycopyrrolate stability range for 48 hr at 25°C	331	C
Hydroxyzine HCl	PF	25 mg/1 mL	RB	0.4 mg/2 mL	Physically compatible. pH in glycopyrrolate stability range for 48 hr at 25°C	331	C

Drugs in Syringe Compatibility (Cont.)

Test Drug	Mfr	Amt	Mfr	Amt	Remarks	Ref	C/I
Lidocaine HCl	ES	10 mg/1 mL	RB	0.2 mg/1 mL	Physically compatible. pH in glycopyrrolate stability range for 48 hr at 25°C	331	C
Lidocaine HCl	ES	20 mg/2 mL	RB	0.2 mg/1 mL	Physically compatible. pH in glycopyrrolate stability range for 48 hr at 25°C	331	C
Lidocaine HCl	ES	10 mg/1 mL	RB	0.4 mg/2 mL	Physically compatible. pH in glycopyrrolate stability range for 48 hr at 25°C	331	C
Lidocaine HCl	ES	20 mg/1 mL	RB	0.2 mg/1 mL	Physically compatible. pH in glycopyrrolate stability range for 48 hr at 25°C	331	C
Lidocaine HCl	ES	40 mg/2 mL	RB	0.2 mg/1 mL	Physically compatible. pH in glycopyrrolate stability range for 48 hr at 25°C	331	C
Lidocaine HCl	ES	20 mg/1 mL	RB	0.4 mg/2 mL	Physically compatible. pH in glycopyrrolate stability range for 48 hr at 25°C	331	C
Meperidine HCl	WI	50 mg/1 mL	RB	0.2 mg/1 mL	Physically compatible. pH in glycopyrrolate stability range for 48 hr at 25°C	331	C
Meperidine HCl	WI	100 mg/2 mL	RB	0.2 mg/1 mL	Physically compatible. pH in glycopyrrolate stability range for 48 hr at 25°C	331	C
Meperidine HCl	WI	50 mg/1 mL	RB	0.4 mg/2 mL	Physically compatible. pH in glycopyrrolate stability range for 48 hr at 25°C	331	C
Methohexital sodium	LI	10 mg/1 mL	RB	0.2 mg/1 mL	Precipitates immediately	331	I
Methohexital sodium	LI	20 mg/2 mL	RB	0.2 mg/1 mL	Precipitates immediately	331	I
Methohexital sodium	LI	10 mg/1 mL	RB	0.4 mg/2 mL	Precipitates immediately	331	I
Midazolam HCl	RC	5 mg/1 mL	RB	0.2 mg/1 mL	Physically compatible for 4 hr at 25°C	1145	C
Morphine sulfate	LI	15 mg/1 mL	RB	0.2 mg/1 mL	Physically compatible. pH in glycopyrrolate stability range for 48 hr at 25°C	331	C
Morphine sulfate	LI	30 mg/2 mL	RB	0.2 mg/1 mL	Physically compatible. pH in glycopyrrolate stability range for 48 hr at 25°C	331	C
Morphine sulfate	LI	15 mg/1 mL	RB	0.4 mg/2 mL	Physically compatible. pH in glycopyrrolate stability range for 48 hr at 25°C	331	C
Nalbuphine HCl	DU	10 mg/1 mL	RB	0.2 mg/1 mL	Physically compatible for 48 hr	128	C
Nalbuphine HCl	DU	20 mg/1 mL	RB	0.2 mg/1 mL	Physically compatible for 48 hr	128	C
Neostigmine methyl-sulfate	RC	0.5 mg/1 mL	RB	0.2 mg/1 mL	Physically compatible. pH in glycopyrrolate stability range for 48 hr at 25°C	331	C
Neostigmine methyl-sulfate	RC	1 mg/2 ml	RB	0.2 mg/1 mL	Physically compatible. pH in glycopyrrolate stability range for 48 hr at 25°C	331	C
Neostigmine methyl-sulfate	RC	0.5 mg/1 mL	RB	0.4 mg/2 mL	Physically compatible. pH in glycopyrrolate stability range for 48 hr at 25°C	331	C
Ondansetron HCl	GW	1 mg/mL[a]	AMR	0.1 mg/mL[a]	Physically compatible. Little loss of either drug in 24 hr at 4 or 23°C	2199	C
Pentazocine lactate	WI	30 mg/1 mL	RB	0.2 mg/1 mL	Precipitates immediately	331	I
Pentazocine lactate	WI	60 mg/2 mL	RB	0.2 mg/1 mL	Precipitates immediately	331	I
Pentazocine lactate	WI	30 mg/1 mL	RB	0.4 mg/2 mL	Precipitates immediately	331	I
Pentobarbital sodium	AB	50 mg/1 mL	RB	0.2 mg/1 mL	Precipitates immediately	331	I
Pentobarbital sodium	AB	100 mg/2 mL	RB	0.2 mg/1 mL	Precipitates immediately	331	I
Pentobarbital sodium	AB	50 mg/1 mL	RB	0.4 mg/2 mL	Precipitates immediately	331	I

Drugs in Syringe Compatibility (Cont.)

Test Drug	Mfr	Amt	Mfr	Amt	Remarks	Ref	C/I
Prochlorperazine edisylate	SKF	5 mg/1 mL	RB	0.2 mg/1 mL	Physically compatible. pH in glycopyrrolate stability range for 48 hr at 25°C	331	C
Prochlorperazine edisylate	SKF	10 mg/2 mL	RB	0.2 mg/1 mL	Physically compatible. pH in glycopyrrolate stability range for 48 hr at 25°C	331	C
Prochlorperazine edisylate	SKF	5 mg/1 mL	RB	0.4 mg/2 mL	Physically compatible. pH in glycopyrrolate stability range for 48 hr at 25°C	331	C
Promethazine HCl	WY	25 mg/1 mL	RB	0.2 mg/1 mL	Physically compatible. pH in glycopyrrolate stability range for 48 hr at 25°C	331	C
Promethazine HCl	WY	50 mg/2 mL	RB	0.2 mg/1 mL	Physically compatible. pH in glycopyrrolate stability range for 48 hr at 25°C	331	C
Promethazine HCl	WY	25 mg/1 mL	RB	0.4 mg/2 mL	Physically compatible. pH in glycopyrrolate stability range for 48 hr at 25°C	331	C
Ranitidine HCl	GL	50 mg/2 mL	RB	0.2 mg/1 mL	Physically compatible for 1 hr at 25°C	978	C
Scopolamine HBr	ES	0.4 mg/1 mL	RB	0.2 mg/1 mL	Physically compatible. pH in glycopyrrolate stability range for 48 hr at 25°C	331	C
Scopolamine HBr	ES	0.8 mg/2 mL	RB	0.2 mg/1 mL	Physically compatible. pH in glycopyrrolate stability range for 48 hr at 25°C	331	C
Scopolamine HBr	ES	0.4 mg/1 mL	RB	0.4 mg/2 mL	Physically compatible. pH in glycopyrrolate stability range for 48 hr at 25°C	331	C
Sodium bicarbonate	AB	75 mg/1 mL	RB	0.2 mg/1 mL	Gas evolves	331	I
Sodium bicarbonate	AB	150 mg/2 mL	RB	0.2 mg/1 mL	Gas evolves	331	I
Sodium bicarbonate	AB	75 mg/1 mL	RB	0.4 mg/2 mL	Gas evolves	331	I
Trimethobenzamide HCl	BE	100 mg/1 mL	RB	0.2 mg/1 mL	Physically compatible. pH in glycopyrrolate stability range for 48 hr at 25°C	331	C
Trimethobenzamide HCl	BE	200 mg/2 mL	RB	0.2 mg/1 mL	Physically compatible. pH in glycopyrrolate stability range for 48 hr at 25°C	331	C
Trimethobenzamide HCl	BE	100 mg/1 mL	RB	0.4 mg/2 mL	Physically compatible. pH in glycopyrrolate stability range for 48 hr at 25°C	331	C

a Tested in sodium chloride 0.9%.

Y-Site Injection Compatibility (1:1 Mixture)

Glycopyrrolate

Test Drug	Mfr	Conc	Mfr	Conc	Remarks	Ref	C/I
Palonosetron HCl	MGI	50 mcg/mL	BA	0.2 mg/mL	Physically compatible. No loss of either drug in 4 hr at room temperature	2773	C
Propofol	ZENa	10 mg/mL	RB	0.2 mg/mL	Physically compatible for 1 hr at 23°C	2066	C

a Test performed using the formulation WITH edetate disodium.

Selected Revisions January 31, 2020. © Copyright, October 1982.
American Society of Health-System Pharmacists, Inc.

Granisetron Hydrochloride
AHFS 56:22.20

Products

Granisetron hydrochloride is available in 1-mL single-use and 4-mL multiple-use vials containing in each mL the equivalent of granisetron 1 mg and sodium chloride 9 mg.[3123] [3124] [3125] [3126] Preservatives and other excipients can vary among products and may include benzyl alcohol,[3125] methyl- and propylparaben,[3123] [3126] and phenol.[3124] Sodium hydroxide and/or hydrochloric acid may have been added to adjust the pH.[3123] [3125] [3126] Specific product labeling should be consulted for additional formulation details.

Preservative-free formulations of the 1-mg/mL concentration in 1-mL single-use vial also are available.[3124]

Granisetron hydrochloride also is available in 1-mL single-use vials containing the equivalent of granisetron 0.1 mg and sodium chloride 9 mg.[3123] [3124] [3125] Excipients can vary among products.[3123] [3124] [3125] [3126] Sodium hydroxide and/or hydrochloric acid may have been added to adjust the pH.[3123] [3125] [3126] Specific product labeling should be consulted for additional formulation details.

pH

From 4 to 6[3123] [3124] [3125] or from 4.4 to 5.[3126]

Equivalency

Granisetron hydrochloride 1.12 mg provides 1 mg of granisetron.[3123] [3124] [3125] [3126]

Administration

Granisetron hydrochloride may be administered intravenously undiluted over 30 seconds or by intravenous infusion over 5 minutes after dilution with sodium chloride 0.9% or dextrose 5%.[3123] [3124] [3125] [3126]

Stability

Granisetron hydrochloride is a clear, colorless injection.[3123] [3124] [3125] [3126] Intact vials should be stored at controlled room temperature and retained in the original carton to protect from light; vials should not be frozen.[3123] [3124] [3125] [3126] The unused portion from a single-use vial should be discarded;[3123] the contents of multiple-use vials should be used within 30 days after initial stopper penetration.[3123] [3124] [3125] [3126] Solutions diluted for infusion in sodium chloride 0.9% or dextrose 5% should be prepared at the time of administration, but have been noted to be stable for at least 24 hours when stored at room temperature under normal lighting conditions.[3123] [3124] [3125] [3126] Solutions should be visually inspected for particulate matter and discoloration prior to administration.[3123] [3124] [3125] [3126]

Syringes

Granisetron hydrochloride (SmithKline Beecham) 0.05, 0.07, and 0.1 mg/mL (as granisetron) in sodium chloride 0.9% and in dextrose 5% was repackaged in polypropylene syringes (Sherwood Medical) (closure unspecified). Little or no granisetron hydrochloride loss occurred after 14 days at 5 and 24°C.[1968]

Granisetron hydrochloride (SmithKline Beecham) 1 mg/mL was repackaged into Plastipak (Becton Dickinson) polypropylene syringes and stored at room temperature exposed to or protected from light and refrigerated at 4°C. Little granisetron hydrochloride loss occurred in 15 days under any of these storage conditions.[2149]

Central Venous Catheter

Granisetron hydrochloride (SmithKline Beecham) 10 mcg/mL in dextrose 5% was found to be compatible with the ARROW-g+ard Blue Plus (Arrow International) chlorhexidine-bearing triple-lumen central catheter. Essentially complete delivery of the drug was found with little or no drug loss occurring. Furthermore, chlorhexidine delivered from the catheter remained at trace amounts with no substantial increase due to the delivery of the drug through the catheter.[2335]

Compatibility Information

Solution Compatibility

Granisetron HCl

Test Soln Name	Mfr	Mfr	Conc/L or %	Remarks	Ref	C/I
Dextrose 5% in sodium chloride 0.45%	BA[b]	SKB	20 mg	Physically compatible. Little loss in 24 hr at 20°C under fluorescent light	1883	C
Dextrose 5% in sodium chloride 0.9%	BA[b]	SKB	20 mg	Physically compatible. Little loss in 24 hr at 20°C under fluorescent light	1883	C
Dextrose 5%	BA[b]	SKB	20 mg	Physically compatible. Little loss in 24 hr at 20°C under fluorescent light	1883	C
Dextrose 5%	BA[a]	SKB	200 mg	Physically compatible. Little loss in 24 hr at 20°C under fluorescent light	1883	C
Dextrose 5%		BE	56[b] and 150[a] mg	Visually compatible. Little loss in 30 days at –20°C then 7 days at 4°C then 3 days at 20°C	1884	C

DOI: 10.37573/9781585286850.188

Solution Compatibility (Cont.)

Test Soln Name	Mfr	Mfr	Conc/L or %	Remarks	Ref	C/I
Dextrose 5%	MG[c]	SKB	20 mg	5% or less loss in 14 days at 4°C	1837	C
Sodium chloride 0.9%	BA[b]	SKB	20 mg	Physically compatible. Little loss in 24 hr at 20°C under fluorescent light	1883	C
Sodium chloride 0.9%	BA[a]	SKB	200 mg	Physically compatible. Little loss in 24 hr at 20°C under fluorescent light	1883	C
Sodium chloride 0.9%		BE	56[b] and 150[a] mg	Visually compatible. Little loss in 30 days at –20°C then 7 days at 4°C then 3 days at 20°C	1884	C
Sodium chloride 0.9%	MG[c]	SKB	20 mg	5% or less drug loss in 7 days at 4°C, but 13% loss in 14 days	1837	C

[a] Tested in polypropylene syringes.

[b] Tested in PVC containers.

[c] Tested in Homepump (Block Medical) elastomeric reservoir pumps.

Additive Compatibility

Granisetron HCl

Test Drug	Mfr	Conc/L or %	Mfr	Conc/L or %	Test Solution	Remarks	Ref	C/I
Butorphanol tartrate	HE	80 mg	NIN	30 and 60 mg	NS[e]	Physically compatible with little to no loss of either drug in 14 days at 4°C protected from light or 48 hr at 25°C in room light	3120	C
Butorphanol tartrate	HE	80 mg	NIN	30 and 60 mg	NS[f]	Physically compatible with little to no loss of either drug in 14 days at 4°C protected from light or 48 hr at 25°C in room light	3120	C
Dexamethasone sodium phosphate	AMR	92 mg	SKB	10 and 40 mg	D5W, NS[a]	Visually compatible. Little loss of either drug in 14 days at 4 and 24°C in dark	1875	C
Dexamethasone sodium phosphate	AMR	660 mg	SKB	10 and 40 mg	D5W, NS[a]	Visually compatible. Little dexamethasone and 8% granisetron loss in 14 days at 4 and 24°C in dark	1875	C
Dexamethasone sodium phosphate	MSD	75 and 345 mg	BE	55 and 51 mg	D5W, NS[a]	Visually compatible. Little loss of either drug in 72 hr at room temperature	1884	C
Dexamethasone sodium phosphate	[d]	100 mg		26 mg	NS	Physically compatible for 24 hr at 25°C in light	2999	C
Fosaprepitant dime-glumine	MSD	1 g		26 mg	NS	Physically compatible for 24 hr at 25°C in light	2999	C
Fosaprepitant dime-glumine	MSD[b]	1 g		26 mg	NS	Physically compatible for 24 hr at 25°C in light	2999	C
Fosaprepitant dime-glumine	MSD[c]	1 g		26 mg	NS	Physically compatible for 24 hr at 25°C in light	2999	C
Methylprednisolone sodium succinate	DAK	2.26 g	BE	56 mg	D5W, NS[a]	Visually compatible. Little loss of either drug in 72 hr at room temperature	1884	C
Methylprednisolone sodium succinate	[d]	700 mg		26 mg		Physically compatible for 24 hr at 25°C in light	2999	C

[a] Tested in PVC containers.

[b] Tested with dexamethasone sodium phosphate 100 mg/L.

[c] Tested with methylprednisolone sodium succinate 700 mg/L.

[d] Tested with fosaprepitant dimeglumine (MSD) 1 g/L.

[e] Tested in polyolefin containers.

[f] Tested in glass containers.

Drugs in Syringe Compatibility

Granisetron HCl

Test Drug	Mfr	Amt	Mfr	Amt	Remarks	Ref	C/I
Dexamethasone sodium phosphate	MSD	0.2 and 1 mg/mL[a]	BE	0.15 mg/mL[a]	Visually compatible. Little loss of either drug in 72 hr at room temperature	1884	C
Methylprednisolone sodium succinate	DAK	6 mg/mL[a]	BE	0.15 mg/mL[a]	Visually compatible. Little loss of either drug in 72 hr at room temperature	1884	C

[a] Diluted with water.

Y-Site Injection Compatibility (1:1 Mixture)

Granisetron HCl

Test Drug	Mfr	Conc	Mfr	Conc	Remarks	Ref	C/I
Acetaminophen	CAD	10 mg/mL	APO, TE	0.1 mg/mL	Physically compatible with less than 10% acetaminophen loss over 4 hr at room temperature	2841, 2844	C
Acetaminophen	CAD	10 mg/mL	WOC	1 mg/mL	Physically compatible with little loss of either drug in 4 hr at 23°C	2901, 2902	C
Acyclovir sodium	BW	7 mg/mL[a]	SKB	0.05 mg/mL[a]	Physically compatible for 4 hr at 23°C	2000	C
Acyclovir sodium	BV	5 mg/mL[b]	RC	1 mg/mL	Crystals form	2794	I
Allopurinol sodium	BW	3 mg/mL[a]	SKB	0.05 mg/mL[a]	Physically compatible for 4 hr at 23°C	2000	C
Amifostine	USB	10 mg/mL[a]	SKB	0.05 mg/mL[a]	Physically compatible for 4 hr at 23°C	2000	C
Amikacin sulfate	AB	5 mg/mL[a]	SKB	0.05 mg/mL[a]	Physically compatible for 4 hr at 23°C	2000	C
Aminophylline	AB	2.5 mg/mL[a]	SKB	0.05 mg/mL[a]	Physically compatible for 4 hr at 23°C	2000	C
Amphotericin B	PH	0.6 mg/mL[a]	SKB	0.05 mg/mL[a]	Large increase in measured turbidity occurs immediately	2000	I
Ampicillin sodium	MAR	20 mg/mL[b]	SKB	0.05 mg/mL[a]	Physically compatible for 4 hr at 23°C	2000	C
Ampicillin sodium–sulbactam sodium	RR	20 mg/mL[b i]	SKB	0.05 mg/mL[a]	Physically compatible for 4 hr at 23°C	2000	C
Amsacrine	NCI	1 mg/mL[a]	SKB	0.05 mg/mL[a]	Physically compatible for 4 hr at 23°C. Precipitate forms in 24 hr	2000	C
Aztreonam	SQ	40 mg/mL[a]	SKB	0.05 mg/mL[a]	Physically compatible for 4 hr at 23°C	2000	C
Bleomycin sulfate	MJ	1 unit/mL[b]	SKB	0.05 mg/mL[a]	Physically compatible for 4 hr at 23°C	2000	C
Bumetanide	RC	0.04 mg/mL[a]	SKB	0.05 mg/mL[a]	Physically compatible for 4 hr at 23°C	2000	C
Buprenorphine HCl	RKC	0.04 mg/mL[a]	SKB	0.05 mg/mL[a]	Physically compatible for 4 hr at 23°C	2000	C
Butorphanol tartrate	APC	0.04 mg/mL[a]	SKB	0.05 mg/mL[a]	Physically compatible for 4 hr at 23°C	2000	C
Calcium gluconate	AB	40 mg/mL[a]	SKB	0.05 mg/mL[a]	Physically compatible for 4 hr at 23°C	2000	C
Carboplatin	BR	1 mg/mL[b]	SKB	1 mg/mL	Physically compatible with little or no loss of either drug in 4 hr at 22°C	1883	C
Carmustine	BMS	1.5 mg/mL[a]	SKB	0.05 mg/mL[a]	Physically compatible for 4 hr at 23°C	2000	C
Cefazolin sodium	SKB	20 mg/mL[a]	SKB	0.05 mg/mL[a]	Physically compatible for 4 hr at 23°C	2000	C
Cefepime HCl	BMS	20 mg/mL[a]	SKB	0.05 mg/mL[a]	Physically compatible for 4 hr at 23°C	2000	C
Cefotaxime sodium	HO	20 mg/mL[a]	SKB	0.05 mg/mL[a]	Physically compatible for 4 hr at 23°C	2000	C
Cefotetan disodium	STU	20 mg/mL[a]	SKB	0.05 mg/mL[a]	Physically compatible for 4 hr at 23°C	2000	C

Y-Site Injection Compatibility (1:1 Mixture) (Cont.)

Test Drug	Mfr	Conc	Mfr	Conc	Remarks	Ref	C/I
Cefoxitin sodium	ME	20 mg/mL[a]	SKB	0.05 mg/mL[a]	Physically compatible for 4 hr at 23°C	2000	C
Ceftaroline fosamil	FOR	2.22 mg/mL[a b c]	CUP	50 mcg/mL[a b c]	Physically compatible for 4 hr at 23°C	2826	C
Ceftazidime	SKB	16.7 mg/mL[b]	SKB	1 mg/mL	Physically compatible with little or no loss of either drug in 4 hr at 22°C	1883	C
Ceftriaxone sodium	RC	20 mg/mL[a]	SKB	0.05 mg/mL[a]	Physically compatible for 4 hr at 23°C	2000	C
Cefuroxime sodium	LI	30 mg/mL[a]	SKB	0.05 mg/mL[a]	Physically compatible for 4 hr at 23°C	2000	C
Chlorpromazine HCl	SCN	2 mg/mL[a]	SKB	0.05 mg/mL[a]	Physically compatible for 4 hr at 23°C	2000	C
Ciprofloxacin	MI	1 mg/mL[a]	SKB	0.05 mg/mL[a]	Physically compatible for 4 hr at 23°C	2000	C
Cisplatin	BR	0.05 mg/mL[b]	SKB	1 mg/mL	Physically compatible with little or no granisetron loss in 4 hr at 22°C	1883	C
Cisplatin	BR	1 mg/mL	SKB	1 mg/mL	Physically compatible with little or no loss of either drug in 4 hr at 22°C	1883	C
Cladribine	ORT	0.015[b] and 0.5[d] mg/mL	SKB	0.05 mg/mL[b]	Physically compatible for 4 hr at 23°C	1969	C
Clindamycin phosphate	AB	10 mg/mL[a]	SKB	0.05 mg/mL[a]	Physically compatible for 4 hr at 23°C	2000	C
Cyclophosphamide	MJ	2 mg/mL[b]	SKB	1 mg/mL	Physically compatible with little loss of either drug in 4 hr at 22°C	1883	C
Cytarabine	UP	2 mg/mL[b]	SKB	1 mg/mL	Physically compatible with little loss of either drug in 4 hr at 22°C	1883	C
Cytarabine	UP	50 mg/mL	SKB	0.05 mg/mL[a]	Physically compatible for 4 hr at 23°C	2000	C
Dacarbazine	MI	1.7 mg/mL[b]	SKB	1 mg/mL	Physically compatible with little loss of either drug in 4 hr at 22°C	1883	C
Dactinomycin	ME	0.01 mg/mL[a]	SKB	0.05 mg/mL[a]	Physically compatible for 4 hr at 23°C	2000	C
Daunorubicin HCl	CHI	1 mg/mL[a]	SKB	0.05 mg/mL[a]	Physically compatible for 4 hr at 23°C	2000	C
Dexamethasone sodium phosphate	ME	0.24 mg/mL[b]	SKB	1 mg/mL	Physically compatible with little or no loss of either drug in 4 hr at 22°C	1883	C
Dexmedetomidine HCl	AB	4 mcg/mL[b]	SKB	50 mcg/mL[b]	Physically compatible for 4 hr at 23°C	2383	C
Diphenhydramine HCl	PD	1 mg/mL[b]	SKB	1 mg/mL	Physically compatible with little loss of either drug in 4 hr at 22°C	1883	C
Diphenhydramine HCl	SCN	2 mg/mL[a]	SKB	0.05 mg/mL[a]	Physically compatible for 4 hr at 23°C	2000	C
Dobutamine HCl	BA	4 mg/mL[a]	SKB	0.05 mg/mL[a]	Physically compatible for 4 hr at 23°C	2000	C
Docetaxel	RPR	0.9 mg/mL[a]	SKB	0.05 mg/mL[a]	Physically compatible for 4 hr at 23°C	2224	C
Dopamine HCl	AB	3.2 mg/mL[a]	SKB	0.05 mg/mL[a]	Physically compatible for 4 hr at 23°C	2000	C
Doripenem	JJ	5 mg/mL[a b]	RC	0.05 mg/mL[a b]	Physically compatible for 4 hr at 23°C	2743	C
Doxorubicin HCl	AD	0.2 mg/mL[b]	SKB	1 mg/mL	Physically compatible with little loss of either drug in 4 hr at 22°C	1883	C
Doxorubicin HCl liposomal	SEQ	0.4 mg/mL[a]	SKB	0.05 mg/mL[a]	Physically compatible for 4 hr at 23°C	2087	C
Doxycycline hyclate	LY	1 mg/mL[a]	SKB	0.05 mg/mL[a]	Physically compatible for 4 hr at 23°C	2000	C

Y-Site Injection Compatibility (1:1 Mixture) (Cont.)

Test Drug	Mfr	Conc	Mfr	Conc	Remarks	Ref	C/I
Droperidol	AB	0.4 mg/mL[a]	SKB	0.05 mg/mL[a]	Physically compatible for 4 hr at 23°C	2000	C
Enalaprilat	MSD	0.1 mg/mL[a]	SKB	0.05 mg/mL[a]	Physically compatible for 4 hr at 23°C	2000	C
Etoposide	BMS	0.4 mg/mL[b]	SKB	1 mg/mL	Physically compatible with little or no loss of either drug in 4 hr at 22°C	1883	C
Etoposide	BR	0.4 mg/mL[a]	SKB	0.05 mg/mL[a]	Physically compatible for 4 hr at 23°C	2000	C
Etoposide phosphate	BR	5 mg/mL[a]	SKB	0.05 mg/mL[a]	Physically compatible for 4 hr at 23°C	2218	C
Famotidine	ME	2 mg/mL[a]	SKB	0.05 mg/mL[a]	Physically compatible for 4 hr at 23°C	2000	C
Fenoldopam mesylate	AB	80 mcg/mL[b]	SKB	50 mcg/mL[b]	Physically compatible for 4 hr at 23°C	2467	C
Filgrastim	AMG	30 mcg/mL[a]	SKB	0.05 mg/mL[a]	Physically compatible for 4 hr at 23°C	2000	C
Floxuridine	RC	3 mg/mL[a]	SKB	0.05 mg/mL[a]	Physically compatible for 4 hr at 23°C	2000	C
Fluconazole	PF	2 mg/mL	SKB	0.05 mg/mL[a]	Physically compatible for 4 hr at 23°C	2000	C
Fludarabine phosphate	BX	1 mg/mL[a]	SKB	0.05 mg/mL[a]	Physically compatible for 4 hr at 23°C	2000	C
Fluorouracil	AD	16 mg/mL[a]	SKB	0.05 mg/mL[a]	Physically compatible for 4 hr at 23°C	1804	C
Fluorouracil	RC	2 mg/mL[b]	SKB	1 mg/mL	Physically compatible with little or no loss of either drug in 4 hr at 22°C	1883	C
Fluorouracil	AD	16 mg/mL[a]	SKB	0.05 mg/mL[a]	Physically compatible for 4 hr at 23°C	2000	C
Furosemide	AB	3 mg/mL[a]	SKB	0.05 mg/mL[a]	Physically compatible for 4 hr at 23°C	1804	C
Furosemide	HO	0.4 mg/mL[b]	SKB	1 mg/mL	Physically compatible with little or no loss of either drug in 4 hr at 22°C	1883	C
Gallium nitrate	FUJ	0.4 mg/mL[a]	SKB	0.05 mg/mL[a]	Physically compatible for 4 hr at 23°C	2000	C
Ganciclovir sodium	SY	20 mg/mL[a]	SKB	0.05 mg/mL[a]	Physically compatible for 4 hr at 23°C	2000	C
Gemcitabine HCl	LI	10 mg/mL[b]	SKB	0.05 mg/mL[b]	Physically compatible for 4 hr at 23°C	2226	C
Gentamicin sulfate	ES	1.5 mg/mL[b]	SKB	1 mg/mL	Physically compatible with little loss of either drug in 4 hr at 22°C	1883	C
Haloperidol lactate	MN	0.2 mg/mL[a]	SKB	0.05 mg/mL[a]	Physically compatible for 4 hr at 23°C	2000	C
Heparin sodium	AB	100 units/mL[a]	SKB	0.05 mg/mL[a]	Physically compatible for 4 hr at 23°C	2000	C
Hetastarch in lactated electrolyte	AB	6%	SKB	0.05 mg/mL[a]	Physically compatible for 4 hr at 23°C	2339	C
Hydrocortisone sodium succinate	AB	1 mg/mL[a]	SKB	0.05 mg/mL[a]	Physically compatible for 4 hr at 23°C	2000	C
Hydromorphone HCl	KN	0.5 mg/mL[b]	SKB	1 mg/mL	Physically compatible with little or no loss of either drug in 4 hr at 22°C	1883	C
Hydromorphone HCl	ES	0.5 mg/mL[a]	SKB	0.05 mg/mL[a]	Physically compatible for 4 hr at 23°C	2000	C
Hydroxyzine HCl	ES	2 mg/mL[a]	SKB	0.05 mg/mL[a]	Physically compatible for 4 hr at 23°C	2000	C
Idarubicin HCl	AD	0.5 mg/mL[a]	SKB	0.05 mg/mL[a]	Physically compatible for 4 hr at 23°C	2000	C
Ifosfamide	MJ	4 mg/mL[b]	SKB	1 mg/mL	Physically compatible with little or no loss of either drug in 4 hr at 22°C	1883	C
Imipenem–cilastatin sodium	ME	10 mg/mL[a i]	SKB	0.05 mg/mL[a]	Physically compatible for 4 hr at 23°C	2000	C

Y-Site Injection Compatibility (1:1 Mixture) (Cont.)

Test Drug	Mfr	Conc	Mfr	Conc	Remarks	Ref	C/I
Leucovorin calcium	IMM	2 mg/mL[a]	SKB	0.05 mg/mL[a]	Physically compatible for 4 hr at 23°C	2000	C
Levoleucovorin calcium	LE	2 mg/mL[a]	SKB	0.05 mg/mL[a]	Physically compatible with no change in measured turbidity or increase in particle content in 4 hr at 23°C	2000	C
Linezolid	PHU	2 mg/mL	SKB	0.05 mg/mL[a]	Physically compatible for 4 hr at 23°C	2264	C
Lorazepam	WY	0.1 mg/mL[b]	SKB	1 mg/mL	Physically compatible with little or no loss of either drug in 4 hr at 22°C	1883	C
Lorazepam	WY	0.1 mg/mL[a]	SKB	0.05 mg/mL[a]	Physically compatible for 4 hr at 23°C	2000	C
Magnesium sulfate	AB	16 mg/mL[b]	SKB	1 mg/mL	Physically compatible with little or no loss of granisetron in 4 hr at 22°C	1883	C
Magnesium sulfate	AB	100 mg/mL[a]	SKB	0.05 mg/mL[a]	Physically compatible for 4 hr at 23°C	2000	C
Mechlorethamine HCl	MSD	0.5 mg/mL[b]	SKB	1 mg/mL	Physically compatible with little or no loss of either drug in 4 hr at 22°C	1883	C
Melphalan HCl	BW	0.1 mg/mL[b]	SKB	0.05 mg/mL[a]	Physically compatible for 4 hr at 23°C	2000	C
Meperidine HCl	WY	4 mg/mL[a]	SKB	0.05 mg/mL[a]	Physically compatible for 4 hr at 23°C	2000	C
Meropenem		50 mg/mL	OM	1 mg/mL	Physically compatible for 4 hr at room temperature	3538	C
Mesna	MJ	4 mg/mL[b]	SKB	1 mg/mL	Physically compatible with little or no loss of either drug in 4 hr at 22°C	1883	C
Methotrexate sodium	CET	12.5 mg/mL[b]	SKB	1 mg/mL	Physically compatible with little or no loss of either drug in 4 hr at 22°C	1883	C
Methylprednisolone sodium succinate	WY	5 mg/mL[a]	SKB	0.05 mg/mL[a]	Physically compatible for 4 hr at 23°C	2000	C
Metoclopramide HCl	AB	5 mg/mL	SKB	0.05 mg/mL[a]	Physically compatible for 4 hr at 23°C	2000	C
Metronidazole	BA	5 mg/mL	SKB	0.05 mg/mL[a]	Physically compatible for 4 hr at 23°C	2000	C
Mitomycin	BMS	0.5 mg/mL	SKB	0.05 mg/mL[a]	Physically compatible for 4 hr at 23°C	2000	C
Mitoxantrone HCl	IMM	0.5 mg/mL[a]	SKB	0.05 mg/mL[a]	Physically compatible for 4 hr at 23°C	2000	C
Morphine sulfate	AST	1 mg/mL[b]	SKB	1 mg/mL	Physically compatible with little or no loss of either drug in 4 hr at 22°C	1883	C
Morphine sulfate	AST	1 mg/mL[a]	SKB	0.05 mg/mL[a]	Physically compatible for 4 hr at 23°C	2000	C
Nalbuphine HCl	AB	10 mg/mL	SKB	0.05 mg/mL[a]	Physically compatible for 4 hr at 23°C	2000	C
Oxaliplatin	SS	0.5 mg/mL[a]	SKB	0.05 mg/mL[a]	Physically compatible for 4 hr at 23°C	2566	C
Paclitaxel	MJ	0.3 mg/mL[b]	SKB	1 mg/mL	Physically compatible with little or no loss of either drug in 4 hr at 22°C	1883	C
Paclitaxel	MJ	1.2 mg/mL[a]	SKB	0.05 mg/mL[a]	Physically compatible for 4 hr at 23°C	2000	C
Pemetrexed disodium	LI	20 mg/mL[b]	RC	0.05 mg/mL[a]	Physically compatible for 4 hr at 23°C	2564	C
Piperacillin sodium–tazobactam sodium	CY[h]	40 mg/mL[a j]	SKB	0.05 mg/mL[a]	Physically compatible for 4 hr at 23°C	2000	C
Potassium chloride	LY	0.04 mEq/mL[b]	SKB	1 mg/mL	Physically compatible with little or no loss of granisetron in 4 hr at 22°C	1883	C
Prochlorperazine edisylate	SCN	0.5 mg/mL[a]	SKB	0.05 mg/mL[a]	Physically compatible for 4 hr at 23°C	2000	C
Promethazine HCl	WY	2 mg/mL[a]	SKB	0.05 mg/mL[a]	Physically compatible for 4 hr at 23°C	2000	C

Y-Site Injection Compatibility (1:1 Mixture) (Cont.)

Test Drug	Mfr	Conc	Mfr	Conc	Remarks	Ref	C/I
Propofol	ZEN[m]	10 mg/mL	SKB	0.05 mg/mL[a]	Physically compatible for 1 hr at 23°C	2066	C
Ranitidine HCl	GL	2 mg/mL[a]	SKB	0.05 mg/mL[a]	Physically compatible for 4 hr at 23°C	2000	C
Sargramostim	IMM	10 mcg/mL[b]	SKB	0.05 mg/mL[a]	Physically compatible for 4 hr at 23°C	2000	C
Sodium bicarbonate	AB	1 mEq/mL	SKB	0.05 mg/mL[a]	Physically compatible for 4 hr at 23°C	1804	C
Sodium bicarbonate	AB	0.33 mEq/mL[b]	SKB	1 mg/mL	Physically compatible with 8% loss of granisetron in 4 hr at 22°C	1883	C
Sodium bicarbonate	AB	1 mEq/mL	SKB	0.05 mg/mL[a]	Physically compatible for 4 hr at 23°C	2000	C
Streptozocin	UP	9.1 mg/mL[b]	SKB	1 mg/mL	Physically compatible with little or no loss of either drug in 4 hr at 22°C	1883	C
Teniposide	BMS	0.1 mg/mL[a]	SKB	0.05 mg/mL[a]	Physically compatible for 4 hr at 23°C	2000	C
Thiotepa	IMM[f]	1 mg/mL[a]	SKB	0.05 mg/mL[a]	Physically compatible for 4 hr at 23°C	1861	C
TNA #218 to #226[g]			SKB	0.05 mg/mL[a]	Visually compatible for 4 hr at 23°C	2215	C
Tobramycin sulfate	AB	5 mg/mL[a]	SKB	0.05 mg/mL[a]	Physically compatible for 4 hr at 23°C	2000	C
Topotecan HCl	SKB	56 mcg/mL[a b]	SKB	20 mcg/mL[a b]	Visually compatible. Little loss of either drug in 4 hr at 22°C	2245	C
TPN #212 to #215[g]			SKB	0.05 mg/mL[a]	Physically compatible for 4 hr at 23°C	2109	C
Trimethoprim–sulfamethoxazole	ES	0.8 mg/mL[a k]	SKB	0.05 mg/mL[a]	Physically compatible for 4 hr at 23°C	2000	C
Vancomycin HCl	AB	10 mg/mL[a]	SKB	0.05 mg/mL[a]	Physically compatible for 4 hr at 23°C	2000	C
Vinblastine sulfate	LI	0.12 mg/mL[a]	SKB	0.05 mg/mL[a]	Physically compatible for 4 hr at 23°C	2000	C
Vincristine sulfate	LI	0.01 and 0.34 mg/mL[b]	SKB	1 mg/mL	Physically compatible with little or no loss of either drug in 4 hr at 22°C	1883	C
Vinorelbine tartrate	BW	1 mg/mL[a]	SKB	0.05 mg/mL[a]	Physically compatible for 4 hr at 23°C	2000	C
Zidovudine	BW	4 mg/mL[a]	SKB	0.05 mg/mL[a]	Physically compatible for 4 hr at 23°C	2000	C

[a] Tested in dextrose 5%.

[b] Tested in sodium chloride 0.9%.

[c] Tested in Ringer's injection, lactated.

[d] Tested in bacteriostatic sodium chloride 0.9% preserved with benzyl alcohol 0.9%.

[e] Granisetron HCl tested in both sodium chloride 0.9% and dextrose 5%.

[f] Lyophilized formulation tested.

[g] Refer to Appendix for the composition of parenteral nutrition solutions. TNA indicates a 3-in-1 admixture, and TPN indicates a 2-in-1 admixture.

[h] Test performed using the formulation WITHOUT edetate disodium.

[i] Ampicillin component. Ampicillin in a 2:1 fixed-ratio concentration with sulbactam.

[j] Piperacillin component. Piperacillin in an 8:1 fixed-ratio concentration with tazobactam.

[k] Trimethoprim component. Trimethoprim in a 1:5 fixed-ratio concentration with sulfamethoxazole.

[l] Not specified whether concentration refers to single component or combined components.

[m] Test performed using the formulation WITH edetate disodium.

Selected Revisions May 1, 2020. © Copyright, October 1996.
American Society of Health-System Pharmacists, Inc.

Haloperidol Lactate
AHFS 28:16.08.08

Products

Haloperidol lactate is available in 1-mL ampuls and vials and 10-mL multiple-dose vials. Each mL of solution contains haloperidol 5 mg (as the lactate) and lactic acid for pH adjustment.[1(2/08)]

pH
From 3 to 3.6[1(2/08)] or 3.8.[17]

Trade Name(s)
Haldol

Administration

Haloperidol lactate should be administered intramuscularly,[1(2/08)] [4] although intravenous administration has been performed.[4] [571] [1258]

Stability

Haloperidol lactate should be stored at controlled room temperature and protected from light; freezing and temperatures above 40°C should be avoided.[1(2/08)] [4]

Central Venous Catheter

Haloperidol lactate (McNeil) 0.2 mg/mL in dextrose 5% was found to be compatible with the ARROWg+ard Blue Plus (Arrow International) chlorhexidine-bearing triple-lumen central catheter. Essentially complete delivery of the drug was found with little or no drug loss occurring. Furthermore, chlorhexidine delivered from the catheter remained at trace amounts with no substantial increase due to the delivery of the drug through the catheter.[2335]

Compatibility Information

Solution Compatibility

Haloperidol lactate

Test Soln Name	Mfr	Mfr	Conc/L or %	Remarks	Ref	C/I
Dextrose 5% in sodium chloride 0.225%	AB	MN	0.1 to 1 g	Visually compatible for 7 days at 21°C	1740	C
Dextrose 5% in sodium chloride 0.225%	AB	MN	2 and 3 g	Precipitate forms in 30 to 60 min	1740	I
Dextrose 5%	TR[a]	MN	100 mg	Physically compatible and stable for 38 days at 24°C	571	C
Dextrose 5%	AB	MN	0.1 to 3 g	Visually compatible for 7 days at 21°C	1740	C
Ringer's injection, lactated	AB	MN	0.1 to 1 g	Visually compatible for 7 days at 21°C	1740	C
Ringer's injection, lactated	AB	MN	2 g	Precipitate forms within 15 min	1740	I
Ringer's injection, lactated	AB	MN	3 g	Precipitate forms immediately	1740	I
Sodium chloride 0.45%	AB	MN	0.1 to 1 g	Visually compatible for 7 days at 21°C	1740	C
Sodium chloride 0.45%	AB	MN	2 g	Precipitate forms within 15 min	1740	I
Sodium chloride 0.45%	AB	MN	3 g	Precipitate forms immediately	1740	I
Sodium chloride 0.9%	AB[b]	MN	2 and 3 g	Slight precipitate forms immediately and becomes much heavier within 15 to 30 min	1523	I
Sodium chloride 0.9%	AB[b]	MN	1 g	Slight precipitate forms immediately and persists through 8 hr	1523	I
Sodium chloride 0.9%	AB[b]	MN	100 and 500 mg	Visually compatible for 8 hr at 21°C under fluorescent light	1523	C
Sodium chloride 0.9%	AB	MN	0.1 to 0.75 g	Visually compatible for 7 days at 21°C	1740	C
Sodium chloride 0.9%	AB	MN	1 to 3 g	Precipitate forms immediately	1740	I

[a] Tested in both glass and PVC containers.

[b] Tested in glass containers.

DOI: 10.37573/9781585286850.189

Additive Compatibility

Haloperidol lactate

Test Drug	Mfr	Conc/L or %	Mfr	Conc/L or %	Test Solution	Remarks	Ref	C/I
Buprenorphine HCl with glycopyrrolate	RKC	84 mg 25 mg	ON	104 mg	NS[a]	Visually compatible with less than 10% loss of any drug in 30 days at 4 and 25°C in the dark	2436	C
Glycopyrrolate with buprenorphine HCl	RKC	25 mg 84 mg	ON	104 mg	NS[a]	Visually compatible with less than 10% loss of any drug in 30 days at 4 and 25°C in the dark	2436	C
Oxycodone HCl	NAP	1 g	JC	125 mg	NS, W	Visually compatible. Under 4% concentration change in 24 hr at 25°C	2600	C
Tramadol HCl	AND	11.18 g	EST	210 mg	NS[b]	Visually compatible for 7 days at 25°C protected from light	2701	C
Tramadol HCl	AND	33.3 g	EST	620 mg	NS[b]	Visually compatible for 7 days at 25°C protected from light	2701	C

[a] Tested in PVC containers.

[b] Tested in elastomeric pump reservoirs (Baxter).

Drugs in Syringe Compatibility

Haloperidol lactate

Test Drug	Mfr	Amt	Mfr	Amt	Remarks	Ref	C/I
Benztropine mesylate	MSD	2 mg	MN	0.25, 0.5, 1 mg	Visually compatible for 24 hr at 21°C	1781	C
Benztropine mesylate	MSD	2 mg	MN	2 mg	Precipitate forms within 4 hr at 21°C	1781	I
Benztropine mesylate	MSD	2 mg	MN	3, 4, 5 mg	Precipitate forms within 15 min at 21°C	1781	I
Benztropine mesylate	MSD	1 mg	MN	0.25 and 0.5 mg	Visually compatible for 24 hr at 21°C	1781	C
Benztropine mesylate	MSD	1 mg	MN	1 to 5 mg	Precipitate forms within 15 min at 21°C	1781	I
Benztropine mesylate	MSD	0.5 mg	MN	0.25 to 5 mg	Precipitate forms within 15 min at 21°C	1781	I
Benztropine mesylate	MSD	2 mg/2 mL	MN	10 mg/2 mL	White precipitate forms within 5 min	1784	I
Buprenorphine HCl with glycopyrrolate	RKC	4 mg 1.2 mg	ON	5 mg	Diluted to 48 mL with NS. Visually compatible with less than 10% loss of any drug in 30 days at 4 and 25°C in the dark	2436	C
Cyclizine lactate	WEL	150 mg/3 mL	SE	1.5 mg/0.3 mL	Diluted with 17 mL of NS. Crystals of cyclizine form within 24 hr at 25°C	1761	I
Cyclizine lactate	WEL	150 mg/3 mL	SE	1.5 mg/0.3 mL	Diluted with 17 mL of D5W or W. Visually compatible for 24 hr at 25°C	1761	C
Cyclizine lactate with diamorphine HCl	WEL BP	16 mg/mL 11 mg/mL	JC	2.2 mg/mL	Physically compatible with less than 10% loss of any drug in 7 days at 23°C	2071	C
Cyclizine lactate with diamorphine HCl	WEL BP	25 mg/mL 16 mg/mL	JC	2.2 mg/mL	Physically compatible with less than 10% loss of any drug in 7 days at 23°C	2071	C
Cyclizine lactate with diamorphine HCl	WEL BP	11 mg/mL 40 mg/mL	JC	2.2 mg/mL	Physically compatible with less than 10% loss of any drug in 7 days at 23°C	2071	C
Cyclizine lactate with diamorphine HCl	WEL BP	13 mg/mL 42 mg/mL	JC	2.1 mg/mL	Physically compatible with less than 10% loss of any drug in 7 days at 23°C	2071	C
Cyclizine lactate with diamorphine HCl	WEL BP	9 mg/mL 55 mg/mL	JC	2.1 mg/mL	Physically compatible with less than 10% loss of any drug in 7 days at 23°C	2071	C

Drugs in Syringe Compatibility (Cont.)

Test Drug	Mfr	Amt	Mfr	Amt	Remarks	Ref	C/I
Cyclizine lactate with diamorphine HCl	WEL BP	13 mg/mL 56 mg/mL	JC	2.1 mg/mL	Physically compatible with less than 10% loss of any drug in 7 days at 23°C	2071	C
Diamorphine HCl	MB	10, 25, 50 mg/1 mL	SE	1.5 mg/1 mL[a]	Physically compatible and diamorphine content retained for 24 hr at room temperature	1454	C
Diamorphine HCl	EV	20 mg/1 mL	SE	2 mg/1 mL	Crystallization with 58% haloperidol loss in 7 days at room temperature	1455	I
Diamorphine HCl	EV	50 and 150 mg/1 mL	SE	5 mg/1 mL	Precipitates immediately	1455	I
Diamorphine HCl	EV	100 mg/8 mL	SE	2.5 mg/8 mL	Physically compatible for 24 hr at room temperature and 7 days at 6°C	1456	C
Diamorphine HCl	HC	20 to 100 mg/mL	SE	0.75 mg/mL	Visually compatible for 48 hr at 5 and 20°C	1672	C
Diamorphine HCl	HC	2 mg/mL	SE	0.75 mg/mL	5% diamorphine loss in 14.8 days at 20°C. Haloperidol stable for 45 days	1672	C
Diamorphine HCl	HC	20 mg/mL	SE	0.75 mg/mL	5% diamorphine loss in 20.7 days at 20°C. Haloperidol stable for 45 days	1672	C
Diamorphine HCl	BP	20, 50, 100 mg/mL	JC	2 and 3 mg/mL	Physically compatible with less than 10% loss of either drug in 7 days at 23°C	2071	C
Diamorphine HCl	BP	20 and 50 mg/mL	JC	4 mg/mL	Physically compatible with less than 10% loss of either drug in 7 days at 23°C	2071	C
Diamorphine HCl with cyclizine lactate	BP WEL	11 mg/mL 16 mg/mL	JC	2.2 mg/mL	Physically compatible with less than 10% loss of any drug in 7 days at 23°C	2071	C
Diamorphine HCl with cyclizine lactate	BP WEL	25 mg/mL 16 mg/mL	JC	2.2 mg/mL	Physically compatible with less than 10% loss of any drug in 7 days at 23°C	2071	C
Diamorphine HCl with cyclizine lactate	BP WEL	40 mg/mL 11 mg/mL	JC	2.2 mg/mL	Physically compatible with less than 10% loss of any drug in 7 days at 23°C	2071	C
Diamorphine HCl with cyclizine lactate	BP WEL	42 mg/mL 13 mg/mL	JC	2.1 mg/mL	Physically compatible with less than 10% loss of any drug in 7 days at 23°C	2071	C
Diamorphine HCl with cyclizine lactate	BP WEL	55 mg/mL 9 mg/mL	JC	2.1 mg/mL	Physically compatible with less than 10% loss of any drug in 7 days at 23°C	2071	C
Diamorphine HCl with cyclizine lactate	BP WEL	56 mg/mL 13 mg/mL	JC	2.1 mg/mL	Physically compatible with less than 10% loss of any drug in 7 days at 23°C	2071	C
Diphenhydramine HCl	ES	100 mg/2 mL	MN	10 mg/2 mL	White precipitate forms within 5 min	1784	I
Diphenhydramine HCl	ES	50 mg/1 mL	MN	5 mg/1 mL	White cloudy precipitate forms in 2 hr at room temperature	1886	I
Glycopyrrolate with buprenorphine HCl	RKC	1.2 mg 4 mg	ON	5 mg	Diluted to 48 mL with NS. Visually compatible with less than 10% loss of any drug in 30 days at 4 and 25°C in the dark	2436	C
Heparin sodium		2500 units/1 mL	JN	5 mg/1 mL	Turbidity or precipitate forms within 5 min	1053	I
Hydromorphone HCl	KN	1[a] and 10 mg/1 mL	MN	1[a], 2[a], 5 mg/1 mL	Visually compatible for 24 hr at 25°C under fluorescent light	1785	C
Hydromorphone HCl	KN	10 and 15 mg/mL	MN	2 mg/mL	White precipitate of haloperidol forms immediately	668	I
Hydroxyzine HCl	ES	100 mg/2 mL	MN	10 mg/2 mL	White precipitate forms within 5 min	1784	I
Ketorolac tromethamine	SY	30 mg/1 mL	SO	5 mg/1 mL	White crystalline precipitate forms immediately	1786	I
Lorazepam	WY	2 mg/1 mL	MN	5 mg/1 mL	Physically compatible and chemically stable for 16 hr at room temperature	1838	C

Drugs in Syringe Compatibility (Cont.)

Test Drug	Mfr	Amt	Mfr	Amt	Remarks	Ref	C/I
Lorazepam	WY	4 mg/1 mL	MN	5 mg/1 mL	Visually compatible with no loss of either drug in 24 hr at 4 and 25°C	260	C
Lorazepam	WY	2 mg/1 mL	MN	5 mg/1 mL	Visually compatible for 4 hr at room temperature	260	C
Morphine sulfate		5 and 10 mg/1 mL[c]	MN	5 mg/1 mL	Cloudiness forms immediately, becoming a crystalline precipitate of haloperidol and parabens	1901	I
Morphine sulfate	ME	20 mg/mL[a]	MN	2 mg/mL	White precipitate of haloperidol forms on mixing	668	I
Oxycodone HCl	NAP	200 mg/20 mL	JC	15 mg/3 mL	Visually compatible. Under 4% concentration change in 24 hr at 25°C	2600	C
Scopolamine butylbromide	BI	2.5, 5, 10 mg/mL		0.3125 mg/mL	Physically compatible. Less than 10% loss of both drugs in 15 days at 4 and 25°C	2521	C
Scopolamine butylbromide	BI	2.5, 5, 10 mg/mL		0.625 mg/mL	Physically compatible. Less than 10% loss of both drugs in 7 days at 4 and 25°C. Over 10% loss of scopolamine in 15 days at both temperatures	2521	C
Scopolamine butylbromide	BI	2.5, 5, 10 mg/mL		1.25 mg/mL	Physically incompatible. Haloperidol precipitates in 15 days at 25°C and 7 days at 4°C	2521	I
Tramadol HCl	GRU	8.33, 16.67, 33.33 mg/mL[d]	EST	0.208 mg/mL[d]	Physically compatible with no loss of either drug in 15 days at 4 and 25°C protected from light	2672	C

[a] Diluted with sterile water for injection.

[b] Morphine sulfate powder dissolved in dextrose 5%.

[c] Morphine sulfate powder dissolved in water.

[d] Diluted with sodium chloride 0.9%.

Y-Site Injection Compatibility (1:1 Mixture)

Haloperidol lactate

Test Drug	Mfr	Conc	Mfr	Conc	Remarks	Ref	C/I
Allopurinol sodium	BW	3 mg/mL[b]	MN	0.2 mg/mL[b]	Immediate turbidity. Crystals in 1 hr	1686	I
Amifostine	USB	10 mg/mL[a]	MN	0.2 mg/mL[a]	Physically compatible for 4 hr at 23°C	1845	C
Amsacrine	NCI	1 mg/mL[a]	MN	0.2 mg/mL[a]	Visually compatible for 4 hr at 22°C	1381	C
Aztreonam	SQ	40 mg/mL[a]	MN	0.2 mg/mL[a]	Physically compatible for 4 hr at 23°C	1758	C
Bivalirudin	TMC	5 mg/mL[a]	MN	0.2 mg/mL[a]	Physically compatible for 4 hr at 23°C	2373	C
Cangrelor tetrasodium	TMC	1 mg/mL[b]		0.2 mg/mL[b]	Physically compatible for 4 hr	3243	C
Ceftaroline fosamil	FOR	2.22 mg/mL[a b f]	BED	0.2 mg/mL[a b f]	Physically compatible for 4 hr at 23°C	2826	C
Cisatracurium besylate	GW	0.1, 2, 5 mg/mL[a]	MN	0.2 mg/mL[a]	Physically compatible for 4 hr at 23°C	2074	C
Cladribine	ORT	0.015[b] and 0.5[c] mg/mL	MN	0.2 mg/mL[b]	Physically compatible for 4 hr at 23°C	1969	C
Dexmedetomidine HCl	AB	4 mcg/mL[b]	MN	0.2 mg/mL[b]	Physically compatible for 4 hr at 23°C	2383	C
Dobutamine HCl	LI	4 mg/mL[a]	MN	0.5[a] and 5 mg/mL	Visually compatible for 24 hr at 21°C	1523	C
Docetaxel	RPR	0.9 mg/mL[a]	MN	0.2 mg/mL[a]	Physically compatible for 4 hr at 23°C	2224	C
Dopamine HCl	DU	1.6 mg/mL[a]	MN	0.5[a] and 5 mg/mL	Visually compatible for 24 hr at 21°C	1523	C

Y-Site Injection Compatibility (1:1 Mixture) (Cont.)

Test Drug	Mfr	Conc	Mfr	Conc	Remarks	Ref	C/I
Doxorubicin HCl liposomal	SEQ	0.4 mg/mL[a]	MN	0.2 mg/mL[a]	Physically compatible for 4 hr at 23°C	2087	C
Etoposide phosphate	BR	5 mg/mL[a]	MN	0.2 mg/mL[a]	Physically compatible for 4 hr at 23°C	2218	C
Famotidine	MSD	0.267 mg/mL[a]	MN	0.5[a] and 5 mg/mL	Visually compatible for 24 hr at 21°C	1523	C
Famotidine	ME	2 mg/mL[b]		0.2 mg/mL[a]	Visually compatible for 4 hr at 22°C	1936	C
Fenoldopam mesylate	AB	80 mcg/mL[b]	APP	0.2 mg/mL[b]	Physically compatible for 4 hr at 23°C	2467	C
Fentanyl citrate	JN	0.025 mg/mL[a]	MN	0.2 mg/mL[a]	Physically compatible for 48 hr at 22°C	1706	C
Filgrastim	AMG	30 mcg/mL[a]	MN	0.2 mg/mL[a]	Physically compatible for 4 hr at 22°C	1687	C
Fluconazole	RR	2 mg/mL	MN	5 mg/mL	Precipitate forms	1407	I
Fludarabine phosphate	BX	1 mg/mL[a]	MN	0.2 mg/mL[a]	Visually compatible for 4 hr at 22°C	1439	C
Foscarnet sodium	AST	24 mg/mL	LY	5 mg/mL	Delayed formation of fine white precipitate	1335	I
Gallium nitrate	FUJ	1 mg/mL[b]	MN	5 mg/mL	Immediate white cloudiness	1673	I
Gemcitabine HCl	LI	10 mg/mL[b]	MN	0.2 mg/mL[b]	Physically compatible for 4 hr at 23°C	2226	C
Granisetron HCl	SKB	0.05 mg/mL[a]	MN	0.2 mg/mL[a]	Physically compatible for 4 hr at 23°C	2000	C
Heparin sodium	OR	25,000 and 50,000 units/250 mL[e i]	MN	5 mg/1 mL[d]	White precipitate forms immediately	779	I
Hetastarch in lactated electrolyte	AB	6%	MN	0.2 mg/mL[a]	Physically compatible for 4 hr at 23°C	2339	C
Hydromorphone HCl	AST	0.5 mg/mL[a]	MN	0.2 mg/mL[a]	Physically compatible for 48 hr at 22°C	1706	C
Lidocaine HCl	AB	4 mg/mL[a]	MN	0.5[a] and 5 mg/mL	Visually compatible for 24 hr at 21°C	1523	C
Linezolid	PHU	2 mg/mL	MN	0.2 mg/mL[a]	Physically compatible for 4 hr at 23°C	2264	C
Lorazepam	WY	0.33 mg/mL[b]	JN	0.5 and 5 mg/mL	Visually compatible for 24 hr at 22°C	1855	C
Melphalan HCl	BW	0.1 mg/mL[b]	MN	0.2 mg/mL[b]	Physically compatible for 3 hr at 22°C	1557	C
Methadone HCl	LI	1 mg/mL[a]	MN	0.2 mg/mL[a]	Physically compatible for 48 hr at 22°C	1706	C
Midazolam HCl	RC	5 mg/mL	JN	0.5 and 5 mg/mL	Visually compatible for 24 hr at 22°C	1855	C
Morphine sulfate	AST	1 mg/mL[a]	MN	0.2 mg/mL[a]	Physically compatible for 48 hr at 22°C	1706	C
Nitroglycerin	DU	0.4 mg/mL[a]	MN	0.5[a] and 5 mg/mL	Visually compatible for 24 hr at 21°C	1523	C
Norepinephrine bitartrate	WI	0.032 mg/mL[a]	MN	0.5[a] and 5 mg/mL	Visually compatible for 24 hr at 21°C	1523	C
Ondansetron HCl	GL	1 mg/mL[b]	LY	0.2 mg/mL[a]	Visually compatible for 4 hr at 22°C	1365	C
Oritavancin diphosphate	TAR	0.8, 1.2, and 2 mg/mL[a]	BED	1 mg/mL[a]	Visually compatible for 4 hr at 20 to 24°C	2928	C
Oxaliplatin	SS	0.5 mg/mL[a]	APP	0.2 mg/mL[a]	Physically compatible for 4 hr at 23°C	2566	C
Paclitaxel	NCI	1.2 mg/mL[a]		0.2 mg/mL[a]	Physically compatible for 4 hr at 22°C	1528	C
Pemetrexed disodium	LI	20 mg/mL[b]	APP	0.2 mg/mL[a]	Physically compatible for 4 hr at 23°C	2564	C
Phenylephrine HCl	WB	0.02 mg/mL[a]	MN	0.5[a] and 5 mg/mL	Visually compatible for 24 hr at 21°C	1523	C
Piperacillin sodium–tazobactam sodium	LE[h]	40 mg/mL[a j]	MN	0.2 mg/mL[a]	White turbidity and particles form immediately	1688	I

Y-Site Injection Compatibility (1:1 Mixture) (Cont.)

Test Drug	Mfr	Conc	Mfr	Conc	Remarks	Ref	C/I
Propofol	ZEN[n]	10 mg/mL	MN	0.2 mg/mL[a]	Physically compatible for 1 hr at 23°C	2066	C
Quinupristin–dalfopristin	PF	2 mg/mL[a k]		0.2 mg/mL[a]	Physically compatible	3229	C
Remifentanil HCl	GW	0.025 and 0.25 mg/mL[b]	MN	0.2 mg/mL[a]	Physically compatible for 4 hr at 23°C	2075	C
Sargramostim	IMM	10 mcg/mL[b]	LY	0.2 mg/mL[b]	Small particles form in 4 hr	1436	I
Sodium nitroprusside	AB	0.2 mg/mL[a]	MN	5 mg/mL	Immediate turbidity. Precipitate in 24 hr at 21°C in fluorescent light	1523	I
Sodium nitroprusside	AB	0.2 mg/mL[a]	MN	0.5 mg/mL[a]	Visually compatible for 24 hr at 21°C	1523	C
Tacrolimus	FUJ	1 mg/mL[b]	SO	2.5 mg/mL[a]	Visually compatible for 24 hr at 25°C	1630	C
Teniposide	BR	0.1 mg/mL[a]	MN	0.2 mg/mL[a]	Physically compatible for 4 hr at 23°C	1725	C
Theophylline	TR	1.6 mg/mL[a]	MN	0.5[a] and 5 mg/mL	Visually compatible for 24 hr at 21°C	1523	C
Thiotepa	IMM[i]	1 mg/mL[b]	MN	0.2 mg/mL[b]	Physically compatible for 4 hr at 23°C	1861	C
Tigecycline	WY	1 mg/mL[b]		0.2 mg/mL[b]	Physically compatible for 4 hr	2714	C
Tigecycline	ACD, WY	[e]	[m]		Stated to be compatible	2915, 3459	C
Tigecycline	FRK		[m]		Stated to be incompatible	3460	I
TNA #218 to #226[g]			MN	0.2 mg/mL[a]	Damage to emulsion occurs immediately with free oil formation possible	2215	I
TPN #189[g]			SE	10 mg/mL	Visually compatible for 24 hr at 22°C	1767	C
TPN #212 to #215[g]			MN	0.2 mg/mL[a]	Physically compatible for 4 hr at 23°C	2109	C
Vinorelbine tartrate	BW	1 mg/mL[b]	MN	0.2 mg/mL[b]	Physically compatible for 4 hr at 22°C	1558	C

[a] Tested in dextrose 5%.

[b] Tested in sodium chloride 0.9%.

[c] Tested in bacteriostatic sodium chloride 0.9% preserved with benzyl alcohol 0.9%.

[d] Injected over one minute.

[e] Tested in both dextrose 5% and sodium chloride 0.9%.

[f] Tested in Ringer's injection, lactated.

[g] Refer to Appendix for the composition of parenteral nutrition solutions. TNA indicates a 3-in-1 admixture, and TPN indicates a 2-in-1 admixture.

[h] Test performed using the formulation WITHOUT edetate disodium.

[i] Lyophilized formulation tested.

[j] Piperacillin component. Piperacillin in an 8:1 fixed-ratio concentration with tazobactam.

[k] Quinupristin and dalfopristin components combined.

[l] Run at 1000 units/hr.

[m] Salt not specified.

[n] Test performed using the formulation WITH edetate disodium.

Selected Revisions January 31, 2020. © Copyright, October 1982. American Society of Health-System Pharmacists, Inc.

Heparin Sodium
AHFS 20:12.04.16

Products

Heparin sodium is available from various manufacturers in concentrations ranging from 1000 to 20,000 units/mL, packaged in sizes ranging from 0.5- to 1-mL ampuls, vials, or prefilled syringes to 30-mL multiple-dose vials. Benzyl alcohol or parabens also may be present as preservatives, and hydrochloric acid and/or sodium hydroxide may have been added to adjust pH. Sodium chloride may have been added to some products for isotonicity. In addition, dilute solutions of 10 and 100 units/mL in 1- to 5-mL disposable syringes and 1- to 30-mL vials are available for use in flushing heparin locks.[4]

Heparin sodium also is available premixed in various concentrations in sodium chloride 0.45 and 0.9% and dextrose 5%.[4]

pH

Heparin sodium injection and heparin lock flush solution are adjusted to pH 5 to 7.5 during manufacturing.[1(3/09) 17]

Osmolality

The osmolality of heparin sodium (Elkins-Sinn) 1000 units/mL was determined to be 384 mOsm/kg by freezing-point depression and 283 mOsm/kg by vapor pressure.[1071]

Commercially available heparin sodium infusion solutions in sodium chloride 0.9% and dextrose 5% have osmolalities of 322 and 270 mOsm/kg, respectively.[4]

Osmolarity

One heparin lock flush solution is reported to have an osmolarity of 392 mOsm/L.[4]

Administration

Heparin sodium may be administered by deep subcutaneous injection, by intermittent intravenous injection either undiluted or diluted in 50 to 100 mL of dextrose 5% or sodium chloride 0.9%, or by continuous intravenous infusion in a liter of compatible solution, preferably using an electronic rate-control device. The container should be inverted at least 6 times after heparin sodium addition to prevent pooling of the heparin. Intramuscular injection should not be used because of pain and hematoma formation.[4]

Care is required when adding heparin sodium to infusion solutions, especially in flexible containers. When heparin sodium was added to a flexible polyvinyl chloride (PVC) container of sodium chloride 0.9% hanging in the use position, pooling of the heparin resulted; 97% of the heparin was delivered in the first 30% of the solution. Repeated inversion and agitation of the containers to effect thorough mixing eliminates this pooling (and the danger of overdosage), yielding an even distribution and a constant delivery concentration.[85]

Stability

Heparin sodium solutions are colorless to slightly yellow.[4] Heparin sodium solution should not be used if it is discolored or contains a precipitate. Heparin sodium should be stored at controlled room temperature[1(3/09) 4] and protected from freezing and temperatures exceeding 40°C.[4 21] In a study of hospital-manufactured heparin sodium 1 unit/mL in sodium chloride 0.9%, full anticoagulant activity was retained for at least 12 months after sterilization by autoclaving and subsequent storage at room temperature exposed to daylight.[675]

pH Effects

A pH profile of heparin sodium 20,000 units/L in dextrose 5% over a pH range of 3.8 to 7.6 did not reveal a loss during the 24-hour study.[21] In another report, heparin sodium in sodium chloride 0.9% was tested at pH 3.2 (adjusted with hydrochloric acid) and 9.2 (adjusted with sodium hydroxide). No loss was noted in 24 hours.[57] However, a pH profile of heparin sodium 660 units/mL, when autoclaved for 10 minutes at 10 pounds/inch² at 115°C, showed loss of activity at pH values above 8.5 and especially below 5.[243]

Syringes

The stability of 50 mL of a 500-unit/mL heparin sodium solution in sodium chloride 0.9% packaged in 50-mL polypropylene syringes was studied. Storage both at room temperature and at 0 to 4°C showed an overall trend to lower activity by about 8% after 3 weeks.

When glass containers were compared to plastic syringes, the glass containers consistently showed lower retained activity in as little as 2 hours after preparation. The possibility of adsorption to glass surfaces was noted[676] but has not been demonstrated.

Heparin sodium 1 unit/mL, prefilled into Injekt (Braun) all-plastic syringes having polyethylene barrels and polypropylene plungers, showed no significant activity loss over 52 weeks at 37°C due to decomposition or sorption. However, plastic syringes with rubber-tipped plungers, such as Plastipak (Becton Dickinson) and Perfusor (Braun), exhibited extra ultraviolet peaks, presumably due to leaching of rubber components.[1491]

Heparin sodium (Leo) 300 units/mL in dextrose 5% or water for injection was drawn into 50-mL polypropylene syringes (Plastipak, Becton Dickinson) and stored for 8 hours at room temperature and 4°C. No loss in either solvent occurred.[1799]

The stability of heparin sodium repackaged in 10-mL polypropylene syringes for use in CADD-Micro syringe pumps was evaluated. 10 mL of heparin sodium 1000 units/mL (Elkins-Sinn) and 40,000 units/mL (Schein) were packaged in the test syringes

DOI: 10.37573/9781585286850.190

and capped. Syringes were stored at a near-body temperature of 30°C for 30 days. Little or no loss of heparin sodium content occurred; actual activity in prolonging blood clotting was not evaluated.[2275]

Sorption

Heparin sodium, BP, 2000 units/2 mL was stored for 18 hours at room temperature in plastic syringes: Brunswick (Sherwood Medical), Plastipak (Becton Dickinson), Steriseal (Needle Industries), and Sabre (Gillette U.K.). The first 3 syringes have polypropylene barrels; the Sabre has a combination polypropylene–polystyrene barrel. No significant loss of heparin occurred due to sorption.[784]

Heparin sodium (Leo) 300 units/mL in dextrose 5% or water for injection was delivered at 4 mL/hr by syringe pump through PVC and polyethylene-lined PVC infusion tubing for 12 hours at room temperature. No loss occurred due to sorption to the polyethylene-lined tubing. However, losses of about 15 to 25% occurred with the PVC tubing and were especially high during the first 15 minutes of infusion.[1799]

Filtration

Heparin sodium (Abbott) 10,000 units/L in dextrose 5% and sodium chloride 0.9% was filtered at 120 mL/hr for 6 hours through a 0.22-μm cellulose ester membrane filter (Ivex-2). No significant loss due to binding to the filter was noted.[533]

Central Venous Catheter

Heparin sodium (Elkins-Sinn) 100 units/mL in dextrose 5% was found to be compatible with the ARROWg+ard Blue Plus (Arrow International) chlorhexidine-bearing triple-lumen central catheter. Essentially complete delivery of the drug was found with little or no drug loss occurring. Furthermore, chlorhexidine delivered from the catheter remained at trace amounts with no substantial increase due to the delivery of the drug through the catheter.[2335]

Compatibility Information

Solution Compatibility

Heparin sodium

Test Soln Name	Mfr	Mfr	Conc/L or %	Remarks	Ref	C/I
Amino acids 4.25%, dextrose 25%	MG	RI	20,000 units	No increase in particulate matter in 24 hr at 5°C	349	C
Dextrose 2.5% in half-strength Ringer's injection	AB	AB	1000 and 4000 units	Physically compatible	3	C
Dextrose 5% in Ringer's injection	AB	AB	1000 and 4000 units	Physically compatible	3	C
Dextrose 5% in half-strength Ringer's injection, lactated	AB	AB	1000 and 4000 units	Physically compatible	3	C
Dextrose 2.5% in Ringer's injection, lactated	AB	AB	1000 and 4000 units	Physically compatible	3	C
Dextrose 5% in Ringer's injection, lactated	AB	AB	1000 and 4000 units	Physically compatible	3	C
Dextrose 5% in Ringer's injection, lactated	TR[a]	UP	10,000 units	Stable for 24 hr at 5°C	282	C
Dextrose 10% in Ringer's injection, lactated	AB	AB	1000 and 4000 units	Physically compatible	3	C
Dextrose 2.5% in sodium chloride 0.45%	AB	AB	1000 and 4000 units	Physically compatible	3	C
Dextrose 2.5% in sodium chloride 0.45%	BA	DB	1000 units	Heparin activity retained for 12 months at 4°C	1914	C
Dextrose 2.5% in sodium chloride 0.9%	AB	AB	1000 and 4000 units	Physically compatible	3	C
Dextrose 5% in sodium chloride 0.225%	AB	AB	1000 and 4000 units	Physically compatible	3	C
Dextrose 5% in sodium chloride 0.45%	AB	AB	1000 and 4000 units	Physically compatible	3	C
Dextrose 5% in sodium chloride 0.45%	TR	AB	20,000 units	No decrease in activity in 24 hr at room temperature	407	C

Solution Compatibility (Cont.)

Test Soln Name	Mfr	Mfr	Conc/L or %	Remarks	Ref	C/I
Dextrose 5% in sodium chloride 0.9%	AB	AB	1000 and 4000 units	Physically compatible	3	C
Dextrose 5% in sodium chloride 0.9%			12,000 units	Physically compatible	74	C
Dextrose 5% in sodium chloride 0.9%			32,000 units	Stable for 24 hr	57	C
Dextrose 5% in sodium chloride 0.9%	AB	AB	20,000 units	Stable for 24 hr	21	C
Dextrose 5% in sodium chloride 0.9%	AB		20,000 units	Stable for 72 hr	46	C
Dextrose 5% in sodium chloride 0.9%	TR[a]	UP	10,000 units	Stable for 24 hr at 5°C	282	C
Dextrose 5% in sodium chloride 0.9%	BA		30,000 units	40% loss in 5 hr at 15, 25, and 35°C. Activity recovered 5 to 7 hr later	674	I
Dextrose 10% in sodium chloride 0.9%	AB	AB	1000 and 4000 units	Physically compatible	3	C
Dextrose 2.5%	AB	AB	1000 and 4000 units	Physically compatible	3	C
Dextrose 5%			12,000 units	Physically compatible	74	C
Dextrose 5%	AB	AB	1000 and 4000 units	Physically compatible	3	C
Dextrose 5%	BP		40,000 units	Stable for 24 hr at 23°C	252	C
Dextrose 5%			32,000 units	Stable for 24 hr	57	C
Dextrose 5%	AB	AB	20,000 units	Stable for 24 hr	21	C
Dextrose 5%	AB		20,000 units	Stable for 72 hr	46	C
Dextrose 5%	TR[b]	OR	20,000 and 40,000 units	Stable for 48 hr at 27°C	254	C
Dextrose 5%	TR[a]	UP	10,000 units	Stable for 24 hr at 5°C	282	C
Dextrose 5%	TR	AS	20,000 units	No decrease in activity in 24 hr at room temperature	407	C
Dextrose 5%		OR	20,000 units	50% loss within 1 hr at 23°C	113	I
Dextrose 5%	MG	UP	10,000 units	30 to 50% activity loss in 6 hr at room temperature. Partial rebound in 24 hr	406	I
Dextrose 5%	BA		30,000 units	65% loss in 5 hr at 15, 25, and 35°C. Activity recovered in 24 to 48 hr	674	I
Dextrose 5%		AH	35,000 units	Apparent temporary 50% loss of heparin activity in 4 hr with recovery in 6 hr at 25°C. Heparin activity then maintained for 14 days at 4°C	900	?
Dextrose 5%	BA	DB	1000 units	Heparin activity retained for 7 days at 22°C	1914	C
Dextrose 5%	BA	DB	10,000 units	Heparin activity retained for 12 months at 22°C	1914	C
Dextrose 5%	BA[b]	BRN	7000 units	Visually compatible with about 5% loss in 24 hr at 22°C but little or no loss at 4°C	2289	C
Dextrose 5%	BRN[d]	BRN	7000 units	Visually compatible with little or no loss in 24 hr at 4 and 22°C	2289	C
Dextrose 10%	AB	AB	1000 and 4000 units	Physically compatible	3	C
Dextrose 10%	MG	UP	10,000 units	40% activity loss in 6 hr at room temperature. Partial rebound at 24 hr	406	I

Solution Compatibility (Cont.)

Test Soln Name	Mfr	Mfr	Conc/L or %	Remarks	Ref	C/I
Dextrose 25%		LY	5000 units	About 6% heparin activity loss in 21 days and 11% loss in 28 days at 4°C	2025	C
Ionosol B in dextrose 5%	AB	AB	1000 and 4000 units	Physically compatible	3	C
Ionosol MB in dextrose 5%	AB	AB	1000 and 4000 units	Physically compatible	3	C
Normosol R	AB	AB	20,000 units	Stable for 24 hr	21	C
Ringer's injection	AB	AB	1000 and 4000 units	Physically compatible	3	C
Ringer's injection, lactated	AB	AB	1000 and 4000 units	Physically compatible	3	C
Ringer's injection, lactated			12,000 units	Physically compatible	74	C
Ringer's injection, lactated	TR[a]	UP	10,000 units	Stable for 24 hr at 5°C	282	C
Ringer's injection, lactated		OR	20,000 units	40% loss within 1 hr at 23°C	113	I
Ringer's injection, lactated	MG	UP	10,000 units	50 to 60% activity loss in 6 hr at room temperature. Partial rebound at 24 hr	406	I
Ringer's injection, lactated		AH	35,000 units	Apparent temporary 50% loss of heparin activity in 4 hr with recovery in 6 hr at 25°C. Heparin activity gradually lost over 14 days	900	?
Sodium chloride 0.45%	AB	AB	1000 and 4000 units	Physically compatible	3	C
Sodium chloride 0.9%			12,000 units	Physically compatible	74	C
Sodium chloride 0.9%	AB	AB	1000 and 4000 units	Physically compatible	3	C
Sodium chloride 0.9%			32,000 units	Stable for 24 hr	57	C
Sodium chloride 0.9%	AB	AB	20,000 units	Stable for 24 hr	21	C
Sodium chloride 0.9%	AB		20,000 units	Stable for 72 hr	46	C
Sodium chloride 0.9%	TR[a]	UP	10,000 units	Stable for 24 hr at 5°C	282	C
Sodium chloride 0.9%	TR[b]	OR	20,000 and 40,000 units	Stable for 48 hr at 27°C	254	C
Sodium chloride 0.9%		AH	35,000 units	Heparin activity stable for 24 hr at 25°C followed by 14 days at 4°C	900	C
Sodium chloride 0.9%	MG	UP	10,000 units	30 to 50% activity loss in 6 hr at room temperature. Partial rebound at 24 hr	406	I
Sodium chloride 0.9%	BA	DB	1000 units	Heparin activity retained for 12 months at 22°C	1914	C
Sodium chloride 0.9%	BA	DB	10,000 units	Heparin activity retained for 12 months at 4 and 22°C	1914	C
Sodium chloride 0.9%		LY	5000 units	Heparin activity retained for 28 days at 4°C	2025	C
Sodium chloride 0.9%	BA[b]	BRN	7000 units	Visually compatible with about 5% loss in 24 hr at 22°C but little or no loss at 4°C	2289	C
Sodium chloride 0.9%	BRN[d]	BRN	7000 units	Visually compatible with little or no loss in 24 hr at 4 and 22°C	2289	C
Sodium lactate ⅙ M		OR	20,000 units	50% loss within 1 hr at 23°C	113	I
TPN #48 to #51[c]		AH	35,000 units	Heparin activity retained for 24 hr at 25°C but significantly decreased after 24 hr	900	C
TPN #205[c]		LY	3000 to 20,000 units	Heparin activity retained for 28 days at 4°C	2025	C

[a] Tested in both glass and PVC containers.

[b] Tested in PVC containers.

[c] Refer to Appendix for the composition of parenteral nutrition solutions. TPN indicates a 2-in-1 admixture.

[d] Tested in polyethylene and glass containers.

Additive Compatibility

Heparin sodium

Test Drug	Mfr	Conc/L or %	Mfr	Conc/L or %	Test Solution	Remarks	Ref	C/I
Alteplase	GEN	0.5 g	ES	40,000 units	NS	Heparin interacts with alteplase. Opalescence forms within 5 min with peak intensity at 4 hr at 25°C. Alteplase clot-lysis activity reduced slightly	1856	I
Amikacin sulfate	BR	5 g	AB	30,000 units	D5LR, D5R, D5S, D5W, D10W, LR, NS, R, SL	Precipitates immediately	294	I
Aminophylline		250 mg		12,000 units	D5W	Physically compatible	74	C
Aminophylline	SE	1 g	UP	4000 units	D5W	Physically compatible	15	C
Amphotericin B	SQ	100 mg	AB	4000 units	D	Physically compatible	21	C
Amphotericin B	SQ	100 mg	UP	4000 units	D5W	Physically compatible	15	C
Amphotericin B	SQ	70 and 140 mg		2000 units	D5W	Bioactivity not affected over 24 hr at 25°C	335	C
Ampicillin sodium		2 g		32,000 units	NS	Physically compatible and heparin activity retained for 24 hr	57	C
Ampicillin sodium	BE	10 g	OR	20,000 units	NS	Both stable for 24 hr at 25°C	113	C
Ampicillin sodium	BR	1 g		12,000 units	D10W, LR, NS	Ampicillin stable for 24 hr at 4°C	87	C
Ampicillin sodium	BR	1 g		12,000 units	D5S	15% ampicillin decomposition in 24 hr at 4°C	87	I
Ampicillin sodium	BR	1 g		12,000 units	D5S, D10W, LR	20 to 25% ampicillin decomposition in 24 hr at 25°C	87	I
Antithymocyte globulin (rabbit)[d]	SGS	200 and 300 mg	ES	2000 units	D5W	Immediate haze and precipitation	2488	I
Antithymocyte globulin (rabbit)[d]	SGS	200 and 300 mg	ES	2000 units	NS	Physically compatible for 24 hr at 23°C	2488	C
Ascorbic acid	UP	500 mg	UP	4000 units	D5W	Physically compatible	15	C
Atracurium besylate	BW	500 mg		40,000 units	D5W	Particles form at 5 and 30°C	1694	I
Bleomycin sulfate	BR	20 and 30 units	RI	10,000 to 200,000 units	NS	Physically compatible and bleomycin activity retained for 1 week at 4°C. Heparin not tested	763	C
Calcium gluconate		1 g		12,000 units	D5W	Physically compatible	74	C
Calcium gluconate	UP	1 g	UP	4000 units	D5W	Physically compatible	15	C
Calcium gluconate	UP	1 g	AB	20,000 units		Physically compatible	21	C
Cefepime HCl	BR	4 g	MG	10,000 and 50,000 units	D5W, NS	Visually compatible with 4% cefepime loss in 24 hr at room temperature and 3% in 7 days at 5°C. No heparin loss	1681	C
Ceftazidime		4 g		10,000 and 50,000 units	D5W, NS	Ceftazidime stable for 24 hr at room temperature and 7 days refrigerated	4	C
Chloramphenicol sodium succinate	PD	500 mg		12,000 units	D5W	Physically compatible	74	C
Chloramphenicol sodium succinate	PD	10 g	UP	4000 units	D5W	Physically compatible	15	C

Additive Compatibility (Cont.)

Test Drug	Mfr	Conc/L or %	Mfr	Conc/L or %	Test Solution	Remarks	Ref	C/I
Chloramphenicol sodium succinate	PD	1 g	AB	20,000 units		Physically compatible	6, 21	C
Ciprofloxacin	BAY	2 g	CP	10,000, 100,000, 1 million units	NS	White precipitate forms immediately	1934	I
Ciprofloxacin	MI	2 g		4100 units	NS	Physically incompatible	888	I
Ciprofloxacin	MI	2 g		8300 units	NS	Physically incompatible	888	I
Clindamycin phosphate	UP	9 g		100,000 units	D5W	Clindamycin stable for 24 hr	101	C
Cloxacillin sodium		2 g		32,000 units	NS	Physically compatible and heparin stable for 24 hr	57	C
Colistimethate sodium	WC	500 mg	AB	20,000 units	D	Physically compatible	21	C
Colistimethate sodium	WC	500 mg	UP	4000 units	D5W	Physically compatible	15	C
Cytarabine	UP	500 mg		10,000 units	NS	Haze formation	174	I
Cytarabine	UP	100 mg		20,000 units	D5W	Haze formation	174	I
Daunorubicin HCl	FA	200 mg	UP	4000 units	D5W	Physically incompatible	15	I
Dimenhydrinate	SE	50 mg		12,000 units	D5W	Physically compatible	74	C
Dimenhydrinate	SE	500 mg	UP	4000 units	D5W	Physically compatible	15	C
Dimenhydrinate	SE	50 mg	AB	20,000 units	D	Physically compatible	21	C
Dobutamine HCl	LI	1 g	ES	40,000 units	D5W, NS	Physically compatible with no color change in 24 hr at 25°C	789	C
Dobutamine HCl	LI	1 g	LY	50,000 units	D5W, NS	Physically compatible for 24 hr at 21°C	812	C
Dobutamine HCl	LI	1 g	ES	5 million units	D5W, NS	Pink discoloration within 6 hr at 21°C	812	I
Dobutamine HCl	LI	1 g	ES	50,000 units	D5W	Precipitate forms within 3 min	841	I
Dobutamine HCl	LI	1.5 g	LY	50,000 units	D5W, NS	Obvious precipitation	1318	I
Dobutamine HCl	LI	900 mg	LY	50,000 units	D5W, W	Physically compatible for 4 hr, but heat of reaction detected by microcalorimetry	1318	I
Dobutamine HCl	LI	900 mg	LY	50,000 units	NS	Physically compatible for 4 hr with no heat of reaction detected by microcalorimetry	1318	C
Dopamine HCl	AS	800 mg	AB	200,000 units	D5W	No dopamine or heparin loss in 24 hr at 25°C	312	C
Enalaprilat	MSD	12 mg	ES	50,000 units	D5Wa	Visually compatible. Little enalaprilat loss in 24 hr at room temperature under fluorescent light. Heparin not tested	1572	C
Epirubicin HCl	PHU					Potential precipitation	3377	I
Eptifibatide	ME	750 mg		24,000 units		Physically compatible and chemically stable for up to 24 hr at 25°C	3049	C
Erythromycin lactobionate	AB	1 g	AB	1500 units		Precipitate forms within 1 hr	20	I
Erythromycin lactobionate	AB	5 g	UP	4000 units	D5W	Physically incompatible	15	I

Additive Compatibility (Cont.)

Test Drug	Mfr	Conc/L or %	Mfr	Conc/L or %	Test Solution	Remarks	Ref	C/I
Erythromycin lactobionate	AB	1.5 g	OR	20,000 units	D5W, NS	Precipitate forms	113	I
Erythromycin lactobionate	AB	1 g	AB	20,000 units		Precipitate forms within 1 hr	21	I
Esmolol HCl	DU	6 g	LY	50,000 units	D5W	Physically compatible with no esmolol loss in 24 hr at room temperature under fluorescent light. Heparin not tested	1358	C
Floxacillin sodium	BE	20 g	WED	20,000 units	NS	Physically compatible for 24 hr at 15 and 30°C. Haze forms in 48 hr at 30°C. No change at 15°C	1479	C
Fluconazole	PF	1 g	BA	50,000 units	D5W	Fluconazole stable for 24 hr at 25°C in fluorescent light. Heparin not tested	1676	C
Flumazenil	RC	20 mg	ES	50,000 units	D5W[a]	Visually compatible. 4% flumazenil loss in 24 hr at 23°C in fluorescent light. Heparin not tested	1710	C
Furosemide	HO	1 g	WED	20,000 units	NS	Physically compatible for 72 hr at 15 and 30°C	1479	C
Gentamicin sulfate		320 mg	BP	20,000 units	D5W, NS	Precipitates immediately	26	I
Gentamicin sulfate	SC	1 g	OR	20,000 units	D5W, NS	Opalescence	113	I
Gentamicin sulfate	ME	88 mg	BRN	1000 to 6000 units	D10W, NS	Activity of both drugs greatly reduced	1570	I
Hydrocortisone sodium succinate		800 mg		32,000 units	NS	Physically compatible and heparin activity retained for 24 hr	57	C
Hydrocortisone sodium succinate	UP	500 mg	UP	4000 units	D5W	Physically incompatible	15	I
Hydrocortisone sodium succinate	UP	100 mg		12,000 units	D5W	Precipitates immediately	74	I
Hydromorphone HCl	KN	20 g	OR	1000 units	D5W[a]	Visually compatible with no loss of hydromorphone in 18 days at 4 and 23°C. Heparin not tested	2410	C
Hydromorphone HCl	KN	5 g	OR	500 units	D5W[a]	Visually compatible with no loss of hydromorphone in 18 days at 4 and 23°C. Heparin not tested	2410	C
Hydromorphone HCl	KN	5 g	OR	8000 units	D5W[a]	Visually compatible with no loss of hydromorphone in 18 days at 4 and 23°C. Heparin not tested	2410	C
Immune globulin human	GRI[f]					Stated to be incompatible	3060	I
Immune globulin human	GRI[g]					Stated to be incompatible	3062	I
Isoproterenol HCl		2 mg		32,000 units	NS	Physically compatible and heparin activity retained for 24 hr	57	C
Isoproterenol HCl	WI	4 mg	AB	20,000 units		Physically compatible	59	C
Lidocaine HCl		4 g		32,000 units	NS	Physically compatible and heparin activity retained for 24 hr	57	C
Lidocaine HCl	AST	2 g	AB	20,000 units		Physically compatible	24	C
Lincomycin HCl	UP	600 mg	AB	20,000 units		Physically compatible	21	C

Additive Compatibility (Cont.)

Test Drug	Mfr	Conc/L or %	Mfr	Conc/L or %	Test Solution	Remarks	Ref	C/I
Magnesium sulfate		130 mEq		50,000 units	NS[b]	Visually compatible with heparin activity retained for 14 days at 24°C under fluorescent light	1908	C
Meropenem	ZEN	1 and 20 g	ES	20,000 units	NS	Visually compatible for 4 hr at room temperature	1994	C
Methyldopa HCl	MSD	1 g	AB	20,000 units	D5W, D10W, D2.5½S, D2.5S, D5¼S, D5½S, D5S, D10S, NS, ½S	Physically compatible	23	C
Methylprednisolone sodium succinate	UP	40 mg		10,000 units	D5S	Clear solution for 24 hr	329	C
Methylprednisolone sodium succinate	UP	125 mg		5000 units	D5S, D5W, LR, R	Clear solution for 24 hr	329	C
Methylprednisolone sodium succinate	UP	25 g		40,000 units	NS	Clear solution for 24 hr	329	C
Mitomycin	BR	167 mg	ES	33,300 units	NS[b]	Visually compatible. 10% mitomycin calculated loss in 21 hr and no decrease in heparin bioactivity at 25°C	1866	I
Mitomycin	BR	167 mg	ES	33,300 units	NS[a]	Visually compatible. 10% mitomycin calculated loss in 25 hr and no decrease in heparin bioactivity at 25°C	1866	C
Mitomycin	BR	500 mg	ES	33,300 units	NS[b]	Visually compatible. 10% mitomycin calculated loss in 42 hr and no decrease in heparin bioactivity at 25°C	1866	C
Mitomycin	BR	500 mg	ES	33,300 units	NS[a]	Visually compatible. 10% mitomycin calculated loss in 61 hr and no decrease in heparin bioactivity at 25°C	1866	C
Nafcillin sodium	WY	500 mg	AB, WY	20,000 units		Physically compatible	27	C
Nafcillin sodium	WY	500 mg	AB	20,000 units		Physically compatible	21	C
Norepinephrine bitartrate	WI	8 mg		12,000 units	D5W	Physically compatible	74	C
Norepinephrine bitartrate	WI	8 mg	AB	20,000 units	D5W, D10W, D2.5½S, D2.5S, D5¼S, D5½S, D5S, D10S, NS, ½S	Physically compatible	77	C
Octreotide acetate	SZ	1.5 mg	ES	1000 units	TPN #120[c]	Little octreotide loss over 48 hr at room temperature in ambient light	1373	C
Penicillin G potassium		1 million units		12,000 units	D5W	Physically compatible	74	C
Penicillin G potassium	SQ	1 million units	AB	20,000 units	D5W	Penicillin stable for 24 hr at 25°C	47	C
Penicillin G potassium	SQ	20 million units	UP	4000 units	D5W	Physically incompatible	15	I
Penicillin G sodium	BE	20 million units	OR	20,000 units	NS	Both stable for 24 hr at 25°C	113	C
Penicillin G sodium	UP	20 million units	UP	4000 units	D5W	Physically incompatible	15	I
Polymyxin B sulfate	BP	20 mg	BP	20,000 units	D5W	Precipitates immediately	26	I
Polymyxin B sulfate	BP	20 mg	BP	20,000 units	NS	Haze develops over 3 hr	26	I
Potassium chloride		3 g		12,000 units	D5W	Physically compatible	74	C
Potassium chloride	AB	40 mEq	AB	20,000 units		Physically compatible	21	C

Additive Compatibility (Cont.)

Test Drug	Mfr	Conc/L or %	Mfr	Conc/L or %	Test Solution	Remarks	Ref	C/I
Potassium chloride		80 mEq		32,000 units	NS	Physically compatible and heparin activity retained for 24 hr	57	C
Promethazine HCl	WY	250 mg	UP	4000 units	D5W	Physically incompatible	15	I
Ranitidine HCl	GL	2 g	ES	10,000 and 40,000 units	D5W, NSª	Physically compatible. 2% ranitidine loss in 48 hr at room temperature in light. Heparin not tested	1361	C
Ranitidine HCl	GL	50 mg	ES	10,000 and 40,000 units	NSª	Physically compatible. No ranitidine loss in 48 hr at room temperature in light. Heparin not tested	1361	C
Ranitidine HCl	GL	50 mg	ES	10,000 and 40,000 units	D5Wª	Physically compatible. 7% ranitidine loss in 24 hr and 12% loss in 48 hr at room temperature in light. Heparin not tested	1361	C
Sodium bicarbonate	AB	2.4 mEqᵉ	AB	20,000 units	D5W	Physically compatible for 24 hr	772	C
Streptomycin sulfate		1 g	AB	20,000 units		Precipitate forms within 1 hr	21	I
Streptomycin sulfate	BP	4 g	BP	20,000 units	D5W, NS	Precipitates immediately	26	I
Teicoplanin	HO	2 g	CPP	20,000 and 40,000 units	D5W, NS	Visually compatible. No loss of teicoplanin and heparin in 24 hr at 25°C	2165	C
Vancomycin HCl	LI	1 g		12,000 units	D5W	Precipitates immediately	74	I
Vancomycin HCl	LE	400 mg	IX	1000 units	TPN #95ᶜ	Physically compatible and vancomycin stable for 8 days at room temperature and under refrigeration	1321	C
Vancomycin HCl	LI	25 mg	ES	100,000 units	NS	Physically compatible. Under 10% vancomycin loss and no heparin loss in 30 days at 28°C and 63 days at 4°C	2542	C
Verapamil HCl	KN	80 mg	ES	20,000 units	D5W, NS	Physically compatible for 24 hr	764	C

ª Tested in PVC containers.

ᵇ Tested in glass containers.

ᶜ Refer to Appendix for the composition of parenteral nutrition solutions. TPN indicates a 2-in-1 admixture.

ᵈ Hydrocortisone sodium succinate (Pharmacia Upjohn) 50 mg/L was also present.

ᵉ One vial of Neut added to a liter of admixture.

ᶠ Test performed using the Gammaked (Grifols) formulation.

ᵍ Test performed using the Gamunex-C (Grifols) formulation.

Drugs in Syringe Compatibility

Heparin sodium

Test Drug	Mfr	Amt	Mfr	Amt	Remarks	Ref	C/I
Amikacin sulfate		100 mg		2500 units/1 mL	Turbidity or precipitate forms within 5 min	1053	I
Aminophylline		240 mg/10 mL		2500 units/1 mL	Physically compatible for at least 5 min	1053	C
Amiodarone HCl	LZ	150 mg/3 mL		2500 units/1 mL	Turbidity or precipitate forms within 5 min	1053	I
Amphotericin B		50 mg		2500 units/1 mL	Physically compatible for at least 5 min	1053	C
Ampicillin sodium		2 g		2500 units/1 mL	Physically compatible for at least 5 min	1053	C
Atropine sulfate		0.5 mg/1 mL		2500 units/1 mL	Physically compatible for at least 5 min	1053	C

Drugs in Syringe Compatibility (Cont.)

Test Drug	Mfr	Amt	Mfr	Amt	Remarks	Ref	C/I
Bleomycin sulfate		1.5 units/0.5 mL		500 units/0.5 mL	Physically compatible for 5 min at room temperature followed by 8 min of centrifugation	980	C
Buprenorphine HCl	BM	300 mg/1 mL		2500 units/1 mL	Visually compatible for at least 5 min	1053	C
Caffeine citrate		20 mg/1 mL	AB	10 units/1 mL	Visually compatible for 4 hr at 25°C	2440	C
Cefazolin sodium		2 g		2500 units/1 mL	Physically compatible for at least 5 min	1053	C
Cefotaxime sodium	HO	2 g		2500 units/1 mL	Physically compatible for at least 5 min	1053	C
Cefotaxime sodium	WW	10 mg/mL	HOS	5000 units/mL	Physically compatible. No cefotaxime loss in 3 days at 4°C. Losses of 7 and 14% in 1 and 2 days at 27°C	2820	C
Cefoxitin sodium	MSD	2 g		2500 units/1 mL	Physically compatible for at least 5 min	1053	C
Chloramphenicol sodium succinate	PD	1 g	AB	20,000 units/1 mL	Physically compatible for at least 30 min	21	C
Chloramphenicol sodium succinate		1 g		2500 units/1 mL	Physically compatible for at least 5 min	1053	C
Chlorpromazine HCl		50 mg/2 mL		2500 units/1 mL	Turbidity or precipitate forms within 5 min	1053	I
Cisplatin		0.5 mg/0.5 mL		500 units/0.5 mL	Physically compatible for 5 min at room temperature followed by 8 min of centrifugation	980	C
Clindamycin phosphate	UP	300 mg		2500 units/1 mL	Physically compatible for at least 5 min	1053	C
Clonazepam	RC	1 mg/2 mL		2500 units/1 mL	Visually compatible for at least 5 min	1053	C
Clonidine HCl	BI	0.15 mg/1 mL		2500 units/1 mL	Visually compatible for at least 5 min	1053	C
Cyclophosphamide		10 mg/0.5 mL		500 units/0.5 mL	Physically compatible for 5 min at room temperature followed by 8 min of centrifugation	980	C
Diazepam		10 mg/2 mL		2500 units/1 mL	Turbidity or precipitate forms within 5 min	1053	I
Digoxin		0.25 mg/1 mL		2500 units/1 mL	Physically compatible for at least 5 min	1053	C
Dimenhydrinate		65 mg/10 mL		2500 units/1 mL	Physically compatible for at least 5 min	1053	C
Dimenhydrinate		10 mg/1 mL		25,000 units/1 mL	Precipitate forms	2569	I
Dobutamine HCl	LI	250 mg/10 mL		2500 units/1 mL	Physically compatible for at least 5 min	1053	C/I
Dopamine HCl		50 mg/5 mL		2500 units/1 mL	Physically compatible for at least 5 min	1053	C
Doxorubicin HCl		1 mg/0.5 mL		500 units/0.5 mL	Precipitates immediately	980	I
Droperidol		1.25 mg/0.5 mL		500 units/0.5 mL	Precipitates immediately	980	I
Droperidol	JN	5 mg/2 mL		2500 units/1 mL	Turbidity or precipitate forms within 5 min	1053	I
Epinephrine HCl		1 mg/1 mL		2500 units/1 mL	Physically compatible for at least 5 min	1053	C
Erythromycin lactobionate	AB	1 g	AB	20,000 units/1 mL	Physically incompatible	21	I
Etomidate	JN	20 mg/10 mL		2500 units/1 mL	Visually compatible for at least 5 min	1053	C
Fentanyl citrate	JN	0.1 mg/2 mL		2500 units/1 mL	Physically compatible for at least 5 min	1053	C
Floxacillin sodium	BE	1 g		2500 units/1 mL	Visually compatible for at least 5 min	1053	C
Fluorouracil		25 mg/0.5 mL		500 units/0.5 mL	Physically compatible for 5 min at room temperature followed by 8 min of centrifugation	980	C
Fluorouracil	DB	500 mg/20 mL	LEO	20,000 units/0.8 mL	Visually compatible with no loss of either drug in 7 days at 25°C and 14 days at 4°C in the dark	2415	C

Drugs in Syringe Compatibility (Cont.)

Test Drug	Mfr	Amt	Mfr	Amt	Remarks	Ref	C/I
Furosemide		5 mg/0.5 mL		500 units/0.5 mL	Physically compatible for 5 min at room temperature followed by 8 min of centrifugation	980	C
Furosemide		20 mg/2 mL		2500 units/1 mL	Physically compatible for at least 5 min	1053	C
Gentamicin sulfate		40 mg		2500 units/1 mL	Turbidity or precipitate forms within 5 min	1053	I
Haloperidol lactate	JN	5 mg/1 mL		2500 units/1 mL	Turbidity or precipitate forms within 5 min	1053	I
Hydromorphone HCl	KN	50 mg/1 mL	OR	10 units/1 mL	White cloudy precipitate	2410	I
Hydromorphone HCl	KN	50 mg/1 mL	LEO	100 units/1 mL	White cloudy precipitate	2410	I
Hydromorphone HCl	KN	50 mg/1 mL	OR	25,000 units/1 mL	White cloudy precipitate	2410	I
Iohexol	WI	64.7%, 5 mL	OR	5000 units/0.5 mL	Physically compatible for at least 2 hr	1438	C
Iopamidol	SQ	61%, 5 mL	OR	5000 units/0.5 mL	Physically compatible for at least 2 hr	1438	C
Iothalamate meglumine	MA	60%, 5 mL	OR	5000 units/0.5 mL	Physically compatible for at least 2 hr	1438	C
Ioxaglate meglumine–ioxaglate sodium	MA	5 mL	OR	5000 units/0.5 mL	Physically compatible for at least 2 hr	1438	C
Leucovorin calcium		5 mg/0.5 mL		500 units/0.5 mL	Physically compatible for 5 min at room temperature followed by 8 min of centrifugation	980	C
Lidocaine HCl	AST	100 mg/5 mL		2500 units/1 mL	Physically compatible for at least 5 min	1053	C
Lincomycin HCl	UP	600 mg/2 mL	AB	20,000 units/1 mL	Physically compatible for at least 30 min	21	C
Meperidine HCl	HO	100 mg/2 mL		2500 units/1 mL	Turbidity or precipitate forms within 5 min	1053	I
Methotrexate sodium		12.5 mg/0.5 mL		500 units/0.5 mL	Physically compatible for 5 min at room temperature followed by 8 min of centrifugation	980	C
Methotrimeprazine HCl		25 mg/1 mL		2500 units/1 mL	Turbidity or precipitate forms within 5 min	1053	I
Metoclopramide HCl		2.5 mg/0.5 mL		500 units/0.5 mL	Physically compatible for 5 min at room temperature followed by 8 min of centrifugation	980	C
Metoclopramide HCl		10 mg/2 mL		2500 units/1 mL	Physically compatible for at least 5 min	1053	C
Metoclopramide HCl	RB	10 mg/2 mL	ES	2000 units/2 mL	Physically compatible for 48 hr at 25°C	1167	C
Metoclopramide HCl	RB	10 mg/2 mL	ES	4000 units/4 mL	Physically compatible for 48 hr at 25°C	1167	C
Metoclopramide HCl	RB	160 mg/32 mL	ES	16,000 units/16 mL	Physically compatible for 48 hr at 25°C	1167	C
Mexiletine HCl	BI	250 mg/10 mL		2500 units/1 mL	Turbidity or precipitate forms within 5 min	1053	I
Midazolam HCl	RC	15 mg/3 mL		2500 units/1 mL	Turbidity or precipitate forms within 5 min	1053	I
Mitomycin		0.25 mg/0.5 mL		500 units/0.5 mL	Physically compatible for 5 min at room temperature followed by 8 min of centrifugation	980	C
Morphine sulfate		1, 2, 5, 10 mg	WY	100 and 200 units	Brought to 5 mL with NS. Physically compatible with no morphine loss in 24 hr at 23°C	985	C
Morphine sulfate		1, 2, 5 mg	WY	100 and 200 units	Brought to 5 mL with W. Physically compatible with no morphine loss in 24 hr at 23°C	985	C
Morphine sulfate		10 mg	WY	100 and 200 units	Brought to 5 mL with W. Immediate haze with precipitate and 5 to 7% morphine loss	985	I
Nafcillin sodium	WY	500 mg	AB	20,000 units/1 mL	Physically compatible for at least 30 min	21	C
Naloxone HCl	DU	0.4 mg/1 mL		2500 units/1 mL	Physically compatible for at least 5 min	1053	C
Neostigmine methyl-sulfate	RC	0.5 mg/1 mL		2500 units/1 mL	Physically compatible for at least 5 min	1053	C

Drugs in Syringe Compatibility (Cont.)

Test Drug	Mfr	Amt	Mfr	Amt	Remarks	Ref	C/I
Nitroglycerin		25 mg/25 mL		2500 units/1 mL	Physically compatible for at least 5 min	1053	C
Pancuronium bromide		4 mg/2 mL		2500 units/1 mL	Physically compatible for at least 5 min	1053	C
Pantoprazole sodium	c	4 mg/1 mL		25,000 units/1 mL	Precipitates within 1 hr	2574	I
Pentazocine lactate	WI	30 mg/1 mL		2500 units/1 mL	Turbidity or precipitate forms within 5 min	1053	I
Phenobarbital sodium		200 mg/1 mL		2500 units/1 mL	Physically compatible for at least 5 min	1053	C
Promethazine HCl		50 mg/2 mL		2500 units/1 mL	Turbidity or precipitate forms within 5 min	1053	I
Ranitidine HCl	GL	50 mg/5 mL		2500 units/1 mL	Visually compatible for at least 5 min	1053	C
Sodium nitroprusside		60 mg/5 mL		2500 units/1 mL	Physically compatible for at least 5 min	1053	C
Streptomycin sulfate		1 g	AB	20,000 units/1 mL	Physically incompatible	21	I
Succinylcholine chloride		100 mg/5 mL		2500 units/1 mL	Physically compatible for at least 5 min	1053	C
Tobramycin sulfate		80 mg/2 mL		10 units/1 mL	Turbidity or fine white precipitate due to formation of an insoluble salt	845	I
Tobramycin sulfate	LI	40 mg		2500 units/1 mL	Turbidity or precipitate forms within 5 min	1053	I
Tramadol HCl	GRU	100 mg/2 mL		2500 units/1 mL	Visually compatible for at least 5 min	1053	C
Trimethoprim–sulfamethoxazole		80 mg/5 mL[b]		2500 units/1 mL	Physically compatible for at least 5 min	1053	C
Vancomycin HCl	LI	500 mg		2500 units/1 mL	Turbidity or precipitate forms within 5 min	1053	I
Verapamil HCl	KN	5 mg/2 mL		2500 units/1 mL	Physically compatible for at least 5 min	1053	C
Vinblastine sulfate		0.5 mg/0.5 mL		500 units/0.5 mL	Physically compatible for 5 min at room temperature followed by 8 min of centrifugation	980	C
Vinblastine sulfate	LI	1 mg/1 mL		200 units/1 mL[a]	Turbidity appears in 2 to 3 min	767	I
Vincristine sulfate		0.5 mg/0.5 mL		500 units/0.5 mL	Physically compatible for 5 min at room temperature followed by 8 min of centrifugation	980	C

[a] Tested in bacteriostatic sodium chloride 0.9%.

[b] Trimethoprim component. Trimethoprim in a 1:5 fixed-ratio concentration with sulfamethoxazole.

[c] Test performed using the formulation WITHOUT edetate disodium.

Y-Site Injection Compatibility (1:1 Mixture)

Heparin sodium

Test Drug	Mfr	Conc	Mfr	Conc	Remarks	Ref	C/I
Acetaminophen	CAD	10 mg/mL	HOS	100 units/mL	Physically compatible with less than 10% acetaminophen loss over 4 hr at room temperature	2841, 2844	C
Acyclovir sodium	BW	5 mg/mL[a]	ES	50 units/mL[a]	Physically compatible for 4 hr at 25°C	1157	C
Acyclovir sodium	BV	5 mg/mL[b]	BD	100 units/mL	Physically compatible	2794	C
Aldesleukin	CHI	33,800 I.U./mL[a]	BA	100 units/mL	Visually compatible with little or no loss of aldesleukin activity	1857	C
Aldesleukin	CHI[r]	a			Visually compatible but aldesleukin activity was variable depending on rate of delivery. Heparin not tested	1890	?
Allopurinol sodium	BW	3 mg/mL[b]	ES	100 units/mL[b]	Physically compatible for 4 hr at 22°C	1686	C
Alteplase	GEN	1 mg/mL	ES	100 units/mL[a]	Haze noted in 24 hr	1340	I

Y-Site Injection Compatibility (1:1 Mixture) (Cont.)

Test Drug	Mfr	Conc	Mfr	Conc	Remarks	Ref	C/I
Amifostine	USB	10 mg/mL[a]	ES	100 units/mL[a]	Physically compatible for 4 hr at 23°C	1845	C
Aminophylline	SE	25 mg/mL	RI	1000 units/L[c]	Physically compatible for 4 hr at room temperature	322	C
Amiodarone HCl				300 units/mL[b]	White precipitate forms upon sequential administration	791	I
Amphotericin B	SQ	0.1 mg/mL[a]	SO	100 units/mL[b]	Turbidity forms in 45 min	1435	I
Ampicillin sodium	BR	25, 50, 100, 125 mg/mL	RI	1000 units/L[c]	Physically compatible for 4 hr at room temperature	322	C
Ampicillin sodium	WY	20 mg/mL[b]	TR	50 units/mL	Visually compatible for 4 hr at 25°C	1793	C
Ampicillin sodium	NOP	10 mg/mL[b]	LEO	10 and 5000 units/mL[b]	Physically compatible with little change in heparin activity in 14 days at 4 and 37°C. Antibiotic not tested	2684	C
Ampicillin sodium–sulbactam sodium	PF	20 mg/mL[b u]	TR	50 units/mL	Visually compatible for 4 hr at 25°C	1793	C
Amsacrine	NCI	1 mg/mL[a]	SO	40 units/mL[a]	Orange precipitate forms immediately	1381	I
Anidulafungin	VIC	0.5 mg/mL[a]	AB	100 units/mL	Physically compatible for 4 hr at 23°C	2617	C
Antithymocyte globulin (rabbit)	SGS	0.2 mg/mL[a]	ES	2 units/mL[a]	Haze and precipitate form immediately	2488	I
Antithymocyte globulin (rabbit)	SGS	0.3 mg/mL[a]	ES	2 units/mL[a]	Haze and precipitate form immediately	2488	I
Antithymocyte globulin (rabbit)	SGS	0.2 mg/mL[b]	ES	2 units/mL[b]	Physically compatible for 4 hr at 23°C	2488	C
Antithymocyte globulin (rabbit)	SGS	0.3 mg/mL[b]	ES	2 units/mL[b]	Physically compatible for 4 hr at 23°C	2488	C
Antithymocyte globulin (rabbit)	SGS	0.2 mg/mL[a b]	ES	100 units/mL	Physically compatible for 4 hr at 23°C	2488	C
Antithymocyte globulin (rabbit)	SGS	0.3 mg/mL[a b]	ES	100 units/mL	Physically compatible for 4 hr at 23°C	2488	C
Atracurium besylate	BW	0.5 mg/mL[a]	SO	40 units/mL[a]	Physically compatible for 24 hr at 28°C	1337	C
Atropine sulfate	BW	0.5 mg/mL	UP	1000 units/L[e]	Physically compatible for 4 hr at room temperature	534	C
Aztreonam	SQ	40 mg/mL[a]	ES	100 units/mL[a]	Physically compatible for 4 hr at 23°C	1758	C
Aztreonam	BV	20 mg/mL[a]	TR	50 units/mL	Visually compatible for 4 hr at 25°C	1793	C
Bivalirudin	TMC	5 mg/mL[a]	AB	100 units/mL	Physically compatible for 4 hr at 23°C	2373	C
Bleomycin sulfate		3 units/mL		1000 units/mL	Drugs injected sequentially in Y-site with no flush. No precipitate seen	980	C
Blinatumomab	AMG	0.125 mcg/mL[b]	PAN	192.3 units/mL[b]	Persistent particulate formation when blinatumomab is added to heparin; not observed when order of mixing was reversed	3405, 3417	?
Blinatumomab	AMG	0.375 mcg/mL[b]	PAN	192.3 units/mL[b]	Persistent particulate formation	3405, 3417	I
Caffeine citrate		20 mg/mL		1 unit/mL[a]	Compatible and stable for 24 hr at room temperature	1(3/09)	C
Calcium gluconate	ES	100 mg/mL	RI	1000 units/L[c]	Physically compatible for 4 hr at room temperature	322	C
Cangrelor tetrasodium	TMC	1 mg/mL[b]		100 units/mL	Physically compatible for 4 hr	3243	C
Caspofungin acetate	ME	0.7 mg/mL[b]	HOS	100 units/mL	Immediate white turbid precipitate forms	2758	I
Caspofungin acetate	ME	0.5 mg/mL[b]	BA	100 units/mL	Fine white crystalline material reported	2766	I
Cefazolin sodium	SKB	20 mg/mL	TR	50 units/mL	Visually compatible for 4 hr at 25°C	1793	C

Y-Site Injection Compatibility (1:1 Mixture) (Cont.)

Test Drug	Mfr	Conc	Mfr	Conc	Remarks	Ref	C/I
Cefazolin sodium	NOP	10 mg/mL[b]	LEO	10 and 5000 units/mL[b]	Physically compatible with little change in heparin activity in 14 days at 4 and 37°C. Antibiotic not tested	2684	C
Cefotetan disodium	STU	40 mg/mL[a]	TR	50 units/mL	Visually compatible for 4 hr at 25°C	1793	C
Ceftaroline fosamil	FOR	2.22 mg/mL[a b k]	HOS	100 units/mL	Physically compatible for 4 hr at 23°C	2826	C
Ceftazidime	LI	20 mg/mL	TR	50 units/mL	Visually compatible for 4 hr at 25°C	1793	C
Ceftazidime–avibactam sodium	ALL	20 mg/mL[z aa]			Physically compatible for up to 4 hr at room temperature	3004	C
Ceftolozane sulfate–tazobactam sodium	CUB	10 mg/mL[f y]	SGT	1000 units/mL	Physically compatible for 2 hr	3262	C
Ceftriaxone sodium	RC	20 mg/mL	TR	50 units/mL	Visually compatible for 4 hr at 25°C	1793	C
Chlorpromazine HCl	SKF	25 mg/mL	UP	1000 units/L[e]	Physically compatible for 4 hr at room temperature	534	C
Chlorpromazine HCl	RPR	0.13 mg/mL[a]	NOV	29.2 units/mL[a]	Visually compatible for 150 min	2244	C
Ciprofloxacin		2 mg/mL		10 units/mL	Turbidity forms rapidly with subsequent white precipitate	1483	I
Ciprofloxacin	MI	2 mg/mL[f]	LY	100 units/mL	Crystals form immediately	1655	I
Ciprofloxacin	BAY	2 mg/mL[b]	CP	10, 100, 1000 units/mL[b]	White precipitate forms immediately	1934	I
Cisatracurium besylate	GW	0.1 and 2 mg/mL[a]	AB	100 units/mL	Physically compatible for 4 hr at 23°C	2074	C
Cisatracurium besylate	GW	5 mg/mL[a]	AB	100 units/mL	White cloudiness forms immediately	2074	I
Cisplatin		1 mg/mL		1000 units/mL	Drugs injected sequentially in Y-site with no flush. No precipitate seen	980	C
Cladribine	ORT	0.015[b] and 0.5[g] mg/mL	WY	100 units/mL[b]	Physically compatible for 4 hr at 23°C	1969	C
Clarithromycin	AB	4 mg/mL[a]	CPP	1000 units/mL[a]	White cloudiness forms immediately	2174	I
Clevidipine butyrate	CHS	0.5 mg/mL		100 units/mL[b]	Physically compatible for 24 hr at 23°C	3334	C
Clindamycin phosphate	UP	12 mg/mL[a]	TR	50 units/mL	Visually compatible for 4 hr at 25°C	1793	C
Cloxacillin sodium	SMX	100 mg/mL	PPC	100 units/mL	Physically compatible for up to 4 hr at room temperature	3245	C
Cyanocobalamin	PD	0.1 mg/mL	UP	1000 units/L[e]	Physically compatible for 4 hr at room temperature	534	C
Cyclophosphamide		20 mg/mL		1000 units/mL	Drugs injected sequentially in Y-site with no flush. No precipitate seen	980	C
Dacarbazine	MI	25 mg/mL[b]	WY	100 units/mL	White precipitate forms immediately[h]	1158	I
Dacarbazine	MI	10 mg/mL[b]	WY	100 units/mL	No observable precipitation[h]	1158	C
Daptomycin	CUB[x]	19.6 mg/mL[b l]	ES	98 units/mL[b l]	Physically compatible with no loss of either drug in 2 hr at 25°C	2553	C
Defibrotide sodium	JAZ	8 mg/mL[b]	SAA	373 units/mL[b]	Visually compatible for 4 hr at room temperature	3149	C
Dexamethasone sodium phosphate	ES	0.08 mg/mL[a]	TR	50 units/mL	Visually compatible for 4 hr at 25°C	1793	C
Dexamethasone sodium phosphate	MSD	4 mg/mL	RI	1000 units/L[c]	Physically compatible for 4 hr at room temperature	322	C
Dexmedetomidine HCl	AB	4 mcg/mL[b]	AB	100 units/mL	Physically compatible for 4 hr at 23°C	2383	C
Diazepam	RC	5 mg/mL	RI	1000 units/L[c]	Immediate haziness and globule formation	322	I
Digoxin	BW	0.25 mg/mL	RI	1000 units/L[c]	Physically compatible for 4 hr at room temperature	322	C

Y-Site Injection Compatibility (1:1 Mixture) (Cont.)

Test Drug	Mfr	Conc	Mfr	Conc	Remarks	Ref	C/I
Diltiazem HCl	MMD	5 mg/mL	LY	20,000 units/mL	Precipitate forms	1807	I
Diltiazem HCl	MMD	1 mg/mL[b]	LY	20,000 units/mL	Visually compatible	1807	C
Diltiazem HCl	MMD	1[b] and 5 mg/mL	SCN	5000 and 10,000 units/mL	Visually compatible	1807	C
Diltiazem HCl	MMD	5 mg/mL	LY, SCN	80 units/mL[f]	Visually compatible	1807	C
Diltiazem HCl	MMD	1 mg/mL[a]	ES	100 units/mL[a]	Visually compatible for 4 hr at 27°C	2062	C
Diphenhydramine HCl	PD	50 mg/mL	UP	1000 units/L[e]	Physically compatible for 4 hr at room temperature	534	C
Dobutamine HCl	LI	4 mg/mL[b]	ES	50 units/mL[b]	Physically compatible for 3 hr	1316	C
Dobutamine HCl	LI	4 mg/mL[a]	ES	50 units/mL[a]	Immediate gross precipitation	1316	I
Dobutamine HCl	LI	1 mg/mL[a]	TR	50 units/mL	Visually compatible for 4 hr at 25°C	1793	C
Dobutamine HCl	LI	4 mg/mL[a]	OR	100 units/mL[a]	Haze and white precipitate form	1877	I
Dobutamine HCl	LI	4 mg/mL[a]	ES	100 units/mL[a]	Precipitate forms in 4 hr at 27°C	2062	I
Docetaxel	RPR	0.9 mg/mL[a]	ES	100 units/mL	Physically compatible for 4 hr at 23°C	2224	C
Dopamine HCl	ACC	40 mg/mL	UP	1000 units/L[e]	Physically compatible for 4 hr at room temperature	534	C
Dopamine HCl	BA	1.6 mg/mL	TR	50 units/mL	Visually compatible for 4 hr at 25°C	1793	C
Dopamine HCl	AB	3.2 mg/mL[a]	ES	100 units/mL[a]	Visually compatible for 4 hr at 27°C	2062	C
Doripenem	JJ	5 mg/mL[a b]	HOS	100 units/mL	Physically compatible for 4 hr at 23°C	2743	C
Doxapram HCl	RB	2 mg/mL[a]	APP	1 unit/mL[t]	Visually compatible for 4 hr at 23°C	2470	C
Doxorubicin HCl		2 mg/mL		1000 units/mL	Drugs injected sequentially in Y-site with no flush. Precipitates immediately	980	I
Doxorubicin HCl liposomal	SEQ	0.4 mg/mL[a]	ES	1000 units/mL[a]	Physically compatible for 4 hr at 23°C	2087	C
Doxycycline hyclate	ES	1 mg/mL[a]	TR	50 units/mL	Visually incompatible within 4 hr at 25°C	1793	I
Droperidol		2.5 mg/mL		1000 units/mL	Drugs injected sequentially in Y-site with no flush. Precipitates immediately	980	I
Droperidol	CR	1.25 mg/mL	UP	1000 units/L[e]	Physically compatible for 4 hr at room temperature	534	C
Edrophonium chloride	RC	10 mg/mL	UP	1000 units/L[e]	Physically compatible for 4 hr at room temperature	534	C
Enalaprilat	MSD	0.05 mg/mL[a b k]	IX	40 units/mL[a]	Physically compatible for 24 hr at room temperature under fluorescent light	1355	C
Epinephrine HCl	AB	0.1 mg/mL	UP	1000 units/L[e]	Physically compatible for 4 hr at room temperature	534	C
Epinephrine HCl	AB	0.02 mg/mL[a]	ES	100 units/mL[a]	Visually compatible for 4 hr at 27°C	2062	C
Eravacycline dihydrochloride	TET	0.6 mg/mL[b]	SGT	1000 units/mL[b]	Physically compatible for 2 hr at room temperature	3532	C
Ertapenem sodium	ME	10 mg/mL[b]	APP	40 and 100 units/mL[a]	Visually compatible with about 4% ertapenem loss in 4 hr	2487	C
Ertapenem sodium	ME	10 mg/mL[b]	APP	50 and 100 units/mL[b]	Visually compatible with about 3% ertapenem loss in 4 hr	2487	C
Erythromycin lactobionate	AB	3.3 mg/mL[b]	TR	50 units/mL	Visually compatible for 4 hr at 25°C	1793	C
Esmolol HCl	DCC	10 mg/mL[a]	IX	40 units/mL[a]	Physically compatible for 24 hr at 22°C	1169	C
Estrogens, conjugated	AY	5 mg/mL	RI	1000 units/L[c]	Physically compatible for 4 hr at room temperature	322	C

Y-Site Injection Compatibility (1:1 Mixture) (Cont.)

Test Drug	Mfr	Conc	Mfr	Conc	Remarks	Ref	C/I
Ethacrynate sodium	MSD	1 mg/mL	RI	1000 units/L[c]	Physically compatible for 4 hr at room temperature	322	C
Etoposide phosphate	BR	5 mg/mL[a]	ES	100 units/mL[a]	Physically compatible for 4 hr at 23°C	2218	C
Famotidine	MSD	0.2 mg/mL[a]	ES	40 units/mL[b]	Physically compatible for 14 hr	1196	C
Famotidine	MSD	0.2 mg/mL[a]	TR	50 units/mL[a]	Physically compatible for 4 hr at 25°C	1188	C
Famotidine	ME	2 mg/mL[b]		40 units/mL[a]	Visually compatible for 4 hr at 22°C	1936	C
Fenoldopam mesylate	AB	80 mcg/mL[b]	AB	100 units/mL	Physically compatible for 4 hr at 23°C	2467	C
Fentanyl citrate	MN	0.05 mg/mL	UP	1000 units/L[e]	Physically compatible for 4 hr at room temperature	534	C
Fentanyl citrate	ES	0.05 mg/mL	ES	100 units/mL[a]	Visually compatible for 4 hr at 27°C	2062	C
Filgrastim	AMG	30 mcg/mL[a]	ES	100 units/mL[a]	Particles and filaments form immediately	1687	I
Fluconazole	RR	2 mg/mL	LY	1000 units/mL	Physically compatible for 24 hr at 25°C	1407	C
Fluconazole	PF	2 mg/mL	TR	50 units/mL	Visually compatible for 4 hr at 25°C	1793	C
Fludarabine phosphate	BX	1 mg/mL[a]	SO, WY	40[a], 100, 1000 units/mL	Visually compatible for 4 hr at 22°C	1439	C
Fluorouracil	RC	50 mg/mL	UP	1000 units/L[e]	Physically compatible for 4 hr at room temperature	534	C
Fluorouracil		50 mg/mL		1000 units/mL	Drugs injected sequentially in Y-site with no flush. No precipitate seen	980	C
Foscarnet sodium	AST	24 mg/mL	ES	1000 units/mL	Physically compatible for 24 hr at room temperature under fluorescent light	1335	C
Foscarnet sodium	AST	24 mg/mL	LY	100 units/mL[f]	Physically compatible for 24 hr at 25°C under fluorescent light	1393	C
Furosemide		10 mg/mL		1000 units/mL	Drugs injected sequentially in Y-site with no flush. No precipitate seen	980	C
Furosemide	HO	10 mg/mL	UP	1000 units/L[e]	Physically compatible for 4 hr at room temperature	534	C
Furosemide	AMR	10 mg/mL	ES	100 units/mL[a]	Visually compatible for 4 hr at 27°C	2062	C
Furosemide	HMR	2.6 mg/mL[a]	NOV	29.2 units/mL[a]	Visually compatible for 150 min	2244	C
Gallium nitrate	FUJ	1 mg/mL[b]	ES	40 units/mL[b]	Visually compatible for 24 hr at 25°C	1673	C
Gemcitabine HCl	LI	10 mg/mL[b]	ES	100 units/mL[b]	Physically compatible for 4 hr at 23°C	2226	C
Gentamicin sulfate	RS	80 mg		[b]	Precipitates immediately	528	I
Gentamicin sulfate	ES	3.2 mg/mL[f]	ES	50 units/mL[f]	Immediate gross haze	1316	I
Gentamicin sulfate	TR	2 mg/mL	TR	50 units/mL	Visually incompatible within 4 hr at 25°C	1793	I
Granisetron HCl	SKB	0.05 mg/mL[a]	AB	100 units/mL[a]	Physically compatible for 4 hr at 23°C	2000	C
Haloperidol lactate	MN	5 mg/1 mL[i]	OR	25,000 and 50,000 units/250 mL[f bb]	White precipitate forms immediately	779	I
Hetastarch in lactated electrolyte	AB	6%	ES	100 units/mL	Physically compatible for 4 hr at 23°C	2339	C
Hydralazine HCl	CI	20 mg/mL	UP	1000 units/L[e]	Physically compatible for 4 hr at room temperature	534	C
Hydrocortisone sodium succinate	UP	2 mg/mL[a]	TR	50 units/mL	Visually compatible for 4 hr at 25°C	1793	C

Y-Site Injection Compatibility (1:1 Mixture) (Cont.)

Test Drug	Mfr	Conc	Mfr	Conc	Remarks	Ref	C/I
Hydrocortisone sodium succinate	UP	125 mg/mL	ES	100 units/mL[f]	Visually compatible for 24 hr at room temperature in test tubes. No precipitate found on filter from Y-site delivery	2063	C
Hydromorphone HCl	KN	1 mg/mL	ES	100 units/mL[a]	Visually compatible for 4 hr at 27°C	2062	C
Hydroxyethyl starch 130/0.4 in sodium chloride 0.9%	FRK	6%	HOS	10 units/mL	Visually compatible for 24 hr at room temperature	2770	C
Hydroxyethyl starch 130/0.4 in sodium chloride 0.9%	FRK	6%	PP	1000, 10,000 units/mL	Visually compatible for 24 hr at room temperature	2770	C
Ibuprofen lysinate	OVA	10 mg/mL	HOS	10 units/mL[a]	Physically compatible for 4 hr at room temperature	3541	C
Ibuprofen lysinate	OVA	10 mg/mL	HOS	10 and 100 units/mL	Physically compatible for 4 hr at room temperature	3541	C
Idarubicin HCl	AD	1 mg/mL[b]	ES, SO	100 and 1000 units/mL	Haze forms immediately and precipitate forms in 12 to 20 min	1525	I
Insulin, regular	LI	0.2 unit/mL[b]	ES	60 units/mL[a]	Physically compatible for 2 hr at 25°C	1395	C
Isavuconazonium sulfate	ASP	1.5 mg/mL[f]	PRP	1000 units/mL[f]	Measured turbidity increases immediately	3263	I
Isoproterenol HCl	WI	0.2 mg/mL	UP	1000 units/L[e]	Physically compatible for 4 hr at room temperature	534	C
Isosorbide dinitrate	RP	10 mg/mL	LEO	300 units/mL[a]	Erratic availability of both drugs delivered through PVC tubing	1799	I
Labetalol HCl	SC	1 mg/mL[a]	IX	40 units/mL[a]	Physically compatible for 24 hr at 18°C	1171	C
Labetalol HCl	GL	5 mg/mL	OR	100 units/mL[a]	Cloudiness with particles forms immediately	1877	I
Labetalol HCl	AH	2 mg/mL[a]	ES	100 units/mL[a]	Visually compatible for 4 hr at 27°C	2062	C
Leucovorin calcium		10 mg/mL		1000 units/mL	Drugs injected sequentially in Y-site with no flush. No precipitate seen	980	C
Levofloxacin	OMN	5 mg/mL[a]	ES	10 units/mL	Cloudy precipitate forms	2233	I
Lidocaine HCl	AST	20 mg/mL	RI	1000 units/L[c]	Physically compatible for 4 hr at room temperature	322	C
Lidocaine HCl	TR	4 mg/mL	TR	50 units/mL	Visually compatible for 4 hr at 25°C	1793	C
Linezolid	PHU	2 mg/mL	ES	1000 units/mL[a]	Physically compatible for 4 hr at 23°C	2264	C
Lorazepam	WY	0.33 mg/mL[b]		417 units/mL	Visually compatible for 24 hr at 22°C	1855	C
Lorazepam	WY	0.5 mg/mL[a]	ES	100 units/mL[a]	Visually compatible for 4 hr at 27°C	2062	C
Magnesium sulfate	AB	500 mg/mL	UP	1000 units/L	Physically compatible for 4 hr at room temperature	534	C
Melphalan HCl	BW	0.1 mg/mL[b]	WY	100 units/mL[b]	Physically compatible for 3 hr at 22°C	1557	C
Meperidine HCl	WY	10 mg/mL[b]	ES	60 units/mL[a]	Physically compatible for 1 hr at 25°C	1338	C
Meropenem	ZEN	1 and 50 mg/mL[b]	ES	1 unit/mL[j]	Visually compatible for 4 hr at room temperature	1994	C
Meropenem		50 mg/mL	SZ	1000 units/mL	Physically compatible for 4 hr at room temperature	3538	C
Meropenem–vaborbactam	TMC	8 mg/mL[b w]	SGT	1000 units/mL[b]	Physically compatible for 3 hr at 20 to 25°C	3380	C
Methotrexate sodium		25 mg/mL		1000 units/mL	Drugs injected sequentially in Y-site with no flush. No precipitate seen	980	C
Methyldopate HCl	ES	5 mg/mL[a]	TR	50 units/mL	Visually compatible for 4 hr at 25°C	1793	C

Y-Site Injection Compatibility (1:1 Mixture) (Cont.)

Test Drug	Mfr	Conc	Mfr	Conc	Remarks	Ref	C/I
Methylergonovine maleate	SZ	0.2 mg/mL	UP	1000 units/L[e]	Physically compatible for 4 hr at room temperature	534	C
Methylprednisolone sodium succinate	UP	2.5 mg/mL[a]	TR	50 units/mL	Visually compatible for 4 hr at 25°C	1793	C
Methylprednisolone sodium succinate	UP	5 mg/mL[b]	ES	100 units/mL[f]	Visually compatible for 24 hr at room temperature in test tubes. No precipitate found on filter from Y-site delivery	2063	C
Metoclopramide HCl		5 mg/mL		1000 units/mL	Drugs injected sequentially in Y-site with no flush. No precipitate seen	980	C
Metoprolol tartrate	BED	1 mg/mL	BA	1000 units/mL[a]	Visually compatible for 24 hr at 19°C	2795	C
Metronidazole	MG	5 mg/mL	TR	50 units/mL	Visually compatible for 4 hr at 25°C	1793	C
Micafungin sodium	ASP	1.5 mg/mL[b]	AB	100 units/mL	Physically compatible for 4 hr at 23°C	2683	C
Midazolam HCl	RC	5 mg/mL		417 units/mL	Visually compatible for 24 hr at 22°C	1855	C
Midazolam HCl	RC	2 mg/mL[a]	ES	100 units/mL[a]	Visually compatible for 4 hr at 27°C	2062	C
Midazolam HCl	RC[d]	15 mg/3 mL		50 units/mL[b]	Clear solution	1053	C
Milrinone lactate	SW	0.2 mg/mL[a]	ES	100 units/mL[a]	Visually compatible for 4 hr at 27°C	2062	C
Milrinone lactate	SW	0.4 mg/mL[a]	ES	100 units/mL[a]	Visually compatible. Little loss of milrinone and heparin in 4 hr at 23°C	2214	C
Mitomycin		0.5 mg/mL		1000 units/mL	Drugs injected sequentially in Y-site with no flush. No precipitate seen	980	C
Morphine sulfate	WY	15 mg/mL	UP	1000 units/L[e]	Physically compatible for 4 hr at room temperature	534	C
Morphine sulfate	WY	0.2 mg/mL[f]	ES	50 units/mL[f]	Physically compatible for 3 hr	1316	C
Morphine sulfate	ES	1 mg/mL[b]	ES	60 units/mL[a]	Physically compatible for 1 hr at 25°C	1338	C
Morphine sulfate	SCN	2 mg/mL[a]	ES	100 units/mL[a]	Visually compatible for 4 hr at 27°C	2062	C
Nafcillin sodium	WY	20 mg/mL[a]	TR	50 units/mL	Visually compatible for 4 hr at 25°C	1793	C
Neostigmine methyl-sulfate	RC	0.5 mg/mL	UP	1000 units/L[e]	Physically compatible for 4 hr at room temperature	534	C
Nesiritide	SCI	50 mcg/mL[a b]		0.1, 1, 10 units/mL	Physically incompatible	2625	I
Nicardipine HCl	WY	1 mg/mL[a]	ES	100 units/mL[a]	Precipitate forms immediately	2062	I
Nicardipine HCl	DCC	0.1 mg/mL[a]	IX	40 units/mL[a]	Visually compatible for 24 hr at room temperature	235	C
Nitroglycerin	BA	0.2 mg/mL	ES	50 units/mL	Visually compatible for 24 hr at 23°C	1794	C
Nitroglycerin	OM	0.2 mg/mL[a]	OR	100 units/mL[a]	Visually compatible for 24 hr at 23°C	1877	C
Nitroglycerin	AB	0.4 mg/mL[a]	ES	100 units/mL[a]	Visually compatible for 4 hr at 27°C	2062	C
Norepinephrine bitartrate	WI	1 mg/mL	UP	1000 units/L[e]	Physically compatible for 4 hr at room temperature	534	C
Norepinephrine bitartrate	AB	0.128 mg/mL[a]	ES	100 units/mL[a]	Visually compatible for 4 hr at 27°C	2062	C
Ondansetron HCl	GL	1 mg/mL[b]	SO	40 units/mL[a]	Visually compatible for 4 hr at 22°C	1365	C
Oritavancin diphosphate	TAR	0.8, 1.2, and 2 mg/mL[a]	ABX	100 units/mL[a]	Haze forms immediately with precipitate after 1 hr	2928	I
Oxacillin sodium	BR	100 mg/mL	UP	1000 units/L[e]	Physically compatible for 4 hr at room temperature	534	C
Oxaliplatin	SS	0.5 mg/mL[a]	AB	100 units/mL	Physically compatible for 4 hr at 23°C	2566	C

Y-Site Injection Compatibility (1:1 Mixture) (Cont.)

Test Drug	Mfr	Conc	Mfr	Conc	Remarks	Ref	C/I
Oxytocin	SZ	1 unit/mL	UP	1000 units/L[e]	Physically compatible for 4 hr at room temperature	534	C
Paclitaxel	NCI	1.2 mg/mL[a]	WY	100 units/mL[a]	Physically compatible for 4 hr at 22°C	1556	C
Palonosetron HCl	MGI	50 mcg/mL	HOS	100 units/mL	Physically compatible. No loss of either drug in 4 hr at room temperature	2771	C
Pancuronium bromide	ES	0.05 mg/mL[a]	SO	40 units/mL[a]	Physically compatible for 24 hr at 28°C	1337	C
Pemetrexed disodium	LI	20 mg/mL[b]	AB	100 units/mL	Physically compatible for 4 hr at 23°C	2564	C
Penicillin G potassium	LI	200,000 units/mL	RI	1000 units/L[c]	Physically compatible for 4 hr at room temperature	322	C
Penicillin G potassium	RR	40,000 units/mL[a]	TR	50 units/mL	Visually compatible for 4 hr at 25°C	1793	C
Pentazocine lactate	WI	30 mg/mL	UP	1000 units/L[e]	Physically compatible for 4 hr at room temperature	534	C
Phenytoin sodium	PD	50 mg/mL	RI	1000 units/L[c]	Immediate crystal formation	322	I
Phenytoin sodium	ES	2 mg/mL[b]	TR	50 units/mL	Cloudy immediately and becomes white precipitate in 4 hr at 25°C	1793	I
Phytonadione	RC	10 mg/mL	UP	1000 units/L[e]	Physically compatible for 4 hr at room temperature	534	C
Piperacillin sodium–tazobactam sodium	LE[q]	40 mg/mL[a v]	ES	100 units/mL[a]	Physically compatible for 4 hr at 22°C	1688	C
Plazomicin sulfate	ACH	24 mg/mL[f]	SGT	1000 units/mL[f]	Cloudy with immediate increase in measured turbidity	3432	I
Potassium chloride	AB	0.2 mEq/mL[a]	TR	50 units/mL	Visually compatible for 4 hr at 25°C	1793	C
Potassium chloride	BRN	0.625 mEq/mL[a]	NOV	29.2 units/mL[a]	Visually compatible for 150 min	2244	C
Procainamide HCl	SQ	100 mg/mL	UP	1000 units/L[e]	Physically compatible for 4 hr at room temperature	534	C
Prochlorperazine edisylate	SKF	5 mg/mL	UP	1000 units/L[e]	Physically compatible for 4 hr at room temperature	534	C
Promethazine HCl	SV	50 mg/mL	UP	1000 units/L[m]	Physically compatible for 4 hr at room temperature	534	C
Promethazine HCl	SV	50 mg/mL	UP	1000 units/L[p]	Clear initially, but cloudiness develops in 4 hr at room temperature	534	I
Propofol	ZEN[cc]	10 mg/mL	ES	100 units/mL[a]	Physically compatible for 1 hr at 23°C	2066	C
Propranolol HCl	AY	1 mg/mL	UP	1000 units/L[e]	Physically compatible for 4 hr at room temperature	534	C
Quinidine gluconate	LI	6 mg/mL[b]	ES	50 units/mL[b]	Physically compatible for 3 hr	1316	C
Quinidine gluconate	LI	6 mg/mL[a]	ES	50 units/mL[a]	Immediate gross haze	1316	I
Ranitidine HCl	GL	0.5 mg/mL	LY	50 units/mL[a]	Physically compatible for 24 hr	1323	C
Ranitidine HCl	GL	1 mg/mL	TR	50 units/mL	Visually compatible for 4 hr at 25°C	1793	C
Ranitidine HCl	GL	1 mg/mL[a]	ES	100 units/mL[a]	Visually compatible for 4 hr at 27°C	2062	C
Remifentanil HCl	GW	0.025 and 0.25 mg/mL[b]	AB	100 units/mL	Physically compatible for 4 hr at 23°C	2075	C
Sargramostim	IMM	10 mcg/mL[b]	WY	100 units/mL	Visually compatible for 4 hr at 22°C	1436	C
Sargramostim	IMM	6[b r] and 15[b] mcg/mL	ES	100 units/mL[f]	Visually compatible for 2 hr	1618	C
Scopolamine HBr	BW	0.86 mg/mL	UP	1000 units/L[e]	Physically compatible for 4 hr at room temperature	534	C
Sodium bicarbonate	BR	75 mg/mL	RI	1000 units/L[c]	Physically compatible for 4 hr at room temperature	322	C
Sodium bicarbonate		1.4%	CH	500 units/mL[b]	Visually compatible for 4 hr at room temperature	1788	C

Y-Site Injection Compatibility (1:1 Mixture) (Cont.)

Test Drug	Mfr	Conc	Mfr	Conc	Remarks	Ref	C/I
Sodium nitroprusside	ES	0.2 mg/mL[a]	TR	50 units/mL	Visually compatible for 4 hr at 25°C protected from light	1793	C
Sodium nitroprusside	RC	0.2 mg/mL[a]	OR	100 units/mL[a]	Visually compatible for 24 hr at 23°C	1877	C
Sodium nitroprusside	RC	1.2 and 3 mg/mL[a]	OR	48, 200, 480 units/mL[s]	Visually compatible for 48 hr at 24°C protected from light	2357	C
Sodium nitroprusside	RC	0.3 mg/mL[a]	OR	480 units/mL[s]	Visually compatible for 48 hr at 24°C protected from light	2357	C
Succinylcholine chloride	BW	20 mg/mL	RI	1000 units/L[c]	Physically compatible for 4 hr at room temperature	322	C
Tacrolimus	FUJ	1 mg/mL[b]	ES	10 units/mL[a]	Visually compatible for 24 hr at 25°C	1630	C
Tedizolid phosphate	CUB	0.8 mg/mL[b]	PRP	1000 units/mL[b]	Physically compatible for 2 hr	3244	C
Telavancin HCl	ASP	7.5 mg/mL[a b]	APP	1000 units/mL	Measured turbidity increased	2830	I
Telavancin HCl	ASP	7.5 mg/mL[k]	APP	1000 units/mL	Physically compatible for 2 hr	2830	C
Theophylline	TR	4 mg/mL	TR	50 units/mL	Visually compatible for 4 hr at 25°C	1793	C
Thiotepa	IMM[n]	1 mg/mL[a]	ES	100 units/mL[a]	Physically compatible for 4 hr at 23°C	1861	C
Tigecycline	WY	1 mg/mL[b]		10 units/mL	Physically compatible for 4 hr	2714	C
Tigecycline	WY	1 mg/mL[b]		100 units/mL[b]	Physically compatible for 4 hr	2714	C
Tirofiban HCl	ME	0.05 mg/mL[a b]	AB	40 units/mL[a]	Physically compatible. No tirofiban or heparin loss in 4 hr at room temperature	2250	C
Tirofiban HCl	ME	0.05 mg/mL[b]	AB	50 units/mL[b]	Physically compatible. No tirofiban or heparin loss in 4 hr at room temperature	2250	C
Tirofiban HCl	ME	0.05 mg/mL[a b]	AB	100 units/mL[a b]	Physically compatible. No tirofiban or heparin loss in 4 hr at room temperature	2250	C
TNA #218 to #226[o]			AB	100 units/mL	Damage to emulsion occurs immediately with free oil formation possible	2215	I
Tobramycin sulfate	LI	3.2 mg/mL[f]	ES	50 units/mL[f]	Immediate gross haze	1316	I
Tobramycin sulfate	LI	0.8 mg/mL[a]	TR	50 units/mL	Visually incompatible within 4 hr at 25°C	1793	I
TPN #189[o]			DB	500 units/mL[b]	Visually compatible for 24 hr at 22°C	1767	C
TPN #212 to #215[o]			AB	100 units/mL	Physically compatible for 4 hr at 23°C	2109	C
Tranexamic acid	PF				Manufacturer states compatible	2887	C
Trimethobenzamide HCl	RC	100 mg/mL	UP	1000 units/L[e]	Physically compatible for 4 hr at room temperature	534	C
Vancomycin HCl	LI	6.6 mg/mL[a]	TR	50 units/mL	Visually incompatible within 4 hr at 25°C	1793	I
Vancomycin HCl	LE	10 mg/mL[b]	ES	100 units/mL[f]	Precipitate forms	2063	I
Vancomycin HCl	PHS	2.5 mg/mL[b]	LEO	10 and 5000 units/mL[b]	Physically compatible with little change in heparin activity in 14 days at 4 and 37°C. Antibiotic not tested	2684	C
Vancomycin HCl	PHS	2 mg/mL[b]	LEO	10 units/mL[b]	Physically compatible with little change in heparin activity in 14 days at 4 and 37°C. Antibiotic not tested	2684	C
Vasopressin	AMR	2 and 4 units/mL[b]	BA	100 units/mL[a]	Physically compatible with vasopressin pushed through a Y-site over 5 sec	2478	C
Vecuronium bromide	OR	0.1 mg/mL[a]	SO	40 units/mL[a]	Physically compatible for 24 hr at 28°C	1337	C
Vecuronium bromide	OR	1 mg/mL	ES	100 units/mL[a]	Visually compatible for 4 hr at 27°C	2062	C
Vinblastine sulfate		1 mg/mL		1000 units/mL	Drugs injected sequentially in Y-site with no flush. No precipitate seen	980	C

Y-Site Injection Compatibility (1:1 Mixture) (Cont.)

Test Drug	Mfr	Conc	Mfr	Conc	Remarks	Ref	C/I
Vincristine sulfate		1 mg/mL		1000 units/mL	Drugs injected sequentially in Y-site with no flush. No precipitate seen	980	C
Vinorelbine tartrate	BW	1 mg/mL[b]	ES	100 units/mL[b]	Physically compatible for 4 hr at 22°C	1558	C
Vinorelbine tartrate	GW	3 mg/mL[b]		100 units/mL[b]	A fine haze forms immediately, becoming cloudy in 15 min	2238	I
Vinorelbine tartrate	GW	2 mg/mL[b]		100 units/mL[b]	Visually compatible for at least 15 min	2238	C
Vinorelbine tartrate	GW	1 mg/mL[b]		100 units/mL[b]	Visually compatible for at least 15 min	2238	C
Vinorelbine tartrate	GW	4 mg/4 mL[b]		100 units/1 mL[b]	Volumes mixed as cited. Visually compatible for at least 15 min	2238	C
Vinorelbine tartrate	GW	8 mg/4 mL[b]		100 units/1 mL[b]	Volumes mixed as cited. Precipitate forms	2238	I
Vinorelbine tartrate	GW	12 mg/4 mL[b]		100 units/1 mL[b]	Volumes mixed as cited. Precipitate forms	2238	I
Zidovudine	BW	4 mg/mL[a]	LY	100 units/mL[a]	Physically compatible for 4 hr at 25°C	1193	C

[a] Tested in dextrose 5%.

[b] Tested in sodium chloride 0.9%.

[c] Tested in combination with hydrocortisone sodium succinate (Upjohn) 100 mg/L in dextrose 5%, sodium chloride 0.9%, and Ringer's injection, lactated.

[d] Given over three minutes into a heparin infusion run at 1 mL/min.

[e] Tested in dextrose 5% in Ringer's injection, dextrose 5% in Ringer's injection, lactated, dextrose 5%, Ringer's injection, lactated, and sodium chloride 0.9%.

[f] Tested in both dextrose 5% and sodium chloride 0.9%.

[g] Tested in bacteriostatic sodium chloride 0.9% preserved with benzyl alcohol 0.9%.

[h] Dacarbazine in intravenous tubing flushed with heparin sodium.

[i] Injected over one minute.

[j] Tested in sterile water for injection.

[k] Tested in Ringer's injection, lactated.

[l] Final concentration after mixing.

[m] Tested in dextrose 5% in Ringer's injection, lactated, dextrose 5%, Ringer's injection, lactated, and sodium chloride 0.9%.

[n] Lyophilized formulation tested.

[o] Refer to Appendix for the composition of parenteral nutrition solutions. TNA indicates a 3-in-1 admixture, and TPN indicates a 2-in-1 admixture.

[p] Tested in dextrose 5% in Ringer's injection.

[q] Test performed using the formulation WITHOUT edetate disodium.

[r] Tested with albumin human 0.1%.

[s] Tested in dextrose 5% in sodium chloride 0.225%.

[t] Tested in sodium chloride 0.45%.

[u] Ampicillin component. Ampicillin in a 2:1 fixed-ratio concentration with sulbactam.

[v] Piperacillin component. Piperacillin in an 8:1 fixed-ratio concentration with tazobactam.

[w] Meropenem component. Meropenem in a 1:1 fixed-ratio concentration with vaborbactam.

[x] Test performed using the Cubicin formulation.

[y] Ceftolozane component. Ceftolozane in a 2:1 fixed-ratio concentration with tazobactam.

[z] Ceftazidime component. Ceftazidime in a 4:1 fixed-ratio concentration with avibactam.

[aa] Tested in both dextrose 5% and Ringer's injection, lactated.

[bb] Run at 1000 units/hr.

[cc] Test performed using the formulation WITH edetate disodium.

Additional Compatibility Information

Parenteral Nutrition Admixtures

In solutions of amino acids 5% and dextrose 5 or 25% with vitamins or trace elements, heparin activity was retained for 24 hours at 25°C. However, the activity fell significantly after 24 hours.[900]

Flocculation of fat emulsion (Kabi-Vitrum) was reported during Y-site administration into a line being used to infuse a parenteral nutrition solution containing both calcium gluconate and heparin sodium. Subsequent evaluation indicated that the combination of calcium gluconate (0.46 and 1.8 mM/125 mL) plus heparin sodium (25 and 100 units/125 mL) in amino acids plus dextrose would induce flocculation of the fat emulsion within 2 to 4 minutes at concentrations that resulted in no visually apparent flocculation in 30 minutes with either agent alone.[1214]

Calcium chloride concentrations of 1 to 20 mM normally result in slow flocculation of fat emulsion 20%, intravenous, over a period of hours. When heparin sodium 5 units/mL was added, the flocculation rate accelerated greatly; a cream layer was observed visually in a few minutes. This effect was not observed when sodium ion was substituted for the divalent calcium.[1406]

Destabilization of fat emulsion (Intralipid 20%) was observed when administered simultaneously with a parenteral nutrition admixture. The damage, detected by viscosity measurement, occurred immediately upon contact at the Y-site. The extent of the destabilization was dependent on the concentration of the heparin and the presence of MVI Pediatric with its surfactant content. In addition to the viscosity changes, phase separation was observed in 2 hours. Parenteral nutrition admixtures containing heparin should never be premixed with fat emulsion as a 3-in-1 total nutrient admixture because of this emulsion destabilization. The damage might be minimized during Y-site co-administration as long as the heparin was kept at a sufficiently low concentration (no visible separation occurred at a heparin concentration of 0.5 unit/mL) and the length of tubing between the Y-site and the patient was minimized.[2282]

However, because the damage to emulsion integrity has been found to occur immediately upon mixing with heparin in the presence of the calcium ions in parenteral nutrition admixtures[1214 2215 2282] and no evaluation and documentation of the clinical safety of using such destabilized emulsions has been performed, use of such damaged emulsions in patients is suspect.

Peritoneal Dialysis Solutions

The activity of heparin 35,000 units/L was evaluated in peritoneal dialysis fluids containing 1.5 and 2.5% dextrose (Dianeal, Travenol). Storage at 25°C resulted in an apparent temporary 50% loss of heparin activity in 4 hours with recovery in 6 hours. Heparin activity was then retained for 14 days at 4°C.[900]

Gentamicin sulfate 10 mg/L with heparin sodium 1000 units/L in Dianeal with dextrose 5% had no significant reduction in gentamicin sulfate concentration or of heparin sodium in 4 to 6 hours.[228] However, a marked reduction in the anticoagulant activity of heparin sodium occurred if opalescence or a precipitate is formed, which results if the undiluted drugs are combined, even if the precipitate redissolves. Heparin activity was retained if one drug was added to a dilute solution of the other and no precipitate formed.[295]

Vancomycin hydrochloride (Lilly) 15 mg/L to 5.3 g/L in Dianeal with dextrose 2.5 or 4.25% was physically compatible with heparin sodium (Organon) 500 to 14,300 units/L for 24 hours at 25°C under fluorescent light. However, a white precipitate formed immediately in combinations of heparin sodium with vancomycin hydrochloride 6.9 to 14.3 g/L.[1322]

Heparin Locks

Heparin locks, weak heparin solutions instilled or "locked" into infusion ports or sets through a resealing latex diaphragm, are useful in providing an established intravenous route for intermittent intravenous injections. To maintain patency, a weak heparin solution is left in the tubing. Concentrations of heparin sodium used have varied from about 10 to 1000 units/mL of sodium chloride 0.9%, with 10 and 100 units/mL being the most common. The volume of dilute heparin sodium in sodium chloride 0.9% usually used to flush the set is 0.2 to 1 mL.[255 256 257 258 405 677 678 901 2119] However, the use of sodium chloride 0.9% instead of a solution containing heparin has been suggested to maintain patency. Studies have found sodium chloride 0.9% to be as effective in maintaining patency as 10- and 100-unit/mL solutions of heparin.[902 903 1109 1266 1267 1268 1269 1639 1640 1641 1656 1839 1959 2003 2119] Other investigators reported that even small amounts of heparin solution are more effective than sodium chloride 0.9% alone.[678 1270 2120 2121]

Evaluations of the use of heparinized solutions as locks or continuous flow solutions to help maintain patency in central venous catheters and arterial catheters have resulted in similarly variable results and recommendations.[2122 2123 2124 2125 2126] Although use of such heparinized solutions has been generally considered a benign technique causing minimal problems, a number of adverse effects have been reported, especially from solutions with a high heparin concentration and/or numerous heparin flushes.[2127 2128 2129 2130 2131 2132]

Vancomycin hydrochloride (Lilly) 25 mcg/mL and heparin sodium (Elkins-Sinn) 100 units/mL in 0.9% sodium chloride injection as a catheter flush solution was evaluated for stability when stored at 4°C for 14 days. The flush solution was visually clear, and vancomycin activity and heparin activity were retained throughout the storage period. However, an additional 24 hours at 37°C to simulate use conditions resulted in losses of both agents ranging from 20 to 37%.[1933]

Vancomycin hydrochloride 25 mcg/mL combined with heparin sodium (Hospira) 10 units/mL in sterile water for injection for use as a lock solution was found to be physically compatible. Little or no vancomycin loss occurred in 3 days at 4°C. However, losses of 8% occurred in 3 days at 27°C and 1 day at 40°C.[2820]

If ciprofloxacin (Sicor) 2 mg/mL was added to this flush solution, a white precipitate appeared within 1 day. Losses of both ciprofloxacin and vancomycin occurred as well.[2820]

A combination of daptomycin (Cubist) 5 mg/mL and heparin sodium (Hospira) 100 units/mL in Ringer's injection, lactated was evaluated for stability as a lock solution stored in 5-mL aliquots in 5-mL polypropylene syringes (Becton Dickinson) at 4 and −20°C.[2978] The solution remained clear and colorless on visual inspection and little or no loss of either drug occurred throughout the 14-day study period.[2978]

Methylprednisolone

The compatibility of methylprednisolone sodium succinate (Upjohn) with heparin sodium added to an auxiliary medication infusion unit has been studied. Primary admixtures were prepared by adding heparin sodium 10,000 units/L to dextrose 5%, dextrose 5% in sodium chloride 0.9%, and Ringer's injection, lactated. Up to 100 mL of the primary admixture was added along with methylprednisolone sodium succinate (Upjohn) to the auxiliary medication infusion unit with the following results:[329]

Selected Revisions May 1, 2020. © Copyright, October 1982. American Society of Health-System Pharmacists, Inc.

Methylprednisolone Sodium Succinate	Heparin Sodium 10,000 units/L of Primary Solution	Results
500 mg	D5S, D5W qs 100 mL	Clear solution for 24 hr
500 mg	LR qs 100 mL or added to 100 mL LR	Clear solution for 6 hr
1000 mg	D5S, D5W qs 100 mL	Clear solution for 6 hr
1000 mg	Added to 100 mL D5W	Clear solution for 24 hr
1000 mg	LR qs 100 mL or added to 100 mL LR	Clear solution for 4 to 6 hr
2000 mg	D5W qs 100 mL	Clear solution for 6 hr
2000 mg	D5S, LR qs 100 mL	Clear solution for 24 hr

Hetastarch in Lactated Electrolyte
AHFS 40:12

Products

Hetastarch 6% in lactated electrolyte is available in 500-mL flexible plastic infusion containers.[2867] Each 100 mL of solution contains hetastarch 6 g, sodium chloride 672 mg, sodium lactate anhydrous 317 mg, dextrose hydrous 99 mg, calcium chloride dihydrate 37 mg, potassium chloride 22 mg, and magnesium chloride hexahydrate 9 mg in water for injection.[2867] The concentrations of electrolytes are shown in Table 1.[2867]

Table 1. Electrolyte composition[2867]

Electrolyte	mEq/L
Sodium	143
Calcium	5
Potassium	3
Magnesium	0.9
Chloride	124
Lactate	28

pH

Approximately 5.9 with negligible buffering capacity.[2867]

Osmolarity

The calculated osmolarity is approximately 307 mOsm/L.[2867]

Tonicity

The injection is an isotonic solution.[2867]

Trade Name(s)

Hextend

Administration

Hetastarch 6% in lactated electrolyte is administered only by intravenous infusion.[2867] The dosage and rate of infusion should be individualized according to the patient's condition and response.[2867] The container is made of polyvinyl chloride (PVC) and is latex free.[2867] The product should be inspected for discoloration and particulate matter prior to use.[2867] If the drug is administered by pressure infusion, all air should be withdrawn or expelled from the container through the medication port prior to infusion.[2867]

Solutions such as this product that contain calcium should not be administered simultaneously with blood through the same set because of the likelihood of coagulation.[2867]

Stability

Intact containers of hetastarch 6% in lactated electrolyte should be stored at 25°C and protected from freezing and excessive heat.[2867] Brief exposure at temperatures up to 40°C does not adversely affect the product.[2867]

Hetastarch 6% in lactated electrolyte is a clear, pale yellow to amber solution.[2867] Prolonged exposure to adverse conditions may result in the formation of a turbid deep brown appearance or crystalline precipitate; such solutions should not be used.[2867]

Compatibility Information

Additive Compatibility

Hetastarch in lactated electrolyte

Test Drug	Mfr	Conc/L or %	Mfr	Conc/L or %	Test Solution	Remarks	Ref	C/I
Tranexamic acid		2 g	HOS	5.88%		No evidence of physical incompatibility over 4 hr	3454	C

Y-Site Injection Compatibility (1:1 Mixture)

Hetastarch in lactated electrolyte

Test Drug	Mfr	Conc	Mfr	Conc	Remarks	Ref	C/I
Alfentanil HCl	TAY	0.125 mg/mL[a]	AB	6%	Physically compatible for 4 hr at 23°C	2339	C
Amikacin sulfate	APC	5 mg/mL[a]	AB	6%	Physically compatible for 4 hr at 23°C	2339	C
Aminophylline	AMR	2.5 mg/mL[a]	AB	6%	Physically compatible for 4 hr at 23°C	2339	C

DOI: 10.37573/9781585286850.191

Y-Site Injection Compatibility (1:1 Mixture) (Cont.)

Test Drug	Mfr	Conc	Mfr	Conc	Remarks	Ref	C/I
Amiodarone HCl	WAY	4 mg/mL[a]	AB	6%	Physically compatible for 4 hr at 23°C	2339	C
Amphotericin B	APC	0.6 mg/mL[a]	AB	6%	Immediate gross precipitation	2339	I
Ampicillin sodium	APC	20 mg/mL[b]	AB	6%	Physically compatible for 4 hr at 23°C	2339	C
Ampicillin sodium–sulbactam sodium	PF	20 mg/mL[b d]	AB	6%	Physically compatible for 4 hr at 23°C	2339	C
Atracurium besylate	GW	0.5 mg/mL[a]	AB	6%	Physically compatible for 4 hr at 23°C	2339	C
Azithromycin	PF	2 mg/mL[a]	AB	6%	Physically compatible for 4 hr at 23°C	2339	C
Aztreonam	BMS	40 mg/mL[a]	AB	6%	Physically compatible for 4 hr at 23°C	2339	C
Bumetanide	OHM	0.04 mg/mL[a]	AB	6%	Physically compatible for 4 hr at 23°C	2339	C
Butorphanol tartrate	APC	0.04 mg/mL[a]	AB	6%	Physically compatible for 4 hr at 23°C	2339	C
Calcium gluconate	FUJ	40 mg/mL[a]	AB	6%	Physically compatible for 4 hr at 23°C	2339	C
Cefazolin sodium	LI	20 mg/mL[a]	AB	6%	Physically compatible for 4 hr at 23°C	2339	C
Cefepime HCl	BMS	20 mg/mL[a]	AB	6%	Physically compatible for 4 hr at 23°C	2339	C
Cefotaxime sodium	HO	20 mg/mL[a]	AB	6%	Physically compatible for 4 hr at 23°C	2339	C
Cefotetan disodium	ZEN	20 mg/mL[a]	AB	6%	Physically compatible for 4 hr at 23°C	2339	C
Cefoxitin sodium	ME	20 mg/mL[a]	AB	6%	Physically compatible for 4 hr at 23°C	2339	C
Ceftazidime	GW	40 mg/mL[a]	AB	6%	Physically compatible for 4 hr at 23°C	2339	C
Cefuroxime sodium	LI	30 mg/mL[a]	AB	6%	Physically compatible for 4 hr at 23°C	2339	C
Chlorpromazine HCl	ES	2 mg/mL[a]	AB	6%	Physically compatible for 4 hr at 23°C	2339	C
Ciprofloxacin	BAY	2 mg/mL[a]	AB	6%	Physically compatible for 4 hr at 23°C	2339	C
Cisatracurium besylate	GW	0.5 mg/mL[a]	AB	6%	Physically compatible for 4 hr at 23°C	2339	C
Clindamycin phosphate	PHU	10 mg/mL[a]	AB	6%	Physically compatible for 4 hr at 23°C	2339	C
Dexamethasone sodium phosphate	APP	1 mg/mL[a]	AB	6%	Physically compatible for 4 hr at 23°C	2339	C
Diazepam	AB	5 mg/mL	AB	6%	White turbidity forms immediately	2339	I
Digoxin	ES	0.25 mg/mL	AB	6%	Physically compatible for 4 hr at 23°C	2339	C
Diltiazem HCl	BA	5 mg/mL	AB	6%	Physically compatible for 4 hr at 23°C	2339	C
Diphenhydramine HCl	SCN	2 mg/mL[a]	AB	6%	Physically compatible for 4 hr at 23°C	2339	C
Dobutamine HCl	AST	4 mg/mL[a]	AB	6%	Physically compatible for 4 hr at 23°C	2339	C
Dolasetron mesylate	HO	2 mg/mL[a]	AB	6%	Physically compatible for 4 hr at 23°C	2339	C
Dopamine HCl	AB	3.2 mg/mL[a]	AB	6%	Physically compatible for 4 hr at 23°C	2339	C
Doxycycline hyclate	APP	1 mg/mL[a]	AB	6%	Physically compatible for 4 hr at 23°C	2339	C
Droperidol	AMR	2.5 mg/mL	AB	6%	Physically compatible for 4 hr at 23°C	2339	C
Enalaprilat	ME	0.1 mg/mL[a]	AB	6%	Physically compatible for 4 hr at 23°C	2339	C
Ephedrine sulfate	TAY	5 mg/mL[a]	AB	6%	Physically compatible for 4 hr at 23°C	2339	C
Epinephrine HCl	AB	0.05 mg/mL[a]	AB	6%	Physically compatible for 4 hr at 23°C	2339	C
Erythromycin lactobionate	AB	5 mg/mL[b]	AB	6%	Physically compatible for 4 hr at 23°C	2339	C

Y-Site Injection Compatibility (1:1 Mixture) (Cont.)

Test Drug	Mfr	Conc	Mfr	Conc	Remarks	Ref	C/I
Esmolol HCl	OHM	10 mg/mL	AB	6%	Physically compatible for 4 hr at 23°C	2339	C
Famotidine	ME	2 mg/mL[a]	AB	6%	Physically compatible for 4 hr at 23°C	2339	C
Fenoldopam mesylate	AB	80 mcg/mL[b]	AB	6%	Physically compatible for 4 hr at 23°C	2467	C
Fentanyl citrate	ES	12.5 mcg/mL[a]	AB	6%	Physically compatible for 4 hr at 23°C	2339	C
Fluconazole	PF	2 mg/mL	AB	6%	Physically compatible for 4 hr at 23°C	2339	C
Furosemide	AMR	3 mg/mL[a]	AB	6%	Physically compatible for 4 hr at 23°C	2339	C
Gentamicin sulfate	SC	5 mg/mL[a]	AB	6%	Physically compatible for 4 hr at 23°C	2339	C
Granisetron HCl	SKB	0.05 mg/mL[a]	AB	6%	Physically compatible for 4 hr at 23°C	2339	C
Haloperidol lactate	MN	0.2 mg/mL[a]	AB	6%	Physically compatible for 4 hr at 23°C	2339	C
Heparin sodium	ES	100 units/mL	AB	6%	Physically compatible for 4 hr at 23°C	2339	C
Hydrocortisone sodium succinate	PHU	1 mg/mL[a]	AB	6%	Physically compatible for 4 hr at 23°C	2339	C
Hydromorphone HCl	AST	0.5 mg/mL[a]	AB	6%	Physically compatible for 4 hr at 23°C	2339	C
Hydroxyzine HCl	ES	2 mg/mL[a]	AB	6%	Physically compatible for 4 hr at 23°C	2339	C
Isoproterenol HCl	AB	0.02 mg/mL[a]	AB	6%	Physically compatible for 4 hr at 23°C	2339	C
Ketorolac tromethamine	AB	15 mg/mL	AB	6%	Physically compatible for 4 hr at 23°C	2339	C
Labetalol HCl	GW	2 mg/mL[a]	AB	6%	Physically compatible for 4 hr at 23°C	2339	C
Levofloxacin	OMN	5 mg/mL[a]	AB	6%	Physically compatible for 4 hr at 23°C	2339	C
Lidocaine HCl	AB	8 mg/mL[a]	AB	6%	Physically compatible for 4 hr at 23°C	2339	C
Lorazepam	OHM	0.5 mg/mL[a]	AB	6%	Physically compatible for 4 hr at 23°C	2339	C
Magnesium sulfate	AST	100 mg/mL[a]	AB	6%	Physically compatible for 4 hr at 23°C	2339	C
Mannitol	BA	15%	AB	6%	Physically compatible for 4 hr at 23°C	2339	C
Meperidine HCl	OHM	4 mg/mL[a]	AB	6%	Physically compatible for 4 hr at 23°C	2339	C
Methylprednisolone sodium succinate	PHU	5 mg/mL[a]	AB	6%	Physically compatible for 4 hr at 23°C	2339	C
Metoclopramide HCl	FAU	5 mg/mL	AB	6%	Physically compatible for 4 hr at 23°C	2339	C
Metronidazole	AB	5 mg/mL	AB	6%	Physically compatible for 4 hr at 23°C	2339	C
Midazolam HCl	RC	1 mg/mL[a]	AB	6%	Physically compatible for 4 hr at 23°C	2339	C
Milrinone lactate	SAN	0.2 mg/mL[a]	AB	6%	Physically compatible for 4 hr at 23°C	2339	C
Morphine sulfate	AST	1 mg/mL[a]	AB	6%	Physically compatible for 4 hr at 23°C	2339	C
Nalbuphine HCl	AST	10 mg/mL	AB	6%	Physically compatible for 4 hr at 23°C	2339	C
Nitroglycerin	AMR	0.4 mg/mL[a]	AB	6%	Physically compatible for 4 hr at 23°C	2339	C
Norepinephrine bitartrate	AB	0.12 mg/mL[a]	AB	6%	Physically compatible for 4 hr at 23°C	2339	C
Ondansetron HCl	GW	1 mg/mL[a]	AB	6%	Physically compatible for 4 hr at 23°C	2339	C
Palonosetron HCl	MGI	50 mcg/mL	HOS	6%	Physically compatible. No palonosetron loss in 4 hr at room temperature	2775	C
Pancuronium bromide	ES	0.1 mg/mL[a]	AB	6%	Physically compatible for 4 hr at 23°C	2339	C
Phenylephrine HCl	OHM	1 mg/mL[a]	AB	6%	Physically compatible for 4 hr at 23°C	2339	C

Y-Site Injection Compatibility (1:1 Mixture) (Cont.)

Test Drug	Mfr	Conc	Mfr	Conc	Remarks	Ref	C/I
Piperacillin sodium–tazobactam sodium	LE[c]	40 mg/mL[a] [e]	AB	6%	Physically compatible for 4 hr at 23°C	2339	C
Potassium chloride	AB	0.1 mEq/mL[a]	AB	6%	Physically compatible for 4 hr at 23°C	2339	C
Procainamide HCl	ES	10 mg/mL[a]	AB	6%	Physically compatible for 4 hr at 23°C	2339	C
Prochlorperazine edisylate	SO	0.5 mg/mL[a]	AB	6%	Physically compatible for 4 hr at 23°C	2339	C
Promethazine HCl	SCN	2 mg/mL[a]	AB	6%	Physically compatible for 4 hr at 23°C	2339	C
Ranitidine HCl	GW	2 mg/mL[a]	AB	6%	Physically compatible for 4 hr at 23°C	2339	C
Rocuronium bromide	OR	1 mg/mL[a]	AB	6%	Physically compatible for 4 hr at 23°C	2339	C
Sodium bicarbonate	AB	1 mEq/mL	AB	6%	Microprecipitate develops rapidly	2339	I
Sodium nitroprusside	OHM	2 mg/mL[a]	AB	6%	Physically compatible for 4 hr at 23°C protected from light	2339	C
Succinylcholine chloride	AB	2 mg/mL[a]	AB	6%	Physically compatible for 4 hr at 23°C	2339	C
Sufentanil citrate	BA	12.5 mcg/mL[a]	AB	6%	Physically compatible for 4 hr at 23°C	2339	C
Theophylline	BA	4 mg/mL[a]	AB	6%	Physically compatible for 4 hr at 23°C	2339	C
Tobramycin sulfate	GNS	5 mg/mL[a]	AB	6%	Physically compatible for 4 hr at 23°C	2339	C
Tranexamic acid		100 mg/mL	HOS	6%	No evidence of physical incompatibility over 4 hr	3454	C
Trimethoprim–sulfamethoxazole	ES	0.8 mg/mL[a] [f]	AB	6%	Physically compatible for 4 hr at 23°C	2339	C
Vancomycin HCl	LI	10 mg/mL[a]	AB	6%	Physically compatible for 4 hr at 23°C	2339	C
Vecuronium bromide	OR	0.2 mg/mL[a]	AB	6%	Physically compatible for 4 hr at 23°C	2339	C
Verapamil HCl	AMR	1.25 mg/mL[a]	AB	6%	Physically compatible for 4 hr at 23°C	2339	C

[a] Tested in dextrose 5%.

[b] Tested in sodium chloride 0.9%.

[c] Test performed using the formulation WITHOUT edetate disodium.

[d] Ampicillin component. Ampicillin in a 2:1 fixed-ratio concentration with sulbactam.

[e] Piperacillin component. Piperacillin in an 8:1 fixed-ratio concentration with tazobactam.

[f] Trimethoprim component. Trimethoprim in a 1:5 fixed-ratio concentration with sulfamethoxazole.

Selected Revisions September 30, 2019. © Copyright, October 2002. American Society of Health-System Pharmacists, Inc.

Hetastarch in Sodium Chloride 0.9%
AHFS 40:12

Products

Hetastarch is available as a 6% (6 g/100 mL) injection in sodium chloride 0.9% in 500-mL plastic containers.[3050] The solution also contains sodium hydroxide for pH adjustment during manufacturing.[3050]

pH

Approximately 5.9.[3050]

Osmolarity

The product has a calculated osmolarity of 309 mOsm/L.[3050]

Sodium Content

Hetastarch 6% in sodium chloride 0.9% provides 77 mEq of sodium per 500-mL container.[3050]

Trade Name(s)

Hespan

Administration

Hetastarch is administered only by intravenous infusion.[3050] The dosage and rate of infusion must be individualized to the patient's condition and response.[3050]

Stability

Hetastarch injection is a clear, pale yellow to amber colloidal solution.[3050] The product should be stored at controlled room temperature and protected from freezing and excessive heat.[3050] Brief exposure to temperatures up to 40°C does not affect stability; however, prolonged storage under adverse conditions may result in the formation of a crystalline precipitate or a change to a deep brown turbid appearance.[3050] Such solutions should not be administered.[3050]

Containers are for single use; any unused portions should be discarded.[3050]

Hetastarch is derived from a waxy starch composed almost entirely of amylopectin.[3050] Amylose has been shown to associate and precipitate over time in solution.[2296] Before hetastarch is used, the colloidal solution should be checked for clarity and particulates and the flexible plastic containers should be squeezed to check for small leaks.[3050]

Compatibility Information

Additive Compatibility

Hetastarch in sodium chloride 0.9%

Test Drug	Mfr	Conc/L or %	Mfr	Conc/L or %	Test Solution	Remarks	Ref	C/I
Ampicillin sodium		4 g		6%	NS	18% loss in 6 hr and 35% in 24 hr at 20°C	834	I
Azacitidine						Stated to be incompatible	3325, 3326	I
Enalaprilat	MSD	25 mg	DU	6%		Physically compatible for 24 hr at room temperature under fluorescent light	1355	C
Fosphenytoin sodium	PD[a]	1, 8, 20 mg PE/mL	MG	6%	NS	Visually compatible with little or no loss in 7 days at 25°C under fluorescent light	2083	C
Oxacillin sodium		4 g		6%		1% oxacillin loss in 24 hr at 20°C	834	C

[a] Concentration of fosphenytoin expressed in milligrams of phenytoin sodium equivalents (PE) per mL.

Y-Site Injection Compatibility (1:1 Mixture)

Hetastarch in sodium chloride 0.9%

Test Drug	Mfr	Conc	Mfr	Conc	Remarks	Ref	C/I
Amikacin sulfate	BR	5 mg/mL[a]	DCC	6%	Small crystals form immediately after mixing and persist for 4 hr	1313	I
Ampicillin sodium	BR	20 mg/mL[a]	DCC	6%	Visually compatible for 4 hr at room temperature	1313	C
Ampicillin sodium	BR	20 mg/mL[a]	DCC	6%	One or two particles in one of five vials. Fine white strands appeared immediately during Y-site infusion	1315	I

DOI: 10.37573/9781585286850.192

Y-Site Injection Compatibility (1:1 Mixture) (Cont.)

Test Drug	Mfr	Conc	Mfr	Conc	Remarks	Ref	C/I
Cefazolin sodium	SKF	20 mg/mL[a]	DCC	6%	Visually compatible for 4 hr at room temperature	1313	C
Cefazolin sodium	SKF	20 mg/mL[a]	DCC	6%	Simulation in vials showed no incompatibility, but white precipitate formed in Y-site during infusion	1315	I
Cefotaxime sodium	HO	20 mg/mL[a]	DCC	6%	Small crystals form immediately after mixing and persist for 4 hr	1313	I
Cefoxitin sodium	MSD	20 mg/mL[a]	DCC	6%	Precipitate in 1 hr at room temperature	1313	I
Clevidipine butyrate	CHS	0.5 mg/mL		6%	Emulsion broke	3334	I
Diltiazem HCl	MMD	5 mg/mL	DU	6%	Visually compatible	1807	C
Doxycycline hyclate	LY	1 mg/mL[a]	DCC	6%	Visually compatible for 4 hr at room temperature	1313	C
Doxycycline hyclate	LY	1 mg/mL[a]	DCC	6%	White particle in one of five tests. No incompatibility during Y-site infusion	1315	?
Enalaprilat	MSD	0.05 mg/mL[b]	DCC	6%	Physically compatible for 24 hr at room temperature under fluorescent light	1355	C
Ertapenem sodium	ME	10 mg/mL[b]	AB	6%	Visually compatible with about 3% ertapenem loss in 8 hr	2487	C
Gentamicin sulfate	TR	0.8 mg/mL[c]	DCC	6%	Precipitates immediately but disappears after 1 hr at room temperature	1313	I
Nicardipine HCl	DCC	0.1 mg/mL[a]	DU	6%	Visually compatible for 24 hr at room temperature	235	C
Ranitidine HCl	GL	0.5 mg/mL[c]	DCC	6%	Visually compatible for 4 hr at room temperature	1313	C
Ranitidine HCl	GL	0.5 mg/mL	DCC	6%	Barely visible particles appeared and disappeared	1314	I
Ranitidine HCl	GL	0.5 mg/mL	DCC	6%	Small white particles and white fiber	1315	I
Theophylline	TR	4 mg/mL[c]	DCC	6%	Precipitates after 2 hr at room temperature	1313	I
Tobramycin sulfate	LI	0.8 mg/mL[c]	DCC	6%	Small crystals form immediately after mixing and persist for 4 hr	1313	I

[a] Tested in dextrose 5%.

[b] Tested in sodium chloride 0.9%.

[c] Tested as the premixed infusion solution.

Additional Compatibility Information

Other Drugs

The manufacturer states that admixtures of 500 to 560 mL of hetastarch 6% in sodium chloride 0.9% with citrate concentrations of up to 2.5% were compatible for 24 hours at room temperature.[3050]

Selected Revisions May 1, 2020. © Copyright, October 1992. American Society of Health-System Pharmacists, Inc.

Hyaluronidase
AHFS 44:00

Products

Hyaluronidase is supplied as a 150-unit/mL solution in 1-mL fill vials. Each mL also contains sodium chloride 8.5 mg, edetate disodium 1 mg, calcium chloride 0.4 mg, and thimerosal not more than 0.1 mg in sodium phosphate buffer.[1(11/05)]

pH
From 6.4 to 7.4.[4]

Osmolality
From 295 to 355 mOsm/kg.[1(11/05)]

Trade Name(s)
Amphadase

Administration

Hyaluronidase is administered subcutaneously, intradermally, or intramuscularly along with other drugs or solutions. The solutions should be isotonic for subcutaneous administration. It should not be administered intravenously.[1(11/05) 4]

Stability

Hyaluronidase injection in intact vials should be stored under refrigeration at 2 to 8°C. It should not be used if it is discolored or contains a precipitate.[4]

Hyaluronidase (Wyeth) 75 units/mL in citric acid/sodium citrate buffer (pH 4.5) was found to lose about 7 to 8% activity in 24 hours at 4 and 23°C. Hyaluronidase activity decreased by 25 to 33% in 48 hours.[1907]

Compatibility Information

Solution Compatibility

Hyaluronidase

Test Soln Name	Mfr	Mfr	Conc/L or %	Remarks	Ref	C/I
Dextrose 2.5% in half-strength Ringer's injection	AB	AB	150 units	Physically compatible	3	C
Dextrose 5% in Ringer's injection	AB	AB	150 units	Physically compatible	3	C
Dextrose 2.5% in Ringer's injection, lactated	AB	AB	150 units	Physically compatible	3	C
Dextrose 5% in half-strength Ringer's injection, lactated	AB	AB	150 units	Physically compatible	3	C
Dextrose 5% in Ringer's injection, lactated	AB	AB	150 units	Physically compatible	3	C
Dextrose 10% in Ringer's injection, lactated	AB	AB	150 units	Physically compatible	3	C
Dextrose 2.5% in sodium chloride 0.45%	AB	AB	150 units	Physically compatible	3	C
Dextrose 2.5% in sodium chloride 0.9%	AB	AB	150 units	Physically compatible	3	C
Dextrose 5% in sodium chloride 0.225%	AB	AB	150 units	Physically compatible	3	C
Dextrose 5% in sodium chloride 0.45%	AB	AB	150 units	Physically compatible	3	C
Dextrose 5% in sodium chloride 0.9%	AB	AB	150 units	Physically compatible	3	C
Dextrose 10% in sodium chloride 0.9%	AB	AB	150 units	Physically compatible	3	C
Dextrose 2.5%	AB	AB	150 units	Physically compatible	3	C
Dextrose 5%	AB	AB	150 units	Physically compatible	3	C
Dextrose 10%	AB	AB	150 units	Physically compatible	3	C
Ionosol B in dextrose 5%	AB	AB	150 units	Physically compatible	3	C
Ionosol MB in dextrose 5%	AB	AB	150 units	Physically compatible	3	C
Ringer's injection	AB	AB	150 units	Physically compatible	3	C

DOI: 10.37573/9781585286850.193

Solution Compatibility (Cont.)

Test Soln Name	Mfr	Mfr	Conc/L or %	Remarks	Ref	C/I
Ringer's injection, lactated	AB	AB	150 units	Physically compatible	3	C
Sodium chloride 0.45%	AB	AB	150 units	Physically compatible	3	C
Sodium chloride 0.9%	AB	AB	150 units	Physically compatible	3	C
Sodium lactate ⅙ M	AB	AB	150 units	Physically compatible	3	C

Additive Compatibility

Hyaluronidase

Test Drug	Mfr	Conc/L or %	Mfr	Conc/L or %	Test Solution	Remarks	Ref	C/I
Amikacin sulfate	BR	5 g	SE	150 units	D5LR, D5R, D5S, D5W, D10W, LR, NS, R, SL	Physically compatible and amikacin stable for 24 hr at 25°C. Hyaluronidase not analyzed	294	C
Sodium bicarbonate	AB	2.4 mEq[a]	WY	150 units	D5W	Physically compatible for 24 hr	772	C

[a] One vial of Neut added to a liter of admixture.

Drugs in Syringe Compatibility

Hyaluronidase

Test Drug	Mfr	Amt	Mfr	Amt	Remarks	Ref	C/I
Hydromorphone HCl	KN	2 mg/mL[a]	WY	150 units/mL[a]	43 and 56% hyaluronidase loss in 24 hr at 4 and 23°C, respectively	1907	I
Hydromorphone HCl	KN	10 and 40 mg/mL[a]	WY	150 units/mL[a]	70 to 82% hyaluronidase loss in 24 hr at 4 and 23°C	1907	I
Iodipamide meglumine		52%, 2 to 40 mL		1 mL[b]	Physically compatible for 48 hr	530	C
Iodipamide meglumine		52%, 1 mL		1 mL[b]	Physically compatible for at least 1 hr but a precipitate forms within 48 hr	530	I
Iothalamate meglumine		60%, 1 to 40 mL		1 mL[b]	Physically compatible for 48 hr	530	C
Pentobarbital sodium	AB	500 mg/10 mL	AB	150 units	Physically compatible	55	C

[a] Mixed in equal quantities.

[b] Concentration unspecified.

Selected Revisions April 9, 2015. © Copyright, October 1982.
American Society of Health-System Pharmacists, Inc.

Hydralazine Hydrochloride
AHFS 24:08.20

Products

Hydralazine hydrochloride is available in 1-mL vials. Each mL of solution contains hydralazine hydrochloride 20 mg, methylparaben 0.65 mg, propylparaben 0.35 mg, and propylene glycol 103.6 mg in water for injection. The pH may have been adjusted with hydrochloric acid and/or sodium hydroxide.[1(1/09)]

pH

From 3.4 to 4.4.[1(1/09)]

Administration

Hydralazine hydrochloride may be administered intramuscularly or as a rapid direct intravenous injection; the manufacturer does not recommend adding the drug to infusion solutions.[1(1/09) 4]

Stability

Hydralazine hydrochloride in intact vials should be stored at controlled room temperature and protected from freezing.[1(1/09) 4] Refrigeration of the intact containers may result in precipitation or crystallization.[593]

Hydralazine hydrochloride undergoes color changes in most infusion solutions. However, it has been stated that color changes within 8 to 12 hours of admixture preparation in solutions stored at 30°C are not indicative of drug losses.[4] The manufacturer does not recommend admixture in infusion solutions.[1(1/09)]

Hydralazine hydrochloride may react with various metals[1(1/09)] to yield discolored solutions, often yellow or pink. One report indicated a pink discoloration in prefilled syringes when the hydralazine hydrochloride had been drawn up through filter needles (Monoject) with a stainless steel filter and stored for up to 12 hours. The reaction is not specific to any one metal. Consequently, contact with metal parts should be minimized, and hydralazine hydrochloride should be prepared just prior to use.[906]

pH Effects

Hydralazine hydrochloride exhibits maximum stability at pH 3.5 and is stable over the pH range of 3 to 5. It undergoes more rapid decomposition as the pH becomes alkaline.[106 466]

Light Effects

Exposure to light increases the rate of hydralazine hydrochloride decomposition during long-term storage. At a concentration of 0.35 mg/mL in sodium chloride 0.9% in glass bottles, 10% decomposition was calculated to occur in 14.4 weeks in the dark and 12.3 weeks under fluorescent light. In PVC containers, decomposition occurs more rapidly; a 10% loss was calculated to occur in 12.8 weeks in the dark and 9.9 weeks under fluorescent light.[1561]

Sorption

Hydralazine hydrochloride 27 mg/L in sodium chloride 0.9% in PVC bags exhibited approximately 10% loss in 1 week at 15 to 20°C due to sorption.[536] However, no loss due to sorption occurred during a 7-hour simulated infusion through an infusion set consisting of a cellulose propionate burette chamber and 170 cm of PVC tubing.[606]

Hydralazine hydrochloride was shown not to exhibit sorption to polyethylene tubing, Silastic tubing, and polypropylene syringes.[606]

Compatibility Information
Solution Compatibility

Hydralazine HCl

Test Soln Name	Mfr	Mfr	Conc/L or %	Remarks	Ref	C/I
Dextrose 2.5% in half-strength Ringer's injection	AB	CI	400 mg	Physically compatible	3	C
Dextrose 5% in Ringer's injection	AB	CI	400 mg	Physically compatible	3	C
Dextrose 2.5% in half-strength Ringer's injection, lactated	AB	CI	400 mg	Physically compatible	3	C
Dextrose 5% in half-strength Ringer's injection, lactated	AB	CI	400 mg	Physically compatible	3	C
Dextrose 2.5% in Ringer's injection, lactated	AB	CI	400 mg	Physically compatible	3	C
Dextrose 5% in Ringer's injection, lactated	AB	CI	400 mg	Physically compatible	3	C

DOI: 10.37573/9781585286850.194

Solution Compatibility (Cont.)

Test Soln Name	Mfr	Mfr	Conc/L or %	Remarks	Ref	C/I
Dextrose 10% in Ringer's injection, lactated	AB	CI	400 mg	Color change	3	I
Dextrose 2.5% in sodium chloride 0.45%	AB	CI	400 mg	Physically compatible	3	C
Dextrose 2.5% in sodium chloride 0.9%	AB	CI	400 mg	Physically compatible	3	C
Dextrose 5% in sodium chloride 0.225%	AB	CI	400 mg	Physically compatible	3	C
Dextrose 5% in sodium chloride 0.45%	AB	CI	400 mg	Physically compatible	3	C
Dextrose 5% in sodium chloride 0.9%	AB	CI	400 mg	Physically compatible	3	C
Dextrose 10% in sodium chloride 0.9%	AB	CI	400 mg	Physically compatible	3	C
Dextrose 2.5%	AB	CI	400 mg	Physically compatible	3	C
Dextrose 5%		CI	40 mg	Yellow color within 1 hr. 4% decomposition in 2 hr and 8% in 3.5 hr	466	I
Dextrose 5%			200 to 400 mg	Progressive yellow discoloration due to hydralazine reaction with dextrose	845	I
Dextrose 5%	TR[a]		350 mg	10% loss in 1 hr at 21°C under fluorescent light. Approximately 11 to 12% loss in 1.5 hr at 21°C in the dark	1561	I
Dextrose 5%	BA	AMR	200 mg	41% loss in 24 hr at 25°C	2644	I
Dextrose 10%	AB	CI	400 mg	Physically compatible	3	C
Ionosol B in dextrose 5%	AB	CI	400 mg	Physically compatible	3	C
Ionosol MB in dextrose 5%	AB	CI	400 mg	Physically compatible	3	C
Ringer's injection	AB	CI	400 mg	Physically compatible	3	C
Ringer's injection, lactated	AB	CI	400 mg	Physically compatible	3	C
Ringer's injection, lactated		CI	40 mg	No decomposition in 2.5 hr	466	C
Sodium chloride 0.45%	AB	CI	400 mg	Physically compatible	3	C
Sodium chloride 0.9%	AB	CI	400 mg	Physically compatible	3	C
Sodium chloride 0.9%		CI	40 mg	No decomposition in 4 days	466	C
Sodium chloride 0.9%			200 to 400 mg	Physically compatible	845	C
Sodium chloride 0.9%	TR[a]		350 mg	6 to 8% loss in 52 days at 21°C under fluorescent light	1561	C
Sodium chloride 0.9%	BA	AMR	200 mg	8% loss in 2 days and 13% loss in 3 days at 25°C	2644	C
Sodium lactate ⅙ M	AB	CI	400 mg	Physically compatible	3	C

[a] Tested in both glass and PVC containers.

Additive Compatibility

Hydralazine HCl

Test Drug	Mfr	Conc/L or %	Mfr	Conc/L or %	Test Solution	Remarks	Ref	C/I
Aminophylline	BP	1 g	BP	80 mg	D5W	Yellow color produced	26	I
Ampicillin sodium	BP	2 g	BP	80 mg	D5W	Yellow color produced	26	I
Chlorothiazide sodium	BP	2 g	BP	80 mg	D5W, NS	Yellow color with precipitate in 3 hr	26	I

Additive Compatibility (Cont.)

Test Drug	Mfr	Conc/L or %	Mfr	Conc/L or %	Test Solution	Remarks	Ref	C/I
Dobutamine HCl	LI	200 mg	CI	200 mg	NS	Physically compatible for 24 hr	552	C
Edetate calcium disodium	RI	4 g	BP	80 mg	D5W	Yellow color produced	26	I
Ethacrynate sodium	MSD	50 mg	CI	20 mg	NS	Altered UV spectra at room temperature	16	I
Hydrocortisone sodium succinate	BP	400 mg	BP	80 mg	D5W	Yellow color produced	26	I
Methohexital sodium	BP	2 g	BP	80 mg	D5W, NS	Yellow color with precipitate in 3 hr	26	I
Nitroglycerin	ACC	400 mg	CI	1 g	D5W[a]	Yellow color. 4% nitroglycerin loss in 48 hr at 23°C. Hydralazine not tested	929	I
Nitroglycerin	ACC	400 mg	CI	1 g	NS[a]	Yellow color. No nitroglycerin loss in 48 hr at 23°C. Hydralazine not tested	929	I
Phenobarbital sodium	BP	800 mg	BP	80 mg	D5W	Yellow color and precipitate in 3 hr	26	I
Verapamil HCl	KN	80 mg	CI	40 mg	D5W, NS	Yellow discoloration	764	I

[a] Tested in glass containers.

Drugs in Syringe Compatibility

Hydralazine HCl

Test Drug	Mfr	Amt	Mfr	Amt	Remarks	Ref	C/I
Pantoprazole sodium	[a]	4 mg/1 mL		20 mg/1 mL	Precipitates within 4 hr	2574	I

[a] Test performed using the formulation WITHOUT edetate disodium.

Y-Site Injection Compatibility (1:1 Mixture)

Hydralazine HCl

Test Drug	Mfr	Conc	Mfr	Conc	Remarks	Ref	C/I
Aminophylline	ES	4 mg/mL[a]	SO	1 mg/mL[a]	Gross color change in 1 hr	1316	I
Aminophylline	ES	4 mg/mL[b]	SO	1 mg/mL[b]	Color change in 1 hr and haze in 3 hr	1316	I
Ampicillin sodium	WY	40 mg/mL[b]	SO	1 mg/mL[a]	Moderate color change in 1 hr	1316	I
Ampicillin sodium	WY	40 mg/mL[b]	SO	1 mg/mL[b]	Moderate color change in 3 hr	1316	I
Caspofungin acetate	ME	0.5 mg/mL[b]	APP	20 mg/mL	Physically compatible with hydralazine HCl i.v. push over 2 to 5 min	2766	C
Cloxacillin sodium	SMX	100 mg/mL	SMX	20 mg/mL	Opaque yellow turbidity forms within 4 hr	3245	I
Furosemide	ES	1 mg/mL[c]	SO	1 mg/mL[c]	Slight color change in 3 hr	1316	I
Heparin sodium	UP	1000 units/L[d]	CI	20 mg/mL	Physically compatible for 4 hr at room temperature	534	C
Hydrocortisone sodium succinate	UP	10 mg/L[d]	CI	20 mg/mL	Physically compatible for 4 hr at room temperature	534	C
Meropenem		50 mg/mL	SMX	20 mg/mL	Yellow-brown color changed occurred immediately	3538	I
Nesiritide	SCI	50 mcg/mL[a b]		20 mg/mL	Physically incompatible	2625	I
Nitroglycerin	LY	0.4 mg/mL[a]	SO	1 mg/mL[a]	Physically compatible for 3 hr	1316	C
Nitroglycerin	LY	0.4 mg/mL[b]	SO	1 mg/mL[b]	Slight precipitate in 3 hr	1316	I

Y-Site Injection Compatibility (1:1 Mixture) (Cont.)

Test Drug	Mfr	Conc	Mfr	Conc	Remarks	Ref	C/I
Potassium chloride	AB	40 mEq/L[d]	CI	20 mg/mL	Physically compatible for 4 hr at room temperature	534	C
Verapamil HCl	LY	0.2 mg/mL[c]	SO	1 mg/mL[c]	Physically compatible for 3 hr	1316	C

[a] Tested in dextrose 5%.

[b] Tested in sodium chloride 0.9%.

[c] Tested in both dextrose 5% and sodium chloride 0.9%.

[d] Tested in dextrose 5% in Ringer's injection, dextrose 5% in Ringer's injection, lactated, dextrose 5%, Ringer's injection, lactated, and sodium chloride 0.9%.

Selected Revisions May 1, 2020. © Copyright, October 1982.
American Society of Health-System Pharmacists, Inc.

Hydrocortisone Sodium Succinate
AHFS 68:04

Products

Hydrocortisone sodium succinate is available in a variety of sizes and containers,[4] including 100-mg conventional vials containing hydrocortisone sodium succinate equivalent to hydrocortisone 100 mg with monobasic sodium phosphate anhydrous 0.8 mg and dibasic sodium phosphate dried 8.73 mg. Reconstitute the vial by adding not more than 2 mL of bacteriostatic water for injection or bacteriostatic sodium chloride injection.[1(5/08)]

Hydrocortisone sodium succinate is also supplied in "Act-O-Vial" containers of 100, 250, 500, and 1000 mg. For the "Act-O-Vial" containers, press the plastic activator down to force the diluent into the lower chamber. Agitate gently to dissolve the drug. When reconstituted, each mL of solution contains:[1(5/08)]

Component	100 mg	250, 500, 1000 mg
Hydrocortisone equivalent (as sodium succinate)	50 mg	125 mg
Monobasic sodium phosphate anhydrous	0.4 mg	1 mg
Dibasic sodium phosphate dried	4.38 mg	11 mg
Benzyl alcohol	~9 mg	~8.3 mg
Water for injection	qs	qs

The pH has been adjusted when necessary with sodium hydroxide.

pH

From 7 to 8.[1(5/08) 4]

Osmolality

The osmolality of hydrocortisone sodium succinate (Abbott) 50 mg/mL was determined to be 292 mOsm/kg by freezing-point depression and 260 mOsm/kg by vapor pressure.[1071]

Sodium Content

Hydrocortisone sodium succinate contains 2.066 mEq of sodium per gram of drug.[846]

Trade Name(s)

Solu-Cortef

Administration

Hydrocortisone sodium succinate may be administered by intramuscular injection, direct intravenous injection over 30 seconds to several minutes, or continuous or intermittent intravenous infusion at a concentration of 0.1 to 1 mg/mL in a compatible infusion solution. Benzyl alcohol-containing products should not be used in premature infants.[1(5/08) 4]

Stability

Hydrocortisone sodium succinate in intact containers should be stored at controlled room temperatures of 20 to 25°C.[1(5/08)] After reconstitution, solutions are stable at controlled room temperature or below if protected from light. The solution should only be used if it is clear. Unused solutions should be discarded after 3 days. Hydrocortisone sodium succinate is heat labile and must not be autoclaved.[1(5/08) 4]

pH Effects

Hydrocortisone sodium succinate is optimally stable at pH 7 to 8. It is stable for 72 hours at pH 6 and for 12 hours at pH 5. More acidic solutions cause precipitation.[41]

Solutions of hydrocortisone buffered to pH 9.1 showed oxidation to 21-dehydrocortisone at rates of 1.6 to 2.8%/hr at 26°C. This rate is 4 or 5 times greater than that observed at pH 6.9 to 7.9.[531]

Freezing Solutions

Hydrocortisone sodium succinate (Upjohn) 500-mg/4-mL reconstituted solution exhibited no loss over 4 weeks when stored frozen.[69]

Intrathecal Injections

In a study of solutions for intrathecal injection, hydrocortisone sodium succinate (Upjohn) was reconstituted to a concentration of 1 mg/mL with Elliott's B solution (295 mOsm/kg, pH 7.3), sodium chloride 0.9% (296 mOsm/kg, pH 7), and Ringer's injection, lactated (258 mOsm/kg, pH 7). In Ringer's injection, lactated and sodium chloride 0.9%, no decomposition was observed in 24 hours at room temperature under fluorescent light or at 30°C. However, in 7 days, approximately 10% decomposition occurred at room temperature and about 15% at 30°C. In Elliott's B solution, hydrocortisone sodium succinate is much less stable. In 24 hours, a 7% loss occurred at room temperature and a 12% loss occurred at 30°C, increasing to 21 and 32%, respectively, at 72 hours. Less than 10% decomposition of this combination occurred in 4 to 8 hours.[327]

In another study, the stability and compatibility of cytarabine (Upjohn), methotrexate (NCI), and hydrocortisone (Upjohn), mixed together in intrathecal injections, were evaluated. Two combinations were tested: (1) cytarabine 50 mg, methotrexate 12 mg (as the sodium salt), and hydrocortisone 25 mg (as the sodium succinate salt); and (2) cytarabine 30 mg, methotrexate 12 mg (as the sodium salt), and hydrocortisone 15 mg (as the sodium succinate salt). Each drug combination was added to 12 mL of Elliott's B solution (NCI), sodium chloride 0.9% (Abbott), dextrose 5% (Abbott), and Ringer's injection, lactated (Abbott) and stored for 24 hours at 25°C. Cytarabine and methotrexate were both chemically stable, with no drug loss after the full 24 hours in all solutions. Hydrocortisone also

DOI: 10.37573/9781585286850.195

was stable in the sodium chloride 0.9%, dextrose 5%, and Ringer's injection, lactated, with about a 2% drug loss. However, in Elliott's B solution, hydrocortisone was significantly less stable, with a 6% loss in the 25-mg concentration over 24 hours. The 15-mg concentration was worse, with a 5% loss in 10 hours and a 13% loss in 24 hours. The higher pH of Elliott's B solution and the lower concentration of hydrocortisone may have been factors in this increased decomposition. All mixtures were physically compatible for 24 hours, but a precipitate formed after several days of storage.[819]

Hydrocortisone sodium succinate (Upjohn) 2 mg/mL diluted in Elliott's B solution (Orphan Medical) was packaged as 20 mL in 30-mL glass vials and 20-mL plastic syringes (Becton Dickinson) with Red Cap (Burron) Luer-lok syringe tip caps. The solution was physically compatible and chemically stable exhibiting about 9% or less loss in 24 hours at 23°C and 7% or less loss in 48 hours at 4°C.[1976]

Bacterially contaminated intrathecal solutions could pose grave risks and, consequently, such solutions should be administered as soon as possible after preparation.[328]

Syringes

Hydrocortisone sodium succinate (Upjohn) 10 mg/mL in sodium chloride 0.9% was packaged in polypropylene syringes (Becton Dickinson) and stored under refrigeration at 5°C and at room temperature of 25°C. The drug solution remained clear throughout the study, and about 2% hydrocortisone loss occurred after 21 days under refrigeration. At room temperature, about 5% loss occurred in 3 days and 10% loss occurred in 7 days. Stability in glass containers was found to be comparable.[2331]

Hydrocortisone sodium succinate (Pharmacia) 50 mg/mL in sterile water for injection packaged in polypropylene syringes (Braun) was visually compatible with calculated shelf lives of 6.8 days at room temperature and 81 days under refrigeration.[2654]

Sorption

Hydrocortisone sodium succinate was shown not to exhibit sorption to polyvinyl chloride (PVC) bags and tubing, polyethylene tubing, Silastic tubing, and polypropylene syringes.[12 536 606]

Filtration

Hydrocortisone sodium succinate (Upjohn) 10 mg/L in dextrose 5% and sodium chloride 0.9% did not display significant sorption to a 0.45-μm cellulose membrane filter (Abbott S-A-I-F) during an 8-hour simulated infusion.[567]

Central Venous Catheter

Hydrocortisone sodium succinate (Abbott) 1 mg/mL in dextrose 5% was found to be compatible with the ARROWg+ard Blue Plus (Arrow International) chlorhexidine-bearing triple-lumen central catheter. Essentially complete delivery of the drug was found with little or no drug loss occurring. Furthermore, chlorhexidine delivered from the catheter remained at trace amounts with no substantial increase due to the delivery of the drug through the catheter.[2335]

Compatibility Information
Solution Compatibility

Hydrocortisone sodium succinate

Test Soln Name	Mfr	Mfr	Conc/L or %	Remarks	Ref	C/I
Dextrose 2.5% in half-strength Ringer's injection	AB	UP	250 mg	Physically compatible	3	C
Dextrose 5% in Ringer's injection	AB	UP	250 mg	Physically compatible	3	C
Dextrose 5% in half-strength Ringer's injection, lactated	AB	UP	250 mg	Physically compatible	3	C
Dextrose 2.5% in Ringer's injection, lactated	AB	UP	250 mg	Physically compatible	3	C
Dextrose 5% in Ringer's injection, lactated	AB	UP	250 mg	Physically compatible	3	C
Dextrose 5% in Ringer's injection, lactated	TR[a]	UP	500 mg	Stable for 24 hr at 5°C	282	C
Dextrose 5% in Ringer's injection, lactated	BA	UP	600 mg	Physically compatible for 24 hr	315	C
Dextrose 10% in Ringer's injection, lactated	AB	UP	250 mg	Physically compatible	3	C
Dextrose 2.5% in sodium chloride 0.45%	AB	UP	250 mg	Physically compatible	3	C
Dextrose 2.5% in sodium chloride 0.9%	AB	UP	250 mg	Physically compatible	3	C
Dextrose 5% in sodium chloride 0.225%	AB	UP	250 mg	Physically compatible	3	C
Dextrose 5% in sodium chloride 0.45%	AB	UP	250 mg	Physically compatible	3	C
Dextrose 5% in sodium chloride 0.9%	AB	UP	250 mg	Physically compatible	3	C

Solution Compatibility (Cont.)

Test Soln Name	Mfr	Mfr	Conc/L or %	Remarks	Ref	C/I
Dextrose 5% in sodium chloride 0.9%		UP	100, 200, 300 mg	Stable for 48 hr	43	C
Dextrose 5% in sodium chloride 0.9%	AB	UP	250 mg	Stable for 48 hr	46	C
Dextrose 5% in sodium chloride 0.9%		UP	100 mg	Physically compatible	74	C
Dextrose 5% in sodium chloride 0.9%	TR[a]	UP	500 mg	Stable for 24 hr at 5°C	282	C
Dextrose 5% in sodium chloride 0.9%	BA	UP	600 mg	Physically compatible for 24 hr	315	C
Dextrose 10% in sodium chloride 0.9%	AB	UP	250 mg	Physically compatible	3	C
Dextrose 2.5%	AB	UP	250 mg	Physically compatible	3	C
Dextrose 5%	AB	UP	250 mg	Physically compatible	3	C
Dextrose 5%	AB	UP	250 mg	Stable for 48 hr	46	C
Dextrose 5%		UP	100 mg	Physically compatible	74	C
Dextrose 5%	TR[a]	UP	500 mg	Stable for 24 hr at 5°C	282	C
Dextrose 5%	BA	UP	600 mg	Physically compatible for 24 hr	315	C
Dextrose 10%	AB	UP	250 mg	Physically compatible	3	C
Dextrose 10%	BA	UP	600 mg	Physically compatible for 24 hr	315	C
Dextrose 20%	BA	UP	600 mg	Physically compatible for 24 hr	315	C
Ionosol B in dextrose 5%	AB	UP	250 mg	Physically compatible	3	C
Ionosol MB in dextrose 5%	AB	UP	250 mg	Physically compatible	3	C
Ringer's injection	AB	UP	250 mg	Physically compatible	3	C
Ringer's injection, lactated	AB	UP	250 mg	Physically compatible	3	C
Ringer's injection, lactated		UP	100 mg	Physically compatible	74	C
Ringer's injection, lactated	TR[a]	UP	500 mg	Stable for 24 hr at 5°C	282	C
Ringer's injection, lactated	BA	UP	600 mg	Physically compatible for 24 hr	315	C
Sodium chloride 0.45%	AB	UP	250 mg	Physically compatible	74	C
Sodium chloride 0.9%	AB	UP	250 mg	Physically compatible	3	C
Sodium chloride 0.9%	AB	UP	250 mg	Stable for 48 hr	46	C
Sodium chloride 0.9%		UP	100 mg	Physically compatible	74	C
Sodium chloride 0.9%	TR[a]	UP	500 mg	Stable for 24 hr at 5°C	282	C
Sodium chloride 0.9%	BA	UP	600 mg	Physically compatible for 24 hr	315	C
Sodium chloride 0.9%	[b]	PH	1 g	Visually compatible. Calculated shelf lives of 7 days at room temperature and 41 days (PVC) and 48 days (polyolefin) under refrigeration	2654	C
Sodium lactate ⅙ M	AB	UP	250 mg	Physically compatible	3	C
Sodium lactate ⅙ M	BA	UP	600 mg	Physically compatible for 24 hr	315	C

[a] Tested in both glass and PVC containers.

[b] Tested in PVC (Baxter) and polyolefin (Fresenius Kabi) containers.

Additive Compatibility

Hydrocortisone sodium succinate

Test Drug	Mfr	Conc/L or %	Mfr	Conc/L or %	Test Solution	Remarks	Ref	C/I
Amikacin sulfate	BR	5 g	UP	200 mg	D5LR, D5R, D5S, D5W, D10W, LR, NS, R, SL	Physically compatible and both stable for 24 hr at 25°C	294	C
Aminophylline		250 mg	UP	100 mg	D5W	Physically compatible	74	C
Aminophylline	SE	1 g	UP	500 mg	D5W	Physically compatible	15	C
Aminophylline	SE	500 mg	UP	100 mg		Physically compatible	6	C
Aminophylline		625 mg		250 mg	D5W	Physically compatible and aminophylline stable for 24 hr at 4 and 30°C. Total hydrocortisone content changed little but substantial ester hydrolysis	521	C
Amphotericin B	SQ	100 mg	UP	500 mg	D5W	Physically compatible	15	C
Amphotericin B	SQ	70 and 140 mg		50 mg	D5W	Bioactivity not significantly affected over 24 hr at 25°C	335	C
Ampicillin sodium	BR	1 g		200 and 400 mg	LR	Ampicillin stable for 24 hr at 25°C	87	C
Ampicillin sodium	BR	1 g		1.8 g	D5S, D5W, D10W, IM, IP, LR, NS	Ampicillin stable for 24 hr at 4°C	87	C
Ampicillin sodium	BR	1 g		50 and 100 mg	LR	14% ampicillin loss in 12 hr at 25°C	87	I
Ampicillin sodium	BR	1 g		1.8 g	D5S, D10W, IM, IP, LR	11 to 28% ampicillin loss in 24 hr at 25°C	87	I
Ampicillin sodium	BE	20 g		200 mg	NS	18% ampicillin loss in 6 hr at 25°C	89	I
Ampicillin sodium	BE	20 g		200 mg	D5W	23% ampicillin loss in 6 hr at 25°C	89	I
Ampicillin sodium	BE	20 g		200 mg	D2.5½S, D2.5S, D5¼S, D5½S, D5S, D10S	32% ampicillin loss in 6 hr at 25°C	89	I
Antithymocyte globulin (rabbit)[c]	SGS	200 and 300 mg	PHU	50 mg	D5W	Immediate haze and precipitation	2488	I
Antithymocyte globulin (rabbit)[c]	SGS	200 and 300 mg	PHU	50 mg	NS	Physically compatible for 24 hr at 23°C	2488	C
Ascorbic acid	UP		UP			Concentration-dependent incompatibility	15	I
Bleomycin sulfate	BR	20 and 30 units	AB	300 mg, 750 mg, 1 g, 2.5 g	NS	60 to 100% loss of bleomycin activity in 1 week at 4°C	763	I
Calcium chloride	UP	1 g	UP	500 mg	D5W	Physically compatible	15	C
Calcium gluconate		1 g	UP	100 mg	D5W	Physically compatible	74	C
Calcium gluconate	UP	1 g	UP	500 mg	D5W	Physically compatible	15	C
Chloramphenicol sodium succinate	PD	500 mg	UP	100 mg	D5W	Physically compatible	74	C
Chloramphenicol sodium succinate	PD	10 g	UP	500 mg	D5W	Physically compatible	15	C
Chloramphenicol sodium succinate	PD	1 g	UP	500 mg		Physically compatible	6	C

Additive Compatibility (Cont.)

Test Drug	Mfr	Conc/L or %	Mfr	Conc/L or %	Test Solution	Remarks	Ref	C/I
Clindamycin phosphate	UP	1.2 g	UP	1 g	W	Clindamycin stable for 24 hr	101	C
Cloxacillin sodium	BE	20 g	GL	200 mg	D5S, D5W, NS	Physically compatible and cloxacillin stable for 24 hr at 25°C	89	C
Colistimethate sodium	WC	500 mg	UP	500 mg	D5W	Physically incompatible	15	I
Cytarabine	UP	360 mg	UP	500 mg	D5S, D10S	Physically compatible for 40 hr	174	C
Cytarabine	UP	360 mg	UP	500 mg	R, SL	Physically incompatible	174	I
Daunorubicin HCl	FA	200 mg	UP	500 mg	D5W	Physically compatible	15	C
Dimenhydrinate	SE	50 mg	UP	100 mg	D5W	Physically compatible	74	C
Dimenhydrinate	SE	500 mg	UP	500 mg	D5W	Physically incompatible	15	I
Dopamine HCl	AS	800 mg	UP	1 g	D5W	No dopamine loss in 18 hr at 25°C	312	C
Erythromycin lactobionate	AB	5 g	UP	500 mg	D5W	Physically compatible	15	C
Erythromycin lactobionate	AB	1 g	UP	250 mg		Physically compatible	20	C
Fat emulsion, intravenous	VT	10%	RS	160 mg		Physically compatible for 24 hr at 8 and 25°C	825	C
Floxacillin sodium	BE	20 g	UP	50 g	NS	Physically compatible for 72 hr at 15 and 30°C	1479	C
Furosemide		200 and 400 mg		1 g	D5W, NS	6 to 8% hydrocortisone loss and 5 to 6% furosemide loss in 24 hr at 25°C	1348	C
Furosemide		200 and 400 mg		300 mg	D5W, NS	6 to 8% hydrocortisone loss in 6 hr and 10 to 14% loss in 24 hr at 25°C. 5 to 6% furosemide loss in 24 hr	1348	I
Furosemide	HO	1 g	UP	50 g	NS	Physically compatible for 72 hr at 15 and 30°C	1479	C
Heparin sodium		32,000 units		800 mg	NS	Physically compatible and heparin activity retained for 24 hr	57	C
Heparin sodium	UP	4000 units	UP	500 mg	D5W	Physically incompatible	15	I
Heparin sodium		12,000 units	UP	100 mg	D5W	Precipitates immediately	74	I
Hydralazine HCl	BP	80 mg	BP	400 mg	D5W	Yellow color produced	26	I
Lidocaine HCl	AST	2 g	UP	250 mg		Physically compatible	24	C
Magnesium sulfate	ES	750 mg	UP	100 mg	AA 3.5%, D 25%	Physically compatible	302	C
Metronidazole	SE	5 g	ES	10 g		No loss of either drug in 7 days at 25°C and 12 days at 5°C	993	C
Mitomycin	BR	1 g	AB	33.3 g	W[b]	Visually compatible. 10% calculated loss of mitomycin in 172 hr and hydrocortisone in 212 hr at 25°C	1866	C
Mitomycin	BR	1 g	AB	33.3 g	W[a]	Visually compatible. 10% calculated loss of mitomycin in 206 hr and hydrocortisone in 218 hr at 25°C	1866	C
Mitomycin	BR	1 g	AB	33.3 g	W[b]	Visually compatible. 10% calculated loss of mitomycin in 1423 hr and hydrocortisone in 176 hr at 4°C	1866	C

Additive Compatibility (Cont.)

Test Drug	Mfr	Conc/L or %	Mfr	Conc/L or %	Test Solution	Remarks	Ref	C/I
Mitomycin	BR	1 g	AB	33.3 g	W[a]	Visually compatible. 10% calculated loss of mitomycin in 820 hr and hydrocortisone in 807 hr at 4°C	1866	C
Mitoxantrone HCl	LE	50 to 200 mg		100 mg to 2 g	D5W, NS[a]	Physically compatible and both drugs stable for 24 hr at room temperature	1293	C
Nafcillin sodium	WY	500 mg	UP	250 mg		Precipitate forms within 1 hr	27	I
Norepinephrine bitartrate	WI	8 mg	UP	100 mg	D5W	Physically compatible	74	C
Penicillin G potassium		1 million units	UP	100 mg	D5W	Physically compatible	74	C
Penicillin G potassium	SQ	20 million units	UP	500 mg	D5W	Physically compatible	15	C
Penicillin G potassium	SQ	5 million units	UP	250 mg	D	Physically compatible	47	C
Penicillin G sodium	UP	20 million units	UP	500 mg	D5W	Physically compatible	15	C
Pentobarbital sodium	AB	1 g	UP	500 mg	D5W	Physically incompatible	15	I
Phenobarbital sodium	WI	200 mg	UP	500 mg	D5W	Physically incompatible	15	I
Polymyxin B sulfate	BW	200 mg	UP	500 mg	D5W	Physically compatible	15	C
Potassium chloride		3 g	UP	100 mg	D5W	Physically compatible	74	C
Promethazine HCl	WY	250 mg	UP	500 mg	D5W	Physically incompatible	15	I
Vancomycin HCl	LI	1 g	UP	100 mg	D5W	Physically compatible	74	C
Verapamil HCl	KN	80 mg	UP	200 mg	D5W, NS	Physically compatible for 24 hr	764	C

[a] Tested in PVC containers.

[b] Tested in glass containers.

[c] Heparin sodium (Elkins-Sinn) 2000 units/L was also present.

Drugs in Syringe Compatibility

Hydrocortisone sodium succinate

Test Drug	Mfr	Amt	Mfr	Amt	Remarks	Ref	C/I
Dimenhydrinate		10 mg/1 mL		125 mg/1 mL	Clear solution	2569	C
Doxapram HCl	RB	400 mg/20 mL	UP	500 mg/2 mL	Immediate turbidity and precipitation	1177	I
Iohexol	WI	64.7%, 5 mL	UP	10 mg/1 mL	Physically compatible for at least 2 hr	1438	C
Iopamidol	SQ	61%, 5 mL	UP	10 mg/1 mL	Physically compatible for at least 2 hr	1438	C
Iothalamate meglumine	MA	60%, 5 mL	UP	10 mg/1 mL	Physically compatible for at least 2 hr	1438	C
Ioxaglate meglumine–ioxaglate sodium	MA	5 mL	UP	10 mg/1 mL	Physically compatible for at least 2 hr	1438	C
Magnesium sulfate	ES	500 mg/mL	UP	100 mg/2 mL	White precipitate formed	302	I
Pantoprazole sodium	[a]	4 mg/1 mL		125 mg/1 mL	Possible precipitate within 15 min	2574	I

[a] Test performed using the formulation WITHOUT edetate disodium.

Y-Site Injection Compatibility (1:1 Mixture)

Hydrocortisone sodium succinate

Test Drug	Mfr	Conc	Mfr	Conc	Remarks	Ref	C/I
Acetaminophen	CAD	10 mg/mL	PF	50 mg/mL	Physically compatible with less than 10% acetaminophen loss over 4 hr at room temperature	2841, 2844	C
Acetaminophen	CAD	10 mg/mL	PF	125 mg/mL	Physically compatible for 4 hr at 23°C	2901, 2902	C
Acyclovir sodium	BW	5 mg/mL[a]	LY	1 mg/mL[a]	Physically compatible for 4 hr at 25°C	1157	C
Allopurinol sodium	BW	3 mg/mL[b]	UP	1 mg/mL[b]	Physically compatible for 4 hr at 22°C	1686	C
Amifostine	USB	10 mg/mL[a]	UP	1 mg/mL[a]	Physically compatible for 4 hr at 23°C	1845	C
Aminophylline	SE	25 mg/mL	UP	100 mg/L[c]	Physically compatible for 4 hr at room temperature	322	C
Ampicillin sodium	BR	25, 50, 100, 125 mg/mL	UP	100 mg/L[c]	Physically compatible for 4 hr at room temperature	322	C
Amsacrine	NCI	1 mg/mL[a]	UP	1 mg/mL[a]	Visually compatible for 4 hr at 22°C	1381	C
Anidulafungin	VIC	0.5 mg/mL[a]	PHU	1 mg/mL[a]	Physically compatible for 4 hr at 23°C	2617	C
Antithymocyte globulin (rabbit)	SGS	0.2 and 0.3 mg/mL[a b]	PHU	0.5 mg/mL[a b]	Physically compatible for 4 hr at 23°C	2488	C
Antithymocyte globulin (rabbit)	SGS	0.2 and 0.3 mg/mL[a b]	PHU	1 mg/mL[a b]	Physically compatible for 4 hr at 23°C	2488	C
Argatroban	GSK	1 mg/mL[b]	PHU	50 mg/mL	Visually compatible for 24 hr at 23°C	2391	C
Atracurium besylate	BW	0.5 mg/mL[a]	AB	1 mg/mL[a]	Physically compatible for 24 hr at 28°C	1337	C
Atropine sulfate	BW	0.5 mg/mL	UP	10 mg/L[d]	Physically compatible for 4 hr at room temperature	534	C
Aztreonam	SQ	40 mg/mL[a]	UP	1 mg/mL[a]	Physically compatible for 4 hr at 23°C	1758	C
Bivalirudin	TMC	5 mg/mL[a]	PHU	1 mg/mL[a]	Physically compatible for 4 hr at 23°C	2373	C
Bivalirudin	TMC	5 mg/mL[a b]	PHU	50 mg/mL	Visually compatible for 6 hr at 23°C	2680	C
Blinatumomab	AMG	0.125 and 0.375 mcg/mL[b]	SRB	0.98 mg/mL[b]	Visually compatible for 12 hr at room temperature	3405, 3417	C
Calcium gluconate	ES	100 mg/mL	UP	100 mg/L[c]	Physically compatible for 4 hr at room temperature	322	C
Cangrelor tetrasodium	TMC	1 mg/mL[b]		1 mg/mL[b]	Physically compatible for 4 hr	3243	C
Caspofungin acetate	ME	0.7 mg/mL[b]	HOS	1 mg/mL[b]	Physically compatible for 4 hr at room temperature	2758	C
Ceftaroline fosamil	FOR	2.22 mg/mL[a b h]	PF	1 mg/mL[a b h]	Physically compatible for 4 hr at 23°C	2826	C
Ceftolozane sulfate–tazobactam sodium	CUB	10 mg/mL[e o]	PF	1 mg/mL[e]	Physically compatible for 2 hr	3262	C
Chlorpromazine HCl	SKF	25 mg/mL	UP	10 mg/L[d]	Physically compatible for 4 hr at room temperature	534	C
Ciprofloxacin	MI	2 mg/mL[e]	UP	50 mg/mL	Transient cloudiness rapidly dissipates. Crystals form in 1 hr at 24°C	1655	I
Cisatracurium besylate	GW	0.1, 2, 5 mg/mL[a]	AB	1 mg/mL[a]	Physically compatible for 4 hr at 23°C	2074	C
Cladribine	ORT	0.015[b] and 0.5[f] mg/mL	UP	1 mg/mL[b]	Physically compatible for 4 hr at 23°C	1969	C
Cloxacillin sodium	SMX	100 mg/mL	NOP	125 mg/mL	Physically compatible for up to 4 hr at room temperature	3245	C

Y-Site Injection Compatibility (1:1 Mixture) (Cont.)

Test Drug	Mfr	Conc	Mfr	Conc	Remarks	Ref	C/I
Cyanocobalamin	PD	0.1 mg/mL	UP	10 mg/L[d]	Physically compatible for 4 hr at room temperature	534	C
Cytarabine	UP	16 mg/mL[b]	UP	125 mg/mL	Visually compatible for 24 hr at room temperature in test tubes. No precipitate found on filter from Y-site delivery	2063	C
Dacarbazine					Pink precipitate forms immediately	524	I
Defibrotide sodium	JAZ	8 mg/mL[b]	UP	1.9 mg/mL[b]	Visually compatible for 4 hr at room temperature	3149	C
Dexamethasone sodium phosphate	MSD	4 mg/mL	UP	100 mg/L[c]	Physically compatible for 4 hr at room temperature	322	C
Dexmedetomidine HCl	HOS	4 mcg/mL[b]			Stated to be compatible	3181	C
Diazepam	RC	5 mg/mL	UP	100 mg/L[c]	Immediate haziness and globule formation	322	I
Digoxin	BW	0.25 mg/mL	UP	100 mg/L[c]	Physically compatible for 4 hr at room temperature	322	C
Diltiazem HCl	MMD	5 mg/mL	UP	50 and 125 mg/mL	Precipitate forms but clears with swirling	1807	?
Diltiazem HCl	MMD	1 mg/mL[b]	UP	50 and 125 mg/mL	Visually compatible	1807	C
Diltiazem HCl	MMD	5 mg/mL	UP	1[b] and 2[a] mg/mL	Visually compatible	1807	C
Diphenhydramine HCl	PD	50 mg/mL	UP	10 mg/L[d]	Physically compatible for 4 hr at room temperature	534	C
Docetaxel	RPR	0.9 mg/mL[a]	AB	1 mg/mL[a]	Physically compatible for 4 hr at 23°C	2224	C
Dopamine HCl	ACC	40 mg/mL	UP	10 mg/L[d]	Physically compatible for 4 hr at room temperature	534	C
Doripenem	JJ	5 mg/mL[a b]	PHU	1 mg/mL[a b]	Physically compatible for 4 hr at 23°C	2743	C
Doxorubicin HCl liposomal	SEQ	0.4 mg/mL[a]	AB	1 mg/mL[a]	Physically compatible for 4 hr at 23°C	2087	C
Droperidol	CR	1.25 mg/mL	UP	10 mg/L[d]	Physically compatible for 4 hr at room temperature	534	C
Edrophonium chloride	RC	10 mg/mL	UP	10 mg/L[d]	Physically compatible for 4 hr at room temperature	534	C
Enalaprilat	MSD	0.05 mg/mL[b]	UP	2 mg/mL[a]	Physically compatible for 24 hr at room temperature under fluorescent light	1355	C
Epinephrine HCl	AB	0.1 mg/mL	UP	10 mg/L[d]	Physically compatible for 4 hr at room temperature	534	C
Esmolol HCl	DCC	10 mg/mL[a]	LY	1 mg/mL[a]	Physically compatible for 24 hr at 22°C	1169	C
Esmolol HCl	MYL	10 mg/mL	PF	1 mg/mL[b]	Physically compatible for 1 hr at 23°C	3533	C
Estrogens, conjugated	AY	5 mg/mL	UP	100 mg/L[c]	Physically compatible for 4 hr at room temperature	322	C
Ethacrynate sodium	MSD	1 mg/mL	UP	100 mg/L[c]	Physically compatible for 4 hr at room temperature	322	C
Etoposide phosphate	BR	5 mg/mL[a]	UP	1 mg/mL[a]	Physically compatible for 4 hr at 23°C	2218	C
Famotidine	MSD	0.2 mg/mL[a]	AB	1 mg/mL[a]	Physically compatible for 4 hr at 25°C	1188	C
Famotidine	MSD	0.2 mg/mL[a]	AB	125 mg/mL	Physically compatible for 14 hr	1196	C
Fenoldopam mesylate	AB	80 mcg/mL[b]	PHU	1 mg/mL[b]	Physically compatible for 4 hr at 23°C	2467	C
Fentanyl citrate	MN	0.05 mg/mL	UP	10 mg/L[d]	Physically compatible for 4 hr at room temperature	534	C
Filgrastim	AMG	30 mcg/mL[a]	UP	1 mg/mL[a]	Physically compatible for 4 hr at 22°C	1687	C
Fludarabine phosphate	BX	1 mg/mL[a]	UP	1 mg/mL[a]	Visually compatible for 4 hr at 22°C	1439	C
Fluorouracil	RC	50 mg/mL	UP	10 mg/L[d]	Physically compatible for 4 hr at room temperature	534	C

Y-Site Injection Compatibility (1:1 Mixture) (Cont.)

Test Drug	Mfr	Conc	Mfr	Conc	Remarks	Ref	C/I
Foscarnet sodium	AST	24 mg/mL	UP	50 mg/mL	Physically compatible for 24 hr at room temperature under fluorescent light	1335	C
Furosemide	HO	10 mg/mL	UP	10 mg/L[d]	Physically compatible for 4 hr at room temperature	534	C
Gallium nitrate	FUJ	1 mg/mL[b]	AB	50 mg/mL	Visually compatible for 24 hr at 25°C	1673	C
Gemcitabine HCl	LI	10 mg/mL[b]	UP	1 mg/mL[b]	Physically compatible for 4 hr at 23°C	2226	C
Granisetron HCl	SKB	0.05 mg/mL[a]	AB	1 mg/mL[a]	Physically compatible for 4 hr at 23°C	2000	C
Heparin sodium	TR	50 units/mL	UP	2 mg/mL[b]	Visually compatible for 4 hr at 25°C	1793	C
Heparin sodium	ES	100 units/mL[e]	UP	125 mg/mL	Visually compatible for 24 hr at room temperature in test tubes. No precipitate found on filter from Y-site delivery	2063	C
Hetastarch in lactated electrolyte	AB	6%	PHU	1 mg/mL[a]	Physically compatible for 4 hr at 23°C	2339	C
Hydralazine HCl	CI	20 mg/mL	UP	10 mg/L[d]	Physically compatible for 4 hr at room temperature	534	C
Idarubicin HCl	AD	1 mg/mL[b]	UP	2[a] and 50 mg/mL	Haze forms immediately and precipitate forms in 20 min	1525	I
Isavuconazonium sulfate	ASP	1.5 mg/mL[e]	PF	1 mg/mL[e]	Physically compatible for 2 hr	3263	C
Isoproterenol HCl	WI	0.2 mg/mL	UP	10 mg/L[d]	Physically compatible for 4 hr at room temperature	534	C
Labetalol HCl	HOS	5 mg/mL	PF	1 mg/mL[b]	Measured turbidity increased	3533	I
Letermovir	ME	[a]		[a]	Physically compatible	3398	C
Lidocaine HCl	AST	20 mg/mL	UP	100 mg/L[c]	Physically compatible for 4 hr at room temperature	322	C
Linezolid	PHU	2 mg/mL	UP	1 mg/mL[a]	Physically compatible for 4 hr at 23°C	2264	C
Lorazepam	WY	0.33 mg/mL[b]	UP	50 mg/mL	Visually compatible for 24 hr at 22°C	1855	C
Magnesium sulfate	AB	500 mg/mL	UP	10 mg/L[d]	Physically compatible for 4 hr at room temperature	534	C
Melphalan HCl	BW	0.1 mg/mL[b]	UP	1 mg/mL[b]	Physically compatible for 3 hr at 22°C	1557	C
Meperidine HCl	AB	10 mg/mL	AB	2 mg/mL[a]	Physically compatible for 4 hr at 25°C	1397	C
Meropenem		50 mg/mL	PF	125 mg/mL	Physically compatible for 4 hr at room temperature	3538	C
Meropenem–vaborbactam	TMC	8 mg/mL[b, p]	PF	1 mg/mL[b]	Physically compatible for 3 hr at 20 to 25°C	3380	C
Methylergonovine maleate	SZ	0.2 mg/mL	UP	10 mg/L[d]	Physically compatible for 4 hr at room temperature	534	C
Metoprolol tartrate	HOS	0.4 mg/mL[b]	PF	1 mg/mL[b]	Physically compatible for 1 hr at 23°C	3533	C
Midazolam HCl	RC	5 mg/mL	UP	50 mg/mL	White precipitate forms immediately	1855	I
Morphine sulfate	WY	15 mg/mL	UP	10 mg/L[d]	Physically compatible for 4 hr at room temperature	534	C
Neostigmine methyl-sulfate	RC	0.5 mg/mL	UP	10 mg/L[d]	Physically compatible for 4 hr at room temperature	534	C
Nicardipine HCl	DCC	0.1 mg/mL[a]	UP	2 mg/mL[a]	Visually compatible for 24 hr at room temperature	235	C
Norepinephrine bitar-trate	WI	1 mg/mL	UP	10 mg/L[d]	Physically compatible for 4 hr at room temperature	534	C
Ondansetron HCl	GL	1 mg/mL[b]	UP	1 mg/mL[a]	Visually compatible for 4 hr at 22°C	1365	C
Oritavancin diphos-phate	TAR	0.8, 1.2, and 2 mg/mL[a]	PF	1 mg/mL[a]	Haze forms immediately with precipitate after 1 hr	2928	I

Y-Site Injection Compatibility (1:1 Mixture) (Cont.)

Test Drug	Mfr	Conc	Mfr	Conc	Remarks	Ref	C/I
Oxacillin sodium	BR	100 mg/mL	UP	10 mg/L[d]	Physically compatible for 4 hr at room temperature	534	C
Oxaliplatin	SS	0.5 mg/mL[a]	PHU	1 mg/mL[a]	Physically compatible for 4 hr at 23°C	2566	C
Oxytocin	SZ	1 unit/mL	UP	10 mg/L[d]	Physically compatible for 4 hr at room temperature	534	C
Paclitaxel	NCI	1.2 mg/mL[a]	AB	1 mg/mL[a]	Physically compatible for 4 hr at 22°C	1556	C
Pancuronium bromide	ES	0.05 mg/mL[a]	AB	1 mg/mL[a]	Physically compatible for 24 hr at 28°C	1337	C
Penicillin G potassium	LI	200,000 units/mL	UP	100 mg/L[c]	Physically compatible for 4 hr at room temperature	322	C
Pentazocine lactate	WI	30 mg/mL	UP	10 mg/L[d]	Physically compatible for 4 hr at room temperature	534	C
Phenytoin sodium	PD	50 mg/mL	UP	100 mg/L[c]	Immediate crystal formation	322	I
Phytonadione	RC	10 mg/mL	UP	10 mg/L[d]	Physically compatible for 4 hr at room temperature	534	C
Piperacillin sodium–tazobactam sodium	LE[k]	40 mg/mL[a m]	UP	1 mg/mL[a]	Physically compatible for 4 hr at 22°C	1688	C
Plazomicin sulfate	ACH	24 mg/mL[e]	PF	1 mg/mL[e]	Physically compatible for 1 hr at 20 to 25°C	3432	C
Procainamide HCl	SQ	100 mg/mL	UP	10 mg/L[d]	Physically compatible for 4 hr at room temperature	534	C
Prochlorperazine edisylate	SKF	5 mg/mL	UP	10 mg/L[d]	Physically compatible for 4 hr at room temperature	534	C
Promethazine HCl	SV	50 mg/mL	UP	10 mg/L[l]	Physically compatible for 4 hr at room temperature	534	C
Promethazine HCl	SV	50 mg/mL	UP	10 mg/L[g]	Clear initially, but cloudiness develops in 4 hr at room temperature	534	I
Propofol	ZEN[q]	10 mg/mL	UP	1 mg/mL[a]	Physically compatible for 1 hr at 23°C	2066	C
Propranolol HCl	AY	1 mg/mL	UP	10 mg/L[d]	Physically compatible for 4 hr at room temperature	534	C
Quinupristin–dalfopristin		2 mg/mL[a n]		1 mg/mL	Reported to be incompatible	3230	I
Remifentanil HCl	GW	0.025 and 0.25 mg/mL[b]	AB	1 mg/mL[a]	Physically compatible for 4 hr at 23°C	2075	C
Sargramostim	IMM	10 mcg/mL[b]	UP	1 mg/mL[b]	Few small particles in 1 hr	1436	I
Scopolamine HBr	BW	0.86 mg/mL	UP	10 mg/L[d]	Physically compatible for 4 hr at room temperature	534	C
Sodium bicarbonate	BR	75 mg/mL	UP	100 mg/L[c]	Physically compatible for 4 hr at room temperature	322	C
Succinylcholine chloride	BW	20 mg/mL	UP	100 mg/L[c]	Physically compatible for 4 hr at room temperature	322	C
Tacrolimus	FUJ	1 mg/mL[b]	AB	50 mg/mL[a]	Visually compatible for 24 hr at 25°C	1630	C
Tedizolid phosphate	CUB	0.8 mg/mL[b]	PF	1 mg/mL[b]	Physically compatible for 2 hr	3244	C
Telavancin HCl	ASP	7.5 mg/mL[a b h]	PF	1 mg/mL[a b h]	Physically compatible for 2 hr	2830	C
Teniposide	BR	0.1 mg/mL[a]	UP	1 mg/mL[a]	Physically compatible for 4 hr at 23°C	1725	C
Theophylline	TR	4 mg/mL	UP	2 mg/mL[a]	Visually compatible for 6 hr at 25°C	1793	C
Thiotepa	IMM[i]	1 mg/mL[a]	UP	1 mg/mL[a]	Physically compatible for 4 hr at 23°C	1861	C
TNA #218 to #226[j]			AB	1 mg/mL[a]	Visually compatible for 4 hr at 23°C	2215	C
TPN #189[j]			UP	50 mg/mL[b]	Visually compatible for 24 hr at 22°C	1767	C
TPN #212 to #215[j]			AB	1 mg/mL[a]	Physically compatible for 4 hr at 23°C	2109	C
Trimethobenzamide HCl	RC	100 mg/mL	UP	10 mg/L[d]	Physically compatible for 4 hr at room temperature	534	C

Y-Site Injection Compatibility (1:1 Mixture) (Cont.)

Test Drug	Mfr	Conc	Mfr	Conc	Remarks	Ref	C/I
Vecuronium bromide	OR	0.1 mg/mL[a]	AB	1 mg/mL[a]	Physically compatible for 24 hr at 28°C	1337	C
Vinorelbine tartrate	BW	1 mg/mL[b]	UP	1 mg/mL[b]	Physically compatible for 4 hr at 22°C	1558	C

[a] Tested in dextrose 5%.

[b] Tested in sodium chloride 0.9%.

[c] Tested in combination with heparin sodium (Riker) 1000 units/L in dextrose 5%, sodium chloride 0.9%, and Ringer's injection, lactated.

[d] Tested in dextrose 5% in Ringer's injection, dextrose 5% in Ringer's injection, lactated, dextrose 5%, Ringer's injection, lactated, and sodium chloride 0.9%.

[e] Tested in both dextrose 5% and sodium chloride 0.9%.

[f] Tested in bacteriostatic sodium chloride 0.9% preserved with benzyl alcohol 0.9%.

[g] Tested in dextrose 5% in Ringer's injection.

[h] Tested in Ringer's injection, lactated.

[i] Lyophilized formulation tested.

[j] Refer to Appendix for the composition of parenteral nutrition solutions. TNA indicates a 3-in-1 admixture, and TPN indicates a 2-in-1 admixture.

[k] Test performed using the formulation WITHOUT edetate disodium.

[l] Tested in dextrose 5% in Ringer's injection, lactated, dextrose 5%, Ringer's injection, lactated, and sodium chloride 0.9%.

[m] Piperacillin component. Piperacillin in an 8:1 fixed-ratio concentration with tazobactam.

[n] Quinupristin and dalfopristin components combined.

[o] Ceftolozane component. Ceftolozane in a 2:1 fixed-ratio concentration with tazobactam.

[p] Meropenem component. Meropenem in a 1:1 fixed-ratio concentration with vaborbactam.

[q] Test performed using the formulation WITH edetate disodium.

Hydromorphone Hydrochloride
AHFS 28:08.08

Products

Hydromorphone hydrochloride is available in prefilled syringes with each mL of the solution containing hydromorphone hydrochloride 1, 2, or 4 mg with sodium citrate 0.2% and citric acid 0.2%.[3302] Although no preservatives have been added to the formulation, residual amounts of sodium metabisulfite, a reagent used in the purification process of the drug, may be present.[3307]

Hydromorphone hydrochloride also is available in ampuls, cartridges, and prefilled syringes with each mL of the solution containing hydromorphone hydrochloride 1, 2, or 4 mg with sodium lactate 5.4 mg and sodium chloride; lactic acid or sodium hydroxide is used for pH adjustment.[3303] Hydromorphone hydrochloride also is available in 1-mL vials and 20-mL multidose vials with each mL of the solution containing hydromorphone hydrochloride 2 mg with edetate disodium 0.5 mg, methylparaben 1.8 mg, and propylparaben 0.2 mg in water for injection; sodium hydroxide and/or hydrochloric acid may have been added to adjust the pH.[3306]

A high potency formulation of hydromorphone hydrochloride is available packaged in ampuls, prefilled syringes, and single-dose vials; each mL of the solution contains 10 mg of hydromorphone hydrochloride with citric acid 0.2% and sodium citrate 0.2%.[3302 3304 3305] Such formulations are noted to have no added preservatives;[3302 3304 3305] however, sodium metabisulfite may be present in some formulations.[3304]

Care should be taken to avoid confusion between the various standard concentrations of hydromorphone hydrochloride and the more concentrated high potency formulation in order to reduce the risk of medication errors.[3302 3304 3305]

pH

From 3.5 to 5.5.[3302 3303 3304 3305 3306]

Trade Name(s)

Dilaudid, Dilaudid-HP

Administration

Hydromorphone hydrochloride may be administered by subcutaneous, intramuscular, or **slow** direct intravenous injection over at least 2 to 3[3302 3303 3304 3305] or 3 to 5 minutes.[3306] Administration by rapid intravenous injection increases the risk of adverse reactions.[3302 3303 3304 3305 3306]

Stability

Hydromorphone hydrochloride products should be stored at controlled room temperature and should be protected from light until time of use.[3302 3303 3304 3305 3306] Hydromorphone hydrochloride should not be stored under refrigeration because of possible precipitation or crystallization. Resolubilization at room temperature or upon warming may be performed without affecting the stability of the drug.[593]

Hydromorphone hydrochloride solution should be visually inspected for particulate matter and discoloration prior to administration.[3302 3303 3304 3305] The solution may develop a slight yellowish discoloration; however, no associated loss of potency has been demonstrated.[3302 3303 3304 3305] If the solution is darker than pale yellow, more than slightly discolored, discolored in any other way, or if it contains a precipitate, it should not be used.[3302 3306] Any unused portions should be discarded.[3302 3303 3304 3305]

Hydromorphone hydrochloride is physically compatible and chemically stable for at least 24 hours in most common large volume parenteral solutions when stored at 25°C protected from light.[3302 3303 3304 3305]

Extemporaneously prepared hydromorphone hydrochloride 10 and 50 mg/mL, stored in 100-mL glass vials or polyvinyl chloride (PVC) bags, exhibited no loss in 42 days at 4 and 23°C.[1394]

Syringes

In 2015, reports of decreased potency of certain drugs (e.g., hydromorphone hydrochloride) stored in Becton Dickinson syringes for extended periods (i.e., exceeding 24 hours) were confirmed by the manufacturer of these syringes; the cause of this change was later identified to be the inclusion of an alternate rubber stopper in the plunger of certain product lots of syringes.[3029 3036 3037 3039 3041 3042] Decreased potency was not observed when the syringes were filled and used promptly.[3037] Use of the alternate stopper was later discontinued and use of the primary stopper in such syringes was resumed; however, Becton Dickinson states that its general-use syringes are cleared by FDA for immediate use in fluid aspiration and injection and that such syringes, regardless of the stopper material, have not been cleared by FDA for use as a closed-container system.[3391]

Hydromorphone hydrochloride (Knoll) 10 mg/mL undiluted and diluted to 0.1 mg/mL in sodium chloride 0.9% was packaged as 3 mL in 10-mL polypropylene infusion pump syringes (Pharmacia Deltec). No loss occurred over 30 days at 30°C.[1967]

Hydromorphone hydrochloride 1.5 and 80 mg/mL in sodium chloride 0.9% packaged as 20 mL in 30-mL polypropylene syringes was evaluated for physical and chemical stability. Sample solutions were stored for 60 days at 4°C protected from light and 23°C exposed to normal fluorescent light. Other sample solutions were stored frozen at −20°C and at elevated temperature of 37°C for 2 days to simulate more extreme conditions during express shipping. About 2 to 5% loss occurred in 60 days at 4 and 23°C. The frozen and 37°C samples exhibited little change in concentration in 2 days. However, samples stored frozen at −20°C exhibited the formation of microparticulates in the thousands per mL, possibly shed by the syringe components.[2377]

DOI: 10.37573/9781585286850.196

Implantable Pumps

The stability of hydromorphone hydrochloride 2 (Dilaudid) and 10 (Dilaudid-HP) mg/mL was evaluated in SynchroMed implantable pumps over 16 weeks at 37°C. Little or no drug loss and no adverse effects on the pumps occurred.[2584]

Central Venous Catheter

Hydromorphone hydrochloride (Knoll) 0.5 mg/mL in dextrose 5% was found to be compatible with the ARROWg+ard Blue Plus (Arrow International) chlorhexidine-bearing triple-lumen central catheter. Essentially complete delivery of the drug was found with little or no drug loss occurring. Furthermore, chlorhexidine delivered from the catheter remained at trace amounts with no substantial increase due to the delivery of the drug through the catheter.[2335]

Compatibility Information

Solution Compatibility

Hydromorphone HCl

Test Soln Name	Mfr	Mfr	Conc/L or %	Remarks	Ref	C/I
Dextrose 5% in Ringer's injection	CU	KN[a]	80 mg	Physically compatible. No loss in 24 hr at 25°C	572	C
Dextrose 5% in Ringer's injection, lactated	MG	KN[a]	80 mg	Physically compatible. No loss in 24 hr at 25°C	572	C
Dextrose 5%	TR[b]	KN[a]	80 mg	Physically compatible. No loss in 24 hr at 25°C	572	C
Dextrose 5%	MG[c]	KN[a]	80 mg	Physically compatible. No loss in 24 hr at 25°C	572	C
Dextrose 5%	[b]	KN	1 and 5 g	No loss in 42 days at 4 and 23°C	1394	C
Dextrose 5% in sodium chloride 0.45%	MG	KN[a]	80 mg	Physically compatible. No loss in 24 hr at 25°C	572	C
Dextrose 5% in sodium chloride 0.9%	MG	KN[a]	80 mg	Physically compatible. No loss in 24 hr at 25°C	572	C
Ringer's injection	MG	KN[a]	80 mg	Physically compatible. No loss in 24 hr at 25°C	572	C
Ringer's injection, lactated	MG	KN[a]	80 mg	Physically compatible. No loss in 24 hr at 25°C	572	C
Sodium chloride 0.45%	MG	KN[a]	80 mg	Physically compatible. No loss in 24 hr at 25°C	572	C
Sodium chloride 0.9%	TR[b]	KN[a]	80 mg	Physically compatible. No loss in 24 hr at 25°C	572	C
Sodium chloride 0.9%	MG[c]	KN[a]	80 mg	Physically compatible. No loss in 24 hr at 25°C	572	C
Sodium chloride 0.9%	[b]	KN	1 and 5 g	No loss in 42 days at 4 and 23°C	1394	C
Sodium chloride 0.9%	AB[b]	KN	20 and 100 mg	Visually compatible. Little or no loss in 72 hr at 24°C under fluorescent light	1870	C
Sodium chloride 0.9%	BA[d]	[e]	1.5 to 80 g	Physically compatible. 2 to 5% hydromorphone loss in 60 days at 4°C protected from light and 23°C under fluorescent light	2377	C
Sodium chloride 0.9%	[f]	BA	200 mg	Under 8% loss in 112 days at 4 and 20°C	2818	C
Sodium lactate ⅙ M	CU	KN[a]	80 mg	Physically compatible. No loss in 24 hr at 25°C	572	C

[a] Both ampul and vial formulations tested.

[b] Tested in PVC containers.

[c] Tested in polyolefin containers.

[d] Tested in polypropylene syringes.

[e] Extemporaneously compounded from hydromorphone hydrochloride powder.

[f] Tested in PCA injectors.

Additive Compatibility

Hydromorphone HCl

Test Drug	Mfr	Conc/L or %	Mfr	Conc/L or %	Test Solution	Remarks	Ref	C/I
Bupivacaine HCl	AB	625 mg and 1.25 g	KN	20 mg	NS[a]	Visually compatible with little or no loss of either drug in 72 hr at 24°C under fluorescent light	1870	C
Bupivacaine HCl	AB	625 mg and 1.25 g	KN	100 mg	NS[a]	Visually compatible with little or no loss of either drug in 72 hr at 24°C under fluorescent light	1870	C
Clonidine HCl	BI	150 mg		25 mg	[b]	No clonidine loss in 35 days at 37°C	2593	C
Fluorouracil	AB	1 g	AST	500 mg	D5W, NS[a]	Physically compatible. Little loss of either drug in 7 days at 32°C and 35 days at 23, 4, and −20°C	1977	C
Fluorouracil	AB	16 g	AST	500 mg	D5W, NS[a]	Physically compatible. Little loss of either drug in 3 days at 32°C, 7 days at 23°C, and 35 days at 4 and −20°C	1977	C
Heparin sodium	OR	1000 units	KN	20 g	D5W[a]	Visually compatible with no loss of hydromorphone in 18 days at 4 and 23°C. Heparin not tested	2410	C
Heparin sodium	OR	500 units	KN	5 g	D5W[a]	Visually compatible with no loss of hydromorphone in 18 days at 4 and 23°C. Heparin not tested	2410	C
Heparin sodium	OR	8000 units	KN	5 g	D5W[a]	Visually compatible with no loss of hydromorphone in 18 days at 4 and 23°C. Heparin not tested	2410	C
Ketamine HCl	SZ	200 mg, 600 mg, 1 g	SZ	200 mg	NS[d]	Visually compatible. Under 10% loss of both drugs in 7 days at 25°C	2799	C
Midazolam HCl	RC	0.1 to 4.5 g	KN	0.5 to 45 g	D5W, NS	Visually compatible for 24 hr at room temperature	2086	C
Midazolam HCl	RC	100 and 500 mg	KN	2 and 20 g	D5W, NS	Visually compatible. Under 7% hydromorphone and midazolam loss in 23 days at 4 and 23°C	2086	C
Ondansetron HCl	GL	100 mg and 1 g	ES	500 mg	NS	Physically compatible. No loss of either drug in 7 days at 32°C or 31 days at 4 and 22°C protected from light	1690	C
Potassium chloride	AST	0.5 and 1 mEq/mL	KN	2 and 20 mg/mL	D5W[a]	Visually compatible with no loss of hydromorphone in 18 days at 4 and 23°C. Potassium chloride not tested	2410	C
Promethazine HCl	ES	300 mg	KN	1 g	NS[a]	Visually compatible for 21 days at 4 and 25°C	1992	C
Verapamil HCl	KN	80 mg	KN	16 mg	D5W, NS	Physically compatible for 24 hr	764	C
Ziconotide acetate	ELN	25 mg[b]	BB	35 g[c]		90% ziconotide retained for 19 days at 37°C. No hydromorphone loss in 25 days	2702	C

[a] Tested in PVC containers.

[b] Tested in SynchroMed implantable pumps.

[c] Hydromorphone HCl powder dissolved in ziconotide acetate injection.

[d] Tested in amber glass and PVC containers.

Drugs in Syringe Compatibility

Hydromorphone HCl

Test Drug	Mfr	Amt	Mfr	Amt	Remarks	Ref	C/I
Ampicillin sodium	AY	250 mg/1 mL	KN	2, 10, 40 mg/1 mL	Visually compatible but 10% loss of ampicillin in 5 hr at room temperature	2082	I
Atropine sulfate	ES	0.4 mg/0.5 mL	KN	4 mg/2 mL[a]	Physically compatible for 30 min	517	C
Bupivacaine HCl	AST	7.5 mg/mL	KN	65 mg/mL	Visually compatible for 30 days at 25°C	1660	C
Cefazolin sodium	SKF	>200 mg/1 mL	KN	2, 10, 40 mg/1 mL	Precipitate forms	2082	I
Cefazolin sodium	SKF	150 mg/1 mL	KN	2, 10, 40 mg/1 mL	Visually compatible with less than 10% loss of each drug in 24 hr at room temperature	2082	C
Ceftazidime	GL	180 mg/1 mL	KN	2, 10, 40 mg/1 mL	Visually compatible with less than 10% loss of either drug in 24 hr at room temperature	2082	C
Chlorpromazine HCl	ES	25 mg/1 mL	KN	4 mg/2 mL[a]	Physically compatible for 30 min	517	C
Cloxacillin sodium	AY	250 mg/1 mL	KN	2, 10, 40 mg/1 mL	Precipitate forms but dissipates with shaking. Under 10% loss of both drugs in 24 hr at room temperature	2082	?
Dexamethasone sodium phosphate	SX	4 mg/mL[b]	KN	2, 10, 40 mg/mL[b]	Visually compatible and both drugs stable for 24 hr at 24°C	1542	C
Dexamethasone sodium phosphate	DB	10 mg/mL[b]	KN	2 and 10 mg/mL[b]	Visually compatible and both drugs stable for 24 hr at 24°C	1542	C
Dexamethasone sodium phosphate	DB	10 mg/mL[b]	KN	40 mg/mL[b]	White turbidity forms immediately	1542	I
Dexamethasone sodium phosphate	DB	7.1 mg/mL[c]	KN	11.6 mg/mL[c]	Visually compatible for 24 hr at 24°C	1542	C
Dexamethasone sodium phosphate	DB	5.5 to 6.6 mg/mL[c]	KN	13.3 to 17.5 mg/mL[c]	Precipitate forms	1542	I
Dexamethasone sodium phosphate	DB	4.75 mg/mL[c]	KN	10.5 mg/mL[c]	Visually compatible for 24 hr at 24°C	1542	C
Dexamethasone sodium phosphate	DB	3 to 4.1 mg/mL[c]	KN	14.75 to 25 mg/mL[c]	Precipitate forms	1542	I
Dexamethasone sodium phosphate	SX	3.34 mg/mL[c]	KN	26.66 mg/mL[c]	Visually compatible for 24 hr at 24°C	1542	C
Diazepam	SX	5 mg/1 mL	KN	2, 10, 40 mg/1 mL	Diazepam precipitate forms immediately due to aqueous dilution	2082	I
Dimenhydrinate	SQ	50 mg/1 mL	KN	2, 10, 40 mg/1 mL	Visually compatible with both drugs stable for 24 hr at 4, 23, and 37°C. Precipitate forms after 24 hr	1776	C
Dimenhydrinate		10 mg/1 mL		50 mg/1 mL	Precipitate forms in about 2 hr	2569	I
Diphenhydramine HCl	PD	50 mg/1 mL	KN	4 mg/2 mL[a]	Physically compatible for 30 min	517	C
Fentanyl citrate	MN	0.05 mg/1 mL	KN	4 mg/2 mL[a]	Physically compatible for 30 min	517	C
Glycopyrrolate	RB	0.2 mg/1 mL	KN	2 mg/1 mL	Physically compatible. pH in glycopyrrolate stability range for 48 hr at 25°C	331	C
Glycopyrrolate	RB	0.2 mg/1 mL	KN	4 mg/2 mL	Physically compatible. pH in glycopyrrolate stability range for 48 hr at 25°C	331	C
Glycopyrrolate	RB	0.4 mg/2 mL	KN	2 mg/1 mL	Physically compatible. pH in glycopyrrolate stability range for 48 hr at 25°C	331	C

Drugs in Syringe Compatibility (Cont.)

Test Drug	Mfr	Amt	Mfr	Amt	Remarks	Ref	C/I
Haloperidol lactate	MN	1[d], 2[d], 5 mg/1 mL	KN	1[d] and 10 mg/1 mL	Visually compatible for 24 hr at 25°C under fluorescent light	1785	C
Haloperidol lactate	MN	2 mg/mL	KN	10 and 15 mg/mL	White precipitate of haloperidol forms immediately	668	I
Heparin sodium	OR	10 units/1 mL	KN	50 mg/1 mL	White cloudy precipitate	2410	I
Heparin sodium	LEO	100 units/1 mL	KN	50 mg/1 mL	White cloudy precipitate	2410	I
Heparin sodium	OR	25,000 units/1 mL	KN	50 mg/1 mL	White cloudy precipitate	2410	I
Hyaluronidase	WY	150 units/mL[e]	KN	2 mg/mL[e]	43 and 56% hyaluronidase loss in 24 hr at 4 and 23°C, respectively	1907	I
Hyaluronidase	WY	150 units/mL[e]	KN	10 and 40 mg/mL[e]	70 to 82% hyaluronidase loss in 24 hr at 4 and 23°C	1907	I
Hydroxyzine HCl	PF	50 mg/1 mL	KN	4 mg/2 mL[a]	Physically compatible for 30 min	517	C
Hydroxyzine HCl	PF	100 mg/2 mL	KN	0.75 mg/0.8 mL	Physically compatible	771	C
Ketamine HCl	SZ	0.2, 0.6, 1 mg/mL[j]	SZ	0.2 mg/mL[j]	Visually compatible. Under 10% loss of both drugs in 7 days at 25°C	2799	C
Ketorolac tromethamine	SY	30 mg/1 mL	KN	10 mg/1 mL	Cloudiness forms immediately but clears with swirling	1785	?
Ketorolac tromethamine	SY	30 mg/1 mL	KN	1 mg/1 mL[d]	Visually compatible for 24 hr at 25°C under fluorescent light	1785	C
Ketorolac tromethamine	SY	15 mg/1 mL[d]	KN	1[d] and 10 mg/1 mL	Visually compatible for 24 hr at 25°C under fluorescent light	1785	C
Lorazepam	WY	4 mg/1 mL	KN	2, 10, 40 mg/1 mL	Visually compatible. 10% lorazepam loss in 6 days at 4°C, 4 days at 23°C, and 24 hr at 37°C. Little hydromorphone loss in 7 days at all temperatures	1776	C
Methotrimeprazine HCl	LE	10 mg/mL	KN	10 mg/mL	Visually compatible with less than 10% loss of either drug in 7 days at 8°C	668	C
Metoclopramide HCl	RB	5 mg/mL	KN	10 and 20 mg/mL	Visually compatible with less than 10% loss of either drug in 7 days at 8°C	668	C
Midazolam HCl	RC	5 mg/1 mL	WB	2 mg/0.5 mL	Physically compatible for 4 hr at 25°C	1145	C
Pantoprazole sodium	i	4 mg/1 mL		10 mg/1 mL	Whitish precipitate forms within 4 hr	2574	I
Pentazocine lactate	WI	30 mg/1 mL	KN	4 mg/2 mL[a]	Physically compatible for 30 min	517	C
Pentobarbital sodium	AB	50 mg/1 mL	KN	4 mg/2 mL[f]	Physically compatible for 30 min	517	C
Pentobarbital sodium	AB	50 mg/1 mL	KN	4 mg/2 mL[g]	Transient precipitate that dissipates after mixing and stays clear for 30 min	517	?
Phenobarbital sodium	AB	120 mg/1 mL	KN	2, 10, 40 mg/1 mL	Precipitate forms immediately but dissipates with shaking. Phenobarbital precipitates after 6 hr at room temperature	2082	I
Phenytoin sodium	AB	50 mg/1 mL	KN	2, 10, 40 mg/1 mL	White precipitate of phenytoin forms immediately	2082	I
Potassium chloride	AST	2 mEq/1 mL	KN	50 mg/1 mL	Visually compatible for 24 hr at room temperature	2410	C
Prochlorperazine edisylate	SKF	5 mg/1 mL	KN	4 mg/2 mL[f]	Precipitates immediately	517	I
Prochlorperazine edisylate	SKF	5 mg/1 mL	KN	4 mg/2 mL[g]	Physically compatible for 30 min	517	C

Drugs in Syringe Compatibility (Cont.)

Test Drug	Mfr	Amt	Mfr	Amt	Remarks	Ref	C/I
Prochlorperazine mesylate	RP	5 mg/1 mL	KN	2, 10, 40 mg/1 mL	Visually compatible. Little or no loss of either drug in 7 days at 4, 23, and 37°C	1776	C
Prochlorperazine mesylate	RP	1.5 mg/mL^i	SX	0.5 mg/mL^i	Physically compatible for 96 hr at room temperature exposed to light	2171	C
Promethazine HCl	WY	50 mg/1 mL	KN	4 mg/2 mL^a	Physically compatible for 30 min	517	C
Promethazine HCl	WY	25 mg/1 mL	KN	4 mg/2 mL^a	Physically compatible for 30 min	517	C
Ranitidine HCl	GL	50 mg/2 mL	PE	2 mg/1 mL	Physically compatible for 1 hr at 25°C	978	C
Salbutamol sulfate	GL	2.5 mg/2.5 mL^b	KN	1 mg/0.5 mL	Physically compatible for 1 hr	1904	C
Scopolamine HBr	BW	0.43 mg/0.5 mL	KN	4 mg/2 mL^a	Physically compatible for 30 min	517	C
Trimethobenzamide HCl	BE	100 mg/1 mL	KN	4 mg/2 mL^a	Physically compatible for 30 min	517	C
Ziconotide acetate	ELN	25 mcg/mL	BB	35 mg/mL^k	No loss of either drug in 25 days at 5°C	2702	C

^{a} Both ampul and vial formulations tested.

^{b} Mixed in equal quantities. Final concentration is one-half the indicated concentration.

^{c} Mixed in varying quantities to yield the final concentrations noted.

^{d} Dilution prepared in sterile water for injection.

^{e} Mixed in equal quantities for testing.

^{f} Vial formulation tested.

^{g} Ampul formulation tested.

^{h} Both preserved (benzyl alcohol 0.9%; benzalkonium chloride 0.01%) and unpreserved sodium chloride 0.9% were used as a diluent.

^{i} Test performed using the formulation WITHOUT edetate disodium.

^{j} Diluted in sodium chloride 0.9%.

^{k} Hydromorphone HCl powder dissolved in ziconotide acetate injection.

Y-Site Injection Compatibility (1:1 Mixture)

Hydromorphone HCl

Test Drug	Mfr	Conc	Mfr	Conc	Remarks	Ref	C/I
Acetaminophen	CAD	10 mg/mL	WW	2 mg/mL	Physically compatible for 4 hr at 23°C	2901, 2902	C
Acetaminophen	CAD	10 mg/mL	HOS	4 mg/mL	Physically compatible with less than 10% acetaminophen loss over 4 hr at room temperature	2841, 2844	C
Acyclovir sodium	BW	5 mg/mL^a	WB	0.04 mg/mL^a	Physically compatible for 4 hr at 25°C	1157	C
Allopurinol sodium	BW	3 mg/mL^b	KN	0.5 mg/mL^b	Physically compatible for 4 hr at 22°C	1686	C
Amifostine	USB	10 mg/mL^a	AST	0.5 mg/mL^a	Physically compatible for 4 hr at 23°C	1845	C
Amikacin sulfate	BR	5 mg/mL^a	WY	0.2 mg/mL^a	Physically compatible for 4 hr at 25°C	987	C
Ampicillin sodium	BR	20 mg/mL^b	WY	0.2 mg/mL^a	Physically compatible for 4 hr at 25°C	987	C
Ampicillin sodium	AY	20^a and 250 mg/mL	KN	2, 10, 40 mg/mL	Visually compatible. Hydromorphone stable for 24 hr. 10% ampicillin loss in 5 hr	1532	I
Amsacrine	NCI	1 mg/mL^a	AST	0.5 mg/mL^a	Visually compatible for 4 hr at 22°C	1381	C
Atropine sulfate	LY	0.4 mg/mL	AST	0.5 mg/mL^a	Physically compatible for 48 hr at 22°C	1706	C

Y-Site Injection Compatibility (1:1 Mixture) (Cont.)

Test Drug	Mfr	Conc	Mfr	Conc	Remarks	Ref	C/I
Aztreonam	SQ	40 mg/mL[a]	KN	0.5 mg/mL[a]	Physically compatible for 4 hr at 23°C	1758	C
Bivalirudin	TMC	5 mg/mL[a]	AST	0.5 mg/mL[a]	Physically compatible for 4 hr at 23°C	2373	C
Cangrelor tetrasodium	TMC	1 mg/mL[b]		0.5[b] and 1[b] mg/mL	Physically compatible for 4 hr	3243	C
Caspofungin acetate	ME	0.7 mg/mL[b]	BA	1 mg/mL[b]	Physically compatible for 4 hr at room temperature	2758	C
Caspofungin acetate	ME	0.5 mg/mL[b]	HOS	1 mg/mL	Physically compatible with hydromorphone HCl i.v. push over 2 to 5 min	2766	C
Cefazolin sodium	SKF	20 mg/mL[a]	WY	0.2 mg/mL[a]	Physically compatible for 4 hr at 25°C	987	C
Cefazolin sodium	SKF	20[a] and 150 mg/mL	KN	2, 10, 40 mg/mL	Visually compatible and both drugs stable for 24 hr	1532	C
Cefazolin sodium	SKF	>200 mg/mL	KN	2, 10, 40 mg/mL	Precipitate forms immediately	1532	I
Cefotaxime sodium	HO	20 mg/mL[a]	WY	0.2 mg/mL[a]	Physically compatible for 4 hr at 25°C	987	C
Cefoxitin sodium	MSD	20 mg/mL[a]	WY	0.2 mg/mL[a]	Physically compatible for 4 hr at 25°C	987	C
Ceftaroline fosamil	FOR	2.22 mg/mL[a b f]	HOS	0.5 mg/mL[a b f]	Physically compatible for 4 hr at 23°C	2826	C
Ceftazidime	GL	40[a] and 180 mg/mL	KN	2, 10, 40 mg/mL	Visually compatible and both drugs stable for 24 hr	1532	C
Ceftolozane sulfate–tazobactam sodium	CUB	10 mg/mL[k l]	AKN	1 mg/mL[k]	Physically compatible for 2 hr	3262	C
Cefuroxime sodium	GL	30 mg/mL[a]	WY	0.2 mg/mL[a]	Physically compatible for 4 hr at 25°C	987	C
Chloramphenicol sodium succinate	LY	20 mg/mL[a]	WY	0.2 mg/mL[a]	Physically compatible for 4 hr at 25°C	987	C
Cisatracurium besylate	GW	0.1, 2, 5 mg/mL[a]	ES	0.5 mg/mL[a]	Physically compatible for 4 hr at 23°C	2074	C
Cladribine	ORT	0.015[b] and 0.5[d] mg/mL	KN	0.5 mg/mL[b]	Physically compatible for 4 hr at 23°C	1969	C
Clevidipine butyrate	CHS	0.5 mg/mL		10 mg/mL	Physically incompatible	3334	I
Clindamycin phosphate	UP	12 mg/mL[a]	WY	0.2 mg/mL[a]	Physically compatible for 4 hr at 25°C	987	C
Cloxacillin sodium	AY	250 mg/mL	KN	2, 10, 40 mg/mL	Turbidity forms but dissipates with shaking and solution remains clear. Both drugs stable for 24 hr	1532	?
Cloxacillin sodium	AY	40 mg/mL[a]	KN	2, 10, 40 mg/mL	Turbidity forms immediately and cloxacillin precipitate develops	1532	I
Cloxacillin sodium	AY	27 mg/mL[a]	KN	2, 10, 40 mg/mL	Turbidity forms immediately	1532	I
Cloxacillin sodium	AY	12 mg/mL[a]	KN	2, 10, 40 mg/mL	Visually compatible for 24 hr; precipitate forms in 96 hr	1532	C
Cloxacillin sodium	SMX	100 mg/mL	SZ	10 mg/mL	Physically compatible for up to 4 hr at room temperature	3245	C
Dexamethasone sodium phosphate	AMR	1 mg/mL[a]	AST	0.5 mg/mL[a]	Physically compatible for 48 hr at 22°C	1706	C
Dexmedetomidine HCl	AB	4 mcg/mL[b]	AST	0.5 mg/mL[b]	Physically compatible for 4 hr at 23°C	2383	C
Diazepam	SX	5 mg/mL	KN	2, 10, 40 mg/mL	Turbidity forms immediately and diazepam precipitate develops	1532	I

Y-Site Injection Compatibility (1:1 Mixture) (Cont.)

Test Drug	Mfr	Conc	Mfr	Conc	Remarks	Ref	C/I
Diazepam	ES	0.5 mg/mL[a]	AST	0.5 mg/mL[a]	Physically compatible for 48 hr at 22°C	1706	C
Diltiazem HCl	MMD	1 mg/mL[a]	KN	1 mg/mL	Visually compatible for 4 hr at 27°C	2062	C
Diphenhydramine HCl	SCN	2 mg/mL[a]	AST	0.5 mg/mL[a]	Physically compatible for 48 hr at 22°C	1706	C
Dobutamine HCl	LI	4 mg/mL[a]	KN	1 mg/mL	Visually compatible for 4 hr at 27°C	2062	C
Docetaxel	RPR	0.9 mg/mL[a]	AST	0.5 mg/mL[a]	Physically compatible for 4 hr at 23°C	2224	C
Dopamine HCl	AB	3.2 mg/mL[a]	KN	1 mg/mL	Visually compatible for 4 hr at 27°C	2062	C
Doripenem	JJ	5 mg/mL[a][b]	BA	1 mg/mL[a][b]	Physically compatible for 4 hr at 23°C	2743	C
Doxorubicin HCl liposomal	SEQ	0.4 mg/mL[a]	ES	0.5 mg/mL[a]	Physically compatible for 4 hr at 23°C	2087	C
Doxycycline hyclate	ES	1 mg/mL[a]	WY	0.2 mg/mL[a]	Physically compatible for 4 hr at 25°C	987	C
Epinephrine HCl	AB	0.02 mg/mL[a]	KN	1 mg/mL	Visually compatible for 4 hr at 27°C	2062	C
Eravacycline dihydrochloride	TET	0.6 mg/mL[b]	AKN	1 mg/mL[b]	Physically compatible for 2 hr at room temperature	3532	C
Erythromycin lactobionate	AB	5 mg/mL[a]	WY	0.2 mg/mL[a]	Physically compatible for 4 hr at 25°C	987	C
Etoposide phosphate	BR	5 mg/mL[a]	ES	0.5 mg/mL[a]	Physically compatible for 4 hr at 23°C	2218	C
Famotidine	ME	2 mg/mL[b]		0.5 mg/mL[a]	Visually compatible for 4 hr at 22°C	1936	C
Fenoldopam mesylate	AB	80 mcg/mL[b]	ES	0.5 mg/mL[b]	Physically compatible for 4 hr at 23°C	2467	C
Fentanyl citrate	ES	0.05 mg/mL	KN	1 mg/mL	Visually compatible for 4 hr at 27°C	2062	C
Filgrastim	AMG	30 mcg/mL[a]	KN	0.5 mg/mL[a]	Physically compatible for 4 hr at 22°C	1687	C
Fludarabine phosphate	BX	1 mg/mL[a]	KN	0.5 mg/mL[a]	Visually compatible for 4 hr at 22°C	1439	C
Foscarnet sodium	AST	24 mg/mL	KN	10 mg/mL	Physically compatible for 24 hr at room temperature under fluorescent light	1335	C
Furosemide	AMR	10 mg/mL	KN	1 mg/mL	Visually compatible for 4 hr at 27°C	2062	C
Gallium nitrate	FUJ	1 mg/mL[b]	WY	4 mg/mL	Precipitate forms in 24 hr at 25°C	1673	I
Gemcitabine HCl	LI	10 mg/mL[b]	AST	0.5 mg/mL[b]	Physically compatible for 4 hr at 23°C	2226	C
Gentamicin sulfate	TR	0.8 mg/mL[a]	WY	0.2 mg/mL[a]	Physically compatible for 4 hr at 25°C	987	C
Granisetron HCl	SKB	1 mg/mL	KN	0.5 mg/mL[b]	Physically compatible with little or no loss of either drug in 4 hr at 22°C	1883	C
Granisetron HCl	SKB	0.05 mg/mL[a]	ES	0.5 mg/mL[a]	Physically compatible for 4 hr at 23°C	2000	C
Haloperidol lactate	MN	0.2 mg/mL[a]	AST	0.5 mg/mL[a]	Physically compatible for 48 hr at 22°C	1706	C
Heparin sodium	ES	100 units/mL[a]	KN	1 mg/mL	Visually compatible for 4 hr at 27°C	2062	C
Hetastarch in lactated electrolyte	AB	6%	AST	0.5 mg/mL[a]	Physically compatible for 4 hr at 23°C	2339	C
Hydroxyethyl starch 130/0.4 in sodium chloride 0.9%	FRK	6%	SZ	0.4[a], 1.2[a], 2 mg/mL	Visually compatible for 24 hr at room temperature	2770	C
Hydroxyzine HCl	WI	4 mg/mL[a]	AST	0.5 mg/mL[a]	Physically compatible for 48 hr at 22°C	1706	C
Isavuconazonium sulfate	ASP	1.5 mg/mL[k]	AKN	1 mg/mL[k]	Physically compatible for 2 hr	3263	C
Ketorolac tromethamine	WY	1 mg/mL[a]	AST	0.5 mg/mL[a]	Physically compatible for 48 hr at 22°C	1706	C
Labetalol HCl	AH	2 mg/mL[a]	KN	1 mg/mL	Visually compatible for 4 hr at 27°C	2062	C
Levofloxacin	OMN	5 mg/mL[a]	HOS	2 mg/mL	Physically compatible	2794	C

Y-Site Injection Compatibility (1:1 Mixture) (Cont.)

Test Drug	Mfr	Conc	Mfr	Conc	Remarks	Ref	C/I
Linezolid	PHU	2 mg/mL	AST	0.5 mg/mL[a]	Physically compatible for 4 hr at 23°C	2264	C
Lorazepam	WY	0.5 mg/mL[a]	KN	1 mg/mL	Visually compatible for 4 hr at 27°C	2062	C
Lorazepam	WY	0.1 mg/mL[a]	AST	0.5 mg/mL[a]	Physically compatible for 48 hr at 22°C	1706	C
Magnesium sulfate	LY	16.7, 33.3, 50, 100 mg/mL[a]	KN	2 mg/mL[a]	Visually compatible for 4 hr at 25°C	1549	C
Melphalan HCl	BW	0.1 mg/mL[b]	KN	0.5 mg/mL[b]	Physically compatible for 3 hr at 22°C	1557	C
Meropenem		50 mg/mL	SZ	10 mg/mL	Physically compatible for 4 hr at room temperature	3538	C
Meropenem–vaborbactam	TMC	8 mg/mL[b m]	AKN	1 mg/mL[b]	Physically compatible for 3 hr at 20 to 25°C	3380	C
Methotrimeprazine HCl	LE	0.2 mg/mL[a]	AST	0.5 mg/mL[a]	Physically compatible for 48 hr at 22°C	1706	C
Metoclopramide HCl	DU	5 mg/mL	AST	0.5 mg/mL[a]	Physically compatible for 48 hr at 22°C	1706	C
Metronidazole	SE	5 mg/mL	WY	0.2 mg/mL[a]	Physically compatible for 4 hr at 25°C	987	C
Micafungin sodium	ASP	1.5 mg/mL[b]	BA	0.5 mg/mL[b]	Physically compatible for 4 hr at 23°C	2683	C
Midazolam HCl	RC	2 mg/mL[a]	KN	1 mg/mL	Visually compatible for 4 hr at 27°C	2062	C
Midazolam HCl	RC	0.2 mg/mL[a]	AST	0.5 mg/mL[a]	Physically compatible for 48 hr at 22°C	1706	C
Milrinone lactate	SW	0.2 mg/mL[a]	KN	1 mg/mL	Visually compatible for 4 hr at 27°C	2062	C
Morphine sulfate	SCN	2 mg/mL[a]	KN	1 mg/mL	Visually compatible for 4 hr at 27°C	2062	C
Nafcillin sodium	WY	20 mg/mL[a]	WY	0.2 mg/mL[a]	Physically compatible for 4 hr at 25°C	987	C
Nicardipine HCl	WY	1 mg/mL[a]	KN	1 mg/mL	Visually compatible for 4 hr at 27°C	2062	C
Nitroglycerin	AB	0.4 mg/mL[a]	KN	1 mg/mL	Visually compatible for 4 hr at 27°C	2062	C
Norepinephrine bitartrate	AB	0.128 mg/mL[a]	KN	1 mg/mL	Visually compatible for 4 hr at 27°C	2062	C
Ondansetron HCl	GL	1 mg/mL[b]	KN	0.5 mg/mL[a]	Visually compatible for 4 hr at 22°C	1365	C
Oxacillin sodium	BE	20 mg/mL[a]	WY	0.2 mg/mL[a]	Physically compatible for 4 hr at 25°C	987	C
Oxaliplatin	SS	0.5 mg/mL[a]	ES	0.5 mg/mL[a]	Physically compatible for 4 hr at 23°C	2566	C
Paclitaxel	NCI	1.2 mg/mL[a]	KN	0.5 mg/mL[a]	Physically compatible for 4 hr at 22°C	1556	C
Palonosetron HCl	MGI	50 mcg/mL	BA	0.5 mg/mL[a]	Physically compatible and no loss of either drug in 4 hr	2720	C
Pemetrexed disodium	LI	20 mg/mL[b]	ES	0.5 mg/mL[a]	Physically compatible for 4 hr at 23°C	2564	C
Penicillin G potassium	PF	100,000 units/mL[a]	WY	0.2 mg/mL[a]	Physically compatible for 4 hr at 25°C	987	C
Phenobarbital sodium	AB	120 mg/mL	KN	2, 10, 40 mg/mL	Turbidity forms but dissipates; phenobarbital precipitates in 6 hr	1532	I
Phenobarbital sodium	WY	2 mg/mL[a]	AST	0.5 mg/mL[a]	Physically compatible for 48 hr at 22°C	1706	C
Phenytoin sodium	AB	50 mg/mL	KN	2, 10, 40 mg/mL	Turbidity forms immediately and phenytoin precipitate develops	1532	I
Phenytoin sodium	ES	2 mg/mL[a b]	AST	0.5 mg/mL[a]	Precipitate forms within 1 hr	1706	I
Piperacillin sodium–tazobactam sodium	LE[e]	40 mg/mL[a i]	ES	0.5 mg/mL[a]	Physically compatible for 4 hr at 22°C	1688	C
Plazomicin sulfate	ACH	24 mg/mL[k]	AKN	1 mg/mL[k]	Physically compatible for 1 hr at 20 to 25°C	3432	C

Y-Site Injection Compatibility (1:1 Mixture) (Cont.)

Test Drug	Mfr	Conc	Mfr	Conc	Remarks	Ref	C/I
Posaconazole	ME	18 mg/mL		10 mg/mL[k]	Physically compatible	2911, 2912	C
Propofol	ZEN[n]	10 mg/mL	AST	0.5 mg/mL[a]	Physically compatible for 1 hr at 23°C	2066	C
Ranitidine HCl	GL	1 mg/mL[a]	KN	1 mg/mL	Visually compatible for 4 hr at 27°C	2062	C
Remifentanil HCl	GW	0.025 and 0.25 mg/mL[b]	ES	0.5 mg/mL[a]	Physically compatible for 4 hr at 23°C	2075	C
Sargramostim	IMM	10 mcg/mL[b]	WI	0.5 mg/mL[b]	Few small particles in 30 min	1436	I
Scopolamine HBr	LY	0.05 mg/mL[a]	AST	0.5 mg/mL[a]	Physically compatible for 48 hr at 22°C	1706	C
Tacrolimus	FUJ	10 and 40 mcg/mL[a]	KN	2 and 0.2 mg/mL[a]	Visually compatible. No loss of either drug in 4 hr at 24°C	2216	C
Tedizolid phosphate	CUB	0.8 mg/mL[b]	AKN	1 mg/mL[b]	Physically compatible for 2 hr	3244	C
Teniposide	BR	0.1 mg/mL[a]	KN	0.5 mg/mL[a]	Physically compatible for 4 hr at 23°C	1725	C
Thiotepa	IMM[g]	1 mg/mL[a]	AST	0.5 mg/mL[a]	Physically compatible for 4 hr at 23°C	1861	C
TNA #218, #220, #221, #223[h]			ES	0.5 mg/mL[a]	Visually compatible for 4 hr at 23°C	2215	C
TNA #219, #222, #224 to #226[h]			ES	0.5 mg/mL[a]	Damage to emulsion occurs immediately with free oil formation possible	2215	I
Tobramycin sulfate	DI	0.8 mg/mL[a]	WY	0.2 mg/mL[a]	Physically compatible for 4 hr at 25°C	987	C
TPN #212 to #215[h]			ES	0.5 mg/mL[a]	Physically compatible for 4 hr at 23°C	2109	C
Trimethoprim–sulfamethox-azole	BW	0.8 mg/mL[a][j]	WY	0.2 mg/mL[a]	Physically compatible for 4 hr at 25°C	987	C
Vancomycin HCl	LI	5 mg/mL[a]	WY	0.2 mg/mL[a]	Physically compatible for 4 hr at 25°C	987	C
Vancomycin HCl	HOS	4 mg/mL[b]	HOS	2 mg/mL	Physically compatible	2794	C
Vecuronium bromide	OR	1 mg/mL	KN	1 mg/mL	Visually compatible for 4 hr at 27°C	2062	C
Vinorelbine tartrate	BW	1 mg/mL[b]	KN	0.5 mg/mL[b]	Physically compatible for 4 hr at 22°C	1558	C

[a] Tested in dextrose 5%.

[b] Tested in sodium chloride 0.9%.

[c] Tested in sterile water for injection.

[d] Tested in bacteriostatic sodium chloride 0.9% preserved with benzyl alcohol 0.9%.

[e] Test performed using the formulation WITHOUT edetate disodium.

[f] Tested in Ringer's injection, lactated.

[g] Lyophilized formulation tested.

[h] Refer to Appendix for the composition of parenteral nutrition solutions. TNA indicates a 3-in-1 admixture, and TPN indicates a 2-in-1 admixture.

[i] Piperacillin component. Piperacillin in an 8:1 fixed-ratio concentration with tazobactam.

[j] Trimethoprim component. Trimethoprim in a 1:5 fixed-ratio concentration with sulfamethoxazole.

[k] Tested in both dextrose 5% and sodium chloride 0.9%.

[l] Ceftolozane component. Ceftolozane in a 2:1 fixed-ratio concentration with tazobactam.

[m] Meropenem component. Meropenem in a 1:1 fixed-ratio concentration with vaborbactam.

[n] Test performed using the formulation WITH edetate disodium.

Hydroxyethyl Starch 130/0.4 in Sodium Chloride 0.9%
AHFS 40:12

Products

Hydroxyethyl starch 130/0.4 is available as a 6% (6 g/100 mL) injection in sodium chloride 0.9% in 500-mL plastic containers.[3453] The solution also contains sodium hydroxide or hydrochloric acid for pH adjustment.[3453]

pH

From 4 to 5.5.[3453]

Osmolarity

The calculated osmolarity is 308 mOsm/L.[3453]

Tonicity

The injection is an isotonic solution.[3453]

Sodium Content

The product provides 77 mEq of sodium per 500-mL container.[3453]

Trade Name(s)

Voluven

Administration

Hydroxyethyl starch 130/0.4 6% in sodium chloride 0.9% is administered only by intravenous infusion.[3453] Any remaining solution in partially used containers should be discarded.[3453] The dosage and rate of infusion should be individualized according to the patient's condition and response.[3453] The container is made of nondiethylhexyl phthalate (non-DEHP) plastic and is latex free.[3453] The container itself does not require a vented intravenous administration set, and the manufacturer states that administration of the drug should not be vented.[3453] The product should be inspected for discoloration and particulate matter prior to use.[3453] If the drug is administered by pressure infusion, air should be withdrawn or expelled from the container through the medication/administration port prior to infusion.[3453]

Stability

Hydroxyethyl starch 130/0.4 6% in sodium chloride 0.9% is a clear to slightly opalescent colorless to slightly yellow colloidal solution.[3453] The product should be stored at 15 to 25°C and should *not* be frozen.[3453] The bag of solution should not be removed from the overwrap until immediately prior to use.[3453] It should only be administered if the solution is clear and free from particles.[3453] The solution should be administered immediately after insertion of the administration set.[3453]

Compatibility Information

Y-Site Injection Compatibility (1:1 Mixture)

Hydroxyethyl starch 130/0.4 in sodium chloride 0.9%

Test Drug	Mfr	Conc	Mfr	Conc	Remarks	Ref	C/I
Ampicillin sodium	NOP	10, 25, 40 mg/mL[a]	FRK	6%	Visually compatible for 24 hr at room temperature	2770	C
Calcium chloride	HOS	20, 40, 80 mg/mL[a]	FRK	6%	Visually compatible for 24 hr at room temperature	2770	C
Calcium gluconate	PP	20, 30, 40 mg/mL[a]	FRK	6%	Visually compatible for 24 hr at room temperature	2770	C
Cefazolin sodium	NOP	20, 30, 40 mg/mL[a]	FRK	6%	Visually compatible for 24 hr at room temperature	2770	C
Ceftriaxone sodium	RC	20, 30, 40 mg/mL[a]	FRK	6%	Visually compatible for 24 hr at room temperature	2770	C
Ciprofloxacin	AB	0.5, 1, 2 mg/mL[a]	FRK	6%	Visually compatible for 24 hr at room temperature	2770	C
Clindamycin phosphate	SZ	6, 12, 24 mg/mL[a]	FRK	6%	Visually compatible for 24 hr at room temperature	2770	C
Dimenhydrinate	SZ	0.5, 0.75, 1 mg/mL[a]	FRK	6%	Visually compatible for 24 hr at room temperature	2770	C
Dobutamine HCl	SZ	1, 2, 4 mg/mL[a]	FRK	6%	Visually compatible for 24 hr at room temperature	2770	C
Dopamine HCl	BMS	0.8, 3.2, 6.4 mg/mL[a]	FRK	6%	Visually compatible for 24 hr at room temperature	2770	C
Epinephrine HCl	BIO	16, 24, 32 mcg/mL[a]	FRK	6%	Color change within 4 hr	2770	I
Esmolol HCl	BA	10 mg/mL[a]	FRK	6%	Visually compatible for 24 hr at room temperature	2770	C
Fentanyl citrate	SZ	20[a], 35[a], 50 mcg/mL	FRK	6%	Visually compatible for 24 hr at room temperature	2770	C

DOI: 10.37573/9781585286850.197

Y-Site Injection Compatibility (1:1 Mixture) (Cont.)

Test Drug	Mfr	Conc	Mfr	Conc	Remarks	Ref	C/I
Furosemide	SZ	1, 1.5, 2 mg/mL[a]	FRK	6%	Visually compatible for 24 hr at room temperature	2770	C
Gentamicin sulfate	SX	1, 3, 5 mg/mL[a]	FRK	6%	Visually compatible for 24 hr at room temperature	2770	C
Heparin sodium	HOS	10 units/mL	FRK	6%	Visually compatible for 24 hr at room temperature	2770	C
Heparin sodium	PP	1000, 10,000 units/mL	FRK	6%	Visually compatible for 24 hr at room temperature	2770	C
Hydromorphone HCl	SZ	0.4[a], 1.2[a], 2 mg/mL	FRK	6%	Visually compatible for 24 hr at room temperature	2770	C
Insulin, regular	NOV	5, 27.5, 50 units/mL[a]	FRK	6%	Visually compatible for 24 hr at room temperature	2770	C
Labetalol HCl	SZ	1.25[a], 2.5[a], 5 mg/mL	FRK	6%	Visually compatible for 24 hr at room temperature	2770	C
Levofloxacin	OMN	1, 2.5, 5 mg/mL[a]	FRK	6%	Visually compatible for 24 hr at room temperature	2770	C
Magnesium sulfate	SZ	125[a], 250[a], 500 mg/mL	FRK	6%	Visually compatible for 24 hr at room temperature	2770	C
Meperidine HCl	SZ	1, 5, 10 mg/mL[a]	FRK	6%	Visually compatible for 24 hr at room temperature	2770	C
Methylprednisolone sodium succinate	NOP	0.25[a], 5[a], 62.5 mg/mL	FRK	6%	Visually compatible for 24 hr at room temperature	2770	C
Metronidazole	HOS	1[a], 2.5[a], 5 mg/mL	FRK	6%	Visually compatible for 24 hr at room temperature	2770	C
Midazolam HCl	SZ	1, 1.5, 2 mg/mL[a]	FRK	6%	Visually compatible for 24 hr at room temperature	2770	C
Morphine sulfate	SZ	1, 5, 10 mg/mL[a]	FRK	6%	Visually compatible for 24 hr at room temperature	2770	C
Moxifloxacin HCl	BAY	0.4[a], 0.8[a], 1.6 mg/mL	FRK	6%	Visually compatible for 24 hr at room temperature	2770	C
Multivitamins	SX	2.5, 5, 10 mL/L[a]	FRK	6%	Visually compatible for 24 hr at room temperature	2770	C
Nitroglycerin	SZ	0.1, 0.25, 0.4 mg/mL[a]	FRK	6%	Visually compatible for 24 hr at room temperature	2770	C
Norepinephrine bitartrate	SZ	6, 8, 64 mcg/mL[a]	FRK	6%	Visually compatible for 24 hr at room temperature	2770	C
Octreotide acetate	NVA	5, 7.5, 10 mcg/mL[a]	FRK	6%	Visually compatible for 24 hr at room temperature	2770	C
Phenytoin sodium	SZ	6, 7.5, 9 mg/mL[a]	FRK	6%	White precipitate forms immediately	2770	I
Potassium chloride	HOS	0.02, 0.4, 0.8 mEq/mL[a]	FRK	6%	Visually compatible for 24 hr at room temperature	2770	C
Potassium phosphates	SX	0.003, 0.0765, 0.15 mmol/mL[a]	FRK	6%	Visually compatible for 24 hr at room temperature	2770	C
Propofol	NOP	2.5[a], 5[a], 10 mg/mL	FRK	6%	Visually compatible for 24 hr at room temperature	2770	C
Sodium bicarbonate	HOS	0.25[a], 0.5[a], 1 mmol/mL	FRK	6%	Visually compatible for 24 hr at room temperature	2770	C
Vasopressin	SZ	0.4, 0.7, 1 unit/mL[a]	FRK	6%	Visually compatible for 24 hr at room temperature	2770	C

[a] Tested in dextrose 5%.

Selected Revisions September 30, 2019. © Copyright, October 2010. American Society of Health-System Pharmacists, Inc.

Hydroxyzine Hydrochloride
AHFS 28:24.92

Products

Hydroxyzine hydrochloride is available as a 25-mg/mL solution in 1-mL vials and 10-mL multiple-dose vials. It also is available as a 50-mg/mL solution in 1- and 2-mL single-dose vials and 10-mL multiple-dose vials. Also present in the solutions are benzyl alcohol 0.9% and sodium hydroxide and/or hydrochloric acid to adjust the pH.[1(11/06) 4]

pH

From 3.5 to 6.[17]

Administration

Hydroxyzine hydrochloride may be administered undiluted by intramuscular injection only, preferably into the upper outer quadrant of the buttock or the midlateral thigh muscles in adults. In children, the midlateral muscles of the thigh are preferred.[1(11/06) 4]

Stability

Hydroxyzine should be stored at controlled room temperature and protected from freezing and excessive temperatures.[1(11/06) 4]

Compatibility Information

Additive Compatibility

Hydroxyzine HCl

Test Drug	Mfr	Conc/L or %	Mfr	Conc/L or %	Test Solution	Remarks	Ref	C/I
Aminophylline	SE	1 g	RR	250 mg	D5W	Physically incompatible	15	I
Chloramphenicol sodium succinate	PD	10 g	RR	250 mg	D5W	Physically incompatible	15	I
Cisplatin	BR	200 mg	LY	500 mg	NS[a]	Physically compatible for 48 hr	1190	C
Cyclophosphamide	AD	1 g	LY	500 mg	D5W[a]	Physically compatible for 48 hr	1190	C
Cytarabine	UP	1 g	LY	500 mg	D5W[a]	Physically compatible for 48 hr	1190	C
Dimenhydrinate	SE	500 mg	RR	250 mg	D5W	Physically compatible	15	C
Etoposide	BR	1 g	LY	500 mg	D5W[a]	Physically compatible for 48 hr	1190	C
Lidocaine HCl	AST	2 g	PF	100 mg		Physically compatible	24	C
Mesna	AW	3 g	LY	500 mg	D5W[a]	Physically compatible for 48 hr	1190	C
Methotrexate sodium	BV	1 and 3 g	LY	500 mg	D5W[a]	Physically compatible for 48 hr	1190	C
Nafcillin sodium	WY	500 mg	PF	100 mg		Physically compatible	27	C
Penicillin G potassium	SQ	20 million units	RR	250 mg	D5W	Physically incompatible	15	I
Penicillin G sodium	UP	20 million units	RR	250 mg	D5W	Physically incompatible	15	I
Pentobarbital sodium	AB	1 g	RR	250 mg	D5W	Physically incompatible	15	I
Phenobarbital sodium	WI	200 mg	RR	250 mg	D5W	Physically incompatible	15	I

[a] Tested in glass containers.

DOI: 10.37573/9781585286850.198

Drugs in Syringe Compatibility

Hydroxyzine HCl

Test Drug	Mfr	Amt	Mfr	Amt	Remarks	Ref	C/I
Atropine sulfate		0.4 mg/1 mL	PF	100 mg/2 mL	Physically compatible	771	C
Atropine sulfate		0.4 mg/1 mL	PF	50 mg/1 mL	Physically compatible	771	C
Atropine sulfate		0.6 mg/1.5 mL	PF	100 mg/4 mL	Physically compatible for at least 15 min	14	C
Atropine sulfate	USP	0.4 mg/0.4 mL	NF	50 mg/1 mL	Hydroxyzine stable for at least 10 days at 3 and 25°C	49	C
Atropine sulfate	ST	0.4 mg/1 mL	PF	50 mg/1 mL	Physically compatible for at least 15 min	326	C
Buprenorphine HCl					Physically and chemically compatible	4	C
Butorphanol tartrate	BR	2 mg/1 mL	PF	50 mg/1 mL	Physically compatible	771	C
Butorphanol tartrate	BR	1 mg/1 mL	PF	100 mg/2 mL	Physically compatible	771	C
Chlorpromazine HCl	PO	50 mg/2 mL	PF	50 mg/1 mL	Physically compatible for at least 15 min	326	C
Chlorpromazine HCl	STS	50 mg/2 mL	ES	100 mg/2 mL	Visually compatible for 60 min	1784	C
Dimenhydrinate	HR	50 mg/1 mL	PF	50 mg/1 mL	Physically incompatible within 15 min	326	I
Diphenhydramine HCl	PD	50 mg/1 mL	PF	50 mg/1 mL	Physically compatible for at least 15 min	326	C
Doxapram HCl	RB	400 mg/20 mL		25 mg/1 mL	Physically compatible with no doxapram loss in 24 hr	1177	C
Droperidol	MN	2.5 mg/1 mL	PF	50 mg/1 mL	Physically compatible for at least 15 min	326	C
Fentanyl citrate	MN	0.05 mg/1 mL	PF	50 mg/1 mL	Physically compatible for at least 15 min	326	C
Fentanyl citrate	CR	0.05 mg/1 mL	PF	50 mg/1 mL	Physically compatible	771	C
Fentanyl citrate	CR	0.05 mg/1 mL	PF	100 mg/2 mL	Physically compatible	771	C
Fluphenazine HCl	LY	5 mg/2 mL	ES	100 mg/2 mL	Visually compatible for 60 min	1784	C
Glycopyrrolate	RB	0.2 mg/1 mL	PF	25 mg/1 mL	Physically compatible. pH in glycopyrrolate stability range for 48 hr at 25°C	331	C
Glycopyrrolate	RB	0.2 mg/1 mL	PF	50 mg/2 mL	Physically compatible. pH in glycopyrrolate stability range for 48 hr at 25°C	331	C
Glycopyrrolate	RB	0.4 mg/2 mL	PF	25 mg/1 mL	Physically compatible. pH in glycopyrrolate stability range for 48 hr at 25°C	331	C
Haloperidol lactate	MN	10 mg/2 mL	ES	100 mg/2 mL	White precipitate forms within 5 min	1784	I
Hydromorphone HCl	KN	4 mg/2 mL	PF	50 mg/1 mL	Physically compatible for 30 min	517	C
Hydromorphone HCl	KN	0.75 mg/0.8 mL	PF	100 mg/2 mL	Physically compatible	771	C
Ketorolac tromethamine	SY	180 mg/6 mL	SO	150 mg/3 mL	Heavy white precipitate forms immediately, separating into two layers over time	1703	I
Lidocaine HCl	AST	2%/2 mL	PF	50 mg/2 mL	Physically compatible	771	C
Lidocaine HCl	AST	2%/2 mL	PF	100 mg/2 mL	Physically compatible	771	C
Meperidine HCl	WI	100 mg/2 mL	PF	50 mg/1 mL	Physically compatible	771	C
Meperidine HCl	WI	50 mg/1 mL	PF	100 mg/2 mL	Physically compatible	771	C
Meperidine HCl	WY	100 mg/1 mL	PF	100 mg/4 mL	Physically compatible for at least 15 min	14	C
Meperidine HCl	WI	50 mg/1 mL	PF	50 mg/1 mL	Physically compatible for at least 15 min	326	C
Methotrimeprazine HCl	LE	20 mg/1 mL	PF	50 mg/1 mL	Physically compatible	771	C

Drugs in Syringe Compatibility (Cont.)

Test Drug	Mfr	Amt	Mfr	Amt	Remarks	Ref	C/I
Methotrimeprazine HCl	LE	10 mg/0.5 mL	PF	100 mg/2 mL	Physically compatible	771	C
Metoclopramide HCl	NO	10 mg/2 mL	PF	50 mg/1 mL	Physically compatible for 15 min at room temperature	565	C
Midazolam HCl	RC	5 mg/1 mL	ES	100 mg/2 mL	Physically compatible for 4 hr at 25°C	1145	C
Morphine sulfate	WY	15 mg/1 mL	PF	100 mg/4 mL	Physically compatible for at least 15 min	14	C
Morphine sulfate	ST	15 mg/1 mL	PF	50 mg/1 mL	Physically compatible for at least 15 min	326	C
Morphine sulfate		10 mg/0.7 mL	PF	50 mg/1 mL	Physically compatible	771	C
Morphine sulfate		5 mg/0.3 mL	PF	100 mg/2 mL	Physically compatible	771	C
Nalbuphine HCl	EN	10 mg/1 mL	PF	50 mg	Physically compatible for 36 hr at 27°C	762	C
Nalbuphine HCl	EN	5 mg/0.5 mL	PF	50 mg	Physically compatible for 36 hr at 27°C	762	C
Nalbuphine HCl	EN	2.5 mg/0.25 mL	PF	50 mg	Physically compatible for 36 hr at 27°C	762	C
Nalbuphine HCl	DU	10 mg/1 mL	PF	25 mg/1 mL	Physically compatible for 48 hr	128	C
Nalbuphine HCl	DU	20 mg/1 mL	PF	25 mg/1 mL	Physically compatible for 48 hr	128	C
Pentazocine lactate	WI	60 mg/2 mL	PF	50 mg/1 mL	Physically compatible	771	C
Pentazocine lactate	WI	30 mg/1 mL	PF	100 mg/2 mL	Physically compatible	771	C
Pentazocine lactate	WI	30 mg/1 mL	PF	100 mg/4 mL	Physically compatible for at least 15 min	14	C
Pentazocine lactate	WI	30 mg/1 mL	PF	50 mg/1 mL	Physically compatible for at least 15 min	326	C
Pentobarbital sodium	WY	100 mg/2 mL	PF	100 mg/4 mL	Precipitate forms within 15 min	14	I
Pentobarbital sodium	AB	50 mg/1 mL	PF	50 mg/1 mL	Physically incompatible within 15 min	326	I
Prochlorperazine edisylate	PO	5 mg/1 mL	PF	50 mg/1 mL	Physically compatible for at least 15 min	326	C
Promethazine HCl	WY	50 mg/2 mL	PF	100 mg/4 mL	Physically compatible for at least 15 min	14	C
Promethazine HCl	PO	50 mg/2 mL	PF	50 mg/1 mL	Physically compatible for at least 15 min	326	C
Ranitidine HCl	GL	50 mg/2 mL	PF	50 mg/1 mL	Immediate white haze that disappears following vortex mixing	978	I
Scopolamine HBr		0.6 mg/1.5 mL	PF	100 mg/4 mL	Physically compatible for at least 15 min	14	C
Scopolamine HBr	ST	0.4 mg/1 mL	PF	50 mg/1 mL	Physically compatible for at least 15 min	326	C
Scopolamine HBr		0.65 mg/1 mL	PF	100 mg/2 mL	Physically compatible	771	C
Scopolamine HBr		0.65 mg/1 mL	PF	50 mg/1 mL	Physically compatible	771	C

Y-Site Injection Compatibility (1:1 Mixture)

Hydroxyzine HCl

Test Drug	Mfr	Conc	Mfr	Conc	Remarks	Ref	C/I
Acetaminophen	CAD	10 mg/mL	ABX	2 mg/mL[b]	Physically compatible with less than 10% acetaminophen loss over 4 hr at room temperature	2841, 2844	C
Allopurinol sodium	BW	3 mg/mL[b]	ES	4 mg/mL[b]	Immediate turbidity and precipitate	1686	I
Amifostine	USB	10 mg/mL[a]	WI	4 mg/mL[a]	Subvisible haze forms immediately	1845	I
Aztreonam	SQ	40 mg/mL[a]	WI	4 mg/mL[a]	Physically compatible for 4 hr at 23°C	1758	C

Y-Site Injection Compatibility (1:1 Mixture) (Cont.)

Test Drug	Mfr	Conc	Mfr	Conc	Remarks	Ref	C/I
Blinatumomab	AMG	0.125 mcg/mL[b]	REN	0.4 mg/mL[b]	Visually compatible for 12 hr at room temperature	3405, 3417	C
Blinatumomab	AMG	0.375 mcg/mL[b]	REN	0.4 mg/mL[b]	Persistent particulate formation when hydroxyzine is added to blinatumomab; not observed when order of mixing was reversed	3405, 3417	?
Ceftaroline fosamil	FOR	2.22 mg/mL[a b h]	ABX	2 mg/mL[a b h]	Physically compatible for 4 hr at 23°C	2826	C
Ciprofloxacin	MI	2 mg/mL[c]	ES	50 mg/mL	Visually compatible for 24 hr at 24°C	1655	C
Cisatracurium besylate	GW	0.1, 2, 5 mg/mL[a]	ES	2 mg/mL[a]	Physically compatible for 4 hr at 23°C	2074	C
Cladribine	ORT	0.015[b] and 0.5[d] mg/mL	ES	4 mg/mL[b]	Physically compatible for 4 hr at 23°C	1969	C
Defibrotide sodium	JAZ	8 mg/mL[b]	REN	0.79 mg/mL[b]	Visually compatible for 4 hr at room temperature	3149	C
Dexmedetomidine HCl	AB	4 mcg/mL[b]	ES	2 mg/mL[b]	Physically compatible for 4 hr at 23°C	2383	C
Docetaxel	RPR	0.9 mg/mL[a]	ES	2 mg/mL[a]	Physically compatible for 4 hr at 23°C	2224	C
Doxorubicin HCl liposomal	SEQ	0.4 mg/mL[a]	ES	2 mg/mL[a]	10-fold increase in particles ≥10 μm in 4 hr	2087	I
Etoposide phosphate	BR	5 mg/mL[a]	ES	4 mg/mL[a]	Physically compatible for 4 hr at 23°C	2218	C
Famotidine	ME	2 mg/mL[b]		4 mg/mL[b]	Visually compatible for 4 hr at 22°C	1936	C
Fenoldopam mesylate	AB	80 mcg/mL[b]	ES	2 mg/mL[b]	Physically compatible for 4 hr at 23°C	2467	C
Fentanyl citrate	JN	0.025 mg/mL[a]	WI	4 mg/mL[a]	Physically compatible for 48 hr at 22°C	1706	C
Filgrastim	AMG	30 mcg/mL[a]	ES	4 mg/mL[a]	Physically compatible for 4 hr at 22°C	1687	C
Fluconazole	RR	2 mg/mL	ES	50 mg/mL	Cloudiness develops	1407	I
Fludarabine phosphate	BX	1 mg/mL[a]	WI	4 mg/mL[a]	Slight haze forms immediately	1439	I
Foscarnet sodium	AST	24 mg/mL	LY	50 mg/mL	Physically compatible for 24 hr at room temperature under fluorescent light	1335	C
Gemcitabine HCl	LI	10 mg/mL[b]	ES	2 mg/mL[b]	Physically compatible for 4 hr at 23°C	2226	C
Granisetron HCl	SKB	0.05 mg/mL[a]	ES	2 mg/mL[a]	Physically compatible for 4 hr at 23°C	2000	C
Hetastarch in lactated electrolyte	AB	6%	ES	2 mg/mL[a]	Physically compatible for 4 hr at 23°C	2339	C
Hydromorphone HCl	AST	0.5 mg/mL[a]	WI	4 mg/mL[a]	Physically compatible for 48 hr at 22°C	1706	C
Linezolid	PHU	2 mg/mL	ES	2 mg/mL[a]	Physically compatible for 4 hr at 23°C	2264	C
Melphalan HCl	BW	0.1 mg/mL[b]	WI	4 mg/mL[b]	Physically compatible for 3 hr at 22°C	1557	C
Meropenem		50 mg/mL	SZ	50 mg/mL	Precipitates immediately	3538	I
Methadone HCl	LI	1 mg/mL[a]	WI	4 mg/mL[a]	Physically compatible for 48 hr at 22°C	1706	C
Morphine sulfate	AST	1 mg/mL[a]	WI	4 mg/mL[a]	Physically compatible for 48 hr at 22°C	1706	C
Ondansetron HCl	GL	1 mg/mL[b]	WI	4 mg/mL[a]	Visually compatible for 4 hr at 22°C	1365	C
Oxaliplatin	SS	0.5 mg/mL[a]	ES	2 mg/mL[a]	Physically compatible for 4 hr at 23°C	2566	C
Paclitaxel	NCI	1.2 mg/mL[a]	ES	4 mg/mL[a]	Normal inherent haze from paclitaxel decreases immediately	1556	I
Pemetrexed disodium	LI	20 mg/mL[b]	APP	2 mg/mL[a]	Physically compatible for 4 hr at 23°C	2564	C

Y-Site Injection Compatibility (1:1 Mixture) (Cont.)

Test Drug	Mfr	Conc	Mfr	Conc	Remarks	Ref	C/I
Piperacillin sodium–tazobactam sodium	LE[g]	40 mg/mL[a i]	WI	4 mg/mL[a]	Haze and particles form immediately	1688	I
Propofol	ZEN[j]	10 mg/mL	ES	2 mg/mL[a]	Physically compatible for 1 hr at 23°C	2066	C
Remifentanil HCl	GW	0.025 and 0.25 mg/mL[b]	ES	2 mg/mL[a]	Physically compatible for 4 hr at 23°C	2075	C
Sargramostim	IMM	10 mcg/mL[b]	ES	4 mg/mL[b]	Slight haze and particles form in 4 hr	1436	I
Teniposide	BR	0.1 mg/mL[a]	WI	4 mg/mL[a]	Physically compatible for 4 hr at 23°C	1725	C
Thiotepa	IMM[e]	1 mg/mL[a]	ES	4 mg/mL[a]	Physically compatible for 4 hr at 23°C	1861	C
TNA #218 to #226[f]			ES	2 mg/mL[a]	Visually compatible for 4 hr at 23°C	2215	C
TPN #212 to #215[f]			ES	2 mg/mL[a]	Physically compatible for 4 hr at 23°C	2109	C
Vinorelbine tartrate	BW	1 mg/mL[b]	ES	4 mg/mL[b]	Physically compatible for 4 hr at 22°C	1558	C

[a] Tested in dextrose 5%.

[b] Tested in sodium chloride 0.9%.

[c] Tested in both dextrose 5% and sodium chloride 0.9%.

[d] Tested in bacteriostatic sodium chloride 0.9% preserved with benzyl alcohol 0.9%.

[e] Lyophilized formulation tested.

[f] Refer to Appendix for the composition of parenteral nutrition solutions. TNA indicates a 3-in-1 admixture, and TPN indicates a 2-in-1 admixture.

[g] Test performed using the formulation WITHOUT edetate disodium.

[h] Tested in Ringer's injection, lactated.

[i] Piperacillin component. Piperacillin in an 8:1 fixed-ratio concentration with tazobactam.

[j] Test performed using the formulation WITH edetate disodium.

Additional Compatibility Information

Chlorpromazine and Meperidine

Chlorpromazine hydrochloride (Elkins-Sinn) 6.25 mg/mL, hydroxyzine hydrochloride (Pfizer) 12.5 mg/mL, and meperidine hydrochloride (Winthrop) 25 mg/mL, in both glass and plastic syringes, were reported to be physically compatible and chemically stable for at least 1 year at 4 and 25°C when protected from light.[989]

Selected Revisions May 1, 2020. © Copyright, October 1982. American Society of Health-System Pharmacists, Inc.

Ibandronate Sodium
AHFS 92:24

Products

Ibandronate sodium is available as a ready-to-use solution in 3-mL prefilled single-use glass syringes (as a kit with a needle and tubing) and vials containing the equivalent of 3 mg of ibandronate as the free acid.[3136][3137] Sodium chloride, sodium acetate, glacial acetic acid, and water for injection also are present in each syringe or vial.[3136][3137]

Equivalency

Ibandronate sodium 3.375 mg as the monohydrate is equivalent to 3 mg of ibandronate as the free acid.[3136][3137]

Trade Name(s)

Boniva

Administration

Ibandronate sodium is administered intravenously over a period of 15 to 30 seconds.[3136][3137] Ibandronate sodium should *not* be administered by any other route of administration; care must be taken to avoid intra-arterial or paravenous administration because such administration may result in tissue damage.[3136][3137] Contents of prefilled syringes should be administered only using the 25-gauge needle provided in the prefilled syringe kit.[3136]

Stability

Ibandronate sodium is a clear, colorless solution.[3136][3137] Intact prefilled syringes and vials should be stored at controlled room temperature.[3136][3137]

Ibandronate sodium solution should be visually inspected for particulate matter or discoloration prior to administration; if particulate matter is present or discoloration occurs, the solution should not be used.[3136][3137] Any unused portion of the solution should be discarded.[3136][3137]

Compatibility Information

Solution Compatibility

Ibandronate sodium

Test Soln Name	Mfr	Mfr	Conc/L or %	Remarks	Ref	C/I
Dextrose 5% in Ringer's injection	GEN, HER			Must not be mixed with calcium-containing solutions	3136, 3137	I
Dextrose 5% in Ringer's injection, lactated	GEN, HER			Must not be mixed with calcium-containing solutions	3136, 3137	I
Ringer's injection	GEN, HER			Must not be mixed with calcium-containing solutions	3136, 3137	I
Ringer's injection, lactated	GEN, HER			Must not be mixed with calcium-containing solutions	3136, 3137	I

DOI: 10.37573/9781585286850.199

Ibuprofen
AHFS 28:08.04.92

Products

Ibuprofen is available as a 100-mg/mL concentrate for injection in single-dose vials containing 800 mg of the drug.[3534] Each mL of the concentrate for injection also contains 78 mg of arginine in water for injection.[3534] **CAUTION: Care should be taken to ensure that the correct drug product, dose, and administration procedures are used and that no confusion with other products (e.g., ibuprofen lysinate [NeoProfen]) occurs.**

The concentrate for injection must be diluted in a compatible diluent prior to administration.[3534] The concentrate for injection should be diluted to a final concentration of 4 mg/mL or less in sodium chloride 0.9%, dextrose 5%, or Ringer's injection, lactated.[3534] For fixed doses of 100, 200, and 400 mg, the manufacturer recommends dilution in at least 100 mL; for fixed doses of 800 mg, the manufacturer recommends dilution in at least 200 mL.[3534] For patients requiring weight-based dosing (e.g., some pediatric patients), the drug should be diluted to a concentration of 4 mg/mL or less.[3534]

Ibuprofen also is available as 4-mg/mL iso-osmotic, ready-to-use solution for infusion in single-dose flexible polypropylene bags containing 800 mg of the drug.[3534] The solution also contains sodium phosphate, sodium hydroxide, and sodium chloride in water for injection.[3534] The ready-to-use solution for infusion is for use only in those for whom ibuprofen doses of 800 mg are intended.[3534]

pH

The pH of both the concentrate for injection and the ready-to-use 4-mg/mL solution for infusion is approximately 7.4.[3534]

Trade Name(s)

Caldolor

Administration

Ibuprofen injection is intended only for intravenous administration.[3534] Solutions of ibuprofen at concentrations of 4 mg/mL or less are administered by intravenous infusion over at least 30 minutes in adults and over at least 10 minutes in pediatric patients.[3534]

Stability

Both the concentrate for injection and the ready-to-use solution for infusion are clear and colorless.[3534] Intact vials and bags should be stored at controlled room temperature.[3534] Unused portions should be discarded.[3534]

Compatibility Information

Solution Compatibility

Ibuprofen

Test Soln Name	Mfr	Mfr	Conc/L or %	Remarks	Ref	C/I
Dextrose 5%		CMB		Stable for up to 24 hr at approximately 20 to 25°C	3534	C
Ringer's injection, lactated		CMB		Stable for up to 24 hr at approximately 20 to 25°C	3534	C
Sodium chloride 0.9%		CMB		Stable for up to 24 hr at approximately 20 to 25°C	3534	C

Y-Site Injection Compatibility (1:1 Mixture)

Ibuprofen

Test Drug	Mfr	Conc	Mfr	Conc	Remarks	Ref	C/I
Esmolol HCl	MYL	10 mg/mL	CMB	4 mg/mL	White cloudy solution forms upon mixing	3533	I
Labetalol HCl	HOS	5 mg/mL	CMB	4 mg/mL	White cloudy solution forms upon mixing	3533	I
Metoprolol tartrate	HOS	0.4 mg/mL[a]	CMB	4 mg/mL	Physically compatible for 1 hr at 23°C	3533	C

[a] Tested in sodium chloride 0.9%.

DOI: 10.37573/9781585286850.200

Ibuprofen Lysinate
AHFS 28:08.04.92

Products

Ibuprofen lysinate is available as a preservative-free solution containing in each mL the L-lysine salt of (±) ibuprofen 17.1 mg (equivalent to ibuprofen 10 mg) with sodium hydroxide or hydrochloric acid to adjust pH during manufacturing in water for injection.[3540] The injection is packaged in single-use 2-mL vials.[3540] **CAUTION: Care should be taken to ensure that the correct drug product, dose, and administration procedures are used and that no confusion with other products (e.g., ibuprofen [Caldolor]) occurs.**

pH

The pH of the solution is adjusted to 7.[3540]

Trade Name(s)

NeoProfen

Administration

Ibuprofen lysinate is administered intravenously using the intravenous port that is nearest the insertion site following dilution of the drug to a suitable volume with dextrose or saline infusion solution.[3540] The drug should be prepared and administered within 30 minutes of preparation by intravenous infusion over 15 minutes taking care to avoid extravasation.[3540]

The manufacturer states that administration of the drug using an umbilical arterial line has not been evaluated.[3540]

Stability

Intact vials of ibuprofen lysinate should be stored at controlled room temperature protected from light.[3540] The manufacturer recommends retaining the vials in their carton until use.[3540]

After dilution to an appropriate volume with dextrose or saline intravenous infusion solution, ibuprofen lysinate should be administered within 30 minutes over a period of 15 minutes.[3540] Any remaining solution in the single-use vials should be discarded because no antimicrobial preservative is present.[3540] The manufacturer recommends not administering ibuprofen lysinate into a line running a total parenteral nutrition (TPN) admixture; the TPN should be interrupted if necessary for 15 minutes both before and after administering ibuprofen lysinate maintaining line patency using dextrose or saline infusion solution.[3540]

Compatibility Information

Solution Compatibility

Ibuprofen lysinate

Test Soln Name	Mfr	Mfr	Conc/L or %	Remarks	Ref	C/I
Dextrose 5%			1 and 4 g	6 to 7% loss occurred in 15 days at 25°C	2610	C
Sodium chloride 0.9%			1 and 4 g	4 to 7% loss occurred in 15 days at 25°C	2610	C

Y-Site Injection Compatibility (1:1 Mixture)

Ibuprofen lysinate

Test Drug	Mfr	Conc	Mfr	Conc	Remarks	Ref	C/I
Amikacin sulfate	HOS	50 mg/mL[a]	OVA	10 mg/mL	Measured turbidity increased immediately and solution became milky white and opaque	3541	I
Amikacin sulfate	HOS	50 mg/mL[b]	OVA	10 mg/mL	Measured turbidity increased immediately and solution became milky white and opaque with particulate matter present	3541	I
Amikacin sulfate	HOS	250 mg/mL	OVA	10 mg/mL	Measured turbidity increased immediately and solution became milky white and opaque with particulate matter present	3541	I
Amino acids	BRN	10%	OVA	10 mg/mL	Measured turbidity increased immediately and solution developed a cloudy haze	3541	I

DOI: 10.37573/9781585286850.201

Y-Site Injection Compatibility (1:1 Mixture) (Cont.)

Test Drug	Mfr	Conc.	Mfr	Conc	Remarks	Ref	C/I
Caffeine citrate	MJ	20 mg/mL	OVA	10 mg/mL	Measured turbidity increased immediately and solution became milky white and opaque with a white precipitate	3541	I
Ceftazidime	GSK	200 mg/mL[c]	OVA	10 mg/mL	Slight turbidity increase	3541	I
Dobutamine HCl	HOS	1 mg/mL[e]	OVA	10 mg/mL	Measured turbidity increased immediately and solution became hazy white with a white precipitate	3541	I
Dopamine HCl	HOS	3.2 mg/mL[e]	OVA	10 mg/mL	Precipitate formed within 4 hr	3541	I
Epinephrine[g]	AMR	8, 64, and 100 mcg/mL[a]	OVA	10 mg/mL	Physically compatible for 4 hr at room temperature	3541	C
Fat emulsion, intravenous	BA	10%	OVA	10 mg/mL	Could not be evaluated because of initial milky white opaque appearance and high turbidity	3541	?
Fat emulsion, intravenous		20%		1.25, 2.5, 5 mg/mL[b]	Physically compatible	3546	C
Furosemide	HOS	10 mg/mL	OVA	10 mg/mL	Physically compatible for 4 hr at room temperature	3541	C
Heparin sodium	HOS	10 units/mL[a]	OVA	10 mg/mL	Physically compatible for 4 hr at room temperature	3541	C
Heparin sodium	HOS	10 and 100 units/mL	OVA	10 mg/mL	Physically compatible for 4 hr at room temperature	3541	C
Insulin, regular	LI	0.1 and 1 unit/mL[b]	OVA	10 mg/mL	Physically compatible for 4 hr at room temperature	3541	C
Isoproterenol HCl	HOS	0.2 mg/mL	OVA	10 mg/mL	Measured turbidity increased immediately and solution became milky white	3541	I
Midazolam HCl	HOS	1 mg/mL[c]	OVA	10 mg/mL	Measured turbidity increased immediately and solution became milky white and opaque	3541	I
Midazolam HCl	HOS	5 mg/mL	OVA	10 mg/mL	Measured turbidity increased immediately and solution became milky white and opaque	3541	I
Morphine sulfate	HOS	0.5 mg/mL[c]	OVA	10 mg/mL	Physically compatible for 4 hr at room temperature	3541	C
Morphine sulfate	HOS	50 mg/mL	OVA	10 mg/mL	Measured turbidity increased immediately and solution became milky white and opaque	3541	I
Phenobarbital sodium	BA	30 mg/mL[c]	OVA	10 mg/mL	Physically compatible for 4 hr at room temperature	3541	C
Phenobarbital sodium	BA	130 mg/mL	OVA	10 mg/mL	Physically compatible for 4 hr at room temperature	3541	C
Potassium chloride	HOS	2 mEq/mL	OVA	10 mg/mL	Physically compatible for 4 hr at room temperature	3541	C
Sodium bicarbonate	HOS	1 mEq/mL	OVA	10 mg/mL	Physically compatible for 4 hr at room temperature	3541	C
TPN #281, #282, #283[f]				1.25 mg/mL[b]	Physically compatible for 4 hr at room temperature	3546	C
TPN #281[f]				2.5 mg/mL[b]	Slightly cloudy, opaque solution formed	3546	I
TPN #282, #283[f]				2.5 mg/mL[b]	Physically compatible for 4 hr at room temperature	3546	C

Y-Site Injection Compatibility (1:1 Mixture) (Cont.)

Test Drug	Mfr	Conc	Mfr	Conc	Remarks	Ref	C/I
TPN #281, #282, #283[f]				5 mg/mL[b]	Cloudy, opaque solution formed with sediment detected after 24 hr	3546	I
Vancomycin HCl	HOS	50 mg/mL[d]	OVA	10 mg/mL	Measured turbidity increased immediately and solution became milky white and opaque	3541	I
Vecuronium bromide	HOS	1 and 2 mg/mL[c]	OVA	10 mg/mL	Measured turbidity increased immediately and solution became milky white and opaque	3541	I

[a] Tested in dextrose 5%.

[b] Tested in sodium chloride 0.9%.

[c] Tested in both dextrose 5% and sodium chloride 0.9%.

[d] Tested in sterile water for injection.

[e] Tested as the premixed infusion solution.

[f] Refer to Appendix for the composition of parenteral nutrition solutions. TNA indicates a 3-in-1 admixture, and TPN indicateds a 2-in-1 admixture.

[g] Salt not specified.

Selected Revisions May 1, 2020. © Copyright, October 2010.
American Society of Health-System Pharmacists, Inc.

Ibutilide Fumarate
AHFS 24:04.04.20

Products

Ibutilide fumarate is available in single-use 10-mL vials containing 1 mg of the drug.[3193] Each mL of solution contains 0.1 mg of ibutilide fumarate and also contains sodium acetate trihydrate 0.189 mg, sodium chloride 8.9 mg, and sodium hydroxide and/or hydrochloric acid to adjust the pH in water for injection.[3193]

Equivalency

Ibutilide fumarate 0.1 mg is equivalent to 0.087 mg of ibutilide as the free base.[3193]

pH

The pH of the 0.1-mg/mL solution has been adjusted to approximately 4.6.[3193]

Tonicity

Ibutilide fumarate injection is isotonic.[3193]

Trade Name(s)

Corvert

Administration

Ibutilide fumarate is administered intravenously as an infusion over 10 minutes.[3193] The drug may be administered undiluted or diluted in 50 mL of dextrose 5% or sodium chloride 0.9%.[3193]

Stability

Ibutilide fumarate injection is a clear, colorless solution.[3193] Intact vials should be stored at controlled room temperature and kept in the carton until use.[3193]

Compatibility Information

Solution Compatibility

Ibutilide fumarate

Test Soln Name	Mfr	Mfr	Conc/L or %	Remarks	Ref	C/I
Dextrose 5%	a	PHU	17 mg	Physically compatible and chemically stable for 24 hr at 15 to 30°C or 48 hr at 2 to 8°C	3193	C
Sodium chloride 0.9%	a	PHU	17 mg	Physically compatible and chemically stable for 24 hr at 15 to 30°C or 48 hr at 2 to 8°C	3193	C

[a] Tested in PVC and polyolefin containers.

Y-Site Injection Compatibility (1:1 Mixture)

Ibutilide fumarate

Test Drug	Mfr	Conc	Mfr	Conc	Remarks	Ref	C/I
Argatroban	SZ	1 mg/mL	PF	0.017 mg/mL[a]	Increased turbidity and pH changes occur within 8 and 5 hr, respectively	3192, 3266	I

[a] Tested in dextrose 5%.

© Copyright, June 2017. American Society of Health-System Pharmacists, Inc.

DOI: 10.37573/9781585286850.202

Idarubicin Hydrochloride
AHFS 10:00

Products

Idarubicin hydrochloride is available as a 1-mg/mL red-orange preservative-free solution in single-use vials containing 5, 10, and 20 mL.[2964][2965] In addition to the drug, each mL also contains glycerin 25 mg in water for injection;[2964][2965] hydrochloric acid[2964] or hydrochloric acid and/or sodium hydroxide[2965] is used to adjust pH.[2964][2965]

pH

The pH of idarubicin hydrochloride has been adjusted to a target of 3.5.[2964][2965]

Tonicity

Idarubicin hydrochloride injection is isotonic.[2964][2965]

Trade Name(s)

Idamycin PFS

Administration

Idarubicin hydrochloride should be administered by slow intravenous injection over 10 to 15 minutes into the tubing of a running infusion of sodium chloride 0.9% or dextrose 5%.[2964][2965] The manufacturer recommends that the tubing be attached to a butterfly needle or other suitable device, inserted preferably into a large vein.[2964][2965] The drug should not be given subcutaneously or intramuscularly, and extravasation should be avoided to prevent severe tissue necrosis.[2964][2965] Care should be exercised during dose preparation to avoid inadvertent skin contact with the drug.[2964][2965]

Stability

Idarubicin hydrochloride in intact vials should be stored under refrigeration at 2 to 8°C and protected from light.[2964][2965] Leaving the vials in the carton until the time of use is recommended.[2964][2965]

Idarubicin hydrochloride (Farmitalia) 0.07 mg/mL diluted in sodium chloride 0.9% and stored at 22°C did not exhibit an antimicrobial effect on the growth of 4 organisms (*Enterococcus faecium, Staphylococcus aureus, Pseudomonas aeruginosa,* and *Candida albicans*) inoculated into the solution. Viability was maintained for periods of 48 to 120 hours. The author recommended that diluted solutions of idarubicin hydrochloride be stored under refrigeration whenever possible and that the potential for microbiological growth be considered when assigning expiration periods.[2160]

pH Effects

Idarubicin hydrochloride in prolonged contact with alkaline solutions will undergo decomposition.[1368][2964][2965]

Light Effects

Dilute solutions (0.01 mg/mL) of idarubicin hydrochloride are light sensitive, undergoing some degradation with exposure to light over periods greater than 6 hours.[1368] However, the manufacturers suggest that no special precautions are necessary to protect freshly prepared solutions for administration.[1369]

Sorption

Idarubicin hydrochloride is compatible with PVC, glass, and polypropylene.[1369]

Compatibility Information
Solution Compatibility

Idarubicin HCl

Test Soln Name	Mfr	Mfr	Conc/L or %	Remarks	Ref	C/I
Dextrose 5% in sodium chloride 0.9%		FA	10 mg	No loss in 72 hr at room temperature protected from light. Less than 10% loss in 6 hr at room temperature exposed to light	1493	C
Dextrose 5%		FA	100 mg	Up to 5% loss in 4 weeks at 25°C in the dark	1007	C
Dextrose 5%		FA	10 mg	No loss in 72 hr at room temperature protected from light. Less than 10% loss in 6 hr at room temperature exposed to light	1493	C
Ringer's injection, lactated		FA	100 mg	Up to 5% loss in 4 weeks at 25°C in the dark	1007	C
Sodium chloride 0.9%		FA	100 mg	Up to 5% loss in 4 weeks at 25°C in the dark	1007	C
Sodium chloride 0.9%		FA	10 mg	No loss in 72 hr at room temperature protected from light. Less than 10% loss in 6 hr at room temperature exposed to light	1493	C

DOI: 10.37573/9781585286850.203

Y-Site Injection Compatibility (1:1 Mixture)

Idarubicin HCl

Test Drug	Mfr	Conc	Mfr	Conc	Remarks	Ref	C/I
Acyclovir sodium	BW	5 mg/mL[b]	AD	1 mg/mL[b]	Haze forms and color changes immediately. Precipitate forms in 12 min	1525	I
Allopurinol sodium	BW	3 mg/mL[b]	AD	0.5 mg/mL[b]	Immediate reddish-purple color. Particles in 1 hr. Total color loss in 24 hr	1686	I
Amifostine	USB	10 mg/mL[a]	AD	0.5 mg/mL[a]	Physically compatible for 4 hr at 23°C	1845	C
Amikacin sulfate	BR	5 mg/mL[a]	AD	1 mg/mL[b]	Visually compatible for 24 hr at 25°C	1525	C
Ampicillin sodium–sulbactam sodium	RR	20 mg/mL[b,g]	AD	1 mg/mL[b]	Haze forms and color changes immediately. Precipitate forms in 20 min	1525	I
Aztreonam	SQ	40 mg/mL[a]	AD	0.5 mg/mL[a]	Physically compatible for 4 hr at 23°C	1758	C
Cefazolin sodium	LI	20 mg/mL[a]	AD	1 mg/mL[b]	Precipitate forms in 1 hr	1525	I
Ceftazidime	LI	20 mg/mL[a]	AD	1 mg/mL[b]	Haze forms in 1 hr	1525	I
Cladribine	ORT	0.015[b] and 0.5[c] mg/mL	AD	0.5 mg/mL[b]	Physically compatible for 4 hr at 23°C	1969	C
Clindamycin phosphate	AST	12 mg/mL[a]	AD	1 mg/mL[b]	Haze and precipitate form immediately	1525	I
Cyclophosphamide	AD	4 mg/mL[a]	AD	1 mg/mL[b]	Visually compatible for 24 hr at 25°C	1525	C
Cytarabine	CET	6 mg/mL[a]	AD	1 mg/mL[b]	Visually compatible for 24 hr at 25°C	1525	C
Dexamethasone sodium phosphate	OR	10 mg/mL	AD	1 mg/mL[b]	Haze forms immediately and precipitate forms in 20 min	1525	I
Dexamethasone sodium phosphate	AMR	0.2 mg/mL[b]	AD	1 mg/mL[b]	Haze forms in 20 min	1525	I
Diphenhydramine HCl	ES	1[a] and 50 mg/mL	AD	1 mg/mL[b]	Visually compatible for 24 hr at 25°C	1525	C
Droperidol	AMR	0.04[a] and 2.5 mg/mL	AD	1 mg/mL[b]	Visually compatible for 24 hr at 25°C	1525	C
Erythromycin lactobionate	ES	2 mg/mL[b]	AD	1 mg/mL[b]	Visually compatible for 24 hr at 25°C	1525	C
Etoposide	BR	0.4 mg/mL[a]	AD	1 mg/mL[b]	Gas forms immediately	1525	I
Etoposide phosphate	BR	5 mg/mL[a]	AD	0.5 mg/mL[a]	Physically compatible for 4 hr at 23°C	2218	C
Filgrastim	AMG	30 mcg/mL[a]	AD	0.5 mg/mL[a]	Physically compatible for 4 hr at 22°C	1687	C
Furosemide	AB	10 mg/mL	AD	1 mg/mL[b]	Precipitate forms immediately	1525	I
Furosemide	AB	0.8 mg/mL[b]	AD	1 mg/mL[b]	Haze forms immediately	1525	I
Gemcitabine HCl	LI	10 mg/mL[b]	AD	0.5 mg/mL[b]	Physically compatible for 4 hr at 23°C	2226	C
Granisetron HCl	SKB	0.05 mg/mL[a]	AD	0.5 mg/mL[a]	Physically compatible for 4 hr at 23°C	2000	C
Heparin sodium	ES, SO	100 and 1000 units/mL	AD	1 mg/mL[b]	Haze forms immediately and precipitate forms in 12 to 20 min	1525	I
Hydrocortisone sodium succinate	UP	2[a] and 50 mg/mL	AD	1 mg/mL[b]	Haze forms immediately and precipitate forms in 20 min	1525	I
Imipenem–cilastatin sodium	MSD	5 mg/mL[b,i]	AD	1 mg/mL[b]	Visually compatible for 12 hr at 25°C in light. Precipitate in 24 hr	1525	C
Lorazepam	WY	2 mg/mL	AD	1 mg/mL[b]	Color changes immediately	1525	I

Y-Site Injection Compatibility (1:1 Mixture) (Cont.)

Test Drug	Mfr	Conc	Mfr	Conc	Remarks	Ref	C/I
Magnesium sulfate	SO	2 mg/mL[b]	AD	1 mg/mL[b]	Visually compatible for 24 hr at 25°C	1525	C
Mannitol	AB	12.5 mg/mL[a]	AD	1 mg/mL[b]	Visually compatible for 24 hr at 25°C	1525	C
Melphalan HCl	BW	0.1 mg/mL[b]	AD	0.5 mg/mL[b]	Physically compatible for 3 hr at 22°C	1557, 1675	C
Meperidine HCl	WY	1[a] and 50 mg/mL	AD	1 mg/mL[b]	Color changes immediately	1525	I
Methotrexate sodium	LE	25 mg/mL	AD	1 mg/mL[b]	Color changes immediately	1525	I
Metoclopramide HCl	SO	5 mg/mL	AD	1 mg/mL[b]	Visually compatible for 24 hr at 25°C	1525	C
Piperacillin sodium–tazobactam sodium	LE[f]	40 mg/mL[a h]	AD	0.5 mg/mL[a]	Immediate increase in haze	1688	I
Potassium chloride	AB	0.03 mEq/mL[b]	AD	1 mg/mL[b]	Visually compatible for 24 hr at 25°C	1525	C
Ranitidine HCl	GL	1 mg/mL[a]	AD	1 mg/mL[b]	Visually compatible for 24 hr at 25°C	1525	C
Sargramostim	IMM	10 mcg/mL[b]	AD	0.5 mg/mL[b]	Physically compatible	1675	C
Sodium bicarbonate	AB	0.09 mEq/mL[a]	AD	1 mg/mL[b]	Haze forms and color changes immediately. Precipitate forms in 20 min	1525	I
Teniposide	BR	0.1 mg/mL[a]	AD	0.5 mg/mL[a]	Unacceptable increase in turbidity	1725	I
Thiotepa	IMM[d]	1 mg/mL[a]	AD	0.5 mg/mL[a]	Physically compatible for 4 hr at 23°C	1861	C
TPN #140[e]			AD	1 mg/mL[b]	Visually compatible for 24 hr at 25°C	1525	C
Vancomycin HCl	AD	4 mg/mL[a]	AD	1 mg/mL[b]	Color changes immediately	1525	I
Vincristine sulfate	AD	1 mg/mL	AD	1 mg/mL[b]	Color changes immediately	1525	I
Vinorelbine tartrate	BW	1 mg/mL[b]	AD	0.5 mg/mL[b]	Physically compatible for 4 hr at 22°C	1558, 1675	C

[a] Tested in dextrose 5%.

[b] Tested in sodium chloride 0.9%.

[c] Tested in bacteriostatic sodium chloride 0.9% preserved with benzyl alcohol 0.9%.

[d] Lyophilized formulation tested.

[e] Refer to Appendix for the composition of parenteral nutrition solutions. TPN indicates a 2-in-1 admixture.

[f] Test performed using the formulation WITHOUT edetate disodium.

[g] Ampicillin component. Ampicillin in a 2:1 fixed-ratio concentration with sulbactam.

[h] Piperacillin component. Piperacillin in an 8:1 fixed-ratio concentration with tazobactam.

[i] Not specified whether concentration refers to single component or combined components.

Selected Revisions July 13, 2015. © Copyright, October 1992.
American Society of Health-System Pharmacists, Inc.

Idarucizumab
AHFS 20:28.92

Products

Idarucizumab is available as a preservative-free solution in single-use vials in packs containing 2 vials.[3094] Each 50-mL vial contains idarucizumab 2.5 g, glacial acetic acid 10.05 mg, poly-sorbate 20 10 mg, sodium acetate trihydrate 147.35 mg, sorbitol 2004.2 mg, and water for injection.[3094]

Idarucizumab should be visually inspected for particulate matter or discoloration prior to administration.[3094]

pH

From 5.3 to 5.7.[3094]

Osmolality

Idarucizumab is isotonic with an osmolality of 270 to 330 mOsm/kg.[3094]

Trade Name(s)

Praxbind

Administration

Idarucizumab should be administered intravenously by infusion or by bolus injection.[3094] For intravenous infusion, each 2.5-g vial should be infused consecutively to total 5 g.[3094] The drug also has been administered as a single infusion of 5 g over 5 minutes in some clinical studies.[3094]

For intravenous bolus injection, a syringe should be used to withdraw and consecutively inject the contents of 2 vials.[3094]

If an existing intravenous line is used for idarucizumab administration, the line must be flushed with sodium chloride 0.9% prior to administration.[3094]

Stability

Intact vials should be stored at 2 to 8°C.[3094] Idarucizumab is a colorless to slightly yellow, clear to slightly opalescent solution.[3094] Vials should not be frozen or shaken.[3094]

Unopened vials of idarucizumab may be stored at 25°C for up to 48 hours when stored in the original package to protect from light or for up to 6 hours when exposed to light.[3094]

Administration of idarucizumab should begin promptly (within 1 hour) once the solution has been withdrawn from the vial.[3094]

DOI: 10.37573/9781585286850.204

Ifosfamide
AHFS 10:00

Products

Ifosfamide is available in vials containing 1 or 3 g of drug. Reconstitute the ifosfamide with 20 or 60 mL of sterile water for injection or bacteriostatic water for injection (parabens or benzyl alcohol), respectively, to yield a 50-mg/mL solution.[1(7/07)]

pH

Approximately 6.[72]

Trade Name(s)

Ifex

Administration

Ifosfamide is administered by slow intravenous infusion over a minimum of 30 minutes diluted to a concentration between 0.6 and 20 mg/mL.[1(7/07)] [4] Ifosfamide also has been administered by continuous intravenous infusion.[4] To prevent bladder toxicity, mesna and at least 2 L/day of fluid should be given.[1(7/07)] [4]

Stability

Intact vials of ifosfamide should be stored at controlled room temperature and protected from temperatures above 30°C.[1(7/07)] Ifosfamide may liquify at temperatures above 35°C.[72]

The reconstituted solution is stated to be chemically and physically stable for 7 days at 30°C and for up to 6 weeks under refrigeration.[4][72] Because of microbiological concerns, the manufacturer recommends storage under refrigeration and use in 24 hours for reconstituted or diluted ifosfamide solutions.[1(7/07)]

Ifosfamide (Boehringer-Ingelheim) 80 mg/mL in sodium chloride 0.9% exhibited about 7% loss in 9 days at 37°C in the dark.[1494]

Reconstitution to an ifosfamide concentration of 100 mg/mL with benzyl alcohol-preserved bacteriostatic water for injection resulted in a turbid mixture, separating into 2 distinct liquid phases. The separate phases dissolved completely, with no loss of drug or preservative, when diluted to about 60 mg/mL or less.[1289]

pH Effects

Ifosfamide exhibits maximum solution stability in the pH range of 4 to 10; the rate of decomposition is essentially the same over this pH range. At pH values less than 4 and above 10, increased rates of decomposition have been observed.[2002][2401]

Syringes

Ifosfamide 0.6 and 20 mg/mL in dextrose 5%, lactated Ringer's injection, sodium chloride 0.9%, and sterile water for injection in polypropylene syringes (Becton Dickinson) is physically and chemically stable for at least 24 hours at 30°C.[1496]

Ambulatory Pumps

Ifosfamide (Asta Medica) 20 mg/mL and mesna (Asta Medica) 20 mg/mL in water for injection were evaluated for stability and compatibility in polyvinyl chloride (PVC) reservoirs for Graseby 9000 ambulatory pumps. The solutions were physically compatible and analysis found about 3% ifosfamide and 9% mesna loss in 7 days at 37°C. About 2% or less loss of both drugs was found after 14 days at 4°C. Furthermore, weight losses due to moisture loss were minimal.[2288]

Compatibility Information

Solution Compatibility

Ifosfamide

Test Soln Name	Mfr	Mfr	Conc/L or %	Remarks	Ref	C/I
Dextrose 5% in Ringer's injection			600 mg and 16 g	Physically compatible. Under 5% loss in 7 days at 30°C and no loss in 6 weeks at 5°C	72	C
Dextrose 5% in sodium chloride 0.9%	b		0.6 to 20 g	Physically compatible and stable for 7 days at 30°C and 6 weeks at 5°C	4	C
Dextrose 5% in sodium chloride 0.9%			600 mg and 16 g	Physically compatible. Under 5% loss in 7 days at 30°C and no loss in 6 weeks at 5°C	72	C
Dextrose 5%	b		0.6 to 20 g	Physically compatible and stable for 7 days at 30°C and 6 weeks at 5°C	4	C
Dextrose 5%			600 mg and 16 g	Physically compatible. Under 5% loss in 7 days at 30°C and no loss in 6 weeks at 5°C	72	C
Ringer's injection, lactated	b		0.6 to 20 g	Physically compatible and stable for 7 days at 30°C and 6 weeks at 5°C	4	C
Ringer's injection, lactated			600 mg and 16 g	Physically compatible. Under 5% loss in 7 days at 30°C and no loss in 6 weeks at 5°C	72	C

DOI: 10.37573/9781585286850.205

Solution Compatibility (Cont.)

Test Soln Name	Mfr	Mfr	Conc/L or %	Remarks	Ref	C/I
Sodium chloride 0.45%			600 mg and 16 g	Physically compatible. Under 5% loss in 7 days at 30°C and no loss in 6 weeks at 5°C	72	C
Sodium chloride 0.9%	b		0.6 to 20 g	Physically compatible and stable for 7 days at 30°C and 6 weeks at 5°C	4	C
Sodium chloride 0.9%			600 mg and 16 g	Physically compatible. Under 5% loss in 7 days at 30°C and no loss in 6 weeks at 5°C	72	C
Sodium chloride 0.9%		BI	80 g	7% loss in 9 days at 37°C in dark	1494	C
Sodium chloride 0.9%	a		10 g	No loss in 8 days at 4 and 25°C protected from light and at 25°C in light	1551	C
Sodium chloride 0.9%	a		20, 40, 80 g	No loss in 8 days at 35°C	1551	C
Sodium lactate ⅙ M			600 mg and 16 g	Physically compatible. Under 5% loss in 7 days at 30°C and no loss in 6 weeks at 5°C	72	C

[a] Tested in PVC containers.

[b] Tested in glass, PVC, and polyolefin containers.

Additive Compatibility

Ifosfamide

Test Drug	Mfr	Conc/L or %	Mfr	Conc/L or %	Test Solution	Remarks	Ref	C/I
Carboplatin		1 g		1 g	W	Both drugs stable for 5 days at room temperature	1379	C
Cisplatin		200 mg		2 g	NS	Both drugs stable for 7 days at room temperature	1379	C
Cisplatin with etoposide		200 mg 200 mg		2 g	NS	All drugs stable for 5 days at room temperature	1379	C
Epirubicin HCl		1 g		2.5 g	NS	Under 10% loss of either drug in 14 days	1379	C
Etoposide		200 mg		2 g	NS	Both drugs stable for 5 days at room temperature	1379	C
Etoposide with cisplatin		200 mg 200 mg		2 g	NS	All drugs stable for 5 days at room temperature	1379	C
Fluorouracil		10 g		2 g	NS	Both drugs stable for 5 days at room temperature	1379	C
Mesna	AW	3.3 g	MJ	3.3 g	D5W, LR	Physically compatible. No ifosfamide loss and about 5% mesna loss in 24 hr at 21°C exposed to light	72	C
Mesna	AW	5 g	MJ	5 g	D5W, LR	Physically compatible. No ifosfamide loss and about 5% mesna loss in 24 hr at 21°C exposed to light	72	C
Mesna	BI	79 g	BI	83.3 g	NS	Little or no ifosfamide loss in 9 days at room temperature and 7% ifosfamide loss in 9 days at 37°C. Mesna not tested	1494	C
Mesna		1.6 g		2.6 g	D5S[a]	No increase in decomposition products in 8 hr at room temperature	1495	C
Mesna	BR	600 mg	BR	600 mg	D5½S, D5W, LR, NS[b]	Both drugs chemically stable for at least 24 hr at room temperature	1496	C
Mesna	AM	20 g	AM	20 g	W[c]	Physically compatible with about 3% ifosfamide loss and 9% mesna loss in 7 days at 37°C. About 2% or less loss of both drugs in 14 days at 4°C	2288	C

[a] Tested in polyethylene containers.

[b] Tested in PVC containers.

[c] Tested in PVC reservoirs for Graseby 9000 ambulatory pumps.

Drugs in Syringe Compatibility

Ifosfamide

Test Drug	Mfr	Amt	Mfr	Amt	Remarks	Ref	C/I
Epirubicin HCl		1 mg/mL[a]		50 mg/mL[a]	Little or no loss of either drug in 28 days at 4 and 20°C	1564	C
Epirubicin HCl with mesna		1 mg/mL 40 mg/mL[a]		50 mg/mL[a]	50% epirubicin loss in 7 days at 4 and 20°C. No loss of other drugs in 7 days	1564	I
Mesna		200 mg/5 mL		250 mg/5 mL	3% ifosfamide loss in 7 days and 12% in 4 weeks at 4°C and room temperature. No mesna loss	1290	C
Mesna		40 mg/mL[a]		50 mg/mL[a]	Little or no loss of either drug in 28 days at 4 and 20°C	1564	C
Mesna with epirubicin HCl		40 mg/mL[a] 1 mg/mL		50 mg/mL[a]	50% epirubicin loss in 7 days at 4 and 20°C. No loss of other drugs in 7 days	1564	I

[a] Diluted in sodium chloride 0.9%.

Y-Site Injection Compatibility (1:1 Mixture)

Ifosfamide

Test Drug	Mfr	Conc	Mfr	Conc	Remarks	Ref	C/I
Allopurinol sodium	BW	3 mg/mL[b]	MJ	25 mg/mL[b]	Physically compatible for 4 hr at 22°C	1686	C
Amifostine	USB	10 mg/mL[a]	MJ	25 mg/mL[a]	Physically compatible for 4 hr at 23°C	1845	C
Anidulafungin	VIC	0.5 mg/mL[a]	BMS	25 mg/mL[a]	Physically compatible for 4 hr at 23°C	2617	C
Aztreonam	SQ	40 mg/mL[a]	MJ	25 mg/mL[a]	Physically compatible for 4 hr at 23°C	1758	C
Caspofungin acetate	ME	0.7 mg/mL[b]	BA	20 mg/mL[b]	Physically compatible for 4 hr at room temperature	2758	C
Doripenem	JJ	5 mg/mL[a b]	BMS	20 mg/mL[a b]	Physically compatible for 4 hr at 23°C	2743	C
Doxorubicin HCl liposomal	SEQ	0.4 mg/mL[a]	MJ	25 mg/mL[a]	Physically compatible for 4 hr at 23°C	2087	C
Etoposide phosphate	BR	5 mg/mL[a]	MJ	25 mg/mL[a]	Physically compatible for 4 hr at 23°C	2218	C
Filgrastim	AMG	30 mcg/mL[a]	MJ	25 mg/mL[a]	Physically compatible for 4 hr at 22°C	1687	C
Fludarabine phosphate	BX	1 mg/mL[a]	MJ	25 mg/mL[a]	Visually compatible for 4 hr at 22°C	1439	C
Gallium nitrate	FUJ	1 mg/mL[b]	MJ	20 mg/mL[b]	Visually compatible for 24 hr at 25°C	1673	C
Gemcitabine HCl	LI	10 mg/mL[b]	MJ	25 mg/mL[b]	Physically compatible for 4 hr at 23°C	2226	C
Granisetron HCl	SKB	1 mg/mL	MJ	4 mg/mL[b]	Physically compatible with little or no loss of either drug in 4 hr at 22°C	1883	C
Linezolid	PHU	2 mg/mL	MJ	25 mg/mL[a]	Physically compatible for 4 hr at 23°C	2264	C
Melphalan HCl	BW	0.1 mg/mL[b]	BR	25 mg/mL[b]	Physically compatible for 3 hr at 22°C	1557	C
Methotrexate sodium		30 mg/mL		36 mg/mL[a]	Visually compatible for 2 hr at room temperature. Yellow precipitate in 4 hr	1788	I
Ondansetron HCl	GL	1 mg/mL[b]	MJ	25 mg/mL[a]	Visually compatible for 4 hr at 22°C	1365	C
Oxaliplatin	SS	0.5 mg/mL[a]	MJ	20 mg/mL[a]	Physically compatible for 4 hr at 23°C	2566	C
Paclitaxel	NCI	1.2 mg/mL[a]	BR	25 mg/mL[a]	Physically compatible for 4 hr at 22°C	1556	C
Palonosetron HCl	MGI	50 mcg/mL	MJ	10 mg/mL[a]	Physically compatible and no loss of either drug in 4 hr	2640	C

Y-Site Injection Compatibility (1:1 Mixture) (Cont.)

Test Drug	Mfr	Conc	Mfr	Conc	Remarks	Ref	C/I
Pemetrexed disodium	LI	20 mg/mL[b]	MJ	20 mg/mL[a]	Physically compatible for 4 hr at 23°C	2564	C
Piperacillin sodium–tazobactam sodium	LE[e]	40 mg/mL[a] [f]	MJ	25 mg/mL[a]	Physically compatible for 4 hr at 22°C	1688	C
Propofol	ZEN[g]	10 mg/mL	MJ	25 mg/mL[a]	Physically compatible for 1 hr at 23°C	2066	C
Sargramostim	IMM	10 mcg/mL[b]	MJ	25 mg/mL[b]	Visually compatible for 4 hr at 22°C	1436	C
Sodium bicarbonate		1.4%		36 mg/mL[a]	Visually compatible for 4 hr at room temperature	1788	C
Teniposide	BR	0.1 mg/mL[a]	MJ	25 mg/mL[a]	Physically compatible for 4 hr at 23°C	1725	C
Thiotepa	IMM[c]	1 mg/mL[a]	MJ	25 mg/mL[a]	Physically compatible for 4 hr at 23°C	1861	C
TNA #218 to #226[d]			MJ	25 mg/mL[a]	Visually compatible for 4 hr at 23°C	2215	C
Topotecan HCl	SKB	56 mcg/mL[a] [b]	MJ	14.28 mg/mL[a] [b]	Visually compatible. Little loss of either drug in 4 hr at 22°C	2245	C
TPN #212 to #215[d]			MJ	25 mg/mL[a]	Physically compatible for 4 hr at 23°C	2109	C
Vinorelbine tartrate	BW	1 mg/mL[b]	MJ	25 mg/mL[b]	Physically compatible for 4 hr at 22°C	1558	C

[a] Tested in dextrose 5%.

[b] Tested in sodium chloride 0.9%.

[c] Lyophilized formulation tested.

[d] Refer to Appendix for the composition of parenteral nutrition solutions. TNA indicates a 3-in-1 admixture, and TPN indicates a 2-in-1 admixture.

[e] Test performed using the formulation WITHOUT edetate disodium.

[f] Piperacillin component. Piperacillin in an 8:1 fixed-ratio concentration with tazobactam.

[g] Test performed using the formulation WITH edetate disodium.

Selected Revisions January 31, 2020. © Copyright, October 1990. American Society of Health-System Pharmacists, Inc.

Imipenem–Cilastatin Sodium
AHFS 8:12.07.08

Products

Imipenem–cilastatin sodium for intravenous use is available as a fixed combination of equal quantities of both drugs. The combination is provided in vials and infusion bottles containing 250 or 500 mg of each drug with sodium bicarbonate 10 or 20 mg, respectively.[1(8/06)]

The contents of a vial should be reconstituted with about 10 mL of a compatible diluent from a 100-mL infusion container and shaken well to form a suspension. Diluents containing benzyl alcohol should not be used to reconstitute the drug for use in neonates and small pediatric patients. The suspension must be transferred to the remaining solution in the infusion container for dilution. The suspension is *not* for direct injection. The procedure is then repeated: a 10-mL aliquot from the admixture is added to the vial and, once again, returned to the infusion admixture. This procedure ensures that all of the vial contents are transferred. The admixture should be agitated until it is clear to yield either a 2.5- or 5-mg/mL concentration, depending on the vial content. The admixture should *not* be heated to aid dissolution.[1(8/06) 4]

ADD-Vantage vials of imipenem–cilastatin sodium should be prepared with 100 mL of dextrose 5% or sodium chloride 0.9% in ADD-Vantage diluent bags.[1(8/06) 4]

The 250- and 500-mg piggyback infusion bottles should be reconstituted with 100 mL of compatible diluent and shaken until clear to yield 2.5- and 5-mg/mL concentrations, respectively.[1(8/06) 4]

Imipenem–cilastatin sodium for intramuscular use is available in vials containing 500 or 750 mg of each component. The vials should be reconstituted with 2 or 3 mL, respectively, of lidocaine hydrochloride 1% (without epinephrine) and agitated to form a suspension. This intramuscular formulation is not for intravenous use.[1(8/06) 4]

pH
The intravenous product is buffered to pH 6.5 to 8.5.[1(8/06)]

Osmolarity
When reconstituted and diluted as directed by the manufacturer, the osmolarity of the intravenous admixture approximates that of the diluent.[4]

Sodium Content
The 250- and 500-mg intravenous vials contain 0.8 mEq (18.8 mg) and 1.6 mEq (37.5 mg) of sodium, respectively. The 500- and 750-mg intramuscular vials contain 1.4 mEq (32 mg) and 2.1 mEq (48 mg) of sodium, respectively.[1(8/06) 4]

Trade Name(s)
Primaxin I.V., Primaxin I.M.

Administration

Imipenem–cilastatin sodium for intravenous use is administered by intermittent intravenous infusion at a concentration not exceeding 5 mg/mL. Infusion periods vary from 20 to 60 minutes, depending on the dose. The intramuscular formulation should be injected deeply into a large muscle mass. Suspensions of either formulation should not be given intravenously.[1(8/06) 4]

Stability

The product should be stored below 25°C.[1(8/06) 4]

Reconstituted as directed, intravenous solutions are colorless to yellow but may become a deeper yellow over time. Intramuscular suspensions are white to light tan. The manufacturer indicates that stability is not affected by color variations within this range,[1(8/06)] but the solutions should be discarded if they darken to brown.[4] Intramuscular suspensions prepared with lidocaine hydrochloride (without epinephrine) should be used within 1 hour.[1(8/06) 4]

In solution, imipenem is substantially less stable than cilastatin and is the determining factor in the overall stability of the combination product. Reconstitution results in solutions that are stable for 4 hours at room temperature or 24 hours under refrigeration at 4°C.[1(8/06)]

Imipenem degradation kinetics were determined for a 2.5-mg/mL solution in sodium chloride 0.9%. The degradation rates were temperature dependent, with a half-life of over 44 hours at 2°C dropping to 6 hours at 25°C and to 2 hours at 37°C. The decomposition was consistent with hydrolysis, and the loss of antimicrobial activity suggests cleavage of the β-lactam ring.[1272]

Concentration Effects
In one study, solutions of imipenem–cilastatin in sterile water for injection at concentrations exceeding 8 g/L (not specified whether concentration refers to single component or combined components) resulted in precipitation.[3105]

pH Effects
Imipenem is inactivated at acidic or alkaline pH but is more stable at neutral pH.[4] The pH range of maximum stability appears to be 6.5 to 7.5, with increasing rates of decomposition occurring as the pH moves away from this range.[1273] At a pH of about 4, the half-life of imipenem is about 35 minutes.[2166]

Freezing Solutions
The manufacturer recommends that imipenem–cilastatin solutions not be frozen.[1(8/06)] At concentrations of 250 and 500 mg/100 mL in sodium chloride 0.9%, imipenem losses of around 15% occurred in 1 week when frozen at –20 and –10°C.[1141] Freezing solutions at

DOI: 10.37573/9781585286850.206

temperatures above –70°C offers no stability advantage over refrigerated storage[1141] and results in decomposition of imipenem in a manner similar to ampicillin.[4]

Effects of Solution Components

Dextrose exerts an adverse effect on the stability of imipenem. Dextrose 5 and 10% reduced the time to 10% decomposition by about one-half compared to sterile water. Sodium chloride content increases imipenem stability because of a positive kinetic salt effect similar to other β-lactam antibiotics. Both lactate and bicarbonate anions attack the β-lactam ring and decrease imipenem stability.[1141]

Elastomeric Reservoir Pumps

Imipenem–cilastatin sodium (Merck) 5 mg/mL in both dextrose 5% and sodium chloride 0.9% was evaluated for binding

potential to natural rubber elastomeric reservoirs (Baxter). Less than 1% binding was found after storage for 2 weeks at 35°C with gentle agitation.[2014]

Central Venous Catheter

Imipenem–cilastatin (MSD) 2 mg/mL in sodium chloride 0.9% was found to be compatible with the ARROWg+ard Blue Plus (Arrow International) chlorhexidine-bearing triple-lumen central catheter. Essentially complete delivery of the drug was found with little or no drug loss occurring. Furthermore, chlorhexidine delivered from the catheter remained at trace amounts with no substantial increase due to the delivery of the drug through the catheter.[2335]

Compatibility Information

Solution Compatibility

Imipenem–cilastatin sodium

Test Soln Name	Mfr	Mfr	Conc/L or %	Remarks	Ref	C/I
Dextrose 5% in Ringer's injection, lactated	AB[a]	MSD	2.5[d] g	8% imipenem loss in 3 hr, 15% in 6 hr at 25°C. 9% loss in 24 hr, 15% in 48 hr at 4°C	1141	I
Dextrose 5% in Ringer's injection, lactated	AB[a]	MSD	5[d] g	14% imipenem loss in 3 hr at 25°C and 13% in 24 hr at 4°C	1141	I
Dextrose 5% in sodium chloride 0.225%	AB[a]	MSD	2.5[d] g	8% imipenem loss in 6 hr and 12% in 9 hr at 25°C. 10% loss in 48 hr at 4°C	1141	I[b]
Dextrose 5% in sodium chloride 0.225%	AB[a]	MSD	5[d] g	5% imipenem loss in 3 hr, 13% in 6 hr at 25°C. 7% loss in 24 hr, 13% in 48 hr at 4°C	1141	I[b]
Dextrose 5% in sodium chloride 0.45%	AB[a]	MSD	2.5[d] g	8% imipenem loss in 6 hr, 11% in 9 hr at 25°C. 9% loss in 48 hr, 13% in 72 hr at 4°C	1141	I[b]
Dextrose 5% in sodium chloride 0.45%	AB[a]	MSD	5[d] g	5% imipenem loss in 3 hr, 11% in 6 hr at 25°C. 6% loss in 24 hr, 13% in 48 hr at 4°C	1141	I[b]
Dextrose 5% in sodium chloride 0.9%	AB[a]	MSD	2.5[d] g	6% imipenem loss in 6 hr, 10% in 9 hr at 25°C. 6% loss in 24 hr, 11% in 48 hr at 4°C	1141	I[b]
Dextrose 5% in sodium chloride 0.9%	AB[a]	MSD	5[d] g	6% imipenem loss in 3 hr, 11% in 6 hr at 25°C. 6% loss in 24 hr, 13% in 48 hr at 4°C	1141	I[b]
Dextrose 5%	AB[a]	MSD	2.5[d] g	5% imipenem loss in 3 hr, 10% in 6 hr at 25°C. 8% loss in 24 hr, 14% in 48 hr at 4°C	1141	I[b]
Dextrose 5%	AB[a]	MSD	5[d] g	6% imipenem loss in 3 hr, 15% in 6 hr at 25°C. 8% loss in 24 hr, 14% in 48 hr at 4°C	1141	I[b]
Dextrose 5%	BA	MSD	5[d] g	Visually compatible. 10% imipenem loss in about 6 hr at 23°C and in 48 hr at 4°C	2166	I[b]
Dextrose 10%	AB[a]	MSD	2.5[d] g	6% imipenem loss in 3 hr, 10% in 6 hr at 25°C. 8% loss in 24 hr, 13% in 48 hr at 4°C	1141	I[b]
Dextrose 10%	AB[a]	MSD	5[d] g	8% imipenem loss in 3 hr and 13% in 6 hr at 25°C. 10% loss in 24 hr at 4°C	1141	I[b]
Normosol M in dextrose 5%	AB[a]	MSD	2.5[d] g	7% imipenem loss in 3 hr, 11% in 6 hr at 25°C. 9% loss in 24 hr, 19% in 48 hr at 4°C	1141	I[b]

Solution Compatibility (Cont.)

Test Soln Name	Mfr	Mfr	Conc/L or %	Remarks	Ref	C/I
Normosol M in dextrose 5%	AB[a]	MSD	5[d] g	8% imipenem loss in 3 hr and 14% in 6 hr at 25°C. 10% loss in 24 hr at 4°C	1141	I[b]
Ringer's injection, lactated	AB[a]	MSD	2.5[d] g	9% imipenem loss in 6 hr, 12% in 9 hr at 25°C. 4% loss in 24 hr, 10% in 48 hr at 4°C	1141	I
Ringer's injection, lactated	AB[a]	MSD	5[d] g	6% imipenem loss in 3 hr, 12% in 6 hr at 25°C. 7% loss in 24 hr, 12% in 48 hr at 4°C	1141	I
Sodium chloride 0.9%	AB[a]	MSD	2.5[d] g	6% imipenem loss in 9 hr at 25°C. 7% loss in 72 hr at 4°C	1141	I[b]
Sodium chloride 0.9%	AB[a]	MSD	5[d] g	8% imipenem loss in 9 hr at 25°C. 7% loss in 48 hr and 11% in 72 hr at 4°C	1141	I[b]
Sodium chloride 0.9%		ME	5[e] g	More than 10% loss by 6, 4, and 3 hr at temperatures of 30, 35, and 40°C, respectively	3109	I
Sodium lactate ⅙ M	AB[a]	MSD	2.5[d] g	13% imipenem loss in 3 hr at 25°C. 8% loss in 24 hr and 15% in 48 hr at 4°C	1141	I
Sodium lactate ⅙ M	AB[a]	MSD	5[d] g	18% imipenem loss in 3 hr at 25°C. 14% loss in 24 hr at 4°C	1141	I
TPN #107[c]			500[e] mg	57% imipenem loss in 24 hr at 21°C	1326	I
TPN #241[c]		MSD	5[d] g	8 to 10% imipenem loss within 30 min at 25°C under fluorescent light	493	I
TPN #242[c]		MSD	5[d] g	8 to 10% imipenem loss within 30 min at 25°C under fluorescent light	493	I

[a] Tested in glass containers.

[b] Incompatible by conventional standards but recommended for dilution of imipenem–cilastatin with use in shorter periods of time.

[c] Refer to Appendix for the composition of parenteral nutrition solutions. TPN indicates a 2-in-1 admixture.

[d] Imipenem component. Imipenem in a 1:1 fixed-ratio concentration with cilastatin.

[e] Not specified whether concentration refers to single component or combined components.

Additive Compatibility

Imipenem–cilastatin sodium

Test Drug	Mfr	Conc/L or %	Mfr	Conc/L or %	Test Solution	Remarks	Ref	C/I
Amoxicillin sodium	MSD	8 g	GSK	4[c] g	NS	Blue discoloration formed in 2 hr. Amoxicillin and imipenem losses of 40 and 72%, respectively, in 12 hr	2800	I
Mannitol	AB[a]	2.5%	MSD	2.5[c] g		9% imipenem loss in 9 hr at 25°C. 7% loss in 48 hr and 11% in 72 hr at 4°C	1141	I[b]
Mannitol	AB[a]	2.5%	MSD	5[c] g		6% imipenem loss in 3 hr and 12% in 6 hr at 25°C. 7% loss in 24 hr and 10% in 48 hr at 4°C	1141	I[b]
Mannitol	AB[a]	5%	MSD	2.5[c] g		6% imipenem loss in 3 hr and 10% in 6 hr at 25°C. 9% loss in 48 hr and 13% in 72 hr at 4°C	1141	I[b]
Mannitol	AB[a]	5%	MSD	5[c] g		7% imipenem loss in 3 hr and 12% in 6 hr at 25°C. 12% loss in 48 hr at 4°C	1141	I[b]
Mannitol	AB[a]	10%	MSD	2.5[c] g		6% imipenem loss in 3 hr and 10% in 6 hr at 25°C. 7% loss in 24 hr and 12% in 48 hr at 4°C	1141	I[b]
Mannitol	AB[a]	10%	MSD	5[c] g		12% imipenem loss in 3 hr at 25°C. 13% loss in 48 hr at 4°C	1141	I[b]
Sodium bicarbonate	AB	5%	MSD	2.5[c] g		43% imipenem loss in 3 hr at 25°C and 52% in 24 hr at 4°C	1141	I

Additive Compatibility (Cont.)

Test Drug	Mfr	Conc/L or %	Mfr	Conc/L or %	Test Solution	Remarks	Ref	C/I
Sodium bicarbonate	AB	5%	MSD	5[c] g		45% imipenem loss in 3 hr at 25°C and 50% in 24 hr at 4°C	1141	I
Tobramycin sulfate		10 mg		100[d] mg	W	Little or no loss of antibiotic activity in 24 hr at 37°C	498	C

[a] Tested in glass containers.

[b] Incompatible by conventional standards but may be used in shorter periods of time.

[c] Imipenem component. Imipenem in a 1:1 fixed-ratio concentration with cilastatin.

[d] Not specified whether concentration refers to single component or combined components.

Y-Site Injection Compatibility (1:1 Mixture)

Imipenem–cilastatin sodium

Test Drug	Mfr	Conc	Mfr	Conc	Remarks	Ref	C/I
Acyclovir sodium	BW	5 mg/mL[a]	MSD	5 mg/mL[b h]	Physically compatible for 4 hr at 25°C	1157	C
Allopurinol sodium	BW	3 mg/mL[b]	MSD	10 mg/mL[b i]	Haze and particles form in 1 hr	1686	I
Amifostine	USB	10 mg/mL[a]	MSD	10 mg/mL[a i]	Physically compatible for 4 hr at 23°C	1845	C
Amiodarone HCl	WY	6 mg/mL[a]	ME	5 mg/mL[a i]	Immediate haze. Becomes yellow in 24 hr	2352	I
Anidulafungin	VIC	0.5 mg/mL[a]	ME	5 mg/mL[b i]	Physically compatible for 4 hr at 23°C	2617	C
Azithromycin	PF	2 mg/mL[b]	ME	5 mg/mL[b g h]	Whitish-yellow microcrystals found	2368	I
Aztreonam	SQ	40 mg/mL[a]	MSD	10 mg/mL[a i]	Physically compatible for 4 hr at 23°C	1758	C
Blinatumomab	AMG	0.125 and 0.375 mcg/mL[b]	PAN	5 mg/mL[b i]	Particles, flakes, thin needles, or haze transiently appears when blinatumomab is added to imipenem–cilastatin; not observed when order of mixing was reversed	3405, 3417	?
Caspofungin acetate	ME	0.7 mg/mL[b]	ME	5 mg/mL[b i]	Physically compatible for 4 hr at room temperature	2758	C
Ceftazidime–avibactam sodium	ALL	20 mg/mL[n o]	[k]		Physically compatible for up to 4 hr at room temperature	3004	C
Ceftolozane sulfate–tazobactam sodium	CUB	10 mg/mL[c l]	FRK	5 mg/mL[c h]	Physically compatible for 2 hr	3247, 3262	C
Cisatracurium besylate	GW	0.1, 2, 5 mg/mL[a]	ME	10 mg/mL[b i]	Physically compatible for 4 hr at 23°C	2074	C
Colistimethate sodium	MIL	1.5 mg/mL[b]	MSD	5 mg/mL[b h]	Visually compatible for 1 hr at 26°C	3335	C
Defibrotide sodium	JAZ	8 mg/mL[b]	PAN	9.94 mg/mL[b h]	Visually compatible for 4 hr at room temperature	3149	C
Diltiazem HCl	MMD	5 mg/mL	MSD	5 mg/mL[c i]	Visually compatible	1807	C
Docetaxel	RPR	0.9 mg/mL[a]	ME	10 mg/mL[b i]	Physically compatible for 4 hr at 23°C	2224	C
Eravacycline dihydrochloride	TET	0.6 mg/mL[b]	FRK	5 mg/mL[b h]	Physically compatible for 2 hr at room temperature	3532	C
Etoposide phosphate	BR	5 mg/mL[a]	ME	10 mg/mL[b i]	Yellow color forms in 4 hr at 23°C	2218	I
Famotidine	MSD	0.2 mg/mL[a]	MSD	10 mg/mL[b i]	Physically compatible for 14 hr	1196	C
Famotidine	ME	2 mg/mL[b]		5 mg/mL[b i]	Visually compatible for 4 hr at 22°C	1936	C
Fat emulsion, intravenous	OTS	20%[q]	MSD	5 mg/mL[a i r]	No change in particle size ≥1.3 μm observed in 24 hr at 25°C in the dark	3452	C
Filgrastim	AMG	30 mcg/mL[a]	MSD	10 mg/mL[a i]	Physically compatible for 4 hr at 22°C	1687	C

Y-Site Injection Compatibility (1:1 Mixture) (Cont.)

Test Drug	Mfr	Conc	Mfr	Conc	Remarks	Ref	C/I
Filgrastim	AMG	40 mcg/mL[a]	ME	5 mg/mL[a h]	16% loss of filgrastim in 4 hr at 25°C. Little imipenem–cilastatin loss	2060	I
Filgrastim	AMG	10 mcg/mL[d]	ME	5 mg/mL[a h]	Visually compatible. Little loss of filgrastim and imipenem–cilastatin in 4 hr at 25°C	2060	C
Fluconazole	RR	2 mg/mL	MSD	10 mg/mL[i]	Precipitates immediately	1407	I
Fludarabine phosphate	BX	1 mg/mL[a]	MSD	5 mg/mL[a i]	Visually compatible for 4 hr at 22°C	1439	C
Foscarnet sodium	AST	24 mg/mL	MSD	10 mg/mL[i]	Physically compatible for 24 hr at room temperature under fluorescent light	1335	C
Foscarnet sodium	AST	24 mg/mL	MSD	5 mg/mL[a i]	Physically compatible for 24 hr at 25°C under fluorescent light	1393	C
Gallium nitrate	FUJ	1 mg/mL[b]	MSD	5 mg/mL[b h]	Precipitates immediately	1673	I
Gemcitabine HCl	LI	10 mg/mL[b]	ME	10 mg/mL[b i]	Yellow-green discoloration forms in 1 hr	2226	I
Granisetron HCl	SKB	0.05 mg/mL[a]	ME	10 mg/mL[a i]	Physically compatible for 4 hr at 23°C	2000	C
Idarubicin HCl	AD	1 mg/mL[b]	MSD	5 mg/mL[b i]	Visually compatible for 12 hr at 25°C in light. Precipitate in 24 hr	1525	C
Insulin, regular	LI	0.2 unit/mL[b]	MSD	4 and 5 mg/mL[b i]	Physically compatible for 2 hr at 25°C	1395	C
Isavuconazonium sulfate	ASP	1.5 mg/mL[c]	PRP	5 mg/mL[c h]	Physically compatible for 2 hr	3263	C
Linezolid	PHU	2 mg/mL	ME	10 mg/mL[b i]	Physically compatible for 4 hr at 23°C	2264	C
Lorazepam	WY	0.33 mg/mL[b]	MSD	5 mg/mL[i]	Yellow precipitate forms in 24 hr	1855	I
Melphalan HCl	BW	0.1 mg/mL[b]	MSD	10 mg/mL[b i]	Physically compatible for 3 hr at 22°C	1557	C
Meperidine HCl	AB	10 mg/mL	MSD	5 mg/mL[a i]	Yellow color forms in 2 hr at 25°C	1397	I
Meropenem		50 mg/mL	HOS	50 mg/mL[h]	Physically compatible for 4 hr at room temperature	3538, 3547	C
Meropenem–vaborbactam	TMC	8 mg/mL[b m]	ME	5 mg/mL[b h]	Physically compatible for 3 hr at 20 to 25°C	3380	C
Midazolam HCl	RC	5 mg/mL	MSD	5 mg/mL[i]	Haze forms in 24 hr	1855	I
Milrinone lactate	SS	0.2 mg/mL[a]	ME	5 mg/mL[b h]	Yellow color darkening in 4 hr at 25°C	2381	I
Ondansetron HCl	GL	1 mg/mL[b]	MSD	5 mg/mL[b i]	Visually compatible for 4 hr at 22°C	1365	C
Plazomicin sulfate	ACH	24 mg/mL[c]	FRK	5 mg/mL[c h]	Physically compatible for 1 hr at 20 to 25°C	3432	C
Propofol	ZEN[p]	10 mg/mL	ME	10 mg/mL[b i]	Physically compatible for 1 hr at 23°C	2066	C
Quinupristin–dalfopristin		2 mg/mL[a j]	[k]	5 mg/mL	Reported to be incompatible	3230	I
Remifentanil HCl	GW	0.025 and 0.25 mg/mL[b]	ME	10 mg/mL[a i]	Physically compatible for 4 hr at 23°C	2075	C
Sargramostim	IMM	10 mcg/mL[b]	MSD	5 mg/mL[b i]	Large particle and clump form in 4 hr	1436	I
Tacrolimus	FUJ	1 mg/mL[b]	MSD	10 mg/mL[b i]	Visually compatible for 24 hr at 25°C	1630	C
Tedizolid phosphate	CUB	0.8 mg/mL[b]	PRP	5 mg/mL[b h]	Physically compatible for 2 hr	3244	C
Telavancin HCl	ASP	7.5 mg/mL[a]	ME	5 mg/mL[a h]	Slight measured turbidity increase	2830	I
Telavancin HCl	ASP	7.5 mg/mL[b]	ME	5 mg/mL[b h]	Physically compatible for 2 hr	2830	C
Teniposide	BR	0.1 mg/mL[a]	MSD	10 mg/mL[b i]	Physically compatible for 4 hr at 23°C	1725	C

Y-Site Injection Compatibility (1:1 Mixture) (Cont.)

Test Drug	Mfr	Conc	Mfr	Conc	Remarks	Ref	C/I
Thiotepa	IMM[e]	1 mg/mL[a]	ME	10 mg/mL[a i]	Physically compatible for 4 hr at 23°C	1861	C
Tigecycline	WY	1 mg/mL[b]		2.5 mg/mL[b h]	Physically compatible for 4 hr	2714, 2917	C
TNA #218[f]			ME	10 mg/mL[b i]	Visually compatible for 4 hr at 23°C	2215	C
TNA #219[f]			ME	10 mg/mL[b i]	Visually compatible for 4 hr at 23°C	2215	C
TNA #220[f]			ME	10 mg/mL[b i]	Visually compatible for 4 hr at 23°C	2215	C
TNA #221[f]			ME	10 mg/mL[b i]	Visually compatible for 4 hr at 23°C	2215	C
TNA #222[f]			ME	10 mg/mL[b i]	Visually compatible for 4 hr at 23°C	2215	C
TNA #223[f]			ME	10 mg/mL[b i]	Visually compatible for 4 hr at 23°C	2215	C
TNA #224[f]			ME	10 mg/mL[b i]	Visually compatible for 4 hr at 23°C	2215	C
TNA #225[f]			ME	10 mg/mL[b i]	Visually compatible for 4 hr at 23°C	2215	C
TNA #226[f]			ME	10 mg/mL[b i]	Visually compatible for 4 hr at 23°C	2215	C
TPN #212[f]			ME	10 mg/mL[b i]	Physically compatible for 4 hr at 23°C	2109	C
TPN #213[f]			ME	10 mg/mL[b i]	Physically compatible for 4 hr at 23°C	2109	C
TPN #214[f]			ME	10 mg/mL[b i]	Physically compatible for 4 hr at 23°C	2109	C
TPN #215[f]			ME	10 mg/mL[b i]	Physically compatible for 4 hr at 23°C	2109	C
Vasopressin	APP	0.2 unit/mL[b]	ME	5 mg/mL[a h]	Physically compatible	2641	C
Vinorelbine tartrate	BW	1 mg/mL[b]	MSD	10 mg/mL[b i]	Physically compatible for 4 hr at 22°C	1558	C
Zidovudine	BW	4 mg/mL[a]	MSD	5 mg/mL[a i]	Physically compatible for 4 hr at 25°C	1193	C

[a] Tested in dextrose 5%.

[b] Tested in sodium chloride 0.9%.

[c] Tested in both dextrose 5% and sodium chloride 0.9%.

[d] Tested in dextrose 5% with albumin human 2 mg/mL.

[e] Lyophilized formulation tested.

[f] Refer to Appendix for the composition of parenteral nutrition solutions. TNA indicates a 3-in-1 admixture, and TPN indicates a 2-in-1 admixture.

[g] Injected via Y-site into an administration set running azithromycin.

[h] Imipenem component. Imipenem in a 1:1 fixed-ratio concentration with cilastatin.

[i] Not specified whether concentration refers to single component or combined components.

[j] Quinupristin and dalfopristin components combined.

[k] Salt not specified.

[l] Ceftolozane component. Ceftolozane in a 2:1 fixed-ratio concentration with tazobactam.

[m] Meropenem component. Meropenem in a 1:1 fixed-ratio concentration with vaborbactam.

[n] Ceftazidime component. Ceftazidime in a 4:1 fixed-ratio concentration with avibactam.

[o] Tested in dextrose 5%, sodium chloride 0.9%, and Ringer's injection, lactated.

[p] Test performed using the formulation WITH edetate disodium.

[q] Run at 25 mL/hr with dextrose 5% run at 83 mL/hr.

[r] Run at 100 mL/hr.

Imipenem–Cilastatin Sodium–Relebactam
AHFS 8:12.07.08

Products

The fixed combination of imipenem–cilastatin sodium–relebactam is available as a powder for injection in single-dose vials containing 1.25 g (imipenem 500 mg [as the monohydrate], cilastatin 500 mg [as the sodium salt], relebactam 250 mg [as the monohydrate]) along with sodium bicarbonate 20 mg to adjust the pH.[3505]

To prepare the fixed combination for administration, infusion bags containing 100 mL of a compatible diluent should be used; if an infusion bag containing 100 mL of a compatible diluent is not available, 100 mL of a compatible diluent may be transferred into an empty infusion bag.[3505] Twenty mL (as two 10-mL aliquots) of the compatible diluent should be removed from the infusion bag.[3505] The contents of one 1.25-g vial should be reconstituted initially with one 10-mL aliquot of the compatible diluent (withdrawn from the infusion bag) and the vial should be shaken well.[3505] The resulting suspension should then be transferred into the infusion bag containing the remaining 80 mL of diluent.[3505] The second 10-mL aliquot of the compatible diluent should then be added to the vial and shaken well to ensure complete transfer of any remaining vial contents; the resulting suspension should be transferred to the infusion bag to total 100 mL and the infusion bag should be agitated until the infusion solution is clear.[3505]

The manufacturer's instructions for preparing various doses of imipenem–cilastatin–relebactam from the infusion solution are as follows:[3505]

For 1.25 g (imipenem 500 mg, cilastatin 500 mg, relebactam 250 mg), do not remove any volume from the prepared infusion bag; the solution delivers a 1.25-g dose in 100 mL.

For 1 g (imipenem 400, cilastatin 400 mg, relebactam 200 mg), remove and discard 20 mL from the prepared infusion bag; the remaining solution (i.e., 80 mL) delivers a 1-g dose.

For 0.75 g (imipenem 300 mg, cilastatin 300 mg, relebactam 150 mg), remove and discard 40 mL from the prepared infusion bag; the remaining solution (i.e., 60 mL) delivers a 0.75-g dose.

For 0.5 g (imipenem 200 mg, cilastatin 200 mg, relebactam 100 mg), remove and discard 60 mL from the prepared infusion bag; the remaining solution (i.e., 40 mL) delivers a 0.5-g dose.

Equivalency

In imipenem–cilastatin sodium–relebactam, cilastatin sodium 531 mg is equivalent to 500 mg of cilastatin.[3505]

pH

Diluted solutions of imipenem–cilastatin–relebactam for infusion have a pH ranging from 6.5 to 7.6.[3505]

Sodium Content

Each 1.25-g vial of this fixed combination contains 37.5 mg (1.6 mEq) of sodium.[3505]

Trade Name(s)

Recarbrio

Administration

Imipenem–cilastatin sodium–relebactam is administered by intravenous infusion over 30 minutes after reconstitution and dilution.[3505]

Stability

Imipenem–cilastatin sodium–relebactam is a white to light yellow lyophilized powder that forms a clear, colorless to yellow solution upon reconstitution and dilution; variations in color within this range do not affect the potency of the product.[3505] Intact vials of imipenem–cilastatin sodium–relebactam should be stored at controlled room temperature.[3505]

Diluted solutions of imipenem–cilastatin–relebactam for infusion should be visually inspected for particulate matter and discoloration prior to administration.[3505] Solutions that are discolored and those in which visible particles are observed should be discarded.[3505]

The diluted solution for infusion is stable for 2 hours at room temperature up to 30°C or for 24 hours at 2 to 8°C.[3505]

Freezing Solutions

The manufacturer states that solution of imipenem–cilastatin sodium–relebactam should not be frozen.[3505]

DOI: 10.37573/9781585286850.207

Compatibility Information

Solution Compatibility

Imipenem–cilastatin sodium–relebactam

Test Soln Name	Mfr	Mfr	Conc/L or %	Remarks	Ref	C/I
Dextrose 5%		ME	5 g[a]	Stable for 2 hr if stored at room temperature up to 30°C or 24 hr if stored at 2 to 8°C	3505	C
Dextrose 5% in sodium chloride 0.225%		ME	5 g[a]	Stable for 2 hr if stored at room temperature up to 30°C or 24 hr if stored at 2 to 8°C	3505	C
Dextrose 5% in sodium chloride 0.45%		ME	5 g[a]	Stable for 2 hr if stored at room temperature up to 30°C or 24 hr if stored at 2 to 8°C	3505	C
Dextrose 5% in sodium chloride 0.9%		ME	5 g[a]	Stable for 2 hr if stored at room temperature up to 30°C or 24 hr if stored at 2 to 8°C	3505	C
Sodium chloride 0.9%		ME	5 g[a]	Stable for 2 hr if stored at room temperature up to 30°C or 24 hr if stored at 2 to 8°C	3505	C

[a] Imipenem component. Imipenem in a 2:2:1 fixed-ratio concentration with cilastatin and relebactam.

Additive Compatibility

Imipenem–cilastatin sodium–relebactam

Test Drug	Mfr	Conc/L or %	Mfr	Conc/L or %	Test Solution	Remarks	Ref	C/I
Propofol			ME		D5W	Physically incompatible	3505	I
Propofol			ME		NS	Physically incompatible	3505	I

Immune Globulin Human
AHFS 80:04

Products

Immune globulin human products may be formulated for intravenous or subcutaneous infusion or for intramuscular injection; the product labeling must be consulted for details on the specific product, including instructions for preparation, administration, and storage.

Immune globulin human products for intravenous administration include: Bivigam (Biotest); Carimune NF (CSL Behring); Flebogamma DIF (5 or 10%, Grifols); Gammagard S/D (Baxter); Gammagard Liquid (Baxter); Gammaked (Grifols); Gammaplex (BPL); Gamunex-C (Grifols); Octagam (5 or 10%, Octapharma); and Privigen (CSL Behring).[3053 3054 3055 3056 3058 3059 3060 3061 3062 3065 3066 3067]

Immune globulin human products intended exclusively for subcutaneous infusion include: Cuvitru (Baxalta), Hizentra (CSL Behring) and HyQvia (Baxter).[3063 3064 3240] In addition, several of the intravenous immune globulin human preparations also may be administered by subcutaneous infusion for certain indications; these products include Gammagard Liquid (Baxter); Gammaked (Grifols); and Gamunex-C (Grifols).[3059 3060 3062]

GamaSTAN S/D (Grifols) immune globulin human is labeled solely for administration by intramuscular injection.[3057]

Immune Globulin Human Products for Intravenous Administration Only

Immune globulin human intravenous is available from a number of manufacturers in both liquid and lyophilized powder forms that are prepared with varying manufacturing processes and excipients, resulting in different physicochemical properties for each formulation.[3075] Protein concentrations of 5 and 10% are available in liquid forms.[3075] Lyophilized preparation vial sizes vary by product, but typically contain between 3 and 12 g of protein.[3054 3058] Lyophilized preparations require reconstitution with the diluents and volumes specified by the manufacturers and typically result in protein concentrations of 3 to 12%.[3054 3058 3075]

Bivigam (Biotest) is available as a 10% solution in 50- and 100-mL single-use vials.[3053] The drug also contains sodium chloride 0.1 to 0.14 M (approximately 5.8 to 8.2 mg/mL), glycine 0.2 to 0.29 M (approximately 15 to 21.8 mg/mL), and polysorbate 80 0.15 to 0.25% in water for injection.[3053] The concentration of IgA present in the formulation does not exceed 200 mcg/mL.[3053]

Carimune NF (CSL Behring) is available as a lyophilized powder in single-use vials containing 3, 6, and 12 g of protein.[3054] The drug should be reconstituted with sodium chloride 0.9%, dextrose 5%, or sterile water for injection in the amounts shown in Table 1.[3054]

Table 1. Reconstitution of Carimune NF[3054]

Target Concentration	Volume of Diluent to be Added		
	3-g Vial	6-g Vial	12-g Vial
3%	100 mL	200 mL	a
6%	50 mL	100 mL	200 mL
9%	33 mL	66 mL	132 mL
12%	25 mL	50 mL	100 mL

a Container not large enough to permit concentration.

Vials of Carimune NF also contain sucrose 1.67 g and less than 20 mg of sodium chloride per gram of protein.[3054] Trace amounts of IgA and IgM are present.[3054]

Flebogamma DIF (Grifols) is available as a 5% solution in 10-, 50-, 100-, 200-, and 400-mL single-use vials[3055] and as a 10% solution in 50-, 100-, and 200-mL single-use vials.[3056] Both strengths contain D-sorbitol 5 g in 100 mL of water for injection, trace amounts of sodium, and no greater than 3 or 6 mg/mL of polyethylene glycol in the 5 or 10% preparations, respectively.[3055 3056] The 5% solutions typically contain less than 50 mcg/mL of IgA,[3055] and the 10% solutions typically contain less than 100 mcg/mL.[3056] Both strengths contain trace amounts of IgM.[3055 3056]

Gammagard S/D (Baxter) is available in a kit containing 5 or 10 g of lyophilized immune globulin human in a single-use bottle, a diluent bottle containing sterile water for injection, a transfer device, and an administration set with an integral airway and a 15-µm filter.[3058] To produce the desired concentration, the powder must be reconstituted with an appropriate amount of the provided diluent.[3058] Before the provided transfer device is attached to the diluent vial, however, the amounts of diluent shown in Table 2 must be *removed* from the vial depending on the target concentration; the amount remaining in the vial is then used to reconstitute the lyophilized immune globulin human using the transfer device.[3058] The manufacturer's prescribing information should be consulted for specific instructions.[3058]

Table 2. Reconstitution of Gammagard S/D[3058]

Target Concentration	Volume of Diluent to be *Removed* from Diluent Vial	
	5-g Vial	10-g Vial
5%	0 mL a	0 mL a
10%	48 mL	96 mL

a Do not remove any diluent from the diluent vial to prepare a 5% solution.

DOI: 10.37573/9781585286850.208

When Gammagard S/D is reconstituted as directed, each mL of the resulting 5% solution also contains sodium chloride 8.5 mg, albumin human 3 mg, glycine 22.5 mg, glucose 20 mg, polyethylene glycol 2 mg, tri-n-butyl phosphate (TNBP) 1 mcg, octoxynol 9 1 mcg, and polysorbate 80 100 mcg.[3058] (A 10% solution contains twice the concentration of these excipients per mL contained in the 5% solution.[3058]) Less than 1 mcg/mL of IgA is present in the 5% solution and less than 2 mcg/mL is present in the 10% solution.[3058] Trace amounts of IgM also are present.[3058]

Gammaplex (BPL) is available as a 5% solution in 50-, 100-, 200-, and 400-mL single-use bottles.[3061] The formulation also contains 5 g D-sorbitol in 100 mL of buffer solution, which contains glycine 0.6 g, sodium acetate 0.2 g, sodium chloride 0.3 g, and polysorbate 80 approximately 5 mg.[3061] IgA is present at a concentration of less than 10 mcg/mL.[3061]

Octagam (Octapharma) 5 and 10% solutions are available in 20-, 50-, 100-, and 200-mL single-use bottles.[3065] [3066] The 5% solution also is available in 500-mL single-use bottles.[3065] To prevent coring, needles larger than 16 gauge should not be used with either strength of the drug.[3065] [3066] Each mL of the 5% formulation also contains maltose 100 mg, octoxynol (TRITON X-100) no greater than 5 mcg, TNBP no greater than 1 mcg, and sodium no greater than 0.03 mmol in water for injection.[3065] Each mL of the 10% formulation also contains maltose 90 mg and sodium no greater than 0.03 mmol.[3066] No greater than 200 mcg/mL of IgA and 100 mcg/mL of IgM are present in the 5% solution.[3065] In the 10% formulation, IgA is present at an average concentration of 106 mcg/mL with even lesser amounts of IgM.[3066]

Privigen (CSL Behring) is available as a 10% solution in 50-, 100-, 200-, and 400-mL single-use vials.[3067] Each mL of the formulation also contains L-proline 0.25 mmol (range: 0.21 to 0.29 mmol) and trace amounts of sodium.[3067] The concentration of IgA present in the formulation does not exceed 25 mcg/mL.[3067]

Immune Globulin Human Products for Intravenous or Subcutaneous Administration

Several immune globulin human preparations (e.g., Gammagard Liquid, Gammaked, and Gamunex-C) may be administered by intravenous or subcutaneous infusion depending on the specific indication.[3059] [3060] [3062]

Gammagard Liquid (Baxter) is available as a 10% solution in 10-, 25-, 50-, 100-, 200-, and 300-mL single-use bottles.[3059] The formulation also contains glycine 0.25 M (approximately 18.8 mg/mL).[3059] IgA is present at an average concentration of 37 mcg/mL; trace amounts of IgM are present.[3059]

Gammaked and Gamunex-C (both manufactured by Grifols) are available as 10% solutions in 10-, 25-, 50-, 100-, and 200-mL single-use vials.[3060] [3062] Gamunex-C also is available in 400-mL single-use vials.[3062] Only 18-gauge needles should be used to penetrate the stopper of Gammaked or Gamunex-C 10-mL vials; for vials containing 25 mL or more, 16-gauge needles or dispensing pins should be used.[3060] [3062] Both products also contain glycine 0.16 to 0.24 M (approximately 12 to 18 mg/mL)

and residual caprylate concentrations no greater than 216 mg/mL (1.3 mmol/L).[3060] [3062] IgA is present at an average concentration of 46 mcg/mL; trace amounts of IgM also are present.[3060] [3062]

Immune Globulin Human Products for Subcutaneous Administration

Some immune globulin human products are intended only for administration by subcutaneous infusion.[3063] [3064] [3240]

Cuvitru (Baxalta) is available as a 20% solution in 5-, 10-, 20-, and 40-mL single-use vials for subcutaneous use only.[3240] Each vial also contains glycine 0.25 M.[3240] IgA is present at an average concentration of 80 mcg/mL.[3240]

Hizentra (CSL Behring) is available as a 20% solution in 5-, 10-, 20-, and 50-mL single-use vials for subcutaneous use only.[3063] Each mL of the formulation also contains L-proline 0.25 mmol (range: 0.21 to 0.29 mmol), polysorbate 80 0.008 to 0.03 mg, and trace amounts of sodium.[3063] The concentration of IgA present in the formulation does not exceed 50 mcg/mL.[3063]

HyQvia (Baxter) is available as a 10% solution in 25-, 50-, 100-, 200-, and 300-mL single-use vials; each vial is packaged with a vial containing recombinant human hyaluronidase 160 units/mL.[3064] The 2 vials should *not* be mixed; they are intended for *sequential* subcutaneous use only.[3064] The immune globulin human vial also contains glycine 0.25 M (approximately 18.8 mg/mL); IgA is present at an average concentration of less than 37 mcg/mL, and trace amounts of IgM also are present.[3064] Each mL of the recombinant human hyaluronidase solution also contains sodium chloride 8.5 mg, sodium phosphate dibasic dihydrate 1.78 mg, human albumin 1 mg, edetate disodium dihydrate 1 mg, and calcium chloride dihydrate 0.4 mg; sodium hydroxide 0.17 mg has been added for pH adjustment.[3064]

Immune Globulin Human Products for Intramuscular Administration

GamaSTAN S/D (Grifols) is available as a 15 to 18% solution in 2- and 10-mL single-use vials for intramuscular use only.[3057] The formulation also contains glycine 0.21 to 0.32 M (approximately 15.8 to 24 mg/mL).[3057] IgA presence and/or concentration is not specified in the prescribing information.[3057]

Reconstitution of Lyophilized Immune Globulin Human

To reconstitute a lyophilized immune globulin human powder, the diluent specified by the manufacturer should be added and then the vial or bottle should be rotated or swirled to dissolve particles.[3054] [3058] Foaming, which has been noted to be very slow to subside in some products,[3054] results from shaking and should be avoided[3054] [3058] because it may impede dissolution.[1499] In general, liquid and reconstituted immune globulin human products should not be shaken.[3053] [3054] [3058] [3059] [3060] [3061] [3062] [3063] [3064] [3067]

Reconstitution of Sandoglobulin (no longer commercially available in the US) with dextrose 5% has resulted in extended dissolution times of 75 and 135 minutes for the 3 and 6% solutions, respectively. With sodium chloride 0.9%, dissolution occurs over a few minutes; exceptional cases take up to 20 minutes.[1498]

pH

Bivigam: From 4 to 4.6.[3053]

Carimune NF: From 6.4 to 6.8.[3054]

Cuvitru: From 4.6 to 5.1.[3240]

Flebogamma DIF: From 5 to 6.[3055 3056]

GamaSTAN: From 6.4 to 7.2.[3057]

Gammagard Liquid: From 4.6 to 5.1.[3059]

Gammagard S/D: From 6.4 to 7.2.[3058]

Gammaked: From 4 to 4.5.[3060]

Gammaplex: From 4.8 to 5.1.[3061]

Gamunex-C: From 4 to 4.5.[3062]

Hizentra: From 4.6 to 5.2.[3063]

HyQvia: From 4.6 to 5.1.[3064]

Octagam 5%: From 5.1 to 6;[3065] Octagam 10%: From 4.5 to 5.[3066]

Privigen: From 4.6 to 5.[3067]

Osmolality

Carimune NF: Following reconstitution of the Carimune NF formulation of immune globulin human to targeted concentrations of 3, 6, 9, or 12%, the calculated osmolality of the solution varied with the diluent used.[3054] (See Table 3.)

Table 3. Calculated osmolality of reconstituted Carimune NF (CSL Behring)[3054]

Diluent	Osmolality (mOsm/kg)			
	Carimune NF 3%	Carimune NF 6%	Carimune NF 9%	Carimune NF 12%
Dextrose 5%	444	636	828	1020
Sodium chloride 0.9%	498	690	882	1074
Sterile water for injection	192	384	576	768

Cuvitru: 280 to 292 mOsm/kg.[3240]

Flebogamma DIF 5 and 10%: 240 to 370 mOsm/kg.[3055 3056]

Gammagard Liquid: 240 to 300 mOsm/kg.[3059]

Gammaked: 258 mOsm/kg.[3060]

Gammaplex: Typically 420 to 500 mOsm/kg.[3061] Not less than 240 mOsm/kg.[3061]

Gamunex-C: 258 mOsm/kg.[3062]

HyQvia: 240 to 300 mOsm/kg.[3064]

Octagam 5 and 10%: 310 to 380 mOsm/kg.[3065 3066]

Privigen: Approximately 320 mOsm/kg (range: 240 to 440 mOsm/kg).[3067]

Trade Name(s)

Bivigam, Carimune NF, Cuvitru, Flebogamma DIF, GamaSTAN S/D, Gammagard Liquid, Gammagard S/D, Gammaked, Gammaplex, Gamunex-C, Hizentra, HyQvia, Octagam, Privigen

Administration

Immune globulin human may be administered by intravenous infusion,[3053 3054 3055 3056 3058 3059 3060 3061 3062 3065 3066 3067] subcutaneous infusion using an infusion pump,[3059 3060 3062 3063 3064] or intramuscular injection.[3057] The route of administration and, where applicable, the rate of infusion depend upon the product selected, the indication for the drug, and patient-specific risk factors.[3053 3054 3055 3056 3057 3058 3059 3060 3061 3062 3063 3064 3065 3066 3067]

For intravenous infusion, a slow initial infusion rate is usually maintained for 10 to 30 minutes prior to gradually (e.g., every 15 to 30 minutes) increasing the rate according to patient tolerance and the product-specific maximum rate.[3053 3054 3055 3056 3059 3060 3061 3062 3065 3066 3067]

For subcutaneous infusion, initial infusion rates range from 5 to 20 mL/hour per site, with product-specific maximum rates and number of infusion sites.[3059 3060 3062 3063 3064 3240] For subcutaneous infusion of HyQvia, a 24-gauge subcutaneous needle set that is labeled for high flow rates should be used.[3064]

GamaSTAN S/D is administered only by intramuscular injection; the drug should *not* be administered subcutaneously or intravenously.[3057]

Stability

Recommended storage conditions vary among the different immune globulin human products.[3075 3076] Typically, intact immune globulin human products are stored either at room temperature, under refrigeration, or some combination of both and have a shelf life of about 24[3055 3056 3058 3059 3061 3065 3066] to 36 months[3059 3060 3062 3067 3240] from the date of manufacture.[3075 3076] Immune globulin human products should not be frozen.[3053 3054 3055 3056 3057 3058 3059 3060 3061 3062 3063 3064 3065 3066 3067 3240] Manufacturers of certain products state that the drug should be kept in the carton to protect from light.[3055 3056 3059 3061 3063 3064 3067 3240] Specific product labeling should be consulted for all storage requirements.

In general, liquid and reconstituted immune globulin human products should not be shaken.[3053 3054 3058 3059 3060 3061 3062 3063 3064 3067 3240]

Containers of immune globulin human are for single use only; partially used containers should be discarded.[3053 3054 3055 3056 3057 3058 3059 3060 3061 3062 3063 3064 3065 3066 3067 3240]

Most immune globulin human solutions are colorless to pale yellow in appearance.[3053 3055 3056 3058 3059 3060 3061 3062 3064 3067 3240] Oxidative reactions may be a cause of yellowish discoloration of intravenous immune globulin human solutions.[3076]

Two immune globulin human products (Gammagard S/D, Baxter and Polygam S/D [no longer commercially available in the US], American Red Cross) for intravenous use were reconstituted with sterile water for injection to concentrations of 50 mg/mL (5%) and 100 mg/mL (10%). Stability of the reconstituted product was evaluated in the original glass vials and also after transfer to PVC bags at 4°C for 48 hours and at 25°C for 12 hours. The visual appearance of the solutions remained acceptable, extremely low amounts of diethylhexyl phthalate (DEHP) plasticizer were leached from the PVC bags, and all tests for protein content and antibody activity indicated that stability was maintained throughout the study under both storage conditions.[2435]

pH Effects

One study evaluated multiple substances (e.g., sugars, polyalcohols, amino acids) for their ability to stabilize dissolved immune globulin G (IgG) molecules to prevent aggregation, dimerization, and fragmentation across a range of pH conditions when stored at 37°C for 90 days.[3076] The lowest percentage of aggregates was observed at weakly acidic conditions (pH 5.3) and the highest percentage of aggregates was observed at the lowest pH tested (i.e., 4.8 for L-lysine and L-ornithine; 4.1 for all other stabilizers tested).[3076] L-Proline, sucrose, and maltose showed good stabilizing effects over the entire pH range tested (4.1 to 6.8); glycine was less effective over this range, and L-lysine and L-ornithine were only marginally stabilizing at pH 6.8.[3076]

In terms of dimerization, L-proline was the most effective stabilizer tested, decreasing the percentage of dimers over the entire pH range tested.[3076] Sucrose also was effective over the entire pH range tested; however, its effects were less robust than those of L-proline.[3076] Glycine, L-lysine, and L-ornithine had negligible effects on dimerization, with glycine being the least effective.[3076] Mannitol and maltose actually increased dimer formation as compared with control solutions of immune globulin not containing a stabilizer.[3076]

The greatest amounts of fragmentation occurred at the lowest pH tested (i.e., 4.1).[3076] No substantial differences in fragmentation were observed among solutions containing L-proline, glycine, or no stabilizer except at a neutral pH of 6.8, where the formulation without stabilizer contained slightly more fragments.[3076] These results suggest that glycine and L-proline have a small inhibitory effect on neutral proteases (e.g., serine proteases).[3076]

Sorption

A stability evaluation of immune globulin human for intravenous use in PVC bags found no loss of activity due to sorption when compared to glass containers.[2435]

Filtration

For details on filtration of immune globulin human products, the product labeling should be consulted; some manufacturers do not make specific recommendations.

Carimune NF (CSL Behring) may be filtered, but filtration is not required.[3054] Filters with pore sizes of 15 μm or larger will be less likely to slow the infusion, especially at higher concentrations.[3054] Antibacterial filters (i.e., 0.2-μm filters) may be used.[3054]

Use of an inline filter with Gammagard Liquid (Baxter) is optional.[3059]

The administration set provided with Gammagard S/D (Baxter) contains an integral airway and a 15-μm filter.[3058] If an alternative administration set is used to administer the drug, an administration set containing a similar filter should be used.[3058]

Inline filtration is not required with Octagam (Octapharma); however, if a filter is used, the pore size should be 0.2 to 200 μm.[3065] [3066]

Plasticizer Leaching

Storage of reconstituted immune globulin human for intravenous use in PVC containers for 48 hours at 4°C and 12 hours at 25°C resulted in very low amounts of leached DEHP plasticizer from undetectable amounts up to a maximum of 86 ng/mL.[2435]

Compatibility Information

Solution Compatibility

Immune globulin human

Test Soln Name	Mfr	Mfr	Conc/L or %	Remarks	Ref	C/I
Dextrose 5%	a	HY[c]	2.5%	Visually compatible with no alteration of IgG concentration or functional activity	1885	C
Dextrose 15%	a	HY[c]	2.5%	Visually compatible with no alteration of IgG concentration or functional activity	1885	C
Dextrose 5% in sodium chloride 0.225%	a	HY[c]	2.5%	Visually compatible with no alteration of IgG concentration or functional activity	1885	C
Sodium chloride 0.9%		GRI[d]		Must not be mixed with sodium chloride 0.9%	3060	I
Sodium chloride 0.9%		GRI[e]		Must not be mixed with sodium chloride 0.9%	3062	I
TPN #194[b]	a	HY[c]	2.5%	Visually compatible with no alteration of IgG concentration or functional activity	1885	C

Solution Compatibility (Cont.)

Test Soln Name	Mfr	Mfr	Conc/L or %	Remarks	Ref	C/I
TPN #195[b]	a	HY[c]	2.5%	Visually compatible with no alteration of IgG concentration or functional activity	1885	C

[a] Tested in PVC containers.

[b] Refer to Appendix for the composition of parenteral nutrition solutions. TPN indicates a 2-in-1 admixture.

[c] Test performed using the lyophilized Gammagard (Baxter-Hyland) formulation.

[d] Test performed using the Gammaked (Grifols) formulation.

[e] Test performed using the Gamunex-C (Grifols) formulation.

Additive Compatibility

Immune globulin human

Test Drug	Mfr	Conc/L or %	Mfr	Conc/L or %	Test Solution	Remarks	Ref	C/I
Heparin sodium			GRI[a]			Stated to be incompatible	3060	I
Heparin sodium			GRI[b]			Stated to be incompatible	3062	I

[a] Test performed using the Gammaked (Grifols) formulation.

[b] Test performed using the Gamunex-C (Grifols) formulation.

Y-Site Injection Compatibility (1:1 Mixture)

Immune globulin human

Test Drug	Mfr	Conc	Mfr	Conc	Remarks	Ref	C/I
Fluconazole	RR	2 mg/mL	CU	50 mg/mL	Physically compatible for 24 hr at 25°C	1407	C
Sargramostim	IMM	6[a b] and 15 mcg/mL[b]	CU	50 mg/mL	Visually compatible for 2 hr	1618	C

[a] With albumin human 0.1%.

[b] Tested in sodium chloride 0.9%.

Additional Compatibility Information

Immune globulin human products are manufactured using differing processes and exhibit differing compatibility and stability characteristics.[3075] All manufacturers recommend using a separate infusion line for administration and not mixing other drugs with immune globulin human.[3053 3054 3055 3056 3058 3059 3060 3061 3062 3063 3064 3065 3066 3067 3240] Pooling of vials of the same product and strength (and where applicable, the same diluent used for reconstitution) into sterile empty infusion containers is acceptable to facilitate the administration of large doses; however, storage requirements and the maximum duration of time allowed from the time of pooling to infusion vary among products.[3053 3054 3055 3056 3058 3059 3060 3061 3062 3064 3065 3066 3067] Specific product labeling should be consulted. Different formulations of immune globulin human from the same or different manufacturers should not be mixed.[3053 3054 3055 3056 3058 3059 3060 3061 3062 3063 3064 3065 3066 3067] The manufacturers make the recommendations cited in Table 4 regarding compatibility with infusion solutions.

Table 4. Immune globulin human products: compatibility with infusion solutions

Product	Remarks	Ref
Bivigam	Do not dilute.	3053
Carimune NF	May be reconstituted with sodium chloride 0.9%, dextrose 5%, or sterile water for injection.	3054
Cuvitru	Do not dilute.	3240
Flebogamma DIF	Do not dilute.	3055, 3056
Gammagard Liquid	May be diluted with dextrose 5%; incompatible for dilution with sodium chloride 0.9%. Line may be flushed with sodium chloride 0.9%.	3059
Gammagard S/D	Reconstitute with sterile water for injection packaged with drug.	3058

Table 4. Immune globulin human products: compatibility with infusion solutions (Cont.)

Product	Remarks	Ref
Gammaked	May be diluted with dextrose 5%; incompatible for dilution with sodium chloride 0.9%. Line may be flushed with either dextrose 5% or sodium chloride 0.9%.	3060
Gamunex-C	May be diluted with dextrose 5%; incompatible for dilution with sodium chloride 0.9%. Line may be flushed with either dextrose 5% or sodium chloride 0.9%.	3062
HyQvia	Line may be flushed with either sodium chloride 0.9% or dextrose 5%.	3064
Octagam	Do not dilute. Line may be flushed with sodium chloride 0.9% or dextrose 5%.	3065, 3066
Privigen	May be diluted with dextrose 5%. Line may be flushed with dextrose 5% or sodium chloride 0.9%.	3067

Selected Revisions April 16, 2018. © Copyright, October 1992. American Society of Health-System Pharmacists, Inc.

Heparin Locks

The manufacturer of Gammaked and Gamunex-C immune globulin human products (Grifols) specifically states that heparin locks through which either drug has been administered should be flushed only with dextrose 5% or sodium chloride 0.9%; heparin should *not* be used to flush the lock.[3060] [3062]

Indomethacin Sodium Trihydrate
AHFS 28:08.04.92

Products

Indomethacin sodium trihydrate is supplied as a lyophilized product in vials containing the equivalent of 1 mg of indomethacin. Reconstitute with 1 or 2 mL of preservative-free sterile water for injection or sodium chloride 0.9% to yield a 1- or 0.5-mg/mL solution, respectively.[1(7/06)]

pH

From 6 to 7.5.[4]

Trade Name(s)

Indocin I.V.

Administration

Indomethacin sodium trihydrate is usually administered by intravenous injection over 20 to 30 minutes, although dilution after reconstitution is not recommended. Extravasation should be avoided.[1(7/06) 4]

Stability

Indomethacin sodium trihydrate is supplied as a white to yellow powder. Color variations have no relationship to indomethacin content. The vials should be stored below 30°C and protected from light.[1(7/06)]

The manufacturer recommends discarding any unused solution because of the absence of an antibacterial preservative.[1(7/06)] However, at 1 mg/mL in sodium chloride 0.9%, the drug is stated to be chemically stable for 16 days at room temperature.[4]

Solutions of indomethacin sodium trihydrate (Abbott and Fujisawa) diluted in sodium chloride 0.9% to a concentration of 0.1 mg/mL were evaluated for visual and chemical stability stored in the original vials. Little or no loss was found after storage for 10 days at 25°C.[2105]

The stability of indomethacin sodium trihydrate (Merck Sharp & Dohme) 0.5 mg/mL reconstituted with sterile water for injection in the original vials and repackaged into 1-mL polypropylene syringes (Sherwood) was reported. The reconstituted solutions were stored at room temperature (about 23°C) exposed to fluorescent light for 12 hours daily and under refrigeration (about 4°C) in the dark. Little or no loss of indomethacin in the refrigerated solutions occurred after 14 days of storage. The solutions stored at room temperature exhibited 9% loss in 10 days. The solutions at both temperatures remained visually clear and colorless throughout the study.[2228]

pH Effects

Reconstitution of indomethacin sodium trihydrate with solutions having pH values below 6 may result in precipitation of free indomethacin.[1(7/06) 4]

Compatibility Information
Solution Compatibility

Indomethacin sodium trihydrate

Test Soln Name	Test Soln Mfr	Mfr	Conc/L or %	Remarks	Ref	C/I
Dextrose 2.5%	BA	MSD	1 g[a]	Visually compatible for 24 hr at 28°C	1527	C
Dextrose 5%	BA	MSD	1 g[a]	Visually compatible for 24 hr at 28°C	1527	C
Dextrose 7.5%	BA	MSD	1 g[a]	Haze forms in 2 hr and precipitate forms in 4 hr	1527	I
Dextrose 10%	BA	MSD	1 g[a]	Haze forms in 2 hr and precipitate forms in 4 hr	1527	I

[a] Tested in sodium chloride 0.9%.

Drugs in Syringe Compatibility

Indomethacin sodium trihydrate

Test Drug	Mfr	Amt	Mfr	Amt	Remarks	Ref	C/I
Pantoprazole sodium	[a]	4 mg/1 mL		0.5 mg/1 mL	Precipitates within 1 hr	2574	I

[a] Test performed using the formulation WITHOUT edetate disodium.

DOI: 10.37573/9781585286850.209

Y-Site Injection Compatibility (1:1 Mixture)

Indomethacin sodium trihydrate

Test Drug	Mfr	Conc	Mfr	Conc	Remarks	Ref	C/I
Amino acids	MG	1 and 2%[c]	MSD	1 mg/mL[b]	Haze forms in 2 hr and white precipitate forms in 4 hr	1527	I
Amino acids	MG	1 and 2%[d]	MSD	1 mg/mL[b]	Haze forms in 30 min and white precipitate forms in 1 hr	1527	I
Calcium gluconate	AMR	100 mg/mL	MSD	1 mg/mL[b]	Fine yellow precipitate forms within 1 hr	1527	I
Dobutamine HCl	LI	1.2 mg/mL[a]	MSD	1 mg/mL[b]	Hazy precipitate forms immediately	1527	I
Dopamine HCl	AB	1.2 mg/mL[a]	MSD	1 mg/mL[b]	Hazy precipitate forms immediately	1527	I
Furosemide	AB	10 mg/mL	MSD	1 mg/mL[b]	Visually compatible for 24 hr at 28°C	1527	C
Gentamicin sulfate		1 mg/mL[a]	MSD	0.5 and 1 mg/mL[a]	White turbidity forms immediately and becomes white flakes in 1 hr	1550	I
Insulin, regular	NOV	1 unit/mL[b]	MSD	1 mg/mL[b]	Visually compatible for 24 hr at 28°C	1527	C
Levofloxacin	OMN	5 mg/mL[a]	ME	1 mg/mL	Cloudy precipitate forms	2233	I
Potassium chloride	AB	0.2 mEq/mL[a]	MSD	1 mg/mL[b]	Visually compatible for 24 hr at 28°C	1527	C
Sodium bicarbonate	AB	0.5 mEq/mL[a]	MSD	1 mg/mL[b]	Visually compatible for 24 hr at 28°C	1527	C
Sodium nitroprusside	AB	0.2 mg/mL[a]	MSD	1 mg/mL[b]	Visually compatible for 24 hr at 28°C	1527	C
Tobramycin sulfate		1 mg/mL[a]	MSD	0.5 and 1 mg/mL[a]	White turbidity forms immediately and becomes white flakes in 1 hr	1550	I

[a] Tested in dextrose 5%.

[b] Tested in sodium chloride 0.9%.

[c] TrophAmine in dextrose 10%.

[d] TrophAmine in sterile water for injection.

Selected Revisions February 1, 2013. © Copyright, October 1994.
American Society of Health-System Pharmacists, Inc.

Infliximab

AHFS 92:36

Products

Infliximab is available as a lyophilized powder in 100-mg preservative-free, single-use vials.[3035] Each vial also contains sucrose 500 mg, polysorbate 80 0.5 mg, monobasic sodium phosphate monohydrate 2.2 mg, and dibasic sodium phosphate dihydrate 6.1 mg.[3035]

Calculate the required number of infliximab vials and the total volume of reconstituted solution needed to provide the appropriate dose.[3035] Each 100-mg vial should be reconstituted by transferring 10 mL of sterile water for injection into the vial using a syringe with 21-gauge or smaller needle, directing the stream of diluent against the vial wall.[3035] The solution should be gently swirled by rotating the vial to dissolve the powder.[3035] Foaming of the solution may occur; the reconstituted solution should be allowed to stand for 5 minutes.[3035] Prolonged or vigorous agitation should be avoided; the vial should *not* be shaken.[3035] The resultant reconstituted solution contains infliximab 10 mg/mL.[3035]

The total volume required of the reconstituted infliximab solution should be further diluted to 250 mL by first removing a volume of diluent (equal to the volume of infliximab solution to be added) from a 250-mL container of sodium chloride 0.9%.[3035] The appropriate dose of the reconstituted solution should then be slowly added to the bottle or bag and gently mixed.[3035] The manufacturer states that solutions other than 0.9% sodium chloride should *not* be used for dilution.[3035] The final concentration of infliximab in the resultant diluted solution should be between 0.4 and 4 mg/mL.[3035]

pH

Reconstituted infliximab solutions have a pH of approximately 7.2.[3035]

Trade Name(s)

Remicade

Administration

Infliximab is administered by intravenous infusion over a period of at least 2 hours.[3035] The diluted solution for infusion *must* be administered through an infusion set with a low-protein-binding inline filter with a pore size of 1.2 μm or smaller.[3035]

Stability

Intact vials of infliximab should be stored at 2 to 8°C.[3035] These unopened vials also may be stored at temperatures not exceeding 30°C with up to 75% relative humidity for a single period of up to 6 months; however, the cartons of such vials must be marked with a new expiration date of 6 months after transfer to these storage conditions.[3035 3077] Vials should be used by the newly marked expiration date or the original expiration date printed on the carton, whichever comes first.[3035 3077] The drug should not be returned to refrigerated storage once it has been removed.[3035 3077]

Results of a stability study of unreconstituted infliximab vials stored at –20°C for 7 days with 3 freeze-thaw cycles followed by storage for up to 28 months at 2 to 8°C did not demonstrate any adverse effects on the biochemical or physical properties of infliximab.[3077] No adverse effects on the biochemical and physical properties of infliximab were observed following exposure of vials of the unreconstituted drug to 50°C for 3 days and return to the recommended temperature range of 2 to 8°C for 28 months; no significant increase in visible particle content was observed following exposure to 50°C for 3 days or at the 28-month time point after exposure.[3077]

Infliximab is a white lyophilized powder that forms an opalescent, colorless to light yellow solution when reconstituted with sterile water for injection.[3035] The solution may develop a few translucent particles because infliximab is a protein.[3035] The drug should be visually inspected for discoloration and particulate matter prior to administration.[3035] The solution should not be used if the lyophilized cake has not fully dissolved or if visibly opaque particles, foreign particles, or discoloration is present.[3035]

The manufacturer states that administration of the drug should begin within 3 hours of reconstitution and dilution to protect against microbiological contamination.[3035 3079]

In studies evaluating the stability of infliximab after reconstitution, the drug was found to remain biochemically and physically stable for 24 hours at room temperature when reconstituted with sterile water for injection, sodium chloride 0.45%, or sodium chloride 0.9%.[3078 3080] Reconstitution of the drug with dextrose 5% resulted in an irreversible reaction detected within 24 hours by changes in the isoelectric focusing banding pattern as compared with the reference standard; reconstitution of the drug with dextrose 5% is not recommended.[3078]

Ikeda et al. studied the stability of infliximab at a concentration of 0.4 mg/mL in sodium chloride 0.9% in PVC bags, which were stored at 4°C for up to 14 days.[3122] An indirect ELISA method was used to determine infliximab activity based on calculated consumption of a known quantity of tumor necrosis factor [TNF; TNF-α] when combined with infliximab.[3122] The authors reported that no loss of infliximab's ability to bind TNF-α was detected at 7 or 14 days.[3122] However, other measures of stability (e.g., physical or chemical analyses or other bioassay results) were not reported in this study;[2812 3122] in addition, the manufacturer stated that the protocols and methods it has used to assess infliximab stability are proprietary and specific to the drug, and it cannot support nor refute the results of this study.[2290]

Plasticizer Leaching

The surfactant (polysorbate 80) contained in the infliximab formulation can leach plasticizer from diethylhexyl phthalate

DOI: 10.37573/9781585286850.210

(DEHP)-plasticized PVC containers and administration sets.[3035] [3081] To eliminate the potential for exposure to DEHP for patients receiving infliximab, the use of DEHP-containing PVC equipment with infliximab was previously restricted; however, potential exposure to DEHP from a dose of infliximab (for a 50- to 70-kg patient) was found to be approximately 50 to 70 times lower than the reference dose for DEHP set by the US Environmental Protection Agency (EPA) based on results of DEHP toxicity studies.[3081] Based on this information, the requirement of using non-PVC administration equipment with infliximab has been removed from the current prescribing information.[3035] [3081]

Filtration

The diluted solution of infliximab for infusion *must* be administered with an infusion set containing a low-protein-binding inline filter with a pore size of 1.2 μm or smaller.[3035]

Compatibility Information

Solution Compatibility

Infliximab

Test Soln Name	Mfr	Mfr	Conc/L or %	Remarks	Ref	C/I
Sodium chloride 0.45%		JN	2.5 g	Physically and biochemically stable for 24 hr at room temperature	3080	C
Sodium chloride 0.9%	a	JN	0.4 to 4 g	Physically and biochemically stable for 24 hr at room temperature	3079	C
Sodium chloride 0.9%	b	JN	0.4 to 4 g	Physically and biochemically stable for 24 hr at room temperature	3079	C
Sodium chloride 0.9%	c	JN	0.4 to 4 g	Physically and biochemically stable for 24 hr at room temperature	3079	C

[a] Tested in polyethylene containers.

[b] Tested in ethyl vinyl acetate (EVA) containers.

[c] Tested in glass containers.

Insulin

AHFS 68:20.08

Products

Regular insulin is available in 10-mL vials and 1.5-mL prefilled syringes and syringe cartridges at a concentration of 100 units/mL. Human insulin is produced using recombinant DNA technology. Regular concentrated insulin (Lilly) also is available in 20-mL vials containing 500 units/mL. Glycerin 1.4 to 1.8% and phenol or cresol 0.1 to 0.25% also may be present.[1(1/08)] [4]

Several modified forms of insulin (Isophane, Lente, etc.) are available, each having a characteristic onset of action, time to peak effect, and duration of action.[4]

Adequately mixing these products is necessary prior to use, but vigorous shaking may entrain air bubbles that could interfere with accurate dosing. Gentle shaking of the vial combined with end-over-end inversion and rolling in the palms has been suggested.[2270]

pH

All regular insulin products have a neutral pH of approximately 7 to 7.8.[4] [261]

Trade Name(s)

Humulin R

Administration

Regular insulin usually is administered by subcutaneous injection into the thighs, arms, buttocks, or abdomen, with sites rotated. Syringes calibrated for the particular concentration of insulin to be given must be used. Regular insulin also may be administered intramuscularly or by intravenous infusion, usually diluted in sodium chloride 0.9%. Regular insulin is the only form of insulin that can be given intravenously.[4]

Care is required when adding insulin to infusion solutions, especially in flexible containers. Adding insulin to a plasma expander carrier solution hanging in the use position resulted in stratification, with the insulin floating to the top. Little insulin was delivered initially, and 87% of the insulin appeared in the last 28% of the solution. Repeated inversion and agitation of the container to effect thorough mixture eliminates this stratification, yielding an even distribution and a constant delivery concentration.[85]

Disposable insulin syringes are usually siliconized. Reuse of disposable plastic insulin syringes (Plastipak Microfine II, Becton Dickinson) has resulted in contamination of vials of insulin with silicone oil, causing a white precipitate and impairment of biological effects and is not recommended. In a test of insulin from several sources, repeated drawing of the insulin into the disposable syringes and then expulsion of it back into the vials introduced substantial amounts of silicone oil; a white precipitate formed within 12 hours at 8°C.[1110]

Stability

Regular insulin should be stored under refrigeration and protected from freezing.[1(1/08)] [4] Although refrigerated storage is required, some manufacturers have stated the drug may be stored at room temperature for 28 to 30 days.[2745] [2769] Freezing of insulin products may alter the protein structure, decreasing concentration.[559] In one study of several insulin products, 1 cycle of freezing for 45 hours followed by slow thawing at 21°C or rapid thawing in a water bath at 37°C did not result in a loss of bioactivity. However, microscopic examination revealed particle aggregation, and some crystal damage had occurred.[680]

The stability of regular insulin (Novo Nordisk) was evaluated under simulated shipping conditions. Sample vials were packaged in both insulated and non-insulated mailers and packaged with either two 12-oz. frozen gel packs for simulated summer mailing or one 12-oz. frozen gel pack for simulated winter shipping. The evaluation was conducted for simulated transit periods ranging from 24 hours to 120 hours (overnight air delivery to ground delivery). Visual inspection found no change in appearance in any of the samples tested. Microscopy found no formation of aggregates. No loss of insulin content occurred in any of the samples with any of the shipping methods and conditions. Size exclusion chromatography found little or no change in high-molecular-weight protein content. The regular insulin remained within USP specifications with all of the shipping methods and time periods studied.[2769]

As with other protein and peptide products, insulin aggregation with possible reduced bioactivity can be a problem. Aggregates have been found to form in a variety of infusion devices and under various storage conditions, including static storage and continuous rotational or reciprocating motion.[1948] [1995] [2406] Aggregation may occur at air-water interfaces. Such interfaces have been generated by turbulence, such as shaking and repeatedly passing insulin through a syringe and needle. With sufficient vigor, both actions can turn the insulin turbid from insoluble aggregates.[1948] In addition, contact with silicone rubber appears to promote insulin aggregation.[1995]

Factors that increase the formation rate of insulin transformation products (such as deamidated insulin, covalent dimers, and higher oligamers) in beef and human insulin products were evaluated during 6 months of storage. A low rate of transformation product appeared at 4°C. Higher temperatures, as might occur when insulin is carried in a shirt pocket or car glove compartment, accelerated this production (especially for human insulin) and also fibril formation. Exposure to light increased the dimer and higher oligamer content. Insulin should not be exposed to direct sunlight or subjected to vibration or extremes of temperature.[1663]

DOI: 10.37573/9781585286850.211

The appearance of transformation products was found to be 2- to 3-fold greater when using polyvinyl chloride (PVC) administration sets compared to polyethylene and polypropylene infusion equipment. Furthermore, use of the PVC sets resulted in up to 30% reduction in the concentration of methylparaben, phenol, and m-cresol preservatives in insulin products.[311]

Regular insulin, containing 100 units/mL, is clear and colorless or almost colorless. The concentrated injection containing 500 units/mL may be straw colored. Discoloration, turbidity, or unusual viscosity indicates deterioration or contamination.[4]

Syringes

It has been stated that neutral regular insulin (and also NPH and Lente insulin) can be stored for 5 to 7 days under refrigeration in either glass or plastic syringes. Mixtures of these insulins also can be stored similarly.[679]

Insulin soluble, BP, 1.6 units/2 mL diluted in sodium chloride 0.9% was stored for 18 hours at room temperature in the following plastic syringes: Brunswick (Sherwood Medical), Plastipak (Becton Dickinson), and Sabre (Gillette U.K.). The first 2 syringes have polypropylene barrels; the Sabre has a combination polypropylene–polystyrene barrel. No significant loss of insulin occurred due to sorption. Significant (but unspecified) losses did occur when the concentration was reduced to 0.2 unit/mL, but the make of syringe did not influence this adsorption.[784]

No apparent degradation or binding occurred for at least 14 days when insulin, USP (Lilly), 100 units/mL was stored under refrigeration in 1-mL polypropylene syringes (Becton Dickinson).[805]

The soluble insulins Velosulin (Nordisk), Actrapid and Human Actrapid (Novo), Humulin S (Lilly), Neusulin (Wellcome), and Quicksol (Boots) in 1-mL 100-unit Plastipak syringes (Becton Dickinson) exhibited no loss in 29 days when stored at 4 and 20°C.[1275]

Regular insulin human (Humulin R, 100 units/mL, Lilly), isophane insulin human (Humulin N, 100 units/mL, Lilly), and the combination product (Humulin N/R 70/30, Lilly) were evaluated for stability packaged in plastic syringes. Test samples of 0.4 mL of each insulin product were drawn into 1-mL polypropylene syringes (Plastipak, Becton Dickinson) and 1-mL polypropylene–ethylene copolymer syringes (Terumo) and stored for 28 days at 4 and 23°C. No loss of insulin from any insulin product occurred in either syringe type. However, the antibacterial preservatives present in the insulin formulations were lost, especially in the polypropylene syringes at room temperature. Storage under refrigeration to slow the loss of preservative as much as possible was recommended.[1124]

Infusion Pumps

Insulin solutions may form highly insoluble polymers. In areas having high shear rates such as the tubing, cannula, and needle, aggregation can lead to blockage. In low shear areas such as the insulin reservoir of implantable pumps, gentle agitation can lead to the formation of a cross-linked gel.[1112]

Sorption

The adsorption of insulin to the surfaces of intravenous infusion solution containers, glass and plastic (including PVC, ethylene vinyl acetate [EVA], polyethylene, and other polyolefins), tubing, and filters has been demonstrated. Estimates of the loss range up to about 80% for the entire infusion apparatus, although varying results using differing test methods, equipment, and procedures have been reported. Estimates of adsorption of around 20 to 30% are common. The percent adsorbed is inversely proportional to the concentration of insulin. Other important factors are the amount of container surface area and the fill volume of the solution. The amount of insulin adsorbed varies directly with the available surface area and indirectly with the ratio of fluid volume to container capacity. The container material is a factor, with glass possibly adsorbing insulin more extensively than some plastics. Other factors influencing the extent of insulin adsorption include the type of solution, type and length of administration set, rate of infusion, temperature, previous exposure of tubing to insulin, and presence of albumin human, whole blood, electrolytes, and other drugs.[266 267 268 269 420 422 423 424 425 426 428 533 681 682 683 684 685 686 687 688 689 690 854 908 909 910 911 912 913 1111 1112 1274 1282 1408 1497 1664 1665 2079 2301]

The adsorption of insulin to container surfaces is an instantaneous process.[267 425 911 912 913] However, the effect of adsorption on the deliverable amount of insulin appears to vary with time. Several investigators reported a dramatic initial drop in delivered insulin followed by a return to higher (although variable) levels. The bulk of the insulin adsorption apparently occurs in the first 30 to 60 minutes. Although flow rate does not influence total insulin binding, the plateau phase of delivered insulin may be reached more quickly at faster infusion rates.[422 424 425 426 428 687 688 689 854 2301]

In a study of insulin loss during simulated delivery to low-birth-weight infants, insulin 0.2 unit/mL was delivered at rates of 0.05 and 0.2 mL/hr through microbore PVC tubing and polyethylene-lined PVC tubing. During the early hours, the amount of insulin delivered through both types of tubing was much reduced, especially at the slower delivery rate. The authors indicated that this loss might contribute to the 14- to 24-hour delays in blood glucose normalization in these infants. The priming of microbore tubing with 5 units/mL of insulin for 20 minutes was suggested to accelerate the achievement of steady-state insulin delivery. The time courses of insulin delivery observed for representative unprimed and primed sets are presented in Table 1.[2301]

Regular human insulin 0.1 unit/mL in sodium chloride 0.9% in VISIV polyolefin bags was tested for 24 hours at room temperature near 23°C. About 35% loss occurred, which is consistent with the drug's potential for adsorption to surfaces.[2660 2792]

Table 1. Approximate amount of insulin delivered through unprimed and primed[a] administration sets[2301]

Set Type	Delivered Insulin (%)				
	1 hr	2 hr	4 hr	8 hr	24 hr
Unprimed	17	11	27	55	100
Primed	70	70	70	100	100

[a] Primed with insulin 5 units/mL for 20 minutes.

The addition of albumin human to infusion solutions helps to reduce the adsorption of insulin. The degree to which albumin human prevents adsorption is uncertain. Reported losses of insulin in albumin-containing solutions have varied from about zero to approximately 30%. However, most work indicates a substantial reduction in insulin adsorption.[266] [267] [268] [269] [418] [428] [683] [684] [685] [908] [909] Other additives such as vitamins, electrolytes, and drugs may also have a similar effect.[425] [909] [914]

Other recommended approaches to avoiding or minimizing adsorption include adding a small amount of the patient's blood to the insulin solution[689] [690] [691] and storing or flushing the administration apparatus with the insulin solution to saturate the set prior to administration.[428] [1111] [2301] Addition of extra insulin to compensate for the losses has also been suggested.[1112] As an alternative, administration of insulin using a syringe pump with a short cannula has been recommended. This procedure will reduce the surface area in relation to the amount of insulin present.[1033]

The clinical significance of this adsorption is uncertain. Some clinical studies indicated no relevant effect on the success of therapy.[415] [427] [685] Some investigators felt that the importance of insulin adsorption to the surfaces of the infusion container and tubing may be a moot point since the dosage is individualized on the basis of blood and urine glucose determinations. Simply adding more insulin may saturate binding sites and yield the desired response.[270] [271] [854] [909]

Still others indicated that the adsorption may indeed be relevant for solutions with an insulin content of less than 100 or 200 units/L.[424] [426] [428] [908] [2301]

If the apparent dose of intravenous insulin is used as the basis for determining the subsequent dose upon discontinuing the intravenous one, then a potential for dosing error exists. The actual amount of insulin being administered could be substantially less than the apparent amount.[533]

Whether one attempts to prevent insulin adsorption or not, it does not appear to be possible to add an amount of insulin to an infusion solution and know precisely what portion of that amount will actually be given to the patient. Monitoring the patient's response to therapy and making the appropriate adjustments on the basis of that response are, therefore, of prime importance.[690] [854] [1664]

Implantable Pumps

Insulin, regular human (Genapol, Hoeschst-Roussel) 400 units/mL with heparin sodium 500 units/mL was evaluated in MIP 2001 implantable pumps (MiniMed) at 37°C for 3 months. The drug solution remained visually clear, but the insulin content dropped to 65% of the initial amount. The activity of heparin declined by even more. Only 45% remained after 3 months. The losses were attributed to the shaking that occurred during use rather than temperature, interaction with pump materials, or interaction of the 2 drugs with each other.[239]

Compatibility Information

Solution Compatibility

Insulin, regular

Test Soln Name	Mfr	Mfr	Conc/L or %	Remarks	Ref	C/I
Sodium chloride 0.9%	HOS[b]	NOV	100 units	35 to 45% loss in 24 hr due to adsorption	2660, 2792	?
Sodium chloride 0.9%	BA[a]	LI	1000 units	10% loss in 1 hr in 50-mL bag and in 4 hr in 250-mL bag	2079	I
TNA #267[c]	[d]	NOV	10 units	40 to 60% loss likely due to sorption	2599	I

[a] Tested in PVC containers.

[b] Tested in VISIV polyolefin containers.

[c] Refer to Appendix for the composition of parenteral nutrition solutions. TPN indicates a 2-in-1 admixture.

[d] Tested in EVA containers.

Additive Compatibility

Insulin, regular

Test Drug	Mfr	Conc/L or %	Mfr	Conc/L or %	Test Solution	Remarks	Ref	C/I
Cytarabine	UP	100 and 500 mg		40 units	D5W	Fine precipitate forms	174	I
Meropenem	ZEN	1 and 20 g	LI	1000 units	NS	Visually compatible for 4 hr at room temperature	1994	C
Octreotide acetate		50 mcg		5 units	TPN	Substantial insulin loss	1377	I

Additive Compatibility (Cont.)

Test Drug	Mfr	Conc/L or %	Mfr	Conc/L or %	Test Solution	Remarks	Ref	C/I
Ranitidine HCl	GL	600 mg	LI	1000 units	NSa	Visually compatible. Little ranitidine loss in 24 hr at ambient temperature but insulin losses of 9% in 4 hr and 14% in 24 hr, presumably due to sorption	2079	I

a Tested in PVC containers.

Drugs in Syringe Compatibility

Insulin, regular

Test Drug	Mfr	Amt	Mfr	Amt	Remarks	Ref	C/I
Pantoprazole sodium	a	4 mg/1 mL		100 units/1 mL	Precipitates within 1 hr	2574	I

a Test performed using the formulation WITHOUT edetate disodium.

Y-Site Injection Compatibility (1:1 Mixture)

Insulin, regular

Test Drug	Mfr	Conc	Mfr	Conc	Remarks	Ref	C/I
Amiodarone HCl	WY	4.8 mg/mLa	LI	1 unit/mLa	Visually compatible for 24 hr at 23°C	1877	C
Ampicillin sodium	WY	20 mg/mLb	LI	0.2 unit/mLb	Physically compatible for 2 hr at 25°C	1395	C
Ampicillin sodium–sulbactam sodium	RR	20 mg/mLb l	LI	0.2 unit/mLb	Physically compatible for 2 hr at 25°C	1395	C
Aztreonam	SQ	20 mg/mL	LI	0.2 unit/mLb	Physically compatible for 2 hr at 25°C	1395	C
Caspofungin acetate	ME	0.7 mg/mLb	NOV	1 unit/mLb	Physically compatible for 4 hr at room temperature	2758	C
Caspofungin acetate	ME	0.5 mg/mLb	NOV	1 unit/mLb	Physically compatible over 60 min	2766	C
Cefazolin sodium	LI	20 mg/mLa	LI	0.2 unit/mLb	Physically compatible for 2 hr at 25°C	1395	C
Cefepime HCl	BMS	120 mg/mLc		100 units/mL	Physically compatible with less than 10% cefepime loss. Insulin not tested	2513	C
Cefotetan disodium	STU	20 and 40 mg/mLa	LI	0.2 unit/mLb	Physically compatible for 2 hr at 25°C	1395	C
Ceftaroline fosamil	FOR	2.22 mg/mLf	NOV	1 unit/mLf	Physically compatible for 4 hr at 23°C	2826	C
Ceftazidime	GSK	120 mg/mLh		100 units/mL	Physically compatible with less than 10% ceftazidime loss. Insulin not tested	2513	C
Ceftolozane sulfate–tazobactam sodium	CUB	10 mg/mLe p	NVN	1 unit/mLe	Physically compatible for 2 hr	3262	C
Cisatracurium besylate	AB	1 mg/mLb	LI	1 unit/mLb	Physically compatible for 1 hr at 23°C	3157	C
Clarithromycin	AB	4 mg/mLa	NOV	4 units/mLa	Visually compatible for 72 hr at both 30 and 17°C	2174	C
Clevidipine butyrate	CHS	0.5 mg/mL		100 units/mL	Physically compatible for 24 hr at 23°C	3334	C

Y-Site Injection Compatibility (1:1 Mixture) (Cont.)

Test Drug	Mfr	Conc	Mfr	Conc	Remarks	Ref	C/I
Cloxacillin sodium	SMX	100 mg/mL	LI	100 units/mL	Physically compatible for up to 4 hr at room temperature	3245	C
Digoxin	ES	0.005 mg/mL[b]	LI	1 unit/mL[b]	Physically compatible for 3 hr	1316	C
Digoxin	ES	0.005 mg/mL[a]	LI	1 unit/mL[a]	Slight haze in 1 hr	1316	I
Diltiazem HCl	BED			100 units/mL	Physically incompatible	2875	I
Dobutamine HCl	LI	4 mg/mL[e]	LI	1 unit/mL[e]	Physically compatible for 3 hr	1316	C
Dopamine HCl	DU	3.2 mg/mL[a]	LI	1 unit/mL[a]	White precipitate forms immediately, dissolves quickly, and reforms in 24 hr at 23°C	1877	I
Doripenem	JJ	5 mg/mL[a b]	NOV	1 unit/mL[a b]	Physically compatible for 4 hr at 23°C	2743	C
Doxapram HCl	RB	2 mg/mL[a]	NOV	1 unit/mL[d]	Visually compatible for 4 hr at 23°C	2470	C
Eravacycline dihydrochloride	TET	0.6 mg/mL[b]	LI	1 unit/mL[b]	Physically compatible for 2 hr at room temperature	3532	C
Esmolol HCl	DU	40 mg/mL[a]	LI	1 unit/mL[a]	Visually compatible for 24 hr at 23°C	1877	C
Famotidine	MSD	0.2 mg/mL[a]	LI	0.03 unit/mL[a]	Physically compatible for 4 hr at 25°C	1188	C
Gentamicin sulfate	TR	1.2 mg/mL[b]	LI	0.2 unit/mL[b]	Physically compatible for 2 hr at 25°C	1395	C
Heparin sodium	ES	60 units/mL[a]	LI	0.2 unit/mL[b]	Physically compatible for 2 hr at 25°C	1395	C
Hydroxyethyl starch 130/0.4 in sodium chloride 0.9%	FRK	6%	NOV	5, 27.5, 50 units/mL[a]	Visually compatible for 24 hr at room temperature	2770	C
Ibuprofen lysinate	OVA	10 mg/mL	LI	0.1 and 1 unit/mL[b]	Physically compatible for 4 hr at room temperature	3541	C
Imipenem–cilastatin sodium	MSD	4 and 5 mg/mL[b m]	LI	0.2 unit/mL[b]	Physically compatible for 2 hr at 25°C	1395	C
Indomethacin sodium trihydrate	MSD	1 mg/mL[b]	NOV	1 unit/mL[b]	Visually compatible for 24 hr at 28°C	1527	C
Isavuconazonium sulfate	ASP	1.5 mg/mL[e]	NVN	1 unit/mL[e]	Physically compatible for 2 hr	3263	C
Labetalol HCl	GL	5 mg/mL	LI	1 unit/mL[a]	Visually compatible for 4 hr. White precipitate forms in 24 hr at 23°C	1877	?
Letermovir	ME	[b]		[b]	Physically compatible	3398	C
Levofloxacin	OMN	5 mg/mL[a]	LI	100 units/mL	Cloudy precipitate forms	2233	I
Levofloxacin	OMN	5 mg/mL[a]	LI	1 unit/mL	Visually compatible for 4 hr at 24°C	2233	C
Magnesium sulfate	LY	40 mg/mL[g]	LI	0.2 unit/mL[b]	Physically compatible for 2 hr at 25°C	1395	C
Meperidine HCl	WY	10 mg/mL[b]	LI	0.2 unit/mL[b]	Physically compatible for 1 hr at 25°C	1338	C
Meperidine HCl	AST	50 mg/mL[a]	LI	0.2 unit/mL[b]	Physically compatible for 2 hr at 25°C	1395	C
Meropenem	ZEN	1 and 50 mg/mL[b]	LI	0.2 unit/mL[h]	Visually compatible for 4 hr at room temperature	1994	C
Meropenem		50 mg/mL	LI	100 units/mL	Physically compatible for 4 hr at room temperature	3538	C
Meropenem–vaborbactam	TMC	8 mg/mL[b n]	LI	1 unit/mL[b]	Physically compatible for 3 hr at 20 to 25°C	3380	C

Y-Site Injection Compatibility (1:1 Mixture) (Cont.)

Test Drug	Mfr	Conc	Mfr	Conc	Remarks	Ref	C/I
Micafungin sodium	ASP	1.5 mg/mL[b]	NOV	1 unit/mL[b]	Increase in haze and microparticulates form in 4 hr	2683	I
Midazolam HCl	RC	1 mg/mL[a]	LI	1 unit/mL[a]	Visually compatible for 24 hr at 23°C	1877	C
Milrinone lactate	SW	0.4 mg/mL[a]	NOV	1 unit/mL[b]	Visually compatible. Little loss of either drug in 4 hr at 23°C	2214	C
Morphine sulfate	ES	1 mg/mL[b]	LI	0.2 unit/mL[b]	Physically compatible for 1 hr at 25°C	1338	C
Morphine sulfate	ES	5 mg/mL[a]	LI	0.2 unit/mL[b]	Physically compatible for 2 hr at 25°C	1395	C
Morphine sulfate	SX	1 mg/mL[a]	LI	1 unit/mL[a]	Visually compatible for 24 hr at 23°C	1877	C
Nafcillin sodium	BA	20 and 40 mg/mL[a]	LI	0.2 unit/mL[b]	Precipitates immediately	1395	I
Nesiritide	SCI	50 mcg/mL[a b]		Up to 100 units/mL	Physically incompatible	2625	I
Nitroglycerin	OM	0.2 mg/mL[a]	LI	1 unit/mL[a]	Visually compatible for 24 hr at 23°C	1877	C
Norepinephrine bitartrate	STR	0.064 mg/mL[a]	LI	1 unit/mL[a]	White precipitate forms immediately	1877	I
Oritavancin diphosphate	TAR	0.8, 1.2, and 2 mg/mL[a]	LI	1 unit/mL[a]	Visually compatible for 4 hr at 20 to 24°C	2928	C
Oxytocin	PD	0.02 unit/mL[i]	LI	0.2 unit/mL[b]	Physically compatible for 2 hr at 25°C	1395	C
Pantoprazole sodium	ALT[c]	0.16 to 0.8 mg/mL[b]	LI	5 to 50 units/mL[a]	Visually compatible for 12 hr at 23°C	2603	C
Pentobarbital sodium	WY	2 mg/mL[e]	LI	1 unit/mL[e]	Physically compatible for 3 hr	1316	C
Plazomicin sulfate	ACH	24 mg/mL[e]	LI	1 unit/mL[e]	Physically compatible for 1 hr at 20 to 25°C	3432	C
Propofol	ZEN[q]	10 mg/mL	NOV	1 unit/mL[a]	Physically compatible for 1 hr at 23°C	2066	C
Quinupristin–dalfopristin		2 mg/mL[a o]		100 units/mL	Reported to be incompatible	3230	I
Ranitidine HCl	GL	1 mg/mL[b]	LI	1 unit/mL[b]	Visually compatible. Little loss of ranitidine in 4 hr but insulin losses of 9% in 1 hr and 20% in 4 hr, presumably due to sorption	2079	I
Sodium bicarbonate	AB	1 mEq/mL	LI	1 unit/mL	Physically compatible for 3 hr	1316	C
Sodium nitroprusside	RC	0.2 mg/mL[a]	LI	1 unit/mL[a]	Visually compatible for 24 hr at 23°C	1877	C
Sodium nitroprusside	RC	1.2 and 3 mg/mL[a]	LI	1 and 2 units/mL[b]	Visually compatible for 48 hr at 24°C protected from light	2357	C
Tacrolimus	FUJ	1 mg/mL[b]	LI	0.1 unit/mL[a]	Visually compatible for 24 hr at 25°C	1630	C
Tedizolid phosphate	CUB	0.8 mg/mL[b]	NVN	1 unit/mL[b]	Physically compatible for 2 hr	3244	C
Terbutaline sulfate	CI	0.02 mg/mL[a]	LI	0.2 unit/mL[b]	Physically compatible for 2 hr at 25°C	1395	C
Tobramycin sulfate	LI	1.6 and 2 mg/mL[a]	LI	0.2 unit/mL[b]	Physically compatible for 2 hr at 25°C	1395	C
TNA #218 to #226[j]			NOV	1 unit/mL[a]	Visually compatible for 4 hr at 23°C	2215	C
TPN #189[j]			NOV	2 units/mL[k]	Visually compatible for 24 hr at 22°C	1767	C
TPN #212 to #215[j]			NOV	1 unit/mL[b]	Physically compatible for 4 hr at 23°C	2109	C

Y-Site Injection Compatibility (1:1 Mixture) (Cont.)

Test Drug	Mfr	Conc	Mfr	Conc	Remarks	Ref	C/I
Vancomycin HCl	LI	4 mg/mL[a]	LI	0.2 unit/mL[b]	Physically compatible for 2 hr at 25°C	1395	C
Vasopressin	APP	0.2 unit/mL[b]	NOV	1 unit/mL[b]	Physically compatible	2641	C

[a] Tested in dextrose 5%.

[b] Tested in sodium chloride 0.9%.

[c] Test performed using the formulation WITHOUT edetate disodium.

[d] Tested in sodium chloride 0.45%.

[e] Tested in both dextrose 5% and sodium chloride 0.9%.

[f] Tested in dextrose 5%, sodium chloride 0.9%, and Ringer's injection, lactated.

[g] Tested in Ringer's injection, lactated.

[h] Tested in sterile water for injection.

[i] Tested in dextrose 5% in Ringer's injection, lactated.

[j] Refer to Appendix for the composition of parenteral nutrition solutions. TNA indicates a 3-in-1 admixture, and TPN indicates a 2-in-1 admixture.

[k] Tested in Haemaccel (Behring).

[l] Ampicillin component. Ampicillin in a 2:1 fixed-ratio concentration with sulbactam.

[m] Not specified whether concentration refers to single component or combined components.

[n] Meropenem component. Meropenem in a 1:1 fixed-ratio concentration with vaborbactam.

[o] Quinupristin and dalfopristin components combined.

[p] Ceftolozane component. Ceftolozane in a 2:1 fixed-ratio concentration with tazobactam.

[q] Test performed using the formulation WITH edetate disodium.

Additional Compatibility Information

Mixing Insulin Products

Mixing of the various types of insulin has been utilized. The following compatibility results have been cited:[1076]

Insulin Types	Compatibility
Regular with NPH	Mixtures are stable in all ratios
Regular with protamine zinc	Stability is unpredictable
Regular with Lente	Reduces activity of regular due to binding to excess zinc
Lente, Semilente, Ultralente	Mixtures are stable in all ratios
Lente, Semilente, Ultralente with phosphate-buffered insulins[a]	Should not be mixed due to precipitation

[a] Includes Humulin BR, NPH, protamine zinc, Velosulin insulins.

It has been stated that neutral regular insulin may be combined with modified insulin in any proportions.[263][264] However, losses of soluble insulins when mixed with zinc and isophane insulins were reported. These losses generally ranged from about 20 to 50% but were as high as 99%, depending on the ratio and sources of the 2 insulins in the mixture. The reaction occurred within the first 90 to 120 seconds after mixing, with no further losses occurring after this time. This phenomenon could explain clinical reports of failure to control postprandial blood sugar levels.[1275]

The loss of solubility when short-acting insulins were mixed in ratios of 1:1, 1:2, 1:3, and 1:5 with long-acting insulins was reported. Iletin II Regular (Lilly) was mixed with Iletin II Lente, NPH, or Ultralente (Lilly). Actrapid (Novo) was mixed with Monotard (Novo). Velosulin (Nordisk) was mixed with Insulatard (Nordisk). The mixtures were centrifuged after storage times of approximately 20 minutes and 75 seconds. The level of soluble short-acting insulin in the supernatant was determined. In a 1:1 ratio, no significant loss of solubility occurred with the Iletin II Lente combination within 20 minutes and with the Actrapid–Monotard combination in 75 seconds. All other combinations, ratios, and time periods had losses ranging from 10 to 75%. The worst losses were experienced with the highest ratios of long-acting insulins and with the longer time period. The method used to prolong insulin action (precipitation) might affect the solubility of the short-acting insulin when admixed.[1156]

The loss of initial hypoglycemic effect when Actrapid HM (Novo) was mixed with Ultratard HM (Novo), an ultralente insulin, for 5 minutes before injection was noted. The authors recommended not mixing the 2 types of insulin to preserve the rapid hypoglycemic effect of regular insulin.[73]

Octreotide

Insulin levels in a 3-L bag of parenteral nutrition solution showed a marked reduction when octreotide 150 mcg was added to the container. Sample parenteral nutrition solutions, with and without octreotide, were prepared with regular insulin 15 units/3-L bag. Subsequent analysis found an insulin level of 3.5 units/L in the plain parenteral nutrition solution, an amount consistent with the losses occurring due to surface adsorption. However, in the parenteral nutrition solution containing octreotide, the insulin level was only 0.6 unit/L. The reason for this potential incompatibility is not known.[1377]

Peritoneal Dialysis Solutions

Insulin 4, 10, 20, and 40 units/L was evaluated in the following Baxter peritoneal dialysis solutions in PVC and Clear-Flex polyolefin containers:

- Dianeal PD-4 with 1.36% dextrose in PVC containers
- Physioneal 40 with 1.36% dextrose in PVC containers
- Physioneal 40 Clear-Flex with 1.36% dextrose in Clear-Flex

In Dianeal PD-4, more than 90% of the insulin concentration remained over 24 hours. The insulin 10, 20, and 40 units/L in Physioneal 40 retained more than 90% of the insulin concentration over 6 hours and more than 80% over 24 hours. The insulin 4 units/L in Physioneal 40 retained more than 90% of the insulin concentration over 3 hours and more than 70% over 24 hours. No difference was found between the results in PVC and Clear-Flex containers.[2647]

Insulin Lispro
AHFS 68:20.08

Products

Insulin lispro is available in vials, cartridges, and pens as a suspension containing in each mL insulin lispro 100 units with glycerin 16 mg, dibasic sodium phosphate 1.88 mg, metacresol 3.15 mg, zinc ion 0.0197 mg (as oxide), a trace of phenol, and sodium hydroxide and/or hydrochloric acid to adjust pH during manufacturing in water for injection.[1(9/07)]

pH

From 7.0 to 7.8.[1(9/07)]

Trade Name(s)

Humalog

Administration

Insulin lispro is an injectable suspension intended for subcutaneous injection including using some external insulin pumps.[1(9/07)]

Stability

Intact vials of insulin lispro should be stored under refrigeration and protected from freezing, excessive heat, and light.[1(9/07)]

Although refrigerated storage is required, the manufacturer has stated the drug may be stored at room temperature for 28 days. Visually inspect insulin lispro before use. Discard if it is cloudy, contains a precipitate, has thickened, or is discolored.[1(9/07)] [2745]

Insulin lispro diluted with Sterile Diluent for Humalog to 10 or 50 units/mL can be used for 28 days refrigerated and for 14 days at room temperatures up to 30°C. If diluting insulin lispro, great care is essential to avoid concentration errors. Insulin lispro in a cartridge or used in an external insulin pump must not be diluted.[1(9/07)]

Insulin lispro cartridges used in D-TRON and D-TRON Plus external pumps should be discarded after seven days and the cartridge adapters and external pump reservoir should be discarded every 48 hours.[1(9/07)]

The physical and chemical stability of insulin lispro 100 units/mL in MiniMed507c, H-TRONplus, and D-TRON CSII insulin infusion devices stored at 37°C and subjected to mechanical shaking at 100 strokes/min was evaluated over 7 days. The insulin lispro solution remained clear and free of aggregation and precipitation, and concentrations remained at 95%.[2638]

Selected Revisions October 1, 2012. © Copyright, October 2010. American Society of Health-System Pharmacists, Inc.

DOI: 10.37573/9781585286850.212

Interferon Alfa-2b
AHFS 8:18.20

Products

Interferon alfa-2b is available as a dry powder for injection in single-use vials containing 10, 18, or 50 million international units packaged with sterile water for injection diluent.[2952]

Select the vial size and dosage form that are appropriate for the intended use of the product.[2952] Only the 10-million international unit dry powder for injection single-use vial is recommended for intralesional use.[2952] The 50-million international unit dry powder for injection single-use vial is used only in the treatment of malignant melanoma or AIDS-related Kaposi's sarcoma.[2952]

For *intramuscular, subcutaneous, or intralesional* use, reconstitute the 10-, 18-, or 50-million international unit dry powder for injection vials with 1 mL of the provided sterile water for injection diluent to yield solutions containing 10, 18, or 50 million international units/mL, respectively.[2952] Direct the stream of diluent at the vial wall.[2953] Gently swirl in a circular motion to dissolve the powder;[2952] [2953] do not shake.[2953] If undissolved powder remains, gently invert the vial until the remainder of the powder is dissolved.[2953]

In addition to the drug, each mL of the reconstituted solutions contains glycine 20 mg, sodium phosphate dibasic 2.3 mg, sodium phosphate monobasic 0.55 mg, and albumin human 1 mg.[2952] These vials contain no preservative.[2952]

For *intravenous infusion*, reconstitute the appropriately sized dry powder for injection vial contents with the diluent provided.[2952] Gently swirl to dissolve the powder;[2952] do not shake.[2953] If undissolved powder remains, gently invert the vial until the remainder of the powder is dissolved.[2953] Withdraw the appropriate dose and add it to 100 mL of sodium chloride 0.9%, ensuring that the final concentration is not less than 10 million international units/100 mL.[2952]

Interferon alfa-2b also is available as a solution for intramuscular, subcutaneous, or intralesional use in multidose vials labeled as containing 18 million international units (22.8 million international units/3.8 mL [i.e., 6 million international units/mL]) or 25 million international units (32 million international units/3.2 mL [i.e., 10 million international units/mL]).[2952] Only the 25-million international unit (32-million international units/3.2 mL [i.e., 10-million international unit/mL]) solution is recommended for intralesional use.[2952] Each mL of solution also contains sodium chloride 7.5 mg, sodium phosphate dibasic 1.8 mg, sodium phosphate monobasic 1.3 mg, edetate disodium 0.1 mg, polysorbate 80 0.1 mg, and metacresol 1.5 mg.[2952] The solution products are albumin-free.[2952]

Interferon alfa-2b solution products are not labeled for intravenous administration.[2952]

Specific Activity

Approximately 2.6 × 10⁸ international units/mg of protein.[2952]

Tonicity

Reconstitution of the 10-million international unit vial with 1 mL of water for injection results in an isotonic solution.[1369]

Trade Name(s)

Intron A

Administration

The administration of interferon alfa-2b is dependent upon the intended use and specific dosage form.[2952] The dry powder products, reconstituted as directed, may be administered by intramuscular and subcutaneous injection or intravenous infusion.[2952] The contents of the 10-million international unit vial, reconstituted as directed, also may be given by intralesional injection.[2952] For intravenous infusions, interferon alfa-2b may be diluted further to a concentration of not less than 10 million international units/100 mL of sodium chloride 0.9% to be infused over 20 minutes.[2952]

The solution products are administered by intramuscular or subcutaneous injection.[2952] The labeled 25-million international unit multidose vial also may be used for intralesional injection.[2952] The solution products are *not* for use in the treatment of malignant melanoma or AIDS-related Kaposi's sarcoma.[2952]

Stability

Interferon alfa-2b dry powder in vials is a white to cream color.[2952] It is not photosensitive.[1369] The reconstituted solution is clear and colorless to light yellow.[2952] Intact vials should be stored under refrigeration at 2 to 8°C,[2952] but have been noted to be stable for up to 28 days at room temperature.[1369] The manufacturer recommends that the reconstituted solution be used immediately, but the solution may be stored under refrigeration for up to 24 hours.[2952]

Interferon alfa-2b solution in multidose vials is clear and colorless.[2952] Intact vials of solution should be stored under refrigeration at 2 to 8°C,[2952] but have been noted to be stable for up to 7 days at or below 25°C.[2961] After opening, vials have been found to be stable for up to 28 days at 2 to 8°C.[2961]

Interferon alfa-2b contains amino acid residues that are susceptible to oxidation.[2961] Although oxidation products might not directly affect cytokine activity, oxidized interferon alfa-2b is prone to aggregation; oxidation catalyzed by metals, in particular, may result in the formation of highly immunogenic aggregates.[2961] Therefore, edetate disodium has been included as a chelating agent in the solution formulation of interferon alfa-2b.[2961]

Interferon alfa-2b (Schering) containing albumin human in the formulation reconstituted with bacteriostatic water for injection and diluted further to 2 million international units/mL with sterile water for injection was stored at 4°C for 21 days in polypropylene centrifuge tubes. Biological activity was retained throughout the study period.[2022]

DOI: 10.37573/9781585286850.213

In another study, the retention of bioactivity by albumin-free interferon alfa-2b 6 million units/mL was compared to samples of that product to which albumin human 1 mg/mL was added and also to the reconstituted product containing albumin human in the formulation. The solutions were packaged as 0.5 mL in polypropylene syringes and stored at 4°C for 42 days. In addition, the albumin-free product was diluted to 2 million units/mL with sterile water for injection and stored in a 60-mL polypropylene syringe under the same conditions. No substantial loss of biological activity was found in any of the samples.[2188]

Sodium chloride 0.9% is recommended for preparation of intravenous infusion admixtures.[2952]

Interferon alfa-2b dry powder is stated to be compatible with sodium chloride 0.9%, Ringer's injection, and Ringer's injection, lactated.[1369] It is stated to be incompatible with dextrose solutions.[1369]

pH Effects

Interferon alfa-2b is most stable between pH 6.9 and 7.5.[1369]

Freezing Solutions

Interferon alfa-2b solutions frozen at −20°C are stated to be stable for 56 days including 4 freeze-thaw cycles.[1369] Frozen solutions stored at −80°C are stable for 1 year.[1369]

Selected Revisions June 1, 2019. © Copyright, October 1998. American Society of Health-System Pharmacists, Inc.

Syringes

Interferon alfa-2b (Intron A, Kirby-Warwick) 3 million units was diluted in 6 mL of sterile water for injection and packaged in 10-mL polypropylene syringes. The samples were stored for 14 days under refrigeration and for 24 hours at 37°C. Analysis found changes indicating interconversion between interferon monomers and possibly oligomer formation. Dilution and packaging in polypropylene syringes was considered to be unsuitable.[744]

Sorption

In general, cytokines are commonly susceptible to adsorption.[2961] Polysorbate 80, incorporated into interferon alfa-2b solution products, inhibits adsorption by competing with proteins for hydrophobic surfaces and interfaces.[2961] The solution dosage forms are albumin-free.[2952] Conversely, albumin human is incorporated into the dry powder dosage forms to minimize adsorption by competing with proteins for surface adsorption sites.[2961]

Iodipamide Meglumine
AHFS 36:68

Products

Iodipamide meglumine is available in 20-mL vials containing an aqueous solution composed of 52% iodipamide meglumine (5.2 g bound iodine/20 mL) with 0.32% sodium citrate buffer and 0.04% edetate disodium.[1(7/06)] [4]

pH

From 6.5 to 7.7.[1(7/06)] [4]

Sodium Content

The 52% solution contains approximately 18.2 mg of sodium per 20 mL.[1(7/06)]

Trade Name(s)

Cholografin Meglumine

Administration

Iodipamide meglumine is administered slowly intravenously only. After warming to body temperature, the 52% injection is injected over 10 minutes.[1(7/06)] [4]

Stability

The solutions may vary from colorless to pale yellow or light amber. Darker solutions should not be used. Crystallization may occur in the 52% solution. To redissolve it, place the vial in hot water and shake gently for several minutes. If cloudiness does not disappear, the solution should not be used.[1(7/06)] [4]

Plastic syringes have been stated to be unsuitable for accommodating radiopaque solutions for any length of time. The plastic is attacked, and the plunger tends to freeze on prolonged storage.[40] However, when iodipamide meglumine (Squibb) 52% was stored in polystyrene syringes (Pharmaseal) at 25 and 37°C, no apparent changes were noted visually or spectrophotometrically over five days.[530]

Iodipamide meglumine solutions should be protected from light and excessive heat.[1(7/06)]

Compatibility Information

Additive Compatibility

Iodipamide meglumine

Test Drug	Mfr	Conc/L or %	Mfr	Conc/L or %	Test Solution	Remarks	Ref	C/I
Diphenhydramine HCl	PD	20 to 200 mg	SQ	52%	NS	Dense putty-like white precipitate forms immediately	309	I

Drugs in Syringe Compatibility

Iodipamide meglumine

Test Drug	Mfr	Amt	Mfr	Amt	Remarks	Ref	C/I
Dimenhydrinate		1 mL[a]		52%, 40 mL	Forms a precipitate initially but clears within 1 hr and remains clear for 48 hr	530	?
Dimenhydrinate		1 mL[a]		52%, 2 to 20 mL	Forms a precipitate initially but clears within 1 hr. Precipitate reforms on standing	530	I
Dimenhydrinate		1 mL[a]		52%, 1 mL	Precipitates immediately	530	I
Diphenhydramine HCl	PD	5 mg/0.1 mL to 50 mg/1 mL	SQ		Dense putty-like white precipitate forms immediately	309	I
Diphenhydramine HCl		1 mL[a]		52%, 1 to 40 mL	Forms a precipitate initially but clears within 1 hr and remains clear for 48 hr	530	?
Hyaluronidase		1 mL[a]		52%, 2 to 40 mL	Physically compatible for 48 hr	530	C

DOI: 10.37573/9781585286850.214

Drugs in Syringe Compatibility (Cont.)

Test Drug	Mfr	Amt	Mfr	Amt	Remarks	Ref	C/I
Hyaluronidase		1 mL[a]		52%, 1 mL	Physically compatible for at least 1 hr but a precipitate forms within 48 hr	530	I
Promethazine HCl		1 mL[a]		52%, 20 to 40 mL	Forms a precipitate initially but clears within 1 hr and remains clear for 48 hr	530	?
Promethazine HCl		1 mL[a]		52%, 1 to 10 mL	Precipitates immediately	530	I

[a] Concentration unspecified.

Y-Site Injection Compatibility (1:1 Mixture)

Iodipamide meglumine

Test Drug	Mfr	Conc	Mfr	Conc	Remarks	Ref	C/I
Gentamicin sulfate			SQ		White precipitate forms immediately downstream to Y-site when given into a set through which gentamicin was administered previously	324	I

Selected Revisions April 9, 2015. © Copyright, October 1982.
American Society of Health-System Pharmacists, Inc.

Iodixanol
AHFS 36:68

Products

Iodixanol is available at 270 mg/mL of organically bound iodine (as 550 mg/mL of iodixanol) with calcium chloride dihydrate 0.074 mg/mL and sodium chloride 1.87 mg/mL. It is also available at 320 mg/mL of organically bound iodine (as 652 mg/mL of iodixanol) with calcium chloride dihydrate 0.044 mg/mL and sodium chloride 1.11 mg/mL. Each mL of the solutions also contains tromethamine 1.2 mg, edetate calcium disodium 0.1 mg, and hydrochloric acid and/or sodium hydroxide to adjust pH. The products are packaged from 50 to 200 mL.[1(5/06)]

pH

Adjusted during manufacturing to pH 7.4 with a range from 6.8 to 7.7 at 22°C.[1(5/06)]

Osmolality

Both concentrations have an osmolality of 290 mOsm/kg.[1(5/06)]

Density

The 270-mg I/mL product has a density of 1.314 g/mL at 20°C and 1.303 g/mL at 37°C. The 320-mg I/mL product has a density of 1.369 g/mL at 20°C and 1.356 g/mL at 37°C.[1(5/06)]

Trade Name(s)

Visipaque

Administration

Iodixanol is administered intravenously and intra-arterially. It is not intended for intrathecal use. The drug may be administered at either body or room temperature.[1(5/06)]

Stability

Intact containers of clear, colorless to pale yellow iodixanol injection should be stored at controlled room temperature and protected from exposure to direct sunlight and from freezing. Discard the product if inadvertently frozen because of possible damage to closure integrity. The foil overwrap on the flexible plastic containers serves as both a moisture and light barrier and should not be removed until immediately before use. Vials and bottles of iodixanol may be stored for up to one month at 37°C in a contrast agent warmer using circulating warm air.[1(5/06)]

Compatibility Information

Y-Site Injection Compatibility (1:1 Mixture)

Iodixanol

Test Drug	Mfr	Conc	Mfr	Conc	Remarks	Ref	C/I
Fenoldopam mesylate	AB	80 mcg/mL[a]	NYC	55%	Physically compatible for 4 hr at 23 and 37°C	2467	C

[a] Tested in sodium chloride 0.9%.

Selected Revisions October 1, 2012. © Copyright, October 2004.
American Society of Health-System Pharmacists, Inc.

DOI: 10.37573/9781585286850.215

Iohexol

AHFS 36:68

Products

Iohexol is available in concentrations ranging from 30.2% (140 mg/mL organically bound iodine) to 75.5% (350 mg/mL organically bound iodine) in numerous vial and bottle sizes from 10 to 250 mL; not all concentrations are available in all sizes. Also present in each mL are tromethamine 1.21 mg, edetate calcium disodium 0.1 mg, and hydrochloric acid or sodium hydroxide to adjust the pH.[1(1/07)]   Table 1 presents the characteristics of iohexol products.

Table 1. Iohexol product characteristics[1(1/07)]

Iohexol Concentration (%)	Iodine Concentration (mg/mL)	Osmolality (mOsm/kg)	Specific Gravity (37°C)
30.2	140	322	1.164
38.8	180	408	1.209
51.8	240	520	1.280
64.7	300	672	1.349
75.5	350	844	1.406

pH

From 6.8 to 7.7.[1(1/07)]

Trade Name(s)

Omnipaque

Administration

Iohexol at appropriate concentrations may be administered intravenously, intra-arterially, intrathecally (except for Omnipaque 350) slowly over one to two minutes, intra-articularly, or directly into selected areas for visualization. Solutions should be warmed to body temperature prior to administration.[1(1/07)]

Stability

Iohexol is colorless to pale yellow. Intact vials should be stored at controlled room temperature and protected from direct exposure to sunlight and freezing. The product should not be used if particulate matter is present. Do not remove the iohexol containers from the moisture- and light-protective foil overwrap until immediately before use.[1(1/07)]

Compatibility Information

Drugs in Syringe Compatibility

Iohexol

Test Drug	Mfr	Amt	Mfr	Amt	Remarks	Ref	C/I
Ampicillin sodium	BR	30 mg/1 mL	WI	64.7%, 5 mL	Physically compatible for at least 2 hr	1438	C
Bupivacaine HCl	AST	0.25 and 0.125%[b], 4 mL		64.7%, 1 mL	Visually compatible with no bupivacaine loss in 24 hr at room temperature. Iohexol not tested	1611	C
Chloramphenicol sodium succinate	PD	33 mg/1 mL	WI	64.7%, 5 mL	Physically compatible for at least 2 hr	1438	C
Diphenhydramine HCl	PD	12.5 mg/0.25 mL	WI	64.7%, 5 mL	Physically compatible for at least 2 hr	1438	C
Epinephrine HCl	PD	1 mg/1 mL	WI	64.7%, 5 mL	Physically compatible for at least 2 hr	1438	C
Gentamicin sulfate	SC	0.8 mg/1 mL	WI	64.7%, 5 mL	Physically compatible for at least 2 hr	1438	C
Heparin sodium	OR	5000 units/0.5 mL	WI	64.7%, 5 mL	Physically compatible for at least 2 hr	1438	C
Hydrocortisone sodium succinate	UP	10 mg/1 mL	WI	64.7%, 5 mL	Physically compatible for at least 2 hr	1438	C
Methylprednisolone sodium succinate	UP	10 mg/1 mL	WI	64.7%, 5 mL	Physically compatible for at least 2 hr	1438	C
Papaverine HCl	LI	30 mg/1 mL	WI	64.7%, 5 mL	Physically compatible for at least 2 hr	1438	C
Protamine sulfate	LI	10 mg/1 mL	WI	64.7%, 5 mL	Physically compatible for at least 2 hr	1438	C

[a] Concentration unspecified.

[b] Diluted 1:1 in sodium chloride 0.9%.

DOI: 10.37573/9781585286850.216

Y-Site Injection Compatibility (1:1 Mixture)

Iohexol

Test Drug	Mfr	Conc	Mfr	Conc	Remarks	Ref	C/I
Fenoldopam mesylate	AB	80 mcg/mL[a]	NYC	51.8%	Physically compatible for 4 hr at 23 and 37°C	2467	C

[a] Tested in sodium chloride 0.9%.

Selected Revisions October 1, 2012. © Copyright, October 1994.
American Society of Health-System Pharmacists, Inc.

Iopamidol
AHFS 36:68

Products

Iopamidol products are available in concentrations ranging from 41% (200 mg/mL organically bound iodine) to 76% (370 mg/mL organically bound iodine) in numerous vial and bottle sizes from 20 to 200 mL; not all concentrations are available in all sizes. Also present in each mL are tromethamine 1 mg, edetate calcium disodium, with hydrochloric acid and/or sodium hydroxide to adjust the pH.[1(3/07)] Table 1 presents the characteristics of iopamidol products.

Table 1. Iopamidol product characteristics[1(3/07)]

Iopamidol Concentration (%)	Iodine Concentration (mg/mL)	Osmolality (mOsm/kg)	Specific Gravity (37°C)
41	200	413	1.227
51	250	524	1.281
61	300	616	1.339
76	370	796	1.405

pH

From 6.5 to 7.5.[1(3/07)]

Trade Name(s)

Isovue

Administration

Iopamidol may be administered intravenously or intra-arterially. Solutions should be warmed to body temperature prior to administration.[1(3/07)]

Stability

Iopamidol injection is colorless to pale yellow. Intact vials should be stored at controlled room temperature and protected from light. If crystals form, they should be dissolved by warming of the vial in hot (60 to 100°C) water for about five minutes and gentle shaking. The vials should cool to body temperature before use. If crystals fail to dissolve, the vials should be discarded.[1(3/07)]

Compatibility Information

Drugs in Syringe Compatibility

Iopamidol

Test Drug	Mfr	Amt	Mfr	Amt	Remarks	Ref	C/I
Ampicillin sodium	BR	30 mg/1 mL	SQ	61%, 5 mL	Physically compatible for at least 2 hr	1438	C
Chloramphenicol sodium succinate	PD	33 mg/1 mL	SQ	61%, 5 mL	Physically compatible for at least 2 hr	1438	C
Diphenhydramine HCl	PD	12.5 mg/0.25 mL	SQ	61%, 5 mL	Physically compatible for at least 2 hr	1438	C
Epinephrine HCl	PD	1 mg/1 mL	SQ	61%, 5 mL	Physically compatible for at least 2 hr	1438	C
Gentamicin sulfate	SC	0.8 mg/1 mL	SQ	61%, 5 mL	Physically compatible for at least 2 hr	1438	C
Heparin sodium	OR	5000 units/0.5 mL	SQ	61%, 5 mL	Physically compatible for at least 2 hr	1438	C
Hydrocortisone sodium succinate	UP	10 mg/1 mL	SQ	61%, 5 mL	Physically compatible for at least 2 hr	1438	C
Methylprednisolone sodium succinate	UP	10 mg/1 mL	SQ	61%, 5 mL	Physically compatible for at least 2 hr	1438	C
Papaverine HCl	LI	30 mg/1 mL	SQ	61%, 5 mL	Physically compatible for at least 2 hr	1438	C
Protamine sulfate	LI	10 mg/1 mL	SQ	61%, 5 mL	Physically compatible for at least 2 hr	1438	C

Y-Site Injection Compatibility (1:1 Mixture)

Iopamidol

Test Drug	Mfr	Conc	Mfr	Conc	Remarks	Ref	C/I
Fenoldopam mesylate	AB	80 mcg/mL[a]	BRD	51%	Physically compatible for 4 hr at 23 and 37°C	2467	C

[a] Tested in sodium chloride 0.9%.

Selected Revisions October 1, 2012. © Copyright, October 1994.
American Society of Health-System Pharmacists, Inc.

DOI: 10.37573/9781585286850.217

Iothalamate Meglumine
AHFS 36:68

Products

Iothalamate meglumine injection is available as a solution in concentrations ranging from 30 to 60% in vials and bottles in a variety of sizes.[3320][3321][3322] Each mL of the 30% solution (Conray 30) contains iothalamate meglumine 300 mg, edetate calcium disodium 0.11 mg, and monobasic sodium phosphate 0.125 mg.[3320] Each mL of the 43% solution (Conray 43) contains iothalamate meglumine 430 mg, edetate calcium disodium 0.11 mg, and monobasic sodium phosphate 0.115 mg.[3321] Each mL of the 60% solution (Conray) contains iothalamate meglumine 600 mg, edetate calcium disodium 0.09 mg, and monobasic sodium phosphate 0.125 mg.[3322]

Iothalamate meglumine also is available as a 17.2% solution for cystography and cystourethrography; this product is not intended for intravascular or intrathecal administration.[3323]

Some examples of iothalamate meglumine products are listed in Table 1.

Table 1. Some representative iothalamate meglumine products[3320][3321][3322][3323]

Iothalamate Meglumine Content (%)	Bound Iodine (mg/mL)	Representative Trade Names
Ureteral solutions (not for intravascular use)		
17.2	81	Cysto-Conray II
Parenteral solutions		
30	141	Conray 30
43	202	Conray 43
60	282	Conray

Sodium Content

Each mL of iothalamate meglumine 30% solution contains approximately 0.04 mg sodium.[3320]

pH

Iothalamate meglumine 43%: From 6.6 to 7.6.[3321]

Iothalamate meglumine 30 and 60%: From 6.5 to 7.7.[3320][3322]

Osmolarity

Iothalamate meglumine 30%: 500 mOsml/L.[3320]

Iothalamate meglumine 43%: 800 mOsml/L.[3321]

Iothalamate meglumine 60%: 1000 mOsml/L.[3322]

Osmolality

Iothalamate meglumine 30, 43, and 60% solutions are hypertonic, having osmolalities of 600, 800, and 1400 mOsm/kg, respectively.[3320][3321][3322]

Trade Name(s)

Conray, Conray 30, Conray 43

Administration

Iothalamate meglumine 30, 43, and 60% solutions may be administered intravenously, intra-arterially, or by injection into pancreatic and biliary ducts, specific to the procedure for which the solution is being employed.[3320][3321][3322] Solutions should be warmed to body temperature prior to administration.[3320][3321][3322] For certain procedures, the manufacturer states that iothalamate meglumine 60% may be diluted with sodium chloride injection or sterile water for injection.[3322]

If a minor reaction occurs during iothalamate meglumine administration, the injection should be slowed or stopped until the reaction has subsided.[3320][3321][3322] If a major reaction occurs, administration of the drug should be discontinued immediately.[3320][3321][3322][3323]

Iothalamate meglumine solutions are *not* indicated for intrathecal administration.[3320][3321][3322][3323] Care must be taken to ensure that the drug is not administered intrathecally.[3320][3321][3322][3323]

Iothalamate meglumine solution 17.2% (Cysto-Conray II) is instilled by gravity flow or syringe into the urinary bladder; this solution should *not* be administered intravascularly or intrathecally.[3323]

Stability

Iothalamate meglumine solutions are clear.[3320][3321][3322] Iothalamate meglumine 30, 43, and 60% solutions should be stored below 30°C.[3320][3321][3322] Crystallization does not occur at room temperature, but exposure to very cold temperatures may result in crystallization of the salt.[3320][3321][3322] If crystallization occurs, the solution should be brought to room temperature; intermittent[3320] or vigorous shaking[3321][3322] also may be necessary to redissolve the crystals. The speed of dissolution may be increased for some products by heating the vials in circulating warm air.[3321][3322]

The manufacturer states that iothalamate meglumine solutions must not be mixed in the same syringe with corticosteroids or antihistamines due to the potential for chemical incompatibility.[3320][3321][3322]

Iothalamate meglumine solution should be visually inspected for particulate matter or discoloration prior to administration.[3320][3321][3322]

pH Effects

Iothalamate meglumine is sensitive to low pH values. At reported pH values of about 2.4 to 2.7, turbidity or frank precipitation may appear in the 60% product.[479]

Light Effects

Iothalamate meglumine solutions are light sensitive and should be protected from strong daylight and direct sunlight.[3320][3321][3322]

DOI: 10.37573/9781585286850.218

Syringes

Iothalamate meglumine 60% was stored in polystyrene syringes (Pharmaseal) at 25 and 37°C. No apparent changes were noted over 5 days.[530]

Syringe material is one of many factors that may contribute to the development of thromboembolic events that have been reported with the use of contrast media in angiographic procedures.[3320 3321 3322] The use of plastic syringes rather than glass has been reported to decrease, but not entirely eliminate, the likelihood of in vitro clotting.[3320 3321 3322]

Compatibility Information

Drugs in Syringe Compatibility

Iothalamate meglumine

Test Drug	Mfr	Amt	Mfr	Amt	Remarks	Ref	C/I
Ampicillin sodium	BR	30 mg/1 mL	MA	60%, 5 mL	Physically compatible for at least 2 hr	1438	C
Chloramphenicol sodium succinate	PD	33 mg/1 mL	MA	60%, 5 mL	Physically compatible for at least 2 hr	1438	C
Dimenhydrinate		50 mg/1 mL[a]		60%, 1 to 40 mL	Physically compatible for 48 hr	530	C
Diphenhydramine HCl		50 mg/1 mL[a]		60%, 1 to 40 mL	Physically compatible for 48 hr	530	C
Diphenhydramine HCl	PD	50 mg/1 mL	MA	60%, 5 mL[a]	No precipitate observed	309	C
Diphenhydramine HCl	PD	12.5 mg/0.25 mL	MA	60%, 5 mL	Physically compatible for at least 2 hr	1438	C
Epinephrine HCl	PD	1 mg/1 mL	MA	60%, 5 mL	Physically compatible for at least 2 hr	1438	C
Gentamicin sulfate	SC	0.8 mg/1 mL	MA	60%, 5 mL	Physically compatible for at least 2 hr	1438	C
Heparin sodium	OR	5000 units/0.5 mL	MA	60%, 5 mL	Physically compatible for at least 2 hr	1438	C
Hyaluronidase		1 mL[a]		60%, 1 to 40 mL	Physically compatible for 48 hr	530	C
Hydrocortisone sodium succinate	UP	10 mg/1 mL	MA	60%, 5 mL	Physically compatible for at least 2 hr	1438	C
Methylprednisolone sodium succinate	UP	10 mg/1 mL	MA	60%, 5 mL	Physically compatible for at least 2 hr	1438	C
Papaverine HCl	LI	30 mg/1 mL	MA	60%, 5 mL	Physically compatible for at least 2 hr	1438	C
Promethazine HCl		1 mL[a]		60%, 1 to 40 mL	Precipitates immediately	530	I
Protamine sulfate	LI	10 mg/1 mL	MA	60%, 5 mL	Physically compatible for at least 2 hr	1438	C

[a] Concentration unspecified.

Selected Revisions February 21, 2018. © Copyright, October 1982. American Society of Health-System Pharmacists, Inc.

Ioxaglate Meglumine–Ioxaglate Sodium
AHFS 36:68

Products

Ioxaglate meglumine 39.3% and ioxaglate sodium 19.6% (Mallinckrodt) is available in containers ranging in size from 20 to 200 mL. Each mL contains ioxaglate meglumine 393 mg, ioxaglate sodium 196 mg, and edetate calcium disodium 0.1 mg. The product provides 32% organically bound iodine.[1(2/05)]

pH
From 6 to 7.6.[1(2/05)]

Osmolality
The osmolality of the product is 600 mOsm/kg.[1(2/05)]

Sodium Content
Each mL provides 0.15 mEq (3.48 mg) of sodium.[1(2/05)]

Trade Name(s)
Hexabrix

Administration

The product may be administered intravenously, intra-arterially, or intra-articularly. It also may be injected or instilled directly into selected areas to be visualized. The solutions should be warmed to body temperature before administration.[1(2/05)]

Stability

The product should be stored below 30°C and protected from freezing and direct exposure to sun or strong daylight. The solution is colorless to pale yellow. Crystallization does not occur at normal room temperatures. If the product is frozen or crystallization occurs, bring it to room temperature and shake vigorously to dissolve all crystals. Warming with circulating warm air is recommended to speed dissolution. Submersion in water is not recommended.[1(2/05)]

Compatibility Information

Drugs in Syringe Compatibility

Ioxaglate meglumine–ioxaglate sodium

Test Drug	Mfr	Amt	Mfr	Amt	Remarks	Ref	C/I
Ampicillin sodium	BR	30 mg/1 mL	MA	5 mL	Physically compatible for at least 2 hr	1438	C
Chloramphenicol sodium succinate	PD	33 mg/1 mL	MA	5 mL	Physically compatible for at least 2 hr	1438	C
Diphenhydramine HCl	PD	12.5 mg/0.25 mL	MA	5 mL	Precipitate forms immediately and persists for at least 2 hr	1438	I
Epinephrine HCl	PD	1 mg/1 mL	MA	5 mL	Physically compatible for at least 2 hr	1438	C
Gentamicin sulfate	SC	0.8 mg/1 mL	MA	5 mL	Transient precipitate clears within 5 min	1438	?
Heparin sodium	OR	5000 units/0.5 mL	MA	5 mL	Physically compatible for at least 2 hr	1438	C
Hydrocortisone sodium succinate	UP	10 mg/1 mL	MA	5 mL	Physically compatible for at least 2 hr	1438	C
Methylprednisolone sodium succinate	UP	10 mg/1 mL	MA	5 mL	Physically compatible for at least 2 hr	1438	C
Papaverine HCl	ME	32 mg/1 mL	MA	5 mL	Precipitate forms immediately and persists for at least 2 hr	1438	I
Papaverine HCl	LI	30 mg/1 mL	MA	3 and 5 mL	White amorphous precipitate forms immediately and persists for 24 hr. If shaken, it dissolves in 20 to 30 min	1437	I
Papaverine HCl	LI	30 mg/2 to 6 mL[a]	MA	5 mL	Precipitate forms	1437	I
Papaverine HCl	LI	30 mg/11 and 16 mL[a]	MA	5 mL	Precipitate forms and then redissolves	1437	?
Papaverine HCl	LI	30 mg/21 mL[a]	MA	5 mL	Physically compatible	1437	C
Papaverine HCl	LI	30 mg/11 mL[a]	MA	15 and 30 mL	Physically compatible	1437	C

DOI: 10.37573/9781585286850.219

Drugs in Syringe Compatibility (Cont.)

Test Drug	Mfr	Amt	Mfr	Amt	Remarks	Ref	C/I
Papaverine HCl	LI	60 mg/12 and 17 mL[a]	MA	5 mL	Precipitate forms	1437	I
Papaverine HCl	LI	60 mg/22 mL[a]	MA	5 mL	Precipitate forms	1437	I
Protamine sulfate	LI	10 mg/1 mL	MA	5 mL	Precipitate forms immediately and persists for at least 2 hr	1438	I

[a] Diluted in sodium chloride 0.9%.

Y-Site Injection Compatibility (1:1 Mixture)

Ioxaglate meglumine–ioxaglate sodium

Test Drug	Mfr	Conc	Mfr	Conc	Remarks	Ref	C/I
Fenoldopam mesylate	AB	80 mcg/mL[a]	MA	39.3% + 19.6%	Physically compatible for 4 hr at 23 and 37°C	2467	C

[a] Tested in sodium chloride 0.9%.

Selected Revisions October 1, 2012. © Copyright, October 1992.
American Society of Health-System Pharmacists, Inc.

Irinotecan Hydrochloride
AHFS 10:00

Products

Irinotecan hydrochloride is available as a concentrate for injection in 2-, 5-, 15-, and 25-mL single-use vials containing 40, 100, 300, and 500 mg of drug, respectively, on the basis of the trihydrate.[3202] [3203] Each mL of solution contains irinotecan hydrochloride trihydrate 20 mg, sorbitol 45 mg, lactic acid 0.9 mg, and hydrochloric acid or sodium hydroxide to adjust the pH in water for injection.[3202] [3203] The product must be diluted prior to use.[3202] [3203]

Irinotecan hydrochloride concentrate for injection should be visually inspected for particulate matter and discoloration in the vial and again once the solution has been drawn from the vial into the syringe.[3202] [3203] Irinotecan hydrochloride concentrate for injection should be diluted to a final concentration of 0.12 to 2.8 mg/mL with dextrose 5% (preferred) or sodium chloride 0.9% prior to administration.[3202] [3203]

CAUTION: Care should be taken to ensure that the correct drug product, dose, and administration procedures are used and that no confusion with other products occurs.

pH

Irinotecan hydrochloride concentrate for injection has a pH from 3 to 4.[3202] [3203] [3204]

Trade Name(s)

Camptosar

Administration

Irinotecan hydrochloride is administered by intravenous infusion over 90 minutes after dilution to a final concentration in the range of 0.12 to 2.8 mg/mL in dextrose 5% (preferred) or sodium chloride 0.9%.[3203] [3203]

As with other toxic drugs, caution should be exercised in the handling and preparation of irinotecan hydrochloride solutions for infusion.[3202] [3203] Manufacturers recommend the use of gloves.[3202] [3203] If skin contact with the drug occurs, the affected area(s) should be washed immediately and thoroughly with soap and water; for mucosal membrane contact, the affected(s) area should be flushed thoroughly with water.[3202] [3203] Extravasation should be avoided.[3202] [3203]

CAUTION: Care should be taken to ensure that the correct drug product, dose, and administration procedures are used and that no confusion with other products occurs.

Stability

Irinotecan hydrochloride injection is a clear pale yellow solution.[3202] [3203] Intact vials should be stored upright at controlled room temperature and in the original carton to protect from light until use.[3202] [3203]

Manufacturers recommend that diluted solutions of irinotecan hydrochloride for infusion should be used immediately or within 4 hours after dilution if stored at room temperature (in dextrose 5% or sodium chloride 0.9%) or 24 hours if stored at 2 to 8°C (in dextrose 5% only).[3202] [3203] Refrigeration of admixtures of the drug prepared with sodium chloride 0.9% should be avoided because of the potential for a low and sporadic incidence of visible particulate formation.[3202] [3203]

Irinotecan hydrochloride (Aventis Pharma) 0.35 mg/mL in sodium chloride 0.9% did not result in the loss of viability of *Staphylococcus aureus*, *Enterococcus faecium*, *Pseudomonas aeruginosa*, and *Candida albicans* within 120 hours at room temperature of 22°C. Diluted solutions should be stored under refrigeration whenever possible, and the potential for microbiological growth should be considered when assigning expiration periods.[2740]

pH Effects

Irinotecan hydrochloride stability is pH dependent. In solution at acidic pH the drug is stable, but neutral and alkaline solutions are problematic. Maximum stability is demonstrated at pH 6 or lower. Increasing solution pH to more than pH 6.5 has resulted in 10% loss in as little as 3 hours. At pH 7.4, decomposition is rapid. Mixing irinotecan hydrochloride with neutral or alkaline drugs and solutions should be avoided.[1881] [2274] [2375]

Light Effects

Irinotecan hydrochloride is subject to photodegradation, including the formation of a precipitate. The structural changes exhibited by the decomposition products would indicate that they are unlikely to be active antineoplastic compounds.[1997] [1998] [2137] Exposure to ultraviolet light for 3 days produced a darkening in the solution color and the formation of a yellow precipitate composed of several decomposition products.[1997] Photodegradation of irinotecan hydrochloride occurs under any pH condition but is accelerated in neutral and alkaline solutions compared with acidic solutions. At pH 10, photodegradation is very rapid; at pH 3 it is much slower. At pH 7, irinotecan 0.34 mg/mL lost 32% in 6 hours exposed to a daylight lamp and 19% exposed to a white fluorescent light. In infusion solutions having neutral pH, irinotecan hydrochloride exposed to lighting (such as that of a medical facility) may have rapid decomposition. Protection from light exposure has been recommended to maintain product quality during administration.[1998] Other researchers have found that unacceptable losses occur within 7 days when exposed to fluorescent light but that light protection during administration is not needed.[2419]

Freezing Solutions

Precipitation may result from freezing irinotecan hydrochloride concentrate for injection and diluted solutions for infusion; freezing should be avoided.[3202] [3203]

DOI: 10.37573/9781585286850.220

Compatibility Information

Solution Compatibility

Irinotecan HCl

Test Soln Name	Mfr	Mfr	Conc/L or %	Remarks	Ref	C/I
Dextrose 5%			0.12 to 2.8 g	Stable for 48 hr at 2 to 8°C protected from light	3202, 3203	C
Dextrose 5%	AB[a]	PH	20 mg	About 9% loss occurred in 24 hr at 25°C	2375	C
Dextrose 5%	LME[a], BA[b]	RPR	2 g	Visually compatible with little or no loss in 2 hr at room temperature and in 4 days refrigerated	2396	C
Dextrose 5%	BA[a b]	RPR	2.8 g	Visually compatible with little or no loss in 24 hr at room temperature in light or dark	2397	C
Dextrose 5%	BA[b]	RPR	0.4, 1, 2.8 g	Visually compatible with no loss in 28 days at both 4 and 25 ° protected from light	2419	C
Sodium chloride 0.9%			0.12 to 2.8 g	Storage at 2 to 8°C not recommended due to potential for visible particulate formation	3202, 3203	I
Sodium chloride 0.9%	AB[a]	PH	20 mg	About 11% loss occurred in 2 hr at 25°C	2375	I
Sodium chloride 0.9%	LME[a], BA[b]	RPR	2 g	Visually compatible with little or no loss in 2 hr at room temperature and in 4 days refrigerated	2396	C
Sodium chloride 0.9%	BA[a b]	RPR	2.8 g	Visually compatible with little or no loss in 24 hr at room temperature in light or dark	2397	C
Sodium chloride 0.9%	BA[b]	RPR	0.4, 1, 2.8 g	Visually compatible with no loss in 28 days at both 4 and 25°C protected from light	2419	C
Sodium chloride 0.9%	BA[b]	RPR	0.4 and 1 g	8 to 10% loss in 7 days and 13 to 17% loss in 14 days at 25°C exposed to light. Color darkens and a precipitate may appear within 4 weeks	2419	C
Sodium chloride 0.9%	BA[b]	RPR	2.8 g	9% loss in 14 days and 15% loss in 21 days at 25°C exposed to light. Color darkens and a precipitate may appear within 4 weeks	2419	C

[a] Tested in glass containers.

[b] Tested in PVC containers.

Additive Compatibility

Irinotecan HCl

Test Drug	Mfr	Conc/L or %	Mfr	Conc/L or %	Test Solution	Remarks	Ref	C/I
Epirubicin HCl	CE	560 mg	RPR	640 mg	NS	UV spectrum changes immediately upon mixing	2670	I

Y-Site Injection Compatibility (1:1 Mixture)

Irinotecan HCl

Test Drug	Mfr	Conc	Mfr	Conc	Remarks	Ref	C/I
Gemcitabine HCl	LI	10 mg/mL[b]	PHU	5 mg/mL[b]	Subvisible haze with green discoloration forms immediately	2226	I
Oxaliplatin	SS	0.5 mg/mL[a]	PHU	1 mg/mL[a]	Physically compatible for 4 hr at 23°C	2566	C

Y-Site Injection Compatibility (1:1 Mixture) (Cont.)

Test Drug	Mfr	Conc	Mfr	Conc	Remarks	Ref	C/I
Palonosetron HCl	MGI	50 mcg/mL	PHU	1 mg/mL[a]	Physically compatible. No palonosetron and 5% irinotecan loss in 4 hr	2609	C
Pemetrexed disodium	LI	20 mg/mL[b]	PHU	1 mg/mL[a]	Color darkening occurs over 4 hr	2564	I

[a] Tested in dextrose 5%.

[b] Tested in sodium chloride 0.9%.

Selected Revisions March 13, 2017. © Copyright, October 1998.
American Society of Health-System Pharmacists, Inc.

Irinotecan Hydrochloride Liposomal
AHFS 10:00

Products

Irinotecan hydrochloride liposomal injection is available in 10-mL single-use vials containing 43 mg of irinotecan as the free base in a white to slightly yellow opaque liposomal dispersion.[3147] Irinotecan is provided inside liposome carriers (approximate diameter 110 nm) in a gelated or precipitated state as the sucrose octasulfate salt.[3147] Liposomes encapsulating irinotecan are composed of distearoyl phosphatidylcholine (DSPC) 6.81 mg/mL, cholesterol 2.22 mg/mL, and methoxy-terminated polyethylene glycol 2000 distearoylphosphatidyl ethanolamine (MPEG-2000-DSPE) 0.12 mg/mL.[3147] Each vial also contains sodium chloride 8.42 mg/mL and hydroxyethylpiperazine ethane sulfonic acid (HEPES) 4.05 mg/mL.[3147]

CAUTION: Care should be taken to ensure that the correct drug product, dose, and administration procedures are used and that no confusion with other products occurs. The manufacturer states that irinotecan hydrochloride liposomal injection *must not* be substituted for other drugs containing irinotecan hydrochloride.[3147]

The appropriate dose of the drug should be withdrawn from the vial and diluted in 500 mL of dextrose 5% or sodium chloride 0.9%.[3147] The diluted solution should be mixed by gentle inversion.[3147]

Tonicity

Irinotecan hydrochloride liposomal injection is isotonic.[3147]

Trade Name(s)

Onivyde

Administration

Irinotecan hydrochloride liposomal injection is administered by intravenous infusion over 90 minutes following dilution in dextrose 5% or sodium chloride 0.9%.[3147] If solutions diluted for infusion have been refrigerated, the solution should be allowed to come to room temperature prior to administration.[3147] Diluted solutions should be protected from light.[3147]

As with other toxic drugs, applicable special handling and disposal procedures for irinotecan hydrochloride liposomal should be followed.[3147]

CAUTION: Care should be taken to ensure that the correct drug product, dose, and administration procedures are used and that no confusion with other products occurs.

Stability

Intact vials of irinotecan hydrochloride liposomal injection should be stored at 2 to 8°C.[3147] Both intact vials and solutions diluted for infusion should be protected from light and should not be frozen.[3147] The manufacturer states that diluted solutions should be used within 4 hours after dilution if stored at room temperature or within 24 hours if refrigerated at 2 to 8°C.[3147] Any unused portions of the solution should be discarded.[3147]

Filtration

Inline filters should *not* be used for administration of irinotecan hydrochloride liposomal injection.[3147]

Compatibility Information
Solution Compatibility

Irinotecan HCl liposomal

Test Soln Name	Mfr	Mfr	Conc/L or %	Remarks	Ref	C/I
Dextrose 5%		MM		Use within 4 hr of preparation when stored at room temperature or 24 hr at 2 to 8°C	3147	C
Sodium chloride 0.9%		MM		Use within 4 hr of preparation when stored at room temperature or 24 hr at 2 to 8°C	3147	C

DOI: 10.37573/9781585286850.221

Iron Dextran
AHFS 20:04.04

Products

Iron dextran injection is available as a dark brown liquid complex of ferric hydroxide and dextran in 2-mL single-dose vials.[3575] Each mL contains the equivalent of 50 mg of elemental iron in sodium chloride approximately 0.9% and water for injection.[3575] Sodium hydroxide and/or hydrochloric acid may have been used to adjust the pH.[3575]

pH

The pH of the solution ranges from 4.5 to 7.[3575]

Trade Name(s)

INFeD

Administration

Iron dextran is administered intravenously and intramuscularly.[3575] With either route of administration, a test dose should be administered prior to the first therapeutic dose.[3575]

Iron dextran may be administered undiluted by slow intravenous injection.[3575] A test dose of 0.5 mL (25 mg of elemental iron) should be administered at a gradual rate over at least 30 seconds prior to the first therapeutic dose of iron dextran.[3575] If no signs or symptoms of anaphylactic-type reactions have occurred after a period of at least one hour has elapsed, the remainder of the initial therapeutic dose (i.e., the therapeutic dose less the test dose) may be administered at a slow, gradual rate of no more than 1 mL (50 mg of elemental iron)/min.[3575]

Iron dextran also may be administered by deep intramuscular injection into the upper outer quadrant of the buttock using a 2- or 3-inch, 19- or 20-gauge needle.[3575] Staining of the skin associated with inadvertent injection or leakage of the drug into the subcutaneous tissue can be minimized by displacing the skin laterally prior to intramuscular injection (i.e., Z-track technique).[3575] A test dose of 0.5 mL (25 mg of elemental iron) should be administered in the buttock prior to the first therapeutic dose of iron dextran.[3575] If no signs or symptoms of anaphylactic-type reactions have occurred after a period of at least one hour has elapsed, the remainder of the initial therapeutic dose (i.e., the therapeutic dose less the test dose) may be administered.[3575] Subsequent injections should be made into alternate buttocks.[3575]

Iron dextran also has been administered by intravenous infusion over 1 to 6 hours after dilution in sodium chloride 0.9% (e.g., 1 g diluted in 250 mL of sodium chloride 0.9% administered over 1 hour).[3576 3577 3578 3579 3580]

Dilution in dextrose 5% results in a greater incidence of pain and phlebitis.[75] The manufacturer recommends not adding iron dextran injection to parenteral nutrition solutions,[3575] especially 3-in-1 mixtures.[1814]

Stability

Intact vials of iron dextran injection should be stored at controlled room temperature.[3575]

Filtration

Iron dextran adsorbs to sterilizing membrane filters composed of cellulose nitrate and acetate combined. An iron dextran solution containing 5 mcg/mL in water was estimated to lose 93% of the iron from the first mL passed through the filter. As more solution was passed through the filter, a decreasing proportion of the iron was adsorbed, indicating that the filter was approaching saturation. The extent of iron adsorption increased in the presence of electrolytes and trace elements. Adsorption can be substantial, especially when small amounts of iron dextran are involved.[918]

Compatibility Information

Solution Compatibility

Iron dextran

Test Soln Name	Mfr	Mfr	Conc/L or %	Remarks	Ref	C/I
TNA #122[a]		FI	50 mg	Lipid oiling out in 18 to 19 hr with formation of yellow-brown layer	1383	I
TNA #159 to #166[a]		FI	2 mg	Physically compatible with no change in particle size distribution in 48 hr at 4 and 25°C	1648	C
TPN #31 to #33[a]		FI	100 mg	Physically compatible with minimal changes to iron dextran and amino acids for 18 hr at room temperature	692	C
TPN #207, #208[a]		SCN	10 mg	Rust-colored precipitate forms in 12 hr at 19°C protected from sunlight	2103	I
TPN #209[a]		SCN	10 mg	Rust-colored precipitate forms in 18 to 24 hr at 19°C protected from sunlight	2103	I

DOI: 10.37573/9781585286850.222

Solution Compatibility (Cont.)

Test Soln Name	Mfr	Mfr	Conc/L or %	Remarks	Ref	C/I
TPN #210[a]		SCN	10 mg	Visually compatible for 48 hr at 19°C protected from sunlight. Trace iron precipitation found after 48 hr	2103	?
TPN #211[a]		SCN	10 mg	Visually compatible for 48 hr at 19°C protected from sunlight. No iron precipitation found after 48 hr	2103	C

[a] Refer to Appendix for the composition of parenteral nutrition solutions. TNA indicates a 3-in-1 admixture, and TPN indicates a 2-in-1 admixture.

Selected Revisions July 1, 2020. © Copyright, October 1982.
American Society of Health-System Pharmacists, Inc.

Iron Sucrose
AHFS 20:04.04

Products

Iron sucrose injection is available as a brown solution in 2.5-, 5-, and 10-mL single-dose (preservative-free) vials containing 50, 100, and 200 mg of elemental iron, respectively.[3551] Each mL of the solution contains 20 mg of elemental iron and 300 mg of sucrose in water for injection.[3551]

pH

Iron sucrose injection has a pH ranging from 10.5 to 11.1.[3551]

Osmolarity

Iron sucrose injection has an osmolarity of 1250 mOsmol/L.[3551]

Trade Name(s)

Venofer

Administration

Iron sucrose is administered only intravenously, as an injection or an infusion.[3551] Stable intravenous access should be insured to avoid extravasation.[3551]

In adults, doses of elemental iron up to 200 mg can be administered undiluted as a slow intravenous injection over 2 to 5 minutes; doses of 100 or 200 mg also may be administered as an intravenous infusion over at least 15 minutes following dilution of the dose in a maximum of 100 mL of sodium chloride 0.9%.[3551] Doses of elemental iron of 300 or 400 mg should be administered as an intravenous infusion over 1.5 or 2.5 hours, respectively, following dilution of the dose in a maximum of 250 mL of sodium chloride 0.9%.[3551] The manufacturer states that there is limited experience with the administration of 500-mg doses of elemental iron as an intravenous infusion over 3.5 to 4 hours following dilution of the dose in a maximum of 250 mL of sodium chloride 0.9%.[3551]

In pediatric patients 2 years of age or older, doses of elemental iron up to 100 mg can be administered undiluted as a slow intravenous injection over 5 minutes or as an intravenous infusion over 5 to 60 minutes following dilution of the dose to an elemental iron concentration of 1 to 2 mg/mL in sodium chloride 0.9%.[3551]

Iron sucrose injection should *not* be diluted to an elemental iron concentration of less than 1 mg/mL.[3551]

Stability

Intact vials of iron sucrose should be stored at controlled room temperature; freezing should be avoided.[3551]

Iron sucrose injection should *not* be diluted to an elemental iron concentration of less than 1 mg/mL.[3551]

Iron sucrose injection should be visually inspected for particulate matter and discoloration prior to administration.[3551] The manufacturer states that iron sucrose injection should not be mixed with other drugs or added to parenteral nutrition solutions for intravenous infusion.[3551]

Syringes

Iron sucrose (American Regent) containing 20 mg/mL of elemental iron undiluted or diluted to concentrations ranging from 2 to 10 mg/mL in sodium chloride 0.9% and stored in plastic syringes was found to be physically and chemically stable for 7 days at 23 to 27°C and 2 to 6°C.[3551]

Compatibility Information

Solution Compatibility

Iron sucrose

Test Soln Name	Mfr	Mfr	Conc/L or %	Remarks	Ref	C/I
Sodium chloride 0.9%	a	AMR	1 to 2 g	Physically and chemically stable for 7 days at 23 to 27°C	3551	C
Sodium chloride 0.9%	b	AMR	1 to 2 g	Physically and chemically stable for 7 days at 23 to 27°C	3551	C

a Tested in PVC containers.

b Tested in non-PVC containers.

© Copyright, July 2020. American Society of Health-System Pharmacists, Inc.

DOI: 10.37573/9781585286850.223

Isavuconazonium Sulfate
AHFS 8:14.08

Products

Isavuconazonium sulfate is a prodrug that is metabolized in vivo to isavuconazole.[3006] Isavuconazonium sulfate is available as a lyophilized powder in single-use (preservative-free) vials containing 372 mg of the drug (equivalent to 200 mg of isavuconazole) and mannitol 96 mg.[3006] Sulfuric acid also is present to adjust the pH.[3006]

Each 372-mg vial of isavuconazonium sulfate should be reconstituted with 5 mL of sterile water for injection and gently shaken to completely dissolve the powder.[3006] The reconstituted solution should be visually inspected for particulate matter and discoloration.[3006] To prepare a 372-mg dose, 5 mL of the reconstituted solution should be withdrawn from the vial and added to an infusion bag containing 250 mL of sodium chloride 0.9% or dextrose 5%, yielding an approximate isavuconazonium sulfate concentration of 1.5 mg/mL.[3006]

Visible translucent to white insoluble particulates of isavuconazole may form in diluted solutions of the drug.[3006] The diluted solution should be gently mixed or rolled to minimize the formation of such particulates.[3006] Any unnecessary vibration or vigorous shaking should be avoided; pneumatic transport systems should *not* be used.[3006] The final diluted solution *must* be administered through a 0.2- to 1.2-µm inline filter to remove isavuconazole particulates.[3006] A reminder sticker regarding the need for an inline filter should be affixed to the infusion bag.[3006]

Trade Name(s)

Cresemba

Administration

Isavuconazonium sulfate should be administered by intravenous infusion over at least 1 hour after dilution in 250 mL of sodium chloride 0.9% or dextrose 5%.[3006] The drug should *not* be administered by intravenous bolus injection.[3006]

The final diluted solution of isavuconazonium sulfate *must* be administered through a 0.2- to 1.2-µm inline filter.[3006] The drug should not be infused with other intravenous medications; if a common infusion line is being used to administer other drugs, the line should be flushed with sodium chloride 0.9% or dextrose 5% prior to and following infusion of isavuconazonium sulfate.[3006]

Stability

Intact vials of isavuconazonium sulfate should be stored under refrigeration at 2 to 8°C.[3006] Isavuconazonium sulfate is a white to yellow powder that forms a clear solution when reconstituted with sterile water for injection.[3006]

The manufacturer states that the reconstituted solution should be used immediately, but may be stored below 25°C for up to 1 hour prior to dilution.[3006] The total time for storage (of the diluted solution in the infusion bag) and the infusion time together should not exceed 6 hours if stored at room temperature or 24 hours if stored at 2 to 8°C.[3006] The infusion solution should *not* be frozen.[3006]

Filtration

The diluted solution for infusion *must* be administered with an infusion set containing a 0.2- to 1.2-µm inline filter to remove insoluble isavuconazole particulates that may form in diluted solutions of the drug.[3006]

Compatibility Information

Solution Compatibility

Isavuconazonium sulfate

Test Soln Name	Mfr	Mfr	Conc/L or %	Remarks	Ref	C/I
Dextrose 5%		ASP	1.5 g	Complete administration within 6 hr of dilution if stored at room temperature or 24 hr if stored at 2 to 8°C	3006	C
Sodium chloride 0.9%		ASP	1.5 g	Complete administration within 6 hr of dilution if stored at room temperature or 24 hr if stored at 2 to 8°C	3006	C

Y-Site Injection Compatibility (1:1 Mixture)

Isavuconazonium sulfate

Test Drug	Mfr	Conc	Mfr	Conc	Remarks	Ref	C/I
Albumin human	CBH	250 mg/mL	ASP	1.5 mg/mL[c]	Measured turbidity increases immediately	3263	I
Amikacin sulfate	HER	5 mg/mL[c]	ASP	1.5 mg/mL[c]	Physically compatible for 2 hr	3263	C

DOI: 10.37573/9781585286850.224

Y-Site Injection Compatibility (1:1 Mixture) (Cont.)

Test Drug	Mfr	Conc	Mfr	Conc	Remarks	Ref	C/I
Amiodarone HCl	APP	2 mg/mL^c	ASP	1.5 mg/mL^c	Physically compatible for 2 hr	3263	C
Amphotericin B	XGN	0.1 mg/mL^a	ASP	1.5 mg/mL^a	Measured turbidity increases immediately	3263	I
Amphotericin B lipid complex	SIG	1 mg/mL^a	ASP	1.5 mg/mL^a	Immediate change in measured turbidity	3263	I
Amphotericin B liposomal	ASP	2 mg/mL^a	ASP	1.5 mg/mL^a	Measured turbidity increases immediately	3263	I
Ampicillin sodium–sulbactam sodium	FRK	20 mg/mL$^{c\ d}$	ASP	1.5 mg/mL^c	Measured turbidity increases immediately with precipitation within 2 hr	3263	I
Anidulafungin	PF	0.77 mg/mL^c	ASP	1.5 mg/mL^c	Physically compatible for 2 hr	3263	C
Azithromycin	APP	2 mg/mL^a	ASP	1.5 mg/mL^a	Measured turbidity increases within 2 hr	3263	I
Azithromycin	APP	2 mg/mL^b	ASP	1.5 mg/mL^b	Physically compatible for 2 hr	3263	C
Aztreonam	APP	20 mg/mL^c	ASP	1.5 mg/mL^c	Physically compatible for 2 hr	3263	C
Bumetanide	HOS	0.25 mg/mL	ASP	1.5 mg/mL^a	Measured turbidity increases within 15 min	3263	I
Bumetanide	HOS	0.25 mg/mL	ASP	1.5 mg/mL^b	Physically compatible for 2 hr	3263	C
Calcium chloride	HOS, AMP	20 mg/mL^c	ASP	1.5 mg/mL^c	Physically compatible for 2 hr	3263	C
Calcium gluconate	APP	20 mg/mL^c	ASP	1.5 mg/mL^c	Physically compatible for 2 hr	3263	C
Caspofungin acetate	ME	0.5 mg/mL^b	ASP	1.5 mg/mL^b	Physically compatible for 2 hr	3263	C
Cefazolin sodium	APO	20 mg/mL^c	ASP	1.5 mg/mL^c	Measured turbidity increases immediately	3263	I
Cefepime HCl	SGT	40 mg/mL^c	ASP	1.5 mg/mL^c	Measured turbidity increases immediately	3263	I
Ceftaroline fosamil	FOR	12 mg/mL^c	ASP	1.5 mg/mL^c	Measured turbidity increases within 1 hr	3263	I
Ceftazidime	HOS	40 mg/mL^c	ASP	1.5 mg/mL^c	Measured turbidity increases immediately	3263	I
Ceftolozane sulfate-tazobactam sodium	CUB	10 mg/mL$^{c\ e}$	ASP	1.5 mg/mL^c	Physically compatible for 2 hr	3262, 3263	C
Ceftriaxone sodium	WOC	20 mg/mL^c	ASP	1.5 mg/mL^c	Measured turbidity increases immediately with precipitation within 1 hr	3263	I
Cefuroxime sodium	COV	30 mg/mL^c	ASP	1.5 mg/mL^c	Measured turbidity increases immediately	3263	I
Ciprofloxacin	HOS	2 mg/mL^c	ASP	1.5 mg/mL^c	Physically compatible for 2 hr	3263	C
Cisatracurium besylate	ABV	0.4 mg/mL^c	ASP	1.5 mg/mL^c	Physically compatible for 2 hr	3263	C
Colistimethate sodium	APP	4.5 mg/mL^c	ASP	1.5 mg/mL^c	Measured turbidity increases immediately	3263	I
Cyclosporine	DRX	5 mg/mL^c	ASP	1.5 mg/mL^c	Immediate change in measured turbidity	3263	I
Daptomycin	CUB^j	10 mg/mL^b	ASP	1.5 mg/mL^b	Physically compatible for 2 hr	3247, 3263	C
Dexamethasone sodium phosphate	FRK	1 mg/mL^c	ASP	1.5 mg/mL^c	Measured turbidity increases within 1 hr	3263	I
Dexmedetomidine HCl	HOS	4 mcg/mL^c	ASP	1.5 mg/mL^c	Physically compatible for 2 hr	3263	C
Digoxin	SZ	0.25 mg/mL	ASP	1.5 mg/mL^c	Physically compatible for 2 hr	3263	C
Diltiazem HCl	AKN	5 mg/mL	ASP	1.5 mg/mL^c	Physically compatible for 2 hr	3263	C
Diphenhydramine HCl	APP	50 mg/mL	ASP	1.5 mg/mL^c	Physically compatible for 2 hr	3263	C
Dobutamine HCl	HOS	4.1 mg/mL^c	ASP	1.5 mg/mL^c	Physically compatible for 2 hr	3263	C
Dopamine HCl	HOS	0.8 mg/mL^c	ASP	1.5 mg/mL^c	Physically compatible for 2 hr	3263	C

Y-Site Injection Compatibility (1:1 Mixture) (Cont.)

Test Drug	Mfr	Conc	Mfr	Conc	Remarks	Ref	C/I
Doripenem	SHI	4.5 mg/mL[c]	ASP	1.5 mg/mL[c]	Physically compatible for 2 hr	3263	C
Doxycycline hyclate	PRP	1 mg/mL[c]	ASP	1.5 mg/mL[c]	Physically compatible for 2 hr	3263	C
Epinephrine[k]	JHP	16 mcg/mL[c]	ASP	1.5 mg/mL[c]	Physically compatible for 2 hr	3247, 3263	C
Eptifibatide	ME	0.75 mg/mL	ASP	1.5 mg/mL[b]	Physically compatible for 2 hr	3263	C
Ertapenem sodium	ME	20 mg/mL[b]	ASP	1.5 mg/mL[b]	Measured turbidity increases within 1 hr	3263	I
Esmolol HCl	MYL, FRK	10 mg/mL	ASP	1.5 mg/mL[c]	Physically compatible for 2 hr	3263	C
Esomeprazole sodium	ASZ	0.8 mg/mL[c]	ASP	1.5 mg/mL[c]	Measured turbidity increases immediately with color changes within 15 to 60 min	3263	I
Famotidine	WW	4 mg/mL[c]	ASP	1.5 mg/mL[c]	Physically compatible for 2 hr	3263	C
Fentanyl citrate	WW	50 mcg/mL	ASP	1.5 mg/mL[c]	Physically compatible for 2 hr	3263	C
Filgrastim	AMG	15 mcg/mL[a]	ASP	1.5 mg/mL[a]	Measured turbidity increases within 15 min	3263	I
Fosphenytoin sodium	WW[i]	25 mg PE/mL[c]	ASP	1.5 mg/mL[c]	Measured turbidity increases immediately	3247, 3263	I
Furosemide	HOS	3 mg/mL[c]	ASP	1.5 mg/mL[c]	Immediate precipitation and increase in measured turbidity	3263	I
Gentamicin sulfate	PPR	5 mg/mL[c]	ASP	1.5 mg/mL[c]	Physically compatible for 2 hr	3263	C
Heparin sodium	PRP	1000 units/mL[c]	ASP	1.5 mg/mL[c]	Measured turbidity increases immediately	3263	I
Hydrocortisone sodium succinate	PF	1 mg/mL[c]	ASP	1.5 mg/mL[c]	Physically compatible for 2 hr	3263	C
Hydromorphone HCl	AKN	1 mg/mL[c]	ASP	1.5 mg/mL[c]	Physically compatible for 2 hr	3263	C
Imipenem–cilastatin sodium	PRP	5 mg/mL[c f]	ASP	1.5 mg/mL[c]	Physically compatible for 2 hr	3263	C
Insulin, regular	NVN	1 unit/mL[c]	ASP	1.5 mg/mL[c]	Physically compatible for 2 hr	3263	C
Labetalol HCl	HOS	2 mg/mL[c]	ASP	1.5 mg/mL[c]	Physically compatible for 2 hr	3263	C
Levofloxacin	AUR	5 mg/mL[c]	ASP	1.5 mg/mL[c]	Physically compatible for 2 hr	3263	C
Lidocaine HCl	APP	8 mg/mL[c]	ASP	1.5 mg/mL[c]	Physically compatible for 2 hr	3263	C
Linezolid	PF	2 mg/mL[a]	ASP	1.5 mg/mL[c]	Physically compatible for 2 hr	3247, 3263	C
Lorazepam	WW	1 mg/mL[c]	ASP	1.5 mg/mL[c]	Physically compatible for 2 hr	3263	C
Magnesium sulfate	HOS	100 mg/mL[c]	ASP	1.5 mg/mL[c]	Physically compatible for 2 hr	3263	C
Mannitol	HOS	20%	ASP	1.5 mg/mL[c]	Physically compatible for 2 hr	3263	C
Meperidine HCl	WW	10 mg/mL[c]	ASP	1.5 mg/mL[c]	Physically compatible for 2 hr	3263	C
Meropenem	PRP	10 mg/mL[c]	ASP	1.5 mg/mL[c]	Measured turbidity increases within 15 min	3263	I
Meropenem–vaborbactam	TMC	8 mg/mL[b l]	ASP	0.8 mg/mL[b]	Measured turbidity increases within 30 min. pH increased by >5 units within 3 hr	3380	I
Mesna	PRP	20 mg/mL[c]	ASP	1.5 mg/mL[c]	Physically compatible for 2 hr	3263	C
Methylprednisolone sodium succinate	PF	20 mg/mL[c]	ASP	1.5 mg/mL[c]	Transient turbidity forms then clears	3263	I
Metoclopramide HCl	TE	0.2 mg/mL[c]	ASP	1.5 mg/mL[c]	Physically compatible for 2 hr	3263	C

Y-Site Injection Compatibility (1:1 Mixture) (Cont.)

Test Drug	Mfr	Conc	Mfr	Conc	Remarks	Ref	C/I
Micafungin sodium	ASP	2 mg/mL[c]	ASP	1.5 mg/mL[c]	Immediate precipitation and increase in measured turbidity	3263	I
Midazolam HCl	APP	1 mg/mL[c]	ASP	1.5 mg/mL[c]	Physically compatible for 2 hr	3263	C
Milrinone lactate	HIK	0.2 mg/mL[c]	ASP	1.5 mg/mL[c]	Physically compatible for 2 hr	3263	C
Morphine sulfate	WW	1 mg/mL[c]	ASP	1.5 mg/mL[c]	Physically compatible for 2 hr	3263	C
Mycophenolate mofetil HCl	GEN	6 mg/mL[a]	ASP	1.5 mg/mL[a]	Physically compatible for 2 hr	3263	C
Naloxone HCl	PPR	0.04 mg/mL[c]	ASP	1.5 mg/mL[c]	Physically compatible for 2 hr	3263	C
Nesiritide	SCI	6 mcg/mL[c]	ASP	1.5 mg/mL[c]	Physically compatible for 2 hr	3263	C
Nicardipine HCl	BA	0.2 mg/mL[c]	ASP	1.5 mg/mL[c]	Physically compatible for 2 hr	3263	C
Nitroglycerin	BA	0.4 mg/mL[c]	ASP	1.5 mg/mL[c]	Physically compatible for 2 hr	3263	C
Norepinephrine bitartrate	HOS	32 mcg/mL[c]	ASP	1.5 mg/mL[c]	Physically compatible for 2 hr	3263	C
Octreotide acetate	FRK	4 mcg/mL[c]	ASP	1.5 mg/mL[c]	Physically compatible for 2 hr	3263	C
Ondansetron HCl	HOS	0.16 mg/mL[c]	ASP	1.5 mg/mL[c]	Physically compatible for 2 hr	3263	C
Pantoprazole sodium	NVP[h]	0.4 mg/mL[c]	ASP	1.5 mg/mL[c]	Measured turbidity increases within 1 hr	3247, 3263	I
Penicillin G potassium	PF	100,000 units/mL[a]	ASP	1.5 mg/mL[a]	Measured turbidity increases within 1 hr	3263	I
Penicillin G potassium	PF	100,000 units/mL[b]	ASP	1.5 mg/mL[b]	Physically compatible for 2 hr	3263	C
Phenylephrine HCl	SZ	1 mg/mL[c]	ASP	1.5 mg/mL[c]	Physically compatible for 2 hr	3263	C
Phenytoin sodium	WW	10 mg/mL[b]	ASP	1.5 mg/mL[b]	Immediate precipitation and increase in measured turbidity	3263	I
Piperacillin sodium–tazobactam sodium	PRP[h]	40 mg/mL[a, g]	ASP	1.5 mg/mL[a]	Measured turbidity increases immediately	3247, 3263	I
Piperacillin sodium–tazobactam sodium	PRP[h]	40 mg/mL[b, g]	ASP	1.5 mg/mL[b]	Physically compatible for 2 hr	3247, 3263	C
Plazomicin sulfate	ACH	24 mg/mL[c]	ASP	0.8 mg/mL[c]	Physically compatible for 1 hr at 20 to 25°C	3432	C
Potassium chloride	HOS	0.1 mEq/mL[c]	ASP	1.5 mg/mL[c]	Physically compatible for 2 hr	3263	C
Potassium phosphates	HOS	0.3 mmol/mL[c]	ASP	1.5 mg/mL[c]	Measured turbidity increases within 1 hr	3263	I
Propofol	PPR	10 mg/mL	ASP	1.5 mg/mL[a]	Immediate formation of free oil layer atop fat plug	3263	I
Ranitidine HCl	ZY	2.5 mg/mL[c]	ASP	1.5 mg/mL[c]	Physically compatible for 2 hr	3263	C
Rocuronium bromide	PRM	5 mg/mL[c]	ASP	1.5 mg/mL[c]	Physically compatible for 2 hr	3263	C
Sodium bicarbonate	HOS	1 mEq/mL	ASP	1.5 mg/mL[c]	Measured turbidity increases within 15 min	3263	I
Sodium nitroprusside	MTN	0.4 mg/mL[c]	ASP	1.5 mg/mL[c]	Physically compatible for 2 hr	3263	C
Sodium phosphates	FRK	0.5 mmol/mL[c]	ASP	1.5 mg/mL[c]	Measured turbidity increases within 1 hr	3263	I
Tacrolimus	ASP	0.02 mg/mL[c]	ASP	1.5 mg/mL[c]	Physically compatible for 2 hr	3263	C
Tedizolid phosphate	CUB	0.8 mg/mL[b]	ASP	1.5 mg/mL[b]	Measured turbidity increases within 15 min	3244, 3263	I
Tigecycline	PF	1 mg/mL[c]	ASP	1.5 mg/mL[c]	Physically compatible for 2 hr	3263	C
Tobramycin sulfate	MYL	5 mg/mL[c]	ASP	1.5 mg/mL[c]	Physically compatible for 2 hr	3263	C

Y-Site Injection Compatibility (1:1 Mixture) (Cont.)

Test Drug	Mfr	Conc	Mfr	Conc	Remarks	Ref	C/I
Vancomycin HCl	HOS	5 mg/mL^c	ASP	1.5 mg/mL^c	Physically compatible for 2 hr	3263	C
Vasopressin	JHP	1 unit/mL^c	ASP	1.5 mg/mL^c	Physically compatible for 2 hr	3263	C
Vecuronium bromide	CRC	1 mg/mL	ASP	1.5 mg/mL^c	Physically compatible for 2 hr	3263	C

^{a} Tested in dextrose 5%.

^{b} Tested in sodium chloride 0.9%.

^{c} Tested in both dextrose 5% and sodium chloride 0.9%.

^{d} Ampicillin component. Ampicillin in a 2:1 fixed-ratio concentration with sulbactam.

^{e} Ceftolozane component. Ceftolozane in a 2:1 fixed-ratio concentration with tazobactam.

^{f} Imipenem component. Imipenem in a 1:1 fixed-ratio concentration with cilastatin.

^{g} Piperacillin component. Piperacillin in an 8:1 fixed-ratio concentration with tazobactam.

^{h} Test performed using the formulation WITH edetate disodium.

^{i} Concentration of fosphenytoin expressed in milligrams of phenytoin sodium equivalents (PE) per mL.

^{j} Test performed using the Cubicin formulation.

^{k} As epinephrine base rather than the salt.

^{l} Meropenem component. Meropenem in a 1:1 fixed-ratio concentration with vaborbactam.

Selected Revisions September 30, 2019. © Copyright, September 2017. American Society of Health-System Pharmacists, Inc.

Isoproterenol Hydrochloride

AHFS 12:12.08.04

Isoprenaline Hydrochloride

Products

Isoproterenol hydrochloride is available at a concentration of 0.2 mg/mL in 1- and 5-mL ampuls.[2903] In addition to the drug, each mL contains sodium chloride 7 mg, sodium citrate dihydrate 2.07 mg, citric acid anhydrous 2.5 mg, edetate disodium 0.2 mg, and hydrochloric acid or sodium hydroxide to adjust the pH in water for injection.[2903]

pH

From 3.5 to 4.5.[2903]

Osmolality

The osmolality of isoproterenol hydrochloride 0.2 mg/mL was determined to be 277 mOsm/kg by freezing-point depression and 293 mOsm/kg by vapor pressure.[1071]

Trade Name(s)

Isuprel

Administration

Isoproterenol hydrochloride may be administered by intravenous infusion; by direct intravenous, intramuscular, or subcutaneous injection; and, in extreme emergencies, by intracardiac injection.[2903] For direct intravenous injection, 1 mL of the 0.2-mg/mL injection should be diluted to 10 mL with sodium chloride 0.9% or dextrose 5% to provide a 20-mcg/mL solution.[2903] Intravenous infusions are prepared by diluting 5 or 10 mL of the 0.2-mg/mL injection in 500 mL of dextrose 5% to yield solutions containing 2 or 4 mcg/mL, respectively.[2903] Intravenous infusion concentrations of up to 20 mcg/mL have been used when fluid restriction is essential.[2903]

For intramuscular, subcutaneous, and intracardiac injection, isoproterenol hydrochloride should be administered undiluted.[2903]

Stability

Isoproterenol hydrochloride injection in intact containers should be stored at controlled room temperature and protected from light.[2903] Ampuls should be kept in opaque containers until use.[2903] The drug should not be used if the solution is pinkish or slightly darker than yellow or if a precipitate is present.[2903] Exposure to air, light, or increased temperature may cause a pink to brownish pink color to develop.[4][975]

Isoproterenol hydrochloride under simulated summer conditions in paramedic vehicles was exposed to temperatures ranging from 26 to 38°C over 4 weeks. Analysis found about 4% loss of the drug in 7 days and 11% loss in 4 weeks.[2562]

pH Effects

The pH of a solution is the primary determinant of catecholamine stability in intravenous admixtures.[527] Isoproterenol hydrochloride 5 mg/L in dextrose 5% was stable for more than 24 hours at 25°C over a pH range of 3.7 to 5.7.[59][3026] However, isoproterenol hydrochloride displayed significant decomposition at a pH value above approximately 6.[48][59][430] If drugs that may raise the pH above 6 are mixed, they should be administered immediately after preparation,[59] or, preferably, administered separately.[24]

Visual inspection for color changes related to decomposition may be inadequate to assess the compatibility of admixtures. In one evaluation with aminophylline stored at 25°C, a color change was not noted until 24 hours had elapsed. However, no intact isoproterenol hydrochloride was present in the admixture at 24 hours.[527]

Filtration

Isoproterenol hydrochloride (Winthrop) 2 mg/L in dextrose 5%, sodium chloride 0.9%, and Ringer's injection, lactated, filtered over 12 hours through a 5-μm stainless steel depth filter (Argyle Filter Connector), a 0.22-μm cellulose ester membrane filter (Ivex-2 Filter Set) and a 0.22-μm polycarbonate membrane filter (In-Sure Filter Set) showed no significant reduction due to binding to the filters.[320]

In another study, isoproterenol hydrochloride (Winthrop) 4 mg/L in dextrose 5% and sodium chloride 0.9% did not display significant sorption to a 0.45-μm cellulose membrane filter (Abbott S-A-I-F) during an 8-hour simulated infusion.[567]

Central Venous Catheter

Isoproterenol hydrochloride (Abbott) 0.02 mg/mL in dextrose 5% was found to be compatible with the ARROWg+ard Blue Plus (Arrow International) chlorhexidine-bearing triple-lumen central catheter. Essentially complete delivery of the drug was found with little or no drug loss occurring. Furthermore, chlorhexidine delivered from the catheter remained at trace amounts with no substantial increase due to the delivery of the drug through the catheter.[2335]

DOI: 10.37573/9781585286850.225

Compatibility Information

Solution Compatibility

Isoproterenol HCl

Test Soln Name	Mfr	Mfr	Conc/L or %	Remarks	Ref	C/I
Amino acids 4.25%, dextrose 25%	MG	WI	2 mg	No increase in particulate matter in 24 hr at 5°C	349	C
Dextrose 5%	AB	BN	2 mg	Physically compatible and chemically stable. 10% decomposition is calculated to occur in 24 hr in the light and 250 hr in the dark at 25°C	527	C
Dextrose 5%		HOS	2 and 4 mg	Manufacturer recommended solution	2903	C

Additive Compatibility

Isoproterenol HCl

Test Drug	Mfr	Conc/L or %	Mfr	Conc/L or %	Test Solution	Remarks	Ref	C/I
Aminophylline	SE	500 mg	BN	2 mg	D5W	At 25°C, 10% isoproterenol decomposition in 2.2 to 2.5 hr in light and dark	527	I
Atracurium besylate	BW	500 mg		4 mg	D5W	Physically compatible and atracurium stable for 24 hr at 5 and 30°C	1694	C
Calcium chloride	UP	1 g	WI	4 mg		Physically compatible	59	C
Dobutamine HCl	LI	1 g	ES	2 mg	D5W, NS	Physically compatible for 24 hr at 21°C	812	C
Floxacillin sodium	BE	20 g	PX	4 mg	D5W	Physically compatible for 24 hr at 15 and 30°C. Haze forms in 48 hr and precipitate forms in 72 hr	1479	C
Furosemide	HO	1 g	PX	4 mg	D5W	Precipitates immediately	1479	I
Heparin sodium		32,000 units		2 mg	NS	Physically compatible and heparin activity retained for 24 hr	57	C
Heparin sodium	AB	20,000 units	WI	4 mg		Physically compatible	59	C
Magnesium sulfate		1 g	WI	4 mg		Physically compatible	59	C
Multivitamins	USV	10 mL	WI	4 mg		Physically compatible	59	C
Potassium chloride	AB	40 mEq	WI	4 mg		Physically compatible	59	C
Ranitidine HCl	GL	50 mg and 2 g		20 mg	D5W	Physically compatible. Ranitidine stable for 24 hr at 25°C. Isoproterenol not tested	1515	C
Sodium bicarbonate	AB	2.4 mEq[a]	BN	1 mg	D5W	Isoproterenol decomposition	772	I
Sodium bicarbonate		5%	WI	5 mg		Isoproterenol decomposition	48	I
Succinylcholine chloride	AB	2 g	WI	4 mg		Physically compatible	59	C
Verapamil HCl	KN	80 mg	BN	10 mg	D5W, NS	Physically compatible for 24 hr	764	C

[a] One vial of Neut added to a liter of admixture.

Drugs in Syringe Compatibility

Isoproterenol HCl

Test Drug	Mfr	Amt	Mfr	Amt	Remarks	Ref	C/I
Caffeine citrate		20 mg/1 mL	SW	0.2 mg/1 mL	Visually compatible for 4 hr at 25°C	2440	C
Pantoprazole sodium	[a]	4 mg/1 mL		0.2 mg/1 mL	Whitish precipitate	2574	I

[a] Test performed using the formulation WITHOUT edetate disodium.

Y-Site Injection Compatibility (1:1 Mixture)

Isoproterenol HCl

Test Drug	Mfr	Conc	Mfr	Conc	Remarks	Ref	C/I
Amiodarone HCl	LZ	4 mg/mL[c]	ES	4 mcg/mL[c]	Physically compatible for 24 hr at 21°C	1032	C
Atracurium besylate	BW	0.5 mg/mL[a]	ES	4 mcg/mL[a]	Physically compatible for 24 hr at 28°C	1337	C
Bivalirudin	TMC	5 mg/mL[a]	AB	20 mcg/mL[a]	Physically compatible for 4 hr at 23°C	2373	C
Cangrelor tetrasodium	TMC	1 mg/mL[b]		20 mcg/mL[b]	Physically compatible for 4 hr	3243	C
Cisatracurium besylate	GW	0.1, 2, 5 mg/mL[a]	AB	0.02 mg/mL[a]	Physically compatible for 4 hr at 23°C	2074	C
Cloxacillin sodium	SMX	100 mg/mL	SZ	0.2 mg/mL	Physically compatible for up to 4 hr at room temperature	3245	C
Dexmedetomidine HCl	AB	4 mcg/mL[b]	AB	20 mcg/mL[b]	Physically compatible for 4 hr at 23°C	2383	C
Famotidine	MSD	0.2 mg/mL[a]	ES	0.004 mg/mL[a]	Physically compatible for 4 hr at 25°C	1188	C
Fenoldopam mesylate	AB	80 mcg/mL[b]	AB	20 mcg/mL[b]	Physically compatible for 4 hr at 23°C	2467	C
Heparin sodium	UP	1000 units/L[d]	WI	0.2 mg/mL	Physically compatible for 4 hr at room temperature	534	C
Hetastarch in lactated electrolyte	AB	6%	AB	0.02 mg/mL[a]	Physically compatible for 4 hr at 23°C	2339	C
Hydrocortisone sodium succinate	UP	10 mg/L[d]	WI	0.2 mg/mL	Physically compatible for 4 hr at room temperature	534	C
Ibuprofen lysinate	OVA	10 mg/mL	HOS	0.2 mg/mL	Measured turbidity increased immediately and solution became milky white	3541	I
Levofloxacin	OMN	5 mg/mL[a]	ES	0.2 mg/mL	Visually compatible for 4 hr at 24°C	2233	C
Meropenem		50 mg/mL	SZ	0.2 mg/mL	Physically compatible for 4 hr at room temperature	3538	C
Milrinone lactate	SW	0.4 mg/mL[a]	ES	8 mcg/mL[a]	Visually compatible. Little loss of either drug in 4 hr at 23°C	2214	C
Pancuronium bromide	ES	0.05 mg/mL[a]	ES	4 mcg/mL[a]	Physically compatible for 24 hr at 28°C	1337	C
Potassium chloride	AB	40 mEq/L[d]	WI	0.2 mg/mL	Physically compatible for 4 hr at room temperature	534	C
Propofol	ZEN[g]	10 mg/mL	AB	0.004 mg/mL[a]	Physically compatible for 1 hr at 23°C	2066	C
Remifentanil HCl	GW	0.025 and 0.25 mg/mL[b]	SW	0.02 mg/mL[a]	Physically compatible for 4 hr at 23°C	2075	C
Sodium nitroprusside	RC	0.3, 1.2, 3 mg/mL[a]	SX	20 mcg/mL[f]	Visually compatible for 48 hr at 24°C protected from light	2357	C
Sodium nitroprusside	RC	1.2 and 3 mg/mL[a]	SX	80 mcg/mL[f]	Visually compatible for 48 hr at 24°C protected from light	2357	C
Tacrolimus	FUJ	1 mg/mL[b]	ES	0.04 mg/mL[a]	Visually compatible for 24 hr at 25°C	1630	C
TNA #73[e]			BR	4 mcg/mL[c]	Visually compatible for 4 hr	1009	C
Vecuronium bromide	OR	0.1 mg/mL[a]	ES	4 mcg/mL[a]	Physically compatible for 24 hr at 28°C	1337	C

[a] Tested in dextrose 5%.

[b] Tested in sodium chloride 0.9%.

[c] Tested in both dextrose 5% and sodium chloride 0.9%.

[d] Tested in dextrose 5% in Ringer's injection, dextrose 5% in Ringer's injection, lactated, dextrose 5%, Ringer's injection, lactated, and sodium chloride 0.9%.

[e] Refer to Appendix for the composition of parenteral nutrition solutions. TNA indicates a 3-in-1 admixture.

[f] Tested in dextrose 5% in sodium chloride 0.225%.

[g] Test performed using the formulation WITH edetate disodium.

Selected Revisions May 1, 2020. © Copyright, October 1982.
American Society of Health-System Pharmacists, Inc.

Isosorbide Dinitrate
AHFS 24:12.08

Products

Isosorbide dinitrate is available as a 0.1% concentrate for injection in 10-mL ampuls and 50- and 100-mL vials and bottles; each mL contains isosorbide dinitrate 1 mg with sodium chloride in water for injection.[3573][3574] Hydrochloric acid and sodium hydroxide may be present to adjust the pH.[3573] The concentrate for injection *must* be diluted prior to intravenous administration.[3573][3574] Manufacturers state that 50 mL (50 mg) of isosorbide dinitrate 0.1% concentrate for injection may be diluted in 450 mL of a compatible infusion solution for a final isosorbide dinitrate concentration of 0.1 mg/mL.[3573][3574] If reduced fluid intake is necessary, 100 mL (100 mg) of isosorbide dinitrate 0.1% concentrate for injection may be diluted to a total volume of 500 mL using a compatible infusion solution for a final isosorbide dinitrate concentration of 0.2 mg/mL; if fluid intake is strictly limited, a 50% dilution of the concentrate for injection (i.e., to a final isosorbide dinitrate concentration of 0.5 mg/mL) is recommended.[3573][3574]

The drug also is available as a 0.05% solution in 50-mL vials and bottles and 10-mL prefilled syringes; each mL contains isosorbide dinitrate 0.5 mg with sodium chloride in water for injection.[3571][3572] Hydrochloric acid and sodium hydroxide also may be present to adjust the pH.[3571]

Sodium Content

Each mL of isosorbide dinitrate 0.05 or 0.1% solution contains 3.54[3571][3572][3573] or 3.6 mg[3574] of sodium.

Trade Name(s)

Isoket, Risordan

Administration

Isosorbide dinitrate is administered by intravenous infusion.[3571][3572][3573][3574] Only the 0.05% solution may be administered undiluted by slow infusion using a syringe pump; alternatively, the 0.05% solution may be diluted in a compatible infusion solution for administration.[3571][3572] The 0.1% concentrate for injection *must* be diluted in a compatible infusion solution prior to intravenous administration.[3573][3574]

Isosorbide dinitrate also may be administered as an intracoronary bolus injection during percutaneous transluminal coronary angioplasty.[3571][3572][3573][3574] Manufacturers recommend a 50% dilution of the 0.1% concentrate for injection (i.e., to a final isosorbide dinitrate concentration of 0.5 mg/mL) if administered by the intracoronary route.[3573][3574]

Stability

Once opened, containers should be used immediately, and any remainder should be discarded.[3571][3572][3573][3574] Specific product labeling should be consulted for additional storage details.

One manufacturer (Merus Labs) states that isosorbide dinitrate diluted in a compatible infusion solution (e.g., sodium chloride [concentration unspecified], dextrose 5 to 30%, Ringer's injection) is physically and chemically stable for 24 hours at 2 to 8°C.[3571][3573] Another manufacturer (Torbay) states that isosorbide dinitrate diluted in sodium chloride (concentration unspecified) or dextrose (concentration unspecified) has been shown to be physically and chemically stable for 72 hours at 25°C when stored protected from light in polypropylene or glass containers.[3572][3574]

Syringes

Isosorbide dinitrate (Rhone-Poulenc) 1 mg/mL was repackaged in polypropylene syringes (Plastipak, Becton Dickinson) and stored for 8 hours at room temperature and 4°C. No loss of drug was found.[1799]

Isosorbide dinitrate (Takeda) 30 mg/50 mL in sodium chloride 0.9% in a 50-mL polypropylene syringe (BD) was physically stable for 48 hours at room temperature.[3545]

Isosorbide dinitrate (Takeda) 0.6 mg/mL in sodium chloride 0.9% in a 50-mL polypropylene syringe (BD) was physically stable with a mean loss of 5.4% in 28 days at 2 to 8°C protected from light.[3570]

Sorption

Isosorbide dinitrate undergoes rapid and extensive sorption to polyvinyl chloride (PVC) and polyamide containers and PVC administration tubing. Studies have reported isosorbide dinitrate losses ranging from about 15 to 50%, depending on concentration, flow rate, contact time, length of tubing, and temperature. The majority of loss occurs at the beginning of contact with the plastic and then declines as saturation occurs. Isosorbide dinitrate also undergoes sorption of about 16 to 26% to cellulose propionate and butadiene styrene burette chambers but only 2% to methacrylate butadiene styrene burette chambers. However, little or no sorption occurs to glass, polyethylene, polybutadiene, nylon, and polypropylene containers and administration equipment. Consequently, glass, polyethylene, polypropylene, polybutadiene, and polytetrafluoroethylene containers and equipment are recommended while PVC, polyurethane, and polyamide are not.[769][782][795][1027][1392][1464][1465][1466][1467][1619][2143][2289][3571][3572][3573][3574]

Filtration

Losses due to sorption of isosorbide dinitrate 250 mg/L in sodium chloride 0.9% delivered at 20 mL/hr through cellulose acetate filters (Sterifix, Ivex HP) were 15 to 26%. Losses to polyamide filters (Pall) were 9 to 13% under the same conditions.[1465]

The loss of isosorbide dinitrate due to sorption to filters extends to filters used in hemodialysis. Isosorbide dinitrate 0.1 mg/mL in sodium chloride 0.9% during simulated hemodialysis using 5 different filter media underwent substantial drug losses from the solution and binding to some of the filters. Losses of approximately 86% with polysulfone (Fresenius), 72% with cellulose acetate (Baxter), 43% with polyacrylonitrile (Hospal), and 12% cuprophan (Gambro) were found. However, with hemophan filters (Gambro), no loss of drug due to sorption occurred.[2138]

DOI: 10.37573/9781585286850.226

Compatibility Information

Solution Compatibility

Isosorbide dinitrate

Test Soln Name	Mfr	Mfr	Conc/L or %	Remarks	Ref	C/I
Dextrose 5%	BA[a]	BRN	20 mg	Visually compatible but 43% loss of drug due to sorption to the PVC container at 22°C and 17% loss at 4°C in 24 hr	2289	I
Dextrose 5%	BRN[b c]	BRN	20 mg	Visually compatible with 2 to 3% loss in 24 hr at 4 and 22°C	2289	C
Dextrose 5%		MER		Physically and chemically stable for 24 hr at 2 to 8°C	3571, 3573	C
Dextrose 10%		MER		Physically and chemically stable for 24 hr at 2 to 8°C	3571, 3573	C
Ringer's injection		MER		Physically and chemically stable for 24 hr at 2 to 8°C	3571, 3573	C
Sodium chloride 0.9%	TR[a], BT[a]		80 mg	38% loss in 24 hr at room temperature	1464	I
Sodium chloride 0.9%	TR[b], BT[c]		80 mg	Physically compatible with little or no loss in 6 hr at room temperature	1464	C
Sodium chloride 0.9%	TR[a]		100 mg	9% loss in 2 hr and 23% loss in 24 hr at 21°C in the dark	1392	I
Sodium chloride 0.9%	[b d]		100 mg	Physically compatible with little or no loss in 24 hr at 21°C in the dark	1392	C
Sodium chloride 0.9%	BA[a]	BRN	20 mg	Visually compatible but 43% loss of drug due to sorption to the PVC container at 22°C and 17% loss at 4°C in 24 hr	2289	I
Sodium chloride 0.9%	BRN[b c]	BRN	20 mg	Visually compatible with 2 to 3% loss in 24 hr at 4 and 22°C	2289	C

[a] Tested in PVC containers.

[b] Tested in glass containers.

[c] Tested in polypropylene containers.

[d] Tested in Clear-Flex polyethylene-lined laminated containers.

Additive Compatibility

Isosorbide dinitrate

Test Drug	Mfr	Conc/L or %	Mfr	Conc/L or %	Test Solution	Remarks	Ref	C/I
Floxacillin sodium	BE	20 g		1 g		Physically compatible for 24 hr at 15 and 30°C. Haze forms in 48 hr and precipitate forms in 72 hr at 30°C. No change at 15°C	1479	C
Furosemide	HO	1 g		1 g		Physically compatible for 72 hr at 15 and 30°C	1479	C

Y-Site Injection Compatibility (1:1 Mixture)

Isosorbide dinitrate

Test Drug	Mfr	Conc	Mfr	Conc	Remarks	Ref	C/I
Cefepime HCl	BMS	120 mg/mL[b]		0.2 mg/mL	Physically compatible with less than 10% cefepime loss. Isosorbide not tested	2513	C
Ceftazidime	GSK	120 mg/mL[b]		0.2 mg/mL	Physically compatible with less than 10% ceftazidime loss. Isosorbide not tested	2513	C
Heparin sodium	LEO	300 units/mL[a]	RP	10 mg/mL	Erratic availability of both drugs delivered through PVC tubing	1799	I

[a] Tested in dextrose 5%.

[b] Tested in sterile water for injection.

Selected Revisions July 1, 2020. © Copyright, October 1992.
American Society of Health-System Pharmacists, Inc.

Ketamine Hydrochloride
AHFS 28:04.92

Products

Ketamine hydrochloride is available in concentrations equivalent to 10, 50, or 100 mg/mL of ketamine in 20-, 10-, or 5-mL multidose vials, respectively.[3116][3117] The injections also contain no more than 0.1 mg/mL of the preservative benzethonium chloride.[3116][3117]

The 10-mg/mL concentration should not be diluted.[3116] However, the 100-mg/mL injection is a concentrate and *must* be diluted prior to intravenous use.[3116][3117] Doses should be diluted with an equal volume of sterile water for injection, dextrose 5%, or sodium chloride 0.9%.[3116][3117]

pH
From 3.5 to 5.5.[3116][3117]

Tonicity
The 10-mg/mL concentration is made isotonic with sodium chloride.[3116]

Osmolality
The osmolalities of ketamine hydrochloride products were determined to be 300 mOsm/kg for the 10-mg/mL concentration and 387 mOsm/kg for the 50-mg/mL concentration.[1233]

Trade Name(s)
Ketalar

Administration

Ketamine hydrochloride may be administered intramuscularly or by slow intravenous injection over 60 seconds.[3116][3117] The 100-mg/mL preparation should not be administered without proper dilution.[3116][3117] For intravenous infusion, a 1- or 2-mg/mL solution may be prepared by adding 500 mg of ketamine to 500 or 250 mL, respectively, of dextrose 5% or sodium chloride 0.9%.[3116][3117]

Diazepam and barbiturates must be administered separately from ketamine hydrochloride and must not be mixed in the same container.[3116][3117]

Stability

Intact vials of ketamine hydrochloride should be stored at controlled room temperature and protected from light.[3116][3117]

Ketamine hydrochloride injection varies from colorless to very slightly yellow.[3117] The drug may darken upon prolonged exposure to light; however, this darkening does not affect potency.[3117] The product should be visually inspected for particulate matter and discoloration prior to administration and should not be used if a precipitate appears.[3117]

Ketamine hydrochloride (Sandoz) prepared at a ketamine concentration of 10 mg/mL diluted in sterile water for injection was packaged in 5-mL glass vials and stored at room temperature with exposure to light for 182 days.[3118] The solution remained clear and without discoloration and less than 4% drug loss occurred.[3118]

Syringes

Ketamine hydrochloride (Abbott) prepared at a ketamine concentration of 10 mg/mL diluted in sterile water for injection was packaged in 1-mL polypropylene tuberculin syringes (Becton Dickinson) and was stored at 25°C.[2431] The drug solution remained clear and no loss occurred in 30 days.[2431]

Ketamine hydrochloride (Fagron) prepared at a ketamine concentration of 1 mg/mL diluted in sodium chloride 0.9% was packaged in polypropylene syringes with tip caps and stored at 4, 25, and 40°C for 12 months.[2779] No visible changes occurred, and drug concentrations remained above 95% at all temperatures.[2779]

Ketamine hydrochloride (Pfizer) undiluted at a ketamine concentration of 50 mg/mL was packaged as 1 mL in 3-mL polypropylene syringes (Terumo).[3194] The syringes were stored at 25°C protected from light for 180 days.[3194] Solutions were physically stable with no substantial changes in pH or optical density throughout the study.[3194] Little loss of the drug occurred in 180 days.[3194]

Ketamine hydrochloride (Pfizer) undiluted at a ketamine concentration of 50 mg/mL was packaged as 1 mL in 3-mL syringes (Becton Dickinson).[3584] The syringes were stored at room temperature for 50 days.[3584] Solutions were physically stable with no substantial changes in pH or spectrophotometric measurements throughout the study.[3584] Less than 10% loss of the drug occurred in 50 days.[3584]

DOI: 10.37573/9781585286850.227

Compatibility Information

Solution Compatibility

Ketamine HCl

Test Soln Name	Mfr	Mfr	Conc/L or %	Remarks	Ref	C/I
Dextrose 5%		PAR	1 and 2 g	Manufacturer-recommended solution	3116	C
Sodium chloride 0.9%		PAR	1 and 2 g	Manufacturer-recommended solution	3116	C
Sodium chloride 0.9%	FRK[a]	PAN	1 g	Physically compatible with little loss in 28 days at 23 to 27° and 7 days at 33°C	3582	C

[a] Tested in PVC containers.

Additive Compatibility

Ketamine HCl

Test Drug	Mfr	Conc/L or %	Mfr	Conc/L or %	Test Solution	Remarks	Ref	C/I
Acetaminophen	BMS	8.2 g	PAN[d e]	123 mg[f]	NS	Physically compatible with less than 5% loss of either drug over 24 hr at 25°C	2842, 2843	C
Butorphanol tartrate	HE	50 mg	QI	1, 2, 4 g	NS[g]	Physically compatible with little to no loss of either drug in 15 days at 4, 25, and 37°C in the dark	3119	C
Butorphanol tartrate	HE	100 mg	QI	1, 2, 4 g	NS[g]	Physically compatible with little to no loss of either drug in 15 days at 4, 25, and 37°C in the dark	3119	C
Butorphanol tartrate	HE	150 mg	QI	1, 2, 4 g	NS[g]	Physically compatible with little to no loss of either drug in 15 days at 4, 25, and 37°C in the dark	3119	C
Droperidol with fentanyl citrate	JN DB	50 mg 10 mg	JN	1 g	NS[a]	Visually compatible. 5% increase in all drugs in 30 days at 4 and 25°C due to water loss	2653	C
Droperidol with fentanyl citrate	JN DB	50 mg 10 mg	JN	1 g	NS[c]	Visually compatible with little loss of the drugs in 30 days at 25°C	2653	C
Fentanyl citrate with droperidol	DB JN	10 mg 50 mg	JN	1 g	NS[a]	Visually compatible. 5% increase in all drugs in 30 days at 4 and 25°C due to water loss	2653	C
Fentanyl citrate with droperidol	DB JN	10 mg 50 mg	JN	1 g	NS[c]	Visually compatible with little loss of the drugs in 30 days at 25°C	2653	C
Hydromorphone HCl	SZ	200 mg	SZ	200 mg, 600 mg, 1 g	NS[a c]	Visually compatible. Under 10% loss of both drugs in 7 days at 25°C	2799	C
Morphine sulfate	SX	1 g	PD	1 g	NS[a]	At least 90% of both drugs retained for 6 days at room temperature	2260	C
Morphine sulfate	SX	25 g	PD	25 g	NS[a]	At least 90% of both drugs retained for 6 days at room temperature	2260	C
Morphine sulfate	SX	25 g	PD	25 g	NS[b]	At least 90% of both drugs retained for 6 days at room temperature	2260	C
Morphine sulfate	AB	2 g	PD	1.33 g	NS	Little loss of either drug in 4 days at room temperature	2786	C
Oxycodone HCl	MUN	400 mg	PAN	40 g	NS[a]	Physically compatible with little to no loss of either drug in 7 days at 22 to 23°C	3585, 3586	C

Additive Compatibility (Cont.)

Test Drug	Mfr	Conc/L or %	Mfr	Conc/L or %	Test Solution	Remarks	Ref	C/I
Oxycodone HCl	MUN	10 g	PAN	100 mg	NS[a]	Physically compatible with little to no loss of either drug in 7 days at 22 to 23°C	3585, 3586	C
Oxycodone HCl	MUN	10 g	PAN	40 g	NS[a]	Physically compatible with little to no loss of either drug in 7 days at 22 to 23°C	3585, 3586	C
Tramadol HCl	GRU	5 g	QI	500 mg	NS[e]	Physically compatible with little loss of either drug in 14 days at 4 and 25°C in the dark	3583	C
Tramadol HCl	GRU	5 g	QI	1 g	NS[e]	Physically compatible with little loss of either drug in 14 days at 4 and 25°C in the dark	3583	C
Tramadol HCl	GRU	5 g	QI	2 g	NS[e]	Physically compatible with little loss of either drug in 14 days at 4 and 25°C in the dark	3583	C

[a] Tested in PVC containers.

[b] Tested in plastic medication cassette reservoirs (Deltec).

[c] Tested in glass containers.

[d] Test performed using the formulation containing chlorobutanol.

[e] Tested in polyolefin containers.

[f] Tested in sodium chloride 0.9%.

[g] Tested in polyolefin containers.

Drugs in Syringe Compatibility

Ketamine HCl

Test Drug	Mfr	Amt	Mfr	Amt	Remarks	Ref	C/I
Bupivacaine HCl with fentanyl citrate	SW JN	1.5 mg/mL 0.01 mg/mL	PD	2 mg/mL	Diluted to 5 mL with NS. Visually compatible with no new GC/MS peaks in 1 hr at room temperature	1956	C
Clonidine HCl with tetracaine HCl	BI SW	0.03 mg/mL 2 mg/mL	PD	2 mg/mL	Diluted to 5 mL with NS. Visually compatible with no new GC/MS peaks in 1 hr at room temperature	1956	C
Dexamethasone sodium phosphate	OR	50 and 600 mg	PF	1 mg	Diluted to 14 mL with NS. Physically compatible with no loss of either drug in 8 days at 4 and 23°C	2677	C
Doxapram HCl	RB	400 mg/20 mL	PD	200 mg/20 mL	Physically compatible with no doxapram loss in 9 hr but 12% loss in 24 hr	1177	I
Fentanyl citrate		40 mcg/mL	PF	1 mg/mL	Diluted in sodium chloride 0.9%. Physically compatible for 96 hr at 25°C	2563	C
Fentanyl citrate with bupivacaine HCl	JN SW	0.01 mg/mL 1.5 mg/mL	PD	2 mg/mL	Diluted to 5 mL with NS. Visually compatible with no new GC/MS peaks in 1 hr at room temperature	1956	C
Hydromorphone HCl	SZ	0.2 mg/mL[a]	SZ	0.2, 0.6, 1 mg/mL[a]	Visually compatible. Under 10% loss of both drugs in 7 days at 25°C	2799	C
Lidocaine HCl	APN	1 g/20 mL	REN	125 mg/2.5 mL	Diluted to 50 mL with NS. Physically compatible with little to no loss of either drug in 48 hr at 28°C protected from light	3587	C
Lidocaine HCl with morphine sulfate	AST ES	2 mg/mL 0.2 mg/mL	PD	2 mg/mL	Diluted to 5 mL with NS. Visually compatible with no new GC/MS peaks in 1 hr at room temperature	1956	C
Meperidine HCl	DB	12 mg/mL	PD	2 mg/mL	Diluted to 50 mL with NS. Visually compatible for 48 hr at 25°C	2059	C
Morphine sulfate	SX	1 mg/mL[a], 10 mg/mL[a]	PD	1 mg/mL[a]	At least 90% of both drugs retained for 6 days at room temperature	2260	C

Drugs in Syringe Compatibility (Cont.)

Test Drug	Mfr	Amt	Mfr	Amt	Remarks	Ref	C/I
Morphine sulfate	SX	25 mg/mL[a]	PD	1 mg/mL[a]	5% morphine loss in 6 days at room temperature. Up to 15% ketamine loss in 2 to 6 days	2260	C
Morphine sulfate	SX	1, 10, 25 mg/mL[a]	PD[a]	10, 25 mg/mL	At least 90% of both drugs retained for 6 days at room temperature	2260	C
Morphine sulfate		1 mg/1 mL		5, 10, 20 mg/1 mL	No substantial change in the concentration of either drug over 4 days	669	C
Morphine sulfate	SZ	2, 5, 10 mg/mL[a]	SZ	2 mg/mL[a]	Physically compatible. Little loss of either drug at 23 and 5°C in 91 days	2797	C
Morphine sulfate with lidocaine HCl	ES AST	0.2 mg/mL 2 mg/mL	PD	2 mg/mL	Diluted to 5 mL with NS. Visually compatible with no new GC/MS peaks in 1 hr at room temperature	1956	C
Oxycodone HCl	MUN	0.4 mg/mL[a]	PAN	40 mg/mL[a]	Physically compatible with little to no loss of either drug in 7 days at 22 to 23°C	3585, 3586	C
Oxycodone HCl	MUN	10 mg/mL[a]	PAN	0.1 mg/mL[a]	Physically compatible with little to no loss of either drug in 7 days at 22 to 23°C	3585, 3586	C
Oxycodone HCl	MUN	10 mg/mL[a]	PAN	40 mg/mL[a]	Physically compatible with little to no loss of either drug in 7 days at 22 to 23°C	3585, 3586	C
Propofol	NOP	50 mg/5 mL	SZ	50 mg/5 mL	Physically compatible. Little loss of either drug in 3 hr at room temperature	2790	C
Propofol	NOP	70 mg/7 mL	SZ	30 mg/3 mL	Physically compatible. Little loss of either drug in 3 hr at room temperature	2790	C
Tetracaine HCl with clonidine HCl	SW BI	2 mg/mL 0.03 mg/mL	PD	2 mg/mL	Diluted to 5 mL with NS. Visually compatible with no new GC/MS peaks in 1 hr at room temperature	1956	C

[a] Diluted in sodium chloride 0.9%.

Y-Site Injection Compatibility (1:1 Mixture)

Ketamine HCl

Test Drug	Mfr	Conc	Mfr	Conc	Remarks	Ref	C/I
Cefepime HCl	BMS	120 mg/mL[a]		10 mg/mL	Physically compatible with less than 10% cefepime loss. Ketamine not tested	2513	C
Ceftazidime	SKB	125 mg/mL		10 mg/mL	Visually compatible with less than 10% loss of ceftazidime in 24 hr. Ketamine not tested	2434	C
Ceftazidime	GSK	120 mg/mL[a]		10 mg/mL	Physically compatible with less than 10% ceftazidime loss. Ketamine not tested	2513	C
Cloxacillin sodium	SMX	100 mg/mL	SZ	50 mg/mL	Physically compatible for up to 4 hr at room temperature	3245	C
Meropenem		50 mg/mL	SZ	50 mg/mL	Precipitates immediately	3538	I
Propofol	ZEN[b]	10 mg/mL	PD	10 mg/mL	Physically compatible for 1 hr at 23°C	2066	C

[a] Tested in sterile water for injection.

[b] Test performed using the formulation WITH edetate disodium.

Selected Revisions July 1, 2020. © Copyright, October 1982.
American Society of Health-System Pharmacists, Inc.

Ketorolac Tromethamine
AHFS 28:08.04.92

Products

Ketorolac tromethamine is available as a 15-mg/mL solution in 1-mL vials and also as a 30-mg/mL solution in 1-mL vials. Ketorolac tromethamine 30 mg/mL is also available in 2-mL vials for intramuscular use. In addition to ketorolac tromethamine, the formulations contain ethanol, sodium chloride, and citric acid in water for injection. The product also contains sodium hydroxide or hydrochloric acid to adjust the pH.[1(6/08)]

pH

From 6.9 to 7.9.[1(6/08) 4]

Tonicity

Both ketorolac tromethamine concentrations are isotonic.[4]

Administration

Ketorolac tromethamine is administered slowly by deep intramuscular injection or by intravenous injection over no less than 15 seconds.[1(6/08) 4] The 60 mg/2 mL injection is for intramuscular use only.[1(6/08)]

Stability

Ketorolac tromethamine injection should be stored at controlled room temperature and protected from light. The injection is clear and has a slight yellow color.[1(6/08) 4] Prolonged exposure to light may result in discoloration of the solution and precipitation.[4] Ketorolac tromethamine is chemically stable over a wide pH range from about pH 3 to 11[499], but precipitation may occur in solutions and with drugs having a relatively low pH.[4]

Compatibility Information
Solution Compatibility

Ketorolac tromethamine

Test Soln Name	Mfr	Mfr	Conc/L or %	Remarks	Ref	C/I
Dextrose 5% in sodium chloride 0.9%	TR[a]	SY	600 mg	Physically compatible. No loss in 48 hr at room temperature	1646	C
Dextrose 5%	TR[b]	SY	600 mg	Physically compatible. No loss in 48 hr at room temperature	1646	C
Dextrose 5%	BA[a]	RC	600 mg	Visually compatible. Little loss in 7 days and 14% loss in 14 days at 25°C. Less than 2% loss in 50 days at 5°C	2095	C
Dextrose 5%	[a]	RC	300 and 600 mg	Visually compatible. Little loss in 21 days at 4 and 23°C	2442	C
Dextrose 5%	[c]	RC	200 mg	Visually compatible. Less than 10% loss after –20°C storage for 90 days, microwave thawing, and storage at 4°C for 60 days	2645	C
Dextrose 5%	BA[c]	RC	100 and 300 mg	Visually compatible. Less than 3% drug loss after 15 days at –20°C then 35 days at 4°C	2707	C
Plasma-Lyte A, pH 7.4	TR[a]	SY	600 mg	Physically compatible. No loss in 48 hr at room temperature	1646	C
Plasma-Lyte A, pH 7.4	TR[b]	SY	60 mg	Physically compatible. No loss in 48 hr at room temperature	1646	C
Ringer's injection	TR[a]	SY	600 mg	Physically compatible. No loss in 48 hr at room temperature	1646	C
Ringer's injection	TR[b]	SY	60 mg	Physically compatible. No loss in 48 hr at room temperature	1646	C
Ringer's injection, lactated	TR[a]	SY	600 mg	Physically compatible. No loss in 48 hr at room temperature	1646	C
Sodium chloride 0.9%	TR[b]	SY	600 mg	Physically compatible. No loss in 48 hr at room temperature	1646	C
Sodium chloride 0.9%	BA[a]	RC	600 mg	Visually compatible. No loss in 35 days at 25°C and in 50 days at 5°C	2095	C

[a] Tested in PVC containers.

[b] Tested in both glass and PVC containers.

[c] Tested in polyolefin containers.

DOI: 10.37573/9781585286850.228

Drugs in Syringe Compatibility

Ketorolac tromethamine

Test Drug	Mfr	Amt	Mfr	Amt	Remarks	Ref	C/I
Cyclizine lactate	WEL	50 mg/mL	RC	30 mg/mL	White precipitate forms	2495	I
Diazepam	ES	15 mg/3 mL	SY	180 mg/6 mL	Visually compatible for 4 hr at 24°C. Increase in absorbance occurs immediately, persists for 30 min, and dissipates by 1 hr	1703	?
Haloperidol lactate	SO	5 mg/1 mL	SY	30 mg/1 mL	White crystalline precipitate forms immediately	1786	I
Hydromorphone HCl	KN	10 mg/1 mL	SY	30 mg/1 mL	Cloudiness forms immediately but clears with swirling	1785	?
Hydromorphone HCl	KN	1 mg/1 mL[a]	SY	30 mg/1 mL	Visually compatible for 24 hr at 25°C under fluorescent light	1785	C
Hydromorphone HCl	KN	1[a] and 10 mg/1 mL	SY	15 mg/1 mL[a]	Visually compatible for 24 hr at 25°C under fluorescent light	1785	C
Hydroxyzine HCl	SO	150 mg/3 mL	SY	180 mg/6 mL	Heavy white precipitate forms immediately, separating into two layers over time	1703	I
Nalbuphine HCl	DU	30 mg/3 mL	SY	180 mg/6 mL	Solid white precipitate forms immediately and settles to bottom	1703	I
Prochlorperazine edisylate	STS	15 mg/3 mL	SY	180 mg/6 mL	Heavy white precipitate forms immediately, separating into two layers over time	1703	I
Promethazine HCl	ES	75 mg/3 mL	SY	180 mg/6 mL	Heavy white precipitate forms immediately, separating into two layers over time	1703	I

[a] Dilutions prepared with sterile water for injection.

Y-Site Injection Compatibility (1:1 Mixture)

Ketorolac tromethamine

Test Drug	Mfr	Conc	Mfr	Conc	Remarks	Ref	C/I
Acetaminophen	CAD	10 mg/mL	WOC	15 mg/mL	Physically compatible with less than 10% acetaminophen loss over 4 hr at room temperature	2841, 2844	C
Acetaminophen	CAD	10 mg/mL	HOS	30 mg/mL	Physically compatible with no loss of either drug in 4 hr at 23°C	2901, 2902	C
Azithromycin	PF	2 mg/mL[b]	AB	15 mg/mL[c]	Amber microcrystals found	2368	I
Cisatracurium besylate	GW	0.1, 2, 5 mg/mL[a]	RC	15 mg/mL[a]	Physically compatible for 4 hr at 23°C	2074	C
Cisatracurium besylate	ABV				Manufacturer states incompatible	2868	I
Dexmedetomidine HCl	AB	4 mcg/mL[b]	AB	15 mg/mL	Physically compatible for 4 hr at 23°C	2383	C
Fenoldopam mesylate	AB	80 mcg/mL[b]	AB	15 mg/mL[b]	Trace haze forms immediately	2467	I
Fentanyl citrate	JN	0.025 mg/mL[a]	WY	1 mg/mL[a]	Physically compatible for 48 hr at 22°C	1706	C
Hetastarch in lactated electrolyte	AB	6%	AB	15 mg/mL	Physically compatible for 4 hr at 23°C	2339	C
Hydromorphone HCl	AST	0.5 mg/mL[a]	WY	1 mg/mL[a]	Physically compatible for 48 hr at 22°C	1706	C
Methadone HCl	LI	1 mg/mL[a]	WY	1 mg/mL[a]	Physically compatible for 48 hr at 22°C	1706	C

Y-Site Injection Compatibility (1:1 Mixture) (Cont.)

Test Drug	Mfr	Conc	Mfr	Conc	Remarks	Ref	C/I
Morphine sulfate	AST	1 mg/mL[a]	WY	1 mg/mL[a]	Physically compatible for 48 hr at 22°C	1706	C
Remifentanil HCl	GW	0.025 and 0.25 mg/mL[b]	RC	15 mg/mL[a]	Physically compatible for 4 hr at 23°C	2075	C

[a] Tested in dextrose 5%.

[b] Tested in sodium chloride 0.9%.

[c] Injected via Y-site into an administration set running azithromycin.

Selected Revisions September 30, 2019. © Copyright, October 1994. American Society of Health-System Pharmacists, Inc.

Labetalol Hydrochloride
AHFS 24:24

Products

Labetalol hydrochloride is available in 20- and 40-mL multiple-dose vials and 4- and 8-mL vials and disposable syringes. Each mL of solution contains labetalol hydrochloride 5 mg, dextrose, anhydrous 45 mg, edetate disodium 0.1 mg, methylparaben 0.8 mg, propylparaben 0.1 mg, and citric acid anhydrous and sodium hydroxide as necessary to adjust pH in water for injection.[1(2/07)]

pH

From 3 to 4.5.[17]

Administration

Labetalol hydrochloride is administered by slow direct intravenous injection, over 2 minutes, or by continuous intravenous infusion at an initial rate of 2 mg/min with subsequent adjustments based on blood pressure response. For continuous infusion, concentrations of 1 mg/mL or 2 mg/3 mL can be made by adding 200 mg (40 mL) to 160 or 250 mL of compatible infusion solution. To facilitate the infusion of labetalol hydrochloride at an accurate rate of administration, a controlled-infusion device, such as a pump, may be used.[1(2/07) 4]

Stability

Labetalol hydrochloride may be stored at room temperature or under refrigeration and should be protected from light and freezing. The solution is clear and colorless to slightly yellow.[1(2/07)]

pH Effects

Labetalol hydrochloride has optimal stability at pH 3 to 4. Addition to an alkaline drug or solution has resulted in precipitate formation.[757 1715 2062]

Compatibility Information

Solution Compatibility

Labetalol HCl

Test Soln Name	Mfr	Mfr	Conc/L or %	Remarks	Ref	C/I
Dextrose 5% in Ringer's injection	TR	SC	1.25 and 3.75 g	Physically compatible and chemically stable for 72 hr at 4 and 25°C	757	C
Dextrose 5% in Ringer's injection, lactated	TR	SC	1.25 and 3.75 g	Physically compatible and chemically stable for 72 hr at 4 and 25°C	757	C
Dextrose 2.5% in sodium chloride 0.45%	TR	SC	1.25 and 3.75 g	Physically compatible and chemically stable for 72 hr at 4 and 25°C	757	C
Dextrose 5% in sodium chloride 0.225%	TR	SC	1.25 and 3.75 g	Physically compatible and chemically stable for 72 hr at 4 and 25°C	757	C
Dextrose 5% in sodium chloride 0.33%	TR	SC	1.25 and 3.75 g	Physically compatible and chemically stable for 72 hr at 4 and 25°C	757	C
Dextrose 5% in sodium chloride 0.9%	TR	SC	1.25 and 3.75 g	Physically compatible and chemically stable for 72 hr at 4 and 25°C	757	C
Dextrose 5%	TR	SC	1.25 and 3.75 g	Physically compatible and chemically stable for 72 hr at 4 and 25°C	757	C
Ringer's injection	TR	SC	1.25 and 3.75 g	Physically compatible and chemically stable for 72 hr at 4 and 25°C	757	C
Ringer's injection, lactated	TR	SC	1.25 and 3.75 g	Physically compatible and chemically stable for 72 hr at 4 and 25°C	757	C
Sodium chloride 0.9%				Physically compatible and stable for 24 hr at room temperature or refrigerated	1(2/07)	C

Additive Compatibility

Labetalol HCl

Test Drug	Mfr	Conc/L or %	Mfr	Conc/L or %	Test Solution	Remarks	Ref	C/I
Sodium bicarbonate	TR	5%	SC	1.25, 2.5, 3.75 g		White precipitate forms within 6 hr after mixing at 4 and 25°C	757	I

DOI: 10.37573/9781585286850.229

Drugs in Syringe Compatibility

Labetalol HCl

Test Drug	Mfr	Amt	Mfr	Amt	Remarks	Ref	C/I
Pantoprazole sodium	a	4 mg/1 mL		5 mg/1 mL	Whitish precipitate	2574	I

[a] Test performed using the formulation WITHOUT edetate disodium.

Y-Site Injection Compatibility (1:1 Mixture)

Labetalol HCl

Test Drug	Mfr	Conc	Mfr	Conc	Remarks	Ref	C/I
Acetaminophen	CAD	10 mg/mL	HOS	5 mg/mL	Physically compatible for 1 hr at 23°C	3533	C
Albumin human	OCT	250 mg/mL	HOS	5 mg/mL	Measured turbidity increased	3533	I
Amikacin sulfate	BR	5 mg/mL[a]	SC	1 mg/mL[a]	Physically compatible for 24 hr at 18°C	1171	C
Aminophylline	ES	1 mg/mL[a]	SC	1 mg/mL[a]	Physically compatible for 24 hr at 18°C	1171	C
Amiodarone HCl	WY	4.8 mg/mL[a]	GL	5 mg/mL	Visually compatible for 24 hr at 23°C	1877	C
Amiodarone HCl	WY	6 mg/mL[a]	BED	5 mg/mL	Visually compatible for 24 hr at 22°C	2352	C
Ampicillin sodium	WY	10 mg/mL[b]	SC	1 mg/mL[a]	Physically compatible for 24 hr at 18°C	1171	C
Bivalirudin	TMC	5 mg/mL[a]	FP	2 mg/mL[a]	Physically compatible for 4 hr at 23°C	2373	C
Butorphanol tartrate	BR	0.04 mg/mL[a]	SC	1 mg/mL[a]	Physically compatible for 24 hr at 18°C	1171	C
Calcium gluconate	AMR	0.23 mEq/mL[a]	SC	1 mg/mL[a]	Physically compatible for 24 hr at 18°C	1171	C
Cangrelor tetrasodium	TMC	1 mg/mL[b]		2[b] and 5 mg/mL	Gross white turbid precipitate forms immediately	3243	I
Cefazolin sodium	LI	10 mg/mL[a]	SC	1 mg/mL[a]	Physically compatible for 24 hr at 18°C	1171	C
Cefepime HCl	APP	40 mg/mL[b]	HOS	5 mg/mL	Slight haze and particulate matter forms immediately	3533	I
Ceftaroline fosamil	FOR	2.22 mg/mL[a]	HOS	5 mg/mL	Increase in measured haze and microparticulates	2826	I
Ceftaroline fosamil	FOR	2.22 mg/mL[b e]	HOS	5 mg/mL	Increase in measured haze	2826	I
Ceftazidime	GL	10 mg/mL[a]	SC	1 mg/mL[a]	Physically compatible for 24 hr at 18°C	1171	C
Ceftolozane sulfate–tazobactam sodium	CUB	10 mg/mL[g h]	HOS	2 mg/mL[g]	Physically compatible for 2 hr	3262	C
Ceftriaxone sodium	RC	20[a b] and 100[c] mg/mL	GL	2.5[c] and 5 mg/mL	Fluffy white precipitate forms immediately	1964	I
Chloramphenicol sodium succinate	PD	10 mg/mL[a]	SC	1 mg/mL[a]	Physically compatible for 24 hr at 18°C	1171	C
Ciprofloxacin	SZ	2 mg/mL	HOS	5 mg/mL	Physically compatible for 1 hr at 23°C	3533	C
Cisatracurium besylate	AB	2 mg/mL	HOS	5 mg/mL	Physically compatible for 1 hr at 23°C	3533	C
Clindamycin phosphate	UP	9 mg/mL[a]	SC	1 mg/mL[a]	Physically compatible for 24 hr at 18°C	1171	C
Clonidine HCl	BI	18 mcg/mL[b]	GSK	1 mg/mL[a b]	Visually compatible	2642	C
Cloxacillin sodium	SMX	100 mg/mL	SZ	5 mg/mL	Precipitates immediately	3245	I
Dexmedetomidine HCl	AB	4 mcg/mL[b]	AB	2 mg/mL[b]	Physically compatible for 4 hr at 23°C	2383	C
Diltiazem HCl	MMD	1 mg/mL[a]	AH	2 mg/mL[a]	Visually compatible for 4 hr at 27°C	2062	C

Y-Site Injection Compatibility (1:1 Mixture) (Cont.)

Test Drug	Mfr	Conc	Mfr	Conc	Remarks	Ref	C/I
Dobutamine HCl	LI	2.5 mg/mL[a]	GL	1 mg/mL[a]	Visually compatible. Little loss of either drug in 4 hr at room temperature	1762	C
Dobutamine HCl	LI	4 mg/mL[a]	GL	5 mg/mL	Visually compatible for 24 hr at 23°C	1877	C
Dobutamine HCl	LI	4 mg/mL[a]	AH	2 mg/mL[a]	Visually compatible for 4 hr at 27°C	2062	C
Dopamine HCl	IMS	1.6 mg/mL[a]	SC	1 mg/mL[a]	Physically compatible for 24 hr at 18°C	1171	C
Dopamine HCl	ES	1.6 mg/mL[a]	GL	1 mg/mL[a]	Visually compatible. Little loss of either drug in 4 hr at room temperature	1762	C
Dopamine HCl	AB	3.2 mg/mL[a]	AH	2 mg/mL[a]	Visually compatible for 4 hr at 27°C	2062	C
Doripenem	JJ	5 mg/mL[a b]	HOS	2 mg/mL[a b]	Physically compatible for 4 hr at 23°C	2743	C
Doripenem	SHI	4.5 mg/mL[b]	HOS	5 mg/mL	Physically compatible for 1 hr at 23°C	3533	C
Enalaprilat	MSD	0.05 mg/mL[b]	GL	1 mg/mL[a]	Physically compatible for 24 hr at room temperature under fluorescent light	1355	C
Epinephrine HCl	AB	0.02 mg/mL[a]	AH	2 mg/mL[a]	Visually compatible for 4 hr at 27°C	2062	C
Epinephrine[k]	AMP	0.128 mg/mL[b]	HOS	5 mg/mL	Physically compatible for 1 hr at 23°C	3533	C
Erythromycin lactobionate	AB	5 mg/mL[a]	SC	1 mg/mL[a]	Physically compatible for 24 hr at 18°C	1171	C
Esmolol HCl	DU	40 mg/mL[a]	GL	5 mg/mL	Visually compatible for 24 hr at 23°C	1877	C
Esomeprazole sodium	ASZ	0.8 mg/mL[b]	HOS	5 mg/mL	Light pink solution forms immediately	3533	I
Famotidine	MSD	0.2 mg/mL[a]	SC	1 mg/mL[a]	Physically compatible for 4 hr at 25°C	1188	C
Fenoldopam mesylate	AB	80 mcg/mL[b]	AB	2 mg/mL[b]	Physically compatible for 4 hr at 23°C	2467	C
Fentanyl citrate	JN	10 mcg/mL[a]	SC	1 mg/mL[a]	Physically compatible for 24 hr at 18°C	1171	C
Fentanyl citrate	ES	0.05 mg/mL	AH	2 mg/mL[a]	Visually compatible for 4 hr at 27°C	2062	C
Furosemide	ES	10 mg/mL[d]	SC	1.6 mg/mL[d]	White precipitate forms immediately	1715	I
Furosemide	AMR	10 mg/mL	AH	2 mg/mL[a]	Precipitate forms immediately	2062	I
Gentamicin sulfate	ES	0.8 mg/mL[a]	SC	1 mg/mL[a]	Physically compatible for 24 hr at 18°C	1171	C
Heparin sodium	IX	40 units/mL[a]	SC	1 mg/mL[a]	Physically compatible for 24 hr at 18°C	1171	C
Heparin sodium	OR	100 units/mL[a]	GL	5 mg/mL	Cloudiness with particles forms immediately	1877	I
Heparin sodium	ES	100 units/mL[a]	AH	2 mg/mL[a]	Visually compatible for 4 hr at 27°C	2062	C
Hetastarch in lactated electrolyte	AB	6%	GW	2 mg/mL[a]	Physically compatible for 4 hr at 23°C	2339	C
Hydrocortisone sodium succinate	PF	1 mg/mL[b]	HOS	5 mg/mL	Measured turbidity increased	3533	I
Hydromorphone HCl	KN	1 mg/mL	AH	2 mg/mL[a]	Visually compatible for 4 hr at 27°C	2062	C
Hydroxyethyl starch 130/0.4 in sodium chloride 0.9%	FRK	6%	SZ	1.25[a], 2.5[a], 5 mg/mL	Visually compatible for 24 hr at room temperature	2770	C
Ibuprofen	CMB	4 mg/mL	HOS	5 mg/mL	White cloudy solution forms upon mixing	3533	I
Insulin, regular	LI	1 unit/mL[a]	GL	5 mg/mL	Visually compatible for 4 hr. White precipitate forms in 24 hr at 23°C	1877	?
Isavuconazonium sulfate	ASP	1.5 mg/mL[g]	HOS	2 mg/mL[g]	Physically compatible for 2 hr	3263	C
Levofloxacin	SGT	5 mg/mL	HOS	5 mg/mL	Physically compatible for 1 hr at 23°C	3533	C

Y-Site Injection Compatibility (1:1 Mixture) (Cont.)

Test Drug	Mfr	Conc	Mfr	Conc	Remarks	Ref	C/I
Levothyroxine sodium	PRP	0.4 mcg/mL[b]	HOS	5 mg/mL	Physically compatible for 1 hr at 23°C	3533	C
Lidocaine HCl	AST	20 mg/mL[a]	SC	1 mg/mL[a]	Physically compatible for 24 hr at 18°C	1171	C
Linezolid	PHU	2 mg/mL	GW	5 mg/mL	Physically compatible for 4 hr at 23°C	2264	C
Lorazepam	WY	0.5 mg/mL[a]	AH	2 mg/mL[a]	Visually compatible for 4 hr at 27°C	2062	C
Magnesium sulfate	LY	10 mg/mL[a]	SC	1 mg/mL[a]	Physically compatible for 24 hr at 18°C	1171	C
Meperidine HCl	AB	10 mg/mL	GL	5 mg/mL	Physically compatible for 4 hr at 25°C	1397	C
Meropenem	NVP	20 mg/mL[b]	HOS	5 mg/mL	Physically compatible for 1 hr at 23°C	3533	C
Meropenem		50 mg/mL	SZ	5 mg/mL	Physically compatible for 4 hr at room temperature	3538	C
Meropenem–vaborbactam	TMC	8 mg/mL[b i]	AKN	2 mg/mL[b]	Physically compatible for 3 hr at 20 to 25°C	3380	C
Metronidazole	SE	5 mg/mL	SC	1 mg/mL[a]	Physically compatible for 24 hr at 18°C	1171	C
Micafungin sodium	ASP	1.5 mg/mL[b]	AB	2 mg/mL[b]	White cloudiness forms immediately	2683	I
Midazolam HCl	RC	1 mg/mL[a]	GL	5 mg/mL	Visually compatible for 24 hr at 23°C	1877	C
Midazolam HCl	RC	2 mg/mL[a]	AH	2 mg/mL[a]	Visually compatible for 4 hr at 27°C	2062	C
Milrinone lactate	SW	0.2 mg/mL[a]	AH	2 mg/mL[a]	Visually compatible for 4 hr at 27°C	2062	C
Morphine sulfate	WY	1 mg/mL[a]	SC	1 mg/mL[a]	Physically compatible for 24 hr at 18°C	1171	C
Morphine sulfate	AB	1 mg/mL[a]	GL	5 mg/mL	Physically compatible for 4 hr at 25°C	1397	C
Morphine sulfate	ES	0.5 mg/mL[a]	GL	1 mg/mL[a]	Visually compatible. Little loss of either drug in 4 hr at room temperature	1762	C
Morphine sulfate	SCN	2 mg/mL[a]	AH	2 mg/mL[a]	Visually compatible for 4 hr at 27°C	2062	C
Nafcillin sodium	BR	10 mg/mL[a]	SC	1 mg/mL[a]	Cloudy precipitate forms immediately	1171	I
Nicardipine HCl	WY	1 mg/mL[a]	AH	2 mg/mL[a]	Visually compatible for 4 hr at 27°C	2062	C
Nicardipine HCl	DCC	0.1 mg/mL[a]	GL	1 mg/mL[a]	Visually compatible for 24 hr at room temperature	235	C
Nitroglycerin	DU	0.2 mg/mL[a]	GL	1 mg/mL[a]	Visually compatible. No labetalol loss and 6% nitroglycerin loss in 4 hr at room temperature	1762	C
Nitroglycerin	OM	0.2 mg/mL[a]	GL	5 mg/mL	Visually compatible for 24 hr at 23°C	1877	C
Nitroglycerin	AB	0.4 mg/mL[a]	AH	2 mg/mL[a]	Visually compatible for 4 hr at 27°C	2062	C
Norepinephrine bitartrate	STR	64 mcg/mL[a]	GL	5 mg/mL	Visually compatible for 24 hr at 23°C	1877	C
Norepinephrine bitartrate	AB	0.128 mg/mL[a]	AH	2 mg/mL[a]	Visually compatible for 4 hr at 27°C	2062	C
Norepinephrine bitartrate	HOS	0.128 mg/mL[b]	HOS	5 mg/mL	Physically compatible for 1 hr at 23°C	3533	C
Oxacillin sodium	BR	10 mg/mL[a]	SC	1 mg/mL[a]	Physically compatible for 24 hr at 18°C	1171	C
Penicillin G potassium	PF	50,000 units/mL[a]	SC	1 mg/mL[a]	Physically compatible for 24 hr at 18°C	1171	C
Plazomicin sulfate	ACH	24 mg/mL[g]	BRK	2 mg/mL[g]	Physically compatible for 1 hr at 20 to 25°C	3432	C
Potassium chloride	IX	0.4 mEq/mL[a]	SC	1 mg/mL[a]	Physically compatible for 24 hr at 18°C	1171	C
Potassium phosphates	LY	0.44 mEq/mL[a]	SC	1 mg/mL[a]	Physically compatible for 24 hr at 18°C	1171	C
Propofol	ZEN[j]	10 mg/mL	AH	5 mg/mL	Physically compatible for 1 hr at 23°C	2066	C
Ranitidine HCl	GL	0.5 mg/mL[a]	SC	1 mg/mL[a]	Physically compatible for 24 hr at 18°C	1171	C

Y-Site Injection Compatibility (1:1 Mixture) (Cont.)

Test Drug	Mfr	Conc	Mfr	Conc	Remarks	Ref	C/I
Ranitidine HCl	GL	0.6 mg/mL[a]	GL	1 mg/mL[a]	Visually compatible. Little ranitidine and 5% labetalol loss in 4 hr at room temperature	1762	C
Ranitidine HCl	GL	1 mg/mL[a]	AH	2 mg/mL[a]	Visually compatible for 4 hr at 27°C	2062	C
Sodium acetate	LY	0.4 mEq/mL[a]	SC	1 mg/mL[a]	Physically compatible for 24 hr at 18°C	1171	C
Sodium nitroprusside	RC	0.2 mg/mL[a]	GL	5 mg/mL	Visually compatible for 24 hr at 23°C	1877	C
Tedizolid phosphate	CUB	0.8 mg/mL[b]	HOS	2 mg/mL[b]	Physically compatible for 2 hr	3244	C
Telavancin HCl	ASP	7.5 mg/mL[a b e]	BED	5 mg/mL[a b e]	Physically compatible for 2 hr	2830	C
Tobramycin sulfate	LI	0.8 mg/mL[a]	SC	1 mg/mL[a]	Physically compatible for 24 hr at 18°C	1171	C
Trimethoprim–sulfamethoxazole	BW	0.8 mg/mL[a f]	SC	1 mg/mL[a]	Physically compatible for 24 hr at 18°C	1171	C
Vancomycin HCl	LE	5 mg/mL[a]	SC	1 mg/mL[a]	Physically compatible for 24 hr at 18°C	1171	C
Vecuronium bromide	OR	1 mg/mL	AH	2 mg/mL[a]	Visually compatible for 4 hr at 27°C	2062	C

[a] Tested in dextrose 5%.

[b] Tested in sodium chloride 0.9%.

[c] Tested in sterile water for injection.

[d] Furosemide 0.5 mL injected in the Y-site port of a running infusion of labetalol hydrochloride in dextrose 5%.

[e] Tested in Ringer's injection, lactated.

[f] Trimethoprim component. Trimethoprim in a 1:5 fixed-ratio concentration with sulfamethoxazole.

[g] Tested in both dextrose 5% and sodium chloride 0.9%.

[h] Ceftolozane component. Ceftolozane in a 2:1 fixed-ratio concentration with tazobactam.

[i] Meropenem component. Meropenem in a 1:1 fixed-ratio concentration with vaborbactam.

[j] Test performed using the formulation WITH edetate disodium.

[k] Salt not specified.

Selected Revisions May 1, 2020. © Copyright, October 1986.
American Society of Health-System Pharmacists, Inc.

Lacosamide
AHFS 28:12.92

Products

Lacosamide is available as a 10-mg/mL solution in 20-mL single-use vials.[3201] Each vial also contains sodium chloride, water for injection, and hydrochloric acid to adjust the pH.[3201] Solutions containing particulate matter or those in which discoloration has occurred should not be used.[3201] Any unused portion should be discarded.[3201]

pH

Lacosamide 10-mg/mL solution has an adjusted pH from 3.5 to 5.[3201]

Trade Name(s)

Vimpat

Administration

Lacosamide is administered intravenously as an infusion either undiluted or diluted in a compatible infusion solution over a period of 15 to 60 minutes.[3201] (See Solution Compatibility.) The manufacturer states that a 30- to 60-minute infusion is preferred when a 15-minute administration is not required.[3201]

Stability

Lacosamide is a clear, colorless solution.[3201] Intact vials should be stored at controlled room temperature and protected from freezing.[3201]

Lacosamide diluted for infusion in a compatible infusion solution should not be stored for more than 4 hours at room temperature.[3201]

Compatibility Information

Solution Compatibility

Lacosamide

Test Soln Name	Mfr	Mfr	Conc/L or %	Remarks	Ref	C/I
Dextrose 5%		UCB		Stable for 4 hr at room temperature	3201	C
Ringer's injection, lactated		UCB		Stable for 4 hr at room temperature	3201	C
Sodium chloride 0.9%		UCB		Stable for 4 hr at room temperature	3201	C

DOI: 10.37573/9781585286850.230

Lefamulin Acetate
AHFS 8:12.28.26

Products

Lefamulin acetate is available as a concentrate for injection in single-dose vials containing 15 mL of the concentrate packaged with a 250-mL bag of 10 mM citrate-buffered sodium chloride 0.9% (pH 5) diluent.[3513] Each mL of the concentrate for injection contains 10 mg of lefamulin (as the acetate) in sodium chloride 0.9%.[3513] Each mL of the diluent contains sodium chloride 9 mg, trisodium citrate dihydrate 2 mg, and citric acid anhydrous 0.615 mg in water for injection.[3513]

To prepare the drug for intravenous infusion, the entire contents of the vial containing the concentrate for injection (i.e., 15 mL [150 mg of lefamulin]) should be transferred to the accompanying diluent bag.[3513]

Equivalency

Lefamulin acetate 168 mg is equivalent to 150 mg of lefamulin.[3513]

pH

The provided 10 mM citrate-buffered sodium chloride 0.9% diluent has a pH ranging from 4.5 to 5.5.[3513]

Osmolality

The provided 10 mM citrate-buffered sodium chloride 0.9% diluent has an osmolality of 280 to 340 mOsm/kg.[3513]

© Copyright, January 2020. American Society of Health-System Pharmacists, Inc.

Sodium Content

The provided 10 mM citrate-buffered sodium chloride 0.9% diluent has a sodium content of 174 mEq/L.[3513]

Trade Name(s)

Xenleta

Administration

Lefamulin acetate is administered intravenously by infusion over 60 minutes following dilution of the concentrate for injection.[3513]

Stability

Both the concentrate for injection and the provided diluent are clear, colorless solutions.[3513] Intact vials of lefamulin acetate should be stored at 2 to 8°C and should *not* be frozen.[3513] The manufacturer states that the accompanying diluent bag should be stored at controlled room temperature;[3513] however, such bags also may be stored at 2 to 25°C.[3518]

Lefamulin acetate diluted in the accompanying citrate-buffered sodium chloride 0.9% diluent can be stored for up to 24 hours at room temperature and up to 48 hours under refrigeration at 2 to 8°C.[3513]

DOI: 10.37573/9781585286850.231

Lenograstim
AHFS 20:16

Products

Lenograstim (rHuG-CSF) is available as a lyophilized powder in single-use vials containing 13.4 million international units (Granocyte-13) or 33.6 million international units (Granocyte-34). In addition to lenograstim, each vial of the product contains mannitol 2.5%, arginine 1%, phenylalanine 1%, methionine 0.1%, polysorbate 20 0.01%, and hydrochloric acid to adjust pH.[38]

Lenograstim vials of either strength should be reconstituted with 1.05 mL of the accompanying water for injection diluent. Gently mix to effect dissolution, usually about 5 seconds. Do not shake the vials vigorously. Both the lenograstim vials and the diluent are overfilled by 5% to permit withdrawal of a full 1 mL of the reconstituted product containing 13.4 or 33.6 million international units.[38]

Units

Each 13.4-million international unit vial contains 105 mcg of lenograstim. Each 33.6-million international unit vial contains 263 mcg of lenograstim.[38]

pH

The reconstituted solution has a pH buffered to 6.5.[38]

Trade Name(s)

Granocyte-13, Granocyte-34

Administration

Lenograstim is administered by subcutaneous injection and intravenous infusion after dilution in sodium chloride 0.9% in glass or polyvinyl chloride (PVC) containers or dextrose 5% in glass containers. Granocyte-13 should not be diluted to a concentration lower than 0.26 million international units/mL (2 mcg/mL); Granocyte-34 should not be diluted to a concentration lower than 0.32 million international units/mL (2.5 mcg/mL). The dilution volume should not exceed 50 mL for each vial of Granocyte-13 and 100 mL for each vial of Granocyte-34.[38]

Stability

Intact vials of lenograstim should be stored at 30°C or below and protected from freezing. When reconstituted as directed, lenograstim is stable for 24 hours under refrigeration. Diluted for administration to concentrations not less than 0.26 million international units/mL (Granocyte-13) or 0.32 million international units/mL (Granocyte-34), lenograstim is stable for up to 24 hours at 5 or 25°C.[38]

At concentrations not less than 0.26 million international units/mL (Granocyte-13) or 0.32 million international units/mL (Granocyte-34), lenograstim is stable for up to 24 hours at 5 or 25°C in sodium chloride 0.9% in both PVC and glass containers and in dextrose 5% in glass containers.[38]

Ambulatory Pumps

The stability of lenograstim (Rhône-Poulenc Rorer) 33.6 million international units (263 mcg) and 67.2 million international units (526 mcg) each in 100 mL of sodium chloride 0.9% filled into Intermate elastomeric infusion devices (Baxter) was evaluated stored at 4°C for 14 days. No loss of lenograstim was found.[2048]

Sorption

Lenograstim prepared in sodium chloride 0.9% is compatible with PVC containers and common administration sets.[38]

Selected Revisions June 1, 2019. © Copyright, October 1998. American Society of Health-System Pharmacists, Inc.

DOI: 10.37573/9781585286850.232

Letermovir
AHFS 8:18.92

Products

Letermovir is available as a 20-mg/mL concentrate for injection in single-dose (preservative-free) vials containing 240 mg (12 mL) or 480 mg (24 mL) of the drug, respectively, packaged in 30-mL vials.[3398] Each mL of concentrate for injection also contains hydroxypropyl-beta-cyclodextrin 150 mg, sodium chloride 3.1 mg, and sodium hydroxide in water for injection.[3398] The amount of sodium hydroxide used to adjust the pH may vary.[3398]

Letermovir concentrate for injection must be diluted prior to administration.[3398] The appropriate volume of the concentrate should be withdrawn from the vial and transferred to an infusion bag containing 250 mL of sodium chloride 0.9% or dextrose 5%.[3398] The diluted solution for infusion should be gently mixed and should *not* be shaken.[3398]

pH

The concentrate for injection has a pH adjusted to approximately 7.5.[3398]

Trade Name(s)

Prevymis

Administration

The entire contents of the intravenous bag containing the diluted solution of letermovir for infusion should be administered as an intravenous infusion at a constant rate over 1 hour through a peripheral catheter or central venous line.[3398] The drug should *not* be administered by intravenous bolus injection.[3398]

Stability

Letermovir concentrate for injection is a clear, colorless solution that forms a clear solution ranging from colorless to yellow upon dilution; variations in color within this range do not affect product quality.[3398] Intact vials should be stored at controlled room temperature in the original carton to protect from light.[3398]

Letermovir concentrate for injection should be visually inspected for particulate matter and discoloration in the vial and again once the solution has been diluted in the intravenous infusion bag; if visible particulates are present or if discoloration occurs, the solution should not be used and should be discarded.[3398] Vials are for single use only; any unused portion should be discarded.[3398]

Sorption

Letermovir is noted to be compatible with polyvinyl chloride (PVC), ethylene vinyl acetate (EVA), and polyolefin (polypropylene and polyethylene) intravenous infusion bags, as well as PVC, polyethylene, polybutadiene, silicone rubber, styrene-butadiene copolymer, styrene-butadiene-styrene copolymer, and polystyrene infusion sets.[3398] Only intravenous infusion bags and infusion sets made of these materials are recommended for use with letermovir.[3398]

Letermovir also is compatible with radiopaque polyurethane catheters; however, the drug is not recommended for use with polyurethane-containing intravenous administration set tubing.[3398]

Plasticizer Leaching

Letermovir is compatible with materials containing plasticizers such as diethylhexyl phthalate (DEHP), trioctyl trimellitate (TOTM), and benzyl butyl phthalate.[3398]

Compatibility Information

Solution Compatibility

Letermovir

Test Soln Name	Mfr	Mfr	Conc/L or %	Remarks	Ref	C/I
Dextrose 5%	a	ME	0.92 and 1.75 g	Complete administration within 24 hr if stored at room temperature or 48 hr if stored at 2 to 8°C	3398	C
Sodium chloride 0.9%	a	ME	0.92 and 1.75 g	Complete administration within 24 hr if stored at room temperature or 48 hr if stored at 2 to 8°C	3398	C

a Tested in PVC, EVA, and polyolefin (polypropylene and polyethylene) containers.

DOI: 10.37573/9781585286850.233

Y-Site Injection Compatibility (1:1 Mixture)

Letermovir

Test Drug	Mfr	Conc	Mfr	Conc	Remarks	Ref	C/I
Amiodarone HCl			ME		Physically incompatible	3398	I
Amphotericin B lipid complex		a	ME	a	Physically compatible	3398	C
Amphotericin B liposomal			ME		Physically incompatible	3398	I
Ampicillin sodium		b	ME	b	Physically compatible	3398	C
Ampicillin sodium–sulbactam sodium		b	ME	b	Physically compatible	3398	C
Anidulafungin		a	ME	a	Physically compatible	3398	C
Aztreonam			ME		Physically incompatible	3398	I
Cefazolin sodium		a	ME	a	Physically compatible	3398	C
Cefepime HCl			ME		Physically incompatible	3398	I
Ceftriaxone sodium		a	ME	a	Physically compatible	3398	C
Ciprofloxacin			ME		Physically incompatible	3398	I
Cyclosporine			ME		Physically incompatible	3398	I
Daptomycin		b	ME	b	Physically compatible	3398	C
Diltiazem HCl			ME		Physically incompatible	3398	I
Doripenem		a	ME	a	Physically compatible	3398	C
Famotidine		a	ME	a	Physically compatible	3398	C
Fentanyl citrate		b	ME	b	Physically compatible	3398	C
Filgrastim			ME		Physically incompatible	3398	I
Fluconazole		b	ME	b	Physically compatible	3398	C
Folic acid		a	ME	a	Physically compatible	3398	C
Furosemide		b	ME	b	Physically compatible	3398	C
Ganciclovir sodium		a	ME	a	Physically compatible	3398	C
Gentamicin sulfate			ME		Physically incompatible	3398	I
Hydrocortisone sodium succinate		a	ME	a	Physically compatible	3398	C
Insulin, regular		b	ME	b	Physically compatible	3398	C
Levofloxacin			ME		Physically incompatible	3398	I
Linezolid			ME		Physically incompatible	3398	I
Lorazepam			ME		Physically incompatible	3398	I
Magnesium sulfate		b	ME	b	Physically compatible	3398	C
Midazolam HCl			ME		Physically incompatible	3398	I
Morphine sulfate		a	ME	a	Physically compatible	3398	C
Mycophenolate mofetil HCl			ME		Physically incompatible	3398	I
Norepinephrine bitartrate		a	ME	a	Physically compatible	3398	C
Pantoprazole sodium	c	a	ME	a	Physically compatible	3398	C
Potassium chloride		a	ME	a	Physically compatible	3398	C

Y-Site Injection Compatibility (1:1 Mixture) (Cont.)

Test Drug	Mfr	Conc	Mfr	Conc	Remarks	Ref	C/I
Potassium phosphates		a	ME	a	Physically compatible	3398	C
Tacrolimus		a	ME	a	Physically compatible	3398	C
Tigecycline		a	ME	a	Physically compatible	3398	C

[a] Tested in dextrose 5%.

[b] Tested in sodium chloride 0.9%.

[c] Presence or absence of edetate disodium not specified.

© Copyright, June 2018. American Society of Health-System Pharmacists, Inc.

Leucovorin Calcium
AHFS 92:12

Products

Leucovorin calcium is available in lyophilized form in vials containing leucovorin 50, 100, 200, 350, and 500 mg as the calcium salt with sodium chloride and sodium hydroxide or hydrochloric acid to adjust the pH. Reconstitute the vials with bacteriostatic water for injection containing benzyl alcohol or sterile water for injection with the volumes indicated in Table 1.[1(1/04)] [4]

Table 1. Recommended reconstitution of leucovorin calcium[1(1/04)] [4]

Vial Size (mg)	Volume of Diluent (mL)	Concentration (mg/mL)
50	5	10
100	10	10
200	20	10
350	17.5	20
500	50	10

Leucovorin calcium is also available at a concentration of 10 mg/mL containing no preservative in vials of 10, 25, and 30 mL.[4]

pH
From 6.5 to 8.5.[17]

Administration

Leucovorin calcium is administered by intramuscular or intravenous injection or infusion at a rate not exceeding 160 mg/min. When doses greater than 10 mg/m² are required, diluents containing benzyl alcohol should not be used for reconstitution.[1(1/04)] [4]

Stability

Leucovorin calcium injection should be stored at room temperature and protected from light.[1(1/04)] [4]

The reconstituted solution of leucovorin calcium is stated to be stable for 7 days. When reconstituted with diluents that contain no preservatives, immediate use is recommended.[1(1/04)]

pH Effects

Leucovorin calcium solutions exhibit good stability at pH 6.5 to 10. The pH of maximum stability was determined to be 7.1 to 7.4. Below pH 6, increased decomposition occurs.[1276]

Central Venous Catheter

Leucovorin calcium (Gensia) 2 mg/mL in dextrose 5% was found to be compatible with the ARROWg+ard Blue Plus (Arrow International) chlorhexidine-bearing triple-lumen central catheter. Essentially complete delivery of the drug was found with little or no drug loss occurring. Furthermore, chlorhexidine delivered from the catheter remained at trace amounts with no substantial increase due to the delivery of the drug through the catheter.[2335]

Compatibility Information
Solution Compatibility

Leucovorin calcium

Test Soln Name	Mfr	Mfr	Conc/L or %	Remarks	Ref	C/I
Dextrose 10% in sodium chloride 0.9%		LE	50 mg	Under 10% loss in 24 hr at room temperature in dark	488	C
Dextrose 5%	TRᵃ	LE	910 mg	Under 10% loss in 24 hr at room temperature	519	C
Dextrose 5%	ᵃ	LE	0.1, 0.5, 1, 1.5 g	Little loss in 4 days at 4 and 23°C in dark	1596	C
Dextrose 5%	MGᵇ		910 mg	Under 10% loss in 24 hr at room temperature in light	1658	C
Dextrose 10%		LE	50 mg	Under 10% loss in 24 hr at room temperature in dark	488	C
Ringer's injection		LE	50 mg	Under 10% loss in 24 hr at room temperature in dark	488	C
Ringer's injection, lactated		LE	50 mg	Under 10% loss in 24 hr at room temperature in dark	488	C
Sodium chloride 0.9%	ᵃ	LE	1 and 1.5 g	Little loss in 4 days at 4 and 23°C in dark	1596	C

DOI: 10.37573/9781585286850.234

Solution Compatibility (Cont.)

Test Soln Name	Mfr	Mfr	Conc/L or %	Remarks	Ref	C/I
Sodium chloride 0.9%	c	LE	0.5 g	Little loss in 4 days at 4 and 23°C in dark	1596	C
Sodium chloride 0.9%	c	LE	0.1 g	9% loss in 4 days at 4 and 23°C in dark	1596	C
Sodium chloride 0.9%	d	LE	0.1 and 0.5 g	Variable losses, up to 24%, in 4 days at 4 and 23°C in dark	1596	I
Sodium chloride 0.9%	b	LE	1 g	Stable for 7 days at 4 and 25°C in dark	1669	C

[a] Tested in both glass and PVC containers.

[b] Tested in both glass and polyolefin containers.

[c] Tested in glass containers.

[d] Tested in PVC containers.

Additive Compatibility

Leucovorin calcium

Test Drug	Mfr	Conc/L or %	Mfr	Conc/L or %	Test Solution	Remarks	Ref	C/I
Cisplatin		200 mg		140 mg	NS	Both drugs stable for 15 days at room temperature protected from light	1379	C
Cisplatin with floxuridine		200 mg 700 mg		140 mg	NS	All drugs stable for 7 days at room temperature	1379	C
Floxuridine	QU	1 g	QU	30 mg	NS	Physically compatible. Stable for 48 hr at 4 and 20°C. No floxuridine and 10% leucovorin loss in 48 hr at 40°C	1317	C
Floxuridine	QU	2 g	QU	240 mg	NS	Physically compatible. Stable for 48 hr at 4 and 20°C. No floxuridine and 7% leucovorin loss in 48 hr at 40°C	1317	C
Floxuridine	QU	4 g	QU	960 mg	NS	Physically compatible. Stable for 48 hr at 4, 20, and 40°C	1317	C
Floxuridine		10 g		200 mg	NS	Both drugs stable for 15 days at room temperature protected from light	1387	C
Floxuridine with cisplatin		700 mg 200 mg		140 mg	NS	All drugs stable for 7 days at room temperature	1379	C
Fluorouracil	AD	16.7 to 46.2 g	LE	1.5 to 13.3 g	a	Subvisible particulates form in all combinations in variable periods from 1 to 4 days at 4, 23, and 32°C	1816	I

[a] Tested with both drugs undiluted and diluted by 25% with dextrose 5%.

Drugs in Syringe Compatibility

Leucovorin calcium

Test Drug	Mfr	Amt	Mfr	Amt	Remarks	Ref	C/I
Bleomycin sulfate		1.5 units/0.5 mL		5 mg/0.5 mL	Physically compatible for 5 min at room temperature followed by 8 min of centrifugation	980	C
Cisplatin		0.5 mg/0.5 mL		5 mg/0.5 mL	Physically compatible for 5 min at room temperature followed by 8 min of centrifugation	980	C
Cyclophosphamide		10 mg/0.5 mL		5 mg/0.5 mL	Physically compatible for 5 min at room temperature followed by 8 min of centrifugation	980	C
Doxorubicin HCl		1 mg/0.5 mL		5 mg/0.5 mL	Physically compatible for 5 min at room temperature followed by 8 min of centrifugation	980	C

Drugs in Syringe Compatibility (Cont.)

Test Drug	Mfr	Amt	Mfr	Amt	Remarks	Ref	C/I
Droperidol		1.25 mg/0.5 mL		5 mg/0.5 mL	Precipitates immediately	980	I
Fluorouracil		25 mg/0.5 mL		5 mg/0.5 mL	Physically compatible for 5 min at room temperature followed by 8 min of centrifugation	980	C
Furosemide		5 mg/0.5 mL		5 mg/0.5 mL	Physically compatible for 5 min at room temperature followed by 8 min of centrifugation	980	C
Heparin sodium		500 units/0.5 mL		5 mg/0.5 mL	Physically compatible for 5 min at room temperature followed by 8 min of centrifugation	980	C
Methotrexate sodium		12.5 mg/0.5 mL		5 mg/0.5 mL	Physically compatible for 5 min at room temperature followed by 8 min of centrifugation	980	C
Metoclopramide HCl		2.5 mg/0.5 mL		5 mg/0.5 mL	Physically compatible for 5 min at room temperature followed by 8 min of centrifugation	980	C
Mitomycin		0.25 mg/0.5 mL		5 mg/0.5 mL	Physically compatible for 5 min at room temperature followed by 8 min of centrifugation	980	C
Vinblastine sulfate		0.5 mg/0.5 mL		5 mg/0.5 mL	Physically compatible for 5 min at room temperature followed by 8 min of centrifugation	980	C
Vincristine sulfate		0.5 mg/0.5 mL		5 mg/0.5 mL	Physically compatible for 5 min at room temperature followed by 8 min of centrifugation	980	C

Y-Site Injection Compatibility (1:1 Mixture)

Leucovorin calcium

Test Drug	Mfr	Conc	Mfr	Conc	Remarks	Ref	C/I
Amifostine	USB	10 mg/mL[a]	LE	2 mg/mL[a]	Physically compatible for 4 hr at 23°C	1845	C
Anidulafungin	VIC	0.5 mg/mL[a]	BED	2 mg/mL[a]	Physically compatible for 4 hr at 23°C	2617	C
Aztreonam	SQ	40 mg/mL[a]	LE	2 mg/mL[a]	Physically compatible for 4 hr at 23°C	1758	C
Bleomycin sulfate		3 units/mL		10 mg/mL	Drugs injected sequentially in Y-site with no flush. No precipitate seen	980	C
Cisplatin		1 mg/mL		10 mg/mL	Drugs injected sequentially in Y-site with no flush. No precipitate seen	980	C
Cladribine	ORT	0.015[b] and 0.5[c] mg/mL	IMM	2 mg/mL[b]	Physically compatible for 4 hr at 23°C	1969	C
Cyclophosphamide		20 mg/mL		10 mg/mL	Drugs injected sequentially in Y-site with no flush. No precipitate seen	980	C
Docetaxel	RPR	0.9 mg/mL[a]	ES	2 mg/mL[a]	Physically compatible for 4 hr at 23°C	2224	C
Doxorubicin HCl		2 mg/mL		10 mg/mL	Drugs injected sequentially in Y-site with no flush. No precipitate seen	980	C
Doxorubicin HCl liposomal	SEQ	0.4 mg/mL[a]	IMM	2 mg/mL[a]	Physically compatible for 4 hr at 23°C	2087	C
Droperidol		2.5 mg/mL		10 mg/mL	Drugs injected sequentially in Y-site with no flush. Precipitates immediately	980	I
Etoposide phosphate	BR	5 mg/mL[a]	IMM	2 mg/mL[a]	Physically compatible for 4 hr at 23°C	2218	C
Filgrastim	AMG	30 mcg/mL[a]	LE	2 mg/mL[a]	Physically compatible for 4 hr at 22°C	1687	C
Fluconazole	RR	2 mg/mL	LE	10 mg/mL	Physically compatible for 24 hr at 25°C	1407	C
Fluorouracil		50 mg/mL		10 mg/mL	Drugs injected sequentially in Y-site with no flush. No precipitate seen	980	C

Y-Site Injection Compatibility (1:1 Mixture) (Cont.)

Test Drug	Mfr	Conc	Mfr	Conc	Remarks	Ref	C/I
Foscarnet sodium	AST	24 mg/mL	QU	10 mg/mL	Cloudy yellow solution	1335	I
Furosemide		10 mg/mL		10 mg/mL	Drugs injected sequentially in Y-site with no flush. No precipitate seen	980	C
Gemcitabine HCl	LI	10 mg/mL[b]	IMM	2 mg/mL[b]	Physically compatible for 4 hr at 23°C	2226	C
Granisetron HCl	SKB	0.05 mg/mL[a]	IMM	2 mg/mL[a]	Physically compatible for 4 hr at 23°C	2000	C
Heparin sodium		1000 units/mL		10 mg/mL	Drugs injected sequentially in Y-site with no flush. No precipitate seen	980	C
Linezolid	PHU	2 mg/mL	GNS	2 mg/mL[a]	Physically compatible for 4 hr at 23°C	2264	C
Methotrexate sodium		25 mg/mL		10 mg/mL	Drugs injected sequentially in Y-site with no flush. No precipitate seen	980	C
Methotrexate sodium		30 mg/mL	LE	10 mg/mL	Visually compatible for 4 hr at room temperature	1788	C
Metoclopramide HCl		5 mg/mL		10 mg/mL	Drugs injected sequentially in Y-site with no flush. No precipitate seen	980	C
Mitomycin		0.5 mg/mL		10 mg/mL	Drugs injected sequentially in Y-site with no flush. No precipitate seen	980	C
Oxaliplatin	SS	0.5 mg/mL[a]	BED	2 mg/mL[a]	Physically compatible for 4 hr at 23°C	2566	C
Pemetrexed disodium	LI	20 mg/mL[b]	SIC	2 mg/mL[a]	Physically compatible for 4 hr at 23°C	2564	C
Piperacillin sodium–tazobactam sodium	LE[f]	40 mg/mL[a g]	LE	2 mg/mL[a]	Physically compatible for 4 hr at 22°C	1688	C
Sodium bicarbonate		1.4%	LE	10 mg/mL	Yellow precipitate forms in 0.5 hr at room temperature	1788	I
Tacrolimus	FUJ	1 mg/mL[b]	ES	10 mg/mL[a]	Visually compatible for 24 hr at 25°C	1630	C
Teniposide	BR	0.1 mg/mL[a]	LE	2 mg/mL[a]	Physically compatible for 4 hr at 23°C	1725	C
Thiotepa	IMM[d]	1 mg/mL[a]	LE	2 mg/mL[a]	Physically compatible for 4 hr at 23°C	1861	C
TNA #218 to #226[e]			IMM	2 mg/mL[a]	Visually compatible for 4 hr at 23°C	2215	C
TPN #212 to #215[e]			IMM	2 mg/mL[a]	Physically compatible for 4 hr at 23°C	2109	C
Vinblastine sulfate		1 mg/mL		10 mg/mL	Drugs injected sequentially in Y-site with no flush. No precipitate seen	980	C
Vincristine sulfate		1 mg/mL		10 mg/mL	Drugs injected sequentially in Y-site with no flush. No precipitate seen	980	C

[a] Tested in dextrose 5%.

[b] Tested in sodium chloride 0.9%.

[c] Tested in bacteriostatic sodium chloride 0.9% preserved with benzyl alcohol 0.9%.

[d] Lyophilized formulation tested.

[e] Refer to Appendix for the composition of parenteral nutrition solutions. TNA indicates a 3-in-1 admixture, and TPN indicates a 2-in-1 admixture.

[f] Test performed using the formulation WITHOUT edetate disodium.

[g] Piperacillin component. Piperacillin in an 8:1 fixed-ratio concentration with tazobactam.

Additional Compatibility Information

Fluorouracil

Several articles reported the chemical stability and physical compatibility of fluorouracil with leucovorin calcium.[505] [980] [1309] [1387] [1817] However, more recent work found substantial amounts of subvisual particles in this drug combination over numerous concentrations when stored at 4, 23, and 32°C. Particulate formation sometimes clogged filters and disrupted multiple-day treatment. Particulate formation began in about 24 hours in most samples, and particles were found in all samples within 7 days. Fluorouracil and leucovorin calcium in the same container can no longer be considered a compatible combination.[1816]

Fluorouracil combined with leucovorin calcium for repeated administration using a Fresenius implanted port resulted in blockage of the pump catheter and necessitated surgical removal of the port. The blockage was caused by precipitation of calcium carbonate in the catheter.[2504]

Selected Revisions December 13, 2018. © Copyright, October 1982. American Society of Health-System Pharmacists, Inc.

Levetiracetam
AHFS 28:12.92

Products

Levetiracetam is available as a 100-mg/mL concentrate for injection in 5-mL single-use vials.[2833] The concentrate must be diluted prior to administration.[2833]

Levetiracetam also is available as a single-use, ready-to-use solution for intravenous infusion containing 500 mg, 1 g, or 1.5 g levetiracetam in 100 mL of sodium chloride in dual-port plastic bags.[2834]

Both the concentrate and the ready-to-use formulations contain water for injection and sodium chloride as well as glacial acetic acid and sodium acetate trihydrate to adjust the pH.[2833] [2834]

pH

Approximately 5.5.[2833] [2834]

Osmolality

Levetiracetam 100-mg/mL concentrate for injection has an osmolality of approximately 950 mOsm/kg.[2835] Following dilution of 500 mg of the concentrate in 100 mL of sodium chloride 0.9%, the solution has an osmolality of approximately 430 mOsm/kg.[2835]

Sodium Content

Ready-to-use solutions of levetiracetam 500 mg, 1 g, and 1.5 g in 100 mL of sodium chloride injection contain 820, 750, and 540 mg of sodium, respectively.[2834]

Trade Name(s)

Keppra

Administration

Levetiracetam concentrate for injection is administered by intravenous infusion over 15 minutes after dilution in 100 mL of a compatible diluent.[2833] If a smaller infusion volume is required (e.g., for pediatric patients or fluid-restricted patients), the final concentration of the diluted solution should not exceed 15 mg/mL.[2833]

Single-use, ready-to-use solutions of levetiracetam should not be further diluted prior to intravenous infusion.[2834] The ready-to-use solution is administered by intravenous infusion over 15 minutes.[2834]

Stability

Levetiracetam concentrate and diluted solutions should be clear and colorless.[2833] [2834] Intact vials of levetiracetam concentrate and ready-to-use bags of levetiracetam in solution in their unopened aluminum overwrap should be stored at controlled room temperature.[2833] [2834] Discolored products or products containing particulate matter should not be used.[2833] [2834] Ready-to-use levetiracetam infusion bags should be used promptly once the aluminum overwrap has been removed.[2834]

The unused contents of an opened vial or a partially used infusion bag should be discarded.[2833] [2834] Storage of levetiracetam diluted for infusion should not exceed 4 hours at 15 to 30°C.[2835]

Syringes

Levetiracetam (Hospira) was diluted to a concentration of 40 mg/mL in sodium chloride 0.9% and packaged as 25 mL in 30-mL polypropylene syringes (Becton Dickinson).[3114] The syringes were stored for 14 days at 2 to 8°C.[3114] Neither changes in color or clarity nor appreciable changes in pH from baseline values occurred.[3114] Samples exhibited a loss of less than 6% of levetiracetam concentration at 14 days.[3114]

Compatibility Information

Solution Compatibility

Levetiracetam

Test Soln Name	Mfr	Mfr	Conc/L or %	Remarks	Ref	C/I
Dextrose 5%	a	UCB		Stable for 4 hr at 15 to 30°C	2833	C
Ringer's injection lactated	a	UCB		Stable for 4 hr at 15 to 30°C	2833	C
Sodium chloride 0.9%	a	UCB		Stable for 4 hr at 15 to 30°C	2833	C
Sodium chloride 0.9%	BA[a]	HOS	40 g	Physically compatible. Less than 6% loss in 14 days at 2 to 8°C	3114	C
Sodium chloride 0.9%	BA[b]	HOS	40 g	Physically compatible. Less than 6% loss in 14 days at 2 to 8°C	3114	C

DOI: 10.37573/9781585286850.235

Solution Compatibility (Cont.)

Test Soln Name	Mfr	Mfr	Conc/L or %	Remarks	Ref	C/I
TNA #279[c]	BRN[d]	SZ	0.4 and 4.8 g	Visually compatible for 7 days at 4°C protected from light	3455	C
TNA #279[c]	BRN[d]	SZ	0.4 and 4.8 g	Visually compatible for 7 days at 23°C	3455	C
TNA #279[c]	BRN[d]	SZ	1.6 g	Visually compatible for 7 days at 4°C protected from light and physically compatible for 7 days at 23°C	3455	C
TNA #279[c]	BRN[d]	SZ	0.4, 1.6, and 4.8 g	Yellowish discoloration forms after 4 days at 37°C	3455	?
TNA #280[c]	BRN[d]	SZ	0.4 and 4.8 g	Visually compatible for 7 days at 4°C protected from light	3455	C
TNA #280[c]	BRN[d]	SZ	0.4 and 4.8 g	Visually compatible for 7 days at 23°C	3455	C
TNA #280[c]	BRN[d]	SZ	1.6 g	Visually compatible for 7 days at 4°C protected from light and physically compatible for 7 days at 23°C	3455	C
TNA #280[c]	BRN[d]	SZ	0.4, 1.6, and 4.8 g	Yellowish discoloration forms after 4 days at 37°C	3455	?

[a] Tested in PVC containers.

[b] Tested in polyolefin containers.

[c] Refer to Appendix for the composition of parenteral nutrition solutions. TNA indicates a 3-in-1 admixture.

[d] Tested in glass containers.

Additive Compatibility

Levetiracetam

Test Drug	Mfr	Conc/L or %	Mfr	Conc/L or %	Test Solution	Remarks	Ref	C/I
Diazepam			UCB		D5W, LR, NS[a]	Stable for 4 hr at 15 to 30°C	2833	C
Lorazepam			UCB		D5W, LR, NS[a]	Stable for 4 hr at 15 to 30°C	2833	C
Valproate sodium			UCB		D5W, LR, NS[a]	Stable for 4 hr at 15 to 30°C	2833	C

[a] Tested in PVC containers.

Selected Revisions September 30, 2019. © Copyright, May 2013.
American Society of Health-System Pharmacists, Inc.

Levocarnitine
AHFS 92:92

Products

Levocarnitine is available as a 200-mg/mL solution in single-use (preservative-free) 5-mL vials containing 1 g of levocarnitine with hydrochloric acid or sodium hydroxide to adjust the pH in water for injection.[3217] [3218]

pH

The pH of the undiluted solution ranges from 6 to 6.5.[3217] [3218]

Trade Name(s)

Carnitor

Administration

Levocarnitine is administered intravenously as a slow bolus injection over 2 to 3 minutes or by infusion.[3217] [3218]

Stability

Intact vials should be stored at controlled room temperature.[3217] [3218] One manufacturer states that vials of the drug should be kept in the carton to protect from light until time of use and that vials should not be frozen.[3218]

Solutions should be visually inspected for particulate matter and discoloration prior to administration.[3217] [3218] Any unused portion should be discarded.[3217] [3218]

Compatibility Information

Solution Compatibility

Levocarnitine

Test Soln Name	Mfr	Mfr	Conc/L or %	Remarks	Ref	C/I
Ringer's injection, lactated	a	SIG	0.5 to 8.06 g	Compatible and stable for up to 24 hr at 25°C	3217, 3239	C
Sodium chloride 0.9%	a	SIG	0.5 to 8.06 g	Compatible and stable for up to 24 hr at 25°C	3217, 3239	C

a Tested in PVC containers.

Y-Site Injection Compatibility (1:1 Mixture)

Levocarnitine

Test Drug	Mfr	Conc	Mfr	Conc	Remarks	Ref	C/I
Cloxacillin sodium	SMX	100 mg/mL	SIG	200 mg/mL	Physically compatible for up to 4 hr at room temperature	3245	C
Meropenem		50 mg/mL	SIG	200 mg/mL	Physically compatible for 4 hr at room temperature	3538	C

Selected Revisions May 1, 2020. © Copyright, June 2017. American Society of Health-System Pharmacists, Inc.

DOI: 10.37573/9781585286850.236

Levofloxacin
AHFS 8:12.18

Products

Levofloxacin is available as a 25-mg/mL preservative-free concentrate for injection in 20-mL (500-mg) and 30-mL (750-mg) single-use vials.[2895] This concentrate must be diluted to a 5-mg/mL solution before administration.[2895] Adding 250 mg (10 mL) to 40 mL of diluent, 500 mg (20 mL) to 80 mL of diluent, or 750 mg (30 mL) to 120 mL of diluent will result in a concentration of 5 mg/mL.[2895]

The drug is also available as premixed infusion solutions of 5 mg/mL in dextrose 5% in 50-mL (250-mg), 100-mL (500-mg), and 150-mL (750-mg) flexible plastic bags.[2895] The premixed infusion solutions in plastic bags are ready to use and require no further dilution.[2895] Sodium hydroxide and hydrochloric acid may have been added to adjust the pH.[2895]

pH

From 3.8 to 5.8.[2895]

The pH of a 5-mg/mL solution in dextrose 5% or sodium chloride 0.9% is about 4.6 to 4.7.[2895] A 5-mg/mL solution had a pH of 4.9 in dextrose 5% in Ringer's injection, lactated, a pH of 5 in Plasma-Lyte 56/dextrose 5%, and a pH of 5.5 in sodium lactate ⅙ M.[2895]

Tonicity

The premixed infusion solutions are nearly isotonic.[2895]

Trade Name(s)

Levaquin

Administration

The 25-mg/mL levofloxacin concentrate must be diluted to 5 mg/mL prior to administration.[2895] Levofloxacin is administered only at a concentration of 5 mg/mL by slow intravenous infusion over at least 60 minutes.[2895] Doses of 750 mg should be administered over 90 minutes.[2895] No other route is recommended.[2895] Rapid infusion or bolus administration must not be used because of the potential for hypotension.[2895]

Stability

Intact vials should be stored at controlled room temperature and protected from light.[2895] The premixed infusion solutions should be stored at or below 25°C and protected from light, freezing, and excessive heat.[2895] A brief exposure to temperatures up to 40°C does not adversely affect the premixed product.[2895] The injection and infusion admixtures are clear and yellow to greenish yellow in appearance.[2895] This color also does not adversely affect the product.[1986][2895] Discard any remaining unused portion of the injection because no preservatives are present.[2895]

Levofloxacin diluted in a compatible diluent to 5 mg/mL is stated to be stable for 72 hours stored at or below 25°C and for 14 days stored at 5°C.[2895]

Levofloxacin may form stable coordination compounds with metal ions.[2895] The chelation potential is greatest with Al^{3+} and declines from Cu^{2+} to Zn^{2+} to Mg^{2+} to Ca^{2+}.[2895]

pH Effects

Levofloxacin has a solubility of 100 mg/mL at pH values ranging from 0.6 to 5.8.[2895] The solubility increases as pH increases up to 6.7, with a maximum solubility of 272 mg/mL.[2895] Above pH 6.7, solubility decreases to a minimum of 50 mg/mL at pH 6.9.[2895]

Freezing Solutions

Levofloxacin 5 mg/mL diluted in a compatible diluent in glass bottles or plastic infusion containers is stable for 6 months frozen at –20°C.[2895] Frozen solutions should be thawed at room temperature or in the refrigerator.[2895] Accelerated thawing using microwaves or hot water immersion is not recommended.[2895] Thawed solutions should not be refrozen.[2895]

Light Effects

Levofloxacin undergoes slow degradation when exposed to ultraviolet light.[2399] Losses have been reported upon long-term light exposure.[2636]

Central Venous Catheter

Levofloxacin (McNeil) 1 mg/mL in dextrose 5% was found to be compatible with the ARROWg+ard Blue Plus (Arrow International) chlorhexidine-bearing triple-lumen central catheter. Essentially complete delivery of the drug was found with little or no drug loss occurring. Furthermore, chlorhexidine delivered from the catheter remained at trace amounts with no substantial increase due to the delivery of the drug through the catheter.[2335]

DOI: 10.37573/9781585286850.237

Compatibility Information

Solution Compatibility

Levofloxacin

Test Soln Name	Mfr	Mfr	Conc/L or %	Remarks	Ref	C/I
Dextrose 5% in Ringer's injection, lactated	BA[a]	OMJ	0.5 and 5 g	Physically compatible. No loss in 3 days at 25°C, 14 days at 5°C, 26 weeks at –20°C, in dark	1986	C
Dextrose 5% in sodium chloride 0.9%	BA[a]	OMJ	0.5 and 5 g	Physically compatible. No loss in 3 days at 25°C, 14 days at 5°C, 26 weeks at –20°C, in dark	1986	C
Dextrose 5%	BA[a]	OMJ	0.5 and 5 g	Physically compatible. No loss in 3 days at 25°C, 14 days at 5°C, 26 weeks at –20°C, in dark	1986	C
Dextrose 5%	BRN	HOS	2.5 g	Visually compatible for 6 hr at 22°C	2894	C
Plasma-Lyte 56 in dextrose 5%	BA[a]	OMJ	0.5 and 5 g	Physically compatible. No loss in 3 days at 25°C, 14 days at 5°C, 26 weeks at –20°C, in dark	1986	C
Sodium chloride 0.9%	BA[a]	OMJ	0.5 and 5 g	Physically compatible. No loss in 3 days at 25°C, 14 days at 5°C, 26 weeks at –20°C, in dark	1986	C
Sodium chloride 0.9%	BRN	HOS	2.5 g	Visually compatible for 6 hr at 22°C	2894	C
Sodium lactate ⅙ M	BA[a]	OMJ	0.5 and 5 g	Physically compatible. <4% loss in 3 days at 25°C, 14 days at 5°C, 26 weeks at –20°C, in dark	1986	C

[a] Tested in PVC containers.

Additive Compatibility

Levofloxacin

Test Drug	Mfr	Conc/L or %	Mfr	Conc/L or %	Test Solution	Remarks	Ref	C/I
Linezolid	PHU	2 g	OMN	5 g	[a]	Physically compatible. Little drug loss in 7 days at 4 and 23°C in dark	2334	C
Mannitol	BA	20%	OMJ	0.5 g		Precipitate forms within a few hours	1986	I
Mannitol	BA	20%	OMJ	5 g		Precipitate forms within 13 weeks at –20°C	1986	I
Mannitol	BA	20%	OMJ	5 g		Physically compatible. <4% loss in 3 days at 25°C, 14 days at 5°C, in dark	1986	C
Micafungin sodium	ASP	0.5 g	HOS	2.5 g	NS	Hazy precipitate forms immediately	2894	I
Sodium bicarbonate	BA[b]	5%	OMJ	0.5 g		Physically compatible. No loss in 3 days at 25°C, 14 days at 5°C, in dark	1986	C
Sodium bicarbonate	BA[b]	5%	OMJ	0.5 g		Precipitate forms within 13 weeks at –20°C	1986	I
Sodium bicarbonate	BA[b]	5%	OMJ	5 g		Physically compatible. No loss in 3 days at 25°C, 14 days at 5°C, 26 weeks at –20°C, in dark	1986	C

[a] Admixed in the linezolid infusion container.

[b] Tested in PVC containers.

Y-Site Injection Compatibility (1:1 Mixture)

Levofloxacin

Test Drug	Mfr	Conc	Mfr	Conc	Remarks	Ref	C/I
Acyclovir sodium	BW	50 mg/mL	OMN	5 mg/mL[a]	Cloudy precipitate forms	2233	I
Alprostadil	UP	0.5 mg/mL	OMN	5 mg/mL[a]	Precipitate forms	2233	I

Y-Site Injection Compatibility (1:1 Mixture) (Cont.)

Test Drug	Mfr	Conc	Mfr	Conc	Remarks	Ref	C/I
Amikacin sulfate	BED	50 mg/mL	OMN	5 mg/mL[a]	Visually compatible for 4 hr at 24°C	2233	C
Aminophylline	AMR	25 mg/mL	OMN	5 mg/mL[a]	Visually compatible for 4 hr at 24°C	2233	C
Ampicillin sodium	MAR	50 mg/mL	OMN	5 mg/mL[a]	Visually compatible for 4 hr at 24°C	2233	C
Anidulafungin	VIC	0.5 mg/mL[a]	OMN	5 mg/mL[a]	Physically compatible for 4 hr at 23°C	2617	C
Azithromycin	PF	2 mg/mL[b]	ORT	5 mg/mL[e]	White and amber microcrystals found	2368	I
Bivalirudin	TMC	5 mg/mL[a]	ORT	5 mg/mL[a]	Physically compatible for 4 hr at 23°C	2373	C
Caffeine citrate		5 mg/mL	OMN	5 mg/mL[a]	Visually compatible for 4 hr at 24°C	2233	C
Cangrelor tetrasodium	TMC	1 mg/mL[b]		5 mg/mL[b]	Physically compatible for 4 hr	3243	C
Caspofungin acetate	ME	0.7 mg/mL[b]	JN	5 mg/mL[b]	Physically compatible for 4 hr at room temperature	2758	C
Caspofungin acetate	ME	0.5 mg/mL[b]	HOS	5 mg/mL[a]	Physically compatible over 60 min	2766	C
Cefotaxime sodium	HO	200 mg/mL	OMN	5 mg/mL[a]	Visually compatible for 4 hr at 24°C	2233	C
Ceftaroline fosamil	FOR	2.22 mg/mL[a b c]	OMN	5 mg/mL[a b c]	Physically compatible for 4 hr at 23°C	2826	C
Ceftazidime–avibactam sodium	ALL	20 mg/mL[k l]			Physically compatible for up to 4 hr at room temperature	3004	C
Ceftolozane sulfate–tazobactam sodium	CUB	10 mg/mL[g i]	CLA	5 mg/mL[g]	Physically compatible for 2 hr	3262	C
Clindamycin phosphate	UP	150 mg/mL	OMN	5 mg/mL[a]	Visually compatible for 4 hr at 24°C	2233	C
Cloxacillin sodium	SMX	100 mg/mL	HOS	5 mg/mL	Physically compatible for up to 4 hr at room temperature	3245	C
Daptomycin	CUB[h]	14.3 mg/mL[b f]	OMN	7.1 mg/mL[b f]	Physically compatible with no loss of either drug in 2 hr at 25°C	2553	C
Dexamethasone sodium phosphate	ES	4 mg/mL	OMN	5 mg/mL[a]	Visually compatible for 4 hr at 24°C	2233	C
Dexmedetomidine HCl	AB	4 mcg/mL[b]	ORT	5 mg/mL[b]	Physically compatible for 4 hr at 23°C	2383	C
Dobutamine HCl	AB	12.5 mg/mL	OMN	5 mg/mL[a]	Visually compatible for 4 hr at 24°C	2233	C
Dopamine HCl	AMR	80 mg/mL	OMN	5 mg/mL[a]	Visually compatible for 4 hr at 24°C	2233	C
Doripenem	JJ	5 mg/mL[a b]	OMN	5 mg/mL[a b]	Physically compatible for 4 hr at 23°C	2743	C
Epinephrine HCl	AB	1 mg/mL	OMN	5 mg/mL[a]	Visually compatible for 4 hr at 24°C	2233	C
Eravacycline dihydro-chloride	TET	0.6 mg/mL[b]	AUR	5 mg/mL[b]	Physically compatible for 2 hr at room temperature	3532	C
Esmolol HCl	MYL	10 mg/mL	SGT	5 mg/mL	Physically compatible for 1 hr at 23°C	3533	C
Fenoldopam mesylate	AB	80 mcg/mL[b]	OMN	5 mg/mL[b]	Physically compatible for 4 hr at 23°C	2467	C
Fentanyl citrate	AB	0.05 mg/mL	OMN	5 mg/mL[a]	Visually compatible for 4 hr at 24°C	2233	C
Furosemide	AST	10 mg/mL	OMN	5 mg/mL[a]	Cloudy precipitate forms	2233	I
Gentamicin sulfate	ES	10 mg/mL	OMN	5 mg/mL[a]	Visually compatible for 4 hr at 24°C	2233	C
Heparin sodium	ES	10 units/mL	OMN	5 mg/mL[a]	Cloudy precipitate forms	2233	I
Hetastarch in lactated electrolyte	AB	6%	OMN	5 mg/mL[a]	Physically compatible for 4 hr at 23°C	2339	C

Y-Site Injection Compatibility (1:1 Mixture) (Cont.)

Test Drug	Mfr	Conc	Mfr	Conc	Remarks	Ref	C/I
Hydromorphone HCl	HOS	2 mg/mL	OMN	5 mg/mL[a]	Physically compatible	2794	C
Hydroxyethyl starch 130/0.4 in sodium chloride 0.9%	FRK	6%	OMN	1, 2.5, 5 mg/mL[a]	Visually compatible for 24 hr at room temperature	2770	C
Indomethacin sodium trihydrate	ME	1 mg/mL	OMN	5 mg/mL[a]	Cloudy precipitate forms	2233	I
Insulin, regular	LI	1 unit/mL	OMN	5 mg/mL[a]	Visually compatible for 4 hr at 24°C	2233	C
Insulin, regular	LI	100 units/mL	OMN	5 mg/mL[a]	Cloudy precipitate forms	2233	I
Isavuconazonium sulfate	ASP	1.5 mg/mL[g]	AUR	5 mg/mL[g]	Physically compatible for 2 hr	3263	C
Isoproterenol HCl	ES	0.2 mg/mL	OMN	5 mg/mL[a]	Visually compatible for 4 hr at 24°C	2233	C
Labetalol HCl	HOS	5 mg/mL	SGT	5 mg/mL	Physically compatible for 1 hr at 23°C	3533	C
Letermovir	ME				Physically incompatible	3398	I
Lidocaine HCl	AB	10 mg/mL[d]	OMN	5 mg/mL[a]	Visually compatible for 4 hr at 24°C	2233	C
Linezolid	PHU	2 mg/mL	ORT	5 mg/mL[a]	Physically compatible for 4 hr at 23°C	2264	C
Lorazepam		2 mg/mL	OMN	5 mg/mL[a]	Visually compatible for 4 hr at 24°C	2233	C
Magnesium sulfate	AMR	20 mg/mL[b]	OMN	5 mg/mL[a]	Physically compatible	2794	C
Meropenem–vaborbactam	TMC	8 mg/mL[b j]	AUB	5 mg/mL[b]	Physically compatible for 3 hr at 20 to 25°C	3380, 3382	C
Metoclopramide HCl	ES	5 mg/mL	OMN	5 mg/mL[a]	Visually compatible for 4 hr at 24°C	2233	C
Metoprolol tartrate	HOS	0.4 mg/mL[b]	SGT	5 mg/mL	Physically compatible for 1 hr at 23°C	3533	C
Morphine sulfate	SW	4 mg/mL	OMN	5 mg/mL[a]	Visually compatible for 4 hr at 24°C	2233	C
Nitroglycerin	AMR	5 mg/mL	OMN	5 mg/mL[a]	Cloudy precipitate forms	2233	I
Norepinephrine bitartrate	HOS	64 mcg/mL[a]	SZ	5 mg/mL	Physically compatible with no loss of either drug in 4 hr at room temperature	3510	C
Oxacillin sodium	APC	167 mg/mL	OMN	5 mg/mL[a]	Visually compatible for 4 hr at 24°C	2233	C
Pancuronium bromide	ES	1 mg/mL	OMN	5 mg/mL[a]	Visually compatible for 4 hr at 24°C	2233	C
Penicillin G sodium	MAR	500,000 units/mL	OMN	5 mg/mL[a]	Visually compatible for 4 hr at 24°C	2233	C
Phenobarbital sodium	ES	130 mg/mL	OMN	5 mg/mL[a]	Visually compatible for 4 hr at 24°C	2233	C
Phenylephrine HCl	AMR	10 mg/mL	OMN	5 mg/mL[a]	Visually compatible for 4 hr at 24°C	2233	C
Plazomicin sulfate	ACH	24 mg/mL[g]	SGT	5 mg/mL[g]	Measured turbidity increases immediately	3432, 3433	I
Posaconazole	ME	18 mg/mL		40 mg/mL[g]	Physically compatible	2911, 2912	C
Potassium chloride	HOS	0.04 mEq/mL[a]	OMN	5 mg/mL[a]	Physically compatible	2794	C
Sodium bicarbonate	AB	0.5 mEq/mL	OMN	5 mg/mL[a]	Visually compatible for 4 hr at 24°C	2233	C
Sodium nitroprusside	ES	10 mg/mL[b]	OMN	5 mg/mL[a]	Fluffy precipitate forms	2233	I
Tedizolid phosphate	CUB	0.8 mg/mL[b]	AUR	5 mg/mL[b]	Physically compatible for 2 hr	3244	C

Y-Site Injection Compatibility (1:1 Mixture) (Cont.)

Test Drug	Mfr	Conc	Mfr	Conc	Remarks	Ref	C/I
Telavancin HCl	ASP	7.5 mg/mL[a b c]	OMN	5 mg/mL[a b c]	Discoloration and measured haze increase	2830	I
Vancomycin HCl	LI	50 mg/mL	OMN	5 mg/mL[a]	Visually compatible for 4 hr at 24°C	2233	C

[a] Tested in dextrose 5%.

[b] Tested in sodium chloride 0.9%.

[c] Tested in Ringer's injection, lactated.

[d] Preservative free.

[e] Injected via Y-site into an administration set running azithromycin.

[f] Final concentration after mixing.

[g] Tested in both dextrose 5% and sodium chloride 0.9%.

[h] Test performed using the Cubicin formulation.

[i] Ceftolozane component. Ceftolozane in a 2:1 fixed-ratio concentration with tazobactam.

[j] Meropenem component. Meropenem in a 1:1 fixed-ratio concentration with vaborbactam.

[k] Ceftazidime component. Ceftazidime in a 4:1 fixed-ratio concentration with avibactam.

[l] Tested in dextrose 5%, sodium chloride 0.9%, and Ringer's injection, lactated.

Selected Revisions May 1, 2020. © Copyright, October 1998.
American Society of Health-System Pharmacists, Inc.

Levoleucovorin Calcium
AHFS 92:12

Products

Levoleucovorin calcium is available as a lyophilized powder in (preservative-free) single-use vials containing the equivalent of 50 or 175 mg of levoleucovorin.[3196] [3343] The 50-mg vial also contains mannitol 50 mg and sodium hydroxide and/or hydrochloric acid to adjust the pH.[3196] The 50-mg vial should be reconstituted only with 5.3 mL of sodium chloride 0.9% to yield a levoleucovorin concentration of 10 mg/mL.[3196] The 175-mg vial also contains mannitol 175 mg and sodium hydroxide and/or hydrochloric acid to adjust the pH.[3343] The 175-mg vial should be reconstituted only with 17.7 mL of sodium chloride 0.9% to yield a levoleucovorin concentration of 10 mg/mL.[3343] Reconstitution with sodium chloride solutions containing a preservative (e.g., benzyl alcohol) has not been studied.[3196] [3343] The reconstituted solution may be immediately diluted in sodium chloride 0.9% or dextrose 5% to a final levoleucovorin concentration of 0.5 to 5 mg/mL.[3196] [3343]

Levoleucovorin calcium also is available as a solution in (preservative-free) single-use vials.[3197] Each 17.5- or 25-mL vial contains 175 or 250 mg, respectively, of levoleucovorin as the calcium salt in sodium chloride 0.83%.[3197] Each vial also contains sodium hydroxide to adjust the pH.[3197] Levoleucovorin calcium injection solution may be further diluted with sodium chloride 0.9% or dextrose 5% to a final concentration of 0.5 mg/mL.[3197]

Equivalency

Levoleucovorin calcium pentahydrate 64 mg is equivalent to levoleucovorin 50 mg.[3196]

Levoleucovorin calcium pentahydrate 222 mg is equivalent to levoleucovorin 175 mg.[3343]

pH

Levoleucovorin calcium injection solution has an adjusted pH ranging from 6.5 to 8.5.[3197]

Trade Name(s)

Fusilev

Administration

Levoleucovorin calcium is administered intravenously by infusion or injection.[3196] [3197] [3343] For certain indications, the manufacturer states that the drug should be administered by slow intravenous injection over at least 3 minutes.[3196] Levoleucovorin calcium should *not* be administered at a rate faster than 160 mg/min due to the calcium content.[3196] [3197] [3343]

Levoleucovorin calcium should *not* be administered intrathecally.[3196] [3197] [3343]

Stability

Intact vials of levoleucovorin calcium lyophilized powder for injection should be stored at controlled room temperature.[3196] [3343] Intact vials of levoleucovorin calcium injection solution should be stored at 2 to 8°C.[3197] Both formulations should be stored in their cartons until use to protect from light.[3196] [3197] [3343]

Reconstituted and/or diluted solutions of levoleucovorin prepared with 50- or 175-mg vials of the lyophilized powder for injection and sodium chloride 0.9% may be stored at room temperature for up to 12 or 24 hours (total), respectively.[3196] [3343] Diluted solutions of levoleucovorin prepared with 50- or 175-mg vials of the lyophilized powder for injection and dextrose 5% may be stored at room temperature for up to 4 hours.[3196] [3343]

Diluted solutions of levoleucovorin prepared with the injection solution and sodium chloride 0.9% or dextrose 5% may be stored at room temperature for up to 4 hours.[3197]

Reconstituted and/or diluted solutions of levoleucovorin should be visually inspected for particulate matter and discoloration prior to administration; if cloudiness or precipitate is observed, solutions should not be used.[3196] [3197] [3343]

Compatibility Information

Solution Compatibility

Levoleucovorin calcium

Test Soln Name	Mfr	Mfr	Conc/L or %	Remarks	Ref	C/I
Dextrose 5%		SP, ACT	0.5 to 5 g	Stable for up to 4 hr at room temperature	3196, 3343	C
Dextrose 5%		SZ	0.5 g	Stable for up to 4 hr at room temperature	3197	C
Sodium chloride 0.9%		SP	0.5 to 5 g	Stable for up to 12 hr at room temperature	3196	C
Sodium chloride 0.9%		ACT[a]	0.5 to 5 g	Stable for up to 24 hr at room temperature	3343	C
Sodium chloride 0.9%		SZ	0.5 g	Stable for up to 4 hr at room temperature	3197	C

[a] Lyophilized formulation (175-mg) tested.

DOI: 10.37573/9781585286850.238

Additive Compatibility

Levoleucovorin calcium

Test Drug	Mfr	Conc/L or %	Mfr	Conc/L or %	Test Solution	Remarks	Ref	C/I
Fluorouracil	AD	16.7 to 46.2 g	CY	1.5 to 13.3 g	a	Subvisible particulates form in all combinations in variable periods from 1 to 4 days at 4, 23, and 32°C	1816	I

[a] Tested both drugs undiluted and diluted by 25% with dextrose 5%.

Y-Site Injection Compatibility (1:1 Mixture)

Levoleucovorin calcium

Test Drug	Mfr	Conc	Mfr	Conc	Remarks	Ref	C/I
Granisetron HCl	SKB	0.05 mg/mL[a]	LE	2 mg/mL[a]	Physically compatible with no change in measured turbidity or increase in particle content in 4 hr at 23°C	2000	C

[a] Tested in dextrose 5%.

Selected Revisions September 30, 2019. © Copyright, June 2017.
American Society of Health-System Pharmacists, Inc.

Levothyroxine Sodium
AHFS 68:36.04

Products

Levothyroxine sodium is available in 100-, 200-, and 500-mcg vials.[2883] Also present in the vials are dibasic sodium phosphate heptahydrate, mannitol, and sodium hydroxide.[2883] Reconstitute vials by adding 5 mL of sodium chloride 0.9%, resulting in solutions containing 20, 40, and 100 mcg/mL, respectively.[2883] Shake well to ensure complete dissolution.[2883]

Administration

Levothyroxine sodium injection may be administered undiluted by intravenous injection.[2883] The drug also has been administered by intramuscular injection,[2885] however the current labeling no longer includes this information.[2883]

Stability

Intact vials should be stored at controlled room temperature and protected from light.[2883] After reconstitution, the drug is stable for 4 hours; however, the manufacturer states that the drug should be used immediately.[2883] Vials are intended for single-use only; unused portions should be discarded.[2883] The manufacturer also states that levothyroxine sodium injection should not be added to intravenous solutions.[2883]

Syringes

Levothyroxine sodium 0.1 mg/mL in sodium chloride 0.9% was packaged as 5 mL in 6-mL polypropylene syringes (Monoject). No loss of drug was found after seven days at 5°C.[2354]

Sorption

In a study of levothyroxine sodium stability in glass, polyolefin, and PVC containers for continuous infusion, delivery of the drug through PVC tubing resulted in 13% loss of drug in glass and polyolefin containers and 18% loss of drug in PVC containers over 1 hour as a result of sorption to the PVC materials.[2884] Levothyroxine sodium concentrations returned to greater than 90% of the initial concentration by 3 hours in all 3 container types and thereafter remained above 90% for the duration of the 24-hour study period.[2884] The use of polyolefin tubing or flushing of a PVC line with levothyroxine solution prior to administration has been suggested to minimize such sorption.[2884]

Compatibility Information

Solution Compatibility

Levothyroxine sodium

Test Soln Name	Mfr	Mfr	Conc/L or %	Remarks	Ref	C/I
Dextrose 5%	BA[b]	PP	1 mg	Physically compatible. Little to no loss in 24 hr at 22°C	2884	C
Dextrose 5%	BA[a]	PP	1 mg	Physically compatible. Less than 10% loss in 24 hr at 22°C	2884	C
Sodium chloride 0.9%	BA[a]	PP	0.4 and 2 mg	Physically compatible. Less than 10% loss in 8 hr at 25°C	2823	C

[a] Tested in PVC containers.

[b] Tested in glass and polyolefin containers.

Y-Site Injection Compatibility (1:1 Mixture)

Levothyroxine sodium

Test Drug	Mfr	Conc	Mfr	Conc	Remarks	Ref	C/I
Esmolol HCl	MYL	10 mg/mL	PRP	0.4 mcg/mL[a]	Physically compatible for 1 hr at 23°C	3533	C
Labetalol HCl	HOS	5 mg/mL	PRP	0.4 mcg/mL[a]	Physically compatible for 1 hr at 23°C	3533	C
Metoprolol tartrate	HOS	0.4 mg/mL[a]	PRP	0.4 mcg/mL[a]	Physically compatible for 1 hr at 23°C	3533	C

[a] Tested in sodium chloride 0.9%.

DOI: 10.37573/9781585286850.239

Lidocaine Hydrochloride
AHFS 24:04.04.08
Lignocaine Hydrochloride

Products

Lidocaine hydrochloride for direct intravenous use is available in concentrations of 10 and 20 mg/mL in ampuls and vials from 5 to 50 mL and in 5-mL prefilled syringes. The drug also is available as 40-, 100-, and 200-mg/mL concentrates for intravenous admixture preparation. The pH of these solutions is adjusted with sodium hydroxide and/or hydrochloric acid. Multiple-dose vials and automatic injection devices also may contain methylparaben and EDTA or sulfites.[4]

Lidocaine hydrochloride also is available premixed in dextrose 5% in concentrations of 0.2, 0.4, and 0.8% (2, 4, and 8 mg/mL, respectively). The solutions are available in container sizes ranging from 250 to 1000 mL.[4]

pH

The pH of the injection is about 6.5 but may range from 5 to 7.[1][4] The premixed infusion solutions in dextrose 5% have a pH of 3 to 7.[4][17]

Osmolality

The osmolalities of lidocaine hydrochloride products were determined to be 296 mOsm/kg for the 10-mg/mL concentration and 352 mOsm/kg for the 20-mg/mL concentration.[1233]

Osmolarity

The commercially available lidocaine hydrochloride 0.2, 0.4, and 0.8% premixed solutions have osmolarities of approximately 266, 281, and 308 mOsm/L, respectively.[4]

Trade Name(s)

Xylocaine

Administration

Lidocaine hydrochloride is administered by direct intravenous injection and continuous intravenous infusion.[4] The drug also may be administered by intramuscular injection.[4][118][119][120] Products containing 40, 100, or 200 mg/mL should not be administered by direct intravenous injection without prior dilution to a 1- or 2-mg/mL (0.1 or 0.2%) solution. Lidocaine hydrochloride products containing preservatives should not be given intravenously. Products containing epinephrine should not be used to treat arrhythmias.[4]

Stability

Lidocaine hydrochloride injection and premixed infusion solutions should be stored at controlled room temperature and protected from excessive heat and freezing.[4]

pH Effects

Although lidocaine hydrochloride is stable across a broad pH range, its pH of maximum stability is 3 to 6.[1277]

Buffering lidocaine hydrochloride injection with sodium bicarbonate has been used to reduce pain on injection. Increasing the pH results in an increased percentage of the drug being present as the unionized base, which is less stable and soluble. Lidocaine base precipitation has been shown to occur at a pH around 7.5 to 7.6.[2409]

The stability of lidocaine hydrochloride 2%, with and without epinephrine hydrochloride, was studied after alkalinization with sodium bicarbonate. Lidocaine hydrochloride alone was alkalinized to pH 7.2, while the lidocaine–epinephrine combination was adjusted to pH 6.5 and also 7.05. The combinations were compatible, and no loss of lidocaine or epinephrine occurred over 6 hours.[1401]

The stability of lidocaine hydrochloride 1% (Elkins-Sinn) buffered with sodium bicarbonate to pH 6.8, 7.2, and 7.4 was evaluated. No loss occurred in 27 days at pH 6.8. At pH 7.2, adequate concentrations were retained for 19 days, but by 27 days, concentrations had fallen to about 88% and a crystalline precipitate formed. At pH 7.4, losses of up to 23% were accompanied by crystalline precipitation between 5 and 15 days.[2407]

Lidocaine hydrochloride is stable when mixed with certain acid-stable drugs such as epinephrine hydrochloride, norepinephrine bitartrate, and isoproterenol hydrochloride. However, its buffering action may raise the pH of intravenous admixtures above 5.5, the maximum pH for stability of the other drugs. The final pH is usually about 6. These drugs begin to deteriorate within several hours. Note: This does not apply to commercial lidocaine–epinephrine combinations, which have the pH adjusted to retain epinephrine.[24]

Syringes

Lidocaine hydrochloride (Abbott) 20 mg/mL was packaged as 10 mL of undiluted injection in 12-mL polypropylene syringes (Becton Dickinson) and stored at 23°C under fluorescent light and 4°C. No lidocaine loss was found after 90 days of storage.[2428]

Lidocaine hydrochloride 2% (20 mg/mL) in auto-injector syringes (Abbott) was evaluated for stability over 45 days under use conditions in paramedic vehicles. Temperatures fluctuated with locations and conditions and ranged from 6.5°C (43.7 °F) to 52°C (125.6 °F) in high desert conditions. No visually apparent changes occurred, and no loss was found.[2548]

Lidocaine hydrochloride under simulated summer conditions in paramedic vehicles was exposed to temperatures ranging from 26 to 38°C over 4 weeks. No loss of the drug occurred.[2562]

Sorption

Lidocaine hydrochloride in solutions with acidic pH was shown not to exhibit sorption to polyvinyl chloride (PVC) bags and tubing, elastomeric pump reservoirs, polyethylene tubing, Silastic tubing, and polypropylene syringes.[12][536][606][2014]

DOI: 10.37573/9781585286850.240

However, in a slightly alkaline (pH 8) cardioplegia solution, the percentage of unionized lidocaine base increased to 58%. This compares to 3% in dextrose 5% and sodium chloride 0.9% at around pH 6. The unionized form is highly lipid soluble and may interact with PVC bags. Storage of the cardioplegia solutions in PVC bags at 22°C resulted in a 12 to 19% lidocaine loss in 2 days and a 65 to 75% loss in 21 days. Degradation was not likely because storage in glass bottles did not result in any lidocaine loss after 21 days at 22°C. Refrigeration of the PVC bags at 4°C slowed the lidocaine loss to 9% or less in 21 days.[776]

Filtration

Lidocaine hydrochloride (Astra) 200 mg/L in dextrose 5% and sodium chloride 0.9% did not display significant sorption to a 0.45-μm cellulose membrane filter (Abbott S-A-I-F) during an 8-hour simulated infusion.[567]

Central Venous Catheter

Lidocaine hydrochloride (Astra) 2 mg/mL in dextrose 5% was found to be compatible with the ARROWg+ard Blue Plus (Arrow International) chlorhexidine-bearing triple-lumen central catheter. Essentially complete delivery of the drug was found with little or no drug loss occurring. Furthermore, chlorhexidine delivered from the catheter remained at trace amounts with no substantial increase due to the delivery of the drug through the catheter.[2335]

Compatibility Information

Solution Compatibility

Lidocaine HCl

Test Soln Name	Mfr	Mfr	Conc/L or %	Remarks	Ref	C/I
Amino acids 4.25%, dextrose 25%	MG	AST	1 g	No increase in particulate matter in 24 hr at 5°C	349	C
Dextrose 5% in Ringer's injection, lactated	TR[a]	AST	1 g	Stable for 24 hr at 5°C	282	C
Dextrose 5% in Ringer's injection, lactated	TR[a]	AST	2 g	Physically compatible. Little loss in 14 days at 25°C	775	C
Dextrose 5% in sodium chloride 0.45%	CU, AB[a]	AST	2 g	Physically compatible. Little loss in 14 days at 25°C	775	C
Dextrose 5% in sodium chloride 0.9%	TR[a]	AST	1 g	Stable for 24 hr at 5°C	282	C
Dextrose 5%	TR[a]	AST	2 g	Physically compatible. No loss in 14 days at 25°C	775	C
Dextrose 5%	AB[a]	ES	515 mg	No loss over 21 days at 20 to 24°C	776	C
Dextrose 5%	TR[a]	AST	1 g	Stable for 24 hr at 5°C	282	C
Dextrose 5%	TR[b]	ES	4 g	Stable for 120 days at 4 and 30°C	543	C
Dextrose 5%	TR[b]	AST	1 and 8 g	Visually compatible. No loss in 48 hr at room temperature	1802	C
Ringer's injection, lactated	TR[a]	AST	1 g	Stable for 24 hr at 5°C	282	C
Ringer's injection, lactated	TR[a]	AST	2 g	Physically compatible. No loss in 14 days at 25°C	775	C
Sodium chloride 0.45%	AB[a]	AST	2 g	Physically compatible. No loss in 14 days at 25°C	775	C
Sodium chloride 0.9%	TR[a]	AST	2 g	Physically compatible. No loss in 14 days at 25°C	775	C
Sodium chloride 0.9%	AB[a]	ES	515 mg	No loss over 21 days at 20 to 24°C	776	C
Sodium chloride 0.9%	BA[c]	AST		Stable for 24 hr	45	C
Sodium chloride 0.9%	TR[a]	AST	1 g	Stable for 24 hr at 5°C	282	C
Sodium chloride 0.9%	TR[b]	AST	1 g	Stable for 24 hr	45	C
Sodium chloride 0.9%	TR[b]	AST	1 and 8 g	Visually compatible. Little loss in 48 hr at room temperature	1802	C

[a] Tested in both glass and PVC containers.

[b] Tested in PVC containers.

[c] Tested in glass containers.

Additive Compatibility

Lidocaine HCl

Test Drug	Mfr	Conc/L or %	Mfr	Conc/L or %	Test Solution	Remarks	Ref	C/I
Alteplase	GEN	0.5 g	AST	4 g	D5W	Visually compatible with no alteplase clot-lysis activity loss in 24 hr at 25°C	1856	C
Alteplase	GEN	0.5 g	AST	4 g	NS	Visually compatible with 7% alteplase clot-lysis activity loss in 24 hr at 25°C	1856	C
Aminophylline	SE	500 mg	AST	2 g		Physically compatible	24	C
Aminophylline	AQ	1 g	AST	2 g	D5W, LR, NS	Physically compatible for 24 hr at 25°C	775	C
Amiodarone HCl	LZ	1.8 g	AB	4 g	D5W, NS[a] [d]	Physically compatible. 9% or less amiodarone loss in 24 hr at 24°C in light	1031	C
Atracurium besylate	BW	500 mg		2 g	D5W	Physically compatible and atracurium stable for 24 hr at 5 and 30°C	1694	C
Calcium chloride	UP	1 g	AST	2 g		Physically compatible	24	C
Calcium gluconate	ES	2 g	AST	2 g	D5W, LR, NS	Physically compatible for 24 hr at 25°C	775	C
Chloramphenicol sodium succinate	PD	1 g	AST	2 g		Physically compatible	24	C
Chlorothiazide sodium	MSD	500 mg	AST	2 g		Physically compatible	24	C
Ciprofloxacin	MI	2 g		1 g	NS	Compatible for 24 hr at 25°C	888	C
Ciprofloxacin	MI	2 g		1.5 g	NS	Compatible for 24 hr at 25°C	888	C/I
Dexamethasone sodium phosphate	MSD	4 mg	AST	2 g		Physically compatible	24	C
Digoxin	ES	1 mg	AST	2 g	D5W, LR, NS	Physically compatible for 24 hr at 25°C	775	C
Diphenhydramine HCl	PD	50 mg	AST	2 g		Physically compatible	24	C
Dobutamine HCl	LI	1 g	ES	4 g	D5W, NS	Visually compatible for 24 hr at 25°C	789	C
Dobutamine HCl	LI	1 g	AST	4 and 10 g	D5W, NS	Physically compatible for 24 hr at 21°C	812	C
Dopamine HCl	AS	800 mg	AST	4 g	D5W[a]	No dopamine or lidocaine loss in 24 hr at 25°C	312	C
Dopamine HCl	ACC	800 mg	AST	2 g	D5W, LR, NS	Physically compatible for 24 hr at 25°C	775	C
Ephedrine sulfate		50 mg	AST	2 g		Physically compatible	24	C
Eptifibatide	ME	750 mg		2 g		Physically compatible and chemically stable for up to 24 hr at 25°C	3049	C
Erythromycin lactobionate	AB	1 g	AST	2 g		Physically compatible	24	C
Fentanyl citrate		2 mg	AST	2.5 g	NS[a]	Physically compatible with no loss of lidocaine or fentanyl at pH 5.8 in 30 days at 4 and 23°C	2305	C
Fentanyl citrate		2 mg	BRN	2.5 g	NS[a]	Physically compatible with little lidocaine loss but 18% fentanyl loss at 23°C and 10% loss at 4°C in 2 days due to sorption at pH 6.7 from higher pH lidocaine product	2305	I
Floxacillin sodium	BE	20 g	ANT	2 g	NS	Physically compatible for 72 hr at 15 and 30°C	1479	C
Flumazenil	RC	20 mg	AB	4 g	D5W[a]	Visually compatible. 4% flumazenil loss in 24 hr at 23°C in fluorescent light. Lidocaine not tested	1710	C
Furosemide	HO	1 g	ANT	2 g	NS	Physically compatible for 72 hr at 15 and 30°C	1479	C

Additive Compatibility (Cont.)

Test Drug	Mfr	Conc/L or %	Mfr	Conc/L or %	Test Solution	Remarks	Ref	C/I
Heparin sodium		32,000 units		4 g	NS	Physically compatible and heparin activity retained for 24 hr	57	C
Heparin sodium	AB	20,000 units	AST	2 g		Physically compatible	24	C
Hydrocortisone sodium succinate	UP	250 mg	AST	2 g		Physically compatible	24	C
Hydroxyzine HCl	PF	100 mg	AST	2 g		Physically compatible	24	C
Methohexital sodium	BP	2 g	BP	2 g	D5W	Precipitates immediately	26	I
Nafcillin sodium	AP	20 g	AST	0.6 g	D5Wa , NSd	Visually compatible. Little nafcillin loss in 48 hr at 23°C. Lidocaine not tested	1806	C
Nitroglycerin	ACC	400 mg	IMS	4 g	D5W, NSe	Physically compatible. No nitroglycerin loss in 48 hr at 23°C. Lidocaine not tested	929	C
Penicillin G potassium	SQ	1 million units	AST	2 g		Physically compatible	24	C
Pentobarbital sodium	AB	500 mg	AST	2 g		Physically compatible	24	C
Phenylephrine HCl	WI	20 mg	AST	2 g		Physically compatible	24	C
Phenytoin sodium	ES	1 g	AST	2 g	D5W, LR, NS	Immediate formation of a white cloudy precipitate	775	I
Potassium chloride	AB	40 mEq	AST	2 g		Physically compatible	24	C
Procainamide HCl	SQ	1 g	AST	2 g	D5W, LR, NS	Physically compatible for 24 hr at 25°C	775	C
Prochlorperazine edisylate	SKF	10 mg	AST	2 g		Physically compatible	24	C
Ranitidine HCl	GL	50 mg and 2 g	AST	1 and 8 g	D5W, NSa	Physically compatible. 3% ranitidine loss in 24 hr at room temperature in light. Lidocaine not tested	1361	C
Ranitidine HCl	GL	50 mg and 2 g		2.5 g	D5W	Physically compatible. Ranitidine stable for 24 hr at 25°C. Lidocaine not tested	1515	C
Ranitidine HCl	GL	50 mg and 2 g	AST	1 and 8 g	D5W, NSa	Visually compatible. Little loss of either drug in 48 hr at room temperature	1802	C
Sodium bicarbonate	AB	40 mEq	AST	2 g		Physically compatible	24	C
Sodium bicarbonate	AB	2.4 mEqc		1 g	D5W	Physically compatible for 24 hr	772	C
Sodium lactate	AB	50 mEq	AST	2 g		Physically compatible	24	C
Theophylline		2 g		380 mg	D5W	Visually compatible with little or no loss of either drug in 48 hr	1909	C
Verapamil HCl	KN	80 mg	IMS	2 g	D5W, NS	Physically compatible for 48 hr	739	C

a Tested in PVC containers.

b Tested in both glass and PVC containers.

c One vial of Neut added to a liter of admixture.

d Tested in polyolefin containers.

e Tested in glass containers.

Drugs in Syringe Compatibility

Lidocaine HCl

Test Drug	Mfr	Amt	Mfr	Amt	Remarks	Ref	C/I
Ampicillin sodium	BE	500 mg		0.5 and 2.5%/1.5 mL	Physically compatible	89	C
Ampicillin sodium	BE	250 mg		0.5 and 2.5%/1.5 mL	Occasional turbidity	89	I
Caffeine citrate		20 mg/1 mL	AB	1%, 1 mL	Visually compatible for 4 hr at 25°C	2440	C
Cefazolin sodium	SKF	1 g	AST	0.5%, 3 mL	Precipitate forms within 3 to 4 hr at 4°C	532	I
Ceftriaxone sodium	RC	450 mg/mL	LY	1%	5% ceftriaxone loss in 8 weeks at −15°C but solution failed the particulate matter test	1824	I
Ceftriaxone sodium	RC	250 and 450 mg/mL	DW	1%	10% ceftriaxone loss in 3 days at 20°C, 7 to 8% loss in 35 days at 4°C, and 4 to 6% loss in 168 days at −20°C. Lidocaine not tested	1991	C
Clonidine HCl with fentanyl citrate	BI JN	0.03 mg/mL 0.01 mg/mL	AST	2 mg/mL	Diluted to 5 mL with NS. Visually compatible with no new GC/MS peaks in 1 hr at room temperature	1956	C
Cloxacillin sodium	BE				Physically compatible	89	C
Fentanyl citrate with clonidine HCl	JN BI	0.01 mg/mL 0.03 mg/mL	AST	2 mg/mL	Diluted to 5 mL with NS. Visually compatible with no new GC/MS peaks in 1 hr at room temperature	1956	C
Glycopyrrolate	RB	0.2 mg/1 mL	ES	10 mg/1 mL	Physically compatible. pH in glycopyrrolate stability range for 48 hr at 25°C	331	C
Glycopyrrolate	RB	0.2 mg/1 mL	ES	20 mg/2 mL	Physically compatible. pH in glycopyrrolate stability range for 48 hr at 25°C	331	C
Glycopyrrolate	RB	0.4 mg/2 mL	ES	10 mg/1 mL	Physically compatible. pH in glycopyrrolate stability range for 48 hr at 25°C	331	C
Glycopyrrolate	RB	0.2 mg/1 mL	ES	20 mg/1 mL	Physically compatible. pH in glycopyrrolate stability range for 48 hr at 25°C	331	C
Glycopyrrolate	RB	0.2 mg/1 mL	ES	40 mg/2 mL	Physically compatible. pH in glycopyrrolate stability range for 48 hr at 25°C	331	C
Glycopyrrolate	RB	0.4 mg/2 mL	ES	20 mg/1 mL	Physically compatible. pH in glycopyrrolate stability range for 48 hr at 25°C	331	C
Heparin sodium		2500 units/1 mL	AST	100 mg/5 mL	Physically compatible for at least 5 min	1053	C
Hydroxyzine HCl	PF	50 mg/2 mL	AST	2%/2 mL	Physically compatible	771	C
Hydroxyzine HCl	PF	100 mg/2 mL	AST	2%/2 mL	Physically compatible	771	C
Ketamine HCl	REN	125 mg/2.5 mL	APN	1 g/20 mL	Diluted to 50 mL with NS. Physically compatible with little to no loss of either drug in 48 hr at 28°C protected from light	3587	C
Ketamine HCl with morphine sulfate	PD ES	2 mg/mL 0.2 mg/mL	AST	2 mg/mL	Diluted to 5 mL with NS. Visually compatible with no new GC/MS peaks in 1 hr at room temperature	1956	C
Metoclopramide HCl	RB	10 mg/2 mL	ES	50 mg/5 mL	Physically compatible for 48 hr at 25°C	1167	C
Metoclopramide HCl	RB	10 mg/2 mL	ES	100 mg/10 mL	Physically compatible for 48 hr at 25°C	1167	C

Drugs in Syringe Compatibility (Cont.)

Test Drug	Mfr	Amt	Mfr	Amt	Remarks	Ref	C/I
Metoclopramide HCl	RB	160 mg/32 mL	ES	50 mg/5 mL	Physically compatible for 48 hr at 25°C	1167	C
Metoclopramide HCl	RB	160 mg/32 mL	ES	100 mg/10 mL	Physically compatible for 48 hr at 25°C	1167	C
Milrinone lactate	STR	5.25 mg/5.25 mL	AB	100 mg/10 mL	Physically compatible. No loss of either drug in 20 min at 23°C	1410	C
Morphine sulfate with ketamine HCl	ES PD	0.2 mg/mL 2 mg/mL	AST	2 mg/mL	Diluted to 5 mL with NS. Visually compatible with no new GC/MS peaks in 1 hr at room temperature	1956	C
Nalbuphine HCl	DU	10 mg/1 mL		40 mg	Physically compatible for 48 hr	128	C
Nalbuphine HCl	DU	20 mg/1 mL		40 mg	Physically compatible for 48 hr	128	C
Pantoprazole sodium	d	4 mg/1 mL		200 mg/1 mL	Precipitates within 4 hr	2574	I
Phenylephrine HCl		0.25%		2%	No loss of either drug in 66 days at 25°C	1278	C
Propofol	ASZd	200 mg/20 mL	ASZ	5 mg/1 mL	Physically compatible for 24 hr	2490	C
Propofol	ASZd	200 mg/20 mL	ASZ	10 mg/1 mL	Physically compatible for 24 hr	2490	C
Propofol	ASZd	200 mg/20 mL	ASZ	20 mg/1 mL	Physically incompatible. Increased fat droplet size and layering in 3 hr	2490	I
Propofol	ASZd	200 mg/20 mL	ASZ	40 mg/2 mL	Physically incompatible. Increased fat droplet size and layering in 3 hr	2490	I
Propofol	ZEN	1%, 20 mL		10 mg	Physically compatible for 6 hr	2543	C
Propofol	ZEN	1%, 20 mL		30 to 50 mg	Increased fat droplet size	2543	I
Sodium bicarbonate	AB	3 mEq/3 mL	ES	2%, 30 mLa	11% lidocaine and 28% epinephrine loss in 1 week at 25°C	1712	I
Sodium bicarbonate	AB	3 mEq/3 mL	ES	2%, 30 mLa	6% lidocaine loss in 4 weeks at 4°C. 12% epinephrine loss in 3 weeks at 4°C	1712	C
Sodium bicarbonate	LY	0.1 mEq/mL	AST	1%a	25% epinephrine loss in 1 week at room temperature. Lidocaine not tested	1713	I
Sodium bicarbonate		0.088 mEq/mL		0.9%	11% lidocaine loss in 7 days at room temperature	1723	C
Sodium bicarbonate	AST	8.4%/2 mL	AST	1 and 1.5%, 20 mLb	Visually compatible for up to 5 hr at room temperature	1724	C
Sodium bicarbonate	AST	8.4%/2 mL	AST	2%, 20 mLb	Haze forms but dissipates with gentle agitation	1724	?
Sodium bicarbonate	AB	4%/4 mL	AST	1 and 1.5%, 20 mLb	Visually compatible for up to 5 hr at room temperature	1724	C
Sodium bicarbonate	AB	4%/4 mL	AST	2%, 20 mLb	Haze forms but dissipates with gentle agitation	1724	?
Sodium bicarbonate		1.4 and 8.4%/1.5 mL	BEL	2%, 20 mLc	8% epinephrine loss in 7 days at room temperature. Lidocaine not tested	1743	C
Sodium bicarbonate		8.4%/1 mL		2%/10 mL	Physically compatible. No loss of lidocaine in 6 hr	1401	C
Sodium bicarbonate		8.4%/1.5 mL		2%, 10 mLa	Physically compatible. No loss of lidocaine or epinephrine in 6 hr	1401	C
Sodium bicarbonate		1.4%/1.5 mL		2%, 10 mLa	Physically compatible. No loss of lidocaine or epinephrine in 6 hr	1401	C

Drugs in Syringe Compatibility (Cont.)

Test Drug	Mfr	Amt	Mfr	Amt	Remarks	Ref	C/I
Sodium bicarbonate		8.4%/1 mL		1%, 10 mLᵃ	Cloudiness in some samples with no epinephrine loss for 72 hr in the dark. Exposed to light and air, precipitation and 20% epinephrine loss in 24 hr. Lidocaine not tested	2408	?
Sodium bicarbonate	HOS	8.4%/0.3 mL	ASZ	1 and 2%, 2.7 mLᵃ	Physically compatible. 10% epinephrine loss in 7 days and 5% lidocaine loss in 28 days at 5°C in dark	2815	C

ᵃ Tested with epinephrine hydrochloride 1:100,000 added.

ᵇ Tested with epinephrine hydrochloride 1:200,000 added.

ᶜ Tested with epinephrine hydrochloride 1:80,000 added.

ᵈ Test performed using the formulation WITHOUT edetate disodium.

Y-Site Injection Compatibility (1:1 Mixture)

Lidocaine HCl

Test Drug	Mfr	Conc	Mfr	Conc	Remarks	Ref	C/I
Acetaminophen	CAD	10 mg/mL	HOS	20 mg/mL	Physically compatible with less than 10% acetaminophen loss over 4 hr at room temperature	2841, 2844	C
Alteplase	GEN	1 mg/mL	AB	8 mg/mLᵃ	Physically compatible for 6 days	1340	C
Amiodarone HCl	LZ	4 mg/mLᶜ	AST	8 mg/mLᶜ	Physically compatible for 24 hr at 21°C	1032	C
Argatroban	SKB	1 mg/mLᵃ	BA	8 mg/mLᵃ	Physically compatible for 24 hr at 23°C	2572	C
Bivalirudin	TMC	5 mg/mLᵃ	AST	10 mg/mLᵃ	Physically compatible for 4 hr at 23°C	2373	C
Cangrelor tetrasodium	TMC	1 mg/mLᵇ		8 mg/mLᵇ	Physically compatible for 4 hr	3243	C
Cefazolin sodium	LI	40 mg/mLᶜ	AB	8 mg/mLᶜ	Physically compatible for 3 hr	1316	C
Ceftaroline fosamil	FOR	2.22 mg/mLᵈ	HOS	10 mg/mL	Physically compatible for 4 hr at 23°C	2826	C
Ceftolozane sulfate–tazobactam sodium	CUB	10 mg/mLᶜ ᵐ	APP	8 mg/mLᶜ	Physically compatible for 2 hr	3262	C
Ciprofloxacin	MI	2 mg/mLᶜ	AB	4ᵃ and 20 mg/mL	Visually compatible for 24 hr at 24°C	1655	C
Cisatracurium besylate	GW	0.1, 2, 5 mg/mLᵃ	AST	8 mg/mLᵃ	Physically compatible for 4 hr at 23°C	2074	C
Clarithromycin	AB	4 mg/mLᵃ	ANT	4 mg/mLᵃ	Visually compatible for 72 hr at both 30 and 17°C	2174	C
Cloxacillin sodium	SMX	100 mg/mL	ALV	1 mg/mL	Physically compatible for up to 4 hr at room temperature	3245	C
Daptomycin	CUBᶩ	16.7 mg/mLᵇ ⁱ	ASZ	3.3 mg/mLᵇ ⁱ	Physically compatible with no loss of either drug in 2 hr at 25°C	2553	C
Dexmedetomidine HCl	AB	4 mcg/mLᵇ	AST	10 mg/mLᵇ	Physically compatible for 4 hr at 23°C	2383	C
Diltiazem HCl	MMD	1 mg/mLᵃ	AST	8 mg/mLᵃ	Visually compatible for 24 hr at 25°C	1530	C
Diltiazem HCl	MMD	1ᵇ and 5 mg/mL	AB	10 mg/mLᵇ	Visually compatible	1807	C
Diltiazem HCl	MMD	5 mg/mL	AB, SCN	4 and 8 mg/mLᵃ	Visually compatible	1807	C
Dobutamine HCl	LI	4 mg/mLᶜ	AB	8 mg/mLᶜ	Physically compatible for 3 hr	1316	C

Y-Site Injection Compatibility (1:1 Mixture) (Cont.)

Test Drug	Mfr	Conc	Mfr	Conc	Remarks	Ref	C/I
Dobutamine HCl with dopamine HCl	LI DCC	4 mg/mL[c] 3.2 mg/mL[c]	AB	8 mg/mL[c]	Physically compatible for 3 hr	1316	C
Dobutamine HCl with nitroglycerin	LI LY	4 mg/mL[c] 0.4 mg/mL[c]	AB	8 mg/mL[c]	Physically compatible for 3 hr	1316	C
Dobutamine HCl with sodium nitroprusside	LI ES	4 mg/mL[c] 0.4 mg/mL[c]	AB	8 mg/mL[c]	Physically compatible for 3 hr	1316	C
Dopamine HCl	DCC	3.2 mg/mL[c]	AB	8 mg/mL[c]	Physically compatible for 3 hr	1316	C
Dopamine HCl with dobutamine HCl	DCC LI	3.2 mg/mL[c] 4 mg/mL[c]	AB	8 mg/mL[c]	Physically compatible for 3 hr	1316	C
Dopamine HCl with nitroglycerin	DCC LY	3.2 mg/mL[c] 0.4 mg/mL[c]	AB	8 mg/mL[c]	Physically compatible for 3 hr	1316	C
Dopamine HCl with sodium nitroprusside	DCC ES	3.2 mg/mL[c] 0.4 mg/mL[c]	AB	8 mg/mL[c]	Physically compatible for 3 hr	1316	C
Enalaprilat	MSD	0.05 mg/mL[b]	AST	4 mg/mL[a]	Physically compatible for 24 hr at room temperature under fluorescent light	1355	C
Etomidate	AB	2 mg/mL	AST	20 mg/mL	Visually compatible for 7 days at 25°C	1801	C
Famotidine	MSD	0.2 mg/mL[a]	TR	4 mg/mL[a]	Physically compatible for 4 hr at 25°C	1188	C
Famotidine	MSD	0.2 mg/mL[a]	LY	1 mg/mL[a]	Physically compatible for 14 hr	1196	C
Fenoldopam mesylate	AB	80 mcg/mL[b]	AST	10 mg/mL[b]	Physically compatible for 4 hr at 23°C	2467	C
Haloperidol lactate	MN	0.5[a] and 5 mg/mL	AB	4 mg/mL[a]	Visually compatible for 24 hr at 21°C	1523	C
Heparin sodium	TR	50 units/mL	TR	4 mg/mL	Visually compatible for 4 hr at 25°C	1793	C
Heparin sodium[k]	RI	1000 units/L[d]	AST	20 mg/mL	Physically compatible for 4 hr at room temperature	322	C
Hetastarch in lactated electrolyte	AB	6%	AB	8 mg/mL[a]	Physically compatible for 4 hr at 23°C	2339	C
Hydrocortisone sodium succinate[f]	UP	100 mg/L[d]	AST	20 mg/mL	Physically compatible for 4 hr at room temperature	322	C
Isavuconazonium sulfate	ASP	1.5 mg/mL[c]	APP	8 mg/mL[c]	Physically compatible for 2 hr	3263	C
Labetalol HCl	SC	1 mg/mL[a]	AST	20 mg/mL[a]	Physically compatible for 24 hr at 18°C	1171	C
Levofloxacin	OMN	5 mg/mL[a]	AB	10 mg/mL[g]	Visually compatible for 4 hr at 24°C	2233	C
Linezolid	PHU	2 mg/mL	AB	10 mg/mL[a]	Physically compatible for 4 hr at 23°C	2264	C
Meropenem		50 mg/mL	ALV	10 mg/mL	Physically compatible for 4 hr at room temperature	3538	C
Meperidine HCl	AB	10 mg/mL	AB	1 mg/mL[a]	Physically compatible for 4 hr at 25°C	1397	C
Meropenem–vaborbactam	TMC	8 mg/mL[b n]	FRK	8 mg/mL[b]	Physically compatible for 3 hr at 20 to 25°C	3380	C
Metoprolol tartrate	BED	1 mg/mL	BA	8 mg/mL[a]	Trace precipitate in 8 hr at 19°C	2795	I
Micafungin sodium	ASP	1.5 mg/mL[b]	AB	10 mg/mL[b]	Physically compatible for 4 hr at 23°C	2683	C

Y-Site Injection Compatibility (1:1 Mixture) (Cont.)

Test Drug	Mfr	Conc	Mfr	Conc	Remarks	Ref	C/I
Morphine sulfate	AB	1 mg/mL	AB	1 mg/mL[a]	Physically compatible for 4 hr at 25°C	1397	C
Nesiritide	SCI	50 mcg/mL[a b]		20 mg/mL	Physically compatible for 4 hr. May be chemically incompatible with nesiritide[j]	2625	?
Nicardipine HCl	DCC	0.1 mg/mL[a]	AST	4 mg/mL[a]	Visually compatible for 24 hr at room temperature	235	C
Nitroglycerin	LY	0.4 mg/mL[c]	AB	8 mg/mL[c]	Physically compatible for 3 hr	1316	C
Nitroglycerin with dobutamine HCl	LY LI	0.4 mg/mL[c] 4 mg/mL[c]	AB	8 mg/mL[c]	Physically compatible for 3 hr	1316	C
Nitroglycerin with dopamine HCl	LY DCC	0.4 mg/mL[c] 3.2 mg/mL[c]	AB	8 mg/mL[c]	Physically compatible for 3 hr	1316	C
Nitroglycerin with sodium nitroprusside	LY ES	0.4 mg/mL[c] 0.4 mg/mL[c]	AB	8 mg/mL[c]	Physically compatible for 3 hr	1316	C
Palonosetron HCl	MGI	50 mcg/mL	AB	10 mg/mL[a]	Physically compatible. No loss of either drug in 4 hr at room temperature	2771	C
Plazomicin sulfate	ACH	24 mg/mL[c]	AUR	8 mg/mL[c]	Physically compatible for 1 hr at 20 to 25°C	3432	C
Potassium chloride		40 mEq/L[d]	AST	20 mg/mL	Physically compatible for 4 hr at room temperature	322	C
Propofol	ZEN°	10 mg/mL	AST	10 mg/mL	Physically compatible for 1 hr at 23°C	2066	C
Remifentanil HCl	GW	0.025 and 0.25 mg/mL[b]	AST	8 mg/mL[a]	Physically compatible for 4 hr at 23°C	2075	C
Sodium nitroprusside	ES	0.4 mg/mL[c]	AB	8 mg/mL[c]	Physically compatible for 3 hr	1316	C
Sodium nitroprusside	RC	1.2 and 3 mg/mL[a]	AST	6 mg/mL[h]	Visually compatible for 48 hr at 24°C protected from light	2357	C
Sodium nitroprusside	RC	0.3, 1.2, 3 mg/mL[a]	AST	20 and 40 mg/mL[h]	Visually compatible for 48 hr at 24°C protected from light	2357	C
Sodium nitroprusside with dobutamine HCl	ES LI	0.4 mg/mL[c] 4 mg/mL[c]	AB	8 mg/mL[c]	Physically compatible for 3 hr	1316	C
Sodium nitroprusside with dopamine HCl	ES DCC	0.4 mg/mL[c] 3.2 mg/mL[c]	AB	8 mg/mL[c]	Physically compatible for 3 hr	1316	C
Sodium nitroprusside with nitroglycerin	ES LY	0.4 mg/mL[c] 0.4 mg/mL[c]	AB	8 mg/mL[c]	Physically compatible for 3 hr	1316	C
Tedizolid phosphate	CUB	0.8 mg/mL[b]	APP	8 mg/mL[b]	Physically compatible for 2 hr	3244	C
Theophylline	TR	4 mg/mL	TR	4 mg/mL	Visually compatible for 6 hr at 25°C	1793	C
Tigecycline	WY	1 mg/mL[b]		200 mg/mL	Physically compatible for 4 hr	2714	C
Tigecycline	ACD, FRK, WY	[c]			Stated to be compatible	2915, 3459, 3460	C
Tirofiban HCl	ME	0.05 mg/mL[a b]	AB	1 and 20 mg/mL[a b]	Physically compatible. Little loss of either drug in 4 hr at room temperature	2250	C

Y-Site Injection Compatibility (1:1 Mixture) (Cont.)

Test Drug	Mfr	Conc	Mfr	Conc	Remarks	Ref	C/I
TNA #73[e]			ES	4 mg/mL[c]	Visually compatible for 4 hr	1009	C
Vasopressin	AMR	2 and 4 units/mL[b]	BA	4 mg/mL[a]	Physically compatible with vasopressin pushed into a Y-site over 5 sec	2478	C

[a] Tested in dextrose 5%.

[b] Tested in sodium chloride 0.9%.

[c] Tested in both dextrose 5% and sodium chloride 0.9%.

[d] Tested in dextrose 5%, sodium chloride 0.9%, and Ringer's injection, lactated.

[e] Refer to Appendix for the composition of parenteral nutrition solutions. TNA indicates a 3-in-1 admixture.

[f] Tested in combination with heparin sodium (Riker) 1000 units/L.

[g] Preservative free.

[h] Tested in dextrose 5% in sodium chloride 0.225%.

[i] Final concentration after mixing.

[j] Nesiritide is incompatible with bisulfite antioxidants used in some drug formulations. The specific formulation of the product to be used should be checked to ensure that no sulfite antioxidants are present.

[k] Tested in combination with hydrocortisone sodium succinate (Upjohn) 100 mg/L

[l] Test performed using the Cubicin formulation.

[m] Ceftolozane component. Ceftolozane sulfate in a 2:1 fixed-ratio concentration with tazobactam sodium.

[n] Meropenem component. Meropenem in a 1:1 fixed-ratio concentration with vaborbactam.

[o] Test performed using the formulation WITH edetate disodium.

Selected Revisions July 1, 2020. © Copyright, October 1982.
American Society of Health-System Pharmacists, Inc.

Lincomycin Hydrochloride
AHFS 8:12.28.20

Products

Lincomycin hydrochloride is available in 2- and 10-mL vials.[3164][3165] Each mL contains lincomycin hydrochloride equivalent to lincomycin 300 mg and benzyl alcohol 9.45 mg.[3164][3165]

pH

From 3 to 5.5.[17]

Trade Name(s)

Lincocin

Administration

Lincomycin hydrochloride may be administered by intramuscular injection, intravenous infusion, or subconjunctival injection.[3164][3165] For intravenous infusion, each gram of lincomycin should be diluted in at least 100 mL of a compatible infusion solution and infused over at least 1 hour at a rate of 1 g per hour.[3164][3165]

Stability

Lincomycin hydrochloride injection should be stored at controlled room temperature.[3164][3165]

pH Effects

The degradation rate for lincomycin hydrochloride was reported to be at a minimum near pH 4; the drug was least stable at pH 2.[3166]

Compatibility Information

Solution Compatibility

Lincomycin HCl

Test Soln Name	Mfr	Mfr	Conc/L or %	Remarks	Ref	C/I
Dextrose 5% in sodium chloride 0.9%		UP	1.2 g	Stable for 24 hr	109	C
Dextrose 5% in sodium chloride 0.9%		PHU, XGN	6 and 10 g	Physically compatible for 24 hr at room temperature	3164, 3165	C
Dextrose 10% in sodium chloride 0.9%		PHU, XGN	6 and 10 g	Physically compatible for 24 hr at room temperature	3164, 3165	C
Dextrose 5%		UP	1.2 g	Stable for 24 hr	109	C
Dextrose 5%		PHU, XGN	6 and 10 g	Physically compatible for 24 hr at room temperature	3164, 3165	C
Dextrose 5%	BRN[a]	PF	600 mg	Less than 10% loss in 31 days at 25°C	3166	C
Dextrose 10%		UP	1.2 g	Stable for 24 hr	109	C
Dextrose 10%		PHU, XGN	6 and 10 g	Physically compatible for 24 hr at room temperature	3164, 3165	C
Dextrose 10%	FRE[a]	PF	600 mg	Little loss in 31 days at 25°C	3166	C
Ringer's injection		PHU, XGN	6 and 10 g	Physically compatible for 24 hr at room temperature	3164, 3165	C
Sodium chloride 0.9%		UP	1.2 g	Stable for 24 hr	109	C
Sodium chloride 0.9%	BA[a]	PF	600 mg	Little loss in 31 days at 25°C	3166	C
Sodium lactate ⅙ M		PHU, XGN	6 and 10 g	Physically compatible for 24 hr at room temperature	3164, 3165	C

[a] Tested in glass containers.

DOI: 10.37573/9781585286850.241

Additive Compatibility

Lincomycin HCl

Test Drug	Mfr	Conc/L or %	Mfr	Conc/L or %	Test Solution	Remarks	Ref	C/I
Amikacin sulfate	BR	5 g	UP	10 g	D5LR, D5R, D5S, D5W, D10W, LR, NS, R, SL	Physically compatible and both stable for 24 hr at 25°C	293	C
Ampicillin sodium			PHU, XGN			Physically compatible for 24 hr at room temperature	3164, 3165	C
Chloramphenicol sodium succinate			PHU, XGN			Physically compatible for 24 hr at room temperature	3164, 3165	C
Cytarabine	UP	500 mg		1, 1.5, 2, 2.4, 3 g		Physically compatible for 48 hr	174	C
Heparin sodium	AB	20,000 units	UP	600 mg		Physically compatible	21	C
Penicillin G potassium	SQ	20 million units	UP	6 g	D5W	Physically compatible	15	C
Penicillin G potassium	SQ	5 million units	UP	600 mg	D	Physically compatible	47	C
Penicillin G sodium	UP	20 million units	UP	6 g	D5W	Physically compatible	15	C
Polymyxin B sulfate			PHU, XGN			Physically compatible for 24 hr at room temperature	3164, 3165	C
Ranitidine HCl	GL	50 mg and 2 g		2.4 g	D5W	Physically compatible. Ranitidine stable for 24 hr at 25°C. Lincomycin not tested	1515	C

Drugs in Syringe Compatibility

Lincomycin HCl

Test Drug	Mfr	Amt	Mfr	Amt	Remarks	Ref	C/I
Ampicillin sodium	AY	500 mg	UP	600 mg/2 mL	Physically incompatible within 1 hr at room temperature	99	I
Ampicillin sodium	AY	500 mg	UP	600 mg/2 mL	Precipitate forms within 1 hr at room temperature	300	I
Cloxacillin sodium	AY	250 mg	UP	600 mg/2 mL	Physically compatible for 1 hr at room temperature	300	C
Cloxacillin sodium	BE	250 mg	UP	600 mg/2 mL	No precipitate or color change within 1 hr at room temperature	99	C
Doxapram HCl	RB	400 mg/20 mL		300 mg/1 mL	Physically compatible with no doxapram loss in 24 hr	1177	C
Heparin sodium	AB	20,000 units/1 mL	UP	600 mg/2 mL	Physically compatible for at least 30 min	21	C
Penicillin G sodium		1 million units	UP	600 mg/2 mL	No precipitate or color change within 1 hr at room temperature	99	C

Selected Revisions March 16, 2017. © Copyright, October 1982.
American Society of Health-System Pharmacists, Inc.

Linezolid
AHFS 8:12.28.24

Products

Linezolid is available as a single-use, ready-to-use solution for infusion in 100-, 200-, and 300-mL flexible plastic containers.[3183] [3184] Each mL of linezolid (Zyvox, Pfizer) ready-to-use solution for infusion provides linezolid 2 mg along with dextrose, sodium citrate, and citric acid in water for injection.[3183] Each mL of linezolid (Hospira) ready-to-use solution for infusion provides linezolid 2 mg along with citric acid anhydrous, sodium chloride, and sodium hydroxide in water for injection.[3184] Sodium hydroxide and/or hydrochloric acid is used to adjust the pH.[3183] [3184]

Tonicity

Linezolid ready-to-use solutions for infusion are isotonic.[3183] [3184]

pH

Linezolid (Zyvox) ready-to-use solution for infusion is adjusted to pH 4.8.[3183]

Linezolid (Hospira) ready-to-use solution for infusion is adjusted to pH 4.4 to 5.2.[3184]

Sodium Content

The sodium concentration of linezolid (Zyvox) ready-to-use solution for infusion is 0.38 mg/mL or 1.7 mEq in a 100-mL bag, 3.3 mEq in a 200-mL bag, and 5 mEq in a 300-mL bag.[3183]

The sodium concentration of linezolid (Hospira) ready-to-use solution for infusion is 3.98 mg/mL or 52 mEq in a 300-mL bag.[3184]

Trade Name(s)

Zyvox

Administration

Linezolid is administered by intravenous infusion over a period of 30 to 120 minutes.[3183] [3184] If a common intravenous line is being used to administer other drugs in addition to linezolid, the line should be flushed with a compatible infusion solution (e.g., sodium chloride 0.9%, dextrose 5%, Ringer's injection, lactated) prior to and following infusion of linezolid.[3183] [3184]

Stability

Linezolid solutions may exhibit a yellow color that can intensify over time without affecting the stability of the drug.[3183] [3184] Intact containers should be kept in their protective overwrap until ready for use, and should be stored at controlled room temperature and protected from light and freezing.[3183] [3184]

Linezolid solutions should be visually inspected for particulate matter prior to administration.[3183] [3184] The manufacturers state that additives should not be mixed with linezolid ready-to-use solution for infusion.[3183] [3184]

Temperature Effects

Linezolid (Pfizer) 2 mg/mL remained stable without noticeable degradation for 72 hours when stored at 70°C.[3514]

Sorption

Linezolid was found to be compatible with common types of intravenous administration sets including diethylhexyl phthalate (DEHP) plasticized PVC, trioctyl trimellitate (TOTM) plasticized PVC, and polyolefin sets. The total dose of linezolid was fully delivered with the delivered concentration remaining constant throughout. In addition, no detectable levels of plasticizer were found in the delivered solutions.[2338]

Compatibility Information

Solution Compatibility

Linezolid

Test Soln Name	Mfr	Mfr	Conc/L or %	Remarks	Ref	C/I
Dextrose 5%	BRN		2 g	Little to no loss in 34 days at 25°C	3514	C
Dextrose 10%			2 g	Little to no loss in 34 days at 25°C	3514	C
Sodium chloride 0.9%	BA		2 g	Little to no loss in 34 days at 25°C	3514	C

DOI: 10.37573/9781585286850.242

Additive Compatibility

Linezolid

Test Drug	Mfr	Conc/L or %	Mfr	Conc/L or %	Test Solution	Remarks	Ref	C/I
Aztreonam	SQ	20 g	PHU	2 g	a	Physically compatible with no linezolid loss in 7 days at 4 and 23°C protected from light. About 9% aztreonam loss at 23°C and less than 4% loss at 4°C in 7 days	2263	C
Cefazolin sodium	APC	10 g	PHU	2 g	a	Physically compatible with 5% or less loss of each drug in 3 days at 23°C and 7 days at 4°C protected from light	2262	C
Ceftazidime	GW	20 g	PHU	2 g	a	Physically compatible with no linezolid loss in 7 days at 4 and 23°C protected from light. Ceftazidime losses of 5% in 24 hr and 12% in 3 days at 23°C and about 3% in 7 days at 4°C	2262	C
Ceftriaxone sodium	RC	10 g	PHU	2 g	a	Physically compatible, but up to 37% ceftriaxone loss in 24 hr at 23°C and 10% loss in 3 days at 4°C	2262	I
Ceftriaxone sodium			PHU, HOS			Stated to be chemically incompatible	3183, 3184	I
Ciprofloxacin	BAY	4 g	PHU	2 g	a	Physically compatible with little or no loss of either drug in 7 days at 23°C protected from light. Refrigeration results in precipitation after 1 day	2334	C
Erythromycin lactobionate	AB	5 g	PHU	2 g	a	Erythromycin loss of 15% in 1 hr and 30% in 4 hr at 23°C. Loss of 45% in 1 day at 4°C	2333	I
Gentamicin sulfate	AB	800 mg	PHU	2 g	a	Physically compatible. Little linezolid loss in 7 days at 4 and 23°C in dark. Gentamicin losses of 5 to 7% in 7 days at 4°C and 8% in 5 days at 23°C	2332	C
Levofloxacin	OMN	5 g	PHU	2 g	a	Physically compatible. Little drug loss in 7 days at 4 and 23°C in dark	2334	C
Tobramycin sulfate	GNS	800 mg	PHU	2 g	a	Physically compatible. Little linezolid loss in 7 days at 4 and 23°C in dark. No tobramycin loss in 7 days at 4°C but losses of 4% in 1 day and 12% in 3 days at 23°C	2332	C
Trimethoprim–sulfamethoxazole	ES	800 mg[b]	PHU	2 g	a	A large amount of white needle-like crystals forms immediately	2333	I

[a] Admixed in the linezolid infusion container.

[b] Trimethoprim component. Trimethoprim in a 1:5 fixed-ratio concentration with sulfamethoxazole.

Y-Site Injection Compatibility (1:1 Mixture)

Linezolid

Test Drug	Mfr	Conc	Mfr	Conc	Remarks	Ref	C/I
Acyclovir sodium	APP	7 mg/mL[a]	PHU	2 mg/mL	Physically compatible for 4 hr at 23°C	2264	C
Alfentanil HCl	TAY	0.5 mg/mL	PHU	2 mg/mL	Physically compatible for 4 hr at 23°C	2264	C
Amikacin sulfate	AB	5 mg/mL[a]	PHU	2 mg/mL	Physically compatible for 4 hr at 23°C	2264	C
Aminophylline	AB	2.5 mg/mL[a]	PHU	2 mg/mL	Physically compatible for 4 hr at 23°C	2264	C

Y-Site Injection Compatibility (1:1 Mixture) (Cont.)

Test Drug	Mfr	Conc	Mfr	Conc	Remarks	Ref	C/I
Amphotericin B	AB	0.6 mg/mL[a]	PHU	2 mg/mL	Yellow precipitate forms within 5 min	2264	I
Amphotericin B			PHU, HOS	2 mg/mL	Stated to be physically incompatible	3183, 3184	I
Ampicillin sodium	APC	20 mg/mL[b]	PHU	2 mg/mL	Physically compatible for 4 hr at 23°C	2264	C
Ampicillin sodium–sulbactam sodium	PF	20 mg/mL[b d]	PHU	2 mg/mL	Physically compatible for 4 hr at 23°C	2264	C
Anidulafungin	VIC	0.5 mg/mL[a]	PH	2 mg/mL	Physically compatible for 4 hr at 23°C	2617	C
Aztreonam	SQ	40 mg/mL[a]	PHU	2 mg/mL	Physically compatible for 4 hr at 23°C	2264	C
Buprenorphine HCl	RKC	0.04 mg/mL[a]	PHU	2 mg/mL	Physically compatible for 4 hr at 23°C	2264	C
Butorphanol tartrate	APC	0.04 mg/mL[a]	PHU	2 mg/mL	Physically compatible for 4 hr at 23°C	2264	C
Calcium gluconate	AMR	40 mg/mL[a]	PHU	2 mg/mL	Physically compatible for 4 hr at 23°C	2264	C
Cangrelor tetrasodium	TMC	1 mg/mL[b]		2 mg/mL	Physically compatible for 4 hr	3243	C
Carboplatin	BR	5 mg/mL[a]	PHU	2 mg/mL	Physically compatible for 4 hr at 23°C	2264	C
Caspofungin acetate	ME	0.7 mg/mL[b]	PHU	2 mg/mL[b]	Physically compatible for 4 hr at room temperature	2758	C
Caspofungin acetate	ME	0.5 mg/mL[b]	PF	2 mg/mL	Physically compatible over 60 min	2766	C
Cefazolin sodium	SKB	20 mg/mL[a]	PHU	2 mg/mL	Physically compatible for 4 hr at 23°C	2264	C
Cefotetan disodium	ZEN	20 mg/mL[a]	PHU	2 mg/mL	Physically compatible for 4 hr at 23°C	2264	C
Cefoxitin sodium	ME	20 mg/mL[a]	PHU	2 mg/mL	Physically compatible for 4 hr at 23°C	2264	C
Ceftazidime	SKB	40 mg/mL[a]	PHU	2 mg/mL	Physically compatible for 4 hr at 23°C	2264	C
Ceftazidime–avibactam sodium	ALL	20 mg/mL[i k]			Physically compatible for up to 4 hr at room temperature	3004	C
Ceftolozane sulfate–tazobactam sodium	CUB	10 mg/mL[g h]	PF	2 mg/mL[a]	Physically compatible for 2 hr	3247, 3262	C
Ceftriaxone sodium	RC	20 mg/mL[a]	PHU	2 mg/mL	Physically compatible for 4 hr at 23°C	2264	C
Cefuroxime sodium	GL	30 mg/mL[a]	PHU	2 mg/mL	Physically compatible for 4 hr at 23°C	2264	C
Chlorpromazine HCl	ES	2 mg/mL[a]	PHU	2 mg/mL	Measured haze level increases immediately	2264	I
Chlorpromazine HCl			PHU, HOS	2 mg/mL	Stated to be physically incompatible	3183, 3184	I
Ciprofloxacin	BAY	1 mg/mL[a]	PHU	2 mg/mL	Physically compatible for 4 hr at 23°C	2264	C
Cisatracurium besylate	GW	2 mg/mL	PHU	2 mg/mL	Physically compatible for 4 hr at 23°C	2264	C
Cisplatin	BR	1 mg/mL	PHU	2 mg/mL	Physically compatible for 4 hr at 23°C	2264	C
Clindamycin phosphate	UP	10 mg/mL[a]	PHU	2 mg/mL	Physically compatible for 4 hr at 23°C	2264	C
Colistimethate sodium	MIL	1.5 mg/mL[b]	PF	2 mg/mL	Visually compatible for 1 hr at 26°C	3335	C
Cyclophosphamide	MJ	10 mg/mL[a]	PHU	2 mg/mL	Physically compatible for 4 hr at 23°C	2264	C
Cyclosporine	SZ	5 mg/mL[a]	PHU	2 mg/mL	Physically compatible for 4 hr at 23°C	2264	C
Cytarabine	BED	50 mg/mL	PHU	2 mg/mL	Physically compatible for 4 hr at 23°C	2264	C
Dexamethasone sodium phosphate	FUJ	1 mg/mL[a]	PHU	2 mg/mL	Physically compatible for 4 hr at 23°C	2264	C
Dexmedetomidine HCl	AB	4 mcg/mL[b]	PHU	2 mg/mL	Physically compatible for 4 hr at 23°C	2383	C

Y-Site Injection Compatibility (1:1 Mixture) (Cont.)

Test Drug	Mfr	Conc	Mfr	Conc	Remarks	Ref	C/I
Diazepam	AB	5 mg/mL	PHU	2 mg/mL	Turbid precipitate forms immediately	2264	I
Diazepam			PHU, HOS	2 mg/mL	Stated to be physically incompatible	3183, 3184	I
Digoxin	ES	0.25 mg/mL	PHU	2 mg/mL	Physically compatible for 4 hr at 23°C	2264	C
Diphenhydramine HCl	ES	2 mg/mL[a]	PHU	2 mg/mL	Physically compatible for 4 hr at 23°C	2264	C
Dobutamine HCl	AST	4 mg/mL[a]	PHU	2 mg/mL	Physically compatible for 4 hr at 23°C	2264	C
Dopamine HCl	AB	3.2 mg/mL[a]	PHU	2 mg/mL	Physically compatible for 4 hr at 23°C	2264	C
Doripenem	JJ	5 mg/mL[a b]	PHU	2 mg/mL	Physically compatible for 4 hr at 23°C	2743	C
Doxorubicin HCl	FUJ	2 mg/mL	PHU	2 mg/mL	Physically compatible for 4 hr at 23°C	2264	C
Doxycycline hyclate	FUJ	1 mg/mL[a]	PHU	2 mg/mL	Physically compatible for 4 hr at 23°C	2264	C
Droperidol	AMR	0.4 mg/mL[a]	PHU	2 mg/mL	Physically compatible for 4 hr at 23°C	2264	C
Enalaprilat	ME	0.1 mg/mL[a]	PHU	2 mg/mL	Physically compatible for 4 hr at 23°C	2264	C
Eravacycline dihydrochloride	TET	0.6 mg/mL[b]	PF	2 mg/mL[l]	Physically compatible for 2 hr at room temperature	3532	C
Erythromycin lactobionate			PHU, HOS	2 mg/mL	Stated to be physically incompatible	3183, 3184	I
Esmolol HCl	OHM	10 mg/mL	PHU	2 mg/mL	Physically compatible for 4 hr at 23°C	2264	C
Etoposide phosphate	BR	5 mg/mL[a]	PHU	2 mg/mL	Physically compatible for 4 hr at 23°C	2264	C
Famotidine	ME	2 mg/mL[a]	PHU	2 mg/mL	Physically compatible for 4 hr at 23°C	2264	C
Fenoldopam mesylate	AB	80 mcg/mL[b]	PHU	2 mg/mL	Physically compatible for 4 hr at 23°C	2467	C
Fentanyl citrate	AB	0.05 mg/mL	PHU	2 mg/mL	Physically compatible for 4 hr at 23°C	2264	C
Fluconazole	RR	2 mg/mL	PHU	2 mg/mL	Physically compatible for 4 hr at 23°C	2264	C
Fluorouracil	PH	16 mg/mL[a]	PHU	2 mg/mL	Physically compatible for 4 hr at 23°C	2264	C
Furosemide	AMR	3 mg/mL[a]	PHU	2 mg/mL	Physically compatible for 4 hr at 23°C	2264	C
Ganciclovir sodium	RC	20 mg/mL[a]	PHU	2 mg/mL	Physically compatible for 4 hr at 23°C	2264	C
Gemcitabine HCl	LI	10 mg/mL[a]	PHU	2 mg/mL	Physically compatible for 4 hr at 23°C	2264	C
Gentamicin sulfate	FUJ	5 mg/mL[a]	PHU	2 mg/mL	Physically compatible for 4 hr at 23°C	2264	C
Granisetron HCl	SKB	0.05 mg/mL[a]	PHU	2 mg/mL	Physically compatible for 4 hr at 23°C	2264	C
Haloperidol lactate	MN	0.2 mg/mL[a]	PHU	2 mg/mL	Physically compatible for 4 hr at 23°C	2264	C
Heparin sodium	ES	1000 units/mL[a]	PHU	2 mg/mL	Physically compatible for 4 hr at 23°C	2264	C
Hydrocortisone sodium succinate	UP	1 mg/mL[a]	PHU	2 mg/mL	Physically compatible for 4 hr at 23°C	2264	C
Hydromorphone HCl	AST	0.5 mg/mL[a]	PHU	2 mg/mL	Physically compatible for 4 hr at 23°C	2264	C
Hydroxyzine HCl	ES	2 mg/mL[a]	PHU	2 mg/mL	Physically compatible for 4 hr at 23°C	2264	C
Ifosfamide	MJ	25 mg/mL[a]	PHU	2 mg/mL	Physically compatible for 4 hr at 23°C	2264	C
Imipenem–cilastatin sodium	ME	10 mg/mL[b f]	PHU	2 mg/mL	Physically compatible for 4 hr at 23°C	2264	C
Isavuconazonium sulfate	ASP	1.5 mg/mL[g]	PF	2 mg/mL[a]	Physically compatible for 2 hr	3247, 3263	C
Labetalol HCl	GW	5 mg/mL	PHU	2 mg/mL	Physically compatible for 4 hr at 23°C	2264	C
Letermovir	ME				Physically incompatible	3398	I
Leucovorin calcium	GNS	2 mg/mL[a]	PHU	2 mg/mL	Physically compatible for 4 hr at 23°C	2264	C

Y-Site Injection Compatibility (1:1 Mixture) (Cont.)

Test Drug	Mfr	Conc	Mfr	Conc	Remarks	Ref	C/I
Levofloxacin	ORT	5 mg/mL[a]	PHU	2 mg/mL	Physically compatible for 4 hr at 23°C	2264	C
Lidocaine HCl	AB	10 mg/mL[a]	PHU	2 mg/mL	Physically compatible for 4 hr at 23°C	2264	C
Lorazepam	WY	0.1 mg/mL[a]	PHU	2 mg/mL	Physically compatible for 4 hr at 23°C	2264	C
Magnesium sulfate	AST	100 mg/mL[a]	PHU	2 mg/mL	Physically compatible for 4 hr at 23°C	2264	C
Mannitol	BA	15%	PHU	2 mg/mL	Physically compatible for 4 hr at 23°C	2264	C
Meperidine HCl	AST	4 mg/mL[a]	PHU	2 mg/mL	Physically compatible for 4 hr at 23°C	2264	C
Meropenem	ZEN	2.5 mg/mL[b]	PHU	2 mg/mL	Physically compatible for 4 hr at 23°C	2264	C
Meropenem		50 mg/mL	TE	2 mg/mL	Physically compatible for 4 hr at room temperature	3538	C
Meropenem–vaborbactam	TMC	8 mg/mL[b i]	PF	2 mg/mL[b]	Physically compatible for 3 hr at 20 to 25°C	3380	C
Mesna	MJ	10 mg/mL[a]	PHU	2 mg/mL	Physically compatible for 4 hr at 23°C	2264	C
Methotrexate sodium	IMM	15 mg/mL[a]	PHU	2 mg/mL	Physically compatible for 4 hr at 23°C	2264	C
Methylprednisolone sodium succinate	AB	5 mg/mL[a]	PHU	2 mg/mL	Physically compatible for 4 hr at 23°C	2264	C
Metoclopramide HCl	FAU	5 mg/mL	PHU	2 mg/mL	Physically compatible for 4 hr at 23°C	2264	C
Metronidazole	BA	5 mg/mL	PHU	2 mg/mL	Physically compatible for 4 hr at 23°C	2264	C
Midazolam HCl	RC	2 mg/mL[a]	PHU	2 mg/mL	Physically compatible for 4 hr at 23°C	2264	C
Mitoxantrone HCl	IMM	0.5 mg/mL[a]	PHU	2 mg/mL	Physically compatible for 4 hr at 23°C	2264	C
Morphine sulfate	AST	1 mg/mL[a]	PHU	2 mg/mL	Physically compatible for 4 hr at 23°C	2264	C
Nalbuphine HCl	AST	10 mg/mL	PHU	2 mg/mL	Physically compatible for 4 hr at 23°C	2264	C
Naloxone HCl	DU	0.4 mg/mL	PHU	2 mg/mL	Physically compatible for 4 hr at 23°C	2264	C
Nicardipine HCl	WAY	1 mg/mL[a]	PHU	2 mg/mL	Physically compatible for 4 hr at 23°C	2264	C
Nitroglycerin	FAU	0.4 mg/mL[a]	PHU	2 mg/mL	Physically compatible for 4 hr at 23°C	2264	C
Ondansetron HCl	GW	1 mg/mL[a]	PHU	2 mg/mL	Physically compatible for 4 hr at 23°C	2264	C
Paclitaxel	MJ	0.6 mg/mL[a]	PHU	2 mg/mL	Physically compatible for 4 hr at 23°C	2264	C
Pentamidine isethionate	FUJ	6 mg/mL[a]	PHU	2 mg/mL	Crystalline precipitate forms in 1 to 4 hr	2264	I
Pentamidine isethionate			PHU, HOS	2 mg/mL	Stated to be physically incompatible	3183, 3184	I
Pentobarbital sodium	AB	5 mg/mL[a]	PHU	2 mg/mL	Physically compatible for 4 hr at 23°C	2264	C
Phenobarbital sodium	WY	5 mg/mL[a]	PHU	2 mg/mL	Physically compatible for 4 hr at 23°C	2264	C
Phenytoin sodium	ES	50 mg/mL	PHU	2 mg/mL	Crystalline precipitate forms immediately	2264	I
Phenytoin sodium			PHU, HOS	2 mg/mL	Stated to be physically incompatible	3183, 3184	I
Piperacillin sodium–tazobactam sodium	LE[c]	40 mg/mL[a e]	PHU	2 mg/mL	Physically compatible for 4 hr at 23°C	2264	C
Plazomicin sulfate	ACH	24 mg/mL[g]	PF	2 mg/mL[g]	Physically compatible for 1 hr at 20 to 25°C	3432	C
Potassium chloride	FUJ	0.1 mEq/mL[a]	PHU	2 mg/mL	Physically compatible for 4 hr at 23°C	2264	C
Prochlorperazine edisylate	SO	0.5 mg/mL[a]	PHU	2 mg/mL	Physically compatible for 4 hr at 23°C	2264	C
Promethazine HCl	SCN	2 mg/mL[a]	PHU	2 mg/mL	Physically compatible for 4 hr at 23°C	2264	C
Propranolol HCl	WAY	1 mg/mL	PHU	2 mg/mL	Physically compatible for 4 hr at 23°C	2264	C

Y-Site Injection Compatibility (1:1 Mixture) (Cont.)

Test Drug	Mfr	Conc	Mfr	Conc	Remarks	Ref	C/I
Ranitidine HCl	GW	2 mg/mL[a]	PHU	2 mg/mL	Physically compatible for 4 hr at 23°C	2264	C
Remifentanil HCl	GW	0.5 mg/mL[a]	PHU	2 mg/mL	Physically compatible for 4 hr at 23°C	2264	C
Sodium bicarbonate	AB	1 mEq/mL	PHU	2 mg/mL	Physically compatible for 4 hr at 23°C	2264	C
Sufentanil citrate	ES	0.05 mg/mL	PHU	2 mg/mL	Physically compatible for 4 hr at 23°C	2264	C
Theophylline	BA	4 mg/mL[a]	PHU	2 mg/mL	Physically compatible for 4 hr at 23°C	2264	C
Tigecycline	WY	1 mg/mL[b]	PF	2 mg/mL	Physically compatible for 4 hr	2714	C
Tobramycin sulfate	AB	5 mg/mL[a]	PHU	2 mg/mL	Physically compatible for 4 hr at 23°C	2264	C
Trimethoprim–sulfamethoxazole			PHU, HOS	2 mg/mL	Stated to be physically incompatible	3183, 3184	I
Vancomycin HCl	FUJ	10 mg/mL[a]	PHU	2 mg/mL	Physically compatible for 4 hr at 23°C	2264	C
Vasopressin	APP	0.2 unit/mL[b]	PHU	2 mg/mL	Physically compatible	2641	C
Vecuronium bromide	OR	1 mg/mL	PHU	2 mg/mL	Physically compatible for 4 hr at 23°C	2264	C
Verapamil HCl	AB	2.5 mg/mL	PHU	2 mg/mL	Physically compatible for 4 hr at 23°C	2264	C
Vincristine sulfate	LI	0.05 mg/mL[a]	PHU	2 mg/mL	Physically compatible for 4 hr at 23°C	2264	C
Zidovudine	GW	4 mg/mL[a]	PHU	2 mg/mL	Physically compatible for 4 hr at 23°C	2264	C

[a] Tested in dextrose 5%.

[b] Tested in sodium chloride 0.9%.

[c] Test performed using the formulation WITHOUT edetate disodium.

[d] Ampicillin component. Ampicillin in a 2:1 fixed-ratio concentration with sulbactam.

[e] Piperacillin component. Piperacillin in an 8:1 fixed-ratio concentration with tazobactam.

[f] Not specified whether concentration refers to single component or combined components.

[g] Tested in both dextrose 5% and sodium chloride 0.9%.

[h] Ceftolozane component. Ceftolozane in a 2:1 fixed-ratio concentration with tazobactam.

[i] Meropenem component. Meropenem in a 1:1 fixed-ratio concentration with vaborbactam.

[j] Ceftazidime component. Ceftazidime in a 4:1 fixed-ratio concentration with avibactam.

[k] Tested in both dextrose 5% and Ringer's injection, lactated.

[l] Tested as the premixed infusion solution.

Additional Compatibility Information

Infusion Solutions

The manufacturers state that linezolid ready-to-use solutions for infusion are compatible with sodium chloride 0.9%, dextrose 5%, and Ringer's injection, lactated.[3183] [3184]

One study found little to no loss of linezolid in Hartmann's solution in 34 days at 25°C.[3514]

Peritoneal Dialysis Solutions

Linezolid 150, 300, and 600 mg/L in Dianeal PD-2 with 1.5 or 4.25% dextrose stored at 37, 25, and 4°C protected from light was physically compatible and exhibited no loss.[2500]

Lorazepam
AHFS 28:24.08

Products

Lorazepam is available in 2- and 4-mg/mL solutions in 1-mL single-use vials and 10-mL multidose vials.[3031] Both concentrations also are available in 1-mL disposable syringe cartridges.[3033] Each mL of lorazepam injection solution also contains 0.18 mL of polyethylene glycol 400 and 2% benzyl alcohol in propylene glycol.[3031] [3033]

For intramuscular use, lorazepam may be injected undiluted.[3031] [3033] For intravenous use, however, lorazepam *must* be diluted immediately prior to injection with an equal volume of a compatible diluent (e.g., sterile water for injection, dextrose 5%).[3031] [3033]

To dilute the dose in a syringe cartridge, all of the air should first be eliminated and the proper volume of a compatible diluent (e.g., sterile water for injection, dextrose 5%) should then be aspirated.[3033] The plunger should then be pulled back slightly to provide some mixing space and the syringe cartridge should be repeatedly and gently inverted to mix the contents.[3033] A similar procedure should be followed for diluting a dose withdrawn from a vial, taking care to repeatedly and gently invert the container until a homogenous solution results.[3031] To avoid air entrapment, neither the syringe cartridge nor the container should be shaken vigorously.[3031] [3033]

Trade Name(s)

Ativan

Administration

Lorazepam may be administered by deep intramuscular injection; alternatively, the drug may be administered by intravenous injection, when diluted immediately prior to use with an equal volume of a compatible diluent (e.g., sterile water for injection, dextrose 5%);[3031] [3033] the volume of the diluent to be added should not exceed the volume of the drug.[3033] Intravenous injection should be made slowly (i.e., at a rate not exceeding 2 mg/min), with frequent aspiration, directly into a vein or into the tubing of a running intravenous infusion.[3031] [3033]

Lorazepam also has been administered by continuous intravenous infusion.[3034]

Care should be taken to ensure that intra-arterial administration or perivascular extravasation do not occur.[3031] [3033]

Stability

Intact vials and syringe cartridges of lorazepam should be refrigerated and stored in the original carton to protect from light.[3031] [3033] One manufacturer had previously stated that the product could be stored for up to 2 weeks at room temperature[1181] and other manufacturers had acknowledged that both physical and chemical stability were acceptable for 60 to 90 days at room temperature;[1674] [2829] however, these recommendations for extended room temperature stability are no longer supported by manufacturers.[3032]

Lorazepam injection solution should be visually inspected for discoloration and particulate matter; if discolored or if a precipitate is present, the solution should not be used.[3031] [3033]

Precipitation

The choice of commercial lorazepam concentration to use in the preparation of dilutions is a critical factor in the physical stability of the dilutions.[2207] [2208] Both the 2- and 4-mg/mL concentrations utilize the same concentrations of solubilizing solvents.[1945] [1981] [2207] [3031] [3033] On admixture, the solvents that keep the aqueous insoluble lorazepam in solution are diluted twice as much using the 4-mg/mL concentration than if the 2-mg/mL were used, resulting in different precipitation potentials for the same concentration of lorazepam.[1945] [1981] [2207] Care should be taken to ensure that the compounding procedure that is to be used for lorazepam admixtures has been demonstrated to result in solutions in which the lorazepam remains soluble.

Lorazepam concentrations up to 0.08 mg/mL have been reported to be physically stable, while occasional precipitate formation in admixtures of lorazepam 0.1 to 0.2 mg/mL has been reported. The precipitate has been observed in both containers and in administration set tubing.[1943] [1979] [1980] In one case, a visible precipitate formed in a lorazepam 0.5-mg/mL admixture in sodium chloride 0.9% in a glass bottle.[1945] However, a 0.5-mg/mL concentration may remain in solution longer if prepared from the 2-mg/mL concentration, yielding a higher concentration of organic solvents in the final admixture.[1981] [2207] Concentrations of 1 and 2 mg/mL have been reported to be physically stable for up to 24 hours, as well as concentrations below 0.08 mg/mL.[1980] [2208] Concentrations in the middle range of 0.08 to 1 mg/mL may be problematic.[1980] In one report, use of lorazepam 2 mg/mL to prepare lorazepam 1-mg/mL admixtures in dextrose 5% or sodium chloride 0.9% was acceptable, but use of the lorazepam 4-mg/mL concentration to prepare the same solutions resulted in almost immediate precipitation.[2207]

Lorazepam solubility in common infusion solutions has been reported (Table 1). Solubility of lorazepam in sodium chloride 0.9% is approximately half that found in the other tested solutions. This result was attributed to the pH of the sodium chloride 0.9% solution (pH 6.3) being essentially the same as the isoelectric point of lorazepam (pH 6.4), where aqueous solubility would be the lowest. Dextrose 5% was the best diluent for lorazepam in this study.[787]

DOI: 10.37573/9781585286850.243

Table 1. Lorazepam equilibrium solubility[787]

Solution	Lorazepam Solubility (mg/mL)	Solution pH
Deionized water	0.054	7.09
Dextrose 5%	0.062	4.41
Ringer's injection, lactated	0.055	7.21
Sodium chloride 0.9%	0.027	6.30

Bacteriostatic Water

Dilution of lorazepam (Wyeth) to 1 mg/mL with bacteriostatic water for injection (bacteriostat unspecified), packaged in glass vials, resulted in lorazepam losses. Losses of about 10% at 4°C and 12% at 22°C occurred in 7 days. Drug precipitated in varying periods after the first week of storage.[1840]

Syringes

Lorazepam (Wyeth) 2 mg/mL was packaged as 3 mL in 10-mL polypropylene infusion pump syringes (Pharmacia Deltec). About 12 to 14% loss occurred in 3 days and 25% loss occurred in 10 days at 5 and 30°C. The authors recommended against storing lorazepam in the syringes for these time periods.[1967]

Lorazepam (Wyeth) 1 mg/mL, prepared from the 2-mg/mL commercial concentration and diluted in dextrose 5% or in sodium chloride 0.9%, was filled as 40 mL in 60-mL polypropylene syringes (Becton Dickinson). The filled syringes were stored at 22°C for 28 hours. Visual inspection found that the solutions remained physically stable, and less than 3% drug loss occurred in this time period.[2208]

The physical and chemical stability of lorazepam (Wyeth-Ayerst) 0.2, 0.5, and 1 mg/mL in dextrose 5% and in sodium chloride 0.9% was evaluated when packaged in polypropylene syringes. When prepared using lorazepam 2 mg/mL, the solutions were found to be physically stable over 24 hours and chemically stable for 48 hours at room temperature. When prepared using lorazepam 4 mg/mL, the solutions consistently precipitated.[2416]

Lorazepam (Pfizer) 4 mg/24 mL in sodium chloride 0.9% in a 30-mL polypropylene syringe (BD) was physically stable for 48 hours at room temperature.[3545]

Sorption

Lorazepam (Wyeth) 2- and 4-mg/mL concentrations were diluted 1:1 using dextrose 5%, sodium chloride 0.9%, and water for injection. A 2-mL sample of each dilution was injected into the Y-sites of administration sets from 5 different manufacturers through which dextrose 5%, sodium chloride 0.9%, Ringer's injection, or Ringer's injection, lactated was flowing at rates of 30 and 125 mL/hr. No differences were found among the various infusion sets, infusion solutions, or flow rates. All effluent solutions were visually acceptable and had no loss of lorazepam.[786]

In another study, lorazepam (Wyeth) 2 mg/50 mL in dextrose 5% was delivered at rates of 600, 200, and 100 mL/hr using an infusion controller fitted with 180 or 350 cm of polyvinyl chloride (PVC) tubing. Lorazepam loss due to sorption was greater with the longer tubing and at slower rates. Losses ranged from a high of 5% (350 cm, 100 mL/hr) to a low of 0.7% (180 cm, 600 mL/hr).[787]

In static sorption studies, lorazepam (Wyeth) 2 mg/50 mL in dextrose 5% was filled into PVC containers in the following amounts: 50 mL into 50-mL bags, 100 mL into 50-mL bags, and 100 mL into 250-mL bags. The bags were stored at 23°C. A rapid initial loss of lorazepam occurred (about 3.9 to 5.8% in the first hour) followed by a slower, approximately constant loss after 8 hours. Cumulative losses of 6 to 8% occurred in about 5 hours in the smaller bags with smaller bag surface area to volume ratios. The solution in the larger bags exhibited over a 10% loss in 2 hours.[787]

Plasticizer Leaching

Lorazepam (Wyeth-Ayerst) 0.1 mg/mL in dextrose 5% did not leach diethylhexyl phthalate (DEHP) plasticizer from 50-mL PVC bags in 24 hours at 24°C.[1683]

Compatibility Information

Solution Compatibility

Lorazepam

Test Soln Name	Mfr	Mfr	Conc/L or %	Remarks	Ref	C/I
Dextrose 5%	BAª	WY	0.1 g	Sorption losses of 11% in 8 hr and 27% in 24 hr at 37°C, 8% in 8 hr and 17% in 24 hr at 24°C, and 3% in 24 hr and 8% in 7 days at 4°C	1684	I
Dextrose 5%	MGᵇ	WY	0.1 g	3% loss in 24 hr and 9% in 72 hr at 37°C, little or no loss in 24 hr and 5% in 7 days at 24°C, and no loss in 7 days at 4 and –20°C	1684	C
Dextrose 5%	ABᶜ	WY	0.16, 0.24, 0.5 g	About 10 to 20% loss due to sorption throughout 24-hr delivery at 24°C under fluorescent light	1858	I
Dextrose 5%	BAª	WY	0.08 g	10 to 17% loss due to sorption in 4 hr at 4°C. 17% loss in 1 hr, increasing to over 30% in 24 hr at 21°C	1873	I
Dextrose 5%	BAª	WY	0.5 g	About 14% loss due to sorption in 4 hr at 21°C	1873	I

Solution Compatibility (Cont.)

Test Soln Name	Mfr	Mfr	Conc/L or %	Remarks	Ref	C/I
Dextrose 5%	BA[a]	WY	1 g	6% sorption loss in 6 hr with no further loss in 24 hr at 25°C	2203	C
Dextrose 5%	AB[e]	WY	1 g	Prepared with 4-mg/mL lorazepam. White precipitate forms in 8 hours at 22°C	2208	I
Dextrose 5%	AB[e]	WY	1 g	Prepared with 2-mg/mL lorazepam. Visually compatible with little loss in 28 hr at 22°C under fluorescent light	2208	C
Dextrose 5%	AB[e]	WY	2 g	Prepared with 4-mg/mL lorazepam. Visually compatible with little loss in 28 hr at 22°C under fluorescent light	2208	C
Dextrose 5%	HOS[f]	BA	200 mg	No loss in 24 hr	2660, 2792	C
Ringer's injection, lactated	BA[a]	WY	0.1 g	Sorption losses of 25% in 8 hr at 37°C, 14% in 8 hr at 24°C, and 5% in 24 hr and 9% in 72 hr at 4°C	1684	I
Ringer's injection, lactated	MG[b]	WY	0.1 g	2% loss in 24 hr and 7% in 72 hr at 37°C, little or no loss in 24 hr and 4% in 7 days at 24°C, and no loss in 7 days at 4°C	1684	C
Sodium chloride 0.9%	[d]		40 mg	Physically compatible with less than 3% loss in 24 hr at 21°C in the dark	1392	C
Sodium chloride 0.9%	BA[a]	WY	0.1 g	Sorption losses of 13% in 8 hr and 29% in 24 hr at 37°C, 8% in 8 hr and 17% in 24 hr at 24°C, and 3% in 24 hr and 8% in 7 days at 4°C	1684	I
Sodium chloride 0.9%	MG[b]	WY	0.1 g	2% loss in 24 hr and 7% in 72 hr at 37°C, little or no loss in 24 hr and 4% in 7 days at 24°C, and no loss in 7 days at 4°C	1684	C
Sodium chloride 0.9%	AB[c]	WY	0.16, 0.24, 0.5 g	About 10 to 20% loss due to sorption throughout 24-hr delivery at 24°C under fluorescent light	1858	I
Sodium chloride 0.9%	BA[a]	WY	0.08 g	8 to 10% sorption loss in 4 hr at 4°C. 17 to 23% loss in 1 hr, increasing to 25 to 30% loss in 4 hr at 21°C	1873	I
Sodium chloride 0.9%	BA[a]	WY	0.5 g	17% or more sorption loss in 4 hr at 21°C	1873	I
Sodium chloride 0.9%	BRN[b]	AB	1 g	No loss in 35 days at −20, 4, and 24°C	2525	C

[a] Tested in PVC containers.

[b] Tested in polyolefin containers.

[c] Tested in PVC and glass containers and delivered through PVC administration sets.

[d] Tested in PVC, glass, and polyethylene-lined laminated containers.

[e] Tested in glass containers.

[f] Tested in VISIV polyolefin containers.

Additive Compatibility

Lorazepam

Test Drug	Mfr	Conc/L or %	Mfr	Conc/L or %	Test Solution	Remarks	Ref	C/I
Dexamethasone sodium phosphate with diphenhydramine HCl and metoclopramide HCl	AMR ES DU	400 mg 2 g 4 g	WY	40 mg	NS[a]	Rapid lorazepam losses of 8, 10, and 15% at 3, 23, and 30°C, respectively, in 24 hr. Other drugs stable for 14 days at all three storage temperatures	1733	I
Diphenhydramine HCl with dexamethasone sodium phosphate and metoclopramide HCl	ES AMR DU	2 g 400 mg 4 g	WY	40 mg	NS[a]	Rapid lorazepam losses of 8, 10, and 15% at 3, 23, and 30°C, respectively, in 24 hr. Other drugs stable for 14 days at all three storage temperatures	1733	I
Levetiracetam	UCB				D5W, LR, NS[b]	Stable for 4 hr at 15 to 30°C	2833	C

Additive Compatibility (Cont.)

Test Drug	Mfr	Conc/L or %	Mfr	Conc/L or %	Test Solution	Remarks	Ref	C/I
Metoclopramide HCl with dexamethasone sodium phosphate and diphenhydramine HCl	DU AMR ES	4 g 400 mg 2 g	WY	40 mg	NS[a]	Rapid lorazepam losses of 8, 10, and 15% at 3, 23, and 30°C, respectively, in 24 hr. Other drugs stable for 14 days at all three storage temperatures	1733	I

[a] Tested in Pharmacia-Deltec PVC pump reservoirs.

[b] Tested in PVC containers.

Drugs in Syringe Compatibility

Lorazepam

Test Drug	Mfr	Amt	Mfr	Amt	Remarks	Ref	C/I
Aripiprazole	BMS	6.75 mg/0.9 mL	HOS	0.2 mg/0.1 mL	Visually compatible for 30 min	2719	C
Aripiprazole	BMS	5.25 mg/0.7 mL	HOS	0.6 mg/0.3 mL	Visually compatible for 30 min	2719	C
Aripiprazole	BMS	3.75 mg/0.5 mL	HOS	1 mg/0.5 mL	Visually compatible for 30 min	2719	C
Aripiprazole	BMS	2.25 mg/0.3 mL	HOS	1.4 mg/0.7 mL	Visually compatible for 30 min	2719	C
Aripiprazole	BMS	0.75 mg/0.1 mL	HOS	1.8 mg/0.9 mL	Visually compatible for 30 min	2719	C
Buprenorphine HCl					Incompatible	4	I
Caffeine citrate		20 mg/1 mL	SW	2 mg/1 mL	Haze forms immediately becoming two layers over time	2440	I
Dimenhydrinate		10 mg/1 mL		4 mg/1 mL	Clear solution	2569	C
Haloperidol lactate	MN	5 mg/1 mL	WY	2 mg/1 mL	Physically compatible and chemically stable for 16 hr at room temperature	1838	C
Haloperidol lactate	MN	5 mg/1 mL	WY	4 mg/1 mL	Visually compatible with no loss of either drug in 24 hr at 4 and 25°C	260	C
Haloperidol lactate	MN	5 mg/1 mL	WY	2 mg/1 mL	Visually compatible for 4 hr at room temperature	260	C
Hydromorphone HCl	KN	2, 10, 40 mg/1 mL	WY	4 mg/1 mL	Visually compatible. 10% lorazepam loss in 6 days at 4°C, 4 days at 23°C, and 24 hr at 37°C. Little hydromorphone loss in 7 days at all temperatures	1776	C
Pantoprazole sodium	[a]	4 mg/1 mL		4 mg/1 mL	Precipitates	2574	I
Ranitidine HCl	GL	50 mg/2 mL	WY	4 mg/1 mL	Poor mixing and layering, which disappears following vortex mixing	978	?

[a] Test performed using the formulation WITHOUT edetate disodium.

Y-Site Injection Compatibility (1:1 Mixture)

Lorazepam

Test Drug	Mfr	Conc	Mfr	Conc	Remarks	Ref	C/I
Acetaminophen	CAD	10 mg/mL	HOS	0.5 mg/mL[b]	Physically compatible with less than 10% acetaminophen loss over 4 hr at room temperature	2841, 2844	C
Acyclovir sodium	BW	5 mg/mL[a]	WY	0.04 mg/mL[a]	Physically compatible for 4 hr at 25°C	1157	C
Albumin human		200 mg/mL	WY	0.33 mg/mL[b]	Visually compatible for 24 hr at 22°C	1855	C

Y-Site Injection Compatibility (1:1 Mixture) (Cont.)

Test Drug	Mfr	Conc	Mfr	Conc	Remarks	Ref	C/I
Aldesleukin	CHI	33,800 I.U./mL[a]	WY	2 mg/mL	Globules form immediately	1857	I
Allopurinol sodium	BW	3 mg/mL[b]	WY	0.1 mg/mL[b]	Physically compatible for 4 hr at 22°C	1686	C
Amifostine	USB	10 mg/mL[a]	WY	0.1 mg/mL[a]	Physically compatible for 4 hr at 23°C	1845	C
Amikacin sulfate	BMS	5 mg/mL	WY	0.33 mg/mL[b]	Visually compatible for 24 hr at 22°C	1855	C
Amiodarone HCl	WY	6 mg/mL[a]	WY	1 mg/mL[a]	Visually compatible for 24 hr at 22°C	2352	C
Amoxicillin sodium	SKB	50 mg/mL	WY	0.33 mg/mL[b]	Visually compatible for 24 hr at 22°C	1855	C
Amoxicillin sodium–clavulanate potassium	SKB	20 mg/mL[i]	WY	0.33 mg/mL[b]	Visually compatible for 24 hr at 22°C	1855	C
Amsacrine	NCI	1 mg/mL[a]	WY	0.1 mg/mL[a]	Visually compatible for 4 hr at 22°C	1381	C
Anakinra	SYN	4 and 36 mg/mL[b]	WY	0.1 mg/mL[b]	Physically compatible with no loss of either drug in 4 hr at 22°C	2512	C
Atracurium besylate	BW	0.5 mg/mL[a]	WY	0.5 mg/mL[a]	Physically compatible for 24 hr at 28°C	1337	C
Aztreonam	SQ	40 mg/mL[a]	WY	0.1 mg/mL[a]	Haze forms within 1 hr	1758	I
Bivalirudin	TMC	5 mg/mL[a]	ESL[a]	0.5 mg/mL	Physically compatible for 4 hr at 23°C	2373	C
Bumetanide	LEO	0.5 mg/mL	WY	0.33 mg/mL[b]	Visually compatible for 24 hr at 22°C	1855	C
Cangrelor tetrasodium	TMC	1 mg/mL[b]		0.5 mg/mL[b]	Physically compatible for 4 hr	3243	C
Caspofungin acetate	ME	0.7 mg/mL[b]	HOS	0.5 mg/mL[b]	Physically compatible for 4 hr at room temperature	2758	C
Cefotaxime sodium	RS	10 mg/mL	WY	0.33 mg/mL[b]	Visually compatible for 24 hr at 22°C	1855	C
Ceftaroline fosamil	FOR	2.22 mg/mL[a b e]	HOS	0.5 mg/mL[a b e]	Physically compatible for 4 hr at 23°C	2826	C
Ceftolozane sulfate–tazobactam sodium	CUB	30 mg/mL[a m]		2 mg/mL	Physically compatible with no loss of either drug in 4 hr at 25°C	2959	C
Ceftolozane sulfate–tazobactam sodium	CUB	30 mg/mL[b m]		2 mg/mL	Physically compatible with no loss of either drug in 24 hr at 25°C	2959	C
Ceftolozane sulfate–tazobactam sodium	CUB	10 mg/mL[m n]	WW	1 mg/mL[n]	Physically compatible for 2 hr	3262	C
Ciprofloxacin	BAY	2 mg/mL	WY	0.33 mg/mL[b]	Visually compatible for 24 hr at 22°C	1855	C
Cisatracurium besylate	GW	0.1, 2, 5 mg/mL[a]	WY	0.5 mg/mL[a]	Physically compatible for 4 hr at 23°C	2074	C
Cladribine	ORT	0.015[b] and 0.5[d] mg/mL	WY	0.1 mg/mL[b]	Physically compatible for 4 hr at 23°C	1969	C
Clonidine HCl	BI	0.015 mg/mL	WY	0.33 mg/mL[b]	Visually compatible for 24 hr at 22°C	1855	C
Cloxacillin sodium	SMX	100 mg/mL	SZ	4 mg/mL	Large particles form within 4 hr	3245	I
Dexamethasone sodium phosphate		4 mg/mL	WY	0.33 mg/mL[b]	Visually compatible for 24 hr at 22°C	1855	C
Dexmedetomidine HCl	AB	4 mcg/mL[b]	ESL	0.5 mg/mL[b]	Physically compatible for 4 hr at 23°C	2383	C
Diltiazem HCl	MMD	5 mg/mL	WY	4 mg/mL	Visually compatible	1807	C
Diltiazem HCl	MMD	1 mg/mL[b]	WY	2 mg/mL[b]	Visually compatible	1807	C
Diltiazem HCl	MMD	1 mg/mL[a]	WY	0.5 mg/mL[a]	Visually compatible for 4 hr at 27°C	2062	C
Dobutamine HCl	LI	4 mg/mL[a]	WY	0.5 mg/mL[a]	Visually compatible for 4 hr at 27°C	2062	C
Docetaxel	RPR	0.9 mg/mL[a]	WY	0.5 mg/mL[a]	Physically compatible for 4 hr at 23°C	2224	C
Dopamine HCl	AB	3.2 mg/mL[a]	WY	0.5 mg/mL[a]	Visually compatible for 4 hr at 27°C	2062	C

Y-Site Injection Compatibility (1:1 Mixture) (Cont.)

Test Drug	Mfr	Conc	Mfr	Conc	Remarks	Ref	C/I
Doripenem	JJ	5 mg/mL[a b]	BED	0.5 mg/mL[a b]	Physically compatible for 4 hr at 23°C	2743	C
Doxorubicin HCl liposomal	SEQ	0.4 mg/mL[a]	WY	0.1 mg/mL[a]	Physically compatible for 4 hr at 23°C	2087	C
Epinephrine HCl	AB	0.02 mg/mL[a]	WY	0.5 mg/mL[a]	Visually compatible for 4 hr at 27°C	2062	C
Erythromycin lactobionate	AB	5 mg/mL	WY	0.33 mg/mL[b]	Visually compatible for 24 hr at 22°C	1855	C
Etomidate	AB	2 mg/mL	WY	2 mg/mL	Visually compatible for 7 days at 25°C	1801	C
Etoposide phosphate	BR	5 mg/mL[a]	WY	0.5 mg/mL[a]	Physically compatible for 4 hr at 23°C	2218	C
Famotidine	ME	2 mg/mL[b]		0.1 mg/mL[a]	Visually compatible for 4 hr at 22°C	1936	C
Fenoldopam mesylate	AB	80 mcg/mL[b]	ES	0.5 mg/mL[b]	Physically compatible for 4 hr at 23°C	2467	C
Fentanyl citrate		0.05 mg/mL	WY	0.33 mg/mL[b]	Visually compatible for 24 hr at 22°C	1855	C
Fentanyl citrate	ES	0.05 mg/mL	WY	0.5 mg/mL[a]	Visually compatible for 4 hr at 27°C	2062	C
Fentanyl citrate	JN	0.025 mg/mL[a]	WY	0.1 mg/mL[a]	Physically compatible for 48 hr at 22°C	1706	C
Filgrastim	AMG	30 mcg/mL[a]	WY	0.1 mg/mL[a]	Physically compatible for 4 hr at 22°C	1687	C
Floxacillin sodium	SKB	50 mg/mL	WY	0.33 mg/mL[b]	White opalescence forms in 4 hr	1855	I
Fluconazole	PF	2 mg/mL	WY	0.33 mg/mL[b]	Visually compatible for 24 hr at 22°C	1855	C
Fludarabine phosphate	BX	1 mg/mL[a]	WY	0.1 mg/mL[a]	Visually compatible for 4 hr at 22°C	1439	C
Foscarnet sodium	AST	24 mg/mL	WY	4 mg/mL	Gas production	1335	I
Foscarnet sodium	AST	24 mg/mL	WY	0.08 mg/mL[a]	Physically compatible for 24 hr at 25°C under fluorescent light	1393	C
Fosphenytoin sodium	PD	1 mg PE/mL[b h]	WY	2 mg/mL	Samples remained clear with no loss of either drug in 8 hr	2223	C
Furosemide	CNF	10 mg/mL	WY	0.33 mg/mL[b]	Visually compatible for 24 hr at 22°C	1855	C
Furosemide	AMR	10 mg/mL	WY	0.5 mg/mL[a]	Visually compatible for 4 hr at 27°C	2062	C
Gallium nitrate	FUJ	1 mg/mL[b]	WY	1 mg/mL[b]	White haze and precipitate form immediately but clear in 30 min	1673	I
Gemcitabine HCl	LI	10 mg/mL[b]	WY	0.5 mg/mL[a]	Physically compatible for 4 hr at 23°C	2226	C
Gentamicin sulfate	CNF	3 mg/mL	WY	0.33 mg/mL[b]	Visually compatible for 24 hr at 22°C	1855	C
Granisetron HCl	SKB	1 mg/mL	WY	0.1 mg/mL[b]	Physically compatible with little or no loss of either drug in 4 hr at 22°C	1883	C
Granisetron HCl	SKB	0.05 mg/mL[a]	WY	0.1 mg/mL[a]	Physically compatible for 4 hr at 23°C	2000	C
Haloperidol lactate	JN	0.5 and 5 mg/mL	WY	0.33 mg/mL[b]	Visually compatible for 24 hr at 22°C	1855	C
Heparin sodium		417 units/mL	WY	0.33 mg/mL[b]	Visually compatible for 24 hr at 22°C	1855	C
Heparin sodium	ES	100 units/mL[a]	WY	0.5 mg/mL[a]	Visually compatible for 4 hr at 27°C	2062	C
Hetastarch in lactated electrolyte	AB	6%	OHM	0.5 mg/mL[a]	Physically compatible for 4 hr at 23°C	2339	C
Hydrocortisone sodium succinate	UP	50 mg/mL	WY	0.33 mg/mL[b]	Visually compatible for 24 hr at 22°C	1855	C
Hydromorphone HCl	KN	1 mg/mL	WY	0.5 mg/mL[a]	Visually compatible for 4 hr at 27°C	2062	C
Hydromorphone HCl	AST	0.5 mg/mL[a]	WY	0.1 mg/mL[a]	Physically compatible for 48 hr at 22°C	1706	C
Idarubicin HCl	AD	1 mg/mL[b]	WY	2 mg/mL	Color changes immediately	1525	I

Y-Site Injection Compatibility (1:1 Mixture) (Cont.)

Test Drug	Mfr	Conc	Mfr	Conc	Remarks	Ref	C/I
Imipenem–cilastatin sodium	MSD	5 mg/mL[l]	WY	0.33 mg/mL[b]	Yellow precipitate forms in 24 hr	1855	I
Isavuconazonium sulfate	ASP	1.5 mg/mL[n]	WW	1 mg/mL[n]	Physically compatible for 2 hr	3263	C
Labetalol HCl	AH	2 mg/mL[a]	WY	0.5 mg/mL[a]	Visually compatible for 4 hr at 27°C	2062	C
Letermovir	ME				Physically incompatible	3398	I
Levofloxacin	OMN	5 mg/mL[a]		2 mg/mL	Visually compatible for 4 hr at 24°C	2233	C
Linezolid	PHU	2 mg/mL	WY	0.1 mg/mL[a]	Physically compatible for 4 hr at 23°C	2264	C
Melphalan HCl	BW	0.1 mg/mL[b]	WY	0.1 mg/mL[b]	Physically compatible for 3 hr at 22°C	1557	C
Meropenem		50 mg/mL	HOS	4 mg/mL	Temperature increased upon mixing	3538	I
Meropenem–vaborbactam	TMC	8 mg/mL[b o]	WW	1 mg/mL[b]	Physically compatible for 3 hr at 20 to 25°C	3380	C
Methadone HCl	LI	1 mg/mL[a]	WY	0.1 mg/mL[a]	Physically compatible for 48 hr at 22°C	1706	C
Metronidazole	BRN	5 mg/mL	WY	0.33 mg/mL[b]	Visually compatible for 24 hr at 22°C	1855	C
Micafungin sodium	ASP	1.5 mg/mL[b]	AB	0.5 mg/mL[b]	Physically compatible for 4 hr at 23°C	2683	C
Midazolam HCl	RC	2 mg/mL[a]	WY	0.5 mg/mL[a]	Visually compatible for 4 hr at 27°C	2062	C
Milrinone lactate	SW	0.2 mg/mL[a]	WY	0.5 mg/mL[a]	Visually compatible for 4 hr at 27°C	2062	C
Milrinone lactate	SW	0.4 mg/mL[a]	WY	0.2 mg/mL[a]	Visually compatible. Little loss of either drug in 4 hr at 23°C	2214	C
Milrinone lactate	SS	0.2 mg/mL[a]	WY	1 mg/mL[a]	Visually compatible for 4 hr at 25°C	2381	C
Milrinone lactate	SS	0.2 mg/mL[a]	WY	2 mg/mL[a]	Visually compatible for 4 hr at 25°C	2381	C
Morphine sulfate	SCN	2 mg/mL[a]	WY	0.5 mg/mL[a]	Visually compatible for 4 hr at 27°C	2062	C
Morphine sulfate	AST	1 mg/mL[a]	WY	0.1 mg/mL[a]	Physically compatible for 48 hr at 22°C	1706	C
Nicardipine HCl	WY	1 mg/mL[a]	WY	0.5 mg/mL[a]	Visually compatible for 4 hr at 27°C	2062	C
Nitroglycerin	AB	0.4 mg/mL[a]	WY	0.5 mg/mL[a]	Visually compatible for 4 hr at 27°C	2062	C
Norepinephrine bitartrate	AB	0.128 mg/mL[a]	WY	0.5 mg/mL[a]	Visually compatible for 4 hr at 27°C	2062	C
Omeprazole sodium	AST	4 mg/mL	WY	0.33 mg/mL[b]	Yellow discoloration forms	1855	I
Ondansetron HCl	GL	1 mg/mL[b]	WY	0.1 mg/mL[a]	Light haze develops immediately	1365	I
Oritavancin diphosphate	TAR	0.8, 1.2, and 2 mg/mL[a]	HOS	1 mg/mL[a]	Visually compatible for 4 hr at 20 to 24°C	2928	C
Oxaliplatin	SS	0.5 mg/mL[a]	ESL	0.5 mg/mL[a]	Physically compatible for 4 hr at 23°C	2566	C
Paclitaxel	NCI	1.2 mg/mL[a]		0.1 mg/mL[a]	Physically compatible for 4 hr at 22°C	1528	C
Palonosetron HCl	MGI	50 mcg/mL	BA	0.5 mg/mL[a]	Physically compatible. No loss of either drug in 4 hr	2608	C
Pancuronium bromide	ES	0.05 mg/mL[a]	WY	0.5 mg/mL[a]	Physically compatible for 24 hr at 28°C	1337	C
Pemetrexed disodium	LI	20 mg/mL[b]	ES	0.5 mg/mL[a]	Physically compatible for 4 hr at 23°C	2564	C
Piperacillin sodium–tazobactam sodium	LE[c]	40 mg/mL[a j]	WY	0.1 mg/mL[a]	Physically compatible for 4 hr at 22°C	1688	C
Plazomicin sulfate	ACH	24 mg/mL[n]	WW	1 mg/mL[n]	Physically compatible for 1 hr at 20 to 25°C	3432	C
Posaconazole	ME	18 mg/mL		1 mg/mL[n]	Physically compatible	2911, 2912	C

Y-Site Injection Compatibility (1:1 Mixture) (Cont.)

Test Drug	Mfr	Conc	Mfr	Conc	Remarks	Ref	C/I
Potassium chloride	BRN	1 mEq/mL	WY	0.33 mg/mL[b]	Visually compatible for 24 hr at 22°C	1855	C
Propofol	ZEN[p]	10 mg/mL	WY	0.1 mg/mL[a]	Physically compatible for 1 hr at 23°C	2066	C
Ranitidine HCl	GL	0.5 mg/mL	WY	0.33 mg/mL[b]	Visually compatible for 24 hr at 22°C	1855	C
Ranitidine HCl	GL	1 mg/mL[a]	WY	0.5 mg/mL[a]	Visually compatible for 4 hr at 27°C	2062	C
Remifentanil HCl	GW	0.025 and 0.25 mg/mL[b]	WY	0.5 mg/mL[a]	Physically compatible for 4 hr at 23°C	2075	C
Sargramostim	IMM	10 mcg/mL[b]	WY	0.1 mg/mL[b]	Slightly bluish haze forms in 1 hr	1436	I
Tacrolimus	FUJ	1 mg/mL[b]	WY	1 mg/mL[a]	Visually compatible for 24 hr at 25°C	1630	C
Tedizolid phosphate	CUB	0.8 mg/mL[b]	WW	1 mg/mL[b]	Physically compatible for 2 hr	3244	C
Teniposide	BR	0.1 mg/mL[a]	WY	0.1 mg/mL[a]	Physically compatible for 4 hr at 23°C	1725	C
Thiotepa	IMM[f]	1 mg/mL[a]	WY	0.1 mg/mL[a]	Physically compatible for 4 hr at 23°C	1861	C
TNA #218 to #226[g]			WY	0.1 mg/mL[a]	Damage to emulsion occurs in 1 hr	2215	I
TPN #212 to #215[g]			WY	0.1 mg/mL[a]	Physically compatible for 4 hr at 23°C	2109	C
Trimethoprim–sulfamethoxazole	RC	0.8 mg/mL[k]	WY	0.33 mg/mL[b]	Visually compatible for 24 hr at 22°C	1855	C
Vancomycin HCl	LI	5 mg/mL	WY	0.33 mg/mL[b]	Visually compatible for 24 hr at 22°C	1855	C
Vecuronium bromide	OR	0.1 mg/mL[a]	WY	0.5 mg/mL[a]	Physically compatible for 24 hr at 28°C	1337	C
Vecuronium bromide	OR	4 mg/mL	WY	0.33 mg/mL[b]	Visually compatible for 24 hr at 22°C	1855	C
Vecuronium bromide	OR	1 mg/mL	WY	0.5 mg/mL[a]	Visually compatible for 4 hr at 27°C	2062	C
Vinorelbine tartrate	BW	1 mg/mL[b]	WY	0.1 mg/mL[b]	Physically compatible for 4 hr at 22°C	1558	C
Zidovudine	BW	4 mg/mL[a]	WY	80 mcg/mL[a]	Physically compatible for 4 hr at 25°C	1193	C

[a] Tested in dextrose 5%.

[b] Tested in sodium chloride 0.9%.

[c] Test performed using the formulation WITHOUT edetate disodium.

[d] Tested in bacteriostatic sodium chloride 0.9% preserved with benzyl alcohol 0.9%.

[e] Tested in Ringer's injection, lactated.

[f] Lyophilized formulation tested.

[g] Refer to Appendix for the composition of parenteral nutrition solutions. TNA indicates a 3-in-1 admixture, and TPN indicates a 2-in-1 admixture.

[h] Concentration expressed in milligrams of phenytoin sodium equivalents (PE) per mL.

[i] Amoxicillin component. Amoxicillin in a 10:1 fixed-ratio concentration with clavulanic acid.

[j] Piperacillin component. Piperacillin in an 8:1 fixed-ratio concentration with tazobactam.

[k] Trimethoprim component. Trimethoprim in a 1:5 fixed-ratio concentration with sulfamethoxazole.

[l] Not specified whether concentration refers to single component or combined components.

[m] Ceftolozane component. Ceftolozane in a 2:1 fixed-ratio concentration with tazobactam.

[n] Tested in both dextrose 5% and sodium chloride 0.9%.

[o] Meropenem component. Meropenem in a 1:1 fixed-ratio concentration with vaborbactam.

[p] Test performed using the formulation WITH edetate disodium.

Selected Revisions July 1, 2020. © Copyright, October 1984.
American Society of Health-System Pharmacists, Inc.

Magnesium Sulfate
AHFS 28:12.92

Products

Magnesium sulfate is available in concentrations of 50, 8, 4, 2, and 1% in a variety of container sizes.[4] The 50% solution provides 500 mg/mL of magnesium sulfate (magnesium 4.06 mEq/mL). The pH of these concentrations may have been adjusted with sodium hydroxide and/or sulfuric acid.[1(7/07)] [4]

Magnesium sulfate is available as 4% (40 mg/mL; 0.325 mEq/mL) and 8% (80 mg/mL; 0.65 mEq/mL) solutions in water for injection. Magnesium sulfate in dextrose 5% is available as 1% (10 mg/mL; 0.081 mEq/mL) and 2% (20 mg/mL; 0.162 mEq/mL).[1(7/07)]

pH

Magnesium sulfate injection has a pH adjusted to 5.5 to 7.[1(7/07)] The premixed infusion solutions have pH values in the range of 3.5 to 6.5.[17]

Osmolarity

The 50% solution has a calculated osmolarity of 4060 mOsm/L.[1(7/07)]

Magnesium sulfate 4 and 8% solutions in water for injection have osmolarities of 325 and 649 mOsm/L, respectively. Magnesium sulfate 1 and 2% solutions in dextrose 5% have osmolarities of 333 and 415 mOsm/L.[1(7/07)]

Administration

Magnesium sulfate may be administered by intramuscular or direct intravenous injection and by continuous or intermittent intravenous infusion. For intravenous injection, a concentration of 20% or less should be used; the rate of injection should not exceed 1.5 mL of a 10% solution (or equivalent) per minute. For intramuscular injection, a 25 or 50% concentration is satisfactory for adults, but dilute to 20% for infants and children.[1(7/07)] [4]

Stability

Magnesium sulfate 50% injection and magnesium sulfate 4 and 8% in water for injection or 1 and 2% in dextrose 5% should be stored at controlled room temperature and protected from freezing.[1(7/07)] [4] Refrigeration of intact ampuls may result in precipitation or crystallization.[593]

Compatibility Information

Solution Compatibility

Magnesium sulfate

Test Soln Name	Mfr	Mfr	Conc/L or %	Remarks	Ref	C/I
Dextrose 5%	MG	AB	40 g	Physically compatible. Stable for 60 days at 0°C	922	C
Ringer's injection, lactated	BA[a][b]	AMR	37 g	Visually compatible. No change in composition in 3 months stored at room temperature	2184	C
Sodium chloride 0.9%	BA[a][b]	AMR	37 g	Visually compatible. No change in composition in 3 months stored at room temperature	2184	C

[a] Tested in glass containers.

[b] Tested in PVC containers.

Additive Compatibility

Magnesium sulfate

Test Drug	Mfr	Conc/L or %	Mfr	Conc/L or %	Test Solution	Remarks	Ref	C/I
Amphotericin B	SQ	40 and 80 mg	IMS	2 and 4 g	D5W	Physically incompatible in 3 hr at 24°C with decreased clarity and development of supernatant	1578	I
Calcium chloride	DB	4 to 20 g	DB	10 to 50 g	D5W, NS	Visible precipitate or microprecipitate forms at room temperature	2597	I
Calcium chloride	DB	2 g	DB	4 g	D5W, NS	No visible precipitate. Microscopic examination was inconclusive	2597	?

DOI: 10.37573/9781585286850.244

Additive Compatibility (Cont.)

Test Drug	Mfr	Conc/L or %	Mfr	Conc/L or %	Test Solution	Remarks	Ref	C/I
Calcium chloride	DB	2 g	DB	2.5 g	TPN #266[c]	No visible precipitate or microprecipitate in 24 hr at room temperature	2597	C
Calcium gluconate	DB	12 to 60 g	DB	10 to 50 g	D5W, NS	Visible precipitate or microprecipitate forms at room temperature	2597	I
Calcium gluconate	DB	6 g	DB	5 g	D5W, NS	No visible precipitate or microprecipitate in 24 hr at room temperature	2597	C
Calcium gluconate	PP	4 g	SZ	4 g	D5W, NS	Physically compatible for 7 days at 5 and 25°C protected from light	2909	C
Calcium gluconate	PP	10 g	SZ	10 g	D5W, NS	Physically compatible for 7 days at 5 and 25°C protected from light	2909	C
Chloramphenicol sodium succinate	PD	10 g	LI	16 mEq	D5W	Physically compatible	15	C
Cisplatin	BR	50 and 200 mg		1 and 2 g	D5½S[a]	Compatible for 48 hr at 25°C and 96 hr at 4°C followed by 48 hr at 25°C	1088	C
Cyclosporine	SZ	2 g	LY	30 g	D5W	Transient turbidity upon preparation. 5% cyclosporine loss in 6 hr and 10% loss in 12 hr at 24°C under fluorescent light	1629	I
Dobutamine HCl	LI	167 mg	ES	83 g	NS	Haze forms between 20 and 24 hr	552	I
Dobutamine HCl	LI	1 g	TO	2 g	D5W, NS	Slightly pink in 24 hr at 25°C	789	I
Heparin sodium		50,000 units		130 mEq	NS[b]	Visually compatible with heparin activity retained for 14 days at 24°C under fluorescent light	1908	C
Hydrocortisone sodium succinate	UP	100 mg	ES	750 mg	AA 3.5%, D 25%	Physically compatible	302	C
Isoproterenol HCl	WI	4 mg		1 g		Physically compatible	59	C
Meropenem	ZEN	1 and 20 g	AST	1 g	NS	Visually compatible for 4 hr at room temperature	1994	C
Methyldopa HCl	MSD	1 g		1 g	D5W, D10W, D2.5½S, D2.5S, D5¼S, D5½S, D5S, D10S, NS, ½S	Physically compatible	23	C
Norepinephrine bitartrate	WI	8 mg		1 g	D5W, D10W, D2.5½S, D2.5S, D5¼S, D5½S, D5S, D10S, NS, ½S	Physically compatible	77	C
Penicillin G potassium	PF	500 mg		1 g	W	5% penicillin loss in 1 day and 13% in 2 days at 24°C	999	C
Penicillin G potassium	PF	500 mg		2 to 8 g	W	7 to 8% penicillin loss in 1 day and 20 to 25% in 2 days at 24°C	999	C
Polymyxin B sulfate	BW	200 mg	LI	16 mEq	D5W	Physically incompatible	15	I
Potassium acetate		25 mmol		10 mmol	TPN	Transient precipitate forms	2266	?
Potassium chloride	BRN	80 mEq	DB	3.9 g	D5W, NS	Visually compatible. Under 5% loss of ions in 24 hr at 22°C	2360	C
Sodium bicarbonate	AB	80 mEq	LI	16 mEq	D5W	Physically incompatible	15	I

Additive Compatibility (Cont.)

Test Drug	Mfr	Conc/L or %	Mfr	Conc/L or %	Test Solution	Remarks	Ref	C/I
Sodium bicarbonate	BA	50 mEq	HOS	1.5 and 15 mEq	d	Physically compatible. No loss of ions for 48 hr at 23°C	2814	C
Verapamil HCl	KN	80 mg	IX	10 g	D5W, NS	Physically compatible for 24 hr	764	C

[a] Tested in PVC containers.

[b] Tested in glass containers.

[c] Refer to Appendix for the composition of parenteral nutrition solutions. TPN indicates a 2-in-1 admixture.

[d] Tested in an extemporaneously-compounded hemofiltration solution.

Drugs in Syringe Compatibility

Magnesium sulfate

Test Drug	Mfr	Amt	Mfr	Amt	Remarks	Ref	C/I
Dimenhydrinate		10 mg/1 mL		500 mg/1 mL	Clear solution	2569	C
Hydrocortisone sodium succinate	UP	100 mg/2 mL	ES	500 mg/mL	White precipitate formed	302	I
Metoclopramide HCl	RB	10 mg/2 mL	ES	500 mg/1 mL	Physically compatible for 48 hr at 25°C	1167	C
Metoclopramide HCl	RB	10 mg/2 mL	ES	1 g/2 mL	Physically compatible for 48 hr at 25°C	1167	C
Metoclopramide HCl	RB	160 mg/32 mL	ES	1 g/2 mL	Physically compatible for 48 hr at 25°C	1167	C
Pantoprazole sodium	[a]	4 mg/1 mL		500 mg/1 mL	Whitish precipitate	2574	I

[a] Test performed using the formulation WITHOUT edetate disodium.

Y-Site Injection Compatibility (1:1 Mixture)

Magnesium sulfate

Test Drug	Mfr	Conc	Mfr	Conc	Remarks	Ref	C/I
Acyclovir sodium	BW	5 mg/mL[a]	LY	20 mg/mL[a]	Physically compatible for 4 hr at 25°C	1157	C
Aldesleukin	CHI	33,800 I.U./mL[a]	LY	20 mg/mL[a]	Visually compatible with little or no loss of aldesleukin activity	1857	C
Amifostine	USB	10 mg/mL[a]	AST	100 mg/mL[a]	Physically compatible for 4 hr at 23°C	1845	C
Amikacin sulfate	BR	5 mg/mL[a]	IX	16.7, 33.3, 66.7, 100 mg/mL[a]	Physically compatible for at least 4 hr at 32°C	813	C
Amiodarone HCl	WY	6 mg/mL[a]	APP	500 mg/mL	Immediate opaque white turbidity becoming thick precipitate in 24 hr at 22°C	2352	I
Amiodarone HCl	WY	6 mg/mL[a]	APP	20 mg/mL[a]	Visually compatible for 24 hr at 22°C	2352	C
Ampicillin sodium	WY	20 mg/mL[b]	IX	16.7, 33.3, 66.7, 100 mg/mL[a]	Physically compatible for at least 4 hr at 32°C	813	C
Aztreonam	SQ	40 mg/mL[a]	AST	100 mg/mL[a]	Physically compatible for 4 hr at 23°C	1758	C
Bivalirudin	TMC	5 mg/mL[a]	APP	100 mg/mL[a]	Physically compatible for 4 hr at 23°C	2373	C
Cangrelor tetrasodium	TMC	1 mg/mL[b]		100 mg/mL[b]	Physically compatible for 4 hr	3243	C
Caspofungin acetate	ME	0.7 mg/mL[b]	AMR	100 mg/mL[b]	Physically compatible for 4 hr at room temperature	2758	C
Caspofungin acetate	ME	0.5 mg/mL[b]	HOS	40 mg/mL	Physically compatible over 60 min	2766	C

Y-Site Injection Compatibility (1:1 Mixture) (Cont.)

Test Drug	Mfr	Conc	Mfr	Conc	Remarks	Ref	C/I
Cefazolin sodium	LI	20 mg/mL[a]	IX	16.7, 33.3, 66.7, 100 mg/mL[a]	Physically compatible for at least 4 hr at 32°C	813	C
Cefotaxime sodium	HO	20 mg/mL[a]	IX	16.7, 33.3, 66.7, 100 mg/mL[a]	Physically compatible for at least 4 hr at 32°C	813	C
Cefoxitin sodium	MSD	20 mg/mL[a]	IX	16.7, 33.3, 66.7, 100 mg/mL[a]	Physically compatible for at least 4 hr at 32°C	813	C
Ceftaroline fosamil	FOR	2.22 mg/mL[a b]	AMR	100 mg/mL[a b]	Physically compatible for 4 hr at 23°C	2826	C
Ceftaroline fosamil	FOR	2.22 mg/mL[f]	AMR	100 mg/mL[f]	Increase in measured haze	2826	I
Ceftazidime–avibactam sodium	ALL	20 mg/mL[o p]			Physically compatible for up to 4 hr at room temperature	3004	C
Ceftolozane sulfate–tazobactam sodium	CUB	10 mg/mL[d m]	APP	100 mg/mL[d]	Physically compatible for 2 hr	3262	C
Chloramphenicol sodium succinate	PD	20 mg/mL[a]	IX	16.7, 33.3, 66.7, 100 mg/mL[a]	Physically compatible for at least 4 hr at 32°C	813	C
Ciprofloxacin	MI	2 mg/mL[a]	LY	50%	Visually compatible for 2 hr at 25°C	1628	C
Ciprofloxacin	MI	2 mg/mL[d]	AB	4 mEq/mL	Precipitate forms in 4 hr in D5W and 1 hr in NS at 24°C	1655	I
Cisatracurium besylate	GW	0.1, 2, 5 mg/mL[a]	AB	100 mg/mL[a]	Physically compatible for 4 hr at 23°C	2074	C
Clindamycin phosphate	UP	12 mg/mL[a]	IX	16.7, 33.3, 66.7, 100 mg/mL[a]	Physically compatible for at least 4 hr at 32°C	813	C
Clonidine HCl	BI	18 mcg/mL[b]	BRN	9.6 mg/mL[a]	Visually compatible	2642	C
Cloxacillin sodium	SMX	100 mg/mL	PPC	500 mg/mL	Physically compatible for up to 4 hr at room temperature	3245	C
Dexmedetomidine HCl	AB	4 mcg/mL[b]	APP	100 mg/mL[b]	Physically compatible for 4 hr at 23°C	2383	C
Dexmedetomidine HCl	HOS, HQS	4 mcg/mL[b]		100 mg/mL	Stated to be compatible	2848, 3179	C
Dobutamine HCl	LI	4 mg/mL[d]	LY	40 mg/mL[d]	Physically compatible for 3 hr	1316	C
Docetaxel	RPR	0.9 mg/mL[a]	AST	100 mg/mL[a]	Physically compatible for 4 hr at 23°C	2224	C
Doripenem	JJ	5 mg/mL[a b]	AMR	100 mg/mL[a b]	Physically compatible for 4 hr at 23°C	2743	C
Doxorubicin HCl liposomal	SEQ	0.4 mg/mL[a]	AST	100 mg/mL[a]	Physically compatible for 4 hr at 23°C	2087	C
Doxycycline hyclate	PF	1 mg/mL[a]	IX	16.7, 33.3, 66.7, 100 mg/mL[a]	Physically compatible for at least 4 hr at 32°C	813	C
Enalaprilat	MSD	0.05 mg/mL[b]	LY	10 mEq/mL[a]	Physically compatible for 24 hr at room temperature under fluorescent light	1355	C
Eravacycline dihydrochloride	TET	0.6 mg/mL[b]	FRK	100 mg/mL[b]	Physically compatible for 2 hr at room temperature	3532	C
Erythromycin lactobionate	AB	5 mg/mL[a]	IX	16.7, 33.3, 66.7, 100 mg/mL[a]	Physically compatible for at least 4 hr at 32°C	813	C
Esmolol HCl	DCC	10 mg/mL[a]	LY	10 mg/mL[a]	Physically compatible for 24 hr at 22°C	1169	C
Etoposide phosphate	BR	5 mg/mL[a]	AST	100 mg/mL[a]	Physically compatible for 4 hr at 23°C	2218	C
Famotidine	MSD	0.2 mg/mL[a]	SO	100 mg/mL[b]	Physically compatible for 14 hr	1196	C
Famotidine	ME	2 mg/mL[b]		100 mg/mL[a]	Visually compatible for 4 hr at 22°C	1936	C
Fenoldopam mesylate	AB	80 mcg/mL[b]	APP	100 mg/mL[b]	Physically compatible for 4 hr at 23°C	2467	C
Fludarabine phosphate	BX	1 mg/mL[a]	SO	100 mg/mL[a]	Visually compatible for 4 hr at 22°C	1439	C

Y-Site Injection Compatibility (1:1 Mixture) (Cont.)

Test Drug	Mfr	Conc	Mfr	Conc	Remarks	Ref	C/I
Gallium nitrate	FUJ	1 mg/mL[b]	AMR	200 mg/mL[b]	Visually compatible for 24 hr at 25°C	1673	C
Gentamicin sulfate	SC	0.8 mg/mL[a]	IX	16.7, 33.3, 66.7, 100 mg/mL[a]	Physically compatible for at least 4 hr at 32°C	813	C
Granisetron HCl	SKB	1 mg/mL	AB	16 mg/mL[b]	Physically compatible with little or no loss of granisetron in 4 hr at 22°C	1883	C
Granisetron HCl	SKB	0.05 mg/mL[a]	AB	100 mg/mL[a]	Physically compatible for 4 hr at 23°C	2000	C
Heparin sodium	UP	1000 units/L[e]	AB	500 mg/mL	Physically compatible for 4 hr at room temperature	534	C
Hetastarch in lactated electrolyte	AB	6%	AST	100 mg/mL[a]	Physically compatible for 4 hr at 23°C	2339	C
Hydrocortisone sodium succinate	UP	10 mg/L[e]	AB	500 mg/mL	Physically compatible for 4 hr at room temperature	534	C
Hydromorphone HCl	KN	2 mg/mL[a]	LY	16.7, 33.3, 50, 100 mg/mL[a]	Visually compatible for 4 hr at 25°C	1549	C
Hydroxyethyl starch 130/0.4 in sodium chloride 0.9%	FRK	6%	SZ	125[a], 250[a], 500 mg/mL	Visually compatible for 24 hr at room temperature	2770	C
Idarubicin HCl	AD	1 mg/mL[b]	SO	2 mg/mL[b]	Visually compatible for 24 hr at 25°C	1525	C
Insulin, regular	LI	0.2 unit/mL[b]	LY	40 mg/mL[f]	Physically compatible for 2 hr at 25°C	1395	C
Isavuconazonium sulfate	ASP	1.5 mg/mL[d]	HOS	100 mg/mL[d]	Physically compatible for 2 hr	3263	C
Labetalol HCl	SC	1 mg/mL[a]	LY	10 mg/mL[a]	Physically compatible for 24 hr at 18°C	1171	C
Letermovir	ME	[b]		[b]	Physically compatible	3398	C
Levofloxacin	OMN	5 mg/mL[a]	AMR	20 mg/mL[b]	Physically compatible	2794	C
Linezolid	PHU	2 mg/mL	AST	100 mg/mL[a]	Physically compatible for 4 hr at 23°C	2264	C
Meperidine HCl	WI	10 mg/mL[a]	LY	16.7, 33.3, 50, 100 mg/mL[a]	Visually compatible for 4 hr at 25°C	1549	C
Meropenem		50 mg/mL	FRK	500 mg/mL	Physically compatible for 4 hr at room temperature	3538	C
Meropenem–vaborbactam	TMC	8 mg/mL[b n]	XGN	100 mg/mL[b]	Physically compatible for 3 hr at 20 to 25°C	3380	C
Metronidazole	SE	5 mg/mL	IX	16.7, 33.3, 66.7, 100 mg/mL[a]	Physically compatible for at least 4 hr at 32°C	813	C
Micafungin sodium	ASP	1.5 mg/mL[b]	AMR	100 mg/mL[b]	Physically compatible for 4 hr at 23°C	2683	C
Milrinone lactate	SW	0.4 mg/mL[a]	SO	40 mg/mL[a]	Visually compatible. No milrinone loss in 4 hr at 23°C	2214	C
Morphine sulfate	ES	1 mg/mL[a]	LY	16.7, 33.3, 50, 100 mg/mL[d]	Visually compatible for 4 hr at 25°C	1549	C
Morphine sulfate	[g]	2 mg/mL[b]	AB	2, 4, 8 mg/mL[b]	Visually compatible for 8 hr at room temperature	1719	C
Nafcillin sodium	WY	20 mg/mL[a]	IX	16.7, 33.3, 66.7, 100 mg/mL[a]	Physically compatible for at least 4 hr at 32°C	813	C
Nicardipine HCl	DCC	0.1 mg/mL[a]	LY	10 mg/mL[a]	Visually compatible for 24 hr at room temperature	235	C
Ondansetron HCl	GL	1 mg/mL[b]	SO	100 mg/mL[a]	Visually compatible for 4 hr at 22°C	1365	C
Oxacillin sodium	BE	20 mg/mL[a]	IX	16.7, 33.3, 66.7, 100 mg/mL[a]	Physically compatible for at least 4 hr at 32°C	813	C
Oxaliplatin	SS	0.5 mg/mL[a]	APP	100 mg/mL[a]	Physically compatible for 4 hr at 23°C	2566	C
Paclitaxel	NCI	1.2 mg/mL[a]	AST	100 mg/mL[a]	Physically compatible for 4 hr at 22°C	1556	C

Y-Site Injection Compatibility (1:1 Mixture) (Cont.)

Test Drug	Mfr	Conc	Mfr	Conc	Remarks	Ref	C/I
Penicillin G potassium	SQ	100,000 units/mL[a]	IX	16.7, 33.3, 66.7, 100 mg/mL[a]	Physically compatible for at least 4 hr at 32°C	813	C
Piperacillin sodium–tazobactam sodium	LE[c]	40 mg/mL[a k]	AST	100 mg/mL[a]	Physically compatible for 4 hr at 22°C	1688	C
Plazomicin sulfate	ACH	24 mg/mL[d]	XGN	100 mg/mL[d]	Physically compatible for 1 hr at 20 to 25°C	3432	C
Potassium chloride	AB	40 mEq/L[e]	AB	500 mg/mL	Physically compatible for 4 hr at room temperature	534	C
Propofol	ZEN[q]	10 mg/mL	AST	100 mg/mL[a]	Physically compatible for 1 hr at 23°C	2066	C
Remifentanil HCl	GW	0.025 and 0.25 mg/mL[b]	AB	100 mg/mL[a]	Physically compatible for 4 hr at 23°C	2075	C
Sargramostim	IMM	10 mcg/mL[b]	LY	100 mg/mL[b]	Visually compatible for 4 hr at 22°C	1436	C
Sodium nitroprusside	RC	0.3, 1.2, 3 mg/mL[a]	SX	0.4 and 0.8 mEq/mL[i]	Visually compatible for 48 hr at 24°C protected from light	2357	C
Tedizolid phosphate	CUB	0.8 mg/mL[b]	HOS	100 mg/mL[b]	Immediate precipitation and increase in measured turbidity	3244	I
Telavancin HCl	ASP	7.5 mg/mL[a b f]	AMR	100 mg/mL[a b f]	Physically compatible for 2 hr	2830	C
Thiotepa	IMM[h]	1 mg/mL[a]	AST	100 mg/mL[a]	Physically compatible for 4 hr at 23°C	1861	C
TNA #218 to #226[i]			AB	100 mg/mL[a]	Visually compatible for 4 hr at 23°C	2215	C
Tobramycin sulfate	DI	0.8 mg/mL[a]	IX	16.7, 33.3, 66.7, 100 mg/mL[a]	Physically compatible for at least 4 hr at 32°C	813	C
TPN #212 to #215[i]			AB	100 mg/mL[a]	Physically compatible for 4 hr at 23°C	2109	C
Trimethoprim–sulfamethoxazole	RC	0.8 mg/mL[a l]	IX	16.7, 33.3, 66.7, 100 mg/mL[a]	Physically compatible for at least 4 hr at 32°C	813	C
Vancomycin HCl	LI	5 mg/mL[a]	IX	16.7, 33.3, 66.7, 100 mg/mL[a]	Physically compatible for at least 4 hr at 32°C	813	C

[a] Tested in dextrose 5%.

[b] Tested in sodium chloride 0.9%.

[c] Test performed using the formulation WITHOUT edetate disodium.

[d] Tested in both dextrose 5% and sodium chloride 0.9%.

[e] Tested in dextrose 5% in Ringer's injection, dextrose 5% in Ringer's injection, lactated, dextrose 5%, Ringer's injection, lactated, and sodium chloride 0.9%.

[f] Tested in Ringer's injection, lactated.

[g] Extemporaneously prepared product.

[h] Lyophilized formulation tested.

[i] Refer to Appendix for the composition of parenteral nutrition solutions. TNA indicates a 3-in-1 admixture, and TPN indicates a 2-in-1 admixture.

[j] Tested in dextrose 5% in sodium chloride 0.225%.

[k] Piperacillin component. Piperacillin in an 8:1 fixed-ratio concentration with tazobactam.

[l] Trimethoprim component. Trimethoprim in a 1:5 fixed-ratio concentration with sulfamethoxazole.

[m] Ceftolozane component. Ceftolozane in a 2:1 fixed-ratio concentration with tazobactam.

[n] Meropenem component. Meropenem in a 1:1 fixed-ratio concentration with vaborbactam.

[o] Ceftazidime component. Ceftazidime in a 4:1 fixed-ratio concentration with avibactam.

[p] Tested in dextrose 5%, sodium chloride 0.9%, and Ringer's injection, lactated.

[q] Test performed using the formulation WITH edetate disodium.

Selected Revisions May 1, 2020. © Copyright, October 1982.
American Society of Health-System Pharmacists, Inc.

Mannitol
AHFS 40:28.12

Products

Mannitol is available in concentrations ranging from 5 to 25%:[1(6/06)] [4]

Concentration	Osmolarity	Available Sizes
5%	275 mOsm/L	1000 mL
10%	550 mOsm/L	500 and 1000 mL
15%	825 mOsm/L	500 mL
20%	1100 mOsm/L	250 and 500 mL
25%	1375 mOsm/L	50 mL

pH

From 4.5 to 7.[1(6/06)] [4]

Trade Name(s)

Osmitrol

Administration

Mannitol is administered by intravenous infusion. An administration set with a filter should be used for infusion solutions containing mannitol 20% or more. The dosage, concentration, and administration rate are dependent on the patient's condition and response.[1(6/06)] [4]

Stability

Mannitol solutions should be stored at controlled room temperature and protected from freezing.[1(6/06)] [4] The solutions are chemically stable. Mannitol 25% was chemically and physically stable after 5 autoclavings at 250°F for 15 minutes. In addition, no extracts or visible particles from the rubber closures were found.[83]

Crystallization

In concentrations of 15% or greater, mannitol may crystallize when exposed to low temperatures.[1(6/06)] [4] [593] Do not use a mannitol solution containing crystals. If such crystallization occurs, the recommended procedure for resolubilization is to heat the mannitol in a dry heat cabinet to 70°C for flexible plastic containers with the overwrap intact or to 80°C for glass containers with vigorous shaking. The use of a water bath is not recommended. Mannitol 25% in glass vials may be autoclaved at 121°C. The solution should cool to body temperature before use.[1(6/06)] [4]

The use of a microwave oven to resolubilize crystallized mannitol in glass ampuls has been suggested. Exposure to microwave radiation followed by shaking satisfactorily resolubilized the crystals in a shorter total time than the water bath and autoclave methods and resulted in no chemical decomposition.[694]

Unfortunately, the use of microwave radiation to solubilize mannitol crystals is a highly risky undertaking. Explosions of mannitol ampuls during microwave exposure have been reported.[695] [697] Such explosions could injure someone as well as ruin the microwave oven. The explosion results from pressure building during the heating of the solution that occurs from the microwave exposure.[696] [697]

One inventive pharmacist redissolved mannitol crystals using a coffeemaker.[1114]

As an alternative to resolubilizing techniques, the use of warming chambers to maintain the solutions in a crystal-free condition has been recommended.[698] [699] [700] Various chambers have been described, including a wooden cabinet,[698] a metal kettle,[699] and even a bun warmer.[700] Storage temperatures of 35 and 50°C have been utilized.[698] [699]

A related but differing effect is seen when supersaturated solutions of mannitol are placed in polyvinyl chloride (PVC) bags. Within a few minutes, a heavy white flocculent precipitate forms. The needle-like crystals in mannitol solutions result from slow undisturbed growth. The white flocculent mannitol precipitate results from contact with the PVC surfaces, which act as nuclei for rapid crystallization of small crystals. Attempts to resolubilize the precipitate with the aid of heat are not fruitful because crystallization may recur in a short time.[432]

Compatibility Information
Additive Compatibility

Mannitol

Test Drug	Mfr	Conc/L or %	Mfr	Conc/L or %	Test Solution	Remarks	Ref	C/I
Amikacin sulfate	BR	250 mg and 5 g	BA	20%		Compatible and stable for 24 hr at 25°C, 60 days at 4°C, 30 days at –15°C	292	C
Aztreonam				50 and 100 g		Manufacturer-recommended solution	2864, 2866	C

DOI: 10.37573/9781585286850.245

Additive Compatibility (Cont.)

Test Drug	Mfr	Conc/L or %	Mfr	Conc/L or %	Test Solution	Remarks	Ref	C/I
Cefoxitin sodium	MSD	1, 2, 10, 20 g		10%		4 to 5% cefoxitin loss in 24 hr and 10 to 11% in 48 hr at 25°C. 2 to 5% cefoxitin loss in 7 days at 5°C	308	C
Ceftriaxone sodium	RC	10 to 40 g		5 and 10%		Less than 10% loss in 24 hr at 25°C	1(6/06)	C
Cisplatin	BR	50 and 200 mg		18.75 g	D5½Sᵃ	Compatible for 48 hr at 25°C and 96 hr at 4°C followed by 48 hr at 25°C	1088	C
Dopamine HCl	AS	800 mg	MG	20%		Under 5% dopamine loss in 48 hr at 25°C	79	C
Ertapenem sodium	ME	10 and 20 g	AB	5%		Precipitate in <1 hr. 15% loss in 20 hr at 25°C. 7% loss in 2 days at 4°C	2487	I
Ertapenem sodium	ME	10 and 20 g	AB	20%		Precipitate in <1 hr. 13% loss in 6 hr at 25°C. 8% loss in 1 day at 4°C	2487	I
Fosphenytoin sodium	PD	2, 8, 20 mg PE/mLᵇ	BAᵃ	20%		Visually compatible with little or no loss in 7 days at 25°C under fluorescent light	2083	C
Furosemide	AB	200, 400, 800 mg	BAᵃ	20%		Visually compatible for 72 hr at 22°C	1803	C
Gentamicin sulfate		120 mg		20%		Physically compatible and gentamicin stable for 24 hr at 25°C	897	C
Imipenem–cilastatin sodium	MSD	2.5ᶠ g	ABᶜ	2.5%		9% imipenem loss in 9 hr at 25°C. 7% loss in 48 hr and 11% in 72 hr at 4°C	1141	Iᵈ
Imipenem–cilastatin sodium	MSD	5ᶠ g	ABᶜ	2.5%		6% imipenem loss in 3 hr and 12% in 6 hr at 25°C. 7% loss in 24 hr and 10% in 48 hr at 4°C	1141	Iᵈ
Imipenem–cilastatin sodium	MSD	2.5ᶠ g	ABᶜ	5%		6% imipenem loss in 3 hr and 10% in 6 hr at 25°C. 9% loss in 48 hr and 13% in 72 hr at 4°C	1141	Iᵈ
Imipenem–cilastatin sodium	MSD	5ᶠ g	ABᶜ	5%		7% imipenem loss in 3 hr and 12% in 6 hr at 25°C. 12% loss in 48 hr at 4°C	1141	Iᵈ
Imipenem–cilastatin sodium	MSD	2.5ᶠ g	ABᶜ	10%		6% imipenem loss in 3 hr and 10% in 6 hr at 25°C. 7% loss in 24 hr and 12% in 48 hr at 4°C	1141	Iᵈ
Imipenem–cilastatin sodium	MSD	5ᶠ g	ABᶜ	10%		12% imipenem loss in 3 hr at 25°C. 13% loss in 48 hr at 4°C	1141	Iᵈ
Levofloxacin	OMJ	0.5 g	BA	20%		Precipitate forms within a few hours	1986	I
Levofloxacin	OMJ	5 g	BA	20%		Precipitate forms within 13 weeks at –20°C	1986	I
Levofloxacin	OMJ	5 g	BA	20%		Physically compatible. <4% loss in 3 days at 25°C, 14 days at 5°C, in dark	1986	C
Meropenem	ZEN	1 g	BAᵃ	2.5%		7 to 8% meropenem loss in 8 hr at 24°C and in 24 hr at 4°C	2089	Iᵈ
Meropenem	ZEN	20 g	BAᵃ	2.5%		7 to 9% meropenem loss in 4 hr at 24°C and 6% loss in 20 hr at 4°C	2089	Iᵈ
Meropenem	ZEN	1 g	BAᵃ	10%		10 to 11% meropenem loss in 4 hr at 24°C and in 20 hr at 4°C	2089	Iᵈ
Meropenem	ZEN	20 g	BAᵃ	10%		10% meropenem loss in 3 hr at 24°C and in 20 hr at 4°C	2089	Iᵈ
Metoclopramide HCl	RB	40 and 100 mg	AB	20%		Physically compatible for 48 hr at room temperature	924	C
Metoclopramide HCl	RB	40 and 100 mg	AB	20%		Physically compatible 48 hr at 25°C	1167	C

Additive Compatibility (Cont.)

Test Drug	Mfr	Conc/L or %	Mfr	Conc/L or %	Test Solution	Remarks	Ref	C/I
Metoclopramide HCl	RB	640 mg and 1.6 g	AB	20%		Physically compatible for 48 hr at 25°C	1167	C
Ondansetron HCl	GL	16 mg	BP[a]	10%		Physically compatible. Stable for 7 days at room temperature in light and at 4°C	1366	C
Sodium bicarbonate	AB	44.6 mEq	AMR	25 g	D5LR, D5¼S, D5½S, D5S, D5W, D10W, NS, ½S[e]	Visually compatible for 24 hr at 24°C	1853, 1973	C
Tobramycin sulfate	LI	200 mg and 1 g		20%		Physically compatible and chemically stable for 48 hr at 25°C	147	C
Tramadol HCl	GRU	0.4 g		20%		Visually compatible with no tramadol loss in 24 hr at room temperature and 4°C	2652	C
Verapamil HCl	KN	80 mg	IX	25 g	D5W, NS	Physically compatible for 24 hr	764	C

[a] Tested in PVC containers.

[b] Concentration expressed in milligrams of phenytoin sodium equivalents (PE) per mL.

[c] Tested in glass containers.

[d] Incompatible by conventional standards but may be used in shorter periods of time.

[e] Tested in polyolefin containers.

[f] Imipenem component. Imipenem in a 1:1 fixed-ratio concentration with cilastatin.

Y-Site Injection Compatibility (1:1 Mixture)

Mannitol

Test Drug	Mfr	Conc	Mfr	Conc	Remarks	Ref	C/I
Acetaminophen	CAD	10 mg/mL	HOS	150 mg/mL	Physically compatible with less than 10% acetaminophen loss over 4 hr at room temperature	2841, 2844	C
Allopurinol sodium	BW	3 mg/mL[b]	BA	15%	Physically compatible for 4 hr at 22°C	1686	C
Amifostine	USB	10 mg/mL[a]	BA	15%	Physically compatible for 4 hr at 23°C	1845	C
Aztreonam	SQ	40 mg/mL[a]	BA	15%	Physically compatible for 4 hr at 23°C	1758	C
Bivalirudin	TMC	5 mg/mL[a]	BA	15%	Physically compatible for 4 hr at 23°C	2373	C
Cangrelor tetrasodium	TMC	1 mg/mL[b]		15%	Physically compatible for 4 hr	3243	C
Ceftaroline fosamil	FOR	2.22 mg/mL[a b h]	HOS	15%	Physically compatible for 4 hr at 23°C	2826	C
Ceftolozane sulfate–tazobactam sodium	CUB	10 mg/mL[i k]	HOS	25%	Physically compatible for 2 hr	3262	C
Cisatracurium besylate	GW	0.1, 2, 5 mg/mL[a]	BA	15%	Physically compatible for 4 hr at 23°C	2074	C
Cladribine	ORT	0.015[b] and 0.5[c] mg/mL	BA	15%	Physically compatible for 4 hr at 23°C	1969	C
Cloxacillin sodium	SMX	100 mg/mL	HOS	250 mg/mL	Physically compatible for up to 4 hr at room temperature	3245	C
Dexmedetomidine HCl	HOS, HQS	4 mcg/mL[b]		20%	Stated to be compatible	2848, 3179	C
Docetaxel	RPR	0.9 mg/mL[a]	BA	15%	Physically compatible for 4 hr at 23°C	2224	C
Doripenem	JJ	5 mg/mL[a b]	HOS	15%	Physically compatible for 4 hr at 23°C	2743	C

Y-Site Injection Compatibility (1:1 Mixture) (Cont.)

Test Drug	Mfr	Conc	Mfr	Conc	Remarks	Ref	C/I
Doxorubicin HCl liposomal	SEQ	0.4 mg/mL[a]	BA	15%	Partial loss of measured natural turbidity	2087	I
Etoposide phosphate	BR	5 mg/mL[a]	BA	15%	Physically compatible for 4 hr at 23°C	2218	C
Fenoldopam mesylate	AB	80 mcg/mL[b]	BA	15%	Physically compatible for 4 hr at 23°C	2467	C
Filgrastim	AMG	30 mcg/mL[a]	BA	15%	Filaments form immediately	1687	I
Fludarabine phosphate	BX	1 mg/mL[a]	BA	15%	Visually compatible for 4 hr at 22°C	1439	C
Fluorouracil	SO	1 and 2 mg/mL[d]		20%	Physically compatible and fluorouracil stable for 24 hr. Mannitol not tested	1526	C
Gallium nitrate	FUJ	1 mg/mL[b]	AB	250 mg/mL	Visually compatible for 24 hr at 25°C	1673	C
Gemcitabine HCl	LI	10 mg/mL[b]	BA	15%	Physically compatible for 4 hr at 23°C	2226	C
Hetastarch in lactated electrolyte	AB	6%	BA	15%	Physically compatible for 4 hr at 23°C	2339	C
Idarubicin HCl	AD	1 mg/mL[b]	AB	12.5 mg/mL[b]	Visually compatible for 24 hr at 25°C	1525	C
Isavuconazonium sulfate	ASP	1.5 mg/mL[j]	HOS	20%	Physically compatible for 2 hr	3263	C
Linezolid	PHU	2 mg/mL	BA	15%	Physically compatible for 4 hr at 23°C	2264	C
Melphalan HCl	BW	0.1 mg/mL[b]	BA	15%	Physically compatible for 3 hr at 22°C	1557	C
Meropenem		50 mg/mL	HOS	250 mg/mL	Physically compatible for 4 hr at room temperature	3538	C
Meropenem–vaborbactam	TMC	8 mg/mL[b l]	HOS	20%	Physically compatible for 3 hr at 20 to 25°C	3380	C
Ondansetron HCl	GL	1 mg/mL[b]	BA	15%	Visually compatible for 4 hr at 22°C	1365	C
Oxaliplatin	SS	0.5 mg/mL[a]	BA	15%	Physically compatible for 4 hr at 23°C	2566	C
Paclitaxel	NCI	1.2 mg/mL[a]	BA	15%	Physically compatible for 4 hr at 22°C	1556	C
Palonosetron HCl	MGI	50 mcg/mL	HOS	15%	Physically compatible. No palonosetron loss in 4 hr at room temperature	2775	C
Pantoprazole sodium	[g]	4 mg/mL		25%	Precipitates	2574	I
Pemetrexed disodium	LI	20 mg/mL[b]	BA	15%	Physically compatible for 4 hr at 23°C	2564	C
Piperacillin sodium–tazobactam sodium	LE[g]	40 mg/mL[a i]	BA	15%	Physically compatible for 4 hr at 22°C	1688	C
Plazomicin sulfate	ACH	24 mg/mL[j]	HOS	20%	Physically compatible for 1 hr at 20 to 25°C	3432	C
Propofol	ZEN[m]	10 mg/mL	BA	15%	Physically compatible for 1 hr at 23°C	2066	C
Remifentanil HCl	GW	0.025 and 0.25 mg/mL[b]	BA	15%	Physically compatible for 4 hr at 23°C	2075	C
Sargramostim	IMM	10 mcg/mL[b]	BA	15%	Visually compatible for 4 hr at 22°C	1436	C
Tedizolid phosphate	CUB	0.8 mg/mL[b]	HOS	20%	Physically compatible for 2 hr	3244	C
Telavancin HCl	ASP	7.5 mg/mL[a b h]	HOS	20%	Physically compatible for 2 hr	2830	C
Teniposide	BR	0.1 mg/mL[a]	BA	15%	Physically compatible for 4 hr at 23°C	1725	C
Thiotepa	IMM[e]	1 mg/mL[b]	BA	15%	Physically compatible for 4 hr at 23°C	1861	C
TNA #218 to #226[f]			BA	15%	Visually compatible for 4 hr at 23°C	2215	C

Y-Site Injection Compatibility (1:1 Mixture) (Cont.)

Test Drug	Mfr	Conc	Mfr	Conc	Remarks	Ref	C/I
TPN #212 to #215[f]			BA	15%	Physically compatible for 4 hr at 23°C	2109	C
Vinorelbine tartrate	BW	1 mg/mL[b]	BA	15%	Physically compatible for 4 hr at 22°C	1558	C

[a] Tested in dextrose 5%.

[b] Tested in sodium chloride 0.9%.

[c] Tested in bacteriostatic sodium chloride 0.9% preserved with benzyl alcohol 0.9%.

[d] Tested in dextrose 5% in sodium chloride 0.45%, dextrose 5%, and sodium chloride 0.9%.

[e] Lyophilized formulation tested.

[f] Refer to Appendix for the composition of parenteral nutrition solutions. TNA indicates a 3-in-1 admixture, and TPN indicates a 2-in-1 admixture.

[g] Test performed using the formulation WITHOUT edetate disodium.

[h] Tested in Ringer's injection, lactated.

[i] Piperacillin component. Piperacillin in an 8:1 fixed-ratio concentration with tazobactam.

[j] Tested in both dextrose 5% and sodium chloride 0.9%.

[k] Ceftolozane component. Ceftolozane in a 2:1 fixed-ratio concentration with tazobactam.

[l] Meropenem component. Meropenem in a 1:1 fixed-ratio concentration with vaborbactam.

[m] Test performed using the formulation WITH edetate disodium.

Selected Revisions May 1, 2020. © Copyright, October 1982.
American Society of Health-System Pharmacists, Inc.

Mechlorethamine Hydrochloride
AHFS 10:00
Mustine Hydrochloride

Products

Mechlorethamine hydrochloride is available in vials containing 10 mg of drug and sodium chloride qs 100 mg. While taking appropriate protective measures, including wearing protective gloves, reconstitute the vial with 10 mL of water for injection or sodium chloride 0.9%. With the needle in the rubber stopper, shake the vial several times to dissolve the drug. The resultant solution contains mechlorethamine hydrochloride 1 mg/mL.[1(10/05)]

pH

The reconstituted solution has a pH of 3 to 5.[1(10/05)] [4]

Trade Name(s)

Mustargen

Administration

Mechlorethamine hydrochloride is administered intravenously or into body cavities.[1(10/05)] [4] The drug is extremely irritating to tissues and should not be given intramuscularly or subcutaneously.[4] For intravenous use, the drug may be injected over a few minutes directly into the vein or into the tubing of a running infusion solution.[1(10/05)] [4] After administration, flushing the vein with about 5 to 10 mL of intravenous solution has been recommended.[4] The drug is a powerful vesicant, and extravasation should be avoided.[1(10/05)] [4] [377] For intracavitary administration, the drug may be diluted up to 100 mL with sodium chloride 0.9%.[1(10/05)] [4]

Spillage of the drug on gloves, etc., can be neutralized by soaking in an aqueous solution containing equal amounts of sodium thiosulfate 5% and sodium bicarbonate 5% for 45 minutes. Unused injection solution also may be neutralized by mixing with an equal volume of the sodium thiosulfate–sodium bicarbonate solution for 45 minutes.[1(10/05)] [1200]

Stability

In dry form, the drug is a light yellow-brown and is stable at temperatures up to 40°C.[4] Solutions decompose on standing and should be prepared immediately before use. The drug is even less stable in neutral or alkaline solutions than in the acidic reconstituted solution. Do not use if the solution is discolored or if water droplets form within the vial before reconstitution. Discard unused portions after neutralization.[1(10/05)] [4]

Because of the rapid decomposition of mechlorethamine hydrochloride in solution, administration in intravenous infusion solutions is not recommended.[4] One report indicated a 7% loss of mechlorethamine in one hour at room temperature when diluted to 0.1 mg/mL in sodium chloride 0.9%.[923] Injecting the drug into the tubing of a running intravenous infusion rather than adding it to the entire volume of the solution minimizes the extent of chemical decomposition.[1(10/05)]

The stability of mechlorethamine hydrochloride (Boots) 1 mg/mL when reconstituted with water for injection or sodium chloride 0.9% in vials and plastic syringes was determined. About an 8 to 10% loss occurred in samples over six hours at 22°C; losses of 4 to 6% occurred in six hours in samples stored at 4°C.[1279]

Immersion of a needle with an aluminum component in mechlorethamine (MSD) 1 mg/mL resulted in no visually apparent reaction after seven days at 24°C.[988]

Freezing Solutions

The stability of mechlorethamine hydrochloride (Boots) 1 mg/mL in water for injection and sodium chloride 0.9% frozen at −20°C was determined. In water for injection, about a 7% loss occurred after 12 weeks; about a 15% loss occurred in eight weeks with sodium chloride 0.9% as the diluent. At a concentration of 10 mg/500 mL in sodium chloride 0.9% in PVC bags, about a 10% loss occurred in eight weeks frozen at −20°C.[1279]

Compatibility Information

Solution Compatibility

Mechlorethamine HCl

Test Soln Name	Test Soln Mfr	Mfr	Conc/L or %	Remarks	Ref	C/I
Dextrose 5%	a	BT	20 mg	10% loss in 5 hr at 22°C. 4% loss in 6 hr at 4°C	1279	I
Sodium chloride 0.9%	a	BT	20 mg	10% loss in 3 hr at 22°C. 10% loss in 4 hr at 4°C	1279	I

a Tested in PVC containers.

DOI: 10.37573/9781585286850.246

Additive Compatibility

Mechlorethamine HCl

Test Drug	Mfr	Conc/L or %	Mfr	Conc/L or %	Test Solution	Remarks	Ref	C/I
Methohexital sodium	BP	2 g	BP	40 mg	D5W, NS	Haze develops over 3 hr	26	I

Y-Site Injection Compatibility (1:1 Mixture)

Mechlorethamine HCl

Test Drug	Mfr	Conc	Mfr	Conc	Remarks	Ref	C/I
Allopurinol sodium	BW	3 mg/mL[b]	MSD	1 mg/mL	Haze and small particles form immediately. Numerous large particles in 4 hr	1686	I
Amifostine	USB	10 mg/mL[a]	MSD	1 mg/mL	Physically compatible for 4 hr at 23°C	1845	C
Aztreonam	SQ	40 mg/mL[a]	MSD	1 mg/mL	Physically compatible for 4 hr at 23°C	1758	C
Filgrastim	AMG	30 mcg/mL[a]	MSD	1 mg/mL	Physically compatible for 4 hr at 22°C	1687	C
Fludarabine phosphate	BX	1 mg/mL[a]	MSD	1 mg/mL	Visually compatible for 4 hr at 22°C	1439	C
Granisetron HCl	SKB	1 mg/mL	MSD	0.5 mg/mL[b]	Physically compatible with little or no loss of either drug in 4 hr at 22°C	1883	C
Melphalan HCl	BW	0.1 mg/mL[b]	MSD	1 mg/mL	Physically compatible for 3 hr at 22°C	1557	C
Ondansetron HCl	GL	1 mg/mL[b]	MSD	1 mg/mL	Visually compatible for 4 hr at 22°C	1365	C
Sargramostim	IMM	10 mcg/mL[b]	MSD	1 mg/mL	Visually compatible for 4 hr at 22°C	1436	C
Teniposide	BR	0.1 mg/mL[a]	MSD	1 mg/mL	Physically compatible for 4 hr at 23°C	1725	C
Vinorelbine tartrate	BW	1 mg/mL[b]	MSD	1 mg/mL	Physically compatible for 4 hr at 22°C	1558	C

[a] Tested in dextrose 5%.

[b] Tested in sodium chloride 0.9%.

Meloxicam
AHFS 28:08.04.92

Products

Meloxicam injection is available as an opaque, pale yellow dispersion in 2-mL single-dose vials containing 1 mL of the dispersion.[3552] Each mL of the dispersion contains 30 mg of meloxicam, as well as sucrose 60 mg, polyvinylpyrrolidone 9 mg, and sodium deoxycholate 3 mg in water for injection.[3552]

Trade Name(s)

Anjeso

Administration

Meloxicam is for intravenous use only.[3552] The drug should be administered as a direct intravenous injection over 15 seconds.[3552]

© Copyright, July 2020. American Society of Health-System Pharmacists, Inc.

Stability

Meloxicam injection is an opaque, pale yellow aqueous dispersion.[3552] Intact vials of the drug should be stored at 15 to 25°C, with excursions permitted from 4 to 30°C.[3552] Vials should be stored in the carton to protect from light.[3552] Freezing should be avoided.[3552]

DOI: 10.37573/9781585286850.247

Melphalan Hydrochloride
AHFS 10:00

Products

Melphalan hydrochloride (generic versions of Alkeran, which is no longer commercially available in the US) is available as a lyophilized powder in single-use or single-dose vials containing the equivalent of 50 mg of melphalan and povidone 20 mg.[3173] [3425] [3426] Each vial is packaged with a 10-mL vial of special diluent containing sodium citrate 0.2 g, propylene glycol 6 mL, alcohol (e.g., ethanol [96%] 0.52 mL,[3173] dehydrated alcohol 0.51 mL,[3425] ethanol [100%] 0.5 mL),[3426] and sterile water for injection.[3173] [3425] [3426] The contents of each vial should be reconstituted by rapidly injecting 10 mL of the special diluent into the vial using a syringe with a 20-gauge or larger needle, and the vial should be shaken vigorously until the solution is clear to yield a 5-mg/mL solution of melphalan; rapid addition of the diluent and subsequent vigorous shaking are important for proper dissolution of the drug.[3173] [3425] [3426] The appropriate dose of the reconstituted solution should be diluted immediately in sodium chloride 0.9% to a concentration not exceeding 0.45 mg/mL.[3173] [3425] [3426]

Melphalan hydrochloride (Evomela, Spectrum) also is available as a lyophilized powder in single-dose vials containing the equivalent of 50 mg of melphalan and betadex sulfobutyl ether sodium 2700 mg as a stabilizing excipient.[3171] [3172] This formulation is propylene glycol-free.[3171] [3172] [3427] The contents of each vial should be reconstituted with 8.6 mL of sodium chloride 0.9% to yield a 5-mg/mL solution of melphalan.[3172] The appropriate dose of the reconstituted solution should be withdrawn from the vial and diluted with sodium chloride 0.9% to a concentration of 0.45 mg/mL.[3172]

Equivalency

Melphalan hydrochloride 56 mg is equivalent to 50 mg of melphalan free base.[3172]

Trade Name(s)

Alkeran, Evomela

Administration

Melphalan hydrochloride is administered intravenously as an infusion.[3172] [3173] [3425] [3426] The manufacturers recommend that the drug be administered slowly into a fast-running intravenous infusion solution via a central venous line or injection port.[3172] [3173]

The final diluted solution of melphalan (generic versions of Alkeran) for infusion is administered over at least 15 minutes (usually 15 to 20 minutes).[3173] [3425] [3426]

The final diluted solution of melphalan (Evomela) for infusion is administered over 15 to 20 minutes or 30 minutes, depending on the indication.[3172]

Extravasation of melphalan hydrochloride may cause local tissue damage and should be avoided.[3172] [3173] [3425] [3426] The drug should *not* be administered by direct injection into a periph-eral vein.[3172] [3173] [3425] [3426] In cases of poor peripheral access, consideration should be given to the use of a central venous line.[3173] [3425] [3426]

As with other toxic drugs, caution should be exercised in the handling and preparation of melphalan hydrochloride and applicable special handling and disposal procedures should be followed.[3172] [3173] [3425] [3426] Some manufacturers recommend the use of gloves as skin reactions may occur with accidental exposure.[3173] [3425] [3426] If skin or mucosal contact with the drug occurs, the affected area(s) should be washed immediately and thoroughly with soap and water.[3173] [3425] [3426]

Stability

Intact vials should be stored at controlled room temperature and protected from light;[3172] [3173] [3425] [3426] some manufacturers recommend storage in the original carton.[3173] [3425]

The solution should be visually inspected for particulate matter and discoloration prior to administration; if particulate matter is present or discoloration occurs, the solution should not be used.[3172] [3173] [3425] [3426]

The reconstituted solution of melphalan (generic versions of Alkeran) should *not* be refrigerated; a precipitate forms in the reconstituted product if stored at 5°C.[3173] [3425] [3426]

Melphalan Hydrochloride (generic versions of Alkeran)

The time between reconstitution and dilution and administration of solutions of melphalan (generic versions of Alkeran) should be minimized.[3173] [3425] [3426] In as little as 30 minutes from reconstitution, a citrate derivative of melphalan has been detected; upon further dilution with sodium chloride 0.9%, nearly 1% of the drug is hydrolyzed every 10 minutes.[3173] [3425] [3426] Manufacturers recommend that administration of melphalan hydrochloride be completed within 60 minutes of reconstitution.[3173] [3425] [3426]

Melphalan Hydrochloride (Evomela, Spectrum)

The manufacturer states that the 5-mg/mL reconstituted solution of Evomela is stable for 1 hour at room temperature or 24 hours under refrigeration at 5°C without any precipitation because of its high solubility.[3172] After dilution of Evomela to a melphalan concentration of 0.45 mg/mL in sodium chloride 0.9%, this formulation is stable for 4 hours at room temperature in addition to the 1 hour at room temperature following reconstitution.[3172]

One study found that a 5-mg/mL reconstituted solution of melphalan (as the Evomela formulation) was stable for 25 hours at room temperature based on experimental trend analysis and for up to 48 hours when stored at 2 to 8°C.[3171] [3427] At 2 to 8°C, the 5-mg/mL reconstituted solution exhibited an antimicrobial effect for up to 72 hours against 8 microorganisms tested in the study (*Aspergillus brasiliensis*, *Candida albicans*, *Bacillus subtilis*, *Escherichia coli*, *Pseudomonas aeruginosa*, *Staphylococcus*

DOI: 10.37573/9781585286850.248

aureus, methicillin-resistant *S. aureus* [MRSA], and vancomycin-resistant *Enterococcus faecalis* [VRE]).[3171] Concentrations of 0.45, 1, and 2 mg/mL diluted in sodium chloride 0.9% were calculated to be stable for a time of 4, 7, and 11 hours, respectively, based on experimental trend analysis.[3171] [3427]

pH Effects

Melphalan is most stable over a pH range of 3 to 7; decomposition increases at pH 9.[971]

Sorption

Melphalan (GlaxoWellcome) 60 mcg/mL in sodium chloride 0.9% exhibited no loss due to sorption in polyethylene, polyvinyl chloride (PVC) containers, and glass containers over 24 hours under refrigeration and 8 hours at room temperature.[2420] [2430]

Filtration

Melphalan 20 mcg/mL in 1 mL of sodium chloride 0.9% was filtered through the following filters; minimal adsorption occurred in all cases:[970]

Filter	Delivered Concentration (% of initial)
Cellulose acetate 0.2 µm (Minisart-N, Sartorius)	99
Polysulfone 0.45 µm (Acrodisc, Gelman)	98
Polytetrafluoroethylene 0.45 µm (Acrodisc-CR, Gelman)	96

Compatibility Information

Solution Compatibility

Melphalan HCl

Test Soln Name	Mfr	Mfr	Conc/L or %	Remarks	Ref	C/I
Dextrose 5%		BW	40 and 400 mg	10% loss in 90 min at 20°C and 36 min at 25°C	971	I
Ringer's injection, lactated		BW	40 and 400 mg	10% loss in 2.9 hr at 20°C and 90 min at 25°C	971	I
Sodium chloride 0.9%			20 mg	4% loss in 6 months at –20°C	970	C
Sodium chloride 0.9%		BW	40 and 400 mg	10% loss in 4.5 hr at 20°C and 2.4 hr at 25°C	971	I[a]
Sodium chloride 0.9%		BW	100 and 450 mg	10% loss in 45 min at 30°C	234	I
Sodium chloride 0.9%		BW	100 mg	10% loss in 3 hr at 20°C	234	I[a]
Sodium chloride 0.9%	b	WEL	200 mg	Visually compatible. 6% loss in 3 hr and 17% in 6 hr at room temperature. 6% loss in 6 hr and 13% in 24 hr at 4°C. No loss in 72 hr at –20°C	1841	I[a]
Sodium chloride 0.9%	b	GSK	0.5 g	More than 10% loss in 1 hr at 5°C protected from light	3174	I
Sodium chloride 0.9%	b	GSK	0.5 and 2 g	Physically compatible. Less than 10% loss in 2 hr at 25°C	3174	I[a]
Sodium chloride 0.9%	b	GSK	2 g	Physically compatible. Less than 10% loss in 24 hr at 5°C protected from light	3174	C
Sodium chloride 0.9%	b	GSK	4 g	Turbidity and discoloration in 4 hr at 5°C protected from light	3174	I
Sodium chloride 0.9%	b	GSK	4 g	Physically compatible. Less than 10% loss in 8 hr at 25°C	3174	C
Sodium chloride 0.9%		SP[c]	450 mg	Stated to be stable for 4 hr at room temperature	3172	C

[a] Incompatible by conventional standards. May be used in shorter time periods.

[b] Tested in PVC containers.

[c] Test performed using the Evomela formulation.

Y-Site Injection Compatibility (1:1 Mixture)

Melphalan HCl

Test Drug	Mfr	Conc	Mfr	Conc	Remarks	Ref	C/I
Acyclovir sodium	BW	7 mg/mL[b]	BW	0.1 mg/mL[b]	Physically compatible for 3 hr at 22°C	1557	C
Amikacin sulfate	BR	5 mg/mL[b]	BW	0.1 mg/mL[b]	Physically compatible for 3 hr at 22°C	1557	C

Y-Site Injection Compatibility (1:1 Mixture) (Cont.)

Test Drug	Mfr	Conc	Mfr	Conc	Remarks	Ref	C/I
Aminophylline	AB	2.5 mg/mL[b]	BW	0.1 mg/mL[b]	Physically compatible for 3 hr at 22°C	1557	C
Amphotericin B	SQ	0.6 mg/mL[a]	BW	0.1 mg/mL[b]	Immediate increase in measured turbidity	1557	I
Amphotericin B	SQ	0.6 mg/mL[a]	BW	0.1 mg/mL[a]	Physically compatible but rapid melphalan loss in D5W precludes use	1557	I
Ampicillin sodium	WY	20 mg/mL[b]	BW	0.1 mg/mL[b]	Physically compatible for 3 hr at 22°C	1557	C
Aztreonam	SQ	40 mg/mL[b]	BW	0.1 mg/mL[b]	Physically compatible for 3 hr at 22°C	1557	C
Bleomycin sulfate	BR	1 unit/mL[b]	BW	0.1 mg/mL[b]	Physically compatible for 3 hr at 22°C	1557	C
Bumetanide	RC	0.04 mg/mL[b]	BW	0.1 mg/mL[b]	Physically compatible for 3 hr at 22°C	1557	C
Buprenorphine HCl	RKC	0.04 mg/mL[b]	BW	0.1 mg/mL[b]	Physically compatible for 3 hr at 22°C	1557	C
Butorphanol tartrate	BR	0.04 mg/mL[b]	BW	0.1 mg/mL[b]	Physically compatible for 3 hr at 22°C	1557	C
Calcium gluconate	AST	40 mg/mL[b]	BW	0.1 mg/mL[b]	Physically compatible for 3 hr at 22°C	1557	C
Carboplatin	BR	5 mg/mL[b]	BW	0.1 mg/mL[b]	Physically compatible for 3 hr at 22°C	1557	C
Carmustine	BR	1.5 mg/mL[b]	BW	0.1 mg/mL[b]	Physically compatible for 3 hr at 22°C	1557	C
Caspofungin acetate	ME	0.7 mg/mL[b]	CAR	1 mg/mL[b]	Physically compatible for 4 hr at room temperature	2758	C
Cefazolin sodium	GEM	20 mg/mL[b]	BW	0.1 mg/mL[b]	Physically compatible for 3 hr at 22°C	1557	C
Cefotaxime sodium	HO	20 mg/mL[b]	BW	0.1 mg/mL[b]	Physically compatible for 3 hr at 22°C	1557	C
Cefotetan disodium	STU	20 mg/mL[b]	BW	0.1 mg/mL[b]	Physically compatible for 3 hr at 22°C	1557	C
Ceftazidime	LI	40 mg/mL[b]	BW	0.1 mg/mL[b]	Physically compatible for 3 hr at 22°C	1557	C
Ceftriaxone sodium	RC	20 mg/mL[b]	BW	0.1 mg/mL[b]	Physically compatible for 3 hr at 22°C	1557	C
Cefuroxime sodium	GL	20 mg/mL[b]	BW	0.1 mg/mL[b]	Physically compatible for 3 hr at 22°C	1557	C
Chlorpromazine HCl	ES	2 mg/mL[b]	BW	0.1 mg/mL[b]	Large increase in measured turbidity occurs within 1 hr and grows over 3 hr	1557	I
Cisplatin	BR	1 mg/mL	BW	0.1 mg/mL[b]	Physically compatible for 3 hr at 22°C	1557	C
Clindamycin phosphate	AB	10 mg/mL[b]	BW	0.1 mg/mL[b]	Physically compatible for 3 hr at 22°C	1557	C
Cyclophosphamide	BR	10 mg/mL[b]	BW	0.1 mg/mL[b]	Physically compatible for 3 hr at 22°C	1557	C
Cytarabine	UP	50 mg/mL	BW	0.1 mg/mL[b]	Physically compatible for 3 hr at 22°C	1557	C
Dacarbazine	MI	4 mg/mL[b]	BW	0.1 mg/mL[b]	Physically compatible for 3 hr at 22°C	1557	C
Dactinomycin	MSD	0.01 mg/mL[b]	BW	0.1 mg/mL[b]	Physically compatible for 3 hr at 22°C	1557	C
Daunorubicin HCl	WY	1 mg/mL[b]	BW	0.1 mg/mL[b]	Physically compatible for 3 hr at 22°C	1557	C
Dexamethasone sodium phosphate	LY	1 mg/mL[b]	BW	0.1 mg/mL[b]	Physically compatible for 3 hr at 22°C	1557	C
Diphenhydramine HCl	WY	2 mg/mL[b]	BW	0.1 mg/mL[b]	Physically compatible for 3 hr at 22°C	1557	C
Doxorubicin HCl	AD	2 mg/mL	BW	0.1 mg/mL[b]	Physically compatible for 3 hr at 22°C	1557	C
Doxycycline hyclate	LY	1 mg/mL[b]	BW	0.1 mg/mL[b]	Physically compatible for 3 hr at 22°C	1557	C
Droperidol	JN	0.4 mg/mL[b]	BW	0.1 mg/mL[b]	Physically compatible for 3 hr at 22°C	1557	C
Enalaprilat	MSD	0.1 mg/mL[b]	BW	0.1 mg/mL[b]	Physically compatible for 3 hr at 22°C	1557	C
Etoposide	BR	0.4 mg/mL[b]	BW	0.1 mg/mL[b]	Physically compatible for 3 hr at 22°C	1557	C

Y-Site Injection Compatibility (1:1 Mixture) (Cont.)

Test Drug	Mfr	Conc	Mfr	Conc	Remarks	Ref	C/I
Famotidine	MSD	2 mg/mL[b]	BW	0.1 mg/mL[b]	Physically compatible for 3 hr at 22°C	1557	C
Filgrastim	AMG	30 mcg/mL[a]	BW	0.1 mg/mL[a]	Physically compatible for 4 hr at 22°C	1687	C
Floxuridine	RC	3 mg/mL[b]	BW	0.1 mg/mL[b]	Physically compatible for 3 hr at 22°C	1557	C
Fluconazole	RR	2 mg/mL	BW	0.1 mg/mL[b]	Physically compatible for 3 hr at 22°C	1557	C
Fludarabine phosphate	BX	1 mg/mL[b]	BW	0.1 mg/mL[b]	Physically compatible for 3 hr at 22°C	1557	C
Fluorouracil	LY	16 mg/mL[b]	BW	0.1 mg/mL[b]	Physically compatible for 3 hr at 22°C	1557	C
Furosemide	AB	3 mg/mL[b]	BW	0.1 mg/mL[b]	Physically compatible for 3 hr at 22°C	1557	C
Gallium nitrate	FUJ	0.4 mg/mL[b]	BW	0.1 mg/mL[b]	Physically compatible for 3 hr at 22°C	1557	C
Ganciclovir sodium	SY	20 mg/mL[b]	BW	0.1 mg/mL[b]	Physically compatible for 3 hr at 22°C	1557	C
Gentamicin sulfate	LY	5 mg/mL[b]	BW	0.1 mg/mL[b]	Physically compatible for 3 hr at 22°C	1557	C
Granisetron HCl	SKB	0.05 mg/mL[a]	BW	0.1 mg/mL[b]	Physically compatible for 4 hr at 23°C	2000	C
Haloperidol lactate	MN	0.2 mg/mL[b]	BW	0.1 mg/mL[b]	Physically compatible for 3 hr at 22°C	1557	C
Heparin sodium	WY	100 units/mL[b]	BW	0.1 mg/mL[b]	Physically compatible for 3 hr at 22°C	1557	C
Hydrocortisone sodium succinate	UP	1 mg/mL[b]	BW	0.1 mg/mL[b]	Physically compatible for 3 hr at 22°C	1557	C
Hydromorphone HCl	KN	0.5 mg/mL[b]	BW	0.1 mg/mL[b]	Physically compatible for 3 hr at 22°C	1557	C
Hydroxyzine HCl	WI	4 mg/mL[b]	BW	0.1 mg/mL[b]	Physically compatible for 3 hr at 22°C	1557	C
Idarubicin HCl	AD	0.5 mg/mL[b]	BW	0.1 mg/mL[b]	Physically compatible for 3 hr at 22°C	1557, 1675	C
Ifosfamide	BR	25 mg/mL[b]	BW	0.1 mg/mL[b]	Physically compatible for 3 hr at 22°C	1557	C
Imipenem–cilastatin sodium	MSD	10 mg/mL[b d]	BW	0.1 mg/mL[b]	Physically compatible for 3 hr at 22°C	1557	C
Lorazepam	WY	0.1 mg/mL[b]	BW	0.1 mg/mL[b]	Physically compatible for 3 hr at 22°C	1557	C
Mannitol	BA	15%	BW	0.1 mg/mL[b]	Physically compatible for 3 hr at 22°C	1557	C
Mechlorethamine HCl	MSD	1 mg/mL	BW	0.1 mg/mL[b]	Physically compatible for 3 hr at 22°C	1557	C
Meperidine HCl	WY	4 mg/mL[b]	BW	0.1 mg/mL[b]	Physically compatible for 3 hr at 22°C	1557	C
Mesna	BR	10 mg/mL[b]	BW	0.1 mg/mL[b]	Physically compatible for 3 hr at 22°C	1557	C
Methotrexate sodium	LE	15 mg/mL[b]	BW	0.1 mg/mL[b]	Physically compatible for 3 hr at 22°C	1557	C
Methylprednisolone sodium succinate	AB	5 mg/mL[b]	BW	0.1 mg/mL[b]	Physically compatible for 3 hr at 22°C	1557	C
Metoclopramide HCl	RB	5 mg/mL	BW	0.1 mg/mL[b]	Physically compatible for 3 hr at 22°C	1557	C
Metronidazole	AB	5 mg/mL	BW	0.1 mg/mL[b]	Physically compatible for 3 hr at 22°C	1557	C
Mitomycin	BR	0.5 mg/mL	BW	0.1 mg/mL[b]	Physically compatible for 3 hr at 22°C	1557	C
Mitoxantrone HCl	LE	0.5 mg/mL[b]	BW	0.1 mg/mL[b]	Physically compatible for 3 hr at 22°C	1557	C
Morphine sulfate	WI	1 mg/mL[b]	BW	0.1 mg/mL[b]	Physically compatible for 3 hr at 22°C	1557	C
Nalbuphine HCl	AST	10 mg/mL	BW	0.1 mg/mL[b]	Physically compatible for 3 hr at 22°C	1557	C
Ondansetron HCl	GL	1 mg/mL[b]	BW	0.1 mg/mL[b]	Physically compatible for 3 hr at 22°C	1557	C
Pentostatin	PD	0.4 mg/mL[b]	BW	0.1 mg/mL[b]	Physically compatible for 3 hr at 22°C	1557	C

Y-Site Injection Compatibility (1:1 Mixture) (Cont.)

Test Drug	Mfr	Conc	Mfr	Conc	Remarks	Ref	C/I
Potassium chloride	AB	0.1 mEq/mL[b]	BW	0.1 mg/mL[b]	Physically compatible for 3 hr at 22°C	1557	C
Prochlorperazine edisylate	SKB	0.5 mg/mL[b]	BW	0.1 mg/mL[b]	Physically compatible for 3 hr at 22°C	1557	C
Promethazine HCl	WY	2 mg/mL[b]	BW	0.1 mg/mL[b]	Physically compatible for 3 hr at 22°C	1557	C
Ranitidine HCl	GL	2 mg/mL[b]	BW	0.1 mg/mL[b]	Physically compatible for 3 hr at 22°C	1557	C
Sodium bicarbonate	AB	1 mEq/mL	BW	0.1 mg/mL[b]	Physically compatible for 3 hr at 22°C	1557	C
Streptozocin	UP	40 mg/mL[b]	BW	0.1 mg/mL[b]	Physically compatible for 3 hr at 22°C	1557	C
Teniposide	BR	0.1 mg/mL[a]	BW	0.1 mg/mL[a]	Physically compatible for 4 hr at 23°C	1725	C
Thiotepa	LE	10 mg/mL[b]	BW	0.1 mg/mL[b]	Physically compatible for 3 hr at 22°C	1557	C
Tobramycin sulfate	LI	5 mg/mL[b]	BW	0.1 mg/mL[b]	Physically compatible for 3 hr at 22°C	1557	C
Trimethoprim–sulfamethoxazole	ES	0.8 mg/mL[b][c]	BW	0.1 mg/mL[b]	Physically compatible for 3 hr at 22°C	1557	C
Vancomycin HCl	LY	10 mg/mL[b]	BW	0.1 mg/mL[b]	Physically compatible for 3 hr at 22°C	1557	C
Vinblastine sulfate	LI	0.12 mg/mL[b]	BW	0.1 mg/mL[b]	Physically compatible for 3 hr at 22°C	1557	C
Vincristine sulfate	LI	0.05 mg/mL[b]	BW	0.1 mg/mL[b]	Physically compatible for 3 hr at 22°C	1557	C
Vinorelbine tartrate	BW	1 mg/mL[b]	BW	0.1 mg/mL[b]	Physically compatible for 4 hr at 22°C	1558	C
Zidovudine	BW	4 mg/mL[b]	BW	0.1 mg/mL[b]	Physically compatible for 3 hr at 22°C	1557	C

[a] Tested in dextrose 5%.

[b] Tested in sodium chloride 0.9%.

[c] Trimethoprim component. Trimethoprim in a 1:5 fixed-ratio concentration with sulfamethoxazole.

[d] Not specified whether concentration refers to single component or combined components.

Selected Revisions September 30, 2019. © Copyright, October 1994. American Society of Health-System Pharmacists, Inc.

Meperidine Hydrochloride

AHFS 28:08.08

Pethidine Hydrochloride

Products

Meperidine hydrochloride is available in concentrations of 10, 25, 50, 75, and 100 mg/mL in a variety of packaging sizes and configurations, including ampuls, vials, and disposable cartridge units.[1(10/06)] Some products also contain an antioxidant such as sodium metabisulfite and antibacterial preservatives such as phenol and metacresol.[4]

pH

The pH is adjusted to 3.5 to 6.[1(10/06)] [4]

Osmolality

The osmolality of meperidine hydrochloride 50 mg/mL was determined to be 302 mOsm/kg.[1233]

Trade Name(s)

Demerol

Administration

Meperidine hydrochloride is administered by intramuscular injection into a large muscle mass. It may also be given subcutaneously or slowly by intravenous injection or infusion in a diluted solution.[1(10/06)] [4] A 10-mg/mL concentration has been recommended for slow intravenous injection. The 10-mg/mL commercial injection does not require further dilution and is for use with a compatible infusion device. Intravenous infusion of a 1-mg/mL concentration has been used to supplement anesthesia.[4]

Stability

Meperidine hydrochloride should be stored at controlled room temperature and protected from light and freezing.[4]

Syringes

Meperidine hydrochloride (Wyeth) 5 and 10 mg/mL in dextrose 5% and sodium chloride 0.9% was packaged in 30-mL Plastipak (Becton Dickinson) syringes capped with Monoject (Sherwood) tip caps. Syringes were stored at 23°C exposed to light and protected from light, 4°C protected from light, and frozen at −20°C protected from light for 12 weeks. Both concentrations at all storage conditions were stable for at least 12 weeks.[1894]

Preservative-free meperidine hydrochloride (Abbott) was diluted to concentrations of 0.25, 1, 10, 20, and 30 mg/mL with dextrose 5% and with sodium chloride 0.9%. The solutions were packaged in 60-mL polypropylene syringes (Becton Dickinson), sealed with Luer lock caps, and stored at 22 and 4°C for 28 days protected from light. The solutions were visually colorless and free of precipitation over the course of the study. Little or no loss of meperidine hydrochloride occurred in either solution at either temperature in 28 days.[2200]

Sorption

Meperidine hydrochloride was shown not to exhibit sorption to PVC bags and tubing, polyethylene tubing, Silastic tubing, and polypropylene syringes.[536] [606]

Central Venous Catheter

Meperidine hydrochloride (Wyeth) 4 mg/mL in dextrose 5% was found to be compatible with the ARROWg+ard Blue Plus (Arrow International) chlorhexidine-bearing triple-lumen central catheter. Essentially complete delivery of the drug was found with little or no drug loss occurring. Furthermore, chlorhexidine delivered from the catheter remained at trace amounts with no substantial increase due to the delivery of the drug through the catheter.[2335]

Compatibility Information

Solution Compatibility

Meperidine HCl

Test Soln Name	Mfr	Mfr	Conc/L or %	Remarks	Ref	C/I
Dextrose 2.5% in half-strength Ringer's injection	AB	WI	100 mg	Physically compatible	3	C
Dextrose 5% in Ringer's injection	AB	WI	100 mg	Physically compatible	3	C
Dextrose 2.5% in Ringer's injection, lactated	AB	WI	100 mg	Physically compatible	3	C
Dextrose 5% in half-strength Ringer's injection, lactated	AB	WI	100 mg	Physically compatible	3	C

DOI: 10.37573/9781585286850.249

Solution Compatibility (Cont.)

Test Soln Name	Mfr	Mfr	Conc/L or %	Remarks	Ref	C/I
Dextrose 5% in Ringer's injection, lactated	AB	WI	100 mg	Physically compatible	3	C
Dextrose 10% in Ringer's injection, lactated	AB	WI	100 mg	Physically compatible	3	C
Dextrose 2.5% in sodium chloride 0.45%	AB	WI	100 mg	Physically compatible	3	C
Dextrose 2.5% in sodium chloride 0.9%	AB	WI	100 mg	Physically compatible	3	C
Dextrose 5% in sodium chloride 0.225%	AB	WI	100 mg	Physically compatible	3	C
Dextrose 5% in sodium chloride 0.45%	AB	WI	100 mg	Physically compatible	3	C
Dextrose 5% in sodium chloride 0.9%	AB	WI	100 mg	Physically compatible	3	C
Dextrose 10% in sodium chloride 0.9%	AB	WI	100 mg	Physically compatible	3	C
Dextrose 2.5%	AB	WI	100 mg	Physically compatible	3	C
Dextrose 5%	AB	WI	100 mg	Physically compatible	3	C
Dextrose 5%	TR[a]	WI	1.2 g	Physically compatible. No loss in 36 hr at 22°C	1000	C
Dextrose 5%		DB	300 mg	Stable for at least 24 hr at 25°C	53	C
Dextrose 10%	AB	WI	100 mg	Physically compatible	3	C
Ionosol B in dextrose 5%	AB	WI	100 mg	Physically compatible	3	C
Ionosol MB in dextrose 5%	AB	WI	100 mg	Physically compatible	3	C
Ringer's injection	AB	WI	100 mg	Physically compatible	3	C
Ringer's injection, lactated	AB	WI	100 mg	Physically compatible	3	C
Sodium chloride 0.18%		DB	300 mg	Stable for at least 24 hr at 25°C	53	C
Sodium chloride 0.45%	AB	WI	100 mg	Physically compatible	3	C
Sodium chloride 0.9%	AB	WI	100 mg	Physically compatible	3	C
Sodium chloride 0.9%	FRE[a]		2.5 g	Visually compatible with little or no loss in 24 days at room temperature	1791	C
Sodium chloride 0.9%		DB	300 mg	Stable for at least 24 hr at 25°C	53	C
Sodium chloride 0.9%	BA	SW	10 g	No loss occurs in 90 days at 37°C in an implantable pump[c]	2246	C
Sodium chloride 0.9%	MAC	AGT	1 and 40 g[d]	Physically compatible with little or no loss in 30 days at room temperature protected from light	2633	C
Sodium lactate ⅙ M	AB	WI	100 mg	Physically compatible	3	C
TPN #71[b]	[a]	WI	100 mg	Physically compatible. No loss in 36 hr at 22°C	1000	C

[a] Tested in PVC containers.

[b] Refer to Appendix for the composition of parenteral nutrition solutions. TPN indicates a 2-in-1 admixture.

[c] Tested in an Infusaid implantable pump.

[d] Tested in Deltec medication cassettes.

Additive Compatibility

Meperidine HCl

Test Drug	Mfr	Conc/L or %	Mfr	Conc/L or %	Test Solution	Remarks	Ref	C/I
Cefazolin sodium	FUJ	10 g		0.5 g	D5W	Visually compatible. 5% loss of each drug in 5 days at 25°C. 5% cefazolin and 7% meperidine loss in 20 days at 4°C	1966	C
Clonidine HCl	BI	3 mg		8 g	NS[a]	Visually compatible with no loss of either drug in 21 days at room temperature	2710	C
Dobutamine HCl	LI	1 g	ES	50 g	D5W, NS	Physically compatible for 24 hr at 21°C	812	C
Eptifibatide	ME	750 mg		10 g		Physically compatible and chemically stable for up to 24 hr at 25°C	3049	C
Floxacillin sodium	BE	20 g	RC	5 g	W	Haze forms immediately and precipitate forms in 5 to 24 hr	1479	I
Furosemide	HO	1 g	RC	5 g	W	Fine precipitate forms immediately	1479	I
Metoclopramide HCl	DW	150 mg	DW	7.35 g	D5W, NS	Visually compatible. Little loss of drugs over 48 hr at 32°C in light or dark	2253	C
Ondansetron HCl	GL	100 mg and 1 g	WY	4 g	NS[a]	Physically compatible. No loss of either drug in 31 days at 4 and 22°C and in 7 days at 32°C	1862	C
Scopolamine HBr		0.43 mg	WI	100 mg		Physically compatible	3	C
Sodium bicarbonate	AB	2.4 mEq[b]	WI	100 mg	D5W	Physically compatible for 24 hr	772	C
Succinylcholine chloride	AB	2 g	WI	100 mg		Physically compatible	3	C
Verapamil HCl	KN	80 mg	WI	150 mg	D5W, NS	Physically compatible for 24 hr	764	C

[a] Tested in PVC containers.

[b] One vial of Neut added to a liter of admixture.

Drugs in Syringe Compatibility

Meperidine HCl

Test Drug	Mfr	Amt	Mfr	Amt	Remarks	Ref	C/I
Atropine sulfate		0.6 mg/1.5 mL	WY	100 mg/1 mL	Physically compatible for at least 15 min	14	C
Atropine sulfate	ST	0.4 mg/1 mL	WI	50 mg/1 mL	Physically compatible for at least 15 min	326	C
Butorphanol tartrate	BR	4 mg/2 mL	WI	50 mg/1 mL	Physically compatible for 30 min at room temperature	566	C
Chlorpromazine HCl	SKF	50 mg/2 mL	WY	100 mg/1 mL	Physically compatible for at least 15 min	14	C
Chlorpromazine HCl	PO	50 mg/2 mL	WI	50 mg/1 mL	Physically compatible for at least 15 min	326	C
Dimenhydrinate	HR	50 mg/1 mL	WI	50 mg/1 mL	Physically compatible for at least 15 min	326	C
Diphenhydramine HCl	PD	50 mg/1 mL	WY	100 mg/1 mL	Physically compatible for at least 15 min	14	C
Diphenhydramine HCl	PD	50 mg/1 mL	WI	50 mg/1 mL	Physically compatible for at least 15 min	326	C
Droperidol	MN	2.5 mg/1 mL	WI	50 mg/1 mL	Physically compatible for at least 15 min	326	C
Fentanyl citrate	MN	0.05 mg/1 mL	WI	50 mg/1 mL	Physically compatible for at least 15 min	326	C

Drugs in Syringe Compatibility (Cont.)

Test Drug	Mfr	Amt	Mfr	Amt	Remarks	Ref	C/I
Glycopyrrolate	RB	0.2 mg/1 mL	WI	50 mg/1 mL	Physically compatible. pH in glycopyrrolate stability range for 48 hr at 25°C	331	C
Glycopyrrolate	RB	0.2 mg/1 mL	WI	100 mg/2 mL	Physically compatible. pH in glycopyrrolate stability range for 48 hr at 25°C	331	C
Glycopyrrolate	RB	0.4 mg/2 mL	WI	50 mg/1 mL	Physically compatible. pH in glycopyrrolate stability range for 48 hr at 25°C	331	C
Heparin sodium		2500 units/1 mL	HO	100 mg/2 mL	Turbidity or precipitate forms within 5 min	1053	I
Hydroxyzine HCl	PF	100 mg/4 mL	WY	100 mg/1 mL	Physically compatible for at least 15 min	14	C
Hydroxyzine HCl	PF	50 mg/1 mL	WI	50 mg/1 mL	Physically compatible for at least 15 min	326	C
Hydroxyzine HCl	PF	50 mg/1 mL	WI	100 mg/2 mL	Physically compatible	771	C
Hydroxyzine HCl	PF	100 mg/2 mL	WI	50 mg/1 mL	Physically compatible	771	C
Ketamine HCl	PD	2 mg/mL	DB	12 mg/mL	Diluted to 50 mL with NS. Visually compatible for 48 hr at 25°C	2059	C
Metoclopramide HCl	NO	10 mg/2 mL	WI	50 mg/1 mL	Physically compatible for 15 min at room temperature	565	C
Metoclopramide HCl	DW	10 mg/2 mL	DW	50 mg/1 mL	Visually compatible. Little loss of either drug over 48 hr at 32°C in light or dark	2253	C
Midazolam HCl	RC	5 mg/1 mL	WB	100 mg/1 mL	Physically compatible for 4 hr at 25°C	1145	C
Morphine sulfate	ST	15 mg/1 mL	WI	50 mg/1 mL	Physically incompatible within 15 min	326	I
Ondansetron HCl	GW	1.33 mg/mL[a]	ES	8.33 mg/mL[a]	Physically compatible. Little loss of either drug in 24 hr at 4 or 23°C	2199	C
Pantoprazole sodium	[b]	4 mg/1 mL		100 mg/1 mL	Yellowish precipitate within 15 min	2574	I
Pentazocine lactate	WI	30 mg/1 mL	WI	50 mg/1 mL	Physically compatible for at least 15 min	326	C
Pentobarbital sodium	WY	100 mg/2 mL	WY	100 mg/1 mL	Precipitate forms within 15 min	14	I
Pentobarbital sodium	AB	500 mg/10 mL	WI	100 mg/2 mL	Physically incompatible	55	I
Pentobarbital sodium	AB	50 mg/1 mL	WI	50 mg/1 mL	Physically incompatible within 15 min	326	I
Prochlorperazine edisylate	SKF		WY	100 mg/1 mL	Physically compatible for at least 15 min	14	C
Prochlorperazine edisylate	PO	5 mg/1 mL	WI	50 mg/1 mL	Physically compatible for at least 15 min	326	C
Promethazine HCl	WY	50 mg/2 mL	WY	100 mg/1 mL	Physically compatible for at least 15 min	14	C
Promethazine HCl	PO	50 mg/2 mL	WI	50 mg/1 mL	Physically compatible for at least 15 min	326	C
Ranitidine HCl	GL	50 mg/2 mL	WI	100 mg/1 mL	Physically compatible for 1 hr at 25°C	978	C
Scopolamine HBr		0.6 mg/1.5 mL	WY	100 mg/1 mL	Physically compatible for at least 15 min	14	C
Scopolamine HBr	ST	0.4 mg/1 mL	WI	50 mg/1 mL	Physically compatible for at least 15 min	326	C

[a] Tested in sodium chloride 0.9%.

[b] Test performed using the formulation WITHOUT edetate disodium.

Y-Site Injection Compatibility (1:1 Mixture)

Meperidine HCl

Test Drug	Mfr	Conc	Mfr	Conc	Remarks	Ref	C/I
Acetaminophen	CAD	10 mg/mL	HOS	50 mg/mL	Physically compatible for 4 hr at 23°C	2901, 2902	C
Acetaminophen	CAD	10 mg/mL	HOS	100 mg/mL	Physically compatible with less than 10% acetaminophen loss over 4 hr at room temperature	2841, 2844	C
Acyclovir sodium	BW	5 mg/mL[a]	WB	1 mg/mL[a]	Physically compatible for 4 hr at 25°C	1157	C
Acyclovir sodium	BW	5 mg/mL[a]	AB	10 mg/mL	White crystalline precipitate forms within 1 hr at 25°C	1397	I
Acyclovir sodium	BW	5 mg/mL[a b]	WY	100 mg/mL	Visually compatible for 24 hr at room temperature in test tubes. No precipitate found on filter from Y-site delivery	2063	C
Allopurinol sodium	BW	3 mg/mL[b]	WY	4 mg/mL[b]	Tiny particles form immediately and increase in number over 4 hr	1686	I
Amifostine	USB	10 mg/mL[a]	WY	4 mg/mL[a]	Physically compatible for 4 hr at 23°C	1845	C
Amikacin sulfate	BR	5 mg/mL[a]	WY	10 mg/mL[a]	Physically compatible for 4 hr at 25°C	987	C
Ampicillin sodium	BR	20 mg/mL[b]	WY	10 mg/mL[a]	Physically compatible for 4 hr at 25°C	987	C
Ampicillin sodium–sulbactam sodium	RR	20 mg/mL[b k]	WY	10 mg/mL[b]	Physically compatible for 1 hr at 25°C	1338	C
Anidulafungin	VIC	0.5 mg/mL[a]	AB	10 mg/mL[a]	Physically compatible for 4 hr at 23°C	2617	C
Aztreonam	SQ	20 mg/mL[a]	AB	10 mg/mL	Physically compatible for 4 hr at 25°C	1397	C
Aztreonam	SQ	40 mg/mL[a]	WY	4 mg/mL[a]	Physically compatible for 4 hr at 23°C	1758	C
Bivalirudin	TMC	5 mg/mL[a]	AST	10 mg/mL[a]	Physically compatible for 4 hr at 23°C	2373	C
Bumetanide	RC	0.25 mg/mL	AB	10 mg/mL	Physically compatible for 4 hr at 25°C	1397	C
Cangrelor tetrasodium	TMC	1 mg/mL[b]		4 mg/mL[b]	Physically compatible for 4 hr	3243	C
Caspofungin acetate	ME	0.7 mg/mL[b]	HOS	10 mg/mL[b]	Physically compatible for 4 hr at room temperature	2758	C
Cefazolin sodium	SKF	20 mg/mL[a]	WY	10 mg/mL[a]	Physically compatible for 4 hr at 25°C	987	C
Cefotaxime sodium	HO	20 mg/mL[a]	WY	10 mg/mL[a]	Physically compatible for 4 hr at 25°C	987	C
Cefotetan disodium	STU	20 and 40 mg/mL[a]	WY	10 mg/mL[b]	Physically compatible for 1 hr at 25°C	1338	C
Cefoxitin sodium	MSD	20 mg/mL[a]	WY	10 mg/mL[a]	Physically compatible for 4 hr at 25°C	987	C
Cefoxitin sodium	MSD	40 mg/mL[a]	WY	10 mg/mL[b]	Physically compatible for 1 hr at 25°C	1338	C
Ceftaroline fosamil	FOR	2.22 mg/mL[a b c]	HOS	10 mg/mL[a b c]	Physically compatible for 4 hr at 23°C	2826	C
Ceftazidime	LI	20 and 40 mg/mL[a]	AB	10 mg/mL	Physically compatible for 4 hr at 25°C	1397	C
Ceftolozane sulfate–tazobactam sodium	CUB	10 mg/mL[p q]	WW	10 mg/mL[p]	Physically compatible for 2 hr	3262	C
Ceftriaxone sodium	RC	20 and 40 mg/mL[a]	AB	10 mg/mL	Physically compatible for 4 hr at 25°C	1397	C
Cefuroxime sodium	GL	30 mg/mL[a]	WY	10 mg/mL[a]	Physically compatible for 4 hr at 25°C	987	C
Chloramphenicol sodium succinate	LY	20 mg/mL[a]	WY	10 mg/mL[a]	Physically compatible for 4 hr at 25°C	987	C
Cisatracurium besylate	GW	0.1, 2, 5 mg/mL[a]	AST	4 mg/mL[a]	Physically compatible for 4 hr at 23°C	2074	C

Y-Site Injection Compatibility (1:1 Mixture) (Cont.)

Test Drug	Mfr	Conc	Mfr	Conc	Remarks	Ref	C/I
Cladribine	ORT	0.015[b] and 0.5[e] mg/mL	WY	4 mg/mL[b]	Physically compatible for 4 hr at 23°C	1969	C
Clindamycin phosphate	UP	12 mg/mL[a]	WY	10 mg/mL[a]	Physically compatible for 4 hr at 25°C	987	C
Dexamethasone sodium phosphate	LY	0.2 mg/mL[a]	AB	10 mg/mL	Physically compatible for 4 hr at 25°C	1397	C
Dexmedetomidine HCl	AB	4 mcg/mL[b]	AST	10 mg/mL[b]	Physically compatible for 4 hr at 23°C	2383	C
Digoxin	BW	0.25 mg/mL	AB	10 mg/mL	Physically compatible for 4 hr at 25°C	1397	C
Diltiazem HCl	MMD	1[b] and 5 mg/mL	WY	100 mg/mL	Visually compatible	1807	C
Diltiazem HCl	MMD	5 mg/mL	WY	10 mg/mL[b]	Visually compatible	1807	C
Diphenhydramine HCl	ES	1[a] and 50 mg/mL	AB	10 mg/mL	Physically compatible for 4 hr at 25°C	1397	C
Dobutamine HCl	LI	1 mg/mL	AB	10 mg/mL	Physically compatible for 4 hr at 25°C	1397	C
Docetaxel	RPR	0.9 mg/mL[a]	AST	4 mg/mL[a]	Physically compatible for 4 hr at 23°C	2224	C
Dopamine HCl	AB	1.6 mg/mL	AB	10 mg/mL	Physically compatible for 4 hr at 25°C	1397	C
Doripenem	JJ	5 mg/mL[a b]	HOS	10 mg/mL[a b]	Physically compatible for 4 hr at 23°C	2743	C
Doxorubicin HCl liposomal	SEQ	0.4 mg/mL[a]	AST	4 mg/mL[a]	Increase in measured turbidity	2087	I
Doxycycline hyclate	ES	1 mg/mL[a]	WY	10 mg/mL[a]	Physically compatible for 4 hr at 25°C	987	C
Droperidol	AMR	2.5 mg/mL[a]	AB	10 mg/mL	Physically compatible for 4 hr at 25°C	1397	C
Erythromycin lactobionate	AB	5 mg/mL[a]	WY	10 mg/mL[a]	Physically compatible for 4 hr at 25°C	987	C
Etoposide phosphate	BR	5 mg/mL[a]	AST	4 mg/mL[a]	Physically compatible for 4 hr at 23°C	2218	C
Famotidine	MSD	0.2 mg/mL[a]	AB	10 mg/mL	Physically compatible for 4 hr at 25°C	1397	C
Famotidine	ME	2 mg/mL[b]		4 mg/mL[a]	Visually compatible for 4 hr at 22°C	1936	C
Fenoldopam mesylate	AB	80 mcg/mL[b]	AB	4 mg/mL[b]	Physically compatible for 4 hr at 23°C	2467	C
Filgrastim	AMG	30 mcg/mL[a]	WY	4 mg/mL[a]	Physically compatible for 4 hr at 22°C	1687	C
Fluconazole	RR	2 mg/mL	AB	10 mg/mL	Physically compatible for 4 hr at 25°C	1397	C
Fludarabine phosphate	BX	1 mg/mL[a]	WI	4 mg/mL[a]	Visually compatible for 4 hr at 22°C	1439	C
Furosemide	ES	0.8 mg/mL[a]	AB	10 mg/mL	Physically compatible for 4 hr at 25°C	1397	C
Furosemide	ES	2.4 mg/mL[a]	AB	10 mg/mL	White cloudiness forms immediately	1397	I
Furosemide	ES	10 mg/mL	AB	10 mg/mL	White precipitate forms immediately	1397	I
Gallium nitrate	FUJ	1 mg/mL[b]	WY	50 mg/mL	Visually compatible for 24 hr at 25°C	1673	C
Gemcitabine HCl	LI	10 mg/mL[b]	AST	4 mg/mL[b]	Physically compatible for 4 hr at 23°C	2226	C
Gentamicin sulfate	TR	0.8 mg/mL[a]	WY	10 mg/mL[a]	Physically compatible for 4 hr at 25°C	987	C
Gentamicin sulfate	ES	1.2 and 2 mg/mL[b]	WY	10 mg/mL[b]	Physically compatible for 1 hr at 25°C	1338	C
Granisetron HCl	SKB	0.05 mg/mL[a]	WY	4 mg/mL[a]	Physically compatible for 4 hr at 23°C	2000	C
Heparin sodium	ES	60 units/mL[a]	WY	10 mg/mL[b]	Physically compatible for 1 hr at 25°C	1338	C
Hetastarch in lactated electrolyte	AB	6%	OHM	4 mg/mL[a]	Physically compatible for 4 hr at 23°C	2339	C
Hydrocortisone sodium succinate	AB	2 mg/mL[a]	AB	10 mg/mL	Physically compatible for 4 hr at 25°C	1397	C

Y-Site Injection Compatibility (1:1 Mixture) (Cont.)

Test Drug	Mfr	Conc	Mfr	Conc	Remarks	Ref	C/I
Hydroxyethyl starch 130/0.4 in sodium chloride 0.9%	FRK	6%	SZ	1, 5, 10 mg/mL[a]	Visually compatible for 24 hr at room temperature	2770	C
Idarubicin HCl	AD	1 mg/mL[b]	WY	1[a] and 50 mg/mL	Color changes immediately	1525	I
Imipenem–cilastatin sodium	MSD	5 mg/mL[a] [n]	AB	10 mg/mL	Yellow color forms in 2 hr at 25°C	1397	I
Insulin, regular	LI	0.2 unit/mL[b]	WY	10 mg/mL[b]	Physically compatible for 1 hr at 25°C	1338	C
Insulin, regular	LI	0.2 unit/mL[b]	AST	50 mg/mL[a]	Physically compatible for 2 hr at 25°C	1395	C
Isavuconazonium sulfate	ASP	1.5 mg/mL[p]	WW	10 mg/mL[p]	Physically compatible for 2 hr	3263	C
Labetalol HCl	GL	5 mg/mL	AB	10 mg/mL	Physically compatible for 4 hr at 25°C	1397	C
Lidocaine HCl	AB	1 mg/mL[a]	AB	10 mg/mL	Physically compatible for 4 hr at 25°C	1397	C
Linezolid	PHU	2 mg/mL	AST	4 mg/mL[a]	Physically compatible for 4 hr at 23°C	2264	C
Magnesium sulfate	LY	16.7, 33.3, 50, 100 mg/mL[a]	WI	10 mg/mL[a]	Visually compatible for 4 hr at 25°C	1549	C
Melphalan HCl	BW	0.1 mg/mL[b]	WY	4 mg/mL[b]	Physically compatible for 3 hr at 22°C	1557	C
Meropenem–vaborbactam	TMC	8 mg/mL[b] [o]	WW	10 mg/mL[b]	Physically compatible for 3 hr at 20 to 25°C	3380	C
Methyldopate HCl	AMR	2.5 mg/mL[a]	AB	10 mg/mL	Physically compatible for 4 hr at 25°C	1397	C
Methylprednisolone sodium succinate	UP	2.5 mg/mL[a]	AB	10 mg/mL	Physically compatible for 4 hr at 25°C	1397	C
Metoclopramide HCl	SN	0.2 mg/mL[a]	AB	10 mg/mL	Physically compatible for 4 hr at 25°C	1397	C
Metoprolol tartrate	CI	1 mg/mL	AB	10 mg/mL	Physically compatible for 4 hr at 25°C	1397	C
Metronidazole	SE	5 mg/mL	WY	10 mg/mL[a]	Physically compatible for 4 hr at 25°C	987	C
Micafungin sodium	ASP	1.5 mg/mL[b]	AB	10 mg/mL[b]	Milky precipitate forms immediately	2683	I
Nafcillin sodium	WY	20 mg/mL[a]	WY	10 mg/mL[a]	Cloudy haze cleared on mixing and remained clear for 4 hr at 25°C	987	?
Nafcillin sodium	WY	20 and 30 mg/mL[a]	WY	10 mg/mL[b]	Cloudy solution formed immediately and persisted for at least 1 hr at 25°C	1338	I
Nesiritide	SCI	50 mcg/mL[a] [b]		100 mg/mL	Physically compatible for 4 hr. May be chemically incompatible with nesiritide[f]	2625	?
Ondansetron HCl	GL	1 mg/mL[b]	WI	4 mg/mL[a]	Visually compatible for 4 hr at 22°C	1365	C
Oxacillin sodium	BE	20 mg/mL[a]	WY	10 mg/mL[a]	Physically compatible for 4 hr at 25°C	987	C
Oxaliplatin	SS	0.5 mg/mL[a]	AB	10 mg/mL[a]	Physically compatible for 4 hr at 23°C	2566	C
Oxytocin	PD	0.02 unit/mL[h]	WY	10 mg/mL[b]	Physically compatible for 1 hr at 25°C	1338	C
Paclitaxel	NCI	1.2 mg/mL[a]	WY	4 mg/mL[a]	Physically compatible for 4 hr at 22°C	1556	C
Palonosetron HCl	MGI	50 mcg/mL	AB	10 mg/mL[a]	Physically compatible. No loss of either drug in 4 hr	2720	C
Pemetrexed disodium	LI	20 mg/mL[b]	AB	10 mg/mL[a]	Physically compatible for 4 hr at 23°C	2564	C
Penicillin G potassium	PF	100,000 units/mL[a]	WY	10 mg/mL[a]	Physically compatible for 4 hr at 25°C	987	C
Piperacillin sodium–tazobactam sodium	LE[d]	40 mg/mL[a] [l]	WY	4 mg/mL[a]	Physically compatible for 4 hr at 22°C	1688	C

Y-Site Injection Compatibility (1:1 Mixture) (Cont.)

Test Drug	Mfr	Conc	Mfr	Conc	Remarks	Ref	C/I
Plazomicin sulfate	ACH	24 mg/mL^p	WW	10 mg/mL^p	Physically compatible for 1 hr at 20 to 25°C	3432	C
Potassium chloride	AB	0.4 mEq/mL^a	AB	10 mg/mL	Physically compatible for 4 hr at 25°C	1397	C
Propofol	ZEN^r	10 mg/mL	WY	4 mg/mL^a	Physically compatible for 1 hr at 23°C	2066	C
Propranolol HCl	WY	1 mg/mL	AB	10 mg/mL	Physically compatible for 4 hr at 25°C	1397	C
Ranitidine HCl	GL	0.5 mg/mL^i	WY	10 mg/mL^b	Physically compatible for 1 hr at 25°C	1338	C
Remifentanil HCl	GW	0.025 and 0.25 mg/mL^b	AST	4 mg/mL^a	Physically compatible for 4 hr at 23°C	2075	C
Sargramostim	IMM	10 mcg/mL^b	WI	4 mg/mL^b	Visually compatible for 4 hr at 22°C	1436	C
Tedizolid phosphate	CUB	0.8 mg/mL^b	WW	10 mg/mL^b	Physically compatible for 2 hr	3244	C
Teniposide	BR	0.1 mg/mL^a	WY	4 mg/mL^a	Physically compatible for 4 hr at 23°C	1725	C
Thiotepa	IMM^j	1 mg/mL^a	WY	4 mg/mL^a	Physically compatible for 4 hr at 23°C	1861	C
TNA #218 to #226^g			AST	4 mg/mL^a	Visually compatible for 4 hr at 23°C	2215	C
Tobramycin sulfate	DI	0.8 mg/mL^a	WY	10 mg/mL^a	Physically compatible for 4 hr at 25°C	987	C
Tobramycin sulfate	LI	1.6, 2, 2.4 mg/mL^a	WY	10 mg/mL^b	Physically compatible for 1 hr at 25°C	1338	C
TPN #131, #132^g			AB	10 mg/mL	Physically compatible for 4 hr at 25°C	1397	C
TPN #189^g			DB	50 mg/mL	Visually compatible for 24 hr at 22°C	1767	C
TPN #212 to #215^g			AST	4 mg/mL^a	Physically compatible for 4 hr at 23°C	2109	C
Trimethoprim–sulfamethoxazole	BW	0.8 mg/mL$^{a\ m}$	WY	10 mg/mL^a	Physically compatible for 4 hr at 25°C	987	C
Vancomycin HCl	LI	5 mg/mL^a	WY	10 mg/mL^a	Physically compatible for 4 hr at 25°C	987	C
Verapamil HCl	DU	2.5 mg/mL	AB	10 mg/mL	Physically compatible for 4 hr at 25°C	1397	C
Vinorelbine tartrate	BW	1 mg/mL^b	WY	4 mg/mL^b	Physically compatible for 4 hr at 22°C	1558	C

^{a} Tested in dextrose 5%.

^{b} Tested in sodium chloride 0.9%.

^{c} Tested in Ringer's injection, lactated.

^{d} Test performed using the formulation WITHOUT edetate disodium.

^{e} Tested in bacteriostatic sodium chloride 0.9% preserved with benzyl alcohol 0.9%.

^{f} Nesiritide is incompatible with bisulfite antioxidants used in some drug formulations. The specific formulation of the product to be used should be checked to ensure that no sulfite antioxidants are present.

^{g} Refer to Appendix for the composition of parenteral nutrition solutions. TNA indicates a 3-in-1 admixture, and TPN indicates a 2-in-1 admixture.

^{h} Tested in dextrose 5% in Ringer's injection, lactated.

^{i} Tested in sodium chloride 0.45%.

^{j} Lyophilized formulation tested.

^{k} Ampicillin component. Ampicillin in a 2:1 fixed-ratio concentration with sulbactam.

^{l} Piperacillin component. Piperacillin in an 8:1 fixed-ratio concentration with tazobactam.

^{m} Trimethoprim component. Trimethoprim in a 1:5 fixed-ratio concentration with sulfamethoxazole.

^{n} Not specified whether concentration refers to single component or combined components.

^{o} Meropenem component. Meropenem in a 1:1 fixed-ratio concentration with vaborbactam.

^{p} Tested in both dextrose 5% and sodium chloride 0.9%.

^{q} Ceftolozane component. Ceftolozane in a 2:1 fixed-ratio concentration with tazobactam.

^{r} Test performed using the formulation WITH edetate disodium.

Additional Compatibility Information

Chlorpromazine and Hydroxyzine

Chlorpromazine hydrochloride (Elkins-Sinn) 6.25 mg/mL, hydroxyzine hydrochloride (Pfizer) 12.5 mg/mL, and meperidine hydrochloride (Winthrop) 25 mg/mL, in both glass and plastic syringes, have been reported to be physically compatible and chemically stable for at least 1 year at 4 and 25°C when protected from light.[989]

Chlorpromazine and Promethazine

Chlorpromazine hydrochloride, meperidine hydrochloride, and promethazine hydrochloride combined as an extemporaneous mixture for preoperative sedation, developed a brownish-yellow color after 2 weeks of storage with protection from light. The discoloration was attributed to the metacresol preservative content of the meperidine hydrochloride product used. Use of meperidine hydrochloride which contains a different preservative resulted in a solution that remained clear and colorless for at least 3 months when protected from light.[1148]

Mepivacaine Hydrochloride
AHFS 72:00

Products

Mepivacaine hydrochloride is available in concentrations of 1, 1.5, and 2%. Methylparaben is incorporated into multiple-dose containers, but single-dose containers may be preservative free. The pH may have been adjusted with sodium hydroxide and/or hydrochloric acid.[1(5/06)] [4]

pH

From 4.5 to 6.8.[1(5/06)] [4]

Osmolality

Mepivacaine hydrochloride injections are isotonic.[1(5/06)]

Trade Name(s)

Carbocaine, Polocaine, Polocaine-MPF

Administration

Mepivacaine hydrochloride may be administered by infiltration and by peripheral or sympathetic nerve block. Mepivacaine hydrochloride *without* preservatives may be administered by epidural block, including caudal anesthesia; forms containing preservatives should not be administered by this route[4].

Stability

Mepivacaine hydrochloride in intact containers should be stored at controlled room temperature and protected from temperatures above 40°C and from freezing. Mepivacaine hydrochloride is resistant to hydrolysis and may be autoclaved repeatedly.[1(5/06)] [4] However, mepivacaine hydrochloride in dental cartridges should not be subjected to autoclaving because of breakdown of the dental cartridge closures.[4]

Syringes

The stability of mepivacaine (salt form unspecified) 10 mg/mL repackaged in polypropylene syringes was evaluated. Little change in concentration was found after four weeks of storage at room temperature not exposed to direct light.[2164]

Compatibility Information

Drugs in Syringe Compatibility

Mepivacaine HCl

Test Drug	Mfr	Amt	Mfr	Amt	Remarks	Ref	C/I
Sodium bicarbonate	AB	4%; 1, 2, 4 mL	AST, WI	1 and 1.5%/20 mL	Precipitate forms within approximately 1 hr	1724	I
Sodium bicarbonate	AST	8.4%; 0.5, 1, 2 mL	AST, WI	1 and 1.5%/20 mL	Precipitate forms within approximately 1 hr	1724	I

Selected Revisions October 1, 2012. © Copyright, October 2000.
American Society of Health-System Pharmacists, Inc.

DOI: 10.37573/9781585286850.250

Meropenem
AHFS 8:12.07.08

Products

Meropenem is available as a dry powder in single-use 20- and 30-mL vials containing 500 mg and 1 g, respectively, of meropenem (as the trihydrate).[3102] Vials also contain anhydrous sodium carbonate.[3102]

For intravenous bolus injection administration, the 500-mg and 1-g vials should be reconstituted with 10 and 20 mL, respectively, of sterile water for injection.[3102] Vials should be shaken to dissolve the vial contents and allowed to stand until the solution is clear.[3102] Each mL of the resultant solution contains approximately 50 mg of meropenem.[3102]

For intravenous infusion administration, vials may be reconstituted directly with a compatible infusion solution.[3102] Alternatively, the appropriate dose of the reconstituted meropenem solution may be transferred to an intravenous container and further diluted with an appropriate infusion solution (e.g., sodium chloride 0.9%, dextrose 5%).[3102]

For intravenous infusion, meropenem also is available in dual-chamber single-use flexible containers containing 500 mg or 1 g of meropenem (as the trihydrate) with sodium carbonate.[3103] The diluent chamber contains 50 mL of sodium chloride 0.9%.[3103] If meropenem doses less than the full dose supplied in the container are needed, the manufacturer states that these containers should not be used.[3103] Specific product labeling should be consulted for instructions on reconstitution (activation) of the dual-chamber container.[3103]

pH

The freshly reconstituted solution has a pH ranging from 7.3 to 8.3.[3102 3103]

Osmolality

Meropenem 500 mg or 1 g in dual-chamber single-use flexible containers has an osmolality of approximately 356 or 417 mOsm/kg, respectively, when activated with the sodium chloride 0.9% diluent.[3103]

Sodium Content

Each gram of meropenem in single-use vials provides 3.92 mEq (90.2 mg) of sodium from the sodium carbonate present in the formulation.[3102]

After reconstitution with the sodium chloride 0.9% diluent, each dual-chamber container of meropenem 500 mg or 1 g provides 10.7 mEq (245.1 mg) or 12.6 mEq (290.2 mg), respectively, of sodium.[3103]

Trade Name(s)

Merrem I.V.

Administration

Meropenem is administered by intravenous bolus injection of 5 to 20 mL over 3 to 5 minutes[3102] or by intravenous infusion diluted in a compatible infusion solution over 15 to 30 minutes.[3102 3103]

Extended infusion strategies for meropenem have been examined in the literature;[2261 2568 3104 3105 3106] however, the poor stability of the drug, particularly at room temperature, typically limits the use of such strategies.[2261 3105]

Stability

Intact vials of meropenem should be stored at a controlled room temperature of 20 to 25°C.[3102] The drug is a white to pale yellow powder that yields a colorless to yellow solution depending on the concentration.[3102]

For intravenous bolus administration, the manufacturer indicates that solutions of meropenem reconstituted in vials with sterile water for injection at concentrations of up to 50 mg/mL are stable for up to 3 hours at temperatures of up to 25°C and for 13 hours at temperatures of up to 5°C.[3102]

For administration by intravenous infusion, meropenem solutions in sodium chloride 0.9% at a concentration of 1 to 20 mg/mL are stated to be stable for 1 hour at temperatures of up to 25°C or 15 hours at temperatures of up to 5°C.[3102] Intravenous infusion solutions prepared in dextrose 5% at these concentrations should be used immediately.[3102]

Unactivated, dual-chamber meropenem containers should be stored at a controlled room temperature of 20 to 25°C.[3103] Once the foil strip has been removed from the drug chamber, the product must be protected from light and used within 7 days or the labeled expiration date, whichever occurs first.[3103] Once reconstituted (activated), the drug should be used within 1 hour if stored at room temperatures of up to 25°C or 15 hours if stored under refrigeration at temperatures of up to 5°C.[3103]

Meropenem 50 mg/mL reconstituted with sodium chloride 0.9% is reported to reach 10% loss in 4.8 hours at 25°C.[2697]

Meropenem (AstraZeneca) 1 g reconstituted with 20 mL of water for injection and diluted with 50 mL of sodium chloride 0.9% was stored in polyvinyl chloride (PVC) infusion bags.[3517] Yellow discoloration was observed after 7 hours in solutions stored at 33°C and after 12 hours in solutions stored at 22°C.[3517]

Concentration Effects

Degradation of meropenem is concentration dependent.[3104 3106 3298] Meropenem has demonstrated improved stability in solution at concentrations of 40 g/L or lower.[3104 3106]

In one study, reconstituting meropenem with sterile water for injection to concentrations exceeding 64 g/L resulted in unacceptably viscous solutions that impeded flow from elastomeric pumps to less than 75% of the nominal flow rate.[3105]

Temperature Effects

Degradation of meropenem also is temperature dependent.[3104 3105 3106] Meropenem has demonstrated improved stability in solution at temperatures less than or equal to 25°C.[3104] [3105] [3106] Meropenem (AstraZeneca) 5 mg/mL in sodium chloride 0.9% exceeded 10% drug loss by 12, 8, and 6 hours at temperatures of 30, 35, and 40°C, respectively.[3109]

Freezing Solutions

Manufacturers state that solutions of meropenem should not be frozen.[3102] [3103]

Syringes

Meropenem (AstraZeneca; Fresenius Kabi; Hospira; Sandoz) was diluted to concentrations of 10, 20, and 40 mg/mL in sodium chloride 0.9% and stored in polypropylene syringes (Becton Dickinson).[3298] Solutions containing meropenem 10 and 20 mg/mL were stable for 12 hours at 25°C; solutions containing meropenem 40 mg/mL were stable for 8 hours at 25°C.[3298]

Central Venous Catheter

Meropenem (Zeneca) 5 mg/mL in sodium chloride 0.9% was found to be compatible with the ARROWg+ard Blue Plus (Arrow International) chlorhexidine-bearing triple-lumen central catheter. Essentially complete delivery of the drug was found with little or no drug loss occurring. Furthermore, chlorhexidine delivered from the catheter remained at trace amounts with no substantial increase due to the delivery of the drug through the catheter.[2335]

Compatibility Information

Solution Compatibility

Meropenem

Test Soln Name	Mfr	Mfr	Conc/L or %	Remarks	Ref	C/I
Dextrose 5% in Ringer's injection, lactated	BA[a]	ZEN	1 g	11% loss in 8 hr at 24°C and 4 to 10% loss in 48 hr at 4°C	2089	I[c]
Dextrose 5% in Ringer's injection, lactated	BA[a]	ZEN	20 g	15% loss in 4 hr at 24°C and 10% loss in 18 hr at 4°C	2089	I[c]
Dextrose 2.5% in sodium chloride 0.45%	BA[a]	ZEN	1 g	10% loss in 6 hr at 24°C and 7% loss in 24 hr at 4°C	2089	I[c]
Dextrose 2.5% in sodium chloride 0.45%	BA[a]	ZEN	20 g	8% loss in 4 hr at 24°C and 7% loss in 24 hr at 4°C	2089	I[c]
Dextrose 5% in sodium chloride 0.225%	BA[a]	ZEN	1 g	10 to 11% loss in 4 hr at 24°C and in 16 hr at 4°C	2089	I[c]
Dextrose 5% in sodium chloride 0.225%	BA[a]	ZEN	20 g	Up to 10% loss in 3 hr at 24°C and 9% loss in 18 hr at 4°C	2089	I[c]
Dextrose 5% in sodium chloride 0.9%	BA[a]	ZEN	1 g	11 to 13% loss in 4 hr at 24°C and in 14 hr at 4°C	2089	I[c]
Dextrose 5% in sodium chloride 0.9%	BA[a]	ZEN	20 g	9 to 11% loss in 3 hr at 24°C and in 14 hr at 4°C	2089	I[c]
Dextrose 5%	BA[a]	ZEN	1 g	9% loss in 4 hr at 24°C and in 14 hr at 4°C	2089	I[c]
Dextrose 5%	BA[b]	ZEN	2.5 g	6 to 7% loss in 4 hr at 24°C and 8 to 10% loss in 24 hr at 4°C	2089	I[c]
Dextrose 5%	BA[a]	ZEN	20 g	11 to 12% loss in 4 hr at 24°C and in 18 hr at 4°C	2089	I[c]
Dextrose 5%	BA[b]	ZEN	50 g	9 to 10% loss in 3 hr at 24°C and in 24 hr at 4°C	2089	I[c]
Dextrose 5%	BA[a i]	ZEN	1 g	10 to 11% loss in 4 hr at 24°C and in 18 hr at 4°C	2089	I[c]
Dextrose 5%	BA[a i]	ZEN	20 g	8 to 10% loss in 3 hr at 24°C and in 18 hr at 4°C	2089	I[c]
Dextrose 5%	BA[a j]	ZEN	1 g	11% loss in 4 hr at 24°C and 9% loss in 18 hr at 4°C	2089	I[c]
Dextrose 5%	BA[a j]	ZEN	20 g	10 to 12% loss in 3 hr at 24°C and 10% loss in 20 hr at 4°C	2089	I[c]
Dextrose 5%	[a]	ZEN	1 g	Visually compatible. Calculated time to 10% loss in 4.5 hr at 23°C, 1.8 days at 4°C, and 1.2 days at −20°C	2492	I
Dextrose 5%	[a]	ZEN	22 g	Visually compatible. Calculated time to 10% loss in 8 hr at 23°C, 2.1 days at 4°C, and 7.8 days at −20°C	2492	I

Solution Compatibility (Cont.)

Test Soln Name	Mfr	Mfr	Conc/L or %	Remarks	Ref	C/I
Dextrose 10%	BA[a]	ZEN	1 g	10 to 12% loss in 3 hr at 24°C and in 8 hr at 4°C	2089	I[c]
Dextrose 10%	BA[a]	ZEN	20 g	9 to 10% loss in 2 hr at 24°C and in 8 hr at 4°C	2089	I[c]
Normosol M in dextrose 5%	AB[a]	ZEN	1 g	5% loss in 8 hr at 24°C and 4% loss in 48 hr at 4°C	2089	I[c]
Normosol M in dextrose 5%	AB[a]	ZEN	20 g	10% loss in 3 hr at 24°C and 7 to 8% loss in 24 hr at 4°C	2089	I[c]
Ringer's injection	BA[a]	ZEN	1 g	6% loss in 10 hr at 24°C and 4 to 5% loss in 48 hr at 4°C	2089	I[c]
Ringer's injection	BA[a]	ZEN	20 g	7% loss in 8 hr at 24°C and 7% loss in 48 hr at 4°C	2089	I[c]
Ringer's injection, lactated	BA[a]	ZEN	1 g	10 to 12% loss in 10 hr at 24°C and 9% loss in 48 hr at 4°C	2089	I[c]
Ringer's injection, lactated	BA[a]	ZEN	20 g	9% loss in 8 hr at 24°C and 7% loss in 48 hr at 4°C	2089	I[c]
Sodium chloride 0.45%	AB[d]	ZEN	5 g	9 to 10% loss in 22 hr at 24°C and 3% loss in 48 hr at 4°C	2089	I[c]
Sodium chloride 0.45%	AB[d]	ZEN	20 g	6 to 8% loss in 10 hr at 24°C and 5 to 6% loss in 48 hr at 4°C	2089	I[c]
Sodium chloride 0.9%	BA[a]	ZEN	1 g	8 to 10% loss in 20 hr at 24°C and 3 to 4% loss in 48 hr at 4°C	2089	I[c]
Sodium chloride 0.9%	BA[b]	ZEN	2.5 g	10% loss in 24 hr at 24°C and 2% loss in 48 hr at 4°C	2089	C
Sodium chloride 0.9%	BA[a]	ZEN	20 g	8% loss in 10 hr at 24°C and 5 to 7% loss in 48 hr at 4°C	2089	I[c]
Sodium chloride 0.9%	BA[b]	ZEN	50 g	9 to 10% loss in 8 hr at 24°C and in 48 hr at 4°C	2089	I[c]
Sodium chloride 0.9%	[e]	ZEN	20 and 30 g	Less than 3% loss in 24 hr when kept at less than 5°C	2261	C
Sodium chloride 0.9%	[h]	ZEN	5 g	Visually compatible. Calculated time to 10% loss was 34 hr at 24°C	2152	C
Sodium chloride 0.9%	[h]	ZEN	5 g	11% loss in 120 hr at 5°C	2152	I
Sodium chloride 0.9%	[h]	ZEN	10 g	Visually compatible. Calculated time to 10% loss was 20 hr at 24°C	2152	C
Sodium chloride 0.9%	[h]	ZEN	10 g	11% loss in 120 hr at 5°C	2152	I
Sodium chloride 0.9%	[a]	ZEN	1 g	Visually compatible. Calculated time to 10% loss in 22 hr at 23°C, 10.7 days at 4°C, and 33.4 days at −20°C	2492	I
Sodium chloride 0.9%	[a]	ZEN	22 g	Visually compatible. Calculated time to 10% loss in 17 hr at 23°C, 4.9 days at 4°C, and 11.4 days at −20°C	2492	I
Sodium chloride 0.9%		ASZ	5 g	6% loss in 8 hr at 20°C and 12% loss in 8 hr at 37°C	2532	C
Sodium chloride 0.9%	[f]	ASZ	30 g	No loss in 24 hr kept in a cold pouch with two freezer packs	2568	C
Sodium chloride 0.9%	[a g]	ZEN	4 g	3 to 4% loss in 168 hr at 5°C	2554	C
Sodium chloride 0.9%	[a g]	ZEN	10 g	2 to 5% loss in 120 hr at 5°C	2554	C
Sodium chloride 0.9%	[a g]	ZEN	20 g	7% loss in 120 hr at 5°C	2554	C
Sodium chloride 0.9%		ASZ	1 to 20 g	Stable for 1 hr at up to 25°C or 15 hr at up to 5°C	3102	C
Sodium chloride 0.9%		ASZ	5 g	More than 10% loss by 12, 8, and 6 hr at temperatures of 30, 35, and 40°C, respectively	3109	I
Sodium chloride 0.9%	[k]		10 g	Less than 10% loss in theoretical concentration in 8 hr at ambient temperature when administered as a continuous infusion	3535	C
Sodium chloride 0.9%	[k]		20 and 40 g	Less than 10% loss in theoretical concentration in 4 hr at ambient temperature when administered as a continuous infusion	3535	C
Sodium lactate ⅙ M	BA[a]	ZEN	1 g	7% loss in 8 hr at 24°C and 6 to 7% loss in 48 hr at 4°C	2089	I[c]

Solution Compatibility (Cont.)

Test Soln Name	Mfr	Mfr	Conc/L or %	Remarks	Ref	C/I
Sodium lactate ⅙ M	BA[a]	ZEN	20 g	9% loss in 8 hr at 24°C and 4 to 5% loss in 24 hr at 4°C	2089	I[c]

[a] Tested in PVC containers.

[b] Tested in glass containers.

[c] Incompatible by conventional standards but recommended for dilution of meropenem with use in shorter periods of time.

[d] Tested in Abbott ADD-Vantage system.

[e] Tested in CADD-Plus medication cassettes.

[f] Tested in Deltec medication cassettes.

[g] Tested in Homepump Eclipse elastomeric pump reservoirs.

[h] Tested in Intermate SV elastomeric pump reservoirs.

[i] Tested with potassium chloride 0.15%.

[j] Tested with sodium bicarbonate 0.02%.

[k] Tested in polypropylene syringes.

Additive Compatibility

Meropenem

Test Drug	Mfr	Conc/L or %	Mfr	Conc/L or %	Test Solution	Remarks	Ref	C/I
Acyclovir sodium	BW	5 g	ZEN	1 g	NS	Visually compatible for 4 hr at room temperature	1994	C
Acyclovir sodium	BW	5 g	ZEN	20 g	NS	Precipitates immediately	1994	I
Aminophylline	AMR	1 g	ZEN	1 and 20 g	NS	Visually compatible for 4 hr at room temperature	1994	C
Amphotericin B	SQ	200 mg	ZEN	1 and 20 g	NS	Precipitate forms	2068	I
Atropine sulfate	ES	40 mg	ZEN	1 and 20 g	NS	Visually compatible for 4 hr at room temperature	1994	C
Ciprofloxacin	SZ[c]	1 g	ASZ[c]	10 g		White precipitate forms	3107	I
Dexamethasone sodium phosphate	MSD	4 g	ZEN	1 and 20 g	NS	Visually compatible for 4 hr at room temperature	1994	C
Dobutamine HCl	LI	1 g	ZEN	1 and 20 g	NS	Visually compatible for 4 hr at room temperature	1994	C
Dopamine HCl	DU	800 mg	ZEN	1 and 20 g	NS	Visually compatible for 4 hr at room temperature	1994	C
Doxycycline hyclate	RR	200 mg	ZEN	1 g	NS	Visually compatible for 4 hr at room temperature	1994	C
Doxycycline hyclate	RR	200 mg	ZEN	20 g	NS	Brown discoloration forms in 1 hr at room temperature	1994	I
Enalaprilat	MSD	50 mg	ZEN	1 and 20 g	NS	Visually compatible for 4 hr at room temperature	1994	C
Fluconazole	RR	2 g	ZEN	1 and 20 g	NS	Visually compatible for 4 hr at room temperature	1994	C
Furosemide	HO	1 g	ZEN	1 and 20 g	NS	Visually compatible for 4 hr at room temperature	1994	C
Gentamicin sulfate	SC	800 mg	ZEN	1 and 20 g	NS	Visually compatible for 4 hr at room temperature	1994	C
Heparin sodium	ES	20,000 units	ZEN	1 and 20 g	NS	Visually compatible for 4 hr at room temperature	1994	C
Insulin, regular	LI	1000 units	ZEN	1 and 20 g	NS	Visually compatible for 4 hr at room temperature	1994	C
Magnesium sulfate	AST	1 g	ZEN	1 and 20 g	NS	Visually compatible for 4 hr at room temperature	1994	C
Mannitol	BA[a]	2.5%	ZEN	1 g		7 to 8% meropenem loss in 8 hr at 24°C and in 24 hr at 4°C	2089	I[b]
Mannitol	BA[a]	2.5%	ZEN	20 g		7 to 9% meropenem loss in 4 hr at 24°C and 6% loss in 20 hr at 4°C	2089	I[b]

Additive Compatibility (Cont.)

Test Drug	Mfr	Conc/L or %	Mfr	Conc/L or %	Test Solution	Remarks	Ref	C/I
Mannitol	BA[a]	10%	ZEN	1 g		10 to 11% meropenem loss in 4 hr at 24°C and in 20 hr at 4°C	2089	I[b]
Mannitol	BA[a]	10%	ZEN	20 g		10% meropenem loss in 3 hr at 24°C and in 20 hr at 4°C	2089	I[b]
Metoclopramide HCl	RB	100 mg	ZEN	1 and 20 g	NS	Visually compatible for 4 hr at room temperature	1994	C
Morphine sulfate	ES	1 g	ZEN	1 and 20 g	NS	Visually compatible for 4 hr at room temperature	1994	C
Multivitamins	AST	50 mL	ZEN	1 and 20 g	NS	Color darkened in 4 hr at room temperature	1994	I
Norepinephrine bitartrate	WI	8 g	ZEN	1 and 20 g	NS	Visually compatible for 4 hr at room temperature	1994	C
Ondansetron HCl	GL	1 g	ZEN	1 g	NS	Visually compatible for 4 hr at room temperature	1994	C
Ondansetron HCl	GL	1 g	ZEN	20 g	NS	White precipitate forms immediately	1994	I
Phenobarbital sodium	ES	200 mg	ZEN	1 and 20 g	NS	Visually compatible for 4 hr at room temperature	1994	C
Ranitidine HCl	GL	100 mg	ZEN	1 and 20 g	NS	Visually compatible for 4 hr at room temperature	1994	C
Sodium bicarbonate	BA	5%	ZEN	1 g		10% meropenem loss in 4 hr at 24°C and 18 hr at 4°C	2089	I[b]
Sodium bicarbonate	BA	5%	ZEN	20 g		9 to 10% meropenem loss in 3 hr at 24°C and 18 hr at 4°C	2089	I[b]
Vancomycin HCl	LI	1 g	ZEN	1 and 20 g	NS	Visually compatible for 4 hr at room temperature	1994	C
Zidovudine	BW	4 g	ZEN	1 g	NS	Visually compatible for 4 hr at room temperature	1994	C
Zidovudine	BW	4 g	ZEN	20 g	NS	Dark yellow discoloration forms in 4 hr at room temperature	1994	I

[a] Tested in PVC containers.

[b] Incompatible by conventional standards but may be used in shorter periods of time.

[c] Tested in glass containers.

Drugs in Syringe Compatibility

Meropenem

Test Drug	Mfr	Amt	Mfr	Amt	Remarks	Ref	C/I
Pantoprazole sodium	[a]	4 mg/1 mL		50 mg/1 mL	Precipitates within 15 min	2574	I

[a] Test performed using the formulation WITHOUT edetate disodium.

Y-Site Injection Compatibility (1:1 Mixture)

Meropenem

Test Drug	Mfr	Conc	Mfr	Conc	Remarks	Ref	C/I
Acetylcysteine	ALV	200 mg/mL		50 mg/mL	Physically compatible for 4 hr at room temperature	3538	C
Acyclovir sodium	BW	5 mg/mL[c]	ZEN	1 mg/mL[b]	Visually compatible for 4 hr at room temperature	1994	C
Acyclovir sodium	BW	5 mg/mL[c]	ZEN	50 mg/mL[b]	Precipitate forms	2068	I
Albumin human	CBH	250 mg/mL		50 mg/mL	Physically compatible for 4 hr at room temperature	3538	C

Y-Site Injection Compatibility (1:1 Mixture) (Cont.)

Test Drug	Mfr	Conc	Mfr	Conc	Remarks	Ref	C/I
Amikacin sulfate	SZ	250 mg/mL		50 mg/mL	Physically compatible for 4 hr at room temperature	3538	C
Aminophylline	AMR	25 mg/mL	ZEN	1 and 50 mg/mL[b]	Visually compatible for 4 hr at room temperature	1994	C
Amiodarone HCl	SZ	50 mg/mL		50 mg/mL	Solution became opaque within 1 hr	3538	I
Amphotericin B	SQ	5 mg/mL	ZEN	1 and 50 mg/mL[b]	Precipitate forms	2068	I
Amphotericin B liposomal	ASP	2 mg/mL[a]		50 mg/mL	Physically compatible for 4 hr at room temperature	3538, 3547	C
Ampicillin sodium	NOP	250 mg/mL		50 mg/mL	Physically compatible for 4 hr at room temperature	3538	C
Anidulafungin	VIC	0.5 mg/mL[a]	ASZ	2.5 mg/mL[b]	Physically compatible for 4 hr at 23°C	2617	C
Atropine sulfate	ES	0.4 mg/mL	ZEN	1 and 50 mg/mL[b]	Visually compatible for 4 hr at room temperature	1994	C
Atropine sulfate	ALV	0.4 mg/mL		50 mg/mL	Physically compatible for 4 hr at room temperature	3538	C
Azithromycin	SMX	100 mg/mL		50 mg/mL	Physically compatible for 4 hr at room temperature	3538	C
Aztreonam	SQ	100 mg/mL		50 mg/mL	Physically compatible for 4 hr at room temperature	3538	C
Benztropine mesylate	OM	1 mg/mL		50 mg/mL	Physically compatible for 4 hr at room temperature	3538	C
Blinatumomab	AMG	0.125 mcg/mL[b]	ARR	8.3 mg/mL[b]	Persistent particulate formation	3405, 3417	I
Blinatumomab	AMG	0.375 mcg/mL[b]	ARR	8.3 mg/mL[b]	Visually compatible for 12 hr at room temperature	3405, 3417	C
Bupivacaine HCl	HOS	5 mg/mL		50 mg/mL	Solution became opaque immediately	3538	I
Caffeine citrate	SGT	20 mg/mL		50 mg/mL	Physically compatible for 4 hr at room temperature	3538	C
Calcium chloride	LIF	100 mg/mL		50 mg/mL	Physically compatible for 4 hr at room temperature	3538	C
Calcium gluconate	AMR	4 mg/mL[c]	ZEN	1 mg/mL[b]	Visually compatible for 4 hr at room temperature	1994	C
Calcium gluconate	AMR	4 mg/mL[c]	ZEN	50 mg/mL[b]	Yellow discoloration forms in 4 hr at room temperature	1994	I
Calcium gluconate	FRK	100 mg/mL		50 mg/mL	Yellow color change occurred within 4 hr	3538	I
Cangrelor tetrasodium	TMC	1 mg/mL[b]		2.5 mg/mL[b]	Physically compatible for 4 hr	3243	C
Caspofungin acetate	ME	0.7 mg/mL[b]	ASZ	2.5 mg/mL[b]	Physically compatible for 4 hr at room temperature	2758	C
Caspofungin acetate	ME	0.5 mg/mL[b]	ASZ	10 mg/mL[b]	Physically compatible over 30 min	2766	C
Caspofungin acetate	ME	0.5 mg/mL		50 mg/mL	Physically compatible for 4 hr at room temperature	3538, 3547	C
Cefazolin sodium	HOS	100 mg/mL		50 mg/mL	Physically compatible for 4 hr at room temperature	3538	C
Cefotaxime sodium	SMX	100 mg/mL		50 mg/mL	Physically compatible for 4 hr at room temperature	3538, 3547	C
Cefoxitin sodium	NOP	100 mg/mL		50 mg/mL	Physically compatible for 4 hr at room temperature	3538	C
Ceftazidime	FRK	100 mg/mL		50 mg/mL	Physically compatible for 4 hr at room temperature	3538	C
Ceftazidime–avibactam sodium	ALL	20 mg/mL[b j]			Physically compatible for up to 4 hr at room temperature	3004	C
Ceftolozane sulfate-tazobactam sodium	CUB	10 mg/mL[g i]	FRK	10 mg/mL[g]	Physically compatible for 2 hr	3262	C
Ceftriaxone sodium	SMX	100 mg/mL		50 mg/mL	Physically compatible for 4 hr at room temperature	3538	C

Y-Site Injection Compatibility (1:1 Mixture) (Cont.)

Test Drug	Mfr	Conc	Mfr	Conc	Remarks	Ref	C/I
Cefuroxime sodium	SMX	100 mg/mL		50 mg/mL	Physically compatible for 4 hr at room temperature	3538	C
Ciprofloxacin[k]	SZ	2 mg/mL		50 mg/mL	Crystallization occurred within 4 hr	3538	I
Clindamycin phosphate	SZ	150 mg/mL		50 mg/mL	Physically compatible for 4 hr at room temperature	3538	C
Cloxacillin sodium	SMX	100 mg/mL	SZ	50 mg/mL	Physically compatible for up to 4 hr at room temperature	3245	C
Cloxacillin sodium	SMX	250 mg/mL		50 mg/mL	Physically compatible for 4 hr at room temperature	3538	C
Colistimethate sodium	MIL	1.5 mg/mL[b]	ASZ	10 mg/mL[b]	Visually compatible for 1 hr at 26°C	3335	C
Colistimethate sodium	SMX	75 mg/mL		50 mg/mL	Physically compatible for 4 hr at room temperature	3538	C
Cyclosporine	BED	1 mg/mL[a]	ASZ	10 mg/mL[b]	Physically compatible	2794	C
Cyclosporine	NVA	5 mg/mL		50 mg/mL	Physically compatible for 4 hr at room temperature	3538	C
Cyclosporine	NVA	50 mg/mL		50 mg/mL	Unacceptably viscous	3538	I
Dexamethasone sodium phosphate	MSD	10 mg/mL[c]	ZEN	1 and 50 mg/mL[b]	Visually compatible for 4 hr at room temperature	1994	C
Dexamethasone sodium phosphate	SZ	4 mg/mL		50 mg/mL	Physically compatible for 4 hr at room temperature	3538	C
Dexmedetomidine HCl	HOS	0.1 mg/mL		50 mg/mL	Physically compatible for 4 hr at room temperature	3538	C
Diazepam	RC	5 mg/mL	ZEN	1 and 50 mg/mL[b]	White precipitate forms immediately	1994	I
Diazepam	SZ	5 mg/mL		50 mg/mL	Precipitates immediately	3538	I
Digoxin	BW	0.25 mg/mL	ZEN	1 and 50 mg/mL[b]	Visually compatible for 4 hr at room temperature	1994	C
Digoxin	SZ	0.25 mg/mL		50 mg/mL	Physically compatible for 4 hr at room temperature	3538	C
Dimenhydrinate	SZ	10 mg/mL		50 mg/mL	Physically compatible for 4 hr at room temperature	3538	C
Diphenhydramine HCl	PD	50 mg/mL	ZEN	1 and 50 mg/mL[b]	Visually compatible for 4 hr at room temperature	1994	C
Diphenhydramine HCl	FRK	50 mg/mL		50 mg/mL	Physically compatible for 4 hr at room temperature	3538	C
Dobutamine HCl	HOS	12.5 mg/mL		50 mg/mL	Precipitation occurred within 4 hr	3538	I
Docetaxel	RPR	0.9 mg/mL[a]	ZEN	20 mg/mL[b]	Physically compatible for 4 hr at 23°C	2224	C
Dopamine HCl	HOS	32 mg/mL[q]		50 mg/mL	Physically compatible for 4 hr at room temperature	3538	C
Doxycycline hyclate	RR	1 mg/mL[c]	ZEN	1 mg/mL[b]	Visually compatible for 4 hr at room temperature	1994	C
Doxycycline hyclate	RR	1 mg/mL[c]	ZEN	50 mg/mL[b]	Amber discoloration forms within 30 min	1994	I
Enalaprilat	MSD	0.05 mg/mL[c]	ZEN	1 and 50 mg/mL[b]	Visually compatible for 4 hr at room temperature	1994	C
Epinephrine HCl	ERF	1 mg/mL		50 mg/mL	Physically compatible for 4 hr at room temperature	3538	C
Eravacycline dihydrochloride	TET	0.3 and 0.6 mg/mL[b]	FRK	20 mg/mL[b]	Measured turbidity increased immediately	3532	I
Ertapenem sodium	ME	100 mg/mL		50 mg/mL	Physically compatible for 4 hr at room temperature	3538	C
Erythromycin lactobionate	AMD	50 mg/mL		50 mg/mL	Physically compatible for 4 hr at room temperature	3538	C
Esmolol HCl	MYL	10 mg/mL	NVP	20 mg/mL[b]	Physically compatible for 1 hr at 23°C	3533	C
Esmolol HCl	BA	10 mg/mL		50 mg/mL	Physically compatible for 4 hr at room temperature	3538	C

Y-Site Injection Compatibility (1:1 Mixture) (Cont.)

Test Drug	Mfr	Conc	Mfr	Conc	Remarks	Ref	C/I
Fentanyl citrate	SZ	50 mcg/mL		50 mg/mL	Physically compatible for 4 hr at room temperature	3538	C
Fluconazole	RR	2 mg/mL	ZEN	1 and 50 mg/mL[b]	Visually compatible for 4 hr at room temperature	1994	C
Fluconazole	SZ	2 mg/mL		50 mg/mL	Physically compatible for 4 hr at room temperature	3538	C
Foscarnet sodium	CLN	24 mg/mL		50 mg/mL	Physically compatible for 4 hr at room temperature	3538	C
Furosemide	HO	10 mg/mL	ZEN	1 and 50 mg/mL[b]	Visually compatible for 4 hr at room temperature	1994	C
Furosemide	OM	10 mg/mL		50 mg/mL	Physically compatible for 4 hr at room temperature	3538	C
Gentamicin sulfate	SC	4 mg/mL[c]	ZEN	1 and 50 mg/mL[b]	Visually compatible for 4 hr at room temperature	1994	C
Gentamicin sulfate	AMS	30 mg/mL[e]	ASZ	10 mg/mL[b]	Physically compatible	2794	C
Gentamicin sulfate	SZ	40 mg/mL		50 mg/mL	Physically compatible for 4 hr at room temperature	3538	C
Granisetron HCl	OM	1 mg/mL		50 mg/mL	Physically compatible for 4 hr at room temperature	3538	C
Heparin sodium	ES	1 unit/mL[c]	ZEN	1 and 50 mg/mL[b]	Visually compatible for 4 hr at room temperature	1994	C
Heparin sodium	SZ	1000 units/mL		50 mg/mL	Physically compatible for 4 hr at room temperature	3538	C
Hydralazine HCl	SMX	20 mg/mL		50 mg/mL	Yellow-brown color change occurred immediately	3538	I
Hydrocortisone sodium succinate	PF	125 mg/mL		50 mg/mL	Physically compatible for 4 hr at room temperature	3538	C
Hydromorphone HCl	SZ	10 mg/mL		50 mg/mL	Physically compatible for 4 hr at room temperature	3538	C
Hydroxyzine HCl	SZ	50 mg/mL		50 mg/mL	Precipitates immediately	3538	I
Imipenem–cilastatin sodium	HOS	50 mg/mL[o]		50 mg/mL	Physically compatible for 4 hr at room temperature	3538, 3547	C
Insulin, regular	LI	0.2 unit/mL[c]	ZEN	1 and 50 mg/mL[b]	Visually compatible for 4 hr at room temperature	1994	C
Insulin, regular	LI	100 units/mL		50 mg/mL	Physically compatible for 4 hr at room temperature	3538	C
Isavuconazonium sulfate	ASP	1.5 mg/mL[g]	PRP	10 mg/mL[g]	Measured turbidity increases within 15 min	3263	I
Isoproterenol HCl	SZ	0.2 mg/mL		50 mg/mL	Physically compatible for 4 hr at room temperature	3538	C
Ketamine HCl	SZ	50 mg/mL		50 mg/mL	Precipitates immediately	3538	I
Labetalol HCl	HOS	5 mg/mL	NVP	20 mg/mL[b]	Physically compatible for 1 hr at 23°C	3533	C
Labetalol HCl	SZ	5 mg/mL		50 mg/mL	Physically compatible for 4 hr at room temperature	3538	C
Levocarnitine	SIG	200 mg/mL		50 mg/mL	Physically compatible for 4 hr at room temperature	3538	C
Lidocaine HCl	ALV	10 mg/mL		50 mg/mL	Physically compatible for 4 hr at room temperature	3538	C
Linezolid	PHU	2 mg/mL	ZEN	2.5 mg/mL[b]	Physically compatible for 4 hr at 23°C	2264	C
Linezolid	TE	2 mg/mL		50 mg/mL	Physically compatible for 4 hr at room temperature	3538	C
Lorazepam	HOS	4 mg/mL		50 mg/mL	Temperature increased upon mixing	3538	I
Magnesium sulfate	FRK	500 mg/mL		50 mg/mL	Physically compatible for 4 hr at room temperature	3538	C
Mannitol	HOS	250 mg/mL		50 mg/mL	Physically compatible for 4 hr at room temperature	3538	C
Methylprednisolone sodium succinate	NOP	62.5 mg/mL		50 mg/mL	Physically compatible for 4 hr at room temperature	3538	C

Y-Site Injection Compatibility (1:1 Mixture) (Cont.)

Test Drug	Mfr	Conc	Mfr	Conc	Remarks	Ref	C/I
Metoclopramide HCl	RB	5 mg/mL	ZEN	1 and 50 mg/mL[b]	Visually compatible for 4 hr at room temperature	1994	C
Metoclopramide HCl	SZ	5 mg/mL		50 mg/mL	Physically compatible for 4 hr at room temperature	3538	C
Metoprolol tartrate	HOS	0.4 mg/mL[b]	NVP	20 mg/mL[b]	Physically compatible for 1 hr at 23°C	3533	C
Metoprolol tartrate	SZ	1 mg/mL		50 mg/mL	Physically compatible for 4 hr at room temperature	3538	C
Metronidazole	HOS	5 mg/mL		50 mg/mL	Physically compatible for 4 hr at room temperature	3538	C
Midazolam[l]	SZ	1 mg/mL		50 mg/mL	Precipitates immediately	3538	I
Milrinone lactate	SS	0.2 mg/mL[a]	ZEN	50 mg/mL[a]	Visually compatible for 4 hr at 25°C	2381	C
Milrinone lactate	FRK	1 mg/mL		50 mg/mL	Physically compatible for 4 hr at room temperature	3538	C
Morphine sulfate	ES	1 mg/mL[c]	ZEN	1 and 50 mg/mL[b]	Visually compatible for 4 hr at room temperature	1994	C
Morphine sulfate	SZ	50 mg/mL		50 mg/mL	Physically compatible for 4 hr at room temperature	3538	C
Multivitamins	SZ			50 mg/mL	Physically compatible for 4 hr at room temperature	3538	C
Naloxone HCl	ALV	0.4 mg/mL		50 mg/mL	Physically compatible for 4 hr at room temperature	3538	C
Nitroglycerin	OM	5 mg/mL		50 mg/mL	Solution became opaque immediately	3538	I
Norepinephrine bitartrate	WI	1 mg/mL	ZEN	1 and 50 mg/mL[b]	Visually compatible for 4 hr at room temperature	1994	C
Norepinephrine bitartrate	SZ	1 mg/mL		50 mg/mL	Physically compatible for 4 hr at room temperature	3538	C
Ondansetron HCl	GL	1 mg/mL[c]	ZEN	1 mg/mL[b]	Visually compatible for 4 hr at room temperature	1994	C
Ondansetron HCl	GL	1 mg/mL[c]	ZEN	50 mg/mL[b]	White precipitate forms immediately	1994	I
Ondansetron HCl	MYL	2 mg/mL		50 mg/mL	Precipitates immediately	3538	I
Oritavancin diphosphate	TAR	0.8, 1.2, and 2 mg/mL[a]	ASZ	10 mg/mL[a]	Haze forms immediately with precipitate after 1 hr	2928	I
Oxytocin	HOS	10 units/mL		50 mg/mL	Physically compatible for 4 hr at room temperature	3538	C
Pantoprazole sodium	SZ[n]	4 mg/mL[b]		50 mg/mL	Physically compatible for 4 hr at room temperature	3538, 3547	C
Penicillin G sodium	FRK	500,000 units/mL		50 mg/mL	Physically compatible for 4 hr at room temperature	3538	C
Phenobarbital sodium	ES	0.32 mg/mL[c]	ZEN	1 and 50 mg/mL[b]	Visually compatible for 4 hr at room temperature	1994	C
Phenytoin sodium	SMX	50 mg/mL		50 mg/mL	Solution became opaque immediately	3538	I
Piperacillin sodium–tazobactam sodium	SMX[n]	200 mg/mL[p]		50 mg/mL	Physically compatible for 4 hr at room temperature	3538, 3547	C
Plazomicin sulfate	ACH	24 mg/mL[g]	FRK	20 mg/mL[g]	Physically compatible for 1 hr at 20 to 25°C	3432	C
Posaconazole	ME	18 mg/mL		1 mg/mL[g]	Physically compatible	2911, 2912	C
Potassium chloride		10 and 40 mEq/L[a]	ZEN	1 mg/mL[a]	Visually compatible. Calculated 10% meropenem loss in 3.3 hr at 23°C	2492	C
Potassium chloride		10 and 40 mEq/L[b]	ZEN	1 mg/mL[a]	Visually compatible. Calculated 10% meropenem loss in 5 hr at 23°C	2492	C
Potassium chloride		10 and 40 mEq/L[a]	ZEN	1 mg/mL[b]	Visually compatible. Calculated 10% meropenem loss in 5.8 hr at 23°C	2492	C

Y-Site Injection Compatibility (1:1 Mixture) (Cont.)

Test Drug	Mfr	Conc	Mfr	Conc	Remarks	Ref	C/I
Potassium chloride		10 and 40 mEq/L[b]	ZEN	1 mg/mL[b]	Visually compatible. Calculated 10% meropenem loss in 22 hr at 23°C	2492	C
Potassium chloride		10 and 40 mEq/L[a]	ZEN	22 mg/mL[a]	Visually compatible. Calculated 10% meropenem loss in 7.7 hr at 23°C	2492	C
Potassium chloride		10 and 40 mEq/L[b]	ZEN	22 mg/mL[a]	Visually compatible. Calculated 10% meropenem loss in 13 hr at 23°C	2492	C
Potassium chloride		10 and 40 mEq/L[a]	ZEN	22 mg/mL[b]	Visually compatible. Calculated 10% meropenem loss in 8 hr at 23°C	2492	C
Potassium chloride		10 and 40 mEq/L[b]	ZEN	22 mg/mL[b]	Visually compatible. Calculated 10% meropenem loss in 20 hr at 23°C	2492	C
Potassium chloride	HOS	2 mEq/mL		50 mg/mL	Physically compatible for 4 hr at room temperature	3538	C
Potassium phosphates	BA	3 mmol/mL		50 mg/mL[b]	Physically compatible for 4 hr at room temperature	3538, 3547	C
Procainamide HCl	SZ	100 mg/mL		50 mg/mL	Physically compatible for 4 hr at room temperature	3538	C
Propranolol HCl	SZ	1 mg/mL		50 mg/mL	Physically compatible for 4 hr at room temperature	3538	C
Quinupristin–dalfopristin		2 mg/mL[a h]		10 mg/mL	Reported to be incompatible	3230	I
Ranitidine HCl	SZ	25 mg/mL		50 mg/mL	Physically compatible for 4 hr at room temperature	3538	C
Rocuronium bromide	SZ	10 mg/mL		50 mg/mL	Physically compatible for 4 hr at room temperature	3538	C
Salbutamol sulfate	GSK	1 mg/mL		50 mg/mL	Physically compatible for 4 hr at room temperature	3538	C
Sodium bicarbonate	HOS	1 mEq/mL		50 mg/mL	Physically compatible for 4 hr at room temperature	3538	C
Sodium nitroprusside	HOS	25 mg/mL		50 mg/mL	Physically compatible for 4 hr at room temperature	3538	C
Sodium phosphates	SZ	3 mmol/mL		50 mg/mL	Gas bubbles evolve within 1 hr	3538, 3547	I
Sufentanil citrate	SZ	50 mcg/mL		50 mg/mL	Physically compatible for 4 hr at room temperature	3538	C
Tedizolid phosphate	CUB	0.8 mg/mL[b]	PRP	10 mg/mL[b]	Physically compatible for 2 hr	3244	C
Telavancin HCl	ASP	7.5 mg/mL[a b f]	ASZ	10 mg/mL[a b f]	Physically compatible for 2 hr	2830	C
TNA #218 to #226[d]			ZEN	20 mg/mL[a]	Visually compatible for 4 hr at 23°C	2215	C
Tobramycin sulfate	FRK	40 mg/mL		50 mg/mL	Physically compatible for 4 hr at room temperature	3538	C
Trimethoprim–sulfamethoxazole	APR	16 mg/mL[m]		50 mg/mL	Physically compatible for 4 hr at room temperature	3538	C
Valproate sodium	ABV	100 mg/mL		50 mg/mL	Physically compatible for 4 hr at room temperature	3538	C
Vancomycin HCl	LI	5 mg/mL[c]	ZEN	1 and 50 mg/mL[b]	Visually compatible for 4 hr at room temperature	1994	C
Vancomycin HCl	SZ	50 mg/mL		50 mg/mL	Precipitates immediately	3538	I
Vasopressin	APP	0.2 unit/mL[b]	ASZ	5 mg/mL[a]	Physically compatible	2641	C
Voriconazole	SZ	10 mg/mL		50 mg/mL	Physically compatible for 4 hr at room temperature	3538	C
Zidovudine	BW	4 mg/mL[c]	ZEN	1 mg/mL[b]	Visually compatible for 4 hr at room temperature	1994	C

Y-Site Injection Compatibility (1:1 Mixture) (Cont.)

Test Drug	Mfr	Conc	Mfr	Conc	Remarks	Ref	C/I
Zidovudine	BW	4 mg/mL[c]	ZEN	50 mg/mL[b]	Yellow color in 4 hr at room temperature	1994	I

[a] Tested in dextrose 5%.

[b] Tested in sodium chloride 0.9%.

[c] Tested in sterile water for injection.

[d] Refer to Appendix for the composition of parenteral nutrition solutions. TNA indicates a 3-in-1 admixture.

[e] Tested in sodium chloride 0.45%.

[f] Tested in Ringer's injection, lactated.

[g] Tested in both dextrose 5% and sodium chloride 0.9%.

[h] Quinupristin and dalfopristin components combined.

[i] Ceftolozane component. Ceftolozane in a 2:1 fixed-ratio concentration with tazobactam.

[j] Ceftazidime component. Ceftazidime in a 4:1 fixed-ratio concentration with avibactam.

[k] Test performed using the lactate salt formulation.

[l] As midazolam base rather than the salt.

[m] Trimethoprim component. Trimethoprim in a 1:5 fixed-ratio concentration with sulfamethoxazole.

[n] Test performed using the formulation WITHOUT edetate disodium.

[o] Imipenem component. Imipenem in a 1:1 fixed-ratio concentration with cilastatin.

[p] Piperacillin component. Piperacillin in an 8:1 fixed-ratio concentration with tazobactam.

[q] Tested as the premixed infusion solution.

Additional Compatibility Information

Peritoneal Dialysis Solutions

Meropenem (AstraZeneca) 1 g in 2 L of Dianeal PD-4 with dextrose 2.5% (Baxter) exhibited 6% drug loss over 6 hours at 37°C.[3108]

Selected Revisions May 1, 2020. © Copyright, October 1998. American Society of Health-System Pharmacists, Inc.

Meropenem–Vaborbactam
AHFS 8:12.07.08

Products

The fixed combination of meropenem–vaborbactam is available as a powder in single-dose (preservative-free) vials containing 2 g (meropenem 1 g [as the trihydrate] plus vaborbactam 1 g) and sodium carbonate 0.575 g.[3379]

The contents of each 2-g vial should be reconstituted with 20 mL of sodium chloride 0.9% (withdrawn from an infusion bag) and mixed gently to dissolve the powder.[3379] The reconstituted solution will have approximate meropenem and vaborbactam concentrations of 50 mg/mL each.[3379] The reconstituted solution is *not* suitable for direct injection.[3379]

The reconstituted solution must be diluted immediately in the infusion bag containing sodium chloride 0.9% from which the volume used for reconstitution of the appropriate dose was withdrawn.[3379] The manufacturer's instructions for preparing various doses of meropenem–vaborbactam from the reconstituted solution are as follows:[3379]

For 4 g (meropenem 2 g plus vaborbactam 2 g), withdraw the entire contents (i.e., approximately 21 mL each) of 2 vials and add to an infusion bag containing 250, 500, or 1000 mL of sodium chloride 0.9% (less the 40 mL used for reconstitution).

For 2 g (meropenem 1 g plus vaborbactam 1 g), withdraw the entire contents (i.e., approximately 21 mL) of 1 vial and add to an infusion bag containing 125, 250, or 500 mL of sodium chloride 0.9% (less the 20 mL used for reconstitution).

For 1 g (meropenem 0.5 g plus vaborbactam 0.5 g), withdraw 10.5 mL and add to an infusion bag containing 70, 125, or 250 mL of sodium chloride 0.9% (less the 20 mL used for reconstitution).

Sodium Content

Each 2-g vial of this fixed combination contains 0.25 g (10.9 mEq) of sodium.[3379]

Trade Name(s)

Vabomere

Administration

The diluted solution of meropenem–vaborbactam for infusion is administered intravenously over 3 hours.[3379] The reconstituted solution is *not* suitable for direct injection.[3379]

Stability

Meropenem–vaborbactam is a white to light yellow powder that forms a colorless to light yellow solution upon both reconstitution and dilution.[3379] Intact vials of meropenem–vaborbactam should be stored at controlled room temperature.[3379]

Diluted solutions of meropenem–vaborbactam for infusion should be visually inspected for particulate matter and discoloration prior to administration.[3379] Administration of the diluted solution for infusion must be completed within 4 hours if stored at room temperature or 22 hours if stored at 2 to 8°C.[3379] Any unused portions should be discarded.[3379]

Meropenem–vaborbactam reconstituted and diluted for infusion demonstrated less than 10% loss of either drug when stored for up to 10 hours at room temperature and for up to 26 hours under refrigeration (5°C); however, a degradation product formation assessment revealed that the solution did not consistently meet impurity limits during this period.[3381]

Compatibility Information

Solution Compatibility

Meropenem–vaborbactam

Test Soln Name	Mfr	Mfr	Conc/L or %	Remarks	Ref	C/I
Sodium chloride 0.9%		MEL	2, 4, 7.15, and 8 g[a]	Complete administration within 4 hr if stored at room temperature or 22 hr if stored at 2 to 8°C	3379	C
Sodium chloride 0.9%	BA[b]	MEL	2 g[a]	Less than 6% loss of either component in 12 hr at 24°C; calculated time to 10% loss was 21.4 hr	3588	C
Sodium chloride 0.9%	BA[b]	MEL	2 g[a]	Less than 9% loss of either component in 5 days at 4°C; calculated time to 10% loss was 175.3 hr	3588	C
Sodium chloride 0.9%	BA[b]	MEL	4 g[a]	Less than 8% loss of either component in 12 hr at 24°C; calculated time to 10% loss was 15.8 hr	3588	C
Sodium chloride 0.9%	BA[b]	MEL	4 g[a]	Less than 7% loss of either component in 6 days at 4°C; calculated time to 10% loss was 223.8 hr	3588	C

DOI: 10.37573/9781585286850.252

Solution Compatibility (Cont.)

Test Soln Name	Mfr	Mfr	Conc/L or %	Remarks	Ref	C/I
Sodium chloride 0.9%	BA[c]	MEL	5.7 g[a]	Less than 8% loss of either component in 12 hr at 24°C; calculated time to 10% loss was 14.8 hr	3588	C
Sodium chloride 0.9%	BA[c]	MEL	5.7 g[a]	Less than 9% loss of either component in 5 days at 4°C; calculated time to 10% loss was 154.5 hr	3588	C
Sodium chloride 0.9%	BA[b]	MEL	8 g[a]	Less than 9% loss of either component in 12 hr at 24°C; calculated time to 10% loss was 14.6 hr	3588	C
Sodium chloride 0.9%	BA[b]	MEL	8 g[a]	Less than 9% loss of either component in 6 days at 4°C; calculated time to 10% loss was 172 hr	3588	C

[a] Meropenem component. Meropenem in a 1:1 fixed-ratio concentration with vaborbactam.

[b] Tested in PVC containers.

[c] Tested in Homepump Eclipse elastomeric pump reservoirs.

Y-Site Injection Compatibility (1:1 Mixture)

Meropenem–vaborbactam

Test Drug	Mfr	Conc	Mfr	Conc	Remarks	Ref	C/I
Albumin human	BXT	250 mg/mL	TMC	8 mg/mL[a i]	Measured turbidity increases immediately	3380	I
Amikacin sulfate	FRK	5 mg/mL[a]	TMC	8 mg/mL[a i]	Physically compatible for 3 hr at 20 to 25°C	3380	C
Amiodarone HCl	APP	2 mg/mL[a]	TMC	8 mg/mL[a i]	Measured turbidity increases immediately. pH increased by >3 units within 3 hr	3380	I
Ampicillin sodium–sulbactam sodium	PF	20 mg/mL[a b]	TMC	8 mg/mL[a i]	Physically compatible for 3 hr at 20 to 25°C	3380	C
Anidulafungin	PF	0.77 mg/mL[a]	TMC	8 mg/mL[a i]	Immediate change in measured turbidity. pH increased by >3 units within 3 hr	3380	I
Azithromycin	FRK	2 mg/mL[a]	TMC	8 mg/mL[a i]	Physically compatible for 3 hr at 20 to 25°C	3380	C
Aztreonam	FRK	20 mg/mL[a]	TMC	8 mg/mL[a i]	Physically compatible for 3 hr at 20 to 25°C	3380	C
Bumetanide	HOS	0.25 mg/mL	TMC	8 mg/mL[a i]	Physically compatible for 3 hr at 20 to 25°C	3380	C
Calcium chloride	HOS	20 mg/mL[a]	TMC	8 mg/mL[a i]	Precipitation and increase in measured turbidity within 30 min. pH increased by >3 units within 3 hr	3380	I
Calcium gluconate	FRK	20 mg/mL[a]	TMC	8 mg/mL[a i]	Physically compatible for 3 hr at 20 to 25°C	3380	C
Caspofungin acetate	ME	0.5 mg/mL[a]	TMC	8 mg/mL[a i]	Measured turbidity increases immediately. pH increased by >2 units within 3 hr	3380	I
Cefazolin sodium	SGT	20 mg/mL[a]	TMC	8 mg/mL[a i]	Physically compatible for 3 hr at 20 to 25°C	3380	C
Cefepime HCl	HOS	40 mg/mL[a]	TMC	8 mg/mL[a i]	Physically compatible for 3 hr at 20 to 25°C	3380	C
Ceftaroline fosamil	FOR	12 mg/mL[a]	TMC	8 mg/mL[a i]	Measured turbidity increases within 30 min. pH increased by >2 units within 3 hr	3380	I
Ceftazidime	SGT	40 mg/mL[a]	TMC	8 mg/mL[a i]	Physically compatible for 3 hr at 20 to 25°C	3380	C
Ceftazidime–avibactam sodium	GSK	40 mg/mL[a c]	TMC	8 mg/mL[a i]	Physically compatible for 3 hr at 20 to 25°C	3380	C
Ceftolozane sulfate–tazobactam sodium	ME	20 mg/mL[a d]	TMC	8 mg/mL[a i]	Physically compatible for 3 hr at 20 to 25°C	3380	C
Ceftriaxone sodium	SGT	20 mg/mL[a]	TMC	8 mg/mL[a i]	Physically compatible for 3 hr at 20 to 25°C	3380	C
Cefuroxime sodium	SGT	30 mg/mL[a]	TMC	8 mg/mL[a i]	Physically compatible for 3 hr at 20 to 25°C	3380	C

Y-Site Injection Compatibility (1:1 Mixture) (Cont.)

Test Drug	Mfr	Conc	Mfr	Conc	Remarks	Ref	C/I
Ciprofloxacin	HOS	2 mg/mL[a]	TMC	8 mg/mL[a i]	Precipitation and increase in measured turbidity within 30 min. pH increased by >3 units within 3 hr	3380, 3382	I
Cisatracurium besylate	ABV	0.4 mg/mL[a]	TMC	8 mg/mL[a i]	Physically compatible for 3 hr at 20 to 25°C	3380	C
Colistimethate sodium	APP	4.5 mg/mL[a]	TMC	8 mg/mL[a i]	Physically compatible for 3 hr at 20 to 25°C	3380	C
Daptomycin	TE	20 mg/mL[a]	TMC	8 mg/mL[a i]	Immediate change in measured turbidity. pH increased by 2 units within 3 hr	3380	I
Dexamethasone sodium phosphate	FRK	1 mg/mL[a]	TMC	8 mg/mL[a i]	Physically compatible for 3 hr at 20 to 25°C	3380	C
Dexmedetomidine HCl	HOS	4 mcg/mL	TMC	8 mg/mL[a i]	Physically compatible for 3 hr at 20 to 25°C	3380	C
Digoxin	SZ	0.25 mg/mL	TMC	8 mg/mL[a i]	Physically compatible for 3 hr at 20 to 25°C	3380	C
Diltiazem HCl	AKN	5 mg/mL	TMC	8 mg/mL[a i]	Physically compatible for 3 hr at 20 to 25°C	3380	C
Diphenhydramine HCl	FRK	50 mg/mL	TMC	8 mg/mL[a i]	Immediate change in measured turbidity with precipitation within 3 hr. pH increased by >2 units within 3 hr	3380	I
Dobutamine HCl	HOS	4.1 mg/mL[a]	TMC	8 mg/mL[a i]	Measured turbidity increases within 1 hr. pH increased by >3 units within 3 hr	3380	I
Dopamine HCl	HOS	0.8 mg/mL[a]	TMC	8 mg/mL[a i]	Physically compatible for 3 hr at 20 to 25°C	3380	C
Doripenem	APO	10 mg/mL[a]	TMC	8 mg/mL[a i]	Physically compatible for 3 hr at 20 to 25°C	3380	C
Doxycycline hyclate	FRK	1 mg/mL[a]	TMC	8 mg/mL[a i]	Physically compatible for 3 hr at 20 to 25°C	3380	C
Epinephrine[e]	HOS	16 mcg/mL[a]	TMC	8 mg/mL[a i]	Physically compatible for 3 hr at 20 to 25°C	3380	C
Eptifibatide	AMB	2 mg/mL	TMC	8 mg/mL[a i]	Physically compatible for 3 hr at 20 to 25°C	3380	C
Eravacycline dihydro-chloride	TET	0.6 mg/mL[a]	FAC	8 mg/mL[a i]	Measured turbidity increased immediately	3532	I
Ertapenem sodium	ME	20 mg/mL[a]	TMC	8 mg/mL[a i]	Physically compatible for 3 hr at 20 to 25°C	3380	C
Esmolol HCl	MYL	10 mg/mL	TMC	8 mg/mL[a i]	Physically compatible for 3 hr at 20 to 25°C	3380	C
Esomeprazole sodium	ASZ	0.8 mg/mL[a]	TMC	8 mg/mL[a i]	Physically compatible for 3 hr at 20 to 25°C	3380	C
Famotidine	FRK	4 mg/mL[a]	TMC	8 mg/mL[a i]	Physically compatible for 3 hr at 20 to 25°C	3380	C
Fentanyl citrate	HOS	50 mcg/mL	TMC	8 mg/mL[a i]	Physically compatible for 3 hr at 20 to 25°C	3380	C
Fosphenytoin sodium	AMB[j]	25 mg/mL[a]	TMC	8 mg/mL[a i]	Physically compatible for 3 hr at 20 to 25°C	3380, 3382	C
Furosemide	CLA	3 mg/mL[a]	TMC	8 mg/mL[a i]	Physically compatible for 3 hr at 20 to 25°C	3380	C
Gentamicin sulfate	FRK	5 mg/mL[a]	TMC	8 mg/mL[a i]	Physically compatible for 3 hr at 20 to 25°C	3380	C
Heparin sodium	SGT	1000 units/mL[a]	TMC	8 mg/mL[a i]	Physically compatible for 3 hr at 20 to 25°C	3380	C
Hydrocortisone sodium succinate	PF	1 mg/mL[a]	TMC	8 mg/mL[a i]	Physically compatible for 3 hr at 20 to 25°C	3380	C
Hydromorphone HCl	AKN	1 mg/mL[a]	TMC	8 mg/mL[a i]	Physically compatible for 3 hr at 20 to 25°C	3380	C
Imipenem–cilastatin sodium	ME	5 mg/mL[a f]	TMC	8 mg/mL[a i]	Physically compatible for 3 hr at 20 to 25°C	3380	C
Insulin, regular	LI	1 unit/mL[a]	TMC	8 mg/mL[a i]	Physically compatible for 3 hr at 20 to 25°C	3380	C
Isavuconazonium sulfate	ASP	0.8 mg/mL[a]	TMC	8 mg/mL[a i]	Measured turbidity increases within 30 min. pH increased by >5 units within 3 hr	3380	I

Y-Site Injection Compatibility (1:1 Mixture) (Cont.)

Test Drug	Mfr	Conc	Mfr	Conc	Remarks	Ref	C/I
Labetalol HCl	AKN	2 mg/mL[a]	TMC	8 mg/mL[a i]	Physically compatible for 3 hr at 20 to 25°C	3380	C
Levofloxacin	AUB	5 mg/mL[a]	TMC	8 mg/mL[a i]	Physically compatible for 3 hr at 20 to 25°C	3380, 3382	C
Lidocaine HCl	FRK	8 mg/mL[a]	TMC	8 mg/mL[a i]	Physically compatible for 3 hr at 20 to 25°C	3380	C
Linezolid	PF	2 mg/mL[a]	TMC	8 mg/mL[a i]	Physically compatible for 3 hr at 20 to 25°C	3380	C
Lorazepam	WW	1 mg/mL[a]	TMC	8 mg/mL[a i]	Physically compatible for 3 hr at 20 to 25°C	3380	C
Magnesium sulfate	XGN	100 mg/mL[a]	TMC	8 mg/mL[a i]	Physically compatible for 3 hr at 20 to 25°C	3380	C
Mannitol	HOS	20%	TMC	8 mg/mL[a i]	Physically compatible for 3 hr at 20 to 25°C	3380	C
Meperidine HCl	WW	10 mg/mL[a]	TMC	8 mg/mL[a i]	Physically compatible for 3 hr at 20 to 25°C	3380	C
Mesna	SGT	20 mg/mL[a]	TMC	8 mg/mL[a i]	Physically compatible for 3 hr at 20 to 25°C	3380	C
Methylprednisolone sodium succinate	SGT	20 mg/mL[a]	TMC	8 mg/mL[a i]	Physically compatible for 3 hr at 20 to 25°C	3380	C
Metoclopramide HCl	TE	0.2 mg/mL[a]	TMC	8 mg/mL[a i]	Physically compatible for 3 hr at 20 to 25°C	3380	C
Metronidazole	BA	5 mg/mL[a]	TMC	8 mg/mL[a i]	Physically compatible for 3 hr at 20 to 25°C	3380	C
Micafungin sodium	ASP	4 mg/mL[a]	TMC	8 mg/mL[a i]	Physically compatible for 3 hr at 20 to 25°C	3380	C
Midazolam HCl	HOS	1 mg/mL[a]	TMC	8 mg/mL[a i]	Measured turbidity increases immediately. pH increased by >4 units within 3 hr	3380	I
Milrinone lactate	WW	0.2 mg/mL[a]	TMC	8 mg/mL[a i]	Physically compatible for 3 hr at 20 to 25°C	3380	C
Morphine sulfate	WW	1 mg/mL[a]	TMC	8 mg/mL[a i]	Physically compatible for 3 hr at 20 to 25°C	3380	C
Naloxone HCl	MYL	0.04 mg/mL[a]	TMC	8 mg/mL[a i]	Physically compatible for 3 hr at 20 to 25°C	3380	C
Nicardipine HCl	EXL	0.1 mg/mL[a]	TMC	8 mg/mL[a i]	Measured turbidity increases immediately. pH increased by >3 units within 3 hr	3380	I
Nitroglycerin	BA	0.4 mg/mL[a]	TMC	8 mg/mL[a i]	Physically compatible for 3 hr at 20 to 25°C	3380	C
Norepinephrine bitartrate	HOS	32 mcg/mL[a]	TMC	8 mg/mL[a i]	Physically compatible for 3 hr at 20 to 25°C	3380	C
Octreotide acetate	FRK	4 mcg/mL[a]	TMC	8 mg/mL[a i]	Physically compatible for 3 hr at 20 to 25°C	3380	C
Ondansetron HCl	HER	0.16 mg/mL[a]	TMC	8 mg/mL[a i]	Immediate precipitation and increase in measured turbidity. pH increased by >4 units within 3 hr	3380	I
Pantoprazole sodium	WY[g]	0.4 mg/mL[a]	TMC	8 mg/mL[a i]	Physically compatible for 3 hr at 20 to 25°C	3380	C
Penicillin G potassium	PF	100,000 units/mL[a]	TMC	8 mg/mL[a i]	Physically compatible for 3 hr at 20 to 25°C	3380	C
Phenylephrine HCl	ECL	1 mg/mL[a]	TMC	8 mg/mL[a i]	Physically compatible for 3 hr at 20 to 25°C	3380	C
Phenytoin sodium	WW	10 mg/mL[a]	TMC	8 mg/mL[a i]	Measured turbidity increases immediately with precipitation within 30 min. pH decreased by >1 unit within 3 hr	3380	I
Piperacillin sodium–tazobactam sodium	FRK[k]	40 mg/mL[a h]	TMC	8 mg/mL[a i]	Physically compatible for 3 hr at 20 to 25°C	3380	C
Plazomicin sulfate	ACH	24 mg/mL[l]	FAC	8 mg/mL[i l]	Physically compatible for 1 hr at 20 to 25°C	3432	C
Potassium chloride	HOS	0.1 mEq/mL[a]	TMC	8 mg/mL[a i]	Physically compatible for 3 hr at 20 to 25°C	3380	C
Potassium phosphates	HOS	0.3 mmol/mL[a]	TMC	8 mg/mL[a i]	Physically compatible for 3 hr at 20 to 25°C	3380	C

Y-Site Injection Compatibility (1:1 Mixture) (Cont.)

Test Drug	Mfr	Conc	Mfr	Conc	Remarks	Ref	C/I
Ranitidine HCl	ZY	2.5 mg/mL[a]	TMC	8 mg/mL[a i]	Physically compatible for 3 hr at 20 to 25°C	3380	C
Rocuronium bromide	MYL	5 mg/mL[a]	TMC	8 mg/mL[a i]	Physically compatible for 3 hr at 20 to 25°C	3380	C
Sodium bicarbonate	HOS	1 mEq/mL	TMC	8 mg/mL[a i]	Physically compatible for 3 hr at 20 to 25°C	3380	C
Sodium phosphates	FRK	0.5 mmol/mL[a]	TMC	8 mg/mL[a i]	Physically compatible for 3 hr at 20 to 25°C	3380	C
Tedizolid phosphate	ME	0.8 mg/mL[a]	TMC	8 mg/mL[a i]	Physically compatible for 3 hr at 20 to 25°C	3380	C
Tigecycline	WY	1 mg/mL[a]	TMC	8 mg/mL[a i]	Physically compatible for 3 hr at 20 to 25°C	3380	C
Tobramycin sulfate	FRK	5 mg/mL[a]	TMC	8 mg/mL[a i]	Physically compatible for 3 hr at 20 to 25°C	3380	C
Vancomycin HCl	FRK	5 mg/mL[a]	TMC	8 mg/mL[a i]	Physically compatible for 3 hr at 20 to 25°C	3380	C
Vasopressin	PAR	1 unit/mL[a]	TMC	8 mg/mL[a i]	Physically compatible for 3 hr at 20 to 25°C	3380	C
Vecuronium bromide	MYL	1 mg/mL	TMC	8 mg/mL[a i]	Physically compatible for 3 hr at 20 to 25°C	3380	C

[a] Tested in sodium chloride 0.9%.

[b] Ampicillin component. Ampicillin in a 2:1 fixed-ratio concentration with sulbactam.

[c] Ceftazidime component. Ceftazidime in a 4:1 fixed-ratio concentration with avibactam.

[d] Ceftolozane component. Ceftolozane in a 2:1 fixed-ratio concentration with tazobactam.

[e] As epinephrine base rather than the salt.

[f] Imipenem component. Imipenem in a 1:1 fixed-ratio concentration with cilastatin.

[g] Test performed using the formulation WITH edetate disodium.

[h] Piperacillin component. Piperacillin in an 8:1 fixed-ratio concentration with tazobactam.

[i] Meropenem component. Meropenem in a 1:1 fixed-ratio concentration with vaborbactam.

[j] Concentration of fosphenytoin expressed in milligrams of phenytoin sodium equivalents (PE) per mL.

[k] Test performed using the formulation WITHOUT edetate disodium.

[l] Tested in both dextrose 5% and sodium chloride 0.9%.

Mesna
AHFS 92:56

Products

Mesna is available as a 100-mg/mL solution in 10-mL multidose vials. Each mL of solution also contains edetate disodium 0.25 mg and sodium hydroxide to adjust the pH. In addition, the multidose vials contain benzyl alcohol 10.4 mg/mL.[1(5/06)]

pH

The pH of mesna injection is stated to be pH 6.5 to 7.3 or pH 7.5 to 8.5, depending on the specific product.[1(5/06)]

Trade Name(s)

Mesnex

Administration

Mesna may be administered by intravenous injection or infusion.[1(5/06)] [4] Infusion is usually performed over 15 to 30 minutes, but continuous infusion has also been utilized.[4] Dilution to a concentration of 20 mg/mL in a compatible solution is recommended for intravenous infusion.[1(5/06)] [4]

Stability

Intact ampuls of mesna should be stored at controlled room temperature. The solution is clear and colorless[1(5/06)] and is not light sensitive.[72] When exposed to oxygen, mesna oxidizes to the disulfide form, dimesna. Unused mesna injection in opened ampuls should be discarded after dose preparation. However, the multidose vials may be stored and used for up to 8 days after initial entry.[1(5/06)]

pH Effects

Mesna and ifosfamide have been found to be stable in combined admixtures.[72] [1380] [1494] [1495] [1496] However, mesna has been found to undergo more extensive decomposition when mixed with ifosfamide in an infusion solution made alkaline with sodium bicarbonate. At pH 8, mesna was stable for 6 hours, but lost about 13% in 24 hours and 23% in 48 hours. Ifosfamide underwent only 6% loss in 24 hours, but lost 14% in 48 hours.[2281]

Syringes

The short-term use of plastic syringes for preparing mesna infusions appears to be satisfactory. However, extended storage of mesna in a plastic and a glass syringe resulted in the formation of dark or thread-like particles and a change in viscosity after 12 hours at room temperature.[72]

Mesna (Asta Pharma) 100 mg/mL was packaged as 10 mL in 20-mL polypropylene syringes (Becton Dickinson). Samples having the air expelled from the syringes were stored at 5, 24, and 35°C, and samples with air drawn into the syringes were stored at 24°C. After 9 days of storage, little or no change in the mesna concentration was found in all samples with no air present. The maximum loss was less than 4% found in the samples stored at 35°C. However, the syringes containing air exhibited 10% loss in 8 days at 24°C. Minimizing the exposure of mesna to air during storage was recommended to slow the formation of dimesna.[2181]

Compatibility Information

Solution Compatibility

Mesna

Test Soln Name	Mfr	Mfr	Conc/L or %	Remarks	Ref	C/I
Dextrose 5% in sodium chloride 0.225%			20 g	Physically and chemically stable for 24 hr at 25°C	1(5/06)	C
Dextrose 5% in sodium chloride 0.45%			20 g	Physically and chemically stable for 24 hr at 25°C	1(5/06)	C
Dextrose 5% in sodium chloride 0.45%		AW	1 g	4% loss in 72 hr at room temperature	72	C
Dextrose 5% in sodium chloride 0.45%		AW	20 g	5% loss in 48 hr at room temperature	72	C
Dextrose 5%			20 g	Physically and chemically stable for 24 hr at 25°C	1(5/06)	C
Dextrose 5%		AW	1 g	5% loss in 24 hr and 13% in 48 hr at room temperature	72	C
Dextrose 5%		AW	20 g	5% loss in 48 hr at room temperature	72	C
Dextrose 5%	BA[a]	BED	10 g	Under 10% loss in 14 days at 25°C and 28 days at 5°C	2810	C
Ringer's injection, lactated			20 g	Physically and chemically stable for 24 hr at 25°C	1(5/06)	C

DOI: 10.37573/9781585286850.253

Solution Compatibility (Cont.)

Test Soln Name	Mfr	Mfr	Conc/L or %	Remarks	Ref	C/I
Ringer's injection, lactated		AW	1 g	4% loss in 24 hr and 11% in 48 hr at room temperature	72	C
Sodium chloride 0.9%			20 g	Physically and chemically stable for 24 hr at 25°C	1(5/06)	C
Sodium chloride 0.9%		AW	1 g	10% loss in 48 hr at room temperature	72	C

[a] Tested in ReadyMed elastomeric pump reservoirs.

Additive Compatibility

Mesna

Test Drug	Mfr	Conc/L or %	Mfr	Conc/L or %	Test Solution	Remarks	Ref	C/I
Carboplatin		1 g		1 g	W	More than 10% carboplatin loss in 24 hr at room temperature	1379	I
Cisplatin		67 mg		3.33 g	NS	Cisplatin not detectable after 1 hr	1291	I
Cisplatin		67 mg		110 mg	NS	Cisplatin weakly detected after 1 hr	1291	I
Cyclophosphamide	AM	10.8 g	AM	3.2 g	D5W	Physically compatible with about 5% loss of both drugs in 24 hr at 22°C. 7% cyclophosphamide loss and 10% mesna loss occurred in 72 hr at 4°C	2486	C
Cyclophosphamide	AM	1.8 g	AM	540 mg	D5W	Physically compatible with about 10% loss of both drugs in 12 hr at 22°C	2486	I
Cyclophosphamide	AM	1.8 g	AM	540 mg	D5W	Physically compatible with about 9% loss of both drugs in 72 hr at 4°C	2486	C
Hydroxyzine HCl	LY	500 mg	AW	3 g	D5W[a]	Physically compatible for 48 hr	1190	C
Ifosfamide	MJ	3.3 g	AW	3.3 g	D5W, LR	Physically compatible. No ifosfamide loss and about 5% mesna loss in 24 hr at 21°C exposed to light	72	C
Ifosfamide	MJ	5 g	AW	5 g	D5W, LR	Physically compatible. No ifosfamide loss and about 5% mesna loss in 24 hr at 21°C exposed to light	72	C
Ifosfamide	BI	83.3 g	BI	79 g	NS	Little or no ifosfamide loss in 9 days at room temperature and 7% ifosfamide loss in 9 days at 37°C. Mesna not tested	1494	C
Ifosfamide		2.6 g		1.6 g	D5S[b]	No increase in decomposition products in 8 hr at room temperature	1495	C
Ifosfamide	BR	600 mg	BR	600 mg	D5½S, D5W, LR, NS[c]	Both drugs chemically stable for at least 24 hr at room temperature	1496	C
Ifosfamide	AM	20 g	AM	20 g	W[d]	Physically compatible with about 3% ifosfamide loss and 9% mesna loss in 7 days at 37°C. About 2% or less loss of both drugs in 14 days at 4°C	2288	C

[a] Tested in glass containers.

[b] Tested in polyethylene containers.

[c] Tested in PVC containers.

[d] Tested in PVC reservoirs for the Graseby 9000 ambulatory pump.

Drugs in Syringe Compatibility

Mesna

Test Drug	Mfr	Amt	Mfr	Amt	Remarks	Ref	C/I
Epirubicin HCl with ifosfamide		1 mg/mL[a] 50 mg/mL[a]		40 mg/mL[a]	50% epirubicin loss in 7 days at 4 and 20°C. No loss of other drugs in 7 days	1564	I
Ifosfamide		250 mg/5 mL		200 mg/5 mL	3% ifosfamide loss in 7 days and 12% in 4 weeks at 4°C and room temperature. No mesna loss	1290	C
Ifosfamide		50 mg/mL[a]		40 mg/mL[a]	Little or no loss of either drug in 28 days at 4 and 20°C	1564	C
Ifosfamide with epirubicin HCl		50 mg/mL[a] 1 mg/mL[a]		40 mg/mL[a]	50% epirubicin loss in 7 days at 4 and 20°C. No loss of other drugs in 7 days	1564	I

[a] Diluted with sodium chloride 0.9%.

Y-Site Injection Compatibility (1:1 Mixture)

Mesna

Test Drug	Mfr	Conc	Mfr	Conc	Remarks	Ref	C/I
Allopurinol sodium	BW	3 mg/mL[b]	MJ	10 mg/mL[b]	Physically compatible for 4 hr at 22°C	1686	C
Amifostine	USB	10 mg/mL[a]	MJ	10 mg/mL[a]	Physically compatible for 4 hr at 23°C	1845	C
Aztreonam	SQ	40 mg/mL[a]	MJ	10 mg/mL[a]	Physically compatible for 4 hr at 23°C	1758	C
Ceftolozane sulfate–tazobactam sodium	CUB	10 mg/mL[h i]	TE	20 mg/mL[h]	Physically compatible for 2 hr	3262	C
Cladribine	ORT	0.015[b] and 0.5[c] mg/mL	MJ	10 mg/mL[b]	Physically compatible for 4 hr at 23°C	1969	C
Defibrotide sodium	JAZ	8 mg/mL[b]	BA	4.76 mg/mL[b]	Visually compatible for 4 hr at room temperature	3149	C
Docetaxel	RPR	0.9 mg/mL[a]	MJ	10 mg/mL[a]	Physically compatible for 4 hr at 23°C	2224	C
Doxorubicin HCl liposomal	SEQ	0.4 mg/mL[a]	MJ	10 mg/mL[a]	Physically compatible for 4 hr at 23°C	2087	C
Etoposide phosphate	BR	5 mg/mL[a]	MJ	10 mg/mL[a]	Physically compatible for 4 hr at 23°C	2218	C
Filgrastim	AMG	30 mcg/mL[a]	MJ	10 mg/mL[a]	Physically compatible for 4 hr at 22°C	1687	C
Fludarabine phosphate	BX	1 mg/mL[a]	BR	10 mg/mL[a]	Visually compatible for 4 hr at 22°C	1439	C
Gallium nitrate	FUJ	1 mg/mL[b]	MJ	20 mg/mL	Visually compatible for 24 hr at 25°C	1673	C
Gemcitabine HCl	LI	10 mg/mL[b]	MJ	10 mg/mL[b]	Physically compatible for 4 hr at 23°C	2226	C
Granisetron HCl	SKB	1 mg/mL	MJ	4 mg/mL[b]	Physically compatible with little or no loss of either drug in 4 hr at 22°C	1883	C
Isavuconazonium sulfate	ASP	1.5 mg/mL[h]	PRP	20 mg/mL[h]	Physically compatible for 2 hr	3263	C
Linezolid	PHU	2 mg/mL	MJ	10 mg/mL[a]	Physically compatible for 4 hr at 23°C	2264	C
Melphalan HCl	BW	0.1 mg/mL[b]	BR	10 mg/mL[b]	Physically compatible for 3 hr at 22°C	1557	C
Meropenem–vaborbactam	TMC	8 mg/mL[b j]	SGT	20 mg/mL[b]	Physically compatible for 3 hr at 20 to 25°C	3380	C
Methotrexate sodium		30 mg/mL		1.8 mg/mL[a]	Visually compatible for 4 hr at room temperature	1788	C
Micafungin sodium	ASP	1.5 mg/mL[b]	APP	20 mg/mL[b]	Physically compatible for 4 hr at 23°C	2683	C

Y-Site Injection Compatibility (1:1 Mixture) (Cont.)

Test Drug	Mfr	Conc	Mfr	Conc	Remarks	Ref	C/I
Ondansetron HCl	GL	1 mg/mL[b]	BR	10 mg/mL[a]	Visually compatible for 4 hr at 22°C	1365	C
Oxaliplatin	SS	0.5 mg/mL[a]	MJ	10 mg/mL[a]	Physically compatible for 4 hr at 23°C	2566	C
Paclitaxel	NCI	1.2 mg/mL[a]	MJ	10 mg/mL[a]	Physically compatible for 4 hr at 22°C	1556	C
Pemetrexed disodium	LI	20 mg/mL[b]	APP	10 mg/mL[a]	Physically compatible for 4 hr at 23°C	2564	C
Piperacillin sodium–tazobactam sodium	LE[f]	40 mg/mL[a g]	MJ	10 mg/mL[a]	Physically compatible for 4 hr at 22°C	1688	C
Plazomicin sulfate	ACH	24 mg/mL[h]	SGT	20 mg/mL[h]	Physically compatible for 1 hr at 20 to 25°C	3432	C
Sargramostim	IMM	10 mcg/mL[b]	MJ	10 mg/mL[b]	Visually compatible for 4 hr at 22°C	1436	C
Sodium bicarbonate		1.4%		1.8 mg/mL[a]	Visually compatible for 4 hr at room temperature	1788	C
Tedizolid phosphate	CUB	0.8 mg/mL[b]	PRP	20 mg/mL[b]	Physically compatible for 2 hr	3244	C
Teniposide	BR	0.1 mg/mL[a]	MJ	10 mg/mL[a]	Physically compatible for 4 hr at 23°C	1725	C
Thiotepa	IMM[d]	1 mg/mL[a]	MJ	10 mg/mL[a]	Physically compatible for 4 hr at 23°C	1861	C
TNA #218 to #226[e]			MJ	10 mg/mL[a]	Visually compatible for 4 hr at 23°C	2215	C
TPN #212 to #215[e]			MJ	10 mg/mL[a]	Physically compatible for 4 hr at 23°C	2109	C
Vinorelbine tartrate	BW	1 mg/mL[b]	MJ	10 mg/mL[b]	Physically compatible for 4 hr at 22°C	1558	C

[a] Tested in dextrose 5%.

[b] Tested in sodium chloride 0.9%.

[c] Tested in bacteriostatic sodium chloride 0.9% preserved with benzyl alcohol 0.9%.

[d] Lyophilized formulation tested.

[e] Refer to Appendix for the composition of parenteral nutrition solutions. TNA indicates a 3-in-1 admixture, and TPN indicates a 2-in-1 admixture.

[f] Test performed using the formulation WITHOUT edetate disodium.

[g] Piperacillin component. Piperacillin in an 8:1 fixed-ratio concentration with tazobactam.

[h] Tested in both dextrose 5% and sodium chloride 0.9%.

[i] Ceftolozane component. Ceftolozane in a 2:1 fixed-ratio concentration with tazobactam.

[j] Meropenem component. Meropenem in a 1:1 fixed-ratio concentration with vaborbactam.

Selected Revisions June 1, 2019. © Copyright, October 1990.
American Society of Health-System Pharmacists, Inc.

Methadone Hydrochloride
AHFS 28:08.08

Products

Methadone hydrochloride is available in 20-mL multidose vials. Each mL of solution contains methadone hydrochloride 10 mg and sodium chloride 0.9% with sodium hydroxide and/or hydrochloric acid to adjust the pH. In addition, the 20-mL vials contain chlorobutanol 0.5%.[1(3/06)]

pH

From 4.5 to 6.5.[1(3/06)]

Administration

Methadone hydrochloride may be administered by subcutaneous, intramuscular, or intravenous injection.[1(3/06)][4]

Stability

Methadone hydrochloride in intact vials should be stored at controlled room temperature and protected from light.[1(3/06)]

Syringes

In 2015, reports of decreased potency of certain drugs (e.g., methadone hydrochloride) stored in Becton Dickinson syringes for extended periods (i.e., exceeding 24 hours) were confirmed by the manufacturer of these syringes; the cause of this change was later identified to be the inclusion of an alternate rubber stopper in the plunger of certain product lots of syringes.[3029][3036][3037][3039][3041][3042] Decreased potency was not observed when the syringes were filled and used promptly.[3037] Use of the alternate stopper was later discontinued and use of the primary stopper in such syringes was resumed; however, Becton Dickinson states that its general-use syringes are cleared by FDA for immediate use in fluid aspiration and injection and that such syringes, regardless of the stopper material, have not been cleared by FDA for use as a closed-container system.[3391]

Compatibility Information

Solution Compatibility

Methadone HCl

Test Soln Name	Mfr	Mfr	Conc/L or %	Remarks	Ref	C/I
Sodium chloride 0.9%	TR[a]	LI	1, 2, 5 g	Little or no loss in 28 days at room temperature exposed to light	1500	C

[a] Tested in PVC containers.

Y-Site Injection Compatibility (1:1 Mixture)

Methadone HCl

Test Drug	Mfr	Conc	Mfr	Conc	Remarks	Ref	C/I
Atropine sulfate	LY	0.4 mg/mL	LI	1 mg/mL[a]	Physically compatible for 48 hr at 22°C	1706	C
Dexamethasone sodium phosphate	AMR	1 mg/mL[a]	LI	1 mg/mL[a]	Physically compatible for 48 hr at 22°C	1706	C
Diazepam	ES	0.5 mg/mL[a]	LI	1 mg/mL[a]	Physically compatible for 48 hr at 22°C	1706	C
Diphenhydramine HCl	SCN	2 mg/mL[a]	LI	1 mg/mL[a]	Physically compatible for 48 hr at 22°C	1706	C
Haloperidol lactate	MN	0.2 mg/mL[a]	LI	1 mg/mL[a]	Physically compatible for 48 hr at 22°C	1706	C
Hydroxyzine HCl	WI	4 mg/mL[a]	LI	1 mg/mL[a]	Physically compatible for 48 hr at 22°C	1706	C
Ketorolac tromethamine	WY	1 mg/mL[a]	LI	1 mg/mL[a]	Physically compatible for 48 hr at 22°C	1706	C
Lorazepam	WY	0.1 mg/mL[a]	LI	1 mg/mL[a]	Physically compatible for 48 hr at 22°C	1706	C
Methotrimeprazine HCl	LE	0.2 mg/mL[a]	LI	1 mg/mL[a]	Physically compatible for 48 hr at 22°C	1706	C

DOI: 10.37573/9781585286850.254

Y-Site Injection Compatibility (1:1 Mixture) (Cont.)

Test Drug	Mfr	Conc	Mfr	Conc	Remarks	Ref	C/I
Metoclopramide HCl	DU	5 mg/mL	LI	1 mg/mL[a]	Physically compatible for 48 hr at 22°C	1706	C
Midazolam HCl	RC	0.2 mg/mL[a]	LI	1 mg/mL[a]	Physically compatible for 48 hr at 22°C	1706	C
Phenobarbital sodium	WY	2 mg/mL[a]	LI	1 mg/mL[a]	Physically compatible for 48 hr at 22°C	1706	C
Phenytoin sodium	ES	2 mg/mL[a][b]	LI	1 mg/mL[a]	Precipitate forms immediately	1706	I
Scopolamine HBr	LY	0.05 mg/mL[a]	LI	1 mg/mL[a]	Physically compatible for 48 hr at 22°C	1706	C

[a] Tested in dextrose 5%.

[b] Tested in sodium chloride 0.9%.

Selected Revisions December 12, 2018. © Copyright, October 1982. American Society of Health-System Pharmacists, Inc.

Methocarbamol
AHFS 12:20.04

Products

Methocarbamol 100 mg/mL is available in 10-mL vials. Also present in the formulation is polyethylene glycol 300 50% in water for injection with sodium hydroxide and/or hydrochloric acid to adjust pH during manufacturing.[1(8/06)]

pH

From 3.5 to 6.0.[1(8/06)]

Tonicity

Methocarbamol injection is hypertonic.[4]

Trade Name(s)

Robaxin

Administration

Methocarbamol injection is administered intramuscularly or intravenously. It should not be given subcutaneously. For intramuscular injection, not more than 5 mL (500 mg) should be given into each gluteal region. Direct intravenous injection should be made slowly at a maximum rate of 3 mL (300 mg) per minute. For intravenous infusion, 1 g of methocarbamol may be diluted in 250 mL of dextrose 5% or sodium chloride 0.9%.[1(8/06)]

Stability

Store at controlled room temperature[1(8/06)] and protect from freezing. Methocarbamol was stable for up to six days when diluted in sterile water for injection, dextrose 5%, or sodium chloride 0.9% to a concentration of 4 mg/mL. Refrigeration of methocarbamol diluted for intravenous infusion to concentrations of 15.4 mg/mL and greater may result in precipitation.[4]

Compatibility Information

Solution Compatibility

Methocarbamol

Test Soln Name	Mfr	Mfr	Conc/L or %	Remarks	Ref	C/I
Dextrose 5% in sodium chloride 0.45%		RB	≤15.4 g	Physically compatible. Stable for 6 days at room temperature	2449	C
Dextrose 5% in sodium chloride 0.45%		RB	>15.4 g	Methocarbamol precipitates	2449	I
Dextrose 5%		RB	≤15.4 g	Physically compatible. Stable for 6 days at room temperature	2449	C
Dextrose 5%		RB	>15.4 g	Methocarbamol precipitates	2449	I
Sodium chloride 0.9%		RB	≤15.4 g	Physically compatible. Stable for 6 days at room temperature	2449	C
Sodium chloride 0.9%		RB	>15.4 g	Methocarbamol precipitates	2449	I

Selected Revisions October 1, 2012. © Copyright, October 2006.
American Society of Health-System Pharmacists, Inc.

DOI: 10.37573/9781585286850.255

Methohexital Sodium
AHFS 28:04.04

Products

Methohexital sodium is available in single-use vials containing methohexital sodium 200 mg with anhydrous sodium carbonate 12 mg and multiple-use vials containing methohexital sodium 500 mg with anhydrous sodium carbonate 30 mg or methohexital sodium 2.5 g with anhydrous sodium carbonate 150 mg.[2926] Recommended diluents are based on the intended route of administration.[2926] Diluents containing bacteriostatic agents should *not* be used.[2926]

To prepare a 1% (10-mg/mL) solution of methohexital sodium for intermittent intravenous injection, reconstitute the 200-mg single-use or the 500-mg multiple-use vials with 20 or 50 mL, respectively, of diluent.[2926] For the 2.5-g multiple-use vial, reconstitute with 15 mL of diluent and further dilute by adding the drug to 235 mL of diluent to total 250 mL.[2926] The preferred diluent for intermittent intravenous injection is sterile water for injection, but dextrose 5% or sodium chloride 0.9% also may be used.[2926]

Initial dilution of the 2.5-g vial results in a yellow solution.[2926] When further diluted to a final concentration of 1%, the solution must be clear and colorless or it should not be used.[2926]

To prepare a 0.2% (2-mg/mL) solution of methohexital sodium for continuous intravenous infusion, reconstitute the 500-mg vial with 15 mL of diluent and further dilute by adding the drug to 235 mL of diluent to total 250 mL.[2926] For continuous intravenous infusion, use only dextrose 5% or sodium chloride 0.9% as a diluent.[2926] Do *not* use sterile water for injection to prepare this concentration for continuous intravenous infusion to avoid extreme hypotonicity.[2926]

To prepare a 5% (50-mg/mL) solution for intramuscular use, reconstitute the 200- or 500-mg vials with 4 or 10 mL, respectively, of diluent.[2926] For the 2.5-g vial, reconstitute with 50 mL of diluent.[2926] No further dilution of the reconstituted solution for intramuscular use is required.[2926] The preferred diluent for intramuscular use is sterile water for injection, but sodium chloride 0.9% also may be used.[2926]

pH

A 0.2% solution in dextrose 5% has a pH of 9.5 to 10.5; a 1% solution in sterile water for injection has a pH of 10 to 11.[2926]

Sodium Content

Methohexital sodium contains 4.652 mEq of sodium per gram of drug; the sodium carbonate provides 1.132 mEq while the balance comes from the drug itself.[869]

Trade Name(s)

Brevital Sodium

Administration

Methohexital sodium is administered intravenously, by intermittent injection at a concentration of 1% or by continuous infusion at a concentration of 0.2%.[2926] Intra-arterial injection and extravasation should be avoided.[2926]

Intramuscular injection of 5% solutions of methohexital sodium has also been described.[2926]

Stability

Intact vials should be stored at controlled room temperature.[2926] Reconstituted solutions of methohexital sodium are stable at room temperature for 24 hours.[2926]

The manufacturer states that Ringer's injection, lactated is incompatible as a diluent; the potential for incompatibility exists between the sodium carbonate in the drug formulation and the calcium ions of the infusion solution.[282] [2926]

pH Effects

Methohexital sodium is alkaline in solution and is incompatible with acidic solutions and phenol-containing solutions.[4]

Methohexital sodium exhibits poor solubility in an acidic medium and may precipitate in solutions containing acidic drugs.[22]

Since solubility is maintained only at relatively high pH, mixing methohexital sodium with acidic solutions is not recommended.[4] Mixed with methohexital sodium, a haze or precipitate forms in 15 minutes with atropine sulfate, in 30 minutes with succinylcholine chloride, and in 60 minutes with scopolamine HBr.[2926]

When barbiturates are mixed with succinylcholine chloride, either free barbiturate precipitates or the succinylcholine chloride is hydrolyzed, depending on the final pH of the admixture.[4] [21] Similarly, atracurium besylate may be inactivated by alkaline solutions, such as barbiturates, and a free acid of the admixed drug may precipitate, depending on the resultant pH of the admixture.[4]

Methohexital sodium may raise the pH of admixture solutions to the alkaline range and, therefore, should not be mixed with drugs that are alkali labile.[4]

Sorption

Methohexital sodium (Lilly) 32 mg/L displayed 7.9% sorption to a PVC plastic test strip in 24 hours.[12] However, another test did not confirm this finding. No significant loss in PVC containers and no difference between glass and PVC containers were found.[282]

DOI: 10.37573/9781585286850.256

Compatibility Information

Solution Compatibility

Methohexital sodium

Test Soln Name	Mfr	Mfr	Conc/L or %	Remarks	Ref	C/I
Dextrose 5% in Ringer's injection, lactated	TR[a]	LI	2 g	Stable for 24 hr at 5°C	282	C
Dextrose 5% in sodium chloride 0.9%	TR[a]	LI	2 g	Stable for 24 hr at 5°C	282	C
Dextrose 5%	TR[a]	LI	2 g	Stable for 24 hr at 5°C	282	C
Ringer's injection, lactated	TR[a]	LI	2 g	Stable for 24 hr at 5°C	282	C
Ringer's injection, lactated		JHP		Stated to be incompatible	2926	I
Sodium chloride 0.9%	TR[a]	LI	2 g	Stable for 24 hr at 5°C	282	C

[a] Tested in both glass and PVC containers.

Additive Compatibility

Methohexital sodium

Test Drug	Mfr	Conc/L or %	Mfr	Conc/L or %	Test Solution	Remarks	Ref	C/I
Chlorpromazine HCl	BP	200 mg	BP	2 g	D5W, NS	Precipitates immediately	26	I
Hydralazine HCl	BP	80 mg	BP	2 g	D5W, NS	Yellow color with precipitate in 3 hr	26	I
Lidocaine HCl	BP	2 g	BP	2 g	D5W	Precipitates immediately	26	I
Mechlorethamine HCl	BP	40 mg	BP	2 g	D5W, NS	Haze develops over 3 hr	26	I
Methyldopate HCl		1 g	BP	2 g	D5W	Haze develops over 3 hr	26	I
Methyldopate HCl		1 g	BP	2 g	NS	Crystals produced	26	I
Prochlorperazine mesylate	BP	100 mg	BP	2 g	D5W	Haze develops over 3 hr	26	I
Promethazine HCl	BP	100 mg	BP	2 g	D5W, NS	Precipitates immediately	26	I
Streptomycin sulfate	BP	4 g	BP	2 g	NS	Crystals produced	26	I

Drugs in Syringe Compatibility

Methohexital sodium

Test Drug	Mfr	Amt	Mfr	Amt	Remarks	Ref	C/I
Glycopyrrolate	RB	0.2 mg/1 mL	LI	10 mg/1 mL	Precipitates immediately	331	I
Glycopyrrolate	RB	0.2 mg/1 mL	LI	20 mg/2 mL	Precipitates immediately	331	I
Glycopyrrolate	RB	0.4 mg/2 mL	LI	10 mg/1 mL	Precipitates immediately	331	I
Scopolamine HBr					Haze forms in 1 hr	4	I

Y-Site Injection Compatibility (1:1 Mixture)

Methohexital sodium

Test Drug	Mfr	Conc	Mfr	Conc	Remarks	Ref	C/I
Fenoldopam mesylate	AB	80 mcg/mL[a]	JP	10 mg/mL[a]	Microparticulates and yellow color form immediately	2467	I

[a] Tested in sodium chloride 0.9%.

Methotrexate Sodium
AHFS 10:00

Products

Methotrexate sodium is available in liquid[2966][2967] and lyophilized dosage forms.[2968]

The liquid dosage forms contain methotrexate sodium equivalent to methotrexate 25 mg/mL and are available in vials of various sizes from 2 to 40 mL.[2966][2967] The products also contain sodium chloride,[2966][2967] and the preserved products contain benzyl alcohol.[2966] The pH has been adjusted during manufacturing with sodium hydroxide and/or hydrochloric acid.[2966][2967]

Methotrexate (as the sodium salt) is available as a lyophilized powder in single-use vials containing 1 g.[2968] The pH may have been adjusted during manufacturing with sodium hydroxide and/or hydrochloric acid.[2968] The 1-g vial requires 19.4 mL of sterile, preservative-free diluent (e.g., dextrose 5%, sodium chloride 0.9%) for reconstitution to yield a 50-mg/mL concentration.[2968]

Methotrexate also is available in prefilled auto-injector syringes for subcutaneous use containing 50 mg/mL in various sizes from 0.15 to 0.6 mL.[2970] Prefilled auto-injector syringes for subcutaneous use also are available containing 7.5, 10, 15, 20 or 25 mg per 0.4 mL.[2969]

pH

The pH of the liquid forms in vials is approximately 8.5.[2966][2967] The pH of the lyophilized form is approximately 8.5 to 8.7.[2968] The pH of the Otrexup and Rasuvo prefilled auto-injector syringes is 8 and 8.5, respectively.[2969][2970]

Tonicity

The liquid forms of methotrexate sodium in vials are isotonic.[2966][2967]

Sodium Content

Methotrexate sodium preservative-free liquid injections in vials contain sodium 0.43, 0.86, 1.72, 2.15, and 8.6 mEq in the 2-, 4-, 8-, 10-, and 40-mL sizes, respectively.[2967] The lyophilized product contains 7 mEq of sodium in the 1-g vial.[2968]

Trade Name(s)

Otrexup, Rasuvo

Administration

Methotrexate sodium may be administered by intramuscular, intra-arterial, subcutaneous, or intrathecal injection, by direct intravenous injection, or by intravenous infusion.[2966][2967][2968][2969][2970] For intrathecal injection, a preservative-free form is diluted to a 1-mg/mL concentration in an appropriate preservative-free diluent (e.g., sodium chloride 0.9%, Elliott's B solution, the patient's own spinal fluid).[4][435][830][2967][2968]

For high-dose regimens, it is recommended that preservative-free forms of methotrexate sodium be used.[241][242][2967][2968]

The manufacturer of the lyophilized powder form of methotrexate sodium states that high doses of methotrexate administered by intravenous infusion are to be diluted in dextrose 5%.[2968] High doses of methotrexate sodium require leucovorin rescue.[2967][2968]

Stability

Store the lyophilized powder and injection vials and the prefilled auto-injector syringes at controlled room temperature with protection from light.[2966][2967][2968][2969][2970] Retain the lyophilized form in its original carton until use.[2968]

For intrathecal injection, the preservative-free dosage forms should be diluted immediately prior to use.[2967] Although reconstitution of the lyophilized vials immediately prior to use is also recommended (because of the absence of antibacterial preservatives),[2968] the reconstituted solution is stable for at least 1 week at room temperature.[234]

Immersion of a needle with an aluminum component in methotrexate sodium (Lederle) 25 mg/mL resulted in the formation of orange crystals on the aluminum surface after 36 hours at 24°C with protection from light.[988]

pH Effects

Methotrexate is most stable between pH 6 and 8. Drugs producing extremes of pH should not be added to methotrexate.[1072][1379]

Freezing Solutions

Methotrexate sodium (Lederle) 50 mg/100 mL in polyvinyl chloride (PVC) bags of dextrose 5% (Travenol) was frozen at −20°C for at least 30 days and thawed by microwave radiation for 2 minutes with no significant change in concentration. Even after 5 repetitions of the freeze–thaw treatment, the methotrexate concentration showed no significant change.[818]

The stability of methotrexate 5 mg, 50 mg, and 1 g in 50 mL of sodium chloride 0.9% in PVC bags frozen at −20°C for up to 12 weeks and thawed in a microwave oven was evaluated. No loss was found in any of the concentrations.[1281]

Light Effects

Photolability, although unrecognized for many years, is a stability problem that is increased by dilution and mixture with sodium bicarbonate.[1202]

In dilute solutions of 0.1 mg/mL, methotrexate is reported to undergo photodegradation on exposure to light. Decomposition of 5 to 8% in 10 days and 11 to 17% in 20 days has been reported. This effect was not observed in the more concentrated solutions of the commercial preparation (25 mg/mL)[433] or in admixtures of methotrexate during short-term light exposure. No significant loss of methotrexate occurred due to light exposure for 4 hours in solutions composed of 5 mg, 50 mg, or 1 g of methotrexate in 50 mL of sodium chloride 0.9% in PVC containers.[1281]

DOI: 10.37573/9781585286850.257

Little methotrexate loss was found from a 1-mg/mL solution in sodium chloride 0.9% in 3 burette drip chambers made of cellulose propionate (Avon A200 standard and A2000 Amberset) and methacrylate butadiene styrene (Avon A2001 Sureset) when exposed to normal mixed daylight and fluorescent lighting conditions for 24 hours. However, in 48 hours about 10 and 12% losses were observed in the A200 and A2001, respectively. With exposure to direct sunlight, an 11% loss occurred in the A200 in 7 hours. No loss occurred when the Amberset or Sureset was wrapped in foil and exposed to either light condition for 48 hours.[1378]

Exposure of methotrexate 1-mg/mL solution in PVC and polybutadiene tubing to mixed daylight and fluorescent light produced significant losses after 8 to 12 hours. The Amberset PVC tubing or foil wrapping for the polybutadiene tubing to protect solutions from light reduced losses to 12 to 16% in 48 hours.[1378]

Methotrexate sodium (R. Bellon), reconstituted to a concentration of 1 mg/mL with sodium chloride 0.9%, was evaluated for stability in translucent containers (Perfupack, Baxter) and 5 opaque containers (green PVC Opafuseur [Bruneau], white EVA Perfu-opaque [Baxter], orange PVC PF170 [Cair], white PVC V86 [Codan], and white EVA Perfecran [Fandre]) when exposed to sunlight for 28 days. Photodegradation was found after storage in the translucent Perfupack. Losses ranged from 18.5 to 27% after 24 hours at a methotrexate sodium concentration of 5 mg/mL. At 1 mg/mL, losses of 4% or less occurred in 24 hours in the opaque containers.[1750]

Intrathecal Injections

In a study of intrathecal injections, preservative-free methotrexate sodium (Ben Venue) was reconstituted to a concentration of 2.5 mg/mL with Elliott's B solution (305 mOsm/kg, pH 7.2), sodium chloride 0.9% injection (303 mOsm/kg, pH 7.6), or Ringer's injection, lactated (270 mOsm/kg, pH 7.6). In all 3 solutions, methotrexate exhibited no change in concentration over 7 days under fluorescent light at 30°C.[327]

In another study, the stability and compatibility of cytarabine (Upjohn), methotrexate (NCI), and hydrocortisone (Upjohn), mixed together in intrathecal injections, were evaluated. Two combinations were tested: (1) cytarabine 50 mg, methotrexate 12 mg (as the sodium salt), and hydrocortisone 25 mg (as the sodium succinate salt); and (2) cytarabine 30 mg, methotrexate 12 mg (as the sodium salt), and hydrocortisone 15 mg (as the sodium succinate salt). Each drug combination was added to 12 mL of Elliott's B solution (NCI), sodium chloride 0.9% (Abbott), dextrose 5% (Abbott), and Ringer's injection, lactated (Abbott) and stored for 24 hours at 25°C. Cytarabine and methotrexate were both chemically stable, with no drug loss after the full 24 hours in all solutions. Hydrocortisone was also stable in the sodium chloride 0.9%, dextrose 5%, and Ringer's injection, lactated with about a 2% drug loss.

However, in Elliott's B solution, hydrocortisone was significantly less stable, with a 6% loss in the 25-mg concentration over 24 hours. The 15-mg concentration was worse, with a 5% loss in 10 hours and a 13% loss in 24 hours. The higher pH of Elliott's B solution and the lower concentration of hydrocortisone may have been factors in this increased decomposition. All mixtures were physically compatible during this study, but a precipitate formed after several days of storage.[819]

Methotrexate sodium (Lederle) 2 mg/mL diluted in Elliott's B solution (Orphan Medical) was packaged as 20 mL in 30-mL glass vials and 20-mL plastic syringes (Becton Dickinson) with Red Cap (Burron) Luer-Lok syringe tip caps. The solution was physically compatible and chemically stable exhibiting little loss during storage for 48 hours at 4 and 23°C.[1976]

Bacterially contaminated intrathecal solutions can pose very grave risks. Consequently, intrathecal solutions should be administered as soon as possible after preparation.[328]

Syringes

Methotrexate (Lederle) 50 mg/mL was stable for up to 8 months when stored in Monoject or Plastipak plastic syringes at 25°C. Because of possible alteration in water vapor permeability, use of Sabre and Steriseal plastic syringes is limited to 70 days at 25°C.[1280]

Methotrexate sodium (Lederle) 2.5 mg/mL was repackaged into 10-mL plastic syringes (Becton Dickinson) and stored at 4 and 25°C for 7 days. No loss of methotrexate was found. Furthermore, no contaminants from the syringes were observed.[1913]

Sorption

Methotrexate sodium 22.5 mg/100 mL and 12 g/500 mL in both dextrose 5% and sodium chloride 0.9% in PVC containers (Macoflex, Macopharma) exhibited no sorption loss during 30 days of storage at 4°C protected from light. Simulated infusion of methotrexate sodium 2.25 g/500 mL in dextrose 5% and sodium chloride 0.9% over 24 hours through opaque PVC infusion sets (Perfecran, Fandre) also showed no sorption loss to the PVC tubing.[1867]

Methotrexate sodium (Medac) 0.36 mg/mL in dextrose 5% and in sodium chloride 0.9% exhibited little or no loss due to sorption in polyethylene, PVC, and glass containers over 72 hours at room and refrigeration temperatures.[2420][2430]

Central Venous Catheter

Methotrexate sodium (Immunex) 2.5 mg/mL in dextrose 5% was found to be compatible with the ARROWg+ard Blue Plus (Arrow International) chlorhexidine-bearing triple-lumen central catheter. Essentially complete delivery of the drug was found with little or no drug loss occurring. Furthermore, chlorhexidine delivered from the catheter remained at trace amounts with no substantial increase due to the delivery of the drug through the catheter.[2335]

Compatibility Information

Solution Compatibility

Methotrexate sodium

Test Soln Name	Mfr	Mfr	Conc/L or %	Remarks	Ref	C/I
Amino acids 4.25%, dextrose 25%	MG	LE	50 mg	No increase in particulate matter in 24 hr at 5°C	349	C
Dextrose 5%	TR[a]	LE	960 mg	Under 10% loss in 24 hr at room temperature	519	C
Dextrose 5%	[b]		225 mg and 24 g	Visually compatible with no loss in 30 days at 4°C protected from light	1867	C
Dextrose 5%				Manufacturer-recommended solution	2967	C
Sodium chloride 0.9%	[a]	FA	1.25 and 12.5 g	Visually compatible with little or no loss in 105 days at 4°C followed by 7 days at 25°C in the dark	1567	C
Sodium chloride 0.9%	[b]		225 mg and 24 g	Visually compatible with no loss in 30 days at 4°C protected from light	1867	C
Sodium chloride 0.9%		APP		Under 10% loss in 24 hr at 21 to 25°C	2966	C
Sodium chloride 0.9%				Manufacturer-recommended solution	2967	C

[a] Tested in both glass and PVC containers.

[b] Tested in PVC containers.

Additive Compatibility

Methotrexate sodium

Test Drug	Mfr	Conc/L or %	Mfr	Conc/L or %	Test Solution	Remarks	Ref	C/I
Bleomycin sulfate	BR	20 and 30 units	LE	250 and 500 mg	NS	About 60% loss of bleomycin activity in 1 week at 4°C	763	I
Cyclophosphamide		1.67 g		25 mg	NS	6.6% cyclophosphamide loss in 14 days at room temperature	1379, 1389	C
Cyclophosphamide with fluorouracil		1.67 g 8.3 g		25 mg	NS	9.3% cyclophosphamide loss in 7 days at room temperature. No loss of other drugs observed	1389	C
Cytarabine	UP	400 mg	LE	200 mg	D5W	Physically compatible. Very little change in UV spectra in 8 hr at room temperature	207	C
Fluorouracil		10 g		30 mg	NS	Both drugs stable for 15 days at room temperature	1379	C
Fluorouracil with cyclophosphamide		8.3 g 1.67 g		25 mg	NS	9.3% cyclophosphamide loss in 7 days at room temperature. No loss of other drugs observed	1389	C
Hydroxyzine HCl	LY	500 mg	BV	1 and 3 g	D5W[a]	Physically compatible for 48 hr	1190	C
Mercaptopurine sodium	BW	1 g	LE	100 mg	D5W	Physically compatible	15	C
Ondansetron HCl	GL	30 and 300 mg	LE	0.5 and 6 g	D5W[b]	Physically compatible with little or no loss of either drug in 48 hr at 23°C	1876	C
Sodium bicarbonate		50 mEq	LE	750 mg	D5W	6% methotrexate loss in 1 week at 5°C in dark. At 23°C in light, 6% loss in 72 hr and 15% in 1 week	465	C

Additive Compatibility (Cont.)

Test Drug	Mfr	Conc/L or %	Mfr	Conc/L or %	Test Solution	Remarks	Ref	C/I
Sodium bicarbonate		50 mEq		2 g		No photodegradation products in 12 hr in room light	433	C
Vincristine sulfate	LI	10 mg	LE	100 mg	D5W	Physically compatible	15	C
Vincristine sulfate	LI	4 mg	LE	8 mg	D5W	Physically compatible. No change in UV spectra in 8 hr at room temperature	207	C

a Tested in glass containers.

b Tested in PVC containers.

Drugs in Syringe Compatibility

Methotrexate sodium

Test Drug	Mfr	Amt	Mfr	Amt	Remarks	Ref	C/I
Bleomycin sulfate		1.5 units/0.5 mL		12.5 mg/0.5 mL	Physically compatible for 5 min at room temperature followed by 8 min of centrifugation	980	C
Cisplatin		0.5 mg/0.5 mL		12.5 mg/0.5 mL	Physically compatible for 5 min at room temperature followed by 8 min of centrifugation	980	C
Cyclophosphamide		10 mg/0.5 mL		12.5 mg/0.5 mL	Physically compatible for 5 min at room temperature followed by 8 min of centrifugation	980	C
Doxapram HCl	RB	400 mg/20 mL		50 mg/20 mL	Physically compatible with 4% doxapram loss in 24 hr	1177	C
Doxorubicin HCl		1 mg/0.5 mL		12.5 mg/0.5 mL	Physically compatible for 5 min at room temperature followed by 8 min of centrifugation	980	C
Droperidol		1.25 mg/0.5 mL		12.5 mg/0.5 mL	Precipitates immediately	980	I
Fluorouracil		25 mg/0.5 mL		12.5 mg/0.5 mL	Physically compatible for 5 min at room temperature followed by 8 min of centrifugation	980	C
Furosemide		5 mg/0.5 mL		12.5 mg/0.5 mL	Physically compatible for 5 min at room temperature followed by 8 min of centrifugation	980	C
Heparin sodium		500 units/0.5 mL		12.5 mg/0.5 mL	Physically compatible for 5 min at room temperature followed by 8 min of centrifugation	980	C
Leucovorin calcium		5 mg/0.5 mL		12.5 mg/0.5 mL	Physically compatible for 5 min at room temperature followed by 8 min of centrifugation	980	C
Metoclopramide HCl		2.5 mg/0.5 mL		12.5 mg/0.5 mL	Physically compatible for 5 min at room temperature followed by 8 min of centrifugation	980	C
Metoclopramide HCl	RB	10 mg/2 mL	LE	50 mg/2 mL	Incompatible. If mixed, use immediately	1167	I
Metoclopramide HCl	RB	160 mg/32 mL	LE	200 mg/8 mL	Incompatible. If mixed, use immediately	1167	I
Mitomycin		0.25 mg/0.5 mL		12.5 mg/0.5 mL	Physically compatible for 5 min at room temperature followed by 8 min of centrifugation	980	C
Vinblastine sulfate		0.5 mg/0.5 mL		12.5 mg/0.5 mL	Physically compatible for 5 min at room temperature followed by 8 min of centrifugation	980	C
Vincristine sulfate		0.5 mg/0.5 mL		12.5 mg/0.5 mL	Physically compatible for 5 min at room temperature followed by 8 min of centrifugation	980	C

Y-Site Injection Compatibility (1:1 Mixture)

Methotrexate sodium

Test Drug	Mfr	Conc	Mfr	Conc	Remarks	Ref	C/I
Allopurinol sodium	BW	3 mg/mLᵇ	LE	15 mg/mLᵇ	Physically compatible for 4 hr at 22°C	1686	C
Amifostine	USB	10 mg/mLᵃ	LE	15 mg/mLᵃ	Physically compatible for 4 hr at 23°C	1845	C
Aztreonam	SQ	40 mg/mLᵃ	LE	15 mg/mLᵃ	Physically compatible for 4 hr at 23°C	1758	C
Bleomycin sulfate		3 units/mL		25 mg/mL	Drugs injected sequentially in Y-site with no flush. No precipitate seen	980	C
Ceftriaxone sodium	RC	100 mg/mL		30 mg/mL	Visually compatible for 4 hr at room temperature	1788	C
Cisplatin		1 mg/mL		25 mg/mL	Drugs injected sequentially in Y-site with no flush. No precipitate seen	980	C
Cyclophosphamide		20 mg/mL		25 mg/mL	Drugs injected sequentially in Y-site with no flush. No precipitate seen	980	C
Cyclophosphamide		20 mg/mLᵃ		30 mg/mL	Visually compatible for 4 hr at room temperature	1788	C
Cytarabine	UP	0.6 mg/mLᵃ		30 mg/mL	Visually compatible for 4 hr at room temperature	1788	C
Daunorubicin HCl	BEL	0.52 mg/mLᵃ		30 mg/mL	Visually compatible for 4 hr at room temperature	1788	C
Dexamethasone sodium phosphate	MSD	4 mg/mL		30 mg/mL	Visually compatible for 2 hr at room temperature. Precipitate forms in 4 hr	1788	I
Doripenem	JJ	5 mg/mLᵃ ᵇ	BED	12.5 mg/mLᵃ ᵇ	Physically compatible for 4 hr at 23°C	2743	C
Doxorubicin HCl		2 mg/mL		25 mg/mL	Drugs injected sequentially in Y-site with no flush. No precipitate seen	980	C
Doxorubicin HCl	FA	0.4 mg/mLᵃ		30 mg/mL	Visually compatible for 4 hr at room temperature	1788	C
Doxorubicin HCl liposomal	SEQ	0.4 mg/mLᵃ	IMM	15 mg/mLᵃ	Physically compatible for 4 hr at 23°C	2087	C
Droperidol		2.5 mg/mL		25 mg/mL	Precipitate forms	977	I
Droperidol		2.5 mg/mL		25 mg/mL	Drugs injected sequentially in Y-site with no flush. Precipitates immediately	980	I
Etoposide	BR	0.6 mg/mLᵇ		30 mg/mL	Visually compatible for 4 hr at room temperature	1788	C
Etoposide phosphate	BR	5 mg/mLᵃ	IMM	15 mg/mLᵃ	Physically compatible for 4 hr at 23°C	2218	C
Filgrastim	AMG	30 mcg/mLᵃ	LE	15 mg/mLᵃ	Physically compatible for 4 hr at 22°C	1687	C
Fludarabine phosphate	BX	1 mg/mLᵃ	CET	15 mg/mLᵃ	Visually compatible for 4 hr at 22°C	1439	C
Fluorouracil		50 mg/mL		25 mg/mL	Drugs injected sequentially in Y-site with no flush. No precipitate seen	980	C
Furosemide		10 mg/mL		25 mg/mL	Drugs injected sequentially in Y-site with no flush. No precipitate seen	980	C
Gallium nitrate	FUJ	1 mg/mLᵇ	LE	25 mg/mLᵇ	Visually compatible for 24 hr at 25°C	1673	C
Gemcitabine HCl	LI	10 mg/mLᵇ	IMM	15 mg/mLᵇ	Precipitate forms immediately, redissolves, but reprecipitates in 15 to 20 min	2226	I
Granisetron HCl	SKB	1 mg/mL	CET	12.5 mg/mLᵇ	Physically compatible with little or no loss of either drug in 4 hr at 22°C	1883	C
Heparin sodium		1000 units/mL		25 mg/mL	Drugs injected sequentially in Y-site with no flush. No precipitate seen	980	C

Y-Site Injection Compatibility (1:1 Mixture) (Cont.)

Test Drug	Mfr	Conc	Mfr	Conc	Remarks	Ref	C/I
Idarubicin HCl	AD	1 mg/mL[b]	LE	25 mg/mL	Color changes immediately	1525	I
Ifosfamide		36 mg/mL[a]		30 mg/mL	Visually compatible for 2 hr at room temperature. Yellow precipitate in 4 hr	1788	I
Leucovorin calcium		10 mg/mL		25 mg/mL	Drugs injected sequentially in Y-site with no flush. No precipitate seen	980	C
Leucovorin calcium	LE	10 mg/mL		30 mg/mL	Visually compatible for 4 hr at room temperature	1788	C
Linezolid	PHU	2 mg/mL	IMM	15 mg/mL[a]	Physically compatible for 4 hr at 23°C	2264	C
Melphalan HCl	BW	0.1 mg/mL[b]	LE	15 mg/mL[b]	Physically compatible for 3 hr at 22°C	1557	C
Mesna		1.8 mg/mL[a]		30 mg/mL	Visually compatible for 4 hr at room temperature	1788	C
Methylprednisolone sodium succinate	UP	20 mg/mL		30 mg/mL	Visually compatible for 4 hr at room temperature	1788	C
Metoclopramide HCl		5 mg/mL		25 mg/mL	Drugs injected sequentially in Y-site with no flush. No precipitate seen	980	C
Midazolam HCl	RC	5 mg/mL		30 mg/mL	Yellow precipitate forms immediately	1788	I
Mitomycin		0.5 mg/mL		25 mg/mL	Drugs injected sequentially in Y-site with no flush. No precipitate seen	980	C
Nalbuphine HCl	DU	10 mg/mL		30 mg/mL	Yellow precipitate forms immediately	1788	I
Ondansetron HCl	GL	1 mg/mL[b]	CET	15 mg/mL[a]	Visually compatible for 4 hr at 22°C	1365	C
Ondansetron HCl	GL	2 mg/mL		30 mg/mL	Visually compatible for 4 hr at room temperature	1788	C
Oxacillin sodium	BR	250 mg/mL		30 mg/mL	Visually compatible for 4 hr at room temperature	1788	C
Oxaliplatin	SS	0.5 mg/mL[a]	BED	12.5 mg/mL[a]	Physically compatible for 4 hr at 23°C	2566	C
Paclitaxel	NCI	1.2 mg/mL[a]		15 mg/mL[a]	Physically compatible for 4 hr at 22°C	1528	C
Piperacillin sodium–tazobactam sodium	LE[c]	40 mg/mL[a h]	LE	15 mg/mL[a]	Physically compatible for 4 hr at 22°C	1688	C
Propofol	ZEN[i]	10 mg/mL	LE	15 mg/mL[a]	White precipitate forms in 1 hr	2066	I
Sargramostim	IMM	10 mcg/mL[b]	CET	15 mg/mL[b]	Visually compatible for 4 hr at 22°C	1436	C
Teniposide	BR	0.1 mg/mL[a]	LE	15 mg/mL[a]	Physically compatible for 4 hr at 23°C	1725	C
Thiotepa	IMM[e]	1 mg/mL[a]	LE	15 mg/mL[a]	Physically compatible for 4 hr at 23°C	1861	C
TNA #218 to #226[d]			IMM	15 mg/mL[a]	Visually compatible for 4 hr at 23°C	2215	C
TPN #212 to #215[d]			LE	15 mg/mL[a]	Substantial loss of natural haze with a microprecipitate	2109	I
Vancomycin HCl	AB	510 mg[f]	LE	[g]	Physically compatible during 1-hr simultaneous infusion	1405	C
Vancomycin HCl		5 mg/mL[a]		30 mg/mL	Visually compatible for 2 hr at room temperature. Yellow precipitate in 4 hr	1788	I
Vinblastine sulfate		1 mg/mL		25 mg/mL	Drugs injected sequentially in Y-site with no flush. No precipitate seen	980	C
Vincristine sulfate		1 mg/mL		25 mg/mL	Drugs injected sequentially in Y-site with no flush. No precipitate seen	980	C
Vincristine sulfate	LI	0.1 mg/mL		30 mg/mL	Visually compatible for 4 hr at room temperature	1788	C

Y-Site Injection Compatibility (1:1 Mixture) (Cont.)

Test Drug	Mfr	Conc	Mfr	Conc	Remarks	Ref	C/I
Vinorelbine tartrate	BW	1 mg/mL[b]	LE	15 mg/mL[b]	Physically compatible for 4 hr at 22°C	1558	C

[a] Tested in dextrose 5%.

[b] Tested in sodium chloride 0.9%.

[c] Test performed using the formulation WITHOUT edetate disodium.

[d] Refer to Appendix for the composition of parenteral nutrition solutions. TNA indicates a 3-in-1 admixture, and TPN indicates a 2-in-1 admixture.

[e] Lyophilized formulation tested.

[f] Infused over one hour simultaneously with methotrexate.

[g] Diluted in dextrose 5%; concentration not cited.

[h] Piperacillin component. Piperacillin in an 8:1 fixed-ratio concentration with tazobactam.

[i] Test performed using the formulation WITH edetate disodium.

Selected Revisions January 31, 2020. © Copyright, October 1982. American Society of Health-System Pharmacists, Inc.

Methotrimeprazine Hydrochloride
AHFS 28:24.92
Levomepromazine Hydrochloride

Products

Methotrimeprazine hydrochloride is available in 1-mL ampuls as a 25-mg/mL (2.5% w/v) solution. The injection also contains ascorbic acid, sodium sulfite, and sodium chloride in water for injection.[38] [115]

pH
From 3 to 5.[17]

Osmolality

Methotrimeprazine hydrochloride injection is an isotonic solution.[38] [115]

Trade Name(s)

Nozinan

Administration

Methotrimeprazine hydrochloride is administered by intramuscular injection or intravenously after dilution with an equal volume of sodium chloride 0.9% immediately before use. It may also be given by continuous subcutaneous infusion diluted with the appropriate volume of sodium chloride 0.9%.[38] [115]

Stability

Methotrimeprazine hydrochloride injection is a clear, colorless solution. It should be stored at controlled room temperature and protected from light. On exposure to light, methotrimeprazine hydrochloride rapidly develops a pink or yellow discoloration; discolored solutions should be discarded. The drug is incompatible with alkaline solutions.[38] [115]

Compatibility Information

Additive Compatibility

Methotrimeprazine HCl

Test Drug	Mfr	Conc/L or %	Mfr	Conc/L or %	Test Solution	Remarks	Ref	C/I
Oxycodone HCl	NAP	1 g		250 mg	NS, W	Visually compatible. Under 4% concentration change in 24 hr at 25°C	2600	C

Drugs in Syringe Compatibility

Methotrimeprazine HCl

Test Drug	Mfr	Amt	Mfr	Amt	Remarks	Ref	C/I
Butorphanol tartrate	BR	4 mg/2 mL		25 mg/1 mL	Physically compatible for 30 min at room temperature	566	C
Diamorphine HCl	MB	50 mg/1 mL	MB	1.25 and 2.5 mg/1 mL[a]	Physically compatible and diamorphine stable for 24 hr at room temperature	1454	C
Heparin sodium		2500 units/1 mL		25 mg/1 mL	Turbidity or precipitate forms within 5 min	1053	I
Hydromorphone HCl	KN	10 mg/mL	LE	10 mg/mL	Visually compatible with less than 10% loss of either drug in 7 days at 8°C	668	C
Hydroxyzine HCl	PF	50 mg/1 mL	LE	20 mg/1 mL	Physically compatible	771	C
Hydroxyzine HCl	PF	100 mg/2 mL	LE	10 mg/0.5 mL	Physically compatible	771	C
Metoclopramide HCl	NO	10 mg/2 mL	RP	10 mg/2 mL	Physically compatible for 15 min at room temperature	565	C
Oxycodone HCl	NAP	200 mg/20 mL		200 mg/8 mL	Visually compatible. Under 4% concentration change in 24 hr at 25°C	2600	C
Ranitidine HCl	GL	50 mg/2 mL	RP	25 mg/1 mL	Immediate white turbidity	978	I

[a] Diluted with sterile water for injection.

DOI: 10.37573/9781585286850.258

Y-Site Injection Compatibility (1:1 Mixture)

Methotrimeprazine HCl

Test Drug	Mfr	Conc	Mfr	Conc	Remarks	Ref	C/I
Fentanyl citrate	JN	0.025 mg/mL[a]	LE	0.2 mg/mL[a]	Physically compatible for 48 hr at 22°C	1706	C
Hydromorphone HCl	AST	0.5 mg/mL[a]	LE	0.2 mg/mL[a]	Physically compatible for 48 hr at 22°C	1706	C
Methadone HCl	LI	1 mg/mL[a]	LE	0.2 mg/mL[a]	Physically compatible for 48 hr at 22°C	1706	C
Morphine sulfate	AST	1 mg/mL[a]	LE	0.2 mg/mL[a]	Physically compatible for 48 hr at 22°C	1706	C

[a] Tested in dextrose 5%.

Methyldopate Hydrochloride
AHFS 24:08.16

Products

Methyldopate hydrochloride is available as a 50-mg/mL solution in 5-mL single-use vials.[3009] Each mL of solution also contains citric acid, anhydrous 5 mg, sodium bisulfite 3.2 mg, monothioglycerol 2 mg, methylparaben 1.5 mg, edetate disodium 0.5 mg, propylparaben 0.2 mg, and sodium hydroxide and/or hydrochloric acid to adjust the pH in water for injection.[3009]

pH

From 3 to 4.2.[17]

Administration

Methyldopate hydrochloride should be diluted and administered by intravenous infusion.[3009] Intramuscular and subcutaneous injections are *not* recommended due to erratic absorption.[3020] The appropriate dose should be added to 100 mL of dextrose 5%;[3009] alternatively, the dose may be administered as 100 mg/10 mL in dextrose 5%.[3009] The diluted dose should be slowly infused over 30 to 60 minutes.[3009]

Stability

Intact vials should be stored at controlled room temperature.[3009] In aqueous solutions, the drug is most stable at acid to neutral pH. Oxidation of the catechol ring is the most important degradation process. The rate of such oxidation increases with increasing oxygen supply, increasing pH, and decreasing drug concentration.[1072]

The pH of infusion solutions containing methyldopate hydrochloride tends to be 7 or less, even when alkaline intravenous infusion solutions are used.[3021] It has been suggested that drugs poorly soluble in acidic media, such as barbiturate salts, be mixed cautiously with methyldopate hydrochloride since its acidity imparts some buffer capacity to intravenous admixtures. Furthermore, it should not be used with drugs known to be acid labile.[23]

Methyldopate hydrochloride oxidation is facilitated in alkaline solutions, yielding inactive, dark-colored compounds.[23 436] At pH 7.8, more than a 5% loss occurred over 24 hours.[437]

Compatibility Information

Solution Compatibility

Methyldopate HCl

Test Soln Name	Mfr	Mfr	Conc/L or %	Remarks	Ref	C/I
Amino acids 4.25%, dextrose 25%	MG	MSD	500 mg	No increase in particulate matter in 24 hr at 5°C	349	C
Dextrose 5% in sodium chloride 0.9%	AB	MSD	1 g	Stable for 24 hr	23	C
Dextrose 5%	AB	MSD	1 g	Stable for 24 hr	23	C
Dextrose 5%	AB	MSD	1 g	Physically compatible. 10% calculated loss in 125 hr at 25°C	527	C
Normosol M in dextrose 5%	AB	MSD	1 g	Stable for 24 hr	23	C
Normosol R	AB	MSD	1 g	Stable for 24 hr	23	C
Ringer's injection	AB	MSD	1 g	Stable for 24 hr	23	C
Sodium chloride 0.9%	AB	MSD	1 g	Stable for 24 hr	23	C

Additive Compatibility

Methyldopate HCl

Test Drug	Mfr	Conc/L or %	Mfr	Conc/L or %	Test Solution	Remarks	Ref	C/I
Aminophylline	SE	500 mg	MSD	1 g	D5W, D10W, D2.5½S, D2.5S, D5¼S, D5½S, D5S, D10S, NS, ½S	Physically compatible	23	C
Aminophylline	SE	500 mg	MSD	1 g	D5W	Physically compatible. At 25°C, 10% methyldopate decomposition in 90 hr	527	C

DOI: 10.37573/9781585286850.259

Additive Compatibility (Cont.)

Test Drug	Mfr	Conc/L or %	Mfr	Conc/L or %	Test Solution	Remarks	Ref	C/I
Amphotericin B		200 mg		1 g	D5W	Haze develops over 3 hr	26	I
Ascorbic acid	AB	1 g	MSD	1 g	D5W, D10W, D2.5½S, D2.5S, D5¼S, D5½S, D5S, D10S, NS, ½S	Physically compatible	23	C
Chloramphenicol sodium succinate	PD	1 g	MSD	1 g	D5W, D10W, D2.5½S, D2.5S, D5¼S, D5½S, D5S, D10S, NS, ½S	Physically compatible	23	C
Diphenhydramine HCl	PD	50 mg	MSD	1 g	D5W, D10W, D2.5½S, D2.5S, D5¼S, D5½S, D5S, D10S, NS, ½S	Physically compatible	23	C
Heparin sodium	AB	20,000 units	MSD	1 g	D5W, D10W, D2.5½S, D2.5S, D5¼S, D5½S, D5S, D10S, NS, ½S	Physically compatible	23	C
Magnesium sulfate		1 g	MSD	1 g	D5W, D10W, D2.5½S, D2.5S, D5¼S, D5½S, D5S, D10S, NS, ½S	Physically compatible	23	C
Methohexital sodium	BP	2 g		1 g	D5W	Haze develops over 3 hr	26	I
Methohexital sodium	BP	2 g		1 g	NS	Crystals produced	26	I
Multivitamins	USV	10 mL	MSD	1 g	D5W, D10W, D2.5½S, D2.5S, D5¼S, D5½S, D5S, D10S, NS, ½S	Physically compatible	23	C
Potassium chloride		40 mEq	MSD	1 g	D5W, D10W, D2.5½S, D2.5S, D5¼S, D5½S, D5S, D10S, NS, ½S	Physically compatible	23	C
Sodium bicarbonate		50 mEq	MSD	1 g	D5W, D10W, D2.5½S, D2.5S, D5¼S, D5½S, D5S, D10S, NS, ½S	Physically compatible	23	C
Sodium bicarbonate	AB	5%	MSD	1 g		Stable for 24 hr	23	C
Succinylcholine chloride	AB	2 g	MSD	1 g	D5W, D10W, D2.5½S, D2.5S, D5¼S, D5½S, D5S, D10S, NS, ½S	Physically compatible	23	C
Verapamil HCl	KN	80 mg	MSD	500 mg	D5W, NS	Physically compatible for 24 hr	764	C

Y-Site Injection Compatibility (1:1 Mixture)

Methyldopate HCl

Test Drug	Mfr	Conc	Mfr	Conc	Remarks	Ref	C/I
Esmolol HCl	DCC	10 mg/mL[a]	MSD	5 mg/mL[a]	Physically compatible for 24 hr at 22°C	1169	C
Heparin sodium	TR	50 units/mL	ES	5 mg/mL[a]	Visually compatible for 4 hr at 25°C	1793	C
Meperidine HCl	AB	10 mg/mL	AMR	2.5 mg/mL[a]	Physically compatible for 4 hr at 25°C	1397	C
Morphine sulfate	AB	1 mg/mL	AMR	2.5 mg/mL[a]	Physically compatible for 4 hr at 25°C	1397	C
Theophylline	TR	4 mg/mL	ES	5 mg/mL[a]	Visually compatible for 6 hr at 25°C	1793	C
TNA #73[c]			MSD	5 mg/mL[a]	Cracked the lipid emulsion	1009	I
TNA #73[c]			MSD	5 mg/mL[b]	Visually compatible for 4 hr	1009	C

[a] Tested in dextrose 5%.

[b] Tested in sodium chloride 0.9%.

[c] Refer to Appendix for the composition of parenteral nutrition solutions. TNA indicates a 3-in-1 admixture.

Selected Revisions January 26, 2016. © Copyright, October 1982. American Society of Health-System Pharmacists, Inc.

Methylene Blue
AHFS 92:12

Products

Methylene blue (ProvayBlue, American Regent) is available in 10-mL single-use ampuls.[3156] Each mL of solution contains 5 mg of methylene blue in water for injection.[3156]

Methylene blue (Akorn) also is available in single-use vials containing 1 or 10 mL of the injection solution.[3158] Each mL of solution contains 10 mg of methylene blue in water for injection and hydrochloric acid and/or sodium hydroxide to adjust the pH when necessary.[3158]

Tonicity

The 5-mg/mL methylene blue solution (ProvayBlue) is hypotonic.[3156]

pH

The 5-mg/mL methylene blue solution (ProvayBlue) has a pH ranging from 3 to 4.5.[3156]

Osmolality

The 5-mg/mL methylene blue solution (ProvayBlue) has an osmolality of 10 to 15 mOsm/kg.[3156]

Trade Name(s)

ProvayBlue

Administration

Methylene blue is administered intravenously very slowly over a period of several minutes[3158] or over 5 to 30 minutes.[3156] Patent venous access should be confirmed prior to administration.[3156] Methylene blue should *not* be administered subcutaneously[3156] [3158] or intrathecally;[3158] intraspinal injection is contraindicated.[3158]

The manufacturer of ProvayBlue states that the drug may be diluted prior to administration in 50 mL of dextrose 5% in order to avoid local pain, particularly in pediatric patients.[3156]

Stability

Methylene blue injection is a clear, dark blue solution.[3156] Intact ampuls and vials should be stored at controlled room temperature.[3156] [3158] The manufacturer of ProvayBlue states that ampuls should be stored in the original container to protect from light and that the drug should not be refrigerated or frozen.[3156]

Methylene blue injection solution should be visually inspected for particulate matter and discoloration prior to administration.[3156] Any unused portion of the solution should be discarded.[3156]

Solutions of methylene blue diluted in dextrose 5% should be used immediately following preparation.[3156] Sodium chloride 0.9% should not be mixed with methylene blue as chloride has been shown to reduce the solubility of the drug.[3156]

Compatibility Information
Solution Compatibility

Methylene blue

Test Soln Name	Mfr	Mfr	Conc/L or %	Remarks	Ref	C/I
Dextrose 5%		AMR		Manufacturer-recommended solution	3156	C
Sodium chloride 0.9%		AMR		Chloride reduces the solubility of methylene blue	3156	I

Selected Revisions July 1, 2020. © Copyright, March 2017. American Society of Health-System Pharmacists, Inc.

DOI: 10.37573/9781585286850.260

Methylergonovine Maleate
AHFS 76:00

Products

Methylergonovine maleate 0.2 mg/mL is available in 1-mL ampuls.[3299] Each mL of solution also contains maleic acid 0.1 mg and sodium chloride 7 mg in water for injection.[3299]

pH

From 2.7 to 3.5.[17]

Trade Name(s)

Methergine

Administration

Methylergonovine maleate is administered intramuscularly.[3299] The drug also may be administered intravenously slowly over no less than 1 minute, in combination with careful blood pressure monitoring, if intravenous administration is considered essential as a life-saving measure; it should *not* be administered routinely by the intravenous route.[3299] Administration of methylergonovine maleate by intra-arterial or periarterial injection must be strictly avoided.[3299]

Stability

Methylergonovine maleate injection is a clear, colorless solution.[3299] Intact ampuls should be stored under refrigeration at 2 to 8°C and protected from light.[3299] The product should be inspected visually for particulate matter and discoloration prior to administration.[3299]

To prevent inadvertent administration of methylergonovine maleate to newborn infants, the ampuls should be stored separately from medications intended for neonatal administration.[3299]

Compatibility Information

Y-Site Injection Compatibility (1:1 Mixture)

Methylergonovine maleate

Test Drug	Mfr	Conc	Mfr	Conc	Remarks	Ref	C/I
Heparin sodium	UP	1000 units/L[a]	SZ	0.2 mg/mL	Physically compatible for 4 hr at room temperature	534	C
Hydrocortisone sodium succinate	UP	10 mg/L[a]	SZ	0.2 mg/mL	Physically compatible for 4 hr at room temperature	534	C

[a] Tested in dextrose 5% in Ringer's injection, dextrose 5% in Ringer's injection, lactated, dextrose 5%, Ringer's injection, lactated, and sodium chloride 0.9%.

Selected Revisions September 28, 2017. © Copyright, October 1982. American Society of Health-System Pharmacists, Inc.

DOI: 10.37573/9781585286850.261

Methylprednisolone Acetate
AHFS 68:04

Products

Methylprednisolone acetate is an injectable suspension that is available in 20-, 40-, and 80-mg/mL concentrations in 5- and 10-mL multiple-dose vials. Each mL contains[1(3/03)] :

Component	Concentration/mL		
Methylprednisolone acetate	20 mg	40 mg	80 mg
Polyethylene glycol 3350	29.5 mg	29.1 mg	28.2 mg
Polysorbate 80	1.97 mg	1.94 mg	1.88 mg
Monobasic sodium phosphate	6.9 mg	6.8 mg	6.59 mg
Dibasic sodium phosphate	1.44 mg	1.42 mg	1.37 mg
Benzyl alcohol	9.3 mg	9.16 mg	8.88 mg
Sodium chloride	to adjust tonicity	to adjust tonicity	to adjust tonicity
Sodium hydroxide and/or hydrochloric acid	qs	qs	qs

Methylprednisolone acetate is also available at concentrations of 40- and 80-mg/mL in 1-mL single-dose vials. Each mL contains[1(3/03)] :

Component	Concentration/mL	
Methylprednisolone acetate	40 mg	80 mg
Polyethylene glycol 3350	29 mg	28 mg
Myristyl-gamma-picolinium chloride	0.195 mg	0.189 mg
Sodium chloride	to adjust tonicity	to adjust tonicity
Sodium hydroxide and/or hydrochloric acid	qs	qs

pH

From 3.5 to 7.0.[1(3/03)]

Trade Name(s)

Depo-Medrol

Administration

Methylprednisolone acetate is administered by intramuscular, intra-articular, intrasynovial, soft tissue, and intralesional injection without dilution. The drug is a suspension that must not be administered intravenously.[1(3/03)]

Stability

The intact vials should be stored at controlled room temperature.[1(3/03)]

Compatibility Information
Drugs in Syringe Compatibility

Methylprednisolone acetate

Test Drug	Mfr	Amt	Mfr	Amt	Remarks	Ref	C/I
Ropivacaine HCl	AST	6 mg/3 mL	PHU	80 mg/2 mL	Little loss of either drug in 30 days at 4 and 24°C in light or dark	2367	C

Selected Revisions October 1, 2012. © Copyright, October 2004. American Society of Health-System Pharmacists, Inc.

DOI: 10.37573/9781585286850.262

Methylprednisolone Sodium Succinate
AHFS 68:04

Products

Methylprednisolone sodium succinate is available in 40-mg (1-mL), 125-mg (2-mL), 500-mg (4-mL), and 1-g (8-mL) dual-chamber containers and 500-mg (8-mL), 1-g (16-mL), and 2-g (30.6-mL) vials with and without diluent. Monobasic sodium phosphate anhydrous, dibasic sodium phosphate dried, and lactose in the 40-mg size are also present. Use only the special diluent or bacteriostatic water for injection with benzyl alcohol to reconstitute the vials. The reconstituted solutions contain the methylprednisolone equivalent (as sodium succinate) of 40, 62.5, 125, or 65.4 mg/mL depending on the vial size and reconstitution volume used.[1(7/04)]

pH

The pH is adjusted to 7 to 8.[1(7/04)] [4]

Osmolarity

The osmolarities of the 40-, 62.5-, 125-, and 65.4-mg/mL concentrations are 500, 400, 440, and 420 mOsm/L, respectively.[1(7/04)]

Osmolality

The osmolality of methylprednisolone sodium succinate was calculated for the following dilutions:[1054]

Diluent	Osmolality (mOsm/kg)	
	50 mL	100 mL
500 mg		
Dextrose 5%	291	275
Sodium chloride 0.9%	317	301
1 g		
Dextrose 5%	318	292
Sodium chloride 0.9%	345	319

Sodium Content

Each gram of methylprednisolone sodium succinate contains 2.01 mEq of sodium.[846]

Trade Name(s)

A-MethaPred, Solu-Medrol

Administration

Methylprednisolone sodium succinate may be administered by intramuscular and direct intravenous injection and by intermittent or continuous intravenous infusion.[1(7/04)] [4] Direct intravenous injection should be performed over at least 1 minute[4] or over several minutes. High-dose therapy is given intravenously over at least 30 minutes.[1(7/04)]

Stability

Intact vials should be stored at controlled room temperature between 20 and 25°C and protected from light. Reconstituted solutions also should be stored between 20 and 25°C and should be used within 48 hours.[1(7/04)]

The drug is subject to both ester hydrolysis and acyl migration. Degradation products include free methylprednisolone, succinate, and methylprednisolone-17-succinate.[1072] Gross decomposition may result in insoluble free methylprednisolone.[2426] The solution should not be used unless it is clear and free of particulate matter.[4]

Methylprednisolone sodium succinate (Upjohn) diluted to a concentration of 4 mg/mL with sterile water for injection and packaged in glass vials was evaluated for stability. The samples stored at 22°C lost 10% in 24 hours while those stored at 4°C lost 6% in 7 days and 17% in 14 days.[1938]

pH Effects

The minimum rate of hydrolysis occurs at pH 3.5. Between pH 3.4 and 7.4, acyl migration is the dominant effect.[1501]

Freezing Solutions

Reconstituted methylprednisolone sodium succinate (Upjohn) 125 mg/2 mL, when stored frozen, exhibited no loss over 4 weeks.[69]

When stored frozen at −20°C, methylprednisolone sodium succinate (Upjohn) 500 mg/108 mL in sodium chloride 0.9% in polyvinyl chloride (PVC) bags exhibited no loss after 12 months followed by microwave thawing. Furthermore, the solution was physically compatible.[1612]

Syringes

Methylprednisolone sodium succinate (Pharmacia & Upjohn) 10 mg/mL in sodium chloride 0.9% was packaged in 10-mL polypropylene syringes (Becton Dickinson) and 12-mL polypropylene syringes (Monoject) and stored at 5 and 25°C. The drug solutions remained clear, and about 10% loss occurred in 7 days at 25°C and about 4% loss in 21 days at 5°C. The losses were comparable to the drug solution stored in a glass flask, indicating sorption to syringe components did not occur.[2340]

Central Venous Catheter

Methylprednisolone sodium succinate (Abbott) 5 mg/mL in dextrose 5% was found to be compatible with the ARROW-g+ard Blue Plus (Arrow International) chlorhexidine-bearing triple-lumen central catheter. Essentially complete delivery of the drug was found with little or no drug loss occurring. Furthermore, chlorhexidine delivered from the catheter remained at trace amounts with no substantial increase due to the delivery of the drug through the catheter.[2335]

Compatibility Information

Solution Compatibility

Methylprednisolone sodium succinate

Test Soln Name	Mfr	Mfr	Conc/L or %	Remarks	Ref	C/I
Amino acids 4.25%, dextrose 25%	MG	UP	250 mg	No increase in particulate matter in 24 hr at 5°C	349	C
Dextrose 5% in sodium chloride 0.45%		UP	5 to 10 g	Physically compatible for at least 4 hr	329	C
Dextrose 5% in sodium chloride 0.9%		UP	80 mg	Physically compatible for 24 hr	329	C
Dextrose 5%	AB	AB	500 mg to 1 g	Physically compatible and chemically stable for 24 hr at 25°C	758	C
Dextrose 5%	AB	AB	1.25 g	Physically compatible for 12 hr at 25°C. Haze from free methylprednisolone possible after 12 hr	758	I
Dextrose 5%	AB	AB	2 to 20 g	Physically compatible for 8 hr at 25°C. Haze from free methylprednisolone possible after 8 hr	758	I
Dextrose 5%	AB	AB	30 g	Physically compatible and chemically stable for 24 hr at 25°C	758	C
Dextrose 5%	TR[a]	UP	400 mg and 1.25 g	Physically compatible with 6 to 8% methylprednisolone 21-succinate ester loss in 24 hr at 24°C	1418	C
Dextrose 5%	TR[a]	UP	40 mg and 2 g	Visually compatible with 4% or less loss in 48 hr at room temperature	1802	C
Dextrose 5%	BA[a], BRN[b]	HO	125 mg	Visually compatible with little or no loss in 24 hr at 4 and 22°C	2289	C
Ringer's injection, lactated		UP	80 mg	Physically compatible for 24 hr	329	C
Sodium chloride 0.9%	AB	AB	500 mg to 30 g	Physically compatible and chemically stable for 24 hr at 25°C	758	C
Sodium chloride 0.9%	TR[a]	UP	40 mg	Visually compatible with 6% loss in 48 hr at room temperature	1802	C
Sodium chloride 0.9%	TR[a]	UP	2 g	Visually compatible with 9% loss in 24 hr and 12% loss in 48 hr at room temperature	1802	C
Sodium chloride 0.9%	BA[a], BRN[b]	HO	125 mg	Visually compatible with little or no loss in 24 hr at 4 and 22°C	2289	C
TNA #237[c]		PHU	25, 63, 125 mg	Physically compatible with no substantial change in lipid particle size. Variable assay results, but <10% change in drug concentration and <8% change in TNA components after 7 days at 4°C, followed by 24 hr at ambient temperature and light	2347	C
TPN #236[c]		PHU	25, 63, 125 mg	Variable assay results, but less than 10% change in drug concentration and less than 12% change in TPN components after 7 days at 4°C, followed by 24 hr at ambient temperature and light	2347	C

[a] Tested in PVC containers.

[b] Tested in polyethylene and glass containers.

[c] Refer to Appendix for the composition of parenteral nutrition solutions. TNA indicates a 3-in-1 admixture, and TPN indicates a 2-in-1 admixture.

Additive Compatibility

Methylprednisolone sodium succinate

Test Drug	Mfr	Conc/L or %	Mfr	Conc/L or %	Test Solution	Remarks	Ref	C/I
Aminophylline		500 mg	UP	40 to 250 mg	D5W, NS	Clear solution for 24 hr	329	C
Aminophylline		1 g	UP	80 mg	D5W	Clear solution for 24 hr	329	C

Additive Compatibility (Cont.)

Test Drug	Mfr	Conc/L or %	Mfr	Conc/L or %	Test Solution	Remarks	Ref	C/I
Aminophylline	SE	500 mg	UP	125 mg		Precipitate forms after 6 hr but within 24 hr	6	I
Aminophylline		1 g	UP	250 mg to 1 g	D5W	Precipitate forms	329	I
Aminophylline		~400 mg	UP	10 to 20 g	D5S, D5W, LR	Yellow color forms	329	I
Aminophylline	SE	1 g	UP	500 mg and 2 g	D5W	Physically compatible. No amino-phylline or methylpredniso-lone alcohol loss in 3 hr at room temperature, but 7 to 10% ester hydrolysis	1022	C
Aminophylline	SE	1 g	UP	500 mg and 2 g	NS	Physically compatible. No amino-phylline or methylpredniso-lone alcohol loss in 3 hr at room temperature, but 12 to 18% ester hydrolysis	1022	C
Calcium gluconate		1 g	UP	40 mg	D5S	Physically incompatible	329	I
Chloramphenicol sodium succinate	PD	1 g	UP	40 mg	D5W	Clear solution for 20 hr	329	C
Chloramphenicol sodium succinate	PD	2 g	UP	80 mg	D5W	Clear solution for 20 hr	329	C
Clindamycin phosphate	UP	1.2 g	UP	500 mg	D5W, W	Clindamycin stable for 24 hr	101	C
Cytarabine	UP	360 mg	UP	250 mg	D5S, D10S, NS	Clear solution for 24 hr	329	C
Cytarabine	UP	360 mg	UP	250 mg	R, SL	Physically incompatible	329	I
Dopamine HCl	AS	800 mg	UP	500 mg	D5W	No dopamine loss in 18 hr at 25°C	312	C
Dopamine HCl	AS	800 mg	UP	500 mg	D5W	Clear solution for 24 hr	329	C
Fosaprepitant dime-glumine	MSD[c]	1 g		700 mg	NS	Physically compatible for 24 hr at 25°C in light	2999	C
Fosaprepitant dime-glumine	MSD[d]	1 g		700 mg	NS	Physically compatible for 24 hr at 25°C in light	2999	C
Fosaprepitant dime-glumine	MSD[e]	1 g		700 mg	NS	Physically compatible for 24 hr at 25°C in light	2999	C
Glycopyrrolate	RB	1.33 mg	UP	250 mg	D5½S	Physically incompatible	329	I
Granisetron HCl	BE	56 mg	DAK	2.26 g	D5W, NS[a]	Visually compatible. Little loss of either drug in 72 hr at room temperature	1884	C
Granisetron HCl	[f]	26 mg		700 mg	NS	Physically compatible for 24 hr at 25°C in light	2999	C
Heparin sodium		5000 units	UP	125 mg	D5S, D5W, LR, R	Clear solution for 24 hr	329	C
Heparin sodium		10,000 units	UP	40 mg	D5S	Clear solution for 24 hr	329	C
Heparin sodium		40,000 units	UP	25 g	NS	Clear solution for 24 hr	329	C
Nafcillin sodium	WY	500 mg	UP	125 mg	D5W	Precipitate forms	329	I
Norepinephrine bitar-trate	WI	8 mg	UP	40 mg	D5S	Physically compatible	329	C
Ondansetron HCl	GSK	160 mg	PH	2.4 g	D5W, NS	Transient turbidity forms then clears. 5% or less loss of either drug in 24 hr at 23°C and 48 hr at 6°C	2643	?

Additive Compatibility (Cont.)

Test Drug	Mfr	Conc/L or %	Mfr	Conc/L or %	Test Solution	Remarks	Ref	C/I
Ondansetron HCl	f	70 mg		700 mg	NS	Physically compatible for 24 hr at 25°C in light	2999	C
Penicillin G potassium		2 to 10 million units	UP	80 mg	D5S, D5W, LR	Clear solution for 24 hr	329	C
Penicillin G sodium		5 million units	UP	125 mg	D5W, LR	Precipitate forms	329	I
Ranitidine HCl	GL	50 mg	UP	40 mg	D5W[a]	Visually compatible with 7% ranitidine loss and no methylprednisolone loss in 48 hr at room temperature	1802	C
Ranitidine HCl	GL	50 mg	UP	2 g	D5W[a]	Visually compatible with 6% ranitidine loss and 10% methylprednisolone loss in 48 hr at room temperature	1802	C
Ranitidine HCl	GL	2 g	UP	40 mg and 2 g	D5W[a]	Visually compatible with no loss of either drug in 48 hr at room temperature	1802	C
Ranitidine HCl	GL	50 mg and 2 g	UP	40 mg and 2 g	NS[a]	Visually compatible with no ranitidine loss and about 10% methylprednisolone loss in 48 hr at room temperature	1802	C
Theophylline	AB	4 g[b]	UP	500 mg and 2 g		Physically compatible. Little theophylline or methylprednisolone alcohol loss in 24 hr at room temperature, but 8% ester hydrolysis	1150	C
Theophylline	AB	400 mg[b]	UP	500 mg and 2 g		Physically compatible. Little theophylline or methylprednisolone alcohol loss in 24 hr at room temperature, but 11% ester hydrolysis	1150	C
Tropisetron HCl	f	43 mg		700 mg	NS	Physically compatible for 24 hr at 25°C in light	2999	C
Verapamil HCl	KN	80 mg	UP	250 mg	D5W, NS	Physically compatible for 24 hr	764	C

[a] Tested in PVC containers.

[b] Tested as the premixed infusion solution.

[c] Tested with granisetron HCl 26 mg/L.

[d] Tested with ondansetron HCl 70 mg/L.

[e] Tested with tropisetron HCl 43 mg/L.

[f] Tested with fosaprepitant dimeglumine (MSD) 1 g/L.

Drugs in Syringe Compatibility

Methylprednisolone sodium succinate

Test Drug	Mfr	Amt	Mfr	Amt	Remarks	Ref	C/I
Doxapram HCl	RB	400 mg/20 mL	UP	40 mg/2 mL	Immediate turbidity and precipitation	1177	I
Granisetron HCl	BE	0.15 mg/mL[a]	DAK	6 mg/mL[a]	Visually compatible. Little loss of either drug in 72 hr at room temperature	1884	C
Iohexol	WI	64.7%, 5 mL	UP	10 mg/1 mL	Physically compatible for at least 2 hr	1438	C
Iopamidol	SQ	61%, 5 mL	UP	10 mg/1 mL	Physically compatible for at least 2 hr	1438	C

Drugs in Syringe Compatibility (Cont.)

Test Drug	Mfr	Amt	Mfr	Amt	Remarks	Ref	C/I
Iothalamate meglumine	MA	60%, 5 mL	UP	10 mg/1 mL	Physically compatible for at least 2 hr	1438	C
Ioxaglate meglumine–ioxaglate sodium	MA	5 mL	UP	10 mg/1 mL	Physically compatible for at least 2 hr	1438	C
Metoclopramide HCl	RB	10 mg/2 mL	ES	62.5 mg/1 mL	Physically compatible for 24 hr at 25°C	1167	C
Metoclopramide HCl	RB	10 mg/2 mL	ES	250 mg/4 mL	Physically compatible for 24 hr at 25°C	1167	C
Metoclopramide HCl	RB	160 mg/32 mL	ES	250 mg/4 mL	Physically compatible for 24 hr at 25°C	1167	C
Pantoprazole sodium	[b]	4 mg/1 mL		62.5 mg/1 mL	Precipitates within 15 min	2574	I

[a] Diluted with water.

[b] Test performed using the formulation WITHOUT edetate disodium.

Y-Site Injection Compatibility (1:1 Mixture)

Methylprednisolone sodium succinate

Test Drug	Mfr	Conc	Mfr	Conc	Remarks	Ref	C/I
Acetaminophen	CAD	10 mg/mL	PF	62.5 mg/mL	Physically compatible for 4 hr at 23°C	2901, 2902	C
Acetaminophen	CAD	10 mg/mL	PF	125 mg/mL	Physically compatible with less than 10% acetaminophen loss over 4 hr at room temperature	2841, 2844	C
Acyclovir sodium	BW	5 mg/mL[a]	LY	0.8 mg/mL[a]	Physically compatible for 4 hr at 25°C	1157	C
Allopurinol sodium	BW	3 mg/mL[b]	AB	5 mg/mL[b]	Haze forms in 1 hr with white precipitate in 24 hr	1686	I
Alprostadil	BED	7.5 mcg/mL[f]	PH	40 mg/mL[e]	Visually compatible for 1 hr	2746	C
Amifostine	USB	10 mg/mL[a]	AB	5 mg/mL[a]	Physically compatible for 4 hr at 23°C	1845	C
Amiodarone HCl	WY	6 mg/mL[a]	PHU	125 mg/mL	Visually compatible for 24 hr at 22°C	2352	C
Amsacrine	NCI	1 mg/mL[a]	UP	5 mg/mL[a]	Immediate orange turbidity and precipitate in 4 hr	1381	I
Anidulafungin	VIC	0.5 mg/mL[a]	PH	5 mg/mL[a]	Physically compatible for 4 hr at 23°C	2617	C
Aztreonam	SQ	40 mg/mL[a]	AB	5 mg/mL[a]	Physically compatible for 4 hr at 23°C	1758	C
Bivalirudin	TMC	5 mg/mL[a]	PHU	5 mg/mL[a]	Physically compatible for 4 hr at 23°C	2373	C
Blinatumomab	AMG	0.125 and 0.375 mcg/mL[b]	MYL	5 mg/mL[b]	Persistent particulate formation when blinatumomab is added to methylprednisolone; not observed when order of mixing was reversed	3405, 3417	?
Cangrelor tetrasodium	TMC	1 mg/mL[b]		5 mg/mL[b]	Physically compatible for 4 hr	3243	C
Caspofungin acetate	ME	0.7 mg/mL[b]	PHU	5 mg/mL[b]	Immediate white turbid precipitate forms	2758	I
Cefepime HCl	BMS	120 mg/mL[j]		50 mg/mL	Physically compatible with less than 10% cefepime loss. Methylprednisolone not tested	2513	C
Ceftaroline fosamil	FOR	2.22 mg/mL[a b g]	PHU	5 mg/mL[a b g]	Physically compatible for 4 hr at 23°C	2826	C
Ceftazidime	GSK	120 mg/mL[j]		50 mg/mL	Physically compatible. Less than 10% ceftazidime loss. Methylprednisolone not tested	2513	C
Ceftolozane sulfate–tazobactam sodium	CUB	10 mg/mL[c m]	PF	20 mg/mL[c]	Physically compatible for 2 hr	3247, 3262	C

Y-Site Injection Compatibility (1:1 Mixture) (Cont.)

Test Drug	Mfr	Conc	Mfr	Conc	Remarks	Ref	C/I
Ciprofloxacin	MI	2 mg/mL[c]	UP	62.5 mg/mL	Transient cloudiness rapidly dissipates. Crystals form in 2 hr at 24°C	1655	I
Cisatracurium besylate	GW	0.1 mg/mL[a]	AB	5 mg/mL[a]	Physically compatible for 4 hr at 23°C	2074	C
Cisatracurium besylate	GW	2 mg/mL[a]	AB	5 mg/mL[a]	Subvisible haze forms immediately	2074	I
Cisatracurium besylate	GW	5 mg/mL[a]	AB	5 mg/mL[a]	Haze forms immediately	2074	I
Cladribine	ORT	0.015[b] and 0.5[d] mg/mL	AB	5 mg/mL[b]	Physically compatible for 4 hr at 23°C	1969	C
Cloxacillin sodium	SMX	100 mg/mL	NOP	62.5 mg/mL	Physically compatible for up to 4 hr at room temperature	3245	C
Cytarabine	UP	16 mg/mL[b]	UP	5 mg/mL[a]	Visually compatible for 24 hr at room temperature in test tubes. No precipitate found on filter from Y-site delivery	2063	C
Defibrotide sodium	JAZ	8 mg/mL[b]	MYL	10 mg/mL[b]	Visually compatible for 4 hr at room temperature	3149	C
Dexmedetomidine HCl	AB	4 mcg/mL[b]	PHU	5 mg/mL[b]	Physically compatible for 4 hr at 23°C	2383	C
Diltiazem HCl	MMD	5 mg/mL	UP	2.5 mg/mL[a]	Cloudiness forms	1807	I
Diltiazem HCl	MMD	5 mg/mL	UP	20 mg/mL[b]	Precipitate forms	1807	I
Diltiazem HCl	MMD	5 mg/mL	UP	62.5 mg/mL	Cloudiness forms but clears with swirling	1807	?
Diltiazem HCl	MMD	1 mg/mL[b]	UP	2.5[a], 20[b], 62.5 mg/mL	Visually compatible	1807	C
Docetaxel	RPR	0.9 mg/mL[a]	PHU	5 mg/mL[a]	Partial loss of measured natural turbidity occurs immediately	2224	I
Dopamine HCl	AB	0.8 mg/mL[a]	UP	5 mg/mL[a]	Visually compatible for 24 hr at room temperature in test tubes. No precipitate found on filter from Y-site delivery	2063	C
Doripenem	JJ	5 mg/mL[a b]	PHU	5 mg/mL[a b]	Physically compatible for 4 hr at 23°C	2743	C
Doxorubicin HCl liposomal	SEQ	0.4 mg/mL[a]	UP	5 mg/mL[a]	Physically compatible for 4 hr at 23°C	2087	C
Enalaprilat	MSD	0.05 mg/mL[b]	UP	0.8 mg/mL[a]	Physically compatible for 24 hr at room temperature under fluorescent light	1355	C
Etoposide phosphate	BR	5 mg/mL[a]	AB	5 mg/mL[a]	Haze with subvisible microparticles forms immediately. Particle content increases fivefold over 4 hr at 23°C	2218	I
Famotidine	MSD	0.2 mg/mL[a]	AB	1 mg/mL[a]	Physically compatible for 4 hr at 25°C	1188	C
Famotidine	MSD	0.2 mg/mL[a]	QU	40 mg/mL	Physically compatible for 14 hr	1196	C
Famotidine	ME	2 mg/mL[b]		5 mg/mL[a]	Visually compatible for 4 hr at 22°C	1936	C
Fenoldopam mesylate	AB	80 mcg/mL[b]	PHU	5 mg/mL[b]	Microparticulates form immediately	2467	I
Filgrastim	AMG	30 mcg/mL[a]	AB	5 mg/mL[a]	Haze, particles, and filaments form immediately	1687	I
Fludarabine phosphate	BX	1 mg/mL[a]	UP	5 mg/mL[a]	Visually compatible for 4 hr at 22°C	1439	C
Gemcitabine HCl	LI	10 mg/mL[b]	AB	5 mg/mL[b]	Gross precipitation occurs immediately	2226	I
Granisetron HCl	SKB	0.05 mg/mL[a]	WY	5 mg/mL[a]	Physically compatible for 4 hr at 23°C	2000	C
Heparin sodium	TR	50 units/mL	UP	2.5 mg/mL[a]	Visually compatible for 4 hr at 25°C	1793	C

Y-Site Injection Compatibility (1:1 Mixture) (Cont.)

Test Drug	Mfr	Conc	Mfr	Conc	Remarks	Ref	C/I
Heparin sodium	ES	100 units/mL[c]	UP	5 mg/mL[a]	Visually compatible for 24 hr at room temperature in test tubes. No precipitate found on filter from Y-site delivery	2063	C
Hetastarch in lactated electrolyte	AB	6%	PHU	5 mg/mL[a]	Physically compatible for 4 hr at 23°C	2339	C
Hydroxyethyl starch 130/0.4 in sodium chloride 0.9%	FRK	6%	NOP	0.25[a], 5[a], 62.5 mg/mL	Visually compatible for 24 hr at room temperature	2770	C
Isavuconazonium sulfate	ASP	1.5 mg/mL[c]	PF	20 mg/mL[c]	Transient turbidity forms then clears	3263	I
Linezolid	PHU	2 mg/mL	AB	5 mg/mL[a]	Physically compatible for 4 hr at 23°C	2264	C
Melphalan HCl	BW	0.1 mg/mL[b]	AB	5 mg/mL[b]	Physically compatible for 3 hr at 22°C	1557	C
Meperidine HCl	AB	10 mg/mL	UP	2.5 mg/mL[a]	Physically compatible for 4 hr at 25°C	1397	C
Meropenem		50 mg/mL	NOP	62.5 mg/mL	Physically compatible for 4 hr at room temperature	3538	C
Meropenem–vaborbactam	TMC	8 mg/mL[b n]	SGT	20 mg/mL[b]	Physically compatible for 3 hr at 20 to 25°C	3380	C
Methotrexate sodium		30 mg/mL	UP	20 mg/mL	Visually compatible for 4 hr at room temperature	1788	C
Metronidazole	MG	5 mg/mL	UP	5 mg/mL[a]	Visually compatible for 24 hr at room temperature in test tubes. No precipitate found on filter from Y-site delivery	2063	C
Midazolam HCl	RC	1 mg/mL[a]	UP	40 mg/mL	Visually compatible for 24 hr at 23°C	1847	C
Milrinone lactate	SS	0.2 mg/mL[a]	PHU	125 mg/mL	Visually compatible for 4 hr at 25°C	2381	C
Morphine sulfate	AB	1 mg/mL	UP	2.5 mg/mL[a]	Physically compatible for 4 hr at 25°C	1397	C
Nicardipine HCl	DCC	0.1 mg/mL[a]	UP	0.8 mg/mL[a]	Visually compatible for 24 hr at room temperature	235	C
Ondansetron HCl	GL	1 mg/mL[b]	UP	5 mg/mL[a]	Light haze develops in 30 min	1365	I
Oxaliplatin	SS	0.5 mg/mL[a]	PHU	5 mg/mL[a]	Physically compatible for 4 hr at 23°C	2566	C
Paclitaxel	NCI	1.2 mg/mL[a]	UP	5 mg/mL[a]	Normal inherent haze from paclitaxel decreases immediately	1556	I
Palonosetron HCl	MGI	50 mcg/mL	PHU	5 mg/mL[a]	Microprecipitate begins to form immediately and becomes visible within 4 hr	2681	I
Pemetrexed disodium	LI	20 mg/mL[b]	PHU	5 mg/mL[a]	Physically compatible for 4 hr at 23°C	2564	C
Piperacillin sodium–tazobactam sodium	LE[k]	40 mg/mL[a l]	AB	5 mg/mL[a]	Physically compatible for 4 hr at 22°C	1688	C
Plazomicin sulfate	ACH	24 mg/mL[c]	SGT	20 mg/mL[c]	Cloudy with immediate increase in measured turbidity; gross sedimentation occurs within 30 min	3432	I
Potassium chloride		40 mEq/L[a]	UP	40 mg/mL	Physically compatible for 4 hr at room temperature	322	C
Potassium chloride		40 mEq/L[b]	UP	40 mg/mL	Physically compatible initially but haze forms in 4 hr at room temperature	322	I
Potassium chloride		40 mEq/L[g]	UP	40 mg/mL	Immediate haze formation	322	I
Propofol	ZEN[o]	10 mg/mL	AB	5 mg/mL[a]	White precipitate forms immediately	2066	I

Y-Site Injection Compatibility (1:1 Mixture) (Cont.)

Test Drug	Mfr	Conc	Mfr	Conc	Remarks	Ref	C/I
Remifentanil HCl	GW	0.025 and 0.25 mg/mL[b]	AB	5 mg/mL[a]	Physically compatible for 4 hr at 23°C	2075	C
Sargramostim	IMM	10 mcg/mL[b]	UP	5 mg/mL[b]	Small amounts of particles and filaments form in 4 hr	1436	I
Sodium bicarbonate		1.4%	UP	20 mg/mL	Visually compatible for 4 hr at room temperature	1788	C
Tacrolimus	FUJ	1 mg/mL[b]	UP	0.8 mg/mL[a]	Visually compatible for 24 hr at 25°C	1630	C
Tedizolid phosphate	CUB	0.8 mg/mL[b]	PF	20 mg/mL[b]	Physically compatible for 2 hr	3244	C
Telavancin HCl	ASP	7.5 mg/mL[a]	PF	5 mg/mL[a]	Slight measured turbidity increase	2830	I
Telavancin HCl	ASP	7.5 mg/mL[b g]	PF	5 mg/mL[b g]	Physically compatible for 2 hr	2830	C
Teniposide	BR	0.1 mg/mL[a]	AB	5 mg/mL[a]	Physically compatible for 4 hr at 23°C	1725	C
Theophylline	TR	4 mg/mL	UP	2.5 mg/mL[a]	Visually compatible for 6 hr at 25°C	1793	C
Thiotepa	IMM[h]	1 mg/mL[a]	AB	5 mg/mL[a]	Physically compatible for 4 hr at 23°C	1861	C
Tigecycline	WY	1 mg/mL[b]		20 mg/mL[b]	Microparticulates form	2714	I
TNA #218 to #226[i]			AB	5 mg/mL[a]	Visually compatible for 4 hr at 23°C	2215	C
Topotecan HCl	SKB	56 mcg/mL[a b]	UP	2.4 mg/mL[a b]	Yellow color forms. Little loss of either drug in 4 hr at 22°C	2245	C
TPN #212[i]			AB	5 mg/mL[a]	Physically compatible for 4 hr at 23°C	2109[i]	C
TPN #213[i]			AB	5 mg/mL[a]	Physically compatible for 4 hr at 23°C	2109	C
TPN #214[i]			AB	5 mg/mL[a]	Physically compatible for 4 hr at 23°C	2109	C
TPN #215[i]			AB	5 mg/mL[a]	Physically compatible for 4 hr at 23°C	2109	C
Vancomycin HCl	LI	10 mg/mL[a]	[p]	50 mg/mL	Physically incompatible	3536	I
Vinorelbine tartrate	BW	1 mg/mL[b]	AB	5 mg/mL[b]	Heavy white precipitate forms immediately	1558	I

[a] Tested in dextrose 5%.

[b] Tested in sodium chloride 0.9%.

[c] Tested in both dextrose 5% and sodium chloride 0.9%.

[d] Tested in bacteriostatic sodium chloride 0.9% preserved with benzyl alcohol 0.9%.

[e] Tested in either dextrose 5% or in sodium chloride 0.9%, but the report did not specify which solution.

[f] Tested in a 1:1 mixture of (1) D5W and D5½S with and without KCl 20 mEq/L, and also (2) D10½S with and without KCl 20 mEq/L, and also (3) D5W and TPN #274 (see Appendix).

[g] Tested in Ringer's injection, lactated.

[h] Lyophilized formulation tested.

[i] Refer to Appendix for the composition of parenteral nutrition solutions. TNA indicates a 3-in-1 admixture, and TPN indicates a 2-in-1 admixture.

[j] Tested in sterile water for injection.

[k] Test performed using the formulation WITHOUT edetate disodium.

[l] Piperacillin component. Piperacillin in an 8:1 fixed-ratio concentration with tazobactam.

[m] Ceftolozane component. Ceftolozane in a 2:1 fixed-ratio concentration with tazobactam.

[n] Meropenem component. Meropenem in a 1:1 fixed-ratio concentration with vaborbactam.

[o] Test performed using the formulation WITH edetate disodium.

[p] Salt not specified.

Additional Compatibility Information

Infusion Solutions

Solution haziness was reported for methylprednisolone sodium succinate admixtures in intravenous fluids.[702][758] Changes in the manufacturing process for bulk methylprednisolone sodium succinate powder have resulted in substantial improvements in admixture clarity and absence of the haze formation that developed previously in solutions of Solu-Medrol.[670][702]

In a study of the turbidity produced by methylprednisolone sodium succinate (Abbott) 500 mg to 30 g/L, turbidity was substantially higher in dextrose 5% than in sodium chloride 0.9%.[758] Another important factor was the concentration of methylprednisolone sodium succinate. Turbidity was generally higher at intermediate concentrations (2 to 15 g/L) than at low (300 mg/L) or high (20 g/L) concentrations.[758]

These differences in the development of turbidity cannot be explained by simple increased ester hydrolysis due to differing pH values and drug concentrations. Rather, the solubility of free methylprednisolone in various concentrations of methylprednisolone sodium succinate has been suggested as the primary factor. The solubility of free methylprednisolone is increased as the concentration of the sodium succinate ester increases. The increased solubilization is believed to overshadow increased formation of free methylprednisolone in concentrations over 10 g/L, preventing or minimizing precipitation and turbidity. Differences in turbidity between the drug in dextrose 5% and sodium chloride 0.9% are believed to result primarily from the electrolyte content of sodium chloride 0.9% and, to a much lesser extent, the pH of the dextrose admixtures. These differences are presumed to affect the solubilizing capacity and reactivity of the ester.[758]

Other Drugs

The compatibility of methylprednisolone sodium succinate (Upjohn) with several drugs added to auxiliary medication infusion units has been studied. Primary admixtures were prepared by adding various drugs to dextrose 5%, dextrose 5% in sodium chloride 0.9%, and Ringer's injection, lactated. Up to 100 mL of the primary admixture was added along with methylprednisolone sodium succinate (Upjohn) to the auxiliary medication infusion unit with the following results:[329]

Methylprednisolone Sodium Succinate	Primary Solution	Result
	Aminophylline 500 mg/L	
500 mg	D5S, D5W qs 100 mL	Clear solution for 24 hr
500 mg	LR qs 100 mL	Clear solution for 24 hr
500 mg	Added to 100 mL LR	Clear solution for 1 hr
1000 mg	D5W qs 100 mL	Yellow solution, clear for 24 hr

Methylprednisolone Sodium Succinate	Primary Solution	Result
1000 mg	D5S qs 100 mL	Yellow solution, clear for 6 hr
1000 mg	Added to 100 mL D5S	Yellow solution, clear for 24 hr
1000 mg	LR qs 100 mL or added to 100 mL LR	Yellow solution, clear for 4 hr
2000 mg	D5S, D5W, LR qs 100 mL	Yellow solution, clear for 24 hr
	Heparin Sodium 10,000 units/L	
500 mg	D5S, D5W qs 100 mL	Clear solution for 24 hr
500 mg	LR qs 100 mL or added to 100 mL LR	Clear solution for 6 hr
1000 mg	D5S, D5W qs 100 mL	Clear solution for 6 hr
1000 mg	Added to 100 mL D5W	Clear solution for 24 hr
1000 mg	LR qs 100 mL or added to 100 mL LR	Clear solution for 4 to 6 hr
2000 mg	D5W qs 100 mL	Clear solution for 6 hr
2000 mg	D5S, LR qs 100 mL	Clear solution for 24 hr
	Potassium Chloride 40 mEq/L	
500 mg	D5S, D5W, LR qs 100 mL	Clear solution for 24 hr
1000 mg	D5W qs 100 mL	Clear solution for 24 hr
1000 mg	D5S, LR qs 100 mL or added to 100 mL D5S, LR	Clear solution for 6 hr
2000 mg	D5S, D5W, LR qs 100 mL	Clear solution for 24 hr
	Sodium Bicarbonate 44.6 mEq/L	
500 mg	D5S, D5W qs 100 mL	Clear solution for 24 hr
500 mg	LR qs 100 mL or added to 100 mL LR	Clear solution for 1 hr
1000 mg	D5W qs 100 mL	Clear solution for 24 hr
1000 mg	D5S qs 100 mL or added to 100 mL D5S	Clear solution for 24 hr
1000 mg	LR qs 100 mL	Clear solution for 1 hr
1000 mg	Added to 100 mL LR	Clear solution for 4 hr
2000 mg	D5S, D5W qs 100 mL	Clear solution for 24 hr
2000 mg	LR qs 100 mL	Clear solution for 30 min
2000 mg	Added to 100 mL LR	Clear solution for 4 hr

Metoclopramide Hydrochloride
AHFS 56:32

Products

Metoclopramide hydrochloride is available in 2-mL ampuls and 2-, 10-, and 30-mL vials. Each mL of solution contains metoclopramide (as the hydrochloride) 5 mg with sodium chloride 8.5 mg and hydrochloric acid and/or sodium hydroxide, if necessary, in water for injection.[1(5/05)]

pH

From 4.5 to 6.5.[1(5/05)] Metoclopramide hydrochloride 1.25, 2.22, and 3.75 mg/mL in sodium chloride 0.9% had pH values of 4.4, 4.1, and 4, respectively.[2161]

Osmolality

The osmolality of metoclopramide hydrochloride 5 mg/mL was determined to be 280 mOsm/kg.[1233] Metoclopramide hydrochloride 1.25, 2.22, and 3.75 mg/mL in sodium chloride 0.9% had osmolalities of 285, 286, and 294 mOsm/kg, respectively.[2161]

Trade Name(s)

Reglan

Administration

Metoclopramide hydrochloride is administered by intramuscular injection, by direct intravenous injection undiluted slowly over 1 or 2 minutes for 10 mg doses of drug, or by intermittent intravenous infusion over 15 minutes diluted in 50 mL of compatible diluent for larger doses.[1(5/05) 4]

Stability

Metoclopramide hydrochloride injection is a clear, colorless solution; it should be stored at controlled room temperature and protected from freezing. The drug is stable over a pH range of 2 to 9. Metoclopramide hydrochloride is photosensitive; protection from light for the product during storage has been recommended.[4] However, the manufacturer no longer recommends light protection for dilutions under normal lighting conditions, stating that they may be stored up to 24 hours.[1(5/05)]

Freezing Solutions

Undiluted metoclopramide hydrochloride (Robins) 5 mg/mL packaged as 3 mL in plastic infusion-pump syringes (MiniMed) fitted with Luer-Lok tip caps (Burron) exhibited microprecipitation that did not redissolve upon warming to room temperature when stored frozen at −20°C for as little as 1 day. The precipitate was not visible with the unaided eye. Freezing is not an acceptable storage method for undiluted metoclopramide hydrochloride injection.[2001]

Syringes

Undiluted metoclopramide hydrochloride (Robins) 5 mg/mL was packaged as 3 mL in plastic infusion-pump syringes (MiniMed) fitted with Luer-Lok tip caps (Burron). Stored for 7 days at 32°C to simulate wearing a portable infusion pump close to the body, metoclopramide hydrochloride was physically stable and little loss occurred. At 23°C, metoclopramide hydrochloride was physically and chemically stable for up to 60 days with little loss occurring. However, large quantities of subvisible particulates formed after that time, making the drug unsuitable for use. Stored under refrigeration at 4°C, metoclopramide hydrochloride remained both physically and chemically stable for up to 90 days.[2001]

Metoclopramide hydrochloride (Solopak) 2.5 mg/mL in sodium chloride 0.9% packaged in polypropylene syringes (Sherwood) was physically stable and exhibited little or no loss in 24 hours stored at 4 and 23°C.[2199]

Central Venous Catheter

Metoclopramide hydrochloride (Abbott) 0.5 mg/mL in dextrose 5% was found to be compatible with the ARROWg+ard Blue Plus (Arrow International) chlorhexidine-bearing triple-lumen central catheter. Essentially complete delivery of the drug was found with little or no drug loss occurring. Furthermore, chlorhexidine delivered from the catheter remained at trace amounts with no substantial increase due to the delivery of the drug through the catheter.[2335]

Compatibility Information
Solution Compatibility

Metoclopramide HCl

Test Soln Name	Mfr	Mfr	Conc/L or %	Remarks	Ref	C/I
Amino acids 2.75%, dextrose 25%, electrolytes	TR	RB	5 and 20 mg	Metoclopramide chemically stable for 72 hr at room temperature	854	C
Dextrose 5% in sodium chloride 0.45%				Compatible for 48 hr at room temperature	1(5/05)	C
Dextrose 5% in sodium chloride 0.45%	TR[a]	RB	200 mg	Physically compatible with 2% loss in 24 hr at 25°C exposed to normal room light	1167	C

DOI: 10.37573/9781585286850.264

Solution Compatibility (Cont.)

Test Soln Name	Mfr	Mfr	Conc/L or %	Remarks	Ref	C/I
Dextrose 5% in sodium chloride 0.45%	TRa	RB	3.2 g	Physically compatible with 4 to 5% loss in 24 hr at 25°C exposed to normal room light	1167	C
Dextrose 5%				Compatible for 24 hr at room temperature	1(5/05)	C
Dextrose 5%	TRa	RB	200 mg	Physically compatible with no loss in 24 hr at 25°C exposed to normal room light	1167	C
Dextrose 5%	TRa	RB	200 mg	9% loss after 2 weeks and 14% loss after 4 weeks frozen at −20°C followed by 24 hr at room temperature	1167	C
Dextrose 5%	TRa	RB	3.2 g	Physically compatible with 5% loss in 24 hr at 25°C exposed to normal room light	1167	C
Dextrose 5%	TRa	RB	3.2 g	11% loss after 1 week and 37% loss after 4 weeks frozen at −20°C followed by 24 hr at room temperature	1167	I
Ringer's injection				Compatible for 48 hr at room temperature	1(5/05)	C
Ringer's injection, lactated				Compatible for 48 hr at room temperature	1(5/05)	C
Sodium chloride 0.9%				Compatible for 48 hr at room temperature	1(5/05)	C
Sodium chloride 0.9%	TRa	RB	200 mg and 3.2 g	No loss after 4 weeks frozen at −20°C followed by 24 hr at room temperature	1167	C
Sodium chloride 0.9%	TRa	RB	200 mg and 3.2 g	Physically compatible with no loss in 24 hr at 25°C exposed to normal room light	1167	C
Sodium chloride 0.9%	BA	BA	500 mg	Physically compatible with no drug loss in 21 days at 25°C	2586	C
TPN #89b		RB	5 mg	Physically compatible with no metoclopramide loss in 24 hr and 10% loss in 48 hr at 25°C	1167b	C
TPN #89b		RB	20 mg	Physically compatible with no metoclopramide loss in 72 hr at 25°C	1167	C
TPN #90b		RB	5 mg	Physically compatible with no metoclopramide loss in 72 hr at 25°C	1167	C
TPN #90b		RB	20 mg	Physically compatible with 3% metoclopramide loss in 72 hr at 25°C	1167	C

a Tested in PVC containers.

b Refer to Appendix for the composition of parenteral nutrition solutions. TPN indicates a 2-in-1 admixture.

Additive Compatibility

Metoclopramide HCl

Test Drug	Mfr	Conc/L or %	Mfr	Conc/L or %	Test Solution	Remarks	Ref	C/I
Clindamycin phosphate	UP	6 g	RB	100 and 200 mg		Physically compatible for 24 hr at 25°C	1167	C
Clindamycin phosphate	UP	3.5 g	RB	1.9 g		Physically compatible for 24 hr at 25°C	1167	C
Clindamycin phosphate	UP	4.4 g	RB	1.2 g		Physically compatible for 24 hr at 25°C	1167	C
Dexamethasone sodium phosphate with lorazepam and diphenhydramine HCl	AMR WY ES	400 mg 40 mg 2 g	DU	4 g	NSa	Rapid lorazepam losses of 8, 10, and 15% at 3, 23, and 30°C, respectively, in 24 hr. Other drugs stable for 14 days at all three storage temperatures	1733	I
Diphenhydramine HCl with dexamethasone sodium phosphate and lorazepam	ES AMR WY	2 g 400 mg 40 mg	DU	4 g	NSa	Rapid lorazepam losses of 8, 10, and 15% at 3, 23, and 30°C, respectively, in 24 hr. Other drugs stable for 14 days at all three storage temperatures	1733	I
Erythromycin lactobionate	AB	4 g	RB	400 mg	NS	Incompatible. If mixed, use immediately	924	I

Additive Compatibility (Cont.)

Test Drug	Mfr	Conc/L or %	Mfr	Conc/L or %	Test Solution	Remarks	Ref	C/I
Erythromycin lactobionate	AB	4.1 g	RB	416 mg		Incompatible. If mixed, use immediately	1167	I
Erythromycin lactobionate	AB	5 g	RB	100 mg	NS	Incompatible. If mixed, use immediately	924	I
Erythromycin lactobionate	AB	3.5 g	RB	1.1 g		Incompatible. If mixed, use immediately	1167	I
Floxacillin sodium	BE	20 g	ANT	1 g	NS	White precipitate forms immediately	1479	I
Fluorouracil	RC	2.5 g	FUJ	100 mg	D5W	10% metoclopramide loss in 6 hr and 27% loss in 24 hr at 25°C. 5% metoclopramide loss in 120 hr at 4°C. 5 and 7% fluorouracil losses in 120 hr at 4 and 25°C, respectively	1780	I
Furosemide	HO	1 g	ANT	1 g	NS	Precipitates immediately	1479	I
Lorazepam with dexamethasone sodium phosphate and diphenhydramine HCl	WY AMR ES	40 mg 400 mg 2 g	DU	4 g	NS[a]	Rapid lorazepam losses of 8, 10, and 15% at 3, 23, and 30°C, respectively, in 24 hr. Other drugs stable for 14 days at all three storage temperatures	1733	I
Mannitol	AB	20%	RB	40 and 100 mg		Physically compatible for 48 hr at room temperature	924	C
Mannitol	AB	20%	RB	40 and 100 mg		Physically compatible for 48 hr at 25°C	1167	C
Mannitol	AB	20%	RB	640 mg and 1.6 g		Physically compatible for 48 hr at 25°C	1167	C
Meperidine HCl	DW	7.35 g	DW	150 mg	D5W, NS	Visually compatible. Little loss of drugs over 48 hr at 32°C in light or dark	2253	C
Meropenem	ZEN	1 and 20 g	RB	100 mg	NS	Visually compatible for 4 hr at room temperature	1994	C
Morphine sulfate	EV	1 g	SKB	500 mg	NS[b]	Visually compatible. Little loss of either drug in 35 days at 22°C and 182 days at 4°C followed by 7 days at 32°C	1939	C
Morphine sulfate	EV	1 g	SKB	500 mg	D5W[c]	Visually compatible. 8% metoclopramide loss in 14 days at 22°C and 98 days at 4°C. No morphine loss	1939	C
Multivitamins	USV	20 mL	RB	20 and 320 mg	NS	Physically compatible for 48 hr at room temperature	924	C
Multivitamins	USV	20 mL	RB	20 and 320 mg	NS	Physically compatible for 48 hr at room temperature	924	C
Oxycodone HCl	NAP	770 mg		1.2 g	NS, W	Visually compatible. Under 4% concentration change in 24 hr at 25°C	2600	C
Potassium acetate	IX	20 mEq	RB	10 and 160 mg	NS	Physically compatible for 48 hr at room temperature	924	C
Potassium chloride	ES	30 mEq	RB	10 and 160 mg	NS	Physically compatible for 48 hr at room temperature	924	C
Potassium phosphates	IX	15 mmol	RB	10 and 160 mg	NS	Physically compatible for 48 hr at room temperature	924	C
Ranitidine HCl	GSK	926 mg	SZ	185 mg		Visually compatible for up to 72 hr at room temperature (about 25°C)	3496	C
Tramadol HCl	AND	1.118 g	SYO	1.11 g	NS[d]	Visually compatible for 7 days at 25°C protected from light	2701	C
Tramadol HCl	AND	3.33 g	SYO	3.33 g	NS[d]	Visually compatible for 7 days at 25°C protected from light	2701	C
Verapamil HCl	KN	80 mg	RB	20 mg	D5W, NS	Physically compatible for 24 hr	764	C

Additive Compatibility (Cont.)

a Tested in Pharmacia-Deltec PVC pump reservoirs.

b Tested in PVC containers.

c Tested in PCA Infusors (Baxter).

d Tested in elastomeric pump reservoirs (Baxter).

Drugs in Syringe Compatibility

Metoclopramide HCl

Test Drug	Mfr	Amt	Mfr	Amt	Remarks	Ref	C/I
Aminophylline	ES	500 mg/20 mL	RB	160 mg/32 mL	Physically compatible for 24 hr at 25°C	1167	C
Aminophylline	ES	80 mg/3.2 mL	RB	10 mg/2 mL	Physically compatible for 24 hr at 25°C	1167	C
Aminophylline	ES	500 mg/20 mL	RB	10 mg/2 mL	Physically compatible for 24 hr at 25°C	1167	C
Ampicillin sodium	BR	250 mg/2.5 mL	RB	10 mg/2 mL	Incompatible. If mixed, use immediately	1167	I
Ampicillin sodium	BR	1 g/10 mL	RB	10 mg/2 mL	Incompatible. If mixed, use immediately	1167	I
Ampicillin sodium	BR	1 g/10 mL	RB	160 mg/32 mL	Incompatible. If mixed, use immediately	1167	I
Ascorbic acid	AB	250 mg/0.5 mL	RB	160 mg/32 mL	Physically compatible for 48 hr at 25°C	1167	C
Ascorbic acid	AB	250 mg/0.5 mL	RB	10 mg/2 mL	Physically compatible for 48 hr at 25°C	1167	C
Atropine sulfate	GL	0.4 mg/1 mL	NO	10 mg/2 mL	Physically compatible for 15 min at room temperature	565	C
Benztropine mesylate	MSD	2 mg/2 mL	RB	160 mg/32 mL	Physically compatible for 48 hr at 25°C	1167	C
Benztropine mesylate	MSD	2 mg/2 mL	RB	10 mg/2 mL	Physically compatible for 48 hr at 25°C	1167	C
Bleomycin sulfate		1.5 units/0.5 mL		2.5 mg/0.5 mL	Physically compatible for 5 min at room temperature followed by 8 min of centrifugation	980	C
Butorphanol tartrate	BR	4 mg/2 mL	NO	10 mg/2 mL	Physically compatible for 30 min at room temperature	566	C
Caffeine citrate		20 mg/1 mL	ES	5 mg/1 mL	Visually compatible for 4 hr at 25°C	2440	C
Calcium gluconate	ES	1 g/10 mL	RB	10 mg/2 mL	Possible precipitate formation	924	I
Calcium gluconate	ES	1 g/10 mL	RB	160 mg/32 mL	Incompatible. If mixed, use immediately	1167	I
Chloramphenicol sodium succinate	PD	250 mg/2.5 mL	RB	10 mg/2 mL	White precipitate forms immediately at 25°C	1167	I
Chloramphenicol sodium succinate	PD	2 g/20 mL	RB	10 mg/2 mL	White precipitate forms immediately at 25°C	1167	I
Chloramphenicol sodium succinate	PD	2 g/20 mL	RB	160 mg/32 mL	White precipitate forms immediately at 25°C	1167	I
Chlorpromazine HCl	MB	25 mg/1 mL	NO	10 mg/2 mL	Physically compatible for 15 min at room temperature	565	C
Cisplatin		0.5 mg/0.5 mL		2.5 mg/0.5 mL	Physically compatible for 5 min at room temperature followed by 8 min of centrifugation	980	C
Cyclophosphamide		10 mg/0.5 mL		2.5 mg/0.5 mL	Physically compatible for 5 min at room temperature followed by 8 min of centrifugation	980	C
Cyclophosphamide	MJ	1 g/50 mL	RB	10 mg/2 mL	Physically compatible for 24 hr at 25°C	1167	C
Cyclophosphamide	MJ	1 g/50 mL	RB	160 mg/32 mL	Physically compatible for 24 hr at 25°C	1167	C
Cyclophosphamide	MJ	40 mg/2 mL	RB	10 mg/2 mL	Physically compatible for 24 hr at 25°C	1167	C

Drugs in Syringe Compatibility (Cont.)

Test Drug	Mfr	Amt	Mfr	Amt	Remarks	Ref	C/I
Cytarabine	UP	500 mg/10 mL	RB	160 mg/32 mL	Physically compatible for 48 hr at 25°C	1167	C
Cytarabine	UP	50 mg/1 mL	RB	10 mg/2 mL	Physically compatible for 48 hr at 25°C	1167	C
Dexamethasone sodium phosphate	ES, MSD	8 mg/2 mL	RB	160 mg/32 mL	Physically compatible for 48 hr at 25°C	1167	C
Dexamethasone sodium phosphate	ES, MSD	8 mg/2 mL	RB	10 mg/2 mL	Physically compatible for 48 hr at 25°C	1167	C
Diamorphine HCl	MB	10, 25, 50 mg/1 mL	BK	5 mg/1 mL	Physically compatible and diamorphine stable for 24 hr at room temperature	1454	C
Diamorphine HCl	EV	50 and 150 mg/1 mL	LA	5 mg/1 mL	Slight discoloration with 8% metoclopramide loss and 9% diamorphine loss in 7 days at room temperature	1455	C
Dimenhydrinate	HR	50 mg/1 mL	NO	10 mg/2 mL	Physically compatible for 15 min at room temperature	565	C
Diphenhydramine HCl	PD	50 mg/1 mL	NO	10 mg/2 mL	Physically compatible for 15 min at room temperature	565	C
Diphenhydramine HCl	PD	40 mg/4 mL	RB	160 mg/32 mL	Physically compatible for 48 hr at 25°C	1167	C
Diphenhydramine HCl	PD	200 mg/20 mL	RB	160 mg/32 mL	Physically compatible for 48 hr at 25°C	1167	C
Diphenhydramine HCl	PD	50 mg/5 mL	RB	10 mg/2 mL	Physically compatible for 48 hr at 25°C	1167	C
Diphenhydramine HCl	PD	250 mg/25 mL	RB	10 mg/2 mL	Physically compatible for 48 hr at 25°C	1167	C
Doxorubicin HCl		1 mg/0.5 mL		2.5 mg/0.5 mL	Physically compatible for 5 min at room temperature followed by 8 min of centrifugation	980	C
Doxorubicin HCl	AD	90 mg/45 mL	RB	160 mg/32 mL	Physically compatible for 48 hr at 25°C	1167	C
Doxorubicin HCl	AD	40 mg/20 mL	RB	10 mg/2 mL	Physically compatible for 48 hr at 25°C	1167	C
Droperidol	MN	2.5 mg/1 mL	NO	10 mg/2 mL	Physically compatible for 15 min at room temperature	565	C
Droperidol		1.25 mg/0.5 mL		2.5 mg/0.5 mL	Physically compatible for 5 min at room temperature followed by 8 min of centrifugation	980	C
Fentanyl citrate	MN	0.05 mg/1 mL	NO	10 mg/2 mL	Physically compatible for 15 min at room temperature	565	C
Fentanyl citrate with midazolam HCl	DB RC	1 mg/20 mL 15 mg/3 mL	AST	20 mg/4 mL	Visually compatible with 7% or less loss of each drug in 10 days at 32°C	2268	C
Fluorouracil		25 mg/0.5 mL		2.5 mg/0.5 mL	Physically compatible for 5 min at room temperature followed by 8 min of centrifugation	980	C
Furosemide		5 mg/0.5 mL		2.5 mg/0.5 mL	Precipitates immediately	980	I
Heparin sodium		500 units/0.5 mL		2.5 mg/0.5 mL	Physically compatible for 5 min at room temperature followed by 8 min of centrifugation	980	C
Heparin sodium		2500 units/1 ml		10 mg/2 mL	Physlcally compatible for at least 5 min	1053	C
Heparin sodium	ES	16,000 units/16 mL	RB	160 mg/32 mL	Physically compatible for 48 hr at 25°C	1167	C
Heparin sodium	ES	2000 units/2 mL	RB	10 mg/2 mL	Physically compatible for 48 hr at 25°C	1167	C
Heparin sodium	ES	4000 units/4 mL	RB	10 mg/2 mL	Physically compatible for 48 hr at 25°C	1167	C
Hydromorphone HCl	KN	10 and 20 mg/mL	RB	5 mg/mL	Visually compatible with less than 10% loss of either drug in 7 days at 8°C	668	C
Hydroxyzine HCl	PF	50 mg/1 mL	NO	10 mg/2 mL	Physically compatible for 15 min at room temperature	565	C
Leucovorin calcium		5 mg/0.5 mL		2.5 mg/0.5 mL	Physically compatible for 5 min at room temperature followed by 8 min of centrifugation	980	C
Lidocaine HCl	ES	50 mg/5 mL	RB	160 mg/32 mL	Physically compatible for 48 hr at 25°C	1167	C

Drugs in Syringe Compatibility (Cont.)

Test Drug	Mfr	Amt	Mfr	Amt	Remarks	Ref	C/I
Lidocaine HCl	ES	100 mg/10 mL	RB	160 mg/32 mL	Physically compatible for 48 hr at 25°C	1167	C
Lidocaine HCl	ES	50 mg/5 mL	RB	10 mg/2 mL	Physically compatible for 48 hr at 25°C	1167	C
Lidocaine HCl	ES	100 mg/10 mL	RB	10 mg/2 mL	Physically compatible for 48 hr at 25°C	1167	C
Magnesium sulfate	ES	1 g/2 mL	RB	160 mg/32 mL	Physically compatible for 48 hr at 25°C	1167	C
Magnesium sulfate	ES	500 mg/1 mL	RB	10 mg/2 mL	Physically compatible for 48 hr at 25°C	1167	C
Magnesium sulfate	ES	1 g/2 mL	RB	10 mg/2 mL	Physically compatible for 48 hr at 25°C	1167	C
Meperidine HCl	WI	50 mg/1 mL	NO	10 mg/2 mL	Physically compatible for 15 min at room temperature	565	C
Meperidine HCl	DW	50 mg/1 mL	DW	10 mg/2 mL	Visually compatible. Little loss of either drug over 48 hr at 32°C in light or dark	2253	C
Methotrexate sodium		12.5 mg/0.5 mL		2.5 mg/0.5 mL	Physically compatible for 5 min at room temperature followed by 8 min of centrifugation	980	C
Methotrexate sodium	LE	200 mg/8 mL	RB	160 mg/32 mL	Incompatible. If mixed, use immediately	1167	I
Methotrexate sodium	LE	50 mg/2 mL	RB	10 mg/2 mL	Incompatible. If mixed, use immediately	1167	I
Methotrimeprazine HCl	RP	10 mg/2 mL	NO	10 mg/2 mL	Physically compatible for 15 min at room temperature	565	C
Methylprednisolone sodium succinate	ES	250 mg/4 mL	RB	160 mg/32 mL	Physically compatible for 24 hr at 25°C	1167	C
Methylprednisolone sodium succinate	ES	62.5 mg/1 mL	RB	10 mg/2 mL	Physically compatible for 24 hr at 25°C	1167	C
Methylprednisolone sodium succinate	ES	250 mg/4 mL	RB	10 mg/2 mL	Physically compatible for 24 hr at 25°C	1167	C
Midazolam HCl	RC	5 mg/1 mL	RB	10 mg/2 mL	Physically compatible for 4 hr at 25°C	1145	C
Midazolam HCl with fentanyl citrate	RC DB	15 mg/3 mL 1 mg/20 mL	AST	20 mg/4 mL	Visually compatible with 7% or less loss of each drug in 10 days at 32°C	2268	C
Mitomycin		0.25 mg/0.5 mL		2.5 mg/0.5 mL	Physically compatible for 5 min at room temperature followed by 8 min of centrifugation	980	C
Morphine sulfate	AH	10 mg/1 mL	NO	10 mg/2 mL	Physically compatible for 15 min at room temperature	565	C
Morphine sulfate	EV	1 mg/mL	SKB	0.5 mg/mL	Diluted with NS. 5% or less loss of both drugs in 35 days at 22°C and 182 days at 4°C followed by 7 days at 32°C	1939	C
Morphine sulfate	ME	25 mg/mL[b]	RB	5 mg/mL	Visually compatible with less than 10% drug loss in 7 days at 8°C	668	C
Ondansetron HCl	GW	1 mg/mL[c]	SO	2.5 mg/mL[c]	Physically compatible. Under 6% ondansetron and under 5% metoclopramide losses in 24 hr at 4 or 23°C	2199	C
Oxycodone HCl	NAP	200 mg/20 mL		100 mg/20 mL	Visually compatible. Under 4% concentration change in 24 hr at 25°C	2600	C
Pantoprazole sodium	[a]	4 mg/1 mL		5 mg/1 mL	Precipitates within 15 min	2574	I
Penicillin G potassium	SQ	250,000 units/1 mL	RB	10 mg/2 mL	Incompatible. If mixed, use immediately	924, 1167	I
Penicillin G potassium	SQ	1 million units/4 mL	RB	10 mg/2 mL	Incompatible. If mixed, use immediately	924, 1167	I
Pentazocine lactate	WI	30 mg/1 mL	NO	10 mg/2 mL	Physically compatible for 15 min at room temperature	565	C
Prochlorperazine edisylate	MB	10 mg/2 mL	NO	10 mg/2 mL	Physically compatible for 15 min at room temperature	565	C

Drugs in Syringe Compatibility (Cont.)

Test Drug	Mfr	Amt	Mfr	Amt	Remarks	Ref	C/I
Promethazine HCl	WY	25 mg/1 mL	NO	10 mg/2 mL	Physically compatible for 15 min at room temperature	565	C
Ranitidine HCl	GL	50 mg/2 mL	RB	10 mg/1 mL	Physically compatible for 1 hr at 25°C	978	C
Scopolamine HBr	ST	0.4 mg/1 mL	NO	10 mg/2 mL	Physically compatible for 15 min at room temperature	565	C
Sodium bicarbonate	AB	100 mEq/100 mL	RB	10 mg/2 mL	Gas evolves	1167	I
Sodium bicarbonate	AB	100 mEq/100 mL	RB	160 mg/32 mL	Gas evolves	1167	I
Vinblastine sulfate		0.5 mg/0.5 mL		2.5 mg/0.5 mL	Physically compatible for 5 min at room temperature followed by 8 min of centrifugation	980	C
Vincristine sulfate		0.5 mg/0.5 mL		2.5 mg/0.5 mL	Physically compatible for 5 min at room temperature followed by 8 min of centrifugation	980	C

[a] Test performed using the formulation WITHOUT edetate disodium.

[b] Tested in sterile water for injection.

[c] Tested in sodium chloride 0.9%.

Y-Site Injection Compatibility (1:1 Mixture)

Metoclopramide HCl

Test Drug	Mfr	Conc	Mfr	Conc	Remarks	Ref	C/I
Acetaminophen	CAD	10 mg/mL	HOS	5 mg/mL	Physically compatible with less than 10% acetaminophen loss over 4 hr at room temperature	2841, 2844	C
Acyclovir sodium	BW	5 mg/mL[a]	ES	0.2 mg/mL[a]	Physically compatible for 4 hr at 25°C	1157	C
Acyclovir sodium	BV	5 mg/mL[b]	SIC	5 mg/mL	Crystals form	2794	I
Aldesleukin	CHI	33,800 I.U./mL[a]	DU	5 mg/mL	Visually compatible with little or no loss of aldesleukin activity	1857	C
Allopurinol sodium	BW	3 mg/mL[b]	DU	5 mg/mL	Heavy white precipitate forms immediately	1686	I
Amifostine	USB	10 mg/mL[a]	ES	5 mg/mL	Physically compatible for 4 hr at 23°C	1845	C
Amsacrine	NCI	1 mg/mL[a]	RB	2.5 mg/mL[a]	Orange turbidity becomes orange precipitate in 1 hr	1381	I
Aztreonam	SQ	40 mg/mL[a]	ES	5 mg/mL	Physically compatible for 4 hr at 23°C	1758	C
Bivalirudin	TMC	5 mg/mL[a]	FAU	5 mg/mL	Physically compatible for 4 hr at 23°C	2373	C
Bleomycin sulfate		3 units/mL		5 mg/mL	Drugs injected sequentially in Y-site with no flush. No precipitate seen	980	C
Cangrelor tetrasodium	TMC	1 mg/mL[b]		5 mg/mL	Physically compatible for 4 hr	3243	C
Ceftaroline fosamil	FOR	2.22 mg/mL[a h e]	HOS	5 mg/mL	Physically compatible for 4 hr at 23°C	2826	C
Ceftolozane sulfate–tazobactam sodium	CUB	10 mg/mL[c k]	TE	0.2 mg/mL[c]	Physically compatible for 2 hr	3247, 3262	C
Ciprofloxacin	MI	2 mg/mL[c]	DU	5 mg/mL	Visually compatible for 24 hr at 24°C	1655	C
Ciprofloxacin	BAY	2 mg/mL[b]		5 mg/mL	Visually compatible. No ciprofloxacin loss in 15 min. Metoclopramide not tested	1934	C
Cisatracurium besylate	GW	0.1, 2, 5 mg/mL[a]	AB	5 mg/mL	Physically compatible for 4 hr at 23°C	2074	C
Cisplatin		1 mg/mL		5 mg/mL	Drugs injected sequentially in Y-site with no flush. No precipitate seen	980	C

Y-Site Injection Compatibility (1:1 Mixture) (Cont.)

Test Drug	Mfr	Conc	Mfr	Conc	Remarks	Ref	C/I
Cladribine	ORT	0.015[b] and 0.5[d] mg/mL	RB	5 mg/mL	Physically compatible for 4 hr at 23°C	1969	C
Clarithromycin	AB	4 mg/mL[a]	ANT	5 mg/mL	Visually compatible for 72 hr at both 30 and 17°C	2174	C
Cloxacillin sodium	SMX	100 mg/mL	SZ	5 mg/mL	Physically compatible for up to 4 hr at room temperature	3245	C
Cyclophosphamide		20 mg/mL		5 mg/mL	Drugs injected sequentially in Y-site with no flush. No precipitate seen	980	C
Dexmedetomidine HCl	AB	4 mcg/mL[b]	FAU	5 mg/mL	Physically compatible for 4 hr at 23°C	2383	C
Diltiazem HCl	MMD	1[b] and 5 mg/mL	RB	5 mg/mL	Visually compatible	1807	C
Diltiazem HCl	MMD	5 mg/mL	RB	0.2 mg/mL[b]	Visually compatible	1807	C
Docetaxel	RPR	0.9 mg/mL[a]	AB	5 mg/mL	Physically compatible for 4 hr at 23°C	2224	C
Doripenem	JJ	5 mg/mL[a b]	HOS	5 mg/mL	Physically compatible for 4 hr at 23°C	2743	C
Doxapram HCl	RB	2 mg/mL[a]	AB	1 mg/mL	Visually compatible for 4 hr at 23°C	2470	C
Doxorubicin HCl		2 mg/mL		5 mg/mL	Drugs injected sequentially in Y-site with no flush. No precipitate seen	980	C
Doxorubicin HCl liposomal	SEQ	0.4 mg/mL[a]	GNS	5 mg/mL	Increase in measured turbidity	2087	I
Droperidol		2.5 mg/mL		5 mg/mL	Drugs injected sequentially in Y-site with no flush. No precipitate seen	980	C
Etoposide phosphate	BR	5 mg/mL[a]	FAU	5 mg/mL	Physically compatible for 4 hr at 23°C	2218	C
Famotidine	MSD	0.2 mg/mL[a]	RB	5 mg/mL	Physically compatible for 14 hr	1196	C
Famotidine	ME	2 mg/mL[b]		5 mg/mL	Visually compatible for 4 hr at 22°C	1936	C
Fenoldopam mesylate	AB	80 mcg/mL[b]	RB	5 mg/mL	Physically compatible for 4 hr at 23°C	2467	C
Fentanyl citrate	JN	0.025 mg/mL[a]	DU	5 mg/mL	Physically compatible for 48 hr at 22°C	1706	C
Filgrastim	AMG	30 mcg/mL[a]	ES	5 mg/mL	Physically compatible for 4 hr at 22°C	1687	C
Fluconazole	RR	2 mg/mL	RB	5 mg/mL	Physically compatible for 24 hr at 25°C	1407	C
Fludarabine phosphate	BX	1 mg/mL[a]	DU	5 mg/mL	Visually compatible for 4 hr at 22°C	1439	C
Fluorouracil		50 mg/mL		5 mg/mL	Drugs injected sequentially in Y-site with no flush. No precipitate seen	980	C
Foscarnet sodium	AST	24 mg/mL	RB	4 mg/mL	Physically compatible for 24 hr at room temperature under fluorescent light	1335	C
Foscarnet sodium	AST	24 mg/mL	RB	2 mg/mL[c]	Physically compatible for 24 hr at 25°C under fluorescent light	1393	C
Furosemide		10 mg/mL		5 mg/mL	Drugs injected sequentially in Y-site with no flush. Precipitates immediately	980	I
Gallium nitrate	FUJ	1 mg/mL[b]	SO	5 mg/mL	Visually compatible for 24 hr at 25°C	1673	C
Gemcitabine HCl	LI	10 mg/mL[b]	FAU	5 mg/mL	Physically compatible for 4 hr at 23°C	2226	C
Granisetron HCl	SKB	0.05 mg/mL[a]	AB	5 mg/mL	Physically compatible for 4 hr at 23°C	2000	C
Heparin sodium		1000 units/mL		5 mg/mL	Drugs injected sequentially in Y-site with no flush. No precipitate seen	980	C
Hetastarch in lactated electrolyte	AB	6%	FAU	5 mg/mL	Physically compatible for 4 hr at 23°C	2339	C

Y-Site Injection Compatibility (1:1 Mixture) (Cont.)

Test Drug	Mfr	Conc	Mfr	Conc	Remarks	Ref	C/I
Hydromorphone HCl	AST	0.5 mg/mL[a]	DU	5 mg/mL	Physically compatible for 48 hr at 22°C	1706	C
Idarubicin HCl	AD	1 mg/mL[b]	SO	5 mg/mL	Visually compatible for 24 hr at 25°C	1525	C
Isavuconazonium sulfate	ASP	1.5 mg/mL[c]	TE	0.2 mg/mL[c]	Physically compatible for 2 hr	3263	C
Leucovorin calcium		10 mg/mL		5 mg/mL	Drugs injected sequentially in Y-site with no flush. No precipitate seen	980	C
Levofloxacin	OMN	5 mg/mL[a]	ES	5 mg/mL	Visually compatible for 4 hr at 24°C	2233	C
Linezolid	PHU	2 mg/mL	FAU	5 mg/mL	Physically compatible for 4 hr at 23°C	2264	C
Melphalan HCl	BW	0.1 mg/mL[b]	RB	5 mg/mL	Physically compatible for 3 hr at 22°C	1557	C
Meperidine HCl	AB	10 mg/mL	SN	0.2 mg/mL[a]	Physically compatible for 4 hr at 25°C	1397	C
Meropenem	ZEN	1 and 50 mg/mL[b]	RB	5 mg/mL	Visually compatible for 4 hr at room temperature	1994	C
Meropenem		50 mg/mL	SZ	5 mg/mL	Physically compatible for 4 hr at room temperature	3538	C
Meropenem–vaborbactam	TMC	8 mg/mL[b i]	TE	0.2 mg/mL[b]	Physically compatible for 3 hr at 20 to 25°C	3380	C
Methadone HCl	LI	1 mg/mL[a]	DU	5 mg/mL	Physically compatible for 48 hr at 22°C	1706	C
Methotrexate sodium		25 mg/mL		5 mg/mL	Drugs injected sequentially in Y-site with no flush. No precipitate seen	980	C
Mitomycin		0.5 mg/mL		5 mg/mL	Drugs injected sequentially in Y-site with no flush. No precipitate seen	980	C
Morphine sulfate	AB	1 mg/mL	SN	0.2 mg/mL[a]	Physically compatible for 4 hr at 25°C	1397	C
Morphine sulfate	AST	1 mg/mL[a]	DU	5 mg/mL	Physically compatible for 48 hr at 22°C	1706	C
Ondansetron HCl	GL	1 mg/mL[b]	DU	5 mg/mL	Visually compatible for 4 hr at 22°C	1365	C
Oxaliplatin	SS	0.5 mg/mL[a]	RB	5 mg/mL	Physically compatible for 4 hr at 23°C	2566	C
Paclitaxel	NCI	1.2 mg/mL[a]		5 mg/mL	Physically compatible for 4 hr at 22°C	1528	C
Palonosetron HCl	MGI	50 mcg/mL	BA	5 mg/mL	Physically compatible. No loss of either drug in 4 hr	2716	C
Pemetrexed disodium	LI	20 mg/mL[b]	RB	5 mg/mL	Physically compatible for 4 hr at 23°C	2564	C
Piperacillin sodium–tazobactam sodium	LE[h]	40 mg/mL[a i]	RB	5 mg/mL	Physically compatible for 4 hr at 22°C	1688	C
Plazomicin sulfate	ACH	24 mg/mL[c]	TE	0.2 mg/mL[c]	Physically compatible for 1 hr at 20 to 25°C	3432	C
Quinupristin–dalfopristin	PF	2 mg/mL[a j]		5 mg/mL[a]	Physically compatible	3229	C
Remifentanil HCl	GW	0.025 and 0.25 mg/mL[b]	AB	5 mg/mL	Physically compatible for 4 hr at 23°C	2075	C
Sargramostim	IMM	10 mcg/mL[b]	DU	5 mg/mL	Visually compatible for 4 hr at 22°C	1436	C
Tacrolimus	FUJ	1 mg/mL[b]	DU	0.2 mg/mL[a]	Visually compatible for 24 hr at 25°C	1630	C
Tedizolid phosphate	CUB	0.8 mg/mL[b]	TE	0.2 mg/mL[b]	Physically compatible for 2 hr	3244	C
Telavancin HCl	ASP	7.5 mg/mL[a b e]	HOS	1 mg/mL	Physically compatible for 2 hr	2830	C
Teniposide	BR	0.1 mg/mL[a]	ES	5 mg/mL	Physically compatible for 4 hr at 23°C	1725	C
Thiotepa	IMM[f]	1 mg/mL[a]	RB	5 mg/mL	Physically compatible for 4 hr at 23°C	1861	C
Tigecycline	WY	1 mg/mL[b]		5 mg/mL	Physically compatible for 4 hr	2714	C

Y-Site Injection Compatibility (1:1 Mixture) (Cont.)

Test Drug	Mfr	Conc	Mfr	Conc	Remarks	Ref	C/I
Tigecycline	ACD, FRK, WY	c	m		Stated to be compatible	2915, 3459, 3460	C
TNA #218 to #226[g]			AB	5 mg/mL	Visually compatible for 4 hr at 23°C	2215	C
Topotecan HCl	SKB	56 mcg/mL[a b]	RB	1.72 mg/mL[a b]	Visually compatible. Little loss of either drug in 4 hr at 22°C	2245	C
TPN #212 to #215[g]			AB	5 mg/mL	Substantial loss of natural haze occurs immediately	2109	I
Vinblastine sulfate		1 mg/mL		5 mg/mL	Drugs injected sequentially in Y-site with no flush. No precipitate seen	980	C
Vincristine sulfate		1 mg/mL		5 mg/mL	Drugs injected sequentially in Y-site with no flush. No precipitate seen	980	C
Vinorelbine tartrate	BW	1 mg/mL[b]	RB	5 mg/mL	Physically compatible for 4 hr at 22°C	1558	C
Zidovudine	BW	4 mg/mL[a]	RB	2 mg/mL[a]	Physically compatible for 4 hr at 25°C	1193	C

[a] Tested in dextrose 5%.

[b] Tested in sodium chloride 0.9%.

[c] Tested in both dextrose 5% and sodium chloride 0.9%.

[d] Tested in bacteriostatic sodium chloride 0.9% preserved with benzyl alcohol 0.9%.

[e] Tested in Ringer's injection, lactated.

[f] Lyophilized formulation tested.

[g] Refer to Appendix for the composition of parenteral nutrition solutions. TNA indicates a 3-in-1 admixture, and TPN indicates a 2-in-1 admixture.

[h] Test performed using the formulation WITHOUT edetate disodium.

[i] Piperacillin component. Piperacillin in an 8:1 fixed-ratio concentration with tazobactam.

[j] Quinupristin and dalfopristin components combined.

[k] Ceftolozane component. Ceftolozane in a 2:1 fixed-ratio concentration with tazobactam.

[l] Meropenem component. Meropenem in a 1:1 fixed-ratio concentration with vaborbactam.

[m] Salt not specified.

Selected Revisions May 1, 2020. © Copyright, October 1982.
American Society of Health-System Pharmacists, Inc.

Metoprolol Tartrate
AHFS 24:24

Products

Metoprolol tartrate is available in 5-mL ampuls, vials, and syringe cartridges.[3542] [3543] Each mL of solution contains 1 mg of metoprolol tartrate and 9 mg of sodium chloride.[3542]

pH

The pH of the injection ranges from 5 to 8.[17]

Administration

Metoprolol tartrate is administered intravenously.[3542]

Stability

Metoprolol tartrate injection should be stored at controlled room temperature in the original carton and protected from light and freezing.[3542]

Metoprolol tartrate under simulated summer conditions in paramedic vehicles was exposed to temperatures ranging from 26 to 38°C over 4 weeks. Analysis found no loss of the drug under these conditions.[2562]

Compatibility Information

Solution Compatibility

Metoprolol tartrate

Test Soln Name	Mfr	Mfr	Conc/L or %	Remarks	Ref	C/I
Dextrose 5%	BA[a]	CI	300 mg	Visually compatible. Little loss in 36 hr at 24°C in light	1679	C
Dextrose 5%			0.5 g	Physically compatible. No loss in 30 hr at room temperature	2728	C
Sodium chloride 0.9%	BA[a]	CI	300 mg	Visually compatible. Little loss in 36 hr at 24°C in light	1679	C
Sodium chloride 0.9%			0.5 g	Physically compatible. No loss in 30 hr at room temperature	2728	C

[a] Tested in PVC containers.

Additive Compatibility

Metoprolol tartrate

Test Drug	Mfr	Conc/L or %	Mfr	Conc/L or %	Test Solution	Remarks	Ref	C/I
Eptifibatide	ME	750 mg		1 g		Physically compatible and chemically stable for up to 24 hr at 25°C	3049	C

Y-Site Injection Compatibility (1:1 Mixture)

Metoprolol tartrate

Test Drug	Mfr	Conc	Mfr	Conc	Remarks	Ref	C/I
Abciximab	LI	36 mcg/mL[a]	AB	1 mg/mL	Visually compatible for 12 hr at 23°C	2374	C
Acetaminophen	CAD	10 mg/mL	HOS	0.4 mg/mL[b]	Physically compatible for 1 hr at 23°C	3533	C
Albumin human	OCT	250 mg/mL	HOS	0.4 mg/mL[b]	Physically compatible for 1 hr at 23°C	3533	C
Alteplase	GEN	1 mg/mL	CI	1 mg/mL	Visually compatible with no alteplase clot-lysis activity loss in 24 hr at 25°C	1856	C
Amiodarone HCl	BIO	1.8 mg/mL[a]	BED	1 mg/mL	Visually compatible for 24 hr at 19°C	2795	C
Argatroban	GSK	1 mg/mL[b]	AB	1 mg/mL	Visually compatible for 24 hr at 23°C	2391	C
Bivalirudin	TMC	5 mg/mL[a][b]	AB	1 mg/mL	Visually compatible for 6 hr at 23°C	2680	C

DOI: 10.37573/9781585286850.265

Y-Site Injection Compatibility (1:1 Mixture) (Cont.)

Test Drug	Mfr	Conc	Mfr	Conc	Remarks	Ref	C/I
Cangrelor tetrasodium	TMC	1 mg/mL[b]		1 mg/mL	Physically compatible for 4 hr	3243	C
Cefepime HCl	APP	40 mg/mL[b]	HOS	0.4 mg/mL[b]	Physically compatible for 1 hr at 23°C	3533	C
Ceftaroline fosamil	FOR	2.22 mg/mL[a b c]	HOS	1 mg/mL	Physically compatible for 4 hr at 23°C	2826	C
Ciprofloxacin	SZ	2 mg/mL	HOS	0.4 mg/mL[b]	Physically compatible for 1 hr at 23°C	3533	C
Cisatracurium besylate	AB	2 mg/mL	HOS	0.4 mg/mL[b]	Physically compatible for 1 hr at 23°C	3533	C
Clevidipine butyrate	CHS	0.5 mg/mL		1 mg/mL	Physically compatible for 24 hr at 23°C	3334	C
Diltiazem HCl	NVP[a]	1 mg/mL	BED	1 mg/mL	Visually compatible for 24 hr at 19°C	2795	C
Doripenem	SHI	4.5 mg/mL[b]	HOS	0.4 mg/mL[b]	Physically compatible for 1 hr at 23°C	3533	C
Epinephrine[d]	AMP	0.128 mg/mL[b]	HOS	0.4 mg/mL[b]	Physically compatible for 1 hr at 23°C	3533	C
Eptifibatide	SC	0.75 mg/mL	BED	1 mg/mL	Visually compatible for 24 hr at 19°C	2795	C
Esomeprazole sodium	ASZ	0.8 mg/mL[b]	HOS	0.4 mg/mL[b]	Physically compatible for 1 hr at 23°C	3533	C
Furosemide	HOS	10 mg/mL	BED	1 mg/mL	Visually compatible for 24 hr at 19°C	2795	C
Heparin sodium	BA	1000 units/mL[a]	BED	1 mg/mL	Visually compatible for 24 hr at 19°C	2795	C
Hydrocortisone sodium succinate	PF	1 mg/mL[b]	HOS	0.4 mg/mL[b]	Physically compatible for 1 hr at 23°C	3533	C
Ibuprofen	CMB	4 mg/mL	HOS	0.4 mg/mL[b]	Physically compatible for 1 hr at 23°C	3533	C
Levofloxacin	SGT	5 mg/mL	HOS	0.4 mg/mL[b]	Physically compatible for 1 hr at 23°C	3533	C
Levothyroxine sodium	PRP	0.4 mcg/mL[b]	HOS	0.4 mg/mL[b]	Physically compatible for 1 hr at 23°C	3533	C
Lidocaine HCl	BA	8 mg/mL[a]	BED	1 mg/mL	Trace precipitate in 8 hr at 19°C	2795	I
Meperidine HCl	AB	10 mg/mL	CI	1 mg/mL	Physically compatible for 4 hr at 25°C	1397	C
Meropenem	NVP	20 mg/mL[b]	HOS	0.4 mg/mL[b]	Physically compatible for 1 hr at 23°C	3533	C
Meropenem		50 mg/mL	SZ	1 mg/mL	Physically compatible for 4 hr at room temperature	3538	C
Milrinone lactate	NVP	0.2 mg/mL[a]	BED	1 mg/mL	Visually compatible for 24 hr at 19°C	2795	C
Morphine sulfate	AB	1 mg/mL	CI	1 mg/mL	Physically compatible for 4 hr at 25°C	1397	C
Nesiritide	SCI	50 mcg/mL[a b]		1 mg/mL	Physically compatible for 4 hr	2625	C
Nesiritide	SCI	6 mcg/mL[a]	BED	1 mg/mL	Trace precipitate in 24 hr at 19°C	2795	I
Nitroglycerin	BA	0.2 mg/mL[a]	BED	1 mg/mL	Trace precipitate in 8 hr at 19°C	2795	I
Norepinephrine bitartrate	HOS	0.128 mg/mL[b]	HOS	0.4 mg/mL[b]	Physically compatible for 1 hr at 23°C	3533	C
Procainamide HCl	HOS	8 mg/mL[b]	BED	1 mg/mL	Visually compatible for 24 hr at 19°C	2795	C
Sodium nitroprusside	HOS	0.4 mg/mL[a]	BED	1 mg/mL	Visually compatible for 24 hr at 19°C	2795	C

[a] Tested in dextrose 5%.

[b] Tested in sodium chloride 0.9%.

[c] Tested in Ringer's injection, lactated.

[d] Salt not specified.

Selected Revisions May 1, 2020. © Copyright, October 1992.
American Society of Health-System Pharmacists, Inc.

Metronidazole
AHFS 8:30.92

Products

Metronidazole 5 mg/mL is available as a ready-to-use solution in 100-mL (500-mg) single-dose polyvinyl chloride (PVC) plastic bags. No dilution or buffering is required. Each bag also contains dibasic sodium phosphate 48 mg, citric acid anhydrous 23 mg, and sodium chloride 790 mg in water for injection.[1(6/08)]

pH

Metronidazole has a pH of 5.5 (ranging from 4.5 to 7).[1(6/08)] [17]

Osmolarity

Metronidazole has an osmolarity of 310 mOsm/L.[1(6/08)]

Sodium Content

Metronidazole contains 14 mEq of sodium from the excipients per 500 mg of metronidazole.[1(6/08)] [4]

Administration

Metronidazole is administered by continuous intravenous infusion or by intermittent intravenous infusion over 1 hour.[1(6/08)] [4]

Stability

Metronidazole is a clear, colorless, ready-to-use solution that should be stored at controlled room temperature and protected from light. It should not be stored under refrigeration.[1(6/08)] [4] Refrigeration may result in crystal formation. However, the crystals redissolve on warming to room temperature.[1115]

Light Effects

Prolonged exposure to light will cause a darkening of the product.[4] However, most manufacturers indicate that short-term exposure to normal room light does not adversely affect metronidazole stability. Direct sunlight should be avoided.[1115]

Sorption

Metronidazole was shown not to exhibit sorption to PVC bags and tubing, polyethylene tubing, Silastic tubing, and polypropylene syringes.[536] [606]

Central Venous Catheter

Metronidazole (Baxter) 5 mg/mL in dextrose 5% was found to be compatible with the ARROWg+ard Blue Plus (Arrow International) chlorhexidine-bearing triple-lumen central catheter. Essentially complete delivery of the drug was found with little or no drug loss occurring. Furthermore, chlorhexidine delivered from the catheter remained at trace amounts with no substantial increase due to the delivery of the drug through the catheter.[2335]

Compatibility Information

Additive Compatibility

Metronidazole

Test Drug	Mfr	Conc/L or %	Mfr	Conc/L or %	Test Solution	Remarks	Ref	C/I
Amoxicillin sodium–clavulanate potassium	BE	20 g[b]	BAY	5 g		Physically compatible with 8% clavulanate loss in 2 hr and 25% loss in 6 hr at 21°C. 7 to 8% amoxicillin and no metronidazole loss in 6 hr at 21°C	1920	I
Ampicillin sodium	BR	20 g	SE	5 g		9% ampicillin loss in 22 hr at 25°C and in 12 days at 5°C. No metronidazole loss	993	C
Aztreonam	SQ	10 and 20 g	MG	5 g		Pink color develops in 12 hr, becoming cherry red in 48 hr at 25°C. Pink color develops in 3 days at 4°C. No loss of either drug detected	1023	I
Cefazolin sodium	LI	10 g	SE	5 g		5% cefazolin loss and no metronidazole loss in 7 days at 25°C. No loss of either drug in 12 days at 5°C	993	C
Cefazolin sodium	LI	10 g	AB	5 g		Visually compatible with no loss of either drug in 72 hr at 8°C	1649	C
Cefepime HCl	BR	4 and 40 g	AB, ES, SE	5 g		4 to 5% cefepime loss in 24 hr at room temperature exposed to light and up to 10% loss in 7 days at 5°C. No metronidazole loss. Orange color develops in 18 hr at room temperature and 24 hr at 5°C	1682	?

DOI: 10.37573/9781585286850.266

Additive Compatibility (Cont.)

Test Drug	Mfr	Conc/L or %	Mfr	Conc/L or %	Test Solution	Remarks	Ref	C/I
Cefepime HCl	BMS	2.5, 5, 10, and 20 g	SCS	5 g	a	Visually compatible. 7 to 9% cefepime loss in 48 hr at 23°C; 2 to 8% cefepime loss in 7 days at 4°C. 7% or less metronidazole loss in 7 days at 4 and 23°C	2324	C
Cefepime HCl	ELN	3.3, 6.6, 10, 20 g	AB	5 g	a	Physically compatible and less than 6% metronidazole loss at 4 and 23°C in 14 days. 2 to 5% cefepime loss in 14 days at 4°C. At 23°C, 10 to 12% cefepime loss in 72 hr	2726	C
Cefotaxime sodium	HO	10 g	AB	5 g		Both drugs stable for 72 hr at 8°C	1547	C
Cefotaxime sodium	HO	10 g	AB	5 g		Visually compatible with 10% cefotaxime loss in 19 hr at 28°C and 8% loss in 96 hr at 5°C. No metronidazole loss in 96 hr at 5 or 28°C	1754	C
Cefoxitin sodium	MSD	30 g	SE	5 g		9% cefoxitin loss in 48 hr at 25°C and 3% in 12 days at 5°C. No metronidazole loss	993	C
Ceftazidime	GL	20 g		5 g		No loss of either drug in 4 hr	1345	C
Ceftazidime	LI	10 g	AB	5 g		Visually compatible with little or no loss of either drug in 72 hr at 8°C	1849	C
Ceftriaxone sodium	RC	10 g	AB	5 g		Visually compatible with little or no loss of either drug in 72 hr at 8°C	1849	C
Ceftriaxone sodium	RC	10 g	BA	5 g		Visually compatible with no metronidazole loss and with 6% ceftriaxone loss in 3 days and 8% in 4 days at 25°C	2101	C
Cefuroxime sodium	GL	7.5 g		5 g		Physically compatible with no loss of either drug in 1 hr	1036	C
Cefuroxime sodium	GL	15 g		5 g		No loss of either drug in 4 hr at 24°C	1376	C
Cefuroxime sodium	GL	7.5 g		5 g		10% cefuroxime loss in 16 days at 4°C and 35 hr at 25°C. No metronidazole loss in 15 days at 4 and 25°C	1565	C
Cefuroxime sodium	GL	7.5 and 15 g	IVX	5 g		Physically compatible. No loss of metronidazole and about 6% cefuroxime loss in 49 days at 5°C	2192	C
Ciprofloxacin		2 g		5 g		No loss of either drug in 4 hr at 24°C	1346	C
Ciprofloxacin	MI	1.6 g	SE	4.2 g		Visually compatible. Both drugs stable for 48 hr at 25°C in light and 4°C in dark	1541	C
Ciprofloxacin		1 g	RPR	2.5 g		Under 3% metronidazole loss in 24 hr at 25°C in light or dark. Ciprofloxacin not tested	2361	C
Ciprofloxacin	BAY	1 g	SCS	2.5 g		Visually compatible. No ciprofloxacin loss in 24 hr at 22°C in light. Metronidazole not tested	2413	C
Floxacillin sodium	BE	10 g		5 g		Physically compatible for 48 hr. Both drugs stable for 1 hr at room temperature	1036	C
Fluconazole	PF	1 g	AB	2.5 g		Visually compatible with no fluconazole loss in 72 hr at 25°C under fluorescent light. Metronidazole not tested	1677	C
Gentamicin sulfate	SC	800 mg and 1.2 g	SE	5 g		Physically compatible with no loss of either drug in 2 days at 18°C. At 4°C, no metronidazole loss but up to 10% gentamicin loss in 7 days	1242	C
Gentamicin sulfate		800 mg	RP	5 g		Visually compatible with no loss of metronidazole in 15 days at 5 and 25°C. 10% gentamicin loss in 63 hr at 25°C and 10.6 days at 5°C	1931	C
Hydrocortisone sodium succinate	ES	10 g	SE	5 g		No loss of either drug in 7 days at 25°C and 12 days at 5°C	993	C

Additive Compatibility (Cont.)

Test Drug	Mfr	Conc/L or %	Mfr	Conc/L or %	Test Solution	Remarks	Ref	C/I
Midazolam HCl	RC	50, 250, 400 mg		5 g	NS	Visually compatible for 4 hr	355	C
Penicillin G potassium	PF	200 million units	SE	5 g		5% penicillin loss in 22 hr and 8% in 72 hr at 25°C. 2% penicillin loss in 12 days at 5°C. No metronidazole loss	993	C
Tobramycin sulfate	LI	1 g	RP	5 g		Visually compatible with no loss of metronidazole in 15 days at 5 and 25°C. 10% tobramycin loss in 73 hr at 25°C and 12.1 days at 5°C	1931	C

a Tested in PVC containers.

b Amoxicillin component. Amoxicillin in a 10:1 fixed-ratio concentration with clavulanic acid.

Y-Site Injection Compatibility (1:1 Mixture)

Metronidazole

Test Drug	Mfr	Conc	Mfr	Conc	Remarks	Ref	C/I
Acyclovir sodium	BW	5 mg/mL[a]	SE	5 mg/mL	Physically compatible for 4 hr at 25°C	1157	C
Allopurinol sodium	BW	3 mg/mL[b]	BA	5 mg/mL	Physically compatible for 4 hr at 22°C	1686	C
Amifostine	USB	10 mg/mL[a]	BA	5 mg/mL	Physically compatible for 4 hr at 23°C	1845	C
Anidulafungin	VIC	0.5 mg/mL[a]	BA	5 mg/mL	Physically compatible for 4 hr at 23°C	2617	C
Aztreonam	SQ	40 mg/mL[a]	BA	5 mg/mL	Orange color forms in 4 hr	1758	I
Bivalirudin	TMC	5 mg/mL[a]	BA	5 mg/mL	Physically compatible for 4 hr at 23°C	2373	C
Blinatumomab	AMG	0.125 mcg/mL[b]	BRN	2.5 mg/mL	Persistent particulate formation when blinatumomab is added to metronidazole; not observed when order of mixing was reversed	3405, 3417	?
Blinatumomab	AMG	0.375 mcg/mL[b]	BRN	2.5 mg/mL	Flakes transiently appear when metronidazole is added to blinatumomab; not observed when order of mixing was reversed	3405, 3417	?
Cangrelor tetrasodium	TMC	1 mg/mL[b]		5 mg/mL	Physically compatible for 4 hr	3243	C
Caspofungin acetate	ME	0.7 mg/mL[b]	BA	5 mg/mL	Physically compatible for 4 hr at room temperature	2758	C
Caspofungin acetate	ME	0.5 mg/mL[b]	BA	5 mg/mL	Physically compatible over 60 min	2766	C
Ceftaroline fosamil	FOR	2.22 mg/mL[a b e]	BA	5 mg/mL	Physically compatible for 4 hr at 23°C	2826	C
Ceftazidime–avibactam sodium	ALL	20 mg/mL[m n]			Physically compatible for up to 4 hr at room temperature	3004	C
Ceftolozane sulfate–tazobactam sodium	CUB	10 mg/mL[j k]	RA	5 mg/mL[i]	Physically compatible for 2 hr	3262	C
Cisatracurium besylate	GW	0.1, 2, 5 mg/mL[a]	AB	5 mg/mL	Physically compatible for 4 hr at 23°C	2074	C
Clarithromycin	AB	4 mg/mL[a]	PRK	5 mg/mL	Visually compatible for 72 hr at both 30 and 17°C	2174	C
Cloxacillin sodium	SMX	100 mg/mL	HOS	5 mg/mL	Physically compatible for up to 4 hr at room temperature	3245	C
Cyclophosphamide	MJ	20 mg/mL[a]	SE	5 mg/mL	Physically compatible for 4 hr at 25°C	1194	C
Defibrotide sodium	JAZ	8 mg/mL[b]	BRN	5 mg/mL	Visually compatible for 4 hr at room temperature	3149	C
Dexmedetomidine HCl	AB	4 mcg/mL[b]	BA	5 mg/mL	Physically compatible for 4 hr at 23°C	2383	C
Diltiazem HCl	MMD	5 mg/mL	SE	5 mg/mL	Visually compatible	1807	C

Y-Site Injection Compatibility (1:1 Mixture) (Cont.)

Test Drug	Mfr	Conc	Mfr	Conc	Remarks	Ref	C/I
Dimenhydrinate		10 mg/mL		5 mg/mL	Clear solution	2569	C
Docetaxel	RPR	0.9 mg/mL[a]	BA	5 mg/mL	Physically compatible for 4 hr at 23°C	2224	C
Dopamine HCl	AB	0.8 mg/mL[a]	MG	5 mg/mL	Visually compatible for 24 hr at room temperature in test tubes. No precipitate found on filter from Y-site delivery	2063	C
Doripenem	JJ	5 mg/mL[a b]	BA	5 mg/mL	Physically compatible for 4 hr at 23°C	2743	C
Doxapram HCl	RB	2 mg/mL[a]	AB	5 mg/mL	Visually compatible for 4 hr at 23°C	2470	C
Doxorubicin HCl liposomal	SEQ	0.4 mg/mL[a]	AB	5 mg/mL	Physically compatible for 4 hr at 23°C	2087	C
Enalaprilat	MSD	0.05 mg/mL[b]	SE	5 mg/mL	Physically compatible for 24 hr at room temperature under fluorescent light	1355	C
Eravacycline dihydrochloride	TET	0.6 mg/mL[b]	BA	5 mg/mL[q]	Physically compatible for 2 hr at room temperature	3532	C
Esmolol HCl	DCC	10 mg/mL[a]	SE	5 mg/mL	Physically compatible for 24 hr at 22°C	1169	C
Etoposide phosphate	BR	5 mg/mL[a]	AB	5 mg/mL	Physically compatible for 4 hr at 23°C	2218	C
Fat emulsion, intravenous	OTS	20%[o]	PF	5 mg/mL[p]	Fine particles increased after preparation and continued to increase over time	3452	I
Fenoldopam mesylate	AB	80 mcg/mL[b]	BA	5 mg/mL	Physically compatible for 4 hr at 23°C	2467	C
Filgrastim	AMG	30 mcg/mL[a]	BA	5 mg/mL	Particles form immediately. Filaments form in 1 hr	1687	I
Fluconazole	RR	2 mg/mL	AB	5 mg/mL	Physically compatible for 24 hr at 25°C	1407	C
Foscarnet sodium	AST	24 mg/mL	AB	5 mg/mL	Physically compatible for 24 hr at room temperature under fluorescent light	1335	C
Foscarnet sodium	AST	24 mg/mL	SE	5 mg/mL	Physically compatible for 24 hr at 25°C under fluorescent light	1393	C
Gemcitabine HCl	LI	10 mg/mL[b]	AB	5 mg/mL	Physically compatible for 4 hr at 23°C	2226	C
Granisetron HCl	SKB	0.05 mg/mL[a]	BA	5 mg/mL	Physically compatible for 4 hr at 23°C	2000	C
Heparin sodium	TR	50 units/mL	MG	5 mg/mL	Visually compatible for 4 hr at 25°C	1793	C
Hetastarch in lactated electrolyte	AB	6%	AB	5 mg/mL	Physically compatible for 4 hr at 23°C	2339	C
Hydromorphone HCl	WY	0.2 mg/mL[a]	SE	5 mg/mL	Physically compatible for 4 hr at 25°C	987	C
Hydroxyethyl starch 130/0.4 in sodium chloride 0.9%	FRK	6%	HOS	1[a], 2.5[a], 5 mg/mL	Visually compatible for 24 hr at room temperature	2770	C
Labetalol HCl	SC	1 mg/mL[a]	SE	5 mg/mL	Physically compatible for 24 hr at 18°C	1171	C
Linezolid	PHU	2 mg/mL	BA	5 mg/mL	Physically compatible for 4 hr at 23°C	2264	C
Lorazepam	WY	0.33 mg/mL[b]	BRN	5 mg/mL	Visually compatible for 24 hr at 22°C	1855	C
Magnesium sulfate	IX	16.7, 33.3, 66.7, 100 mg/mL[a]	SE	5 mg/mL	Physically compatible for at least 4 hr at 32°C	813	C
Melphalan HCl	BW	0.1 mg/mL[b]	AB	5 mg/mL	Physically compatible for 3 hr at 22°C	1557	C

Y-Site Injection Compatibility (1:1 Mixture) (Cont.)

Test Drug	Mfr	Conc	Mfr	Conc	Remarks	Ref	C/I
Meperidine HCl	WY	10 mg/mL[a]	SE	5 mg/mL	Physically compatible for 4 hr at 25°C	987	C
Meropenem		50 mg/mL	HOS	5 mg/mL	Physically compatible for 4 hr at room temperature	3538	C
Meropenem–vaborbactam	TMC	8 mg/mL[b i]	BA	5 mg/mL[b]	Physically compatible for 3 hr at 20 to 25°C	3380	C
Methylprednisolone sodium succinate	UP	5 mg/mL[a]	MG	5 mg/mL	Visually compatible for 24 hr at room temperature in test tubes. No precipitate found on filter from Y-site delivery	2063	C
Midazolam HCl	RC	1 mg/mL[a]	BA	5 mg/mL	Visually compatible for 24 hr at 23°C	1847	C
Midazolam HCl	RC	5 mg/mL	BRN	5 mg/mL	Visually compatible for 24 hr at 22°C	1855	C
Milrinone lactate	SS	0.2 mg/mL[a]	AB	5 mg/mL	Visually compatible for 4 hr at 25°C	2381	C
Morphine sulfate	WI	1 mg/mL[a]	SE	5 mg/mL	Physically compatible for 4 hr at 25°C	987	C
Nicardipine HCl	DCC	0.1 mg/mL[a]	SE	5 mg/mL	Visually compatible for 24 hr at room temperature	235	C
Oritavancin diphosphate	TAR	0.8 and 1.2 mg/mL[a]	HOS	5 mg/mL[h]	Visually compatible for 4 hr at 20 to 24°C	2928	C
Oritavancin diphosphate	TAR	2 mg/mL[a]	HOS	5 mg/mL[h]	Fine particles form immediately	2928	I
Palonosetron HCl	MGI	50 mcg/mL	BA	5 mg/mL	Physically compatible. No loss of either drug in 4 hr at room temperature	2765	C
Pemetrexed disodium	LI	20 mg/mL[b]	BA	5 mg/mL	Color darkening and brownish discoloration occur immediately	2564	I
Piperacillin sodium–tazobactam sodium	LE[f]	40 mg/mL[a g]	BA	5 mg/mL	Physically compatible for 4 hr at 22°C	1688	C
Plazomicin sulfate	ACH	24 mg/mL[j]	BA	5 mg/mL[j]	Physically compatible for 1 hr at 20 to 25°C	3432	C
Quinupristin–dalfopristin		2 mg/mL[a i]		5 mg/mL	Reported to be incompatible	3230	I
Remifentanil HCl	GW	0.025 and 0.25 mg/mL[b]	AB	5 mg/mL	Physically compatible for 4 hr at 23°C	2075	C
Sargramostim	IMM	10 mcg/mL[b]	MG	5 mg/mL	Visually compatible for 4 hr at 22°C	1436	C
Tacrolimus	FUJ	1 mg/mL[b]	AB	5 mg/mL	Visually compatible for 24 hr at 25°C	1630	C
Tedizolid phosphate	CUB	0.8 mg/mL[b]	BA	5 mg/mL[b]	Physically compatible for 2 hr	3244	C
Teniposide	BR	0.1 mg/mL[a]	BA	5 mg/mL	Physically compatible for 4 hr at 23°C	1725	C
Theophylline	TR	4 mg/mL	MG	5 mg/mL	Visually compatible for 6 hr at 25°C	1793	C
Thiotepa	IMM[c]	1 mg/mL[a]	BA	5 mg/mL	Physically compatible for 4 hr at 23°C	1861	C
TNA #218 to #226[d]			AB	5 mg/mL	Visually compatible for 4 hr at 23°C	2215	C
TPN #189[d]			DB	5 mg/mL	Visually compatible for 24 hr at 22°C	1767[d]	C
TPN #203, #204[d]			AB	5 mg/mL	Visually compatible for 2 hr at 23°C	1974	C
TPN #212 to #215[d]			SCS	5 mg/mL	Physically compatible for 4 hr at 23°C	2109	C
Vasopressin	APP	0.2 unit/mL[b]	AB	5 mg/mL	Physically compatible	2641	C
Vinorelbine tartrate	BW	1 mg/mL[b]	BA	5 mg/mL	Physically compatible for 4 hr at 22°C	1558	C

Y-Site Injection Compatibility (1:1 Mixture) (Cont.)

[a] Tested in dextrose 5%.

[b] Tested in sodium chloride 0.9%.

[c] Lyophilized formulation tested.

[d] Refer to Appendix for the composition of parenteral nutrition solutions. TNA indicates a 3-in-1 admixture, and TPN indicates a 2-in-1 admixture.

[e] Tested in Ringer's injection, lactated.

[f] Test performed using the formulation WITHOUT edetate disodium

[g] Piperacillin component. Piperacillin in an 8:1 fixed-ratio concentration with tazobactam.

[h] Tested undiluted.

[i] Quinupristin and dalfopristin components combined.

[j] Tested in both dextrose 5% and sodium chloride 0.9%.

[k] Ceftolozane component. Ceftolozane in a 2:1 fixed-ratio concentration with tazobactam.

[l] Meropenem component. Meropenem in a 1:1 fixed-ratio concentration with vaborbactam.

[m] Ceftazidime component. Ceftazidime in a 4:1 fixed-ratio concentration with avibactam.

[n] Tested in dextrose 5%, sodium chloride 0.9%, and Ringer's injection, lactated.

[o] Run at 25 mL/hr with dextrose 5% run at 83 mL/hr.

[p] Run at 100 mL/hr.

[q] Tested as the premixed infusion solution.

Selected Revisions July 1, 2020. © Copyright, October 1982.
American Society of Health-System Pharmacists, Inc.

Mexiletine Hydrochloride
AHFS 24:04.04.08

Products

Mexiletine hydrochloride is available as a 25-mg/mL solution in 10-mL (250-mg) ampuls. The product also contains sodium chloride and water for injection.[38]

Trade Name(s)

Mexitil

Administration

Mexiletine hydrochloride is administered intravenously. It should never be given as a bolus. A loading dose is given by intravenous injection at a rate of 1 mL (25 mg) per minute. This is followed by intravenous infusion of a 500-mg/500 mL (1-mg/mL) dilution in a suitable infusion solution. The initial infusion rate of the first 250 mL of the admixture is 4 mL/min over the first hour followed by infusion of the next 250 mL at 2 mL/min over the next two hours. Maintenance is performed using a 250-mg/500 mL (0.5-mg/mL) dilution administered at a rate of 1 mL/min.[38]

Stability

Mexiletine hydrochloride injection is a clear, colorless solution that should be stored below 25°C and protected from light. Dilutions for infusion are stable for up to eight hours.[38]

Compatibility Information

Solution Compatibility

Mexiletine HCl

Test Soln Name	Mfr	Mfr	Conc/L or %	Remarks	Ref	C/I
Dextrose 5%				Compatible for 8 hr	38	C
Sodium chloride 0.9%[a]				Compatible for 8 hr	38	C
Sodium lactate ⅙ M				Compatible for 8 hr	38	C

[a] Tested with and without potassium chloride 0.3 and 0.6% present.

Drugs in Syringe Compatibility

Mexiletine HCl

Test Drug	Mfr	Amt	Mfr	Amt	Remarks	Ref	C/I
Heparin sodium		2500 units/1 mL	BI	250 mg/10 mL	Turbidity or precipitate forms within 5 min	1053	I

Selected Revisions October 1, 2012. © Copyright, October 2002.
American Society of Health-System Pharmacists, Inc.

DOI: 10.37573/9781585286850.267

Micafungin Sodium
AHFS 8:14.16

Products

Micafungin sodium is available in vials containing 50 and 100 mg of drug with lactose 200 mg and citric acid and/or sodium hydroxide added during manufacturing to adjust pH.[2893] Reconstitute the 50- or 100-mg vials with 5 mL of sodium chloride 0.9% or dextrose 5%, resulting in solutions containing micafungin sodium 10 or 20 mg/mL, respectively.[2893] Diluents containing a bacteriostatic agent should not be used for reconstitution.[2893] To minimize foaming, gently swirl the vials to dissolve the contents.[2893] Do not shake vigorously.[2893]

pH

From 5 to 7.[2893]

Trade Name(s)

Mycamine

Administration

Micafungin sodium is diluted in 100 mL of sodium chloride 0.9% or dextrose 5% and administered by intravenous infusion over 1 hour.[2893] Existing infusion lines should be flushed with sodium chloride 0.9% prior to starting the micafungin sodium infusion.[2893]

Stability

Store intact vials at controlled room temperature.[2893] When reconstituted as directed, the manufacturer indicates that micafungin sodium is stable for up to 24 hours at room temperature in the original container.[2893] However, the drug does not contain a preservative, and the manufacturer recommends discarding partially used vials.[2893] Micafungin sodium diluted for infusion is stable for up to 24 hours at room temperature when protected from light.[2893]

Light Effects

The manufacturer states that micafungin sodium dilutions should be protected from light but that covering tubing and drip chambers is not necessary.[2893]

Syringes

Micafungin sodium (Astellas) reconstituted with and further diluted in sodium chloride 0.9% to a concentration of 0.5 or 1 mg/mL and stored in 3 different polypropylene syringes demonstrated physical and chemical stability for 15 days stored at 25°C with 60% relative humidity in the dark.[3273]

Compatibility Information

Solution Compatibility

Micafungin sodium

Test Soln Name	Mfr	Mfr	Conc/L or %	Remarks	Ref	C/I
Dextrose 5%		ASP	0.5, 1, 1.5 g	Manufacturer-recommended solution	2893	C
Dextrose 5%	BRN	ASP	0.5 g	Visually compatible for 6 hr at 22°C protected from light	2894	C
Sodium chloride 0.9%		ASP	0.5, 1, 1.5 g	Manufacturer-recommended solution	2893	C
Sodium chloride 0.9%	BRN	ASP	0.5 g	Visually compatible for 6 hr at 22°C protected from light	2894	C

Additive Compatibility

Micafungin sodium

Test Drug	Mfr	Conc/L or %	Mfr	Conc/L or %	Test Solution	Remarks	Ref	C/I
Levofloxacin	HOS	2.5 g	ASP	0.5 g	NS	Hazy precipitate forms immediately	2894	I

DOI: 10.37573/9781585286850.268

Y-Site Injection Compatibility (1:1 Mixture)

Micafungin sodium

Test Drug	Mfr	Conc	Mfr	Conc	Remarks	Ref	C/I
Albumin human	ZLB	25%	ASP	1.5 mg/mL[b]	Immediate increase in measured haze	2683	I
Aminophylline	AMR	2.5 mg/mL[b]	ASP	1.5 mg/mL[b]	Physically compatible for 4 hr at 23°C	2683	C
Amiodarone HCl	BA	4 mg/mL[b]	ASP	1.5 mg/mL[b]	Gross milky white precipitate forms	2683	I
Bumetanide	BED	40 mcg/mL[b]	ASP	1.5 mg/mL[b]	Physically compatible for 4 hr at 23°C	2683	C
Calcium chloride	AB	40 mg/mL[b]	ASP	1.5 mg/mL[b]	Physically compatible for 4 hr at 23°C	2683	C
Calcium gluconate	AMR	40 mg/mL[b]	ASP	1.5 mg/mL[b]	Physically compatible for 4 hr at 23°C	2683	C
Cangrelor tetrasodium	TMC	1 mg/mL[b]		1.5 mg/mL[b]	Physically compatible for 4 hr	3243	C
Carboplatin	BA	5 mg/mL[b]	ASP	1.5 mg/mL[b]	Physically compatible for 4 hr at 23°C	2683	C
Ceftolozane sulfate–tazobactam sodium	CUB	10 mg/mL[d e]	ASP	2 mg/mL[d]	Physically compatible for 2 hr	3262	C
Cisatracurium besylate	AB	0.5 mg/mL[b]	ASP	1.5 mg/mL[b]	Gross precipitate forms immediately	2683	I
Cyclosporine	BED	5 mg/mL[b]	ASP	1.5 mg/mL[b]	Physically compatible for 4 hr at 23°C	2683	C
Diltiazem HCl	BA	5 mg/mL	ASP	1.5 mg/mL[b]	Gross precipitate forms immediately	2683	I
Dobutamine HCl	AB	4 mg/mL[b]	ASP	1.5 mg/mL[b]	Gross precipitate forms immediately	2683	I
Dopamine HCl	AMR	3.2 mg/mL[b]	ASP	1.5 mg/mL[b]	Physically compatible for 4 hr at 23°C	2683	C
Doripenem	JJ	5 mg/mL[a b]	ASP	1.5 mg/mL[a b]	Physically compatible for 4 hr at 23°C	2743	C
Epinephrine HCl	AB	50 mcg/mL[b]	ASP	1.5 mg/mL[b]	Microparticulates form in 4 hr	2683	I
Eptifibatide	SC	0.75 mg/mL	ASP	1.5 mg/mL[b]	Physically compatible for 4 hr at 23°C	2683	C
Eravacycline dihydrochloride	TET	0.6 mg/mL[b]	ASP	4 mg/mL[b]	Measured turbidity increased immediately; pH increased by >2 units within 60 min	3532	I
Esmolol HCl	BA	10 mg/mL[b]	ASP	1.5 mg/mL[b]	Physically compatible for 4 hr at 23°C	2683	C
Etoposide	SIC	0.4 mg/mL[b]	ASP	1.5 mg/mL[b]	Physically compatible for 4 hr at 23°C	2683	C
Fat emulsion, intravenous	OTS	20%[g]	ASP	0.25 mg/mL[a h]	No change in particle size ≥1.3 µm observed in 24 hr at 25°C in the dark	3452	C
Fenoldopam mesylate	BA	80 mcg/mL[b]	ASP	1.5 mg/mL[b]	Physically compatible for 4 hr at 23°C	2683	C
Furosemide	AMR	3 mg/mL[b]	ASP	1.5 mg/mL[b]	Physically compatible for 4 hr at 23°C	2683	C
Heparin sodium	AB	100 units/mL	ASP	1.5 mg/mL[b]	Physically compatible for 4 hr at 23°C	2683	C
Hydromorphone HCl	BA	0.5 mg/ml[b]	ASP	1.5 mg/mL[b]	Physically compatible for 4 hr at 23°C	2683	C
Insulin, regular	NOV	1 unit/mL[b]	ASP	1.5 mg/mL[b]	Increase in haze and microparticulates form in 4 hr	2683	I
Isavuconazonium sulfate	ASP	1.5 mg/mL[d]	ASP	2 mg/mL[d]	Immediate precipitation and increase in measured turbidity	3263	I
Labetalol HCl	AB	2 mg/mL[b]	ASP	1.5 mg/mL[b]	White cloudiness forms immediately	2683	I
Lidocaine HCl	AB	10 mg/mL[b]	ASP	1.5 mg/mL[b]	Physically compatible for 4 hr at 23°C	2683	C
Lorazepam	AB	0.5 mg/mL[b]	ASP	1.5 mg/mL[b]	Physically compatible for 4 hr at 23°C	2683	C

Y-Site Injection Compatibility (1:1 Mixture) (Cont.)

Test Drug	Mfr	Conc	Mfr	Conc	Remarks	Ref	C/I
Magnesium sulfate	AMR	100 mg/mL[b]	ASP	1.5 mg/mL[b]	Physically compatible for 4 hr at 23°C	2683	C
Meperidine HCl	AB	10 mg/mL[b]	ASP	1.5 mg/mL[b]	Milky precipitate forms immediately	2683	I
Meropenem–vaborbactam	TMC	8 mg/mL[b f]	ASP	4 mg/mL[b]	Physically compatible for 3 hr at 20 to 25°C	3380	C
Mesna	APP	20 mg/mL[b]	ASP	1.5 mg/mL[b]	Physically compatible for 4 hr at 23°C	2683	C
Midazolam HCl	APP	2 mg/mL[b]	ASP	1.5 mg/mL[b]	Gross precipitate forms immediately	2683	I
Milrinone lactate	BED	0.2 mg/mL[b]	ASP	1.5 mg/mL[b]	Physically compatible for 4 hr at 23°C	2683	C
Morphine sulfate	APP	15 mg/mL	ASP	1.5 mg/mL[b]	White precipitate forms immediately	2683	I
Mycophenolate mofetil HCl	RC	6 mg/mL[a]	ASP	1.5 mg/mL[b]	White precipitate forms immediately	2683	I
Nesiritide	SCI	6 mcg/mL[a]	ASP	1.5 mg/mL[b]	Microparticulates form immediately	2683	I
Nicardipine HCl	ESP	1 mg/mL[b]	ASP	1.5 mg/mL[b]	Precipitate forms immediately	2683	I
Nitroglycerin	AMR	0.4 mg/mL[b]	ASP	1.5 mg/mL[b]	Physically compatible for 4 hr at 23°C	2683	C
Norepinephrine bitartrate	BED	0.128 mg/mL[b]	ASP	1.5 mg/mL[b]	Physically compatible for 4 hr at 23°C	2683	C
Octreotide acetate	NVA	5 mcg/mL[b]	ASP	1.5 mg/mL[b]	Microparticulates form in 4 hr	2683	I
Ondansetron HCl	GSK	1 mg/mL[b]	ASP	1.5 mg/mL[b]	White precipitate forms immediately	2683	I
Phenylephrine HCl	BA	1 mg/mL[b]	ASP	1.5 mg/mL[b]	Physically compatible for 4 hr at 23°C	2683	C
Phenytoin sodium	HOS	50 mg/mL	ASP	1.5 mg/mL[b]	Measured haze increases within 1 hr	2683	I
Plazomicin sulfate	ACH	24 mg/mL[d]	ASP	4 mg/mL[d]	Cloudy with gross sedimentation and immediate increase in measured turbidity	3432	I
Posaconazole	ME	18 mg/mL		0.2 mg/mL[d]	Physically compatible	2911, 2912	C
Potassium chloride	AB	0.1 mEq/mL[b]	ASP	1.5 mg/mL[b]	Physically compatible for 4 hr at 23°C	2683	C
Potassium phosphates	APP	0.5 mmol/mL[b]	ASP	1.5 mg/mL[b]	Physically compatible for 4 hr at 23°C	2683	C
Rocuronium bromide	OR	1 mg/mL[b]	ASP	1.5 mg/mL[b]	White precipitate forms immediately	2683	I
Sodium nitroprusside	AB	2 mg/mL[b]	ASP	1.5 mg/mL[b]	Physically compatible for 4 hr at 23°C protected from light	2683	C
Sodium phosphates	AMR	0.5 mmol/mL[b]	ASP	1.5 mg/mL[b]	Physically compatible for 4 hr at 23°C	2683	C
Tacrolimus	FUJ	20 mcg/mL[b]	ASP	1.5 mg/mL[b]	Physically compatible for 4 hr at 23°C	2683	C
Tedizolid phosphate	CUB	0.8 mg/mL[b]	ASP	2 mg/mL[b]	Physically compatible for 2 hr	3244	C
Telavancin HCl	ASP	7.5 mg/mL[a b]	ASP	5 mg/mL[a b]	Visible haze forms	2830	I
Theophylline	AB	4 mg/mL	ASP	1.5 mg/mL[b]	Physically compatible for 4 hr at 23°C	2683	C
TPN #268[c]			ASP	1.5 mg/mL[b]	Physically compatible for 4 hr at 23°C	2683	C
Vasopressin	AMR	1 unit/mL	ASP	1.5 mg/mL[b]	Physically compatible for 4 hr at 23°C	2683	C
Vecuronium bromide	BED	1 mg/mL	ASP	1.5 mg/mL[b]	White precipitate forms immediately	2683	I

Y-Site Injection Compatibility (1:1 Mixture) (Cont.)

ᵃ Tested in dextrose 5%.

ᵇ Tested in sodium chloride 0.9%.

ᶜ Refer to Appendix for the composition of parenteral nutrition solutions. TPN indicates a 2-in-1 admixture.

ᵈ Tested in both dextrose 5% and sodium chloride 0.9%.

ᵉ Ceftolozane component. Ceftolozane in a 2:1 fixed-ratio concentration with tazobactam.

ᶠ Meropenem component. Meropenem in a 1:1 fixed-ratio concentration with vaborbactam.

ᵍ Run at 25 mL/hr with dextrose 5% run at 83 mL/hr.

ʰ Run at 100 mL/hr.

Selected Revisions May 1, 2020. © Copyright, October 2008.
American Society of Health-System Pharmacists, Inc.

Midazolam Hydrochloride
AHFS 28:24.08

Products

Midazolam hydrochloride is available at concentrations equivalent to midazolam 1 and 5 mg/mL in packages containing 1, 2, 5, or 10 mL of solution.[3206 3590 3591 3592] The drug also is available in a 100-mL pharmacy bulk package at a concentration equivalent to midazolam 5 mg/mL.[3250] Formulations generally also contain sodium chloride 0.8%.[3206 3250 3590 3591 3592] Some formulations contain disodium edetate 0.01%, with or without benzyl alcohol 1%.[3206 3250 3590] Preservative-free formulations of midazolam hydrochloride also are available.[3591 3592] The pH of both the preservative-containing and preservative-free formulations of the injection is adjusted with hydrochloric acid and, if necessary, sodium hydroxide.[3206 3250 3590 3591 3592]

Midazolam hydrochloride (Seizalam) also is available at a concentration equivalent to midazolam 5 mg/mL in multidose vials containing 10 mL labeled only for intramuscular administration.[3593] Each mL also contains sodium chloride 0.8%, disodium edetate 0.01%, and benzyl alcohol 1%.[3593] The pH of the injection is adjusted with hydrochloric acid and, if necessary, sodium hydroxide.[3593]

pH

The pH of the injection (Hospira) is approximately 3;[3590 3591 3592] pH ranges including 3 also have been reported for other products.[3206 3250]

The pH of the injection (Seizalam) labeled only for intramuscular administration is approximately 3.[3593]

Midazolam (Roche) 0.625, 1.25, and 1.67 mg/mL in sodium chloride 0.9% had pH values of 3.6, 3.4, and 3.4, respectively.[2161]

Osmolality

Midazolam (Roche) 0.625, 1.25, and 1.67 mg/mL in sodium chloride 0.9% had osmolalities of 274, 262, and 259 mOsm/kg, respectively.[2161]

Trade Name(s)

Versed, Seizalam

Administration

Midazolam hydrochloride is administered intramuscularly by injection deep into a large muscle mass or intravenously by slow intermittent injection in incremental doses or by continuous infusion.[3590 3591 3592] Use of the 1-mg/mL concentration or dilution of the 1- or 5-mg/mL concentration is recommended to facilitate slower injection.[3590 3591 3592] While the 5-mg/mL concentration is recommended for dilution for continuous intravenous infusion, both the 1- and 5-mg/mL concentrations may be diluted with sodium chloride 0.9% or dextrose 5%.[3590 3591 3592]

Administration of midazolam hydrochloride by rapid intravenous injection should be avoided, especially in neonatal and non-neonatal pediatric populations.[3590 3591 3592]

Intra-arterial injection and extravasation should be avoided.[3590 3591 3592]

Midazolam hydrochloride (Seizalam) is labeled only for intramuscular administration, specifically into the mid-outer thigh (i.e., vastus lateralis muscle).[3593]

Stability

Intact vials and cartridges should be stored at controlled room temperature.[3590 3591 3592 3593]

pH Effects

Midazolam hydrochloride is highly water soluble at pH 4 or less; at higher pH values, increased lipid solubility occurs.[1145] The rate of photodecomposition increases with increasing pH from 1.3 to 6.4.[1944]

Light Effects

Exposure of the commercially available injection (Roche) to sunlight for 4 months resulted in the yellowing of the solution in 1 month and a midazolam loss of about 8% in 4 months.[1944]

Syringes

In 2015, reports of decreased potency of certain drugs (e.g., midazolam hydrochloride) stored in Becton Dickinson syringes for extended periods (i.e., exceeding 24 hours) were confirmed by the manufacturer of these syringes; the cause of this change was later identified to be the inclusion of an alternate rubber stopper in the plunger of certain product lots of syringes.[3029 3036 3037 3039 3041 3042] Decreased potency was not observed when the syringes were filled and used promptly.[3037] Use of the alternate stopper was later discontinued and use of the primary stopper in such syringes was resumed; however, Becton Dickinson states that its general-use syringes are cleared by FDA for immediate use in fluid aspiration and injection and that such syringes, regardless of the stopper material, have not been cleared by FDA for use as a closed-container system.[3391]

Midazolam hydrochloride (Roche) prepared at a midazolam concentration of 2 mg/mL in sodium chloride 0.9% was packaged as 3 mL in 10-mL polypropylene infusion pump syringes (Pharmacia Deltec). Little or no loss occurred during 10 days of storage at 5 and 30°C.[1967]

Midazolam hydrochloride (Roche) prepared at a midazolam concentration of 3 mg/mL in sodium chloride 0.9% exhibited no visual changes and had losses of 6.5% at 20°C and 8.7% at 32°C in polypropylene syringes (Terumo) and of 8.9% at 32°C in glass vials after 13 days.[1595]

The stability of midazolam (salt form unspecified) 1 mg/mL repackaged in polypropylene syringes was evaluated. Little change in concentration was found after 4 weeks of storage at room temperature not exposed to direct light.[2164]

Midazolam hydrochloride (Roche) at a midazolam concentration of 5 mg/mL was packaged as 10 mL in 12-mL polypropylene syringes (Sherwood). No loss occurred in 36 days stored at 25°C protected from light.[2088]

DOI: 10.37573/9781585286850.269

Compatibility Information

Solution Compatibility

Midazolam HCl

Test Soln Name	Mfr	Mfr	Conc/L or %	Remarks	Ref	C/I
Dextrose 5% in sodium chloride 0.9%	GRI	RC	0.1 and 0.5 g	8 to 10% loss in 24 hr at ambient temperature	1868	C
Dextrose 5% in sodium chloride 0.9%	GRI	RC	1 g	4% loss in 24 hr at ambient temperature. 10% calculated loss in 54 hr	1868	C
Dextrose 5%	MG[b]	RC	0.5 g	Visually compatible. No loss in 30 days at 23°C in the dark or at 4°C	1717	C
Dextrose 5%	[c]	RC	30 mg	No loss in 72 hr at 20°C	1798	C
Dextrose 5%	AB	RC	0.1 and 0.5 g	Visually compatible. No loss in 3 hr at 24°C	1852	C
Dextrose 5%	GRI	RC	0.1, 0.5, 1 g	3 to 5% loss in 24 hr at ambient temperature. 10% calculated loss in 63 to 112 hr	1868	C
Dextrose 5%	BA[a i]	RC	0.1 and 0.5 g	13% loss in 24 hr at ambient temperature. 10% calculated loss in 20 hr	1868	I
Dextrose 5%	BA[a i]	RC	1 g	7% loss in 24 hr at ambient temperature. 10% calculated loss in 35 hr	1868	C
Dextrose 5%	BA[g]	RC	500 mg	Visually compatible. No loss in 36 days at 4, 25, and 40°C protected from light	2088	C
Dextrose 5%	BA[a], BRN[g h]	RC	35 mg	Visually compatible. 4 to 6% loss in 24 hr at 4 and 22°C	2289	C
Dextrose 5%	[g]	RC	100 and 500 mg	Visually compatible for 4 hr	355	C
Dextrose 5%	BA[a]	HOS	1 g	Little to no loss in 27 days at 20 to 25°C in fluorescent light or amber bags and at 3 to 4°C	3274	C
Dextrose 5%	[b]	HOS	1 g	Little to no loss in 27 days at 20 to 25°C in fluorescent light or amber bags and at 3 to 4°C	3274	C
Dextrose 5%		HOS	500 mg	Compatible for 24 hr	3590, 3591	C
Ringer's injection, lactated	GRI	RC	0.1 g	10% calculated loss in 2 hr at ambient temperature	1868	I
Ringer's injection, lactated	GRI	RC	0.5 g	10% calculated loss in 6 hr at ambient temperature	1868	I
Ringer's injection, lactated	GRI	RC	1 g	10% calculated loss in 10 hr at ambient temperature	1868	I
Ringer's injection, lactated	[g]	RC	100 and 500 mg	Visually compatible for 4 hr	355	C
Ringer's injection, lactated		HOS	500 mg	Compatible for 4 hr	3590, 3591	C
Sodium chloride 0.9%	[d]	RC	40 mg	Physically compatible. No loss in 24 hr at 21°C in the dark	1392	C
Sodium chloride 0.9%	MG[b]	RC	0.5 g	Visually compatible. No loss in 30 days at 23°C in the dark or at 4°C	1717	C
Sodium chloride 0.9%	[c]	RC	30 mg	No loss in 72 hr at 20°C	1798	C
Sodium chloride 0.9%	BA[a]	RC	1 g[e]	Visually compatible. 5% or less loss in 10 days at 23°C both in light and dark	1859	C
Sodium chloride 0.9%	BA[a]	RC	1 g	Visually compatible. 4 to 6% loss in 49 days at 4 and 20°C in light and at 20°C in dark	1863	C
Sodium chloride 0.9%	GRI	RC	0.1, 0.5, 1 g	8 to 10% loss in 24 hr at ambient temperature	1868	C

Solution Compatibility (Cont.)

Test Soln Name	Mfr	Mfr	Conc/L or %	Remarks	Ref	C/I
Sodium chloride 0.9%	BA[g]	RC	500 mg	Visually compatible. No loss in 36 days at 4, 25, and 40°C protected from light	2088	C
Sodium chloride 0.9%	BA[a], BRN[g h]	RC	35 mg	Visually compatible. 4 to 6% loss in 24 hr at 4 and 22°C	2289	C
Sodium chloride 0.9%	[g]	RC	100 and 500 mg	Visually compatible for 4 hr	355	C
Sodium chloride 0.9%	BA	RC	300, 600, 900 mg	Visually compatible. No loss in 48 hr at room temperature	2531	C
Sodium chloride 0.9%	BA[k]	MYL	1 g	Physically compatible with less than 3% loss in 1 year at 2 to 8°C and –25 to –15°C	3589	C
Sodium chloride 0.9%	BA[k]	MYL	1 g	Physically compatible with less than 10% loss in 90 days at 23 to 27°C and 55 to 65% relative humidity	3589	C
Sodium chloride 0.9%	BA[j]	MYL	1 g	Physically compatible with less than 4% loss in 1 year at 2 to 8°C and –25 to –15°C	3589	C
Sodium chloride 0.9%	BA[j]	MYL	1 g	Physically compatible with less than 10% loss in 180 days at 23 to 27°C and 55 to 65% relative humidity	3589	C
Sodium chloride 0.9%		HOS	500 mg	Compatible for 24 hr	3590, 3591	C
TPN #174 to #176[f]		RC	600 mg to 1 g	Precipitates immediately	1624	I
TPN #174 to #176[f]		RC	100 and 500 mg	Visually compatible with no midazolam loss and less than 10% loss of any amino acid in 5 hr at 22°C	1624	C

[a] Tested in PVC containers.

[b] Tested in polyolefin containers.

[c] Tested in both glass and PVC containers.

[d] Tested in PVC, glass, and polyethylene-lined laminated containers.

[e] Also contained benzyl alcohol 1%.

[f] Refer to Appendix for the composition of parenteral nutrition solutions. TPN indicates a 2-in-1 admixture.

[g] Tested in glass containers.

[h] Tested in polyethylene containers.

[i] Tested with potassium chloride 0.15%.

[j] Tested in cyclic olefin copolymer (COC) containers.

[k] Tested in polypropylene syringes.

Additive Compatibility

Midazolam HCl

Test Drug	Mfr	Conc/L or %	Mfr	Conc/L or %	Test Solution	Remarks	Ref	C/I
Aminophylline		720 mg	RC	50 mg	NS	Visually compatible for 4 hr	355	C
Aminophylline		720 mg	RC	250 mg	NS	Transient precipitate that dissipates	355	?
Aminophylline		720 mg	RC	400 mg	NS	Precipitate forms immediately	355	I
Amoxicillin sodium	BE	10 g	RC	50 and 250 mg	NS	Transient precipitate	355	?
Amoxicillin sodium	BE	10 g	RC	400 mg	NS	Precipitate forms immediately	355	I
Cefuroxime sodium	GL	7.5 g	RC	50, 250, 400 mg	NS	Visually compatible for 4 hr	355	C

Additive Compatibility (Cont.)

Test Drug	Mfr	Conc/L or %	Mfr	Conc/L or %	Test Solution	Remarks	Ref	C/I
Ciprofloxacin	BAY	2 g	RC	200 mg	D5W	Visually compatible. No ciprofloxacin loss in 24 hr at 22°C in light. Midazolam not tested	2413	C
Eptifibatide	ME	750 mg		1 g		Physically compatible and chemically stable for up to 24 hr at 25°C	3049	C
Furosemide		80 mg	RC	50 and 250 mg	NS	Visually compatible for 4 hr	355	C
Gentamicin sulfate	EX	800 mg	RC	50, 250, 400 mg	NS	Visually compatible for 4 hr	355	C
Hydromorphone HCl	KN	0.5 to 45 g	RC	0.1 to 4.5 g	D5W, NS	Visually compatible for 24 hr at room temperature	2086	C
Hydromorphone HCl	KN	2 and 20 g	RC	100 and 500 mg	D5W, NS	Visually compatible. Under 7% hydromorphone and midazolam loss in 23 days at 4 and 23°C	2086	C
Metronidazole		5 g	RC	50, 250, 400 mg	NS	Visually compatible for 4 hr	355	C
Oxycodone HCl	NAP	830 mg	RC	830 mg	NS, W	Visually compatible. Under 4% concentration change in 24 hr at 25°C	2600	C
Ranitidine HCl	GL	400 mg	RC	50 and 250 mg	NS	Visually compatible for 4 hr	355	C
Sodium bicarbonate	b	5%	RC	100 mg		Transient precipitation upon mixing	355	?
Sodium bicarbonate	b	5%	RC	500 mg		Precipitation upon mixing	355	I
Tramadol HCl	AND	11.18 g	RC	500 mg	NS[a]	Visually compatible for 7 days at 25°C protected from light	2701	C
Tramadol HCl	AND	33.3 g	RC	1.5 g	NS[a]	Visually compatible for 7 days at 25°C protected from light	2701	C

[a] Tested in elastomeric pump reservoirs (Baxter).

[b] Tested in glass containers.

Drugs in Syringe Compatibility

Midazolam HCl

Test Drug	Mfr	Amt	Mfr	Amt	Remarks	Ref	C/I
Alfentanil HCl	JN	0.5 mg/mL	RC	0.2 mg/mL[a]	Visually compatible. 8% midazolam and 2% alfentanil loss in 3 weeks at 20°C in light. No alfentanil loss and 7% midazolam loss in 4 weeks at 6°C in dark	2133	C
Atracurium besylate	BW	10 mg/mL		5 mg/mL	Physically compatible and atracurium stable for 24 hr at 5 and 30°C	1694	C
Atropine sulfate	IX	0.4 mg/1 mL	RC	5 mg/1 mL	Physically compatible for 4 hr at 25°C	1145	C
Buprenorphine HCl	NE	0.3 mg/1 mL	RC	5 mg/1 mL	Physically compatible for 4 hr at 25°C	1145	C
Butorphanol tartrate	BR	2 mg/1 mL	RC	5 mg/1 mL	Physically compatible for 4 hr at 25°C	1145	C
Chlorpromazine HCl	SKF	50 mg/2 mL	RC	5 mg/1 mL	Physically compatible for 4 hr at 25°C	1145	C
Dexamethasone sodium phosphate	DB	2 mg/8 mL	RC	2.5 mg/8 mL	Diluted in NS. Visually clear. No dexamethasone loss in 48 hr. Midazolam losses over 10% beyond 24 hr at room temperature	2531	C

Drugs in Syringe Compatibility (Cont.)

Test Drug	Mfr	Amt	Mfr	Amt	Remarks	Ref	C/I
Dexamethasone sodium phosphate	DB	2 mg/8 mL	RC	5 mg/8 mL	Diluted in NS. Visually clear. No dexamethasone loss in 48 hr. Midazolam losses were 7% in 48 hr at room temperature	2531	C
Dexamethasone sodium phosphate	DB	4 mg/8 mL	RC	5 mg/8 mL	Diluted in NS. Cloudiness forms immediately	2531	I
Dexamethasone sodium phosphate	DB	4 mg/8 mL	RC	7.5 mg/8 mL	Diluted in NS. Cloudiness forms immediately	2531	I
Dexamethasone sodium phosphate	DB	2 mg/8 mL	RC	7.5 mg/8 mL	Diluted in NS. Crystals form in some samples within 24 hr	2531	I
Diamorphine HCl	EV	10 mg	RC	10[b] and 75[c] mg	Visually compatible. 10% diamorphine and no midazolam loss in 15.9 days at 22°C	1792	C
Diamorphine HCl	EV	500 mg	RC	10[b] and 75[c] mg	Visually compatible. 10% diamorphine and no midazolam loss in 22.2 days at 22°C	1792	C
Dimenhydrinate	SE	50 mg/1 mL	RC	5 mg/1 mL	White precipitate forms immediately	1145	I
Diphenhydramine HCl	ES	50 mg/1 mL	RC	5 mg/1 mL	Physically compatible for 4 hr at 25°C	1145	C
Droperidol	JN	2.5 mg/1 mL	RC	5 mg/1 mL	Physically compatible for 4 hr at 25°C	1145	C
Fentanyl citrate	ES	0.1 mg/2 mL	RC	5 mg/1 mL	Physically compatible for 4 hr at 25°C	1145	C
Fentanyl citrate	DB	12.5 mcg/mL[a]	RC	0.625 and 0.938 mg/mL[a]	Visually compatible. Little fentanyl loss. 7 and 9% midazolam loss in 7 days at 5 and 22°C, respectively	2202	C
Fentanyl citrate	DB	37.5 mcg/mL[a]	RC	0.625 mg/mL[a]	Visually compatible. No fentanyl loss. 5 and 8% midazolam loss in 7 days at 5 and 22°C, respectively	2202	C
Fentanyl citrate	DB	37.5 mcg/mL[a]	RC	0.938 mg/mL[a]	Visually compatible. Little fentanyl loss. 7 and 9% midazolam loss in 7 days at 5 and 22°C, respectively	2202	C
Fentanyl citrate	DB	33.3 mcg/mL[a]	RC	0.278 and 0.833 mg/mL[a]	Visually compatible. No fentanyl loss. 5 and 7% midazolam loss in 7 days at 5 and 22°C, respectively	2202	C
Fentanyl citrate with metoclopramide HCl	DB AST	1 mg/20 mL 20 mg/4 mL	RC	15 mg/3 mL	Visually compatible with 7% or less loss of each drug in 10 days at 32°C	2268	C
Glycopyrrolate	RB	0.2 mg/1 mL	RC	5 mg/1 mL	Physically compatible for 4 hr at 25°C	1145	C
Heparin sodium		2500 units/1 mL	RC	15 mg/3 mL	Turbidity or precipitate forms within 5 min	1053	I
Hydromorphone HCl	WB	2 mg/0.5 mL	RC	5 mg/1 mL	Physically compatible for 4 hr at 25°C	1145	C
Hydroxyzine HCl	ES	100 mg/2 mL	RC	5 mg/1 mL	Physically compatible for 4 hr at 25°C	1145	C
Meperidine HCl	WB	100 mg/1 mL	RC	5 mg/1 mL	Physically compatible for 4 hr at 25°C	1145	C
Metoclopramide HCl	RB	10 mg/2 mL	RC	5 mg/1 mL	Physically compatible for 4 hr at 25°C	1145	C
Metoclopramide HCl with fentanyl citrate	AST DB	20 mg/4 mL 1 mg/20 mL	RC	15 mg/3 mL	Visually compatible with 7% or less loss of each drug in 10 days at 32°C	2268	C
Morphine sulfate	WB	10 mg/1 mL	RC	5 mg/1 mL	Physically compatible for 4 hr at 25°C	1145	C
Morphine sulfate		5 and 10 mg/1 mL[d]	RC	5 mg/1 mL	Visually compatible. 9% or less morphine and 8% or less midazolam loss in 14 days at 22°C in dark. Microprecipitate may form, requiring filtration	1901	C
Morphine sulfate		5 and 10 mg/1 mL[e]	RC	5 mg/1 mL	Visually compatible. 8% or less morphine and 3% or less midazolam loss in 14 days at 22°C protected from light. Microprecipitate may form, requiring filtration	1901	C

Drugs in Syringe Compatibility (Cont.)

Test Drug	Mfr	Amt	Mfr	Amt	Remarks	Ref	C/I
Nalbuphine HCl	DU	10 mg/1 mL	RC	5 mg/1 mL	Physically compatible for 4 hr at 25°C	1145	C
Ondansetron HCl	GW	1.33 mg/mL[a]	RC	1.66 mg/mL[a]	Physically compatible. Under 4% ondansetron and under 7% midazolam losses in 24 hr at 4 or 23°C	2199	C
Oxycodone HCl	NAP	200 mg/20 mL	RC	100 mg/20 mL	Visually compatible. Under 4% concentration change in 24 hr at 25°C	2600	C
Pantoprazole sodium	[f]	4 mg/1 mL		5 mg/1 mL	Precipitates immediately	2574	I
Pentobarbital sodium	WY	100 mg/2 mL	RC	5 mg/1 mL	White precipitate forms immediately	1145	I
Prochlorperazine edisylate	SKF	10 mg/2 mL	RC	5 mg/1 mL	White precipitate forms immediately	1145	I
Promethazine HCl	WY	25 mg/1 mL	RC	5 mg/1 mL	Physically compatible for 4 hr at 25°C	1145	C
Ranitidine HCl	GL	50 mg/2 mL	RC	5 mg/1 mL	White precipitate forms immediately	1145	I
Scopolamine HBr	BW	0.43 mg/0.5 mL	RC	5 mg/1 mL	Physically compatible for 4 hr at 25°C	1145	C
Trimethobenzamide HCl	BE	200 mg/2 mL	RC	5 mg/1 mL	Physically compatible for 4 hr at 25°C	1145	C

[a] Diluted with sodium chloride 0.9%.

[b] Diluted with sterile water to 15 mL.

[c] Diamorphine hydrochloride constituted with midazolam injection.

[d] Morphine sulfate powder dissolved in dextrose 5%.

[e] Morphine sulfate powder dissolved in water and sodium chloride 0.9%.

[f] Test performed using the formulation WITHOUT edetate disodium.

Y-Site Injection Compatibility (1:1 Mixture)

Midazolam HCl

Test Drug	Mfr	Conc	Mfr	Conc	Remarks	Ref	C/I
Abciximab	LI	36 mcg/mL[a]	BED	2 mg/mL	Visually compatible for 12 hr at 23°C	2374	C
Acetaminophen	CAD	10 mg/mL	ABX, BED	5 mg/mL	Physically compatible with less than 10% acetaminophen loss over 4 hr at room temperature	2841, 2844	C
Acetaminophen	CAD	10 mg/mL	HOS	5 mg/mL	Physically compatible for 4 hr at 23°C	2901, 2902	C
Albumin human		200 mg/mL	RC	5 mg/mL	White precipitate forms immediately	1855	I
Amikacin sulfate	BMS	5 mg/mL	RC	5 mg/mL	Visually compatible for 24 hr at 22°C	1855	C
Amiodarone HCl	WY	4.8 mg/mL[a]	RC	1 mg/mL[a]	Visually compatible for 24 hr at 23°C	1877	C
Amiodarone HCl	WY	6 mg/mL[a]	RC	1 mg/mL[a]	Visually compatible for 24 hr at 22°C	2352	C
Amoxicillin sodium	SKB	50 mg/mL	RC	5 mg/mL	White precipitate forms immediately	1855	I
Amoxicillin sodium–clavulanate potassium	SKB	20 mg/mL[k]	RC	5 mg/mL	White precipitate forms immediately	1855	I
Ampicillin sodium	WY	20 mg/mL[b]	RC	1 mg/mL[a]	Haze forms immediately	1847	I
Anidulafungin	VIC	0.5 mg/mL[a]	BA	1 mg/mL[a]	Physically compatible for 4 hr at 23°C	2617	C
Argatroban	GSK	1 mg/mL[b]	AB	2 mg/mL	Visually compatible for 24 hr at 23°C	2391	C
Atracurium besylate	BW	0.5 mg/mL[a]	RC	0.05 mg/mL[a]	Physically compatible for 24 hr at 28°C	1337	C

Y-Site Injection Compatibility (1:1 Mixture) (Cont.)

Test Drug	Mfr	Conc	Mfr	Conc	Remarks	Ref	C/I
Atracurium besylate	GW	1 and 5 mg/mL[a]	RC	0.1 mg/mL[a]	Visually compatible with no loss of either drug in 3 hr at 25°C	2112	C
Atracurium besylate	GW	5 mg/mL[a]	RC	0.5 mg/mL[a]	Visually compatible with no loss of either drug in 3 hr at 25°C	2112	C
Atracurium besylate	GW	1 mg/mL[a]	RC	0.5 mg/mL[a]	Visually compatible with no loss of midazolam and 4% loss of atracurium in 3 hr at 25°C	2112	C
Bivalirudin	TMC	5 mg/mL[a]	BA	1 mg/mL[a]	Physically compatible for 4 hr at 23°C	2373	C
Bivalirudin	TMC	5 mg/mL[a b]	AB	2 mg/mL	Visually compatible for 6 hr at 23°C	2680	C
Bumetanide	LEO	0.5 mg/mL	RC	5 mg/mL	White precipitate forms immediately	1855	I
Butorphanol tartrate	BR	[f]	RC	[f]	Crystalline midazolam precipitate forms	2144	I
Calcium gluconate	FUJ	100 mg/mL	RC	1 mg/mL[a]	Visually compatible for 24 hr at 23°C	1847	C
Cangrelor tetrasodium	TMC	1 mg/mL[b]		1 mg/mL[b]	Physically compatible for 4 hr	3243	C
Cangrelor tetrasodium	TMC	1 mg/mL[b]		5 mg/mL	Cloudy white precipitate with particulates appears immediately	3243	I
Caspofungin acetate	ME	0.7 mg/mL[b]	APP	2 mg/mL[b]	Physically compatible for 4 hr at room temperature	2758	C
Cefazolin sodium	MAR	20 mg/mL[a]	RC	1 mg/mL[a]	Visually compatible for 24 hr at 23°C	1847	C
Cefepime HCl	BMS	120 mg/mL[c]		5 mg/mL	Over 10% cefepime loss occurs in 1 hr	2513	I
Cefotaxime sodium	HO	20 mg/mL[a]	RC	1 mg/mL[a]	Visually compatible for 24 hr at 23°C	1847	C
Cefotaxime sodium	RS	10 mg/mL	RC	5 mg/mL	Visually compatible for 24 hr at 22°C	1855	C
Ceftaroline fosamil	FOR	2.22 mg/mL[a b d]	BV	2 mg/mL[a b d]	Physically compatible for 4 hr at 23°C	2826	C
Ceftazidime	LI	20 mg/mL[a]	RC	1 mg/mL[a]	Haze forms in 1 hr	1847	I
Ceftazidime	SKB	125 mg/mL		5 mg/mL	Precipitates immediately	2434	I
Ceftazidime	GSK	120 mg/mL[c]		5 mg/mL	Precipitates	2513	I
Ceftolozane sulfate–tazobactam sodium	CUB	10 mg/mL[n o]	APP	1 mg/mL[n]	Physically compatible for 2 hr	3262	C
Cefuroxime sodium	LI	15 mg/mL[a]	RC	1 mg/mL[a]	Particles form in 8 hr	1847	I
Ciprofloxacin	BAY	2 mg/mL	RC	5 mg/mL	Visually compatible for 24 hr at 22°C	1855	C
Cisatracurium besylate	GW	0.1, 2, 5 mg/mL[a]	RC	1 mg/mL[a]	Physically compatible for 4 hr at 23°C	2074	C
Clindamycin phosphate	UP	9 mg/mL[a]	RC	1 mg/mL[a]	Visually compatible for 24 hr at 23°C	1847	C
Clonidine HCl	BI	0.015 mg/mL	RC	5 mg/mL	Orange color in 24 hr at 22°C	1855	I
Clonidine HCl	BI	18 mcg/mL[b]	ALP	1 mg/mL	Visually compatible	2642	C
Cloxacillin sodium	SMX	100 mg/mL	PPC	5 mg/mL	Precipitates immediately	3245	I
Defibrotide sodium	JAZ	8 mg/mL[b]	PAN	5 mg/mL	A fine and transient suspension forms within 2.5 hr only when midazolam HCl added to defibrotide; not observed when order of mixing was reversed	3149	?
Dexamethasone sodium phosphate	ES	4 mg/mL	RC	1 mg/mL[a]	Immediate haze. Precipitate in 8 hr	1847	I
Dexamethasone sodium phosphate		4 mg/mL	RC	5 mg/mL	White precipitate forms immediately	1855	I
Dexmedetomidine HCl	HOS	4 mcg/mL[b]			Stated to be compatible	3181	C

Y-Site Injection Compatibility (1:1 Mixture) (Cont.)

Test Drug	Mfr	Conc	Mfr	Conc	Remarks	Ref	C/I
Digoxin	BW	0.1 mg/mL	RC	1 mg/mL[a]	Visually compatible for 24 hr at 23°C	1847	C
Diltiazem HCl	MMD	1 mg/mL[a]	RC	2 mg/mL[a]	Visually compatible for 4 hr at 27°C	2062	C
Dobutamine HCl	GNS	2 mg/mL[a]	RC	1 mg/mL[a]	Particles form in 8 hr	1847	I
Dobutamine HCl	LI	4 mg/mL[a]	RC	1 mg/mL[a]	Visually compatible for 24 hr at 23°C	1877	C
Dobutamine HCl	LI	4 mg/mL[a]	RC	2 mg/mL[a]	Visually compatible for 4 hr at 27°C	2062	C
Dopamine HCl	AB	1.6 mg/mL[a]	RC	1 mg/mL[a]	Visually compatible for 24 hr at 23°C	1847	C
Dopamine HCl	DU	3.2 mg/mL[a]	RC	1 mg/mL[a]	Visually compatible for 24 hr at 23°C	1877	C
Dopamine HCl	AB	3.2 mg/mL[a]	RC	2 mg/mL[a]	Visually compatible for 4 hr at 27°C	2062	C
Doripenem	JJ	5 mg/mL[a b]	BED	2 mg/mL[a b]	Physically compatible for 4 hr at 23°C	2743	C
Epinephrine HCl	AB	0.02 mg/mL[a]	RC	2 mg/mL[a]	Visually compatible for 4 hr at 27°C	2062	C
Eravacycline dihydro-chloride	TET	0.6 mg/mL[b]	HOS	1 mg/mL[b]	Physically compatible for 2 hr at room temperature	3532	C
Erythromycin lactobi-onate	AB	5 mg/mL	RC	5 mg/mL	Visually compatible for 24 hr at 22°C	1855	C
Esmolol HCl	DU	40 mg/mL[a]	RC	1 mg/mL[a]	Visually compatible for 24 hr at 23°C	1877	C
Etomidate	AB	2 mg/mL	RC	5 mg/mL	Visually compatible for 7 days at 25°C	1801	C
Famotidine	MSD	0.2 mg/mL[a]	RC	0.15 mg/mL[a]	Physically compatible for 4 hr at 25°C	1188	C
Famotidine	ME	2 mg/mL[b]		1.5 mg/mL[a]	Visually compatible for 4 hr at 22°C	1936	C
Fenoldopam mesylate	AB	80 mcg/mL[b]	APP	1 mg/mL[b]	Physically compatible for 4 hr at 23°C	2467	C
Fentanyl citrate	ES	0.05 mg/mL	RC	1 mg/mL[a]	Visually compatible for 24 hr at 23°C	1847	C
Fentanyl citrate	JN	0.02 mg/mL[a]	RC	0.1 and 0.5 mg/mL[a]	Visually compatible. No midazolam and 4% fentanyl loss in 3 hr at 24°C	1852	C
Fentanyl citrate	JN	0.04 mg/mL[a]	RC	0.1 and 0.5 mg/mL[a]	Visually compatible with no loss of either drug in 3 hr at 24°C	1852	C
Fentanyl citrate		0.05 mg/mL	RC	5 mg/mL	Visually compatible for 24 hr at 22°C	1855	C
Fentanyl citrate	ES	0.05 mg/mL	RC	2 mg/mL[a]	Visually compatible for 4 hr at 27°C	2062	C
Fentanyl citrate	JN	0.025 mg/mL[a]	RC	0.2 mg/mL[a]	Physically compatible for 48 hr at 22°C	1706	C
Floxacillin sodium	SKB	50 mg/mL	RC	5 mg/mL	White precipitate forms immediately	1855	I
Fluconazole	RR	2 mg/mL	RC	5 mg/mL	Physically compatible for 24 hr at 25°C	1407	C
Fluconazole	PF	2 mg/mL	RC	5 mg/mL	Visually compatible for 24 hr at 22°C	1855	C
Foscarnet sodium	AST	24 mg/mL	RC	5 mg/mL	Gas production	1335	I
Fosphenytoin sodium	PD	1 mg PE/mL[b g]	RC	2 mg/mL[b]	Midazolam base precipitates immediately	2223	I
Furosemide	AST	10 mg/mL	RC	1 mg/mL[a]	Immediate haze. Precipitate in 2 hr	1847	I
Furosemide	CNF	10 mg/mL	RC	5 mg/mL	White precipitate forms immediately	1855	I
Furosemide	AMR	10 mg/mL	RC	2 mg/mL[a]	Precipitate forms immediately	2062	I
Gentamicin sulfate	ES	10 mg/mL	RC	1 mg/mL[a]	Visually compatible for 24 hr at 23°C	1847	C
Gentamicin sulfate	CNF	3 mg/mL	RC	5 mg/mL	Visually compatible for 24 hr at 22°C	1855	C
Haloperidol lactate	JN	0.5 and 5 mg/mL	RC	5 mg/mL	Visually compatible for 24 hr at 22°C	1855	C
Heparin sodium		417 units/mL	RC	5 mg/mL	Visually compatible for 24 hr at 22°C	1855	C

Y-Site Injection Compatibility (1:1 Mixture) (Cont.)

Test Drug	Mfr	Conc	Mfr	Conc	Remarks	Ref	C/I
Heparin sodium	ES	100 units/mL[a]	RC	2 mg/mL[a]	Visually compatible for 4 hr at 27°C	2062	C
Heparin sodium		50 units/mL[b]	RC[h]	15 mg/3 mL	Clear solution	1053	C
Hetastarch in lactated electrolyte	AB	6%	RC	1 mg/mL[a]	Physically compatible for 4 hr at 23°C	2339	C
Hydrocortisone sodium succinate	UP	50 mg/mL	RC	5 mg/mL	White precipitate forms immediately	1855	I
Hydromorphone HCl	KN	1 mg/mL	RC	2 mg/mL[a]	Visually compatible for 4 hr at 27°C	2062	C
Hydromorphone HCl	AST	0.5 mg/mL[a]	RC	0.2 mg/mL[a]	Physically compatible for 48 hr at 22°C	1706	C
Hydroxyethyl starch 130/0.4 in sodium chloride 0.9%	FRK	6%	SZ	1, 1.5, 2 mg/mL[a]	Visually compatible for 24 hr at room temperature	2770	C
Ibuprofen lysinate	OVA	10 mg/mL	HOS	1 mg/mL[n]	Measured turbidity increased immediately and solution became milky white and opaque	3541	I
Ibuprofen lysinate	OVA	10 mg/mL	HOS	5 mg/mL	Measured turbidity increased immediately and solution became milky white and opaque	3541	I
Imipenem–cilastatin sodium	MSD	5 mg/mL[m]	RC	5 mg/mL	Haze forms in 24 hr	1855	I
Insulin, regular	LI	1 unit/mL[a]	RC	1 mg/mL[a]	Visually compatible for 24 hr at 23°C	1877	C
Isavuconazonium sulfate	ASP	1.5 mg/mL[n]	APP	1 mg/mL[n]	Physically compatible for 2 hr	3263	C
Labetalol HCl	GL	5 mg/mL	RC	1 mg/mL[a]	Visually compatible for 24 hr at 23°C	1877	C
Labetalol HCl	AH	2 mg/mL[a]	RC	2 mg/mL[a]	Visually compatible for 4 hr at 27°C	2062	C
Letermovir	ME				Physically incompatible	3398	I
Linezolid	PHU	2 mg/mL	RC	2 mg/mL[a]	Physically compatible for 4 hr at 23°C	2264	C
Lorazepam	WY	0.5 mg/mL[a]	RC	2 mg/mL[a]	Visually compatible for 4 hr at 27°C	2062	C
Meropenem		50 mg/mL	SZ[r]	1 mg/mL	Precipitates immediately	3538	I
Meropenem–vaborbactam	TMC	8 mg/mL[b p]	HOS	1 mg/mL[b]	Measured turbidity increases immediately. pH increased by >4 units within 3 hr	3380	I
Methadone HCl	LI	1 mg/mL[a]	RC	0.2 mg/mL[a]	Physically compatible for 48 hr at 22°C	1706	C
Methotrexate sodium		30 mg/mL	RC	5 mg/mL	Yellow precipitate forms immediately	1788	I
Methylprednisolone sodium succinate	UP	40 mg/mL	RC	1 mg/mL[a]	Visually compatible for 24 hr at 23°C	1847	C
Metronidazole	BA	5 mg/mL	RC	1 mg/mL[a]	Visually compatible for 24 hr at 23°C	1847	C
Metronidazole	BRN	5 mg/mL	RC	5 mg/mL	Visually compatible for 24 hr at 22°C	1855	C
Micafungin sodium	ASP	1.5 mg/mL[b]	APP	2 mg/mL[b]	Gross precipitate forms immediately	2683	I
Milrinone lactate	SW	0.2 mg/mL[a]	RC	2 mg/mL[a]	Visually compatible for 4 hr at 27°C	2062	C
Milrinone lactate	SW	0.4 mg/mL[a]	RC	1 mg/mL	Visually compatible. Little loss of either drug in 4 hr at 23°C	2214	C
Morphine sulfate	AST	1 mg/mL[a]	RC	0.2 mg/mL[a]	Physically compatible for 48 hr at 22°C	1706	C
Morphine sulfate	ES	0.25 mg/mL[a]	RC	0.1 and 0.5 mg/mL[a]	Visually compatible with no loss of either drug in 3 hr at 24°C	1789	C
Morphine sulfate	ES	1 mg/mL[a]	RC	0.1 and 0.5 mg/mL[a]	Visually compatible with no loss of either drug in 3 hr at 24°C	1789	C
Morphine sulfate	SX	1 mg/mL[a]	RC	1 mg/mL[a]	Visually compatible for 24 hr at 23°C	1877	C

Y-Site Injection Compatibility (1:1 Mixture) (Cont.)

Test Drug	Mfr	Conc	Mfr	Conc	Remarks	Ref	C/I
Morphine sulfate	SCN	2 mg/mL[a]	RC	2 mg/mL[a]	Visually compatible for 4 hr at 27°C	2062	C
Nafcillin sodium	WY	20 mg/mL[a]	RC	1 mg/mL[a]	Immediate haze. Particles in 4 hr	1847	I
Nicardipine HCl	WY	1 mg/mL[a]	RC	2 mg/mL[a]	Visually compatible for 4 hr at 27°C	2062	C
Nitroglycerin	SO	0.2 mg/mL[a]	RC	1 mg/mL[a]	Visually compatible for 24 hr at 23°C	1847	C
Nitroglycerin	OM	0.2 mg/mL[a]	RC	1 mg/mL[a]	Visually compatible for 24 hr at 23°C	1877	C
Nitroglycerin	AB	0.4 mg/mL[a]	RC	2 mg/mL[a]	Visually compatible for 4 hr at 27°C	2062	C
Norepinephrine bitartrate	STR	0.064 mg/mL[a]	RC	1 mg/mL[a]	Visually compatible for 24 hr at 23°C	1877	C
Norepinephrine bitartrate	AB	0.128 mg/mL[a]	RC	2 mg/mL[a]	Visually compatible for 4 hr at 27°C	2062	C
Omeprazole sodium	AST	4 mg/mL	RC	5 mg/mL	Brown color then precipitate	1855	I
Oritavancin diphosphate	TAR	0.8, 1.2, and 2 mg/mL[a]	BA	1 mg/mL[a]	Visually compatible for 4 hr at 20 to 24°C	2928	C
Palonosetron HCl	MGI	50 mcg/mL	BA	2 mg/mL[a]	Physically compatible. No loss of either drug in 4 hr	2608	C
Pancuronium bromide	ES	0.05 mg/mL[a]	RC	0.05 mg/mL[a]	Physically compatible for 24 hr at 28°C	1337	C
Pantoprazole sodium	ALT[j]	0.16 to 0.8 mg/mL[b]	SX	1 to 2 mg/mL[a]	Discoloration and reddish-brown precipitate form	2603	I
Pantoprazole sodium	ALT[j]	8 mg/mL	RC	0.1 mg/mL	Yellow color forms immediately	2727	I
Pantoprazole sodium	WY[q], AUR[q]				Stated to be incompatible	2850, 3358	I
Pantoprazole sodium	WW[j]				Stated to be incompatible	3357	I
Plazomicin sulfate	ACH	24 mg/mL[n]	HOS	1 mg/mL[n]	Physically compatible for 1 hr at 20 to 25°C	3432	C
Posaconazole	ME	18 mg/mL		1 mg/mL[n]	Physically compatible	2912	C
Potassium chloride	BRN	1 mEq/mL	RC	5 mg/mL	Visually compatible for 24 hr at 22°C	1855	C
Propofol	STU	2 mg/mL	RC	5 mg/mL	Oil droplets form within 7 days at 25°C. No visible change in 24 hr	1801	?
Propofol	ZEN[q]	10 mg/mL	RC	2 mg/mL[a]	Physically compatible for 1 hr at 23°C	2066	C
Ranitidine HCl	GL	0.5 mg/mL	RC	5 mg/mL	Visually compatible for 24 hr at 22°C	1855	C
Ranitidine HCl	GL	1 mg/mL[a]	RC	2 mg/mL[a]	Visually compatible for 4 hr at 27°C	2062	C
Remifentanil HCl	GW	0.025 and 0.25 mg/mL[b]	RC	1 mg/mL[a]	Physically compatible for 4 hr at 23°C	2075	C
Sodium bicarbonate		1.4%	RC	5 mg/mL	White precipitate forms immediately	1788	I
Sodium bicarbonate	IMS	1 mEq/mL	RC	1 mg/mL[a]	Immediate haze. Precipitate in 2 hr	1847	I
Sodium nitroprusside	ES	0.2 mg/mL[a]	RC	1 mg/mL[a]	Visually compatible for 24 hr at 23°C	1847	C
Sodium nitroprusside	RC	0.2 mg/mL[a]	RC	1 mg/mL[a]	Visually compatible for 24 hr at 23°C	1877	C
Sodium nitroprusside	RC	1.2 and 3 mg/mL[a]	RC	1.2 and 2.4 mg/mL[i]	Visually compatible for 48 hr at 24°C protected from light	2357	C
Sodium nitroprusside	RC	0.3, 1.2, 3 mg/mL[a]	RC	5 mg/mL[i]	Visually compatible for 48 hr at 24°C protected from light	2357	C
Tedizolid phosphate	CUB	0.8 mg/mL[b]	APP	1 mg/mL[b]	Physically compatible for 2 hr	3244	C
Theophylline	BA	1.6 mg/mL[a]	RC	1 mg/mL[a]	Visually compatible for 24 hr at 23°C	1847	C

Y-Site Injection Compatibility (1:1 Mixture) (Cont.)

Test Drug	Mfr	Conc	Mfr	Conc	Remarks	Ref	C/I
Tirofiban HCl	ME	50 mcg/mL[a b]	RC	5 and 0.05[a b] mg/mL	Physically compatible. No loss of either drug in 4 hr at 23°C	2356	C
TNA #218 to #226[e]			RC	2 mg/mL[a]	Damage to emulsion occurs immediately with free oil formation possible	2215	I
Tobramycin sulfate	LI	10 mg/mL	RC	1 mg/mL[a]	Visually compatible for 24 hr at 23°C	1847	C
TPN #189[e]			RC	5 mg/mL	White haze and precipitate form immediately. Crystals form in 24 hr	1767	I
TPN #212 to #215[e]			RC	2 mg/mL[a]	White cloudiness forms rapidly	2109	I
Trimethoprim–sulfame-thoxazole	RC	0.8 mg/mL[l]	RC	5 mg/mL	White precipitate forms immediately	1855	I
Vancomycin HCl	LI	5 mg/mL[a]	RC	1 mg/mL[a]	Visually compatible for 24 hr at 23°C	1847	C
Vancomycin HCl	LI	5 mg/mL	RC	5 mg/mL	Visually compatible for 24 hr at 22°C	1855	C
Vecuronium bromide	OR	0.1 mg/mL[a]	RC	0.05 mg/mL[a]	Physically compatible for 24 hr at 28°C	1337	C
Vecuronium bromide	OR	4 mg/mL	RC	5 mg/mL	Visually compatible for 24 hr at 22°C	1855	C
Vecuronium bromide	OR	1 mg/mL	RC	2 mg/mL[a]	Visually compatible for 4 hr at 27°C	2062	C

[a] Tested in dextrose 5%.

[b] Tested in sodium chloride 0.9%.

[c] Tested in sterile water for injection.

[d] Tested in Ringer's injection, lactated.

[e] Refer to Appendix for the composition of parenteral nutrition solutions. TNA indicates a 3-in-1 admixture, and TPN indicates a 2-in-1 admixture.

[f] Concentration unspecified.

[g] Concentration expressed in milligrams of phenytoin sodium equivalents (PE) per mL.

[h] Given over three minutes into a heparin infusion run at 1 mL/min.

[i] Tested in dextrose 5% in sodium chloride 0.225%.

[j] Test performed using the formulation WITHOUT edetate disodium.

[k] Amoxicillin component. Amoxicillin in a 10:1 fixed-ratio concentration with clavulanic acid.

[l] Trimethoprim component. Trimethoprim in a 1:5 fixed-ratio concentration with sulfamethoxazole.

[m] Not specified whether concentration refers to single component or combined components.

[n] Tested in both dextrose 5% and sodium chloride 0.9%.

[o] Ceftolozane component. Ceftolozane in a 2:1 fixed-ratio concentration with tazobactam.

[p] Meropenem component. Meropenem in a 1:1 fixed-ratio concentration with vaborbactam.

[q] Test performed using the formulation WITH edetate disodium.

[r] As midazolam base rather than the salt.

Additional Compatibility Information

Other Drugs

One manufacturer (Hospira) states that midazolam hydrochloride may be administered in the same syringe as atropine sulfate, meperidine hydrochloride, morphine sulfate, and scopolamine hydrobromide.[3590 3591 3592]

Milrinone Lactate
AHFS 24:04.08

Products

Milrinone lactate is available as a solution containing the equivalent of milrinone 1 mg/mL in 10-, 20-, and 50-mL single-dose vials. Each mL also contains dextrose, anhydrous, 47 mg in water for injection. Lactic acid or sodium hydroxide may have been used to adjust the pH. The total lactic acid concentration may vary between 0.95 and 1.29 mg/mL. The 1-mg/mL concentration must be diluted for use.[1(9/07)]

Milrinone lactate is also available as a ready-to-use solution in 100- and 200-mL flexible polyvinyl chloride (PVC) containers at a concentration equivalent to milrinone 0.2 mg/mL (200 mcg/mL). The solution has a nominal lactic acid concentration of 0.282 mg/mL and also contains dextrose, anhydrous 49.4 mg/mL.[1(9/07)]

pH

From 3.2 to 4.[1(9/07)]

Administration

Milrinone lactate is administered intravenously. For maintenance administration by continuous intravenous infusion, milrinone lactate in vials is diluted in a compatible diluent, usually to 200 mcg/mL. The premixed 200-mcg/mL infusion in flexible plastic containers need not be diluted for use. When milrinone lactate is administered by continuous infusion, the use of a calibrated electronic infusion device is recommended.[1(9/07)]

Stability

Milrinone lactate solutions are colorless to pale yellow. The 1-mg/mL concentration should be stored at controlled room temperature and protected from freezing. The 0.2-mg/mL concentration in PVC containers should be stored at room temperature of 25°C and should be protected from freezing and exposure to excessive heat. Brief exposure to temperatures up to 40°C does not adversely affect the product.[1(9/07)]

Compatibility Information

Solution Compatibility

Milrinone lactate

Test Soln Name	Mfr	Mfr	Conc/L or %	Remarks	Ref	C/I
Dextrose 5%	c	WI	200 mg	Physically compatible. Stable for 72 hr at room temperature in light or dark	1468	C
Dextrose 5%	a	SW	0.2 g	Visually compatible. Little loss after 14 days at 23°C in light and at 4°C	2106	C
Dextrose 5%	BAª	SW	0.4, 0.6, 0.8 g	Visually compatible. Little loss after 14 days at 23°C and at 4°C	2107	C
Dextrose 5%	BAª	SW	0.4 g	Visually compatible. No loss after 7 days at 23°C under fluorescent light	2214	C
Dextrose 5%	BAᵈ	GH	600 mg	Physically compatible with little to no loss in 7 days at 4°C, followed by 24 hr at 25°C and an additional 24 hr at 35°C	3597	C
Ringer's injection, lactated	BAª	SW	0.4 g	Visually compatible. 3% loss after 7 days at 23°C under fluorescent light	2214	C
Sodium chloride 0.45%	c	WI	200 mg	Physically compatible. Stable for 72 hr at room temperature in light or dark	1468	C
Sodium chloride 0.45%	BAª	SW	0.4 g	Visually compatible. No loss after 7 days at 23°C under fluorescent light	2214	C
Sodium chloride 0.9%	c	WI	200 mg	Physically compatible. Stable for 72 hr at room temperature in light or dark	1468	C
Sodium chloride 0.9%	a	SW	0.2 g	Visually compatible. Little loss after 14 days at 23°C in light and at 4°C	2106	C
Sodium chloride 0.9%	MGᵇ	SW	0.4, 0.6, 0.8 g	Visually compatible. Little loss after 14 days at 23 and 4°C	2107	C
Sodium chloride 0.9%	BAª	SW	0.4 g	Visually compatible. No loss after 7 days at 23°C under fluorescent light	2214	C

DOI: 10.37573/9781585286850.270

Solution Compatibility (Cont.)

Test Soln Name	Mfr	Mfr	Conc/L or %	Remarks	Ref	C/I
Sodium chloride 0.9%	BA[d]	GH	600 mg	Physically compatible with little to no loss in 7 days at 4°C, followed by 24 hr at 25°C and an additional 24 hr at 35°C	3597	C

[a] Tested in PVC containers.

[b] Tested in polyolefin containers.

[c] Tested in glass (Abbott), Accumed (McGaw), and PVC (Travenol) containers.

[d] Tested in a medication cassette reservoir.

Additive Compatibility

Milrinone lactate

Test Drug	Mfr	Conc/L or %	Mfr	Conc/L or %	Test Solution	Remarks	Ref	C/I
Procainamide HCl	SQ	2 and 4 g	WI	200 mg	D5W	3% procainamide loss in 1 hr and 11% in 4 hr at 23°C. No milrinone loss	1191	I
Quinidine gluconate	LI	16 g	WI	200 mg	D5W	Physically compatible with no loss of either drug in 4 hr at 23°C	1191	C

Drugs in Syringe Compatibility

Milrinone lactate

Test Drug	Mfr	Amt	Mfr	Amt	Remarks	Ref	C/I
Atropine sulfate	IX	2 mg/2 mL	STR	5.25 mg/5.25 mL	Physically compatible. No loss of either drug in 20 min at 23°C	1410	C
Calcium chloride	AB	3 g/30 mL	STR	5.25 mg/5.25 mL	Physically compatible. No milrinone loss in 20 min at 23°C	1410	C
Digoxin	BW	0.5 mg/2 mL	WI	3.5 mg/3.5 mL	Brought to 10-mL total volume with D5W. Physically compatible with no loss of either drug in 4 hr at 23°C	1191	C
Epinephrine HCl	AB	0.5 mg/0.5 mL	STR	5.25 mg/5.25 mL	Physically compatible. No loss of either drug in 20 min at 23°C	1410	C
Furosemide	LY	40 mg/4 mL	WI	3.5 mg/3.5 mL	Brought to 10-mL total volume with D5W. Precipitates immediately	1191	I
Lidocaine HCl	AB	100 mg/10 mL	STR	5.25 mg/5.25 mL	Physically compatible. No loss of either drug in 20 min at 23°C	1410	C
Morphine sulfate	WI	40 mg/5 mL	STR	5.25 mg/5.25 mL	Physically compatible. No loss of either drug in 20 min at 23°C	1410	C
Propranolol HCl	AY	3 mg/3 mL	WI	3.5 mg/3.5 mL	Brought to 10-mL total volume with D5W. Physically compatible with no loss of either drug in 4 hr at 23°C	1191	C
Sodium bicarbonate	AB	3.75 g/50 mL	STR	5.25 mg/5.25 mL	Physically compatible. No milrinone loss in 20 min at 23°C	1410	C
Verapamil HCl	KN	10 mg/4 mL	WI	3.5 mg/3.5 mL	Brought to 10-mL total volume with D5W. Physically compatible with no loss of either drug in 4 hr at 23°C	1191	C

Y-Site Injection Compatibility (1:1 Mixture)

Milrinone lactate

Test Drug	Mfr	Conc	Mfr	Conc	Remarks	Ref	C/I
Acyclovir sodium	APP	7 mg/mL[a]	SS	0.2 mg/mL[a]	Visually compatible for 4 hr at 25°C	2381	C
Amikacin sulfate	AB	5 mg/mL[a]	SS	0.2 mg/mL[a]	Visually compatible for 4 hr at 25°C	2381	C
Amiodarone HCl	WY	6 mg/mL[a]	SAN	0.4 mg/mL[a]	Visually compatible for 24 hr at 22°C	2352	C
Ampicillin sodium	APO	100 mg/mL[b]	SS	0.2 mg/mL[a]	Visually compatible for 4 hr at 25°C	2381	C

Y-Site Injection Compatibility (1:1 Mixture) (Cont.)

Test Drug	Mfr	Conc	Mfr	Conc	Remarks	Ref	C/I
Argatroban	SKB	1 mg/mL[a]	NVP	0.4 mg/mL[a]	Physically compatible for 24 hr at 23°C	2572	C
Atracurium besylate	BW	1 mg/mL[a]	SW	0.4 mg/mL[a]	Visually compatible with little or no loss of either drug in 4 hr at 23°C	2214	C
Bivalirudin	TMC	5 mg/mL[a]	SAN	0.2 mg/mL[a]	Physically compatible for 4 hr at 23°C	2373	C
Bumetanide	RC	0.25 mg/mL	SW	0.4 mg/mL[a]	Visually compatible with little or no loss of either drug in 4 hr at 23°C	2214	C
Calcium chloride	AMR	20 mg/mL[a]	SS	0.2 mg/mL[a]	Visually compatible for 4 hr at 25°C	2381	C
Calcium gluconate	LY	0.465 mEq/mL	SW	0.4 mg/mL[a]	Visually compatible with no loss of milrinone in 4 hr at 23°C	2214	C
Calcium gluconate	AMR	50 mg/mL[a]	SS	0.2 mg/mL[a]	Visually compatible for 4 hr at 25°C	2381	C
Cangrelor tetrasodium	TMC	1 mg/mL[b]		0.2 mg/mL[b]	Physically compatible for 4 hr	3243	C
Caspofungin acetate	ME	0.7 mg/mL[b]	BA	0.2 mg/mL[b]	Physically compatible for 4 hr at room temperature	2758	C
Cefazolin sodium	APO	100 mg/mL[a]	SS	0.2 mg/mL[a]	Visually compatible for 4 hr at 25°C	2381	C
Cefepime HCl	BMS	100 mg/mL	SS	0.2 mg/mL[a]	Visually compatible for 4 hr at 25°C	2381	C
Cefotaxime sodium	HO	150 mg/mL[a]	SS	0.2 mg/mL[a]	Visually compatible for 4 hr at 25°C	2381	C
Ceftaroline fosamil	FOR	2.22 mg/mL[a b e]	BED	0.2 mg/mL[a b e]	Physically compatible for 4 hr at 23°C	2826	C
Ceftazidime	GW	100 mg/mL[a]	SS	0.2 mg/mL[a]	Visually compatible for 4 hr at 25°C	2381	C
Ceftolozane sulfate–tazo-bactam sodium	CUB	10 mg/mL[j k]	APP	0.2 mg/mL[j]	Physically compatible for 2 hr	3262	C
Cefuroxime sodium	LI	100 mg/mL[a]	SS	0.2 mg/mL[a]	Visually compatible for 4 hr at 25°C	2381	C
Ciprofloxacin	BAY	2 mg/mL	SS	0.2 mg/mL[a]	Visually compatible for 4 hr at 25°C	2381	C
Clevidipine butyrate	CHS	0.5 mg/mL		0.5 mg/mL[a]	Physically incompatible	3334	I
Clindamycin phosphate	PHU	18 mg/mL[a]	SS	0.2 mg/mL[a]	Visually compatible for 4 hr at 25°C	2381	C
Cloxacillin sodium	SMX	100 mg/mL	PPC	1 mg/mL	Physically compatible for up to 4 hr at room temperature	3245	C
Dexamethasone sodium phosphate	ES	10 mg/mL[a]	SS	0.2 mg/mL[a]	Visually compatible for 4 hr at 25°C	2381	C
Dexmedetomidine HCl	AB	4 mcg/mL[b]	SAN	0.2 mg/mL[b]	Physically compatible for 4 hr at 23°C	2383	C
Digoxin	BW	0.25 mg/mL	WI	200 mcg/mL[a]	Physically compatible with no loss of either drug in 4 hr at 23°C	1191	C
Diltiazem HCl	MMD	1 mg/mL[a]	SW	0.2 mg/mL[a]	Visually compatible for 4 hr at 27°C	2062	C
Diltiazem HCl	MMD	1 mg/mL[a]	SW	0.4 mg/mL[a]	Visually compatible with little loss of either drug in 4 hr at 23°C	2214	C
Dobutamine HCl	LI	4 mg/mL[a]	SW	0.2 mg/mL[a]	Visually compatible for 4 hr at 27°C	2062	C
Dobutamine HCl	GEN	8 mg/mL[a]	SW	0.4 mg/mL[a]	Visually compatible. Little loss of either drug in 4 hr at 23°C	2214	C
Dopamine HCl	AB	3.2 mg/mL[a]	SW	0.2 mg/mL[a]	Visually compatible for 4 hr at 27°C	2062	C
Dopamine HCl	SO	6.4 mg/mL[a]	SW	0.4 mg/mL[a]	Visually compatible. Little loss of either drug in 4 hr at 23°C	2214	C
Doripenem	JJ	5 mg/mL[a b]	BA	0.2 mg/mL[a b]	Physically compatible for 4 hr at 23°C	2743	C
Epinephrine HCl	AB	0.02 mg/mL[a]	SW	0.2 mg/mL[a]	Visually compatible for 4 hr at 27°C	2062	C

Y-Site Injection Compatibility (1:1 Mixture) (Cont.)

Test Drug	Mfr	Conc	Mfr	Conc	Remarks	Ref	C/I
Epinephrine HCl	AB	0.064 mg/mL[a]	SW	0.4 mg/mL[a]	Visually compatible. Little loss of either drug in 4 hr at 23°C	2214	C
Fenoldopam mesylate	AB	80 mcg/mL[b]	SAN	0.2 mg/mL[b]	Physically compatible for 4 hr at 23°C	2467	C
Fentanyl citrate	ES	0.05 mg/mL	SW	0.2 mg/mL[a]	Visually compatible for 4 hr at 27°C	2062	C
Fentanyl citrate	ES	50 mcg/mL	SW	0.4 mg/mL[a]	Visually compatible. Little loss of either drug in 4 hr at 23°C	2214	C
Furosemide	LY	10 mg/mL	WI	200 mcg/mL[a]	Precipitates immediately	1191	I
Furosemide	AMR	10 mg/mL	SW	0.2 mg/mL[a]	Precipitate forms in 4 hr at 27°C	2062	I
Gentamicin sulfate	APP	10 mg/mL[a]	SS	0.2 mg/mL[a]	Visually compatible for 4 hr at 25°C	2381	C
Heparin sodium	ES	100 units/mL[a]	SW	0.2 mg/mL[a]	Visually compatible for 4 hr at 27°C	2062	C
Heparin sodium	ES	100 units/mL[a]	SW	0.4 mg/mL[a]	Visually compatible. Little loss of milrinone and heparin in 4 hr at 23°C	2214	C
Hetastarch in lactated electrolyte	AB	6%	SAN	0.2 mg/mL[a]	Physically compatible for 4 hr at 23°C	2339	C
Hydromorphone HCl	KN	1 mg/mL	SW	0.2 mg/mL[a]	Visually compatible for 4 hr at 27°C	2062	C
Imipenem–cilastatin sodium	ME	5 mg/mL[b h]	SS	0.2 mg/mL[a]	Yellow color darkening in 4 hr at 25°C	2381	I
Insulin, regular human	NOV	1 unit/mL[b]	SW	0.4 mg/mL[a]	Visually compatible. Little loss of either drug in 4 hr at 23°C	2214	C
Isavuconazonium sulfate	ASP	1.5 mg/mL[i]	HIK	0.2 mg/mL[i]	Physically compatible for 2 hr	3263	C
Isoproterenol HCl	ES	8 mcg/mL[a]	SW	0.4 mg/mL[a]	Visually compatible. Little loss of either drug in 4 hr at 23°C	2214	C
Labetalol HCl	AH	2 mg/mL[a]	SW	0.2 mg/mL[a]	Visually compatible for 4 hr at 27°C	2062	C
Lorazepam	WY	0.5 mg/mL[a]	SW	0.2 mg/mL[a]	Visually compatible for 4 hr at 27°C	2062	C
Lorazepam	WY	0.2 mg/mL[a]	SW	0.4 mg/mL[a]	Visually compatible. Little loss of either drug in 4 hr at 23°C	2214	C
Lorazepam	WY	1 mg/mL[a]	SS	0.2 mg/mL[a]	Visually compatible for 4 hr at 25°C	2381	C
Lorazepam	WY	2 mg/mL[a]	SS	0.2 mg/mL[a]	Visually compatible for 4 hr at 25°C	2381	C
Magnesium sulfate	SO	40 mg/mL[a]	SW	0.4 mg/mL[a]	Visually compatible. No milrinone loss in 4 hr at 23°C	2214	C
Meropenem	ZEN	50 mg/mL[a]	SS	0.2 mg/mL[a]	Visually compatible for 4 hr at 25°C	2381	C
Meropenem		50 mg/mL	FRK	1 mg/mL	Physically compatible for 4 hr at room temperature	3538	C
Meropenem–vaborbactam	TMC	8 mg/mL[b i]	WW	0.2 mg/mL[b]	Physically compatible for 3 hr at 20 to 25°C	3380	C
Methylprednisolone sodium succinate	PHU	125 mg/mL	SS	0.2 mg/mL[a]	Visually compatible for 4 hr at 25°C	2381	C
Metoprolol tartrate	BED	1 mg/mL	NVP	0.2 mg/mL[a]	Visually compatible for 24 hr at 19°C	2795	C
Metronidazole	AB	5 mg/mL	SS	0.2 mg/mL[a]	Visually compatible for 4 hr at 25°C	2381	C
Micafungin sodium	ASP	1.5 mg/mL[b]	BED	0.2 mg/mL[b]	Physically compatible for 4 hr at 23°C	2683	C
Midazolam HCl	RC	2 mg/mL[a]	SW	0.2 mg/mL[a]	Visually compatible for 4 hr at 27°C	2062	C
Midazolam HCl	RC	1 mg/mL	SW	0.4 mg/mL[a]	Visually compatible. Little loss of either drug in 4 hr at 23°C	2214	C

Y-Site Injection Compatibility (1:1 Mixture) (Cont.)

Test Drug	Mfr	Conc	Mfr	Conc	Remarks	Ref	C/I
Morphine sulfate	SCN	2 mg/mL[a]	SW	0.2 mg/mL[a]	Visually compatible for 4 hr at 27°C	2062	C
Morphine sulfate	AST	1 mg/mL[a]	SW	0.4 mg/mL[a]	Visually compatible. Little loss of either drug in 4 hr at 23°C	2214	C
Morphine sulfate	FAU	25 mg/mL[a]	SS	0.2 mg/mL[a]	Visually compatible for 4 hr at 25°C	2381	C
Nesiritide	SCI	50 mcg/mL[a b]		1 mg/mL	Physically compatible for 4 hr	2625	C
Nicardipine HCl	WY	1 mg/mL[a]	SW	0.2 mg/mL[a]	Visually compatible for 4 hr at 27°C	2062	C
Nitroglycerin	AB	0.4 mg/mL[a]	SW	0.2 mg/mL[a]	Visually compatible for 4 hr at 27°C	2062	C
Nitroglycerin	SO	0.8 mg/mL[a]	SW	0.4 mg/mL[a]	Visually compatible. Little loss of either drug in 4 hr at 23°C	2214	C
Norepinephrine bitartrate	AB	0.128 mg/mL[a]	SW	0.2 mg/mL[a]	Visually compatible for 4 hr at 27°C	2062	C
Norepinephrine bitartrate	SW	0.064 mg/mL[a]	SW	0.4 mg/mL[a]	Visually compatible. Little loss of either drug in 4 hr at 23°C	2214	C
Oxacillin sodium	APO	100 mg/mL[a]	SS	0.2 mg/mL[a]	Visually compatible for 4 hr at 25°C	2381	C
Pancuronium bromide	GNS	1 mg/mL	SW	0.4 mg/mL[a]	Visually compatible. Little loss of either drug in 4 hr at 23°C	2214	C
Piperacillin sodium–tazobactam sodium	LE[c]	200 mg/mL[g]	SS	0.2 mg/mL[a]	Visually compatible for 4 hr at 25°C	2381	C
Plazomicin sulfate	ACH	24 mg/mL[j]	WW	0.2 mg/mL[j]	Physically compatible for 1 hr at 20 to 25°C	3432	C
Potassium chloride	AB	1 mEq/mL[a]	SW	0.4 mg/mL[a]	Visually compatible. No milrinone loss in 4 hr at 23°C	2214	C
Procainamide HCl	SQ	2 and 4 mg/mL[a]	WI	350 mcg/mL[a]	3 to 6% procainamide loss in 1 hr and 10 to 13% in 4 hr at 23°C. No milrinone loss	1191	I
Propofol	ZEN	10 mg/mL	SW	0.4 mg/mL[a]	Little loss of either drug in 4 hr at 23°C	2214	C
Propranolol HCl	AY	1 mg/mL[a]	WI	200 mcg/mL[a]	Physically compatible with no loss of either drug in 4 hr at 23°C	1191	C
Quinidine gluconate	LI	16 mg/mL[a]	WI	350 mcg/mL[a]	Physically compatible with no loss of either drug in 4 hr at 23°C	1191	C
Ranitidine HCl	GL	1 mg/mL[a]	SW	0.2 mg/mL[a]	Visually compatible for 4 hr at 27°C	2062	C
Ranitidine HCl	GL	2 mg/mL[a]	SW	0.4 mg/mL[a]	Visually compatible. Little loss of either drug in 4 hr at 23°C	2214	C
Rocuronium bromide	OR	2 mg/mL[a]	SW	0.4 mg/mL[a]	Visually compatible. Little loss of either drug in 4 hr at 23°C	2214	C
Sodium bicarbonate	AB	1 mEq/mL	SW	0.4 mg/mL[a]	Visually compatible with 4% loss of milrinone in 4 hr at 23°C	2214	C
Sodium nitroprusside	AB	0.8 mg/mL[a]	SW	0.4 mg/mL[a]	Visually compatible. Little loss of either drug in 4 hr at 23°C protected from light	2214	C
Sodium nitroprusside	RC	0.3, 1.2, 3 mg/mL[a]	SW	0.1[f], 0.4[f], 1 mg/mL	Visually compatible for 48 hr at 24°C protected from light	2357	C
Tedizolid phosphate	CUB	0.8 mg/mL[b]	HIK	0.2 mg/mL[b]	Physically compatible for 2 hr	3244	C
Telavancin HCl	ASP	7.5 mg/mL[a b e]	BED	0.2 mg/mL[a b e]	Physically compatible for 2 hr	2830	C
Theophylline	AB	1.6 mg/mL[a]	SW	0.4 mg/mL[a]	Visually compatible. Little loss of either drug in 4 hr at 23°C	2214	C
Tobramycin sulfate	LI	10 mg/mL[a]	SS	0.2 mg/mL[a]	Visually compatible for 4 hr at 25°C	2381	C

Y-Site Injection Compatibility (1:1 Mixture) (Cont.)

Test Drug	Mfr	Conc	Mfr	Conc	Remarks	Ref	C/I
Torsemide	BM	10 mg/mL	SW	0.4 mg/mL[a]	Visually compatible. Little loss of either drug in 4 hr at 23°C	2214	C
TPN #217[d]			SW	0.4 mg/mL[a]	Visually compatible with no loss of milrinone in 4 hr at 23°C	2214	C
TPN #243, #244[d]			SS	0.2 mg/mL[a]	Visually compatible for 4 hr at 25°C	2381	C
Vancomycin HCl	OR	5 mg/mL[a]	SS	0.2 mg/mL[a]	Visually compatible for 4 hr at 25°C	2381	C
Vasopressin	AMR	2 and 4 units/mL[b]	AB	0.2 mg/mL[a]	Physically compatible with vasopressin pushed through a Y-site over 5 sec	2478	C
Vecuronium bromide	OR	1 mg/mL	SW	0.2 mg/mL[a]	Visually compatible for 4 hr at 27°C	2062	C
Vecuronium bromide	OR	1 mg/mL	SW	0.4 mg/mL[a]	Visually compatible. Little loss of either drug in 4 hr at 23°C	2214	C
Verapamil HCl	KN	2.5 mg/mL[a]	WI	200 mcg/mL[a]	Physically compatible with no loss of either drug in 4 hr at 23°C	1191	C

[a] Tested in dextrose 5%.

[b] Tested in sodium chloride 0.9%.

[c] Test performed using the formulation WITHOUT edetate disodium.

[d] Refer to Appendix for the composition of parenteral nutrition solutions. TPN indicates a 2-in-1 admixture.

[e] Tested in Ringer's injection, lactated.

[f] Tested in dextrose 5% in sodium chloride 0.225%.

[g] Piperacillin component. Piperacillin in an 8:1 fixed-ratio concentration with tazobactam.

[h] Imipenem component. Imipenem in a 1:1 fixed-ratio concentration with cilastatin.

[i] Meropenem component. Meropenem in a 1:1 fixed-ratio concentration with vaborbactam.

[j] Tested in both dextrose 5% and sodium chloride 0.9%.

[k] Ceftolozane component. Ceftolozane in a 2:1 fixed-ratio concentration with tazobactam.

Selected Revisions July 1, 2020. © Copyright, October 1992.
American Society of Health-System Pharmacists, Inc.

Minocycline Hydrochloride
AHFS 8:12.24

Products

Minocycline hydrochloride is available as a yellow to amber lyophilized powder in single-use vials containing the equivalent of 100 mg of minocycline with 269 mg of magnesium sulfate heptahydrate (2.2 mEq of magnesium) and sodium hydroxide to adjust the pH.[3226]

The 100-mg vial should be reconstituted with 5 mL of sterile water for injection to yield a solution containing minocycline 20 mg/mL.[3226][3269] The reconstituted solution should be further diluted immediately in 100 to 1000 mL of dextrose 5%, dextrose 5% in sodium chloride 0.9%, or sodium chloride 0.9%; alternatively, the reconstituted solution may be diluted in 250 to 1000 mL of Ringer's injection, lactated (see Stability).[3226][3232]

pH

The pH of the reconstituted solution ranges from 4.5 to 5.[3226] When diluted in a compatible infusion solution, the pH usually ranges from 4.5 to 6.[3226]

Trade Name(s)

Minocin

Administration

Minocycline hydrochloride is administered by intravenous infusion over 60 minutes following dilution in a compatible infusion solution.[3226] If a common infusion line is being used to administer other drugs in addition to minocycline hydrochloride, the line should be flushed with a compatible infusion solution prior to and following infusion of minocycline.[3226]

Stability

Intact vials should be stored at controlled room temperature.[3226]

Upon dilution in an infusion bag containing a compatible solution, minocycline is stable for up to 4 hours at room temperature or up to 24 hours at 2 to 8°C.[3226]

Although minocycline hydrochloride is noted to be stable at certain concentrations in Ringer's injection, lactated, the drug should not be mixed with other calcium-containing solutions, especially neutral or alkaline solutions, due to the potential for precipitation.[3226] Unused portions should be discarded.[3226]

pH Effects

A precipitate may form if minocycline hydrochloride is diluted in neutral or alkaline solutions.[3226]

Compatibility Information

Solution Compatibility

Minocycline HCl

Test Soln Name	Mfr	Mfr	Conc/L or %	Remarks	Ref	C/I
Dextrose 5% in sodium chloride 0.9%		TMC		Stable for up to 4 hr at room temperature or up to 24 hr at 2 to 8°C	3226, 3232	C
Dextrose 5%		TMC		Stable for up to 4 hr at room temperature or up to 24 hr at 2 to 8°C	3226, 3232	C
Ringer's injection, lactated		TMC		Stable for up to 4 hr at room temperature or up to 24 hr at 2 to 8°C	3226	C
Sodium chloride 0.9%		TMC		Stable for up to 4 hr at room temperature or up to 24 hr at 2 to 8°C	3226, 3232	C

Additive Compatibility

Minocycline HCl

Test Drug	Mfr	Conc/L or %	Mfr	Conc/L or %	Test Solution	Remarks	Ref	C/I
Doxapram HCl	WW					8% doxapram loss in 3 hr and 13% loss in 6 hr	3220	I

DOI: 10.37573/9781585286850.271

Y-Site Injection Compatibility (1:1 Mixture)

Minocycline HCl

Test Drug	Mfr	Conc	Mfr	Conc	Remarks	Ref	C/I
Fat emulsion, intravenous	OTS	20%[b]	PF	1 mg/mL[a c]	Coarsening of particle diameter observed immediately after preparation	3452	I

[a] Tested in dextrose 5%.

[b] Run at 25 mL/hr with dextrose 5% run at 83 mL/hr.

[c] Run at 100 mL/hr.

Selected Revisions September 30, 2019. © Copyright, June 2017. American Society of Health-System Pharmacists, Inc.

Mitomycin
AHFS 10:00

Products

Mitomycin is available in 5-, 20-, and 40-mg vials with mannitol 10, 40, and 80 mg, respectively. Reconstitute the 5-mg vials with 10 mL, the 20-mg vials with 40 mL, and the 40-mg vials with 80 mL of sterile water for injection and shake to aid dissolution. Allow to stand at room temperature if dissolution does not take place immediately. The reconstituted solution contains 500 mcg/mL of mitomycin.[1(10/06) 4]

pH

From 6 to 8.[4]

Administration

Mitomycin is administered intravenously through a functioning intravenous catheter. Extravasation should be avoided because cellulitis, ulceration, and sloughing may occur. It has been recommended that mitomycin be administered through the tubing of a running infusion solution to avoid this problem.[1(10/06) 4]

In the event of spills or leaks, Bristol-Myers Squibb recommends the use of sodium hypochlorite 5% (household bleach) or potassium permanganate 1% to inactivate mitomycin.[1200]

Stability

Intact vials should be stored at controlled room temperature and protected from light. Temperatures exceeding 40°C should be avoided. Reconstituted solutions are stable for two weeks stored under refrigeration or for one week at room temperature.[1(10/06) 4]

Mitomycin (Kyowa) 0.6 and 0.8 mg/mL in water for injection exhibited 10% loss in seven days at 21°C in the dark. When stored at 4°C in the dark, the 0.6-mg/mL concentration lost 7% in seven days. Although exhibiting no loss in 24 hours when stored at 4°C in the dark, the 0.8-mg/mL concentration developed a fine, pink, needle-like precipitate in three days. At a higher concentration of 1 mg/mL in water for injection similar results were obtained. Refrigeration resulted in fine, pink, needle-like precipitate formation in 24 hours. The 1-mg/mL concentration stored at 21°C exposed to fluorescent light exhibited 6% loss in 24 hours and developed the fine, pink, needle-like precipitate in four days. Stored at a higher temperature of 25°C in the dark, losses of 6% in 24 hours and 10% in seven days were found with no precipitate forming.[1503]

pH Effects

Mitomycin is very stable in solution at a neutral pH but undergoes more rapid decomposition at acidic and basic pH.[1119 1203 1204 1866]

The decomposition is complex and pH dependent, producing different decomposition products in acidic and basic solutions.[1119 1283 1284] The pH of maximum stability is approximately pH 7.[1072 1203 1204 1379] At pH 7, a 10% mitomycin loss occurs in seven days at room temperature.[1072] At a concentration of 0.05 mg/mL in dextrose 5% buffered to pH 7.8 with a mixture of phosphates, mitomycin was stable for 15 days at room temperature and over 120 days when refrigerated.[1118]

Both pH and storage temperature are important to mitomycin stability. Mitomycin (150 to 600 mcg/mL) stability was tested in pH 6, 7, and 8 buffer solutions. The drug was less stable at pH 6 than at pH 7 and especially pH 8. At pH 6, drug losses of around 96 and 41% occurred at room temperature and under refrigeration, respectively, over 28 days. However, mitomycin was more stable at pH 7 and 8. Drug losses when stored under refrigeration for 28 days were about 10 to 20% in this pH range.[2651]

Temperature Effects

Heating mitomycin 0.6 mg/mL in sodium chloride 0.9% to 100°C resulted in a 24% drug loss in 30 minutes and a 58% loss in one hour.[1285]

Freezing Solutions

Mitomycin 0.6 mg/mL in sodium chloride 0.9% crystallized out of solution when frozen at −20°C. The particles did not redissolve after thawing in a microwave oven. Freezing to −30°C, below the eutectic temperature, resulted in no loss of mitomycin during four weeks of storage, microwave thawing, and refreezing at −30°C for another four weeks.[1285]

Light Effects

The stability of mitomycin is not adversely affected by the presence or absence of normal fluorescent light.[1503]

Syringes

Mitomycin (Bristol-Myers Squibb) reconstituted to a concentration of 0.5 mg/mL with sterile water was repackaged in 1-mL polypropylene tuberculin syringes (Sherwood). Syringes were stored at both 5 and 25°C protected from light. About 7% mitomycin loss occurred in 11 days at 25°C and about 8% loss in 42 days at 5°C.[2179]

Filtration

Mitomycin 10 to 75 mcg/mL exhibited little or no loss due to sorption to either cellulose nitrate/cellulose acetate ester (Millex OR) or Teflon (Millex FG) filters.[1415 1416]

DOI: 10.37573/9781585286850.272

Compatibility Information

Solution Compatibility

Mitomycin

Test Soln Name	Mfr	Mfr	Conc/L or %	Remarks	Ref	C/I
Dextrose 3.3% in sodium chloride 0.3%		BR	50 mg	10% loss in 1.6 hr at 25°C	1205	I
Dextrose 5%			20 and 40 mg	Stable for 3 hr at room temperature	1(10/06)	C
Dextrose 5%	TR[a]	BR	400 mg	10% loss in 1 or 2 hr at room temperature	519	I
Dextrose 5%	TR[b]	CH	50 mg	Violet color appeared in 4 hr and intensified over 12 hr. 74% loss in 12 hr at 28°C in light and 33% in 12 hr at 5°C in dark	1118	I
Dextrose 5%		BR	50 mg	10% loss in 2.6 hr at 25°C	1205	I
Dextrose 5%	MG[c]	BR	20 mg	10% loss in 3 hr at 25°C	1866	I
Dextrose 5%	MG[c]	BR	40 mg	10% loss in 24 hr at 4°C	1866	C
Dextrose 5%	TR[b]	BR	20 mg	10% loss in 7 hr at 25°C	1866	I
Dextrose 5%	TR[b]	BR	40 mg	10% loss in 23 hr at 4°C	1866	C
Ringer's injection, lactated		BR	50 mg	10% loss in 43 hr at 25°C	1205	C
Ringer's injection, lactated	MG[c]	BR	20 mg	10% loss in 143 hr at 25°C	1866	C
Ringer's injection, lactated	MG[c]	BR	40 mg	10% loss in 480 hr at 4°C	1866	C
Ringer's injection, lactated	TR[b]	BR	20 mg	10% loss in 142 hr at 25°C	1866	C
Ringer's injection, lactated	TR[b]	BR	40 mg	10% loss in 370 hr at 4°C	1866	C
Sodium chloride 0.45%	[a d]	KY	600 mg	6 to 8% loss in 7 days at 4°C in the dark	1503	C
Sodium chloride 0.6%	[b d]	KY	400 mg	9% loss in 7 days at 4°C in the dark	1503	C
Sodium chloride 0.9%			20 and 40 mg	Stable for 12 hr at room temperature	1(10/06)	C
Sodium chloride 0.9%	TR[a]	BR	400 mg	Under 10% loss in 24 hr at room temperature	519	C
Sodium chloride 0.9%	TR[b]	CH	50 mg	Violet color appeared in 4 hr and intensified over 12 hr. 10% loss in 12 hr at 5°C in dark	1118	I
Sodium chloride 0.9%		BR	50 mg	10% loss in 5 days at 25°C	1205	C
Sodium chloride 0.9%	[a]	KY	600 mg	5% loss in 24 hr and 9% in 4 days at 4°C in dark	1503	C
Sodium chloride 0.9%	MG[c]	BR	40 mg	10% loss in 128 hr at 4°C	1866	C
Sodium chloride 0.9%	TR[b]	BR	40 mg	10% loss in 126 hr at 4°C	1866	C
Sodium lactate ⅙ M			20 and 40 mg	Stable for 24 hr at room temperature	1(10/06)	C

[a] Tested in both glass and PVC containers.

[b] Tested in PVC containers.

[c] Tested in glass containers.

[d] Prepared from sodium chloride 0.9% and water for injection.

Additive Compatibility

Mitomycin

Test Drug	Mfr	Conc/L or %	Mfr	Conc/L or %	Test Solution	Remarks	Ref	C/I
Bleomycin sulfate	BR	20 and 30 units	BR	10 mg	NS	20% loss of bleomycin activity in 1 week at 4°C	763	I

Additive Compatibility (Cont.)

Test Drug	Mfr	Conc/L or %	Mfr	Conc/L or %	Test Solution	Remarks	Ref	C/I
Bleomycin sulfate	BR	20 and 30 units	BR	50 mg	NS	52% loss of bleomycin activity in 1 week at 4°C	763	I
Dexamethasone sodium phosphate	LY	5 g	BR	100 mg	NS[a]	Visually compatible. 10% calculated loss of mitomycin in 68 hr and dexamethasone in 250 hr at 25°C	1866	C
Dexamethasone sodium phosphate	LY	5 g	BR	100 mg	NS[b]	Visually compatible. 10% calculated loss of mitomycin in 91 hr and dexamethasone in 154 hr at 25°C	1866	C
Dexamethasone sodium phosphate	LY	5 g	BR	100 mg	NS[a]	Visually compatible. 10% calculated loss of mitomycin in 211 hr and dexamethasone in 98 hr at 4°C	1866	C
Dexamethasone sodium phosphate	LY	5 g	BR	100 mg	NS[b]	Visually compatible. 10% calculated loss of mitomycin in 238 hr and dexamethasone in 355 hr at 4°C	1866	C
Heparin sodium	ES	33,300 units	BR	167 mg	NS[a]	Visually compatible. 10% mitomycin calculated loss in 21 hr and no decrease in heparin bioactivity at 25°C	1866	I
Heparin sodium	ES	33,300 units	BR	167 mg	NS[b]	Visually compatible. 10% mitomycin calculated loss in 25 hr and no decrease in heparin bioactivity at 25°C	1866	C
Heparin sodium	ES	33,300 units	BR	500 mg	NS[a]	Visually compatible. 10% mitomycin calculated loss in 42 hr and no decrease in heparin bioactivity at 25°C	1866	C
Heparin sodium	ES	33,300 units	BR	500 mg	NS[b]	Visually compatible. 10% mitomycin calculated loss in 61 hr and no decrease in heparin bioactivity at 25°C	1866	C
Hydrocortisone sodium succinate	AB	33.3 g	BR	1 g	W[a]	Visually compatible. 10% calculated loss of mitomycin in 172 hr and hydrocortisone in 212 hr at 25°C	1866	C
Hydrocortisone sodium succinate	AB	33.3 g	BR	1 g	W[b]	Visually compatible. 10% calculated loss of mitomycin in 206 hr and hydrocortisone in 218 hr at 25°C	1866	C
Hydrocortisone sodium succinate	AB	33.3 g	BR	1 g	W[a]	Visually compatible. 10% calculated loss of mitomycin in 1423 hr and hydrocortisone in 176 hr at 4°C	1866	C
Hydrocortisone sodium succinate	AB	33.3 g	BR	1 g	W[b]	Visually compatible. 10% calculated loss of mitomycin in 820 hr and hydrocortisone in 807 hr at 4°C	1866	C

[a] Tested in glass containers.

[b] Tested in PVC containers.

Drugs in Syringe Compatibility

Mitomycin

Test Drug	Mfr	Amt	Mfr	Amt	Remarks	Ref	C/I
Bleomycin sulfate		1.5 units/0.5 mL		0.25 mg/0.5 mL	Physically compatible for 5 min at room temperature followed by 8 min of centrifugation	980	C
Cisplatin		0.5 mg/0.5 mL		0.25 mg/0.5 mL	Physically compatible for 5 min at room temperature followed by 8 min of centrifugation	980	C

Drugs in Syringe Compatibility (Cont.)

Test Drug	Mfr	Amt	Mfr	Amt	Remarks	Ref	C/I
Cisplatin with doxorubicin HCl	BMS BED	50 mg 25 mg	BMS	5 mg	Brought to a 5-mL final volume with NS. Visually compatible but more than 10% loss of mitomycin in 4 hr at 25°C. At 4°C, less than 10% loss of all three drugs in 12 hr, but about 16% mitomycin loss in 24 hr	2423	I
Cyclophosphamide		10 mg/0.5 mL		0.25 mg/0.5 mL	Physically compatible for 5 min at room temperature followed by 8 min of centrifugation	980	C
Doxorubicin HCl		1 mg/0.5 mL		0.25 mg/0.5 mL	Physically compatible for 5 min at room temperature followed by 8 min of centrifugation	980	C
Doxorubicin HCl with cisplatin	BED BMS	25 mg 50 mg	BMS	5 mg	Brought to a 5-mL final volume with NS. Visually compatible but more than 10% loss of mitomycin in 4 hr at 25°C. At 4°C, less than 10% loss of all three drugs in 12 hr, but about 16% mitomycin loss in 24 hr	2423	I
Droperidol		1.25 mg/0.5 mL		0.25 mg/0.5 mL	Physically compatible for 5 min at room temperature followed by 8 min of centrifugation	980	C
Fluorouracil		25 mg/0.5 mL		0.25 mg/0.5 mL	Physically compatible for 5 min at room temperature followed by 8 min of centrifugation	980	C
Furosemide		5 mg/0.5 mL		0.25 mg/0.5 mL	Physically compatible for 5 min at room temperature followed by 8 min of centrifugation	980	C
Heparin sodium		500 units/0.5 mL		0.25 mg/0.5 mL	Physically compatible for 5 min at room temperature followed by 8 min of centrifugation	980	C
Leucovorin calcium		5 mg/0.5 mL		0.25 mg/0.5 mL	Physically compatible for 5 min at room temperature followed by 8 min of centrifugation	980	C
Methotrexate sodium		12.5 mg/0.5 mL		0.25 mg/0.5 mL	Physically compatible for 5 min at room temperature followed by 8 min of centrifugation	980	C
Metoclopramide HCl		2.5 mg/0.5 mL		0.25 mg/0.5 mL	Physically compatible for 5 min at room temperature followed by 8 min of centrifugation	980	C
Vinblastine sulfate		0.5 mg/0.5 mL		0.25 mg/0.5 mL	Physically compatible for 5 min at room temperature followed by 8 min of centrifugation	980	C
Vincristine sulfate		0.5 mg/0.5 mL		0.25 mg/0.5 mL	Physically compatible for 5 min at room temperature followed by 8 min of centrifugation	980	C

Y-Site Injection Compatibility (1:1 Mixture)

Mitomycin

Test Drug	Mfr	Conc	Mfr	Conc	Remarks	Ref	C/I
Amifostine	USB	10 mg/mL[a]	BR	0.5 mg/mL	Physically compatible for 4 hr at 23°C	1845	C
Aztreonam	SQ	40 mg/mL[a]	BMS	0.5 mg/mL	Reddish-purple color forms in 4 hr	1758	I
Bleomycin sulfate		3 units/mL		0.5 mg/mL	Drugs injected sequentially in Y-site with no flush. No precipitate seen	980	C
Caspofungin acetate	ME	0.7 mg/mL[b]	BED	0.5 mg/mL[b]	Physically compatible for 4 hr at room temperature	2758	C
Cisplatin		1 mg/mL		0.5 mg/mL	Drugs injected sequentially in Y-site with no flush. No precipitate seen	980	C
Cyclophosphamide		20 mg/mL		0.5 mg/mL	Drugs injected sequentially in Y-site with no flush. No precipitate seen	980	C
Doxorubicin HCl		2 mg/mL		0.5 mg/mL	Drugs injected sequentially in Y-site with no flush. No precipitate seen	980	C

Y-Site Injection Compatibility (1:1 Mixture) (Cont.)

Test Drug	Mfr	Conc	Mfr	Conc	Remarks	Ref	C/I
Droperidol		2.5 mg/mL		0.5 mg/mL	Drugs injected sequentially in Y-site with no flush. No precipitate seen	980	C
Etoposide phosphate	BR	5 mg/mL[a]	BR	0.5 mg/mL	Color changed from light blue to reddish purple in 4 hr at 23°C	2218	I
Filgrastim	AMG	30 mcg/mL[a]	BR	0.5 mg/mL	Color changes to reddish purple in 1 hr	1687	I
Fluorouracil		50 mg/mL		0.5 mg/mL	Drugs injected sequentially in Y-site with no flush. No precipitate seen	980	C
Furosemide		10 mg/mL		0.5 mg/mL	Drugs injected sequentially in Y-site with no flush. No precipitate seen	980	C
Gemcitabine HCl	LI	10 mg/mL[b]	BR	0.5 mg/mL	Reddish-purple color forms in 1 hr	2226	I
Granisetron HCl	SKB	0.05 mg/mL[a]	BMS	0.5 mg/mL	Physically compatible for 4 hr at 23°C	2000	C
Heparin sodium		1000 units/mL		0.5 mg/mL	Drugs injected sequentially in Y-site with no flush. No precipitate seen	980	C
Leucovorin calcium		10 mg/mL		0.5 mg/mL	Drugs injected sequentially in Y-site with no flush. No precipitate seen	980	C
Melphalan HCl	BW	0.1 mg/mL[b]	BR	0.5 mg/mL	Physically compatible for 3 hr at 22°C	1557	C
Methotrexate sodium		25 mg/mL		0.5 mg/mL	Drugs injected sequentially in Y-site with no flush. No precipitate seen	980	C
Metoclopramide HCl		5 mg/mL		0.5 mg/mL	Drugs injected sequentially in Y-site with no flush. No precipitate seen	980	C
Ondansetron HCl	GL	1 mg/mL[b]	BR	0.5 mg/mL	Visually compatible for 4 hr at 22°C	1365	C
Piperacillin sodium–tazobactam sodium	LE[d]	40 mg/mL[a e]	BR	0.5 mg/mL	Blue color darkens in 4 hr, becoming reddish purple in 24 hr	1688	I
Sargramostim	IMM	10 mcg/mL[b]	BR	0.5 mg/mL	Slight haze in 30 min	1436	I
Teniposide	BR	0.1 mg/mL[a]	BR	0.5 mg/mL	Physically compatible for 4 hr at 23°C	1725	C
Thiotepa	IMM[c]	1 mg/mL[a]	BMS	0.5 mg/mL	Physically compatible for 4 hr at 23°C	1861	C
Topotecan HCl	SKB	56 mcg/mL[a b]	BR	84 mcg/mL[a b]	Pale purple color forms immediately becoming a dark pinkish-lavender in 4 hr. 15 to 20% mitomycin loss in 4 hr at 22°C	2245	I
Vinblastine sulfate		1 mg/mL		0.5 mg/mL	Drugs injected sequentially in Y-site with no flush. No precipitate seen	980	C
Vincristine sulfate		1 mg/mL		0.5 mg/mL	Drugs injected sequentially in Y-site with no flush. No precipitate seen	980	C
Vinorelbine tartrate	BW	1 mg/mL[b]	BR	0.5 mg/mL	Reddish-purple color in 1 hr	1558	I

[a] Tested in dextrose 5%.

[b] Tested in sodium chloride 0.9%.

[c] Lyophilized formulation tested.

[d] Test performed using the formulation WITHOUT edetate disodium.

[e] Piperacillin component. Piperacillin in an 8:1 fixed-ratio concentration with tazobactam.

Selected Revisions May 28, 2014. © Copyright, October 1982.
American Society of Health-System Pharmacists, Inc.

Mitoxantrone Hydrochloride
AHFS 10:00

Products

Mitoxantrone hydrochloride is supplied as a concentrate for injection in multidose vials.[2948] [2949] The concentrate must be diluted prior to administration.[2948] [2949] Each mL of the dark blue aqueous concentrate contains mitoxantrone 2 mg (as the hydrochloride salt), sodium chloride 0.8%, sodium acetate 0.005%, and acetic acid 0.046%.[2948] [2949] Some products also contain sodium metabisulfite 0.01%.[2949]

pH

From 3 to 4.5.[2948] [2949]

Sodium Content

Each mL contains sodium 0.14 mEq.[2948] [2949]

Administration

Mitoxantrone hydrochloride concentrate for injection must be diluted for use.[2948] [2949] The drug is administered by intravenous infusion after dilution to at least 50 mL in dextrose 5% or sodium chloride 0.9%.[2948] [2949] The drug may be further diluted in dextrose 5%; sodium chloride 0.9%; or dextrose 5% in sodium chloride 0.9%.[2948] [2949] Mitoxantrone hydrochloride is administered over about 5 to 15 minutes as a short intravenous infusion or 24 hours by continuous intravenous infusion.[2948] [2949] The drug should be administered into the tubing of a freely running intravenous solution of sodium chloride 0.9% or dextrose 5%.[2948] [2949] The tubing should be attached to a butterfly needle or other suitable device, inserted preferentially into a large vein.[2948] [2949] The drug should not be given over less than 3 minutes.[2948] [2949]

Mitoxantrone hydrochloride should *not* be administered by other routes (e.g., subcutaneous, intramuscular, intra-arterial, intrathecal).[2948] [2949]

Stability

Intact vials of the dark blue concentrate for injection should be stored upright at controlled room temperature and protected from freezing.[2948] [2949] Refrigeration of the concentrate may cause a precipitate, which redissolves upon warming to room temperature.[72] [1369]

The manufacturers indicate that mitoxantrone hydrochloride concentrate remaining in partially used vials may be stored for up to 7 days at 15 or 20 to 25°C and up to 14 days under refrigeration but should not be frozen.[2948] [2949]

Combining heparin with mitoxantrone hydrochloride may result in precipitate formation.[1293] [2948] [2949]

pH Effects

The pH range of maximum stability is 2 to 4.5; the solution was unstable when the pH was increased to 7.4.[1379]

Light Effects

Mitoxantrone hydrochloride is not photolabile. Exposure of the product to direct sunlight for 1 month caused no change in its appearance or concentration.[72] [1293]

Syringes

Mitoxantrone hydrochloride 0.2 mg/mL in sodium chloride 0.9% in polypropylene syringes (Braun Omnifix) is reported to be stable for 28 days at 4 and 20°C.[1564] Mitoxantrone hydrochloride 0.2 mg/mL in water for injection in polypropylene syringes is reported to be stable for 14 days at 4 and 20°C and for 24 hours at 37°C.[1369]

Mitoxantrone hydrochloride (Lederle) 2 mg/mL in glass vials and drawn into 12-mL plastic syringes (Monoject) exhibited no visual changes and little or no loss when stored for 42 days at 4 and 23°C. Potential extractable materials from the syringes were not detectable during the study period.[1593]

Sorption

Mitoxantrone hydrochloride (Lederle) 1 mg/mL in sodium chloride 0.9% exhibited no loss due to sorption to polyvinyl chloride (PVC) and polyethylene administration lines during simulated infusion at 0.875 mL/hr for 2.5 hours via a syringe pump.[1795]

Filtration

Although binding of mitoxantrone hydrochloride to filters has been reported,[1249] [1415] [1416] one manufacturer stated that filtration of mitoxantrone hydrochloride through a 0.22-μm filter (Millipore) resulted in no loss.[1293]

Mitoxantrone hydrochloride (Lederle) 1 mg/mL in sodium chloride 0.9%, during simulated infusion at 0.875 mL/hr for 2.5 hours via a syringe pump, exhibited no loss due to sorption to cellulose acetate (Minisart 45, Sartorius), polysulfone (Acrodisc 45, Gelman), and nylon (Posidyne ELD96, Pall) filters.[1795]

DOI: 10.37573/9781585286850.273

Compatibility Information

Solution Compatibility

Mitoxantrone HCl

Test Soln Name	Mfr	Mfr	Conc/L or %	Remarks	Ref	C/I
Dextrose 5% in sodium chloride 0.9%	a	LE	20 to 500 mg	Physically compatible. At least 90% retained for 48 hr at room temperature	1293	C
Dextrose 5%	a	LE	20 to 500 mg	Physically compatible. At least 90% retained for 7 days at room temperature and under refrigeration	72, 1293	C
Dextrose 5%		LE	5 mg	Physically compatible. No loss in 48 hr	72	C
Sodium chloride 0.9%	a	LE	20 to 500 mg	Physically compatible. At least 90% retained for 7 days at room temperature and under refrigeration	72, 1293	C
Sodium chloride 0.9%	b	LE	20 to 500 mg	Physically compatible. At least 90% retained for 48 hr at room temperature	1293	C
Sodium chloride 0.9%		LE	5 mg	Physically compatible. No loss in 48 hr	72	C

[a] Tested in PVC containers.

[b] Tested in glass containers.

Additive Compatibility

Mitoxantrone HCl

Test Drug	Mfr	Conc/L or %	Mfr	Conc/L or %	Test Solution	Remarks	Ref	C/I
Cyclophosphamide	AD	10 g	LE	500 mg	D5W	Visually compatible. Mitoxantrone stable for 24 hr at room temperature. Cyclophosphamide not tested	1531	C
Cytarabine	UP	500 mg	LE	500 mg	D5W	Visually compatible. Mitoxantrone stable for 24 hr at room temperature. Cytarabine not tested	1531	C
Etoposide	BR	500 mg	LE	50 mg	NS	Visually compatible with no loss of either drug in 22 hr at room temperature	2271	C
Fluorouracil		25 g	LE	500 mg	D5W	Visually compatible. Mitoxantrone stable for 24 hr at room temperature. Fluorouracil not tested	1531	C
Hydrocortisone sodium succinate		100 mg to 2 g	LE	50 to 200 mg	D5W, NS[a]	Physically compatible and both drugs stable for 24 hr at room temperature	1293	C
Potassium chloride		50 mEq	LE	500 mg	D5W	Visually compatible. Mitoxantrone stable for 24 hr at room temperature	1531	C

[a] Tested in PVC containers.

Y-Site Injection Compatibility (1:1 Mixture)

Mitoxantrone HCl

Test Drug	Mfr	Conc	Mfr	Conc	Remarks	Ref	C/I
Allopurinol sodium	BW	3 mg/mL[b]	LE	0.5 mg/mL[b]	Physically compatible for 4 hr at 22°C	1686	C
Amifostine	USB	10 mg/mL[a]	LE	0.5 mg/mL[a]	Physically compatible for 4 hr at 23°C	1845	C
Aztreonam	SQ	40 mg/mL[a]	LE	0.5 mg/mL[a]	Heavy precipitate forms in 1 hr	1758	I
Cladribine	ORT	0.015[b] and 0.5[c] mg/mL	LE	0.5 mg/mL[b]	Physically compatible for 4 hr at 23°C	1969	C
Doxorubicin HCl liposomal	SEQ	0.4 mg/mL[a]	IMM	0.5 mg/mL[a]	Partial loss of measured natural turbidity	2087	I

Y-Site Injection Compatibility (1:1 Mixture) (Cont.)

Test Drug	Mfr	Conc	Mfr	Conc	Remarks	Ref	C/I
Etoposide	BR	20 mg/mL	LE	2 mg/mL	Visually compatible with no loss of either drug in 22 hr at room temperature	2271	C
Etoposide phosphate	BR	5 mg/mL[a]	IMM	0.5 mg/mL[a]	Physically compatible for 4 hr at 23°C	2218	C
Filgrastim	AMG	30 mcg/mL[a]	LE	0.5 mg/mL[a]	Physically compatible for 4 hr at 22°C	1687	C
Fludarabine phosphate	BX	1 mg/mL[a]	LE	0.5 mg/mL[a]	Visually compatible for 4 hr at 22°C	1439	C
Gemcitabine HCl	LI	10 mg/mL[b]	IMM	0.5 mg/mL[b]	Physically compatible for 4 hr at 23°C	2226	C
Granisetron HCl	SKB	0.05 mg/mL[a]	IMM	0.5 mg/mL[a]	Physically compatible for 4 hr at 23°C	2000	C
Linezolid	PHU	2 mg/mL	IMM	0.5 mg/mL[a]	Physically compatible for 4 hr at 23°C	2264	C
Melphalan HCl	BW	0.1 mg/mL[b]	LE	0.5 mg/mL[b]	Physically compatible for 3 hr at 22°C	1557	C
Ondansetron HCl	GL	1 mg/mL[b]	LE	0.5 mg/mL[a]	Visually compatible for 4 hr at 22°C	1365	C
Oxaliplatin	SS	0.5 mg/mL[a]	IMM	0.5 mg/mL[a]	Physically compatible for 4 hr at 23°C	2566	C
Paclitaxel	NCI	1.2 mg/mL[a]	LE	0.5 mg/mL[a]	Normal inherent haze from paclitaxel decreases immediately	1556	I
Pemetrexed disodium	LI	20 mg/mL[b]	IMM	0.5 mg/mL[a]	Dark-blue precipitate forms immediately	2564	I
Piperacillin sodium–tazobactam sodium	LE[f]	40 mg/mL[a g]	LE	0.5 mg/mL[a]	Haze and particles form immediately. Large particles form in 4 hr	1688	I
Propofol	ZEN[h]	10 mg/mL	IMM	0.5 mg/mL[a]	Particles form immediately	2066	I
Sargramostim	IMM	10 mcg/mL[b]	LE	0.5 mg/mL[b]	Visually compatible for 4 hr at 22°C	1436	C
Teniposide	BR	0.1 mg/mL[a]	LE	0.5 mg/mL[a]	Physically compatible for 4 hr at 23°C	1725	C
Thiotepa	IMM[d]	1 mg/mL[a]	IMM	0.5 mg/mL[a]	Physically compatible for 4 hr at 23°C	1861	C
TNA #218 to #226[e]			IMM	0.5 mg/mL[a]	Visually compatible for 4 hr at 23°C	2215	C
TPN #212 to #215[e]			IMM	0.5 mg/mL[a]	Substantial loss of natural haze occurs immediately	2109	I
Vinorelbine tartrate	BW	1 mg/mL[b]	LE	0.5 mg/mL[b]	Physically compatible for 4 hr at 22°C	1558	C

[a] Tested in dextrose 5%.

[b] Tested in sodium chloride 0.9%.

[c] Tested in bacteriostatic sodium chloride 0.9% preserved with benzyl alcohol 0.9%.

[d] Lyophilized formulation tested.

[e] Refer to Appendix for the composition of parenteral nutrition solutions. TNA indicates a 3-in-1 admixture, and TPN indicates a 2-in-1 admixture.

[f] Test performed using the formulation WITHOUT edetate disodium.

[g] Piperacillin component. Piperacillin in an 8:1 fixed-ratio concentration with tazobactam.

[h] Test performed using the formulation WITH edetate disodium.

Selected Revisions January 31, 2020. © Copyright, October 1990. American Society of Health-System Pharmacists, Inc.

Morphine Sulfate
AHFS 28:08.08

Products

Morphine sulfate is available in a variety of concentrations (e.g., ranging from 0.5 to 50 mg/mL), packages (e.g., vials, ampuls, cartridges, syringes, patient-controlled analgesia [PCA] vials, auto-injectors), and sizes.[3484] [3485] [3486] [3487] [3488] [3489] [3490] [3491] Some formulations are preservative free and may be labeled for epidural and intrathecal administration.[3484] [3485] [3486] Other morphine products may contain various preservatives, antioxidants, and buffers, including edetate disodium, sodium metabisulfite, benzyl alcohol, and citric acid;[3487] [3488] [3489] [3490] [3491] specific product labeling should be consulted for additional formulation details and labeled routes of administration of each product.

Morphine also is available in some countries as the hydrochloride and tartrate salts.

pH

The pH of many morphine sulfate products falls within the range of 2.5 to 6.5,[3484] [3487] [3489] [3491] with some products exhibiting a more narrow pH range of 2.5 to 4[3488] or a pH of 4.5;[3485] [3486] specific product labeling should be consulted for the pH of a specific product.

Morphine sulfate (David Bull) 7.5 mg/mL in sodium chloride 0.9% had a pH of 3.5.[2161]

Osmolality

Morphine sulfate (David Bull) 7.5 mg/mL in sodium chloride 0.9% had an osmolality of 236 mOsm/kg.[2161]

Trade Name(s)

Astramorph PF, Duramorph, Infumorph, Mitigo

Administration

Morphine sulfate may be administered by slow, direct intravenous injection[3488] [3490] or by intramuscular[3489] [3490] or subcutaneous injection; the drug also may be given by slow intravenous injection or continuous intravenous infusion after dilution.[3491] For continuous intravenous infusion using an infusion pump, one manufacturer recommends a final morphine sulfate concentration of 0.2 to 1 mg/mL in dextrose 5%;[3491] more concentrated solutions also have been used. Some products containing no preservatives may be labeled for intrathecal or epidural administration.[3484] [3485] [3486]

Some higher-concentration morphine sulfate products (e.g., 10, 25, or 50 mg/mL) are not recommended for subcutaneous, intramuscular, intravenous, or neuraxial injection of individual doses; such products may be labeled for intraspinal administration (with or without dilution) using a continuous microinfusion device[3485] [3486] or for continuous intravenous infusion only after dilution using an infusion pump.[3491]

Stability

Intact containers should be stored in the carton at controlled room temperature and protected from freezing and light.[3484] [3485] [3486] [3487] [3488] [3489] [3490] [3491] Manufacturers state that the products should not be heat sterilized[3484] [3485] [3486] [3487] [3488] [3491] or autoclaved.[3490] Morphine sulfate darkens with age and upon prolonged exposure to light;[3488] [3490] [3491] the injection should not be used if it is darker than pale yellow in color or if is discolored in any other way.[3484] [3485] [3486] [3487] [3490] [3491]

Undiluted morphine sulfate 10 mg/mL, stored in 100-mL glass vials and polyvinyl chloride (PVC) bags, exhibited no loss in 30 days at 23°C.[1394]

Morphine sulfate (Wyeth) 1 mg/mL in bacteriostatic sodium chloride 0.9% containing benzyl alcohol 0.9%, when stored in glass vials with protection from light, exhibited no loss at 4°C and a 4% loss at 22°C after 91 days.[1583]

Morphine sulfate 15 mg/mL and 2 mg/mL diluted with sterile water for injection stored at 4 and 24°C in 200-mL PVC bags (Baxter) was stable at both temperatures with little loss in 15 days.[1504]

Morphine sulfate under simulated summer conditions in paramedic vehicles was exposed to 26 to 38°C over 4 weeks. No drug loss occurred under these conditions.[2562]

Morphine sulfate 1 mg/mL compounded in sodium chloride 0.9% was packaged in 100-mL polypropylene infusion bags and was autoclaved at 121°C for 20 minutes for sterilization. No visible precipitation appeared and microparticulate levels remained acceptable in all samples when stored at 25°C for 3 years and at 30 and 40°C for 6 months. No evidence of evaporation was found in the samples, and no loss of morphine sulfate occurred in any of the solutions throughout the study. While PVC bags cannot be autoclaved and exhibit excessive loss of water through evaporation upon storage, polypropylene bags can be successfully used for compounding bags of morphine sulfate solutions with 3-year stability for use in patient-controlled analgesia.[2665]

pH Effects

Morphine sulfate is relatively stable at acidic pH, especially below pH 4, but degradation increases greatly at neutral or basic pH. Degradation is often accompanied by a yellow to brown discoloration in the normally colorless solution.[1072] [2170]

Morphine sulfate stability at a low concentration of 2 mg/mL in an admixture with ketamine hydrochloride in sodium chloride 0.9% with the pH adjusted over a range of pH 5.5 to 7.5 was stored at room temperature over 4 days. No difference in physical or chemical drug stability was observed among the samples.[2786]

DOI: 10.37573/9781585286850.274

However, at higher concentrations of morphine at pH values of 6.4 and above, precipitation may occur. Morphine sulfate at about 18 mg/mL mixed with ketamine hydrochloride exhibited a pH near 4.85. Adjusting the pH higher with sodium bicarbonate injection up to pH 5.9 resulted in mixtures that were clear over 24 hours at 21°C. However, adjusting to pH 6.2 resulted in precipitation within 2 hours. Adjusting to pH 6.4 and above resulted in immediate precipitation.[2787]

Freezing Solutions

Manufacturers state that morphine sulfate products should not be frozen.[3484 3485 3486 3487 3488 3489 3490 3491]

Morphine sulfate (Lilly) 1 and 2 mg/mL in dextrose 5% and sodium chloride 0.9% in PVC bags exhibited no loss during 14 weeks of frozen storage at −20°C.[1286]

Syringes

In 2015, reports of decreased potency of certain drugs (e.g., morphine sulfate) stored in Becton Dickinson syringes for extended periods (i.e., exceeding 24 hours) were confirmed by the manufacturer of these syringes; the cause of this change was later identified to be the inclusion of an alternate rubber stopper in the plunger of certain product lots of syringes.[3029 3036 3037 3039 3041 3042] Decreased potency was not observed when the syringes were filled and used promptly.[3037] Use of the alternate stopper was later discontinued and use of the primary stopper in such syringes was resumed; however, Becton Dickinson states that its general-use syringes are cleared by FDA for immediate use in fluid aspiration and injection and that such syringes, regardless of the stopper material, have not been cleared by FDA for use as a closed-container system.[3391]

Prefilled into plastic syringes with syringe caps (Braun), morphine sulfate is stated to remain within acceptable limits of degradation for at least 69 days at room temperature.[982]

In another study, less than a 3% loss of morphine sulfate occurred in 12 weeks when stored in plastic syringes at 22°C and exposed to light. A smaller loss occurred when the morphine sulfate was stored at 3°C with light protection.[1287]

Morphine sulfate (Lilly) 1 and 5 mg/mL in dextrose 5% and sodium chloride 0.9% was packaged in 30-mL Plastipak (Becton Dickinson) syringes capped with Monoject (Sherwood) tip caps. Syringes were stored at 23°C in light and dark, 4°C protected from light, and frozen at −20°C protected from light for 12 weeks. Both concentrations at all 3 temperatures were stable for at least 6 weeks when protected from light. However, the samples stored at 23°C exposed to light were stable for 1 week, but developed unacceptable losses after that.[1894]

Morphine sulfate 2 mg/mL in sodium chloride 0.9% was packaged in 50-mL (Becton Dickinson) and 30-mL (Becton Dickinson and Sherwood) polypropylene syringes for use in patient-controlled analgesia and in stoppered glass vials. The samples were stored at room temperature in the dark for 6 weeks. Little loss of morphine sulfate occurred in the 50-mL syringes and the glass vials in 6 weeks. About 5% loss occurred when packaged in both Becton Dickinson and Sherwood 30-mL syringes. Addition

of sodium metabisulfite 0.1% as an antioxidant increased the rate of drug loss up to 10% in 2 weeks.[2040]

Morphine sulfate 5 mg/mL in sodium chloride 0.9% and 50 mg/mL in sterile water for injection and also in sodium chloride 0.9% packaged as 20 mL in 30-mL polypropylene syringes were stored for 60 days at 4°C protected from light and 23°C exposed to normal fluorescent light. Other solutions were stored frozen at −20°C and at elevated temperature of 37°C for 2 days to simulate more extreme conditions during express shipping. Little or no morphine sulfate loss occurred in the 50-mg/mL samples stored for 60 days at 4 and 23°C even though slight yellow discoloration occurred after 30 days. The 5-mg/mL samples stored at 4 and 23°C exhibited about 4 to 5% loss in 60 days. The frozen and 37°C samples exhibited little or no change in morphine sulfate concentration in 2 days. However, samples of the 50-mg/mL concentration stored at −20 and 4°C and samples of the 5-mg/mL concentration stored frozen at −20°C precipitated upon low temperature storage. Although the precipitate redissolved upon warming at 37°C for several hours, large amounts of microparticulates in the tens of thousands per mL remained, possibly shed by the syringe components.[2376]

Ambulatory Pumps

Walker et al. reported the stability of undiluted morphine sulfate (Sabex) 50 and 25 mg/mL, with and without sodium metabisulfite preservative, in portable infusion pump cassettes (Pharmacia) stored at 4 and 23°C.[1505] At both concentrations with and without sodium metabisulfite at 4 and 23°C, samples remained clear and colorless.[1505] Morphine sulfate losses of less than 10% were found during 31 days of storage.[1505]

Stiles et al. studied the stability of undiluted morphine sulfate 25 and 15 mg/mL in pump reservoirs (Pharmacia Deltec) stored at 5°C in the dark and 25°C for 30 days.[1507] After the initial storage period, the solutions were subsequently stored at 37°C and pumped at a flow rate of 0.4 mL/hr for 3 days to simulate patient use.[1507] No color change or precipitation occurred in any sample.[1507] Little to no losses were detected; in fact, increased concentrations were observed, especially at room temperature.[1507] The concentration increases were attributed to water evaporation during storage.[1507] The authors recommended a maximum storage of 30 days under refrigeration and 14 days at room temperature because of the evaporation.[1507]

Elastomeric Reservoir Pumps

Morphine sulfate 15 mg/mL and 2 mg/mL diluted with sterile water for injection was stored at 4 and 24°C in Intermate 200 (Infusion Systems) and Infusor (Baxter) disposable elastomeric infusion devices.[1504] In the Intermate 200 with 100 mL of morphine sulfate solution, little or no loss occurred in 15 days at either 4 or 24°C and even at 31°C (simulating use next to a patient's skin or clothing).[1504] In the Infusor, with 50 mL, losses of 5% or more were observed in 12 days in some containers.[1504]

Morphine sulfate 0.5 mg/mL in both dextrose 5% and sodium chloride 0.9% was evaluated for binding potential to natural rubber elastomeric reservoirs (Baxter). No binding was found after storage for 2 weeks at 35°C with gentle agitation.[2014]

Morphine sulfate 2 and 10 mg/mL is reported to be physically and chemically stable in Accufuser Plus silicone balloon infusers when stored at room temperature and refrigerated. Little or no loss of morphine sulfate occurred in 40 days.[2678]

Implantable Pumps

Morphine sulfate 10 mg/mL was filled into a VIP 30 implantable infusion pump (Fresenius) and associated capillary tubing and stored at 37°C. No morphine loss and no contamination from components of pump materials occurred during 8 weeks of storage.[1903]

Morphine sulfate (Infumorph) 20 mg/mL with clonidine hydrochloride (Boehringer Ingelheim) 50 mcg/mL and morphine sulfate 2 mg/mL with clonidine hydrochloride 1.84 mg/mL were evaluated in SynchroMed EL (Medtronic) implantable pumps with silicone elastomer intrathecal catheters at 37°C for 3 months. No visible incompatibilities were observed; delivered concentrations of both drugs were in the range of 94 to 99.6% throughout the study. Furthermore, no impairment of mechanical performance of the pump or any of its components was found.[2477]

An admixture of bupivacaine hydrochloride 25 mg/mL, clonidine hydrochloride 2 mg/mL, and morphine sulfate 50 mg/mL in sterile water for injection was reported to be physically and chemically stable for 90 days at 37°C in SynchroMed implantable pumps. Little or no loss of any of the drugs was found.[2585]

Clonidine hydrochloride and morphine sulfate powders were dissolved in ziconotide acetate (Elan) injection to yield concentrations of 2 and 35 mg/mL and 25 mcg/mL, respectively. Stored at 37°C, 11% ziconotide loss in 7 days, 4% clonidine loss in 20 days, and no morphine loss in 28 days occurred.[2752]

Other Devices

The stability of 2 intrathecal solutions of morphine sulfate 10 mg/mL in sodium chloride 0.9% (isobaric) and 5 mg/mL in dextrose 7% in water (hyperbaric) was evaluated. The solutions were stored at 4 and 37°C in glass ampuls and pump reservoirs composed of silicone rubber reinforced with polyester (Cordis Europa). No precipitation or discoloration and no loss of morphine sulfate or increase in degradation products occurred in the solutions in glass ampuls after 2 months at either temperature. However, in the pump reservoirs, the isobaric solution in sodium chloride 0.9% developed a yellow color. Furthermore, a decomposition product, pseudomorphine, was detectable in 3 days and increased to 1% in 1 month at 37°C. This level was 20 times that of the pseudomorphine found in the hyperbaric dextrose 7% in water solution under the same conditions. The decomposition was attributed to dissolved oxygen, ethylene oxide sterilant, and silicone rubber.[1508]

Central Venous Catheter

Morphine sulfate (Astra) 1 mg/mL in dextrose 5% was found to be compatible with the ARROWg+ard Blue Plus (Arrow International) chlorhexidine-bearing triple-lumen central catheter. Essentially complete delivery of the drug was found with little or no drug loss occurring. Furthermore, chlorhexidine delivered from the catheter remained at trace amounts with no substantial increase due to the delivery of the drug through the catheter.[2335]

Compatibility Information

Solution Compatibility

Morphine sulfate

Test Soln Name	Mfr	Mfr	Conc/L or %	Remarks	Ref	C/I
Dextrose 2.5% in half-strength Ringer's injection	AB		16.2 mg	Physically compatible	3	C
Dextrose 5% in Ringer's injection	AB		16.2 mg	Physically compatible	3	C
Dextrose 2.5% in Ringer's injection, lactated	AB		16.2 mg	Physically compatible	3	C
Dextrose 5% in half-strength Ringer's injection, lactated	AB		16.2 mg	Physically compatible	3	C
Dextrose 5% in Ringer's injection, lactated	AB		16.2 mg	Physically compatible	3	C
Dextrose 10% in Ringer's injection, lactated	AB		16.2 mg	Physically compatible	3	C
Dextrose 2.5% in sodium chloride 0.45%	AB		16.2 mg	Physically compatible	3	C
Dextrose 2.5% in sodium chloride 0.9%	AB		16.2 mg	Physically compatible	3	C

Solution Compatibility (Cont.)

Test Soln Name	Mfr	Mfr	Conc/L or %	Remarks	Ref	C/I
Dextrose 5% in sodium chloride 0.225%	AB		16.2 mg	Physically compatible	3	C
Dextrose 5% in sodium chloride 0.45%	AB		16.2 mg	Physically compatible	3	C
Dextrose 5% in sodium chloride 0.9%	AB		16.2 mg	Physically compatible	3	C
Dextrose 10% in sodium chloride 0.9%	AB		16.2 mg	Physically compatible	3	C
Dextrose 2.5%	AB		16.2 mg	Physically compatible	3	C
Dextrose 5%	AB		16.2 mg	Physically compatible	3	C
Dextrose 5%	TR[a]	LI	1.2 g	Physically compatible. No loss in 36 hr at 22°C	1000	C
Dextrose 5%	TR[b]	AB, AH	40 and 400 mg	Physically compatible with little or no loss in 7 days at 23 and 4°C	1349	C
Dextrose 5%	[a]	AH	5 g	No loss in 30 days at 23°C	1394	C
Dextrose 5%	[g]	SX	10 g	Visually compatible. Less than 10% loss in 31 days at 4 and 23°C	1505	C
Dextrose 10%	AB		16.2 mg	Physically compatible	3	C
Ionosol B in dextrose 5%	AB		16.2 mg	Physically compatible	3	C
Ionosol MB in dextrose 5%	AB		16.2 mg	Physically compatible	3	C
Ringer's injection	AB		16.2 mg	Physically compatible	3	C
Ringer's injection, lactated	AB		16.2 mg	Physically compatible	3	C
Sodium chloride 0.45%	AB		16.2 mg	Physically compatible	3	C
Sodium chloride 0.9%	AB		16.2 mg	Physically compatible	3	C
Sodium chloride 0.9%	TR[b]	AB, AH	40 and 400 mg	Physically compatible with little or no loss in 7 days at 23 and 4°C	1349	C
Sodium chloride 0.9%	[a]	AH	5 g	No loss in 30 days at 23°C	1394	C
Sodium chloride 0.9%	AB[a]	SCN	100 and 500 mg	Visually compatible with no loss in 72 hr at 24°C under fluorescent light	2058	C
Sodium chloride 0.9%	[e]	PHS	1 and 10 g	Visually compatible. No loss in 16 days at 32°C in the dark. 4% concentration increase consistent with slight evaporation	2254	C
Sodium chloride 0.9%	[f]	CNF	0.5, 1.5, 2.5 g	Visually compatible. No loss in 60 days at 32°C. 8% concentration increase was due to evaporation	1312	C
Sodium chloride 0.9%	[g]	SX	10 g	Visually compatible. Less than 10% loss in 31 days at 4 and 23°C	1505	C
Sodium chloride 0.9%	[h]		0.5, 15, 30 g[i]	No loss in 14 days at 5°C. Slight concentration increase at 37°C due to evaporation. Light brown color after 5 days at 37°C	1506	C
Sodium chloride 0.9%	[h]		60 g[i]	At 37°C, slight concentration increase in 14 days due to evaporation. Light brown color in 5 days	1506	C
Sodium chloride 0.9%	[h]		60 g[i]	At 5°C, morphine precipitates in 4 days with over 40% loss	1506	I
Sodium chloride 0.9%	[e]	ES	1 and 5 g	Visually compatible for 30 days at 5 and 25°C. Increased concentration due to evaporation. Maximum storage of 30 days at 5°C and 14 days at 25°C	1507	C
Sodium chloride 0.9%	BA[j]	[i]	5 g	Physically compatible. 4 to 5% loss in 60 days at 23°C in light and at 4°C in dark	2376	C

Solution Compatibility (Cont.)

Test Soln Name	Mfr	Mfr	Conc/L or %	Remarks	Ref	C/I
Sodium chloride 0.9%	BA[j]	i	50 g	Physically compatible. Little loss in 60 days at 23°C in light. Yellow color not indicative of decomposition	2376	C
Sodium chloride 0.9%	BA[j]	i	50 g	At 4°C, morphine sulfate precipitates but redissolves on warming leaving tens of thousands of microparticulates. Little loss in 60 days at 4°C	2376	?
Sodium chloride 0.9%	MAC[e]	AGT	1 and 40 g	Physically compatible. No loss in 30 days at room temperature protected from light. Concentration increase due to water loss	2633	C
Sodium chloride 0.9%	BA[k]	ANT	2 and 3 g	Physically compatible. Little drug loss in 60 days at 4 and 25°C. Less than 2.5% loss of moisture during storage	2628	C
Sodium lactate ⅙ M	AB		16.2 mg	Physically compatible	3	C
Sterile water for injection	BA[c]	i	50 g	Physically compatible. Little loss in 60 days at 23°C in light. Yellow color not indicative of decomposition	2376	C
Sterile water for injection	BA[c]	i	50 g	At 4°C, morphine sulfate precipitates but redissolves on warming leaving tens of thousands of microparticulates. Little loss in 60 days at 4°C	2376	?
TPN #71[d]	a	LI	100 mg	Physically compatible and no morphine loss in 36 hr at 22°C	1000	C

[a] Tested in PVC containers.

[b] Tested in both glass and PVC containers.

[c] Note: Not suitable for large-volume infusion.

[d] Refer to Appendix for the composition of parenteral nutrition solutions. TPN indicates a 2-in-1 admixture.

[e] Tested in Pharmacia or SIMS Deltec medication cassette reservoirs.

[f] Tested in Pharmacia Deltec PVC/Kalex phthalate ester medication cassette reservoirs.

[g] Tested in Pharmacia cassette reservoirs.

[h] Tested in Cormed III Kalex reservoirs.

[i] Prepared from morphine sulfate powder.

[j] Tested in polypropylene syringes.

[k] Tested in ANAPA Plus (E-WHA International) ambulatory infusion device and PEGA (Pegasus) sets.

Additive Compatibility

Morphine sulfate

Test Drug	Mfr	Conc/L or %	Mfr	Conc/L or %	Test Solution	Remarks	Ref	C/I
Alteplase	GEN	0.5 g	WY	1 g	NS	Visually compatible with 5 to 8% alteplase clot-lysis activity loss in 24 hr at 25°C	1856	C
Atracurium besylate	BW	500 mg		1 g	D5W	Physically compatible and atracurium stable for 24 hr at 5 and 30°C	1694	C
Baclofen	CI	200 mg	DB	1 and 1.5 g	NS[d]	Physically compatible. Little loss of either drug in 30 days at 37°C	1911	C
Baclofen	CI	800 mg	DB	1 g	NS[d]	Physically compatible. Little baclofen loss and less than 7% morphine loss in 29 days at 37°C	1911	C
Baclofen	CI	800 mg	DB	1.5 g	NS[d]	Physically compatible. Little loss of either drug in 30 days at 37°C	1911	C
Baclofen	CI	1.5 g	DB	7.5 g	NS[d]	Physically compatible. Little loss of either drug in 30 days at 37°C	2170	C

Additive Compatibility (Cont.)

Test Drug	Mfr	Conc/L or %	Mfr	Conc/L or %	Test Solution	Remarks	Ref	C/I
Baclofen	CI	1 g	DB	15 g	NS[d]	Physically compatible. Little loss of either drug in 30 days at 37°C	2170	C
Baclofen	CI	200 mg	DB	21 g	NS[d]	Physically compatible. 7% baclofen loss and little morphine loss in 30 days at 37°C	2170	C
Bupivacaine HCl	AST	3 g		1 g	[b]	Little loss of either drug in 30 days at 18°C	1932	C
Bupivacaine HCl	AB	625 mg and 1.25 g	SCN	100 mg	NS[b]	Visually compatible. No loss of either drug in 72 hr at 24°C in light	2058	C
Bupivacaine HCl	AB	625 mg and 1.25 g	SCN	500 mg	NS[b]	Visually compatible. No loss of either drug in 72 hr at 24°C in light	2058	C
Dobutamine HCl	LI	1 g	ES	5 g	D5W, NS	Physically compatible for 24 hr at 21°C	812	C
Eptifibatide	ME	750 mg		1 g		Physically compatible and chemically stable for up to 24 hr at 25°C	3049	C
Floxacillin sodium	BE	20 g	EV	1 g	W	Haze forms in 24 hr and precipitate forms in 48 hr at 30°C. No change at 15°C	1479	I
Fluconazole	PF	1 g	ES	0.25 g	D5W[b]	Fluconazole stable for 24 hr at 25°C in fluorescent light. Morphine not tested	1676	C
Fluorouracil	AB	1 and 16 g	AST	1 g	D5W, NS[b]	Subvisible morphine precipitate forms immediately, becoming grossly visible within 24 hr. Morphine losses of 60 to 80% occur within 1 day	1977	I
Furosemide	HO	1 g	EV	1 g	W	Physically compatible for 72 hr at 15 and 30°C	1479	C
Ketamine HCl	PD	1 g	SX	1 g	NS[b]	At least 90% of both drugs retained for 6 days at room temperature	2260	C
Ketamine HCl	PD	25 g	SX	25 g	NS[b]	At least 90% of both drugs retained for 6 days at room temperature	2260	C
Ketamine HCl	PD	25 g	SX	25 g	NS[e]	At least 90% of both drugs retained for 6 days at room temperature	2260	C
Ketamine HCl	PD	1.33 g	AB	2 g	NS	Little loss of either drug in 4 days at room temperature	2786	C
Meropenem	ZEN	1 and 20 g	ES	1 g	NS	Visually compatible for 4 hr at room temperature	1994	C
Metoclopramide HCl	SKB	500 mg	EV	1 g	NS[b]	Visually compatible. Little loss of either drug in 35 days at 22°C and 182 days at 4°C followed by 7 days at 32°C	1939	C
Metoclopramide HCl	SKB	500 mg	EV	1 g	D5W[c]	Visually compatible. 8% metoclopramide loss in 14 days at 22°C and 98 days at 4°C. No morphine loss	1939	C
Naloxone HCl	SZ	4 mg	BA	1 g[h]	[b]	Physically compatible with less than 10% loss of either drug in 3 days at 22°C and 30 days at 4°C	3492	C
Naloxone HCl	SZ	12.5 mg	BA	1 g[h]	[b]	Physically compatible with less than 10% loss of either drug in 3 days at 22°C and 30 days at 4°C	3492	C
Naloxone HCl	SZ	25 mg	BA	1 g[h]	[b]	Physically compatible with less than 10% loss of either drug in 3 days at 22°C and 30 days at 4°C	3492	C
Ondansetron HCl	GL	100 mg and 1 g	AST	1 g	NS[b]	Physically compatible. No ondansetron loss and 5% or less morphine loss in 7 days at 32°C or 31 days at 4 and 22°C protected from light	1690	C
Ropivacaine HCl	ASZ	1 g	AST	20 mg	NS[f]	Physically compatible. Little loss of either drug in 30 days at 30°C in the dark	2433	C

Additive Compatibility (Cont.)

Test Drug	Mfr	Conc/L or %	Mfr	Conc/L or %	Test Solution	Remarks	Ref	C/I
Ropivacaine HCl	ASZ	2 g	AST	20 and 100 mg	f	Physically compatible. Little loss of either drug in 30 days at 30°C in the dark	2433	C
Ropivacaine HCl	FRKⁱ	6 g	CDM	2 g	NSⁱ	Visually compatible and chemically stable for up to 14 days at 21°C	3493	C
Succinylcholine chloride	AB	2 g		16.2 mg		Physically compatible	3	C
Verapamil HCl	KN	80 mg	KN	30 mg	D5W, NS	Physically compatible for 24 hr	764	C
Ziconotide acetate	ELN	25 mgª	BB	35 gᵍ		90% ziconotide retained for 8 days at 37°C. No morphine loss in 17 days	2702	C
Ziconotide acetate	ELN	25 mgª	BB	20 gᵍ		90% ziconotide retained for 19 days at 37°C. No morphine loss in 28 days	2713	C
Ziconotide acetate	ELN	25 mgª	BB	10 gᵍ		10% ziconotide loss in 34 days. No morphine loss in 60 days at 37°C	2780	C
Ziconotide acetate	ELN	25 mgª	BB	20 gᵍ		10% ziconotide loss in 19 days. No morphine loss in 28 days at 37°C	2780	C
Ziconotide acetate	EIᵏ	200 mg	CDM	2 g	NSⁱ	Visually compatible and chemically stable for up to 14 days at 21°C	3493	C

ª Tested in SynchroMed II implantable pumps.

ᵇ Tested in PVC containers.

ᶜ Tested in PCA Infusors (Baxter).

ᵈ Tested in glass containers.

ᵉ Tested in Deltec plastic medication cassette reservoirs.

ᶠ Tested in polypropylene bags (Mark II Polybags).

ᵍ Morphine sulfate powder dissolved in ziconotide acetate injection.

ʰ Tested as the premixed infusion solution.

ⁱ Tested in polyolefin containers.

ʲ Tested with ziconotide acetate (EI) 200 mg/L.

ᵏ Tested with ropivacaine HCl (FRK) 6 g/L.

Drugs in Syringe Compatibility

Morphine sulfate

Test Drug	Mfr	Amt	Mfr	Amt	Remarks	Ref	C/I
Alfentanil HCl	ASZ	55 mcg/mLᵉ	DB	0.8 mg/mLᵉ	No loss of either drug in 182 days at room temperature or refrigerated	2527	C
Atropine sulfate		0.6 mg/1.5 mL	WY	15 mg/1 mL	Physically compatible for at least 15 min	14	C
Atropine sulfate	ST	0.4 mg/1 mL	ST	15 mg/1 mL	Physically compatible for at least 15 min	326	C
Bupivacaine HCl	AST	3 mg/mL		1 mg/mL	Little loss of either drug in 30 days at 18°C	1932	C
Bupivacaine HCl	ᵍ	2.5 mg/mLᵉ	ᵍ	5 mg/mLᵉ	Physically compatible. Little morphine or bupivacaine loss in 60 days at 23°C in fluorescent light and at 4°C	2378	C
Bupivacaine HCl	ᵍ	2.5 mg/mLᵉ	ᵍ	5 mg/mLᵉ	Little or no loss of either drug in 2 days at 37°C	2378	C
Bupivacaine HCl	ᵍ	2.5 mg/mLᵉ	ᵍ	5 mg/mLᵉ	Formation of large amounts of microparticulates upon thawing following little or no loss of either drug in 2 days at −20°C	2378	I

Drugs in Syringe Compatibility (Cont.)

Test Drug	Mfr	Amt	Mfr	Amt	Remarks	Ref	C/I
Bupivacaine HCl	g	25 mg/mL[a]	g	50 mg/mL[a]	Physically compatible. Little morphine or bupivacaine loss in 60 days at 23°C in fluorescent light and at 4°C in dark. Slight yellow discoloration at 23°C not indicative of decomposition	2378	C
Bupivacaine HCl	g	25 mg/mL[a]	g	50 mg/mL[a]	Little or no loss of either drug in 2 days at 37°C	2378	C
Bupivacaine HCl	g	25 mg/mL[a]	g	50 mg/mL[a]	Formation of large amounts of microparticulates upon thawing following little or no loss of either drug in 2 days at −20°C	2378	I
Bupivacaine HCl with clonidine HCl	SW BI	1.5 mg/mL 0.03 mg/mL	ES	0.2 mg/mL	Diluted to 5 mL with NS. Visually compatible with no new GC/MS peaks in 1 hr at room temperature	1956	C
Butorphanol tartrate	BR	4 mg/2 mL	AH	15 mg/1 mL	Physically compatible for 30 min at room temperature	566	C
Caffeine citrate		20 mg/1 mL	SW	4 mg/1 mL	Visually compatible for 4 hr at 25°C	2440	C
Chlorpromazine HCl	SKF	50 mg/2 mL	WY	15 mg/1 mL	Physically compatible for at least 15 min	14	C
Chlorpromazine HCl	PO	50 mg/2 mL	ST	15 mg/1 mL	Physically compatible for at least 15 min	326	C
Clonidine HCl	FUJ	100 mcg/1 mL	ES	10 mg/1 mL	Physically and chemically stable for 14 days at room temperature	2069	C
Clonidine HCl	g	0.25 mg/mL[e]	g	5 mg/mL[e]	Physically compatible. Little morphine or clonidine loss in 60 days at 23°C in light and at 4°C in dark	2380	C
Clonidine HCl	g	4 mg/mL[c]	g	50 mg/mL[a]	Physically compatible. Little morphine or clonidine loss in 60 days at 23°C in light and at 4°C in dark. Slight yellow discoloration at 23°C not indicative of decomposition	2380	C
Clonidine HCl with bupivacaine HCl	BI SW	0.03 mg/mL 1.5 mg/mL	ES	0.2 mg/mL	Diluted to 5 mL with NS. Visually compatible with no new GC/MS peaks in 1 hr at room temperature	1956	C
Dimenhydrinate	HR	50 mg/1 mL	ST	15 mg/1 mL	Physically compatible for at least 15 min	326	C
Diphenhydramine HCl	PD	50 mg/1 mL	WY	15 mg/1 mL	Physically compatible for at least 15 min	14	C
Diphenhydramine HCl	PD	50 mg/1 mL	ST	15 mg/1 mL	Physically compatible for at least 15 min	326	C
Droperidol	MN	2.5 mg/1 mL	ST	15 mg/1 mL	Physically compatible for at least 15 min	326	C
Fentanyl citrate	MN	0.05 mg/1 mL	ST	15 mg/1 mL	Physically compatible for at least 15 min	326	C
Glycopyrrolate	RB	0.2 mg/1 mL	LI	15 mg/1 mL	Physically compatible. pH in glycopyrrolate stability range for 48 hr at 25°C	331	C
Glycopyrrolate	RB	0.2 mg/1 mL	LI	30 mg/2 mL	Physically compatible. pH in glycopyrrolate stability range for 48 hr at 25°C	331	C
Glycopyrrolate	RB	0.4 mg/2 mL	LI	15 mg/1 mL	Physically compatible. pH in glycopyrrolate stability range for 48 hr at 25°C	331	C
Haloperidol lactate	MN	5 mg/1 mL		5 and 10 mg/1 mL[c]	Cloudiness forms immediately, becoming a crystalline precipitate of haloperidol and parabens	1901	I
Haloperidol lactate	MN	2 mg/mL	ME	20 mg/mL[a]	White precipitate of haloperidol forms on mixing	668	I
Heparin sodium	WY	100 and 200 units		1, 2, 5, 10 mg	Brought to 5 mL with NS. Physically compatible with no morphine loss in 24 hr at 23°C	985	C
Heparin sodium	WY	100 and 200 units		1, 2, 5 mg	Brought to 5 mL with W. Physically compatible with no morphine loss in 24 hr at 23°C	985	C
Heparin sodium	WY	100 and 200 units		10 mg	Brought to 5 mL with W. Immediate haze with precipitate and 5 to 7% morphine loss	985	I
Hydroxyzine HCl	PF	100 mg/4 mL	WY	15 mg/1 mL	Physically compatible for at least 15 min	14	C

Drugs in Syringe Compatibility (Cont.)

Test Drug	Mfr	Amt	Mfr	Amt	Remarks	Ref	C/I
Hydroxyzine HCl	PF	50 mg/1 mL	ST	15 mg/1 mL	Physically compatible for at least 15 min	326	C
Hydroxyzine HCl	PF	50 mg/1 mL		10 mg/0.7 mL	Physically compatible	771	C
Hydroxyzine HCl	PF	100 mg/2 mL		5 mg/0.3 mL	Physically compatible	771	C
Ketamine HCl	PD	1 mg/mL^e	SX	1 mg/mL^e, 10 mg/mL^e	At least 90% of both drugs retained for 6 days at room temperature	2260	C
Ketamine HCl	PD	1 mg/mL^e	SX	25 mg/mL^e	5% morphine loss in 6 days at room temperature. Up to 15% ketamine loss in 2 to 6 days	2260	C
Ketamine HCl	PD	10, 25 mg/mL^e	SX	1, 10, 25 mg/mL^e	At least 90% of both drugs retained for 6 days at room temperature	2260	C
Ketamine HCl		5, 10, 20 mg/1 mL		1 mg/1 mL	No substantial change in the concentration of either drug over 4 days	669	C
Ketamine HCl	SZ	2 mg/mL^e	SZ	2, 5, 10 mg/mL^e	Physically compatible. Little loss of either drug at 23 and 5°C in 91 days	2797	C
Ketamine HCl with lidocaine HCl	PD AST	2 mg/mL 2 mg/mL	ES	0.2 mg/mL	Diluted to 5 mL with NS. Visually compatible with no new GC/MS peaks in 1 hr at room temperature	1956	C
Lidocaine HCl with ketamine HCl	AST PD	2 mg/mL 2 mg/mL	ES	0.2 mg/mL	Diluted to 5 mL with NS. Visually compatible with no new GC/MS peaks in 1 hr at room temperature	1956	C
Meperidine HCl	WI	50 mg/1 mL	ST	15 mg/1 mL	Physically incompatible within 15 min	326	I
Metoclopramide HCl	NO	10 mg/2 mL	AH	10 mg/1 mL	Physically compatible for 15 min at room temperature	565	C
Metoclopramide HCl	SKB	0.5 mg/mL	EV	1 mg/mL	Diluted with NS. 5% or less loss of both drugs in 35 days at 22°C and 182 days at 4°C followed by 7 days at 32°C	1939	C
Metoclopramide HCl	RB	5 mg/mL	ME	25 mg/mL^a	Visually compatible with less than 10% drug loss in 7 days at 8°C	668	C
Midazolam HCl	RC	5 mg/1 mL	WB	10 mg/1 mL	Physically compatible for 4 hr at 25°C	1145	C
Midazolam HCl	RC	5 mg/1 mL		5 and 10 mg/1 mL^c	Visually compatible. 9% or less morphine and 8% or less midazolam loss in 14 days at 22°C in dark. Microprecipitate may form, requiring filtration	1901	C
Midazolam HCl	RC	5 mg/1 mL		5 and 10 mg/1 mL^d	Visually compatible. 8% or less morphine and 3% or less midazolam loss in 14 days at 22°C protected from light. Microprecipitate may form, requiring filtration	1901	C
Milrinone lactate	STR	5.25 mg/5.25 mL	WI	40 mg/5 mL	Physically compatible. No loss of either drug in 20 min at 23°C	1410	C
Ondansetron HCl	GW	1.33 mg/mL^e	ES	2.67 mg/mL^e	Physically compatible. Under 5% ondansetron and under 4% morphine losses in 24 hr at 4 or 23°C	2199	C
Pantoprazole sodium	^{b}	4 mg/1 mL		50 mg/1 mL	Yellowish precipitate	2574	I
Pentazocine lactate	WI	30 mg/1 mL	ST	15 mg/1 mL	Physically compatible for at least 15 min	326	C
Pentobarbital sodium	AB	500 mg/10 mL		16.2 mg/1 mL	Physically compatible	55	C
Pentobarbital sodium	WY	100 mg/2 mL	WY	15 mg/1 mL	Precipitate forms within 15 min	14	I
Pentobarbital sodium	AB	50 mg/1 mL	ST	15 mg/1 mL	Physically incompatible within 15 min	326	I
Prochlorperazine edisylate	SKF		WY	15 mg/1 mL	Physically compatible for at least 15 min	14	C
Prochlorperazine edisylate	PO	5 mg/1 mL	ST	15 mg/1 mL	Physically compatible for at least 15 min	326	C

Drugs in Syringe Compatibility (Cont.)

Test Drug	Mfr	Amt	Mfr	Amt	Remarks	Ref	C/I
Prochlorperazine edisylate	ES, SKF	10 mg/2 mL	WB	10 mg/1 mL	Precipitates immediately, probably due to phenol in morphine formulation	1006	I
Prochlorperazine edisylate	SKF	5 mg/1 mL	WY	8, 10, 15 mg/1 mL	Physically compatible for 24 hr at 25°C	1086	C
Promethazine HCl	WY	50 mg/2 mL	WY	15 mg/1 mL	Physically compatible for at least 15 min	14	C
Promethazine HCl	PO	50 mg/2 mL	ST	15 mg/1 mL	Physically compatible for at least 15 min	326	C
Promethazine HCl	WY	12.5 mg	WY	8 mg	Cloudiness develops	98	I
Ranitidine HCl	GL	50 mg/2 mL	AH	10 mg/1 mL	Physically compatible for 1 hr at 25°C	978	C
Ropivacaine HCl	FRK[i]	7.5 mg/mL[e]	CDM	3.5 mg/mL[e]	Visually compatible and chemically stable for up to 3 day at 5°C	3493	C
Ropivacaine HCl	FRK[i]	7.5 mg/mL[e]	CDM	3.5 mg/mL[e]	Chemically unstable after 6 hr at 21 and 31°C	3493	I
Salbutamol sulfate	GL	2.5 mg/2.5 mL[f]	AB	5 mg/0.5 mL	Physically compatible for 1 hr	1904	C
Scopolamine HBr		0.6 mg/1.5 mL	WY	15 mg/1 mL	Physically compatible for at least 15 min	14	C
Scopolamine HBr	ST	0.4 mg/1 mL	ST	15 mg/1 mL	Physically compatible for at least 15 min	326	C
Scopolamine HBr	BP	5 mg/5 mL	BP	500 mg/5 mL	Little scopolamine loss in 14 days at room temperature or 37°C. Morphine not tested	1609	C
Ziconotide acetate	ELN	25 mcg/mL	BB	35 mg/mL[h]	No loss of either drug in 17 days at 5°C	2702	C
Ziconotide acetate	EI[j]	1 mcg/mL[e]	CDM	3.5 mg/mL[e]	Visually compatible and chemically stable for up to 3 days at 5°C	3493	C
Ziconotide acetate	EI[j]	1 mcg/mL[e]	CDM	3.5 mg/mL[e]	Chemically unstable after 6 hr at 21 and 31°C	3493	I

[a] Tested in sterile water for injection.

[b] Test performed using the formulation WITHOUT edetate disodium.

[c] Morphine sulfate powder dissolved in dextrose 5%.

[d] Morphine sulfate powder dissolved in water and sodium chloride 0.9%.

[e] Tested in sodium chloride 0.9%.

[f] Both preserved (benzyl alcohol 0.9%; benzalkonium chloride 0.01%) and unpreserved sodium chloride 0.9% were used as a diluent.

[g] Extemporaneously compounded from bulk drug powders.

[h] Morphine sulfate powder dissolved in ziconotide acetate injection.

[i] Tested with ziconotide acetate (EI) 1 mcg/mL.

[j] Tested with ropivacaine HCl (FRK) 7.5 mg/mL.

Y-Site Injection Compatibility (1:1 Mixture)

Morphine sulfate

Test Drug	Mfr	Conc	Mfr	Conc	Remarks	Ref	C/I
Acetaminophen	CAD	10 mg/mL	BA	15 mg/mL	Physically compatible with less than 10% acetaminophen loss over 4 hr at room temperature	2841, 2844	C
Acetaminophen	CAD	10 mg/mL	WW	15 mg/mL	Physically compatible for 4 hr at 23°C	2901, 2902	C
Acyclovir sodium	BW	5 mg/mL[a]	WB	0.08 mg/mL[a]	Physically compatible for 4 hr at 25°C	1157	C
Acyclovir sodium	BW	5 mg/mL[a]	AB	1 mg/mL	Precipitate forms in 2 hr at 25°C	1397	I
Allopurinol sodium	BW	3 mg/mL[b]	WI	1 mg/mL[b]	Physically compatible for 4 hr at 22°C	1686	C
Amifostine	USB	10 mg/mL[a]	AST	1 mg/mL[a]	Physically compatible for 4 hr at 23°C	1845	C

Y-Site Injection Compatibility (1:1 Mixture) (Cont.)

Test Drug	Mfr	Conc	Mfr	Conc	Remarks	Ref	C/I
Amikacin sulfate	BR	5 mg/mL[a]	WI	1 mg/mL[a]	Physically compatible for 4 hr at 25°C	987	C
Aminophylline	ES	4 mg/mL[c]	WY	0.2 mg/mL[c]	Physically compatible for 3 hr	1316	C
Amiodarone HCl	WY	4.8 mg/mL[a]	SX	1 mg/mL[a]	Visually compatible for 24 hr at 23°C	1877	C
Amiodarone HCl	WY	6 mg/mL[a]	WY	1 mg/mL[a]	Visually compatible for 24 hr at 22°C	2352	C
Amiodarone HCl	WY	6 mg/mL[a]	WY	10 mg/mL	Visually compatible for 24 hr at 22°C	2352	C
Ampicillin sodium	BR	20 mg/mL[b]	WI	1 mg/mL[a]	Physically compatible for 4 hr at 25°C	987	C
Ampicillin sodium–sulbactam sodium	RR	20 mg/mL[b r]	ES	1 mg/mL[b]	Physically compatible for 1 hr at 25°C	1338	C
Amsacrine	NCI	1 mg/mL[a]	ES	1 mg/mL[a]	Visually compatible for 4 hr at 22°C	1381	C
Anidulafungin	VIC	0.5 mg/mL[a]	ES	15 mg/mL	Physically compatible for 4 hr at 23°C	2617	C
Argatroban	GSK	1 mg/mL[b]	ES	10 mg/mL	Visually compatible for 24 hr at 23°C	2391	C
Atracurium besylate	BW	0.5 mg/mL[a]	WY	1 mg/mL[a]	Physically compatible for 24 hr at 28°C	1337	C
Atropine sulfate	LY	0.4 mg/mL	AST	1 mg/mL[a]	Physically compatible for 48 hr at 22°C	1706	C
Azithromycin	PF	2 mg/mL[b]	WY	1 mg/mL[q]	White microcrystals found	2368	I
Aztreonam	SQ	20 mg/mL[a]	AB	1 mg/mL	Physically compatible for 4 hr at 25°C	1397	C
Aztreonam	SQ	40 mg/mL[a]	AST	1 mg/mL[a]	Physically compatible for 4 hr at 23°C	1758	C
Bivalirudin	TMC	5 mg/mL[a]	AST	1 mg/mL[a]	Physically compatible for 4 hr at 23°C	2373	C
Bivalirudin	TMC	5 mg/mL[a b]	ES	10 mg/mL	Visually compatible for 6 hr at 23°C	2680	C
Bumetanide	RC	0.25 mg/mL	AB	1 mg/mL	Physically compatible for 4 hr at 25°C	1397	C
Calcium chloride	AB	4 mg/mL[c]	WY	0.2 mg/mL[c]	Physically compatible for 3 hr	1316	C
Cangrelor tetrasodium	TMC	1 mg/mL[b]		1 mg/mL[b]	Physically compatible for 4 hr	3243	C
Caspofungin acetate	ME	0.7 mg/mL[b]	BA	15 mg/mL	Physically compatible for 4 hr at room temperature	2758	C
Caspofungin acetate	ME	0.5 mg/mL[b]	HOS	2 mg/mL	Physically compatible with morphine sulfate i.v. push over 2 to 5 min	2766	C
Cefazolin sodium	SKF	20 mg/mL[a]	WI	1 mg/mL[a]	Physically compatible for 4 hr at 25°C	987	C
Cefepime HCl	BMS	120 mg/mL[d]		1 mg/mL	Physically compatible with less than 10% cefepime loss. Morphine not tested	2513	C
Cefotaxime sodium	HO	20 mg/mL[a]	WI	1 mg/mL[a]	Physically compatible for 4 hr at 25°C	987	C
Cefotetan disodium	STU	20 and 40 mg/mL[a]	ES	1 mg/mL[b]	Physically compatible for 1 hr at 25°C	1338	C
Cefoxitin sodium	MSD	20 mg/mL[a]	WI	1 mg/mL[a]	Physically compatible for 4 hr at 25°C	987	C
Cefoxitin sodium	MSD	40 mg/mL[a]	ES	1 mg/mL[b]	Physically compatible for 1 hr at 25°C	1338	C
Ceftaroline fosamil	FOR	2.22 mg/mL[a b i]	BA	15 mg/mL	Physically compatible for 4 hr at 23°C	2826	C
Ceftazidime	LI	20 and 40 mg/mL[a]	AB	1 mg/mL	Physically compatible for 4 hr at 25°C	1397	C
Ceftazidime	GSK	120 mg/mL[d]		1 mg/mL	Physically compatible with less than 10% ceftazidime loss. Morphine not tested	2513	C
Ceftolozane sulfate–tazobactam sodium	CUB	30 mg/mL[a v]		1 mg/mL	Physically compatible with no loss of either drug in 4 hr at 25°C	2959	C

Y-Site Injection Compatibility (1:1 Mixture) (Cont.)

Test Drug	Mfr	Conc	Mfr	Conc	Remarks	Ref	C/I
Ceftolozane sulfate–tazobactam sodium	CUB	30 mg/mL[b v]		1 mg/mL	Physically compatible with no loss of either drug in 24 hr at 25°C	2959	C
Ceftolozane sulfate–tazobactam sodium	CUB	10 mg/mL[c v]	WW	1 mg/mL[c]	Physically compatible for 2 hr	3262	C
Ceftriaxone sodium	RC	20 and 40 mg/mL[a]	AB	1 mg/mL	Physically compatible for 4 hr at 25°C	1397	C
Cefuroxime sodium	GL	30 mg/mL[a]	WI	1 mg/mL[a]	Physically compatible for 4 hr at 25°C	987	C
Chloramphenicol sodium succinate	LY	20 mg/mL[a]	WI	1 mg/mL[a]	Physically compatible for 4 hr at 25°C	987	C
Cisatracurium besylate	GW	0.1, 2, 5 mg/mL[a]	AST	1 mg/mL[a]	Physically compatible for 4 hr at 23°C	2074	C
Cladribine	ORT	0.015[b] and 0.5[e] mg/mL	AST	1 mg/mL[b]	Physically compatible for 4 hr at 23°C	1969	C
Clindamycin phosphate	UP	12 mg/mL[a]	WI	1 mg/mL[a]	Physically compatible for 4 hr at 25°C	987	C
Cloxacillin sodium	SMX	100 mg/mL	SZ	50 mg/mL	Precipitates immediately	3245	I
Dexamethasone sodium phosphate	LY	0.2 mg/mL[a]	AB	1 mg/mL	Physically compatible for 4 hr at 25°C	1397	C
Dexamethasone sodium phosphate	AMR	1 mg/mL[a]	AST	1 mg/mL[a]	Physically compatible for 48 hr at 22°C	1706	C
Dexmedetomidine HCl	HOS	4 mcg/mL[b]			Stated to be compatible	3181	C
Diazepam	ES	0.5 mg/mL[a]	AST	1 mg/mL[a]	Physically compatible for 48 hr at 22°C	1706	C
Digoxin	BW	0.25 mg/mL	AB	1 mg/mL	Physically compatible for 4 hr at 25°C	1397	C
Diltiazem HCl	MMD	1[b] and 5 mg/mL	SCN	15 mg/mL	Visually compatible	1807	C
Diltiazem HCl	MMD	5 mg/mL	SCN	0.4 mg/mL[b]	Visually compatible	1807	C
Diltiazem HCl	MMD	1 mg/mL[a]	SCN	2 mg/mL[a]	Visually compatible for 4 hr at 27°C	2062	C
Diphenhydramine HCl	SCN	2 mg/mL[a]	AST	1 mg/mL[a]	Physically compatible for 48 hr at 22°C	1706	C
Dobutamine HCl	LI	4 mg/mL[a]	SCN	2 mg/mL[a]	Visually compatible for 4 hr at 27°C	2062	C
Docetaxel	RPR	0.9 mg/mL[a]	ES	1 mg/mL[a]	Physically compatible for 4 hr at 23°C	2224	C
Dopamine HCl	AB	1.6 mg/mL[a]	AB	1 mg/mL	Physically compatible for 4 hr at 25°C	1397	C
Dopamine HCl	AB	3.2 mg/mL[a]	SCN	2 mg/mL[a]	Visually compatible for 4 hr at 27°C	2062	C
Doripenem	JJ	5 mg/mL[a b]	BA	15 mg/mL	Physically compatible for 4 hr at 23°C	2743	C
Doxorubicin HCl liposomal	SEQ	0.4 mg/mL[a]	ES	1 mg/mL[a]	Partial loss of measured natural turbidity	2087	I
Doxycycline hyclate	ES	1 mg/mL[a]	WI	1 mg/mL[a]	Physically compatible for 4 hr at 25°C	987	C
Enalaprilat	MSD	0.05 mg/mL[b]	WY	0.2 mg/mL[a]	Physically compatible for 24 hr at room temperature under fluorescent light	1355	C
Epinephrine HCl	AB	0.02 mg/mL[a]	SCN	2 mg/mL[a]	Visually compatible for 4 hr at 27°C	2062	C
Eravacycline dihydrochloride	TET	0.6 mg/mL[b]	WW	1 mg/mL[b]	Physically compatible for 2 hr at room temperature	3532	C
Erythromycin lactobionate	AB	5 mg/mL[a]	WI	1 mg/mL[a]	Physically compatible for 4 hr at 25°C	987	C
Esmolol HCl	DCC	1 g/100 mL[f]	ES	15 mg/1 mL	Physically compatible when morphine is injected in Y-site[d]	1168	C
Esmolol HCl	DCC	10 mg/mL[f]	ES	15 mg/mL	Physically compatible. No drug loss in 8 hr at room temperature in light	1168	C

Y-Site Injection Compatibility (1:1 Mixture) (Cont.)

Test Drug	Mfr	Conc	Mfr	Conc	Remarks	Ref	C/I
Etomidate	AB	2 mg/mL	ES	10 mg/mL	Visually compatible for 7 days at 25°C	1801	C
Etoposide phosphate	BR	5 mg/mL[a]	ES	1 mg/mL[a]	Physically compatible for 4 hr at 23°C	2218	C
Famotidine	MSD	0.2 mg/mL[a]	ES	0.2 mg/mL[a]	Physically compatible for 4 hr at 25°C	1188	C
Famotidine	MSD	0.2 mg/mL[a]	AB	1 mg/mL	Physically compatible for 4 hr at 25°C	1397	C
Famotidine	ME	2 mg/mL[b]		1 mg/mL[a]	Visually compatible for 4 hr at 22°C	1936	C
Fenoldopam mesylate	AB	80 mcg/mL[b]	ES	1 mg/mL[b]	Physically compatible for 4 hr at 23°C	2467	C
Fentanyl citrate	ES	0.05 mg/mL	SCN	2 mg/mL[a]	Visually compatible for 4 hr at 27°C	2062	C
Filgrastim	AMG	30 mcg/mL[a]	WY	1 mg/mL[a]	Physically compatible for 4 hr at 22°C	1687	C
Fluconazole	RR	2 mg/mL	IMS	25 mg/mL	Physically compatible for 24 hr at 25°C	1407	C
Fluconazole	RR	2 mg/mL	AB	1 mg/mL	Physically compatible for 4 hr at 25°C	1397	C
Fludarabine phosphate	BX	1 mg/mL[a]	WI	1 mg/mL[a]	Visually compatible for 4 hr at 22°C	1439	C
Foscarnet sodium	AST	24 mg/mL	IMS	1 mg/mL	Physically compatible for 24 hr at room temperature under fluorescent light	1335	C
Foscarnet sodium	AST	24 mg/mL	ES	1 mg/mL[c]	Physically compatible for 24 hr at 25°C under fluorescent light	1393	C
Foscarnet sodium	AST	24 mg/mL	ES	5[b] and 15 mg/mL	Visually compatible for 24 hr at 23°C under fluorescent light	1529	C
Furosemide	ES	0.8[a], 2.4[a], 10 mg/mL	AB	1 mg/mL	White precipitate in 1 hr at 25°C	1397	I
Furosemide	AMR	10 mg/mL	SCN	2 mg/mL[a]	Visually compatible for 4 hr at 27°C	2062	C
Gallium nitrate	FUJ	1 mg/mL[b]	SCN	1 mg/mL[b]	Precipitate forms in 24 hr at 25°C	1673	I
Gemcitabine HCl	LI	10 mg/mL[b]	ES	1 mg/mL[b]	Physically compatible for 4 hr at 23°C	2226	C
Gentamicin sulfate	TR	0.8 mg/mL[a]	WI	1 mg/mL[a]	Physically compatible for 4 hr at 25°C	987	C
Gentamicin sulfate	ES	1.2 and 2 mg/mL[b]	ES	1 mg/mL[b]	Physically compatible for 1 hr at 25°C	1338	C
Granisetron HCl	SKB	1 mg/mL	AST	1 mg/mL[b]	Physically compatible with little or no loss of either drug in 4 hr at 22°C	1883	C
Granisetron HCl	SKB	0.05 mg/mL[a]	AST	1 mg/mL[a]	Physically compatible for 4 hr at 23°C	2000	C
Haloperidol lactate	MN	0.2 mg/mL[a]	AST	1 mg/mL[a]	Physically compatible for 48 hr at 22°C	1706	C
Heparin sodium	UP	1000 units/L[h]	WY	15 mg/mL	Physically compatible for 4 hr at room temperature	534	C
Heparin sodium	ES	50 units/mL[c]	WY	0.2 mg/mL[c]	Physically compatible for 3 hr	1316	C
Heparin sodium	ES	60 units/mL[a]	ES	1 mg/mL[b]	Physically compatible for 1 hr at 25°C	1338	C
Heparin sodium	ES	100 units/mL[a]	SCN	2 mg/mL[a]	Visually compatible for 4 hr at 27°C	2062	C
Hetastarch in lactated electrolyte	AB	6%	AST	1 mg/mL[a]	Physically compatible for 4 hr at 23°C	2339	C
Hydrocortisone sodium succinate	UP	10 mg/L[f]	WY	15 mg/mL	Physically compatible for 4 hr at room temperature	534	C
Hydromorphone HCl	KN	1 mg/mL	SCN	2 mg/mL[a]	Visually compatible for 4 hr at 27°C	2062	C

Y-Site Injection Compatibility (1:1 Mixture) (Cont.)

Test Drug	Mfr	Conc	Mfr	Conc	Remarks	Ref	C/I
Hydroxyethyl starch 130/0.4 in sodium chloride 0.9%	FRK	6%	SZ	1, 5, 10 mg/mL[a]	Visually compatible for 24 hr at room temperature	2770	C
Hydroxyzine HCl	WI	4 mg/mL[a]	AST	1 mg/mL[a]	Physically compatible for 48 hr at 22°C	1706	C
Ibuprofen lysinate	OVA	10 mg/mL	HOS	0.5 mg/mL[c]	Physically compatible for 4 hr at room temperature	3541	C
Ibuprofen lysinate	OVA	10 mg/mL	HOS	50 mg/mL	Measured turbidity increased immediately and solution became milky white and opaque	3541	I
Insulin, regular	LI	0.2 unit/mL[b]	ES	1 mg/mL[b]	Physically compatible for 1 hr at 25°C	1338	C
Insulin, regular	LI	0.2 unit/mL[b]	ES	5 mg/mL[b]	Physically compatible for 2 hr at 25°C	1395	C
Insulin, regular	LI	1 unit/mL[a]	SX	1 mg/mL[a]	Visually compatible for 24 hr at 23°C	1877	C
Isavuconazonium sulfate	ASP	1.5 mg/mL[c]	WW	1 mg/mL[c]	Physically compatible for 2 hr	3263	C
Ketorolac tromethamine	WY	1 mg/mL[a]	AST	1 mg/mL[a]	Physically compatible for 48 hr at 22°C	1706	C
Labetalol HCl	SC	1 mg/mL[a]	WY	1 mg/mL[a]	Physically compatible for 24 hr at 18°C	1171	C
Labetalol HCl	GL	5 mg/mL	AB	1 mg/mL	Physically compatible for 4 hr at 25°C	1397	C
Labetalol HCl	GL	1 mg/mL[a]	ES	0.5 mg/mL[a]	Visually compatible. Little loss of either drug in 4 hr at room temperature	1762	C
Labetalol HCl	AH	2 mg/mL[a]	SCN	2 mg/mL[a]	Visually compatible for 4 hr at 27°C	2062	C
Letermovir	ME	[a]		[a]	Physically compatible	3398	C
Levofloxacin	OMN	5 mg/mL[a]	SW	4 mg/mL	Visually compatible for 4 hr at 24°C	2233	C
Lidocaine HCl	AB	1 mg/mL[a]	AB	1 mg/mL	Physically compatible for 4 hr at 25°C	1397	C
Linezolid	PHU	2 mg/mL	AST	1 mg/mL[a]	Physically compatible for 4 hr at 23°C	2264	C
Lorazepam	WY	0.5 mg/mL[a]	SCN	2 mg/mL[a]	Visually compatible for 4 hr at 27°C	2062	C
Lorazepam	WY	0.1 mg/mL[a]	AST	1 mg/mL[a]	Physically compatible for 48 hr at 22°C	1706	C
Magnesium sulfate	LY	16.7, 33.3, 50, 100 mg/mL[a]	ES	1 mg/mL[a]	Visually compatible for 4 hr at 25°C	1549	C
Magnesium sulfate	AB	2, 4, 8 mg/mL[b]	j	2 mg/mL[b]	Visually compatible for 8 hr at room temperature	1719	C
Melphalan HCl	BW	0.1 mg/mL[b]	WI	1 mg/mL[b]	Physically compatible for 3 hr at 22°C	1557	C
Meropenem	ZEN	1 and 50 mg/mL[b]	ES	1 mg/mL[d]	Visually compatible for 4 hr at room temperature	1994	C
Meropenem		50 mg/mL	SZ	50 mg/mL	Physically compatible for 4 hr at room temperature	3538	C
Meropenem–vaborbactam	TMC	8 mg/mL[b,u]	WW	1 mg/mL[b]	Physically compatible for 3 hr at 20 to 25°C	3380	C
Methotrimeprazine HCl	LE	0.2 mg/mL[a]	AST	1 mg/mL[a]	Physically compatible for 48 hr at 22°C	1706	C
Methyldopate HCl	AMR	2.5 mg/mL[a]	AB	1 mg/mL	Physically compatible for 4 hr at 25°C	1397	C
Methylprednisolone sodium succinate	UP	2.5 mg/mL[a]	AB	1 mg/mL	Physically compatible for 4 hr at 25°C	1397	C
Metoclopramide HCl	SN	0.2 mg/mL[a]	AB	1 mg/mL	Physically compatible for 4 hr at 25°C	1397	C
Metoclopramide HCl	DU	5 mg/mL	AST	1 mg/mL[a]	Physically compatible for 48 hr at 22°C	1706	C
Metoprolol tartrate	CI	1 mg/mL	AB	1 mg/mL	Physically compatible for 4 hr at 25°C	1397	C

Y-Site Injection Compatibility (1:1 Mixture) (Cont.)

Test Drug	Mfr	Conc	Mfr	Conc	Remarks	Ref	C/I
Metronidazole	SE	5 mg/mL	WI	1 mg/mL[a]	Physically compatible for 4 hr at 25°C	987	C
Micafungin sodium	ASP	1.5 mg/mL[b]	APP	15 mg/mL	White precipitate forms immediately	2683	I
Midazolam HCl	RC	0.2 mg/mL[a]	AST	1 mg/mL[a]	Physically compatible for 48 hr at 22°C	1706	C
Midazolam HCl	RC	0.1 and 0.5 mg/mL[a]	ES	0.25 mg/mL[a]	Visually compatible with no loss of either drug in 3 hr at 24°C	1789	C
Midazolam HCl	RC	0.1 and 0.5 mg/mL[a]	ES	1 mg/mL[a]	Visually compatible with no loss of either drug in 3 hr at 24°C	1789	C
Midazolam HCl	RC	1 mg/mL[a]	SX	1 mg/mL[a]	Visually compatible for 24 hr at 23°C	1877	C
Midazolam HCl	RC	2 mg/mL[a]	SCN	2 mg/mL[a]	Visually compatible for 4 hr at 27°C	2062	C
Milrinone lactate	SW	0.2 mg/mL[a]	SCN	2 mg/mL[a]	Visually compatible for 4 hr at 27°C	2062	C
Milrinone lactate	SW	0.4 mg/mL[a]	AST	1 mg/mL[a]	Visually compatible. Little loss of either drug in 4 hr at 23°C	2214	C
Milrinone lactate	SS	0.2 mg/mL[a]	FAU	25 mg/mL[a]	Visually compatible for 4 hr at 25°C	2381	C
Nafcillin sodium	WY	20 mg/mL[a]	WI	1 mg/mL[a]	Physically compatible for 4 hr at 25°C	987	C
Nafcillin sodium	WY	30 mg/mL[a]	ES	1 mg/mL[b]	Physically compatible for 1 hr at 25°C	1338	C
Nesiritide	SCI	50 mcg/mL[a b]		15 mg/mL	Physically compatible for 4 hr. May be chemically incompatible with nesiritide[k]	2625	?
Nicardipine HCl	WY	1 mg/mL[a]	SCN	2 mg/mL[a]	Visually compatible for 4 hr at 27°C	2062	C
Nicardipine HCl	DCC	0.1 mg/mL[a]	WY	0.2 mg/mL[a]	Visually compatible for 24 hr at room temperature	235	C
Nitroglycerin	AB	0.4 mg/mL[a]	SCN	2 mg/mL[a]	Visually compatible for 4 hr at 27°C	2062	C
Norepinephrine bitartrate	STR	0.064 mg/mL[a]	SX	1 mg/mL[a]	Visually compatible for 24 hr at 23°C	1877	C
Norepinephrine bitartrate	AB	0.128 mg/mL[a]	SCN	2 mg/mL[a]	Visually compatible for 4 hr at 27°C	2062	C
Ondansetron HCl	GL	1 mg/mL[b]	WI	1 mg/mL[a]	Visually compatible for 4 hr at 22°C	1365	C
Oritavancin diphosphate	TAR	0.8, 1.2, and 2 mg/mL[a]	HOS	1 mg/mL[a]	Visually compatible for 4 hr at 20 to 24°C	2928	C
Oxacillin sodium	BE	20 mg/mL[a]	WI	1 mg/mL[a]	Physically compatible for 4 hr at 25°C	987	C
Oxaliplatin	SS	0.5 mg/mL[a]	ES	15 mg/mL	Physically compatible for 4 hr at 23°C	2566	C
Oxytocin	PD	0.02 unit/mL[m]	ES	1 mg/mL[b]	Physically compatible for 1 hr at 25°C	1338	C
Paclitaxel	NCI	1.2 mg/mL[a]	WY	1 mg/mL[a]	Physically compatible for 4 hr at 22°C	1556	C
Palonosetron HCl	MGI	50 mcg/mL	BA	15 mg/mL	Physically compatible. No loss of either drug in 4 hr	2720	C
Pancuronium bromide	ES	0.05 mg/mL[a]	WY	1 mg/mL[a]	Physically compatible for 24 hr at 28°C	1337	C
Pantoprazole sodium	ALT[l]	0.16 to 0.8 mg/mL[b]	AB	1 to 10 mg/mL[a]	Visually compatible for 12 hr at 23°C	2603	C
Pemetrexed disodium	LI	20 mg/mL[b]	ES	15 mg/mL	Physically compatible for 4 hr at 23°C	2564	C
Penicillin G potassium	PF	100,000 units/mL[a]	WI	1 mg/mL[a]	Physically compatible for 4 hr at 25°C	987	C
Phenobarbital sodium	WY	2 mg/mL[a]	AST	1 mg/mL[a]	Physically compatible for 48 hr at 22°C	1706	C
Phenytoin sodium	ES	2 mg/mL[a b]	AST	1 mg/mL[a]	Precipitate forms after 1 hr	1706	I
Piperacillin sodium–tazobactam sodium	LE[l]	40 mg/mL[a s]	WY	1 mg/mL[a]	Physically compatible for 4 hr at 22°C	1688	C

Y-Site Injection Compatibility (1:1 Mixture) (Cont.)

Test Drug	Mfr	Conc	Mfr	Conc	Remarks	Ref	C/I
Plazomicin sulfate	ACH	24 mg/mL^c	WW	1 mg/mL^c	Physically compatible for 1 hr at 20 to 25°C	3432	C
Posaconazole	ME	18 mg/mL		1 mg/mL^c	Physically compatible	2911, 2912	C
Potassium chloride	AB	40 mEq/L^f	WY	15 mg/mL	Physically compatible for 4 hr at room temperature	534	C
Propofol	ZEN^x	10 mg/mL	AST	1 mg/mL^a	Physically compatible for 1 hr at 23°C	2066	C
Propranolol HCl	WY	1 mg/mL	AB	1 mg/mL	Physically compatible for 4 hr at 25°C	1397	C
Ranitidine HCl	GL	0.5 mg/mL^n	ES	1 mg/mL^b	Physically compatible for 1 hr at 25°C	1338	C
Ranitidine HCl	GL	1 mg/mL^a	SCN	2 mg/mL^a	Visually compatible for 4 hr at 27°C	2062	C
Remifentanil HCl	GW	0.025 and 0.25 mg/mL^b	AST	1 mg/mL^a	Physically compatible for 4 hr at 23°C	2075	C
Sargramostim	IMM	10 mcg/mL^b	WI	1 mg/mL^b	Slight haze and particles in 1 hr	1436	I
Scopolamine HBr	LY	0.05 mg/mL^a	AST	1 mg/mL^a	Physically compatible for 48 hr at 22°C	1706	C
Sodium bicarbonate	AB	1 mEq/mL	WY	0.2 mg/mL^c	Physically compatible for 3 hr	1316	C
Sodium nitroprusside	RC	0.2 mg/mL^a	SX	1 mg/mL^a	Visually compatible for 24 hr at 23°C	1877	C
Sodium nitroprusside	RC	0.3, 1.2, 3 mg/mL^a	AB	0.5 mg/mL^g	Visually compatible for 48 hr at 24°C protected from light	2357	C
Sodium nitroprusside	RC	1.2 and 3 mg/mL^a	AB	1 mg/mL^g	Visually compatible for 48 hr at 24°C protected from light	2357	C
Tacrolimus	FUJ	10 and 40 mcg/mL^b	SCN	1 and 3 mg/mL^b	Visually compatible. No loss of either drug in 4 hr at 24°C	2216	C
Tedizolid phosphate	CUB	0.8 mg/mL^b	WW	1 mg/mL^b	Physically compatible for 2 hr	3244	C
Teniposide	BR	0.1 mg/mL^a	AST	1 mg/mL^a	Physically compatible for 4 hr at 23°C	1725	C
Thiotepa	IMM^o	1 mg/mL^a	AST	1 mg/mL^a	Physically compatible for 4 hr at 23°C	1861	C
Tigecycline	ACD, FRK, WY	^{c}	^{w}		Stated to be compatible	2915, 3459, 3460	C
Tirofiban HCl	ME	50 mcg/mL$^{a\,b}$	ES	0.1 and 1 mg/mL^a	Physically compatible. No loss of either drug in 4 hr at 23°C	2356	C
TNA #218 to #226^p			ES	1 mg/mL^a	Visually compatible for 4 hr at 23°C	2215	C
TNA #218 to #226^p			ES	15 mg/mL	Damage to emulsion occurs immediately with free oil formation possible	2215	I
Tobramycin sulfate	DI	0.8 mg/mL^a	WI	1 mg/mL^a	Physically compatible for 4 hr at 25°C	987	C
Tobramycin sulfate	LI	1.6, 2, 2.4 mg/mL^a	ES	1 mg/mL^b	Physically compatible for 1 hr at 25°C	1338	C
TPN #131, #132^p			AB	1 mg/mL	Physically compatible for 4 hr at 25°C	1397	C
TPN #189^p			DB	30 mg/mL	Visually compatible for 24 hr at 22°C	1767	C
TPN #203, #204^p			ES	1 mg/mL	Visually compatible for 2 hr at 23°C	1974	C
TPN #212 to #215^p			AST	1 mg/mL^a	Physically compatible for 4 hr at 23°C	2109	C
Trimethoprim–sulfamethoxazole	BW	0.8 mg/mL$^{a\,t}$	WI	1 mg/mL^a	Physically compatible for 4 hr at 25°C	987	C
Vancomycin HCl	LI	5 mg/mL^a	WI	1 mg/mL^a	Physically compatible for 4 hr at 25°C	987	C

Y-Site Injection Compatibility (1:1 Mixture) (Cont.)

Test Drug	Mfr	Conc	Mfr	Conc	Remarks	Ref	C/I
Vecuronium bromide	OR	0.1 mg/mL[a]	WY	1 mg/mL[a]	Physically compatible for 24 hr at 28°C	1337	C
Vecuronium bromide	OR	1 mg/mL	SCN	2 mg/mL[a]	Visually compatible for 4 hr at 27°C	2062	C
Vinorelbine tartrate	BW	1 mg/mL[b]	WI	1 mg/mL[b]	Physically compatible for 4 hr at 22°C	1558	C
Zidovudine	BW	4 mg/mL[a]	ES	1 mg/mL[a]	Physically compatible for 4 hr at 25°C	1193	C

[a] Tested in dextrose 5%.

[b] Tested in sodium chloride 0.9%.

[c] Tested in both dextrose 5% and sodium chloride 0.9%.

[d] Tested in sterile water for injection.

[e] Tested in bacteriostatic sodium chloride 0.9% preserved with benzyl alcohol 0.9%.

[f] Tested in dextrose 5% in sodium chloride 0.9%.

[g] Tested in dextrose 5% in sodium chloride 0.225%.

[h] Tested in dextrose 5% in Ringer's injection, dextrose 5% in Ringer's injection, lactated, dextrose 5%, Ringer's injection, lactated, and sodium chloride 0.9%.

[i] Tested in Ringer's injection, lactated.

[j] Extemporaneously prepared product.

[k] Nesiritide is incompatible with bisulfite antioxidants used in some drug formulations. The specific formulation of the product to be used should be checked to ensure that no sulfite antioxidants are present.

[l] Test performed using the formulation WITHOUT edetate disodium.

[m] Tested in dextrose 5% in Ringer's injection, lactated.

[n] Tested in sodium chloride 0.45%.

[o] Lyophilized formulation tested.

[p] Refer to Appendix for the composition of parenteral nutrition solutions. TNA indicates a 3-in-1 admixture, and TPN indicates a 2-in-1 admixture.

[q] Injected via Y-site into an administration set running azithromycin.

[r] Ampicillin component. Ampicillin in a 2:1 fixed-ratio concentration with sulbactam.

[s] Piperacillin component. Piperacillin in an 8:1 fixed-ratio concentration with tazobactam.

[t] Trimethoprim component. Trimethoprim in a 1:5 fixed-ratio concentration with sulfamethoxazole.

[u] Meropenem component. Meropenem in a 1:1 fixed-ratio concentration with vaborbactam.

[v] Ceftolozane component. Ceftolozane in a 2:1 fixed-ratio concentration with tazobactam.

[w] Salt not specified.

[x] Test performed using the formulation WITH edetate disodium.

Additional Compatibility Information

Bupivacaine

Bupivacaine hydrochloride 25 mg/mL admixed with morphine sulfate 50 mg/mL in sterile water for injection appeared to prevent the formation of precipitation that occurs with morphine sulfate 50 mg/mL alone when refrigerated.[2378]

Bupivacaine hydrochloride 2.5 mg/mL admixed with morphine sulfate 5 mg/mL in sodium chloride 0.9% and bupivacaine hydrochloride 25 mg/mL admixed with morphine sulfate 50 mg/mL in sterile water for injection exhibited little or no loss of either drug in 60 days at 4 and 23°C. The slight yellow discoloration that appeared in the high concentration samples was not indicative of drug decomposition. Samples stored for 2 days at 37°C and frozen for 2 days at −20°C resulted in little or no loss of either drug. However, the frozen samples upon thawing exhibited the formation of large amounts of microparticulates numbering in the thousands per mL, possibly shed by the syringe components.[2378]

Clonidine Hydrochloride

Clonidine hydrochloride (Fujisawa) 100 mcg/mL and morphine sulfate (Elkins-Sinn) 10 mg/mL were mixed in equal quantities, transferred to flint glass vials with rubber stoppers, and stored for 14 days at controlled room temperature protected from light. The solutions remained clear and colorless with no increase in particulate content. Little or no change in the concentration of either drug occurred.[2069]

Clonidine hydrochloride 0.25 mg/mL admixed with morphine sulfate 5 mg/mL in sodium chloride 0.9% and clonidine hydrochloride 4 mg/mL admixed with morphine sulfate 50 mg/mL in sterile water for injection exhibited little or no loss of either drug at 4 and 23°C. The slight yellow discoloration that appeared in the high concentration samples was not indicative of drug decomposition. Samples stored for 2 days at 37°C and frozen for 2 days at −20°C resulted in little or no loss of either drug. However, a precipitate formed in the frozen samples as freezing occurred and in the refrigerated high concentration samples after 2 to 4 days. Upon warming to room temperature the precipitate redissolved, but the samples exhibited large amounts of undissolved microparticulates numbering in the thousands per mL remaining in the solutions, possibly shed by the syringe components.[2380]

Moxifloxacin Hydrochloride
AHFS 8:12.18

Products

Moxifloxacin hydrochloride (Avelox, Merck) is available as a single-use (preservative-free), premixed, ready-to-use solution of moxifloxacin 400 mg in 250 mL of sodium chloride 0.8% in a flexible container.[3175] Hydrochloric acid and/or sodium hydroxide may have been added to adjust the pH.[3175] No further dilution of the solution is necessary.[3175]

Moxifloxacin hydrochloride (Fresenius Kabi) also is available as a single-use, premixed, ready-to-use solution of moxifloxacin 400 mg in a flexible plastic (Freeflex) container.[3176] Each 250-mL bag also contains sodium acetate trihydrate 1702.5 mg and disodium sulfate 2840 mg in water for injection.[3176] Sulfuric acid may have been added to adjust the pH.[3176]

Equivalency

Moxifloxacin hydrochloride 437.5 mg is equivalent to moxifloxacin 400 mg.[3176]

pH

The pH of moxifloxacin hydrochloride (Avelox) solution is from 4.1 to 4.6.[3175] The pH of moxifloxacin hydrochloride (Fresenius Kabi) solution is from 5 to 6.[3176]

Sodium Content

Each 250 mL of moxifloxacin hydrochloride (Avelox, Merck) solution contains approximately 34.2 mEq (787 mg) of sodium.[3175]

Each 250 mL of moxifloxacin hydrochloride (Fresenius Kabi) solution contains approximately 52.5 mEq (1207 mg) of sodium.[3176]

Trade Name(s)

Avelox

Administration

Moxifloxacin hydrochloride is administered intravenously by slow infusion over 60 minutes.[3175][3176] The solution may be infused directly or through a Y-type infusion set.[3175][3176] The solution must *not* be infused rapidly or as a bolus; it also is not intended for intra-arterial, intramuscular, intrathecal, intraperitoneal, or subcutaneous administration.[3175][3176]

Moxifloxacin hydrochloride should not be infused simultaneously through a line being used to administer other drugs.[3175][3176] If a common intravenous line is being used to administer other drugs in addition to moxifloxacin hydrochloride, the infusion line should be flushed prior to and following infusion of moxifloxacin hydrochloride solution with a compatible infusion solution.[3175][3176]

Stability

Moxifloxacin hydrochloride injection is a clear yellow solution.[3175][3176] One manufacturer notes that this yellow color is not affected by nor indicative of the stability of the product.[3175]

Intact containers of moxifloxacin hydrochloride should be stored at controlled room temperature.[3175][3176] The solution should not be refrigerated because precipitation may result.[3175][3176] Because of light sensitivity, moxifloxacin hydrochloride (Fresenius Kabi) solution should be stored in its overwrap until immediately prior to use.[3176]

Moxifloxacin hydrochloride solution should be visually inspected for particulate matter and discoloration prior to administration; if particulate matter is present or discoloration occurs, the solution should not be used.[3175][3176] Any unused portion of the solution should be discarded.[3175][3176]

Compatibility Information
Solution Compatibility

Moxifloxacin HCl

Test Soln Name	Mfr	Mfr	Conc/L or %	Remarks	Ref	C/I
Dextrose 5%		ME, FRK	a	Compatible	3175, 3176	C
Dextrose 10%		ME, FRK	a	Compatible	3175, 3176	C
Ringer's injection, lactated		ME, FRK	a	Compatible	3175, 3176	C
Sodium chloride 0.9%		ME, FRK	a	Compatible	3175, 3176	C

a Combined in ratios from 1:10 to 10:1.

DOI: 10.37573/9781585286850.275

Y-Site Injection Compatibility (1:1 Mixture)

Moxifloxacin HCl

Test Drug	Mfr	Conc	Mfr	Conc	Remarks	Ref	C/I
Cangrelor tetrasodium	TMC	1 mg/mL[b]		1.6 mg/mL	Physically compatible for 4 hr	3243	C
Ceftaroline fosamil	FOR	2.22 mg/mL[a b c]	BAY	1.6 mg/mL	Physically compatible for 4 hr at 23°C	2826	C
Doripenem	JJ	5 mg/mL[a b]	BAY	1.6 mg/mL	Physically compatible for 4 hr at 23°C	2743	C
Hydroxyethyl starch 130/0.4 in sodium chloride 0.9%	FRK	6%	BAY	0.4[a], 0.8[a], 1.6 mg/mL	Visually compatible for 24 hr at room temperature	2770	C
Norepinephrine bitartrate	HOS	64 mcg/mL[a]	ME	1.6 mg/mL	Physically compatible with little to no loss of either drug in 4 hr at room temperature	3510	C
Vasopressin	APP	0.2 unit/mL[b]	BAY	1.6 mg/mL	Physically compatible	2641	C

[a] Tested in dextrose 5%.

[b] Tested in sodium chloride 0.9%.

[c] Tested in Ringer's injection, lactated.

Additional Compatibility Information

Peritoneal Dialysis Solutions

Moxifloxacin hydrochloride 25 mg/mL in 2 peritoneal dialysis solutions was evaluated for stability. No color change or precipitation occurred. In Dianeal PD1 1.36% and 3.86%, moxifloxacin hydrochloride lost 2% and 9%, respectively, in 14 days at 4°C, and 3% and 11%, respectively, in 7 days at 25°C. Losses at 37°C were higher. In Dianeal PD1 1.36%, 10% loss occurred in 3 days; in Dianeal PD1 3.86%, 7% loss occurred in 12 hours and 13% loss occurred in 24 hours.[2712]

Selected Revisions January 31, 2020. © Copyright, October 2010. American Society of Health-System Pharmacists, Inc.

Multivitamins
AHFS 88:28

Products

Multivitamin products for parenteral administration are available in a variety of compositions and sizes. The following products are representative formulations.

M.V.I. Adult is available as a package of 2 vials (labeled Vial 1 and Vial 2) that are prepared for use by transferring the contents of Vial 1 into Vial 2 and mixing gently. After mixing, the product contains:[1(5/07)]

Ascorbic acid	200 mg
Vitamin A (retinol)	1 mg
Vitamin D (ergocalciferol)	5 mcg
Thiamine (as hydrochloride)	6 mg
Riboflavin (as 5'-phosphate sodium)	3.6 mg
Pyridoxine hydrochloride	6 mg
Niacinamide	40 mg
Dexpanthenol	15 mg
Vitamin E (dl-α tocopheryl acetate)	10 mg
Vitamin K	150 mcg
Folic acid	600 mcg
Biotin	60 mcg
Vitamin B_{12} (cyanocobalamin)	5 mcg

The product also contains propylene glycol 30%, polysorbate 80 1.4%, citric acid, and sodium hydroxide and/or hydrochloric acid in water for injection. The concentrated vitamins must be diluted for use; do not give undiluted.[1(5/07)]

M.V.I.-12 has the same vitamin content as M.V.I. Adult except for the absence of vitamin K.[1(5/07)]

M.V.I. Pediatric is available as a lyophilized powder in vials containing a single dose. Each single dose contains:[1(5/07)]

Ascorbic acid	80 mg
Vitamin A (retinol)	0.7 mg
Vitamin D (ergocalciferol)	10 mcg
Thiamine (as hydrochloride)	1.2 mg
Riboflavin (as 5'-phosphate sodium)	1.4 mg
Pyridoxine (as hydrochloride)	1 mg
Niacinamide	17 mg
Dexpanthenol	5 mg

Vitamin E (dl-alpha tocopheryl acetate)	7 mg
Biotin	20 mcg
Folic acid	140 mcg
Cyanocobalamin	1 mcg
Phytonadione	200 mcg

M.V.I. Pediatric also contains, in each vial, mannitol 375 mg, polysorbate 80 50 mg, polysorbate 20 0.8 mg, butylated hydroxytoluene 58 mcg, butylated hydroxyanisole 14 mcg, and sodium hydroxide for pH adjustment.[1(5/07)]

Reconstitute the single-dose vial with 5 mL of sterile water for injection, dextrose 5%, or sodium chloride 0.9% and swirl gently. The solution is ready within 3 minutes. This solution must be further diluted for use; do not give it undiluted.[1(5/07)]

Administration

Multivitamin infusion preparations are administered by intravenous infusion only. They should not be given by direct intravenous injection. M.V.I. Adult is diluted in not less than 500 mL but preferably 1000 mL of intravenous infusion solution for administration. M.V.I. Pediatric should be added to at least 100 mL of a compatible intravenous infusion solution for administration.[1(5/07)]

Stability

Multivitamin products for infusion should be stored under refrigeration and protected from light. Since some of the vitamins, especially A, D, and riboflavin, are light sensitive, light protection is necessary. After reconstitution of M.V.I. Pediatric, use of the product without delay is recommended. However, if this is not possible, the manufacturer permits use within a maximum of 4 hours from the initial penetration of the closure.[1(5/07)]

Light Effects

The effects of photoirradiation on a FreAmine II–dextrose 10% parenteral nutrition solution containing 1 mL/500 mL of multivitamins (USV) were evaluated. During simulated continuous administration to an infant at 0.156 mL/min, the amino acids were stable when the bottle, infusion tubing, and collection bottle were shielded with foil. Only 20 cm of tubing in the incubator was exposed to light. However, if the flow was stopped, marked reductions in methionine (40%), tryptophan (44%), and histidine (22%) occurred in the solution exposed to light for 24 hours. In a similar solution without vitamins, only the tryptophan concentration decreased. The difference was attributed to the presence of riboflavin, a photosensitizer. The authors recommended administering the multivitamins separately and shielding from light.[833]

DOI: 10.37573/9781585286850.276

The stability of 5 B vitamins was studied over 8 hours in representative parenteral nutrition solutions exposed to fluorescent light, indirect sunlight, or direct sunlight. One 5-mL vial of multivitamin concentrate (Lyphomed) and 1 mg of folic acid (Lederle) were added to a liter of parenteral nutrition solution composed of amino acids 4.25% and dextrose 25% (Travenol) with standard electrolytes and trace elements. The 5 B vitamins were stable for 8 hours at room temperature when exposed to fluorescent light. In addition, folic acid and niacinamide were stable over 8 hours in direct or indirect sunlight. Exposure to indirect sunlight appeared to have little or no effect on thiamine hydrochloride and pyridoxine hydrochloride in 8 hours, but riboflavin-5'-phosphate lost 47%. Direct sunlight caused a 26% loss of thiamine hydrochloride and an 86% loss of pyridoxine hydrochloride in 8 hours. A 4-hour exposure of riboflavin-5'-phosphate to direct sunlight resulted in a 98% loss.[842]

A parenteral nutrition solution in glass bottles exposed to sunlight was studied. Vitamin A decomposed rapidly, losing more than 50% in 3 hours. The decomposition could be slowed by covering the bottle with a light-resistant vinyl bag, resulting in about a 25% loss in 3 hours. Vitamin E was stable in the parenteral nutrition solution in glass bottles exposed to sunlight, with no loss occurring during 6 hours of exposure.[1040]

Vitamin A rapidly and significantly decomposes when exposed to daylight. The extent and rate of loss were dependent on the degree of exposure to daylight which, in turn, depended on various factors such as the direction of the radiation, time of day, and climatic conditions. Delivery of less than 10% of the expected amount was reported.[1047] In controlled light experiments, the decomposition initially progressed exponentially. Subsequently, the rate of decomposition slowed. This result was attributed to a protective effect of the degradation products on the remaining vitamin A. The presence of amino acids provided greater protection. Compared to degradation rates in dextrose 5%, decomposition was reduced by up to 50% in some amino acid mixtures.[1048]

The stability of several water-soluble vitamins in dextrose 5% and sodium chloride 0.9% in polyvinyl chloride (PVC) and Clear-Flex containers was evaluated. Thiamine, riboflavin, ascorbic acid, and folic acid were stable at 23°C when protected from light, exhibiting 10% or less loss in 24 hours. When exposed to light, thiamine and folic acid were stable but ascorbic acid was reduced by approximately 50 to 65% and riboflavin was completely lost.[1509]

The stability of phytonadione in a TPN solution containing amino acids 2%, dextrose 12.5%, "standard" electrolytes, and M.V.I. Pediatric over 24 hours while exposed to light was evaluated. Vitamin loss was about 7% in 4 hours and 27% in 24 hours. Some loss was attributed to the light sensitivity of the phytonadione.[1815]

Substantial loss of retinol all-*trans* palmitate and phytonadione was reported from both TPN and TNA admixtures due to exposure to sunlight. In 3 hours of exposure to sunlight, essentially total loss of retinol and 50% loss of phytonadione had occurred. The presence or absence of lipids did not affect stability. In contrast, tocopherol concentrations remained

essentially unchanged by exposure to sunlight through 12 hours. The container material used to store the nutrition admixtures affected the concentration of the vitamins as well. Losses were greatest (10 to 25%) in PVC containers and were slightly better in EVA and glass containers.[2049]

Sorption

The following vitamins did not reveal significant sorption to a PVC plastic test strip in 24 hours:[12]

Ascorbic acid
Niacinamide
Pyridoxine hydrochloride
Riboflavin
Thiamine hydrochloride
Vitamin D
Vitamin E acetate

Riboflavin was shown not to exhibit sorption to PVC bags and tubing, polyethylene tubing, Silastic tubing, and polypropylene syringes.[536 606]

Vitamin A (as the acetate) (Sigma) 7.5 mg/L displayed 66.7% sorption to a PVC plastic test strip in 24 hours. The presence of dextrose 5% and sodium chloride 0.9% increased the extent of the sorption.[12]

In another report, vitamin A acetate 3 mg/L displayed 78% sorption to 200-mL PVC containers after 24 hours at 25°C with gentle shaking. The sorption was increased by 10% in sodium chloride 0.9% and by 20% in dextrose 5%.[133]

However, vitamin A delivery is also reduced in glass intravenous containers. At a concentration of 10,000 units/L in glass and PVC plastic containers protected from light with aluminum foil, 77 and 71%, respectively, of the vitamin A were delivered over a 10-hour period. Without light protection, 61% was delivered from glass and 49% from PVC plastic containers over a 10-hour period.[290]

In another test using multivitamin infusion (USV), 1 ampul per liter of sodium chloride 0.9% in glass and PVC plastic containers not protected from light, 69.4 and 67.9% of the vitamin A were delivered from glass and PVC containers, respectively, over a 10-hour period. The amount of vitamin A was constant over the test period.[282]

The delivery of vitamins A, D, and E from a parenteral nutrition solution composed of 3% amino acid solution (Pharmacia) in dextrose 10% with electrolytes, trace elements, vitamin K, folate, and vitamin B_{12} was evaluated. To this solution was added 6 mL of multivitamin infusion (USV). The solution was prepared in PVC bags (Travenol), and administration was simulated through a fluid chamber (Buretrol) and infusion tubing with a 0.5-μm filter at 10 mL/hr. During the first 60 to 90 minutes, minimal delivery of the vitamins occurred. This was followed by a rise and plateau in the delivered vitamins, which were attributed to an increasing saturation of adsorptive binding sites in the tubing. The total amounts delivered over 24 hours were 31% for vitamin A, 68% for vitamin D, and 64% for vitamin E. Sorption of the vitamins was found in the PVC bag, fluid chamber, and tubing. Decomposition was not a factor.[836]

A patient receiving 3000 international units of retinol daily in a parenteral nutrition solution experienced 2 episodes of night blindness. The pharmacy prepared the parenteral nutrition solution in 1-L PVC bags in weekly batches and stored them at 4°C in the dark until use. A subsequent in vitro study showed losses of vitamin A of 23 and 77% in 3- and 14-day periods, respectively, under these conditions. About 30% of the lost vitamin A could be extracted from the PVC bag.[1038]

Vitamin A was lost from multivitamin infusion (USV) in a neonatal parenteral nutrition solution. The solution was prepared in colorless glass bottles and run through an administration set with a burette (Travenol). The total loss of vitamin A was 75% in 24 hours, with about 16% as decomposition in the glass bottle. The decomposition was not noticeable during the first 12 hours, but then vitamin A levels fell rather precipitously to about one-third of the initial amount. The balance of the loss, averaging about 59%, occurred during transit through the administration set. Removal of the inline filter and treatment of the set with albumin human had no effect on vitamin A delivery. Increasing three- to fourfold the amount of vitamin A was suggested to compensate for the losses.[1039]

A 50% loss of vitamin A from a bottle of parenteral nutrition solution prepared with multivitamin infusion (USV) after 5.5 hours of infusion was noted. The amount delivered through an Ivex-2 filter set was only 6.3% of the added amount. Similar quantities were found after 20 hours of infusion. Vitamin A binding to the infusion bottles and tubing was confirmed.[704]

Solutions containing multivitamin infusion (USV) spiked with ³H-labeled retinol in intravenous tubing protected from light and agitated to simulate flow for 5 hours were evaluated. About half of the vitamin A was lost in 30 minutes, and 88 to 96% was lost in 5 hours.[1049]

The stability of vitamin E (alpha-tocopherol acetate from M.V.I.-1000 or Soluzyme) and selenium (from Selepen) in amino acids (Abbott) and dextrose in PVC bags was studied. Exposure to fluorescent light and room temperature (23°C) for 24 hours and simulated infusion at 50 mL/hr for 8 hours through a Medlon TPN administration set with a 0.22-μm filter did not affect the concentrations of vitamin E and selenium.[1224]

The stability of numerous vitamins in parenteral nutrition solutions composed of amino acids (Kabi-Vitrum), dextrose 30%, and fat emulsion 20% (Kabi-Vitrum) in a 2:1:1 ratio with electrolytes, trace elements, and both fat- and water-soluble vitamins was reported. The admixtures were stored in darkness at 2 to 8°C for 96 hours with no significant loss of retinyl palmitate, alpha-tocopherol, thiamine mononitrate, sodium riboflavin-5'-phosphate, pyridoxine hydrochloride, nicotinamide, folic acid, biotin, sodium pantothenate, and cyanocobalamin. Sodium ascorbate and its biologically active degradation product, dehydroascorbic acid, totaled 59 and 42% of the nominal starting concentration at 24 and 96 hours, respectively.[1225]

When the admixture was subjected to simulated infusion over 24 hours at 20°C, either exposed to room light or light protected, or stored for 6 days in the dark under refrigeration and then subjected to the same simulated infusion, once again the retinyl palmitate, alpha-tocopherol, and sodium riboflavin-5'-phosphate did not undergo significant loss. However, sodium ascorbate and its degradation product, dehydroascorbic acid, had initial combined concentrations of 51 to 65% of the nominal initial concentration, with further declines during infusion. Light protection did not significantly alter the loss of total ascorbic acid.[1225]

Neonatal parenteral nutrition solutions containing multivitamin infusion prepared in bags were delivered at 10 mL/hr through Buretrol sets (Travenol). The bags and sets were protected from light. About 26% of the vitamin A was lost before the flow was started. At 10 mL/hr, about 67% was lost from the effluent. More rapid flow reduced the extent of loss. Analysis of clinical samples of parenteral nutrition solutions showed losses of 21 to 57% after 20 hours. Because losses after 5 hours were of the same magnitude, it was concluded that the loss occurs rapidly and is not due to decomposition.[1049]

Retinol losses of 40% occurred in 2 hours and 60% in 5 hours from parenteral nutrition solutions pumped at 10 mL/hr through standard infusion sets at room temperature. The retinol concentration in the bottle remained constant while the retinol in the effluent decreased. Antioxidants had no effect. Much of the vitamin A was recoverable from the tubing.[1050]

To minimize the importance of this sorption, Allwood suggested using vitamin A palmitate instead of acetate; he stated that vitamin A palmitate does not sorb to PVC. However, this does not alter the problem of degradation from exposure to light.[1033]

Plasticizer Leaching

Multivitamins (Lyphomed) 1 mL in 50 mL of dextrose 5% leached insignificant amounts of diethylhexyl phthalate (DEHP) plasticizer due to the surfactant polysorbate 80 in the formulation. This finding is consistent with the low surfactant concentration (0.032%) in the admixture solution.[1683]

Compatibility Information

Solution Compatibility

Multivitamins

Test Soln Name	Mfr	Mfr	Conc/L or %	Remarks	Ref	C/I
Amino acids 2%, dextrose 12.5%, electrolytes		ROR	5 mL[b]	7% phytonadione loss in 4 hr and 27% loss in 24 hr under ambient temperature and light	1815	I
Amino acids 4.25%, dextrose 25%	TR	USV	1 vial	No thiamine loss in 22 hr at 30°C	843	C

Solution Compatibility (Cont.)

Test Soln Name	Mfr	Mfr	Conc/L or %	Remarks	Ref	C/I
Amino acids 4.25%, dextrose 25%	MG[c d]	LY	10 mL	All vitamins stable for 24 hr at 4°C	926	C
Amino acids 2.5%, dextrose 25%	AB[c d]	LY	10 mL	All vitamins stable for 24 hr at 4°C	926	C
Dextrose 5% in Ringer's injection, lactated	BA	USV	20 mL	Physically compatible for 24 hr	315	C
Dextrose 5% in sodium chloride 0.9%	BA	USV	20 mL	Physically compatible for 24 hr	315	C
Dextrose 5% in sodium chloride 0.9%	[b]	LY	10 mL	All vitamins stable for 24 hr at 4°C	926	C
Dextrose 5%	BA	USV	20 mL	Physically compatible for 24 hr	315	C
Dextrose 5%	TR[c]	RC	4 mL[a]	8% or less thiamine loss in 24 hr at 23°C	774	C
Dextrose 5%	[d]	LY	10 mL	All vitamins stable for 24 hr at 4°C	926	C
Dextrose 10%	BA	USV	20 mL	Physically compatible for 24 hr	315	C
Dextrose 10%	TR[c]	RC	4 mL[a]	5% or less thiamine loss in 24 hr at 23°C	774	C
Dextrose 10%	MG[d]	RC	4 mL[a]	11% or less thiamine loss in 24 hr at 23°C	774	C
Dextrose 20%	BA	USV	20 mL	Physically compatible for 24 hr	315	C
Ringer's injection, lactated	BA	USV	20 mL	Physically compatible for 24 hr	315	C
Ringer's injection, lactated	TR[c]	RC	4 mL[a]	5% or less thiamine loss in 24 hr at 23°C	774	C
Sodium chloride 0.9%	BA	USV	20 mL	Physically compatible for 24 hr	315	C
Sodium chloride 0.9%	TR[c]	RC	4 mL[a]	Thiamine losses of 6 to 11% in 24 hr at 23°C	774	C
Sodium lactate ⅙ M	BA	USV	20 mL	Physically compatible for 24 hr	315	C

[a] Berocca Parenteral Nutrition.

[b] M.V.I. Pediatric.

[c] Tested in both glass and PVC containers.

[d] Tested in polyolefin containers.

Additive Compatibility

Multivitamins

Test Drug	Mfr	Conc/L or %	Mfr	Conc/L or %	Test Solution	Remarks	Ref	C/I
Cefoxitin sodium	MSD	10 g	USV	50 mL[a]	W	5% cefoxitin loss in 24 hr and 10% in 48 hr at 25°C; 3% in 48 hr at 5°C	308	C
Fat emulsion, intravenous	VT	10%	USV	4 mL		Physically compatible for 48 hr at 4°C and room temperature	32	C
Fat emulsion, intravenous	KA	10%	KA			Physically compatible for 24 hr at 26°C. Little loss of most vitamins; up to 52% ascorbate loss	2050	C
Isoproterenol HCl	WI	4 mg	USV	10 mL		Physically compatible	59	C
Meropenem	ZEN	1 and 20 g	AST	50 mL	NS	Color darkened in 4 hr at room temperature	1994	I
Methyldopate HCl	MSD	1 g	USV	10 mL	D5W, D10W, D2.5½S, D2.5S, D5¼S, D5½S, D5S, D10S, NS, ½S	Physically compatible	23	C

Additive Compatibility (Cont.)

Test Drug	Mfr	Conc/L or %	Mfr	Conc/L or %	Test Solution	Remarks	Ref	C/I
Metoclopramide HCl	RB	20 and 320 mg	USV	20 mL[b]	NS	Physically compatible for 48 hr at room temperature	924	C
Metoclopramide HCl	RB	20 and 320 mg	USV	20 mL[c]	NS	Physically compatible for 48 hr at room temperature	924	C
Norepinephrine bitartrate	WI	8 mg	USV	10 mL	D5W, D10W, D2.5½S, D2.5S, D5¼S, D5½S, D5S, D10S, NS, ½S	Physically compatible	77	C
Sodium bicarbonate	AB	4.8 mEq[d]	USV	10 mL	D5W	Physically compatible for 24 hr	772	C
Verapamil HCl	KN	80 mg	USV	10 mL	D5W, NS	Physically compatible for 24 hr	764	C

[a] Concentrate.

[b] M.V.I.

[c] M.V.I.-12.

[d] Two vials of Neut added to a liter of admixture.

Y-Site Injection Compatibility (1:1 Mixture)

Multivitamins

Test Drug	Mfr	Conc	Mfr	Conc	Remarks	Ref	C/I
Acyclovir sodium	BW	5 mg/mL[a]	LY	0.01 mL/mL[a]	Physically compatible for 4 hr at 25°C	1157	C
Ampicillin sodium	AY	1 g/50 mL[a][b]	USV	5 mL/L[a]	Physically compatible for 24 hr at room temperature	323	C
Cefazolin sodium	SKF	1 g/50 mL[a]	USV	5 mL/L[a]	Physically compatible for 24 hr at room temperature	323	C
Ceftaroline fosamil	FOR	2.22 mg/mL[a][b][g]	BA	5 mL/L[a][b][g]	Physically compatible for 4 hr at 23°C	2826	C
Clindamycin phosphate	UP	600 mg/100 mL[a]	USV	5 mL/L[a]	Physically compatible for 24 hr at room temperature	323	C
Cloxacillin sodium	SMX	100 mg/mL	SZ		Physically compatible for up to 4 hr at room temperature	3245	C
Diltiazem HCl	MMD	5 mg/mL		[c]	Visually compatible	1807	C
Erythromycin lactobionate	AB	500 mg/250 mL[b]	USV	5 mL/L[a]	Physically compatible for 24 hr at room temperature	323	C
Fludarabine phosphate	BX	1 mg/mL[a]	ROR	0.01 mL/mL[a]	Visually compatible for 4 hr at 22°C	1439	C
Gentamicin sulfate	SC	80 mg/100 mL[a]	USV	5 mL/L[a]	Physically compatible for 24 hr at room temperature	323	C
Hydroxyethyl starch 130/0.4 in sodium chloride 0.9%	FRK	6%	SX	2.5, 5, 10 mL/L[a]	Visually compatible for 24 hr at room temperature	2770	C
Meropenem		50 mg/mL	SZ		Physically compatible for 4 hr at room temperature	3538	C
Pantoprazole sodium	[f]	4 mg/mL	SX		Precipitates within 1 hr	2574	I
Tacrolimus	FUJ	1 mg/mL[b]	LY	0.001 mL/mL[a]	Visually compatible for 24 hr at 25°C	1630	C

Y-Site Injection Compatibility (1:1 Mixture) (Cont.)

Test Drug	Mfr	Conc	Mfr	Conc	Remarks	Ref	C/I
TPN #189[d]			ROR	[e]	Visually compatible for 24 hr at 22°C	1767	C

[a] Tested in dextrose 5%.

[b] Tested in sodium chloride 0.9%.

[c] Concentration unspecified.

[d] Refer to Appendix for the composition of parenteral nutrition solutions. TPN indicates a 2-in-1 admixture.

[e] M.V.I.-12.

[f] Test performed using the formulation WITHOUT edetate disodium.

[g] Tested in Ringer's injection, lactated.

Additional Compatibility Information

Parenteral Nutrition Solutions

In a parenteral nutrition solution composed of amino acids, dextrose, electrolytes, trace elements, and multivitamins in PVC bags stored at 4 and 25°C, vitamin A rapidly deteriorated to 10% of the initial concentration in 8 hours at 25°C when exposed to light. The decomposition was slowed by light protection and refrigeration, with a loss of about 25% in 4 days. Folic acid concentration dropped 40% initially on admixture and then remained relatively constant for 28 days of storage. About 35% of the ascorbic acid was lost in 39 hours at 25°C when exposed to light. The loss was reduced to a negligible amount in 4 days by refrigeration and light protection. Thiamine content dropped by 50% initially but then remained unchanged over 120 hours of storage.[1063]

The stability of ascorbic acid in parenteral nutrition solutions, with and without fat emulsion, was studied. Both with and without fat emulsion, the total vitamin C content (ascorbic acid plus dehydroascorbic acid) remained above 90% for 12 hours when the solutions were exposed to fluorescent light and for 24 hours when they were protected from light. When stored in a cool dark place, the solutions were stable for 7 days.[1227]

Samples from 24 1-L and four 2-L parenteral nutrition solutions, containing 1 vial each of multivitamin concentrate (USV), were evaluated for thiamine hydrochloride content 48 and 72 hours after mixing. The parenteral nutrition solutions contained amino acids 2.75 to 5%, dextrose 15 to 25%, and electrolytes. Thiamine hydrochloride was stable in all of the solutions tested in spite of approximately 0.05% sulfite content.[843]

The vitamins in Cernevit (Baxter) diluted in three 2-in-1 parenteral nutrition admixtures were tested for stability over 48 hours. Nearly all of the vitamins retained their initial concentrations. However, ascorbic acid exhibited losses of about 5%, 13%, and 17% in TPNs with dextrose concentrations of 10, 15, and 25%, respectively.[2796]

Erythromycin

Erythromycin 5 mg/mL as the lactobionate in pH 8 buffer was combined with riboflavin in concentrations varying from 1 mg/mL to 20 mcg/mL. On exposure to light for 4 hours, almost total decomposition of the erythromycin occurred, with only 4 to 12% remaining. Protection from light resulted in 12 to 25% decomposition. When no riboflavin was present, 10% or less decomposition of the erythromycin occurred. It was concluded that a photodynamic decomposition reaction was taking place.[564]

Penicillin G

The times to 10% decomposition of combinations of penicillin G potassium buffered with multivitamin infusion concentrate in dextrose 5% and sodium chloride 0.9% have been calculated on the pH of the admixture:[304]

Penicillin G Potassium	Multivitamin Infusion Concentrate	pH	Time to 10% Decomposition
1 million units/L	1 mL/L	5.1	6.51 hr
1 million units/L	5 mL/L	4.9	4.56 hr
3 million units/L	1 mL/L	5.4	13.54 hr
3 million units/L	5 mL/L	5.0	6.38 hr
5 million units/L	1 mL/L	5.7	22.01 hr
5 million units/L	5 mL/L	5.1	6.51 hr
10 million units/L	1 mL/L	5.9	over 24 hr
10 million units/L	5 mL/L	5.4	13.54 hr

Selected Revisions May 1, 2020. © Copyright, October 1982. American Society of Health-System Pharmacists, Inc.

Mycophenolate Mofetil Hydrochloride
AHFS 92:44

Products

Mycophenolate mofetil hydrochloride is available as a lyophilized powder in vials containing 500 mg of mycophenolate mofetil along with polysorbate 80 25 mg and citric acid 5 mg.[3516] [3519] Sodium hydroxide may have been added during manufacturing to adjust pH.[3516] [3519]

Manufacturers recommend the use of dextrose 5% for reconstitution and dilution of the drug.[3516] [3519] Individuals who handle or prepare mycophenolate mofetil hydrochloride solutions should use care and take precautions to avoid contact with the drug solution.[3516] [3519] Each vial should be reconstituted with 14 mL of dextrose 5% and gently shaken to dissolve the drug.[3516] [3519] The reconstituted solution must be further diluted with dextrose 5% to yield a solution with a final mycophenolate mofetil concentration of 6 mg/mL.[3516] [3519] The volumes of dextrose 5% to be used for the dilution of 1- and 1.5-g doses of the reconstituted solution are 140 and 210 mL, respectively.[3516] [3519] The solution should be inspected for particulate matter and discoloration.[3516] [3519]

pH

The pH of the reconstituted solution ranges from 2.4 to 4.1[3516] or 2.7 to 4.1.[3519]

Trade Name(s)

CellCept

Administration

Mycophenolate mofetil hydrochloride is administered by slow intravenous infusion over a minimum of 2 hours into either a central line or peripheral vein.[3516] [3519] The drug should *not* be administered by rapid or bolus administration.[3516] [3519]

Stability

Mycophenolate mofetil hydrochloride is a white to off-white lyophilized powder that forms slightly yellow solution upon reconstitution and dilution.[3516] [3519] Intact vials of the drug should be stored at controlled room temperature[3519] or at 25°C with excursions permitted from 15 to 30°C.[3516] Dextrose 5% is the manufacturer-recommended diluent for reconstitution and dilution of mycophenolate mofetil hydrochloride; all other solutions are stated to be incompatible.[3516] [3519] Reconstituted solutions and solution diluted for infusion also may be kept at 25°C.[3516] [3519] Manufacturers indicate that administration of the diluted drug should begin within 4 hours after reconstitution and dilution of the drug.[3516] [3519]

Freezing Solutions

Mycophenolate mofetil (Hoffmann-La Roche, Accord) 1, 4, and 10 mg/mL in polypropylene bags of dextrose 5% (Grifols) was stable for 35 days when frozen at −15 to −25°C.[3520]

Sorption

Mycophenolate mofetil (Hoffmann-La Roche, Accord) 1, 4, and 10 mg/mL prepared with dextrose 5% using a closed-system transfer device (CSTD) (Equashield) demonstrated negligible amounts of sorption to the CSTD.[3520]

Compatibility Information
Solution Compatibility

Mycophenolate mofetil HCl

Test Soln Name	Mfr	Mfr	Conc/L or %	Remarks	Ref	C/I
Dextrose 5%	MAC[a]	RC	1, 5, 10 g	Physically compatible. No loss in 7 days at 4 and 25°C	2394	C
Dextrose 5%		GEN, ZYD	6 g	Initiate administration within 4 hr after reconstitution and dilution	3516, 3519	C
Dextrose 5%	GRI[b]	RC, ACD	1 and 4 g	Physically and chemically stable for 35 days at 2 to 8°C and 14 days at 23 to 27°C	3520	C
Dextrose 5%	GRI[b]	RC	10 g	Physically and chemically stable for 35 days at 2 to 8°C and 14 days at 23 to 27°C	3520	C
Dextrose 5%	GRI[b]	ACD	10 g	Physically and chemically stable for 35 days at 2 to 8°C and 21 days at 23 to 27°C	3520	C

[a] Tested in PVC containers.

[b] Tested in polypropylene containers.

DOI: 10.37573/9781585286850.277

Y-Site Injection Compatibility (1:1 Mixture)

Mycophenolate mofetil HCl

Test Drug	Mfr	Conc	Mfr	Conc	Remarks	Ref	C/I
Anidulafungin	VIC	0.5 mg/mL[a]	RC	6 mg/mL[a]	Physically compatible for 4 hr at 23°C	2617	C
Cangrelor tetrasodium	TMC	1 mg/mL[b]		6 mg/mL[a]	Gross white turbid precipitate forms immediately	3243	I
Caspofungin acetate	ME	0.7 mg/mL[b]	RC	6 mg/mL[b]	Physically compatible for 4 hr at room temperature	2758	C
Cefepime HCl		20 mg/mL[a]	RC	5.9 mg/mL[a]	Physically compatible with no mycophenolate mofetil loss in 4 hr	2738	C
Ceftolozane sulfate–tazobactam sodium	CUB	10 mg/mL[a][c]	GEN	6 mg/mL[a]	Physically compatible for 2 hr	3262	C
Cyclosporine	BED	1 mg/mL[a]	RC	5.9 mg/mL[a]	Effervescence reported. No mycophenolate mofetil loss in 4 hr	2738	?
Defibrotide sodium	JAZ	8 mg/mL[b]	RC	11.9 mg/mL[a]	Solution became milky white and opaque	3149	I
Dopamine HCl	AMR	4 mg/mL[a]	RC	5.9 mg/mL[a]	Physically compatible and 4% mycophenolate mofetil loss in 4 hr	2738	C
Isavuconazonium sulfate	ASP	1.5 mg/mL[a]	GEN	6 mg/mL[a]	Physically compatible for 2 hr	3263	C
Letermovir	ME				Physically incompatible	3398	I
Micafungin sodium	ASP	1.5 mg/mL[b]	RC	6 mg/mL[a]	White precipitate forms immediately	2683	I
Norepinephrine bitartrate		1 mg/mL[a]	RC	5.9 mg/mL[a]	Physically compatible and 2% mycophenolate mofetil loss in 4 hr	2738	C
Tacrolimus	FUJ	0.02 mg/mL[a]	RC	5.9 mg/mL[a]	Physically compatible and 2% mycophenolate mofetil loss in 4 hr	2738	C
Vancomycin HCl		10 mg/mL[a]	RC	5.9 mg/mL[a]	Physically compatible and 3% mycophenolate mofetil loss in 4 hr	2738	C

[a] Tested in dextrose 5%.

[b] Tested in sodium chloride 0.9%.

[c] Ceftolozane component. Ceftolozane in a 2:1 fixed-ratio concentration with tazobactam.

Selected Revisions January 31, 2020. © Copyright, October 2004. American Society of Health-System Pharmacists, Inc.

Nafcillin Sodium
AHFS 8:12.16.12

Products

Nafcillin sodium is available in vials containing the equivalent of 1 and 2 g of nafcillin.[4] Reconstitute the 1-g vial with 3.4 mL and the 2-g vial with 6.6 mL of sterile water for injection, sodium chloride 0.9%, or bacteriostatic water for injection containing parabens or benzyl alcohol. The solution then contains nafcillin sodium equivalent to nafcillin 250 mg/mL with sodium citrate buffer. The final volumes of the 1- and 2-g vials are 4 and 8 mL, respectively.[4]

A 10-g pharmacy bulk vial is also available and is reconstituted with 93 mL of sterile water for injection or sodium chloride 0.9% to yield a 100-mg/mL solution with sodium citrate buffer 4 mg/mL.[4]

Nafcillin sodium is also available as frozen premixed solutions containing 1 and 2 g of nafcillin per minibag in dextrose 3.6% or 2%, respectively.[1(2/07)]

pH

The pH of the reconstituted solution and frozen premixed solution is 6 to 8.5.[4]

Osmolality

The osmolality of nafcillin sodium 250 mg/mL in sterile water for injection was 709 mOsm/kg by freezing-point depression and 665 mOsm/kg by vapor pressure.[1071]

The frozen premixed solutions have an osmolality of 300 mOsm/kg.[4]

The osmolality of nafcillin sodium (Wyeth) 40 mg/mL was determined to be 403 mOsm/kg in dextrose 5% and 402 mOsm/kg in sodium chloride 0.9%.[1375]

The osmolality of nafcillin sodium was calculated for the following dilutions[1054]:

Diluent	Osmolality (mOsm/kg)	
	50 mL	100 mL
2 g		
Dextrose 5%	399	334
Sodium chloride 0.9%	425	361
3 g		
Dextrose 5%	458	371
Sodium chloride 0.9%	485	398

The following maximum nafcillin sodium concentrations were recommended to achieve osmolalities suitable for peripheral infusion in fluid-restricted patients[1180]:

Diluent	Maximum Concentration (mg/mL)	Osmolality (mOsm/kg)
Dextrose 5%	71	491
Sodium chloride 0.9%	64	470
Sterile water for injection	128	319

Sodium Content

Each gram of nafcillin sodium with sodium citrate buffer contains 2.9 mEq (66 mg) of sodium.[4 27]

Administration

Nafcillin sodium may be administered intramuscularly by deep intragluteal injection, by direct intravenous injection, or by intermittent intravenous infusion. For direct intravenous injection, the dose should be diluted with 15 to 30 mL of sterile water for injection or sodium chloride 0.45 or 0.9% and given over five to 10 minutes into the tubing of a running intravenous infusion. Intermittent intravenous infusion in a concentration between 2 and 40 mg/mL should be administered slowly, over 30 to 60 minutes.[4]

Stability

Intact containers should be stored at controlled room temperature or lower.[4] When reconstituted to a concentration of 250 mg/mL, nafcillin sodium is stable for three days at room temperature or seven days when refrigerated at 2 to 8°C.[4 27] At concentrations of 2 to 40 mg/mL, nafcillin sodium is stable for 24 hours at room temperature or 96 hours under refrigeration.[4]

Commercially available frozen premixed nafcillin sodium solutions, thawed at room temperature or under refrigeration, are stable for 72 hours at 25°C and 21 days at 5°C.[4]

The activity of nafcillin 100 mg/L was evaluated in peritoneal dialysis fluids containing dextrose 1.5 or 4.25% (Dianeal 137, Travenol). Storage at 25°C resulted in no loss of antimicrobial activity in 24 hours.[515]

The stability of nafcillin sodium (Wyeth) 100 mg/L in peritoneal dialysis solutions (Dianeal 137 and PD2) with heparin sodium 500 units/L was evaluated. About 98% activity remained after 24 hours at 25°C.[1228]

DOI: 10.37573/9781585286850.278

pH Effects

The stability of nafcillin sodium is pH dependent, with a maximum stability at pH 6 and a preferred range of pH 5 to 8. Drug decomposition is increased as pH values vary from this range. Additives that may result in a final pH of above 8 or below 5 should not be mixed with nafcillin sodium.[27]

Freezing Solutions

At a concentration of 250 mg/mL in sterile water for injection and frozen at –20°C, the drug is stable for up to three months.[27][123]

In one study, however, when nafcillin sodium (Wyeth) 1 g/4 mL was frozen at –20°C in glass syringes (Hy-Pod), the drug was stable for nine months.[532]

In another study, nafcillin sodium (Wyeth) 1 g/50 mL of dextrose 5% in PVC bags frozen at –20°C for 30 days and then thawed by exposure to ambient temperature or microwave radiation showed no evidence of precipitation or color change but had a 2 to 3% loss. Subsequent storage of the admixture at room temperature for 24 hours also yielded physically compatible solutions with no additional loss of activity.[555]

Syringes

Nafcillin sodium (Apothecon) 10 mg/mL in sodium chloride 0.9% was packaged in 10-mL polypropylene syringes (Becton Dickinson) and stored at 5 and 25°C. The solutions remained clear under refrigeration for 44 days and at room temperature for seven days. A yellow color developed after 14 days at room temperature. About 2% loss of nafcillin sodium occurred after seven days and 18% loss in 14 days at 25°C. Under refrigeration, 1% loss occurred after 44 days. Stability in glass containers was comparable.[2325]

Ambulatory Pumps

Nafcillin sodium (Marsam) 20 mg/mL in sterile water for injection in PVC portable pump reservoirs (Pharmacia Deltec) exhibited no loss in three days stored at 25°C and in 14 days at 5°C. However, at a concentration of 120 mg/mL, 6% loss was found in three days at 25°C, and 2% loss occurred in 14 days at 5°C.[2080]

Nafcillin sodium 40 and 50 mg/mL in sodium chloride 0.9% precipitated in as little as one day at the simulated ambulatory use temperature of 35°C. At 20 mg/mL, precipitation appeared in three days. When stored at room temperature, no precipitation appeared at any concentration in three days.[2664]

Compatibility Information

Solution Compatibility

Nafcillin sodium

Test Soln Name	Mfr	Mfr	Conc/L or %	Remarks	Ref	C/I
Dextrose 5% in Ringer's injection	AB	WY	2 and 30 g	Physically compatible and stable for 24 hr at 25°C	27	C
Dextrose 5% in half-strength Ringer's injection, lactated	AB	WY	2 and 30 g	Physically compatible	27	C
Dextrose 5% in Ringer's injection, lactated	AB	WY	2 and 30 g	Physically compatible	27	C
Dextrose 5% in sodium chloride 0.225%	AB	WY	2 and 30 g	Physically compatible	27	C
Dextrose 5% in sodium chloride 0.45%			2 to 40 g	Under 10% loss in 24 hr at room temperature and 96 hr refrigerated	4	C
Dextrose 5% in sodium chloride 0.45%	AB	WY	2 and 30 g	Physically compatible and stable for 24 hr at 25°C	27	C
Dextrose 5% in sodium chloride 0.9%	AB	WY	2 and 30 g	Physically compatible and stable for 24 hr at 25°C	27	C
Dextrose 5%			2 to 40 g	Under 10% loss in 24 hr at room temperature and 96 hr refrigerated	4	C
Dextrose 5%		WY	1 g	Stable for 24 hr	109	C
Dextrose 5%	AB	WY	2 and 30 g	Physically compatible and stable for 24 hr at 25°C	27	C
Dextrose 5%	TR[a]	WY	20 g	Physically compatible and stable for 24 hr at room temperature	555	C
Dextrose 5%	TR[a]	WY	20 g	About 10% loss in 7 days at 24°C and 8% loss in 15 days at 4°C	336	C
Dextrose 10% in sodium chloride 0.9%	AB	WY	2 and 30 g	Physically compatible	27	C
Dextrose 10%	AB	WY	2 and 30 g	Physically compatible	27	C
Ionosol T in dextrose 5%	AB	WY	2 and 30 g	Physically compatible	27	C

Solution Compatibility (Cont.)

Test Soln Name	Mfr	Mfr	Conc/L or %	Remarks	Ref	C/I
Normosol M in dextrose 5%	AB	WY	2 and 30 g	Physically compatible and stable for 24 hr at 25°C	27	C
Normosol R	AB	WY	2 and 30 g	Physically compatible	27	C
Normosol R in dextrose 5%	AB	WY	2 and 30 g	Physically compatible	27	C
Ringer's injection			2 to 40 g	Under 10% loss in 24 hr at room temperature and 96 hr refrigerated	4	C
Ringer's injection	AB	WY	2 and 30 g	Physically compatible and stable for 24 hr at 25°C	27	C
Ringer's injection, lactated	AB	WY	2 and 30 g	Physically compatible and stable for 24 hr at 25°C	27	C
Sodium chloride 0.9%			2 to 40 g	Under 10% loss in 24 hr at room temperature and 96 hr refrigerated	4	C
Sodium chloride 0.9%		WY	1 g	Stable for 24 hr	109	C
Sodium chloride 0.9%	AB	WY	2 and 30 g	Physically compatible and stable for 24 hr at 25°C	27	C
Sodium chloride 0.9%	AB[c]	WY	80 g	5% or less loss with 24-hr storage at 5°C then 48 hr at 30°C	1779	C
Sodium chloride 0.9%	TR[a]	WY	20 g	About 6% loss in 3 days at 24°C and 6% loss in 24 days at 4°C	336	C
Sodium lactate ⅙ M			2 to 40 g	Under 10% loss in 24 hr at room temperature and 96 hr refrigerated	4	C
Sodium lactate ⅙ M	AB	WY	2 and 30 g	Physically compatible and stable for 24 hr at 25°C	27	C
TPN #107[b]			1 and 2 g	Nafcillin activity retained for 24 hr at 21°C	1326	C

[a] Tested in PVC containers.

[b] Refer to Appendix for the composition of parenteral nutrition solutions. TPN indicates a 2-in-1 admixture.

[c] Tested in portable pump reservoirs (Pharmacia Deltec).

Additive Compatibility

Nafcillin sodium

Test Drug	Mfr	Conc/L or %	Mfr	Conc/L or %	Test Solution	Remarks	Ref	C/I
Aminophylline	SE	500 mg	WY	30 g	D5W	Nafcillin retained for 24 hr at 25°C	27	C
Aminophylline	SE	500 mg	WY	2 g	D5W	14% nafcillin loss in 24 hr at 25°C	27	I
Ascorbic acid	UP	500 mg	WY	5 g	D5W	Physically incompatible	15	I
Aztreonam	SQ	20 g	BR	20 g	D5W, NS[a]	Cloudiness and precipitate form. 7% aztreonam and 11% nafcillin loss in 24 hr at room temperature	1028	I
Bleomycin sulfate	BR	20 and 30 units	BR	2.5 g	NS	Substantial loss of bleomycin activity in 1 week at 4°C	763	I
Chloramphenicol sodium succinate	PD	1 g	WY	500 mg		Physically compatible	27	C
Chlorothiazide sodium	MSD	500 mg	WY	500 mg		Physically compatible	27	C
Cytarabine	UP	100 mg		4 g	D5W	Heavy crystalline precipitation	174	I
Dexamethasone sodium phosphate	MSD	4 mg	WY	500 mg		Physically compatible	27	C
Dextran 40	PH	10%	WY	2 and 30 g	D5W	Physically compatible and stable for 24 hr at 25°C	27	C
Diphenhydramine HCl	PD	50 mg	WY	500 mg		Physically compatible	27	C
Ephedrine sulfate		50 mg	WY	500 mg		Physically compatible	27	C

Additive Compatibility (Cont.)

Test Drug	Mfr	Conc/L or %	Mfr	Conc/L or %	Test Solution	Remarks	Ref	C/I
Gentamicin sulfate		75 mg		1 g	TPN #107[b]	10% gentamicin loss in 24 hr at 21°C	1326	I
Heparin sodium	AB, WY	20,000 units	WY	500 mg		Physically compatible	27	C
Heparin sodium	AB	20,000 units	WY	500 mg		Physically compatible	21	C
Hydrocortisone sodium succinate	UP	250 mg	WY	500 mg		Precipitate forms within 1 hr	27	I
Hydroxyzine HCl	PF	100 mg	WY	500 mg		Physically compatible	27	C
Lidocaine HCl	AST	0.6 g	AP	20 g	D5W[a], NS[c]	Visually compatible. Little nafcillin loss in 48 hr at 23°C. Lidocaine not tested	1806	C
Methylprednisolone sodium succinate	UP	125 mg	WY	500 mg	D5W	Precipitate forms	329	I
Potassium chloride	TR	40 mEq	WY	30 g	NS	Nafcillin stable for 24 hr at 25°C	27	C
Potassium chloride	AB	40 mEq	WY	500 mg		Physically compatible	27	C
Prochlorperazine edisylate	SKF	10 mg	WY	500 mg		Physically compatible	27	C
Sodium bicarbonate	AB	40 mEq	WY	500 mg		Physically compatible	27	C
Sodium lactate	AB	50 mEq	WY	500 mg		Physically compatible	27	C
Verapamil HCl	KN	80 mg	WY	4 g	D5W, NS	Physically compatible for 24 hr	764	C
Verapamil HCl	SE	[d]	WY	40 g	D5W, NS	Cloudy solution clears with agitation	1166	?

[a] Tested in PVC containers.

[b] Refer to Appendix for the composition of parenteral nutrition solutions. TPN indicates a 2-in-1 admixture.

[c] Tested in polyolefin containers.

[d] Final concentration unspecified.

Drugs in Syringe Compatibility

Nafcillin sodium

Test Drug	Mfr	Amt	Mfr	Amt	Remarks	Ref	C/I
Heparin sodium	AB	20,000 units/1 mL	WY	500 mg	Physically compatible for at least 30 min	21	C

Y-Site Injection Compatibility (1:1 Mixture)

Nafcillin sodium

Test Drug	Mfr	Conc	Mfr	Conc	Remarks	Ref	C/I
Acyclovir sodium	BW	5 mg/mL[a]	WY	20 mg/mL[a]	Physically compatible for 4 hr at 25°C	1157	C
Atropine sulfate		0.4 mg/mL	WY	33 mg/mL[b]	No precipitation	547	C
Caspofungin acetate	ME	0.7 mg/mL[b]	SZ	20 mg/mL[b]	Transient turbidity becomes white precipitate	2758	I
Cyclophosphamide	MJ	20 mg/mL[a]	WY	20 mg/mL[a]	Physically compatible for 4 hr at 25°C	1194	C
Diazepam		5 mg/mL	WY	33 mg/mL[b]	No precipitation	547	C
Diltiazem HCl	MMD	5 mg/mL	WY	10 mg/mL[b]	Cloudiness forms and persists	1807	I
Diltiazem HCl	MMD	5 mg/mL	WY	200 mg/mL[b]	Cloudiness forms but clears with swirling	1807	?

Y-Site Injection Compatibility (1:1 Mixture) (Cont.)

Test Drug	Mfr	Conc	Mfr	Conc	Remarks	Ref	C/I
Diltiazem HCl	MMD	1 mg/mL[b]	WY	10 and 200 mg/mL[b]	Visually compatible	1807	C
Droperidol		2.5 mg/mL	WY	33 mg/mL[b]	Precipitate forms, probably free nafcillin	547	I
Enalaprilat	MSD	0.05 mg/mL[b]	BR	10 mg/mL[a]	Physically compatible for 24 hr at room temperature under fluorescent light	1355	C
Esmolol HCl	DCC	10 mg/mL[a]	BR	10 mg/mL[a]	Physically compatible for 24 hr at 22°C	1169	C
Famotidine	MSD	0.2 mg/mL[a]	WY	15 mg/mL[b]	Physically compatible for 14 hr	1196	C
Fentanyl citrate		0.05 mg/mL	WY	33 mg/mL[b]	No precipitation	547	C
Fluconazole	RR	2 mg/mL	BR	20 mg/mL	Physically compatible for 24 hr at 25°C	1407	C
Foscarnet sodium	AST	24 mg/mL	BR	20 mg/mL[c]	Physically compatible for 24 hr at 25°C under fluorescent light	1393	C
Heparin sodium	TR	50 units/mL	WY	20 mg/mL[a]	Visually compatible for 4 hr at 25°C	1793	C
Hydromorphone HCl	WY	0.2 mg/mL[a]	WY	20 mg/mL[a]	Physically compatible for 4 hr at 25°C	987	C
Insulin, regular	LI	0.2 unit/mL[b]	BA	20 and 40 mg/mL[a]	Precipitates immediately	1395	I
Labetalol HCl	SC	1 mg/mL[a]	BR	10 mg/mL[a]	Cloudy precipitate forms immediately	1171	I
Magnesium sulfate	IX	16.7, 33.3, 66.7, 100 mg/mL[a]	WY	20 mg/mL[a]	Physically compatible for at least 4 hr at 32°C	813	C
Meperidine HCl	WY	10 mg/mL[a]	WY	20 mg/mL[a]	Cloudy haze cleared on mixing and remained clear for 4 hr at 25°C	987	?
Meperidine HCl	WY	10 mg/mL[b]	WY	20 and 30 mg/mL[a]	Cloudy solution formed immediately and persisted for at least 1 hr at 25°C	1338	I
Midazolam HCl	RC	1 mg/mL[a]	WY	20 mg/mL[a]	Immediate haze. Particles in 4 hr	1847	I
Morphine sulfate	WI	1 mg/mL[a]	WY	20 mg/mL[a]	Physically compatible for 4 hr at 25°C	987	C
Morphine sulfate	ES	1 mg/mL[b]	WY	30 mg/mL[a]	Physically compatible for 1 hr at 25°C	1338	C
Nalbuphine HCl		10 mg/mL	WY	33 mg/mL[b]	Precipitate forms, probably free nafcillin	547	I
Nicardipine HCl	DCC	0.1 mg/mL[a]	BR	10 mg/mL[a]	Visually compatible for 24 hr at room temperature	235	C
Pentazocine lactate		30 mg/mL	WY	33 mg/mL[b]	Precipitate forms, probably free nafcillin	547	I
Propofol	ZEN[j]	10 mg/mL	MAR	20 mg/mL[a]	Physically compatible for 1 hr at 23°C	2066	C
Theophylline	TR	4 mg/mL	WY	20 mg/mL[a]	Visually compatible for 6 hr at 25°C	1793	C
TNA #218 to #226[d]			BE, APC	20 mg/mL[a]	Visually compatible for 4 hr at 23°C	2215	C
TPN #54[d]				250 mg/mL	Physically compatible and nafcillin activity retained over 6 hr at 22°C	1045	C
TPN #61[d]		[e]	WY	250 mg/1 mL[f]	Physically compatible	1012	C
TPN #61[d]		[g]	WY	1.5 g/6 mL[f]	Physically compatible	1012	C
TPN #212 to #215[d]			BE	20 mg/mL[a]	Physically compatible for 4 hr at 23°C	2109	C
Vancomycin HCl	AB	20 mg/mL[a]	BE	250 mg/mL[i]	Transient precipitate forms followed by a visibly hazy solution	2189	I
Vancomycin HCl	AB	20 mg/mL[a]	BE	10 and 50 mg/mL[b]	Gross white precipitate forms immediately	2189	I
Vancomycin HCl	AB	20 mg/mL[a]	BE	1 mg/mL[b]	Physically compatible for 4 hr at 23°C	2189	C
Vancomycin HCl	AB	2 mg/mL[a]	BE	10[b], 50[b], 250[i] mg/mL	Subvisible measured haze forms immediately	2189	I

Y-Site Injection Compatibility (1:1 Mixture) (Cont.)

Test Drug	Mfr	Conc	Mfr	Conc	Remarks	Ref	C/I
Vancomycin HCl	AB	2 mg/mL[a]	BE	1 mg/mL[b]	Physically compatible for 4 hr at 23°C	2189	C
Verapamil HCl		[h]			White milky precipitate forms immediately	840, 1303	I
Verapamil HCl	SE	2.5 mg/mL	WY	40 mg/mL[c]	White precipitate forms immediately. 20% of verapamil precipitated	1166	I
Zidovudine	BW	4 mg/mL[a]	BR	20 mg/mL[a]	Physically compatible for 4 hr at 25°C	1193	C

[a] Tested in dextrose 5%.

[b] Tested in sodium chloride 0.9%.

[c] Tested in both dextrose 5% and sodium chloride 0.9%.

[d] Refer to Appendix for the composition of parenteral nutrition solutions. TNA indicates a 3-in-1 admixture, and TPN indicates a 2-in-1 admixture.

[e] Run at 21 mL/hr.

[f] Given over five minutes by syringe pump.

[g] Run at 94 mL/hr.

[h] Injected into a line being used to infuse nafcillin sodium.

[i] Tested in sterile water for injection.

[j] Test performed using the formulation WITH edetate disodium.

Selected Revisions January 31, 2020. © Copyright, October 1982. American Society of Health-System Pharmacists, Inc.

Nalbuphine Hydrochloride
AHFS 28:08.12

Products

Nalbuphine hydrochloride is available as a 10-mg/mL solution in 1-mL ampuls and 10-mL vials and as a 20-mg/mL solution in 1-mL ampuls and 10-mL vials. Each mL of solution in vials also contains sodium citrate hydrous 0.94%, citric acid anhydrous 1.26%, methyl- and propylparabens 0.2%, and hydrochloric acid to adjust pH. The 10-mg/mL solution contains sodium chloride 0.225%. The ampul formulation contains no parabens.[1(6/06)]

pH

The pH is adjusted to about 3.5 to 3.7.[1(6/06)]

Administration

Nalbuphine hydrochloride is administered by subcutaneous, intramuscular, or intravenous injection.[1(6/06) 4]

Stability

Intact vials and ampuls should be protected from excessive light and stored at 15 to 30°C.[1(6/06) 4]

Central Venous Catheter

Nalbuphine hydrochloride (Astra) 1 mg/mL in dextrose 5% was found to be compatible with the ARROWg+ard Blue Plus (Arrow International) chlorhexidine-bearing triple-lumen central catheter. Essentially complete delivery of the drug was found with little or no drug loss occurring. Furthermore, chlorhexidine delivered from the catheter remained at trace amounts with no substantial increase due to the delivery of the drug through the catheter.[2335]

Compatibility Information

Solution Compatibility

Nalbuphine HCl

Test Soln Name	Mfr	Mfr	Conc/L or %	Remarks	Ref	C/I
Dextrose 5% in sodium chloride 0.9%		DU	3.3 to 10 g	Physically compatible for 48 hr	128	C
Dextrose 10%		DU	3.3 to 10 g	Physically compatible for 48 hr	128	C
Ringer's injection, lactated		DU	3.3 to 10 g	Physically compatible for 48 hr	128	C
Sodium chloride 0.9%		DU	3.3 to 10 g	Physically compatible for 48 hr	128	C

Drugs in Syringe Compatibility

Nalbuphine HCl

Test Drug	Mfr	Amt	Mfr	Amt	Remarks	Ref	C/I
Atropine sulfate	WY	0.2 mg	EN	10 mg/1 mL	Physically compatible for 36 hr at 27°C	762	C
Atropine sulfate	WY	0.2 mg	EN	5 mg/0.5 mL	Physically compatible for 36 hr at 27°C	762	C
Atropine sulfate	WY	0.5 mg	EN	10 mg/1 mL	Physically compatible for 36 hr at 27°C	762	C
Atropine sulfate	WY	0.5 mg	EN	5 mg/0.5 mL	Physically compatible for 36 hr at 27°C	762	C
Atropine sulfate		0.4 and 1 mg	DU	10 mg/1 mL	Physically compatible for 48 hr	128	C
Atropine sulfate		0.4 and 1 mg	DU	20 mg/1 mL	Physically compatible for 48 hr	128	C
Diazepam	RC	5 mg/1 mL	EN	10 mg/1 mL	Immediate milky precipitate that persists for 36 hr at 27°C	762	I
Diazepam	RC	5 mg/1 mL	EN	5 mg/0.5 mL	Immediate milky precipitate that clears upon shaking. Clear for 36 hr at 27°C	762	?
Diazepam	RC	5 mg/1 mL	EN	2.5 mg/0.25 mL	Immediate milky precipitate that clears upon shaking. Clear for 36 hr at 27°C	762	?
Diazepam	RC	10 mg/2 mL	DU	10 mg/1 mL	Physically incompatible	128	I

DOI: 10.37573/9781585286850.279

Drugs in Syringe Compatibility (Cont.)

Test Drug	Mfr	Amt	Mfr	Amt	Remarks	Ref	C/I
Diazepam	RC	10 mg/2 mL	DU	20 mg/1 mL	Physically incompatible	128	I
Diphenhydramine HCl	PD	50 mg/1 mL	DU	10 mg/1 mL	Physically compatible for 48 hr	128	C
Diphenhydramine HCl	PD	50 mg/1 mL	DU	20 mg/1 mL	Physically compatible for 48 hr	128	C
Droperidol	JN	5 mg/2 mL	EN	5 mg/0.5 mL	Physically compatible for 36 hr at 27°C	762	C
Droperidol	JN	2.5 mg/1 mL	EN	10 mg/1 mL	Physically compatible for 36 hr at 27°C	762	C
Droperidol	JN	2.5 mg/1 mL	EN	5 mg/0.5 mL	Physically compatible for 36 hr at 27°C	762	C
Droperidol	JN	5 mg/2 mL	DU	10 mg/1 mL	Physically compatible for 48 hr	128	C
Droperidol	JN	5 mg/2 mL	DU	20 mg/1 mL	Physically compatible for 48 hr	128	C
Glycopyrrolate	RB	0.2 mg/1 mL	DU	10 mg/1 mL	Physically compatible for 48 hr	128	C
Glycopyrrolate	RB	0.2 mg/1 mL	DU	20 mg/1 mL	Physically compatible for 48 hr	128	C
Hydroxyzine HCl	PF	50 mg	EN	10 mg/1 mL	Physically compatible for 36 hr at 27°C	762	C
Hydroxyzine HCl	PF	50 mg	EN	5 mg/0.5 mL	Physically compatible for 36 hr at 27°C	762	C
Hydroxyzine HCl	PF	50 mg	EN	2.5 mg/0.25 mL	Physically compatible for 36 hr at 27°C	762	C
Hydroxyzine HCl	PF	25 mg/1 mL	DU	10 mg/1 mL	Physically compatible for 48 hr	128	C
Hydroxyzine HCl	PF	25 mg/1 mL	DU	20 mg/1 mL	Physically compatible for 48 hr	128	C
Ketorolac tromethamine	SY	180 mg/6 mL	DU	30 mg/3 mL	Solid white precipitate forms immediately and settles to bottom	1703	I
Lidocaine HCl		40 mg	DU	10 mg/1 mL	Physically compatible for 48 hr	128	C
Lidocaine HCl		40 mg	DU	20 mg/1 mL	Physically compatible for 48 hr	128	C
Midazolam HCl	RC	5 mg/1 mL	DU	10 mg/1 mL	Physically compatible for 4 hr at 25°C	1145	C
Pentobarbital sodium	WY	50 mg/1 mL	EN	10 mg/1 mL	Immediate white milky precipitate that persists for 36 hr at 27°C	762	I
Pentobarbital sodium	WY	50 mg/1 mL	EN	2.5 mg/0.25 mL	Immediate white milky precipitate that clears upon vigorous shaking	762	I
Pentobarbital sodium	WY	50 mg/1 mL	EN	5 mg/0.5 mL	Immediate white milky precipitate that persists for 36 hr at 27°C	762	I
Prochlorperazine edisylate	WY	5 mg/1 mL	EN	10 mg/1 mL	Physically compatible for 36 hr at 27°C	762	C
Prochlorperazine edisylate	WY	5 mg/1 mL	EN	5 mg/0.5 mL	Physically compatible for 36 hr at 27°C	762	C
Prochlorperazine edisylate	WY	5 mg/1 mL	EN	2.5 mg/0.25 mL	Physically compatible for 36 hr at 27°C	762	C
Prochlorperazine edisylate	SKF	10 mg/2 mL	DU	10 mg/1 mL	Physically compatible for 48 hr	128	C
Prochlorperazine edisylate	SKF	10 mg/2 mL	DU	20 mg/1 mL	Physically compatible for 48 hr	128	C
Promethazine HCl	ES	25 mg	EN	10 mg/1 mL	Physically compatible for 36 hr at 27°C	762	C
Promethazine HCl	ES	25 mg	EN	5 mg/0.5 mL	Physically compatible for 36 hr at 27°C	762	C
Promethazine HCl	ES	12.5 mg	EN	10 mg/1 mL	Physically compatible for 36 hr at 27°C	762	C
Promethazine HCl	WY	25 and 50 mg	DU	10 mg/1 mL	Physically incompatible	128	I

Drugs in Syringe Compatibility (Cont.)

Test Drug	Mfr	Amt	Mfr	Amt	Remarks	Ref	C/I
Promethazine HCl	WY	25 and 50 mg	DU	20 mg/1 mL	Physically incompatible	128	I
Promethazine HCl	WY	25 mg/1 mL	DU	10 mg/1 mL	White flocculent precipitate forms immediately	1184	I
Promethazine HCl	ES	25 mg/1 mL	DU	10 mg/1 mL	Physically compatible for 24 hr at room temperature	1184	C
Ranitidine HCl	GL	50 mg/2 mL	EN	10 mg/1 mL	Physically compatible for 1 hr at 25°C	978	C
Scopolamine HBr	BW	0.86 mg/1 mL	EN	10 mg/1 mL	Physically compatible for 36 hr at 27°C	762	C
Scopolamine HBr	BW	0.86 mg/1 mL	EN	5 mg/0.5 mL	Physically compatible for 36 hr at 27°C	762	C
Scopolamine HBr	BW	0.43 mg/0.5 mL	EN	10 mg/1 mL	Physically compatible for 36 hr at 27°C	762	C
Scopolamine HBr		0.4 mg	DU	10 mg/1 mL	Physically compatible for 48 hr	128	C
Scopolamine HBr		0.4 mg	DU	20 mg/1 mL	Physically compatible for 48 hr	128	C
Trimethoben-zamide HCl	BE	100 mg/1 mL	EN	10 mg/1 mL	Physically compatible for 36 hr at 27°C	762	C
Trimethoben-zamide HCl	BE	100 mg/1 mL	EN	5 mg/0.5 mL	Physically compatible for 36 hr at 27°C	762	C
Trimethoben-zamide HCl	BE	100 mg/1 mL	EN	2.5 mg/0.25 mL	Physically compatible for 36 hr at 27°C	762	C
Trimethoben-zamide HCl		200 mg/2 mL	DU	10 mg/1 mL	Physically compatible for 48 hr	128	C
Trimethoben-zamide HCl		200 mg/2 mL	DU	20 mg/1 mL	Physically compatible for 48 hr	128	C

Y-Site Injection Compatibility (1:1 Mixture)

Nalbuphine HCl

Test Drug	Mfr	Conc	Mfr	Conc	Remarks	Ref	C/I
Acetaminophen	CAD	10 mg/mL	HOS	10 mg/mL	Physically compatible with little or no loss of either drug in 4 hr at 23°C	2901, 2902	C
Acetaminophen	CAD	10 mg/mL	HOS	20 mg/mL	Physically compatible with less than 10% acetamino-phen loss over 4 hr at room temperature	2841, 2844	C
Acyclovir sodium	BV	5 mg/mL[b]	HOS	10 mg/mL	Physically compatible	2794	C
Allopurinol sodium	BW	3 mg/mL[b]	DU	10 mg/mL	Particles in 1 hr. Crystals in 4 hr	1686	I
Amifostine	USB	10 mg/mL[a]	AST	10 mg/mL	Physically compatible for 4 hr at 23°C	1845	C
Aztreonam	SQ	40 mg/mL[a]	AST	10 mg/mL	Physically compatible for 4 hr at 23°C	1758	C
Bivalirudin	TMC	5 mg/mL[a]	AST	10 mg/mL	Physically compatible for 4 hr at 23°C	2373	C
Blinatumomab	AMG	0.125 mcg/mL[b]	MYL	1 mg/mL[b]	Persistent particulate formation	3405, 3417	I
Blinatumomab	AMG	0.375 mcg/mL[b]	MYL	1 mg/mL[b]	Flakes transiently appear when blinatumomab is added to nalbuphine; not observed when order of mixing was reversed	3405, 3417	?
Cangrelor tetrasodium	TMC	1 mg/mL[b]		10 mg/mL	Physically compatible for 4 hr	3243	C
Cisatracurium besylate	GW	0.1, 2, 5 mg/mL[a]	AST	10 mg/mL	Physically compatible for 4 hr at 23°C	2074	C
Cladribine	ORT	0.015[b] and 0.5[c] mg/mL	AST	10 mg/mL	Physically compatible for 4 hr at 23°C	1969	C
Defibrotide sodium	JAZ	8 mg/mL[b]	MYL	2 mg/mL[b]	Visually compatible for 4 hr at room temperature	3149	C

Y-Site Injection Compatibility (1:1 Mixture) (Cont.)

Test Drug	Mfr	Conc	Mfr	Conc	Remarks	Ref	C/I
Dexmedetomidine HCl	AB	4 mcg/mL[b]	AST	10 mg/mL	Physically compatible for 4 hr at 23°C	2383	C
Docetaxel	RPR	0.9 mg/mL[a]	AST	10 mg/mL	Increase in measured subvisible turbidity occurs immediately	2224	I
Etoposide phosphate	BR	5 mg/mL[a]	AST	10 mg/mL	Physically compatible for 4 hr at 23°C	2218	C
Fenoldopam mesylate	AB	80 mcg/mL[b]	EN	10 mg/mL	Physically compatible for 4 hr at 23°C	2467	C
Filgrastim	AMG	30 mcg/mL[a]	DU	10 mg/mL	Physically compatible for 4 hr at 22°C	1687	C
Fludarabine phosphate	BX	1 mg/mL[a]	DU	10 mg/mL	Visually compatible for 4 hr at 22°C	1439	C
Gemcitabine HCl	LI	10 mg/mL[b]	AST	10 mg/mL	Physically compatible for 4 hr at 23°C	2226	C
Granisetron HCl	SKB	0.05 mg/mL[a]	AB	10 mg/mL	Physically compatible for 4 hr at 23°C	2000	C
Hetastarch in lactated electrolyte	AB	6%	AST	10 mg/mL	Physically compatible for 4 hr at 23°C	2339	C
Linezolid	PHU	2 mg/mL	AST	10 mg/mL	Physically compatible for 4 hr at 23°C	2264	C
Melphalan HCl	BW	0.1 mg/mL[b]	AST	10 mg/mL	Physically compatible for 3 hr at 22°C	1557	C
Methotrexate sodium		30 mg/mL	DU	10 mg/mL	Yellow precipitate forms immediately	1788	I
Nafcillin sodium	WY	33 mg/mL[b]		10 mg/mL	Precipitate forms, probably free nafcillin	547	I
Oxaliplatin	SS	0.5 mg/mL[a]	EN	10 mg/mL	Physically compatible for 4 hr at 23°C	2566	C
Paclitaxel	NCI	1.2 mg/mL[a]	AST	10 mg/mL	Physically compatible for 4 hr at 22°C	1556	C
Pemetrexed disodium	LI	20 mg/mL[b]	EN	10 mg/mL	White precipitate forms immediately	2564	I
Piperacillin sodium–tazobactam sodium	LE[f]	40 mg/mL[a g]	DU	10 mg/mL	Heavy white turbidity forms immediately. Particles form in 4 hr	1688	I
Propofol	ZEN[h]	10 mg/mL	AB	10 mg/mL	Physically compatible for 1 hr at 23°C	2066	C
Remifentanil HCl	GW	0.025 and 0.25 mg/mL[b]	AST	10 mg/mL	Physically compatible for 4 hr at 23°C	2075	C
Sargramostim	IMM	10 mcg/mL[b]	DU	10 mg/mL	Haze and filament form	1436	I
Sodium bicarbonate		1.4%	DU	10 mg/mL	Gas evolves	1788	I
Teniposide	BR	0.1 mg/mL[a]	DU	10 mg/mL	Physically compatible for 4 hr at 23°C	1725	C
Thiotepa	IMM[d]	1 mg/mL[a]	AST	10 mg/mL	Physically compatible for 4 hr at 23°C	1861	C
TNA #218 to #226[e]			AB, AST	10 mg/mL	Damage to emulsion occurs immediately with free oil formation possible	2215	I
TPN #212 to #215[e]			AB	10 mg/mL	Physically compatible for 4 hr at 23°C	2109	C
Vinorelbine tartrate	BW	1 mg/mL[b]	AST	10 mg/mL	Physically compatible for 4 hr at 22°C	1558	C

[a] Tested in dextrose 5%.

[b] Tested in sodium chloride 0.9%.

[c] Tested in bacteriostatic sodium chloride 0.9% preserved with benzyl alcohol 0.9%.

[d] Lyophilized formulation tested.

[e] Refer to Appendix for the composition of parenteral nutrition solutions. TNA indicates a 3-in-1 admixture, and TPN indicates a 2-in-1 admixture.

[f] Test performed using the formulation WITHOUT edetate disodium.

[g] Piperacillin component. Piperacillin in an 8:1 fixed-ratio concentration with tazobactam.

[h] Test performed using the formulation WITH edetate disodium.

Selected Revisions January 31, 2020. © Copyright, October 1984. American Society of Health-System Pharmacists, Inc.

Naloxone Hydrochloride
AHFS 28:10

Products

Naloxone hydrochloride is available in the following formulations:[1(6/06)]

Component	Preserved (mg/mL)		Paraben-Free (mg/mL)		
Naloxone HCl	1	0.4	1	0.4	0.02
Sodium chloride	8.35	8.6	9	9	9
Methyl- and propylparabens (9:1)	2	2	0	0	0
Sizes (mL)	10	10	2	1	2

pH

The pH is adjusted during manufacturing with hydrochloric acid to a target pH of 3 to 4[1(6/06)] with a range of 3 to 6.5.[17]

Osmolality

The osmolality of the 0.02-mg/mL concentration was determined to be 293 mOsm/kg by freezing-point depression and 289 mOsm/kg by vapor pressure.[1071]

The osmolality of naloxone hydrochloride 0.4 mg/mL was determined to be 301 mOsm/kg.[1233]

Trade Name(s)

Narcan

Administration

Naloxone hydrochloride may be administered by subcutaneous, intramuscular, or intravenous injection or by continuous intravenous infusion. Solutions for continuous intravenous infusion may be prepared as 2 mg/500 mL (4 mcg/mL) of sodium chloride 0.9% or dextrose 5%.[1(6/06) 4]

Stability

Naloxone hydrochloride should be stored at room temperature and protected from excessive light. Naloxone hydrochloride should not be mixed with bisulfite, sulfite, or long-chain or high molecular weight anions or any solution with an alkaline pH.[1(6/06) 4]

Naloxone hydrochloride under simulated summer conditions in paramedic vehicles was exposed to 26 to 38°C over 4 weeks. Analysis found no loss of the drug under these conditions.[2562]

Syringes

Naloxone hydrochloride (Astra) 0.133 mg/mL in sodium chloride 0.9% packaged in polypropylene syringes (Sherwood) was physically stable and exhibited little or no loss in 24 hours stored at 4 and 23°C.[2199]

Compatibility Information

Solution Compatibility

Naloxone HCl

Test Soln Name	Mfr	Mfr	Conc/L or %	Remarks	Ref	C/I
Dextrose 5%			4 mg	Discard after 24 hr	1(6/06)	C
Sodium chloride 0.9%			4 mg	Discard after 24 hr	1(6/06)	C

Additive Compatibility

Naloxone HCl

Test Drug	Mfr	Conc/L or %	Mfr	Conc/L or %	Test Solution	Remarks	Ref	C/I
Morphine sulfate	BA	1 g[b]	SZ	4 mg	[a]	Physically compatible with less than 10% loss of either drug in 3 days at 22°C and 30 days at 4°C	3492	C
Morphine sulfate	BA	1 g[b]	SZ	12.5 mg	[a]	Physically compatible with less than 10% loss of either drug in 3 days at 22°C and 30 days at 4°C	3492	C
Morphine sulfate	BA	1 g[b]	SZ	25 mg	[a]	Physically compatible with less than 10% loss of either drug in 3 days at 22°C and 30 days at 4°C	3492	C
Verapamil HCl	KN	80 mg	EN	0.8 mg	D5W, NS	Physically compatible for 24 hr	764	C

[a] Tested in PVC containers.

[b] Tested as the premixed infusion solution.

DOI: 10.37573/9781585286850.280

Drugs in Syringe Compatibility

Naloxone HCl

Test Drug	Mfr	Amt	Mfr	Amt	Remarks	Ref	C/I
Dimenhydrinate		10 mg/1 mL		0.4 mg/1 mL	Clear solution	2569	C
Heparin sodium		2500 units/1 mL	DU	0.4 mg/1 mL	Physically compatible for at least 5 min	1053	C
Ondansetron HCl	GW	1.33 mg/mL[a]	AST	0.133 mg/mL[a]	Physically compatible. Under 6% ondansetron and under 5% naloxone losses in 24 hr at 4 or 23°C	2199	C
Pantoprazole sodium	[b]	4 mg/1 mL		0.4 mg/1 mL	Precipitates within 4 hr	2574	I

[a] Tested in sodium chloride 0.9%.

[b] Test performed using the formulation WITHOUT edetate disodium.

Y-Site Injection Compatibility (1:1 Mixture)

Naloxone HCl

Test Drug	Mfr	Conc	Mfr	Conc	Remarks	Ref	C/I
Blinatumomab	AMG	0.125 mcg/mL[b]	MYL	0.2 mg/mL[b]	Particles, flakes, thin needles, or haze transiently appears when naloxone is added to blinatumomab; not observed when order of mixing was reversed	3405, 3417	?
Blinatumomab	AMG	0.375 mcg/mL[b]	MYL	0.2 mg/mL[b]	Visually compatible for 12 hr at room temperature	3405, 3417	C
Ceftolozane sulfate–tazobactam sodium	CUB	10 mg/mL[c d]	MYL	0.04 mg/mL[c]	Physically compatible for 2 hr	3262	C
Cloxacillin sodium	SMX	100 mg/mL	SZ	0.4 mg/mL	Physically compatible for up to 4 hr at room temperature	3245	C
Defibrotide sodium	JAZ	8 mg/mL[b]	MYL	0.4 mg/mL	Visually compatible for 4 hr at room temperature	3149	C
Fenoldopam mesylate	AB	80 mcg/mL[b]	AB	0.4 mg/mL[b]	Physically compatible for 4 hr at 23°C	2467	C
Isavuconazonium sulfate	ASP	1.5 mg/mL[c]	PPR	0.04 mg/mL[c]	Physically compatible for 2 hr	3263	C
Linezolid	PHU	2 mg/mL	DU	0.4 mg/mL	Physically compatible for 4 hr at 23°C	2264	C
Meropenem		50 mg/mL	ALV	0.4 mg/mL	Physically compatible for 4 hr at room temperature	3538	C
Meropenem–vaborbactam	TMC	8 mg/mL[b e]	MYL	0.04 mg/mL[b]	Physically compatible for 3 hr at 20 to 25°C	3380	C
Plazomicin sulfate	ACH	24 mg/mL[c]	MYL	0.04 mg/mL[c]	Physically compatible for 1 hr at 20 to 25°C	3432	C
Propofol	ZEN	10 mg/mL	AST	0.4 mg/mL	Physically compatible for 1 hr at 23°C	2066	C
Tedizolid phosphate	CUB	0.8 mg/mL[h]	PPR	0.04 mg/mL[b]	Physically compatible for 2 hr	3244	C

[a] Tested in dextrose 5%.

[b] Tested in sodium chloride 0.9%.

[c] Tested in both dextrose 5% and sodium chloride 0.9%.

[d] Ceftolozane component. Ceftolozane in a 2:1 fixed-ratio concentration with tazobactam.

[e] Meropenem component. Meropenem in a 1:1 fixed-ratio concentration with vaborbactam.

Selected Revisions May 1, 2020. © Copyright, October 1982.
American Society of Health-System Pharmacists, Inc.

Neostigmine Methylsulfate
AHFS 12:04

Products

Neostigmine methylsulfate is available in concentrations of 0.5 and 1 mg/mL in 10-mL vials with methyl- and propylparabens 0.2%.[1(6/06)]

pH

The pH is adjusted to near 5.9 with a range of 5 to 6.5.[1(6/06) 17]

Administration

Neostigmine methylsulfate may be administered intramuscularly, subcutaneously, or slowly intravenously.[1(6/06) 4]

Stability

Neostigmine methylsulfate in intact containers should be stored at controlled room temperature and protected from light, freezing, and temperatures of 40°C or more.[1(6/06) 4]

Syringes

In 2015, reports of decreased potency of certain drugs (e.g., neostigmine methylsulfate) stored in Becton Dickinson syringes for extended periods (i.e., exceeding 24 hours) were confirmed by the manufacturer of these syringes; the cause of this change was later identified to be the inclusion of an alternate rubber stopper in the plunger of certain product lots of syringes.[3029 3036 3037 3039 3041 3042] Decreased potency was not observed when the syringes were filled and used promptly.[3037] Use of the alternate stopper was later discontinued and use of the primary stopper in such syringes was resumed; however, Becton Dickinson states that its general-use syringes are cleared by FDA for immediate use in fluid aspiration and injection and that such syringes, regardless of the stopper material, have not been cleared by FDA for use as a closed-container system.[3391]

The stability of neostigmine 0.5 mg/mL repackaged in polypropylene syringes was evaluated. Little concentration change was found after 4 weeks of storage at room temperature not exposed to direct light.[2164]

Neostigmine methylsulfate (Elkins-Sinn) 0.167 mg/mL in sodium chloride 0.9% packaged in polypropylene syringes (Sherwood) was physically stable and exhibited no loss in 24 hours stored at 4 and 23°C.[2199]

Undiluted neostigmine methylsulfate (American Pharmaceutical Partners) 1 mg/mL was packaged in 6-mL polypropylene syringes (Becton Dickinson) and stored at 23°C in fluorescent light and at 4°C for 90 days. The drug remained physically stable and under 2% loss occurred.[2425]

Compatibility Information

Drugs in Syringe Compatibility

Neostigmine methylsulfate

Test Drug	Mfr	Amt	Mfr	Amt	Remarks	Ref	C/I
Glycopyrrolate	RB	0.2 mg/1 mL	RC	0.5 mg/1 mL	Physically compatible. pH in glycopyrrolate stability range for 48 hr at 25°C	331	C
Glycopyrrolate	RB	0.2 mg/1 mL	RC	1 mg/2 mL	Physically compatible. pH in glycopyrrolate stability range for 48 hr at 25°C	331	C
Glycopyrrolate	RB	0.4 mg/2 mL	RC	0.5 mg/1 mL	Physically compatible. pH in glycopyrrolate stability range for 48 hr at 25°C	331	C
Heparin sodium		2500 units/1 mL	RC	0.5 mg/1 mL	Physically compatible for at least 5 min	1053	C
Ondansetron HCl	GW	1.33 mg/mL[a]	ES	0.167 mg/mL[a]	Physically compatible. Under 3% ondansetron and under 5% neostigmine losses in 24 hr at 4 or 23°C	2199	C
Pentobarbital sodium	AB	500 mg/10 mL	RC	0.5 mg/1 mL	Physically compatible	55	C

[a] Tested in sodium chloride 0.9%.

Y-Site Injection Compatibility (1:1 Mixture)

Neostigmine methylsulfate

Test Drug	Mfr	Conc	Mfr	Conc	Remarks	Ref	C/I
Heparin sodium	UP	1000 units/L[a]	RC	0.5 mg/mL	Physically compatible for 4 hr at room temperature	534	C
Hydrocortisone sodium succinate	UP	10 mg/L[a]	RC	0.5 mg/mL	Physically compatible for 4 hr at room temperature	534	C

DOI: 10.37573/9781585286850.281

Y-Site Injection Compatibility (1:1 Mixture) (Cont.)

Test Drug	Mfr	Conc	Mfr	Conc	Remarks	Ref	C/I
Palonosetron HCl	MGI	50 mcg/mL	BA	0.5 mg/mL	Physically compatible. No loss of either drug in 4 hr	2772	C
Potassium chloride	AB	40 mEq/L[a]	RC	0.5 mg/mL	Physically compatible for 4 hr at room temperature	534	C

[a] Tested in dextrose 5% in Ringer's injection, dextrose 5% in Ringer's injection, lactated, dextrose 5%, Ringer's injection, lactated, and sodium chloride 0.9%.

Selected Revisions June 1, 2019. © Copyright, October 1982.
American Society of Health-System Pharmacists, Inc.

Nesiritide
AHFS 24:12.92

Products

Nesiritide is available in 1.5-mg single-use vials containing 1.58 mg of nesiritide with mannitol 20 mg, citric acid monohydrate 2.1 mg, and sodium citrate dihydrate 2.94 mg.[1(1/07)]

Reconstitute nesiritide using 5 mL of solution from a 250-mL plastic intravenous infusion container of dextrose 5%, sodium chloride 0.9%, dextrose 5% in sodium chloride 0.45%, or dextrose 5% in sodium chloride 0.225%, yielding a nesiritide concentration of 0.32 mg/mL. Gently rock the vial to aid dissolution making sure all surfaces, including the stopper, are in contact with the diluent; do not shake the vial. The reconstituted solution should be clear and colorless. Add the entire contents of the vial into the 250-mL plastic infusion solution container and invert several times to yield a nesiritide infusion concentration of 6 mcg/mL.[1(1/07)]

Trade Name(s)

Natrecor

Administration

Nesiritide is administered by an initial intravenous injection drawn from the intravenous infusion solution and given over about 1 minute followed by continuous intravenous infusion. The intravenous tubing should be primed with 5 mL of the solution before connecting to the patient's access port and before administering the initial bolus dose or beginning the infusion.[1(1/07)]

Stability

Intact vials should be stored below 25°C in the original carton to protect from light. Protect the vials from freezing.[1(1/07)]

The manufacturer states that the reconstituted nesiritide should be used within 24 hours stored between 2 and 25°C because no antimicrobial preservative is present.[1(1/07)]

Nesiritide is incompatible with sodium metabisulfite and other bisulfite antioxidants used in some drug formulations. The specific formulation of the product to be used should be checked to ensure that no sulfite antioxidants are present. Drugs that contain sulfite antioxidants should not be administered into the same intravenous infusion line as nesiritide. The line should be flushed between administration of the incompatible drugs and nesiritide.[1(1/07) 2625]

Sorption

The official product labeling states that nesiritide may bind to heparin-coated administration catheters decreasing the delivery of nesiritide to the patient and that heparin-coated administration lines must not be used to administer nesiritide.[1(1/07)]

However, a study of nesiritide delivery through unprimed PVC and polyethylene tubing, a polyurethane central catheter, and a heparin-coated PVC catheter found little alteration of the delivered concentration. About 94 to 98% of the drug was delivered through these devices compared to 98% through primed PVC tubing alone.[2646]

Compatibility Information

Y-Site Injection Compatibility (1:1 Mixture)

Nesiritide

Test Drug	Mfr	Conc	Mfr	Conc	Remarks	Ref	C/I
Amiodarone HCl		50 mg/mL	SCI	50 mcg/mL[a b]	Physically compatible for 4 hr	2625	C
Argatroban	SKB	1 mg/mL[a]	SCI	6 mcg/mL[a]	Physically compatible for 24 hr at 23°C	2572	C
Bumetanide		0.25 mg/mL	SCI	50 mcg/mL[a b]	Physically incompatible	2625	I
Digoxin		0.25 mg/mL	SCI	50 mcg/mL[a b]	Physically compatible for 4 hr	2625	C
Diltiazem HCl		5 mg/mL	SCI	50 mcg/mL[a b]	Physically compatible for 4 hr	2625	C
Dobutamine HCl		12.5 mg/mL	SCI	50 mcg/mL[a b]	Physically compatible for 4 hr. May be chemically incompatible with nesiritide[c]	2625	?
Dopamine HCl		80 mg/mL	SCI	50 mcg/mL[a b]	Physically compatible for 4 hr. May be chemically incompatible with nesiritide[c]	2625	?
Enalaprilat		1.25 mg/mL	SCI	50 mcg/mL[a b]	Physically incompatible	2625	I
Epinephrine HCl		1 mg/mL	SCI	50 mcg/mL[a b]	Physically compatible for 4 hr. May be chemically incompatible with nesiritide[c]	2625	?
Ethacrynate sodium		1 mg/mL	SCI	50 mcg/mL[a b]	Physically incompatible	2625	I

DOI: 10.37573/9781585286850.282

Y-Site Injection Compatibility (1:1 Mixture) (Cont.)

Test Drug	Mfr	Conc	Mfr	Conc	Remarks	Ref	C/I
Fentanyl citrate		0.05 mg/mL	SCI	50 mcg/mL[a][b]	Physically compatible for 4 hr	2625	C
Furosemide		10 mg/mL	SCI	50 mcg/mL[a][b]	Physically incompatible	2625	I
Heparin sodium		0.1, 1, 10 units/mL	SCI	50 mcg/mL[a][b]	Physically incompatible	2625	I
Hydralazine HCl		20 mg/mL	SCI	50 mcg/mL[a][b]	Physically incompatible	2625	I
Insulin, regular		Up to 100 units/mL	SCI	50 mcg/mL[a][b]	Physically incompatible	2625	I
Isavuconazonium sulfate	ASP	1.5 mg/mL[d]	SCI	6 mcg/mL[d]	Physically compatible for 2 hr	3263	C
Lidocaine HCl		20 mg/mL	SCI	50 mcg/mL[a][b]	Physically compatible for 4 hr. May be chemically incompatible with nesiritide[c]	2625	?
Meperidine HCl		100 mg/mL	SCI	50 mcg/mL[a][b]	Physically compatible for 4 hr. May be chemically incompatible with nesiritide[c]	2625	?
Metoprolol tartrate		1 mg/mL	SCI	50 mcg/mL[a][b]	Physically compatible for 4 hr	2625	C
Metoprolol tartrate	BED	1 mg/mL	SCI	6 mcg/mL[a]	Trace precipitate in 24 hr at 19°C	2795	I
Micafungin sodium	ASP	1.5 mg/mL[b]	SCI	6 mcg/mL[a]	Microparticulates form immediately	2683	I
Milrinone lactate		1 mg/mL	SCI	50 mcg/mL[a][b]	Physically compatible for 4 hr	2625	C
Morphine sulfate		15 mg/mL	SCI	50 mcg/mL[a][b]	Physically compatible for 4 hr. May be chemically incompatible with nesiritide[c]	2625	?
Nicardipine HCl		2.5 mg/mL	SCI	50 mcg/mL[a][b]	Physically compatible for 4 hr	2625	C
Nitroglycerin		0.2 mg/mL	SCI	50 mcg/mL[a][b]	Physically compatible for 4 hr	2625	C
Norepinephrine bitartrate		1 mg/mL	SCI	50 mcg/mL[a][b]	Physically compatible for 4 hr. May be chemically incompatible with nesiritide[c]	2625	?
Phenylephrine HCl		10 mg/mL	SCI	50 mcg/mL[a][b]	Physically compatible for 4 hr. May be chemically incompatible with nesiritide[c]	2625	?
Procainamide HCl		500 mg/mL	SCI	50 mcg/mL[a][b]	Physically compatible for 4 hr. May be chemically incompatible with nesiritide[c]	2625	?
Propranolol HCl		1 mg/mL	SCI	50 mcg/mL[a][b]	Physically compatible for 4 hr	2625	C
Quinidine gluconate		80 mg/mL	SCI	50 mcg/mL[a][b]	Physically compatible for 4 hr	2625	C
Sodium nitroprusside		5 mg/mL	SCI	50 mcg/mL[a][b]	Physically compatible for 4 hr	2625	C
Torsemide		10 mg/mL	SCI	50 mcg/mL[a][b]	Physically compatible for 4 hr	2625	C
Verapamil HCl		2.5 mg/mL	SCI	50 mcg/mL[a][b]	Physically compatible for 4 hr	2625	C

[a] Tested in dextrose 5%.

[b] Tested in sodium chloride 0.9%.

[c] Nesiritide is incompatible with bisulfite antioxidants used in some drug formulations. The specific formulation of the product to be used should be checked to ensure that no sulfite antioxidants are present.

[d] Tested in both dextrose 5% and sodium chloride 0.9%.

Selected Revisions September 29, 2017. © Copyright, October 2008. American Society of Health-System Pharmacists, Inc.

Nicardipine Hydrochloride
AHFS 24:28.08

Products

Nicardipine hydrochloride is available as a 2.5-mg/mL concentrate for injection in 10-mL ampuls. Each mL also contains sorbitol 48 mg, citric acid monohydrate 0.525 mg, and sodium hydroxide 0.09 mg in water for injection. Additional citric acid and/or sodium hydroxide may have been added to adjust solution pH.[1(1/06)]

pH

Buffered to pH 3.5.[1(1/06)]

Trade Name(s)

Cardene I.V.

Administration

Nicardipine hydrochloride concentrate for injection must be diluted for use. It is administered as a slow continuous intravenous infusion at a concentration of 0.1 mg/mL. The infusion is prepared by adding 10 mL of nicardipine hydrochloride (25 mg) to 240 mL of compatible infusion solution, making 250 mL of a 0.1-mg/mL solution. If nicardipine hydrochloride is administered via a peripheral vein, the infusion site should be changed every 12 hours to avoid venous irritation.[1(1/06) 4]

Stability

Intact ampuls of the clear, yellow solution should be stored at controlled room temperature and protected from light. Freezing does not adversely affect the product, but exposure to elevated temperatures should be avoided.[1(1/06)]

Light Effects

Deliberate exposure of a 0.1-mg/mL nicardipine hydrochloride solution to daylight resulted in about 8% loss in 7 hours and 21% loss in 14 hours. Protection from light may be considered.[2193]

Sorption

Nicardipine hydrochloride (Dupont Merck) 50 and 500 mg/L in a variety of infusion solutions in polyvinyl chloride (PVC) containers showed a decline in concentration due to sorption to the plastic. Losses were rapid in Ringer's injection, lactated with up to 42% lost in 24 hours. The concentrations were stable in glass containers.[1380]

Compatibility Information

Solution Compatibility

Nicardipine HCl

Test Soln Name	Mfr	Mfr	Conc/L or %	Remarks	Ref	C/I
Dextrose 5% in Ringer's injection, lactated	MG[a]	DME	50 and 500 mg	Physically compatible. 7% loss in 7 days at room temperature in light	1380	C
Dextrose 5% in Ringer's injection, lactated	TR[b]	DME	500 mg	Physically compatible. 7% loss in 24 hr at room temperature in light	1380	C
Dextrose 5% in Ringer's injection, lactated	TR[b]	DME	50 mg	Physically compatible. 11% loss in 24 hr at room temperature in light	1380	I
Dextrose 5% in sodium chloride 0.45%	a b		100 mg	Stable for 24 hr at room temperature	1(1/06)	C
Dextrose 5% in sodium chloride 0.45%	MG[a]	DME	50 and 500 mg	Physically compatible. Little loss in 7 days at room temperature in light	1380	C
Dextrose 5% in sodium chloride 0.45%	TR[b]	DME	50 and 500 mg	Physically compatible. 9% loss in 72 hr at room temperature in light	1380	C
Dextrose 5% in sodium chloride 0.9%	a b		100 mg	Stable for 24 hr at room temperature	1(1/06)	C
Dextrose 5% in sodium chloride 0.9%	MG[a]	DME	50 and 500 mg	Physically compatible. Little loss in 7 days at room temperature in light	1380	C
Dextrose 5% in sodium chloride 0.9%	TR[b]	DME	50 and 500 mg	Physically compatible. 7% loss in 7 days at room temperature in light	1380	C
Dextrose 5%	a b		100 mg	Stable for 24 hr at room temperature	1(1/06)	C
Dextrose 5%	MG[a]	DME	50 and 500 mg	Physically compatible. Little loss in 7 days at room temperature in light	1380	C

DOI: 10.37573/9781585286850.283

Solution Compatibility (Cont.)

Test Soln Name	Mfr	Mfr	Conc/L or %	Remarks	Ref	C/I
Dextrose 5%	TR[b]	DME	500 mg	Physically compatible. 6% loss in 7 days at room temperature in light	1380	C
Dextrose 5%	TR[b]	DME	50 mg	Physically compatible. 13% loss in 24 hr at room temperature in light	1380	I
Ringer's injection, lactated				Incompatible	1(1/06)	I
Ringer's injection, lactated	MG[a]	DME	50 and 500 mg	Physically compatible. Little loss in 7 days at room temperature in light	1380	C
Ringer's injection, lactated	TR[b]	DME	500 mg	Physically compatible. 15% loss in 24 hr at room temperature in light	1380	I
Ringer's injection, lactated	TR[b]	DME	50 mg	Physically compatible. 42% loss in 24 hr at room temperature in light	1380	I
Sodium chloride 0.45%	a b		100 mg	Stable for 24 hr at room temperature	1(1/06)	C
Sodium chloride 0.45%	MG[a]	DME	50 and 500 mg	Physically compatible. Little loss in 7 days at room temperature in light	1380	C
Sodium chloride 0.45%	TR[b]	DME	500 mg	Physically compatible. 3% loss in 7 days at room temperature in light	1380	C
Sodium chloride 0.45%	TR[b]	DME	50 mg	Physically compatible. 11% loss in 24 hr at room temperature in light	1380	I
Sodium chloride 0.9%	a b		100 mg	Stable for 24 hr at room temperature	1(1/06)	C
Sodium chloride 0.9%	MG[a]	DME	50 and 500 mg	Physically compatible. Little loss in 7 days at room temperature in light	1380	C
Sodium chloride 0.9%	TR[b]	DME	50 and 500 mg	Physically compatible. 8% loss in 72 hr at room temperature in light	1380	C

[a] Tested in glass containers.

[b] Tested in PVC containers.

Additive Compatibility

Nicardipine HCl

Test Drug	Mfr	Conc/L or %	Mfr	Conc/L or %	Test Solution	Remarks	Ref	C/I
Potassium chloride	ES	40 mEq	DME	50 and 500 mg	D5W[a]	Physically compatible. Little loss in 7 days at room temperature in light	1380	C
Potassium chloride	ES	40 mEq	DME	50 and 500 mg	D5W[b]	Physically compatible. 12% loss in 7 days at room temperature in light	1380	C
Sodium bicarbonate	TR[a]	5%	DME	50 and 500 mg		Precipitate forms immediately	1380	I

[a] Tested in glass containers.

[b] Tested in PVC containers.

Y-Site Injection Compatibility (1:1 Mixture)

Nicardipine HCl

Test Drug	Mfr	Conc	Mfr	Conc	Remarks	Ref	C/I
Amikacin sulfate	BR	2 mg/mL[a]	DCC	0.1 mg/mL[a]	Visually compatible for 24 hr at room temperature	235	C
Aminophylline	ES	1 mg/mL[a]	DCC	0.1 mg/mL[a]	Visually compatible for 24 hr at room temperature	235	C
Ampicillin sodium	BR	10 mg/mL[a b]	DCC	0.1 mg/mL[a b]	Turbidity forms immediately	235	I

Y-Site Injection Compatibility (1:1 Mixture) (Cont.)

Test Drug	Mfr	Conc	Mfr	Conc	Remarks	Ref	C/I
Ampicillin sodium–sulbactam sodium	PF	10 mg/mL[a b d]	DCC	0.1 mg/mL[a b]	Turbidity forms immediately	235	I
Aztreonam	SQ	10 mg/mL[a]	DCC	0.1 mg/mL[a]	Visually compatible for 24 hr at room temperature	235	C
Butorphanol tartrate	BR	0.4 mg/mL[a]	DCC	0.1 mg/mL[a]	Visually compatible for 24 hr at room temperature	235	C
Calcium gluconate	ES	0.092 mEq/mL[a]	DCC	0.1 mg/mL[a]	Visually compatible for 24 hr at room temperature	235	C
Cefazolin sodium	SKF	20 mg/mL[a]	DCC	0.1 mg/mL[a]	Visually compatible for 24 hr at room temperature	235	C
Cefepime HCl	BMS	120 mg/mL[c]		1 mg/mL	Precipitates	2513	I
Ceftazidime	GL	10 mg/mL[a]	DCC	0.1 mg/mL[a]	Visually compatible for 24 hr at room temperature	235	C
Ceftazidime	SKB	125 mg/mL		1 mg/mL	Precipitates immediately	2434	I
Ceftazidime	GSK	120 mg/mL[c]		1 mg/mL	Precipitates	2513	I
Ceftolozane sulfate–tazobactam sodium	CUB	10 mg/mL[f g]	EXL	0.1 mg/mL[f]	Immediate gross precipitation and increase in measured turbidity	3247, 3262	I
Chloramphenicol sodium succinate	PD	10 mg/mL[a]	DCC	0.1 mg/mL[a]	Visually compatible for 24 hr at room temperature	235	C
Cisatracurium besylate	AB	1 mg/mL[b]	CRC	0.5 mg/mL[b]	Physically compatible for 1 hr at 23°C	3157	C
Clevidipine butyrate	CHS	0.5 mg/mL		0.1 mg/mL[c]	pH shifted outside of specified pH range for clevidipine within 24 hr	3334	?
Clindamycin phosphate	UP	9 mg/mL[a]	DCC	0.1 mg/mL[a]	Visually compatible for 24 hr at room temperature	235	C
Defibrotide sodium	JAZ	8 mg/mL[b]	AGT	0.5 mg/mL[b]	Small particles form in 4 hr	3149	I
Dextran 40 in dextrose 5%	TR	10%	DCC	0.1 mg/mL[a]	Visually compatible for 24 hr at room temperature	235	C
Diltiazem HCl	MMD	1 mg/mL[a]	WY	1 mg/mL[a]	Visually compatible for 4 hr at 27°C	2062	C
Dobutamine HCl	LI	4 mg/mL[a]	WY	1 mg/mL[a]	Visually compatible for 4 hr at 27°C	2062	C
Dobutamine HCl	LI	1 mg/mL[a]	DCC	0.1 mg/mL[a]	Visually compatible for 24 hr at room temperature	235	C
Dopamine HCl	AB	3.2 mg/mL[a]	WY	1 mg/mL[a]	Visually compatible for 4 hr at 27°C	2062	C
Dopamine HCl	IMS	1.6 mg/mL[a]	DCC	0.1 mg/mL[a]	Visually compatible for 24 hr at room temperature	235	C
Enalaprilat	MSD	0.05 mg/mL[b]	DU	0.1 mg/mL[a]	Physically compatible for 24 hr at room temperature under fluorescent light	1355	C
Enalaprilat	MSD	0.5 mg/mL[a]	DCC	0.1 mg/mL[a]	Visually compatible for 24 hr at room temperature	235	C
Epinephrine HCl	AB	0.02 mg/mL[a]	WY	1 mg/mL[a]	Visually compatible for 4 hr at 27°C	2062	C
Eravacycline dihydrochloride	TET	0.6 mg/mL[b]	EXL	0.1 mg/mL[b]	Physically compatible for 2 hr at room temperature	3532	C
Erythromycin lactobionate	AB	5 mg/mL[a]	DCC	0.1 mg/mL[a]	Visually compatible for 24 hr at room temperature	235	C
Esmolol HCl	DU	10 mg/mL[a]	DCC	0.1 mg/mL[a]	Visually compatible for 24 hr at room temperature	235	C
Famotidine	MSD	0.2 mg/mL[a]	DCC	0.1 mg/mL[a]	Visually compatible for 24 hr at room temperature	235	C
Fenoldopam mesylate	AB	80 mcg/mL[b]	WAY	1 mg/mL[b]	Physically compatible for 4 hr at 23°C	2467	C
Fentanyl citrate	ES	0.05 mg/mL	WY	1 mg/mL[a]	Visually compatible for 4 hr at 27°C	2062	C
Fentanyl citrate	ES	2 mcg/mL[a]	DCC	0.1 mg/mL[a]	Visually compatible for 24 hr at room temperature	235	C
Furosemide	AMR	10 mg/mL	WY	1 mg/mL[a]	Precipitate forms immediately	2062	I
Gentamicin sulfate	ES	0.8 mg/mL[a]	DCC	0.1 mg/mL[a]	Visually compatible for 24 hr at room temperature	235	C
Heparin sodium	ES	100 units/mL[a]	WY	1 mg/mL[a]	Precipitate forms immediately	2062	I

Y-Site Injection Compatibility (1:1 Mixture) (Cont.)

Test Drug	Mfr	Conc	Mfr	Conc	Remarks	Ref	C/I
Heparin sodium	IX	40 units/mL[a]	DCC	0.1 mg/mL[a]	Visually compatible for 24 hr at room temperature	235	C
Hetastarch in sodium chloride 0.9%	DU	6%	DCC	0.1 mg/mL[a]	Visually compatible for 24 hr at room temperature	235	C
Hydrocortisone sodium succinate	UP	2 mg/mL[a]	DCC	0.1 mg/mL[a]	Visually compatible for 24 hr at room temperature	235	C
Hydromorphone HCl	KN	1 mg/mL	WY	1 mg/mL[a]	Visually compatible for 4 hr at 27°C	2062	C
Isavuconazonium sulfate	ASP	1.5 mg/mL[f]	BA	0.2 mg/mL[f]	Physically compatible for 2 hr	3263	C
Labetalol HCl	AH	2 mg/mL[a]	WY	1 mg/mL[a]	Visually compatible for 4 hr at 27°C	2062	C
Labetalol HCl	GL	1 mg/mL[a]	DCC	0.1 mg/mL[a]	Visually compatible for 24 hr at room temperature	235	C
Lidocaine HCl	AST	4 mg/mL[a]	DCC	0.1 mg/mL[a]	Visually compatible for 24 hr at room temperature	235	C
Linezolid	PHU	2 mg/mL	WAY	1 mg/mL[a]	Physically compatible for 4 hr at 23°C	2264	C
Lorazepam	WY	0.5 mg/mL[a]	WY	1 mg/mL[a]	Visually compatible for 4 hr at 27°C	2062	C
Magnesium sulfate	LY	10 mg/mL[a]	DCC	0.1 mg/mL[a]	Visually compatible for 24 hr at room temperature	235	C
Meropenem–vaborbactam	TMC	8 mg/mL[b h]	EXL	0.1 mg/mL[b]	Measured turbidity increases immediately. pH increased by >3 units within 3 hr	3380	I
Methylprednisolone sodium succinate	UP	0.8 mg/mL[a]	DCC	0.1 mg/mL[a]	Visually compatible for 24 hr at room temperature	235	C
Metronidazole	SE	5 mg/mL	DCC	0.1 mg/mL[a]	Visually compatible for 24 hr at room temperature	235	C
Micafungin sodium	ASP	1.5 mg/mL[b]	ESP	1 mg/mL[b]	Precipitate forms immediately	2683	I
Midazolam HCl	RC	2 mg/mL[a]	WY	1 mg/mL[a]	Visually compatible for 4 hr at 27°C	2062	C
Milrinone lactate	SW	0.2 mg/mL[a]	WY	1 mg/mL[a]	Visually compatible for 4 hr at 27°C	2062	C
Morphine sulfate	SCN	2 mg/mL[a]	WY	1 mg/mL[a]	Visually compatible for 4 hr at 27°C	2062	C
Morphine sulfate	WY	0.2 mg/mL[a]	DCC	0.1 mg/mL[a]	Visually compatible for 24 hr at room temperature	235	C
Nafcillin sodium	BR	10 mg/mL[a]	DCC	0.1 mg/mL[a]	Visually compatible for 24 hr at room temperature	235	C
Nesiritide	SCI	50 mcg/mL[a b]		2.5 mg/mL	Physically compatible for 4 hr	2625	C
Nitroglycerin	AB	0.4 mg/mL[a]	WY	1 mg/mL[a]	Visually compatible for 4 hr at 27°C	2062	C
Norepinephrine bitartrate	AB	0.128 mg/mL[a]	WY	1 mg/mL[a]	Visually compatible for 4 hr at 27°C	2062	C
Penicillin G potassium	PF	50,000 units/mL[a]	DCC	0.1 mg/mL[a]	Visually compatible for 24 hr at room temperature	235	C
Plazomicin sulfate	ACH	24 mg/mL[f]	EXL	0.1 mg/mL[f]	Physically compatible for 1 hr at 20 to 25°C	3432	C
Potassium chloride	LY	0.4 mEq/mL[a]	DCC	0.1 mg/mL[a]	Visually compatible for 24 hr at room temperature	235	C
Potassium phosphates	LY	0.44 mEq/mL[a]	DCC	0.1 mg/mL[a]	Visually compatible for 24 hr at room temperature	235	C
Ranitidine HCl	GL	1 mg/mL[a]	WY	1 mg/mL[a]	Visually compatible for 4 hr at 27°C	2062	C
Ranitidine HCl	GL	0.5 mg/mL[a]	DCC	0.1 mg/mL[a]	Visually compatible for 24 hr at room temperature	235	C
Sodium acetate	LY	0.4 mEq/mL[a]	DCC	0.1 mg/mL[a]	Visually compatible for 24 hr at room temperature	235	C
Sodium nitroprusside	LY	0.2 mg/mL[a]	DCC	0.1 mg/mL[a]	Visually compatible for 24 hr at room temperature	235	C
Tedizolid phosphate	CUB	0.8 mg/mL[b]	BA	0.2 mg/mL[b]	Immediate precipitation and increase in measured turbidity	3244	I
Tobramycin sulfate	LI	0.8 mg/mL[a]	DCC	0.1 mg/mL[a]	Visually compatible for 24 hr at room temperature	235	C

Y-Site Injection Compatibility (1:1 Mixture) (Cont.)

Test Drug	Mfr	Conc	Mfr	Conc	Remarks	Ref	C/I
Trimethoprim–sulfamethoxazole	QU	0.16 mg/mL[a] [e]	DCC	0.1 mg/mL[a]	Visually compatible for 24 hr at room temperature	235	C
Vancomycin HCl	LE	5 mg/mL[a]	DCC	0.1 mg/mL[a]	Visually compatible for 24 hr at room temperature	235	C
Vecuronium bromide	OR	1 mg/mL	WY	1 mg/mL[a]	Visually compatible for 4 hr at 27°C	2062	C

[a] Tested in dextrose 5%.

[b] Tested in sodium chloride 0.9%.

[c] Tested in sterile water for injection.

[d] Ampicillin component. Ampicillin in a 2:1 fixed-ratio concentration with sulbactam.

[e] Trimethoprim component. Trimethoprim in a 1:5 fixed-ratio concentration with sulfamethoxazole.

[f] Tested in both dextrose 5% and sodium chloride 0.9%.

[g] Ceftolozane component. Ceftolozane in a 2:1 fixed-ratio concentration with tazobactam.

[h] Meropenem component. Meropenem in a 1:1 fixed-ratio concentration with vaborbactam.

Selected Revisions May 1, 2020. © Copyright, October 1998.
American Society of Health-System Pharmacists, Inc.

Nimodipine
AHFS 24:28.08

Products

Nimodipine 0.02% (0.2 mg/mL) is available in 50-mL brown glass vials and 250-mL brown glass bottles. The product also contains ethanol 20% (w/v), polyethylene glycol 400, sodium citrate, citric acid, and water for injection.[38][115]

Administration

Nimodipine is given by intravenous infusion via a central catheter;[38][115] use of an infusion pump has been recommended.[115] Intracisternal instillation has also been described.[115] The drug must not be added to an infusion bag or bottle. For administration, nimodipine injection is drawn into a 50-mL syringe and connected to a three-way stopcock and polyethylene tube that permits simultaneous administration of the nimodipine and a co-infusion running at a rate of 40 mL/hr. Dextrose 5%, sodium chloride 0.9%, lactated Ringer's injection, lactated Ringer's injection with magnesium, dextran 40, mannitol 10%, albumin human 5%, and hetastarch 6% in sodium chloride 0.9% have been recommended for use as the co-infusion solution.[38][115]

Stability

Nimodipine injection is a clear yellow solution. Intact containers of the drug should be stored at or below 25°C. The drug is light sensitive and should be stored in the light-protective container within the carton that is supplied with the product. Nimodipine should not be added to infusion solution bags or bottles or mixed with other drugs. The 250-mL bottles are intended for single use only and should be pierced only once. Once pierced, the bottle should be used for no longer than 25 hours regardless of whether all of the solution has been administered.[38][115]

Light Effects

Nimodipine is light sensitive. The drug drawn into a syringe for administration must be protected from direct sunlight during administration but is stable for up to 10 hours exposed to diffuse daylight and artificial light. The 250-mL infusion bottle should also be protected from direct sunlight at all times. Opaque coverings for infusion pumps and tubing or black, brown, yellow, or red infusion lines can be used when needed.[38][115]

Sorption

Nimodipine reacts with PVC equipment but is compatible with polyethylene and polypropylene containers, syringes, and administration sets as well as glass containers.[38][115]

Nimodipine (Bayer) 0.01 mg/mL in dextrose 5% and sodium chloride 0.9% packaged in PVC, polyethylene, and glass containers exhibited only 3 to 5% loss in glass and polyethylene containers but 94% loss due to sorption in PVC containers when stored at 4 and 22°C for 24 hours protected from light.[2289]

Compatibility Information

Solution Compatibility

Nimodipine

Test Soln Name	Mfr	Mfr	Conc/L or %	Remarks	Ref	C/I
Dextrose 5%	BA[a]	BAY	10 mg	Visually compatible. 94% loss to PVC at 22°C and 81% loss at 4°C in 24 hr	2289	I
Dextrose 5%	BRN[b][c]	BAY	10 mg	Visually compatible. 3 to 5% loss in 24 hr at 4 and 22°C	2289	C
Sodium chloride 0.9%	BA[a]	BAY	10 mg	Visually compatible. 94% loss to PVC at 22°C and 81% loss at 4°C in 24 hr	2289	I
Sodium chloride 0.9%	BRN[b][c]	BAY	10 mg	Visually compatible. 3 to 5% loss in 24 hr at 4 and 22°C	2289	C

[a] Tested in PVC containers.

[b] Tested in glass containers.

[c] Tested in polyethylene containers.

DOI: 10.37573/9781585286850.284

Nitroglycerin

AHFS 24:12.08

Products

Nitroglycerin injection is available in a 5-mg/mL concentration in 5- and 10-mL vials. The product also contains ethanol 30% and propylene glycol 30% in water for injection. The pH may have been adjusted during manufacture with sodium hydroxide and/or hydrochloric acid. Nitroglycerin injection must be diluted before use.[1(10/06)] [4]

Nitroglycerin is available premixed in dextrose 5% at concentrations of 100, 200, and 400 mcg/mL in 250- and 500-mL containers. The Baxter premixed infusions contain propylene glycol and ethanol with citric acid as a buffer and sodium hydroxide and/or hydrochloric acid, if necessary, to adjust the pH during manufacturing. The Hospira premixed infusions also contain propylene glycol (but no ethanol) and nitric acid to adjust pH during manufacturing.[1(10/06)]

pH

The concentrate for injection has a pH of 3 to 6.5.[1(10/06)] [4] The Baxter premixed infusion solution has a pH of 4 (range 3 to 5). The Hospira premixed infusion solution also has a pH of about 4 but with a range of 3 to 6.5.[1(10/06)]

Osmolarity

The osmolarities of the nitroglycerin premixed infusion solutions in dextrose 5% vary by manufacturer but are all within the normal range for infusions:[1(10/06)]

Nitroglycerin Concentration	Osmolarity (mOsm/L)	
	Hospira	Baxter
100 mcg/mL	265	428
200 mcg/mL	277	440
400 mcg/mL	301	465

Administration

Nitroglycerin injection is administered by intravenous infusion after dilution in dextrose 5% or sodium chloride 0.9% contained in glass bottles, using an infusion control device. The use of filters should be avoided. Various concentrations and administration rates are utilized, depending on the fluid requirements of the patient and the duration of therapy. An initial concentration of 50 to 100 mcg/mL, with adjustment to the concentration if necessary, has been recommended. The concentration should not exceed 400 mcg/mL.[1(10/06)] [4]

Because of nitroglycerin sorption into polyvinyl chloride (PVC) plastic, dosing is higher with standard PVC administration sets and should be reduced when nonabsorbing administration sets are used.[4]

Inaccurate nitroglycerin dosing may occur with nonabsorbing high-density polyethylene plastic administration sets. Such tubing is less pliable than PVC and may not work well with some infusion control devices designed for PVC tubing, resulting in overinfusion.[729] [730] [731] [1120]

Stability

Nitroglycerin injections are practically colorless and stable in the intact containers. The solutions are not explosive. Storage should be at controlled room temperature; the containers should be protected from freezing.[1(10/06)] [4] Exposure to light, even high intensity light, does not adversely affect nitroglycerin stability.[506] [510] [928] [930] [1941]

pH Effects

The rate of nitroglycerin hydrolysis becomes significant at low pH values and is also quite rapid in alkaline solutions.[933] In neutral to weakly acidic solutions, the drug is stable. No loss was observed over 136 days at room temperature at pH 3 to 5.[1072]

Syringes

Plastic syringes having polypropylene barrels and polyethylene plungers (Pharma-Plast) and all-glass containers were compared in an investigation of the possible sorption of nitroglycerin. After 24 hours of storage of aqueous nitroglycerin solutions (concentrations unspecified), no drug loss was found in either the plastic syringes or glass containers. The authors indicated that these plastic syringes could be substituted for glass syringes for use with syringe pumps.[782]

Nitroglycerin (DuPont) (concentration unspecified) was filled into 3-mL plastic syringes (Becton Dickinson, Sherwood Monoject, and Terumo) and stored at −20, 4, and 25°C in the dark. Nitroglycerin losses in 1 day ranged from 10 to 15% at 25°C, to 2 to 3% at 4°C, to 2% or less at −20°C. Long-term storage for 7 days at 4°C and 30 days at −20°C resulted in losses of 5 to 7% and 2% or less, respectively. The losses were presumably due to sorption to surfaces and/or the elastomeric plunger.[1562]

Nitroglycerin (DuPont) 50 mg/50 mL in dextrose 5% exhibited no change in appearance and about a 3.6% loss when stored in 60-mL plastic syringes (Becton Dickinson) for 24 hours at 25°C.[1579]

Nitroglycerin concentrate 5 mg/mL from 4 manufacturers (Abbott, DuPont, Goldline, Marion) was filled as 10 mL in 10-mL glass syringes (Becton Dickinson) and in 10-mL (Becton Dickinson) and 12-mL (Monoject) polypropylene plastic syringes. No loss of nitroglycerin content occurred in 23 hours when stored at 25°C protected from light. Mean nitroglycerin concentrations were greater than 99% and were the same for both the glass and plastic syringes.[2055]

Nitroglycerin 110 mcg/mL prepared from nitroglycerin 100 mcg/mL in dextrose 5% injection (Hospira) and nitroglycerin 5 mg/mL

DOI: 10.37573/9781585286850.285

injection (American Regent) and packaged as 10.1 mL in 12-mL polypropylene syringes (Terumo) was tested for stability at a controlled room temperature of 23 to 27°C protected from light.[2976] The solution exhibited no change in appearance and about an 8% loss at 14 days; calculated time to 10% loss was 24 days.[2976]

Sorption

Nitroglycerin readily undergoes sorption to many soft plastics, especially PVC which is commonly used to make infusion solution bags and intravenous tubing.

Plastics such as polyethylene and polypropylene generally do not absorb nitroglycerin. Consequently, it is recommended that only infusion solution containers made from glass or a plastic known to be compatible with nitroglycerin (i.e., polyolefin) be used for mixing infusions.

To circumvent the significant loss to PVC tubing, use of the special high-density polyethylene administration sets provided by the various nitroglycerin injection manufacturers is recommended. Nitroglycerin is not significantly sorbed to these special sets, but the rate of loss to conventional PVC sets is significant (40 to 80%), although not constant nor self-limiting. Many factors including flow rate, concentration, and length of the set affect the extent of sorption. The greatest amount of sorption occurs early in the infusion. A slow rate of flow and long tubing length increase the loss. Simple calculations or corrections cannot be applied to this complex phenomenon to determine or control the actual amount of nitroglycerin delivered through PVC tubing.[1(10/06) 4 503 506 508 509 510 511 721 723 724 725 726 727 728 769 770 797 930 931 932 934 943 1027 1121 1122 1392 1510 1511 1512 1796 2143 2289 2660 2792]

In addition to PVC bags and infusion tubing, nitroglycerin has been demonstrated to undergo similar sorption to cellulose propionate drip chambers,[725 931 1027 1512] polystyrolbutadiene burettes,[1512] PVC pulmonary artery catheters[937] and central venous pressure catheters (Intracath, Deseret),[938] a polyurethane sponge used to defoam blood in a bubble oxygenator,[939] a silicone rubber membrane in a membrane oxygenator,[940] an infusion pump cassette (Accuset C-924, IMED),[941] and silicone rubber microbore intravenous infusion tubing.[942]

However, the clinical importance of the sorption to PVC has been questioned because nitroglycerin administration is titrated to clinical response, not in a fixed dosage.[1120 1123 2015 2016 2054] A 25 to 35% loss to PVC tubing was reported at rates of nitroglycerin administration of 80 and 60 mcg/min, respectively. Polyethylene tubing delivered essentially 100% of the nitroglycerin. Nevertheless, there was no statistically significant difference in physiologic response in patients when a variety of parameters were evaluated. The type of tubing used does not influence the ultimate hemodynamic responses significantly, because even the PVC delivered a significant amount of the drug. It was advised that physiologic endpoints be monitored in patients on intravenous nitroglycerin.[1120]

A number of similar results were also reported.[2015 2016 2054] Adequate clinical response was achieved using PVC containers and tubing. However, changes in patient hemodynamic status could occur if containers for nitroglycerin infusions were changed during the treatment course; switching from PVC to glass or vice versa could require substantial adjustment in the rate of administration to achieve a similar clinical response.[2016]

Filtration

Some filters absorb nitroglycerin and should be avoided.[4] Filtration of 250 mL of a 485-mcg/mL aqueous solution through 3 different 142-mm, 0.2-μm filters was performed. A loss of 55% resulted with the Gelman GA filter composed of cellulose triacetate. Losses of only 5% occurred with a Millipore GS filter (a mixture of cellulose acetate and cellulose nitrate), and 2% losses occurred with a Gelman Tuffryn filter (a high-temperature aromatic polymer).[724]

In one study, a filter material specially treated with a proprietary agent was evaluated for a possible reduction in nitroglycerin binding. Nitroglycerin (Abbott) 62.5 mg/250 mL in dextrose 5% and in sodium chloride 0.9% was run through an administration set with a treated 0.22-μm cellulose ester inline filter at a rate of 3 mL/min. Cumulative nitroglycerin losses of less than 6% occurred from 200 mL of either solution. However, equilibrium binding studies showed no significant differences in drug affinity between treated and untreated filter material in either solution.[904] Ivex integral filter and extension sets use the treated filter material.[1074]

Compatibility Information

Solution Compatibility

Nitroglycerin

Test Soln Name	Mfr	Mfr	Conc/L or %	Remarks	Ref	C/I
Dextrose 5% in Ringer's injection, lactated	MG[c d]	ACC	200 and 400 mg	Physically compatible. Little or no loss after 28 days at 4°C and room temperature	928	C
Dextrose 5% in sodium chloride 0.45%	MG[c d]	ACC	200 and 400 mg	Physically compatible. Little or no loss after 28 days at 4°C and room temperature	928	C
Dextrose 5% in sodium chloride 0.9%	MG[c d]	ACC	200 and 400 mg	Physically compatible. Little or no loss after 28 days at 4°C and room temperature	928	C
Dextrose 5%	[c]	LI[c]	32 mg	Negligible loss over 24 hr at room temperature	510	C

Solution Compatibility (Cont.)

Test Soln Name	Mfr	Mfr	Conc/L or %	Remarks	Ref	C/I
Dextrose 5%	c	a	100 mg	1% loss in 24 hr at room temperature	509	C
Dextrose 5%	TR[c]		50 mg	Little change in 2 hr	508	C
Dextrose 5%	TR[c]	a	465 mg	8% loss in 24 hr and 13% in 50 hr at room temperature	506	C
Dextrose 5%	c	a	35 mg	Little loss after 70 days at room temperature or under refrigeration	503	C
Dextrose 5%	MG[c]	ACC	50 mg	0 to 3% loss in 48 hr at 4 and 25°C	721	C
Dextrose 5%	MG[d]	ACC	50 mg	1 to 6% loss in 48 hr at 4 and 25°C	721	C
Dextrose 5%	MG[c]	a	50 mg	Stable for 48 hr at 4 and 25°C	724	C
Dextrose 5%	c		100 mg	Little or no loss in 8 hr	726	C
Dextrose 5%	ON[c d]	a	90 mg	No precipitate and negligible loss in 24 hr at 25°C	797	C
Dextrose 5%	MG[c d]	ACC	200 and 400 mg	Physically compatible. Little loss after 28 days at 4°C and room temperature	928	C
Dextrose 5%	TR[c]	a	200 mg	No loss after 52 hr at 29°C	930	C
Dextrose 5%	c		200 to 800 mg	Physically compatible. 4% loss in 24 hr in light	1412	C
Dextrose 5%	c		250 mg	3% loss in 24 hr at 6, 20, and 40°C in light or dark	1512	C
Dextrose 5%	TR[b]	LI	32 mg	50% loss in 24 hr at room temperature	510	I
Dextrose 5%	TR[b]		50 mg	Almost 50% loss in 2 hr	508	I
Dextrose 5%	TR[b]	a	465 mg	Over 50% loss in 8 hr and 83% in 50 hr at room temperature	506	I
Dextrose 5%	b	a	35 mg	10% loss in 1 hr. In 7 days, 55% loss at room temperature and 30% under refrigeration	503	I
Dextrose 5%	TR[b]	ACC	50 mg	44% loss in 48 hr at 4°C and 70% loss at 25°C	721	I
Dextrose 5%	TR[b]	a	50 mg	43% loss at 4°C and 64% at 25°C in 24 hr	724	I
Dextrose 5%	TR[b]	a	100 and 500 mg	50% loss in 24 hr at 20 to 24°C	725	I
Dextrose 5%	TR[b]		100 mg	20% loss in 1 hr and 35% in 8 hr	726	I
Dextrose 5%	b	a	90 mg	No precipitate but 10% loss in 3 hr and 27% loss in 24 hr at 25°C	797	I
Dextrose 5%	BA[c]	AMR	800 mg	No loss in 24 hr at 23°C	2085	C
Dextrose 5%	BA[b]	PB	10 mg	Visually compatible. 66% loss at 22°C and 33% at 4°C in 24 hr	2289	I
Dextrose 5%	BRN[c d]	PB	10 mg	Visually compatible. No loss in 24 hr at 4 and 22°C	2289	C
Dextrose 5%	HOS[e]	AMR	400 mg	Less than 2% loss in 24 hr	2660, 2792	C
Ringer's injection, lactated	MG[c d]	ACC	200 and 400 mg	Physically compatible. Little loss after 28 days at 4°C and room temperature	928	C
Sodium chloride 0.45%	MG[c d]	ACC	200 and 400 mg	Physically compatible. Little loss after 28 days at 4°C and room temperature	928	C
Sodium chloride 0.9%	TR[c]	a	465 mg	8% loss in 24 hr and 13% in 50 hr at room temperature	506	C
Sodium chloride 0.9%	c	a	35 to 87 mg	Little loss after 70 days at room temperature or under refrigeration	503	C
Sodium chloride 0.9%	MG[c]	ACC	50 mg	5% loss in 48 hr at 4 and 25°C	721	C

Solution Compatibility (Cont.)

Test Soln Name	Mfr	Mfr	Conc/L or %	Remarks	Ref	C/I
Sodium chloride 0.9%	MG[d]	ACC	50 mg	No loss in 48 hr at 4 and 25°C	721	C
Sodium chloride 0.9%	[c]	[a]	200 mg	No loss in 24 hr and 5% loss in 3 months at room temperature or under refrigeration	722	C
Sodium chloride 0.9%	[c]	[a]	3.6 to 95 mg	Little loss in 48 hr at 35°C	723	C
Sodium chloride 0.9%	[c]	[a]	0.2 mg	10% loss in 24 hr and 13% in 48 hr at 35°C	723	C
Sodium chloride 0.9%	MG[c]	[a]	50 mg	Stable for 48 hr at 4 and 25°C	724	C
Sodium chloride 0.9%	ON[c d]	[a]	90 mg	No precipitate. 2 to 3% loss in 24 hr at 25°C	797	C
Sodium chloride 0.9%	MG[c d]	ACC	200 and 400 mg	Physically compatible. Little loss after 28 days at 4°C and room temperature	928	C
Sodium chloride 0.9%	TR[c]	[a]	200 mg	No loss after 52 hr at 29°C	930	C
Sodium chloride 0.9%	[c]		200 to 800 mg	Physically compatible. 8% or less loss in 24 hr exposed to light	1412	C
Sodium chloride 0.9%	[c d]		100 mg	Physically compatible. 2 to 5% loss in 24 hr at 21°C in the dark	1392	C
Sodium chloride 0.9%	[c]		250 mg	4% loss at 6°C and 7% loss at 40°C in 6 hr; no further loss in 24 hr	1512	C
Sodium chloride 0.9%	TR[b]	[a]	465 mg	Over 50% loss in 8 hr and 83% in 50 hr at room temperature	506	I
Sodium chloride 0.9%	TR[b]	ACC	50 mg	38% loss in 48 hr at 4°C and 68% at 25°C	721	I
Sodium chloride 0.9%	TR[b]	[a]	50 mg	45% loss at 4°C and 54% at 25°C in 24 hr	724	I
Sodium chloride 0.9%	TR[b]	[a]	100 and 500 mg	50% loss in 24 hr at 20 to 24°C	725	I
Sodium chloride 0.9%	[b]	[a]	90 mg	No precipitate but 10% loss in 3 hr and 28% loss in 24 hr at 25°C	797	I
Sodium chloride 0.9%	TR[b]	[a]	200 mg	38 to 44% loss in 8 hr at 29°C. At 6°C, 14% loss in 8 hr	930	I
Sodium chloride 0.9%	[b]		100 mg	10% loss in 1 hr and 51% loss in 24 hr at 21°C in the dark	1392	I
Sodium chloride 0.9%	[c]	PD	50, 125, 200 mg	About 14% loss in 8 hr at 24°C	1510	I
Sodium chloride 0.9%	ON[c d]	ON	100 mg	Visually compatible. No loss in 24 hr at 21°C	1796	C
Sodium chloride 0.9%	ON[b]	ON	100 mg	Visually compatible. 50% loss in 24 hr and 75% loss in 120 hr at 21°C	1796	I
Sodium chloride 0.9%	BA[b]	PB	10 mg	Visually compatible. 66% loss in 24 hr at 4 and 22°C	2289	I
Sodium chloride 0.9%	BRN[c d]	PR	10 mg	Visually compatible. 4 to 5% loss in 24 hr at 4 and 22°C	2289	C
Sodium lactate ⅙ M	MG[c d]	ACC	200 and 400 mg	Physically compatible. Little loss after 28 days at 4°C and room temperature in glass and polyolefin containers	928	C

[a] An extemporaneous preparation was tested.

[b] Tested in PVC containers.

[c] Tested in glass containers.

[d] Tested in polyolefin containers.

[e] Tested in VISIV polyolefin containers.

Additive Compatibility

Nitroglycerin

Test Drug	Mfr	Conc/L or %	Mfr	Conc/L or %	Test Solution	Remarks	Ref	C/I
Alteplase	GEN	0.5 g	ACC	400 mg	D5W, NS	Visually compatible with 2% or less clot-lysis activity loss in 24 hr at 25°C	1856	C
Aminophylline	IX	1 g	ACC	400 mg	D5W[a]	Physically compatible with 4% nitroglycerin loss in 24 hr and 6% loss in 48 hr at 23°C. Aminophylline not tested	929	C
Aminophylline	IX	1 g	ACC	400 mg	NS[a]	Physically compatible with no nitroglycerin loss in 24 hr and 5% loss in 48 hr at 23°C. Aminophylline not tested	929	C
Dobutamine HCl	LI	1 g	AB	120 mg	D5W, NS	Physically compatible for 24 hr at 21°C	812	C
Dobutamine HCl	LI	500 mg	ACC	100 mg	D5S	Stable with no loss of either drug after 24 hr at 25°C. Pink color after 4 hr	990	C
Dobutamine HCl with sodium nitroprusside		2 to 8 g 200 to 800 mg		200 to 800 mg	D5W[a]	Pink color with small amount of dark brown precipitate and 11 to 19% nitroglycerin loss in 24 hr exposed to light	1412	I
Dobutamine HCl with sodium nitroprusside		2 to 8 g 200 to 800 mg		200 to 800 mg	NS[a]	Pink color with 8% or less loss for any drug for 24 hr exposed to light	1412	C
Dopamine HCl	ACC	800 mg	ACC	400 mg	D5W, NS[a]	Physically compatible with little or no nitroglycerin loss in 48 hr at 23°C. Dopamine not tested	929	C
Enalaprilat	MSD	12 mg	DU	200 mg	D5W[a]	Visually compatible. 4% enalaprilat loss in 24 hr at room temperature in light. Nitroglycerin not tested	1572	C
Eptifibatide	ME	750 mg		400 mg		Physically compatible and chemically stable for up to 24 hr at 25°C	3049	C
Furosemide	HO	1 g	ACC	400 mg	D5W[a]	Physically compatible with no nitroglycerin loss in 48 hr at 23°C. Furosemide not tested	929	C
Furosemide	HO	1 g	ACC	400 mg	NS[a]	Physically compatible with 3% nitroglycerin loss in 48 hr at 23°C. Furosemide not tested	929	C
Hydralazine HCl	CI	1 g	ACC	400 mg	D5W[a]	Yellow color. 4% nitroglycerin loss in 48 hr at 23°C. Hydralazine not tested	929	I
Hydralazine HCl	CI	1 g	ACC	400 mg	NS[a]	Yellow color. No nitroglycerin loss in 48 hr at 23°C. Hydralazine not tested	929	I
Lidocaine HCl	IMS	4 g	ACC	400 mg	D5W, NS[a]	Physically compatible. No nitroglycerin loss in 48 hr at 23°C. Lidocaine not tested	929	C
Phenytoin sodium	PD	1 g	ACC	400 mg	D5W, NS[a]	Phenytoin crystals in 24 hr. 3 to 4% nitroglycerin loss in 24 hr and 9% in 48 hr at 23°C. Phenytoin not tested	929	I
Sodium nitroprusside with dobutamine HCl		200 to 800 mg 2 to 8 g		200 to 800 mg	D5W[a]	Pink color with small amount of dark brown precipitate and 11 to 19% nitroglycerin loss in 24 hr exposed to light	1412	I
Sodium nitroprusside with dobutamine HCl		200 to 800 mg 2 to 8 g		200 to 800 mg	NS[a]	Pink color with 8% or less loss for any drug for 24 hr exposed to light	1412	C
Verapamil HCl	KN	80 mg	ACC	100 mg	D5W, NS	Physically compatible for 24 hr	764	C

[a] Tested in glass containers.

Drugs in Syringe Compatibility

Nitroglycerin

Test Drug	Mfr	Amt	Mfr	Amt	Remarks	Ref	C/I
Caffeine citrate		20 mg/1 mL	SO	5 mg/1 mL	White precipitate forms immediately becoming two layers over time	2440	I
Heparin sodium		2500 units/1 mL		25 mg/25 mL	Physically compatible for at least 5 min	1053	C
Pantoprazole sodium	[a]	4 mg/1 mL		5 mg/1 mL	Precipitates	2574	I

[a] Test performed using the formulation WITHOUT edetate disodium.

Y-Site Injection Compatibility (1:1 Mixture)

Nitroglycerin

Test Drug	Mfr	Conc	Mfr	Conc	Remarks	Ref	C/I
Alteplase	GEN	1 mg/mL	DU	0.2 mg/mL[a]	Haze noted in 24 hr	1340	I
Amiodarone HCl	LZ	4 mg/mL[c]	AB	0.24 mg/mL[c]	Physically compatible for 24 hr at 21°C	1032	C
Argatroban	SKB	1 mg/mL[a]	BA	0.2 mg/mL[a]	Physically compatible for 24 hr at 23°C	2572	C
Atracurium besylate	BW	0.5 mg/mL[a]	SO	0.4 mg/mL[a]	Physically compatible for 24 hr at 28°C	1337	C
Bivalirudin	TMC	5 mg/mL[a]	AMR	0.4 mg/mL[a]	Physically compatible for 4 hr at 23°C	2373	C
Cangrelor tetrasodium	TMC	1 mg/mL[b]		0.4 mg/mL[b]	Physically compatible for 4 hr	3243	C
Ceftolozane sulfate–tazobactam sodium	CUB	10 mg/mL[c h]	BA	0.4 mg/mL[c]	Physically compatible for 2 hr	3262	C
Cisatracurium besylate	GW	0.1, 2, 5 mg/mL[a]	DU	0.4 mg/mL[a]	Physically compatible for 4 hr at 23°C	2074	C
Clevidipine butyrate	CHS	0.5 mg/mL		0.4 mg/mL[a]	Physically compatible for 24 hr at 23°C	3334	C
Clonidine HCl	BI	18 mcg/mL[b]	NYC	0.4 mg/mL[a]	Visually compatible	2642	C
Cloxacillin sodium	SMX	100 mg/mL	OM	5 mg/mL	Large particles form within 4 hr	3245	I
Dexmedetomidine HCl	AB	4 mcg/mL[b]	AMR	0.4 mg/mL[b]	Physically compatible for 4 hr at 23°C	2383	C
Diltiazem HCl	MMD	1 mg/mL[a]	DU	0.032 mg/mL[a]	Visually compatible for 24 hr at 25°C	1530	C
Diltiazem HCl	MMD	1[b] and 5 mg/mL	DU	400 mcg/mL[b]	Visually compatible	1807	C
Diltiazem HCl	MMD	5 mg/mL	DU	400 mcg/mL[a]	Visually compatible	1807	C
Diltiazem HCl	MMD	1 mg/mL[a]	AB	0.4 mg/mL[a]	Visually compatible for 4 hr at 27°C	2062	C
Dobutamine HCl	LI	4 mg/mL[c]	LY	0.4 mg/mL[c]	Physically compatible for 3 hr	1316	C
Dobutamine HCl	LI	4 mg/mL[a]	AB	0.4 mg/mL[a]	Visually compatible for 4 hr at 27°C	2062	C
Dobutamine HCl with dopamine HCl	LI DCC	4 mg/mL[c] 3.2 mg/mL[c]	LY	0.4 mg/mL[c]	Physically compatible for 3 hr	1316	C
Dobutamine HCl with lidocaine HCl	LI AB	4 mg/mL[c] 8 mg/mL[c]	LY	0.4 mg/mL[c]	Physically compatible for 3 hr	1316	C
Dobutamine HCl with sodium nitroprusside	LI ES	4 mg/mL[c] 0.4 mg/mL[c]	LY	0.4 mg/mL[c]	Physically compatible for 3 hr	1316	C
Dopamine HCl	DCC	3.2 mg/mL[c]	LY	0.4 mg/mL[c]	Physically compatible for 3 hr	1316	C
Dopamine HCl	AB	3.2 mg/mL[a]	AB	0.4 mg/mL[a]	Visually compatible for 4 hr at 27°C	2062	C
Dopamine HCl with dobutamine HCl	DCC LI	3.2 mg/mL[c] 4 mg/mL[c]	LY	0.4 mg/mL[c]	Physically compatible for 3 hr	1316	C

Y-Site Injection Compatibility (1:1 Mixture) (Cont.)

Test Drug	Mfr	Conc	Mfr	Conc	Remarks	Ref	C/I
Dopamine HCl with lidocaine HCl	DCC AB	3.2 mg/mL[c] 8 mg/mL[c]	LY	0.4 mg/mL[c]	Physically compatible for 3 hr	1316	C
Dopamine HCl with sodium nitroprusside	DCC ES	3.2 mg/mL[c] 0.4 mg/mL[c]	LY	0.4 mg/mL[c]	Physically compatible for 3 hr	1316	C
Epinephrine HCl	AB	0.02 mg/mL[a]	AB	0.4 mg/mL[a]	Visually compatible for 4 hr at 27°C	2062	C
Esmolol HCl	DU	40 mg/mL[a]	OM	0.2 mg/mL[a]	Visually compatible for 24 hr at 23°C	1877	C
Famotidine	MSD	0.2 mg/mL[a]	IMS	0.8 mg/mL[a]	Physically compatible for 4 hr at 25°C	1188	C
Famotidine	MSD	0.2 mg/mL[a]	PD	85 mcg/mL[b]	Physically compatible for 14 hr	1196	C
Fenoldopam mesylate	AB	80 mcg/mL[b]	AMR	0.4 mg/mL[b]	Physically compatible for 4 hr at 23°C	2467	C
Fentanyl citrate	ES	0.05 mg/mL	AB	0.4 mg/mL[a]	Visually compatible for 4 hr at 27°C	2062	C
Fluconazole	RR	2 mg/mL	AMR	0.2 mg/mL[a]	Visually compatible for 24 hr at 28°C under fluorescent light	1760	C
Furosemide	AMR	10 mg/mL	AB	0.4 mg/mL[a]	Visually compatible for 4 hr at 27°C	2062	C
Furosemide	AMR	10 mg/mL	BA	0.1 mg/mL[e]	Precipitation occurs immediately	2725	I
Furosemide	AMR	10 mg/mL	AMR	0.1 mg/mL[a]	Physically compatible for 48 hr at room temperature	2725	C
Haloperidol lactate	MN	0.5[a] and 5 mg/mL	DU	0.4 mg/mL[a]	Visually compatible for 24 hr at 21°C	1523	C
Heparin sodium	ES	50 units/mL	BA	0.2 mg/mL	Visually compatible for 24 hr at 23°C	1794	C
Heparin sodium	OR	100 units/mL[a]	OM	0.2 mg/mL[a]	Visually compatible for 24 hr at 23°C	1877	C
Heparin sodium	ES	100 units/mL[a]	AB	0.4 mg/mL[a]	Visually compatible for 4 hr at 27°C	2062	C
Hetastarch in lactated electrolyte	AB	6%	AMR	0.4 mg/mL[a]	Physically compatible for 4 hr at 23°C	2339	C
Hydralazine HCl	SO	1 mg/mL[a]	LY	0.4 mg/mL[a]	Physically compatible for 3 hr	1316	C
Hydralazine HCl	SO	1 mg/mL[b]	LY	0.4 mg/mL[b]	Slight precipitate in 3 hr	1316	I
Hydromorphone HCl	KN	1 mg/mL	AB	0.4 mg/mL[a]	Visually compatible for 4 hr at 27°C	2062	C
Hydroxyethyl starch 130/0.4 in sodium chloride 0.9%	FRK	6%	SZ	0.1, 0.25, 0.4 mg/mL[a]	Visually compatible for 24 hr at room temperature	2770	C
Insulin, regular	LI	1 unit/mL[a]	OM	0.2 mg/mL[a]	Visually compatible for 24 hr at 23°C	1877	C
Isavuconazonium sulfate	ASP	1.5 mg/mL[c]	BA	0.4 mg/mL[c]	Physically compatible for 2 hr	3263	C
Labetalol HCl	GL	1 mg/mL[a]	DU	0.2 mg/mL[a]	Visually compatible. No labetalol loss and 6% nitroglycerin loss in 4 hr at room temperature	1762	C
Labetalol HCl	GL	5 mg/mL	OM	0.2 mg/mL[a]	Visually compatible for 24 hr at 23°C	1877	C
Labetalol HCl	AH	2 mg/mL[a]	AB	0.4 mg/mL[a]	Visually compatible for 4 hr at 27°C	2062	C
Levofloxacin	OMN	5 mg/mL[a]	AMR	5 mg/mL	Cloudy precipitate forms	2233	I
Lidocaine HCl	AB	8 mg/mL[c]	LY	0.4 mg/mL[c]	Physically compatible for 3 hr	1316	C
Lidocaine HCl with dobutamine HCl	AB LI	8 mg/mL[c] 4 mg/mL[c]	LY	0.4 mg/mL[c]	Physically compatible for 3 hr	1316	C
Lidocaine HCl with dopamine HCl	AB DCC	8 mg/mL[c] 3.2 mg/mL[c]	LY	0.4 mg/mL[c]	Physically compatible for 3 hr	1316	C

Y-Site Injection Compatibility (1:1 Mixture) (Cont.)

Test Drug	Mfr	Conc	Mfr	Conc	Remarks	Ref	C/I
Lidocaine HCl with sodium nitroprusside	AB ES	8 mg/mL[c] 0.4 mg/mL[c]	LY	0.4 mg/mL[c]	Physically compatible for 3 hr	1316	C
Linezolid	PHU	2 mg/mL	FAU	0.4 mg/mL[a]	Physically compatible for 4 hr at 23°C	2264	C
Lorazepam	WY	0.5 mg/mL[a]	AB	0.4 mg/mL[a]	Visually compatible for 4 hr at 27°C	2062	C
Meropenem		50 mg/mL	OM	5 mg/mL	Solution became opaque immediately	3538	I
Meropenem–vaborbactam	TMC	8 mg/mL[b i]	BA	0.4 mg/mL[b]	Physically compatible for 3 hr at 20 to 25°C	3380	C
Metoprolol tartrate	BED	1 mg/mL	BA	0.2 mg/mL[a]	Trace precipitate in 8 hr at 19°C	2795	I
Micafungin sodium	ASP	1.5 mg/mL[b]	AMR	0.4 mg/mL[b]	Physically compatible for 4 hr at 23°C	2683	C
Midazolam HCl	RC	1 mg/mL[a]	SO	0.2 mg/mL[a]	Visually compatible for 24 hr at 23°C	1847	C
Midazolam HCl	RC	1 mg/mL[a]	OM	0.2 mg/mL[a]	Visually compatible for 24 hr at 23°C	1877	C
Midazolam HCl	RC	2 mg/mL[a]	AB	0.4 mg/mL[a]	Visually compatible for 4 hr at 27°C	2062	C
Milrinone lactate	SW	0.2 mg/mL[a]	AB	0.4 mg/mL[a]	Visually compatible for 4 hr at 27°C	2062	C
Milrinone lactate	SW	0.4 mg/mL[a]	SO	0.8 mg/mL[a]	Visually compatible. Little loss of either drug in 4 hr at 23°C	2214	C
Morphine sulfate	SCN	2 mg/mL[a]	AB	0.4 mg/mL[a]	Visually compatible for 4 hr at 27°C	2062	C
Nesiritide	SCI	50 mcg/mL[a b]		0.2 mg/mL	Physically compatible for 4 hr	2625	C
Nicardipine HCl	WY	1 mg/mL[a]	AB	0.4 mg/mL[a]	Visually compatible for 4 hr at 27°C	2062	C
Norepinephrine bitartrate	AB	0.128 mg/mL[a]	AB	0.4 mg/mL[a]	Visually compatible for 4 hr at 27°C	2062	C
Oritavancin diphosphate	TAR	0.8, 1.2, and 2 mg/mL[a]	AMR	0.4 mg/mL[a]	Visually compatible for 4 hr at 20 to 24°C	2928	C
Pancuronium bromide	ES	0.05 mg/mL[a]	SO	0.4 mg/mL[a]	Physically compatible for 24 hr at 28°C	1337	C
Pantoprazole sodium	ALT[d]	0.16 to 0.8 mg/mL[b]	SX	0.1 to 0.4 mg/mL[a]	Visually compatible for 12 hr at 23°C	2603	C
Plazomicin sulfate	ACH	24 mg/mL[c]	BA	0.4 mg/mL[c]	Physically compatible for 1 hr at 20 to 25°C	3432	C
Propofol	ZEN[j]	10 mg/mL	DU	0.4 mg/mL[a]	Physically compatible for 1 hr at 23°C	2066	C
Ranitidine HCl	GL	0.5 mg/mL	SO	0.2 mg/mL[a]	Physically compatible for 24 hr	1323	C
Ranitidine HCl	GL	1 mg/mL[a]	AB	0.4 mg/mL[a]	Visually compatible for 4 hr at 27°C	2062	C
Remifentanil HCl	GW	0.025 and 0.25 mg/mL[b]	DU	0.4 mg/mL[a]	Physically compatible for 4 hr at 23°C	2075	C
Sodium nitroprusside	ES	0.4 mg/mL[c]	LY	0.4 mg/mL[c]	Physically compatible for 3 hr	1316	C
Sodium nitroprusside	RC	1.2 and 3 mg/mL[a]	SX	0.4 and 1.5 mg/mL[g]	Visually compatible for 48 hr at 24°C protected from light	2357	C
Sodium nitroprusside with dobutamine HCl	ES LI	0.4 mg/mL[c] 4 mg/mL[c]	LY	0.4 mg/mL[c]	Physically compatible for 3 hr	1316	C
Sodium nitroprusside with dopamine HCl	ES DCC	0.4 mg/mL[c] 3.2 mg/mL[c]	LY	0.4 mg/mL[c]	Physically compatible for 3 hr	1316	C
Sodium nitroprusside with lidocaine HCl	ES AB	0.4 mg/mL[c] 8 mg/mL[c]	LY	0.4 mg/mL[c]	Physically compatible for 3 hr	1316	C
Tacrolimus	FUJ	1 mg/mL[b]	DU	0.1 mg/mL[a]	Visually compatible for 24 hr at 25°C	1630	C
Tedizolid phosphate	CUB	0.8 mg/mL[b]	BA	0.4 mg/mL[b]	Physically compatible for 2 hr	3244	C
Theophylline	TR	4 mg/mL	LY	0.2 mg/mL[a]	Visually compatible for 6 hr at 25°C	1793	C

Y-Site Injection Compatibility (1:1 Mixture) (Cont.)

Test Drug	Mfr	Conc	Mfr	Conc	Remarks	Ref	C/I
Tirofiban HCl	ME	50 mcg/mL[a][b]	AB	0.1 and 0.4 mg/mL	Physically compatible. No loss of either drug in 4 hr at 23°C	2356	C
TNA #218 to #226[f]			DU	0.4 mg/mL[a]	Visually compatible for 4 hr at 23°C	2215	C
TPN #212 to #215[f]			DU	0.4 mg/mL[a]	Physically compatible for 4 hr at 23°C	2109	C
Vasopressin	AMR	2 and 4 units/mL[b]	BA	0.2 mg/mL[a]	Physically compatible with vasopressin pushed through a Y-site over 5 sec	2478	C
Vecuronium bromide	OR	0.1 mg/mL[a]	SO	0.4 mg/mL[a]	Physically compatible for 24 hr at 28°C	1337	C
Vecuronium bromide	OR	1 mg/mL	AB	0.4 mg/mL[a]	Visually compatible for 4 hr at 27°C	2062	C

[a] Tested in dextrose 5%.

[b] Tested in sodium chloride 0.9%.

[c] Tested in both dextrose 5% and sodium chloride 0.9%.

[d] Test performed using the formulation WITHOUT edetate disodium.

[e] Tested using Baxter Healthcare premixed nitroglycerin infusion in dextrose 5% with citrate buffer.

[f] Refer to Appendix for the composition of parenteral nutrition solutions. TNA indicates a 3-in-1 admixture, and TPN indicates a 2-in-1 admixture.

[g] Tested in dextrose 5% in sodium chloride 0.225%.

[h] Ceftolozane component. Ceftolozane in a 2:1 fixed-ratio concentration with tazobactam.

[i] Meropenem component. Meropenem in a 1:1 fixed-ratio concentration with vaborbactam.

[j] Test performed using the formulation WITH edetate disodium.

Selected Revisions May 1, 2020. © Copyright, October 1982.
American Society of Health-System Pharmacists, Inc.

Norepinephrine Bitartrate
AHFS 12:12.12
Noradrenaline Acid Tartrate

Products

Norepinephrine bitartrate is available as 1 mg/mL of norepinephrine base in 4-mL vials. Each mL of solution also contains sodium metabisulfite 0.2 mg and sodium chloride for isotonicity in water for injection.[1(6/07)]

pH

From 3 to 4.5.[1(6/07) 77]

Tonicity

Norepinephrine bitartrate injection is adjusted to isotonicity with sodium chloride.[1(6/07)]

Trade Name(s)

Levophed

Administration

Norepinephrine bitartrate is administered by intravenous infusion into a large vein, using a pump or other flow rate control device. Extravasation may cause tissue damage and should be avoided. A 4-mcg/mL dilution of norepinephrine base for infusion is usually prepared by adding 4 mg of base (4 mL) to 1000 mL of dextrose 5% with or without sodium chloride. The concentration and infusion rate depend on the patient's requirements.[1(6/07) 4]

Stability

Norepinephrine bitartrate in intact containers should be stored at controlled room temperature and protected from light.[1(6/07) 4] Dextrose 5% and dextrose 5% in sodium chloride 0.9% are the recommended diluents for infusion because their dextrose content provides protection against significant drug loss due to oxidation. The drug gradually darkens upon exposure to light or air and must not be used if it is discolored or has a precipitate.[4]

pH Effects

Norepinephrine bitartrate is stable at pH 3.6 to 6 in dextrose 5%.[48 77] The pH of a solution is the primary determinant of catecholamine stability in intravenous admixtures.[527] At a concentration of 5 mg/L in dextrose 5% at pH 6.5, norepinephrine bitartrate loses 5% in 6 hours; at pH 7.5, it loses 5% in 4 hours.[77] The rate of loss also increases with exposure to increasing temperatures.[1929]

Caution should be employed in mixing additives that may result in a final pH above 6 since norepinephrine bitartrate is alkali labile.[6 24 77]

Visual inspection for color change may be inadequate to assess compatibility of admixtures. In one evaluation with aminophylline stored at 25°C, a color change was not noted until 48 hours had elapsed. However, no intact norepinephrine bitartrate was present in the admixture at 48 hours.[527]

Syringes

Norepinephrine bitartrate (Aguettant) 0.24 mg/mL in sodium chloride 0.9% was packaged in 50-mL polypropylene syringes (Becton Dickinson) and stored at 2 to 8°C with light protection.[3508] Solutions were physically stable with less than 10% loss in 30 days.[3508]

Norepinephrine bitartrate 0.5 and 1.16 mg/mL in dextrose 5% was packaged as 48 mL in 50-mL clear polypropylene and amber polypropylene syringes (Becton Dickinson) and stored at 20 to 25°C.[3509] Solutions both with and without light protection were physically stable with little to no loss of drug in 48 hours.[3509]

Noradrenaline (as the tartrate salt) (Aguettant) 6 mg/50 mL and 12 mg/50 mL in sodium chloride 0.9% in a 50-mL polypropylene syringe (BD) was physically stable for 48 hours at room temperature.[3545]

Filtration

Norepinephrine bitartrate 4 mg/L in dextrose 5% and sodium chloride 0.9% was filtered at a rate of 120 mL/hr for 6 hours through a 0.22-μm cellulose ester membrane filter (Ivex-2). No significant drug loss due to binding to the filter was noted.[533]

Central Venous Catheter

Norepinephrine bitartrate 0.1 mg/mL in dextrose 5% was found to be compatible with the ARROWg+ard Blue Plus (Arrow International) chlorhexidine-bearing triple-lumen central catheter. Essentially complete delivery of the drug was found with little or no drug loss occurring. Furthermore, chlorhexidine delivered from the catheter remained at trace amounts with no substantial increase due to the delivery of the drug through the catheter.[2335]

Compatibility Information

Solution Compatibility

Norepinephrine bitartrate

Test Soln Name	Mfr	Mfr	Conc/L or %	Remarks	Ref	C/I
Amino acids 4.25%, dextrose 25%	MG	WI	4 mg	No increase in particulate matter in 24 hr at 5°C	349	C
Dextrose 5% in sodium chloride 0.9%		WI	8 mg	Physically compatible	74	C

DOI: 10.37573/9781585286850.286

Solution Compatibility (Cont.)

Test Soln Name	Mfr	Mfr	Conc/L or %	Remarks	Ref	C/I
Dextrose 5%		WI	8 mg	Physically compatible	74	C
Dextrose 5%	AB	WI	8 mg	Physically compatible. 10% calculated loss in 2500 hr at 25°C	527	C
Dextrose 5%	TR[a]	WI	4 and 8 mg	2 to 4% loss in 24 hr at room temperature exposed to light	1163	C
Dextrose 5%	BA[a]	WI	16 mg	5% loss in 47.2 days at 5°C in the dark	1610	C
Dextrose 5%	BA[a]	WI	40 mg	5% loss in 87.7 days at 5°C in the dark	1610	C
Dextrose 5%	TR[a]	RC	4 and 8 mg	Visually compatible. No loss in 48 hr at room temperature	1802	C
Dextrose 5%	BA[a]	SW	42 mg	No loss in 24 hr at 23°C in the dark	2085	C
Dextrose 5%	[a]	SX	4 and 16 mg	Less than 4% loss in 7 days at 20°C	2776	C
Dextrose 5%	BA[a]	SZ	64.5 mg	Little loss in 61 days at 4 and 23°C protected from light	2813	C
Ringer's injection, lactated		WI	8 mg	Physically compatible	74	C
Sodium chloride 0.9%		WI	8 mg	Physically compatible	74	C
Sodium chloride 0.9%	TR[a]	WI	4 and 8 mg	2% loss in 24 hr at room temperature in light	1163	C
Sodium chloride 0.9%	[a]	SX	4 and 16 mg	Less than 3% loss in 7 days at 20°C	2776	C
Sodium chloride 0.9%	HOS[a]	SZ	64.5 mg	Less than 10% loss in 61 days at 4 and 23°C protected from light	2813	C

[a] Tested in PVC containers.

Additive Compatibility

Norepinephrine bitartrate

Test Drug	Mfr	Conc/L or %	Mfr	Conc/L or %	Test Solution	Remarks	Ref	C/I
Amikacin sulfate	BR	5 g	WI	8 mg	D5LR, D5R, D5S, D5W, D10W, LR, NS, R, SL	Physically compatible and both stable for 24 hr at 25°C	294	C
Aminophylline	SE	500 mg	WI	8 mg	D5W	10% norepinephrine loss in 3.6 hr at 25°C	527	I
Calcium chloride	UP	1 g	WI	8 mg	D5W, D10W, D2.5½S, D2.5S, D5¼S, D5½S, D5S, D10S, NS, ½S	Physically compatible	77	C
Calcium gluconate		1 g	WI	8 mg	D5W	Physically compatible	74	C
Ciprofloxacin	BAY	2 g	SW	64 mg	D5W	Visually compatible. No ciprofloxacin loss in 24 hr at 22°C in light. Norepinephrine not tested	2413	C
Dimenhydrinate	SE	50 mg	WI	8 mg	D5W	Physically compatible	74	C
Dobutamine HCl	LI	1 g	BN	32 mg	D5W, NS	Physically compatible for 24 hr at 21°C	812	C
Heparin sodium		12,000 units	WI	8 mg	D5W	Physically compatible	74	C
Heparin sodium	AB	20,000 units	WI	8 mg	D5W, D10W, D2.5½S, D2.5S, D5¼S, D5½S, D5S, D10S, NS, ½S	Physically compatible	77	C
Hydrocortisone sodium succinate	UP	100 mg	WI	8 mg	D5W	Physically compatible	74	C

Additive Compatibility (Cont.)

Test Drug	Mfr	Conc/L or %	Mfr	Conc/L or %	Test Solution	Remarks	Ref	C/I
Magnesium sulfate		1 g	WI	8 mg	D5W, D10W, D2.5½S, D2.5S, D5¼S, D5½S, D5S, D10S, NS, ½S	Physically compatible	77	C
Meropenem	ZEN	1 and 20 g	WI	8 g	NS	Visually compatible for 4 hr at room temperature	1994	C
Methylprednisolone sodium succinate	UP	40 mg	WI	8 mg	D5S	Physically compatible	329	C
Multivitamins	USV	10 mL	WI	8 mg	D5W, D10W, D2.5½S, D2.5S, D5¼S, D5½S, D5S, D10S, NS, ½S	Physically compatible	77	C
Potassium chloride		3 g	WI	8 mg	D5W	Physically compatible	74	C
Potassium chloride	AB	40 mEq	WI	8 mg	D5W, D10W, D2.5½S, D2.5S, D5¼S, D5½S, D5S, D10S, NS, ½S	Physically compatible	77	C
Ranitidine HCl	GL	50 mg	WI	4 and 8 mg	D5W, NS[a]	Physically compatible. 2 to 6% ranitidine loss in 48 hr at room temperature in light. Norepinephrine not tested	1361	C
Ranitidine HCl	GL	50 mg		4 mg	D5W	Physically compatible. Ranitidine stable for 24 hr at 25°C. Norepinephrine not tested	1515	C
Ranitidine HCl	GL	50 mg	RC	4 and 8 mg	D5W[a]	Visually compatible. 5 to 7% ranitidine loss and little norepinephrine loss in 48 hr at room temperature	1802	C
Ranitidine HCl	GL	2 g	RC	4 mg	D5W[a]	Visually compatible. 7% norepinephrine loss in 4 hr and 13% in 12 hr at room temperature. No ranitidine loss in 48 hr	1802	I
Ranitidine HCl	GL	2 g	RC	8 mg	D5W[a]	Visually compatible. 6% norepinephrine loss in 12 hr and 11% in 24 hr at room temperature. No ranitidine loss in 48 hr	1802	I
Sodium bicarbonate	AB	80 mEq	WI	2 mg	D5W	Physically incompatible	15	I
Sodium bicarbonate	AB	2.4 mEq[b]	BN	8 mg	D5W	Norepinephrine decomposition	772	I
Succinylcholine chloride	AB	2 g	WI	8 mg	D5W, D10W, D2.5½S, D2.5S, D5¼S, D5½S, D5S, D10S, NS, ½S	Physically compatible	77	C
Verapamil HCl	KN	80 mg	BN	8 mg	D5W, NS	Physically compatible for 24 hr	764	C

[a] Tested in PVC containers.

[b] One vial of Neut added to a liter of admixture.

Drugs in Syringe Compatibility

Norepinephrine bitartrate

Test Drug	Mfr	Amt	Mfr	Amt	Remarks	Ref	C/I
Pantoprazole sodium	[a]	4 mg/1 mL		1 mg/1 mL	Precipitates within 15 min	2574	I

[a] Test performed using the formulation WITHOUT edetate disodium.

Y-Site Injection Compatibility (1:1 Mixture)

Norepinephrine bitartrate

Test Drug	Mfr	Conc	Mfr	Conc	Remarks	Ref	C/I
Amiodarone HCl	LZ	4 mg/mL[c]	BN	64 mcg/mL[c]	Physically compatible for 24 hr at 21°C	1032	C
Angiotensin II acetate	LJ	5 and 10 mcg/mL[b]			Stated to be compatible	3430	C
Anidulafungin	VIC	0.5 mg/mL[a]	BED	0.12 mg/mL[a]	Physically compatible for 4 hr at 23°C	2617	C
Argatroban	GSK	1 mg/mL[b]	AB	1 mg/mL	Visually compatible for 24 hr at 23°C	2391	C
Bivalirudin	TMC	5 mg/mL[a]	AB	0.12 mg/mL[a]	Physically compatible for 4 hr at 23°C	2373	C
Cangrelor tetrasodium	TMC	1 mg/mL[b]		120 mcg/mL[b]	Physically compatible for 4 hr	3243	C
Caspofungin acetate	ME	0.7 mg/mL[b]	BED	0.128 mg/mL[b]	Physically compatible for 4 hr at room temperature	2758	C
Ceftaroline fosamil	FOR	2.22 mg/mL[a b i]	BED	0.128 mg/mL[a b i]	Physically compatible for 4 hr at 23°C	2826	C
Ceftazidime–avibactam sodium	ALL	20 mg/mL[l m]			Physically compatible for up to 4 hr at room temperature	3004	C
Ceftolozane sulfate–tazobactam sodium	CUB	30 mg/mL[c j]		32 mcg/mL	Physically compatible with no loss of either drug in 4 hr at 25°C	2959	C
Ceftolozane sulfate–tazobactam sodium	CUB	10 mg/mL[c j]	HOS	32 mcg/mL[c]	Physically compatible for 2 hr	3262	C
Cisatracurium besylate	GW	0.1, 2, 5 mg/mL[a]	SW	0.12 mg/mL[a]	Physically compatible for 4 hr at 23°C	2074	C
Clonidine HCl	BI	18 mcg/mL[b]	APO	20 mcg/mL[a]	Visually compatible	2642	C
Cloxacillin sodium	SMX	100 mg/mL	SZ	1 mg/mL	Physically compatible for up to 4 hr at room temperature	3245	C
Dexmedetomidine HCl	AB	4 mcg/mL[b]	AB	0.12 mg/mL[b]	Physically compatible for 4 hr at 23°C	2383	C
Diltiazem HCl	MMD	1 mg/mL[a]	WI	0.12 mg/mL[a]	Visually compatible for 24 hr at 25°C	1530	C
Diltiazem HCl	MMD	1 mg/mL[a]	AB	0.128 mg/mL[a]	Visually compatible for 4 hr at 27°C	2062	C
Dobutamine HCl	LI	4 mg/mL[a]	AB	0.128 mg/mL[a]	Visually compatible for 4 hr at 27°C	2062	C
Dopamine HCl	DU	3.2 mg/mL[a]	STR	0.064 mg/mL[a]	Visually compatible for 24 hr at 23°C	1877	C
Dopamine HCl	AB	3.2 mg/mL[a]	AB	0.128 mg/mL[a]	Visually compatible for 4 hr at 27°C	2062	C
Doripenem	JJ	5 mg/mL[a b]	BED	0.128 mg/mL[a b]	Physically compatible for 4 hr at 23°C	2743	C
Epinephrine HCl	AB	0.02 mg/mL[a]	AB	0.128 mg/mL[a]	Visually compatible for 4 hr at 27°C	2062	C
Eravacycline dihydrochloride	TET	0.6 mg/mL[b]	CLA	32 mcg/mL[b]	Physically compatible for 2 hr at room temperature	3532	C
Esmolol HCl	DU	40 mg/mL[a]	STR	0.064 mg/mL[a]	Visually compatible for 24 hr at 23°C	1877	C
Esmolol HCl	MYL	10 mg/mL	HOS	0.128 mg/mL[b]	Physically compatible for 1 hr at 23°C	3533	C
Famotidine	MSD	0.2 mg/mL[a]	WI	0.004 mg/mL[a]	Physically compatible for 4 hr at 25°C	1188	C
Fenoldopam mesylate	AB	80 mcg/mL[b]	AB	0.12 mg/mL[b]	Physically compatible for 4 hr at 23°C	2467	C
Fentanyl citrate	ES	0.05 mg/mL	AB	0.128 mg/mL[a]	Visually compatible for 4 hr at 27°C	2062	C
Furosemide	AMR	10 mg/mL	AB	0.128 mg/mL[a]	Visually compatible for 4 hr at 27°C	2062	C
Haloperidol lactate	MN	0.5[a] and 5 mg/mL	WI	0.032 mg/mL[a]	Visually compatible for 24 hr at 21°C	1523	C
Heparin sodium	UP	1000 units/L[d]	WI	1 mg/mL	Physically compatible for 4 hr at room temperature	534	C
Heparin sodium	ES	100 units/mL[a]	AB	0.128 mg/mL[a]	Visually compatible for 4 hr at 27°C	2062	C

Y-Site Injection Compatibility (1:1 Mixture) (Cont.)

Test Drug	Mfr	Conc	Mfr	Conc	Remarks	Ref	C/I
Hetastarch in lactated electrolyte	AB	6%	AB	0.12 mg/mL[a]	Physically compatible for 4 hr at 23°C	2339	C
Hydrocortisone sodium succinate	UP	10 mg/L[d]	WI	1 mg/mL	Physically compatible for 4 hr at room temperature	534	C
Hydromorphone HCl	KN	1 mg/mL	AB	0.128 mg/mL[a]	Visually compatible for 4 hr at 27°C	2062	C
Hydroxyethyl starch 130/0.4 in sodium chloride 0.9%	FRK	6%	SZ	6, 8, 64 mcg/mL[a]	Visually compatible for 24 hr at room temperature	2770	C
Insulin, regular	LI	1 unit/mL[a]	STR	0.064 mg/mL[a]	White precipitate forms immediately	1877	I
Isavuconazonium sulfate	ASP	1.5 mg/mL[c]	HOS	32 mcg/mL[c]	Physically compatible for 2 hr	3263	C
Labetalol HCl	GL	5 mg/mL	STR	64 mcg/mL[a]	Visually compatible for 24 hr at 23°C	1877	C
Labetalol HCl	AH	2 mg/mL[a]	AB	0.128 mg/mL[a]	Visually compatible for 4 hr at 27°C	2062	C
Labetalol HCl	HOS	5 mg/mL	HOS	0.128 mg/mL[b]	Physically compatible for 1 hr at 23°C	3533	C
Letermovir	ME	[a]		[a]	Physically compatible	3398	C
Levofloxacin	SZ	5 mg/mL	HOS	64 mcg/mL[a]	Physically compatible with no loss of either drug in 4 hr at room temperature	3510	C
Lorazepam	WY	0.5 mg/mL[a]	AB	0.128 mg/mL[a]	Visually compatible for 4 hr at 27°C	2062	C
Meropenem	ZEN	1 and 50 mg/mL[b]	WI	1 mg/mL	Visually compatible for 4 hr at room temperature	1994	C
Meropenem		50 mg/mL	SZ	1 mg/mL	Physically compatible for 4 hr at room temperature	3538	C
Meropenem–vaborbactam	TMC	8 mg/mL[b k]	HOS	32 mcg/mL[b]	Physically compatible for 3 hr at 20 to 25°C	3380	C
Metoprolol tartrate	HOS	0.4 mg/mL[b]	HOS	0.128 mg/mL[b]	Physically compatible for 1 hr at 23°C	3533	C
Micafungin sodium	ASP	1.5 mg/mL[b]	BED	0.128 mg/mL[b]	Physically compatible for 4 hr at 23°C	2683	C
Midazolam HCl	RC	1 mg/mL[a]	STR	0.064 mg/mL[a]	Visually compatible for 24 hr at 23°C	1877	C
Midazolam HCl	RC	2 mg/mL[a]	AB	0.128 mg/mL[a]	Visually compatible for 4 hr at 27°C	2062	C
Milrinone lactate	SW	0.2 mg/mL[a]	AB	0.128 mg/mL[a]	Visually compatible for 4 hr at 27°C	2062	C
Milrinone lactate	SW	0.4 mg/mL[a]	SW	0.064 mg/mL[a]	Visually compatible. Little loss of either drug in 4 hr at 23°C	2214	C
Morphine sulfate	SX	1 mg/mL[a]	STR	0.064 mg/mL[a]	Visually compatible for 24 hr at 23°C	1877	C
Morphine sulfate	SCN	2 mg/mL[a]	AB	0.128 mg/mL[a]	Visually compatible for 4 hr at 27°C	2062	C
Moxifloxacin	ME	1.6 mg/mL	HOS	64 mcg/mL[a]	Physically compatible with little to no loss of either drug in 4 hr at room temperature	3510	C
Mycophenolate mofetil HCl	RC	5.9 mg/mL[a]		1 mg/mL[a]	Physically compatible and 2% myco-phenolate mofetil loss in 4 hr	2738	C
Nesiritide	SCI	50 mcg/mL[a b]		1 mg/mL	Physically compatible for 4 hr. May be chemically incompatible with nesiritide[g]	2625	?
Nicardipine HCl	WY	1 mg/mL[a]	AB	0.128 mg/mL[a]	Visually compatible for 4 hr at 27°C	2062	C
Nitroglycerin	AB	0.4 mg/mL[a]	AB	0.128 mg/mL[a]	Visually compatible for 4 hr at 27°C	2062	C
Oritavancin diphosphate	TAR	0.8, 1.2, and 2 mg/mL[a]	BED	0.12 mg/mL[a]	Visually compatible for 4 hr at 20 to 24°C	2928	C
Pantoprazole sodium	ALT[h]	0.16 to 0.8 mg/mL[b]	SX	6 to 8 mcg/mL[a]	Visually compatible for 12 hr at 23°C	2603	C
Pantoprazole sodium	ALT[h]	0.16 mg/mL[b]	SX	64 mcg/mL[a]	Visually compatible for 12 hr at 23°C	2603	C

Y-Site Injection Compatibility (1:1 Mixture) (Cont.)

Test Drug	Mfr	Conc	Mfr	Conc	Remarks	Ref	C/I
Pantoprazole sodium	ALT[h]	0.4 to 0.8 mg/mL[b]	SX	64 mcg/mL[a]	Turns cloudy upon mixing	2603	I
Plazomicin sulfate	ACH	24 mg/mL[c]	CLA	32 mcg/mL[c]	Physically compatible for 1 hr at 20 to 25°C	3432	C
Posaconazole	ME	18 mg/mL		0.004 mg/mL[c]	Physically compatible	2911, 2912	C
Potassium chloride	AB	40 mEq/L[d]	WI	1 mg/mL	Physically compatible for 4 hr at room temperature	534	C
Propofol	ZEN[o]	10 mg/mL	AB	0.016 mg/mL[a]	Physically compatible for 1 hr at 23°C	2066	C
Ranitidine HCl	GL	1 mg/mL[a]	AB	0.128 mg/mL[a]	Visually compatible for 4 hr at 27°C	2062	C
Remifentanil HCl	GW	0.025 and 0.25 mg/mL[b]	SW	0.12 mg/mL[a]	Physically compatible for 4 hr at 23°C	2075	C
Sodium nitroprusside	RC	0.3, 1.2, 3 mg/mL[a]	SX	0.03, 0.12, 3 mg/mL[f]	Visually compatible for 48 hr at 24°C protected from light	2357	C
Tedizolid phosphate	CUB	0.8 mg/mL[b]	HOS	32 mcg/mL[b]	Physically compatible for 2 hr	3244	C
Telavancin HCl	ASP	7.5 mg/mL[a b i]	BED	0.128 mg/mL[a b i]	Physically compatible for 2 hr	2830	C
Tigecycline	ACD, FRK, WY	[c]	[n]		Stated to be compatible	2915, 3459, 3460	C
TNA #73[e]			BN	8 mcg/mL[c]	Visually compatible for 4 hr	1009	C
TPN #212 to #215[e]			AB	16 mcg/mL[a]	Physically compatible for 4 hr at 23°C	2109	C
Vasopressin	AMR	2 and 4 units/mL[b]	AB	4 mcg/mL[b]	Physically compatible with vasopressin pushed through a Y-site over 5 sec	2478	C
Vasopressin	APP	0.2 unit/mL[b]	GNS	16 mcg/mL[b]	Physically compatible	2641	C
Vasopressin	APP	0.2 unit/mL[b]	AB	4 mcg/mL[b]	Physically compatible	2641	C
Vecuronium bromide	OR	1 mg/mL	AB	0.128 mg/mL[a]	Visually compatible for 4 hr at 27°C	2062	C

[a] Tested in dextrose 5%.

[b] Tested in sodium chloride 0.9%.

[c] Tested in both dextrose 5% and sodium chloride 0.9%.

[d] Tested in dextrose 5% in Ringer's injection, dextrose 5% in Ringer's injection, lactated, dextrose 5%, Ringer's injection, lactated, and sodium chloride 0.9%.

[e] Refer to Appendix for the composition of parenteral nutrition solutions. TNA indicates a 3-in-1 admixture, and TPN indicates a 2-in-1 admixture.

[f] Tested in dextrose 5% in sodium chloride 0.225%.

[g] Nesiritide is incompatible with bisulfite antioxidants used in some drug formulations. The specific formulation of the product to be used should be checked to ensure that no sulfite antioxidants are present.

[h] Test performed using the formulation WITHOUT edetate disodium.

[i] Tested in Ringer's injection, lactated.

[j] Ceftolozane component. Ceftolozane in a 2:1 fixed-ratio concentration with tazobactam.

[k] Meropenem component. Meropenem in a 1:1 fixed-ratio concentration with vaborbactam.

[l] Ceftazidime component. Ceftazidime in a 4:1 fixed-ratio concentration with avibactam.

[m] Tested in dextrose 5%, sodium chloride 0.9%, and Ringer's injection, lactated.

[n] Salt not specified.

[o] Test performed using the formulation WITH edetate disodium.

Selected Revisions May 1, 2020. © Copyright, October 1982.
American Society of Health-System Pharmacists, Inc.

Octreotide Acetate
AHFS 68:29.04

Products

Octreotide acetate injection is available in 1-mL ampuls containing 0.05 mg (50 mcg), 0.1 mg (100 mcg), and 0.5 mg (500 mcg) of octreotide and in 5-mL multiple-dose vials containing 0.2 mg (200 mcg) and 1 mg (1000 mcg) of octreotide in each mL.[1(1/09)]

The Sandostatin (Sandoz) products also contain in each mL lactic acid 3.4 mg, mannitol 45 mg, phenol 5 mg (vial only), and sodium bicarbonate to adjust pH in water for injection.[1(1/09)]

Octreotide acetate (Bedford) has a differing formulation. In addition to the octreotide acetate, the Bedford formulation in ampuls and multidose vials contains in each mL L-lactic acid 3 mg and sodium chloride 7 mg with sodium hydroxide for pH adjustment in water for injection. The multidose vials also contain phenol 5 mg/mL as a preservative.[1(1/09)]

pH

From 3.9 to 4.5.[1(1/09)]

Trade Name(s)

Sandostatin

Administration

Octreotide acetate injection usually is administered by subcutaneous injection in the smallest volume that will deliver the dose. Subcutaneous injection sites should be rotated. Multiple subcutaneous injections at the same site within a short time should be avoided. Administration by intravenous injection over 3 minutes or by infusion over 15 to 30 minutes after further dilution with 50 to 200 mL of dextrose 5% or sodium chloride 0.9% also has been recommended.[1(1/09) 4] NOTE: Do not confuse octreotide acetate injection with the injectable depot suspension product, which cannot be given by these routes of administration.[1(1/09)]

Stability

Octreotide acetate injection is a clear solution. Ampuls and vials should be stored under refrigeration and protected from light. However, octreotide acetate injection can be stored at room temperature for up to 14 days when protected from light.[1(1/09) 4]

The manufacturers state that octreotide acetate injection should not be added to total parenteral nutrition solutions because of the formation of a glycosyl octreotide conjugate that may decrease the product's efficacy,[1(1/09)] although the clinical value of this administration approach has been debated.[2136]

Syringes

The stability of octreotide acetate injection (Sandoz) 0.2 mg/mL packaged as 1 mL in 3-mL polypropylene syringes sealed with tip caps (Becton Dickinson) was evaluated at 3 and 23°C both exposed to and protected from normal room light. No octreotide acetate loss was found in 29 days stored at 3°C protected from light, but about 7 to 9% loss occurred in 15 to 22 days exposed to light. At 23°C, the drug was less stable. Although results were variable, more than 10% loss occurred in about 2 weeks. Maximum storage of 1 week at 23°C, whether protected from light or not, was recommended.[2020]

In a similar study, the stability of octreotide acetate injection (Sandoz) 0.2 mg/mL was evaluated for 60 days stored at 5 and −20°C (light conditions unspecified). The undiluted octreotide acetate injection was packaged as 1 mL in 3-mL polypropylene syringes (Terumo) and sealed with a cap. A loss of about 6% at both storage conditions after 60 days was found.[2021]

Sorption

The manufacturer indicates that octreotide, a peptide, has the potential for adsorption to plastic and, possibly, glass.[1540] However, the drug was not adsorbed to glass infusion bottles or a polyvinyl chloride (PVC) administration set at a concentration of 5 mcg/mL in sodium chloride 0.9%.[1371]

Compatibility Information

Solution Compatibility

Octreotide acetate

Test Soln Name	Mfr	Mfr	Conc/L or %	Remarks	Ref	C/I
Sodium chloride 0.9%	TR[a]	SZ	1.5 mg	Little octreotide loss over 48 hr at room temperature in ambient room light	1373	C
TNA #139[b]	c	SZ	450 mcg	Physically compatible with no change in lipid particle size in 48 hr at 22°C under fluorescent light and 7 days at 4°C. Octreotide activity highly variable	1540	?
TPN #119, #120[b]	a	SZ	1.5 mg	Little octreotide loss over 48 hr at room temperature in ambient room light	1373	C

[a] Tested in PVC containers.

[b] Refer to Appendix for the composition of parenteral nutrition solutions. TNA indicates a 3-in-1 admixture, and TPN indicates a 2-in-1 admixture.

[c] Tested in both glass and ethylene vinyl acetate (EVA) containers.

DOI: 10.37573/9781585286850.287

Additive Compatibility

Octreotide acetate

Test Drug	Mfr	Conc/L or %	Mfr	Conc/L or %	Test Solution	Remarks	Ref	C/I
Fat emulsion, intravenous	KV	10%	SZ	1.5 mg		Octreotide content unstable	1373	I
Heparin sodium	ES	1000 units	SZ	1.5 mg	TPN #120[a]	Little octreotide loss over 48 hr at room temperature in ambient light	1373	C
Insulin, regular		5 units		50 mcg	TPN	Substantial insulin loss	1377	I

[a] Refer to Appendix for the composition of parenteral nutrition solutions. TPN indicates a 2-in-1 admixture.

Drugs in Syringe Compatibility

Octreotide acetate

Test Drug	Mfr	Amt	Mfr	Amt	Remarks	Ref	C/I
Diamorphine HCl	EV	50 mg/8 mL[a]	NVA	300 mcg/8 mL[a]	Visually compatible with no octreotide loss in 48 hr. Diamorphine not tested	2709	C
Diamorphine HCl	EV	50 mg/8 mL[a]	NVA	600 mcg/8 mL[a]	Visually compatible with no octreotide loss in 48 hr. Diamorphine not tested	2709	C
Diamorphine HCl	EV	50 mg/8 mL[a]	NVA	900 mcg/8 mL[a]	Visually compatible with 1% octreotide loss in 48 hr. Diamorphine not tested	2709	C
Diamorphine HCl	EV	100 mg/8 mL[a]	NVA	300 mcg/8 mL[a]	Visually compatible with 4% octreotide loss in 48 hr. Diamorphine not tested	2709	C
Diamorphine HCl	EV	100 mg/8 mL[a]	NVA	600 mcg/8 mL[a]	Visually compatible with 6% octreotide loss in 48 hr. Diamorphine not tested	2709	C
Diamorphine HCl	EV	100 mg/8 mL[a]	NVA	900 mcg/8 mL[a]	Visually compatible with 5% octreotide loss in 48 hr. Diamorphine not tested	2709	C
Diamorphine HCl	EV	200 mg/8 mL[a]	NVA	600 mcg/8 mL[a]	Visually compatible with 6% octreotide loss in 48 hr. Diamorphine not tested	2709	C
Dimenhydrinate		10 mg/1 mL		0.5 mg/1 mL	Precipitate forms in about 1 hr	2569	I
Pantoprazole sodium	[b]	4 mg/1 mL		0.5 mcg/1 mL	Precipitates	2574	I

[a] Tested in sterile water for injection.

[b] Test performed using the formulation WITHOUT edetate disodium.

Y-Site Injection Compatibility (1:1 Mixture)

Octreotide acetate

Test Drug	Mfr	Conc	Mfr	Conc	Remarks	Ref	C/I
Ceftolozane sulfate–tazobactam sodium	CUB	10 mg/mL[e] [f]	APP, FRK	4 mcg/mL[e]	Physically compatible for 2 hr	3262	C
Eravacycline dihydrochloride	TET	0.6 mg/mL[b]	FRK	4 mcg/mL[b]	Physically compatible for 2 hr at room temperature	3532	C
Hydroxyethyl starch 130/0.4 in sodium chloride 0.9%	FRK	6%	NVA	5, 7.5, 10 mcg/mL[a]	Visually compatible for 24 hr at room temperature	2770	C
Isavuconazonium sulfate	ASP	1.5 mg/mL[e]	FRK	4 mcg/mL[e]	Physically compatible for 2 hr	3263	C
Meropenem–vaborbactam	TMC	8 mg/mL[b] [g]	FRK	4 mcg/mL[b]	Physically compatible for 3 hr at 20 to 25°C	3380	C
Micafungin sodium	ASP	1.5 mg/mL[b]	NVA	5 mcg/mL[b]	Microparticulates form in 4 hr	2683	I

Y-Site Injection Compatibility (1:1 Mixture) (Cont.)

Test Drug	Mfr	Conc	Mfr	Conc	Remarks	Ref	C/I
Pantoprazole sodium	ALT[c]	0.16 to 0.4 mg/mL[b]	NVA	5 to 10 mcg/mL[a]	Yellow discoloration forms	2603	I
Pantoprazole sodium	ALT[c]	0.8 mg/mL[b]	NVA	7.5 to 10 mcg/mL[a]	Yellow discoloration forms	2603	I
Pantoprazole sodium	ALT[c]	0.8 mg/mL[b]	NVA	5 mcg/mL[a]	Visually compatible for 12 hr at 23°C	2603	C
Plazomicin sulfate	ACH	24 mg/mL[e]	FRK	4 mcg/mL[e]	Physically compatible for 1 hr at 20 to 25°C	3432	C
TNA #218 to #226[d]			SZ	0.01 mg/mL[a]	Visually compatible for 4 hr at 23°C	2215	C
TPN #212 to #215[d]			SZ	0.01 mg/mL[a]	Physically compatible for 4 hr at 23°C	2109	C

[a] Tested in dextrose 5%.

[b] Tested in sodium chloride 0.9%.

[c] Test performed using the formulation WITHOUT edetate disodium.

[d] Refer to Appendix for the composition of parenteral nutrition solutions. TNA indicates a 3-in-1 admixture, and TPN indicates a 2-in-1 admixture.

[e] Tested in both dextrose 5% and sodium chloride 0.9%.

[f] Ceftolozane component. Ceftolozane in a 2:1 fixed-ratio concentration with tazobactam.

[g] Meropenem component. Meropenem in a 1:1 fixed-ratio concentration with vaborbactam.

Selected Revisions May 1, 2020. © Copyright, October 1992.
American Society of Health-System Pharmacists, Inc.

Omadacycline Tosylate
AHFS 8:12.24.04

Products

Omadacycline tosylate is available in single-dose vials as a cake of lyophilized powder containing the equivalent of 100 mg of omadacycline and 100 mg of sucrose in each vial.[3435] Each 100-mg vial should be reconstituted with 5 mL of sterile water for injection.[3435] Vials should be swirled gently and then left to stand until the cake has dissolved completely and any foam has dispersed; vials should not be shaken.[3435] The reconstituted solution should be visually inspected for particulate matter and discoloration prior to further dilution.[3435] If necessary, vials may be inverted and swirled gently to dissolve any remaining powder.[3435]

The appropriate dose of the reconstituted solution should be further diluted immediately (within 1 hr) to a volume of 100 mL with sodium chloride 0.9% or dextrose 5% to a final omadacycline concentration of 1 or 2 mg/mL.[3435] The diluted solution should be visually inspected for particulate matter and discoloration prior to administration.[3435]

Equivalency

Omadacycline tosylate 131 mg is equivalent to 100 mg of omadacycline.[3435]

Trade Name(s)

Nuzyra

Administration

Omadacycline tosylate is administered by intravenous infusion through a dedicated intravenous line or through a Y-site after reconstitution and further dilution; 100-mg doses should be infused over 30 minutes and 200-mg doses should be infused over 60 minutes.[3435] If a common infusion line is being used to administer other drugs in addition to omadacycline tosylate, the line should be flushed with sodium chloride 0.9% or dextrose 5% prior to and following infusion of omadacycline tosylate.[3435] Omadacycline tosylate must not be administered through the same intravenous line with any solution containing multivalent cations (e.g., calcium, magnesium).[3435]

Stability

Omadacycline tosylate is a yellow to dark orange powder that forms a yellow to dark orange solution upon reconstitution.[3435] Intact vials should be stored at controlled room temperature.[3435] The reconstituted solution of omadacycline should be diluted immediately (within 1 hour).[3435] The diluted solution in sodium chloride 0.9% or dextrose 5% should be used within 12 hours if stored at room temperature (not exceeding 25°C) or within 48 hours if stored at 2 to 8°C.[3435] If the diluted solution has been stored under refrigeration, it should be removed from the refrigerator and kept at room temperature in an upright (vertical) position for 60 minutes prior to use.[3435]

Freezing Solutions

The manufacturer states that diluted solutions of omadacycline should not be frozen.[3435]

Compatibility Information

Solution Compatibility

Omadacycline tosylate

Test Soln Name	Mfr	Mfr	Conc/L or %	Remarks	Ref	C/I
Dextrose 5%		PTK	1 and 2 g	Use within 12 hr if stored at room temperature up to 25°C or 48 hr if stored at 2 to 8°C	3435	C
Sodium chloride 0.9%		PTK	1 and 2 g	Use within 12 hr if stored at room temperature up to 25°C or 48 hr if stored at 2 to 8°C	3435	C

Additional Compatibility Information

Infusion Solutions

Omadacycline tosylate must not be administered through the same intravenous line with any solution containing multivalent cations (e.g., calcium, magnesium).[3435]

DOI: 10.37573/9781585286850.288

Omeprazole Sodium
AHFS 56:28.36

Products

Omeprazole *for infusion* is available as a powder in vials containing 40 mg of the drug as the sodium salt[3408] [3409] or 40 mg of the drug as the base.[3410] Each vial of the drug also contains disodium edetate and sodium hydroxide for pH adjustment.[3408] [3409] [3410] Each 40-mg vial of omeprazole should be reconstituted with 5 mL of solution withdrawn from a 100-mL infusion bag or bottle of sodium chloride 0.9% or dextrose 5% and then mixed thoroughly until all of the powder has dissolved.[3408] [3409] [3410] The reconstituted solution should then be transferred back into the same 100-mL infusion bag or bottle from which the solution used for reconstitution was withdrawn.[3408] [3409] [3410]

Omeprazole *for injection* is available as a powder in vials containing 40 mg of the drug as the sodium salt with an accompanying ampul containing 10 mL of solvent.[3411] Each vial of the drug also contains sodium hydroxide.[3411] The solvent contains citric acid monohydrate and polyethylene glycol 400 in water for injection.[3411] Each 40-mg vial of omeprazole should be reconstituted only with 10 mL of the provided solvent; no other solvents should be used.[3411]

Equivalency

Omeprazole sodium 42.6 mg is equivalent to 40 mg of omeprazole.[3408]

pH

The pH of omeprazole (Azevedos) 0.4-mg/mL solution (reconstituted from omeprazole sodium) in dextrose 5% and sodium chloride 0.9% ranges from 8.9 to 9.5 and from 9.3 to 10.3, respectively.[3408]

The pH of omeprazole (Sandoz) 0.4-mg/mL solution (reconstituted from omeprazole sodium) in dextrose 5% or sodium chloride 0.9% ranges from 9 to 10.5.[3409]

The pH of a reconstituted solution of 40 mg of omeprazole (Sandoz) (reconstituted from omeprazole sodium) prepared with 10 mL of accompanying solvent is about 8.6.[3411]

Osmolality

The osmolality of omeprazole (Sandoz) 0.4-mg/mL solution (reconstituted from omeprazole sodium) in dextrose 5% or sodium chloride 0.9% is 297 or 282 mOsm/kg, respectively.[3409]

Administration

Omeprazole is administered by intravenous infusion[3408] [3409] [3410] or by intravenous injection,[3411] depending upon the product used.

After omeprazole *for infusion* is reconstituted and diluted to 100 mL with sodium chloride 0.9% or dextrose 5%, it should be administered as a 20- to 30-minute intravenous infusion.[3408] [3409] [3410]

After omeprazole *for injection* is reconstituted with the accompanying solvent, it should be administered as a slow intravenous injection over at least 2.5 minutes at a maximum rate of 4 mL/min.[3411]

Stability

Intact containers of omeprazole *for infusion* and omeprazole *for injection* (and accompanying solvent) generally should be stored at temperatures not exceeding 25°C in the outer carton to protect from light.[3408] [3409] [3410] [3411]

Stability of omeprazole solutions varies depending upon which product is used; specific product labeling should be consulted.[3408] [3409] [3410] [3411]

When stored at temperatures that do not exceed 25°C, omeprazole solutions *for infusion* are reportedly stable for 12 hours when prepared with sodium chloride 0.9%,[3408] [3409] for 6 hours when prepared with dextrose 5%,[3408] [3409] or for 6 hours in either solution;[3410] when stored at 2 to 8°C, one product has been reported as stable for 24 hours in either solution.[3409]

Omeprazole *for injection* reconstituted with the accompanying solvent is stable for up to 4 hours when stored at temperatures below 25°C.[3411]

Light Effects

Intact containers of omeprazole, omeprazole sodium, and solvent, when provided, should be stored in their outer carton to protect from light.[3408] [3409] [3410] [3411] At least one manufacturer states that vials may be exposed to normal indoor light outside of the box for up to 24 hours.[3408]

Reconstituted omeprazole (AstraZeneca) has been reported to develop an unacceptable discoloration indicating decomposition within 6 hours at room temperature when exposed to light.[2507]

Compatibility Information

Solution Compatibility

Omeprazole sodium

Test Soln Name	Mfr	Mfr	Conc/L or %	Remarks	Ref	C/I
Dextrose 5%	BA	PH	400 mg	Physically compatible. 10% loss occurs in 2.5 days at 22°C in light	2696	C
Dextrose 5%		SZ	400 mg	Stable for 6 hr below 25°C or 24 hr at 2 to 8°C	3409	C

DOI: 10.37573/9781585286850.289

Solution Compatibility (Cont.)

Test Soln Name	Mfr	Mfr	Conc/L or %	Remarks	Ref	C/I
Dextrose 5%		AZV	400 mg	Stable for 6 hr at 25°C	3408	C
Sodium chloride 0.9%	BA	PH	400 mg	Physically compatible. 10% loss occurs in 8 days at 22°C in light	2696, 3082	C
Sodium chloride 0.9%		SZ	400 mg	Stable for 12 hr below 25°C or 24 hr at 2 to 8°C	3409	C
Sodium chloride 0.9%		AZV	400 mg	Stable for 12 hr at 25°C	3408	C

Y-Site Injection Compatibility (1:1 Mixture)

Omeprazole sodium

Test Drug	Mfr	Conc	Mfr	Conc	Remarks	Ref	C/I
Lorazepam	WY	0.33 mg/mL[b]	AST	4 mg/mL	Yellow discoloration forms	1855	I
Midazolam HCl	RC	5 mg/mL	AST	4 mg/mL	Brown color then precipitate	1855	I
Tigecycline	ACD, FRK, WY		[c]		Stated to be incompatible	2915, 3459, 3460	I

[a] Tested in dextrose 5%.

[b] Tested in sodium chloride 0.9%.

[c] Salt not specified.

Selected Revisions January 31, 2020. © Copyright, October 2000. American Society of Health-System Pharmacists, Inc.

Ondansetron Hydrochloride
AHFS 56:22.20

Products

Ondansetron hydrochloride is available in 20-mL multiple-dose vials and 2-mL single-dose vials.[2836] [2837] Each mL of solution in multiple-dose vials contains ondansetron (as the hydrochloride dihydrate) 2 mg with sodium chloride 8.3 mg, citric acid monohydrate 0.5 mg, sodium citrate dihydrate 0.25 mg, methylparaben 1.2 mg, and propylparaben 0.15 mg in water for injection.[2836] [2837] Each mL of solution in single-dose vials contains ondansetron (as the hydrochloride dihydrate) 2 mg with sodium chloride 9 mg, citric acid monohydrate 0.5 mg, and sodium citrate dihydrate 0.25 mg in water for injection.[2836]

pH

From 3.3 to 4.[2836]

Trade Name(s)

Zofran

Administration

Ondansetron hydrochloride is administered by intravenous infusion over 15 minutes after further dilution with 50 mL of sodium chloride 0.9% or dextrose 5%.[2836] [2837] By intravenous injection, it is administered undiluted over at least 30 seconds and preferably over 2 to 5 minutes.[2836] [2837]

Ondansetron hydrochloride also has been administered intramuscularly *without* dilution.[2836] [2837]

Stability

Ondansetron hydrochloride is a clear, colorless solution.[2836] [2837] It should be stored at 2 to 30°C and protected from light.[2836] [2837] Although ondansetron hydrochloride is unstable under intense light, it is stable for about 1 month in daylight with added fluorescent light.[1366] Ondansetron occasionally may precipitate at the stopper/vial interface in vials that are stored upright; the potency and safety of ondansetron are not affected.[2836] [2837] If a precipitate is observed, the drug may be resolubilized by vigorously shaking the vial.[2836] [2837]

Ondansetron hydrochloride (Glaxo) 0.03 and 0.3 mg/mL in dextrose 5% or sodium chloride 0.9% was stable when frozen at −20°C, exhibiting a 10% or less loss in 3 months.[1642]

pH Effects

The natural pH of ondansetron hydrochloride solutions is about 4.5 to 4.6.[1366] [1367] The pH of commercially available ondansetron solution has been adjusted with citric acid monohydrate and sodium citrate dihydrate to the range of 3.3 to 4.[2836] [2837] If the pH is increased, a precipitate of ondansetron free base has been reported to develop at pH 5.7[1366] and pH 7.[1513] Redissolution of the ondansetron precipitate occurs at pH 6.2 when titrated with hydrochloric acid.[1513] Precipitation by combination with alkaline drugs has been observed.[1365] [1513]

Syringes

The stability of ondansetron hydrochloride undiluted at 2 mg/mL and diluted in dextrose 5% and sodium chloride 0.9% at 1, 0.5, and 0.25 mg/mL packaged in polypropylene syringes was reported. Representative syringes were stored at 24°C for 48 hours, 4°C for 14 days, and frozen at −20°C for 90 days. Visually, the solutions exhibited no precipitate or color or clarity changes. Ondansetron hydrochloride concentrations in all samples remained above 90%; most samples were above 95%. Sequentially storing sample syringes for 90 days at −20°C followed by 14 days at 4°C followed by 48 hours at 24°C did not alter the stability.[2056]

When diluted with compatible infusion solutions, ondansetron hydrochloride is stable for up to 7 days at room temperature or under refrigeration in Plastipak syringes with syringe caps.[1366]

Filtration

Ondansetron hydrochloride (Glaxo) 0.03 and 0.2 mg/mL (30 and 200 mcg/mL) in sodium chloride 0.9% was delivered over 15 minutes through 5 different 0.2-μm inline filters: Continu-Flo Solution Set (Baxter, 2C5561S), Filtered Extension Sets (Burron, PFE-2007 and FE-2024), Universal Primary infusion set (IVAC, 52023), and Ivex-HP Filterset-SL (Abbott, 4524). Little or no ondansetron loss was found.[1678]

Central Venous Catheter

Ondansetron hydrochloride (Glaxo Wellcome) 0.2 mg/mL in dextrose 5% was found to be compatible with the ARROW-g+ard Blue Plus (Arrow International) chlorhexidine-bearing triple-lumen central catheter. Essentially complete delivery of the drug was found with little or no drug loss occurring. Furthermore, chlorhexidine delivered from the catheter remained at trace amounts with no substantial increase due to the delivery of the drug through the catheter.[2335]

DOI: 10.37573/9781585286850.290

Compatibility Information

Solution Compatibility

Ondansetron HCl

Test Soln Name	Mfr	Mfr	Conc/L or %	Remarks	Ref	C/I
Dextrose 5% in sodium chloride 0.45%		CLA, GSK		Stable for 48 hr at room temperature in light	2836, 2837	C
Dextrose 5% in sodium chloride 0.9%		CLA, GSK		Stable for 48 hr at room temperature in light	2836, 2837	C
Dextrose 5%		CLA, GSK		Stable for 48 hr at room temperature in light	2836, 2837	C
Dextrose 5%	BP[a]	GL	16 and 80 mg	Physically compatible and stable for 7 days at room temperature in light and at 4°C	1366	C
Dextrose 5%		GL	24 and 96 mg	Visually compatible. No loss in 14 days at 24°C or 14 days at 5°C then 2 days at 24°C	1560	C
Dextrose 5%	BA[a]	GL	30 and 300 mg	Visually compatible with 5% or less loss in 48 hr at 25°C or 14 days at 5°C	1642	C
Dextrose 5%	MG[b]	GL	0.03 and 0.3 g	Visually compatible with no loss in 14 days at 4°C in light	1722	C
Dextrose 5% with potassium chloride 0.3%	BP[a]	GL	16 mg	Physically compatible and stable for 7 days at room temperature in light and at 4°C	1366	C
Ringer's injection	BP[a]	GL	16 mg	Physically compatible and stable for 7 days at room temperature in light and at 4°C	1366	C
Ringer's injection, lactated		GL	24 and 96 mg	Visually compatible. No loss in 14 days at 24°C or 14 days at 5°C then 2 days at 24°C	1560	C
Sodium chloride 0.9%		CLA, GSK		Stable for 48 hr at room temperature in light	2836, 2837	C
Sodium chloride 0.9%	BP[a]	GL	16 and 80 mg	Physically compatible and stable for 7 days at room temperature in light and at 4°C	1366	C
Sodium chloride 0.9%		GL	24 and 96 mg	Visually compatible. No loss in 14 days at 24°C or 14 days at 5°C then 2 days at 24°C	1560	C
Sodium chloride 0.9%	BA[c]	GL	240 mg	No loss in 24 hr at 30°C or 30 days at 3°C then 24 hr at 30°C	1553	C
Sodium chloride 0.9%	BA[a]	GL	30 and 300 mg	Visually compatible with 4% or less loss in 48 hr at 25°C or 14 days at 5°C	1642	C
Sodium chloride 0.9%	MG[b]	GL	0.03 and 0.3 g	Visually compatible with no loss in 14 days at 4°C in light	1722	C
Sodium chloride 0.9%	BA[a]	CER	100 mg	Visually compatible. 6 to 7% loss after 30 days at 4°C then 2 days at 23°C	1882	C
Sodium chloride 0.9%	BA[a]	CER	200, 400, 640 mg	Visually compatible. Up to 4% loss after 30 days at 4°C then 2 days at 23°C	1882	C
Sodium chloride 0.9%	AGT[a]	GL	80 mg	Visually compatible with 4% loss in 120 days at 4 and −20°C	2405	C
Sodium chloride 0.9% with potassium chloride 0.3%	BP[a]	GL	16 mg	Physically compatible and stable for 7 days at room temperature in light and at 4°C	1366	C
TNA #190[d]		GL	0.03 and 0.3 g	Physically compatible with no loss in 48 hr at 24°C in light	1766	C

[a] Tested in PVC containers.

[b] Tested in a Kraton polymer elastomeric infusion device (Homepump, Block).

[c] Tested in a medication cassette reservoir (Pharmacia Deltec CADD-1).

[d] Refer to Appendix for the composition of parenteral nutrition solutions. TNA indicates a 3-in-1 admixture.

Additive Compatibility

Ondansetron HCl

Test Drug	Mfr	Conc/L or %	Mfr	Conc/L or %	Test Solution	Remarks	Ref	C/I
Cisplatin	BR	485 mg	GL	1.031 g	NS[a]	Physically compatible. Little loss of drugs in 24 hr at 4°C then 7 days at 30°C	1846	C
Cisplatin	BR	219 mg	GL	479 mg	NS[b]	Physically compatible. Little loss of drugs in 7 days at 4°C then 24 hr at 30°C	1846	C
Cyclophosphamide	MJ	300 mg	GL	50 mg	D5W[a], NS[a]	Visually compatible with 9 to 10% cyclophosphamide loss and no ondansetron loss in 5 days at 24°C. No loss of either drug in 8 days at 4°C	1812	C
Cyclophosphamide	MJ	2 g	GL	400 mg	D5W[a], NS[a]	Visually compatible with 10% cyclophosphamide loss and no ondansetron loss in 5 days at 24°C. No loss of either drug in 8 days at 4°C	1812	C
Cytarabine	UP	200 mg	GL	30 and 300 mg	D5W[a]	Physically compatible with little loss of either drug in 48 hr at 23°C	1876	C
Cytarabine	UP	40 g	GL	30 and 300 mg	D5W[a]	Physically compatible with little loss of either drug in 48 hr at 23°C	1876	C
Dacarbazine	MI	1 g	GL	30 and 300 mg	D5W[a]	Physically compatible with little loss of ondansetron in 48 hr at 23°C. 8 to 12% dacarbazine loss in 24 hr and 20% loss in 48 hr at 23°C	1876	C
Dacarbazine	MI	3 g	GL	30 and 300 mg	D5W[a]	Physically compatible with little loss of ondansetron in 48 hr at 23°C. 8% dacarbazine loss in 24 hr and 15% loss in 48 hr at 23°C	1876	C
Dacarbazine with doxorubicin HCl	LY AD	8 g 800 mg	GL	640 mg	D5W[a]	Visually compatible. Under 10% ondansetron and doxorubicin loss in 24 hr at 30°C and 7 days at 4°C then 24 hr at 30°C. Dacarbazine stable for 8 hr but 13% loss in 24 hr	2092	I
Dacarbazine with doxorubicin HCl	LY AD	8 g 800 mg	GL	640 mg	D5W[b]	Visually compatible. Under 10% loss of all drugs in 24 hr at 30°C and 7 days at 4°C then 24 hr at 30°C	2092	C
Dacarbazine with doxorubicin HCl	LY AD	20 g 1.5 g	GL	640 mg	D5W[a b]	Visually compatible. Under 10% loss of all drugs in 24 hr at 30°C and 7 days at 4°C then 24 hr at 30°C	2092	C
Dexamethasone sodium phosphate		20 and 40 mg	GL	48 mg	D5W, NS	Visually compatible for 24 hr at 22°C	1608	C
Dexamethasone sodium phosphate		200 and 400 mg	GL	160 mg	NS	Visually compatible for 24 hr at 22°C	1608	C
Dexamethasone sodium phosphate	ES	200 mg	CER	100 mg	NS[a]	Visually compatible. No dexamethasone and 8% ondansetron loss in 30 days at 4°C then 2 days at 23°C	1882	C
Dexamethasone sodium phosphate	ES	400 mg	CER	100 and 200 mg	NS[a]	Visually compatible. No dexamethasone and 7 to 10% ondansetron loss in 30 days at 4°C then 2 days at 23°C	1882	C
Dexamethasone sodium phosphate	ES	200 mg	CER	200, 400, 640 mg	NS[a]	Visually compatible. No dexamethasone and 5% ondansetron loss in 30 days at 4°C then 2 days at 23°C	1882	C
Dexamethasone sodium phosphate	ES	400 mg	CER	400 and 640 mg	NS[a]	Visually compatible. No dexamethasone and 3% ondansetron loss in 30 days at 4°C then 2 days at 23°C	1882	C
Dexamethasone sodium phosphate	ES	200 and 400 mg	CER	640 mg	D5W[c]	Visually compatible. 7% dexamethasone and no ondansetron loss in 30 days at 4°C then 2 days at 23°C	1882	C
Dexamethasone sodium phosphate	MSD	400 mg	GL	150 mg	NS[a]	Visually compatible. 4% or less loss of either drug in 28 days at 4 and 22°C	2084	C

Additive Compatibility (Cont.)

Test Drug	Mfr	Conc/L or %	Mfr	Conc/L or %	Test Solution	Remarks	Ref	C/I
Dexamethasone sodium phosphate	MSD	400 mg	GL	150 mg	D5W[a]	Visually compatible. 4% or less loss of either drug in 28 days at 4°C. 10% ondansetron loss in 3 days at 22°C	2084	C
Dexamethasone sodium phosphate	MSD	230 mg	GL	750 mg	NS[a]	Visually compatible. 4% or less loss of either drug in 28 days at 4°C. 10% ondansetron loss in 7 days at 22°C	2084	C
Dexamethasone sodium phosphate	MSD	230 mg	GL	750 mg	D5W[a]	Visually compatible. Up to 13% ondansetron loss in 3 days at 4 and 22°C	2084	?
Dexamethasone sodium phosphate	OR	100 mg	GSK	80 mg	D5W[d]	Visually compatible. Under 3% ondansetron and 8% dexamethasone loss when frozen for 3 months then stored refrigerated for 30 days	2822	C
Dexamethasone sodium phosphate	[g]	100 mg		70 mg	NS	Physically compatible for 24 hr at 25°C in light	2999	C
Doxorubicin HCl	MJ	100 mg and 2 g	GL	30 and 300 mg	D5W[a]	Physically compatible with little loss of either drug in 48 hr at 23°C	1876	C
Doxorubicin HCl with dacarbazine	AD LY	800 mg 8 g	GL	640 mg	D5W[a]	Visually compatible. Under 10% ondansetron and doxorubicin loss in 24 hr at 30°C and 7 days at 4°C then 24 hr at 30°C. Dacarbazine stable for 8 hr but 13% loss in 24 hr	2092	I
Doxorubicin HCl with dacarbazine	AD LY	800 mg 8 g	GL	640 mg	D5W[b]	Visually compatible. Under 10% loss of all drugs in 24 hr at 30°C and 7 days at 4°C then 24 hr at 30°C	2092	C
Doxorubicin HCl with dacarbazine	AD LY	1.5 g 20 g	GL	640 mg	D5W[a b]	Visually compatible. Under 10% loss of all drugs in 24 hr at 30°C and 7 days at 4°C then 24 hr at 30°C	2092	C
Doxorubicin HCl with vincristine sulfate	AD LI	400 mg 14 mg	GL	480 mg	D5W[b]	Visually compatible. Under 10% loss of all drugs in 5 days at 4°C then 24 hr at 30°C	2092	C
Doxorubicin HCl with vincristine sulfate	AD LI	800 mg 28 mg	GL	960 mg	D5W[a]	Visually compatible. Under 10% loss of all drugs after 120 hr at 30°C	2092	C
Etoposide	BR	100 mg	GL	30 and 300 mg	D5W[a]	Physically compatible. Little or no loss of ondansetron in 48 hr at 23°C. 4% etoposide loss in 24 hr and 6% loss in 48 hr at 23°C	1876	C
Etoposide	BR	400 mg	GL	30 and 300 mg	D5W[a]	Physically compatible with little or no loss of either drug in 48 hr at 23°C	1876	C
Fluconazole with ranitidine HCl	RR GL	2 g 500 mg	GL	100 mg	[a]	Visually compatible with no loss of any drug in 4 hr	1730	C
Fosaprepitant dimeglumine	MSD	1 g		70 mg	NS	Physically compatible for 24 hr at 25°C in light	2999	C
Fosaprepitant dimeglumine	MSD[e]	1 g		70 mg	NS	Physically compatible for 24 hr at 25°C in light	2999	C
Fosaprepitant dimeglumine	MSD[f]	1 g		70 mg	NS	Physically compatible for 24 hr at 25°C in light	2999	C
Hydromorphone HCl	ES	500 mg	GL	100 mg and 1 g	NS	Physically compatible. No loss of either drug in 7 days at 32°C or 31 days at 4 and 22°C protected from light	1690	C
Mannitol	BP[a]	10%	GL	16 mg		Physically compatible. Stable for 7 days at room temperature in light and at 4°C	1366	C
Meperidine HCl	WY	4 g	GL	100 mg and 1 g	NS[a]	Physically compatible. No loss of either drug in 31 days at 4 and 22°C and in 7 days at 32°C	1862	C
Meropenem	ZEN	1 g	GL	1 g	NS	Visually compatible for 4 hr at room temperature	1994	C
Meropenem	ZEN	20 g	GL	1 g	NS	White precipitate forms immediately	1994	I

Additive Compatibility (Cont.)

Test Drug	Mfr	Conc/L or %	Mfr	Conc/L or %	Test Solution	Remarks	Ref	C/I
Methotrexate sodium	LE	0.5 and 6 g	GL	30 and 300 mg	D5W[a]	Physically compatible with little or no loss of either drug in 48 hr at 23°C	1876	C
Methylprednisolone sodium succinate	PH	2.4 g	GSK	160 mg	D5W, NS	Transient turbidity forms then clears. 5% or less loss of either drug in 24 hr at 23°C and 48 hr at 6°C	2643	?
Methylprednisolone sodium succinate	g	700 mg		70 mg	NS	Physically compatible for 24 hr at 25°C in light	2999	C
Morphine sulfate	AST	1 g	GL	100 mg and 1 g	NS	Physically compatible. No ondansetron loss and 5% or less morphine loss in 7 days at 32°C or 31 days at 4 and 22°C protected from light	1690	C
Ranitidine HCl with fluconazole	GL RR	500 mg 2 g	GL	100 mg	[a]	Visually compatible with no loss of any drug in 4 hr	1730	C
Tramadol HCl	GRU	400 mg	GL	1.6 mg	NS	Visually compatible with about 7% tramadol loss in 24 hr at room temperature	2652	C
Vincristine sulfate with doxorubicin HCl	LI AD	14 mg 400 mg	GL	480 mg	D5W[b]	Visually compatible. Under 10% loss of all drugs in 5 days at 4°C then 24 hr at 30°C	2092	C
Vincristine sulfate with doxorubicin HCl	LI AD	28 mg 800 mg	GL	960 mg	D5W[a]	Visually compatible. Under 10% loss of all drugs after 120 hr at 30°C	2092	C

[a] Tested in PVC containers.

[b] Tested in polyisoprene reservoirs (Travenol Infusors).

[c] Tested in ondansetron hydrochloride ready-to-use CR3 polyester bags.

[d] Tested in polyolefin containers.

[e] Tested with dexamethasone sodium phosphate 100 mg/L.

[f] Tested with methylprednisolone sodium phosphate 700 mg/L.

[g] Tested with fosaprepitant dimeglumine (MSD) 1 g/L.

Drugs in Syringe Compatibility

Ondansetron HCl

Test Drug	Mfr	Amt	Mfr	Amt	Remarks	Ref	C/I
Alfentanil HCl	JN	0.167 mg/mL[b]	GW	1.33 mg/mL[b]	Physically compatible. Little loss of either drug in 24 hr at 4 or 23°C	2199	C
Atropine sulfate	GNS	0.133 mg/mL[b]	GW	1.33 mg/mL[b]	Physically compatible. Under 6% ondansetron and under 7% atropine losses in 24 hr at 4 or 23°C	2199	C
Dexamethasone sodium phosphate	ES	0.33 and 0.67 mg/mL[a]	CER	0.17 mg/mL[a]	Visually compatible. No loss of either drug in 30 days at 4°C then 2 days at 23°C	1882	C
Dexamethasone sodium phosphate	ES	0.5 mg/mL[a]	CER	0.25 mg/mL[a]	Visually compatible. No loss of either drug in 30 days at 4°C then 2 days at 23°C	1882	C
Dexamethasone sodium phosphate	ES	1 mg/mL[a]	CER	0.25 mg/mL[a]	Visually compatible for 3 days at 4°C. Precipitation of ondansetron observed at 7 days as opaque white ring	1882	C
Dexamethasone sodium phosphate	ES	0.33 and 0.67 mg/mL[a]	CER	0.33 mg/mL[a]	Visually compatible. No loss of either drug in 30 days at 4°C then 2 days at 23°C	1882	C
Dexamethasone sodium phosphate	ES	0.5 mg/mL[a]	CER	0.5 mg/mL[a]	Visually compatible. No loss of either drug in 30 days at 4°C then 2 days at 23°C	1882	C
Dexamethasone sodium phosphate	ES	1 mg/mL[a]	CER	0.5 mg/mL[a]	Visually compatible for 3 days at 4°C. Precipitation of ondansetron observed at 5 days as opaque white ring	1882	C

Drugs in Syringe Compatibility (Cont.)

Test Drug	Mfr	Amt	Mfr	Amt	Remarks	Ref	C/I
Dexamethasone sodium phosphate	ES	0.33 and 0.67 mg/mL[a]	CER	0.67 mg/mL[a]	Visually compatible. No loss of either drug in 30 days at 4°C then 2 days at 23°C	1882	C
Dexamethasone sodium phosphate	ES	0.33 mg/mL[a]	CER	1.07 mg/mL[a]	Visually compatible. No loss of either drug in 30 days at 4°C then 2 days at 23°C	1882	C
Dexamethasone sodium phosphate	ES	0.67 mg/mL[a]	CER	1.07 mg/mL[a]	Heavy white precipitate in 72 hr at 4°C. 25 to 30% loss of both drugs	1882	I
Dexamethasone sodium phosphate	OM[c]	4 mg/1 mL		4 mg/2 mL	Physically incompatible within 3 min	2767	I
Dexamethasone sodium phosphate	[d]	4 mg/1 mL		4 mg/2 mL	Physically compatible	2767	C
Droperidol	AMR	1.25 mg/mL[b]	GW	1 mg/mL[b]	Droperidol precipitates at 4°C. At 23°C, little or no loss of either drug in 8 hr, but droperidol precipitates after that time	2199	I
Fentanyl citrate	ES	16.7 mcg/mL[b]	GW	1.33 mg/mL[b]	Physically compatible. Little loss of either drug in 24 hr at 4 or 23°C	2199	C
Glycopyrrolate	AMR	0.1 mg/mL[b]	GW	1 mg/mL[b]	Physically compatible. Little loss of either drug in 24 hr at 4 or 23°C	2199	C
Meperidine HCl	ES	8.33 mg/mL[b]	GW	1.33 mg/mL[b]	Physically compatible. Little loss of either drug in 24 hr at 4 or 23°C	2199	C
Metoclopramide HCl	SO	2.5 mg/mL[b]	GW	1 mg/mL[b]	Physically compatible. Under 6% ondansetron and under 5% metoclopramide losses in 24 hr at 4 or 23°C	2199	C
Midazolam HCl	RC	1.66 mg/mL[b]	GW	1.33 mg/mL[b]	Physically compatible. Under 4% ondansetron and under 7% midazolam losses in 24 hr at 4 or 23°C	2199	C
Morphine sulfate	ES	2.67 mg/mL[b]	GW	1.33 mg/mL[b]	Physically compatible. Under 5% ondansetron and under 4% morphine losses in 24 hr at 4 or 23°C	2199	C
Naloxone HCl	AST	0.133 mg/mL[b]	GW	1.33 mg/mL[b]	Physically compatible. Under 6% ondansetron and under 5% naloxone losses in 24 hr at 4 or 23°C	2199	C
Neostigmine methyl-sulfate	ES	0.167 mg/mL[b]	GW	1.33 mg/mL[b]	Physically compatible. Under 3% ondansetron and under 5% neostigmine losses in 24 hr at 4 or 23°C	2199	C
Propofol	STU	1 and 5 mg/mL[b]	GW	1 mg/mL[b]	Physically compatible. Little loss of either drug in 4 hr at 23°C	2199	C

[a] Diluted with sodium chloride 0.9% drawn into a syringe prior to drugs to yield the concentrations cited.

[b] Tested in sodium chloride 0.9%.

[c] Contained benzyl alcohol as a preservative.

[d] Contained parabens as preservatives.

Y-Site Injection Compatibility (1:1 Mixture)

Ondansetron HCl

Test Drug	Mfr	Conc	Mfr	Conc	Remarks	Ref	C/I
Acetaminophen	CAD	10 mg/mL	WOC	2 mg/mL	Physically compatible with little or no loss of either drug in 4 hr at 23°C	2901, 2902	C
Acetaminophen	CAD	10 mg/mL	WW	2 mg/mL	Physically compatible with less than 10% acetaminophen loss over 4 hr at room temperature	2841, 2844	C
Acyclovir sodium	BW	7 mg/mL[a]	GL	1 mg/mL[b]	Precipitates immediately	1365	I

Y-Site Injection Compatibility (1:1 Mixture) (Cont.)

Test Drug	Mfr	Conc	Mfr	Conc	Remarks	Ref	C/I
Aldesleukin	CHI	33,800 I.U./mL[a]	GL	0.7 mg/mL[a]	Visually compatible with little or no loss of aldesleukin activity	1857	C
Aldesleukin	CHI	5 to 40 mcg/mL[k]	GL		Visually compatible. Aldesleukin activity retained if each drug infused at a similar rate. Ondansetron not tested	1890	C
Allopurinol sodium	BW	3 mg/mL[b]	GL	1 mg/mL[b]	Immediate turbidity becoming precipitate	1686	I
Amifostine	USB	10 mg/mL[a]	GL	1 mg/mL[a]	Physically compatible for 4 hr at 23°C	1845	C
Amikacin sulfate	BR	5 mg/mL[a]	GL	1 mg/mL[b]	Visually compatible for 4 hr at 22°C	1365	C
Aminophylline	AMR	2.5 mg/mL[a]	GL	1 mg/mL[b]	Immediate turbidity and precipitation	1365	I
Amphotericin B	SQ	0.6 mg/mL[a]	GL	1 mg/mL[a]	Immediate yellow turbid precipitate	1365	I
Ampicillin sodium	BR	20 mg/mL[b]	GL	1 mg/mL[b]	Immediate turbidity and precipitation	1365	I
Ampicillin sodium–sulbactam sodium	RR	20 mg/mL[b i]	GL	1 mg/mL[b]	Immediate turbidity and precipitation	1365	I
Amsacrine	NCI	1 mg/mL[a]	GL	1 mg/mL[a]	Orange precipitate forms within 30 min	1365	I
Azithromycin	PF	2 mg/mL[b]	GW	2 mg/mL[j]	Visually compatible	2368	C
Aztreonam	SQ	40 mg/mL[a]	GL	1 mg/mL[b]	Visually compatible for 4 hr at 22°C	1365	C
Aztreonam	SQ	40 mg/mL[a]	GL	0.03 and 0.3 mg/mL[a]	Visually compatible with little loss of either drug in 4 hr at 25°C	1732	C
Aztreonam	SQ	40 mg/mL[a]	GL	1 mg/mL[a]	Physically compatible for 4 hr at 23°C	1758	C
Bleomycin sulfate	BR	1 unit/mL[b]	GL	1 mg/mL[b]	Visually compatible for 4 hr at 22°C	1365	C
Carboplatin	BR	5 mg/mL[a]	GL	1 mg/mL[b]	Visually compatible for 4 hr at 22°C	1365	C
Carboplatin		0.18 to 9.9 mg/mL	GL	16 to 160 mcg/mL	Physically compatible when carboplatin given over 10 to 60 min via Y-site	1366	C
Carmustine	BR	1.5 mg/mL[a]	GL	1 mg/mL[b]	Visually compatible for 4 hr at 22°C	1365	C
Caspofungin acetate	ME	0.5 mg/mL[b]	BED	2 mg/mL	Physically compatible with ondansetron HCl i.v. push over 2 to 5 min	2766	C
Cefazolin sodium	LEM	20 mg/mL[a]	GL	1 mg/mL[b]	Visually compatible for 4 hr at 22°C	1365	C
Cefazolin sodium	LI	20 mg/mL[a]	GL	0.03 and 0.3 mg/mL[a]	Visually compatible with little loss of either drug in 4 hr at 25°C	1732	C
Cefotaxime sodium	HO	20 mg/mL[a]	GL	1 mg/mL[b]	Visually compatible for 4 hr at 22°C	1365	C
Cefoxitin sodium	MSD	20 mg/mL[a]	GL	1 mg/mL[b]	Visually compatible for 4 hr at 22°C	1365	C
Ceftaroline fosamil	FOR	2.22 mg/mL[a b i]	WOC	1 mg/mL[a b i]	Physically compatible for 4 hr at 23°C	2826	C
Ceftazidime	GL	40 mg/mL[a]	GL	1 mg/mL[b]	Visually compatible for 4 hr at 22°C	1365	C
Ceftazidime		100 to 200 mg/mL	GL	16 to 160 mcg/mL	Physically compatible when ceftazidime given as 5-min bolus via Y-site	1366	C
Ceftazidime	LI	40 mg/mL[a]	GL	0.03 and 0.3 mg/mL[a]	Visually compatible with less than 10% loss of either drug in 4 hr at 25°C	1732	C
Ceftolozane sulfate-tazobactam sodium	CUB	10 mg/mL[p q]	HOS	0.16 mg/mL[p]	Physically compatible for 2 hr	3262	C
Cefuroxime sodium	LI	30 mg/mL[a]	GL	1 mg/mL[b]	Visually compatible for 4 hr at 22°C	1365	C

Y-Site Injection Compatibility (1:1 Mixture) (Cont.)

Test Drug	Mfr	Conc	Mfr	Conc	Remarks	Ref	C/I
Chlorpromazine HCl	ES	2 mg/mL[a]	GL	1 mg/mL[b]	Visually compatible for 4 hr at 22°C	1365	C
Cisatracurium besylate	GW	0.1, 2, 5 mg/mL[a]	CER	1 mg/mL[a]	Physically compatible for 4 hr at 23°C	2074	C
Cisplatin	BR	1 mg/mL	GL	1 mg/mL[b]	Visually compatible for 4 hr at 22°C	1365	C
Cisplatin		0.48 mg/mL	GL	16 to 160 mcg/mL	Physically compatible when cisplatin given over 1 to 8 hr via Y-site	1366	C
Cladribine	ORT	0.015[b] and 0.5[d] mg/mL	CER	1 mg/mL[b]	Physically compatible for 4 hr at 23°C	1969	C
Clindamycin phosphate	LY	10 mg/mL[a]	GL	1 mg/mL[b]	Visually compatible for 4 hr at 22°C	1365	C
Cloxacillin sodium	SMX	100 mg/mL	SZ	2 mg/mL	Physically compatible for up to 4 hr at room temperature	3245	C
Cyclophosphamide	MJ	10 mg/mL[a]	GL	1 mg/mL[b]	Visually compatible for 4 hr at 22°C	1365	C
Cyclophosphamide		20 mg/mL	GL	16 to 160 mcg/mL	Physically compatible when cyclophosphamide given as 5-min bolus via Y-site	1366	C
Cytarabine	UP	50 mg/mL	GL	1 mg/mL[b]	Visually compatible for 4 hr at 22°C	1365	C
Dacarbazine	MI	4 mg/mL[a]	GL	1 mg/mL[b]	Visually compatible for 4 hr at 22°C	1365	C
Dactinomycin	MSD	0.01 mg/mL[a]	GL	1 mg/mL[b]	Visually compatible for 4 hr at 22°C	1365	C
Daunorubicin HCl	WY	2 mg/mL[a]	GL	1 mg/mL[b]	Visually compatible for 4 hr at 22°C	1365	C
Defibrotide sodium	JAZ	8 mg/mL[b]	ACD	0.16 mg/mL[b]	Visually compatible for 4 hr at room temperature	3149	C
Dexamethasone sodium phosphate	MSD	1 mg/mL[a]	GL	1 mg/mL[b]	Visually compatible for 4 hr at 22°C	1365	C
Dexmedetomidine HCl	AB	4 mcg/mL[b]	GW	1 mg/mL[b]	Physically compatible for 4 hr at 23°C	2383	C
Diphenhydramine HCl	PD	2 mg/mL[a]	GL	1 mg/mL[b]	Visually compatible for 4 hr at 22°C	1365	C
Docetaxel	RPR	0.9 mg/mL[a]	GW	1 mg/mL[a]	Physically compatible for 4 hr at 23°C	2224	C
Dopamine HCl	AB	0.8 mg/mL[a]	GL	0.32 mg/mL[c]	Visually compatible for 24 hr at room temperature in test tubes. No precipitate found on filter from Y-site delivery	2063	C
Doripenem	JJ	5 mg/mL[a b]	WOC	1 mg/mL[a b]	Physically compatible for 4 hr at 23°C	2743	C
Doxorubicin HCl	CET	2 mg/mL	GL	1 mg/mL[b]	Visually compatible for 4 hr at 22°C	1365	C
Doxorubicin HCl		2 mg/mL	GL	16 to 160 mcg/mL	Physically compatible when doxorubicin given as 5-min bolus via Y-site	1366	C
Doxorubicin HCl liposomal	SEQ	0.4 mg/mL[a]	CER	1 mg/mL[a]	Physically compatible for 4 hr at 23°C	2087	C
Doxycycline hyclate	ES	1 mg/mL[a]	GL	1 mg/mL[b]	Visually compatible for 4 hr at 22°C	1365	C
Droperidol	JN	0.4 mg/mL[a]	GL	1 mg/mL[b]	Visually compatible for 4 hr at 22°C	1365	C
Etoposide	BR	0.4 mg/mL[a]	GL	1 mg/mL[b]	Visually compatible for 4 hr at 22°C	1365	C
Etoposide		0.144 to 0.25 mg/mL	GL	16 to 160 mcg/mL	Physically compatible when etoposide given over 30 to 60 min via Y-site	1366	C

Y-Site Injection Compatibility (1:1 Mixture) (Cont.)

Test Drug	Mfr	Conc	Mfr	Conc	Remarks	Ref	C/I
Etoposide phosphate	BR	5 mg/mL[a]	GW	1 mg/mL[a]	Physically compatible for 4 hr at 23°C	2218	C
Famotidine	MSD	2 mg/mL[a]	GL	1 mg/mL[b]	Visually compatible for 4 hr at 22°C	1365	C
Fenoldopam mesylate	AB	80 mcg/mL[b]	GW	1 mg/mL[b]	Physically compatible for 4 hr at 23°C	2467	C
Filgrastim	AMG	30 mcg/mL[a]	GL	1 mg/mL[a]	Physically compatible for 4 hr at 22°C	1687	C
Floxuridine	RC	3 mg/mL[a]	GL	1 mg/mL[b]	Visually compatible for 4 hr at 22°C	1365	C
Fluconazole	PF	2 mg/mL	GL	1 mg/mL[b]	Visually compatible for 4 hr at 22°C	1365	C
Fluconazole	RR	2 mg/mL[b]	GL	0.03 and 0.3 mg/mL[a]	Visually compatible. Little loss of either drug in 4 hr at 25°C in light	1732	C
Fluconazole	RR	2 mg/mL	GL	0.03, 0.1, 0.3 mg/mL[a b]	Visually compatible. Little loss of both drugs in 4 hr. 5% or less loss of both in 12 hr at room temperature	2168	C
Fludarabine phosphate	BX	1 mg/mL[a]	GL	0.5 mg/mL[a]	Visually compatible for 4 hr at 22°C	1439	C
Fluorouracil	SO	16 mg/mL[a]	GL	1 mg/mL[b]	Precipitates immediately	1365	I
Fluorouracil		≤0.8 mg/mL	GL	16 to 160 mcg/mL	Physically compatible when fluorouracil given at 20 mL/hr via Y-site	1366	C
Furosemide	AB	3 mg/mL[a]	GL	1 mg/mL[b]	Immediate turbidity and precipitation	1365	I
Gallium nitrate	FUJ	1 mg/mL[b]	GL	0.3 mg/mL[b]	Visually compatible for 24 hr at 25°C	1673	C
Ganciclovir sodium	SY	20 mg/mL[a]	GL	1 mg/mL[b]	Immediate turbidity and precipitation	1365	I
Gemcitabine HCl	LI	10 mg/mL[b]	GW	1 mg/mL[b]	Physically compatible for 4 hr at 23°C	2226	C
Gentamicin sulfate	ES	5 mg/mL[a]	GL	1 mg/mL[b]	Visually compatible for 4 hr at 22°C	1365	C
Haloperidol lactate	LY	0.2 mg/mL[a]	GL	1 mg/mL[b]	Visually compatible for 4 hr at 22°C	1365	C
Heparin sodium	SO	40 units/mL[a]	GL	1 mg/mL[b]	Visually compatible for 4 hr at 22°C	1365	C
Hetastarch in lactated electrolyte	AB	6%	GW	1 mg/mL[a]	Physically compatible for 4 hr at 23°C	2339	C
Hydrocortisone sodium succinate	UP	1 mg/mL[a]	GL	1 mg/mL[b]	Visually compatible for 4 hr at 22°C	1365	C
Hydromorphone HCl	KN	0.5 mg/mL[a]	GL	1 mg/mL[b]	Visually compatible for 4 hr at 22°C	1365	C
Hydroxyzine HCl	WI	4 mg/mL[a]	GL	1 mg/mL[b]	Visually compatible for 4 hr at 22°C	1365	C
Ifosfamide	MJ	25 mg/mL[a]	GL	1 mg/mL[b]	Visually compatible for 4 hr at 22°C	1365	C
Imipenem–cilastatin sodium	MSD	5 mg/mL[b n]	GL	1 mg/mL[b]	Visually compatible for 4 hr at 22°C	1365	C
Isavuconazonium sulfate	ASP	1.5 mg/mL[p]	HOS	0.16 mg/mL[p]	Physically compatible for 2 hr	3263	C
Linezolid	PHU	2 mg/mL	GW	1 mg/mL[a]	Physically compatible for 4 hr at 23°C	2264	C
Lorazepam	WY	0.1 mg/mL[a]	GL	1 mg/mL[b]	Light haze develops immediately	1365	I
Magnesium sulfate	SO	100 mg/mL[a]	GL	1 mg/mL[b]	Visually compatible for 4 hr at 22°C	1365	C

Y-Site Injection Compatibility (1:1 Mixture) (Cont.)

Test Drug	Mfr	Conc	Mfr	Conc	Remarks	Ref	C/I
Mannitol	BA	15%	GL	1 mg/mL[b]	Visually compatible for 4 hr at 22°C	1365	C
Mechlorethamine HCl	MSD	1 mg/mL	GL	1 mg/mL[b]	Visually compatible for 4 hr at 22°C	1365	C
Melphalan HCl	BW	0.1 mg/mL[b]	GL	1 mg/mL[b]	Physically compatible for 3 hr at 22°C	1557	C
Meperidine HCl	WI	4 mg/mL[a]	GL	1 mg/mL[b]	Visually compatible for 4 hr at 22°C	1365	C
Meropenem	ZEN	1 mg/mL[b]	GL	1 mg/mL[c]	Visually compatible for 4 hr at room temperature	1994	C
Meropenem	ZEN	50 mg/mL[b]	GL	1 mg/mL[c]	White precipitate forms immediately	1994	I
Meropenem		50 mg/mL	MYL	2 mg/mL	Precipitates immediately	3538	I
Meropenem–vaborbactam	TMC	8 mg/mL[b o]	HER	0.16 mg/mL[b]	Immediate precipitation and increase in measured turbidity. pH increased by >4 units within 3 hr	3380	I
Mesna	BR	10 mg/mL[a]	GL	1 mg/mL[b]	Visually compatible for 4 hr at 22°C	1365	C
Methotrexate sodium	CET	15 mg/mL[a]	GL	1 mg/mL[b]	Visually compatible for 4 hr at 22°C	1365	C
Methotrexate sodium		30 mg/mL	GL	2 mg/mL	Visually compatible for 4 hr at room temperature	1788	C
Methylprednisolone sodium succinate	UP	5 mg/mL[a]	GL	1 mg/mL[b]	Light haze develops in 30 min	1365	I
Metoclopramide HCl	DU	5 mg/mL	GL	1 mg/mL[b]	Visually compatible for 4 hr at 22°C	1365	C
Micafungin sodium	ASP	1.5 mg/mL[b]	GSK	1 mg/mL[b]	White precipitate forms immediately	2683	I
Mitomycin	BR	0.5 mg/mL	GL	1 mg/mL[b]	Visually compatible for 4 hr at 22°C	1365	C
Mitoxantrone HCl	LE	0.5 mg/mL[a]	GL	1 mg/mL[b]	Visually compatible for 4 hr at 22°C	1365	C
Morphine sulfate	WI	1 mg/mL[a]	GL	1 mg/mL[b]	Visually compatible for 4 hr at 22°C	1365	C
Oxaliplatin	SS	0.5 mg/mL[a]	GW	1 mg/mL[a]	Physically compatible for 4 hr at 23°C	2566	C
Paclitaxel	NCI	1.2 mg/mL[a]	GL	0.5 mg/mL[a]	Physically compatible for 4 hr at 22°C	1556	C
Paclitaxel	BR	0.3 mg/mL[a]	GL	0.03 and 0.3 mg/mL[a]	Visually compatible with no loss of either drug in 4 hr at 23°C	1741	C
Paclitaxel	BR	1.2 mg/mL[a]	GL	0.03 and 0.3 mg/mL[a]	Visually compatible with no loss of either drug in 4 hr at 23°C	1741	C
Paclitaxel with ranitidine HCl	BR GL	1.2 mg/mL[a] 2 mg/mL[a]	GL	0.3 mg/mL[a]	Visually compatible with no loss of any drug in 4 hr at 23°C	1741	C
Pemetrexed disodium	LI	20 mg/mL[b]	GSK	1 mg/mL[a]	Trace haze and microparticulates form immediately. White cloudy precipitate forms in 4 hr	2564	I
Pentostatin	NCI	0.4 mg/mL[b]	GL	1 mg/mL[b]	Visually compatible for 4 hr at 22°C	1365	C
Piperacillin sodium–tazobactam sodium	LE[h]	40 mg/mL[a m]	GL	1 mg/mL[a]	Physically compatible for 4 hr at 22°C	1688	C
Piperacillin sodium–tazobactam sodium	LE[h]	40 mg/mL[b m]	GL	0.03, 0.1, 0.3 mg/mL[b]	Visually compatible with no loss of any component in 4 hr	1752	C
Piperacillin sodium–tazobactam sodium	LE[h]	80 mg/mL[b m]	GL	0.03, 0.1, 0.3 mg/mL[b]	Visually compatible with no loss of any component in 4 hr	1752	C

Y-Site Injection Compatibility (1:1 Mixture) (Cont.)

Test Drug	Mfr	Conc	Mfr	Conc	Remarks	Ref	C/I
Plazomicin sulfate	ACH	24 mg/mL[p]	HER	0.16 mg/mL[p]	Physically compatible for 1 hr at 20 to 25°C	3432	C
Potassium chloride	AB	0.1 mEq/mL[a]	GL	1 mg/mL[b]	Visually compatible for 4 hr at 22°C	1365	C
Prochlorperazine edisylate	SKF	0.5 mg/mL[a]	GL	1 mg/mL[b]	Visually compatible for 4 hr at 22°C	1365	C
Promethazine HCl	ES	2 mg/mL[a]	GL	1 mg/mL[b]	Visually compatible for 4 hr at 22°C	1365	C
Ranitidine HCl	GL	2 mg/mL[a]	GL	1 mg/mL[b]	Visually compatible for 4 hr at 22°C	1365	C
Ranitidine HCl	GL	0.5 mg/mL[a]	GL	0.03, 0.1, 0.3 mg/mL[a]	Visually compatible with no loss of either drug in 4 hr	1730	C
Ranitidine HCl	GL	2 mg/mL[a]	GL	0.03, 0.1, 0.3 mg/mL[a]	Visually compatible with no loss of either drug in 4 hr	1730	C
Ranitidine HCl with paclitaxel	GL BR	2 mg/mL[a] 1.2 mg/mL[a]	GL	0.3 mg/mL[a]	Visually compatible with no loss of any drug in 4 hr at 23°C	1741	C
Remifentanil HCl	GW	0.025 and 0.25 mg/mL[b]	CER	1 mg/mL[a]	Physically compatible for 4 hr at 23°C	2075	C
Sargramostim	IMM	10 mcg/mL[b]	GL	0.5 mg/mL[b]	Filaments form in 30 to 60 min	1436	I
Sodium acetate		0.1 and 1 mEq/mL[a]	GL	0.1 mg/mL[a]	Physically compatible for 4 hr at room temperature	1661	C
Sodium bicarbonate		0.05 mmol/mL[e]	GL	0.32 mg/mL[a]	White precipitate forms immediately	1513	I
Sodium bicarbonate		0.1 mEq/mL[a]	GL	0.1 mg/mL[a]	Visible particles in 30 to 60 min at room temperature	1661	I
Sodium bicarbonate		1.4%	GL	2 mg/mL	Heavy white precipitate forms immediately	1788	I
Streptozocin	UP	30 mg/mL[a]	GL	1 mg/mL[b]	Visually compatible for 4 hr at 22°C	1365	C
Sugammadex sodium	ME	100 mg/mL		2 mg/mL	Particles form in 1 hr	3111, 3115	I
Tedizolid phosphate	CUB	0.8 mg/mL[b]	HOS	0.16 mg/mL[b]	Physically compatible for 2 hr	3244	C
Telavancin HCl	ASP	7.5 mg/mL[a b i]	BA	1 mg/mL[a b i]	Physically compatible for 2 hr	2830	C
Teniposide	BR	0.1 mg/mL[a]	GL	1 mg/mL[b]	Visually compatible for 4 hr at 22°C	1365	C
Teniposide	BR	0.1 mg/mL[a]	GL	1 mg/mL[a]	Physically compatible for 4 hr at 23°C	1725	C
Thiotepa	IMM[f]	1 mg/mL[a]	GL	1 mg/mL[a]	Physically compatible for 4 hr at 23°C	1861	C
TNA #218 to #226[g]			CER	1 mg/mL[a]	Damage to emulsion occurs immediately with free oil formation possible	2215	I
Topotecan HCl	SKB	56 mcg/mL[a b]	CER	0.48 mg/mL[a b]	Visually compatible. Little loss of either drug in 4 hr at 22°C	2245	C
TPN #212 to #215[g]			GL	1 mg/mL[a]	Physically compatible for 4 hr at 23°C	2109	C
Vancomycin HCl	LI	10 mg/mL[a]	GL	1 mg/mL[b]	Visually compatible for 4 hr at 22°C	1365	C
Vinblastine sulfate	LY	0.12 mg/mL[a]	GL	1 mg/mL[b]	Visually compatible for 4 hr at 22°C	1365	C
Vincristine sulfate	LY	0.05 mg/mL[a]	GL	1 mg/mL[b]	Visually compatible for 4 hr at 22°C	1365	C

Y-Site Injection Compatibility (1:1 Mixture) (Cont.)

Test Drug	Mfr	Conc	Mfr	Conc	Remarks	Ref	C/I
Vinorelbine tartrate	BW	1 mg/mL[b]	GL	1 mg/mL[b]	Physically compatible for 4 hr at 22°C	1558	C
Zidovudine	BW	4 mg/mL[a]	GL	1 mg/mL[b]	Visually compatible for 4 hr at 22°C	1365	C

[a] Tested in dextrose 5%.

[b] Tested in sodium chloride 0.9%.

[c] Tested in sterile water for injection.

[d] Tested in bacteriostatic sodium chloride 0.9% preserved with benzyl alcohol 0.9%.

[e] Tested in dextrose 5% with potassium chloride 0.02 mM/mL.

[f] Lyophilized formulation tested.

[g] Refer to Appendix for the composition of parenteral nutrition solutions. TNA indicates a 3-in-1 admixture, and TPN indicates a 2-in-1 admixture.

[h] Test performed using the formulation WITHOUT edetate disodium.

[i] Tested in Ringer's injection, lactated.

[j] Injected via Y-site into an administration set running azithromycin.

[k] Tested with albumin human 0.1%.

[l] Ampicillin component. Ampicillin in a 2:1 fixed-ratio concentration with sulbactam.

[m] Piperacillin component. Piperacillin in an 8:1 fixed-ratio concentration with tazobactam.

[n] Not specified whether concentration refers to single component or combined components.

[o] Meropenem component. Meropenem in a 1:1 fixed-ratio concentration with vaborbactam.

[p] Tested in both dextrose 5% and sodium chloride 0.9%.

[q] Ceftolozane component. Ceftolozane in a 2:1 fixed-ratio concentration with tazobactam.

Selected Revisions May 1, 2020. © Copyright, October 1992.
American Society of Health-System Pharmacists, Inc.

Oritavancin Diphosphate
AHFS 8:12.28.16

Products

Oritavancin is available as a lyophilized powder in single-use (unpreserved) vials containing oritavancin diphosphate equivalent to oritavancin 400 mg as the free base and mannitol.[2927] Phosphoric acid has been added to adjust the pH.[2927]

Each vial should be reconstituted with 40 mL of sterile water for injection to yield a solution containing oritavancin 10 mg/mL.[2927] To avoid foaming, each vial should be gently swirled until the contents are completely dissolved.[2927] Vials contain a calculated excess (equivalent to a total of 405 mg of oritavancin) so that when reconstituted as directed, 400 mg of the drug can be withdrawn from the vial.[2927]

To prepare a 1.2-g dose, 120 mL should be removed from a 1-L intravenous bag of dextrose 5% and discarded.[2927] From each of 3 reconstituted vials of oritavancin, 40 mL should be withdrawn and transferred to the dextrose 5% bag to bring the total bag volume to 1 L, yielding a final concentration of oritavancin 1.2 mg/mL.[2927]

Equivalency

Oritavancin diphosphate 449 mg is equivalent to 405 mg of oritavancin free base.[2927]

pH

From 3.1 to 4.3.[2927]

Trade Name(s)

Orbactiv

Administration

Oritavancin is administered by intravenous infusion over 3 hours after dilution only in dextrose 5%.[2927] If a common infusion line is being used to administer other drugs in addition to oritavancin, the line should be flushed with dextrose 5% prior to and following infusion of oritavancin.[2927] Administration of the diluted drug over 3 hours is intended to minimize the risk of infusion-related reactions; however, interruption of the infusion or reduction in the rate of infusion may be necessary if such reactions occur.[2927]

Stability

Oritavancin diphosphate is a white to off-white powder that forms a clear, colorless to pale yellow solution when reconstituted with sterile water for injection and when further diluted in dextrose 5%.[2927] Intact vials of oritavancin diphosphate should be stored at controlled room temperature.[2927]

The manufacturer states that the diluted solution should be used within 6 hours of preparation when stored at room temperature or within 12 hours when refrigerated at 2 to 8°C.[2927] The total time for storage (the reconstituted drug in the vial and the diluted solution in the infusion bag) and the infusion time together should not exceed 6 hours if stored at room temperature or 12 hours if stored under refrigeration.[2927]

pH Effects

Oritavancin may be incompatible with drugs formulated at a basic or neutral pH.[2927]

Compatibility Information

Solution Compatibility

Oritavancin diphosphate

Test Soln Name	Mfr	Mfr	Conc/L or %	Remarks	Ref	C/I
Dextrose 5%		MEL	1.2 g	Complete administration within 6 hr after reconstitution and dilution if stored at room temperature or 12 hr if stored at 2 to 8°C	2927	C
Sodium chloride 0.9%		MEL		Stated to be incompatible	2927	I

Y-Site Injection Compatibility (1:1 Mixture)

Oritavancin diphosphate

Test Drug	Mfr	Conc	Mfr	Conc	Remarks	Ref	C/I
Aminophylline	AMR	1 mg/mL[a]	TAR	0.8, 1.2, and 2 mg/mL[a]	Haze or precipitate forms immediately	2928	I
Amphotericin B	XGN	0.1 mg/mL[a]	TAR	0.8, 1.2, and 2 mg/mL[a]	Slight haze forms immediately	2928	I
Aztreonam	BMS	20 mg/mL[a]	TAR	0.8, 1.2, and 2 mg/mL[a]	Precipitate forms immediately	2928	I
Bumetanide	HOS	0.1 mg/mL[a]	TAR	0.8, 1.2, and 2 mg/mL[a]	Haze forms immediately with precipitate after 30 min	2928	I

DOI: 10.37573/9781585286850.291

Y-Site Injection Compatibility (1:1 Mixture) (Cont.)

Test Drug	Mfr	Conc	Mfr	Conc	Remarks	Ref	C/I
Calcium gluconate	AMR	40 mg/mL[a]	TAR	0.8, 1.2, and 2 mg/mL[a]	Visually compatible for 4 hr at 20 to 24°C	2928	C
Ciprofloxacin	HOS[d]	2 mg/mL[a]	TAR	0.8, 1.2, and 2 mg/mL[a]	Visually compatible for 4 hr at 20 to 24°C	2928	C
Clindamycin phosphate	HOS	12 mg/mL[a]	TAR	0.8, 1.2, and 2 mg/mL[a]	Haze forms immediately with precipitate after 30 to 60 min	2928	I
Dexmedetomidine HCl	HOS	4 mcg/mL[a]	TAR	0.8, 1.2, and 2 mg/mL[a]	Visually compatible for 4 hr at 20 to 24°C	2928	C
Dobutamine HCl	HOS	4 mg/mL[a]	TAR	0.8, 1.2, and 2 mg/mL[a]	Visually compatible for 4 hr at 20 to 24°C	2928	C
Dopamine HCl	HOS	3.2 mg/mL[a]	TAR	0.8, 1.2, and 2 mg/mL[a]	Visually compatible for 4 hr at 20 to 24°C	2928	C
Epinephrine HCl	HOS	40 mcg/mL[a]	TAR	0.8, 1.2, and 2 mg/mL[a]	Visually compatible for 4 hr at 20 to 24°C	2928	C
Famotidine	BED	0.2 mg/mL[a]	TAR	0.8, 1.2, and 2 mg/mL[a]	Visually compatible for 4 hr at 20 to 24°C	2928	C
Fentanyl citrate	HOS	50 mcg/mL[b]	TAR	0.8, 1.2, and 2 mg/mL[a]	Visually compatible for 4 hr at 20 to 24°C	2928	C
Fluconazole	BED	2 mg/mL[a]	TAR	0.8, 1.2, and 2 mg/mL[a]	Visually compatible for 4 hr at 20 to 24°C	2928	C
Furosemide	AMR	5 mg/mL[a]	TAR	0.8, 1.2, and 2 mg/mL[a]	Haze forms immediately with precipitate after 30 min	2928	I
Gentamicin sulfate	ABX	5 mg/mL[a]	TAR	0.8, 1.2, and 2 mg/mL[a]	Visually compatible for 4 hr at 20 to 24°C	2928	C
Haloperidol lactate	BED	1 mg/mL[a]	TAR	0.8, 1.2, and 2 mg/mL[a]	Visually compatible for 4 hr at 20 to 24°C	2928	C
Heparin sodium	ABX	100 units/mL[a]	TAR	0.8, 1.2, and 2 mg/mL[a]	Haze forms immediately with precipitate after 1 hr	2928	I
Hydrocortisone sodium succinate	PF	1 mg/mL[a]	TAR	0.8, 1.2, and 2 mg/mL[a]	Haze forms immediately with precipitate after 1 hr	2928	I
Insulin	LI	1 unit/mL[a]	TAR	0.8, 1.2, and 2 mg/mL[a]	Visually compatible for 4 hr at 20 to 24°C	2928	C
Lorazepam	HOS	1 mg/mL[a]	TAR	0.8, 1.2, and 2 mg/mL[a]	Visually compatible for 4 hr at 20 to 24°C	2928	C
Meropenem	ASZ	10 mg/mL[a]	TAR	0.8, 1.2, and 2 mg/mL[a]	Haze forms immediately with precipitate after 1 hr	2928	I
Metronidazole	HOS	5 mg/mL[b]	TAR	0.8 and 1.2 mg/mL[a]	Visually compatible for 4 hr at 20 to 24°C	2928	C/I
Metronidazole	HOS	5 mg/mL[b]	TAR	2 mg/mL[a]	Fine particles form immediately	2928	I
Midazolam HCl	BA	1 mg/mL[a]	TAR	0.8, 1.2, and 2 mg/mL[a]	Visually compatible for 4 hr at 20 to 24°C	2928	C
Morphine sulfate	HOS	1 mg/mL[a]	TAR	0.8, 1.2, and 2 mg/mL[a]	Visually compatible for 4 hr at 20 to 24°C	2928	C
Nitroglycerin	AMR	0.4 mg/mL[a]	TAR	0.8, 1.2, and 2 mg/mL[a]	Visually compatible for 4 hr at 20 to 24°C	2928	C
Norepinephrine bitartrate	BED	0.12 mg/mL[a]	TAR	0.8, 1.2, and 2 mg/mL[a]	Visually compatible for 4 hr at 20 to 24°C	2928	C
Pancuronium bromide	SIC	0.1 mg/mL[a]	TAR	0.8, 1.2, and 2 mg/mL[a]	Visually compatible for 4 hr at 20 to 24°C	2928	C
Phenylephrine HCl	PNT	0.2 mg/mL[a]	TAR	0.8, 1.2, and 2 mg/mL[a]	Visually compatible for 4 hr at 20 to 24°C	2928	C
Phenytoin sodium	HOS	6 mg/mL[a]	TAR	0.8, 1.2, and 2 mg/mL[a]	Haze forms immediately	2928	I
Potassium chloride	HOS	0.2 mEq/mL[a]	TAR	0.8, 1.2, and 2 mg/mL[a]	Visually compatible for 4 hr at 20 to 24°C	2928	C
Ranitidine HCl	BED	2 mg/mL[a]	TAR	0.8, 1.2, and 2 mg/mL[a]	Visually compatible for 4 hr at 20 to 24°C	2928	C

Y-Site Injection Compatibility (1:1 Mixture) (Cont.)

Test Drug	Mfr	Conc	Mfr	Conc	Remarks	Ref	C/I
Sodium bicarbonate	HOS	1 mEq/mL[b]	TAR	0.8, 1.2, and 2 mg/mL[a]	Haze forms immediately but disappears with shaking	2928	?
Sodium nitroprusside	HOS	0.4 mg/mL[a]	TAR	0.8, 1.2, and 2 mg/mL[a]	Haze forms immediately with precipitate after 1 hr	2928	I
Tobramycin sulfate	SIC	5 mg/mL[a]	TAR	0.8, 1.2, and 2 mg/mL[a]	Visually compatible for 4 hr at 20 to 24°C	2928	C
Trimethoprim–sulfamethoxazole	SIC[c]	0.8 mg/mL[a]	TAR	0.8, 1.2, and 2 mg/mL[a]	Haze and particles form immediately with precipitate after 1 hr	2928	I

[a] Tested in dextrose 5%.

[b] Tested undiluted.

[c] Trimethoprim component. Trimethoprim in a 1:5 fixed-ratio concentration with sulfamethoxazole.

[d] Test performed using the lactate salt formulation.

Selected Revisions July 2, 2018. © Copyright, April 2015. American Society of Health-System Pharmacists, Inc.

Oxacillin Sodium
AHFS 8:12.16.12

Products

Oxacillin sodium is available in vials containing the equivalent of oxacillin 1 and 2 g. A 10-g hospital bulk package also is available. The products contain dibasic sodium phosphate 20 mg/g of drug.[4]

For intramuscular use, reconstitute the 1-g vials with 5.7 mL and the 2-g vials with 11.5 mL of sterile water for injection or sodium chloride 0.45 or 0.9% and shake until a clear solution is obtained. A 250-mg/1.5 mL (167-mg/mL) solution results.[4]

For direct intravenous injection, reconstitute the 1- or 2-g vials with 10 or 20 mL, respectively, of sterile water for injection, sodium chloride 0.45%, or sodium chloride 0.9% and shake until a clear solution is obtained to yield a 100-mg/mL concentration.[4]

The 10-g hospital bulk package is reconstituted with 93 mL of sterile water for injection to yield a 100-mg/mL solution.[4]

Frozen premixed solutions of oxacillin 1 g/50 mL in dextrose 3% and 2 g/50 mL in dextrose 0.6% are also available. The solutions also contain sodium citrate buffer and hydrochloric acid and/or sodium hydroxide to adjust the pH.[1(2/07) 4]

pH

From 6 to 8.5.[17] At 10 g/L in dextrose 5%, the pH has been variously reported as 7.4[149] and 7.94.[153] At this concentration in sodium chloride 0.9%, the pH has been reported as 7.73.[153]

Osmolality

The osmolality of oxacillin sodium 250 mg/1.5 mL in sterile water for injection was 596 mOsm/kg by freezing-point depression and 657 mOsm/kg by vapor pressure.[1071]

The osmolality of oxacillin sodium 50 mg/mL was 381 mOsm/kg in dextrose 5% and 396 mOsm/kg in sodium chloride 0.9%.[1375]

The osmolality of oxacillin sodium was calculated for the following dilutions:[1054]

Diluent	Osmolality (mOsm/kg)	
	50 mL	100 mL
1 g		
Dextrose 5%	326	295
Sodium chloride 0.9%	353	321
2 g		
Dextrose 5%	379	329
Sodium chloride 0.9%	406	356

The following maximum oxacillin sodium concentrations have been recommended to achieve osmolalities suitable for peripheral infusion in fluid-restricted patients:[1180]

Diluent	Maximum Concentration (mg/mL)	Osmolality (mOsm/kg)
Dextrose 5%	59	530
Sodium chloride 0.9%	53	519
Sterile water for injection	106	422

The frozen premixed solutions are iso-osmotic, having an osmolality of about 300 mOsm/kg.[4]

Sodium Content

Each gram of oxacillin sodium powder contains approximately 2.5 to 3.1 mEq of sodium.[4]

Administration

Oxacillin sodium may be administered by deep intramuscular injection, direct intravenous injection, or by continuous or intermittent intravenous infusion. By direct intravenous injection, the dose should be given over a 10-minute period. To minimize vein irritation, intravenous injections should be made as slowly as possible. For intermittent infusion, the drug should be further diluted with a compatible solution to a concentration of 0.5 to 40 mg/mL.[4]

Stability

Oxacillin sodium in intact vials should be stored at controlled room temperature. After reconstitution, oxacillin sodium is stable for 3 days at room temperature and for 1 week under refrigeration at concentrations used for intramuscular or direct intravenous injection. The reconstituted hospital bulk package is stable for 24 hours at room temperature.[4]

The frozen premixed injection is stable at –20°C for at least 90 days after shipping. The frozen premixed infusions should be thawed at room temperature or under refrigeration and should not be refrozen after being thawed. The thawed solutions are stated to be stable for 48 hours at room temperature and 21 days under refrigeration.[4]

Freezing Solutions

Oxacillin sodium, 500 mg/2.5 mL and 1 g/5 mL in sterile water for injection in glass and plastic syringes and 200 mg/mL in the original vial, was frozen at –20°C. Adequate stability was maintained over 3 months.[303]

DOI: 10.37573/9781585286850.292

In another study, oxacillin sodium 1 g/100 mL of dextrose 5% in polyvinyl chloride (PVC) bags was frozen at –20°C for 30 days. The bags were then thawed by exposure to ambient temperature or microwave radiation. The solutions had no precipitation or color change and no drug loss. Subsequent storage at room temperature for 24 hours yielded a physically compatible solution, which exhibited a 3 to 4% loss.[554]

Syringes

Oxacillin sodium (Bristol) 8.33, 16.7, and 33.3 mg/mL in dextrose 5% and in sodium chloride 0.9% packaged in plastic syringes was reported to be stable for 24 hours at room temperature, 8 days refrigerated, and 30 days frozen at –20°C.[31]

Ambulatory Pumps

The stability of oxacillin sodium 120 mg/mL in sterile water for injection was evaluated in PVC portable infusion pump reservoirs (Pharmacia Deltec). No oxacillin loss in 3 days at 25°C and 5% loss in 14 days at 5°C was found.[2080]

Sorption

Little loss due to sorption of oxacillin sodium (Bristol) 1 g/100 mL in dextrose 5% and sodium chloride 0.9% in trilayer solution bags (Bieffe Medital) composed of polyethylene, polyamide, and polypropylene occurred in 2 hours. Similarly, no loss was found during a 1-hour simulated infusion.[1918]

Compatibility Information

Solution Compatibility

Oxacillin sodium

Test Soln Name	Mfr	Mfr	Conc/L or %	Remarks	Ref	C/I
Amino acids 4.25%, dextrose 25%	MG	BR	500 mg	No increase in particulate matter in 24 hr at 5°C	349	C
Dextrose 5% in Ringer's injection, lactated	TR[a]	BR	1 g	Stable for 24 hr at 5°C	282	C
Dextrose 5% in sodium chloride 0.45%			10 to 30 g	Stable for 24 hr at 25°C, 4 days at 4°C, and 30 days at –20°C	1(2/07)	C
Dextrose 5% in sodium chloride 0.9%			0.5 to 2 g	Under 10% loss in 6 hr at room temperature	1(2/07)	C
Dextrose 5% in sodium chloride 0.9%	TR[a]	BR	1 g	Stable for 24 hr at 5°C	282	C
Dextrose 5% in sodium chloride 0.9%		BR	2 g	12% decomposition in 12 hr and 14% in 24 hr	109	I
Dextrose 5%			10 to 30 g	Stable for 4 days at 4°C and 30 days at –20°C	1(2/07)	C
Dextrose 5%			0.5 to 2 g	Stable for 6 hr at room temperature	1(2/07)	C
Dextrose 5%		BR	2 g	Stable for 24 hr	109	C
Dextrose 5%		BR	1, 10, 50 g	4 to 9% decomposition in 24 hr at 23°C	153	C
Dextrose 5%	TR[a]	BR	1 g	Stable for 24 hr at 5°C	282	C
Dextrose 5%	TR[b]	BR	10 g	Physically compatible with 8% loss in 24 hr at room temperature	554	C
Dextrose 5%			4 g	8% loss in 6 hr and 14% loss in 24 hr at room temperature	768	I
Dextrose 5%	[b]	BR	20 g	No drug loss during 2-hr storage and 1-hr simulated infusion	1774	C
Dextrose 10%		BR	2 g	Stable for 24 hr	109	C
Ringer's injection, lactated			0.5 to 2 g	Stable for 6 hr at room temperature	1(2/07)	C
Ringer's injection, lactated			10 to 30 g	Stable for 4 days at 4°C and 30 days at –20°C	1(2/07)	C
Ringer's injection, lactated	TR[a]	BR	1 g	Stable for 24 hr at 5°C	282	C
Sodium chloride 0.9%			10 to 100 g	Stable for 4 days at 25°C, 7 days at 4°C, and 30 days at –20°C	1(2/07)	C
Sodium chloride 0.9%		BR	2 g	Stable for 24 hr	109	C

Solution Compatibility (Cont.)

Test Soln Name	Mfr	Mfr	Conc/L or %	Remarks	Ref	C/I
Sodium chloride 0.9%		BR	1, 10, 50 g	2 to 4% decomposition in 24 hr at 23°C	153	C
Sodium chloride 0.9%	TR[a]	BR	1 g	Stable for 24 hr at 5°C	282	C
Sodium chloride 0.9%			4 g	10% loss in 8 hr and 12% loss in 24 hr at room temperature	768	I
Sodium chloride 0.9%	[b]	BR	20 g	No drug loss during 2-hr storage and 1-hr simulated infusion	1774	C
Sodium lactate ⅙ M			10 to 30 g	Stable for 24 hr at 25°C, 4 days at 4°C, and 30 days at −20°C	1(2/07)	C

[a] Tests performed in both glass and PVC containers.

[b] Tested in PVC containers.

Additive Compatibility

Oxacillin sodium

Test Drug	Mfr	Conc/L or %	Mfr	Conc/L or %	Test Solution	Remarks	Ref	C/I
Amikacin sulfate	BR	5 g	BR	2 g	D5LR, D5R, D5S, D5W, D10W, LR, NS, R	Physically compatible and both stable for 24 hr at 25°C	293	C
Amikacin sulfate	BR	5 g	BR	2 g	NR, SL	Oxacillin stable for 8 hr at 25°C. Over 10% loss in 24 hr	293	I
Chloramphenicol sodium succinate	PD	500 mg	BR	500 mg	D5S, D5W	Therapeutic availability maintained	110	C
Chloramphenicol sodium succinate	PD	1 g	BR	2 g	D5S, D5W	Therapeutic availability maintained	110	C
Chloramphenicol sodium succinate	PD	1 g	BR	2 g		Physically compatible	6	C
Cytarabine	UP	100 mg		2 g	D5W	pH outside stability range for oxacillin	174	I
Dextran 40		10%		4 g	D5W	3% loss in 24 hr at 20°C	834	C
Dopamine HCl	AS	800 mg	BR	2 g	D5W	No dopamine and 2% oxacillin loss in 24 hr at 25°C	312	C
Hetastarch in sodium chloride 0.9%		6%		4 g		1% oxacillin loss in 24 hr at 20°C	834	C
Potassium chloride		20, 40, 80 mEq	BR	1, 2.5, 4 g	D5S, D5W	Therapeutic availability maintained	110	C
Verapamil HCl	KN	80 mg	BR	4 g	D5W, NS	Physically compatible for 24 hr	764	C
Verapamil HCl	SE	[a]	BR	40 g	D5W, NS	Cloudy solution clears with agitation	1166	?

[a] Final concentration unspecified.

Drugs in Syringe Compatibility

Oxacillin sodium

Test Drug	Mfr	Amt	Mfr	Amt	Remarks	Ref	C/I
Caffeine citrate		20 mg/1 mL	APC	50 mg/1 mL	White precipitate forms immediately becoming two layers over time	2440	I

Y-Site Injection Compatibility (1:1 Mixture)

Oxacillin sodium

Test Drug	Mfr	Conc	Mfr	Conc	Remarks	Ref	C/I
Acyclovir sodium	BW	5 mg/mL[a]	BE	20 mg/mL[a]	Physically compatible for 4 hr at 25°C	1157	C
Cyclophosphamide	MJ	20 mg/mL[a]	BE	20 mg/mL[a]	Physically compatible for 4 hr at 25°C	1194	C
Diltiazem HCl	MMD	1[b] and 5 mg/mL		100 mg/mL[b]	Visually compatible	1807	C
Diltiazem HCl	MMD	5 mg/mL		10 mg/mL[b]	Visually compatible	1807	C
Doxapram HCl	RB	2 mg/mL[a]	APO	20 mg/mL[a]	Visually compatible for 4 hr at 23°C	2470	C
Famotidine	MSD	0.2 mg/mL[a]	BE	20 mg/mL[b]	Physically compatible for 14 hr	1196	C
Fluconazole	RR	2 mg/mL	BE	40 mg/mL	Physically compatible for 24 hr at 25°C	1407	C
Foscarnet sodium	AST	24 mg/mL	BR	40 mg/mL	Physically compatible for 24 hr at room temperature under fluorescent light	1335	C
Foscarnet sodium	AST	24 mg/mL	BE	20 mg/mL[c]	Physically compatible for 24 hr at 25°C under fluorescent light	1393	C
Heparin sodium	UP	1000 units/L[d]	BR	100 mg/mL	Physically compatible for 4 hr at room temperature	534	C
Hydrocortisone sodium succinate	UP	10 mg/L[d]	BR	100 mg/mL	Physically compatible for 4 hr at room temperature	534	C
Hydromorphone HCl	WY	0.2 mg/mL[a]	BE	20 mg/mL[a]	Physically compatible for 4 hr at 25°C	987	C
Labetalol HCl	SC	1 mg/mL[a]	BR	10 mg/mL[a]	Physically compatible for 24 hr at 18°C	1171	C
Levofloxacin	OMN	5 mg/mL[a]	APC	167 mg/mL	Visually compatible for 4 hr at 24°C	2233	C
Magnesium sulfate	IX	16.7, 33.3, 66.7, 100 mg/mL[a]	BE	20 mg/mL[a]	Physically compatible for at least 4 hr at 32°C	813	C
Meperidine HCl	WY	10 mg/mL[a]	BE	20 mg/mL[a]	Physically compatible for 4 hr at 25°C	987	C
Methotrexate sodium		30 mg/mL	BR	250 mg/mL	Visually compatible for 4 hr at room temperature	1788	C
Milrinone lactate	SS	0.2 mg/mL[a]	APO	100 mg/mL[a]	Visually compatible for 4 hr at 25°C	2381	C
Morphine sulfate	WI	1 mg/mL[a]	BE	20 mg/mL[a]	Physically compatible for 4 hr at 25°C	987	C
Potassium chloride	AB	40 mEq/L[d]	BR	100 mg/mL	Physically compatible for 4 hr at room temperature	534	C
Sodium bicarbonate		1.4%	BR	250 mg/mL	Gas evolves	1788	I
Tacrolimus	FUJ	1 mg/mL[b]	BR	40 mg/mL[a]	Visually compatible for 24 hr at 25°C	1630	C
TNA #73[e]		32.5 mL[f]	BE	20 mg/mL[a]	Visually compatible for 4 hr at 25°C	1008	C
TPN #54[e]				100 and 150 mg/mL	Physically compatible with 88 to 94% oxacillin activity retained over 6 hr at 22°C	1045	C
TPN #61[e]		[g]	BE	250 mg/1.5 mL[h]	Physically compatible	1012	C
TPN #61[e]		[i]	BE	1.5 g/9 mL[h]	Physically compatible	1012	C
Vancomycin HCl	HOS	10 mg/mL[a]	AUR	20 mg/mL[j]	Precipitates immediately	3477	I
Verapamil HCl	SE	2.5 mg/mL	BR	40 mg/mL[c]	White precipitate forms immediately. 39% of verapamil precipitated	1166	I

Y-Site Injection Compatibility (1:1 Mixture) (Cont.)

Test Drug	Mfr	Conc	Mfr	Conc	Remarks	Ref	C/I
Zidovudine	BW	4 mg/mL[a]	BR	20 mg/mL[a]	Physically compatible for 4 hr at 25°C	1193	C

[a] Tested in dextrose 5%.

[b] Tested in sodium chloride 0.9%.

[c] Tested in both dextrose 5% and sodium chloride 0.9%.

[d] Tested in dextrose 5% in Ringer's injection, dextrose 5% in Ringer's injection, lactated, dextrose 5%, Ringer's injection, lactated, and sodium chloride 0.9%.

[e] Refer to Appendix for the composition of parenteral nutrition solutions. TNA indicates a 3-in-1 admixture, and TPN indicates a 2-in-1 admixture.

[f] A 32.5-mL sample of parenteral nutrition solution mixed with 50 mL of antibiotic solution.

[g] Run at 21 mL/hr.

[h] Given over five minutes by syringe pump.

[i] Run at 94 mL/hr.

[j] Tested in sterile water for injection.

Selected Revisions September 30, 2019. © Copyright, October 1982. American Society of Health-System Pharmacists, Inc.

Oxaliplatin
AHFS 10:00

Products

Oxaliplatin is available as a 5-mg/mL concentrated solution in 10-, 20-, and 40-mL single-use vials.[2852][2853]

Oxaliplatin is also available in single-use vials containing 50 or 100 mg of lyophilized drug and lactose monohydrate as an excipient.[2854] Reconstitute the 50- or 100-mg vials with 10 or 20 mL, respectively, of water for injection or dextrose 5%.[2854]

Trade Name(s)

Eloxatin

Administration

For intravenous infusion, both the concentrated injection and the reconstituted solution must be diluted in 250 to 500 mL of dextrose 5% prior to administration.[2852][2853][2854] Chloride-containing solutions must *not* be used for reconstitution[2854] or dilution.[2852][2853][2854]

Oxaliplatin is administered by intravenous infusion over 2 hours.[2852][2853][2854]

Contact of oxaliplatin solutions with aluminum in needles or metal parts of administration equipment should be avoided.[2852][2853][2854] Aluminum has caused degradation of some platinum compounds.[2852][2853][2854]

Stability

Intact vials of both formulations are stored at controlled room temperature.[2852][2853][2854] Protect vials of the concentrated solution from light by storing in the outer carton, and do not freeze.[2852][2853] Vials of the lyophilized formulation and solutions diluted for infusion do not require light protection.[2852][2853][2854]

Following reconstitution of the lyophilized oxaliplatin formulation in the original vial, the resulting solution may be stored up to 24 hours under refrigeration.[2854]

After final dilution of either formulation for administration in 250 to 500 mL of dextrose 5%, the manufacturers indicate that the drug is stable for six hours at room temperature or for 24 hours under refrigeration.[2852][2853][2854] However, Sanofi stated that oxaliplatin diluted in dextrose 5% for infusion was stable for 24 hours at room temperature; at a concentration of 3 g/L, the drug was stated to be stable for at least five days at room temperature.[2623]

pH Effects

Oxaliplatin is incompatible with alkaline drugs and solutions and should not be mixed with or administered simultaneously with them.[2852][2853][2854] Administration lines should be flushed with dextrose 5% prior to administering any other medication.[2852][2853][2854]

Compatibility Information

Solution Compatibility

Oxaliplatin

Test Soln Name	Mfr	Mfr	Conc/L or %	Remarks	Ref	C/I
Dextrose 5%	KA[a]	SAA	700 mg	Visually compatible and 5% or less drug loss in 30 days refrigerated or at room temperature	2744	C
Dextrose 5%	KA[b]	AVE	250 mg	Visually compatible and less than 4% drug loss in 90 days refrigerated or at room temperature	2782	C
Dextrose 5%	FRK[b], MAC[c], BRN[d]	SAA	200 mg and 1.3 g	Physically compatible with 2% or less drug loss in 14 days at 4 and 20°C	2855	C

[a] Tested in Macoflex N polyolefin containers.

[b] Tested in FreeFlex polyolefin containers.

[c] Tested in Macoflex PVC containers.

[d] Tested in Ecoflac polyethylene containers.

DOI: 10.37573/9781585286850.293

Y-Site Injection Compatibility (1:1 Mixture)

Oxaliplatin

Test Drug	Mfr	Conc	Mfr	Conc	Remarks	Ref	C/I
Bumetanide	BA	0.04 mg/mL[a]	SS	0.5 mg/mL[a]	Physically compatible for 4 hr at 23°C	2566	C
Buprenorphine HCl	RKC	0.04 mg/mL[a]	SS	0.5 mg/mL[a]	Physically compatible for 4 hr at 23°C	2566	C
Butorphanol tartrate	APO	0.04 mg/mL[a]	SS	0.5 mg/mL[a]	Physically compatible for 4 hr at 23°C	2566	C
Calcium gluconate	APP	40 mg/mL[a]	SS	0.5 mg/mL[a]	Physically compatible for 4 hr at 23°C	2566	C
Carboplatin	BR	5 mg/mL[a]	SS	0.5 mg/mL[a]	Physically compatible for 4 hr at 23°C	2566	C
Chlorpromazine HCl	ES	2 mg/mL[a]	SS	0.5 mg/mL[a]	Physically compatible for 4 hr at 23°C	2566	C
Cyclophosphamide	MJ	10 mg/mL[a]	SS	0.5 mg/mL[a]	Physically compatible for 4 hr at 23°C	2566	C
Dexamethasone sodium phosphate	AMR	1 mg/mL[a]	SS	0.5 mg/mL[a]	Physically compatible for 4 hr at 23°C	2566	C
Diazepam	AB	5 mg/mL	SS	0.5 mg/mL[a]	Gross white turbidity forms immediately	2566	I
Diphenhydramine HCl	ES	2 mg/mL[a]	SS	0.5 mg/mL[a]	Physically compatible for 4 hr at 23°C	2566	C
Dobutamine HCl	BED	4 mg/mL[a]	SS	0.5 mg/mL[a]	Physically compatible for 4 hr at 23°C	2566	C
Docetaxel	AVE	2 mg/mL[a]	SS	0.5 mg/mL[a]	Physically compatible for 4 hr at 23°C	2566	C
Dolasetron mesylate	AVE	2 mg/mL[a]	SS	0.5 mg/mL[a]	Physically compatible for 4 hr at 23°C	2566	C
Dopamine HCl	AB	3.2 mg/mL[a]	SS	0.5 mg/mL[a]	Physically compatible for 4 hr at 23°C	2566	C
Doxorubicin HCl	APP	1 mg/mL[a]	SS	0.5 mg/mL[a]	Physically compatible for 4 hr at 23°C	2566	C
Droperidol	AB	2.5 mg/mL	SS	0.5 mg/mL[a]	Physically compatible for 4 hr at 23°C	2566	C
Enalaprilat	BA	0.1 mg/mL[a]	SS	0.5 mg/mL[a]	Physically compatible for 4 hr at 23°C	2566	C
Epirubicin HCl	PHU	0.5 mg/mL[a]	SS	0.5 mg/mL[a]	Physically compatible for 4 hr at 23°C	2566	C
Etoposide phosphate	BR	5 mg/mL[a]	SS	0.5 mg/mL[a]	Physically compatible for 4 hr at 23°C	2566	C
Famotidine	ESL	2 mg/mL[a]	SS	0.5 mg/mL[a]	Physically compatible for 4 hr at 23°C	2566	C
Fentanyl citrate	AB	0.05 mg/mL[a]	SS	0.5 mg/mL[a]	Physically compatible for 4 hr at 23°C	2566	C
Furosemide	AMR	3 mg/mL[a]	SS	0.5 mg/mL[a]	Physically compatible for 4 hr at 23°C	2566	C
Gemcitabine HCl	LI	10 mg/mL[a]	SS	0.5 mg/mL[a]	Physically compatible for 4 hr at 23°C	2566	C
Granisetron HCl	SKB	0.05 mg/mL[a]	SS	0.5 mg/mL[a]	Physically compatible for 4 hr at 23°C	2566	C
Haloperidol lactate	APP	0.2 mg/mL[a]	SS	0.5 mg/mL[a]	Physically compatible for 4 hr at 23°C	2566	C
Heparin sodium	AB	100 units/mL	SS	0.5 mg/mL[a]	Physically compatible for 4 hr at 23°C	2566	C
Hydrocortisone sodium succinate	PHU	1 mg/mL[a]	SS	0.5 mg/mL[a]	Physically compatible for 4 hr at 23°C	2566	C
Hydromorphone HCl	ES	0.5 mg/mL[a]	SS	0.5 mg/mL[a]	Physically compatible for 4 hr at 23°C	2566	C
Hydroxyzine HCl	ES	2 mg/mL[a]	SS	0.5 mg/mL[a]	Physically compatible for 4 hr at 23°C	2566	C
Ifosfamide	MJ	20 mg/mL[a]	SS	0.5 mg/mL[a]	Physically compatible for 4 hr at 23°C	2566	C
Irinotecan HCl	PHU	1 mg/mL[a]	SS	0.5 mg/mL[a]	Physically compatible for 4 hr at 23°C	2566	C
Leucovorin calcium	BED	2 mg/mL[a]	SS	0.5 mg/mL[a]	Physically compatible for 4 hr at 23°C	2566	C
Lorazepam	ESL	0.5 mg/mL[a]	SS	0.5 mg/mL[a]	Physically compatible for 4 hr at 23°C	2566	C

Y-Site Injection Compatibility (1:1 Mixture) (Cont.)

Test Drug	Mfr	Conc	Mfr	Conc	Remarks	Ref	C/I
Magnesium sulfate	APP	100 mg/mL[a]	SS	0.5 mg/mL[a]	Physically compatible for 4 hr at 23°C	2566	C
Mannitol	BA	15%	SS	0.5 mg/mL[a]	Physically compatible for 4 hr at 23°C	2566	C
Meperidine HCl	AB	10 mg/mL[a]	SS	0.5 mg/mL[a]	Physically compatible for 4 hr at 23°C	2566	C
Mesna	MJ	10 mg/mL[a]	SS	0.5 mg/mL[a]	Physically compatible for 4 hr at 23°C	2566	C
Methotrexate sodium	BED	12.5 mg/mL[a]	SS	0.5 mg/mL[a]	Physically compatible for 4 hr at 23°C	2566	C
Methylprednisolone sodium succinate	PHU	5 mg/mL[a]	SS	0.5 mg/mL[a]	Physically compatible for 4 hr at 23°C	2566	C
Metoclopramide HCl	RB	5 mg/mL	SS	0.5 mg/mL[a]	Physically compatible for 4 hr at 23°C	2566	C
Mitoxantrone HCl	IMM	0.5 mg/mL[a]	SS	0.5 mg/mL[a]	Physically compatible for 4 hr at 23°C	2566	C
Morphine sulfate	ES	15 mg/mL	SS	0.5 mg/mL[a]	Physically compatible for 4 hr at 23°C	2566	C
Nalbuphine HCl	EN	10 mg/mL	SS	0.5 mg/mL[a]	Physically compatible for 4 hr at 23°C	2566	C
Ondansetron HCl	GW	1 mg/mL[a]	SS	0.5 mg/mL[a]	Physically compatible for 4 hr at 23°C	2566	C
Paclitaxel	MJ	0.6 mg/mL[a]	SS	0.5 mg/mL[a]	Physically compatible for 4 hr at 23°C	2566	C
Palonosetron HCl	MGI	50 mcg/mL	SS	0.5 mg/mL[a]	Physically compatible. No loss of either drug in 4 hr	2579	C
Potassium chloride	APP	0.1 mEq/mL[a]	SS	0.5 mg/mL[a]	Physically compatible for 4 hr at 23°C	2566	C
Prochlorperazine edisylate	SKB	0.5 mg/mL[a]	SS	0.5 mg/mL[a]	Physically compatible for 4 hr at 23°C	2566	C
Promethazine HCl	ES	2 mg/mL[a]	SS	0.5 mg/mL[a]	Physically compatible for 4 hr at 23°C	2566	C
Ranitidine HCl	GW	2 mg/mL[a]	SS	0.5 mg/mL[a]	Physically compatible for 4 hr at 23°C	2566	C
Theophylline	AB	4 mg/mL	SS	0.5 mg/mL[a]	Physically compatible for 4 hr at 23°C	2566	C
Topotecan HCl	SKB	0.1 mg/mL[a]	SS	0.5 mg/mL[a]	Physically compatible for 4 hr at 23°C	2566	C
Verapamil HCl	AB	1.25 mg/mL[a]	SS	0.5 mg/mL[a]	Physically compatible for 4 hr at 23°C	2566	C
Vincristine sulfate	FAU	0.05 mg/mL[a]	SS	0.5 mg/mL[a]	Physically compatible for 4 hr at 23°C	2566	C
Vinorelbine tartrate	GW	1 mg/mL[a]	SS	0.5 mg/mL[a]	Physically compatible for 4 hr at 23°C	2566	C

[a] Tested in dextrose 5%.

Additional Compatibility Information

Infusion Solutions

Stability of oxaliplatin (Accord) 0.1 mg/mL in dextrose 5% (Braun), sodium chloride 0.9% (Braun), Ringer's injection, lactated (Braun), Dianeal PD-4 with dextrose 1.36% (Baxter), and phosphate buffer (pH 7.4) 0.14 M at 42°C was evaluated for use of the drug as hyperthermic intraperitoneal chemotherapy.[3524]

Less than 10% oxaliplatin loss occurred in 2 hours in dextrose 5%.[3524] In phosphate buffer and Dianeal PD-4 with dextrose 1.36%, drug losses of less than 10% occurred within 30 minutes; however, losses exceeded 10% by 2 hours.[3524] In Ringer's injection, lactated and sodium chloride 0.9%, the solutions with the greatest chloride ion concentrations, drugs losses exceeded 10% as early as 30 minutes and losses of 18 and 21%, respectively, occurred within 2 hours.[3524]

Selected Revisions January 31, 2020. © Copyright, October 2006. American Society of Health-System Pharmacists, Inc.

Oxycodone Hydrochloride
AHFS 28:08.08

Products

Oxycodone hydrochloride is available as a 10-mg/mL injection (equivalent to 9 mg of oxycodone base per mL) in 1- and 2-mL ampuls. Also present in the formulation are citric acid monohydrate, sodium citrate, sodium chloride, and hydrochloric acid and/or sodium hydroxide to adjust pH in water for injection.[38]

Administration

Oxycodone hydrochloride is administered by subcutaneous or intravenous injection or infusion. For infusion, the drug may be diluted to a concentration of 1 mg/mL in dextrose 5% or sodium chloride 0.9%.[38]

Stability

Intact vials should be stored at controlled room temperature. The ampuls should be used immediately upon opening; unused portions should be discarded immediately. The manufacturer states that oxycodone hydrochloride diluted for infusion is stable for 24 hours under refrigeration.[38]

Compatibility Information

Solution Compatibility

Oxycodone HCl

Test Soln Name	Mfr	Mfr	Conc/L or %	Remarks	Ref	C/I
Dextrose 5%	BA[b]		5 and 50 g	Visually compatible with little or no loss in 35 days at 4 and 24°C	2590	C
Dextrose 5%	BA[a]	NAP	1 g	Visually compatible with less than 4% change in concentration in 14 days at 4 and 25°C	2600	C
Dextrose 5%	BA[b c]	NAP	1 g	Visually compatible with less than 4% change in concentration in 7 days at 4 and 25°C	2600	C
Dextrose 5%	[b]	MUN	1 g	Visually compatible. No drug loss in 28 days at 25°C	2827	C
Sodium chloride 0.9%	BA[b]		5 and 50 g	Visually compatible with little or no loss in 35 days at 4 and 24°C	2590	C
Sodium chloride 0.9%	BA[a]	NAP	1 g	Visually compatible with less than 4% change in concentration in 14 days at 4 and 25°C	2600	C
Sodium chloride 0.9%	BA[b c]	NAP	1 g	Visually compatible with less than 4% change in concentration in 7 days at 4 and 25°C	2600	C
Sodium chloride 0.9%	[b]	MUN	1 g	Visually compatible. No drug loss in 28 days at 25°C	2827	C

[a] Tested in glass containers.

[b] Tested in PVC containers.

[c] Tested in EVA containers.

Additive Compatibility

Oxycodone HCl

Test Drug	Mfr	Conc/L or %	Mfr	Conc/L or %	Test Solution	Remarks	Ref	C/I
Cyclizine lactate	GW	1 g	NAP	1 g	NS	Crystals form in a few hours	2600	I
Cyclizine lactate	GW	1 g	NAP	1 g	W	Visually compatible. Under 4% concentration change in 24 hr at 25°C	2600	C
Cyclizine lactate	GW	500 mg	NAP	1 g	NS	Crystals form in a few hours	2600	I
Cyclizine lactate	GW	500 mg	NAP	1 g	W	Visually compatible. Under 4% concentration change in 24 hr at 25°C	2600	C

DOI: 10.37573/9781585286850.294

Additive Compatibility (Cont.)

Test Drug	Mfr	Conc/L or %	Mfr	Conc/L or %	Test Solution	Remarks	Ref	C/I
Dexamethasone sodium phosphate	FAU	0.8 g	NAP	0.8 g	NS, W	Visually compatible. Under 4% concentration change in 24 hr at 25°C	2600	C
Haloperidol lactate	JC	125 mg	NAP	1 g	NS, W	Visually compatible. Under 4% concentration change in 24 hr at 25°C	2600	C
Ketamine HCl	PAN	40 g	MUN	400 mg	NS[a]	Physically compatible with little to no loss of either drug in 7 days at 22 to 23°C	3585, 3586	C
Ketamine HCl	PAN	100 mg	MUN	10 g	NS[a]	Physically compatible with little to no loss of either drug in 7 days at 22 to 23°C	3585, 3586	C
Ketamine HCl	PAN	40 g	MUN	10 g	NS[a]	Physically compatible with little to no loss of either drug in 7 days at 22 to 23°C	3585, 3586	C
Methotrimeprazine HCl		250 mg	NAP	1 g	NS, W	Visually compatible. Under 4% concentration change in 24 hr at 25°C	2600	C
Metoclopramide HCl		1.2 g	NAP	770 mg	NS, W	Visually compatible. Under 4% concentration change in 24 hr at 25°C	2600	C
Midazolam HCl	RC	830 mg	NAP	830 mg	NS, W	Visually compatible. Under 4% concentration change in 24 hr at 25°C	2600	C
Prochlorperazine mesylate		600 mg	NAP	1 g	NS, W	Substantial change in prochlorperazine concentration in 24 hr at 25°C	2600	I
Scopolamine butylbromide	BI	1 g	NAP	1 g	NS, W	Visually compatible. Under 4% concentration change in 24 hr at 25°C	2600	C
Scopolamine HBr		30 mg	NAP	1 g	NS, W	Visually compatible. Under 4% concentration change in 24 hr at 25°C	2600	C

[a] Tested in PVC containers.

Drugs in Syringe Compatibility

Oxycodone HCl

Test Drug	Mfr	Amt	Mfr	Amt	Remarks	Ref	C/I
Cyclizine lactate	GW	150 mg/3 mL	NAP	200 mg/20 mL	Crystals form in 5 hr	2600	I
Cyclizine lactate	GW	50 mg/1 mL	NAP	70 mg/7 mL	Crystals form in 5 hr	2600	I
Cyclizine lactate	GW	50 mg/1 mL	NAP	100 mg/10 mL	Visually compatible. Under 4% concentration change in 24 hr at 25°C	2600	C
Cyclizine lactate	GW	50 mg/1 mL	NAP	150 mg/15 mL	Visually compatible. Under 4% concentration change in 24 hr at 25°C	2600	C
Cyclizine lactate	GW	50 mg/1 mL	NAP	200 mg/20 mL	Visually compatible. Under 4% concentration change in 24 hr at 25°C	2600	C
Cyclizine lactate	GW	100 mg/2 mL	NAP	200 mg/20 mL	Visually compatible. Under 4% concentration change in 24 hr at 25°C	2600	C
Dexamethasone sodium phosphate	FAU	40 mg/10 mL	NAP	200 mg/20 mL	Visually compatible. Under 4% concentration change in 24 hr at 25°C	2600	C
Haloperidol lactate	JC	15 mg/3 mL	NAP	200 mg/20 mL	Visually compatible. Under 4% concentration change in 24 hr at 25°C	2600	C
Ketamine HCl	PAN	40 mg/mL[a]	MUN	0.4 mg/mL[a]	Physically compatible with little to no loss of either drug in 7 days at 22 to 23°C	3585, 3586	C
Ketamine HCl	PAN	0.1 mg/mL[a]	MUN	10 mg/mL[a]	Physically compatible with little to no loss of either drug in 7 days at 22 to 23°C	3585, 3586	C

Drugs in Syringe Compatibility (Cont.)

Test Drug	Mfr	Amt	Mfr	Amt	Remarks	Ref	C/I
Ketamine HCl	PAN	40 mg/mL[a]	MUN	10 mg/mL[a]	Physically compatible with little to no loss of either drug in 7 days at 22 to 23°C	3585, 3586	C
Methotrimeprazine HCl		200 mg/8 mL	NAP	200 mg/20 mL	Visually compatible. Under 4% concentration change in 24 hr at 25°C	2600	C
Metoclopramide HCl		100 mg/20 mL	NAP	200 mg/20 mL	Visually compatible. Under 4% concentration change in 24 hr at 25°C	2600	C
Midazolam HCl	RC	100 mg/20 mL	NAP	200 mg/20 mL	Visually compatible. Under 4% concentration change in 24 hr at 25°C	2600	C
Prochlorperazine mesylate		12.5 mg/1 mL	NAP	200 mg/20 mL	Substantial change in prochlorperazine concentration in 24 hr at 25°C	2600	I
Scopolamine butylbromide	BI	60 mg/3 mL	NAP	200 mg/20 mL	Visually compatible. Under 4% concentration change in 24 hr at 25°C	2600	C
Scopolamine HBr		2.4 mg/6 mL	NAP	200 mg/20 mL	Visually compatible. Under 4% concentration change in 24 hr at 25°C	2600	C

[a] Diluted in sodium chloride 0.9%.

Selected Revisions July 1, 2020. © Copyright, October 2006.
American Society of Health-System Pharmacists, Inc.

Oxytocin
AHFS 76:00

Products

Oxytocin is available in 1-mL single-use vials and 10-, 30-, and 50-mL multiple-dose vials.[2856][2857][2858] Each mL contains oxytocin 10 units with chlorobutanol 0.5%.[2856][2857][2858] Acetic acid may have been added to adjust the pH during manufacture.[4][2856][2857][2858]

Units

One unit of oxytocin is equivalent to 2 to 2.2 mcg of pure oxytocin.[4]

pH

The pH range is from 3 to 5.[17][2858]

Trade Name(s)

Pitocin

Administration

Oxytocin is administered by intravenous infusion using an infusion control device;[4] the drug may also be administered by intramuscular injection,[2856][2857][2858] although intramuscular injection is usually not recommended for induction or augmentation of labor because the drug's effects are unpredictable and difficult to control.[4]

For intravenous administration, the injection should be diluted to a usual concentration of 10 milliunits/mL by adding 10 units (1 mL) to 1000 mL of Ringer's injection, lactated, or sodium chloride 0.9%.[4][2856][2857][2858] A higher concentration range of 10 to 40 milliunits/mL in sodium chloride 0.9% or dextrose 5% has been cited for select indications.[2856][2857][2858]

Stability

Oxytocin injection should be stored at controlled room temperature[2856][2857][2858] and protected from freezing.[2858] Do not use the solution if it is discolored or contains a precipitate.[4][2856][2857][2858] Discard unused portions of the drug.[2857][2858]

Oxytocin appears to be rapidly decomposed in the presence of sodium bisulfite.[333]

Filtration

Oxytocin (Parke-Davis) 25 units/100 mL in dextrose 5% and sodium chloride 0.9% was filtered at about 3 mL/min through a 0.22-µm cellulose ester membrane filter (Ivex-2). At this concentration, 25 times higher than normally used, oxytocin appeared to bind initially to the filter from the sodium chloride 0.9% solution. Results in dextrose 5% were equivocal. From these data, it is not possible to draw a definite conclusion regarding substantial binding of oxytocin during normal usage.[533]

Compatibility Information

Solution Compatibility

Oxytocin

Test Soln Name	Mfr	Mfr	Conc/L or %	Remarks	Ref	C/I
Dextrose 2.5% in half-strength Ringer's injection	AB	PD	5 units	Physically compatible	3	C
Dextrose 5% in Ringer's injection	AB	PD	5 units	Physically compatible	3	C
Dextrose 2.5% in Ringer's injection, lactated	AB	PD	5 units	Physically compatible	3	C
Dextrose 5% in half-strength Ringer's injection, lactated	AB	PD	5 units	Physically compatible	3	C
Dextrose 5% in Ringer's injection, lactated	AB	PD	5 units	Physically compatible	3	C
Dextrose 10% in Ringer's injection, lactated	AB	PD	5 units	Physically compatible	3	C
Dextrose 2.5% in sodium chloride 0.45%	AB	PD	5 units	Physically compatible	3	C
Dextrose 2.5% in sodium chloride 0.9%	AB	PD	5 units	Physically compatible	3	C
Dextrose 5% in sodium chloride 0.225%	AB	PD	5 units	Physically compatible	3	C
Dextrose 5% in sodium chloride 0.45%	AB	PD	5 units	Physically compatible	3	C
Dextrose 5% in sodium chloride 0.9%	AB	PD	5 units	Physically compatible	3	C

DOI: 10.37573/9781585286850.295

Solution Compatibility (Cont.)

Test Soln Name	Mfr	Mfr	Conc/L or %	Remarks	Ref	C/I
Dextrose 10% in sodium chloride 0.9%	AB	PD	5 units	Physically compatible	3	C
Dextrose 2.5%	AB	PD	5 units	Physically compatible	3	C
Dextrose 5%	AB	PD	5 units	Physically compatible	3	C
Dextrose 5%		CN	10.4 units	Stable for at least 6 hr at room temperature	333	C
Dextrose 5%	BAª	APP	80 units	Physically compatible with little or no loss of oxytocin in 90 days at 23°C protected from light	2671	C
Dextrose 10%	AB	PD	5 units	Physically compatible	3	C
Ionosol B in dextrose 5%	AB	PD	5 units	Physically compatible	3	C
Ionosol MB in dextrose 5%	AB	PD	5 units	Physically compatible	3	C
Ringer's injection	AB	PD	5 units	Physically compatible	3	C
Ringer's injection, lactated	AB	PD	5 units	Physically compatible	3	C
Ringer's injection, lactated	BAª	APP	80 units	Physically compatible with little or no loss of oxytocin in 28 days at 23°C protected from light. Microprecipitate forms and loss of oxytocin occurs after that time	2671	C
Ringer's injection, lactated	BAª	APP	20 units	Highly variable results. Oxytocin concentrations after 31 days of 99% at 4°C and 106% at 25°C. Physical stability not evaluated	2688	?
Ringer's injection, lactated	BAª	APP	60 units	Highly variable results. Oxytocin concentrations after 31 days of 91% at 4°C and 108% at 25°C. Physical stability not evaluated	2688	?
Sodium chloride 0.45%	AB	PD	5 units	Physically compatible	3	C
Sodium chloride 0.9%	AB	PD	5 units	Physically compatible	3	C
Sodium chloride 0.9%	BAª	APP	80 units	Physically compatible with little or no loss of oxytocin in 90 days at 23°C protected from light	2671	C
Sodium lactate ⅙ M	AB	PD	5 units	Physically compatible	3	C

ª Tested in PVC containers.

Additive Compatibility

Oxytocin

Test Drug	Mfr	Conc/L or %	Mfr	Conc/L or %	Test Solution	Remarks	Ref	C/I
Chloramphenicol sodium succinate	PD	1 g	PD	5 units		Physically compatible	6	C
Sodium bicarbonate	AB	2.4 mEqª	PD	5 units	D5W	Physically compatible for 24 hr	772	C
Verapamil HCl	KN	80 mg	SZ	40 units	D5W, NS	Physically compatible for 24 hr	764	C

ª One vial of Neut added to a liter of admixture.

Drugs in Syringe Compatibility

Oxytocin

Test Drug	Mfr	Amt	Mfr	Amt	Remarks	Ref	C/I
Dimenhydrinate		10 mg/1 mL		10 units/1 mL	Precipitate forms	2569	I
Pantoprazole sodium	ª	4 mg/1 mL		10 units/1 mL	Orange precipitate	2574	I

ª Test performed using the formulation WITHOUT edetate disodium.

Y-Site Injection Compatibility (1:1 Mixture)

Oxytocin

Test Drug	Mfr	Conc	Mfr	Conc	Remarks	Ref	C/I
Cloxacillin sodium	SMX	100 mg/mL	PPC	10 units/mL	Physically compatible for up to 4 hr at room temperature	3245	C
Heparin sodium	UP	1000 units/L[d]	SZ	1 unit/mL	Physically compatible for 4 hr at room temperature	534	C
Hydrocortisone sodium succinate	UP	10 mg/L[d]	SZ	1 unit/mL	Physically compatible for 4 hr at room temperature	534	C
Insulin, regular	LI	0.2 unit/mL[b]	PD	0.02 unit/mL[c]	Physically compatible for 2 hr at 25°C	1395	C
Meperidine HCl	WY	10 mg/mL[b]	PD	0.02 unit/mL[c]	Physically compatible for 1 hr at 25°C	1338	C
Meropenem		50 mg/mL	HOS	10 units/mL	Physically compatible for 4 hr at room temperature	3538	C
Morphine sulfate	ES	1 mg/mL[b]	PD	0.02 unit/mL[c]	Physically compatible for 1 hr at 25°C	1338	C
Potassium chloride	AB	40 mEq/L[d]	SZ	1 unit/mL	Physically compatible for 4 hr at room temperature	534	C
Zidovudine	GSK	2 mg/mL[a]	NVA	10 milliunits/mL[a]	Visually compatible with no zidovudine loss in 6 hr at 20°C	2491	C
Zidovudine	GSK	4 mg/mL[a]	NVA	10 milliunits/mL[a]	Visually compatible with no zidovudine loss in 6 hr at 20°C	2491	C

[a] Tested in dextrose 5%.

[b] Tested in sodium chloride 0.9%.

[c] Tested in dextrose 5% in Ringer's injection, lactated.

[d] Tested in dextrose 5% in Ringer's injection, dextrose 5% in Ringer's injection, lactated, dextrose 5%, Ringer's injection, lactated, and sodium chloride 0.9%.

Selected Revisions May 1, 2020. © Copyright, October 1982.
American Society of Health-System Pharmacists, Inc.

Paclitaxel
AHFS 10:00

Products

Paclitaxel is available as a 6-mg/mL non-aqueous concentrate for injection in 5-, 16.7-, 25-, and 50-mL multidose vials.[3338 3339 3341] In most formulations, each mL of the concentrate for injection also contains polyoxyl 35 castor oil (Cremophor EL; polyoxyethylated castor oil) surfactant 527 mg and dehydrated alcohol 396 mg.[3338 3339] Some formulations also incorporate citric acid anhydrous 2 mg/mL.[3339] The concentrate for injection must be diluted prior to administration.[3338 3339]

CAUTION: Care should be taken to ensure that the correct drug product, dose, and administration procedures are used and that no confusion with other products occurs. Although Abraxane, an albumin-bound paclitaxel suspension also exists,[3219] it is sufficiently different from conventional solvent-formulated paclitaxel that extrapolating information to or from it would be inappropriate.

pH

The pH of paclitaxel (WG Critical Care) diluted for infusion ranges from 3 to 7.[3342]

Trade Name(s)

Taxol

Administration

Paclitaxel is administered by intravenous infusion.[3338 3339] The concentrate must be diluted to a final paclitaxel concentration of 0.3 to 1.2 mg/mL in dextrose 5%, sodium chloride 0.9%, dextrose 5% in sodium chloride 0.9%, or dextrose 5% in Ringer's injection.[3338 3339] Manufacturers note that the Chemo Dispensing Pin device or other similar devices with spikes should *not* be used with paclitaxel vials because they can cause the stopper to collapse, thereby resulting in loss of solution sterility.[3338 3339]

Administration of the diluted solution over 3 or 24 hours is often recommended, depending upon the indication and the specific regimen used.[3338 3339] An inline filter with a pore size not greater than 0.22 μm should be used for administration of the diluted solution.[3338 3339] Intravenous solution containers and administration sets used should be free of the plasticizer diethylhexyl phthalate (DEHP) that may be leached from polyvinyl chloride (PVC) infusion bags or sets.[3338 3339] Diluted paclitaxel solutions preferably should be stored in glass, polypropylene, or polyolefin containers and administered through polyethylene-lined administration sets.[3338 3339] The infusion site should be monitored closely for possible infiltration during administration.[3338 3339]

As with other toxic drugs, caution should be exercised in the handling of paclitaxel.[3338 3339] The use of impervious gloves is always advised when handling vials of the drug.[3338 3339] If skin contact with paclitaxel occurs, the exposed area should be washed immediately and thoroughly with soap and water.[3338 3339]

For mucous membrane contact, the exposed area should be flushed thoroughly with water.[3338 3339] Procedures for the proper disposal of paclitaxel should be considered.[3338 3339]

Use of self-venting sets spiked into glass bottles of paclitaxel admixtures has occasionally resulted in solution dripping from the air vent. Presumably, the surfactant content wetted the hydrophobic filter, allowing the solution to drip.[1843] In another observation, the spikes of administration sets were made sufficiently slippery by surfactant in the paclitaxel formulation that the spike slipped out after it had been seated through the rubber bung of the glass bottle. The admixture also leaked due to a poor seal. The authors recommend use of non-PVC plastic solution containers to avoid the problem.[2052]

CAUTION: Care should be taken to ensure that the correct drug product, dose, and administration procedures are used and that no confusion with other products occurs.

Stability

Paclitaxel is a clear, colorless to slightly yellow viscous solution.[3338 3339] Intact vials should be stored at controlled room temperature in the original package to protect from light.[3338 3339] Stability is not adversely affected by refrigeration or freezing.[3338 3339] Refrigeration may result in the precipitation of formulation components; however, warming to room temperature redissolves the material and does not adversely affect the product.[3338 3339] If the solution remains cloudy or an insoluble precipitate is noted, the product should be discarded.[3338 3339] Diluted paclitaxel solutions should be visually inspected for particulate matter and discoloration prior to administration.[3338 3339]

Paclitaxel 0.7 mg/mL diluted in sodium chloride 0.9% did not exhibit an antimicrobial effect on the growth of 3 of 4 organisms (*Enterococcus faecium*, *Staphylococcus aureus*, *Pseudomonas aeruginosa*, and *Candida albicans*) inoculated into the solution. *S. aureus* remained viable for 4 hours. *E. faecium* and *P. aeruginosa* remained viable for 48 hours, and *C. albicans* remained viable to the end of the study at 120 hours. Diluted solutions of paclitaxel should be stored under refrigeration whenever possible, and the potential for microbiological growth should be considered when assigning expiration periods.[2160]

Turbidity

Paclitaxel is a clear, colorless to slightly yellow viscous solution.[3338 3339] After dilution in an infusion solution, the drug may exhibit haziness because of the surfactant content of the formulation.[1528 3338 3339]

Precipitation

Although after dilution in specified infusion solutions, paclitaxel is physically and chemically stable for up to 27 hours[3338 3339] or longer,[1746 1842 2708] precipitation has occurred irregularly and unpredictably. Such precipitation occurs within the recommended range of 0.3 to 1.2 mg/mL and at lower paclitaxel

DOI: 10.37573/9781585286850.296

concentrations. These precipitates have been observed in the infusion tubing distal to the pump chamber.[1716] Although precipitation of insoluble drugs in an aqueous medium is a foregone conclusion, the time to precipitation is irregular. It may be accelerated by the presence or formation of crystallization nuclei, agitation, and contact with incompatible drugs or materials.[1374] [1521] Since the mechanism of this irregular precipitation has not been identified,[1739] vigilance throughout the infusion of paclitaxel is required.

Sorption

No paclitaxel loss due to sorption to containers or sets has been observed.[1520 2230 2231 2232]

Plasticizer Leaching

Contact of undiluted paclitaxel concentrate with plasticized PVC equipment and devices is not recommended.[3338 3339] With use of infusion bags and tubing that are free of DEHP plasticizer and the elimination of PVC precision flow regulators, a reduction in leached DEHP of up to 96% has been reported.[2679]

Paclitaxel vehicle equivalent to paclitaxel 1.2 mg/mL in dextrose 5% in VISIV polyolefin bags was tested at room temperature near 23°C for 24 hours. No plastic components leached within the 24-hour study period.[2660 2792]

Paclitaxel itself does not contribute to the extraction of the plasticizer DEHP.[1520] However, the surfactant, Cremophor EL, in the paclitaxel formulation extracts DEHP from PVC containers and sets. The amount of DEHP extracted increases with time and drug concentration.[1520 1683 2146] Consequently, the use of DEHP-plasticized PVC containers and sets is not recommended for infusion of paclitaxel solutions.[3338 3339] Instead, manufacturers recommend the use of glass, polypropylene, or polyolefin containers and non-PVC containing administration sets (e.g., polyethylene-lined administration sets).[3338 3339]

The use of inline filters that incorporate short PVC-coated inlet and outlet tubing (e.g., Ivex-2) has not resulted in a substantial amount of DEHP leaching.[3338 3339]

A study was performed on the compatibility of paclitaxel 0.3- and 1.2-mg/mL infusions with various non-PVC infusion sets. The paclitaxel infusions were run through the study sets, and the effluent was then analyzed for leached DEHP plasticizer. The following sets had significant and unacceptable amounts of leached DEHP: Baxter vented nitroglycerin (2C7552S), Baxter vented basic solution (1C8355S), McGaw Horizon pump vented nitroglycerin (V7450), and McGaw Intelligent pump vented nitroglycerin (V7150). Although these sets were largely non-PVC, their highly plasticized pumping segments contributed the DEHP. The administration and extension sets cited in Tables 1 and 2 exhibited no more leached DEHP than the Ivex-2 filter set specified in the product labeling.[1843]

Table 1. Administration sets compatible with paclitaxel infusions by manufacturer[1843]

Abbott	LifeCare 5000 Plum PVC specialty set (11594)
Abbott	Life Shield anesthesia pump set OL with cartridge (13503)
Abbott	LifeCare model 4P specialty set, non-PVC (11434)
Abbott	Omni-Flow universal primary intravenous pump short minibore patient line (40527)
Baxter	Vented volumetric pump nitroglycerin set (2C1042)
Block Medical	Verifuse nonvented administration set with 0.22-μm filter, check valve, injection site, and non-DEHP PVC tubing (V021015)
I-Flow	Vivus-4000 polyethylene-lined infusion set (5000-784)
IMED	Standard PVC set (9215)
IMED	Closed-system non-PVC fluid path nonvented quick-spike administration set (9635)
IMED	Non-PVC set with inline filter (9986)
IMED	Gemini 20 nonvented primary administration set for nitroglycerin and emulsions (2262)
IVAC	Universal set with low-sorbing tubing (52053, 59953, and S75053)
Ivion/Medex	WalkMed spike set (SP-06) with pump set (PS-401, PS-360, FPS-560, or FPX-560)
Siemens	Reduced-PVC full set MiniMed Uni-Set macrobore (28-60-190)

Table 2. Extension sets compatible with paclitaxel infusions by manufacturer[1843]

Abbott	Ivex-HP filter set (4524)
Abbott	Ivex-2 filter set (2679)
Becton Dickinson	Intima intravenous catheter placement set (38-6918-1)
Becton Dickinson	J-loop connector (38-1252-2)
Becton Dickinson	E-Z infusion set shorty (38-53741)
Becton Dickinson	E-Z infusion set (38-53121)
Baxter	Polyethylene-lined extension set with 0.22-μm air-eliminating filter (1C8363)
Braun	0.2-μm filter extension set (FE-2012L)
Braun	Small-bore 0.2-μm filter extension set (PFE-2007)
Braun	Whin-winged extension set with 90° Huber needle (HW-2267)
Braun	Whin extension set with Y-site and Huber needle (HW-2276 YHR)
Braun	Y-extension set with valve (ET-08-YL)
Braun	Small-bore extension set with T-fitting (ET-04T)
Braun	Small-bore extension set with reflux valve (ET-116L)
Gish Biomedical	VasTack noncoring portal-access needle system (VT-2022)
IMED	0.2-μm add-on filter set (9400 XL)
IVAC	Spec-Sets extension set with 0.22-μm inline filter (C20028 and C20350)

Table 2. Extension sets compatible with paclitaxel infusions by manufacturer[1843] (Cont.)

Ivion/Medex	Extension set with 0.22-μm filter (IV4A07-IV3)
PALL	SetSaver extended-life disposable set with 0.2-μm filter (ELD-96P and ELD-96LL)
PALL	SetSaver extended-life disposable microbore extension tubing with 0.2-μm Posidyne filter (ELD-96LYL and ELD-96LYLN)
Pfizer/Strato Medical	Lifeport vascular-access system infusion set with Y-site (LPS 3009)

Paclitaxel 0.3 and 1.2 mg/mL was prepared in PVC bags in dextrose 5% and in sodium chloride 0.9%. Leaching of the plasticizer was found to be time and concentration dependent; however, there was little difference between the 2 infusion solutions. After storage for 8 hours at 21°C, leached DEHP in the range from 73 to 108 mcg/mL was found for the 1.2-mg/mL concentration and from 21 to 30 mcg/mL for the 0.3-mg/mL concentration. During a simulated 1-hour infusion using DEHP plasticized administration sets, the amount of leached DEHP did not exceed 18 mcg/mL at the 0.3-mg/mL paclitaxel concentration, but resulted in a maximum of 114 mcg/mL at the 1.2-mg/mL paclitaxel concentration.[1825]

DEHP plasticizer leaching from PVC containers and administration sets and the amount of DEHP leached was reported to depend on surfactant concentration and length of contact period. Authors also reported leaching of up to 30 mg of DEHP per dose from Flo-Gard Low Adsorption Sets (Baxter), a set with a reduced amount of PVC present in its construction.[2146]

In 1996, an acceptability limit of no more than 5 parts per million (5 mcg/mL) for DEHP plasticizer released from PVC-containing devices (e.g., containers, administration sets, other equipment) was proposed based on a review of metabolic and toxicologic considerations.[2185] FDA later evaluated the safety of DEHP exposure by comparing doses of DEHP received by patients undergoing various medical procedures with a defined tolerable intake value of DEHP, a value that was based upon the results of selected critical toxicity studies in experimental animals.[3100] Based on the results of the safety assessment, FDA concluded that there is little risk posed by exposure to the amount of DEHP released from PVC bags used to store and administer drugs that require an excipient for solubilization *when label instructions for preparation and administration are followed.*[3100] However, such conclusions do not take into account increased risk for adverse effects from DEHP exposure in certain patients (e.g., critically ill male neonates or infants, male infants less than 1 year of age, male offspring of pregnant or breast-feeding women undergoing certain medical treatments) or potential adverse effects related to aggregate exposure for patients exposed to multiple medical devices, procedures, or intravenous medications known to leach DEHP, for which there are varying levels of concern.[3100] [3101]

Two reduced-phthalate administration sets for the Acclaim (Abbott) pump were evaluated. Administration set model 11993-48 (Abbott) is composed of polyethylene tubing but has

a DEHP-plasticized pumping segment. Administration set model L-12060 (Abbott) is composed of tris(2-ethylhexyl)trimellitate (TOTM)-plasticized PVC tubing and a DEHP-plasticized pumping segment. Paclitaxel diluent at concentrations equivalent to 0.3 and 1.2 mg/mL in dextrose 5% delivered rapidly over 3 hours at 23°C did not leach detectable levels of TOTM from model L-12060 or DEHP from either set. Similarly, slow delivery over 4 days of the 0.3-mg/mL concentration yielded detectable but not quantifiable amounts of plasticizer. However, slow delivery of the equivalent of 1.2 mg/mL over 4 days yielded large but variable amounts of DEHP from both sets; DEHP concentrations ranged from 30 to 150 mcg/mL. Consequently, these 2 reduced-phthalate sets are suitable for short-term delivery up to 3 hours of paclitaxel at concentrations up to 1.2 mg/mL. However, these sets should not be used for slow delivery of paclitaxel.[2198]

Paclitaxel vehicle equivalent to paclitaxel 0.3 and 1.2 mg/mL in dextrose 5% did not leach TOTM plasticizer from a TOTM-plasticized PVC set (SoloPak) during simulated 3-hour administration. During extremely slow delivery at 5.2 mL/hr for 4 days, no detectable TOTM was found in the 0.3-mg/mL equivalent concentration, and only a barely detectable, unquantifiable amount of TOTM was found with the 1.2-mg/mL equivalent solution.[2232]

Paclitaxel 0.3 and 1.2 mg/mL in dextrose 5% or in sodium chloride 0.9% in ethylene vinyl acetate (EVA) containers was found to leach an unknown material stored at 25 and 32°C for 24 hours.[2182]

Filtration

The manufacturer recommends the use of an inline filter with a pore size not greater than 0.22 μm for administration of diluted paclitaxel.[3338] [3339] No substantial loss of paclitaxel due to filtration through an inline 0.22-μm filter has occurred during simulated delivery.[1520] [3338] [3339]

The acceptability of the 0.22-μm IV Express Filter Unit (Millipore) for the administration of paclitaxel was evaluated. Paclitaxel vehicle equivalent to paclitaxel 1.2 mg/mL (for plasticizer leaching) and paclitaxel 0.3 mg/mL (for sorption potential) in 500 mL of dextrose 5% in polyolefin containers was delivered through the filter units over a 3-hour period at a rate of 167 mL/hr at about 23°C to simulate paclitaxel administration. No leached plasticizer and no loss of paclitaxel due to sorption was found.[2231]

Central Venous Catheter

The acceptability of the Arrow-Howes triple-lumen, 7 French, 30-cm polyurethane central catheter (Arrow International) for the administration of paclitaxel was evaluated. Paclitaxel vehicle equivalent to paclitaxel 0.3 and 1.2 mg/mL (for catheter component leaching) and paclitaxel 0.3 mg/mL (for sorption potential) were prepared in polyolefin bags of dextrose 5%. The solutions were delivered through the polyurethane central venous catheters for periods of 3 hours and of 24 hours at 23°C to simulate rapid and slow administration. No leached catheter components were found in the effluent solution and no loss of paclitaxel occurred.[2230]

Compatibility Information

Solution Compatibility

Paclitaxel

Test Soln Name	Mfr	Mfr	Conc/L or %.	Remarks	Ref	C/I
Dextrose 5% in Ringer's injection	h	WG, HOS	0.3 to 1.2 g	Physically and chemically stable for up to 27 hr at 25°C	3338, 3339	C
Dextrose 5% in sodium chloride 0.9%	h	WG, HOS	0.3 to 1.2 g	Physically and chemically stable for up to 27 hr at 25°C	3338, 3339	C
Dextrose 5%	MG, TR[a]	NCI	0.3, 0.6, 0.9 g	Visually compatible. No loss in 12 hr at 22°C	1520	C
Dextrose 5%	MG[b]	NCI	0.6 g	Visually compatible. No loss in 25 hr at 22°C	1520	C
Dextrose 5%	MG, TR[c]	NCI	1.2 g	Visually compatible. No loss in 12 hr at 22°C	1520	C
Dextrose 5%		BR	0.2 to 0.58 g	Fluffy, white precipitate forms occasionally in administration set just distal to pump chamber	1716	I
Dextrose 5%	MG[b]	BR	0.1 and 1 g	Physically compatible. Stable for 3 days at 4, 22, and 32°C. Crystals after 3 days	1746	C
Dextrose 5%	MG[b]	BR	0.3 and 1.2 g	Physically compatible and chemically stable for 48 hr at 22°C	1842	C
Dextrose 5%	BA[d]	FAU	0.3 and 1.2 g	Physically compatible. Stable for 3 days at 25 and 32°C. Unknown material leached from EVA container by 24 hr	2182	?
Dextrose 5%	BA[b], BRN[b], FRE[b], MAC[b]	BMS	0.3 and 1.2 g	Physically compatible with less than 5% loss in 72 hr at 37°C in the dark	2669	C
Dextrose 5%	BRN[e]	BMS	0.4 and 1.2 g	Physically compatible. Little loss in 5 days at 23 and 4°C. Precipitation occurred after this	2673	C
Dextrose 5%	BA[f]	TE	0.3 g	Chemically stable until precipitation. Precipitate after 3 days at 25°C and 13 days at 5°C	2708	C
Dextrose 5%	BRN[e]	TE	0.3 g	Chemically stable until precipitation. Precipitate found after 3 days at 25°C and 18 days at 5°C	2708	C
Dextrose 5%	BRN[g]	TE	0.3 g	Chemically stable until precipitation. Precipitate found after 7 days at 25°C and 20 days at 5°C	2708	C
Dextrose 5%	BA[f]	TE	1.2 g	Chemically stable until precipitation. Precipitate found after 3 days at 25°C and 10 days at 5°C	2708	C
Dextrose 5%	BRN[e]	TE	1.2 g	Chemically stable until precipitation. Precipitate found after 3 days at 25°C and 12 days at 5°C	2708	C
Dextrose 5%	BRN[g]	TE	1.2 g	Chemically stable until precipitation. Precipitate found after 7 days at 25°C and 10 days at 5°C	2708	C
Dextrose 5%	FRK[b]	MAY	0.3 g	Chemically stable for 8 days at 25°C and 28 days at 5°C; then precipitation	2729	C
Dextrose 5%	FRK[b]	MAY	0.75 g	Chemically stable for 4 days at 25°C and 20 days at 5°C; then precipitation	2729	C
Dextrose 5%	FRK[b]	MAY	1.2 g	Chemically stable for 4 days at 25°C and 12 days at 5°C; then precipitation	2729	C
Dextrose 5%	h	WG, HOS	0.3 to 1.2 g	Physically and chemically stable for up to 27 hr at 25°C	3338, 3339	C
Sodium chloride 0.9%	MG, TR[a]	NCI	0.3, 0.6, 0.9, 1.2 g	Visually compatible. No loss over 12 hr at 22°C	1520	C
Sodium chloride 0.9%	MG[b]	NCI	0.6 and 1.2 g	Visually compatible. No loss over 26 hr at 22°C	1520	C
Sodium chloride 0.9%	MG[b]	BR	0.1 and 1 g	Physically compatible. Stable for 3 days at 4, 22, and 32°C. Crystals after 3 days	1746	C

Solution Compatibility (Cont.)

Test Soln Name	Mfr	Mfr	Conc/L or %	Remarks	Ref	C/I
Sodium chloride 0.9%	MG[b]	BR	0.3 and 1.2 g	Physically compatible and chemically stable for 48 hr at 22°C	1842	C
Sodium chloride 0.9%	BA[d]	FAU	0.3 and 1.2 g	Physically compatible. Stable for 3 days at 25 and 32°C. Unknown material leached from EVA container by 24 hr	2182	?
Sodium chloride 0.9%	BA[b], BRN[b], FRE[b], MAC[b]	BMS	0.3 and 1.2 g	Physically compatible with less than 5% loss in 72 hr at 37°C in the dark	2669	C
Sodium chloride 0.9%	BA[f]	TE	0.3 g	Chemically stable until precipitation. Precipitate found after 3 days at 25°C and 13 days at 5°C	2708	C
Sodium chloride 0.9%	BRN[e]	TE	0.3 g	Chemically stable until precipitation. Precipitate found after 3 days at 25°C and 16 days at 5°C	2708	C
Sodium chloride 0.9%	BRN[g]	TE	0.3 g	Chemically stable until precipitation. Precipitate found after 3 days at 25°C and 13 days at 5°C	2708	C
Sodium chloride 0.9%	BA[f]	TE	1.2 g	Chemically stable until precipitation. Precipitate found after 3 days at 25°C and 9 days at 5°C	2708	C
Sodium chloride 0.9%	BRN[e]	TE	1.2 g	Chemically stable until precipitation. Precipitate found after 3 days at 25°C and 12 days at 5°C	2708	C
Sodium chloride 0.9%	BRN[g]	TE	1.2 g	Chemically stable until precipitation. Precipitate found after 5 days at 25°C and 8 days at 5°C	2708	C
Sodium chloride 0.9%	FRK[b]	MAY	0.3 g	Chemically stable for 6 days at 25°C and 28 days at 5°C; then precipitation	2729	C
Sodium chloride 0.9%	FRK[b]	MAY	0.75 g	Chemically stable for 6 days at 25°C and 20 days at 5°C; then precipitation	2729	C
Sodium chloride 0.9%	FRK[b]	MAY	1.2 g	Chemically stable for 4 days at 25°C and 12 days at 5°C; then precipitation	2729	C
Sodium chloride 0.9%	[h]	WG, HOS	0.3 to 1.2 g	Physically and chemically stable for up to 27 hr at 25°C	3338, 3339	C

[a] Tested in both glass and PVC containers.

[b] Tested in polyolefin containers.

[c] Tested in glass, PVC, and polyolefin containers.

[d] Tested in Baxter ethylene vinyl acetate (EVA) containers.

[e] Tested in ECOFLAC low-density polyethylene plastic containers.

[f] Tested in polyolefin containers.

[g] Tested in glass containers.

[h] Tested in glass, polypropylene, and polyolefin containers.

Additive Compatibility

Paclitaxel

Test Drug	Mfr	Conc/L or %	Mfr	Conc/L or %	Test Solution	Remarks	Ref	C/I
Carboplatin	BMS	2 g	BMS	300 mg and 1.2 g	NS	No paclitaxel loss but carboplatin losses of less than 2, 5, and 6 to 7% at 4, 24, and 32°C, respectively, in 24 hr. Physically compatible for 24 hr but microparticles of paclitaxel form after 3 to 5 days	2094	C
Carboplatin	BMS	2 g	BMS	300 mg and 1.2 g	D5W	No paclitaxel and carboplatin loss at 4, 24, and 32°C in 24 hr. Physically compatible for 24 hr but microparticles of paclitaxel form after 3 to 5 days	2094	C

Additive Compatibility (Cont.)

Test Drug	Mfr	Conc/L or %	Mfr	Conc/L or %	Test Solution	Remarks	Ref	C/I
Cisplatin	BMS	200 mg	BMS	300 mg	NS	No paclitaxel loss and cisplatin losses of 1, 4, and 5% at 4, 24, and 32°C, respectively, in 24 hr. Physically compatible for 24 hr but microparticles of paclitaxel form after 3 to 5 days	2094	C
Cisplatin	BMS	200 mg	BMS	1.2 g	NS	No paclitaxel loss but cisplatin losses of 10, 19, and 22% at 4, 24, and 32°C, respectively, in 24 hr. Physically compatible for 24 hr but microparticles of paclitaxel form after 3 to 5 days	2094	I
Doxorubicin HCl	PH	200 mg	BMS	300 mg	D5W, NS	Visually compatible for 1 day with microprecipitation in 3 to 5 days and gross precipitation in 7 days at 4, 23, and 32°C in the dark. No paclitaxel and under 8% doxorubicin loss in 7 days	2247	C
Doxorubicin HCl	PH	200 mg	BMS	1.2 g	D5W, NS	Visually compatible for 1 day with microprecipitation in 3 to 5 days and gross precipitation in 7 days at 4, 23, and 32°C in the dark. No paclitaxel and less than 7% doxorubicin loss in 7 days	2247	C

Y-Site Injection Compatibility (1:1 Mixture)

Paclitaxel

Test Drug	Mfr	Conc	Mfr	Conc	Remarks	Ref	C/I
Acyclovir sodium	BW	7 mg/mL[a]	NCI	1.2 mg/mL[a]	Physically compatible for 4 hr at 22°C	1556	C
Amikacin sulfate	BR	5 mg/mL[a]	NCI	1.2 mg/mL[a]	Physically compatible for 4 hr at 22°C	1556	C
Aminophylline	AB	2.5 mg/mL[a]	NCI	1.2 mg/mL[a]	Physically compatible for 4 hr at 22°C	1556	C
Amphotericin B	SQ	0.6 mg/mL[a]	NCI	1.2 mg/mL[a]	Immediate increase in measured turbidity followed by separation into two layers in 24 hr at 22°C	1556	I
Ampicillin sodium–sulbactam sodium	RR	20 mg/mL[b f]	NCI	1.2 mg/mL[a]	Physically compatible for 4 hr at 22°C	1556	C
Anidulafungin	VIC	0.5 mg/mL[a]	MJ	0.6 mg/mL[a]	Physically compatible for 4 hr at 23°C	2617	C
Bleomycin sulfate	MJ	1 unit/mL[a]	NCI	1.2 mg/mL[a]	Physically compatible for 4 hr at 22°C	1556	C
Butorphanol tartrate	BR	0.04 mg/mL[a]	NCI	1.2 mg/mL[a]	Physically compatible for 4 hr at 22°C	1556	C
Calcium chloride	AST	20 mg/mL[a]	NCI	1.2 mg/mL[a]	Physically compatible for 4 hr at 22°C	1556	C
Carboplatin		5 mg/mL[a]	NCI	1.2 mg/mL[a]	Physically compatible for 4 hr at 22°C	1528	C
Cefotetan disodium	STU	20 mg/mL[a]	NCI	1.2 mg/mL[a]	Physically compatible for 4 hr at 22°C	1556	C
Ceftazidime	LI	40 mg/mL[a]	NCI	1.2 mg/mL[a]	Physically compatible for 4 hr at 22°C	1556	C
Ceftriaxone sodium	RC	20 mg/mL[a]	NCI	1.2 mg/mL[a]	Physically compatible for 4 hr at 22°C	1556	C
Chlorpromazine HCl	ES	2 mg/mL[a]	NCI	1.2 mg/mL[a]	Normal inherent haze from paclitaxel decreases immediately	1556	I
Cisplatin		1 mg/mL	NCI	1.2 mg/mL[a]	Physically compatible for 4 hr at 22°C	1528	C
Cladribine	ORT	0.015[b] and 0.5[c] mg/mL	BR	0.6 mg/mL[b]	Physically compatible for 4 hr at 23°C	1969	C
Cyclophosphamide		10 mg/mL[a]	NCI	1.2 mg/mL[a]	Physically compatible for 4 hr at 22°C	1528	C

Y-Site Injection Compatibility (1:1 Mixture) (Cont.)

Test Drug	Mfr	Conc	Mfr	Conc	Remarks	Ref	C/I
Cytarabine		50 mg/mL	NCI	1.2 mg/mL[a]	Physically compatible for 4 hr at 22°C	1528	C
Dacarbazine	MI	4 mg/mL[a]	NCI	1.2 mg/mL[a]	Physically compatible for 4 hr at 22°C	1556	C
Dexamethasone sodium phosphate		1 mg/mL[a]	NCI	1.2 mg/mL[a]	Physically compatible for 4 hr at 22°C	1528	C
Diphenhydramine HCl		2 mg/mL[a]	NCI	1.2 mg/mL[a]	Physically compatible for 4 hr at 22°C	1528	C
Doripenem	JJ	5 mg/mL[a b]	MAY	0.6 mg/mL[a b]	Physically compatible for 4 hr at 23°C	2743	C
Doxorubicin HCl		2 mg/mL	NCI	1.2 mg/mL[a]	Physically compatible for 4 hr at 22°C	1528	C
Doxorubicin HCl liposomal	SEQ	0.4 mg/mL[a]	MJ	0.6 mg/mL[a]	Partial loss of measured natural turbidity	2087	I
Droperidol	JN	0.4 mg/mL[a]	NCI	1.2 mg/mL[a]	Physically compatible for 4 hr at 22°C	1556	C
Etoposide		0.4 mg/mL[a]	NCI	1.2 mg/mL[a]	Physically compatible for 4 hr at 22°C	1528	C
Etoposide phosphate	BR	5 mg/mL[a]	MJ	1.2 mg/mL[a]	Physically compatible for 4 hr at 23°C	2218	C
Famotidine	MSD	2 mg/mL[a]	NCI	1.2 mg/mL[a]	Physically compatible for 4 hr at 22°C	1556	C
Floxuridine	RC	3 mg/mL[a]	NCI	1.2 mg/mL[a]	Physically compatible for 4 hr at 22°C	1556	C
Fluconazole	RR	2 mg/mL	NCI	1.2 mg/mL[a]	Physically compatible for 4 hr at 22°C	1556	C
Fluconazole	PF	2 mg/mL	BR	0.3 and 1.2 mg/mL[a]	Visually compatible. No loss of either drug in 4 hr at 23°C	1790	C
Fluorouracil		16 mg/mL[a]	NCI	1.2 mg/mL[a]	Physically compatible for 4 hr at 22°C	1528	C
Furosemide	AST	3 mg/mL[a]	NCI	1.2 mg/mL[a]	Physically compatible for 4 hr at 22°C	1556	C
Ganciclovir sodium	SY	20 mg/mL[a]	NCI	1.2 mg/mL[a]	Physically compatible for 4 hr at 22°C	1556	C
Gemcitabine HCl	LI	10 mg/mL[b]	MJ	1.2 mg/mL[a]	Physically compatible for 4 hr at 23°C	2226	C
Gentamicin sulfate	ES	5 mg/mL[a]	NCI	1.2 mg/mL[a]	Physically compatible for 4 hr at 22°C	1556	C
Granisetron HCl	SKB	1 mg/mL	MJ	0.3 mg/mL[b]	Physically compatible with little or no loss of either drug in 4 hr at 22°C	1883	C
Granisetron HCl	SKB	0.05 mg/mL[a]	MJ	1.2 mg/mL[a]	Physically compatible for 4 hr at 23°C	2000	C
Haloperidol lactate		0.2 mg/mL[a]	NCI	1.2 mg/mL[a]	Physically compatible for 4 hr at 22°C	1528	C
Heparin sodium	WY	100 units/mL[a]	NCI	1.2 mg/mL[a]	Physically compatible for 4 hr at 22°C	1556	C/I
Hydrocortisone sodium succinate	AB	1 mg/mL[a]	NCI	1.2 mg/mL[a]	Physically compatible for 4 hr at 22°C	1556	C
Hydromorphone HCl	KN	0.5 mg/mL[a]	NCI	1.2 mg/mL[a]	Physically compatible for 4 hr at 22°C	1556	C
Hydroxyzine HCl	ES	4 mg/mL[a]	NCI	1.2 mg/mL[a]	Normal inherent haze from paclitaxel decreases immediately	1556	I
Ifosfamide	BR	25 mg/mL[a]	NCI	1.2 mg/mL[a]	Physically compatible for 4 hr at 22°C	1556	C
Linezolid	PHU	2 mg/mL	MJ	0.6 mg/mL[a]	Physically compatible for 4 hr at 23°C	2264	C
Lorazepam		0.1 mg/mL[a]	NCI	1.2 mg/mL[a]	Physically compatible for 4 hr at 22°C	1528	C
Magnesium sulfate	AST	100 mg/mL[a]	NCI	1.2 mg/mL[a]	Physically compatible for 4 hr at 22°C	1556	C
Mannitol	BA	15%	NCI	1.2 mg/mL[a]	Physically compatible for 4 hr at 22°C	1556	C
Meperidine HCl	WY	4 mg/mL[a]	NCI	1.2 mg/mL[a]	Physically compatible for 4 hr at 22°C	1556	C
Mesna	MJ	10 mg/mL[a]	NCI	1.2 mg/mL[a]	Physically compatible for 4 hr at 22°C	1556	C

Y-Site Injection Compatibility (1:1 Mixture) (Cont.)

Test Drug	Mfr	Conc	Mfr	Conc	Remarks	Ref	C/I
Methotrexate sodium		15 mg/mL[a]	NCI	1.2 mg/mL[a]	Physically compatible for 4 hr at 22°C	1528	C
Methylprednisolone sodium succinate	UP	5 mg/mL[a]	NCI	1.2 mg/mL[a]	Normal inherent haze from paclitaxel decreases immediately	1556	I
Metoclopramide HCl		5 mg/mL	NCI	1.2 mg/mL[a]	Physically compatible for 4 hr at 22°C	1528	C
Mitoxantrone HCl	LE	0.5 mg/mL[a]	NCI	1.2 mg/mL[a]	Normal inherent haze from paclitaxel decreases immediately	1556	I
Morphine sulfate	WY	1 mg/mL[a]	NCI	1.2 mg/mL[a]	Physically compatible for 4 hr at 22°C	1556	C
Nalbuphine HCl	AST	10 mg/mL	NCI	1.2 mg/mL[a]	Physically compatible for 4 hr at 22°C	1556	C
Ondansetron HCl	GL	0.5 mg/mL[a]	NCI	1.2 mg/mL[a]	Physically compatible for 4 hr at 22°C	1556	C
Ondansetron HCl	GL	0.03 and 0.3 mg/mL[a]	BR	0.3 mg/mL[a]	Visually compatible with no loss of either drug in 4 hr at 23°C	1741	C
Ondansetron HCl	GL	0.03 and 0.3 mg/mL[a]	BR	1.2 mg/mL[a]	Visually compatible with no loss of either drug in 4 hr at 23°C	1741	C
Ondansetron HCl with ranitidine HCl	GL GL	0.3 mg/mL[a] 2 mg/mL[a]	BR	1.2 mg/mL[a]	Visually compatible with no loss of any drug in 4 hr at 23°C	1741	C
Oxaliplatin	SS	0.5 mg/mL[a]	MJ	0.6 mg/mL[a]	Physically compatible for 4 hr at 23°C	2566	C
Palonosetron HCl	MGI	50 mcg/mL	MJ	1.2 mg/mL[a]	Physically compatible. Little loss of either drug in 4 hr	2533	C
Pemetrexed disodium	LI	20 mg/mL[b]	MJ	0.6 mg/mL[a]	Physically compatible for 4 hr at 23°C	2564	C
Pentostatin	NCI	0.4 mg/mL[b]	NCI	1.2 mg/mL[a]	Physically compatible for 4 hr at 22°C	1556	C
Potassium chloride	AB	0.1 mEq/mL[a]	NCI	1.2 mg/mL[a]	Physically compatible for 4 hr at 22°C	1556	C
Prochlorperazine edisylate		0.5 mg/mL[a]	NCI	1.2 mg/mL[a]	Physically compatible for 4 hr at 22°C	1528	C
Propofol	ZEN[g]	10 mg/mL	MJ	1.2 mg/mL[a]	Physically compatible for 1 hr at 23°C	2066	C
Ranitidine HCl		2 mg/mL[a]	NCI	1.2 mg/mL[a]	Physically compatible for 4 hr at 22°C	1528	C
Ranitidine HCl	GL	0.5 and 2 mg/mL[a]	BR	0.3 and 1.2 mg/mL[a]	Visually compatible. No loss of either drug in 4 hr at 23°C	1741	C
Ranitidine HCl with ondansetron HCl	GL GL	2 mg/mL[a] 0.3 mg/mL[a]	BR	1.2 mg/mL[a]	Visually compatible with no loss of any drug in 4 hr at 23°C	1741	C
Sodium bicarbonate	LY	1 mEq/mL	NCI	1.2 mg/mL[a]	Physically compatible for 4 hr at 22°C	1556	C
Thiotepa	IMM[d]	1 mg/mL[a]	MJ	0.6 mg/mL[a]	Physically compatible for 4 hr at 23°C	1861	C
TNA #218 to #226[e]			MJ	1.2 mg/mL[a]	Visually compatible for 4 hr at 23°C	2215	C
Topotecan HCl	SKB	56 mcg/mL[a b]	MJ	0.54 mg/mL[a b]	Visually compatible. Little loss of either drug in 4 hr at 22°C	2245	C
TPN #212 to #215[e]			MJ	1.2 mg/mL[a]	Physically compatible for 4 hr at 23°C	2109	C
Vancomycin HCl		10 mg/mL[a]	NCI	1.2 mg/mL[a]	Physically compatible for 4 hr at 22°C	1528	C
Vinblastine sulfate	LI	0.12 mg/mL[b]	NCI	1.2 mg/mL[a]	Physically compatible for 4 hr at 22°C	1556	C
Vincristine sulfate	LI	0.05 mg/mL[a]	NCI	1.2 mg/mL[a]	Physically compatible for 4 hr at 22°C	1556	C

Y-Site Injection Compatibility (1:1 Mixture) (Cont.)

Test Drug	Mfr	Conc	Mfr	Conc	Remarks	Ref	C/I
Zidovudine	BW	4 mg/mL[a]	NCl	1.2 mg/mL[a]	Physically compatible for 4 hr at 22°C	1556	C

[a] Tested in dextrose 5%.

[b] Tested in sodium chloride 0.9%.

[c] Tested in bacteriostatic sodium chloride 0.9% preserved with benzyl alcohol 0.9%.

[d] Lyophilized formulation tested.

[e] Refer to Appendix for the composition of parenteral nutrition solutions. TNA indicates a 3-in-1 admixture, and TPN indicates a 2-in-1 admixture.

[f] Ampicillin component. Ampicillin in a 2:1 fixed-ratio concentration with sulbactam.

[g] Test performed using the formulation WITH edetate disodium.

Selected Revisions January 31, 2020. © Copyright, October 1994. American Society of Health-System Pharmacists, Inc.

Paclitaxel (albumin-bound)
AHFS 10:00

Products

Albumin-bound paclitaxel is available as a white to yellow lyophilized powder or cake in single-use vials.[3219] Each vial contains 100 mg of paclitaxel formulated as albumin-bound nanoparticles (mean particle size of approximately 130 nm).[3219] Each vial contains human albumin 900 mg with sodium caprylate and sodium acetyltryptophanate.[3219]

CAUTION: Care should be taken to ensure that the correct drug product, dose, and administration procedures are used and that no confusion with other products occurs. Albumin-bound paclitaxel should not be substituted for or with other paclitaxel formulations.[3219]

The lyophilized powder or cake should be reconstituted by slowly (over at least 1 minute) injecting 20 mL of sodium chloride 0.9%, directing the stream of diluent onto the inside wall of the vial.[3219] The diluent should *not* be injected directly onto the lyophilized powder or cake as this will result in foaming.[3219] After injection of the full volume of the diluent, the vial should be allowed to stand for at least 5 minutes to ensure proper wetting of the powder or cake, after which point the vial should be gently swirled and/or inverted slowly for at least 2 minutes until complete powder or cake dissolution has occurred.[3219] Foam generation should be avoided; if foaming or clumping occurs, the reconstituted suspension should stand for at least 15 minutes until the foaming subsides.[3219]

The reconstituted albumin-bound paclitaxel suspension should be milky, homogenous, and free of visible particulates.[3219] If particulates are visible or settling occurs, the vial should be inverted gently again to ensure resuspension prior to use.[3219] If precipitates are observed, the suspension should be discarded.[3219]

Each mL of the reconstituted suspension contains 5 mg of paclitaxel.[3219] The appropriate dose of the drug should be withdrawn from the vial and injected into an empty plasticized polyvinyl chloride (PVC) container or a PVC or non-PVC type intravenous bag.[3219]

The use of medical devices (e.g., syringes, intravenous bags) containing silicone oil as a lubricant in the preparation and administration of albumin-bound paclitaxel may result in the formation of proteinaceous strands.[3219] Following transfer of the reconstituted suspension into the intravenous bag, the suspension should be visually inspected prior to administration; the suspension should be discarded if proteinaceous strands have formed or if particulate matter or discoloration is observed.[3219]

Trade Name(s)

Abraxane

Administration

Albumin-bound paclitaxel suspension is administered by intravenous infusion over 30 or 30 to 40 minutes, depending upon the indication.[3219] The manufacturer states that limiting the infusion time to 30 minutes reduces the possibility of infusion-related reactions.[3219]

Extravasation of albumin-bound paclitaxel has been reported.[3219] The infusion site should be monitored closely for possible infiltration during administration.[3219]

As with other toxic drugs, caution should be exercised in the handling of albumin-bound paclitaxel.[3219] Manufacturers recommend the use of gloves.[3219] If skin contact with the lyophilized powder or cake or the reconstituted suspension occurs, the affected area(s) should be washed immediately and thoroughly with soap and water since tingling, burning, and redness may occur following topical exposure; for mucosal membrane contact, the affected area(s) should be flushed thoroughly with water.[3219] Procedures for the proper disposal of albumin-bound paclitaxel should be considered.[3219]

CAUTION: Care should be taken to ensure that the correct drug product, dose, and administration procedures are used and that no confusion with other products occurs.

Stability

Intact vials should be stored at 20 to 25°C in the original package to protect from bright light; neither freezing nor refrigeration of the vials is noted to adversely affect stability.[3219]

Reconstituted albumin-bound paclitaxel suspension prepared in the vial should be used immediately, but may be stored for a maximum of 24 hours at 2 to 8°C when replaced in the original carton to protect from bright light.[3219] Reconstituted albumin-bound paclitaxel suspension transferred to an infusion bag also should be used immediately, but may be stored for a maximum of 24 hours at 2 to 8°C when protected from bright light.[3219] The time after reconstitution in the vial and after transfer to an infusion bag together should not exceed a combined time of 24 hours at 2 to 8°C; however, this refrigerated storage time may be followed by additional storage of the infusion bag at ambient temperature (approximately 25°C) and lighting conditions for a maximum of 4 hours.[3219]

Vials are for single use only; unused portions should be discarded.[3219]

Plasticizer Leaching

Use of diethylhexyl phthalate (DEHP)-free containers or administration sets is *not* required for the preparation or administration of albumin-bound paclitaxel suspension.[3219]

DOI: 10.37573/9781585286850.297

Palonosetron Hydrochloride
AHFS 56:22.20

Products

Palonosetron is available as a 50-mcg/mL solution in 5-mL (0.25-mg) and 1.5-mL (0.075-mg) single-use vials containing palonosetron hydrochloride equivalent to palonosetron as the free base.[2870] Each mL of solution also contains mannitol 41.5 mg, disodium edetate, and citrate buffer in water for injection.[2870]

Equivalency

Palonosetron hydrochloride 0.28 mg is equivalent to 0.25 mg of palonosetron as the free base.[2870]

pH

From 4.5 to 5.5.[2870]

Tonicity

Palonosetron hydrochloride injection is isotonic.[2870]

Trade Name(s)

Aloxi

Administration

Palonosetron hydrochloride injection is administered intravenously without dilution.[2870]

In adults, a dose should be administered over 10 or 30 seconds, depending upon the indication.[2870] Pediatric doses should be infused over 15 minutes.[2870]

The manufacturer states that the infusion line should be flushed with sodium chloride 0.9% prior to and following administration of palonosetron hydrochloride injection.[2870]

Stability

Palonosetron hydrochloride injection is a clear, colorless solution.[2870] Intact vials of palonosetron hydrochloride injection should be stored at controlled room temperature and should be protected from light and freezing.[2870]

Palonosetron hydrochloride injection should be visually inspected for particulate matter or discoloration prior to administration.[2870]

Compatibility Information
Solution Compatibility

Palonosetron HCl

Test Soln Name	Mfr	Mfr	Conc/L or %	Remarks	Ref	C/I
Dextrose 5% in Ringer's injection, lactated	BA[a]	MGI	5 and 30 mg	Physically compatible. Stable for 48 hr at 23°C in light and 14 days at 4°C	2535	C
Dextrose 5% in sodium chloride 0.45%	BA[a]	MGI	5 and 30 mg	Physically compatible. Stable for 48 hr at 23°C in light and 14 days at 4°C	2535	C
Dextrose 5%	BA[a]	MGI	5 and 30 mg	Physically compatible. Stable for 48 hr at 23°C in light and 14 days at 4°C	2535	C
Sodium chloride 0.9%	BA[a]	MGI	5 and 30 mg	Physically compatible. Stable for 48 hr at 23°C in light and 14 days at 4°C	2535	C

[a] Tested in PVC containers.

Additive Compatibility

Palonosetron HCl

Test Drug	Mfr	Conc/L or %	Mfr	Conc/L or %	Test Solution	Remarks	Ref	C/I
Dexamethasone sodium phosphate	AMR	200 and 400 mg	MGI	5 mg	D5W, NS[a]	Physically compatible. Little loss of either drug in 48 hr at 23°C in light and 14 days at 4°C	2552	C
Rolapitant HCl	TES	1.7 g	EI	2.6 mg	[b]	Physically compatible. Little to no loss of either drug in 48 hr at 20 to 25°C and 7 days at 2 to 8°C protected from light	3373	C

[a] Tested in PVC containers.

[b] Tested in cyclic olefin copolymer (COC) and glass containers.

DOI: 10.37573/9781585286850.298

Drugs in Syringe Compatibility

Palonosetron HCl

Test Drug	Mfr	Amt	Mfr	Amt	Remarks	Ref	C/I
Dexamethasone sodium phosphate	AMR	3.3 mg/5 mL[a][b]	MGI	0.25 mg/5 mL	Physically compatible. Little loss of either drug in 48 hr at 23°C in light and 14 days at 4°C	2552	C

[a] Tested in dextrose 5%.

[b] Tested in sodium chloride 0.9%.

Y-Site Injection Compatibility (1:1 Mixture)

Palonosetron HCl

Test Drug	Mfr	Conc	Mfr	Conc	Remarks	Ref	C/I
Ampicillin sodium–sulbactam sodium	RR	20 mg/mL[b][c]	MGI	50 mcg/mL	Physically compatible and no loss of either drug in 4 hr at room temperature	2749	C
Atropine sulfate	AMR	0.4 mg/mL	MGI	50 mcg/mL	Physically compatible and no loss of either drug in 4 hr at room temperature	2771	C
Carboplatin	BMS	5 mg/mL[a]	MGI	50 mcg/mL	Physically compatible. No palonosetron and 2% carboplatin loss in 4 hr	2579	C
Cefazolin sodium	WAT	20 mg/mL[a]	MGI	50 mcg/mL	Physically compatible and no loss of either drug in 4 hr at room temperature	2749	C
Cefotetan disodium	ASZ	20 mg/mL[b]	MGI	50 mcg/mL	Physically compatible and no loss of either drug in 4 hr at room temperature	2749	C
Cisatracurium besylate	AB	0.5 mg/mL[a]	MGI	50 mcg/mL	Physically compatible with no loss of either drug in 4 hr at room temperature	2764	C
Cisplatin	BMS	0.5 mg/mL[b]	MGI	50 mcg/mL	Physically compatible. No palonosetron and 5% cisplatin loss in 4 hr	2579	C
Cyclophosphamide	MJ	10 mg/mL[a]	MGI	50 mcg/mL	Physically compatible and no loss of either drug in 4 hr	2640	C
Dacarbazine	BV	4 mg/mL[a]	MGI	50 mcg/mL	Physically compatible and no loss of either drug in 4 hr	2681	C
Docetaxel	AVE	0.8 mg/mL[a]	MGI	50 mcg/mL	Physically compatible and no loss of either drug in 4 hr	2533	C
Famotidine	BED	2 mg/mL[a]	MGI	50 mcg/mL	Physically compatible and no loss of either drug in 4 hr at room temperature	2771	C
Fentanyl citrate	AB	50 mcg/mL	MGI	50 mcg/mL	Physically compatible and no loss of either drug in 4 hr	2720	C
Fluorouracil	APP	16 mg/mL[a]	MGI	50 mcg/mL	Physically compatible and no loss of either drug in 4 hr	2627	C
Gemcitabine HCl	LI	10 mg/mL[a]	MGI	50 mcg/mL	Physically compatible and no loss of either drug in 4 hr	2627	C
Gentamicin sulfate	APP	5 mg/mL[a]	MGI	50 mcg/mL	Physically compatible. No loss of either drug in 4 hr at room temperature	2765	C
Glycopyrrolate	BA	0.2 mg/mL	MGI	50 mcg/mL	Physically compatible. No loss of either drug in 4 hr at room temperature	2773	C
Heparin sodium	HOS	100 units/mL	MGI	50 mcg/mL	Physically compatible. No loss of either drug in 4 hr at room temperature	2771	C
Hetastarch in lactated electrolyte	HOS	6%	MGI	50 mcg/mL	Physically compatible. No palonosetron loss in 4 hr at room temperature	2775	C
Hydromorphone HCl	BA	0.5 mg/mL[a]	MGI	50 mcg/mL	Physically compatible and no loss of either drug in 4 hr	2720	C
Ifosfamide	MJ	10 mg/mL[a]	MGI	50 mcg/mL	Physically compatible and no loss of either drug in 4 hr	2640	C

Y-Site Injection Compatibility (1:1 Mixture) (Cont.)

Test Drug	Mfr	Conc	Mfr	Conc	Remarks	Ref	C/I
Irinotecan HCl	PHU	1 mg/mL[a]	MGI	50 mcg/mL	Physically compatible. No palonosetron and 5% irinotecan loss in 4 hr	2609	C
Lidocaine HCl	AB	10 mg/mL[a]	MGI	50 mcg/mL	Physically compatible. No loss of either drug in 4 hr at room temperature	2771	C
Lorazepam	BA	0.5 mg/mL[a]	MGI	50 mcg/mL	Physically compatible. No loss of either drug in 4 hr	2608	C
Mannitol	HOS	15%	MGI	50 mcg/mL	Physically compatible. No palonosetron loss in 4 hr at room temperature	2775	C
Meperidine HCl	AB	10 mg/mL[a]	MGI	50 mcg/mL	Physically compatible. No loss of either drug in 4 hr	2720	C
Methylprednisolone sodium succinate	PHU	5 mg/mL[a]	MGI	50 mcg/mL	Microprecipitate begins to form immediately and becomes visible within 4 hr	2681	I
Metoclopramide HCl	BA	5 mg/mL	MGI	50 mcg/mL	Physically compatible. No loss of either drug in 4 hr	2716	C
Metronidazole	BA	5 mg/mL	MGI	50 mcg/mL	Physically compatible. No loss of either drug in 4 hr at room temperature	2765	C
Midazolam HCl	BA	2 mg/mL[a]	MGI	50 mcg/mL	Physically compatible. No loss of either drug in 4 hr	2608	C
Morphine sulfate	BA	15 mg/mL	MGI	50 mcg/mL	Physically compatible. No loss of either drug in 4 hr	2720	C
Neostigmine methylsulfate	BA	0.5 mg/mL	MGI	50 mcg/mL	Physically compatible. No loss of either drug in 4 hr	2772	C
Oxaliplatin	SS	0.5 mg/mL[a]	MGI	50 mcg/mL	Physically compatible. No loss of either drug in 4 hr	2579	C
Paclitaxel	MJ	1.2 mg/mL[a]	MGI	50 mcg/mL	Physically compatible. Little loss of either drug in 4 hr	2533	C
Potassium chloride	AB	0.1 mEq/mL[a]	MGI	50 mcg/mL	Physically compatible. No loss of either drug in 4 hr at room temperature	2771	C
Promethazine HCl	PAD	2 mg/mL[a]	MGI	50 mcg/mL	Physically compatible. No loss of either drug in 4 hr	2716	C
Rocuronium bromide	BA	1 mg/mL[a]	MGI	50 mcg/mL	Physically compatible and no loss of either drug in 4 hr at room temperature	2764	C
Succinylcholine chloride	SZ	2 mg/mL[a]	MGI	50 mcg/mL	Physically compatible and no loss of either drug in 4 hr at room temperature	2764	C
Sufentanil citrate	HOS	12.5 mcg/mL[a]	MGI	50 mcg/mL	Physically compatible. No loss of either drug in 4 hr	2720	C
Topotecan HCl	GSK	0.1 mg/mL[a]	MGI	50 mcg/mL	Physically compatible. Little loss of either drug in 4 hr	2609	C
Vancomycin HCl	HOS	5 mg/mL[a]	MGI	50 mcg/mL	Physically compatible and no loss of either drug in 4 hr at room temperature	2765	C
Vecuronium bromide	BED	1 mg/mL	MGI	50 mcg/mL	Physically compatible and no loss of either drug in 4 hr at room temperature	2764	C

[a] Tested in dextrose 5%.

[b] Tested in sodium chloride 0.9%.

[c] Ampicillin component. Ampicillin in a 2:1 fixed-ratio concentration with sulbactam.

Selected Revisions April 12, 2018. © Copyright, October 2006.
American Society of Health-System Pharmacists, Inc.

Pamidronate Disodium
AHFS 92:24

Products

Pamidronate disodium is available as a concentrate for injection in 10-mL vials containing 30, 60, or 90 mg pamidronate disodium in 10 mL water for injection.[2846][2847] Each mL of solution also contains mannitol 47, 40, or 37.5 mg, respectively, and phosphoric acid and/or sodium hydroxide to adjust the pH.[2846][2847]

Pamidronate disodium is also available as a lyophilized powder in vials containing 30 or 90 mg of the drug.[2847] Reconstitute 30- or 90-mg vial with 10 mL sterile water for injection to yield solutions containing 3 or 9 mg/mL, respectively, of pamidronate disodium.[2847] Each mL of the resulting 3- or 9-mg/mL pamidronate disodium solution also contains mannitol 47 or 37.5 mg, respectively, and phosphoric acid for pH adjustment.[2847]

pH

The injection concentrate has a pH of 6 to 7.[2846][2847]

The pH of the lyophilized product is adjusted to 6.5 prior to lyophilization.[2847] After reconstitution, the pH is 6 to 7.4.[2847]

Trade Name(s)

Aredia

Administration

Pamidronate disodium concentrate or reconstituted solution is administered by intravenous infusion over 2 to 24 hours after dilution in 250 to 1000 mL of a compatible diluent.[2846][2847]

Stability

Intact vials of pamidronate disodium concentrate and lyophilized powder for injection should be stored at controlled room temperature.[2846][2847]

After the lyophilized pamidronate disodium powder for injection has been reconstituted as directed, the manufacturer states that the drug may be stored under refrigeration for up to 24 hours.[2847]

Compatibility Information

Solution Compatibility

Pamidronate disodium

Test Soln Name	Mfr	Mfr	Conc/L or %	Remarks	Ref	C/I
Dextrose 5% in Ringer's injection		HOS, BED		Must not be mixed with calcium-containing solutions	2846, 2847	I
Dextrose 5% in Ringer's injection, lactated		HOS, BED		Must not be mixed with calcium-containing solutions	2846, 2847	I
Dextrose 5%		HOS, BED	60 and 90 mg	Stated to be stable for 24 hours at room temperature	2846, 2847	C
Dextrose 5%		HOS, BED	180 and 360 mg	Manufacturer-recommended solution	2846, 2847	C
Ringer's injection		HOS, BED		Must not be mixed with calcium-containing solutions	2846, 2847	I
Ringer's injection, lactated		HOS, BED		Must not be mixed with calcium-containing solutions	2846, 2847	I
Sodium chloride 0.45%		HOS, BED	60 and 90 mg	Stated to be stable for 24 hours at room temperature	2846, 2847	C
Sodium chloride 0.45%		HOS, BED	180 and 360 mg	Manufacturer-recommended solution	2846, 2847	C
Sodium chloride 0.9%		HOS, BED	60 and 90 mg	Stated to be stable for 24 hours at room temperature	2846, 2847	C
Sodium chloride 0.9%		HOS, BED	180 and 360 mg	Manufacturer-recommended solution	2846, 2847	C

DOI: 10.37573/9781585286850.299

Pancuronium Bromide
AHFS 12:20.20

Products

Pancuronium bromide is available in 2- and 5-mL vials containing 2 mg/mL of drug.[2871] It is also available in 10-mL vials at a concentration of 1 mg/mL.[2871 2872] Each mL (Hospira) also contains sodium acetate anhydrous 1.2 mg, benzyl alcohol 1%, and sodium chloride to adjust for isotonicity.[2872] Each mL (Teva) also contains sodium acetate anhydrous 2 mg, benzyl alcohol 1%, sodium chloride 4 mg for isotonicity, and water for injection.[2871] Acetic acid and/or sodium hydroxide is added to adjust the pH.[2871 2872]

pH

The solution has been adjusted to pH 3.8 to 4.2 by the manufacturer.[2871 2872]

Osmolality

The osmolality of pancuronium bromide (Organon) 1 mg/mL was determined to be 277 mOsm/kg by freezing-point depression and 273 mOsm/kg by vapor pressure.[1071]

The osmolality of pancuronium bromide 2 mg/mL was determined to be 338 mOsm/kg.[1233]

Administration

Pancuronium bromide is administered intravenously.[2871 2872]

Stability

Pancuronium bromide should be stored under refrigeration at 2 to 8°C.[2871 2872] However, the manufacturer indicates that the drug is stable for 6 months at room temperature.[853 1181 1433 2871 2872]

Sorption

The manufacturer indicates that pancuronium bromide in compatible infusion solutions does not undergo sorption to glass or plastic containers during short-term storage over 48 hours.[2871 2872] However, the drug may exhibit sorption to plastic containers with prolonged contact.[4]

Compatibility Information

Solution Compatibility

Pancuronium bromide

Test Soln Name	Mfr	Mfr	Conc/L or %	Remarks	Ref	C/I
Dextrose 5% in sodium chloride 0.45%				No loss in 48 hr	1(10/06)	C
Dextrose 5% in sodium chloride 0.9%				No loss in 48 hr	1(10/06)	C
Dextrose 5%				No loss in 48 hr	2871, 2872	C
Ringer's injection, lactated				No loss in 48 hr	2871, 2872	C
Sodium chloride 0.9%				No loss in 48 hr	2871, 2872	C

Additive Compatibility

Pancuronium bromide

Test Drug	Mfr	Conc/L or %	Mfr	Conc/L or %	Test Solution	Remarks	Ref	C/I
Ciprofloxacin	BAY	1.6 g	OR	200 mg	D5W	Visually compatible with no loss of ciprofloxacin in 24 hr at 22°C under fluorescent light. Pancuronium not tested	2413	C
Verapamil HCl	KN	80 mg	OR	8 mg	D5W, NS	Physically compatible for 24 hr	764	C

DOI: 10.37573/9781585286850.300

Drugs in Syringe Compatibility

Pancuronium bromide

Test Drug	Mfr	Amt	Mfr	Amt	Remarks	Ref	C/I
Caffeine citrate		20 mg/1 mL	GNS	1 mg/1 mL	Visually compatible for 4 hr at 25°C	2440	C
Heparin sodium		2500 units/1 mL		4 mg/2 mL	Physically compatible for at least 5 min	1053	C
Pantoprazole sodium	a	4 mg/1 mL		2 mg/1 mL	Orange precipitate	2574	I

a Test performed using the formulation WITHOUT edetate disodium.

Y-Site Injection Compatibility (1:1 Mixture)

Pancuronium bromide

Test Drug	Mfr	Conc	Mfr	Conc	Remarks	Ref	C/I
Aminophylline	AB	1 mg/mLᵃ	ES	0.05 mg/mLᵃ	Physically compatible for 24 hr at 28°C	1337	C
Cefazolin sodium	LY	10 mg/mLᵃ	ES	0.05 mg/mLᵃ	Physically compatible for 24 hr at 28°C	1337	C
Cefuroxime sodium	GL	7.5 mg/mLᵃ	ES	0.05 mg/mLᵃ	Physically compatible for 24 hr at 28°C	1337	C
Dexmedetomidine HCl	HOS	4 mcg/mLᵇ			Stated to be compatible	3181	C
Diazepam	ES	5 mg/mL	ES	0.05 mg/mLᵃ	Cloudy solution forms immediately	1337	I
Dobutamine HCl	LI	1 mg/mLᵃ	ES	0.05 mg/mLᵃ	Physically compatible for 24 hr at 28°C	1337	C
Dopamine HCl	SO	1.6 mg/mLᵃ	ES	0.05 mg/mLᵃ	Physically compatible for 24 hr at 28°C	1337	C
Epinephrine HCl	AB	4 mcg/mLᵃ	ES	0.05 mg/mLᵃ	Physically compatible for 24 hr at 28°C	1337	C
Esmolol HCl	DCC	10 mg/mLᵃ	ES	0.05 mg/mLᵃ	Physically compatible for 24 hr at 28°C	1337	C
Etomidate	AB	2 mg/mL	GNS	2 mg/mL	Visually compatible for 7 days at 25°C	1801	C
Fenoldopam mesylate	AB	80 mcg/mLᵇ	BA	0.1 mg/mLᵇ	Physically compatible for 4 hr at 23°C	2467	C
Fentanyl citrate	ES	10 mcg/mLᵃ	ES	0.05 mg/mLᵃ	Physically compatible for 24 hr at 28°C	1337	C
Fluconazole	RR	2 mg/mL	GNS	0.5 mg/mLᵇ	Visually compatible for 24 hr at 28°C under fluorescent light	1760	C
Gentamicin sulfate	ES	2 mg/mLᵃ	ES	0.05 mg/mLᵃ	Physically compatible for 24 hr at 28°C	1337	C
Heparin sodium	SO	40 units/mLᵃ	ES	0.05 mg/mLᵃ	Physically compatible for 24 hr at 28°C	1337	C
Hetastarch in lactated electrolyte	AB	6%	ES	0.1 mg/mLᵃ	Physically compatible for 4 hr at 23°C	2339	C
Hydrocortisone sodium succinate	AB	1 mg/mLᵃ	ES	0.05 mg/mLᵃ	Physically compatible for 24 hr at 28°C	1337	C
Isoproterenol HCl	ES	4 mcg/mL	ES	0.05 mg/mLᵃ	Physically compatible for 24 hr at 28°C	1337	C
Levofloxacin	OMN	5 mg/mLᵃ	ES	1 mg/mL	Visually compatible for 4 hr at 24°C	2233	C
Lorazepam	WY	0.5 mg/mLᵃ	ES	0.05 mg/mLᵃ	Physically compatible for 24 hr at 28°C	1337	C
Midazolam HCl	RC	0.05 mg/mLᵃ	ES	0.05 mg/mLᵃ	Physically compatible for 24 hr at 28°C	1337	C
Milrinone lactate	SW	0.4 mg/mLᵃ	GNS	1 mg/mL	Visually compatible. Little loss of either drug in 4 hr at 23°C	2214	C
Morphine sulfate	WY	1 mg/mLᵃ	ES	0.05 mg/mLᵃ	Physically compatible for 24 hr at 28°C	1337	C
Nitroglycerin	SO	0.4 mg/mLᵃ	ES	0.05 mg/mLᵃ	Physically compatible for 24 hr at 28°C	1337	C

Y-Site Injection Compatibility (1:1 Mixture) (Cont.)

Test Drug	Mfr	Conc	Mfr	Conc	Remarks	Ref	C/I
Oritavancin diphosphate	TAR	0.8, 1.2, and 2 mg/mL[a]	SIC	0.1 mg/mL[a]	Visually compatible for 4 hr at 20 to 24°C	2928	C
Propofol	STU	2 mg/mL	GNS	2 mg/mL	Oil droplets form within 7 days at 25°C. No visible change in 24 hr	1801	?
Propofol	ZEN[d]	10 mg/mL	AST	1 mg/mL	Physically compatible for 1 hr at 23°C	2066	C
Ranitidine HCl	GL	0.5 mg/mL[a]	ES	0.05 mg/mL[a]	Physically compatible for 24 hr at 28°C	1337	C
Sodium nitroprusside	ES	0.2 mg/mL[a]	ES	0.05 mg/mL[a]	Physically compatible for 24 hr at 28°C	1337	C
Trimethoprim–sulfamethoxazole	ES	0.64 mg/mL[a c]	ES	0.05 mg/mL[a]	Physically compatible for 24 hr at 28°C	1337	C
Vancomycin HCl	ES	5 mg/mL[a]	ES	0.05 mg/mL[a]	Physically compatible for 24 hr at 28°C	1337	C

[a] Tested in dextrose 5%.

[b] Tested in sodium chloride 0.9%.

[c] Trimethoprim component. Trimethoprim in a 1:5 fixed-ratio concentration with sulfamethoxazole.

[d] Test performed using the formulation WITH edetate disodium.

Selected Revisions January 31, 2020. © Copyright, October 1986. American Society of Health-System Pharmacists, Inc.

Pantoprazole Sodium
AHFS 56:28.36

Products

Pantoprazole sodium is available as a lyophilized powder in single-dose vials containing pantoprazole 40 mg as the sodium salt with edetate disodium 1 mg and sodium hydroxide to adjust pH during manufacturing.[2850][3358]

Pantoprazole sodium also is available as a lyophilized powder in single-dose vials containing pantoprazole 40 mg as the sodium salt with sodium hydroxide to adjust pH during manufacturing.[3357]

Reconstitute a 40-mg vial with 10 mL of sodium chloride 0.9% to a concentration of 4 mg/mL.[2850][3357][3358] For intravenous infusion, 1 vial (40 mg) of the reconstituted drug solution may be diluted with 100 mL or 2 vials (80 mg) may be diluted with 80 mL of sodium chloride 0.9%, dextrose 5%, or Ringer's injection, lactated to yield concentrations of about 0.4 or 0.8 mg/mL, respectively.[2850][3357][3358]

pH

The pH of the reconstituted solution ranges from 9 to 10.5 [2850][3358] or from 9.5 to 11.5.[3357]

Equivalency

Pantoprazole sodium 45.1 mg provides 40 mg of pantoprazole.[2850][3357][3358]

Trade Name(s)

Protonix I.V.

Administration

Pantoprazole sodium injection reconstituted as directed to a concentration of 4 mg/mL may be administered by intravenous infusion over a period of at least 2 minutes.[2850][3357][3358] The reconstituted solution also may be diluted in a compatible infusion solution to a concentration of about 0.4 or 0.8 mg/mL and administered by intravenous infusion over about 15 minutes.[2850][3357][3358] Manufacturers state that pantoprazole sodium injection is only for intravenous infusion and that other parenteral routes of administration are not recommended.[2850][3357][3358]

The drug also has been administered as an intravenous bolus, followed by continuous intravenous infusion administered at a rate of 8 mg/hr.[3359][3360]

Pantoprazole sodium injection should be administered intravenously through a dedicated intravenous line or Y-site.[2850][3357][3358] The intravenous line used to administer the drug should be flushed with dextrose 5%, sodium chloride 0.9%, or Ringer's injection, lactated prior to and following pantoprazole sodium administration.[2850][3357][3358]

Administration of pantoprazole sodium formulations containing edetate disodium has been associated with thrombophlebitis.[2850][3358]

Caution should be used when formulations of pantoprazole sodium injection containing edetate disodium are co-administered intravenously with other drugs containing EDTA.[2850][3358] (See Stability.)

Stability

Intact vials of pantoprazole sodium should be stored at controlled room temperature and should be protected from light during storage.[2850][3357][3358]

After reconstitution as directed, pantoprazole sodium injection may be stored for up to 6 hours at room temperature before dilution or 24 hours at room temperature if administered without dilution.[2850][3357][3358] Manufacturers note that the reconstituted[2850][3357][3358] and diluted solutions[3357] should not be frozen.

After dilution in a compatible infusion solution, the drug must be used within 24 hours from the time of initial reconstitution when stored at room temperature.[2850][3357][3358]

Reconstituted and diluted solutions of pantoprazole sodium should be visually inspected for particulate matter and discoloration prior to and during administration.[2850][3357][3358] Protection from light exposure is not required for reconstituted or diluted solutions.[2850][3357][3358]

Some formulations of pantoprazole sodium injection contain edetate disodium, the salt form of EDTA.[2850][3358] Edetate disodium may chelate metal ions (e.g., zinc), and therefore some formulations of pantoprazole sodium injection may not be compatible with products containing zinc.[2850][3358] Caution should be used when formulations of the drug containing edetate disodium are co-administered intravenously with other drugs containing EDTA.[2850][3358]

Pantoprazole sodium admixtures prepared for infusion did not undergo discoloration over 24 hours at room temperature when exposed to light;[2507] however, solutions have been noted to develop a slight yellow shade that is more apparent in more highly concentrated solutions over periods of up to 28 days.[2851] This color change did not appear to be associated with decomposition of the drug.[2851]

pH Effects

The stability of pantoprazole in solution is pH dependent; the rate of degradation of the drug increases with decreasing pH.[2850][3357][3358]

Syringes

Reconstituted pantoprazole sodium (Wyeth) 4 mg/mL in sodium chloride 0.9% in polypropylene syringes (Terumo) has been found to be physically and chemically stable for at least 96 hours at room temperature of 24°C when exposed to light and when refrigerated at 4°C.[2656]

DOI: 10.37573/9781585286850.301

Compatibility Information
Solution Compatibility

Pantoprazole sodium

Test Soln Name	Mfr	Mfr	Conc/L or %	Remarks	Ref	C/I
Dextrose 5%		WY[b], AUR[b]	400 or 800 mg	Use within 24 hr after reconstitution when stored at room temperature	2850, 3358	C
Dextrose 5%		WW[a]	400 or 800 mg	Use within 24 hr after reconstitution when stored at room temperature	3357	C
Dextrose 5%	BA	PH[a]	400 mg	Physically compatible. 10% loss occurs in 4 days at 22°C in light	2696	C
Dextrose 5%	BA	ALT[b]	160 mg	10% loss in 24 hr at 23°C. 5% loss in 14 days and 11% in 21 days at 4°C	2798	C
Dextrose 5%	BA	ALT[b]	800 mg	9% loss in 4 days at 23°C. Little loss in 21 days at 4°C	2798	C
Dextrose 5%	d	SZ[a]	400 mg	5% loss in 2 days at room temperature with exposure to light; 4% loss in 14 days under refrigeration protected from light	2851	C
Dextrose 5%	d	SZ[a]	800 mg	7% loss in 3 days at room temperature with exposure to light; 8% loss in 28 days under refrigeration protected from light	2851	C
Ringer's injection, lactated		WY[b], AUR[b]	400 or 800 mg	Use within 24 hr after reconstitution when stored at room temperature	2850, 3358	C
Ringer's injection, lactated		WW[a]	400 or 800 mg	Use within 24 hr after reconstitution when stored at room temperature	3357	C
Sodium chloride 0.9%	AB	WY[b]	4 g	Physically and chemically stable for 96 hr at 24°C in light and 4°C	2656	C
Sodium chloride 0.9%	BA	PH[a]	400 mg	Physically compatible. Less than 10% loss occurs in 10 days at 22°C in light	2696, 3082	C
Sodium chloride 0.9%	HOS	ALT[b]	160 mg	6% loss in 48 hr and 11% in 4 days at 23°C. 5% loss in 21 days at 4°C	2798	C
Sodium chloride 0.9%	HOS	ALT[b]	800 mg	4% loss in 7 days and 11% in 9 days at 23°C. Little loss in 21 days at 4°C	2798	C
Sodium chloride 0.9%	d	SZ[a]	400 mg	5% loss in 3 days at room temperature with exposure to light; 4% loss in 28 days under refrigeration protected from light	2851	C
Sodium chloride 0.9%	d	SZ[a]	800 mg	5% loss in 3 days at room temperature with exposure to light; 5% loss in 28 days under refrigeration protected from light	2851	C
Sodium chloride 0.9%		WY[b], AUR[b]	400 or 800 mg	Use within 24 hr after reconstitution when stored at room temperature	2850, 3358	C
Sodium chloride 0.9%		WW[a]	400 or 800 mg	Use within 24 hr after reconstitution when stored at room temperature	3357	C
TPN #275[c]		ALT[b]	13.3 mg	Yellow color and losses of 12% in 3 hr at room temperature in dark	2789	I

[a] Test performed using the formulation WITHOUT edetate disodium.

[b] Test performed using the formulation WITH edetate disodium.

[c] Refer to Appendix for the composition of parenteral nutrition solutions. TPN indicates a 2-in-1 admixture.

[d] Tested in PVC containers.

Drugs in Syringe Compatibility

Pantoprazole sodium

Test Drug	Mfr	Amt	Mfr	Amt	Remarks	Ref	C/I
Acetazolamide sodium		100 mg/1 mL	a	4 mg/1 mL	Clear solution	2574	C
Acyclovir sodium		50 mg/1 mL	a	4 mg/1 mL	Precipitates within 4 hr	2574	I
Alprostadil		0.5 mg/1 mL	a	4 mg/1 mL	Clear solution	2574	C
Amikacin sulfate		250 mg/1 mL	a	4 mg/1 mL	Precipitates	2574	I

Drugs in Syringe Compatibility (Cont.)

Test Drug	Mfr	Amt	Mfr	Amt	Remarks	Ref	C/I
Aminophylline		50 mg/1 mL	a	4 mg/1 mL	Clear solution	2574	C
Amiodarone HCl		50 mg/1 mL	a	4 mg/1 mL	Precipitates	2574	I
Amphotericin B		5 mg/1 mL	a	4 mg/1 mL	Opacity within 1 hr	2574	I
Ampicillin sodium		250 mg/1 mL	a	4 mg/1 mL	Clear solution	2574	C
Atropine sulfate		0.4 mg/1 mL	a	4 mg/1 mL	Incompatible after 4 hr	2574	I
Caffeine citrate		10 mg/1 mL	a	4 mg/1 mL	Precipitates	2574	I
Calcium chloride		100 mg/1 mL	a	4 mg/1 mL	Precipitates	2574	I
Calcium gluconate		100 mg/1 mL	a	4 mg/1 mL	Precipitates	2574	I
Cefazolin sodium		100 mg/1 mL	a	4 mg/1 mL	Precipitates immediately	2574	I
Cefotaxime sodium		100 mg/1 mL	a	4 mg/1 mL	Precipitates immediately	2574	I
Cefoxitin sodium		100 mg/1 mL	a	4 mg/1 mL	Precipitates immediately	2574	I
Ceftazidime		100 mg/1 mL	a	4 mg/1 mL	Precipitates immediately	2574	I
Cefuroxime sodium		100 mg/1 mL	a	4 mg/1 mL	Precipitates immediately	2574	I
Chlorpromazine HCl		25 mg/1 mL	a	4 mg/1 mL	Precipitates immediately	2574	I
Ciprofloxacin		2 mg/1 mL	a	4 mg/1 mL	Precipitates immediately	2574	I
Clindamycin phosphate		150 mg/1 mL	a	4 mg/1 mL	Precipitates within 1 hr	2574	I
Cloxacillin sodium		100 mg/1 mL	a	4 mg/1 mL	Precipitates immediately	2574	I
Cyclosporine		50 mg/1 mL	a	4 mg/1 mL	Precipitates	2574	I
Dexamethasone sodium phosphate		10 mg/1 mL	a	4 mg/1 mL	Precipitates immediately	2574	I
Diazepam		5 mg/1 mL	a	4 mg/1 mL	Red precipitate forms immediately	2574	I
Digoxin		0.05 mg/1 mL	a	4 mg/1 mL	Precipitates within 4 hr	2574	I
Dimenhydrinate		50 mg/1 mL	a	4 mg/1 mL	White precipitate	2574	I
Diphenhydramine HCl		50 mg/1 mL	a	4 mg/1 mL	Precipitates immediately	2574	I
Dobutamine HCl		12.5 mg/1 mL	a	4 mg/1 mL	White precipitate forms within 1 hr	2574	I
Dopamine HCl		40 mg/1 mL	a	4 mg/1 mL	Whitish precipitate forms within 1 hr	2574	I
Enalaprilat		1.25 mg/1 mL	a	4 mg/1 mL	Precipitate forms within 1 hr	2574	I
Epinephrine HCl		1 mg/1 mL	a	4 mg/1 mL	Precipitates	2574	I
Estrogens, conjugated		5 mg/1 mL	a	4 mg/1 mL	Possible precipitate within 1 hr	2574	I
Fentanyl citrate		50 mcg/1 mL	a	4 mg/1 mL	Possible precipitate within 15 min	2574	I
Fluconazole		2 mg/1 mL	a	4 mg/1 mL	Possible precipitate within 4 hr	2574	I
Furosemide		10 mg/1 mL	a	4 mg/1 mL	Possible precipitate within 15 min	2574	I
Gentamicin sulfate		40 mg/1 mL	a	4 mg/1 mL	Whitish precipitate	2574	I
Heparin sodium		25,000 units/1 mL	a	4 mg/1 mL	Precipitates within 1 hr	2574	I
Hydralazine HCl		20 mg/1 mL	a	4 mg/1 mL	Precipitates within 4 hr	2574	I
Hydrocortisone sodium succinate		125 mg/1 mL	a	4 mg/1 mL	Possible precipitate within 15 min	2574	I

Drugs in Syringe Compatibility (Cont.)

Test Drug	Mfr	Amt	Mfr	Amt	Remarks	Ref	C/I
Hydromorphone HCl		10 mg/1 mL	a	4 mg/1 mL	Whitish precipitate forms within 4 hr	2574	I
Indomethacin sodium trihydrate		0.5 mg/1 mL	a	4 mg/1 mL	Precipitates within 1 hr	2574	I
Insulin, regular		100 units/1 mL	a	4 mg/1 mL	Precipitates within 1 hr	2574	I
Isoproterenol HCl		0.2 mg/1 mL	a	4 mg/1 mL	Whitish precipitate	2574	I
Labetalol HCl		5 mg/1 mL	a	4 mg/1 mL	Whitish precipitate	2574	I
Lidocaine HCl		200 mg/1 mL	a	4 mg/1 mL	Precipitates within 4 hr	2574	I
Lorazepam		4 mg/1 mL	a	4 mg/1 mL	Precipitates	2574	I
Magnesium sulfate		500 mg/1 mL	a	4 mg/1 mL	Whitish precipitate	2574	I
Meperidine HCl		100 mg/1 mL	a	4 mg/1 mL	Yellowish precipitate within 15 min	2574	I
Meropenem		50 mg/1 mL	a	4 mg/1 mL	Precipitates within 15 min	2574	I
Methylprednisolone sodium succinate		62.5 mg/1 mL	a	4 mg/1 mL	Precipitates within 15 min	2574	I
Metoclopramide HCl		5 mg/1 mL	a	4 mg/1 mL	Precipitates within 15 min	2574	I
Midazolam HCl		5 mg/1 mL	a	4 mg/1 mL	Precipitates immediately	2574	I
Morphine sulfate		50 mg/1 mL	a	4 mg/1 mL	Yellowish precipitate	2574	I
Naloxone HCl		0.4 mg/1 mL	a	4 mg/1 mL	Precipitates within 4 hr	2574	I
Nitroglycerin		5 mg/1 mL	a	4 mg/1 mL	Precipitates	2574	I
Norepinephrine bitartrate		1 mg/1 mL	a	4 mg/1 mL	Precipitates within 15 min	2574	I
Octreotide acetate		0.5 mcg/1 mL	a	4 mg/1 mL	Precipitates	2574	I
Oxytocin		10 units/1 mL	a	4 mg/1 mL	Orange precipitate	2574	I
Pancuronium bromide		2 mg/1 mL	a	4 mg/1 mL	Orange precipitate	2574	I
Penicillin G sodium		500,000 units/1 mL	a	4 mg/1 mL	Clear solution	2574	C
Phenobarbital sodium		120 mg/1 mL	a	4 mg/1 mL	Precipitates within 4 hr	2574	I
Phenytoin sodium		50 mg/1 mL	a	4 mg/1 mL	Precipitates within 1 hr	2574	I
Piperacillin sodium–tazobactam sodium	a	200 mg/1 mL[b]	a	4 mg/1 mL	Precipitates within 1 hr	2574	I
Potassium chloride		2 mEq/1 mL	a	4 mg/1 mL	Clear solution	2574	C
Potassium phosphates		4 mmol/1 mL	a	4 mg/1 mL	Precipitates	2574	I
Procainamide HCl		100 mg/1 mL	a	4 mg/1 mL	Clear solution	2574	C
Prochlorperazine edisylate		5 mg/1 mL	a	4 mg/1 mL	Yellowish precipitate forms	2574	I
Propofol		10 mg/1 mL	a	4 mg/1 mL	No change seen	2574	?
Propranolol HCl		1 mg/1 mL	a	4 mg/1 mL	Precipitates	2574	I
Ranitidine HCl		25 mg/1 mL	a	4 mg/1 mL	Possible precipitate within 4 hr	2574	I
Salbutamol[d]		1 mg/1 mL	a	4 mg/1 mL	Precipitates immediately	2574	I
Sodium bicarbonate		1 mEq/1 mL	a	4 mg/1 mL	Precipitates after 1 hr	2574	I
Sodium nitroprusside		10 mg/1 mL	a	4 mg/1 mL	Precipitates within 15 min	2574	I

Drugs in Syringe Compatibility (Cont.)

Test Drug	Mfr	Amt	Mfr	Amt	Remarks	Ref	C/I
Tobramycin sulfate		40 mg/1 mL	a	4 mg/1 mL	Precipitates immediately	2574	I
Trimethoprim–sulfamethoxazole		16 mg/1 mL[c]	a	4 mg/1 mL	Possible precipitate within 1 hr	2574	I
Vancomycin HCl		50 mg/1 mL	a	4 mg/1 mL	Clear solution	2574	C
Vecuronium bromide		1 mg/1 mL	a	4 mg/1 mL	Precipitates	2574	I
Verapamil HCl		2.5 mg/1 mL	a	4 mg/1 mL	Whitish precipitate	2574	I
Zidovudine		10 mg/1 mL	a	4 mg/1 mL	Clear solution	2574	C

[a] Test performed using the formulation WITHOUT edetate disodium.

[b] Piperacillin component. Piperacillin in an 8:1 fixed-ratio concentration with tazobactam.

[c] Trimethoprim component. Trimethoprim in a 1:5 fixed-ratio concentration with sulfamethoxazole.

[d] Salt not specified.

Y-Site Injection Compatibility (1:1 Mixture)

Pantoprazole sodium

Test Drug	Mfr	Conc	Mfr	Conc	Remarks	Ref	C/I
Ampicillin sodium	NVP	10 to 40 mg/mL[a]	ALT[c]	0.16 to 0.8 mg/mL[b]	Visually compatible for 12 hr at 23°C	2603	C
Anidulafungin	VIC	0.5 mg/mL[a]	WAY[c]	0.4 mg/mL[a]	Physically compatible for 4 hr at 23°C	2617	C
Blinatumomab	AMG	0.125 mcg/mL[b]	ARR[f]	0.8 mg/mL[b]	Visually compatible for 12 hr at room temperature	3405, 3417	C
Blinatumomab	AMG	0.375 mcg/mL[b]	ARR[f]	0.8 mg/mL[b]	Particles, flakes, thin needles, or haze transiently appears when pantoprazole is added to blinatumomab; not observed when order of mixing was reversed	3405, 3417	?
Cangrelor tetrasodium	TMC	1 mg/mL[b]		0.4 mg/mL[b]	Physically compatible for 4 hr	3243	C
Caspofungin acetate	ME	0.7 mg/mL[b]	WY[d]	0.4 mg/mL[b]	Physically compatible for 4 hr at room temperature	2758	C
Caspofungin acetate	ME	0.5 mg/mL[b]	WY[d]	0.4 mg/mL[b]	White particles reported	2766	I
Cefazolin sodium	NOP	20 to 40 mg/mL[a]	ALT[c]	0.16 to 0.8 mg/mL[b]	Visually compatible for 12 hr at 23°C	2603	C
Ceftaroline fosamil	FOR	2.22 mg/mL[a b e]	WY[d]	0.4 mg/mL[a b e]	Physically compatible for 4 hr at 23°C	2826	C
Ceftolozane sulfate–tazobactam sodium	CUB	10 mg/mL[g h]	PF[d]	0.4 mg/mL[g]	Physically compatible for 2 hr	3247, 3262	C
Ceftriaxone sodium	RC	20 to 40 mg/mL[a]	ALT[c]	0.16 to 0.8 mg/mL[b]	Visually compatible for 12 hr at 23°C	2603	C
Cisatracurium besylate	AB	1 mg/mL[b]	PF	0.8 mg/mL[b f]	Increase in measured turbidity	3157	I
Cloxacillin sodium	SMX	100 mg/mL	SZ[f]	4 mg/mL	Physically compatible for up to 4 hr at room temperature	3245	C
Defibrotide sodium	JAZ	8 mg/mL[b]	TAK	1.6 mg/mL[b]	Visually compatible for 4 hr at room temperature	3149	C
Dimenhydrinate	AST	0.5 to 1 mg/mL[a]	ALT[c]	0.16 to 0.8 mg/mL[b]	Visually compatible for 12 hr at 23°C	2603	C
Dobutamine HCl	LI	1 to 4 mg/mL[a]	ALT[c]	0.16 to 0.8 mg/mL[b]	Cloudiness forms over time	2603	I

Y-Site Injection Compatibility (1:1 Mixture) (Cont.)

Test Drug	Mfr	Conc	Mfr	Conc	Remarks	Ref	C/I
Dopamine HCl	DU	0.8 to 3.2 mg/mL[a]	ALT[c]	0.16 to 0.8 mg/mL[b]	Visually compatible for 12 hr at 23°C	2603	C
Doripenem	JJ	5 mg/mL[a b]	WY[d]	0.4 mg/mL[a b]	Physically compatible for 4 hr at 23°C	2743	C
Epinephrine HCl	AB	16 to 32 mcg/mL[a]	ALT[c]	0.16 to 0.8 mg/mL[b]	Visually compatible for 12 hr at 23°C	2603	C
Eravacycline dihydro-chloride	TET	0.6 mg/mL[b]	PF	0.4 mg/mL[b]	Physically compatible for 2 hr at room temperature	3532	C
Esmolol HCl	BA	10 to 20 mg/mL[a]	ALT[c]	0.16 to 0.8 mg/mL[b]	Discoloration and reddish-brown precipitate form	2603	I
Furosemide	SX	1 to 2 mg/mL[a]	ALT[c]	0.16 to 0.8 mg/mL[b]	Visually compatible for 12 hr at 23°C	2603	C
Insulin, regular	LI	5 to 50 units/mL[a]	ALT[c]	0.16 to 0.8 mg/mL[b]	Visually compatible for 12 hr at 23°C	2603	C
Isavuconazonium sulfate	ASP	1.5 mg/mL[g]	NVP[d]	0.4 mg/mL[g]	Measured turbidity increases within 1 hr	3247, 3263	I
Letermovir	ME	[a]	[f]	[a]	Physically compatible	3398	C
Mannitol		25%	[c]	4 mg/mL	Precipitates	2574	I
Meropenem		50 mg/mL	SZ[c]	4 mg/mL[b]	Physically compatible for 4 hr at room temperature	3538, 3547	C
Meropenem–vabor-bactam	TMC	8 mg/mL[b i]	WY[d]	0.4 mg/mL[b]	Physically compatible for 3 hr at 20 to 25°C	3380	C
Midazolam HCl	SX	1 to 2 mg/mL[a]	ALT[c]	0.16 to 0.8 mg/mL[b]	Discoloration and reddish-brown precipitate form	2603	I
Midazolam HCl	RC	0.1 mg/mL	ALT[c]	8 mg/mL	Yellow color forms immediately	2727	I
Midazolam HCl			WY[d], AUR[d]		Stated to be incompatible	2850, 3358	I
Midazolam HCl			WW[c]		Stated to be incompatible	3357	I
Morphine sulfate	AB	1 to 10 mg/mL[a]	ALT[c]	0.16 to 0.8 mg/mL[b]	Visually compatible for 12 hr at 23°C	2603	C
Multivitamins	SX		[c]	4 mg/mL	Precipitates within 1 hr	2574	I
Nitroglycerin	SX	0.1 to 0.4 mg/mL[a]	ALT[c]	0.16 to 0.8 mg/mL[b]	Visually compatible for 12 hr at 23°C	2603	C
Norepinephrine bitar-trate	SX	6 to 8 mcg/mL[a]	ALT[c]	0.16 to 0.8 mg/mL[b]	Visually compatible for 12 hr at 23°C	2603	C
Norepinephrine bitar-trate	SX	64 mcg/mL[a]	ALT[c]	0.16 mg/mL[b]	Visually compatible for 12 hr at 23°C	2603	C
Norepinephrine bitar-trate	SX	64 mcg/mL[a]	ALT[c]	0.4 to 0.8 mg/mL[b]	Turns cloudy upon mixing	2603	I
Octreotide acetate	NVA	5 to 10 mcg/mL[a]	ALT[c]	0.16 to 0.4 mg/mL[b]	Yellow discoloration forms	2603	I
Octreotide acetate	NVA	7.5 to 10 mcg/mL[a]	ALT[c]	0.8 mg/mL[b]	Yellow discoloration forms	2603	I
Octreotide acetate	NVA	5 mcg/mL[a]	ALT[c]	0.8 mg/mL[b]	Visually compatible for 12 hr at 23°C	2603	C
Plazomicin sulfate	ACH	24 mg/mL[g]	WGC[j]	0.4 mg/mL[f g]	Physically compatible for 1 hr at 20 to 25°C	3432	C
Potassium chloride	AST	20 to 210 mEq/L[a]	ALT[c]	0.16 to 0.8 mg/mL[b]	Visually compatible for 12 hr at 23°C	2603	C
Tedizolid phosphate	CUB	0.8 mg/mL[b]	NVP[d]	0.4 mg/mL[b]	Physically compatible for 2 hr	3244, 3247	C
Telavancin HCl	ASP	7.5 mg/mL[a b e]	WY[d]	0.4 mg/mL[a b e]	Physically compatible for 2 hr	2830	C
Vancomycin HCl	ME	40 mg/mL	ALT[c]	8 mg/mL	Color change after 10 hr	2727	I

Y-Site Injection Compatibility (1:1 Mixture) (Cont.)

Test Drug	Mfr	Conc	Mfr	Conc	Remarks	Ref	C/I
Vasopressin	FER	0.4 to 1 unit/mL[a]	ALT[c]	0.16 to 0.8 mg/mL[b]	Visually compatible for 12 hr at 23°C	2603	C

[a] Tested in dextrose 5%

[b] Tested in sodium chloride 0.9%.

[c] Test performed using the formulation WITHOUT edetate disodium.

[d] Test performed using the formulation WITH edetate disodium.

[e] Tested in Ringer's injection, lactated.

[f] Presence or absence of edetate disodium not specified.

[g] Tested in both dextrose 5% and sodium chloride 0.9%.

[h] Ceftolozane component. Ceftolozane in a 2:1 fixed-ratio concentration with tazobactam.

[i] Meropenem component. Meropenem in a 1:1 fixed-ratio concentration with vaborbactam.

[j] Salt not specified.

Papaverine Hydrochloride
AHFS 24:12.92

Products

Papaverine hydrochloride is available in 2-mL single-dose ampuls and vials and 10-mL multiple-dose vials. Each mL of solution contains 30 mg of papaverine as the hydrochloride.[1(2/06)] [4] The multiple-dose vials also contain edetate disodium 0.005%, chlorobutanol 0.5%, and sodium hydroxide to adjust the pH.[1(2/06)] The single-dose containers are preservative free.[4]

pH

Not below 3.[17]

Administration

Papaverine hydrochloride may be administered by intramuscular or slow intravenous injection over one to two minutes.[1(2/06)] [4]

Stability

Papaverine hydrochloride injection should be stored at controlled room temperature and protected from light, temperatures of 40°C or higher, and from freezing.[1(2/06)] [4] It should not be refrigerated because of a reduction in solubility with possible precipitation.[593] The solutions should be clear and colorless to pale yellow.[1(2/06)] The yellow discoloration of papaverine hydrochloride injection does not appear to be related to drug decomposition. Analysis of a yellow injection found nearly 100% of the drug. Furthermore, yellow discoloration is not produced by intentional degradation from boiling with acid or base.[1996]

Compatibility Information

Solution Compatibility

Papaverine HCl

Test Soln Name	Mfr	Mfr	Conc/L or %	Remarks	Ref	C/I
Dextrose 2.5% in half-strength Ringer's injection	AB		96 mg	Physically compatible	3	C
Dextrose 5% in Ringer's injection	AB		96 mg	Physically compatible	3	C
Dextrose 2.5% in sodium chloride 0.45%	AB		96 mg	Physically compatible	3	C
Dextrose 2.5% in sodium chloride 0.9%	AB		96 mg	Physically compatible	3	C
Dextrose 5% in sodium chloride 0.225%	AB		96 mg	Physically compatible	3	C
Dextrose 5% in sodium chloride 0.45%	AB		96 mg	Physically compatible	3	C
Dextrose 5% in sodium chloride 0.9%	AB		96 mg	Physically compatible	3	C
Dextrose 10% in sodium chloride 0.9%	AB		96 mg	Physically compatible	3	C
Dextrose 2.5%	AB		96 mg	Physically compatible	3	C
Dextrose 5%	AB		96 mg	Physically compatible	3	C
Dextrose 10%	AB		96 mg	Physically compatible	3	C
Ionosol B in dextrose 5%	AB		96 mg	Physically compatible	3	C
Ionosol MB in dextrose 5%	AB		96 mg	Physically compatible	3	C
Ringer's injection	AB		96 mg	Physically compatible	3	C
Ringer's injection, lactated				Precipitation occurs	4	I
Sodium chloride 0.45%	AB		96 mg	Physically compatible	3	C
Sodium chloride 0.9%	AB		96 mg	Physically compatible	3	C
Sodium lactate ⅙ M	AB		96 mg	Physically compatible	3	C

DOI: 10.37573/9781585286850.302

Additive Compatibility

Papaverine HCl

Test Drug	Mfr	Conc/L or %	Mfr	Conc/L or %	Test Solution	Remarks	Ref	C/I
Theophylline		2 g		160 mg	D5W	Visually compatible with little or no loss of either drug in 48 hr	1909	C

Drugs in Syringe Compatibility

Papaverine HCl

Test Drug	Mfr	Amt	Mfr	Amt	Remarks	Ref	C/I
Iohexol	WI	64.7%, 5 mL	LI	30 mg/1 mL	Physically compatible for at least 2 hr	1438	C
Iopamidol	SQ	61%, 5 mL	LI	30 mg/1 mL	Physically compatible for at least 2 hr	1438	C
Iothalamate meglumine	MA	60%, 5 mL	LI	30 mg/1 mL	Physically compatible for at least 2 hr	1438	C
Ioxaglate meglumine–ioxaglate sodium	MA	5 mL	ME	32 mg/1 mL	Precipitate forms immediately and persists for at least 2 hr	1438	I
Ioxaglate meglumine–ioxaglate sodium	MA	3 and 5 mL	LI	30 mg/1 mL	White amorphous precipitate forms immediately and persists for 24 hr. If shaken, it dissolves in 20 to 30 min	1437	I
Ioxaglate meglumine–ioxaglate sodium	MA	5 mL	LI	30 mg/2 to 6 mL[a]	Precipitate forms	1437	I
Ioxaglate meglumine–ioxaglate sodium	MA	5 mL	LI	30 mg/11 and 16 mL[a]	Precipitate forms and then redissolves	1437	?
Ioxaglate meglumine–ioxaglate sodium	MA	5 mL	LI	30 mg/21 mL[a]	Physically compatible	1437	C
Ioxaglate meglumine–ioxaglate sodium	MA	15 and 30 mL	LI	30 mg/11 mL[a]	Physically compatible	1437	C
Ioxaglate meglumine–ioxaglate sodium	MA	5 mL	LI	60 mg/12 and 17 mL[a]	Precipitate forms	1437	I
Ioxaglate meglumine–ioxaglate sodium	MA	5 mL	LI	60 mg/22 mL[a]	Precipitate forms	1437	I
Phentolamine mesylate	BV, CI	0.5 mg/mL[b]	LI	30 mg/mL	Physically compatible. Little papaverine loss at 5 and 25°C. 1 to 3% phentolamine loss at 5°C and 4 to 5% at 25°C in 30 days	1161	C

[a] Diluted in sodium chloride 0.9%.

[b] Reconstituted with the papaverine hydrochloride injection.

Selected Revisions February 21, 2018. © Copyright, October 1982. American Society of Health-System Pharmacists, Inc.

Pemetrexed Disodium
AHFS 10:00

Products

Pemetrexed disodium is available in single-dose vials containing 100 or 500 mg of pemetrexed as the disodium salt.[3396] Vials also contain mannitol 106 or 500 mg, respectively.[3396] Hydrochloric acid and/or sodium hydroxide may have been added to adjust pH.[3396]

Each 100- or 500-mg vial of pemetrexed should be reconstituted with 4.2 or 20 mL, respectively, of sodium chloride 0.9% (without preservatives) and swirled gently until the powder is completely dissolved to yield a 25-mg/mL solution.[3396] Calcium-containing solutions should not be used for reconstitution.[3396] The reconstituted solution should be visually inspected for particulate matter and discoloration prior to dilution; if particulate matter is present, the vial should be discarded.[3396] The appropriate dose of the reconstituted solution must be diluted with additional sodium chloride 0.9% (without preservatives) to achieve a total volume of 100 mL.[3396]

Equivalency

Pemetrexed disodium 139.8 mg as the heptahydrate is equivalent to 100 mg of pemetrexed.[3396] Pemetrexed disodium 699 mg as the heptahydrate is equivalent to 500 mg of pemetrexed.[3396]

Trade Name(s)

Alimta

Administration

Pemetrexed disodium diluted for infusion should be administered by intravenous infusion over 10 minutes.[3396]

As with other toxic drugs, caution should be exercised in the handling and preparation of pemetrexed and applicable special handling and disposal procedures should be followed.[3396]

Stability

Pemetrexed disodium is a white to light-yellow or green-yellow powder that forms a clear, colorless to yellow or green-yellow solution upon reconstitution.[3396] Intact vials of pemetrexed disodium should be stored at controlled room temperature.[3396] The reconstituted solution and the diluted solution for infusion may be stored for up to 24 hours after reconstitution at 2 to 8°C.[3396] Any unused portions should be discarded.[3396]

Pemetrexed (Lilly) 9 mg/mL in sodium chloride 0.9% did not result in the loss of viability of *Pseudomonas aeruginosa* within 120 hours at room temperature of 22°C. A slight antimicrobial effect against *Staphylococcus aureus* was reported after 120 hours at room temperature; this slight effect cannot be regarded as sufficient for patient protection from growth of this microorganism. Diluted solutions should be stored under refrigeration whenever possible, and the potential for microbiological growth should be considered when assigning expiration periods.[2740]

Pemetrexed (Lilly) 25 mg/mL reconstituted with sodium chloride 0.9% was reported to be stable for 48 hours at 23°C exposed to or protected from light and for 31 days at 4°C exhibiting little or no drug loss when packaged in polypropylene syringes (Becton Dickinson) with Red Cap tip seals (Burron).[2676]

Freezing Solutions

Pemetrexed (Lilly) 2 to 20 mg/mL in dextrose 5% and also in sodium chloride 0.9% frozen at −20°C in polyvinyl chloride (PVC) bags developed substantial amounts of microparticulates, up to 30,000/mL, at all time points in the study up to 90 days. Especially concerning was the presence of hundreds of particles of 10 μm and larger, which may adversely impact patient safety. Although little loss of the drug occurred, the formation of such large quantities of microparticulates made the solutions unacceptable for use. The microparticulates that formed appeared to be related to the PVC containers because upon repeating the study in glass laboratory vessels, few microparticulates appeared.[2693]

Compatibility Information
Solution Compatibility

Pemetrexed disodium

Test Soln Name	Mfr	Mfr	Conc/L or %	Remarks	Ref	C/I
Dextrose 5%	BA[a]	LI	2, 10, 20 g	Physically compatible for 48 hr at 23°C. At 4°C, microprecipitation occurs after 24 hr. No loss in 48 hr at 23°C and in 31 days at 4°C	2689	C
Sodium chloride 0.9%		LI		May be stored for up to 24 hr after reconstitution at 2 to 8°C	3396	C

DOI: 10.37573/9781585286850.303

dtype.

Solution Compatibility (Cont.)

Test Soln Name	Mfr	Mfr	Conc/L or %	Remarks	Ref	C/I
Sodium chloride 0.9%	BA[a]	LI	2, 10, 20 g	Physically compatible for 48 hr at 23°C. At 4°C, microprecipitation occurs after 24 hr. No loss in 48 hr at 23°C and in 31 days at 4°C	2689	C
Sodium chloride 0.9%	MAC[a]	LI	5 g	About 5% loss in 28 days at 2 to 8°C. No visible precipitation, but possible microprecipitation not evaluated	2733	?

[a] Tested in PVC containers.

Y-Site Injection Compatibility (1:1 Mixture)

Pemetrexed disodium

Test Drug	Mfr	Conc	Mfr	Conc	Remarks	Ref	C/I
Acyclovir sodium	APP	7 mg/mL[a]	LI	20 mg/mL[b]	Physically compatible for 4 hr at 23°C	2564	C
Amifostine	MDI	10 mg/mL[b]	LI	20 mg/mL[b]	Physically compatible for 4 hr at 23°C	2564	C
Amikacin sulfate	APC	5 mg/mL[a]	LI	20 mg/mL[b]	Physically compatible for 4 hr at 23°C	2564	C
Aminophylline	AB	2.5 mg/mL[a]	LI	20 mg/mL[b]	Physically compatible for 4 hr at 23°C	2564	C
Amphotericin B	PHT	0.6 mg/mL[a]	LI	20 mg/mL[b]	Yellow precipitate forms immediately	2564	I
Ampicillin sodium	APC	20 mg/mL[b]	LI	20 mg/mL[b]	Physically compatible for 4 hr at 23°C	2564	C
Ampicillin sodium–sulbactam sodium	LE	20 mg/mL[b c]	LI	20 mg/mL[b]	Physically compatible for 4 hr at 23°C	2564	C
Aztreonam	BMS	40 mg/mL[a]	LI	20 mg/mL[b]	Physically compatible for 4 hr at 23°C	2564	C
Bumetanide	BA	0.04 mg/mL[a]	LI	20 mg/mL[b]	Physically compatible for 4 hr at 23°C	2564	C
Buprenorphine HCl	RKB	0.04 mg/mL[a]	LI	20 mg/mL[b]	Physically compatible for 4 hr at 23°C	2564	C
Butorphanol tartrate	BMS	0.04 mg/mL[a]	LI	20 mg/mL[b]	Physically compatible for 4 hr at 23°C	2564	C
Calcium gluconate	APP	40 mg/mL[a]	LI	20 mg/mL[b]	White microparticulates form within 4 hr	2564	I
Carboplatin	BMS	5 mg/mL[a]	LI	20 mg/mL[b]	Physically compatible for 4 hr at 23°C	2564	C
Cefazolin sodium	GVA	20 mg/mL[a]	LI	20 mg/mL[b]	Slight color darkening occurs over 4 hr	2564	I
Cefotaxime sodium	APP	20 mg/mL[a]	LI	20 mg/mL[b]	Slight color darkening occurs over 4 hr	2564	I
Cefotetan disodium	ASZ	20 mg/mL[a]	LI	20 mg/mL[b]	Color darkening and brownish discoloration occur immediately	2564	I
Cefoxitin sodium	APP	20 mg/mL[a]	LI	20 mg/mL[b]	Immediate brown discoloration	2564	I
Ceftazidime	GW	40 mg/mL[a]	LI	20 mg/mL[b]	Color darkening and brownish discoloration occur over 4 hr	2564	I
Ceftriaxone sodium	RC	20 mg/mL[a]	LI	20 mg/mL[b]	Physically compatible for 4 hr at 23°C	2564	C
Cefuroxime sodium	GSK	30 mg/mL[a]	LI	20 mg/mL[b]	Physically compatible for 4 hr at 23°C	2564	C
Chlorpromazine HCl	ES	2 mg/mL[a]	LI	20 mg/mL[b]	Cloudy precipitate forms immediately	2564	I
Ciprofloxacin	BAY	2 mg/mL[a]	LI	20 mg/mL[b]	Slight color darkening occurs over 4 hr	2564	I
Cisplatin	BMS	0.5 mg/mL[b]	LI	20 mg/mL[b]	Physically compatible for 4 hr at 23°C	2564	C
Clindamycin phosphate	PHU	10 mg/mL[a]	LI	20 mg/mL[b]	Physically compatible for 4 hr at 23°C	2564	C
Cyclophosphamide	MJ	10 mg/mL[a]	LI	20 mg/mL[b]	Physically compatible for 4 hr at 23°C	2564	C
Cytarabine	PHU	50 mg/mL	LI	20 mg/mL[b]	Physically compatible for 4 hr at 23°C	2564	C

Y-Site Injection Compatibility (1:1 Mixture) (Cont.)

Test Drug	Mfr	Conc	Mfr	Conc	Remarks	Ref	C/I
Dexamethasone sodium phosphate	AMR	1 mg/mL[a]	LI	20 mg/mL[b]	Physically compatible for 4 hr at 23°C	2564	C
Dexrazoxane HCl	PHU	5 mg/mL[a]	LI	20 mg/mL[b]	Physically compatible for 4 hr at 23°C	2564	C
Diphenhydramine HCl	ES	2 mg/mL[a]	LI	20 mg/mL[b]	Physically compatible for 4 hr at 23°C	2564	C
Dobutamine HCl	AB	4 mg/mL[a]	LI	20 mg/mL[b]	White cloudy precipitate with microparticulates forms immediately	2564	I
Docetaxel	AVE	0.8 mg/mL[a]	LI	20 mg/mL[b]	Physically compatible for 4 hr at 23°C	2564	C
Dopamine HCl	AB	3.2 mg/mL[a]	LI	20 mg/mL[b]	Physically compatible for 4 hr at 23°C	2564	C
Doxorubicin HCl	BED	1 mg/mL[a]	LI	20 mg/mL[b]	Dark-red discoloration forms immediately	2564	I
Doxycycline hyclate	APP	1 mg/mL[a]	LI	20 mg/mL[b]	Cloudy precipitate forms immediately	2564	I
Droperidol	AB	2.5 mg/mL	LI	20 mg/mL[b]	Gross white precipitate forms immediately	2564	I
Enalaprilat	BED	0.1 mg/mL[a]	LI	20 mg/mL[b]	Physically compatible for 4 hr at 23°C	2564	C
Famotidine	ESL	2 mg/mL[a]	LI	20 mg/mL[b]	Physically compatible for 4 hr at 23°C	2564	C
Fluconazole	PF	2 mg/mL	LI	20 mg/mL[b]	Physically compatible for 4 hr at 23°C	2564	C
Fluorouracil	APP	16 mg/mL[a]	LI	20 mg/mL[b]	Physically compatible for 4 hr at 23°C	2564	C
Ganciclovir sodium	RC	20 mg/mL[a]	LI	20 mg/mL[b]	Physically compatible for 4 hr at 23°C	2564	C
Gemcitabine HCl	LI	10 mg/mL[a]	LI	20 mg/mL[b]	Cloudy precipitate forms immediately	2564	I
Gentamicin sulfate	AB	5 mg/mL[a]	LI	20 mg/mL[b]	Gross white precipitate forms immediately	2564	I
Granisetron HCl	RC	0.05 mg/mL[a]	LI	20 mg/mL[b]	Physically compatible for 4 hr at 23°C	2564	C
Haloperidol lactate	APP	0.2 mg/mL[a]	LI	20 mg/mL[b]	Physically compatible for 4 hr at 23°C	2564	C
Heparin sodium	AB	100 units/mL	LI	20 mg/mL[b]	Physically compatible for 4 hr at 23°C	2564	C
Hydromorphone HCl	ES	0.5 mg/mL[a]	LI	20 mg/mL[b]	Physically compatible for 4 hr at 23°C	2564	C
Hydroxyzine HCl	APP	2 mg/mL[a]	LI	20 mg/mL[b]	Physically compatible for 4 hr at 23°C	2564	C
Ifosfamide	MJ	20 mg/mL[a]	LI	20 mg/mL[b]	Physically compatible for 4 hr at 23°C	2564	C
Irinotecan HCl	PHU	1 mg/mL[a]	LI	20 mg/mL[b]	Color darkening occurs over 4 hr	2564	I
Leucovorin calcium	SIC	2 mg/mL[a]	LI	20 mg/mL[b]	Physically compatible for 4 hr at 23°C	2564	C
Lorazepam	ES	0.5 mg/mL[a]	LI	20 mg/mL[b]	Physically compatible for 4 hr at 23°C	2564	C
Mannitol	BA	15%	LI	20 mg/mL[b]	Physically compatible for 4 hr at 23°C	2564	C
Meperidine HCl	AB	10 mg/mL[a]	LI	20 mg/mL[b]	Physically compatible for 4 hr at 23°C	2564	C
Mesna	APP	10 mg/mL[a]	LI	20 mg/mL[b]	Physically compatible for 4 hr at 23°C	2564	C
Methylprednisolone sodium succinate	PHU	5 mg/mL[a]	LI	20 mg/mL[b]	Physically compatible for 4 hr at 23°C	2564	C
Metoclopramide HCl	RB	5 mg/mL	LI	20 mg/mL[b]	Physically compatible for 4 hr at 23°C	2564	C
Metronidazole	BA	5 mg/mL	LI	20 mg/mL[b]	Color darkening and brownish discoloration occur immediately	2564	I
Mitoxantrone HCl	IMM	0.5 mg/mL[a]	LI	20 mg/mL[b]	Dark-blue precipitate forms immediately	2564	I
Morphine sulfate	ES	15 mg/mL	LI	20 mg/mL[b]	Physically compatible for 4 hr at 23°C	2564	C
Nalbuphine HCl	EN	10 mg/mL	LI	20 mg/mL[b]	White precipitate forms immediately	2564	I

Y-Site Injection Compatibility (1:1 Mixture) (Cont.)

Test Drug	Mfr	Conc	Mfr	Conc	Remarks	Ref	C/I
Ondansetron HCl	GSK	1 mg/mL[a]	LI	20 mg/mL[b]	Trace haze and microparticulates form immediately. White cloudy precipitate forms in 4 hr	2564	I
Paclitaxel	MJ	0.6 mg/mL[a]	LI	20 mg/mL[b]	Physically compatible for 4 hr at 23°C	2564	C
Potassium chloride	APP	0.1 mEq/mL[a]	LI	20 mg/mL[b]	Physically compatible for 4 hr at 23°C	2564	C
Prochlorperazine edisylate	SKB	0.5 mg/mL[a]	LI	20 mg/mL[b]	Cloudy precipitate forms immediately	2564	I
Promethazine HCl	SIC	0.5 mg/mL[a]	LI	20 mg/mL[b]	Physically compatible for 4 hr at 23°C	2564	C
Ranitidine HCl	GSK	2 mg/mL[a]	LI	20 mg/mL[b]	Physically compatible for 4 hr at 23°C	2564	C
Sodium bicarbonate	AB	1 mEq/mL	LI	20 mg/mL[b]	Physically compatible for 4 hr at 23°C	2564	C
Tobramycin sulfate	AB	5 mg/mL[a]	LI	20 mg/mL[b]	White precipitate forms immediately	2564	I
Topotecan HCl	GSK	0.1 mg/mL[a]	LI	20 mg/mL[b]	Color darkening occurs immediately	2564	I
Trimethoprim–sulfame-thoxazole	ES	0.8 mg/mL[a] [d]	LI	20 mg/mL[b]	Physically compatible for 4 hr at 23°C	2564	C
Vancomycin HCl	AB	10 mg/mL[a]	LI	20 mg/mL[b]	Physically compatible for 4 hr at 23°C	2564	C
Vinblastine sulfate	APP	0.12 mg/mL[a]	LI	20 mg/mL[b]	Physically compatible for 4 hr at 23°C	2564	C
Vincristine sulfate	SIC	0.05 mg/mL[a]	LI	20 mg/mL[b]	Physically compatible for 4 hr at 23°C	2564	C
Zidovudine	GSK	4 mg/mL[a]	LI	20 mg/mL[b]	Physically compatible for 4 hr at 23°C	2564	C

[a] Tested in dextrose 5%.

[b] Tested in sodium chloride 0.9%.

[c] Ampicillin component. Ampicillin in a 2:1 fixed-ratio concentration with sulbactam.

[d] Trimethoprim component. Trimethoprim in a 1:5 fixed-ratio concentration with sulfamethoxazole.

Selected Revisions December 12, 2018. © Copyright, October 2006. American Society of Health-System Pharmacists, Inc.

Penicillin G Potassium
AHFS 8:12.16.04
Benzylpenicillin Potassium

Products

Penicillin G potassium is available in vial sizes of 5 million and 20 million units.[1(2/08)] The commercial products contain sodium citrate and citric acid as buffers. Depending on the route of administration, reconstitute the vials with sterile water for injection, dextrose 5%, or sodium chloride 0.9%. The recommended reconstitution volumes may vary slightly among manufacturers; the amount of diluent recommended by the manufacturer should be used for reconstitution. To reconstitute the product, loosen the powder in the vials. While holding the vial horizontally, rotate it and add the diluent slowly, directing the stream against the wall of the vial. Shake the vial vigorously. When the required volume of solvent is greater than the capacity of the vial, a portion of the total volume of diluent may be added to the vial first to dissolve the drug. The resulting solution should then be withdrawn and mixed with the remainder of the needed diluent in a larger container.[1(2/08) 4]

Penicillin G potassium is also available as frozen premixed infusion solutions of 1, 2, and 3 million units in 50 mL of dextrose 4, 2.3, and 0.7%, respectively. The products also contain sodium citrate buffer; hydrochloric acid and/or sodium hydroxide may have been used to adjust the pH during manufacture.[1(2/08)]

Units

Each milligram of penicillin G potassium has 1440 to 1680 USP units. Each milligram of the powder for injection (which contains sodium citrate buffer) has 1355 to 1595 USP units.[4]

pH

The reconstituted powder for injection has a pH of 6 to 8.5.[1(2/08)] The frozen premixed infusion solutions have a pH of 5.5 to 8.[1(2/08) 4]

Osmolality

The frozen premixed penicillin G potassium infusion solutions are iso-osmotic with an osmolality of 300 mOsm/kg.[1(2/08)]

The osmolality of penicillin G potassium (Pfizer) 250,000 units/mL in sterile water for injection was determined to be 776 mOsm/kg by freezing-point depression and 767 mOsm/kg by vapor pressure.[1071] Another report cited the osmolality of this concentration as 749 mOsm/kg.[50]

The osmolality of penicillin G potassium 50,000 units/mL was 402 mOsm/kg in dextrose 5% and 414 mOsm/kg in sodium chloride 0.9%. At 100,000 units/mL, the osmolality was 535 mOsm/kg in dextrose 5% and 554 mOsm/kg in sodium chloride 0.9%.[1375]

The osmolality of penicillin G potassium was calculated for the following dilutions:[1054]

Diluent	Osmolality (mOsm/kg)	
	50 mL	100 mL
3 million units		
Dextrose 5%	411	340
Sodium chloride 0.9%	437	367
5 million units		
Dextrose 5%	501	394
Sodium chloride 0.9%	527	420

The following maximum penicillin G potassium concentrations were recommended to achieve osmolalities suitable for peripheral infusion in fluid-restricted patients:[1180]

Diluent	Maximum Concentration (units/mL)	Osmolality (mOsm/kg)
Dextrose 5%	81,568	566
Sodium chloride 0.9%	73,455	545
Sterile water for injection	147,205	513

Sodium and Potassium Content

Penicillin G potassium contains, in each million units, 1.7 mEq of potassium and 0.3 mEq of sodium.[1(2/08)]

Administration

NOTE: Do not confuse other forms of penicillin G with penicillin G potassium.

Penicillin G potassium is administered by intramuscular injection or continuous or intermittent intravenous infusion. It may also be administered by intrathecal, intra-articular, and intrapleural injections and other local instillations. Vials containing 20 million units are intended for intravenous administration. For intramuscular injections, concentrations of up to 100,000 units/mL will cause a minimum of discomfort. Higher concentrations may be used when needed.[1(2/08) 4]

In high doses, intravenous administration should be performed slowly to avoid electrolyte imbalance from the potassium content. For daily doses of 10 million units or more, the drug may be diluted in 1 or 2 L of infusion solution and administered in a 24-hour period. By intermittent intravenous infusion, one-fourth or one-sixth of the daily dose may be given over 1 to 2 hours and repeated every 6 to 4 hours, respectively. Divided doses are generally infused over 15 to 30 minutes in children and neonates.[4]

DOI: 10.37573/9781585286850.304

Stability

The drug powder is stable at room temperature. After reconstitution, the drug is stable for 7 days under refrigeration.[1(2/08)] [4]

However, penicillin G potassium 500,000 units/mL was stored at room temperature and 4°C. After 24 hours at room temperature, a new compound formed, which increased by 72 hours. Storage at 4°C substantially reduced the rate of formation. Although the activity of penicillin G potassium was retained over the time period, its potential as an antigen may change due to formation of polymers or conjugation products that may cause allergic reactions. It was recommended that the drug be freshly prepared before use or refrigerated during storage.[785]

Another study found increased formation of specific antipenicillin antibodies in patients administered aged penicillin solutions, not only at room temperature, but also 4°C. The causative antigens were degradation or transformation products of penicillin G. Freshly prepared solutions did not seem to be immunogenic.[946]

pH Effects

The stability of penicillin G potassium 500,000 units/mL is greatest at pH 7.[160] Penicillin G activity rapidly declines at pH 5.5 and below and at pH values above 8.[47]

Penicillin G potassium is both an acid- and alkali-labile drug. It should not be mixed with drugs that may result in a final pH outside of its stability range of pH 5.5 to 8.[47] Unfortunately, the citrate buffer is of little value in the presence of strongly acidic or alkaline drugs.[48]

The times to 10% decomposition of combinations of penicillin G potassium buffered with multivitamin infusion concentrate in dextrose 5% and sodium chloride 0.9% have been calculated on the basis of the final pH of the admixture:[304]

Penicillin G Potassium	Multivitamin Infusion Concentrate	pH	Time to 10% Decomposition
1 million units/L	1 mL/L	5.1	6.51 hr
1 million units/L	5 mL/L	4.9	4.56 hr
3 million units/L	1 mL/L	5.4	13.54 hr
3 million units/L	5 mL/L	5	6.38 hr
5 million units/L	1 mL/L	5.7	22.01 hr
5 million units/L	5 mL/L	5.1	6.51 hr
10 million units/L	1 mL/L	5.9	over 24 hr
10 million units/L	5 mL/L	5.4	13.54 hr

Freezing Solutions

Frozen premixed infusion solutions of penicillin G potassium are stable for at least 90 days from shipping stored at −20°C. The frozen solutions should be thawed at room temperature or under refrigeration and, once thawed, should not be refrozen. Thawing should not be performed using a warm water bath or microwave radiation. Thawed solutions are stated to be stable for 24 hours at room temperature and for 14 days under refrigeration.[4]

Penicillin G potassium 1 million units/100 mL of dextrose 5% in polyvinyl chloride (PVC) bags was frozen at −20°C for 30 days and then thawed by exposure to ambient temperature or microwave radiation. No evidence of precipitation or color change was observed, and a 3 to 4% loss was reported. The thawed solution at room temperature was physically compatible and exhibited no further loss over 24 hours.[554]

A fivefold increase in particles of 2 to 60 μm was produced by freezing and thawing penicillin G potassium (Squibb) 2 million units/100 mL of dextrose 5% (Travenol). The constituted drug was filtered through a 0.45-μm filter into PVC bags of solution and frozen for 7 days at −20°C. Thawing was performed at 29°C for 12 hours. Although the total number of particles increased significantly, no particles greater than 60 μm were observed; the solutions complied with USP standards for particle sizes and numbers in large volume parenteral solutions.[822]

Penicillin G potassium 1 million units/50 mL of sodium chloride 0.9% lost 5% in 16 days and 7% in 25 days when frozen at −7°C. However, samples of the same solution stored at 4°C showed similar results, indicating a lack of advantage for frozen storage.[1035]

Ambulatory Pumps

The stability of penicillin G potassium 100,000 and 200,000 units/mL in sterile water for injection was evaluated in PVC portable pump reservoirs (Pharmacia Deltec). A 6% loss occurred in 3 days at 25°C. The 200,000-unit/mL concentration was also tested stored at 5°C. A 3% loss occurred in 14 days.[2080]

Elastomeric Reservoir Pumps

Penicillin G potassium (Pfizer) 40,000 units/mL in both dextrose 5% and sodium chloride 0.9% was evaluated for binding potential to natural rubber elastomeric reservoirs (Baxter). No binding was found after storage for 2 weeks at 35°C with gentle agitation.[2014]

Filtration

Filtering penicillin G potassium (Pfizer) through 5-μm stainless steel and 0.22-μm cellulose ester inline filters resulted in no significant reduction in activity under conditions of varying doses, temperatures, flow rates, and administration methods.[167]

Compatibility Information
Solution Compatibility

Penicillin G potassium

Test Soln Name	Mfr	Mfr	Conc/L or %	Remarks	Ref	C/I
Amino acids 4.25%, dextrose 25%	MG	LI	1 million units[b]	No increase in particulate matter in 24 hr at 5°C	349	C
Amino acids 4.25%, dextrose 25%	MG	LI	1 million units[b]	No increase in particulate matter in 24 hr at 5°C	349	C
Dextrose 2.5% in half-strength Ringer's injection	AB		1 million units[b]	Physically compatible	3	C
Dextrose 5% in Ringer's injection	AB		1 million units[b]	Physically compatible	3	C
Dextrose 5% in half-strength Ringer's injection, lactated	AB		1 million units[b]	Physically compatible	3	C
Dextrose 2.5% in Ringer's injection, lactated	AB		1 million units[b]	Physically compatible	3	C
Dextrose 5% in Ringer's injection, lactated	AB		1 million units[b]	Physically compatible	3	C
Dextrose 5% in Ringer's injection, lactated	TR[c]	SQ	10 million units[b]	Stable for 24 hr at 5°C	282	C
Dextrose 10% in Ringer's injection, lactated	AB		1 million units[b]	Physically compatible	3	C
Dextrose 2.5% in sodium chloride 0.45%	AB		1 million units[b]	Physically compatible	3	C
Dextrose 2.5% in sodium chloride 0.9%	AB		1 million units[b]	Physically compatible	3	C
Dextrose 5% in sodium chloride 0.225%	AB		1 million units[b]	Physically compatible	3	C
Dextrose 5% in sodium chloride 0.45%	AB		1 million units[b]	Physically compatible	3	C
Dextrose 5% in sodium chloride 0.9%	AB		1 million units[b]	Physically compatible	3	C
Dextrose 5% in sodium chloride 0.9%	MG	SQ	5 million units[b]	Stable for 24 hr at 4 and 25°C	105	C
Dextrose 5% in sodium chloride 0.9%		SQ	2 million units[b]	Stable for 24 hr	109	C
Dextrose 5% in sodium chloride 0.9%	AB, BA, CU	[a]	5 million units[b]	Stable for 48 hr at 25°C	164	C
Dextrose 5% in sodium chloride 0.9%			1 million units[b]	Physically compatible	74	C
Dextrose 5% in sodium chloride 0.9%	TR[c]	SQ	10 million units[b]	Stable for 24 hr at 5°C	282	C
Dextrose 10% in sodium chloride 0.9%	AB		1 million units[b]	Physically compatible	3	C
Dextrose 2.5%	AB		1 million units[b]	Physically compatible	3	C
Dextrose 5%	AB		1 million units[b]	Physically compatible	3	C
Dextrose 5%			10 million units[b]	No decomposition in 12 hr	165	C
Dextrose 5%			100 million units[b]	7.5% decomposition in 48 hr at 25°C and none at 5°C	141	C
Dextrose 5%	MG	SQ	5 million units[b]	Stable for 24 hr at 4 and 25°C	105	C
Dextrose 5%		SQ	2 million units[b]	Stable for 24 hr	109	C
Dextrose 5%		[a]	900,000 units	Stable for 24 hr at 25°C	48	C
Dextrose 5%			1 million units[b]	Physically compatible	74	C
Dextrose 5%	TR[c]	SQ	10 million units[b]	Stable for 24 hr at 5°C	282	C

Solution Compatibility (Cont.)

Test Soln Name	Mfr	Mfr	Conc/L or %	Remarks	Ref	C/I
Dextrose 5%	BA[c], TR	AY	40 million units[b]	Stable for 24 hr at 5 and 22°C	298	C
Dextrose 5%	TR[d]	SQ	10 million units[b]	Physically compatible. 5% loss in 24 hr at room temperature	554	C
Dextrose 10%	AB		1 million units[b]	Physically compatible	3	C
Dextrose 10%	MG	SQ	5 million units[b]	Stable for 24 hr at 4 and 25°C	105	C
Dextrose 10%		SQ	2 million units[b]	Stable for 24 hr	109	C
Isolyte M in dextrose 5%	MG	SQ	5 million units[b]	Stable for 24 hr at 4 and 25°C	105	C
Isolyte P in dextrose 5%	MG	SQ	5 million units[b]	Stable for 24 hr at 4 and 25°C	105	C
Ionosol B in dextrose 5%	AB		1 million units[b]	Physically compatible	3	C
Ionosol MB in dextrose 5%	AB		1 million units[b]	Physically compatible	3	C
Ringer's injection	AB		1 million units[b]	Physically compatible	3	C
Ringer's injection, lactated	AB		1 million units[b]	Physically compatible	3	C
Ringer's injection, lactated	MG	SQ	5 million units[b]	Stable for 24 hr at 4 and 25°C	105	C
Ringer's injection, lactated			1 million units[b]	Physically compatible	74	C
Ringer's injection, lactated	TR[c]	SQ	10 million units[b]	Stable for 24 hr at 5°C	282	C
Sodium chloride 0.45%	AB		1 million units[b]	Physically compatible	3	C
Sodium chloride 0.9%	AB		1 million units[b]	Physically compatible	3	C
Sodium chloride 0.9%			100 million units[b]	Stable for 48 hr at 5°C	141	C
Sodium chloride 0.9%	MG	SQ	5 million units[b]	Stable for 24 hr at 4 and 25°C	105	C
Sodium chloride 0.9%		SQ	2 million units[b]	Stable for 24 hr	109	C
Sodium chloride 0.9%	AB, BA, CU	[a]	5 million units[b]	Stable for 48 hr at 25°C	164	C
Sodium chloride 0.9%			1 million units[b]	Physically compatible	74	C
Sodium chloride 0.9%	TR[c]	SQ	10 million units[b]	Stable for 24 hr at 5°C	282	C
Sodium chloride 0.9%	BA[c], TR	AY	40 million units[b]	Stable for 24 hr at 5 and 22°C	298	C
Sodium chloride 0.9%	TR[d]	PD	20 million units[b]	5% loss at 24°C and no loss at 4°C in 4 days	1035	C
TPN #21[e]		SQ	5 million units[b]	Activity retained for 24 hr at 4 and 25°C	87	C
TPN #22[e]		AY	25 million units[b]	Physically compatible with no loss of activity in 24 hr at 22°C in dark	837	C
TPN #107[e]			2 g	Activity retained for 24 hr at 21°C	1326	C

[a] Indicate a buffered preparation.

[b] Million units.

[c] Tested in both glass and PVC containers.

[d] Tested in PVC containers.

[e] Refer to Appendix for the composition of parenteral nutrition solutions. TPN indicates a 2-in-1 admixture.

Additive Compatibility

Penicillin G potassium

Test Drug	Mfr	Conc/L or %	Mfr	Conc/L or %	Test Solution	Remarks	Ref	C/I
Amikacin sulfate	BR	5 g	LI	20 million units	D5LR, D5R, D5S, D5W, D10W, LR, NS, R, SL	Physically compatible and both stable for 24 hr at 25°C	293	C
Aminophylline	SE	500 mg	a	900,000 units	D5W	22% penicillin loss in 6 hr at 25°C	48	I
Aminophylline	SE	500 mg	SQ	1 million units	D5W	44% penicillin loss in 24 hr at 25°C	47	I
Amphotericin B		200 mg	BP	10 million units	D5W	Haze develops over 3 hr	26	I
Amphotericin B	SQ	50 mg	SQ	5 million units		Precipitate forms within 1 hr	47	I
Amphotericin B	SQ	100 mg	SQ	20 million units	D5W	Physically incompatible	15	I
Ascorbic acid	AB	1 g		1 million units		Physically compatible	3	C
Ascorbic acid	PD	500 mg	SQ	10 million units	D5W	1% penicillin loss in 8 hr	166	C
Calcium chloride	UP	1 g	SQ	20 million units	D5W	Physically compatible	15	C
Calcium gluconate	UP	1 g	SQ	20 million units	D5W	Physically compatible	15	C
Calcium gluconate		1 g		1 million units	D5W	Physically compatible	74	C
Chloramphenicol sodium succinate	PD	10 g	SQ	20 million units	D5W	Physically compatible	15	C
Chloramphenicol sodium succinate	PD	1 g	SQ	5 million units		Physically compatible	47	C
Chloramphenicol sodium succinate	PD	500 mg	SQ	1 million units	D5S, D5W	Therapeutic availability maintained	110	C
Chloramphenicol sodium succinate	PD	1 g	SQ	5 and 10 million units	D5S, D5W	Therapeutic availability maintained	110	C
Chloramphenicol sodium succinate	PD	1 g		1 million units		Physically compatible	3	C
Chloramphenicol sodium succinate	PD	1 g	SQ	10 million units		Physically compatible	6	C
Chlorpromazine HCl	BP	200 mg	BP	10 million units	NS	Haze develops over 3 hr	26	I
Colistimethate sodium	WC	500 mg	SQ	20 million units	D5W	Physically compatible	15	C
Colistimethate sodium	WC	500 mg	SQ	5 million units	D	Physically compatible	47	C
Dextran 40		10%		6 million units	D5W	34% loss in 24 hr at 20°C	834	I
Dimenhydrinate	SE	50 mg		1 million units	D5W	Physically compatible	74	C
Diphenhydramine HCl	PD	80 mg	SQ	20 million units	D5W	Physically compatible	15	C
Diphenhydramine HCl	PD	50 mg	SQ	1 million units	D5W	Physically compatible. Penicillin stable for 24 hr at 25°C	47	C
Dopamine HCl	AS	800 mg	LI	20 million units	D5W	14% penicillin loss in 24 hr at 25°C. Dopamine stable for 24 hr	78	I
Ephedrine sulfate		50 mg		1 million units		Physically compatible	3	C
Ephedrine sulfate	AB	50 mg	SQ	5 million units		Physically compatible	47	C
Erythromycin lactobi-onate	AB	5 g	SQ	20 million units	D5W	Physically compatible	15	C

Additive Compatibility (Cont.)

Test Drug	Mfr	Conc/L or %	Mfr	Conc/L or %	Test Solution	Remarks	Ref	C/I
Erythromycin lactobionate	AB	1 g	SQ	5 million units		Physically compatible	20, 47	C
Erythromycin lactobionate	AB	1 g		1 million units		Physically compatible	3	C
Heparin sodium		12,000 units		1 million units	D5W	Physically compatible	74	C
Heparin sodium	AB	20,000 units	SQ	1 million units	D5W	Penicillin stable for 24 hr at 25°C	47	C
Heparin sodium	UP	4000 units	SQ	20 million units	D5W	Physically incompatible	15	I
Hydrocortisone sodium succinate	UP	500 mg	SQ	20 million units	D5W	Physically compatible	15	C
Hydrocortisone sodium succinate	UP	250 mg	SQ	5 million units	D	Physically compatible	47	C
Hydrocortisone sodium succinate	UP	100 mg		1 million units	D5W	Physically compatible	74	C
Hydroxyzine HCl	RR	250 mg	SQ	20 million units	D5W	Physically incompatible	15	I
Lidocaine HCl	AST	2 g	SQ	1 million units		Physically compatible	24	C
Lincomycin HCl	UP	6 g	SQ	20 million units	D5W	Physically compatible	15	C
Lincomycin HCl	UP	600 mg	SQ	5 million units	D	Physically compatible	47	C
Magnesium sulfate		1 g	PF	500 mg	W	5% penicillin loss in 1 day and 13% in 2 days at 24°C	999	C
Magnesium sulfate		2 to 8 g	PF	500 mg	W	7 to 8% penicillin loss in 1 day and 20 to 25% in 2 days at 24°C	999	C
Methylprednisolone sodium succinate	UP	80 mg		2 to 10 million units	D5S, D5W, LR	Clear solution for 24 hr	329	C
Metronidazole	SE	5 g	PF	200 million units		5% penicillin loss in 22 hr and 8% in 72 hr at 25°C. 2% penicillin loss in 12 days at 5°C. No metronidazole loss	993	C
Pentobarbital sodium	AB	500 mg	a	900,000 units	D5W	17% penicillin loss in 6 hr at 25°C	48	I
Pentobarbital sodium	AB	500 mg	SQ	1 million units	D5W	42% penicillin loss in 24 hr at 25°C	47	I
Polymyxin B sulfate	BW	200 mg	SQ	20 million units	D5W	Physically compatible	15	C
Polymyxin B sulfate	BW	200 mg	SQ	5 million units	D	Physically compatible	47	C
Potassium chloride		20 mEq	SQ	1 million units	D5S, D5W	Therapeutic availability maintained	110	C
Potassium chloride		40 mEq	SQ	5 million units	D5S, D5W	Therapeutic availability maintained	110	C
Potassium chloride	AB	40 mEq	SQ	5 million units		Physically compatible	47	C
Prochlorperazine edisylate	SKF	10 mg	SQ	5 million units	D5W	Physically compatible. Penicillin stable for 24 hr at 25°C	47	C
Prochlorperazine edisylate	SKF	10 mg	a	900,000 units	D5W	Penicillin stable for 24 hr at 25°C	48	C
Prochlorperazine mesylate	BP	100 mg	BP	10 million units	NS	Haze develops over 3 hr	26	I
Promethazine HCl	WY	100 mg	SQ	5 million units		Physically compatible	47	C
Promethazine HCl	WY	100 mg		1 million units		Physically compatible	3	C
Promethazine HCl	WY	250 mg	SQ	20 million units	D5W	Physically incompatible	15	I

Additive Compatibility (Cont.)

Test Drug	Mfr	Conc/L or %	Mfr	Conc/L or %	Test Solution	Remarks	Ref	C/I
Ranitidine HCl	GL	50 mg and 2 g		24 million units	D5W, NS	Physically compatible. Ranitidine stable for 24 hr at 25°C. Penicillin not tested	1515	C
Sodium bicarbonate		0.5 and 0.75 g	SQ	1 million units	D5W	Penicillin loss at 20°C due to pH	135	I
Sodium bicarbonate		3.75 g	a	900,000 units	D5W	26% penicillin loss in 24 hr at 25°C	48	I
Sodium bicarbonate	AB	3.75 g	SQ	1 million units	D5W	26% penicillin loss in 24 hr at 25°C	47	I
Sodium bicarbonate	AB	2.4 mEq[b]		100 million units	D5W	Physically compatible for 24 hr	772	C
Tranexamic acid	PF					Manufacturer states incompatible	2887	I
Verapamil HCl	KN	80 mg	SQ	10 million units	D5W, NS	Physically compatible for 24 hr	764	C
Verapamil HCl	SE	c	PD	62.5 g	D5W, NS	Physically compatible for 24 hr at 21°C under fluorescent light	1166	C

[a] Indicate a buffered preparation.

[b] One vial of Neut added to a liter of admixture.

[c] Final concentration unspecified.

Drugs in Syringe Compatibility

Penicillin G potassium

Test Drug	Mfr	Amt	Mfr	Amt	Remarks	Ref	C/I
Metoclopramide HCl	RB	10 mg/2 mL	SQ	250,000 units/1 mL	Incompatible. If mixed, use immediately	924, 1167	I
Metoclopramide HCl	RB	10 mg/2 mL	SQ	1 million units/4 mL	Incompatible. If mixed, use immediately	924, 1167	I

Y-Site Injection Compatibility (1:1 Mixture)

Penicillin G potassium

Test Drug	Mfr	Conc	Mfr	Conc	Remarks	Ref	C/I
Acyclovir sodium	BW	5 mg/mL[a]	PF	40,000 units/mL[a]	Physically compatible for 4 hr at 25°C	1157	C
Amiodarone HCl	LZ	4 mg/mL[c]	PF	100,000 units/mL[c]	Physically compatible for 4 hr at room temperature	1444	C
Ceftolozane sulfate–tazobactam sodium	CUB	10 mg/mL[c I]	PF	100,000 units/mL[c]	Physically compatible for 2 hr	3262	C
Cyclophosphamide	MJ	20 mg/mL[a]	PF	100,000 units/mL[a]	Physically compatible for 4 hr at 25°C	1194	C
Diltiazem HCl	MMD	1[b] and 5 mg/mL	RR	1 million units/mL	Visually compatible	1807	C
Diltiazem HCl	MMD	5 mg/mL	RR	100,000 units/mL[b]	Visually compatible	1807	C
Enalaprilat	MSD	0.05 mg/mL[b]	PF	50,000 units/mL[a]	Physically compatible for 24 hr at room temperature under fluorescent light	1355	C
Esmolol HCl	DCC	10 mg/mL[a]	PF	50,000 units/mL[a]	Physically compatible for 24 hr at 22°C	1169	C
Fluconazole	RR	2 mg/mL	RR	100,000 units/mL	Physically compatible for 24 hr at 25°C	1407	C
Foscarnet sodium	AST	24 mg/mL	SQ	100,000 units/mL	Physically compatible for 24 hr at room temperature under fluorescent light	1335	C

Y-Site Injection Compatibility (1:1 Mixture) (Cont.)

Test Drug	Mfr	Conc	Mfr	Conc	Remarks	Ref	C/I
Heparin sodium	TR	50 units/mL	RR	40,000 units/mL[b]	Visually compatible for 4 hr at 25°C	1793	C
Heparin sodium[j]	RI	1000 units/L[d]	LI	200,000 units/mL	Physically compatible for 4 hr at room temperature	322	C
Hydrocortisone sodium succinate[k]	UP	100 mg/L[d]	LI	200,000 units/mL	Physically compatible for 4 hr at room temperature	322	C
Hydromorphone HCl	WY	0.2 mg/mL[a]	PF	100,000 units/mL[a]	Physically compatible for 4 hr at 25°C	987	C
Isavuconazonium sulfate	ASP	1.5 mg/mL[a]	PF	100,000 units/mL[a]	Measured turbidity increases within 1 hr	3263	I
Isavuconazonium sulfate	ASP	1.5 mg/mL[b]	PF	100.000 units/mL[b]	Physically compatible for 2 hr	3263	C
Labetalol HCl	SC	1 mg/mL[a]	PF	50,000 units/mL[a]	Physically compatible for 24 hr at 18°C	1171	C
Magnesium sulfate	IX	16.7, 33.3, 66.7, 100 mg/mL[a]	SQ	100,000 units/mL[a]	Physically compatible for at least 4 hr at 32°C	813	C
Meperidine HCl	WY	10 mg/mL[a]	PF	100,000 units/mL[a]	Physically compatible for 4 hr at 25°C	987	C
Meropenem–vabor-bactam	TMC	8 mg/mL[b m]	PF	100,000 units/mL[b]	Physically compatible for 3 hr at 20 to 25°C	3380	C
Morphine sulfate	WI	1 mg/mL[a]	PF	100,000 units/mL[a]	Physically compatible for 4 hr at 25°C	987	C
Nicardipine HCl	DCC	0.1 mg/mL[a]	PF	50,000 units/mL[a]	Visually compatible for 24 hr at room temperature	235	C
Plazomicin sulfate	ACH	24 mg/mL[c]	PF	100,000 units/mL[c]	Physically compatible for 1 hr at 20 to 25°C	3432	C
Potassium chloride		40 mEq/L[d]	LI	200,000 units/mL	Physically compatible for 4 hr at room temperature	322	C
Tacrolimus	FUJ	1 mg/mL[b]	BR	100,000 units/mL[a]	Visually compatible for 24 hr at 25°C	1630	C
Tedizolid phosphate	CUB	0.8 mg/mL[b]	PF	100,000 units/mL[b]	Immediate change in measured turbidity	3244	I
Theophylline	TR	4 mg/mL	RR	40,000 units/mL[b]	Visually compatible for 6 hr at 25°C	1793	C
TNA #73[e]		32.5 mL[f]	SQ	40,000 units/mL[a]	Visually compatible for 4 hr at 25°C	1008	C
TPN #54[e]				320,000 and 500,000 units/mL	Physically compatible and 88% penicillin activity retained over 6 hr at 22°C	1045	C
TPN #61[e]		[g]	PF	200,000 units/ 2 mL[h]	Physically compatible	1012	C
TPN #61[e]		[i]	PF	1.2 million units/1.2 mL[h]	Physically compatible	1012	C
TPN #189[e]				300 mg/mL[b]	Visually compatible for 24 hr at 22°C	1767	C
TPN #203, #204[e]			MAR	500,000 units/mL	Visually compatible for 2 hr at 23°C	1974	C

Y-Site Injection Compatibility (1:1 Mixture) (Cont.)

Test Drug	Mfr	Conc	Mfr	Conc	Remarks	Ref	C/I
Verapamil HCl	SE	2.5 mg/mL	PD	62.5 mg/mL[c]	Physically compatible for 15 min at 21°C	1166	C

[a] Tested in dextrose 5%.

[b] Tested in sodium chloride 0.9%.

[c] Tested in both dextrose 5% and sodium chloride 0.9%.

[d] Tested in dextrose 5%, Ringer's injection, lactated, and sodium chloride 0.9%.

[e] Refer to Appendix for the composition of parenteral nutrition solutions. TNA indicates a 3-in-1 admixture, and TPN indicates a 2-in-1 admixture.

[f] A 32.5-mL sample of parenteral nutrition solution mixed with 50 mL of antibiotic solution.

[g] Run at 21 mL/hr.

[h] Given over five minutes by syringe pump.

[i] Run at 94 mL/hr.

[j] Tested in combination with hydrocortisone sodium succinate (Upjohn) 100 mg/L.

[k] Tested in combination with heparin sodium (Riker) 1000 units/L.

[l] Ceftolozane component. Ceftolozane in a 2:1 fixed-ratio concentration with tazobactam.

[m] Meropenem component. Meropenem in a 1:1 fixed-ratio concentration with vaborbactam.

Additional Compatibility Information

Peritoneal Dialysis Solutions

The activity of penicillin G 6 mg/L was evaluated in peritoneal dialysis fluids containing dextrose 1.5 and 4.25% (Dianeal 137, Travenol). Storage at 25°C resulted in about a 25% loss of antimicrobial activity in 24 hours. The loss of activity was attributed to the pH (5.2) of the dialysis fluids.[515]

However, penicillin G potassium (Parke-Davis) 500,000 units/L in peritoneal dialysis concentrate (Travenol) containing dextrose 30% with and without heparin sodium 2500 units/L underwent substantial reduction in activity within as little as 10 minutes.[273]

Selected Revisions June 1, 2019. © Copyright, October 1982. American Society of Health-System Pharmacists, Inc.

Penicillin G Sodium
AHFS 8:12.16.04
Benzylpenicillin Sodium

Products

Penicillin G sodium is available in vials containing 5 million units of drug with sodium citrate and citric acid as buffers. Depending on the route of administration, reconstitute the vials with sterile water for injection, dextrose 5%, or sodium chloride 0.9%; reconstitution of the 5 million-unit vial with 3 or 8 mL of diluent results in a final concentration of 1 million or 500,000 units/mL, respectively. Loosen the powder in the vial; while holding the vial horizontally, rotate it, and add the diluent slowly, directing the stream against the wall of the vial. Shake the vial vigorously.[1(11/06) 4]

Units

Each milligram of penicillin G sodium has 1500 to 1750 USP units. Each milligram of the powder for injection (which contains sodium citrate buffer) has 1420 to 1667 USP units.[4]

pH

From 5 to 7.5.[1(11/06)]

Osmolality

Penicillin G sodium 250,000 units/mL in sterile water for injection has an osmolality of 795 mOsm/kg.[50]

The osmolality of penicillin G sodium was calculated for the following dilutions:[1054]

Diluent	Osmolality (mOsm/kg)	
	50 mL	100 mL
3 million units		
Dextrose 5%	413	341
Sodium chloride 0.9%	439	368
5 million units		
Dextrose 5%	502	394
Sodium chloride 0.9%	529	421

The following maximum penicillin G sodium concentrations were recommended to achieve osmolalities suitable for peripheral infusion in fluid-restricted patients:[1180]

Diluent	Maximum Concentration (units/mL)	Osmolality (mOsm/kg)
Dextrose 5%	85,383	573
Sodium chloride 0.9%	76,891	563
Sterile water for injection	154,091	545

Sodium Content

Penicillin G sodium contains 1.68 mEq of sodium per million units.[1(11/06)]

Administration

NOTE: Do not confuse other forms of penicillin G with penicillin G sodium.

Penicillin G sodium is administered by intramuscular injection or by continuous or intermittent intravenous infusion. For intramuscular injections, concentrations of up to 100,000 units/mL will cause a minimum of discomfort. Higher concentrations may be used when needed. In high doses, intravenous administration should be performed slowly to avoid electrolyte imbalance from the sodium content. For daily doses of 10 million units or more, the drug may be diluted in 1 or 2 L of infusion solution and administered in a 24-hour period. By intermittent intravenous infusion, one-fourth or one-sixth of the daily dose may be given over 1 to 2 hours and repeated every 6 to 4 hours, respectively. Divided doses are generally infused over 15 to 30 minutes in children and neonates.[4]

Stability

The dry powder may be stored at controlled room temperature. After reconstitution, solutions may be stored for 3 days[1(11/06)] to 7 days[4] under refrigeration. Intravenous infusions containing this drug are stable at room temperature for at least 24 hours.[4]

The activity of penicillin G 6 mg/L was evaluated in peritoneal dialysis fluids containing dextrose 1.5 and 4.25% (Dianeal 137, Travenol). Storage at 25°C resulted in about a 25% loss of antimicrobial activity in 24 hours. The loss of activity was attributed to the pH (5.2) of the dialysis fluids.[515]

pH Effects

At 25°C, the maximum stability of penicillin G sodium is attained at pH 6.8,[131] but little difference in the rate of decomposition occurs in the pH range of 6.5 to 7.5.[1947] Not more than 10% loss occurs in 24 hours in a pH range of 5.4 to 8.5.[131] Unbuffered penicillin G sodium injection 12 and 48 mg/mL in sodium chloride 0.9% had an initial pH between 5.4 and 5.8. A 7% loss occurred in 2 days in samples stored at 5°C. However, reconstituting with citrate buffers having pH values of 6.5, 7, and 7.5 resulted in great stability improvement. At these same concentrations in sodium chloride 0.9% in minibags stored at 5°C, losses of 5 to 7% occurred in 28 days and 10% in 56 days.[1671]

Freezing Solutions

It has been shown that penicillin G sodium in concentrations of 1 to 10%, buffered to pH 6.85, loses not more than 1% in 1 month when frozen at −20°C.[99] Another report stated that solutions

DOI: 10.37573/9781585286850.305

of penicillin G sodium at a concentration of 50,000 units/mL in water, sodium chloride 0.9%, and 0.05 M citrate buffer and also at a concentration of 500,000 units/mL with sodium citrate 15 mg are stable for at least 12 weeks when frozen at −25°C. At −5°C in the citrate buffer, the rate of decomposition is considerably higher than at either −25 or 5°C.[156]

Penicillin G sodium 2.5 million units/50 mL of dextrose 5% in PVC containers was physically compatible and stable for 39 days frozen at −20°C. Subsequent thawing and storage at 4°C resulted in a 3 to 4% loss in 10 to 15 days and up to a 10% loss in 31 days.[1125]

Little penicillin G sodium loss occurred in a solution containing 180,000 units/mL in sterile water for injection in PVC and glass containers after 30 days at −20°C. Subsequent thawing and storage for 4 days at 5°C, followed by 24 hours at 37°C to simulate the use of a portable infusion pump, resulted in about a 12 to 16% penicillin loss.[1391]

Ambulatory Pumps

The stability of penicillin G sodium 100,000 and 200,000 units/mL in sterile water for injection was evaluated in PVC portable pump reservoirs (Pharmacia Deltec). A 4 to 6% loss occurred in 3 days at 25°C.[2080]

Compatibility Information

Solution Compatibility

Penicillin G sodium

Test Soln Name	Mfr	Mfr	Conc/L or %	Remarks	Ref	C/I
Dextrose 5%		KA	6 million units[a]	Stable for 24 hr at 25°C	131	C
Dextrose 5%		BE	20 million units[a]	25% loss in 24 hr at 25°C	113	I
Dextrose 5%			4 million units[a] [b]	7% loss in 6 hr and 29% in 24 hr at room temperature	768	I
Dextrose 5%	TR[c]	AY	50 million units[a]	No loss in 39 days at −20°C. Then up to 10% loss in 31 days at 5°C	1125	C
Dextrose 5%	BA[c]	TE	2.5 million units[a]	Physically compatible with less than 10% loss in 28 days at 5°C	2981	C
Dextrose 5%	BA[f]	TE	2.5 million units[a]	Physically compatible with less than 10% loss in 28 days at 5°C	2981	C
Dextrose 5%	BA[c]	TE	50 million units[a]	Physically compatible with less than 10% loss in 28 days at 5°C	2981	C
Dextrose 5%	BA[f]	TE	50 million units[a]	Physically compatible with less than 10% loss in 28 days at 5°C	2981	C
Sodium chloride 0.9%		KA	20 million units[a]	Stable for 24 hr at 25°C	131	C
Sodium chloride 0.9%			4 million units[a] [b]	10% loss in 8 hr and 16% in 24 hr at room temperature	768	I
Sodium chloride 0.9%	TR[c]	GL	20 and 80 million units[a]	In unbuffered solution. 7 to 8% loss in 48 hr and 18% in 96 hr at 5°C	1671	C
Sodium chloride 0.9%	TR[c]	GL	20 million units[a]	Reconstituted with citrate buffer (pH 6.5 to 7.5). 5% loss in 28 days and 10% in 56 days at 5°C	1671	C
Sodium chloride 0.9%	BA[e]	CSL	133 million units[a]	Losses of 10% in 13 hr at 22°C and 5 hr at 36°C. More than 10% loss in 7 days at 4°C	2547	I
Sodium chloride 0.9%	BA[c]	TE	2.5 million units[a]	Physically compatible with less than 10% loss in 21 days at 5°C	2981	C
Sodium chloride 0.9%	BA[f]	TE	2.5 million units[a]	Physically compatible with less than 10% loss in 21 days at 5°C	2981	C
Sodium chloride 0.9%	BA[c]	TE	50 million units[a]	Physically compatible with less than 10% loss in 28 days at 5°C	2981	C
Sodium chloride 0.9%	BA[f]	TE	50 million units[a]	Physically compatible with less than 10% loss in 28 days at 5°C	2981	C
TPN #107[d]			2 g	Activity retained for 24 hr at 21°C	1326	C

[a] Million units.

[b] An unbuffered preparation was specified.

[c] Tested in PVC containers.

[d] Refer to Appendix for the composition of parenteral nutrition solutions. TPN indicates a 2-in-1 admixture.

[e] Tested in IntraVia polypropylene containers.

[f] Tested in Intermate elastomeric pump reservoirs.

Additive Compatibility

Penicillin G sodium

Test Drug	Mfr	Conc/L or %	Mfr	Conc/L or %	Test Solution	Remarks	Ref	C/I
Amphotericin B	SQ	100 mg	UP	20 million units	D5W	Physically incompatible	15	I
Amphotericin B		200 mg	BP	10 million units	D5W	Haze develops over 3 hr	26	I
Bleomycin sulfate	BR	20 and 30 units	SQ	2 million units	NS	77% loss of bleomycin activity in 1 week at 4°C	763	I
Bleomycin sulfate	BR	20 and 30 units	SQ	5 million units	NS	41% loss of bleomycin activity in 1 week at 4°C	763	I
Calcium chloride	UP	1 g	UP	20 million units	D5W	Physically compatible	15	C
Calcium gluconate	UP	1 g	UP	20 million units	D5W	Physically compatible	15	C
Chloramphenicol sodium succinate	PD	10 g	UP	20 million units	D5W	Physically compatible	15	C
Chlorpromazine HCl	BP	200 mg	BP	10 million units	NS	Haze develops over 3 hr	26	I
Colistimethate sodium	WC	500 mg	UP	20 million units	D5W	Physically compatible	15	C
Cytarabine	UP	200 mg		2 million units	D5W	pH outside stability range for penicillin G	174	I
Dextran 40	PH	10%	KA	6 million units		Stable for 24 hr at 25°C	131	C
Diphenhydramine HCl	PD	80 mg	UP	20 million units	D5W	Physically compatible	15	C
Erythromycin lactobionate	AB	5 g	UP	20 million units	D5W	Physically compatible	15	C
Gentamicin sulfate	RS	160 mg	GL	13 and 40 million units	D5¼S, D5W, NS	Gentamicin stable for 24 hr at room temperature	157	C
Heparin sodium	OR	20,000 units	BE	20 million units	NS	Both stable for 24 hr at 25°C	113	C
Heparin sodium	UP	4000 units	UP	20 million units	D5W	Physically incompatible	15	I
Hydrocortisone sodium succinate	UP	500 mg	UP	20 million units	D5W	Physically compatible	15	C
Hydroxyzine HCl	RR	250 mg	UP	20 million units	D5W	Physically incompatible	15	I
Lincomycin HCl	UP	6 g	UP	20 million units	D5W	Physically compatible	15	C
Methylprednisolone sodium succinate	UP	125 mg		5 million units	D5W, LR	Precipitate forms	329	I
Polymyxin B sulfate	BW	200 mg	UP	20 million units	D5W	Physically compatible	15	C
Potassium chloride		40 mEq	KA	6 million units	D5W	Penicillin stable for 48 hr at 25°C	131	C
Potassium chloride		40 mEq	KA	5 million units	IS10	pH outside stability range for penicillin	131	I
Prochlorperazine mesylate	BP	100 mg	BP	10 million units	NS	Haze develops over 3 hr	26	I
Promethazine HCl	WY	250 mg	UP	20 million units	D5W	Physically incompatible	15	I
Ranitidine HCl	GL	100 mg		2.4 million units	D5W	Physically compatible for 24 hr at ambient temperature in light	1151	C
Tranexamic acid	PF					Manufacturer states incompatible	2887	I
Verapamil HCl	KN	80 mg	SQ	10 million units	D5W, NS	Physically compatible for 24 hr	764	C

Drugs in Syringe Compatibility

Penicillin G sodium

Test Drug	Mfr	Amt	Mfr	Amt	Remarks	Ref	C/I
Chloramphenicol sodium succinate	PD	250 and 400 mg/1.5 mL		1 million units	No precipitate or color change within 1 hr at room temperature	99	C
Chloramphenicol sodium succinate	PD	250 and 400 mg/2 mL		1 million units	No precipitate or color change within 1 hr at room temperature	99	C
Colistimethate sodium	PX	40 mg/2 mL		1 million units	No precipitate or color change within 1 hr at room temperature	99	C
Dimenhydrinate		10 mg/1 mL		500,000 units/1 mL	Clear solution	2569	C
Gentamicin sulfate		80 mg/2 mL		1 million units	No precipitate or color change within 1 hr at room temperature	99	C
Lincomycin HCl	UP	600 mg/2 mL		1 million units	No precipitate or color change within 1 hr at room temperature	99	C
Pantoprazole sodium	a	4 mg/1 mL		500,000 units/1 mL	Clear solution	2574	C
Polymyxin B sulfate	BW	25 mg/1.5 to 2 mL		1 million units	No precipitate or color change within 1 hr at room temperature	99	C
Streptomycin sulfate		1 g/2 mL		1 million units	No precipitate or color change within 1 hr at room temperature	99	C

a Test performed using the formulation WITHOUT edetate disodium.

Y-Site Injection Compatibility (1:1 Mixture)

Penicillin G sodium

Test Drug	Mfr	Conc	Mfr	Conc	Remarks	Ref	C/I
Clarithromycin	AB	4 mg/mL[a]	BRT	24 mg/mL[a]	Visually compatible for 72 hr at both 30 and 17°C	2174	C
Cloxacillin sodium	SMX	100 mg/mL	PPC	500,000 units/mL	Physically compatible for up to 4 hr at room temperature	3245	C
Levofloxacin	OMN	5 mg/mL[a]	MAR	500,000 units/mL	Visually compatible for 4 hr at 24°C	2233	C
Meropenem		50 mg/mL	FRK	500,000 units/mL	Physically compatible for 4 hr at room temperature	3538	C
TPN #54[e]				320,000 and 500,000 units/mL	Physically compatible and 88% penicillin activity retained over 6 hr at 22°C	1045	C
TPN #61[e]		b	PF	200,000 units/2 mL[c]	Physically compatible	1012	C
TPN #61[e]		d	PF	1.2 million units/12 mL[c]	Physically compatible	1012	C
TPN #189[e]				300 mg/mL[f]	Visually compatible for 24 hr at 22°C	1767	C

a Tested in dextrose 5%.

b Run at 21 mL/hr.

c Given over five minutes by syringe pump.

d Run at 94 mL/hr.

e Refer to Appendix for the composition of parenteral nutrition solutions. TPN indicates a 2-in-1 admixture.

f Tested in sodium chloride 0.9%.

Selected Revisions May 1, 2020. © Copyright, October 1982.
American Society of Health-System Pharmacists, Inc.

Pentamidine Isethionate
AHFS 8:30.92

Products

Pentamidine isethionate is available as a lyophilized powder in single-dose vials containing 300 mg of the salt.[3311] For intramuscular injection, the vial contents should be reconstituted with 3 mL of sterile water for injection at 22 to 30°C.[3311] For intravenous administration, the vial contents should be reconstituted with 3 to 5 mL of sterile water for injection or dextrose 5% at 22 to 30°C; then the dose should be withdrawn from the vial and further diluted in 50 to 250 mL of dextrose 5% for administration.[3311]

Sodium chloride 0.9% should *not* be used initially to reconstitute pentamidine isethionate because precipitation will occur.[3311]

pH

From 4.5 to 7.5.[3312]

Equivalency

Pentamidine isethionate 1.74 mg is equivalent to pentamidine 1 mg.[3315][3316] Care should be taken to clarify upon which moiety (i.e., salt or base) a dosage is expressed and to ensure that no confusion exists with other pentamidine salts.[3314][3315][3316]

Trade Name(s)

Pentam 300

Administration

Pentamidine isethionate injection may be administered by intravenous infusion or deep intramuscular injection.[3311] Regardless of the route of administration, patients receiving the drug should be in the supine position and their blood pressure should be monitored closely during administration and several times thereafter until the blood pressure has stabilized.[3311]

For intravenous infusion, the calculated dose should be diluted in 50 to 250 mL of dextrose 5% prior to administration and infused over 60 to 120 minutes.[3311] The drug should *not* be administered by rapid intravenous injection or infusion.[3311]

Extravasation of pentamidine isethionate may cause ulceration, tissue necrosis, and/or sloughing at the site of injection.[3311] The intravenous needle or catheter must be properly positioned and closely observed throughout administration.[3311] If extravasation occurs, the injection should be discontinued immediately and restarted in another vein.[3311]

Stability

Intact vials of powder should be stored at controlled room temperature and protected from light.[3311]

Reconstituted solutions prepared with sterile water for injection are stable for 48 hours in the original vial at room temperature if protected from light.[3311] Reconstituted solutions should be stored at 22 to 30°C to avoid crystallization.[3311] Solutions for intravenous infusion prepared in dextrose 5% containing pentamidine isethionate 1 and 2.5 mg/mL are stable for up to 24 hours at room temperature.[3311] Because no preservative is present, the manufacturer recommends discarding any remaining solution.[3311]

Solutions should be visually inspected for particulate matter and discoloration prior to administration.[3311]

Pentamidine isethionate (Fresenius Kabi) 0.8 to 98 mg/mL in sterile water for injection in polyvinyl chloride (PVC) bags and glass vials has been reported to be stable for 30 days at 4°C.[3312]

Freezing Solutions

The manufacturer states that pentamidine isethionate solutions should be stored at 22 to 30°C to avoid crystallization.[3311]

Pentamidine isethionate (Fresenius Kabi) 1 to 30 mg/mL in dextrose 5% and sterile water for injection in PVC bags has been reported to be stable for 90 days at −20°C.[3312] Pentamidine isethionate (Fresenius Kabi) 0.8 to 2.5 mg/mL in dextrose 5% in PVC bags has been reported to be stable for 120 days at −20°C.[3312]

Pentamidine isethionate (Fresenius Kabi) 0.8 to 98 mg/mL in dextrose 5% and sterile water for injection in glass vials has been reported to be stable for 90 days at −20°C.[3312]

Syringes

Pentamidine isethionate (Fresenius Kabi) 0.8 to 97 mg/mL in dextrose 5% and sterile water for injection packaged in disposable plastic syringes has been reported to be stable for 30 days at 4°C and 120 days at −20°C.[3312]

Elastomeric Reservoir Pumps

Pentamidine isethionate (Fujisawa) 3 mg/mL in dextrose 5% and 2 mg/mL in sodium chloride 0.9% was evaluated for binding potential to natural rubber elastomeric reservoirs.[2014] No binding was found after storage for 2 weeks at 35°C with gentle agitation.[2014]

Sorption

One study that demonstrated stability of pentamidine isethionate (Lyphomed) 1 or 2 mg/mL in dextrose 5% or sodium chloride 0.9% for 48 hours at 22 to 26°C in PVC bags also demonstrated losses of 2 or 10% when 2-mg/mL solutions in dextrose 5% or sodium chloride 0.9%, respectively, were infused through a PVC infusion set, potentially suggesting adsorption of the drug to the set.[1142]

DOI: 10.37573/9781585286850.306

Compatibility Information

Solution Compatibility

Pentamidine isethionate

Test Soln Name	Mfr	Mfr	Conc/L or %	Remarks	Ref	C/I
Dextrose 5%	TRª	LY	1 g	Physically compatible with 3% loss in 48 hr at 24°C under fluorescent light	1142	C
Dextrose 5%	TRª	LY	2 g	Physically compatible with 1% loss in 48 hr at 24°C under fluorescent light	1142	C
Dextrose 5%	TRª	MB	2 g	Physically compatible with little or no loss in 24 hr at 20°C	1311	C
Dextrose 5%	a	FRK	0.8 to 98 g	Reported to be stable for 30 days at 4°C	3312	C
Dextrose 5%	b	FRK	0.8 to 98 g	Reported to be stable for 30 days at 4°C	3312	C
Sodium chloride 0.9%	TRª	LY	1 g	Physically compatible with 2% loss in 48 hr at 24°C under fluorescent light	1142	C
Sodium chloride 0.9%	TRª	LY	2 g	Physically compatible with no loss in 48 hr at 24°C under fluorescent light	1142	C
Sodium chloride 0.9%	TRª	MB	2 g	Physically compatible with little or no loss in 24 hr at 20°C	1311	C

ª Tested in PVC containers.

ᵇ Tested in glass containers.

Y-Site Injection Compatibility (1:1 Mixture)

Pentamidine isethionate

Test Drug	Mfr	Conc	Mfr	Conc	Remarks	Ref	C/I
Aldesleukin	CHI	33,800 I.U./mLª	FUJ	6 mg/mLª	Aldesleukin bioactivity inhibited	1857	I
Cefazolin sodium	SKB	20 mg/mLª	FUJ	3 mg/mLª	Cloudy precipitation forms immediately	1880	I
Cefotaxime sodium	HO	20 mg/mLª	FUJ	3 mg/mLª	Fine precipitate forms immediately	1880	I
Cefoxitin sodium	ME	20 mg/mLᶜ	FUJ	3 mg/mLª	Immediate cloudy precipitation	1880	I
Ceftazidime	LI	20 mg/mLª	FUJ	3 mg/mLª	Fine precipitate forms immediately	1880	I
Ceftriaxone sodium	RC	20 mg/mLª	FUJ	3 mg/mLª	Heavy white precipitate forms immediately	1880	I
Diltiazem HCl	MMD	5 mg/mL	LY	6 and 30 mg/mLª	Visually compatible	1807	C
Fluconazole	RR	2 mg/mL	LY	6 mg/mL	Cloudiness develops	1407	I
Foscarnet sodium	AST	24 mg/mL	LY	6 mg/mL	Precipitates immediately	1335	I
Foscarnet sodium	AST	24 mg/mL	LY	6 mg/mLª ᵇ	Pentamidine crystals form immediately	1393	I
Linezolid	PHU	2 mg/mL	FUJ	6 mg/mLª	Crystalline precipitate forms in 1 to 4 hr	2264	I
Linezolid	PHU, HOS	2 mg/mL			Stated to be physically incompatible	3183, 3184	I
Zidovudine	BW	4 mg/mLª	LY	6 mg/mLª	Physically compatible for 4 hr at 25°C	1193	C

ª Tested in dextrose 5%.

ᵇ Tested in sodium chloride 0.9%.

ᶜ Tested in dextrose 4%.

Selected Revisions September 29, 2017. © Copyright, October 1988. American Society of Health-System Pharmacists, Inc.

Pentazocine Lactate
AHFS 28:08.12

Products

Pentazocine lactate is supplied in 1-mL ampuls, 1- and 2-mL syringe cartridges, and 10-mL multiple-dose vials. Each mL of solution contains[1(10/06)]:

Component	Ampul	Cartridge Unit	Vial
Pentazocine (as lactate)	30 mg	30 mg	30 mg
Sodium chloride	2.8 mg	2.2 mg	1.5 mg
Acetone sodium bisulfite		1 mg	2 mg
Methylparaben			1 mg
Water for injection	qs 1 mL	qs 1 mL	qs 1 mL

pH

The pH is adjusted to 4 to 5 with lactic acid or sodium hydroxide.[1(10/06)]

Osmolality

The osmolality of pentazocine lactate 30 mg/mL was determined to be 307 mOsm/kg.[1233]

Trade Name(s)

Talwin

Administration

Pentazocine lactate may be administered by intramuscular, subcutaneous, or intravenous injection. For repeated administration, intramuscular injection with constant rotation of the injection sites should be used. Subcutaneous injection should be used only when necessary because of possible tissue damage.[1(10/06)] [4]

Stability

Pentazocine lactate injection should be stored at controlled room temperature[1(10/06)] and protected from temperatures of 40°C or above and from freezing. Pentazocine lactate is incompatible with alkaline substances.[4]

Syringes

Pentazocine lactate (Winthrop) 30 mg/1 mL, repackaged in 3-mL clear glass syringes (Hy-Pod) and stored at 25°C, exhibited no significant changes in pH, physical appearance, or drug concentration during 360 days of storage.[535]

Compatibility Information

Additive Compatibility

Pentazocine lactate

Test Drug	Mfr	Conc/L or %	Mfr	Conc/L or %	Test Solution	Remarks	Ref	C/I
Aminophylline	SE	1 g	WI	300 mg	D5W	Physically incompatible	15	I
Pentobarbital sodium	AB	1 g	WI	300 mg	D5W	Physically incompatible	15	I
Phenobarbital sodium	WI	200 mg	WI	300 mg	D5W	Physically incompatible	15	I
Sodium bicarbonate	AB	80 mEq	WI	300 mg	D5W	Physically incompatible	15	I

Drugs in Syringe Compatibility

Pentazocine lactate

Test Drug	Mfr	Amt	Mfr	Amt	Remarks	Ref	C/I
Atropine sulfate		0.6 mg/1.5 mL	WI	30 mg/1 mL	Physically compatible for at least 15 min	14	C
Atropine sulfate	ST	0.4 mg/1 mL	WI	30 mg/1 mL	Physically compatible for at least 15 min	326	C
Butorphanol tartrate	BR	4 mg/2 mL	WI	30 mg/1 mL	Physically compatible for 30 min at room temperature	566	C
Chlorpromazine HCl	SKF	50 mg/2 mL	WI	30 mg/1 mL	Physically compatible for at least 15 min	14	C
Chlorpromazine HCl	PO	50 mg/2 mL	WI	30 mg/1 mL	Physically compatible for at least 15 min	326	C

DOI: 10.37573/9781585286850.307

Drugs in Syringe Compatibility (Cont.)

Test Drug	Mfr	Amt	Mfr	Amt	Remarks	Ref	C/I
Dimenhydrinate	HR	50 mg/1 mL	WI	30 mg/1 mL	Physically compatible for at least 15 min	326	C
Diphenhydramine HCl	PD	50 mg/1 mL	WI	30 mg/1 mL	Physically compatible for at least 15 min	326	C
Droperidol	MN	2.5 mg/1 mL	WI	30 mg/1 mL	Physically compatible for at least 15 min	326	C
Fentanyl citrate	MN	0.05 mg/1 mL	WI	30 mg/1 mL	Physically compatible for at least 15 min	326	C
Glycopyrrolate	RB	0.2 mg/1 mL	WI	30 mg/1 mL	Precipitates immediately	331	I
Glycopyrrolate	RB	0.2 mg/1 mL	WI	60 mg/2 mL	Precipitates immediately	331	I
Glycopyrrolate	RB	0.4 mg/2 mL	WI	30 mg/1 mL	Precipitates immediately	331	I
Heparin sodium		2500 units/1 mL	WI	30 mg/1 mL	Turbidity or precipitate forms within 5 min	1053	I
Hydromorphone HCl	KN	4 mg/2 mL	WI	30 mg/1 mL	Physically compatible for 30 min	517	C
Hydroxyzine HCl	PF	100 mg/4 mL	WI	30 mg/1 mL	Physically compatible for at least 15 min	14	C
Hydroxyzine HCl	PF	50 mg/1 mL	WI	30 mg/1 mL	Physically compatible for at least 15 min	326	C
Hydroxyzine HCl	PF	50 mg/1 mL	WI	60 mg/2 mL	Physically compatible	771	C
Hydroxyzine HCl	PF	100 mg/2 mL	WI	30 mg/1 mL	Physically compatible	771	C
Meperidine HCl	WI	50 mg/1 mL	WI	30 mg/1 mL	Physically compatible for at least 15 min	326	C
Metoclopramide HCl	NO	10 mg/2 mL	WI	30 mg/1 mL	Physically compatible for 15 min at room temperature	565	C
Morphine sulfate	ST	15 mg/1 mL	WI	30 mg/1 mL	Physically compatible for at least 15 min	326	C
Pentobarbital sodium	WY	100 mg/2 mL	WI	30 mg/1 mL	Precipitate forms within 15 min	14	I
Pentobarbital sodium	AB	50 mg/1 mL	WI	30 mg/1 mL	Physically incompatible within 15 min	326	I
Prochlorperazine edisylate	PO	5 mg/1 mL	WI	30 mg/1 mL	Physically compatible for at least 15 min	326	C
Promethazine HCl	WY	50 mg/2 mL	WI	30 mg/1 mL	Physically compatible for at least 15 min	14	C
Promethazine HCl	PO	50 mg/2 mL	WI	30 mg/1 mL	Physically compatible for at least 15 min	326	C
Ranitidine HCl	GL	50 mg/2 mL	WI	60 mg/2 mL	Physically compatible for 1 hr at 25°C	978	C
Scopolamine HBr		0.6 mg/1.5 mL	WI	30 mg/1 mL	Physically compatible for at least 15 min	14	C
Scopolamine HBr	ST	0.4 mg/1 mL	WI	30 mg/1 mL	Physically compatible for at least 15 min	326	C

Y-Site Injection Compatibility (1:1 Mixture)

Pentazocine lactate

Test Drug	Mfr	Conc	Mfr	Conc	Remarks	Ref	C/I
Heparin sodium	UP	1000 units/L[a]	WI	30 mg/mL	Physically compatible for 4 hr at room temperature	534	C
Hydrocortisone sodium succinate	UP	10 mg/L[a]	WI	30 mg/mL	Physically compatible for 4 hr at room temperature	534	C
Nafcillin sodium	WY	33 mg/mL[b]		30 mg/mL	Precipitate forms, probably free nafcillin	547	I
Potassium chloride	AB	40 mEq/L[a]	WI	30 mg/mL	Physically compatible for 4 hr at room temperature	534	C

[a] Tested in dextrose 5% in Ringer's injection, dextrose 5% in Ringer's injection, lactated, dextrose 5%, Ringer's injection, lactated, and sodium chloride 0.9%.

[b] Tested in sodium chloride 0.9%.

Selected Revisions October 1, 2012. © Copyright, October 1982.
American Society of Health-System Pharmacists, Inc.

Pentobarbital Sodium
AHFS 28:24.04

Products

Pentobarbital sodium 50 mg/mL is available in 20- and 50-mL multiple-dose vials. Each mL of solution also contains propylene glycol 40% (v/v), alcohol 10%, and hydrochloric acid and/or sodium hydroxide to adjust pH in water for injection.[1(3/07)]

pH

Adjusted to approximately 9.5;[1(3/07)] range 9 to 10.5.[17]

Trade Name(s)

Nembutal

Administration

Pentobarbital sodium may be administered by deep intramuscular injection into a large muscle or by slow intravenous injection. The rate of intravenous administration should not exceed 50 mg/min. No more than 5 mL of solution (250 mg) should be injected intramuscularly at any one site.[1(3/07) 4]

Stability

Intact vials of pentobarbital sodium should be stored at controlled room temperature and protected from excessive heat and freezing. Brief exposures to temperatures up to 40°C does not adversely affect the product.[1(3/07)]

Aqueous solutions of pentobarbital sodium are not stable. The commercially available pentobarbital sodium in a propylene glycol vehicle is more stable. In an acidic medium, pentobarbital sodium may precipitate.[4] No solution containing a precipitate or that is cloudy should be used.[1(3/07) 4]

Pentobarbital sodium may raise the pH of admixture solutions to the alkaline range and, therefore, should not be mixed with alkali-labile drugs.[47]

Syringes

Pentobarbital sodium 50 mg/mL was packaged in 1-mL glass and polypropylene syringes and 3-mL polypropylene syringes (Becton Dickinson) and stored at 25°C. No loss occurred in 31 days.[2429]

Sorption

Pentobarbital sodium did not undergo sorption to a polyvinyl chloride (PVC) plastic test strip or PVC infusion solution bag.[12 770]

Plasticizer Leaching

Pentobarbital sodium 2 mg/mL in dextrose 5% did not leach diethylhexyl phthalate (DEHP) plasticizer from 50-mL PVC bags in 24 hours at 24°C.[1683]

Filtration

Pentobarbital sodium 600 mg/L and 1.25 g/L in dextrose 5% and also sodium chloride 0.9% was filtered through a 0.45-µm filter. The delivered concentration did not decrease.[754]

Compatibility Information

Solution Compatibility

Pentobarbital sodium

Test Soln Name	Mfr	Mfr	Conc/L or %	Remarks	Ref	C/I
Dextrose 2.5% in half-strength Ringer's injection	AB	AB	500 mg	Physically compatible	3	C
Dextrose 5% in Ringer's injection	AB	AB	500 mg	Physically compatible	3	C
Dextrose 2.5% in Ringer's injection, lactated	AB	AB	500 mg	Physically compatible	3	C
Dextrose 5% in half-strength Ringer's injection, lactated	AB	AB	500 mg	Physically compatible	3	C
Dextrose 5% in Ringer's injection, lactated	AB	AB	500 mg	Physically compatible	3	C
Dextrose 10% in Ringer's injection, lactated	AB	AB	500 mg	Physically compatible	3	C
Dextrose 2.5% in sodium chloride 0.45%	AB	AB	500 mg	Physically compatible	3	C
Dextrose 2.5% in sodium chloride 0.9%	AB	AB	500 mg	Physically compatible	3	C
Dextrose 5% in sodium chloride 0.225%	AB	AB	500 mg	Physically compatible	3	C
Dextrose 5% in sodium chloride 0.45%	AB	AB	500 mg	Physically compatible	3	C

DOI: 10.37573/9781585286850.308

Solution Compatibility (Cont.)

Test Soln Name	Mfr	Mfr	Conc/L or %	Remarks	Ref	C/I
Dextrose 5% in sodium chloride 0.9%	AB	AB	500 mg	Physically compatible	3	C
Dextrose 10% in sodium chloride 0.9%	AB	AB	500 mg	Physically compatible	3	C
Dextrose 2.5%	AB	AB	500 mg	Physically compatible	3	C
Dextrose 5%	AB	AB	500 mg	Physically compatible	3	C
Dextrose 5%	MG[a]	AB	600 mg and 1.25 g	Physically compatible and chemically stable for 12-hr study period	754	C
Dextrose 5%	BA[b]	AB	4 and 8 g	Visually compatible with no loss in 24 hr	1590	C
Dextrose 5%	BA[b]	AB	>8 g	Occasional visible precipitation	1590	I
Dextrose 10%	AB	AB	500 mg	Physically compatible	3	C
Ionosol B in dextrose 5%	AB	AB	500 mg	Physically compatible	3	C
Ionosol MB in dextrose 5%	AB	AB	500 mg	Physically compatible	3	C
Ringer's injection	AB	AB	500 mg	Physically compatible	3	C
Ringer's injection, lactated	AB	AB	500 mg	Physically compatible	3	C
Sodium chloride 0.45%	AB	AB	500 mg	Physically compatible	3	C
Sodium chloride 0.9%	AB	AB	500 mg	Physically compatible	3	C
Sodium chloride 0.9%	MG[a]	AB	600 mg and 1.25 g	Physically compatible and chemically stable for 12-hr study period	754	C
Sodium chloride 0.9%	BA[b]	AB	4 and 8 g	Visually compatible with no loss in 24 hr	1590	C
Sodium chloride 0.9%	BA[b]	AB	>8 g	Occasional visible precipitation	1590	I
Sodium chloride 0.9%	BA	AB	10 g	Crystals form in less than 24 hr at 25°C	2429	I
Sodium lactate ⅙ M	AB	AB	500 mg	Physically compatible	3	C

[a] Tested in polyolefin containers.

[b] Tested in PVC containers.

Additive Compatibility

Pentobarbital sodium

Test Drug	Mfr	Conc/L or %	Mfr	Conc/L or %	Test Solution	Remarks	Ref	C/I
Amikacin sulfate	BR	5 g	AB	100 mg	D5LR, D5R, D5S, D5W, D10W, LR, NS, R, SL	Physically compatible and both stable for 24 hr at 25°C	294	C
Aminophylline		500 mg	AB	500 mg		Physically compatible	3	C
Aminophylline	SE	500 mg	AB	500 mg		Physically compatible	6	C
Aminophylline	SE	1 g	AB	1 g	D5W	Physically compatible	15	C
Calcium chloride	UP	1 g	AB	1 g	D5W	Physically compatible	15	C
Chloramphenicol sodium succinate	PD	1 g	AB	200 mg		Physically compatible	6	C
Dimenhydrinate	SE	500 mg	AB	1 g	D5W	Physically compatible	15	C
Ephedrine sulfate	LI	250 mg	AB	1 g	D5W	Physically incompatible	15	I

Additive Compatibility (Cont.)

Test Drug	Mfr	Conc/L or %	Mfr	Conc/L or %	Test Solution	Remarks	Ref	C/I
Erythromycin lactobionate	AB	1 g	AB	500 mg		Physically compatible. Erythromycin stable for 24 hr at 25°C	20	C
Hydrocortisone sodium succinate	UP	500 mg	AB	1 g	D5W	Physically incompatible	15	I
Hydroxyzine HCl	RR	250 mg	AB	1 g	D5W	Physically incompatible	15	I
Lidocaine HCl	AST	2 g	AB	500 mg		Physically compatible	24	C
Penicillin G potassium	[a]	900,000 units	AB	500 mg	D5W	17% penicillin loss in 6 hr at 25°C	48	I
Penicillin G potassium	SQ	1 million units	AB	500 mg	D5W	42% penicillin loss in 24 hr at 25°C	47	I
Pentazocine lactate	WI	300 mg	AB	1 g	D5W	Physically incompatible	15	I
Promethazine HCl	WY	250 mg	AB	1 g	D5W	Physically incompatible	15	I
Sodium bicarbonate	AB	80 mEq	AB	1 g	D5W	Physically incompatible	15	I
Succinylcholine chloride						Pentobarbital precipitates or succinylcholine hydrolyzes	4	I
Verapamil HCl	KN	80 mg	AB	200 mg	D5W, NS	Physically compatible for 24 hr	764	C

[a] A buffered preparation was specified.

Drugs in Syringe Compatibility

Pentobarbital sodium

Test Drug	Mfr	Amt	Mfr	Amt	Remarks	Ref	C/I
Aminophylline		500 mg/2 mL	AB	500 mg/10 mL	Physically compatible	55	C
Atropine sulfate		0.6 mg/1.5 mL	WY	100 mg/2 mL	Physically compatible for at least 15 min	14	C
Atropine sulfate	ST	0.4 mg/1 mL	AB	50 mg/1 mL	Physically compatible for at least 15 min	326	C
Atropine sulfate	LI	0.6 mg/1.5 mL	AB	100 mg/2 mL	Precipitate forms in 24 hr at room temperature	542	I
Butorphanol tartrate	BR	4 mg/2 mL	AB	50 mg/1 mL	Precipitates immediately	761	I
Chlorpromazine HCl	SKF	50 mg/2 mL	AB	500 mg/10 mL	Physically incompatible	55	I
Chlorpromazine HCl	SKF	50 mg/2 mL	WY	100 mg/2 mL	Precipitate forms within 15 min	14	I
Chlorpromazine HCl	PO	50 mg/2 mL	AB	50 mg/1 mL	Physically incompatible within 15 min	326	I
Dimenhydrinate	SE	50 mg/1 mL	AB	500 mg/10 mL	Physically incompatible	55	I
Dimenhydrinate	HR	50 mg/1 mL	AB	50 mg/1 mL	Physically incompatible within 15 min	326	I
Diphenhydramine HCl	PD	50 mg/1 mL	WY	100 mg/2 mL	Precipitate observed within 15 min	14	I
Diphenhydramine HCl	PD	50 mg/1 mL	AB	500 mg/10 mL	Physically incompatible	55	I
Diphenhydramine HCl	PD	50 mg/1 mL	AB	50 mg/1 mL	Physically incompatible within 15 min	326	I
Droperidol	MN	2.5 mg/1 mL	AB	50 mg/1 mL	Physically incompatible within 15 min	326	I
Ephedrine sulfate		50 mg/1 mL	AB	500 mg/10 mL	Physically compatible	55	C
Fentanyl citrate	MN	0.05 mg/1 mL	AB	50 mg/1 mL	Physically incompatible within 15 min	326	I
Glycopyrrolate	RB	0.2 mg/1 mL	AB	50 mg/1 mL	Precipitates immediately	331	I
Glycopyrrolate	RB	0.4 mg/2 mL	AB	50 mg/1 mL	Precipitates immediately	331	I

Drugs in Syringe Compatibility (Cont.)

Test Drug	Mfr	Amt	Mfr	Amt	Remarks	Ref	C/I
Glycopyrrolate	RB	0.2 mg/1 mL	AB	100 mg/2 mL	Precipitates immediately	331	I
Hyaluronidase	AB	150 units	AB	500 mg/10 mL	Physically compatible	55	C
Hydromorphone HCl	KN	4 mg/2 mLª	AB	50 mg/1 mL	Physically compatible for 30 min	517	C
Hydromorphone HCl	KN	4 mg/2 mLᵇ	AB	50 mg/1 mL	Transient precipitate that dissipates after mixing and stays clear for 30 min	517	?
Hydroxyzine HCl	PF	100 mg/4 mL	WY	100 mg/2 mL	Precipitate forms within 15 min	14	I
Hydroxyzine HCl	PF	50 mg/1 mL	AB	50 mg/1 mL	Physically incompatible within 15 min	326	I
Meperidine HCl	WI	100 mg/2 mL	AB	500 mg/10 mL	Physically incompatible	55	I
Meperidine HCl	WY	100 mg/1 mL	WY	100 mg/2 mL	Precipitate forms within 15 min	14	I
Meperidine HCl	WI	50 mg/1 mL	AB	50 mg/1 mL	Physically incompatible within 15 min	326	I
Midazolam HCl	RC	5 mg/1 mL	WY	100 mg/2 mL	White precipitate forms immediately	1145	I
Morphine sulfate		16.2 mg/1 mL	AB	500 mg/10 mL	Physically compatible	55	C
Morphine sulfate	WY	15 mg/1 mL	WY	100 mg/2 mL	Precipitate forms within 15 min	14	I
Morphine sulfate	ST	15 mg/1 mL	AB	50 mg/1 mL	Physically incompatible within 15 min	326	I
Nalbuphine HCl	EN	10 mg/1 mL	WY	50 mg/1 mL	Immediate white milky precipitate that persists for 36 hr at 27°C	762	I
Nalbuphine HCl	EN	2.5 mg/0.25 mL	WY	50 mg/1 mL	Immediate white milky precipitate that clears upon vigorous shaking	762	I
Nalbuphine HCl	EN	5 mg/0.5 mL	WY	50 mg/1 mL	Immediate white milky precipitate that persists for 36 hr at 27°C	762	I
Neostigmine methylsulfate	RC	0.5 mg/1 mL	AB	500 mg/10 mL	Physically compatible	55	C
Pentazocine lactate	WI	30 mg/1 mL	WY	100 mg/2 mL	Precipitate forms within 15 min	14	I
Pentazocine lactate	WI	30 mg/1 mL	AB	50 mg/1 mL	Physically incompatible within 15 min	326	I
Prochlorperazine edisylate	SKF	10 mg/2 mL	AB	500 mg/10 mL	Physically incompatible	55	I
Prochlorperazine edisylate	SKF		WY	100 mg/2 mL	Precipitate forms within 15 min	14	I
Prochlorperazine edisylate	PO	5 mg/1 mL	AB	50 mg/1 mL	Physically incompatible within 15 min	326	I
Promethazine HCl	WY	100 mg/4 mL	AB	500 mg/10 mL	Physically incompatible	55	I
Promethazine HCl	WY	50 mg/2 mL	WY	100 mg/2 mL	Precipitate forms within 15 min	14	I
Promethazine HCl	PO	50 mg/2 mL	AB	50 mg/1 mL	Physically incompatible within 15 min	326	I
Ranitidine HCl	GL	50 mg/5 mL	AB	100 mg	Precipitates immediately	1151	I
Scopolamine HBr		0.6 mg/1.5 mL	WY	100 mg/2 mL	Physically compatible for at least 15 min	14	C
Scopolamine HBr		0.13 mg/0.26 mL	AB	500 mg/10 mL	Physically compatible	55	C
Scopolamine HBr	ST	0.4 mg/1 mL	AB	50 mg/1 mL	Physically compatible for at least 15 min	326	C
Sodium bicarbonate		3.75 g/50 mL	AB	500 mg/10 mL	Physically compatible	55	C

ª Vial formulation was tested.

ᵇ Ampul formulation was tested.

Y-Site Injection Compatibility (1:1 Mixture)

Pentobarbital sodium

Test Drug	Mfr	Conc	Mfr	Conc	Remarks	Ref	C/I
Acyclovir sodium	BW	5 mg/mL[a]	WY	2 mg/mL[a]	Physically compatible for 4 hr at 25°C	1157	C
Fenoldopam mesylate	AB	80 mcg/mL[b]	AB	5 mg/mL[b]	Trace haze and microparticulates form immediately	2467	I
Insulin, regular	LI	1 unit/mL[b]	WY	2 mg/mL[b]	Physically compatible for 3 hr	1316	C
Linezolid	PHU	2 mg/mL	AB	5 mg/mL[a]	Physically compatible for 4 hr at 23°C	2264	C
Propofol	ZEN[d]	10 mg/mL	WY	5 mg/mL[a]	Physically compatible for 1 hr at 23°C	2066	C
TNA #218 to #226[c]			AB	5 mg/mL[a]	Damage to emulsion occurs immediately with free oil formation possible	2215	I
TPN #212 to #215[c]			AB	5 mg/mL[a]	Physically compatible for 4 hr at 23°C	2109	C

[a] Tested in dextrose 5%.

[b] Tested in sodium chloride 0.9%.

[c] Refer to Appendix for the composition of parenteral nutrition solutions. TNA indicates a 3-in-1 admixture, and TPN indicates a 2-in-1 admixture.

[d] Test performed using the formulation WITH edetate disodium.

Selected Revisions January 31, 2020. © Copyright, October 1982. American Society of Health-System Pharmacists, Inc.

Pentostatin

AHFS 10:00

Products

Pentostatin is available as a lyophilized powder in vials containing 10 mg of drug. Also present are 50 mg of mannitol and sodium hydroxide or hydrochloric acid to adjust the pH. Reconstitute the vial contents with 5 mL of sterile water for injection and shake well to yield a 2-mg/mL solution.[1(8/07)]

pH

From 7 to 8.5.[1(8/07)]

Trade Name(s)

Nipent

Administration

Pentostatin is administered intravenously by injection over five minutes or by infusion over 20 to 30 minutes when diluted in 25 to 50 mL of dextrose 5% or sodium chloride 0.9%. Adequate hydration is necessary prior to administering pentostatin. Administration of 500 to 1000 mL of dextrose 5% in sodium chloride 0.45% or similar solution prior to drug administration with an additional 500 mL of dextrose 5% or similar solution after drug administration is recommended.[1(8/07)] [4]

Stability

The manufacturer recommends that pentostatin be stored under refrigeration,[1(8/07)] but other information indicates that the drug in intact vials is stable for at least three years at room temperature.[234]

The white to off-white powder yields a colorless solution when reconstituted. The manufacturer states that reconstituted pentostatin solutions are stable at room temperature for up to eight hours only because of the absence of antibacterial preservatives.[1(8/07)] Other information indicates that the reconstituted solution is stable for 72 hours at room temperature, exhibiting a 2 to 4% loss.[234] [1453]

Pentostatin (Parke-Davis) 0.03 mg/mL diluted in sodium chloride 0.9% and stored at 22°C did not exhibit a substantial antimicrobial effect on the growth of four organisms (*Enterococcus faecium*, *Staphylococcus aureus*, *Pseudomonas aeruginosa*, and *Candida albicans*) inoculated into the solution. *C. albicans* maintained viability for 24 hours, and the others were viable for 48 to 120 hours. The author recommended that diluted solutions of pentostatin be stored under refrigeration whenever possible and that the potential for microbiological growth be considered when assigning expiration periods.[2160]

pH Effects

Pentostatin displays greater decomposition under acidic conditions compared to alkaline conditions. The pH range of maximum stability is about 6.5 to 11.5. At pH 6 to 8, hydrolysis is not sensitive to the ionic strength of the solution.[1453]

Sorption

Pentostatin does not undergo sorption to PVC containers or administration sets at concentrations between 0.18 and 0.33 mg/mL in dextrose 5% or sodium chloride 0.9%.[1(8/07)]

Compatibility Information

Solution Compatibility

Pentostatin

Test Soln Name	Mfr	Mfr	Conc/L or %	Remarks	Ref	C/I
Dextrose 5%		NCI	20 mg	2% loss in 24 hr and 8 to 10% in 48 hr at room temperature. No loss in 96 hr refrigerated	234	C
Dextrose 5%	TR[a], BA[b]	NCI	20 mg	10% loss in 54 hr at 23°C	1453	C
Dextrose 5%	TR[a], BA[b]	NCI	2 mg	10% loss in 11 hr at 23°C	1453	I
Ringer's injection, lactated		NCI	20 mg	Up to 4% loss in 48 hr at room temperature	234	C
Sodium chloride 0.9%		NCI	20 mg	Up to 4% loss in 48 hr at room temperature. No loss in 96 hr under refrigeration	234	C
Sodium chloride 0.9%	AB[a], BA[b]	NCI	20 mg	1 to 4% loss in about 49 hr at 23°C	1453	C
Sodium chloride 0.9%	AB[a], BA[b]	NCI	2 mg	3 to 6% loss in 48 hr at 23°C	1453	C

[a] Tested in glass containers.

[b] Tested in PVC containers.

DOI: 10.37573/9781585286850.309

Y-Site Injection Compatibility (1:1 Mixture)

Pentostatin

Test Drug	Mfr	Conc	Mfr	Conc	Remarks	Ref	C/I
Fludarabine phosphate	BX	1 mg/mL[a]	NCI	0.4 mg/mL[b]	Visually compatible for 4 hr at 22°C	1439	C
Melphalan HCl	BW	0.1 mg/mL[b]	PD	0.4 mg/mL[b]	Physically compatible for 3 hr at 22°C	1557	C
Ondansetron HCl	GL	1 mg/mL[b]	NCI	0.4 mg/mL[b]	Visually compatible for 4 hr at 22°C	1365	C
Paclitaxel	NCI	1.2 mg/mL[a]	NCI	0.4 mg/mL[b]	Physically compatible for 4 hr at 22°C	1556	C
Sargramostim	IMM	10 mcg/mL[b]	NCI	0.4 mg/mL[b]	Visually compatible for 4 hr at 22°C	1436	C

[a] Tested in dextrose 5%.

[b] Tested in sodium chloride 0.9%.

Selected Revisions October 1, 2012. © Copyright, October 1992.
American Society of Health-System Pharmacists, Inc.

Peramivir
AHFS 8:18.28

Products

Peramivir injection is available as a concentrate in single-use vials containing peramivir 10 mg/mL (on the anhydrous basis) in sodium chloride 0.9%.[2960] Sodium hydroxide and/or hydrochloric acid may have been added to adjust the pH.[2960]

pH

From 5.5 to 8.5.[2960]

Tonicity

Peramivir injection is isotonic.[2960]

Trade Name(s)

Rapivab

Administration

Peramivir is administered by intravenous infusion over 15 to 30 minutes after dilution of the injection concentrate to a maximum of 100 mL with a compatible infusion solution.[2960] (See Solution Compatibility.)

Stability

Peramivir injection concentrate should be clear and colorless.[2960] Intact vials should be stored at controlled room temperature and retained in the original carton.[2960]

Visually inspect peramivir injection for particulate matter or discoloration prior to use.[2960]

Single-use vials of peramivir do not contain any preservatives.[2960] Diluted solutions should be used immediately or stored for up to 24 hours under refrigeration; any unused portion should be discarded after 24 hours.[2960] If refrigerated, diluted solutions should be allowed to come to room temperature and then administered immediately.[2960]

Sorption

Peramivir injection is stated to be compatible with materials commonly used for administration (e.g., PVC bags, PVC-free bags, polypropylene syringes, polyethylene tubing).[2960]

Compatibility Information

Solution Compatibility

Peramivir

Test Soln Name	Mfr	Mfr	Conc/L or %	Remarks	Ref	C/I
Dextrose 5%		BCT		Manufacturer-recommended solution	2960	C
Ringer's injection, lactated		BCT		Manufacturer-recommended solution	2960	C
Sodium chloride 0.45%		BCT		Manufacturer-recommended solution	2960	C
Sodium chloride 0.9%		BCT		Manufacturer-recommended solution	2960	C

DOI: 10.37573/9781585286850.310

Pertuzumab
AHFS 10:00

Products

Pertuzumab is available as a preservative-free solution at a concentration of 30 mg/mL in 420-mg single-use vials.[3091] Each vial also contains L-histidine acetate 20 mM, sucrose 120 mM, and polysorbate 20 0.02%.[3091]

Vials of pertuzumab should be visually inspected for particulate matter and discoloration.[3091] To prepare a solution for infusion, the appropriate dose of the solution should be diluted in 250 mL of sodium chloride 0.9% in a polyvinyl chloride (PVC) or polyolefin bag; dextrose 5% should *not* be used.[3091] The infusion bag should be gently inverted to mix the diluted solution.[3091] The diluted solution should not be shaken.[3091]

pH
6.[3091]

Trade Name(s)
Perjeta

Administration

Pertuzumab is administered only by intravenous infusion following dilution in 250 mL of sodium chloride 0.9%.[3091] Doses of 840 mg should be infused over 60 minutes; doses of 420 mg should be infused over 30 to 60 minutes.[3091] Pertuzumab should *not* be administered by intravenous push or bolus injection.[3091]

Stability

Intact vials of pertuzumab should be stored at 2 to 8°C in the outer carton to protect from light until time of use.[3091] The drug should not be frozen or shaken.[3091]

The manufacturer recommends that diluted solutions of pertuzumab be used immediately once prepared; however, diluted solutions may be stored at 2 to 8°C for up to 24 hours when prepared as directed.[3091] The manufacturer states that pertuzumab should not be mixed with other drugs.[3091]

Compatibility Information

Solution Compatibility

Pertuzumab

Test Soln Name	Mfr	Mfr	Conc/L or %	Remarks	Ref	C/I
Sodium chloride 0.9%	a	GEN	1.6 and 3 g	Stable for up to 24 hr at 2 to 8°C	3091	C
Sodium chloride 0.9%	b	GEN	1.6 and 3 g	Stable for up to 24 hr at 2 to 8°C	3091	C
Sodium chloride 0.9%	BRN[b]	GEN	1.6 g	Stable for up to 24 hr at 30°C	3090	C
Sodium chloride 0.9%	BRN[b]	GEN	3 g	Stable for up to 24 hr at 5 and 30°C	3090	C
Sodium chloride 0.9%	BA[a]	GEN	3 g	Stable for up to 24 hr at 5 and 30°C	3090	C

[a] Tested in PVC containers.

[b] Tested in polyolefin containers.

Additive Compatibility

Pertuzumab

Test Drug	Mfr	Conc/L or %	Mfr	Conc/L or %	Test Solution	Remarks	Ref	C/I
Trastuzumab	GEN	1.5 g	GEN	1.5 g	NS[a]	Compatible and stable for up to 24 hr at 30°C	3090	C
Trastuzumab	GEN	2.3 g	GEN	2.7 g	NS[b]	Compatible and stable for up to 24 hr at 5 and 30°C	3090	C

[a] Tested in polyolefin containers.

[b] Tested in polyolefin and PVC containers.

DOI: 10.37573/9781585286850.311

Phenobarbital Sodium
AHFS 28:12.04

Products

Phenobarbital sodium injection is available in various dosage forms and sizes, including 30, 60, 65, and 130 mg/mL, from several manufacturers. The product formulations also contain ethanol 10%, propylene glycol 67.8 to 75%, and water for injection. Some products also contain benzyl alcohol 1.5% as a preservative.[1(2/08)] [4]

pH

The USP cites the official pH range as 9.2 to 10.2.[17]

Osmolality

The osmolality of phenobarbital sodium 65 mg/mL was 15,570 mOsm/kg by freezing-point depression and 9285 mOsm/kg by vapor pressure.[1071] The osmolality of phenobarbital sodium 200 mg/mL was 10,800 mOsm/kg.

The osmolality of phenobarbital sodium 100 mg was calculated for the following dilutions:[1054]

Diluent	Osmolality (mOsm/kg)	
	50 mL	100 mL
Dextrose 5%	296	289
Sodium chloride 0.9%	325	317

Trade Name(s)

Luminal Sodium

Administration

Phenobarbital sodium is administered by intramuscular injection into a large muscle and slow intravenous injection. The commercial injection is highly alkaline and may cause local tissue damage. Do not administer subcutaneously. When given intravenously, the rate of injection should not exceed 60 mg/min.[1(2/08)] [4]

Stability

Phenobarbital sodium injection in intact containers should be stored at controlled room temperature and protected from light.[1(2/08)]

Phenobarbital sodium under simulated summer conditions in paramedic vehicles was exposed to temperatures ranging from 26 to 38°C over 4 weeks. Analysis found no loss of the drug under these conditions.[2562]

Phenobarbital sodium is not generally considered stable in aqueous solutions.[4] However, a test of phenobarbital sodium 10% (w/v) in aqueous solution showed 7% decomposition in 4 weeks when stored at 20°C. There was no measurable decomposition in 8 weeks with storage at −25°C.[233]

In addition, the stability of phenobarbital sodium diluted to a 10-mg/mL concentration in sodium chloride 0.9% for use in infants was studied. When stored at 4°C, the dilution was physically compatible with no loss of drug over 28 days.[1294]

Phenobarbital may precipitate from solutions of phenobarbital sodium, depending on the concentration and acidic pH.[4] No solution containing a precipitate or that is more than slightly discolored should be used.[1(2/08)] [4]

Phenobarbital sodium may raise the pH of admixture solutions to the alkaline range and, therefore, should not be mixed with alkali-labile drugs.[47]

Plasticizer Leaching

Phenobarbital sodium 6 mg/mL in dextrose 5% did not leach diethylhexyl phthalate (DEHP) plasticizer from 50-mL polyvinyl chloride (PVC) bags in 24 hours at 24°C.[1683]

Filtration

Phenobarbital sodium 130 mg/L in dextrose 5%, sodium chloride 0.9%, and Ringer's injection, lactated filtered over 12 hours through a 5-μm stainless steel depth filter (Argyle Filter Connector), a 0.22-μm cellulose ester membrane filter (Ivex-2 Filter Set), and a 0.22-μm polycarbonate membrane filter (In-Sure Filter Set), showed no loss due to binding to the filters.[320]

Compatibility Information

Solution Compatibility

Phenobarbital sodium

Test Soln Name	Mfr	Mfr	Conc/L or %	Remarks	Ref	C/I
Dextrose 2.5% in half-strength Ringer's injection	AB		320 mg	Physically compatible	3	C
Dextrose 5% in Ringer's injection	AB		320 mg	Physically compatible	3	C

DOI: 10.37573/9781585286850.312

Solution Compatibility (Cont.)

Test Soln Name	Mfr	Mfr	Conc/L or %	Remarks	Ref	C/I
Dextrose 2.5% in Ringer's injection, lactated	AB		320 mg	Physically compatible	3	C
Dextrose 5% in half-strength Ringer's injection, lactated	AB		320 mg	Physically compatible	3	C
Dextrose 5% in Ringer's injection, lactated	AB		320 mg	Physically compatible	3	C
Dextrose 10% in Ringer's injection, lactated	AB		320 mg	Physically compatible	3	C
Dextrose 2.5% in sodium chloride 0.45%	AB		320 mg	Physically compatible	3	C
Dextrose 2.5% in sodium chloride 0.9%	AB		320 mg	Physically compatible	3	C
Dextrose 5% in sodium chloride 0.225%	AB		320 mg	Physically compatible	3	C
Dextrose 5% in sodium chloride 0.45%	AB		320 mg	Physically compatible	3	C
Dextrose 5% in sodium chloride 0.9%	AB		320 mg	Physically compatible	3	C
Dextrose 10% in sodium chloride 0.9%	AB		320 mg	Physically compatible	3	C
Dextrose 2.5%	AB		320 mg	Physically compatible	3	C
Dextrose 5%	AB		320 mg	Physically compatible	3	C
Dextrose 10%	AB		320 mg	Physically compatible	3	C
Ionosol B in dextrose 5%	AB		320 mg	Physically compatible	3	C
Ionosol MB in dextrose 5%	AB		320 mg	Physically compatible	3	C
Ringer's injection	AB		320 mg	Physically compatible	3	C
Ringer's injection, lactated	AB		320 mg	Physically compatible	3	C
Sodium chloride 0.45%	AB		320 mg	Physically compatible	3	C
Sodium chloride 0.9%	AB		320 mg	Physically compatible	3	C
Sodium lactate ⅙ M	AB		320 mg	Physically compatible	3	C

Additive Compatibility

Phenobarbital sodium

Test Drug	Mfr	Conc/L or %	Mfr	Conc/L or %	Test Solution	Remarks	Ref	C/I
Amikacin sulfate	BR	5 g	LI	300 mg	D5LR, D5R, D5S, D5W, D10W, LR, NS, R, SL	Physically compatible and both stable for 24 hr at 25°C	294	C
Aminophylline	SE	500 mg	AB	100 mg		Physically compatible	6	C
Aminophylline	SE	1 g	WI	200 mg	D5W	Physically compatible	15	C
Calcium chloride	UP	1 g	WI	200 mg	D5W	Physically compatible	15	C
Calcium gluconate	UP	1 g	WI	200 mg	D5W	Physically compatible	15	C
Chlorpromazine HCl	BP	200 mg	BP	800 mg	D5W, NS	Precipitates immediately	26	I
Colistimethate sodium	WC	500 mg	WI	200 mg	D5W	Physically compatible	15	C
Dimenhydrinate	SE	500 mg	WI	200 mg	D5W	Physically compatible	15	C
Ephedrine sulfate	LI	250 mg	WI	200 mg	D5W	Physically incompatible	15	I
Hydralazine HCl	BP	80 mg	BP	800 mg	D5W	Yellow color and precipitate in 3 hr	26	I
Hydrocortisone sodium succinate	UP	500 mg	WI	200 mg	D5W	Physically incompatible	15	I

Additive Compatibility (Cont.)

Test Drug	Mfr	Conc/L or %	Mfr	Conc/L or %	Test Solution	Remarks	Ref	C/I
Hydroxyzine HCl	RR	250 mg	WI	200 mg	D5W	Physically incompatible	15	I
Meropenem	ZEN	1 and 20 g	ES	200 mg	NS	Visually compatible for 4 hr at room temperature	1994	C
Pentazocine lactate	WI	300 mg	WI	200 mg	D5W	Physically incompatible	15	I
Polymyxin B sulfate	BW	200 mg	WI	200 mg	D5W	Physically compatible	15	C
Prochlorperazine mesylate	BP	100 mg	BP	800 mg	D5W	Haze develops over 3 hr	26	I
Prochlorperazine mesylate	BP	100 mg	BP	800 mg	NS	Precipitates immediately	26	I
Promethazine HCl	WY	250 mg	WI	200 mg	D5W	Physically incompatible	15	I
Promethazine HCl	BP	100 mg	BP	800 mg	D5W	Haze develops over 3 hr	26	I
Promethazine HCl	BP	100 mg	BP	800 mg	NS	Precipitates immediately	26	I
Succinylcholine chloride						Phenobarbital precipitates or succinylcholine hydrolyzes	4	I
Verapamil HCl	KN	80 mg	ES	260 mg	D5W, NS	Physically compatible for 24 hr	764	C

Drugs in Syringe Compatibility

Phenobarbital sodium

Test Drug	Mfr	Amt	Mfr	Amt	Remarks	Ref	C/I
Caffeine citrate		20 mg/1 mL	ES	130 mg/1 mL	Visually compatible for 4 hr at 25°C	2440	C
Heparin sodium		2500 units/1 mL		200 mg/1 mL	Physically compatible for at least 5 min	1053	C
Hydromorphone HCl	KN	2, 10, 40 mg/1 mL	AB	120 mg/1 mL	Precipitate forms immediately but dissipates with shaking. Phenobarbital precipitates after 6 hr at room temperature	2082	I
Pantoprazole sodium	a	4 mg/1 mL		120 mg/1 mL	Precipitates within 4 hr	2574	I
Ranitidine HCl	GL	50 mg/2 mL	AB	120 mg/1 mL	Immediate white haze	978	I

[a] Test performed using the formulation WITHOUT edetate disodium.

Y-Site Injection Compatibility (1:1 Mixture)

Phenobarbital sodium

Test Drug	Mfr	Conc	Mfr	Conc	Remarks	Ref	C/I
Doripenem	JJ	5 mg/mL[a b]	BA	5 mg/mL[a b]	Physically compatible for 4 hr at 23°C	2743	C
Doxapram HCl	RB	2 mg/mL[a]	ES	10 mg/mL[b]	Visually compatible for 4 hr at 23°C	2470	C
Enalaprilat	MSD	1.25 mg/mL	WY	0.32 mg/mL[a b]	Physically compatible for 4 hr at 21°C	1409	C
Fentanyl citrate	JN	0.025 mg/mL[a]	WY	2 mg/mL[a]	Physically compatible for 48 hr at 22°C	1706	C
Fosphenytoin sodium	PD[e]	10 mg PE/mL[b]		130 mg/mL	Visually compatible with no loss of either drug in 8 hr at room temperature	2212	C
Hydromorphone HCl	KN	2, 10, 40 mg/mL	AB	120 mg/mL	Turbidity forms but dissipates; phenobarbital precipitates in 6 hr	1532	I

Y-Site Injection Compatibility (1:1 Mixture) (Cont.)

Test Drug	Mfr	Conc	Mfr	Conc	Remarks	Ref	C/I
Hydromorphone HCl	AST	0.5 mg/mL[a]	WY	2 mg/mL[a]	Physically compatible for 48 hr at 22°C	1706	C
Ibuprofen lysinate	OVA	10 mg/mL	BA	30 mg/mL[g]	Physically compatible for 4 hr at room temperature	3541	C
Ibuprofen lysinate	OVA	10 mg/mL	BA	130 mg/mL	Physically compatible for 4 hr at room temperature	3541	C
Levofloxacin	OMN	5 mg/mL[a]	ES	130 mg/mL	Visually compatible for 4 hr at 24°C	2233	C
Linezolid	PHU	2 mg/mL	WY	5 mg/mL[a]	Physically compatible for 4 hr at 23°C	2264	C
Meropenem	ZEN	1 and 50 mg/mL[b]	ES	0.32 mg/mL[c]	Visually compatible for 4 hr at room temperature	1994	C
Methadone HCl	LI	1 mg/mL[a]	WY	2 mg/mL[a]	Physically compatible for 48 hr at 22°C	1706	C
Morphine sulfate	AST	1 mg/mL[a]	WY	2 mg/mL[a]	Physically compatible for 48 hr at 22°C	1706	C
Propofol	ZEN[f]	10 mg/mL	WY	5 mg/mL[a]	Physically compatible for 1 hr at 23°C	2066	C
TNA #218 to #226[d]			WY	5 mg/mL[a]	Damage to emulsion occurs immediately with free oil formation possible	2215	I
TPN #212 to #215[d]			WY	5 mg/mL[a]	Physically compatible for 4 hr at 23°C	2109	C

[a] Tested in dextrose 5%.

[b] Tested in sodium chloride 0.9%.

[c] Tested in sterile water for injection.

[d] Refer to Appendix for the composition of parenteral nutrition solutions. TNA indicates a 3-in-1 admixture, and TPN indicates a 2-in-1 admixture.

[e] Concentration of fosphenytoin expressed in milligrams of phenytoin sodium equivalents (PE) per mL.

[f] Test performed using the formulation WITH edetate disodium.

[g] Tested in both dextrose 5% and sodium chloride 0.9%.

Selected Revisions May 1, 2020. © Copyright, October 1982.
American Society of Health-System Pharmacists, Inc.

Phentolamine Mesylate

AHFS 12:16.04.04

Products

Phentolamine mesylate is available in vials containing 5 mg of drug with 25 mg of mannitol as a lyophilized powder. Reconstitution with 1 mL of sterile water for injection results in a 5-mg/mL solution.[1(4/06)] [4]

pH

From 4.5 to 6.5.[4]

Administration

Phentolamine mesylate may be administered by intramuscular or intravenous injection.[1(4/06)] [4]

Stability

The intact vials should be stored at controlled room temperature.[1(4/06)] [4] Although the manufacturer recommends that reconstituted solutions be used immediately and not stored,[1(4/06)] other information indicates that such solutions are stable for 48 hours at room temperature and one week at 2 to 8°C.[4]

Sorption

Phentolamine mesylate was shown not to exhibit sorption to PVC bags and tubing, polyethylene tubing, Silastic tubing, and polypropylene syringes.[536] [606]

Compatibility Information

Additive Compatibility

Phentolamine mesylate

Test Drug	Mfr	Conc/L or %	Mfr	Conc/L or %	Test Solution	Remarks	Ref	C/I
Dobutamine HCl	LI	1 g	CI	20 mg	D5W, NS	Physically compatible for 24 hr at 21°C	812	C
Verapamil HCl	KN	80 mg	RC	10 mg	D5W, NS	Physically compatible for 24 hr	764	C

Drugs in Syringe Compatibility

Phentolamine mesylate

Test Drug	Mfr	Amt	Mfr	Amt	Remarks	Ref	C/I
Papaverine HCl	LI	30 mg/mL	BV, CI	0.5 mg/mL[a]	Physically compatible. Little papaverine loss at 5 and 25°C. 1 to 3% phentolamine loss at 5°C and 4 to 5% at 25°C in 30 days	1161	C

[a] Constituted with the papaverine hydrochloride injection.

Y-Site Injection Compatibility (1:1 Mixture)

Phentolamine mesylate

Test Drug	Mfr	Conc	Mfr	Conc	Remarks	Ref	C/I
Amiodarone HCl	LZ	4 mg/mL[a b]	CI	0.04 mg/mL[a b]	Physically compatible for 24 hr at 21°C under fluorescent light	1032	C

[a] Tested in dextrose 5%.

[b] Tested in sodium chloride 0.9%.

Selected Revisions October 1, 2012. © Copyright, October 1982.
American Society of Health-System Pharmacists, Inc.

DOI: 10.37573/9781585286850.313

Phenylephrine Hydrochloride
AHFS 12:12.04

Products

Phenylephrine hydrochloride is available as a 1% solution in 1-mL single-use vials and 5- and 10-mL pharmacy bulk vials.[3051] [3052] Each mL of solution contains phenylephrine hydrochloride 10 mg with sodium citrate dihydrate 4 mg, citric acid monohydrate 1 mg, sodium chloride 3.5 mg, and sodium metabisulfite 2 mg in water for injection.[3051] [3052] The pH may have been adjusted with sodium hydroxide and/or hydrochloric acid during manufacturing.[3051] [3052]

Pharmacy bulk vials should only be used in the preparation of solutions for continuous infusion.[3052]

pH

The 10% solution of phenylephrine (West-Ward) has a pH ranging from 3 to 6.5.[3051] The 10% solution of Vazculep has a pH ranging from 3.5 to 5.5.[3052]

Trade Name(s)

Vazculep

Administration

Phenylephrine hydrochloride is administered by intravenous bolus injection or by continuous intravenous infusion.[3051] [3052] For intravenous bolus injection, a 100-mcg/mL solution from which the bolus injection is withdrawn should be prepared by diluting 1 mL (10 mg) of phenylephrine hydrochloride with 99 mL of dextrose 5% or sodium chloride 0.9%.[3051] [3052] For continuous intravenous infusion, 1 mL (10 mg) of phenylephrine hydrochloride should be added to 500 mL of dextrose 5% or sodium chloride 0.9% to yield a final concentration of 20 mcg/mL.[3051] [3052]

Stability

Intact vials of phenylephrine hydrochloride should be stored at controlled room temperature and protected from light by storing in the original carton until time of use.[3051] [3052]

The diluted solution should be visually inspected for particulate matter and discoloration prior to use; the solution should not be used if it is colored or cloudy or contains particulate matter.[3051] [3052]

Once the closure of the pharmacy bulk vial has been penetrated with a suitable sterile transfer set or dispensing set that allows the measured dispensing of the vial contents, the vial should not be re-entered, and dispensing from the vial should be completed within 4 hours.[3052] Any unused portion should be discarded.[3052]

Phenylephrine hydrochloride was stable for 84 days at 60°C in a 250-mg/100-mL concentration in sterile water for injection.[132]

Phenylephrine hydrochloride in dextrose 5% is stated to be stable for at least 48 hours at pH 3.5 to 7.5.[4]

Syringes

Phenylephrine hydrochloride (Gensia Sicor) 0.1 mg/mL packaged in polypropylene plastic syringes fitted with tip seals and stored at 23 to 25°C in fluorescent light and at 3 to 5°C and at −20°C in the dark for 30 days exhibited no precipitation, cloudiness, or color change and virtually no loss of drug.[2737]

Central Venous Catheter

Phenylephrine hydrochloride (Ohmeda) 1 mg/mL in dextrose 5% was found to be compatible with the ARROWg+ard Blue Plus (Arrow International) chlorhexidine-bearing triple-lumen central catheter. Essentially complete delivery of the drug was found with little or no drug loss occurring. Furthermore, chlorhexidine delivered from the catheter remained at trace amounts with no substantial increase due to the delivery of the drug through the catheter.[2335]

Compatibility Information
Solution Compatibility

Phenylephrine HCl

Test Soln Name	Mfr	Mfr	Conc/L or %	Remarks	Ref	C/I
Dextrose 2.5% in half-strength Ringer's injection	AB	WI	1 mg	Physically compatible	3	C
Dextrose 5% in Ringer's injection	AB	WI	1 mg	Physically compatible	3	C
Dextrose 2.5% in Ringer's injection, lactated	AB	WI	1 mg	Physically compatible	3	C
Dextrose 5% in half-strength Ringer's injection, lactated	AB	WI	1 mg	Physically compatible	3	C

DOI: 10.37573/9781585286850.314

Solution Compatibility (Cont.)

Test Soln Name	Mfr	Mfr	Conc/L or %	Remarks	Ref	C/I
Dextrose 5% in Ringer's injection, lactated	AB	WI	1 mg	Physically compatible	3	C
Dextrose 10% in Ringer's injection, lactated	AB	WI	1 mg	Physically compatible	3	C
Dextrose 2.5% in sodium chloride 0.45%	AB	WI	1 mg	Physically compatible	3	C
Dextrose 2.5% in sodium chloride 0.9%	AB	WI	1 mg	Physically compatible	3	C
Dextrose 5% in sodium chloride 0.225%	AB	WI	1 mg	Physically compatible	3	C
Dextrose 5% in sodium chloride 0.45%	AB	WI	1 mg	Physically compatible	3	C
Dextrose 5% in sodium chloride 0.9%	AB	WI	1 mg	Physically compatible	3	C
Dextrose 10% in sodium chloride 0.9%	AB	WI	1 mg	Physically compatible	3	C
Dextrose 2.5%	AB	WI	1 mg	Physically compatible	3	C
Dextrose 5%	AB	WI	1 mg	Physically compatible	3	C
Dextrose 5%		WW	20 and 100 mg	Stable for 4 hr at room temperature or 24 hr under refrigeration	3051	C
Dextrose 5%		ECL	20 and 100 mg	Stable for 4 hr at room temperature or 24 hr under refrigeration	3052	C
Dextrose 10%	AB	WI	1 mg	Physically compatible	3	C
Ionosol B in dextrose 5%	AB	WI	1 mg	Physically compatible	3	C
Ionosol MB in dextrose 5%	AB	WI	1 mg	Physically compatible	3	C
Ringer's injection	AB	WI	1 mg	Physically compatible	3	C
Ringer's injection, lactated	AB	WI	1 mg	Physically compatible	3	C
Sodium chloride 0.45%	AB	WI	1 mg	Physically compatible	3	C
Sodium chloride 0.9%		WI	2.5 g	Stable for 24 hr at 22°C	132	C
Sodium chloride 0.9%	AB	WI	1 mg	Physically compatible	3	C
Sodium chloride 0.9%	BA[a]	BA	100 and 200 mg	Physically compatible with no loss in 14 days at 25°C	2524	C
Sodium chloride 0.9%	BA[a]	SZ	200 and 400 mg	Physically compatible with less than 5% loss in 60 days at room temperature in light	2963	C
Sodium chloride 0.9%		WW	20 and 100 mg	Stable for 4 hr at room temperature or 24 hr under refrigeration	3051	C
Sodium chloride 0.9%		ECL	20 and 100 mg	Stable for 4 hr at room temperature or 24 hr under refrigeration	3052	C
Sodium lactate ⅙ M	AB	WI	1 mg	Physically compatible	3	C

[a] Tested in PVC containers.

Additive Compatibility

Phenylephrine HCl

Test Drug	Mfr	Conc/L or %	Mfr	Conc/L or %	Test Solution	Remarks	Ref	C/I
Chloramphenicol sodium succinate[b]	PD	500 mg	WI	2.5 g	D5W, NS	Phenylephrine stable for 24 hr at 22°C	132	C
Dobutamine HCl	LI	1 g	WI	20 mg	D5W, NS	Physically compatible for 24 hr at 21°C	812	C
Lidocaine HCl	AST	2 g	WI	20 mg		Physically compatible	24	C

Additive Compatibility (Cont.)

Test Drug	Mfr	Conc/L or %	Mfr	Conc/L or %	Test Solution	Remarks	Ref	C/I
Potassium chloride	AB	40 mEq	WI	2.5 g	D5W	Phenylephrine stable for 24 hr at 22°C	132	C
Sodium bicarbonate	AB	2.4 mEq[a]	WI	10 mg	D5W	Physically compatible for 24 hr	772	C
Sodium bicarbonate		5%	WI	20 mg		Stable for 24 hr at 25°C	48	C

[a] One vial of Neut added to a liter of admixture.

[b] Tested both with and without sodium bicarbonate 7.5 g/L.

Drugs in Syringe Compatibility

Phenylephrine HCl

Test Drug	Mfr	Amt	Mfr	Amt	Remarks	Ref	C/I
Caffeine citrate		20 mg/1 mL	ES	10 mg/1 mL	Visually compatible for 4 hr at 25°C	2440	C
Lidocaine HCl		2%		0.25%	No loss of either drug in 66 days at 25°C	1278	C

Y-Site Injection Compatibility (1:1 Mixture)

Phenylephrine HCl

Test Drug	Mfr	Conc	Mfr	Conc	Remarks	Ref	C/I
Amiodarone HCl	LZ	4 mg/mL[a][b]	WI	0.04 mg/mL[a][b]	Physically compatible for 24 hr at 21°C	1032	C
Angiotensin II acetate	LJ	5 and 10 mcg/mL[b]			Stated to be compatible	3430	C
Anidulafungin	VIC	0.5 mg/mL[a]	BA	1 mg/mL[a]	Physically compatible for 4 hr at 23°C	2617	C
Argatroban	GSK	1 mg/mL[b]	AMR	10 mg/mL	Visually compatible for 24 hr at 23°C	2391	C
Bivalirudin	TMC	5 mg/mL[a]	AMR	1 mg/mL[a]	Physically compatible for 4 hr at 23°C	2373	C
Bivalirudin	TMC	5 mg/mL[a][b]	AMR	10 mg/mL	Visually compatible for 6 hr at 23°C	2680	C
Cangrelor tetrasodium	TMC	1 mg/mL[b]		1 mg/mL[b]	Physically compatible for 4 hr	3243	C
Caspofungin acetate	ME	0.7 mg/mL[b]	BA	1 mg/mL[b]	Physically compatible for 4 hr at room temperature	2758	C
Ceftazidime–avibactam sodium	ALL	20 mg/mL[h][i]			Physically compatible for up to 4 hr at room temperature	3004	C
Ceftolozane sulfate–tazobactam sodium	CUB	10 mg/mL[e][f]	WW	1 mg/mL[e]	Physically compatible for 2 hr	3262	C
Cisatracurium besylate	GW	0.1, 2, 5 mg/mL[a]	GNS	1 mg/mL[a]	Physically compatible for 4 hr at 23°C	2074	C
Dexmedetomidine HCl	HOS	4 mcg/mL[b]			Stated to be compatible	3181	C
Doripenem	JJ	5 mg/mL[a][b]	GNS	1 mg/mL[a][b]	Physically compatible for 4 hr at 23°C	2743	C
Eravacycline dihydro-chloride	TET	0.6 mg/mL[b]	AVD	1 mg/mL[b]	Physically compatible for 2 hr at room temperature	3532	C
Etomidate	AB	2 mg/mL	ES	10 mg/mL	Visually compatible for 7 days at 25°C	1801	C
Famotidine	MSD	0.2 mg/mL[a]	WI	0.02 mg/mL[a]	Physically compatible for 4 hr at 25°C	1188	C
Fenoldopam mesylate	AB	80 mcg/mL[b]	AMR	1 mg/mL[b]	Physically compatible for 4 hr at 23°C	2467	C
Furosemide	AB	4 mg/mL[a][b]	BA	0.64 mg/mL[a][b]	Precipitates in 5 to 15 min	2687	I
Haloperidol lactate	MN	0.5[a] and 5 mg/mL	WB	0.02 mg/mL[a]	Visually compatible for 24 hr at 21°C	1523	C

Y-Site Injection Compatibility (1:1 Mixture) (Cont.)

Test Drug	Mfr	Conc	Mfr	Conc	Remarks	Ref	C/I
Hetastarch in lactated electrolyte	AB	6%	OHM	1 mg/mL[a]	Physically compatible for 4 hr at 23°C	2339	C
Isavuconazonium sulfate	ASP	1.5 mg/mL[e]	SZ	1 mg/mL[e]	Physically compatible for 2 hr	3263	C
Levofloxacin	OMN	5 mg/mL[a]	AMR	10 mg/mL	Visually compatible for 4 hr at 24°C	2233	C
Meropenem–vaborbactam	TMC	8 mg/mL[b g]	ECL	1 mg/mL[b]	Physically compatible for 3 hr at 20 to 25°C	3380	C
Micafungin sodium	ASP	1.5 mg/mL[b]	BA	1 mg/mL[b]	Physically compatible for 4 hr at 23°C	2683	C
Nesiritide	SCI	50 mcg/mL[a b]		10 mg/mL	Physically compatible for 4 hr. May be chemically incompatible with nesiritide[c]	2625	?
Oritavancin diphosphate	TAR	0.8, 1.2, and 2 mg/mL[a]	PNT	0.2 mg/mL[a]	Visually compatible for 4 hr at 20 to 24°C	2928	C
Plazomicin sulfate	ACH	24 mg/mL[e]	AVD	1 mg/mL[e]	Physically compatible for 1 hr at 20 to 25°C	3432	C
Propofol	STU	2 mg/mL	ES	10 mg/mL	Yellow discoloration forms within 7 days at 25°C. No visible change in 24 hr	1801	?
Propofol	ZEN[j]	10 mg/mL	ES	0.1 mg/mL[a]	Physically compatible for 1 hr at 23°C	2066	C
Remifentanil HCl	GW	0.025 and 0.25 mg/mL[b]	AMR	1 mg/mL[a]	Physically compatible for 4 hr at 23°C	2075	C
Tedizolid phosphate	CUB	0.8 mg/mL[b]	SZ	1 mg/mL[b]	Physically compatible for 2 hr	3244	C
Telavancin HCl	ASP	7.5 mg/mL[a b d]	SZ	1 mg/mL[a b d]	Physically compatible for 2 hr	2830	C
Vasopressin	AMR	2 and 4 units/mL[b]	AMR	40 mcg/mL[b]	Physically compatible with vasopressin pushed through a Y-site over 5 sec	2478	C
Zidovudine	BW	4 mg/mL[a]	WI	1 mg/mL[a]	Physically compatible for 4 hr at 25°C	1193	C

[a] Tested in dextrose 5%.

[b] Tested in sodium chloride 0.9%.

[c] Nesiritide is incompatible with bisulfite antioxidants used in some drug formulations. The specific formulation of the product to be used should be checked to ensure that no sulfite antioxidants are present.

[d] Tested in Ringer's injection, lactated.

[e] Tested in both dextrose 5% and sodium chloride 0.9%.

[f] Ceftolozane component. Ceftolozane in a 2:1 fixed-ratio concentration with tazobactam.

[g] Meropenem component. Meropenem in a 1:1 fixed-ratio concentration with vaborbactam.

[h] Ceftazidime component. Ceftazidime in a 4:1 fixed-ratio concentration with avibactam.

[i] Tested in dextrose 5%, sodium chloride 0.9%, and Ringer's injection, lactated.

[j] Test performed using the formulation WITH edetate disodium.

Selected Revisions May 1, 2020. © Copyright, October 1982.
American Society of Health-System Pharmacists, Inc.

Phenytoin Sodium
AHFS 28:12.12

Products

Phenytoin sodium is available as a 50-mg/mL solution in 2- and 5-mL single-dose vials.[3376] Each mL of solution also contains propylene glycol 40% (v/v) and alcohol 10% (v/v) in water for injection.[3376] Sodium hydroxide may have been added to adjust the pH.[3376]

CAUTION: Care should be taken to avoid confusion between phenytoin sodium and fosphenytoin sodium to prevent dosing errors.[3280]

pH

From 10 to 12.3.[3376]

Osmolality

The osmolality of phenytoin sodium 50 mg/mL was 9740 mOsm/kg by freezing-point depression and 6175 mOsm/kg by vapor pressure.[1071] Another report indicated that the osmolality was 3035 mOsm/kg by freezing-point depression.[1233]

The osmolality of phenytoin sodium 500 mg in 50 and 100 mL of sodium chloride 0.9% was calculated to be 336 and 312 mOsm/kg, respectively.[1054]

Administration

Phenytoin sodium is preferably administered intravenously, directly into a large peripheral or central vein through a large-gauge catheter.[3376] Prior to administration, patency of the intravenous catheter should be tested with a flush of sodium chloride.[3376] Following each intravenous administration of phenytoin sodium, the same catheter used to administer the drug should be flushed with sodium chloride to avoid irritation caused by the alkalinity of the phenytoin sodium formulation.[3376]

For the treatment of status epilepticus, a loading dose of phenytoin sodium should be administered intravenously slowly.[3376] For adults, the manufacturer recommends administration of phenytoin sodium at a rate not exceeding 50 mg/min.[3376] For pediatric patients, the manufacturer recommends administration of phenytoin sodium at a rate not exceeding 1 to 3 mg/kg/min or 50 mg/min, whichever is slower.[3376] The intramuscular route of administration should not be used in the treatment of status epilepticus.[3376]

For non-emergent indications, phenytoin sodium should be administered more slowly, either as a loading dose or by intermittent intravenous infusion.[3376] When administered as an intravenous infusion, phenytoin sodium solution should be diluted in sodium chloride 0.9% to a final phenytoin sodium concentration no less than 5 mg/mL.[3376] Administration of phenytoin sodium solution diluted in sodium chloride 0.9% should begin immediately after dilution through an inline filter with a pore size of 0.22 to 0.55 μm.[3376]

Although phenytoin sodium also may be administered by intramuscular injection, it can cause pain, necrosis, and abscess formation at the injection site and can result in erratic or delayed absorption of the drug.[3376] The manufacturer states that the drug generally should not be administered intramuscularly because of these risks.[3376] In addition, the intramuscular route of administration should not be used in the treatment of status epilepticus.[3376]

Purple glove syndrome, characterized by edema, discoloration, and pain distal to the site of infusion, has been reported following intravenous administration of phenytoin sodium through a peripheral vein and may or may not be associated with extravasation.[3376]

Stability

Intact vials should be stored at controlled room temperature.[3376] If the undiluted solution is refrigerated or frozen, a precipitate may form; however, this precipitate will dissolve upon standing at room temperature.[3376] On dissolution of the precipitate, the product is still suitable for use.[3376] Also, a faint yellow color, which has no effect on concentration, may sometimes develop in the injection.[3376]

Phenytoin sodium solution diluted for infusion should not be refrigerated.[3376] Infusion of phenytoin sodium solution diluted in sodium chloride 0.9% should begin immediately after dilution and must be completed within 1 to 4 hours after preparation.[3376]

Phenytoin sodium solution should be visually inspected for particulate matter and discoloration prior to administration.[3376] Any unused portions should be discarded.[3376]

Precipitation

The solubility of phenytoin sodium is such that crystallization or precipitation may result if the special vehicle is altered or the pH is lowered.[62 63 613] Unfortunately, direct intravenous injection of phenytoin sodium is inconvenient due to limitations on the rate of administration, and rapid administration increases the risk of severe adverse cardiovascular effects.[3376] In spite of the caveat against dilution, some clinicians have advocated the infusion of phenytoin sodium[443 448 611 947 948 949 950 1295] or administration into the tubing of a running infusion solution.[63 65 338 445]

There are a number of reports of phenytoin crystallization in infusion solutions within varying periods after dilution. While the time to crystal formation may be variable and difficult to predict, crystal formation is nonetheless inevitable.[65 66 305 306 447 449 450 451 708 709 710 1421]

The relationship of phenytoin sodium solubility to various solution characteristics was explored. It was noted that the effect of the special solvent system could be disregarded in dilutions of 1:5 or more. The pH of the admixture was stated to be the primary determinant of the occurrence or absence of crystallization. With a given solution, the pH is dependent on the volume of dilution, with a lower pH resulting from greater dilution. Phenytoin becomes less soluble in aqueous solution

DOI: 10.37573/9781585286850.315

as the pH drops. Equations for predicting the compatibility of phenytoin sodium in admixture solutions were presented, but it was noted that it is not possible to predict the time required to develop precipitation.[713]

Although some may feel that infusion of phenytoin sodium is, perhaps, too dangerous to perform clinically,[452] others indicate that such administration may be feasible provided proper precautions are taken such as using a suitable vehicle (i.e., sodium chloride 0.9% or Ringer's injection, lactated), using a sufficiently concentrated solution, starting the infusion immediately after preparation and completing administration within a relatively short time, using a 0.22-μm inline filter, and watching the admixture very carefully.[305 306 453 611 612 613 708 709 710 947 948 949 950 1295]

Phenytoin may precipitate if the injection is mixed with dextrose or dextrose-containing solutions; mixing with these solutions should be avoided.[3376] Such precipitation has been found to occlude catheters. Instilling 5 mL of 8.4% sodium bicarbonate injection at 15- to 30-minute intervals has cleared catheters occluded with phenytoin precipitate. The sodium bicarbonate apparently raised the pH enough to result in dissolution of a sufficient amount of the phenytoin precipitate to reopen the catheter;[2299 2300] however, the safety is uncertain because it is not known if some of the precipitated phenytoin is delivered into the bloodstream upon opening the occlusion.

Sorption

Phenytoin sodium was shown not to exhibit sorption to polyvinyl chloride (PVC) bags and tubing, polyethylene tubing, Silastic tubing, and polypropylene syringes.[536 606]

Plasticizer Leaching

Phenytoin sodium 10 mg/mL in sodium chloride 0.9% did not leach diethylhexyl phthalate (DEHP) plasticizer from 50-mL PVC bags in 24 hours at 24°C.[1683]

Filtration

The manufacturer recommends the use of an inline filter with a pore size of 0.22 to 0.55 μm for administration of phenytoin sodium solution diluted for infusion.[3376]

Phenytoin sodium 250 mg/5 mL was filtered at a rate of 1 mL/min through a 5-μm stainless steel depth filter (Argyle Filter Connector). No reduction due to binding to the filter was observed.[320]

Compatibility Information

Solution Compatibility

Phenytoin sodium

Test Soln Name	Mfr	Mfr	Conc/L or %	Remarks	Ref	C/I
Dextrose 5% in sodium chloride 0.9%	TR	PD	1 g	Visible crystals in minutes. 21% crystallized in 8 hr and 38% in 24 hr	306	I
Dextrose 5%	TR	PD	1 g	Visible crystals in minutes. 15% crystallized in 8 hr and 36% in 24 hr	306	I
Dextrose 5%	TR	PD	4.6, 9.2, 18.4 g	Crystal formation. Erratic concentrations through 0.2-μm filter over 24 hr at 29°C	305	I
Dextrose 5%	MG	PD	1 g	No precipitate or drug loss in 8 hr at room temperature. Precipitate forms within 24 hr with 15% drug	446	I
Dextrose 5%	TR	PD	1 g	Crystal formation in 1 hr	450, 451	I
Dextrose 5%	AB	PD	1 g	Visible crystals in less than 12 min. 18% loss of phenytoin in 14 hr and 22% in 24 hr	452	I
Dextrose 5%			1 g	10% of phenytoin removed by filtration in 2 hr and 15 to 18% in 4 hr	453	I
Dextrose 5%		PD	670 mg to 4 g	Phenytoin crystals within 5 to 25 min. Reduced phenytoin concentration	708	I
Dextrose 5%	AB, CU, MG, TR	ES, PD	0.4 to 4.55 g	Visible precipitate in 10 to 60 min with drug loss in 20 to 45 min	710	I
Dextrose 5%	TR	PD	1, 1.5, 2, 4, 10 g	Visible crystals in 30 min. 12 to 20% crystallized in 4 hr	951	I
Ringer's injection, lactated	TR	PD	4.6, 9.2, 18.4 g	Crystal formation. Erratic concentration through 0.2-μm filter over 24 hr at 29°C	305	I
Ringer's injection, lactated	TR	PD	1 g	Visible crystals in 6 to 9 hr. Approximately 0.8% crystallized in 8 hr and 7% in 24 hr	306	I

Solution Compatibility (Cont.)

Test Soln Name	Mfr	Mfr	Conc/L or %	Remarks	Ref	C/I
Ringer's injection, lactated	TR	ES, PD	0.4 to 4.55 g	No drug loss for 12 to 24 hr at 23°C. Inconsistent precipitate	710	I
Sodium chloride 0.45%	TR	PD	4.6, 9.2, 18.4 g	Crystal formation. Under 10% drug loss through 0.2-μm filter over 24 hr at 29°C	305	I
Sodium chloride 0.9%		PD	1 to 10 g	Phenytoin crystal formation in 20 to 30 min	63	I
Sodium chloride 0.9%		PD	200 mg to 10 g	Phenytoin crystal formation in 30 min	65, 447	I
Sodium chloride 0.9%		PD	2 and 4 g	Phenytoin crystal formation in 10 to 15 min	66	I
Sodium chloride 0.9%	TR	PD	1 g	Visible crystals in 6 to 9 hr. Approximately 0.8% crystallized in 8 hr and 7% in 24 hr	306	I
Sodium chloride 0.9%	TR	PD	4.6, 9.2, 18.4 g	Crystal formation. Under 10% drug loss through 0.2-μm filter over 24 hr at 29°C	305	I
Sodium chloride 0.9%			1 g	10% of phenytoin removed by filtration in 4 hr	453	I
Sodium chloride 0.9%		PD	670 mg to 4 g	No crystals observed during 1-hr study period	708	C
Sodium chloride 0.9%	TR	PD	1 to 10 g	Crystals formed in unfiltered solutions in 18 hr. Filtered solutions stored at 6°C had no crystals and no reduction in phenytoin in 24 hr	709	I
Sodium chloride 0.9%	TR	ES, PD	0.4 to 4.55 g	No reduction in phenytoin for 8 to 24 hr at 23°C. Inconsistent precipitate	710	I
Sodium chloride 0.9%	TR	PD	1, 1.5, 2, 4, 10 g	Visible precipitation appeared in some samples in 3 hr	951	I
Sodium chloride 0.9%	TR	PD	9.2 and 18.4 g	Physically compatible for 2 hr. Filtration did not reduce drug concentration	1514	C
Sodium chloride 0.9%	TR	ES, LY, SO	9.2 and 18.4 g	Microcrystals formed repeatedly, but inconsistently, over 2 hr. Filtration did not reduce drug concentration	1514	?
Sodium chloride 0.9%		WW		Manufacturer-recommended solution	3376	C

Additive Compatibility

Phenytoin sodium

Test Drug	Mfr	Conc/L or %	Mfr	Conc/L or %	Test Solution	Remarks	Ref	C/I
Amikacin sulfate	BR	5 g	PD	250 mg	D5LR, D5R, D5S, D5W, D10W, LR, NS, R, SL	Precipitates immediately	294	I
Dobutamine HCl	LI	1 g	ES	1 g	D5W, NS	White precipitate forms within 5 to 10 min	789	I
Dobutamine HCl	LI	1 g	AHP	25 g	D5W, NS	White precipitate forms rapidly, with brown solution in 6 hr at 21°C	812	I
Fat emulsion, intravenous	VT	10%	PD	1 g		Phenytoin crystal precipitation	32	I
Lidocaine HCl	AST	2 g	ES	1 g	D5W, LR, NS	Immediate formation of a white cloudy precipitate	775	I
Nitroglycerin	ACC	400 mg	PD	1 g	D5W, NS[a]	Phenytoin crystals in 24 hr. 3 to 4% nitroglycerin loss in 24 hr and 9% in 48 hr at 23°C. Phenytoin not tested	929	I
Verapamil HCl	KN	80 mg	PD	500 mg	D5W, NS	Physically compatible for 48 hr	739	C

[a] Tested in glass containers.

Drugs in Syringe Compatibility

Phenytoin sodium

Test Drug	Mfr	Amt	Mfr	Amt	Remarks	Ref	C/I
Hydromorphone HCl	KN	2, 10, 40 mg/1 mL	AB	50 mg/1 mL	White precipitate of phenytoin forms immediately	2082	I
Pantoprazole sodium	a	4 mg/1 mL		50 mg/1 mL	Precipitates within 1 hr	2574	I

a Test performed using the formulation WITHOUT edetate disodium.

Y-Site Injection Compatibility (1:1 Mixture)

Phenytoin sodium

Test Drug	Mfr	Conc	Mfr	Conc	Remarks	Ref	C/I
Cefepime HCl	BMS	120 mg/mL[h]		50 mg/mL	Precipitates	2513	I
Ceftazidime	GSK	120 mg/mL[h]		50 mg/mL	Precipitates	2513	I
Ceftolozane sulfate–tazobactam sodium	CUB	10 mg/mL[b j]	WW	10 mg/mL[b]	Immediate gross precipitation and increase in measured turbidity	3262	I
Ciprofloxacin	MI	2 mg/mL[c]	PD	50 mg/mL	Immediate crystal formation	1655	I
Clarithromycin	AB	4 mg/mL[a]	ANT	20 mg/mL[a]	White cloudy precipitate in 1 hr at both 30 and 17°C	2174	I
Cloxacillin sodium	SMX	100 mg/mL	SZ	50 mg/mL	Precipitates within 1 hr	3245	I
Diltiazem HCl	MMD	1 mg/mL[b]	PD	50 mg/mL	Precipitate forms	1807	I
Enalaprilat	MSD	1.25 mg/mL	PD	1 mg/mL[b]	Crystalline precipitate forms immediately	1409	I
Esmolol HCl	DCC	10 mg/mL[a]	IX	1 mg/mL[a]	Physically compatible for 24 hr at 22°C	1169	C
Famotidine	MSD	0.2 mg/mL[a]	PD	50 mg/mL	Physically compatible for 14 hr	1196	C
Fenoldopam mesylate	AB	80 mcg/mL[b]	ES	50 mg/mL	Microcrystals and yellowish darkening form immediately	2467	I
Fentanyl citrate	JN	0.025 mg/mL[a]	ES	2 mg/mL[a b]	Precipitate forms within 1 hr	1706	I
Fluconazole	RR	2 mg/mL	PD	50 mg/mL	Physically compatible for 24 hr at 25°C	1407	C
Heparin sodium	TR	50 units/mL	ES	2 mg/mL[b]	Cloudy immediately and becomes white precipitate in 4 hr at 25°C	1793	I
Heparin sodium[i]	RI	1000 units/L[d]	PD	50 mg/mL	Immediate crystal formation	322	I
Hydrocortisone sodium succinate[g]	UP	100 mg/L[d]	PD	50 mg/mL	Immediate crystal formation	322	I
Hydromorphone HCl	KN	2, 10, 40 mg/mL	AB	50 mg/mL	Turbidity forms immediately and phenytoin precipitate develops	1532	I
Hydromorphone HCl	AST	0.5 mg/mL[a]	ES	2 mg/mL[a b]	Precipitate forms within 1 hr	1706	I
Hydroxyethyl starch 130/0.4 in sodium chloride 0.9%	FRK	6%	SZ	6, 7.5, 9 mg/mL[a]	White precipitate forms immediately	2770	I
Isavuconazonium sulfate	ASP	1.5 mg/mL[b]	WW	10 mg/mL[b]	Immediate precipitation and increase in measured turbidity	3263	I
Linezolid	PHU	2 mg/mL	ES	50 mg/mL	Crystalline precipitate forms immediately	2264	I
Linezolid	PHU, HOS	2 mg/mL			Stated to be physically incompatible	3183, 3184	I

Y-Site Injection Compatibility (1:1 Mixture) (Cont.)

Test Drug	Mfr	Conc	Mfr	Conc	Remarks	Ref	C/I
Meropenem		50 mg/mL	SMX	50 mg/mL	Solution became opaque immediately	3538	I
Meropenem–vaborbactam	TMC	8 mg/mL[b k]	WW	10 mg/mL[b]	Measured turbidity increases immediately with precipitation within 30 min. pH decreased by >1 unit within 3 hr	3380	I
Methadone HCl	LI	1 mg/mL[a]	ES	2 mg/mL[a b]	Precipitate forms immediately	1706	I
Micafungin sodium	ASP	1.5 mg/mL[b]	HOS	50 mg/mL	Measured haze increases within 1 hr	2683	I
Morphine sulfate	AST	1 mg/mL[a]	ES	2 mg/mL[a b]	Precipitate forms after 1 hr	1706	I
Oritavancin diphosphate	TAR	0.8, 1.2, and 2 mg/mL[a]	HOS	6 mg/mL[a]	Haze forms immediately	2928	I
Plazomicin sulfate	ACH	24 mg/mL[b]	WW	10 mg/mL[b]	Cloudy with immediate increase in measured turbidity; pH decreased by nearly 3 units within 30 min	3432	I
Potassium chloride		40 mEq/L[a]	PD	50 mg/mL	Immediate formation of phenytoin crystals	322	I
Potassium chloride		40 mEq/L[e]	PD	50 mg/mL	Crystals in 4 hr at room temperature	322	I
Propofol	ZEN[i]	10 mg/mL	ES	50 mg/mL	Needle-like crystals form immediately	2066	I
Tacrolimus	FUJ	1 mg/mL[b]	ES	5 mg/mL[a]	Visually compatible for 4 hr at 25°C. White haze forms by 24 hr	1630	C
Tedizolid phosphate	CUB	0.8 mg/mL[b]	WW	10 mg/mL[b]	Measured turbidity increases immediately	3244	I
Theophylline	TR	4 mg/mL	ES	2 mg/mL[b]	Immediately cloudy. Dense precipitate in 6 hr at 25°C	1793	I
TPN #189[f]			PD	50 mg/mL	Heavy white precipitate forms immediately	1767	I
Vancomycin HCl	LI	10 mg/mL[a]	m	50 mg/mL	Physically incompatible	3536	I
Vasopressin	APP	0.2 unit/mL[b]	ES	50 mg/mL	Crystals form immediately	2641	I

[a] Tested in dextrose 5%.

[b] Tested in sodium chloride 0.9%.

[c] Tested in both dextrose 5% and sodium chloride 0.9%.

[d] Tested in dextrose 5%, Ringer's injection, lactated, and sodium chloride 0.9%.

[e] Tested in both Ringer's injection, lactated and sodium chloride 0.9%.

[f] Refer to Appendix for the composition of parenteral nutrition solutions. TPN indicates a 2-in-1 admixture.

[g] Tested in combination with heparin sodium (Riker) 1000 units/L.

[h] Tested in sterile water for injection.

[i] Tested in combination with hydrocortisone sodium succinate (Upjohn) 100 mg/L.

[j] Ceftolozane component. Ceftolozane in a 2:1 fixed-ratio concentration with tazobactam.

[k] Meropenem component. Meropenem in a 1:1 fixed-ratio concentration with vaborbactam.

[l] Test performed using the formulation WITH edetate disodium.

[m] Salt not specified.

Selected Revisions May 1, 2020. © Copyright, October 1982.
American Society of Health-System Pharmacists, Inc.

Phytonadione
AHFS 88:24
Phytomenadione

Products

Phytonadione is available as a 2-mg/mL aqueous dispersion in 0.5-mL ampuls and as a 10-mg/mL aqueous dispersion in 1-mL ampuls and 5-mL vials. Each mL also contains polyoxyethylated fatty acid 70 mg, dextrose 37.5 mg, and benzyl alcohol 0.9% in water for injection.[1(8/06)]

pH

The USP cites the official pH range as 3.5 to 7.[17] Phytonadione (Hospira) has a pH of 5 to 7.[1(8/06)]

Osmolality

The osmolality of phytonadione 10 mg/mL was 325 mOsm/kg by freezing-point depression and 303 mOsm/kg by vapor pressure.[1071]

Administration

The intramuscular or subcutaneous routes are preferred for phytonadione. If intravenous injection is unavoidable, phytonadione may be given by direct intravenous injection at a rate not exceeding 1 mg/min or by intravenous infusion.[1(8/06) 4]

Stability

Phytonadione injection is available as an essentially clear yellow liquid. Phytonadione is photosensitive and should be protected from light at all times.[1(8/06) 4] When dilutions are indicated, administration should start immediately after mixing with the diluent; unused portions of the dilution, as well as unused contents of the ampul, should be discarded.[4]

Light Effects

A study of phytonadione in intravenous solutions showed 50% decomposition in 15 days under fluorescent light and 43 to 63%

in three hours on exposure to sunlight.[463] A 10 to 15% loss occurs over 24 hours on exposure to fluorescent light or sunlight.[854] It has been recommended that infusion solutions containing phytonadione require wrapping the container with aluminum foil or other opaque material for light protection.[4]

The loss of phytonadione (Roche) 0.05 to 0.1 mg/mL from solutions in glass and polypropylene containers unprotected or packaged in light-protective overwraps when exposed to neon light and daylight was evaluated. Losses approached 80% in one day unprotected from light exposure. A brown polyethylene light protection bag provided the best protection, yielding no phytonadione loss during a seven-day exposure period. A white "light-tight" light-protective overwrap and a black plastic waste disposal bag failed to protect the phytonadione completely. In the black bag, phytonadione losses of over 30% occurred in seven days; the white light-protective overwrap was worse, allowing loss of nearly half of the phytonadione in one day. Substantial differences in light protection are afforded by the different materials and the efficacy of purported light-protection barriers for light-sensitive drugs should be validated prior to use.[1923]

Substantial loss of phytonadione from both TPN and TNA admixtures due to exposure to sunlight was reported. In three hours of exposure to sunlight, 50% loss of phytonadione had occurred. The presence or absence of lipids did not affect stability.[2049]

Filtration

The manufacturer states that phytonadione passes through an inline filter with negligible loss occurring.[854]

Compatibility Information
Solution Compatibility

Phytonadione

Test Soln Name	Mfr	Mfr	Conc/L or %	Remarks	Ref	C/I
Amino acids 2%, dextrose 12.5%		ROR	5 mL	7% phytonadione loss in 4 hr and 27% loss in 24 hr under ambient temperature and light	1815	I
Amino acids 4.25%, dextrose 25%	MG	MSD	10 mg	No increase in particulate matter in 24 hr at 4°C	349	C
Dextrose 2.5% in half-strength Ringer's injection	AB	AB	50 mg	Physically compatible	3	C
Dextrose 5% in Ringer's injection	AB	AB	50 mg	Physically compatible	3	C

DOI: 10.37573/9781585286850.316

Solution Compatibility (Cont.)

Test Soln Name	Mfr	Mfr	Conc/L or %	Remarks	Ref	C/I
Dextrose 5% in half-strength Ringer's injection, lactated	AB	AB	50 mg	Physically compatible	3	C
Dextrose 2.5% in Ringer's injection, lactated	AB	AB	50 mg	Physically compatible	3	C
Dextrose 5% in Ringer's injection, lactated	AB	AB	50 mg	Physically compatible	3	C
Dextrose 10% in Ringer's injection, lactated	AB	AB	50 mg	Physically compatible	3	C
Dextrose 2.5% in sodium chloride 0.45%	AB	AB	50 mg	Physically compatible	3	C
Dextrose 2.5% in sodium chloride 0.9%	AB	AB	50 mg	Physically compatible	3	C
Dextrose 5% in sodium chloride 0.225%	AB	AB	50 mg	Physically compatible	3	C
Dextrose 5% in sodium chloride 0.45%	AB	AB	50 mg	Physically compatible	3	C
Dextrose 5% in sodium chloride 0.9%	AB	AB	50 mg	Physically compatible	3	C
Dextrose 10% in sodium chloride 0.9%	AB	AB	50 mg	Physically compatible	3	C
Dextrose 2.5%	AB	AB	50 mg	Physically compatible	3	C
Dextrose 5%	AB	AB	50 mg	Physically compatible	3	C
Dextrose 10%	AB	AB	50 mg	Physically compatible	3	C
Ionosol B in dextrose 5%	AB	AB	50 mg	Physically compatible	3	C
Ionosol MB in dextrose 5%	AB	AB	50 mg	Physically compatible	3	C
Ringer's injection	AB	AB	50 mg	Physically compatible	3	C
Ringer's injection, lactated	AB	AB	50 mg	Physically compatible	3	C
Sodium chloride 0.45%	AB	AB	50 mg	Physically compatible	3	C
Sodium chloride 0.9%	AB	AB	50 mg	Physically compatible	3	C
Sodium lactate ⅙ M	AB	AB	50 mg	Physically compatible	3	C

Additive Compatibility

Phytonadione

Test Drug	Mfr	Conc/L or %	Mfr	Conc/L or %	Test Solution	Remarks	Ref	C/I
Amikacin sulfate	BR	5 g	MSD	200 mg	D5LR, D5R, D5S, D5W, D10W, LR, NS, R, SL	Physically compatible and amikacin stable for 24 hr at 25°C. Phytonadione not analyzed	294	C
Chloramphenicol sodium succinate	PD	1 g	MSD	50 mg		Physically compatible	6	C
Ranitidine HCl	GL	50 mg and 2 g		100 mg	D5W	Ranitidine stable for only 6 hr at 25°C. Phytonadione not tested	1515	I
Sodium bicarbonate	AB	2.4 mEq[a]	MSD	10 mg	D5W	Physically compatible for 24 hr	772	C

[a] One vial of Neut added to a liter of admixture.

Drugs in Syringe Compatibility

Phytonadione

Test Drug	Mfr	Amt	Mfr	Amt	Remarks	Ref	C/I
Doxapram HCl	RB	400 mg/20 mL		10 mg/1 mL	Physically compatible with no doxapram loss in 24 hr	1177	C

Y-Site Injection Compatibility (1:1 Mixture)

Phytonadione

Test Drug	Mfr	Conc	Mfr	Conc	Remarks	Ref	C/I
Ampicillin sodium	WY	40 mg/mL[b]	MSD	0.4 mg/mL[c]	Physically compatible for 3 hr	1316	C
Dobutamine HCl	LI	4 mg/mL[c]	MSD	0.4 mg/mL[c]	Slight haze in 3 hr	1316	I
Epinephrine HCl	ES	0.032 mg/mL[c]	MSD	0.4 mg/mL[c]	Physically compatible for 3 hr	1316	C
Famotidine	MSD	0.2 mg/mL[a]	MSD	2 mg/mL	Physically compatible for 14 hr	1196	C
Heparin sodium	UP	1000 units/L[d]	RC	10 mg/mL	Physically compatible for 4 hr at room temperature	534	C
Hydrocortisone sodium succinate	UP	10 mg/L[d]	RC	10 mg/mL	Physically compatible for 4 hr at room temperature	534	C
Potassium chloride	AB	40 mEq/L[d]	RC	10 mg/mL	Physically compatible for 4 hr at room temperature	534	C

[a] Tested in dextrose 5%.

[b] Tested in sodium chloride 0.9%

[c] Tested in both dextrose 5% and sodium chloride 0.9%.

[d] Tested in dextrose 5% in Ringer's injection, dextrose 5% in Ringer's injection, lactated, dextrose 5%, Ringer's injection, lactated, and sodium chloride 0.9%.

Selected Revisions January 24, 2014. © Copyright, October 1982. American Society of Health-System Pharmacists, Inc.

Piperacillin Sodium–Tazobactam Sodium
AHFS 8:12.16.16

Products

The fixed combination of piperacillin sodium–tazobactam sodium is available as a lyophilized powder in preservative-free single-dose and ADD-Vantage vials containing 2.25 g (piperacillin 2 g plus tazobactam 250 mg), 3.375 g (piperacillin 3 g plus tazobactam 375 mg), or 4.5 g (piperacillin 4 g plus tazobactam 500 mg) as the sodium salts.[2918 2919 2921] The drug is also available in a pharmacy bulk package containing 40.5 g (piperacillin 36 g plus tazobactam 4.5 g) as the sodium salts.[2918 2920]

Generic piperacillin sodium–tazobactam sodium and Zosyn (Wyeth) products are *not* identical.[2922 2932] In 2006, all Zosyn products were reformulated to contain edetate disodium dihydrate (EDTA) as a metal chelator and sodium citrate as a buffering agent; these excipients were added to address issues with sporadic batch failures associated with excessive particulate matter related to commercially available diluents and solutions with acidic pH and the presence of trace amounts of zinc ions.[2922 2932] Other piperacillin sodium–tazobactam sodium products do not contain EDTA, sodium citrate, or any other excipients.[2919 2920 2921] These formulation differences between Zosyn products and other piperacillin sodium–tazobactam sodium products have been demonstrated to result in some differing compatibilities with certain solutions (e.g., Ringer's injection, lactated).[2922 2932 2985] Therefore, results of compatibility tests for one formulation cannot be extrapolated to another.[2922 2932] (See Solution Compatibility.)

Each 2.25, 3.375, or 4.5 g (combined components) single-dose vial should be reconstituted with 10, 15, or 20 mL, respectively, of sterile water for injection, sodium chloride 0.9%, bacteriostatic water for injection or bacteriostatic sodium chloride 0.9% (preserved with benzyl alcohol or parabens), or dextrose 5% and should be swirled until dissolved.[2918 2921] The contents of each single-dose vial should then be diluted in 50 to 150 mL of a compatible infusion solution; however, if sterile water for injection is used as the diluent, the maximum recommended volume per dose is 50 mL.[2918 2921]

ADD-Vantage vials of piperacillin sodium–tazobactam sodium should be prepared with 50 or 100 mL of dextrose 5% or sodium chloride 0.9% in ADD-Vantage diluent bags.[2919]

The 40.5-g pharmacy bulk package should be reconstituted with 152 mL of sterile water for injection, sodium chloride 0.9%, bacteriostatic water for injection or bacteriostatic sodium chloride 0.9% (preserved with benzyl alcohol or parabens), or dextrose 5% and should be shaken until dissolved; the resulting solution contains piperacillin 200 mg/mL plus tazobactam 25 mg/mL.[2918 2920] The reconstituted pharmacy bulk package solution must be diluted further in a compatible infusion solution; the recommended volume per dose is 50 to 100 mL;[2918 2920 2922] however, if sterile water for injection is used as the diluent, the maximum recommended volume per dose is 50 mL.[2918 2920 2922]

Piperacillin sodium–tazobactam sodium (Zosyn, Wyeth) also is available as a frozen iso-osmotic premixed injection in single-dose Galaxy containers containing piperacillin 40 mg/mL plus tazobactam 5 mg/mL or piperacillin 60 mg/mL plus tazobactam 7.5 mg/mL, as well as EDTA and sodium citrate dihydrate, in water for injection.[2918 2922] Dextrose hydrous is added to adjust the osmolality, and sodium bicarbonate and hydrochloric acid are used to adjust the pH.[2918 2922]

pH

Zosyn (Wyeth) products: From 5.5 to 6.8.[2918 2922]

Sodium Content

Zosyn (Wyeth) products contain 2.79 mEq (64 mg) of sodium per gram of piperacillin in the combination product.[2918]

Generic piperacillin sodium–tazobactam sodium products contain 2.35 mEq (54 mg) of sodium per gram of piperacillin in the combination product.[2919 2920 2921]

Trade Name(s)

Zosyn

Administration

Piperacillin–tazobactam solution for infusion prepared from single-dose vials or the pharmacy bulk package should be administered by intravenous infusion over at least 30 minutes after dilution in a compatible diluent to provide a recommended volume per dose of 50 to 150 mL.[2918 2920 2921] Such solutions for infusion prepared using single-dose vials or the pharmacy bulk package also can be infused using ambulatory infusion pumps.[2918 2920 2921]

Piperacillin sodium–tazobactam sodium (Zosyn, Wyeth) frozen iso-osmotic premixed injection in single-dose Galaxy containers should be thawed (see Stability: Freezing Solutions), and the solution should be administered by intravenous infusion over at least 30 minutes.[2918]

Use of extended infusion strategies (e.g., infusion over 4 hours) for piperacillin–tazobactam has been described in the literature.[2934] In such circumstances, however, careful attention must be paid to the possibility of incomplete dose administration resulting from drug loss through tubing residuals.[2934] Such loss is a function of both the concentration of the solution being infused and the residual volume of the specific tubing used for administration.[2934]

Stability

The white to off-white[2918 2920 2921] or yellowish[2919] piperacillin sodium–tazobactam sodium lyophilized powder in intact vials should be stored at controlled room temperature.[2918 2919 2920 2921]

Single-dose vials of the solution should be used immediately after reconstitution.[2918 2921] Any remaining unused portion

DOI: 10.37573/9781585286850.317

should be discarded after 24 hours at room temperature or 48 hours under refrigeration at 2 to 8°C.[2918 2921] Vials should NOT be frozen after reconstitution.[2918 2919 2921]

The entire contents of the reconstituted pharmacy bulk package also should be used immediately after reconstitution.[2918 2920] Manufacturers' recommendations differ on the duration that the bulk pharmacy package may be stored at room temperature following reconstitution;[2918 2920] the specific product labeling should be consulted in such situations. Pharmacy bulk vials should NOT be frozen after reconstitution.[2918 2920]

After dilution in compatible infusion solutions, the drug is stable for up to 24 hours at room temperature or 1 week under refrigeration.[2918 2920 2921] Glass and plastic (including syringes, intravenous solution bags, and tubing) do not affect stability.[2918 2919 2920 2921]

Solutions prepared using the ADD-Vantage vials are stable for up to 24 hours at room temperature.[2919] These solutions should not be refrigerated nor frozen following reconstitution.[2919]

Concentration Effects

In one study, piperacillin plus tazobactam dissolved in sterile water for injection to concentrations greater than 128 plus 16 g/L, respectively, resulted in unacceptably viscous solutions that impeded flow from elastomeric pumps to less than 75% of the nominal flow rate.[3105]

Freezing Solutions

The commercially available, premixed frozen injection in single-dose Galaxy containers should be stored at or below –20°C.[2918] Thaw at room temperature or under refrigeration but not in a warm water bath or by microwave radiation.[2918] Thawed solutions should not be refrozen.[2918] After thawing, the solutions are stable for 24 hours at room temperature or 14 days refrigerated.[2918]

Piperacillin 80 mg/mL plus tazobactam 10 mg/mL in polyvinyl chloride (PVC) bags of dextrose 5% and sodium chloride 0.9% was frozen at –15°C for 30 days and thawed by microwave radiation for 45 seconds with no loss of either component.[1768]

Piperacillin 150 mg/mL plus tazobactam 18.75 mg/mL and piperacillin 200 mg/mL plus tazobactam 25 mg/mL in dextrose 5% and sodium chloride 0.9% were drawn as 20-mL aliquots into polypropylene syringes (Becton Dickinson). The syringes were frozen at –15°C for 30 days and then stored at 4°C for 7 days with no loss of either component.[1768]

Piperacillin 40 mg/mL plus tazobactam 5 mg/mL in dextrose 5% lost less than 3% after 3 months stored at –20°C. After microwave thawing, refrigerated storage resulted in 10% loss in 35 days.[2614]

Syringes

Piperacillin 150 mg/mL plus tazobactam 18.75 mg/mL and piperacillin 200 mg/mL plus tazobactam 25 mg/mL in dextrose 5% and sodium chloride 0.9% were drawn as 20-mL aliquots into polypropylene syringes (Becton Dickinson). The syringes were stored at 25°C for 1 day and at 4°C for 7 days with no loss of either drug in the dextrose 5% samples. Similarly, no tazobactam loss occurred in the sodium chloride 0.9% solutions. However, piperacillin losses of 7% in 1 day at 25°C and 4% in 7 days at 4°C were found in the sodium chloride 0.9% solutions.[1768]

Ambulatory Pumps

Infusion solutions prepared from single-dose vials and the bulk product have been shown to be stable for up to 12 hours at room temperature in an ambulatory infusion pump.[2918 2920 2921 2922] Each dose was diluted to 25 or 37.5 mL, and stability was not affected.[2918 2920 2921]

Central Venous Catheter

Piperacillin 10 mg/mL plus tazobactam 1.25 mg/mL (Lederle) in dextrose 5% was found to be compatible with the ARROW-g+ard Blue Plus (Arrow International) chlorhexidine-bearing triple-lumen central catheter. Essentially complete delivery of the drug was found with little or no drug loss occurring. Furthermore, chlorhexidine delivered from the catheter remained at trace amounts with no substantial increase due to the delivery of the drug through the catheter.[2335]

Compatibility Information

Solution Compatibility

Piperacillin sodium–tazobactam sodium

Test Soln Name	Mfr	Mfr	Conc/L or %	Remarks	Ref	C/I
Dextrose 5%		WY[d]	13.3 to 80[e] g	Compatible	2918	C
Dextrose 5%		[c]	13.3 to 80[e] g	Compatible	2920, 2921	C
Dextrose 5%	HOS	HOS[c]	20 to 80[e] g	Stable up to 24 hours at room temperature	2919	C
Dextrose 5%	BA[a]	WY[d]	20[e], 80[e] g	Visually compatible. Little loss of either drug in 28 days at 5°C then 72 hr at 23°C in light	2806	C
Ringer's injection, lactated		[c]		Incompatible	2920, 2921	I

Solution Compatibility (Cont.)

Test Soln Name	Mfr	Mfr	Conc/L or %	Remarks	Ref	C/I
Ringer's injection, lactated	WY[d]			Compatible only via Y-site administration	2918, 2985	C
Sodium chloride 0.9%		WY[d]	13.3 to 80[e] g	Compatible	2918	C
Sodium chloride 0.9%		[c]	13.3 to 80[e] g	Compatible	2920, 2921	C
Sodium chloride 0.9%	HOS	HOS[c]	20 to 80[e] g	Stable up to 24 hours at room temperature	2919	C
Sodium chloride 0.9%	BA[a]	WY[c]	40[e] g	Calculated 10% loss in 5.8 days at 7°C and 3.8 days at room temperature in light	2667	C
Sodium chloride 0.9%	BA[b]	WY[c]	40[e] g	Calculated 10% loss in 17.7 days at 7°C and 2.8 days at room temperature in light	2667	C
Sodium chloride 0.9%	BA[a]	WY[d]	20[e], 80[e] g	Visually compatible. 5% tazobactam and 2% piperacillin loss in 28 days at 5°C then 72 hr at 23°C in light	2806	C
Sodium chloride 0.9%	[f]	[g] [h]	80 g[e]	Less than 10% loss in theoretical concentration in 12 hr at ambient temperature when administered as a continuous infusion	3535	C

[a] Tested in PVC containers.

[b] Tested in polyolefin containers.

[c] Test performed using the formulation WITHOUT edetate disodium.

[d] Test performed using the formulation WITH edetate disodium.

[e] Piperacillin component. Piperacillin in an 8:1 fixed-ratio concentration with tazobactam.

[f] Tested in polypropylene syringes.

[g] Salt not specified.

[h] Presence or absence of edetate disodium not specified.

Additive Compatibility

Piperacillin sodium–tazobactam sodium

Test Drug	Mfr	Conc/L or %	Mfr	Conc/L or %	Test Solution	Remarks	Ref	C/I
Vancomycin HCl	HOS	2.9 g	SZ[b]	8.6[a] g	NS	Visually compatible for up to 5 days at room temperature	2935	C
Vancomycin HCl	HOS	2.9 g	APO[b]	11.4[a] g	NS	Visually compatible for up to 5 days at room temperature	2935	C

[a] Piperacillin component. Piperacillin in an 8:1 fixed-ratio concentration with tazobactam.

[b] Test performed using the formulation WITHOUT edetate disodium.

Drugs in Syringe Compatibility

Piperacillin sodium–tazobactam sodium

Test Drug	Mfr	Amt	Mfr	Amt	Remarks	Ref	C/I
Dimenhydrinate		10 mg/1 mL	[a]	200 mg/1 mL[b]	Clear solution	2569	C
Pantoprazole sodium	[a]	4 mg/1 mL	[a]	200 mg/1 mL[b]	Precipitates within 1 hr	2574	I

[a] Test performed using the formulation WITHOUT edetate disodium.

[b] Piperacillin component. Piperacillin in an 8:1 fixed-ratio concentration with tazobactam.

Y-Site Injection Compatibility (1:1 Mixture)

Piperacillin sodium–tazobactam sodium

Test Drug	Mfr	Conc	Mfr	Conc	Remarks	Ref	C/I
Acetaminophen	CAD	10 mg/mL	WY	89 mg/mL[i]	Physically compatible with less than 2% loss of either drug in 4 hr at 23°C	2901, 2902	C
Acyclovir sodium	BW	7 mg/mL[a]	LE[g]	40 mg/mL[a i]	Particles form in 1 hr	1688	I
Amikacin sulfate		1.75 to 7.5 mg/mL	WY[h]	26.7 to 40 mg/mL[a b i]	Compatible	2918, 2922	C
Amikacin sulfate		1.75 to 7.5 mg/mL	[g]		Stated to be compatible	2919, 2920, 2921, 2985	C
Aminophylline	AB	2.5 mg/mL[a]	LE[g]	40 mg/mL[a i]	Physically compatible for 4 hr at 22°C	1688	C
Amiodarone HCl	WY	6 mg/mL[a]	LE[g]	60 mg/mL[a i]	White haze in 24 hr at 22°C	2352	I
Amphotericin B	SQ	0.6 mg/mL[a]	LE[g]	40 mg/mL[a i]	Yellow precipitate forms immediately	1688	I
Anidulafungin	VIC	0.5 mg/mL[a]	LE[g]	40 mg/mL[a i]	Physically compatible for 4 hr at 23°C	2617	C
Azithromycin	PF	2 mg/mL[b]	LE[g]	100 mg/mL[b f i]	White microcrystals found	2368	I
Aztreonam	SQ	40 mg/mL[a]	LE[g]	40 mg/mL[a i]	Physically compatible for 4 hr at 22°C	1688	C
Bivalirudin	TMC	5 mg/mL[a]	LE[g]	40 mg/mL[a i]	Physically compatible for 4 hr at 23°C	2373	C
Bleomycin sulfate	BR	1 unit/mL[b]	LE[g]	40 mg/mL[a i]	Physically compatible for 4 hr at 22°C	1688	C
Bumetanide	RC	0.04 mg/mL[a]	LE[g]	40 mg/mL[a i]	Physically compatible for 4 hr at 22°C	1688	C
Buprenorphine HCl	RKC	0.04 mg/mL[a]	LE[g]	40 mg/mL[a i]	Physically compatible for 4 hr at 22°C	1688	C
Butorphanol tartrate	BR	0.04 mg/mL[a]	LE[g]	40 mg/mL[a i]	Physically compatible for 4 hr at 23°C	1688	C
Calcium gluconate	AMR	40 mg/mL[a]	LE[g]	40 mg/mL[a i]	Physically compatible for 4 hr at 22°C	1688	C
Cangrelor tetrasodium	TMC	1 mg/mL[b]		40 mg/mL[b i]	Physically compatible for 4 hr	3243	C
Carboplatin	BR	5 mg/mL[a]	LE[g]	40 mg/mL[a i]	Physically compatible for 4 hr at 22°C	1688	C
Carmustine	BR	1.5 mg/mL[a]	LE[g]	40 mg/mL[a i]	Physically compatible for 4 hr at 22°C	1688	C
Caspofungin acetate	ME	0.7 mg/mL[b]	WY[h]	40 mg/mL[b i]	Immediate white turbid precipitate forms	2758	I
Caspofungin acetate	ME	0.5 mg/mL[b]	WY[m]	80 mg/mL[b i]	Black particles reported	2766	I
Ceftolozane sulfate–tazobactam sodium	CUB	10 mg/mL[p q]	WY[h]	40 mg/mL[i p]	Physically compatible for 2 hr	3247, 3262	C
Chlorpromazine HCl	RU	2 mg/mL[a]	LE[g]	40 mg/mL[a i]	Heavy white turbidity forms immediately. White precipitate forms in 4 hr	1688	I
Cisatracurium besylate	GW	0.1 and 2 mg/mL[a]	CY[g]	40 mg/mL[a i]	Physically compatible for 4 hr at 23°C	2074	C
Cisatracurium besylate	GW	5 mg/mL[a]	CY[g]	40 mg/mL[a i]	Particles and subvisible haze within 4 hr	2074	I
Cisplatin	BR	1 mg/mL	LE[g]	40 mg/mL[a i]	Haze and particles form in 1 hr	1688	I
Clindamycin phosphate	AB	10 mg/mL[a]	LE[g]	40 mg/mL[a i]	Physically compatible for 4 hr at 22°C	1688	C
Cloxacillin sodium	SMX	100 mg/mL	SZ[m]	200 mg/mL[i]	Physically compatible for up to 4 hr at room temperature	3245	C
Colistimethate sodium	MIL	1.5 mg/mL[b]	ASZ[m]	40 mg/mL[b i]	Visually compatible for 1 hr at 26°C	3335	C
Cyclophosphamide	MJ	10 mg/mL[a]	LE[g]	40 mg/mL[a i]	Physically compatible for 4 hr at 22°C	1688	C
Cytarabine	SCN	50 mg/mL	LE[g]	40 mg/mL[a i]	Physically compatible for 4 hr at 22°C	1688	C

Y-Site Injection Compatibility (1:1 Mixture) (Cont.)

Test Drug	Mfr	Conc	Mfr	Conc	Remarks	Ref	C/I
Dacarbazine	MI	4 mg/mL[a]	LE[g]	40 mg/mL[a i]	Turbidity and particles form immediately and increase over 4 hr	1688	I
Daunorubicin HCl	WY	1 mg/mL[a]	LE[g]	40 mg/mL[a i]	Turbidity increases immediately	1688	I
Dexamethasone sodium phosphate	LY	1 mg/mL[a]	LE[g]	40 mg/mL[a i]	Physically compatible for 4 hr at 22°C	1688	C
Dexmedetomidine HCl	AB	4 mcg/mL[b]	LE[g]	40 mg/mL[b i]	Physically compatible for 4 hr at 23°C	2383	C
Diphenhydramine HCl	WY	2 mg/mL[a]	LE[g]	40 mg/mL[a i]	Physically compatible for 4 hr at 22°C	1688	C
Dobutamine HCl	LI	4 mg/mL[a]	LE[g]	40 mg/mL[a i]	Heavy white turbidity forms immediately	1688	I
Docetaxel	RPR	0.9 mg/mL[a]	CY[g]	40 mg/mL[a i]	Physically compatible for 4 hr at 23°C	2224	C
Dopamine HCl	AST	3.2 mg/mL[a]	LE[g]	40 mg/mL[a i]	Physically compatible for 4 hr at 22°C	1688	C
Doxorubicin HCl	CET	2 mg/mL	LE[g]	40 mg/mL[a i]	Turbidity forms immediately	1688	I
Doxorubicin HCl liposomal	SEQ	0.4 mg/mL[a]	CY[g]	40 mg/mL[a i]	Partial loss of measured natural turbidity	2087	I
Doxycycline hyclate	ES	1 mg/mL[a]	LE[g]	40 mg/mL[a i]	Heavy white turbidity forms immediately	1688	I
Droperidol	JN	0.4 mg/mL[a]	LE[g]	40 mg/mL[a i]	Heavy white turbidity with white precipitate forms immediately	1688	I
Enalaprilat	MSD	0.1 mg/mL[a]	LE[g]	40 mg/mL[a i]	Physically compatible for 4 hr at 22°C	1688	C
Eravacycline dihydrochloride	TET	0.6 mg/mL[b]	FRK[g]	40 mg/mL[b i]	Physically compatible for 2 hr at room temperature	3532	C
Etoposide	BR	0.4 mg/mL[a]	LE[g]	40 mg/mL[a i]	Physically compatible for 4 hr at 22°C	1688	C
Etoposide phosphate	BR	5 mg/mL[a]	LE[g]	40 mg/mL[b i]	Physically compatible for 4 hr at 23°C	2218	C
Famotidine	MSD	2 mg/mL[a]	LE[g]	40 mg/mL[a i]	Particles form immediately	1688	I
Fenoldopam mesylate	AB	80 mcg/mL[b]	LE[g]	40 mg/mL[b i]	Physically compatible for 4 hr at 23°C	2467	C
Floxuridine	RC	3 mg/mL[a]	LE[g]	40 mg/mL[a i]	Physically compatible for 4 hr at 22°C	1688	C
Fluconazole	RR	2 mg/mL	LE[g]	40 mg/mL[a i]	Physically compatible for 4 hr at 22°C	1688	C
Fludarabine phosphate	BX	1 mg/mL[a]	LE[g]	40 mg/mL[a i]	Physically compatible for 4 hr at 22°C	1688	C
Fluorouracil	LY	16 mg/mL[a]	LE[g]	40 mg/mL[a i]	Physically compatible for 4 hr at 22°C	1688	C
Furosemide	AB	3 mg/mL[a]	LE[g]	40 mg/mL[a i]	Physically compatible for 4 hr at 22°C	1688	C
Gallium nitrate	FUJ	0.4 mg/mL[a]	LE[g]	40 mg/mL[a i]	Physically compatible for 4 hr at 22°C	1688	C
Ganciclovir sodium	SY	20 mg/mL[a]	LE[g]	40 mg/mL[a i]	Large crystals form in 1 hr and become heavy white precipitate in 4 hr	1688	I
Gemcitabine HCl	LI	10 mg/mL[b]	LE[g]	40 mg/mL[b i]	Cloudiness forms immediately, becoming flocculent precipitate in 1 hr	2226	I
Gentamicin sulfate		0.7 to 3.32 mg/mL	WY[h]	26.7 to 40 mg/mL[a b i]	Compatible	2918, 2922	C
Gentamicin sulfate		0.7 to 3.32 mg/mL	WY[h]	40 mg/mL[i k]	Compatible	2918, 2922	C
Gentamicin sulfate		0.7 to 3.32 mg/mL	WY[h]	60 mg/mL[i k]	Incompatible	2918, 2922	I
Gentamicin sulfate		0.7 to 3.32 mg/mL	[g]		Stated to be compatible	2919, 2920, 2921, 2985	C

Y-Site Injection Compatibility (1:1 Mixture) (Cont.)

Test Drug	Mfr	Conc	Mfr	Conc	Remarks	Ref	C/I
Granisetron HCl	SKB	0.05 mg/mL[a]	CY[g]	40 mg/mL[a i]	Physically compatible for 4 hr at 23°C	2000	C
Haloperidol lactate	MN	0.2 mg/mL[a]	LE[g]	40 mg/mL[a i]	White turbidity and particles form immediately	1688	I
Heparin sodium	ES	100 units/mL[a]	LE[g]	40 mg/mL[a i]	Physically compatible for 4 hr at 22°C	1688	C
Hetastarch in lactated electrolyte	AB	6%	LE[g]	40 mg/mL[a i]	Physically compatible for 4 hr at 23°C	2339	C
Hydrocortisone sodium succinate	UP	1 mg/mL[a]	LE[g]	40 mg/mL[a i]	Physically compatible for 4 hr at 22°C	1688	C
Hydromorphone HCl	ES	0.5 mg/mL[a]	LE[g]	40 mg/mL[a i]	Physically compatible for 4 hr at 22°C	1688	C
Hydroxyzine HCl	WI	4 mg/mL[a]	LE[g]	40 mg/mL[a i]	Haze and particles form immediately	1688	I
Idarubicin HCl	AD	0.5 mg/mL[a]	LE[g]	40 mg/mL[a i]	Immediate increase in haze	1688	I
Ifosfamide	MJ	25 mg/mL[a]	LE[g]	40 mg/mL[a i]	Physically compatible for 4 hr at 22°C	1688	C
Isavuconazonium sulfate	ASP	1.5 mg/mL[a]	PRP[h]	40 mg/mL[a i]	Measured turbidity increases immediately	3247, 3263	I
Isavuconazonium sulfate	ASP	1.5 mg/mL[b]	PRP[h]	40 mg/mL[b i]	Physically compatible for 2 hr	3247, 3263	C
Leucovorin calcium	LE	2 mg/mL[a]	LE[g]	40 mg/mL[a i]	Physically compatible for 4 hr at 22°C	1688	C
Linezolid	PHU	2 mg/mL	LE[g]	40 mg/mL[a i]	Physically compatible for 4 hr at 23°C	2264	C
Lorazepam	WY	0.1 mg/mL[a]	LE[g]	40 mg/mL[a i]	Physically compatible for 4 hr at 22°C	1688	C
Magnesium sulfate	AST	100 mg/mL	LE[g]	40 mg/mL[a i]	Physically compatible for 4 hr at 22°C	1688	C
Mannitol	BA	15%	LE[g]	40 mg/mL[a i]	Physically compatible for 4 hr at 22°C	1688	C
Meperidine HCl	WY	4 mg/mL[a]	LE[g]	40 mg/mL[a i]	Physically compatible for 4 hr at 22°C	1688	C
Meropenem		50 mg/mL	SMX[g]	200 mg/mL[i]	Physically compatible for 4 hr at room temperature	3538, 3547	C
Meropenem–vaborbactam	TMC	8 mg/mL[b r]	FRK[g]	40 mg/mL[b i]	Physically compatible for 3 hr at 20 to 25°C	3380	C
Mesna	MJ	10 mg/mL[a]	LE[g]	40 mg/mL[a i]	Physically compatible for 4 hr at 22°C	1688	C
Methotrexate sodium	LE	15 mg/mL[a]	LE[g]	40 mg/mL[a i]	Physically compatible for 4 hr at 22°C	1688	C
Methylprednisolone sodium succinate	AB	5 mg/mL[a]	LE[g]	40 mg/mL[a i]	Physically compatible for 4 hr at 22°C	1688	C
Metoclopramide HCl	RB	5 mg/mL	LE[g]	40 mg/mL[a i]	Physically compatible for 4 hr at 22°C	1688	C
Metronidazole	BA	5 mg/mL	LE[g]	40 mg/mL[a i]	Physically compatible for 4 hr at 22°C	1688	C
Milrinone lactate	SS	0.2 mg/mL[a]	LE[g]	200 mg/mL[i]	Visually compatible for 4 hr at 25°C	2381	C
Mitomycin	BR	0.5 mg/mL	LE[g]	40 mg/mL[a i]	Blue color darkens in 4 hr, becoming reddish purple in 24 hr	1688	I
Mitoxantrone HCl	LE	0.5 mg/mL[a]	LE[g]	40 mg/mL[a i]	Haze and particles form immediately. Large particles form in 4 hr	1688	I
Morphine sulfate	WY	1 mg/mL[a]	LE[g]	40 mg/mL[a i]	Physically compatible for 4 hr at 22°C	1688	C
Nalbuphine HCl	DU	10 mg/mL	LE[g]	40 mg/mL[a i]	Heavy white turbidity forms immediately. Particles form in 4 hr	1688	I
Ondansetron HCl	GL	1 mg/mL[a]	LE[g]	40 mg/mL[a i]	Physically compatible for 4 hr at 22°C	1688	C

Y-Site Injection Compatibility (1:1 Mixture) (Cont.)

Test Drug	Mfr	Conc	Mfr	Conc	Remarks	Ref	C/I
Ondansetron HCl	GL	0.03, 0.1, 0.3 mg/mL[b]	LE[g]	40 mg/mL[b i]	Visually compatible with no loss of any component in 4 hr	1752	C
Ondansetron HCl	GL	0.03, 0.1, 0.3 mg/mL[b]	LE[g]	80 mg/mL[b i]	Visually compatible with no loss of any component in 4 hr	1752	C
Plazomicin sulfate	ACH	24 mg/mL[p]	FRK[g]	40 mg/mL[i p]	Physically compatible for 1 hr at 20 to 25°C	3432	C
Potassium chloride	AB	0.1 mEq/mL[a]	LE[g]	40 mg/mL[a i]	Physically compatible for 4 hr at 22°C	1688	C
Prochlorperazine edisylate	SCN	0.5 mg/mL[a]	LE[g]	40 mg/mL[a i]	White turbidity forms immediately	1688	I
Promethazine HCl	SCN	2 mg/mL[a]	LE[g]	40 mg/mL[a i]	Heavy white turbidity forms immediately. Particles form in 4 hr	1688	I
Quinupristin–dalfopristin		2 mg/mL[a n]	[o]		Reported to be incompatible	3230	I
Ranitidine HCl	GL	2 mg/mL[a]	LE[g]	40 mg/mL[a i]	Physically compatible for 4 hr at 22°C	1688	C
Ranitidine HCl	GL	0.5 and 2 mg/mL[b]	LE[g]	80 mg/mL[b i]	Visually compatible. Little loss of any component in 4 hr at 23°C	1759	C
Ranitidine HCl	GL	0.5 and 2 mg/mL[b]	LE[g]	40 mg/mL[b i]	Visually compatible. Little loss of ranitidine and tazobactam in 4 hr at 23°C. Piperacillin not tested	1759	C
Remifentanil HCl	GW	0.025 and 0.25 mg/mL[b]	CY[g]	40 mg/mL[a i]	Physically compatible for 4 hr at 23°C	2075	C
Sargramostim	HO	10 mcg/mL[a]	LE[g]	40 mg/mL[a i]	Physically compatible for 4 hr at 22°C	1688	C
Sodium bicarbonate	AB	1 mEq/mL	LE[g]	40 mg/mL[a i]	Physically compatible for 4 hr at 22°C	1688	C
Streptozocin	UP	40 mg/mL[a]	LE[g]	40 mg/mL[a i]	Particles form in 1 hr	1688	I
Tedizolid phosphate	CUB	0.8 mg/mL[b]	PRP[h]	40 mg/mL[b i]	Physically compatible for 2 hr	3244, 3247	C
Telavancin HCl	ASP	7.5 mg/mL[a b e]	WY[h]	40 mg/mL[a b e i]	Physically compatible for 2 hr	2830	C
Thiotepa	LE	1 mg/mL[a]	LE[g]	40 mg/mL[a i]	Physically compatible for 4 hr at 22°C	1688	C
Tigecycline	WY	1 mg/mL[b]		3 mg/mL[b i]	Physically compatible for 4 hr	2714	C
Tigecycline	ACD, WY	[p]	[h o]		Stated to be compatible	2915, 3459	C
TNA #218 to #226[c]			LE[g]	40 mg/mL[a i]	Visually compatible for 4 hr at 23°C	2215	C
Tobramycin sulfate			WY[h]		Incompatible	2918	I
Tobramycin sulfate			[g]		Incompatible	2919, 2920, 2921	I
TPN #212 to #215[c]			CY[g]	40 mg/mL[a i]	Physically compatible for 4 hr at 23°C	2109	C
Trimethoprim–sulfamethoxazole	ES	0.8 mg/mL[a j]	LE[g]	40 mg/mL[a i]	Physically compatible for 4 hr at 22°C	1688	C
Vancomycin HCl	AB	10 mg/mL[a]	LE[g]	40 mg/mL[a i]	White turbidity forms immediately and white precipitate forms in 4 hr	1688	I
Vancomycin HCl	AB	20 mg/mL[a]	LE[g]	200 mg/mL[d i]	Transient precipitate forms	2189	?
Vancomycin HCl	AB	20 mg/mL[a]	LE[g]	10, 50 mg/mL[a i]	Gross white precipitate forms immediately	2189	I
Vancomycin HCl	AB	20 mg/mL[a]	LE[g]	1 mg/mL[a i]	Physically compatible for 4 hr at 23°C	2189	C

Y-Site Injection Compatibility (1:1 Mixture) (Cont.)

Test Drug	Mfr	Conc	Mfr	Conc	Remarks	Ref	C/I
Vancomycin HCl	AB	2 mg/mL[a]	LE[g]	1[a i], 10[a i], 50[a i], 200[d i] mg/mL	Physically compatible for 4 hr at 23°C	2189	C
Vancomycin HCl	APP	4 mg/mL[d]	SZ[g]	30 mg/mL[d i l]	Physically compatible for 5 days at 25°C	2935, 3474	C
Vancomycin HCl	APP	4 mg/mL[d]	SZ[g]	40 mg/mL[d i l]	Physically compatible for 5 days at 25°C	2935	C
Vancomycin HCl	APP	10 mg/mL[a]	HOS[g]	100 mg/mL[d i]	Transient precipitate clears within 15 seconds	2933	?
Vancomycin HCl	APP	2 mg/mL[b]	APP[g]	16, 30, 40, 80, 100 mg/mL[b i]	Physically compatible for up to 4 hr	3476	C
Vancomycin HCl	APP	4 mg/mL[a]	APP[g]	16, 30, 40 mg/mL[a i]	Physically compatible for up to 4 hr	3476	C
Vancomycin HCl	APP	4 mg/mL[a]	APP[g]	80, 100 mg/mL[a i]	White precipitate forms only when piperacillin–tazobactam added to vancomycin; not observed when order of mixing was reversed	3476	I
Vancomycin HCl	APP	5 mg/mL[b]	APP[g]	16, 30, 40, 80, 100 mg/mL[b i]	Physically compatible for up to 4 hr	3476	C
Vancomycin HCl	APP	8 mg/mL[a]	APP[g]	16 mg/mL[a i]	Persistent white precipitate forms	3476	I
Vancomycin HCl	APP	8 mg/mL[a]	APP[g]	30, 40, 80, 100 mg/mL[a i]	Immediate white cloudiness forms, then dissipates	3476	?
Vancomycin HCl	APP	10 mg/mL[b]	APP[g]	16, 30 mg/mL[b i]	Physically compatible for up to 4 hr	3476	C
Vancomycin HCl	APP	10 mg/mL[b]	APP[g]	40 mg/mL[b i]	White precipitate forms only when piperacillin–tazobactam added to vancomycin; not observed when order of mixing was reversed	3476	I
Vancomycin HCl	APP	10 mg/mL[b]	APP[g]	80, 100 mg/mL[b i]	Immediate white cloudiness forms, then dissipates	3476	?
Vancomycin HCl	APP	4 mg/mL[b]	HOS[g]	30, 40, 44.4, 53.3, 60, 71.1, 80 mg/mL[b i]	Physically compatible for 24 hr at 21 to 25°C	3478	C
Vancomycin HCl	APP	5 mg/mL[b]	HOS[g]	30, 40, 44.4, 53.3, 60, 71.1, 80 mg/mL[b i]	Physically compatible for 24 hr at 21 to 25°C	3478	C
Vancomycin HCl	APP	5, 8, 9 mg/mL[b]	BA[h]	60 mg/mL[i k]	Physically compatible for 24 hr at 21 to 25°C	3478	C
Vancomycin HCl	APP	5 mg/mL[b]	WY[h]	30, 53.3, 80 mg/mL[i]	Physically compatible for 24 hr at 21 to 25°C	3478	C
Vancomycin HCl	APP	6 mg/mL[b]	HOS[g]	30, 40, 44.4, 53.3, 60, 71.1, 80 mg/mL[b i]	Physically compatible for 24 hr at 21 to 25°C	3478	C
Vancomycin HCl	APP	7 mg/mL[b]	HOS[g]	30, 40, 44.4, 53.3, 60, 71.1, 80 mg/mL[b i]	Physically compatible for 24 hr at 21 to 25°C	3478	C
Vancomycin HCl	APP	8 mg/mL[b]	HOS[g]	30, 40, 44.4, 53.3, 60 mg/mL[b i]	Physically compatible for 24 hr at 21 to 25°C	3478	C
Vancomycin HCl	APP	8 mg/mL[b]	HOS[g]	71.1, 80 mg/mL[b i]	Transient and reversible precipitate forms	3478	?
Vancomycin HCl	APP	8 mg/mL[b]	WY[h]	30, 53.3, 80 mg/mL[i]	Physically compatible for 24 hr at 21 to 25°C	3478	C
Vancomycin HCl	APP	10 mg/mL[b]	HOS[g]	30, 40, 44.4, 53.3, 60, 71.1, 80 mg/mL[b i]	Transient and reversible precipitate forms	3478	?

Y-Site Injection Compatibility (1:1 Mixture) (Cont.)

Test Drug	Mfr	Conc	Mfr	Conc	Remarks	Ref	C/I
Vancomycin HCl	APP	12 mg/mL[b]	HOS[g]	30, 40, 44.4, 53.3, 60, 71.1, 80 mg/mL[b i]	Irreversible precipitate forms	3478	I
Vancomycin HCl	BA	5 mg/mL[k]	BA[h]	60 mg/mL[i k]	Physically compatible for 24 hr at 21 to 25°C	3478	C
Vancomycin HCl	BA	5 mg/mL[k]	WY[h]	30, 53.3, 80 mg/mL[i]	Physically compatible for 24 hr at 21 to 25°C	3478	C
Vancomycin HCl	HOS	5 mg/mL[a]	SZ[g]	28 mg/mL[a i]	Physically compatible for up to 24 hr at room temperature with no loss of anti-microbial activity	3480	C
Vancomycin HCl	HOS	10, 15, 20 mg/mL[a]	SZ[g]	28 mg/mL[a i]	Physically incompatible	3480	I
Vancomycin HCl	BA	5 mg/mL[k]	PF[h]	60 mg/mL[i k]	No evidence of physical incompatibility via simulated Y-site infusion; however, a white precipitate forms during actual Y-site infusion	3481	?
Vancomycin HCl	LI	10 mg/mL[a]	[m o]	200 mg/mL[s]	Physically incompatible	3536	I
Vasopressin	APP	0.2 unit/mL[b]	WY[g]	100 mg/mL[i]	Physically compatible	2641	C
Vinblastine sulfate	LI	0.12 mg/mL[a]	LE[g]	40 mg/mL[a i]	Physically compatible for 4 hr at 22°C	1688	C
Vincristine sulfate	LI	0.05 mg/mL[a]	LE[g]	40 mg/mL[a i]	Physically compatible for 4 hr at 22°C	1688	C
Zidovudine	BW	4 mg/mL[a]	LE[g]	40 mg/mL[a i]	Physically compatible for 4 hr at 22°C	1688	C

[a] Tested in dextrose 5%.

[b] Tested in sodium chloride 0.9%.

[c] Refer to Appendix for the composition of parenteral nutrition solutions. TNA indicates a 3-in-1 admixture, and TPN indicates a 2-in-1 admixture.

[d] Tested in sterile water for injection.

[e] Tested in Ringer's injection, lactated.

[f] Injected via Y-site into an administration set running azithromycin.

[g] Test performed using the formulation WITHOUT edetate disodium.

[h] Test performed using the formulation WITH edetate disodium.

[i] Piperacillin component. Piperacillin in an 8:1 fixed-ratio concentration with tazobactam.

[j] Trimethoprim component. Trimethoprim in a 1:5 fixed-ratio concentration with sulfamethoxazole.

[k] Tested as the premixed infusion solution.

[l] If sterile water for injection is used as the diluent, manufacturers recommend a maximum volume per dose of 50 mL.

[m] Presence or absence of edetate disodium not specified.

[n] Quinupristin and dalfopristin components combined.

[o] Salt not specified.

[p] Tested in both dextrose 5% and sodium chloride 0.9%.

[q] Ceftolozane component. Ceftolozane in a 2:1 fixed-ratio concentration with tazobactam.

[r] Meropenem component. Meropenem in a 1:1 fixed-ratio concentration with vaborbactam.

[s] Not specified whether concentration refers to single component or combined components.

Additional Compatibility Information

Infusion Solutions

Piperacillin–tazobactam (Zosyn, Wyeth) containing EDTA is compatible with Ringer's injection, lactated solution only for Y-site administration.[2918] Formulations of the drug that do *not* contain EDTA are incompatible with Ringer's injection, lactated solution.[2919 2920 2921]

Peritoneal Dialysis Solutions

The physical and chemical stability of piperacillin plus tazobactam (without EDTA) at concentrations of 200 plus 25 mcg/mL, respectively, were evaluated in Dianeal PD-2 with dextrose 1.5% and Dianeal PD-2 with dextrose 4.25%. Samples were stored at 4°C for 14 days, 23°C for 7 days, and 37°C for 1 day. The samples were physically and chemically stable. Little or no loss of either component occurred in the 4°C samples throughout the 14-day period. At 23°C, losses of each component were in the range of 3 to 6% in 7 days. The 1-day losses at 37°C were similarly small.[2018]

Selected Revisions May 1, 2020. © Copyright, October 1994. American Society of Health-System Pharmacists, Inc.

Plazomicin Sulfate
AHFS 8:12.02

Products

Plazomicin sulfate is available in a concentration equivalent to plazomicin base 50 mg/mL in 10-mL single-dose (preservative-free) vials.[3431] Each vial also contains sodium hydroxide for pH adjustment and water for injection.[3431] The appropriate dose of plazomicin solution should be diluted in sodium chloride 0.9% or Ringer's injection, lactated to achieve a final volume of 50 mL.[3431]

pH
Adjusted to 6.5.[3431]

Trade Name(s)
Zemdri

Administration

Plazomicin sulfate is administered by intravenous infusion over 30 minutes after dilution in sodium chloride 0.9% or Ringer's injection, lactated.[3431]

Stability

Intact vials of plazomicin sulfate should be stored under refrigeration at 2 to 8°C.[3431] Plazomicin sulfate injection is a clear, colorless to yellow solution.[3431] The manufacturer states that the solution may become yellow, but that this change does not indicate a decrease in potency.[3431]

The manufacturer states that a solution of plazomicin diluted for infusion in sodium chloride 0.9% or Ringer's injection, lactated to concentrations of 2.5 to 45 mg/mL is stable for up to 24 hours at room temperature.[3431]

Compatibility Information

Solution Compatibility

Plazomicin sulfate

Test Soln Name	Mfr	Mfr	Conc/L or %	Remarks	Ref	C/I
Ringer's injection, lactated		ACH	2.5 to 45 g	Stable for 24 hr at room temperature	3431	C
Sodium chloride 0.9%		ACH	2.5 to 45 g	Stable for 24 hr at room temperature	3431	C

Y-Site Injection Compatibility (1:1 Mixture)

Plazomicin sulfate

Test Drug	Mfr	Conc	Mfr	Conc	Remarks	Ref	C/I
Albumin human	BXT	250 mg/mL	ACH	24 mg/mL[c]	Measured turbidity increases immediately	3432	I
Amiodarone HCl	MYL	2 mg/mL[c]	ACH	24 mg/mL[c]	Measured turbidity increases immediately; pH increased by >1 unit within 30 min	3432	I
Amphotericin B	XGN	0.1 mg/mL[a]	ACH	24 mg/mL[a]	Measured turbidity increases immediately	3432	I
Ampicillin sodium–sulbactam sodium	AUR	20 mg/mL[c d]	ACH	24 mg/mL[c]	Physically compatible for 1 hr at 20 to 25°C	3432	C
Anidulafungin	PF	0.77 mg/mL[c]	ACH	24 mg/mL[c]	Measured turbidity increases within 15 min; pH increased by >1 unit within 30 min	3432	I
Azithromycin	PF	2 mg/mL[c]	ACH	24 mg/mL[c]	Physically compatible for 1 hr at 20 to 25°C	3432	C
Aztreonam	FRK	20 mg/mL[c]	ACH	24 mg/mL[c]	Physically compatible for 1 hr at 20 to 25°C	3432	C
Bumetanide	HOS	0.25 mg/mL	ACH	24 mg/mL[c]	Physically compatible for 1 hr at 20 to 25°C	3432	C

DOI: 10.37573/9781585286850.318

Y-Site Injection Compatibility (1:1 Mixture) (Cont.)

Test Drug	Mfr	Conc	Mfr	Conc	Remarks	Ref	C/I
Calcium chloride	HOS	20 mg/mL[c]	ACH	24 mg/mL[c]	White particulates form within 1 hr; pH increased by >1 unit within 30 min	3432	I
Calcium gluconate	FRK	20 mg/mL[c]	ACH	24 mg/mL[c]	Physically compatible for 1 hr at 20 to 25°C	3432	C
Caspofungin acetate	ME	0.5 mg/mL[b]	ACH	24 mg/mL[b]	Physically compatible for 1 hr at 20 to 25°C	3432	C
Cefazolin sodium	SGT	20 mg/mL[c]	ACH	24 mg/mL[c]	Physically compatible for 1 hr at 20 to 25°C	3432	C
Cefepime HCl	WG	40 mg/mL[c]	ACH	24 mg/mL[c]	Physically compatible for 1 hr at 20 to 25°C	3432	C
Cefoxitin sodium	FRK	20 mg/mL[c]	ACH	24 mg/mL[c]	Physically compatible for 1 hr at 20 to 25°C	3432	C
Ceftaroline fosamil	FAC	12 mg/mL[c]	ACH	24 mg/mL[c]	Physically compatible for 1 hr at 20 to 25°C	3432	C
Ceftazidime	SGT	40 mg/mL[c]	ACH	24 mg/mL[c]	Physically compatible for 1 hr at 20 to 25°C	3432	C
Ceftazidime–avibactam sodium	GSK	40 mg/mL[c e]	ACH	24 mg/mL[c]	Physically compatible for 1 hr at 20 to 25°C	3432	C
Ceftolozane sulfate–tazobactam sodium	ME	20 mg/mL[c f]	ACH	24 mg/mL[c]	Physically compatible for 1 hr at 20 to 25°C	3432	C
Ceftriaxone sodium	HOS	20 mg/mL[c]	ACH	24 mg/mL[c]	Physically compatible for 1 hr at 20 to 25°C	3432	C
Cefuroxime sodium	HIK	30 mg/mL[c]	ACH	24 mg/mL[c]	Physically compatible for 1 hr at 20 to 25°C	3432	C
Ciprofloxacin	CLA	2 mg/mL[c]	ACH	24 mg/mL[c]	Physically compatible for 1 hr at 20 to 25°C	3432	C
Cisatracurium besylate	ABV	0.4 mg/mL[c]	ACH	24 mg/mL[c]	Physically compatible for 1 hr at 20 to 25°C	3432	C
Colistimethate sodium	PAR	4.5 mg/mL[c]	ACH	24 mg/mL[c]	Physically compatible for 1 hr at 20 to 25°C	3432	C
Daptomycin	TE	20 mg/mL[b]	ACH	24 mg/mL[b]	Measured turbidity increases immediately	3432	I
Dexamethasone sodium phosphate	FRK	1 mg/mL[c]	ACH	24 mg/mL[c]	Physically compatible for 1 hr at 20 to 25°C	3432	C
Dexmedetomidine HCl	HOS	4 mcg/mL	ACH	24 mg/mL[c]	Physically compatible for 1 hr at 20 to 25°C	3432	C
Digoxin	WW	0.25 mg/mL	ACH	24 mg/mL[c]	Physically compatible for 1 hr at 20 to 25°C	3432	C
Diltiazem HCl	AKN	5 mg/mL	ACH	24 mg/mL[c]	Physically compatible for 1 hr at 20 to 25°C	3432	C
Diphenhydramine HCl	FRK	50 mg/mL	ACH	24 mg/mL[c]	Physically compatible for 1 hr at 20 to 25°C	3432	C
Dobutamine HCl	HOS	4.1 mg/mL[c]	ACH	24 mg/mL[c]	Physically compatible for 1 hr at 20 to 25°C	3432	C
Dopamine HCl	HOS	0.8 mg/mL[c]	ACH	24 mg/mL[c]	Physically compatible for 1 hr at 20 to 25°C	3432	C
Doripenem	SHI	10 mg/mL[c]	ACH	24 mg/mL[c]	Physically compatible for 1 hr at 20 to 25°C	3432	C
Doxycycline hyclate	FRK	1 mg/mL[c]	ACH	24 mg/mL[c]	Physically compatible for 1 hr at 20 to 25°C	3432	C
Epinephrine[i]	HOS	16 mcg/mL[c]	ACH	24 mg/mL[c]	Physically compatible for 1 hr at 20 to 25°C	3432	C
Eptifibatide	ME	2 mg/mL	ACH	24 mg/mL[b]	Physically compatible for 1 hr at 20 to 25°C	3432	C
Ertapenem sodium	ME	20 mg/mL[b]	ACH	24 mg/mL[b]	Physically compatible for 1 hr at 20 to 25°C	3432	C
Esmolol HCl	MYL	10 mg/mL	ACH	24 mg/mL[c]	Physically compatible for 1 hr at 20 to 25°C	3432	C
Esomeprazole sodium	ASZ	0.8 mg/mL[c]	ACH	24 mg/mL[c]	Measured turbidity increases within 1 hr; pH decreased by nearly 3 units within 30 min	3432	I
Famotidine	FRK	4 mg/mL[c]	ACH	24 mg/mL[c]	Physically compatible for 1 hr at 20 to 25°C	3432	C
Fentanyl citrate	WW	50 mcg/mL	ACH	24 mg/mL[c]	Physically compatible for 1 hr at 20 to 25°C	3432	C
Fluconazole	SGT	2 mg/mL[c]	ACH	24 mg/mL[c]	Physically compatible for 1 hr at 20 to 25°C	3432	C
Fosphenytoin sodium	AMB	25 mg/mL[c g]	ACH	24 mg/mL[c]	Physically compatible for 1 hr at 20 to 25°C	3432	C

Y-Site Injection Compatibility (1:1 Mixture) (Cont.)

Test Drug	Mfr	Conc	Mfr	Conc	Remarks	Ref	C/I
Furosemide	CLA	3 mg/mL[c]	ACH	24 mg/mL[c]	Physically compatible for 1 hr at 20 to 25°C	3432	C
Heparin sodium	SGT	1000 units/mL[c]	ACH	24 mg/mL[c]	Cloudy with immediate increase in measured turbidity	3432	I
Hydrocortisone sodium succinate	PF	1 mg/mL[c]	ACH	24 mg/mL[c]	Physically compatible for 1 hr at 20 to 25°C	3432	C
Hydromorphone HCl	AKN	1 mg/mL[c]	ACH	24 mg/mL[c]	Physically compatible for 1 hr at 20 to 25°C	3432	C
Imipenem–cilastatin sodium	FRK	5 mg/mL[c h]	ACH	24 mg/mL[c]	Physically compatible for 1 hr at 20 to 25°C	3432	C
Insulin, regular	LI	1 unit/mL[c]	ACH	24 mg/mL[c]	Physically compatible for 1 hr at 20 to 25°C	3432	C
Isavuconazonium sulfate	ASP	0.8 mg/mL[c]	ACH	24 mg/mL[c]	Physically compatible for 1 hr at 20 to 25°C	3432	C
Labetalol HCl	BRK	2 mg/mL[c]	ACH	24 mg/mL[c]	Physically compatible for 1 hr at 20 to 25°C	3432	C
Levofloxacin	SGT	5 mg/mL[c]	ACH	24 mg/mL[c]	Measured turbidity increases immediately	3432, 3433	I
Lidocaine HCl	AUR	8 mg/mL[c]	ACH	24 mg/mL[c]	Physically compatible for 1 hr at 20 to 25°C	3432	C
Linezolid	PF	2 mg/mL[c]	ACH	24 mg/mL[c]	Physically compatible for 1 hr at 20 to 25°C	3432	C
Lorazepam	WW	1 mg/mL[c]	ACH	24 mg/mL[c]	Physically compatible for 1 hr at 20 to 25°C	3432	C
Magnesium sulfate	XGN	100 mg/mL[c]	ACH	24 mg/mL[c]	Physically compatible for 1 hr at 20 to 25°C	3432	C
Mannitol	HOS	20%	ACH	24 mg/mL[c]	Physically compatible for 1 hr at 20 to 25°C	3432	C
Meperidine HCl	WW	10 mg/mL[c]	ACH	24 mg/mL[c]	Physically compatible for 1 hr at 20 to 25°C	3432	C
Meropenem	FRK	20 mg/mL[c]	ACH	24 mg/mL[c]	Physically compatible for 1 hr at 20 to 25°C	3432	C
Meropenem–vaborbactam	FAC	8 mg/mL[c i]	ACH	24 mg/mL[c]	Physically compatible for 1 hr at 20 to 25°C	3432	C
Mesna	SGT	20 mg/mL[c]	ACH	24 mg/mL[c]	Physically compatible for 1 hr at 20 to 25°C	3432	C
Methylprednisolone sodium succinate	SGT	20 mg/mL[c]	ACH	24 mg/mL[c]	Cloudy with immediate increase in measured turbidity; gross sedimentation occurs within 30 min	3432	I
Metoclopramide HCl	TE	0.2 mg/mL[c]	ACH	24 mg/mL[c]	Physically compatible for 1 hr at 20 to 25°C	3432	C
Metronidazole	BA	5 mg/mL[c]	ACH	24 mg/mL[c]	Physically compatible for 1 hr at 20 to 25°C	3432	C
Micafungin sodium	ASP	4 mg/mL[c]	ACH	24 mg/mL[c]	Cloudy with gross sedimentation and immediate increase in measured turbidity	3432	I
Midazolam HCl	HOS	1 mg/mL[c]	ACH	24 mg/mL[c]	Physically compatible for 1 hr at 20 to 25°C	3432	C
Milrinone lactate	WW	0.2 mg/mL[c]	ACH	24 mg/mL[c]	Physically compatible for 1 hr at 20 to 25°C	3432	C
Morphine sulfate	WW	1 mg/mL[c]	ACH	24 mg/mL[c]	Physically compatible for 1 hr at 20 to 25°C	3432	C
Naloxone HCl	MYL	0.04 mg/mL[c]	ACH	24 mg/mL[c]	Physically compatible for 1 hr at 20 to 25°C	3432	C
Nicardipine HCl	EXL	0.1 mg/mL[c]	ACH	24 mg/mL[c]	Physically compatible for 1 hr at 20 to 25°C	3432	C
Nitroglycerin	BA	0.4 mg/mL[c]	ACH	24 mg/mL[c]	Physically compatible for 1 hr at 20 to 25°C	3432	C
Norepinephrine bitartrate	CLA	32 mcg/mL[c]	ACH	24 mg/mL[c]	Physically compatible for 1 hr at 20 to 25°C	3432	C
Octreotide acetate	FRK	4 mcg/mL[c]	ACH	24 mg/mL[c]	Physically compatible for 1 hr at 20 to 25°C	3432	C
Ondansetron HCl	HER	0.16 mg/mL[c]	ACH	24 mg/mL[c]	Physically compatible for 1 hr at 20 to 25°C	3432	C

Y-Site Injection Compatibility (1:1 Mixture) (Cont.)

Test Drug	Mfr	Conc	Mfr	Conc	Remarks	Ref	C/I
Pantoprazole[m]	WGC	0.4 mg/mL[c j]	ACH	24 mg/mL[c]	Physically compatible for 1 hr at 20 to 25°C	3432	C
Penicillin G potassium	PF	100,000 units/mL[c]	ACH	24 mg/mL[c]	Physically compatible for 1 hr at 20 to 25°C	3432	C
Phenylephrine HCl	AVD	1 mg/mL[c]	ACH	24 mg/mL[c]	Physically compatible for 1 hr at 20 to 25°C	3432	C
Phenytoin sodium	WW	10 mg/mL[b]	ACH	24 mg/mL[b]	Cloudy with immediate increase in measured turbidity; pH decreased by nearly 3 units within 30 min	3432	I
Piperacillin sodium–tazobactam sodium	FRK[n]	40 mg/mL[c k]	ACH	24 mg/mL[c]	Physically compatible for 1 hr at 20 to 25°C	3432	C
Potassium chloride	APP	0.1 mEq/mL[c]	ACH	24 mg/mL[c]	Physically compatible for 1 hr at 20 to 25°C	3432	C
Potassium phosphates	FRK	0.3 mmol/mL[c]	ACH	24 mg/mL[c]	Physically compatible for 1 hr at 20 to 25°C	3432	C
Propofol	SGT	10 mg/mL[a]	ACH	24 mg/mL[a]	Immediate formation of free oil layer atop fat plug	3432	I
Ranitidine HCl	ZY	2.5 mg/mL[c]	ACH	24 mg/mL[c]	Physically compatible for 1 hr at 20 to 25°C	3432	C
Rocuronium bromide	XGN	5 mg/mL[c]	ACH	24 mg/mL[c]	Physically compatible for 1 hr at 20 to 25°C	3432	C
Sodium bicarbonate	HOS	1 mEq/mL	ACH	24 mg/mL[c]	Physically compatible for 1 hr at 20 to 25°C	3432	C
Sodium nitroprusside	SGT	0.4 mg/mL[a]	ACH	24 mg/mL[a]	Physically compatible for 1 hr at 20 to 25°C	3432	C
Sodium phosphates	FRK	0.5 mmol/mL[c]	ACH	24 mg/mL[c]	Physically compatible for 1 hr at 20 to 25°C	3432	C
Tedizolid phosphate	ME	0.8 mg/mL[b]	ACH	24 mg/mL[b]	Physically compatible for 1 hr at 20 to 25°C	3432	C
Tigecycline	PF	1 mg/mL[c]	ACH	24 mg/mL[c]	Physically compatible for 1 hr at 20 to 25°C	3432	C
Vancomycin HCl	FRK	5 mg/mL[c]	ACH	24 mg/mL[c]	Physically compatible for 1 hr at 20 to 25°C	3432	C
Vasopressin	PAR	1 unit/mL[c]	ACH	24 mg/mL[c]	Physically compatible for 1 hr at 20 to 25°C	3432	C
Vecuronium bromide	TE	1 mg/mL	ACH	24 mg/mL[c]	Physically compatible for 1 hr at 20 to 25°C	3432	C

[a] Tested in dextrose 5%.

[b] Tested in sodium chloride 0.9%.

[c] Tested in both dextrose 5% and sodium chloride 0.9%.

[d] Ampicillin component. Ampicillin in a 2:1 fixed-ratio concentration with sulbactam.

[e] Ceftazidime component. Ceftazidime in a 4:1 fixed-ratio concentration with avibactam.

[f] Ceftolozane component. Ceftolozane in a 2:1 fixed-ratio concentration with tazobactam.

[g] Concentration of fosphenytoin expressed in milligrams of phenytoin sodium equivalents (PE) per mL.

[h] Imipenem component. Imipenem in a 1:1 fixed-ratio concentration with cilastatin.

[i] Meropenem component. Meropenem in a 1:1 fixed-ratio concentration with vaborbactam.

[j] Presence or absence of edetate disodium not specified.

[k] Piperacillin component. Piperacillin in an 8:1 fixed-ratio concentration with tazobactam.

[l] As epinephrine base rather than the salt.

[m] Salt not specified.

[n] Test performed using the formulation WITHOUT edetate disodium.

© Copyright, June 2019. American Society of Health-System Pharmacists, Inc.

Polymyxin B Sulfate
AHFS 8:12.28.28

Products

Polymyxin B sulfate is available as a powder in vials containing 500,000 units of polymyxin B.[3162] [3163] For intramuscular injection, the 500,000-unit vial should be reconstituted with 2 mL of sterile water for injection, sodium chloride 0.9%, or procaine hydrochloride 1%.[3162] [3163] For intravenous infusion, 500,000 units of polymyxin B should be reconstituted by dissolving the drug in 300 to 500 mL of dextrose 5%.[3162] [3163] For intrathecal administration, the 500,000-unit vial should be reconstituted with 10 mL of sodium chloride 0.9%.[3162] [3163]

Units

Each milligram of pure polymyxin base is equivalent to 10,000 units.[3162] [3163] Each microgram of pure polymyxin base is equivalent to 10 units.[3162] [3163]

Administration

Polymyxin B sulfate is administered intravenously by continuous infusion, intrathecally, or intramuscularly.[3162] [3163] Although poly-myxin B sulfate may be administered by intramuscular injection, this route is not recommended due to severe injection site pain, particularly in infants and children.[3162] [3163]

Stability

Intact vials should be stored at controlled room temperature and retained in the carton until time of use to protect from light.[3162] [3163] Aqueous solutions of polymyxin B sulfate may be stored under refrigeration for up to 12 months without a significant loss of potency; however, it is recommended that unused, refrigerated portions of the reconstituted solution be discarded after 72 hours.[3162] [3163]

pH Effects

The pH of maximum stability of polymyxin B is 3.4.[2422] In the pH range of 2 to 7, pH has little effect on the rate of decomposition; however, as pH values become more alkaline, solutions are less stable and the rate of decomposition increases markedly.[1946] [2422] [3162] [3163]

Compatibility Information

Solution Compatibility

Polymyxin B sulfate

Test Soln Name	Mfr	Mfr	Conc/L or %	Remarks	Ref	C/I
Sodium chloride 0.9%	HOS	APP, BED, XGN	56 to 78 mg	Under 10% loss in 24 hr at 4 and 25°C	2816	C
TPN #52, #53[a]		NOV	40 mg	Physically compatible with no polymyxin loss in 24 hr at 29°C	440	C

[a] Refer to Appendix for the composition of parenteral nutrition solutions. TPN indicates a 2-in-1 admixture.

Additive Compatibility

Polymyxin B sulfate

Test Drug	Mfr	Conc/L or %	Mfr	Conc/L or %	Test Solution	Remarks	Ref	C/I
Amikacin sulfate	BR	5 g	BW	200 mg	D5LR, D5R, D5S, D5W, D10W, LR, NS, R, SL	Physically compatible and amikacin stable for 24 hr at 25°C. Polymyxin not analyzed	293	C
Amphotericin B		200 mg	BP	20 mg	D5W	Haze develops over 3 hr	26	I
Ascorbic acid	UP	500 mg	BW	200 mg	D5W	Physically compatible	15	C
Chloramphenicol sodium succinate	PD	10 g	BW	200 mg	D5W	Physically incompatible	15	I
Chloramphenicol sodium succinate	PD	10 g	BW	200 mg		Precipitate forms within 1 hr	6	I

DOI: 10.37573/9781585286850.319

Additive Compatibility (Cont.)

Test Drug	Mfr	Conc/L or %	Mfr	Conc/L or %	Test Solution	Remarks	Ref	C/I
Chlorothiazide sodium	BP	2 g	BP	20 mg	D5W	Yellow color produced	26	I
Colistimethate sodium	WC	500 mg	BW	200 mg	D5W	Physically compatible	15	C
Diphenhydramine HCl	PD	80 mg	BW	200 mg	D5W	Physically compatible	15	C
Erythromycin lactobionate	AB	5 g	BW	200 mg	D5W	Physically compatible	15	C
Heparin sodium	BP	20,000 units	BP	20 mg	D5W	Precipitates immediately	26	I
Heparin sodium	BP	20,000 units	BP	20 mg	NS	Haze develops over 3 hr	26	I
Hydrocortisone sodium succinate	UP	500 mg	BW	200 mg	D5W	Physically compatible	15	C
Lincomycin HCl	PHU, XGN					Physically compatible for 24 hr at room temperature	3164, 3165	C
Magnesium sulfate	LI	16 mEq	BW	200 mg	D5W	Physically incompatible	15	I
Penicillin G potassium	SQ	20 million units	BW	200 mg	D5W	Physically compatible	15	C
Penicillin G potassium	SQ	5 million units	BW	200 mg	D	Physically compatible	47	C
Penicillin G sodium	UP	20 million units	BW	200 mg	D5W	Physically compatible	15	C
Phenobarbital sodium	WI	200 mg	BW	200 mg	D5W	Physically compatible	15	C
Ranitidine HCl	GL	50 mg and 2 g		1 million units	D5W	Physically compatible. Ranitidine stable for 24 hr at 25°C. Polymyxin B not tested	1515	C

Drugs in Syringe Compatibility

Polymyxin B sulfate

Test Drug	Mfr	Amt	Mfr	Amt	Remarks	Ref	C/I
Ampicillin sodium	AY	500 mg	BW	25 mg/1.5 mL	Physically compatible for 1 hr at room temperature	300	C
Ampicillin sodium	AY	250 mg	BW	25 mg/1.5 mL	Precipitate forms within 1 hr at room temperature	300	I
Cloxacillin sodium	BE	250 mg	BE	250,000 units/1.5 to 2 mL	Physically incompatible within 1 hr at room temperature	99	I
Penicillin G sodium		1 million units	BW	25 mg/1.5 to 2 mL	No precipitate or color change within 1 hr at room temperature	99	C

Y-Site Injection Compatibility (1:1 Mixture)

Polymyxin B sulfate

Test Drug	Mfr	Conc	Mfr	Conc	Remarks	Ref	C/I
Esmolol HCl	DCC	10 mg/mL[a]	PF	0.005 unit/mL[a]	Physically compatible for 24 hr at 22°C	1169	C

[a] Tested in dextrose 5%.

Selected Revisions January 4, 2017. © Copyright, October 1982.
American Society of Health-System Pharmacists, Inc.

Posaconazole
AHFS 8:14.08

Products

Posaconazole is available as an 18-mg/mL concentrate for injection in single-use vials containing 300 mg of the drug.[2911] The concentrate must be diluted prior to administration.[2911] Also present in each vial are betadex sulfobutyl ether sodium 6.68 g, edetate disodium 3 mg, hydrochloric acid and sodium hydroxide to adjust the pH, and water for injection.[2911]

pH
The pH is adjusted to 2.6.[2911]

Trade Name(s)
Noxafil

Administration

Single-use vials contain posaconazole concentrate for injection that is administered only by slow intravenous infusion after diluting 16.7 mL (300 mg) of the concentrate in an intravenous bag or bottle containing a sufficient volume of a compatible infusion solution to yield a solution containing 1 to 2 mg/mL.[2911] Prior to dilution, the vials should be allowed to come to room temperature.[2911] The diluted solution must only be administered using a 0.22-µm polyethersulfone or polyvinylidene difluoride inline filter.[2911]

Posaconazole is administered by slow intravenous infusion over approximately 90 minutes through a central venous line (e.g., central venous catheter, peripherally inserted central catheter).[2911] In certain circumstances (i.e., in anticipation of central venous line placement or while the central venous line is being replaced or is being used for another treatment), a *single* dose of posaconazole may be administered through a peripheral venous catheter over approximately 30 minutes.[2911] If multiple doses of the drug are needed, a central line should be used; repeated administration of posaconazole through a peripheral venous catheter has been associated with thrombophlebitis.[2911] Posaconazole should *not* be administered as a bolus intravenous injection.[2911]

Stability

Posaconazole concentrate for injection is a clear, colorless to yellow solution.[2911] Intact vials of posaconazole should be stored under refrigeration at 2 to 8°C.[2911] The injection contains no preservatives and is for single use.[2911] Any unused portions should be discarded.[2911]

After dilution, the resulting posaconazole solution also ranges from colorless to yellow; variations in color within this range do not affect product quality.[2911] Diluted solutions should be visually inspected for particulate matter prior to administration.[2911] Diluted solutions of posaconazole for infusion should be used immediately; admixtures not used immediately may be stored under refrigeration for up to 24 hours.[2911]

Filtration
The concentrate for injection diluted for infusion must be administered through a 0.22-µm polyethersulfone or polyvinylidene difluoride inline filter.[2911]

Compatibility Information
Solution Compatibility

Posaconazole

Test Soln Name	Mfr	Mfr	Conc/L or %	Remarks	Ref	C/I
Dextrose 5% in Ringer's injection, lactated		ME		Stated to be incompatible	2911	I
Dextrose 5% in sodium chloride 0.45%		ME	1 to 2 g	Stated to be stable for up to 24 hr under refrigeration	2911	C
Dextrose 5% in sodium chloride 0.9%		ME	1 to 2 g	Stated to be stable for up to 24 hr under refrigeration	2911	C
Dextrose 5%		ME	1 to 2 g	Stated to be stable for up to 24 hr under refrigeration	2911	C
Ringer's injection, lactated		ME		Stated to be incompatible	2911	I
Sodium chloride 0.45%		ME	1 to 2 g	Stated to be stable for up to 24 hr under refrigeration	2911	C
Sodium chloride 0.9%		ME	1 to 2 g	Stated to be stable for up to 24 hr under refrigeration	2911	C

DOI: 10.37573/9781585286850.320

Additive Compatibility

Posaconazole

Test Drug	Mfr	Conc/L or %	Mfr	Conc/L or %	Test Solution	Remarks	Ref	C/I
Potassium chloride		a	ME	1 to 2 g	D5W	Stated to be stable for up to 24 hr under refrigeration	2911	C
Sodium bicarbonate		b	ME			Stated to be incompatible	2911	I

a Final potassium chloride concentration not specified.

b Final sodium bicarbonate concentration not specified.

Y-Site Injection Compatibility (1:1 Mixture)

Posaconazole

Test Drug	Mfr	Conc	Mfr	Conc	Remarks	Ref	C/I
Amikacin sulfate		5 mg/mLa	ME	18 mg/mL	Physically compatible	2911, 2912	C
Caspofungin acetate		0.28 mg/mLa	ME	18 mg/mL	Physically compatible	2911, 2912	C
Ciprofloxacin		2 mg/mLa	ME	18 mg/mL	Physically compatible	2911, 2912	C
Daptomycin		20 mg/mLa	ME	18 mg/mL	Physically compatible	2911, 2912	C
Dobutamine HCl		5 mg/mLa	ME	18 mg/mL	Physically compatible	2911, 2912	C
Famotidine		4 mg/mLa	ME	18 mg/mL	Physically compatible	2911, 2912	C
Fentanyl citrate		0.05 mg/mLa	ME	18 mg/mL	Physically compatible	2912	C
Filgrastim		6 mcg/mLa	ME	18 mg/mL	Physically compatible	2911, 2912	C
Gentamicin sulfate		1.6 mg/mLa	ME	18 mg/mL	Physically compatible	2911, 2912	C
Hydromorphone HCl		10 mg/mLa	ME	18 mg/mL	Physically compatible	2911, 2912	C
Levofloxacin		40 mg/mLa	ME	18 mg/mL	Physically compatible	2911, 2912	C
Lorazepam		1 mg/mLa	ME	18 mg/mL	Physically compatible	2911, 2912	C
Meropenem		1 mg/mLa	ME	18 mg/mL	Physically compatible	2911, 2912	C
Micafungin sodium		0.2 mg/mLa	ME	18 mg/mL	Physically compatible	2911, 2912	C
Midazolam HCl		1 mg/mLa	ME	18 mg/mL	Physically compatible	2912	C
Morphine sulfate		1 mg/mLa	ME	18 mg/mL	Physically compatible	2911, 2912	C
Norepinephrine bitartrate		0.004 mg/mLa	ME	18 mg/mL	Physically compatible	2911, 2912	C
Potassium chloride		0.04 mEq/mLa	ME	18 mg/mL	Physically compatible	2911, 2912	C
Vancomycin HCl		5 mg/mLa	ME	18 mg/mL	Physically compatible	2911, 2912	C
Voriconazole		5 mg/mLa	ME	18 mg/mL	Physically compatible	2912	C

a Tested in both dextrose 5% and sodium chloride 0.9%.

Selected Revisions June 9, 2016. © Copyright, January 2015.
American Society of Health-System Pharmacists, Inc.

Potassium Acetate
AHFS 40:12

Products

Potassium acetate additive solution is available in 20-, 50-, and 100-mL single-dose vials at a concentration of 2 mEq/mL in water for injection. Each mL provides potassium acetate 196 mg. It is also available in 50-mL vials at a concentration of 4 mEq/mL in water for injection. Each mL provides 392 mg of potassium acetate. The pH of the solutions may have been adjusted with acetic acid when necessary. These concentrated solutions must be diluted for administration.[1(9/06)]

pH

The pH of potassium acetate additive solution has been stated to be approximately 7.1 to 7.7[4] with a range of 5.5 to 8.[1(9/06)]

Osmolarity

The osmolarity of the 2-mEq/mL solution is 4000 mOsm/L and the 4-mEq/mL solution is 8000 mOsm/L.[1(9/06)]

Administration

Potassium acetate is administered as a dilute solution by slow intravenous infusion. It must not be administered undiluted.[1(9/06)][4] In most cases, the maximum recommended concentration is 40 mEq/L. Solutions generally may be infused at a rate up to 20 mEq/hr.[4]

Stability

Potassium acetate additive solution should be stored at room temperature and protected from freezing. It should not be administered unless the solution is clear.[1(9/06)]

Compatibility Information

Additive Compatibility

Potassium acetate

Test Drug	Mfr	Conc/L or %	Mfr	Conc/L or %	Test Solution	Remarks	Ref	C/I
Magnesium sulfate		10 mmol		25 mmol	TPN	Transient precipitate forms	2266	?
Metoclopramide HCl	RB	10 and 160 mg	IX	20 mEq	NS	Physically compatible for 48 hr at room temperature	924	C

Y-Site Injection Compatibility (1:1 Mixture)

Potassium acetate

Test Drug	Mfr	Conc	Mfr	Conc	Remarks	Ref	C/I
Ciprofloxacin	MI	2 mg/mL[a]	LY	2 mEq/mL	Visually compatible for 2 hr at 25°C	1628	C

[a] Tested in dextrose 5%.

Selected Revisions October 1, 2012. © Copyright, October 1988. American Society of Health-System Pharmacists, Inc.

DOI: 10.37573/9781585286850.321

Potassium Chloride
AHFS 40:12

Products

Potassium chloride is available as concentrated solutions of 1.5 and 2 mEq/mL in 10-, 20-, 30-, and 40-mEq sizes in water for injection in ampuls, vials, and syringes. It is also available in a 30-mL (60-mEq) multiple-dose vial containing methylparaben 0.05% and propylparaben 0.005% as preservatives and 250-mL pharmacy bulk packages. The pH may have been adjusted with hydrochloric acid and if necessary potassium hydroxide during manufacture. The concentrated solutions must be diluted for use.[1(5/06)]

Potassium chloride is also available premixed in infusion solutions in concentrations of 10, 20, 30, and 40 mEq/L.[4]

pH

The pH is usually near 4.6 with a range from 4 to 8.[1(5/06) 17]

Osmolarity

The injections are very hypertonic; the 2-mEq/mL concentration has an osmolarity of 4000 mOsm/L. The injection must be diluted for use.[1(5/06)]

Osmolality

The osmolality of potassium chloride (Abbott) 2 mEq/mL was determined to be 4355 mOsm/kg by freezing-point depression and 3440 mOsm/kg by vapor pressure.[1071]

The osmolality of a potassium chloride 7.5% solution was determined to be 1895 mOsm/kg.[1233]

Administration

Potassium chloride in the concentrated injections must be diluted before slow intravenous administration. Mix potassium chloride injection thoroughly with the infusion solution before administration. The usual maximum concentration is 40 mEq/L. Extravasation should be avoided.[1(5/06) 4]

Great care is required when adding potassium chloride to infusion solutions, whether in flexible plastic containers or in rigid bottles. Adding potassium chloride to running infusion solutions hanging in the use position, especially in flexible containers, has resulted in the pooling of potassium chloride and a resultant high-concentration bolus of the drug being administered to patients, with serious and even fatal consequences. Attempts to mix adequately the potassium chloride in flexible containers by squeezing the container in the hanging position were unsuccessful. It is recommended that drugs be admixed with solutions in flexible containers when positioned with the injection arm of the container uppermost. With both rigid bottles and flexible containers, subsequent repeated inversion and agitation to effect thorough mixture are necessary.[85 130 454 455 456 714 715 1127 1778 2151]

Stability

The solution should be stored at controlled room temperature and used only if it is clear.[1(5/06)]

Potassium chloride injection 80 mEq/L added to dextrose 5% contained in glass bottles results in a leaching of precipitates consisting of silica and alumina.[129]

Compatibility Information
Solution Compatibility

Potassium chloride

Test Soln Name	Mfr	Mfr	Conc/L or %	Remarks	Ref	C/I
Dextrose 2.5% in half-strength Ringer's injection	AB	AB	160 mEq	Physically compatible	3	C
Dextrose 5% in Ringer's injection	AB	AB	160 mEq	Physically compatible	3	C
Dextrose 5% in half-strength Ringer's injection, lactated	AB	AB	160 mEq	Physically compatible	3	C
Dextrose 2.5% in Ringer's injection, lactated	AB	AB	160 mEq	Physically compatible	3	C
Dextrose 5% in Ringer's injection, lactated	AB	AB	160 mEq	Physically compatible	3	C
Dextrose 5% in Ringer's injection, lactated	BA	LI	80 mEq	Physically compatible for 24 hr	315	C
Dextrose 10% in Ringer's injection, lactated	AB	AB	160 mEq	Physically compatible	3	C
Dextrose 2.5% in sodium chloride 0.45%	AB	AB	160 mEq	Physically compatible	3	C

DOI: 10.37573/9781585286850.322

Solution Compatibility (Cont.)

Test Soln Name	Mfr	Mfr	Conc/L or %	Remarks	Ref	C/I
Dextrose 2.5% in sodium chloride 0.9%	AB	AB	160 mEq	Physically compatible	3	C
Dextrose 5% in sodium chloride 0.225%	AB	AB	160 mEq	Physically compatible	3	C
Dextrose 5% in sodium chloride 0.45%	AB	AB	160 mEq	Physically compatible	3	C
Dextrose 5% in sodium chloride 0.9%	AB	AB	160 mEq	Physically compatible	3	C
Dextrose 5% in sodium chloride 0.9%			3 g	Physically compatible	74	C
Dextrose 5% in sodium chloride 0.9%	BA	LI	80 mEq	Physically compatible for 24 hr	315	C
Dextrose 10% in sodium chloride 0.9%	AB	AB	160 mEq	Physically compatible	3	C
Dextrose 2.5%	AB	AB	160 mEq	Physically compatible	3	C
Dextrose 5%			3 g	Physically compatible	74	C
Dextrose 5%	AB	AB	160 mEq	Physically compatible	3	C
Dextrose 5%	BA	LI	80 mEq	Physically compatible for 24 hr	315	C
Dextrose 10%	AB	AB	160 mEq	Physically compatible	3	C
Dextrose 10%	BA	LI	80 mEq	Physically compatible for 24 hr	315	C
Dextrose 20%	BA	LI	80 mEq	Physically compatible for 24 hr	315	C
Ionosol B in dextrose 5%	AB	AB	160 mEq	Physically compatible	3	C
Ionosol MB in dextrose 5%	AB	AB	160 mEq	Physically compatible	3	C
Ringer's injection	AB	AB	160 mEq	Physically compatible	3	C
Ringer's injection			3 g	Physically compatible	74	C
Ringer's injection, lactated	AB	AB	160 mEq	Physically compatible	3	C
Ringer's injection, lactated	BA	LI	80 mEq	Physically compatible for 24 hr	315	C
Sodium chloride 0.45%	AB	AB	160 mEq	Physically compatible	3	C
Sodium chloride 0.9%			3 g	Physically compatible	74	C
Sodium chloride 0.9%	AB	AB	160 mEq	Physically compatible	3	C
Sodium chloride 0.9%	BA	LI	80 mEq	Physically compatible for 24 hr	315	C
Sodium lactate ⅙ M	AB	AB	160 mEq	Physically compatible	3	C
Sodium lactate ⅙ M	BA	LI	80 mEq	Physically compatible for 24 hr	315	C

Additive Compatibility

Potassium chloride

Test Drug	Mfr	Conc/L or %	Mfr	Conc/L or %	Test Solution	Remarks	Ref	C/I
Amikacin sulfate	BR	5 g	LI	3 g	D5LR, D5R, D5S, D5W, D10W, LR, NS, R, SL	Physically compatible and both stable for 24 hr at 25°C	294	C
Aminophylline		250 mg	AB	3 g	D5W	Physically compatible	74	C
Aminophylline	SE	500 mg	AB	40 mEq		Physically compatible	6	C
Amiodarone HCl	LZ	1.8 g	AB	40 mEq	D5W, NS[a]	Physically compatible. No amiodarone loss in 24 hr at 24°C in light	1031	C

Additive Compatibility (Cont.)

Test Drug	Mfr	Conc/L or %	Mfr	Conc/L or %	Test Solution	Remarks	Ref	C/I
Amphotericin B		200 mg	BP	4 g	D5W	Haze develops over 3 hr	26	I
Amphotericin B	SQ	100 mg	AB	100 mEq	D5W	Physically incompatible	15	I
Atracurium besylate	BW	500 mg		80 mEq	D5W	Physically compatible and atracurium stable for 24 hr at 5 and 30°C	1694	C
Calcium gluconate		1 g		3 g	D5W	Physically compatible	74	C
Cefepime HCl	BR	4 g	AB	10 and 40 mEq	D5W, NS	Visually compatible with 2% cefepime loss in 24 hr at room temperature or 7 days at 5°C	1681	C
Ceftazidime		4 g		10 and 40 mEq	D5W, NS	Ceftazidime stable for 24 hr at room temperature and 7 days refrigerated	4	C
Chloramphenicol sodium succinate	PD	500 mg		3 g	D5W	Physically compatible	74	C
Chloramphenicol sodium succinate	PD	1 g	AB	40 mEq		Physically compatible	6	C
Chloramphenicol sodium succinate	PD	500 mg and 1 g		20 and 40 mEq	D2.5½S, D5W	Therapeutic availability maintained	110	C
Ciprofloxacin	MI	2 g		40 mEq	NS	Compatible for 24 hr at 25°C	888	C
Ciprofloxacin	BAY	2 g	AB	40 mEq	NS	Visually compatible with little or no ciprofloxacin loss in 24 hr at 25°C	1934	C
Ciprofloxacin	BAY	2 g	LY	2.9 g	D5W	Visually compatible with no loss of ciprofloxacin in 24 hr at 22°C under fluorescent light. Potassium chloride not tested	2413	C
Clindamycin phosphate	UP	600 mg		40 mEq	D5½S	Physically compatible and clindamycin stable for 24 hr at room temperature	104	C
Clindamycin phosphate	UP	600 mg		100 mEq	D5W, NS	Physically compatible	101	C
Clindamycin phosphate	UP	6 g		400 mEq	D5½S	Clindamycin stable for 24 hr	101	C
Cloxacillin sodium	AST	2.25 g		60 mEq	D5W	10% cloxacillin loss in 48 hr at 25°C	1476	C
Cytarabine	UP	2 g		100 mEq	D5S	Physically compatible. Stable for 8 days	174	C
Cytarabine	UP	170 mg		80 mEq	D5S	Physically compatible for 24 hr	174	C
Dimenhydrinate	SE	50 mg		3 g	D5W	Physically compatible	74	C
Dobutamine HCl	LI	1 g	ES	160 mEq	D5W, NS	Slightly pink in 24 hr at 25°C	789	I
Dobutamine HCl	LI	1 g	AB	20 mEq	D5W, NS	Physically compatible for 24 hr at 21°C	812	C
Dopamine HCl	AS	800 mg	MG		D5W	No dopamine loss in 24 hr at 25°C	312	C
Enalaprilat	MSD	12 mg	AB	3 g	D5Wᵃ	Visually compatible. Little enalaprilat loss in 24 hr at room temperature in light	1572	C
Eptifibatide	ME	50 and 250 mg		40 mEq	NRD5W	Physically compatible and chemically stable for up to 24 hr at 25°C	3049	C
Eptifibatide	ME	75 and 375 mg		40 mEq	NRD5W	Physically compatible and chemically stable for up to 24 hr at 25°C	3049	C
Eptifibatide	ME	50 and 250 mg		40 mEq	NS	Physically compatible and chemically stable for up to 24 hr at 25°C	3049	C
Eptifibatide	ME	75 and 375 mg		40 mEq	NS	Physically compatible and chemically stable for up to 24 hr at 25°C	3049	C

Additive Compatibility (Cont.)

Test Drug	Mfr	Conc/L or %	Mfr	Conc/L or %	Test Solution	Remarks	Ref	C/I
Eptifibatide	ME	50 and 250 mg		60 mEq	NRD5W	Physically compatible and chemically stable for up to 24 hr at 25°C	3049	C
Eptifibatide	ME	75 and 375 mg		60 mEq	NRD5W	Physically compatible and chemically stable for up to 24 hr at 25°C	3049	C
Eptifibatide	ME	50 and 250 mg		60 mEq	NS	Physically compatible and chemically stable for up to 24 hr at 25°C	3049	C
Eptifibatide	ME	75 and 375 mg		60 mEq	NS	Physically compatible and chemically stable for up to 24 hr at 25°C	3049	C
Erythromycin lactobionate	AB	1 g	AB	40 mEq		Physically compatible	20	C
Fat emulsion, intravenous	VT	10%		100 mEq		Physically compatible for 48 hr at 4°C and room temperature	32	C
Fat emulsion, intravenous	CU	10%		100 mEq		No change in 24 hr at room temperature, but lipid coalescence in 48 hr	656	C
Fat emulsion, intravenous	CU	10%		200 mEq		Coalescence with surface creaming in 4 hr at room temperature. Oil globules on surface at 48 hr	656	I
Fat emulsion, intravenous	VT	10%	DB	4 g		Lipid coalescence in 24 hr at 8 and 25°C	825	I
Floxacillin sodium	BE	20 g	ANT	40 mmol	W	Physically compatible for 72 hr at 15 and 30°C	1479	C
Fluconazole	PF	1 g	AB	10 mEq	D5W[a]	Fluconazole stable for 24 hr at 25°C in fluorescent light	1676	C
Foscarnet sodium	AST	12 g		20 to 120 mmol	NS	Foscarnet concentrations of 93 to 99% were maintained for at least 65 hr	2156	C
Fosphenytoin sodium	PD	1, 8, 20 mg PE/mL[c]	BA	20 and 40 mEq	D5½S[a]	Visually compatible with little or no loss in 7 days at 25°C under fluorescent light	2083	C
Furosemide	HO	1 g	ANT	40 mmol	W	Physically compatible for 72 hr at 15 and 30°C	1479	C
Heparin sodium		12,000 units		3 g	D5W	Physically compatible	74	C
Heparin sodium	AB	20,000 units	AB	40 mEq		Physically compatible	21	C
Heparin sodium		32,000 units		80 mEq	NS	Physically compatible and heparin activity retained for 24 hr	57	C
Hydrocortisone sodium succinate	UP	100 mg		3 g	D5W	Physically compatible	74	C
Hydromorphone HCl	KN	2 and 20 mg/mL	AST	0.5 and 1 mEq/mL	D5W[a]	Visually compatible with no loss of hydromorphone in 18 days at 4 and 23°C. Potassium chloride not tested	2410	C
Isoproterenol HCl	WI	4 mg	AB	40 mEq		Physically compatible	59	C
Lidocaine HCl	AST	2 g	AB	40 mEq		Physically compatible	24	C
Magnesium sulfate	DB	3.9 g	BRN	80 mEq	D5W, NS	Visually compatible. Under 5% loss of ions in 24 hr at 22°C	2360	C
Methyldopate HCl	MSD	1 g		40 mEq	D5W, D10W, D2.5½S, D2.5S, D5¼S, D5½S, D5S, D10S, NS, ½S	Physically compatible	23	C

Additive Compatibility (Cont.)

Test Drug	Mfr	Conc/L or %	Mfr	Conc/L or %	Test Solution	Remarks	Ref	C/I
Metoclopramide HCl	RB	10 and 160 mg	ES	30 mEq	NS	Physically compatible for 48 hr at room temperature	924	C
Mitoxantrone HCl	LE	500 mg		50 mEq	D5W	Visually compatible. Mitoxantrone stable for 24 hr at room temperature	1531	C
Nafcillin sodium	WY	500 mg	AB	40 mEq		Physically compatible	27	C
Nafcillin sodium	WY	30 g	TR	40 mEq	NS	Nafcillin stable for 24 hr at 25°C	27	C
Nicardipine HCl	DME	50 and 500 mg	ES	40 mEq	D5W[b]	Physically compatible. Little loss in 7 days at room temperature in light	1380	C
Nicardipine HCl	DME	50 and 500 mg	ES	40 mEq	D5W[a]	Physically compatible. 12% loss in 7 days at room temperature in light	1380	C
Norepinephrine bitartrate	WI	8 mg		3 g	D5W	Physically compatible	74	C
Norepinephrine bitartrate	WI	8 mg	AB	40 mEq	D5W, D10W, D2.5½S, D2.5S, D5¼S, D5½S, D5S, D10S, NS, ½S	Physically compatible	77	C
Oxacillin sodium	BR	1, 2.5, 4 g		20, 40, 80 mEq	D5S, D5W	Therapeutic availability maintained	110	C
Penicillin G potassium	SQ	5 million units	AB	40 mEq		Physically compatible	47	C
Penicillin G potassium	SQ	5 million units		40 mEq	D5S, D5W	Therapeutic availability maintained	110	C
Penicillin G potassium	SQ	1 million units		20 mEq	D5S, D5W	Therapeutic availability maintained	110	C
Penicillin G sodium	KA	6 million units		40 mEq	D5W	Penicillin stable for 48 hr at 25°C	131	C
Penicillin G sodium	KA	5 million units		40 mEq	IS10	pH outside stability range for penicillin	131	I
Phenylephrine HCl	WI	2.5 g	AB	40 mEq	D5W	Phenylephrine stable for 24 hr at 22°C	132	C
Posaconazole	ME	1 to 2 g		e	D5W	Stated to be stable for up to 24 hr under refrigeration	2911	C
Ranitidine HCl	GL	2 g	LY	10 and 60 mEq	D5W, NS[a]	Physically compatible. 2% ranitidine loss in 48 hr at room temperature in light	1361	C
Ranitidine HCl	GL	50 mg	LY	10 and 60 mEq	NS[a]	Physically compatible. No ranitidine loss in 48 hr at room temperature in light	1361	C
Ranitidine HCl	GL	50 mg	LY	10 and 60 mEq	D5W[a]	Physically compatible. 7% ranitidine loss in 48 hr at room temperature in light	1361	C
Ranitidine HCl	GL	50 mg and 2 g		80 mEq	D5S, D5W, NS	Physically compatible. Ranitidine stable for 24 hr at 25°C	1515	C
Sodium bicarbonate	AB	2.4 mEq[d]		120 mEq	D5W	Physically compatible for 24 hr	772	C
Vancomycin HCl	LI	1 g		3 g	D5W	Physically compatible	74	C
Verapamil HCl	KN	80 mg	TR	80 mEq	D5W, NS	Physically compatible for 24 hr	764	C

[a] Tested in PVC containers.

[b] Tested in glass containers.

[c] Concentration expressed in milligrams of phenytoin sodium equivalents (PE) per mL.

[d] One vial of Neut added to a liter of admixture.

[e] Final potassium chloride concentration not specified.

Drugs in Syringe Compatibility

Potassium chloride

Test Drug	Mfr	Amt	Mfr	Amt	Remarks	Ref	C/I
Dimenhydrinate		10 mg/1 mL		2 mEq/1 mL	Precipitate forms in about 1 hr	2569	I
Hydromorphone HCl	KN	50 mg/1 mL	AST	2 mEq/1 mL	Visually compatible for 24 hr at room temperature	2410	C
Pantoprazole sodium	a	4 mg/1 mL		2 mEq/1 mL	Clear solution	2574	C

[a] Test performed using the formulation WITHOUT edetate disodium.

Y-Site Injection Compatibility (1:1 Mixture)

Potassium chloride

Test Drug	Mfr	Conc	Mfr	Conc	Remarks	Ref	C/I
Acetaminophen	CAD	10 mg/mL	HOS, BED	0.1 mEq/mL[b]	Physically compatible with less than 10% acetaminophen loss over 4 hr at room temperature	2841, 2844	C
Acyclovir sodium	BW	5 mg/mL[a]	IX	0.04 mEq/mL[a]	Physically compatible for 4 hr at 25°C	1157	C
Aldesleukin	CHI	33,800 I.U./mL[a]	AB	0.2 mEq/mL	Visually compatible with little or no loss of aldesleukin activity	1857	C
Aldesleukin	CHI	a p			Loss of aldesleukin activity	1890	I
Allopurinol sodium	BW	3 mg/mL[b]	AB	0.1 mEq/mL[b]	Physically compatible for 4 hr at 22°C	1686	C
Amifostine	USB	10 mg/mL[a]	AB	0.1 mEq/mL[a]	Physically compatible for 4 hr at 23°C	1845	C
Aminophylline	SE	25 mg/mL		40 mEq/L[c]	Physically compatible for 4 hr at room temperature	322	C
Amiodarone HCl	LZ	4 mg/mL[d]	AB	0.04 mEq/mL[d]	Physically compatible for 24 hr at 21°C	1032	C
Ampicillin sodium	BR	25, 50, 100, 125 mg/mL		40 mEq/L[c]	Physically compatible for 4 hr at room temperature	322	C
Anidulafungin	VIC	0.5 mg/mL[a]	APP	0.1 mEq/mL[a]	Physically compatible for 4 hr at 23°C	2617	C
Atropine sulfate	BW	0.5 mg/mL	AB	40 mEq/L[f]	Physically compatible for 4 hr at room temperature	534	C
Azithromycin	PF	2 mg/mL[b]	BA	20 mEq/L[n]	White microcrystals found	2368	I
Aztreonam	SQ	40 mg/mL[a]	AB	0.1 mEq/mL[a]	Physically compatible for 4 hr at 23°C	1758	C
Bivalirudin	TMC	5 mg/mL[a]	APP	0.1 mEq/mL[a]	Physically compatible for 4 hr at 23°C	2373	C
Blinatumomab	AMG	0.125 mcg/mL[b]	AGT	0.0249 mg/mL[b]	Flakes transiently appear when blinatumomab is added to potassium chloride; not observed when order of mixing was reversed	3405, 3417	?
Blinatumomab	AMG	0.375 mcg/mL[b]	AGT	0.0249 mg/mL[b]	Persistent particulate formation when blinatumomab is added to potassium chloride; not observed when order of mixing was reversed	3405, 3417	?
Calcium gluconate	ES	100 mg/mL		40 mEq/L[c]	Physically compatible for 4 hr at room temperature	322	C
Cangrelor tetrasodium	TMC	1 mg/mL[b]		0.1 mEq/mL[b]	Physically compatible for 4 hr	3243	C
Caspofungin acetate	ME	0.7 mg/mL[b]	APP	0.1 mEq/mL[b]	Physically compatible for 4 hr at room temperature	2758	C

Y-Site Injection Compatibility (1:1 Mixture) (Cont.)

Test Drug	Mfr	Conc	Mfr	Conc	Remarks	Ref	C/I
Caspofungin acetate	ME	0.5 mg/mL[b]	BA	0.04 mEq/mL[b]	Physically compatible over 60 min	2766	C
Ceftaroline fosamil	FOR	2.22 mg/mL[c]	HOS	0.1 mEq/mL[c]	Physically compatible for 4 hr at 23°C	2826	C
Ceftazidime–avibactam sodium	ALL	20 mg/mL[i v]		0.4 mEq/mL	Physically compatible for up to 4 hr at room temperature	3004	C
Ceftolozane sulfate–tazobactam sodium	CUB	10 mg/mL[d t]	HOS	0.1 mEq/mL[d]	Physically compatible for 2 hr	3262	C
Chlorpromazine HCl	SKF	25 mg/mL	AB	40 mEq/L[f]	Physically compatible for 4 hr at room temperature	534	C
Chlorpromazine HCl	RPR	0.13 mg/mL[a]	BRN	0.625 mEq/mL[a]	Visually compatible for 150 min	2244	C
Ciprofloxacin	MI	2 mg/mL[d]	LY	0.04 mEq/mL	Visually compatible for 24 hr at 24°C	1655	C
Ciprofloxacin	MI	2 mg/mL[a]	AMR	2 mEq/mL	Visually compatible for 2 hr at 25°C	1628	C
Cisatracurium besylate	GW	0.1, 2, 5 mg/mL[a]	AB	0.1 mEq/mL[a]	Physically compatible for 4 hr at 23°C	2074	C
Cladribine	ORT	0.015[b] and 0.5[h] mg/mL	AB	0.1 mEq/mL[b]	Physically compatible for 4 hr at 23°C	1969	C
Clarithromycin	AB	4 mg/mL[a]	ANT	0.08 mmol/mL[a]	Visually compatible for 72 hr at both 30 and 17°C	2174	C
Clevidipine butyrate	CHS	0.5 mg/mL		[b]	Physically compatible for 24 hr at 23°C	3334	C
Clonidine HCl	BI	18 mcg/mL[b]	BRN	1 mEq/mL	Visually compatible	2642	C
Cloxacillin sodium	SMX	100 mg/mL	HOS	2 mEq/mL	Physically compatible for up to 4 hr at room temperature	3245	C
Cyanocobalamin	PD	0.1 mg/mL	AB	40 mEq/L[f]	Physically compatible for 4 hr at room temperature	534	C
Dexamethasone sodium phosphate	MSD	4 mg/mL		40 mEq/L[c]	Physically compatible for 4 hr at room temperature	322	C
Dexmedetomidine HCl	AB	4 mcg/mL[b]	AB	0.1 mEq/mL[b]	Physically compatible for 4 hr at 23°C	2383	C
Dexmedetomidine HCl	HOS, HQS	4 mcg/mL[b]		0.04 mEq/mL	Stated to be compatible	2848, 3179	C
Diazepam	RC	5 mg/mL		40 mEq/L[c]	Immediate haziness and globule formation	322	I
Digoxin	BW	0.25 mg/mL		40 mEq/L[c]	Physically compatible for 4 hr at room temperature	322	C
Diltiazem HCl	MMD	5 mg/mL	LY	0.08[a] and 2 mEq/mL	Visually compatible	1807	C
Diphenhydramine HCl	PD	50 mg/mL	AB	40 mEq/L[f]	Physically compatible for 4 hr at room temperature	534	C
Dobutamine HCl	LI	4 mg/mL[d]	AB	0.06 mEq/mL[d]	Physically compatible for 3 hr	1316	C
Docetaxel	RPR	0.9 mg/mL[a]	AB	0.1 mEq/mL[a]	Physically compatible for 4 hr at 23°C	2224	C
Dopamine HCl	ACC	40 mg/mL	AB	40 mEq/L[f]	Physically compatible for 4 hr at room temperature	534	C
Doripenem	JJ	5 mg/mL[a b]	APP	0.1 mEq/mL[a b]	Physically compatible for 4 hr at 23°C	2743	C
Doxorubicin HCl liposomal	SEQ	0.4 mg/mL[a]	AB	0.1 mEq/mL[a]	Physically compatible for 4 hr at 23°C	2087	C

Y-Site Injection Compatibility (1:1 Mixture) (Cont.)

Test Drug	Mfr	Conc	Mfr	Conc	Remarks	Ref	C/I
Droperidol	CR	1.25 mg/mL	AB	40 mEq/L[f]	Physically compatible for 4 hr at room temperature	534	C
Edrophonium chloride	RC	10 mg/mL	AB	40 mEq/L[f]	Physically compatible for 4 hr at room temperature	534	C
Enalaprilat	MSD	0.05 mg/mL[b]	LY	0.4 mEq/mL[a]	Physically compatible for 24 hr at room temperature under fluorescent light	1355	C
Epinephrine HCl	AB	0.1 mg/mL	AB	40 mEq/L[f]	Physically compatible for 4 hr at room temperature	534	C
Ergotamine tartrate	SZ	0.5 mg/mL	AB	40 mEq/L[f]	Crystal formation and brown discoloration in 4 hr at room temperature	534	I
Ertapenem sodium	ME	10 mg/mL[b]	AB	0.01 and 0.04 mEq/mL[g]	Visually compatible with about 2% ertapenem loss in 4 hr	2487	C
Esmolol HCl	DCC	10 mg/mL[a]	IX	0.4 mEq/mL[a]	Physically compatible for 24 hr at 22°C	1169	C
Estrogens, conjugated	AY	5 mg/mL		40 mEq/L[c]	Physically compatible for 4 hr at room temperature	322	C
Ethacrynate sodium	MSD	1 mg/mL		40 mEq/L[c]	Physically compatible for 4 hr at room temperature	322	C
Etoposide phosphate	BR	5 mg/mL[a]	AB	0.1 mEq/mL[a]	Physically compatible for 4 hr at 23°C	2218	C
Famotidine	MSD	0.2 mg/mL[a]	AB	0.04 mEq/mL[a]	Physically compatible for 4 hr at 25°C	1188	C
Famotidine	ME	2 mg/mL[b]		0.1 mEq/mL[a]	Visually compatible for 4 hr at 22°C	1936	C
Fenoldopam mesylate	AB	80 mcg/mL[b]	APP	0.1 mEq/mL[b]	Physically compatible for 4 hr at 23°C	2467	C
Fentanyl citrate	MN	0.05 mg/mL	AB	40 mEq/L[f]	Physically compatible for 4 hr at room temperature	534	C
Filgrastim	AMG	30 mcg/mL[a]	AB	0.1 mEq/mL[a]	Physically compatible for 4 hr at 22°C	1687	C
Fludarabine phosphate	BX	1 mg/mL[a]	AB	0.1 mEq/mL[a]	Visually compatible for 4 hr at 22°C	1439	C
Fluorouracil	RC	50 mg/mL	AB	40 mEq/L[f]	Physically compatible for 4 hr at room temperature	534	C
Furosemide	HO	10 mg/mL	AB	40 mEq/L[f]	Physically compatible for 4 hr at room temperature	534	C
Furosemide	HMR	2.6 mg/mL[a]	BRN	0.625 mEq/mL[a]	Visually compatible for 150 min	2244	C
Gallium nitrate	FUJ	1 mg/mL[b]	AB	0.3 mEq/mL[b]	Visually compatible for 24 hr at 25°C	1673	C
Gemcitabine HCl	LI	10 mg/mL[b]	AB	0.1 mEq/mL[b]	Physically compatible for 4 hr at 23°C	2226	C
Gentamicin sulfate	AMS	30 mg/mL[e]	BA	0.02 mEq/mL[o]	Physically compatible	2794	C
Granisetron HCl	SKB	1 mg/mL	LY	0.04 mEq/mL[b]	Physically compatible with little or no loss of granisetron in 4 hr at 22°C	1883	C
Heparin sodium	TR	50 units/mL	AB	0.2 mEq/mL[a]	Visually compatible for 4 hr at 25°C	1793	C
Heparin sodium	NOV	29.2 units/mL[a]	BRN	0.625 mEq/mL[a]	Visually compatible for 150 min	2244	C
Hetastarch in lactated electrolyte	AB	6%	AB	0.1 mEq/mL[a]	Physically compatible for 4 hr at 23°C	2339	C
Hydralazine HCl	CI	20 mg/mL	AB	40 mEq/L[f]	Physically compatible for 4 hr at room temperature	534	C

Y-Site Injection Compatibility (1:1 Mixture) (Cont.)

Test Drug	Mfr	Conc	Mfr	Conc	Remarks	Ref	C/I
Hydroxyethyl starch 130/0.4 in sodium chloride 0.9%	FRK	6%	HOS	0.02, 0.4, 0.8 mEq/mL[a]	Visually compatible for 24 hr at room temperature	2770	C
Ibuprofen lysinate	OVA	10 mg/mL	HOS	2 mEq/mL	Physically compatible for 4 hr at room temperature	3541	C
Idarubicin HCl	AD	1 mg/mL[b]	AB	0.03 mEq/mL[b]	Visually compatible for 24 hr at 25°C	1525	C
Indomethacin sodium trihydrate	MSD	1 mg/mL[b]	AB	0.2 mEq/mL[a]	Visually compatible for 24 hr at 28°C	1527	C
Isavuconazonium sulfate	ASP	1.5 mg/mL[d]	HOS	0.1 mEq/mL[d]	Physically compatible for 2 hr	3263	C
Isoproterenol HCl	WI	0.2 mg/mL	AB	40 mEq/L[f]	Physically compatible for 4 hr at room temperature	534	C
Labetalol HCl	SC	1 mg/mL[a]	IX	0.4 mEq/mL[a]	Physically compatible for 24 hr at 18°C	1171	C
Letermovir	ME	[a]		[a]	Physically compatible	3398	C
Levofloxacin	OMN	5 mg/mL[a]	HOS	0.04 mEq/mL[a]	Physically compatible	2794	C
Lidocaine HCl	AST	20 mg/mL		40 mEq/L[c]	Physically compatible for 4 hr at room temperature	322	C
Linezolid	PHU	2 mg/mL	FUJ	0.1 mEq/mL[a]	Physically compatible for 4 hr at 23°C	2264	C
Lorazepam	WY	0.33 mg/mL[b]	BRN	1 mEq/mL	Visually compatible for 24 hr at 22°C	1855	C
Magnesium sulfate	AB	500 mg/mL	AB	40 mEq/L[f]	Physically compatible for 4 hr at room temperature	534	C
Melphalan HCl	BW	0.1 mg/mL[b]	AB	0.1 mEq/mL[b]	Physically compatible for 3 hr at 22°C	1557	C
Meperidine HCl	AB	10 mg/mL	AB	0.4 mEq/mL[a]	Physically compatible for 4 hr at 25°C	1397	C
Meropenem	ZEN	1 mg/mL[a]		10 and 40 mEq/L[a]	Visually compatible. Calculated 10% meropenem loss in 3.3 hr at 23°C	2492	C
Meropenem	ZEN	1 mg/mL[a]		10 and 40 mEq/L[b]	Visually compatible. Calculated 10% meropenem loss in 5 hr at 23°C	2492	C
Meropenem	ZEN	1 mg/mL[b]		10 and 40 mEq/L[a]	Visually compatible. Calculated 10% meropenem loss in 5.8 hr at 23°C	2492	C
Meropenem	ZEN	1 mg/mL[b]		10 and 40 mEq/L[b]	Visually compatible. Calculated 10% meropenem loss in 22 hr at 23°C	2492	C
Meropenem	ZEN	22 mg/mL[a]		10 and 40 mEq/L[a]	Visually compatible. Calculated 10% meropenem loss in 7.7 hr at 23°C	2492	C
Meropenem	ZEN	22 mg/mL[a]		10 and 40 mEq/L[b]	Visually compatible. Calculated 10% meropenem loss in 13 hr at 23°C	2492	C
Meropenem	ZEN	22 mg/mL[b]		10 and 40 mEq/L[a]	Visually compatible. Calculated 10% meropenem loss in 8 hr at 23°C	2492	C
Meropenem	ZEN	22 mg/mL[b]		10 and 40 mEq/L[b]	Visually compatible. Calculated 10% meropenem loss in 20 hr at 23°C	2492	C
Meropenem		50 mg/mL	HOS	2 mEq/mL	Physically compatible for 4 hr at room temperature	3538	C
Meropenem–vaborbactam	TMC	8 mg/mL[b, u]	HOS	0.1 mEq/mL[b]	Physically compatible for 3 hr at 20 to 25°C	3380	C
Methylprednisolone sodium succinate	UP	40 mg/mL		40 mEq/L[a]	Physically compatible for 4 hr at room temperature	322	C

Y-Site Injection Compatibility (1:1 Mixture) (Cont.)

Test Drug	Mfr	Conc	Mfr	Conc	Remarks	Ref	C/I
Methylprednisolone sodium succinate	UP	40 mg/mL		40 mEq/L[b]	Physically compatible initially but haze forms in 4 hr at room temperature	322	I
Methylprednisolone sodium succinate	UP	40 mg/mL		40 mEq/L[i]	Immediate haze formation	322	I
Micafungin sodium	ASP	1.5 mg/mL[b]	AB	0.1 mEq/mL[b]	Physically compatible for 4 hr at 23°C	2683	C
Midazolam HCl	RC	5 mg/mL	BRN	1 mEq/mL	Visually compatible for 24 hr at 22°C	1855	C
Milrinone lactate	SW	0.4 mg/mL[a]	AB	1 mEq/mL[a]	Visually compatible. No milrinone loss in 4 hr at 23°C	2214	C
Morphine sulfate	WY	15 mg/mL	AB	40 mEq/L[f]	Physically compatible for 4 hr at room temperature	534	C
Neostigmine methyl-sulfate	RC	0.5 mg/mL	AB	40 mEq/L[f]	Physically compatible for 4 hr at room temperature	534	C
Nicardipine HCl	DCC	0.1 mg/mL[a]	LY	0.4 mEq/mL[a]	Visually compatible for 24 hr at room temperature	235	C
Norepinephrine bitar-trate	WI	1 mg/mL	AB	40 mEq/L[f]	Physically compatible for 4 hr at room temperature	534	C
Ondansetron HCl	GL	1 mg/mL[b]	AB	0.1 mEq/mL[a]	Visually compatible for 4 hr at 22°C	1365	C
Oritavancin diphosphate	TAR	0.8, 1.2, and 2 mg/mL[a]	HOS	0.2 mEq/mL[a]	Visually compatible for 4 hr at 20 to 24°C	2928	C
Oxacillin sodium	BR	100 mg/mL	AB	40 mEq/L[f]	Physically compatible for 4 hr at room temperature	534	C
Oxaliplatin	SS	0.5 mg/mL[a]	APP	0.1 mEq/mL[a]	Physically compatible for 4 hr at 23°C	2566	C
Oxytocin	SZ	1 unit/mL	AB	40 mEq/L[f]	Physically compatible for 4 hr at room temperature	534	C
Paclitaxel	NCI	1.2 mg/mL[a]	AB	0.1 mEq/mL[a]	Physically compatible for 4 hr at 22°C	1556	C
Palonosetron HCl	MGI	50 mcg/mL	AB	0.1 mEq/mL[a]	Physically compatible. No loss of either drug in 4 hr at room temperature	2771	C
Pantoprazole sodium	ALT[q]	0.16 to 0.8 mg/mL[b]	AST	20 to 210 mEq/L[a]	Visually compatible for 12 hr at 23°C	2603	C
Pemetrexed disodium	LI	20 mg/mL[b]	APP	0.1 mEq/mL[a]	Physically compatible for 4 hr at 23°C	2564	C
Penicillin G potassium	LI	200,000 units/mL		40 mEq/L[c]	Physically compatible for 4 hr at room temperature	322	C
Pentazocine lactate	WI	30 mg/mL	AB	40 mEq/L[f]	Physically compatible for 4 hr at room temperature	534	C
Phenytoin sodium	PD	50 mg/mL		40 mEq/L[a]	Immediate formation of phenytoin crystals	322	I
Phenytoin sodium	PD	50 mg/mL		40 mEq/L[b i]	Crystals in 4 hr at room temperature	322	I
Phytonadione	RC	10 mg/mL	AB	40 mEq/L[f]	Physically compatible for 4 hr at room temperature	534	C
Piperacillin sodium–tazobactam sodium	LE[q]	40 mg/mL[a r]	AB	0.1 mEq/mL[a]	Physically compatible for 4 hr at 22°C	1688	C
Plazomicin sulfate	ACH	24 mg/mL[d]	APP	0.1 mEq/mL[d]	Physically compatible for 1 hr at 20 to 25°C	3432	C
Posaconazole	ME	18 mg/mL		0.04 mEq/mL[d]	Physically compatible	2911, 2912	C

Y-Site Injection Compatibility (1:1 Mixture) (Cont.)

Test Drug	Mfr	Conc	Mfr	Conc	Remarks	Ref	C/I
Procainamide HCl	SQ	100 mg/mL	AB	40 mEq/L[f]	Physically compatible for 4 hr at room temperature	534	C
Prochlorperazine edisylate	SKF	5 mg/mL	AB	40 mEq/L[f]	Physically compatible for 4 hr at room temperature	534	C
Promethazine HCl	SV	50 mg/mL	AB	40 mEq/L[j]	Clear initially, but cloudiness develops in 4 hr at room temperature	534	I
Promethazine HCl	SV	50 mg/mL	AB	40 mEq/L[k]	Physically compatible for 4 hr at room temperature	534	C
Propofol	ZEN[w]	10 mg/mL	AB	0.1 mEq/mL[a]	Physically compatible for 1 hr at 23°C	2066	C
Propranolol HCl	AY	1 mg/mL	AB	40 mEq/L[f]	Physically compatible for 4 hr at room temperature	534	C
Quinupristin–dalfo-pristin	PF	2 mg/mL[a s]		0.04 mEq/mL[a]	Physically compatible	3229	C
Remifentanil HCl	GW	0.025 and 0.25 mg/mL[b]	AB	0.1 mEq/mL[a]	Physically compatible for 4 hr at 23°C	2075	C
Sargramostim	IMM	10 mcg/mL[b]	AB	0.1 mEq/mL[b]	Visually compatible for 4 hr at 22°C	1436	C
Scopolamine HBr	BW	0.86 mg/mL	AB	40 mEq/L[f]	Physically compatible for 4 hr at room temperature	534	C
Sodium bicarbonate	BR	75 mg/mL		40 mEq/L[c]	Physically compatible for 4 hr at room temperature	322	C
Sodium nitroprusside	RC	0.3, 1.2, 3 mg/mL[a]	AST	0.04 and 0.5 mEq/mL[o]	Visually compatible for 48 hr at 24°C protected from light	2357	C
Succinylcholine chloride	BW	20 mg/mL		40 mEq/L[c]	Physically compatible for 4 hr at room temperature	322	C
Tacrolimus	FUJ	1 mg/mL[b]	AB	2 mEq/mL	Visually compatible for 24 hr at 25°C	1630	C
Tedizolid phosphate	CUB	0.8 mg/mL[b]	HOS	0.1 mEq/mL[b]	Physically compatible for 2 hr	3244	C
Telavancin HCl	ASP	7.5 mg/mL[c]	HOS	0.1 mEq/mL[c]	Physically compatible for 2 hr	2830	C
Teniposide	BR	0.1 mg/mL[a]	AB	0.1 mEq/mL[a]	Physically compatible for 4 hr at 23°C	1725	C
Theophylline	TR	4 mg/mL	AB	0.2 mEq/mL[a]	Visually compatible for 6 hr at 25°C	1793	C
Thiotepa	IMM[l]	1 mg/mL[a]	AMR	0.1 mEq/mL[a]	Physically compatible for 4 hr at 23°C	1861	C
Tigecycline	WY	1 mg/mL[b]		0.3 mEq/mL[b]	Physically compatible for 4 hr	2714	C
Tigecycline	ACD, FRK, WY	[d]			Stated to be compatible	2915, 3459, 3460	C
Tirofiban HCl	ME	0.05 mg/mL[a b]	AB	0.01 and 0.04 mEq/mL[a b]	Physically compatible. No tirofiban loss in 4 hr at room temperature	2250	C
TNA #218 to #226[m]			AB	0.1 mEq/mL[a]	Visually compatible for 4 hr at 23°C	2215	C
TPN #189[m]			AST	30 mg/mL[b]	Visually compatible for 24 hr at 22°C	1767	C
TPN #212 to #215[m]			AB	0.1 mEq/mL[a]	Physically compatible for 4 hr at 23°C	2109	C
Trimethobenzamide HCl	RC	100 mg/mL	AB	40 mEq/L[f]	Physically compatible for 4 hr at room temperature	534	C
Vinorelbine tartrate	BW	1 mg/mL[b]	AB	0.1 mEq/mL[b]	Physically compatible for 4 hr at 22°C	1558	C

Y-Site Injection Compatibility (1:1 Mixture) (Cont.)

Test Drug	Mfr	Conc	Mfr	Conc	Remarks	Ref	C/I
Zidovudine	BW	4 mg/mL[a]	IMS	0.67 mEq/mL[a]	Physically compatible for 4 hr at 25°C	1193	C

[a] Tested in dextrose 5%.

[b] Tested in sodium chloride 0.9%.

[c] Tested in dextrose 5%, sodium chloride 0.9%, and Ringer's injection, lactated.

[d] Tested in both dextrose 5% and sodium chloride 0.9%.

[e] Tested in sodium chloride 0.45%.

[f] Tested in dextrose 5% in Ringer's injection, dextrose 5% in Ringer's injection, lactated, dextrose 5%, Ringer's injection, lactated, and sodium chloride 0.9%.

[g] Tested in sterile water for injection.

[h] Tested in bacteriostatic sodium chloride 0.9% preserved with benzyl alcohol 0.9%.

[i] Tested in Ringer's injection, lactated.

[j] Tested in dextrose 5% in Ringer's injection.

[k] Tested in dextrose 5% in Ringer's injection, lactated, dextrose 5%, Ringer's injection, lactated, and sodium chloride 0.9%.

[l] Lyophilized formulation tested.

[m] Refer to Appendix for the composition of parenteral nutrition solutions. TNA indicates a 3-in-1 admixture, and TPN indicates a 2-in-1 admixture.

[n] Tested in dextrose 5% in sodium chloride 0.45%.

[o] Tested in dextrose 5% in sodium chloride 0.225%.

[p] Tested with albumin human 0.1%.

[q] Test performed using the formulation WITHOUT edetate disodium.

[r] Piperacillin component. Piperacillin in an 8:1 fixed-ratio concentration with tazobactam.

[s] Quinupristin and dalfopristin components combined.

[t] Ceftolozane component. Ceftolozane in a 2:1 fixed-ratio concentration with tazobactam.

[u] Meropenem component. Meropenem in a 1:1 fixed-ratio concentration with vaborbactam.

[v] Ceftazidime component. Ceftazidime in a 4:1 fixed-ratio concentration with avibactam.

[w] Test performed using the formulation WITH edetate disodium.

Additional Compatibility Information

Methylprednisolone

The compatibility of methylprednisolone sodium succinate (Upjohn) with potassium chloride added to an auxiliary medication infusion unit has been studied. Primary admixtures were prepared by adding potassium chloride 40 mEq/L to dextrose 5%, dextrose 5% in sodium chloride 0.9%, and Ringer's injection, lactated. The primary admixture was added along with methylprednisolone sodium succinate (Upjohn) to the auxiliary medication infusion unit with the following results:[329]

Methylprednisolone Sodium Succinate	Potassium Chloride 40 mEq/L Primary Solution	Results
500 mg	D5S, D5W, LR qs 100 mL	Clear solution for 24 hr
1000 mg	D5W qs 100 mL	Clear solution for 24 hr
1000 mg	D5S, LR qs 100 mL	Clear solution for 6 hr
2000 mg	D5S, D5W, LR qs 100 mL	Clear solution for 24 hr

Selected Revisions May 1, 2020. © Copyright, October 1982. American Society of Health-System Pharmacists, Inc.

Potassium Phosphates

AHFS 40:12

Products

Potassium phosphates is available as a concentrate for injection in 5- or 15-mL single-dose vials and in a 50-mL pharmacy bulk package.[3594 3595 3596] The concentrate for injection must be diluted for use.[3594 3595 3596]

Each mL of the Fresenius Kabi and Hospira products contains monobasic potassium phosphate 224 mg and dibasic potassium phosphate 236 mg in water for injection.[3594 3596] The phosphate concentration of the concentrate for injection is 3 mmol/mL, and the potassium concentration is 4.4 mEq/mL.[3594 3596]

Each mL of the CMP Pharma product contains monobasic potassium phosphate 175 mg and dibasic potassium phosphate 300 mg in water for injection.[3595] The phosphate concentration of the concentrate for injection is 3 mmol/mL, and the potassium concentration is 4.7 mEq/mL.[3595]

The relationship between milliequivalents and millimoles of phosphate is expressed in the following equation:

(mEq phosphate = mmol phosphate × valence)

However, the average valence of phosphate changes with changes in pH. Consequently, it is necessary to specify a pH before the valence, and therefore the milliequivalents, can be determined. To avoid this problem, it has been suggested that doses of phosphate be expressed in terms of millimoles, which is independent of valence.[178 716 717 718] Alternatively, the dose may be expressed in terms of milligrams of phosphorus: 1 millimole of phosphorus equals 31 mg.[205 717 3594 3595 3596]

pH

Potassium phosphates injection (Fresenius Kabi) is stated to have a pH of 6 to 7.[3594]

Potassium phosphates injection (CMP Pharma) is stated to have a pH of 6.5 to 7.5.[3595]

Osmolarity

The calculated osmolarity of potassium phosphates injection (Fresenius Kabi, Hospira) is 7.4 mOsm/mL.[3594 3596]

The calculated osmolarity of potassium phosphates injection (CMP Pharma) is 7.7 mOsm/mL.[3595]

Aluminum Content

Potassium phosphates injection (Fresenius Kabi) contains no more than 2000 mcg of aluminum per L.[3594]

Potassium phosphates injection (CMP Pharma) contains no more than 15,000 mcg of aluminum per L.[3595]

Potassium phosphates injection (Hospira) contains no more than 31,000 mcg of aluminum per L.[3596]

Administration

Potassium phosphates injection is administered by intravenous infusion *only* after dilution or admixing in a larger volume of fluid;

the concentrate for injection is *not* for direct infusion.[3594 3595 3596] Administration of undiluted or insufficiently diluted potassium phosphates injection and administration by rapid infusion (e.g., over 1 to 3 hours) or by bolus or rapid intravenous push has resulted in serious and sometimes fatal adverse effects.[3594 3595]

When the drug is used diluted in intravenous fluids for the correction of hypophosphatemia in *adults and pediatric patients 12 years or age or older*, the appropriate dose of potassium phosphates should be diluted to a total volume of 100 to 250 mL in sodium chloride 0.9% or dextrose 5%.[3594 3595] For *peripheral venous administration*, Fresenius Kabi states that the maximum recommended concentration is 6.8 mmol of phosphate/100 mL and the maximum recommended rate of administration is 6.8 mmol of phosphate/hr.[3594] For *peripheral venous administration*, CMP Pharma states that the maximum recommended concentration is 6.4 mmol of phosphate/100 mL and the maximum recommended rate of administration is 6.4 mmol of phosphate/hr.[3595] For *central venous administration*, manufacturers state that the maximum recommended concentration is 18 mmol of phosphate/100 mL and the maximum recommended rate of administration is 15 mmol of phosphate/hr.[3594 3595]

When the drug is used diluted in intravenous fluids for the correction of hypophosphatemia in *pediatric patients less than 12 years of age*, the appropriate dose of potassium phosphates should be diluted in the smallest recommended volume, taking into consideration the daily fluid requirements and the maximum concentrations recommended for peripheral and central venous administration.[3594] For *peripheral venous administration*, the manufacturer states that the maximum recommended concentration is 0.27 mmol of phosphate/10 mL.[3594] For *central venous administration*, the manufacturer states that the maximum recommended concentration is 0.55 mmol of phosphate/10 mL.[3594]

When the drug is used in parenteral nutrition admixtures, the appropriate dose of potassium phosphates injection should be added to the parenteral nutrition solution *after* the addition of amino acids, dextrose, and electrolyte solutions and *prior* to the addition of fat emulsion, if included.[3594 3595] Selection of the peripheral or central venous route depends upon the osmolarity of the final infusate.[3594 3595] Manufacturers state that solutions with an osmolarity of 900 mOsm/L or more must be infused through a central vein.[3594 3595]

The infusion set and catheter should be checked periodically during administration for precipitates.[3594 3595] Peripheral venous administration of the diluted and admixed drug can cause thrombophlebitis.[3594 3595] If thrombophlebitis develops, the catheter should be removed as soon as possible and appropriate treatment should be initiated.[3594 3595]

Stability

Potassium phosphates injection is a clear and colorless solution.[3594 3595 3596] Intact vials of potassium phosphates injection (Fresenius

DOI: 10.37573/9781585286850.323

Kabi, Hospira) should be stored at controlled room temperature.[3594] [3596] Intact vials of potassium phosphates injection (CMP Pharma) should be stored at 2 to 8°C and should not be frozen.[3595]

Solutions should be visually inspected for particulate matter and discoloration prior to and after dilution, and again prior to administration of the diluted solution for infusion or admixture.[3594] [3595] [3596]

Fresenius Kabi states that diluted solutions of potassium phosphates for infusion in dextrose 5% and sodium chloride 0.9% are stable for 4 hours at 20 to 25°C and 14 days at 2 to 8°C.[3594] CMP Pharma states that diluted solutions of potassium phosphates for infusion in dextrose 5% and sodium chloride 0.9% are stable for 48 hours at 20 to 25°C and 2 to 8°C.[3595]

Manufacturers state that parenteral nutrition admixtures to which potassium phosphates injection has been added should be inspected both after mixing and prior to administration to ensure that precipitates have not formed and that the emulsion has not separated, in the case that fat emulsion has been added.[3594] [3595] Parenteral nutrition admixtures to which potassium phosphates injection has been added should be used promptly after mixing.[3594] [3595] Any storage of the admixtures should be limited to no longer than 24 hours at 2 to 8°C protected from light.[3594] [3595] After removal from refrigeration, admixtures should be allowed to come to room temperature and should be used promptly, with completion of the infusion within 24 hours.[3594] [3595] Any admixture remaining after that time should be discarded.[3594] [3595]

Unused portions of single-dose vials should be discarded.[3594] [3595] [3596] The pharmacy bulk package should be discarded within 4 hours of initial entry.[3594]

Compatibility Information

Solution Compatibility

Potassium phosphates

Test Soln Name	Mfr	Mfr	Conc/L or %	Remarks	Ref	C/I
Dextrose 5% in Ringer's injection	AB	AB	160 mEq[a]	Haze or precipitate forms within 1 hr	3	I
Dextrose 2.5% in half-strength Ringer's injection, lactated	AB	AB	160 mEq[a]	Haze or precipitate forms within 24 hr	3	I
Dextrose 5% in Ringer's injection, lactated	AB	AB	160 mEq[a]	Haze or precipitate forms within 24 hr	3	I
Dextrose 5% in sodium chloride 0.9%	AB	AB	160 mEq[a]	Physically compatible	3	C
Dextrose 5% in sodium chloride 0.45%	AB	AB	160 mEq[a]	Physically compatible	3	C
Dextrose 5% in sodium chloride 0.225%	AB	AB	160 mEq[a]	Physically compatible	3	C
Dextrose 2.5% in sodium chloride 0.9%	AB	AB	160 mEq[a]	Physically compatible	3	C
Dextrose 2.5% in sodium chloride 0.45%	AB	AB	160 mEq[a]	Physically compatible	3	C
Dextrose 10% in sodium chloride 0.9%	AB	AB	160 mEq[a]	Haze or precipitate forms within 24 hr	3	I
Dextrose 2.5%	AB	AB	160 mEq[a]	Physically compatible	3	C
Dextrose 5%	AB	AB	160 mEq[a]	Physically compatible	3	C
Dextrose 5%		FRK		Stable for 4 hr at 20 to 25°C and 14 days at 2 to 8°C	3594	C
Dextrose 5%		CMP		Stable for 48 hr at 2 to 8°C and 20 to 25°C	3595	C
Dextrose 10%	AB	AB	160 mEq[a]	Physically compatible	3	C
Ionosol B in dextrose 5%	AB	AB	160 mEq[a]	Physically compatible	3	C
Ionosol MB in dextrose 5%	AB	AB	160 mEq[a]	Physically compatible	3	C
Ringer's injection	AB	AB	160 mEq[a]	Haze or precipitate forms within 1 hr	3	I
Ringer's injection, lactated	AB	AB	160 mEq[a]	Haze or precipitate forms within 24 hr	3	I
Sodium chloride 0.45%	AB	AB	160 mEq[a]	Physically compatible	3	C
Sodium chloride 0.9%	AB	AB	160 mEq[a]	Physically compatible	3	C

Solution Compatibility (Cont.)

Test Soln Name	Mfr	Mfr	Conc/L or %	Remarks	Ref	C/I
Sodium chloride 0.9%		FRK		Stable for 4 hr at 20 to 25°C and 14 days at 2 to 8°C	3594	C
Sodium chloride 0.9%		CMP		Stable for 48 hr at 2 to 8°C and 20 to 25°C	3595	C
Sodium lactate ⅙ M	AB	AB	160 mEq[a]	Physically compatible	3	C

[a] Not specified whether concentration refers to potassium or phosphates content.

Additive Compatibility

Potassium phosphates

Test Drug	Mfr	Conc/L or %	Mfr	Conc/L or %	Test Solution	Remarks	Ref	C/I
Calcium chloride						Compatibility dependent on solubility and concentration and is not entirely predictable. See the monograph discussion under Additional Compatibility Information	1777, 2803	?
Calcium gluconate						Compatibility dependent on solubility and concentration and is not entirely predictable. See the monograph discussion under Additional Compatibility Information	1777, 2803	?
Ciprofloxacin		2 g		60 mg	D5W	Precipitation occurs	671	I
Dobutamine HCl	LI	200 mg	AB	100 mmol	NS	Small particles form after 1 hr. White precipitate noted after 15 hr	552	I
Metoclopramide HCl	RB	10 and 160 mg	IX	15 mmol	NS	Physically compatible for 48 hr at room temperature	924	C
Verapamil HCl	KN	80 mg	AB	88 mEq	D5W, NS	Physically compatible for 24 hr	764	C

Drugs in Syringe Compatibility

Potassium phosphates

Test Drug	Mfr	Amt	Mfr	Amt	Remarks	Ref	C/I
Pantoprazole sodium	a	4 mg/1 mL		4 mmol/1 mL	Precipitates	2574	I

[a] Test performed using the formulation WITHOUT edetate disodium.

Y-Site Injection Compatibility (1:1 Mixture)

Potassium phosphates

Test Drug	Mfr	Conc	Mfr	Conc	Remarks	Ref	C/I
Amiodarone HCl	WY	6 mg/mL[a]	APP[a]	0.12 mmol/mL	Immediate white cloudiness	2352	I
Caspofungin acetate	ME	0.7 mg/mL[b]	APP	0.5 mmol/mL[b]	Immediate white turbid precipitate forms	2758	I
Ceftaroline fosamil	FOR	2.22 mg/mL[a]	HOS	0.5 mmol/mL[a]	Increase in measured haze and microparticulates	2826	I
Ceftaroline fosamil	FOR	2.22 mg/mL[b e]	HOS	0.5 mmol/mL[b e]	Increase in measured haze	2826	I
Ceftazidime–avibactam sodium	ALL	20 mg/mL[f i]			Physically compatible for up to 4 hr at room temperature	3004	C
Ceftolozane sulfate–tazobactam sodium	CUB	10 mg/mL[f g]	HOS	0.3 mmol/mL[f]	Physically compatible for 2 hr	3262	C

Y-Site Injection Compatibility (1:1 Mixture) (Cont.)

Test Drug	Mfr	Conc	Mfr	Conc	Remarks	Ref	C/I
Cloxacillin sodium	SMX	100 mg/mL	PPC	3 mmol/mL	Large particles form within 4 hr	3245	I
Diltiazem HCl	MMD	5 mg/mL	AMR	0.015 mmol/mL	Visually compatible	1807	C
Doripenem	JJ	5 mg/mL[a b]	APP	0.5 mmol/mL[a b]	Measured haze increases after 1 hr	2743	I
Enalaprilat	MSD	0.05 mg/mL[b]	LY	0.44 mEq/mL[a]	Physically compatible for 24 hr at room temperature under fluorescent light	1355	C
Esmolol HCl	DCC	10 mg/mL[a]	LY	0.44 mEq/mL[a]	Physically compatible for 24 hr at 22°C	1169	C
Famotidine	MSD	0.2 mg/mL[a]	LY	0.03 mmol/mL[b]	Physically compatible for 14 hr	1196	C
Hydroxyethyl starch 130/0.4 in sodium chloride 0.9%	FRK	6%	SX	0.003, 0.0765, 0.15 mmol/mL[a]	Visually compatible for 24 hr at room temperature	2770	C
Isavuconazonium sulfate	ASP	1.5 mg/mL[f]	HOS	0.3 mmol/mL[f]	Measured turbidity increases within 1 hr	3263	I
Labetalol HCl	SC	1 mg/mL[a]	LY	0.44 mEq/mL[a]	Physically compatible for 24 hr at 18°C	1171	C
Letermovir	ME	[a]		[a]	Physically compatible	3398	C
Meropenem		50 mg/mL	BA	3 mmol/mL	Physically compatible for 4 hr at room temperature	3538, 3547	C
Meropenem–vaborbactam	TMC	8 mg/mL[b h]	HOS	0.3 mmol/mL[b]	Physically compatible for 3 hr at 20 to 25°C	3380	C
Micafungin sodium	ASP	1.5 mg/mL[b]	APP	0.5 mmol/mL[b]	Physically compatible for 4 hr at 23°C	2683	C
Nicardipine HCl	DCC	0.1 mg/mL[a]	LY	0.44 mEq/mL[a]	Visually compatible for 24 hr at room temperature	235	C
Plazomicin sulfate	ACH	24 mg/mL[f]	FRK	0.3 mmol/mL[f]	Physically compatible for 1 hr at 20 to 25°C	3432	C
Sodium nitroprusside	RC	0.3, 1.2, 3 mg/mL[a]	AB	0.3 mmol/mL[d]	Visually compatible for 48 hr at 24°C protected from light	2357	C
Tedizolid phosphate	CUB	0.8 mg/mL[b]	HOS	0.3 mmol/mL[b]	Physically compatible for 2 hr	3244	C
Telavancin HCl	ASP	7.5 mg/mL[a b e]	AMR	0.5 mEq/mL[a b e]	Physically compatible for 2 hr	2830	C
TNA #218[c]			AB	3 mmol/mL	Damage to emulsion occurs immediately with free oil formation possible	2215	I
TNA #219[c]			AB	3 mmol/mL	Damage to emulsion occurs immediately with free oil formation possible	2215	I
TNA #220[c]			AB	3 mmol/mL	Damage to emulsion occurs immediately with free oil formation possible	2215	I
TNA #221[c]			AB	3 mmol/mL	Damage to emulsion occurs immediately with free oil formation possible	2215	I
TNA #222[c]			AB	3 mmol/mL	Damage to emulsion occurs immediately with free oil formation possible	2215	I
TNA #223[c]			AB	3 mmol/mL	Damage to emulsion occurs immediately with free oil formation possible	2215	I
TNA #224[c]			AB	3 mmol/mL	Damage to emulsion occurs immediately with free oil formation possible	2215	I
TNA #225[c]			AB	3 mmol/mL	Damage to emulsion occurs immediately with free oil formation possible	2215	I
TNA #226[c]			AB	3 mmol/mL	Damage to emulsion occurs immediately with free oil formation possible	2215	I

Y-Site Injection Compatibility (1:1 Mixture) (Cont.)

Test Drug	Mfr	Conc	Mfr	Conc	Remarks	Ref	C/I
TPN #212[c]			AB	3 mmol/mL	Increased turbidity forms immediately	2109	I
TPN #213[c]			AB	3 mmol/mL	Increased turbidity forms immediately	2109	I
TPN #214[c]			AB	3 mmol/mL	Increased turbidity forms immediately	2109	I
TPN #215[c]			AB	3 mmol/mL	Increased turbidity forms immediately	2109	I

[a] Tested in dextrose 5%.

[b] Tested in sodium chloride 0.9%.

[c] Refer to Appendix for the composition of parenteral nutrition solutions. TNA indicates a 3-in-1 admixture, and TPN indicates a 2-in-1 admixture.

[d] Tested in dextrose 5% in sodium chloride 0.225%.

[e] Tested in Ringer's injection, lactated.

[f] Tested in both dextrose 5% and sodium chloride 0.9%.

[g] Ceftolozane component. Ceftolozane in a 2:1 fixed-ratio concentration with tazobactam.

[h] Meropenem component. Meropenem in a 1:1 fixed-ratio concentration with vaborbactam.

[i] Ceftazidime component. Ceftazidime in a 4:1 fixed-ratio concentration with avibactam.

Additional Compatibility Information

Infusion Solutions

Potassium phosphates injection diluted for infusion should not be infused with calcium-containing intravenous fluids.[3594 3595]

Calcium and Phosphate

UNRECOGNIZED CALCIUM PHOSPHATE PRECIPITATION IN A 3-IN-1 PARENTERAL NUTRITION MIXTURE RESULTED IN PATIENT DEATH.

The potential for the formation of a calcium phosphate precipitate in parenteral nutrition solutions is well studied and documented,[1771 1777] but the information is complex and difficult to apply to the clinical situation.[1770 1772 1777] The incorporation of fat emulsion in 3-in-1 parenteral nutrition solutions obscures any precipitate that is present which has led to substantial debate on the dangers associated with 3-in-1 parenteral nutrition mixtures and when or if the danger to the patient is warranted therapeutically.[1770 1771 1772 2031 2032 2033 2034 2035 2036] Because such precipitation may be life-threatening to patients,[2037 2291] FDA issued a Safety Alert containing the following recommendations:[1769]

1. "The amounts of phosphorus and of calcium added to the admixture are critical. The solubility of the added calcium should be calculated from the volume at the time the calcium is added. It should not be based upon the final volume.

    Some amino acid injections for TPN admixtures contain phosphate ions (as a phosphoric acid buffer). These phosphate ions and the volume at the time the phosphate is added should be considered when calculating the concentration of phosphate additives. Also, when adding calcium and phosphate to an admixture, the phosphate should be added first.

    The line should be flushed between the addition of any potentially incompatible components.
2. A lipid emulsion in a 3-in-1 admixture obscures the presence of a precipitate. Therefore, if a lipid emulsion is needed, either (1) use a 2-in-1 admixture with the lipid infused separately, or (2) if a 3-in-1 admixture is medically necessary, then add the calcium before the lipid emulsion and according to the recommendations in number 1 above.

    If the amount of calcium or phosphate which must be added is likely to cause a precipitate, some or all of the calcium should be administered separately. Such separate infusions must be properly diluted and slowly infused to avoid serious adverse events related to the calcium.
3. When using an automated compounding device, the above steps should be considered when programming the device. In addition, automated compounders should be maintained and operated according to the manufacturer's recommendations.

    Any printout should be checked against the programmed admixture and weight of components.
4. During the mixing process, pharmacists who mix parenteral nutrition admixtures should periodically agitate the admixture and check for precipitates. Medical or home care personnel who start and monitor these infusions should carefully inspect for the presence of precipitates both before and during infusion. Patients and care givers should be trained to visually inspect for signs of precipitation. They also should be advised to stop the infusion and seek medical assistance if precipitates are noted.
5. A filter should be used when infusing either central or peripheral parenteral nutrition admixtures. At this time, data have not been submitted to document which size filter is most effective in trapping precipitates.

Standards of practice vary, but the following is suggested: a 1.2-μm air-eliminating filter for lipid-containing admixtures and a 0.22-μm air-eliminating filter for non-lipid-containing admixtures.

6. Parenteral nutrition admixtures should be administered within the following time frames: if stored at room temperature, the infusion should be started within 24 hours after mixing; if stored at refrigerated temperatures, the infusion should be started within 24 hours of rewarming. Because warming parenteral nutrition admixtures may contribute to the formation of precipitates, once administration begins, care should be taken to avoid excessive warming of the admixture.

Persons administering home care parenteral nutrition admixtures may need to deviate from these time frames. Pharmacists who initially prepare these admixtures should check a reserve sample for precipitates over the duration and under the conditions of storage.

7. If symptoms of acute respiratory distress, pulmonary emboli, or interstitial pneumonitis develop, the infusion should be stopped immediately and thoroughly checked for precipitates. Appropriate medical interventions should be instituted. Home care personnel and patients should immediately seek medical assistance."[1769]

Calcium Phosphate Precipitation Fatalities

Fatal cases of paroxysmal respiratory failure in 2 previously healthy women receiving peripheral vein parenteral nutrition were reported. The patients experienced sudden cardiopulmonary arrest consistent with pulmonary emboli. The authors used in vitro simulations and an animal model to conclude that unrecognized calcium phosphate precipitation in a 3-in-1 total nutrition admixture caused the fatalities. The precipitation resulted during compounding by introducing calcium and phosphate near to one another in the compounding sequence and prior to complete fluid addition. This resulted in a temporarily high concentration of the drugs and precipitation of calcium phosphate. Observation of the precipitate was obscured by the incorporation of 20% fat emulsion, intravenous, into the nutrition mixture. No filter was used during infusion of the fatal nutrition admixtures.[2037]

In a follow-up retrospective review, 5 patients were identified who had respiratory distress associated with the infusion of the 3-in-1 admixtures at around the same time. Four of these 5 patients died, although the cause of death could be definitively determined for only 2.[2291]

Calcium and Phosphate Conditional Compatibility

Calcium salts are conditionally compatible with phosphate in parenteral nutrition solutions. The incompatibility is dependent on a solubility and concentration phenomenon and is not entirely predictable. Precipitation may occur during compounding or at some time after compounding is completed.

NOTE: Some amino acids solutions inherently contain calcium and phosphate, which must be considered in any projection of compatibility.

The compatibility of calcium and phosphate in several parenteral nutrition formulas for newborn infants was evaluated. Calcium gluconate 10% (Cutter) and potassium phosphate (Abbott) were used to achieve concentrations of 2.5 to 100 mEq/L of calcium and 2.5 to 100 mmol/L of phosphorus added. The parenteral nutrition solutions evaluated were as shown in Table 1. The results were reported as graphic depictions.

Table 1. Parenteral nutrition solutions evaluated[609]

Component	Solution Number			
	#1	#2	#3	#4
FreAmine III	4%	2%	1%	1%
Dextrose	25%	20%	10%	10%
pH	6.3	6.4	6.6	7.0[a]

[a] Adjusted with sodium hydroxide.

The pH dependence of the phosphate–calcium precipitation has been noted. Dibasic calcium phosphate is very insoluble, while monobasic calcium phosphate is relatively soluble. At low pH, the soluble monobasic form predominates; but as the pH increases, more dibasic phosphate becomes available to bind with calcium and precipitate. Therefore, the lower the pH of the parenteral nutrition solution, the more calcium and phosphate can be solubilized. Once again, the effects of temperature were observed. As the temperature is increased, more calcium ion becomes available and more dibasic calcium phosphate is formed. Therefore, temperature increases will increase the amount of precipitate.[609]

Similar calcium and phosphate solubility curves were reported for neonatal parenteral nutrition solutions using TrophAmine (McGaw) 2, 1.5, and 0.8% as the sources of amino acids. The solutions also contained dextrose 10%, with cysteine and pH adjustment being used in some admixtures. Calcium and phosphate solubility followed the patterns reported previously.[609] A slightly greater concentration of phosphate could be used in some mixtures, but this finding was not consistent.[1024]

Using a similar study design, 6 neonatal parenteral nutrition solutions based on Aminosyn-PF (Abbott) 2, 1.5, and 0.8%, with and without added cysteine hydrochloride and dextrose 10% were studied. Calcium concentrations ranged from 2.5 to 50 mEq/L, and phosphate concentrations ranged from 2.5 to 50 mmol/L. Solutions sat for 18 hours at 25°C and then were warmed to 37°C in a water bath to simulate the clinical situation of warming prior to infusion into a child. Solubility curves were markedly different than those for TrophAmine in the previous study.[1024] Solubilities were reported to decrease by 15 mEq/L for calcium and 15 mmol/L for phosphate. The solutions remained clear during room temperature storage, but crystals often formed on warming to 37°C.[1211]

However, these data were questioned. The similarities between the Aminosyn-PF and TrophAmine products were noted, and little difference was found in calcium and phosphate solubilities in a preliminary report.[1212] In the full report,[1213] parenteral nutrition solutions containing Aminosyn-PF or TrophAmine 1 or 2.5% with dextrose 10 or 25%, respectively, plus electrolytes and trace metals, with or without cysteine hydrochloride, were evaluated under the same conditions. Calcium concentrations ranged from 2.5 to 50 mEq/L, and phosphate concentrations ranged from 5 to 50 mmol/L. In contrast to the previous results,[1024] the solubility curves were very similar for the Aminosyn-PF and TrophAmine parenteral nutrition solutions but very different from those of the previous Aminosyn-PF study.[1211] The authors again showed that the solubility of calcium and phosphate is greater in solutions containing higher concentrations of amino acids and dextrose.[1213]

Calcium and phosphate solubility curves for TrophAmine 1 and 2% with dextrose 10% and electrolytes, vitamins, heparin, and trace elements were reported. Calcium concentrations ranged from 10 to 60 mEq/L, and phosphorus concentrations ranged from 10 to 40 mmol/L. Calcium and phosphate solubilities were assessed by analysis of the calcium concentrations and followed patterns similar to those reported previously.[608] [609] The higher percentage of amino acids (TrophAmine 2%) permitted a slightly greater solubility of calcium and phosphate, especially in the 10 to 50-mEq/L and 10 to 35-mmol/L ranges, respectively.[1614]

The maximal product of the amount of calcium (as gluconate) times phosphate (as potassium) that can be added to a parenteral nutrition solution, composed of amino acids 1% (Travenol) and dextrose 10%, for preterm infants was reported. Turbidity was observed on initial mixing when the solubility product was around 115 to 130 mmol² (mmol squared) or greater. After storage at 7°C for 20 hours, visible precipitates formed at solubility products of 130 mmol² (mmol squared) or greater. If the solution was administered through a barium-impregnated silicone rubber catheter, crystalline precipitates obstructed the catheters in 12 hours at a solubility product of 100 mmol² (mmol squared) and in 10 days at 79 mmol² (mmol squared), much lower than the in vitro results.[1041]

The solubility of calcium and phosphorus in neonatal parenteral nutrition solutions composed of amino acids (Abbott) 1.25 and 2.5% with dextrose 5 and 10%, respectively, was evaluated. Also present were multivitamins and trace elements. The solutions contained calcium (as gluconate) in amounts ranging from 25 to 200 mg/100 mL. The phosphorus (as potassium phosphate) concentrations evaluated ranged from 25 to 150 mg/100 mL. If calcium gluconate was added first, cloudiness occurred immediately. If potassium phosphate was added first, substantial quantities could be added with no precipitate formation in 48 hours at 4°C (Table 2). However, if stored at 22°C, the solutions were stable for only 24 hours, and all contained precipitates after 48 hours.[1210]

Table 2. Maximum calcium and phosphorus concentrations physically compatible for 48 hours at 4°C[1210]

Calcium (mg/100 mL)	Phosphorus (mg/100 mL)	
	Amino Acids 1.25% + Dextrose 5%[a]	Amino Acids 2.5% + Dextrose 10%[a]
200[b]	50	75

Calcium (mg/100 mL)	Phosphorus (mg/100 mL)	
	Amino Acids 1.25% + Dextrose 5%[a]	Amino Acids 2.5% + Dextrose 10%[a]
150	50	100
100	75	100
50	100	125
25	150[b]	150[b]

[a] Plus multivitamins and trace elements.

[b] Maximum concentration tested.

The physical compatibility of calcium gluconate 10 to 40 mEq/L and potassium phosphates 10 to 40 mmol/L in 3 neonatal parenteral nutrition solutions (TPN #123 to #125 in Appendix), alone and with retrograde administration of aminophylline 7.5 mg diluted with 1.5 mL of sterile water for injection was reported. Contact of the alkaline aminophylline solution with the parenteral nutrition solutions resulted in the precipitation of calcium phosphate at much lower concentrations than were compatible in the parenteral nutrition solutions alone.[1404]

The maximum allowable concentrations of calcium and phosphate in a 3-in-1 parenteral nutrition mixture for children (TNA #192 in Appendix) reported. Added calcium was varied from 1.5 to 150 mmol/L, while added phosphate was varied from 21 to 300 mmol/L. The mixtures were stable for 48 hours at 22 and 37°C as long as the pH was not greater than 5.7, the calcium concentration was below 16 mmol/L, the phosphate concentration was below 52 mmol/L, and the product of the calcium and phosphate concentrations was below 250 mmol²/L² (mmol squared per liter squared).[1773]

Additional calcium and phosphate solubility curves were reported for specialty parenteral nutrition solutions based on NephrAmine and also HepatAmine at concentrations of 0.8, 1.5, and 2% as the sources of amino acids. The solutions also contained dextrose 10%, with cysteine and pH adjustment to simulate addition of fat emulsion used in some admixtures. Calcium and phosphate solubility followed the hyperbolic patterns previously reported.[609] Temperature, time, and pH affected calcium and phosphate solubility, with pH having the greatest effect.[2038]

The maximum sodium phosphate concentrations were reported for given amounts of calcium gluconate that could be admixed in parenteral nutrition solutions containing TrophAmine in varying quantities (with cysteine hydrochloride 40 mg/g of amino acid) and dextrose 10%. The solutions also contained magnesium sulfate 4 mEq/L, potassium acetate 24 mEq/L, sodium chloride 32 mEq/L, pediatric multivitamins, and trace elements. The presence of cysteine hydrochloride reduces the solution pH and increases the amount of calcium and phosphate that can be incorporated before precipitation occurs. The results of this study cannot be safely extrapolated to TPN solutions with compositions other than the ones tested. The admixtures were compounded with the sodium phosphate added last after thorough mixing of all other components. The authors noted that this is not the preferred order of mixing (usually phosphate is added first and thoroughly mixed before adding calcium last); however, they believed this reversed order of mixing would provide a margin of error in cases in which the proper order is not followed. After compounding, the solutions were stored for 24 hours at 40°C. The maximum calcium and phosphate amounts that could be mixed in the various solutions were reported tabularly and are shown in Table 3.[2039] However, these results are not entirely consistent with another study. See Table 4.

Table 3. Maximum amount of phosphate (as sodium) (mmol/L) not resulting in precipitation.[2039] See CAUTION below.[a]

| Calcium (as Gluconate) | Amino Acid (as TrophAmine) with Cysteine HCl 40 mg/g of Amino Acid | | | | |
	0%	0.4%	1%	2%	3%
9.8 mEq/L	0	27	42	60	66
14.7 mEq/L	0	15	18	30	36
19.6 mEq/L	0	6	15	27	30
29.4 mEq/L	0	3	6	21	24

[a] CAUTION: The results cannot be safely extrapolated to other solutions. See text.

The temperature dependence of the calcium–phosphate precipitation has resulted in the occlusion of a subclavian catheter by a solution apparently free of precipitation. The parenteral nutrition solution consisted of FreAmine III 500 mL, dextrose 70% 500 mL, sodium chloride 50 mEq, sodium phosphate 40 mmol, potassium acetate 10 mEq, potassium phosphate 40 mmol, calcium gluconate 10 mEq, magnesium sulfate 10 mEq, and Shil's trace metals solution 1 mL. Although there was no evidence of precipitation in the bottle, tubing and pump cassette, and filter (all at approximately 26°C) during administration, the occluded catheter and Vicra Loop Lock (next to the patient's body at 37°C) had numerous crystals identified as calcium phosphate. In vitro, this parenteral nutrition solution had a precipitate in 12 hours at 37°C but was clear for 24 hours at 26°C.[610]

Similarly, a parenteral nutrition solution that was clear and free of particulates after 2 weeks under refrigeration developed a precipitate in 4 to 6 hours when stored at room temperature. When the solution was warmed in a 37°C water bath, precipitation occurred in 1 hour. Administration of the solution before the precipitate was noticed led to interstitial pneumonitis due to deposition of calcium phosphate crystals.[1427]

Calcium phosphate precipitation phenomena was evaluated in a series of parenteral nutrition admixtures composed of dextrose 22%, amino acids (FreAmine III) 2.7%, and fat emulsion (Abbott) 0, 1, and 3.2%. Incorporation of calcium gluconate 19 to 24 mEq/L and phosphate (as sodium) 22 to 28 mmol/L resulted in visible precipitation in the fat-free admixtures. New precipitate continued to form over 14 days, even after repeated filtrations of the solutions through 0.2-μm filters. The presence of the amino acids increased calcium and phosphate solubility, compared with simple aqueous solutions. However, the incorporation of the fat emulsion did not result in a statistically significant increase in calcium and phosphate solubility. The

authors noted that the kinetics of calcium phosphate precipitate formation do not appear to be entirely predictable; both transient and permanent precipitation can occur either during the compounding process or at some time afterward. Because calcium phosphate precipitation can be very dangerous clinically, the use of inline filters was recommended. The authors suggested that the filters should have a porosity appropriate to the parenteral nutrition admixture—1.2 μm for fat-containing and 0.2 or 0.45 μm for fat-free nutrition mixtures.[2061]

Laser particle analysis was used to evaluate the formation of calcium phosphate precipitation in pediatric TPN solutions containing TrophAmine in concentrations ranging from 0.5 to 3% with dextrose 10% and also containing L-cysteine hydrochloride 1 g/L. The solutions also contained in each liter sodium chloride 20 mEq, sodium acetate 20 mEq, magnesium sulfate 3 mEq, trace elements 3 mL, and heparin sodium 500 units. The presence of L-cysteine hydrochloride reduces the solution pH and increases the amount of calcium and phosphate that can be incorporated before precipitation occurs. The results of this study cannot be safely extrapolated to TPN solutions with compositions other than the ones tested. The maximum amount of phosphate that was incorporated without the appearance of a measurable increase in particulates in 24 hours at 37°C for each of the amino acids concentrations is shown in Table 4.[2196] These results are not entirely consistent with previous results.[2039] See above. The use of more sensitive electronic particle measurement for the formation of subvisible particulates in this study may contribute to the differences in the results.

Table 4. Maximum amount of phosphate (as potassium) (mmol/L) not resulting in precipitation.[2196] See CAUTION below.[a]

| Calcium (as Gluconate) (mEq/L) | Amino Acid (as TrophAmine) plus Cysteine HCl 1 g/L | | | | | |
	0.5%	1%	1.5%	2%	2.5%	3%
10	22	28	38	38	38	43
14	18	18	18	38	38	43
19	18	18	18	33	33	38
24	12	18	18	22	28	28
28	12	18	18	18	18	18
33	12	12	12	12	12	12
37	12	12	12	12	12	12
41	9	9	9	12	12	12
45	0	9	9	12	12	12
49	0	9	9	9	12	12
53	0	9	9	9	9	9

[a] CAUTION: The results cannot be safely extrapolated to solutions with formulas other than the ones tested. See text.

Calcium and phosphate compatibility was evaluated in a series of adult formula parenteral nutrition admixtures composed of FreAmine III, in concentrations ranging from 1 to 5% (TPN #258 through #262). The solutions also contained dextrose ranging from 15% up to 25%. Also present were sodium chloride, potassium chloride, and magnesium sulfate in common amounts. Cysteine hydrochloride was added in an amount of 25 mg/g of amino acids from FreAmine III to reduce the pH by about 0.5 pH unit and thereby increase the amount of calcium and phosphates that can be added to the TPN admixtures as has been done with pediatric parenteral nutrition admixtures. Phosphates as the potassium salts and calcium as the gluconate salt were added in variable quantities to determine the maximum amounts of calcium and phosphates that could be added to the test admixtures. The samples were evaluated at 23 and 37°C over 48 hours by visual inspection in ambient light and using a Tyndall beam and electronic measurement of turbidity and microparticulates. The addition of the cysteine hydrochloride resulted in an increase of calcium and phosphates solubility of about 30% by lowering the solution pH 0.5 pH unit. The boundaries between the compatible and incompatible concentrations were presented graphically as hyperbolic curves.[2469]

The presence of magnesium in solutions may also influence the reaction between calcium and phosphate, including the nature and extent of precipitation.[158][159]

The interaction of calcium and phosphate in parenteral nutrition solutions is a complex phenomenon. Various factors have been identified as playing a role in the solubility or precipitation of a given combination, including:[608][609][1042][1063][1404][1427][2778]

1. Concentration of calcium
2. Salt form of calcium
3. Concentration of phosphate
4. Concentration of amino acids
5. Amino acids composition
6. Concentration of dextrose
7. Temperature of solution
8. pH of solution
9. Presence of other additives
10. Order of mixing

Enhanced precipitate formation would be expected from such factors as high concentrations of calcium and phosphate, increases in solution pH, decreased amino acid concentrations, increases in temperature, addition of calcium prior to the phosphate, lengthy standing times or slow infusion rates, and use of calcium as the chloride salt.[854]

Even if precipitation does not occur in the container, it has been reported that crystallization of calcium phosphate may occur in a Silastic infusion pump chamber or tubing if the rate of administration is slow, as for premature infants. Water vapor may be transmitted outward and be replaced by air rapidly enough to produce supersaturation.[202] Several other cases of catheter occlusion have been reported.[610][1427][1428][1429]

Pralidoxime Chloride
AHFS 92:12

Products

Pralidoxime chloride is available as a dry powder in 1-g vials with sodium hydroxide to adjust pH during manufacturing. Reconstitute with 20 mL of sterile water for injection to yield 50 mg/mL. For intravenous infusion, a concentration of 10 to 20 mg/mL in sodium chloride 0.9% is recommended. For intramuscular injection when intravenous administration is not feasible, reconstitute each vial with 3.3 mL of sterile water for injection to yield 300 mg/mL.[1(6/08)]

Pralidoxime chloride is also available as 600 mg/2 mL in autoinjectors. Also present in the formulation are benzyl alcohol 20 mg/mL and glycine 11.26 mg/mL in water for injection.[1(6/08)]

pH

Vials: From 3.5 to 4.5. Autoinjectors: From 2 to 3.[1(6/08)]

Administration

Pralidoxime chloride in vials is given by intravenous infusion at a concentration of 10 to 20 mg/mL in sodium chloride 0.9%. If necessary, the 50-mg/mL reconstituted drug may be given by slow intravenous injection over not less than five minutes. For intramuscular injection when intravenous administration is not feasible, a 300-mg/mL concentration may be used. Pralidoxime chloride in the autoinjectors is intended for intramuscular administration only.[1(6/08)]

Stability

Pralidoxime chloride vials should be stored at controlled room temperature. Autoinjectors should be stored at room temperature and protected from freezing.[1(6/08)]

Compatibility Information

Solution Compatibility

Pralidoxime chloride

Test Soln Name	Mfr	Mfr	Conc/L or %	Remarks	Ref	C/I
Sodium chloride 0.9%		MMT	8 and 10 g	Physically compatible with less than 10% loss in 28 days at −20, 4, 25, and 50°C	2685	C

Selected Revisions October 1, 2012. © Copyright, October 2008. American Society of Health-System Pharmacists, Inc.

DOI: 10.37573/9781585286850.324

Procainamide Hydrochloride
AHFS 24:04.04.04

Products

Procainamide hydrochloride is available in 10-mL multidose vials providing 100 mg/mL or 2-mL multidose vials providing 500 mg/mL.[3400] Each mL of solution in the 10-mL vial also contains methylparaben 1 mg and sodium metabisulfite 0.8 mg in water for injection.[3400] Each mL of solution in the 2-mL vial also contains methylparaben 1 mg and sodium metabisulfite 1.8 mg in water for injection.[3400] In both vial sizes, the solution also may contain hydrochloric acid and/or sodium hydroxide to adjust the pH.[3400]

Procainamide hydrochloride also is available in single-dose, prefilled 10-mL syringes providing 100 mg/mL.[3401] Prefilled syringes are intended only for use in the preparation of intravenous infusion solutions.[3401] Each mL of solution also contains benzyl alcohol 9 mg and sodium bisulfite 0.9 mg in water for injection.[3401] The solution also may contain hydrochloric acid and/or sodium hydroxide to adjust the pH.[3401]

pH

Procainamide hydrochloride injection solution has a pH adjusted to 5 (ranges from 4 to 6).[3400] [3401]

Administration

Procainamide hydrochloride may be administered by intramuscular or direct intravenous injection or intravenous infusion.[3400] [3401] Manufacturers recommend that procainamide hydrochloride injection solution be diluted to a final volume with dextrose 5% prior to intravenous use in order to facilitate control of the administration rate.[3400] [3401]

If procainamide hydrochloride is administered as a direct injection into a vein or into the tubing of an established intravenous line, the drug should be administered slowly, and the rate of administration should not exceed 50 mg/min.[3400] [3401] Alternatively, a loading infusion may be administered.[3400] [3401] To prepare a 20-mg/mL initial loading infusion, 1 g of procainamide hydrochloride should be diluted to 50 mL with dextrose 5% for intravenous administration at a rate of 1 mL/min for 25 to 30 minutes.[3400] [3401]

Maintenance infusions of 2 mg/mL or 4 mg/mL (for fluid-restricted patients) should be prepared by diluting 1 g of procainamide hydrochloride to 500 or 250 mL, respectively, with dextrose 5%.[3400] [3401] Intravenous infusions with a final concentration of 2 mg/mL may be administered at a rate of 1 to 3 mL/min; infusions with a final concentration of 4 mg/mL may be administered at a rate of 0.5 to 1.5 mL/min.[3400] [3401]

Stability

Intact vials and prefilled syringes of procainamide hydrochloride should be stored at controlled room temperature.[3400] [3401] Intact containers are packaged using nitrogen.[3400] [3401] Injection of air into the vial causes the solution to darken.[40] Sulfites (e.g., sodium metabisulfite) are included in the formulation primarily to prevent discoloration that occurs as a result of oxidation of p-aminobenzoic acid, a degradation product of procainamide hydrochloride.[1916] The injection solution is initially colorless, but may turn slightly yellow over time.[3400] [3401] Solutions that appear darker than a light amber color or are otherwise discolored should not be used.[3400] [3401]

Procainamide hydrochloride forms α- and β-glucosylamine compounds with dextrose.[1896] The reaction proceeds rapidly, with about 10% procainamide loss in dextrose 5% occurring in about 5 hours and 30% loss in 24 hours at 25°C.[1896] Equilibrium is achieved with about 62% of the procainamide present as glucosylamines.[1896] The bioavailability, activity, and metabolic fate of these compounds is not known.[546] [1896] The α- and β-glucosylamine compounds that form are reversible,[1422] [1896] although the extent of reversibility in plasma has been questioned.[2051] The rate and extent of complex formation are dependent on the dextrose concentration and the solution pH but are independent of the procainamide hydrochloride concentration.[1422] In dextrose concentrations ranging from 1 to 5%, the extent of procainamide complex formation ranged from 6% in 2 days in dextrose 1% up to 35[1422] to 60%[1896] in dextrose 5%. Lowering the pH from the normal 4.5 to 1.4 with 0.01 N hydrochloric acid completely prevented complex formation.[1422] Similarly, increasing the solution pH to 8 is reported to block complexation.[1423] Maximum complex formation occurred at pH 3 to 5[1423] or 4 to 5.2,[1358] the natural pH of procainamide hydrochloride admixtures in dextrose 5%. The clinical importance of this complexation, if any, is uncertain.

Procainamide hydrochloride (Sandoz) 100 mg/mL repackaged in clear glass vials exhibited less than 10% loss in 193 days stored at 23°C when exposed to light and 5°C when protected from light.[3402] All solutions of procainamide hydrochloride stored at 23°C exposed to light exhibited an increase or darkening of yellow color; however, the 100-mg/mL solution stored in glass vials exhibited a more intense color as compared with 3-mg/mL solutions diluted in sodium chloride 0.9% stored in polyvinyl chloride (PVC) bags.[3402] Solutions stored in either container at 5°C and protected from light did not exhibit such color changes.[3402]

Sorption

Procainamide hydrochloride was shown not to exhibit sorption to PVC bags and tubing, polyethylene tubing, Silastic tubing, and polypropylene syringes.[536] [606]

DOI: 10.37573/9781585286850.325

Compatibility Information

Solution Compatibility

Procainamide HCl

Test Soln Name	Mfr	Mfr	Conc/L or %	Remarks	Ref	C/I
Dextrose 5% in sodium chloride 0.9%	MG[a b]	SQ	4 g	17% loss at room temperature and 5% loss at 4°C in 24 hr	522	I
Dextrose 5%		HOS, IMS	2, 4, and 20 g	Manufacturer-recommended solution	3400, 3401	C
Dextrose 5%[c]	BA[b]	ASC	4 and 8 g	10% or less loss in 24 hr at room temperature and under refrigeration	1327	C
Dextrose 5%	TR[a]	SQ	1 g	No loss in 8 hr but 12% loss in 24 hr at room temperature	545	I
Dextrose 5%	BA[b]	ASC	4 and 8 g	12 to 14% loss in 12 hr at room temperature. 6 to 10% loss in 24 hr under refrigeration	1327	I
Dextrose 5%	TR	ES	4 g	24% loss in 24 hr at room temperature in light	1358	I
Dextrose 5%		LY	4 and 10 g	Physically compatible with 14 to 15% loss in 4 hr at 22°C	1419	I
Dextrose 5%	AB	SQ	2 g	10% loss in 5 hr and 30% loss in 24 hr at 25°C due to reaction with dextrose	1896	I
Sodium chloride 0.45%		LY	4 and 10 g	Physically compatible with no loss in 4 hr at 22°C	1419	C
Sodium chloride 0.9%	TR[a]	SQ	1 g	No decomposition in 24 hr at room temperature	545	C
Sodium chloride 0.9%	BA[b]	SZ	3 g	Less than 10% loss in 193 days at 23°C exposed to light. Slightly increased concentration, likely due to evaporation, after 28 days, and increase in yellow color	3402	C
Sodium chloride 0.9%	BA[b]	SZ	3 g	Less than 10% loss in 193 days at 5°C protected from light	3402	C

[a] Tested in glass containers.

[b] Tested in PVC containers.

[c] Adjusted to approximately pH 7.5 with sodium bicarbonate 8.4%.

Additive Compatibility

Procainamide HCl

Test Drug	Mfr	Conc/L or %	Mfr	Conc/L or %	Test Solution	Remarks	Ref	C/I
Amiodarone HCl	LZ	1.8 g	SQ	4 g	D5W, NS[a]	Physically compatible. 5% or less amiodarone loss in 24 hr at 24°C in light	1031	C
Atracurium besylate	BW	500 mg		4 g	D5W	Physically compatible and atracurium stable for 24 hr at 5 and 30°C	1694	C
Dobutamine HCl	LI	1 g	SQ	1 g	D5W, NS	Physically compatible with no color change in 24 hr at 25°C	789	C
Dobutamine HCl	LI	1 g	AHP	4 and 50 g	D5W, NS	Physically compatible for 24 hr at 21°C	812	C
Esmolol HCl	DU	6 g	ES	4 g	D5W	43% procainamide loss in 24 hr at room temperature under fluorescent light	1358	I
Ethacrynate sodium	MSD	50 mg	SQ	1 g	NS	Altered UV spectra at room temperature	16	I
Flumazenil	RC	20 mg	ES	4 g	D5W[b]	Visually compatible. No flumazenil loss in 24 hr at 23°C in fluorescent light. Procainamide not tested	1710	C
Lidocaine HCl	AST	2 g	SQ	1 g	D5W, LR, NS	Physically compatible for 24 hr at 25°C	775	C

Additive Compatibility (Cont.)

Test Drug	Mfr	Conc/L or %	Mfr	Conc/L or %	Test Solution	Remarks	Ref	C/I
Milrinone lactate	WI	200 mg	SQ	2 and 4 g	D5W	3% procainamide loss in 1 hr and 11% in 4 hr at 23°C. No milrinone loss	1191	I
Verapamil HCl	KN	80 mg	SQ	2 g	D5W, NS	Physically compatible for 48 hr	739	C

[a] Tested in both polyolefin and PVC containers.

[b] Tested in PVC containers.

Drugs in Syringe Compatibility

Procainamide HCl

Test Drug	Mfr	Amt	Mfr	Amt	Remarks	Ref	C/I
Pantoprazole sodium	[a]	4 mg/1 mL		100 mg/1 mL	Clear solution	2574	C

[a] Test performed using the formulation WITHOUT edetate disodium.

Y-Site Injection Compatibility (1:1 Mixture)

Procainamide HCl

Test Drug	Mfr	Conc	Mfr	Conc	Remarks	Ref	C/I
Amiodarone HCl	LZ	4 mg/mL[c]	AHP	8 mg/mL[c]	Physically compatible for 24 hr at 21°C	1032	C
Argatroban	SZ	1 mg/mL	HOS	4 mg/mL[a]	Physically compatible for up to 5 hr at 19 to 24°C in ambient light and 28 to 40% relative humidity	3192	C
Bivalirudin	TMC	5 mg/mL[a]	ES	10 mg/mL[a]	Physically compatible for 4 hr at 23°C	2373	C
Cangrelor tetrasodium	TMC	1 mg/mL[b]		10 mg/mL[b]	Physically compatible for 4 hr	3243	C
Cisatracurium besylate	GW	0.1, 2, 5 mg/mL[a]	ES	10 mg/mL[a]	Physically compatible for 4 hr at 23°C	2074	C
Dexmedetomidine HCl	AB	4 mcg/mL[b]	ES	10 mg/mL[b]	Physically compatible for 4 hr at 23°C	2383	C
Diltiazem HCl	MMD	5 mg/mL	ES	500 mg/mL	Cloudiness forms but clears within 2 min	1807	?
Diltiazem HCl	MMD	1 mg/mL[b]	ES	50 mg/mL[a]	Visually compatible	1807	C
Diltiazem HCl	MMD	5 mg/mL	ES	2 mg/mL[a]	Visually compatible	1807	C
Famotidine	MSD	0.2 mg/mL[a]	ASC	5 mg/mL[a]	Physically compatible for 4 hr at 25°C	1188	C
Fenoldopam mesylate	AB	80 mcg/mL[b]	ES	10 mg/mL[b]	Physically compatible for 4 hr at 23°C	2467	C
Heparin sodium	UP	1000 units/L[e]	SQ	100 mg/mL	Physically compatible for 4 hr at room temperature	534	C
Hetastarch in lactated electrolyte	AB	6%	ES	10 mg/mL[a]	Physically compatible for 4 hr at 23°C	2339	C
Hydrocortisone sodium succinate	UP	10 mg/L[e]	SQ	100 mg/mL	Physically compatible for 4 hr at room temperature	534	C
Meropenem		50 mg/mL	SZ	100 mg/mL	Physically compatible for 4 hr at room temperature	3538	C
Metoprolol tartrate	BED	1 mg/mL	HOS	8 mg/mL[b]	Visually compatible for 24 hr at 19°C	2795	C
Milrinone lactate	WI	350 mcg/mL[a]	SQ	2 and 4 mg/mL[a]	3 to 6% procainamide loss in 1 hr and 10 to 13% in 4 hr at 23°C. No milrinone loss	1191	I

Y-Site Injection Compatibility (1:1 Mixture) (Cont.)

Test Drug	Mfr	Conc	Mfr	Conc	Remarks	Ref	C/I
Nesiritide	SCI	50 mcg/mL[a][b]		500 mg/mL	Physically compatible for 4 hr. May be chemically incompatible with nesiritide[d]	2625	?
Potassium chloride	AB	40 mEq/L[e]	SQ	100 mg/mL	Physically compatible for 4 hr at room temperature	534	C
Ranitidine HCl	GL	0.5 mg/mL	BA	4 mg/mL[a]	Physically compatible for 24 hr	1323	C
Remifentanil HCl	GW	0.025 and 0.25 mg/mL[b]	ES	10 mg/mL[a]	Physically compatible for 4 hr at 23°C	2075	C
Sodium nitroprusside	RC	0.3, 1.2, 3 mg/mL[a]	SX	6, 20, 40 mg/mL[b]	Visually compatible for 48 hr at 24°C protected from light	2357	C
Vasopressin	AMR	2 and 4 units/mL[b]	AB	4 mg/mL[b]	Physically compatible with vasopressin pushed through a Y-site over 5 sec	2478	C

[a] Tested in dextrose 5%.

[b] Tested in sodium chloride 0.9%.

[c] Tested in both dextrose 5% and sodium chloride 0.9%.

[d] Nesiritide is incompatible with bisulfite antioxidants used in some drug formulations. The specific formulation of the product to be used should be checked to ensure that no sulfite antioxidants are present.

[e] Tested in dextrose 5% in Ringer's injection, dextrose 5% in Ringer's injection, lactated, dextrose 5%, Ringer's injection, lactated, and sodium chloride 0.9%.

Selected Revisions May 1, 2020. © Copyright, October 1982.
American Society of Health-System Pharmacists, Inc.

Prochlorperazine Edisylate
AHFS 28:16.08.24

Products

Prochlorperazine 5 mg/mL (as edisylate) is available in 2-mL vials and 10-mL multiple-dose vials. Each mL of solution also contains sodium biphosphate 5 mg, sodium tartrate 12 mg, sodium saccharin 0.9 mg, and benzyl alcohol 0.75% in water for injection.[1(2/08)]

pH

From 4.2 to 6.2.[1(2/08)]

Administration

Prochlorperazine edisylate may be given intramuscularly deep into the upper outer quadrant of the buttock. It also may be given by direct intravenous injection at a rate not exceeding 5 mg/min. It can be given undiluted or diluted in a compatible diluent. It should not be given as a bolus intravenous injection.[1(2/08)] [4] For intravenous infusion, dilution of 20 mg in a liter of compatible infusion solution is recommended.[4] Because the drug causes local irritation, subcutaneous injection is not recommended.[1(2/08)] [4]

Stability

Intact containers should be stored at controlled room temperature and protected from temperatures of 40°C or more and from freezing. Solutions of prochlorperazine edisylate are light sensitive and, therefore, should be protected from light. A slightly yellow solution has not had its concentration altered. However, a markedly discolored solution should be discarded.[1(2/08)] [4]

Dilution of prochlorperazine edisylate to a 1-mg/mL concentration with bacteriostatic sodium chloride 0.9% containing methyl- and propylparabens resulted in a distinctly cloudy solution. This cloudiness did not occur when sodium chloride 0.9% preserved with benzyl alcohol was used for the dilution.[752]

Light Effects

Prochlorperazine edisylate (Wyeth) 20 mg/L in dextrose 5% exhibited about 20% loss in 2 hours at room temperature when exposed to light. More rapid and extensive decomposition occurred when sodium chloride 0.9% was used as the diluent.[2412]

Filtration

Prochlorperazine edisylate (SKF) 5 mg/L in dextrose 5% and sodium chloride 0.9% did not display significant sorption to a 0.45-μm cellulose membrane filter.[567]

Central Venous Catheter

Prochlorperazine edisylate (SoloPak) 0.5 mg/mL in dextrose 5% was found to be compatible with the ARROWg+ard Blue Plus (Arrow International) chlorhexidine-bearing triple-lumen central catheter. Essentially complete delivery of the drug was found with little or no drug loss occurring. Furthermore, chlorhexidine delivered from the catheter remained at trace amounts with no substantial increase due to the delivery of the drug through the catheter.[2335]

Compatibility Information

Solution Compatibility

Prochlorperazine edisylate

Test Soln Name	Mfr	Mfr	Conc/L or %	Remarks	Ref	C/I
Dextrose 2.5% in half-strength Ringer's injection	AB	SKF	10 mg	Physically compatible	3	C
Dextrose 5% in Ringer's injection	AB	SKF	10 mg	Physically compatible	3	C
Dextrose 2.5% in Ringer's injection, lactated	AB	SKF	10 mg	Physically compatible	3	C
Dextrose 5% in half-strength Ringer's injection, lactated	AB	SKF	10 mg	Physically compatible	3	C
Dextrose 5% in Ringer's injection, lactated	AB	SKF	10 mg	Physically compatible	3	C
Dextrose 10% in Ringer's injection, lactated	AB	SKF	10 mg	Physically compatible	3	C
Dextrose 2.5% in sodium chloride 0.45%	AB	SKF	10 mg	Physically compatible	3	C
Dextrose 2.5% in sodium chloride 0.9%	AB	SKF	10 mg	Physically compatible	3	C
Dextrose 5% in sodium chloride 0.225%	AB	SKF	10 mg	Physically compatible	3	C
Dextrose 5% in sodium chloride 0.45%	AB	SKF	10 mg	Physically compatible	3	C

DOI: 10.37573/9781585286850.326

Solution Compatibility (Cont.)

Test Soln Name	Mfr	Mfr	Conc/L or %	Remarks	Ref	C/I
Dextrose 5% in sodium chloride 0.9%	AB	SKF	10 mg	Physically compatible	3	C
Dextrose 10% in sodium chloride 0.9%	AB	SKF	10 mg	Physically compatible	3	C
Dextrose 2.5%	AB	SKF	10 mg	Physically compatible	3	C
Dextrose 5%	AB	SKF	10 mg	Physically compatible	3	C
Dextrose 10%	AB	SKF	10 mg	Physically compatible	3	C
Ionosol B in dextrose 5%	AB	SKF	10 mg	Physically compatible	3	C
Ionosol MB in dextrose 5%	AB	SKF	10 mg	Physically compatible	3	C
Ringer's injection	AB	SKF	10 mg	Physically compatible	3	C
Ringer's injection, lactated	AB	SKF	10 mg	Physically compatible	3	C
Sodium chloride 0.45%	AB	SKF	10 mg	Physically compatible	3	C
Sodium chloride 0.9%	AB	SKF	10 mg	Physically compatible	3	C
Sodium lactate ⅙ M	AB	SKF	10 mg	Physically compatible	3	C

Additive Compatibility

Prochlorperazine edisylate

Test Drug	Mfr	Conc/L or %	Mfr	Conc/L or %	Test Solution	Remarks	Ref	C/I
Amikacin sulfate	BR	5 g	SKF	20 mg	D5LR, D5R, D5S, D5W, D10W, LR, NS, R, SL	Physically compatible and both stable for 24 hr at 25°C	294	C
Aminophylline	SE	1 g	SKF	100 mg	D5W	Physically incompatible	15	I
Ascorbic acid	UP	500 mg	SKF	100 mg	D5W	Physically compatible	15	C
Calcium gluconate	UP	1 g	SKF	100 mg	D5W	Physically compatible	15	C
Chloramphenicol sodium succinate	PD	10 g	SKF	100 mg	D5W	Physically incompatible	15	I
Dexamethasone sodium phosphate	MSD	20 mg	SKF	100 mg	D5W	Physically compatible	15	C
Dimenhydrinate	SE	500 mg	SKF	100 mg	D5W	Physically compatible	15	C
Erythromycin lactobionate	AB	1 g	SKF	10 mg		Physically compatible. Erythromycin stable for 24 hr at 25°C	20	C
Ethacrynate sodium	MSD	80 mg	SKF	20 mg	NS	Little alteration of UV spectra within 8 hr at room temperature	16	C
Floxacillin sodium	BE	20 g	MB	1.25 g	W	Precipitates immediately	1479	I
Furosemide	HO	1 g	MB	1.25 g	W	Yellow precipitate forms immediately	1479	I
Lidocaine HCl	AST	2 g	SKF	10 mg		Physically compatible	24	C
Nafcillin sodium	WY	500 mg	SKF	10 mg		Physically compatible	27	C
Penicillin G potassium	SQ	5 million units	SKF	10 mg	D5W	Physically compatible. Penicillin stable for 24 hr at 25°C	47	C
Penicillin G potassium	[a]	900,000 units	SKF	10 mg	D5W	Penicillin stable for 24 hr at 25°C	48	C

Additive Compatibility (Cont.)

Test Drug	Mfr	Conc/L or %	Mfr	Conc/L or %	Test Solution	Remarks	Ref	C/I
Sodium bicarbonate	AB	2.4 mEq[b]	SKF	10 mg	D5W	Physically compatible for 24 hr	772	C

[a] A buffered preparation was specified.

[b] One vial of Neut added to a liter of admixture.

Drugs in Syringe Compatibility

Prochlorperazine edisylate

Test Drug	Mfr	Amt	Mfr	Amt	Remarks	Ref	C/I
Atropine sulfate		0.6 mg/1.5 mL	SKF		Physically compatible for at least 15 min	14	C
Atropine sulfate	ST	0.4 mg/1 mL	PO	5 mg/1 mL	Physically compatible for at least 15 min	326	C
Butorphanol tartrate	BR	4 mg/2 mL	MB	5 mg/1 mL	Physically compatible for 30 min at room temperature	566	C
Chlorpromazine HCl	SKF	50 mg/2 mL	SKF		Physically compatible for at least 15 min	14	C
Chlorpromazine HCl	PO	50 mg/2 mL	PO	5 mg/1 mL	Physically compatible for at least 15 min	326	C
Diamorphine HCl	MB	10, 25, 50 mg/1 mL	MB	1.25 mg/1 mL[a]	Physically compatible and diamorphine content retained for 24 hr at room temperature	1454	C
Dimenhydrinate	HR	50 mg/1 mL	PO	5 mg/1 mL	Physically incompatible within 15 min	326	I
Diphenhydramine HCl	PD	50 mg/1 mL	PO	5 mg/1 mL	Physically compatible for at least 15 min	326	C
Droperidol	MN	2.5 mg/1 mL	PO	5 mg/1 mL	Physically compatible for at least 15 min	326	C
Fentanyl citrate	MN	0.05 mg/1 mL	PO	5 mg/1 mL	Physically compatible for at least 15 min	326	C
Glycopyrrolate	RB	0.2 mg/1 mL	SKF	5 mg/1 mL	Physically compatible. pH in glycopyrrolate stability range for 48 hr at 25°C	331	C
Glycopyrrolate	RB	0.2 mg/1 mL	SKF	10 mg/2 mL	Physically compatible. pH in glycopyrrolate stability range for 48 hr at 25°C	331	C
Glycopyrrolate	RB	0.4 mg/2 mL	SKF	5 mg/1 mL	Physically compatible. pH in glycopyrrolate stability range for 48 hr at 25°C	331	C
Hydromorphone HCl	KN	4 mg/2 mL[b]	SKF	5 mg/1 mL	Precipitates immediately	517	I
Hydromorphone HCl	KN	4 mg/2 mL[c]	SKF	5 mg/1 mL	Physically compatible for 30 min	517	C
Hydroxyzine HCl	PF	50 mg/1 mL	PO	5 mg/1 mL	Physically compatible for at least 15 min	326	C
Ketorolac tromethamine	SY	180 mg/6 mL	STS	15 mg/3 mL	Heavy white precipitate forms immediately, separating into two layers over time	1703	I
Meperidine HCl	WY	100 mg/1 mL	SKF		Physically compatible for at least 15 min	14	C
Meperidine HCl	WI	50 mg/1 mL	PO	5 mg/1 mL	Physically compatible for at least 15 min	326	C
Metoclopramide HCl	NO	10 mg/2 mL	MB	10 mg/2 mL	Physically compatible for 15 min at room temperature	565	C
Midazolam HCl	RC	5 mg/1 mL	SKF	10 mg/2 mL	White precipitate forms immediately	1145	I
Morphine sulfate	WY	15 mg/1 mL	SKF		Physically compatible for at least 15 min	14	C
Morphine sulfate	ST	15 mg/1 mL	PO	5 mg/1 mL	Physically compatible for at least 15 min	326	C
Morphine sulfate	WB	10 mg/1 mL	ES, SKF	10 mg/2 mL	Precipitates immediately, probably due to phenol in morphine formulation	1006	I

Drugs in Syringe Compatibility (Cont.)

Test Drug	Mfr	Amt	Mfr	Amt	Remarks	Ref	C/I
Morphine sulfate	WY	8, 10, 15 mg/1 mL	SKF	5 mg/1 mL	Physically compatible for 24 hr at 25°C	1086	C
Nalbuphine HCl	EN	10 mg/1 mL	WY	5 mg/1 mL	Physically compatible for 36 hr at 27°C	762	C
Nalbuphine HCl	EN	5 mg/0.5 mL	WY	5 mg/1 mL	Physically compatible for 36 hr at 27°C	762	C
Nalbuphine HCl	EN	2.5 mg/0.25 mL	WY	5 mg/1 mL	Physically compatible for 36 hr at 27°C	762	C
Nalbuphine HCl	DU	10 mg/1 mL	SKF	10 mg/2 mL	Physically compatible for 48 hr	128	C
Nalbuphine HCl	DU	20 mg/1 mL	SKF	10 mg/2 mL	Physically compatible for 48 hr	128	C
Pantoprazole sodium	d	4 mg/1 mL		5 mg/1 mL	Yellowish precipitate forms	2574	I
Pentazocine lactate	WI	30 mg/1 mL	PO	5 mg/1 mL	Physically compatible for at least 15 min	326	C
Pentobarbital sodium	WY	100 mg/2 mL	SKF		Precipitate forms within 15 min	14	I
Pentobarbital sodium	AB	500 mg/10 mL	SKF	10 mg/2 mL	Physically incompatible	55	I
Pentobarbital sodium	AB	50 mg/1 mL	PO	5 mg/1 mL	Physically incompatible within 15 min	326	I
Promethazine HCl	PO	50 mg/2 mL	PO	5 mg/1 mL	Physically compatible for at least 15 min	326	C
Ranitidine HCl	GL	50 mg/2 mL	RP	10 mg/2 mL	Physically compatible for 1 hr at 25°C	978	C
Scopolamine HBr		0.6 mg/1.5 mL	SKF		Physically compatible for at least 15 min	14	C
Scopolamine HBr	ST	0.4 mg/1 mL	PO	5 mg/1 mL	Physically compatible for at least 15 min	326	C

[a] Diluted with sterile water for injection.

[b] The vial formulation was tested.

[c] The ampul formulation was tested.

[d] Test performed using the formulation WITHOUT edetate disodium.

Y-Site Injection Compatibility (1:1 Mixture)

Prochlorperazine edisylate

Test Drug	Mfr	Conc	Mfr	Conc	Remarks	Ref	C/I
Acetaminophen	CAD	10 mg/mL	BED	5 mg/mL	Physically compatible with less than 10% acetaminophen loss over 4 hr at room temperature	2841, 2844	C
Aldesleukin	CHI	33,800 I.U./mL[a]	SKB	5 mg/mL	Aldesleukin bioactivity inhibited	1857	I
Allopurinol sodium	BW	3 mg/mL[b]	SKB	0.5 mg/mL[b]	Heavy turbidity forms immediately	1686	I
Amifostine	USB	10 mg/mL[a]	SN	0.5 mg/mL[a]	Immediate increase in measured haze	1845	I
Amsacrine	NCI	1 mg/mL[a]	SKF	0.5 mg/mL[a]	Visually compatible for 4 hr at 22°C	1381	C
Aztreonam	SQ	40 mg/mL[a]	ES	0.5 mg/mL[a]	Haze and tiny particles form within 4 hr	1758	I
Bivalirudin	TMC	5 mg/mL[a]	SKB	0.5 mg/mL[a]	Gross white precipitate forms immediately	2373	I
Calcium gluconate	AMR	10 mg/mL[b]	SCN	5 mg/mL	Visually compatible for 24 hr at room temperature	2063	C
Cangrelor tetrasodium	TMC	1 mg/mL[b]		0.5 mg/mL[b]	Gross white turbid precipitate forms immediately	3243	I
Cisatracurium besylate	GW	0.1, 2, 5 mg/mL[a]	SO	0.5 mg/mL[a]	Physically compatible for 4 hr at 23°C	2074	C
Cladribine	ORT	0.015[b] and 0.5[d] mg/mL	SCN	0.5 mg/mL[b]	Physically compatible for 4 hr at 23°C	1969	C

Y-Site Injection Compatibility (1:1 Mixture) (Cont.)

Test Drug	Mfr	Conc	Mfr	Conc	Remarks	Ref	C/I
Dexmedetomidine HCl	AB	4 mcg/mL[b]	SKB	0.5 mg/mL[b]	Physically compatible for 4 hr at 23°C	2383	C
Docetaxel	RPR	0.9 mg/mL[a]	SO	0.5 mg/mL[a]	Physically compatible for 4 hr at 23°C	2224	C
Doxorubicin HCl liposomal	SEQ	0.4 mg/mL[a]	SO	0.5 mg/mL[a]	Physically compatible for 4 hr at 23°C	2087	C
Etoposide phosphate	BR	5 mg/mL[a]	ES	0.5 mg/mL[a]	White cloudy solution forms immediately with precipitate in 4 hr	2218	I
Fenoldopam mesylate	AB	80 mcg/mL[b]	SKB	0.5 mg/mL[b]	Trace haze forms in 4 hr	2467	I
Filgrastim	AMG	30 mcg/mL[a]	SCN	0.5 mg/mL[a]	Particles form immediately. Filaments form in 1 hr	1687	I
Fluconazole	RR	2 mg/mL	SKF	5 mg/mL	Physically compatible for 24 hr at 25°C	1407	C
Fludarabine phosphate	BX	1 mg/mL[a]	WY	0.5 mg/mL[a]	Slight haze forms within 30 min	1439	I
Foscarnet sodium	AST	24 mg/mL	SKF	5 mg/mL	Cloudy brown solution	1335	I
Gallium nitrate	FUJ	1 mg/mL[b]	SCN	5 mg/mL	Precipitates immediately	1673	I
Gemcitabine HCl	LI	10 mg/mL[b]	SCN	0.5 mg/mL[b]	Subvisible haze forms immediately	2226	I
Granisetron HCl	SKB	0.05 mg/mL[a]	SCN	0.5 mg/mL[a]	Physically compatible for 4 hr at 23°C	2000	C
Heparin sodium	UP	1000 units/L[e]	SKF	5 mg/mL	Physically compatible for 4 hr at room temperature	534	C
Hetastarch in lactated electrolyte	AB	6%	SO	0.5 mg/mL[a]	Physically compatible for 4 hr at 23°C	2339	C
Hydrocortisone sodium succinate	UP	10 mg/L[e]	SKF	5 mg/mL	Physically compatible for 4 hr at room temperature	534	C
Linezolid	PHU	2 mg/mL	SO	0.5 mg/mL[a]	Physically compatible for 4 hr at 23°C	2264	C
Melphalan HCl	BW	0.1 mg/mL[b]	SKB	0.5 mg/mL[b]	Physically compatible for 3 hr at 22°C	1557	C
Ondansetron HCl	GL	1 mg/mL[b]	SKF	0.5 mg/mL[a]	Visually compatible for 4 hr at 22°C	1365	C
Oxaliplatin	SS	0.5 mg/mL[a]	SKB	0.5 mg/mL[a]	Physically compatible for 4 hr at 23°C	2566	C
Paclitaxel	NCI	1.2 mg/mL[a]		0.5 mg/mL[a]	Physically compatible for 4 hr at 22°C	1528	C
Pemetrexed disodium	LI	20 mg/mL[b]	SKB	0.5 mg/mL[a]	Cloudy precipitate forms immediately	2564	I
Piperacillin sodium–tazobactam sodium	LE[f]	40 mg/mL[a h]	SCN	0.5 mg/mL[a]	White turbidity forms immediately	1688	I
Potassium chloride	AB	40 mEq/L[e]	SKF	5 mg/mL	Physically compatible for 4 hr at room temperature	534	C
Propofol	ZEN[i]	10 mg/mL	SCN	0.5 mg/mL[a]	Physically compatible for 1 hr at 23°C	2066	C
Remifentanil HCl	GW	0.025 and 0.25 mg/mL[b]	SO	0.5 mg/mL[a]	Physically compatible for 4 hr at 23°C	2075	C
Sargramostim	IMM	10 mcg/mL[b]	ES	0.5 mg/mL[b]	Visually compatible for 4 hr at 22°C	1436	C
Teniposide	BR	0.1 mg/mL[a]	SCN	0.5 mg/mL[a]	Physically compatible for 4 hr at 23°C	1725	C
Thiotepa	IMM[g]	1 mg/mL[a]	SCN	0.5 mg/mL[a]	Physically compatible for 4 hr at 23°C	1861	C
TNA #218 to #226[c]			SCN, SO	0.5 mg/mL[a]	Visually compatible for 4 hr at 23°C	2215	C

Y-Site Injection Compatibility (1:1 Mixture) (Cont.)

Test Drug	Mfr	Conc	Mfr	Conc	Remarks	Ref	C/I
Topotecan HCl	SKB	56 mcg/mL[a][b]	SKB	0.192 mg/mL[a][b]	Visually compatible. Little loss of either drug in 4 hr at 22°C	2245	C
TPN #212 to #215[c]			SCN	0.5 mg/mL[a]	Physically compatible for 4 hr at 23°C	2109	C
Vinorelbine tartrate	BW	1 mg/mL[b]	SKB	0.5 mg/mL[b]	Physically compatible for 4 hr at 22°C	1558	C

[a] Tested in dextrose 5%.

[b] Tested in sodium chloride 0.9%.

[c] Refer to Appendix for the composition of parenteral nutrition solutions. TNA indicates a 3-in-1 admixture, and TPN indicates a 2-in-1 admixture.

[d] Tested in bacteriostatic sodium chloride 0.9% preserved with benzyl alcohol 0.9%.

[e] Tested in dextrose 5% in Ringer's injection, dextrose 5% in Ringer's injection, lactated, dextrose 5%, Ringer's injection, lactated, and sodium chloride 0.9%.

[f] Test performed using the formulation WITHOUT edetate disodium.

[g] Lyophilized formulation tested.

[h] Piperacillin component. Piperacillin in an 8:1 fixed-ratio concentration with tazobactam.

[i] Test performed using the formulation WITH edetate disodium.

Selected Revisions January 31, 2020. © Copyright, October 1982. American Society of Health-System Pharmacist, Inc.

Prochlorperazine Mesylate
AHFS 28:16.08.24

Products

Prochlorperazine mesylate injection is available in 1- and 2-mL glass ampuls. Each mL of solution contains prochlorperazine mesylate 12.5 mg with sodium sulfite, sodium metabisulfite, sodium chloride, ethanolamine, and water for injection.[38][115]

Trade Name(s)

Stemetil

Administration

Prochlorperazine mesylate injection is given by deep intramuscular injection.[38][115]

Stability

Intact ampuls should be stored at controlled room temperature and protected from light. Exposure to light results in discoloration. Discolored injection should be discarded.[38][115]

Compatibility Information

Additive Compatibility

Prochlorperazine mesylate

Test Drug	Mfr	Conc/L or %	Mfr	Conc/L or %	Test Solution	Remarks	Ref	C/I
Aminophylline	BP	1 g	BP	100 mg	D5W, NS	Precipitates immediately	26	I
Amphotericin B		200 mg	BP	100 mg	D5W	Haze develops over 3 hr	26	I
Ampicillin sodium	BP	2 g	BP	100 mg	D5W, NS	Precipitates immediately	26	I
Chloramphenicol sodium succinate	BP	4 g	BP	100 mg	NS	Haze develops over 3 hr	26	I
Chlorothiazide sodium	BP	2 g	BP	100 mg	D5W	Precipitates immediately	26	I
Chlorothiazide sodium	BP	2 g	BP	100 mg	NS	Haze develops over 3 hr	26	I
Methohexital sodium	BP	2 g	BP	100 mg	D5W	Haze develops over 3 hr	26	I
Oxycodone HCl	NAP	1 g		600 mg	NS, W	Substantial change in prochlorperazine concentration in 24 hr at 25°C	2600	I
Penicillin G potassium	BP	10 million units	BP	100 mg	NS	Haze develops over 3 hr	26	I
Penicillin G sodium	BP	10 million units	BP	100 mg	NS	Haze develops over 3 hr	26	I
Phenobarbital sodium	BP	800 mg	BP	100 mg	D5W	Haze develops over 3 hr	26	I
Phenobarbital sodium	BP	800 mg	BP	100 mg	NS	Precipitates immediately	26	I

Drugs in Syringe Compatibility

Prochlorperazine mesylate

Test Drug	Mfr	Amt	Mfr	Amt	Remarks	Ref	C/I
Hydromorphone HCl	KN	2, 10, 40 mg/1 mL	RP	5 mg/1 mL	Visually compatible. Little or no loss of either drug in 7 days at 4, 23, and 37°C	1776	C
Hydromorphone HCl	SX	0.5 mg/mL[a]	RP	1.5 mg/mL[a]	Physically compatible for 96 hr at room temperature exposed to light	2171	C
Ketoprofen		50 mg/mL		12.5 mg/mL	White precipitate forms but then disappears	2495	?
Oxycodone HCl	NAP	200 mg/20 mL		12.5 mg/1 mL	Substantial change in prochlorperazine concentration in 24 hr at 25°C	2600	I

[a] Diluted in sodium chloride 0.9%.

DOI: 10.37573/9781585286850.327

Y-Site Injection Compatibility (1:1 Mixture)

Prochlorperazine mesylate

Test Drug	Mfr	Conc	Mfr	Conc	Remarks	Ref	C/I
Clarithromycin	AB	4 mg/mL[a]	ANT	12.5 mg/mL	Visually compatible for 72 hr at both 30 and 17°C	2174	C

[a] Tested in dextrose 5%.

Promethazine Hydrochloride
AHFS 28:24.92

Products

Promethazine hydrochloride is available in vials, ampuls, and syringe cartridges in concentrations of 25 and 50 mg/mL. Each mL also contains disodium edetate 0.1 mg, calcium chloride 0.04 mg, sodium metabisulfite 0.25 mg, phenol 5 mg, and acetic acid-sodium acetate buffer in water for injection.[1(12/06)]

pH

From 4 to 5.5.[1(12/06)]

Osmolality

The osmolality of promethazine hydrochloride 25 mg/mL was determined to be 291 mOsm/kg.[1233]

Administration

Promethazine hydrochloride is administered preferably by deep intramuscular injection. It should not be given subcutaneously or intra-arterially. If given by intravenous injection, a concentration not exceeding 25 mg/mL should be given into the tubing of a running infusion solution at a rate not exceeding 25 mg/min.[1(12/06)] [4] Extravasation should be avoided.[4] [2312]

Stability

Store at controlled room temperature and protect from freezing and light. Inspect prior to administration for particulate matter formation and discoloration; discard if particulate matter or discoloration is observed.[1(12/06)] [4] Promethazine hydrochloride exhibits increasing stability with decreasing pH.[1072]

Syringes

Promethazine hydrochloride 25 mg/mL repackaged in 3-mL amber glass syringes (Hy-Pod) and stored at 25°C exhibited no changes in pH or appearance over 360 days. A possible reduction in concentration to 95% of initial was noted.[535]

Sorption

Promethazine hydrochloride (May & Baker) 8 mg/L in sodium chloride 0.9% (Travenol) in polyvinyl chloride (PVC) bags exhibited only about 5% sorption to the plastic during 1 week of storage at room temperature (15 to 20°C). However, when the solution was buffered from its initial pH of 5 to 7.4, approximately 59% of the drug was lost in 1 week due to sorption.[536]

In another study, promethazine hydrochloride (May & Baker) 8 mg/L in sodium chloride 0.9% exhibited a cumulative 22% loss due to sorption during a 7-hour simulated infusion through an infusion set (Travenol) consisting of a cellulose propionate burette chamber and 170 cm of PVC tubing. Both the burette and the tubing contributed to the loss. The extent of sorption was found to be independent of concentration.[606]

The drug was also tested as a simulated infusion over at least 1 hour by a syringe pump system. A glass syringe on a syringe pump was fitted with 20 cm of polyethylene tubing or 50 cm of Silastic tubing. Only 5% of the drug was lost with the polyethylene tubing, but a cumulative loss of 72% occurred during the 1-hour infusion through the Silastic tubing.[606]

A 25-mL aliquot of promethazine hydrochloride (May & Baker) 8 mg/L in sodium chloride 0.9% was stored in all-plastic syringes composed of polypropylene barrels and polyethylene plungers for 24 hours at room temperature in the dark. No loss due to sorption occurred.[606]

Central Venous Catheter

Promethazine hydrochloride (Schein) 2 mg/mL in dextrose 5% was found to be compatible with the ARROWg+ard Blue Plus (Arrow International) chlorhexidine-bearing triple-lumen central catheter. Essentially complete delivery of the drug was found with little or no drug loss occurring. Furthermore, chlorhexidine delivered from the catheter remained at trace amounts with no substantial increase due to the delivery of the drug through the catheter.[2335]

Compatibility Information

Solution Compatibility

Promethazine HCl

Test Soln Name	Mfr	Mfr	Conc/L or %	Remarks	Ref	C/I
Dextrose 2.5% in half-strength Ringer's injection	AB	WY	100 mg	Physically compatible	3	C
Dextrose 5% in Ringer's injection	AB	WY	100 mg	Physically compatible	3	C
Dextrose 2.5% in Ringer's injection, lactated	AB	WY	100 mg	Physically compatible	3	C
Dextrose 5% in half-strength Ringer's injection, lactated	AB	WY	100 mg	Physically compatible	3	C
Dextrose 5% in Ringer's injection, lactated	AB	WY	100 mg	Physically compatible	3	C
Dextrose 10% in Ringer's injection, lactated	AB	WY	100 mg	Physically compatible	3	C

DOI: 10.37573/9781585286850.328

Solution Compatibility (Cont.)

Test Soln Name	Mfr	Mfr	Conc/L or %	Remarks	Ref	C/I
Dextrose 2.5% in sodium chloride 0.45%	AB	WY	100 mg	Physically compatible	3	C
Dextrose 2.5% in sodium chloride 0.9%	AB	WY	100 mg	Physically compatible	3	C
Dextrose 5% in sodium chloride 0.225%	AB	WY	100 mg	Physically compatible	3	C
Dextrose 5% in sodium chloride 0.45%	AB	WY	100 mg	Physically compatible	3	C
Dextrose 5% in sodium chloride 0.9%	AB	WY	100 mg	Physically compatible	3	C
Dextrose 10% in sodium chloride 0.9%	AB	WY	100 mg	Physically compatible	3	C
Dextrose 2.5%	AB	WY	100 mg	Physically compatible	3	C
Dextrose 5%	AB	WY	100 mg	Physically compatible	3	C
Dextrose 10%	AB	WY	100 mg	Physically compatible	3	C
Ionosol B in dextrose 5%	AB	WY	100 mg	Physically compatible	3	C
Ionosol MB in dextrose 5%	AB	WY	100 mg	Physically compatible	3	C
Ringer's injection	AB	WY	100 mg	Physically compatible	3	C
Ringer's injection, lactated	AB	WY	100 mg	Physically compatible	3	C
Sodium chloride 0.45%	AB	WY	100 mg	Physically compatible	3	C
Sodium chloride 0.9%	AB	WY	100 mg	Physically compatible	3	C
Sodium chloride 0.9%	a		100 mg	Physically compatible with little or no drug loss in 24 hr at 21°C in the dark	1392	C
Sodium lactate ⅙ M	AB	WY	100 mg	Physically compatible	3	C

a Tested in PVC, glass, and polyethylene-lined laminated containers.

Additive Compatibility

Promethazine HCl

Test Drug	Mfr	Conc/L or %	Mfr	Conc/L or %	Test Solution	Remarks	Ref	C/I
Amikacin sulfate	BR	5 g	WY	100 mg	D5LR, D5R, D5S, D5W, D10W, LR, NS, R, SL	Physically compatible and both stable for 24 hr at 25°C	294	C
Aminophylline	SE	1 g	WY	250 mg	D5W	Physically incompatible	15	I
Aminophylline	BP	1 g	BP	100 mg	D5W, NS	Precipitates immediately	26	I
Ascorbic acid	UP	500 mg	WY	250 mg	D5W	Physically compatible	15	C
Cefazolin sodium	LI	10 g	ES	250 mg	D5W	Cloudiness forms then dissipates	1753	?
Cefotetan disodium	ZEN	10 g	ES	250 mg	D5W	Precipitates immediately	1753	I
Chloramphenicol sodium succinate	PD	10 g	WY	250 mg	D5W	Physically incompatible	15	I
Chlorothiazide sodium	BP	2 g	BP	100 mg	D5W, NS	Precipitates immediately	26	I
Floxacillin sodium	BE	20 g	MB	5 g	W	White precipitate forms immediately	1479	I
Furosemide	HO	1 g	MB	5 g	W	White precipitate forms immediately	1479	I
Heparin sodium	UP	4000 units	WY	250 mg	D5W	Physically incompatible	15	I
Hydrocortisone sodium succinate	UP	500 mg	WY	250 mg	D5W	Physically incompatible	15	I

Additive Compatibility (Cont.)

Test Drug	Mfr	Conc/L or %	Mfr	Conc/L or %	Test Solution	Remarks	Ref	C/I
Hydromorphone HCl	KN	1 g	ES	300 mg	NS[a]	Visually compatible for 21 days at 4 and 25°C	1992	C
Methohexital sodium	BP	2 g	BP	100 mg	D5W, NS	Precipitates immediately	26	I
Penicillin G potassium	SQ	20 million units	WY	250 mg	D5W	Physically incompatible	15	I
Penicillin G potassium		1 million units	WY	100 mg		Physically compatible	3	C
Penicillin G potassium	SQ	5 million units	WY	100 mg		Physically compatible	47	C
Penicillin G sodium	UP	20 million units	WY	250 mg	D5W	Physically incompatible	15	I
Pentobarbital sodium	AB	1 g	WY	250 mg	D5W	Physically incompatible	15	I
Phenobarbital sodium	WI	200 mg	WY	250 mg	D5W	Physically incompatible	15	I
Phenobarbital sodium	BP	800 mg	BP	100 mg	D5W	Haze develops over 3 hr	26	I
Phenobarbital sodium	BP	800 mg	BP	100 mg	NS	Precipitates immediately	26	I

[a] Tested in PVC containers.

Drugs in Syringe Compatibility

Promethazine HCl

Test Drug	Mfr	Amt	Mfr	Amt	Remarks	Ref	C/I
Atropine sulfate		0.6 mg/1.5 mL	WY	50 mg/2 mL	Physically compatible for at least 15 min	14	C
Atropine sulfate	ST	0.4 mg/1 mL	PO	50 mg/2 mL	Physically compatible for at least 15 min	326	C
Buprenorphine HCl					Physically and chemically compatible	4	C
Butorphanol tartrate	BR	4 mg/2 mL	WY	25 mg/1 mL	Physically compatible for 30 min at room temperature	566	C
Cefotetan disodium	ZEN	50 mg/5 mL[a]	ES	25 mg/1 mL	White precipitate, resembling cottage cheese, forms immediately	1753	I
Chlorpromazine HCl	PO	50 mg/2 mL	PO	50 mg/2 mL	Physically compatible for at least 15 min	326	C
Dimenhydrinate	HR	50 mg/1 mL	PO	50 mg/2 mL	Physically incompatible within 15 min	326	I
Dimenhydrinate		10 mg/1 mL		25 mg/1 mL	Solution discolors	2569	I
Diphenhydramine HCl	PD	50 mg/1 mL	WY	50 mg/2 mL	Physically compatible for at least 15 min	14	C
Diphenhydramine HCl	PD	50 mg/1 mL	PO	50 mg/2 mL	Physically compatible for at least 15 min	326	C
Droperidol	MN	2.5 mg/1 mL	PO	50 mg/2 mL	Physically compatible for at least 15 min	326	C
Fentanyl citrate	MN	0.05 mg/1 mL	PO	50 mg/2 mL	Physically compatible for at least 15 min	326	C
Glycopyrrolate	RB	0.2 mg/1 mL	WY	25 mg/1 mL	Physically compatible. pH in glycopyrrolate stability range for 48 hr at 25°C	331	C
Glycopyrrolate	RB	0.2 mg/1 mL	WY	50 mg/2 mL	Physically compatible. pH in glycopyrrolate stability range for 48 hr at 25°C	331	C
Glycopyrrolate	RB	0.4 mg/2 mL	WY	25 mg/1 mL	Physically compatible. pH in glycopyrrolate stability range for 48 hr at 25°C	331	C
Heparin sodium		2500 units/1 mL		50 mg/2 mL	Turbidity or precipitate forms within 5 min	1053	I

Drugs in Syringe Compatibility (Cont.)

Test Drug	Mfr	Amt	Mfr	Amt	Remarks	Ref	C/I
Hydromorphone HCl	KN	4 mg/2 mL	WY	50 mg/1 mL	Physically compatible for 30 min	517	C
Hydromorphone HCl	KN	4 mg/2 mL	WY	25 mg/1 mL	Physically compatible for 30 min	517	C
Hydroxyzine HCl	PF	100 mg/4 mL	WY	50 mg/2 mL	Physically compatible for at least 15 min	14	C
Hydroxyzine HCl	PF	50 mg/1 mL	PO	50 mg/2 mL	Physically compatible for at least 15 min	326	C
Iodipamide meglumine		52%, 20 to 40 mL		1 mL[b]	Forms a precipitate initially but clears within 1 hr and remains clear for 48 hr	530	?
Iodipamide meglumine		52%, 1 to 10 mL		1 mL[b]	Precipitates immediately	530	I
Iothalamate meglumine		60%, 1 to 40 mL		1 mL[b]	Precipitates immediately	530	I
Ketorolac tromethamine	SY	180 mg/6 mL	ES	75 mg/3 mL	Heavy white precipitate forms immediately, separating into two layers over time	1703	I
Meperidine HCl	WY	100 mg/1 mL	WY	50 mg/2 mL	Physically compatible for at least 15 min	14	C
Meperidine HCl	WI	50 mg/1 mL	PO	50 mg/2 mL	Physically compatible for at least 15 min	326	C
Metoclopramide HCl	NO	10 mg/2 mL	WY	25 mg/1 mL	Physically compatible for 15 min at room temperature	565	C
Midazolam HCl	RC	5 mg/1 mL	WY	25 mg/1 mL	Physically compatible for 4 hr at 25°C	1145	C
Morphine sulfate	WY	15 mg/1 mL	WY	50 mg/2 mL	Physically compatible for at least 15 min	14	C
Morphine sulfate	ST	15 mg/1 mL	PO	50 mg/2 mL	Physically compatible for at least 15 min	326	C
Morphine sulfate	WY	8 mg	WY	12.5 mg	Cloudiness develops	98	I
Nalbuphine HCl	EN	10 mg/1 mL	ES	25 mg	Physically compatible for 36 hr at 27°C	762	C
Nalbuphine HCl	EN	5 mg/0.5 mL	ES	25 mg	Physically compatible for 36 hr at 27°C	762	C
Nalbuphine HCl	EN	10 mg/1 mL	ES	12.5 mg	Physically compatible for 36 hr at 27°C	762	C
Nalbuphine HCl	DU	10 mg/1 mL	WY	25 and 50 mg	Physically incompatible	128	I
Nalbuphine HCl	DU	20 mg/1 mL	WY	25 and 50 mg	Physically incompatible	128	I
Nalbuphine HCl	DU	10 mg/1 mL	WY	25 mg/1 mL	White flocculent precipitate forms immediately	1184	I
Nalbuphine HCl	DU	10 mg/1 mL	ES	25 mg/1 mL	Physically compatible for 24 hr at room temperature	1184	C
Pentazocine lactate	WI	30 mg/1 mL	WY	50 mg/2 mL	Physically compatible for at least 15 min	14	C
Pentazocine lactate	WI	30 mg/1 mL	PO	50 mg/2 mL	Physically compatible for at least 15 min	326	C
Pentobarbital sodium	AB	500 mg/10 mL	WY	100 mg/4 mL	Physically incompatible	55	I
Pentobarbital sodium	WY	100 mg/2 mL	WY	50 mg/2 mL	Precipitate forms within 15 min	14	I
Pentobarbital sodium	AB	50 mg/1 mL	PO	50 mg/2 mL	Physically incompatible within 15 min	326	I
Prochlorperazine edisylate	PO	5 mg/1 mL	PO	50 mg/2 mL	Physically compatible for at least 15 min	326	C
Ranitidine HCl	GL	50 mg/2 mL	RP	25 mg/1 mL	Physically compatible for 1 hr at 25°C	978	C
Ranitidine HCl	GL	50 mg/5 mL	RP	25 mg	Physically compatible for 4 hr	1151	C
Scopolamine HBr		0.6 mg/1.5 mL	WY	50 mg/2 mL	Physically compatible for at least 15 min	14	C
Scopolamine HBr	ST	0.4 mg/1 mL	PO	50 mg/2 mL	Physically compatible for at least 15 min	326	C

[a] Tested in dextrose 5%.

[b] Concentration unspecified.

Y-Site Injection Compatibility (1:1 Mixture)

Promethazine HCl

Test Drug	Mfr	Conc	Mfr	Conc	Remarks	Ref	C/I
Aldesleukin	CHI	33,800 I.U./mL[a]	ES	25 mg/mL	Aldesleukin bioactivity inhibited	1857	I
Allopurinol sodium	BW	3 mg/mL[b]	WY	2 mg/mL[b]	Immediate turbidity. Particles in 4 hr	1686	I
Amifostine	USB	10 mg/mL[a]	ES	2 mg/mL[a]	Physically compatible for 4 hr at 23°C	1845	C
Amsacrine	NCI	1 mg/mL[a]	ES	2 mg/mL[a]	Visually compatible for 4 hr at 22°C	1381	C
Aztreonam	SQ	40 mg/mL[a]	SCN	2 mg/mL[a]	Physically compatible for 4 hr at 23°C	1758	C
Bivalirudin	TMC	5 mg/mL[a]	ES	2 mg/mL[a]	Physically compatible for 4 hr at 23°C	2373	C
Cangrelor tetrasodium	TMC	1 mg/mL[b]		2 mg/mL[b]	Gross white turbid precipitate forms immediately	3243	I
Cefazolin sodium	LI	10 mg/mL[a]	ES	25 mg/mL	Cloudiness forms then dissipates	1753	?
Cefotetan disodium	ZEN	10 mg/mL[a]	ES	25 mg/mL	White precipitate forms immediately despite flushing of line with NS	1753	I
Ceftaroline fosamil	FOR	2.22 mg/mL[a b h]	SIC	2 mg/mL[a b h]	Physically compatible for 4 hr at 23°C	2826	C
Ciprofloxacin	MI	2 mg/mL[a b]	ES	25 mg/mL	Visually compatible for 24 hr at 24°C	1655	C
Cisatracurium besylate	GW	0.1, 2, 5 mg/mL[a]	ES	2 mg/mL[a]	Physically compatible for 4 hr at 23°C	2074	C
Cladribine	ORT	0.015[b] and 0.5[d] mg/mL	SCN	2 mg/mL[b]	Physically compatible for 4 hr at 23°C	1969	C
Cloxacillin sodium	SMX	100 mg/mL	SZ	25 mg/mL	Precipitates immediately	3245	I
Dexmedetomidine HCl	AB	4 mcg/mL[b]	ES	2 mg/mL[b]	Physically compatible for 4 hr at 23°C	2383	C
Docetaxel	RPR	0.9 mg/mL[a]	SCN	2 mg/mL[a]	Physically compatible for 4 hr at 23°C	2224	C
Doxorubicin HCl liposomal	SEQ	0.4 mg/mL[a]	ES	2 mg/mL[a]	Increase in measured turbidity	2087	I
Etoposide phosphate	BR	5 mg/mL[a]	SCN	2 mg/mL[a]	Physically compatible for 4 hr at 23°C	2218	C
Fenoldopam mesylate	AB	80 mcg/mL[b]	ES	2 mg/mL[b]	Physically compatible for 4 hr at 23°C	2467	C
Filgrastim	AMG	30 mcg/mL[a]	SCN	2 mg/mL[a]	Physically compatible for 4 hr at 22°C	1687	C
Fluconazole	RR	2 mg/mL	ES	50 mg/mL	Physically compatible for 24 hr at 25°C	1407	C
Fludarabine phosphate	BX	1 mg/mL[a]	WY	2 mg/mL[a]	Visually compatible for 4 hr at 22°C	1439	C
Foscarnet sodium	AST	24 mg/mL	ES	50 mg/mL	Gas production	1335	I
Gemcitabine HCl	LI	10 mg/mL[b]	SCN	2 mg/mL[b]	Physically compatible for 4 hr at 23°C	2226	C
Granisetron HCl	SKB	0.05 mg/mL[a]	WY	2 mg/mL[a]	Physically compatible for 4 hr at 23°C	2000	C
Heparin sodium	UP	1000 units/L[f]	SV	50 mg/mL	Physically compatible for 4 hr at room temperature	534	C
Heparin sodium	UP	1000 units/L[g]	SV	50 mg/mL	Clear initially, but cloudiness develops in 4 hr at room temperature	534	I
Hetastarch in lactated electrolyte	AB	6%	SCN	2 mg/mL[a]	Physically compatible for 4 hr at 23°C	2339	C
Hydrocortisone sodium succinate	UP	10 mg/L[f]	SV	50 mg/mL	Physically compatible for 4 hr at room temperature	534	C
Hydrocortisone sodium succinate	UP	10 mg/L[g]	SV	50 mg/mL	Clear initially, but cloudiness develops in 4 hr at room temperature	534	I
Linezolid	PHU	2 mg/mL	SCN	2 mg/mL[a]	Physically compatible for 4 hr at 23°C	2264	C

Y-Site Injection Compatibility (1:1 Mixture) (Cont.)

Test Drug	Mfr	Conc	Mfr	Conc	Remarks	Ref	C/I
Melphalan HCl	BW	0.1 mg/mL[b]	WY	2 mg/mL[b]	Physically compatible for 3 hr at 22°C	1557	C
Ondansetron HCl	GL	1 mg/mL[b]	ES	2 mg/mL[a]	Visually compatible for 4 hr at 22°C	1365	C
Oxaliplatin	SS	0.5 mg/mL[a]	ES	2 mg/mL[a]	Physically compatible for 4 hr at 23°C	2566	C
Palonosetron HCl	MGI	50 mcg/mL	PAD	2 mg/mL[a]	Physically compatible. No loss of either drug in 4 hr	2716	C
Pemetrexed disodium	LI	20 mg/mL[b]	SIC	0.5 mg/mL[a]	Physically compatible for 4 hr at 23°C	2564	C
Piperacillin sodium-tazobactam sodium	LE[c]	40 mg/mL[a j]	SCN	2 mg/mL[a]	Heavy white turbidity forms immediately. Particles form in 4 hr	1688	I
Potassium chloride	AB	40 mEq/L[f]	SV	50 mg/mL	Physically compatible for 4 hr at room temperature	534	C
Potassium chloride	AB	40 mEq/L[g]	SV	50 mg/mL	Clear initially, but cloudiness develops in 4 hr at room temperature	534	I
Remifentanil HCl	GW	0.025 and 0.25 mg/mL[b]	SCN	2 mg/mL[a]	Physically compatible for 4 hr at 23°C	2075	C
Sargramostim	IMM	10 mcg/mL[b]	ES	2 mg/mL[b]	Visually compatible for 4 hr at 22°C	1436	C
Teniposide	BR	0.1 mg/mL[a]	WY	2 mg/mL[a]	Physically compatible for 4 hr at 23°C	1725	C
Thiotepa	IMM[i]	1 mg/mL[a]	WY	2 mg/mL[a]	Physically compatible for 4 hr at 23°C	1861	C
TNA #218 to #226[e]			SCN	2 mg/mL[a]	Visually compatible for 4 hr at 23°C	2215	C
TPN #212, #214[e]			SCN	2 mg/mL[a]	Physically compatible for 4 hr at 23°C	2109	C
TPN #213, #215[e]			SCN	2 mg/mL[a]	Amber discoloration forms in 4 hr	2109	I
Vinorelbine tartrate	BW	1 mg/mL[b]	ES	2 mg/mL[b]	Physically compatible for 4 hr at 22°C	1558	C

[a] Tested in dextrose 5%.

[b] Tested in sodium chloride 0.9%.

[c] Test performed using the formulation WITHOUT edetate disodium.

[d] Tested in bacteriostatic sodium chloride 0.9% preserved with benzyl alcohol 0.9%.

[e] Refer to Appendix for the composition of parenteral nutrition solutions. TNA indicates a 3-in-1 admixture, and TPN indicates a 2-in-1 admixture.

[f] Tested in dextrose 5% in Ringer's injection, lactated, dextrose 5%, Ringer's injection, lactated, and sodium chloride 0.9%.

[g] Tested in dextrose 5% in Ringer's injection.

[h] Tested in Ringer's injection, lactated.

[i] Lyophilized formulation tested.

[j] Piperacillin component. Piperacillin in an 8:1 fixed-ratio concentration with tazobactam.

Additional Compatibility Information

Chlorpromazine and Meperidine

Chlorpromazine hydrochloride, meperidine hydrochloride, and promethazine hydrochloride combined as an extemporaneous mixture for preoperative sedation, developed a brownish-yellow color after 2 weeks of storage with protection from light. The discoloration was attributed to the metacresol preservative content of the meperidine hydrochloride product used. Use of meperidine hydrochloride which contains a different preservative resulted in a solution that remained clear and colorless for at least 3 months when protected from light.[1148]

Selected Revisions December 13, 2018. © Copyright, October 1982. American Society of Health-System Pharmacists, Inc.

Propofol
AHFS 28:04.92

Products

Propofol is available as a ready-to-use oil-in-water emulsion in 20-, 50-, and 100-mL vials.[3499 3500 3501 3502 3503] Each mL contains propofol 10 mg along with soybean oil 100 mg, glycerol 22.5 mg, egg lecithin or phospholipids 12 mg, and sodium hydroxide to adjust the pH.[3499 3500 3501 3502 3503] Propofol products are not identical.[3499 3500 3501 3502 3503] Diprivan products contain disodium edetate 0.05 mg/mL (0.005%) as an antimicrobial agent.[3499] Generic propofol formulations may contain benzyl alcohol 1.5 mg/mL,[3500] benzyl alcohol 1.5 mg/mL and sodium benzoate 0.7 mg/mL,[3501] sodium metabisulfite 0.25 mg/mL,[3502] or sodium benzoate 1 mg/mL[3503] as an antimicrobial agent. Additionally, Diprivan and some generic propofol formulations have differing pH values (see Products: pH), which also may contribute to differing compatibility results among the products.[2336]

Compatibility information for propofol with other drugs established using the Diprivan formulation should not be extrapolated to generic propofol products because of formulation differences.[2336]

pH

Diprivan has a pH ranging from 7 to 8.5.[3499]

The metabisulfite-containing formulation of propofol has a pH ranging from 4.5 to 6.6.[3502] The benzyl alcohol-containing formulation has a pH ranging from 5.5 to 7.4.[3500] The benzyl alcohol- and sodium benzoate-containing formulation and the sodium benzoate-containing formulations both have a pH ranging from 6 to 8.5.[3501 3503]

Tonicity

Propofol 10 mg/mL injectable emulsion is isotonic.[3499 3500 3501 3502 3503]

Trade Name(s)

Diprivan

Administration

Before use, propofol should be shaken well.[3499 3500 3501 3502 3503] Propofol is administered by intravenous injection or infusion; if necessary, propofol may be diluted with dextrose 5% to a concentration not less than 2 mg/mL.[3499 3500 3501 3502 3503]

Numerous outbreaks of serious postoperative infections have resulted from inadvertent contamination of propofol.[1930 3499 3500 3501 3502 3503] The contamination resulted from risky preparation practices and lapses in aseptic technique.[1930] The lipid base supports microbiological growth.[1930 3499 3500 3501 3502 3503] The disodium edetate, sodium metabisulfite, or benzyl alcohol and/or sodium benzoate in the formulations can retard the growth of microorganisms for up to 12 hours, but the products can still support growth and are not antimicrobially preserved.[3499 3500 3501 3502 3503] Strict aseptic procedures are required during handling.[3499 3500 3501 3502 3503]

Stability

Propofol injection is a white, oil-in-water emulsion.[3499 3500 3501 3502 3503] Intact containers should be stored at 4 to 25°C[3499 3500 3502 3503] or 20 to 25°C.[3501] Vials should not be frozen.[3499 3500 3501 3502 3503] The emulsion should not be used if there is evidence of excessive creaming or aggregation, if large droplets are visible, or if other forms of phase separation indicating compromised stability are present.[3499 3500 3501 3502 3503]

Because propofol undergoes oxidative degradation when exposed to oxygen, intact containers are packaged under nitrogen to avoid oxygen exposure.[3499 3500 3501 3502 3503] Whether propofol is administered directly from the vial or drawn into a syringe, administration should begin immediately and should be completed within 12 hours after the vial is spiked.[3499 3500 3501 3502 3503] The tubing and any unused propofol should be discarded after 12 hours.[3499 3500 3501 3502 3503]

Propofol formulated with sodium metabisulfite antioxidant is subject to a differing decomposition reaction compared with the edetate-containing Diprivan formulation. Exposure to air results in the formation of a yellow discoloration in about 6 to 7 hours, which does not occur with Diprivan. The yellow discoloration is a result of the formation of oxidized propofol dimer quinone from sulfite radicals that form in the generic product and may be associated with increased adverse effects. This oxidation product does not form in Diprivan containing edetate.[2344 2575 2576] Stability information for propofol established using the Diprivan formulation should not be extrapolated to generic formulations.[2336 2344]

The physical stability of both Diprivan and propofol containing sodium metabisulfite was evaluated. The formulation differences, principally pH, resulted in a much higher zeta potential for Diprivan, making it a more rugged emulsion and less subject to damage from physical agitation and thermal insult. Physical agitation resulted in no increase in fat droplet size in Diprivan after 16 hours, but a substantial increase in fat droplets larger than 5 μm occurred in as little as 4 hours in the sodium metabisulfite-containing formulation.[2445]

One benzyl alcohol-containing formulation of propofol had the same pH as Diprivan (pH 7 to 8.5) and exhibited the same degree of ruggedness and resistance to emulsion disruption as Diprivan.[2659]

In another study, propofol (Diprivan) was again reported to be a more rugged emulsion than the generic formulation containing sodium metabisulfite. Diprivan had a very low quantity of fat globules exceeding 5 μm throughout its shelf life. The sodium metabisulfite-containing formulation formed much greater amounts of globules of 5 μm or larger within a few months after manufacture and well before the expiration date. This 5-μm or larger globule size is an important threshold because globules of this size may occlude capillaries and lead to embolic syndrome. The safety of using this sodium metabisulfite-containing formulation of propofol, especially as the product nears its expiration date, was questioned.[2589]

DOI: 10.37573/9781585286850.329

Propofol emulsion is a single-access product and can support the growth of microorganisms.[1930 3499 3500 3501 3502 3503] In one study, propofol strongly supported the growth of *Escherichia coli* and *Candida albicans*.[2411] Strict adherence to proper aseptic procedures, including disinfecting the vial stopper with isopropyl alcohol 70%, is required.[3499 3500 3501 3502 3503] Use of the drug within 6 hours has been recommended.[2411]

Plastic and Glass Containers

Diluted in dextrose 5%, propofol has been shown to be more stable in glass than in plastic containers; manufacturers indicate that only 95% of the drug remains after only 2 hours of a running infusion in plastic (material unspecified).[3499 3500 3501 3502 3503]

Syringes

Propofol (Diprivan) 10 mg/mL was repackaged into 60-mL polypropylene syringes (Monoject, Sherwood Medical) and stored at 23°C under fluorescent light and at 4°C protected from light. No visually apparent changes occurred to the emulsion under either storage condition. Propofol losses were 7% in 5 days and 12% in 7 days in the room-temperature samples. No propofol losses occurred in 13 days in the refrigerated samples.[1984]

Propofol (Diprivan) 1% was repackaged into 2- and 10-mL Plastipak (Becton Dickinson) and 2-mL Injekt (B. Braun) plastic syringes and was stored at 5°C. Propofol losses were about 7 to 8% in the Plastipak syringes and about 2% in the Injekt syringes after 28 days of refrigerated storage.[2118]

Sorption

Propofol (Diprivan) injection was diluted to 2 mg/mL with dextrose 5% and stored in polyvinyl chloride (PVC) tubing (Kendall-McGaw). A propofol loss exceeding 31% occurred after static storage for 2 hours. In simulated infusions using the same initial concentration, administration through 72-inch PVC administration sets at a rate of 1.75 mL/min resulted in an average propofol loss of 7.7% over the 2-hour period.[2057]

When tested undiluted at 10 mg/mL, propofol (Diprivan) sorption to administration tubing composed principally of PVC did not represent a substantial portion of the total amount of drug delivered. Any losses that did occur were within the error of the method and were not clinically relevant.[2297]

Propofol (Diprivan) was delivered at rates of 1 and 10 mL/hr through PVC tubing. Little loss occurred at the higher rate of delivery. However, at the slower rate, up to 6% propofol loss due to sorption occurred.[2468]

Plasticizer Leaching

As happens with surfactant-containing drug formulations, propofol emulsion also has been shown to leach diethylhexyl phthalate (DEHP) plasticizer from PVC equipment such as administration sets. The use of non-PVC administration sets has been recommended.[2424]

Filtration

When filtration is clinically appropriate, manufacturers recommend that propofol be administered with caution only through a filter with a pore size of 5 μm or greater, unless the filter has demonstrated no effects on flow and/or breakdown of the emulsion.[3499 3500 3501 3502 3503] Continuous monitoring for restricted flow and/or emulsion breakdown is necessary if a filter is used.[3499 3500 3501 3502 3503] Filters with a pore size less than 5 μm should not be used.[3499 3500 3501 3502 3503]

Propofol (Diprivan) 1% 10 mL filtered through a 5-μm filter needle (Burron Medical) underwent no loss.[2057]

Compatibility Information

Solution Compatibility

Propofol

Test Soln Name	Mfr	Mfr	Conc/L or %	Remarks	Ref	C/I
Dextrose 5% in Ringer's injection, lactated		FRK[a]		Compatible via Y-site administration	3499	C
Dextrose 5% in Ringer's injection, lactated		b		Compatible via Y-site administration	3500, 3501, 3502, 3503	C
Dextrose 5% in sodium chloride 0.2%		FRK[a]		Compatible via Y-site administration	3499	C
Dextrose 5% in sodium chloride 0.2%		b		Compatible via Y-site administration	3500, 3501, 3502, 3503	C
Dextrose 5% in sodium chloride 0.45%		FRK[a]		Compatible via Y-site administration	3499	C
Dextrose 5% in sodium chloride 0.45%		b		Compatible via Y-site administration	3500, 3501, 3502, 3503	C
Dextrose 5%		FRK[a]		Compatible	3499	C
Dextrose 5%		b		Compatible	3500, 3501, 3502, 3503	C
Ringer's injection, lactated		FRK[a]		Compatible via Y-site administration	3499	C
Ringer's injection, lactated		b		Compatible via Y-site administration	3500, 3501, 3502, 3503	C

[a] Test performed using the formulation WITH edetate disodium.

[b] Test performed using the formulation WITHOUT edetate disodium.

Additive Compatibility

Propofol

Test Drug	Mfr	Conc/L or %	Mfr	Conc/L or %	Test Solution	Remarks	Ref	C/I
Imipenem–cilastatin sodium–relebactam	ME				D5W	Physically incompatible	3505	I
Imipenem–cilastatin sodium–relebactam	ME				NS	Physically incompatible	3505	I

Drugs in Syringe Compatibility

Propofol

Test Drug	Mfr	Amt	Mfr	Amt	Remarks	Ref	C/I
Ketamine HCl	SZ	50 mg/5 mL	NOP	50 mg/5 mL	Physically compatible. Little loss of either drug in 3 hr at room temperature	2790	C
Ketamine HCl	SZ	30 mg/3 mL	NOP	70 mg/7 mL	Physically compatible. Little loss of either drug in 3 hr at room temperature	2790	C
Lidocaine HCl	ASZ	5 mg/1 mL	ASZ[a]	200 mg/20 mL	Physically compatible for 24 hr	2490	C
Lidocaine HCl	ASZ	10 mg/1 mL	ASZ[a]	200 mg/20 mL	Physically compatible for 24 hr	2490	C
Lidocaine HCl	ASZ	20 mg/1 mL	ASZ[a]	200 mg/20 mL	Physically incompatible. Increased fat droplet size and layering in 3 hr	2490	I
Lidocaine HCl	ASZ	40 mg/2 mL	ASZ[a]	200 mg/20 mL	Physically incompatible. Increased fat droplet size and layering in 3 hr	2490	I
Lidocaine HCl		10 mg	ZEN	1%, 20 mL	Physically compatible for 6 hr	2543	C
Lidocaine HCl		30 to 50 mg	ZEN	1%, 20 mL	Increased fat droplet size	2543	I
Ondansetron HCl	GW	1 mg/mL[b]	STU	1 and 5 mg/mL[b]	Physically compatible. Little loss of either drug in 4 hr at 23°C	2199	C
Pantoprazole sodium	[a]	4 mg/1 mL		10 mg/1 mL	No change seen	2574	?
Remifentanil HCl	GL	1.25 mg/1.25 mL	ASZ	487.5 mg/48.75 mL	Separation and layering of the drugs occurred with syringes stored in an upright vertical position	3504	I
Remifentanil HCl	GL	2.5 mg/2.5 mL	ASZ	475 mg/47.5 mL	Separation and layering of the drugs occurred with syringes stored in an upright vertical position	3504	I
Remifentanil HCl	GL	5 mg/5 mL	ASZ	450 mg/45 mL	Separation and layering of the drugs occurred with syringes stored in an upright vertical position	3504	I

[a] Test performed using the formulation WITHOUT edetate disodium.

[b] Tested in sodium chloride 0.9%.

Y-Site Injection Compatibility (1:1 Mixture)

Propofol

Test Drug	Mfr	Conc	Mfr	Conc	Remarks	Ref	C/I
Acyclovir sodium	BW	7 mg/mL[a]	ZEN[h]	10 mg/mL	Physically compatible for 1 hr at 23°C	2066	C
Alfentanil HCl	JN	0.5 mg/mL	ZEN[h]	10 mg/mL	Physically compatible for 1 hr at 23°C	2066	C
Amikacin sulfate	DU	5 mg/mL[a]	ZEN[h]	10 mg/mL	Immediate precipitate and yellow color	2066	I
Aminophylline	AMR	2.5 mg/mL[a]	ZEN[h]	10 mg/mL	Physically compatible for 1 hr at 23°C	2066	C
Amphotericin B	APC	0.6 mg/mL[a]	ZEN[h]	10 mg/mL	Gel-like precipitate forms immediately	2066	I
Ampicillin sodium	WY	20 mg/mL[b]	ZEN[h]	10 mg/mL	Physically compatible for 1 hr at 23°C	2066	C

Y-Site Injection Compatibility (1:1 Mixture) (Cont.)

Test Drug	Mfr	Conc	Mfr	Conc	Remarks	Ref	C/I
Ascorbic acid	AB	500 mg/mL	STU	2 mg/mL	No visible change in 24 hr at 25°C. Yellow color forms within 7 days	1801	?
Atracurium besylate	BW	10 mg/mL	STU	2 mg/mL	Oil droplets form within 24 hr, followed by phase separation at 25°C	1801	I
Atracurium besylate	BW	10 mg/mL	ZEN[h]	10 mg/mL	Emulsion broke and oiled out	2066	I
Atracurium besylate		10 mg/mL	ASZ[h]	10 mg/mL	Emulsion disruption upon mixing	2336	I
Atracurium besylate		10 mg/mL	BA[i]	10 mg/mL	Emulsion disruption upon mixing	2336	I
Atracurium besylate		5 mg/mL	ASZ[h]	10 mg/mL	Emulsion disruption upon mixing	2336	I
Atracurium besylate		5 mg/mL	BA[i]	10 mg/mL	Emulsion disruption upon mixing	2336	I
Atracurium besylate		0.5 mg/mL[a]	BA[i]	10 mg/mL	Emulsion disruption upon mixing	2336	I
Atracurium besylate		0.5 mg/mL[a]	ASZ[h]	10 mg/mL	Physically compatible	2336	C
Atropine sulfate	GNS	0.4 mg/mL	STU	2 mg/mL	Oil droplets form within 7 days at 25°C. No visible change in 24 hr	1801	?
Atropine sulfate	AST	0.1 mg/mL[a]	ZEN[h]	10 mg/mL	Physically compatible for 1 hr at 23°C	2066	C
Aztreonam	SQ	40 mg/mL[a]	ZEN[h]	10 mg/mL	Physically compatible for 1 hr at 23°C	2066	C
Bumetanide	RC	0.04 mg/mL[a]	ZEN[h]	10 mg/mL	Physically compatible for 1 hr at 23°C	2066	C
Buprenorphine HCl	RKC	0.04 mg/mL[a]	ZEN[h]	10 mg/mL	Physically compatible for 1 hr at 23°C	2066	C
Butorphanol tartrate	APC	0.04 mg/mL[a]	ZEN[h]	10 mg/mL	Physically compatible for 1 hr at 23°C	2066	C
Calcium chloride	AST	40 mg/mL[a]	ZEN[h]	10 mg/mL	White precipitate forms in 1 hr	2066	I
Calcium gluconate	AMR	40 mg/mL[a]	ZEN[h]	10 mg/mL	Physically compatible for 1 hr at 23°C	2066	C
Cangrelor tetrasodium	TMC	1 mg/mL[b]		10 mg/mL[b]	Physically compatible for 4 hr	3243	C
Carboplatin	BR	5 mg/mL[a]	ZEN[h]	10 mg/mL	Physically compatible for 1 hr at 23°C	2066	C
Cefazolin sodium	MAR	20 mg/mL[a]	ZEN[h]	10 mg/mL	Physically compatible for 1 hr at 23°C	2066	C
Cefepime HCl	BMS	120 mg/mL[c]		1 mg/mL	Precipitates	2513	I
Cefotaxime sodium	HO	20 mg/mL[a]	ZEN[h]	10 mg/mL	Physically compatible for 1 hr at 23°C	2066	C
Cefotetan disodium	STU	20 mg/mL[a]	ZEN[h]	10 mg/mL	Physically compatible for 1 hr at 23°C	2066	C
Cefoxitin sodium	ME	20 mg/mL[a]	ZEN[h]	10 mg/mL	Physically compatible for 1 hr at 23°C	2066	C
Ceftaroline fosamil	FOR	2.22 mg/mL[a b c]	HOS[i]	10 mg/mL	Physically compatible for 4 hr at 23°C	2826	C
Ceftazidime	SKB	40 mg/mL[a]	ZEN[h]	10 mg/mL	Physically compatible for 1 hr at 23°C	2066	C
Ceftazidime	SKB	125 mg/mL		1 mg/mL	Physically incompatible	2434	I
Ceftazidime	GSK	120 mg/mL		1 mg/mL	Precipitates	2513	I
Ceftolozane sulfate–tazobactam sodium	CUB	10 mg/mL[g f]	FRK[h]	10 mg/mL	Immediate formation of free oil layer atop fat plug	3262	I
Ceftriaxone sodium	RC	20 mg/mL[a]	ZEN[h]	10 mg/mL	Physically compatible for 1 hr at 23°C	2066	C
Cefuroxime sodium	LI	30 mg/mL[a]	ZEN[h]	10 mg/mL	Physically compatible for 1 hr at 23°C	2066	C
Chlorpromazine HCl	SCN	2 mg/mL[a]	ZEN[h]	10 mg/mL	Physically compatible for 1 hr at 23°C	2066	C
Cisatracurium besylate	GW	5 mg/mL	ASZ[h]	10 mg/mL	Emulsion disruption upon mixing	2336	I
Cisatracurium besylate	GW	5 mg/mL	BA[i]	10 mg/mL	Emulsion disruption upon mixing	2336	I

Y-Site Injection Compatibility (1:1 Mixture) (Cont.)

Test Drug	Mfr	Conc	Mfr	Conc	Remarks	Ref	C/I
Cisatracurium besylate	GW	0.5 mg/mL[a]	BA[i]	10 mg/mL	Emulsion disruption upon mixing	2336	I
Cisatracurium besylate	GW	0.5 mg/mL[a]	ASZ[h]	10 mg/mL	Physically compatible	2336	C
Cisatracurium besylate	ABV		[h]		Manufacturer states incompatible	2868	I
Cisplatin	BR	1 mg/mL	ZEN[h]	10 mg/mL	Physically compatible for 1 hr at 23°C	2066	C
Clevidipine butyrate	CHS	0.5 mg/mL		10 mg/mL	Physically compatible for 24 hr at 23°C	3334	C
Clindamycin phosphate	AST	10 mg/mL[a]	ZEN[h]	10 mg/mL	Physically compatible for 1 hr at 23°C	2066	C
Cyclophosphamide	MJ	10 mg/mL[a]	ZEN[h]	10 mg/mL	Physically compatible for 1 hr at 23°C	2066	C
Cyclosporine	SZ	5 mg/mL[a]	ZEN[h]	10 mg/mL	Physically compatible for 1 hr at 23°C	2066	C
Cytarabine	CHI	50 mg/mL	ZEN[h]	10 mg/mL	Physically compatible for 1 hr at 23°C	2066	C
Dexamethasone sodium phosphate	AMR	1 mg/mL[a]	ZEN[h]	10 mg/mL	Physically compatible for 1 hr at 23°C	2066	C
Dexmedetomidine HCl	AB	4 mcg/mL[b]	ASZ[h]	10 mg/mL	Physically compatible for 4 hr at 23°C	2383	C
Diazepam	ES	5 mg/mL	ZEN[h]	10 mg/mL	Emulsion broke and oiled out	2066	I
Diphenhydramine HCl	SCN	2 mg/mL[a]	ZEN[h]	10 mg/mL	Physically compatible for 1 hr at 23°C	2066	C
Dobutamine HCl	LI	4 mg/mL[a]	ZEN[h]	10 mg/mL	Physically compatible for 1 hr at 23°C	2066	C
Dopamine HCl	AST	3.2 mg/mL[a]	ZEN[h]	10 mg/mL	Physically compatible for 1 hr at 23°C	2066	C
Doripenem	JJ	5 mg/mL[a b]	BED	10 mg/mL	Precipitation forms immediately	2743	I
Doxycycline hyclate	LY	1 mg/mL[a]	ZEN[h]	10 mg/mL	Physically compatible for 1 hr at 23°C	2066	C
Droperidol	JN	0.4 mg/mL[a]	ZEN[h]	10 mg/mL	Physically compatible for 1 hr at 23°C	2066	C
Enalaprilat	MSD	0.1 mg/mL[a]	ZEN[h]	10 mg/mL	Physically compatible for 1 hr at 23°C	2066	C
Ephedrine sulfate	AB	5 mg/mL[a]	ZEN[h]	10 mg/mL	Physically compatible for 1 hr at 23°C	2066	C
Epinephrine HCl	AMR	0.1 mg/mL	ZEN[h]	10 mg/mL	Physically compatible for 1 hr at 23°C	2066	C
Eravacycline dihydro-chloride	TET	0.3 and 0.6 mg/mL[b]	FRK[h]	10 mg/mL	Physically incompatible; pH decreased by >1 unit within 60 min	3532	I
Esmolol HCl	OHM	10 mg/mL	ZEN[h]	10 mg/mL	Physically compatible for 1 hr at 23°C	2066	C
Famotidine	ME	2 mg/mL[a]	ZEN[h]	10 mg/mL	Physically compatible for 1 hr at 23°C	2066	C
Fenoldopam mesylate	AB	80 mcg/mL[b]	ASZ[h]	10 mg/mL	Physically compatible for 4 hr at 23°C	2467	C
Fentanyl citrate	AB	0.05 mg/mL	ZEN[h]	10 mg/mL	Physically compatible for 1 hr at 23°C	2066	C
Fluconazole	PF	2 mg/mL[a]	ZEN[h]	10 mg/mL	Physically compatible for 1 hr at 23°C	2066	C
Fluorouracil	AD	16 mg/mL[a]	ZEN[h]	10 mg/mL	Physically compatible for 1 hr at 23°C	2066	C
Furosemide	AB	3 mg/mL[a]	ZEN[h]	10 mg/mL	Physically compatible for 1 hr at 23°C	2066	C
Ganciclovir sodium	SY	20 mg/mL[a]	ZEN[h]	10 mg/mL	Physically compatible for 1 hr at 23°C	2066	C
Gentamicin sulfate	ES	5 mg/mL[a]	ZEN[h]	10 mg/mL	White precipitate forms immediately	2066	I
Glycopyrrolate	RB	0.2 mg/mL	ZEN[h]	10 mg/mL	Physically compatible for 1 hr at 23°C	2066	C
Granisetron HCl	SKB	0.05 mg/mL[a]	ZEN[h]	10 mg/mL	Physically compatible for 1 hr at 23°C	2066	C
Haloperidol lactate	MN	0.2 mg/mL[a]	ZEN[h]	10 mg/mL	Physically compatible for 1 hr at 23°C	2066	C
Heparin sodium	ES	100 units/mL[a]	ZEN[h]	10 mg/mL	Physically compatible for 1 hr at 23°C	2066	C

Y-Site Injection Compatibility (1:1 Mixture) (Cont.)

Test Drug	Mfr	Conc	Mfr	Conc	Remarks	Ref	C/I
Hydrocortisone sodium succinate	UP	1 mg/mL[a]	ZEN[h]	10 mg/mL	Physically compatible for 1 hr at 23°C	2066	C
Hydromorphone HCl	AST	0.5 mg/mL[a]	ZEN[h]	10 mg/mL	Physically compatible for 1 hr at 23°C	2066	C
Hydroxyethyl starch 130/0.4 in sodium chloride 0.9%	FRK	6%	NOP	2.5[a], 5[a], 10 mg/mL	Visually compatible for 24 hr at room temperature	2770	C
Hydroxyzine HCl	ES	2 mg/mL[a]	ZEN[h]	10 mg/mL	Physically compatible for 1 hr at 23°C	2066	C
Ifosfamide	MJ	25 mg/mL[a]	ZEN[h]	10 mg/mL	Physically compatible for 1 hr at 23°C	2066	C
Imipenem–cilastatin sodium	ME	10 mg/mL[b e]	ZEN[h]	10 mg/mL	Physically compatible for 1 hr at 23°C	2066	C
Insulin	NOV	1 unit/mL[a]	ZEN[h]	10 mg/mL	Physically compatible for 1 hr at 23°C	2066	C
Isavuconazonium sulfate	ASP	1.5 mg/mL[a]	PPR	10 mg/mL	Immediate formation of free oil layer atop fat plug	3263	I
Isoproterenol HCl	AB	0.004 mg/mL[a]	ZEN[h]	10 mg/mL	Physically compatible for 1 hr at 23°C	2066	C
Ketamine HCl	PD	10 mg/mL	ZEN[h]	10 mg/mL	Physically compatible for 1 hr at 23°C	2066	C
Labetalol HCl	AH	5 mg/mL	ZEN[h]	10 mg/mL	Physically compatible for 1 hr at 23°C	2066	C
Lidocaine HCl	AST	10 mg/mL	ZEN[h]	10 mg/mL	Physically compatible for 1 hr at 23°C	2066	C
Lorazepam	WY	0.1 mg/mL[a]	ZEN[h]	10 mg/mL	Physically compatible for 1 hr at 23°C	2066	C
Magnesium sulfate	AST	100 mg/mL[a]	ZEN[h]	10 mg/mL	Physically compatible for 1 hr at 23°C	2066	C
Mannitol	BA	15%	ZEN[h]	10 mg/mL	Physically compatible for 1 hr at 23°C	2066	C
Meperidine HCl	WY	4 mg/mL[a]	ZEN[h]	10 mg/mL	Physically compatible for 1 hr at 23°C	2066	C
Methotrexate sodium	LE	15 mg/mL[a]	ZEN[h]	10 mg/mL	White precipitate forms in 1 hr	2066	I
Methylprednisolone sodium succinate	AB	5 mg/mL[a]	ZEN[h]	10 mg/mL	White precipitate forms immediately	2066	I
Midazolam HCl	RC	5 mg/mL	STU	2 mg/mL	Oil droplets form within 7 days at 25°C. No visible change in 24 hr	1801	?
Midazolam HCl	RC	2 mg/mL[a]	ZEN[h]	10 mg/mL	Physically compatible for 1 hr at 23°C	2066	C
Milrinone lactate	SW	0.4 mg/mL[a]	ZEN	10 mg/mL	Little loss of either drug in 4 hr at 23°C	2214	C
Mitoxantrone HCl	IMM	0.5 mg/mL[a]	ZEN[h]	10 mg/mL	Particles form immediately	2066	I
Morphine sulfate	AST	1 mg/mL[a]	ZEN[h]	10 mg/mL	Physically compatible for 1 hr at 23°C	2066	C
Nafcillin sodium	MAR	20 mg/mL[a]	ZEN[h]	10 mg/mL	Physically compatible for 1 hr at 23°C	2066	C
Nalbuphine HCl	AB	10 mg/mL	ZEN[h]	10 mg/mL	Physically compatible for 1 hr at 23°C	2066	C
Naloxone HCl	AST	0.4 mg/mL	ZEN[h]	10 mg/mL	Physically compatible for 1 hr at 23°C	2066	C
Nitroglycerin	DU	0.4 mg/mL[a]	ZEN[h]	10 mg/mL	Physically compatible for 1 hr at 23°C	2066	C
Norepinephrine bitartrate	AB	0.016 mg/mL[a]	ZEN[h]	10 mg/mL	Physically compatible for 1 hr at 23°C	2066	C
Paclitaxel	MJ	1.2 mg/mL[a]	ZEN[h]	10 mg/mL	Physically compatible for 1 hr at 23°C	2066	C
Pancuronium bromide	GNS	2 mg/mL	STU	2 mg/mL	Oil droplets form within 7 days at 25°C. No visible change in 24 hr	1801	?
Pancuronium bromide	AST	1 mg/mL	ZEN[h]	10 mg/mL	Physically compatible for 1 hr at 23°C	2066	C

Y-Site Injection Compatibility (1:1 Mixture) (Cont.)

Test Drug	Mfr	Conc	Mfr	Conc	Remarks	Ref	C/I
Pentobarbital sodium	WY	5 mg/mL[a]	ZEN[h]	10 mg/mL	Physically compatible for 1 hr at 23°C	2066	C
Phenobarbital sodium	WY	5 mg/mL[a]	ZEN[h]	10 mg/mL	Physically compatible for 1 hr at 23°C	2066	C
Phenylephrine HCl	ES	10 mg/mL	STU	2 mg/mL	Yellow discoloration forms within 7 days at 25°C. No visible change in 24 hr	1801	?
Phenylephrine HCl	ES	0.1 mg/mL[a]	ZEN[h]	10 mg/mL	Physically compatible for 1 hr at 23°C	2066	C
Phenytoin sodium	ES	50 mg/mL	ZEN[h]	10 mg/mL	Needle-like crystals form immediately	2066	I
Plazomicin sulfate	ACH	24 mg/mL[a]	SGT[i]	10 mg/mL[a]	Immediate formation of free oil layer atop fat plug	3432	I
Potassium chloride	AB	0.1 mEq/mL[a]	ZEN[h]	10 mg/mL	Physically compatible for 1 hr at 23°C	2066	C
Prochlorperazine edisylate	SCN	0.5 mg/mL[a]	ZEN[h]	10 mg/mL	Physically compatible for 1 hr at 23°C	2066	C
Propranolol HCl	SO	1 mg/mL	ZEN[h]	10 mg/mL	Physically compatible for 1 hr at 23°C	2066	C
Ranitidine HCl	GL	2 mg/mL[a]	ZEN[h]	10 mg/mL	Physically compatible for 1 hr at 23°C	2066	C
Scopolamine HBr	LY	0.4 mg/mL	ZEN[h]	10 mg/mL	Physically compatible for 1 hr at 23°C	2066	C
Sodium bicarbonate	AB	1 mEq/mL	ZEN[h]	10 mg/mL	Physically compatible for 1 hr at 23°C	2066	C
Sodium nitroprusside	ES	0.4 mg/mL[a]	ZEN[h]	10 mg/mL	Physically compatible for 1 hr at 23°C	2066	C
Succinylcholine chloride	AB	20 mg/mL	ZEN[h]	10 mg/mL	Physically compatible for 1 hr at 23°C	2066	C
Sufentanil citrate	JN	0.05 mg/mL	ZEN[h]	10 mg/mL	Physically compatible for 1 hr at 23°C	2066	C
Telavancin HCl	ASP	7.5 mg/mL[a]	APP[h]	10 mg/mL	Physically compatible for 2 hr	2830	C
Telavancin HCl	ASP	7.5 mg/mL[b c]	APP[h]	10 mg/mL	Emulsion broke and oiled out	2830	I
Tigecycline	ACD, WY	[g]			Stated to be compatible	2915, 3459	C
Tigecycline	FRK	[a]			Stated to be compatible	3460	C
Tobramycin sulfate	AB	5 mg/mL[a]	ZEN[h]	10 mg/mL	Precipitate forms immediately	2066	I
TPN #186[d]			STU	500 mg	Physically compatible but 28% propofol loss in 5 hr at 22°C	1805	I
TPN #186[d]			STU	2 and 3 g	Physically compatible and 6% or less propofol loss in 5 hr at 22°C	1805	C
TPN #187[d]			STU	500 mg	Physically compatible and 6% or less propofol loss in 5 hr at 22°C	1805	C
TPN #187[d]			STU	2 and 3 g	Physically compatible and 6% or less propofol loss in 5 hr at 22°C	1805	C
TPN #188[d]			STU	500 mg	Physically compatible and 6% or less propofol loss in 5 hr at 22°C	1805	C
TPN #188[d]			STU	2 and 3 g	Physically compatible and 6% or less propofol loss in 5 hr at 22°C	1805	C
Vancomycin HCl	AB	10 mg/mL[a]	ZEN[h]	10 mg/mL	Physically compatible for 1 hr at 23°C	2066	C
Vancomycin HCl		10 mg/mL[a]	BA[i]	10 mg/mL	Emulsion disruption within 1 to 4 hr at room temperature	2336	I
Vancomycin HCl		10 mg/mL[a]	ASZ[h]	10 mg/mL	Physically compatible for up to 30 days at room temperature	2336	C
Vancomycin HCl	LI	10 mg/mL[a]	[j]	1 mg/mL	Physically incompatible	3536	I

Y-Site Injection Compatibility (1:1 Mixture) (Cont.)

Test Drug	Mfr	Conc	Mfr	Conc	Remarks	Ref	C/I
Vecuronium bromide	OR	1 mg/mL	ZEN[h]	10 mg/mL	Physically compatible for 1 hr at 23°C	2066	C
Verapamil HCl	AMR	2.5 mg/mL	ZEN[h]	10 mg/mL	Physically compatible for 1 hr at 23°C	2066	C

[a] Tested in dextrose 5%.

[b] Tested in sodium chloride 0.9%.

[c] Tested in Ringer's injection, lactated.

[d] Refer to Appendix for the composition of parenteral nutrition solutions. TPN indicates a 2-in-1 admixture.

[e] Not specified whether concentration refers to single component or combined components.

[f] Ceftolozane component. Ceftolozane in a 2:1 fixed-ratio concentration with tazobactam.

[g] Tested in both dextrose 5% and sodium chloride 0.9%.

[h] Test performed using the formulation WITH edetate disodium.

[i] Test performed using the formulation WITHOUT edetate disodium.

[j] Presence or absence of edetate disodium not specified.

Selected Revisions May 1, 2020. © Copyright, October 1996.
American Society of Health-System Pharmacists, Inc.

Propranolol Hydrochloride
AHFS 24:24

Products

Propranolol hydrochloride is available in 1-mL ampuls containing 1 mg of the drug with citric acid to adjust the pH in water for injection.[1(9/06)]

pH

From 2.8 to 4.[1(9/06)]

Osmolality

The osmolality of propranolol hydrochloride 1 mg/mL was determined to be 12 mOsm/kg.[1233]

Trade Name(s)

Inderal

Administration

Propranolol hydrochloride is administered by intravenous injection at a rate not exceeding 1 mg/min for life-threatening arrhythmias or those occurring during anesthesia.[1(9/06) 4]

Stability

Propranolol hydrochloride should be stored at controlled room temperature around 25°C and protected from light, freezing, or excessive heat.[1(9/06) 4] Solutions of the drug have maximum stability at pH 3 and decompose rapidly at alkaline pH. Decomposition in aqueous solutions is accompanied by a lowered pH and discoloration. Solutions fluoresce at pH 4 to 5.[4]

Sorption

Propranolol hydrochloride was shown not to exhibit sorption to polyvinyl chloride (PVC) bags and tubing, polyolefin containers, polyethylene tubing, Silastic tubing, and polypropylene syringes.[536 606 746]

Compatibility Information

Solution Compatibility

Propranolol HCl

Test Soln Name	Mfr	Mfr	Conc/L or %	Remarks	Ref	C/I
Dextrose 5% in sodium chloride 0.45%	AB[a], TR[a]	AY	0.5 and 20 mg	Physically compatible and chemically stable for 24 hr at room temperature	746	C
Dextrose 5% in sodium chloride 0.45%	MG[b]	AY	0.5 and 20 mg	Physically compatible and chemically stable for 24 hr at room temperature	746	C
Dextrose 5% in sodium chloride 0.9%	AB[a], TR[a]	AY	0.5 and 20 mg	Physically compatible and chemically stable for 24 hr at room temperature	746	C
Dextrose 5% in sodium chloride 0.9%	MG[b]	AY	0.5 and 20 mg	Physically compatible and chemically stable for 24 hr at room temperature	746	C
Dextrose 5%	AB[a], TR[a]	AY	0.5 and 20 mg	Physically compatible and chemically stable for 24 hr at room temperature	746	C
Dextrose 5%	MG[b]	AY	0.5 and 20 mg	Physically compatible and chemically stable for 24 hr at room temperature	746	C
Ringer's injection, lactated	AB[a], TR[a]	AY	0.5 and 20 mg	Physically compatible and chemically stable for 24 hr at room temperature	746	C
Ringer's injection, lactated	MG[b]	AY	0.5 and 20 mg	Physically compatible and chemically stable for 24 hr at room temperature	746	C
Sodium chloride 0.45%		LY	500 mg	Physically compatible with no loss in 4 hr at 22°C	1419	C
Sodium chloride 0.9%	AB[a], TR[a]	AY	0.5 and 20 mg	Physically compatible and chemically stable for 24 hr at room temperature	746	C
Sodium chloride 0.9%	MG[b]	AY	0.5 and 20 mg	Physically compatible and chemically stable for 24 hr at room temperature	746	C

[a] Tested in PVC containers.

[b] Tested in polyolefin containers.

DOI: 10.37573/9781585286850.330

Additive Compatibility

Propranolol HCl

Test Drug	Mfr	Conc/L or %	Mfr	Conc/L or %	Test Solution	Remarks	Ref	C/I
Dobutamine HCl	LI	1 g	AY	50 mg	D5W, NS	Physically compatible for 24 hr at 21°C	812	C
Verapamil HCl	KN	80 mg	AY	4 mg	D5W, NS	Physically compatible for 24 hr	764	C

Drugs in Syringe Compatibility

Propranolol HCl

Test Drug	Mfr	Amt	Mfr	Amt	Remarks	Ref	C/I
Milrinone lactate	WI	3.5 mg/3.5 mL	AY	3 mg/3 mL	Brought to 10-mL total volume with D5W. Physically compatible with no loss of either drug in 4 hr at 23°C	1191	C
Pantoprazole sodium	a	4 mg/1 mL		1 mg/1 mL	Precipitates	2574	I

[a] Test performed using the formulation WITHOUT edetate disodium.

Y-Site Injection Compatibility (1:1 Mixture)

Propranolol HCl

Test Drug	Mfr	Conc	Mfr	Conc	Remarks	Ref	C/I
Alteplase	GEN	1 mg/mL	AY	1 mg/mL	Visually compatible. 2% clot-lysis activity loss in 24 hr at 25°C	1856	C
Clevidipine butyrate	CHS	0.5 mg/mL		1 mg/mL	Physically incompatible	3334	I
Cloxacillin sodium	SMX	100 mg/mL	SZ	1 mg/mL	Physically compatible for up to 4 hr at room temperature	3245	C
Fenoldopam mesylate	AB	80 mcg/mL[b]	WAY	1 mg/mL	Physically compatible for 4 hr at 23°C	2467	C
Heparin sodium	UP	1000 units/L[c]	AY	1 mg/mL	Physically compatible for 4 hr at room temperature	534	C
Hydrocortisone sodium succinate	UP	10 mg/L[c]	AY	1 mg/mL	Physically compatible for 4 hr at room temperature	534	C
Linezolid	PHU	2 mg/mL	WAY	1 mg/mL	Physically compatible for 4 hr at 23°C	2264	C
Meperidine HCl	AB	10 mg/mL	WY	1 mg/mL	Physically compatible for 4 hr at 25°C	1397	C
Meropenem		50 mg/mL	SZ	1 mg/mL	Physically compatible for 4 hr at room temperature	3538	C
Milrinone lactate	WI	200 mcg/mL[a]	AY	1 mg/mL	Physically compatible with no loss of either drug in 4 hr at 23°C	1191	C
Morphine sulfate	AB	1 mg/mL	WY	1 mg/mL	Physically compatible for 4 hr at 25°C	1397	C
Nesiritide	SCI	50 mcg/mL[a][b]		1 mg/mL	Physically compatible for 4 hr	2625	C
Potassium chloride	AB	40 mEq/L[c]	AY	1 mg/mL	Physically compatible for 4 hr at room temperature	534	C
Propofol	ZEN[d]	10 mg/mL	SO	1 mg/mL	Physically compatible for 1 hr at 23°C	2066	C
Tacrolimus	FUJ	1 mg/mL[b]	AY	1 mg/mL	Visually compatible for 24 hr at 25°C	1630	C
Tirofiban HCl	ME	50 mcg/mL[a][b]	WAY	1 mg/mL	Physically compatible. No loss of either drug in 4 hr at 23°C	2356	C

[a] Tested in dextrose 5%.

[b] Tested in sodium chloride 0.9%.

[c] Tested in dextrose 5% in Ringer's injection, dextrose 5% in Ringer's injection, lactated, dextrose 5%, Ringer's injection, lactated, and sodium chloride 0.9%.

[d] Test performed using the formulation WITH edetate disodium.

Selected Revisions May 1, 2020. © Copyright, October 1982.
American Society of Health-System Pharmacists, Inc.

Protamine Sulfate
AHFS 20:28.08

Products

Protamine sulfate is available in 5- and 25-mL vials. Each mL contains protamine sulfate 10 mg with sodium chloride 0.9% and sodium phosphate and/or sulfuric acid to adjust the pH.[1(1/08)]

pH

From 6 to 7.[1(1/08)]

Osmolality

The osmolality of protamine sulfate 10 mg/mL was determined to be 290 mOsm/kg by freezing-point depression and 292 mOsm/kg by vapor pressure.[1071]

Administration

Protamine sulfate 10 mg/mL is administered by slow intravenous injection undiluted. No more than 50 mg should be administered in any 10-minute period. It has also been given by intravenous infusion after dilution in sodium chloride 0.9% or dextrose 5%.[1(1/08)] [4]

Stability

Protamine sulfate should be stored under refrigeration; freezing should be avoided.[1(1/08)] However, protamine sulfate has been stated to be stable for 10 days[1433] to 2 weeks[853] at room temperature.

Protamine sulfate is incompatible with some antibiotics including cephalosporins and penicillins.[1(1/08)]

Filtration

Protamine sulfate (Fournier Freres) 0.2 mg/mL in dextrose 5% and sodium chloride 0.9% was filtered through a 0.22-μm cellulose ester membrane filter (Ivex-HP, Millipore) over 6 hours. No significant drug loss due to binding to the filter was noted.[1034]

Compatibility Information

Additive Compatibility

Protamine sulfate

Test Drug	Mfr	Conc/L or %	Mfr	Conc/L or %	Test Solution	Remarks	Ref	C/I
Ranitidine HCl	GL	50 mg and 2 g		500 mg	D5W	Physically compatible. Ranitidine stable for 24 hr at 25°C. Protamine not tested	1515	C
Verapamil HCl	KN	80 mg	LI	100 mg	D5W, NS	Physically compatible for 24 hr	764	C

Drugs in Syringe Compatibility

Protamine sulfate

Test Drug	Mfr	Amt	Mfr	Amt	Remarks	Ref	C/I
Iohexol	WI	64.7%, 5 mL	LI	10 mg/1 mL	Physically compatible for at least 2 hr	1438	C
Iopamidol	SQ	61%, 5 mL	LI	10 mg/1 mL	Physically compatible for at least 2 hr	1438	C
Iothalamate meglumine	MA	60%, 5 mL	LI	10 mg/1 mL	Physically compatible for at least 2 hr	1438	C
Ioxaglate meglumine–ioxaglate sodium	MA	5 mL	LI	10 mg/1 mL	Precipitate forms immediately and persists for at least 2 hr	1438	I

Y-Site Injection Compatibility (1:1 Mixture)

Protamine sulfate

Test Drug	Mfr	Conc	Mfr	Conc	Remarks	Ref	C/I
Sugammadex sodium	ME	100 mcg/mL[a]	LI	50 mcg/mL[a]	Precipitates immediately	3113	I

[a] Tested in sodium chloride 0.9%.

Selected Revisions June 14, 2016. © Copyright, October 1986.
American Society of Health-System Pharmacists, Inc.

DOI: 10.37573/9781585286850.331

Prothrombin Complex Concentrate (Human)
AHFS 20:28.16

Products

Prothrombin complex concentrate (human) is available in a kit as a lyophilized powder in single-use (preservative-free) vials.[3182] Each kit contains a vial of prothrombin complex concentrate (human) with a nominal concentration of 500 or 1000 units packaged with 20 or 40 mL, respectively, of sterile water for injection, a Mix2Vial filter transfer set, and an alcohol swab.[3182] Each vial of prothrombin complex concentrate (human) contains coagulation factors II, VII, IX, and X, and antithrombotic proteins C and S.[3182] Vials also contain antithrombin III, heparin, albumin human, sodium chloride, sodium citrate, hydrochloric acid, and sodium hydroxide as excipients.[3182]

Prothrombin complex concentrate (human) (Kcentra, CSL Behring) ingredient composition per vial

Ingredient	Prothrombin complex concentrate (human) nominal 500-unit vial	Prothrombin complex concentrate (human) nominal 1000-unit vial
Total protein	120 to 280 mg	240 to 560 mg
Factor II	380 to 800 units	760 to 1600 units
Factor VII	200 to 500 units	400 to 1000 units
Factor IX	400 to 620 units	800 to 1240 units
Factor X	500 to 1020 units	1000 to 2040 units
Protein C	420 to 820 units	840 to 1640 units
Protein S	240 to 680 units	480 to 1360 units
Heparin	8 to 40 units	16 to 80 units
Antithrombin III	4 to 30 units	8 to 60 units
Albumin human	40 to 80 mg	80 to 160 mg
Sodium chloride	60 to 120 mg	120 to 240 mg
Sodium citrate	40 to 80 mg	80 to 160 mg
Hydrochloric acid	Small amounts	Small amounts
Sodium hydroxide	Small amounts	Small amounts

The actual amount of coagulation factor and antithrombotic protein units contained in each vial is printed on the vial carton.[3182] The actual amount of factor IX units contained in each vial also is printed on the vial label.[3182]

© Copyright, March 2017. American Society of Health-System Pharmacists, Inc.

Vials of prothrombin complex concentrate (human) and provided diluent should be allowed to come to room temperature prior to reconstitution.[3182] The nominal 500- or 1000-unit vial should be reconstituted with 20 or 40 mL, respectively, of sterile water for injection.[3182] The Mix2Vial filter transfer set provided in each kit should be used for reconstitution; specific product labeling should be consulted for additional preparation details.[3182] Vials should be gently swirled until the contents have completely dissolved and should not be shaken.[3182] The reconstituted contents of multiple vials may be pooled for patients requiring doses exceeding those provided in a single vial; however, a separate, unused Mix2Vial filter transfer set should be used for the reconstitution of each vial.[3182] When reconstituted as directed, the final concentration of factor IX units in each vial will range from 20 to 31 units/mL.[3182]

Trade Name(s)

Kcentra

Administration

Prothrombin complex concentrate (human) is administered by intravenous infusion at a rate of 0.12 mL/kg/min (approximately 3 factor IX units/kg/min) up to a maximum rate of 8.4 mL/min (approximately 210 factor IX units/min).[3182] If the reconstituted solution has been stored under refrigeration or cooled, the solution should be warmed to 20 to 25°C prior to administration.[3182]

Prothrombin complex concentrate (human) should be infused through a separate line from other medications.[3182] Blood should not enter the syringe containing the drug due to the possibility of fibrin clot formation.[3182]

Stability

Intact vials should be stored at 2 to 25°C and kept in the original carton to protect from light.[3182] Vials should not be frozen.[3182] Prothrombin complex concentrate (human) reconstituted as directed with sterile water for injection is a colorless, clear to slightly opalescent solution.[3182]

Reconstituted solutions should be visually inspected for particulate matter and discoloration prior to administration; solutions that are cloudy or those containing deposits should not be used.[3182] Reconstituted solutions may be stored at 2 to 25°C; however, solutions should be used promptly and must be used within 4 hours following reconstitution.[3182] Any unused portion should be discarded.[3182]

DOI: 10.37573/9781585286850.332

Pyridoxine Hydrochloride
AHFS 88:08

Products

Pyridoxine hydrochloride 100 mg/mL is available in 1-, 10-, and 30-mL multiple-dose vials. Antimicrobial preservatives, such as benzyl alcohol 1.5% or chlorobutanol 0.5%, may also be present. Sodium hydroxide and/or hydrochloric acid may have been used to adjust pH.[1(6/06)] [4]

pH

From 2 to 3.8.[1(6/06)] [4]

Osmolality

The osmolality of pyridoxine hydrochloride 100 mg/mL was determined to be 870 mOsm/kg by freezing-point depression and 852 mOsm/kg by vapor pressure.[1071]

Administration

Pyridoxine hydrochloride may be administered by intramuscular, subcutaneous, or intravenous injection.[4]

Compatibility Information

Drugs in Syringe Compatibility

Pyridoxine HCl

Test Drug	Mfr	Amt	Mfr	Amt	Remarks	Ref	C/I
Doxapram HCl	RB	400 mg/20 mL		10 mg/1 mL	Physically compatible with 6% doxapram loss in 24 hr	1177	C

Additional Compatibility Information

Parenteral Nutrition Solutions

The stability of pyridoxine hydrochloride 15 mg/L was studied in representative parenteral nutrition solutions exposed to fluorescent light, indirect sunlight, and direct sunlight for eight hours. One 5-mL vial of multivitamin concentrate (Lyphomed) containing 15 mg of pyridoxine hydrochloride and also 1 mg of folic acid (Lederle) was added to a liter of parenteral nutrition solution composed of amino acids 4.25%–dextrose 25% (Travenol) with standard electrolytes and trace elements. Pyridoxine hydrochloride was stable over the eight-hour study at room temperature under fluorescent light and indirect sunlight.

Stability

The product should be stored at controlled room temperature and protected from freezing and from light.[1(6/06)] [4]

Because pyridoxine hydrochloride is photosensitive and degrades slowly when exposed to light, protection from light has been recommended.[4]

Syringes

Pyridoxine hydrochloride 100 mg/mL was stable for six months at room temperature packaged in 5-, 10-, and 20-mL polypropylene syringes (Becton Dickinson).[2692]

Sorption

Pyridoxine hydrochloride (Sigma) 40 mg/L did not display significant sorption to a PVC plastic test strip in 24 hours.[12]

However, eight hours of exposure to direct sunlight caused an 86% loss of pyridoxine hydrochloride.[842]

The stability of numerous vitamins in parenteral nutrition solutions composed of amino acids (Kabi-Vitrum), dextrose 30%, and fat emulsion 20% (Kabi-Vitrum) in a 2:1:1 ratio with electrolytes, trace elements, and both fat- and water-soluble vitamins was reported. The admixtures were stored in darkness at 2 to 8°C for 96 hours with no significant loss of pyridoxine hydrochloride.[1225]

The vitamins in Cernevit (Baxter) diluted in three 2-in-1 parenteral nutrition admixtures were tested for stability over 48 hours. Most of the other vitamins, including pyridoxine hydrochloride, retained their initial concentrations.[2796]

Selected Revisions October 1, 2012. © Copyright, October 1982. American Society of Health-System Pharmacists, Inc.

DOI: 10.37573/9781585286850.333

Quinidine Gluconate
AHFS 24:04.04.04

Products

Quinidine gluconate is available in 10-mL vials. Each mL contains 80 mg of drug with edetate disodium 0.005% and phenol 0.25% in water for injection. D-gluconic acid delta-lactone may have been added to adjust the pH.[1(9/06)]

Equivalency

Quinidine gluconate 800 mg is equivalent to 500 mg of anhydrous quinidine.[1(9/06)]

pH

Quinidine gluconate injection has a pH of 5.5 to 7.[4]

Administration

Quinidine gluconate injection may be given by intermittent or continuous intravenous administration.[4] For intravenous administration in treating arrhythmias, 800 mg (10 mL) is diluted with 40 mL of dextrose 5% for a total of 50 mL to yield a 16-mg/mL solution. The drug has also been given by intramuscular injection, but this route is not recommended because of variable absorption.[1(9/06) 4]

For the treatment of malaria, continuous and intermittent infusion regimens have been used. A loading dose is prepared as a dilution in 250 mL of sodium chloride 0.9% and given as a one- or two-hour (continuous regimen) or four-hour (intermittent regimen) infusion.[4]

Infusions of quinidine gluconate must be delivered slowly at a rate no faster than 0.25 mg/kg/min, preferably using a volumetric pump to control the rate of administration.[1(9/06)]

Stability

Quinidine gluconate should be stored at controlled room temperature.[1(9/06)] Quinidine salts slowly discolor on exposure to light, acquiring a brownish tint. Only clear, colorless solutions are suitable for injection.[4]

Sorption

A substantial loss of quinidine (as the gluconate) was noted due to sorption to PVC containers and administration sets. Quinidine gluconate 6 mg/mL in dextrose 5% in 100-mL PVC bags (Baxter) exhibited about 5 to 7% loss. Administration of the solution over 30 minutes through 112-inch PVC administration sets (Gemini, IMED) resulted in an additional loss of over 30% of the quinidine gluconate from the delivered solution. Losses totaled over 40% for both bag and catheter. Use of a glass syringe on a syringe pump and a winged administration catheter having only 12 inches of PVC tubing reduced the loss to about 3%.[2005]

In two studies, quinidine (as the sulfate) was shown not to exhibit sorption to PVC bags and tubing, polyethylene tubing, Silastic tubing, and polypropylene syringes.[536 606]

Compatibility Information
Solution Compatibility

Quinidine gluconate

Test Soln Name	Mfr	Mfr	Conc/L or %	Remarks	Ref	C/I
Dextrose 5%			16 g	Stable for 24 hr at room temperature and 48 hr refrigerated	4	C

Additive Compatibility

Quinidine gluconate

Test Drug	Mfr	Conc/L or %	Mfr	Conc/L or %	Test Solution	Remarks	Ref	C/I
Amiodarone HCl	LZ	1.8 g	LI	1 g	D5W[a]	Milky precipitation. 13% amiodarone loss in 6 hr and 23% in 24 hr at 24°C in light	1031	I
Amiodarone HCl	LZ	1.8 g	LI	1 g	D5W[b]	Milky precipitation. No amiodarone loss in 24 hr at 24°C in light	1031	I
Amiodarone HCl	LZ	1.8 g	LI	1 g	NS[a]	Physically compatible. 13% amiodarone loss in 24 hr at 24°C in light	1031	I
Amiodarone HCl	LZ	1.8 g	LI	1 g	NS[b]	Physically compatible. No amiodarone loss in 24 hr at 24°C in light	1031	C
Atracurium besylate	BW	500 mg		8.3 g	D5W	Particles form and atracurium unstable at 5 and 30°C	1694	I

DOI: 10.37573/9781585286850.334

Additive Compatibility (Cont.)

Test Drug	Mfr	Conc/L or %	Mfr	Conc/L or %	Test Solution	Remarks	Ref	C/I
Milrinone lactate	WI	200 mg	LI	16 g	D5W	Physically compatible with no loss of either drug in 4 hr at 23°C	1191	C
Ranitidine HCl	GL	50 mg and 2 g		3.2 g	D5W	Physically compatible. Ranitidine stable for 24 hr at 25°C. Quinidine not tested	1515	C
Verapamil HCl	KN	80 mg	LI	800 mg	D5W, NS	Physically compatible for 48 hr	739	C

[a] Tested in PVC containers.

[b] Tested in polyolefin containers.

Y-Site Injection Compatibility (1:1 Mixture)

Quinidine gluconate

Test Drug	Mfr	Conc	Mfr	Conc	Remarks	Ref	C/I
Diazepam	ES	0.2 mg/mL[a b]	LI	6 mg/mL[a b]	Physically compatible for 3 hr	1316	C
Furosemide	ES	4 mg/mL[a b]	LI	6 mg/mL[a b]	Immediate gross precipitation	1316	I
Heparin sodium	ES	50 units/mL[b]	LI	6 mg/mL[b]	Physically compatible for 3 hr	1316	C
Heparin sodium	ES	50 units/mL[a]	LI	6 mg/mL[a]	Immediate gross haze	1316	I
Milrinone lactate	WI	350 mcg/mL[a]	LI	16 mg/mL[a]	Physically compatible with no loss of either drug in 4 hr at 23°C	1191	C
Nesiritide	SCI	50 mcg/mL[a b]		80 mg/mL	Physically compatible for 4 hr	2625	C

[a] Tested in dextrose 5%.

[b] Tested in sodium chloride 0.9%.

Selected Revisions October 1, 2012. © Copyright, October 1982.
American Society of Health-System Pharmacists, Inc.

Quinupristin–Dalfopristin
AHFS 8:12.28.32

Products

Quinupristin–dalfopristin is available as a lyophilized powder in single-dose vials containing a total of 500 mg of the two pristinamycin derivatives (quinupristin 150 mg and dalfopristin 350 mg).[3229] The 500-mg vial should be reconstituted with 5 mL of dextrose 5% or sterile water for injection and gently swirled (without shaking) to facilitate dissolution while limiting foam formation.[3229] The reconstituted solution should be allowed to sit for a few minutes until all of the foam has dissipated and a clear 100-mg/mL solution has formed; this solution must be diluted for administration.[3229]

The appropriate dose of quinupristin–dalfopristin should be added to an infusion bag containing 250 mL of dextrose 5%.[3229] For central line administration, 100 mL of dextrose 5% may be used for dilution.[3229]

Diluted solutions of quinupristin–dalfopristin for infusion should be visually inspected for particulate matter prior to administration.[3229]

Trade Name(s)

Synercid

Administration

Quinupristin–dalfopristin is administered by intravenous infusion over 60 minutes following dilution of the reconstituted solution in dextrose 5%; other infusion rates are not recommended.[3229] An infusion pump or device may be used to control the rate of infusion.[3229]

If moderate-to-severe venous irritation occurs during peripheral administration of the reconstituted solution diluted in 250 mL of dextrose 5%, consideration should be given to increasing the infusion volume to 500 or 750 mL, changing the infusion site, or infusing through a peripherally inserted central catheter (PICC) or central venous catheter.[3229]

If a common infusion line is used for the intermittent infusion of quinupristin–dalfopristin and other drugs, the manufacturer recommends flushing the line with dextrose 5% prior to and following administration of quinupristin–dalfopristin.[3229] The vein also should be flushed with dextrose 5% following completion of peripheral administration of the drug in order to minimize venous irritation; the vein should *not* be flushed with sodium chloride or heparin after drug administration.[3229]

Stability

Intact vials of quinupristin–dalfopristin should be stored under refrigeration.[3229] Although refrigerated storage is required, one manufacturer has stated that the drug may be stored at room temperature for 7 days.[2745] Because no antimicrobial preservative is present, the manufacturer recommends dilution of the reconstituted solution within 30 minutes.[3229] Quinupristin–dalfopristin diluted for infusion in dextrose 5% is stated to be stable for 5 hours at room temperature and 54 hours at 2 to 8°C.[3229]

Use of sodium chloride-containing solutions for dilution or flushing is not recommended because of incompatibility.[3229]

Freezing Solutions

Diluted solutions of quinupristin–dalfopristin for infusion should not be frozen.[3229]

Compatibility Information

Solution Compatibility

Quinupristin–dalfopristin

Test Soln Name	Mfr	Mfr	Conc/L or %	Remarks	Ref	C/I
Dextrose 5%		PF		Stable for 5 hr at room temperature and 54 hr at 2 to 8°C	3229	C
Sodium chloride 0.45%		PF		Stated to be incompatible	3229	I
Sodium chloride 0.9%		PF		Stated to be incompatible	3229	I

Y-Site Injection Compatibility (1:1 Mixture)

Quinupristin–dalfopristin

Test Drug	Mfr	Conc	Mfr	Conc	Remarks	Ref	C/I
Acyclovir[d]		5 mg/mL		2 mg/mL[a c]	Reported to be incompatible	3230	I
Anidulafungin	VIC	0.5 mg/mL[a]	AVE	5 mg/mL[a c]	Physically compatible for 4 hr at 23°C	2617	C

DOI: 10.37573/9781585286850.335

Y-Site Injection Compatibility (1:1 Mixture) (Cont.)

Test Drug	Mfr	Conc	Mfr	Conc	Remarks	Ref	C/I
Aminophylline		2.5 mg/mL		2 mg/mL[a] [c]	Reported to be incompatible	3230	I
Amphotericin B		0.6 mg/mL		2 mg/mL[a] [c]	Reported to be incompatible	3230	I
Aztreonam		20 mg/mL[a]	PF	2 mg/mL[a] [c]	Physically compatible	3229	C
Cangrelor tetrasodium	TMC	1 mg/mL[b]		5 mg/mL[b] [c]	Gross white turbid precipitate with fluffy particulates forms immediately	3243	I
Caspofungin acetate	ME	0.7 mg/mL[b]	MON	5 mg/mL[b] [c]	Physically compatible for 4 hr at room temperature	2758	C
Cefotaxime[d]		20 mg/mL		2 mg/mL[a] [c]	Reported to be incompatible	3230	I
Ceftazidime		20 mg/mL		2 mg/mL[a] [c]	Reported to be incompatible	3230	I
Ciprofloxacin		1 mg/mL[a]	PF	2 mg/mL[a] [c]	Physically compatible	3229	C
Digoxin		0.25 mg/mL		2 mg/mL[a] [c]	Reported to be incompatible	3230	I
Dobutamine[d]		4 mg/mL		2 mg/mL[a] [c]	Reported to be incompatible	3230	I
Dopamine[d]		2.2 mg/mL		2 mg/mL[a] [c]	Reported to be incompatible	3230	I
Erythromycin lactobionate		5 mg/mL		2 mg/mL[a] [c]	Reported to be incompatible	3230	I
Fenoldopam mesylate	AB	80 mcg/mL[b]	AVE	5 mg/mL[b] [c]	Physically compatible for 4 hr at 23°C	2467	C
Fluconazole		2 mg/mL	PF	2 mg/mL[a] [c]	Physically compatible	3229	C
Furosemide		3 mg/mL		2 mg/mL[a] [c]	Reported to be incompatible	3230	I
Gentamicin[d]		3 mg/mL		2 mg/mL[a] [c]	Reported to be incompatible	3230	I
Haloperidol lactate		0.2 mg/mL[a]	PF	2 mg/mL[a] [c]	Physically compatible	3229	C
Hydrocortisone sodium succinate		1 mg/mL		2 mg/mL[a] [c]	Reported to be incompatible	3230	I
Imipenem–cilastatin[d]		5 mg/mL		2 mg/mL[a] [c]	Reported to be incompatible	3230	I
Insulin, regular		100 units/mL		2 mg/mL[a] [c]	Reported to be incompatible	3230	I
Meropenem		10 mg/mL		2 mg/mL[a] [c]	Reported to be incompatible	3230	I
Metoclopramide HCl		5 mg/mL[a]	PF	2 mg/mL[a] [c]	Physically compatible	3229	C
Metronidazole		5 mg/mL		2 mg/mL[a] [c]	Reported to be incompatible	3230	I
Piperacillin–tazobactam[d]				2 mg/mL[a] [c]	Reported to be incompatible	3230	I
Potassium chloride		0.04 mEq/mL[a]	PF	2 mg/mL[a] [c]	Physically compatible	3229	C

[a] Tested in dextrose 5%.

[b] Tested in sodium chloride 0.9%.

[c] Quinupristin and dalfopristin components combined.

[d] Salt not specified.

Selected Revisions December 12, 2018. © Copyright, October 2004. American Society of Health-System Pharmacists, Inc.

Ranitidine Hydrochloride
AHFS 56:28.12

Products

Ranitidine hydrochloride is available in 2-mL single-dose vials,[3497] [3512] 6-mL multiple-dose vials,[3497] [3512] and 40-mL pharmacy bulk packages.[3498] Each mL of solution contains ranitidine (as the hydrochloride) 25 mg, phenol 5 mg, dibasic sodium phosphate 2.4 mg, and monobasic potassium phosphate 0.96 mg.[3497 3498 3512]

Equivalency

Ranitidine hydrochloride 28 mg is approximately equivalent to 25 mg of ranitidine.[3497 3498]

pH

The pH of the injection solution ranges from 6.7 to 7.3.[3497 3498]

Osmolality

The osmolality of ranitidine hydrochloride 10 mg/mL was determined to be 59 mOsm/kg.[1233]

The osmolality of ranitidine hydrochloride (Glaxo) 1 mg/mL was 260 mOsm/kg in dextrose 5% and 302 mOsm/kg in sodium chloride 0.9%.[1375] At 2 mg/mL, the osmolality was 257 mOsm/kg in dextrose 5% and 294 mOsm/kg in sodium chloride 0.9%.[1375]

Trade Name(s)

Zantac

Administration

Ranitidine hydrochloride is administered intravenously after dilution.[3497 3497 3512] For intravenous injection, 50 mg should be diluted to a total volume of at least 20 mL (i.e., to a concentration no greater than 2.5 mg/mL) with a compatible infusion solution and administered over at least 5 minutes.[3497 3498 3512] For intermittent intravenous infusion, 50 mg should be diluted to a total volume of at least 100 mL (i.e., to a concentration no greater than 0.5 mg/mL) with a compatible infusion solution and infused over at least 15 to 20 minutes.[3497 3498 3512] For continuous intravenous infusion, ranitidine hydrochloride also should be diluted in a compatible infusion solution (e.g., 150 mg in 250 mL); for some indications where administration by continuous infusion is recommended, the manufacturers recommend dilution to a concentration no greater than 2.5 mg/mL.[3497 3498 3512]

Ranitidine hydrochloride also is administered intramuscularly.[3497 3498 3512] Dilution of the drug is not required for intramuscular administration.[3497 3498 3512]

Stability

Ranitidine hydrochloride injection should be stored between 4 and 25°C[3497 3498] or 20 and 25°C[3512] with excursions permitted to 30°C.[3497] Vials should be protected from light and excessive heat.[3497 3498 3512] Brief exposure to temperatures up to 40°C will not adversely affect the stability of the injection.[3497 3512] However, ranitidine hydrochloride injection has been reported to form an unacceptable brown discoloration if stored at 40°C or higher for several months.[2505] The product is a clear, colorless to yellow solution.[3497 3498 3512] Manufacturers note that the yellow color of the undiluted drug may intensify over time without adversely affecting the potency of the product.[3497 3498 3512]

Ranitidine hydrochloride (Glaxo) diluted to a concentration of 2.5 mg/mL with preserved sterile water for injection and repackaged in 30-mL glass vials was stored at 4°C for 91 days.[1965] Approximately 5% loss occurred after 91 days of storage under refrigeration.[1965]

Ranitidine hydrochloride (GlaxoSmithKline) 25 mg/mL was repackaged as 2.2 mL in glass vials and stored for 6 months at 5°C protected from light and 25°C both protected from and exposed to light.[3495] While solutions were colorless to slightly yellow initially, some samples turned more yellow over time, and this change was especially apparent in samples exposed to light.[3495] Color changes were not associated with a decrease in ranitidine concentration, and little loss of the drug occurred in 6 months at any of the storage conditions tested.[3495]

Freezing Solutions

Manufacturers state that the drug should be protected from freezing.[3497 3498 3512]

Ranitidine hydrochloride (Glaxo) 0.5, 1, and 2 mg/mL in dextrose 5% and sodium chloride 0.9% in polyvinyl chloride (PVC) bags showed no change in appearance or concentration when frozen for 30 days at −30°C.[1143] An additional 14 days of refrigerated storage at 4°C for these previously frozen solutions also resulted in no loss.[1143] At a concentration of 2 mg/mL in dextrose 5% and sodium chloride 0.9% in PVC containers, no change in appearance or drug loss occurred after 100 days of storage at −30°C.[1143]

The stability of ranitidine hydrochloride (Glaxo) 0.5, 1, and 2 mg/mL in several infusion fluids frozen at −20°C for 60 days followed by 7 days at 23°C or 14 days at 4°C was studied. In dextrose 5% in sodium chloride 0.45%, dextrose 5%, dextrose 10%, and sodium chloride 0.9%, ranitidine was physically compatible and chemically stable, retaining more than 90% of the initial concentration under these storage conditions. However, in dextrose 5% in Ringer's injection, lactated, the thawed solutions were slightly yellow with ranitidine hydrochloride losses of 25, 16, and 9% at 0.5, 1, and 2 mg/mL, respectively.[1516]

Ranitidine hydrochloride (Glaxo) 1.5 mg/mL in dextrose 5% or in sodium chloride 0.9% was packaged in PVC infusion pump reservoirs. The reservoirs were stored at −20°C for 30 days. The frozen solutions were then thawed by storing at 3°C for 24 hours followed by 24 hours at 30°C to simulate use conditions. No loss was found.[1865]

DOI: 10.37573/9781585286850.336

Syringes

Ranitidine hydrochloride (Glaxo) was diluted to a concentration of 2.5 mg/mL with preserved sterile water for injection and repackaged in 10-mL polypropylene syringes (Becton Dickinson).[1965] Approximately 6% loss occurred after 91 days of storage at 4°C.[1965] Freshly prepared syringes and syringes initially stored at 4°C for 91 days also were stored at 22°C for 72 hours.[1965] No loss was found in the freshly prepared syringes, and about 2% additional loss was found in syringes initially stored under refrigeration for 91 days.[1965]

Ranitidine hydrochloride (GlaxoSmithKline) 5 mg/mL in sodium chloride 0.9% repackaged as 5 mL in polypropylene syringes (Becton Dickinson) exhibited less than 10% loss after storage for 91 days at 5°C protected from light and at 25°C both protected from light and exposed to light.[3495] While solutions were colorless to slightly yellow initially, some samples turned more yellow over time, and this change was especially apparent in certain samples (e.g., those exposed to light, undiluted 25-mg/mL samples).[3495] Such color changes were not associated with a decrease in ranitidine concentration.[3495]

Filtration

Filtration of ranitidine hydrochloride (Glaxo) 0.25, 0.5, and 2.5 mg/mL in sodium chloride 0.9% through 0.2-μm polysulfone filters (IVS Set-P Supor Filter, Codan) at a rate of 4 mL/hr for 5 hours did not result in any loss of drug due to sorption to the filter.[2229]

Central Venous Catheter

Ranitidine hydrochloride (Glaxo Wellcome) 0.2 mg/mL in dextrose 5% was found to be compatible with the ARROW-g+ard Blue Plus (Arrow International) chlorhexidine-bearing triple-lumen central catheter. Essentially complete delivery of the drug was found with little or no drug loss occurring. Furthermore, chlorhexidine delivered from the catheter remained at trace amounts with no substantial increase due to the delivery of the drug through the catheter.[2335]

Compatibility Information

Solution Compatibility

Ranitidine HCl

Test Soln Name	Mfr	Mfr	Conc/L or %	Remarks	Ref	C/I
Dextrose 5% in Ringer's injection, lactated	TR[a]	GL	50 mg	15% loss in 2 days at room temperature in light	1362	I
Dextrose 5% in Ringer's injection, lactated	TR[a]	GL	500 mg, 1 g, 2 g	Physically compatible. Up to 5% loss in 7 days at 23°C and 8% loss in 30 days at 4°C	1516	C
Dextrose 5% in sodium chloride 0.45%	TR[a]	GL	50 mg	10% loss in 7 days at room temperature in light	1362	C
Dextrose 5% in sodium chloride 0.45%	TR[a]	GL	500 mg, 1 g, 2 g	Physically compatible. Up to 5% loss in 7 days at 23°C and 8% loss in 30 days at 4°C	1516	C
Dextrose 5%		TEL		Stable for 48 hr at room temperature	3497, 3498	C
Dextrose 5%	TR[a]	GL	1 g	Little or no loss in 10 days at 4°C	1143	C
Dextrose 5%	TR[a]		1 g	Physically compatible. 8% loss in 18 days at 25°C and 3% loss in 66 days at 5°C	1342	C
Dextrose 5%	TR[a]	GL	1 g	Physically compatible. No loss in 92 days at 4°C	1350	C
Dextrose 5%	TR[a]	GL	50 mg and 2 g	Physically compatible. 6% or less loss in 48 hr at room temperature in light	1361	C
Dextrose 5%	TR[a]	GL	500 mg, 1 g, 2 g	5% or less loss in 28 days at room temperature in light	1362	C
Dextrose 5%	TR[a]	GL	50 mg	10% loss in 7 days at room temperature in light	1362	C
Dextrose 5%	TR[a]	GL	500 mg, 1 g, 2 g	Physically compatible. Up to 5% loss in 7 days at 23°C and 6% loss in 30 days at 4°C	1516	C
Dextrose 5%	MG	GL	441 mg	Visually compatible. No loss after 30 days at −20°C then 10 days at 4°C	1539	C
Dextrose 5%	TR[a]	GL	50 mg and 2 g	Visually compatible. 6% or less loss in 48 hr at room temperature	1802	C
Dextrose 5%	AB[a]	GL	1.5 g	Little loss in 24 hr at 30°C and for 7 days at 3°C then 24 hr at 30°C	1865	C

Solution Compatibility (Cont.)

Test Soln Name	Mfr	Mfr	Conc/L or %	Remarks	Ref	C/I
Dextrose 5%	BA[a]	GW	250 mg	Visually compatible. 5% or less loss in 24 hr at 4 and 22°C	2289	C
Dextrose 5%	BRN[b]	GW	250 mg	Visually compatible. 5% or less loss in 24 hr at 4 and 22°C	2289	C
Dextrose 10%		TEL		Stable for 48 hr at room temperature	3497, 3498	C
Dextrose 10%	TR[a]	GL	50 mg	7% loss in 2 days at room temperature in light	1362	C
Dextrose 10%	TR[a]	GL	500 mg, 1 g, 2 g	Physically compatible. Up to 4% loss in 7 days at 23°C and 8% loss in 30 days at 4°C	1516	C
Ringer's injection, lactated		TEL		Stable for 48 hr at room temperature	3497, 3498	C
Sodium chloride 0.9%		TEL		Stable for 48 hr at room temperature	3497, 3498	C
Sodium chloride 0.9%	TR	GL	50 and 100 mg	No loss in 48 hr at 24°C in light	1010	C
Sodium chloride 0.9%	TR[a]	GL	1 g	Little loss in 10 days at 4°C	1143	C
Sodium chloride 0.9%	TR[a]		1 g	Physically compatible with no loss in 18 days at 25°C and in 66 days at 5°C	1342	C
Sodium chloride 0.9%	TR[a]	GL	1 g	Physically compatible. No loss in 92 days at 4°C	1350	C
Sodium chloride 0.9%	TR	GL	50 mg	Physically compatible. No loss in 48 hr at 25°C	1360	C
Sodium chloride 0.9%	TR	GL	100 mg	Physically compatible. No loss in 48 hr at 25°C and refrigerated for 24 hr then 24 hr at 25°C	1360	C
Sodium chloride 0.9%	TR[a]	GL	50 mg and 2 g	Physically compatible. No loss in 48 hr at room temperature in light	1361	C
Sodium chloride 0.9%	TR[a]	GL	50 mg to 2 g	3% or less loss in 28 days at room temperature in light	1362	C
Sodium chloride 0.9%	TR[a]	GL	500 mg, 1 g, 2 g	Physically compatible. No loss in 7 days at 23°C and 3% loss in 30 days at 4°C	1516	C
Sodium chloride 0.9%	TR[a]	GL	50 mg and 2 g	Visually compatible. Little loss in 48 hr at room temperature	1802	C
Sodium chloride 0.9%	AB[a]	GL	1.5 g	Little loss in 24 hr at 30°C and for 7 days at 3°C then 24 hr at 30°C	1865	C
Sodium chloride 0.9%	BA[a]	GL	0.6 and 1 g	Visually compatible. Little loss in 24 hr at ambient temperature	2079	C
Sodium chloride 0.9%	BA[a]	GW	250 mg	Visually compatible. 5% or less loss in 24 hr at 4 and 22°C	2289	C
Sodium chloride 0.9%	BRN[b]	GW	250 mg	Visually compatible. 5% or less loss in 24 hr at 4 and 22°C	2289	C
TNA #92[d]	[c]	GL	50 and 100 mg	7 to 10% ranitidine loss in 12 hr and 20 to 28% loss in 24 hr at 23°C in light	1183	I
TNA #118[d]		GL	50 and 100 mg	Physically compatible. 6 to 10% ranitidine loss in 36 hr under refrigeration and at 25°C	1360	C
TNA #197 to #200[d]		GL	75 mg	Physically compatible with 7% or less ranitidine loss in 24 hr at 22°C in light. About 15% loss in 48 hr	1921	C
TNA #245[d]			200 mg	No ranitidine loss and no lipid change in 24 hr at room temperature	486	C
TNA #246[d]		GL	72 mg	Less than 7% ranitidine loss and no change in emulsion integrity in 14 days at 4°C	501	C
TPN #58[d]		GL	83, 167, 250 mg	10% ranitidine loss in 48 hr at 23°C	997	C
TPN #59, #60[d]	[a]	GL	50 and 100 mg	No color change and 7 to 9% ranitidine loss in 24 hr at 24°C in light. Amino acids unaffected. Darkened color and 10 to 12% ranitidine loss in 48 hr	1010	C

Solution Compatibility (Cont.)

Test Soln Name	Mfr	Mfr	Conc/L or %	Remarks	Ref	C/I
TPN #117[d]		GL	50 and 100 mg	Physically compatible and 5% ranitidine loss in 48 hr refrigerated and at 25°C	1360	C
TPN #196[d]		GL	75 mg	Physically compatible with 7% or less ranitidine loss in 24 hr at 22°C in light. About 12% loss in 48 hr	1921	C
TPN #247[d]		GL	72 mg	2% ranitidine loss in 14 days at 4°C	501	C

[a] Tested in PVC containers.

[b] Tested in polyethylene and glass containers.

[c] Tested in ethylene vinyl acetate containers.

[d] Refer to Appendix for the composition of parenteral nutrition solutions. TNA indicates a 3-in-1 admixture, and TPN indicates a 2-in-1 admixture.

Additive Compatibility

Ranitidine HCl

Test Drug	Mfr	Conc/L or %	Mfr	Conc/L or %	Test Solution	Remarks	Ref	C/I
Acetazolamide sodium		5 g	GL	50 mg and 2 g	D5W	Physically compatible. Ranitidine stable for 24 hr at 25°C. Acetazolamide not tested	1515	C
Amikacin sulfate	BR	1 g	GL	100 mg	D5W	Physically compatible for 24 hr at ambient temperature in light	1151	C
Amikacin sulfate		2.5 g	GL	50 mg and 2 g	D5W	Physically compatible. Ranitidine stable for 24 hr at 25°C. Amikacin not tested	1515	C
Aminophylline	ES	500 mg and 2 g	GL	50 mg and 2 g	D5W, NS[a]	Physically compatible. 4% or less ranitidine loss in 24 hr at room temperature in light. Aminophylline not tested	1361	C
Aminophylline	ES	0.5 and 2 g	GL	50 mg and 2 g	D5W, NS[a]	Visually compatible. Little loss of either drug in 48 hr at room temperature	1802	C
Amphotericin B	SQ	200 mg	GL	100 mg	D5W	Color change and particle formation	1151	I
Ampicillin sodium		2 g	GL	100 mg	D5W	Physically compatible for 24 hr at ambient temperature under fluorescent light. Ampicillin instability is determining factor	1151	?
Ampicillin sodium		1 g	GL	50 mg and 2 g	NS	Physically compatible. Ranitidine stable for 24 hr at 25°C. Ampicillin not tested	1515	C
Atracurium besylate	BW	500 mg		500 mg	D5W	Atracurium unstable due to high pH	1694	I
Cefazolin sodium		2 g	GL	100 mg	D5W	Color change within 24 hr	1151	?
Cefazolin sodium		1 g	GL	50 mg and 2 g	D5W	Ranitidine stable for only 6 hr at 25°C. Cefazolin not tested	1515	I
Cefoxitin sodium		10 g	GL	50 mg and 2 g	D5W	Ranitidine stable for only 4 hr at 25°C. Cefoxitin not tested	1515	I
Ceftazidime	GL	10 g	GL	500 mg	D2.5½S	8% ranitidine loss in 4 hr and 37% loss in 24 hr at 22°C	1632	I
Cefuroxime sodium	GL	1.5 g	GL	100 mg	D5W	Color change in 24 hr at ambient temperature in light	1151	?
Cefuroxime sodium		6 g	GL	50 mg and 2 g	D5W	Ranitidine stable for only 6 hr at 25°C. Cefuroxime not tested	1515	I
Chloramphenicol sodium succinate		2 g	GL	100 mg	D5W	Physically compatible for 24 hr at ambient temperature	1151	C

Additive Compatibility (Cont.)

Test Drug	Mfr	Conc/L or %	Mfr	Conc/L or %	Test Solution	Remarks	Ref	C/I
Chlorothiazide sodium		5 g	GL	50 mg and 2 g	D5W	Physically compatible. Ranitidine stable for 24 hr at 25°C. Chlorothiazide not tested	1515	C
Ciprofloxacin	BAY	2 g	GL	500 mg and 1 g	NS	Visually compatible. Little ciprofloxacin loss in 24 hr at 25°C. Ranitidine not tested	1934	C
Clindamycin phosphate	UP	1.2 g	GL	100 mg	D5W	Color change and gas formation	1151	I
Clindamycin phosphate		1.2 g	GL	50 mg and 2 g	D5W, NS	Physically compatible. Ranitidine stable for 24 hr at 25°C. Clindamycin not tested	1515	C
Colistimethate sodium		1.5 g	GL	50 mg and 2 g	D5W	Physically compatible. Ranitidine stable for 24 hr at 25°C. Colistimethate not tested	1515	C
Dexamethasone sodium phosphate		40 mg	GL	50 mg and 2 g	D5W	Physically compatible. Ranitidine stable for 24 hr at 25°C. Dexamethasone not tested	1515	C
Digoxin		2.5 mg	GL	50 mg and 2 g	D5W	Physically compatible. Ranitidine stable for 24 hr at 25°C. Digoxin not tested	1515	C
Dobutamine HCl	LI	250 mg and 1 g	GL	2 g	D5W, NS[a]	Physically compatible. No ranitidine loss in 48 hr at room temperature in light. Dobutamine not tested	1361	C
Dobutamine HCl	LI	250 mg and 1 g	GL	50 mg	D5W[a]	Physically compatible. 7% ranitidine loss in 48 hr at room temperature in light. Dobutamine not tested	1361	C
Dobutamine HCl	LI	250 mg and 1 g	GL	50 mg	NS[a]	Physically compatible. No ranitidine loss in 48 hr at room temperature in light. Dobutamine not tested	1361	C
Dobutamine HCl	LI	0.25 and 1 g	GL	50 mg and 2 g	D5W, NS[a]	Visually compatible. Little loss of either drug in 48 hr at room temperature	1802	C
Dopamine HCl	ES	400 mg and 3.2 g	GL	50 mg and 2 g	D5W, NS[a]	Physically compatible. 6% ranitidine loss in 48 hr at room temperature in light. Dopamine not tested	1361	C
Dopamine HCl	ES	0.4 and 3.2 g	GL	50 mg and 2 g	D5W, NS[a]	Visually compatible. No dopamine and 7% ranitidine loss in 48 hr at room temperature	1802	C
Doxycycline hyclate	PF	200 mg	GL	100 mg	D5W	Physically compatible for 24 hr at ambient temperature in light	1151	C
Epinephrine HCl		50 mg	GL	50 mg and 2 g	D5W	Physically compatible. Ranitidine stable for 24 hr at 25°C. Epinephrine not tested	1515	C
Erythromycin lactobionate		5 g	GL	50 mg and 2 g	NS	Physically compatible. Ranitidine stable for 24 hr at 25°C. Erythromycin not tested	1515	C
Ethacrynate sodium		500 mg	GL	50 mg and 2 g	D5W	Ranitidine stable for only 6 hr at 25°C. Ethacrynate not tested	1515	I
Fat emulsion, intravenous	KV	10%	GL	50 and 100 mg		Physically compatible. 4% or less ranitidine loss in 48 hr at 25°C in light or dark	1360	C
Floxacillin sodium	BE	20 g	GL	500 mg	NS	Physically compatible for 72 hr at 15 and 30°C	1479	C
Fluconazole with ondansetron HCl	RR GL	2 g 100 mg	GL	500 mg	[a]	Visually compatible with no loss of any drug in 4 hr	1730	C
Flumazenil	RC	20 mg	GL	300 mg	D5W[a]	Visually compatible. 3% flumazenil loss in 24 hr at 23°C in light. Ranitidine not tested	1710	C
Furosemide	HO	1 g	GL	500 mg	NS	Physically compatible for 72 hr at 15 and 30°C	1479	C
Furosemide		400 mg	GL	50 mg and 2 g	D5W	Physically compatible. Ranitidine stable for 24 hr at 25°C. Furosemide not tested	1515	C

Additive Compatibility (Cont.)

Test Drug	Mfr	Conc/L or %	Mfr	Conc/L or %	Test Solution	Remarks	Ref	C/I
Gentamicin sulfate		160 mg	GL	100 mg	D5W	Physically compatible for 24 hr at ambient temperature in light	1151	C
Gentamicin sulfate		80 mg	GL	50 mg and 2 g	D5W, NS	Physically compatible. Ranitidine stable for 24 hr at 25°C. Gentamicin not tested	1515	C
Heparin sodium	ES	10,000 and 40,000 units	GL	2 g	D5W, NS[a]	Physically compatible. 2% ranitidine loss in 48 hr at room temperature in light. Heparin not tested	1361	C
Heparin sodium	ES	10,000 and 40,000 units	GL	50 mg	NS[a]	Physically compatible. No ranitidine loss in 48 hr at room temperature in light. Heparin not tested	1361	C
Heparin sodium	ES	10,000 and 40,000 units	GL	50 mg	D5W[a]	Physically compatible. 7% ranitidine loss in 24 hr and 12% loss in 48 hr at room temperature in light. Heparin not tested	1361	C
Insulin, regular	LI	1000 units	GL	600 mg	NS[a]	Visually compatible. Little ranitidine loss in 24 hr at ambient temperature but insulin losses of 9% in 4 hr and 14% in 24 hr, presumably due to sorption	2079	I
Isoproterenol HCl		20 mg	GL	50 mg and 2 g	D5W	Physically compatible. Ranitidine stable for 24 hr at 25°C. Isoproterenol not tested	1515	C
Lidocaine HCl	AST	1 and 8 g	GL	50 mg and 2 g	D5W, NS[a]	Physically compatible. 3% ranitidine loss in 24 hr at room temperature in light. Lidocaine not tested	1361	C
Lidocaine HCl		2.5 g	GL	50 mg and 2 g	D5W	Physically compatible. Ranitidine stable for 24 hr at 25°C. Lidocaine not tested	1515	C
Lidocaine HCl	AST	1 and 8 g	GL	50 mg and 2 g	D5W, NS[a]	Visually compatible. Little loss of either drug in 48 hr at room temperature	1802	C
Lincomycin HCl		2.4 g	GL	50 mg and 2 g	D5W	Physically compatible. Ranitidine stable for 24 hr at 25°C. Lincomycin not tested	1515	C
Meropenem	ZEN	1 and 20 g	GL	100 mg	NS	Visually compatible for 4 hr at room temperature	1994	C
Methylprednisolone sodium succinate	UP	40 mg	GL	50 mg	D5W[a]	Visually compatible with 7% ranitidine loss and no methylprednisolone loss in 48 hr at room temperature	1802	C
Methylprednisolone sodium succinate	UP	2 g	GL	50 mg	D5W[a]	Visually compatible with 6% ranitidine loss and 10% methylprednisolone loss in 48 hr at room temperature	1802	C
Methylprednisolone sodium succinate	UP	40 mg and 2 g	GL	2 g	D5W[a]	Visually compatible with no loss of either drug in 48 hr at room temperature	1802	C
Methylprednisolone sodium succinate	UP	40 mg and 2 g	GL	50 mg and 2 g	NS[a]	Visually compatible with no ranitidine loss and about 10% methylprednisolone loss in 48 hr at room temperature	1802	C
Metoclopramide HCl	SZ	185 mg	GSK	926 mg	NS	Visually compatible for up to 72 hr at room temperature (about 25°C)	3496	C
Midazolam HCl	RC	50 and 250 mg	GL	400 mg	NS	Visually compatible for 4 hr	355	C
Norepinephrine bitartrate	WI	4 and 8 mg	GL	50 mg	D5W, NS[a]	Physically compatible. 2 to 6% ranitidine loss in 48 hr at room temperature in light. Norepinephrine not tested	1361	C
Norepinephrine bitartrate		4 mg	GL	50 mg	D5W	Physically compatible. Ranitidine stable for 24 hr at 25°C. Norepinephrine not tested	1515	C
Norepinephrine bitartrate	RC	4 and 8 mg	GL	50 mg	D5W[a]	Visually compatible. 5 to 7% ranitidine loss and little norepinephrine loss in 48 hr at room temperature	1802	C
Norepinephrine bitartrate	RC	4 mg	GL	2 g	D5W[a]	Visually compatible. 7% norepinephrine loss in 4 hr and 13% in 12 hr at room temperature. No ranitidine loss in 48 hr	1802	I

Additive Compatibility (Cont.)

Test Drug	Mfr	Conc/L or %	Mfr	Conc/L or %	Test Solution	Remarks	Ref	C/I
Norepinephrine bitartrate	RC	8 mg	GL	2 g	D5W[a]	Visually compatible. 6% norepinephrine loss in 12 hr and 11% in 24 hr at room temperature. No ranitidine loss in 48 hr	1802	I
Ondansetron HCl with fluconazole	GL RR	100 mg 2 g	GL	500 mg	[a]	Visually compatible with no loss of any drug in 4 hr	1730	C
Penicillin G potassium		24 million units	GL	50 mg and 2 g	D5W, NS	Physically compatible. Ranitidine stable for 24 hr at 25°C. Penicillin not tested	1515	C
Penicillin G sodium		2.4 million units	GL	100 mg	D5W	Physically compatible for 24 hr at ambient temperature in light	1151	C
Phytonadione		100 mg	GL	50 mg and 2 g	D5W	Ranitidine stable for only 6 hr at 25°C. Phytonadione not tested	1515	I
Polymyxin B sulfate		1 million units	GL	50 mg and 2 g	D5W	Physically compatible. Ranitidine stable for 24 hr at 25°C. Polymyxin B not tested	1515	C
Potassium chloride	LY	10 and 60 mEq	GL	2 g	D5W, NS[a]	Physically compatible. 2% ranitidine loss in 48 hr at room temperature in light	1361	C
Potassium chloride	LY	10 and 60 mEq	GL	50 mg	NS[a]	Physically compatible. No ranitidine loss in 48 hr at room temperature in light	1361	C
Potassium chloride	LY	10 and 60 mEq	GL	50 mg	D5W[a]	Physically compatible. 7% ranitidine loss in 48 hr at room temperature in light	1361	C
Potassium chloride		80 mEq	GL	50 mg and 2 g	D5S, D5W, NS	Physically compatible. Ranitidine stable for 24 hr at 25°C	1515	C
Protamine sulfate		500 mg	GL	50 mg and 2 g	D5W	Physically compatible. Ranitidine stable for 24 hr at 25°C. Protamine not tested	1515	C
Quinidine gluconate		3.2 g	GL	50 mg and 2 g	D5W	Physically compatible. Ranitidine stable for 24 hr at 25°C. Quinidine not tested	1515	C
Sodium bicarbonate		5%				Stable for 48 hr at room temperature	3497, 3498	C
Sodium nitroprusside	RC	50 and 400 mg	GL	2 g	D5W, NS[a]	Physically compatible. No ranitidine loss in 48 hr at room temperature light protected. Nitroprusside not tested	1361	C
Sodium nitroprusside	RC	50 and 400 mg	GL	50 mg	NS[a]	Physically compatible. No ranitidine loss in 48 hr at room temperature light protected. Nitroprusside not tested	1361	C
Sodium nitroprusside	RC	50 and 400 mg	GL	50 mg	D5W[a]	Physically compatible with 7% or less ranitidine loss in 48 hr protected from light. Nitroprusside not tested	1361	C
Sodium nitroprusside		50 mg and 1 g	GL	50 mg and 2 g	D5W, NS	Physically compatible. Both drugs stable for 48 hr at room temperature protected from light	1515	C
Sodium nitroprusside		100 mg	GL	50 mg and 2 g	D5W	Physically compatible. Ranitidine stable for 24 hr at 25°C. Sodium nitroprusside not tested	1515	C
Sodium nitroprusside	RC	50 and 400 mg	GL	50 mg and 2 g	D5W[a]	Visually compatible. 7% ranitidine and 8% nitroprusside loss in 48 hr at room temperature protected from light	1802	C
Sodium nitroprusside	RC	50 and 400 mg	GL	50 mg and 2 g	NS[a]	Visually compatible. No loss of either drug in 48 hr at room temperature protected from light	1802	C
Tobramycin sulfate	DI	200 mg	GL	100 mg	D5W	Physically compatible for 24 hr at ambient temperature in light	1151	C
Tramadol HCl	GRU	400 mg	AB	0.5 g	NS	Visually compatible with little or no tramadol loss in 24 hr at room temperature	2652	C

Additive Compatibility (Cont.)

Test Drug	Mfr	Conc/L or %	Mfr	Conc/L or %	Test Solution	Remarks	Ref	C/I
Vancomycin HCl	DI	1 g	GL	100 mg	D5W	Physically compatible for 24 hr at ambient temperature in light	1151	C
Vancomycin HCl		5 g	GL	50 mg and 2 g	D5W	Physically compatible. Ranitidine stable for 24 hr at 25°C. Vancomycin not tested	1515	C
Zidovudine	GSK	2 g	GSK	500 mg	NS	Physically compatible with no loss of either drug in 24 hr at 4 and 23°C	2523	C
Zidovudine	GSK	2 g	GSK	500 mg	D5W	Physically compatible. Up to 8% ranitidine loss at 23°C and 2% at 4°C in 24 hr. Zidovudine losses of 5 to 6% in 24 hr at 4 and 23°C	2523	C

ª Tested in PVC containers.

Drugs in Syringe Compatibility

Ranitidine HCl

Test Drug	Mfr	Amt	Mfr	Amt	Remarks	Ref	C/I
Atropine sulfate	GL	0.4 mg/1 mL	GL	50 mg/2 mL	Physically compatible for 1 hr at 25°C	978	C
Chlorpromazine HCl	RP	25 mg/1 mL	GL	50 mg/2 mL	Physically compatible for 1 hr at 25°C	978	C
Chlorpromazine HCl	RP	25 mg	GL	50 mg/5 mL	Gas formation	1151	I
Cyclizine lactate	CA	50 mg/1 mL	GL	50 mg/2 mL	Physically compatible for 1 hr at 25°C	978	C
Dexamethasone sodium phosphate	ME	4 mg	GL	50 mg/5 mL	Physically compatible for 4 hr at ambient temperature under fluorescent light	1151	C
Diazepam	RC	10 mg/2 mL	GL	50 mg/2 mL	Immediate white haze that disappears following vortex mixing	978	?
Diazepam		10 mg	GL	50 mg/5 mL	Physically compatible for 4 hr at ambient temperature under fluorescent light	1151	C
Dimenhydrinate	HR	50 mg/1 mL	GL	50 mg/2 mL	Physically compatible for 1 hr at 25°C	978	C
Diphenhydramine HCl	PD	50 mg/1 mL	GL	50 mg/2 mL	Physically compatible for 1 hr at 25°C	978	C
Dobutamine HCl	LI	25 mg	GL	50 mg/5 mL	Physically compatible for 4 hr at ambient temperature under fluorescent light	1151	C
Dopamine HCl		40 mg	GL	50 mg/5 mL	Physically compatible for 4 hr at ambient temperature under fluorescent light	1151	C
Fentanyl citrate	JN	0.1 mg/2 mL	GL	50 mg/2 mL	Physically compatible for 1 hr at 25°C	978	C
Glycopyrrolate	RB	0.2 mg/1 mL	GL	50 mg/2 mL	Physically compatible for 1 hr at 25°C	978	C
Heparin sodium		2500 units/1 mL	GL	50 mg/5 mL	Visually compatible for at least 5 min	1053	C
Hydromorphone HCl	PE	2 mg/1 mL	GL	50 mg/2 mL	Physically compatible for 1 hr at 25°C	978	C
Hydroxyzine HCl	PF	50 mg/1 mL	GL	50 mg/2 mL	Immediate white haze that disappears following vortex mixing	978	I
Lorazepam	WY	4 mg/1 mL	GL	50 mg/2 mL	Poor mixing and layering, which disappears following vortex mixing	978	?
Meperidine HCl	WI	100 mg/1 mL	GL	50 mg/2 mL	Physically compatible for 1 hr at 25°C	978	C
Methotrimeprazine HCl	RP	25 mg/1 mL	GL	50 mg/2 mL	Immediate white turbidity	978	I
Metoclopramide HCl	RB	10 mg/1 mL	GL	50 mg/2 mL	Physically compatible for 1 hr at 25°C	978	C
Midazolam HCl	RC	5 mg/1 mL	GL	50 mg/2 mL	White precipitate forms immediately	1145	I

Drugs in Syringe Compatibility (Cont.)

Test Drug	Mfr	Amt	Mfr	Amt	Remarks	Ref	C/I
Morphine sulfate	AH	10 mg/1 mL	GL	50 mg/2 mL	Physically compatible for 1 hr at 25°C	978	C
Nalbuphine HCl	EN	10 mg/1 mL	GL	50 mg/2 mL	Physically compatible for 1 hr at 25°C	978	C
Pantoprazole sodium	a	4 mg/1 mL		25 mg/1 mL	Possible precipitate within 4 hr	2574	I
Pentazocine lactate	WI	60 mg/2 mL	GL	50 mg/2 mL	Physically compatible for 1 hr at 25°C	978	C
Pentobarbital sodium	AB	100 mg	GL	50 mg/5 mL	Precipitates immediately	1151	I
Phenobarbital sodium	AB	120 mg/1 mL	GL	50 mg/2 mL	Immediate white haze	978	I
Prochlorperazine edisylate	RP	10 mg/2 mL	GL	50 mg/2 mL	Physically compatible for 1 hr at 25°C	978	C
Promethazine HCl	RP	25 mg/1 mL	GL	50 mg/2 mL	Physically compatible for 1 hr at 25°C	978	C
Promethazine HCl	RP	25 mg	GL	50 mg/5 mL	Physically compatible for 4 hr	1151	C
Scopolamine HBr	AB	0.4 mg/1 mL	GL	50 mg/2 mL	Physically compatible for 1 hr at 25°C	978	C
Scopolamine HBr		0.5 mg	GL	50 mg/5 mL	Physically compatible for 4 hr at ambient temperature under fluorescent light	1151	C

a Test performed using the formulation WITHOUT edetate disodium.

Y-Site Injection Compatibility (1:1 Mixture)

Ranitidine HCl

Test Drug	Mfr	Conc	Mfr	Conc	Remarks	Ref	C/I
Acetaminophen	CAD	10 mg/mL	BED	1 mg/mL[c]	Physically compatible for 4 hr at 23°C	2901, 2902	C
Acyclovir sodium	BW	5 mg/mL[a]	GL	1 mg/mL[a]	Physically compatible for 4 hr at 25°C	1157	C
Aldesleukin	CHI	33,800 I.U./mL[a]	AB	1 mg/mL[c]	Visually compatible with little or no loss of aldesleukin activity	1857	C
Allopurinol sodium	BW	3 mg/mL[b]	GL	2 mg/mL[b]	Physically compatible for 4 hr at 22°C	1686	C
Amifostine	USB	10 mg/mL[a]	GL	2 mg/mL[a]	Physically compatible for 4 hr at 23°C	1845	C
Aminophylline	LY	4 mg/mL[a]	GL	0.5 mg/mL	Physically compatible for 24 hr	1323	C
Amsacrine	NCI	1 mg/mL[a]	GL	2 mg/mL[a]	Visually compatible for 4 hr at 22°C	1381	C
Anidulafungin	VIC	0.5 mg/mL[a]	GSK	2 mg/mL[a]	Physically compatible for 4 hr at 23°C	2617	C
Atracurium besylate	BW	0.5 mg/mL[a]	GL	0.5 mg/mL[a]	Physically compatible for 24 hr at 28°C	1337	C
Aztreonam	SQ	16.7 mg/mL[b]	GL	1 mg/mL[b]	No loss of either drug in 4 hr at 22°C	1632	C
Aztreonam	SQ	40 mg/mL[a]	GL	2 mg/mL[a]	Physically compatible for 4 hr at 23°C	1758	C
Bivalirudin	TMC	5 mg/mL[a]	GW	2 mg/mL[a]	Physically compatible for 4 hr at 23°C	2373	C
Cangrelor tetrasodium	TMC	1 mg/mL[b]		2[b] and 5[b] mg/mL	Physically compatible for 4 hr	3243	C
Cefazolin sodium	FUJ	20 mg/mL[b]	GL	1 mg/mL[b]	Visually compatible with little loss of either drug in 4 hr at 25°C	2259	C
Cefazolin sodium	FUJ	20 mg/mL[b]	GL	1 mg/mL[b]	Visually compatible with no cefazolin loss and 3% ranitidine loss in 4 hr	2362	C
Cefoxitin sodium	BAN	20 mg/mL[b]	GL	1 mg/mL[b]	Visually compatible. No cefoxitin loss. Under 8% ranitidine loss in 4 hr at 25°C	2259	C
Cefoxitin sodium	BAN	20 mg/mL[b]	GL	1 mg/mL[b]	Visually compatible with no cefoxitin loss and 7% ranitidine loss in 4 hr	2362	C

Y-Site Injection Compatibility (1:1 Mixture) (Cont.)

Test Drug	Mfr	Conc	Mfr	Conc	Remarks	Ref	C/I
Ceftaroline fosamil	FOR	2.22 mg/mL[a b d]	BED	2 mg/mL[a b d]	Physically compatible for 4 hr at 23°C	2826	C
Ceftazidime	GL	20 mg/mL[a]	GL	1 mg/mL[b]	8% ranitidine loss and no ceftazidime loss in 4 hr at 22°C	1632	C
Ceftolozane sulfate–tazobactam sodium	CUB	10 mg/mL[e k]	ZY	2.5 mg/mL[e]	Physically compatible for 2 hr	3262	C
Ciprofloxacin	MI	2 mg/mL[e]	GL	0.5 mg/mL[e]	Visually compatible for 24 hr at 24°C	1655	C
Cisatracurium besylate	GW	0.1, 2, 5 mg/mL[a]	GL	2 mg/mL[a]	Physically compatible for 4 hr at 23°C	2074	C
Cladribine	ORT	0.015[b] and 0.5[f] mg/mL	GL	2 mg/mL[b]	Physically compatible for 4 hr at 23°C	1969	C
Clarithromycin	AB	4 mg/mL[a]	GW	5 mg/mL[a]	Visually compatible for 72 hr at both 30 and 17°C	2174	C
Cloxacillin sodium	SMX	100 mg/mL	GSK	25 mg/mL	Physically compatible for up to 4 hr at room temperature	3245	C
Dexmedetomidine HCl	AB	4 mcg/mL[b]	GW	2 mg/mL[b]	Physically compatible for 4 hr at 23°C	2383	C
Diltiazem HCl	MMD	1[b] and 5 mg/mL	GL	25 mg/mL	Visually compatible	1807	C
Diltiazem HCl	MMD	5 mg/mL	GL	0.5[c] and 1[b] mg/mL	Visually compatible	1807	C
Diltiazem HCl	MMD	1 mg/mL[a]	GL	1 mg/mL[a]	Visually compatible for 4 hr at 27°C	2062	C
Dobutamine HCl	LI	1 mg/mL[a]	GL	0.5 mg/mL[n]	Physically compatible for 24 hr	1323	C
Dobutamine HCl	LI	4 mg/mL[a]	GL	1 mg/mL[a]	Visually compatible for 4 hr at 27°C	2062	C
Docetaxel	RPR	0.9 mg/mL[a]	GL	2 mg/mL[a]	Physically compatible for 4 hr at 23°C	2224	C
Dopamine HCl	ES	1.6 mg/mL[a]	GL	0.5 mg/mL[n]	Physically compatible for 24 hr	1323	C
Dopamine HCl	AB	3.2 mg/mL[a]	GL	1 mg/mL[a]	Visually compatible for 4 hr at 27°C	2062	C
Doripenem	JJ	5 mg/mL[a b]	BED	2 mg/mL[a b]	Physically compatible for 4 hr at 23°C	2743	C
Doxapram HCl	RB	2 mg/mL[a]	GSK	5 mg/mL[a]	Visually compatible for 4 hr at 23°C	2470	C
Doxorubicin HCl liposomal	SEQ	0.4 mg/mL[a]	GL	2 mg/mL[a]	Physically compatible for 4 hr at 23°C	2087	C
Enalaprilat	MSD	0.05 mg/mL[b]	GL	0.5 mg/mL[a]	Physically compatible for 24 hr at room temperature under fluorescent light	1355	C
Epinephrine HCl	AB	0.02 mg/mL[a]	GL	1 mg/mL[a]	Visually compatible for 4 hr at 27°C	2062	C
Esmolol HCl	DCC	10 mg/mL[a]	GL	0.5 mg/mL[a]	Physically compatible for 24 hr at 22°C	1169	C
Etoposide phosphate	BR	5 mg/mL[a]	GL	2 mg/mL[a]	Physically compatible for 4 hr at 23°C	2218	C
Fenoldopam mesylate	AB	80 mcg/mL[b]	GW	2 mg/mL[b]	Physically compatible for 4 hr at 23°C	2467	C
Fentanyl citrate	ES	0.05 mg/mL	GL	1 mg/mL[a]	Visually compatible for 4 hr at 27°C	2062	C
Filgrastim	AMG	30 mcg/mL[a]	GL	2 mg/mL[a]	Physically compatible for 4 hr at 22°C	1687	C
Fluconazole	RR	2 mg/mL[b]	GL	0.5 and 2 mg/mL[a]	Visually compatible. No loss of either drug in 4 hr	1730	C
Fludarabine phosphate	BX	1 mg/mL[a]	GL	2 mg/mL[a]	Visually compatible for 4 hr at 22°C	1439	C
Foscarnet sodium	AST	24 mg/mL	GL	2 mg/mL[e]	Physically compatible for 24 hr at 25°C under fluorescent light	1393	C
Furosemide	AMR	10 mg/mL	GL	1 mg/mL[a]	Visually compatible for 4 hr at 27°C	2062	C
Gallium nitrate	FUJ	1 mg/mL[b]	GL	2.5 mg/mL[b]	Visually compatible for 24 hr at 25°C	1673	C

Y-Site Injection Compatibility (1:1 Mixture) (Cont.)

Test Drug	Mfr	Conc	Mfr	Conc	Remarks	Ref	C/I
Gemcitabine HCl	LI	10 mg/mL[b]	GL	2 mg/mL[b]	Physically compatible for 4 hr at 23°C	2226	C
Granisetron HCl	SKB	0.05 mg/mL[a]	GL	2 mg/mL[a]	Physically compatible for 4 hr at 23°C	2000	C
Heparin sodium	LY	50 units/mL[a]	GL	0.5 mg/mL	Physically compatible for 24 hr	1323	C
Heparin sodium	TR	50 units/mL	GL	1 mg/mL	Visually compatible for 4 hr at 25°C	1793	C
Heparin sodium	ES	100 units/mL[a]	GL	1 mg/mL[a]	Visually compatible for 4 hr at 27°C	2062	C
Hetastarch in lactated electrolyte	AB	6%	GW	2 mg/mL[a]	Physically compatible for 4 hr at 23°C	2339	C
Hetastarch in sodium chloride 0.9%	DCC	6%	GL	0.5 mg/mL[n]	Visually compatible for 4 hr at room temperature	1313	C
Hetastarch in sodium chloride 0.9%	DCC	6%	GL	0.5 mg/mL	Barely visible particles appeared and disappeared	1314	I
Hetastarch in sodium chloride 0.9%	DCC	6%	GL	0.5 mg/mL	Small white particles and white fiber	1315	I
Hydromorphone HCl	KN	1 mg/mL	GL	1 mg/mL[a]	Visually compatible for 4 hr at 27°C	2062	C
Idarubicin HCl	AD	1 mg/mL[b]	GL	1 mg/mL[a]	Visually compatible for 24 hr at 25°C	1525	C
Insulin, regular	LI	1 unit/mL[b]	GL	1 mg/mL[b]	Visually compatible. Little loss of ranitidine in 4 hr but insulin losses of 9% in 1 hr and 20% in 4 hr, presumably due to sorption	2079	I
Isavuconazonium sulfate	ASP	1.5 mg/mL[e]	ZY	2.5 mg/mL[e]	Physically compatible for 2 hr	3263	C
Labetalol HCl	SC	1 mg/mL[a]	GL	0.5 mg/mL[a]	Physically compatible for 24 hr at 18°C	1171	C
Labetalol HCl	GL	1 mg/mL[a]	GL	0.6 mg/mL[a]	Visually compatible. Little ranitidine and 5% labetalol loss in 4 hr at room temperature	1762	C
Labetalol HCl	AH	2 mg/mL[a]	GL	1 mg/mL[a]	Visually compatible for 4 hr at 27°C	2062	C
Linezolid	PHU	2 mg/mL	GW	2 mg/mL[a]	Physically compatible for 4 hr at 23°C	2264	C
Lorazepam	WY	0.33 mg/mL[b]	GL	0.5 mg/mL	Visually compatible for 24 hr at 22°C	1855	C
Lorazepam	WY	0.5 mg/mL[a]	GL	1 mg/mL[a]	Visually compatible for 4 hr at 27°C	2062	C
Melphalan HCl	BW	0.1 mg/mL[b]	GL	2 mg/mL[b]	Physically compatible for 3 hr at 22°C	1557	C
Meperidine HCl	WY	10 mg/mL[b]	GL	0.5 mg/mL[c]	Physically compatible for 1 hr at 25°C	1338	C
Meropenem		50 mg/mL	SZ	25 mg/mL	Physically compatible for 4 hr at room temperature	3538	C
Meropenem–vaborbactam	TMC	8 mg/mL[b l]	ZY	2.5 mg/mL[b]	Physically compatible for 3 hr at 20 to 25°C	3380	C
Midazolam HCl	RC	5 mg/mL	GL	0.5 mg/mL	Visually compatible for 24 hr at 22°C	1855	C
Midazolam HCl	RC	2 mg/mL[a]	GL	1 mg/mL[a]	Visually compatible for 4 hr at 27°C	2062	C
Milrinone lactate	SW	0.2 mg/mL[a]	GL	1 mg/mL[a]	Visually compatible for 4 hr at 27°C	2062	C
Milrinone lactate	SW	0.4 mg/mL[a]	GL	2 mg/mL[a]	Visually compatible. Little loss of either drug in 4 hr at 23°C	2214	C
Morphine sulfate	ES	1 mg/mL[b]	GL	0.5 mg/mL[c]	Physically compatible for 1 hr at 25°C	1338	C
Morphine sulfate	SCN	2 mg/mL[a]	GL	1 mg/mL[a]	Visually compatible for 4 hr at 27°C	2062	C
Nicardipine HCl	DCC	0.1 mg/mL[a]	GL	0.5 mg/mL[a]	Visually compatible for 24 hr at room temperature	235	C
Nicardipine HCl	WY	1 mg/mL[a]	GL	1 mg/mL[a]	Visually compatible for 4 hr at 27°C	2062	C
Nitroglycerin	SO	0.2 mg/mL[a]	GL	0.5 mg/mL	Physically compatible for 24 hr	1323	C

Y-Site Injection Compatibility (1:1 Mixture) (Cont.)

Test Drug	Mfr	Conc	Mfr	Conc	Remarks	Ref	C/I
Nitroglycerin	AB	0.4 mg/mL[a]	GL	1 mg/mL[a]	Visually compatible for 4 hr at 27°C	2062	C
Norepinephrine bitar-trate	AB	0.128 mg/mL[a]	GL	1 mg/mL[a]	Visually compatible for 4 hr at 27°C	2062	C
Ondansetron HCl	GL	1 mg/mL[b]	GL	2 mg/mL[a]	Visually compatible for 4 hr at 22°C	1365	C
Ondansetron HCl	GL	0.03, 0.1, 0.3 mg/mL[a]	GL	0.5 mg/mL[a]	Visually compatible with no loss of either drug in 4 hr	1730	C
Ondansetron HCl	GL	0.03, 0.1, 0.3 mg/mL[a]	GL	2 mg/mL[a]	Visually compatible with no loss of either drug in 4 hr	1730	C
Ondansetron HCl with paclitaxel	GL BR	0.3 mg/mL[a] 1.2 mg/mL[a]	GL	2 mg/mL[a]	Visually compatible with no loss of any drug in 4 hr at 23°C	1741	C
Oritavancin diphos-phate	TAR	0.8, 1.2, and 2 mg/mL[a]	BED	2 mg/mL[a]	Visually compatible for 4 hr at 20 to 24°C	2928	C
Oxaliplatin	SS	0.5 mg/mL[a]	GW	2 mg/mL[a]	Physically compatible for 4 hr at 23°C	2566	C
Paclitaxel	NCI	1.2 mg/mL[a]		2 mg/mL[a]	Physically compatible for 4 hr at 22°C	1528	C
Paclitaxel	BR	0.3 and 1.2 mg/mL[a]	GL	0.5 and 2 mg/mL[a]	Visually compatible. No loss of either drug in 4 hr at 23°C	1741	C
Paclitaxel with ondansetron HCl	BR GL	1.2 mg/mL[a] 0.3 mg/mL[a]	GL	2 mg/mL[a]	Visually compatible with no loss of any drug in 4 hr at 23°C	1741	C
Pancuronium bromide	ES	0.05 mg/mL[a]	GL	0.5 mg/mL[a]	Physically compatible for 24 hr at 28°C	1337	C
Pemetrexed disodium	LI	20 mg/mL[b]	GSK	2 mg/mL[a]	Physically compatible for 4 hr at 23°C	2564	C
Piperacillin sodium–tazobactam sodium	LE[g]	40 mg/mL[a h]	GL	2 mg/mL[a]	Physically compatible for 4 hr at 22°C	1688	C
Piperacillin sodium–tazobactam sodium	LE[g]	80 mg/mL[b h]	GL	0.5 and 2 mg/mL[b]	Visually compatible. Little loss of any component in 4 hr at 23°C	1759	C
Piperacillin sodium–tazobactam sodium	LE[g]	40 mg/mL[b h]	GL	0.5 and 2 mg/mL[b]	Visually compatible. Little loss of ranitidine and tazobactam in 4 hr at 23°C. Piperacillin not tested	1759	C
Plazomicin sulfate	ACH	24 mg/mL[e]	ZY	2.5 mg/mL[e]	Physically compatible for 1 hr at 20 to 25°C	3432	C
Procainamide HCl	BA	4 mg/mL[a]	GL	0.5 mg/mL	Physically compatible for 24 hr	1323	C
Propofol	ZEN[m]	10 mg/mL	GL	2 mg/mL[a]	Physically compatible for 1 hr at 23°C	2066	C
Remifentanil HCl	GW	0.025 and 0.25 mg/mL[b]	GL	2 mg/mL[a]	Physically compatible for 4 hr at 23°C	2075	C
Sargramostim	IMM	10 mcg/mL[b]	GL	2 mg/mL[b]	Visually compatible for 4 hr at 22°C	1436	C
Sugammadex sodium	ME	100 mg/mL		25 mg/mL	Particles form in 1 hr	3111, 3115	I
Tacrolimus	FUJ	1 mg/mL[b]	GL	25 mg/mL	Visually compatible for 24 hr at 25°C	1630	C
Tedizolid phosphate	CUB	0.8 mg/mL[b]	ZY	2.5 mg/mL[b]	Physically compatible for 2 hr	3244	C
Telavancin HCl	ASP	7.5 mg/mL[a b d]	BED	2 mg/mL[a b d]	Physically compatible for 2 hr	2830	C
Teniposide	BR	0.1 mg/mL[a]	GL	2 mg/mL[a]	Physically compatible for 4 hr at 23°C	1725	C
Theophylline	TR	4 mg/mL	GL	1 mg/mL	Visually compatible for 6 hr at 25°C	1793	C
Thiotepa	IMM[i]	1 mg/mL[a]	GL	2 mg/mL[a]	Physically compatible for 4 hr at 23°C	1861	C
Tigecycline	WY	1 mg/mL[b]		0.6 mg/mL[b]	Physically compatible for 4 hr	2714	C
Tigecycline	ACD, FRK, WY	[e]			Stated to be compatible	2915, 3459, 3460	C

Y-Site Injection Compatibility (1:1 Mixture) (Cont.)

Test Drug	Mfr	Conc	Mfr	Conc	Remarks	Ref	C/I
TNA #218 to #226[j]			GL	2 mg/mL[a]	Visually compatible for 4 hr at 23°C	2215	C
TPN #189[j]			GL	2.5 mg/mL[b]	Visually compatible for 24 hr at 22°C	1767	C
TPN #203, #204[j]			GL	25 mg/mL	Visually compatible for 2 hr at 23°C	1974	C
TPN #212 to #215[j]			GL	2 mg/mL[a]	Physically compatible for 4 hr at 23°C	2109	C
Vecuronium bromide	OR	0.1 mg/mL[a]	GL	0.5 mg/mL[a]	Physically compatible for 24 hr at 28°C	1337	C
Vecuronium bromide	OR	1 mg/mL	GL	1 mg/mL[a]	Visually compatible for 4 hr at 27°C	2062	C
Vinorelbine tartrate	BW	1 mg/mL[b]	GL	2 mg/mL[b]	Physically compatible for 4 hr at 22°C	1558	C
Zidovudine	BW	4 mg/mL[a]	GL	1 mg/mL[a]	Physically compatible for 4 hr at 25°C	1193	C

[a] Tested in dextrose 5%.

[b] Tested in sodium chloride 0.9%.

[c] Tested in sodium chloride 0.45%.

[d] Tested in Ringer's injection, lactated.

[e] Tested in both dextrose 5% and sodium chloride 0.9%.

[f] Tested in bacteriostatic sodium chloride 0.9% preserved with benzyl alcohol 0.9%.

[g] Test performed using the formulation WITHOUT edetate disodium.

[h] Piperacillin component. Piperacillin in an 8:1 fixed-ratio concentration with tazobactam.

[i] Lyophilized formulation tested.

[j] Refer to Appendix for the composition of parenteral nutrition solutions. TNA indicates a 3-in-1 admixture, and TPN indicates a 2-in-1 admixture.

[k] Ceftolozane component. Ceftolozane in a 2:1 fixed-ratio concentration with tazobactam.

[l] Meropenem component. Meropenem in a 1:1 fixed-ratio concentration with vaborbactam.

[m] Test performed using the formulation WITH edetate disodium.

[n] Tested as the premixed infusion solution.

Selected Revisions May 1, 2020. © Copyright, October 1988.
American Society of Health-System Pharmacists, Inc.

Rasburicase
AHFS 44:00

Products

Rasburicase is available as a lyophilized powder in single-use vials containing 1.5 or 7.5 mg of the drug.[3135] Each 1.5-mg vial also contains mannitol 10.6 mg, L-alanine 15.9 mg, and dibasic sodium phosphate in the range of 12.6 to 14.3 mg.[3135] Each 7.5-mg vial also contains mannitol 53 mg, L-alanine 79.5 mg, and dibasic sodium phosphate in the range of 63 to 71.5 mg.[3135] Each 1.5- or 7.5-mg vial of rasburicase is packaged with an ampul of special diluent containing 1 or 5 mL of water for injection, respectively, and poloxamer 188 1 or 5 mg, respectively.[3135]

The 1.5- and 7.5-mg vials of rasburicase must be reconstituted with 1 and 5 mL of the provided special diluent, respectively, for a solution with a final rasburicase concentration of 1.5 mg/mL.[3135] Vials should be gently swirled until the contents are dissolved and should not be shaken or mixed so vigorously as to form a vortex.[3135] Reconstituted solutions should be visually inspected for particulate matter prior to administration; if particulate matter is present or discoloration occurs, the solution should be discarded.[3135] The appropriate dose of rasburicase should be withdrawn from the vial of reconstituted solution and further diluted in an infusion bag containing sodium chloride 0.9% to achieve a final total volume of 50 mL in the infusion bag.[3135]

Trade Name(s)

Elitek

Administration

Rasburicase is administered intravenously as an infusion over 30 minutes following dilution of the reconstituted solution.[3135] Rasburicase should be infused through a separate line, or, if a common infusion line is being used to administer other drugs in addition to rasburicase, the line should be flushed with at least 15 mL of sodium chloride 0.9% prior to and following infusion of rasburicase.[3135] Rasburicase should *not* be administered by bolus injection.[3135]

Stability

Rasburicase is a white to off-white powder.[3135] Intact vials of rasburicase and accompanying ampuls of special diluent should be stored at 2 to 8°C and protected from light and freezing.[3135]

The reconstituted solution or solutions diluted for infusion in sodium chloride 0.9% should be stored at 2 to 8°C; reconstituted and diluted solutions should be discarded 24 hours after reconstitution.[3135]

Filtration

Filters should not be used during reconstitution or infusion of rasburicase.[3135]

Compatibility Information

Solution Compatibility

Rasburicase

Test Soln Name	Mfr	Mfr	Conc/L or %	Remarks	Ref	C/I
Sodium chloride 0.9%		SAA		Stated to be stable for 24 hr at 2 to 8°C	3135	C

Y-Site Injection Compatibility (1:1 Mixture)

Rasburicase

Test Drug	Mfr	Conc	Mfr	Conc	Remarks	Ref	C/I
Blinatumomab	AMG	0.125 mcg/mL[a]	SAA	0.15 mg/mL[a]	Persistent particulate formation when blinatumomab is added to rasburicase; not observed when order of mixing was reversed	3405, 3417	?
Blinatumomab	AMG	0.375 mcg/mL[a]	SAA	0.15 mg/mL[a]	Flakes transiently appear when rasburicase is added to blinatumomab; not observed when order of mixing was reversed	3405, 3417	?

[a] Tested in sodium chloride 0.9%.

DOI: 10.37573/9781585286850.337

Remdesivir
AHFS 8:18.32

Products

Remdesivir is available in 2 different formulations: a lyophilized powder and a concentrate for injection.[3581] The lyophilized powder is available in single-dose (preservative-free) vials packaged under vacuum containing 100 mg of remdesivir and 3 g of betadex sulfobutyl ether sodium.[3581] Vials also may contain hydrochloric acid and/or sodium hydroxide for pH adjustment.[3581]

The contents of each 100-mg vial of lyophilized powder should be reconstituted only with 19 mL of sterile water for injection using an appropriately-sized syringe and needle; vials should be discarded if the vacuum does not draw the diluent into the vial.[3581] Immediately after adding the sterile water for injection, vials should be shaken for 30 seconds, then the contents allowed to settle for 2 to 3 minutes.[3581] If the contents are not completely dissolved, the vial should be shaken again for 30 seconds and the contents allowed to settle for 2 to 3 minutes.[3581] This procedure should be repeated as necessary until the contents of the vial are completely dissolved and a clear solution results.[3581] The vial should be discarded if the contents are not completely dissolved.[3581] The resulting reconstituted solution has a remdesivir concentration of 5 mg/mL.[3581] The reconstituted solution must be diluted in sodium chloride 0.9% prior to administration.[3581] The reconstituted solution should be visually inspected for particulate matter and discoloration prior to dilution.[3581] The reconstituted solution should be used to prepare the diluted solution for infusion.[3581]

For *adults and pediatric patients 12 years of age or older and weighing at least 40 kg*, loading and maintenance doses of remdesivir must be diluted in either 100- or 250-mL bags of sodium chloride 0.9% after first removing and discarding a volume of infusion fluid equal to the volume of the appropriate dose of the reconstituted solution to be added.[3581]

Remdesivir also is available as a 5-mg/mL concentrate for injection in single-dose (preservative-free) vials containing 20 mL of the concentrate for injection.[3581] Vials contain 6 g of betadex sulfobutyl ether sodium and water for injection; hydrochloric acid and/or sodium hydroxide also may be present to adjust the pH.[3581] The concentrate for injection must be diluted only in sodium chloride 0.9% prior to administration.[3581] Prior to dilution, the vials should be allowed to come to room temperature (20 to 25°C).[3581] Vials should be visually inspected to ensure that the container closure is free of defects and that the solution is free of particulate matter and discoloration.[3581]

For *adults and pediatric patients 12 years of age or older and weighing at least 40 kg*, loading and maintenance doses of remdesivir must be diluted in 250-mL bags of sodium chloride 0.9% after first removing and discarding a volume of infusion fluid equal to the volume of the appropriate dose of the concentrate for injection to be added.[3581] To withdraw the concentrate

for injection from the vial, the plunger rod of an appropriately sized syringe should be pulled back to fill the syringe with approximately 10 mL of air.[3581] The air should be injected into the vial above the level of the solution.[3581] The vial should then be inverted in order to withdraw the appropriate dose of the concentrate for injection; withdrawal of the final 5 mL of solution remaining in the vial requires more force.[3581] After adding the concentrate for injection to the infusion bag, the bag should be gently inverted 20 times to mix the solution; the bag should not be shaken.[3581]

Information on use of the drug in populations not described in the product labeling may be available at www.FDA.gov.

Trade Name(s)

Veklury

Administration

Remdesivir must be administered by intravenous infusion only; the drug should *not* be administered by any other route.[3581] Remdesivir solutions prepared as directed in sodium chloride 0.9% should be infused over 30 to 120 minutes.[3581]

Stability

The lyophilized formulation of remdesivir is a white to off-white to yellow powder that forms a clear solution upon reconstitution.[3581] Intact vials of remdesivir lyophilized powder should be stored below 30°C.[3581] The reconstituted solution should be used immediately after preparation to prepare the diluted solution for infusion.[3581]

Remdesivir concentrate for injection is a clear, colorless to yellow solution free of visible particulates.[3581] Intact vials of remdesivir concentrate for injection should be stored at 2 to 8°C; however, intact vials may be stored at room temperature (20 to 25°C) for up to 12 hours prior to dilution.[3581]

Because no preservatives are present in either formulation, any unused solution remaining in a vial after preparation of the diluted solution for infusion should be discarded.[3581] The diluted solution for infusion should be visually inspected for particulate matter and discoloration prior to administration; if particulate matter is present or discoloration occurs, the diluted solution for infusion should be discarded.[3581] Diluted solutions for infusion may be stored for up to 24 hours at room temperature (20 to 25°C) or 48 hours at 2 to 8°C; however, the manufacturer recommends always administering the diluted solution for infusion immediately after preparation when possible.[3581] The manufacturer also recommends that diluted solutions for infusion prepared with either formulation should be administered within the same day as dilution.[3581]

The manufacturer states that remdesivir should not be administered simultaneously with any other drugs.[3581]

DOI: 10.37573/9781585286850.338

Compatibility Information

Solution Compatibility

Remdesivir

Test Soln Name	Mfr	Mfr	Conc/L or %	Remarks	Ref	C/I
Sodium chloride 0.9%		GIL		Stated to be stable for 24 hr at 20 to 25°C and for 48 hr at 2 to 8°C	3581	C

Remifentanil Hydrochloride
AHFS 28:08.08

Products

Remifentanil hydrochloride is available as a lyophilized powder in single-dose (preservative-free) vials containing 1, 2, or 5 mg of remifentanil base present as the hydrochloride.[3463] Each vial also contains glycine 15 mg and hydrochloric acid for pH adjustment.[3463] The contents of the vials should be reconstituted using 1 mL of a compatible diluent for each milligram of remifentanil base; vials should be shaken well to dissolve the powder, yielding a reconstituted solution with an approximate remifentanil concentration of 1 mg/mL.[3463] The reconstituted solution should be further diluted in a compatible diluent to a recommended final remifentanil concentration of 20, 25, 50, or 250 mcg/mL prior to administration.[3463] Remifentanil hydrochloride should *not* be administered without dilution.[3463]

pH

The reconstituted solution has a pH ranging from 2.5 to 3.5.[3463]

Trade Name(s)

Ultiva

Administration

Remifentanil hydrochloride is administered intravenously only.[3463] Administration of the drug by the epidural or intrathecal route is contraindicated due to the presence of glycine in the formulation.[3463]

Single intravenous doses may be administered over 30 to 60 seconds.[3463] Remifentanil hydrochloride also may be administered by continuous intravenous infusion using an infusion device.[3463] The manufacturer recommends that injection or infusion of the drug be made at or near the venous cannula and that all tubing be cleared at the time the infusion is discontinued.[3463] Bolus doses and continuous infusion should not be administered simultaneously to spontaneously breathing patients.[3463]

Stability

Remifentanil hydrochloride is a white to off-white lyophilized powder that forms a clear, colorless solution upon reconstitution.[3463] Intact vials should be stored between 2 and 25°C.[3463]

The solution should be visually inspected for particulate matter and discoloration prior to administration; if particulate matter is present or discoloration occurs, the solution should not be used.[3463] Vials are for single dose and do not contain preservatives; unused portions should be discarded.[3463]

Syringes

In 2015, reports of decreased potency of certain drugs (e.g., remifentanil hydrochloride) stored in Becton Dickinson syringes for extended periods (i.e., exceeding 24 hours) were confirmed by the manufacturer of these syringes; the cause of this change was later identified to be the inclusion of an alternate rubber stopper in the plunger of certain product lots of syringes.[3029 3036 3037 3039 3041 3042] Decreased potency was not observed when the syringes were filled and used promptly.[3037] Use of the alternate stopper was later discontinued and use of the primary stopper in such syringes was resumed; however, Becton Dickinson states that its general-use syringes are cleared by FDA for immediate use in fluid aspiration and injection and that such syringes, regardless of the stopper material, have not been cleared by FDA for use as a closed-container system.[3391]

Compatibility Information

Solution Compatibility

Remifentanil HCl

Test Soln Name	Mfr	Mfr	Conc/L or %	Remarks	Ref	C/I
Dextrose 5% in Ringer's injection, lactated		MYL	20, 25, 50, and 250 mg	Compatible and stable for 24 hr	3463	C
Dextrose 5% in sodium chloride 0.9%		MYL	20, 25, 50, and 250 mg	Compatible and stable for 24 hr	3463	C
Dextrose 5%		MYL	20, 25, 50, and 250 mg	Compatible and stable for 24 hr	3463	C
Ringer's injection, lactated		MYL	20, 25, 50 and 250 mg	Stable for 4 hr	3463	C
Sodium chloride 0.45%		MYL	20, 25, 50, and 250 mg	Compatible and stable for 24 hr	3463	C
Sodium chloride 0.9%		MYL	20, 25, 50, and 250 mg	Compatible and stable for 24 hr	3463	C

DOI: 10.37573/9781585286850.339

Drugs in Syringe Compatibility

Remifentanil HCl

Test Drug	Mfr	Amt	Mfr	Amt	Remarks	Ref	C/I
Propofol	ASZ	487.5 mg/48.75 mL	GL	1.25 mg/1.25 mL	Separation and layering of the drugs occurred with syringes stored in an upright vertical position	3504	I
Propofol	ASZ	475 mg/47.5 mL	GL	2.5 mg/2.5 mL	Separation and layering of the drugs occurred with syringes stored in an upright vertical position	3504	I
Propofol	ASZ	450 mg/45 mL	GL	5 mg/5 mL	Separation and layering of the drugs occurred with syringes stored in an upright vertical position	3504	I

Y-Site Injection Compatibility (1:1 Mixture)

Remifentanil HCl

Test Drug	Mfr	Conc	Mfr	Conc	Remarks	Ref	C/I
Acyclovir sodium	BW	7 mg/mL[a]	GW	0.025 and 0.25 mg/mL[b]	Physically compatible for 4 hr at 23°C	2075	C
Alfentanil HCl	JN	0.125 mg/mL[a]	GW	0.025 and 0.25 mg/mL[b]	Physically compatible for 4 hr at 23°C	2075	C
Amikacin sulfate	AB	5 mg/mL[a]	GW	0.025 and 0.25 mg/mL[b]	Physically compatible for 4 hr at 23°C	2075	C
Aminophylline	AB	2.5 mg/mL[a]	GW	0.025 and 0.25 mg/mL[b]	Physically compatible for 4 hr at 23°C	2075	C
Amphotericin B	PHT	0.6 mg/mL[a]	GW	0.025 mg/mL[a]	Physically compatible for 4 hr at 23°C	2075	C
Amphotericin B	PHT	0.6 mg/mL[a]	GW	0.25 mg/mL[a]	Yellow precipitate forms immediately	2075	I
Ampicillin sodium	SKB	20 mg/mL[b]	GW	0.025 and 0.25 mg/mL[b]	Physically compatible for 4 hr at 23°C	2075	C
Ampicillin sodium–sulbactam sodium	RR	20 mg/mL[b f]	GW	0.025 and 0.25 mg/mL[b]	Physically compatible for 4 hr at 23°C	2075	C
Aztreonam	SQ	40 mg/mL[a]	GW	0.025 and 0.25 mg/mL[b]	Physically compatible for 4 hr at 23°C	2075	C
Bumetanide	RC	0.04 mg/mL[a]	GW	0.025 and 0.25 mg/mL[b]	Physically compatible for 4 hr at 23°C	2075	C
Buprenorphine HCl	RKC	0.04 mg/mL[a]	GW	0.025 and 0.25 mg/mL[b]	Physically compatible for 4 hr at 23°C	2075	C
Butorphanol tartrate	APC	0.04 mg/mL[a]	GW	0.025 and 0.25 mg/mL[b]	Physically compatible for 4 hr at 23°C	2075	C
Calcium gluconate	AB	40 mg/mL[a]	GW	0.025 and 0.25 mg/mL[b]	Physically compatible for 4 hr at 23°C	2075	C
Cefazolin sodium	SKB	20 mg/mL[a]	GW	0.025 and 0.25 mg/mL[b]	Physically compatible for 4 hr at 23°C	2075	C
Cefepime HCl	BMS	120 mg/mL[c]		0.2 mg/mL	Physically compatible with less than 10% cefepime loss. Remifentanil not tested	2513	C
Cefotaxime sodium	HO	20 mg/mL[a]	GW	0.025 and 0.25 mg/mL[b]	Physically compatible for 4 hr at 23°C	2075	C
Cefotetan disodium	ZEN	20 mg/mL[a]	GW	0.025 and 0.25 mg/mL[b]	Physically compatible for 4 hr at 23°C	2075	C
Cefoxitin sodium	ME	20 mg/mL[a]	GW	0.025 and 0.25 mg/mL[b]	Physically compatible for 4 hr at 23°C	2075	C
Ceftaroline fosamil	FOR	2.22 mg/mL[a b e]	HOS	0.25 mg/mL[a b e]	Physically compatible for 4 hr at 23°C	2826	C
Ceftazidime	GSK	120 mg/mL[c]		0.2 mg/mL	Physically compatible with less than 10% ceftazidime loss. Remifentanil not tested	2513	C
Ceftriaxone sodium	RC	20 mg/mL[a]	GW	0.025 and 0.25 mg/mL[b]	Physically compatible for 4 hr at 23°C	2075	C
Cefuroxime sodium	LI	30 mg/mL[a]	GW	0.025 and 0.25 mg/mL[b]	Physically compatible for 4 hr at 23°C	2075	C
Chlorpromazine HCl	SCN	2 mg/mL[a]	GW	0.025 mg/mL[b]	Slight haze forms in 1 hr	2075	I
Chlorpromazine HCl	SCN	2 mg/mL[a]	GW	0.25 mg/mL[b]	Physically compatible for 4 hr at 23°C	2075	C

Y-Site Injection Compatibility (1:1 Mixture) (Cont.)

Test Drug	Mfr	Conc	Mfr	Conc	Remarks	Ref	C/I
Ciprofloxacin	BAY	1 mg/mL[a]	GW	0.025 and 0.25 mg/mL[b]	Physically compatible for 4 hr at 23°C	2075	C
Cisatracurium besylate	GW	2 mg/mL[a]	GW	0.025 and 0.25 mg/mL[b]	Physically compatible for 4 hr at 23°C	2075	C
Clindamycin phosphate	AST	10 mg/mL[a]	GW	0.025 and 0.25 mg/mL[b]	Physically compatible for 4 hr at 23°C	2075	C
Dexamethasone sodium phosphate	FUJ	2 mg/mL[a]	GW	0.025 and 0.25 mg/mL[b]	Physically compatible for 4 hr at 23°C	2075	C
Dexmedetomidine HCl	AB	4 mcg/mL[b]	AB	0.25 mg/mL[b]	Physically compatible for 4 hr at 23°C	2383	C
Diazepam	ES	5 mg/mL	GW	0.025 and 0.25 mg/mL[b]	White turbidity forms immediately	2075	I
Diazepam	ES	0.25 mg/mL[a]	GW	0.025 and 0.25 mg/mL[b]	Physically compatible for 4 hr at 23°C	2075	C
Digoxin	ES	0.25 mg/mL	GW	0.025 and 0.25 mg/mL[b]	Physically compatible for 4 hr at 23°C	2075	C
Diphenhydramine HCl	SCN	2 mg/mL[a]	GW	0.025 and 0.25 mg/mL[b]	Physically compatible for 4 hr at 23°C	2075	C
Dobutamine HCl	LI	4 mg/mL[a]	GW	0.025 and 0.25 mg/mL[b]	Physically compatible for 4 hr at 23°C	2075	C
Dopamine HCl	AB	3.2 mg/mL[a]	GW	0.025 and 0.25 mg/mL[b]	Physically compatible for 4 hr at 23°C	2075	C
Doxycycline hyclate	FUJ	1 mg/mL[a]	GW	0.025 and 0.25 mg/mL[b]	Physically compatible for 4 hr at 23°C	2075	C
Droperidol	AST	2.5 mg/mL	GW	0.025 and 0.25 mg/mL[b]	Physically compatible for 4 hr at 23°C	2075	C
Enalaprilat	ME	0.1 mg/mL[a]	GW	0.025 and 0.25 mg/mL[b]	Physically compatible for 4 hr at 23°C	2075	C
Epinephrine HCl	AMR	0.05 mg/mL[a]	GW	0.025 and 0.25 mg/mL[b]	Physically compatible for 4 hr at 23°C	2075	C
Esmolol HCl	OHM	10 mg/mL[a]	GW	0.025 and 0.25 mg/mL[b]	Physically compatible for 4 hr at 23°C	2075	C
Famotidine	MSD	2 mg/mL[a]	GW	0.025 and 0.25 mg/mL[b]	Physically compatible for 4 hr at 23°C	2075	C
Fenoldopam mesylate	AB	80 mcg/mL[b]	AB	0.2 mg/mL[b]	Physically compatible for 4 hr at 23°C	2467	C
Fentanyl citrate	ES	12.5 mcg/mL[a]	GW	0.025 and 0.25 mg/mL[b]	Physically compatible for 4 hr at 23°C	2075	C
Fluconazole	RR	2 mg/mL	GW	0.025 and 0.25 mg/mL[b]	Physically compatible for 4 hr at 23°C	2075	C
Furosemide	AMR	3 mg/mL[a]	GW	0.025 and 0.25 mg/mL[b]	Physically compatible for 4 hr at 23°C	2075	C
Ganciclovir sodium	SY	20 mg/mL[a]	GW	0.025 and 0.25 mg/mL[b]	Physically compatible for 4 hr at 23°C	2075	C
Gentamicin sulfate	ES	5 mg/mL[a]	GW	0.025 and 0.25 mg/mL[b]	Physically compatible for 4 hr at 23°C	2075	C
Haloperidol lactate	MN	0.2 mg/mL[a]	GW	0.025 and 0.25 mg/mL[b]	Physically compatible for 4 hr at 23°C	2075	C
Heparin sodium	AB	100 units/mL	GW	0.025 and 0.25 mg/mL[b]	Physically compatible for 4 hr at 23°C	2075	C
Hydrocortisone sodium succinate	AB	1 mg/mL[a]	GW	0.025 and 0.25 mg/mL[b]	Physically compatible for 4 hr at 23°C	2075	C
Hydromorphone HCl	ES	0.5 mg/mL[a]	GW	0.025 and 0.25 mg/mL[b]	Physically compatible for 4 hr at 23°C	2075	C
Hydroxyzine HCl	ES	2 mg/mL[a]	GW	0.025 and 0.25 mg/mL[b]	Physically compatible for 4 hr at 23°C	2075	C
Imipenem–cilastatin sodium	ME	10 mg/mL[a i]	GW	0.025 and 0.25 mg/mL[b]	Physically compatible for 4 hr at 23°C	2075	C
Isoproterenol HCl	SW	0.02 mg/mL[a]	GW	0.025 and 0.25 mg/mL[b]	Physically compatible for 4 hr at 23°C	2075	C
Ketorolac tromethamine	RC	15 mg/mL[a]	GW	0.025 and 0.25 mg/mL[b]	Physically compatible for 4 hr at 23°C	2075	C
Lidocaine HCl	AST	8 mg/mL[a]	GW	0.025 and 0.25 mg/mL[b]	Physically compatible for 4 hr at 23°C	2075	C
Linezolid	PHU	2 mg/mL	GW	0.5 mg/mL[a]	Physically compatible for 4 hr at 23°C	2264	C
Lorazepam	WY	0.5 mg/mL[a]	GW	0.025 and 0.25 mg/mL[b]	Physically compatible for 4 hr at 23°C	2075	C
Magnesium sulfate	AB	100 mg/mL[a]	GW	0.025 and 0.25 mg/mL[b]	Physically compatible for 4 hr at 23°C	2075	C

Y-Site Injection Compatibility (1:1 Mixture) (Cont.)

Test Drug	Mfr	Conc	Mfr	Conc	Remarks	Ref	C/I
Mannitol	BA	15%	GW	0.025 and 0.25 mg/mL[b]	Physically compatible for 4 hr at 23°C	2075	C
Meperidine HCl	AST	4 mg/mL[a]	GW	0.025 and 0.25 mg/mL[b]	Physically compatible for 4 hr at 23°C	2075	C
Methylprednisolone sodium succinate	AB	5 mg/mL[a]	GW	0.025 and 0.25 mg/mL[b]	Physically compatible for 4 hr at 23°C	2075	C
Metoclopramide HCl	AB	5 mg/mL	GW	0.025 and 0.25 mg/mL[b]	Physically compatible for 4 hr at 23°C	2075	C
Metronidazole	AB	5 mg/mL	GW	0.025 and 0.25 mg/mL[b]	Physically compatible for 4 hr at 23°C	2075	C
Midazolam HCl	RC	1 mg/mL[a]	GW	0.025 and 0.25 mg/mL[b]	Physically compatible for 4 hr at 23°C	2075	C
Morphine sulfate	AST	1 mg/mL[a]	GW	0.025 and 0.25 mg/mL[b]	Physically compatible for 4 hr at 23°C	2075	C
Nalbuphine HCl	AST	10 mg/mL	GW	0.025 and 0.25 mg/mL[b]	Physically compatible for 4 hr at 23°C	2075	C
Nitroglycerin	DU	0.4 mg/mL[a]	GW	0.025 and 0.25 mg/mL[b]	Physically compatible for 4 hr at 23°C	2075	C
Norepinephrine bitartrate	SW	0.12 mg/mL[a]	GW	0.025 and 0.25 mg/mL[b]	Physically compatible for 4 hr at 23°C	2075	C
Ondansetron HCl	CER	1 mg/mL[a]	GW	0.025 and 0.25 mg/mL[b]	Physically compatible for 4 hr at 23°C	2075	C
Phenylephrine HCl	AMR	1 mg/mL[a]	GW	0.025 and 0.25 mg/mL[b]	Physically compatible for 4 hr at 23°C	2075	C
Piperacillin sodium–tazobactam sodium	CY[d]	40 mg/mL[a, g]	GW	0.025 and 0.25 mg/mL[b]	Physically compatible for 4 hr at 23°C	2075	C
Potassium chloride	AB	0.1 mEq/mL[a]	GW	0.025 and 0.25 mg/mL[b]	Physically compatible for 4 hr at 23°C	2075	C
Procainamide HCl	ES	10 mg/mL[a]	GW	0.025 and 0.25 mg/mL[b]	Physically compatible for 4 hr at 23°C	2075	C
Prochlorperazine edisylate	SO	0.5 mg/mL[a]	GW	0.025 and 0.25 mg/mL[b]	Physically compatible for 4 hr at 23°C	2075	
Promethazine HCl	SCN	2 mg/mL[a]	GW	0.025 and 0.25 mg/mL[b]	Physically compatible for 4 hr at 23°C	2075	C
Ranitidine HCl	GL	2 mg/mL[a]	GW	0.025 and 0.25 mg/mL[b]	Physically compatible for 4 hr at 23°C	2075	C
Sodium bicarbonate	AB	1 mEq/mL	GW	0.025 and 0.25 mg/mL[b]	Physically compatible for 4 hr at 23°C	2075	C
Sufentanil citrate	ES	0.0125 mg/mL[a]	GW	0.025 and 0.25 mg/mL[b]	Physically compatible for 4 hr at 23°C	2075	C
Theophylline	AB	3.2 mg/mL[a]	GW	0.025 and 0.25 mg/mL[b]	Physically compatible for 4 hr at 23°C	2075	C
Tobramycin sulfate	AB	5 mg/mL[a]	GW	0.025 and 0.25 mg/mL[b]	Physically compatible for 4 hr at 23°C	2075	C
Trimethoprim–sulfamethoxazole	ES	0.8 mg/mL[a, h]	GW	0.025 and 0.25 mg/mL[b]	Physically compatible for 4 hr at 23°C	2075	C
Vancomycin HCl	AB	10 mg/mL[a]	GW	0.025 and 0.25 mg/mL[b]	Physically compatible for 4 hr at 23°C	2075	C
Zidovudine	BW	4 mg/mL[a]	GW	0.025 and 0.25 mg/mL[b]	Physically compatible for 4 hr at 23°C	2075	C

[a] Tested in dextrose 5%.

[b] Tested in sodium chloride 0.9%.

[c] Tested in sterile water for injection.

[d] Test performed using the formulation WITHOUT edetate disodium.

[e] Tested in Ringer's injection, lactated.

[f] Ampicillin component. Ampicillin in a 2:1 fixed-ratio concentration with sulbactam.

[g] Piperacillin component. Piperacillin in an 8:1 fixed-ratio concentration with tazobactam.

[h] Trimethoprim component. Trimethoprim in a 1:5 fixed-ratio concentration with sulfamethoxazole.

[i] Not specified whether concentration refers to single component or combined components.

Additional Compatibility Information

Other Drugs

The manufacturer states that remifentanil hydrochloride (Ultiva, Mylan) has been shown to be compatible with propofol (Diprivan, Fresenius Kabi) when the 2 drugs are coadministered into a running intravenous administration set.[3463]

Selected Revisions January 31, 2020. © Copyright, October 2000. American Society of Health-System Pharmacists, Inc.

Reteplase
AHFS 20:12.20

Products

Reteplase is available as a lyophilized powder in 10.4-unit (18.1-mg) vials; the slight overfill is to ensure that 10 units of drug can be delivered. The vials are packaged with sterile water for injection diluent in kits containing 2 vials of drug and diluent along with syringes, needles, alcohol swabs, and dispensing pins and in half-kits with a single vial of drug and diluent with a dispensing pin. Each vial also contains tranexamic acid 8.32 mg, dipotassium hydrogen phosphate 136.24 mg, phosphoric acid 51.27 mg, sucrose 364 mg, and polysorbate 80 5.2 mg.[1(11/06)]

Reconstitute the reteplase vials using the diluent and dispensing pin provided. Other solutions should not be used to reconstitute the drug. Swirl gently to dissolve the drug yielding a 1-unit/mL solution. Do not shake. If slight foaming occurs, the vials should be allowed to stand for several minutes to dissipate large bubbles.[1(11/06) 4]

pH

The reconstituted solution has a pH from 5.7 to 6.3.[1(11/06)]

Trade Name(s)

Retavase

Administration

Reteplase is administered intravenously as a double bolus injection, each injection delivered over 2 minutes. The second injection is given 30 minutes after completion of the first injection. The manufacturer recommends no other drugs be administered in the line used to deliver reteplase.[1(11/06)]

Stability

Intact packages should be stored between 2 and 25°C. The boxes should stay sealed until use to protect from light. Because no antimicrobial preservatives are present, the manufacturer recommends reconstitution immediately before use. The colorless reconstituted solution may be used for up to 4 hours after reconstitution when stored between 2 and 30°C.[1(11/06)]

Reteplase is incompatible with heparin sodium. If mixed in the same container or run into the same line as heparin sodium, a solid or semisolid mass may form. However, heparin sodium may be administered sequentially with reteplase into the same line used to deliver reteplase if the line is adequately flushed with sodium chloride 0.9% or dextrose 5% both before and after reteplase administration.[1(11/06)]

Compatibility Information

Y-Site Injection Compatibility (1:1 Mixture)

Reteplase

Test Drug	Mfr	Conc	Mfr	Conc	Remarks	Ref	C/I
Bivalirudin	TMC	5 mg/mL[a]	CEN	1 unit/mL[a]	Small aggregates form immediately	2373	I
Cangrelor tetrasodium	TMC	1 mg/mL[b]		1 unit/mL	Cloudy white precipitate with fluffy particulates forms immediately	3243	I

[a] Tested in dextrose 5%.

[b] Tested in sodium chloride 0.9%.

Selected Revisions September 29, 2017. © Copyright, October 2004. American Society of Health-System Pharmacists, Inc.

DOI: 10.37573/9781585286850.340

Rifampin
AHFS 8:16.04

Products

Rifampin is available as a lyophilized powder in vials containing rifampin 600 mg, sodium formaldehyde sulfoxylate 10 mg, and sodium hydroxide to adjust the pH. Reconstitute with 10 mL of sterile water for injection; swirl gently to dissolve the vial contents for a 60-mg/mL solution.[1(7/08)]

Trade Name(s)

Rifadin I.V.

Administration

Rifampin is administered by intravenous infusion. It must not be given intramuscularly or subcutaneously, and extravasation should be avoided. The reconstituted solution may be diluted in 500 mL of dextrose 5% or sodium chloride 0.9% and infused over three hours. Alternatively, the desired dose may be diluted in 100 mL and administered over 30 minutes.[1(7/08)] [4]

Stability

Rifampin powder is reddish brown. Intact vials should be stored at room temperature and protected from excessive heat and light. The reconstituted solution is stable for 24 hours at room temperature.[1(7/08)]

Compatibility Information

Solution Compatibility

Rifampin

Test Soln Name	Mfr	Mfr	Conc/L or %	Remarks	Ref	C/I
Dextrose 5%				Use within 4 hr	1(7/08)	C
Dextrose 5%	AB	MMD	6 g	Gelatinous precipitate after overnight room temperature storage	1543	I
Dextrose 5%	AB	MMD	1.2 g	Clear with no visible precipitation over 3 hr	1543	C
Dextrose 5%	BA[a]	MMD	0.1 g	Brownish color in 4 hr. 5% rifampin loss in 8 hr and 17% loss in 24 hr at 24°C. 8% loss in 3 days at 4°C	1559	I[b]
Sodium chloride 0.9%				Use within 24 hr	1(7/08)	C
Sodium chloride 0.9%	BA[a]	MMD	0.1 g	Brownish color in 4 hr. 7% rifampin loss in 8 hr and 13% loss in 24 hr at 24°C. 7% loss in 3 days at 4°C	1559	I[b]

[a] Tested in PVC containers.

[b] Incompatible by conventional standards. May be used in shorter time periods.

Y-Site Injection Compatibility (1:1 Mixture)

Rifampin

Test Drug	Mfr	Conc	Mfr	Conc	Remarks	Ref	C/I
Diltiazem HCl	MMD	1[a] and 5 mg/mL	MMD	6 mg/mL[a]	Precipitate forms	1807	I
Tramadol HCl	GRU	8.33 mg/mL	AVE	6 mg/mL	Immediate red-orange turbid precipitate	2727	I

[a] Tested in sodium chloride 0.9%.

Selected Revisions July 30, 2015. © Copyright, October 1994. American Society of Health-System Pharmacists, Inc.

DOI: 10.37573/9781585286850.341

Rituximab
AHFS 10:00

Products

Rituximab is available as a preservative-free 10-mg/mL concentrate solution in 100- and 500-mg single-use vials.[3083] Each mL also contains polysorbate 80 0.7 mg, sodium chloride 9 mg, sodium citrate dihydrate 7.35 mg, and water for injection.[3083]

Before preparing a solution for intravenous infusion, rituximab vials should be visually inspected for particulate matter or discoloration; vials should not be used if particulates or discoloration is present.[3083] The appropriate dose of rituximab should be withdrawn and diluted in an infusion bag containing sodium chloride 0.9% or dextrose 5% to yield a final concentration of 1 to 4 mg/mL.[3083] The bag should be gently inverted to mix the solution.[3083] Any unused portion remaining in the vial should be discarded.[3083]

pH

6.5.[3083]

Osmolality

Rituximab is nearly isotonic with an osmolality of approximately 360 mOsm/kg.[3085]

Trade Name(s)

Rituxan, MabThera

Administration

Rituximab is administered only by intravenous infusion after dilution in dextrose 5% or sodium chloride 0.9%.[3083] The drug should *not* be administered by intravenous push or bolus injection.[3083] Patients should receive appropriate premedications as indicated.[3083]

The first infusion should be initiated at a rate of 50 mg/hr.[3083] In the absence of infusion toxicity, the rate may be increased every 30 minutes in increments of 50 mg/hr to a maximum rate of 400 mg/hr.[3083] Subsequent standard infusions may be initiated at 100 mg/hr and, in the absence of infusion toxicity, the rate may be increased every 30 minutes in increments of 100 mg/hr to a maximum rate of 400 mg/hr.[3083] Certain patients treated for specific indications may be eligible for a 90-minute subsequent infusion (i.e., 20% of the dose administered over 30 minutes followed by the remaining 80% administered over 60 minutes); specific product labeling should be consulted for additional administration details.[3083]

Stability

Rituximab concentrate is a clear, colorless solution.[3083] Intact vials are stable at 2 to 8°C.[3083] Vials should be protected from direct sunlight and should not be frozen or shaken.[3083]

Rituximab solutions diluted for infusion may be stored for 24 hours at 2 to 8°C.[3083] Diluted solutions have demonstrated stability for an additional 24 hours at room temperature; however, since such solutions do not contain a preservative, the manufacturer recommends that diluted solutions be stored under refrigeration at 2 to 8°C.[3083]

Sorption

No incompatibilities have been observed with rituximab and bags composed of polyvinyl chloride (PVC) or polyethylene.[3083] The manufacturer states that the use of containers other than those made of PVC or polyethylene (e.g., evacuated glass bottles) with rituximab has not been evaluated and is therefore not recommended.[3085]

Filtration

Use of an inline filter is not required for administration of rituximab-containing solutions.[3085] Based on the results of a study evaluating the effects of using a 0.2-μm inline filter to administer various concentrations of diluted rituximab, inadvertent use of an inline filter is not expected to be problematic.[3085]

Compatibility Information

Solution Compatibility

Rituximab

Test Soln Name	Mfr	Mfr	Conc/L or %	Remarks	Ref	C/I
Dextrose 5%	a	GEN	1 to 4 g	Stable for 24 hr at 2 to 8°C followed by 24 hr at room temperature	3083	C
Sodium chloride 0.9%	a	GEN	1 to 4 g	Stable for 24 hr at 2 to 8°C followed by 24 hr at room temperature	3083	C
Sodium chloride 0.9%	FRK[b]	RC	1 g	Stable for 6 months at 4°C protected from light based on physicochemical tests and direct cytotoxicity assay	3084	C

[a] Tested in PVC and polyethylene containers.

[b] Tested in Freeflex polyolefin containers.

DOI: 10.37573/9781585286850.342

Rocuronium Bromide
AHFS 12:20.20

Products

Rocuronium bromide is available in 5- and 10-mL vials. Each mL contains rocuronium bromide 10 mg with sodium acetate 2 mg, sodium chloride for isotonicity, and acetic acid and/or sodium hydroxide to adjust the pH.[1(9/08)]

pH

Adjusted during manufacture to pH 4.[1(9/08)]

Tonicity

The injection is isotonic.[1(9/08)]

Trade Name(s)

Zemuron

Administration

Rocuronium bromide is administered intravenously only by rapid intravenous injection or by intravenous infusion when admixed in an appropriate intravenous infusion solution. Infusion rates should be individualized for each patient according to the requirements and response.[1(9/08)] [4]

Stability

Intact vials of rocuronium bromide should be stored under refrigeration at 2 to 8°C and protected from freezing. Intact vials stored at room temperature should be used within 60 days. Opened vials should be used within 30 days.[1(9/08)]

Syringes

In 2015, reports of decreased potency of certain drugs (e.g., rocuronium bromide) stored in Becton Dickinson syringes for extended periods (i.e., exceeding 24 hours) were confirmed by the manufacturer of these syringes; the cause of this change was later identified to be the inclusion of an alternate rubber stopper in the plunger of certain product lots of syringes.[3029 3036 3037 3039 3041 3042] Decreased potency was not observed when the syringes were filled and used promptly.[3037] Use of the alternate stopper was later discontinued and use of the primary stopper in such syringes was resumed; however, Becton Dickinson states that its general-use syringes are cleared by FDA for immediate use in fluid aspiration and injection and that such syringes, regardless of the stopper material, have not been cleared by FDA for use as a closed-container system.[3391]

Compatibility Information

Solution Compatibility

Rocuronium bromide

Test Soln Name	Mfr	Mfr	Conc/L or %	Remarks	Ref	C/I
Dextrose 5% in sodium chloride 0.9%				Compatible and stable for 24 hr	1(9/08)	C
Dextrose 5%				Compatible and stable for 24 hr	1(9/08)	C
Ringer's injection, lactated				Compatible and stable for 24 hr	1(9/08)	C
Sodium chloride 0.9%				Compatible and stable for 24 hr	1(9/08)	C

Y-Site Injection Compatibility (1:1 Mixture)

Rocuronium bromide

Test Drug	Mfr	Conc	Mfr	Conc	Remarks	Ref	C/I
Ceftolozane sulfate–tazobactam sodium	CUB	10 mg/mL[c d]	HOS	5 mg/mL[c]	Physically compatible for 2 hr	3262	C
Cloxacillin sodium	SMX	100 mg/mL	ME	10 mg/mL	Precipitates immediately	3245	I
Dexmedetomidine HCl	AB	4 mcg/mL[b]	OR	1 mg/mL[b]	Physically compatible for 4 hr at 23°C	2383	C
Fenoldopam mesylate	AB	80 mcg/mL[b]	OR	1 mg/mL[b]	Physically compatible for 4 hr at 23°C	2467	C
Hetastarch in lactated electrolyte	AB	6%	OR	1 mg/mL[a]	Physically compatible for 4 hr at 23°C	2339	C
Isavuconazonium sulfate	ASP	1.5 mg/mL[c]	PRM	5 mg/mL[c]	Physically compatible for 2 hr	3263	C
Meropenem		50 mg/mL	SZ	10 mg/mL	Physically compatible for 4 hr at room temperature	3538	C

DOI: 10.37573/9781585286850.343

Y-Site Injection Compatibility (1:1 Mixture) (Cont.)

Test Drug	Mfr	Conc	Mfr	Conc	Remarks	Ref	C/I
Meropenem–vaborbactam	TMC	8 mg/mL[b] [e]	MYL	5 mg/mL[b]	Physically compatible for 3 hr at 20 to 25°C	3380	C
Micafungin sodium	ASP	1.5 mg/mL[b]	OR	1 mg/mL[b]	White precipitate forms immediately	2683	I
Milrinone lactate	SW	0.4 mg/mL[a]	OR	2 mg/mL[a]	Visually compatible. Little loss of either drug in 4 hr at 23°C	2214	C
Palonosetron HCl	MGI	50 mcg/mL	BA	1 mg/mL[a]	Physically compatible and no loss of either drug in 4 hr at room temperature	2764	C
Plazomicin sulfate	ACH	24 mg/mL[c]	XGN	5 mg/mL[c]	Physically compatible for 1 hr at 20 to 25°C	3432	C
Tedizolid phosphate	CUB	0.8 mg/mL[b]	PRM	5 mg/mL[b]	Physically compatible for 2 hr	3244	C

[a] Tested in dextrose 5%.

[b] Tested in sodium chloride 0.9%.

[c] Tested in both dextrose 5% and sodium chloride 0.9%.

[d] Ceftolozane component. Ceftolozane in a 2:1 fixed-ratio concentration with tazobactam.

[e] Meropenem component. Meropenem in a 1:1 fixed-ratio concentration with vaborbactam.

Selected Revisions May 1, 2020. © Copyright, October 2002.
American Society of Health-System Pharmacists, Inc.

Rolapitant Hydrochloride
AHFS 56:22.32

Products

Rolapitant hydrochloride is available as a ready-to-use emulsion in single-dose vials that contain 166.5 mg of rolapitant as the free base in 92.5 mL of the emulsion.[3370] [3371] Each mL of the injectable emulsion contains rolapitant 1.8 mg, dibasic sodium phosphate anhydrous 2.8 mg, medium-chain triglycerides 11 mg, polyoxyl 15 hydroxystearate 44 mg, sodium chloride 6.2 mg, and soybean oil 6.5 mg in water for injection.[3370] The injectable emulsion also may contain hydrochloric acid and/or sodium hydroxide to adjust the pH.[3370]

Equivalency

Rolapitant hydrochloride 185 mg is equivalent to 166.5 mg of rolapitant as the free base.[3370] [3372]

pH

From 7 to 8.[3370]

Trade Name(s)

Varubi

Administration

For rolapitant doses of 166.5 mg (92.5 mL), the dose should be administered by inserting a conventional vented intravenous infusion set directly into the septum of the 100-mL vial.[3370] [3371] (See Stability: Compatible Administration Sets.)

Rolapitant hydrochloride injectable emulsion should be administered by intravenous infusion over 30 minutes using an infusion pump.[3370] [3371]

The manufacturer states that the injectable emulsion should *not* be diluted.[3370] (See Additional Compatibility Information.)

Stability

Rolapitant hydrochloride injectable emulsion is translucent and white with some opalescence.[3370] The emulsion is homogenous and does not require shaking.[3370] Intact vials should be stored at controlled room temperature.[3370]

Vials should be inspected for particulate matter and discoloration prior to administration; if particulate matter is present or discoloration has occurred, the vial should be discarded.[3370] Vials also should not be used if contamination is suspected.[3370] Once the vial stopper has been punctured for administration, infusion of the drug should begin immediately.[3370]

Compatible Administration Sets

Rolapitant hydrochloride injectable emulsion was found to be compatible with the administration sets listed in Table 1 for 20 hours at 2 to 8°C, followed by 2 or 8 hours at ambient conditions.[3371] Admixtures of rolapitant hydrochloride with dexamethasone sodium phosphate or palonosetron hydrochloride also were found to be compatible with the administration sets listed in Table 1 for 7 hours at 20 to 25°C followed by 20 hours at 2 to 8°C.[3372] [3373]

Table 1. Administration sets compatible with rolapitant hydrochloride injectable emulsion[3371] [3372] [3373]

Manufacturer	Administration Set
CareFusion	Smartsite low-sorbing diethylhexyl phthalate (DEHP)- and latex-free polyethylene secondary set (10014881)
	Polyvinyl chloride (PVC) (with DEHP) latex-free secondary set (72213N)
Codan	DEHP- and latex-free PVC and polyethylene universal intravenous administration set (A415N)
Medline Industries	DEHP- and latex-free PVC intravenous secondary set with hanger folded extension (DYNDTN1540A)

Compatibility Information
Solution Compatibility

Rolapitant HCl

Test Soln Name	Mfr	Mfr	Conc/L or %	Remarks	Ref	C/I
Dextrose 5% in Ringer's injection, lactated	BRN		1.8 g	Physically compatible and chemically stable for up to 6 hr at room temperature	3371	C
Dextrose 5%	PNN		1.8 g	Physically compatible and chemically stable for up to 6 hr at room temperature	3371	C
Ringer's injection, lactated	HOS		1.8 g	Physically compatible and chemically stable for up to 6 hr at room temperature	3371	C
Sodium chloride 0.9%	PNN		1.8 g	Physically compatible and chemically stable for up to 6 hr at room temperature	3371	C

DOI: 10.37573/9781585286850.344

Additive Compatibility

Rolapitant HCl

Test Drug	Mfr	Conc/L or %	Mfr	Conc/L or %	Test Solution	Remarks	Ref	C/I
Dexamethasone sodium phosphate	APP	105.3 mg	TES	1.8 g	a	Physically compatible. No loss of either drug in 6 hr at 20 to 25°C	3372	C
Dexamethasone sodium phosphate	APP	205.1 mg	TES	1.7 g	a	Physically compatible. No loss of either drug in 6 hr at 20 to 25°C	3372	C
Palonosetron HCl	EI	2.6 mg	TES	1.7 g	a	Physically compatible. Little to no loss of either drug in 48 hr at 20 to 25°C and 7 days at 2 to 8°C protected from light	3373	C

[a] Tested in cyclic olefin copolymer (COC) and glass containers.

Additional Compatibility Information

Infusion Solutions

The manufacturer states that rolapitant hydrochloride inject-able emulsion should not be diluted; however, the drug may be administered via Y-site connection with sodium chloride 0.9%; dextrose 5%; dextrose 5% in Ringer's injection, lactated; and Ringer's injection, lactated.[3370]

Ropivacaine Hydrochloride
AHFS 72:00

Products

Ropivacaine hydrochloride is available in concentrations of 2 mg/mL (0.2%), 5 mg/mL (0.5%), 7.5 mg/mL (0.75%), and 10 mg/mL (1%) along with sodium chloride for isotonicity and sodium hydroxide and/or hydrochloric acid for pH adjustment in water for injection. The products are packaged in single-dose glass vials and in polypropylene plastic ampuls designed to fit Luer-lock and Luer-slip syringes. The 2-mg/mL concentration is also available in 100 and 200-mL infusion bottles. Sterile-Pak products should be selected when a container having a sterile outside is required.[1(4/06)]

pH

From 4 to 6.5.[404]

Tonicity

Ropivacaine hydrochloride injections are isotonic.[1(4/06)]

Specific Gravity

The specific gravities of ropivacaine hydrochloride injections range from 1.002 to 1.005 at 25°C.[1(4/06)]

Trade Name(s)

Naropin

Administration

Ropivacaine hydrochloride is administered parenterally by lumbar epidural injection or infusion, by thoracic epidural infusion, by injection for nerve block, and by infiltration.[1(4/06)]

Stability

Intact containers of ropivacaine hydrochloride should be stored at controlled room temperature. The single-dose containers have no antimicrobial preservatives. The manufacturer recommends that any remaining solution in an opened container be discarded promptly. The continuous infusion bottles should not be left in place for more than 24 hours.[1(4/06)]

Autoclaving

Ropivacaine hydrochloride in glass containers is stable during one autoclaving to sterilize the container.[1(4/06)]

pH Effects

The solubility of ropivacaine hydrochloride is reduced above pH 6. Consequently, contact with alkaline solutions may result in precipitation.[1(4/06)]

Compatibility Information

Additive Compatibility

Ropivacaine HCl

Test Drug	Mfr	Conc/L or %	Mfr	Conc/L or %	Test Solution	Remarks	Ref	C/I
Clonidine HCl	BI	5 and 50 mg	ASZ	1 g	NS[a]	Physically compatible. No loss of either drug in 30 days at 30°C in the dark	2433	C
Clonidine HCl	BI	5 mg	ASZ	2 g	[a]	Physically compatible. No loss of either drug in 30 days at 30°C in the dark	2433	C
Diamorphine HCl		25 mg	ASZ	2 g	[d]	No ropivacaine and 10% diamorphine loss in 70 days at 4°C and 28 days at 21°C	2517	C
Fentanyl citrate	JN	1 mg	ASZ	1 g	NS[a]	Physically compatible. No loss of either drug in 30 days at 30°C in the dark	2433	C
Fentanyl citrate	JN	1 and 10 mg	ASZ	2 g	[a]	Physically compatible. No loss of either drug in 30 days at 30°C in the dark	2433	C
Fentanyl citrate	CUR	3 mg	ASZ	1.5 g	NS[b c]	Physically compatible. No loss of either drug in 51 days at 20 and 4°C	2498	C
Fentanyl citrate	CUR	3 mg	ASZ	1.5 g	NS[d]	Physically compatible. No loss of either drug in 7 days at 20 and 4°C	2498	C
Morphine sulfate	AST	20 mg	ASZ	1 g	NS[a]	Physically compatible. Little loss of either drug in 30 days at 30°C in the dark	2433	C
Morphine sulfate	AST	20 and 100 mg	ASZ	2 g	[a]	Physically compatible. Little loss of either drug in 30 days at 30°C in the dark	2433	C

DOI: 10.37573/9781585286850.345

Additive Compatibility (Cont.)

Test Drug	Mfr	Conc/L or %	Mfr	Conc/L or %	Test Solution	Remarks	Ref	C/I
Morphine sulfate	CDM[f]	2 g	FRK	6 g	NS[e]	Visually compatible and chemically stable for up to 14 days at 21°C	3493	C
Sufentanil citrate	JN	0.4 mg	ASZ	1 g	NS[a]	Physically compatible. No loss of either drug in 30 days at 30°C in the dark	2433	C
Sufentanil citrate	JN	0.4 and 4 mg	ASZ	2 g	[a]	Physically compatible. No loss of either drug in 30 days at 30°C in the dark	2433	C
Sufentanil citrate	JC	0.5, 0.75, 1 mg	ASZ	2 mg	NS[b d]	Physically compatible with no major sufentanil loss in 96 hr at 25°C. Ropivacaine not tested	2506	C
Ziconotide acetate	EI[g]	200 mg	FRK	6 g	NS[e]	Visually compatible and chemically stable for up to 14 days at 21°C	3493	C

[a] Tested in polypropylene bags (Mark II Polybags).

[b] Tested in glass containers.

[c] Tested in ethylene vinyl acetate (EVA) containers.

[d] Tested in PVC containers.

[e] Tested in polyolefin containers.

[f] Tested with ziconotide acetate (EI) 200 mg/L.

[g] Tested with morphine sulfate (CDM) 2 g/L.

Drugs in Syringe Compatibility

Ropivacaine HCl

Test Drug	Mfr	Amt	Mfr	Amt	Remarks	Ref	C/I
Diamorphine HCl		45 mg	ASZ	10 g	No ropivacaine loss and 10% diamorphine loss in 30 days at 4°C and 16 days at 21°C	2517	C
Methylprednisolone acetate	PHU	80 mg/2 mL	AST	6 mg/3 mL	Little loss of either drug in 30 days at 4 and 24°C in light or dark	2367	C
Morphine sulfate	CDM[a]	3.5 mg/mL[c]	FRK	7.5 mg/mL[c]	Visually compatible and chemically stable for up to 3 days at 5°C	3493	C
Morphine sulfate	CDM[a]	3.5 mg/mL[c]	FRK	7.5 mg/mL[c]	Chemically unstable after 6 hr at 21 and 31°C	3493	I
Ziconotide acetate	EI[b]	1 mcg/mL[c]	FRK	7.5 mg/mL[c]	Visually compatible and chemically stable for up to 3 days at 5°C	3493	C
Ziconotide acetate	EI[b]	1 mcg/mL[c]	FRK	7.5 mg/mL[c]	Chemically unstable after 6 hr at 21 and 31°C	3493	I

[a] Tested with ziconotide acetate (EI) 1 mcg/mL.

[b] Tested with morphine sulfate (CDM) 3.5 mg/mL.

[c] Tested in sodium chloride 0.9%.

Selected Revisions January 31, 2020. © Copyright, October 2004. American Society of Health-System Pharmacists, Inc.

Salbutamol Sulfate
AHFS 12:12.08.12

Products

Salbutamol sulfate injection is available as a solution in 1-mL ampuls.[3598] [3600] Each mL contains 500 mcg of salbutamol as the sulfate, as well as sodium chloride, sodium hydroxide, and sulfuric acid in water for injection.[3598] [3600]

Salbutamol sulfate also is available as a concentrate for injection in 5-mL ampuls for use in infusions following dilution.[3599] [3600] Each mL contains 1 mg of salbutamol as the sulfate, as well as sodium chloride, sodium hydroxide, and sulfuric acid in water for injection.[3599] [3600] This concentrate for injection must be diluted in a suitable infusion solution prior to administration.[3599] [3600]

pH

The pH of both the injection and the concentrate for injection (GlaxoSmithKline New Zealand) is adjusted to 3.5.[3600]

Tonicity

Both salbutamol sulfate injection and concentrate for injection are isotonic.[3598] [3599] [3600]

Trade Name(s)

Salbumol, Ventolin

Administration

Salbutamol sulfate injection is administered by subcutaneous, intramuscular, or slow intravenous injection.[3598] [3600] A 50-mcg/mL salbutamol concentration (e.g., 250 mcg diluted in 5 mL) is suitably dilute for slow intravenous injection; the 500-mcg/mL concentration has been diluted with sterile water for injection to achieve the 50-mcg/mL concentration.[3598] [3600]

Salbutamol sulfate concentrate for injection is used to prepare intravenous infusion solutions of the drug; it should *not* be administered undiluted.[3599] [3600] The concentrate for injection should be diluted to a concentration of 10, 20, or 200 mcg/mL, depending upon the indication and infusion method (e.g., syringe pump), with a compatible infusion solution.[3599] [3600] Recommended infusion solutions may vary based on the indication; consult specific labeling for details.[3598] [3599] [3600]

Stability

Salbutamol sulfate injection and concentrate for injection are clear, colorless or pale straw-colored solutions.[3598] [3599] [3600] The intact containers should be stored below 30°C and protected from light (e.g., by storing in the outer container).[3598] [3599] [3600]

Syringes

Salbutamol sulfate (GlaxoSmithKline) prepared at a salbutamol concentration of 3 mg/50 mL in sodium chloride 0.9% in a 50-mL polypropylene syringe (Becton Dickinson) was physically stable for 48 hours at room temperature.[3545]

Salbutamol sulfate (GlaxoSmithKline) prepared at a salbutamol concentration of 0.06 mg/mL in sodium chloride 0.9% in a 50-mL polypropylene syringe (Becton Dickinson) was physically and chemically stable for 30 days at 2 to 8°C protected from light.[3601]

Compatibility Information

Solution Compatibility

Salbutamol sulfate

Test Soln Name	Mfr	Mfr	Conc/L or %	Remarks	Ref	C/I
Dextrose 5%		GSK		Discard 24 hr after preparation	3599, 3600	C
Sodium chloride 0.9%		GSK		Discard 24 hr after preparation	3599, 3600	C

Drugs in Syringe Compatibility

Salbutamol sulfate

Test Drug	Mfr	Amt	Mfr	Amt	Remarks	Ref	C/I
Dimenhydrinate		10 mg/1 mL	c	1 mg/1 mL	Precipitate forms	2569	I
Hydromorphone HCl	KN	1 mg/0.5 mL	GL	2.5 mg/2.5 mL[a]	Physically compatible for 1 hr	1904	C
Morphine sulfate	AB	5 mg/0.5 mL	GL	2.5 mg/2.5 mL[a]	Physically compatible for 1 hr	1904	C

DOI: 10.37573/9781585286850.346

Drugs in Syringe Compatibility (Cont.)

Test Drug	Mfr	Amt	Mfr	Amt	Remarks	Ref	C/I
Pantoprazole sodium	b	4 mg/1 mL	c	1 mg/1 mL	Precipitates immediately	2574	I

[a] Both preserved (benzyl alcohol 0.9%; benzalkonium chloride 0.01%) and unpreserved sodium chloride 0.9% were used as a diluent.

[b] Test performed using the formulation WITHOUT edetate disodium.

[c] Salt not specified.

Y-Site Injection Compatibility (1:1 Mixture)

Salbutamol sulfate

Test Drug	Mfr	Conc	Mfr	Conc	Remarks	Ref	C/I
Cloxacillin sodium	SMX	100 mg/mL	GSK	1 mg/mL	Physically compatible for up to 4 hr at room temperature	3245	C
Meropenem		50 mg/mL	GSK	1 mg/mL	Physically compatible for 4 hr at room temperature	3538	C

Additional Compatibility Information

Infusion Solutions

Manufacturers state that recommended diluents for salbutamol sulfate are limited to sodium chloride (concentration unspecified), sodium chloride and dextrose (concentrations unspecified), dextrose (concentration unspecified), and sterile water for injection.[3598 3599 3600]

Selected Revisions July 1, 2020. © Copyright, October 1998. American Society of Health-System Pharmacists, Inc.

Sargramostim
AHFS 20:16
GM-CSF

Products

Sargramostim is available in single-dose vials labeled as containing 250 mcg. Reconstitute the vial with 1 mL of sterile water for injection or bacteriostatic water for injection containing benzyl alcohol 0.9% directed at the sides of the vial. Gently swirl to avoid foaming during dissolution, and do not shake. Each mL of the reconstituted solution contains sargramostim 250 mcg, mannitol 40 mg, sucrose 10 mg, and tromethamine 1.2 mg.[1(4/08)] [4] The contents of vials reconstituted with different diluents should not be mixed.[1(4/08)]

Sargramostim is also available as a preserved liquid formulation in 1-mL vials containing in each mL sargramostim 500 mcg along with mannitol 40 mg, sucrose 10 mg, tromethamine 1.2 mg, and benzyl alcohol 1.1% as an antimicrobial preservative.[1(4/08)] [4]

Specific Activity

The specific activity is approximately 5.6×10^6 units per milligram.[1(4/08)]

pH

From 7.1 to 7.7.[1(4/08)] [17]

Trade Name(s)

Leukine

Administration

Sargramostim may be administered by subcutaneous injection undiluted or by intravenous infusion usually over 2 to 4 hours after dilution in sodium chloride 0.9%.[1(4/08)] For infusion concentrations below 10 mcg/mL, albumin human at a final concentration of 0.1% should be added to the intravenous solution prior to the addition of sargramostim to prevent adsorption.[1(4/08)]

The preparations containing benzyl alcohol (Leukine liquid, and lyophilized Leukine reconstituted with bacteriostatic water for injection containing benzyl alcohol) should not be used in neonates.[1(4/08)]

Stability

Intact vials, reconstituted solutions, and sargramostim diluted in sodium chloride 0.9% should be stored under refrigeration. Solutions should be protected from freezing and should not be shaken. The liquid formulation is a clear, colorless solution. The white lyophilized powder forms a clear, colorless solution on reconstitution. The manufacturer recommends administration within 6 hours following reconstitution with sterile water for injection and/or dilution in an infusion solution and discarding any unused solution. When reconstituted with bacteriostatic water for injection preserved with benzyl alcohol 0.9%, the manufacturer states that the solution may be stored for up to 20 days under refrigeration.[1(4/08)]

Other information indicates that sargramostim reconstituted with sterile water for injection or bacteriostatic water for injection is stable for 30 days at 25°C or under refrigeration.[226]

Syringes

Sargramostim 250 mcg and 500 mcg reconstituted with 1 mL of bacteriostatic water for injection with benzyl alcohol 0.9% and repackaged in 1-mL tuberculin syringes (Becton Dickinson) is stated to be stable for 14 days when stored under refrigeration.[226]

Sorption

Sargramostim will adsorb to containers and tubing if the concentration is below 10 mcg/mL. Albumin human 0.1% should be added to the intravenous solution to prevent this.[1(4/08)]

Filtration

Sargramostim should not be infused through an inline filter because of possible absorption.[1(4/08)] [4]

Compatibility Information

Solution Compatibility

Sargramostim

Test Soln Name	Mfr	Mfr	Conc/L or %	Remarks	Ref	C/I
Sodium chloride 0.9%			10 mg	Use within 6 hr	1(4/08)	C

DOI: 10.37573/9781585286850.347

Y-Site Injection Compatibility (1:1 Mixture)

Sargramostim

Test Drug	Mfr	Conc	Mfr	Conc	Remarks	Ref	C/I
Acyclovir sodium	BW	7 mg/mL[b]	IMM	10 mcg/mL[b]	Few small white particles form in 4 hr	1436	I
Amikacin sulfate	BR	5 mg/mL[b]	IMM	10 mcg/mL[b]	Visually compatible for 4 hr at 22°C	1436	C
Aminophylline	ES	2.5 mg/mL[b]	IMM	10 mcg/mL[b]	Visually compatible for 4 hr at 22°C	1436	C
Amphotericin B	SQ	0.6 mg/mL[a]	IMM	10 mcg/mL[b]	Yellow precipitate forms immediately	1436	I
Amphotericin B	SQ	0.6 mg/mL[a]	IMM	10 mcg/mL[a]	Visually compatible for 4 hr at 22°C	1436	C
Ampicillin sodium	BR	20 mg/mL[b]	IMM	10 mcg/mL[b]	Few small particles form in 4 hr	1436	I
Ampicillin sodium–sulbactam sodium	RR	20 mg/mL[b g]	IMM	10 mcg/mL[b]	Few small particles form in 4 hr	1436	I
Amsacrine	NCI	1 mg/mL[a]	IMM	10 mcg/mL[a]	Visually compatible for 4 hr at 22°C	1436	C
Amsacrine	NCI	1 mg/mL[a]	IMM	10 mcg/mL[b]	Haze and yellow precipitate form	1436	I
Aztreonam	SQ	40 mg/mL[b]	IMM	10 mcg/mL[b]	Visually compatible for 4 hr at 22°C	1436	C
Aztreonam	SQ	40 mg/mL[a]	IMM	10 mcg/mL[b]	Physically compatible for 4 hr at 23°C	1758	C
Bleomycin sulfate	MJ	1 unit/mL[b]	IMM	10 mcg/mL[b]	Visually compatible for 4 hr at 22°C	1436	C
Butorphanol tartrate	BR	0.04 mg/mL[b]	IMM	10 mcg/mL[b]	Visually compatible for 4 hr at 22°C	1436	C
Calcium gluconate	AMR	40 mg/mL[b]	IMM	10 mcg/mL[b]	Visually compatible for 4 hr at 22°C	1436	C
Carboplatin	BR	5 mg/mL[b]	IMM	10 mcg/mL[b]	Visually compatible for 4 hr at 22°C	1436	C
Carmustine	BR	1.5 mg/mL[b]	IMM	10 mcg/mL[b]	Visually compatible for 4 hr at 22°C	1436	C
Cefazolin sodium	LEM	20 mg/mL[b]	IMM	10 mcg/mL[b]	Visually compatible for 4 hr at 22°C	1436	C
Cefotaxime sodium	HO	20 mg/mL[b]	IMM	10 mcg/mL[b]	Visually compatible for 4 hr at 22°C	1436	C
Cefotetan disodium	STU	20 mg/mL[b]	IMM	10 mcg/mL[b]	Visually compatible for 4 hr at 22°C	1436	C
Ceftazidime	GL	40 mg/mL[b]	IMM	10 mcg/mL[b]	Particles and filaments form in 4 hr	1436	I
Ceftazidime	LI	40 mg/mL[d]	IMM	6[b e] and 15[b] mcg/mL	Visually compatible for 2 hr	1618	C
Ceftriaxone sodium	RC	20 mg/mL[b]	IMM	10 mcg/mL[b]	Visually compatible for 4 hr at 22°C	1436	C
Cefuroxime sodium	GL	30 mg/mL[b]	IMM	10 mcg/mL[b]	Visually compatible for 4 hr at 22°C	1436	C
Chlorpromazine HCl	ES	2 mg/mL[b]	IMM	10 mcg/mL[b]	Slight haze forms immediately	1436	I
Cisplatin	BR	1 mg/mL	IMM	10 mcg/mL[b]	Visually compatible for 4 hr at 22°C	1436	C
Clindamycin phosphate	LY	10 mg/mL[b]	IMM	10 mcg/mL[b]	Visually compatible for 4 hr at 22°C	1436	C
Cyclophosphamide	MJ	10 mg/mL[b]	IMM	10 mcg/mL[b]	Visually compatible for 4 hr at 22°C	1436	C
Cyclosporine	SZ	5 mg/mL[b]	IMM	6[b e] and 15[b] mcg/mL	Visually compatible for 2 hr	1618	C
Cytarabine	SCN	50 mg/mL	IMM	10 mcg/mL[b]	Visually compatible for 4 hr at 22°C	1436	C
Dacarbazine	MI	4 mg/mL[b]	IMM	10 mcg/mL[b]	Visually compatible for 4 hr at 22°C	1436	C
Dactinomycin	MSD	0.01 mg/mL[b]	IMM	10 mcg/mL[b]	Visually compatible for 4 hr at 22°C	1436	C
Dexamethasone sodium phosphate	ES	1 mg/mL[b]	IMM	10 mcg/mL[b]	Visually compatible for 4 hr at 22°C	1436	C
Diphenhydramine HCl	RU	1 mg/mL[b]	IMM	10 mcg/mL[b]	Visually compatible for 4 hr at 22°C	1436	C

Y-Site Injection Compatibility (1:1 Mixture) (Cont.)

Test Drug	Mfr	Conc	Mfr	Conc	Remarks	Ref	C/I
Dopamine HCl	DU	1.6 mg/mL[d]	IMM	6[b][e] and 15[b] mcg/mL	Visually compatible for 2 hr	1618	C
Doxorubicin HCl	CET	2 mg/mL	IMM	10 mcg/mL[b]	Visually compatible for 4 hr at 22°C	1436	C
Doxycycline hyclate	LY	1 mg/mL[b]	IMM	10 mcg/mL[b]	Visually compatible for 4 hr at 22°C	1436	C
Droperidol	DU	0.4 mg/mL[b]	IMM	10 mcg/mL[b]	Visually compatible for 4 hr at 22°C	1436	C
Etoposide	BR	0.4 mg/mL[b]	IMM	10 mcg/mL[b]	Visually compatible for 4 hr at 22°C	1436	C
Famotidine	MSD	2 mg/mL	IMM	10 mcg/mL[b]	Visually compatible for 4 hr at 22°C	1436	C
Fentanyl citrate	ES	50 mcg/mL	IMM	6[b][e] and 15[b] mcg/mL	Visually compatible for 2 hr	1618	C
Floxuridine	RC	3 mg/mL[b]	IMM	10 mcg/mL[b]	Visually compatible for 4 hr at 22°C	1436	C
Fluconazole	RR	2 mg/mL	IMM	10 mcg/mL[b]	Visually compatible for 4 hr at 22°C	1436	C
Fluorouracil	SO	16 mg/mL	IMM	10 mcg/mL[b]	Visually compatible for 4 hr at 22°C	1436	C
Furosemide	AB	3 mg/mL[b]	IMM	10 mcg/mL[b]	Visually compatible for 4 hr at 22°C	1436	C
Ganciclovir sodium	SY	20 mg/mL[b]	IMM	10 mcg/mL[b]	Small particles form in 4 hr	1436	I
Gentamicin sulfate	SO	5 mg/mL[a]	IMM	10 mcg/mL[b]	Visually compatible for 4 hr at 22°C	1436	C
Granisetron HCl	SKB	0.05 mg/mL[a]	IMM	10 mcg/mL[b]	Physically compatible for 4 hr at 23°C	2000	C
Haloperidol lactate	LY	0.2 mg/mL[b]	IMM	10 mcg/mL[b]	Small particles form in 4 hr	1436	I
Heparin sodium	WY	100 units/mL[b]	IMM	10 mcg/mL[b]	Visually compatible for 4 hr at 22°C	1436	C
Heparin sodium	ES	100 units/mL[d]	IMM	6[b][e] and 15[b] mcg/mL	Visually compatible for 2 hr	1618	C
Hydrocortisone sodium succinate	UP	1 mg/mL[b]	IMM	10 mcg/mL[b]	Few small particles in 1 hr	1436	I
Hydromorphone HCl	WI	0.5 mg/mL[b]	IMM	10 mcg/mL[b]	Few small particles in 30 min	1436	I
Hydroxyzine HCl	ES	4 mg/mL[b]	IMM	10 mcg/mL[b]	Slight haze and particles form in 4 hr	1436	I
Idarubicin HCl	AD	0.5 mg/mL[b]	IMM	10 mcg/mL[b]	Physically compatible	1675	C
Ifosfamide	MJ	25 mg/mL[b]	IMM	10 mcg/mL[b]	Visually compatible for 4 hr at 22°C	1436	C
Imipenem–cilastatin sodium	MSD	5 mg/mL[b][j]	IMM	10 mcg/mL[b]	Large particle and clump form in 4 hr	1436	I
Immune globulin human	CU	50 mg/mL	IMM	6[b][e] and 15[b] mcg/mL	Visually compatible for 2 hr	1618	C
Lorazepam	WY	0.1 mg/mL[b]	IMM	10 mcg/mL[b]	Slightly bluish haze forms in 1 hr	1436	I
Magnesium sulfate	LY	100 mg/mL[b]	IMM	10 mcg/mL[b]	Visually compatible for 4 hr at 22°C	1436	C
Mannitol	BA	15%	IMM	10 mcg/mL[b]	Visually compatible for 4 hr at 22°C	1436	C
Mechlorethamine HCl	MSD	1 mg/mL	IMM	10 mcg/mL[b]	Visually compatible for 4 hr at 22°C	1436	C
Meperidine HCl	WI	4 mg/mL[b]	IMM	10 mcg/mL[b]	Visually compatible for 4 hr at 22°C	1436	C
Mesna	MJ	10 mg/mL[b]	IMM	10 mcg/mL[b]	Visually compatible for 4 hr at 22°C	1436	C
Methotrexate sodium	CET	15 mg/mL[b]	IMM	10 mcg/mL[b]	Visually compatible for 4 hr at 22°C	1436	C
Methylprednisolone sodium succinate	UP	5 mg/mL[b]	IMM	10 mcg/mL[b]	Small amounts of particles and filaments form in 4 hr	1436	I
Metoclopramide HCl	DU	5 mg/mL[b]	IMM	10 mcg/mL[b]	Visually compatible for 4 hr at 22°C	1436	C
Metronidazole	MG	5 mg/mL	IMM	10 mcg/mL[b]	Visually compatible for 4 hr at 22°C	1436	C

Y-Site Injection Compatibility (1:1 Mixture) (Cont.)

Test Drug	Mfr	Conc	Mfr	Conc	Remarks	Ref	C/I
Mitomycin	BR	0.5 mg/mL	IMM	10 mcg/mL[b]	Slight haze in 30 min	1436	I
Mitoxantrone HCl	LE	0.5 mg/mL[b]	IMM	10 mcg/mL[b]	Visually compatible for 4 hr at 22°C	1436	C
Morphine sulfate	WI	1 mg/mL[b]	IMM	10 mcg/mL[b]	Slight haze and particles in 1 hr	1436	I
Nalbuphine HCl	DU	10 mg/mL	IMM	10 mcg/mL[b]	Haze and filament form	1436	I
Ondansetron HCl	GL	0.5 mg/mL[b]	IMM	10 mcg/mL[b]	Filaments form in 30 to 60 min	1436	I
Pentostatin	NCI	0.4 mg/mL[b]	IMM	10 mcg/mL[b]	Visually compatible for 4 hr at 22°C	1436	C
Piperacillin sodium–tazobactam sodium	LE[c]	40 mg/mL[a h]	HO	10 mcg/mL[a]	Physically compatible for 4 hr at 22°C	1688	C
Potassium chloride	AB	0.1 mEq/mL[b]	IMM	10 mcg/mL[b]	Visually compatible for 4 hr at 22°C	1436	C
Prochlorperazine edisylate	ES	0.5 mg/mL[b]	IMM	10 mcg/mL[b]	Visually compatible for 4 hr at 22°C	1436	C
Promethazine HCl	ES	2 mg/mL[b]	IMM	10 mcg/mL[b]	Visually compatible for 4 hr at 22°C	1436	C
Ranitidine HCl	GL	2 mg/mL[b]	IMM	10 mcg/mL[b]	Visually compatible for 4 hr at 22°C	1436	C
Sodium bicarbonate	LY	1 mEq/mL	IMM	10 mcg/mL[b]	Small amount of particles forms in 4 hr	1436	I
Teniposide	BR	0.1 mg/mL[b]	IMM	10 mcg/mL[b]	Visually compatible for 4 hr at 22°C	1436	C
Tobramycin sulfate	LI	5 mg/mL[b]	IMM	10 mcg/mL[b]	Particles and filaments form in 4 hr	1436	I
TPN #133[f]			IMM	10 mcg/mL[b]	Visually compatible for 4 hr at 22°C	1436	C
TPN #181[f]			IMM	6[b e] and 15[b] mcg/mL	Visually compatible for 2 hr	1618	C
Trimethoprim–sulfamethoxazole	ES	0.8 mg/mL[b i]	IMM	10 mcg/mL[b]	Visually compatible for 4 hr at 22°C	1436	C
Vancomycin HCl	LI	10 mg/mL[b]	IMM	10 mcg/mL[b]	Visually compatible for 4 hr at 22°C	1436	C
Vancomycin HCl	LI	20 mg/mL[d]	IMM	15 mcg/mL[b]	Visually compatible for 2 hr	1618	C
Vancomycin HCl	LI	20 mg/mL[d]	IMM	6 mcg/mL[b e]	Haze forms within 15 min and increases due to vancomycin incompatibility with albumin human	1618, 1701	I
Vinblastine sulfate	LY	0.12 mg/mL[b]	IMM	10 mcg/mL[b]	Visually compatible for 4 hr at 22°C	1436	C
Vincristine sulfate	LY	0.05 mg/mL[b]	IMM	10 mcg/mL[b]	Visually compatible for 4 hr at 22°C	1436	C
Zidovudine	BW	4 mg/mL[b]	IMM	10 mcg/mL[b]	Visually compatible for 4 hr at 22°C	1436	C

[a] Tested in dextrose 5%.

[b] Tested in sodium chloride 0.9%.

[c] Test performed using the formulation WITHOUT edetate disodium.

[d] Tested in both dextrose 5% and sodium chloride 0.9%.

[e] Tested with 0.1% albumin human added.

[f] Refer to Appendix for the composition of parenteral nutrition solutions. TPN indicates a 2-in-1 admixture.

[g] Ampicillin component. Ampicillin in a 2:1 fixed-ratio concentration with sulbactam.

[h] Piperacillin sodium component. Piperacillin sodium in an 8:1 fixed-ratio concentration tazobactam sodium,

[i] Trimethoprim component. Trimethoprim in a 1:5 fixed-ratio concentration with sulfamethoxazole.

[j] Not specified whether concentration refers to single component or combined components.

Selected Revisions December 12, 2018. © Copyright, October 1992. American Society of Health-System Pharmacists, Inc.

Scopolamine Butylbromide
AHFS 12:08.08

Products

Scopolamine butylbromide 20 mg/mL with sodium chloride in water for injection is available in 1-mL ampuls.[115]

Trade Name(s)

Buscopan, Scoburen

Administration

Scopolamine butylbromide is administered by intramuscular or subcutaneous injection or slowly intravenously. Dextrose 5% and sodium chloride 0.9% are recommended for dilution if needed.[115]

Stability

Scopolamine butylbromide injection is a clear, colorless or nearly colorless solution. Intact containers should be stored below 30°C and protected from light.[115]

Compatibility Information

Additive Compatibility

Scopolamine butylbromide

Test Drug	Mfr	Conc/L or %	Mfr	Conc/L or %	Test Solution	Remarks	Ref	C/I
Floxacillin sodium	BE	20 g	BI	2 g	W	Physically compatible for 24 hr at 15 and 30°C. Precipitate forms in 48 hr at 30°C. No change in 48 hr at 15°C	1479	C
Furosemide	HO	1 g	BI	2 g	W	Physically compatible for 72 hr at 15 and 30°C	1479	C
Oxycodone HCl	NAP	1 g	BI	1 g	NS, W	Visually compatible. Under 4% concentration change in 24 hr at 25°C	2600	C
Tramadol HCl	AND	11.18 g	BI	1.68 g	NS[a]	Visually compatible for 7 days at 25°C protected from light	2701	C
Tramadol HCl	AND	5 g	BI	5 g	NS[a]	Visually compatible for 7 days at 25°C protected from light	2701	C

[a] Tested in elastomeric pump reservoirs (Baxter).

Drugs in Syringe Compatibility

Scopolamine butylbromide

Test Drug	Mfr	Amt	Mfr	Amt	Remarks	Ref	C/I
Diamorphine HCl	EV	50 and 150 mg/1 mL	BI	20 mg/1 mL	Physically compatible with no scopolamine loss and 4% diamorphine loss in 7 days at room temperature	1455	C
Haloperidol lactate		0.3125 mg/mL	BI	2.5, 5, 10 mg/mL	Physically compatible. Less than 10% loss of both drugs in 15 days at 4 and 25°C	2521	C
Haloperidol lactate		0.625 mg/mL	BI	2.5, 5, 10 mg/mL	Physically compatible. Less than 10% loss of both drugs in 7 days at 4 and 25°C. Over 10% loss of scopolamine in 15 days at both temperatures	2521	C
Haloperidol lactate		1.25 mg/mL	BI	2.5, 5, 10 mg/mL	Physically incompatible. Haloperidol precipitates in 15 days at 25°C and 7 days at 4°C	2521	I

DOI: 10.37573/9781585286850.348

Drugs in Syringe Compatibility (Cont.)

Test Drug	Mfr	Amt	Mfr	Amt	Remarks	Ref	C/I
Oxycodone HCl	NAP	200 mg/20 mL	BI	60 mg/3 mL	Visually compatible. Under 4% concentration change in 24 hr at 25°C	2600	C
Tramadol HCl	GRU	8.33, 16.67, 33.33 mg/mL[a]	BI	3.33, 4.99, 6.67 mg/mL[a]	Physically compatible with no loss of tramadol HCl and about 5 to 6% loss of scopolamine butyl-bromide in 15 days at 4 and 25°C protected from light	2632	C

[a] Diluted with sodium chloride 0.9%.

Selected Revisions October 1, 2012. © Copyright, October 2002.
American Society of Health-System Pharmacists, Inc.

Scopolamine Hydrobromide
AHFS 12:08.08
Hyoscine Hydrobromide

Products

Scopolamine hydrobromide is available in 1-mL multiple-dose vials containing 0.4- and 1-mg/mL concentrations. Also present in the products are methylparaben 0.18% and propylparaben 0.02%. Hydrobromic acid may have been used to adjust the pH.[1(6/06) 4]

pH

From 3.5 to 6.5.[1(6/06) 4]

Osmolality

The osmolality of scopolamine hydrobromide 0.5 mg/mL was determined to be 303 mOsm/kg.[1233]

Administration

Scopolamine hydrobromide may be administered subcutaneously, intramuscularly, or intravenously by direct intravenous injection after dilution with sterile water for injection.[1(6/06) 4]

Stability

The product should be stored at controlled room temperature and protected from light.[1(6/06)] Scopolamine hydrobromide is stated to be incompatible with alkalies.[4] Scopolamine hydrobromide decomposition is primarily due to hydrolysis below pH 3 and to both hydrolysis and inversion about the chiral carbon above pH 3. The minimum rate of decomposition occurs at pH 3.5.[1072]

Compatibility Information

Additive Compatibility

Scopolamine HBr

Test Drug	Mfr	Conc/L or %	Mfr	Conc/L or %	Test Solution	Remarks	Ref	C/I
Meperidine HCl	WI	100 mg		0.43 mg		Physically compatible	3	C
Oxycodone HCl	NAP	1 g		30 mg	NS, W	Visually compatible. Under 4% concentration change in 24 hr at 25°C	2600	C
Succinylcholine chloride	AB	2 g		0.43 mg		Physically compatible	3	C

Drugs in Syringe Compatibility

Scopolamine HBr

Test Drug	Mfr	Amt	Mfr	Amt	Remarks	Ref	C/I
Atropine sulfate	ST	0.4 mg/1 mL	ST	0.4 mg/1 mL	Physically compatible for at least 15 min	326	C
Buprenorphine HCl					Physically and chemically compatible	4	C
Butorphanol tartrate	BR	4 mg/2 mL	ST	0.4 mg/1 mL	Physically compatible for 30 min at room temperature	566	C
Chlorpromazine HCl	SKF	50 mg/2 mL		0.6 mg/1.5 mL	Physically compatible for at least 15 min	14	C
Chlorpromazine HCl	PO	50 mg/2 mL	ST	0.4 mg/1 mL	Physically compatible for at least 15 min	326	C
Diamorphine HCl	MB	10, 25, 50 mg/1 mL	EV	60 mcg/1 mL[a]	Physically compatible and diamorphine stable for 24 hr at room temperature	1454	C
Diamorphine HCl	EV	50 and 150 mg/1 mL	EV	0.4 mg/1 mL	Physically compatible with 7% diamorphine loss in 7 days at room temperature	1455	C
Dimenhydrinate	HR	50 mg/1 mL	ST	0.4 mg/1 mL	Physically compatible for at least 15 min	326	C
Diphenhydramine HCl	PD	50 mg/1 mL	ST	0.4 mg/1 mL	Physically compatible for at least 15 min	326	C

DOI: 10.37573/9781585286850.349

Drugs in Syringe Compatibility (Cont.)

Test Drug	Mfr	Amt	Mfr	Amt	Remarks	Ref	C/I
Droperidol	MN	2.5 mg/1 mL	ST	0.4 mg/1 mL	Physically compatible for at least 15 min	326	C
Fentanyl citrate	MN	100 mcg/1 mL		0.6 mg/1.5 mL	Physically compatible for at least 15 min	14	C
Fentanyl citrate	MN	0.05 mg/1 mL	ST	0.4 mg/1 mL	Physically compatible for at least 15 min	326	C
Glycopyrrolate	RB	0.2 mg/1 mL	ES	0.4 mg/1 mL	Physically compatible. pH in glycopyrrolate stability range for 48 hr at 25°C	331	C
Glycopyrrolate	RB	0.2 mg/1 mL	ES	0.8 mg/2 mL	Physically compatible. pH in glycopyrrolate stability range for 48 hr at 25°C	331	C
Glycopyrrolate	RB	0.4 mg/2 mL	ES	0.4 mg/1 mL	Physically compatible. pH in glycopyrrolate stability range for 48 hr at 25°C	331	C
Hydromorphone HCl	KN	4 mg/2 mL	BW	0.43 mg/0.5 mL	Physically compatible for 30 min	517	C
Hydroxyzine HCl	PF	100 mg/4 mL		0.6 mg/1.5 mL	Physically compatible for at least 15 min	14	C
Hydroxyzine HCl	PF	50 mg/1 mL	ST	0.4 mg/1 mL	Physically compatible for at least 15 min	326	C
Hydroxyzine HCl	PF	100 mg/2 mL		0.65 mg/1 mL	Physically compatible	771	C
Hydroxyzine HCl	PF	50 mg/1 mL		0.65 mg/1 mL	Physically compatible	771	C
Meperidine HCl	WY	100 mg/1 mL		0.6 mg/1.5 mL	Physically compatible for at least 15 min	14	C
Meperidine HCl	WI	50 mg/1 mL	ST	0.4 mg/1 mL	Physically compatible for at least 15 min	326	C
Methohexital sodium					Haze forms in 1 hr	4	I
Metoclopramide HCl	NO	10 mg/2 mL	ST	0.4 mg/1 mL	Physically compatible for 15 min at room temperature	565	C
Midazolam HCl	RC	5 mg/1 mL	BW	0.43 mg/0.5 mL	Physically compatible for 4 hr at 25°C	1145	C
Morphine sulfate	WY	15 mg/1 mL		0.6 mg/1.5 mL	Physically compatible for at least 15 min	14	C
Morphine sulfate	ST	15 mg/1 mL	ST	0.4 mg/1 mL	Physically compatible for at least 15 min	326	C
Morphine sulfate	BP	500 mg/5 mL	BP	5 mg/5 mL	Little scopolamine loss in 14 days at room temperature or 37°C. Morphine not tested	1609	C
Nalbuphine HCl	EN	10 mg/1 mL	BW	0.86 mg/1 mL	Physically compatible for 36 hr at 27°C	762	C
Nalbuphine HCl	EN	5 mg/0.5 mL	BW	0.86 mg/1 mL	Physically compatible for 36 hr at 27°C	762	C
Nalbuphine HCl	EN	10 mg/1 mL	BW	0.43 mg/0.5 mL	Physically compatible for 36 hr at 27°C	762	C
Nalbuphine HCl	DU	10 mg/1 mL		0.4 mg	Physically compatible for 48 hr	128	C
Nalbuphine HCl	DU	20 mg/1 mL		0.4 mg	Physically compatible for 48 hr	128	C
Oxycodone HCl	NAP	200 mg/20 mL		2.4 mg/6 mL	Visually compatible. Under 4% concentration change in 24 hr at 25°C	2600	C
Pentazocine lactate	WI	30 mg/1 mL		0.6 mg/1.5 mL	Physically compatible for at least 15 min	14	C
Pentazocine lactate	WI	30 mg/1 mL	ST	0.4 mg/1 mL	Physically compatible for at least 15 min	326	C
Pentobarbital sodium	AB	500 mg/10 mL		0.13 mg/0.26 mL	Physically compatible	55	C
Pentobarbital sodium	WY	100 mg/2 mL		0.6 mg/1.5 mL	Physically compatible for at least 15 min	14	C
Pentobarbital sodium	AB	50 mg/1 mL	ST	0.4 mg/1 mL	Physically compatible for at least 15 min	326	C
Prochlorperazine edisylate	SKF			0.6 mg/1.5 mL	Physically compatible for at least 15 min	14	C
Prochlorperazine edisylate	PO	5 mg/1 mL	ST	0.4 mg/1 mL	Physically compatible for at least 15 min	326	C

Drugs in Syringe Compatibility (Cont.)

Test Drug	Mfr	Amt	Mfr	Amt	Remarks	Ref	C/I
Promethazine HCl	WY	50 mg/2 mL		0.6 mg/1.5 mL	Physically compatible for at least 15 min	14	C
Promethazine HCl	PO	50 mg/2 mL	ST	0.4 mg/1 mL	Physically compatible for at least 15 min	326	C
Ranitidine HCl	GL	50 mg/2 mL	AB	0.4 mg/1 mL	Physically compatible for 1 hr at 25°C	978	C
Ranitidine HCl	GL	50 mg/5 mL		0.5 mg	Physically compatible for 4 hr at ambient temperature under fluorescent light	1151	C

[a] Diluted with sterile water for injection.

Y-Site Injection Compatibility (1:1 Mixture)

Scopolamine HBr

Test Drug	Mfr	Conc	Mfr	Conc	Remarks	Ref	C/I
Fentanyl citrate	JN	0.025 mg/mL[a]	LY	0.05 mg/mL[a]	Physically compatible for 48 hr at 22°C	1706	C
Heparin sodium	UP	1000 units/L[b]	BW	0.86 mg/mL	Physically compatible for 4 hr at room temperature	534	C
Hydrocortisone sodium succinate	UP	10 mg/L[b]	BW	0.86 mg/mL	Physically compatible for 4 hr at room temperature	534	C
Hydromorphone HCl	AST	0.5 mg/mL[a]	LY	0.05 mg/mL[a]	Physically compatible for 48 hr at 22°C	1706	C
Methadone HCl	LI	1 mg/mL[a]	LY	0.05 mg/mL[a]	Physically compatible for 48 hr at 22°C	1706	C
Morphine sulfate	AST	1 mg/mL[a]	LY	0.05 mg/mL[a]	Physically compatible for 48 hr at 22°C	1706	C
Potassium chloride	AB	40 mEq/L[b]	BW	0.86 mg/mL	Physically compatible for 4 hr at room temperature	534	C
Propofol	ZEN[c]	10 mg/mL	LY	0.4 mg/mL	Physically compatible for 1 hr at 23°C	2066	C

[a] Tested in dextrose 5%.

[b] Tested in dextrose 5% in Ringer's injection, lactated, dextrose 5% in Ringer's injection, dextrose 5%, Ringer's injection, lactated, and sodium chloride 0.9%.

[c] Test performed using the formulation WITH edetate disodium.

Selected Revisions January 31, 2020. © Copyright, October 1982. American Society of Health-System Pharmacists, Inc.

Sodium Acetate
AHFS 40:08

Products

Sodium acetate is available as a 16.4% solution in 20-, 50-, 100-, and 250-mL vials. Each mL of solution contains 2 mEq of sodium acetate in water for injection. Sodium acetate is also available as a 32.8% solution in 50- and 100-mL vials. Each mL of solution contains 4 mEq of sodium acetate in water for injection. The pH may have been adjusted with acetic acid.[1(9/06)]

pH

From 6 to 7.[1(9/06) 17]

Osmolarity

Sodium acetate injection is very hypertonic and must be diluted for use. The 2-mEq/mL concentration has a calculated osmolarity of 4 mOsm/mL, and the 4-mEq/mL concentration has a calculated osmolarity of 8 mOsm/mL.[1(9/06)]

Administration

Sodium acetate is administered by slow intravenous infusion after addition to a larger volume of fluid. It must not be given undiluted.[1(9/06)]

Stability

The product should be stored at controlled room temperature and protected from freezing and excessive heat. Discarding the vials four hours after initial entry has been recommended.[1(9/06)]

Compatibility Information

Y-Site Injection Compatibility (1:1 Mixture)

Sodium acetate

Test Drug	Mfr	Conc	Mfr	Conc	Remarks	Ref	C/I
Enalaprilat	MSD	0.05 mg/mL[b]	LY	0.4 mEq/mL[a]	Physically compatible for 24 hr at room temperature under fluorescent light	1355	C
Esmolol HCl	DCC	10 mg/mL[a]	LY	0.4 mEq/mL[a]	Physically compatible for 24 hr at 22°C	1169	C
Labetalol HCl	SC	1 mg/mL[a]	LY	0.4 mEq/mL[a]	Physically compatible for 24 hr at 18°C	1171	C
Nicardipine HCl	DCC	0.1 mg/mL[a]	LY	0.4 mEq/mL[a]	Visually compatible for 24 hr at room temperature	235	C
Ondansetron HCl	GL	0.1 mg/mL[a]		0.1 and 1 mEq/mL[a]	Physically compatible for 4 hr at room temperature	1661	C

[a] Tested in dextrose 5%.

[b] Tested in sodium chloride 0.9%.

Selected Revisions October 1, 2012. © Copyright, October 1990.
American Society of Health-System Pharmacists, Inc.

DOI: 10.37573/9781585286850.350

Sodium Bicarbonate
AHFS 40:08

Products

Sodium bicarbonate injection is available from various manufacturers in vials and syringes as an aqueous solution in concentrations of 4.2, 7.5, and 8.4%.[3223] [3224] Carbon dioxide may have been added to some products to adjust the pH.[3224]

Concentration	Bicarbonate (and Sodium) Concentration	Total Container Content	Osmolarity
8.4%	1 mEq/mL	10 mEq/10 mL	2000 mOsm/L
8.4%	1 mEq/mL	50 mEq/50 mL	2000 mOsm/L
7.5%	0.892 mEq/mL	44.6 mEq/50 mL	1790 mOsm/L
4.2%	0.5 mEq/mL	5 mEq/10 mL	1000 mOsm/L

Sodium bicarbonate 4% neutralizing additive solution (Neut, Hospira) is available in 5-mL single-dose vials.[3225] Each mL of solution provides 0.48 mEq of bicarbonate and sodium and 2 mg of edetate disodium anhydrous.[3225] Sodium bicarbonate neutralizing additive solution is used to raise the pH of acidic solutions.[3225]

Equivalency

Each 84 mg of sodium bicarbonate provides 1 mEq of sodium and bicarbonate ions.[3223] [3224]

pH

From 7 to 8.5.[3223] [3224] [3225]

Administration

Sodium bicarbonate is administered intravenously, either undiluted or diluted in other fluids.[3223] [3224] [3225] It also has been administered subcutaneously if diluted to isotonicity (1.5%).[2043]

Stability

Sodium bicarbonate injection should be stored at controlled room temperature.[3223] [3224] [3225] A solution that is unclear or that contains a precipitate should not be used.[3223] [3224]

Sodium bicarbonate injection under simulated summer conditions in paramedic vehicles was exposed to temperatures ranging from 26 to 38°C over 4 weeks. Analysis found no loss of the drug under these conditions.[2562]

Combining sodium bicarbonate with acids in aqueous solutions results in the liberation of carbon dioxide gas.[2248] The bubbles can evolve to a sufficient quantity to cause effervescence.[2248]

The stability of sodium bicarbonate 7.5% in polypropylene syringes is inversely related to the storage temperature.[136] Estimates of room temperature stability range from 1 week[137] to 1 month.[136] Refrigeration may increase the stability to 60[137] to 90 days.[136] Stability also may be increased by refrigerating the sodium bicarbonate injection and the syringes before preparation, rinsing the syringes twice with refrigerated sterile water for injection, minimizing the contact of the solution with the air by expelling the air from the syringes, and taping the plunger in place to minimize its movement from escaping carbon dioxide.[137]

pH Effects

Drugs such as sodium bicarbonate that may raise the pH of an admixture above 6 may cause significant decomposition of alkali-labile drugs.[59] [77] [79]

The change in pH that occurs when 5 mL of sodium bicarbonate 4% additive solution (Neut, Abbott) is added to a liter of 5 common infusion solutions (Travenol) was reported:[1129]

Solution	Initial pH	pH after Neut Added	pH Increase
Dextrose 5%	4.4	7.5	3.1
Dextrose 10%	3.9	7.1	3.2
Ringer's injection	5.6	7.5	1.9
Sodium chloride 0.45%	5.6	7.8	2.2
Sodium chloride 0.9%	5.5	7.6	2.2

Compatibility Information
Solution Compatibility

Sodium bicarbonate

Test Soln Name	Mfr	Mfr	Conc/L or %	Remarks	Ref	C/I
Dextrose 2.5% in half-strength Ringer's injection	AB		3.75 g	Physically compatible	3	C
Dextrose 5% in Ringer's injection	AB		3.75 g	Physically compatible	3	C

DOI: 10.37573/9781585286850.351

Solution Compatibility (Cont.)

Test Soln Name	Mfr	Mfr	Conc/L or %	Remarks	Ref	C/I
Dextrose 5% in half-strength Ringer's injection, lactated	AB		3.75 g	Physically compatible	3	C
Dextrose 2.5% in Ringer's injection, lactated	AB		3.75 g	Physically compatible	3	C
Dextrose 5% in Ringer's injection, lactated	AB		3.75 g	Physically compatible	3	C
Dextrose 5% in Ringer's injection, lactated	AB	AB	80 mEq	Physically incompatible	15	I
Dextrose 10% in Ringer's injection, lactated	AB		3.75 g	Physically compatible	3	C
Dextrose 2.5% in sodium chloride 0.45%	AB		3.75 g	Physically compatible	3	C
Dextrose 2.5% in sodium chloride 0.9%	AB		3.75 g	Physically compatible	3	C
Dextrose 5% in sodium chloride 0.225%	AB		3.75 g	Physically compatible	3	C
Dextrose 5% in sodium chloride 0.45%	AB		3.75 g	Physically compatible	3	C
Dextrose 5% in sodium chloride 0.9%	AB		3.75 g	Physically compatible	3	C
Dextrose 5% in sodium chloride 0.9%	TR[a]	AB	4 g	Stable for 24 hr at 5°C	282	C
Dextrose 10% in sodium chloride 0.9%	AB		3.75 g	Physically compatible	3	C
Dextrose 2.5%	AB		3.75 g	Physically compatible	3	C
Dextrose 5%	AB		3.75 g	Physically compatible	3	C
Dextrose 5%	TR[a]	AB	4 g	Stable for 24 hr at 5°C	282	C
Dextrose 5%	BRN[c]	HOS	50, 100, 150 mEq	Physically compatible. Bicarbonate and pH remained stable over 7 days at 4 and 24°C	2817	C
Dextrose 10%	AB		3.75 g	Physically compatible	3	C
Ionosol B in dextrose 5%	AB		3.75 g	Physically compatible	3	C
Ionosol MB in dextrose 5%	AB		3.75 g	Physically compatible	3	C
Ringer's injection	AB		3.75 g	Physically compatible	3	C
Ringer's injection, lactated	AB		3.75 g	Physically compatible	3	C
Ringer's injection, lactated	AB	AB	80 mEq	Physically incompatible	15	I
Sodium chloride 0.45%	AB		3.75 g	Physically compatible	3	C
Sodium chloride 0.9%	AB		3.75 g	Physically compatible	3	C
Sodium chloride 0.9%	TR[a]	AB	4 g	Stable for 24 hr at 5°C	282	C
Sodium lactate ⅙ M	AB		3.75 g	Physically compatible	3	C
TNA #66 to #68[b]			100 mEq	Physically compatible with 10% or less carbon dioxide loss and unchanged pH in 7 days at 25°C protected from light	1011	C

Solution Compatibility (Cont.)

Test Soln Name	Mfr	Mfr	Conc/L or %	Remarks	Ref	C/I
TNA #67[b]			100 mEq	Physically compatible with 10% or less carbon dioxide loss and unchanged pH in 7 days at 25°C protected from light	1011	C
TNA #68[b]			100 mEq	Physically compatible with 10% or less carbon dioxide loss and unchanged pH in 7 days at 25°C protected from light	1011	C
TPN #62[b]			50 and 150 mEq	Physically compatible with 10% or less carbon dioxide loss and unchanged pH in 7 days at 25°C protected from light	1011	C
TPN #63[b]			50 and 150 mEq	Physically compatible with 10% or less carbon dioxide loss and unchanged pH in 7 days at 25°C protected from light	1011	C
TPN #64[b]			50 and 150 mEq	Physically compatible with 10% or less carbon dioxide loss and unchanged pH in 7 days at 25°C protected from light	1011	C
TPN #65[b]			50 and 150 mEq	Physically compatible with 10% or less carbon dioxide loss and unchanged pH in 7 days at 25°C protected from light	1011	C

[a] Tested in both glass and PVC containers.

[b] Refer to Appendix for the composition of parenteral nutrition solutions. TNA indicates a 3-in-1 admixture, and TPN indicates a 2-in-1 admixture.

[c] Tested in polyolefin containers.

Additive Compatibility

Sodium bicarbonate

Test Drug	Mfr	Conc/L or %	Mfr	Conc/L or %	Test Solution	Remarks	Ref	C/I
Amikacin sulfate	BR	5 g	BR	15 g	D5LR, D5R, D5S, D5W, D10W, LR, NS, R, SL	Physically compatible and both stable for 24 hr at 25°C	294	C
Aminophylline	SE	1 g	AB	80 mEq	D5W	Physically compatible	15	C
Aminophylline	SE	500 mg	AB	40 mEq		Physically compatible	6	C
Amoxicillin sodium		10, 20, 50 g		2.74%		9% amoxicillin loss in 6 and 4 hr at 10 and 20 g/L, respectively, and 15% loss in 4 hr at 50 g/L at 25°C	1469	I
Amoxicillin sodium		10, 20, 50 g		8.4%		10 and 13% amoxicillin loss in 4 hr at 10 and 20 g/L, respectively, and 17% loss in 3 hr at 50 g/L at 25°C	1469	I
Amphotericin B	SQ	50 mg	AB	2.4 mEq[a]	D5W	Physically compatible for 24 hr	772	C
Ampicillin sodium	AY	2 and 4 g		1.4%		10% ampicillin loss in 6 hr at room temperature	99	I
Ampicillin sodium	BAY	15 g		1.4%		10% ampicillin loss in 10 hr at 25°C	604	I
Ampicillin sodium	BAY	2 g		1.4%		10% ampicillin loss in 17 hr at 25°C	604	I
Ampicillin sodium	BAY	5 g		1.4%		10% ampicillin loss in 14 hr at 25°C	604	I
Amsacrine	NCI			2 mEq	D5W	Amsacrine chemically stable for 96 hr at room temperature	234	C
Ascorbic acid	UP	500 mg	AB	80 mEq	D5W	Physically incompatible	15	I

Additive Compatibility (Cont.)

Test Drug	Mfr	Conc/L or %	Mfr	Conc/L or %	Test Solution	Remarks	Ref	C/I
Atropine sulfate		0.4 mg	AB	2.4 mEq[a]	D5W	Physically compatible for 24 hr	772	C
Azacitidine						Stated to be incompatible	3325, 3326	I
Calcium chloride	UP		AB		D5W	Conditionally compatible depending on concentrations	15	?
Calcium chloride		1 g	AB	2.4 mEq[a]	D5W	Physically compatible for 24 hr	772	C
Calcium gluconate	UP		AB		D5W	Conditionally compatible depending on concentrations	15	?
Carboplatin		1 g		200 mmol		13% carboplatin loss in 24 hr at 27°C	1379	I
Carmustine	BR	100 mg	AB	100 mEq	D5W, NS	10% carmustine loss in 15 min and 27% in 90 min	523	I
Cefoxitin sodium	MSD	1 g	AB	200 mg	W	5 to 6% cefoxitin loss in 24 hr and 11 to 12% in 48 hr at 25°C. 2 to 3% loss in 7 days at 5°C	308	C
Ceftazidime	GL	20 g		4.2%		11% ceftazidime loss in 24 hr at 25°C. 3% loss in 48 hr at 4°C	1136	C
Ceftriaxone sodium	RC	10 to 40 g		5%		Less than 10% loss in 24 hr at 25°C	1(3/06)	C
Chloramphenicol sodium succinate	PD	10 g	AB	80 mEq	D5W	Physically compatible	15	C
Chloramphenicol sodium succinate	PD	1 g	AB	80 mEq		Physically compatible	6	C
Ciprofloxacin	MI	2 g		[i]	D5W	Physically incompatible	888	I
Ciprofloxacin	BAY	2 g	AST	4 g	D5W	Precipitates immediately	2413	I
Cisplatin		50 and 500 mg		5%		Bright gold precipitate forms in 8 to 24 hr at 25°C	635	I
Clindamycin phosphate	UP	1.2 g		44 mEq	D5S, D5W	Clindamycin stable for 24 hr	101	C
Cytarabine	UP	200 mg and 1 g	AB	50 mEq	D5W[b]	Physically compatible with no cytarabine loss in 7 days at 8 and 22°C	748	C
Cytarabine	UP	200 mg	AB	50 mEq	D5¼S[b c]	Physically compatible with no cytarabine loss in 7 days at 8 and 22°C	748	C
Dobutamine HCl	LI	1 g	MG	5%		Cloudy brown with precipitate in 3 hr at 25°C. 18% dobutamine loss in 24 hr	789	I
Dobutamine HCl	LI	1 g	IX	500 mEq	D5W, NS	White precipitate in 6 hr at 21°C	812	I
Dopamine HCl	AS	800 mg	MG	5%		Color change 5 min after mixing	79	I
Doxapram HCl	WW					Precipitation or gas formation	3220	I
Epinephrine HCl		4 mg	AB	2.4 mEq[a]	D5W	Epinephrine inactivated	772	I
Epinephrine HCl		4 mg		5%		Epinephrine rapidly decomposes. 58% loss immediately after mixing	48	I
Ertapenem sodium	ME	10 and 20 g	AB	5%		Visually compatible. 11% loss in 3 hr at 25°C. 16 to 19% loss in 1 day at 4°C	2487	I
Erythromycin lactobionate	AB	1 g	AB	3.75 g		Physically compatible. Erythromycin stable for 24 hr at 25°C	20	C
Erythromycin lactobionate	AB	1 g	AB	2.4 mEq[a]	D5W	Physically compatible for 24 hr	772	C

Additive Compatibility (Cont.)

Test Drug	Mfr	Conc/L or %	Mfr	Conc/L or %	Test Solution	Remarks	Ref	C/I
Esmolol HCl	ACC	10 g	MG[c]	5%		Visually compatible. 5 and 8% esmolol losses in 7 days at 4 and 27°C, respectively	1831	C
Fat emulsion, intravenous	VT	10%	BR	7.5 g		Physically compatible for 48 hr at 4°C and room temperature	32	C
Fat emulsion, intravenous	VT	10%		3.4 g		Lipid coalescence in 24 hr at 8 and 25°C	825	I
Furosemide	HO	1 g	IMS	8.4%		Physically compatible for 72 hr at 15 and 30°C	1479	C
Heparin sodium	AB	20,000 units	AB	2.4 mEq[a]	D5W	Physically compatible for 24 hr	772	C
Hyaluronidase	WY	150 units	AB	2.4 mEq[a]	D5W	Physically compatible for 24 hr	772	C
Imipenem–cilastatin sodium	MSD	2.5[j] g	AB	5%		43% imipenem loss in 3 hr at 25°C and 52% in 24 hr at 4°C	1141	I
Imipenem–cilastatin sodium	MSD	5[j] g	AB	5%		45% imipenem loss in 3 hr at 25°C and 50% in 24 hr at 4°C	1141	I
Isoproterenol HCl	WI	5 mg		5%		Isoproterenol decomposition	48	I
Isoproterenol HCl	BN	1 mg	AB	2.4 mEq[a]	D5W	Isoproterenol decomposition	772	I
Labetalol HCl	SC	1.25, 2.5, 3.75 g	TR	5%		White precipitate forms within 6 hr after mixing at 4 and 25°C	757	I
Levofloxacin	OMJ	0.5 g	BA	5%[b]		Physically compatible. No loss in 3 days at 25°C, 14 days at 5°C, in dark	1986	C
Levofloxacin	OMJ	0.5 g	BA	5%[b]		Precipitate forms within 13 weeks at –20°C	1986	I
Levofloxacin	OMJ	5 g	BA	5%[b]		Physically compatible. No loss in 3 days at 25°C, 14 days at 5°C, 26 weeks at –20°C, in dark	1986	C
Lidocaine HCl	AST	2 g	AB	40 mEq		Physically compatible	24	C
Lidocaine HCl		1 g	AB	2.4 mEq[a]	D5W	Physically compatible for 24 hr	772	C
Magnesium sulfate	LI	16 mEq	AB	80 mEq	D5W	Physically incompatible	15	I
Magnesium sulfate	HOS	1.5 and 15 mEq	BA	50 mEq	[h]	Physically compatible. No loss of ions for 48 hr at 23°C	2814	C
Mannitol	AMR	25 g	AB	44.6 mEq	D5LR, D5¼S, D5½S, D5S, D5W, D10W, NS, ½S[d]	Visually compatible for 24 hr at 24°C	1853, 1973	C
Meperidine HCl	WI	100 mg	AB	2.4 mEq[a]	D5W	Physically compatible for 24 hr	772	C
Meropenem	ZEN	1 g	BA	5%		10% meropenem loss in 4 hr at 24°C and 18 hr at 4°C	2089	I[g]
Meropenem	ZEN	20 g	BA	5%		9 to 10% meropenem loss in 3 hr at 24°C and 18 hr at 4°C	2089	I[g]
Methotrexate sodium		2 g		50 mEq		No photodegradation products in 12 hr in room light	433	C
Methotrexate sodium	LE	750 mg		50 mEq	D5W	6% methotrexate loss in 1 week at 5°C in dark. At 23°C in light, 6% loss in 72 hr and 15% in 1 week	465	C

Additive Compatibility (Cont.)

Test Drug	Mfr	Conc/L or %	Mfr	Conc/L or %	Test Solution	Remarks	Ref	C/I
Methyldopate HCl	MSD	1 g		50 mEq	D5W, D10W, D2.5½S, D2.5S, D5¼S, D5½S, D5S, D10S, NS, ½S	Physically compatible	23	C
Methyldopate HCl	MSD	1 g	AB	5%		Stable for 24 hr	23	C
Midazolam HCl	RC	100 mg	c	5%		Transient precipitation upon mixing	355	?
Midazolam HCl	RC	500 mg	c	5%		Precipitation upon mixing	355	I
Multivitamins	USV	10 mL	AB	4.8 mEq[e]	D5W	Physically compatible for 24 hr	772	C
Nafcillin sodium	WY	500 mg	AB	40 mEq		Physically compatible	27	C
Nicardipine HCl	DME	50 and 500 mg	TR[c]	5%		Precipitate forms immediately	1380	I
Norepinephrine bitartrate	WI	2 mg	AB	80 mEq	D5W	Physically incompatible	15	I
Norepinephrine bitartrate	BN	8 mg	AB	2.4 mEq[a]	D5W	Norepinephrine decomposition	772	I
Oxytocin	PD	5 units	AB	2.4 mEq[a]	D5W	Physically compatible for 24 hr	772	C
Penicillin G potassium		100 million units	AB	2.4 mEq[a]	D5W	Physically compatible for 24 hr	772	C
Penicillin G potassium	SQ	1 million units	AB	3.75 g	D5W	26% penicillin loss in 24 hr at 25°C	47	I
Penicillin G potassium	SQ	1 million units		0.5 and 0.75 g	D5W	Penicillin loss at 20°C due to pH	135	I
Penicillin G potassium	f	900,000 units		3.75 g	D5W	26% penicillin loss in 24 hr at 25°C	48	I
Pentazocine lactate	WI	300 mg	AB	80 mEq	D5W	Physically incompatible	15	I
Pentobarbital sodium	AB	1 g	AB	80 mEq	D5W	Physically incompatible	15	I
Phenylephrine HCl	WI	10 mg	AB	2.4 mEq[a]	D5W	Physically compatible for 24 hr	772	C
Phenylephrine HCl	WI	20 mg		5%		Stable for 24 hr at 25°C	48	C
Phytonadione	MSD	10 mg	AB	2.4 mEq[a]	D5W	Physically compatible for 24 hr	772	C
Posaconazole	ME			i		Stated to be incompatible	2911	I
Potassium chloride		120 mEq	AB	2.4 mEq[a]	D5W	Physically compatible for 24 hr	772	C
Prochlorperazine edisylate	SKF	10 mg	AB	2.4 mEq[a]	D5W	Physically compatible for 24 hr	772	C
Ranitidine HCl				5%		Stable for 48 hr at room temperature	3497, 3498	C
Succinylcholine chloride	AB	1 g	AB	2.4 mEq[a]	D5W	Succinylcholine decomposition	772	I
Verapamil HCl	KN	80 mg	BR	89.2 mEq	D5W, NS	Physically compatible for 24 hr	764	C
Voriconazole	PF, SZ			4.2%		Voriconazole slightly decomposes at room temperature	3233, 3348	I

Additive Compatibility (Cont.)

Test Drug	Mfr	Conc/L or %	Mfr	Conc/L or %	Test Solution	Remarks	Ref	C/I
Voriconazole	XGN			4.2%		Voriconazole slightly decomposes at room temperature	3347	I

[a] One vial of Neut added to a liter of admixture.

[b] Tested in PVC containers.

[c] Tested in glass containers.

[d] Tested in polyolefin containers.

[e] Two vials of Neut added to a liter of admixture.

[f] A buffered preparation was specified.

[g] Incompatible by conventional standards but may be used in shorter periods of time.

[h] Tested in an extemporaneously-compounded hemofiltration solution.

[i] Final sodium bicarbonate concentration not specified.

[j] Imipenem component. Imipenem in a 1:1 fixed-ratio concentration with cilastatin.

Drugs in Syringe Compatibility

Sodium bicarbonate

Test Drug	Mfr	Amt	Mfr	Amt	Remarks	Ref	C/I
Bupivacaine HCl	AST, WI	0.25, 0.5[a], 0.75%[a], 20 mL	AB	4%, 0.05 to 0.6 mL	Precipitate forms in 1 to 2 min up to 2 hr at lowest amount of bicarbonate	1724	I
Bupivacaine HCl	BEL	0.5%[b], 20 mL		1.4%, 1.5 mL	No epinephrine loss in 7 days at room temperature. Bupivacaine not tested	1743	C
Bupivacaine HCl	BEL	0.5%[b], 20 mL		4.2 and 8.4%, 1.5 mL	5 to 7% epinephrine loss in 7 days at room temperature. Bupivacaine not tested	1743	C
Caffeine citrate		20 mg/1 mL	AST	4.2%, 1 mL	Visually compatible for 4 hr at 25°C	2440	C
Dimenhydrinate		10 mg/1 mL		1 mEq/1 mL	Precipitates immediately	2569	I
Glycopyrrolate	RB	0.2 mg/1 mL	AB	75 mg/1 mL	Gas evolves	331	I
Glycopyrrolate	RB	0.2 mg/1 mL	AB	150 mg/2 mL	Gas evolves	331	I
Glycopyrrolate	RB	0.4 mg/2 mL	AB	75 mg/1 mL	Gas evolves	331	I
Lidocaine HCl	ES	2%[c], 30 mL	AB	3 mEq/3 mL	11% lidocaine and 28% epinephrine loss in 1 week at 25°C	1712	I
Lidocaine HCl	ES	2%[c], 30 mL	AB	3 mEq/3 mL	6% lidocaine loss in 4 weeks at 4°C. 12% epinephrine loss in 3 weeks at 4°C	1712	C
Lidocaine HCl	AST	1%[c]	LY	0.1 mEq/mL	25% epinephrine loss in 1 week at room temperature. Lidocaine not tested	1713	I
Lidocaine HCl		0.9%		0.088 mEq/mL	11% lidocaine loss in 7 days at room temperature	1723	C
Lidocaine HCl	AST	1 and 1.5%[a], 20 mL	AST	8.4%/2 mL	Visually compatible for up to 5 hr at room temperature	1724	C
Lidocaine HCl	AST	2%[a], 20 mL	AST	8.4%/2 mL	Haze forms but dissipates with gentle agitation	1724	?
Lidocaine HCl	AST	1 and 1.5%[a], 20 mL	AB	4%/4 mL	Visually compatible for up to 5 hr at room temperature	1724	C
Lidocaine HCl	AST	2%[a], 20 mL	AB	4%/4 mL	Haze forms but dissipates with gentle agitation	1724	?
Lidocaine HCl	BEL	2%[d], 20 mL		1.4 and 8.4%/1.5 mL	8% epinephrine loss in 7 days at room temperature. Lidocaine not tested	1743	C

Drugs in Syringe Compatibility (Cont.)

Test Drug	Mfr	Amt	Mfr	Amt	Remarks	Ref	C/I
Lidocaine HCl		2%/10 mL		8.4%/1 mL	Physically compatible. No loss of lidocaine in 6 hr	1401	C
Lidocaine HCl		2%ᶜ, 10 mL		8.4%/1.5 mL	Physically compatible. No loss of lidocaine or epinephrine in 6 hr	1401	C
Lidocaine HCl		2%ᶜ, 10 mL		1.4%/1.5 mL	Physically compatible. No loss of lidocaine or epinephrine in 6 hr	1401	C
Lidocaine HCl		1%ᶜ, 10 mL		8.4%/1 mL	Cloudiness in some samples with no epinephrine loss for 72 hr in the dark. Exposed to light and air, precipitation and 20% epinephrine loss in 24 hr. Lidocaine not tested	2408	?
Lidocaine HCl	ASZ	1 and 2%ᶜ, 2.7 mL	HOS	8.4%/0.3 mL	Physically compatible. 10% epinephrine loss in 7 days and 5% lidocaine loss in 28 days at 5°C in dark	2815	C
Mepivacaine HCl	AST, WI	1 and 1.5%/20 mL	AST	8.4%; 0.5, 1, 2 mL	Precipitate forms within approximately 1 hr	1724	I
Mepivacaine HCl	AST, WI	1 and 1.5%/20 mL	AB	4%; 1, 2, 4 mL	Precipitate forms within approximately 1 hr	1724	I
Metoclopramide HCl	RB	10 mg/2 mL	AB	100 mEq/100 mL	Gas evolves	1167	I
Metoclopramide HCl	RB	160 mg/32 mL	AB	100 mEq/100 mL	Gas evolves	1167	I
Milrinone lactate	STR	5.25 mg/5.25 mL	AB	3.75 g/50 mL	Physically compatible. No milrinone loss in 20 min at 23°C	1410	C
Pantoprazole sodium	ᵉ	4 mg/1 mL		1 mEq/1 mL	Precipitates after 1 hr	2574	I
Pentobarbital sodium	AB	500 mg/10 mL		3.75 g/50 mL	Physically compatible	55	C

ᵃ Tested with and without epinephrine hydrochloride 1:200,000 added.

ᵇ Tested with epinephrine hydrochloride 1:200,000 added.

ᶜ Tested with epinephrine hydrochloride 1:100,000 added.

ᵈ Tested with epinephrine hydrochloride 1:80,000 added.

ᵉ Test performed using the formulation WITHOUT edetate disodium.

Y-Site Injection Compatibility (1:1 Mixture)

Sodium bicarbonate

Test Drug	Mfr	Conc	Mfr	Conc	Remarks	Ref	C/I
Acyclovir sodium	BW	5 mg/mLᵃ	IX	0.5 mEq/mLᵃ	Physically compatible for 4 hr at 25°C	1157	C
Allopurinol sodium	BW	3 mg/mLᵇ	AB	1 mEq/mL	Small and large crystals form in 1 hr	1686	I
Amifostine	USB	10 mg/mLᵃ	AST	1 mEq/mL	Physically compatible for 4 hr at 23°C	1845	C
Amiodarone HCl	WY	3 mg/mLᵃ	AB	1 mEq/mL	Precipitate forms immediately	1851	I
Amiodarone HCl	WY	6 mg/mLᵃ	AB	1 mEq/mL	Translucent haze in 1 hr	2352	I
Anidulafungin	VIC	0.5 mg/mLᵃ	APP	1 mEq/mL	Haze increases immediately and microparticulates occur in 4 hr	2617	I
Aztreonam	SQ	40 mg/mLᵃ	AB	1 mEq/mL	Physically compatible for 4 hr at 23°C	1758	C
Bivalirudin	TMC	5 mg/mLᵃ	AMR	1 mEq/mL	Physically compatible for 4 hr at 23°C	2373	C
Calcium chloride	AB	4 mg/mLᵈ	AB	1 mEq/mL	Slight haze or precipitate in 1 hr	1316	I

Y-Site Injection Compatibility (1:1 Mixture) (Cont.)

Test Drug	Mfr	Conc	Mfr	Conc	Remarks	Ref	C/I
Cangrelor tetrasodium	TMC	1 mg/mL[b]		1 mEq/mL	Physically compatible for 4 hr	3243	C
Ceftaroline fosamil	FOR	2.22 mg/mL[h]	HOS	1 mEq/mL	Physically compatible for 4 hr at 23°C	2826	C
Ceftazidime–avibactam sodium	ALL	20 mg/mL[a q]			Physically compatible for up to 4 hr at room temperature	3004	C
Ceftolozane sulfate–tazobactam sodium	CUB	10 mg/mL[d o]	HOS	1 mEq/mL	Physically compatible for 2 hr	3262	C
Ceftriaxone sodium	RC	100 mg/mL		1.4%	Visually compatible for 4 hr at room temperature	1788	C
Ciprofloxacin	MI	2 mg/mL[a]	AB	1 mEq/mL	Visually compatible for 24 hr at 24°C	1655	C
Ciprofloxacin	MI	2 mg/mL[b]	AB	1 mEq/mL	Very fine crystals form in 20 min in NS	1655	I
Ciprofloxacin	MI	2 mg/mL[a]	AB	1 mEq/mL	Physically compatible for 4 hr at 23°C	1869	C
Ciprofloxacin	MI	2 mg/mL[a]	AB	0.1 mEq/mL[a]	Subvisible haze forms immediately. Crystalline precipitate in 4 hr at 23°C	1869	I
Ciprofloxacin	BAY	1 and 2 mg/mL[a]	AB	1 and 0.75[a] mEq/mL	Physically compatible for 4 hr at 23°C	2065	C
Ciprofloxacin	BAY	1 mg/mL[b]	AB	1 and 0.75[b] mEq/mL	Physically compatible for 4 hr at 23°C	2065	C
Ciprofloxacin	BAY	2 mg/mL[b]	AB	1 and 0.75[b] mEq/mL	Particles form immediately, becoming more numerous over 4 hr at 23°C	2065	I
Ciprofloxacin	BAY	1 and 2 mg/mL[a]	AB	0.5, 0.25, 0.1 mEq/mL[a]	Particles form immediately, becoming more numerous over 4 hr at 23°C	2065	I
Ciprofloxacin	BAY	1 mg/mL[b]	AB	0.5, 0.25, 0.1 mEq/mL[b]	Particles form immediately, becoming more numerous over 4 hr at 23°C	2065	I
Ciprofloxacin	BAY	2 mg/mL[b]	AB	0.5, 0.25, 0.1 mEq/mL[b]	Precipitate forms immediately	2065	I
Cisatracurium besylate	GW	0.1 mg/mL[a]	AB	1 mEq/mL	Physically compatible for 4 hr at 23°C	2074	C
Cisatracurium besylate	GW	2 mg/mL[a]	AB	1 mEq/mL	Subvisible brown color and haze in 1 hr	2074	I
Cisatracurium besylate	GW	5 mg/mL[a]	AB	1 mEq/mL	Subvisible haze forms immediately with brown color and turbidity in 4 hr	2074	I
Cladribine	ORT	0.015[b] and 0.5[f] mg/mL	AB	1 mEq/mL	Physically compatible for 4 hr at 23°C	1969	C
Cloxacillin sodium	SMX	100 mg/mL	HOS	84 mg/mL	Physically compatible for up to 4 hr at room temperature	3245	C
Cyclophosphamide		20 mg/mL[a]		1.4%	Visually compatible for 4 hr at room temperature	1788	C
Cytarabine	UP	0.6 mg/mL[a]		1.4%	Visually compatible for 4 hr at room temperature	1788	C
Daunorubicin HCl	BEL	0.52 mg/mL[a]		1.4%	Visually compatible for 4 hr at room temperature	1788	C
Dexamethasone sodium phosphate	MSD	4 mg/mL		1.4%	Visually compatible for 4 hr at room temperature	1788	C
Dexmedetomidine HCl	AB	4 mcg/mL[b]	AMR	1 mEq/mL	Physically compatible for 4 hr at 23°C	2383	C
Diltiazem HCl	MMD	5 mg/mL	LY	1 mEq/mL	Precipitate forms	1807	I
Diltiazem HCl	MMD	1 mg/mL[b]	LY	1 mEq/mL	Visually compatible	1807	C

Y-Site Injection Compatibility (1:1 Mixture) (Cont.)

Test Drug	Mfr	Conc	Mfr	Conc	Remarks	Ref	C/I
Diltiazem HCl	MMD	5 mg/mL	AMR	0.05 mEq/mL[a]	Visually compatible	1807	C
Docetaxel	RPR	0.9 mg/mL[a]	AB	1 mEq/mL	Physically compatible for 4 hr at 23°C	2224	C
Doripenem	JJ	5 mg/mL[a b]	HOS	1 mEq/mL	Physically compatible for 4 hr at 23°C	2743	C
Doxorubicin HCl	FA	0.4 mg/mL[a]		1.4%	Visually compatible for 2 hr at room temperature	1788	C
Doxorubicin HCl liposomal	SEQ	0.4 mg/mL[a]	AB	1 mEq/mL	Partial loss of measured natural turbidity	2087	I
Eravacycline dihydrochloride	TET	0.3 and 0.6 mg/mL[b]	FRK	1 mEq/mL	Measured turbidity increased immediately	3532	I
Etoposide	BR	0.6 mg/mL[b]		1.4%	Visually compatible for 4 hr at room temperature	1788	C
Etoposide phosphate	BR	5 mg/mL[a]	AB	1 mEq/mL	Physically compatible for 4 hr at 23°C	2218	C
Famotidine	MSD	0.2 mg/mL[a]	AB	1 mEq/mL	Physically compatible for 4 hr at 25°C	1188	C
Fenoldopam mesylate	AB	80 mcg/mL[b]	APP	1 mEq/mL	Trace haze and microparticulates form immediately with turbidity in 4 hr	2467	I
Filgrastim	AMG	30 mcg/mL[a]	AB	1 mEq/mL	Physically compatible for 4 hr at 22°C	1687	C
Fludarabine phosphate	BX	1 mg/mL[a]	AB	1 mEq/mL	Visually compatible for 4 hr at 22°C	1439	C
Gallium nitrate	FUJ	1 mg/mL[b]	AB	1 mEq/mL	Visually compatible for 24 hr at 25°C	1673	C
Gemcitabine HCl	LI	10 mg/mL[b]	AB	1 mEq/mL	Physically compatible for 4 hr at 23°C	2226	C
Granisetron HCl	SKB	0.05 mg/mL[a]	AB	1 mEq/mL	Physically compatible for 4 hr at 23°C	1804	C
Granisetron HCl	SKB	1 mg/mL	AB	0.33 mEq/mL[b]	Physically compatible with 8% loss of granisetron in 4 hr at 22°C	1883	C
Granisetron HCl	SKB	0.05 mg/mL[a]	AB	1 mEq/mL	Physically compatible for 4 hr at 23°C	2000	C
Heparin sodium	CH	500 units/mL[b]		1.4%	Visually compatible for 4 hr at room temperature	1788	C
Heparin sodium[g]	RI	1000 units/L[h]	BR	75 mg/mL	Physically compatible for 4 hr at room temperature	322	C
Hetastarch in lactated electrolyte	AB	6%	AB	1 mEq/mL	Microprecipitate develops rapidly	2339	I
Hydrocortisone sodium succinate[e]	UP	100 mg/L[h]	BR	75 mg/mL	Physically compatible for 4 hr at room temperature	322	C
Hydroxyethyl starch 130/0.4 in sodium chloride 0.9%	FRK	6%	HOS	0.25[a], 0.5[a], 1 mmol/mL	Visually compatible for 24 hr at room temperature	2770	C
Ibuprofen lysinate	OVA	10 mg/mL	HOS	1 mEq/mL	Physically compatible for 4 hr at room temperature	3541	C
Idarubicin HCl	AD	1 mg/mL[b]	AB	0.09 mEq/mL[a]	Haze forms and color changes immediately. Precipitate forms in 20 min	1525	I
Ifosfamide		36 mg/mL[a]		1.4%	Visually compatible for 4 hr at room temperature	1788	C
Indomethacin sodium trihydrate	MSD	1 mg/mL[b]	AB	0.5 mEq/mL[a]	Visually compatible for 24 hr at 28°C	1527	C
Insulin, regular	LI	1 unit/mL[d]	AB	1 mEq/mL	Physically compatible for 3 hr	1316	C
Isavuconazonium sulfate	ASP	1.5 mg/mL[d]	HOS	1 mEq/mL	Measured turbidity increases within 15 min	3263	I

Y-Site Injection Compatibility (1:1 Mixture) (Cont.)

Test Drug	Mfr	Conc	Mfr	Conc	Remarks	Ref	C/I
Leucovorin calcium	LE	10 mg/mL		1.4%	Yellow precipitate forms in 0.5 hr at room temperature	1788	I
Levofloxacin	OMN	5 mg/mL[a]	AB	0.5 mEq/mL	Visually compatible for 4 hr at 24°C	2233	C
Linezolid	PHU	2 mg/mL	AB	1 mEq/mL	Physically compatible for 4 hr at 23°C	2264	C
Melphalan HCl	BW	0.1 mg/mL[b]	AB	1 mEq/mL	Physically compatible for 3 hr at 22°C	1557	C
Meropenem		50 mg/mL	HOS	1 mEq/mL	Physically compatible for 4 hr at room temperature	3538	C
Meropenem–vaborbactam	TMC	8 mg/mL[b p]	HOS	1 mEq/mL	Physically compatible for 3 hr at 20 to 25°C	3380	C
Mesna		1.8 mg/mL[a]		1.4%	Visually compatible for 4 hr at room temperature	1788	C
Methylprednisolone sodium succinate	UP	20 mg/mL		1.4%	Visually compatible for 4 hr at room temperature	1788	C
Midazolam HCl	RC	5 mg/mL		1.4%	White precipitate forms immediately	1788	I
Midazolam HCl	RC	1 mg/mL[a]	IMS	1 mEq/mL	Immediate haze. Precipitate in 2 hr	1847	I
Milrinone lactate	SW	0.4 mg/mL[a]	AB	1 mEq/mL	Visually compatible with 4% loss of milrinone in 4 hr at 23°C	2214	C
Morphine sulfate	WY	0.2 mg/mL[d]	AB	1 mEq/mL	Physically compatible for 3 hr	1316	C
Nalbuphine HCl	DU	10 mg/mL		1.4%	Gas evolves	1788	I
Ondansetron HCl	GL	0.32 mg/mL[a]		0.05 mmol/mL[i]	White precipitate forms immediately	1513	I
Ondansetron HCl	GL	0.1 mg/mL[a]		0.1 mEq/mL[a]	Visible particles in 30 to 60 min at room temperature	1661	I
Ondansetron HCl	GL	2 mg/mL		1.4%	Heavy white precipitate forms immediately	1788	I
Oritavancin diphosphate	TAR	0.8, 1.2, and 2 mg/mL[a]	HOS	1 mEq/mL[n]	Haze forms immediately but disappears with shaking	2928	?
Oxacillin sodium	BR	250 mg/mL		1.4%	Gas evolves	1788	I
Paclitaxel	NCI	1.2 mg/mL[a]	LY	1 mEq/mL	Physically compatible for 4 hr at 22°C	1556	C
Pemetrexed disodium	LI	20 mg/mL[b]	AB	1 mEq/mL	Physically compatible for 4 hr at 23°C	2564	C
Piperacillin sodium–tazobactam sodium	LE[l]	40 mg/mL[a m]	AB	1 mEq/mL	Physically compatible for 4 hr at 22°C	1688	C
Plazomicin sulfate	ACH	24 mg/mL[d]	HOS	1 mEq/mL	Physically compatible for 1 hr at 20 to 25°C	3432	C
Potassium chloride		40 mEq/L[h]	BR	75 mg/mL	Physically compatible for 4 hr at room temperature	322	C
Propofol	ZEN[r]	10 mg/mL	AB	1 mEq/mL	Physically compatible for 1 hr at 23°C	2066	C
Remifentanil HCl	GW	0.025 and 0.25 mg/mL[b]	AB	1 mEq/mL	Physically compatible for 4 hr at 23°C	2075	C
Sargramostim	IMM	10 mcg/mL[b]	LY	1 mEq/mL	Small amount of particles forms in 4 hr	1436	I
Tacrolimus	FUJ	1 mg/mL[b]	AB	1 mEq/mL	Visually compatible for 24 hr at 25°C	1630	C
Tedizolid phosphate	CUB	0.8 mg/mL[b]	HOS	1 mEq/mL	Physically compatible for 2 hr	3244	C
Telavancin HCl	ASP	7.5 mg/mL[h]	HOS	1 mEq/mL	Physically compatible for 2 hr	2830	C
Teniposide	BR	0.1 mg/mL[a]	AB	1 mEq/mL	Physically compatible for 4 hr at 23°C	1725	C

Y-Site Injection Compatibility (1:1 Mixture) (Cont.)

Test Drug	Mfr	Conc	Mfr	Conc	Remarks	Ref	C/I
Thiotepa	IMM[j]	1 mg/mL[a]	AB	1 mEq/mL	Physically compatible for 4 hr at 23°C	1861	C
TNA #218 to #226[k]			AB	1 mEq/mL	Visually compatible for 4 hr at 23°C	2215	C
TPN #212, #214[k]			AB	1 mEq/mL	Microprecipitate in 1 hr	2109	I
TPN #213, #215[k]			AB	1 mEq/mL	Physically compatible for 4 hr at 23°C	2109	C
Vancomycin HCl		5 mg/mL[a]		1.4%	Visually compatible for 4 hr at room temperature	1788	C
Vasopressin	APP	0.2 unit/mL[b]	AB	0.15 mEq/mL[b]	Physically compatible	2641	C
Verapamil HCl	SE	5 mg/2 mL		88 mEq/L[c]	Crystalline precipitate forms when verapamil injected into infusion line	839	I
Vincristine sulfate	LI	0.1 mg/mL		1.4%	White precipitate forms in 30 min at room temperature	1788	I
Vinorelbine tartrate	BW	1 mg/mL[b]	AB	1 mEq/mL	Tiny particles and haze form immediately. Large particles in 4 hr at 22°C	1558	I

[a] Tested in dextrose 5%.

[b] Tested in sodium chloride 0.9%.

[c] Tested in sodium chloride 0.45%.

[d] Tested in both dextrose 5% and sodium chloride 0.9%.

[e] Tested in combination with heparin sodium (Riker) 1000 units/L.

[f] Tested in bacteriostatic sodium chloride 0.9% preserved with benzyl alcohol 0.9%.

[g] Tested in combination with hydrocortisone sodium succinate (Upjohn) 100 mg/L.

[h] Tested in dextrose 5%, sodium chloride 0.9%, and Ringer's injection, lactated.

[i] Tested in dextrose 5% with potassium chloride 0.02 mM/mL.

[j] Lyophilized formulation tested.

[k] Refer to Appendix for the composition of parenteral nutrition solutions. TNA indicates a 3-in-1 admixture, and TPN indicates a 2-in-1 admixture.

[l] Test performed using the formulation WITHOUT edetate disodium.

[m] Piperacillin component. Piperacillin in an 8:1 fixed-ratio concentration with tazobactam.

[n] Tested undiluted.

[o] Ceftolozane component. Ceftolozane in a 2:1 fixed-ratio concentration with tazobactam.

[p] Meropenem component. Meropenem in a 1:1 fixed-ratio concentration with vaborbactam.

[q] Ceftazidime component. Ceftazidime in a 4:1 fixed-ratio concentration with avibactam.

[r] Test performed using the formulation WITH edetate disodium.

Additional Compatibility Information

Methylprednisolone

The compatibility of methylprednisolone sodium succinate (Upjohn) with sodium bicarbonate added to an auxiliary medication infusion unit has been studied. Primary admixtures were prepared by adding sodium bicarbonate 44.6 mEq/L to dextrose 5%, dextrose 5% in sodium chloride 0.9%, and Ringer's injection, lactated. Up to 100 mL of the primary admixture was added along with methylprednisolone sodium succinate (Upjohn) to the auxiliary medication infusion unit with the following results:[329]

Methylprednisolone Sodium Succinate	Sodium Bicarbonate 44.6 mEq/L Primary Solution	Results
500 mg	D5S, D5W qs 100 mL	Clear solution for 24 hr
500 mg	LR qs 100 mL or added to 100 mL LR	Clear solution for 1 hr
1000 mg	D5W qs 100 mL	Clear solution for 24 hr
1000 mg	D5S qs 100 mL or added to 100 mL D5S	Clear solution for 24 hr
1000 mg	LR qs 100 mL	Clear solution for 1 hr
1000 mg	Added to 100 mL LR	Clear solution for 4 hr
2000 mg	D5S, D5W qs 100 mL	Clear solution for 24 hr
2000 mg	LR qs 100 mL	Clear solution for 30 min
2000 mg	Added to 100 mL LR	Clear solution for 4 hr

Selected Revisions May 1, 2020. © Copyright, October 1982. American Society of Health-System Pharmacists, Inc.

Sodium Chloride
AHFS 40:12

Products

Sodium chloride additive solution is available in various size containers in concentrations of 14.6 and 23.4%. The 14.6% concentration contains sodium chloride 146 mg/mL and provides 2.5 mEq/mL of sodium and chloride ions. The 23.4% concentration contains sodium chloride 234 mg/mL and provides 4 mEq/mL of sodium and chloride ions.[1(2/06)]

NOTE: Do not confuse these high concentration additive solutions with other sodium chloride products with lower concentrations.

Sodium chloride 0.45 and 0.9% infusion solutions are available in a variety of sizes from 25 to 1000 mL. The 0.45 and 0.9% concentrations provide 77 and 154 mEq of sodium and chloride per liter, respectively.[1(2/06) 4]

pH

From 4.5 to 7.[17]

Osmolarity

Sodium chloride additive solutions are very hypertonic and must be diluted for use. The osmolarities of the 14.6 and 23.4% concentrations have been calculated to be about 5000 and 8000 mOsm/L, respectively.[4] The osmolality of the 14.6% concentration was determined to be 5370 mOsm/kg by freezing-point depression and 4783 mOsm/kg by vapor pressure.[1071] A 0.9% sodium chloride solution is isotonic, having an osmolarity of 308 mOsm/L. A 0.45% sodium chloride solution is hypotonic, having a calculated osmolarity of 154 mOsm/L.[4]

Administration

Sodium chloride additive solutions of 14.6 and 23.4% are administered by intravenous infusion only after dilution in a larger volume of fluid.[4] Dextrose 5% has been recommended for this dilution.[1(2/06)] When concentrations of 3 or 5% are indicated, these hypertonic solutions should be administered into a large vein, at a rate not exceeding 100 mL/hr. Infiltration should be avoided.[4]

Stability

Sodium chloride additive solution should be stored at controlled room temperature and protected from excessive heat and freezing.[1(2/06)]

Elastomeric Reservoir Pumps

Sodium chloride 0.9% (Baxter) 250 mL was filled into Intermate LV 250 (Baxter) elastomeric infusion devices and stored at 5 and 23°C for 90 days. The solution remained visually compatible with no change in pH and sodium or chloride concentration and less than 0.1% water loss.[1993]

Compatibility Information
Solution Compatibility

Sodium chloride

Test Soln Name	Mfr	Mfr	Conc/L or %	Remarks	Ref	C/I
Dextrose 2.5% in half-strength Ringer's injection	AB	AB	200 mEq	Physically compatible	3	C
Dextrose 5% in Ringer's injection	AB	AB	200 mEq	Physically compatible	3	C
Dextrose 2.5% in Ringer's injection, lactated	AB	AB	200 mEq	Physically compatible	3	C
Dextrose 5% in half-strength Ringer's injection, lactated	AB	AB	200 mEq	Physically compatible	3	C
Dextrose 5% in Ringer's injection, lactated	AB	AB	200 mEq	Physically compatible	3	C
Dextrose 10% in Ringer's injection, lactated	AB	AB	200 mEq	Physically compatible	3	C
Dextrose 2.5% in sodium chloride 0.45%	AB	AB	200 mEq	Physically compatible	3	C
Dextrose 2.5% in sodium chloride 0.9%	AB	AB	200 mEq	Physically compatible	3	C
Dextrose 5% in sodium chloride 0.225%	AB	AB	200 mEq	Physically compatible	3	C
Dextrose 5% in sodium chloride 0.45%	AB	AB	200 mEq	Physically compatible	3	C
Dextrose 5% in sodium chloride 0.9%	AB	AB	200 mEq	Physically compatible	3	C
Dextrose 10% in sodium chloride 0.9%	AB	AB	200 mEq	Physically compatible	3	C
Dextrose 2.5%	AB	AB	200 mEq	Physically compatible	3	C
Dextrose 5%	AB	AB	200 mEq	Physically compatible	3	C

DOI: 10.37573/9781585286850.352

Solution Compatibility (Cont.)

Test Soln Name	Mfr	Mfr	Conc/L or %	Remarks	Ref	C/I
Dextrose 10%	AB	AB	200 mEq	Physically compatible	3	C
Ionosol B in dextrose 5%	AB	AB	200 mEq	Physically compatible	3	C
Ionosol MB in dextrose 5%	AB	AB	200 mEq	Physically compatible	3	C
Ringer's injection	AB	AB	200 mEq	Physically compatible	3	C
Ringer's injection, lactated	AB	AB	200 mEq	Physically compatible	3	C
Sodium chloride 0.45%	AB	AB	200 mEq	Physically compatible	3	C
Sodium chloride 0.9%	AB	AB	200 mEq	Physically compatible	3	C
Sodium lactate ⅙ M	AB	AB	200 mEq	Physically compatible	3	C

Additive Compatibility

Sodium chloride

Test Drug	Mfr	Conc/L or %	Mfr	Conc/L or %	Test Solution	Remarks	Ref	C/I
Fat emulsion, intravenous	CU	10%		100 mEq		No change for 24 hr at room temperature, but lipid coalescence in 48 hr	656	C
Fat emulsion, intravenous	CU	10%		200 mEq		Lipid coalescence with surface creaming in 4 hr at room temperature. Oil globules on surface at 48 hr	656	I

Y-Site Injection Compatibility (1:1 Mixture)

Sodium chloride

Test Drug	Mfr	Conc	Mfr	Conc	Remarks	Ref	C/I
Ciprofloxacin	MI	2 mg/mL[a]	AMR	4 mEq/mL	Visually compatible for 2 hr at 25°C	1628	C

[a] Tested in dextrose 5%.

Selected Revisions June 1, 2019. © Copyright, October 1982.
American Society of Health-System Pharmacists, Inc.

Sodium Ferric Gluconate Complex
AHFS 20:04.04

Products

Sodium ferric gluconate complex is available as a deep red solution in single-use 5-mL vials containing 62.5 mg of elemental iron as the sodium salt of a ferric ion carbohydrate complex.[3007] Each mL of solution also contains sucrose 195 mg (approximately 20% w/v) and benzyl alcohol 9 mg in water for injection.[3007]

pH

From 7.7 to 9.7.[3007]

Trade Name(s)

Ferrlecit

Administration

Sodium ferric gluconate complex is administered as an intravenous infusion over 1 hour after dilution of the dose in 100 or 25 mL of sodium chloride 0.9% for adult or pediatric patients, respectively.[3007] In adult patients, the drug also may be administered undiluted by slow intravenous injection at a rate no faster than 12.5 mg/min.[3007]

Stability

Intact vials of sodium ferric gluconate complex should be stored at controlled room temperature.[3007] Freezing should be avoided.[3007]

Diluted solutions of sodium ferric gluconate complex should be visually inspected for particulate matter and discoloration prior to use.[3007] Diluted solutions of sodium ferric gluconate complex should be used immediately.[3007]

In one study, sodium ferric gluconate complex was diluted in 100 mL of sodium chloride 0.9% to concentrations of 0.625 and 1.25 mg/mL of elemental iron.[3008] Spectrophotometric evaluation showed that the elemental iron concentration in the solutions was stable for at least 1 day at room temperature and at least 7 days at 2 to 8°C.[3008] Additionally, no substantial changes in the apparent molecular weight of sodium ferric gluconate complex were noted to have occurred during these time periods.[3008]

Syringes

Undiluted sodium ferric gluconate complex containing 12.5 mg/mL of elemental iron was packaged as 10 mL in 10-mL syringes with capped needles.[3008] Spectrophotometric evaluation showed that the elemental iron concentration was stable for at least 1 day at room temperature and at least 3 days at 2 to 8°C.[3008] Additionally, no substantial changes in the apparent molecular weight of sodium ferric gluconate complex were noted to have occurred during these time periods.[3008]

Compatibility Information

Solution Compatibility

Sodium ferric gluconate complex

Test Soln Name	Mfr	Mfr	Conc/L or %	Remarks	Ref	C/I
Sodium chloride 0.9%		SAA	1.25 and 5 g[a]	Manufacturer-recommended solution	3007	C

[a] Concentration expressed in terms of elemental iron.

DOI: 10.37573/9781585286850.353

Sodium Lactate
AHFS 40:08

Products

Sodium lactate additive solution is available in 10-mL vials. Each mL of solution contains 5 mEq of sodium lactate. The 10-mL vial contains a total of 50 mEq each of Na^+ and lactate ion (5.6 g of sodium lactate). The pH is adjusted with hydrochloric acid, lactic acid, or sodium hydroxide if necessary.[1(10/06) 4]

Sodium lactate ⅙ M (1.9%) infusion solution is available in 500- and 1000-mL containers. It provides 167 mEq of sodium and lactate per liter.[4]

pH

From 6 to 7.3.[1(10/06) 17]

Osmolality

Sodium lactate additive solution is very hypertonic and must be diluted for use. The osmolarity was calculated to be about 10,000 mOsm/L.[1(10/06)] The osmolality was determined to be 11,490 mOsm/kg by freezing-point depression and 10,665 mOsm/kg by vapor pressure.[1071]

Sodium lactate ⅙ M (1.9%) is approximately isotonic with a calculated osmolarity of 330 mOsm/L.[4]

Administration

Sodium lactate additive solution is administered by intravenous infusion only after dilution in a larger volume of fluid. A ⅙ M (1.9%) solution may be prepared by diluting 50 mEq of the additive solution to 300 mL with a nonelectrolyte solution or sterile water for injection. Sodium lactate ⅙ M infusion solution does not require dilution prior to use. The rate of infusion should not exceed 300 mL/hr in adults.[1(10/06) 4]

Stability

Sodium lactate additive solution should be stored at controlled room temperature and protected from freezing and excessive temperatures of 40°C or more.[1(10/06) 4]

Compatibility Information

Solution Compatibility

Sodium lactate

Test Soln Name	Mfr	Mfr	Conc/L or %	Remarks	Ref	C/I
Dextrose 2.5% in half-strength Ringer's injection	AB	AB	200 mEq	Physically compatible	3	C
Dextrose 5% in Ringer's injection	AB	AB	200 mEq	Physically compatible	3	C
Dextrose 2.5% in Ringer's injection, lactated	AB	AB	200 mEq	Physically compatible	3	C
Dextrose 5% in half-strength Ringer's injection, lactated	AB	AB	200 mEq	Physically compatible	3	C
Dextrose 5% in Ringer's injection, lactated	AB	AB	200 mEq	Physically compatible	3	C
Dextrose 10% in Ringer's injection, lactated	AB	AB	200 mEq	Physically compatible	3	C
Dextrose 2.5% in sodium chloride 0.45%	AB	AB	200 mEq	Physically compatible	3	C
Dextrose 2.5% in sodium chloride 0.9%	AB	AB	200 mEq	Physically compatible	3	C
Dextrose 5% in sodium chloride 0.225%	AB	AB	200 mEq	Physically compatible	3	C
Dextrose 5% in sodium chloride 0.45%	AB	AB	200 mEq	Physically compatible	3	C
Dextrose 5% in sodium chloride 0.9%	AB	AB	200 mEq	Physically compatible	3	C
Dextrose 10% in sodium chloride 0.9%	AB	AB	200 mEq	Physically compatible	3	C
Dextrose 2.5%	AB	AB	200 mEq	Physically compatible	3	C
Dextrose 5%	AB	AB	200 mEq	Physically compatible	3	C
Dextrose 10%	AB	AB	200 mEq	Physically compatible	3	C
Ionosol B in dextrose 5%	AB	AB	200 mEq	Physically compatible	3	C
Ionosol MB in dextrose 5%	AB	AB	200 mEq	Physically compatible	3	C

DOI: 10.37573/9781585286850.354

Solution Compatibility (Cont.)

Test Soln Name	Mfr	Mfr	Conc/L or %	Remarks	Ref	C/I
Ringer's injection	AB	AB	200 mEq	Physically compatible	3	C
Ringer's injection, lactated	AB	AB	200 mEq	Physically compatible	3	C
Sodium chloride 0.45%	AB	AB	200 mEq	Physically compatible	3	C
Sodium chloride 0.9%	AB	AB	200 mEq	Physically compatible	3	C

Additive Compatibility

Sodium lactate

Test Drug	Mfr	Conc/L or %	Mfr	Conc/L or %	Test Solution	Remarks	Ref	C/I
Lidocaine HCl	AST	2 g	AB	50 mEq		Physically compatible	24	C
Nafcillin sodium	WY	500 mg	AB	50 mEq		Physically compatible	27	C

Selected Revisions March 26, 2013. © Copyright, October 1982.
American Society of Health-System Pharmacists, Inc.

Sodium Nitroprusside
AHFS 24:08.20

Products

Sodium nitroprusside is available in 2-mL single-dose amber vials as a concentrate for injection with each mL containing the equivalent of 25 mg of sodium nitroprusside dihydrate in sterile water for injection.[3282] The concentrate for injection must be further diluted in 250 to 1000 mL of dextrose 5% prior to administration.[3282] The diluted solution for infusion should be protected from light using the provided opaque sleeve, aluminum foil, or another opaque material.[3282] The manufacturers state that covering the infusion drip chamber and tubing is not necessary.[3282]

Sodium nitroprusside also is available as a ready-to-use solution in 100-mL single-use (unpreserved) amber vials containing sodium nitroprusside 50 mg in 100 mL of sodium chloride 0.9%.[3283] The ready-to-use solution in the amber vial should be stored in the carton until use to protect from light[3283] but does not require light protection during administration.[3290]

pH

The pH of a 1-mg/mL solution in dextrose 5% was reported to be 4.2 (Roche)[1579] or 4.74 to 4.94 (Valeant).[3284]

Sodium Content

Contains sodium 0.335 mEq/50 mg of drug.[846]

Trade Name(s)

Nipride RTU, Nitropress

Administration

Sodium nitroprusside is administered only as an intravenous infusion as the ready-to-use solution[3283] or after proper dilution of the concentrate for injection in 250 to 1000 mL of dextrose 5%.[3282] The concentrate for injection is not suitable for direct injection.[3282] A volumetric infusion pump must be used to administer sodium nitroprusside;[3283] the solution for infusion should not be infused through an ordinary intravenous apparatus regulated only by gravity and mechanical clamps.[3282]

Infusion of sodium nitroprusside should be initiated at a rate of 0.3 mcg/kg/min with an upward titration every few minutes until the desired effect is achieved or the maximum recommended infusion rate of 10 mcg/kg/min has been reached.[3282] [3283] Manufacturers state that infusion at the maximum rate of 10 mcg/kg/min should be limited to less than 10 minutes.[3282] [3283] The maximum recommended infusion rate for patients with severe renal impairment and anuric patients is less than 3 mcg/kg/min and 1 mcg/kg/min, respectively.[3282] [3283]

Stability

Sodium nitroprusside is colorless to reddish-brown[3283] or faint brownish in color.[3282] Intact vials should be stored at controlled room temperature and retained in the original carton until use to protect from light.[3282] [3283]

Sodium nitroprusside protected from light has been reported to be stable for 12 to 24 hours,[93] [460] [1296] [1579] [3282] to 48 hours,[958] to 13 days,[95] or even longer.[94] [458] [459] [732]

Sodium nitroprusside solutions for infusion should be inspected for particulate matter and discoloration prior to administration; any solution that is discolored or in which particulate matter is visible should not be used.[3282] [3283] Sodium nitroprusside may be inactivated and/or rapidly degraded by reactions with trace contaminants, forming highly colored reaction products (usually blue, green, or bright red).[3282] [3283] Such solutions should not be used.[3282] [3283] It is, therefore, recommended that no other drug be added to sodium nitroprusside solutions.[3282] [3283]

Dextrose 5% is the recommended infusion solution for admixture of the concentrate for injection[90] [91] [3282] although it turns blue more rapidly than the drug in saline solution.[732]

Sodium nitroprusside 1 mg/mL in 6 solutions in PVC bags was evaluated for production of cyanide, produced by sodium nitroprusside degradation from exposure to 300 foot-candles of light for 72 hours. The solutions tested included 3 nonelectrolyte solutions (dextrose 5%; dextrose 10%; distilled water) and 3 electrolyte solutions (sodium chloride 0.9%; Ringer's injection, lactated; dextrose 5% in Ringer's injection, lactated). There was no difference in the amount of cyanide produced among the solutions throughout the first 24 hours. However, the electrolyte solutions exhibited statistically significant lower mean cyanide ion concentrations (about 2 to 5 ppm) than the nonelectrolyte solutions (about 7 to 9 ppm). These levels of cyanide are an order of magnitude greater than in light-protected solutions. It was concluded that electrolyte solutions may be preferable to dextrose 5% for sodium nitroprusside administration and that all doses should be prepared as freshly as possible and protected from light.[2023]

Temperature Effects

Sodium nitroprusside solutions are heat sensitive. Autoclaving a solution of 100 mg/250 mL in dextrose 5% at 115°C for 30 minutes results in decomposition to a pale blue-green precipitate.[458] It has been stated that autoclaving is less deleterious than even moderate exposure to light.[94]

Light Effects

Solutions of sodium nitroprusside exhibit a color variously described as faint brownish,[3282] brown,[90] red-brown,[3283] brownish-pink,[91] light orange,[95] and straw.[92] These solutions are highly sensitive to light.[3282] Exposure to light causes decomposition, resulting in a highly colored solution of light yellow,[1579] orange,[92] dark brown,[91] or blue.[90] [91] [92] A blue color indicates almost complete degradation.[92]

The rate of decomposition of sodium nitroprusside when exposed to light is dependent on such factors as the wavelength and intensity of light, temperature, infusion fluid, pH, and container material. The amount of loss occurring in the

DOI: 10.37573/9781585286850.355

administration tubing can be affected additionally by the nature and thickness of the tubing wall, duration of light exposure, volume of fluid, and flow rate.[1297]

In one study, sodium nitroprusside 0.01% in both water and dextrose 5% in glass bottles exhibited 9 to 10% decomposition in 2 hours and 18 to 20% decomposition in 4 hours on exposure to fluorescent light. No decomposition was detected in either solution in 24 hours when protected from light. In PVC bags, even greater decomposition occurred on exposure to light.[460]

In another study, 10-mg/mL aqueous solutions of sodium nitroprusside lost 3% in 24 hours on exposure to fluorescent light and 10% in 24 hours when exposed to both fluorescent light and indirect daylight. At a concentration of 200 mg/L in infusion solutions, exposure to bright daylight increased the loss to approximately 15 to 30% in 5 hours. The rate of breakdown was related to the amount of illumination. When the containers were protected from light by wrapping with foil, no decomposition was observed in infusion solutions for 7 days at room temperature and for 2 years at 10 mg/mL in glass tubes at room temperature or 4°C.[732]

The rate of decomposition of sodium nitroprusside (David Bull Laboratories) 1 mg/mL in dextrose 5% was studied when exposed to fluorescent light and natural daylight. The solutions were stored at 23°C in the burette chambers of an amber light-protective set, a clear colorless set, and a clear set covered with a foil overwrap. With exposure to fluorescent light, losses in the clear burette chamber totaled 11% in 150 minutes and 100% in 24 hours. Both the amber and foil-wrapped clear sets sustained virtually no loss in 4 hours and about a 3 to 4% loss in 24 hours. Natural daylight caused a more rapid drug loss in the unprotected burette; essentially all drug was lost in 30 to 150 minutes, depending on the daylight intensity. The amber set slowed the degradation rate, but 32% was still lost in 2 hours with exposure to intense direct sunlight.[1296]

Solutions of sodium nitroprusside prepared from the concentrate for injection should be protected from light by wrapping the container with the provided opaque sleeve, aluminum foil, or another opaque material.[90][91][1297][3282] The container should be wrapped as soon as practical without delaying therapy.[959] Amber plastic bags, which are often used for light protection, have been stated not to provide sufficient protection for sodium nitroprusside against photodegradation. Only opaque materials should be used.[733]

The effect of the light exposure that sodium nitroprusside infusions receive while flowing through a 3-m long PVC infusion set tubing was evaluated. Sodium nitroprusside infusions in dextrose 5%, sodium chloride 0.9%, and Ringer's injection, lactated, were studied for 24 and 8 hours at flow rates of 10 and 50 mL/hr, respectively. The delivered amount of sodium nitroprusside was not reduced.[958]

The stability of sodium nitroprusside (Roche) 100 mcg/mL in dextrose 5% was studied when delivered through tubing exposed to normal room light. No degradation occurred in the infusion container wrapped in foil, but concentration differences in the delivered solution of about 2% were noted at each time point sampled over the 5-hour study. When the effects of different light sources on a 50-mcg/mL solution in dextrose 5% were compared, about a 7% loss occurred on exposure to fluorescent light for 6 hours, but a 32% loss occurred in 1 hour on exposure to direct sunlight.[1131]

The stability of sodium nitroprusside (Roche) 0.5 and 1.67 mg/mL in dextrose 5% administered by a syringe pump system was evaluated. In polypropylene syringes (Sherwood Medical) exposed to both artificial light and daylight, sodium nitroprusside losses after 24 hours were 26 and 18.7% at 0.5 and 1.67 mg/mL, respectively. The level of free cyanide exceeded 2 mcg/mL. The time to 10% decomposition was about 4 hours. Syringes wrapped in foil exhibited less than a 5% loss in 24 hours. A comparison of the decomposition occurring in the delivery tubing showed that about 10.3 and 3.7% were lost from the 0.5- and 1.67-mg/mL concentrations, respectively, when delivered by pumps at 3 mL/hr through tubing exposed to the light. Wrapping the line with foil prevented any decomposition over the 24-hour study.[1130]

Sodium nitroprusside (Roche) 50 mg/50 mL in dextrose 5% exhibited no change in appearance and no loss when stored for 24 hours at 25°C in 60-mL plastic syringes (Becton Dickinson) wrapped in foil;[1579] however, if the syringes were not wrapped in foil for light protection, the solution turned yellow in 12 hours and had approximately 11, 17, and 22% losses in 6, 12, and 24 hours, respectively.[1579]

Syringes

Sodium nitroprusside (Valeant) 1 mg/mL in dextrose 5% packaged as 6.25 mL in 20-mL polypropylene syringes (Becton Dickinson) and wrapped in aluminum foil was physically and chemically stable for 9 days when stored at 4°C.[3284]

Sorption

Sodium nitroprusside was shown not to exhibit sorption to PVC bags and tubing, polyethylene tubing, Silastic tubing, and polypropylene syringes.[536][606][1131]

Compatibility Information

Solution Compatibility

Sodium nitroprusside

Test Soln Name	Mfr	Mfr	Conc/L or %	Remarks	Ref	C/I
Dextrose 5%			100 mg	No decomposition in 24 hr protected from light	460	C
Dextrose 5%			100 mg	9 to 10% decomposition in 2 hr exposed to light	460	I

Solution Compatibility (Cont.)

Test Soln Name	Mfr	Mfr	Conc/L or %	Remarks	Ref	C/I
Dextrose 5%	TR		200 mg	No decomposition in 7 days at room temperature in foil-wrapped bottles	732	C
Dextrose 5%	TR		200 mg	14 to 16% decomposition in 5 hr exposed to bright daylight	732	I
Dextrose 5%	TR[a]		88 mg	18% loss in 24 hr when bag was exposed to both daylight and fluorescent light	732	I
Dextrose 5%	TR	RC	165 mg	4% loss in 65 min in bright daylight	732	I
Dextrose 5%	AB[b]	RC	50 and 100 mg	No decomposition in 48 hr in foil-wrapped bottles and bags at room temperature	958	C
Dextrose 5%	MG	RC	50 mg	Little or no loss over 6 days at room temperature protected from light	1131	C
Dextrose 5%	MG	RC	50 mg	10% loss in 7 hr at room temperature exposed to fluorescent light. 32% loss in 1 hr exposed to direct sunlight	1131	I
Dextrose 5%	BT[c]	DB	100 mg	11% loss in 2.5 hr and 100% in 24 hr at 23°C under fluorescent light. 100% loss in 0.5 to 2.5 hr in daylight	1296	I
Dextrose 5%	BT[c]	DB	100 mg	3 to 4% loss in 24 hr at 23°C protected from light with foil wrapping or amber light-protective set	1296	C
Dextrose 5%	BT[c]	DB	100 mg	32% loss in 2 hr at 23°C in intense daylight in amber light-protective set	1296	I
Dextrose 5%	[d]		200 to 800 mg	Physically compatible with 7% or less loss in 24 hr exposed to light	1412	C
Dextrose 5%	TR[a]	RC	50 and 400 mg	Visually compatible with little or no drug loss in 48 hr at room temperature	1802	C
Ringer's injection, lactated	AB[b]	RC	50 and 100 mg	No decomposition in 48 hr in foil-wrapped bottles and bags at room temperature	958	C
Sodium chloride 0.9%	TR		200 mg	No decomposition in 7 days at room temperature in foil-wrapped bottles	732	C
Sodium chloride 0.9%	TR		200 mg	24 to 28% decomposition in 5 hr exposed to bright daylight	732	I
Sodium chloride 0.9%	TR		289 mg	4% loss in 3 hr exposed to both daylight and fluorescent light	732	I
Sodium chloride 0.9%	TR		206 mg	2% loss in 60 min exposed to both daylight and fluorescent light	732	I
Sodium chloride 0.9%	TR		183 mg	1% loss in 2 hr in fluorescent light only	732	I
Sodium chloride 0.9%	AB[b]	RC	50 and 100 mg	No decomposition in 48 hr in foil-wrapped bottles and bags at room temperature	958	C
Sodium chloride 0.9%	[d]		200 to 800 mg	Physically compatible with 8% or less loss in 24 hr exposed to light	1412	C
Sodium chloride 0.9%	TR[a]	RC	50 and 400 mg	Visually compatible with little or no drug loss in 48 hr at room temperature	1802	C

[a] Tested in PVC containers.

[b] Tested in both glass and PVC containers.

[c] Tested in burette chambers of administration sets.

[d] Tested in glass containers.

Additive Compatibility

Sodium nitroprusside

Test Drug	Mfr	Conc/L or %	Mfr	Conc/L or %	Test Solution	Remarks	Ref	C/I
Atracurium besylate	BW	500 mg		2 g	D5W	Physically incompatible. Haze, particles, and yellow color form	1694	I
Dobutamine HCl with nitroglycerin		2 to 8 g 200 to 800 mg		200 to 800 mg	D5W[a]	Pink color with small amount of dark brown precipitate and 11 to 19% nitroglycerin loss in 24 hr exposed to light	1412	I
Dobutamine HCl with nitroglycerin		2 to 8 g 200 to 800 mg		200 to 800 mg	NS[a]	Pink color with 8% or less loss for any drug for 24 hr exposed to light	1412	C
Enalaprilat	MSD	12 mg	ES	1 g	D5W[b]	Visually compatible. Little enalaprilat loss in 24 hr at room temperature under fluorescent light. Sodium nitroprusside not tested	1572	C
Nitroglycerin with dobutamine HCl		200 to 800 mg 2 to 8 g		200 to 800 mg	D5W[a]	Pink color with small amount of dark brown precipitate and 11 to 19% nitroglycerin loss in 24 hr exposed to light	1412	I
Nitroglycerin with dobutamine HCl		200 to 800 mg 2 to 8 g		200 to 800 mg	NS[a]	Pink color with 8% or less loss for any drug for 24 hr exposed to light	1412	C
Ranitidine HCl	GL	2 g	RC	50 and 400 mg	D5W, NS[b]	Physically compatible. No ranitidine loss in 48 hr at room temperature light protected. Nitroprusside not tested	1361	C
Ranitidine HCl	GL	50 mg	RC	50 and 400 mg	NS[b]	Physically compatible. No ranitidine loss in 48 hr at room temperature light protected. Nitroprusside not tested	1361	C
Ranitidine HCl	GL	50 mg	RC	50 and 400 mg	D5W[b]	Physically compatible with 7% or less ranitidine loss in 48 hr protected from light. Nitroprusside not tested	1361	C
Ranitidine HCl	GL	50 mg and 2 g		50 mg and 1 g	D5W, NS	Physically compatible. Both drugs stable for 48 hr at room temperature protected from light	1515	C
Ranitidine HCl	GL	50 mg and 2 g		100 mg	D5W	Physically compatible. Ranitidine stable for 24 hr at 25°C. Sodium nitroprusside not tested	1515	C
Ranitidine HCl	GL	50 mg and 2 g	RC	50 and 400 mg	D5W[a]	Visually compatible. 7% ranitidine and 8% nitroprusside loss in 48 hr at room temperature protected from light	1802	C
Ranitidine HCl	GL	50 mg and 2 g	RC	50 and 400 mg	NS[a]	Visually compatible. No loss of either drug in 48 hr at room temperature protected from light	1802	C
Sodium thiosulfate	AMR	1.8 g	HOS	180 mg	D5W, NS	Physically compatible with less than 10% loss of either drug in 48 hr at room temperature protected from light	2825	C
Verapamil HCl	KN	80 mg	RC	100 mg	D5W, NS	Physically compatible for 24 hr	764	C

[a] Tested in glass containers.

[b] Tested in PVC containers.

Drugs in Syringe Compatibility

Sodium nitroprusside

Test Drug	Mfr	Amt	Mfr	Amt	Remarks	Ref	C/I
Caffeine citrate		20 mg/1 mL	ES	25 mg/1 mL	Visually compatible for 4 hr at 25°C	2440	C
Heparin sodium		2500 units/1 mL		60 mg/5 mL	Physically compatible for at least 5 min	1053	C
Pantoprazole sodium	a	4 mg/1 mL		10 mg/1 mL	Precipitates within 15 min	2574	I

[a] Test performed using the formulation WITHOUT edetate disodium.

Y-Site Injection Compatibility (1:1 Mixture)

Sodium nitroprusside

Test Drug	Mfr	Conc	Mfr	Conc	Remarks	Ref	C/I
Alprostadil	UP	2 mcg/mL[a]	RC	0.3, 1.2, 3 mg/mL[a]	Visually compatible for 48 hr at 24°C protected from light	2357	C
Alprostadil	UP	10 mcg/mL[a]	RC	0.3, 1.2, 3 mg/mL[a]	Visually compatible for 48 hr at 24°C protected from light	2357	C
Amiodarone HCl	WY	6 mg/mL[a]	BA	0.4 mg/mL[a]	Visually compatible for 24 hr at 22°C	2352	C
Amiodarone HCl	WAY	1.5 mg/mL[a]	RC	0.3 mg/mL[a]	Cloudy precipitate forms within 4 hr at 24°C protected from light	2357	I
Amiodarone HCl	WAY	1.5 mg/mL[a]	RC	1.2 and 3 mg/mL[a]	Cloudy precipitate forms immediately	2357	I
Amiodarone HCl	WAY	6 and 15 mg/mL[a]	RC	0.3 mg/mL[a]	Visually compatible for 48 hr at 24°C protected from light	2357	C
Amiodarone HCl	WAY	6 and 15 mg/mL[a]	RC	1.2 and 3 mg/mL[a]	Cloudy precipitate forms immediately	2357	I
Argatroban	SKB	1 mg/mL[a]	AB	0.2 mg/mL[a]	Physically compatible for 24 hr at 23°C	2572	C
Atracurium besylate	BW	0.5 mg/mL[a]	ES	0.2 mg/mL[a]	Physically compatible for 24 hr at 28°C	1337	C
Bivalirudin	TMC	5 mg/mL[a]	BA	2 mg/mL[a]	Physically compatible for 4 hr at 23°C protected from light	2373	C
Calcium chloride	AST	0.4 and 1.36 mEq/mL[d]	RC	0.3, 1.2, 3 mg/mL[a]	Visually compatible for 48 hr at 24°C protected from light	2357	C
Calcium chloride	AST	0.8 mEq/mL[d]	RC	1.2 and 3 mg/mL[a]	Visually compatible for 48 hr at 24°C protected from light	2357	C
Cangrelor tetrasodium	TMC	1 mg/mL[b]		2 mg/mL[b]	Physically compatible for 4 hr	3243	C
Ceftolozane sulfate–tazobactam sodium	CUB	10 mg/mL[c f]	MTN	0.4 mg/mL[c]	Physically compatible for 2 hr	3262	C
Cisatracurium besylate	GW	0.1 mg/mL[a]	AB	2 mg/mL[a]	Physically compatible for 4 hr at 23°C protected from light	2074	C
Cisatracurium besylate	GW	2 and 5 mg/mL[a]	AB	2 mg/mL[a]	White cloudiness forms immediately	2074	I
Clevidipine butyrate	CHS	0.5 mg/mL		2 mg/mL[a]	Physically compatible for 24 hr at 23°C	3334	C
Cloxacillin sodium	SMX	100 mg/mL	HOS	25 mg/mL	Physically compatible for up to 4 hr at room temperature	3245	C
Dexmedetomidine HCl	AB	4 mcg/mL[b]	BA	2 mg/mL[b]	Physically compatible for 4 hr at 23°C protected from light	2383	C
Diltiazem HCl	MMD	5 mg/mL	AB	0.2 mg/mL[a]	Visually compatible	1807	C
Dobutamine HCl	LI	4 mg/mL[c]	ES	0.4 mg/mL[c]	Physically compatible for 3 hr	1316	C

Y-Site Injection Compatibility (1:1 Mixture) (Cont.)

Test Drug	Mfr	Conc	Mfr	Conc	Remarks	Ref	C/I
Dobutamine HCl	LI	1.5 mg/mL[d]	RC	0.3, 1.2, 3 mg/mL[a]	Visually compatible for 48 hr at 24°C protected from light	2357	C
Dobutamine HCl	LI	6 mg/mL[d]	RC	1.2 and 3 mg/mL[a]	Color darkening occurs over 48 hr at 24°C protected from light	2357	?
Dobutamine HCl	LI	12.5 mg/mL[d]	RC	0.3 and 1.2 mg/mL[a]	Visually compatible for 48 hr at 24°C protected from light	2357	C
Dobutamine HCl	LI	12.5 mg/mL[d]	RC	3 mg/mL[a]	Color darkening occurs over 48 hr at 24°C protected from light	2357	?
Dobutamine HCl with dopamine HCl	LI DCC	4 mg/mL[c] 3.2 mg/mL[c]	ES	0.4 mg/mL[c]	Physically compatible for 3 hr	1316	C
Dobutamine HCl with lidocaine HCl	LI AB	4 mg/mL[c] 8 mg/mL[c]	ES	0.4 mg/mL[c]	Physically compatible for 3 hr	1316	C
Dobutamine HCl with nitroglycerin	LI LY	4 mg/mL[c] 0.4 mg/mL[c]	ES	0.4 mg/mL[c]	Physically compatible for 3 hr	1316	C
Dopamine HCl	DCC	3.2 mg/mL[c]	ES	0.4 mg/mL[c]	Physically compatible for 3 hr	1316	C
Dopamine HCl	DU	1.5, 6, 15 mg/mL[d]	RC	0.3, 1.2, 3 mg/mL[a]	Visually compatible for 48 hr at 24°C protected from light	2357	C
Dopamine HCl with dobutamine HCl	DCC LI	3.2 mg/mL[c] 4 mg/mL[c]	ES	0.4 mg/mL[c]	Physically compatible for 3 hr	1316	C
Dopamine HCl with lidocaine HCl	DCC AB	3.2 mg/mL[c] 8 mg/mL[c]	ES	0.4 mg/mL[c]	Physically compatible for 3 hr	1316	C
Dopamine HCl with nitroglycerin	DCC LY	3.2 mg/mL[c] 0.4 mg/mL[c]	ES	0.4 mg/mL[c]	Physically compatible for 3 hr	1316	C
Enalaprilat	MSD	0.05 mg/mL[b]	LY	0.2 mg/mL[a]	Physically compatible for 24 hr at room temperature protected from light	1355	C
Epinephrine HCl	AB	0.03, 0.12, 0.3 mg/mL[d]	RC	1.2 and 3 mg/mL[a]	Visually compatible for 48 hr at 24°C protected from light	2357	C
Esmolol HCl	DU	40 mg/mL[a]	RC	0.2 mg/mL[a]	Visually compatible for 24 hr at 23°C	1877	C
Famotidine	MSD	0.2 mg/mL[a]	ES	0.2 mg/mL[a]	Physically compatible for 4 hr at 25°C protected from light	1188	C
Furosemide	SX	1.2[d] and 10 mg/mL	RC	0.3, 1.2, 3 mg/mL[a]	Visually compatible for 48 hr at 24°C protected from light	2357	C
Furosemide	SX	5 mg/mL[a]	RC	1.2 and 3 mg/mL[a]	Visually compatible for 48 hr at 24°C protected from light	2357	C
Haloperidol lactate	MN	5 mg/mL	AB	0.2 mg/mL[a]	Immediate turbidity. Precipitate in 24 hr at 21°C in fluorescent light	1523	I
Haloperidol lactate	MN	0.5 mg/mL[a]	AB	0.2 mg/mL[a]	Visually compatible for 24 hr at 21°C	1523	C
Heparin sodium	TR	50 units/mL	ES	0.2 mg/mL[a]	Visually compatible for 4 hr at 25°C protected from light	1793	C
Heparin sodium	OR	100 units/mL[a]	RC	0.2 mg/mL[a]	Visually compatible for 24 hr at 23°C	1877	C
Heparin sodium	OR	48, 200, 480 units/mL[d]	RC	1.2 and 3 mg/mL[a]	Visually compatible for 48 hr at 24°C protected from light	2357	C
Heparin sodium	OR	480 units/mL[d]	RC	0.3 mg/mL[a]	Visually compatible for 48 hr at 24°C protected from light	2357	C
Hetastarch in lactated electrolyte	AB	6%	OHM	2 mg/mL[a]	Physically compatible for 4 hr at 23°C protected from light	2339	C

Y-Site Injection Compatibility (1:1 Mixture) (Cont.)

Test Drug	Mfr	Conc	Mfr	Conc	Remarks	Ref	C/I
Indomethacin sodium trihydrate	MSD	1 mg/mL[b]	AB	0.2 mg/mL[a]	Visually compatible for 24 hr at 28°C	1527	C
Insulin, regular	LI	1 unit/mL[a]	RC	0.2 mg/mL[a]	Visually compatible for 24 hr at 23°C	1877	C
Insulin, regular	LI	1 and 2 units/mL[b]	RC	1.2 and 3 mg/mL[a]	Visually compatible for 48 hr at 24°C protected from light	2357	C
Isavuconazonium sulfate	ASP	1.5 mg/mL[c]	MTN	0.4 mg/mL[c]	Physically compatible for 2 hr	3263	C
Isoproterenol HCl	SX	20 mcg/mL[d]	RC	0.3, 1.2, 3 mg/mL[a]	Visually compatible for 48 hr at 24°C protected from light	2357	C
Isoproterenol HCl	SX	80 mcg/mL[d]	RC	1.2 and 3 mg/mL[a]	Visually compatible for 48 hr at 24°C protected from light	2357	C
Labetalol HCl	GL	5 mg/mL	RC	0.2 mg/mL[a]	Visually compatible for 24 hr at 23°C	1877	C
Levofloxacin	OMN	5 mg/mL[a]	ES	10 mg/mL[b]	Fluffy precipitate forms	2233	I
Lidocaine HCl	AB	8 mg/mL[c]	ES	0.4 mg/mL[c]	Physically compatible for 3 hr	1316	C
Lidocaine HCl	AST	6 mg/mL[d]	RC	1.2 and 3 mg/mL[a]	Visually compatible for 48 hr at 24°C protected from light	2357	C
Lidocaine HCl	AST	20 and 40 mg/mL[d]	RC	0.3, 1.2, 3 mg/mL[a]	Visually compatible for 48 hr at 24°C protected from light	2357	C
Lidocaine HCl with dobutamine HCl	AB LI	8 mg/mL[c] 4 mg/mL[c]	ES	0.4 mg/mL[c]	Physically compatible for 3 hr	1316	C
Lidocaine HCl with dopamine HCl	AB DCC	8 mg/mL[c] 3.2 mg/mL[c]	ES	0.4 mg/mL[c]	Physically compatible for 3 hr	1316	C
Lidocaine HCl with nitroglycerin	AB LY	8 mg/mL[c] 0.4 mg/mL[a]	ES	0.4 mg/mL[c]	Physically compatible for 3 hr	1316	C
Magnesium sulfate	SX	0.4 and 0.8 mEq/mL[d]	RC	0.3, 1.2, 3 mg/mL[a]	Visually compatible for 48 hr at 24°C protected from light	2357	C
Meropenem		50 mg/mL	HOS	25 mg/mL	Physically compatible for 4 hr at room temperature	3538	C
Metoprolol tartrate	BED	1 mg/mL	HOS	0.4 mg/mL[a]	Visually compatible for 24 hr at 19°C	2795	C
Micafungin sodium	ASP	1.5 mg/mL[b]	AB	2 mg/mL[b]	Physically compatible for 4 hr at 23°C protected from light	2683	C
Midazolam HCl	RC	1 mg/mL[a]	ES	0.2 mg/mL[a]	Visually compatible for 24 hr at 23°C	1847	C
Midazolam HCl	RC	1 mg/mL[a]	RC	0.2 mg/mL[a]	Visually compatible for 24 hr at 23°C	1877	C
Midazolam HCl	RC	1.2 and 2.4 mg/mL[d]	RC	1.2 and 3 mg/mL[a]	Visually compatible for 48 hr at 24°C protected from light	2357	C
Midazolam HCl	RC	5 mg/mL[d]	RC	0.3, 1.2, 3 mg/mL[a]	Visually compatible for 48 hr at 24°C protected from light	2357	C
Milrinone lactate	SW	0.4 mg/mL[a]	AB	0.8 mg/mL[a]	Visually compatible. Little loss of either drug in 4 hr at 23°C protected from light	2214	C
Milrinone lactate	SW	0.1[d], 0.4[d], 1 mg/mL	RC	0.3, 1.2, 3 mg/mL[a]	Visually compatible for 48 hr at 24°C protected from light	2357	C
Morphine sulfate	SX	1 mg/mL[a]	RC	0.2 mg/mL[a]	Visually compatible for 24 hr at 23°C	1877	C
Morphine sulfate	AB	0.5 mg/mL[d]	RC	0.3, 1.2, 3 mg/mL[a]	Visually compatible for 48 hr at 24°C protected from light	2357	C
Morphine sulfate	AB	1 mg/mL[d]	RC	1.2 and 3 mg/mL[a]	Visually compatible for 48 hr at 24°C protected from light	2357	C

Y-Site Injection Compatibility (1:1 Mixture) (Cont.)

Test Drug	Mfr	Conc	Mfr	Conc	Remarks	Ref	C/I
Nesiritide	SCI	50 mcg/mL[a][b]		5 mg/mL	Physically compatible for 4 hr	2625	C
Nicardipine HCl	DCC	0.1 mg/mL[a]	LY	0.2 mg/mL[a]	Visually compatible for 24 hr at room temperature	235	C
Nitroglycerin	LY	0.4 mg/mL[c]	ES	0.4 mg/mL[c]	Physically compatible for 3 hr	1316	C
Nitroglycerin	SX	0.4 and 1.5 mg/mL[d]	RC	1.2 and 3 mg/mL[a]	Visually compatible for 48 hr at 24°C protected from light	2357	C
Nitroglycerin with dobutamine HCl	LY LI	0.4 mg/mL[c] 4 mg/mL[c]	ES	0.4 mg/mL[c]	Physically compatible for 3 hr	1316	C
Nitroglycerin with dopamine HCl	LY DCC	0.4 mg/mL[c] 3.2 mg/mL[c]	ES	0.4 mg/mL[c]	Physically compatible for 3 hr	1316	C
Nitroglycerin with lidocaine HCl	LY AB	0.4 mg/mL[c] 8 mg/mL[c]	ES	0.4 mg/mL[c]	Physically compatible for 3 hr	1316	C
Norepinephrine bitartrate	SX	0.03, 0.12, 3 mg/mL[d]	RC	0.3, 1.2, 3 mg/mL[a]	Visually compatible for 48 hr at 24°C protected from light	2357	C
Oritavancin diphosphate	TAR	0.8, 1.2, and 2 mg/mL[a]	HOS	0.4 mg/mL[a]	Haze forms immediately with precipitate after 1 hr	2928	I
Pancuronium bromide	ES	0.05 mg/mL[a]	ES	0.2 mg/mL[a]	Physically compatible for 24 hr at 28°C	1337	C
Plazomicin sulfate	ACH	24 mg/mL[a]	SGT	0.4 mg/mL[a]	Physically compatible for 1 hr at 20 to 25°C	3432	C
Potassium chloride	AST	0.04 and 0.5 mEq/mL[d]	RC	0.3, 1.2, 3 mg/mL[a]	Visually compatible for 48 hr at 24°C protected from light	2357	C
Potassium phosphates	AB	0.3 mmol/mL[d]	RC	0.3, 1.2, 3 mg/mL[a]	Visually compatible for 48 hr at 24°C protected from light	2357	C
Procainamide HCl	SX	6, 20, 40 mg/mL[b]	RC	0.3, 1.2, 3 mg/mL[a]	Visually compatible for 48 hr at 24°C protected from light	2357	C
Propofol	ZEN[g]	10 mg/mL	ES	0.4 mg/mL[a]	Physically compatible for 1 hr at 23°C	2066	C
Tacrolimus	FUJ	1 mg/mL[b]	ES	0.004 mg/mL[a]	Visually compatible for 24 hr at 25°C	1630	C
Theophylline	TR	4 mg/mL	ES	0.2 mg/mL[a]	Visually compatible for 6 hr at 25°C protected from light	1793	C
TNA #218[e]			AB	0.4 mg/mL[a]	Visually compatible for 4 hr at 23°C protected from light	2215	C
TNA #219[e]			AB	0.4 mg/mL[a]	Visually compatible for 4 hr at 23°C protected from light	2215	C
TNA #220[e]			AB	0.4 mg/mL[a]	Visually compatible for 4 hr at 23°C protected from light	2215	C
TNA #221[e]			AB	0.4 mg/mL[a]	Visually compatible for 4 hr at 23°C protected from light	2215	C
TNA #222[e]			AB	0.4 mg/mL[a]	Visually compatible for 4 hr at 23°C protected from light	2215	C
TNA #223[e]			AB	0.4 mg/mL[a]	Visually compatible for 4 hr at 23°C protected from light	2215	C
TNA #224[e]			AB	0.4 mg/mL[a]	Visually compatible for 4 hr at 23°C protected from light	2215	C
TNA #225[e]			AB	0.4 mg/mL[a]	Visually compatible for 4 hr at 23°C protected from light	2215	C
TNA #226[e]			AB	0.4 mg/mL[a]	Visually compatible for 4 hr at 23°C protected from light	2215	C

Y-Site Injection Compatibility (1:1 Mixture) (Cont.)

Test Drug	Mfr	Conc	Mfr	Conc	Remarks	Ref	C/I
TPN #212[e]			AB	0.4 mg/mL[a]	Physically compatible for 4 hr at 23°C protected from light	2109	C
TPN #213[e]			AB	0.4 mg/mL[a]	Physically compatible for 4 hr at 23°C protected from light	2109	C
TPN #214[e]			AB	0.4 mg/mL[a]	Physically compatible for 4 hr at 23°C protected from light	2109	C
TPN #215[e]			AB	0.4 mg/mL[a]	Physically compatible for 4 hr at 23°C protected from light	2109	C
Vecuronium bromide	OR	0.1 mg/mL[a]	ES	0.2 mg/mL[a]	Physically compatible for 24 hr at 28°C	1337	C

[a] Tested in dextrose 5%.

[b] Tested in sodium chloride 0.9%.

[c] Tested in both dextrose 5% and sodium chloride 0.9%.

[d] Tested in dextrose 5% in sodium chloride 0.225%.

[e] Refer to Appendix for the composition of parenteral nutrition solutions. TNA indicates a 3-in-1 admixture, and TPN indicates a 2-in-1 admixture.

[f] Ceftolozane component. Ceftolozane in a 2:1 fixed-ratio concentration with tazobactam.

[g] Test performed using the formulation WITH edetate disodium.

Selected Revisions May 1, 2020. © Copyright, October 1982.
American Society of Health-System Pharmacists, Inc.

ASHP INJECTABLE DRUG INFORMATION

Sodium Phosphates
AHFS 40:12

Products

Sodium phosphates additive solution is available in 5-, 15-, and 50-mL vials.[1(6/06)] Each mL contains monobasic sodium phosphate monohydrate 276 mg and dibasic sodium phosphate anhydrous 142 mg.[3301] The phosphorus concentration is 3 mmol/mL (93 mg/mL), and the sodium content is 4 mEq/mL (92 mg/mL).[3301] Aluminum also is present.[3301] The additive solution is a concentrate and must be diluted for use.[3301]

pH

From 5 to 6.[3301]

Osmolarity

The osmolar concentration of sodium phosphates additive solution is calculated to be 7 mOsm/mL.[3301]

Administration

Sodium phosphates additive solution must be diluted and thoroughly mixed in a larger volume of fluid before use.[3301]

Stability

Sodium phosphates additive solution should be stored at controlled room temperature.[3301] The solution should be inspected for discoloration or particulate matter prior to use and should be used only if it is clear.[3301] The injection contains no antimicrobial agent or bacteriostat.[3301] Any unused portions should be discarded.[3301]

Compatibility Information

Solution Compatibility

Sodium phosphates

Test Soln Name	Mfr	Mfr	Conc/L or %	Remarks	Ref	C/I
Dextrose 5%	BA[a]	SZ	30 mmol	Physically compatible and chemically stable for 63 days at 23°C. Calculated time to 10% loss of sodium and phosphate 59.2 and 185.1 days, respectively	3275, 3276	C
Dextrose 5%	BA[a]	SZ	30 mmol	Physically compatible and chemically stable for 63 days at 4°C. Calculated time to 10% loss of sodium and phosphate 68.7 and 287.3 days, respectively	3275, 3276	C
Dextrose 5%	BA[a]	SZ	150 mmol	Physically compatible and chemically stable for 63 days at 23°C. Calculated time to 10% loss of sodium and phosphate 69.2 and 87.9 days, respectively	3275, 3276	C
Dextrose 5%	BA[a]	SZ	150 mmol	Physically compatible and chemically stable for 63 days at 4°C. Calculated time to 10% loss of sodium and phosphate 186.1 and 213.2 days, respectively	3275, 3276	C
Sodium chloride 0.9%	BA[a]	SZ	30 mmol	Physically compatible and chemically stable for 63 days at 23°C. Calculated time to 10% loss of sodium and phosphate 246 and 180.1 days, respectively	3275, 3276	C
Sodium chloride 0.9%	BA[a]	SZ	30 mmol	Physically compatible and chemically stable for 63 days at 4°C. Calculated time to 10% loss of sodium and phosphate 469 and 251.2 days, respectively	3275, 3276	C
Sodium chloride 0.9%	BA[a]	SZ	150 mmol	Physically compatible and chemically stable for 63 days at 23°C. Calculated time to 10% loss of sodium and phosphate 102.4 and 75.8 days, respectively	3275, 3276	C
Sodium chloride 0.9%	BA[a]	SZ	150 mmol	Physically compatible and chemically stable for 63 days at 4°C. Calculated time to 10% loss of sodium and phosphate 355.7 and 224 days, respectively	3275, 3276	C

[a] Tested in PVC containers.

DOI: 10.37573/9781585286850.356

Additive Compatibility

Sodium phosphates

Test Drug	Mfr	Conc/L or %	Mfr	Conc/L or %	Test Solution	Remarks	Ref	C/I
Calcium chloride						Compatibility dependent on solubility and concentration and is not entirely predictable. See the monograph discussion under Additional Compatibility Information	1777, 2803	?
Calcium gluconate						Compatibility dependent on solubility and concentration and is not entirely predictable. See the monograph discussion under Additional Compatibility Information	1777, 2803	?

Y-Site Injection Compatibility (1:1 Mixture)

Sodium phosphates

Test Drug	Mfr	Conc	Mfr	Conc	Remarks	Ref	C/I
Amiodarone HCl	WY	6 mg/mL[a]	APP	0.12 mmol/mL[a]	Immediate white cloudiness	2352	I
Ceftaroline fosamil	FOR	2.22 mg/mL[a b e]	HOS	0.5 mmol/mL[a b e]	Increase in measured haze	2826	I
Ceftolozane sulfate–tazobactam sodium	CUB	10 mg/mL[f g]	HOS	0.5 mmol/mL[f]	Physically compatible for 2 hr	3262	C
Ciprofloxacin	BAY	2 mg/mL[a]	AB	3 mmol/mL	Microcrystals form in 1 hr at 23°C	1972	I
Ciprofloxacin	BAY	2 mg/mL[c]	AB	3 mmol/mL	White crystalline precipitate forms immediately	1971, 1972	I
Doripenem	JJ	5 mg/mL[a b]	AMR	0.5 mmol/mL[a b]	Physically compatible for 4 hr at 23°C	2743	C
Isavuconazonium sulfate	ASP	1.5 mg/mL[f]	FRK	0.5 mmol/mL[f]	Measured turbidity increases within 1 hr	3263	I
Meropenem		50 mg/mL	SZ	3 mmol/mL	Gas bubbles evolve within 1 hr	3538, 3547	I
Meropenem–vaborbactam	TMC	8 mg/mL[b h]	FRK	0.5 mmol/mL[b]	Physically compatible for 3 hr at 20 to 25°C	3380	C
Micafungin sodium	ASP	1.5 mg/mL[b]	AMR	0.5 mmol/mL[b]	Physically compatible for 4 hr at 23°C	2683	C
Plazomicin sulfate	ACH	24 mg/mL[f]	FRK	0.5 mmol/mL[f]	Physically compatible for 1 hr at 20 to 25°C	3432	C
Tedizolid phosphate	CUB	0.8 mg/mL[b]	FRE	0.5 mmol/mL[b]	Physically compatible for 2 hr	3244	C
Telavancin HCl	ASP	7.5 mg/mL[a b e]	HOS	0.5 mmol/mL[a b e]	Physically compatible for 2 hr	2830	C
TNA #218[d]			AB	3 mmol/mL	Damage to emulsion occurs immediately with free oil formation possible	2215	I
TNA #219[d]			AB	3 mmol/mL	Damage to emulsion occurs immediately with free oil formation possible	2215	I
TNA #220[d]			AB	3 mmol/mL	Damage to emulsion occurs immediately with free oil formation possible	2215	I
TNA #221[d]			AB	3 mmol/mL	Damage to emulsion occurs immediately with free oil formation possible	2215	I
TNA #222[d]			AB	3 mmol/mL	Damage to emulsion occurs immediately with free oil formation possible	2215	I
TNA #223[d]			AB	3 mmol/mL	Damage to emulsion occurs immediately with free oil formation possible	2215	I
TNA #224[d]			AB	3 mmol/mL	Damage to emulsion occurs immediately with free oil formation possible	2215	I
TNA #225[d]			AB	3 mmol/mL	Damage to emulsion occurs immediately with free oil formation possible	2215	I

Y-Site Injection Compatibility (1:1 Mixture) (Cont.)

Test Drug	Mfr	Conc	Mfr	Conc	Remarks	Ref	C/I
TNA #226[d]			AB	3 mmol/mL	Damage to emulsion occurs immediately with free oil formation possible	2215	I
TPN #212[d]			AB	3 mmol/mL	Increased turbidity forms immediately	2109	I
TPN #213[d]			AB	3 mmol/mL	Increased turbidity forms immediately	2109	I
TPN #214[d]			AB	3 mmol/mL	Increased turbidity forms immediately	2109	I
TPN #215[d]			AB	3 mmol/mL	Increased turbidity forms immediately	2109	I

[a] Tested in dextrose 5%.

[b] Tested in sodium chloride 0.9%.

[c] Tested in both sodium chloride 0.9% and 0.45%.

[d] Refer to Appendix for the composition of parenteral nutrition solutions. TNA indicates a 3-in-1 admixture, and TPN indicates a 2-in-1 admixture.

[e] Tested in Ringer's injection, lactated.

[f] Tested in both dextrose 5% and sodium chloride 0.9%.

[g] Ceftolozane component. Ceftolozane in a 2:1 fixed-ratio concentration with tazobactam.

[h] Meropenem component. Meropenem in a 1:1 fixed-ratio concentration with vaborbactam.

Additional Compatibility Information

Calcium and Phosphate

Phosphates may be incompatible with metal ions such as magnesium and calcium. A number of studies using potassium phosphate have been performed. For additional information, refer to the potassium phosphate monograph.

UNRECOGNIZED CALCIUM PHOSPHATE PRECIPITATION IN A 3-IN-1 PARENTERAL NUTRITION MIXTURE RESULTED IN PATIENT DEATH.

The potential for the formation of a calcium phosphate precipitate in parenteral nutrition solutions is well studied and documented,[1771 1777] but the information is complex and difficult to apply to the clinical situation.[1770 1772 1777] The incorporation of fat emulsion in 3-in-1 parenteral nutrition solutions obscures any precipitate that is present, which has led to substantial debate on the dangers associated with 3-in-1 parenteral nutrition mixtures and when or if the danger to the patient is warranted therapeutically.[1770 1771 1772 2031 2032 2033 2034 2035 2036] Because such precipitation may be life-threatening to patients,[2037 2291] FDA issued a Safety Alert containing the following recommendations:[1769]

1. "The amounts of phosphorus and of calcium added to the admixture are critical. The solubility of the added calcium should be calculated from the volume at the time the calcium is added. It should not be based upon the final volume.

   Some amino acid injections for TPN admixtures contain phosphate ions (as a phosphoric acid buffer). These phosphate ions and the volume at the time the phosphate is added should be considered when calculating the concentration of phosphate additives. Also, when adding calcium and phosphate to an admixture, the phosphate should be added first.

   The line should be flushed between the addition of any potentially incompatible components.

2. A lipid emulsion in a 3-in-1 admixture obscures the presence of a precipitate. Therefore, if a lipid emulsion is needed, either (1) use a 2-in-1 admixture with the lipid infused separately, or (2) if a 3-in-1 admixture is medically necessary, then add the calcium before the lipid emulsion and according to the recommendations in number 1 above.

   If the amount of calcium or phosphate which must be added is likely to cause a precipitate, some or all of the calcium should be administered separately. Such separate infusions must be properly diluted and slowly infused to avoid serious adverse events related to the calcium.

3. When using an automated compounding device, the above steps should be considered when programming the device. In addition, automated compounders should be maintained and operated according to the manufacturer's recommendations.

   Any printout should be checked against the programmed admixture and weight of components.

4. During the mixing process, pharmacists who mix parenteral nutrition admixtures should periodically agitate the admixture and check for precipitates. Medical or home care personnel who start and monitor these infusions should carefully inspect for the presence of precipitates both before and during infusion. Patients and care givers should be trained to visually inspect for signs of precipitation. They also should be advised to stop the infusion and seek medical assistance if precipitates are noted.

5. A filter should be used when infusing either central or peripheral parenteral nutrition admixtures. At this time, data have not been submitted to document which size filter is most effective in trapping precipitates.

   Standards of practice vary, but the following is suggested: a 1.2-μm air-eliminating filter for lipid-containing admixtures and a 0.22-μm air-eliminating filter for non-lipid-containing admixtures.

6. Parenteral nutrition admixtures should be administered within the following time frames: if stored at room temperature, the infusion should be started within 24 hours after mixing; if stored at refrigerated temperatures, the infusion should be started within 24 hours of rewarming. Because warming parenteral nutrition admixtures may contribute to the formation of precipitates, once administration begins, care should be taken to avoid excessive warming of the admixture.

Persons administering home care parenteral nutrition admixtures may need to deviate from these time frames. Pharmacists who initially prepare these admixtures should check a reserve sample for precipitates over the duration and under the conditions of storage.

7. If symptoms of acute respiratory distress, pulmonary emboli, or interstitial pneumonitis develop, the infusion should be stopped immediately and thoroughly checked for precipitates. Appropriate medical interventions should be instituted. Home care personnel and patients should immediately seek medical assistance."[1769]

Calcium Phosphate Precipitation Fatalities

Fatal cases of paroxysmal respiratory failure in 2 previously healthy women receiving peripheral vein parenteral nutrition were reported. The patients experienced sudden cardiopulmonary arrest consistent with pulmonary emboli. The authors used in vitro simulations and an animal model to conclude that unrecognized calcium phosphate precipitation in a 3-in-1 total nutrition admixture caused the fatalities. The precipitation resulted during compounding by introducing calcium and phosphate near to one another in the compounding sequence and prior to complete fluid addition. This resulted in a temporarily high concentration of the drugs and precipitation of calcium phosphate. Observation of the precipitate was obscured by the incorporation of 20% fat emulsion, intravenous, into the nutrition mixture. No filter was used during infusion of the fatal nutrition admixtures.[2037]

In a follow-up retrospective review, 5 patients were identified who had respiratory distress associated with the infusion of the 3-in-1 admixtures at around the same time. Four of these 5 patients died, although the cause of death could be definitively determined for only 2.[2291]

Calcium and Phosphate Conditional Compatibility

Calcium salts are conditionally compatible with phosphates in parenteral nutrition solutions. The incompatibility is dependent on a solubility and concentration phenomenon and is not entirely predictable. Precipitation may occur during compounding or at some time after compounding is completed.

NOTE: Some amino acid solutions inherently contain calcium and phosphate, which must be considered in any projection of compatibility.

A study determined the maximum concentrations of calcium (as chloride and gluconate) and phosphate that can be maintained without precipitation in a parenteral nutrition solution consisting of FreAmine II 4.25% and dextrose 25% for 24 hours at 30°C. It was noted that the amino acids in parenteral nutrition solutions form soluble complexes with calcium and phosphate,

reducing the available free calcium and phosphate that can form insoluble precipitates. The concentration of calcium available for precipitation is greater with the chloride salt compared to the gluconate salt, at least in part because of differences in dissociation characteristics. Consequently, a greater concentration of calcium gluconate than calcium chloride can be mixed with sodium phosphate.[608]

In addition to the concentrations of phosphate and calcium and the salt form of the calcium, the concentration of amino acids and the time and temperature of storage altered the formation of calcium phosphate in parenteral nutrition solutions. As the temperature was increased, the incidence of precipitate formation also increased. This finding was attributed, at least in part, to a greater degree of dissociation of the calcium and phosphate complexes and the decreased solubility of calcium phosphate. Therefore, a solution possibly may be stored at 4°C with no precipitation, but on warming to room temperature a precipitate will form over time.[608]

The solubility characteristics of calcium and phosphate in pediatric parenteral nutrition solutions composed of Aminosyn 0.5, 2, and 4% with dextrose 10 to 25% were reported. Also present were electrolytes and vitamins. Sodium phosphate was added sequentially in phosphorus concentrations from 10 to 30 mmol/L. Calcium gluconate was added last in amounts ranging from 1 to 10 g/L. The solutions were stored at 25°C for 30 hours and examined visually and microscopically for precipitation. The authors found that higher concentrations of Aminosyn increased the solubility of calcium and phosphate. Precipitation occurred at lower calcium and phosphate concentrations in the 0.5% solution compared to the 2 and 4% solutions. For example, at a phosphorus concentration of 30 mmol/L, precipitation occurred at calcium gluconate concentrations of about 1, 2, and 4 g/L in the 0.5, 2, and 4% Aminosyn mixtures, respectively. Similarly, at a calcium gluconate concentration of 8 g/L and above, precipitation occurred at phosphorus concentrations of about 13, 17, and 22 mmol/L in the 0.5, 2, and 4% solutions, respectively. The dextrose concentration did not appear to affect the calcium and phosphate solubility significantly.[1042]

The maximum allowable concentrations of calcium and phosphate in a 3-in-1 parenteral nutrition mixture for children (TNA #192 in Appendix) were reported. Added calcium was varied from 1.5 to 150 mmol/L, and added phosphate was varied from 21 to 300 mmol/L. These mixtures were stable for 48 hours at 22 and 37°C as long as the pH was not greater than 5.7, the calcium concentration was below 16 mmol/L, the phosphate concentration was below 52 mmol/L, and the product of the calcium and phosphate concentrations was below 250 mmol^2/L^2 (mmol squared per liter squared).[1773]

Additional calcium and phosphate solubility curves were reported for specialty parenteral nutrition solutions based on NephrAmine and also HepatAmine at concentrations of 0.8, 1.5, and 2% as the sources of amino acids. The solutions also contained dextrose 10%, with cysteine and pH adjustment to simulate addition of fat emulsion used in some admixtures. Calcium and phosphate solubility followed the hyperbolic patterns previously reported.[609] Temperature, time, and pH affected calcium and phosphate solubility, with pH having the greatest effect.[2038]

The maximum sodium phosphate concentrations were reported for given amounts of calcium gluconate that could be admixed in parenteral nutrition solutions containing TrophAmine in varying quantities (with cysteine hydrochloride 40 mg/g of amino acid) and dextrose 10%. The solutions also contained magnesium sulfate 4 mEq/L, potassium acetate 24 mEq/L, sodium chloride 32 mEq/L, pediatric multivitamins, and trace elements. The presence of cysteine hydrochloride reduces the solution pH and increases the amount of calcium and phosphate that can be incorporated before precipitation occurs. The results of this study cannot be safely extrapolated to TPN solutions with compositions other than the ones tested. The admixtures were compounded with the sodium phosphate added last after thorough mixing of all other components. The authors noted that this is not the preferred order of mixing (usually phosphate is added first and thoroughly mixed before adding calcium last); however, they believed this reversed order of mixing would provide a margin of error in cases in which the proper order is not followed. After compounding, the solutions were stored for 24 hours at 40°C. The maximum calcium and phosphate amounts that could be mixed in the various solutions were reported tabularly and are shown in Table 1.[2039] However, these results are not entirely consistent with another study.[2196]

Table 1. Maximum amount of phosphate (as sodium) (mmol/L) not resulting in precipitation.[2039] See CAUTION below.[a]

Calcium (as Gluconate)	Amino Acid (as TrophAmine) plus Cysteine HCl 40 mg/g of Amino Acid				
	0%	0.4%	1%	2%	3%
9.8 mEq/L	0	27	42	60	66
14.7 mEq/L	0	15	18	30	36
19.6 mEq/L	0	6	15	27	30
29.4 mEq/L	0	3	6	21	24

[a] CAUTION: The results cannot be safely extrapolated to solutions with formulas other than the ones tested. See text.

Calcium phosphate precipitation phenomena was evaluated in a series of parenteral nutrition admixtures composed of dextrose 22%, amino acids (FreAmine III) 2.7%, and fat emulsion (Abbott) 0, 1, and 3.2%. Incorporation of calcium gluconate 19 to 24 mEq/L and phosphate (as sodium) 22 to 28 mmol/L resulted in visible precipitation in the fat-free admixtures. New precipitate continued to form over 14 days, even after repeated filtrations of the solutions through 0.2-μm filters. The presence of the amino acids increased calcium and phosphate solubility, compared with simple aqueous solutions. However, the incorporation of the fat emulsion did not result in a statistically significant increase in calcium and phosphate solubility. The authors noted that the kinetics of calcium phosphate precipitate formation do not appear to be entirely predictable; both transient and permanent precipitation can occur either during the compounding process or at some time afterward. Because calcium phosphate precipitation can be very dangerous clinically, the use of inline filters was recommended. The authors suggested that the filters should have a porosity appropriate to the parenteral nutrition admixture—1.2 μm for fat-containing and 0.2 or 0.45 μm for fat-free nutrition mixtures.[2061]

A 2-mL fluid barrier of dextrose 5% in a microbore retrograde infusion set failed to prevent precipitation when used between calcium gluconate 200 mg/2 mL and sodium phosphate 0.3 mmol/0.1 mL.[1385]

A 2-in-1 parenteral nutrition admixture with final concentrations of TrophAmine 0.5%, dextrose 5%, L-cysteine hydrochloride 40 mg/g of amino acids, calcium gluconate 60 mg/100 mL, and sodium phosphates 46.5 mg/mL was found to result in visible precipitation of calcium phosphate within 30 hours stored at 23 to 27°C. Despite the presence of the acidifying L-cysteine hydrochloride, precipitation occurred at clinically utilized amounts of calcium and phosphates.[2622]

The presence of magnesium in solutions may also influence the reaction between calcium and phosphate, including the nature and extent of precipitation.[158 159]

The interaction of calcium and phosphate in parenteral nutrition solutions is a complex phenomenon. Various factors have been identified as playing a role in the solubility or precipitation of a given combination, including[608 609 1042 1063 1427 2778]:

1. Concentration of calcium
2. Salt form of calcium
3. Concentration of phosphate
4. Concentration of amino acids
5. Amino acids composition
6. Concentration of dextrose
7. Temperature of solution
8. pH of solution
9. Presence of other additives
10. Order of mixing

Enhanced precipitate formation would be expected from such factors as high concentrations of calcium and phosphate, increases in solution pH, decreased amino acid concentrations, increases in temperature, addition of calcium prior to phosphate, lengthy standing times or slow infusion rates, and use of calcium as the chloride salt.[854]

Sodium Thiosulfate
AHFS 92:12

Products

Sodium thiosulfate is available as a 250-mg/mL (25%) solution in 50-mL (12.5-g) vials alone[3092] or packaged with sodium nitrite injection as a kit (Nithiodote®).[3093] Each mL of solution also contains boric acid 2.8 mg and potassium chloride 4.4 mg.[3092 3093] The pH of the solution has been adjusted with boric acid and/or sodium hydroxide.[3092 3093] The drug also may contain trace impurities of sodium sulfite.[3092 3093]

pH

From 7.5 to 9.5.[3092 3093]

Trade Name(s)

Nithiodote

Administration

Sodium thiosulfate is administered by slow intravenous injection.[3092 3093]

Stability

Intact vials of sodium thiosulfate should be stored at controlled room temperature and protected from direct light and freezing.[3092 3093]

Compatibility Information

Additive Compatibility

Sodium thiosulfate

Test Drug	Mfr	Conc/L or %	Mfr	Conc/L or %	Test Solution	Remarks	Ref	C/I
Sodium nitroprusside	HOS	180 mg	AMR	1.8 g	D5W, NS	Physically compatible with less than 10% loss of either drug in 48 hr at room temperature protected from light	2825	C

Additional Compatibility Information

Hydroxocobalamin

The manufacturer of sodium thiosulfate states that the drug should not be administered simultaneously into the same intravenous infusion line as hydroxocobalamin; chemical incompatibility has been reported between these drugs.[3092]

Sodium Nitrite

The manufacturer of sodium thiosulfate states that no chemical incompatibility has been reported between sodium nitrite and sodium thiosulfate when these drugs have been administered sequentially through the same intravenous infusion line.[3092]

Other Cyanide Antidotes

If cyanide antidotes other than sodium nitrite are to be administered to patients receiving sodium thiosulfate, the manufacturer recommends that the drugs not be administered concurrently into the same intravenous infusion line.[3092]

DOI: 10.37573/9781585286850.357

Somatropin
AHFS 68:28

Products

Somatropin derived from *Escherichia coli* is available in vials and cartridges in sizes ranging from 1.5 to 24 mg, depending on the specific product. Each milligram represents about three units of activity. The commercially available dosage forms are variable in components and concentrations; care should be taken to follow the directions for the specific product being used. Most products are supplied in dry form requiring reconstitution using a diluent that is supplied with the product. Manufacturers' specific reconstitution instructions for each product should be followed. For products in vials, the specified amount of the diluent is injected into the somatropin container, aiming the stream at the container wall. The drug is reconstituted by gentle swirling using a rotary motion for most products but vigorous swirling for two minutes for Nutropin Depot. Vial inversion is recommended for reconstitution of Norditropin. Shaking is not recommended for any product and may damage the product.[1]

Norditropin Cartridges and Nutropin AQ are available as liquid injections not requiring dilution for use.[1]

Somatropin derived from mammalian cells (Saizen; Serostim) is available in vials in varying sizes from 4 to 8.8 mg, depending on the specific product. The manufacturer's specific reconstitution instructions for each product using the diluents provided should be followed. The specified amount of the diluent is injected into the somatropin container, aiming the stream at the container wall. The drug is dissolved by gentle swirling using a rotary motion, *not* shaking. Shaking is not recommended for any product and may damage the protein.[1]

pH

The pH values cited by the manufacturers are as follows[1]:

Products	pH
Genotropin	about 6.7
Humatrope	about 7.5
Norditropin	about 7.3
Nutropin	about 7.4
Nutropin AQ	about 6.0
Saizen	6.5 to 8.5
Serostim	7.4 to 8.5

Trade Name(s)

Norditropin, Nutropin AQ, Nutropin Depot, Saizen, Serostim

Administration

Somatropin products are usually administered by subcutaneous injection. Humatrope and Saizen may also be administered intramuscularly.[1]

Stability

Intact containers of somatropin products derived from *E. coli* should be stored under refrigeration and protected from freezing. Genotropin and Norditropin should also be protected from light during storage. Most somatropin products result in clear solutions when reconstituted correctly. Shaking may result in cloudiness, rendering the products unacceptable for use. Reconstituted Nutropin Depot is a thick, milky suspension.[1]

Stability after reconstitution is variable among the products and depends on whether a preservative-containing diluent is used. See Table 1. Unpreserved reconstituted products of Genotropin and Humatrope should be stored under refrigeration and used within 24 hours. Nutropin Depot suspension should be used immediately upon reconstitution, discarding any unused remainder. Products reconstituted with the specified preserved diluents are stable for longer periods. After reconstitution with the appropriate preserved diluent, Norditropin and Nutropin are stable for 14 days, Genotropin for 21 days, and Humatrope for 28 days stored under refrigeration. Nutropin AQ is stable for 28 days after initial stopper penetration when stored under refrigeration.[1]

Intact containers of somatropin products derived from mammalian cells should be stored at controlled room temperature. Saizen reconstituted with the preserved diluent provided is stable for 14 days after reconstitution when stored under refrigeration. Serostim reconstituted with the unpreserved diluent provided is stable for 24 hours stored under refrigeration. Freezing of reconstituted solutions should be avoided.[1]

Table 1. Recommended stability periods for somatropin products using diluents with and without preservatives and stored under refrigeration[1]

Product	Stability Period
Diluent with Preservative	
Genotropin 5.8 and 13.8 mg	21 days
Humatrope	28 days
Norditropin	14 days
Nutropin	14 days
Nutropin AQ	28 days[a]
Saizen	14 days
Diluent without Preservative	
Genotropin 1.5 mg	24 hr
Humatrope	24 hr
Serostim	24 hr

[a] Period after initial penetration of the vial stopper of this liquid product.

DOI: 10.37573/9781585286850.358

Syringes

Somatropin (Humatrope) was reconstituted to concentrations of 1 and 3.33 mg/mL with the accompanying diluent; the diluent contains glycerin 1.7% and *m*-cresol 0.3% as a preservative. The reconstituted product at each concentration was packaged in 1-mL plastic syringes with barrels composed of polypropylene (Becton Dickinson) or propylene–ethylene copolymer (Terumo) and capped and stored under refrigeration at about 5°C for 28 days. Little or no loss of somatropin occurred stored in either syringe. The solutions remained visually acceptable for 28 days in the polypropylene syringes, but an unacceptable turbidity formed within 21 days in the propylene–ethylene copolymer syringes, which became a precipitate by 28 days. The preservative, *m*-cresol, concentrations fell up to 4% but remained above the minimum acceptable concentration. Somatropin should be stored no more than 14 days at 5°C in propylene–ethylene copolymer syringes. Storage up to 28 days was acceptable in the polypropylene syringes.[2210]

Selected Revisions October 1, 2012. © Copyright, October 2002. American Society of Health-System Pharmacists, Inc.

Sterile Water for Injection
AHFS 96:00

Products

Sterile water for injection is available in ampuls, vials, and plastic bags in sizes ranging from 5 mL to 5 L. This diluent is a pharmaceutical aid that contains no antimicrobial preservative or any other solute but must have drugs or other solutes added prior to administration.[1(2/08)]

pH

From 5 to 7.[1(2/08)]

Osmolality

Sterile water for injection has an osmolality of 0 mOsm/kg. It is incompatible with blood and will cause hemolysis if administered intravenously in sufficient quantity.[1(2/08)]

Administration

Sterile water for injection is intended for use as a pharmaceutical aid in dissolving or diluting drugs for subcutaneous, intramuscular, and intravenous injection. It must not be administered intravenously without the addition of a sufficient amount of drugs or other solutes to provide adequate osmolality to make the solution approximately isotonic.[1(2/08)] Death and injury have resulted from hemolysis caused by intravenous administration of a sufficient volume of sterile water for injection and other low-osmolality solutions.[4 1942 2072 2073 2481 2482]

For patient safety, medical orders for large volumes of sterile water for injection, especially plastic bags of any size, without the addition of sufficient drug or solute to render the solutions approximately isotonic (about 308 mOsm/kg) should not be permitted. Immediate consultation with the prescriber or referral to the institutional medical peer review process may be necessary to avoid possible patient harm. Large-volume containers of sterile water for injection should be stored only in pharmacies and not in patient care areas. Suitable warnings near the stored product and computer system alerts should remind staff that sterile water for injection is for diluent use only.[2481]

Stability

The intact single-use containers of sterile water for injection should be stored at controlled room temperature.[1(2/08)]

Selected Revisions July 1, 2020. © Copyright, October 2004. American Society of Health-System Pharmacists, Inc.

DOI: 10.37573/9781585286850.359

Streptomycin Sulfate
AHFS 8:12.02

Products

Streptomycin sulfate is available as a lyophilized powder for injection in vials containing 1 g of drug with no preservatives. Reconstitute with 4.2, 3.2, or 1.8 mL of sterile water for injection to yield solutions containing 200, 250, or 400 mg/mL, respectively.[4]

pH

The reconstituted injection at a concentration of 200 mg/mL has a pH of 4.5 to 7.[1(8/08) 4]

Administration

Streptomycin sulfate is administered by deep intramuscular injection well within the body of a relatively large muscle, such as the upper outer quadrant of the buttock in adults or the midlateral thigh in adults or children. Injection sites should be alternated.[1(8/08) 4] Intravenous injection is not recommended[4], although it has been performed.[1603]

Stability

Intact vials of streptomycin sulfate lyophilized powder should be stored at controlled room temperature and protected from light.[1(8/08) 4]

Reconstituted solutions of streptomycin sulfate are stated to be stable for one week at room temperature and protected from light. However, no preservatives are present and the possibility of microbiological contamination must be considered.[1(8/08) 4]

Compatibility Information

Additive Compatibility

Streptomycin sulfate

Test Drug	Mfr	Conc/L or %	Mfr	Conc/L or %	Test Solution	Remarks	Ref	C/I
Amphotericin B		200 mg	BP	4 g	D5W	Haze develops over 3 hr	26	I
Bleomycin sulfate	BR	20 and 30 units	PF	4 g	NS	Physically compatible and bleomycin activity retained for 1 week at 4°C. Streptomycin not tested	763	C
Heparin sodium	AB	20,000 units		1 g		Precipitate forms within 1 hr	21	I
Heparin sodium	BP	20,000 units	BP	4 g	D5W, NS	Precipitates immediately	26	I
Methohexital sodium	BP	2 g	BP	4 g	NS	Crystals produced	26	I

Drugs in Syringe Compatibility

Streptomycin sulfate

Test Drug	Mfr	Amt	Mfr	Amt	Remarks	Ref	C/I
Ampicillin sodium	AY	500 mg		1 g/2 mL	No precipitate or color change within 1 hr at room temperature	99	C
Ampicillin sodium	AY	500 mg	BP	1 g/2 mL	Physically compatible for 1 hr at room temperature	300	C
Ampicillin sodium	AY	500 mg	BP	1 g/1.5 mL	Syrupy solution forms	300	I
Cloxacillin sodium	BE	250 mg		1 g/2 mL	No precipitate or color change within 1 hr at room temperature	99	C
Cloxacillin sodium	AY	250 mg	BP	1 g/1.5 mL	Syrupy solution forms	300	I
Cloxacillin sodium	AY	250 mg	BP	1 g/2 mL	Physically compatible for 1 hr at room temperature	300	C
Cloxacillin sodium	AY	250 mg	BP	750 mg/1.5 mL	Precipitate forms within 1 hr at room temperature	300	I
Heparin sodium	AB	20,000 units/1 mL		1 g	Physically incompatible	21	I
Penicillin G sodium		1 million units		1 g/2 mL	No precipitate or color change within 1 hr at room temperature	99	C

DOI: 10.37573/9781585286850.360

Y-Site Injection Compatibility (1:1 Mixture)

Streptomycin sulfate

Test Drug	Mfr	Conc	Mfr	Conc	Remarks	Ref	C/I
Esmolol HCl	DCC	10 mg/mL[a]	PF	10 mg/mL[a]	Physically compatible for 24 hr at 22°C	1169	C

[a] Tested in dextrose 5%.

Selected Revisions October 1, 2012. © Copyright, October 1982.
American Society of Health-System Pharmacists, Inc.

Streptozocin
AHFS 10:00

Products

Streptozocin is available in single-dose vials containing 1 g of drug and 220 mg of citric acid anhydrous. Sodium hydroxide may have been used to adjust the pH.[1(5/07)]

Reconstitute with 9.5 mL of sodium chloride 0.9% or dextrose 5% to provide a 100-mg/mL solution.[1(5/07) 4]

pH

From 3.5 to 4.5.[1(5/07)]

Trade Name(s)

Zanosar

Administration

Streptozocin may be administered by rapid intravenous injection or intravenous infusion over 15 minutes to six hours.[1(5/07) 4]

Stability

Intact vials containing a pale yellow powder should be refrigerated and protected from light.[1(5/07) 4]

The pale gold reconstituted solution is stable for 48 hours at room temperature or 96 hours under refrigeration.[4] However, the manufacturer recommends use within 12 hours because the product does not contain an antibacterial preservative.[1(5/07) 4]

Streptozocin (Upjohn) 3 mg/mL in sodium chloride 0.9% did not support the growth of *Staphylococcus aureus*, *Enterococcus faecium*, *Pseudomonas aeruginosa*, and *Candida albicans* with loss of viability over 24 hours at room temperature. Even so, admixtures should be stored under refrigeration whenever possible, and the potential for microbiological growth should be considered when assigning expiration periods.[2740]

Filtration

Streptozocin 10 to 200 mcg/mL exhibited no loss due to sorption to either cellulose nitrate/cellulose acetate ester (Millex OR) or Teflon (Millex FG) filters.[1415 1416]

Compatibility Information

Solution Compatibility

Streptozocin

Test Soln Name	Mfr	Mfr	Conc/L or %	Remarks	Ref	C/I
Dextrose 5%			2 g	Stable for 48 hr at room temperature and 96 hr refrigerated	4	C
Sodium chloride 0.9%			2 g	Stable for 48 hr at room temperature and 96 hr refrigerated	4	C

Y-Site Injection Compatibility (1:1 Mixture)

Streptozocin

Test Drug	Mfr	Conc	Mfr	Conc	Remarks	Ref	C/I
Allopurinol sodium	BW	3 mg/mL[b]	UP	40 mg/mL[b]	Haze and small particles in 1 hr	1686	I
Amifostine	USB	10 mg/mL[a]	UP	40 mg/mL[a]	Physically compatible for 4 hr at 23°C	1845	C
Aztreonam	SQ	40 mg/mL[a]	UP	40 mg/mL[a]	Red color forms in 1 hr	1758	I
Etoposide phosphate	BR	5 mg/mL[a]	UP	40 mg/mL[a]	Physically compatible for 4 hr at 23°C	2218	C
Filgrastim	AMG	30 mcg/mL[a]	UP	40 mg/mL[a]	Physically compatible for 4 hr at 22°C	1687	C
Gemcitabine HCl	LI	10 mg/mL[b]	UP	40 mg/mL[b]	Physically compatible for 4 hr at 23°C	2226	C
Granisetron HCl	SKB	1 mg/mL	UP	9.1 mg/mL[b]	Physically compatible with little or no loss of either drug in 4 hr at 22°C	1883	C
Melphalan HCl	BW	0.1 mg/mL[b]	UP	40 mg/mL[b]	Physically compatible for 3 hr at 22°C	1557	C

DOI: 10.37573/9781585286850.361

Y-Site Injection Compatibility (1:1 Mixture) (Cont.)

Test Drug	Mfr	Conc	Mfr	Conc	Remarks	Ref	C/I
Ondansetron HCl	GL	1 mg/mL[b]	UP	30 mg/mL[a]	Visually compatible for 4 hr at 22°C	1365	C
Piperacillin sodium–tazobactam sodium	LE[d]	40 mg/mL[a e]	UP	40 mg/mL[a]	Particles form in 1 hr	1688	I
Teniposide	BR	0.1 mg/mL[a]	UP	40 mg/mL[a]	Physically compatible for 4 hr at 23°C	1725	C
Thiotepa	IMM[c]	1 mg/mL[a]	UP	40 mg/mL[a]	Physically compatible for 4 hr at 23°C	1861	C
Vinorelbine tartrate	BW	1 mg/mL[b]	UP	40 mg/mL[b]	Physically compatible for 4 hr at 22°C	1558	C

[a] Tested in dextrose 5%.

[b] Tested in sodium chloride 0.9%.

[c] Lyophilized formulation tested.

[d] Test performed using the formulation WITHOUT edetate disodium.

[e] Piperacillin component. Piperacillin in an 8:1 fixed-ratio concentration with tazobactam.

Selected Revisions May 28, 2014. © Copyright, October 1994.
American Society of Health-System Pharmacists, Inc.

Succinylcholine Chloride
AHFS 12:20.20

Products

Succinylcholine chloride is available in a concentration of 20 mg/mL in 5- and 10-mL multiple-dose vials and 5-mL syringes. The vials are preserved with parabens or benzyl alcohol and may contain sodium chloride for isotonicity and hydrochloric acid for pH adjustment. Succinylcholine chloride is also available in higher concentrations of 50 mg/mL in 10-mL ampuls and 100 mg/mL in 10-mL single-dose vials.[1(4/08)] [4]

pH

From 3 to 4.5.[1(4/08)] [4]

Osmolality

The osmolality of succinylcholine chloride 50 mg/mL was determined to be 409 mOsm/kg.[1233]

Trade Name(s)

Anectine, Quelicin

Administration

Succinylcholine chloride is usually administered by direct intermittent intravenous injection or intravenous infusion. For continuous intravenous infusion, a 1- to 2-mg/mL (0.1 to 0.2%) solution is prepared, usually in 250 to 1000 mL of compatible fluid. If necessary, when a suitable vein is inaccessible, a maximum of 150 mg of the drug may be administered by deep intramuscular injection, preferably high into the deltoid muscle.[1(4/08)] [4]

Stability

Commercially available injections of succinylcholine chloride should be stored at 2 to 8°C to retard loss.[1(4/08)] [4] Succinylcholine chloride injection in the original unopened containers is stated in the labeling to be stable for 14 days at room temperature.[1(4/08)] [1433]

Studies indicate that succinylcholine chloride injection in original unopened containers may be stable at room temperature for longer periods. The manufacturer of Quelicin has stated that the drug was stable for 3 months at temperatures up to 25°C.[1239] [2745] More recently, Hospira has stated that Quelicin is stable only for 30 days at room temperature.[2783]

Research studies have also looked at the stability of succinylcholine chloride above refrigeration temperature. In one study, storage for 7 days at 40°C followed by storage at 25°C for four weeks was used to simulate the worst case of shipping followed by storage on an emergency cart. Calculated loss at room temperature was 1%/week; at 40°C, it was 3.2%/week. Therefore, the loss was estimated to be about 7% under such conditions.[960]

In another study, similar results were found. The decomposition rate of succinylcholine chloride was dependent on both concentration and temperature. The calculated degradation rates at room temperature were all higher for the 50-mg/mL concentration (2.1%/month) compared to the 20-mg/mL injection (1.2%/month). The time to 10% decomposition on an emergency cart was about 4.8 months for the 50-mg/mL concentration and was about 8.3 months for the 20-mg/mL concentration. Refrigeration cut the decomposition rates to 0.3 and 0.18% per month, respectively.[2742]

However, a somewhat shorter time to 10% decomposition at room temperature has also been reported. Commercial vials of succinylcholine chloride 20 mg/mL (Quelicin) stored at room temperature were found to decompose about 10 to 11% drug in 6 months. The authors recommended limiting room temperature storage to not more than 6 months.[2763]

After dilution of succinylcholine chloride to a concentration of 1 or 2 mg/mL in sodium chloride 0.9%, the drug is stated to be chemically stable for 4 weeks at 5°C and 1 week at 25°C. However, use within 24 hours of preparation is recommended along with discarding any unused solution.[1(4/08)] [4]

pH Effects

Succinylcholine chloride is unstable in alkaline solutions[1(4/08)] [4] and decomposes in solutions with a pH greater than 4.5.[4] The pH of maximum stability was found to be 3.75 to 4.50.[960]

In combination with barbiturates, either free barbituric acid will precipitate or the succinylcholine chloride will be hydrolyzed, depending on the final pH of the admixture.[1(4/08)] [4] [21] Succinylcholine chloride should not be mixed with barbiturates in the same syringe or given simultaneously through the same needle.[1(4/08)]

Syringes

Succinylcholine chloride (Abbott) 20 mg/mL was packaged in both glass and polypropylene syringes (Becton Dickinson) sealed with rubber luer-tip caps (Becton Dickinson). The syringes were stored for 45 days at 4°C, 22°C and 50% relative humidity, and 37°C and 85% relative humidity. At 4°C, there was little or no succinylcholine chloride loss after 45 days in either glass or plastic syringes. At 22°C and 50% relative humidity, about a 5% loss occurred in 45 days. However, at 37°C and 85% relative humidity, the drug concentration fell below the acceptable USP limit after about 30 days.[1209]

Succinylcholine chloride (Burroughs Wellcome) 20 mg/mL in dextrose 5% and in sodium chloride 0.9% (Baxter) was packaged as 10 mL in 12-mL plastic syringes (Monoject) and wrapped in aluminum foil. Little or no loss of succinylcholine chloride occurred during 107 days of storage at 5°C. At 25°C, about 5 to 6% loss occurred in 100 days. Samples at an elevated temperature of 40°C were stable through 22 days with only 3 to 4% loss but exhibited 12 to 14% loss at 63 days.[1892]

DOI: 10.37573/9781585286850.362

Succinylcholine chloride (Abbott) 20 mg/mL was packaged as 8 mL of undiluted injection in 12-mL polypropylene syringes (Becton Dickinson) and was stored at 4°C and 25°C exposed to fluorescent light. The injection remained visually clear at both temperatures. Little or no loss of succinylcholine chloride occurred in 90 days when stored at 4°C. However, at 25°C losses of about 6, 10, and 12% occurred in 45, 60, and 90 days, respectively.[2438]

Syringes prefilled with succinylcholine chloride injection for emergency use have been reported to freeze upon storage under refrigeration. Care should be taken to make sure that refrigerators are operating within compendial temperature ranges to ensure the availability of stored drugs in emergencies.[2698] [2699]

Compatibility Information

Solution Compatibility

Succinylcholine chloride

Test Soln Name	Mfr	Mfr	Conc/L or %	Remarks	Ref	C/I
Dextrose 2.5% in half-strength Ringer's injection	AB	AB	2 g	Physically compatible	3	C
Dextrose 5% in Ringer's injection	AB	AB	2 g	Physically compatible	3	C
Dextrose 5% in half-strength Ringer's injection, lactated	AB	AB	2 g	Physically compatible	3	C
Dextrose 2.5% in Ringer's injection, lactated	AB	AB	2 g	Physically compatible	3	C
Dextrose 5% in Ringer's injection, lactated	AB	AB	2 g	Physically compatible	3	C
Dextrose 5% in Ringer's injection, lactated	TR[a]	TR	1 g	Stable for 24 hr at 5°C	282	C
Dextrose 10% in Ringer's injection, lactated	AB	AB	2 g	Physically compatible	3	C
Dextrose 2.5% in sodium chloride 0.45%	AB	AB	2 g	Physically compatible	3	C
Dextrose 2.5% in sodium chloride 0.9%	AB	AB	2 g	Physically compatible	3	C
Dextrose 5% in sodium chloride 0.225%	AB	AB	2 g	Physically compatible	3	C
Dextrose 5% in sodium chloride 0.45%	AB	AB	2 g	Physically compatible	3	C
Dextrose 5% in sodium chloride 0.9%	AB	AB	2 g	Physically compatible	3	C
Dextrose 5% in sodium chloride 0.9%	TR[a]	TR	1 g	Stable for 24 hr at 5°C	282	C
Dextrose 10% in sodium chloride 0.9%	AB	AB	2 g	Physically compatible	3	C
Dextrose 2.5%	AB	AB	2 g	Physically compatible	3	C
Dextrose 5%	AB	AB	2 g	Physically compatible	3	C
Dextrose 5%	TR[a]	TR	1 g	Stable for 24 hr at 5°C	282	C
Dextrose 10%	AB	AB	2 g	Physically compatible	3	C
Ionosol B in dextrose 5%	AB	AB	2 g	Physically compatible	3	C
Ionosol MB in dextrose 5%	AB	AB	2 g	Physically compatible	3	C
Ringer's injection	AB	AB	2 g	Physically compatible	3	C
Ringer's injection, lactated	AB	AB	2 g	Physically compatible	3	C
Ringer's injection, lactated	TR[a]	TR	1 g	Stable for 24 hr at 5°C	282	C
Sodium chloride 0.45%	AB	AB	2 g	Physically compatible	3	C
Sodium chloride 0.9%	AB	AB	2 g	Physically compatible	3	C
Sodium chloride 0.9%	TR[a]	TR	1 g	Stable for 24 hr at 5°C	282	C
Sodium lactate ⅙ M	AB	AB	2 g	Physically compatible	3	C

[a] Tested in both glass and PVC containers.

Additive Compatibility

Succinylcholine chloride

Test Drug	Mfr	Conc/L or %	Mfr	Conc/L or %	Test Solution	Remarks	Ref	C/I
Amikacin sulfate	BR	5 g	SQ	2 g	D5LR, D5R, D5S, D5W, D10W, LR, NS, R, SL	Physically compatible and both stable for 24 hr at 25°C	294	C
Isoproterenol HCl	WI	4 mg	AB	2 g		Physically compatible	59	C
Meperidine HCl	WI	100 mg	AB	2 g		Physically compatible	3	C
Methyldopate HCl	MSD	1 g	AB	2 g	D5W, D10W, D2.5½S, D2.5S, D5¼S, D5½S, D5S, D10S, NS, ½S	Physically compatible	23	C
Morphine sulfate		16.2 mg	AB	2 g		Physically compatible	3	C
Norepinephrine bitartrate	WI	8 mg	AB	2 g	D5W, D10W, D2.5½S, D2.5S, D5¼S, D5½S, D5S, D10S, NS, ½S	Physically compatible	77	C
Pentobarbital sodium						Pentobarbital precipitates or succinylcholine hydrolyzes	4	I
Phenobarbital sodium						Phenobarbital precipitates or succinylcholine hydrolyzes	4	I
Scopolamine HBr		0.43 mg	AB	2 g		Physically compatible	3	C
Sodium bicarbonate	AB	2.4 mEq[a]	AB	1 g	D5W	Succinylcholine decomposition	772	I

[a] One vial of Neut added to a liter of admixture.

Drugs in Syringe Compatibility

Succinylcholine chloride

Test Drug	Mfr	Amt	Mfr	Amt	Remarks	Ref	C/I
Heparin sodium		2500 units/1 mL		100 mg/5 mL	Physically compatible for at least 5 min	1053	C

Y-Site Injection Compatibility (1:1 Mixture)

Succinylcholine chloride

Test Drug	Mfr	Conc	Mfr	Conc	Remarks	Ref	C/I
Dexmedetomidine HCl	HOS	4 mcg/mL[b]			Stated to be compatible	3181	C
Etomidate	AB	2 mg/mL	AB	20 mg/mL	Visually compatible for 7 days at 25°C	1801	C
Heparin sodium[d]	RI	1000 units/L[a b c]	BW	20 mg/mL	Physically compatible for 4 hr at room temperature	322	C
Hetastarch in lactated electrolyte	AB	6%	AB	2 mg/mL[a]	Physically compatible for 4 hr at 23°C	2339	C
Hydrocortisone sodium succinate[e]	UP	100 mg/L[a b c]	BW	20 mg/mL	Physically compatible for 4 hr at room temperature	322	C
Palonosetron HCl	MGI	50 mcg/mL	SZ	2 mg/mL[a]	Physically compatible and no loss of either drug in 4 hr at room temperature	2764	C
Potassium chloride		40 mEq/L[a b c]	BW	20 mg/mL	Physically compatible for 4 hr at room temperature	322	C

Y-Site Injection Compatibility (1:1 Mixture) (Cont.)

Test Drug	Mfr	Conc	Mfr	Conc	Remarks	Ref	C/I
Propofol	ZEN[f]	10 mg/mL	AB	20 mg/mL	Physically compatible for 1 hr at 23°C	2066	C

[a] Tested in dextrose 5%.

[b] Tested in sodium chloride 0.9%.

[c] Tested in Ringer's injection, lactated.

[d] Tested in combination with hydrocortisone sodium succinate (Upjohn) 100 mg/L.

[e] Tested in combination with heparin sodium (Riker) 1000 units/L.

[f] Test performed using the formulation WITH edetate disodium.

Selected Revisions January 31, 2020. © Copyright, October 1982. American Society of Health-System Pharmacists, Inc.

Sufentanil Citrate
AHFS 28:08.08

Products

Sufentanil citrate is available as a preservative-free aqueous injection in 1-, 2-, and 5-mL ampuls and vials. Each mL of solution contains sufentanil citrate equivalent to 50 mcg of sufentanil base.[1(7/07)]

pH

From 3.5 to 6.[1(7/07)]

Trade Name(s)

Sufenta

Administration

Sufentanil citrate is administered intravenously by slow injection or infusion. For labor and delivery, it may be administered epidurally. The drug has also been given intramuscularly.[1(7/07)] [4]

Stability

Sufentanil citrate is a stable, clear, aqueous, preservative-free injection. The product should be stored at controlled room temperature and protected from light.[1(7/07)] [4]

pH Effects

Sufentanil citrate is hydrolyzed in acidic solutions. A 5-mcg/mL solution with a pH greater than 3 lost less than 1% in 48 weeks at 90°C. However, at a pH of less than 2, the drug loss was 14% at 60°C and 32% at 90°C in 48 weeks.[1755]

Freezing Solutions

Sufentanil citrate (Janssen) 5 mcg/mL in sodium chloride 0.9% became nonhomogeneous and difficult to restore to homogeneity when frozen at −20°C.[1755]

Syringes

Sufentanil citrate (Janssen) 2 mcg/mL in sodium chloride 0.9% was packaged in 50-mL polypropylene syringes (Omnifix, B. Braun) and stored at 21°C. Less than 10% sufentanil loss occurred in 24 hours.[2201]

Ambulatory Pumps

Sufentanil citrate 50 mcg/mL was evaluated in CADD-1 and CADD-PRIZM medication cassettes. About 4% drug loss occurred in 14 days at room and refrigeration temperatures.[2717]

Sorption

Sufentanil citrate (Janssen) demonstrated loss from solutions in concentrations from 1 to 20 mcg/mL due to sorption to polyvinyl chloride (PVC)/Kalex 3000 reservoirs for use with CADD pumps (Pharmacia Deltec) and administration tubing.[790]

Sufentanil citrate (Janssen) 2 mcg/mL in sodium chloride 0.9% was delivered from 50-mL polypropylene syringes (Omnifix, B. Braun) by a syringe pump (JMS-Syringe-Pump Model SP-100, Japan Medical Supply Company) through polyethylene extension sets (Original-Perfusor-Leitung, Type PE, B. Braun) or PVC extension sets (Original-Perfusor-Leitung, Type N, B. Braun), 0.2-μm epidural filters (Sterifix, B. Braun), and epidural catheters (Perifix, B. Braun) over 24 hours. The pump, syringes, and extension sets were kept at 21°C while the filters and epidural catheters were kept at 36°C. Running at 1 mL/hr, the delivered sufentanil concentration using PVC tubing was about 7 to 10% below the theoretical concentration throughout 24 hours. Using polyethylene tubing, losses were about 16% initially but the concentration returned to expected levels within 1 to 2 hours and remained stable throughout the 24-hour delivery.[2201]

Filtration

Sufentanil citrate (Janssen) 50 mcg/10 mL in sodium chloride 0.9% was evaluated for drug loss when administered through filters or epidural catheters; 2.5-g cellulose acetate/cellulose nitrate 0.2-μm filters (Millex, Millipore) were utilized. Approximately 20% of the sufentanil was lost to the void volume and/or adsorption. This loss should be considered when a new filter is used.[1667]

Sufentanil citrate (Janssen) 2 mcg/mL in sodium chloride 0.9% delivered at 1 mL/hr through 0.2-μm epidural filters (Sterifix, B. Braun) during the first hour was 83% of the theoretical concentration and remained at reduced concentrations of 85 to 89% of theoretical through at least 6 hours. By 24 hours the concentration was near 96% of theoretical. The authors attributed the lower concentrations to sorption of sufentanil onto the filter.[2201]

In addition, sufentanil citrate (Janssen) demonstrated varying amounts of loss from solutions in concentrations ranging from 1 to 20 mcg/mL due to sorption to several filters including Millex-OR, Minisart NML, Schleicher & Schuell FP 30/3, and Sterifix EF.[790]

Sufentanil citrate was found to undergo sorption to 0.22-μm polyamide epidural filters (Perifix, Braun Melsungen). Delivery of a 5-mcg/mL solution through the filter resulted in nearly total loss of the drug from the first mL. 3 mL had to be passed through the filter before the delivered drug concentration was near the original concentration.[2545]

DOI: 10.37573/9781585286850.363

Compatibility Information

Solution Compatibility

Sufentanil citrate

Test Soln Name	Mfr	Mfr	Conc/L or %	Remarks	Ref	C/I
Dextrose 5%	a	JN	5 mg	10% loss in 30 days at 32°C and little loss in 30 days at 4°C	1756	C
Dextrose 5%	HOS[d]	AKN, BA	5 mg	No loss in 24 hr	2660, 2792	C
Sodium chloride 0.9%	a	JN	20 mg	10 and 18% losses in 24 hr at 26 and 37°C, respectively, due to sorption. 5% loss in 10 days at 5°C	1751	I
Sodium chloride 0.9%	a	JN	5 mg	13% loss in 2 days at 32°C due to sorption. Little loss in 25 days at 4°C. Precipitate in 6 days	1755	I
Sodium chloride 0.9%	FRE[b]	JN	5 mg	No loss in 21 days at 4 and 32°C	1755	C
Sodium chloride 0.9%	c	JN	5 mg	No loss in 21 days at 4 and 32°C	1755	C
Sodium chloride 0.9%	a	JN	5 mg	Visually compatible. 11% loss in 48 hr at 32°C. 5% loss in 48 hr when buffered to pH 4.6	2042	C
Sodium chloride 0.9%	AB	AB	1 mg	Visually compatible with little drug loss in 23 days at 4°C and in 3 days at 21°C	2550	C

[a] Tested in PVC/Kalex 3000 (phthalate ester) CADD pump reservoirs.

[b] Tested in glass containers.

[c] Tested in high-density polyethylene containers.

[d] Tested in VISIV polyolefin containers.

Additive Compatibility

Sufentanil citrate

Test Drug	Mfr	Conc/L or %	Mfr	Conc/L or %	Test Solution	Remarks	Ref	C/I
Bupivacaine HCl		3 g	JN	20 mg	NS[a]	5% sufentanil loss and no bupivacaine loss in 10 days at 5, 26, and 37°C	1751	C
Bupivacaine HCl	AST	2 g	JN	5 mg	NS[a]	9% sufentanil loss and 5% bupivacaine loss in 30 days at 32°C. No loss of either drug in 30 days at 4°C	1756	C
Bupivacaine HCl	AST	2 g	JN	5 mg	NS[a]	Buffered with pH 4.6 citrate buffer. Visually compatible with no loss of either drug in 48 hr at 32°C	2042	C
Bupivacaine HCl	AST	40 mg	JN	12 mg	NS[b]	Visually compatible with no loss of either drug in 43 days at 4 and 25°C	2455	C
Ropivacaine HCl	ASZ	1 g	JN	0.4 mg	NS[c]	Physically compatible. No loss of either drug in 30 days at 30°C in the dark	2433	C
Ropivacaine HCl	ASZ	2 g	JN	0.4 and 4 mg	c	Physically compatible. No loss of either drug in 30 days at 30°C in the dark	2433	C
Ropivacaine HCl	ASZ	2 mg	JC	0.5, 0.75, 1 mg	NS[d e]	Physically compatible with no major sufentanil loss in 96 hr at 25°C. Ropivacaine not tested	2506	C

Additive Compatibility (Cont.)

Test Drug	Mfr	Conc/L or %	Mfr	Conc/L or %	Test Solution	Remarks	Ref	C/I
Ziconotide acetate	ELN	25 mg[f]	BB	1 g[g]		10% ziconotide loss in 33 days. No sufentanil loss in 40 days at 37°C	2772	C

[a] Tested in PVC/Kalex 3000 (phthalate ester) CADD pump reservoirs.

[b] Tested in PVC containers.

[c] Tested in polypropylene bags (Mark II Polybags).

[d] Tested in glass containers.

[e] Tested in PVC containers.

[f] Tested in SynchroMed II implantable pumps.

[g] Drug powder dissolved in ziconotide acetate injection.

Drugs in Syringe Compatibility

Sufentanil citrate

Test Drug	Mfr	Amt	Mfr	Amt	Remarks	Ref	C/I
Atracurium besylate	BW	10 mg/mL		50 mcg/mL	Physically compatible and atracurium stable for 24 hr at 5 and 30°C	1694	C

Y-Site Injection Compatibility (1:1 Mixture)

Sufentanil citrate

Test Drug	Mfr	Conc	Mfr	Conc	Remarks	Ref	C/I
Acetaminophen	CAD	10 mg/mL	BA, HOS	50 mcg/mL	Physically compatible with less than 10% acetaminophen loss over 4 hr at room temperature	2841, 2844	C
Bivalirudin	TMC	5 mg/mL[a]	ES	50 mcg/mL	Physically compatible for 4 hr at 23°C	2373	C
Cangrelor tetrasodium	TMC	1 mg/mL[b]		12.5 mcg/mL[b]	Physically compatible for 4 hr	3243	C
Cefepime HCl	BMS	120 mg/mL[c]		5 mcg/mL	Physically compatible with less than 10% cefepime loss. Sufentanil not tested	2513	C
Ceftazidime	SKB	125 mg/mL		50 mcg/mL	Visually compatible with less than 10% loss of ceftazidime in 24 hr. Sufentanil not tested	2434	C
Ceftazidime	GSK	120 mg/mL[c]		5 mcg/mL	Physically compatible with less than 10% ceftazidime loss. Sufentanil not tested	2513	C
Cisatracurium besylate	GW	0.1, 2, 5 mg/mL[a]	ES	0.0125 mg/mL[a]	Physically compatible for 4 hr at 23°C	2074	C
Cloxacillin sodium	SMX	100 mg/mL	SZ	50 mcg/mL	Physically compatible for up to 4 hr at room temperature	3245	C
Dexmedetomidine HCl	AB	4 mcg/mL[b]	AB	50 mcg/mL	Physically compatible for 4 hr at 23°C	2383	C
Etomidate	AB	2 mg/mL	JN	0.05 mg/mL	Visually compatible for 7 days at 25°C	1801	C
Fenoldopam mesylate	AB	80 mcg/mL[b]	BA	12.5 mcg/mL[b]	Physically compatible for 4 hr at 23°C	2467	C

Y-Site Injection Compatibility (1:1 Mixture) (Cont.)

Test Drug	Mfr	Conc	Mfr	Conc	Remarks	Ref	C/I
Hetastarch in lactated electrolyte	AB	6%	BA	12.5 mcg/mL[a]	Physically compatible for 4 hr at 23°C	2339	C
Linezolid	PHU	2 mg/mL	ES	0.05 mg/mL	Physically compatible for 4 hr at 23°C	2264	C
Meropenem		50 mg/mL	SZ	50 mcg/mL	Physically compatible for 4 hr at room temperature	3538	C
Palonosetron HCl	MGI	50 mcg/mL	HOS	12.5 mcg/mL[a]	Physically compatible. No loss of either drug in 4 hr	2720	C
Propofol	ZEN[d]	10 mg/mL	JN	0.05 mg/mL	Physically compatible for 1 hr at 23°C	2066	C
Remifentanil HCl	GW	0.025 and 0.25 mg/mL[b]	ES	0.0125 mg/mL[a]	Physically compatible for 4 hr at 23°C	2075	C

[a] Tested in dextrose 5%.

[b] Tested in sodium chloride 0.9%.

[c] Tested in sterile water for injection.

[d] Test performed using the formulation WITH edetate disodium.

Selected Revisions May 1, 2020. © Copyright, October 1996.
American Society of Health-System Pharmacists, Inc.

Sugammadex Sodium
AHFS 92:12

Products

Sugammadex is available as a 100-mg/mL solution in 2- and 5-mL single-use vials as the sodium salt.[3111] The solution also contains hydrochloric acid and/or sodium hydroxide for pH adjustment.[3111]

pH

The pH is adjusted to a range of 7 to 8.[3111]

Osmolality

The osmolality of sugammadex sodium 100-mg/mL solution is within the range of 300 to 500 mOsm/kg.[3111]

Trade Name(s)

Bridion

Administration

Sugammadex should be administered intravenously as a single bolus injection over 10 seconds into an existing intravenous line.[3111] The intravenous line should be adequately flushed with a compatible infusion solution (e.g., sodium chloride 0.9%) prior to and following administration of sugammadex.[3111]

Stability

Sugammadex injection is a clear, colorless to slightly yellow-brown solution.[3111] Intact vials of the drug should be stored at controlled room temperature and protected from light.[3111] Vials not protected from light should be used within 5 days.[3111]

Compatibility Information

Solution Compatibility

Sugammadex sodium

Test Soln Name	Mfr	Mfr	Conc/L or %	Remarks	Ref	C/I
Dextrose 2.5% in sodium chloride 0.45%		ME	10 g	Physically compatible and chemically stable for 48 hr at 5 and 25°C	3115	C
Dextrose 5% in sodium chloride 0.9%		ME	10 g	Physically compatible and chemically stable for 48 hr at 5 and 25°C	3115	C
Dextrose 5%		ME	10 g	Physically compatible and chemically stable for 48 hr at 5 and 25°C	3115	C
Isolyte P in dextrose 5%		ME	10 g	Physically compatible and chemically stable for 48 hr at 5 and 25°C	3115	C
Ringer's injection		ME	10 g	Physically compatible and chemically stable for 48 hr at 5 and 25°C	3115	C
Ringer's injection, lactated		ME	10 g	Physically compatible and chemically stable for 48 hr at 5 and 25°C	3115	C
Sodium chloride 0.9%		ME	10 g	Physically compatible and chemically stable for 48 hr at 5 and 25°C	3115	C

Y-Site Injection Compatibility (1:1 Mixture)

Sugammadex sodium

Test Drug	Mfr	Conc	Mfr	Conc	Remarks	Ref	C/I
Amiodarone[a]		50 mg/mL		100 mg/mL	Precipitates immediately	3112	I
Dobutamine[a]		12.5 mg/mL		100 mg/mL	Precipitates immediately	3112	I
Ondansetron HCl		2 mg/mL	ME	100 mg/mL	Particles form in 1 hr	3111, 3115	I
Protamine sulfate	LI	50 mcg/mL[b]	ME	100 mcg/mL[b]	Precipitates immediately	3113	I

DOI: 10.37573/9781585286850.364

Y-Site Injection Compatibility (1:1 Mixture) (Cont.)

Test Drug	Mfr	Conc	Mfr	Conc	Remarks	Ref	C/I
Ranitidine HCl		25 mg/mL	ME	100 mg/mL	Particles form in 1 hr	3111, 3115	I
Verapamil HCl		2.5 mg/mL	ME	100 mg/mL	Particles form in 2 hr	3111, 3115	I

ª Salt not specified.

ᵇ Tested in sodium chloride 0.9%.

Selected Revisions June 14, 2016. © Copyright, June 2016.
American Society of Health-System Pharmacists, Inc.

Sumatriptan Succinate
AHFS 28:32.28

Products

Sumatriptan succinate is available at a concentration of 6 mg/0.5 mL with sodium chloride 3.5 mg/0.5 mL in water for injection in single-dose vials and prefilled syringes. The drug is also available at a concentration of 4 mg/0.5 mL with sodium chloride 3.8 mg/0.5 mL in water for injection in prefilled syringes.[1(11/06)]

pH

Approximately 4.2 to 5.3.[1(11/06)]

Osmolality

The solution is nearly isotonic with an osmolality of 291 mOsm/kg.[1(11/06)]

Trade Name(s)

Imitrex

Administration

Sumatriptan succinate is administered subcutaneously. It should not be given by other routes of administration.[1(11/06)]

Selected Revisions October 1, 2012. © Copyright, October 2002. American Society of Health-System Pharmacists, Inc.

Stability

Intact containers of sumatriptan succinate should be stored between 2 and 30°C and protected from light. The injection is a clear, colorless to light yellow solution.[1(11/06)]

Syringes

The stability of sumatriptan succinate (Glaxo Wellcome) 12 mg/mL packaged as 1 mL of solution drawn into 1-mL polypropylene tuberculin syringes was evaluated stored under refrigeration and at room temperature of 25°C both exposed to and protected from fluorescent light. The room temperature samples were evaluated over 24 hours while the refrigerated samples were evaluated over 72 hours. No visible indications of physical instability were observed, and no loss of sumatriptan was found.[2276]

DOI: 10.37573/9781585286850.365

Tacrolimus
AHFS 92:44

Products

Tacrolimus concentrate for injection is available in 1-mL ampuls containing the equivalent of 5 mg of anhydrous tacrolimus per mL.[3127] In addition to tacrolimus, each mL contains polyoxyl 60 hydrogenated castor oil (surfactant) 200 mg and dehydrated alcohol, USP, 80% (v/v).[1683 3127] The product is a concentrate that must be diluted in sodium chloride 0.9% or dextrose 5% prior to administration.[3127]

Trade Name(s)

Prograf

Administration

Tacrolimus is administered only by continuous intravenous infusion following dilution to a final concentration of 0.004 to 0.02 mg/mL (4 to 20 mcg/mL) in sodium chloride 0.9% or dextrose 5%.[3127] Intravenous solution containers should be composed of glass or polyethylene; polyvinyl chloride (PVC) containers should be avoided due to potential leaching of diethylhexyl phthalate (DEHP) plasticizer and decreased stability of the drug.[3127] For more dilute solutions of tacrolimus, non-PVC tubing also should be used to minimize the potential for significant drug adsorption onto the tubing.[3127]

Stability

Intact ampuls should be stored at temperatures between 5 and 25°C.[3127] Diluted solutions for infusion in glass or polyethylene containers should be discarded after 24 hours.[3127] Solutions should be visually inspected for particulate matter and discoloration prior to administration.[3127]

Tacrolimus exhibits a minimum rate of decomposition at pH values between 2 and 6; the rate of decomposition increases substantially at higher pH values[1926] and is unstable above pH 9.[2216] The manufacturer recommends that tacrolimus not be mixed with or even co-infused with solutions having a pH of 9 or greater (e.g., solutions containing acyclovir or ganciclovir).[3127]

Syringes

Tacrolimus (Fujisawa) 100 mcg/mL in sodium chloride 0.9% was packaged as 20 mL in 30-mL plastic syringes (Becton Dickinson) and stored at 24°C exposed to normal room light and protected from light. No decrease in tacrolimus concentration was found after storage for 24 hours.[1864]

Sorption

Tacrolimus (Fujisawa) 100 mcg/mL in dextrose 5% was delivered through PVC anesthesia extension tubing (Abbott), PVC intravenous administration set tubing (Venoset, Abbott), and fat emulsion tubing (Abbott). The delivered solutions had no loss of tacrolimus using the PVC administration set tubing and the fat emulsion tubing and only 2.5% drug loss from the PVC anesthesia extension tubing.[1864]

Tacrolimus 50 mcg/mL delivered through 100 cm of PVC tubing at a rate of 5 mL/hr resulted in the delivery of 76% of the tacrolimus concentration. No loss due to sorption occurred when the tacrolimus solution was delivered through polyolefin tubing.[2452]

Plasticizer Leaching

Parenteral products containing a large amount of surfactant in the formulation, such as tacrolimus injection, will extract the plasticizer DEHP from PVC containers and administration sets.[1683 3127] Consequently, use of PVC containers with tacrolimus should be avoided.[3127] Instead, glass or polyethylene containers and PVC-free tubing are recommended.[1683 3127]

Tacrolimus 50 mcg/mL delivered through 100 cm of PVC tubing at a rate of 5 mL/hr leached 12 mcg/mL of DEHP into the drug solution. No plasticizer leached when the tacrolimus solution was delivered through similar polyolefin tubing.[2452]

Tacrolimus 0.02 mg/mL in dextrose 5% in VISIV polyolefin bags was tested at room temperature near 23°C for 24 hours. No leached plastic components were found within the 24-hour study period.[2660 2792]

Compatibility Information

Solution Compatibility

Tacrolimus

Test Soln Name	Mfr	Mfr	Conc/L or %	Remarks	Ref	C/I
Dextrose 5%	f	ASP	4 to 20 mg	Stable for 24 hr	3127	C
Dextrose 5%	AB[a]	FUJ	100 mg	5 to 8% loss in 48 hr at 24°C	1864	C
Dextrose 5%	AB[b]	FUJ	100 mg	15% loss in 6 hr and 19% loss in 24 hr at 24°C	1864	I
Dextrose 5%	BRN[e]	ASP	10 mg	Physically compatible. No loss in 20 hr at 2 to 8°C followed by 28 hr at 20 to 25°C	3128	C

DOI: 10.37573/9781585286850.366

Solution Compatibility (Cont.)

Test Soln Name	Mfr	Mfr	Conc/L or %	Remarks	Ref	C/I
Dextrose 5%	BRN[e]	ASP	1, 10, 100 mg	Physically compatible. Little to no loss in 48 hr at 20 to 25°C	3128	C
Sodium chloride 0.9%	[f]	ASP	4 to 20 mg	Stable for 24 hr	3127	C
Sodium chloride 0.9%	BA[c]	FUJ	10 mg	Visually compatible with 4% loss in 48 hr	1854	C
Sodium chloride 0.9%	AB[c]	FUJ	100 mg	10 to 12% loss in 24 hr at 24°C	1864	C
Sodium chloride 0.9%	AB[b]	FUJ	100 mg	12% loss in 6 hr and 16% loss in 24 hr at 24°C	1864	I
Sodium chloride 0.9%	BRN[e]	ASP	1 mg	Physically compatible. 6% loss in 24 hr at 20 to 25°C	3128, 3129	C
Sodium chloride 0.9%	BRN[e]	ASP	10 mg	Physically compatible. Little to no loss in 20 hr at 2 to 8°C followed by 28 hr at 20 to 25°C	3128	C
Sodium chloride 0.9%	BRN[e]	ASP	10 and 100 mg	Physically compatible. No loss in 48 hr at 20 to 25°C	3128	C
Sodium chloride 0.9%	BRN[g]	ASP	2, 4, and 8 mg	Physically compatible. Less than 10% loss in 9 days at 23°C in light and 4°C in dark	3277	C
TPN #201[d]	[c]	FUJ	100 mg	Visually compatible with no loss in 24 hr at 24°C	1922	C

[a] Tested in glass and polyolefin containers.

[b] Tested in PVC containers.

[c] Tested in glass containers.

[d] Refer to Appendix for the composition of parenteral nutrition solutions. TPN indicates a 2-in-1 admixture.

[e] Tested in polyolefin containers.

[f] Tested in glass and polyethylene containers.

[g] Tested in Excel non-DEHP non-PVC containers.

Y-Site Injection Compatibility (1:1 Mixture)

Tacrolimus

Test Drug	Mfr	Conc	Mfr	Conc	Remarks	Ref	C/I
Acyclovir sodium			FUJ		Significant tacrolimus loss within 15 min	191	I
Aminophylline	ES	2 mg/mL[a]	FUJ	1 mg/mL[b]	Visually compatible for 24 hr at 25°C	1630	C
Amphotericin B	LY	5 mg/mL[a]	FUJ	1 mg/mL[c]	Visually compatible for 24 hr at 25°C	1630	C
Ampicillin sodium	WY	20 mg/mL[a]	FUJ	1 mg/mL[b]	Visually compatible for 24 hr at 25°C	1630	C
Ampicillin sodium–sulbactam sodium	RR	33.3 mg/mL[a e]	FUJ	1 mg/mL[b]	Visually compatible for 24 hr at 25°C	1630	C
Anidulafungin	VIC	0.5 mg/mL[a]	FUJ	20 mcg/mL[a]	Physically compatible for 4 hr at 23°C	2617	C
Benztropine mesylate	MSD	1 mg/mL[a]	FUJ	1 mg/mL[b]	Visually compatible for 24 hr at 25°C	1630	C
Calcium gluconate	ES	100 mg/mL	FUJ	1 mg/mL[b]	Visually compatible for 24 hr at 25°C	1630	C
Caspofungin acetate	ME	0.7 mg/mL[b]	AST	0.02 mg/mL[b]	Physically compatible for 4 hr at room temperature	2758	C
Cefazolin sodium	BR	40 mg/mL[a]	FUJ	1 mg/mL[b]	Visually compatible for 24 hr at 25°C	1630	C
Cefotetan disodium	STU	40 mg/mL[a]	FUJ	1 mg/mL[b]	Visually compatible for 24 hr at 25°C	1630	C
Ceftazidime	GL	20 mg/mL[a]	FUJ	1 mg/mL[b]	Visually compatible for 24 hr at 25°C	1630	C
Ceftazidime	GW	40 and 200 mg/mL[a]	FUJ	10 and 40 mcg/mL[a]	Visually compatible with no loss of either drug in 4 hr at 24°C	2216	C

Y-Site Injection Compatibility (1:1 Mixture) (Cont.)

Test Drug	Mfr	Conc	Mfr	Conc	Remarks	Ref	C/I
Ceftolozane sulfate–tazobactam sodium	CUB	10 mg/mL[h i]	ASP	0.02 mg/mL[h]	Physically compatible for 2 hr	3262	C
Ceftriaxone sodium	RC	40 mg/mL[a]	FUJ	1 mg/mL[b]	Visually compatible for 24 hr at 25°C	1630	C
Cefuroxime sodium	LI	30 mg/mL[a]	FUJ	1 mg/mL[b]	Visually compatible for 24 hr at 25°C	1630	C
Chloramphenicol sodium succinate	PD	20 mg/mL[a]	FUJ	1 mg/mL[b]	Visually compatible for 24 hr at 25°C	1630	C
Ciprofloxacin	MI	1 mg/mL[a]	FUJ	1 mg/mL[b]	Visually compatible for 24 hr at 25°C	1630	C
Clindamycin phosphate	ES	12 mg/mL[a]	FUJ	1 mg/mL[b]	Visually compatible for 24 hr at 25°C	1630	C
Dexamethasone sodium phosphate	ES	4 mg/mL[a]	FUJ	1 mg/mL[b]	Visually compatible for 24 hr at 25°C	1630	C
Digoxin	WY	0.25 mg/mL	FUJ	1 mg/mL[b]	Visually compatible for 24 hr at 25°C	1630	C
Diphenhydramine HCl	ES	1 mg/mL[a]	FUJ	1 mg/mL[b]	Visually compatible for 24 hr at 25°C	1630	C
Dobutamine HCl	LI	1 mg/mL[a]	FUJ	1 mg/mL[b]	Visually compatible for 24 hr at 25°C	1630	C
Dopamine HCl	ES	1.6 mg/mL[a]	FUJ	1 mg/mL[b]	Visually compatible for 24 hr at 25°C	1630	C
Doripenem	JJ	5 mg/mL[a b]	ASP	0.02 mg/mL[a b]	Physically compatible for 4 hr at 23°C	2743	C
Doxycycline hyclate	RR	5 mg/mL[a]	FUJ	1 mg/mL[b]	Visually compatible for 24 hr at 25°C	1630	C
Erythromycin lactobionate	AB	20 mg/mL[a]	FUJ	1 mg/mL[b]	Visually compatible for 24 hr at 25°C	1630	C
Esmolol HCl	DU	10 mg/mL[a]	FUJ	1 mg/mL[b]	Visually compatible for 24 hr at 25°C	1630	C
Fluconazole	RR	2 mg/mL[a]	FUJ	1 mg/mL[b]	Visually compatible for 24 hr at 25°C	1630	C
Fluconazole	PF	0.5 and 1.5 mg/mL[b]	FUJ	5 and 20 mcg/mL[b]	Visually compatible. No loss of either drug in 3 hr at 24°C	2236	C
Furosemide	ES	10 mg/mL	FUJ	1 mg/mL[b]	Visually compatible for 24 hr at 25°C	1630	C
Ganciclovir sodium			FUJ		Significant tacrolimus loss within 15 min	191	I
Gentamicin sulfate	SCN	4 mg/mL[a]	FUJ	1 mg/mL[b]	Visually compatible for 24 hr at 25°C	1630	C
Haloperidol lactate	SO	2.5 mg/mL[a]	FUJ	1 mg/mL[b]	Visually compatible for 24 hr at 25°C	1630	C
Heparin sodium	ES	10 units/mL[a]	FUJ	1 mg/mL[b]	Visually compatible for 24 hr at 25°C	1630	C
Hydrocortisone sodium succinate	AB	50 mg/mL[a]	FUJ	1 mg/mL[b]	Visually compatible for 24 hr at 25°C	1630	C
Hydromorphone HCl	KN	2 and 0.2 mg/mL[a]	FUJ	10 and 40 mcg/mL[a]	Visually compatible. No loss of either drug in 4 hr at 24°C	2216	C
Imipenem–cilastatin sodium	MSD	10 mg/mL[b g]	FUJ	1 mg/mL[b]	Visually compatible for 24 hr at 25°C	1630	C
Insulin, regular	LI	0.1 unit/mL[a]	FUJ	1 mg/mL[b]	Visually compatible for 24 hr at 25°C	1630	C
Isavuconazonium sulfate	ASP	1.5 mg/mL[h]	ASP	0.02 mg/mL[h]	Physically compatible for 2 hr	3263	C
Isoproterenol HCl	ES	0.04 mg/mL[a]	FUJ	1 mg/mL[b]	Visually compatible for 24 hr at 25°C	1630	C
Letermovir	ME	[a]		[a]	Physically compatible	3398	C
Leucovorin calcium	ES	10 mg/mL[a]	FUJ	1 mg/mL[b]	Visually compatible for 24 hr at 25°C	1630	C
Lorazepam	WY	1 mg/mL[a]	FUJ	1 mg/mL[b]	Visually compatible for 24 hr at 25°C	1630	C

Y-Site Injection Compatibility (1:1 Mixture) (Cont.)

Test Drug	Mfr	Conc	Mfr	Conc	Remarks	Ref	C/I
Methylprednisolone sodium succinate	UP	0.8 mg/mL[a]	FUJ	1 mg/mL[b]	Visually compatible for 24 hr at 25°C	1630	C
Metoclopramide HCl	DU	0.2 mg/mL[a]	FUJ	1 mg/mL[b]	Visually compatible for 24 hr at 25°C	1630	C
Metronidazole	AB	5 mg/mL	FUJ	1 mg/mL[b]	Visually compatible for 24 hr at 25°C	1630	C
Micafungin sodium	ASP	1.5 mg/mL[b]	FUJ	20 mcg/mL[b]	Physically compatible for 4 hr at 23°C	2683	C
Morphine sulfate	SCN	1 and 3 mg/mL[b]	FUJ	10 and 40 mcg/mL[b]	Visually compatible. No loss of either drug in 4 hr at 24°C	2216	C
Multivitamins	LY	0.001 mL/mL[a]	FUJ	1 mg/mL[b]	Visually compatible for 24 hr at 25°C	1630	C
Mycophenolate mofetil HCl	RC	5.9 mg/mL[a]	FUJ	0.02 mg/mL[a]	Physically compatible and 2% mycophenolate mofetil loss in 4 hr	2738	C
Nitroglycerin	DU	0.1 mg/mL[a]	FUJ	1 mg/mL[b]	Visually compatible for 24 hr at 25°C	1630	C
Oxacillin sodium	BR	40 mg/mL[a]	FUJ	1 mg/mL[b]	Visually compatible for 24 hr at 25°C	1630	C
Penicillin G potassium	BR	100,000 units/mL[a]	FUJ	1 mg/mL[b]	Visually compatible for 24 hr at 25°C	1630	C
Phenytoin sodium	ES	5 mg/mL[a]	FUJ	1 mg/mL[b]	Visually compatible for 4 hr at 25°C. White haze forms by 24 hr	1630	C
Potassium chloride	AB	2 mEq/mL	FUJ	1 mg/mL[b]	Visually compatible for 24 hr at 25°C	1630	C
Propranolol HCl	AY	1 mg/mL	FUJ	1 mg/mL[b]	Visually compatible for 24 hr at 25°C	1630	C
Ranitidine HCl	GL	25 mg/mL	FUJ	1 mg/mL[b]	Visually compatible for 24 hr at 25°C	1630	C
Sodium bicarbonate	AB	1 mEq/mL	FUJ	1 mg/mL[b]	Visually compatible for 24 hr at 25°C	1630	C
Sodium nitroprusside	ES	0.004 mg/mL[a]	FUJ	1 mg/mL[b]	Visually compatible for 24 hr at 25°C	1630	C
Tedizolid phosphate	CUB	0.8 mg/mL[b]	ASP	0.02 mg/mL[b]	Physically compatible for 2 hr	3244	C
TNA #218 to #226[d]			FUJ	1 mg/mL[a]	Visually compatible for 4 hr at 23°C	2215	C
Tobramycin sulfate	BR	40 mg/mL	FUJ	1 mg/mL[b]	Visually compatible for 24 hr at 25°C	1630	C
TPN #212 to #215[d]			FUJ	1 mg/mL[a]	Physically compatible for 4 hr at 23°C	2109	C
Trimethoprim–sulfamethoxazole	RC	1.6 mg/mL[a f]	FUJ	1 mg/mL[b]	Visually compatible for 24 hr at 25°C	1630	C
Vancomycin HCl	LI	5 mg/mL[a]	FUJ	1 mg/mL[b]	Visually compatible for 24 hr at 25°C	1630	C

[a] Tested in dextrose 5%.

[b] Tested in sodium chloride 0.9%.

[c] Diluted with sterile water for injection.

[d] Refer to Appendix for the composition of parenteral nutrition solutions. TNA indicates a 3-in-1 admixture, and TPN indicates a 2-in-1 admixture.

[e] Ampicillin component. Ampicillin in a 2:1 fixed-ratio concentration with sulbactam.

[f] Trimethoprim component. Trimethoprim in a 1:5 fixed-ratio concentration with sulfamethoxazole.

[g] Not specified whether concentration refers to single component or combined components.

[h] Tested in both dextrose 5% and sodium chloride 0.9%.

[i] Ceftolozane component. Ceftolozane in a 2:1 fixed-ratio concentration with tazobactam.

Selected Revisions June 20, 2018. © Copyright, October 1996.
American Society of Health-System Pharmacists, Inc.

Tedizolid Phosphate
AHFS 8:12.28.24

Products

Tedizolid phosphate is a prodrug that is metabolized in vivo to tedizolid.[2913] Tedizolid phosphate is available as a lyophilized powder or cake in single-use (unpreserved) vials containing 200 mg of the drug and mannitol 105 mg.[2913] Sodium hydroxide and hydrochloric acid also are present in minimal quantities to adjust the pH.[2913]

Reconstitute the 200-mg vial with 4 mL of sterile water for injection.[2913] Gently swirl the vial to aid dissolution and let stand until the cake has completely dissolved and any foam has disappeared.[2913] To minimize foaming, avoid vigorous agitation or shaking during and after reconstitution.[2913] Inspect the vial to ensure that the solution contains no particulate matter and that no undissolved cake or powder remains attached to the vial wall; if undissolved drug remains, invert the vial and gently swirl to dissolve the remainder.[2913]

Do not invert the vial during withdrawal of the dose; instead, keeping the vial in the upright position, use a syringe with an appropriately sized needle to withdraw 4 mL of the reconstituted solution from the bottom corner of the tilted vial.[2913] Dilute the reconstituted solution only in 250 mL of sodium chloride 0.9%.[2913] Invert the bag gently to mix; do not shake because foaming may occur.[2913]

Trade Name(s)

Sivextro

Administration

Tedizolid phosphate is administered by intravenous infusion over 1 hour after dilution of the reconstituted solution in 250 mL of sodium chloride 0.9%.[2913] If a common infusion line is being used to administer other drugs, the line should be flushed with sodium chloride 0.9% prior to and following infusion of tedizolid phosphate.[2913] Tedizolid is incompatible with any solutions that contain divalent cations (e.g., calcium, magnesium).[2913]

Stability

Intact vials of tedizolid phosphate should be stored at controlled room temperature.[2913] Tedizolid phosphate is a white to off-white powder that forms a clear, colorless to pale yellow solution when reconstituted with sterile water for injection and when further diluted in sodium chloride 0.9%.[2913] The manufacturer states that the reconstituted drug and the diluted solution may be stored under refrigeration or at room temperature.[2913] The total time from reconstitution to dilution to administration should not exceed 24 hours.[2913]

Filtration

Tedizolid phosphate (Cubist) was filtered through a 0.22-μm inline filter.[2914] No significant loss in potency or changes in appearance or impurity levels were observed.[2914]

Compatibility Information

Solution Compatibility

Tedizolid phosphate

Test Soln Name	Mfr	Mfr	Conc/L or %	Remarks	Ref	C/I
Dextrose 5% in Ringer's injection		CUB		Must not be mixed with calcium-containing solutions	2913	I
Dextrose 5% in Ringer's injection, lactated		CUB		Must not be mixed with calcium-containing solutions	2913	I
Dextrose 5%	BA	CUB	200 mg	Stable up to 26 hours at room temperature	2914	?
Dextrose 5%	BRN	CUB	200 mg	Stable up to 26 hours at room temperature	2914	?
Dextrose 5%	BA	CUB	1.6 g	Increase in particulates over 26 hours at room temperature	2914	?
Dextrose 5%	BRN	CUB	1.6 g	Increase in particulates over 26 hours at room temperature	2914	?
Ringer's injection		CUB		Must not be mixed with calcium-containing solutions	2913	I
Ringer's injection, lactated		CUB		Must not be mixed with calcium-containing solutions	2913	I
Sodium chloride 0.9%		CUB	800 mg	Stated to be stable up to 24 hours at room temperature or at 2 to 8°C	2913	C

DOI: 10.37573/9781585286850.367

Y-Site Injection Compatibility (1:1 Mixture)

Tedizolid phosphate

Test Drug	Mfr	Conc	Mfr	Conc	Remarks	Ref	C/I
Albumin human	CBH	250 mg/mL	CUB	0.8 mg/mL[b]	Measured turbidity increases immediately	3244	I
Amikacin sulfate	HER	5 mg/mL[b]	CUB	0.8 mg/mL[b]	Physically compatible for 2 hr	3244	C
Amiodarone HCl	APP	2 mg/mL[b]	CUB	0.8 mg/mL[b]	Physically compatible for 2 hr	3244	C
Ampicillin sodium–sulbactam sodium	FRK	20 mg/mL[b c]	CUB	0.8 mg/mL[b]	Physically compatible for 2 hr	3244	C
Anidulafungin	PF	0.77 mg/mL[b]	CUB	0.8 mg/mL[b]	Physically compatible for 2 hr	3244	C
Azithromycin	APP	2 mg/mL[b]	CUB	0.8 mg/mL[b]	Physically compatible for 2 hr	3244	C
Aztreonam	APP	20 mg/mL[b]	CUB	0.8 mg/mL[b]	Physically compatible for 2 hr	3244	C
Bumetanide	HOS	0.25 mg/mL	CUB	0.8 mg/mL[b]	Physically compatible for 2 hr	3244	C
Calcium chloride	HOS	20 mg/mL[b]	CUB	0.8 mg/mL[b]	Immediate precipitation and increase in measured turbidity	3244	I
Calcium gluconate	APP	20 mg/mL[b]	CUB	0.8 mg/mL[b]	Immediate precipitation and increase in measured turbidity	3244	I
Caspofungin acetate	ME	0.5 mg/mL[b]	CUB	0.8 mg/mL[b]	Immediate precipitation and increase in measured turbidity	3244	I
Cefazolin sodium	APO	20 mg/mL[b]	CUB	0.8 mg/mL[b]	Physically compatible for 2 hr	3244	C
Cefepime HCl	SGT	40 mg/mL[b]	CUB	0.8 mg/mL[b]	Physically compatible for 2 hr	3244	C
Ceftaroline fosamil	FOR	12 mg/mL[b]	CUB	0.8 mg/mL[b]	Measured turbidity increases after 15 min	3244	I
Ceftazidime	SZ	40 mg/mL[b]	CUB	0.8 mg/mL[b]	Physically compatible for 2 hr	3244	C
Ceftazidime–avibactam sodium	ALL	20 mg/mL[a l]			Physically compatible for up to 4 hr at room temperature	3004	C
Ceftolozane sulfate–tazobactam sodium	CUB	10 mg/mL[b d]	CUB	0.8 mg/mL[b]	Physically compatible for 2 hr	3244, 3262	C
Ceftriaxone sodium	WOC	20 mg/mL[b]	CUB	0.8 mg/mL[b]	Physically compatible for 2 hr	3244	C
Cefuroxime sodium	COV	30 mg/mL[b]	CUB	0.8 mg/mL[b]	Physically compatible for 2 hr	3244	C
Ciprofloxacin	HOS	2 mg/mL[b]	CUB	0.8 mg/mL[b]	Physically compatible for 2 hr	3244	C
Cisatracurium besylate	ABV	0.4 mg/mL[b]	CUB	0.8 mg/mL[b]	Physically compatible for 2 hr	3244	C
Colistimethate sodium	APP	4.5 mg/mL[b]	CUB	0.8 mg/mL[b]	Physically compatible for 2 hr	3244	C
Cyclosporine	DRX	5 mg/mL[b]	CUB	0.8 mg/mL[b]	Immediate change in measured turbidity	3244	I
Daptomycin	CUB[i]	10 mg/mL[b]	CUB	0.8 mg/mL[b]	Physically compatible for 2 hr	3244	C
Dexamethasone sodium phosphate	FRK	1 mg/mL[b]	CUB	0.8 mg/mL[b]	Physically compatible for 2 hr	3244	C
Dexmedetomidine HCl	HOS	4 mcg/mL[b]	CUB	0.8 mg/mL[b]	Physically compatible for 2 hr	3244	C
Digoxin	SZ	0.25 mg/mL	CUB	0.8 mg/mL[b]	Physically compatible for 2 hr	3244	C
Diltiazem HCl	AKN	5 mg/mL	CUB	0.8 mg/mL[b]	Physically compatible for 2 hr	3244	C
Diphenhydramine HCl	APP	50 mg/mL	CUB	0.8 mg/mL[b]	Measured turbidity increases within 2 hr	3244	I
Dobutamine HCl	HOS	4.1 mg/mL[b]	CUB	0.8 mg/mL[b]	Immediate precipitation and increase in measured turbidity	3244	I
Dopamine HCl	HOS	0.8 mg/mL[b]	CUB	0.8 mg/mL[b]	Physically compatible for 2 hr	3244	C
Doripenem	SHI	5 mg/mL[b]	CUB	0.8 mg/mL[b]	Physically compatible for 2 hr	3244	C
Doxycycline hyclate	PRP	1 mg/mL[b]	CUB	0.8 mg/mL[b]	Measured turbidity increases immediately	3244	I

Y-Site Injection Compatibility (1:1 Mixture) (Cont.)

Test Drug	Mfr	Conc	Mfr	Conc	Remarks	Ref	C/I
Epinephrine[j]	JHP	16 mcg/mL[b]	CUB	0.8 mg/mL[b]	Physically compatible for 2 hr; however, mean pH change >1 unit within 2 hr	3244, 3247	?
Eptifibatide	ME	0.75 mg/mL	CUB	0.8 mg/mL[b]	Physically compatible for 2 hr	3244	C
Ertapenem sodium	ME	20 mg/mL[b]	CUB	0.8 mg/mL[b]	Physically compatible for 2 hr	3244	C
Esmolol HCl	BA	10 mg/mL	CUB	0.8 mg/mL[b]	Measured turbidity increases immediately	3244	I
Esomeprazole sodium	ASZ	0.8 mg/mL[b]	CUB	0.8 mg/mL[b]	Physically compatible for 2 hr	3244	C
Famotidine	WW	4 mg/mL[b]	CUB	0.8 mg/mL[b]	Physically compatible for 2 hr	3244	C
Fentanyl citrate	WW	50 mcg/mL	CUB	0.8 mg/mL[b]	Physically compatible for 2 hr	3244	C
Fosphenytoin sodium	WW	25 mg PE/mL[b h]	CUB	0.8 mg/mL[b]	Physically compatible for 2 hr	3244, 3247	C
Furosemide	HOS	3 mg/mL[b]	CUB	0.8 mg/mL[b]	Physically compatible for 2 hr	3244	C
Gentamicin sulfate	PRP	5 mg/mL[b]	CUB	0.8 mg/mL[b]	Measured turbidity increases immediately	3244	I
Heparin sodium	PRP	1000 units/mL[b]	CUB	0.8 mg/mL[b]	Physically compatible for 2 hr	3244	C
Hydrocortisone sodium succinate	PF	1 mg/mL[b]	CUB	0.8 mg/mL[b]	Physically compatible for 2 hr	3244	C
Hydromorphone HCl	AKN	1 mg/mL[b]	CUB	0.8 mg/mL[b]	Physically compatible for 2 hr	3244	C
Imipenem–cilastatin sodium	PRP	5 mg/mL[b e]	CUB	0.8 mg/mL[b]	Physically compatible for 2 hr	3244	C
Insulin, regular	NVN	1 unit/mL[b]	CUB	0.8 mg/mL[b]	Physically compatible for 2 hr	3244	C
Isavuconazonium sulfate	ASP	1.5 mg/mL[b]	CUB	0.8 mg/mL[b]	Measured turbidity increases within 15 min	3244, 3263	I
Labetalol HCl	HOS	2 mg/mL[b]	CUB	0.8 mg/mL[b]	Physically compatible for 2 hr	3244	C
Levofloxacin	AUR	5 mg/mL[b]	CUB	0.8 mg/mL[b]	Physically compatible for 2 hr	3244	C
Lidocaine HCl	APP	8 mg/mL[b]	CUB	0.8 mg/mL[b]	Physically compatible for 2 hr	3244	C
Lorazepam	WW	1 mg/mL[b]	CUB	0.8 mg/mL[b]	Physically compatible for 2 hr	3244	C
Magnesium sulfate	HOS	100 mg/mL[b]	CUB	0.8 mg/mL[b]	Immediate precipitation and increase in measured turbidity	3244	I
Mannitol	HOS	20%	CUB	0.8 mg/mL[b]	Physically compatible for 2 hr	3244	C
Meperidine HCl	WW	10 mg/mL[b]	CUB	0.8 mg/mL[b]	Physically compatible for 2 hr	3244	C
Meropenem	PRP	10 mg/mL[b]	CUB	0.8 mg/mL[b]	Physically compatible for 2 hr	3244	C
Meropenem–vaborbactam	TMC	8 mg/mL[b k]	ME	0.8 mg/mL[b]	Physically compatible for 3 hr at 20 to 25°C	3380	C
Mesna	PRP	20 mg/mL[b]	CUB	0.8 mg/mL[b]	Physically compatible for 2 hr	3244	C
Methylprednisolone sodium succinate	PF	20 mg/mL[b]	CUB	0.8 mg/mL[b]	Physically compatible for 2 hr	3244	C
Metoclopramide HCl	TE	0.2 mg/mL[b]	CUB	0.8 mg/mL[b]	Physically compatible for 2 hr	3244	C
Metronidazole	BA	5 mg/mL[b]	CUB	0.8 mg/mL[b]	Physically compatible for 2 hr	3244	C
Micafungin sodium	ASP	2 mg/mL[b]	CUB	0.8 mg/mL[b]	Physically compatible for 2 hr	3244	C
Midazolam HCl	APP	1 mg/mL[b]	CUB	0.8 mg/mL[b]	Physically compatible for 2 hr	3244	C
Milrinone lactate	HIK	0.2 mg/mL[b]	CUB	0.8 mg/mL[b]	Physically compatible for 2 hr	3244	C
Morphine sulfate	WW	1 mg/mL[b]	CUB	0.8 mg/mL[b]	Physically compatible for 2 hr	3244	C

Y-Site Injection Compatibility (1:1 Mixture) (Cont.)

Test Drug	Mfr	Conc	Mfr	Conc	Remarks	Ref	C/I
Naloxone HCl	PPR	0.04 mg/mL[b]	CUB	0.8 mg/mL[b]	Physically compatible for 2 hr	3244	C
Nicardipine HCl	BA	0.2 mg/mL[b]	CUB	0.8 mg/mL[b]	Immediate precipitation and increase in measured turbidity	3244	I
Nitroglycerin	BA	0.4 mg/mL[b]	CUB	0.8 mg/mL[b]	Physically compatible for 2 hr	3244	C
Norepinephrine bitartrate	HOS	32 mcg/mL[b]	CUB	0.8 mg/mL[b]	Physically compatible for 2 hr	3244	C
Ondansetron HCl	HOS	0.16 mg/mL[b]	CUB	0.8 mg/mL[b]	Physically compatible for 2 hr	3244	C
Pantoprazole sodium	NVP[f]	0.4 mg/mL[b]	CUB	0.8 mg/mL[b]	Physically compatible for 2 hr	3244, 3247	C
Penicillin G potassium	PF	100,000 units/mL[b]	CUB	0.8 mg/mL[b]	Immediate change in measured turbidity	3244	I
Phenylephrine HCl	SZ	1 mg/mL[b]	CUB	0.8 mg/mL[b]	Physically compatible for 2 hr	3244	C
Phenytoin sodium	WW	10 mg/mL[b]	CUB	0.8 mg/mL[b]	Measured turbidity increases immediately	3244	I
Piperacillin sodium–tazobactam sodium	PRP[f]	40 mg/mL[b g]	CUB	0.8 mg/mL[b]	Physically compatible for 2 hr	3244, 3247	C
Plazomicin sulfate	ACH	24 mg/mL[b]	ME	0.8 mg/mL[b]	Physically compatible for 1 hr at 20 to 25°C	3432	C
Potassium chloride	HOS	0.1 mEq/mL[b]	CUB	0.8 mg/mL[b]	Physically compatible for 2 hr	3244	C
Potassium phosphates	HOS	0.3 mmol/mL[b]	CUB	0.8 mg/mL[b]	Physically compatible for 2 hr	3244	C
Ranitidine HCl	ZY	2.5 mg/mL[b]	CUB	0.8 mg/mL[b]	Physically compatible for 2 hr	3244	C
Rocuronium bromide	PRM	5 mg/mL[b]	CUB	0.8 mg/mL[b]	Physically compatible for 2 hr	3244	C
Sodium bicarbonate	HOS	1 mEq/mL	CUB	0.8 mg/mL[b]	Physically compatible for 2 hr	3244	C
Sodium phosphates	FRE	0.5 mmol/mL[b]	CUB	0.8 mg/mL[b]	Physically compatible for 2 hr	3244	C
Tacrolimus	ASP	0.02 mg/mL[b]	CUB	0.8 mg/mL[b]	Physically compatible for 2 hr	3244	C
Tigecycline	PF	1 mg/mL[b]	CUB	0.8 mg/mL[b]	Physically compatible for 2 hr	3244	C
Tobramycin sulfate	MYL	5 mg/mL[b]	CUB	0.8 mg/mL[b]	Measured turbidity increases immediately	3244	I
Vancomycin HCl	HOS	5 mg/mL[b]	CUB	0.8 mg/mL[b]	Physically compatible for 2 hr	3244	C
Vasopressin	JHP	1 unit/mL[b]	CUB	0.8 mg/mL[b]	Physically compatible for 2 hr	3244	C
Vecuronium bromide	CRC	1 mg/mL	CUB	0.8 mg/mL[b]	Physically compatible for 2 hr	3244	C

[a] Tested in dextrose 5%.

[b] Tested in sodium chloride 0.9%.

[c] Ampicillin component. Ampicillin in a 2:1 fixed-ratio concentration with sulbactam.

[d] Ceftolozane component. Ceftolozane in a 2:1 fixed-ratio concentration with tazobactam.

[e] Imipenem component. Imipenem in a 1:1 fixed-ratio concentration with cilastatin.

[f] Test performed using the formulation WITH edetate disodium.

[g] Piperacillin component. Piperacillin in an 8:1 fixed-ratio concentration with tazobactam.

[h] Concentration of fosphenytoin expressed in milligrams of phenytoin sodium equivalents (PE) per mL.

[i] Test performed using the Cubicin formulation.

[j] As epinephrine base rather than the salt.

[k] Meropenem component. Meropenem in a 1:1 fixed-ratio concentration with vaborbactam.

[l] Ceftazidime component. Ceftazidime in a 4:1 fixed-ratio concentration with avibactam sodium.

Teicoplanin
AHFS 8:12.28.16

Products

Teicoplanin is available as a lyophilized powder in single-use vials containing teicoplanin 100, 200, or 400 mg.[3412 3413 3414 3415 3416] Each vial also contains sodium chloride and sodium hydroxide to adjust the pH.[3412 3413 3414 3415 3416] Some vials of teicoplanin are packaged with an accompanying ampul of water for injection for use as a diluent.[3413 3414 3416]

To prepare teicoplanin for injection or infusion, the 100-mg vials should be reconstituted with 1.7 mL[3415] and most 200- and 400-mg vials should be reconstituted with 3.14 mL of sterile water for injection, either from a separate vial or from the accompanying ampul of diluent, when provided; the diluent should be injected slowly down the side of the vial wall.[3412 3413 3414 3415] Vials should be rolled gently until the powder is completely dissolved and should not be shaken.[3412 3413 3414 3415 3416] Care should be taken to avoid the formation of foam; if foam develops, the solution should be allowed to stand for 15 minutes until it subsides.[3412 3413 3414 3415 3416] The resulting reconstituted solutions contain teicoplanin 100 mg/1.5 mL, 200 mg/3 mL, or 400 mg/3 mL.[3412 3413 3414 3415 3416] Errors in reconstitution can result in the formation of a stable foam and the delivery of doses that are smaller than intended.[3413 3414 3416] Reconstituted teicoplanin solutions should be extracted slowly from the vial using a syringe (e.g., a 5-mL syringe with a 23-gauge needle).[3412 3413 3414 3415 3416]

The reconstituted solution may be administered by direct injection without further dilution or administered as an intravenous infusion after dilution in a compatible infusion solution.[3412 3413 3414 3415 3416] Most manufacturers recommend dilution of the reconstituted solution in sodium chloride 0.9%, Ringer's injection, Ringer's injection, lactated, dextrose 5 or 10%, dextrose 4% in sodium chloride 0.18%, or dextrose 5% in sodium chloride 0.45%.[3412 3413 3414 3415 3416] Some manufacturers also state that teicoplanin can be prepared in compounded sodium lactate solution[3413 3414] and Hartmann's solution.[3416] Specific product labeling should be consulted.

Equivalency

Each milligram of teicoplanin is equivalent to not less than 1000 international units.[3412 3414 3415]

pH

The pH of teicoplanin (Sanofi-Aventis) 133.3-mg/mL reconstituted solution ranges from 7.2 to 7.8.[3414]

Tonicity

Teicoplanin (Sanofi-Aventis) 133.3-mg/mL reconstituted solution is isotonic.[3414]

Trade Name(s)

Targocid

Administration

Teicoplanin may be administered after reconstitution either intramuscularly, with a maximum of 3 mL in a single site, or by direct intravenous injection over 3 to 5 minutes.[3412 3413 3414 3416] The drug also may be administered as an intravenous infusion over 30 minutes after dilution in a compatible infusion solution.[3412 3413 3414 3415 3416] Only intravenous infusion should be used to administer the drug in neonates.[3412 3415]

Teicoplanin should not be administered intraventricularly.[3412 3413 3414 3415 3416] Safety and efficacy of administration of teicoplanin by the intrathecal route has not been evaluated.[3413 3416]

Manufacturers state that teicoplanin should not be admixed with aminoglycosides due to incompatibility.[3412 3413 3414 3415 3416] Some manufacturers state that administration of teicoplanin must occur separately from other parenteral antibiotics if combination therapy is used.[3412 3415]

Stability

Intact vials of teicoplanin should be stored below 25°C.[3414 3415 3416] Reconstituted and diluted solutions of teicoplanin ideally should be used immediately after preparation, but may be stored under refrigeration at 2 to 8°C for at least 24 hours;[3412 3413 3414 3415 3416] specific product labeling should be consulted. Several manufacturers state that teicoplanin should not be stored in syringes.[3413 3414 3416]

Teicoplanin forms dextrose aldehyde adducts when diluted in dextrose-containing solutions. Equilibrium is reached faster at room temperature (7 days) than with refrigerated storage (30 days). The equilibrium concentration of the adduct is directly related to the dextrose concentration. The reaction is reversible with dilution.[2046]

The stability of catheter flush solutions composed of teicoplanin 133 mg/mL in water for injection, or heparin sodium 10 units/mL or 100 units/mL, was evaluated in Hickman catheters at 25°C over 24 hours. No decomposition products formed, and no loss was found. Indeed, a small (11%) increase in teicoplanin concentration was observed which was attributed to loss of water.[2165]

Syringes

Several manufacturers state that teicoplanin should not be stored in syringes.[3413 3414 3416]

DOI: 10.37573/9781585286850.368

Compatibility Information

Solution Compatibility

Teicoplanin

Test Soln Name	Mfr	Mfr	Conc/L or %	Remarks	Ref	C/I
Dextrose 5% in sodium chloride 0.45%		SAA, GLT		Chemically and physically stable for 24 hr at 2 to 8°C	3412, 3415	C
Dextrose 5%	BAᵃ	HO	2 g	Visually compatible. No loss in 24 hr at 25°C	2165	C
Dextrose 5%	BAᵇ	HO	4 g	Visually compatible. 10% loss in 6 days at 4°C	2364	C
Dextrose 5%		SAA, GLT		Chemically and physically stable for 24 hr at 2 to 8°C	3412, 3415	C
Dextrose 5%		SAA		Use within 24 hr when stored at 4°C	3413	C
Dextrose 10%		SAA, GLT		Chemically and physically stable for 24 hr at 2 to 8°C	3412, 3415	C
Ringer's injection		SAA, GLT		Chemically and physically stable for 24 hr at 2 to 8°C	3412, 3415	C
Ringer's injection, lactated		SAA, GLT		Chemically and physically stable for 24 hr at 2 to 8°C	3412, 3415	C
Sodium chloride 0.9%	BAᵃ	HO	2 g	Visually compatible. No loss in 24 hr at 25°C	2165	C
Sodium chloride 0.9%		SAA, GLT		Chemically and physically stable for 24 hr at 2 to 8°C	3412, 3415	C
Sodium chloride 0.9%		SAA		Stable for up to 7 days at 4°C or 24 hr at room temperature	3413	C

ᵃ Tested in glass containers.

ᵇ Tested in PVC containers.

Additive Compatibility

Teicoplanin

Test Drug	Mfr	Conc/L or %	Mfr	Conc/L or %	Test Solution	Remarks	Ref	C/I
Heparin sodium	CPP	20,000 and 40,000 units	HO	2 g	D5W, NS	Visually compatible. No loss of teicoplanin and heparin in 24 hr at 25°C	2165	C

Y-Site Injection Compatibility (1:1 Mixture)

Teicoplanin

Test Drug	Mfr	Conc	Mfr	Conc	Remarks	Ref	C/I
Blinatumomab	AMG	0.125 mcg/mLᵇ	SAA	4 mg/mLᵃ	Persistent particulate formation when blinatumomab is added to teicoplanin; flakes transiently appeared when order of mixing was reversed	3405, 3417	I
Blinatumomab	AMG	0.375 mcg/mLᵇ	SAA	4 mg/mLᵃ	Persistent particulate formation when blinatumomab is added to teicoplanin; not observed when order of mixing was reversed	3405, 3417	?
Ciprofloxacin	BAY	2 mg/mLᵇ	GRP	60 mg/mL	White precipitate forms immediately but disappears with shaking	1934	?
Defibrotide sodium	JAZ	8 mg/mLᵇ	SAA	125 mg/mL	Visually compatible for 4 hr at room temperature	3149	C
Fat emulsion, intravenous	OTS	20%ᶜ	SAN	2 mg/mLᵃ ᵈ	No change in particle size ≥1.3 μm observed in 24 hr at 25°C in the dark	3452	C

ᵃ Tested in dextrose 5%.

ᵇ Tested in sodium chloride 0.9%.

ᶜ Run at 25 mL/hr with dextrose 5% run at 83 mL/hr.

ᵈ Run at 100 mL/hr.

Additional Compatibility Information

Peritoneal Dialysis Solutions

Some manufacturers state that teicoplanin can be administered in peritoneal dialysis solutions containing 1.36 or 3.86% dextrose.[3412][3415]

Teicoplanin (Marion Merrell Dow) 0.025 mg/mL in Dianeal PD-2 with dextrose 1.5% in polyvinyl chloride (PVC) containers was physically and chemically stable for 24 hours at 25°C exposed to light, exhibiting no loss; additional storage for 8 hours at 37°C resulted in losses of 6% or less. Under refrigeration at 4°C protected from light, no loss occurred in 7 days. Additional storage for 16 hours at 25°C followed by 8 hours at 37°C resulted in about 7% loss.[1989]

Ceftazidime (Glaxo) 0.1 mg/mL admixed with teicoplanin (Marion Merrell Dow) 0.025 mg/mL in Dianeal PD-2 with dextrose 1.5% in PVC containers did not result in a stable mixture. Large (but variable) teicoplanin losses generally in the 20% range were noted in as little as 2 hours at 25°C exposed to light. Ceftazidime losses of about 9% occurred in 16 hours. Refrigeration and protection from light of the peritoneal dialysis admixture reduced losses of both drugs to negligible levels. Even so, admixing these 2 drugs was not recommended because of the high levels of teicoplanin loss at room temperature.[1989]

Teicoplanin (Merrell Dow) 25 mg/L in Dianeal 137 with dextrose 1.36% (Baxter) was evaluated for stability over 42 days. Stored at 4°C, teicoplanin retained stability with a loss of less than 5% in 42 days. At 20°C, 10% loss occurred in about 25 days with 17% loss in 42 days. At an elevated temperature of 37°C, a much greater rate of decomposition occurs with over 40% loss occurring in 42 days.[2145]

Manufacturers state that teicoplanin should not be admixed with aminoglycosides due to incompatibility;[3412][3413][3414][3415][3416] however, several manufacturers state that the drugs *are* compatible when combined in dialysis fluid.[3412][3415] Specific product labeling should be consulted.

Selected Revisions September 30, 2019. © Copyright, October 1998. American Society of Health-System Pharmacists, Inc.

Telavancin Hydrochloride
AHFS 8:12.28.16

Products

Telavancin hydrochloride is available as a lyophilized powder in single-use vials containing telavancin 250 and 750 mg as the hydrochloride.[2831] Also present are hydroxypropyl-beta-cyclo-dextrin, mannitol, and sodium hydroxide and hydrochloric acid to adjust pH.[2831]

The 250-mg vial should be reconstituted with 15 mL and the 750-mg vial with 45 mL of dextrose 5%, sterile water for injection, or sodium chloride 0.9% and mixed thoroughly to yield a telavancin concentration of 15 mg/mL.[2831] To minimize foaming during reconstitution, allow the vacuum of the vial to draw the diluent from the syringe into the vial; do not forcefully inject the diluent.[2831] Any vial that does not have a vacuum should be discarded.[2831] Dissolution may occasionally require up to 20 minutes.[2831] Do not forcefully shake the vial or the diluted solution in the infusion bag.[2831]

pH
From 4 to 5.[2831]

Trade Name(s)
Vibativ

Administration

Telavancin is administered by intravenous infusion over 60 minutes after dilution in a compatible infusion solution.[2831] For telavancin doses of 150 to 800 mg, dilution in 100 to 250 mL is recommended.[2831] For doses outside this range, dilution to a concentration of 0.6 to 8 mg/mL is recommended.[2831] The manufacturer recommends dilution in dextrose 5%; sodium chloride 0.9%; or Ringer's injection, lactated.[2831]

Stability

Intact vials of telavancin hydrochloride should be stored under refrigeration.[2831] The reconstituted drug in the vial and the diluted solution in the infusion bag should be used within 12 hours if stored at room temperature or 7 days if stored under refrigeration.[2831][3097] The total time for the reconstituted drug in the vial and the diluted solution in the infusion bag together should not exceed 12 hours at room temperature or 7 days under refrigeration.[2831][3097]

Freezing Solutions

The manufacturer states that the diluted solution of telavancin in the infusion bag can be stored at −30 to −10°C for up to 32 days.[2831] Telavancin (Ben Venue) 0.6 and 8 mg/mL diluted in sodium chloride 0.9% or dextrose 5% in polyvinyl chloride (PVC) and non-PVC infusion bags and stored at −20°C exhibited less than 10% loss of the drug during the 32-day study period.[3096] The authors recommended that solutions be brought to room temperature without any assistance (e.g., sonication, hot water bath) and used immediately after thawing, or within 12 hours at room temperature; thawed solutions should not be refrozen.[3096]

Compatibility Information

Solution Compatibility

Telavancin HCl

Test Soln Name	Mfr	Mfr	Conc/L or %	Remarks	Ref	C/I
Dextrose 5%		ASP		Use within 12 hr at room temperature or 7 days refrigerated	2831	C
Dextrose 5%	BA[a]	BV	0.6 and 8 g	Stable for 12 hr in ambient conditions or 7 days at 2 to 8°C without light	3097	C
Dextrose 5%	BA[a]	BV	0.6 and 8 g	Less than 10% loss in 32 days at −20°C	3096	C
Dextrose 5%	BRN[b]	BV	0.6 and 8 g	Less than 10% loss in 32 days at −20°C	3096	C
Ringer's injection, lactated		ASP		Use within 12 hr at room temperature or 7 days refrigerated	2831	C
Ringer's injection, lactated	BA[a]	BV	0.6 and 8 g	Stable for 12 hr in ambient conditions or 7 days at 2 to 8°C without light	3097	C
Sodium chloride 0.9%		ASP		Use within 12 hr at room temperature or 7 days refrigerated	2831	C
Sodium chloride 0.9%	BA[a]	BV	0.6 and 8 g	Stable for 12 hr in ambient conditions or 7 days at 2 to 8°C without light	3097	C
Sodium chloride 0.9%	BA[a]	BV	0.6 and 8 g	Less than 10% loss in 32 days at −20°C	3096	C
Sodium chloride 0.9%	BRN[b]	BV	0.6 and 8 g	Less than 10% loss in 32 days at −20°C	3096	C

[a] Tested in PVC containers.

[b] Tested in non-PVC containers.

DOI: 10.37573/9781585286850.369

Y-Site Injection Compatibility (1:1 Mixture)

Telavancin HCl

Test Drug	Mfr	Conc	Mfr	Conc	Remarks	Ref	C/I
Amphotericin B	XGN	0.1 mg/mL[a]	ASP	7.5 mg/mL[a]	Increase in measured turbidity	2830	I
Amphotericin B lipid complex	ENZ	1 mg/mL[a]	ASP	7.5 mg/mL[a]	Physically compatible for 2 hr	2830	C
Amphotericin B liposomal	ASP	1 mg/mL[a]	ASP	7.5 mg/mL[a]	Increase in measured turbidity	2830	I
Ampicillin sodium–sulbactam sodium	BA	20 mg/mL[a b c e]	ASP	7.5 mg/mL[a b c]	Physically compatible for 2 hr	2830	C
Azithromycin	APP	2 mg/mL[a b c]	ASP	7.5 mg/mL[a b c]	Physically compatible for 2 hr	2830	C
Calcium gluconate	APP	40 mg/mL[a b c]	ASP	7.5 mg/mL[a b c]	Physically compatible for 2 hr	2830	C
Caspofungin acetate	ME	0.5 mg/mL[b]	ASP	7.5 mg/mL[b]	Physically compatible for 2 hr	2830	C
Cefepime HCl	SAG	40 mg/mL[a b c]	ASP	7.5 mg/mL[a b c]	Physically compatible for 2 hr	2830	C
Ceftazidime	HOS	40 mg/mL[a b c]	ASP	7.5 mg/mL[a b c]	Physically compatible for 2 hr	2830	C
Ceftriaxone sodium	HOS	20 mg/mL[a b]	ASP	7.5 mg/mL[a b]	Physically compatible for 2 hr	2830	C
Ciprofloxacin	HOS	2 mg/mL[a]	ASP	7.5 mg/mL[a]	Physically compatible for 2 hr	2830	C
Colistimethate sodium	PAD	4.5 mg/mL[a]	ASP	7.5 mg/mL[a]	Visible turbidity formed	2830	I
Colistimethate sodium	PAD	4.5 mg/mL[b c]	ASP	7.5 mg/mL[b c]	Physically compatible for 2 hr	2830	C
Cyclosporine	BED	5 mg/mL[b c]	ASP	7.5 mg/mL[b c]	Increase in measured turbidity	2830	I
Cyclosporine	BED	5 mg/mL[a]	ASP	7.5 mg/mL[a]	Physically compatible for 2 hr	2830	C
Dexamethasone sodium phosphate	AMR	1 mg/mL[a b c]	ASP	7.5 mg/mL[a b c]	Physically compatible for 2 hr	2830	C
Digoxin	BA	0.25 mg/mL	ASP	7.5 mg/mL[a b c]	Visible turbidity formed	2830	I
Diltiazem HCl	BED	5 mg/mL	ASP	7.5 mg/mL[a b c]	Physically compatible for 2 hr	2830	C
Dobutamine HCl	HOS	4 mg/mL[a b c]	ASP	7.5 mg/mL[a b c]	Physically compatible for 2 hr	2830	C
Dopamine HCl	HOS	3.2 mg/mL[a b c]	ASP	7.5 mg/mL[a b c]	Physically compatible for 2 hr	2830	C
Doripenem	OMN	10 mg/mL[a b]	ASP	7.5 mg/mL[a b]	Physically compatible for 2 hr	2830	C
Doxycycline hyclate	APP	1 mg/mL[a b c]	ASP	7.5 mg/mL[a b c]	Physically compatible for 2 hr	2830	C
Ertapenem sodium	ME	20 mg/mL[b]	ASP	7.5 mg/mL[b]	Physically compatible for 2 hr	2830	C
Esomeprazole sodium	ASZ	0.4 mg/mL[a b c]	ASP	7.5 mg/mL[a b c]	Discoloration and increase in measured turbidity	2830	I
Famotidine	BED	2 mg/mL[a b c]	ASP	7.5 mg/mL[a b c]	Physically compatible for 2 hr	2830	C
Fluconazole	SAG	2 mg/mL[b]	ASP	7.5 mg/mL[b]	Physically compatible for 2 hr	2830	C
Furosemide	HOS	3 mg/mL[a b c]	ASP	7.5 mg/mL[a b c]	Immediate precipitation	2830	I
Gentamicin sulfate	HOS	5 mg/mL[a b c]	ASP	7.5 mg/mL[a b c]	Physically compatible for 2 hr	2830	C
Heparin sodium	APP	1000 units/mL	ASP	7.5 mg/mL[a b]	Measured turbidity increased	2830	I
Heparin sodium	APP	1000 units/mL	ASP	7.5 mg/mL[c]	Physically compatible for 2 hr	2830	C
Hydrocortisone sodium succinate	PF	1 mg/mL[a b c]	ASP	7.5 mg/mL[a b c]	Physically compatible for 2 hr	2830	C
Imipenem–cilastatin sodium	ME	5 mg/mL[a g]	ASP	7.5 mg/mL[a]	Slight measured turbidity increase	2830	I
Imipenem–cilastatin sodium	ME	5 mg/mL[b g]	ASP	7.5 mg/mL[b]	Physically compatible for 2 hr	2830	C
Labetalol HCl	BED	5 mg/mL[a b c]	ASP	7.5 mg/mL[a b c]	Physically compatible for 2 hr	2830	C

Y-Site Injection Compatibility (1:1 Mixture) (Cont.)

Test Drug	Mfr	Conc	Mfr	Conc	Remarks	Ref	C/I
Levofloxacin	OMN	5 mg/mL[a b c]	ASP	7.5 mg/mL[a b c]	Discoloration and measured haze increase	2830	I
Magnesium sulfate	AMR	100 mg/mL[a b c]	ASP	7.5 mg/mL[a b c]	Physically compatible for 2 hr	2830	C
Mannitol	HOS	20%	ASP	7.5 mg/mL[a b c]	Physically compatible for 2 hr	2830	C
Meropenem	ASZ	10 mg/mL[a b c]	ASP	7.5 mg/mL[a b c]	Physically compatible for 2 hr	2830	C
Methylprednisolone sodium succinate	PF	5 mg/mL[a]	ASP	7.5 mg/mL[a]	Slight measured turbidity increase	2830	I
Methylprednisolone sodium succinate	PF	5 mg/mL[b c]	ASP	7.5 mg/mL[b c]	Physically compatible for 2 hr	2830	C
Metoclopramide HCl	HOS	1 mg/mL	ASP	7.5 mg/mL[a b c]	Physically compatible for 2 hr	2830	C
Micafungin sodium	ASP	5 mg/mL[a b]	ASP	7.5 mg/mL[a b]	Visible haze forms	2830	I
Milrinone lactate	BED	0.2 mg/mL[a b c]	ASP	7.5 mg/mL[a b c]	Physically compatible for 2 hr	2830	C
Norepinephrine bitartrate	BED	0.128 mg/mL[a b c]	ASP	7.5 mg/mL[a b c]	Physically compatible for 2 hr	2830	C
Ondansetron HCl	BA	1 mg/mL[a b c]	ASP	7.5 mg/mL[a b c]	Physically compatible for 2 hr	2830	C
Pantoprazole sodium	WY[d]	0.4 mg/mL[a b c]	ASP	7.5 mg/mL[a b c]	Physically compatible for 2 hr	2830	C
Phenylephrine HCl	SZ	1 mg/mL[a b c]	ASP	7.5 mg/mL[a b c]	Physically compatible for 2 hr	2830	C
Piperacillin sodium–tazobactam sodium	WY[d]	40 mg/mL[a b c f]	ASP	7.5 mg/mL[a b c]	Physically compatible for 2 hr	2830	C
Potassium chloride	HOS	0.1 mEq/mL[a b c]	ASP	7.5 mg/mL[a b c]	Physically compatible for 2 hr	2830	C
Potassium phosphates	AMR	0.5 mEq/mL[a b c]	ASP	7.5 mg/mL[a b c]	Physically compatible for 2 hr	2830	C
Propofol	APP[d]	10 mg/mL	ASP	7.5 mg/mL[a]	Physically compatible for 2 hr	2830	C
Propofol	APP[d]	10 mg/mL	ASP	7.5 mg/mL[b c]	Emulsion broke and oiled out	2830	I
Ranitidine HCl	BED	2 mg/mL[a b c]	ASP	7.5 mg/mL[a b c]	Physically compatible for 2 hr	2830	C
Sodium bicarbonate	HOS	1 mEq/mL	ASP	7.5 mg/mL[a b c]	Physically compatible for 2 hr	2830	C
Sodium phosphates	HOS	0.5 mmol/mL[a b c]	ASP	7.5 mg/mL[a b c]	Physically compatible for 2 hr	2830	C
Tigecycline	WY	1 mg/mL[a b c]	ASP	7.5 mg/mL[a b c]	Physically compatible for 2 hr	2830	C
Tobramycin sulfate	HOS	5 mg/mL[a b]	ASP	7.5 mg/mL[a b]	Physically compatible for 2 hr	2830	C
Vasopressin	AMR	1 unit/mL[a b c]	ASP	7.5 mg/mL[a b c]	Physically compatible for 2 hr	2830	C

[a] Tested in dextrose 5%.

[b] Tested in sodium chloride 0.9%.

[c] Tested in Ringer's injection, lactated.

[d] Test performed using the formulation WITH edetate disodium.

[e] Ampicillin component. Ampicillin in a 2:1 fixed-ratio concentration with sulbactam.

[f] Piperacillin component. Piperacillin in an 8:1 fixed-ratio concentration with tazobactam.

[g] Imipenem component. Imipenem in a 1:1 fixed-ratio concentration with cilastatin.

Selected Revisions January 31, 2020. © Copyright, January 2012.
American Society of Health-System Pharmacists, Inc.

Temozolomide
AHFS 10:00

Products

Temozolomide is available as a lyophilized powder in single-use vials containing 100 mg of the drug.[3145] Each vial also contains mannitol 600 mg, L-threonine 160 mg, polysorbate 80 120 mg, sodium citrate dihydrate 235 mg, and hydrochloric acid 160 mg.[3145]

Vials containing temozolomide should be allowed to reach room temperature prior to reconstitution.[3145] Each 100-mg vial of temozolomide should be reconstituted with 41 mL of sterile water for injection to yield a solution with a final temozolomide concentration of 2.5 mg/mL.[3145] Vials should be gently swirled until the contents are dissolved; vials should not be shaken.[3145] The reconstituted solution should be visually inspected; if particulate matter is visible, the solution should not be used.[3145] Up to 40 mL may be withdrawn from each reconstituted vial and transferred to an empty 250-mL infusion bag to make up the total dose.[3145] The reconstituted solution should *not* be further diluted.[3145]

Trade Name(s)

Temodar

Administration

Temozolomide is administered only by intravenous infusion over 90 minutes using an infusion pump.[3145] Infusion over a period of time other than 90 minutes may result in suboptimal dosing.[3145]

Temozolomide should be infused through a separate line, or, if a common infusion line is being used to administer other drugs, the line should be flushed (e.g., with sodium chloride 0.9%) prior to and following infusion of temozolomide.[3145]

As with other toxic drugs, temozolomide should be prepared and administered with care.[3145] Vials of the drug should *not* be opened.[3145] Protective measures (e.g., the use of gloves and eye protection) should be taken to avoid inadvertent contact with or inhalation of the drug in the case of breakage of the vial or other accidental spillage.[3145] Applicable disposal procedures for the drug should be followed.[3145]

Stability

Temozolomide is a white to light tan or light pink powder.[3145] Intact vials of temozolomide should be stored at 2 to 8°C.[3145]

The reconstituted solution should be stored at room temperature (i.e., 25°C).[3145] The total time from reconstitution through completion of administration should not exceed 14 hours.[3145]

pH Effects

Temozolomide is stable at acidic pH (less than 5) and is alkali labile.[3145]

Additional Compatibility Information

Infusion Solutions

The manufacturer states that temozolomide solution may be administered in the same intravenous infusion line only with sodium chloride 0.9%.[3145]

DOI: 10.37573/9781585286850.370

Temsirolimus
AHFS 10:00

Products

Temsirolimus is available in a 2-vial kit: the first single-use vial contains temsirolimus concentrate for injection and the second single-use vial contains 1.8 mL of special diluent.[3205] Each vial of temsirolimus concentrate for injection contains temsirolimus 25 mg/mL, dehydrated alcohol 39.5% (w/v), dl-alpha-tocopherol 0.075% (w/v), propylene glycol 50.3% (w/v), and anhydrous citric acid 0.0025% (w/v).[3205] Each vial of special diluent contains polysorbate 80 40% (w/v), polyethylene glycol 400 42.8% (w/v), and dehydrated alcohol 19.9% (w/v).[3205] Both the temsirolimus concentrate for injection vial and the accompanying diluent vial contain an overfill.[3205]

Preparation of the final diluted solution for infusion from this 2-vial kit requires a 2-step dilution procedure prior to administration.[3205] Step 1 is the preparation of the *initial* diluted solution, which is then further diluted to the *final* diluted solution for infusion in step 2.[3205] During handling and preparation of temsirolimus admixtures, the drug should be protected from excessive room light and sunlight.[3205]

To prepare the initial diluted solution (step 1), 1.8 mL of the special diluent should be withdrawn from the vial of accompanying diluent and added to the vial of temsirolimus concentrate for injection.[3205] Each vial of diluted temsirolimus concentrate for injection should be mixed well by inverting the vial.[3205] This initial diluted solution is a clear to slightly turbid, colorless to light yellow solution, essentially free from visual particulates, having a temsirolimus concentration of 10 mg/mL (30 mg/3 mL) and an alcohol content of 35.2%.[3205] The vial should be allowed to stand for a sufficient time to allow air bubbles created during mixing to subside.[3205]

To prepare the final diluted solution (step 2), the appropriate dose of the temsirolimus 10-mg/mL initial diluted solution should be withdrawn from the vial and added to a glass or plastic (e.g., polypropylene, polyolefin) container of 250 mL of sodium chloride 0.9%.[3205] The final diluted solution for infusion should be mixed by inversion of the infusion container; excessive shaking should be avoided as it may cause foaming.[3205] Solutions should be visually inspected for particulate matter and discoloration prior to administration.[3205]

Trade Name(s)

Torisel

Administration

Temsirolimus is administered as an intravenous infusion over 30 to 60 minutes, preferably using an infusion pump, to patients who have been adequately premedicated to control adverse effects.[3205] To minimize patient exposure to the diethylhexyl phthalate (DEHP) plasticizer, the final diluted solution for infusion should be administered using non-DEHP plasticized non-polyvinyl chloride (non-PVC) (e.g., polyethylene-lined) administration sets containing an appropriate filter.[3205] (See Filtration.) If a PVC administration set must be used, it should not contain DEHP.[3205]

Stability

Intact vials of temsirolimus concentrate for injection and special diluent contained in the kit should be stored at 2 to 8°C and protected from light.[3205]

Temsirolimus concentrate for injection is a clear, colorless to light yellow solution.[3205] The initial diluted solution is stable for up to 24 hours at temperatures less than 25°C.[3205] Once the initial diluted solution has been further diluted with sodium chloride 0.9% to the final diluted solution for infusion, administration should be completed within 6 hours of preparation of the final diluted solution for infusion.[3205] The final diluted solution for infusion should be protected from excessive room light and sunlight.[3205]

pH Effects

Temsirolimus is degraded by both acids and bases; combinations of temsirolimus with agents capable of affecting the solution pH should be avoided.[3205]

Light Effects

Temsirolimus is light sensitive.[3214] Intact vials, as well as the final diluted solution for infusion, should be protected from light.[3205] The drug also should be protected from excessive room light and sunlight during handling and preparation of temsirolimus admixtures.[3205]

Temsirolimus diluted for infusion in polypropylene containers protected from light was infused through a 1.85-m length of non-DEHP PVC-lined intravenous infusion tubing (Intrafix Safe Set, B. Braun) either protected from room light (with aluminum foil) or unprotected over a period of 45 minutes at room temperature.[3214] No substantial degradation of temsirolimus was noted following simulated infusion of the diluted solution through tubing with or without light exposure.[3214]

Plasticizer Leaching

Polysorbate 80 contained in the temsirolimus initial diluted solution and the final diluted solution for infusion can increase the rate at which plasticizer is leached from DEHP-plasticized PVC containers and administration sets.[3205] The duration of contact of the diluted drug with PVC during preparation and administration of the drug should be considered.[3205] To minimize patient exposure to the plasticizer, the final diluted solution for infusion should be stored in glass or plastic (e.g., polypropylene, polyolefin) containers and infused using polyethylene-lined administration sets.[3205] If a PVC administration set must be used, it should not contain DEHP.[3205]

Filtration

The manufacturer recommends the use of an inline polyethersulfone filter with a pore size not exceeding 5 μm for administration.[3205] If the available administration set does not contain an inline filter, an endline polyethersulfone filter should be added to the set prior to drug administration.[3205] Different endline filters ranging in pore size from 0.2 to 5 μm may be used; however, the manufacturer does not recommend the use of both an inline and endline filter.[3205]

DOI: 10.37573/9781585286850.371

Compatibility Information

Solution Compatibility

Temsirolimus

Test Soln Name	Mfr	Mfr	Conc/L or %	Remarks	Ref	C/I
Sodium chloride 0.9%	a	WY		Complete administration within 6 hr of preparation of the final diluted solution for infusion	3205	C
Sodium chloride 0.9%	FRE[b]	WY	100 mg	Less than 5% loss in 4 days at 4°C and 3 days at 20°C protected from light	3214	C

[a] Tested in glass, polypropylene, and polyolefin containers.

[b] Tested in polypropylene containers.

© Copyright, June 2017. American Society of Health-System Pharmacists, Inc.

Teniposide

AHFS 10:00

VM-26

Products

Teniposide is available in 5-mL ampuls containing 50 mg of drug. Each mL of solution contains teniposide 10 mg, benzyl alcohol 30 mg, *N,N*-dimethylacetamide (DMA) 60 mg, polyoxyethylated castor oil (Cremophor EL) 500 mg, and dehydrated alcohol 42.7% (v/v). The pH is adjusted with maleic acid. The product is a concentrate that must be diluted for use.[1(6/06)]

pH

Approximately 5.[1(6/06)]

Trade Name(s)

Vumon

Administration

Teniposide is administered by slow intravenous infusion over at least 30 to 60 minutes after dilution in dextrose 5% or sodium chloride 0.9% to a final concentration of 0.1, 0.2, 0.4, or 1 mg/mL.[1(6/06)] Extended infusions of 0.1- and 0.2-mg/mL solutions over 24 hours have resulted in precipitation.[1(6/06) 1502 1521] The intravenous solution containers and sets used to administer teniposide should not contain the plasticizer diethylhexyl phthalate (DEHP). Extravasation should be avoided because of local tissue irritation and phlebitis.[1(6/06) 4]

Heparin sodium can cause precipitation of teniposide. Administration apparatus should be thoroughly flushed before and after teniposide administration with dextrose 5% or sodium chloride 0.9%.[1(6/06) 1502]

Contact of the undiluted teniposide concentrate with plastic equipment and devices during preparation has resulted in softening of the plastic, cracking, and leakage. Damage to plastic equipment has not been reported with diluted solutions.[1(6/06)]

Stability

The teniposide concentrate is clear[1(6/06)] but may exhibit a slight opalescence when diluted in infusion solutions due to the surfactant content.[234]

Intact ampuls should be stored under refrigeration in the original package to protect from light. Teniposide stability is not adversely affected by freezing[1(6/06)] or exposure to normal room fluorescent light during administration.[1374]

The manufacturer does not recommend refrigeration of teniposide diluted in infusion solutions.[1(6/06)]

Precipitation

Although teniposide is chemically stable for at least 24 hours, precipitation from aqueous solutions has occurred irregularly and unpredictably even at 0.1 and 0.2 mg/mL, the lowest recommended concentrations.[1(6/06) 1502 1521] The precipitation rate depends on the formation of crystallization nuclei. Precipitation then proceeds rapidly. The formation of crystallization nuclei may be accelerated by agitation, contact with incompatible drugs or material surfaces, and, possibly, other factors.[1374 1502 1521] The manufacturer recommends avoiding an inordinate amount of agitation during preparation, minimizing storage time prior to administration, and avoiding contact with other drugs and solutions. Even the compatibility of teniposide infusions with some infusion set materials and pumps cannot be assured.[1(6/06) 1502 1521]

Sorption

No teniposide loss due to sorption to polyvinyl chloride (PVC) containers has been observed.[1374 2053]

Plasticizer Leaching

The surfactant, Cremophor EL, in the teniposide formulation leaches the plasticizer DEHP from PVC containers and sets. The amount leached increases with time and drug concentration and is similar for sodium chloride 0.9% and dextrose 5%. The use of non-PVC containers, such as glass bottles and polyolefin bags, and non-PVC administration sets, such as lipid administration sets and nitroglycerin sets, is recommended.[1(6/06)]

Teniposide (Bristol) 0.1 mg/mL in dextrose 5% leached relatively large amounts of DEHP from PVC bags due to the Cremophor EL surfactant in the formulation. After 8 hours at 24°C, the DEHP concentration in 50-mL bags of infusion solution was as much as 7.5 mcg/mL; it continued to increase through 24 hours to 22.2 mcg/mL. This finding is consistent with the surfactant concentration (1%) of the final admixture solution. The actual amount of DEHP leached from PVC containers and administration sets may vary in clinical situations, depending on surfactant concentration, bag size, and contact time.[1683]

Substantial leaching of DEHP plasticizer was reported from PVC bags of dextrose 5% and sodium chloride 0.9% and PVC administration sets by teniposide admixtures containing 0.4 mg/mL of the drug due to the Cremophor EL surfactant used in the formulation. DEHP levels increased throughout the 1-hour infusion time to over 20 mcg/mL from both the bags and sets. There was no difference in plasticizer leaching between the 2 infusion solutions. Storage of the teniposide 0.4-mg/mL admixtures for 48 hours at both 4 and 24°C resulted in substantially greater DEHP leaching. DEHP concentrations ranged from about 60 mcg/mL in the refrigerated samples to over 200 mcg/mL (a total of 52 mg) in the room temperature samples. The actual amount of DEHP a patient will receive is dependent on a number of factors, including Cremophor EL concentration, storage temperature, and contact time. No plasticizer was leached from glass bottles or polyolefin infusion containers. To minimize plasticizer leaching if PVC containers and sets must be used, it is recommended that teniposide admixtures be used immediately after preparation and administered over no more than 1 hour.[2053]

DOI: 10.37573/9781585286850.372

In 1996, an acceptability limit of no more than 5 parts per million (5 mcg/mL) for DEHP plasticizer released from PVC-containing devices (e.g., containers, administration sets, other equipment) was proposed based on a review of metabolic and toxicologic considerations.[2185] FDA later evaluated the safety of DEHP exposure by comparing doses of DEHP received by patients undergoing various medical procedures with a defined tolerable intake value of DEHP, a value that was based upon the results of selected critical toxicity studies in experimental animals.[3100] Based on the results of the safety assessment, FDA concluded that there is little risk posed by exposure to the amount of DEHP released from PVC bags used to store and administer drugs that require an excipient for solubilization *when label instructions for*

preparation and administration are followed.[3100] However, such conclusions do not take into account increased risk for adverse effects from DEHP exposure in certain patients (e.g., critically ill male neonates or infants, male infants less than 1 year of age, male offspring of pregnant or breast-feeding women undergoing certain medical treatments) or potential adverse effects related to aggregate exposure for patients exposed to multiple medical devices, procedures, or intravenous medications known to leach DEHP, for which there are varying levels of concern.[3100] [3101]

Teniposide 0.1 mg/mL in dextrose 5% in VISIV polyolefin bags was tested at room temperature near 23°C for 24 hours. No leached plastic components were found within the 24-hour study period.[2660] [2792]

Compatibility Information

Solution Compatibility

Teniposide

Test Soln Name	Mfr	Mfr	Conc/L or %	Remarks	Ref	C/I
Dextrose 5%			100, 200, 400 mg	Stable for 24 hr at room temperature	1(6/06)	C
Dextrose 5%			1 g	May precipitate in 4 hr	1(6/06)	?
Dextrose 5%	a	BR	400 mg	Physically compatible. 6% loss in 4 days at 21°C in light or dark	1374	C
Ringer's injection, lactated	a	BR	400 mg	Physically compatible. 3% loss in 4 days at 21°C in light or dark	1374	C
Sodium chloride 0.9%			100, 200, 400 mg	Stable for 24 hr at room temperature	1(6/06)	C
Sodium chloride 0.9%			1 g	May precipitate in 4 hr	1(6/06)	?
Sodium chloride 0.9%	b	BR	400 mg	Physically compatible. 4% loss in 4 days at 21°C in light or dark	1374	C
Sodium chloride 0.9%	a	BR	500, 600, 700 mg	Physically compatible for 4 days at 21°C	1374	C

a Tested in glass containers.

b Tested in both glass and PVC containers.

Y-Site Injection Compatibility (1:1 Mixture)

Teniposide

Test Drug	Mfr	Conc	Mfr	Conc	Remarks	Ref	C/I
Acyclovir sodium	BW	7 mg/mL[a]	BR	0.1 mg/mL[a]	Physically compatible for 4 hr at 23°C	1725	C
Allopurinol sodium	BW	3 mg/mL[a]	BR	0.1 mg/mL[a]	Physically compatible for 4 hr at 23°C	1725	C
Amifostine	USB	10 mg/mL[a]	BR	0.1 mg/mL[a]	Physically compatible for 4 hr at 23°C	1845	C
Amikacin sulfate	BR	5 mg/mL[a]	BR	0.1 mg/mL[a]	Physically compatible for 4 hr at 23°C	1725	C
Aminophylline	AB	2.5 mg/mL[a]	BR	0.1 mg/mL[a]	Physically compatible for 4 hr at 23°C	1725	C
Amphotericin B	SQ	0.6 mg/mL[a]	BR	0.1 mg/mL[a]	Physically compatible for 4 hr at 23°C	1725	C
Ampicillin sodium	WY	20 mg/mL[b]	BR	0.1 mg/mL[a]	Physically compatible for 4 hr at 23°C	1725	C
Ampicillin sodium–sulbactam sodium	RR	20 mg/mL[b] [d]	BR	0.1 mg/mL[a]	Physically compatible for 4 hr at 23°C	1725	C
Aztreonam	SQ	40 mg/mL[a]	BR	0.1 mg/mL[a]	Physically compatible for 4 hr at 23°C	1725, 1758	C
Bleomycin sulfate	BR	1 unit/mL[b]	BR	0.1 mg/mL[a]	Physically compatible for 4 hr at 23°C	1725	C

Y-Site Injection Compatibility (1:1 Mixture) (Cont.)

Test Drug	Mfr	Conc	Mfr	Conc	Remarks	Ref	C/I
Bumetanide	RC	0.04 mg/mL[a]	BR	0.1 mg/mL[a]	Physically compatible for 4 hr at 23°C	1725	C
Buprenorphine HCl	RKC	0.04 mg/mL[a]	BR	0.1 mg/mL[a]	Physically compatible for 4 hr at 23°C	1725	C
Butorphanol tartrate	BR	0.04 mg/mL[a]	BR	0.1 mg/mL[a]	Physically compatible for 4 hr at 23°C	1725	C
Calcium gluconate	AMR	40 mg/mL[a]	BR	0.1 mg/mL[a]	Physically compatible for 4 hr at 23°C	1725	C
Carboplatin	BR	5 mg/mL[a]	BR	0.1 mg/mL[a]	Physically compatible for 4 hr at 23°C	1725	C
Carmustine	BR	1.5 mg/mL[a]	BR	0.1 mg/mL[a]	Physically compatible for 4 hr at 23°C	1725	C
Cefazolin sodium	MAR	20 mg/mL[a]	BR	0.1 mg/mL[a]	Physically compatible for 4 hr at 23°C	1725	C
Cefotaxime sodium	HO	20 mg/mL[a]	BR	0.1 mg/mL[a]	Physically compatible for 1 hr at 23°C	1725	C
Cefotetan disodium	STU	20 mg/mL[a]	BR	0.1 mg/mL[a]	Physically compatible for 4 hr at 23°C	1725	C
Cefoxitin sodium	MSD	20 mg/mL[a]	BR	0.1 mg/mL[a]	Physically compatible for 4 hr at 23°C	1725	C
Ceftazidime	LI	40 mg/mL[a]	BR	0.1 mg/mL[a]	Physically compatible for 4 hr at 23°C	1725	C
Ceftriaxone sodium	RC	20 mg/mL[a]	BR	0.1 mg/mL[a]	Physically compatible for 4 hr at 23°C	1725	C
Cefuroxime sodium	GL	20 mg/mL[a]	BR	0.1 mg/mL[a]	Physically compatible for 4 hr at 23°C	1725	C
Chlorpromazine HCl	SCN	2 mg/mL[a]	BR	0.1 mg/mL[a]	Physically compatible for 4 hr at 23°C	1725	C
Ciprofloxacin	MI	2 mg/mL[a]	BR	0.1 mg/mL[a]	Physically compatible for 4 hr at 23°C	1725	C
Cisplatin	BR	1 mg/mL	BR	0.1 mg/mL[a]	Physically compatible for 4 hr at 23°C	1725	C
Cladribine	ORT	0.015[b] and 0.5[c] mg/mL	BR	0.1 mg/mL[b]	Physically compatible for 4 hr at 23°C	1969	C
Clindamycin phosphate	AST	10 mg/mL[a]	BR	0.1 mg/mL[a]	Physically compatible for 4 hr at 23°C	1725	C
Cyclophosphamide	MJ	10 mg/mL[a]	BR	0.1 mg/mL[a]	Physically compatible for 4 hr at 23°C	1725	C
Cytarabine	CET	50 mg/mL	BR	0.1 mg/mL[a]	Physically compatible for 4 hr at 23°C	1725	C
Dacarbazine	MI	4 mg/mL[a]	BR	0.1 mg/mL[a]	Physically compatible for 4 hr at 23°C	1725	C
Dactinomycin	MSD	0.01 mg/mL[a]	BR	0.1 mg/mL[a]	Physically compatible for 4 hr at 23°C	1725	C
Daunorubicin HCl	WY	1 mg/mL[a]	BR	0.1 mg/mL[a]	Physically compatible for 4 hr at 23°C	1725	C
Dexamethasone sodium phosphate	LY	1 mg/mL[a]	BR	0.1 mg/mL[a]	Physically compatible for 4 hr at 23°C	1725	C
Diphenhydramine HCl	ES	2 mg/mL[a]	BR	0.1 mg/mL[a]	Physically compatible for 4 hr at 23°C	1725	C
Doxorubicin HCl	CET	2 mg/mL	BR	0.1 mg/mL[a]	Physically compatible for 4 hr at 23°C	1725	C
Doxycycline hyclate	LY	1 mg/mL[a]	BR	0.1 mg/mL[a]	Physically compatible for 4 hr at 23°C	1725	C
Droperidol	JN	0.4 mg/mL[a]	BR	0.1 mg/mL[a]	Physically compatible for 4 hr at 23°C	1725	C
Enalaprilat	MSD	0.1 mg/mL[a]	BR	0.1 mg/mL[a]	Physically compatible for 4 hr at 23°C	1725	C
Etoposide	BR	0.4 mg/mL[a]	BR	0.1 mg/mL[a]	Physically compatible for 4 hr at 23°C	1725	C
Etoposide phosphate	BR	5 mg/mL[a]	BR	0.1 mg/mL[a]	Physically compatible for 4 hr at 23°C	2218	C
Famotidine	MSD	2 mg/mL[a]	BR	0.1 mg/mL[a]	Physically compatible for 4 hr at 23°C	1725	C
Floxuridine	RC	3 mg/mL[a]	BR	0.1 mg/mL[a]	Physically compatible for 4 hr at 23°C	1725	C
Fluconazole	RR	2 mg/mL	BR	0.1 mg/mL[a]	Physically compatible for 4 hr at 23°C	1725	C
Fludarabine phosphate	BX	1 mg/mL[a]	BR	0.1 mg/mL[a]	Physically compatible for 4 hr at 23°C	1725	C
Fluorouracil	AD	16 mg/mL[a]	BR	0.1 mg/mL[a]	Physically compatible for 4 hr at 23°C	1725	C

Y-Site Injection Compatibility (1:1 Mixture) (Cont.)

Test Drug	Mfr	Conc	Mfr	Conc	Remarks	Ref	C/I
Furosemide	AB	3 mg/mL[a]	BR	0.1 mg/mL[a]	Physically compatible for 4 hr at 23°C	1725	C
Gallium nitrate	FUJ	0.4 mg/mL[a]	BR	0.1 mg/mL[a]	Physically compatible for 4 hr at 23°C	1725	C
Ganciclovir sodium	SY	20 mg/mL[a]	BR	0.1 mg/mL[a]	Physically compatible for 4 hr at 23°C	1725	C
Gemcitabine HCl	LI	10 mg/mL[b]	BR	0.1 mg/mL[a]	Physically compatible for 4 hr at 23°C	2226	C
Gentamicin sulfate	LY	5 mg/mL[a]	BR	0.1 mg/mL[a]	Physically compatible for 4 hr at 23°C	1725	C
Granisetron HCl	SKB	0.05 mg/mL[a]	BMS	0.1 mg/mL[a]	Physically compatible for 4 hr at 23°C	2000	C
Haloperidol lactate	MN	0.2 mg/mL[a]	BR	0.1 mg/mL[a]	Physically compatible for 4 hr at 23°C	1725	C
Hydrocortisone sodium succinate	UP	1 mg/mL[a]	BR	0.1 mg/mL[a]	Physically compatible for 4 hr at 23°C	1725	C
Hydromorphone HCl	KN	0.5 mg/mL[a]	BR	0.1 mg/mL[a]	Physically compatible for 4 hr at 23°C	1725	C
Hydroxyzine HCl	WI	4 mg/mL[a]	BR	0.1 mg/mL[a]	Physically compatible for 4 hr at 23°C	1725	C
Idarubicin HCl	AD	0.5 mg/mL[a]	BR	0.1 mg/mL[a]	Unacceptable increase in turbidity	1725	I
Ifosfamide	MJ	25 mg/mL[a]	BR	0.1 mg/mL[a]	Physically compatible for 4 hr at 23°C	1725	C
Imipenem–cilastatin sodium	MSD	10 mg/mL[b f]	BR	0.1 mg/mL[a]	Physically compatible for 4 hr at 23°C	1725	C
Leucovorin calcium	LE	2 mg/mL[a]	BR	0.1 mg/mL[a]	Physically compatible for 4 hr at 23°C	1725	C
Lorazepam	WY	0.1 mg/mL[a]	BR	0.1 mg/mL[a]	Physically compatible for 4 hr at 23°C	1725	C
Mannitol	BA	15%	BR	0.1 mg/mL[a]	Physically compatible for 4 hr at 23°C	1725	C
Mechlorethamine HCl	MSD	1 mg/mL	BR	0.1 mg/mL[a]	Physically compatible for 4 hr at 23°C	1725	C
Melphalan HCl	BW	0.1 mg/mL[a]	BR	0.1 mg/mL[a]	Physically compatible for 4 hr at 23°C	1725	C
Meperidine HCl	WY	4 mg/mL[a]	BR	0.1 mg/mL[a]	Physically compatible for 4 hr at 23°C	1725	C
Mesna	MJ	10 mg/mL[a]	BR	0.1 mg/mL[a]	Physically compatible for 4 hr at 23°C	1725	C
Methotrexate sodium	LE	15 mg/mL[a]	BR	0.1 mg/mL[a]	Physically compatible for 4 hr at 23°C	1725	C
Methylprednisolone sodium succinate	AB	5 mg/mL[a]	BR	0.1 mg/mL[a]	Physically compatible for 4 hr at 23°C	1725	C
Metoclopramide HCl	ES	5 mg/mL	BR	0.1 mg/mL[a]	Physically compatible for 4 hr at 23°C	1725	C
Metronidazole	BA	5 mg/mL	BR	0.1 mg/mL[a]	Physically compatible for 4 hr at 23°C	1725	C
Mitomycin	BR	0.5 mg/mL	BR	0.1 mg/mL[a]	Physically compatible for 4 hr at 23°C	1725	C
Mitoxantrone HCl	LE	0.5 mg/mL[a]	BR	0.1 mg/mL[a]	Physically compatible for 4 hr at 23°C	1725	C
Morphine sulfate	AST	1 mg/mL[a]	BR	0.1 mg/mL[a]	Physically compatible for 4 hr at 23°C	1725	C
Nalbuphine HCl	DU	10 mg/mL	BR	0.1 mg/mL[a]	Physically compatible for 4 hr at 23°C	1725	C
Ondansetron HCl	GL	1 mg/mL[b]	BR	0.1 mg/mL[a]	Visually compatible for 4 hr at 22°C	1365	C
Ondansetron HCl	GL	1 mg/mL[a]	BR	0.1 mg/mL[a]	Physically compatible for 4 hr at 23°C	1725	C
Potassium chloride	AB	0.1 mEq/mL[a]	BR	0.1 mg/mL[a]	Physically compatible for 4 hr at 23°C	1725	C
Prochlorperazine edisylate	SCN	0.5 mg/mL[a]	BR	0.1 mg/mL[a]	Physically compatible for 4 hr at 23°C	1725	C
Promethazine HCl	WY	2 mg/mL[a]	BR	0.1 mg/mL[a]	Physically compatible for 4 hr at 23°C	1725	C
Ranitidine HCl	GL	2 mg/mL[a]	BR	0.1 mg/mL[a]	Physically compatible for 4 hr at 23°C	1725	C
Sargramostim	IMM	10 mcg/mL[b]	BR	0.1 mg/mL[b]	Visually compatible for 4 hr at 22°C	1436	C
Sodium bicarbonate	AB	1 mEq/mL	BR	0.1 mg/mL[a]	Physically compatible for 4 hr at 23°C	1725	C

Y-Site Injection Compatibility (1:1 Mixture) (Cont.)

Test Drug	Mfr	Conc	Mfr	Conc	Remarks	Ref	C/I
Streptozocin	UP	40 mg/mL[a]	BR	0.1 mg/mL[a]	Physically compatible for 4 hr at 23°C	1725	C
Thiotepa	LE	1 mg/mL[a]	BR	0.1 mg/mL[a]	Physically compatible for 4 hr at 23°C	1725	C
Tobramycin sulfate	LI	5 mg/mL[a]	BR	0.1 mg/mL[a]	Physically compatible for 4 hr at 23°C	1725	C
Trimethoprim–sulfamethoxazole	ES	0.8 mg/mL[a] [e]	BR	0.1 mg/mL[a]	Physically compatible for 4 hr at 23°C	1725	C
Vancomycin HCl	AB	10 mg/mL[a]	BR	0.1 mg/mL[a]	Physically compatible for 4 hr at 23°C	1725	C
Vinblastine sulfate	LI	0.12 mg/mL[a]	BR	0.1 mg/mL[a]	Physically compatible for 4 hr at 23°C	1725	C
Vincristine sulfate	LI	0.05 mg/mL[a]	BR	0.1 mg/mL[a]	Physically compatible for 4 hr at 23°C	1725	C
Vinorelbine tartrate	BW	1 mg/mL[a]	BR	0.1 mg/mL[a]	Physically compatible for 4 hr at 23°C	1725	C
Zidovudine	BW	4 mg/mL[a]	BR	0.1 mg/mL[a]	Physically compatible for 4 hr at 23°C	1725	C

[a] Tested in dextrose 5%.

[b] Tested in sodium chloride 0.9%.

[c] Tested in bacteriostatic sodium chloride 0.9% preserved with benzyl alcohol 0.9%.

[d] Ampicillin component. Ampicillin in a 2:1 fixed-ratio concentration with sulbactam.

[e] Trimethoprim component. Trimethoprim in a 1:5 fixed-ratio concentration with sulfamethoxazole.

[f] Not specified whether concentration refers to single component or combined components.

Selected Revisions December 12, 2018. © Copyright, October 1994. American Society of Health-System Pharmacists, Inc.

Tenoxicam
AHFS 28:08.04

Products

Tenoxicam is available as a lyophilized powder for injection in vials containing 20 and 40 mg of drug. Also present in the vials are mannitol, ascorbic acid, disodium edetate, tromethamine, and sodium hydroxide or hydrochloric acid. The lyophilized powder should be reconstituted using the 2-mL ampuls of sterile water for injection provided for that purpose.[38][115]

Trade Name(s)

Mobiflex, Tilcotil

Administration

Tenoxicam is administered by intramuscular[38][115] or intravenous bolus injection.[38][115] Addition to infusion solutions is not recommended.[38][115]

Stability

The greenish-yellow lyophilized powder in intact vials should be stored at controlled room temperature at or below 25°C[38] to 30°C[115] and protected from freezing. The drug is stable for 24 hours after reconstitution, but administration immediately after preparation is recommended. It should not be added to infusion solutions because of the possibility of precipitation.[38][115]

Compatibility Information

Additive Compatibility

Tenoxicam

Test Drug	Mfr	Conc/L or %	Mfr	Conc/L or %	Test Solution	Remarks	Ref	C/I
Cefazolin sodium	FUJ	5 g	RC	200 mg	D5W	Visually compatible with less than 10% loss of both drugs in 48 hr at 25°C and in 72 hr at 4°C in the dark	2441	C
Ceftazidime	LI	5 g	RC	200 mg	D5W[a]	Visually compatible for up to 72 hr with yellow discoloration. 10% loss of ceftazidime in 96 hr and of tenoxicam in 168 hr at 4 and 25°C	2557	C
Ceftazidime	LI	5 g	RC	200 mg	D5W[b]	Visually compatible with about 10% loss of both drugs in 168 hr at 4 and 25°C	2557	C

[a] Tested in PVC containers.

[b] Tested in glass containers.

Selected Revisions October 1, 2012. © Copyright, October 2004.
American Society of Health-System Pharmacists, Inc.

DOI: 10.37573/9781585286850.373

Terbutaline Sulfate
AHFS 12:12.08.12

Products

Terbutaline sulfate is available in 1-mL ampuls. Each mL contains terbutaline sulfate 1 mg, sodium chloride for isotonicity, and hydrochloric acid to adjust the pH.[1(3/04)]

pH

The pH is adjusted to 3 to 5.[1(3/04)] [4]

Osmolality

The injection is isotonic.[1(3/04)]

Administration

Terbutaline sulfate injection is administered subcutaneously only, usually into the lateral deltoid area.[1(3/04)] [4] Intravenous administration is not recommended by the manufacturer[1(3/04)] but has been used in selected patients with careful monitoring.[4]

Stability

Although relatively stable compared to corresponding catecholamines[738], terbutaline sulfate is nonetheless sensitive to light and excessive heat. The injection should be stored at controlled room temperature and protected from light and freezing. Discolored solutions should not be used.[1(3/04)] [4] Terbutaline sulfate is stated to be stable over the pH range of 1 to 7.[4]

Syringes

The stability of terbutaline sulfate (Geigy) 1 mg/mL was studied packaged in polypropylene syringes (Becton Dickinson) fitted with luer-tip caps (Becton Dickinson). The samples were stored at 4°C in the dark, 25°C in the dark, and 25°C with exposure to fluorescent light. Samples stored in the dark at both temperatures were stable, exhibiting a 5 to 6% drug loss in 60 days. The 25°C samples exposed to light showed a 5% loss in 28 days and an 11% loss in 60 days with a yellow discoloration.[1298]

The stability of terbutaline sulfate (Geigy) 1 mg/mL repackaged in syringes was evaluated. A 0.25-mL sample was drawn into each plastic tuberculin syringe (Becton Dickinson) and sealed with a luer-tip cap (Becton Dickinson). Samples were stored at 4 and 24°C with exposure to light and light protection. Little difference was reported in the terbutaline sulfate content among the four storage conditions. Drug losses of 5% or less were observed after seven weeks of storage. Although no discoloration was reported, it may not have been observed in the small sample present in the tuberculin syringe.[1299]

Compatibility Information

Solution Compatibility

Terbutaline sulfate

Test Soln Name	Mfr	Mfr	Conc/L or %	Remarks	Ref	C/I
Dextrose 5%	AB	CI	4 mg	Physically compatible. Calculated 10% loss in 328 hr at 25°C in light	527	C
Dextrose 5%	TR[a]	MRD	30 mg	Under 10% loss in 7 days at 25°C in light	1133	C
Sodium chloride 0.45%	TR[a]	MRD	30 mg	Under 5% loss in 7 days at 25°C in light or at 4°C	1133	C
Sodium chloride 0.9%	TR[a]	MRD	30 mg	Under 6% loss in 7 days at 25°C in light	1133	C
Sodium chloride 0.9%	BA[a]	NVA	100 mg	Solution remained clear with no loss in 23 days at 25°C	2551	C

[a] Tested in PVC containers.

Additive Compatibility

Terbutaline sulfate

Test Drug	Mfr	Conc/L or %	Mfr	Conc/L or %	Test Solution	Remarks	Ref	C/I
Aminophylline	SE	500 mg	CI	4 mg	D5W	Physically compatible. At 25°C, 10% terbutaline loss in 44 hr in light	527	C
Bleomycin sulfate	BR	20 and 30 units	GG	7.5 mg	NS	36% loss of bleomycin activity in 1 week at 4°C	763	I

DOI: 10.37573/9781585286850.374

Drugs in Syringe Compatibility

Terbutaline sulfate

Test Drug	Mfr	Amt	Mfr	Amt	Remarks	Ref	C/I
Doxapram HCl	RB	400 mg/20 mL		0.2 mg/1 mL	Physically compatible with 6% doxapram loss in 24 hr	1177	C

Y-Site Injection Compatibility (1:1 Mixture)

Terbutaline sulfate

Test Drug	Mfr	Conc	Mfr	Conc	Remarks	Ref	C/I
Insulin, regular	LI	0.2 unit/mL[b]	CI	0.02 mg/mL[a]	Physically compatible for 2 hr at 25°C	1395	C

[a] Tested in dextrose 5%.

[b] Tested in sodium chloride 0.9%.

Selected Revisions October 1, 2012. © Copyright, October 1982.
American Society of Health-System Pharmacists, Inc.

Tetracaine Hydrochloride
AHFS 72:00

Products

Tetracaine hydrochloride is available as a preservative-free solution in a concentration of 10 mg/mL (1%) in 2-mL ampules. The product also contains sodium chloride and hydrochloric acid and/or sodium hydroxide to adjust pH in water for injection.[1(4/06)]

Pontocaine brand of tetracaine hydrochloride 10 mg/mL also contains acetone sodium bisulfite.[4]

Tetracaine hydrochloride hyperbaric solutions are available in concentrations of 0.2 and 0.3% in dextrose 6%.[4]

pH

Tetracaine hydrochloride injection has a pH ranging from 3.2 to 6.0.[1(4/06)] Reconstituted tetracaine hydrochloride powder has a pH ranging from 5 to 6 after reconstitution.[4]

Tonicity

Tetracaine hydrochloride 10-mg/mL injection is isotonic.[1(4/06)]

Trade Name(s)

Pontocaine Hydrochloride

Administration

Tetracaine hydrochloride injection is used for prolonged spinal anesthesia. The injection is isobaric having a specific gravity of 1.0060 to 1.0074 at 25°C, which is very similar to spinal fluid. A hyperbaric solution of tetracaine hydrochloride may be prepared by diluting the 10-mg/mL injection in dextrose 10%.[1(4/06) 4]

Tetracaine hydrochloride powder for injection dissolved in spinal fluid is slightly hyperbaric. A hypobaric solution with a specific gravity of 1.000 at 25°C may be prepared by dissolving the tetracaine hydrochloride powder in sterile water for injection at a concentration of 0.1%. A hyperbaric solution of tetracaine hydrochloride may be prepared by dissolving the powder in dextrose 10% to yield a 10-mg/mL solution. The resulting solution is further diluted with an equal volume of cerebrospinal fluid to yield 5 mg/mL of tetracaine hydrochloride and dextrose.[4]

Stability

Tetracaine hydrochloride injection in intact vials should be stored under refrigeration and protected from light. Freezing should be avoided. The injection should not be used if crystals, cloudiness, or discoloration is present.[1(4/06) 4]

Tetracaine hydrochloride 10-mg/mL injection and tetracaine hydrochloride powder in intact containers can be autoclaved at 121°C for 15 minutes to sterilize the exterior of the ampuls. However, autoclaving may increase the occurrence of crystal formation. Ampuls that have been autoclaved but are not used must be discarded and may not be returned to stock.[1(4/06) 4]

Tetracaine hydrochloride in aqueous solutions undergoes hydrolysis slowly that results in the formation of p-butylaminobenzoic acid crystals. Solutions containing crystals should not be used.[4]

Tetracaine hydrochloride stability in aqueous solution was evaluated. Accelerated degradation at elevated temperatures led to a determination that tetracaine hydrochloride in aqueous solution was stable for at least 12 months at 25°C with about 96% remaining. After two years, the concentration had declined to about 89%.[2453] When stored under refrigeration at 4 to 6°C, no loss of tetracaine hydrochloride was detected after 365 days of storage.[2705]

pH Effects

Tetracaine hydrochloride is unstable in both acidic and alkaline media. The pH of maximum stability was found to be 3.8.[2666 2705] Tetracaine hydrochloride mixed with alkali hydroxides or carbonates results in the precipitation of tetracaine base as an oily liquid.[4]

Compatibility Information
Drugs in Syringe Compatibility

Tetracaine HCl

Test Drug	Mfr	Amt	Mfr	Amt	Remarks	Ref	C/I
Clonidine HCl with ketamine HCl	BI PD	0.03 mg/mL 2 mg/mL	SW	2 mg/mL	Diluted to 5 mL with NS. Visually compatible with no new GC/MS peaks in 1 hr at room temperature	1956	C
Ketamine HCl with clonidine HCl	PD BI	2 mg/mL 0.03 mg/mL	SW	2 mg/mL	Diluted to 5 mL with NS. Visually compatible with no new GC/MS peaks in 1 hr at room temperature	1956	C

Selected Revisions October 1, 2012. © Copyright, October 2008. American Society of Health-System Pharmacists, Inc.

DOI: 10.37573/9781585286850.375

Theophylline

AHFS 86:16

Products

Theophylline is available in concentrations ranging from 0.8 to 4 mg/mL (expressed as anhydrous theophylline) premixed in dextrose 5%.[1(7/08)]

pH

From 3.5 to 6.5.[1(7/08)]

Osmolality

Theophylline premixed in dextrose 5% products have osmolalities in the range of 255 to 275 mOsm/kg.[1(7/08)]

Administration

Theophylline may be administered by continuous or intermittent intravenous infusion. Slow administration, not exceeding 20 mg/min, has been recommended. Loading doses are usually given over 20 to 30 minutes.[1(7/08)]

Stability

Theophylline injection should be stored at controlled room temperature and protected from freezing. Avoid excessive heat.[1(7/08)]

At a concentration of 1 g/L in dextrose 5%, theophylline was stable during autoclaving for 20 minutes at 120°C. No decrease in the theophylline content was detected.[1173]

Compatibility Information

Additive Compatibility

Theophylline

Test Drug	Mfr	Conc/L or %	Mfr	Conc/L or %	Test Solution	Remarks	Ref	C/I
Ascorbic acid		1.9 g		2 g	D5W	Yellow discoloration. 8% ascorbic acid loss in 6 hr and 15% in 24 hr. No theophylline loss	1909	I
Cefepime HCl	BR	4 g	BA	800 mg	D5W	Visually compatible. 3% cefepime loss in 24 hr at room temperature and 7 days at 5°C. No theophylline loss	1681	C
Ceftriaxone sodium	RC	40 g	BA[a]	4 g		Yellow color forms immediately. 14% ceftriaxone loss and no theophylline loss in 24 hr	1727	I
Chlorpromazine HCl		200 mg		2 g	D5W	Visually compatible. 7% chlorpromazine and no theophylline loss in 48 hr	1909	C
Fluconazole	PF	1 g	BA	0.4 g	D5W	Fluconazole stable for 72 hr at 25°C in fluorescent light. Theophylline not tested	1676	C
Furosemide		330 mg		2 g	D5W	Visually compatible. Little theophylline and 10% furosemide loss in 48 hr	1909	C
Lidocaine HCl		380 mg		2 g	D5W	Visually compatible with little or no loss of either drug in 48 hr	1909	C
Methylprednisolone sodium succinate	UP	500 mg and 2 g	AB	4 g[b]		Physically compatible. Little theophylline or methylprednisolone alcohol loss in 24 hr at room temperature, but 8% ester hydrolysis	1150	C
Methylprednisolone sodium succinate	UP	500 mg and 2 g	AB	400 mg[b]		Physically compatible. Little theophylline or methylprednisolone alcohol loss in 24 hr at room temperature, but 11% ester hydrolysis	1150	C
Papaverine HCl		160 mg		2 g	D5W	Visually compatible with little or no loss of either drug in 48 hr	1909	C
Verapamil HCl	KN	100 and 400 mg	AB	400 mg and 4 g	D5W	Physically compatible. Little loss of either drug in 24 hr at 24°C in light	1172	C

[a] Tested in PVC containers.

[b] Tested as the premixed infusion solution.

DOI: 10.37573/9781585286850.376

Y-Site Injection Compatibility (1:1 Mixture)

Theophylline

Test Drug	Mfr	Conc	Mfr	Conc	Remarks	Ref	C/I
Acyclovir sodium	BW	5 mg/mL[a]	TR	1.6 mg/mL[a]	Physically compatible for 4 hr at 25°C	1157	C
Ampicillin sodium	WY	20 mg/mL[b]	TR	4 mg/mL	Visually compatible for 6 hr at 25°C	1793	C
Ampicillin sodium–sulbactam sodium	PF	20 mg/mL[b e]	TR	4 mg/mL	Visually compatible for 6 hr at 25°C	1793	C
Aztreonam	BV	20 mg/mL[a]	TR	4 mg/mL	Visually compatible for 6 hr at 25°C	1793	C
Bivalirudin	TMC	5 mg/mL[a]	BA	4 mg/mL[a]	Physically compatible for 4 hr at 23°C	2373	C
Cangrelor tetrasodium	TMC	1 mg/mL[b]		1.6 mg/mL	Physically compatible for 4 hr	3243	C
Cefazolin sodium	SKB	20 mg/mL	TR	4 mg/mL	Visually compatible for 6 hr at 25°C	1793	C
Cefepime HCl	BMS	120 mg/mL[d]		20 mg/mL	Over 25% cefepime loss in 1 hr	2513	I
Cefotetan disodium	STU	40 mg/mL[a]	TR	4 mg/mL	Visually compatible for 6 hr at 25°C	1793	C
Ceftazidime	LI	20 mg/mL	TR	4 mg/mL	Visually compatible for 6 hr at 25°C	1793	C
Ceftazidime	GSK	120 mg/mL[d]		20 mg/mL	Over 25% ceftazidime loss in 1 hr	2513	I
Ceftriaxone sodium	RC	20 mg/mL	TR	4 mg/mL	Visually compatible for 6 hr at 25°C	1793	C
Cisatracurium besylate	GW	0.1, 2, 5 mg/mL[a]	AB	3.2 mg/mL	Physically compatible for 4 hr at 23°C	2074	C
Clindamycin phosphate	UP	12 mg/mL[a]	TR	4 mg/mL	Visually compatible for 6 hr at 25°C	1793	C
Clonidine HCl	BI	18 mcg/mL[b]	ASZ	1 mg/mL	Visually compatible	2642	C
Dexamethasone sodium phosphate	ES	0.08 mg/mL[a]	TR	4 mg/mL	Visually compatible for 6 hr at 25°C	1793	C
Dexmedetomidine HCl	AB	4 mcg/mL[b]	AB	4 mg/mL[a]	Physically compatible for 4 hr at 23°C	2383	C
Diltiazem HCl	MMD	5 mg/mL	AB	0.8 mg/mL[a]	Visually compatible	1807	C
Dobutamine HCl	LI	1 mg/mL[a]	TR	4 mg/mL	Visually compatible for 6 hr at 25°C	1793	C
Dopamine HCl	BA	1.6 mg/mL	TR	4 mg/mL	Visually compatible for 6 hr at 25°C	1793	C
Doxycycline hyclate	ES	1 mg/mL[a]	TR	4 mg/mL	Visually compatible for 6 hr at 25°C	1793	C
Erythromycin lactobionate	AB	3.3 mg/mL[b]	TR	4 mg/mL	Visually compatible for 6 hr at 25°C	1793	C
Famotidine	MSD	0.2 mg/mL[a]	TR	1.6 mg/mL[a]	Physically compatible for 4 hr at 25°C	1188	C
Fenoldopam mesylate	AB	80 mcg/mL[b]	BA	4 mg/mL[a]	Physically compatible for 4 hr at 23°C	2467	C
Fluconazole	RR	2 mg/mL	AMR	1.6 mg/mL[a]	Visually compatible for 24 hr at 28°C under fluorescent light	1760	C
Fluconazole	PF	2 mg/mL	TR	4 mg/mL	Visually compatible for 6 hr at 25°C	1793	C
Gentamicin sulfate	TR	2 mg/mL	TR	4 mg/mL	Visually compatible for 6 hr at 25°C	1793	C
Haloperidol lactate	MN	0.5[a] and 5 mg/mL	TR	1.6 mg/mL[a]	Visually compatible for 24 hr at 21°C	1523	C
Heparin sodium	TR	50 units/mL	TR	4 mg/mL	Visually compatible for 4 hr at 25°C	1793	C
Hetastarch in lactated electrolyte	AB	6%	BA	4 mg/mL[a]	Physically compatible for 4 hr at 23°C	2339	C
Hetastarch in sodium chloride 0.9%	DCC	6%	TR	4 mg/mL[c]	Precipitates after 2 hr at room temperature	1313	I
Hydrocortisone sodium succinate	UP	2 mg/mL[a]	TR	4 mg/mL	Visually compatible for 6 hr at 25°C	1793	C
Lidocaine HCl	TR	4 mg/mL	TR	4 mg/mL	Visually compatible for 6 hr at 25°C	1793	C
Linezolid	PHU	2 mg/mL	BA	4 mg/mL[a]	Physically compatible for 4 hr at 23°C	2264	C

Y-Site Injection Compatibility (1:1 Mixture) (Cont.)

Test Drug	Mfr	Conc	Mfr	Conc	Remarks	Ref	C/I
Methyldopate HCl	ES	5 mg/mL[a]	TR	4 mg/mL	Visually compatible for 6 hr at 25°C	1793	C
Methylprednisolone sodium succinate	UP	2.5 mg/mL[a]	TR	4 mg/mL	Visually compatible for 6 hr at 25°C	1793	C
Metronidazole	MG	5 mg/mL	TR	4 mg/mL	Visually compatible for 6 hr at 25°C	1793	C
Micafungin sodium	ASP	1.5 mg/mL[b]	AB	4 mg/mL	Physically compatible for 4 hr at 23°C	2683	C
Midazolam HCl	RC	1 mg/mL[a]	BA	1.6 mg/mL[a]	Visually compatible for 24 hr at 23°C	1847	C
Milrinone lactate	SW	0.4 mg/mL[a]	AB	1.6 mg/mL[a]	Visually compatible. Little loss of either drug in 4 hr at 23°C	2214	C
Nafcillin sodium	WY	20 mg/mL[a]	TR	4 mg/mL	Visually compatible for 6 hr at 25°C	1793	C
Nitroglycerin	LY	0.2 mg/mL[a]	TR	4 mg/mL	Visually compatible for 6 hr at 25°C	1793	C
Oxaliplatin	SS	0.5 mg/mL[a]	AB	4 mg/mL	Physically compatible for 4 hr at 23°C	2566	C
Penicillin G potassium	RR	40,000 units/mL[a]	TR	4 mg/mL	Visually compatible for 6 hr at 25°C	1793	C
Phenytoin sodium	ES	2 mg/mL[b]	TR	4 mg/mL	Immediately cloudy. Dense precipitate in 6 hr at 25°C	1793	I
Potassium chloride	AB	0.2 mEq/mL[a]	TR	4 mg/mL	Visually compatible for 6 hr at 25°C	1793	C
Ranitidine HCl	GL	1 mg/mL	TR	4 mg/mL	Visually compatible for 6 hr at 25°C	1793	C
Remifentanil HCl	GW	0.025 and 0.25 mg/mL[b]	AB	3.2 mg/mL[a]	Physically compatible for 4 hr at 23°C	2075	C
Sodium nitroprusside	ES	0.2 mg/mL[a]	TR	4 mg/mL	Visually compatible for 6 hr at 25°C protected from light	1793	C
Tigecycline	WY	1 mg/mL[b]		1.6 mg/mL[a]	Physically compatible for 4 hr	2714	C
Tigecycline	ACD, FRK, WY	[f]			Stated to be compatible	2915, 3459, 3460	C
Tobramycin sulfate	LI	0.8 mg/mL[a]	TR	4 mg/mL	Visually compatible for 6 hr at 25°C	1793	C
Vancomycin HCl	LI	6.6 mg/mL[a]	TR	4 mg/mL	Visually compatible for 6 hr at 25°C	1793	C
Vancomycin HCl	LI	10 mg/mL[a]		20 mg/mL	Physically incompatible	3536	I

[a] Tested in dextrose 5%.

[b] Tested in sodium chloride 0.9%.

[c] Tested as the premixed infusion solution.

[d] Tested in sterile water for injection.

[e] Ampicillin component. Ampicillin in a 2:1 fixed-ratio concentration with sulbactam.

[f] Tested in both dextrose 5% and sodium chloride 0.9%.

Selected Revisions May 1, 2020. © Copyright, October 1990.
American Society of Health-System Pharmacists, Inc.

Thiamine Hydrochloride
AHFS 88:08

Products

Thiamine hydrochloride is available in a concentration of 100 mg/mL in 1- and 2-mL vials. Each mL of solution may also contain chlorobutanol 0.5% as an antibacterial preservative and monothioglycerol 0.5%. Sodium hydroxide and/or hydrochloric acid may be added to adjust the pH.[1(6/06)] [4]

pH

From 2.5 to 4.5.[1(6/06)] [17]

Administration

Thiamine hydrochloride injection may be administered by intramuscular or slow intravenous injection. An intradermal test dose has been recommended for patients with suspected thiamine sensitivity.[1(6/06)] [4]

Stability

Thiamine hydrochloride in intact containers should be stored at controlled room temperature and protected from light and freezing.[1(6/06)] [4]

Thiamine hydrochloride under simulated summer conditions in paramedic vehicles was exposed to temperatures ranging from 26 to 38°C over four weeks. Analysis found no loss of the drug under these conditions.[2562]

Thiamine hydrochloride is stated to be incompatible with oxidizing and reducing agents.[4] In solutions with sulfites or

bisulfites, it is rapidly inactivated.[52] [1072] [1925] Oxidation of thiamine hydrochloride results in the formation of the highly blue-colored and biologically inactive compound thiochrome.[734] [1072]

pH Effects

Thiamine hydrochloride is stable in acid solutions, losing activity very slowly at pH 4 or less. It is maximally stable at pH 2.[1072] Thiamine hydrochloride is unstable in neutral or alkaline solutions.[1(6/06)] [4] [1072]

Syringes

Thiamine hydrochloride (Lilly) 100 mg/mL was repackaged in glass syringes (Glaspak), back-fill glass syringes (Hy-Pod), and plastic syringes (Stylex). Half of the syringes were filled with thiamine hydrochloride injection filtered through 5-μm stainless steel depth filters (Extemp filter pin), and the rest were filled with unfiltered drug. The syringes containing 1 mL of thiamine hydrochloride injection were stored protected from light (amber UV-light-inhibiting plastic bags) at 22 to 24°C for 84 days. No color changes were observed, and changes in pH were minimal. Furthermore, no differences between filtered or unfiltered samples occurred, with all solutions retaining approximately 100% over the 84 days.[734]

Sorption

Thiamine hydrochloride (Merck) 30 mg/L did not display significant sorption to a PVC plastic test strip in 24 hours.[12]

Compatibility Information

Solution Compatibility

Thiamine HCl

Test Soln Name	Mfr	Mfr	Conc/L or %	Remarks	Ref	C/I
Dextrose 2.5% in half-strength Ringer's injection	AB		100 mg	Physically compatible	3	C
Dextrose 5% in Ringer's injection	AB		100 mg	Physically compatible	3	C
Dextrose 2.5% in Ringer's injection, lactated	AB		100 mg	Physically compatible	3	C
Dextrose 5% in half-strength Ringer's injection, lactated	AB		100 mg	Physically compatible	3	C
Dextrose 5% in Ringer's injection, lactated	AB		100 mg	Physically compatible	3	C
Dextrose 10% in Ringer's injection, lactated	AB		100 mg	Physically compatible	3	C
Dextrose 2.5% in sodium chloride 0.45%	AB		100 mg	Physically compatible	3	C
Dextrose 2.5% in sodium chloride 0.9%	AB		100 mg	Physically compatible	3	C
Dextrose 5% in sodium chloride 0.225%	AB		100 mg	Physically compatible	3	C
Dextrose 5% in sodium chloride 0.45%	AB		100 mg	Physically compatible	3	C
Dextrose 5% in sodium chloride 0.9%	AB		100 mg	Physically compatible	3	C

DOI: 10.37573/9781585286850.377

Solution Compatibility (Cont.)

Test Soln Name	Mfr	Mfr	Conc/L or %	Remarks	Ref	C/I
Dextrose 10% in sodium chloride 0.9%	AB		100 mg	Physically compatible	3	C
Dextrose 2.5%	AB		100 mg	Physically compatible	3	C
Dextrose 5%	AB		100 mg	Physically compatible	3	C
Dextrose 10%	AB		100 mg	Physically compatible	3	C
Ionosol B in dextrose 5%	AB		100 mg	Physically compatible	3	C
Ionosol MB in dextrose 5%	AB		100 mg	Physically compatible	3	C
Ringer's injection	AB		100 mg	Physically compatible	3	C
Ringer's injection, lactated	AB		100 mg	Physically compatible	3	C
Sodium chloride 0.45%	AB		100 mg	Physically compatible	3	C
Sodium chloride 0.9%	AB		100 mg	Physically compatible	3	C
Sodium lactate ⅙ M	AB		100 mg	Physically compatible	3	C

Drugs in Syringe Compatibility

Thiamine HCl

Test Drug	Mfr	Amt	Mfr	Amt	Remarks	Ref	C/I
Doxapram HCl	RB	400 mg/20 mL		10 mg/2 mL	Physically compatible with 6% doxapram loss in 24 hr	1177	C

Y-Site Injection Compatibility (1:1 Mixture)

Thiamine HCl

Test Drug	Mfr	Conc	Mfr	Conc	Remarks	Ref	C/I
Famotidine	MSD	0.2 mg/mL[a]	ES	100 mg/mL	Physically compatible for 14 hr	1196	C

[a] Tested in dextrose 5%.

Additional Compatibility Information

Parenteral Nutrition Solutions

The stability of thiamine hydrochloride 50 mg/L was studied in representative parenteral nutrition solutions exposed to fluorescent light, indirect sunlight, and direct sunlight for eight hours. One 5-mL vial of multivitamin concentrate (Lyphomed) containing 50 mg of thiamine hydrochloride and also 1 mg of folic acid (Lederle) were added to a liter of parenteral nutrition solution composed of amino acids 4.25%–dextrose 25% (Travenol) with standard electrolytes and trace elements. Thiamine hydrochloride was stable over the eight-hour study period at room temperature under fluorescent light and indirect sunlight, but direct sunlight caused a 26% loss.[842]

A 50% initial drop in thiamine concentration immediately after admixture of multivitamins in a parenteral nutrition solution composed of amino acids, dextrose, electrolytes, and trace elements in PVC bags was reported. The thiamine concentration then remained relatively constant for 120 hours when stored at both 4 and 25°C.[1063]

The stability of numerous vitamins in parenteral nutrition solutions composed of amino acids (Kabi-Vitrum), dextrose 30%, and fat emulsion 20% (Kabi-Vitrum) in a 2:1:1 ratio with electrolytes, trace elements, and both fat- and water-soluble vitamins was reported. The admixtures were stored in darkness at 2 to 8°C for 96 hours with no significant loss of thiamine mononitrate.[1225]

The stability of several vitamins from M.V.I.-12 (Armour) admixed in parenteral nutrition solutions composed of different amino acid products, with or without Intralipid 10%, when stored in glass bottles and PVC bags at 25 and 5°C for 48 hours was reported. Thiamine hydrochloride was stable in the parenteral nutrition solutions prepared with amino acid products without bisulfite.[1431]

The stability of several vitamins following admixture (as M.V.I-12) with four different amino acid products (Novamine, Neopham, FreAmine III, Travasol) with or without Intralipid when stored in glass bottles or PVC bags at 25°C for 48 hours was reported. Exposure to high intensity phototherapy light did not affect thiamine.[487]

The stability of thiamine hydrochloride from a multiple vitamin product in dextrose 5% and sodium chloride 0.9% in PVC and ClearFlex containers was evaluated. Thiamine hydrochloride was stable at 23°C when exposed to or protected from light, exhibiting losses of 11% or less in 24 hours.[1509]

The degradation of vitamins A, B₁, C, and E from Cernevit (Roche) multivitamins in NuTRIflex Lipid Plus (B. Braun) admixtures prepared in ethylene vinyl acetate (EVA) bags and in multilayer bags was evaluated. After storage for up to 72 hours at 4, 21, and 40°C, greater vitamin losses occurred in the EVA bags. Thiamine hydrochloride losses were 25%. In the multilayer bags (presumably a better barrier to oxygen transfer), losses were less. Thiamine hydrochloride losses were 10%.[2618]

The vitamins in Cernevit (Baxter) diluted in three 2-in-1 parenteral nutrition admixtures were tested for stability over 48 hours. Most of the other vitamins, including thiamine hydrochloride, retained their initial concentrations.[2796]

Selected Revisions March 26, 2013. © Copyright, October 1982. American Society of Health-System Pharmacists, Inc.

Thiotepa
AHFS 10:00

Products

Thiotepa is available as a lyophilized powder in single-dose vials containing 15 or 100 mg of the drug.[3367] The contents of the 15- or 100-mg vials should be reconstituted with 1.5 or 10 mL, respectively, of sterile water for injection and mixed manually by repeated inversions.[3367] Each mL of the reconstituted solutions contains 10 mg of thiotepa.[3367] The reconstituted solution should be diluted in an infusion bag with an appropriate volume of sodium chloride 0.9% (e.g., 500 mL for thiotepa doses of 250 to 500 mg; 1000 mL for thiotepa doses exceeding 500 mg) to achieve a solution with a final thiotepa concentration of 0.5 to 1 mg/mL.[3367]

Thiotepa also is available as a lyophilized powder in single-dose vials labeled as containing 15 mg of the drug.[3368] The vial contents should be reconstituted with 1.5 mL of sterile water for injection.[3368] Vials contain a slight overfill to allow for a withdrawable volume of about 1.4 mL (about 14.7 mg) of the reconstituted solution with an approximate concentration of 10.4 mg/mL.[3368] The appropriate dose of the reconstituted solution should be diluted with sodium chloride 0.9% prior to administration.[3368]

pH

The pH of the reconstituted solution of thiotepa has a range of approximately 5.5 to 7.5.[3367] [3368]

Tonicity

Reconstitution with sterile water for injection results in a hypotonic solution; the reconstituted solution should be diluted in sodium chloride 0.9% prior to use.[3367] [3368]

Solutions of thiotepa at concentrations of 0.5 and 1 mg/mL in sodium chloride 0.9% are nearly isotonic; solutions of thiotepa at concentrations of 3 and 5 mg/mL in sodium chloride 0.9% are hypotonic.[2006]

Osmolality

The osmolalities of thiotepa 0.5 and 1 mg/mL in sodium chloride 0.9% are 277 and 269 mOsm/kg, respectively.[2006]

Trade Name(s)

Tepadina

Administration

Thiotepa is administered by rapid intravenous administration or intravenous infusion or by the intracavitary or intravesical route.[3367] [3368]

The final diluted solution of thiotepa must be filtered prior to administration.[3367] [3368] (See Filtration.)

As with other toxic drugs, caution should be exercised in the handling and preparation of thiotepa.[3367] [3368] The use of gloves has been recommended as skin reactions may occur with accidental exposure.[3368] If skin contact with the solution occurs, the exposed area(s) should be washed thoroughly with soap and water; for mucosal membrane contact, the exposed area(s) should be flushed thoroughly with water.[3367] [3368] Procedures for the proper disposal of thiotepa should be considered.[3367]

Stability

Thiotepa is a white powder that forms a clear solution upon reconstitution.[3367] One manufacturer notes that reconstituted solutions free of particulate matter may exhibit opalescence; however, such solutions still may be diluted for administration.[3367]

Intact vials should be stored at 2 to 8°C.[3367] [3368] One manufacturer (West-Ward) states that thiotepa should be protected from light at all times.[3368] Another manufacturer (Amneal Biosciences) states that thiotepa should not be frozen.[3367]

The reconstituted solution of thiotepa is stable at 2 to 8°C for 8 hours.[3367] [3368] Diluted solutions for infusion should be used immediately;[3367] [3368] however, one manufacturer has stated that diluted solutions for infusion are stable for 24 hours at 2 to 8°C or 4 hours at 25°C.[3367]

Thiotepa may undergo polymerization forming insoluble derivatives.[1369] Solutions should be visually inspected for particulate matter and discoloration prior to administration; diluted solutions should be used only if free of visible particulate matter.[3367] [3368]

Thiotepa is stable in alkaline media, but unstable in acidic media,[3367] [3368] undergoing increased rates of hydrolysis.[1389]

Syringes

Thiotepa reconstituted to a concentration of 10 mg/mL with sterile water for injection was found to be stable for 24 hours under refrigeration at 8°C and at room temperature of 23°C in both the original vials and transferred to plastic syringes.[2006]

Filtration

One manufacturer of thiotepa (Tepadina, Amneal Biosciences) recommends filtration of the diluted solution for infusion through an infusion set containing a 0.2-μm inline filter.[3367] Another manufacturer of thiotepa (West-Ward) recommends filtration of the diluted solution for infusion through a 0.22-μm filter (i.e., polysulfone membrane [Sterile Aerodisc, Gelman] or triton-free mixed ester of cellulose/polyvinyl chloride [PVC] [Millex-GS, Millipore]) to eliminate haze; solutions that remain opaque or precipitate after such filtration should not be used.[3368] Filtration of thiotepa does not alter potency.[3367] [3368]

Thiotepa 10 to 300 mcg/mL exhibited no loss due to sorption to either cellulose nitrate/cellulose acetate ester (Millex OR) or Teflon (Millex FG) filters.[1415] [1416]

DOI: 10.37573/9781585286850.378

Compatibility Information

Solution Compatibility

Thiotepa

Test Soln Name	Mfr	Mfr	Conc/L or %	Remarks	Ref	C/I
Dextrose 5%	BA[a] , MG[b]	IMM	0.5 g	Physically stable. Losses of 10% or less in 8 hr at 4 and 23°C and 17% in 24 hr	2007	I
Dextrose 5%	BA[a] , MG[b]	IMM	5 g	Physically stable with losses of less than 10% in 14 days at 4°C and in 3 days at 23°C	2007	C
Sodium chloride 0.9%	BA[a]	IMM	1 and 3 g	Physically stable with 7 to 10% loss in 24 hr at 25°C and 4% or less in 48 hr at 4°C	2077	C
Sodium chloride 0.9%	BA[a]	IMM	0.5 g	Physically stable but up to 7% loss in 8 hr with substantial chloro-adduct formation. Up to 13% loss in 24 hr at 25°C	2077	I
Sodium chloride 0.9%	BA[a]	IMM	0.5 g	Physically stable with 4% or less loss in 48 hr at 8°C	2077	C
Sodium chloride 0.9%		AMB	0.5 to 1 g	Stable for 24 hr at 2 to 8°C or 4 hr at 25°C	3367	C

[a] Tested in PVC containers.

[b] Tested in polyolefin containers.

Additive Compatibility

Thiotepa

Test Drug	Mfr	Conc/L or %	Mfr	Conc/L or %	Test Solution	Remarks	Ref	C/I
Cisplatin		200 mg		1 g	NS	Yellow precipitation	1379	I

Y-Site Injection Compatibility (1:1 Mixture)

Thiotepa

Test Drug	Mfr	Conc	Mfr	Conc	Remarks	Ref	C/I
Acyclovir sodium	BW	7 mg/mL[a]	IMM[c]	1 mg/mL[a]	Physically compatible for 4 hr at 23°C	1861	C
Allopurinol sodium	BW	3 mg/mL[b]	LE[d]	1 mg/mL[c]	Physically compatible for 4 hr at 22°C	1686	C
Amifostine	USB	10 mg/mL[a]	LE[d]	1 mg/mL[a]	Physically compatible for 4 hr at 23°C	1845	C
Amikacin sulfate	DU	5 mg/mL[a]	IMM[c]	1 mg/mL[a]	Physically compatible for 4 hr at 23°C	1861	C
Aminophylline	AMR	2.5 mg/mL[a]	IMM[c]	1 mg/mL[a]	Physically compatible for 4 hr at 23°C	1861	C
Amphotericin B	APC	0.6 mg/mL[a]	IMM[c]	1 mg/mL[a]	Physically compatible for 4 hr at 23°C	1861	C
Ampicillin sodium	WY	20 mg/mL[b]	IMM[c]	1 mg/mL[a]	Physically compatible for 4 hr at 23°C	1861	C
Ampicillin sodium–sulbactam sodium	RR	20 mg/mL[b g]	IMM[c]	1 mg/mL[a]	Physically compatible for 4 hr at 23°C	1861	C
Aztreonam	SQ	40 mg/mL[a]	LE[d]	1 mg/mL[a]	Physically compatible for 4 hr at 23°C	1758	C
Aztreonam	SQ	40 mg/mL[a]	IMM[c]	1 mg/mL[a]	Physically compatible for 4 hr at 23°C	1861	C
Bleomycin sulfate	MJ	1 unit/mL[b]	IMM[c]	1 mg/mL[a]	Physically compatible for 4 hr at 23°C	1861	C
Bumetanide	RC	0.04 mg/mL[a]	IMM[c]	1 mg/mL[a]	Physically compatible for 4 hr at 23°C	1861	C
Buprenorphine HCl	RKC	0.04 mg/mL[a]	IMM[c]	1 mg/mL[a]	Physically compatible for 4 hr at 23°C	1861	C
Butorphanol tartrate	APC	0.04 mg/mL[a]	IMM[c]	1 mg/mL[a]	Physically compatible for 4 hr at 23°C	1861	C
Calcium gluconate	AMR	40 mg/mL[a]	IMM[c]	1 mg/mL[a]	Physically compatible for 4 hr at 23°C	1861	C

Y-Site Injection Compatibility (1:1 Mixture) (Cont.)

Test Drug	Mfr	Conc	Mfr	Conc	Remarks	Ref	C/I
Carboplatin	BMS	5 mg/mL[a]	IMM[c]	1 mg/mL[a]	Physically compatible for 4 hr at 23°C	1861	C
Carmustine	BMS	1.5 mg/mL[a]	IMM[c]	1 mg/mL[a]	Physically compatible for 4 hr at 23°C	1861	C
Cefazolin sodium	MAR	20 mg/mL[a]	IMM[c]	1 mg/mL[a]	Physically compatible for 4 hr at 23°C	1861	C
Cefotaxime sodium	HO	20 mg/mL[a]	IMM[c]	1 mg/mL[a]	Physically compatible for 1 hr at 23°C	1861	C
Cefotetan disodium	STU	20 mg/mL[a]	IMM[c]	1 mg/mL[a]	Physically compatible for 4 hr at 23°C	1861	C
Cefoxitin sodium	ME	20 mg/mL[a]	IMM[c]	1 mg/mL[a]	Physically compatible for 4 hr at 23°C	1861	C
Ceftazidime	LI	40 mg/mL[a]	IMM[c]	1 mg/mL[a]	Physically compatible for 4 hr at 23°C	1861	C
Ceftriaxone sodium	RC	20 mg/mL[a]	IMM[c]	1 mg/mL[a]	Physically compatible for 4 hr at 23°C	1861	C
Cefuroxime sodium	LI	30 mg/mL[a]	IMM[c]	1 mg/mL[a]	Physically compatible for 4 hr at 23°C	1861	C
Chlorpromazine HCl	SCN	2 mg/mL[a]	IMM[c]	1 mg/mL[a]	Physically compatible for 4 hr at 23°C	1861	C
Ciprofloxacin	MI	1 mg/mL[a]	IMM[c]	1 mg/mL[a]	Physically compatible for 4 hr at 23°C	1861	C
Cisplatin	BMS	1 mg/mL	IMM[c]	1 mg/mL[a]	White cloudiness appears in 4 hr at 23°C	1861	I
Clindamycin phosphate	AST	10 mg/mL[a]	IMM[c]	1 mg/mL[a]	Physically compatible for 4 hr at 23°C	1861	C
Cyclophosphamide	MJ	10 mg/mL[a]	IMM[c]	1 mg/mL[a]	Physically compatible for 4 hr at 23°C	1861	C
Cytarabine	CET	50 mg/mL	IMM[c]	1 mg/mL[a]	Physically compatible for 4 hr at 23°C	1861	C
Dacarbazine	MI	4 mg/mL[a]	IMM[c]	1 mg/mL[a]	Physically compatible for 4 hr at 23°C	1861	C
Dactinomycin	ME	0.01 mg/mL[a]	IMM[c]	1 mg/mL[a]	Physically compatible for 4 hr at 23°C	1861	C
Daunorubicin HCl	WY	1 mg/mL[a]	IMM[c]	1 mg/mL[a]	Physically compatible for 4 hr at 23°C	1861	C
Dexamethasone sodium phosphate	AMR	1 mg/mL[a]	IMM[c]	1 mg/mL[a]	Physically compatible for 4 hr at 23°C	1861	C
Diphenhydramine HCl	WY	2 mg/mL[a]	IMM[c]	1 mg/mL[a]	Physically compatible for 4 hr at 23°C	1861	C
Dobutamine HCl	LI	4 mg/mL[a]	IMM[c]	1 mg/mL[a]	Physically compatible for 4 hr at 23°C	1861	C
Dopamine HCl	AST	3.2 mg/mL[a]	IMM[c]	1 mg/mL[a]	Physically compatible for 4 hr at 23°C	1861	C
Doxorubicin HCl	CHI	2 mg/mL	IMM[c]	1 mg/mL[a]	Physically compatible for 4 hr at 23°C	1861	C
Doxycycline hyclate	LY	1 mg/mL[a]	IMM[c]	1 mg/mL[a]	Physically compatible for 4 hr at 23°C	1861	C
Droperidol	JN	0.4 mg/mL[a]	IMM[c]	1 mg/mL[a]	Physically compatible for 4 hr at 23°C	1861	C
Enalaprilat	ME	0.1 mg/mL[a]	IMM[c]	1 mg/mL[a]	Physically compatible for 4 hr at 23°C	1861	C
Etoposide	BR	0.4 mg/mL[a]	IMM[c]	1 mg/mL[a]	Physically compatible for 4 hr at 23°C	1861	C
Etoposide phosphate	BR	5 mg/mL[a]	IMM[c]	1 mg/mL[a]	Physically compatible for 4 hr at 23°C	2218	C
Famotidine	ME	2 mg/mL[a]	IMM[c]	1 mg/mL[a]	Physically compatible for 4 hr at 23°C	1861	C
Filgrastim	AMG	30 mcg/mL[a]	LE[d]	1 mg/mL[a]	Particles and filaments form immediately	1687	I
Floxuridine	RC	3 mg/mL[a]	IMM[c]	1 mg/mL[a]	Physically compatible for 4 hr at 23°C	1861	C
Fluconazole	RR	2 mg/mL	IMM[c]	1 mg/mL[a]	Physically compatible for 4 hr at 23°C	1861	C
Fludarabine phosphate	BX	1 mg/mL[a]	IMM[c]	1 mg/mL[a]	Physically compatible for 4 hr at 23°C	1861	C
Fluorouracil	AD	16 mg/mL[a]	IMM[c]	1 mg/mL[a]	Physically compatible for 4 hr at 23°C	1861	C
Furosemide	AMR	3 mg/mL[a]	IMM[c]	1 mg/mL[a]	Physically compatible for 4 hr at 23°C	1861	C
Gallium nitrate	FUJ	0.4 mg/mL[a]	IMM[c]	1 mg/mL[a]	Physically compatible for 4 hr at 23°C	1861	C

Y-Site Injection Compatibility (1:1 Mixture) (Cont.)

Test Drug	Mfr	Conc	Mfr	Conc	Remarks	Ref	C/I
Ganciclovir sodium	SY	20 mg/mL[a]	IMM[c]	1 mg/mL[a]	Physically compatible for 4 hr at 23°C	1861	C
Gemcitabine HCl	LI	10 mg/mL[b]	IMM[c]	1 mg/mL[b]	Physically compatible for 4 hr at 23°C	2226	C
Gentamicin sulfate	ES	5 mg/mL[a]	IMM[c]	1 mg/mL[a]	Physically compatible for 4 hr at 23°C	1861	C
Granisetron HCl	SKB	0.05 mg/mL[a]	IMM[c]	1 mg/mL[a]	Physically compatible for 4 hr at 23°C	1861	C
Haloperidol lactate	MN	0.2 mg/mL[a]	IMM[c]	1 mg/mL[a]	Physically compatible for 4 hr at 23°C	1861	C
Heparin sodium	ES	100 units/mL[a]	IMM[c]	1 mg/mL[a]	Physically compatible for 4 hr at 23°C	1861	C
Hydrocortisone sodium succinate	UP	1 mg/mL[a]	IMM[c]	1 mg/mL[a]	Physically compatible for 4 hr at 23°C	1861	C
Hydromorphone HCl	AST	0.5 mg/mL[a]	IMM[c]	1 mg/mL[a]	Physically compatible for 4 hr at 23°C	1861	C
Hydroxyzine HCl	ES	4 mg/mL[a]	IMM[c]	1 mg/mL[a]	Physically compatible for 4 hr at 23°C	1861	C
Idarubicin HCl	AD	0.5 mg/mL[a]	IMM[c]	1 mg/mL[a]	Physically compatible for 4 hr at 23°C	1861	C
Ifosfamide	MJ	25 mg/mL[a]	IMM[c]	1 mg/mL[a]	Physically compatible for 4 hr at 23°C	1861	C
Imipenem–cilastatin sodium	ME	10 mg/mL[a j]	IMM[c]	1 mg/mL[a]	Physically compatible for 4 hr at 23°C	1861	C
Leucovorin calcium	LE	2 mg/mL[a]	IMM[c]	1 mg/mL[a]	Physically compatible for 4 hr at 23°C	1861	C
Lorazepam	WY	0.1 mg/mL[a]	IMM[c]	1 mg/mL[a]	Physically compatible for 4 hr at 23°C	1861	C
Magnesium sulfate	AST	100 mg/mL[a]	IMM[c]	1 mg/mL[a]	Physically compatible for 4 hr at 23°C	1861	C
Mannitol	BA	15%	IMM[c]	1 mg/mL[a]	Physically compatible for 4 hr at 23°C	1861	C
Melphalan HCl	BW	0.1 mg/mL[b]	LE[d]	10 mg/mL[b]	Physically compatible for 3 hr at 22°C	1557	C
Meperidine HCl	WY	4 mg/mL[a]	IMM[c]	1 mg/mL[a]	Physically compatible for 4 hr at 23°C	1861	C
Mesna	MJ	10 mg/mL[a]	IMM[c]	1 mg/mL[a]	Physically compatible for 4 hr at 23°C	1861	C
Methotrexate sodium	LE	15 mg/mL[a]	IMM[c]	1 mg/mL[a]	Physically compatible for 4 hr at 23°C	1861	C
Methylprednisolone sodium succinate	AB	5 mg/mL[a]	IMM[c]	1 mg/mL[a]	Physically compatible for 4 hr at 23°C	1861	C
Metoclopramide HCl	RB	5 mg/mL	IMM[c]	1 mg/mL[a]	Physically compatible for 4 hr at 23°C	1861	C
Metronidazole	BA	5 mg/mL	IMM[c]	1 mg/mL[a]	Physically compatible for 4 hr at 23°C	1861	C
Mitomycin	BMS	0.5 mg/mL	IMM[c]	1 mg/mL[a]	Physically compatible for 4 hr at 23°C	1861	C
Mitoxantrone HCl	IMM	0.5 mg/mL[a]	IMM[c]	1 mg/mL[a]	Physically compatible for 4 hr at 23°C	1861	C
Morphine sulfate	AST	1 mg/mL[a]	IMM[c]	1 mg/mL[a]	Physically compatible for 4 hr at 23°C	1861	C
Nalbuphine HCl	AST	10 mg/mL	IMM[c]	1 mg/mL[a]	Physically compatible for 4 hr at 23°C	1861	C
Ondansetron HCl	GL	1 mg/mL[a]	IMM[c]	1 mg/mL[a]	Physically compatible for 4 hr at 23°C	1861	C
Paclitaxel	MJ	0.6 mg/mL[a]	IMM[c]	1 mg/mL[a]	Physically compatible for 4 hr at 23°C	1861	C
Piperacillin sodium–tazobactam sodium	LE[e]	40 mg/mL[a h]	LE[d]	1 mg/mL[a]	Physically compatible for 4 hr at 22°C	1688	C
Potassium chloride	AMR	0.1 mEq/mL[a]	IMM[c]	1 mg/mL[a]	Physically compatible for 4 hr at 23°C	1861	C
Prochlorperazine edisylate	SCN	0.5 mg/mL[a]	IMM[c]	1 mg/mL[a]	Physically compatible for 4 hr at 23°C	1861	C
Promethazine HCl	WY	2 mg/mL[a]	IMM[c]	1 mg/mL[a]	Physically compatible for 4 hr at 23°C	1861	C
Ranitidine HCl	GL	2 mg/mL[a]	IMM[c]	1 mg/mL[a]	Physically compatible for 4 hr at 23°C	1861	C

Y-Site Injection Compatibility (1:1 Mixture) (Cont.)

Test Drug	Mfr	Conc	Mfr	Conc	Remarks	Ref	C/I
Sodium bicarbonate	AB	1 mEq/mL	IMM[c]	1 mg/mL[a]	Physically compatible for 4 hr at 23°C	1861	C
Streptozocin	UP	40 mg/mL[a]	IMM[c]	1 mg/mL[a]	Physically compatible for 4 hr at 23°C	1861	C
Teniposide	BR	0.1 mg/mL[a]	LE[d]	1 mg/mL[a]	Physically compatible for 4 hr at 23°C	1725	C
Tobramycin sulfate	LI	5 mg/mL[a]	IMM[c]	1 mg/mL[a]	Physically compatible for 4 hr at 23°C	1861	C
TPN #193[f]			IMM[c]	1 mg/mL[a]	Physically compatible for 4 hr at 23°C	1861	C
Trimethoprim–sulfamethoxazole	ES	0.8 mg/mL[a] [i]	IMM[c]	1 mg/mL[a]	Physically compatible for 4 hr at 23°C	1861	C
Vancomycin HCl	AB	10 mg/mL[a]	IMM[c]	1 mg/mL[a]	Physically compatible for 4 hr at 23°C	1861	C
Vinblastine sulfate	LI	0.12 mg/mL[a]	IMM[c]	1 mg/mL[a]	Physically compatible for 4 hr at 23°C	1861	C
Vincristine sulfate	LI	0.05 mg/mL[a]	IMM[c]	1 mg/mL[a]	Physically compatible for 4 hr at 23°C	1861	C
Vinorelbine tartrate	BW	1 mg/mL[b]	LE[d]	10 mg/mL[b]	Immediate cloudiness with particles	1558	I
Zidovudine	BW	4 mg/mL[a]	IMM[c]	1 mg/mL[a]	Physically compatible for 4 hr at 23°C	1861	C

[a] Tested in dextrose 5%.

[b] Tested in sodium chloride 0.9%.

[c] Lyophilized formulation tested.

[d] Powder fill formulation tested.

[e] Test performed using the formulation WITHOUT edetate disodium.

[f] Refer to Appendix for the composition of parenteral nutrition solutions. TPN indicates a 2-in-1 admixture.

[g] Ampicillin component. Ampicillin in a 2:1 fixed-ratio concentration with sulbactam.

[h] Piperacillin sodium component. Piperacillin sodium in an 8:1 fixed-ratio concentration with sulfamethoxazole.

[i] Trimethoprim component. Trimethoprim in a 1:5 fixed-ratio concentration with sulfamethoxazole.

[j] Not specified whether concentration refers to single component versus combined components.

Tigecycline
AHFS 8:12.24.12

Products

Several different formulations of tigecycline are available and excipients vary among them.[2915] [3459] [3460] Some formulation differences have been demonstrated to result in some differing compatibilities.[2951] [3459] [3460]

Tigecycline is available as a 50-mg orange lyophilized powder or cake in single-dose (unpreserved) vials containing lactose monohydrate 100 mg (Tygacil, Wyeth),[2915] maltose monohydrate 100 mg (Accord),[3459] or arginine 82.6 mg (Fresenius Kabi).[3460] In each formulation, the pH is adjusted with hydrochloric acid and, if necessary, sodium hydroxide.[2915] [3459] [3460]

Each 50-mg vial should be reconstituted with 5.3 mL of sodium chloride 0.9%; dextrose 5%; or Ringer's injection, lactated.[2915] [3459] [3460] The vials contain an excess of drug, and this reconstitution volume yields a reconstituted solution with a tigecycline concentration of 10 mg/mL.[2915] [3459] [3460] Vials should be swirled gently until the drug has dissolved.[2915] [3459] [3460] The reconstituted solution must be further diluted prior to administration.[2915] [3459] [3460] The appropriate volume of the reconstituted solution should be withdrawn from the vial(s) and transferred to a 100-mL infusion bag of sodium chloride 0.9%; dextrose 5%; or Ringer's injection, lactated to yield a solution for infusion with a maximum tigecycline concentration of 1 mg/mL.[2915] [3459] [3460] The reconstituted solution should be yellow to orange; the solution should be discarded if it does not have the correct color.[2915] [3459] [3460]

Trade Name(s)

Tygacil

Administration

Tigecycline is administered by intravenous infusion over 30 to 60 minutes only after dilution of the reconstituted solution.[2915] [3459] [3460]

The diluted solution for infusion may be administered through a dedicated intravenous line or through a Y-site.[2915] [3459] [3460] If a common infusion line is being used to administer other drugs in addition to tigecycline, the manufacturer states that the line should be flushed prior to and following infusion of tigecycline with sodium chloride 0.9%; dextrose 5%; or Ringer's injection, lactated.[2915] [3459] [3460] The solution used for flushing should be compatible both with tigecycline and with any other drug administered via the line.[2915] [3459] [3460]

Stability

Intact vials of tigecycline should be stored at controlled room temperature.[2915] [3459] [3460] The reconstituted solution of tigecycline may be stored at room temperature (not exceeding 25°C) for up to 24 hours (up to 6 hours as the reconstituted solution in the vial with the remaining time in the infusion bag).[2915] [3459] [3460] If storage conditions after reconstitution exceed 25°C, the drug should be diluted as directed and used immediately.[2915] [3459] [3460] If further diluted immediately after reconstitution, a solution diluted for infusion in sodium chloride 0.9% or dextrose 5% may be stored for up to 48 hours at 2 to 8°C.[2915] [3459] [3460]

The reconstituted solution should be yellow to orange; solutions should be inspected for particulate matter and discoloration (e.g., the formation of a green or black discoloration).[2915] [3459] [3460] Discolored solutions should be discarded.[2915] [3459] [3460]

Compatibility Information
Solution Compatibility

Tigecycline

Test Soln Name	Mfr	Mfr	Conc/L or %	Remarks	Ref	C/I
Dextrose 5%		WY	1 g	Physically compatible for 4 hr	2714	C
Dextrose 5%		ACD, FRK, WY	0.5 and 1 g	Stable for up to 48 hr at 2 to 8°C	2915, 3459, 3460	C
Dextrose 5% in Ringer's injection, lactated		WY	1 g	Physically compatible for 4 hr	2714	C
Dextrose 5% in sodium chloride 0.9%		WY	1 g	Physically compatible for 4 hr	2714	C
Plasma-Lyte 56 in dextrose 5%	BA	WY	1 g	Physically compatible for 4 hr	2714	C
Ringer's injection, lactated		WY	1 g	Physically compatible for 4 hr	2714	C
Ringer's injection, lactated		ACD, FRK, WY		Stated to be compatible	2915, 3459, 3460	C
Sodium chloride 0.9%		ACD, FRK, WY	0.5 and 1 g	Stable for up to 48 hr at 2 to 8°C	2915, 3459, 3460	C

DOI: 10.37573/9781585286850.379

Y-Site Injection Compatibility (1:1 Mixture)

Tigecycline

Test Drug	Mfr	Conc	Mfr	Conc	Remarks	Ref	C/I
Amikacin sulfate		5 mg/mL[b]	WY	1 mg/mL[b]	Physically compatible for 4 hr	2714	C
Amikacin[k]			ACD, FRK, WY	[h]	Stated to be compatible	2915, 3459, 3460	C
Amphotericin B		2 mg/mL[a]	WY	1 mg/mL[b]	Immediate cloudiness with particulates in 1 hr	2714	I
Amphotericin B			ACD, FRK, WY		Stated to be incompatible	2915, 3459, 3460	I
Amphotericin B lipid complex	ENZ	2 mg/mL[a]	WY	1 mg/mL[b]	Incompatible with sodium chloride diluent	2714	I
Amphotericin B lipid complex			ACD, FRK, WY		Stated to be incompatible	2915, 3459, 3460	I
Azithromycin		2 mg/mL[b]	WY	1 mg/mL[b]	Physically compatible for 4 hr	2714	C
Aztreonam		20 mg/mL[b]	WY	1 mg/mL[b]	Physically compatible for 4 hr	2714	C
Cangrelor tetrasodium	TMC	1 mg/mL[b]		1 mg/mL[b]	Physically compatible for 4 hr	3243	C
Cefepime HCl	ELN	40 mg/mL[b]	WY	1 mg/mL[b]	Physically compatible for 4 hr	2714	C
Cefotaxime sodium		40 mg/mL[b]	WY	1 mg/mL[b]	Physically compatible for 4 hr	2714	C
Ceftazidime		40 mg/mL[b]	WY	1 mg/mL[b]	Physically compatible for 4 hr	2714	C
Ceftolozane sulfate–tazobactam sodium	CUB	10 mg/mL[h i]	PF	1 mg/mL[h]	Physically compatible for 2 hr	3262	C
Ceftriaxone sodium		40 mg/mL[b]	WY	1 mg/mL[b]	Physically compatible for 4 hr	2714	C
Chlorpromazine HCl		1 mg/mL[b]	WY	1 mg/mL[b]	Precipitates immediately	2714	I
Ciprofloxacin		1 mg/mL[b]	WY	1 mg/mL[b]	Physically compatible for 4 hr	2714	C
Diazepam			ACD, FRK, WY		Stated to be incompatible	2915, 3459, 3460	I
Dobutamine HCl		0.2 and 1 mg/mL[b]	WY	1 mg/mL[b]	Physically compatible for 4 hr	2714	C
Dobutamine[k]			ACD, FRK, WY	[h]	Stated to be compatible	2915, 3459, 3460	C
Dopamine HCl		1.6 mg/mL[b]	WY	1 mg/mL[b]	Physically compatible for 4 hr	2714	C
Dopamine HCl			ACD, FRK, WY	[h]	Stated to be compatible	2915, 3459, 3460	C
Doripenem	JJ	5 mg/mL[a b]	WY	1 mg/mL[a b]	Physically compatible for 4 hr at 23°C	2743	C
Epinephrine HCl		4 mcg/mL[b]	WY	1 mg/mL[b]	Physically compatible for 4 hr	2714	C
Ertapenem sodium		20 mg/mL[b]	WY	1 mg/mL[b]	Physically compatible for 4 hr	2714	C
Esomeprazole[k]			ACD, FRK, WY		Stated to be incompatible	2915, 3459, 3460	I
Fluconazole		2 mg/mL	WY	1 mg/mL[b]	Physically compatible for 4 hr	2714	C
Gentamicin sulfate		1.4 mg/mL[b]	WY	1 mg/mL[b]	Physically compatible for 4 hr	2714	C
Gentamicin[k]			ACD, FRK, WY	[h]	Stated to be compatible	2915, 3459, 3460	C
Haloperidol lactate		0.2 mg/mL[b]	WY	1 mg/mL[b]	Physically compatible for 4 hr	2714	C
Haloperidol[k]			ACD, WY	[h]	Stated to be compatible	2915, 3459	C
Haloperidol[k]			FRK		Stated to be incompatible	3460	I

Y-Site Injection Compatibility (1:1 Mixture) (Cont.)

Test Drug	Mfr	Conc	Mfr	Conc	Remarks	Ref	C/I
Heparin sodium		10 units/mL	WY	1 mg/mL[b]	Physically compatible for 4 hr	2714	C
Heparin sodium		100 units/mL[b]	WY	1 mg/mL[b]	Physically compatible for 4 hr	2714	C
Imipenem–cilastatin sodium		2.5 mg/mL[b g]	WY	1 mg/mL[b]	Physically compatible for 4 hr	2714, 2917	C
Isavuconazonium sulfate	ASP	1.5 mg/mL[h]	PF	1 mg/mL[h]	Physically compatible for 2 hr	3263	C
Letermovir	ME	[a]		[a]	Physically compatible	3398	C
Lidocaine HCl		200 mg/mL	WY	1 mg/mL[b]	Physically compatible for 4 hr	2714	C
Lidocaine HCl			ACD, FRK, WY	[h]	Stated to be compatible	2915, 3459, 3460	C
Linezolid	PF	2 mg/mL	WY	1 mg/mL[b]	Physically compatible for 4 hr	2714	C
Meropenem–vaborbactam	TMC	8 mg/mL[b j]	WY	1 mg/mL[b]	Physically compatible for 3 hr at 20 to 25°C	3380	C
Methylprednisolone sodium succinate		20 mg/mL[b]	WY	1 mg/mL[b]	Microparticulates form	2714	I
Metoclopramide HCl		5 mg/mL	WY	1 mg/mL[b]	Physically compatible for 4 hr	2714	C
Metoclopramide[k]			ACD, FRK, WY	[h]	Stated to be compatible	2915, 3459, 3460	C
Morphine[k]			ACD, FRK, WY	[h]	Stated to be compatible	2915, 3459, 3460	C
Norepinephrine[k]			ACD, FRK, WY	[h]	Stated to be compatible	2915, 3459, 3460	C
Omeprazole[k]			ACD, FRK, WY		Stated to be incompatible	2915, 3459, 3460	I
Piperacillin sodium–tazobactam sodium	[c]	3 mg/mL[b e]	WY	1 mg/mL[b]	Physically compatible for 4 hr	2714	C
Piperacillin–tazobactam[k]	[f]		ACD, WY	[h]	Stated to be compatible	2915, 3459	C
Plazomicin sulfate	ACH	24 mg/mL[h]	PF	1 mg/mL[h]	Physically compatible for 1 hr at 20 to 25°C	3432	C
Potassium chloride		0.3 mEq/mL[b]	WY	1 mg/mL[b]	Physically compatible for 4 hr	2714	C
Potassium chloride			ACD, FRK, WY	[h]	Stated to be compatible	2915, 3459, 3460	C
Propofol			ACD, WY	[h]	Stated to be compatible	2915, 3459	C
Propofol			FRK	[a]	Stated to be compatible	3460	C
Ranitidine HCl		0.6 mg/mL[b]	WY	1 mg/mL[b]	Physically compatible for 4 hr	2714	C
Ranitidine HCl			ACD, FRK, WY	[h]	Stated to be compatible	2915, 3459, 3460	C
Tedizolid phosphate	CUB	0.8 mg/mL[b]	PF	1 mg/mL[b]	Physically compatible for 2 hr	3244	C
Telavancin HCl	ASP	7.5 mg/mL[a b d]	WY	1 mg/mL[a b d]	Physically compatible for 2 hr	2830	C
Theophylline		1.6 mg/mL[a]	WY	1 mg/mL[b]	Physically compatible for 4 hr	2714	C
Theophylline			ACD, FRK, WY	[h]	Stated to be compatible	2915, 3459, 3460	C
Tobramycin sulfate		2.5 mg/mL[b]	WY	1 mg/mL[b]	Physically compatible for 4 hr	2714	C
Tobramycin[k]			ACD, FRK, WY	[h]	Stated to be compatible	2915, 3459, 3460	C

Y-Site Injection Compatibility (1:1 Mixture) (Cont.)

Test Drug	Mfr	Conc	Mfr	Conc	Remarks	Ref	C/I
Vancomycin HCl		5 mg/mL[b]	WY	1 mg/mL[b]	Physically compatible for 4 hr	2714	C
Voriconazole	PF	2 mg/mL[b]	WY	1 mg/mL[b]	Microparticulates form	2714	I

[a] Tested in dextrose 5%.

[b] Tested in sodium chloride 0.9%.

[c] Test performed using the formulation WITHOUT edetate disodium.

[d] Tested in Ringer's injection, lactated.

[e] Piperacillin component. Piperacillin in an 8:1 fixed-ratio concentration with tazobactam.

[f] Test performed using the formulation WITH edetate disodium.

[g] Imipenem component. Imipenem in a 1:1 fixed-ratio concentration with cilastatin.

[h] Tested in both dextrose 5% and sodium chloride 0.9%.

[i] Ceftolozane component. Ceftolozane in a 2:1 fixed-ratio concentration with tazobactam.

[j] Meropenem component. Meropenem in a 1:1 fixed-ratio concentration with vaborbactam.

[k] Salt not specified.

Additional Compatibility Information

Peritoneal Dialysis Solutions

Tigecycline (Pfizer) was evaluated for stability in Dianeal PD-4 with dextrose 1.5% (Baxter) and Extraneal with icodextrin 7.5% (Baxter) at a concentration of 2 mg/L with bags stored at 4, 25, and 37°C.[3195] The drug also was evaluated for stability in 2-compartment pH-neutral Balance with dextrose 1.5% (Fresenius).[3195] Bags of 2-compartment pH-neutral Balance with dextrose 1.5% contained tigecycline 4 mg/L in the non-dextrose (i.e., buffer solution) compartment for storage at 4 and 25°C; for bags intended for storage at 37°C, the initial concentration of tigecycline in the non-dextrose compartment also was 4 mg/L; however, the 2 compartments were combined immediately prior to storage at 37°C for a final tigecycline concentration of 2 mg/L.[3195] No color change or precipitation was noted on visual assessment and no meaningful pH changes occurred.[3195] In Dianeal PD-4 with dextrose 1.5% and Extraneal with icodextrin 7.5%, tigecycline loss was 5 and 4%, respectively, in 14 days at 4°C; 7 and 9%, respectively, in 3 days at 25°C; and 4 and 4%, respectively, in 12 hours at 37°C.[3195] In pH-neutral Balance with dextrose 1.5%, tigecycline loss was 6% in 7 days at 4°C, 8% in 3 days at 25°C, and 6% in 8 hours at 37°C.[3195]

Selected Revisions January 31, 2020. © Copyright, October 2008. American Society of Health-System Pharmacists, Inc.

Tirofiban Hydrochloride
AHFS 20:12.18

Products

Tirofiban hydrochloride is available premixed as a ready-to-use solution for infusion in 100- and 250-mL (IntraVia) plastic containers. Each mL of the ready-to-use infusion provides tirofiban 0.05 mg (50 mcg) as the hydrochloride monohydrate along with sodium chloride 9 mg, sodium citrate dihydrate 0.54 mg, citric acid anhydrous 0.032 mg, and sodium hydroxide and/or hydrochloric acid to adjust pH in water for injection.[1(10/07)]

pH

From 5.5 to 6.5.[1(10/07)]

Osmolality

The osmolality of tirofiban hydrochloride premixed infusion solution is approximately 300 mOsm/kg.[4]

Trade Name(s)

Aggrastat

Administration

Tirofiban hydrochloride is administered only by intravenous infusion. The premixed infusion solution is ready to use and does not require dilution.[1(10/07)]

Stability

Tirofiban hydrochloride ready-to-use infusion is clear and colorless. Intact plastic containers should be stored at controlled room temperature of 25°C, with temperature excursions in the range of 15 to 30°C permitted, and protected from light and freezing.[1(10/07)]

Compatibility Information

Solution Compatibility

Tirofiban HCl

Test Soln Name	Mfr	Mfr	Conc/L or %	Remarks	Ref	C/I
Dextrose 5% in sodium chloride 0.45%	AB[a]	ME	50 mg	Visually compatible. No loss in 24 hr at 23°C in light	2249	C
Dextrose 5%	BA[a]	ME	50 mg	Visually compatible. No loss in 24 hr at 23°C in light	2249	C
Sodium chloride 0.9%	AB[a]	ME	50 mg	Visually compatible. No loss in 24 hr at 23°C in light	2249	C
Sodium chloride 0.9%	[b]	MSD	50 mg	Visually compatible. No loss in 30 days at room temperature	2355	C

[a] Tested in PVC containers.

[b] Tested in glass and polyethylene containers.

Y-Site Injection Compatibility (1:1 Mixture)

Tirofiban HCl

Test Drug	Mfr	Conc	Mfr	Conc	Remarks	Ref	C/I
Amiodarone HCl	WY	6 mg/mL[a]	ME	0.25 mg/mL[a]	Visually compatible for 24 hr at 22°C	2352	C
Argatroban	GSK	1 mg/mL[a b c]	ME	0.05 mg/mL[c]	Physically compatible with no loss of either drug in 4 hr at 23°C	2630	C
Atropine sulfate	APP	0.4 mg/mL	ME	50 mcg/mL[a b]	Physically compatible with no loss of either drug in 4 hr at 23°C	2356	C
Atropine sulfate	AMR	1 mg/mL	ME	50 mcg/mL[a b]	Physically compatible with no loss of either drug in 4 hr at 23°C	2356	C
Bivalirudin	TMC	5 mg/mL[a]	ME	50 mcg/mL[a]	Physically compatible for 4 hr at 23°C	2373	C
Cangrelor tetrasodium	TMC	1 mg/mL[b]		50 mcg/mL	Physically compatible for 4 hr	3243	C
Diazepam	ES	5 mg/mL	ME	50 mcg/mL[a b]	Precipitate forms immediately	2356	I

DOI: 10.37573/9781585286850.380

Y-Site Injection Compatibility (1:1 Mixture) (Cont.)

Test Drug	Mfr	Conc	Mfr	Conc	Remarks	Ref	C/I
Dobutamine HCl	AB	0.25 and 5 mg/mL[a b]	ME	50 mcg/mL[a b]	Physically compatible with no loss of either drug in 4 hr at 23°C	2356	C
Dopamine HCl	AMR	0.2 and 3.2 mg/mL[a b]	ME	0.05 mg/mL[a b]	Physically compatible. Little loss of either drug in 4 hr at room temperature	2250	C
Epinephrine HCl	AMR	2 and 100 mcg/mL[a b]	ME	50 mcg/mL[a b]	Physically compatible. No loss of either drug in 4 hr at 23°C	2356	C
Famotidine	ME	2 and 4 mg/mL[a]	ME	0.05 mg/mL[b]	Physically compatible. Little loss of either drug in 4 hr at room temperature	2250	C
Famotidine	ME	2 and 4 mg/mL[b]	ME	0.05 mg/mL[a]	Physically compatible. Little loss of either drug in 4 hr at room temperature	2250	C
Furosemide	AB	0.5[a b] and 10 mg/mL	ME	50 mcg/mL[a b]	Physically compatible with no loss of either drug in 4 hr at 23°C	2356	C
Heparin sodium	AB	40 units/mL[a]	ME	0.05 mg/mL[a b]	Physically compatible. No tirofiban or heparin loss in 4 hr at room temperature	2250	C
Heparin sodium	AB	50 units/mL[b]	ME	0.05 mg/mL[b]	Physically compatible. No tirofiban or heparin loss in 4 hr at room temperature	2250	C
Heparin sodium	AB	100 units/mL[a b]	ME	0.05 mg/mL[a b]	Physically compatible. No tirofiban or heparin loss in 4 hr at room temperature	2250	C
Lidocaine HCl	AB	1 and 20 mg/mL[a b]	ME	0.05 mg/mL[a b]	Physically compatible. Little loss of either drug in 4 hr at room temperature	2250	C
Midazolam HCl	RC	5 and 0.05[a b] mg/mL	ME	50 mcg/mL[a b]	Physically compatible. No loss of either drug in 4 hr at 23°C	2356	C
Morphine sulfate	ES	0.1 and 1 mg/mL[a]	ME	50 mcg/mL[a b]	Physically compatible. No loss of either drug in 4 hr at 23°C	2356	C
Nitroglycerin	AB	0.1 and 0.4 mg/mL	ME	50 mcg/mL[a b]	Physically compatible. No loss of either drug in 4 hr at 23°C	2356	C
Potassium chloride	AB	0.01 and 0.04 mEq/mL[a b]	ME	0.05 mg/mL[a b]	Physically compatible. No tirofiban loss in 4 hr at room temperature	2250	C
Propranolol HCl	WAY	1 mg/mL	ME	50 mcg/mL[a b]	Physically compatible. No loss of either drug in 4 hr at 23°C	2356	C

[a] Tested in dextrose 5%.

[b] Tested in sodium chloride 0.9%.

[c] Mixed argatroban:tirofiban hydrochloride 1:1 and 8:1.

Selected Revisions September 29, 2017. © Copyright, October 2001. American Society of Health-System Pharmacists, Inc.

Tobramycin Sulfate
AHFS 8:12.02

Products

Tobramycin sulfate is available in a concentration equivalent to tobramycin base 40 mg/mL in 2-mL vials as well as 50-mL bulk vials. It is also available as a pediatric injection containing tobramycin sulfate equivalent to tobramycin base 10 mg/mL in 2-, 6-, and 8-mL vials. In addition to tobramycin sulfate, other components may be present in the formulations including varying amounts of sodium metabisulfite, and disodium edetate 0.1 mg in water for injection. Phenol 5 mg is present in some formulations. Sodium hydroxide and/or sulfuric acid may have been added during manufacture for pH adjustment.[1(9/08)]

Tobramycin sulfate is also available premixed in sodium chloride 0.9% in 0.8-mg/mL (80 mg) and 1.2-mg/mL (60 mg) concentrations.[4]

Tobramycin sulfate is also available in a pharmacy bulk package as a dry powder in vials containing the equivalent of tobramycin 1.2 g.[1(9/08)] The vial contents should be diluted with 30 mL of sterile water for injection to yield a 40-mg/mL solution. The reconstituted solution is intended to be diluted in a suitable intravenous infusion solution for administration.[4]

pH

The pH of the injection is adjusted to 3 to 6.5.[1(9/08)]

Osmolality

The osmolality of tobramycin sulfate 10 mg/mL was 133 mOsm/kg by freezing-point depression and 213 mOsm/kg by vapor pressure.[1071]

The osmolality of tobramycin sulfate 1 mg/mL was 254 mOsm/kg in dextrose 5% and 288 mOsm/kg in sodium chloride 0.9%. At 2.5 mg/mL, the osmolality was 261 mOsm/kg in dextrose 5% and 283 mOsm/kg in sodium chloride 0.9%.[1375]

The osmolality of tobramycin sulfate 80 mg was calculated for the following dilutions:[1054]

Diluent	Osmolality (mOsm/kg)	
	50 mL	100 mL
Dextrose 5%	289	285
Sodium chloride 0.9%	319	315

Osmolarity

The premixed products in sodium chloride 0.9% have an osmolarity of approximately 316 mOsm/kg.[4]

Sodium Content

The premixed products contain about 15.4 mEq of sodium per 100 mL of solution.[4]

Administration

Tobramycin sulfate may be administered by intramuscular injection or intermittent intravenous infusion. Intramuscular doses should be withdrawn only from multiple-dose vials; alternatively, the commercial prefilled syringes may be used. When given by intravenous infusion, the dose should be added to 50 to 100 mL of infusion solution and administered over 20 to 60 minutes. In children, the volume should be proportionately less but should allow an infusion period of 20 to 60 minutes. Infusion periods should not be less than 20 minutes; such shorter periods could result in excessive peak serum concentrations.[1(9/08) 4]

Stability

Tobramycin sulfate is stable at room temperature. Intact containers should be stored at controlled room temperature between 15 and 30°C; premixed infusion solutions may be stored at temperatures up to 25°C. Freezing and excessive temperatures above 40°C should be avoided. The injections should not be used if they are discolored. The manufacturer recommends use of the 40-mg/mL reconstituted solution within 24 hours when stored at room temperature or 96 hours if refrigerated.[1(9/08) 4] Tobramycin sulfate is stable for several weeks at pH 1 to 11 at temperatures from 5 to 27°C. It can be autoclaved without loss.[145]

Freezing Solutions

Tobramycin sulfate reconstituted to a concentration of 40 mg/mL and immediately frozen in the original container is stable for up to 12 weeks when stored at −10 to −20°C.[4]

Tobramycin sulfate (Lilly) 160 mg/50 mL of dextrose 5% in polyvinyl chloride (PVC) bags frozen at −20°C for 30 days and then thawed by exposure to ambient temperature or microwave radiation was evaluated. The solutions showed no evidence of precipitation or color change and showed 6% or less loss. Subsequent storage of the admixture at room temperature for 24 hours also yielded a physically compatible solution which exhibited little or no additional loss.[555]

Tobramycin sulfate (Dista) 120 mg/50 mL in dextrose 5% and sodium chloride 0.9% in PVC bags lost 9% activity in 28 days when frozen at −20°C.[981]

Minibags of tobramycin sulfate in dextrose 5% or sodium chloride 0.9%, frozen at −20°C for up to 35 days, were thawed at room temperature and in a microwave oven, with care taken that the thawed solution temperature never exceeded 25°C. No significant differences in tobramycin sulfate concentrations occurred between the 2 thawing methods.[1192]

Syringes

Samples of a 40-mg/mL solution of tobramycin sulfate (Lilly) from a reconstituted 1.2-g vial were stored in Monoject plastic syringes at both 25 and 4°C. After 2 months, no significant change in concentration was detected in samples at either storage temperature. The authors did note that the manufacturer does not recommend storage in plastic syringes because of possible incompatibility with the plunger heads.[736]

DOI: 10.37573/9781585286850.381

Tobramycin sulfate (Dista) 120 mg diluted with 1 mL of sodium chloride 0.9% to a final volume of 4 mL was stable (less than a 10% loss) when stored in polypropylene syringes (Becton Dickinson) for 48 hours at 25°C under fluorescent light.[1159]

Elastomeric Reservoir Pumps

Tobramycin sulfate (Lilly) 0.8 mg/mL in both dextrose 5% and sodium chloride 0.9% was evaluated for binding potential to natural rubber elastomeric reservoirs (Baxter). No binding was found after storage for 2 weeks at 35°C with gentle agitation.[2014]

Sorption

Tobramycin sulfate was shown not to exhibit sorption to PVC bags and tubing, polyethylene tubing, Silastic tubing, and polypropylene syringes.[536] [606]

Tobramycin sulfate (Qualimed) 1.5 mg/mL in dextrose 5% and in sodium chloride 0.9% was packaged in PVC bags (Macropharma) and in multilayer bags composed of polyethylene, polyamide, and polypropylene (Bieffe Medital). The solutions were delivered through PVC administration sets (Abbott) over 1 hour and evaluated for drug loss. No loss due to sorption to any of the plastic materials was found.[2269]

Filtration

Tobramycin sulfate (Lilly) 0.3 mg/mL in dextrose 5% and sodium chloride 0.9% was filtered through a 0.22-μm cellulose ester membrane filter (Ivex-HP, Millipore) over 6 hours. No significant drug loss due to binding to the filter was noted.[1034]

Tobramycin sulfate 5 and 10 mg/55 mL in dextrose 5% and sodium chloride 0.9% filtered over 20 minutes through a 0.22-μm cellulose ester filter set (Ivex-2, Millipore) was evaluated. Little or no binding of the drug to the filter occurred.[1003]

No significant loss due to sorption to a 0.22-μm cellulose ester filter (Continu-Flo 2C0252s, Travenol) occurred from a solution containing tobramycin sulfate (Dista) 80 mg/100 mL of dextrose 5% administered over 30 minutes. No difference in drug recovery was found between filtered and unfiltered solutions. However, 10% or more of the solution may remain in the tubing unless the sets are flushed.[1132]

Central Venous Catheter

Tobramycin sulfate (Lilly) 1 mg/mL in dextrose 5% was found to be compatible with the ARROWg+ard Blue Plus (Arrow International) chlorhexidine-bearing triple-lumen central catheter. Essentially complete delivery of the drug was found with little or no drug loss occurring. Furthermore, chlorhexidine delivered from the catheter remained at trace amounts with no substantial increase due to the delivery of the drug through the catheter.[2335]

Compatibility Information

Solution Compatibility

Tobramycin sulfate

Test Soln Name	Mfr	Mfr	Conc/L or %	Remarks	Ref	C/I
Amino acids 4.25%, dextrose 25%	MG	LI	80 mg	No increase in particulate matter in 24 hr at 25°C	349	C
Dextrose 5% in sodium chloride 0.9%	TR[a]	LI	200 mg and 1 g	Physically compatible and chemically stable for 48 hr at 25°C. Not more than 7% loss occurs	147	C
Dextrose 5%	TR[a]	LI	200 mg and 1 g	Physically compatible and chemically stable for 48 hr at 25°C. Not more than 4% loss occurs	147	C
Dextrose 5%	TR[a]	LI	3.2 g	Physically compatible and no loss in 24 hr at room temperature	555	C
Dextrose 5%		LI	1 and 5 g	Physically compatible with no loss of activity in 60 min at room temperature	984	C
Dextrose 5%	AB[a]	DI	1.2 g	Visually compatible and stable for 48 hr at 25°C under fluorescent light and 4°C in the dark	1541	C
Dextrose 10%	TR[a]	LI	200 mg and 1 g	Physically compatible and chemically stable for 48 hr at 25°C. Not more than 4% loss occurs	147	C
Dextrose 10%	SO	LI	60 mg/21.5 mL[b]	Visually compatible with little or no tobramycin loss in 30 days at 5°C in the dark	1731	C
Dextrose 10%	SO	LI	60 mg/18.5 mL[b]	Visually compatible with little or no tobramycin loss in 30 days at 5°C in the dark	1731	C
Dextrose 10%	SO	LI	120 mg/23 mL[b]	Visually compatible with little or no tobramycin loss in 30 days at 5°C in the dark	1731	C
Dextrose 10%	SO	LI	120 mg/20 mL[b]	Visually compatible with little or no tobramycin loss in 30 days at 5°C in the dark	1731	C

Solution Compatibility (Cont.)

Test Soln Name	Mfr	Mfr	Conc/L or %	Remarks	Ref	C/I
Isolyte E in dextrose 5%	MG	LI	1 g	12% loss in 24 hr at 25°C. Stable for 4 hr	147	I
Isolyte M in dextrose 5%	MG	LI	200 mg and 1 g	12% loss in 24 hr at 25°C. Stable for 4 hr	147	I
Isolyte P in dextrose 5%	MG	LI	200 mg and 1 g	12% loss in 24 hr at 25°C. Stable for 4 hr	147	I
Normosol M in dextrose 5%	AB	LI	200 mg and 1 g	Physically compatible and chemically stable for 24 hr at 25°C. Not more than 10% loss occurs	147	C
Normosol R	AB	LI	200 mg and 1 g	Physically compatible and chemically stable for 24 hr at 25°C	147	C
Normosol R in dextrose 5%	AB	LI	200 mg and 1 g	Physically compatible and chemically stable for 24 hr at 25°C. Not more than 8% loss occurs	147	C
Normosol R, pH 7.4	AB	LI	200 mg and 1 g	Physically compatible and chemically stable for 24 hr at 25°C	147	C
Ringer's injection	TR[a]	LI	200 mg and 1 g	Physically compatible and chemically stable for 24 hr at 25°C	147	C
Ringer's injection, lactated		LI	200 mg and 1 g	Physically compatible and chemically stable for 24 hr at 25°C	147	C
Sodium chloride 0.9%	TR[a]	LI	200 mg and 1 g	Physically compatible and chemically stable for 48 hr at 25°C	147	C
Sodium chloride 0.9%	AB[a]	DI	1.2 g	Visually compatible and stable for 48 hr at 25°C under fluorescent light and 4°C in the dark	1541	C
Sodium chloride 0.9%	AB[c]	MAR	1 and 10 g	Little loss in 3 days at 25°C and 14 days at 5°C in PVC	2080	C
Sodium lactate ⅙ M		LI	200 mg and 1 g	Physically compatible and chemically stable for 48 hr at 25°C	147	C

[a] Tested in PVC containers.

[b] Tested in glass vials as a concentrate.

[c] Tested in PVC portable pump reservoirs (Pharmacia Deltec).

Additive Compatibility

Tobramycin sulfate

Test Drug	Mfr	Conc/L or %	Mfr	Conc/L or %	Test Solution	Remarks	Ref	C/I
Aztreonam	SQ	10 and 20 g	LI	200 and 800 mg	D5W, NS	Little or no loss of either drug in 48 hr at 25°C and 7 days at 4°C	1023	C
Bleomycin sulfate	BR	20 and 30 units	LI	500 mg	NS	Physically compatible and bleomycin activity retained for 1 week at 4°C. Tobramycin not tested	763	C
Calcium gluconate		16 g	LI	5 g	D5W	Physically compatible. No tobramycin loss in 60 min at room temperature	984	C
Calcium gluconate		33 g	LI	1 g	D5W	Physically compatible. No tobramycin loss in 60 min at room temperature	984	C
Cefepime HCl	BR	40 g	AB	0.4 g	D5W, NS	Cloudiness forms immediately	1682	I
Cefepime HCl	BR	2.5 g	AB	2 g	D5W, NS	Cloudiness forms immediately	1682	I
Cefoxitin sodium	MSD	5 g	LI	400 mg	D5S	5% cefoxitin loss in 24 hr and 11% in 48 hr at 25°C. 3% in 48 hr at 5°C. 8% tobramycin loss in 24 hr and 37% in 48 hr at 25°C. 3% in 48 hr at 5°C	308	C

Additive Compatibility (Cont.)

Test Drug	Mfr	Conc/L or %	Mfr	Conc/L or %	Test Solution	Remarks	Ref	C/I
Ciprofloxacin	MI	1.6 g	LI	1 g	D5W, NS	Visually compatible and both drugs stable for 48 hr at 25°C under fluorescent light and 4°C in the dark	1541	C
Ciprofloxacin	BAY	2 g	LI	1.6 g	D5W	Visually compatible with no loss of ciprofloxacin in 24 hr at 22°C under fluorescent light. Tobramycin not tested	2413	C
Clindamycin phosphate	UP	18 g	DI	2.4 g	D5W[a]	8% tobramycin lost in 14 days and 17% in 28 days at −20°C. Clindamycin stable	981	C
Clindamycin phosphate	UP	18 g	DI	2.4 g	NS[a]	Both drugs stable for 28 days frozen at −20°C	981	C
Clindamycin phosphate	UP	9 g	DI	1 g	D5W, NS[b]	Physically compatible and both drugs stable for 48 hr at room temperature exposed to light and for 1 week frozen	174	C
Clindamycin phosphate	UP	9 g	DI	1.2 g	D5W[c]	Physically compatible and clindamycin stable for 28 days frozen. 8% tobramycin loss in 14 days and 17% in 28 days	174	C
Clindamycin phosphate	UP	9 g	DI	1.2 g	NS[c]	Physically compatible and both drugs stable for 28 days frozen	174	C
Dextran 40	TR	10%	LI	200 mg and 1 g	D5W	Physically compatible and stable for 24 hr at 25°C. Not more than 9% loss	147	C
Floxacillin sodium	BE	20 g	LI	8 g	NS	White precipitate forms in 7 hr	1479	I
Furosemide	HO	1 g	LI	8 g	NS	Physically compatible for 72 hr at 15 and 30°C	1479	C
Furosemide	HO	800 mg	DI	1.6 g	D5W, NS	Transient cloudiness then physically compatible for 24 hr at 21°C	876	?
Imipenem–cilastatin sodium		100[e] mg		10 mg	W	Little or no loss of antibiotic activity in 24 hr at 37°C	498	C
Linezolid	PHU	2 g	GNS	800 mg	[d]	Physically compatible. Little linezolid loss in 7 days at 4 and 23°C in dark. No tobramycin loss in 7 days at 4°C but losses of 4% in 1 day and 12% in 3 days at 23°C	2332	C
Mannitol		20%	LI	200 mg and 1 g		Physically compatible and chemically stable for 48 hr at 25°C	147	C
Metronidazole	RP	5 g	LI	1 g		Visually compatible with no loss of metronidazole in 15 days at 5 and 25°C. 10% tobramycin loss in 73 hr at 25°C and 12.1 days at 5°C	1931	C
Ranitidine HCl	GL	100 mg	DI	200 mg	D5W	Physically compatible for 24 hr at ambient temperature in light	1151	C
Verapamil HCl	KN	80 mg	LI	160 mg	D5W, NS	Physically compatible for 24 hr	764	C

[a] Tested in PVC containers.

[b] Tested in both glass and PVC containers.

[c] Tested in glass containers.

[d] Admixed in the linezolid infusion container.

[e] Not specified whether concentration refers to single component or combined components.

Drugs in Syringe Compatibility

Tobramycin sulfate

Test Drug	Mfr	Amt	Mfr	Amt	Remarks	Ref	C/I
Clindamycin phosphate	UP	900 mg/6 mL	DI	120 mg/4 mL[a]	Cloudy white precipitate forms immediately and changes to gel-like precipitate	1159	I
Dimenhydrinate		10 mg/1 mL		40 mg/1 mL	Clear solution	2569	C
Doxapram HCl	RB	400 mg/20 mL		60 mg/1.5 mL	Physically compatible with no doxapram loss in 24 hr	1177	C
Heparin sodium		10 units/1 mL		80 mg/2 mL	Turbidity or fine white precipitate due to formation of an insoluble salt	845	I
Heparin sodium		2500 units/1 mL	LI	40 mg	Turbidity or precipitate forms within 5 min	1053	I
Pantoprazole sodium	[b]	4 mg/1 mL		40 mg/1 mL	Precipitates immediately	2574	I

[a] Diluted to 4 mL with 1 mL of sodium chloride 0.9%.

[b] Test performed using the formulation WITHOUT edetate disodium.

Y-Site Injection Compatibility (1:1 Mixture)

Tobramycin sulfate

Test Drug	Mfr	Conc	Mfr	Conc	Remarks	Ref	C/I
Acyclovir sodium	BW	5 mg/mL[a]	DI	1.6 mg/mL[a]	Physically compatible for 4 hr at 25°C	1157	C
Allopurinol sodium	BW	3 mg/mL[b]	LI	5 mg/mL[b]	Haze and crystals form in 1 hr	1686	I
Alprostadil	BED	7.5 mcg/mL[s n]	LI	1 mg/mL[r]	Visually compatible for 1 hr	2746	C
Amifostine	USB	10 mg/mL[a]	LI	5 mg/mL[a]	Physically compatible for 4 hr at 23°C	1845	C
Amiodarone HCl	LZ	4 mg/mL[c]	LI	0.8 mg/mL[c]	Physically compatible for 4 hr at room temperature	1444	C
Amiodarone HCl	WY	6 mg/mL[a]	LI	5 mg/mL[a]	Visually compatible for 24 hr at 22°C	2352	C
Amsacrine	NCI	1 mg/mL[a]	LI	5 mg/mL[a]	Visually compatible for 4 hr at 22°C	1381	C
Anidulafungin	VIC	0.5 mg/mL[a]	AB	5 mg/mL[a]	Physically compatible for 4 hr at 23°C	2617	C
Azithromycin	PF	2 mg/mL[b]		21 mg/mL[p]	White microcrystals found	2368	I
Aztreonam	SQ	40 mg/mL[a]	LI	5 mg/mL[a]	Physically compatible for 4 hr at 23°C	1758	C
Bivalirudin	TMC	5 mg/mL[a]	GNS	5 mg/mL[a]	Physically compatible for 4 hr at 23°C	2373	C
Cangrelor tetrasodium	TMC	1 mg/mL[b]		5 mg/mL[b]	Gross white turbid precipitate forms immediately	3243	I
Caspofungin acetate	ME	0.7 mg/mL[b]	SIC	5 mg/mL[b]	Physically compatible for 4 hr at room temperature	2758	C
Cefepime HCl	BMS	120 mg/mL[q]		6 mg/mL	Physically compatible with less than 10% cefepime loss. Tobramycin not tested	2513	C
Ceftaroline fosamil	FOR	2.22 mg/mL[a b o]	SIC	5 mg/mL[a b o]	Physically compatible for 4 hr at 23°C	2826	C
Ceftazidime	SKB	125 mg/mL		0.6 mg/mL	Visually compatible with less than 10% loss of both drugs in 1 hr	2434	C
Ceftazidime	GSK	120 mg/mL[q]		6 mg/mL	Physically compatible with less than 10% ceftazidime loss. Tobramycin not tested	2513	C
Ceftazidime–avibactam sodium	ALL	20 mg/mL[x y]	[z]		Physically compatible for up to 4 hr at room temperature	3004	C
Ceftolozane sulfate–tazobactam sodium	CUB	10 mg/mL[c v]	MYL	5 mg/mL[c]	Physically compatible for 2 hr	3262	C

Y-Site Injection Compatibility (1:1 Mixture) (Cont.)

Test Drug	Mfr	Conc	Mfr	Conc	Remarks	Ref	C/I
Ciprofloxacin	MI	1 mg/mL[a]	LI	1.6 mg/mL[c]	Physically compatible for 24 hr at 22°C	1189	C
Cisatracurium besylate	GW	0.1, 2, 5 mg/mL[a]	AB	5 mg/mL[a]	Physically compatible for 4 hr at 23°C	2074	C
Cloxacillin sodium	SMX	100 mg/mL	SZ	40 mg/mL	Precipitates immediately	3245	I
Cyclophosphamide	MJ	20 mg/mL[a]	DI	0.8 mg/mL[a]	Physically compatible for 4 hr at 25°C	1194	C
Defibrotide sodium	JAZ	8 mg/mL[b]	ERM	10 mg/mL	Solution immediately became milky white, opaque or opalescent; precipitate formed within 2.5 hr	3149	I
Dexmedetomidine HCl	AB	4 mcg/mL[b]	GNS	5 mg/mL[b]	Physically compatible for 4 hr at 23°C	2383	C
Diltiazem HCl	MMD	5 mg/mL	LI	2.4[b] and 40 mg/mL	Visually compatible	1807	C
Docetaxel	RPR	0.9 mg/mL[a]	LI	5 mg/mL[a]	Physically compatible for 4 hr at 23°C	2224	C
Doripenem	JJ	5 mg/mL[a b]	SIC	5 mg/mL[a b]	Physically compatible for 4 hr at 23°C	2743	C
Doxorubicin HCl liposomal	SEQ	0.4 mg/mL[a]	AB	5 mg/mL[a]	Physically compatible for 4 hr at 23°C	2087	C
Enalaprilat	MSD	0.05 mg/mL[b]	LI	0.8 mg/mL[a]	Physically compatible for 24 hr at room temperature under fluorescent light	1355	C
Eravacycline dihydrochloride	TET	0.6 mg/mL[b]	FRK	5 mg/mL[b]	Physically compatible for 2 hr at room temperature	3532	C
Esmolol HCl	DCC	10 mg/mL[a]	LI	0.8 mg/mL[a]	Physically compatible for 24 hr at 22°C	1169	C
Etoposide phosphate	BR	5 mg/mL[a]	LI	5 mg/mL[a]	Physically compatible for 4 hr at 23°C	2218	C
Fenoldopam mesylate	AB	80 mcg/mL[b]	LI	5 mg/mL[b]	Physically compatible for 4 hr at 23°C	2467	C
Filgrastim	AMG	30 mcg/mL[a]	LI	5 mg/mL[a]	Physically compatible for 4 hr at 22°C	1687	C
Filgrastim	AMG	10[d] and 40[a] mcg/mL	LI	1.6 mg/mL[a]	Visually compatible. Little loss of filgrastim and tobramycin in 4 hr at 25°C	2060	C
Fluconazole	RR	2 mg/mL	LI	40 mg/mL	Physically compatible for 24 hr at 25°C	1407	C
Fludarabine phosphate	BX	1 mg/mL[a]	LI	5 mg/mL[a]	Visually compatible for 4 hr at 22°C	1439	C
Foscarnet sodium	AST	24 mg/mL	LI	40 mg/mL	Physically compatible for 24 hr at room temperature under fluorescent light	1335	C
Furosemide	HO	10 mg/mL	DI	1.6 mg/mL[c]	Physically compatible for 24 hr at 21°C	876	C
Gemcitabine HCl	LI	10 mg/mL[b]	LI	5 mg/mL[b]	Physically compatible for 4 hr at 23°C	2226	C
Granisetron HCl	SKB	0.05 mg/mL[a]	AB	5 mg/mL[a]	Physically compatible for 4 hr at 23°C	2000	C
Heparin sodium	ES	50 units/mL[c]	LI	3.2 mg/mL[c]	Immediate gross haze	1316	I
Heparin sodium	TR	50 units/mL	LI	0.8 mg/mL[a]	Visually incompatible within 4 hr at 25°C	1793	I
Hetastarch in lactated electrolyte	AB	6%	GNS	5 mg/mL[a]	Physically compatible for 4 hr at 23°C	2339	C
Hetastarch in sodium chloride 0.9%	DCC	6%	LI	0.8 mg/mL[e]	Small crystals form immediately after mixing and persist for 4 hr	1313	I
Hydromorphone HCl	WY	0.2 mg/mL[a]	DI	0.8 mg/mL[a]	Physically compatible for 4 hr at 25°C	987	C
Indomethacin sodium trihydrate	MSD	0.5 and 1 mg/mL[a]		1 mg/mL[a]	White turbidity forms immediately and becomes white flakes in 1 hr	1550	I
Insulin, regular	LI	0.2 unit/mL[b]	LI	1.6 and 2 mg/mL[a]	Physically compatible for 2 hr at 25°C	1395	C

Y-Site Injection Compatibility (1:1 Mixture) (Cont.)

Test Drug	Mfr	Conc	Mfr	Conc	Remarks	Ref	C/I
Isavuconazonium sulfate	ASP	1.5 mg/mL[c]	MYL	5 mg/mL[c]	Physically compatible for 2 hr	3263	C
Labetalol HCl	SC	1 mg/mL[a]	LI	0.8 mg/mL[a]	Physically compatible for 24 hr at 18°C	1171	C
Linezolid	PHU	2 mg/mL	AB	5 mg/mL[a]	Physically compatible for 4 hr at 23°C	2264	C
Magnesium sulfate	IX	16.7, 33.3, 66.7, 100 mg/mL[a]	DI	0.8 mg/mL[a]	Physically compatible for at least 4 hr at 32°C	813	C
Melphalan HCl	BW	0.1 mg/mL[b]	LI	5 mg/mL[b]	Physically compatible for 3 hr at 22°C	1557	C
Meperidine HCl	WY	10 mg/mL[a]	DI	0.8 mg/mL[a]	Physically compatible for 4 hr at 25°C	987	C
Meperidine HCl	WY	10 mg/mL[b]	LI	1.6, 2, 2.4 mg/mL[a]	Physically compatible for 1 hr at 25°C	1338	C
Meropenem		50 mg/mL	FRK	40 mg/mL	Physically compatible for 4 hr at room temperature	3538	C
Meropenem–vaborbactam	TMC	8 mg/mL[b w]	FRK	5 mg/mL[b]	Physically compatible for 3 hr at 20 to 25°C	3380	C
Midazolam HCl	RC	1 mg/mL[a]	LI	10 mg/mL	Visually compatible for 24 hr at 23°C	1847	C
Milrinone lactate	SS	0.2 mg/mL[a]	LI	10 mg/mL[a]	Visually compatible for 4 hr at 25°C	2381	C
Morphine sulfate	WI	1 mg/mL[a]	DI	0.8 mg/mL[a]	Physically compatible for 4 hr at 25°C	987	C
Morphine sulfate	ES	1 mg/mL[b]	LI	1.6, 2, 2.4 mg/mL[a]	Physically compatible for 1 hr at 25°C	1338	C
Nicardipine HCl	DCC	0.1 mg/mL[a]	LI	0.8 mg/mL[a]	Visually compatible for 24 hr at room temperature	235	C
Oritavancin diphosphate	TAR	0.8, 1.2, and 2 mg/mL[a]	SIC	5 mg/mL[a]	Visually compatible for 4 hr at 20 to 24°C	2928	C
Pemetrexed disodium	LI	20 mg/mL[b]	AB	5 mg/mL[a]	White precipitate forms immediately	2564	I
Piperacillin sodium–tazobactam sodium	WY[u]				Incompatible	2918	I
Piperacillin sodium–tazobactam sodium	[t]				Incompatible	2919, 2920, 2921	I
Propofol	ZEN[u]	10 mg/mL	AB	5 mg/mL[a]	Precipitate forms immediately	2066	I
Remifentanil HCl	GW	0.025 and 0.25 mg/mL[b]	AB	5 mg/mL[a]	Physically compatible for 4 hr at 23°C	2075	C
Sargramostim	IMM	10 mcg/mL[b]	LI	5 mg/mL[b]	Particles and filaments form in 4 hr	1436	I
Tacrolimus	FUJ	1 mg/mL[b]	BR	40 mg/mL	Visually compatible for 24 hr at 25°C	1630	C
Tedizolid phosphate	CUB	0.8 mg/mL[b]	MYL	5 mg/mL[b]	Measured turbidity increases immediately	3244	I
Telavancin HCl	ASP	7.5 mg/mL[a b]	HOS	5 mg/mL[a b]	Physically compatible for 2 hr	2830	C
Teniposide	BR	0.1 mg/mL[a]	LI	5 mg/mL[a]	Physically compatible for 4 hr at 23°C	1725	C
Theophylline	TR	4 mg/mL	LI	0.8 mg/mL[a]	Visually compatible for 6 hr at 25°C	1793	C
Thiotepa	IMM[c]	1 mg/mL[a]	LI	5 mg/mL[a]	Physically compatible for 4 hr at 23°C	1861	C
Tigecycline	WY	1 mg/mL[b]		2.5 mg/mL[b]	Physically compatible for 4 hr	2714	C
Tigecycline	ACD, FRK, WY	[c]	[z]		Stated to be compatible	2915, 3459, 3460	C

Y-Site Injection Compatibility (1:1 Mixture) (Cont.)

Test Drug	Mfr	Conc	Mfr	Conc	Remarks	Ref	C/I
TNA #73[g]		32.5 mL[h]	LI	1.6 mg/mL[a]	Visually compatible for 4 hr at 25°C	1008	C
TNA #97[g]			LI	40 mg/mL	Physically compatible and tobramycin content retained for 6 hr at 21°C	1324	C
TNA #98[g]			LI	40 mg/mL	Physically compatible and tobramycin content retained for 6 hr at 21°C	1324	C
TNA #99[g]			LI	40 mg/mL	Physically compatible and tobramycin content retained for 6 hr at 21°C	1324	C
TNA #100[g]			LI	40 mg/mL	Physically compatible and tobramycin content retained for 6 hr at 21°C	1324	C
TNA #101[g]			LI	40 mg/mL	Physically compatible and tobramycin content retained for 6 hr at 21°C	1324	C
TNA #102[g]			LI	40 mg/mL	Physically compatible and tobramycin content retained for 6 hr at 21°C	1324	C
TNA #103[g]			LI	40 mg/mL	Physically compatible and tobramycin content retained for 6 hr at 21°C	1324	C
TNA #104[g]			LI	40 mg/mL	Physically compatible and tobramycin content retained for 6 hr at 21°C	1324	C
TNA #218[g]			AB	5 mg/mL[a]	Visually compatible for 4 hr at 23°C	2215	C
TNA #219[g]			AB	5 mg/mL[a]	Visually compatible for 4 hr at 23°C	2215	C
TNA #220[g]			AB	5 mg/mL[a]	Visually compatible for 4 hr at 23°C	2215	C
TNA #221[g]			AB	5 mg/mL[a]	Visually compatible for 4 hr at 23°C	2215	C
TNA #222[g]			AB	5 mg/mL[a]	Visually compatible for 4 hr at 23°C	2215	C
TNA #223[g]			AB	5 mg/mL[a]	Visually compatible for 4 hr at 23°C	2215	C
TNA #224[g]			AB	5 mg/mL[a]	Visually compatible for 4 hr at 23°C	2215	C
TNA #225[g]			AB	5 mg/mL[a]	Visually compatible for 4 hr at 23°C	2215	C
TNA #226[g]			AB	5 mg/mL[a]	Visually compatible for 4 hr at 23°C	2215	C
TPN #54[g]				20 mg/mL	Physically compatible and tobramycin activity retained over 6 hr at 22°C	1045	C
TPN #61[g]		[i]	DI	12.5 mg/1.25 mL[j]	Physically compatible	1012	C
TPN #61[g]		[k]	DI	75 mg/1.9 mL[j]	Physically compatible	1012	C
TPN #91[g]		[l]	LI	5 mg[m]	Physically compatible	1170	C
TPN #212[g]			AB	5 mg/mL[a]	Physically compatible for 4 hr at 23°C	2109	C
TPN #213[g]			AB	5 mg/mL[a]	Physically compatible for 4 hr at 23°C	2109	C
TPN #214[g]			AB	5 mg/mL[a]	Physically compatible for 4 hr at 23°C	2109	C
TPN #215[g]			AB	5 mg/mL[a]	Physically compatible for 4 hr at 23°C	2109	C

Y-Site Injection Compatibility (1:1 Mixture) (Cont.)

Test Drug	Mfr	Conc	Mfr	Conc	Remarks	Ref	C/I
Vinorelbine tartrate	BW	1 mg/mL[b]	LI	5 mg/mL[b]	Physically compatible for 4 hr at 22°C	1558	C
Zidovudine	BW	4 mg/mL[a]	LI	2 mg/mL[a]	Physically compatible for 4 hr at 25°C	1193	C

[a] Tested in dextrose 5%.

[b] Tested in sodium chloride 0.9%.

[c] Tested in both dextrose 5% and sodium chloride 0.9%.

[d] Tested in dextrose 5% with albumin human 2 mg/mL.

[e] Tested as the premixed infusion solution.

[f] Lyophilized formulation tested.

[g] Refer to Appendix for the composition of parenteral nutrition solutions. TNA indicates a 3-in-1 admixture, and TPN indicates a 2-in-1 admixture.

[h] A 32.5-mL sample of parenteral nutrition solution mixed with 50 mL of antibiotic solution.

[i] Run at 21 mL/hr.

[j] Given over 30 minutes by syringe pump.

[k] Run at 94 mL/hr.

[l] Run at 10 mL/hr.

[m] Given over one hour by syringe pump.

[n] Tested in a 1:1 mixture of dextrose 5% and TPN #274 (see Appendix).

[o] Tested in Ringer's injection, lactated.

[p] Injected via Y-site into an administration set running azithromycin.

[q] Tested in sterile water for injection.

[r] Tested in either dextrose 5% or in sodium chloride 0.9%, but the report did not specify which solution.

[s] Tested in a 1:1 mixture of (1) dextrose 5% and dextrose 5% in sodium chloride 0.45% with and without potassium chloride 20 mEq/L and also in (2) dextrose 10% in sodium chloride 0.45% with and without potassium chloride 20 mEq/L.

[t] Test performed using the formulation WITHOUT edetate disodium.

[u] Test performed using the formulation WITH edetate disodium.

[v] Ceftolozane component. Ceftolozane in a 2:1 fixed-ratio concentration with tazobactam.

[w] Meropenem component. Meropenem in a 1:1 fixed-ratio concentration with vaborbactam.

[x] Ceftazidime component. Ceftazidime in a 4:1 fixed-ratio concentration with avibactam.

[y] Tested in both dextrose 5% and Ringer's injection, lactated.

[z] Salt not specified.

Additional Compatibility Information

Peritoneal Dialysis Solutions

Tobramycin base (Lilly) 3 and 10 mg/L in peritoneal dialysis concentrate with dextrose 50% (McGaw) retained about 50 to 60% of initial activity in 7 hours and about 15 to 30% in 24 hours at room temperature.[1044]

The stability of tobramycin sulfate (Lilly) 10 mg/L in peritoneal dialysis solutions (Dianeal 137 and PD-2) with heparin sodium 500 units/L was evaluated. Approximately 102 ± 20% activity remained after 24 hours at 25°C.[1228]

In another study, the stability of tobramycin sulfate (Lilly) was evaluated in peritoneal dialysis concentrates containing dextrose 30 and 50% (Dianeal) as well as in a diluted solution containing dextrose 2.5%. The tobramycin sulfate concentrations were 100 and 160 mg/L in the peritoneal dialysate concentrates

and 5 and 8 mg/L in the diluted solution. Tobramycin sulfate was found to be stable in the diluted peritoneal dialysis solution for at least 24 hours at 23°C. However, greater decomposition occurred in the concentrates, with a 10% loss in as little as 9 to 15 hours.[1229]

The retention of antimicrobial activity of tobramycin sulfate (Lilly) 120 mg/L alone and with vancomycin hydrochloride (Lilly) 1 g/L was evaluated in Dianeal PD-2 (Travenol) with dextrose 1.5%. Little or no loss of either antibiotic occurred in 8 hours at 37°C. Tobramycin sulfate alone retained activity for at least 48 hours at 4 and 25°C. With vancomycin hydrochloride, the activity of both antibiotics was retained for up to 48 hours; however, the authors recommended refrigeration at 4°C for storage longer than 24 hours.[1414]

Ceftazidime (Fortaz) 125 mg/L and tobramycin sulfate (Lilly) 8 mg/L in Dianeal PD-2 with dextrose 2.5% (Baxter) were visually compatible and chemically stable. After 16 hours of storage at 25°C under fluorescent light, the loss of both drugs was less than 3%. Additional storage for 8 hours at 37°C, to simulate the maximum peritoneal dwell time, showed tobramycin sulfate concentrations of 96% and ceftazidime concentrations of 92 to 96%.[1652]

Tobramycin sulfate (Lilly) 25 mcg/mL combined separately with the cephalosporins cefazolin sodium (Lilly) and cefoxitin (MSD) at a concentration of 125 mcg/mL in peritoneal dialysis solution (Dianeal 1.5%) exhibited enhanced rates of lethality to *Staphylococcus aureus*, *Escherichia coli*, and *Pseudomonas aeruginosa* compared to any of the drugs alone.[1623]

β-Lactam Antibiotics

In common with other aminoglycoside antibiotics, tobramycin sulfate activity may be impaired by the β-lactam antibiotics. The inactivation is dependent on concentration, temperature, and time of exposure.[68 497 498 574 575 654 740 814 816 817 832 824 973 1005 1052 1420]

The clinical significance of these interactions appears to be primarily confined to patients with renal failure.[218 334 361 364 616 737 816 847 952] Literature reports of greatly reduced aminoglycoside levels in such patients have appeared frequently.[363 365 366 367 614 666 962] In addition, the interaction may be clinically important if assays for aminoglycoside levels in serum are sufficiently delayed.[576 618 735 824 832 847 1052]

Most authors believe that in vitro mixing of penicillins with aminoglycoside antibiotics should be avoided but that clinical use of the drugs in combination can be of great value. It is generally recommended that the drugs be given separately in such combined therapy.[157 218 222 224 361 364 368 369 370]

Topotecan Hydrochloride

AHFS 10:00

Products

Topotecan hydrochloride is available in vials containing 4 mg of topotecan base (present as the hydrochloride) as a lyophilized powder. Reconstitute with 4 mL of sterile water for injection to yield a 1-mg/mL topotecan solution. In addition to topotecan hydrochloride, each mL of the reconstituted solution contains mannitol 12 mg and tartaric acid 5 mg. Hydrochloric acid and sodium hydroxide may have been used during manufacture to adjust the pH. The reconstituted solution must be diluted for use.[1(10/07)]

pH

From 2.5 to 3.5.[1(10/07)]

Trade Name(s)

Hycamtin

Administration

Topotecan hydrochloride is administered by intravenous infusion over 30 minutes after dilution in 50 to 250 mL of either sodium chloride 0.9% or dextrose 5%. Extravasation should be avoided; local reactions including erythema and bruising may result.[1(10/07) 4]

As for other toxic drugs, topotecan hydrochloride should be prepared and administered using protective measures to avoid inadvertent contact with the drug. The use of gloves, protective clothing, and vertical laminar flow hoods or biological safety cabinets is recommended. If skin contact with the drug does occur, wash the area thoroughly with soap and water. For mucous membrane contact, flush thoroughly with water. Disposal should also be performed safely to avoid inadvertent exposure.[1(10/07) 4]

Stability

Topotecan hydrochloride in intact vials should be stored in the original cartons at controlled room temperature and protected from light. The lyophilized drug is a light yellow to greenish powder. The reconstituted solution is yellow to yellow-green in color.[1(10/07)] The reconstituted solution should be inspected for particulate matter in the vial and again in the transferring syringe prior to preparing admixtures. As for all parenteral products, the admixtures should also be inspected for particulate matter and discoloration prior to administration.[4]

Reconstituted topotecan hydrochloride is stated to be stable for 24 hours at 20 to 25°C exposed to ambient light.[4] However, the manufacturer recommends use immediately after reconstitution because the product contains no antibacterial preservative.[1(10/07)]

Other information indicates the reconstituted drug may be stable for longer periods. Vials of reconstituted topotecan hydrochloride at a concentration of 1 mg/mL were stored at 5, 25, and 30°C both upright and inverted for 28 days. The solutions remained visually clear with no change in color, and little or no loss of topotecan hydrochloride occurred at any condition.[2211]

Topotecan hydrochloride 1 mg/mL reconstituted with sterile water for injection was physically and chemically stable for 28 days at 4 and 25°C protected from light. No loss of topotecan was found, and no visible precipitation or color change occurred.[2243]

Whether any antimicrobial effect of topotecan hydrochloride exists is uncertain but could be concentration dependent. Two studies that have been performed seem to have different results, perhaps due to the very different topotecan hydrochloride concentrations being tested.

Topotecan hydrochloride 0.01 mg/mL diluted in sodium chloride 0.9% and stored at 22°C did not exhibit an antimicrobial effect on the growth of 4 organisms (*Enterococcus faecium*, *Staphylococcus aureus*, *Pseudomonas aeruginosa*, and *Candida albicans*) inoculated into the solution. The author recommended that diluted solutions of topotecan hydrochloride be stored under refrigeration whenever possible and that the potential for microbiological growth be considered when assigning expiration periods.[2160]

Topotecan hydrochloride 1 mg/mL reconstituted with sterile water did not support the growth of 5 organisms inoculated into the solution. The USP Preservative Effectiveness Test found that *Pseudomonas aeruginosa*, *Staphylococcus aureus*, and *Escherichia coli* were not viable after 16 hours, 24 hours, and 28 days, respectively. *Candida albicans* and *Aspergillus niger* did not lose viability but did not exhibit growth during the test.[2211]

pH Effects

Topotecan hydrochloride has a pH near 3 maintained with tartaric acid to ensure adequate solubility of greater than 2.5 mg/mL. The solubility decreases as the pH increases, becoming virtually insoluble at pH 4.5.[1747] Hydrolysis of the topotecan hydrochloride lactone ring is known to occur at pH values above 4.[2140]

DOI: 10.37573/9781585286850.382

Compatibility Information

Solution Compatibility

Topotecan HCl

Test Soln Name	Mfr	Mfr	Conc/L or %	Remarks	Ref	C/I
Dextrose 5%	BA[a], MG[b], MG[c]	SKB	50 mg	Visually compatible. No loss in 24 hr at 24°C in light and 7 days at 5°C in dark	2140	C
Dextrose 5%	BA[a]	SKB	25 mg	Visually compatible. No loss in 24 hr at 24°C in light and 7 days at 5°C in dark	2140	C
Dextrose 5%	BA[a]	SKB	10, 25, 50 mg	Visually compatible. Little loss in 28 days at 4 and 25°C in dark	2243	C
Dextrose 5%	BA[d]	SKB	10, 25, 50 mg	Visually compatible. Little loss in 28 days at 4 and 25°C in dark followed by 5 days at 37°C	2243	C
Sodium chloride 0.9%	BA[a], MG[b], MG[c]	SKB	50 mg	Visually compatible. No loss in 24 hr at 24°C in light and 7 days at 5°C in dark	2140	C
Sodium chloride 0.9%	BA[a]	SKB	25 mg	Visually compatible. No loss in 24 hr at 24°C in light and 7 days at 5°C in dark	2140	C
Sodium chloride 0.9%	BA[a]	SKB	10, 25, 50 mg	Visually compatible. Little loss in 28 days at 4 and 25°C in dark	2243	C
Sodium chloride 0.9%	BA[d]	SKB	10, 25, 50 mg	Visually compatible. Little loss in 28 days at 4 and 25°C in dark followed by 5 days at 37°C	2243	C
Sodium chloride 0.9%	BA[a]	SKB	10 mg	Visually compatible. 10% loss due to photodegradation in 17 days at room temperature in mixed daylight and fluorescent light	2243	C

[a] Tested in PVC containers.

[b] Tested in polyolefin containers.

[c] Tested in glass containers.

[d] Tested in elastomeric infusion devices (Infusors LV 2, Baxter)

Y-Site Injection Compatibility (1:1 Mixture)

Topotecan HCl

Test Drug	Mfr	Conc	Mfr	Conc	Remarks	Ref	C/I
Carboplatin	BR	0.9 mg/mL[a b]	SKB	56 mcg/mL[a b]	Visually compatible. Little loss of either drug in 4 hr at 22°C	2245	C
Cisplatin	BR	0.168 mg/mL[b]	SKB	56 mcg/mL[b]	Visually compatible. Little loss of either drug in 4 hr at 22°C	2245	C
Cyclophosphamide	MJ	20 mg/mL	SKB	56 mcg/mL[a b]	Visually compatible. Little loss of either drug in 4 hr at 22°C	2245	C
Dexamethasone sodium phosphate	RU	4 mg/mL	SKB	56 mcg/mL[b]	Haze and color change to intense yellow occur immediately	2245	I
Doxorubicin HCl	PH	2 mg/mL	SKB	56 mcg/mL[a b]	Visually compatible. Little loss of either drug in 4 hr at 22°C	2245	C
Etoposide	BR	0.4 mg/mL[a b]	SKB	56 mcg/mL[a b]	Visually compatible. Little loss of either drug in 4 hr at 22°C	2245	C
Fluorouracil	RC	50 mg/mL	SKB	56 mcg/mL[b]	Immediate haze and yellow color	2245	I
Gemcitabine HCl	LI	10 mg/mL[b]	SKB	0.1 mg/mL[b]	Physically compatible for 4 hr at 23°C	2226	C
Granisetron HCl	SKB	20 mcg/mL[a b]	SKB	56 mcg/mL[a b]	Visually compatible. Little loss of either drug in 4 hr at 22°C	2245	C
Ifosfamide	MJ	14.28 mg/mL[a b]	SKB	56 mcg/mL[a b]	Visually compatible. Little loss of either drug in 4 hr at 22°C	2245	C
Methylprednisolone sodium succinate	UP	2.4 mg/mL[a b]	SKB	56 mcg/mL[a b]	Yellow color forms. Little loss of either drug in 4 hr at 22°C	2245	C
Metoclopramide HCl	RB	1.72 mg/mL[a b]	SKB	56 mcg/mL[a b]	Visually compatible. Little loss of either drug in 4 hr at 22°C	2245	C

Y-Site Injection Compatibility (1:1 Mixture) (Cont.)

Test Drug	Mfr	Conc	Mfr	Conc	Remarks	Ref	C/I
Mitomycin	BR	84 mcg/mL[a][b]	SKB	56 mcg/mL[a][b]	Pale purple color forms immediately becoming a dark pinkish-lavender in 4 hr. 15 to 20% mitomycin loss in 4 hr at 22°C	2245	I
Ondansetron HCl	CER	0.48 mg/mL[a][b]	SKB	56 mcg/mL[a][b]	Visually compatible. Little loss of either drug in 4 hr at 22°C	2245	C
Oxaliplatin	SS	0.5 mg/mL[a]	SKB	0.1 mg/mL[a]	Physically compatible for 4 hr at 23°C	2566	C
Paclitaxel	MJ	0.54 mg/mL[a][b]	SKB	56 mcg/mL[a][b]	Visually compatible. Little loss of either drug in 4 hr at 22°C	2245	C
Palonosetron HCl	MGI	50 mcg/mL	GSK	0.1 mg/mL[a]	Physically compatible. Little loss of either drug in 4 hr	2609	C
Pemetrexed disodium	LI	20 mg/mL[b]	GSK	0.1 mg/mL[a]	Color darkening occurs immediately	2564	I
Prochlorperazine edisylate	SKB	0.192 mg/mL[a][b]	SKB	56 mcg/mL[a][b]	Visually compatible. Little loss of either drug in 4 hr at 22°C	2245	C
Vincristine sulfate	LI	1 mg/mL	SKB	56 mcg/mL[a][b]	Visually compatible. Little loss of either drug in 4 hr at 22°C	2245	C

[a] Tested in dextrose 5%.

[b] Tested in sodium chloride 0.9%.

Torsemide
AHFS 40:28.08

Products

Torsemide is available in 2- and 5-mL single-use vials.[3010] Each mL of solution contains torsemide 10 mg along with polyethylene glycol 400, tromethamine, water for injection, and sodium hydroxide if needed to adjust the pH during manufacture.[3010]

pH

Above 8.3.[3010]

Administration

Torsemide is administered intravenously either slowly as a bolus over 2 minutes or as a continuous infusion.[3010] If a common intravenous line is being used to administer other drugs in addition to torsemide, the line should be flushed with sodium chloride 0.9% prior to and following administration of torsemide.[3010]

Stability

Intact vials of torsemide should be stored at controlled room temperature and protected from freezing.[3010]

Torsemide injection solution should be visually inspected for discoloration and particulate matter prior to infusion; if either is present, the solution should not be used.[3010]

Compatibility Information

Solution Compatibility

Torsemide

Test Soln Name	Mfr	Mfr	Conc/L or %	Remarks	Ref	C/I
Dextrose 5%			0.1 to 0.8 g	Stable for 24 hr at room temperature	3010	C
Dextrose 5%	AB[a]	BM	200 mg	6% loss in 72 hr at 24°C	2108	C
Dextrose 5%	AB[a]	BM	5 g	3% loss in 72 hr at 24°C	2108	C
Sodium chloride 0.45%			0.1 to 0.4 g	Stable for 24 hr at room temperature	3010	C
Sodium chloride 0.9%			0.1 to 0.8 g	Stable for 24 hr at room temperature	3010	C

[a] Tested in PVC containers.

Y-Site Injection Compatibility (1:1 Mixture)

Torsemide

Test Drug	Mfr	Conc	Mfr	Conc	Remarks	Ref	C/I
Milrinone lactate	SW	0.4 mg/mL[a]	BM	10 mg/mL	Visually compatible. Little loss of either drug in 4 hr at 23°C	2214	C
Nesiritide	SCI	50 mcg/mL[a b]		10 mg/mL	Physically compatible for 4 hr	2625	C

[a] Tested in dextrose 5%.

[b] Tested in sodium chloride 0.9%.

Selected Revisions January 26, 2016. © Copyright, October 2000. American Society of Health-System Pharmacists, Inc.

DOI: 10.37573/9781585286850.383

Trabectedin

AHFS 10:00

Products

Trabectedin is available as a lyophilized powder in single-use vials containing 1 mg of the drug.[3177] Each vial also contains potassium dihydrogen phosphate 27.2 mg, sucrose 400 mg, and phosphoric acid and potassium hydroxide to adjust the pH.[3177] Each vial should be reconstituted with 20 mL of sterile water for injection to yield a solution containing trabectedin 0.05 mg/mL.[3177] Vials should be shaken until the powder has completely dissolved.[3177] The reconstituted solution should be visually inspected for particulate matter and discoloration prior to dilution; if particulate matter is present or discoloration occurs, the solution should not be used.[3177] The appropriate dose of the reconstituted solution should be withdrawn from the vial immediately after reconstitution and diluted in 500 mL of sodium chloride 0.9% or dextrose 5%.[3177]

pH

The reconstituted solution of trabectedin has a pH from 3.6 to 4.2.[3177]

Trade Name(s)

Yondelis

Administration

Trabectedin is administered as an intravenous infusion over 24 hours through a central venous line following dilution of the reconstituted solution in 500 mL of sodium chloride 0.9% or dextrose 5%.[3177] Trabectedin should be administered using an infusion set with a 0.2-µm polyethersulfone inline filter.[3177]

As with other toxic drugs, applicable special handling and disposal procedures for trabectedin should be followed.[3177]

Extravasation of trabectedin resulting in tissue necrosis and requiring debridement may occur; trabectedin should be administered through a central venous line.[3177]

Stability

Trabectedin is a white to off-white powder or cake that forms a clear, colorless to pale brownish-yellow solution when reconstituted with sterile water for injection.[3177] Intact vials should be stored under refrigeration at 2 to 8°C.[3177]

The reconstituted solution should be diluted immediately following reconstitution.[3177] Both the reconstituted solution and the drug diluted for infusion were found to be physically compatible and chemically stable for up to 30 hours when stored at room temperature in ambient light or under refrigeration.[3178] The total time from reconstitution and dilution through completion of administration should not exceed 30 hours; any unused portion of the reconstituted solution or the drug diluted for infusion should be discarded after that time.[3177]

Sorption

Trabectedin diluted for infusion is noted to be compatible with Type I colorless glass vials; polyvinylchloride (PVC) and polyethylene bags and tubing; polyethylene and polypropylene mixture bags; polyethersulfone inline filters; titanium, platinum, or plastic ports; silicone and polyurethane catheters; and pumps having contact surfaces made of PVC, polyethylene, or a combination of polyethylene and polypropylene.[3177]

Filtration

The diluted solution for infusion should be administered through an infusion set with a 0.2-µm polyethersulfone inline filter.[3177]

Compatibility Information

Solution Compatibility

Trabectedin

Test Soln Name	Mfr	Mfr	Conc/L or %	Remarks	Ref	C/I
Dextrose 5%	a	JN		Complete administration within 30 hr after reconstitution if stored at room temperature in ambient light or under refrigeration	3177, 3178	C
Sodium chloride 0.9%	a	JN		Complete administration within 30 hr after reconstitution if stored at room temperature in ambient light or under refrigeration	3177, 3178	C

a Tested in PVC, glass, and polyethylene containers.

DOI: 10.37573/9781585286850.384

Tramadol Hydrochloride
AHFS 28:08.08

Products

Tramadol hydrochloride is available as a 50-mg/mL aqueous solution in 1- and 2-mL (50- and 100-mg) ampuls. Sodium acetate and water for injection are also present in the formulation.[38][115]

Trade Name(s)

Contramal, Topalgic, Tramal, Zamadol, Zydol

Administration

Tramadol hydrochloride is administered intramuscularly, by direct intravenous injection slowly over 2 to 3 minutes, or by intravenous infusion after dilution.[38][115]

Stability

Tramadol hydrochloride is a clear, colorless solution. The intact ampuls should be stored below 30°C.[38][115]

Exposure to or protection from light did not affect the stability of tramadol hydrochloride 0.5- and 4-mg/mL infusion solutions in dextrose 5% or sodium chloride 0.9%.[434]

Freezing Solutions

Tramadol hydrochloride (Searle) 1 mg/mL in dextrose 5% in polyvinyl chloride (PVC) bags was stored frozen at −20°C for 120 days, microwave thawed, and stored refrigerated at 4°C for 60 days. No visual changes and 5% loss of tramadol hydrochloride was found.[2450][2526]

Compatibility Information

Solution Compatibility

Tramadol HCl

Test Soln Name	Mfr	Mfr	Conc/L or %	Remarks	Ref	C/I
Dextrose 5%		MUN		Physically compatible and chemically stable for 5 days	38	C
Dextrose 5%	a	MUN	0.5 and 4 g	Visually compatible. No loss in 14 days at 4°C and 7 days at room temperature or 40°C	434	C
Dextrose 5%	BA[a]	GRU	0.4 g	Visually compatible with no loss in 24 hr at room temperature and 4°C	2652	C
Ringer's injection, lactated		MUN		Physically compatible and chemically stable for 5 days	38	C
Ringer's injection, lactated		GRU	0.4 g	Visually compatible with no loss in 24 hr at room temperature and 4°C	2652	C
Sodium chloride 0.9%		MUN		Physically compatible and chemically stable for 5 days	38	C
Sodium chloride 0.9%	a	MUN	0.5 and 4 g	Visually compatible with little or no loss in 14 days at 4°C and 7 days at room temperature. 3 to 5% loss in 7 days at 40°C	434	C
Sodium chloride 0.9%	BA[a]	GRU	0.4 g	Visually compatible with no loss in 24 hr at room temperature and 4°C	2652	C

[a] Tested in PVC containers.

Additive Compatibility

Tramadol HCl

Test Drug	Mfr	Conc/L or %	Mfr	Conc/L or %	Test Solution	Remarks	Ref	C/I
Acyclovir sodium	WEL	5 g	GRU	400 mg	NS	Precipitation and 20% tramadol loss in 1 hr	2652	I
Ampicillin sodium–sulbactam sodium	PF	20[b] g	GRU	400 mg	NS	Visually compatible with up to 9% tramadol loss in 24 hr at room temperature	2652	C
Clindamycin phosphate	AB	6 g	GRU	400 mg	NS	Tramadol losses of 20% in 4 hr at room temperature with precipitate	2652	I

DOI: 10.37573/9781585286850.385

Additive Compatibility (Cont.)

Test Drug	Mfr	Conc/L or %	Mfr	Conc/L or %	Test Solution	Remarks	Ref	C/I
Dexamethasone sodium phosphate	ME	440 mg	AND	11.18 g	NS[a]	Visually compatible for 7 days at 25°C protected from light	2701	C
Dexamethasone sodium phosphate	ME	1.33 g	AND	33.3 g	NS[a]	Visually compatible for 7 days at 25°C protected from light	2701	C
Haloperidol lactate	EST	210 mg	AND	11.18 g	NS[a]	Visually compatible for 7 days at 25°C protected from light	2701	C
Haloperidol lactate	EST	620 mg	AND	33.3 g	NS[a]	Visually compatible for 7 days at 25°C protected from light	2701	C
Ketamine HCl	QI	500 mg	GRU	5 g	NS[c]	Physically compatible with little loss of either drug in 14 days at 4 and 25°C in the dark	3583	C
Ketamine HCl	QI	1 g	GRU	5 g	NS[c]	Physically compatible with little loss of either drug in 14 days at 4 and 25°C in the dark	3583	C
Ketamine HCl	QI	2 g	GRU	5 g	NS[c]	Physically compatible with little loss of either drug in 14 days at 4 and 25°C in the dark	3583	C
Mannitol		20%	GRU	0.4 g		Visually compatible with no tramadol loss in 24 hr at room temperature and 4°C	2652	C
Metoclopramide HCl	SYO	1.11 g	AND	1.118 g	NS[a]	Visually compatible for 7 days at 25°C protected from light	2701	C
Metoclopramide HCl	SYO	3.33 g	AND	3.33 g	NS[a]	Visually compatible for 7 days at 25°C protected from light	2701	C
Midazolam HCl	RC	500 mg	AND	11.18 g	NS[a]	Visually compatible for 7 days at 25°C protected from light	2701	C
Midazolam HCl	RC	1.5 g	AND	33.3 g	NS[a]	Visually compatible for 7 days at 25°C protected from light	2701	C
Ondansetron HCl	GL	1.6 mg	GRU	400 mg	NS	Visually compatible with about 7% tramadol loss in 24 hr at room temperature	2652	C
Ranitidine HCl	AB	0.5 g	GRU	400 mg	NS	Visually compatible with little or no tramadol loss in 24 hr at room temperature	2652	C
Scopolamine butylbromide	BI	1.68 g	AND	11.18 g	NS[a]	Visually compatible for 7 days at 25°C protected from light	2701	C
Scopolamine butylbromide	BI	5 g	AND	5 g	NS[a]	Visually compatible for 7 days at 25°C protected from light	2701	C

[a] Tested in elastomeric pump reservoirs (Baxter).

[b] Ampicillin component. Ampicillin in a 2:1 fixed-ratio concentration with sulbactam.

[c] Tested in polyolefin containers.

Drugs in Syringe Compatibility

Tramadol HCl

Test Drug	Mfr	Amt	Mfr	Amt	Remarks	Ref	C/I
Dexamethasone sodium phosphate	ME	3.33, 1.67, 1.33, 0.33 mg/mL[a]	GRU	33.33, 16.66, 8.33 mg/mL[a]	Physically compatible and both drugs chemically stable for 5 days at 25°C protected from light	2747	C
Haloperidol lactate	EST	0.208 mg/mL[a]	GRU	8.33, 16.67, 33.33 mg/mL[a]	Physically compatible with no loss of either drug in 15 days at 4 and 25°C protected from light	2672	C
Heparin sodium		2500 units/1 mL	GRU	100 mg/2 mL	Visually compatible for at least 5 min	1053	C

Drugs in Syringe Compatibility (Cont.)

Test Drug	Mfr	Amt	Mfr	Amt	Remarks	Ref	C/I
Scopolamine butylbromide	BI	3.33, 4.99, 6.67 mg/mL[a]	GRU	8.33, 16.67, 33.33 mg/mL[a]	Physically compatible with no loss of tramadol HCl and about 5 to 6% loss of scopolamine butylbromide in 15 days at 4 and 25°C protected from light	2632	C

[a] Tested in sodium chloride 0.9%.

Y-Site Injection Compatibility (1:1 Mixture)

Tramadol HCl

Test Drug	Mfr	Conc	Mfr	Conc	Remarks	Ref	C/I
Rifampin	AVE	6 mg/mL	GRU	8.33 mg/mL	Immediate red-orange turbid precipitate	2727	I

Selected Revisions July 1, 2020. © Copyright, October 2000.
American Society of Health-System Pharmacists, Inc.

Tranexamic Acid
AHFS 20:28.16

Products

Tranexamic acid is available in 10-mL ampuls and vials.[2886] [2888] Each mL contains 100 mg tranexamic acid in water for injection.[2886] [2888]

pH

From 6.5 to 8.[2886] [2888]

Trade Name(s)

Cyklokapron

Administration

The manufacturer recommends that tranexamic acid be administered by slow intravenous injection at a rate that does not exceed 100 mg/min.[2886] [2888]

The drug also has been administered as a loading dose infused over 10 minutes, followed by an infusion administered over 8 hours.[2889] [2890] [2891]

Stability

Intact vials and ampuls should be stored at controlled room temperature[2886] [2888] and protected from light and freezing.[2887]

The solution does not contain any preservative and is for single use.[2887] [2888] Any unused product should be discarded.[2887]

The manufacturer recommends that solutions for infusion be prepared on the same day that they are to be used.[2886] [2888]

In one study, antifibrinolytic activity of tranexamic acid was retained after ampuls were stored at temperatures ranging from −20 to 50°C for up to 12 weeks; however, all ampuls stored at −20°C were visibly cracked within 1 week.[2988]

Compatibility Information

Solution Compatibility

Tranexamic acid

Test Soln Name	Mfr	Mfr	Conc/L or %	Remarks	Ref	C/I
Dextrose 5%	a b c	PF	10 and 20 g	Stable up to 24 hr at 5°C in dark, room temperature in light, and 30°C and 75% relative humidity in dark	2887	C
Sodium chloride 0.9%	b c	PF	10 and 20 g	Stable 7 days at 5°C in dark, room temperature in light, and 30°C and 75% relative humidity in dark	2887	C
Sodium chloride 0.9%	a	PF	10 and 20 g	Stable 24 hr at room temperature in light and 30°C and 75% relative humidity in dark	2887	C
Sodium chloride 0.9%	a	PF	10 and 20 g	Stable up to 7 days at 5°C in dark	2887	C
Sodium chloride 0.9%	BRN d	MYL	15.4 g	Physically compatible with less than 10% loss in 90 days at 20 to 25°C and 2 to 8°C protected from light	2987	C
Sodium chloride 0.9%	BA a	MYL	20 g	Physically compatible with less than 10% loss in 180 days at 20 to 25°C protected from light	2987	C
Ringer's injection	b	PF	10 and 20 g	Stable up to 7 days at 5°C in dark, room temperature in light, and 30°C and 75% relative humidity in dark	2887	C

a Tested in glass containers.

b Tested in PVC containers.

c Tested in polyethylene and polypropylene containers.

d Tested in polyethylene-polypropylene copolymer PAB bags.

DOI: 10.37573/9781585286850.386

Additive Compatibility

Tranexamic acid

Test Drug	Mfr	Conc/L or %	Mfr	Conc/L or %	Test Solution	Remarks	Ref	C/I
Dextran 40			PF			Manufacturer-recommended solution	2887	C
Hetastarch in lactated electrolyte	HOS	5.88%		2 g		No evidence of physical incompatibility over 4 hr	3454	C
Penicillin G potassium			PF			Manufacturer states incompatible	2887	I
Penicillin G sodium			PF			Manufacturer states incompatible	2887	I

Drugs in Syringe Compatibility

Tranexamic acid

Test Drug	Mfr	Amt	Mfr	Amt	Remarks	Ref	C/I
Doxapram HCl	RB	400 mg/20 mL		250 mg/5 mL	5% doxapram loss in 9 hr and 12% in 24 hr	1177	I

Y-Site Injection Compatibility (1:1 Mixture)

Tranexamic acid

Test Drug	Mfr	Conc	Mfr	Conc	Remarks	Ref	C/I
Blinatumomab	AMG	0.125 mcg/mL[b]	SAA	100 mg/mL	Haze or flakes transiently appear	3405, 3417	?
Blinatumomab	AMG	0.375 mcg/mL[b]	SAA	100 mg/mL	Persistent particulate formation when blinatumomab is added to tranexamic acid; not observed when order of mixing was reversed	3405, 3417	?
Clevidipine butyrate	CHS	0.5 mg/mL		20 mg/mL[a]	Physically compatible for 24 hr at 23°C	3334	C
Defibrotide sodium	JAZ	8 mg/mL[b]	SAA	100 mg/mL	Visually compatible for 4 hr at room temperature	3149	C
Heparin sodium			PF		Manufacturer states compatible	2887	C
Hetastarch in lactated electrolyte	HOS	6%		100 mg/mL	No evidence of physical incompatibility over 4 hr	3454	C

[a] Tested in dextrose 5%.

[b] Tested in sodium chloride 0.9%.

Selected Revisions September 30, 2019. © Copyright, August 2015. American Society of Health-System Pharmacists, Inc.

Trastuzumab
AHFS 10:00

Products

Trastuzumab is available as a lyophilized powder in multiple-use vials containing 440 mg of the drug with α,α-trehalose dihydrate 400 mg, L-histidine hydrochloride 9.9 mg, L-histidine 6.4 mg, and polysorbate 20 1.8 mg; the vial is sealed under a vacuum.[3086] Each vial of trastuzumab is packaged with a 20-mL vial of bacteriostatic water for injection diluent containing benzyl alcohol 1.1% as a preservative.[3086]

CAUTION: Care should be taken to ensure that the correct drug product is prepared and that no confusion with other products (e.g., ado-trastuzumab emtansine) occurs.[3086] Each vial of trastuzumab should be reconstituted with 20 mL of the provided bacteriostatic water for injection to yield a multiple-use solution containing trastuzumab 21 mg/mL.[3086] The drug also may be reconstituted with 20 mL of sterile water for injection (without preservative) to yield a single-use solution containing trastuzumab 21 mg/mL.[3086] The diluent should be slowly injected into the vial, directing the stream of diluent into the lyophilized cake.[3086] The vial should be swirled gently to aid reconstitution; shaking should be avoided.[3086] The vial should be allowed to stand undisturbed for approximately 5 minutes as slight foaming of the product may occur upon reconstitution.[3086] The reconstituted solution should be visually inspected for particulate matter and discoloration; the solution should be free of visible particulates.[3086]

The appropriate dose of the reconstituted solution should be diluted in 250 mL of sodium chloride 0.9% in a polyvinyl chloride (PVC) or polyethylene bag;[3086] dextrose 5% should *not* be used due to the potential risk of protein aggregation.[3086][3088] The infusion bag should be gently inverted to mix the diluted solution.[3086]

pH

The pH of the reconstituted solution is approximately 6.[3086]

Trade Name(s)

Herceptin

Administration

CAUTION: Care should be taken to ensure that the correct drug product is administered and that no confusion with other products (e.g., ado-trastuzumab emtansine) occurs.[3086] Trastuzumab is administered only by intravenous infusion following reconstitution and further dilution in 250 mL of sodium chloride 0.9%.[3086] The drug should be infused over 30 to 90 minutes depending upon previous trastuzumab exposure and the indication for the drug in the specific patient.[3086] Trastuzumab should *not* be administered by intravenous push or bolus injection.[3086]

Stability

Intact vials of trastuzumab are stable at 2 to 8°C.[3086] Trastuzumab is a white to pale yellow lyophilized powder that forms a clear to slightly opalescent and colorless to pale yellow solution upon reconstitution.[3086]

When reconstituted with the provided bacteriostatic water for injection diluent, vials of the reconstituted multiple-use solution are stable for 28 days if stored at 2 to 8°C; any solution remaining after 28 days should be discarded.[3086] Vials of trastuzumab reconstituted with unpreserved sterile water for injection should be used immediately; any unused portions should be discarded.[3086] The manufacturer states that trastuzumab should not be mixed with other drugs.[3086]

Diluted trastuzumab infusion solutions should be stored at 2 to 8°C for no longer than 24 hours prior to use.[3086] Although trastuzumab solutions diluted to concentrations of 0.4, 1, or 4 mg/mL (diluent unspecified) were reported to be physically stable with no change in monomer concentration for up to 28 days when stored at 2 to 8°C, biological activity was not reported in this study.[3089]

Reconstituted solutions or solutions diluted for infusion should not be frozen.[3086]

Temperature Effects

In a study evaluating the physical stability of trastuzumab, solutions containing trastuzumab (Roche) 0.4 or 4 mg/mL (diluent unspecified) showed no increase in particle size up to a temperature of 65°C.[3089] At 75°C, the solutions became turbid, suggesting the formation of insoluble aggregates; following centrifugation, particle size analysis also revealed soluble aggregates within the clear supernatant.[3089] Additional spectrophotometric evaluation showed a loss of ordered structure of the drug at temperatures of 75°C.[3089]

Filtration

Use of an inline filter was not required for administration of trastuzumab-containing solutions in clinical studies.[3087] The manufacturer makes no recommendations regarding filtration of the drug.[3086]

DOI: 10.37573/9781585286850.387

Compatibility Information

Solution Compatibility

Trastuzumab

Test Soln Name	Mfr	Mfr	Conc/L or %	Remarks	Ref	C/I
Sodium chloride 0.9%	a	GEN		Stable for 24 hr at 2 to 8°C	3086	C
Sodium chloride 0.9%	b	GEN		Stable for 24 hr at 2 to 8°C	3086	C
Sodium chloride 0.9%	BRN[c]	GEN	1.5 g	Stable for up to 24 hr at 30°C	3090	C
Sodium chloride 0.9%	BRN[c]	GEN	2.5 g	Stable for up to 24 hr at 5 and 30°C	3090	C
Sodium chloride 0.9%	BA[a]	GEN	2.5 g	Stable for up to 24 hr at 5 and 30°C	3090	C

[a] Tested in PVC containers.

[b] Tested in polyethylene containers.

[c] Tested in polyolefin containers.

Additive Compatibility

Trastuzumab

Test Drug	Mfr	Conc/L or %	Mfr	Conc/L or %	Test Solution	Remarks	Ref	C/I
Pertuzumab	GEN	1.5 g	GEN	1.5 g	NS[a]	Compatible and stable for up to 24 hr at 30°C	3090	C
Pertuzumab	GEN	2.7 g	GEN	2.3 g	NS[b]	Compatible and stable for up to 24 hr at 5 and 30°C	3090	C

[a] Tested in polyolefin containers.

[b] Tested in polyolefin and PVC containers.

Treprostinil Sodium
AHFS 48:48

Products

Treprostinil is available as 1-, 2.5-, 5-, and 10-mg/mL (as sodium) in 20-mL multiple-dose vials. Each mL also contains sodium chloride 5.3 mg (except the 10-mg/mL concentration which contains 4 mg), metacresol 3 mg, and sodium citrate 6.3 mg in water for injection. Sodium hydroxide and/or hydrochloridic acid may have been added during manufacturing to adjust the pH.[1(9/08)]

pH

From 6.0 to 7.2.[1(9/08)]

Trade Name(s)

Remodulin

Administration

Treprostinil sodium is preferably administered by continuous subcutaneous infusion using a syringe pump designed for subcutaneous administration. The drug may also be administered via a central venous catheter only after dilution in sterile water for injection, sodium chloride 0.9%, or Flolan special diluent using an intravenous infusion pump. The subcutaneous or intravenous infusion pump must have a reservoir made of polypropylene, polyvinyl chloride, or glass.[1(9/08)]

Stability

Intact vials should be stored at controlled room temperature. The drug is stable at room temperature and neutral pH. The manufacturer recommends using the vials for no more than 14 days after initial stopper penetration. The undiluted drug is stable for up to 72 hours at 37°C during administration in syringe reservoirs. The manufacturer states that after dilution in sterile water for injection, sodium chloride 0.9%, or Flolan special diluent, the drug is stable for 48 hours at 37°C at concentrations as low as 4 mcg/mL.[1(9/08)]

Using proper technique to penetrate the vial stopper with a needle, limiting the number of punctures of a vial stopper to 10, and using a Clave Connector Multidose Vial Adapter were shown to reduce the amount of particulate matter from the stopper that was found upon multiple-day use of treprostinil sodium 1- and 10-mg/mL vials and to be within the USP limit for such particulate matter over the 30-day test period. No loss of treprostinil sodium occurred during this period as well. Improper needle technique and numerous stopper penetrations were found to result in unacceptable particulate matter from the vial stopper.[2611]

Syringes

The chemical and physical stability of undiluted treprostinil sodium (United Therapeutics) 1, 2.5, 5, and 10 mg/mL was evaluated packaged in 3-mL MiniMed plastic syringe pump reservoirs sealed with plastic tip caps. The samples were stored at 37, 23, 4, and −20°C for 60 days. The samples were clear and colorless, and treprostinil was stable at all four storage temperatures, exhibiting concentrations of 95% or more over 60 days.[2528]

Compatibility Information

Solution Compatibility

Treprostinil sodium

Test Soln Name	Mfr	Mfr	Conc/L or %	Remarks	Ref	C/I
Dextrose 5%	BA[a]	UT	4 mcg/mL	Treprostinil loss of 15 to 20% in 24 to 48 hr at 40°C. Up to 70% loss of metacresol preservative	2476	I
Dextrose 5%	BA[a]	UT	20 and 130 mcg/mL	Treprostinil loss of 5% or less in 48 hr at 40°C. Up to 70% loss of metacresol preservative	2476	C
Sodium chloride 0.9%	BA[a]	UT	4 and 130 mcg/mL	Little or no treprostinil loss in 48 hr at 40°C. Up to 70% loss of metacresol preservative	2476	C

[a] Tested in medication cassette reservoirs (SIMS-Deltec).

Selected Revisions October 1, 2012. © Copyright, October 2004.
American Society of Health-System Pharmacists, Inc.

DOI: 10.37573/9781585286850.388

Trimethobenzamide Hydrochloride
AHFS 56:22.08

Products

Trimethobenzamide hydrochloride 100 mg/mL is available in 2-mL single-dose and 20-mL multiple-dose vials. Each mL of solution also contains sodium citrate, citric acid, and sodium hydroxide to adjust pH. Some products may contain edetate disodium. The multiple-dose vials also contain phenol 0.45%.[1(6/09)]

pH

The official pH range is 4.5 to 5.5.[17] The manufacturer indicates the actual pH is approximately 5.[1(6/09)]

Trade Name(s)

Tigan

Administration

Trimethobenzamide hydrochloride is administered by intramuscular injection deep into the upper outer quadrant of the gluteal region. Intravenous injection is not recommended.[1(6/09)] [4]

Stability

Trimethobenzamide hydrochloride should be stored at controlled room temperature and protected from freezing.[1(6/09)] [4]

Compatibility Information

Drugs in Syringe Compatibility

Trimethobenzamide HCl

Test Drug	Mfr	Amt	Mfr	Amt	Remarks	Ref	C/I
Glycopyrrolate	RB	0.2 mg/1 mL	BE	100 mg/1 mL	Physically compatible. pH in glycopyrrolate stability range for 48 hr at 25°C	331	C
Glycopyrrolate	RB	0.2 mg/1 mL	BE	200 mg/2 mL	Physically compatible. pH in glycopyrrolate stability range for 48 hr at 25°C	331	C
Glycopyrrolate	RB	0.4 mg/2 mL	BE	100 mg/1 mL	Physically compatible. pH in glycopyrrolate stability range for 48 hr at 25°C	331	C
Hydromorphone HCl	KN	4 mg/2 mL	BE	100 mg/1 mL	Physically compatible for 30 min	517	C
Midazolam HCl	RC	5 mg/1 mL	BE	200 mg/2 mL	Physically compatible for 4 hr at 25°C	1145	C
Nalbuphine HCl	EN	10 mg/1 mL	BE	100 mg/1 mL	Physically compatible for 36 hr at 27°C	762	C
Nalbuphine HCl	EN	5 mg/0.5 mL	BE	100 mg/1 mL	Physically compatible for 36 hr at 27°C	762	C
Nalbuphine HCl	EN	2.5 mg/0.25 mL	BE	100 mg/1 mL	Physically compatible for 36 hr at 27°C	762	C
Nalbuphine HCl	DU	10 mg/1 mL		200 mg/2 mL	Physically compatible for 48 hr	128	C
Nalbuphine HCl	DU	20 mg/1 mL		200 mg/2 mL	Physically compatible for 48 hr	128	C

Y-Site Injection Compatibility (1:1 Mixture)

Trimethobenzamide HCl

Test Drug	Mfr	Conc	Mfr	Conc	Remarks	Ref	C/I
Heparin sodium	UP	1000 units/L[a]	RC	100 mg/mL	Physically compatible for 4 hr at room temperature	534	C
Hydrocortisone sodium succinate	UP	10 mg/L[a]	RC	100 mg/mL	Physically compatible for 4 hr at room temperature	534	C
Potassium chloride	AB	40 mEq/L[a]	RC	100 mg/mL	Physically compatible for 4 hr at room temperature	534	C

[a] Tested in dextrose 5% in Ringer's injection, dextrose 5% in Ringer's injection, lactated, dextrose 5%, Ringer's injection, lactated, and sodium chloride 0.9%.

DOI: 10.37573/9781585286850.389

Trimethoprim–Sulfamethoxazole
AHFS 8:12.20
Co-trimoxazole

Products

Trimethoprim–sulfamethoxazole 16 + 80 mg/mL is available as a concentrate in 5-, 10-, and 30-mL vials. Each mL also contains propylene glycol, ethyl alcohol, diethanolamine, benzyl alcohol, sodium metabisulfite, and sodium hydroxide to adjust pH in water for injection.[1(9/08)]

pH

From 9.5 to 10.5.[1(9/08)]

Osmolality

The osmolalities of trimethoprim–sulfamethoxazole (Burroughs Wellcome) in concentrations of 0.8 + 4, 1.1 + 5.5, and 1.6 + 8 mg/mL in dextrose 5% were determined to be 541, 669, and 798 mOsm/kg, respectively. At 1.6 + 8 mg/mL in sodium chloride 0.9%, the osmolality was determined to be 833 mOsm/kg.[1375]

Trade Name(s)

Bactrim

Administration

Trimethoprim–sulfamethoxazole is administered by intravenous infusion only after dilution in dextrose 5%. The drug should not be injected intramuscularly. Infusion over 60 to 90 minutes is recommended; rapid or direct intravenous injection must not be used. It is recommended that each 5 mL be diluted in 125 mL or, if fluid restriction is required, in 75 mL of dextrose 5%. Infusion admixtures should be inspected for cloudiness or crystallization before and during administration.[1(9/08) 4]

Stability

Trimethoprim–sulfamethoxazole in intact vials should be stored at controlled room temperature and not refrigerated. The multiple-dose vials should be used within 48 hours of initial entry.[1(9/08)]

The solubility of trimethoprim in aqueous solutions is partially dependent on the pH of the solution. Trimethoprim is a weak base, and its solubility is lower in solutions with a more alkaline pH.[553]

Precipitation occurs in the diluted infusion solution in varying time periods, depending on the final concentration. For dilutions of 5 mL per 125 mL of dextrose 5% (trimethoprim 640 mg/L, sulfamethoxazole 3.2 g/L), use within 6 hours is recommended.[1(9/08)] However, precipitation within 4 hours has been observed at this concentration.[553] For dilutions of 5 mL per 100 mL of dextrose 5% (trimethoprim 800 mg/L, sulfamethoxazole 4 g/L), use within 4 hours is recommended. For dilutions of 5 mL per 75 mL of dextrose 5% (trimethoprim 1.067 g/L, sulfamethoxazole 5.33 g/L), use within 2 hours is recommended. All infusions should be inspected carefully and watched closely for turbidity and precipitation. Infusion admixtures in dextrose 5% should not be refrigerated.[1(9/08) 4]

The nature of the precipitate that forms from 7 infusion solutions containing trimethoprim–sulfamethoxazole (Roche) was evaluated. In all cases, the sulfamethoxazole concentrations were within 5% of expected values, but the trimethoprim concentrations dropped to about 30% of the initial values. Further evaluation of the solid phases showed them to be trimethoprim alone or with trimethoprim monohydrate.[1895]

Syringes

Undiluted trimethoprim–sulfamethoxazole (Elkins-Sinn) 16 + 80 mg/mL was stored in polypropylene syringes (Becton Dickinson) for 2.5 days at room temperature. The syringes were exposed to fluorescent light during the day but kept in the dark at night. No loss was observed.[1582]

Sorption

Trimethoprim was shown not to exhibit sorption to polyvinyl chloride (PVC) bags and tubing, polyethylene tubing, Silastic tubing, and polypropylene syringes.[536 606]

Plasticizer Leaching

Trimethoprim–sulfamethoxazole (Elkins-Sinn) 0.8 + 4 mg/mL in dextrose 5% did not leach diethylhexyl phthalate (DEHP) plasticizer from 50-mL PVC bags in 24 hours at 24°C.[1683]

Filtration

Filtration of dilutions of trimethoprim–sulfamethoxazole (Roche), ranging from 1:25 (v/v) to 1:10 (v/v) in several common intravenous infusion solutions, did not appear to result in loss of either drug because of sorption to the filter. Filtration of a visibly precipitated solution resulted in a substantial loss of trimethoprim.[747]

Trimethoprim–sulfamethoxazole (Roche) 1.88 mg/mL in dextrose 5% and sodium chloride 0.9% was filtered through a 0.22-µm cellulose ester membrane filter (Ivex-HP, Millipore) over 6 hours. No significant drug loss due to binding to the filter was noted.[1034]

DOI: 10.37573/9781585286850.390

Compatibility Information

Solution Compatibility

Trimethoprim–sulfamethoxazole

Test Soln Name	Mfr	Mfr	Conc/L or %	Remarks	Ref	C/I
Dextrose 5% in sodium chloride 0.45%	AB	RC	640[d] mg	Physically compatible. 6% trimethoprim loss and little sulfamethoxazole loss in 24 hr at 25°C	747	C
Dextrose 5% in sodium chloride 0.45%	AB	RC	800[d] mg	Physically compatible. 4% trimethoprim loss and little sulfamethoxazole loss in 24 hr at 25°C	747	C
Dextrose 5%	AB	RC	640[d] mg	Physically compatible. Little trimethoprim and sulfamethoxazole loss in 24 hr at 25°C	747	C
Dextrose 5%	AB	RC	800[d] mg	Physically compatible. Little trimethoprim and sulfamethoxazole loss in 24 hr at 25°C	747	C
Dextrose 5%	TR	RC	640[d] mg	Admixture clear and colorless for 4 hr at 22°C. Turbidity and precipitation appear after this time. 5% trimethoprim loss in 4 hr and 28% in 24 hr. About 1% sulfamethoxazole loss in 24 hr	553	I[a]
Dextrose 5%	TR	RC	1.6[d] g	Admixture clear and colorless for 2 hr at 22°C. Turbidity and precipitation appear after this time. 5% trimethoprim loss in 2 hr and 64% in 24 hr. About 3% sulfamethoxazole loss in 24 hr	553	I[a]
Dextrose 5%	TR	RC	3.2[d] g	Rapid precipitation and 32% trimethoprim loss in 1 hr. 9% sulfamethoxazole loss in 24 hr	553	I
Dextrose 5%	AB[b]	BW, RC	640[d] mg	Physically compatible. Little trimethoprim and sulfamethoxazole loss in 48 hr at 24°C	1201	C
Dextrose 5%	AB[b]	BW, RC	800[d] mg	Physically compatible. Little or no trimethoprim and sulfamethoxazole loss in 24 hr at 24°C. Precipitate in 48 hr	1201	C
Dextrose 5%	AB[b]	BW, RC	1.07[d] g	Physically compatible. Little or no trimethoprim and sulfamethoxazole loss in 4 hr at 24°C. Precipitate in 8 hr	1201	I[a]
Dextrose 5%	AB[b]	BW, RC	1.6[d] g	Precipitate forms as early as 2 hr at 24°C. Up to 75% trimethoprim loss in 4 hr	1201	I
Dextrose 5%	BA[b]	ES	1.08[d] g	4 of 20 samples precipitated. No loss of trimethoprim in 24 hr at 23°C. Sulfamethoxazole not tested	2536	I
Dextrose 5%	BA[c]	ES	1.08[d] g	Physically compatible. No loss of trimethoprim in 24 hr at 23°C. Sulfamethoxazole not tested	2536	C
Dextrose 5%	BA[b]	ES	1.6[d] g	4 of 20 samples precipitated. No loss of trimethoprim in 24 hr at 23°C. Sulfamethoxazole not tested	2536	I
Dextrose 5%	BA[c]	ES	1.6[d] g	Physically compatible. No loss of trimethoprim in 24 hr at 23°C. Sulfamethoxazole not tested	2536	C
Dextrose 5%	BA[c]	HOS	640[d] mg	Physically compatible with no loss of either drug in 4 hr at 20 to 22°C	3522	C
Dextrose 5%	BA[c]	HOS	800[d] mg	Physically compatible with little to no loss of either drug in 4 hr at 20 to 22°C	3522	C
Dextrose 5%	BA[c]	HOS	1.07[d] g	Increase in particle formation observed by microscopic analysis after 1 hr at 20 to 22°C	3522	?
Dextrose 5%	BA[c]	HOS	1.6[d] g	Microscopic analysis revealed the presence of particles immediately upon dilution; visual analysis demonstrated the formation of particles adherent to the walls of the infusion bag within 1.5 hr	3522	I
Ringer's injection, lactated	AB	RC	640[d] mg	Physically compatible. 4% trimethoprim loss and little sulfamethoxazole loss in 24 hr at 25°C	747	C

Solution Compatibility (Cont.)

Test Soln Name	Mfr	Mfr	Conc/L or %	Remarks	Ref	C/I
Ringer's injection, lactated	AB	RC	800[d] mg	Physically compatible. Little trimethoprim loss and 4% sulfamethoxazole loss in 24 hr at 25°C	747	C
Sodium chloride 0.45%	AB	RC	640[d] mg	Physically compatible. Little trimethoprim and sulfamethoxazole loss in 24 hr at 25°C	747	C
Sodium chloride 0.45%	AB	RC	800[d] mg	Physically compatible. 4% trimethoprim loss and little sulfamethoxazole loss in 24 hr at 25°C	747	C
Sodium chloride 0.9%	AB	RC	640[d] mg	Physically compatible. 5% trimethoprim loss and 4% sulfamethoxazole loss in 24 hr at 25°C	747	C
Sodium chloride 0.9%	AB	RC	800[d] mg	Physically compatible. Little trimethoprim and sulfamethoxazole loss in 24 hr at 25°C	747	C
Sodium chloride 0.9%	TR	RC	640[d] mg	Admixture clear and colorless for 4 hr at 22°C. Turbidity and precipitation appear after this time. 1% trimethoprim loss in 4 hr and 36% in 24 hr. No sulfamethoxazole loss in 24 hr	553	I[a]
Sodium chloride 0.9%	TR	RC	1.6[d] g	Admixture clear and colorless for 1 to 2 hr at 22°C. Turbidity appears after this time. 15% trimethoprim loss in 2 hr and 76% in 24 hr. 5% sulfamethoxazole loss in 24 hr	553	I
Sodium chloride 0.9%	TR	RC	3.2[d] g	Rapid precipitation and 74% trimethoprim loss in 1 hr. 6% sulfamethoxazole loss in 24 hr	553	I
Sodium chloride 0.9%	AB[b]	BW, RC	640[d] mg	Physically compatible. Little trimethoprim and sulfamethoxazole loss in 48 hr at 24°C	1201	C
Sodium chloride 0.9%	AB[b]	BW, RC	800[d] mg	Physically compatible. Little trimethoprim and sulfamethoxazole loss in 14 hr at 24°C. Precipitate forms within 24 hr	1201	I[a]
Sodium chloride 0.9%	AB[b]	BW, RC	1.07[d] g	Physically compatible. Little trimethoprim and sulfamethoxazole loss in 2 hr at 24°C. Precipitate forms within 4 hr	1201	I[a]
Sodium chloride 0.9%	AB[b]	BW, RC	1.6[d] g	Precipitate forms as early as 2 hr at 24°C. Up to 18% trimethoprim loss in 4 hr	1201	I
Sodium chloride 0.9%	[b]	BW	1.6[d] g	Precipitate forms in 1.5 hr at 20°C. 10% trimethoprim loss in 1.5 hr, 21% loss in 3 hr, and 60% loss in 24 hr	1555	I
Sodium chloride 0.9%	BA[b]	ES	1.08[d] g	2 of 20 samples precipitated. 4% loss of trimethoprim in 24 hr at 23°C. Sulfamethoxazole not tested	2536	I
Sodium chloride 0.9%	BA[c]	ES	1.08[d] g	Physically compatible. No loss of trimethoprim in 24 hr at 23°C. Sulfamethoxazole not tested	2536	C
Sodium chloride 0.9%	BA[b]	ES	1.6[d] g	14 of 20 samples precipitated. 4% loss of trimethoprim in 24 hr at 23°C. Sulfamethoxazole not tested	2536	I
Sodium chloride 0.9%	BA[c]	ES	1.6[d] g	Physically compatible. No loss of trimethoprim in 24 hr at 23°C. Sulfamethoxazole not tested	2536	C

[a] Incompatible by conventional standards. May be used in shorter time periods.

[b] Tested in glass containers.

[c] Tested in PVC containers.

[d] Trimethoprim component. Trimethoprim in a 1:5 fixed-ratio concentration with sulfamethoxazole.

Additive Compatibility

Trimethoprim–sulfamethoxazole

Test Drug	Mfr	Conc/L or %	Mfr	Conc/L or %	Test Solution	Remarks	Ref	C/I
Fluconazole	PF	1 g	ES	0.4[b] g	D5W	Delayed cloudiness and precipitation. No fluconazole loss in 72 hr at 25°C under fluorescent light	1677	I
Linezolid	PHU	2 g	ES	800[b] mg	[a]	A large amount of white needle-like crystals forms immediately	2333	I
Verapamil HCl	KN	80 mg	BW	160[b] mg	D5W, NS	Transient precipitate	764	I

[a] Admixed in the linezolid infusion container.

[b] Trimethoprim component. Trimethoprim in a 1:5 fixed-ratio concentration with sulfamethoxazole.

Drugs in Syringe Compatibility

Trimethoprim–sulfamethoxazole

Test Drug	Mfr	Amt	Mfr	Amt	Remarks	Ref	C/I
Dimenhydrinate		10 mg/1 mL		16 mg/1 mL[b]	Clear solution	2569	C
Heparin sodium		2500 units/1 mL		80 mg/5 mL[b]	Physically compatible for at least 5 min	1053	C
Pantoprazole sodium	[a]	4 mg/1 mL		16 mg/1 mL[b]	Possible precipitate within 1 hr	2574	I

[a] Test performed using the formulation WITHOUT edetate disodium.

[b] Trimethoprim component. Trimethoprim in a 1:5 fixed-ratio concentration with sulfamethoxazole.

Y-Site Injection Compatibility (1:1 Mixture)

Trimethoprim–sulfamethoxazole

Test Drug	Mfr	Conc	Mfr	Conc	Remarks	Ref	C/I
Acyclovir sodium	BW	5 mg/mL[a]	RC	0.8 mg/mL[a g]	Physically compatible for 4 hr at 25°C	1157	C
Aldesleukin	CHI	33,800 I.U./mL[a]	BW	1.6 mg/mL[a g]	Visually compatible with little or no loss of aldesleukin activity	1857	C
Allopurinol sodium	BW	3 mg/mL[b]	ES	0.8 mg/mL[b g]	Physically compatible for 4 hr at 22°C	1686	C
Amifostine	USB	10 mg/mL[a]	ES	0.8 mg/mL[a g]	Physically compatible for 4 hr at 23°C	1845	C
Anidulafungin	VIC	0.5 mg/mL[a]	ES	0.8 mg/mL[a g]	Physically compatible for 4 hr at 23°C	2617	C
Atracurium besylate	BW	0.5 mg/mL[a]	ES	0.64 mg/mL[a g]	Physically compatible for 24 hr at 28°C	1337	C
Aztreonam	SQ	40 mg/mL[a]	ES	0.8 mg/mL[a g]	Physically compatible for 4 hr at 23°C	1758	C
Bivalirudin	TMC	5 mg/mL[a]	GNS	0.8 mg/mL[a g]	Physically compatible for 4 hr at 23°C	2373	C
Blinatumomab	AMG	0.125 mcg/mL[b]	RC	3.2 mg/mL[b j]	Visually compatible for 12 hr at room temperature	3405, 3417	C
Blinatumomab	AMG	0.375 mcg/mL[b]	RC	3.2 mg/mL[b j]	Persistent particulate formation when trimethoprim–sulfamethoxazole is added to blinatumomab; flakes transiently appeared when order of mixing was reversed	3405, 3417	I
Cangrelor tetrasodium	TMC	1 mg/mL[b]		0.8[g i] and 1.6[g i] mg/mL	Physically compatible for 4 hr	3243	C
Caspofungin acetate	ME	0.7 mg/mL[b]	SIC	0.8 mg/mL[b g]	Immediate white turbid precipitate forms	2758	I
Ceftaroline fosamil	FOR	2.22 mg/mL[a b f]	SIC	0.8 mg/mL[a b f g]	Physically compatible for 4 hr at 23°C	2826	C

Y-Site Injection Compatibility (1:1 Mixture) (Cont.)

Test Drug	Mfr	Conc	Mfr	Conc	Remarks	Ref	C/I
Cisatracurium besylate	GW	0.1 mg/mL[a]	ES	0.8 mg/mL[a g]	Physically compatible for 4 hr at 23°C	2074	C
Cisatracurium besylate	GW	2 mg/mL[a]	ES	0.8 mg/mL[a g]	Subvisible haze forms in 1 hr	2074	I
Cisatracurium besylate	GW	5 mg/mL[a]	ES	0.8 mg/mL[a g]	Subvisible haze forms immediately	2074	I
Cloxacillin sodium	SMX	100 mg/mL	APT	16 mg/mL[g]	Large particles form immediately and within 4 hr	3245	I
Cyclophosphamide	MJ	20 mg/mL[a]	BW	0.8 mg/mL[a g]	Physically compatible for 4 hr at 25°C	1194	C
Defibrotide sodium	JAZ	8 mg/mL[b]	RC	0.64 mg/mL[b g]	Visually compatible for 4 hr at room temperature	3149	C
Dexmedetomidine HCl	AB	4 mcg/mL[b]	GNS	0.8 mg/mL[b g]	Physically compatible for 4 hr at 23°C	2383	C
Diltiazem HCl	MMD	5 mg/mL	BW, RC	0.21, 0.63 mg/mL[a g]	Visually compatible	1807	C
Docetaxel	RPR	0.9 mg/mL[a]	ES	0.8 mg/mL[a g]	Physically compatible for 4 hr at 23°C	2224	C
Doxorubicin HCl liposomal	SEQ	0.4 mg/mL[a]	ES	0.8 mg/mL[a g]	Physically compatible for 4 hr at 23°C	2087	C
Enalaprilat	MSD	0.05 mg/mL[b]	QU	0.16 mg/mL[a g]	Physically compatible for 24 hr at room temperature under fluorescent light	1355	C
Esmolol HCl	DCC	10 mg/mL[a]	BW	0.64 mg/mL[a g]	Physically compatible for 24 hr at 22°C	1169	C
Etoposide phosphate	BR	5 mg/mL[a]	ES	0.8 mg/mL[a g]	Physically compatible for 4 hr at 23°C	2218	C
Fat emulsion, intravenous	OTS	20%[k]	CHU	0.76 mg/mL[a g l]	No change in particle size ≥1.3 μm observed in 24 hr at 25°C in the dark	3452	C
Fenoldopam mesylate	AB	80 mcg/mL[b]	ES	0.8 mg/mL[b g]	Physically compatible for 4 hr at 23°C	2467	C
Filgrastim	AMG	30 mcg/mL[a]	ES	0.8 mg/mL[a g]	Physically compatible for 4 hr at 22°C	1687	C
Fluconazole	RR	2 mg/mL[g]	BW	16 mg/mL	Viscous gel-like substance forms	1407	I
Fludarabine phosphate	BX	1 mg/mL[a]	ES	0.8 mg/mL[a g]	Visually compatible for 4 hr at 22°C	1439	C
Foscarnet sodium	AST	24 mg/mL	RC	16 mg/mL[g]	Precipitates immediately and gas production	1335	I
Foscarnet sodium	AST	24 mg/mL	BW	0.53 mg/mL[a g]	Physically compatible for 24 hr at 25°C under fluorescent light	1393	C
Gallium nitrate	FUJ	1 mg/mL[b]	ES	0.8 mg/mL[b g]	Visually compatible for 24 hr at 25°C	1673	C
Gemcitabine HCl	LI	10 mg/mL[b]	ES	0.8 mg/mL[b g]	Physically compatible for 4 hr at 23°C	2226	C
Granisetron HCl	SKB	0.05 mg/mL[a]	ES	0.8 mg/mL[a g]	Physically compatible for 4 hr at 23°C	2000	C
Hetastarch in lactated electrolyte	AB	6%	ES	0.8 mg/mL[a g]	Physically compatible for 4 hr at 23°C	2339	C
Hydromorphone HCl	WY	0.2 mg/mL[a]	BW	0.8 mg/mL[a g]	Physically compatible for 4 hr at 25°C	987	C
Labetalol HCl	SC	1 mg/mL[a]	BW	0.8 mg/mL[a g]	Physically compatible for 24 hr at 18°C	1171	C
Linezolid	PHU, HOS	2 mg/mL			Stated to be physically incompatible	3183, 3184	I
Lorazepam	WY	0.33 mg/mL[b]	RC	0.8 mg/mL[g]	Visually compatible for 24 hr at 22°C	1855	C
Magnesium sulfate	IX	16.7, 33.3, 66.7, 100 mg/mL[a]	RC	0.8 mg/mL[a g]	Physically compatible for at least 4 hr at 32°C	813	C
Melphalan HCl	BW	0.1 mg/mL[b]	ES	0.8 mg/mL[b g]	Physically compatible for 3 hr at 22°C	1557	C
Meperidine HCl	WY	10 mg/mL[a]	BW	0.8 mg/mL[a g]	Physically compatible for 4 hr at 25°C	987	C
Meropenem		50 mg/mL	APR	16 mg/mL[g]	Physically compatible for 4 hr at room temperature	3538	C

Y-Site Injection Compatibility (1:1 Mixture) (Cont.)

Test Drug	Mfr	Conc	Mfr	Conc	Remarks	Ref	C/I
Midazolam HCl	RC	5 mg/mL	RC	0.8 mg/mL[g]	White precipitate forms immediately	1855	I
Morphine sulfate	WI	1 mg/mL[a]	BW	0.8 mg/mL[a] [g]	Physically compatible for 4 hr at 25°C	987	C
Nicardipine HCl	DCC	0.1 mg/mL[a]	QU	0.16 mg/mL[a] [g]	Visually compatible for 24 hr at room temperature	235	C
Oritavancin diphosphate	TAR	0.8, 1.2, and 2 mg/mL[a]	SIC	0.8 mg/mL[a] [g]	Haze and particles form immediately with precipitate after 1 hr	2928	I
Pancuronium bromide	ES	0.05 mg/mL[a]	ES	0.64 mg/mL[a] [g]	Physically compatible for 24 hr at 28°C	1337	C
Pemetrexed disodium	LI	20 mg/mL[b]	ES	0.8 mg/mL[a] [g]	Physically compatible for 4 hr at 23°C	2564	C
Piperacillin sodium–tazobactam sodium	LE[e]	40 mg/mL[a] [h]	ES	0.8 mg/mL[a] [g]	Physically compatible for 4 hr at 22°C	1688	C
Remifentanil HCl	GW	0.025 and 0.25 mg/mL[b]	ES	0.8 mg/mL[a] [g]	Physically compatible for 4 hr at 23°C	2075	C
Sargramostim	IMM	10 mcg/mL[b]	ES	0.8 mg/mL[b] [g]	Visually compatible for 4 hr at 22°C	1436	C
Tacrolimus	FUJ	1 mg/mL[b]	RC	1.6 mg/mL[a] [g]	Visually compatible for 24 hr at 25°C	1630	C
Teniposide	BR	0.1 mg/mL[a]	ES	0.8 mg/mL[a] [g]	Physically compatible for 4 hr at 23°C	1725	C
Thiotepa	IMM[c]	1 mg/mL[a]	ES	0.8 mg/mL[a] [g]	Physically compatible for 4 hr at 23°C	1861	C
TNA #218 to #226[d]			ES	0.8 mg/mL[a] [g]	Visually compatible for 4 hr at 23°C	2215	C
TPN #212 to #215[d]			ES	0.8 mg/mL[a] [g]	Physically compatible for 4 hr at 23°C	2109	C
Vecuronium bromide	OR	0.1 mg/mL[a]	ES	0.64 mg/mL[a] [g]	Physically compatible for 24 hr at 28°C	1337	C
Vinorelbine tartrate	BW	1 mg/mL[b]	ES	0.8 mg/mL[b] [g]	Heavy white turbidity forms immediately, developing particles in 1 hr	1558	I
Zidovudine	BW	4 mg/mL[a]	BW	0.53 mg/mL[a] [g]	Physically compatible for 4 hr at 25°C	1193	C

[a] Tested in dextrose 5%.

[b] Tested in sodium chloride 0.9%.

[c] Lyophilized formulation tested.

[d] Refer to Appendix for the composition of parenteral nutrition solutions. TNA indicates a 3-in-1 admixture, and TPN indicates a 2-in-1 admixture.

[e] Test performed using the formulation WITHOUT edetate disodium.

[f] Tested in Ringer's injection, lactated.

[g] Trimethoprim component. Trimethoprim in a 1:5 fixed-ratio concentration with sulfamethoxazole.

[h] Piperacillin component. Piperacillin in an 8:1 fixed-ratio concentration with tazobactam.

[i] Tested in both dextrose 5% and sodium chloride 0.9%.

[j] Not specified whether concentration refers to single component or combined components.

[k] Run at 25 mL/hr with dextrose 5% run at 83 mL/hr.

[l] Run at 100 mL/hr.

Selected Revisions May 1, 2020. © Copyright, October 1982.
American Society of Health-System Pharmacists, Inc.

Tropisetron Hydrochloride
AHFS 56:22.20

Products

Tropisetron hydrochloride is available as an aqueous solution in 2- and 5-mL ampuls. Each mL of solution provides 1 mg of tropisetron (present as 1.13 mg of the hydrochloride). Also present in the formulation are acetic acid, sodium acetate, sodium chloride, and water for injection.[38] [115]

Trade Name(s)

Navoban

Administration

Tropisetron hydrochloride is administered either as a slow intravenous injection over not less than 30 seconds for a 2-mg dose[38] [115] or 1 minute for a 5-mg dose[115] or as an intravenous infusion over 15 minutes.[38]

Stability

Tropisetron hydrochloride injection is a colorless or faintly brown-yellow solution. Intact ampuls should be stored at room temperature.[38]

Syringes

Tropisetron hydrochloride (Sandoz) 1 mg/mL was packaged in polypropylene syringes (Becton Dickinson) and stored under refrigeration at 4°C and at room temperature (about 23°C) exposed to daylight and protected from light for 15 days. About 4% loss of tropisetron hydrochloride occurred in 15 days under any of the storage conditions.[2298]

Sorption

The manufacturer indicates that tropisetron hydrochloride solutions are compatible with both glass and PVC containers and infusion sets.[38]

Compatibility Information

Solution Compatibility

Tropisetron HCl

Test Soln Name	Mfr	Mfr	Conc/L or %	Remarks	Ref	C/I
Dextrose 5%		SZ	50 mg	Compatible and stable for 24 hr refrigerated	38	C
Dextrose 5%	AGT[a], BFM[b]	SZ	50 mg	Visually compatible with no loss in 90 days at 4 and –20°C	470	C
Dextrose 5%	BA[a], BRN[c]	SZ	50 mg	10% or less change in concentration in 15 days at 4 and 23°C in light or dark	2298	C
Ringer's injection		SZ	50 mg	Compatible and stable for 24 hr refrigerated	38	C
Sodium chloride 0.9%		SZ	50 mg	Compatible and stable for 24 hr refrigerated	38	C
Sodium chloride 0.9%	AGT[a], BFM[b]	SZ	50 mg	Visually compatible with no loss in 90 days at 4 and –20°C	470	C
Sodium chloride 0.9%	BA[a], BRN[c]	SZ	50 mg	10% or less change in concentration in 15 days at 4 and 23°C in light or dark	2298	C

[a] Tested in PVC containers.

[b] Tested in three-layer (Clear-Flex) laminate containers having a polyethylene inner surface.

[c] Tested in glass and polyethylene containers.

DOI: 10.37573/9781585286850.391

Additive Compatibility

Tropisetron HCl

Test Drug	Mfr	Conc/L or %	Mfr	Conc/L or %	Test Solution	Remarks	Ref	C/I
Butorphanol tartrate	HE	80 mg	COM	50 mg	NS[d]	Physically compatible with little to no loss of either drug in 14 days at 4 and 25°C in the dark	3121	C
Butorphanol tartrate	HE	80 mg	COM	50 mg	NS[e]	Physically compatible with little to no loss of either drug in 14 days at 4 and 25°C in the dark	3121	C
Dexamethasone sodium phosphate	[c]	100 mg		43 mg	NS	Physically compatible for 24 hr at 25°C in light	2999	C
Fosaprepitant dimeglumine	MSD[a]	1 g		43 mg	NS	Physically compatible for 24 hr at 25°C in light	2999	C
Fosaprepitant dimeglumine	MSD[b]	1 g		43 mg	NS	Physically compatible for 24 hr at 25°C in light	2999	C
Methylprednisolone sodium succinate	[c]	700 mg		43 mg	NS	Physically compatible for 24 hr at 25°C in light	2999	C

[a] Tested with dexamethasone sodium phosphate 100 mg/L.

[b] Tested with methylprednisolone sodium succinate 700 mg/L.

[c] Tested with fosaprepitant dimeglumine (MSD) 1 g/L.

[d] Tested in polyolefin containers.

[e] Tested in glass containers.

Selected Revisions May 19, 2016. © Copyright, October 2000.
American Society of Health-System Pharmacists, Inc.

Valproate Sodium
AHFS 28:12.92

Products

Valproate sodium is available in 5-mL single-dose (preservative-free) vials.[3423] Each mL of solution contains valproate sodium equivalent to valproic acid 100 mg and edetate disodium 0.4 mg in water for injection.[3423] Sodium hydroxide and/or hydrochloric acid are used to adjust pH during manufacture.[3423] The solution should be diluted for use.[3423]

pH

Adjusted to 7.6.[3423]

Trade Name(s)

Depacon

Administration

Valproate sodium is intended for intravenous use only.[3423] The manufacturer recommends that the drug be administered as an intravenous infusion over 60 minutes at a rate that does not exceed 20 mg/min following dilution of the appropriate dose in at least 50 mL of a compatible infusion solution.[3423] (See Solution Compatibility.) For many indications, the manufacturer also recommends that total daily dosages exceeding 250 mg be administered in divided doses.[3423]

The manufacturer states that there is limited experience with infusion of valproate sodium over less than 60 minutes or at rates of infusion exceeding 20 mg/min.[3423] In a safety study, a more rapid infusion of a single dose of the drug over 5 to 10 minutes (1.5 to 3 mg/kg/min) was used.[3423] More rapid infusion rates (e.g., 3 to 6 mg/kg/min) of sometimes larger doses (e.g., loading dose) also have been used in other studies or are recommended in some guidelines for certain indications.[3438 3439 3440 3441 3442 3443] While patients in such studies generally tolerated such infusions well,[3423 3439 3440 3441 3442 3443] the manufacturer states that rapid infusion of valproate sodium has been associated with an increase in adverse reactions.[3423]

Stability

Valproate sodium injection is a clear, colorless solution.[3423] Intact vials should be stored at controlled room temperature of 15 to 30°C.[3423] Because no antibacterial preservatives are present in the formulation, any unused solution remaining in a vial after entry should be discarded.[3423]

Syringes

Valproate sodium (Sanofi) 20 mg/mL in sodium chloride 0.9% packaged in 40-mL polypropylene syringes (BD) was physically and chemically stable for 30 days stored at 2 to 8°C protected from light.[3523]

Valproate sodium (Mylan) 600 mg/50 mL in sodium chloride 0.9% in a 50-mL polypropylene syringe (BD) was physically stable for 48 hours at room temperature.[3545]

Compatibility Information

Solution Compatibility

Valproate sodium

Test Soln Name	Mfr	Mfr	Conc/L or %	Remarks	Ref	C/I
Dextrose 5%	a	ABV		Physically compatible and chemically stable for up to 24 hr at 15 to 30°C	3423	C
Dextrose 5%	GRI[b]	SW	1.6 g	Under 10% loss in 6 days at room temperature	2287	C
Ringer's injection, lactated	a	ABV		Physically compatible and chemically stable for up to 24 hr at 15 to 30°C	3423	C
Ringer's injection, lactated	GRI[b]	SW	1.6 g	Under 10% loss in 6 days at room temperature	2287	C
Sodium chloride 0.9%	a	ABV		Physically compatible and chemically stable for up to 24 hr at 15 to 30°C	3423	C
Sodium chloride 0.9%	GRI[b]	SW	1.6 g	Under 10% loss in 6 days at room temperature	2287	C

[a] Tested in PVC and glass containers.

[b] Tested in glass, polyethylene (polyolefin), and PVC containers.

DOI: 10.37573/9781585286850.392

Additive Compatibility

Valproate sodium

Test Drug	Mfr	Conc/L or %	Mfr	Conc/L or %	Test Solution	Remarks	Ref	C/I
Dobutamine HCl	BA	1 g	WW	4.5 g	a	Physically compatible for 24 hr at 22 to 25°C in ambient light and 34 to 38% relative humidity	3424	C
Dopamine HCl	BA	800 mg	WW	4.5 g	a	Physically compatible for 24 hr at 22 to 25°C in ambient light and 34 to 38% relative humidity	3424	C
Levetiracetam					D5W, LR, NS[a]	Stable for 4 hr at 15 to 30°C	2833	C

[a] Tested in PVC containers.

Y-Site Injection Compatibility (1:1 Mixture)

Valproate sodium

Test Drug	Mfr	Conc	Mfr	Conc	Remarks	Ref	C/I
Cefepime HCl	BMS	120 mg/mL[b]		100 mg/mL	Physically compatible. Under 10% cefepime loss. Valproate not tested	2513	C
Ceftazidime	SKB	125 mg/mL		100 mg/mL	Physically compatible. Under 10% ceftazidime loss. Valproate not tested	2434	C
Ceftazidime	GSK	120 mg/mL[b]		100 mg/mL	Physically compatible. Under 10% ceftazidime loss. Valproate not tested	2513	C
Cloxacillin sodium	SMX	100 mg/mL	AB	100 mg/mL	Physically compatible for up to 4 hr at room temperature	3245	C
Meropenem		50 mg/mL	ABV	100 mg/mL	Physically compatible for 4 hr at room temperature	3538	C
Vancomycin HCl	LI	10 mg/mL[a]		100 mg/mL	Physically incompatible	3536	I

[a] Tested in dextrose 5%.

[b] Tested in sterile water for injection.

Selected Revisions May 1, 2020. © Copyright, October 2002.
American Society of Health-System Pharmacists, Inc.

Vancomycin Hydrochloride
AHFS 8:12.28.16

Products

Vancomycin hydrochloride is available in single-dose vials containing drug equivalent to 250 mg, 500 mg, 750 mg, 1 g, 1.25 g, and 1.5 g of vancomycin base, and pharmacy bulk packages containing drug equivalent to 5, 10, and 100 g of vancomycin base.[3464 3465 3466 3467 3468 3469] To reconstitute single-use vials, 5 mL of sterile water for injection should be added for each 250 mg of vancomycin lyophilized powder contained in the vial (e.g., add 15 mL of sterile water to reconstitute a 750-mg vial of vancomycin) to yield a solution with a vancomycin concentration of 50 mg/mL.[3464 3465 3466] Pharmacy bulk packages containing 5 g of vancomycin should be reconstituted with 100 mL of sterile water for injection to yield a solution with a vancomycin concentration of 50 mg/mL.[3467 3468] Pharmacy bulk packages containing 10 or 100 g of vancomycin should be reconstituted with 95 or 950 mL, respectively, of sterile water for injection to yield a solution with a vancomycin concentration of 100 mg/mL.[3467 3469] The appropriate dose of the reconstituted solution prepared from single-dose vials must be further diluted in a compatible diluent to achieve a final vancomycin concentration of 5 mg/mL (e.g., 500 mg in at least 100 mL, 750 mg in at least 150 mL, 1 g in at least 200 mL).[3464 3465 3466] The appropriate dose of the reconstituted solution prepared from pharmacy bulk packages must be further diluted in at least 100 mL of a compatible diluent;[3467 3468 3469] some manufacturers state that doses of 1 g must be diluted in at least 200 mL of a compatible diluent.[3467 3468] Manufacturers state that vancomycin concentrations of no more than 5 mg/mL are recommended in adults.[3464 3465 3466 3467 3468 3471 3472] More concentrated vancomycin solutions (i.e., up to 10 mg/mL) may be considered for use in selected patients (e.g., fluid-restricted patients); however, use of such solutions increases the risk of infusion-related adverse effects.[3464 3465 3466]

Vancomycin hydrochloride is available in ADD-Vantage vials containing drug equivalent to 500 mg, 750 mg, and 1 g of vancomycin base.[3472] ADD-Vantage vials containing 500 mg of vancomycin should be prepared with *at least* 100 mL of dextrose 5% or sodium chloride 0.9% in ADD-Vantage diluent bags; ADD-Vantage vials containing 750 mg or 1 g of vancomycin should be prepared *only* with 250 mL of dextrose 5% or sodium chloride 0.9% in ADD-Vantage diluent bags.[3472] The manufacturer states that the use of ADD-Vantage vials is indicated only when doses reflecting the full strength of the available products are determined to be appropriate; if vancomycin doses of 500 mg, 750 mg, or 1 g are not appropriate (e.g., in neonates, infants, and pediatric patients requiring doses less than 500 mg), conventional vials of vancomycin hydrochloride should be used.[3472]

Vancomycin hydrochloride also is available in several ready-to-use formulations.[3470 3471] Vancomycin hydrochloride is available as a frozen iso-osmotic premixed injection in single-dose Galaxy containers containing the equivalent of 500 mg, 750 mg, and 1 g of vancomycin base in 100, 150, and 200 mL, respectively, of dextrose 5% or sodium chloride 0.9%.[3470] Each 100 mL of the premixed solution also contains either 5 g of dextrose hydrous or 0.9 g of sodium chloride, and the pH may have been adjusted with hydrochloric acid and/or sodium hydroxide.[3470] Vancomycin hydrochloride is available as a premixed injection in single-dose bags containing the equivalent of 500 mg, 1 g, 1.5 g, and 2 g of vancomycin base in 100, 200, 300, and 400 mL, respectively.[3471] Each 100 mL of the premixed solution also contains polyethylene glycol (PEG) 400 1.8 mL, N-acetyl-D-alanine (NADA) 1.36 g, and L-lysine hydrochloride (monochloride) 1.26 g in water for injection; hydrochloric acid and sodium hydroxide are used for pH adjustment.[3471] The PEG- and NADA-containing formulation should *not* be used in certain patients (e.g., pregnant women, patients younger than 1 month of age, pediatric patients 1 month of age or older requiring less than the entire dose of a single-dose flexible bag).[3471]

pH

A 50- or 100-mg/mL reconstituted solution of vancomycin prepared with sterile water for injection has a pH ranging from 2.5 to 4.5.[3464 3466 3467 3468 3469]

Premixed infusion solutions of vancomycin (Baxter) 5 mg/mL in dextrose 5% or sodium chloride 0.9% have a pH ranging from 3 to 5.[3470]

Premixed infusion solutions of vancomycin (Xellia) 5 mg/mL have a pH ranging from 4.5 to 5.5.[3471]

Osmolality

Vancomycin hydrochloride (Lilly) prepared at a vancomycin concentration of 50 mg/mL in sterile water for injection has an osmolality of 57 mOsm/kg.[50]

The osmolality of vancomycin hydrochloride (Lederle) prepared at a vancomycin concentration of 5 mg/mL was determined to be 249 mOsm/kg in dextrose 5% and 291 mOsm/kg in sodium chloride 0.9%.[1375]

The osmolality of vancomycin hydrochloride (Sandoz) prepared at a vancomycin concentration of 62.5 mg/mL was determined to be 363 to 383 mOsm/kg in dextrose 5% and 337 to 351 mOsm/kg in sodium chloride 0.9%.[3603] The osmolality of vancomycin hydrochloride (Sandoz) prepared at a vancomycin concentration of 83.3 mg/mL was determined to be 379 to 409 mOsm/kg in dextrose 5% and 362 to 378 mOsm/kg in sodium chloride 0.9%.[3603]

Osmolarity

The osmolarity of premixed infusion solutions of vancomycin (Xellia) 5 mg/mL ranges from 350 to 475 mOsmol/L.[3471]

Administration

Vancomycin hydrochloride is administered by intravenous infusion.[3464 3465 3466 3467 3468 3469 3470 3471 3472] The reconstituted solution must be diluted in a compatible infusion solution prior to administration.[3464 3465 3466 3467 3468 3469] The drug is extremely irritating to tissue and may cause necrosis; therefore, it should not be given by intramuscular injection and extravasation should be avoided during intravenous administration.[3464 3465 3466 3467 3468 3469 3470 3471 3472] The frequency and severity of thrombophlebitis can be minimized by administering the drug slowly, using dilute solutions of 2.5 to 5 mg/mL, and rotating venous access sites.[3464 3465 3466 3467 3468 3469 3470 3471 3472]

Manufacturers recommend intermittent intravenous infusion as the preferred method of administration.[3464 3466 3467 3468 3469 3470 3472] Some manufacturers recommend that the drug be administered over a period of at least 60 minutes in adults.[3465 3471] Other manufacturers state that administration rates of no more than 10 mg/min are recommended in adults or that the drug should be administered at a rate no faster than 10 mg/min or over a period of at least 60 minutes, whichever is longer.[3464 3466 3467 3468 3469 3470 3472] In pediatric patients, the drug should be administered over a period of at least 60 minutes;[3464 3465 3466 3467 3468 3469 3470 3471 3472] in neonates, the drug should be administered over a period of 60 minutes.[3464 3465 3466 3467 3468 3469 3470 3472]

Vancomycin hydrochloride (Baxter) frozen iso-osmotic premixed injection in single-dose Galaxy containers should be thawed (see Stability: Freezing Solutions), and the solution should be administered by intravenous infusion.[3470]

Stability

Vancomycin hydrochloride is a lyophilized powder that varies in color from white or off white to light tan, tan, buff, or brownish.[3464 3465 3467 3468 3469] Intact vials and pharmacy bulk packages should be stored at controlled room temperature.[3464 3465 3466 3467 3468 3469] Manufacturers indicate that after reconstitution, single-dose vials of vancomycin hydrochloride may be stored in a refrigerator for 14 days with no significant loss of potency;[3464 3465 3466] other information has indicated that the drug also is stable in solution for 14 days at room temperature.[141]

Intact ADD-Vantage vials of vancomycin hydrochloride should be stored at controlled room temperature.[3472] Solutions prepared using the ADD-Vantage vials may be stored in a refrigerator 14 days for with no significant loss of potency.[3472]

pH Effects

In the pH range of 2 to 10, vancomycin hydrochloride degradation occurs principally via deamidation.[1927] Vancomycin hydrochloride has been reported to be most stable at pH 3 to 5[141] and at pH 5.5,[1927] with relatively pH-independent decomposition in the range of 3 to 8.[1927] The stability of a 1-mg/mL concentration was evaluated in buffer solutions having pH values of 1.4, 5.6, and 7.1 at 24°C. Little or no loss occurred in 24 hours in any solution. However, the pH 1.4 buffer had a 19% loss in 5 days, the pH 5.6 buffer had a 10% loss in 17 days, and the pH 7.1 buffer had an 11% loss in 5 days.[1134]

In an accelerated study at 66°C, the half-life of vancomycin B (the largest component of the commercial product) was 400 minutes in a phosphate buffer with a pH of 2.2 and 650 minutes in a phosphate buffer with a pH of 7.[1354]

Vancomycin hydrochloride has a low pH and may cause chemical or physical instability when mixed with other drugs, especially drugs with an alkaline pH.[873 3464 3465 3466 3467 3468 3469 3471 3472]

The concentration dependency of compatibility or incompatibility of vancomycin hydrochloride mixed with or administered simultaneously with a number of penicillins and cephalosporins has been demonstrated.[2189] Vancomycin hydrochloride is variably compatible with drugs having neutral to mildly alkaline pH, including cephalosporins and penicillins. The compatibility may depend on a number of factors including concentration of each drug, dilution vehicle, actual pH of solutions, and completeness of mixing during administration. Combinations that are compatible when well mixed may result in precipitation if only partially mixed, presumably due to regionally different concentrations and pH values. If attempting to administer vancomycin hydrochloride with another drug product, care should be taken to ensure that the specific combination and concentrations are compatible under the exact administration conditions to be used. An inline filter should be used as a final safety measure.[2189]

Freezing Solutions

The commercially available, premixed frozen injection of vancomycin hydrochloride in single-dose Galaxy containers should be stored in a freezer capable of maintaining the temperature at or below −20°C.[3470] Frozen product containers should be handled with care since they may be fragile in the frozen state.[3470] Freezing of the solution may cause components of the solution to precipitate, but this precipitate will dissolve at room temperature, apparently without affecting potency.[3470] Solutions should be thawed at room temperature (25°C) or under refrigeration (5°C).[3470] Solutions should not be subject to force thawing (e.g., by immersion in water baths or microwaving).[3470] Thawed solutions should not be refrozen.[3470] After the thawed solution has reached room temperature, the solution should be agitated.[3470] The manufacturer indicates that thawed solutions remain chemically stable for 72 hours at room temperature (25°C) or 30 days refrigerated (5°C).[3470]

Vancomycin hydrochloride (Lilly) prepared at a vancomycin concentration of 5 mg/mL in dextrose 5% or sodium chloride 0.9% exhibited no loss after 63 days of storage when frozen at −10°C. However, neither did a loss occur in the same time period when the solution was stored at 5°C.[1134]

In one study, vancomycin hydrochloride (Lilly) prepared at a vancomycin concentration of 5 mg/mL in dextrose 5% was stored frozen at −20°C for 105 days. After thawing in a microwave, the samples were stored for 56 more days under refrigeration. The samples remained clear and had no color change. In addition, no loss of vancomycin occurred throughout the entire test period.[2682]

Syringes

The stability of vancomycin hydrochloride (Lilly) prepared at a vancomycin concentration of 5 mg/mL in dextrose concentrations ranging from 5 to 30% and packaged in plastic syringes was studied. The syringes were stored at 4°C for 24 hours followed by 2 hours at room temperature. Little change in the concentration occurred.[1301]

The stability of vancomycin hydrochloride (Lilly) reconstituted to a vancomycin concentration of 10 mg/mL with sterile water for injection, dextrose 5%, and sodium chloride 0.9% repackaged into plastic syringes was studied. Five mL of the solutions were filled into 3-piece Plastipak (Becton Dickinson) and 2-piece Injekt (Braun) syringes that were then sealed with Luer-Lok hubs (Vigon) and stored at 4 and 25°C for 84 days. Under refrigeration, vancomycin hydrochloride prepared with all 3 solutions and packaged in both kinds of syringes was physically and chemically stable for the 84-day period; losses were 4% or less.[1893] However, stored at 25°C in the Plastipak syringes, 10% loss occurred in about 47 days in water, 55 days in dextrose 5%, and 62 days in sodium chloride 0.9%. In the Injekt syringes, stability was less; 10% loss occurred in 29 days in water, 33 days in dextrose 5%, and 34 days in sodium chloride 0.9%. In addition, a degradation product appeared as a white flocculent precipitate in all room temperature samples after about 8 weeks of storage.[1893]

Vancomycin hydrochloride prepared at a vancomycin concentration of 5 mg/mL in dextrose 5% and in sodium chloride 0.9% packaged in polypropylene syringes (Becton Dickinson) exhibited less than 10% loss in 14 days at room temperature and in 6 months under refrigeration. Refrigerated solutions warmed to room temperature were stable for 48 hours.[2730]

Vancomycin hydrochloride (Mylan) prepared at a vancomycin concentration of 2 g/48 mL in dextrose 5% and in sodium chloride 0.9% packaged in polypropylene syringes (Terumo) was physically and chemically stable for up to 48 hours at an ambient temperature ranging from 18 to 25°C.[3602]

No visual or subvisual changes were noted in polypropylene syringes containing vancomycin hydrochloride prepared at vancomycin concentrations of 40, 50, 58.8, 71, and 83.3 mg/mL in sodium chloride 0.9% in 24 hours at room temperature and 83.3 mg/mL in both sodium chloride 0.9% and dextrose 5% in 48 hours at room temperature.[3603]

Vancomycin hydrochloride (Sandoz) prepared at a vancomycin concentration of 3 g/48 mL in dextrose 5% and packaged in 50-mL polypropylene Plastipak (Becton Dickinson) syringes exhibited little loss in 24 hours at 20 to 25°C with no degradation products, change in pH, or visible modifications noted.[3603] Syringes prepared at a vancomycin concentration of 4 g/48 mL in dextrose 5% exhibited a slight yellow color change and little loss in 6 hours at 20 to 25°C.[3603] While the concentration of vancomycin in one of the 3 syringes (tested in triplicate) dropped below 90% of the initial concentration at 24 hours, the concentration in that syringe measured well above 90% of the initial concentration at 48 hours.[3603] Authors attributed these results to a technical problem likely related to the multiple dilutions required to achieve the desired theoretical concentration of the drug and concluded that the drug was physically and chemically stable for 48 hours at 20 to 25°C.[3603]

Vancomycin hydrochloride (Sandoz) prepared at a vancomycin concentration of 3 g/48 mL in sodium chloride 0.9% and packaged in 50-mL polypropylene Plastipak (Becton Dickinson) syringes exhibited little loss in 48 hours at 20 to 25°C without any physical changes noted.[3603] Syringes prepared at a vancomycin concentration of 4 g/48 mL in sodium chloride 0.9%

exhibited little loss in 24 hours at 20 to 25°C, but a precipitate was observed after 48 hours of storage.[3603]

Elastomeric Reservoir Pumps

Vancomycin hydrochloride (Lilly) prepared at a vancomycin concentration of 10 mg/mL in both dextrose 5% and sodium chloride 0.9% was evaluated for binding potential to natural rubber elastomeric reservoirs (Baxter). No binding was found after storage for 2 weeks at 35°C with gentle agitation.[2014]

Implantable Pumps

Vancomycin hydrochloride (Lilly) prepared at a vancomycin concentration of 1 mg/mL in water in an implantable pump (Infusaid model 100) was incubated in a water bath at 37°C for 28 days. Vancomycin losses were substantial, with about 25% loss in 7 days and 40% loss in 28 days. At the end of the test period, a colloidal precipitate also was found in the pumps.[1302]

Sorption

Vancomycin hydrochloride (Lilly) prepared at a vancomycin concentration of 15 mg/mL in dextrose 5% is reported to undergo substantial sorption to Teflon tubing used in an automatic dilutor (Syva). The vancomycin hydrochloride was apparently released from the tubing into subsequent solutions resulting in vancomycin toxicity.[2153]

Vancomycin hydrochloride prepared at a vancomycin concentration of 10 mg/mL with heparin sodium 5000 units/mL as an antibiotic lock in polyurethane central hemodialysis catheters lost about 50% of the antibiotic over 72 hours at 37°C. The loss was attributed to sorption to the catheters, although precipitation is also possible. Nevertheless, the reduced antibiotic concentration (about 5 mg/mL) remained effective against common microorganisms in catheter-related bacteremia in hemodialysis patients.[2515 2516]

Plasticizer Leaching

Vancomycin hydrochloride (Qualimed Laboratories) prepared at a vancomycin concentration of 8 mg/mL in dextrose 5% and sodium chloride 0.9% in polyvinyl chloride (PVC) containers (Macropharma) did not leach detectable amounts of diethylhexyl phthalate (DEHP) plasticizer during simulated administration over 24 hours. If any DEHP was present, the concentration was less than 1 mcg/mL, the limit of detection in this study.[2148]

Filtration

Vancomycin hydrochloride (Lilly) prepared at a vancomycin concentration of 2 mg/mL in dextrose 5% or sodium chloride 0.9% was filtered through a 0.22-μm cellulose ester filter (Ivex-HP, Millipore) over 6 hours. No significant drug loss due to binding to the filter was noted.[1034]

Central Venous Catheter

Vancomycin hydrochloride (Fujisawa) prepared at a vancomycin concentration of 2 mg/mL in dextrose 5% was found to be compatible with the ARROWg+ard Blue Plus (Arrow International) chlorhexidine-bearing triple-lumen central catheter. Essentially complete delivery of the drug was found with little or no drug loss occurring. Furthermore, chlorhexidine delivered from the catheter remained at trace amounts with no substantial increase due to the delivery of the drug through the catheter.[2335]

Compatibility Information

Solution Compatibility

Vancomycin HCl

Test Soln Name	Mfr	Mfr	Conc/L or %	Remarks	Ref	C/I
Dextrose 5% in Ringer's injection, lactated		FRK, HOS	4 g	May be stored for 96 hr refrigerated	3464, 3466	C
Dextrose 5% in Ringer's injection, lactated		MYL	5 g	May be stored for 96 hr refrigerated	3465	C
Dextrose 5% in sodium chloride 0.9%		FRK, HOS	4 g	May be stored for 96 hr refrigerated	3464, 3466	C
Dextrose 5% in sodium chloride 0.9%		MYL	5 g	May be stored for 96 hr refrigerated	3465	C
Dextrose 5% in sodium chloride 0.9%		LI	1 g	Physically compatible	74	C
Dextrose 5%		FRK, HOS	4 g	May be stored for 14 days refrigerated	3464, 3466	C
Dextrose 5%		MYL	5 g	May be stored for 14 days refrigerated	3465	C
Dextrose 5%		LI	1 g	Physically compatible	74	C
Dextrose 5%		LI	5 g	Stable for 7 days at 5 and 25°C	141	C
Dextrose 5%	TR[a]	LI	5 g	Physically compatible and stability for 24 hr at room temperature	518	C
Dextrose 5%	TR[b]	LI	5 g	Physically compatible with no loss in 7 days and 5% loss in 17 days at 24°C. In glass containers, no loss in 63 days at 5°C	1134	C
Dextrose 5%	TR	LI	4 and 5 g	Physically compatible with 8% loss in 17 days at 23°C and 11% loss in 30 days at 4°C	1354	C
Dextrose 5%	AB[e]	AB	20 and 40 g	Little loss in 96 hr at 25°C and in 30 days at 5°C	2097	C
Dextrose 5%	[a]	QLM	8 g	Visually compatible and no loss during a 24 hr simulated infusion at 22°C	2148	C
Dextrose 5%	[a]	QLM	5 g	Visually compatible and no loss during a 1 hr simulated infusion at 22°C	2148	C
Dextrose 5%	[a]	QLM	5 g	Visually compatible and no loss during storage for 48 hr at 22°C in light and 7 days at 4°C in dark	2148	C
Dextrose 5%	BA[a]	LI	5 and 10 g	Visually compatible with less than 3% loss in 58 days at 4°C	2252	C
Dextrose 5%	BA[f]	QLM	2 g	Visually compatible with no loss at 4°C and 4 to 6% loss at room temperature in 48 hr	2278	C
Dextrose 5%	BA[g]	HOS	1 and 5 g	Under 10% loss in 7 days at 23°C and 31 days at 4°C	2819	C
Dextrose 5%	BA[h]	GSK	10 g	Physically and chemically stable for 23 days at 2 to 8°C	3479	C
Dextrose 5%	BA[h]	MYL	10 g	Physically and chemically stable for 43 days at 2 to 8°C	3479	C
Dextrose 10%		LI	5 g	Physically compatible	143	C
Isolyte E		FRK, HOS	4 g	May be stored for 96 hr refrigerated	3464, 3466	C
Normosol M in dextrose 5%		FRK, HOS	4 g	May be stored for 96 hr refrigerated	3464, 3466	C
Ringer's injection, lactated		FRK, HOS	4 g	May be stored for 96 hr refrigerated	3464, 3466	C

Solution Compatibility (Cont.)

Test Soln Name	Mfr	Mfr	Conc/L or %	Remarks	Ref	C/I
Ringer's injection, lactated		MYL	5 g	May be stored for 96 hr refrigerated	3465	C
Ringer's injection, lactated		LI	5 g	Physically compatible	143	C
Ringer's injection, lactated		LI	1 g	Physically compatible	74	C
Sodium chloride 0.9%		FRK, HOS	4 g	May be stored for 14 days refrigerated	3464, 3466	C
Sodium chloride 0.9%		MYL	5 g	May be stored for 14 days refrigerated	3465	C
Sodium chloride 0.9%		LI	5 g	Stable for at least 7 days at 5 and 25°C	141	C
Sodium chloride 0.9%		LI	1 g	Physically compatible	74	C
Sodium chloride 0.9%	TR[a]	LI	5 g	Physically compatible and stable for 24 hr at room temperature	518	C
Sodium chloride 0.9%	TR[b]	LI	5 g	Physically compatible with no loss in 7 days and 5% loss in 17 days at 24°C. In glass containers, no loss in 63 days at 5°C	1134	C
Sodium chloride 0.9%	TR	LI	4 and 5 g	Physically compatible with 9% loss in 24 days at 23°C and 5 to 6% loss in 30 days at 4°C	1354	C
Sodium chloride 0.9%	AB[c]	ES	10 g	Little loss with 24-hr storage at 5°C followed by 24-hr simulated administration at 30°C via portable pump	1779	C
Sodium chloride 0.9%	[a]	QLM	8 g	Visually compatible and no loss during a 24 hr simulated infusion at 22°C	2148	C
Sodium chloride 0.9%	[a]	QLM	5 g	Visually compatible and no loss during a 1 hr simulated infusion at 22°C	2148	C
Sodium chloride 0.9%	[a]	QLM	5 g	Visually compatible and no loss during storage for 48 hr at 22°C in light and 7 days at 4°C in dark	2148	C
Sodium chloride 0.9%	BA[f]	QLM	2 g	Visually compatible with no loss at 4°C and at room temperature in 48 hr	2278	C
Sodium chloride 0.9%	HOS[g]	HOS	1 and 5 g	Under 10% loss in 7 days at 23°C and 31 days at 4°C	2819	C
Sodium lactate ⅙ M		LI	5 g	Physically compatible	143	C
TPN #95, #96[d]		LE	400 mg	Physically compatible and no vancomycin loss for 8 days at room temperature and refrigerated	1321	C
TPN #105, #106[d]		LI	1 and 6 g	Physically compatible with little or no vancomycin loss in 4 hr at 22°C	1325	C
TPN #107[d]			200 mg	Activity retained for 24 hr at 21°C	1326	C
TPN #202[a d]		LI	500 mg and 1 g	Visually compatible and activity retained for 35 days at 4°C plus 24 hr at 22°C	1933	C

[a] Tested in PVC containers.

[b] Tested in both glass and PVC containers.

[c] Tested in portable pump reservoirs (Pharmacia Deltec).

[d] Refer to Appendix for the composition of parenteral nutrition solutions. TPN indicates a 2-in-1 admixture.

[e] Tested in SIMS Deltec Medication Cassette reservoirs.

[f] Tested in PVC, polyolefin, and glass containers.

[g] Tested in Accufusor reservoirs.

[h] Tested in polyolefin containers.

Additive Compatibility

Vancomycin HCl

Test Drug	Mfr	Conc/L or %	Mfr	Conc/L or %	Test Solution	Remarks	Ref	C/I
Amikacin sulfate	BR	5 g	LI	2 g	D5LR, D5R, D5S, D5W, D10W, LR, NS, R, SL	Physically compatible and amikacin stable for 24 hr at 25°C. Vancomycin not tested	293	C
Aminophylline		250 mg	LI	1 g	D5W	Physically compatible	74	C
Aminophylline	SE	1 g	LI	5 g	D5W	Physically incompatible	15	I
Atracurium besylate	BW	500 mg		5 g	D5W	Physically compatible and atracurium stable for 24 hr at 5 and 30°C	1694	C
Aztreonam	SQ	40 g	AB	10 g	D5W, NS	Immediate microcrystalline precipitate. Turbidity and precipitate over 24 hr	1848	I
Aztreonam	SQ	4 g	AB	1 g	D5W	Physically compatible. Little loss of either drug in 31 days at 4°C. 10% aztreonam loss in 14 days at 23°C and 7 days at 32°C	1848	C
Aztreonam	SQ	4 g	AB	1 g	NS	Physically compatible. Little loss of either drug in 31 days at 4°C. 8% aztreonam loss in 31 days at 23°C and 7 days at 32°C	1848	C
Calcium gluconate		1 g	LI	1 g	D5W	Physically compatible	74	C
Cefepime HCl	BR	4 g	LI	5 g	D5W, NS	4% cefepime loss in 24 hr at room temperature in light and 2% loss in 7 days at 5°C. No vancomycin loss. Cloudiness in 5 days at 5°C	1682	C
Cefepime HCl	BR	40 g	LI	1 g	D5W, NS	4% cefepime loss in 24 hr at room temperature in light and 2% loss in 7 days at 5°C. No vancomycin loss and no cloudiness	1682	C
Chloramphenicol sodium succinate	PD	10 g	LI	5 g	D5W	Physically incompatible	15	I
Dimenhydrinate	SE	50 mg	LI	1 g	D5W	Physically compatible	74	C
Famotidine	YAM	200 mg	AB	5 g	D5W[b]	Visually compatible. 9% vancomycin and 6% famotidine loss in 14 days at 25°C. At 4°C, 4% loss of both drugs in 14 days	2111	C
Fusidate sodium	LEO	500 mg		25 g	D2.5½S, D2.5S, D5¼S, D5½S, D5S, D10S	Physically incompatible	1800	I
Heparin sodium		12,000 units	LI	1 g	D5W	Precipitates immediately	74	I
Heparin sodium	IX	1000 units	LE	400 mg	TPN #95[a]	Physically compatible and vancomycin stable for 8 days at room temperature and under refrigeration	1321	C
Heparin sodium	ES	100,000 units	LI	25 mg	NS	Physically compatible. Under 10% vancomycin loss and no heparin loss in 30 days at 28°C and 63 days at 4°C	2542	C
Hydrocortisone sodium succinate	UP	100 mg	LI	1 g	D5W	Physically compatible	74	C
Meropenem	ZEN	1 and 20 g	LI	1 g	NS	Visually compatible for 4 hr at room temperature	1994	C

Additive Compatibility (Cont.)

Test Drug	Mfr	Conc/L or %	Mfr	Conc/L or %	Test Solution	Remarks	Ref	C/I
Piperacillin sodium–tazobactam sodium	SZ[d]	8.6[c] g	HOS	2.9 g	NS	Visually compatible for up to 5 days at room temperature	2935	C
Piperacillin sodium–tazobactam sodium	APO[d]	11.4[c] g	HOS	2.9 g	NS	Visually compatible for up to 5 days at room temperature	2935	C
Potassium chloride		3 g	LI	1 g	D5W	Physically compatible	74	C
Ranitidine HCl	GL	100 mg	DI	1 g	D5W	Physically compatible for 24 hr at ambient temperature in light	1151	C
Ranitidine HCl	GL	50 mg and 2 g		5 g	D5W	Physically compatible. Ranitidine stable for 24 hr at 25°C. Vancomycin not tested	1515	C
Verapamil HCl	KN	80 mg	LI	1 g	D5W, NS	Physically compatible for 24 hr	764	C

[a] Refer to Appendix for the composition of parenteral nutrition solutions. TPN indicates a 2-in-1 admixture.

[b] Tested in methyl-methacrylate-butadiene-styrene plastic containers.

[c] Piperacillin component. Piperacillin in an 8:1 fixed-ratio concentration with tazobactam.

[d] Test performed using the formulation WITHOUT edetate disodium.

Drugs in Syringe Compatibility

Vancomycin HCl

Test Drug	Mfr	Amt	Mfr	Amt	Remarks	Ref	C/I
Caffeine citrate		20 mg/1 mL	LI	50 mg/1 mL	Visually compatible for 4 hr at 25°C	2440	C
Dimenhydrinate		10 mg/1 mL		50 mg/1 mL	Precipitate forms	2569	I
Heparin sodium		2500 units/1 mL	LI	500 mg	Turbidity or precipitate forms within 5 min	1053	I
Pantoprazole sodium	[a]	4 mg/1 mL		50 mg/1 mL	Clear solution	2574	C

[a] Test performed using the formulation WITHOUT edetate disodium.

Y-Site Injection Compatibility (1:1 Mixture)

Vancomycin HCl

Test Drug	Mfr	Conc	Mfr	Conc	Remarks	Ref	C/I
Acetaminophen	CAD	10 mg/mL	HOS	5 mg/mL[b]	Physically compatible with little or no loss of either drug in 4 hr at 23°C	2901, 2902	C
Acyclovir sodium	BW	5 mg/mL[a]	LI	5 mg/mL[a]	Physically compatible for 4 hr at 25°C	1157	C
Albumin human		0.1 and 1%[b]		20 mg/mL[a]	Heavy turbidity forms immediately and precipitate develops subsequently	1701	I
Aldesleukin	CHI[q]	[a]			Visually compatible. Aldesleukin activity retained. Vancomycin not tested	1890	C
Allopurinol sodium	BW	3 mg/mL[b]	LY	10 mg/mL[b]	Physically compatible for 4 hr at 22°C	1686	C
Alprostadil	BED	7.5 mcg/mL[p e]	LI	5 mg/mL[s]	Visually compatible for 1 hr	2746	C
Amifostine	USB	10 mg/mL[a]	AB	10 mg/mL[a]	Physically compatible for 4 hr at 23°C	1845	C
Amiodarone HCl	LZ	4 mg/mL[c]	LI	5 mg/mL[c]	Physically compatible for 4 hr at room temperature	1444	C

Y-Site Injection Compatibility (1:1 Mixture) (Cont.)

Test Drug	Mfr	Conc	Mfr	Conc	Remarks	Ref	C/I
Amiodarone HCl	WY	6 mg/mL[a]	APP	4 mg/mL[a]	Visually compatible for 24 hr at 22°C	2352	C
Amiodarone HCl	WY	6 mg/mL[a]	APP	10 mg/mL[a]	Visually compatible for 24 hr at 22°C	2352	C
Ampicillin sodium	SKB	250 mg/mL[d]	AB	20 mg/mL[a]	Transient precipitate forms	2189	?
Ampicillin sodium	SKB	1, 10, 50 mg/mL[b]	AB	20 mg/mL[a]	Physically compatible for 4 hr at 23°C	2189	C
Ampicillin sodium	SKB	1[b], 10[b], 50[b], 250[d] mg/mL	AB	2 mg/mL[a]	Physically compatible for 4 hr at 23°C	2189	C
Ampicillin sodium–sulbactam sodium	PF	250 mg/mL[d t]	AB	20 mg/mL[a]	Transient precipitate forms	2189	?
Ampicillin sodium–sulbactam sodium	PF	1, 10, 50 mg/mL[b t]	AB	20 mg/mL[a]	Physically compatible for 4 hr at 23°C	2189	C
Ampicillin sodium–sulbactam sodium	PF	1[b t], 10[b t], 50[b t], 250[d t] mg/mL	AB	2 mg/mL[a]	Physically compatible for 4 hr at 23°C	2189	C
Amsacrine	NCI	1 mg/mL[a]	LI	10 mg/mL[a]	Visually compatible for 4 hr at 22°C	1381	C
Anidulafungin	VIC	0.5 mg/mL[a]	APP	10 mg/mL[a]	Physically compatible for 4 hr at 23°C	2617	C
Atracurium besylate	BW	0.5 mg/mL[a]	ES	5 mg/mL[a]	Physically compatible for 24 hr at 28°C	1337	C
Aztreonam	SQ	200 mg/mL[b]	LI	67 mg/mL[b]	White granular precipitate forms immediately in tubing when given sequentially	1364	I
Aztreonam	SQ	40 mg/mL[a]	AB	10 mg/mL[a]	Physically compatible for 4 hr at 23°C	1758	C
Bivalirudin	TMC	5 mg/mL[a]	AB	10 mg/mL[a]	Gross white precipitate forms immediately	2373	I
Cangrelor tetrasodium	TMC	1 mg/mL[b]		10 mg/mL[b]	Physically compatible for 4 hr	3243	C
Caspofungin acetate	ME	0.7 mg/mL[b]	HOS	10 mg/mL[b]	Physically compatible for 4 hr at room temperature	2758	C
Caspofungin acetate	ME	0.5 mg/mL[b]	HOS	4 mg/mL[b]	Physically compatible over 60 min	2766	C
Cefazolin sodium	SKB	200 mg/mL[d]	AB	20 mg/mL[a]	Transient precipitate forms	2189	?
Cefazolin sodium	SKB	10 and 50 mg/mL[a]	AB	20 mg/mL[a]	Gross white precipitate forms immediately	2189	I
Cefazolin sodium	SKB	1 mg/mL[a]	AB	20 mg/mL[a]	Physically compatible for 4 hr at 23°C	2189	C
Cefazolin sodium	SKB	200 mg/mL[d]	AB	2 mg/mL[a]	Physically compatible for 4 hr at 23°C	2189	C
Cefazolin sodium	SKB	50 mg/mL[a]	AB	2 mg/mL[a]	Subvisible haze forms immediately	2189	I
Cefazolin sodium	SKB	1 and 10 mg/mL[a]	AB	2 mg/mL[a]	Physically compatible for 4 hr at 23°C	2189	C
Cefepime HCl	BMS	120 mg/mL[d]		30 mg/mL	Physically compatible with less than 10% cefepime loss. Vancomycin not tested	2513	C
Cefepime HCl	APO	20 mg/mL[b]	NVP	4 mg/mL[b]	Samples from 4-hr cefepime and 1-hr vancomycin infusions physically compatible during infusion and after 24 hr at 22.5°C in dark. Cefepime chemically stable during infusion and after 12 hr at 22.5°C in dark; vancomycin not measured using an assay noted to be stability indicating	3475	C
Cefepime HCl	APO	20 mg/mL[a]	NVP	5 mg/mL[a]	Samples from 4-hr cefepime and 1-hr vancomycin infusions physically compatible during infusion and after 24 hr at 22.5°C in dark. Cefepime chemically stable during infusion and after 12 hr at 22.5°C in dark; vancomycin not measured using an assay noted to be stability indicating	3475	C

Y-Site Injection Compatibility (1:1 Mixture) (Cont.)

Test Drug	Mfr	Conc	Mfr	Conc	Remarks	Ref	C/I
Cefepime HCl	APO	20 mg/mL[a]	NVP	4 mg/mL[b]	Samples from 4-hr cefepime and 1-hr vancomycin infusions physically compatible during infusion and after 24 hr at 22.5°C in dark. Cefepime chemically stable during infusion and after 12 hr at 22.5°C in dark; vancomycin not measured using an assay noted to be stability indicating	3475	C
Cefepime HCl	APO	20 mg/mL[b]	NVP	5 mg/mL[a]	Samples from 4-hr cefepime and 1-hr vancomycin infusions physically compatible during infusion and after 24 hr at 22.5°C in dark. Cefepime chemically stable during infusion and after 12 hr at 22.5°C in dark; vancomycin not measured using an assay noted to be stability indicating	3475	C
Cefotaxime sodium		100 mg/mL[d]		12.5, 25, 30, 50 mg/mL[d]	White precipitate forms immediately	1721	I
Cefotaxime sodium		100 mg/mL[d]		5 mg/mL[d]	No precipitate visually observed over 7 days at room temperature, but nonvisible incompatibility cannot be ruled out	1721	?
Cefotaxime sodium	HO	200 mg/mL[d]	AB	20 mg/mL[a]	Transient precipitate forms	2189	?
Cefotaxime sodium	HO	50 mg/mL[a]	AB	20 mg/mL[a]	White cloudiness forms immediately	2189	I
Cefotaxime sodium	HO	1 and 10 mg/mL[a]	AB	20 mg/mL[a]	Physically compatible for 4 hr at 23°C	2189	C
Cefotaxime sodium	HO	1[a], 10[a], 50[a], 200[d] mg/mL	AB	2 mg/mL[a]	Physically compatible for 4 hr at 23°C	2189	C
Cefotetan disodium	ZEN	200 mg/mL[d]	AB	20 mg/mL[a]	Transient precipitate forms followed by white precipitate in 4 hr	2189	I
Cefotetan disodium	ZEN	10 and 50 mg/mL[a]	AB	20 mg/mL[a]	Gross white precipitate forms immediately	2189	I
Cefotetan disodium	ZEN	1 mg/mL[a]	AB	20 mg/mL[a]	Subvisible haze forms immediately. White precipitate in 4 hr	2189	I
Cefotetan disodium	ZEN	1[a], 10[a], 50[a], 200[d] mg/mL	AB	2 mg/mL[a]	Physically compatible for 4 hr at 23°C	2189	C
Cefoxitin sodium	ME	180 mg/mL[d]	AB	20 mg/mL[a]	Transient precipitate forms	2189	?
Cefoxitin sodium	ME	50 mg/mL[a]	AB	20 mg/mL[a]	Immediate gross white precipitate	2189	I
Cefoxitin sodium	ME	10 mg/mL[a]	AB	20 mg/mL[a]	Visible haze forms in 4 hr at 23°C	2189	I
Cefoxitin sodium	ME	1 mg/mL[a]	AB	20 mg/mL[a]	Physically compatible for 4 hr at 23°C	2189	C
Cefoxitin sodium	ME	1[a], 10[a], 50[a], 180[d] mg/mL	AB	2 mg/mL[a]	Physically compatible for 4 hr at 23°C	2189	C
Ceftazidime		50 mg/mL[d]		10 mg/mL[a]	Precipitates immediately	873	I
Ceftazidime	SKB	10[a], 50[a], 200[d] mg/mL	AB	20 mg/mL[a]	Gross white precipitate forms immediately	2189	I
Ceftazidime	SKB	1 mg/mL[a]	AB	20 mg/mL[a]	Physically compatible for 4 hr at 23°C	2189	C
Ceftazidime	SKB	1[a], 10[a], 50[a], 200[d] mg/mL	AB	2 mg/mL[a]	Physically compatible for 4 hr at 23°C	2189	C
Ceftazidime	SKB	125 mg/mL		30 mg/mL	Precipitates immediately	2434	I
Ceftazidime	GSK	120 mg/mL[d]		30 mg/mL	Precipitates	2513	I
Ceftazidime		125 mg/mL	LI	10 mg/mL[a]	Physically incompatible	3536	I

Y-Site Injection Compatibility (1:1 Mixture) (Cont.)

Test Drug	Mfr	Conc	Mfr	Conc	Remarks	Ref	C/I
Ceftazidime–avibactam sodium	FOR	8 mg/mL[a cc]	HOS	5, 10, 15, 20 mg/mL[a]	Physically incompatible	3480	I
Ceftazidime–avibactam sodium	FOR	20 mg/mL[a cc]	HOS	5 mg/mL[a]	Physically compatible for up to 24 hr at room temperature with no loss of antimicrobial activity	3480	C
Ceftazidime–avibactam sodium	FOR	20 mg/mL[a cc]	HOS	10, 15, 20 mg/mL[a]	Physically incompatible	3480	I
Ceftazidime–avibactam sodium	FOR	40 mg/mL[a cc]	HOS	5, 10 mg/mL[a]	Physically compatible for up to 24 hr at room temperature with no loss of antimicrobial activity	3480	C
Ceftazidime–avibactam sodium	FOR	40 mg/mL[a cc]	HOS	15, 20 mg/mL[a]	Physically incompatible	3480	I
Ceftolozane sulfate–tazobactam sodium	CUB	10 mg/mL[c x]	APP	5 mg/mL[c]	Physically compatible for 2 hr	3262	C
Ceftolozane sulfate–tazobactam sodium	ME	15 mg/mL[a x]	HOS	5, 10 mg/mL[a]	Physically compatible for up to 24 hr at room temperature with no loss of antimicrobial activity	3480	C
Ceftolozane sulfate–tazobactam sodium	ME	15 mg/mL[a x]	HOS	15, 20 mg/mL[a]	Physically incompatible	3480	I
Ceftriaxone sodium	RC	100 mg/mL	LI	20 mg/mL	White precipitate forms immediately	1398	I
Ceftriaxone sodium	RC	250 mg/mL[d]	AB	20 mg/mL[a]	Transient precipitate forms	2189	?
Ceftriaxone sodium	RC	10 and 50 mg/mL[a]	AB	20 mg/mL[a]	Gross white precipitate forms immediately	2189	I
Ceftriaxone sodium	RC	1 mg/mL[a]	AB	20 mg/mL[a]	Subvisible haze forms immediately	2189	I
Ceftriaxone sodium	RC	1[a], 10[a], 50[a], 250[d] mg/mL	AB	2 mg/mL[a]	Physically compatible for 4 hr at 23°C	2189	C
Cefuroxime sodium	GW	150 mg/mL[d]	AB	20 mg/mL[a]	Transient precipitate forms followed by a subvisible haze	2189	I
Cefuroxime sodium	GW	50 mg/mL[a]	AB	20 mg/mL[a]	Gross white precipitate forms immediately	2189	I
Cefuroxime sodium	GW	10 mg/mL[a]	AB	20 mg/mL[a]	Subvisible haze forms immediately	2189	I
Cefuroxime sodium	GW	1 mg/mL[a]	AB	20 mg/mL[a]	Physically compatible for 4 hr at 23°C	2189	C
Cefuroxime sodium	GW	1[a], 10[a], 50[a], 150[d] mg/mL	AB	2 mg/mL[a]	Physically compatible for 4 hr at 23°C	2189	C
Cisatracurium besylate	GW	0.1, 2, 5 mg/mL[a]	AB	10 mg/mL[a]	Physically compatible for 4 hr at 23°C	2074	C
Clarithromycin	AB	4 mg/mL[a]	DB	10 mg/mL[a]	Visually compatible for 72 hr at both 30 and 17°C	2174	C
Cloxacillin sodium	SMX	100 mg/mL	PPC	50 mg/mL	Precipitates immediately	3245	I
Cloxacillin sodium	SMX	0.8[b] and 1.25[b] mg/mL	PPC	0.3 mg/mL[b]	Visually compatible for up to 1 hr at 25°C	3246	C
Cloxacillin sodium	SMX	23.75 mg/mL[b]	PPC	0.5 mg/mL[b]	Visually compatible for up to 1 hr at 25°C	3246	C
Cloxacillin sodium	SMX	1.25[b] and 1.75[b] mg/mL	PPC	0.6 mg/mL[b]	Visually compatible for up to 1 hr at 25°C	3246	C
Cloxacillin sodium	SMX	1.25[b] and 3.4[b] mg/mL	PPC	1.3 mg/mL[b]	Visually compatible for up to 1 hr at 25°C	3246	C
Cloxacillin sodium	SMX	0.8[b], 1.75[b], 3.4[b], and 6.8[b] mg/mL	PPC	2 mg/mL[b]	Visually compatible for up to 1 hr at 25°C	3246	C
Cloxacillin sodium	SMX	12.5[b] and 20[b] mg/mL	PPC	2 mg/mL[b]	White, gel-like precipitate forms immediately	3246	I
Cloxacillin sodium	SMX	1.25 mg/mL[b]	PPC	2.5 mg/mL[b]	White, gel-like precipitate forms within 1 hr	3246	I

Y-Site Injection Compatibility (1:1 Mixture) (Cont.)

Test Drug	Mfr	Conc	Mfr	Conc	Remarks	Ref	C/I
Cloxacillin sodium	SMX	6.8 mg/mL[b]	PPC	2.5 mg/mL[b]	White, gel-like precipitate forms immediately	3246	I
Cloxacillin sodium	SMX	1.25[b] and 12.5[b] mg/mL	PPC	5 mg/mL[b]	White, gel-like precipitate forms immediately	3246	I
Cloxacillin sodium	SMX	5 mg/mL[b]	PPC	8 mg/mL[b]	White, gel-like precipitate forms immediately	3246	I
Cloxacillin sodium	SMX	1.25 mg/mL[b]	PPC	9.5 mg/mL[b]	White, gel-like precipitate forms immediately	3246	I
Colistimethate sodium	MIL	1.5 mg/mL[b]	SIA	10 mg/mL[b]	Visually compatible for 1 hr at 26°C	3335	C
Cyclophosphamide	MJ	20 mg/mL[a]	LI	5 mg/mL[a]	Physically compatible for 4 hr at 25°C	1194	C
Defibrotide sodium	JAZ	8 mg/mL[b]	MYL	10.4 mg/mL[b]	Solution became milky white and opalescent. Precipitate formed within 1 hr when defibrotide added to vancomycin HCl, but developed immediately when order of mixing was reversed	3149	I
Dexmedetomidine HCl	AB	4 mcg/mL[b]	AB	10 mg/mL[b]	Physically compatible for 4 hr at 23°C	2383	C
Diltiazem HCl	MMD	5 mg/mL	LI	5 and 50 mg/mL[b]	Visually compatible	1807	C
Docetaxel	RPR	0.9 mg/mL[a]	LI	10 mg/mL[a]	Physically compatible for 4 hr at 23°C	2224	C
Doripenem	JJ	5 mg/mL[a b]	HOS	10 mg/mL[a b]	Physically compatible for 4 hr at 23°C	2743	C
Doxapram HCl	RB	2 mg/mL[a]	APP	5 mg/mL[a]	Visually compatible for 4 hr at 23°C	2470	C
Doxorubicin HCl liposomal	SEQ	0.4 mg/mL[a]	AB	10 mg/mL[a]	Physically compatible for 4 hr at 23°C	2087	C
Enalaprilat	MSD	0.05 mg/mL[b]	LE	5 mg/mL[a]	Physically compatible for 24 hr at room temperature under fluorescent light	1355	C
Eravacycline dihydrochloride	TET	0.6 mg/mL[b]	AVG	5 mg/mL[b]	Physically compatible for 2 hr at room temperature	3532	C
Esmolol HCl	DCC	10 mg/mL[a]	LE	5 mg/mL[a]	Physically compatible for 24 hr at 22°C	1169	C
Etoposide phosphate	BR	5 mg/mL[a]	LI	10 mg/mL[a]	Physically compatible for 4 hr at 23°C	2218	C
Fat emulsion, intravenous	OTS	20%[y]	SHI	5 mg/mL[a z]	Fine particles increased after preparation and continued to increase over time	3452	I
Fenoldopam mesylate	AB	80 mcg/mL[b]	APP	10 mg/mL[b]	Physically compatible for 4 hr at 23°C	2467	C
Filgrastim	AMG	30 mcg/mL[a]	AB	10 mg/mL[a]	Physically compatible for 4 hr at 22°C	1687	C
Floxacillin[dd]		250 mg/mL	LI	10 mg/mL[a]	Physically incompatible	3536	I
Fluconazole	RR	2 mg/mL	LY	20 mg/mL	Physically compatible for 24 hr at 25°C	1407	C
Fludarabine phosphate	BX	1 mg/mL[a]	LI	10 mg/mL[a]	Visually compatible for 4 hr at 22°C	1439	C
Foscarnet sodium	AST	24 mg/mL	LE	20 mg/mL	Precipitates immediately	1335	I
Foscarnet sodium	AST	24 mg/mL	LE	15 mg/mL[c]	Physically compatible for 24 hr at 25°C under fluorescent light	1393	C
Foscarnet sodium	AST	24 mg/mL	LE	10 mg/mL[b]	Visually compatible for 24 hr at room temperature. No precipitate found	2063	C
Furosemide		10 mg/mL	LI	10 mg/mL[a]	Physically incompatible	3536	I
Gallium nitrate	FUJ	1 mg/mL[b]	AB	5 mg/mL[b]	Visually compatible for 24 hr at 25°C	1673	C
Gemcitabine HCl	LI	10 mg/mL[b]	LI	10 mg/mL[b]	Physically compatible for 4 hr at 23°C	2226	C
Granisetron HCl	SKB	0.05 mg/mL[a]	AB	10 mg/mL[a]	Physically compatible for 4 hr at 23°C	2000	C

Y-Site Injection Compatibility (1:1 Mixture) (Cont.)

Test Drug	Mfr	Conc	Mfr	Conc	Remarks	Ref	C/I
Heparin sodium	TR	50 units/mL	LI	6.6 mg/mL[a]	Visually incompatible within 4 hr at 25°C	1793	I
Heparin sodium	ES	100 units/mL[c]	LE	10 mg/mL[b]	Precipitate forms	2063	I
Heparin sodium	LEO	10 and 5000 units/mL[b]	PHS	2.5 mg/mL[b]	Physically compatible with little change in heparin activity in 14 days at 4 and 37°C. Antibiotic not tested	2684	C
Heparin sodium	LEO	10 units/mL[b]	PHS	2 mg/mL[b]	Physically compatible with little change in heparin activity in 14 days at 4 and 37°C. Antibiotic not tested	2684	C
Hetastarch in lactated electrolyte	AB	6%	LI	10 mg/mL[a]	Physically compatible for 4 hr at 23°C	2339	C
Hydromorphone HCl	WY	0.2 mg/mL[a]	LI	5 mg/mL[a]	Physically compatible for 4 hr at 25°C	987	C
Hydromorphone HCl	HOS	2 mg/mL	HOS	4 mg/mL[b]	Physically compatible	2794	C
Ibuprofen lysinate	OVA	10 mg/mL	HOS	50 mg/mL[d]	Measured turbidity increased immediately and solution became milky white and opaque	3541	I
Idarubicin HCl	AD	1 mg/mL[b]	AD	4 mg/mL[a]	Color changes immediately	1525	I
Insulin, regular	LI	0.2 unit/mL[b]	LI	4 mg/mL[a]	Physically compatible for 2 hr at 25°C	1395	C
Isavuconazonium sulfate	ASP	1.5 mg/mL[c]	HOS	5 mg/mL[c]	Physically compatible for 2 hr	3263	C
Labetalol HCl	SC	1 mg/mL[a]	LE	5 mg/mL[a]	Physically compatible for 24 hr at 18°C	1171	C
Levofloxacin	OMN	5 mg/mL[a]	LI	50 mg/mL	Visually compatible for 4 hr at 24°C	2233	C
Linezolid	PHU	2 mg/mL	FUJ	10 mg/mL[a]	Physically compatible for 4 hr at 23°C	2264	C
Lorazepam	WY	0.33 mg/mL[b]	LI	5 mg/mL	Visually compatible for 24 hr at 22°C	1855	C
Magnesium sulfate	IX	16.7, 33.3, 66.7, 100 mg/mL[a]	LI	5 mg/mL[a]	Physically compatible for at least 4 hr at 32°C	813	C
Melphalan HCl	BW	0.1 mg/mL[b]	LY	10 mg/mL[b]	Physically compatible for 3 hr at 22°C	1557	C
Meperidine HCl	WY	10 mg/mL[a]	LI	5 mg/mL[a]	Physically compatible for 4 hr at 25°C	987	C
Meropenem	ZEN	1 and 50 mg/mL[b]	LI	5 mg/mL[d]	Visually compatible for 4 hr at room temperature	1994	C
Meropenem		50 mg/mL	SZ	50 mg/mL	Precipitates immediately	3538	I
Meropenem–vabor-bactam	TMC	8 mg/mL[b v]	FRK	5 mg/mL[b]	Physically compatible for 3 hr at 20 to 25°C	3380	C
Methotrexate sodium	LE	[a f]	AB	510 mg[g]	Physically compatible during 1-hr simultaneous infusion	1405	C
Methotrexate sodium		30 mg/mL		5 mg/mL[a]	Visually compatible for 2 hr at room temperature. Yellow precipitate in 4 hr	1788	I
Methylprednisolone[dd]		50 mg/mL	LI	10 mg/mL[a]	Physically incompatible	3536	I
Midazolam HCl	RC	1 mg/mL[a]	LI	5 mg/mL[a]	Visually compatible for 24 hr at 23°C	1847	C
Midazolam HCl	RC	5 mg/mL	LI	5 mg/mL	Visually compatible for 24 hr at 22°C	1855	C
Milrinone lactate	SS	0.2 mg/mL[a]	OR	5 mg/mL[a]	Visually compatible for 4 hr at 25°C	2381	C
Morphine sulfate	WI	1 mg/mL[a]	LI	5 mg/mL[a]	Physically compatible for 4 hr at 25°C	987	C
Mycophenolate mofetil HCl	RC	5.9 mg/mL[a]		10 mg/mL[a]	Physically compatible and 3% mycophenolate mofetil loss in 4 hr	2738	C

Y-Site Injection Compatibility (1:1 Mixture) (Cont.)

Test Drug	Mfr	Conc	Mfr	Conc	Remarks	Ref	C/I
Nafcillin sodium	BE	250 mg/mL[d]	AB	20 mg/mL[a]	Transient precipitate forms followed by a visibly hazy solution	2189	I
Nafcillin sodium	BE	10 and 50 mg/mL[b]	AB	20 mg/mL[a]	Gross white precipitate forms immediately	2189	I
Nafcillin sodium	BE	1 mg/mL[b]	AB	20 mg/mL[a]	Physically compatible for 4 hr at 23°C	2189	C
Nafcillin sodium	BE	10[b], 50[b], 250[d] mg/mL	AB	2 mg/mL[a]	Subvisible measured haze forms immediately	2189	I
Nafcillin sodium	BE	1 mg/mL[b]	AB	2 mg/mL[a]	Physically compatible for 4 hr at 23°C	2189	C
Nicardipine HCl	DCC	0.1 mg/mL[a]	LE	5 mg/mL[a]	Visually compatible for 24 hr at room temperature	235	C
Ondansetron HCl	GL	1 mg/mL[b]	LI	10 mg/mL[a]	Visually compatible for 4 hr at 22°C	1365	C
Oxacillin sodium	AUR	20 mg/mL[d]	HOS	10 mg/mL[a]	Precipitates immediately	3477	I
Paclitaxel	NCI	1.2 mg/mL[a]		10 mg/mL[a]	Physically compatible for 4 hr at 22°C	1528	C
Palonosetron HCl	MGI	50 mcg/mL	HOS	5 mg/mL[a]	Physically compatible and no loss of either drug in 4 hr at room temperature	2765	C
Pancuronium bromide	ES	0.05 mg/mL[a]	ES	5 mg/mL[a]	Physically compatible for 24 hr at 28°C	1337	C
Pantoprazole sodium	ALT[r]	8 mg/mL	ME	40 mg/mL	Color change after 10 hr	2727	I
Pemetrexed disodium	LI	20 mg/mL[b]	AB	10 mg/mL[a]	Physically compatible for 4 hr at 23°C	2564	C
Phenytoin[dd]		50 mg/mL	LI	10 mg/mL[a]	Physically incompatible	3536	I
Piperacillin sodium–tazobactam sodium	LE[r]	40 mg/mL[a u]	AB	10 mg/mL[a]	White turbidity forms immediately and white precipitate forms in 4 hr	1688	I
Piperacillin sodium–tazobactam sodium	LE[r]	200 mg/mL[d u]	AB	20 mg/mL[a]	Transient precipitate forms	2189	?
Piperacillin sodium–tazobactam sodium	LE[r]	10 and 50 mg/mL[a u]	AB	20 mg/mL[a]	Gross white precipitate forms immediately	2189	I
Piperacillin sodium–tazobactam sodium	LE[r]	1 mg/mL[a u]	AB	20 mg/mL[a]	Physically compatible for 4 hr at 23°C	2189	C
Piperacillin sodium–tazobactam sodium	LE[r]	1[a u], 10[a u], 50[a u], 200[d u] mg/mL	AB	2 mg/mL[a]	Physically compatible for 4 hr at 23°C	2189	C
Piperacillin sodium–tazobactam sodium	SZ[r]	30 mg/mL[d u w]	APP	4 mg/mL[d]	Physically compatible for 5 days at 25°C	2935, 3474	C
Piperacillin sodium–tazobactam sodium	SZ[r]	40 mg/mL[d u w]	APP	4 mg/mL[d]	Physically compatible for 5 days at 25°C	2935	C
Piperacillin sodium–tazobactam sodium	HOS[r]	100 mg/mL[d u]	APP	10 mg/mL[a]	Transient precipitate clears within 15 seconds	2933	?
Piperacillin sodium–tazobactam sodium	APP[r]	16, 30, 40, 80, 100 mg/mL[b u]	APP	2 mg/mL[b]	Physically compatible for up to 4 hr	3476	C
Piperacillin sodium–tazobactam sodium	APP[r]	16, 30, 40 mg/mL[a u]	APP	4 mg/mL[a]	Physically compatible for up to 4 hr	3476	C
Piperacillin sodium–tazobactam sodium	APP[r]	80, 100 mg/mL[a u]	APP	4 mg/mL[a]	White precipitate forms only when piperacillin–tazobactam added to vancomycin; not observed when order of mixing was reversed	3476	I
Piperacillin sodium–tazobactam sodium	APP[r]	16, 30, 40, 80, 100 mg/mL[b u]	APP	5 mg/mL[b]	Physically compatible for up to 4 hr	3476	C

Y-Site Injection Compatibility (1:1 Mixture) (Cont.)

Test Drug	Mfr	Conc	Mfr	Conc	Remarks	Ref	C/I
Piperacillin sodium–tazobactam sodium	APP[r]	16 mg/mL[a u]	APP	8 mg/mL[a]	Persistent white precipitate forms	3476	I
Piperacillin sodium–tazobactam sodium	APP[r]	30, 40, 80, 100 mg/mL[a u]	APP	8 mg/mL[a]	Immediate white cloudiness forms, then dissipates	3476	?
Piperacillin sodium–tazobactam sodium	APP[r]	16, 30 mg/mL[b u]	APP	10 mg/mL[b]	Physically compatible for up to 4 hr	3476	C
Piperacillin sodium–tazobactam sodium	APP[r]	40 mg/mL[b u]	APP	10 mg/mL[b]	White precipitate forms only when piperacillin–tazobactam added to vancomycin; not observed when order of mixing was reversed	3476	I
Piperacillin sodium–tazobactam sodium	APP[r]	80, 100 mg[b u]	APP	10 mg/mL[b]	Immediate white cloudiness forms, then dissipates	3476	?
Piperacillin sodium–tazobactam sodium	HOS[r]	30, 40, 44.4, 53.3, 60, 71.1, 80 mg/mL[b u]	APP	4 mg/mL[b]	Physically compatible for 24 hr at 21 to 25°C	3478	C
Piperacillin sodium–tazobactam sodium	HOS[r]	30, 40, 44.4, 53.3, 60, 71.1, 80 mg/mL[b u]	APP	5 mg/mL[b]	Physically compatible for 24 hr at 21 to 25°C	3478	C
Piperacillin sodium–tazobactam sodium	BA[aa]	60 mg/mL[u bb]	APP	5, 8, 9 mg/mL[b]	Physically compatible for 24 hr at 21 to 25°C	3478	C
Piperacillin sodium–tazobactam sodium	WY[aa]	30, 53.3, 80 mg/mL[u]	APP	5 mg/mL[b]	Physically compatible for 24 hr at 21 to 25°C	3478	C
Piperacillin sodium–tazobactam sodium	HOS[r]	30, 40, 44.4, 53.3, 60, 71.1, 80 mg/mL[b u]	APP	6 mg/mL[b]	Physically compatible for 24 hr at 21 to 25°C	3478	C
Piperacillin sodium–tazobactam sodium	HOS[r]	30, 40, 44.4, 53.3, 60, 71.1, 80 mg/mL[b u]	APP	7 mg/mL[b]	Physically compatible for 24 hr at 21 to 25°C	3478	C
Piperacillin sodium–tazobactam sodium	HOS[r]	30, 40, 44.4, 53.3, 60 mg/mL[b u]	APP	8 mg/mL[b]	Physically compatible for 24 hr at 21 to 25°C	3478	C
Piperacillin sodium–tazobactam sodium	HOS[r]	71.1, 80 mg/mL[b u]	APP	8 mg/mL[b]	Transient and reversible precipitate forms	3478	?
Piperacillin sodium–tazobactam sodium	WY[aa]	30, 53.3, 80 mg/mL[u]	APP	8 mg/mL[b]	Physically compatible for 24 hr at 21 to 25°C	3478	C
Piperacillin sodium–tazobactam sodium	HOS[r]	30, 40, 44.4, 53.3, 60, 71.1, 80 mg/mL[b u]	APP	10 mg/mL[b]	Transient and reversible precipitate forms	3478	?
Piperacillin sodium–tazobactam sodium	HOS[r]	30, 40, 44.4, 53.3, 60, 71.1, 80 mg/mL[b u]	APP	12 mg/mL[b]	Irreversible precipitate forms	3478	I
Piperacillin sodium–tazobactam sodium	BA[aa]	60 mg/mL[u bb]	BA	5 mg/mL[bb]	Physically compatible for 24 hr at 21 to 25°C	3478	C
Piperacillin sodium–tazobactam sodium	WY[aa]	30, 53.3, 80 mg/mL[u]	BA	5 mg/mL[bb]	Physically compatible for 24 hr at 21 to 25°C	3478	C
Piperacillin sodium–tazobactam sodium	SZ[r]	28 mg/mL[a u]	HOS	5 mg/mL[a]	Physically compatible for up to 24 hr at room temperature with no loss of antimicrobial activity	3480	C
Piperacillin sodium–tazobactam sodium	SZ[r]	28 mg/mL[a u]	HOS	10, 15, 20 mg/mL[a]	Physically incompatible	3480	I

Y-Site Injection Compatibility (1:1 Mixture) (Cont.)

Test Drug	Mfr	Conc °	Mfr	Conc	Remarks	Ref	C/I
Piperacillin sodium–tazobactam sodium	PF[aa]	60 mg/mL[u bb]	BA	5 mg/mL[bb]	No evidence of physical incompatibility via simulated Y-site infusion; however, a white precipitate forms during actual Y-site infusion	3481	?
Piperacillin–tazobactam[dd]	[ee]	200 mg/mL[ff]	LI	10 mg/mL[a]	Physically incompatible	3536	I
Plazomicin sulfate	ACH	24 mg/mL[c]	FRK	5 mg/mL[c]	Physically compatible for 1 hr at 20 to 25°C	3432	C
Posaconazole	ME	18 mg/mL		5 mg/mL[c]	Physically compatible	2911, 2912	C
Propofol	ZEN[aa]	10 mg/mL	AB	10 mg/mL[a]	Physically compatible for 1 hr at 23°C	2066	C
Propofol	BA[r]	10 mg/mL		10 mg/mL[a]	Emulsion disruption within 1 to 4 hr at room temperature	2336	I
Propofol	ASZ[aa]	10 mg/mL		10 mg/mL[a]	Physically compatible for up to 30 days at room temperature	2336	C
Propofol	[ee]	1 mg/mL	LI	10 mg/mL[a]	Physically incompatible	3536	I
Remifentanil HCl	GW	0.025 and 0.25 mg/mL[b]	AB	10 mg/mL[a]	Physically compatible for 4 hr at 23°C	2075	C
Sargramostim	IMM	10 mcg/mL[b]	LI	10 mg/mL[b]	Visually compatible for 4 hr at 22°C	1436	C
Sargramostim	IMM	15 mcg/mL[b]	LI	20 mg/mL[c]	Visually compatible for 2 hr	1618	C
Sargramostim	IMM	6 mcg/mL[b h]	LI	20 mg/mL[c]	Haze forms within 15 min and increases due to vancomycin incompatibility with albumin human	1618, 1701	I
Sodium bicarbonate		1.4%		5 mg/mL[a]	Visually compatible for 4 hr at room temperature	1788	C
Tacrolimus	FUJ	1 mg/mL[b]	LI	5 mg/mL[a]	Visually compatible for 24 hr at 25°C	1630	C
Tedizolid phosphate	CUB	0.8 mg/mL[b]	HOS	5 mg/mL[b]	Physically compatible for 2 hr	3244	C
Teniposide	BR	0.1 mg/mL[a]	AB	10 mg/mL[a]	Physically compatible for 4 hr at 23°C	1725	C
Theophylline	TR	4 mg/mL	LI	6.6 mg/mL[a]	Visually compatible for 6 hr at 25°C	1793	C
Theophylline		20 mg/mL	LI	10 mg/mL[a]	Physically incompatible	3536	I
Thiotepa	IMM[i]	1 mg/mL[a]	AB	10 mg/mL[a]	Physically compatible for 4 hr at 23°C	1861	C
Tigecycline	WY	1 mg/mL[b]		5 mg/mL[b]	Physically compatible for 4 hr	2714	C
TNA #218 to #226[j]			AB	10 mg/mL[a]	Visually compatible for 4 hr at 23°C	2215	C
TPN #61[j]		[k]	LI	50 mg/1 mL[l]	Physically compatible	1012	C
TPN #61[j]		[m]	LI	300 mg/6 mL[l]	Physically compatible	1012	C
TPN #91[j]		[n]	LI	30 mg[o]	Physically compatible	1170	C
TPN #189[j]			DB	10 mg/mL[b]	Visually compatible for 24 hr at 22°C	1767	C
TPN #212 to #215[j]			AB	10 mg/mL[a]	Physically compatible for 4 hr at 23°C	2109	C
Valproate sodium		100 mg/mL	LI	10 mg/mL[a]	Physically incompatible	3536	I
Vecuronium bromide	OR	0.1 mg/mL[a]	ES	5 mg/mL[a]	Physically compatible for 24 hr at 28°C	1337	C

Y-Site Injection Compatibility (1:1 Mixture) (Cont.)

Test Drug	Mfr	Conc	Mfr	Conc	Remarks	Ref	C/I
Vinorelbine tartrate	BW	1 mg/mL[b]	LY	10 mg/mL[b]	Physically compatible for 4 hr at 22°C	1558	C
Zidovudine	BW	4 mg/mL[a]	LI	15 mg/mL[a]	Physically compatible for 4 hr at 25°C	1193	C

[a] Tested in dextrose 5%.

[b] Tested in sodium chloride 0.9%.

[c] Tested in both dextrose 5% and sodium chloride 0.9%.

[d] Tested in sterile water for injection.

[e] Tested in a 1:1 mixture of dextrose 5% and TPN #274 (see Appendix).

[f] Concentration unspecified.

[g] Infused over one hour simultaneously with methotrexate.

[h] Tested with 0.1% albumin human added.

[i] Lyophilized formulation tested.

[j] Refer to Appendix for the composition of parenteral nutrition solutions. TNA indicates a 3-in-1 admixture, and TPN indicates a 2-in-1 admixture.

[k] Run at 21 mL/hr.

[l] Given over 30 minutes by syringe pump.

[m] Run at 94 mL/hr.

[n] Run at 10 mL/hr.

[o] Given over one hour by syringe pump.

[p] Tested in a 1:1 mixture of (1) dextrose 5% and dextrose 5% in sodium chloride 0.45% with and without potassium chloride 20 mEq/L and also in (2) dextrose 10% in sodium chloride 0.45% with and without potassium chloride 20 mEq/L.

[q] Tested with albumin human 0.1%.

[r] Test performed using the formulation WITHOUT edetate disodium.

[s] Tested in either dextrose 5% or in sodium chloride 0.9%, but the report did not specify which solution.

[t] Ampicillin component. Ampicillin in a 2:1 fixed-ratio concentration with sulbactam.

[u] Piperacillin component. Piperacillin in an 8:1 fixed-ratio concentration with tazobactam.

[v] Meropenem component. Meropenem in a 1:1 fixed-ratio concentration with vaborbactam.

[w] If sterile water for injection is used as the diluent, manufacturers recommend a maximum volume per dose of 50 mL.

[x] Ceftolozane component. Ceftolozane in a 2:1 fixed-ratio concentration with tazobactam.

[y] Run at 25 mL/hr with dextrose 5% run at 83 mL/hr.

[z] Run at 100 mL/hr.

[aa] Test performed using the formulation WITH edetate disodium.

[bb] Tested as the premixed infusion solution.

[cc] Ceftazidime component. Ceftazidime in a 4:1 fixed-ratio concentration with avibactam.

[dd] Salt not specified.

[ee] Presence or absence of edetate disodium not specified.

[ff] Not specified whether concentration refers to single component or combined components.

Additional Compatibility Information

Peritoneal Dialysis Solutions

Reports have revealed that administration of sterile vancomycin by the intraperitoneal route during continuous ambulatory peritoneal dialysis (CAPD) has resulted in a syndrome of chemical peritonitis, ranging from a cloudy dialysate alone to a cloudy dialysate accompanied by variable degrees of abdominal pain and fever.[3464 3465 3466 3467 3468 3469] Manufacturers state that the safety and efficacy of vancomycin administered by the intraperitoneal route have not been established by adequate and well-controlled trials.[3464 3465 3466 3467 3468 3469]

The activity of vancomycin 15 mg/L was evaluated in peritoneal dialysis fluids containing dextrose 1.5 or 4.25% (Dianeal 137, Travenol). Storage at 25°C resulted in virtually no loss of antimicrobial activity in 24 hours.[515]

Vancomycin hydrochloride (Lilly) prepared at vancomycin concentrations of 10 and 50 mg/L in peritoneal dialysis concentrate with dextrose 50% (McGaw) retained 93 to 100% of its initial activity after 24 hours of storage at room temperature.[1044]

The stability of vancomycin hydrochloride (Lilly) prepared at a vancomycin concentration of 20 mg/L in peritoneal dialysis solutions (Dianeal 137 and PD-2) with heparin sodium 500 units/L was evaluated. Approximately 95 ± 12% activity remained after 24 hours at 25°C.[1228]

Vancomycin hydrochloride (Lilly) prepared at a vancomycin concentration of 15 mg/L to 5.3 g/L in Dianeal with dextrose 2.5 or 4.25% was physically compatible with heparin sodium (Organon) 500 to 14,300 units/L for 24 hours at 25°C under fluorescent light. However, a white precipitate formed immediately in combinations of heparin sodium with vancomycin hydrochloride 6.9 to 14.3 g/L.[1322]

The retention of antimicrobial activity of vancomycin hydrochloride (Lilly) prepared at a vancomycin concentration of 1 g/L alone and with each of two aminoglycosides, gentamicin sulfate (SoloPak) prepared at a gentamicin concentration of 120 mg/L and tobramycin sulfate (Lilly) prepared at a tobramycin concentration of 120 mg/L, in Dianeal PD-2 (Travenol) with dextrose 1.5% was evaluated. Little or no loss of any antibiotic occurred in 8 hours at 37°C. Vancomycin hydrochloride alone retained activity for at least 48 hours at 4 and 25°C. In combination with gentamicin sulfate and tobramycin sulfate, antimicrobial activity of both vancomycin and the aminoglycosides was retained for up to 48 hours. However, refrigeration at 4°C was recommended for storage periods greater than 24 hours.[1414]

The stability of vancomycin hydrochloride (Lilly) prepared at a vancomycin concentration of 25 mg/L in Dianeal 137 (Baxter) with dextrose 1.36 and 3.86%, while protected from direct sunlight, was evaluated. At both dextrose concentrations, less than 4% vancomycin was lost in 42 days at 4°C. At 20°C, a 5% or less loss occurred in 28 days. At 37°C, a 10% loss occurred in 6 to 7 days.[1654]

Vancomycin hydrochloride (Lilly) prepared at a vancomycin concentration of 1 mg/mL admixed with ceftazidime (Lilly) 0.5 mg/mL in Dianeal PD-2 (Baxter) with 1.5% and also 4.25% dextrose was evaluated for compatibility and stability. Samples were stored under fluorescent light at 4 and 24°C for 24 hours and at 37°C for 12 hours. No precipitation or other change was observed by visual inspection in any sample. No loss of either drug was found in the samples stored at 4°C and no loss of vancomycin and about 4 to 5% ceftazidime loss were found in the samples stored at 24°C in 24 hours. Vancomycin losses of 3% or less and ceftazidime loss of about 6% were found in the samples stored at 37°C for 12 hours. No difference in stability was found between samples at either dextrose concentration.[2217]

Vancomycin hydrochloride (Lederle) prepared at a vancomycin concentration of 0.05 mg/mL in Dianeal PD-2 with dextrose 1.5% with or without heparin sodium 1 unit/mL in PVC bags was chemically stable for up to 6 days at 4°C (about 3 to 5% loss) and 25°C (up to 7% loss) and 5 days at body temperature of 37°C.[866]

The addition of ceftazidime (Glaxo) 0.1 mg/mL to this peritoneal dialysis solution demonstrated a somewhat reduced stability with the ceftazidime being the defining component. The ceftazidime was chemically stable for up to 6 days at 4°C (about 3% loss), 3 days at 25°C (about 9 to 10% loss), and 12 hours at body temperature of 37°C with the vancomycin exhibiting less loss throughout.[866]

Vancomycin hydrochloride (Lederle) prepared at a vancomycin concentration of 25 mcg/mL in Delflex peritoneal dialysis solution bags with 2.5% dextrose (Fresenius) was stable with little loss occurring in 14 days refrigerated and at room temperature.[2573]

Gentamicin sulfate (American Pharmaceutical Partners) prepared at a gentamicin concentration of 8 mcg/mL with vancomycin hydrochloride (Lederle) prepared at a vancomycin concentration of 25 mcg/mL in Delflex peritoneal dialysis solution bags with 2.5% dextrose (Fresenius) was stable with little or no loss of either drug occurring in 14 days refrigerated and at room temperature.[2573]

Vancomycin hydrochloride (Abbott) prepared at a vancomycin concentration of 1 mg/mL in icodextrin 7.5% PD (Baxter) was tested for stability at 5, 24, and 37°C. The solutions remained clear and colorless. Little or no loss at 5°C and about 3% loss at 24°C after 7 days of storage was found. At 37°C, about 6% loss occurred in 24 hours.[2650]

Vancomycin hydrochloride (Hospira) prepared at a vancomycin concentration of 1 g/L in Extraneal with icodextrin 7.5% (Baxter) peritoneal dialysis solution bags exhibited less than 10% loss in 14 days at 25 and 4°C and 2 days at 37°C.[3537] Vancomycin hydrochloride (Hospira) prepared at a vancomycin concentration of 1 g/L with gentamicin sulfate (Pfizer) prepared at a gentamicin concentration of 20 mg/L in Extraneal with icodextrin 7.5% (Baxter) peritoneal dialysis solution bags exhibited less than 10% loss of either drug in 14 days at 25 and 4°C and 7% loss of vancomycin and 3% loss of gentamicin in 4 days at 37°C.[3537]

Heparin Locks

Vancomycin hydrochloride (Lilly) prepared at a vancomycin concentration of 25 mcg/mL and heparin sodium (Elkins-Sinn) 100 units/mL in sodium chloride 0.9% as a catheter flush solution were evaluated for stability when stored at 4°C for 14 days. The flush solution was visually clear, and the vancomycin activity and heparin activity were retained throughout the storage period. However, an additional 24 hours at 37°C to simulate use conditions resulted in losses of both agents ranging from 20 to 37%.[1933]

Vancomycin hydrochloride (Lilly) prepared at a vancomycin concentration of 25 mcg/mL and preservative-free heparin sodium (Elkins-Sinn) 100 units/mL in sodium chloride 0.9% in 2-mL glass vials for use as a central catheter flush solution were evaluated for compatibility and stability at 4 and 28°C. Visual inspection found no evidence of color change or particulate formation throughout the study. Heparin activity remained unchanged for 100 days. Acceptable vancomycin levels were maintained for 30 days at 28°C and for 63 days at 4°C. However, unacceptable losses occurred after those times. The activity of both drugs was unaffected by the presence of the other when compared to the activity of single drug controls.[2542]

Vancomycin hydrochloride prepared at a vancomycin concentration of 25 mcg/mL combined with heparin sodium (Hospira) 10 units/mL in sterile water for injection for use as a lock solution was found to be physically compatible. Little or no vancomycin loss occurred in 3 days at 4°C. However, losses of 8% occurred in 3 days at 27°C and 1 day at 40°C.[2820] When ciprofloxacin (Sicor) 2 mg/mL was added to this flush solution, a white precipitate appeared within 1 day. Losses of both ciprofloxacin and vancomycin occurred as well.[2820]

Sodium Citrate Locks

The physical compatibility of catheter lock solutions prepared with sodium citrate 4% anticoagulant solution (Baxter) and vancomycin (manufacturer unspecified) 5, 10, and 20 mg/mL was evaluated.[3482] Solutions were stored 22 to 23°C and at 37°C in a water bath, both exposed to light and in the dark.[3482] No evidence of physical incompatibility was observed throughout the 48-hour study period in admixtures of sodium citrate with vancomycin concentrations of 5 and 10 mg/mL.[3482] However, admixtures containing sodium citrate and vancomycin 20 mg/mL demonstrated spectrophotometric evidence of incompatibility in each of the 4 storage conditions, with demonstrated turbidity as assessed by absorbance.[3482]

The physical compatibility, chemical stability, and antimicrobial activity of catheter lock solutions prepared with sodium citrate 4% anticoagulant solution (Fenwal) combined with vancomycin (manufacturer unspecified) 5 and 10 mg/mL and either gentamicin (Hospira) 1 mg/mL or ethanol 40% (v/v) were evaluated.[3473] [3483] Solutions were stored at 25 and 37°C, both with and without light.[3473] All solutions remained visually clear and demonstrated mean pH changes of 0.1 or less from baseline at 72 hours, with the exception of the admixture containing sodium citrate 4% with vancomycin 5 mg/mL and ethanol 40%, which developed slight turbidity after 48 hours in all 4 storage conditions.[3473] Spectrophotometric evaluation demonstrated mean gentamicin and vancomycin concentrations in the range of 95 to 105% of initial concentrations at 72 hours; similarly, antimicrobial activity of gentamicin and vancomycin at 72 hours was calculated to range between 95 and 106% of baseline based on disk diffusion methodology.[3473]

Vasopressin
AHFS 68:28

Products

Vasopressin is available in 1-mL vials.[3000] Each mL of solution contains vasopressin 20 units, chlorobutanol 0.5%, water for injection, and acetic acid to adjust the pH.[3000]

pH

From 3.4 to 3.6.[3000]

Trade Name(s)

Vasostrict

Administration

Vasopressin injection is administered by intravenous infusion.[3000] The drug should be diluted to a concentration of 0.1 or 1 unit/mL in sodium chloride 0.9% or dextrose 5% and inspected for particulate matter and discoloration prior to use.[3000]

The drug also has been administered by intramuscular or subcutaneous injection;[3002] however, approved labeling no longer includes information on these routes.[3000]

Stability

Intact vials should be stored under refrigeration at 2 to 8°C and protected from freezing.[3000] Intact vials removed from refrigeration can be stored at 20 to 25°C for up to 12 months or until the manufacturer's original expiration date (whichever is shorter) at any time within the labeled shelf life.[3000] [3001]

Vials should be discarded 48 hours after initial puncture.[3000] Following dilution, unused solutions should be discarded after 18 hours at room temperature or 24 hours under refrigeration.[3000]

Compatibility Information

Solution Compatibility

Vasopressin

Test Soln Name	Mfr	Mfr	Conc/L or %	Remarks	Ref	C/I
Dextrose 5%		PAR	100 and 1000 units	Stable for 18 hr if stored at room temperature or 24 hr if stored under refrigeration	3000	C
Dextrose 5%		PAR	200 units	Less than 10% loss over 26 hr at 22°C	3001	C
Sodium chloride 0.9%		PAR	100 and 1000 units	Stable for 18 hr if stored at room temperature or 24 hr if stored under refrigeration	3000	C

Additive Compatibility

Vasopressin

Test Drug	Mfr	Conc/L or %	Mfr	Conc/L or %	Test Solution	Remarks	Ref	C/I
Verapamil HCl	KN	80 mg	PD	40 units	D5W, NS	Physically compatible for 24 hr	764	C

Y-Site Injection Compatibility (1:1 Mixture)

Vasopressin

Test Drug	Mfr	Conc	Mfr	Conc	Remarks	Ref	C/I
Amiodarone HCl	WY	6 mg/mL[a]	AMR	0.2 unit/mL[b]	Visually compatible for 24 hr at 22°C	2352	C
Amiodarone HCl	WY	1.5 mg/mL[a]	AMR	2 and 4 units/mL[b]	Physically compatible with vasopressin pushed through a Y-site over 5 sec	2478	C
Angiotensin II acetate	LJ	5 and 10 mcg/mL[b]			Stated to be compatible	3430	C

DOI: 10.37573/9781585286850.394

Y-Site Injection Compatibility (1:1 Mixture) (Cont.)

Test Drug	Mfr	Conc	Mfr	Conc	Remarks	Ref	C/I
Argatroban	SKB	1 mg/mL[a]	AMR	0.4 unit/mL[a]	Physically compatible for 24 hr at 23°C	2572	C
Caspofungin acetate	ME	0.5 mg/mL[b]	APP	0.2 unit/mL[b]	Physically compatible	2641	C
Ceftaroline fosamil	FOR	2.22 mg/mL[a b e]	APP	1 unit/mL[a b e]	Physically compatible for 4 hr at 23°C	2826	C
Ceftazidime–avibactam sodium	ALL	20 mg/mL[k l]			Physically compatible for up to 4 hr at room temperature	3004	C
Ceftolozane sulfate–tazobactam sodium	CUB	10 mg/mL[h i]	JHP	1 unit/mL[h]	Physically compatible for 2 hr	3262	C
Ciprofloxacin	BAY	2 mg/mL[a]	APP	0.2 unit/mL[b]	Physically compatible	2641	C
Cisatracurium besylate	AB	1 mg/mL[b]	AMR	1 unit/mL[b]	Physically compatible for 1 hr at 23°C	3157	C
Diltiazem HCl	NVP	1 mg/mL[b]	AMR	2 and 4 units/mL[b]	Physically compatible with vasopressin pushed through a Y-site over 5 sec	2478	C
Dobutamine HCl	AB	4.2 mg/mL[a]	AMR	2 and 4 units/mL[b]	Physically compatible with vasopressin pushed through a Y-site over 5 sec	2478	C
Dopamine HCl	AMR	4.2 mg/mL[a]	AMR	2 and 4 units/mL[b]	Physically compatible with vasopressin pushed through a Y-site over 5 sec	2478	C
Dopamine HCl	BA	3.2 mg/mL[a]	APP	0.2 unit/mL[b]	Physically compatible	2641	C
Epinephrine HCl	AMR	4 mcg/mL[b]	AMR	2 and 4 units/mL[b]	Physically compatible with vasopressin pushed through a Y-site over 5 sec	2478	C
Eravacycline dihydrochloride	TET	0.6 mg/mL[b]	PAR	1 unit/mL[b]	Physically compatible for 2 hr at room temperature	3532	C
Fluconazole	PF	2 mg/mL	APP	0.2 unit/mL[b]	Physically compatible	2641	C
Furosemide	AB	4 mg/mL[a b]	APP	0.4 unit/mL[a b]	Precipitates in 5 to 15 min	2687	I
Gentamicin sulfate	APP	1.2 mg/mL[c]	APP	0.2 unit/mL[b]	Physically compatible	2641	C
Heparin sodium	BA	100 units/mL[a]	AMR	2 and 4 units/mL[b]	Physically compatible with vasopressin pushed through a Y-site over 5 sec	2478	C
Hydroxyethyl starch 130/0.4 in sodium chloride 0.9%	FRK	6%	SZ	0.4, 0.7, 1 unit/mL[a]	Visually compatible for 24 hr at room temperature	2770	C
Imipenem–cilastatin sodium	ME	5 mg/mL[a g]	APP	0.2 unit/mL[b]	Physically compatible	2641	C
Insulin, regular	NOV	1 unit/mL[b]	APP	0.2 unit/mL[b]	Physically compatible	2641	C
Isavuconazonium sulfate	ASP	1.5 mg/mL[h]	JHP	1 unit/mL[h]	Physically compatible for 2 hr	3263	C
Lidocaine HCl	BA	4 mg/mL[a]	AMR	2 and 4 units/mL[b]	Physically compatible with vasopressin pushed into a Y-site over 5 sec	2478	C
Linezolid	PHU	2 mg/mL	APP	0.2 unit/mL[b]	Physically compatible	2641	C
Meropenem	ASZ	5 mg/mL[a]	APP	0.2 unit/mL[b]	Physically compatible	2641	C
Meropenem–vaborbactam	TMC	8 mg/mL[b j]	PAR	1 unit/mL[b]	Physically compatible for 3 hr at 20 to 25°C	3380	C
Metronidazole	AB	5 mg/mL	APP	0.2 unit/mL[b]	Physically compatible	2641	C
Micafungin sodium	ASP	1.5 mg/mL[b]	AMR	1 unit/mL	Physically compatible for 4 hr at 23°C	2683	C

Y-Site Injection Compatibility (1:1 Mixture) (Cont.)

Test Drug	Mfr	Conc	Mfr	Conc	Remarks	Ref	C/I
Milrinone lactate	AB	0.2 mg/mL[a]	AMR	2 and 4 units/mL[b]	Physically compatible with vasopressin pushed through a Y-site over 5 sec	2478	C
Moxifloxacin HCl	BAY	1.6 mg/mL	APP	0.2 unit/mL[b]	Physically compatible	2641	C
Nitroglycerin	BA	0.2 mg/mL[a]	AMR	2 and 4 units/mL[b]	Physically compatible with vasopressin pushed through a Y-site over 5 sec	2478	C
Norepinephrine bitartrate	AB	4 mcg/mL[b]	AMR	2 and 4 units/mL[b]	Physically compatible with vasopressin pushed through a Y-site over 5 sec	2478	C
Norepinephrine bitartrate	GNS	16 mcg/mL[b]	APP	0.2 unit/mL[b]	Physically compatible	2641	C
Norepinephrine bitartrate	AB	4 mcg/mL[b]	APP	0.2 unit/mL[b]	Physically compatible	2641	C
Pantoprazole sodium	ALT[d]	0.16 to 0.8 mg/mL[b]	FER	0.4 to 1 unit/mL[a]	Visually compatible for 12 hr at 23°C	2603	C
Phenylephrine HCl	AMR	40 mcg/mL[b]	AMR	2 and 4 units/mL[b]	Physically compatible with vasopressin pushed through a Y-site over 5 sec	2478	C
Phenytoin sodium	ES	50 mg/mL	APP	0.2 unit/mL[b]	Crystals form immediately	2641	I
Piperacillin sodium–tazobactam sodium	WY[d]	100 mg/mL[f]	APP	0.2 unit/mL[b]	Physically compatible	2641	C
Plazomicin sulfate	ACH	24 mg/mL[h]	PAR	1 unit/mL[h]	Physically compatible for 1 hr at 20 to 25°C	3432	C
Procainamide HCl	AB	4 mg/mL[b]	AMR	2 and 4 units/mL[b]	Physically compatible with vasopressin pushed through a Y-site over 5 sec	2478	C
Sodium bicarbonate	AB	0.15 mEq/mL[c]	APP	0.2 unit/mL[b]	Physically compatible	2641	C
Tedizolid phosphate	CUB	0.8 mg/mL[b]	JHP	1 unit/mL[b]	Physically compatible for 2 hr	3244	C
Telavancin HCl	ASP	7.5 mg/mL[a b e]	AMR	1 unit/mL[a b e]	Physically compatible for 2 hr	2830	C
Voriconazole	PF	3 mg/mL[c]	APP	0.2 unit/mL[b]	Physically compatible	2641	C

[a] Tested in dextrose 5%.

[b] Tested in sodium chloride 0.9%.

[c] Tested in sodium chloride 0.45%.

[d] Test performed using the formulation WITHOUT edetate disodium.

[e] Tested in Ringer's injection, lactated.

[f] Piperacillin component. Piperacillin in an 8:1 fixed-ratio concentration with tazobactam.

[g] Imipenem component. Imipenem in a 1:1 fixed-ratio concentration with cilastatin.

[h] Tested in both dextrose 5% and sodium chloride 0.9%.

[i] Ceftolozane component. Ceftolozane in a 2:1 fixed-ratio concentration with tazobactam.

[j] Meropenem component. Meropenem in a 1:1 fixed-ratio concentration with vaborbactam.

[k] Ceftazidime component. Ceftazidime in a 4:1 fixed-ratio concentration with avibactam.

[l] Tested in dextrose 5%, sodium chloride 0.9%, and Ringer's injection, lactated.

Selected Revisions May 1, 2020. © Copyright, October 1988.
American Society of Health-System Pharmacists, Inc.

Vecuronium Bromide
AHFS 12:20.20

Products

Vecuronium bromide is available in 10-mg vials as a lyophilized cake, both with and without accompanying bacteriostatic water for injection with benzyl alcohol 0.9% for use as a diluent. It also is available in 20-mg vials without a diluent. The vials also contain citric acid anhydrous, mannitol, and sodium phosphate dibasic anhydrous. Sodium hydroxide and/or phosphoric acid also may be present to adjust the pH.[1(7/07)]

The 10- and 20-mg vials should be reconstituted with 10 and 20 mL, respectively, of the accompanying bacteriostatic water for injection or sterile water for injection to yield a 1-mg/mL solution.[1(7/07)] [4] The bacteriostatic water for injection, which contains benzyl alcohol 0.9%, is not for use in newborns.[1(7/07)]

pH

From 3.5 to 4.5.[1(7/07)]

Osmolality

The osmolality of vecuronium bromide 4 mg/mL was determined to be 292 mOsm/kg.[1233]

Administration

Vecuronium bromide may be administered by rapid intravenous injection or by intravenous infusion using an infusion control device at a concentration of 0.1 to 0.2 mg/mL in a compatible solution. It should not be administered intramuscularly.[4]

Stability

Vecuronium bromide should be stored at room temperature and protected from light. The reconstituted solution is clear and colorless. When reconstituted with bacteriostatic water for injection, the solution may be used for up to 5 days when stored at room temperature or under refrigeration. When reconstituted with sterile water for injection, the vial is a single-use container and should be stored under refrigeration and used within 24 hours.[1(7/07)]

pH Effects

Vecuronium bromide is unstable in the presence of bases and should not be combined with alkaline drugs or simultaneously administered through the same line as an alkaline solution.[4]

Syringes

Vecuronium bromide 1 mg/mL in sterile water for injection and packaged in plastic syringes was found to be stable with no loss of drug for 21 days at room temperature and refrigerated.[2735]

Compatibility Information

Solution Compatibility

Vecuronium bromide

Test Soln Name	Mfr	Mfr	Conc/L or %	Remarks	Ref	C/I
Dextrose 5% in sodium chloride 0.9%				Compatible and stable for 24 hr	1(7/07)	C
Dextrose 5%				Compatible and stable for 24 hr	1(7/07)	C
Ringer's injection, lactated				Compatible and stable for 24 hr	1(7/07)	C
Sodium chloride 0.9%				Compatible and stable for 24 hr	1(7/07)	C

Additive Compatibility

Vecuronium bromide

Test Drug	Mfr	Conc/L or %	Mfr	Conc/L or %	Test Solution	Remarks	Ref	C/I
Ciprofloxacin	BAY	1.6 g	OR	200 mg	D5W	Visually compatible with no loss of ciprofloxacin in 24 hr at 22°C under fluorescent light. Vecuronium not tested	2413	C

DOI: 10.37573/9781585286850.395

Drugs in Syringe Compatibility

Vecuronium bromide

Test Drug	Mfr	Amt	Mfr	Amt	Remarks	Ref	C/I
Pantoprazole sodium	a	4 mg/1 mL		1 mg/1 mL	Precipitates	2574	I

a Test performed using the formulation WITHOUT edetate disodium.

Y-Site Injection Compatibility (1:1 Mixture)

Vecuronium bromide

Test Drug	Mfr	Conc	Mfr	Conc	Remarks	Ref	C/I
Alprostadil	BED	7.5 mcg/mL[d f]	OR	1 mg/mL[e]	Visually compatible for 1 hr	2746	C
Aminophylline	AB	1 mg/mL[a]	OR	0.1 mg/mL[a]	Physically compatible for 24 hr at 28°C	1337	C
Amiodarone HCl	WY	6 mg/mL[a]	OR	1 mg/mL[a]	Visually compatible for 24 hr at 22°C	2352	C
Cefazolin sodium	LY	10 mg/mL[a]	OR	0.1 mg/mL[a]	Physically compatible for 24 hr at 28°C	1337	C
Ceftazidime–avibactam sodium	ALL	20 mg/mL[k l]			Physically compatible for up to 4 hr at room temperature	3004	C
Ceftolozane sulfate–tazobactam sodium	CUB	10 mg/mL[h i]	SUN	1 mg/mL[h]	Physically compatible for 2 hr	3262	C
Cefuroxime sodium	GL	7.5 mg/mL[a]	OR	0.1 mg/mL[a]	Physically compatible for 24 hr at 28°C	1337	C
Clarithromycin	AB	4 mg/mL[a]	OR	2 mg/mL[a]	Visually compatible for 72 hr at both 30 and 17°C	2174	C
Dexmedetomidine HCl	HOS	4 mcg/mL[b]			Stated to be compatible	3181	C
Diazepam	ES	5 mg/mL[a]	OR	0.1 mg/mL[a]	Cloudy solution forms immediately	1337	I
Diltiazem HCl	MMD	1 mg/mL[a]	OR	1 mg/mL	Visually compatible for 4 hr at 27°C	2062	C
Dobutamine HCl	LI	1 mg/mL[a]	OR	0.1 mg/mL[a]	Physically compatible for 24 hr at 28°C	1337	C
Dobutamine HCl	LI	4 mg/mL[a]	OR	1 mg/mL	Visually compatible for 4 hr at 27°C	2062	C
Dopamine HCl	SO	1.6 mg/mL[a]	OR	0.1 mg/mL[a]	Physically compatible for 24 hr at 28°C	1337	C
Dopamine HCl	AB	3.2 mg/mL[a]	OR	1 mg/mL	Visually compatible for 4 hr at 27°C	2062	C
Epinephrine HCl	AB	4 mcg/mL[a]	OR	0.1 mg/mL[a]	Physically compatible for 24 hr at 28°C	1337	C
Epinephrine HCl	AB	0.02 mg/mL[a]	OR	1 mg/mL	Visually compatible for 4 hr at 27°C	2062	C
Eravacycline dihydro-chloride	TET	0.6 mg/mL[b]	TE	1 mg/mL	Physically compatible for 2 hr at room temperature	3532	C
Esmolol HCl	DCC	10 mg/mL[a]	OR	0.1 mg/mL[a]	Physically compatible for 24 hr at 28°C	1337	C
Etomidate	AB	2 mg/mL	OR	1 mg/mL	Slight turbidity and white particles form	1801	I
Fenoldopam mesylate	AB	80 mcg/mL[b]	ES	0.2 mg/mL[b]	Physically compatible for 4 hr at 23°C	2467	C
Fentanyl citrate	ES	10 mcg/mL[a]	OR	0.1 mg/mL[a]	Physically compatible for 24 hr at 28°C	1337	C
Fentanyl citrate	ES	0.05 mg/mL	OR	1 mg/mL	Visually compatible for 4 hr at 27°C	2062	C
Fluconazole	RR	2 mg/mL	OR	1 mg/mL[a]	Visually compatible for 24 hr at 28°C under fluorescent light	1760	C
Furosemide	AMR	10 mg/mL	OR	1 mg/mL	Precipitate forms immediately	2062	I
Gentamicin sulfate	ES	2 mg/mL[a]	OR	0.1 mg/mL[a]	Physically compatible for 24 hr at 28°C	1337	C

Y-Site Injection Compatibility (1:1 Mixture) (Cont.)

Test Drug	Mfr	Conc	Mfr	Conc	Remarks	Ref	C/I
Heparin sodium	SO	40 units/mL[a]	OR	0.1 mg/mL[a]	Physically compatible for 24 hr at 28°C	1337	C
Heparin sodium	ES	100 units/mL[a]	OR	1 mg/mL	Visually compatible for 4 hr at 27°C	2062	C
Hetastarch in lactated electrolyte	AB	6%	OR	0.2 mg/mL[a]	Physically compatible for 4 hr at 23°C	2339	C
Hydrocortisone sodium succinate	AB	1 mg/mL[a]	OR	0.1 mg/mL[a]	Physically compatible for 24 hr at 28°C	1337	C
Hydromorphone HCl	KN	1 mg/mL	OR	1 mg/mL	Visually compatible for 4 hr at 27°C	2062	C
Ibuprofen lysinate	OVA	10 mg/mL	HOS	1 and 2 mg/mL[h]	Measured turbidity increased immediately and solution became milky white and opaque	3541	I
Isavuconazonium sulfate	ASP	1.5 mg/mL[h]	CRC	1 mg/mL	Physically compatible for 2 hr	3263	C
Isoproterenol HCl	ES	4 mcg/mL[a]	OR	0.1 mg/mL[a]	Physically compatible for 24 hr at 28°C	1337	C
Labetalol HCl	AH	2 mg/mL[a]	OR	1 mg/mL	Visually compatible for 4 hr at 27°C	2062	C
Linezolid	PHU	2 mg/mL	OR	1 mg/mL	Physically compatible for 4 hr at 23°C	2264	C
Lorazepam	WY	0.5 mg/mL[a]	OR	0.1 mg/mL[a]	Physically compatible for 24 hr at 28°C	1337	C
Lorazepam	WY	0.33 mg/mL[a]	OR	4 mg/mL	Visually compatible for 24 hr at 22°C	1855	C
Lorazepam	WY	0.5 mg/mL[a]	OR	1 mg/mL	Visually compatible for 4 hr at 27°C	2062	C
Meropenem–vaborbactam	TMC	8 mg/mL[b][j]	MYL	1 mg/mL	Physically compatible for 3 hr at 20 to 25°C	3380	C
Micafungin sodium	ASP	1.5 mg/mL[b]	BED	1 mg/mL	White precipitate forms immediately	2683	I
Midazolam HCl	RC	0.05 mg/mL[a]	OR	0.1 mg/mL[a]	Physically compatible for 24 hr at 28°C	1337	C
Midazolam HCl	RC	5 mg/mL	OR	4 mg/mL	Visually compatible for 24 hr at 22°C	1855	C
Midazolam HCl	RC	2 mg/mL[a]	OR	1 mg/mL	Visually compatible for 4 hr at 27°C	2062	C
Milrinone lactate	SW	0.2 mg/mL[a]	OR	1 mg/mL	Visually compatible for 4 hr at 27°C	2062	C
Milrinone lactate	SW	0.4 mg/mL[a]	OR	1 mg/mL	Visually compatible. Little loss of either drug in 4 hr at 23°C	2214	C
Morphine sulfate	WY	1 mg/mL[a]	OR	0.1 mg/mL[a]	Physically compatible for 24 hr at 28°C	1337	C
Morphine sulfate	SCN	2 mg/mL[a]	OR	1 mg/mL	Visually compatible for 4 hr at 27°C	2062	C
Nicardipine HCl	WY	1 mg/mL[a]	OR	1 mg/mL	Visually compatible for 4 hr at 27°C	2062	C
Nitroglycerin	SO	0.4 mg/mL[a]	OR	0.1 mg/mL[a]	Physically compatible for 24 hr at 28°C	1337	C
Nitroglycerin	AB	0.4 mg/mL[a]	OR	1 mg/mL	Visually compatible for 4 hr at 27°C	2062	C
Norepinephrine bitartrate	AB	0.128 mg/mL[a]	OR	1 mg/mL	Visually compatible for 4 hr at 27°C	2062	C
Palonosetron HCl	MGI	50 mcg/mL	BED	1 mg/mL	Physically compatible and no loss of either drug in 4 hr at room temperature	2764	C
Plazomicin sulfate	ACH	24 mg/mL[h]	TE	1 mg/mL	Physically compatible for 1 hr at 20 to 25°C	3432	C
Propofol	ZEN[m]	10 mg/mL	OR	1 mg/mL	Physically compatible for 1 hr at 23°C	2066	C
Ranitidine HCl	GL	0.5 mg/mL[a]	OR	0.1 mg/mL[a]	Physically compatible for 24 hr at 28°C	1337	C
Ranitidine HCl	GL	1 mg/mL[a]	OR	1 mg/mL	Visually compatible for 4 hr at 27°C	2062	C

Y-Site Injection Compatibility (1:1 Mixture) (Cont.)

Test Drug	Mfr	Conc	Mfr	Conc	Remarks	Ref	C/I
Sodium nitroprusside	ES	0.2 mg/mL[a]	OR	0.1 mg/mL[a]	Physically compatible for 24 hr at 28°C	1337	C
Tedizolid phosphate	CUB	0.8 mg/mL[b]	CRC	1 mg/mL	Physically compatible for 2 hr	3244	C
TPN #189[c]			OR	2 mg/mL[b]	Visually compatible for 24 hr at 22°C	1767	C
Trimethoprim–sulfamethoxazole	ES	0.64 mg/mL[a][g]	OR	0.1 mg/mL[a]	Physically compatible for 24 hr at 28°C	1337	C
Vancomycin HCl	ES	5 mg/mL[a]	OR	0.1 mg/mL[a]	Physically compatible for 24 hr at 28°C	1337	C

[a] Tested in dextrose 5%.

[b] Tested in sodium chloride 0.9%.

[c] Refer to Appendix for the composition of parenteral nutrition solutions. TPN indicates a 2-in-1 admixture.

[d] Tested in a 1:1 mixture of dextrose 5% and TPN #274 (see Appendix).

[e] Tested in either dextrose 5% or in sodium chloride 0.9%, but the report did not specify which solution.

[f] Tested in a 1:1 mixture of (1) dextrose 5% and dextrose 5% in sodium chloride 0.45% with and without potassium chloride 20 mEq/L and also in (2) dextrose 10% in sodium chloride 0.45% with and without potassium chloride 20 mEq/L.

[g] Trimethoprim component. Trimethoprim in a 1:5 fixed-ratio concentration with sulfamethoxazole.

[h] Tested in both dextrose 5% and sodium chloride 0.9%.

[i] Ceftolozane component. Ceftolozane in a 2:1 fixed-ratio concentration with tazobactam.

[j] Meropenem component. Meropenem in a 1:1 fixed-ratio concentration with vaborbactam.

[k] Ceftazidime component. Ceftazidime in a 4:1 fixed-ratio concentration with avibactam.

[l] Tested in dextrose 5%, sodium chloride 0.9%, and Ringer's injection, lactated.

[m] Test performed using the formulation WITH edetate disodium.

Selected Revisions May 1, 2020. © Copyright, October 1992.
American Society of Health-System Pharmacists, Inc.

Verapamil Hydrochloride
AHFS 24:28.92

Products

Verapamil hydrochloride is available in single-dose containers including 2-mL ampuls, vials, and syringes and in 4-mL vials and syringes. Each mL contains verapamil hydrochloride 2.5 mg with sodium chloride 8.5 mg in water for injection. Hydrochloric acid may have been used to adjust pH during manufacture.[1(7/06)]

pH

From 4 to 6.5.[1(7/06)]

Osmolality

The osmolality of verapamil hydrochloride 2.5 mg/mL was determined to be 290 mOsm/kg.[1233]

Administration

Verapamil hydrochloride is administered slowly intravenously. Direct intravenous injection should be performed over at least 2 minutes and at least 3 minutes in older patients.[1(7/06)] [4] Intravenous infusion has also been performed.[4]

Stability

Verapamil hydrochloride should be stored at controlled room temperature and protected from light.[1(7/06)] Freezing should be avoided.[4] It is physically compatible in solution over a pH range of 3 to 6 but may precipitate in solutions having a pH greater than 6[1(7/06)] [4] or 7.[1384]

Verapamil hydrochloride under simulated summer conditions in paramedic vehicles was exposed to temperatures ranging from 26 to 38°C over 4 weeks. Analysis found no loss of the drug under these conditions.[2562]

Compatibility Information

Solution Compatibility

Verapamil HCl

Test Soln Name	Mfr	Mfr	Conc/L or %	Remarks	Ref	C/I
Dextrose 5% in Ringer's injection	MG	KN	40 mg	Physically compatible and chemically stable for 48 hr at 25°C protected from light	548	C
Dextrose 5% in Ringer's injection, lactated	MG	KN	40 mg	Physically compatible and chemically stable for 24 hr at 25°C protected from light	548	C
Dextrose 5% in sodium chloride 0.45%	MG	KN	40 mg	Physically compatible and chemically stable for 24 hr at 25°C protected from light	548	C
Dextrose 5% in sodium chloride 0.9%	MG	KN	40 mg	Physically compatible and chemically stable for 24 hr at 25°C protected from light	548	C
Dextrose 5%	CU	KN	40 mg	Physically compatible and chemically stable for 48 hr at 25°C protected from light	548	C
Dextrose 5%	MG[a]	KN	40 mg	Physically compatible and chemically stable for 24 hr at 25°C protected from light	548	C
Dextrose 5%	TR[b]	KN	40 mg	Physically compatible and chemically stable for 24 hr at 25°C protected from light	548	C
Dextrose 5%	TR[b]	KN	160 mg	Physically compatible. No loss in 7 days at 24°C	811	C
Dextrose 5%	AB	KN	100 and 400 mg	Physically compatible. No loss in 24 hr at 24°C under fluorescent light	1198	C
Ringer's injection	MG	KN	40 mg	Physically compatible and chemically stable for 24 hr at 25°C protected from light	548	C

DOI: 10.37573/9781585286850.396

Solution Compatibility (Cont.)

Test Soln Name	Mfr	Mfr	Conc/L or %	Remarks	Ref	C/I
Ringer's injection, lactated	MG	KN	40 mg	Physically compatible and chemically stable for 24 hr at 25°C protected from light	548	C
Sodium chloride 0.45%	MG	KN	40 mg	Physically compatible and chemically stable for 24 hr at 25°C protected from light	548	C
Sodium chloride 0.45%		LY	1.25 and 2 g	Physically compatible with no drug loss in 4 hr at 22°C	1419	C
Sodium chloride 0.9%	CU	KN	40 mg	Physically compatible and chemically stable for 48 hr at 25°C protected from light	548	C
Sodium chloride 0.9%	MG[a]	KN	40 mg	Physically compatible and chemically stable for 24 hr at 25°C protected from light	548	C
Sodium chloride 0.9%	TR[b]	KN	40 mg	Physically compatible and chemically stable for 24 hr at 25°C protected from light	548	C
Sodium chloride 0.9%	TR[b]	KN	160 mg	Physically compatible. Little loss in 7 days at 24°C	811	C
Sodium lactate ⅙ M	MG	KN	40 mg	Physically compatible and chemically stable for 48 hr at 25°C protected from light	548	C

[a] Tested in polyolefin containers.

[b] Tested in PVC containers.

Additive Compatibility

Verapamil HCl

Test Drug	Mfr	Conc/L or %	Mfr	Conc/L or %	Test Solution	Remarks	Ref	C/I
Albumin human	ARC	25 g	KN	80 mg	D5W, NS	Cloudiness develops within 8 hr	764	I
Amikacin sulfate	BR	2 g	KN	80 mg	D5W, NS	Physically compatible for 24 hr	764	C
Aminophylline	SE+	1 g	KN	80 mg	D5W, NS	Transient precipitate clears rapidly, then clear for 48 hr	739	?
Aminophylline	SE	1 g	KN	400 mg	D5W	Visible turbidity forms immediately. Filtration removes all verapamil	1198	I
Aminophylline	SE	1 g	KN	100 mg	D5W	Visually clear, but precipitate found by microscopic examination. Filtration removes all verapamil	1198	I
Amiodarone HCl	LZ	1.8 g	KN	50 mg	D5W, NS[a]	Physically compatible. 8% or less amiodarone loss in 24 hr at 24°C in light	1031	C
Amphotericin B	SQ	100 mg	KN	80 mg	D5W	Physically incompatible after 8 hr	764	I
Amphotericin B	SQ	100 mg	KN	80 mg	NS	Immediate physical incompatibility	764	I
Ampicillin sodium	BR	4 g	KN	80 mg	D5W, NS	Physically compatible for 24 hr	764	C
Ampicillin sodium	WY	40 g	SE	[b]	D5W, NS	Cloudy solution clears with agitation	1166	?
Ascorbic acid	LI	1 g	KN	80 mg	D5W, NS	Physically compatible for 24 hr	764	C
Atropine sulfate	IX	0.8 mg	KN	80 mg	D5W, NS	Physically compatible for 24 hr	764	C
Calcium chloride	ES	2 g	KN	80 mg	D5W, NS	Physically compatible for 24 hr	764	C
Calcium gluconate	IX	2 g	KN	80 mg	D5W, NS	Physically compatible for 48 hr	739	C
Cefazolin sodium	SKF	2 g	KN	80 mg	D5W, NS	Physically compatible for 24 hr	764	C
Cefotaxime sodium	HO	4 g	KN	80 mg	D5W, NS	Physically compatible for 24 hr	764	C
Cefoxitin sodium	MSD	4 g	KN	80 mg	D5W, NS	Physically compatible for 24 hr	764	C

Additive Compatibility (Cont.)

Test Drug	Mfr	Conc/L or %	Mfr	Conc/L or %	Test Solution	Remarks	Ref	C/I
Chloramphenicol sodium succinate	PD	2 g	KN	80 mg	D5W, NS	Physically compatible for 24 hr	764	C
Clindamycin phosphate	UP	1.2 g	KN	80 mg	D5W, NS	Physically compatible for 24 hr	764	C
Dexamethasone sodium phosphate	MSD	40 mg	KN	80 mg	D5W, NS	Physically compatible for 24 hr	764	C
Dextran 40	TR	10%	KN	80 mg	NS	Physically compatible for 24 hr	764	C
Diazepam	RC	20 mg	KN	80 mg	D5W, NS	Physically compatible for 24 hr	764	C
Digoxin	BW	2 mg	KN	80 mg	D5W, NS	Physically compatible for 48 hr	739	C
Dobutamine HCl	LI	500 mg	KN	80 mg	D5W, NS	Slight pink color develops after 24 hr because of dobutamine oxidation	764	I
Dobutamine HCl	LI	250 mg	KN	160 mg	D5W	No loss of either drug in 48 hr at 24°C or 7 days at 5°C. Transient pink color	811	C
Dobutamine HCl	LI	250 mg	KN	160 mg	NS	Pink color and no verapamil and 3% dobutamine loss in 48 hr at 24°C. At 5°C, no loss of either drug in 7 days	811	C
Dobutamine HCl	LI	1 g	KN	1.25 g	D5W, NS	Physically compatible for 24 hr at 21°C	812	C
Dopamine HCl	ES	400 mg	KN	80 mg	D5W, NS	Physically compatible for 24 hr	764	C
Epinephrine HCl	PD	2 mg	KN	80 mg	D5W, NS	Physically compatible for 24 hr	764	C
Eptifibatide	ME	750 mg		2.5 g		Physically compatible and chemically stable for up to 24 hr at 25°C	3049	C
Erythromycin lactobionate	AB	2 g	KN	80 mg	D5W, NS	Physically compatible for 24 hr	764	C
Floxacillin sodium	BE	20 g	AB	500 mg	NS	Haze and precipitate form in 24 hr at 30°C. No change at 15°C	1479	I
Furosemide	HO	200 mg	KN	80 mg	D5W, NS	Physically compatible for 24 hr	764	C
Furosemide	HO	1 g	AB	500 mg	NS	Slight precipitate forms but dissipates	1479	?
Gentamicin sulfate	SC	160 mg	KN	80 mg	D5W, NS	Physically compatible for 24 hr	764	C
Heparin sodium	ES	20,000 units	KN	80 mg	D5W, NS	Physically compatible for 24 hr	764	C
Hydralazine HCl	CI	40 mg	KN	80 mg	D5W, NS	Yellow discoloration	764	I
Hydrocortisone sodium succinate	UP	200 mg	KN	80 mg	D5W, NS	Physically compatible for 24 hr	764	C
Hydromorphone HCl	KN	16 mg	KN	80 mg	D5W, NS	Physically compatible for 24 hr	764	C
Isoproterenol HCl	BN	10 mg	KN	80 mg	D5W, NS	Physically compatible for 24 hr	764	C
Lidocaine HCl	IMS	2 g	KN	80 mg	D5W, NS	Physically compatible for 48 hr	739	C
Magnesium sulfate	IX	10 g	KN	80 mg	D5W, NS	Physically compatible for 24 hr	764	C
Mannitol	IX	25 g	KN	80 mg	D5W, NS	Physically compatible for 24 hr	764	C
Meperidine HCl	WI	150 mg	KN	80 mg	D5W, NS	Physically compatible for 24 hr	764	C
Methyldopate HCl	MSD	500 mg	KN	80 mg	D5W, NS	Physically compatible for 24 hr	764	C
Methylprednisolone sodium succinate	UP	250 mg	KN	80 mg	D5W, NS	Physically compatible for 24 hr	764	C
Metoclopramide HCl	RB	20 mg	KN	80 mg	D5W, NS	Physically compatible for 24 hr	764	C

Additive Compatibility (Cont.)

Test Drug	Mfr	Conc/L or %	Mfr	Conc/L or %	Test Solution	Remarks	Ref	C/I
Morphine sulfate	KN	30 mg	KN	80 mg	D5W, NS	Physically compatible for 24 hr	764	C
Multivitamins	USV	10 mL	KN	80 mg	D5W, NS	Physically compatible for 24 hr	764	C
Nafcillin sodium	WY	4 g	KN	80 mg	D5W, NS	Physically compatible for 24 hr	764	C
Nafcillin sodium	WY	40 g	SE	b	D5W, NS	Cloudy solution clears with agitation	1166	?
Naloxone HCl	EN	0.8 mg	KN	80 mg	D5W, NS	Physically compatible for 24 hr	764	C
Nitroglycerin	ACC	100 mg	KN	80 mg	D5W, NS	Physically compatible for 24 hr	764	C
Norepinephrine bitartrate	BN	8 mg	KN	80 mg	D5W, NS	Physically compatible for 24 hr	764	C
Oxacillin sodium	BR	4 g	KN	80 mg	D5W, NS	Physically compatible for 24 hr	764	C
Oxacillin sodium	BR	40 g	SE	b	D5W, NS	Cloudy solution clears with agitation	1166	?
Oxytocin	SZ	40 units	KN	80 mg	D5W, NS	Physically compatible for 24 hr	764	C
Pancuronium bromide	OR	8 mg	KN	80 mg	D5W, NS	Physically compatible for 24 hr	764	C
Penicillin G potassium	SQ	10 million units	KN	80 mg	D5W, NS	Physically compatible for 24 hr	764	C
Penicillin G potassium	PD	62.5 g	SE	b	D5W, NS	Physically compatible for 24 hr at 21°C under fluorescent light	1166	C
Penicillin G sodium	SQ	10 million units	KN	80 mg	D5W, NS	Physically compatible for 24 hr	764	C
Pentobarbital sodium	AB	200 mg	KN	80 mg	D5W, NS	Physically compatible for 24 hr	764	C
Phenobarbital sodium	ES	260 mg	KN	80 mg	D5W, NS	Physically compatible for 24 hr	764	C
Phentolamine mesylate	RC	10 mg	KN	80 mg	D5W, NS	Physically compatible for 24 hr	764	C
Phenytoin sodium	PD	500 mg	KN	80 mg	D5W, NS	Physically compatible for 48 hr	739	C
Potassium chloride	TR	80 mEq	KN	80 mg	D5W, NS	Physically compatible for 24 hr	764	C
Potassium phosphates	AB	88 mEq	KN	80 mg	D5W, NS	Physically compatible for 24 hr	764	C
Procainamide HCl	SQ	2 g	KN	80 mg	D5W, NS	Physically compatible for 48 hr	739	C
Propranolol HCl	AY	4 mg	KN	80 mg	D5W, NS	Physically compatible for 24 hr	764	C
Protamine sulfate	LI	100 mg	KN	80 mg	D5W, NS	Physically compatible for 24 hr	764	C
Quinidine gluconate	LI	800 mg	KN	80 mg	D5W, NS	Physically compatible for 48 hr	739	C
Sodium bicarbonate	BR	89.2 mEq	KN	80 mg	D5W, NS	Physically compatible for 24 hr	764	C
Sodium nitroprusside	RC	100 mg	KN	80 mg	D5W, NS	Physically compatible for 24 hr	764	C
Theophylline	AB	400 mg and 4 g	KN	100 and 400 mg	D5W	Physically compatible. Little loss of either drug in 24 hr at 24°C in light	1172	C
Tobramycin sulfate	LI	160 mg	KN	80 mg	D5W, NS	Physically compatible for 24 hr	764	C
Trimethoprim–sulfamethoxazole	BW	160c mg	KN	80 mg	D5W, NS	Transient precipitate	764	I
Vancomycin HCl	LI	1 g	KN	80 mg	D5W, NS	Physically compatible for 24 hr	764	C
Vasopressin	PD	40 units	KN	80 mg	D5W, NS	Physically compatible for 24 hr	764	C

a Tested in both polyolefin and PVC containers.

b Final concentration unspecified.

c Trimethoprim component. Trimethoprim in a 1:5 fixed-ratio concentration with sulfamethoxazole.

Drugs in Syringe Compatibility

Verapamil HCl

Test Drug	Mfr	Amt	Mfr	Amt	Remarks	Ref	C/I
Dimenhydrinate		10 mg/1 mL		2.5 mg/1 mL	Clear solution	2569	C
Heparin sodium		2500 units/1 mL	KN	5 mg/2 mL	Physically compatible for at least 5 min	1053	C
Milrinone lactate	WI	3.5 mg/3.5 mL	KN	10 mg/4 mL	Brought to 10-mL total volume with D5W. Physically compatible with no loss of either drug in 4 hr at 23°C	1191	C
Pantoprazole sodium	a	4 mg/1 mL		2.5 mg/1 mL	Whitish precipitate	2574	I

a Test performed using the formulation WITHOUT edetate disodium.

Y-Site Injection Compatibility (1:1 Mixture)

Verapamil HCl

Test Drug	Mfr	Conc	Mfr	Conc	Remarks	Ref	C/I
Albumin human	HY	250 mg/mLa	LY	0.2 mg/mLa	Slight haze in 1 hr	1316	I
Albumin human	HY	250 mg/mLb	LY	0.2 mg/mLb	Slight haze in 3 hr	1316	I
Ampicillin sodium	WY	40 mg/mLc	SE	2.5 mg/mL	White precipitate forms immediately. 91% of verapamil precipitated	1166	I
Argatroban	GSK	1 mg/mLb	AMR	2.5 mg/mL	Visually compatible for 24 hr at 23°C	2391	C
Bivalirudin	TMC	5 mg/mLa	AB	1.25 mg/mLa	Physically compatible for 4 hr at 23°C	2373	C
Bivalirudin	TMC	5 mg/mLa b	AMR	2.5 mg/mL	Visually compatible for 6 hr at 23°C	2680	C
Cangrelor tetrasodium	TMC	1 mg/mLb		1.25b and 2.5 mg/mL	Physically compatible for 4 hr	3243	C
Ciprofloxacin	MI	2 mg/mLc	KN	2.5 mg/mL	Visually compatible for 24 hr at 24°C	1655	C
Clarithromycin	AB	4 mg/mLa	BKN	2.5 mg/mL	Visually compatible for 72 hr at both 30 and 17°C	2174	C
Clonidine HCl	BI	18 mcg/mLb	AB	2.5 mg/mL	Visually compatible	2642	C
Dexmedetomidine HCl	AB	4 mcg/mLb	AB	1.25 mg/mLb	Physically compatible for 4 hr at 23°C	2383	C
Dobutamine HCl	LI	4 mg/mLc	LY	0.2 mg/mLc	Physically compatible for 3 hr	1316	C
Dopamine HCl				e	Physically compatible	840	C
Famotidine	MSD	0.2 mg/mLa	KN	0.1 mg/mLa	Physically compatible for 4 hr at 25°C	1188	C
Fenoldopam mesylate	AB	80 mcg/mLb	AB	1.25 mg/mLb	Physically compatible for 4 hr at 23°C	2467	C
Hetastarch in lactated electrolyte	AB	6%	AMR	1.25 mg/mLa	Physically compatible for 4 hr at 23°C	2339	C
Hydralazine HCl	SO	1 mg/mLc	LY	0.2 mg/mLc	Physically compatible for 3 hr	1316	C
Linezolid	PHU	2 mg/mL	AB	2.5 mg/mL	Physically compatible for 4 hr at 23°C	2264	C
Meperidine HCl	AB	10 mg/mL	DU	2.5 mg/mL	Physically compatible for 4 hr at 25°C	1397	C
Milrinone lactate	WI	200 mcg/mLa	KN	2.5 mg/mLa	Physically compatible with no loss of either drug in 4 hr at 23°C	1191	C
Nafcillin sodium				f	White milky precipitate forms immediately	840, 1303	I
Nafcillin sodium	WY	40 mg/mLc	SE	2.5 mg/mL	White precipitate forms immediately. 20% of verapamil precipitated	1166	I

Y-Site Injection Compatibility (1:1 Mixture) (Cont.)

Test Drug	Mfr	Conc	Mfr	Conc	Remarks	Ref	C/I
Nesiritide	SCI	50 mcg/mL[a][b]		2.5 mg/mL	Physically compatible for 4 hr	2625	C
Oxacillin sodium	BR	40 mg/mL[c]	SE	2.5 mg/mL	White precipitate forms immediately. 39% of verapamil precipitated	1166	I
Oxaliplatin	SS	0.5 mg/mL[a]	AB	1.25 mg/mL[a]	Physically compatible for 4 hr at 23°C	2566	C
Penicillin G potassium	PD	62.5 mg/mL[c]	SE	2.5 mg/mL	Physically compatible for 15 min at 21°C	1166	C
Propofol	ZEN[g]	10 mg/mL	AMR	2.5 mg/mL	Physically compatible for 1 hr at 23°C	2066	C
Sodium bicarbonate		88 mEq/L[d]	SE	5 mg/2 mL	Crystalline precipitate forms when verapamil injected into infusion line	839	I
Sugammadex sodium	ME	100 mg/mL		2.5 mg/mL	Particles form in 2 hr	3111, 3115	I

[a] Tested in dextrose 5%.

[b] Tested in sodium chloride 0.9%.

[c] Tested in both dextrose 5% and sodium chloride 0.9%.

[d] Tested in sodium chloride 0.45%.

[e] Injected into a line being used to infuse dopamine hydrochloride in dextrose 5% in sodium chloride 0.33% with potassium chloride 20 mEq.

[f] Injected into a line being used to infuse nafcillin sodium.

[g] Test performed using the formulation WITH edetate disodium.

Selected Revisions January 31, 2020. © Copyright, October 1982. American Society of Health-System Pharmacists, Inc.

Vinblastine Sulfate

AHFS 10:00

Products

Vinblastine sulfate is available as a 1-mg/mL solution with benzyl alcohol 0.9% in 10-mL vials.[2946] Each mL also contains sodium chloride 9 mg and water for injection.[2946]

pH

The pH of the vinblastine sulfate injection is 3.5 to 5.[2946]

Administration

Vinblastine sulfate is administered intravenously only.[2946] It should not be given by any other route.[2946] If the drug is prepared in a syringe, a sticker, which is provided in the vinblastine sulfate package, must be affixed directly to the syringe containing the individual dose stating:

FOR INTRAVENOUS USE ONLY – FATAL IF GIVEN BY OTHER ROUTES.[2946]

In addition, the syringe containing the prepared dose must be enclosed in an overwrap, which is labeled:

DO NOT REMOVE COVERING UNTIL MOMENT OF INJECTION.

FOR INTRAVENOUS USE ONLY – FATAL IF GIVEN BY OTHER ROUTES.[2946]

Vinblastine sulfate may be administered over about 1 minute either directly into a vein or into the tubing of a running infusion solution.[2946] The dose of vinblastine sulfate should not be diluted in larger amounts of intravenous fluid (e.g., 100 to 250 mL) or administered over longer time periods (e.g., 30 to 60 minutes) since this frequently increases vein irritation and the chances of extravasation.[2946] Extravasation should be avoided.[2946]

In the event of spills or leaks, sodium hypochlorite 5% (household bleach) has been used to inactivate vinblastine sulfate.[1200]

Stability

The vials should be refrigerated to ensure extended stability.[2946] Room temperature stability of intact vials of a Lilly product was variously reported to be at least 1 month[853] and only 14 days,[1433] while a Lyphomed product was reported to be stable for up to 3 months[1181] and for less than 2 months.[1433]

Vinblastine sulfate 0.015 and 0.5 mg/mL in sodium chloride 0.9% did not inhibit the growth of deliberately inoculated *Staphylococcus epidermidis* (10^6 to 10^7 CFU/mL) during 21 days at 35°C (representing near body temperature).[1659]

Immersion of a needle with an aluminum component in vinblastine sulfate 1 mg/mL resulted in no visually apparent reaction after 7 days at 24°C.[988]

pH Effects

Maximum stability for vinblastine sulfate in aqueous solutions was determined to be from pH 2 to 4. Vinblastine sulfate in solution at pH 3 retained 90% after 39 days at 20°C.[1307]

Vinblastine sulfate in solutions having a pH above 6 may form a precipitate of vinblastine base.[1369]

Freezing Solutions

Vinblastine sulfate (Lilly) 20 mcg/mL in dextrose 5%, Ringer's injection, lactated, and sodium chloride 0.9% underwent no degradation after 4 weeks when frozen at −20°C.[1195]

Light Effects

It is recommended that vials be protected from light and stored in the outer carton until the time of use.[2946]

The effects of light exposure on a 1.197-mg/mL vinblastine sulfate solution in sterile water for injection were studied. Samples at 25°C were exposed to indirect incandescent (not fluorescent) light intermittently for 12 hours each day; another group was exposed to direct incandescent light intermittently for 12 hours daily with at least 2 additional hours of exposure to sunlight. A third group of samples at 30°C was exposed to continuous direct incandescent light. Both groups of samples exposed directly to light showed substantial losses of vinblastine sulfate. Samples exposed to continuous direct light sustained a 10% loss in about 1 day and a 71% loss in 14 days. Samples intermittently exposed to direct light and sunlight sustained a 10% loss in 8 days and a 23% loss in 15 days. However, samples exposed to intermittent indirect light showed no drug loss in 70 days.[1306]

Under 6% vinblastine loss occurred in 48 hours from a 3-mcg/mL solution in sodium chloride 0.9% contained as a static solution in polybutadiene tubing when exposed to normal mixed daylight and fluorescent light. It was concluded that photodegradation is not a problem with vinblastine sulfate under these conditions.[1378]

Syringes

Vinblastine sulfate (David Bull Laboratories) 1 mg/mL in polypropylene syringes was stable for 31 days at 8°C and for at least 23 days at 21°C in the dark; little or no loss occurred.[1566]

Vinblastine sulfate (Lilly) 1 mg/mL in sodium chloride 0.9% was packaged in polypropylene syringes (Plastipak, Becton Dickinson) and stored at 25°C protected from light. No vinblastine sulfate loss was found after storage for 30 days.[2155]

Elastomeric Reservoir Pumps

Vinblastine sulfate 0.2 mg/mL in both dextrose 5% and sodium chloride 0.9% was evaluated for binding potential to natural rubber elastomeric reservoirs (Baxter). Less than 1% binding was found after storage for 2 weeks at 35°C with gentle agitation.[2014]

Implantable Pumps

Vinblastine sulfate (Lilly) 1 mg/mL in bacteriostatic sodium chloride 0.9% was evaluated for stability in an implantable pump (Infusaid model 400). In this in vitro assessment, a 24% vinblastine loss occurred in 24 hours at 37°C with mild agitation. In 12 days, the loss totaled 48%. In comparison, control

DOI: 10.37573/9781585286850.397

solutions in glass vials had no drug loss in 24 hours and a 20% loss in 12 days at 37°C. The authors believed that this indicated an interaction of vinblastine with some component of the Infu-said model 400, rendering it unsuitable for administration with this infusion device.[767]

Sorption

The stability of vinblastine sulfate (Lilly) 3 mcg/mL in methacry-late butadiene styrene (Avon A2001 Sureset) and cellulose propi-onate (Avon A200 standard and A2000 Amberset) when exposed to normal mixed daylight and fluorescent light for up to 48 hours was evaluated. A maximum vinblastine loss of about 5% resulted in the Sureset, with as little as a 2.25% loss occurring with foil wrapping. However, significant losses occurred in both cellulose propionate burettes in 24 hours, and losses of 15 to 20% occurred in 48 hours. The vinblastine sulfate solution in the polybutadiene tubing of the Sureset showed no more than a 6% drug loss with or without light protection. However, in the polyvinyl chloride (PVC) tubing of the standard or Amberset, losses were significant within 4 hours; at 48 hours, losses were 42 to 44%.[1378]

Vinblastine sulfate (Lilly) 10 mg/250 mL in dextrose 5% or sodium chloride 0.9%, in PVC bags at 22°C with protection from light, was infused over 2 hours at 2.08 mL/min through PVC sets. No loss due to sorption was found.[1631]

Vinblastine sulfate (Lederle) 250 mcg/mL in sodium chloride 0.9% exhibited no loss due to sorption to PVC and polyethylene administration lines during simulated infusions at 0.875 mL/hr for 2.5 hours via a syringe pump.[1795]

Filtration

Vinblastine sulfate (Lilly) 10 mg/50 mL in dextrose 5% and sodium chloride 0.9%, filtered at a rate of about 3 mL/min through a 0.22-µm cellulose ester membrane filter (Ivex-2), showed no significant reduction due to binding to the filter.[533]

Vinblastine sulfate 10 to 300 mcg/mL exhibited no loss due to sorption to either cellulose nitrate/cellulose acetate ester (Millex OR) or Teflon (Millex FG) filters.[1415 1416]

Vinblastine sulfate (Lederle) 250 mcg/mL in sodium chloride 0.9% exhibited no loss due to sorption to cellulose acetate (Minisart 45, Sartorius) and polysulfone (Acrodisc 45, Gelman) filters. However, a 10 to 20% loss due to sorption occurred during the first 30 to 60 minutes of infusion through nylon filters (Nylaflo, Gelman, and Utipore, Pall). About a 30% loss was found during the first hour using a positively-charged nylon filter (Posidyne ELD96, Pall). The delivered concentrations gradually returned to the full concentrations within 2 to 2.5 hours.[1795]

Central Venous Catheter

Vinblastine sulfate (Lilly) 0.12 mg/mL in dextrose 5% was found to be compatible with the ARROWg+ard Blue Plus (Arrow International) chlorhexidine-bearing triple-lumen central catheter. Essentially complete delivery of the drug was found with little or no drug loss occurring. Furthermore, chlorhexidine delivered from the catheter remained at trace amounts with no substantial increase due to the delivery of the drug through the catheter.[2335]

Compatibility Information

Solution Compatibility

Vinblastine sulfate

Test Soln Name	Mfr	Mfr	Conc/L or %	Remarks	Ref	C/I
Dextrose 5%	TR[a]	LI	170 mg	Under 10% loss in 24 hr at room temperature	519	C
Dextrose 5%		LI	20 mg	Physically compatible with little loss in 21 days at 4 and 25°C in the dark	1195	C
Dextrose 5%	[b]	LI	100 mg	8% loss in 7 days at 4°C protected from light	1631	C
Dextrose 5%	MG[c]		170 mg	Under 10% loss in 24 hr at room temperature exposed to light	1658	C
Ringer's injection, lactated		LI	20 mg	Physically compatible with 2 to 3% drug loss in 21 days at 4 and 25°C in the dark	1195	C
Sodium chloride 0.9%		LI	20 mg	Physically compatible with little loss in 21 days at 4 and 25°C in the dark	1195	C
Sodium chloride 0.9%	[b]	LI	100 mg	No loss in 7 days at 4°C protected from light	1631	C
Sodium chloride 0.9%	[d]		50 mg	5% loss at 23°C and 3% loss at 4°C in 21 days protected from light	2256	C

[a] Tested in both glass and PVC containers.

[b] Tested in PVC containers.

[c] Tested in both glass and polyolefin containers.

[d] Tested in glass containers.

Additive Compatibility

Vinblastine sulfate

Test Drug	Mfr	Conc/L or %	Mfr	Conc/L or %	Test Solution	Remarks	Ref	C/I
Bleomycin sulfate	BR	20 and 30 units	LI	10 and 100 mg	NS	Physically compatible and bleomycin activity retained for 1 week at 4°C. Vinblastine not tested	763	C
Doxorubicin HCl	AD	500 mg	LI	75 mg	NS[a]	Physically compatible for 10 days at 8, 25, and 32°C. Assays highly erratic	838	?
Doxorubicin HCl	AD	1.5 g	LI	150 mg	NS[a]	Physically compatible for 10 days at 8, 25, and 32°C. Assays highly erratic	838	?

[a] Tested in PVC containers.

Drugs in Syringe Compatibility

Vinblastine sulfate

Test Drug	Mfr	Amt	Mfr	Amt	Remarks	Ref	C/I
Bleomycin sulfate		1.5 units/0.5 mL		0.5 mg/0.5 mL	Physically compatible for 5 min at room temperature followed by 8 min of centrifugation	980	C
Cisplatin		0.5 mg/0.5 mL		0.5 mg/0.5 mL	Physically compatible for 5 min at room temperature followed by 8 min of centrifugation	980	C
Cyclophosphamide		10 mg/0.5 mL		0.5 mg/0.5 mL	Physically compatible for 5 min at room temperature followed by 8 min of centrifugation	980	C
Doxorubicin HCl	AD	45 mg/22.5 mL	LI	4.5 mg/4.5 mL	Brought to 30-mL total volume with NS. Physically compatible for 10 days at 8, 25, and 32°C. Assays highly erratic	838	?
Doxorubicin HCl	AD	15 mg/7.5 mL	LI	2.25 mg/2.25 mL	Brought to 30-mL total volume with NS. Physically compatible for 10 days at 8, 25, and 32°C. Assays highly erratic	838	?
Doxorubicin HCl		1 mg/0.5 mL		0.5 mg/0.5 mL	Physically compatible for 5 min at room temperature followed by 8 min of centrifugation	980	C
Droperidol		1.25 mg/0.5 mL		0.5 mg/0.5 mL	Physically compatible for 5 min at room temperature followed by 8 min of centrifugation	980	C
Fluorouracil		25 mg/0.5 mL		0.5 mg/0.5 mL	Physically compatible for 5 min at room temperature followed by 8 min of centrifugation	980	C
Furosemide		5 mg/0.5 mL		0.5 mg/0.5 mL	Precipitates immediately	980	I
Heparin sodium		200 units/1 mL[a]	LI	1 mg/1 mL	Turbidity appears in 2 to 3 min	767	I
Heparin sodium		500 units/0.5 mL		0.5 mg/0.5 mL	Physically compatible for 5 min at room temperature followed by 8 min of centrifugation	980	C
Leucovorin calcium		5 mg/0.5 mL		0.5 mg/0.5 mL	Physically compatible for 5 min at room temperature followed by 8 min of centrifugation	980	C
Methotrexate sodium		12.5 mg/0.5 mL		0.5 mg/0.5 mL	Physically compatible for 5 min at room temperature followed by 8 min of centrifugation	980	C
Metoclopramide HCl		2.5 mg/0.5 mL		0.5 mg/0.5 mL	Physically compatible for 5 min at room temperature followed by 8 min of centrifugation	980	C
Mitomycin		0.25 mg/0.5 mL		0.5 mg/0.5 mL	Physically compatible for 5 min at room temperature followed by 8 min of centrifugation	980	C
Vincristine sulfate		0.5 mg/0.5 mL		0.5 mg/0.5 mL	Physically compatible for 5 min at room temperature followed by 8 min of centrifugation	980	C

[a] Tested in bacteriostatic sodium chloride 0.9%.

Y-Site Injection Compatibility (1:1 Mixture)

Vinblastine sulfate

Test Drug	Mfr	Conc	Mfr	Conc	Remarks	Ref	C/I
Allopurinol sodium	BW	3 mg/mL[b]	LI	0.12 mg/mL[b]	Physically compatible for 4 hr at 22°C	1686	C
Amifostine	USB	10 mg/mL[a]	LI	0.12 mg/mL[a]	Physically compatible for 4 hr at 23°C	1845	C
Aztreonam	SQ	40 mg/mL[a]	LI	0.12 mg/mL[a]	Physically compatible for 4 hr at 23°C	1758	C
Bleomycin sulfate		3 units/mL		1 mg/mL	Drugs injected sequentially in Y-site with no flush. No precipitate seen	980	C
Cisplatin		1 mg/mL		1 mg/mL	Drugs injected sequentially in Y-site with no flush. No precipitate seen	980	C
Cyclophosphamide		20 mg/mL		1 mg/mL	Drugs injected sequentially in Y-site with no flush. No precipitate seen	980	C
Doxorubicin HCl		2 mg/mL		1 mg/mL	Drugs injected sequentially in Y-site with no flush. No precipitate seen	980	C
Doxorubicin HCl liposomal	SEQ	0.4 mg/mL[a]	FAU	0.12 mg/mL[a]	Physically compatible for 4 hr at 23°C	2087	C
Droperidol		2.5 mg/mL		1 mg/mL	Drugs injected sequentially in Y-site with no flush. No precipitate seen	980	C
Etoposide phosphate	BR	5 mg/mL[a]	FAU	0.12 mg/mL[a]	Physically compatible for 4 hr at 23°C	2218	C
Filgrastim	AMG	30 mcg/mL[a]	LI	0.12 mg/mL[a]	Physically compatible for 4 hr at 22°C	1687	C
Fludarabine phosphate	BX	1 mg/mL[a]	LY	0.12 mg/mL[a]	Visually compatible for 4 hr at 22°C	1439	C
Fluorouracil		50 mg/mL		1 mg/mL	Drugs injected sequentially in Y-site with no flush. No precipitate seen	980	C
Furosemide		10 mg/mL		1 mg/mL	Drugs injected sequentially in Y-site with no flush. Precipitates immediately	980	I
Gemcitabine HCl	LI	10 mg/mL[b]	FAU	0.12 mg/mL[b]	Physically compatible for 4 hr at 23°C	2226	C
Granisetron HCl	SKB	0.05 mg/mL[a]	LI	0.12 mg/mL[a]	Physically compatible for 4 hr at 23°C	2000	C
Heparin sodium		1000 units/mL		1 mg/mL	Drugs injected sequentially in Y-site with no flush. No precipitate seen	980	C
Leucovorin calcium		10 mg/mL		1 mg/mL	Drugs injected sequentially in Y-site with no flush. No precipitate seen	980	C
Melphalan HCl	BW	0.1 mg/mL[b]	LI	0.12 mg/mL[b]	Physically compatible for 3 hr at 22°C	1557	C
Methotrexate sodium		25 mg/mL		1 mg/mL	Drugs injected sequentially in Y-site with no flush. No precipitate seen	980	C
Metoclopramide HCl		5 mg/mL		1 mg/mL	Drugs injected sequentially in Y-site with no flush. No precipitate seen	980	C
Mitomycin		0.5 mg/mL		1 mg/mL	Drugs injected sequentially in Y-site with no flush. No precipitate seen	980	C
Ondansetron HCl	GL	1 mg/mL[b]	LY	0.12 mg/mL[a]	Visually compatible for 4 hr at 22°C	1365	C
Paclitaxel	NCI	1.2 mg/mL[a]	LI	0.12 mg/mL[b]	Physically compatible for 4 hr at 22°C	1556	C
Pemetrexed disodium	LI	20 mg/mL[b]	APP	0.12 mg/mL[a]	Physically compatible for 4 hr at 23°C	2564	C

Y-Site Injection Compatibility (1:1 Mixture) (Cont.)

Test Drug	Mfr	Conc	Mfr	Conc	Remarks	Ref	C/I
Piperacillin sodium–tazobactam sodium	LE[d]	40 mg/mL[a][e]	LI	0.12 mg/mL[a]	Physically compatible for 4 hr at 22°C	1688	C
Sargramostim	IMM	10 mcg/mL[b]	LY	0.12 mg/mL[b]	Visually compatible for 4 hr at 22°C	1436	C
Teniposide	BR	0.1 mg/mL[a]	LI	0.12 mg/mL[a]	Physically compatible for 4 hr at 23°C	1725	C
Thiotepa	IMM[c]	1 mg/mL[a]	LI	0.12 mg/mL[a]	Physically compatible for 4 hr at 23°C	1861	C
Vincristine sulfate		1 mg/mL		1 mg/mL	Drugs injected sequentially in Y-site with no flush. No precipitate seen	980	C
Vinorelbine tartrate	BW	1 mg/mL[b]	LI	0.12 mg/mL[b]	Physically compatible for 4 hr at 22°C	1558	C

[a] Tested in dextrose 5%.

[b] Tested in sodium chloride 0.9%.

[c] Lyophilized formulation tested.

[d] Test performed using the formulation WITHOUT edetate disodium.

[e] Piperacillin component. Piperacillin in an 8:1 fixed-ratio concentration with tazobactam.

Selected Revisions December 13, 2018. © Copyright, October 1982. American Society of Health-System Pharmacists, Inc.

Vincristine Sulfate
AHFS 10:00

Products

Vincristine sulfate is available as a preservative-free solution in a 1-mg/mL concentration with mannitol 100 mg/mL and sulfuric acid or sodium hydroxide to adjust pH during manufacturing.[2947] The ready-to-use solution is available in 1- and 2-mL single-dose vials.[2947] CAUTION: Care should be taken to ensure that the correct drug product, dose, and administration procedures are used and that no confusion with other products occurs.

pH

The official pH range is 3.5 to 5.5.[17] A narrower range of pH 4 to 5 has been cited by a manufacturer.[2947]

Administration

CAUTION: Care should be taken to ensure that the correct drug product, dose, and administration procedures are used and that no confusion with other products occurs.

Vincristine sulfate is administered intravenously only.[2947] It should not be given by any other route.[2947] Vincristine sulfate should be diluted with a suitable infusion solution in a flexible plastic container and prominently labeled "for intravenous use only" to reduce the risk of fatal medication errors due to the incorrect route of administration.[2947] If the drug is prepared in a syringe, a sticker is provided in the vincristine sulfate package that must be affixed directly to the syringe containing the individual dose that states:

FOR INTRAVENOUS USE ONLY – FATAL IF GIVEN BY OTHER ROUTES.[2947]

In addition, the syringe containing the prepared dose must be enclosed in an overwrap that is labeled:

DO NOT REMOVE COVERING UNTIL MOMENT OF INJECTION.[2947]

FOR INTRAVENOUS USE ONLY – FATAL IF GIVEN BY OTHER ROUTES.[2947]

The drug should be administered over 1 minute either directly into a vein or into the tubing of a running infusion solution.[2947] It also has been diluted and administered as an intermittent or continuous intravenous infusion.[4] Extravasation should be avoided.[2947]

In the event of spills or leaks, sodium hypochlorite 5% (household bleach) has been used to inactivate vincristine sulfate.[1200]

Stability

The ready-to-use solution should be stored under refrigeration, kept upright, and protected from light.[2947] Unused drug solution should be discarded.[2947] The pH range of maximum stability is 4 to 6.[1195] Precipitation may occur at alkaline pH values.[1369] Vincristine sulfate should not be added to solutions that would raise or lower the pH outside the 3.5 to 5.5 range.[2947] Only dextrose or sodium chloride 0.9% are recommended.[2947]

Admixtures containing doxorubicin hydrochloride, etoposide phosphate, and vincristine sulfate in a variety of concentration combinations in sodium chloride 0.9% were unable to pass the USP test for antimicrobial growth effectiveness. Mixtures of these drugs are not "self-preserving" and will permit microbial growth.[2343]

Immersion of a needle with an aluminum component in vincristine sulfate 1 mg/mL resulted in no visually apparent reaction after 7 days at 24°C.[988]

Freezing Solutions

Vincristine sulfate (Lilly) 20 mcg/mL in dextrose 5%; Ringer's injection, lactated; and sodium chloride 0.9% underwent no degradation after 4 weeks when frozen at −20°C.[1195]

Syringes

Vincristine sulfate (Lilly) 0.5, 1, 2, and 3 mg diluted to 20 mL with sodium chloride 0.9% and packaged in 30-mL polypropylene syringes (Becton Dickinson) was stored for 7 days at 4°C followed by 2 days at 23°C. All samples remained physically compatible with no increase in measured turbidity or particle content. No loss occurred after 7 days at 4°C and not more than 5% loss after 2 additional days at room temperature.[2350]

Sorption

Vincristine sulfate 2 mg/250 mL in dextrose 5% or sodium chloride 0.9% in polyvinyl chloride (PVC) bags at 22°C with protection from light was infused over 2 hours at 2.08 mL/min through PVC sets. No loss due to sorption was found.[1631]

Vincristine sulfate 25 mcg/mL in sodium chloride 0.9% exhibited no loss due to sorption to a polyethylene administration line (Vygon) during simulated infusions at 0.875 mL/hr for 2.5 hours via a syringe pump. However, about a 9% loss of delivered concentration due to sorption occurred during the first hour using a PVC administration line (Baxter). The delivered concentration returned to the full concentration within 1.5 hours.[1795]

Filtration

Vincristine sulfate (Lilly) 1 mg/50 mL in dextrose 5% and sodium chloride 0.9% was filtered at about 3 mL/min through a 0.22-μm cellulose ester membrane filter (Ivex-2). Losses of vincristine sulfate due to binding to the filters were noted in both solutions. In dextrose 5%, about 6.5% of the vincristine sulfate was bound; about 12% of the drug was lost from the sodium chloride 0.9% solution.[533]

In static equilibrium experiments, 100 mg of 0.22-μm cellulose ester membrane filter (Ivex-2) was soaked in 25 mL of vincristine sulfate (Lilly) 10 and 20 mcg/mL in both dextrose 5% and sodium chloride 0.9%. The higher concentration exhibited about 20 to 30% binding to the filter in 24 to 48 hours. The lower concentration had about 30 to 45% binding in the same period.[533]

DOI: 10.37573/9781585286850.398

A filter material specially treated with a proprietary agent was evaluated for a reduction in vincristine sulfate binding. Vincristine sulfate (Lilly) 1 mg/50 mL in dextrose 5% and sodium chloride 0.9% was run through an administration set with a treated 0.22-μm cellulose ester inline filter at a rate of 3 mL/min. Cumulative vincristine sulfate losses of about 1% occurred from both solutions compared to the much higher losses previously reported for untreated cellulose ester filter material. Furthermore, equilibrium binding studies showed 5- and 7-fold reductions in binding from dextrose 5% and sodium chloride 0.9%, respectively.[904] All Abbott Ivex integral filter and extension sets use this treated filter material.[1074]

Vincristine sulfate 1.5 mg/3 mL was injected through a 0.2-μm nylon, air-eliminating, filter (Ultipor, Pall) to evaluate the effect of filtration on simulated intravenous push delivery. About 90% of the drug was delivered through the filter after flushing with 10 mL of sodium chloride 0.9%.[809]

Vincristine sulfate 10 to 200 mcg/mL exhibited a 10 to 15% loss due to sorption to both cellulose nitrate/cellulose acetate ester (Millex OR) and Teflon (Millex FG) filters.[1415][1416]

Vincristine sulfate (David Bull Laboratories) 250 mcg/mL in sodium chloride 0.9% exhibited little loss due to sorption to cellulose acetate (Minisart 45, Sartorius) and polysulfone (Acrodisc 45, Gelman) filters. However, a 5 to 20% loss due to sorption occurred during the first 30 to 60 minutes of infusion through nylon filters (Nylaflo, Gelman, and Utipore, Pall). About a 20 to 25% loss was found during the first hour using a nylon filter (Posidyne ELD96, Pall). The delivered concentrations gradually returned to the full concentrations within 2 to 2.5 hours.[1795]

Central Venous Catheter

Vincristine sulfate (Lilly) 0.05 mg/mL in dextrose 5% was found to be compatible with the ARROWg+ard Blue Plus (Arrow International) chlorhexidine-bearing triple-lumen central catheter. Essentially complete delivery of the drug was found with little or no drug loss occurring. Furthermore, chlorhexidine delivered from the catheter remained at trace amounts with no substantial increase due to the delivery of the drug through the catheter.[2335]

Compatibility Information
Solution Compatibility

Vincristine sulfate

Test Soln Name	Mfr	Mfr	Conc/L or %	Remarks	Ref	C/I
Dextrose 5%	TR[a]	LI	16.7 mg	No loss in 24 hr at room temperature	806	C
Dextrose 5%		LI	20 mg	Physically compatible. 5% loss in 21 days at 4 and 25°C in dark	1195	C
Dextrose 5%	b	LI	20 mg	Little loss in 7 days at 4°C in dark	1631	C
Dextrose 5%	MG, TR[c]		20 mg	Under 10% loss in 24 hr at room temperature in light	1658	C
Ringer's injection, lactated		LI	20 mg	Physically compatible. Little loss in 21 days at 4 and 25°C in dark	1195	C
Sodium chloride 0.9%		LI	20 mg	Physically compatible. Little loss in 21 days at 4 and 25°C in dark	1195	C
Sodium chloride 0.9%	b	LI	20 mg	8% or less loss in 7 days at 4°C in dark	1631	C
Sodium chloride 0.9%		APP	1.5 to 80 mg	Stable up to 24 hr protected from light or 8 hr under normal light at 25°C	2947	C
Sodium chloride 0.9%	BA[b]	LI	10, 20, 40, 60, 80, 120 mg	Physically compatible. No loss after 7 days at 4°C followed by 2 days at 23°C	2350	C

[a] Tested in both glass and PVC containers.

[b] Tested in PVC containers.

[c] Tested in glass, polyolefin, and PVC containers.

Additive Compatibility

Vincristine sulfate

Test Drug	Mfr	Conc/L or %	Mfr	Conc/L or %	Test Solution	Remarks	Ref	C/I
Bleomycin sulfate	BR	20 and 30 units	LI	50 and 100 mg	NS	Physically compatible and bleomycin activity retained for 1 week at 4°C. Vincristine not tested	763	C
Cytarabine	UP	16 mg	LI	4 mg	D5W	Physically compatible. No alteration in UV spectra in 8 hr at room temperature	207	C
Doxorubicin HCl	FA	1.4 g	LI	33 mg	D5½S, NS	Visually compatible. Less than 10% loss of both drugs for 14 days at 25, 30, and 37°C	1030	C
Doxorubicin HCl	FA	1.88 and 2.37 g	LI	50 mg	D5½S, NS	Visually compatible. Less than 10% loss of both drugs for 14 days at 25 and 30°C. Up to 16% doxorubicin loss at 37°C in 14 days	1030	C
Doxorubicin HCl	NYC	1.67 g	LI	36 mg	NS[a b]	Visually compatible and both drugs stable for 7 days at 4°C then 4 days at 37°C	1874	C
Doxorubicin HCl	PHU	2 g	FAU	200 mg	W[c]	Physically compatible. No loss of either drug in 7 days at 37°C. 4% loss of both drugs in 14 days at 4°C	2288	C
Doxorubicin HCl	PHC	1.4 g	PHC	33 mg	D5½S	Physically compatible. Little loss of either drug in 14 days at 4 and 25°C. 12% loss of both drugs at 37°C	2674	C
Doxorubicin HCl	PHC	1.4 g	PHC	33 mg	NS	Physically compatible. Little loss of either drug in 14 days at 4 and 25°C. 4% loss of both drugs at 37°C	2674	C
Doxorubicin HCl	PHC	1.4 g	PHC	53 mg	D5½S	Physically compatible. Little loss of either drug in 14 days at 4 and 25°C. 8% loss of both drugs at 37°C	2674	C
Doxorubicin HCl	PHC	1.4 g	PHC	53 mg	NS	Physically compatible. Little loss of either drug in 14 days at 4 and 25°C. 9% loss of both drugs at 37°C	2674	C
Doxorubicin HCl with etoposide	PHU BMS	40 mg 200 mg	LI	1.6 mg	NS[d]	Visually compatible. All drugs stable for 72 hr at 30°C in the dark	2239	C
Doxorubicin HCl with etoposide	PHU BMS	25 mg 125 mg	LI	1 mg	NS[d]	Visually compatible. All drugs stable for 96 hr at 24°C in light or dark	2239	C
Doxorubicin HCl with etoposide	PHU BMS	35 mg 175 mg	LI	1.4 mg	NS[d]	Visually compatible. All drugs stable for 96 hr at 24°C in light or dark	2239	C
Doxorubicin HCl with etoposide	PHU BMS	50 mg 250 mg	LI	2 mg	NS[d]	Visually compatible. All drugs stable for 48 hr at 24°C in light or dark. Etoposide precipitate in 72 hr	2239	C
Doxorubicin HCl with etoposide	PHU BMS	70 mg 350 mg	LI	2.8 mg	NS[d]	Visually compatible. All drugs stable for 24 hr at 24°C in light or dark. Etoposide precipitate in 36 hr	2239	C
Doxorubicin HCl with etoposide	PHU BMS	100 mg 500 mg	LI	4 mg	NS[d]	Etoposide precipitate formed in 12 hr at 24°C in light or dark	2239	I
Doxorubicin HCl with etoposide phosphate	PHU BMS	120 mg 600 mg	LI	5 mg	NS[d]	Physically compatible. Little loss of any drug in 124 hr at 4 and 40°C	2343	C
Doxorubicin HCl with etoposide phosphate	PHU BMS	240 mg 1.2 g	LI	10 mg	NS[d]	Physically compatible. Little loss of any drug in 124 hr at 4 and 40°C	2343	C

Additive Compatibility (Cont.)

Test Drug	Mfr	Conc/L or %	Mfr	Conc/L or %	Test Solution	Remarks	Ref	C/I
Doxorubicin HCl with etoposide phosphate	PHU BMS	400 mg 2 g	LI	16 mg	NSd	Physically compatible. Under 4% loss of any drug in 124 hr at 4 and 40°C	2343	C
Doxorubicin HCl with ondansetron HCl	AD GL	400 mg 480 mg	LI	14 mg	D5Wb	Visually compatible. Under 10% loss of all drugs in 5 days at 4°C then 24 hr at 30°C	2092	C
Doxorubicin HCl with ondansetron HCl	AD GL	800 mg 960 mg	LI	28 mg	D5Wa	Visually compatible. Under 10% loss of all drugs after 120 hr at 30°C	2092	C
Etoposide with doxorubicin HCl	BMS PHU	200 mg 40 mg	LI	1.6 mg	NSd	Visually compatible. All drugs stable for 72 hr at 30°C in the dark	2239	C
Etoposide with doxorubicin HCl	BMS PHU	125 mg 25 mg	LI	1 mg	NSd	Visually compatible. All drugs stable for 96 hr at 24°C in light or dark	2239	C
Etoposide with doxorubicin HCl	BMS PHU	175 mg 35 mg	LI	1.4 mg	NSd	Visually compatible. All drugs stable for 96 hr at 24°C in light or dark	2239	C
Etoposide with doxorubicin HCl	BMS PHU	250 mg 50 mg	LI	2 mg	NSd	Visually compatible. All drugs stable for 48 hr at 24°C in light or dark. Etoposide precipitate in 72 hr	2239	C
Etoposide with doxorubicin HCl	BMS PHU	350 mg 70 mg	LI	2.8 mg	NSd	Visually compatible. All drugs stable for 24 hr at 24°C in light or dark. Etoposide precipitate in 36 hr	2239	C
Etoposide with doxorubicin HCl	BMS PHU	500 mg 100 mg	LI	4 mg	NSd	Etoposide precipitate formed in 12 hr at 24°C in light or dark	2239	I
Etoposide phosphate with doxorubicin HCl	BMS PHU	600 mg 120 mg	LI	5 mg	NSd	Physically compatible. Little loss of any drug in 124 hr at 4 and 40°C	2343	C
Etoposide phosphate with doxorubicin HCl	BMS PHU	1.2 g 240 mg	LI	10 mg	NSd	Physically compatible. Little loss of any drug in 124 hr at 4 and 40°C	2343	C
Etoposide phosphate with doxorubicin HCl	BMS PHU	2 g 400 mg	LI	16 mg	NSd	Physically compatible. Under 4% loss of any drug in 124 hr at 4 and 40°C	2343	C
Fluorouracil	RC	10 mg	LI	4 mg	D5W	Physically compatible. No alteration in UV spectra in 8 hr at room temperature	207	C
Methotrexate sodium	LE	100 mg	LI	10 mg	D5W	Physically compatible	15	C
Methotrexate sodium	LE	8 mg	LI	4 mg	D5W	Physically compatible. No change in UV spectra in 8 hr at room temperature	207	C
Ondansetron HCl with doxorubicin HCl	GL AD	480 mg 400 mg	LI	14 mg	D5Wb	Visually compatible. Under 10% loss of all drugs in 5 days at 4°C then 24 hr at 30°C	2092	C
Ondansetron HCl with doxorubicin HCl	GL AD	960 mg 800 mg	LI	28 mg	D5Wa	Visually compatible. Under 10% loss of all drugs after 120 hr at 30°C	2092	C

a Tested in PVC containers.

b Tested in polyisoprene infusion pump reservoirs.

c Tested in PVC reservoirs for the Graseby 9000 ambulatory pumps.

d Tested in polyolefin-lined plastic bags.

Drugs in Syringe Compatibility

Vincristine sulfate

Test Drug	Mfr	Amt	Mfr	Amt	Remarks	Ref	C/I
Bleomycin sulfate		1.5 units/0.5 mL		0.5 mg/0.5 mL	Physically compatible for 5 min at room temperature followed by 8 min of centrifugation	980	C
Cisplatin		0.5 mg/0.5 mL		0.5 mg/0.5 mL	Physically compatible for 5 min at room temperature followed by 8 min of centrifugation	980	C
Cyclophosphamide		10 mg/0.5 mL		0.5 mg/0.5 mL	Physically compatible for 5 min at room temperature followed by 8 min of centrifugation	980	C
Doxapram HCl	RB	400 mg/20 mL		1 mg/10 mL	Physically compatible with 7% doxapram loss in 24 hr	1177	C
Doxorubicin HCl		1 mg/0.5 mL		0.5 mg/0.5 mL	Physically compatible for 5 min at room temperature followed by 8 min of centrifugation	980	C
Droperidol		1.25 mg/0.5 mL		0.5 mg/0.5 mL	Physically compatible for 5 min at room temperature followed by 8 min of centrifugation	980	C
Fluorouracil		25 mg/0.5 mL		0.5 mg/0.5 mL	Physically compatible for 5 min at room temperature followed by 8 min of centrifugation	980	C
Furosemide		5 mg/0.5 mL		0.5 mg/0.5 mL	Precipitates immediately	980	I
Heparin sodium		500 units/0.5 mL		0.5 mg/0.5 mL	Physically compatible for 5 min at room temperature followed by 8 min of centrifugation	980	C
Leucovorin calcium		5 mg/0.5 mL		0.5 mg/0.5 mL	Physically compatible for 5 min at room temperature followed by 8 min of centrifugation	980	C
Methotrexate sodium		12.5 mg/0.5 mL		0.5 mg/0.5 mL	Physically compatible for 5 min at room temperature followed by 8 min of centrifugation	980	C
Metoclopramide HCl		2.5 mg/0.5 mL		0.5 mg/0.5 mL	Physically compatible for 5 min at room temperature followed by 8 min of centrifugation	980	C
Mitomycin		0.25 mg/0.5 mL		0.5 mg/0.5 mL	Physically compatible for 5 min at room temperature followed by 8 min of centrifugation	980	C
Vinblastine sulfate		0.5 mg/0.5 mL		0.5 mg/0.5 mL	Physically compatible for 5 min at room temperature followed by 8 min of centrifugation	980	C

Y-Site Injection Compatibility (1:1 Mixture)

Vincristine sulfate

Test Drug	Mfr	Conc	Mfr	Conc	Remarks	Ref	C/I
Allopurinol sodium	BW	3 mg/mL[b]	LI	0.05 mg/mL[b]	Physically compatible for 4 hr at 22°C	1686	C
Amifostine	USB	10 mg/mL[a]	LI	0.05 mg/mL[a]	Physically compatible for 4 hr at 23°C	1845	C
Anidulafungin	VIC	0.5 mg/mL[a]	FAU	50 mcg/mL[a]	Physically compatible for 4 hr at 23°C	2617	C
Aztreonam	SQ	40 mg/mL[a]	LI	0.05 mg/mL[a]	Physically compatible for 4 hr at 23°C	1758	C
Bleomycin sulfate		3 units/mL		1 mg/mL	Drugs injected sequentially in Y-site with no flush. No precipitate seen	980	C
Caspofungin acetate	ME	0.7 mg/mL[b]	MAY	0.05 mg/mL[b]	Physically compatible for 4 hr at room temperature	2758	C
Cisplatin		1 mg/mL		1 mg/mL	Drugs injected sequentially in Y-site with no flush. No precipitate seen	980	C
Cladribine	ORT	0.015[b] and 0.5[c] mg/mL	LI	0.05 mg/mL[b]	Physically compatible for 4 hr at 23°C	1969	C

Y-Site Injection Compatibility (1:1 Mixture) (Cont.)

Test Drug	Mfr	Conc	Mfr	Conc	Remarks	Ref	C/I
Cyclophosphamide		20 mg/mL		1 mg/mL	Drugs injected sequentially in Y-site with no flush. No precipitate seen	980	C
Doxorubicin HCl		2 mg/mL		1 mg/mL	Drugs injected sequentially in Y-site with no flush. No precipitate seen	980	C
Doxorubicin HCl liposomal	SEQ	0.4 mg/mL[a]	FAU	0.05 mg/mL[a]	Physically compatible for 4 hr at 23°C	2087	C
Droperidol		2.5 mg/mL		1 mg/mL	Drugs injected sequentially in Y-site with no flush. No precipitate seen	980	C
Etoposide phosphate	BR	5 mg/mL[a]	FAU	0.05 mg/mL[a]	Physically compatible for 4 hr at 23°C	2218	C
Filgrastim	AMG	30 mcg/mL[a]	LI	0.05 mg/mL[a]	Physically compatible for 4 hr at 22°C	1687	C
Fludarabine phosphate	BX	1 mg/mL[a]	LY	1 mg/mL[a]	Visually compatible for 4 hr at 22°C	1439	C
Fluorouracil		50 mg/mL		1 mg/mL	Drugs injected sequentially in Y-site with no flush. No precipitate seen	980	C
Furosemide		10 mg/mL		1 mg/mL	Drugs injected sequentially in Y-site with no flush. Precipitates immediately	980	I
Gemcitabine HCl	LI	10 mg/mL[b]	FAU	0.05 mg/mL[b]	Physically compatible for 4 hr at 23°C	2226	C
Granisetron HCl	SKB	1 mg/mL	LI	0.01 and 0.34 mg/mL[b]	Physically compatible with little or no loss of either drug in 4 hr at 22°C	1883	C
Heparin sodium		1000 units/mL		1 mg/mL	Drugs injected sequentially in Y-site with no flush. No precipitate seen	980	C
Idarubicin HCl	AD	1 mg/mL[b]	AD	1 mg/mL	Color changes immediately	1525	I
Leucovorin calcium		10 mg/mL		1 mg/mL	Drugs injected sequentially in Y-site with no flush. No precipitate seen	980	C
Linezolid	PHU	2 mg/mL	LI	0.05 mg/mL[a]	Physically compatible for 4 hr at 23°C	2264	C
Melphalan HCl	BW	0.1 mg/mL[b]	LI	0.05 mg/mL[b]	Physically compatible for 3 hr at 22°C	1557	C
Methotrexate sodium		25 mg/mL		1 mg/mL	Drugs injected sequentially in Y-site with no flush. No precipitate seen	980	C
Methotrexate sodium		30 mg/mL	LI	0.1 mg/mL	Visually compatible for 4 hr at room temperature	1788	C
Metoclopramide HCl		5 mg/mL		1 mg/mL	Drugs injected sequentially in Y-site with no flush. No precipitate seen	980	C
Mitomycin		0.5 mg/mL		1 mg/mL	Drugs injected sequentially in Y-site with no flush. No precipitate seen	980	C
Ondansetron HCl	GL	1 mg/mL[b]	LY	0.05 mg/mL[a]	Visually compatible for 4 hr at 22°C	1365	C
Oxaliplatin	SS	0.5 mg/mL[a]	FAU	0.05 mg/mL[a]	Physically compatible for 4 hr at 23°C	2566	C
Paclitaxel	NCI	1.2 mg/mL[a]	LI	0.05 mg/mL[a]	Physically compatible for 4 hr at 22°C	1556	C
Pemetrexed disodium	LI	20 mg/mL[b]	SIC	0.05 mg/mL[a]	Physically compatible for 4 hr at 23°C	2564	C
Piperacillin sodium–tazobactam sodium	LE[e]	40 mg/mL[a f]	LI	0.05 mg/mL[a]	Physically compatible for 4 hr at 22°C	1688	C
Sargramostim	IMM	10 mcg/mL[b]	LY	0.05 mg/mL[b]	Visually compatible for 4 hr at 22°C	1436	C
Sodium bicarbonate		1.4%	LI	0.1 mg/mL	White precipitate forms in 30 min at room temperature	1788	I

Y-Site Injection Compatibility (1:1 Mixture) (Cont.)

Test Drug	Mfr	Conc	Mfr	Conc	Remarks	Ref	C/I
Teniposide	BR	0.1 mg/mL[a]	LI	0.05 mg/mL[a]	Physically compatible for 4 hr at 23°C	1725	C
Thiotepa	IMM[d]	1 mg/mL[a]	LI	0.05 mg/mL[a]	Physically compatible for 4 hr at 23°C	1861	C
Topotecan HCl	SKB	56 mcg/mL[a b]	LI	1 mg/mL	Visually compatible. Little loss of either drug in 4 hr at 22°C	2245	C
Vinblastine sulfate		1 mg/mL		1 mg/mL	Drugs injected sequentially in Y-site with no flush. No precipitate seen	980	C
Vinorelbine tartrate	BW	1 mg/mL[b]	LI	0.05 mg/mL[b]	Physically compatible for 4 hr at 22°C	1558	C

[a] Tested in dextrose 5%.

[b] Tested in sodium chloride 0.9%.

[c] Tested in bacteriostatic sodium chloride 0.9% preserved with benzyl alcohol 0.9%.

[d] Lyophilized formulation tested.

[e] Test performed using the formulation WITHOUT edetate disodium.

[f] Piperacillin component. Piperacillin in an 8:1 fixed-ratio concentration with tazobactam.

Selected Revisions December 13, 2018. © Copyright, October 1982. American Society of Health-System Pharmacists, Inc.

Vincristine Sulfate Liposomal
AHFS 10:00

Products

Vincristine sulfate liposomal injection is prepared from a kit containing single-use vials of vincristine sulfate solution (5 mg/5 mL), sphingomyelin-cholesterol liposome suspension (1 mL), and sodium phosphate solution (25 mL).[3024] **CAUTION: Care should be taken to ensure that the correct drug product, dose, and administration procedures are used and that no confusion with other products occurs.**

When prepared as directed from the kit components, the resultant product is a white to off-white translucent suspension containing liposome-encapsulated vincristine sulfate 0.16 mg/mL (i.e., 5 mg in a total volume of 31 mL of suspension).[3024] Each vial of vincristine sulfate liposomal injection prepared from the kit components also contains mannitol 500 mg, sphingomyelin 73.5 mg, cholesterol 29.5 mg, sodium citrate 36 mg, citric acid 38 mg, sodium phosphate 355 mg, and sodium chloride 225 mg in 31 mL of suspension.[3024] Over 95% of the vincristine sulfate in the resulting liposomal suspension is provided inside liposome carriers (mean diameter 100 nm), which are composed of sphingomyelin and cholesterol.[3024]

To prepare vincristine sulfate liposomal injection, a water bath should be prepared and maintained *outside* of the sterile area using equipment provided by the manufacturer (i.e., water bath, calibrated thermometer and timer).[3024] The depth of the water bath should be at least 8 cm and the temperature of the water bath should be maintained at 63 to 67°C throughout the preparation procedure.[3024] All steps required to mix and dilute the product should be performed *inside* the sterile area.[3024]

Each vial of the kit should be visually inspected for particulate matter and discoloration prior to use whenever solution and container permit; vials should not be used if a precipitate or foreign matter is present.[3024] A venting needle (or other suitable venting device) with a 0.2-μm filter should be inserted into the vial of sodium phosphate solution, taking care to position the venting needle well above the liquid level of the solution prior to addition of the other components.[3024] One mL should be withdrawn from the vial of sphingomyelin-cholesterol liposome injection and transferred to the vial containing sodium phosphate solution.[3024] Five mL of solution should then be withdrawn from the vial containing vincristine sulfate and transferred to the vial containing the sodium phosphate and sphingomyelin-cholesterol liposome components.[3024] The venting needle should then be removed from the sodium phosphate vial and the vial should be gently inverted 5 times to mix the 3 components; shaking should be avoided.[3024]

After confirming that the temperature of the water bath has warmed to 63 to 67°C, the neck of the sodium phosphate vial containing the mixture of the 3 components should be fitted with the flotation ring and transferred from the sterile area to the water bath.[3024] The vial should remain in the water bath for 10 minutes; the temperature of the water bath and duration of flotation should be closely monitored using the manufacturer-provided calibrated thermometer and electronic timer.[3024] After 10 minutes, the vial should be removed from the water bath using tongs to prevent burns, and the flotation ring should be removed from the vial.[3024] The start time and temperature and the end time and temperature should be recorded on the provided vincristine sulfate liposomal injection overlabel immediately after the vial is placed into the water bath and upon removal, respectively.[3024] The vial exterior should be dried with a clean paper towel upon removal from the water bath, and the vincristine sulfate liposomal injection overlabel should be affixed.[3024] The vial should be gently inverted another 5 times to mix the contents; shaking should be avoided.[3024] The resultant vincristine sulfate liposomal injection should be allowed to equilibrate to controlled room temperature (i.e., 15 to 30°C) for at least 30 minutes.[3024]

Vincristine sulfate liposomal injection must be diluted in an appropriate infusion solution (i.e., dextrose 5% or sodium chloride 0.9%) before administration.[3024] A volume equivalent to the volume of the appropriate dose of vincristine sulfate liposomal should be withdrawn from a 100-mL infusion bag of dextrose 5% or sodium chloride 0.9% prior to addition of the drug.[3024] The appropriate dose of vincristine sulfate liposomal injection should then be transferred to the infusion bag to yield a final volume of 100 mL; the infusion bag label supplied by the drug's manufacturer should be completed and affixed to the bag.[3024]

Specific product labeling should be consulted for additional details on the preparation process for liposomal vincristine sulfate injection.[3024] Deviations from temperature control, timing, and preparation instructions may affect encapsulation of vincristine sulfate into the liposomes.[3024] In the case of such deviations, the manufacturer recommends discarding the components of the kit and using a new kit to prepare vincristine sulfate liposomal injection.[3024]

Trade Name(s)

Marqibo

Administration

Vincristine sulfate liposomal injection is administered by intravenous infusion over 1 hour only after preparation of the liposomal suspension as directed (see Products), followed by dilution in dextrose 5% or sodium chloride 0.9%.[3024] **The manufacturer states that the drug is fatal if given by other routes.[3024] Death has occurred with intrathecal use; such use is contraindicated.[3024]**

CAUTION: Care should be taken to ensure that the correct drug product, dose, and administration procedures are used and that no confusion with other products occurs.

DOI: 10.37573/9781585286850.399

Stability

All intact vials of vincristine sulfate injection solution, sphingo-myelin-cholesterol liposome injection suspension, and sodium phosphate injection solution contained in the kit used in the preparation of vincristine sulfate liposomal injection should be stored at 2 to 8°C and should not be frozen.[3024]

Following constitution, vincristine sulfate liposomal injection should be stored at 15 to 30°C for no more than 12 hours.[3024] Once diluted in the infusion bag, administration of diluted vincristine sulfate liposomal injection should be completed within 12 hours of *initiation* of vincristine sulfate liposomal injection preparation.[3024]

Filtration

Although a venting needle (or other suitable venting device) with a 0.2-μm filter should be used in the preparation of vincristine sulfate liposomal injection, inline filters should *not* be used during administration.[3024]

Compatibility Information

Solution Compatibility

Vincristine sulfate liposomal

Test Soln Name	Mfr	Mfr	Conc/L or %	Remarks	Ref	C/I
Dextrose 5%		TAL		Complete administration within 12 hr of *initiation* of preparation	3024	C
Sodium chloride 0.9%		TAL		Complete administration within 12 hr of *initiation* of preparation	3024	C

Vinorelbine Tartrate
AHFS 10:00

Products

Vinorelbine tartrate is available in a 10-mg/mL concentration in water for injection in 1- and 5-mL single-use vials. No preservatives or other additives are present.[1(7/05)]

Vinorelbine tartrate should be diluted with a compatible diluent for administration. Because skin reactions may occur, gloves should be worn during preparation.[1(7/05)]

pH

The injection has a pH of approximately 3.5.[1(7/05)]

Administration

Vinorelbine tartrate is administered intravenously, after dilution, from a syringe (at a concentration of 1.5 to 3 mg/mL) or infusion solution minibag (at a concentration of 0.5 to 2 mg/mL) over 6 to 10 minutes into the side port of a free-flowing infusion solution closest to the infusion container. After administration, 75 to 125 mL of solution should be used as a flush. Extravasation should be avoided due to tissue irritation, necrosis, and thrombophlebitis.[1(7/05)] A literature review for the period 1966 through 2004 did not find a statistically significant difference in the rate of venous irritation from 1- to 2-minute intravenous pushes and 6- to 10-minute intravenous infusions.[2637]

Intrathecal injection of vinca alkaloids has resulted in death. When vinorelbine tartrate is dispensed in a syringe containing an individual dose, the syringe must be labeled with this statement:[1(7/05)]

WARNING – FOR IV USE ONLY. FATAL if given intrathecally.

Stability

Vinorelbine tartrate injection is a colorless to pale yellow clear solution. Intact vials should be refrigerated at 2 to 8°C and protected from light (by storage in the carton) and freezing. Intact vials are stable at room temperature (up to 25°C) for 72 hours.[1(7/05)]

When diluted to 1.5 to 3 mg/mL in polypropylene syringes or to 0.5 to 2 mg/mL in polyvinyl chloride (PVC) infusion containers, vinorelbine tartrate is stable for 24 hours at 5 to 30°C with exposure to normal room light.[1(7/05)]

Vinorelbine tartrate 0.1 mg/mL diluted in sodium chloride 0.9% and stored at 22°C did not exhibit an antimicrobial effect on the growth of 4 organisms (*Enterococcus faecium*, *Staphylococcus aureus*, *Pseudomonas aeruginosa*, and *Candida albicans*) inoculated into the solution. The author recommended that diluted solutions of vinorelbine tartrate be stored under refrigeration whenever possible and that the potential for microbiological growth be considered when assigning expiration periods.[2160]

Sorption

Vinorelbine tartrate was shown not to exhibit sorption to PVC bags and tubing as well as polyethylene and glass containers.[1631] [2420] [2430]

Compatibility Information
Solution Compatibility

Vinorelbine tartrate

Test Soln Name	Mfr	Mfr	Conc/L or %	Remarks	Ref	C/I
Dextrose 5% in sodium chloride 0.45%			0.5 to 2 g	Stable for 24 hr at 5 to 30°C in light	1(7/05)	C
Dextrose 5%			0.5 to 3 g	Stable for 24 hr at 5 to 30°C in light	1(7/05)	C
Dextrose 5%	a		500 mg	Little loss in 7 days at 4°C in dark	1631	C
Dextrose 5%	a	GW	0.5 and 2 g	Visually compatible. 6% or less loss in 120 hr at 24°C in light	2213	C
Ringer's injection			0.5 to 2 g	Stable for 24 hr at 5 to 30°C in light	1(7/05)	C
Ringer's injection, lactated			0.5 to 2 g	Stable for 24 hr at 5 to 30°C in light	1(7/05)	C
Sodium chloride 0.45%			0.5 to 2 g	Stable for 24 hr at 5 to 30°C in light	1(7/05)	C
Sodium chloride 0.9%			0.5 to 3 g	Stable for 24 hr at 5 to 30°C in light	1(7/05)	C
Sodium chloride 0.9%	a		500 mg	4% loss in 3 days and 14% loss in 7 days at 4°C protected from light	1631	C
Sodium chloride 0.9%	a	GW	0.5 and 2 g	Visually compatible. 3% or less loss in 120 hr at 24°C in light	2213	C

a Tested in PVC containers.

DOI: 10.37573/9781585286850.400

Y-Site Injection Compatibility (1:1 Mixture)

Vinorelbine tartrate

Test Drug	Mfr	Conc	Mfr	Conc	Remarks	Ref	C/I
Acyclovir sodium	BW	7 mg/mL[b]	BW	1 mg/mL[b]	Immediate white precipitate	1558	I
Allopurinol sodium	BW	3 mg/mL[b]	BW	1 mg/mL[b]	Immediate white precipitate	1686	I
Amikacin sulfate	BR	5 mg/mL[b]	BW	1 mg/mL[b]	Physically compatible for 4 hr at 22°C	1558	C
Aminophylline	AB	2.5 mg/mL[b]	BW	1 mg/mL[b]	Visible haze with large particles in 1 hr	1558	I
Amphotericin B	SQ	0.6 mg/mL[a][b]	BW	1 mg/mL[b]	Yellow precipitate forms immediately	1558	I
Ampicillin sodium	WY	20 mg/mL[b]	BW	1 mg/mL[b]	Tiny particles form immediately. White particles in turbidity in 1 hr	1558	I
Aztreonam	SQ	40 mg/mL[b]	BW	1 mg/mL[b]	Physically compatible for 4 hr at 23°C	1558	C
Bleomycin sulfate	BR	1 unit/mL[b]	BW	1 mg/mL[b]	Physically compatible for 4 hr at 22°C	1558	C
Bumetanide	RC	0.04 mg/mL[b]	BW	1 mg/mL[b]	Physically compatible for 4 hr at 22°C	1558	C
Buprenorphine HCl	RKC	0.04 mg/mL[b]	BW	1 mg/mL[b]	Physically compatible for 4 hr at 22°C	1558	C
Butorphanol tartrate	BR	0.04 mg/mL[b]	BW	1 mg/mL[b]	Physically compatible for 4 hr at 22°C	1558	C
Calcium gluconate	AMR	40 mg/mL[b]	BW	1 mg/mL[b]	Physically compatible for 4 hr at 22°C	1558	C
Carboplatin	BR	5 mg/mL[b]	BW	1 mg/mL[b]	Physically compatible for 4 hr at 22°C	1558	C
Carmustine	BR	1.5 mg/mL[b]	BW	1 mg/mL[b]	Physically compatible for 4 hr at 22°C	1558	C
Cefazolin sodium	GEM	20 mg/mL[b]	BW	1 mg/mL[b]	Measured turbidity increases immediately	1558	I
Cefotaxime sodium	HO	20 mg/mL[b]	BW	1 mg/mL[b]	Physically compatible for 4 hr at 22°C	1558	C
Cefotetan disodium	STU	20 mg/mL[b]	BW	1 mg/mL[b]	Tiny particles form immediately. Turbidity in 4 hr	1558	I
Ceftazidime	LI	40 mg/mL[b]	BW	1 mg/mL[b]	Physically compatible for 4 hr at 22°C	1558	C
Ceftriaxone sodium	RC	20 mg/mL[b]	BW	1 mg/mL[b]	Tiny particles form immediately, becoming more numerous in 4 hr at 22°C	1558	I
Cefuroxime sodium	GL	20 mg/mL[b]	BW	1 mg/mL[b]	Large increase in measured turbidity occurs immediately	1558	I
Chlorpromazine HCl	RU	2 mg/mL[b]	BW	1 mg/mL[b]	Physically compatible for 4 hr at 22°C	1558	C
Cisplatin	BR	1 mg/mL	BW	1 mg/mL[b]	Physically compatible for 4 hr at 22°C	1558	C
Clindamycin phosphate	AB	10 mg/mL[b]	BW	1 mg/mL[b]	Physically compatible for 4 hr at 22°C	1558	C
Cyclophosphamide	MJ	10 mg/mL[b]	BW	1 mg/mL[b]	Physically compatible for 4 hr at 22°C	1558	C
Cytarabine	CET	50 mg/mL	BW	1 mg/mL[b]	Physically compatible for 4 hr at 22°C	1558	C
Dacarbazine	MI	4 mg/mL[b]	BW	1 mg/mL[b]	Physically compatible for 4 hr at 22°C	1558	C
Dactinomycin	MSD	0.01 mg/mL[b]	BW	1 mg/mL[b]	Physically compatible for 4 hr at 22°C	1558	C
Daunorubicin HCl	WY	1 mg/mL[b]	BW	1 mg/mL[b]	Physically compatible for 4 hr at 22°C	1558	C
Dexamethasone sodium phosphate	LY	1 mg/mL[b]	BW	1 mg/mL[b]	Physically compatible for 4 hr at 22°C	1558	C
Diphenhydramine HCl	ES	2 mg/mL[b]	BW	1 mg/mL[b]	Physically compatible for 4 hr at 22°C	1558	C
Doxorubicin HCl	CET	2 mg/mL	BW	1 mg/mL[b]	Physically compatible for 4 hr at 22°C	1558	C
Doxorubicin HCl liposomal	SEQ	0.4 mg/mL[a]	BW	1 mg/mL[a]	Physically compatible for 4 hr at 23°C	2087	C

Y-Site Injection Compatibility (1:1 Mixture) (Cont.)

Test Drug	Mfr	Conc	Mfr	Conc	Remarks	Ref	C/I
Doxycycline hyclate	ES	1 mg/mL[b]	BW	1 mg/mL[b]	Physically compatible for 4 hr at 22°C	1558	C
Droperidol	JN	0.4 mg/mL[b]	BW	1 mg/mL[b]	Physically compatible for 4 hr at 22°C	1558	C
Enalaprilat	MSD	0.1 mg/mL[b]	BW	1 mg/mL[b]	Physically compatible for 4 hr at 22°C	1558	C
Etoposide	BR	0.4 mg/mL[b]	BW	1 mg/mL[b]	Physically compatible for 4 hr at 22°C	1558	C
Famotidine	MSD	2 mg/mL[b]	BW	1 mg/mL[b]	Physically compatible for 4 hr at 22°C	1558	C
Filgrastim	AMG	30 mcg/mL[a]	BW	1 mg/mL[b]	Physically compatible for 4 hr at 22°C	1687	C
Floxuridine	RC	3 mg/mL[b]	BW	1 mg/mL[b]	Physically compatible for 4 hr at 22°C	1558	C
Fluconazole	RR	2 mg/mL	BW	1 mg/mL[b]	Physically compatible for 4 hr at 22°C	1558	C
Fludarabine phosphate	BX	1 mg/mL[b]	BW	1 mg/mL[b]	Physically compatible for 4 hr at 22°C	1558	C
Fluorouracil	RC	16 mg/mL[b]	BW	1 mg/mL[b]	Heavy white precipitate forms immediately	1558	I
Furosemide	ES	3 mg/mL[b]	BW	1 mg/mL[b]	Heavy white precipitate forms immediately	1558	I
Gallium nitrate	FUJ	0.4 mg/mL[b]	BW	1 mg/mL[b]	Physically compatible for 4 hr at 22°C	1558	C
Ganciclovir sodium	SY	20 mg/mL[b]	BW	1 mg/mL[b]	Turbid precipitate forms immediately	1558	I
Gemcitabine HCl	LI	10 mg/mL[b]	GW	1 mg/mL[b]	Physically compatible for 4 hr at 23°C	2226	C
Gentamicin sulfate	ES	5 mg/mL[b]	BW	1 mg/mL[b]	Physically compatible for 4 hr at 22°C	1558	C
Granisetron HCl	SKB	0.05 mg/mL[a]	BW	1 mg/mL[a]	Physically compatible for 4 hr at 23°C	2000	C
Haloperidol lactate	MN	0.2 mg/mL[b]	BW	1 mg/mL[b]	Physically compatible for 4 hr at 22°C	1558	C
Heparin sodium	ES	100 units/mL[b]	BW	1 mg/mL[b]	Physically compatible for 4 hr at 22°C	1558	C
Heparin sodium		100 units/mL[b]	GW	3 mg/mL[b]	A fine haze forms immediately, becoming cloudy in 15 min	2238	I
Heparin sodium		100 units/mL[b]	GW	2 mg/mL[b]	Visually compatible for at least 15 min	2238	C
Heparin sodium		100 units/mL[b]	GW	1 mg/mL[b]	Visually compatible for at least 15 min	2238	C
Heparin sodium		100 units/1 mL[b]	GW	4 mg/4 mL[b]	Volumes mixed as cited. Visually compatible for at least 15 min	2238	C
Heparin sodium		100 units/1 mL[b]	GW	8 mg/4 mL[b]	Volumes mixed as cited. Precipitate forms	2238	I
Heparin sodium		100 units/1 mL[b]	GW	12 mg/4 mL[b]	Volumes mixed as cited. Precipitate forms	2238	I
Hydrocortisone sodium succinate	UP	1 mg/mL[b]	BW	1 mg/mL[b]	Physically compatible for 4 hr at 22°C	1558	C
Hydromorphone HCl	KN	0.5 mg/mL[b]	BW	1 mg/mL[b]	Physically compatible for 4 hr at 22°C	1558	C
Hydroxyzine HCl	ES	4 mg/mL[b]	BW	1 mg/mL[b]	Physically compatible for 4 hr at 22°C	1558	C
Idarubicin HCl	AD	0.5 mg/mL[b]	BW	1 mg/mL[b]	Physically compatible for 4 hr at 22°C	1558, 1675	C
Ifosfamide	MJ	25 mg/mL[b]	BW	1 mg/mL[b]	Physically compatible for 4 hr at 22°C	1558	C
Imipenem–cilastatin sodium	MSD	10 mg/mL[b d]	BW	1 mg/mL[b]	Physically compatible for 4 hr at 22°C	1558	C
Lorazepam	WY	0.1 mg/mL[b]	BW	1 mg/mL[b]	Physically compatible for 4 hr at 22°C	1558	C
Mannitol	BA	15%	BW	1 mg/mL[b]	Physically compatible for 4 hr at 22°C	1558	C
Mechlorethamine HCl	MSD	1 mg/mL	BW	1 mg/mL[b]	Physically compatible for 4 hr at 22°C	1558	C

Y-Site Injection Compatibility (1:1 Mixture) (Cont.)

Test Drug	Mfr	Conc	Mfr	Conc	Remarks	Ref	C/I
Melphalan HCl	BW	0.1 mg/mL[b]	BW	1 mg/mL[b]	Physically compatible for 4 hr at 22°C	1558	C
Meperidine HCl	WY	4 mg/mL[b]	BW	1 mg/mL[b]	Physically compatible for 4 hr at 22°C	1558	C
Mesna	MJ	10 mg/mL[b]	BW	1 mg/mL[b]	Physically compatible for 4 hr at 22°C	1558	C
Methotrexate sodium	LE	15 mg/mL[b]	BW	1 mg/mL[b]	Physically compatible for 4 hr at 22°C	1558	C
Methylprednisolone sodium succinate	AB	5 mg/mL[b]	BW	1 mg/mL[b]	Heavy white precipitate forms immediately	1558	I
Metoclopramide HCl	RB	5 mg/mL	BW	1 mg/mL[b]	Physically compatible for 4 hr at 22°C	1558	C
Metronidazole	BA	5 mg/mL	BW	1 mg/mL[b]	Physically compatible for 4 hr at 22°C	1558	C
Mitomycin	BR	0.5 mg/mL	BW	1 mg/mL[b]	Reddish-purple color in 1 hr	1558	I
Mitoxantrone HCl	LE	0.5 mg/mL[b]	BW	1 mg/mL[b]	Physically compatible for 4 hr at 22°C	1558	C
Morphine sulfate	WI	1 mg/mL[b]	BW	1 mg/mL[b]	Physically compatible for 4 hr at 22°C	1558	C
Nalbuphine HCl	AST	10 mg/mL	BW	1 mg/mL[b]	Physically compatible for 4 hr at 22°C	1558	C
Ondansetron HCl	GL	1 mg/mL[b]	BW	1 mg/mL[b]	Physically compatible for 4 hr at 22°C	1558	C
Oxaliplatin	SS	0.5 mg/mL[a]	GW	1 mg/mL[a]	Physically compatible for 4 hr at 23°C	2566	C
Potassium chloride	AB	0.1 mEq/mL[b]	BW	1 mg/mL[b]	Physically compatible for 4 hr at 22°C	1558	C
Prochlorperazine edisylate	SKB	0.5 mg/mL[b]	BW	1 mg/mL[b]	Physically compatible for 4 hr at 22°C	1558	C
Promethazine HCl	ES	2 mg/mL[b]	BW	1 mg/mL[b]	Physically compatible for 4 hr at 22°C	1558	C
Ranitidine HCl	GL	2 mg/mL[b]	BW	1 mg/mL[b]	Physically compatible for 4 hr at 22°C	1558	C
Sodium bicarbonate	AB	1 mEq/mL	BW	1 mg/mL[b]	Tiny particles and haze form immediately. Large particles in 4 hr at 22°C	1558	I
Streptozocin	UP	40 mg/mL[b]	BW	1 mg/mL[b]	Physically compatible for 4 hr at 22°C	1558	C
Teniposide	BR	0.1 mg/mL[a]	BW	1 mg/mL[a]	Physically compatible for 4 hr at 23°C	1725	C
Thiotepa	LE	10 mg/mL[b]	BW	1 mg/mL[b]	Immediate cloudiness with particles	1558	I
Tobramycin sulfate	LI	5 mg/mL[b]	BW	1 mg/mL[b]	Physically compatible for 4 hr at 22°C	1558	C
Trimethoprim–sulfame-thoxazole	ES	0.8 mg/mL[b c]	BW	1 mg/mL[b]	Heavy white turbidity forms immediately, developing particles in 1 hr	1558	I
Vancomycin HCl	LY	10 mg/mL[b]	BW	1 mg/mL[b]	Physically compatible for 4 hr at 22°C	1558	C
Vinblastine sulfate	LI	0.12 mg/mL[b]	BW	1 mg/mL[b]	Physically compatible for 4 hr at 22°C	1558	C
Vincristine sulfate	LI	0.05 mg/mL[b]	BW	1 mg/mL[b]	Physically compatible for 4 hr at 22°C	1558	C
Zidovudine	BW	4 mg/mL[b]	BW	1 mg/mL[b]	Physically compatible for 4 hr at 22°C	1558	C

[a] Tested in dextrose 5%.

[b] Tested in sodium chloride 0.9%.

[c] Trimethoprim component. Trimethoprim in a 1:5 fixed-ratio concentration with sulfamethoxazole.

[d] Not specified whether concentration refers to single component or combined components.

Selected Revisions December 12, 2018. © Copyright, October 1996. American Society of Health-System Pharmacists, Inc.

Vitamin A
AHFS 88:04

Products

Vitamin A 50,000 international units/mL is available in 2-mL single-dose vials. Each mL also contains polysorbate 80, chlorobutanol, citric acid, and sodium hydroxide to adjust pH.[1(4/05)]

pH

From 6.5 to 7.1.[4]

Trade Name(s)

Aquasol A Parenteral

Administration

Vitamin A is administered intramuscularly.[1(4/05)] [4] Intravenous administration is not recommended.[1(4/05)]

Stability

Vitamin A is a light yellow to amber or red oil. It is sensitive to, and should be protected from, light and air.[4] Intact vials should be stored under refrigeration and protected from light and freezing.[1(4/05)] [4] Although refrigerated storage is required, the manufacturer has stated the drug may be stored at room temperature for 4 weeks.[2745]

The stability of retinol palmitate and tocopherols (δ, γ, and α) in 3-in-1 admixtures of amino acids 4%, dextrose 10%, fat emulsion 3% (Intralipid, Liposyn, and ClinOleic), various electrolytes, vitamins, and trace elements in ethylene vinyl acetate (EVA) bags over 3 days at 4, 25, and 37°C was determined. Retinol palmitate was unstable at room temperature with 33 and 50% degradation at 24 and 72 hours after compounding, respectively. Refrigeration of the admixture reduced the degradation to 29% at 72 hours.[2460]

The degradation of vitamins A, B₁, C, and E from Cernevit (Roche) multivitamins was evaluated in NuTRIflex Lipid Plus (B. Braun) admixtures prepared in ethylene vinyl acetate (EVA) bags and in multilayer bags. After storage for up to 72 hours at 4, 21, and 40°C, greater vitamin losses occurred in the EVA bags. Vitamin A (retinyl palmitate) losses were 20%. In the multilayer bags (presumably a better barrier to oxygen transfer), vitamin A (retinyl palmitate) losses were 5%.[2618]

The vitamins in Cernevit (Baxter) diluted in three 2-in-1 parenteral nutrition admixtures were tested for stability over 48 hours. Most of the other vitamins, including vitamin A, retained their initial concentrations.[2796]

Light Effects

A parenteral nutrition solution in glass bottles exposed to sunlight was evaluated. Vitamin A decomposed rapidly, losing more than 50% in 3 hours. The decomposition could be slowed to approximately a 25% loss in 3 hours by covering the bottle with a light-resistant vinyl bag.[1040]

Vitamin A was rapidly and significantly decomposed when exposed to daylight. The extent and rate of loss were dependent on the degree of exposure to daylight which, in turn, depended on various factors such as the direction of the radiation, time of day, and climatic conditions. Delivery of less than 10% of the expected amount was reported.[1047] In controlled light experiments, the decomposition initially progressed exponentially. Subsequently, the rate of decomposition slowed. This result was attributed to a protective effect of the degradation products on the remaining vitamin A. The presence of amino acids provided greater protection. Compared to degradation rates in dextrose 5%, decomposition was reduced by up to 50% in some amino acid mixtures.[1048]

In a parenteral nutrition solution composed of amino acids, dextrose, electrolytes, trace elements, and multivitamins in polyvinyl chloride (PVC) bags stored at 4 and 25°C, vitamin A rapidly deteriorated to 10% of the initial concentration in 8 hours at 25°C while exposed to light. The decomposition was slowed by light protection and refrigeration, with a loss of about 25% in 4 days.[1063]

Substantial loss of retinol all-trans palmitate was reported from both TPN and TNA admixtures due to exposure to sunlight. In 3 hours' exposure to sunlight, essentially total loss of retinol had occurred. The presence or absence of lipids did not affect stability. The container material used to store the nutrition admixtures affected the concentration of the vitamins as well. Losses were greatest in PVC containers and were slightly better in EVA and glass containers.[2049]

The photodegradation of vitamin A in 2-in-1 (Synthamin 9, Glucose 20%) and 3-in-1 (Synthamin 9, Glucose 20%, Intralipid 20%, electrolytes, vitamins, trace elements) admixtures was reported after exposure to 6 hours of indirect daylight. The compounded admixtures were prepared in multilayer bags protected from light and stored at 5°C for a minimum of 5 days. The same admixtures were prepared in EVA bags 24 hours prior to use with vitamins added prior to study. Vitamin A decreased to 60 to 80% of the initial concentrations in 2 to 6 hours. The type of bag had no influence on the photodegradation of vitamin A. Despite fat emulsion, no significant light protection was noted with the 3-in-1 admixture. The authors concluded that light protection can minimize vitamin A losses.[2459]

Sorption

Vitamin A (as the acetate) (Sigma) 7.5 mg/L displayed 66.7% sorption to a PVC plastic test strip in 24 hours. The presence of dextrose 5% and sodium chloride 0.9% increased the extent of sorption.[12]

Vitamin A acetate displayed 78% sorption to 200-mL PVC containers after 24 hours at 25°C with gentle shaking. The initial concentration was 3 mg/L. The sorption was increased by approximately 10% in sodium chloride 0.9% and by 20% in dextrose 5%.[133]

DOI: 10.37573/9781585286850.401

However, vitamin A delivery is also reduced in glass intravenous containers. At a concentration of 10,000 units/L in glass and PVC plastic containers protected from light with aluminum foil, 77 and 71%, respectively, of the vitamin A were delivered in 10 hours. Without light protection, 61% was delivered from glass and 49% from PVC plastic containers over a 10-hour period.[290]

In another test using multivitamin infusion (USV), 1 ampul/L of sodium chloride 0.9% in glass and PVC containers not protected from light, 69.4 and 67.9% of the vitamin A were delivered from the glass and PVC containers, respectively, in 10 hours. The amount of vitamin A was constant over this test period, not decreasing with time.[282]

The delivery of vitamins A, D, and E from a parenteral nutrition solution composed of 3% amino acid solution (Pharmacia) in dextrose 10% with electrolytes, trace elements, vitamin K, folate, and vitamin B_{12} was evaluated. To this solution was added 6 mL of multivitamin infusion (USV). The solution was prepared in PVC bags (Travenol), and administration was simulated through a fluid chamber (Buretrol) and infusion tubing with a 0.5-μm filter at 10 mL/hr. During the first 60 to 90 minutes, minimal delivery of the vitamins occurred. Then a rise and a plateau in the delivered vitamins followed and were attributed to an increasing saturation of adsorptive binding sites in the tubing. Total amounts delivered over 24 hours were: vitamin A, 31%; vitamin D, 68%; and vitamin E, 64%. Sorption of the vitamins was found in the PVC bag, fluid chamber, and tubing. Decomposition was not a factor.[836]

A patient receiving 3000 international units of retinol daily in a parenteral nutrition solution nevertheless experienced 2 episodes of night blindness. The pharmacy prepared the parenteral nutrition solution in 1-L PVC bags in weekly batches and stored them at 4°C in the dark until use. A subsequent in vitro study showed losses of vitamin A of 23 and 77% in 3- and 14-day periods, respectively, under these conditions. About 30% of the lost vitamin A could be extracted from the PVC bag.[1038]

Losses of vitamin A from neonatal parenteral nutrition solutions containing multivitamins (USV) was reported. The solution was prepared in colorless glass bottles and run through an administration set with a burette (Travenol). The total loss of vitamin A was 75% in 24 hours, with about 16% as decomposition in the glass bottle. The decomposition was not noticeable during the first 12 hours, but then vitamin A levels fell rather precipitously to about one-third of the initial amount. The balance of the loss, averaging about 59%, occurred during transit through the administration set. Removal of the inline filter and treatment of the set with albumin had no effect on vitamin A delivery. The authors recommended a three- to fourfold increase in the amount of vitamin A to compensate for the losses.[1039]

A 50% loss of vitamin A was noted from a bottle of parenteral nutrition solution prepared with multivitamin infusion (USV) after 5.5 hours of infusion. The amount delivered through an Ivex-2 filter set was only 6.3% of the added amount. Similar quantities were found after 20 hours of infusion. A reduced light exposure and use of ^{3}H-labeled vitamin A confirmed binding to the infusion bottles and tubing.[704]

Solutions containing multivitamins (USV) spiked with ^{3}H-labeled retinol in intravenous tubing protected from light and agitated to simulate flow for 5 hours were evaluated. About half of the vitamin A was lost in 30 minutes, and 88 to 96% was lost in 5 hours. Hexane rinses and radioactivity determinations on the tubing accounted for the decrease in radioactivity.[1049]

Neonatal parenteral nutrition solutions containing multivitamins prepared in bags were delivered at 10 mL/hr through Buretrol sets (Travenol). The bags and sets were protected from light. About 26% of the vitamin A was lost before the flow was started. At 10 mL/hr, about 67% was lost from the effluent. More rapid flow reduced the extent of loss. Analysis of clinical samples of parenteral nutrition solutions showed losses of 21 to 57% after 20 hours. Because losses after 5 hours were of the same magnitude, the authors concluded that the loss occurs rapidly and is not due to gradual decomposition.[1049]

The stability of numerous vitamins in parenteral nutrition solutions composed of amino acids (Kabi-Vitrum), dextrose 30%, and fat emulsion 20% (Kabi-Vitrum) in a 2:1:1 ratio with electrolytes, trace elements, and both fat- and water-soluble vitamins was reported. The admixtures were stored in darkness at 2 to 8°C for 96 hours with no significant loss of retinyl palmitate.[1225]

When the admixture was subjected to simulated infusion over 24 hours at 20°C, either exposed to room light or light protected, or stored for 6 days in the dark under refrigeration and then subjected to the same simulated infusion, once again the retinyl palmitate did not undergo significant loss.[1225]

Retinol losses of 40% occurred in 2 hours and 60% in 5 hours from parenteral nutrition solutions pumped at 10 mL/hr through standard infusion sets at room temperature. The retinol concentration in the bottle remained constant while the retinol in the effluent decreased. Antioxidants had no effect. Much of the vitamin A was recoverable from hexane washings of the tubing.[1050]

The stability of several vitamins from M.V.I.-12 (Armour) admixed in parenteral nutrition solutions composed of different amino acid products, with or without Intralipid 10%, when stored in glass bottles and PVC bags at 25 and 5°C for 48 hours was reported. No vitamin A was lost from any formula in glass bottles, but samples in PVC containers lost as much as 35 and 60% at 5 and 25°C, respectively, in 48 hours.[1431]

The stability of vitamin A was studied in 2 parenteral nutrition solutions. In TPN #172 (see Appendix), a 10% loss of vitamin A palmitate occurred in about 20 days in PVC bags while no loss occurred in Buretrol chambers in 21 days at 30°C with exposure to normal ward light. In TPN #173 (see Appendix), a 10% loss of vitamin A palmitate occurred in about 12 days in both glass and PVC containers at 2 to 8°C with protection from light.[1606]

The effects of the fat emulsion concentration on vitamin A stability in several parenteral nutrition solutions were evaluated. Vitamin A palmitate was not absorbed into PVC containers from Intralipid 10%. Among TPN solutions with lower Intralipid contents, no correlation existed between the fat emulsion content and the extent of vitamin A loss during refrigerated storage. The fat emulsion content afforded vitamin A some protection from decomposition due to light exposure at 30°C.[1607]

The quantity of retinol delivered from an M.V.I.-containing 2-in-1 parenteral nutrition solution and when M.V.I. was added to Intralipid 10% was evaluated during simulated administration through a PVC administration set. The parenteral nutrition solution was composed of amino acids 2.8%, dextrose 10%, and standard electrolytes; M.V.I. was added to yield a nominal retinol concentration of 455 mcg/150 mL. Retinol losses were about 80% of the admixed amount after being delivered through the PVC set. When M.V.I. was added to Intralipid 10% in a retinol concentration of 455 mcg/20 mL, retinol losses were reduced to about 10% of the admixed amount. The fat emulsion provided retinol protection from sorption to the PVC administration set.[2027]

Substantially higher amounts of retinol were found to be delivered using polyolefin administration set tubing than with PVC tubing during simulated neonatal intensive care administration. Retinol was added to a 2-in-1 parenteral nutrition solution (TPN #206) in concentrations of 25 and 50 international units/mL and run at 4 and 10 mL/hr through 3-meter lengths of polyolefin (MiniMed) and PVC (Baxter) intravenous extension set tubing protected from light and passed through a 37°C water bath. Delivered quantities of retinol varied from 19 to 74% through the PVC tubing and 47 to 87% through the polyolefin tubing. The loss of retinol to the PVC tubing appeared to be saturable. Even so, the use of polyolefin tubing increases the amount of retinol delivered during simulated neonatal administration.[2028]

To minimize the importance of sorption, use vitamin A palmitate, which does not sorb as extensively to PVC,[1033][1606][2026] instead of the acetate. However, this change does not alter the problem of degradation from exposure to light. Alternatively, an excess of vitamin A could be used.[1033]

Plasticizer Leaching

Vitamin A leached significant amounts of diethylhexyl phthalate (DEHP) plasticizer from PVC bags and administration set tubing.[1621]

Voriconazole
AHFS 8:14.08

Products

Voriconazole is available as a lyophilized powder in single-use (preservative-free) vials containing 200 mg of voriconazole with 3.2 g of sulfobutyl ether β-cyclodextrin sodium[3233][3348] or hydroxypropyl β-cyclodextrin[3347] and bearing a vacuum.[3233][3347][3348] Vial contents should be reconstituted with 19 mL of sterile water for injection, and the vial should be shaken until all of the powder is dissolved to yield 20 mL of a voriconazole 10-mg/mL solution.[3233][3347][3348] A 20-mL standard (non-automated) syringe should be used for reconstitution to ensure that the exact amount of sterile water for injection is added; the vial should be discarded if the vacuum does not draw the diluent into the vial.[3233][3347][3348]

The reconstituted solution is a concentrate that must be diluted in a compatible solution to a concentration of 0.5 to 5 mg/mL prior to intravenous administration.[3233][3347][3348] In order to achieve a final concentration in this range, the manufacturer recommends that a volume be removed from the infusion bag or bottle that is at least equivalent to the volume of drug to be added prior to addition of the drug.[3233][3347][3348]

Trade Name(s)
Vfend I.V.

Administration

Voriconazole is administered by intravenous infusion in a compatible infusion solution at a concentration between 0.5 and 5 mg/mL over 1 to 2 hours at a maximum rate of 3 mg/kg/hr.[3233][3347][3348] Voriconazole should *not* be administered as an intravenous bolus injection.[3233][3347][3348]

Stability

Voriconazole is available as a lyophilized white to off-white cake or powder.[3233][3347][3348] Intact vials should be stored at controlled room temperature.[3233][3347][3348] Voriconazole powder reconstituted as directed is chemically and physically stable for 24 hours at 2 to 8°C; however, because no antimicrobial preservative is present, the manufacturer recommends that the drug be used immediately after reconstitution.[3233][3347][3348] Voriconazole solutions should be visually inspected for particulate matter and discoloration prior to administration.[3233][3347][3348] Vials of voriconazole are intended for single use, and any remaining drug should be discarded.[3233][3347][3348]

Compatibility Information
Solution Compatibility

Voriconazole

Test Soln Name	Mfr	Mfr	Conc/L or %	Remarks	Ref	C/I
Dextrose 5% in Ringer's injection, lactated		PF, SZ	0.5 to 5 g	Manufacturer-recommended solution	3233, 3348	C
Dextrose 5% in Ringer's injection, lactated		XGN	0.5 to 5 g	Manufacturer-recommended solution	3347	C
Dextrose 5% in sodium chloride 0.45%		PF, SZ	0.5 to 5 g	Manufacturer-recommended solution	3233, 3348	C
Dextrose 5% in sodium chloride 0.45%		XGN	0.5 to 5 g	Manufacturer-recommended solution	3347	C
Dextrose 5% in sodium chloride 0.9%		PF, SZ	0.5 to 5 g	Manufacturer-recommended solution	3233, 3348	C
Dextrose 5% in sodium chloride 0.9%		XGN	0.5 to 5 g	Manufacturer-recommended solution	3347	C
Dextrose 5%[c]		PF, SZ	0.5 to 5 g	Manufacturer-recommended solution	3233, 3348	C
Dextrose 5%[c]		XGN	0.5 to 5 g	Manufacturer-recommended solution	3347	C
Dextrose 5%	[a]	PF	4 g	Visually compatible. 3% loss in 15 days at 4°C	2662	C
Dextrose 5%	MAC[b]	PF	2 g	Visually compatible. 9% loss in 6 days at 4°C and in 5 days at 25°C	2694	C
Dextrose 5%	[a]	PF	0.5 g	About 13% loss in 2 days at 19 to 24°C	3349	I
Dextrose 5%	[a]	PF	0.5 g	Physically compatible. Less than 10% loss in 9 days at 4 to 7°C	3349	C

DOI: 10.37573/9781585286850.402

Solution Compatibility (Cont.)

Test Soln Name	Mfr	Mfr	Conc/L or %	Remarks	Ref	C/I
Dextrose 5%	BA[d]	PF	2 g	Physically and chemically stable for 96 hr at 4°C and 4 hr at 25 and 35°C	3521	C
Ringer's injection, lactated		PF, SZ	0.5 to 5 g	Manufacturer-recommended solution	3233, 3348	C
Ringer's injection, lactated		XGN	0.5 to 5 g	Manufacturer-recommended solution	3347	C
Sodium chloride 0.45%		PF, SZ	0.5 to 5 g	Manufacturer-recommended solution	3233, 3348	C
Sodium chloride 0.45%		XGN	0.5 to 5 g	Manufacturer-recommended solution	3347	C
Sodium chloride 0.9%		PF, SZ	0.5 to 5 g	Manufacturer-recommended solution	3233, 3348	C
Sodium chloride 0.9%		XGN	0.5 to 5 g	Manufacturer-recommended solution	3347	C
Sodium chloride 0.9%	MAC[b]	PF	2 g	No loss over 32 days at 4°C	2624	C
Sodium chloride 0.9%	MAC[b]	PF	2 g	Visually compatible. No loss at 4°C and 5% loss at 25°C in 8 days	2694	C
Sodium chloride 0.9%	[a]	PF	0.5 g	About 12% loss in 2 days at 19 to 24°C	3349	I
Sodium chloride 0.9%	[a]	PF	0.5 g	Physically compatible. Less than 10% loss in 7 days at 4 to 7°C	3349	C
Sodium chloride 0.9%	BA[d]	PF	2 g	Physically and chemically stable for 96 hr at 4°C and 4 hr at 25 and 35°C	3521	C

[a] Tested in PVC containers.

[b] Tested in polyolefin containers.

[c] Tested with and without potassium chloride 20 mEq present.

[d] Tested in Intermate SV elastomeric pump reservoirs.

Additive Compatibility

Voriconazole

Test Drug	Mfr	Conc/L or %	Mfr	Conc/L or %	Test Solution	Remarks	Ref	C/I
Sodium bicarbonate		4.2%	PF, SZ			Voriconazole slightly decomposes at room temperature	3233, 3348	I
Sodium bicarbonate		4.2%	XGN			Voriconazole slightly decomposes at room temperature	3347	I

Y-Site Injection Compatibility (1:1 Mixture)

Voriconazole

Test Drug	Mfr	Conc	Mfr	Conc	Remarks	Ref	C/I
Anidulafungin	VIC	0.5 mg/mL[a]	PF	4 mg/mL[a]	Physically compatible for 4 hr at 23°C	2617	C
Cangrelor tetrasodium	TMC	1 mg/mL[b]		4 mg/mL[b]	Physically compatible for 4 hr	3243	C
Caspofungin acetate	ME	0.7 mg/mL[b]	PF	4 mg/mL[b]	Physically compatible for 4 hr at room temperature	2758	C
Caspofungin acetate	ME	0.5 mg/mL[b]	PF	2 mg/mL[b]	Physically compatible over 60 min	2766	C
Ceftaroline fosamil	FOR	2.22 mg/mL[a b d]	PF	4 mg/mL[a b d]	Physically compatible for 4 hr at 23°C	2826	C
Cloxacillin sodium	SMX	100 mg/mL	PF	10 mg/mL	Physically compatible for up to 4 hr at room temperature	3245	C

Y-Site Injection Compatibility (1:1 Mixture) (Cont.)

Test Drug	Mfr	Conc	Mfr	Conc	Remarks	Ref	C/I
Doripenem	JJ	5 mg/mL[a][b]	PF	4 mg/mL[a][b]	Physically compatible for 4 hr at 23°C	2743	C
Meropenem		50 mg/mL	SZ	10 mg/mL	Physically compatible for 4 hr at room temperature	3538	C
Posaconazole	ME	18 mg/mL		5 mg/mL[e]	Physically compatible	2912	C
Tigecycline	WY	1 mg/mL[b]	PF	2 mg/mL[b]	Microparticulates form	2714	I
Vasopressin	APP	0.2 unit/mL[b]	PF	3 mg/mL[c]	Physically compatible	2641	C

[a] Tested in dextrose 5%.

[b] Tested in sodium chloride 0.9%.

[c] Tested in sodium chloride 0.45%.

[d] Tested in Ringer's injection, lactated.

[e] Tested in both dextrose 5% and sodium chloride 0.9%.

Additional Compatibility Information

Other Drugs

Manufacturers state that voriconazole must not be infused concomitantly with any short-term infusion of concentrated electrolytes, even if the infusions are running in separate intravenous lines or cannulas. Voriconazole may be infused at the same time as other intravenous solutions containing nonconcentrated electrolytes, but still must be infused through a separate line.[3233][3347][3348]

Parenteral Nutrition Solutions

Manufacturers state that voriconazole may be infused at the same time as parenteral nutrition solutions, but must be infused through a separate line. If a multiple-lumen catheter is used, the parenteral nutrition solution must be administered through a different port than the one used for voriconazole administration.[3233][3347][3348]

Selected Revisions May 1, 2020. © Copyright, October 2008. American Society of Health-System Pharmacists, Inc.

Ziconotide Acetate
AHFS 28:08.92

Products

Ziconotide acetate is available as a 100-mcg/mL solution in 1- and 5-mL single-use vials and as a 25-mcg/mL solution in 20-mL single-use vials.[3167] The formulation also contains L-methionine and sodium chloride excipients, but is preservative free.[3167]

pH

From 4 to 5.[3167]

Osmolarity

Ziconotide acetate in sodium chloride 0.9% at concentrations ranging from 0.25 to 1 mcg/mL had an osmolarity of 308 mOsm/L.[3170]

Trade Name(s)

Prialt

Administration

Ziconotide acetate is administered intrathecally either undiluted (using the 25-mcg/mL solution) or diluted (using the 100-mcg/mL solution) using a programmable implanted variable-rate microinfusion device or an external microinfusion device and catheter.[3167] The 100-mcg/mL solution must be diluted only in preservative-free sodium chloride 0.9%; saline solutions containing preservatives are *not* appropriate for intrathecal drug administration.[3167] Once an appropriate dose has been established, the 100-mcg/mL solution may be administered undiluted.[3167]

The drug is intended for use only with the Medtronic SynchroMed II Infusion System or the CADD-Micro Ambulatory Infusion Pump.[3167]

When using the Medtronic SynchroMed II Infusion System, only the undiluted 25-mcg/mL solution should be used for the initial priming of a new pump.[3167] Three 2-mL rinses of the internal surfaces of the new pump should be performed using the undiluted 25-mcg/mL solution.[3167] After performing the initial rinses of a new pump, only the undiluted 25-mcg/mL solution should be used for the first fill of the pump.[3167] The new pump should be refilled within 14 days of the first fill in order to ensure appropriate dose administration because of initial losses of the drug due to both sorption to titanium internal surfaces and dilution in the residual space of the pump.[3167] Losses resulting from these 2 factors do not occur upon subsequent refill.[3167] For subsequent refills, the pumps should be filled at least every 84 days if the drug is used undiluted or at least every 40 days if the drug is diluted.[3167] The remaining pump contents should be emptied prior to refilling.[3167] A Medtronic refill kit should be used to ensure aseptic transfer of the drug solution into the pump.[3167] The pump manufacturer's manual should be consulted for specific instructions and precautions on rinsing the reservoir, initial filling of the reservoir, refilling the reservoir, and programming the infusion system.[3167]

When using the CADD-Micro Ambulatory Infusion Pump, the pump initially should be filled with ziconotide acetate solution that has been diluted in preservative-free sodium chloride 0.9% to a concentration of 5 mcg/mL.[3167] The pump manufacturer's manual should be consulted for specific instructions and precautions on initial filling of the reservoir, refilling the reservoir or replacing the drug cartridge, and operation of the pump.[3167]

Ziconotide acetate injection is *not* intended for intravenous administration.[3167]

Stability

Intact vials of ziconotide acetate should be stored under refrigeration and protected from light and freezing.[3167] Ziconotide acetate diluted in preservative-free sodium chloride 0.9% may be stored at 2 to 8°C for up to 24 hours prior to beginning the infusion.[3167]

pH Effects

In a study evaluating the influence of pH and temperature on the stability of ziconotide, admixtures of ziconotide acetate, morphine sulfate, and ropivacaine hydrochloride were prepared in a range of concentrations and stored in syringes (Plastipak, BD) at 4 or 20°C or Medtronic SynchroMed II pumps at 37°C.[3168] The resulting pH of the admixtures was influenced by the morphine concentration and the storage temperature.[3168] Admixtures with lower morphine concentrations resulted in a higher pH; admixtures stored at lower temperatures resulted in a lower pH.[3168] Ziconotide prepared in admixtures with lower morphine concentrations and stored at 37°C demonstrated improved ziconotide stability.[3168] Admixtures with a pH exceeding 4.5 demonstrated improved ziconotide stability compared with admixtures with a pH less than 4.5.[3168]

Ambulatory Pumps

Ziconotide acetate is intended for use with the CADD-Micro Ambulatory Infusion Pump.[3167]

Implantable Pumps

Ziconotide acetate is intended for use with the Medtronic SynchroMed II Infusion System.[3167] The manufacturer of ziconotide states that the initial fill of a new pump with 25 mcg/mL of undiluted solution expires in 14 days; subsequent refills with undiluted 25- or 100-mcg/mL solutions of the drug expire in 84 days.[3167] Refills using diluted solutions prepared from the 100-mcg/mL formulation of the drug expire in 40 days.[3167]

In November 2012, Medtronic Neuromodulation warned that intermittent or permanent pump motor stalling due to corrosion has occurred in SynchroMed infusion systems after use of unapproved drugs and drug formulations (i.e., drugs not listed in the device's labeling, including admixtures, compounded drugs, and unapproved drug concentrations).[3169] Medtronic has confirmed through returned product analysis and in vitro testing that such

DOI: 10.37573/9781585286850.403

permanent pump motor stalling has been caused by admixtures containing drugs such as baclofen, bupivacaine, clonidine, fentanyl, hydromorphone, morphine, and sufentanil.[3169] Some antimicrobial or antioxidant preservatives (e.g., sodium metabisulfite) are known to cause pump damage, while some admixtures may have increased the rates of permeation of corrosive agents; admixtures with a pH of 3 or less and those requiring additives to maintain the solubility of a particular concentration also may not be compatible with the infusion system.[3169] Pump problems from previous use of an unapproved drug formulation may persist even if an approved drug formulation is used subsequently.[3169] Medtronic states that only those drugs and drug formulations for which the SynchroMed infusion system is approved should be used to minimize the potential for damage to the internal pump components.[3169]

Clonidine hydrochloride and morphine sulfate powders were dissolved in ziconotide acetate (Elan) injection to yield concentrations of 2 and 35 mg/mL and 25 mcg/mL, respectively.[2752] Stored at 37°C in Medtronic SynchroMed II pumps, 11% ziconotide loss in 7 days, 4% clonidine loss in 20 days, and no morphine loss in 28 days occurred.[2752]

Compatibility Information

Additive Compatibility

Ziconotide acetate

Test Drug	Mfr	Conc/L or %	Mfr	Conc/L or %	Test Solution	Remarks	Ref	C/I
Bupivacaine HCl	BB	5 g[b]	ELN	25 mg[a]		90% ziconotide retained for 22 days at 37°C. No bupivacaine loss in 30 days	2751	C
Clonidine HCl	BB	2 g[b]	ELN	25 mg[a]		No loss of either drug in 28 days at 37°C	2703	C
Fentanyl citrate	BB	1 g[b]	ELN	25 mg[a]		10% ziconotide loss in 26 days. No fentanyl loss in 40 days at 37°C	2772	C
Hydromorphone HCl	BB	35 g[b]	ELN	25 mg[a]		90% ziconotide retained for 19 days at 37°C. No hydromorphone loss in 25 days	2702	C
Morphine sulfate	BB	35 g[b]	ELN	25 mg[a]		90% ziconotide retained for 8 days at 37°C. No morphine loss in 17 days	2702	C
Morphine sulfate	BB	20 g[b]	ELN	25 mg[a]		90% ziconotide retained for 19 days at 37°C. No morphine loss in 28 days	2713	C
Morphine sulfate	BB	20 g[b]	ELN	25 mg[a]		10% ziconotide loss in 19 days. No morphine loss in 28 days at 37°C	2780	C
Morphine sulfate	BB	10 g[b]	ELN	25 mg[a]		10% ziconotide loss in 34 days. No morphine loss in 60 days at 37°C	2780	C
Morphine sulfate	CDM [d]	2 g	EI	200 mg	NS[c]	Visually compatible and chemically stable for up to 14 days at 21°C	3493	C
Ropivacaine HCl	FRK[e]	6 g	EI	200 mg	NS[c]	Visually compatible and chemically stable for up to 14 days at 21°C	3493	C
Sufentanil citrate	BB	1 g[b]	ELN	25 mg[a]		10% ziconotide loss in 33 days. No sufentanil loss in 40 days at 37°C	2772	C

[a] Tested in SynchroMed II implantable pumps.

[b] Drug powder dissolved in ziconotide acetate injection.

[c] Tested in polyolefin containers.

[d] Tested with ropivacaine HCl (FRK) 6 g/L.

[e] Tested with morphine sulfate (CDM) 2 g/L.

Drugs in Syringe Compatibility

Ziconotide acetate

Test Drug	Mfr	Amt	Mfr	Amt	Remarks	Ref	C/I
Clonidine HCl	BB	2 mg/mL[a]	ELN	25 mcg/mL	No loss of either drug in 28 days at 5°C	2703	C
Hydromorphone HCl	BB	35 mg/mL[a]	ELN	25 mcg/mL	No loss of either drug in 25 days at 5°C	2702	C
Morphine sulfate	BB	35 mg/mL[a]	ELN	25 mcg/mL	No loss of either drug in 17 days at 5°C	2702	C
Morphine sulfate	CDM[b]	3.5 mg/mL[d]	EI	1 mcg/mL[d]	Visually compatible and chemically stable for up to 3 days at 5°C	3493	C
Morphine sulfate	CDM[b]	3.5 mg/mL[d]	EI	1 mcg/mL[d]	Chemically unstable after 6 hr at 21 and 31°C	3493	I
Ropivacaine HCl	FRK[c]	7.5 mg/mL[d]	EI	1 mcg/mL[d]	Visually compatible and chemically stable for up to 3 days at 5°C	3493	C
Ropivacaine HCl	FRK[c]	7.5 mg/mL[d]	EI	1 mcg/mL[d]	Chemically unstable after 6 hr at 21 and 31°C	3493	I

[a] Drug powder dissolved in ziconotide acetate injection.

[b] Tested with ropivacaine HCl (FRK) 7.5 mg/mL.

[c] Tested with morphine sulfate (CDM) 3.5 mg/mL.

[d] Tested in sodium chloride 0.9%.

Selected Revisions January 31, 2020. © Copyright, October 2008. American Society of Health-System Pharmacists, Inc.

Zidovudine
AHFS 8:18.08.20

Products

Zidovudine is available in 20-mL single-use vials. Each mL of solution contains zidovudine 10 mg in water for injection. Hydrochloric acid and/or sodium hydroxide may be present to adjust the pH.[1(10/06)]

pH

Approximately 5.5.[1(10/06)]

Trade Name(s)

Retrovir

Administration

Zidovudine must be diluted in dextrose 5% to a concentration no greater than 4 mg/mL prior to administration. The drug is administered by intravenous infusion at a constant rate over 1 hour.[1(10/06)] [4] Zidovudine also has been administered by continuous intravenous infusion.[4] Intramuscular injection, intravenous bolus, and rapid intravenous infusion should be avoided.[1(10/06)] [4]

Stability

Intact vials of zidovudine should be stored at 15 to 25°C and protected from light.[1(10/06)]

Central Venous Catheter

Zidovudine (Glaxo Wellcome) 1 mg/mL in dextrose 5% was found to be compatible with the ARROWg+ard Blue Plus (Arrow International) chlorhexidine-bearing triple-lumen central catheter. Essentially complete delivery of the drug was found with little or no drug loss occurring. Furthermore, chlorhexidine delivered from the catheter remained at trace amounts with no substantial increase due to the delivery of the drug through the catheter.[2335]

Compatibility Information

Solution Compatibility

Zidovudine

Test Soln Name	Mfr	Mfr	Conc/L or %	Remarks	Ref	C/I
Dextrose 5%				Stable for 24 hr at room temperature and 48 hr refrigerated. Use within 8 hr at room temperature and 24 hr refrigerated recommended	1(10/06)	C
Dextrose 5%	a	BW	4 g	Physically compatible. No loss in 8 days at 4 and 25°C	1411	C
Sodium chloride 0.9%	a	BW	4 g	Physically compatible. No loss in 8 days at 4 and 25°C	1411	C

a Tested in PVC containers.

Additive Compatibility

Zidovudine

Test Drug	Mfr	Conc/L or %	Mfr	Conc/L or %	Test Solution	Remarks	Ref	C/I
Dobutamine HCl	AB	1 g	GW	2 g	D5W	No more than 5% loss for either drug at 23°C and 2% loss at 4°C in 24 hr	2489	C
Dobutamine HCl	AB	1 g	GW	2 g	NS	No more than 4% loss for either drug at 23°C and 2% loss at 4°C in 24 hr	2489	C
Meropenem	ZEN	1 g	BW	4 g	NS	Visually compatible for 4 hr at room temperature	1994	C
Meropenem	ZEN	20 g	BW	4 g	NS	Dark yellow discoloration forms in 4 hr at room temperature	1994	I

DOI: 10.37573/9781585286850.404

Additive Compatibility (Cont.)

Test Drug	Mfr	Conc/L or %	Mfr	Conc/L or %	Test Solution	Remarks	Ref	C/I
Ranitidine HCl	GSK	500 mg	GSK	2 g	NS	Physically compatible with no loss of either drug in 24 hr at 4 and 23°C	2523	C
Ranitidine HCl	GSK	500 mg	GSK	2 g	D5W	Physically compatible. Up to 8% ranitidine loss at 23°C and 2% at 4°C in 24 hr. Zidovudine losses of 5 to 6% in 24 hr at 4 and 23°C	2523	C

Drugs in Syringe Compatibility

Zidovudine

Test Drug	Mfr	Amt	Mfr	Amt	Remarks	Ref	C/I
Pantoprazole sodium	a	4 mg/1 mL		10 mg/1 mL	Clear solution	2574	C

a Test performed using the formulation WITHOUT edetate disodium.

Y-Site Injection Compatibility (1:1 Mixture)

Zidovudine

Test Drug	Mfr	Conc	Mfr	Conc	Remarks	Ref	C/I
Acyclovir sodium	BW	7 mg/mLa	BW	4 mg/mLa	Physically compatible for 4 hr at 25°C	1193	C
Allopurinol sodium	BW	3 mg/mLb	BW	4 mg/mLb	Physically compatible for 4 hr at 22°C	1686	C
Amifostine	USB	10 mg/mLa	BW	4 mg/mLa	Physically compatible for 4 hr at 23°C	1845	C
Amikacin sulfate	BR	4 mg/mLa	BW	4 mg/mLa	Physically compatible for 4 hr at 25°C	1193	C
Amphotericin B	SQ	600 mcg/mLa	BW	4 mg/mLa	Physically compatible for 4 hr at 25°C	1193	C
Anidulafungin	VIC	0.5 mg/mLa	GSK	4 mg/mLa	Physically compatible for 4 hr at 23°C	2617	C
Aztreonam	SQ	40 mg/mLa	BW	4 mg/mLa	Physically compatible for 4 hr at 25°C	1193	C
Aztreonam	SQ	40 mg/mLa	BW	4 mg/mLa	Physically compatible for 4 hr at 23°C	1758	C
Ceftazidime	GL	20 mg/mLa	BW	4 mg/mLa	Physically compatible for 4 hr at 25°C	1193	C
Ceftriaxone sodium	RC	20 mg/mLa	BW	4 mg/mLa	Physically compatible for 4 hr at 25°C	1193	C
Cisatracurium besylate	GW	0.1, 2, 5 mg/mLa	BW	4 mg/mLa	Physically compatible for 4 hr at 23°C	2074	C
Clindamycin phosphate	UP	12 mg/mLa	BW	4 mg/mLa	Physically compatible for 4 hr at 25°C	1193	C
Dexamethasone sodium phosphate	ES	0.16 mg/mLa	BW	4 mg/mLa	Physically compatible for 4 hr at 25°C	1193	C
Dobutamine HCl	LI	5 mg/mLa	BW	4 mg/mLa	Physically compatible for 4 hr at 25°C	1193	C
Docetaxel	RPR	0.9 mg/mLa	GW	4 mg/mLa	Physically compatible for 4 hr at 23°C	2224	C
Dopamine HCl	AB	1.6 mg/mLa	BW	4 mg/mLa	Physically compatible for 4 hr at 25°C	1193	C
Doripenem	JJ	5 mg/mLa b	GSK	4 mg/mLa b	Physically compatible for 4 hr at 23°C	2743	C
Doxorubicin HCl liposomal	SEQ	0.4 mg/mLa	BW	4 mg/mLa	Physically compatible for 4 hr at 23°C	2087	C
Erythromycin lactobionate	AB	20 mg/mLa c	BW	4 mg/mLa	Physically compatible for 4 hr at 25°C	1193	C
Etoposide phosphate	BR	5 mg/mLa	BW	4 mg/mLa	Physically compatible for 4 hr at 23°C	2218	C

Y-Site Injection Compatibility (1:1 Mixture) (Cont.)

Test Drug	Mfr	Conc	Mfr	Conc	Remarks	Ref	C/I
Filgrastim	AMG	30 mcg/mL[a]	BW	4 mg/mL[a]	Physically compatible for 4 hr at 22°C	1687	C
Fluconazole	RR	2 mg/mL	BW	10 mg/mL	Physically compatible for 24 hr at 25°C	1407	C
Fludarabine phosphate	BX	1 mg/mL[a]	BW	4 mg/mL[a]	Visually compatible for 4 hr at 22°C	1439	C
Gemcitabine HCl	LI	10 mg/mL[b]	GW	4 mg/mL[b]	Physically compatible for 4 hr at 23°C	2226	C
Gentamicin sulfate	IMS	2 mg/mL[a]	BW	4 mg/mL[a]	Physically compatible for 4 hr at 25°C	1193	C
Granisetron HCl	SKB	0.05 mg/mL[a]	BW	4 mg/mL[a]	Physically compatible for 4 hr at 23°C	2000	C
Heparin sodium	LY	100 units/mL[a]	BW	4 mg/mL[a]	Physically compatible for 4 hr at 25°C	1193	C
Imipenem–cilastatin sodium	MSD	5 mg/mL[a j]	BW	4 mg/mL[a]	Physically compatible for 4 hr at 25°C	1193	C
Linezolid	PHU	2 mg/mL	GW	4 mg/mL[a]	Physically compatible for 4 hr at 23°C	2264	C
Lorazepam	WY	80 mcg/mL[a]	BW	4 mg/mL[a]	Physically compatible for 4 hr at 25°C	1193	C
Melphalan HCl	BW	0.1 mg/mL[b]	BW	4 mg/mL[b]	Physically compatible for 3 hr at 22°C	1557	C
Meropenem	ZEN	1 mg/mL[b]	BW	4 mg/mL[d]	Visually compatible for 4 hr at room temperature	1994	C
Meropenem	ZEN	50 mg/mL[b]	BW	4 mg/mL[d]	Yellow color in 4 hr at room temperature	1994	I
Metoclopramide HCl	RB	2 mg/mL[a]	BW	4 mg/mL[a]	Physically compatible for 4 hr at 25°C	1193	C
Morphine sulfate	ES	1 mg/mL[a]	BW	4 mg/mL[a]	Physically compatible for 4 hr at 25°C	1193	C
Nafcillin sodium	BR	20 mg/mL[a]	BW	4 mg/mL[a]	Physically compatible for 4 hr at 25°C	1193	C
Ondansetron HCl	GL	1 mg/mL[b]	BW	4 mg/mL[a]	Visually compatible for 4 hr at 22°C	1365	C
Oxacillin sodium	BR	20 mg/mL[a]	BW	4 mg/mL[a]	Physically compatible for 4 hr at 25°C	1193	C
Oxytocin	NVA	10 milliunits/mL[a]	GSK	2 mg/mL[a]	Visually compatible with no zidovudine loss in 6 hr at 20°C	2491	C
Oxytocin	NVA	10 milliunits/mL[a]	GSK	4 mg/mL[a]	Visually compatible with no zidovudine loss in 6 hr at 20°C	2491	C
Paclitaxel	NCI	1.2 mg/mL[a]	BW	4 mg/mL[a]	Physically compatible for 4 hr at 22°C	1556	C
Pemetrexed disodium	LI	20 mg/mL[b]	GSK	4 mg/mL[a]	Physically compatible for 4 hr at 23°C	2564	C
Pentamidine isethionate	LY	6 mg/mL[a]	BW	4 mg/mL[a]	Physically compatible for 4 hr at 25°C	1193	C
Phenylephrine HCl	WI	1 mg/mL[a]	BW	4 mg/mL[a]	Physically compatible for 4 hr at 25°C	1193	C
Piperacillin sodium–tazo-bactam sodium	LE[g]	40 mg/mL[a h]	BW	4 mg/mL[a]	Physically compatible for 4 hr at 22°C	1688	C
Potassium chloride	IMS	0.67 mEq/mL[a]	BW	4 mg/mL[a]	Physically compatible for 4 hr at 25°C	1193	C
Ranitidine HCl	GL	1 mg/mL[a]	BW	4 mg/mL[a]	Physically compatible for 4 hr at 25°C	1193	C
Remifentanil HCl	GW	0.025 and 0.25 mg/mL[b]	BW	4 mg/mL[a]	Physically compatible for 4 hr at 23°C	2075	C
Sargramostim	IMM	10 mcg/mL[b]	BW	4 mg/mL[b]	Visually compatible for 4 hr at 22°C	1436	C
Teniposide	BR	0.1 mg/mL[a]	BW	4 mg/mL[a]	Physically compatible for 4 hr at 23°C	1725	C
Thiotepa	IMM[e]	1 mg/mL[a]	BW	4 mg/mL[a]	Physically compatible for 4 hr at 23°C	1861	C
TNA #218 to #226[f]			GW	4 mg/mL[a]	Visually compatible for 4 hr at 23°C	2215	C

Y-Site Injection Compatibility (1:1 Mixture) (Cont.)

Test Drug	Mfr	Conc	Mfr	Conc	Remarks	Ref	C/I
Tobramycin sulfate	LI	2 mg/mL[a]	BW	4 mg/mL[a]	Physically compatible for 4 hr at 25°C	1193	C
TPN #212 to #215[f]			BW	4 mg/mL[a]	Physically compatible for 4 hr at 23°C	2109	C
Trimethoprim–sulfamethox-azole	BW	0.53 mg/mL[a] [i]	BW	4 mg/mL[a]	Physically compatible for 4 hr at 25°C	1193	C
Vancomycin HCl	LI	15 mg/mL[a]	BW	4 mg/mL[a]	Physically compatible for 4 hr at 25°C	1193	C
Vinorelbine tartrate	BW	1 mg/mL[b]	BW	4 mg/mL[b]	Physically compatible for 4 hr at 22°C	1558	C

[a] Tested in dextrose 5%.

[b] Tested in sodium chloride 0.9%.

[c] Sodium bicarbonate 2.5 mEq added to adjust pH.

[d] Tested in sterile water for injection.

[e] Lyophilized formulation tested.

[f] Refer to Appendix for the composition of parenteral nutrition solutions. TNA indicates a 3-in-1 admixture, and TPN indicates a 2-in-1 admixture.

[g] Test performed using the formulation WITHOUT edetate disodium.

[h] Piperacillin component. Piperacillin in an 8:1 fixed-ratio concentration with tazobactam.

[i] Trimethoprim component. Trimethoprim in a 1:5 fixed-ratio concentration with sulfamethoxazole.

[j] Not specified whether concentration refers to single component or combined components.

Selected Revisions December 13, 2018. © Copyright, October 1992. American Society of Health-System Pharmacists, Inc.

Ziv-aflibercept

AHFS 10:00

Products

Ziv-aflibercept is available as a 25-mg/mL concentrate for injection in single-use vials containing 100 or 200 mg of the drug.[2877] Each vial also contains polysorbate 20 0.1%, sodium chloride 100 mM, sodium citrate 5 mM, sodium phosphate 5 mM, and sucrose 20% in water for injection.[2877] The concentrate must be diluted before administration.[2877]

pH

6.2[2877]

Trade Name(s)

Zaltrap

Administration

Ziv-aflibercept is administered by intravenous infusion over one hour following dilution in a compatible diluent to a concentration of 0.6 to 8 mg/mL.[2877] The diluted drug should be administered through a 0.2- or 0.22-μm inline polyethersulfone filter.[2877] [2878] Ziv-aflibercept should *not* be administered as a bolus or push intravenous injection.[2877]

Stability

Ziv-aflibercept concentrate is a clear, colorless to pale yellow solution.[2877] Intact vials should be stored under refrigeration and kept in the original outer carton to protect from light.[2877]

Visually inspect ziv-aflibercept before use.[2877] Discard if the solution is cloudy, contains particles, or is discolored.[2877]

Single-use vials of ziv-aflibercept do not contain any preservatives.[2877] After the appropriate dose has been withdrawn from the vial upon initial puncture, the vial should not be re-entered, and any unused portion should be discarded.[2877]

Diluted solutions of ziv-aflibercept should be prepared in infusion containers composed of either PVC (containing either diethylhexyl phthalate [DEHP] or trioctyl trimellitate [TOTM]) or polyolefin (e.g., polypropylene, polyethylene).[2877] [2878] Ziv-aflibercept should *not* be prepared in infusion containers composed of ethylene vinyl acetate (EVA).[2878]

Diluted solutions of ziv-aflibercept should be used immediately.[2878] Admixtures not used immediately should be refrigerated for up to 4 hours.[2877] Any unused portion remaining in the infusion bag following administration should be discarded.[2877]

Light Effects

Ziv-aflibercept concentrate is light sensitive.[2878] Vials of the concentrate should be stored in the original outer carton to protect from light.[2877] The manufacturer does not specify a need for protecting the diluted solution from light.[2878]

Sorption

No substantial changes in the quality or potency of the drug were noted when diluted solutions of ziv-aflibercept (0.6 to 8 mg/mL) were tested with infusion sets composed of DEHP-plasticized PVC, TOTM-plasticized PVC, polyethylene-lined PVC, or polypropylene.[2877] [2878] Infusion sets composed of polyurethane also were found to be compatible.[2877] [2878]

Filtration

For ziv-aflibercept administration, the manufacturer recommends the use of either a 0.2- or 0.22-μm inline polyethersulfone filter.[2878] Filters composed of polyvinylidene fluoride or nylon were noted to facilitate adsorption during stability testing[2878] and should not be used.[2877]

Compatibility Information

Solution Compatibility

Ziv-aflibercept

Test Soln Name		Mfr	Mfr	Conc/L or %	Remarks	Ref	C/I
Dextrose 5%	a		SAA	600 mg to 8 g	Compatible and stable for 4 hr under refrigeration	2877	C
Sodium chloride 0.9%	a		SAA	600 mg to 8 g	Compatible and stable for 4 hr under refrigeration	2877	C

a Tested in PVC and polyolefin containers.

DOI: 10.37573/9781585286850.405

Zoledronic Acid

AHFS 92:24

Products

Zoledronic acid is available as a ready-to-use solution in single-use bottles[3140] and bags[3142 3143] and as a concentrate for injection in 5-mL single-use vials[3140] containing the equivalent of 4 mg of zoledronic acid.[3140 3142 3143]

Each 100-mL bottle of zoledronic acid (Zometa®; Novartis) ready-to-use solution also contains mannitol 5100 mg and sodium citrate 24 mg in water for injection;[3140] 100-mL bags of ready-to-use solution from other manufacturers also contain sodium chloride 900 mg, mannitol 220 mg, and sodium citrate 24 mg to adjust the pH in water for injection.[3142 3143] Some bottles and bags also contain overfill.[3140 3142]

Vials of zoledronic acid concentrate for injection also contain mannitol 220 mg and sodium citrate 24 mg in water for injection.[3140] The appropriate dose of the concentrate must be withdrawn from the vial and diluted in 100 mL of sodium chloride 0.9% or dextrose 5% immediately prior to administration.[3140] Vials contain overfill to allow for withdrawal of 5 mL of concentrate.[3140]

Zoledronic acid also is available as a lyophilized powder in single-use vials containing the equivalent of 4 mg zoledronic acid.[3141] Each vial also contains mannitol 220 mg and sodium citrate dihydrate to adjust the pH.[3141] Each vial is packaged with an ampul of diluent containing 5 mL of sterile water for injection.[3141] The powder should be reconstituted by adding 5 mL of the diluent to the vial.[3141] Once the vial contents are completely dissolved, the appropriate dose of the resulting concentrate should be withdrawn from the vial with a syringe and further diluted in 100 mL of sodium chloride 0.9% or dextrose 5%.[3141]

Zoledronic acid also is available as a ready-to-use solution in single-use 100-mL bottles[3139] or bags[3144] containing the equivalent of 5 mg of zoledronic acid.[3139 3144] Each bottle or bag also contains mannitol 4950 mg and sodium citrate 30 mg.[3139 3144]

Equivalency

Zoledronic acid 4.264 mg as the monohydrate is equivalent to 4 mg of zoledronic acid.[3140 3141] Zoledronic acid 5.33 mg as the monohydrate is equivalent to 5 mg of zoledronic acid.[3139]

pH

Ready-to-use solutions of zoledronic acid 4 mg in 100 mL (Sagent) have a pH from 5.5 to 6.5.[3142] Ready-to-use solutions of zoledronic acid 5 mg in 100 mL have a pH from 6 to 7.[3139]

The reconstituted zoledronic acid concentrate for injection has a pH from 5.7 to 6.7.[3141]

Trade Name(s)

Reclast, Zometa

Administration

Zoledronic acid concentrate for injection (commercially available or prepared by reconstituting the lyophilized powder) must be diluted prior to administration.[3140 3141]

Ready-to-use solutions may be administered directly without further preparation.[3140 3142] To prepare reduced doses of zoledronic acid (Zometa®) using the 4-mg ready-to-use solution, 12, 18, or 25 mL of the solution should be withdrawn from the container and discarded to yield a zoledronic acid dose of 3.5, 3.3, or 3 mg, respectively; a volume equal to that removed should then be replaced with sodium chloride 0.9% or dextrose 5%.[3140] Another manufacturer (Hospira) recommends that such volumes be removed from the 4-mg container of ready-to-use solution using an intravenous bag transfer device and discarded and that the premixed bag then be labeled to reflect the final drug content and total fluid volume remaining in the container.[3143] The manufacturers of the 5-mg ready-to-use solutions of zoledronic acid do not provide recommendations for preparation of reduced doses.[3139 3144]

Zoledronic acid solution is administered intravenously over a period of at least 15 minutes.[3139 3140 3141] If solutions for infusion have been refrigerated, the solution should be allowed to come to room temperature prior to administration.[3139 3140 3141]

Zoledronic acid should be infused through a separate vented infusion line.[3139 3140 3141] The manufacturers of Reclast® (Novartis) and those of corresponding generic formulations recommend that the line should be flushed with at least 10 mL of sodium chloride 0.9% following infusion of zoledronic acid solution.[3139 3144] Zoledronic acid solution must not be mixed with or allowed to contact calcium or any other solutions containing divalent cations (e.g., Ringer's injection, lactated).[3139 3140 3141]

Stability

Most intact vials, bottles, and bags should be stored at controlled room temperature.[3139 3140 3141] Intact ampuls of the diluent provided with the lyophilized powder also should be stored at controlled room temperature.[3141] One manufacturer (Hospira) recommends that the ready-to-use solution of zoledronic acid 4 mg in 100-mL bags be stored at temperatures not exceeding 30°C and not be frozen.[3143] Specific product labeling should be consulted for additional storage details.

If not used immediately after dilution, solutions diluted for infusion and reduced doses prepared from a ready-to-use bottle should be stored at 2 to 8°C.[3140 3141] The total time from reconstitution and/or dilution to completion of administration should not exceed 24 hours.[3140 3141]

Zoledronic acid solution should be visually inspected for particulate matter and discoloration prior to administration.[3139 3140 3141] Bottles, bags, and vials are for single-use only; any unused portions of the solution should be discarded.[3143 3144]

Syringes

To avoid inadvertent injection, undiluted zoledronic acid concentrate for injection (whether commercially available or prepared by reconstituting lyophilized powder) should not be stored in syringes.[3140 3141]

Compatibility Information

Solution Compatibility

Zoledronic acid

Test Soln Name	Mfr	Mfr	Conc/L or %	Remarks	Ref	C/I
Dextrose 5% in Ringer's injection				Must not be mixed with calcium-containing solutions	3140, 3141	I
Dextrose 5% in Ringer's injection, lactated				Must not be mixed with calcium-containing solutions	3140, 3141	I
Dextrose 5%		NVA		Complete administration within 24 hr of dilution if stored at 2 to 8°C	3140	C
Dextrose 5%		CRC		Complete administration within 24 hour of reconstitution if stored at 2 to 8°C	3141	C
Ringer's injection				Must not be mixed with calcium-containing solutions	3140, 3141	I
Ringer's injection, lactated				Must not be mixed with calcium-containing solutions	3140, 3141	I
Sodium chloride 0.9%		NVA		Complete administration within 24 hr of dilution if stored at 2 to 8°C	3140	C
Sodium chloride 0.9%		CRC		Complete administration within 24 hr of reconstitution if stored at 2 to 8°C	3141	C

Appendix: Parenteral Nutrition Formulas

The following tables summarize the composition of the total parenteral nutrition mixtures that are referenced throughout the *Handbook on Injectable Drugs*. Each unique formula that has been tested for stability and/or compatibility characteristics, alone or in combination with other drugs, is described and assigned a code number. These code numbers are used in the drug monographs to denote the

TNA (3-in-1) or TPN (2-in-1) formulation being discussed (i.e., TPN #183, TPN #184, etc.). The TNA and TPN formulations are described as completely as possible from the original published sources.

The consolidation of the formulations into a single appendix is designed to avoid unnecessary repetition and to facilitate comparisons among different mixtures.

Component	Mfr	Concentration per Liter #21	#22	#23	#24
Amino acids	MG	200 mL			
Amino acids 8.5% with electrolytes	TR		500 mL	500 mL	500 mL
Dextrose 50%		400 mL		500 mL	500 mL
Dextrose 33.3% in water			500 mL		
Phosphate		15 mEq[a]	30 mEq		30 mEq[a]
Acetate		15 mEq[a]	67.5 mEq		
Calcium gluconate		2 g	9 mEq	1 g	
Calcium chloride			7.2 mEq		
Potassium chloride			70 mEq		20 mEq
Sodium chloride		40 mEq	55 mEq		60 mEq
Magnesium sulfate		8.1 mEq			
Multivitamins		10 mL			
Multivitamin concentrate				5 mL	
Water for injection		qs 1000 mL			
Trace elements			present		

[a] *Potassium salt.*

Component	Mfr	Concentration per Liter #25	#26	#27	#28	#29	#30
Amino acids (Aminosyn)	AB	3.5%			1%		
Amino acids (FreAmine III)	MG		4.25%			1%	
Amino acids (Travasol)	TR			4.25%			1%
Dextrose		25%	25%	25%	25%	25%	25%
Sodium phosphate	AB	10 mmol	10 mmol	10 mmol	10 mmol	10 mmol	10 mmol
Multivitamins (M.V.I.-12)	USV	10 mL	10 mL	10 mL	10 mL	10 mL	10 mL
Multielectrolyte concentrate[a]	SE	25 mL	25 mL	25 mL	25 mL	25 mL	25 mL
Trace mineral injection[b]		3.5 mL	3.5 mL	3.5 mL	3.5 mL	3.5 mL	3.5 mL

[a] *Each 25 mL provides: sodium, 25 mEq; potassium, 40.5 mEq; calcium, 5 mEq; magnesium, 8 mEq; chloride, 33.5 mEq; acetate, 40.6 mEq; and gluconate, 5 mEq.*

[b] *Each 3.5 mL provides: zinc, 2 mg; copper, 1 mg; manganese, 0.5 mg; and chromium, 10 mcg.*

DOI: 10.37573/9781585286850.407

Component		Concentration per Liter						
		#31	#32	#33	#34	#35	#36	#37
Amino acids	TR	4.2%	4.2%	4.2%	4.2%	4.2%	4.2%	4.2%
Dextrose		25%	25%	25%	25%	25%	25%	25%
Sodium		29 mEq	29 mEq	29 mEq	29 mEq	69 mEq	69 mEq	69 mEq
Potassium		25 mEq	25 mEq	25 mEq	25 mEq	46 mEq	46 mEq	46 mEq
Calcium		9 mEq	9 mEq	9 mEq	4.5 mEq	9.5 mEq	9.5 mEq	9.5 mEq
Magnesium		4 mEq	4 mEq	4 mEq	4 mEq	12 mEq	12 mEq	12 mEq
Phosphorus		388 mg	388 mg	388 mg	388 mg	388 mg	388 mg	388 mg
Chloride		29 mEq	29 mEq	29 mEq	29 mEq	103 mEq	103 mEq	103 mEq
Acetate		63 mEq	63 mEq	63 mEq	63 mEq	63 mEq	63 mEq	63 mEq
Trace elements			a b	a		a b	a b	a b
Multivitamins	USV			10 mL			5 mL	5 mL
Vitamin B complex with C plus folic acid (Soluzyme)	UP			5 mL				5 mL

a *Trace elements: selenium, 120 mcg; chromium, 2 mcg; zinc, 3 mg; and manganese, 0.7 mg.*

b *Trace elements: iodine, 120 mcg; and copper, 1 mg.*

Component	Concentration per Liter			
	#48	#49	#50	#51
Amino acids	5%	5%	5%	5%
Dextrose	5%	5%	25%	25%
Vitamins	present		present	
Trace elements		present		present

Component	Mfr	Concentration per Liter				
		#52	#53	#54	#55	#56
Amino acids	VT	7%	2.3%			
Amino acids	AB			1.5%		
Amino acids (FreAmine III)	MG				3%	3%
Dextrose			6.5%	15%	25%	25%
Fructose		10%	3.2%			
Sodium		50 mmol	16.2 mmol	a	35 mEq	35 mEq
Potassium		20 mmol	18.4 mmol	a		
Calcium		2.5 mmol	4.9 mmol	300 mg	5 mEq[b]	5 mEq[b]
Magnesium		1.5 mmol	2.1 mmol		8 mEq	8 mEq
Phosphorus				155 mg		
Phosphate			12.1 mmol[c]		40 mEq[d]	40 mEq[d]
Chloride		55 mmol	17.8 mmol	e	35 mEq	35 mEq
Laevulate calcium			9.8 mmol			
Folic acid				0.5 mg		
Cyanocobalamin				f		
Phytonadione				0.2 mg		
Multivitamins			present	4 mL		10 mL
Vitamin B complex with C (Berocca-C)				0.2 mL		

[a] Adjusted to provide 2.5 mEq/kg/day.

[b] Present as the gluconate.

[c] Anion not specified.

[d] Present as the potassium salt.

[e] Adjusted to provide 5 mEq/kg/day.

[f] Present but concentration not specified.

Component	Mfr	Concentration per Liter				
		#57	#58[a]	#59	#60	#61
Amino acids	MG	2.125%	4.25%			
Amino acids	TR			2.125%		
Amino acids	AB				3%	
Amino acids with electrolytes	TR			4.25%		
Dextrose		10%	25%	25%	25%	20%
Sodium		40 mEq	100 mmol	50 mEq	50 mEq	30 mEq
Potassium		30 mEq	60 to 80 mmol			25 mEq
Calcium		15 mEq	5 mmol	5 mEq	5 mEq	15 mEq
Magnesium		12.5 mEq	5 mmol	5 mEq	5 mEq	10 mEq
Phosphorus		6 mmol	10 mmol	465 mg	465 mg	15 mmol
Chloride		40 mEq	100 mmol	50 mEq	50 mEq	
Heparin sodium			1000 units	500 units	500 units	
Phytonadione				1 mg	1 mg	
Multivitamins			10 mL	10 mL	10 mL	2 mL
Multivitamin concentrate		2 mL				
Iron			1 mg			
Trace elements		present	present	present	present	present

[a] Concentration per 1200 mL.

Component	Mfr	Component Amounts						
		#62	#63	#64	#65	#66	#67	#68
Amino acids 8.5% (FreAmine III)	MG	500 mL	500 mL			500 mL		
Amino acids 5.4% (Nephramine)	MG			500 mL			500 mL	
Amino acids 5.2% (Aminosyn RF)	AB				500 mL			500 mL
Dextrose 50%	MG	500 mL	500 mL	500 mL	500 mL	500 mL	500 mL	500 mL
Hyperlyte (electrolyte) concentrate	MG		25 mL					
Fat emulsion 10%, intravenous	CU					500 mL	500 mL	500 mL
Multivitamins (M.V.I.-12)	USV	a	a	a	a	a	a	a

[a] Tested both with and without multivitamins.

Component	Mfr	Component Amounts		
		#69	#70	#71
Amino acids 8.5% (FreAmine II)	MG	1000 mL		
Amino acids 8.5% with electrolytes	TR			1500 mL[a]
Amino acids 7%	AB		500 mL	
Dextrose 50%		500 mL	500 mL	1500 mL
Dextrose 20% with electrolyte pattern A	TR	500 mL[b]		
Dextrose 20%		500 mL		
Sodium chloride 0.9%		500 mL		
Potassium chloride		20 mmol		
Calcium gluconate 10%				30 mL
Multivitamins		1 ampul		10 mL
Multivitamin concentrate			5 mL	
Folic acid		1 mg	0.25, 0.5, 0.75, 1 mg	
Trace elements				present

[a] Each 1500 mL provides: sodium, 105 mEq; potassium, 90 mEq; magnesium, 15 mEq; chloride, 105 mEq; acetate, 203 mEq; and phosphate, 45 mmol.

[b] Each 500 mL provides: magnesium, 14 mmol; calcium, 13 mmol; chloride, 54 mmol; acetate, 0.08 mmol; zinc, 0.04 mmol; and manganese, 0.02 mmol.

Component	Mfr	Component Amounts			
		#72	#73	#74	#75
Amino acids 10%	TR	750 mL	750 mL		
Amino acids 8.5%	TR			500 mL	
Amino acids 8.5%	MG				500 mL
Dextrose 70%		429 mL	429 mL		300 mL
Dextrose 50%				500 mL	
Fat emulsion 20%, intravenous	TR	225 mL	225 mL		
Sterile water for injection		24.2 mL	15 mL		300 mL
Calcium gluconate 10%		20 mL	20 mL		
Calcium gluceptate					8 mEq
Sodium phosphate			15 mmol		
Potassium phosphate		20 mmol		30 mEq	18 mEq
Potassium chloride		30 mEq	40 mEq	20 mEq	20 mEq
Magnesium sulfate 50%		2 mL	2 mL		8 mEq
Sodium chloride		60 mEq	60 mEq	40 mEq	60 mEq
Sodium acetate					5 mEq
Heparin sodium			6000 units		
Multivitamins		10 mL	10 mL		
Trace elements		present	present		

Component	Mfr	Concentration per Liter		
		#86	#87	#88
Amino acids (Aminosyn)	AB	2.5%	4.25%	5%
Dextrose		10%	25%	35%
Calcium		4.5 mEq	4.5 mEq	4.5 mEq
Magnesium		5 mEq	5 mEq	5 mEq
Potassium		23 mEq	40 mEq	40 mEq
Sodium		47 mEq	35 mEq	35 mEq
Acetate		82 mEq	74.5 mEq	74.5 mEq
Chloride		35 mEq	52.5 mEq	52.5 mEq
Phosphorus		9 mmol	12 mmol	12 mmol
Heparin sodium		1000 units	1000 units	1000 units
Insulin		a	a	a

[a] *Insulin 10 to 40 units/L.*

Component	Concentration per Liter	
	#89	#90
Amino acids (Travasol)	4.25%	
Amino acids with electrolytes (Travasol with electrolytes)		4.25%
Dextrose	25%	25%

Component	Mfr	Concentration per 100 mL #91	Concentration per 2 L #92
Amino acids 10%		1.6 mL	
Nitrogen (from amino acids)	PFM		14 g
Dextrose 5%		15 mL	
Dextrose 50%			500 mL
Fat emulsion 20%, intravenous	KA		500 mL
Sodium		3 mEq	150 mEq
Potassium		2.2 mEq	120 mEq
Calcium		1 mEq	15 mEq
Magnesium		0.3 mEq	30 mEq
Phosphate		0.5 mmol	30 mmol
Chloride		2.5 mEq	150 mEq
Sulfate			30 mEq
Acetate			90 mEq
Pediatric multivitamins		5 mL	
Multivitamins			present
Trace elements		a	present
Heparin sodium		100 units	
Water for injection			qs 2000 mL

a Trace elements: zinc, 600 mcg; copper, 40 mcg; manganese, 10 mcg; and chromium, 0.4 mcg.

Component	Mfr	Concentration per Liter #93	#94	#95	#96
Amino acids	TR	4.25%	4.25%		
Amino acids	AB			3%	3%
Dextrose		25%	25%	20%	20%
Potassium chloride		15 mEq	15 mEq	25 mEq	25 mEq
Sodium chloride		15 mEq	15 mEq	30 mEq	30 mEq
Calcium gluconate		4.7 mEq	4.7 mEq	15 mEq	15 mEq
Magnesium sulfate		4.05 mEq	4.05 mEq	10 mEq	10 mEq
Potassium phosphate		5 mEq	5 mEq	15 mmol	15 mmol
Sodium phosphate		10 mEq	10 mEq		
Zinc		1.5 mg	1.5 mg	3 mg	3 mg
Manganese		150 mcg	150 mcg	50 mcg	50 mcg
Chromium		6 mcg	6 mcg	2 mcg	2 mcg
Selenium		30 mcg	30 mcg		
Copper			600 mcg	200 mcg	200 mcg
Multivitamins	LY			2 mL	2 mL
Heparin sodium	IX			1000 units	

Component	Mfr	Milliliters per Container							
		#97	#98	#99	#100	#101	#102	#103	#104
Amino acids 8.5% (FreAmine III)	MG	10	10	10	10	75	75	75	75
Dextrose 70%		89	36	89	36	89	36	89	36
Fat emulsion 20%, intravenous (Intralipid)	KV	5	5	75	75	5	5	50	50
Sterile water qs ad		250	250	250	250	250	250	250	250
Other components		a	a	a	a	a	a	a	a

a *Each TNA admixture also contained: sodium, 25 mEq; potassium, 25 mEq; calcium, 5 mEq; magnesium, 25 mEq; chloride, 30 mEq; acetate, 7.5 mEq; lactate, 10.5 mEq; phosphate, 1.5 mmol; multivitamins (M.V.I. Pediatric), 2.5 mL; trace elements; and heparin sodium, 250 units.*

Component	Mfr	Concentration per Liter			
		#105	#106	#107	#108
Amino acids	TR	1.65%	4.25%	1.5%	1.5%
Dextrose		10%	10%	15%	15%
Sodium		21 mEq	35 mEq		
Potassium		18 mEq	30 mEq		
Magnesium		3 mEq	5 mEq		
Calcium		15 mEq	10 mEq		
Phosphate		10 mmol	15 mmol		
Chloride		21 mEq	35 mEq		
Acetate		30 mEq	68 mEq		
Pediatric multivitamins		1 mL	1 mL		
Trace elements		0.1 mL	0.1 mL		
Unspecified electrolytes and vitamins				present	present

Component	Mfr	#109	#110	#111	#112	#113
		Concentration per Liter				
Amino acids (FreAmine III)	MG	4.25%	2%	4.25%	2.125%	
Amino acids (Travasol)	TR					4.25%
Fat emulsion 20%, intravenous (Intralipid)	KV			200 mL	125 mL	
Dextrose		25%	25%	20%	25%	25%
Sodium		50 mEq	50 mEq	50 mEq	50 mEq	35 mEq
Potassium		40 mEq	40 mEq	40 mEq	40 mEq	30 mEq
Chloride		40 mEq	40 mEq	a	a	35 mEq
Phosphorus		13 mmol	13 mmol	6 mmol	6 mmol	15 mmol
Acetate		31 mEq	31 mEq	a	a	70.5 mEq
Calcium		16.7 mEq	16.7 mEq	10 mEq	10 mEq	4.7 mEq
Magnesium		10 mEq	10 mEq	5 mEq	5 mEq	5 mEq
Multivitamins		4 mL	4 mL	3.33 mL	3.33 mL	
Trace elements		present	present	present	present	present
Heparin sodium		1000 units	1000 units	1000 units	1000 units	
Sterile water		qs	qs	qs	qs	

a Not cited.

Component	#114	#115	#116	#117	#118
	Concentration per Liter				
Nitrogen (from amino acids)	7 g				
Amino acids (Travasol)		4.2%	4.2%	4.5%	3.7%
Dextrose	12.5%	4.2%	21%	22.7%	18.5%
Fat emulsion, intravenous	50 g a				3.7%
Sodium	75 mEq	66.7 mmol	66.7 mmol	40.9 mEq	45 mEq
Potassium	60 mEq	50 mmol	50 mmol	36.4 mEq	40 mEq
Magnesium	15 mEq	4.16 mmol	4.16 mmol	7.3 mEq	8 mEq
Calcium	7.5 mEq	4.16 mmol	4.16 mmol	4.5 mEq	5 mEq
Chloride	75 mEq	66.7 mmol	66.7 mmol	48.2 mEq	53 mEq
Phosphorus	15 mmol	8.3 mmol	8.3 mmol	13.6 mmol	15 mmol
Sulfate	15 mEq				
Acetate	45 mEq	90.8 mmol	90.8 mmol	76.4 mEq	84 mEq
Trace elements	present	present	present		
Multivitamins	present	8.3 mL	8.3 mL		
Sterile water for injection	qs				
Iron		833 mcg	833 mcg		
Heparin sodium		1000 units	1000 units		

a Both Intralipid (long-chain triglycerides) and MCT/LCT (medium- and long-chain triglycerides) tested.

Component	Mfr	Concentration per Liter						
		#119	#120	#121	#122	#123	#124	#125
Amino acids		4.25%	4.25%	5%	5%	1%	2%	
Amino acids (TrophAmine)	MG							2%
Dextrose		35%	35%	20%	14.3%	10%	10%	10%
Fat emulsion					5.7%			
Sodium chloride		50 mEq	50 mEq	20 mEq	4 mEq	16 mEq	16 mEq	16 mEq
Potassium chloride				20 mEq	30 mEq	5 mEq	5 mEq	5 mEq
Potassium phosphate		30 mEq	30 mEq		3 mmol	10 to 40 mmol	10 to 40 mmol	10 to 40 mmol
Magnesium sulfate		10 mEq	10 mEq	8 mEq	12 mEq	4 mEq	4 mEq	4 mEq
Calcium gluconate		4.7 mEq	4.7 mEq	4.8 mEq	4 mEq	10 to 40 mEq	10 to 40 mEq	10 to 40 mEq
Sodium phosphates				20 mEq				
Sodium acetate					20 mEq	10 mEq	10 mEq	10 mEq
Cysteine HCl								1 g
Mixed electrolytes	LY				27 mL			
Trace Elements		1 mL	1 mL	present	3 mL			
Heparin sodium			1000 units					
Multivitamins				10 mL	10 mL			
Phytonadione					1 mg			
Cimetidine HCl					1 g			

Component	Mfr	Concentration per Liter						
		#126	#127	#128	#129	#130	#131	#132	#133
Amino acids (Aminosyn II)	AB	2%	3.3%	3.6%	3.6%	5%	3.5%	3.5%	
Amino acids (Travasol)	TR								4.25%
Dextrose		14.8%	3.3%	23.3%	20.8%	10%	25%	25%	25%
Fat emulsion, intravenous (Liposyn II)	AB	1.2%	3.3%	3.3%	2%	7.1%			
Sodium		39.5 mEq	51.7 mEq	48.4 mEq	96.3 mEq	49.4 mEq	33.6 mEq	33.6 mEq	75 mEq
Potassium		27 mEq	13.3 mEq	21.4 mEq	60 mEq	78.6 mEq	35.6 mEq	35.6 mEq	20 mEq
Calcium		6.6 mEq	3 mEq	6.7 mEq	10 mEq	13.4 mEq	4.5 mEq	4.5 mEq	9.6 mEq
Magnesium		3.2 mEq	3.3 mEq	10 mEq	12 mEq	14.5 mEq	5 mEq	5 mEq	10 mEq
Phosphate		5.5 mmol	10 mmol	10 mmol	15 mmol	21.4 mmol	12 mmol	12 mmol	10 mEq
Chloride		57.9 mEq	23.3 mEq	40 mEq	80 mEq	73.9 mEq	35 mEq	35 mEq	85 mEq
Acetate		21.9 mEq	43.6 mEq	23.9 mEq	65.8 mEq	35.9 mEq	35.7 mEq	35.7 mEq	
Trace elements		present	present	present	present	present		present	3 mL
Multivitamins (M.V.I.-12)								present	10 mL

Component	Mfr	Concentration per Liter						
		#134	#135	#136	#137	#138	#139	#140
Amino acids (Travasol)		5.8%	5.8%	5.8%	5.8%	5.8%	4.26%	6%
Dextrose	BA	23.7%	23.7%	23.7%	23.7%	23.7%	17.5%	25%
Fat emulsion, intravenous (Intralipid)	KV		3%	5%			3%	
Fat emulsion, intravenous (Liposyn II)	AB				3%	5%		
Potassium chloride		54.2 mEq	54.2 mEq	54.2 mEq	54.2 mEq	54.2 mEq	40.2 mEq	30 mEq
Sodium chloride		108 mEq	108 mEq	108 mEq	108 mEq	108 mEq	80.5 mEq	110 mEq
Calcium gluconate 10%		13.6 mL	13.6 mL	13.6 mL	13.6 mL	13.6 mL	4.65 mEq	10 mL
Magnesium sulfate 50%		1.4 mL	1.4 mL	1.4 mL	1.4 mL	1.4 mL	4 mEq	4 mL
Potassium phosphate		20.3 mmol	20.3 mmol	20.3 mmol	20.3 mmol	20.3 mmol	45 mmol	
Multivitamins		6.8 mL	6.8 mL	6.8 mL	6.8 mL	6.8 mL	5 mL	1 vial
Trace elements		present	present	present	present	present	present	present
Phytonadione								1 mg

Component	Mfr	Concentration per Liter			
		#141	#142	#143	#144
Amino acids	AB		2.5%	5%	
Amino acids (Travasol)	TR				4.25%
Dextrose		25%	25%	25%	25%
Sodium				50 mEq	22.5 mEq
Potassium			40 mEq	40 mEq	20 mEq
Magnesium			5 mEq	5 mEq	2.85 mEq
Calcium			5 mEq	5 mEq	4.25 mEq
Phosphorus			15 mmol	15 mmol	15.75 mmol
Chloride			58 mEq	58 mEq	17 mEq
Acetate					58 mEq
Multivitamins			10 mL	10 mL	
Trace elements			1 mL	1 mL	present
Heparin sodium	UP		500 units	500 units	
Sterile water for injection					qs

Component	Mfr	Concentration per Liter			
		#145	#146	#147	#148
Amino acids (Travasol)	BA	5%			
Amino acids	AB		5%	2.5%	1%
Dextrose		15%	25%	25%	25%
Sodium		45 mEq	35 mEq	35 mEq	35 mEq
Potassium		15 mEq	40 mEq	40 mEq	40 mEq
Chloride		20 mEq	35 mEq	35 mEq	35 mEq
Phosphorus		16 mmol	12 mmol	12 mmol	12 mmol
Acetate		81 mEq	82 mEq	82 mEq	82 mEq
Calcium		20 mEq	9 mEq	9 mEq	9 mEq
Magnesium			5 mEq	5 mEq	5 mEq

Component		Component Amounts									
		#149	#150	#151	#152	#153	#154	#155	#156	#157	#158
Amino acids 10% (TrophAmine)		50 mL	50 mL	50 mL	50 mL	350 mL	350 mL	350 mL	350 mL	50 mL	350 mL
Dextrose		10%	10%	10%	10%	25%	25%	25%	25%	25%	25%
Fat emulsion 20%, intravenous[a]		25 mL	25 mL	70 mL	70 mL	25 mL	25 mL	70 mL	70 mL	100 mL	100 mL
Sodium		25 mEq	100 mEq	25 mEq	100 mEq	25 mEq	100 mEq	25 mEq	100 mEq	100 mEq	100 mEq
Potassium		15 mEq	80 mEq	15 mEq	80 mEq	15 mEq	80 mEq	15 mEq	80 mEq	80 mEq	80 mEq
Chloride		25 mEq	100 mEq	25 mEq	100 mEq	25 mEq	100 mEq	25 mEq	100 mEq	100 mEq	100 mEq
Calcium		7 mEq	18 mEq	7 mEq	18 mEq	7 mEq	18 mEq	7 mEq	18 mEq	18 mEq	18 mEq
Magnesium		2.5 mEq	13 mEq	2.5 mEq	13 mEq	2.5 mEq	13 mEq	2.5 mEq	13 mEq	13 mEq	13 mEq
Phosphate		3.4 mmol	9 mmol	3.4 mmol	9 mmol	3.4 mmol	9 mmol	3.4 mmol	9 mmol	9 mmol	9 mmol
Trace elements		present	present	present	present	present	present	present	present	present	present
Multivitamins (M.V.I. Pediatric)		5 mL	5 mL	5 mL	5 mL	5 mL	5 mL	5 mL	5 mL	5 mL	5 mL
Heparin		1000 units	1000 units	1000 units	1000 units	1000 units	1000 units	1000 units	1000 units	1000 units	1000 units

[a] Intralipid 20%, Liposyn II 20%, and Nutrilipid 20% were each tested.

Component	Mfr	#159	#160	#161	#162	#163	#164	#165	#166
Amino acids 5.5% with electrolytes (Travasol)	BA	100 mL	100 mL	400 mL	400 mL	400 mL	400 mL	100 mL	100 mL
Fat emulsion 20%, intravenous (Intralipid)	KV	100 mL		200 mL		100 mL		200 mL	
Fat emulsion 20%, intravenous (Liposyn II)	AB		100 mL		200 mL		100 mL		200 mL
Heparin sodium 1000 units/mL	ES	5 mL	5 mL	5 mL	5 mL	5 mL	5 mL	5 mL	5 mL
Dextrose 10%			795 mL	795 mL				695 mL	695 mL
Dextrose 20%				395 mL	395 mL	495 mL	495 mL		

Component	#167	#168	#169	#170	#171	#172	#173
Aminoplex 12			500 mL		1000 mL		
Aminoplex 24	500 mL	500 mL	500 mL	500 mL			
Vamin glucose							1000 mL
Lipofundin S 20%	500 mL	500 mL	500 mL	500 mL	500 mL		
Fat emulsion 10%, intravenous (Intralipid)						300 mL	
Glucoplex 1000	1000 mL						
Glucoplex 1600		1000 mL	1000 mL		500 mL		
Dextrose 5%					1000 mL		
Dextrose 50%				500 mL			1000 mL
Potassium chloride 15%		37.5 mL		10 mL			
Potassium phosphate 17%	20 mL	20 mL	20 mL	20 mL	10 mL		
Sodium chloride 30%		27 mL		15 mL			
Addamel	10 mL	10 mL	10 mL	10 mL	10 mL		10 mL
Soluvit						7.5 mL	
Vitalipid infant						15 mL	
Pancebrin							10 mL

Component	Mfr	Concentration per Liter					
		#174	#175	#176	#177	#178	#179
Amino acids	AB	25 g	50 g	15 g			
Amino acids	TR				3%		
Nitrogen						7.9 g	7 g
Dextrose		125 g	250 g	100 g	5%	100 g	125 g
Fat emulsion, intravenous (Intralipid)	KV					50 g	5 g
TPN II electrolytes	AB	20 mL	20 mL				
Sodium		26.3 mEq	37.5 mEq	40 mEq	46 mEq	24 mmol	75 mEq
Potassium		35.5 mEq	40 mEq	50 mEq	40 mEq	12.5 mmol	60 mEq
Magnesium		5 mEq	5 mEq	10 mEq	8 mEq	2.5 mmol	15 mEq
Calcium		9 mEq	4.5 mEq	10 mEq	5 mEq		7.5 mEq
Phosphorus		12 mmol	45 mmol	5 mmol	12 mmol	4.5 mmol	15 mmol
Chloride		35 mEq	35 mEq	47.6 mEq	57 mEq	7 mmol	75 mEq
Acetate		25 mEq	43 mEq	31.8 mEq	61 mEq	40.5 mmol	45 mEq
Gluconate					10 mEq		
Sulfate					10 mEq		15 mEq
Trace elements			present	present	present	present	present
Multivitamins (M.V.I. Pediatric)		3 mL		3 mL			
Multivitamins (M.V.I. 9+3)			10 mL				
Multivitamins						present	present
					10 mL		
Vitamin K			5 mg				
Heparin sodium		1000 units	1000 units	1000 units	1000 units		
Sterile water qs ad		1000 mL	1000 mL	1000 mL		1000 mL	1000 mL

Component	Component Amounts	
	#180	#181
Amino acids 10%	1000 mL	400 mL
Dextrose 50%	500 mL	500 mL
Fat emulsion 20%, intravenous (Intralipid)	500 mL	
Sodium	40 mmol	41 mEq
Potassium	70 mmol	22.7 mEq
Calcium	4.6 mmol	5 mEq
Magnesium	5 mmol	5 mEq
Phosphorus	17.5 mmol	12 mmol
Chloride	120 mmol	30 mEq
Acetate	45 mmol	89 mEq
Trace elements		present
Multivitamins		10 mL

Component	Mfr	Concentration per Liter #182
Amino acids	KV	5%
Dextrose		25%
Fat emulsion, intravenous (Intralipid)	KV	2.25%
Potassium phosphate		10 mmol
Potassium chloride		45 mEq
Sodium chloride		75 mEq
Magnesium sulfate		8 mEq
Calcium gluconate		47 mg
Trace elements		present
Multivitamins		5 mL
Sterile water qs ad		1000 mL

Component	Mfr	Component Amounts						
		#183	#184	#185	#186ᵃ	#187ᵇ	#188ᶜ	#189
Amino acids (Aminosyn II)	AB	1%	2.5%	5%				
Amino acids (Aminosyn)	AB				15 g	25 g	50 g	
Amino acids 10% with electrolytes								500 mL
(Synthamin 17 with electrolytes)								
Dextrose	AB	10%	10%	25%	125 g	125 g	250 g	
Dextrose 50%								500 mL
TPN II electrolytes						1 mL	1 mL	
Calcium		9 mEq	4.4 mEq	5 mEq	1 mEq	9 mEq	4.5 mEq	2.2 mmol
Magnesium		5 mEq	5 mEq	5 mEq	1 mEq	5 mEq	5 mEq	2.5 mmol
Potassium		27 mEq	18 mEq	40 mEq	5 mEq	30 mEq	40 mEq	42.5 mmol
Sodium		24 mEq	38 mEq	42 mEq	4 mEq	35 mEq	37.65 mEq	45 mmol
Phosphorus		6 mmol	9 mmol	15 mmol	2 mmol	6 mmol	12 mmol	15 mmol
Chloride		35 mEq	35 mEq	43 mEq	5.7 mEq	46.9 mEq	39.4 mEq	55.65 mmol
Acetate		22 mEq	25 mEq	38 mEq	11.1 mEq	25.6 mEq	43.5 mEq	81.25 mmol
Gluconate					1.1 mEq	2.5 mEq	0.05 mEq	
Sulfate					1.1 mEq			
Trace elements		1 mL	1 mL	1 mL	0.6 mL	1 mL	1 mL	present
Multivitamins (M.V.I. Pediatric)	AST				3 mL	3 mL		
Multivitamins (M.V.I. 9+3)	AST						10 mL	
Heparin sodium	ES				1000 units	1000 units	1000 units	
Sterile water					qs	qs	qs	

ᵃ Neonatal formula.

ᵇ Pediatric formula.

ᶜ Adult formula.

Component	Mfr	Component Amounts		
		#190	#191	#192
Amino acids (Aminosyn II 15%)	AB	333 mL		
Amino acids (Azonutril 25)			500 mL	
Amino acids				17 g
Dextrose 70%		500 mL		
Dextrose 50%			250 mL	
Dextrose 30%			750 mL	
Dextrose				42.4 g
Fat emulsion 20%, intravenous (Intralipid)			500 mL	24.2 g
Fat emulsion 20%, intravenous (Liposyn II)	AB	400 mL		
Sterile water		133 mL		
Sodium				55.7 mmol
Potassium				19.4 mmol
Magnesium				2.3 mmol
Calcium				1.5 to 150 mmol
Phosphate				21 to 300 mmol
Unspecified electrolytes		present		
Vitamins		present		present
Trace elements			present	present

Component	Mfr	Component Amounts
		#193
Amino acids 10%	CL	1000 mL
Dextrose 50%	CL	750 mL
Sodium chloride	AB	140 mEq
Potassium phosphates	AB	20 mmol
Calcium gluconate		4.8 mEq
Magnesium sulfate		40 mEq
Multivitamins	AST	10 mL
Trace elements	LY	3 mL
Famotidine		40 mg

	Concentration per Liter	
Component	**#194**	**#195**
Amino acids	2.2%	2.2%
Dextrose	12.5%	20%
Sodium chloride	26 mEq	26 mEq
Potassium phosphates	15 mmol	15 mmol
Calcium gluconate	25 mEq	25 mEq
Magnesium sulfate	8 mEq	8 mEq
Potassium chloride	2 mEq	2 mEq
Heparin sodium	1000 units	1000 units
Cysteine	660 mg	660 mg
Trace elements	present	present
Multivitamins	20 mL	20 mL

		Concentration per Liter				
Component	**Mfr**	**#196**	**#197**	**#198**	**#199**	**#200**
Amino acids	BA	6%	6%	6%	6%	6%
Dextrose	BA	24%	24%	24%	24%	24%
Intralipid	KV		3%	5%		
Liposyn II	AB				3%	5%
Sodium chloride	LY	108 mEq	108 mEq	108 mEq	108 mEq	108 mEq
Potassium phosphates	AB	20 mmol	20 mmol	20 mmol	20 mmol	20 mmol
Calcium gluconate	LY	6.3 mEq	6.3 mEq	6.3 mEq	6.3 mEq	6.3 mEq
Magnesium sulfate	AST	5.6 mEq	5.6 mEq	5.6 mEq	5.6 mEq	5.6 mEq
Potassium chloride	AB	54 mEq	54 mEq	54 mEq	54 mEq	54 mEq
Trace elements	SO	present	present	present	present	present
Multivitamins	AR	6.8 mL	6.8 mL	6.8 mL	6.8 mL	6.8 mL

Component	Mfr	Concentration per Liter			
		#201	#202	#203[a]	#204[b]
Amino acids	BA	4.25%			
Amino acids	AB		4.25%		
Amino acids (TrophAmine)	MG			2%	3%
Dextrose		25%	25%	10%	20%
Sodium		35 mEq	35 mEq	38 mEq	77 mEq
Potassium		30 mEq	30 mEq	20 mEq	40 mEq
Calcium		5 mEq	9.4 mEq	600 mg	600 mg
Magnesium		3 mEq	10 mEq	2.5 mEq	2.5 mEq
Chloride		47 mEq	[c]	38 mEq	77 mEq
Phosphate		14.3 mEq	15 mmol	400 mg	400 mg
Acetate		67 mEq	50 mEq	29 mEq	58 mEq
L-Cysteine				200 mg	300 mg
Trace elements			present	present	present
Multivitamins			present	present	present
Heparin					500 units

[a] Calculated quantities from a pediatric peripheral line formula.

[b] Calculated quantities from a pediatric central line formula.

[c] Unspecified.

Component	Mfr	Concentration per Liter	
		#205	#206
Amino acids	BA	5%	
Aminosyn	AB		2.125%
Dextrose		25%	20%
Intralipid	KA		
Liposyn II	AB		
Sodium chloride		75 mEq	30 mEq
Potassium chloride		60 mEq	30 mEq
Potassium phosphates		20 mmol	
Sodium phosphates			15 mmol
Calcium gluconate		10 mEq	14 mEq
Magnesium sulfate		10 mEq	50 mg
Trace elements		present	present
Multivitamins			
Heparin sodium		3000 to 20,000 units	

Component	Mfr	Concentration per Liter				
		#207	#208	#209	#210	#211
Amino acids (TrophAmine)	MG	0.5%	1%	1.5%	2%	2.5%
Dextrose		10%	10%	10%	10%	10%
Sodium chloride		20 mEq	20 mEq	20 mEq	20 mEq	20 mEq
Sodium acetate		10 mEq	10 mEq	10 mEq	10 mEq	10 mEq
Potassium acetate		5 mEq	5 mEq	5 mEq	5 mEq	5 mEq
Potassium phosphates		10 mmol	10 mmol	10 mmol	10 mmol	10 mmol
Calcium gluconate		20 mEq	20 mEq	20 mEq	20 mEq	20 mEq
Magnesium sulfate		4 mEq	4 mEq	4 mEq	4 mEq	4 mEq
Trace elements	FUJ	a	a	a	a	a
Multivitamins	AST	b	b	b	b	b
Heparin sodium		1000 units	1000 units	1000 units	1000 units	1000 units
L-Cysteine[c]		200 mg	400 mg	600 mg	800 mg	1 g

[a] Tested with and without trace elements (Neotrace, Fujisawa).

[b] Tested with and without multivitamins (M.V.I. Pediatric, Astra) 3.5 mL/L.

[c] 40 mg/g of protein.

Component	Mfr	Concentration per Liter				
		#212	#213	#214	#215	#216[a]
Amino acids (Aminosyn II)	AB	3.5%		4.25%		
Amino acids (FreAmine III)	MG		3.5%		4.25%	
Amino acids (Travasol)	BA					0.5 to 5%
Dextrose		5%	5%	25%	25%	10 to 20%
Sterile water for injection		516.8 mL	516.75 mL	161 mL	158.6 mL	q.s.
Potassium phosphates		3.5 mmol	b	15 mmol	5.75 mmol[c]	0 to 20 mEq K[d]
Sodium chloride		25 mEq	37.5 mEq	25 mEq	40 mEq	0 to 44 mEq
Sodium acetate						0 to 40 mEq
Potassium chloride		35 mEq	40 mEq	18 mEq	25 mEq	0 to 20 mEq
Magnesium sulfate		8 mEq	8 mEq	8 mEq	8 mEq	4 mEq
Calcium gluconate		9.3 mEq	5 mEq	9.15 mEq	7.5 mEq	19.2 to 28.8 mEq
Multivitamins	AST	10 mL	10 mL	10 mL	10 mL	14 mL
Trace elements		present	present	present	present	present
Heparin sodium	ES					500 units
Ranitidine (as HCl)	GL					0 to 84 mg

[a] Forty parenteral nutrition formulations within the ranges cited were tested. Specific formulations were not reported.

[b] No phosphates added. Phosphates from FreAmine III formulation yielded 3.5 mmol/L.

[c] Added phosphates indicated. All phosphates from addition plus FreAmine III formulation totaled 10 mmol/L.

[d] Reported as potassium concentration.

Component	Mfr	Concentration per Liter			
		#217	#218	#219	#220
Amino acids		5%			
Amino acids	MG		3%	3%	
Amino acids	AB				3%
Dextrose		25%	5%	5%	5%
Intralipid	KA		2%		
Liposyn II	AB			2%	
Liposyn III	AB				2%
Sodium		50 mEq	43 mEq	43 mEq	41.6 mEq
Potassium		40 mEq	40 mEq	40 mEq	40 mEq
Chloride		58 mEq	45 mEq	45 mEq	35 mEq
Phosphorus		15 mmol	7.5 mmol	7.5 mmol	15 mmol
Calcium		5 mEq	5 mEq	5 mEq	9.15 mEq
Magnesium		8 mEq	8 mEq	8 mEq	8 mEq
Acetate			51.7 mEq	51.7 mEq	42 mEq
Heparin sodium		1000 units			
Multivitamins		10 mL	10 mL	10 mL	10 mL
Phytonadione		1 mg			
Trace elements		2 mL	1 mL	1 mL	1 mL
Sterile water for injection			qs	qs	qs

Component	Mfr	Concentration per Liter					
		#221	#222	#223	#224	#225	#226
Amino acids	MG	4.9%	4.9%			6%	6%
Amino acids	AB			4.9%	6%		
Dextrose		20%	20%	20%	11%	10.7%	10.7%
Intralipid	KA		3.5%				4%
Liposyn II	AB	3.5%				4%	
Liposyn III	AB			3.5%	4%		
Sodium		39.8 mEq	39.8 mEq	39.7 mEq	45 mEq	45 mEq	45 mEq
Potassium		40 mEq	40 mEq	40 mEq	40 mEq	40.2 mEq	40.2 mEq
Calcium		7.5 mEq	7.5 mEq	9.15 mEq	9.15 mEq	7.5 mEq	7.5 mEq
Magnesium		8 mEq	8 mEq	8 mEq	8 mEq	8 mEq	8 mEq
Chloride		45 mEq	45 mEq	35 mEq	35 mEq	51 mEq	51 mEq
Acetate		67.7 mEq	67.7 mEq	45 mEq	53.2 mEq	78.4 mEq	78.4 mEq
Phosphate		10 mmol	10 mmol	15 mmol	15 mmol	10 mmol	10 mmol
Multivitamins		10 mL	10 mL	10 mL	10 mL	10 mL	10 mL
Trace elements		1 mL	1 mL	1 mL	1 mL	1 mL	1 mL

Component	Mfr	Concentration per Liter				
		#227	#228	#229	#230	#231
Aminosyn II	AB	2%	3.5%	4.25%	4.25%	5%
Dextrose	AB	10%	10%	15%	25%	25%
Sodium (as chloride)	AB	40 mEq	40 mEq	70 mEq	70 mEq	70 mEq
Potassium (as chloride)	AB	20 mEq	20 mEq	50 mEq	50 mEq	50 mEq
Magnesium (as sulfate)	AB	8 mEq	8 mEq	12 mEq	12 mEq	12 mEq
Phosphates (as potassium)	AB	up to 40 mmol	up to 40 mmol	up to 40 mmol	up to 40 mmol	up to 40 mmol
Calcium (as acetate)	AB	up to 40 mEq	up to 40 mEq	up to 40 mEq	up to 40 mEq	up to 40 mEq

Component	Mfr	Component Amounts					
		#232	#233	#234	#235	#236	#237
Synthamin 17		500 mL	500 mL	500 mL	500 mL		
Vaminolact	FRE					150 mL	150 mL
Dextrose 50%		500 mL	500 mL	500 mL	500 mL	180 mL	154 mL
Sterile water for injection		500 mL	500 mL	500 mL	500 mL		
Intralipid 20%		500 mL	500 mL	500 mL	500 mL		
Medialipide	BRN						50 mL
Albumin, human		100 mL	100 mL	200 mL	200 mL		
Sodium chloride 10%						6.08 mL	6.08 mL
Potassium chloride 10%						18.66 mL	18.66 mL
Calcium chloride			7 mmol		7 mmol		
Calcium gluconate/glucoheptonate						16.1 mL	16.1 mL
Magnesium sulfate			10 mmol		10 mmol		
Magnesium sulfate 15%						1.64 mL	1.64 mL
Phosphorus (Phocytan)						14.56 mL	14.56 mL
Vitamins (Soluvit)						5 mL	5 mL
Trace elements, pediatric (OEP)						10 mL	10 mL

Component	Mfr	Component Amounts		
		#238	#239	#240
Aminoplex 12	GEI	200 mL		
FreAmine III	FRE		200 mL	
Vamin 14	PH			200 mL
Dextrose 20%	BA	300 mL	300 mL	300 mL
Addiphos	PH	4 mL	4 mL	4 mL
Additrace	PH	2 mL	2 mL	2 mL

Component	Mfr	Concentration per Liter	
		#241	#242
Aminosyn	AB	4.25%	5%
Dextrose		25%	25%
Calcium		4.5 mEq	4.5 mEq
Magnesium		5 mEq	5 mEq
Potassium		40 mEq	40 mEq
Sodium		35 mEq	35 mEq
Acetate		74.5 mEq	74.5 mEq
Chloride		52.5 mEq	52.5 mEq
Phosphorus		12 mmol	12 mmol
Heparin sodium		1000 units	1000 units

Component	Concentration per Liter		
	#243	#244	#245
Amino acids (Aminosyn)	4%		
Amino acids (TrophAmine)		3%	
Nitrogen			0.8%
Dextrose	20%	20%	12.5%
Fat emulsion			5%
Sodium chloride	93 mEq	48 mEq	20 mEq
Potassium (from acetate and phosphate)	60 mEq	40 mEq	35 mEq
Calcium (as gluconate)	330 mg	600 mg	4.6 mEq
Chloride			60 mEq
Acetate			22.5 mEq
Magnesium sulfate	8 mEq	4.3 mEq	5 mEq
Trace elements (pediatric)	3 mL	3 mL	
L-Cysteine HCl (40 mg/g amino acids)		1.2 g	
Multivitamin injection (M.V.I. Pediatric)	5 mL	5 mL	present
Heparin sodium	500 units	500 units	

Component	Concentration per Liter	
	#246	#247
Amino acids (Aminoplasmal L10)	1000 mL	1000 mL
Dextrose 37.5% with electrolytes	500 mL	500 mL
Dextrose 10%	500 mL	500 mL
Fat emulsion (Lipofundin-S 20%)	500 mL	
Sterile water for injection		500 mL
Calcium gluconate	2.5 mmol	2.5 mmol
Magnesium sulfate	2 mmol	2 mmol
Addamel	10 mL	10 mL
Potassium phosphate	20 mL[a]	20 mL[a]
Sodium chloride 30%	8 mL	8 mL
Folic acid	15 mg	15 mg
Multivitamins	present	present
Trace elements	present	present

[a] Provided potassium 20 mEq and phosphate 10 mmol.

Component	Concentration per Liter	
	#248	#249
Amino acids (Aminotripa 2)	3.3%	
Amino Acids (Unicaliq N)		3%
Dextrose	19.4%	17.5%
Sodium	38.9 mEq	40 mEq
Potassium	30 mEq	27 mEq
Magnesium	5.6 mEq	6 mEq
Calcium	5.6 mEq	6 mEq
Chloride	38.9 mEq	59 mEq
Sulfate	5.6 mEq	
Acetate	60 mEq	10 mEq
Gluconate	5.6 mEq	6 mEq
Citrate	12.2 mEq	
L-Malate		17 mEq
L-Lactate		35 mEq
Phosphorus	206.7 mg	250 mg
Zinc	11.1 mcmol	20 mcmol

Component	Concentration per Liter							
	#250	#251	#252	#253	#254	#255	#256	#257
Aminosyn II	4%	4%	3.7%	3.7%	2.8%	2.8%	2.5%	2.5%
Dextrose	17.6%	17.6%	16.1%	16.1%	17.6%	17.6%	16.1%	16.1%
Liposyn II	6.0%		5.5%		6.0%		5.5%	
Intralipid		6.0%		5.5%		6.0%		5.5%
Sodium chloride			104 mEq	104 mEq			109 mEq	109 mEq
Potassium chloride			47 mEq	47 mEq			47 mEq	47 mEq
Potassium acetate			43 mEq	43 mEq			43 mEq	43 mEq
Sodium phosphates			11 mmol	11 mmol			11 mmol	11 mmol
Magnesium sulfate			6 mEq	6 mEq			6 mEq	6 mEq
Calcium gluconate			5.1 mEq	5.1 mEq			5 mEq	5 mEq
Sterile water for injection	qs	qs	qs	qs	qs	qs	qs	qs

Component	Concentration per Liter				
	#258	#259	#260	#261	#262
FreAmine III	1%	2%	3%	4%	5%
Dextrose	15%	15%	25%	25%	25%
Cysteine HCl	250 mg	500 mg	750 mg	1 g	1.25 g
Sodium chloride	40 mEq	40 mEq	40 mEq	70 mEq	70 mEq
Potassium chloride	20 mEq	20 mEq	20 mEq	50 mEq	50 mEq
Magnesium sulfate	8 mEq	8 mEq	8 mEq	12 mEq	12 mEq
Sterile water for injection	qs	qs	qs	qs	qs

Component	Concentration per Liter				
	#263	#264	#265	#266	#267
Travasol 10%	267 mL				
Fravasol 10%		250 mL			
Livaframine 10%			250 mL		
Synthamin 10%				500 mL	
Amino acids 17%					1000 mL
Dextrose 70%	347 mL				
Dextrose 50%				500 mL	500 mL
Dextrose 10%		250 mL	250 mL		
Sterile water for injection	367 mL				
Fat emulsion 20%					500 mL
Sodium	36.6 mEq		5 mmoL		
Potassium	26.6 mEq				
Calcium	5 mEq				
Chloride	50 mEq	20 mmoL	4.5 mmoL		
Acetate		41 mmoL	31 mmoL		
Phosphate	9 mmoL		5 mmoL		
Trace elements	present				

Component	Concentration per Liter
	#268
Aminosyn 15%	29.75 mL
Dextrose 70%	37.5 mL
Sterile water for injection	33.65 mL
Sodium chloride	4.7 mEq
Potassium chloride	2.1 mEq
Potassium phosphates	1.05 mmol
Magnesium sulfate	80 mg
Calcium gluconate	137 mg

Component	Concentration per Liter				
	#269	#270	#271	#272	#273
Amino acids (Aminoplasmal 16%)	7.12%	7.34%	7.49%	7.6%	7.68%
Dextrose 70%	19.69%	20.35%	20.82%	21.0%	21.32%
Fat emulsion 20% (Lipofundin MCT)	2.49%	2.54%	2.58%	2.68%	2.69%
Sodium	118.6 mEq	97.8 mEq	83.3 mEq	72.4 mEq	64 mEq
Potassium	71.2 mEq	58.7 mEq	49.9 mEq	43.5 mEq	38.4 mEq
Calcium	11.9 mEq	9.8 mEq	8.3 mEq	7.2 mEq	6.4 mEq
Magnesium	11.9 mEq	9.8 mEq	8.3 mEq	7.2 mEq	6.4 mEq
Phosphate	28.5 mmol	23.5 mmol	19.9 mmol	17.4 mmol	15.4 mmol
Chloride	118.6 mEq	97.8 mEq	83.3 mmol	72.4 mEq	64.0 mEq
Trace elements	3.6 mL	2.9 mL	2.5 mL	2.2 mL	1.9 mL
Multivitamins	11.9 mL	9.8 mL	8.3 mL	7.2 mL	6.4 mL

Component	Concentration per Liter	
	#274	#275
TrophAmine	3.75%	
Amino acids		3.6%
Dextrose	17.5%	10.6%
Sodium	25 mEq	36 mEq
Potassium	19 mEq	25.5 mEq
Calcium	19 mEq	6.4 mEq
Magnesium	3.8 mEq	6.4 mEq
Phosphates	12.5 mEq	5.5 mmol
Acetate	25 mEq	70 mEq
M.V.I.-Pediatric	52 mL	
Trace elements (pediatric)	2.5 mL	
Ranitidine HCl	73 mL	

Component	Concentration per Liter
	#276
Aminosyn	4.25%
Dextrose	25%
Sterile water for injection	97.68 mL
Sodium chloride	50 mEq
Potassium chloride	40 mEq
Potassium phosphates	10 mmol
Magnesium sulfate	8 mEq
Calcium chloride and gluconate	10 mEq

		Component Amounts	
Component	Mfr	#277	#278
Amino acids (Neonutrin 15%)	FRK	500 mL	500 mL
Dextrose 40% (Ardeanutrisol)	ARD	500 mL	500 mL
Fat emulsion 20% (Smoflipid)	FRK	250 mL	
Fat emulsion 20% (Lipoplus)	BRN		250 mL
Sodium chloride 10%	ARD	10 mL	10 mL
Potassium chloride 7.45%	ARD	10 mL	10 mL
Calcium gluconate 10%	HB	10–40 mL	10–40 mL
Magnesium sulfate 10%	HB	10–40 mL	10–40 mL
Potassium phosphate 13.6%		10–40 mL	10–40 mL
Trace elements (Addamel N)	FRK	10 mL	10 mL

[a] Trace elements: chromium, copper, iron, manganese, iodine, fluorine, molybdenum, selenium, and zinc.

	Component Amounts	
Component	#279[a]	#280[b]
Amino acids 14%	250 mL	
Amino acids 14.36%		250 mL
Dextrose 39.6%	250 mL	250 mL
Fat emulsion 20%	125 mL	125 mL
Sodium	33.5 mmol	33.5 mmol
Potassium	23.5 mmol	23.5 mmol
Magnesium	2.65 mmol	2.65 mmol
Calcium	2.65 mmol	2.65 mmol
Zinc	0.02 mmol	0.02 mmol
Chloride	30 mmol	30 mmol
Acetate	30 mmol	30 mmol
Phosphate	10 mmol	10 mmol

[a] Available as a 3-chamber bag of NuTRIflex Lipid Special (Braun) in a fixed volume and concentration with no additional additives.

[b] Available as a 3-chamber bag of NuTRIflex Omega Special (Braun) in a fixed volume and concentration with no additional additives.

Component	Concentration per Liter		
	#281	#282	#283
Amino acids (Primene)	3.3%	3%	3%
Nitrogen	4.95 g	4.5 g	4.5 g
Dextrose	10%	10%	7.5%
Sodium	15 mmol	33 mmol	33 mmol
Potassium		22 mmol	22 mmol
Chloride	9.3 mmol	13.5 mmol	13.5 mmol
Calcium	12 mmol	12 mmol	12 mmol
Magnesium	1.5 mmol	1.5 mmol	1.5 mmol
Phosphate	10 mmol	10 mmol	10 mmol
Acetate	5 mmol	40 mmol	40 mmol
Zinc		3.26 mg	3.26 mg
Selenium		20 mcg	20 mcg
Iodide		8 mcg	8 mcg
Heparin sodium	500 units	500 units	500 units

Selected Revisions September 30, 2019. © Copyright, October 2006. American Society of Health-System Pharmacists, Inc.

References

1. Package insert (for brands listed after the nonproprietary name heading in a monograph; date of package insert given as part of citation)

2. Physicians' desk reference. 63rd ed. Montvale, NJ: Thomson PDR; 2009.

3. Kirkland WD, Jones RW, Ellis JR et al. Compatibility studies of parenteral admixtures. *Am J Hosp Pharm*. 1961; 18:694–9.

4. McEvoy GK, ed. AHFS drug information 2011. Bethesda, MD: American Society of Health-System Pharmacists; 2011.

5. Sweetman SC, ed. Martindale: the complete drug reference. 37th aed. London, England: The Pharmaceutical Press; 2011.

6. Parker EA. Staphcillin injection. *Am J Hosp Pharm*. 1970; 27:67–8.

7. Parker EA. Compatibility digest. *Am J Hosp Pharm*. 1970; 27:672–3.

8. Trissel LA. Trissel's stability of compounded formulations. 4th ed. Washington, DC: American Pharmacists Association; 2009.

9. Patel JA, Phillips GL. Guide to physical compatibility of intravenous drug admixtures. *Am J Hosp Pharm*. 1966; 23:409–11.

10. Bogash RC. Compatibilities and incompatibilities of some parenteral medication. *Bull Am Soc Hosp Pharm*. 1955; 12:445–8.

11. Dunworth RD, Kenna FR. Preliminary report: incompatibility of combinations of medications in intravenous solutions. *Am J Hosp Pharm*. 1965; 22:190–1.

12. Moorhatch P, Chiou WL. Interactions between drugs and plastic intravenous fluid bags, part i: sorption studies on 17 drugs. *Am J Hosp Pharm*. 1974; 31:72–8.

13. Levin HJ, Fieber RA. Stability data for Tubex filled by hospital pharmacists. *Hosp Pharm*. 1973; 8:310–1.

14. Powers S. Incompatibilities of pre-op medications. *Hosp Formul Manage*. 1970; 5:22.

15. Intravenous additive incompatibilities. Bethesda, MD: Pharmacy Department, National Institutes of Health; 1970 Jan.

16. Cantania PN, King JC. Physico-chemical incompatibilities of selected cardiovascular and psychotherapeutic agents with sodium ethacrynate. *Am J Hosp Pharm*. 1972; 29:141–6.

17. *USP-NF* Online: 2020 U.S. Pharmacopeia National Formulary USP 42 NF 37. Rockville, MD: The United States Pharmacopeial Convention; 2020. www.uspnf.com. Updated 2019 Jun 3. Accessed 2020 Jun 5.

18. Kramer W, Inglott A. Some physical and chemical incompatibilities of drugs for i.v. administration. *Drug Intell Clin Pharm*. 1971; 5:211–28.

19. McEvoy GK, ed. American hospital formulary service drug information. Bethesda, MD: American Society of Health-System Pharmacists; prior editions.

20. Parker EA. Compatibility digest. *Am J Hosp Pharm*. 1969; 26:412–3.

21. Parker EA. Compatibility digest. *Am J Hosp Pharm*. 1969; 26:653–5.

22. Parker EA. Compatibility digest. *Am J Hosp Pharm*. 1970; 27:327–9.

23. Parker EA. Compatibility digest. *Am J Hosp Pharm*. 1974; 31:1076.

24. Parker EA. Compatibility digest. *Am J Hosp Pharm*. 1971; 28:805.

25. Souney PF, Solomon MA. Visual compatibility of cimetidine hydrochloride with common preoperative injectable medications. *Am J Hosp Pharm*. 1984; 41:1840–1.

26. Riley BB. Incompatibilities in intravenous solutions. *J Hosp Pharm*. 1970; 28:228–40.

27. Parker EA, Levin HJ. Compatibility digest. *Am J Hosp Pharm*. 1975; 32:943–4.

28. Misgen R. Compatibilities and incompatibilities of some intravenous solution admixtures. *Am J Hosp Pharm*. 1965; 22:92–4.

32. Frank JT. Intralipid compatibility study. *Drug Intell Clin Pharm*. 1973; 7:351–2.

33. Yeo MT, Gazzaniga AB, Bartlett RH et al. Total intravenous nutrition experience with fat emulsions and hypertonic glucose. *Arch Surg*. 1973; 106:792–6.

34. Melly MA, Meng HC. Microbial growth in lipid emulsions used in parenteral nutrition. *Arch Surg*. 1975; 110:1479–81.

35. Deitel M, Kaminsky V. Total nutrition by peripheral vein—the lipid system. *Can Med Assoc J*. 1974; 111:152–4.

36. Cashore WJ, Sedaghatian MR. Nutritional supplements with intravenously administered lipid, protein hydrolysate, and glucose in small premature infants. *Pediatrics*. 1975; 56:8–16.

37. Lynn B. Intralipid compatibility study. *Drug Intell Clin Pharm*. 1974; 8:75.

38. Electronic Medicines Compendium. London, England: Datapharm Communications Ltd.

39. Fortner CL, Grove WR, Bowie D et al. Fat emulsion vehicle for intravenous administration of an aqueous insoluble drug. *Am J Hosp Pharm*. 1975; 32:582–4.

40. Riffkin C. Incompatibilities of manufactured parenteral products. *Am J Hosp Pharm*. 1963; 20:19–22.

41. Edward M. pH—an important factor in the compatibility of additives in intravenous therapy. *Am J Hosp Pharm*. 1967; 24:440–9.

42. Turner FE, King JC. Spectrophotometric analysis of intravenous admixtures containing metaraminol and corticosteroids. *Am J Hosp Pharm*. 1970; 27:540–7.

43. Anderson RW, Latiolais CJ. Physico-chemical incompatibilities of parenteral admixtures—Aramine and Solu-Cortef. *Am J Hosp Pharm*. 1973; 30:128–33.

44. Smith MC. The dextrans. *Am J Hosp Pharm*. 1965; 22:273–5.

45. Stokes TF, Sumner ED. Particulate contamination and stability of three additives in 0.9% sodium chloride injection in plastic and glass large-volume containers. *Am J Hosp Pharm*. 1975; 32:821–6.

46. Parker EA. Solution additive chemical incompatibility study. *Am J Hosp Pharm*. 1967; 24:434–9.

47. Parker EA. Compatibility digest. *Am J Hosp Pharm*. 1969; 26:543–4.

DOI: 10.37573/9781585286850.408

48. Parker EA. Parenteral incompatibilities. *Hosp Pharm*. 1969; 4:14–22.

49. Beatrice MG, Stanaszek WF, Allen LV et al. Physicochemical stability of a preanesthetic mixture of hydroxyzine hydrochloride and atropine sulfate. *Am J Hosp Pharm*. 1975; 32:1133–7.

50. Leff RD, Roberts RJ. Effect of intravenous fluid and drug solution coadministration on final-infusate osmolality, specific gravity, and pH. *Am J Hosp Pharm*. 1982; 39:468–71.

51. Crevar GE, Slotnick IJ. A note on the stability of actinomycin D. *J Pharm Pharmacol*. 1964; 16:429.

52. Coles CLJ, Lees KA. Additives to intravenous fluids. *Pharm J*. 1971; 206:153–4.

53. Rudd L. Pethidine stability in intravenous solutions. *Med J Aust*. 1978; 2:34.

54. Webb JW. A pH pattern for i.v. additives. *Am J Hosp Pharm*. 1969; 26:31–5.

55. Jones RW, Stanko GL. Pharmaceutical compatibilities of Pentothal and Nembutal. *Am J Hosp Pharm*. 1961; 18:700–4.

56. Turco SJ, Sherman NE, Zagar L et al. Stability of aminophylline in 5% dextrose in water. *Hosp Pharm*. 1975; 10:374–5.

57. Hodby ED, Hirsch J. Influence of drugs upon the anticoagulant activity of heparin. *Can Med Assoc J*. 1972; 106:562–4.

58. Pamperl H, Kleinberger G. Morphologic changes of Intralipid 20% liposomes in all-in-one solutions during prolonged storage. *Infusiontherapie*. 1982; 9:86–91.

59. Parker EA. Compatibility digest. *Am J Hosp Pharm*. 1974; 31:775.

60. Wolfert RR, Cox RM. Room temperature stability of drug products labeled for refrigerated storage. *Am J Hosp Pharm*. 1975; 32:585–7.

61. Anon. Intravenous fat. *Lancet*. 1976; 1:1059–60.

62. Sachtler G. Dilantin for i.v. use. *Drug Intell Clin Pharm*. 1973; 7:418.

63. Burke WA. I.V. drug incompatibilities—Dilantin. *Am J IV Ther*. 1975; 2:16–8.

64. Baldwin J, Amerson AB. Intramuscular use of diphenylhydantoin. *Am J Hosp Pharm*. 1973; 30:837–8.

65. Tobias DC, Kellick KA. Dilantin for i.v. use. *Drug Intell Clin Pharm*. 1973; 7:418.

66. Chan NL. Dilantin for i.v. use. *Drug Intell Clin Pharm*. 1973; 7:419.

67. Ammar HO, Salama HA. Studies on the stability of injectable solutions of some phenothiazines, part i: effect of pH and buffer systems. *Pharmazie*. 1975; 30:368–9.

68. Pickering LK, Rutherford I. Effect of concentration and time upon inactivation of tobramycin, gentamicin, netilmicin, and amikacin by azlocillin, carbenicillin, mecillinam, mezlocillin, and piperacillin. *J Pharmacol Exp Ther*. 1981; 217:345–9.

69. Ho NFH, Goeman JA. Prediction of pharmaceutical stability of parenteral solutions. *Drug Intell Clin Pharm*. 1970; 4:69–71.

72. Trissel LA, Davignon JP, Kleinman LM, et al. NCI investigational drugs pharmaceutical data. Bethesda, MD: National Cancer Institute; 1988.

73. Muhlhauser I, Broermann C, Tsotsalas M et al. Miscibility of human and bovine ultralente insulin with soluble insulin. *BMJ*. 1984; 289:1656–7.

74. Grant HR. Compatibilities of intravenous admixtures. *Hosp Pharmacist*. 94 (Mar-Apr) 1962; 15:67–70.

75. Hanson DB, Hendeles L. Guide to total dose intravenous iron dextran therapy. *Am J Hosp Pharm*. 1974; 31:592–5.

76. Duke AB, Kelleher J. Serum iron and iron binding capacity after total dose infusion of iron-dextran for iron deficiency anaemia in pregnancy. *J Obstet Gynaecol Br Commonw*. 1974; 81(11):895–900.

77. Parker EA. Compatibility digest. *Am J Hosp Pharm*. 1975; 32:214.

78. Gardella LA, Kesler H, Carter JE et al. Intropin (dopamine hydrochloride) intravenous admixture compatibility, part ii: stability with some commonly used antibiotics in 5% dextrose injection. *Am J Hosp Pharm*. 1976; 33:537–40.

79. Gardella LA, Zaroslinski JF. Intropin (dopamine hydrochloride) intravenous admixture compatibility, part i: stability with common intravenous fluids. *Am J Hosp Pharm*. 1975; 32:575–8.

80. Garnett W. Diluents for antineoplastic drugs. *Drug Intell Clin Pharm*. 1971; 5:261.

81. Landersjo L, Stjernstrom G. Studies on the stability and compatibility of drugs in infusion fluids V. Effect of lactate and metal ions on the stability of benzylpenicillin. *Acta Pharm Suec*. 1978; 15:161–8.

82. Notari RE, Chin ML. Arabinosylcytosine stability in aqueous solutions: pH profile and shelf life predictions. *J Pharm Sci*. 1972; 61:1189–96.

83. Murty BSR, Kapoor JN. Properties of mannitol injection (25%) after repeated autoclavings. *Am J Hosp Pharm*. 1975; 32:826–7.

84. Rosch JM, Pazin GJ, Fireman P. Reduction of amphotericin B nephrotoxicity with mannitol. *JAMA*. 1976; 235:1995–6.

85. Bergman N, Vellar ID. Potential life-threatening variations of drug concentrations in intravenous infusion systems—potassium chloride, insulin, and heparin. *Med J Aust*. 1982; 2:270–2.

86. Parker EA. Compatibility digest. *Am J Hosp Pharm*. 1970; 27:492–3.

87. Feigen RD, Moss KS. Antibiotic stability in solutions used for intravenous nutrition and fluid therapy. *Pediatrics*. 1973; 51:1016–26.

88. Zost ED, Yanchick VA. Compatibility and stability of disodium carbenicillin in combination with other drugs and large volume parenteral solutions. *Am J Hosp Pharm*. 1972; 29:135–40.

89. Lynn B. Recent work on parenteral penicillins. *J Hosp Pharm*. 1971; 29:183–194.

90. Tourville J. Sodium nitroprusside. *Drug Intell Clin Pharm*. 1975; 9:361–4.

91. Anon. Editorial: Sodium nitroprusside in anaesthesia. *Br Med J*. 1975; 2:524–5.

92. Hargrave RE. Degradation of solutions of sodium nitroprusside. *J Hosp Pharm*. 1974; 32:188–9.

93. Anon. Sodium nitroprusside for hypertensive crisis. *Med Lett Drugs Ther*. 1975; 17:82–3.

94. Anderson RA, Rae W. Stability of sodium nitroprusside solutions. *Aust J Pharm Sci NS1*. 1972; (July):45–6.

95. Schumacher GE. Sodium nitroprusside injection. *Am J Hosp Pharm*. 1966; 23:532.

96. Cruz JE, Maness DD, Yakatan GJ. Kinetics and mechanism of hydrolysis of furosemide. *Int J Pharm*. 1979; 2:275–81.

97. Thomas R. Meperidine HCl and heparin sodium precipitation. *Hosp Pharm*. 1979; 2:275–81.

98. Fleischer NM. Promethazine hydrochloride-morphine sulfate incompatibility. *Am J Hosp Pharm*. 1973; 30:665.

99. Lynn B. Pharmaceutical aspects of semi-synthetic penicillins. *J Hosp Pharm*. 1970; 28:71–86.

100. Meisler JM, Skolaut MW. Extemporaneous sterile compounding in intravenous additives. *Am J Hosp Pharm*. 1966; 23:557–63.

101. Guthaus MR (Medical Services, The Upjohn Company, Kalamazoo, MI): Personal communication; 1973 Aug 9.

102. HamLin WE, Riebe KW, Scothorn WW, et al. Pharmacy profile of cleocin phosphate. Presented at 10th annual ASHP midyear clinical meeting. Washington, DC: 1975 Dec 11.

103. Riebe KW, Oesterling TO. Parenteral development of clindamycin-2–phosphate. *Bull Parenter Drug Assoc*. 1972; 26:139–45.

104. Therapeutic profile: cleocin phosphate. Kalamazoo, MI: The Upjohn Company; 1973.

105. Wyatt RG, Okamato GA. Stability of antibiotics in parenteral solutions. *Pediatrics*. 1972; 49:22–9.

106. Halasi S, Nairn JD. Stability studies of hydralazine hydrochloride in aqueous solutions. *J Parenter Sci Technol*. 1990; 44:30–4.

107. Whiting DA. Treatment of chromoblastomycosis with local concentrations of amphotericin B. *Br J Dermatol*. 1967; 79:345–51.

108. Kirschenbaum BE, Latiolais CJ. Injectable medications—a guide to stability and reconstitution. New York, NY: McMahon Group; 1993.

109. Bair JN, Carew DP. Therapeutic availability of antibiotics in parenteral solutions. *Bull Parenter Drug Assoc*. 1965; 19:153–63.

110. Dancey JW, Carew DP. Availability of antibiotics in combination with other additives in intravenous solutions. *Am J Hosp Pharm*. 1966; 23:543–51.

111. Prasad VK, Granatek AP. Physical compatibility and chemical stability of cephapirin sodium in combination with antibiotics and large-volume parenteral solutions, part i. *Curr Ther Res Clin Exp*. 1974; 16:505–39.

112. Lynn B. Carbenicillin plus gentamicin. *Lancet*. 1971; 1:654.

113. Jacobs J, Kletter D, Superstine E et al. Intravenous infusions of heparin and penicillins. *J Clin Pathol*. 1973; 26:742–6.

114. Lynn B. Penicillin instability in infusions. *Br Med J*. 1971; 1:174.

115. Information for health professionals. Wellington, New Zealand: New Zealand Medicines and Medical Devices Safety Authority.

117. McEvoy GK, ed. American hospital formulary service drug information 95. Bethesda, MD: American Society of Health-System Pharmacists; 1995.

118. Harrison DC. Practical guidelines for the use of lidocaine. Prevention and treatment of cardiac arrhythmias. *JAMA*. 1975; 233:1202–4.

119. Collinsworth K. Clinical pharmacology of lidocaine as an antiarrhythmic drug. *West J Med*. 1976; 124:36–43.

120. Anon. Prophylactic use of lidocaine in myocardial infarction. *Med Lett Drugs Ther*. 1976; 18:1–2.

121. Dundee JW, Gamble JA, Assaf RA. Plasma diazepam levels following intramuscular injection by nurses and doctors. *Lancet*. 1974; 2:1461.

123. Tortorici MP. Stability data on frozen i.m. and i.v. solutions. *Pharm Times*. 1975; 41:68–72.

124. Barbara AC, Clemente C. Physical incompatibility of sulfonamide compounds and polyionic solutions. *N Engl J Med*. 1966; 274:1316–7.

125. Brooke D, Bequette RJ. Chemical stability of cyclophosphamide in parenteral solutions. *Am J Hosp Pharm*. 1973; 30:134–7.

126. Brooke D, Scott JA. Effect of briefly heating cyclophosphamide solutions. *Am J Hosp Pharm*. 1975; 32:44–5.

127. Gallelli JF. Stability studies of drugs used in intravenous solutions, part i. *Am J Hosp Pharm*. 1967; 24:425–33.

128. Dupont Pharmaceuticals. Nubain, physical compatibility. Wilmington, DE; undated.

129. Kramer W, Tanja JJ. Precipitates found in admixtures of potassium chloride and dextrose 5% in water. *Am J Hosp Pharm*. 1970; 27:548–53.

130. Lawson DH. Clinical use of potassium supplements. *Am J Hosp Pharm*. 1975; 32:708–11.

131. Lundgren P, Landersjo L. Studies on the stability and compatibility of drugs in infusion fluids, ii: factors affecting the stability of benzylpenicillin. *Acta Pharm Suec*. 1970; 7:509–26.

132. Weber CR, Gupta VD. Stability of phenylephrine hydrochloride in intravenous solutions. *J Hosp Pharm*. 1970; 28:200–8.

133. Chiou WL, Moorhatch P. Interaction between vitamin A and plastic intravenous fluid bags. *J Am Med Assoc*. 1973; 223:328.

134. Komesaroff D, Field JE. Pancuronium bromide: a new non-depolarizing muscle relaxant. *Med J Aust*. 1969; 1:908–11.

135. Simberkoff MS, Thomas L, McGregor D et al. Inactivation of penicillins by carbohydrate solutions at alkaline pH. *N Engl J Med*. 1970; 283:116–9.

136. Hicks CI, Gallardo JPB. Stability of sodium bicarbonate injection stored in polypropylene syringes. *Am J Hosp Pharm*. 1972; 29:210–6.

137. DeLuca PP, Kowalski RJ. Problems arising from the transfer of sodium bicarbonate injection from ampuls to plastic disposable syringes. *Am J Hosp Pharm*. 1972; 29:217–22.

138. D'Arcy PF, Thompson KM. Stability of chlorpromazine hydrochloride added to intravenous infusion fluids. *Pharm J*. 1973; 210:28.

139. Nahata MC, Zingarelli JR, Hipple TF. Stability of caffeine injection stored in plastic and glass syringes. *DICP*. 1989; 23:1035.

140. Murabito AS (Smith Kline & French Laboratories, Philadelphia, PA): Personal communication; 1986 Dec 15.

141. Mann JM, Coleman DL. Stability of parenteral solutions of sodium cephalothin, cephaloridine, potassium penicillin G (buffered), and vancomycin HCl. *Am J Hosp Pharm.* 1971; 28:760–3.

142. Appleby DH, John JF. Effect of peritoneal dialysis solution on the antimicrobial activity of cephalosporins. *Nephron.* 1982; 30:341–4.

143. Upshaw MD (Medical Information Services, Eli Lilly and Company, Indianapolis, IN): Personal communication; 1972 Jan 10.

144. Gallelli JF, MacLowry JD. Stability of antibiotics in parenteral solutions. *Am J Hosp Pharm.* 1969; 26:630–5.

145. Dienstag JL, Neu HC. Tobramycin: new aminoglycoside antibiotic. *Clin Med.* 1975; 82:13–9.

146. Struhar M, Heinrich J. K sorpcii pentoxifyllinu na infuznu supravu Luer. *Farm Obz.* 1988; 57:405–10.

147. Bergstrom RF, Fites AL. Stability of parenteral solutions of tobramycin sulfate. *Am J Hosp Pharm.* 1975; 32:887–8.

148. Huber RC, Riffkin C. Inline final filters for removing particles from amphotericin B infusions. *Am J Hosp Pharm.* 1975; 32:173–6.

149. Rebagay T, Rapp R, Bivins B et al. Residues in antibiotic preparations, i: scanning electron microscopic studies of surface topography. *Am J Hosp Pharm.* 1976; 33:433–43.

150. Gallelli JF. Assay and stability of amphotericin B in aqueous solutions. *Drug Intell.* 1967; 1:102–5.

151. Piecoro JJ, Goodman NL, Wheeler WE et al. Particulate matter in reconstituted amphotericin B and assay of filtered solutions of amphotericin B. *Am J Hosp Pharm.* 1975; 32:381–4.

152. Gotz V, Simon W. Inline filtration of amphotericin B infusions. *Am J Hosp Pharm.* 1975; 32:458.

153. Chatterji D, Hiranaka PK. Stability of sodium oxacillin in intravenous solutions. *Am J Hosp Pharm.* 1975; 32:1130–2.

154. Facts and Comparisons, Inc. Drug facts and comparisons. St. Louis, MO; 2003.

155. Parodi JF. Stability of frozen antibiotic solutions in Viaflex infusion containers. *Hosp Pharm.* 1976; 11:178–9.

156. Larsen SS. Studies on stability of drugs in frozen systems. IV. The stability of benzylpenicillin sodium in frozen aqueous solutions. *Dan Tidsskr Farm.* 1971; 45:307–16.

157. Noone P, Pattison JR. Therapeutic implications of interaction of gentamicin and penicillins. *Lancet.* 1971; 2:575–8.

158. Boulet M, Marier JR. Effect of magnesium on formation of calcium phosphate precipitates. *Arch Biochem Biophys.* 1962; 96:629–36.

159. van den Berg L, Soliman FS. Composition and pH changes during freezing of solutions containing calcium and magnesium phosphate. *Cryobiology.* 1969; 6:10–4.

160. Ong JTH, Kostenbauder HB. Effect of self-association on rate of penicillin G degradation in concentrated aqueous solutions. *J Pharm Sci.* 1975; 64:1378–80.

161. Shoup LK, Thur MP. Stability of frozen buffered penicillin G potassium injection. *Hosp Formul Manage.* 1968; 3:38–9.

162. Boylan JC, Simmons JL. Stability of frozen solutions of sodium cephalothin and cephaloridine. *Am J Hosp Pharm.* 1972; 29:687–9.

163. Grant NH, Clark DE. Imidazole- and base-catalyzed hydrolysis of penicillin in frozen systems. *J Am Chem Soc.* 1961; 83:4476–7.

164. Lindsay RE, Hem SL. Dosage form for potassium penicillin G intravenous infusion solutions. *Drug Devel Commun.* 1974–5; 1:211–222.

165. Im S, Latiolais CJ. Physico-chemical incompatibilities of parenteral admixtures—penicillin and tetracyclines. *Am J Hosp Pharm.* 1966; 23:333–43.

166. Pfeifer HJ, Webb JW. Compatibility of penicillin and ascorbic acid injection. *Am J Hosp Pharm.* 1976; 33:448–50.

167. Rusmin S, DeLuca PP. Effect of inline filtration on the potency of potassium penicillin G. *Bull Parenter Drug Assoc.* 1976; 30:64–71.

168. Stolar MH, Carlin HS. Effect of freezing on the stability of sodium methicillin injection. *Am J Hosp Pharm.* 1968; 25:32–5.

169. Lynn B. Stability of methicillin in dextrose solutions at alkaline pH. *J Hosp Pharm.* 1972; 30:81–3.

170. Lynn B. Pharmaceutics of the semi-synthetic penicillins. *Chem Drug.* 1967; 187:134–6.

171. Lynn B. Inactivation of methicillin in dextrose solutions at alkaline pH. *N Engl J Med.* 1971; 285:690.

172. Mattson CJ, Clark ST, Colangelo A. Stability of clindamycin phosphate in plastic syringes. Presented at 20th annual ASHP midyear clinical meeting. New Orleans, LA: 1985 Dec.

173. Clark ST, Colangelo A. Stability of clindamycin phosphate in plastic syringes. Presented at 20th annual ASHP midyear clinical meeting. New Orleans, LA: 1985 Dec.

174. Cohon MS (Drug Information Services, Upjohn Company, Kalamazoo, MI): Personal communications; 1986 Dec 12, 1988 Jan 27, 1988 Feb 3.

176. Owen RT (UK Medical Information Section, The Wellcome Foundation Ltd., Cheshire, England): Personal communication; 1993 Aug 19.

177. Lesson LJ, Weidenheimer JF. Stability of tetracycline and riboflavin. *J Pharm Sci.* 1969; 58:355–7.

178. Turco SJ, Burke WA. Methods of ordering and use of intravenous phosphate (mEq vs mM). *Hosp Pharm.* 322, 326 (Aug) 1975; 10:320.

179. Pinkus TF, Jeffrey LP. Incompatibility of calcium and phosphate in parenteral alimentation solutions. *Am J IV Ther.* 1976; 3:22–4.

180. Kaminski MV, Harris DF, Collin CF et al. Electrolyte compatibility in synthetic amino acid hyperalimentation solution. *Am J Hosp Pharm.* 1974; 31:244–6.

181. Schlicht JR. Adjustments in etoposide infusion flow rates when using controllers. *Am J Hosp Pharm.* 1990; 47:2656.

182. FASS, Karolinska Institutet, Huddinge, Sweden. Available at edu.ofa.ki.effica/

183. Lee FA, Gwinn JL. Roentgen patterns of extravasation of calcium gluconate in the tissues of the neonate. *J Pediatr.* 1975; 86:598–601.

184. Weiss Y, Ackerman C. Localized necrosis of scalp in neonates due to calcium gluconate infusions: a cautionary note. *Pediatrics.* 1975; 56:1084–6.

185. Ramamurthy RS, Harris V. Subcutaneous calcium deposition in the neonate associated with intravenous administration of calcium gluconate. *Pediatrics*. 1975; 55:802–6.

186. Laegeler WL, Tio JM. Stability of certain amino acids in a parenteral nutrition solution. *Am J Hosp Pharm*. 1974; 31:776–9.

187. Kleinman LM, Tangrea JA, Gallelli JF et al. Stability of solutions of essential amino acids. *Am J Hosp Pharm*. 1973; 30:1054–7.

188. Rowlands DA. Compatibility of calcium and phosphate in amino acids solution. *Am J Hosp Pharm*. 1975; 32:360.

189. Saudek EC (The Upjohn Company): Personal communication; 1973 Jan 3.

190. Rowlands DA, Wilkinson WR. Storage stability of mixed hyperalimentation solutions. *Am J Hosp Pharm*. 1973; 30:436–8.

191. Aro R (Senior Clinical Research Associate, Fujisawa USA): Personal communication, February 22, 1994.

192. Rodriguez Penin I, Yanez Gonzalez A, Camba Rodriguez A et al. Estabilidad de la mezcla morfina-midazolam en un dispositivo de infusion continua. *Farm Hosp*. 1991; 15:407–9.

193. Nahata MC, Zingarelli JR, Durrell DE. Stability of caffeine injection in intravenous admixtures and parenteral nutrition solutions. *DICP*. 1989; 23:466–7.

194. Hull RL. Use of trace elements in intravenous hyperalimentation solutions. *Am J Hosp Pharm*. 1974; 31:759–61.

195. Johnson C, Cloyd J. Parenteral hyperalimentation. *Drug Intell Clin Pharm*. 1975; 9:493–9.

196. Hankins DA, Riella MC, Scribner BH et al. Whole blood trace element concentrations during total parenteral nutrition. *Surgery*. 1976; 79:674–7.

197. Hamann MA. Trace element requirements in hyperalimentation. *Am J Hosp Pharm*. 1974; 31:1035.

198. Hull RL. Trace element requirements in hyperalimentation. *Am J Hosp Pharm*. 1974; 31:1038.

199. Heird WC, Winters RW. Total intravenous alimentation in pediatric patients. *South Med J*. 1975; 68:1173–6.

200. Baker JA, Kirkman H, Woodley C et al. Computer-assisted pediatric hyperalimentation. *Am J Hosp Pharm*. 1974; 31:752–8.

201. Parish R. Hyperalimentation procedures. *Am J Hosp Pharm*. 1974; 31:1160.

202. Pomerance HH, Rader RE. Crystal formation: a new complication of total parenteral nutrition. *Pediatrics*. 1973; 52:864–6.

203. Bohart RD, Ogawa G. An observation on the stability of cis-dichlorodiammineplatinum (II): a caution regarding its administration. *Cancer Treat Rep*. 1979; 63:2117–8.

204. Prestayko AW, Cadiz M. Incompatibility of aluminum-containing iv administration equipment with cis-dichlorodiammineplatinum (II) administration. *Cancer Treat Rep*. 1979; 63:2118–9.

205. Shils ME. Minerals in total parenteral nutrition. *Drug Intell Clin Pharm*. 1972; 6:385–93.

206. Flack HL, Gans JA, Serlick SE et al. The current status of parenteral hyperalimentation. *Am J Hosp Pharm*. 1971; 28:326–35.

207. McRae MP, King JC. Compatibility of antineoplastic, antibiotic, and corticosteroid drugs in intravenous admixtures. *Am J Hosp Pharm*. 1976; 33:1010–3.

208. Warren E, Synder RJ, Thompson CO et al. Stability of ampicillin in intravenous solutions. *Mayo Clin Proc*. 1972; 47:34–5.

209. Raffanti EF, King JC. Effect of pH on the stability of sodium ampicillin solutions. *Am J Hosp Pharm*. 1974; 31:745–51.

210. Savello DR, Shangraw RF. Stability of sodium ampicillin solutions in the frozen and liquid states. *Am J Hosp Pharm*. 1971; 28:754–9.

211. Jacobs J, Nathan I, Superstine E et al. Ampicillin and carbenicillin stability in commonly used infusion solutions. *Drug Intell Clin Pharm*. 1970; 4:204–8.

212. Hiranaka P, Frazier AG. Stability of sodium ampicillin in aqueous solutions. *Am J Hosp Pharm*. 1972; 29:321–2.

213. Stratton M, Sandmann BJ. Stability studies of ampicillin sodium in intravenous fluids using optical activity. *Bull Parenter Drug Assoc*. 1975; 29:286–95.

214. Pincock RE, Kiovsky TE. Kinetics of reactions in frozen solutions. *J Chem Educ*. 1966; 43:358–60.

215. Hou JP, Poole JW. Kinetics and mechanism of degradation of ampicillin in solution. *J Pharm Sci*. 1969; 58:447–54.

216. Shils ME, Wright WL, Turnbull A et al. Long-term parenteral nutrition through an external arteriovenous shunt. *N Engl J Med*. 1970; 283:341–4.

217. Zia H, Tehrani M. Kinetics of carbenicillin degradation in aqueous solutions. *Can J Pharm Sci*. 1974; 9:112–7.

218. Riff LJ, Jackson GG. Laboratory and clinical conditions for gentamicin inactivation by carbenicillin. *Arch Intern Med*. 1972; 130:887–91.

219. McLaughlin JE, Reeves DS. Clinical and laboratory evidence for inactivation of gentamicin by carbenicillin. *Lancet*. 1971; 1:261–4.

220. Klastersky J. Carbenicillin plus gentamicin. *Lancet*. 1971; 1:653–4.

221. Levison ME, Kaye D. Carbenicillin plus gentamicin. *Lancet*. 1971; 2:45–6.

222. Eykyn S, Phillips I. Gentamicin plus carbenicillin. *Lancet*. 1971; 1:545–6.

223. Riff L, Jackson GG. Gentamicin plus carbenicillin. *Lancet*. 1971; 1:592.

224. Zost ED, Yanchick VA. Stability of gentamicin in combination with carbenicillin. *Am J Hosp Pharm*. 1972; 29:388–90.

225. Jacoby GA. Carbenicillin and gentamicin. *N Engl J Med*. 1971; 284:1096–8.

226. Kleinberg ML (Professional Services, Immunex, Seattle, WA): Personal communication; 1993 Jun 14.

227. Baldini JT (Professional Services, Schering Laboratories, Kenilworth, NJ): Personal communication; 1972 Feb 11.

228. Koup JR, Gerbracht L. Combined use of heparin and gentamicin in peritoneal dialysis solutions. *Drug Intell Clin Pharm*. 1975; 9:388.

229. Reeves DS, Bywater MJ, Wise R et al. Availability of three antibiotics after intramuscular injection into thigh and buttock. *Lancet*. 1974; 2:1421–2.

230. Jackson GG. Gentamicin. *Practitioner*. 1967; 198:855–66.

231. Preskey D, Kayes JB. Stability of sulfadiazine sodium as used in admixture with intravenous infusion fluids. *J Clin Pharm*. 1976; 1:39–48.

232. Physicians' desk reference. 49th ed. Oradell, NJ: Medical Economics Company; 1995.

233. Larsen SS, Jensen VG. Studies on stability of drugs in frozen systems. II. The stabilities of hexobarbital sodium and phenobarbital sodium in frozen aqueous solutions. *Dan Tidsskr Farm*. 1970; 44:21–31.

234. NCI investigational drugs pharmaceutical data. Bethesda, MD: National Cancer Institute; 1988, 1990, 1994.

235. Halpern NA, Colucci RD, Alicea M et al. The compatibility of nicardipine hydrochloride injection with various ICU medications during simulated Y-site injection. *Int J Clin Pharmacol Ther Toxicol*. 1989; 27:250–4.

236. Anon. Kidney toxicity—main source of methotrexate complications. *J Am Med Assoc*. 1975; 223:1036–7.

237. Baker MBC Hospital Products Division, Abbott Laboratories, Abbott Park, Illinois: Personal Communication; 2003 Aug 27.

238. Hoeprich PD, Huston AC. Stability of four antifungal antimicrobics in vitro. *J Infect Dis*. 1978; 137:87–93.

239. Selam JL, Lord P, van Antwerp WP et al. Heparin addition to insulin in implantable pumps to prevent catheter obstruction. *Diabetes Care*. 1989; 12:38–9.

240. Wang DP. Stability of procaine in aqueous systems. *Analyst*. 1983; 108:851–6.

241. Lapidas B. Cautions regarding the preparation of high-dose methotrexate infusions. *Am J Hosp Pharm*. 1976; 33:760.

242. Pelsor FR. Cautions regarding the preparation of high-dose methotrexate infusions. *Am J Hosp Pharm*. 1976; 33:760.

243. Pritchard J. Stability of heparin solutions. *J Pharm Pharmacol*. 1964; 16:487–9.

244. Turco SJ. I.V. drug incompatibilities—heparin sodium USP. *Am J IV Ther*. 1976; 3:16–9.

245. Kakkar VV, Corrigan TP. Prevention of fatal postoperative pulmonary embolism by low doses of heparin: an international multicentre trial. *Lancet*. 1975; 2:45–51.

246. Sherry S. Low-dose heparin prophylaxis for postoperative venous thromboembolism. *N Engl J Med*. 1975; 293:300–2.

247. Gallus AS, Hirsch J, O'Brien SE et al. Prevention of venous thrombosis with small, subcutaneous doses of heparin. *JAMA*. 1976; 235:1980–2.

248. Hopefl AW. Low-dose heparin for the prevention of venous thromboembolism. *Hosp Pharm*. 1976; 11:223.

249. Wessler S. Heparin as an antithrombotic agent. Low-dose prophylaxis. *JAMA*. 1976; 236:389–91.

250. Erdi A, Kakkar VV, Thomas DP et al. Effect of low-dose subcutaneous heparin on whole-blood viscosity. *Lancet*. 1976; 2:342–4.

251. Hadgraft JW. Adding drugs to intravenous infusions. *Lancet*. 1970; 2:1254.

252. Stock SL, Warner N. Heparin in acid solutions. *Br Med J*. 1971; 3:307.

253. Chessells JM, Braithwaite TA. Dextrose and sorbitol as diluents for continuous intravenous heparin infusion. *Br Med J*. 1972; 2:81–2.

254. Mitchell JF, Barger RC. Heparin stability in 5% dextrose and 0.9% sodium chloride. *Am J Hosp Pharm*. 1976; 33:540–2.

255. Thomas RB, Salter FJ. Heparin locks: their advantages and disadvantages. *Hosp Formul*. 1975; 10:536–8.

256. Deeb EN, DiMattia PE. The key question: how much heparin in the lock?. *Am J IV Ther*. 1976; 3:22–6.

257. DeFina E. How we use heparin locks. *Am J IV Ther*. 33 (Dec-Jan) 1976; 3:27.

258. Hanson RL, Grant AM. Heparin-lock maintenance with ten units of sodium heparin in one milliliter of normal saline solution. *Surg Gynecol Obstet*. 1976; 142:373–6.

259. Rebagay T, DeLuca PP. Residues in antibiotic preparations, ii: effect of pH on the nature and level of particulate matter in sodium cephalothin intravenous solutions. *Am J Hosp Pharm*. 1976; 33:443–8.

260. Albano D (Manager Drug Information, Wyeth-Ayerst). Personal Communication; 1994 Jan 5.

261. Hopefl AW. Room temperature stability of drug products. *Am J Hosp Pharm*. 1975; 32:1084.

262. Barger RC. Room temperature stability of drug products. *Am J Hosp Pharm*. 1975; 32:1089.

263. Rosenbloom AL. Advances in commercial insulin preparations. *Am J Dis Child*. 1974; 128:631–3.

264. Rosenberg JM, Simon WA, Sangkachand P et al. Mixing insulin preparations. *Hosp Pharm*. 1976; 11:186.

265. Shainfeld FJ. Errors in insulin doses due to the design of insulin syringes. *Pediatrics*. 1975; 56:302–3.

266. Weisenfeld S, Podolsky S, Goldsmith L et al. Adsorption of insulin to infusion bottles and tubing. *Diabetes*. 1968; 17:766–71.

267. Petty C, Cunningham NL. Insulin adsorption by glass infusion bottles, polyvinylchloride infusion containers, and intravenous tubing. *Anesthesiology*. 1974; 40:400–4.

268. Kraegen EW, Lazarus L, Meler H et al. Carrier solutions for low-level intravenous insulin infusion. *Br Med J*. 1975; 3:464–6.

269. Semple P, Ratcliffe JG. Carrier solutions for low-level intravenous insulin infusion. *Br Med J*. 1975; 4:228–9.

270. Hays DP, Mehl B. I.V. drug incompatibilities—insulin. *Am J IV Ther*. 1976; 3:30–2.

271. Owen JA. The insulin revolution. *Hosp Formul*. 1976; 11:343.

272. Galloway JA (Medical Research Division, Eli Lilly and Company, Indianapolis, IN): Personal communication; 1967 Aug 29.

273. Rubin J, Humphries J, Smith G et al. Antibiotic activity in peritoneal dialysate. *Am J Kidney Dis*. 1983; 3:205–8.

274. De Vroe C, De Muynck C, Remon JP et al. The availability of diltiazem: a study on the sorption by intravenous delivery systems and on the stability of the drug. *J Pharm Pharmacol*. 1989; 41:273–5.

275. Kochevar M, Fry LK. Insulin and dead space volume. *Drug Intell Clin Pharm*. 1974; 8:33–4.

276. Bornstein M, Thomas PN, Coleman DL et al. Stability of parenteral solutions of cefazolin sodium. *Am J Hosp Pharm*. 1974; 31:296–98.

277. Carone SM, Bornstein M, Coleman DL et al. Stability of frozen solutions of cefazolin sodium. *Am J Hosp Pharm*. 1976; 33:639–41.

278. Royston DA (Consumer Technical Services, Eli Lilly and Company, Indianapolis, IN): Personal communication; 1976 Feb 19.

279. Brudney N, Eustace BT. Some formulations and compatibility problems with dimenhydrinate (Gravol). *Can Pharm J.* 1963; 96:470–1.

280. Acred P, Brown DM, Knudsen ET et al. New semi-synthetic penicillin active against pseudomonas pyocyanea. *Nature (London).* 1967; 215:25–30.

281. Schwartz MA, Buckwalter FH. Pharmaceutics of penicillin. *J Pharm Sci.* 1962; 51:1119–28.

282. Thur MP (Parenteral Products, Travenol Laboratories, Deerfield, IL): Personal communication; 1976 Sep 20.

283. Ziemba LJ (Medical Information, ICI Pharmaceuticals Group, Wilmington, DE): Personal communication; 1990 Mar 15.

284. Yamana T, Tsuji A. Comparative stability of cephalosporins in aqueous solution: kinetics and mechanisms of degradation. *J Pharm Sci.* 1976; 65:1563–74.

285. Kleinman LM, Davignon JP, Cradock JC et al. Investigational drug information. *Drug Intell Clin Pharm.* 1976; 10:48–9.

286. Chang SY, Evans TL. The stability of melphalan in the presence of chloride ion. *J Pharm Pharmacol.* 1979; 31:853–4.

287. Mitenko PA, Ogilvie RI. Rational intravenous doses of theophylline. *N Engl J Med.* 1973; 289:600–3.

288. Simons FER, Pierson WE. Current status of the use of intravenously administered aminophylline. *South Med J.* 1975; 68:802–4.

289. Weinberger MW, Matthay RA, Ginchansky EJ et al. Intravenous aminophylline dosage. Use of serum theophylline measurement for guidance. *JAMA.* 1976; 235:2110–3.

290. Nedich RL. Vitamin A absorption from plastic IV bags. *JAMA.* 1973; 224:1531–2.

291. Kaplan MA, Coppola WP, Nunning BC et al. Pharmaceutical properties and stability of amikacin, part i. *Curr Ther Res Clin Exp.* 1976; 20:352–8.

292. Nunning BC, Granatek AP. Physical compatibility and chemical stability of amikacin sulfate in large-volume parenteral solutions, part ii. *Curr Ther Res Clin Exp.* 1976; 20:359–68.

293. Nunning BC, Granatek AP. Physical compatibility and chemical stability of amikacin sulfate in combination with antibiotics in large-volume parenteral solutions, part iii. *Curr Ther Res Clin Exp.* 1976; 20:369–416.

294. Nunning BC, Granatek AP. Physical compatibility and chemical stability of amikacin sulfate in combination with non-antibiotic drugs in large-volume parenteral solutions, part iv. *Curr Ther Res Clin Exp.* 1976; 20:417–91.

295. Koup JR, Gerbracht L. Reduction in heparin activity by gentamicin. *Drug Intell Clin Pharm.* 1975; 9:568.

296. McKinley JD (M.D. Anderson Hospital and Tumor Institute, Houston, TX): Personal communication; 1976 Aug 23.

297. Weiner B, McNeely DJ, Kluge RM et al. Stability of gentamicin sulfate injection following unit dose repackaging. *Am J Hosp Pharm.* 1976; 33:1254–9.

298. Dinel BA, Ayotte DL, Behme RJ et al. Comparative stability of antibiotic admixtures in minibags and minibottles. *Drug Intell Clin Pharm.* 1977; 11:226–39.

299. Dinel BA, Ayotte DL, Behme RJ et al. Stability of antibiotic admixtures frozen in minibags. *Drug Intell Clin Pharm.* 1977; 11:542–8.

300. Lynn B. Pharmaceutics of the semi-synthetic penicillins. *Chem Drug.* 1967; 187:157–60.

301. Stanaszek WF, Pan IH. Analysis of hydroxyzine hydrochloride, meperidine hydrochloride and atropine sulfate in glass and plastic syringes. *Am J Hosp Pharm.* 1978; 35:1084–7.

302. Fraser GL. Incompatibility of magnesium sulfate and hydrocortisone sodium succinate. *Am J Hosp Pharm.* 1978; 35:783.

303. Kresel JJ, McDermott JS, Huffer LM et al. Stability of carbenicillin and oxacillin frozen in syringes. *Am J Hosp Pharm.* 1978; 35:310–2.

304. Manning RE. Predicted expiration times for penicillin G in combination with multivitamin injections. *Am J Hosp Pharm.* 1976; 33:870.

305. Cloyd JC, Bosch DE. Concentration-time profile of phenytoin after admixture with small volumes of intravenous fluids. *Am J Hosp Pharm.* 1978; 35:45–8.

306. Bauman JL, Siepler JK. Phenytoin crystallization in intravenous fluids. *Drug Intell Clin Pharm.* 1977; 11:646–9.

307. Ashwin J, Lynn B. Ampicillin stability in saline or dextrose infusions. *Pharm J.* 1975; 214:487–9.

308. O'Brien MJ, Portnoff JB. Cefoxitin sodium compatibility with intravenous infusions and additives. *Am J Hosp Pharm.* 1979; 36:33–8.

309. Stevens JS. Incompatibility of diphenhydramine hydrochloride (Benadryl) with meglumine iodipamide (Cholografin). *Radiology.* 1975; 117:224–5.

310. Petrick RJ, Wolleben JE. Stability of frozen solutions of doxycycline hyclate for injection. *Am J Hosp Pharm.* 1978; 35:1386–7.

311. Melberg SG, Havelund S, Villumsen J et al. Insulin compatibility with polymer materials used in external pump infusion systems. *Diabet Med.* 1988; 5:243–7.

312. Gardella LA, Kesler H, Amann A et al. Intropin (dopamine hydrochloride) intravenous admixture compatibility, part 3: stability with miscellaneous additives. *Am J Hosp Pharm.* 1978; 35:581–4.

313. Schuetz DH, King JC. Compatibility and stability of electrolytes, vitamins and antibiotics in combination with 8% amino acids solution. *Am J Hosp Pharm.* 1978; 35:33–44.

314. El-Nakeeb MA, Souccar N. Inactivation of various antibiotics by some vitamins. *Can J Pharm Sci.* 1976; 11:85–9.

315. Dixon FW, Weshalek J. Physical compatibility of nine drugs in various intavenous solutions. *Am J Hosp Pharm.* 1972; 29:822–3.

316. Earhart RH. Instability of cis-dichlorodiammineplatinum in dextrose solution. *Cancer Treat Rep.* 1978; 62:1105–6.

317. Greene RF, Chatterji DC, Hiranaka PK et al. Stability of cisplatin in aqueous solution. *Am J Hosp Pharm.* 1979; 36:38–43.

318. Morrison RA, Oseekey KB. 5-Fluorouracil and methotrexate sodium: an admixture incompatibility?. *Am J Hosp Pharm.* 1978; 35:15.

319. King JC. 5-Fluorouracil and methotrexate sodium: an admixture incompatibility?. *Am J Hosp Pharm.* 1978; 35:18.

320. Rusmin S, Welton S, DeLuca P et al. Effect of inline filtration on the potency of drugs administered intravenously. *Am J Hosp Pharm.* 1977; 34:1071–4.

321. Morris ME. Compatibility and stability of diazepam injection following dilution with intravenous fluids. *Am J Hosp Pharm.* 1978; 35:669–72.

322. Allen LV, Levinson RS. Compatibility of various admixtures with secondary additives at Y-injection sites of intravenous administration sets. *Am J Hosp Pharm.* 1977; 34:939–43.

323. Arnold TR, Eder J. Compatibility of primary-piggyback solution combinations. *Am J Hosp Pharm.* 1978; 35:249–50.

324. Jansen JR. Volume control sets and incompatibilities. *Am J Hosp Pharm.* 1975; 32:1225.

325. Aisenstein A, Kahn S. Study of the stability of some frozen antibiotics. *Hosp Pharm.* 1969; 4:17–21.

326. Parker WA. Physical compatibilities of preanesthetic medications. *Can J Hosp Pharm.* 1976; 29:91–2.

327. Cradock JC, Kleinman LM. Evaluation of some pharmaceutical aspects of intrathecal methotrexate sodium, cytarabine and hydrocortisone sodium succinate. *Am J Hosp Pharm.* 1978; 35:402–6.

328. Sarubbi FA, Wilson B, Lee M et al. Nosocomial meningitis and bacteremia due to contaminated amphotericin B. *JAMA.* 1978; 239:416–8.

329. The Upjohn Company. Solu-Medrol IV admixture, dilution, and compatibility information. 1978 Aug.

330. Parker WA, Morris ME. Incompatibility of diazepam injection in plastic intravenous bags. *Am J Hosp Pharm.* 1979; 36:505–7.

331. Ingallinera T, Kapadia AJ, Hagman D et al. Compatibility of glycopyrrolate injection with commonly used infusion solutions and additives. *Am J Hosp Pharm.* 1979; 36:508–10.

332. Bateman NE, Graham MD. Solubility of an ephedrine-phenobarbitone complex in water. *Australas J Pharm.* 1967; 48:S68–9.

333. Chang CH, Ashford WR, Ives DAJ et al. Stability of oxytocin in various infusion solutions. *Can J Hosp Pharm.* 1972; 25:152.

334. Lynn B. Administration of carbenicillin and ticarcillin—pharmaceutical aspects. *Eur J Cancer.* 1973; 9:425–33.

335. Block ER, Bennett JE. Stability of amphotericin B in infusion bottles. *Antimicrob Agents Chemother.* 1973; 4:648–9.

336. Gupta VD, Stewart KR. Quantitation of carbenicillin disodium, cefazolin sodium, cephalothin sodium, nafcillin sodium, and ticarcillin disodium by high-pressure liquid chromatography. *J Pharm Sci.* 1980; 69:1264–7.

337. Anon. Label changes on albumin—a reminder. *FDA Drug Bull.* 1978; 8:32.

338. Knoppert DC, Freeman D, Webb D. Stability of ceftizoxime in 5 percent dextrose and 0.9 percent sodium chloride. *Can J Hosp Pharm.* 1993; 46:13–6.

339. Koup JR, Schentag JJ, Vance JW et al. System for clinical pharmacokinetic monitoring of theophylline therapy. *Am J Hosp Pharm.* 1976; 33:949–56.

340. Jusko WJ, Koup JR, Vance JW et al. Intravenous theophylline therapy: nomogram guidelines. *Ann Intern Med.* 1977; 86:400–4.

341. Travenol Laboratories. Product information on Travasol. Deerfield, IL; 1994 Jan.

342. McGaw Laboratories. Product information on FreAmine III. Irvine, CA; 1991 Sep.

343. Odne MAL, Lee SC. Rationale for adding trace elements to total parenteral nutrient solutions—a brief review. *Am J Hosp Pharm.* 1978; 35:1057–9.

344. Jeejeebhoy KN, Langer B, Tsallas G et al. Total parenteral nutrition at home: studies in patients surviving 4 months to 5 years. *Gastroenterology.* 1976; (Dec):943–53.

345. Hull RL, Cassidy D. Trace element deficiencies during total parenteral nutrition. *Drug Intell Clin Pharm.* 1977; 11:536–41.

346. Shils ME. More on trace elements in total parenteral nutrition solutions. *Am J Hosp Pharm.* 1975; 32:141–2.

347. Okada A, Takagi Y, Itakura T et al. Skin lesions during intravenous hyperalimentation: zinc deficiency. *Surgery.* 1976; 80:629–35.

348. Matoi JR, Jeffreys LP. Formulation of a trace element solution for long-term parenteral nutrition. *Am J Hosp Pharm.* 1978; 35:165–8.

349. Athanikar N, Boyer B, Deamer R et al. Visual compatibility of 30 additives with a parenteral nutrient solution. *Am J Hosp Pharm.* 1979; 36:511–3.

350. Finlayson JS. The birth and demise of "salt-poor" albumin. *Am J Hosp Pharm.* 1978; 35:898–900.

351. Winsnes M, Jeppsson R. Diazepam adsorption to infusion sets and plastic syringes. *Acta Anaesthesiol Scand.* 1981; 25:93–6.

352. Bonner DP, Mechlinski W, Schaffner CP. Stability studies with amphotericin B and amphotericin B methyl ester. *J Antibiot.* 1975; 28:132–5.

353. Shadomy S, Brummer DL. Light sensitivity of prepared solutions of amphotericin B. *Am Rev Resp Dis.* 1973; 107:303–4.

354. Fields BT Jr, Bates JH, Abernathy RS. Effect of rapid intravenous infusion on serum concentrations of amphotericin B. *Appl Microbiol.* 1971; 22:615–7.

355. Janknegt R, van den Berg T, de Jong M et al. Compatibility study with midazolam. *Ziekenhuisfarmacie.* 1986; 2:45–5.

356. Arbuthnot R, Dullea A. Controlling thrombophlebitis from amphotericin B. *Am J Hosp Pharm.* 1978; 35:129.

357. Rosch JM, Pazin G. Mannitol and amphotericin B. *JAMA.* 1977; 237:27.

358. Moore DE, Sithipitaks V. Photolytic degradation of frusemide. *J Pharm Pharmacol.* 1983; 35:489–93.

359. Roberts JR. Cutaneous and subcutaneous complications of calcium infusions. *JACEP.* 1977; 6:16–20.

360. Smith Kline & French Laboratories. Product information on Tagamet. Philadelphia, PA; 1978 Oct.

361. Winters RE, Chow AW, Hecht RH et al. Combined use of gentamicin and carbenicillin. *Ann Intern Med.* 1971; 75:925–7.

362. Waitz JA, Drube CG, Moss EL et al. Biological aspects of the interaction between gentamicin and carbenicillin. *J Antibiot.* 1972; 25:219–25.

363. Ervin FR, Bullock WE. Inactivation of gentamicin by penicillins in patients with renal failure. *Antimicrob Agents Chemother.* 1976; 9:1004–11.

364. Peterson CD, Kaatz BL. Ticarcillin and carbenicillin. *Drug Intell Clin Pharm*. 1977; 11:482–6.

365. Davies M, Morgan JR. Interactions of carbenicillin and ticarcillin with gentamicin. *Antimicrob Agents Chemother*. 1975; 7:431–4.

366. Weibert R, Keane W, Shapiro F. Carbenicillin inactivation of aminoglycosides in patients with severe renal failure. *Trans Am Soc Artif Int Organs*. 1976; 22:439–43.

367. Weibert RT, Keane WF. Carbenicillin-gentamicin interaction in acute renal failure. *Am J Hosp Pharm*. 1977; 34:1137–9.

368. Bodey GP, Feld R. β-Lactam antibiotics alone or in combination with gentamicin for therapy of gram-negative bacillary infections in neutropenic patients. *Am J Med Sci*. 1976; 271:179–86.

369. Schimpff S, Satterlee W, Young UM et al. Empiric therapy with carbenicillin and gentamicin for febrile patients with cancer and granulocytopenia. *N Engl J Med*. 1971; 284:1061–5.

370. Hendeles L. Are carbenicillin and gentamicin synergists or antagonists? *Hosp Pharm*. 1972; (Sep)7:297–8.

371. Kole-James A. Electrolyte content of common intravenous solutions and antibiotics. *Hosp Pharm*. 1977; 12:394.

372. Donnelly RF, Tirona RG. Stability of citrated caffeine injectable solution in glass vials. *Am J Hosp Pharm*. 1994; 51:512–4.

373. Turco SJ, Hasan I. Comparison of features of Kefzol and Ancef. *Hosp Pharm*. 1976; 11:482.

374. Vukovich RA, Sugerman AA. Effect of 2% procaine hydrochloride solution on the bioavailability of cephradine after intramuscular injection. *Curr Ther Res Clin Exp*. 1975; 18:711–9.

375. Stennett DJ, Simonson W. Effect of membrane filtration on 10–mg/mL cefazolin admixtures. *Am J Hosp Pharm*. 1979; 36:657–60.

376. Klink PR, Frable RA, Bornstein M. Stability of mandol in parenteral fluids, frozen solutions and admixtures containing other drugs. Presented at 13th annual ASHP midyear clinical meeting. San Antonio, TX: 1978 Dec.

377. Henney JE, Von Hoff DD, Rozencweig M et al. Thrombophlebitic potential of intravenous cytotoxic agents. *Drug Intell Clin Pharm*. 1977; 11:266–7.

378. Sillers BR. Irritant properties of diazepam. *Br Dent J*. 1968; 124:295.

379. Roche Products Ltd. Irritant properties of diazepam—reply. *Br Dent J*. 1968; 124:295.

380. Friedenberg W, Barker JD Jr. Intravenous diazepam administration. *JAMA*. 1973; 224:901–2.

381. Jusko WJ, Gretch M, Gassett R. Precipitation of diazepam from intravenous preparationsi. *JAMA*. 1973; 225:176.

382. Kortilla K, Sothman A. Polyethylene glycol as a solvent for diazepam: bioavailability and clinical effects after intramuscular administration, comparison of oral, intramuscular and rectal administration, and precipitation from intravenous solutions. *Acta Pharmacol Toxicol (Copenh)*. 1976; 39:104–17.

383. Hillestad L, Hansen T, Melsome H et al. Diazepam metabolism in normal man I. Serum concentrations and clinical effects after intravenous, intramuscular and oral administration. *Clin Pharmacol Ther*. 1974; 16:479–84.

384. Assaf RA, Dundee JW, Gamble JA. The influence of the route of administration on the clinical action of diazepam. *Anaesthesia*. 1975; 30:152–8.

385. Baxter MT, McKenzie DD. Dilution of diazepam in intravenous fluids. *Am J Hosp Pharm*. 1977; 34:124.

386. Thong YH, Abramson DC. Continuous infusion of diazepam in infants with severe recurrent convulsions. *Med Ann DC*. 1974; 43:63–5.

387. Khalid MS, Schultz H. Treatment and management of emergency status epilepticus. *Epilepsia*. 1976; 17:73–6.

388. Gibberd FB. Diseases of the central nervous system—epilepsy. *Br Med J*. 1975; 4:270–2.

389. Kawathekar P, Anusuya SR, Sriniwas P et al. Diazepam (Calmpose) in eclampsia: a preliminary report of 16 cases. *Curr Ther Res Clin Exp*. 1973; 15:845–55.

390. Baskett TF, Bradford CR. Active management of severe pre-eclampsia. *Can Med Assoc J*. 1973; 109:1209–11.

391. Prensky AL, Raff MC, Moore MJ et al. Intravenous diazepam in the treatment of prolonged seizure activity. *N Engl J Med*. 1967; 276:779–84.

392. Tehrani JB, Cavanaugh A. Diazepam infusion in the treatment of tetanus. *Drug Intell Clin Pharm*. 1977; 11:491.

393. McLean WN. Safety of diazepam infusion questioned. *Drug Intell Clin Pharm*. 1977; 11:690.

394. Trissel LA, Kleinman LM, Davignon JP et al. Investigational drug information—daunorubicin hydrochloride and streptozotocin. *Drug Intell Clin Pharm*. 1978; 12:404–6.

395. Elsberry VA, Grangeia JM, Giorgianni SJ et al. The lipid phase in TPN. *Am J IV Ther*. 1977; 4:22–8.

396. Belin RP, Bivins BA, Jona JZ et al. Fat overload with a 10% soybean oil emulsion. *Arch Surg*. 1976; 111:1391–3.

397. McNiff BL. Clinical use of 10% soybean oil emulsion. *Am J Hosp Pharm*. 1977; 34:1080–6.

398. Roche Laboratories, Nutley, NJ: Personal communication.

399. McGaw Laboratories. McGaw compatibility studies: a preliminary report. Irvine, CA; 1978.

400. Bundgaard H, Norgaard T, Nielsen NM. Photodegradation and hydrolysis of furosemide and furosemide esters in aqueous solutions. *Int J Pharm*. 1988; 42:217–24.

401. Kresel JJ, Smith AL. Stability of gentamicin in plastic syringes. *Am J Hosp Pharm*. 1977; 34:570.

402. McNeely DJ, Weiner B, Stewart RB et al. Stability of gentamicin in plastic syringes. *Am J Hosp Pharm*. 1977; 34:570.

403. Chrai SS, Ambrosio TJ. Gentamicin sulfate injection repackaging in syringes. *Am J Hosp Pharm*. 1977; 34:920.

404. Davis SM (Medical Information Manager, Astra Zeneca, Wilmington, Delaware): Personal communication, August 21, 2003.

405. Sohn C, Cupit GC. Concentration of heparin in heparin-locks. *Drug Intell Clin Pharm*. 1978; 12:112.

406. Okuno T, Nelson CA. Anticoagulant activity of heparin in intravenous fluids. *J Clin Pathol*. 1975; 28:494–7.

407. Joy RT, Hyneck ML, Berardi RR et al. Effect of pH on the stability of heparin in 5% dextrose solutions. *Am J Hosp Pharm*. 1979; 36:618–21.

408. Brown J, Stead K. Anti-human lymphocyte globulin-heparin precipitate. *Drug Intell Clin Pharm.* 1976; 10:654.

409. Raab WP, Windisch J. Antagonism of neomycin by heparin. Further observations on the anaphylactoid activity of neomycin. *Arzneimittelforschung.* 1973; 23:1326–8.

410. Stella VJ. A case for prodrugs: Fosphenytoin. *Adv Drug Del Rev.* 1996; 19:311–30.

411. Dupuis LL, Wong B. Stability of propafenone hydrochloride in i.v. solutions. *Am J Health-Syst Pharm.* 1997; 54:1293–5.

412. Dupuis LL, Trope A, Giesbrecht E et al. Compatibility and stability of propafenone hydrochloride with five critical-care medications. *Can J Hosp Pharm.* 1998; 51:55–7.

413. Storvick WO, Henry HJ. Effect of storage temperature on stability of commercial insulin preparations. *Diabetes.* 1968; 17:499–502.

414. Jackson RL, Storvick WO, Hollinden CS et al. Neutral regular insulin. *Diabetes.* 1972; 21:235–45.

415. Page MM, Alberti KGMM, Greenwood R et al. Treatment of diabetic coma with continuous low-dose infusion of insulin. *Br Med J.* 1974; 2:687–90.

416. Kidson W, Casey J, Kraegen E et al. Treatment of severe diabetes mellitus by insulin infusion. *Br Med J.* 1974; 2:691–94.

417. Semple PF, White C. Continuous intravenous infusion of small doses of insulin in treatment of diabetic ketoacidosis. *Br Med J.* 1974; 2:694–8.

418. Campbell LV, Lazarus L, Casey JH et al. Routine use of low-dose intravenous insulin infusion in severe hyperglycaemia. *Med J Aust.* 1976; 2:519–22.

419. Martin MM, Martin ALA. Continuous low-dose infusion of insulin in the treatment of diabetic ketoacidosis in children. *J Pediatr.* 1976; 89:560–4.

420. Drop SLS, Duval-Arnould BJM, Gober AE et al. Low-dose intravenous insulin infusion versus subcutaneous insulin injection: A controlled comparative study of diabetic ketoacidosis. *Pediatrics.* 1977; 59:733–8.

421. Fisher JN, Shahshahani MN. Diabetic ketoacidosis: low-dose insulin therapy by various routes. *N Engl J Med.* 1977; 297:238–41.

422. Goldberg NJ, Levin SR. Insulin adsorption to an inline membrane filter. *N Engl J Med.* 1978; 298:1480.

423. Kristofferson J, Skobba TJ. Adsorption of insulin to infusion equipment. *Nor Farm Tidsskr.* 1977; 85:220–4.

424. Hirsch JI, Fratkin MJ, Wood JH et al. Clinical significance of insulin adsorption by polyvinyl chloride infusion systems. *Am J Hosp Pharm.* 1977; 34:583–8.

425. Weber SS, Wood WA. Availability of insulin from parenteral nutrient solutions. *Am J Hosp Pharm.* 1977; 34:353–7.

426. Whalen FJ, LeCain WK. Availability of insulin from continuous low-dose insulin infusions. *Am J Hosp Pharm.* 1979; 36:330–7.

427. Clarke BF, Campbell IW, Fraser DM et al. Direct addition of small doses of insulin to intravenous infusion in severe uncontrolled diabetes. *Br Med J.* 1977; 2:1395–6.

428. Peterson L, Caldwell J. Insulin adsorbance to polyvinyl chloride surfaces with implications for constant-infusion therapy. *Diabetes.* 1976; 25:72–4.

429. Sadeghi A, Mehrbanpour J, Behmard S et al. A trial of total dose infusion iron therapy as an outpatient procedure in rural Iranian villages (a three month follow-up). *Curr Ther Res Clin Exp.* 1976; 19:595–602.

430. Leach JK, Strickland RD, Millis DL et al. Biological activity of dilute isoproterenol solution stored for long periods in plastic bags. *Am J Hosp Pharm.* 1977; 34:709–12.

431. Browning ML. IM MgSO$_4$ ampuls for IV use. *Hosp Pharm.* 1976; 11:325.

432. Epperson E, Nedich RL. Mannitol crystallization in plastic containers. *Am J Hosp Pharm.* 1978; 35:1337.

433. Chatterji DC, Gallelli JF. Thermal and photolytic decomposition of methotrexate in aqueous solutions. *J Pharm Sci.* 1978; 67:526–31.

434. Muller HJ, Berg J. Stabilitatsstudie zu tramadolhydrochlorid im PVC-infusionbeutel. *Krankenhauspharmazie.* 1997; 18:75–9.

435. Duttera MJ, Gallelli JF, Kleinman LM et al. Intrathecal methotrexate. *Lancet.* 1972; 2:540.

436. Hartshorn EA. Oxidation of methyldopate hydrochloride in alkaline media. *Am J Hosp Pharm.* 1975; 32:244.

437. Parker EA. Oxidation of methyldopate hydrochloride in alkaline media. *Am J Hosp Pharm.* 1975; 32:244.

438. Hartline JV, Zachman RD. Vitamin A delivery in total parenteral nutrition solution. *Pediatrics.* 1976; 58:448–51.

439. Sina A, Youssef MK, Kassem AA et al. Stability of oxytetracycline in solutions and injections. *Can J Pharm Sci.* 1974; 9:44–9.

440. Colding H, Anderson GE. Stability of antibiotics and amino acids in two synthetic L-amino acid solutions commonly used for total parenteral nutrition in children. *Antimicrob Agents Chemother.* 1978; 13:555–8.

441. Schneider E (Knoll AG, Milan, Italy): Personal communication; 2000 Feb 25.

442. Perrier D, Rapp R, Young B et al. Maintenance of therapeutic phenytoin plasma levels via intramuscular administration. *Ann Intern Med.* 1976; 85:318–21.

443. Sellers EM, Kalant H. Alcohol intoxication and withdrawal. *N Engl J Med.* 1976; 294:757–62.

444. Nahata MC. Formulation of caffeine injection for i.v. administration. *Am J Hosp Pharm.* 1987; 44:1308, 1312.

445. Anon. Intravenous phenytoin. *N Engl J Med.* 1976; 295:1078.

446. Anon. Intravenous phenytoin. *N Engl J Med.* 1976; 295:1078.

447. Frank JT. Author's response. *Drug Intell Clin Pharm.* 1973; 7:419.

448. Woo E, Greenblatt DJ. Choosing the right phenytoin dosage. *Drug Ther.* 1977; 7:131–9.

449. Bighley LD, Wille J. Mixing of additives in glass and plastic intravenous fluid containers. *Am J Hosp Pharm.* 1974; 31:736–9.

450. Schondelmeyer S, Gatlin L. Intravenous phenytoin (concluded). *N Engl J Med.* 1977; 296:111.

451. Bauman JL, Siepler JK. Intravenous phenytoin (concluded). *N Engl J Med.* 1977; 296:111.

452. Sistare F, Greene R. Phenytoin crystallization in intravenous fluids. *Drug Intell Clin Pharm.* 1978; 12:120.

453. Biberdorf RI, Spurbeck GH. Phenytoin in IV fluids: results endorsed. *Drug Intell Clin Pharm.* 1978; 12:300–1.

454. Williams RHP. Potassium overdosage: a potential hazard of non-rigid parenteral fluid containers. *Br Med J*. 1973; 1:714–5.

455. Woodside W, King JA. Addition of potassium to non-rigid plastic intravenous infusion containers: a potential hazard. *J Hosp Pharm*. 1973; 31:192–4.

456. Lankton JW, Siler JN. Hyperkalemia after administration of potassium from nonrigid parenteral-fluid containers. *Anesthesiology*. 1973; 39:660–1.

457. Vrabel RB, Amerson AB. Reconstitution of sodium nitroprusside. *Am J Hosp Pharm*. 1975; 32:140–1.

458. Challen RG. Stability of sodium nitroprusside solutions. *Australas J Pharm*. 1967; 48:S110.

459. Martin T, Patel JA. Determination of sodium nitroprusside in aqueous solution. *Am J Hosp Pharm*. 1969; 26:51–3.

460. Frank MJ, Johnson JB. Spectrophotometric determination of sodium nitroprusside and its photodegradation products. *J Pharm Sci*. 1976; 65:44–8.

461. Ammar HO. Stability of injection solutions of vitamin B_1. *Pharmazie*. 1976; 31:373–4.

462. Anon. Correction: sodium in ticarcillin and carbenicillin. *Med Lett Drugs Ther*. 1977; 19:28.

463. Yamaji A, Yasuko F, Okuda H et al. Photodegradation of vitamin K^1 and vitamin K^2 injections in preservation and in intravenous admixtures. *J Nippon Hosp Pharm Assoc Sci Ed*. 1978; 4:7–11.

464. Kobayashi NH, King JC. Compatibility of common additives in protein hydrolysate/dextrose solutions. *Am J Hosp Pharm*. 1977; 34:589–94.

465. Humphreys A, Marty JJ, Gooey SL et al. Stability of methotrexate in an intravenous fluid. *Aust J Hosp Pharm*. 1978; 8:66–7.

466. Clayton SK. Stability of intravenous additive preparations; studies on hydralazine as an additive. *J Clin Pharm*. 1978; 2:247–56.

467. Anon. Mixing chlorpromazine and morphine. *Br Med J*. 1974; 3:681.

468. Crapper JB. Mixing chlorpromazine and morphine. *Br Med J*. 1975; 1:33.

469. Baird GM, Willoughby MLN. Photodegradation of dacarbazine. *Lancet*. 1978; 2:681.

470. Georget S, Vigneron J, Blaise N et al. Stability of refrigerated and frozen solutions of tropisetron in either polyvinylchloride or polyolefin infusion bags. *J Clin Pharm Ther*. 1997; 22:257–60.

471. Bergman HD. Cefamandole. *Drug Intell Clin Pharm*. 1979; 13:144–9.

472. Indelicato JM, Wilham WL. Conversion of cefamandole nafate to cefamandole sodium. *J Pharm Sci*. 1976; 65:1175–8.

473. Palmer MA, Fraterrigo CC. Production of carbon dioxide gas after reconstitution of cefamandole nafate. *Am J Hosp Pharm*. 1979; 36:596–7.

474. Klink PR, McKeechan CW. Production of carbon dioxide gas after reconstitution of cefamandole nafate. *Am J Hosp Pharm*. 1979; 36:597.

475. Bornstein M, Klink PR, Farrell BT et al. Stability of frozen solutions of cefamandole nafate. *Am J Hosp Pharm,*. 1980; 37:98–101.

476. Buckles J, Walters V. Stability of amitriptyline hydrochloride in aqueous solution. *J Clin Pharm*. 1976; 1:107–12.

477. Enever RP, Po ALW, Millard BJ et al. Decomposition of amitriptyline hydrochloride in aqueous solution: identification of decomposition products. *J Pharm Sci*. 1975; 64:1497–9.

478. Enever RP, Po ALW. Factors influencing decomposition rate of amitriptyline hydrochloride in aqueous solution. *J Pharm Sci*. 1977; 66:1087–9.

479. Holman BL, Dewanjee MK. Potential pH incompatibility of pharmacological and isotopic adjuncts to arteriography. *Radiology*. 1974; 110:722–3.

480. Kawilarang CRT, Georghiou K. The effect of additives on the physical properties of a phospholipid-stabilized soybean oil emulsion. *J Clin Hosp Pharm*. 1980; 5:151–60.

481. Bristol Laboratories. Stadol Q&A. Syracuse, NY; 1978 Nov:7.

482. Jacobs RS. Calcitonin-Salmon. *Drug Intell Clin Pharm*. 1975; 9:557–9.

483. Nahata MC, Zingarelli J, Durrell DE. Stability of caffeine citrate injection in intravenous admixtures and parenteral nutrition solutions. *J Clin Pharm Ther*. 1989; 14:53–5.

484. Davignon JP, Yang KW, Wood HB et al. Formulation of three nitrosoureas for intravenous use. *Cancer Chemother Rep 3*. 1973; 4(3):7–11.

485. Buckles J, Walters V. Stability of imipramine hydrochloride solutions. *J Clin Pharm*. 1976; 1:113–8.

486. Andreu A, Garcia B, Pastor C et al. Estudio de la estabilidad *in vitro* de la ranitidine i.v. en una solucion de nutricion parenteral total conteniendo lipidos. *Nutr Hosp*. 1988; 3:50–5.

487. Smith JL, Canham JE, Wells PA. Effect of phototherapy light, sodium bisulfite, and pH on vitamin stability in total parenteral nutrition admixtures. *J Parenter Enteral Nutr*. 1988; 12:394–402.

488. Lauper RD. Leucovorin calcium administration and preparation. *Am J Hosp Pharm*. 1978; 35:377.

489. Tavoloni N, Guarino AM. Photolytic degradation of adriamycin. *J Pharm Pharmacol*. 1980; 32:860–2.

490. Black CD, Popovich NG. Stability of intravenous fat emulsions. *Arch Surg*. 1980; 115:891.

491. Bacon L. A review of two safety factors in the use of paraldehyde. *J R Coll Gen Pract*. 1980; 30:622–4.

492. Horton JK, Stevens MFG. Search for drug interactions between the antitumor agent DTIC and other cytotoxic agents. *J Pharm Pharmacol*. 1979; 31(Suppl):64P.

493. Zaccardelli DS, Krcmarik CS, Wolk R et al. Stability of imipenem and cilastatin sodium in total parenteral nutrient solution. *JPEN J Parenter Enteral Nutr*. 1990; 14:306–309.

494. Kuehnle C, Moore TD. Sodium chloride residue provides potential for drug incompatibilities. *Am J Hosp Pharm*. 1979; 36:881.

495. Trissel LA, Kleinman LM, Cradock JC et al. Investigational drug information—ifosfamide and semustine. *Drug Intell Clin Pharm*. 1979; 13:340–3.

496. Horton JK, Stevens MFG. A new light on the photodecomposition of the antitumour drug DTIC. *J Pharm Pharmacol*. 1981; 33:808–11.

497. Earp CM, Barriere SL. The lack of inactivation of tobramycin by cefazolin, cefamandole, and moxalactam in vitro. *Drug Intell Clin Pharm*. 1985; 19:677–9.

498. Elliott TSJ, Eley A, Cowlishaw A. Stability of tobramycin in combination with selected new beta-lactam antibiotics. *J Antimicrob Chemother*. 1986; 17:680–1.

499. Gu L, Chiang HS, Becker A. Kinetics and mechanisms of the autoxidation of ketorolac tromethamine in aqueous solution. *Int J Pharm*. 1988; 41:95–104.

500. Brown AF, Harvey DA, Hoddinott DJ. Freeze thaw stability of ceftazidime. *Br J Parenter Ther*. 1985; 6:43–5.

501. Grimble GK, Hunjan MK, Payne-James JJ et al. Zantac and TPN. *Br J Intensive Care*. 1991; 32:7.

502. Vieth R, Ledermann SE, Kooh SW et al. Losses of calcitrol to peritoneal dialysis bags and tubing. *Peritoneal Dial Int*. 1989; 9:277–80.

503. McNiff BL, McNiff EF. Potency and stability of extemporaneous nitroglycerin infusions. *Am J Hosp Pharm*. 1979; 36:173–7.

504. Giamarellou H, Mavroudis K, Petrikkos G et al. In vitro and in vivo interactions of recent cephalosporins with gentamicin and amikacin. *Chemioterapia*. 1984; 3:183–7.

505. Milano G, Etienne MC, Cassuto-Viguier E et al. Long-term stability of 5-fluorouracil and folinic acid admixtures. *Eur J Cancer*. 1993; 29A:129–32.

506. Sturek JK, Sokolski TD, Winsley WT et al. Stability of nitroglycerin injection determined by gas chromatography. *Am J Hosp Pharm*. 1978; 35:537–41.

507. Fung HL. Potency and stability of extemporaneously prepared nitroglycerin intravenous solutions (editorial). *Am J Hosp Pharm*. 1978; 35:528–9.

508. Grouthamel WG, Dorsch B, Shangraw R. Loss of nitroglycerin from plastic intravenous bags. *N Engl J Med*. 1978; 299:262.

509. Cossum PA, Galbraith AJ, Roberts MS et al. Loss of nitroglycerin from intravenous infusion sets. *Lancet*. 1978; 2:349–50.

510. Boylan JC, Robison RL. Stability of nitroglycerin solutions in Viaflex plastic containers. *Am J Hosp Pharm*. 1978; 35:1031.

511. Ludwig DJ, Ueda CT. Apparent stability of nitroglycerin in dextrose 5% in water. *Am J Hosp Pharm*. 1978; 35:541–4.

512. Brillaud AR. Interaction of platinol (cisplatin) and the metal aluminum. Syracuse, NY: Bristol Laboratories; 1979 Jul.

513. Baxter Healthcare, Clintec Nutrition Division, Product information on Intralipid 10% and 20%. Deerfield IL; 2007 Apr.

515. Sewell DL, Golper TA. Stability of antimicrobial agents in peritoneal dialysate. *Antimicrob Agents Chemother*. 1982; 21:528–9.

516. El-Mallakh R. Incompatibilities with cimetidine hydrochloride injection. *Am J Hosp Pharm*. 1979; 36:1024.

517. Cutie MR. Letters. *Hosp Formul*. 1980; 15:502–3.

518. Tung EC, Gurwich EL, Sula JA et al. Stability of five antibiotics in plastic intravenous solution containers of dextrose and sodium chloride. *Drug Intell Clin Pharm*. 1980; 14:848–50.

519. Benvenuto JA, Anderson RW, Kerkof K et al. Stability and compatibility of antitumor agents in glass and plastic containers. *Am J Hosp Pharm*. 1981; 38:1914–8.

520. Jhunjhunwala VP, Bhalla HL. Compatibility of mephentermine sulfate with hydrocortisone sodium succinate or aminophylline in 5% dextrose injection. *Am J Hosp Pharm*. 1981; 38:1922–4.

521. Jhunjhunwala VP, Bhalla HL. Compatibility of aminophylline with hydrocortisone sodium succinate or dexamethasone sodium phosphate in 5% dextrose injection. *Am J Hosp Pharm*. 1981; 38:900–1.

522. Lee YC, Malick AW, Amann AH et al. Bretylium tosylate intravenous admixture compatibility. II. Dopamine, lidocaine, procainamide and nitroglycerin. *Am J Hosp Pharm*. 1981; 38:183–7.

523. Colvin M, Hartner J. Stability of carmustine in the presence of sodium bicarbonate. *Am J Hosp Pharm*. 1980; 37:677–8.

524. Dorr RT. Incompatibilities with parenteral anticancer drugs. *Am J IV Ther*. 45, 46, 52 (Feb-Mar) 1979; 6:42.

525. Das Gupta V, Stewart KR. Stability of cefamandole nafate and cefoxitin sodium solutions. *Am J Hosp Pharm*. 1981; 38:875–9.

526. Poochikian GK, Cradock JC. Stability of anthracycline antitumor agents in four infusion fluids. *Am J Hosp Pharm*. 1981; 38:483–6.

527. Newton DW, Fung EYY. Stability of five catecholamines and terbutaline sulfate in 5% dextrose injection in the absence and presence of aminophylline. *Am J Hosp Pharm*. 1981; 38:1314–9.

528. Neil JM. A rational approach to intravenous additives. *Proc Guild*. 1979; 7:3–33.

529. Otterman GE, Samuelson DW. Incompatibility between carbenicillin injection and promethazine injection. *Am J Hosp Pharm*. 1979; 36:1156.

530. Marshall TR, Ling IT, Follis G et al. Pharmacological incompatibility of contrast media with various drugs and agents. *Radiology*. 1965; 84:536–9.

531. Monder C. Stability of corticosteroids in aqueous solutions. *Endocrinology*. 1968; 82:318–26.

532. Kleinberg ML, Stauffer GL, Prior RB et al. Stability of antibiotics frozen and stored in disposable hypodermic syringes. *Am J Hosp Pharm*. 1980; 37:1087–8.

533. Butler LD, Munson JM. Effect of inline filtration on the potency of low-dose drugs. *Am J Hosp Pharm*. 1980; 37:935–41.

534. Allen LV, Stiles ML. Compatibility of various admixtures with secondary additives at Y-injection sites of intravenous administration sets. Part 2. *Am J Hosp Pharm*. 1981; 38:380–1.

535. Kleinberg, ML, Stauffer GL et al. Stability of five liquid drug products after unit dose repackaging. *Am J Hosp Pharm*. 1980; 37:680–2.

536. Kowaluk EA, Roberts MS, Blackburn HD et al. Interactions between drugs and polyvinyl chloride infusion bags. *Am J Hosp Pharm*. 1981; 38:1308–14.

537. Zatz L, Sethia P. Stability of refrigerated aminophylline in 5% dextrose in water: a 96–hour study. *Hosp Pharm*. 1981; 16:548.

538. Scott KR, Bell AF. Drug interactions I: Folic acid and calcium gluconate. *J Pharm Sci*. 1980; 69:234.

539. Jurgens RW, DeLuca PP. Compatibility of amphotericin B with certain large-volume parenterals. *Am J Hosp Pharm*. 1981; 38:377–8.

540. Gotz VP, Mar DD. Compatibility of amphotericin B with drugs used to reduce adverse reactions. *Am J Hosp Pharm*. 1981; 38:378–9.

541. Lee YC, Baaske DM, Amann AH et al. Bretylium tosylate intravenous admixture compatibility. I. Stability in common large-volume parenteral solutions. *Am J Hosp Pharm*. 1980; 37:803–8.

542. Yuhas EM, Lofton FT, Baldinus JG et al. Cimetidine hydrochloride compatibility with preoperative medications. *Am J Hosp Pharm*. 1981; 38:1173–4.

543. Smith FM, Nuessle NO. Stability of lidocaine hydrochloride in 5% dextrose injection in plastic bags. *Am J Hosp Pharm*. 1981; 38:1745–7.

544. Finch ME. Sodium thiopental in 5% dextrose in lactated Ringer's precipitate. *Hosp Pharm*. 1979; 14:559–60.

545. Kirschenbaum HL, Lesko LJ, Mendes RW et al. Stability of procainamide in 0.9% sodium chloride or dextrose 5% in water. *Am J Hosp Pharm*. 1979; 36:1464–5.

546. Baaske DM, Malick AW. Stability of procainamide hydrochloride in dextrose solutions. *Am J Hosp Pharm*. 1980; 37:1050–2.

547. Jeglum EL, Winter E. Nafcillin sodium incompatibility with acidic solutions. *Am J Hosp Pharm*. 1981; 38:462.

548. Cutie MR, Lordi NG. Compatibility of verapamil hydrochloride injection in commonly used large-volume parenterals. *Am J Hosp Pharm*. 1980; 37:675–6.

549. Rosenberg HA, Dougherty JT, Mayron D et al. Cimetidine hydrochloride compatibility I: Chemical aspects and room temperature stability in intravenous infusion fluids. *Am J Hosp Pharm*. 1980; 37:390–3.

550. Yuhas EM, Lofton FT, Mayron D et al. Cimetidine hydrochloride compatibility II: Room temperature stability in intravenous infusion fluids. *Am J Hosp Pharm*. 1981; 38:879–81.

551. Yuhas EM, Lofton FT, Rosenberg HA et al. Cimetidine hydrochloride compatibility III: Room temperature stability in drug admixtures. *Am J Hosp Pharm*. 1981; 38:1919–22.

552. Dahlin PA, Paredes SM. Visual compatibility of dobutamine with seven parenteral drug products. *Am J Hosp Pharm*. 1980; 37:460.

553. Lesko LJ, Marion A, Ericson J et al. Stability of trimethoprim-sulfamethoxazole injection in two infusion fluids. *Am J Hosp Pharm*. 1981; 38:1004–6.

554. Holmes CJ, Ausman RK, Walter CW et al. Activity of antibiotic admixtures subjected to different freeze-thaw treatments. *Drug Intell Clin Pharm*. 1980; 14:353–7.

555. Holmes CJ, Ausman RK, Kundsin RB et al. Effect of freezing and microwave thawing on the stability of six antibiotic admixtures in plastic bags. *Am J Hosp Pharm*. 1982; 39:104–8.

556. Boddapati S, Yang K. Physiochemical properties of aminophylline-dextrose injection admixtures. *Am J Hosp Pharm*. 1982; 39:108–12.

557. Canton EM, Baluch WM. Effect of freezing on particle formation in three antibiotic injections. *Am J Hosp Pharm*. 1982; 39:124–5.

558. Chaudry IA, Bruey KP, Hurlburt LE et al. Compatibility of netilmicin sulfate injection with commonly used intravenous injections and additives. *Am J Hosp Pharm*. 1981; 38:1737–42.

559. Cutie MR. Effects of cold and freezing temperatures on pharmaceutical dosage forms. *US Pharmacist*. 1979; 4:38–40.

560. Gove L, Walls ADF. Mixing parenteral nutrition products. *Pharm J*. 1979; 223:587.

561. Lauder AD. Mixing parenteral nutrition products. *Pharm J*. 1979; 223:587.

562. Hardin TC, Clibon U. Stability of 5-fluorouracil in a crystalline amino acid solution. *Am J IV Ther Clin Nutr*. 1982; 9:39–40.

563. Yamaji A, Fujii Y, Kurata Y et al. Stability of pyridoxine hydrochloride in infusion solution under practical circumstances in wards. *Yakuzaigaku*. 1980; 40:143–50.

564. Dony J, Devleeschouwer MJ. Etude de la degradation photochimique de macrolides en presence de riboflavine. *J Pharm Belg*. 1976; 31:479–84.

565. Parker WA, Shearer CA. Metoclopramide compatibility. *Can J Hosp Pharm*. 1979; 32:38.

566. Parker WA. Compatibility of perphenazine and butorphanol admixtures. *Can J Hosp Pharm*. 1980; 33:152.

567. Stiles ML, Allen LV. Retention of drugs during inline filtration of parenteral solutions. *Infusion*. 1979; 3:67–9.

568. Somani P, Leathem WD, Barlow AL. Safflower oil emulsion: single and multiple infusions with or without added heparin in normal human volunteers. *JPEN J Parenter Enteral Nutr*. 1980; 4:307–11.

569. Rubin M, Bilik R, Gruenewald Z et al. Use of 5-micron filter in administering 'all-in-one' mixtures for total parenteral nutrition. *Clin Nutr*. 1985; 4:163–8.

570. Moore RA, Feldman S, Treuting J et al. Cimetidine and parenteral nutrition. *JPEN J Parenter Enteral Nutr*. 1981; 5:61–3.

571. Das Gupta V, Stewart KR. Stability of haloperidol in 5% dextrose injection. *Am J Hosp Pharm*. 1982; 39:292–4.

572. Cutie MR, Waranis R. Compatibility of hydromorphone hydrochloride in large-volume parenterals. *Am J Hosp Pharm*. 1982; 39:307–8.

573. Mirtallo JM, Caryer K, Schneider PJ et al. Growth of bacteria and fungi in parenteral nutrition solutions containing albumin. *Am J Hosp Pharm*. 1981; 38:1907–10.

574. Holt HA, Broughall JM, McCarthy MM et al. Interactions between aminoglycoside antibiotics and carbenicillin or ticarcillin. *Infection*. 1976; 4:107–9.

575. Pickering LK, Gearhart P. Effect of time and concentration upon interaction between gentamicin, tobramycin, netilmicin, or amikacin and carbenicillin or ticarcillin. *Antimicrob Agents Chemother*. 1979; 15:592–6.

576. Pieper JA, Vidal RA. Animal model distinguishing in vitro from in vivo carbenicillin-aminoglycoside interactions. *Antimicrob Agents Chemother*. 1980; 18:604–9.

577. Sturgeon RJ, Athanikar NK, Henry RS et al. Titratable acidities of crystalline amino acid admixtures. *Am J Hosp Pharm*. 1980; 37:388–90.

578. Ausman RK, Kerkhof K, Holmes CJ et al. Frozen storage and microwave thawing of parenteral nutrition solutions in plastic containers. *Drug Intell Clin Pharm.* 1981; 15:440–3.

579. Tortorici MP, Fearing D, Inman M et al. Photoreaction involving essential amino acid injection. *Am J Hosp Pharm.* 1978; 35:1030.

580. West KR, Sansom LN, Cosh DG et al. Some aspects of the stability of parenteral nutrition solutions. *Pharm Acta Helv.* 1976; 51(1):19–22.

581. Jurgens RW, Henry RS. Amino acid stability in a mixed parenteral nutrition solution. *Am J Hosp Pharm.* 1981; 38:1358–9.

582. Mirtallo JM, Rogers KR, Johnson JA et al. Stability of amino acids and the availability of acid in total parenteral nutrition solutions containing hydrochloric acid. *Am J Hosp Pharm.* 1981; 38:1729–31.

583. Rusho WJ, Standish R. A comparison of crystalline amino acid solutions for total parenteral nutrition. *Hosp Formul.* 1981; 16:29–33.

584. Anon. Guidelines for essential trace element preparations for parenteral use. A statement by an expert panel. AMA Department of Foods and Nutrition. *JAMA.* 1979; 241:2051–54.

585. Freund H, Atamian S, Fischer JE. Chromium deficiency during total parenteral nutrition. *JAMA.* 1979; 241:496–8.

586. Heller RM, Kirchner SG, O'Neill JA et al. Skeletal changes of copper deficiency in infants receiving prolonged total parenteral nutrition. *J Pediatr.* 1978; 92:947–9.

587. Moran DM, Russo J. Zinc deficiency dermatitis accompanying parenteral nutrition supplemented with trace elements. *Clin Pharm.* 1982; 1:169–76.

588. Askari A, Long CL, Blakemore WS. Zinc, copper, and parenteral nutrition in cancer. A review. *JPEN J Parenter Enteral Nutr.* 1980; 4:561–71.

589. Wolman SL, Anderson GH, Marliss EB et al. Zinc in total parenteral nutrition: requirements and metabolic effects. *Gastroenterology.* 1979; 76:458–67.

590. Fliss DM, Lamy PP. Trace elements and total parenteral nutrition. *Hosp Formul.* 1979; 14:698–717.

591. Schneider PJ. Total parenteral nutrition: Part II: What goes into parenteral nutrition solutions?. *J Postgrad Pharm (Hosp Ed).* 1979; 1:18–27.

592. Isaacs JW, Millikan WJ, Stackhouse J et al. Parenteral nutrition of adults with a 900 milliosmolar solution via peripheral veins. *Am J Clin Nutr.* 1977; 30:552–9.

593. Romankiewicz JA, McManus J, Gotz VP et al. Medications not to be refrigerated. *Am J Hosp Pharm.* 1979; 36:1541–5.

594. Swerling R. Dilution of oral and intravenous aminophylline preparations. *Am J Hosp Pharm.* 1981; 38:1359–60.

595. Alcorn BT, Barnes SG. Pharmacy-initiated intravenous infusion guidelines. *Hosp Pharm.* 1982; 17:60–76.

596. Bowtle WJ, Heasman MJ, Prince AP et al. Compatibility of the cephalosporin, cefamandole nafate, with injections. *Int J Pharm.* 1980; 4:263–5.

597. Anon. I.V. dosage guidelines for theophylline products. *FDA Drug Bull.* 1980; 10:4–5.

598. Tipple M, Shadomy S. Availability of active amphotericin B after filtration through membrane filters. *Am Rev Resp Dis.* 1977; 115:879–81.

599. Maddux MS, Barriere SL. A review of complications of amphotericin B therapy: recommendations for prevention and management. *Drug Intell Clin Pharm.* 1980; 14:177–81.

600. Lufter CH, Ball WD. Activity of amphotericin B after filtration. *Drug Intell Clin Pharm.* 1980; 14:719.

601. Kuchinskas EJ, Levy GN. Comparative stabilities of ampicillin and hetacillin in aqueous solutions. *J Pharm Sci.* 1972; 61:727–9.

602. Schwartz MA, Hayton WL. Relative stability of hetacillin and ampicillin in solution. *J Pharm Sci.* 1972; 61:906–9.

603. Bundgaard H. Polymerization of penicillins: kinetics and mechanism of di- and polymerization of ampicillin in aqueous solution. *Acta Pharm Suec.* 1976; 13:9–26.

604. Stjernstrom G, Olson OT, Nyqvist H et al. Studies on the stability and compatibility of drugs in infusion fluids 6. Factors affecting the stability of ampicillin. *Acta Pharm Suec.* 1978; 15:33–50.

605. Johnson CA, Porter WA. Compatibility of azathioprine sodium with intravenous fluids. *Am J Hosp Pharm.* 1981; 38:871–5.

606. Kowaluk EA, Roberts MS. Interactions between drugs and intravenous delivery systems. *Am J Hosp Pharm.* 1982; 39:460–7.

607. Bryan CK, Darby MH. Bretylium tosylate: a review. *Am J Hosp Pharm.* 1979; 36:1189–92.

608. Henry RS, Jurgens RW, Sturgeon R et al. Compatibility of calcium chloride and calcium gluconate with sodium phosphate in a mixed TPN solution. *Am J Hosp Pharm.* 1980; 37:673–4.

609. Eggert LD, Rusho WJ, MacKay MW et al. Calcium and phosphorus compatibility in parenteral nutrition solutions for neonates. *Am J Hosp Pharm.* 1982; 39:49–53.

610. Robinson LA, Wright BT. Central venous catheter occlusion caused by body-heat-mediated calcium phosphate precipitation. *Am J Hosp Pharm.* 1982; 39:120–1.

611. Tuttle CB. Guidelines for phenytoin infusions. *Can J Hosp Pharm.* 1984; 37:137–9.

612. Stewart P, Lourwood D. Guidelines for the administration of a phenytoin loading dose via IVPB. *Hosp Pharm.* 1986; 21:1003–4.

613. Goldschmied S. An evaluation of the stability and safety of phenytoin infusion. *NY State J Pharm.* 1987; 7:45–7.

614. Kradjan WA, Burger R. In vivo inactivation of gentamicin by carbenicillin and ticarcillin. *Arch Intern Med.* 1980; 140:1668–70.

615. Young LS, Decker G. Inactivation of gentamicin by carbenicillin in the urinary tract. *Chemotherapy.* 1974; 20:212–20.

616. Henderson JL, Polk RE. In vitro inactivation of gentamicin, tobramycin, and netilmicin by carbenicillin, azlocillin, or mezlocillin. *Am J Hosp Pharm.* 1981; 38:1167–70.

617. Flournoy DJ. Inactivation of netilmicin by carbenicillin. *Infection.* 1978; 6:241.

618. Russo ME. Penicillin-aminoglycoside inactivation: another possible mechanism of interaction. *Am J Hosp Pharm.* 1980; 37:702–4.

619. Laskar PA, Ayres JW. Degradation of carmustine in aqueous media. *J Pharm Sci.* 1977; 66:1073–6.

620. Cardi V, Willcox GS. Reconstituting cefamandole and protecting from light. *Am J Hosp Pharm.* 1980; 37:334.

621. Kaiser GV, Gorman M. Cefamandole—a review of chemistry and microbiology. *J Infect Dis*. 1978; 137:S10–S16.

622. Wold JS, Joost RR, Black HR et al. Hydrolysis of cefamandole nafate to cefamandole in vivo. *J Infect Dis*. 1978; 137:S17–S24.

623. Palmer MA, Fraterrigo CC. Clarification of "explosive-like" reaction occurring when reconstituted cefamandole nafate was stored in syringes. *Am J Hosp Pharm*. 1979; 36:1025.

624. Fites AL. Reconstituting cefamandole and protecting from light. *Am J Hosp Pharm*. 1980; 37:334.

625. Foster TS, Shrewsbury RP, Coonrod JD. Bioavailability and pain study of cefamandole nafate. *J Clin Pharmacol*. 1980; 20:526–33.

626. Indelicato JM, Stewart BA. Formylation of glucose by cefamandole nafate at alkaline pH. *J Pharm Sci*. 1980; 69:1183–8.

627. Tomecko GW, Kleinberg ML, Latiolais CL et al. Stability of cefazolin sodium admixtures in plastic bags after thawing by microwave radiation. *Am J Hosp Pharm*. 1980; 37:211–5.

628. Janousek JP, Minisci MP. An evaluation of cefazolin sodium injection in an IV piggyback bottle. *Infusion*. 1978; 2:67–73.

629. Stiles ML. Effect of microwave radiation on the stability of frozen cefoxitin sodium solution in plastic bags. *Am J Hosp Pharm*. 1981; 38:1743–5.

630. Oberholtzer ER, Brenner GS. Cefoxitin sodium: solution and solid state chemical stability studies. *J Pharm Sci*. 1979; 68:863–6.

631. Bray RJ, Davies PA. The stability of preservative-free morphine in plastic syringes. *Anaesthesia*. 1986; 41:294–5.

632. Walker SE, Paton TW, Fabian TM et al. Stability and sterility of cimetidine admixtures frozen in minibags. *Am J Hosp Pharm*. 1981; 38:881–3.

633. Cohen MR. Error 148—More on cisplatin storage. *Hosp Pharm*. 1980; 15:158–9.

634. LeRoy AF. Some quantitative data on cis-dichlorodiammineplatinum (II) species in solution. *Cancer Treat Rep*. 1979; 63:231–3.

635. Hincal AA, Long DF. Cis-platin stability in aqueous parenteral vehicles. *J Parenter Drug Assoc*. 1979; 33:107–16.

636. Mariani EP, Southard BJ, Woolever JT, et al. Physical compatibility and chemical stability of cisplatin in various diluents and in large-volume parenteral solutions. In: Cisplatin current status and new developments. New York, NY: Academic Press; 1980:305–16.

637. Repta AJ, Long DF. cis-Dichlorodiammineplatinum (II) stability in aqueous vehicles. *Cancer Treat Rep*. 1979; 63:229–30.

638. Gamble JA, Dundee JW, Assaf RA. Plasma diazepam levels after single dose oral and intramuscular administration. *Anaesthesia*. 1975; 30:164–9.

639. Langdon DE, Harlan JR, Bailey RL. Thrombophlebitis with diazepam used intravenously. *JAMA*. 1973; 223:184–5.

640. Dam M, Christiansen J. Diazepam: intravenous infusion in the treatment of status epilepticus. *Acta Neurol Scand*. 1976; 54:278–80.

641. Huber JW, Raymond GG. Additional conclusions on diazepam injectable precipitate: GC-MS confirmation. *Clin Toxicol*. 1979; 14:439–44.

642. Raymond G, Huber JW. Identification of injectable Valium precipitate. *Drug Intell Clin Pharm*. 1979; 13:612.

643. Newton DW, Driscoll DF, Goudreau JL et al. Solubility characteristics of diazepam in aqueous admixture solutions: theory and practice. *Am J Hosp Pharm*. 1981; 38:179–82.

644. Mason NA, Cline S, Hyneck ML et al. Factors affecting diazepam infusion: solubility, administration-set composition, and flow rate. *Am J Hosp Pharm*. 1981; 38:1449–54.

645. MacKichan J, Duffner PK. Adsorption of diazepam to plastic tubing. *N Engl J Med*. 1979; 301:332–3.

646. Parker WA, MacCara ME. Compatibility of diazepam with intravenous fluid containers and administration sets. *Am J Hosp Pharm*. 1980; 37:496–500.

647. Cloyd JC, Vezeau C. Availability of diazepam from plastic containers. *Am J Hosp Pharm*. 1980; 37:492–6.

648. Cloyd JC. Diluting diazepam injection. *Am J Hosp Pharm*. 1981; 38:32.

649. Dasta JF, Brier K. Loss of diazepam to drug delivery systems. *Am J Hosp Pharm*. 1980; 37:1176.

650. Boatman JA, Johnson JB. A four-stage approach to new-drug development. *Pharm Tech*. 1981; 5:46–56.

651. Martin CM. Chemical incompatibility of Renografin 76 and protamine sulfate. *Am Heart J*. 1976; 91:675–7.

652. Hoffman DM, Grossano DD, Damin L et al. Stability of refrigerated and frozen solutions of doxorubicin hydrochloride. *Am J Hosp Pharm*. 1979; 36:1536–8.

653. Gardiner WA. Possible incompatibility of doxorubicin hydrochloride with aluminum. *Am J Hosp Pharm*. 1981; 38:1276.

654. Pfaller MA, Granich GG, Valdes R et al. Comparative study of the ability of four aminoglycoside assay techniques to detect the inactivation of aminoglycosides by beta-lactam antibiotics. *Diagn Microbiol Infect Dis*. 1984; 2:93–100.

655. Hospira Inc. Product information on Liposyn III 10%, 20%, and 30%. Lake Forest, IL; 2005 Aug/Sep.

656. Black CD, Popovich NG. Study of intravenous emulsion compatibility: effects of dextrose, amino acids and selected electrolytes. *Drug Intell Clin Pharm*. 1981; 15:184–93.

657. Black CD, Popovich NG. Comment on intravenous emulsion compatibility. *Drug Intell Clin Pharm*. 1981; 15:908–9.

658. Pelham LD. Rational use of intravenous fat emulsions. *Am J Hosp Pharm*. 1981; 38:198–208.

659. Solussol C. Long-term parenteral nutrition: an artificial gut. *Int Surg*. 1976; 61:266–70.

660. Wretlind A. Current status of intralipid and other fat emulsions. In: Fat emulsion in parenteral nutrition. Chicago, IL: American Medical Association; 1975:109–19.

661. Higbee KC, Lamy PP. Use of Intralipid in neonates and infants. *Hosp Formul*. (Feb) 1980; 15:117–9, 122, 127.

662. Kleinberg ML, Stauffer GL. Effect of microwave radiation on redissolving precipitated matter in fluorouracil injection. *Am J Hosp Pharm*. 1980; 37:678–9.

663. Driessen O, deVos D. Adsorption of fluorouracil on glass surfaces. *J Pharm Sci*. 1978; 67:1494–5.

664. Ghanekar AG, Das Gupta V. Stability of furosemide in aqueous systems. *J Pharm Sci*. 1978; 67:808–11.

665. McLaughlin JE, Reeves DS. Gentamicin plus carbenicillin. *Lancet*. 1971; 1:864–5.

666. Young LS, Decker G. Inactivation of gentamicin by carbenicillin in the urinary tract. *Chemotherapy*. 1974; 20:212–20.

667. Murillo J, Standiford HC, Schimpff SC et al. Gentamicin and ticarcillin serum levels. *JAMA*. 1979; 241:2401–3.

668. Storey P, Hill HH, St. Louis RH, et al. Subcutaneous infusions for control of cancer symptoms. *J Pain Symptom Manag*. 1990; 5:33–41.

669. Edwards ND, Fletcher A, Cole JR et al. Combined infusions of morphine and ketamine for postoperative pain in elderly patients. *Anaesthesia*. 1993; 48:124–7.

670. Dormarunno CG (Associate Medical Information Scientist, Medical and Drug Information, Pharmacia Corp., Kalamazoo, MI): Personal communication; 2002 Mar 21.

671. Liles S (Department of Pharmacy, Christ Hospital, Cincinnati, OH): Personal communication; 2002 Feb 20.

672. Hayes DM, Reilly RM. The pharmaceutical stability of deferoxamine mesylate. *Can J Hosp Pharm*. 1994; 47:9–14.

673. Downie G, McRae N. Leaching of plasticizers by fat emulsion from polyvinyl chloride. *Br J Parenter Ther*. 1985; 6:142–4.

674. Anderson W, Harthill JE, Couper IA et al. Heparin stability in dextrose solutions [proceedings]. *J Pharm Pharmacol*. 1977; 29:31P.

675. Bowie HM, Haylor V. Stability of heparin in sodium chloride solution. *J Clin Pharm*. 1978; 3:211–4.

676. Tunbridge LJ, Lloyd JV, Penhall RK et al. Stability of diluted heparin sodium stored in plastic syringes. *Am J Hosp Pharm*. 1981; 38:1001–4.

677. Deeb EN, DiMattia PE. Standardization of heparin-lock maintenance solution. *N Engl J Med*. 1976; 294:448.

678. Holford NHG, Vozeh S, Coates P et al. More on heparin lock. *N Engl J Med*. 1977; 296:1300–1.

679. Lynch CL, Linder GE. Frequently asked questions about insulin. *Hosp Pharm*. 1980; 15:213–4.

680. Graham DT, Pomeroy AR. Effects of freezing on commercial insulin suspensions. *Int J Pharm*. 1978; 1:315–22.

681. Hill JB. Adsorption of insulin to glass. *Proc Soc Exp Biol Med*. 1959; 102:75–7.

682. Hill JB. The adsorption of I^{131}-insulin to glass. *Endocrinology*. 1959; 65:515–7.

683. Wiseman R, Baltz BE. Prevention of insulin-I^{131} adsorption to glass. *Endocrinology*. 1961; 68:354–6.

684. Sonksen PH, Ellis JP, Lowy C et al. Quantitative evaluation of the relative efficiency of gelatine and albumin in preventing insulin adsorption to glass. *Diabetologia*. 1965; 1:208–10.

685. Suess V, Froesch ER. Zur therapie des coma diabeticum: quantitative bedeutung des insulinuerlusts am infusionsbesteck. *Schweizer Med Wochanschr*. 1975; 105:1315–8.

686. Okamoto H, Kikuchi T. Adsorption of insulin to infusion bottles and plastic intravenous tubing. *Yakuzaigaku*. 1979; 39:107–11.

687. Wingert TD, Levin SR. Insulin adsorption to an air-eliminating inline filter. *Am J Hosp Pharm*. 1981; 38:382–3.

688. Hirsch JI, Wood JH. Insulin adsorption to polyolefin infusion bottles and polyvinyl chloride administration sets. *Am J Hosp Pharm*. 1981; 38:995–7.

689. Kerchner J, Cocaluca DM. Effect of whole blood on insulin adsorption onto intravenous infusion systems. *Am J Hosp Pharm*. 1980; 37:1323–5.

690. Galloway JA, Bressler R. Insulin treatment in diabetes. *Med Clin N Am*. 1978; 62:663–80.

691. Anon. Letter: Carrier solutions for low-level intravenous insulin infusion. *Br Med J*. 1976; 1:151–2.

692. Wan KK, Tsallas G. Dilute iron dextran formulation for addition to parenteral nutrient solutions. *Am J Hosp Pharm*. 1980; 37:206–10.

693. Bornstein M, Lo AY, Thomas PN et al. Moxalactam disodium compatibility with intramuscular and intravenous diluents. *Am J Hosp Pharm*. 1982; 39:1495–8.

694. Kleinberg ML, Latiolais CJ. Use of a microwave oven to redissolve crystallized mannitol injection (25%) in ampuls. *Hosp Pharm*. 1979; 14:391–2.

695. Hanson GG. Microwave oven explosion. *Hosp Pharm*. 1979; 14:612.

696. Kleinberg ML, Latiolais CJ. Microwave oven explosion. *Hosp Pharm*. 1979; 14:612.

697. Kana MJ. Microwave oven explosion. *Hosp Pharm*. 1980; 15:104.

698. Post RE, Stephen SP. A warming cabinet for storing mannitol ampuls. *Hosp Pharm*. 1975; 10:102–3.

699. Scott KR, Bell AF, Thomas AJ. Warming kettle for storing mannitol injection. *Am J Hosp Pharm*. 1980; 37:16.

700. Herring P. Keeping mannitol in solution. *Hosp Pharm*. 1980; 15:530–1.

701. Church JJ. Continuous narcotic infusions for relief of postoperative pain. *Br Med J*. 1979; 1:977–9.

702. Townsend RJ, Puchala AH. Stability of methylprednisolone sodium succinate in small volumes of 5% dextrose and 0.9% sodium chloride injections. *Am J Hosp Pharm*. 1981; 38:1319–22.

703. Knutsen CV, Epps DR, McCormick DC et al. Total nutrient admixture guidelines. *Drug Intell Clin Pharm*. 1984; 18:253–4.

704. Riggle MA, Brandt RB. Decomposition of TPN solutions. *J Pediatr*. 1982; 100:670.

705. Freund HR, Rimon B, Muggia-Sullam M, et al. The "All in one" system for TPN causes increased rates of catheter blockade. *J Parenter Enteral Nutr*. 1986; 10:543.

706. Cohen MR. Hazard warning—Flagyl IV (metronidazole hydrochloride) product reconstitution. *Hosp Pharm*. 1981; 16:398.

707. Little GB, Boylan JC. I.V. Flagyl reacts with aluminum. *Hosp Pharm*. 1981; 16:627.

708. Carmichael RR, Mahoney CD. Solubility and stability of phenytoin sodium when mixed with intravenous solutions. *Am J Hosp Pharm*. 1980; 37:95–8.

709. Salem RB, Yost RL, Torosian G et al. Investigation of the crystallization of phenytoin in normal saline. *Drug Intell Clin Pharm*. 1980; 14:605–8.

710. Pfeifle CE, Adler DS. Phenytoin sodium solubility in three intravenous solutions. *Am J Hosp Pharm*. 1981; 38:358–2.

712. Gupta VD, Stewart KR. Stability of cefuroxime sodium in some aqueous buffered solutions and intravenous admixtures. *J Clin Hosp Pharm*. 1986; 11:47–54.

713. Newton DW, Kluza RB. Prediction of phenytoin solubility in intravenous admixtures: physicochemical theory. *Am J Hosp Pharm*. 1980; 37:1647–51.

714. Cohen MR. Make sure your nurses mix drug additions to infusing I.V. solutions. *Hosp Pharm*. 1981; 16:164.

715. Schuna A, Nappi J, Kolstad J. Potassium pooling in non-rigid parenteral fluid containers. *J Parenter Drug Assoc*. 1979; 33:184–6.

716. McCloskey WW, Jeffrey LP. Rational ordering of phosphate supplements. *Hosp Pharm*. 1979; 14:486–7.

717. Herman JJ. Phosphate: its valence and methods of quantification in parenteral solutions. *Drug Intell Clin Pharm*. 1979; 13:579–85.

718. Benderev K. Hypophosphatemia and phosphorus supplementation. *Hosp Pharm*. 1980; 15:611–3.

719. Swerling R. Use and preparation of cardioplegic solutions in cardiac surgery. *Hosp Pharm*. 1980; 15:497–503.

720. Loucas SP, Mehl B, Maager P et al. Stability of procaine HCl in a buffered cardioplegia formulation. *Am J Hosp Pharm*. 1981; 38:1924–8.

721. Amann AH, Baaske DM. Plastic i.v. container for nitroglycerin. *Am J Hosp Pharm*. 1980; 37:618.

722. Cacace LG, Harralson A, Clougherty T. Stability of NTG. *Am Heart J*. 1979; 97:817–8.

723. Yuen PH, Denman SL, Sokoloski TD et al. Loss of nitroglycerin from aqueous solution into plastic intravenous delivery systems. *J Pharm Sci*. 1979; 68:1163–6.

724. Baaske DM, Amann AH, Wagenknecht DM et al. Nitroglycerin compatibility with intravenous fluid filters, containers, and administration sets. *Am J Hosp Pharm*. 1980; 37:201–5.

725. Roberts MS, Cossum PA, Galbraith AJ et al. Availability of nitroglycerin from parenteral solutions. *J Pharm Pharmacol*. 1980; 32:237–44.

726. Christiansen H, Skobba TJ, Andersen R et al. Nitroglycerin infusion—factors influencing the concentration of nitroglycerin available to the patient. *J Clin Hosp Pharm*. 1980; 5:209–15.

727. Sokoloski TD, Wu CC. Rapid adsorptive loss of nitroglycerin from aqueous solution to plastic. *Int J Pharm*. 1980; 6:63–76.

728. Baaske DM, Amann AH, Karnatz NN et al. Administration set for use with intravenous nitroglycerin. *Am J Hosp Pharm*. 1982; 39:121–2.

729. Little LA, Hatheway GJ. Problems with administration devices for commercially available nitroglycerin injection. *Am J Hosp Pharm*. 1982; 39:400.

730. Schad RF, Jennings R. Problems with administration devices for commercially available nitroglycerin injection. *Am J Hosp Pharm*. 1982; 39:400.

731. Turco SJ. Problems with administration devices for commercially available nitroglycerin injection. *Am J Hosp Pharm*. 1982; 39:977.

732. Vesey CJ, Batistoni GA. Determination and stability of sodium nitroprusside in aqueous solutions (determination and stability of SNP). *J Clin Pharm*. 1977; 2:105–7.

733. Milewski B, Jones D. Photodecomposition. *Hosp Pharm*. 1981; 16:178.

734. Nolly RJ, Stach PE, Latiolais CJ et al. Stability of thiamine hydrochloride repackaged in disposable syringes. *Am J Hosp Pharm*. 1982; 39:471–4.

735. Polk RE, Kline BJ. Mail order tobramycin serum levels: low values caused by ticarcillin. *Am J Hosp Pharm*. 1980; 37:920.

736. Seitz DJ, Archambault JR, Kresel JJ et al. Stability of tobramycin sulfate in plastic syringes. *Am J Hosp Pharm*. 1980; 37:1614–5.

737. Levison ME, Knight R. In vitro evaluation of tobramycin, a new aminoglycoside antibiotic. *Antimicrob Agents Chemother*. 1972; 1:381–4.

738. Svensson LA. Stressed oxidative degradation of terbutaline in aqueous solution. *Acta Pharm Suec*. 1972; 9:141–6.

739. Cutie MR. Compatibility of verapamil with other additives. *Am J Hosp Pharm*. 1981; 38:231.

740. Lederle Laboratories. Hospital formulary monograph—Pipracil. Wayne, NJ; 1981 Nov.

741. Chan KK, Giannini DD, Staroscik JA et al. 5-Azacytidine hydrolysis kinetics measured by high-pressure liquid chromatography and ^{13}C-NMR spectroscopy. *J Pharm Sci*. 1979; 68:807–12.

742. Rubin M, Bilik R, Aserin A et al. Catheter obstruction: analysis of filter content of total nutrient admixture. *J Parenter Enteral Nutr*. 1989; 13:641–3.

743. Flora KP, Smith SL. Application of a simple high-performance liquid chromatographic method for the determination of melphalan in the presence of its hydrolysis products. *J Chromatogr*. 1979; 177:91–7.

744. Palmer AJ, Sewell GJ, Rowland CG. Qualitative studies on ;ga-interferon-2b in prolonged continuous infusion regimes using gradient elution high-performance liquid chromatography. *J Clin Pharm Ther*. 1988; 13:225–31.

745. Morris ME, Parker WA. Compatibility of chlordiazepoxide HCl injection following dilution. *Can J Pharm Sci*. 1981; 16:43–5.

746. Cummings DS, Park MK. Compatibility of propranolol hydrochloride injection with intravenous infusion fluids in plastic containers. *Am J Hosp Pharm*. 1982; 39:1685–7.

747. Deans KW, Lang JR. Stability of trimethoprim-sulfamethoxazole injection in five infusion fluids. *Am J Hosp Pharm*. 1982; 39:1681–4.

748. Munson JW, Kubiak EJ. Cytosine arabinoside stability in intravenous admixtures with sodium bicarbonate and in plastic syringes. *Drug Intell Clin Pharm*. 1982; 16:765–7.

749. Kirschenbaum HL, Aronoff W, Perentesis GP et al. Stability of dobutamine hydrochloride in selected large-volume parenterals. *Am J Hosp Pharm*. 1982; 39:1923–5.

750. Ray JB, Newton DW, Nye MT et al. Droperidol stability in intravenous admixtures. *Am J Hosp Pharm*. 1983; 40:94–7.

751. Das Gupta V, Stewart KR. Stability of cefotaxime sodium and moxalactam disodium in 5% dextrose and 0.9% sodium chloride injections. *Am J IV Ther Clin Nutr*. 27–9 (Jan) 1983; 10:20.

752. Jett S, Eng SS. Prochlorperazine edisylate incompatibility. *Am J Hosp Pharm*. 1983; 40:210.

753. Porter WR, Johnson CA, Cohon MS et al. Compatibility and stability of clindamycin phosphate with intravenous fluids. *Am J Hosp Pharm*. 1983; 40:91–4.

754. Hittel WP, Iafrate RP, Karnes HT et al. Stability of pentobarbital sodium in 5% dextrose injection and 0.9% sodium chloride injection. *Am J Hosp Pharm*. 1983; 40:294–6.

755. Niemiec PW, Vanderveen TW, Hohenwarter MW et al. Stability of aminophylline injection in three parenteral nutrition solutions. *Am J Hosp Pharm*. 1983; 40:428–32.

756. Perentesis GP, Piltz GW, Kirschenbaum HL et al. Stability and visual compatibility of bretylium tosylate with selected large-volume parenterals and additives. *Am J Hosp Pharm*. 1983; 40:1010–2.

757. Yuen PC, Taddei CR, Wyka BE et al. Compatibility and stability of labetalol hydrochloride in commonly used intravenous solutions. *Am J Hosp Pharm*. 1983; 40:1007–9.

758. Pyter RA, Hsu LCC. Stability of methylprednisolone sodium succinate in 5% dextrose and 0.9% sodium chloride injection. *Am J Hosp Pharm*. 1983; 40:1329–33.

759. Gannon PM, Sesin GP. Stability of cytarabine following repackaging in plastic syringes and glass containers. *Am J IV Ther Clin Nutr*. 1983; 10:11–6.

760. Sesin GP, Millette LA. Stability study of 5-fluorouracil following repackaging in plastic disposable syringes and multidose vials. *Am J IV Ther Clin Nutr*. 29–30 (Sep) 1982; 9:23–5.

761. Parker WA. Compatibility of perphenazine and butorphanol admixtures. *Can J Hosp Pharm*. 1981; 34:38.

762. Jump WG, Plaza VM. Compatibility of nalbuphine hydrochloride with other preoperative medications. *Am J Hosp Pharm*. 1982; 39:841–3.

763. Dorr RT, Peng YM, Alberts DS. Bleomycin compatibility with selected intravenous medications. *J Med*. 1982; 13(1-:2):121–30.

764. Cutie MR. Compatibility of verapamil hydrochloride injection with commonly used additives. *Am J Hosp Pharm*. 1983; 40:1205–7.

765. Shively CD, Redford A. Flagyl I.V., drug-drug physical compatibility. *Am J IV Ther Clin Nutr*. 1981; 8:9–16.

766. Souney PF, Steele L. Effect of vitamin B complex and ascorbic acid on the antimicrobial activity of cefazolin sodium. *Am J Hosp Pharm*. 1982; 39:840–1.

767. Keller JH, Ensminger WD. Stability of cancer chemotherapeutic agents in a totally implanted drug delivery system. *Am J Hosp Pharm*. 1982; 39:1321–3.

768. Rodanelli R, Comelli M, Pascale W et al. Clinical pharmacology of some antibiotics: problems relating to their intravenous use in hospitals. *Farmaco Ed Prat*. 1982; 37:185–8.

769. Kowaluk EA, Roberts MS. Drug loss in polyolefin infusion systems. *Am J Hosp Pharm*. 1983; 40:118–9.

770. Illum L, Bundgaard H. Sorption of drugs by plastic infusion bags. *Int J Pharm*. 1982; 10:339–51.

771. Pfizer Laboratories. Vistaril IM, table of physical compatibilities. New York, NY; 1979 Jul.

772. Abbott Laboratories. Package insert on Neut. North Chicago, IL; 1988 Oct.

773. Jhunjhuowala VP, Bhalla HL. Sodium ampicillin: its stability in some large volume parenteral solutions. *Indian J Hosp Pharm*. 1981; 8:55–7.

774. Scheiner JM, Araujo MM. Thiamine destruction by sodium bisulfite in infusion solutions. *Am J Hosp Pharm*. 1981; 38:1911–3.

775. Kirschenbaum HL, Aronoff W, Perentesis GP et al. Stability and compatibility of lidocaine hydrochloride with selected large-volume parenterals and drug additives. *Am J Hosp Pharm*. 1982; 39:1013–5.

776. Lackner TE, Baldus D, Butler CD et al. Lidocaine stability in cardioplegic solution stored in glass bottles and polyvinyl chloride bags. *Am J Hosp Pharm*. 1983; 40:97–101.

777. Russell WJ, Meyer-Witting M. The stability of atracurium in clinical practice. *Anaesth Intens Care*. 1990; 18:550–2.

778. Shank WA, Coupal JJ. Stability of digoxin in common large-volume injections. *Am J Hosp Pharm*. 1982; 39:844–6.

779. Solomon DA, Nasinnyk KK. Compatibility of haloperidol lactate and heparin sodium. *Am J Hosp Pharm*. 1982; 39:843–4.

780. Elliott GT, McKenzie MW, Curry SH et al. Stability of cimetidine hydrochloride in admixtures after microwave thawing. *Am J Hosp Pharm*. 1983; 40:1002–6.

781. Tsallas G, Allen LC. Stability of cimetidine hydrochloride in parenteral nutrition solutions. *Am J Hosp Pharm*. 1982; 39:484–5.

782. Roberts MS, Cossum PA, Kowaluk EA et al. Plastic syringes and intravenous infusions. *Med J Aust*. 1981; 2:580–1.

783. Das Gupta V, Stewart KR. Effect of tobramycin on the stability of carbenicillin disodium. *Am J Hosp Pharm*. 1983; 40:1013–6.

784. Simmons A, Allwood MC. Sorption to plastic syringes of drugs administered by syringe pump. *J Clin Hosp Pharm*. 1981; 6:71–3.

785. Nicholas E, Hess G. Degradation of penicillin, ticarcillin and carbenicillin resulting from storage of unit doses. *N Engl J Med*. 1982; 306:547–8.

786. Carpenter JP, Gomez EA. Administration of lorazepam injection through intravenous tubing. *Am J Hosp Pharm*. 1981; 38:1514–6.

787. Newton DW, Narducci WA, Leet WA et al. Lorazepam solubility in and sorption from intravenous admixture solutions. *Am J Hosp Pharm*. 1983; 40:424–7.

788. Frable RA, Klink PR, Engel GL et al. Stability of cefamandole nafate injection with parenteral solutions and additives. *Am J Hosp Pharm*. 1982; 39:622–7.

789. Kirschenbaum HL, Aronoff W, Piltz GW et al. Compatibility and stability of dobutamine hydrochloride with large-volume parenterals and selected additives. *Am J Hosp Pharm*. 1983; 40:1690–1.

790. Bosch EH, van Doorne H, Brouwers JRBJ et al. Vermindering van het sufentanilgehalte bij de bereiding en tijdens het gebruik van een epidurale toedieningsvorm. Een orienterend onderzoek. *Ziekenhuisfarmacie*. 1993; 9:97–101.

791. Cairns CJ. Incompatibility of amiodarone. *Pharm J*. 1986; 236:68.

792. Roney JV (Scientific Services, Hoechst-Roussel Pharmaceuinticals, Somerville, NJ): Personal communication; 1983 Dec 4.

793. Berge SM, Henderson NL. Kinetics and mechanism of degradation of cefotaxime sodium in aqueous solution. *J Pharm Sci*. 1983; 72:59–63.

794. Smith FM, Nuessle NO. Stability of diazepam injection repackaged in glass unit-dose syringes. *Am J Hosp Pharm*. 1982; 39:1687–90.

795. Cossum PA, Roberts MS. Availability of isosorbide dinitrate, diazepam and chlormethiazole from I.V. delivery systems. *Eur J Clin Pharmacol.* 1981; 19:181–5.

796. Smith A, Bird G. Compatibility of diazepam with infusion fluids and their containers. *J Clin Hosp Pharm.* 1982; 7:181–6.

797. Yliruusi JK, Sothmann AG, Laine RH et al. Sorptive loss of diazepam and nitroglycerin from solutions to three types of containers. *Am J Hosp Pharm.* 1982; 39:1018–21.

798. Kuhlman J, Abshagen U. Cleavage of glycosidic bonds of digoxin and derivatives as function of pH and time. *Naunyn Schmiedebergs Arch Pharmacol.* 1973; 276:149–56.

799. Gault MH, Charles JD, Sugden DL et al. Hydrolysis of digoxin by acid. *J Pharm Pharmacol.* 1977; 29:27–32.

800. Sternson LA, Shaffer RD. Kinetics of digoxin stability in aqueous solution. *J Pharm Sci.* 1978; 67:327–30.

801. Khalil SA, El-Masry S. Instability of digoxin in acid medium using a nonisotopic method. *J Pharm Sci.* 1978; 67:1358–60.

802. Fagerman KE, Dean RE. Daily digoxin administration in parenteral nutrition solution. *Am J Hosp Pharm.* 1981; 38:1955.

803. Patterson MJ, Tjokrosetio R. Stability of adrenaline injection BP following resterilization. *Aust J Hosp Pharm.* 1981; 11:21–2.

804. Nazeravich DR, Otlen NHH. Effect of inline filtration on delivery of gentamicin at a slow infusion rate. *Am J Hosp Pharm.* 1983; 40:1961–4.

805. Zell M, Paone RP. Stability of insulin in plastic syringes. *Am J Hosp Pharm.* 1983; 40:637–8.

806. Benvenuto JA. Errors in oncolytic agent stability study. *Am J Hosp Pharm.* 1983; 40:1628.

807. Bisaillon S, Sarrazin R. Compatibility of several antibiotics or hydrocortisone when added to metronidazole solution for intravenous infusion. *J Parenter Sci Technol.* 1983; 37:129–132.

808. Gove L. Antibiotic interactions. *Pharm J.* 1983; 231:233.

809. Ennis CE, Merritt RJ, Neff DN. In vitro study of in line filtration of medications commonly administered to pediatric cancer patients. *JPEN J Parenter Enteral Nutr.* 1983; 7:156–8.

810. Buxton PC, Conduit SM. Stability of parentrovite in infusion fluids. *Br J IV Ther.* 1983; 4:5.

811. Das Gupta V, Stewart KR. Stability of dobutamine hydrochloride and verapamil hydrochloride in 0.9% sodium chloride and 5% dextrose injections. *Am J Hosp Pharm.* 1984; 41:686–9.

812. Hasegawa GR, Eder JF. Visual compatibility of dobutamine hydrochloride with other injectable drugs. *Am J Hosp Pharm.* 1984; 41:949–51.

813. Souney PF, Colucci RD, Mariani G et al. Compatibility of magnesium sulfate solutions with various antibiotics during simulated Y-site injection. *Am J Hosp Pharm.* 1984; 41:323–4.

814. Lundergan FS, Lombardi TP, Neilan GE et al. Stability of tobramycin sulfate mixed with oxacillin sodium and nafcillin sodium in human serum. *Am J Hosp Pharm.* 1984; 41:144–5.

815. Parker WA. Physical compatibility update of preoperative medications. *Hosp Pharm.* 1984; 19:475–8.

816. Hale DC, Jenkins R. In-vitro inactivation of aminoglycoside antibiotics by piperacillin and carbenicillin. *Am J Clin Pathol.* 1980; 74:316–9.

817. Rank DM, Packer AM. In vitro inactivation of tobramycin by penicillins. *Am J Hosp Pharm.* 1984; 41:1187–8.

818. Karlsen J, Thonnesen HH, Olsen IR et al. Stability of cytotoxic intravenous solutions subjected to freeze-thaw treatment. *Nor Pharm Acta.* 1983; 45:61–7.

819. Cheung YW, Vishnuvajjala BR. Stability of cytarabine, methotrexate sodium, and hydrocortisone sodium succinate admixtures. *Am J Hosp Pharm.* 1984; 41:1802–6.

820. Bundgaard H, Larsen C. Influence of carbohydrates and polyhydric alcohols on the stability of cephalosporins in aqueous solution. *Int J Pharm.* 1983; 16:319–25.

821. Hamilton G. Adverse reactions to intravenous pyelography contrast agents. *Can Med Assoc J.* 1983; 129:405–6.

822. Miller B, Pesko L. Effect of freezing on particulate matter concentrations in five antibiotic solutions. *Am J IV Ther Clin Nutr.* 1984; 11:19–22.

823. Wagman GH, Bailey JV. Binding of aminoglycoside antibiotics to filtration materials. *Antimicrob Agents Chemother.* 1975; 7:316–319.

824. Tindula RJ, Ambrose PJ. Aminoglycoside inactivation by penicillins and cephalosporins and its impact on drug-level monitoring. *Drug Intell Clin Pharm.* 1983; 17:906–8.

825. Gillies IR. Physical stability of Intralipid following drug addition. *Aust J Hosp Pharm.* 1980; 10:118–20.

826. Hardin TC, Clibon U, Page CP et al. Compatibility of 5-fluorouracil and total parenteral nutrition solutions. *JPEN J Parenter Enteral Nutr.* 1982; 6:163–5.

827. Gaj E, Sesin GP. Evaluation of growth of five microorganisms in doxorubicin and floxuridine media. *Pharm Manufacturing.* 1984; 1:52–3.

828. Gaj E, Griffin RE. Evaluation of growth of six microorganisms in fluorouracil, bacteriostatic sodium chloride 0.9% and sodium chloride 0.9% media. *Hosp Pharm.* 1983; 18:348–9.

829. Turco SJ. Drug adsorption to membrane filters. *Am J IV Ther Clin Nutr.* 1982; 9:6.

830. Robinson WA, Krebs LU. The "real stuff" for intrathecal injection during leukaemia therapy. *Lancet.* 1982; 1:283.

831. Frear RS. Cefoperazone-aminoglycoside incompatibility. *Am J Hosp Pharm.* 1983; 40:564.

832. O'Bey KA, Jim LK, Gee JP et al. Temperature dependence of the stability of tobramycin mixed with penicillins in human serum. *Am J Hosp Pharm.* 1982; 39:1005–8.

833. Bhatia J, Mims LC. Effect of phototherapy on amino acid solutions containing multivitamins. *J Pediatr.* 1980; 96:284–6.

834. Koshiro A, Fujita T. Interaction of penicillins with the components of plasma expanders. *Drug Intell Clin Pharm.* 1983; 17:351–6.

835. Szucsova S, Slana M. Stability of infusion mixtures of 5% glucose solution with injection solutions. *Farm Obzor.* 1983; 52:209–13.

836. Gillis J, Jones G, Pencharz P. Delivery of vitamins A, D, and E in total parenteral nutrition solutions. *JPEN J Parenter Enteral Nutr.* 1983; 7:11–4.

837. Farago S. Compatibility of antibiotics and other drugs in total parenteral nutrition solutions. *Can J Hosp Pharm.* 1983; 36:43–51.

838. Gaj E, Sesin GP. Compatibility of doxorubicin hydrochloride and vinblastine sulfate—stability of a solution stored in Cormed reservoir bags or Monoject plastic syringes. *Am J IV Ther Clin Nutr.* 13–14, 19–20 (May) 1984; 11:8–9.

839. Bar-Or D, Kulig K, Marx JA et al. Precipitation of verapamil. *Ann Intern Med.* 1982; 97:619.

840. Tucker R, Gentile JF. Precipitation of verapamil with nafcillin. *Am J Hosp Pharm.* 1984; 41:2588.

841. Hasegawa GR, Eder JF. Dobutamine-heparin mixture inadvisable. *Am J Hosp Pharm.* 1984; 41:2588.

842. Chen MF, Boyce HW, Triplett L. Stability of the B vitamins in mixed parenteral nutrition solution. *JPEN J Parenter Enteral Nutr.* 1983; 7:462–4.

843. Bowman BB, Nguyen P. Stability of thiamin in parenteral nutrition solutions. *JPEN J Parenter Enteral Nutr.* 1983; 7:567–8.

844. Newton DW. Physicochemical determinants of incompatibility and instability in injectable drug solutions and admixtures. *Am J Hosp Pharm.* 1978; 35:1213–22.

845. Newton DW. Physicochemical determinants of incompatibility and instability of drugs for injection and infusion. In: Trissel LA. Handbook on injectable drugs. 3rd ed. Bethesda, MD: American Society of Hospital Pharmacists; 1983:XI-XXI.

846. Raymond G, Day P. Sodium content of commonly administered intravenous drugs. *Hosp Pharm.* 1982; 17:560–1.

847. Rich DS. Recent information about inactivation of aminoglycosides by carbenicillin and ticarcillin: clinical implications. *Hosp Pharm.* 1983; 18:41–3.

848. Lawrence RI, Flukes WK, Rust VJ et al. Total parenteral nutrition using a combined nutrient solution. *Aust J Hosp Pharm.* 1981; 11:540–2.

849. Davis SS, Galloway M. Total parenteral nutrition. *Pharm J.* 1983; 6 (Jan 1 & 8):230.

850. Travenol Laboratories. 3-in-1 admixture guide from Travenol. 1983 Nov.

851. Chan JC, Malekzadeh M, Hurley H. pH and titratable acidity of amino acid mixtures used in hyperalimentation. *JAMA.* 1972; 220:1119–20.

852. Kirk B, Sprake JM. Stability of aminophylline. *Br J IV Ther.* (Nov) 1982; 3:4, 6, 8.

853. Vogenberg FR, Souney PF. Stability guidelines for routinely refrigerated drug products. *Am J Hosp Pharm.* 1983; 40:101–2.

854. Niemiec PW, Vanderveen TW. Compatibility considerations in parenteral nutrient solutions. *Am J Hosp Pharm.* 1984; 41:893–911.

855. Irving JD, Reynolds PV. Disposable syringe danger. *Lancet.* 1966; 1:362.

856. Salter F (Bristol-Myers Squibb, Princeton, NJ): Personal communication; 1991 Feb 27.

857. Hopefl AW. Clinical use of intravenous acyclovir. *Drug Intell Clin Pharm.* 1983; 17:623–8.

858. Larsen C, Bundgaard H. Polymerization of penicillins VI. Time-course of formation of antigenic di- and polymerization products in aqueous ampicillin sodium solutions. *Arch Pharm Chemi Sci Ed.* 1977; 5:201–9.

859. Carthy BJ, Hill GT. Some aspects of the analysis and stability of atracurium besylate. *Anal Proc.* 1983; 20:177–9.

860. D'Arcy PF. Comment on handling of anticancer drugs. *Drug Intell Clin Pharm.* 1984; 18:417.

861. Adams J, Wilson JP. Instability of bleomycin in plastic containers. *Am J Hosp Pharm.* 1982; 39:1636.

862. Levin VA, Zackheim HS. Stability of carmustine for topical application. *Arch Dermatol.* 1982; 118:450–1.

863. Chan KK, Zackheim HS. Stability of nitrosourea solutions. *Arch Dermatol.* 1973; 107:298.

864. Teil SM, Arwood LL. Stability of gentamicin and cefamandole in serum. *Am J Hosp Pharm.* 1982; 39:485–6.

865. Portnoff JB, Henley MW. Development of sodium cefoxitin as a dosage form. *J Parenter Sci Technol.* 1983; 37:180–5.

866. Vaughan LM, Poon CY. Stability of ceftazidime and vancomycin alone and in combination in heparinized and nonheparinized peritoneal dialysis solution. *Ann Pharmacother.* 1994; 28:572–6.

867. Muller RH, Heinemann S. Fat emulsions for parenteral nutrition. IV. Lipofundin MCT/LCT regimens for total parenteral nutrition (TPN) with high electrolyte load. *Int J Pharm.* 1994; 107:121–32.

868. Sorkin EM, Darvey DC. Review of cimetidine drug interactions. *Drug Intell Clin Pharm.* 1983; 17:110–20.

869. Raymond G, Day P. Multiple sources of sodium in injectable drugs. *Drug Intell Clin Pharm.* 1982; 16:703.

870. Eshaque M, McKay MJ. D-Mannitol platinum complexes. *Wadley Med Bull.* 1977; 7:338–48.

871. Ferguson DE. Degradation of clindamycin in frozen admixtures. *Am J Hosp Pharm.* 1982; 39:1156.

872. Ausman RK, Holmes CJ, Kundsin RB et al. Degradation of clindamycin in frozen admixtures. *Am J Hosp Pharm.* 1982; 39:1156.

873. Cairns CJ, Robertson J. Incompatibility of ceftazidime and vancomycin. *Pharm J.* 1987; 238:577.

874. Sandoz. Sandimmune—pharmacy fact sheet. East Hanover, NJ; 1983 Nov.

875. Senholzi CS, Kerus MP. Crystal formation after reconstituting cefazolin sodium with 0.9% sodium chloride injection. *Am J Hosp Pharm.* 1985; 42:129–30.

876. Thompson DF, Allen LV, Desai SR et al. Compatibility of furosemide with aminoglycoside admixtures. *Am J Hosp Pharm.* 1985; 42:116–9.

877. Geary TG, Akood MA, Jensen JB. Characteristics of chloroquine binding to glass and plastic. *Am J Trop Med Hyg.* 1983; 32:19–23.

878. Yayon A, Ginsburg A. A method for the measurement of chloroquin uptake in erythrocytes. *Anal Biochem.* 1980; 107:332–6.

879. D'Arcy PF. Drug interactions with medical plastics. *Drug Intell Clin Pharm.* 1983; 17:726–31.

880. Kowaluk EA, Roberts MS. Factors affecting the availability of diazepam stored in plastic bags and administered through intravenous sets. *Am J Hosp Pharm.* 1983; 40:417–23.

881. Kasahara K, Ruiz-Torres A. Einwirkung der verdauungssafe auf die bestandigkeit des digoxin-und digitoxin-molekuls. *Klin Wochenschr*. 1969; 47:1109–11.

882. Berman W, Whitman V, Marks KH et al. Inadvertent overadministration of digoxin to low-birth-weight infants. *J Pediatr*. 1978; 92:1024–5.

883. Berman W, Dubynsky O, Whitman V et al. Digoxin therapy in low-birth-weight infants with patent ductus arteriosus. *J Pediatr*. 1978; 93:652–5.

884. Hajratwala BR. Stability of prostaglandins. *Aust J Pharm Sci*. 1975; NS5(Jun):39–41.

885. Roseman TJ, Sims B. Stability of prostaglandins. *Am J Hosp Pharm*. 1973; 30:236–9.

886. Gupta VD, Stewart KR. Stability of cefsulodin in aqueous buffered solutions and some intravenous admixtures. *J Clin Hosp Pharm*. 1984; 9:21–7.

887. Williamson MJ, Luce JK. Doxorubicin hydrochloride-aluminum interaction. *Am J Hosp Pharm*. 1983; 40:214.

888. Chin TH (Professional Services, Miles Inc., West Haven, CT): Personal communication; 1993 Dec 3.

889. Hausrani PK, Davis SS. Preparation and properties of sterile intravenous emulsions. *J Parenter Sci Technol*. 1983; 37:145–50.

890. Gray MS, Singleton WS. Creaming of phosphatide stabilized fat emulsions by electrolyte solutions. *J Pharm Sci*. 1967; 56:1429–31.

891. Knutsen C, Miller P. Compatibility, stability, and effect of mixing 10% fat emulsion in TPN solutions. *JPEN J Parenter Enteral Nutr*. 1981; 5:579.

892. Burnham WR, Hansrani PK, Knott CE et al. Stability of a fat emulsion based intravenous feeding mixture. *Int J Pharm*. 1983; 13:9–22.

893. Hardin TC. Complex parenteral nutrition solutions: II. Addition of fat emulsions. *Nutr Supp Serv*. 1983; 3:50–51.

894. Quebbeman EJ, Hamid AAR, Hoffman NE et al. Stability of fluorouracil in plastic containers used for continuous infusion at home. *Am J Hosp Pharm*. 1984; 41:1153–6.

895. Barker A, Hebron BS, Beck PR et al. Folic acid and total parenteral nutrition. *JPEN J Parenter Enteral Nutr*. 1984; 8:3–8.

896. Louie N, Stennett DJ. Stability of folic acid in 25% dextrose, 3.5% amino acids, and multivitamin solution. *JPEN J Parenter Enteral Nutr*. 1984; 8:421–6.

897. Koshiro A, Oie S, Harima Y et al. Compatibility of gentamicin sulfate injection in parenteral solutions. *Jap J Hosp Pharm*. 1982; 7:377–80.

898. Godefroid RJ. Intravenous gentamicin dilution requirements. *Am J Hosp Pharm*. 1982; 39:1457.

899. Godefroid RJ. Comment on IV guidelines. *Drug Intell Clin Pharm*. 1984; 18:925.

900. Matthews H. Heparin anticoagulant activity in intravenous fluids utilising a chromagenic substrate assay method. *Aust J Hosp Pharm*. 1982; 12:S17–S22.

901. Turco SJ. Heparin locks. *Am J IV Ther Clin Nutr*. 1983; 10:9.

902. Swerling R: Normal saline or dilute heparin for heparin lock flush? *Infusion*. 1982; 6:123–124.

903. Epperson EL. Efficacy of 0.9% sodium chloride injection with and without heparin for maintaining indwelling intermittent injection sites. *Clin Pharm*. 1984; 3:626–9.

904. Kanke M, Eubanks JL. Binding of selected drugs to a "treated" inline filter. *Am J Hosp Pharm*. 1983; 40:1323–8.

905. Anderson W, Harthill JE. Anticoagulant activity of heparins in dextrose solutions. *J Pharm Pharmacol*. 1982; 34:90–6.

906. Enderlin G. Discoloration of hydralazine injection. *Am J Hosp Pharm*. 1984; 41:634.

907. Pingel M, Volund A. Stability of insulin preparations. *Diabetes*. 1972; 21:805–13.

908. Weber SS, Wood WA. Insulin adsorption controversy. *Drug Intell Clin Pharm*. 1976; 10:232–3.

909. Schildt B, Ahlgren T, Berghem L et al. Adsorption of insulin by infusion materials. *Acta Anaesthesiol Scand*. 1978; 22:556–62.

910. Mitrano FP, Newton DW. Factors affecting insulin adherence to type I glass bottles. *Am J Hosp Pharm*. 1982; 39:1491–5.

911. Twardowski ZJ, Nolph KD, McGary TJ et al. Insulin binding to plastic bags: a methodologic study. *Am J Hosp Pharm*. 1983; 40:575–9.

912. Twardowski ZJ, Nolph KD, McGary TJ et al. Nature of insulin binding to plastic bags. *Am J Hosp Pharm*. 1983; 40:579–82.

913. Twardowski ZJ, Nolph KD, McGary TJ et al. Influence of temperature and time on insulin adsorption to plastic bags. *Am J Hosp Pharm*. 1983; 40:583–6.

914. Sato S, Ebert CD. Prevention of insulin self-association and surface adsorption. *J Pharm Sci*. 1983; 72:228–32.

915. Phillips NC, Lauper RD. Review of etoposide. *Clin Pharm*. 1983; 2:112–9.

916. McCollam PL, Garrison TJ. Etoposide: A new chemotherapeutic agent. *Am J IV Ther Clin Nutr*. 27–28 (Mar) 1984; 11:24.

917. Stroup JW, Mighton-Eryou LM. Expiry date guidelines for a centralized IV admixture service. *Can J Hosp Pharm*. 1986; 39:57–9.

918. Bishop BG. Adsorption of iron-dextran on membrane filters. *NZ Pharm*. 1981; 1:49.

919. Reed MD, Bertino JS. Use of intravenous iron dextran injection in children receiving total parenteral nutrition. *Am J Dis Child*. 1981; 135:829–31.

920. Halpin TC. Use of intravenous iron dextran in sick patients receiving TPN. *Nutr Supp Serv*. 1982; 2:19–20.

921. Shimada A. Adverse reactions to total-dose infusion of iron dextran. *Clin Pharm*. 1982; 1:248–9.

922. Thompson DF, Shimanek M. Stability of sterility study with magnesium sulfate admixtures. *Infusion*. 86 (May-June) 1983; 7:83.

923. Ausman RK, Crevar GE, Hagedorn H et al. Studies in the pharmacodynamics of mechlorethamine and AB100. *J Am Med Assoc*. 1961; 178:143–6.

924. A.H. Robins Pharmaceutical Division. Compatibility chart for reglan injectable 5 mg/mL. Richmond, VA; 1983 Oct.

925. Bonati M, Gaspari F, D'Aranno V et al. Physicochemical and analytical characteristics of amiodarone. *J Pharm Sci*. 1984; 73:829–31.

926. Feroz RM, Puppala S, Chaudhry MA, et al. Compatibility of M.V.C. 9+3 (multivitamin concentrate for infusion) in different large volume parenteral solutions. LyphoMed, Inc., 1984.

927. Alam AS. Identification of labetalol precipitate. *Am J Hosp Pharm*. 1984; 41:74.

928. Wagenknecht DM, Baaske DM, Alam AS et al. Stability of nitroglycerin solutions in polyolefin and glass containers. *Am J Hosp Pharm*. 1984; 41:1807–11.

929. Klamerus KJ, Ueda CT. Stability of nitroglycerin in intravenous admixtures. *Am J Hosp Pharm*. 1984; 41:303–5.

930. Scheife AH, Grisafe JA. Stability of intravenous nitroglycerin solutions. *J Pharm Sci*. 1982; 71:55–9.

931. Ingram JK, Miller JD. Plastic absorption adsorption of nitroglycerin solution. *Anesthesiology*. 1979; 51:S132.

932. Mathot F, Bonnard J, Hans P et al. Les perfusions de nitroglycerine: Etude de l'absorption par differents materiaux plastiques. *J Pharm Belg*. 1980; 35:389–93.

933. Sokoloski TD, Wu CC. Nitroglycerin stability: effects on bioavailability, assay and biological dissolution. *J Clin Hosp Pharm*. 1981; 6:227–32.

934. Cawello VW, Bonn R. Bioverfugbarkeitseinflusse durch die wahl des infusionsmaterials bei der therapie mit nitroglycerin. *Arzneimittelforschung*. 1983; 33:595–7.

935. Rock CM, Gull J. Reducing IV-nitroglycerin loss to an intravenous administration set by preliminary preparation. *Am J IV Ther Clin Nutr*. 40–42 (Oct) 1982; 9:36.

936. Nix DE, Tharpe WN. Effects of presaturation on nitroglycerin delivery by polyvinyl chloride infusion sets. *Am J Hosp Pharm*. 1984; 41:1835–7.

937. Jacobi J, Dasta JF, Reilley TE et al. Loss of nitroglycerin to pulmonary artery delivery systems. *Am J Hosp Pharm*. 1983; 40:1980–2.

938. Jacobi J, Dasta JF, Wu LS et al. Loss of nitroglycerin to central venous pressure catheter. *Drug Intell Clin Pharm*. 1982; 16:331–2.

939. Dasta JF, Jacobi J, Sokolowski TD et al. Loss of nitroglycerin to cardiopulmonary bypass apparatus. *Crit Care Med*. 1983; 11:50–2.

940. Dasta JF, Jacobi J, Sokoloski TD et al. Extraction of nitroglycerin by a membrane oxygenator. *J Extra-Corp Tech*. 1983; 15:101–3.

941. St. Peter JV, Cochran TG. Nitroglycerin loss from intravenous solutions administered with a volumetric infusion pump. *Am J Hosp Pharm*. 1982; 39:1328–30.

942. Hola ET. Loss of nitroglycerin during microinfusion. *Am J Hosp Pharm*. 1984; 41:142–4.

943. Yacobi A, Amann AH. Pharmaceutical considerations of nitroglycerin. *Drug Intell Clin Pharm*. 1983; 17:255–63.

944. Malick AW, Amann AH, Baaske DM et al. Loss of nitroglycerin from solutions to intravenous plastic containers: a theoretical treatment. *J Pharm Sci*. 1981; 70:798–800.

945. Amann AH, Baaske DM. Loss of nitroglycerin from intravenous administration sets during infusion: a theoretical treatment. *J Pharm Sci*. 1982; 71:473–4.

946. Neftel KA, Walti M, Spengler H et al. Effect of storage of penicillin G solutions on sensitization to penicillin G after intravenous administration. *Lancet*. 1982; 1:986–8.

947. Salem RB, Wilder BJ, Yost RL et al. Rapid infusion of phenytoin sodium loading doses. *Am J Hosp Pharm*. 1981; 38:354–7.

948. Gannaway WL, Wilding DC, Siepler JK et al. Clinical use of intravenous phenytoin sodium infusions. *Clin Pharm*. 1983; 2:135–8.

949. Boike SC, Rybak MJ, Tintinalli JE et al. Evaluation of a method for intravenous phenytoin infusion. *Clin Pharm*. 1983; 2:444–6.

950. Earnest MP, Marx JA, Drury LR. Complications of intravenous phenytoin for acute treatment of seizures. *JAMA*. 1983; 249:762–5.

951. Giacona N, Bauman JL. Crystallization of three phenytoin preparations in intravenous solutions. *Am J Hosp Pharm*. 1982; 39:630–4.

952. Lau A, Lee M, Flascha S et al. Effect of piperacillin on tobramycin pharmacokinetics in patients with normal renal function. *Antimicrob Agents Chemother*. 1983; 24:533–7.

953. Autian J, Dhorda CN. Evaluation of disposable plastic syringes as to physical incompatibilities with parenteral products. *Am J Hosp Pharm*. 1959; 16:176–9.

954. Addy DP, Alesbury P. Paraldehyde and plastic syringes. *Br Med J*. 1978; 2:1434.

955. Fenton-May V, Lee F. Paraldehyde and plastic syringes. *Br Med J*. 1978; 2:1166.

956. Evans RJ. Effect of paraldehyde on disposable syringes and needles. *Lancet*. 1961; 2:1451.

957. Johnson CE, Vigoreaux JA. Compatibility of paraldehyde with plastic syringes and needle hubs. *Am J Hosp Pharm*. 1984; 41:306–8.

958. Mahony C, Brown JE, Starget WW et al. In vitro stability of sodium nitroprusside solutions for intravenous administration. *J Pharm Sci*. 1984; 73:838–9.

959. Fricker MP, Swerling R. Sodium nitroprusside reconstitution and administration. *Infusion*. 1981; 5:56.

960. Boehm JJ, Dutton DM. Shelf life of unrefrigerated succinylcholine chloride injection. *Am J Hosp Pharm*. 1984; 41:300–2.

961. Roach M. IV tetracycline. *Pharm J*. 1978; 220:143.

962. Chow MS, Qwintiliani R, Nightingale CH. In vivo inactivation of tobramycin by ticarcillin. A case report. *JAMA*. 1982; 247:658–9.

963. Baumgartner TG, Russell WL. Intravenous trimethoprim-sulfamethoxazole administration alert. *Am J IV Ther Clin Nutr*. 1983; 10:14–5.

964. Hiskey CF, Bullock E. Spectrophotometric study of aqueous solutions of warfarin sodium. *J Pharm Sci*. 1962; 51:43–6.

965. Nahata MC. Stability of ceftriaxone sodium in intravenous solutions. *Am J Hosp Pharm*. 1983; 40:2193–4.

966. Smith BR. Effect of storage temperature and time on stability of cefmenoxime, ceftriaxone, and cefotetan in 5% dextrose injection. *Am J Hosp Pharm*. 1983; 40:1024–5.

967. Vishnuvajjala BR, Cradock JC. Compatibility of plastic infusion devices with diluted *N*-methylformamide and *N,N*-dimethylacetamide. *Am J Hosp Pharm*. 1984; 41:1160–3.

968. Godefroid RJ. Vindesine: A new antineoplastic drug. *Cancer Chemother Update*. 1984; 2:4–7.

969. Cheung YW, Vishnuvajjala BR, Morris NL et al. Stability of azacitidine in infusion fluids. *Am J Hosp Pharm*. 1984; 41:1156–9.

970. Bosanquet AG. Stability of melphalan solutions during preparation and storage. *J Pharm Sci.* 1985; 74:348–51.

971. Tabibi SE, Cradock JC. Stability of melphalan in infusion fluids. *Am J Hosp Pharm.* 1984; 41:1380–2.

972. Teresi M, Allison J. Interaction between vancomycin and ticarcillin. *Am J Hosp Pharm.* 1985; 42:2420.

973. Jorgensen JH, Crawford SA. Selective inactivation of aminoglycosides by newer beta-lactam antibiotics. *Curr Ther Res Clin Exp.* 1982; 32:25–35.

974. Bhatia J, Steginck LD, Ziegler EE. Riboflavin enhances photo-oxidation of amino acids under simulated clinical conditions. *JPEN J Parenter Enteral Nutr.* 1983; 7:277–9.

975. Smith G, Hasson K. Effects of ascorbic acid and disodium edetate on the stability of isoprenaline hydrochloride injection. *J Clin Hosp Pharm.* 1984; 9:209–15.

976. Hutchinson SM. Heparin and aminoglycosides instability. *Drug Intell Clin Pharm.* 1986; 20:886.

977. Johnston-Early A, McKenzie MA, Krasnow SH et al. Drug trapping in intravenous infusion side arms. *JAMA.* 1984; 252:2392.

978. Parker WA. Physical compatibility of ranitidine HCl with preoperative injectable medications. *Can J Hosp Pharm.* 1985; 38:160–1.

979. Das Gupta V, Stewart KR. Chemical stabilities of cefamandole nafate and metronidazole when mixed together for intravenous infusion. *J Clin Hosp Pharm.* 1985; 10:379–83.

980. Cohen MH, Johnston-Early A, Hood MA et al. Drug precipitation within iv tubing: a potential hazard of chemotherapy administration. *Cancer Treat Rep.* 1985; 69:1325–6.

981. Marble DA, Bosso JA. Compatibility of clindamycin phosphate with amikacin sulfate at room temperature and with gentamicin sulfate and tobramycin sulfate under frozen conditions. *Drug Intell Clin Pharm.* 1986; 20:960–3.

982. Gove LF, Gordon NH, Miller J et al. Pre-filled syringes for self-administration of epidural opiates. *Pharm J.* 1985; 234:378–9.

983. Bosso JA, Townsend RJ. Stability of clindamycin phosphate and ceftizoxime sodium, cefoxitin sodium, cefamandole nafate, or cefazolin sodium in two intravenous solutions. *Am J Hosp Pharm.* 1985; 42:2211–4.

984. Nahata MC, Durrell DE. Stability of tobramycin sulfate in admixtures with calcium gluconate. *Am J Hosp Pharm.* 1985; 42:1987–8.

985. Baker DE, Yost GS, Craig VL et al. Compatibility of heparin sodium and morphine sulfate. *Am J Hosp Pharm.* 1985; 42:1352–5.

986. Carlson GH, Matzke GR. Particle formation of third-generation cephalosporin injections. *Am J Hosp Pharm.* 1985; 42:1578–9.

987. Nieves-Cordero AL, Luciw HM. Compatibility of narcotic analgesic solutions with various antibiotics during simulated Y-site injection. *Am J Hosp Pharm.* 1985; 42:1108–9.

988. Ogawa GS, Young R. Dispensing-pin problems. *Am J Hosp Pharm.* 1985; 42:1042.

989. Conklin CA, Kerege JF. Stability of an analgesic-sedative combination in glass and plastic single-dose syringes. *Am J Hosp Pharm.* 1985; 42:339–42.

990. Thompson M, Smith M, Gragg R et al. Stability of nitroglycerin and dobutamine in 5% dextrose and 0.9% sodium chloride injection. *Am J Hosp Pharm.* 1985; 42:361–2.

991. Rhodes RS, Rhodes PJ. Stability of meperidine hydrochloride, promethazine hydrochloride, and atropine sulfate in plastic syringes. *Am J Hosp Pharm.* 1985; 42:112–5.

992. Kiel D, Connolly BJ. Visual compatibility of amrinone lactate with various i.v. secondary additives. *Parenterals.* (May-June) 1985; 3:1, 5–6.

993. Das Gupta V, Stewart KR. Chemical stabilities of hydrocortisone sodium succinate and several antibiotics when mixed with metronidazole injection for intravenous infusion. *J Parenter Sci Technol.* 1985; 39:145–8.

994. Foley PT, Bosso JA, Bair JN et al. Compatibility of clindamycin phosphate with cefotaxime sodium or netilmicin sulfate in small-volume admixtures. *Am J Hosp Pharm.* 1985; 42:839–43.

995. Mansur JM, Abramowitz PW, Lerner SA et al. Stability and cost analysis of clindamycin-gentamicin admixtures given every eight hours. *Am J Hosp Pharm.* 1985; 42:332–5.

996. Quock JR, Sakai RI. Stability of cytarabine in a parenteral nutrient solution. *Am J Hosp Pharm.* 1985; 42:592–4.

997. Walker SE, Bayliff CD. Stability of ranitidine hydrochloride in total parenteral nutrient solution. *Am J Hosp Pharm.* 1985; 42:590–2.

998. Baptista RJ, Palumbo JD, Tahan SR et al. Stability of cimetidine hydrochloride in a total nutrient admixture. *Am J Hosp Pharm.* 1985; 42:2208–10.

999. Das Gupta V, Stewart KR. pH-Dependent effect of magnesium sulfate on the stability of penicillin G potassium solution. *Am J Hosp Pharm.* 1985; 42:598–602.

1000. Macias JM, Martin WJ. Stability of morphine sulfate and meperidine hydrochloride in a parenteral nutrient formulation. *Am J Hosp Pharm.* 1985; 42:1087–94.

1001. James MJ, Riley CM. Stability of intravenous admixtures of aztreonam and ampicillin. *Am J Hosp Pharm.* 1985; 42:1095–110.

1002. James MJ, Riley CM. Stability of intravenous admixtures of aztreonam and clindamycin phosphate. *Am J Hosp Pharm.* 1985; 42:1984–6.

1003. Thompson DF, Thompson GD. Effect of inline filtration on pediatric doses of gentamicin and tobramycin. *Infusion.* 1984; 8:31–2.

1004. Alexander SR, Arena R. Predicting calcium phosphate precipitation in premature infant parenteral nutrition solutions. *Hosp Pharm.* 1985; 20:656–8.

1005. Spruill WJ, McCall CY. In vitro inactivation of tobramycin by cephalosporins. *Am J Hosp Pharm.* 1985; 42:2506–9.

1006. Stevenson JG, Patriarca C. Incompatibility of morphine sulfate and prochlorperazine edisylate in syringes. *Am J Hosp Pharm.* 1985; 42:2651.

1007. Beijnen JH, Rosing H, deVries PA et al. Stability of anthracycline antitumor agents in infusion fluids. *J Parenter Sci Technol.* 1985; 39:220–2.

1008. Baptista RJ, Lawrence RW. Compatibility of total nutrient admixtures and secondary antibiotic infusions. *Am J Hosp Pharm.* 1985; 42:362–3.

1009. Baptista RJ, Dumas GJ, Bistrian BR et al. Compatibility of total nutrient admixtures and secondary cardiovascular medications. *Am J Hosp Pharm.* 1985; 42:777–8.

1010. Bullock L, Parks RB, Lampasona V et al. Stability of raniti-dine hydrochloride and amino acids in parenteral nutrient solutions. *Am J Hosp Pharm.* 1985; 42:2683–7.

1011. Henann NE, Jacks TT. Compatibility and availability of sodium bicarbonate in total parenteral nutrient solutions. *Am J Hosp Pharm.* 1985; 42:2718–20.

1012. Watson D. Piggyback compatibility of antibiotics with pediatric parenteral nutrition solutions. *JPEN J Parenter Enteral Nutr.* 1985; 9:220–4.

1013. Turner SA. Stability and clinical use of intravenous admix-tures containing lipid emulsion. *Pharm J.* 1985; 234:799–800.

1014. El Eini D, Knott CE. Stability of iv lipid emulsions. *Pharm J.* 1985; 235:170.

1015. Hobbiss JH. Stability of iv lipid emulsions. *Pharm J.* 1985; 235:170.

1016. Allwood MC. Drop size of infusions containing fat emul-sion. *Br J Parenter Ther.* 1984; 5:113–4.

1017. Iliano L, Delanghe M, van Den Baviere H et al. Effect of electrolytes in the presence of some trace elements on the stability of all-in-one emulsion mixtures for total paren-teral nutrition. *J Clin Hosp Pharm.* 1984; 9:87–93.

1018. Whateley TL, Steele G, Urwin J et al. Particle size stability of Intralipid and mixed total parenteral nutrition mixtures. *J Clin Hosp Pharm.* 1984; 9:113–26.

1019. Harrie KR, Jacob M, McCormick D et al. Comparison of total nutrient admixture stability using two intravenous fat emulsions, Soyacal and Intralipid 20%. *JPEN J Parenter Enteral Nutr.* 1986; 10:381–7.

1020. Riley CM, James MJ. Stability of intravenous admixtures containing aztreonam and cefazolin. *Am J Hosp Pharm.* 1986; 43:925–7.

1021. Kuhn RJ, Nahata MC. Stability of netilmicin sulfate in admixtures with calcium gluconate and aminophylline. *Am J Hosp Pharm.* 1986; 43:1241–2.

1022. Johnson CE, Cohen IA, Craft DA et al. Compatibility of aminophylline and methylprednisolone sodium succi-nate intravenous admixtures. *Am J Hosp Pharm.* 1986; 43:1482–5.

1023. Bell RG, Lipford LC, Massanari MJ et al. Stability of intrave-nous admixtures of aztreonam and cefoxitin, gentamicin, metronidazole, or tobramycin. *Am J Hosp Pharm.* 1986; 43:1444–53.

1024. Fitzgerald KA, MacKay MW. Calcium and phosphate solu-bility in neonatal parenteral nutrient solutions containing TrophAmine. *Am J Hosp Pharm.* 1986; 43:88–93.

1025. Sayeed FA, Johnson HW, Sukumaran KB et al. Stability of Liposyn II fat emulsion in total nutrient admixtures. *Am J Hosp Pharm.* 1986; 43:1230–5.

1026. Marble DA, Bosso JA. Stability of clindamycin phosphate with aztreonam, ceftazidime sodium, ceftriaxone sodium, or piperacillin sodium in two intravenous solutions. *Am J Hosp Pharm.* 1986; 43:1732–6.

1027. Lee MG. Sorption of four drugs to polyvinyl chloride and polybutadiene intravenous administration sets. *Am J Hosp Pharm.* 1986; 43:1945–50.

1028. Riley CM, Lipford LC. Interaction of aztreonam with nafcillin in intravenous admixtures. *Am J Hosp Pharm.* 1986; 43:2221–4.

1029. Walker PC, Kaufmann RE. Compatibility of cefazolin and gentamicin in peritoneal dialysis solutions. *Drug Intell Clin Pharm.* 1986; 20:697–700.

1030. Beijnen JH, Neef C, Menwissen OJAT et al. Stability of intravenous admixtures of doxorubicin and vincristine. *Am J Hosp Pharm.* 1986; 43:3022–7.

1031. Campbell S, Nolan PE, Bliss M et al. Stability of amiodarone hydrochloride in admixtures with other injectable drugs. *Am J Hosp Pharm.* 1986; 43:917–21.

1032. Hasegawa GR, Eder JF. Visual compatibility of amiodarone hydrochloride injection with other injectable drugs. *Am J Hosp Pharm.* 1984; 41:1379–80.

1033. Allwood MC. Sorption of drugs to intravenous delivery systems. *Pharm Int.* 1983; 4:83–5.

1034. Khue NV, Jung L. Study of the retention of child-dose drugs on cellulose ester membranes during inline intrave-nous filtration. *S-T-P-Pharma.* 1985; 1:201–7.

1035. Das Gupta V, Shah KA. Stability of ampicillin sodium and penicillin G potassium solutions using high-pressure liquid chromatography. *Can J Pharm Sci.* 1981; 16:61–5.

1036. Janknegt R, Neil MJLE. De verenigbaarheid van antimicro-biele middelen in infusievloeistoffen. *Pharm Weekbl.* 1985; 120:638–40.

1037. Bouma J, Beijnen JH, Bult A et al. Anthracycline anti-tumor agents, a review of physicochemical, analytical and stability properties. *Pharm Weekbl [Sci].* 1986; 8:109–33.

1038. Howard L, Chu R, Feman S et al. Vitamin A deficiency from long-term parenteral nutrition. *Ann Intern Med.* 1980; 93:576–7.

1039. Shenai JP, Stahlman MT. Vitamin A delivery from paren-teral alimentation solution. *J Pediatr.* 1981; 99:661–3.

1040. Kishi H, Yamaji A, Kataoka K et al. Vitamin A and E require-ments during total parenteral nutrition. *JPEN J Parenter Enteral Nutr.* 1981; 5:420–3.

1041. Knight P, Heer D, Abdenour G. CaxP and Ca/P in the paren-teral feeding of preterm infants. *JPEN J Parenter Enteral Nutr.* 1983; 7:110–4.

1042. Poole RK, Rupp CA, Kerner JA Jr. Calcium and phosphorus in neonatal parenteral nutrition solutions. *JPEN J Parenter Enteral Nutr.* 1983; 7:358–60.

1043. Ritschel WA, Alcorn GJ, Streng WH et al. Cimetidine-the-ophylline complex formation. *Methods Find Exp Clin Phar-macol.* 1983; 5:55–8.

1044. Glew RH, Pavuk RA. Stability of vancomycin and amino-glycoside antibiotics in peritoneal dialysis concentrate. *Nephron.* 1981; 28:241–3.

1045. Kamen BA, Gunther N, Sowinsky N et al. Analysis of anti-biotic stability in a parenteral nutrition solution. *Pediatr Infect Dis.* 1985; 4:387–9.

1046. Baumgartner TG, Sitren HS, Hall J et al. Stability of urokinase in parenteral nutrition solutions. *Nutr Supp Serv.* 1985; 5:41–3.

1047. Allwood MC. Influence of light on vitamin A degradation during administration. *Clin Nutr.* 1982; 1:63–70.

1048. Allwood MC, Plane JH. Degradation of vitamin A exposed to ultraviolet radiation. *Int J Pharm.* 1984; 19:207–13.

1049. Riggle MA, Brandt RB. Decrease of available vitamin A in parenteral nutrition solutions. *JPEN J Parenter Enteral Nutr.* 1986; 10:388–92.

1050. McKenna MC, Bieri JC. Loss of vitamin A from total parenteral nutrition (TPN) solutions. *Fed Proc.* 1980; 39:561.

1051. Bryant CA, Neufeld NJ. Differences in vitamin A content of enteral feeding solutions following exposure to a polyvinyl chloride enteral feeding system. *JPEN J Parenter Enteral Nutr.* 1982; 6:403–5.

1052. Riff LJ, Thomason JL. Comparative aminoglycoside inactivation by beta-lactam antibiotics—effect of cephalosporin and six penicillins on five aminoglycosides. *J Antibiot (Tokyo).* 1982; 35:850–7.

1053. Schutz VH, Schroder F. Heparin-natrium kompatibilitat bei gleichzeitiger applikation anderer pharmaka. *Krankenhauspharmazie.* 1985; 6:7–11.

1054. Wermeling DP, Rapp RP, DeLuca PP et al. Osmolality of small-volume intravenous admixtures. *Am J Hosp Pharm.* 1985; 42:1739–44.

1055. Johnston SJ. Stability of tryptophan in total parenteral nutrient solutions. *Am J Hosp Pharm.* 1986; 43:1424.

1056. Allwood MC. Factors influencing the stability of ascorbic acid in total parenteral nutrition infusions. *J Clin Hosp Pharm.* 1984; 9:75–85.

1057. Parr MD, Bertch KE. Amino acid stability and microbial growth in total parenteral nutrient solutions. *Am J Hosp Pharm.* 1985; 42:2688–91.

1058. Nordfjeld K, Rasmussen M. Storage of mixtures for total parenteral nutrition: long-term stability of a total parenteral nutrition mixture. *J Clin Hosp Pharm.* 1983; 8:265–74.

1059. Nordfjeld K, Pedersen JL, Rasmussen M et al. Storage of mixtures for total parenteral nutrition III. Stability of vitamins in TPN mixtures. *J Clin Hosp Pharm.* 1984; 9:293–301.

1060. Das Gupta V. Stability of vitamins in total parenteral nutrient solutions. *Am J Hosp Pharm.* 1986; 43:2132.

1061. Allwood MC. Stability of vitamins in total parenteral nutrient solutions. *Am J Hosp Pharm.* 1986; 43:2138.

1062. Louie N. Stability of vitamins in total parenteral nutrient solutions. *Am J Hosp Pharm.* 1986; 43:2138.

1063. Shine B, Farwell JA. Stability and compatibility in parenteral nutrition solutions. *Br J Parenter Ther.* 44–46, 50 (Mar) 1984; 5:4.

1064. Pamperl H, Kleinberger G. Stability of intravenous fat emulsions. *Arch Surg.* 1982; 117:859–860.

1065. Hardy G, Cotter R, Dawe R. The stability and comparative clearance of TPN mixtures with lipid. In: Johnson ID, ed. Advances in Clinical Nutrition: Selected Proceedings of the 2nd International Symposium. Lancaster, England: MTP Press; 1983:241–60.

1066. Hardy G, Klim RA. Stability studies of parenteral nutrition mixtures with lipids. *JPEN J Parenter Enteral Nutr.* 1981; 5:569.

1067. Jeppsson RI, Sjoberg B. Compatibility of parenteral nutrition solutions when mixed in a plastic bag. *Clin Nutr.* 1984; 2:149–58.

1068. Parry VA, Harrie KR. Effect of various nutrient ratios on the emulsion stability of total nutrient admixtures. *Am J Hosp Pharm.* 1986; 43:3017–22.

1069. Bettner FS, Stennett DJ. Effects of pH, temperature, concentration, and time on particle counts in lipid-con-

taining total parenteral nutrition admixtures. *JPEN J Parenter Enteral Nutr.* 1986; 10:375–80.

1070. Schneider PJ. Three-in-one TPN formulations. *Infusion.* (May-June) 1984; 8:94–5, 101.

1071. Ernst JA, Williams JM, Glick MR et al. Osmolality of substances used in the intensive care nursery. *Pediatrics.* 1983; 72:347–52.

1072. Connors KA, Amidon GL, Stella VJ. Chemical stability of pharmaceuticals: a handbook for pharmacists. New York: John Wiley & Sons; 1986.

1073. Bosanquet AG. Stability of solutions of antineoplastic agents during preparation and storage for in vitro assays II. Assay methods, adriamycin and the other antitumor antibiotics. *Cancer Chemother Pharmacol.* 1986; 17:1–10.

1074. Grant AM (Medical Affairs, Abbott Laboratories, Abbott Park, IL): Personal communication; 1987 Mar 23.

1075. Bornstein M, Templeton RJ. Crystal formation after reconstituting cefazolin sodium with 0.9% sodium chloride injection. *Am J Hosp Pharm.* 1985; 42:2436.

1076. White JR, Campbell RK. Guide to mixing insulins. *Hosp Pharm.* 1991; 26:1046–48.

1077. Das Gupta V. Stability of cefotaxime sodium as determined by high-performance liquid chromatography. *J Pharm Sci.* 1984; 73:565–7.

1078. Carlson GH, Matzke GR. Particle formation of ceftizoxime sodium injections. *Am J Hosp Pharm.* 1985; 42:2651–2.

1079. Swenson E, Gooch WM. Visual compatibility of ceftizoxime sodium in four electrolyte injections. *Am J Hosp Pharm.* 1986; 43:2242–4.

1080. Barbero JR, Marino EL. Accelerated stability studies on Rocephin by high-efficiency liquid chromatography. *Int J Pharm.* 1984; 19:199–206.

1081. Smith RC. Overfill in cefuroxime sodium vials. *Am J Hosp Pharm.* 1985; 42:1045–6.

1082. Smith RC. No more overfill in cefuroxime sodium vials. *Am J Hosp Pharm.* 1986; 43:2154.

1083. DeVane CL, Wailand LA. Stability of chlorpromazine in five milliliter vials. *Can J Hosp Pharm.* 1984; 37:9.

1084. Mu-Chow KJ, Baptista RJ. Cost-effectiveness of parenteral nutrient solutions containing cimetidine hydrochloride. *Am J Hosp Pharm.* 1984; 41:1321.

1085. Parasrampuria J, Das Gupta V. Stability of acetazolamide sodium in 5% dextrose or 0.9% sodium chloride injection. *Am J Hosp Pharm.* 1987; 44:358–60.

1086. Zuber DE. Compatibility of morphine sulfate injections and prochlorperazine edisylate injections. *Am J Hosp Pharm.* 1987; 44:67.

1087. Cheung YW, Cradock JC, Vishnuvajjala BR et al. Stability of cisplatin, iproplatin, carboplatin, and tetraplatin in commonly used intravenous infusion solutions. *Am J Hosp Pharm.* 1987; 44:124–30.

1088. LaFollette JM, Arbus MH. Stability of cisplatin admixtures in polyvinyl chloride bags. *Am J Hosp Pharm.* 1985; 42:2652.

1089. Hussain AA, Haddadin M. Reaction of cis-platinum with sodium bisulfite. *J Pharm Sci.* 1980; 69:364.

1090. Kirk B, Melia CD, Wilson JV et al. Chemical stability of cyclophosphamide injection. *Br J Parenter Ther.* 1984; 5:90–7.

1091. Ptachcinski RJ, Logue LW, Burckart GJ et al. Stability and availability of cyclosporine in 5% dextrose injection or 0.9% sodium chloride injection. *Am J Hosp Pharm.* 1986; 43:94–7.

1092. Venkataramanan R, Burckart GJ, Ptachcinski RJ et al. Leaching of diethylhexyl phthalate from polyvinyl chloride bags into intravenous cyclosporine solution. *Am J Hosp Pharm.* 1986; 43:2800–2.

1093. Stevens MF, Peatey L. Photodegradation of solutions of the antitumour drug DTIC [proceedings]. *J Pharm Pharmacol.* 1978; 30(Suppl):47P.

1094. Williams BA, Tritton TR. Photoinactivation of anthracyclines. *Photochem Photobiol.* 1981; 34:131–4.

1095. Maloney TJ. Dilution of diazepam injection prior to intravenous administration. *Aust J Hosp Pharm.* 1983; 13:79.

1096. Hancock BG, Black CD. Effect of polyethylene-lined administration set on the availability of diazepam injection. *Am J Hosp Pharm.* 1985; 42:335–9.

1097. Yliruusi JK, Uotila JA. Effect of tubing length on adsorption of diazepam to polyvinyl chloride administration sets. *Am J Hosp Pharm.* 1986; 43:2789–94.

1098. Yliruusi JK, Uotila JA. Effect of flow rate and type of i.v. container on adsorption of diazepam to i.v. administration systems. *Am J Hosp Pharm.* 1986; 43:2795–9.

1099. Bell HE, Bertino JS. Constant diazepam infusion in the treatment of continuous seizure activity. *Drug Intell Clin Pharm.* 1984; 18:965–70.

1100. Dandurand KR, Stennett DJ. Stability of dopamine hydrochloride exposed to blue-light phototherapy. *Am J Hosp Pharm.* 1985; 42:595–7.

1101. Pluta PL, Morgan PK. Stability of erythromycin in intravenous admixtures. *Am J Hosp Pharm.* 1986; 43:2732.

1102. Deitel M, Faksa M, Kaminsky VM et al. Growth of microorganisms in soybean oil emulsion and clinical implications. *Int Surg.* 1979; 64:27–32.

1103. Keammerer D, Mayhall CG, Hall GO et al. Microbial growth patterns in intravenous fat emulsions. *Am J Hosp Pharm.* 1983; 40:1650–3.

1104. Kim CH, Lewis DE. Bacterial and fungal growth in intravenous fat emulsions. *Am J Hosp Pharm.* 1983; 40:2159–61.

1105. Allwood MC. Release of DEHP plasticizer into fat emulsion from iv administration sets. *Pharm J.* 1985; 235:600.

1106. Driscoll DF, Baptista RJ, Bistrian BR et al. Practical considerations regarding the use of total nutrient admixtures. *Am J Hosp Pharm.* 1986; 43:416–9.

1107. Morgan DE, Bergdale S. Effect of syringe-pump position on infusion of fat emulsion with a primary solution. *Am J Hosp Pharm.* 1985; 42:1110–1.

1108. Neil JM, Fell AF. Evaluation of the stability of frusemide in intravenous infusions by reversed-phase high-performance liquid chromatography. *Int J Pharm.* 1984; 22:105–26.

1109. Dean T, Ridley P. Use of 0.9% sodium chloride injection without heparin for maintaining indwelling intermittent injection sites. *Clin Pharm.* 1985; 4:488.

1110. Chantelau EA, Berger M. Pollution of insulin with silicone oil, a hazard of disposable plastic syringes. *Lancet.* 1985; 1:1459.

1111. Furberg H, Jensen AK. Effect of pretreatment with 0.9% sodium chloride or insulin solutions on the delivery of insulin from an infusion system. *Am J Hosp Pharm.* 1986; 43:2209–13.

1112. Kane M, Jay M. Binding of insulin to a continuous ambulatory peritoneal dialysis system. *Am J Hosp Pharm.* 1986; 43:81–8.

1113. Hutchinson KG. Assessment of gelling in insulin solutions for infusion pumps. *J Pharm Pharmacol.* 1985; 37:528–31.

1114. Kamerman B. Dissolving mannitol crystals. *Hosp Pharm.* 1985; 20:360.

1115. Cano SB, Glogiewicz FL. Storage requirements for metronidazole injection. *Am J Hosp Pharm.* 1986; 43:2983.

1116. Schell KH, Copland JR. Metronidazole hydrochloride-aluminum interaction. *Am J Hosp Pharm.* 1985; 42:1040.

1117. Struthers BJ, Parr RJ. Clarifying the metronidazole hydrochloride-aluminum interaction. *Am J Hosp Pharm.* 1985; 42:2660.

1118. Quebbeman EJ, Hoffman NE, Ausman RK et al. Stability of mitomycin admixtures. *Am J Hosp Pharm.* 1985; 42:1750–4.

1119. Edwards D, Selkirk AB. Determination of the stability of mitomycin C by high-performance liquid chromatography. *Int J Pharm.* 1979; 4:21–6.

1120. Young JB, Pratt CM, Farmer JA et al. Specialized delivery systems for intravenous nitroglycerin. Are they necessary?. *Am J Med.* 1984; 76:27–37.

1121. Nix DE, Tharpe WN. Intravenous nitroglycerin delivery: dynamics and cost considerations. *Hosp Pharm.* 1985; 20:230–2.

1122. Schaber DE, Uden DL. Nitroglycerin adsorption to a combination polyvinyl chloride, polyethylene intravenous administration set. *Drug Intell Clin Pharm.* 1985; 19:572–5.

1123. Mendel S, Green JA. Comment: Nitroglycerin iv tubing adsorption. *Drug Intell Clin Pharm.* 1985; 19:946–7.

1124. Tarr BD, Campbell RK. Stability and sterility of biosynthetic human insulin stored in plastic insulin syringes for 28 days. *Am J Hosp Pharm.* 1991; 48:2631–4.

1125. Rayani S, Fakhreddin J. Stability of penicillin G sodium in 5% dextrose in water minibags after freezing. *Can J Hosp Pharm.* 1985; 38:162–3.

1126. Das Gupta V, Davis DD. Stability of piperacillin sodium in dextrose 5% and sodium chloride 0.9% injections. *Am J IV Ther Clin Nutr.* (Feb) 1984; 11:14–5, 18–19.

1127. Deardorff DL, Schmidt CN. Mixing additives by squeezing plastic bags. *Am J Hosp Pharm.* 1985; 42:533–4.

1128. Synave R, Vergote A. Stability of procaine hydrochloride in a cardioplegic solution containing bicarbonate. *J Clin Hosp Pharm.* 1985; 10:385–8.

1129. Raymond G, DeGennaro M. Effect of Neut on the pH of some commercially available intravenous solutions. *Infusion.* 1985; 9:144–6.

1130. Sewell GJ, Forbes DR. Stability of sodium nitroprusside infusion during the administration by motorized syringe-pump. *J Clin Hosp Pharm.* 1985; 10:351–60.

1131. Baaske DM, Smith MD, Karnatz N et al. High-performance liquid chromatographic determination of sodium nitroprusside. *J Chromatogr.* 1981; 212:339–46.

1132. Elenbaas JK, Lander RD. Effect of inline filtration on tobramycin delivery. *Drug Intell Clin Pharm.* 1985; 19:122–5.

1133. Mehta J, Searcy CJ. Stability of terbutaline sulfate admixtures stored in polyvinyl chloride bags. *Am J Hosp Pharm.* 1986; 43:1760–2.

1134. Das Gupta V, Stewart KR. Stability of vancomycin hydrochloride in 5% dextrose and 0.9% sodium chloride injections. *Am J Hosp Pharm.* 1986; 43:1729–31.

1135. Hazlet TK, Tankersley DL. Possible incompatibilities with immune globulin for i.v. use. *Am J Hosp Pharm.* 1993; 50:654, 659–60.

1136. Richardson BL, Woodford JD, Andrews GD. Pharmacy of ceftazidime. *J Antimicrob Chemother.* 1981; 8:233–6.

1137. Cox ME, Roesner M. Production of carbon dioxide gas after reconstitution of ceftazidime. *Am J Hosp Pharm.* 1986; 43:1422.

1138. Fites AL. Production of carbon dioxide gas after reconstitution of ceftazidime. *Am J Hosp Pharm.* 1986; 43:1422–3.

1139. Marwaha RK, Johnson BF. Simple stability-indicating assay for histamine solutions. *Am J Hosp Pharm.* 1985; 42:1568–71.

1140. Marwaha RK, Johnson BF. Long-term stability study of histamine in sterile bronchoprovocation solutions. *Am J Hosp Pharm.* 1986; 43:380–3.

1141. Bigley FP, Forsyth RJ. Compatibility of imipenem–cilastatin sodium with commonly used intravenous solutions. *Am J Hosp Pharm.* 1986; 43:2803–9.

1142. De NC, Alam AS. Stability of pentamidine isethionate in 5% dextrose and 0.9% sodium chloride injections. *Am J Hosp Pharm.* 1986; 43:1486–8.

1143. Lampasona V, Mullins RE. Stability of ranitidine admixtures frozen and refrigerated in minibags. *Am J Hosp Pharm.* 1986; 43:921–5.

1144. Gralla RJ, Tyson LB, Kris MG et al. Management of chemotherapy-induced nausea and vomiting. *Med Clinics N Am.* 1987; 71:289–301.

1145. Forman JK, Souney PF. Visual compatibility of midazolam hydrochloride with common preoperative injectable medications. *Am J Hosp Pharm.* 1987; 44:2298–9.

1146. Thompson DF, Thompson GD. Visual compatibility of esmolol hydrochloride and furosemide in 5% dextrose or 0.9% sodium chloride injections. *Am J Hosp Pharm.* 1987; 44:2740.

1147. Ahmed I, Day P. Stability of cefazolin sodium in various artificial tear solutions and aqueous vehicles. *Am J Hosp Pharm.* 1987; 44:2287–90.

1148. McSherry TJ. Incompatibility between chlorpromazine and metacresol. *Am J Hosp Pharm.* 1987; 44:1574.

1149. Tebbett IR, Melrose E. Stability of promazine as an intravenous infusion. *Pharm J.* 1986; 237:172.

1150. Johnson CE, Cohen IA, Michelini TJ et al. Compatibility of premixed theophylline and methylprednisolone sodium succinate intravenous admixtures. *Am J Hosp Pharm.* 1987; 44:1620–4.

1151. Marti E, Cervera P. Compatibility of ranitidine hydrochloride with other injectable pharmaceuticals in common use. *Rev Assoc Esp Farm Hosp.* 1985; 9:169–72.

1152. Navarro JN, Aznar MT, Ruiz MD et al. Stability of 5-fluorouracil in large volume intravenous solutions. *Rev Assoc Esp Farm Hosp.* 1985; 9:69–72.

1153. Biondi L, Nairn JG. Stability of 5-fluorouracil and flucytosine in parenteral solutions. *Can J Hosp Pharm.* 1986; 39:60–3.

1154. Parr MD, Barton SD, Haver VM et al. Cyclosporine binding to components in medication administration sets. *Drug Intell Clin Pharm.* 1988; 22:173–4.

1155. Gasca M, Fanikos J. Visual compatibility of perphenazine with various antimicrobials during simulated Y-site injection. *Am J Hosp Pharm.* 1987; 44:574–5.

1156. Nolte MS, Poon V, Grodsky GM et al. Reduced solubility of short-acting soluble insulins when mixed with longer-acting insulins. *Diabetes.* 1983; 32:1177–81.

1157. Forman JK, Lachs JR. Visual compatibility of acyclovir sodium with commonly used intravenous drugs during simulated Y-site injection. *Am J Hosp Pharm.* 1987; 44:1408–9.

1158. Nelson RW, Young R. Visual incompatibility of dacarbazine and heparin. *Am J Hosp Pharm.* 1987; 44:2028.

1159. Zbrozek AS, Marble DA, Bosso JA et al. Compatibility and stability of clindamycin phosphate-aminoglycoside combinations within polypropylene syringes. *Drug Intell Clin Pharm.* 1987; 21:806–10.

1160. Perry M, Khalidi N. Stability of penicillins in total parenteral nutrient solution. *Am J Hosp Pharm.* 1987; 44:1625–8.

1161. Tu YH, Allen LV. Stability of papaverine hydrochloride and phentolamine mesylate in injectable mixtures. *Am J Hosp Pharm.* 1987; 44:2524–7.

1162. Seargeant LE, Kobrinsky NL, Sus CJ et al. In vitro stability and compatibility of daunorubicin, cytarabine, and etoposide. *Cancer Treat Rep.* 1987; 71:1189–92.

1163. Baumgartner TG, Knudsen AK, Dunn AJ et al. Norepinephrine stability in saline solutions. *Hosp Pharm.* (Jan) 1988; 23:44, 49, 59.

1164. Marble DA, Bosso JA. Compatibility of clindamycin phosphate with aztreonam in polypropylene syringes and with cefoperazone sodium, cefonicid sodium, and cefuroxime sodium in partial-fill glass bottles. *Drug Intell Clin Pharm.* 1988; 22:54–7.

1165. Welty TE, Cloyd JC. Delivery of paraldehyde in 5% dextrose and 0.9% sodium chloride injections through polyvinyl chloride i.v. sets and burettes. *Am J Hosp Pharm.* 1988; 45:131–5.

1166. Thompson DF, Stiles ML, Allen LV et al. Compatibility of verapamil hydrochloride with penicillin admixtures during simulated Y-site injection. *Am J Hosp Pharm.* 1988; 45:142–5.

1167. Pesko LJ, Arend KA, Hagman DE et al. Physical compatibility and stability of metoclopramide injection. *Parenterals.* (Dec-Jan) 1988; 5:1–3, 6–8.

1168. Karnatz NN, Wong J, Kesler H et al. Compatibility of esmolol hydrochloride with morphine sulfate and fentanyl citrate during simulated Y-site administration. *Am J Hosp Pharm.* 1988; 45:368–71.

1169. Colucci RD, Cobuzzi LE. Visual compatibility of esmolol hydrochloride and various injectable drugs during simulated Y-site injection. *Am J Hosp Pharm.* 1988; 45:630–2.

1170. Schilling CG. Compatibility of drugs with a heparin-containing neonatal total parenteral nutrient solution. *Am J Hosp Pharm.* 1988; 45:313–4.

1171. Colucci RD, Cobuzzi LE. Visual compatibility of labetalol hydrochloride injection with various injectable drugs during simulated Y-site injection. *Am J Hosp Pharm.* 1988; 45:1357–8.

1172. Johnson CE, Lloyd CW, Aviles AI et al. Compatibility of premixed theophylline and verapamil intravenous admixtures. *Am J Hosp Pharm.* 1988; 45:609–12.

1173. Askerud L, Finholt P. Intravenous infusion of theophylline in 5% dextrose solution—formulation and stability. *Medd Nor Farm Selsk.* 1981; 43:17–24.

1174. Morgan GJ, McClellan JD. Stability of a heparin urokinase mixture. *Br J Parenter Ther.* 1987; 8:89.

1175. Garren KW, Repta AJ. Incompatibility of cisplatin and Reglan injectable. *Int J Pharm.* 1985; 24:91–9.

1176. Sanburg AL, Lyndon RC. Effects of freezing, long-term storage and microwave thawing on the stability of three antibiotics reconstituted in minibags. *Aust J Hosp Pharm.* 1987; 17:31–4.

1177. Murase S, Ochiai K, Aoki M et al. Study on compatibility of dopram with other drugs. *Jap J Hosp Pharm.* 1987; 13:244–60.

1178. Borst DL, Sesin GP. Stability of selected beta-lactam antibiotics stored in plastic syringes. *NITA.* 1987; 10:368–72.

1179. Roberts DE, Cross MD, Thomas PH et al. Azlocillin-aminoglycoside combinations in CAPD fluid. *Br J Pharm Pract.* 1987; 9:98–9.

1180. Robinson DC, Cookson TL. Concentration guidelines for parenteral antibiotics in fluid-restricted patients. *Drug Intell Clin Pharm.* 1987; 21:985–9.

1181. Sterchele JA. Update on stability guidelines for routinely refrigerated drug products. *Am J Hosp Pharm.* 1987; 44:2698.

1182. Dahl JM, Roche VF. Visual compatibility of cibenzoline succinate with commonly used acute care medications. *Am J Hosp Pharm.* 1987; 44:1123–5.

1183. Cano SM, Montoro JB, Pastor C et al. Stability of ranitidine hydrochloride in total nutrient admixtures. *Am J Hosp Pharm.* 1988; 45:1100–2.

1184. Jimenez MD. Visual compatibility of nalbuphine hydrochloride and promethazine hydrochloride. *Am J Hosp Pharm.* 1988; 45:1278.

1185. Pereira-Rosario R, Utamura T. Interaction of heparin sodium and dopamine hydrochloride in admixtures studied by microcalorimetry. *Am J Hosp Pharm.* 1988; 45:1350–2.

1186. Baptista RJ, Mitrano FP. Stability and compatibility of cimetidine hydrochloride and aminophylline in dextrose 5% in water injection. *Drug Intell Clin Pharm.* 1988; 22:592–3.

1187. Holmes CJ, Kubey WY. Viability of microorganisms in fluorouracil and cisplatin small-volume injections. *Am J Hosp Pharm.* 1988; 45:1089–91.

1188. Jay GT, Fanikos J. Visual compatibility of famotidine with commonly used critical-care medications during simulated Y-site injection. *Am J Hosp Pharm.* 1988; 45:1556–7.

1189. Tucker DR, Sieradzan R. Visual compatibility of ciprofloxacin lactate with five broad-spectrum antimicrobial agents during simulated Y-site injection. *Am J Hosp Pharm.* 1988; 45:1910–1.

1190. Marquardt ED. Visual compatibility of hydroxyzine hydrochloride with various antineoplastic agents. *Am J Hosp Pharm.* 1988; 45:2127.

1191. Riley CM. Stability of milrinone and digoxin, furosemide, procainamide hydrochloride, propranolol hydrochloride, quinidine gluconate, or verapamil hydrochloride in 5% dextrose injection. *Am J Hosp Pharm.* 1988; 45:2079–91.

1192. Awang DV, Graham KC. Microwave thawing of frozen drug solutions. *Am J Hosp Pharm.* 1987; 44:2256.

1193. Bashaw ED, Amantea MA, Minor JR et al. Visual compatibility of zidovudine with other injectable drugs during simulated Y-site administration. *Am J Hosp Pharm.* 1988; 45:2532–3.

1194. Souney PF, Fanikos J. Compatibility of cyclophosphamide solution with antibiotics during simulated Y-site injection. *Parenterals.* (Aug-Sep) 1988; 6:1, 2, 8.

1195. Beijnen JH, Vendrig DEMM. Stability of Vinca alkaloid anticancer drugs in three commonly used infusion fluids. *J Parenter Sci Technol.* 1989; 43:84–7.

1196. Fong PA, Ward J. Visual compatibility of intravenous famotidine with selected drugs. *Am J Hosp Pharm.* 1989; 46:125–6.

1197. Karnatz NN, Wong J, Baaske DM et al. Stability of esmolol hydrochloride and sodium nitroprusside in intravenous admixtures. *Am J Hosp Pharm.* 1989; 46:101–4.

1198. Johnson CE, Lloyd CW, Mesaros JL et al. Compatibility of aminophylline and verapamil in intravenous admixtures. *Am J Hosp Pharm.* 1989; 46:97–100.

1199. Parti R, Wolf W. Caveats with respect to storage of cisplatin and fluorouracil admixtures. *Am J Hosp Pharm.* 1989; 46:259.

1200. Johnson EG, Janosik JE. Manufacturer's recommendations for handling spilled antineoplastic agents. *Am J Hosp Pharm.* 1989; 46:318–9.

1201. Jarosinski PF, Kennedy PF. Stability of concentrated trimethoprim-sulfamethoxazole admixtures. *Am J Hosp Pharm.* 1989; 46:732–7.

1202. Bosanquet AG. Stability of solutions of antineoplastic agents during preparation and storage for in vitro assays III. Antimetabolites, tubulin-binding agents, platinum drugs, amsacrine, L-asparaginase, interferons, steroids and other miscellaneous antitumor agents. *Cancer Chemother Pharmacol.* 1989; 23:197–207.

1203. Beijnen JH, Underberg WJM. Degradation of mitomycin C in acidic solution. *Int J Pharm.* 1985; 24:219–29.

1204. Beijnen JH, den Hartigh J. Quantitative aspects of the degradation of mitomycin C in alkaline solution. *J Pharm Biomed Anal.* 1985; 3:59–69.

1205. Beijnen JH, Rosing H. Stability of mitomycins in infusion fluids. *Arch Pharm Chemi Sci Ed.* 1985; 13:58–66.

1206. Janssen MJH, Crommelin DJA, Storm G et al. Doxorubicin decomposition on storage. Effect of pH, type of buffer and liposome encapsulation. *Int J Pharm.* 1985; 23:1–11.

1207. Beijnen JH, van der Houwen OAGJ, Voskuilen MCH, et al. Aspects of the degradation kinetics of daunorubicin in aqueous solution. In: Beijnen JH, ed. Chemical stability of mitomycin and anthracycline antineoplastic drugs. Utrecht, The Netherlands: Drukkerij Elkinkwijk BV; 1986:245–60.

1208. Beijnen JH, van der Houwen OAGJ. Aspects of the degradation kinetics of doxorubicin in aqueous solution. *Int J Pharm.* 1986; 32:123–31.

1209. Fritz BL, Lockhart HE. Chemical stability of selected pharmaceuticals repackaged in glass and plastic. *Pharm Tech.* (Nov) 1988; 12:44, 46, 48, 50–2.

1210. Venkataraman PS, Brissie EO. Stability of calcium and phosphorus in neonatal parenteral nutrition solutions. *J Pediatr Gastroenterol Nutr.* 1983; 2:640–3.

1211. Fitzgerald KA, MacKay MW. Calcium and phosphate solubility in neonatal parenteral nutrient solutions containing Aminosyn PF. *Am J Hosp Pharm.* 1987; 44:1396–1400.

1212. Mikrut BA. Calcium and phosphate solubility in neonatal parenteral nutrient solutions containing Aminosyn PF or TrophAmine. *Am J Hosp Pharm.* 1987; 44:2702–4.

1213. Lenz GT, Mikrut BA. Calcium and phosphate solubility in neonatal parenteral nutrient solutions containing Aminosyn-PF or TrophAmine. *Am J Hosp Pharm.* 1988; 45:2367–71.

1214. Raupp P, von Kries R, Schmidt E et al. Incompatibility between fat emulsion and calcium plus heparin in parenteral nutrition of premature babies. *Lancet.* 1988; 1:700.

1215. Waller DJ, Smith SR. Use of infusion devices with total nutrient admixtures. *Am J Hosp Pharm.* 1987; 44:1570.

1216. Gilbert M, Gallagher SC, Eads M et al. Microbial growth patterns in a total parenteral nutrition formulation containing lipid emulsion. *JPEN J Parenter Enteral Nutr.* 1986; 10:494–7.

1217. Barat AC, Harrie K, Jacob M et al. Effect of amino acid solutions on total nutrient admixture stability. *JPEN J Parenter Enteral Nutr.* 1987; 11:384–8.

1218. Cripps AL. Stability studies on total parenteral nutrition mixtures containing fat emulsions. *Br J Pharm Pract.* 1984; 6:187–95.

1219. Davis SS, Galloway M. Studies on fat emulsions in combined nutrition solutions. *J Clin Hosp Pharm.* 1986; 11:33–45.

1220. Ang SD, Canham JE, Daly JM. Parenteral infusion with an admixture of amino acids, dextrose, and fat emulsion solution: compatibility and clinical safety. *JPEN J Parenter Enteral Nutr.* 1987; 11:23–7.

1221. du Plessis J, Van Wyk CJ. The stability of parenteral fat emulsions in nutrition admixtures. *J Clin Pharm Ther.* 1987; 12:307–18.

1222. Sayeed FA, Tripp MG, Sukumaran KB et al. Stability of total nutrient admixtures using various intravenous fat emulsions. *Am J Hosp Pharm.* 1987; 44:2271–80.

1223. Sayeed FA, Tripp MG, Sukumaran KB et al. Stability of various total nutrient admixture formulations using Liposyn II and Aminosyn II. *Am J Hosp Pharm.* 1987; 44:2280–6.

1224. McGee CD, Mascarenhas MG, Ostro MJ et al. Selenium and vitamin E stability in parenteral solutions. *JPEN J Parenter Enteral Nutr.* 1985; 9:568–70.

1225. Dahl GB, Jeppsson RI. Vitamin stability in a TPN mixture stored in an EVA plastic bag. *J Clin Hosp Pharm.* 1986; 11:271–9.

1226. Shenkin A, Fraser WD, McLelland AJ et al. Maintenance of vitamin and trace element status in intravenous nutrition using a complete nutritive mixture. *JPEN J Parenter Enteral Nutr.* 1987; 11:238–42.

1227. Yamaoka K, Nakajima Y, Okinaga S et al. Variation by combination of hyperalimentation with fat emulsion. *Jap J Hosp Pharm.* 1987; 13:211–5.

1228. Sewell DL, Golper TA, Brown SD et al. Stability of single and combination antimicrobial agents in various peritoneal dialysates in the presence of insulin and heparin. *Am J Kidney Dis.* 1983; 3:209–12.

1229. Nance KS, Matzke GR. Stability of gentamicin and tobramycin in concentrate solutions for automated peritoneal dialysis. *Am J Nephrol.* 1984; 4:240–3.

1230. Das Gupta V, Parasrampuria J. Quantitation of acetazolamide in pharmaceutical dosage forms using high-performance liquid chromatography. *Drug Dev Ind Pharm.* 1987; 13:147–57.

1231. Boak LR. Aminophylline stability. *Can J Hosp Pharm.* 1987; 40:155.

1232. Moore BR, Tindula R. Incompatibility between amphotericin B and evacuated i.v. containers. *Am J Hosp Pharm.* 1987; 44:1312.

1233. Bretschneider H. Osmolalities of commercially supplied drugs often used in anesthesia. *Anaesth Analg.* 1987; 66:361–2.

1234. Odgers C. Drug/nutrient interactions and incompatibilities complicating TPN. *N.Z. Pharm.* 1986; 6:64–8.

1235. Kedzierewicz F, Finance C, Nicolas A et al. Etude comparative de la stabilite de solutions de carbenicilline en fonction de la temperature. Interet du cycle congelation-decongelation au four a micro-ondes. *Pharm Acta Helv.* 1987; 62:109–15.

1236. Arbus MH. Room temperature stability guidelines for carmustine. *Am J Hosp Pharm.* 1988; 45:531.

1237. Frederiksson K, Lundgren P. Stability of carmustine—kinetics and compatibility during administration. *Acta Pharm Suec.* 1986; 23:115–24.

1238. Sewell GJ, Riley CM. The stability of carboplatin in ambulatory continuous infusion regimes. *J Clin Pharm Ther.* 1987; 12:427–32.

1239. Ross MB. Additional stability guidelines for routinely refrigerated drug products. *Am J Hosp Pharm.* 1988; 45:1498–9.

1240. Goodell JA, Harry DJ, Low JR. More on production of a carbon dioxide gas after reconstitution of ceftazidime. *Am J Hosp Pharm.* 1987; 44:510.

1241. Savello DR. More on production of carbon dioxide gas after reconstitution of ceftazidime. *Am J Hosp Pharm.* 1987; 44:512.

1242. Rovers JP, Menielly G, Souney PF et al. The use of stability-indicating assays to determine the in vitro compatibility and stability of metronidazole/gentamicin admixtures. *Can J Hosp Pharm.* 1989; 42:143–6.

1243. Walker SE, Dranitsaris G. Stability of reconstituted ceftriaxone in dextrose and saline solutions. *Can J Hosp Pharm.* 1987; 40:161–6.

1244. Martinez-Pancheco R, Vila-Jato JL. Effect of different factors on stability of ceftriaxone in solution. *Farmaco Ed Prat.* 1987; 42:131–7.

1245. Kedzierewicz F, Finance C, Nicolas A et al. Stability of parenteral ceftriaxone disodium solutions in frozen and liquid states: effect of freezing and microwave thawing. *J Pharm Sci.* 1989; 78:73–7.

1246. Kristjansson F, Sternson LA. An investigation on possible oligomer formation in pharmaceutical formulations of cisplatin. *Int J Pharm.* 1988; 41:67–74.

1247. Anon. High-dose Maxolon mixes with cisplatin. *Pharm J.* 1985; 234:593.

1248. Kirk B. The evaluation of a light-protective giving set. The photosensitivity of intravenous dacarbazine solutions. *Br J Parenter Ther.* (May-June) 1987; 8:78, 81–2, 85–6.

1249. Bosanquet AG. Stability of solutions of antineoplastic agents during preparation and storage for in vitro assays. General considerations, the nitrosoureas and alkylating agents. *Cancer Chemother Pharmacol.* 1985; 14:83–95.

1250. Beijnen JH, Potman RP, van Ooijen RD et al. Structure elucidation and characterization of daunorubicin degradation products. *Int J Pharm.* 1987; 34:247–57.

1251. Haronikova K, Pikulikova Z, Kral L et al. Sorption of diazepam on the surface of the plastic infusion unit, part 2. *Farm Obz.* 1986; 55:485–94.

1252. Mathot F, Bonnard J, Paris P et al. Influence des materiaux de perfusion sur les solutions de diazepam. *J Pharm Belg.* 1982; 37:153–6.

1253. Murphy A, Maltby S. Dissolution time, on reconstitution, of a new parenteral formulation of doxorubicin (Doxorubicin Rapid Dissolution). *Int J Pharm.* 1987; 38:257–9.

1254. Baumann TJ, Smythe MA, Kaufmann K et al. Dissolution times of Adriamycin and Adriamycin RDF. *Am J Hosp Pharm.* 1988; 45:1667.

1255. Vogelzang NJ, Ruane M. Phase I trial of an implanted battery-powered, programmable drug delivery system for continuous doxorubicin administration. *J Clin Oncol.* 1985; 3:407–14.

1256. Keusters L, Stolk LML, Umans R et al. Stability of solutions of doxorubicin and epirubicin in plastic minibags for intravesical use after storage at -20 °C and thawing by microwave radiation. *Pharm Weekbl [Sci].* 1986; 8:194–7.

1257. Williamson M, Luce JK. Microwave thawing of doxorubicin hydrochloride admixtures not recommended. *Am J Hosp Pharm.* 1987; 44:505.

1258. Adams S, Fernandez F. Intravenous use of haloperidol. *Hosp Pharm.* 1987; 22:306–7.

1259. Thoma K, Struve M. Untersuchungen zur photo- und thermostabilitat von adrenalin-losungen. *Pharm Acta Helv.* 1986; 61:2–9.

1260. David LM. Phlebitis with intravenous erythromycin. *Am J Hosp Pharm.* 1987; 44:732.

1261. Schwinghammer TL, Reilly M. Cracking of ABS plastic devices used to infuse undiluted etoposide injection. *Am J Hosp Pharm.* 1988; 45:1277.

1262. Beijnen JH, Holthuis JJM, Kerkdijk HG et al. Degradation kinetics of etoposide in aqueous solution. *Int J Pharm.* 1988; 41:169–78.

1263. Brown DH, Simkover RA. Maximum hang times for i.v. fat emulsions. *Am J Hosp Pharm.* 1987; 44:282.

1264. Allwood MC. The release of phthalate ester plasticizer from intravenous administration sets into fat emulsion. *Int J Pharm.* 1986; 29:233–6.

1265. Nahata MC, Hipple TF. Stability of gentamicin diluted in 0.9% sodium chloride injection in glass syringes. *Hosp Pharm.* 1987; 22:1131–2.

1266. Dunn DL, Lenihan SF. The case for the saline flush. *Am J Nurs.* 1987; 87:7989.

1267. Shearer J. Normal saline flush versus dilute heparin flush. A study of peripheral intermittent I.V. devices. *NITA.* 1987; 10:425–7.

1268. Hamilton RA, Plis JM, Clay C et al. Heparin sodium versus 0.9% sodium chloride injection for maintaining patency of indwelling intermittent infusion devices. *Clin Pharm.* 1988; 7:439–43.

1269. Lombardi TP, Gundersen B, Zammett LO et al. Efficacy of 0.9% sodium chloride injection with or without heparin sodium for maintaining patency of intravenous catheters in children. *Clin Pharm.* 1988; 7:832–6.

1270. Cyganski JM, Donahue JM. The case for the heparin flush. *Am J Nurs.* 1987; 87:796–7.

1271. Bullock LS, Fitzgerald JF, Glick MR. Stability of famotidine in minibags refrigerated and/or frozen. *DICP.* 1989; 23:132–5.

1272. Swanson DJ, DeAngelis C, Smith IL et al. Degradation kinetics of imipenem in normal saline and human serum. *Antimicrob Agents Chemother.* 1986; 29:936–7.

1273. Smith GB, Schoenewaldt EF. Stability of N-formimidoylthienamycin in aqueous solution. *J Pharm Sci.* 1981; 70:272–6.

1274. McElnay JC, Elliott DS. Binding of human insulin to burette administration sets. *Int J Pharm.* 1987; 36:199–203.

1275. Adams PS, Haines-Nutt RF. Stability of insulin mixtures in disposable plastic insulin syringes. *J Pharm Pharmacol.* 1987; 39:158–63.

1276. Mozzi G, Conegliani B, Lomi R et al. Stabilita del calcio folinato in soluzioni acquose in funzione del pH e delta temperatura. *Boll Chim Farm.* 1986; 125:424–8.

1277. Powell MF. Stability of lidocaine in aqueous solution: effect of temperature, pH, buffer, and metal ions on amide hydrolysis. *Pharm Res.* 1987; 4:42–5.

1278. Das Gupta V, Stewart KR. Chemical stabilities of lignocaine hydrochloride and phenylephrine hydrochloride in aqueous solution. *J Clin Hosp Pharm.* 1986; 11:449–52.

1279. Kirk B. Stability of reconstituted mustine injection BP during storage. *Br J Parenter Ther.* (July-Aug) 1986; 7:86–7, 90–2.

1280. Wright MP, Newton JM. Stability of methotrexate injection in prefilled, plastic disposable syringes. *Int J Pharm.* 1988; 45:237–44.

1281. Dyvik O, Grislingaas AL, Tonnesen HH et al. Methotrexate in infusion solutions—a stability test for the hospital pharmacy. *J Clin Hosp Pharm.* 1986; 11:343–8.

1282. Cabeza Barrera J, Bautista Paloma J, Garcia de Pesquera F et al. Disminucion de la adsorcion de insulina a los envases de nutricion parenteral. *Rev Assoc Esp Farm Hosp.* 1988; 12:251–4.

1283. Beijnen JH, Fokkens RH, Rosing H et al. Degradation of mitomycin C in acid phosphate and acetate buffer solutions. *Int J Pharm.* 1986; 32:111–21.

1284. Beijnen JH, Lingeman H, Van Munster HA et al. Mitomycin antitumor agents: a review of their physico-chemical and analytical properties and stability. *J Pharm Biomed Anal.* 1986; 4:275–95.

1285. Stolk LML, Fruijtier A. Stability after freezing and thawing of solutions of mitomycin C in plastic minibags for intravesical use. *Pharm Weekbl [Sci].* 1986; 8:286–8.

1286. Depiero D, Rekhi GS, Souney PF et al. Stability of morphine sulfate solutions frozen in polyvinyl chloride intravenous bags. *Pharm Pract News.* (Oct) 1987; 14:1, 39–40.

1287. Hung CT, Young M. Stability of morphine solutions in plastic syringes determined by reversed-phase ion-pair liquid chromatography. *J Pharm Sci.* 1988; 77:719–23.

1288. Visor GC, Lin LH, Jackson SE et al. Stability of ganciclovir sodium (DHPG sodium) in 5% dextrose or 0.9% sodium chloride injections. *Am J Hosp Pharm.* 1986; 43:2810–2.

1289. Behme RJ, Brooke D, Kensler TT et al. Incompatibility of ifosfamide with benzyl-alcohol-preserved bacteriostatic water for injection. *Am J Hosp Pharm.* 1988; 45:627–8.

1290. Rowland CG, Bradford E, Adams P et al. Infusion of ifosfamide plus mesna. *Lancet.* 1984; 2:468.

1291. Bristol-Myers Oncology Division. Product information on Mesnex (Mesna). Evansville, IN; 1989 Jun.

1292. Dorr RT. Mesnex dosing and administration guide. Evansville, IN: Bristol-Myers Company; 1989.

1293. Lederle Laboratories, American Cyanamid Company. Product information on Novantrone. Pearl River, NY; 1988.

1294. Nahata MC, Hipple TF. Stability of phenobarbital sodium diluted in 0.9% sodium chloride injection. *Am J Hosp Pharm.* 1986; 43:384–5.

1295. Dela Cruz FG, Kanter MZ, Fischer JH et al. Efficacy of individualized phenytoin sodium loading doses administered by intravenous infusion. *Clin Pharm.* 1988; 7:219–24.

1296. Davidson SW, Lyall D. Sodium nitroprusside stability in light-protective administration sets. *Pharm J.* 1987; 239:599–601.

1297. Saunders A. Stability and light sensitivity of sodium nitroprusside infusions. *Aust J Hosp Pharm.* 1986; 16:55–6.

1298. Glascock JC, DiPiro JT, Cadwallader DE et al. Stability of terbutaline sulfate repackaged in disposable plastic syringes. *Am J Hosp Pharm.* 1987; 44:2291–3.

1299. Raymond GG. Stability of terbutaline sulfate injection stored in plastic tuberculin syringes. *Drug Intell Clin Pharm.* 1988; 22:303–5.

1300. Das Gupta V, Gardner SN, Jalowsky CM et al. Chemical stability of thiopental sodium injection in disposable plastic syringes. *J Clin Pharm Ther.* 1987; 12:339–42.

1301. Nahata MC, Miller MA. Stability of vancomycin hydrochloride in various concentrations of dextrose injection. *Am J Hosp Pharm.* 1987; 44:802–4.

1302. Greenberg RN, Saeed AMK, Kennedy DJ et al. Instability of vancomycin in Infusaid drug pump model 100. *Antimicrob Agents Chemother.* 1987; 31:610–1.

1303. Tucker R, Gentile JF. Precipitation of verapamil in an intravenous line. *Ann Intern Med.* 1984; 101:880.

1304. Patel SD, Yalkowsky SH. Development of an intravenous formulation for the antiviral drug 9-(beta-D-arabinofuranosyl)-adenine. *J Parenter Sci Technol.* 1987; 41:15–20.

1305. Stolk LML, Huisman W, Nordemann HD et al. Formulation of a stable vidarabine infusion fluid. *Pharm Weekbl [Sci].* 1983; 5:57–60.

1306. Black J, Buechter DD. Stability of vinblastine sulfate when exposed to light. *Drug Intell Clin Pharm.* 1988; 22:634–6.

1307. Vendrig DEMM, Smeets BPGH, Beijnen JH et al. Degradation kinetics of vinblastine sulphate in aqueous solutions. *Int J Pharm.* 1988; 43:131–8.

1308. Cartwight-Shamoon JM, McElnay JC. Examination of sorption and photodegradation of amsacrine during storage in intravenous burette administration sets. *Int J Pharm.* 1988; 42:41–6.

1309. Milano G, Etienne MC, Cassuto-Viguier E et al. Long-term stability of 5-fluorouracil and folinic acid admixtures. *Eur J Cancer.* 1992; 29A:129–32.

1310. Kraynak MA. Pharmaceutical aspects of docetaxel. *Am J Health-Syst Pharm.* 1997; 54:S7–S10.

1311. Leigh PH, Buddle GC. Pentamidine infusion stability. *Br J Pharm Pract.* 1988; 10:22–3.

1312. Roos PJ, Glerum JH, Meilink JW. Stability of morphine hydrochloride in a portable pump reservoir. *Pharm Weekbl Sci.* 1992; 14:23–6.

1313. Wohlford JG, Fowler MD. Visual compatibility of hetastarch with injectable critical-care drugs. *Am J Hosp Pharm.* 1989; 46:995–6.

1314. Wohlford JG. Clarification of visual compatibility of hetastarch and ranitidine hydrochloride. *Am J Hosp Pharm.* 1989; 46:1772.

1315. Wohlford JG, Wright JC. More information on the visual compatibility of hetastarch with injectable critical-care drugs. *Am J Hosp Pharm.* 1990; 47:297–8.

1316. Dasta JF, Hale KN, Stauffer GL et al. Comparison of visual and turbidimetric methods for determining short-term compatibility of intravenous critical-care drugs. *Am J Hosp Pharm.* 1988; 45:2361–6.

1317. Smith JA, Morris A, Duafala ME et al. Stability of floxuridine and leucovorin calcium admixtures for intraperitoneal administration. *Am J Hosp Pharm.* 1989; 46:985–9.

1318. Perrin JH, Pereira-Rosario R. The interaction of dobutamine hydrochloride and heparin sodium in parenteral fluids. *Drug Dev Indust Pharm.* 1988; 14:1617–22.

1319. Lesko AB, Sesin GP. Ceftizoxime stability in iv solutions. *DICP, Ann Pharmacother.* 617–618 (July-Aug) 1989; 23:615.

1320. Mitrano FP, Baptista RJ. Stability of cimetidine HCl and copper sulfate in a TPN solution. *DICP, Ann Pharmacother.* 1989; 23:429–30.

1321. Schilling CG, Watson DM, McCoy HG et al. Stability and delivery of vancomycin hydrochloride when admixed in a total parenteral nutrition solution. *JPEN J Parenter Enteral Nutr.* 1989; 13:63–4.

1322. Strong DK, Ho W. Visual compatibility of vancomycin and heparin in peritoneal dialysis solutions. *Am J Hosp Pharm.* 1989; 46:1832–3.

1323. Chilvers MR, Lysne JM. Visual compatibility of ranitidine hydrochloride with commonly used critical-care medications. *Am J Hosp Pharm.* 1989; 46:2057–8.

1324. Bullock L, Clark JH, Fitzgerald JF et al. The stability of amikacin, gentamicin, and tobramycin in total nutrient admixtures. *JPEN J Parenter Enteral Nutr*. 1989; 13:505–9.

1325. Nahata MC. Stability of vancomycin hydrochloride in total parenteral nutrient solutions. *Am J Hosp Pharm*. 1989; 46:2055–7.

1326. Fox AS, Boyer KM. Antibiotic stability in a pediatric parenteral alimentation solution. *J Pediatr*. 1988; 112:813–7.

1327. Raymond GG, Reed MT, Teagarden JR et al. Stability of procainamide hydrochloride in neutralized 5% dextrose injection. *Am J Hosp Pharm*. 1988; 45:2513–7.

1328. Zbrozek AS, Marble DA. Compatibility and stability of cefazolin sodium, clindamycin phosphate, and gentamicin sulfate in two intravenous solutions. *Drug Intell Clin Pharm*. 1988; 22:873–5.

1329. Stewart CF, Hampton EM. Stability of cisplatin and etoposide in intravenous admixtures. *Am J Hosp Pharm*. 1989; 46:1400–4.

1330. Shea BF, Ptachcinski RJ, O'Neill S et al. Stability of cyclosporine in 5% dextrose injection. *Am J Hosp Pharm*. 1989; 46:2053–5.

1331. Bullock L, Fitzgerald JF, Glick MR et al. Stability of famotidine 20 and 40 mg/L and amino acids in total parenteral nutrient solutions. *Am J Hosp Pharm*. 1989; 46:2321–5.

1332. Bullock L, Fitzgerald JF. Stability of famotidine 20 and 50 mg/L in total nutrient admixtures. *Am J Hosp Pharm*. 1989; 46:2326–9.

1333. Montoro JB, Pou L, Salvador P et al. Stability of famotidine 20 and 40 mg/L in total nutrient admixtures. *Am J Hosp Pharm*. 1989; 46:2329–32.

1334. DiStefano JE, Mitrano FP, Baptista RJ et al. Long-term stability of famotidine 20 mg/L in a total parenteral nutrient solution. *Am J Hosp Pharm*. 1989; 46:2333–5.

1335. Lor E, Takagi J. Visual compatibility of foscarnet with other injectable drugs. *Am J Hosp Pharm*. 1990; 47:157–9.

1336. Scott SM. Incompatibility of cefoperazone and promethazine. *Am J Hosp Pharm*. 1990; 47:519.

1337. Savitsky ME. Visual compatibility of neuromuscular blocking agents with various injectable drugs during simulated Y-site injection. *Am J Hosp Pharm*. 1990; 47:820–1.

1338. Smythe MA, Patel MA. Visual compatibility of narcotic analgesics with selected intravenous admixtures. *Am J Hosp Pharm*. 1990; 47:819–20.

1339. Stewart CF, Fleming RA. Compatibility of cisplatin and fluorouracil in 0.9% sodium chloride injection. *Am J Hosp Pharm*. 1990; 47:1373–7.

1340. Lee CY, Mauro VF. Visual and spectrophotometric determination of compatibility of alteplase and streptokinase with other injectable drugs. *Am J Hosp Pharm*. 1990; 47:606–8.

1341. Gupta VD, Bethea C. Chemical stabilities of cefoperazone sodium and ceftazidime in 5% dextrose and 0.9% sodium chloride injections. *J Clin Pharm Ther*. 1988; 13:199–205.

1342. Gupta VD, Parasrampuria J. Chemical stabilities of famotidine and ranitidine hydrochloride in intravenous admixtures. *J Clin Pharm Ther*. 1988; 13:329–34.

1343. Gupta VD, Pramar Y. Stability of acyclovir sodium in dextrose and sodium chloride injections. *J Clin Pharm Ther*. 1989; 14:451–6.

1344. Underberg WJM, Koomen JM. Stability of famotidine in commonly used nutritional infusion fluids. *J Parenter Sci Technol*. 1988; 42:94–7.

1345. Messerschmidt W. Pharmazeutische kompatibilitat von ceftazidim und metronidazol. *Pharm Ztg*. 1990; 135:36–8.

1346. Messerschmidt W. Kompatibilitat von ciprofloxacin und metronidazol in mischinfusionen. *Pharm Ztg*. 1988; 133:26.

1347. Murdoch JM, Garner ST. Calcium gluconate compatibility. *Pharm J*. 1989; 242:634.

1348. Stoberski P, Zakrzewski Z. Bandanie stabilnosci furosemidu i soli sodowej hemibursztynianu hydrokortyzonu metoda RP-HPLC w wybranych plynach infuzyjnych. *Farm Pol*. 1988; 44:398–401.

1349. Veechio M, Walker SE, Iazzetta J et al. The stability of morphine intravenous infusion solutions. *Can J Hosp Pharm*. 1988; 41:5–9.

1350. Walker SE, Kirby K. Stability of ranitidine hydrochloride admixtures refrigerated in polyvinyl chloride minibags. *Can J Hosp Pharm*. 1988; 41:105–8.

1351. Gupta VD, Parasrampuria J, Bethea C et al. Stability of clindamycin phosphate in dextrose and saline solutions. *Can J Hosp Pharm*. 1989; 42:109–12.

1352. Walker SE, Iazzetta J, Lau DWC et al. Famotidine stability in total parenteral nutrient solutions. *Can J Hosp Pharm*. 1989; 42:97–103.

1353. Walker SE, Dranitsaris G. Ceftazidime stability in normal saline and dextrose 5% in water. *Can J Hosp Pharm*. 1988; 41:65–71.

1354. Walker SE, Birkhans B. Stability of intravenous vancomycin. *Can J Hosp Pharm*. 1988; 41:233–8.

1355. Halpern NA, Colucci RD, Alicea M et al. Visual compatibility of enalaprilat with commonly used critical care medications during simulated Y-site injection. *Int J Clin Pharmacol Ther Toxicol*. 1989; 27:294–7.

1356. Allen LV Jr, Stiles ML. Stability of fentanyl citrate in 0.9% sodium chloride solution in portable infusion pumps. *Am J Hosp Pharm*. 1990; 47:1572–4.

1357. Kowalski SR, Gourlay GK. Stability of fentanyl citrate in glass and plastic containers and in a patient-controlled delivery system. *Am J Hosp Pharm*. 1990; 47:1584–7.

1358. Schaaf LJ, Robinson DH, Vogel GJ et al. Stability of esmolol hydrochloride in the presence of aminophylline, bretylium tosylate, heparin sodium, and procainamide hydrochloride. *Am J Hosp Pharm*. 1990; 47:1567–71.

1359. Rosenberg LS, Hostetler CK, Wagenknecht DM et al. An accurate prediction of the pH change due to degradation: correction for a "produced" secondary buffering system. *Pharm Res*. 1988; 5:514–7.

1360. Williams MF, Hak LJ. In vitro evaluation of the stability of ranitidine hydrochloride in total parenteral nutrient mixtures. *Am J Hosp Pharm*. 1990; 47:1574–9.

1361. Galante LJ, Stewart JT, Warren FW et al. Stability of ranitidine hydrochloride with eight medications in intravenous admixtures. *Am J Hosp Pharm*. 1990; 47:1606–10.

1362. Galante LJ, Stewart JT, Warren FW et al. Stability of ranitidine hydrochloride at dilute concentration in intravenous infusion fluids at room temperature. *Am J Hosp Pharm*. 1990; 47:1580–4.

1363. Marquardt ED. Visual compatibility of tolazoline hydrochloride with various medications during simulated Y-site injection. *Am J Hosp Pharm.* 1990; 47:1802–3.

1364. Chandler SW, Folstad J. Aztreonam-vancomycin incompatibility. *Am J Hosp Pharm.* 1990; 47:1970.

1365. Trissel LA, Tramonte SM. Visual compatibility of ondansetron hydrochloride with other selected drugs during simulated Y-site injection. *Am J Hosp Pharm.* 1991; 48:988–92.

1366. Leak RE, Woodford JD. Pharmaceutical development of ondansetron injection. *Eur J Cancer Clin Oncol.* 1989; 25(Suppl 1):S67–S69.

1367. Mackinnon JW, Collin DT. The chemistry of ondansetron. *Eur J Cancer Clin Oncol.* 1989; 25(Suppl 1):S61.

1368. Adria Laboratories. Idamycin—hospital formulary product information form. Columbus, OH; 1990 Oct 19.

1369. Allwood M, Stanley A, Wright P. The cytotoxics handbook. 4th ed. Oxford, England: Radcliffe Medical Press; 2002.

1370. Genentech, Inc. Avastin® (bevacizumab) injection prescribing information. South San Francisco, CA; 2019 Jun.

1371. Sandoz Laboratories. Sandostatin—compatibility between octreotide in the infusion and the giving set/container. Basle, Switzerland; 1986 Apr 3.

1372. Bakri SJ, Snyder MR, Pulido JS et al. Six-month stability of bevacizumab (Avastin) binding to vascular endothelial growth factor after withdrawal into a syringe and refrigeration or freezing. *Retina.* 2006 May-Jun; 26:519–22.

1373. Marchiarullo M. Stability of octreotide in various infusion supplies. East Hanover, NJ: Sandoz Pharmaceuticals Corporation; 1990 Mar 20.

1374. Beijnen JH, Beijnen-Bandhoe AU, Dubbelman AC et al. Chemical and physical stability of etoposide and teniposide in commonly used infusion fluids. *J Parenter Sci Technol.* 1991; 45:108–12.

1375. Santiero ML, Sagraves R. Osmolality of small-volume i.v. admixtures for pediatric patients. *Am J Hosp Pharm.* 1990; 47:1359–64.

1376. Messerschmidt W. Kompatibilitat von cefuroxim mit metronidazole. *Krankenhauspharmazie.* 1987; 8:45–7.

1377. Rosen GH. Potential incompatibility of insulin and octreotide in total parenteral nutrient solutions. *Am J Hosp Pharm.* 1989; 46:1128.

1378. McElnay JC, Elliott DS, Cartwright-Shamoon J et al. Stability of methotrexate and vinblastine in burette administration sets. *Int J Pharm.* 1988; 47:239–47.

1379. Williams DA. Stability and compatibility of admixtures of antineoplastic drugs. In: Lokich JJ, ed. Cancer chemotherapy by infusion. 2nd ed. Chicago, IL: Precept Press; 1990:52–73.

1380. Baaske DM, DeMay JF, Latona CA et al. Stability of nicardipine hydrochloride in intravenous solutions. *Am J Health-Syst Pharm.* 1996; 53:1701–5.

1381. Trissel LA, Chandler SW. Visual compatibility of amsacrine with selected drugs during simulated Y-site injection. *Am J Hosp Pharm.* 1990; 47:2525–8.

1382. Townsend RS. In vitro inactivation of gentamicin by ampicillin. *Am J Hosp Pharm.* 1989; 46:2250–1.

1383. Vaughn LM, Small C. Incompatibility of iron dextran and a total nutrient admixture. *Am J Hosp Pharm.* 1990; 47:1745–6.

1384. Cutie MR. Verapamil precipitation. *Ann Intern Med.* 1983; 98:672.

1385. Garner SS, Wiest DB. Compatibility of drugs separated by a fluid barrier in a retrograde intravenous infusion system. *Am J Hosp Pharm.* 1990; 47:604–6.

1386. Lokich J, Anderson N, Bern M et al. Combined floxuridine and cisplatin in a 14–day infusion. *Cancer.* 1988; 62:2309–12.

1387. Anderson N, Lokich J, Bern M et al. A phase I clinical trial of combined fluoropyrimidines with leucovorin in a 14–day infusion. *Cancer.* 1989; 63:233–7.

1388. Lokich J, Anderson N, Bern M et al. Etoposide admixed with cisplatin. *Cancer.* 1989; 63:818–21.

1389. Lokich J, Bern M, Anderson N et al. Cyclophosphamide, methotrexate, and 5-fluorouracil in a three-drug admixture. *Cancer.* 1989; 63:822–4.

1390. Anderson N, Lokich J, Bern M et al. Combined 5-fluorouracil and floxuridine administered as a 14–day infusion. *Cancer.* 1989; 63:825–7.

1391. Stiles ML, Tu YH. Stability of cefazolin sodium, cefoxitin sodium, ceftazidime, and penicillin G sodium in portable pump reservoirs. *Am J Hosp Pharm.* 1989; 46:1408–12.

1392. Martens HJ, De Goede PN. Sorption of various drugs in polyvinyl chloride, glass, and polyethylene-lined infusion containers. *Am J Hosp Pharm.* 1990; 47:369–73.

1393. Baltz JK, Kennedy P, Minor JR et al. Visual compatibility of foscarnet with other injectable drugs during simulated Y-site administration. *Am J Hosp Pharm.* 1990; 47:2075–7.

1394. Walker SE, Coons C, Matte D et al. Hydromorphone and morphine stability in portable infusion pump casettes and minibags. *Can J Hosp Pharm.* 1988; 41:177–82.

1395. Smythe M, Malouf E. Visual compatibility of insulin with secondary intravenous drugs in admixtures. *Am J Hosp Pharm.* 1991; 48:125–6.

1396. Tu YH, Stiles ML. Stability of fentanyl citrate and bupivacaine hydrochloride in portable pump reservoirs. *Am J Hosp Pharm.* 1990; 47:2037–40.

1397. Pugh CB, Pabis DJ. Visual compatibility of morphine sulfate and meperidine hydrochloride with other injectable drugs during simulated Y-site injection. *Am J Hosp Pharm.* 1991; 48:123–5.

1398. Pritts D, Hancock D. Incompatibility of ceftriaxone with vancomycin. *Am J Hosp Pharm.* 1991; 48:77.

1399. DeMuynck C, De Vroe C, Remon JP et al. Binding of drugs to end-line filters: a study of four commonly administered drugs in intensive care units. *J Clin Pharm Ther.* 1988; 13:335–40.

1400. Aki H, Sawai N, Yamamoto K et al. Structural confirmation of ampicillin polymers formed in aqueous solution. *Pharm Res.* 1991; 8:119–22.

1401. Bonhomme L, Postaire E, Touratier S et al. Chemical stability of lignocaine (lidocaine) and adrenaline (epinephrine) in pH-adjusted parenteral solutions. *J Clin Pharm Ther.* 1988; 13:257–61.

1402. Lee DKT, Lee A. Compatibility of cefoperazone sodium and furosemide in 5% dextrose injection. *Am J Hosp Pharm.* 1991; 48:108–10.

1403. Lee DKT, Wang DP. Compatibility of cefoperazone sodium and cimetidine hydrochloride in 5% dextrose injection. *Am J Hosp Pharm*. 1991; 48:111–3.

1404. Kirkpatrick AE, Holcome BJ. Effect of retrograde aminophylline administration on calcium and phosphate solubility in neonatal total parenteral nutrient solutions. *Am J Hosp Pharm*. 1989; 46:2496–500.

1405. Seay R, Bostrom B. Apparent compatibility of methotrexate and vancomycin. *Am J Hosp Pharm*. 1990; 47:2656.

1406. Johnson OL, Washington C, Davis SS et al. The destabilization of parenteral feeding emulsions by heparin. *Int J Pharm*. 1989; 53:237–40.

1407. Lor E, Sheybani T. Visual compatibility of fluconazole with commonly used injectable drugs during simulated Y-site administration. *Am J Hosp Pharm*. 1991; 48:744–6.

1408. Tol A, Quik RFP. Adsorption of human and porcine insulins to intravenous administration sets. *Pharm Weekbl [Sci]*. 1988; 10:213–6.

1409. Thompson DF, Allen LV Jr. Visual compatibility of enalaprilat with selected intravenous medications during simulated Y-site injection. *Am J Hosp Pharm*. 1990; 47:2530–1.

1410. Wilson TD, Forde MD. Stability of milrinone and epinephrine, atropine sulfate, lidocaine hydrochloride, or morphine sulfate injection. *Am J Hosp Pharm*. 1990; 47:2504–7.

1411. Lam NP, Kennedy PE, Jarosinski PF et al. Stability of zidovudine in 5% dextrose injection and 0.9% sodium chloride injection. *Am J Hosp Pharm*. 1991; 48:280–2.

1412. Horrow JC, Digregorio GJ, Barbieri EJ et al. Intravenous infusions of nitroprusside, dobutamine, and nitroglycerin are compatible. *Crit Care Med*. 1990; 18:858–61.

1413. Halstead DC, Guzzo J, Giardina JA et al. In vitro bactericidal activities of gentamicin, cefazolin, and imipenem in peritoneal dialysis fluids. *Antimicrob Agents Chemother*. 1989; 33:1553–6.

1414. Drake JM, Myre SA, Staneck JL et al. Antimicrobial activity of vancomycin, gentamicin, and tobramycin in peritoneal dialysis solution. *Am J Hosp Pharm*. 1990; 47:1604–6.

1415. Pavlik EJ, van Nagell JR, Hanson MB et al. Sensitivity to anticancer agents in vitro: standardizing the cytotoxic response and characterizing the sensitivities of a reference cell line. *Gynecol Oncol*. 1982; 14:243–61.

1416. Pavlik EJ, Kenady DE, van Nagell JR et al. Properties of anticancer agents relevant to in vitro determinations of human tumor cell sensitivity. *Cancer Chemother Pharmacol*. 1983; 11:8–15.

1417. Gora ML, Seth S, Visconti JA et al. Stability of dobutamine hydrochloride in peritoneal dialysis solutions. *Am J Hosp Pharm*. 1991; 48:1234–7.

1418. Strom JG Jr, Miller SW. Stability and compatibility of methylprednisolone sodium succinate and cimetidine hydrochloride in 5% dextrose injection. *Am J Hosp Pharm*. 1991; 48:1237–41.

1419. Riley CM, Junkin P. Stability of amrinone and digoxin, procainamide hydrochloride, propranolol hydrochloride, sodium bicarbonate, potassium chloride, or verapamil hydrochloride in intravenous admixtures. *Am J Hosp Pharm*. 1991; 48:1245–52.

1420. Pennell AT, Allington DR. Effect of ceftazidime, cefotaxime, and cefoperazone on serum tobramycin concentrations. *Am J Hosp Pharm*. 1991; 48:520–2.

1421. Collins JL, Lutz RJ. In vitro study of simultaneous infusion of incompatible drugs in multilumen catheters. *Heart Lung*. 1991; 20:271–7.

1422. Gupta VD. Complexation of procainamide with dextrose. *J Pharm Sci*. 1982; 71:994–6.

1423. Gupta VD. Complexation of procainamide with hydroxide-containing compounds. *J Pharm Sci*. 1983; 72:205–7.

1424. Parasrampuria J, Gupta VD. Preformulation studies of acetazolamide: effect of pH, two buffer species, ionic strength, and temperature on its stability. *J Pharm Sci*. 1989; 78:855–7.

1425. Frazin BS. Maximal dilution of activase. *Am J Hosp Pharm*. 1990; 47:1016.

1426. Tripp MG. Automated 3–in–1 admixture compounding: a comparative study of simultaneous versus sequential pumping of core substrates on admixture stability. *Hosp Pharm*. 1990; 25:1090–3.

1427. Knowles JB, Cusson G, Smith M et al. Pulmonary deposition of calcium phosphate crystals as a complication of home total parenteral nutrition. *JPEN J Parenter Enteral Nutr*. 1989; 13:209–13.

1428. Knight PJ, Buchanan S. Calcium and phosphate requirements of preterm infants who require prolonged hyperalimentation. *J Am Med Assoc*. 1980; 243:1244–6.

1429. Stennett DJ, Gerwick WH, Egging PK et al. Precipitate analysis from an indwelling total parenteral nutrition catheter. *JPEN J Parenter Enteral Nutr*. 1988; 12:88–92.

1430. Mazur HI, Stennett DJ, Egging PK. Extraction of diethylhexylphthalate from total nutrient solution-containing polyvinyl chloride bags. *JPEN J Parenter Enteral Nutr*. 1989; 13:59–62.

1431. Smith JL, Canham JE, Kirkland WD et al. Effect of Intralipid, amino acids, container, temperature, and duration of storage on vitamin stability in total parenteral nutrition admixtures. *JPEN J Parenter Enteral Nutr*. 1988; 12:478–83.

1432. Tripp MG, Menon SK. Stability of total nutrient admixtures in a dual-chamber flexible container. *Am J Hosp Pharm*. 1990; 47:2496–503.

1433. Dalton-Bunnow MF, Halvacks FJ. Update on room-temperature stability of drug products labeled for refrigerated storage. *Am J Hosp Pharm*. 1990; 47:2522–4.

1434. Kintzel PE, Kennedy PE. Stability of amphotericin B in 5% dextrose injection at concentrations used for administration through a central venous line. *Am J Hosp Pharm*. 1991; 48:283–5.

1435. Rice JK. Visual compatibility of amphotericin B and flush solutions. *Am J Hosp Pharm*. 1989; 46:2461.

1436. Trissel LA, Bready BB, Kwan JW et al. The visual compatibility of sargramostim with selected chemotherapeutic drugs, anti-infectives, and other drugs during simulated Y-site injection. *Am J Hosp Pharm*. 1992; 49:402–6.

1437. Pilla TJ, Beshany SE. Incompatibility of hexabrix and papaverine. *Am J Roentgenol*. 1986; 146:1300–1.

1438. Irving HD, Burbridge BE. Incompatibility of contrast agents with intravascular medications. *Radiology*. 1989; 173:91–2. [IDIS 307908]

1439. Trissel LA, Parks NPT. Visual compatibility of fludarabine phosphate with antineoplastic drugs, anti-infectives, and other selected drugs during simulated Y-site injection. *Am J Hosp Pharm.* 1991; 48:2186–9.

1440. Tidy PJ, Sewell GJ, Jeffries TM. Microwave freeze-thaw studies on azlocillin infusion. *Pharm J.* 1988; 241:R22–R23.

1441. Koberda M, Zieske PA, Raghavan NV et al. Stability of bleomycin sulfate reconstituted in 5% dextrose injection or 0.9% sodium chloride injection stored in glass vials or polyvinyl chloride containers. *Am J Hosp Pharm.* 1990; 47:2528–9.

1442. Datapharm Publications Ltd. ABPI compendium of data sheets and summaries of product characteristics 1999/2000. London, England; 1999.

1443. Weir SJ, Szucs Myers VA, Bengston KD et al. Sorption of amiodarone to polyvinyl chloride infusion bags and administration sets. *Am J Hosp Pharm.* 1985; 42:2679–83.

1444. Benedict MK, Roche VF, Banakar UV et al. Visual compatibility of amiodarone hydrochloride with various antimicrobial agents during simulated Y-site injection. *Am J Hosp Pharm.* 1988; 45:1117–8.

1445. Capps PA, Robertson AL. Influence of amiodarone injection on delivery rate of intravenous fluids. *Pharm J.* 1985; 234:14–5.

1446. Tsuei SE, Nation RL. Sorption of chlormethiazole by intravenous infusion giving sets. *Eur J Clin Pharmacol.* 1980; 18:333–8.

1447. Lingam S, Bertwistle H, Elliston HM et al. Problems with intravenous chlormethiazole (Heminevrin) in status epilepticus. *Br Med J.* 1980; 280:155–6.

1448. Beaumont IM. Stability study of aqueous solutions of diamorphine and morphine using HPLC. *Pharm J.* 1982; 229:39–41.

1449. Kleinberg ML, Duafala ME, Nacov C et al. Stability of heroin hydrochloride in infusion devices and containers for intravenous administration. *Am J Hosp Pharm.* 1990; 47:377–81.

1450. Jones VA, Hanks GW. New portable infusion pump for prolonged subcutaneous administration of opiod analgesics in patients with advanced cancer. *BMJ.* 1986; 292:1496.

1451. Jones VA, Hoskin PJ, Omar OA, et al. Diamorphine stability in aqueous solution for subcutaneous infusion. *Abs Br Soc Pharmacol Meet.* 1986; 66(Dec)

1452. Omar OA, Hoskin PJ, Johnston A et al. Diamorphine stability in aqueous solution for subcutaneous infusion. *J Pharm Pharmacol.* 1989; 41:275–7.

1453. Al-Razzak LA, Benedetti AE, Waugh WN et al. Chemical stability of pentostatin (NSC-218321), a cytotoxic and immunosuppressive agent. *Pharm Res.* 1990; 7:452–60.

1454. Allwood MC. Diamorphine mixed with antiemetic drugs in plastic syringes. *Br J Pharm Prac.* 1984; 6:88–90.

1455. Regnard C, Pashley S. Anti-emetic/diamorphine mixture compatibility in infusion pumps. *Br J Pharm Pract.* 1986; 8:218–20.

1456. Collins AJ, Abathell JA, Holmes SG et al. Stability of diamorphine hydrochloride with haloperidol in prefilled syringes for continuous subcutaneous administration. *J Pharm Pharmacol.* 1986; 38(S):51P.

1457. Page J, Hudson SA. Diamorphine hydrochloride compatibility with saline. *Pharm J.* 1982; 228:238–9.

1458. Kirk B, Hain WR. Diamorphine injection BP incompatibility. *Pharm J.* 1985; 235:171.

1459. Jones V, Murphy A. Solubility of diamorphine. *Pharm J.* 1985; 235:426.

1460. Wood MJ, Irwin WJ, Scott DK. Stability of doxorubicin, daunorubicin and epirubicin in plastic syringes and minibags. *J Clin Pharm Ther.* 1990; 15:279–89.

1461. Targett PL, Keefe PA. Stability of two concentrations of morphine tartrate in 10 mL polypropylene syringes. *Aust J Hosp Pharm.* 1997; 27:452–4.

1462. Keusters L, Stolk LML, Umans R et al. Stability of solutions of doxorubicin and epirubicin in plastic minibags for intravesical use after storage at -20 °C and thawing by microwave radiation. *Pharm Weekbl [Sci].* 1986; 8:194–7.

1463. Wood MJ, Irwin WJ. Photodegradation of doxorubicin, daunorubicin, and epirubicin measured by high-performance liquid chromatography. *J Clin Pharm Ther.* 1990; 35:291–300.

1464. Lee MG, Fenton-May V. Absorption of isosorbide dinitrate by PVC infusion bags and administration sets. *J Clin Hosp Pharm.* 1981; 6:209–11.

1465. DeMuynck C, Remon JP, Colardyn F. The sorption of isosorbide dinitrate to intravenous delivery systems. *J Pharm Pharmacol.* 1988; 40:601–4.

1466. Struhar M, Mandak M, Heinrich J et al. Sorption of isosorbide dinitrate on infusion sets. *Farm Obz.* 1989; 58:443–6.

1467. Allwood MC. Sorption of parenteral nitrates during administration with a syringe pump and extension set. *Int J Pharm.* 1987; 39:183–6.

1468. Wilson TD, Forde isoMD, Crain AVR et al. Stability of milrinone in 0.45% sodium chloride, 0.9% sodium chloride, or 5% dextrose injections. *Am J Hosp Pharm.* 1986; 43:2218–20.

1469. Cook B, Hill SA. The stability of amoxycillin sodium in intravenous infusion fluids. *J Clin Hosp Pharm.* 1982; 7:245–50.

1470. Concannon J, Lovitt H, Ramage M et al. Stability of aqueous solutions of amoxicillin sodium in the frozen and liquid states. *Am J Hosp Pharm.* 1986; 43:3027–30.

1471. McDonald C, Sunderland VB, Lau H et al. The stability of amoxicillin sodium in normal saline and glucose (5%) solutions in the liquid and frozen states. *J Clin Pharm Ther.* 1989; 14:45–52.

1472. McDonald C, Sunderland VB, Marshall CA et al. Freezing rates of 50–mL infusion bags and some implications for drug stability as shown with amoxycillin. *Aust J Hosp Pharm.* 1989; 19:194–7.

1473. Janknegt R, Schrouff GGM, Hooymans PM et al. Quinolones and penicillins incompatibility. *DICP, Ann Pharmacother.* 1989; 23:91–2.

1474. Ashwin J, Lynn B. Stability and administration of intravenous Augmentin. *Pharm J.* 1987; 238:116–8.

1475. Lynn B. The stability and administration of intravenous penicillins. *Br J IV Ther.* 1981; 2:22–39.

1476. Landersjo L, Kallstrand G. Studies on the stability and compatibility of drugs in infusion fluids III. Factors affecting the stability of cloxacillin. *Acta Pharm Suec.* 1974; 11:563–80.

1477. Bundgaard H, Ilver K. Kinetics of degradation of cloxacillin sodium in aqueous solution. *Dansk Tidsskr Farm.* 1970; 44:365–80.

1478. Brown AF, Harvey DA, Hoddinott DJ et al. Freeze-thaw stability of antibiotics used in an IV additive service. *Br J Parenter Ther.* 1986; 7:42–4.

1479. Beatson C, Taylor A. A physical compatibility study of frusemide and flucloxacillin injections. *Br J Pharm Pract.* 1987; 9:223–6.

1480. Nahata MC, Ahalt PA. Stability of cefazolin sodium in peritoneal dialysis solutions. *Am J Hosp Pharm.* 1991; 48:291–2.

1481. Paap CM, Nahata MC. Stability of cefotaxime in two peritoneal dialysis solutions. *Am J Hosp Pharm.* 1990; 47:147–50.

1482. Mehta AC, McCarty M. The chemical stability of cephradine injection solutions. *Intensive Ther Clin Monit.* 1988; 9:195–6.

1483. Lyall D, Blythe J. Ciprofloxacin lactate infusion. *Pharm J.* 1987; 238:290.

1484. Veljkovic VB, Lazic ML. Stability of bottled dextran solutions with respect to insoluble particle formations: a review. *Pharmazie.* 1989; 44:305–10.

1485. Veljkovic VB, Lazic ML. Mechanism of insoluble particle formation in bottled dextran solutions. *Pharmazie.* 1988; 43:840–2.

1486. Shea BF, Souney PF. Stability of famotidine frozen in polypropylene syringes. *Am J Hosp Pharm.* 1990; 47:2073–4.

1487. Bullock LS, Fitzgerald JF. Stability of intravenous famotidine stored in polyvinyl-chloride syringes. *DICP, Ann Pharmacother.* 1989; 23:588–90.

1488. Thomas SMB. Stability of Intralipid in a parenteral nutrition solution. *Aust J Hosp Pharm.* 1987; 17:115–7.

1489. Stiles ML, Allen LV Jr. Stability of fluorouracil administered through four portable infusion pumps. *Am J Hosp Pharm.* 1989; 46:2036–40.

1490. Tu YH, Stiles ML, Allen LV Jr et al. Stability study of gentamicin sulfate administered via Pharmacia Deltec CADD-VT pump. *Hosp Pharm.* 1990; 25:843–5.

1491. Parkinson R, Wilson JV, Ross M et al. Stability of low-dosage heparin in pre-filled syringes. *Br J Pharm Pract.* 1989; 11:34.

1492. Menzies AR, Benoliel DM. The effects of autoclaving on the physical properties and biological activity of parenteral heparin preparations. *J Pharm Pharmacol.* 1989; 41:512–6.

1493. Farmitalia Carlo Erba. Stability of 4–demethoxydaunorubicin hydrochloride reconstituted solutions with water for injections, sodium chloride, dextrose, and sodium chloride with dextrose injections. Milan, Italy; 1986 Jun.

1494. Radford JA, Margison JM, Swindell R et al. The stability of ifosfamide in aqueous solution and its suitability for continuous 7–day infusion by ambulatory pump. *Cancer Chemother Pharmacol.* 1990; 26:144–6.

1495. Shaw IC, Rose JWP. Infusion of ifosfamide plus mesna. *Lancet.* 1984; 1:1353–4.

1496. Bristol-Myers Oncology. Product information on IFEX (ifosfamide). Evansville, IN; 1990 Feb.

1497. Doglietto GB, Bellantone R, Bossola M et al. Insulin adsorption to three-liter ethylen vinyl acetate bags during 24–hour infusion. *JPEN J Parenter Enteral Nutr.* 1989; 13:539–41.

1498. Donnelly RF. Immune globulin solubility in 5% dextrose injection. *Am J Hosp Pharm.* 1990; 47:1976.

1499. Prouix SM. Reconstitution of intravenous immunoglobulins. *Hosp Pharm.* 1987; 22:1133–4.

1500. Denson DD, Crews JC, Grummich KW et al. Stability of methadone hydrochloride in 0.9% sodium chloride injection in single-dose plastic containers. *Am J Hosp Pharm.* 1991; 48:515–7.

1501. Anderson BD, Taphouse V. Initial rate studies of hydrolysis and acyl migration in methylprednisolone 21–hemisuccinate and 17–hemisuccinate. *J Pharm Sci.* 1981; 70:181–6.

1502. Bogardus JB, Kaplan MA. Precipitation of teniposide during infusion. *Am J Hosp Pharm.* 1990; 47:518.

1503. Beijnen JH, van Gijn R. Chemical stability of the antitumor drug mitomycin C in solutions for intravesical installation. *J Parenter Sci Technol.* 1990; 44:332–5.

1504. Duafala ME, Kleinberg ML, Nacov C et al. Stability of morphine sulfate in infusion devices and containers for intravenous administration. *Am J Hosp Pharm.* 1990; 47:143–6.

1505. Walker SE, Iazetta J. Stability of sulfite free high potency morphine sulfate solutions in portable infusion pump casettes. *Can J Hosp Pharm.* (Oct) 1989; 42:195–200, 218–9.

1506. Altman L, Hopkins RJ, Ahmed S et al. Stability of morphine sulfate in Cormed III (Kalex) intravenous bags. *Am J Hosp Pharm.* 1990; 47:2040–2.

1507. Stiles ML, Tu YH. Stability of morphine sulfate in portable pump reservoirs during storage and simulated administration. *Am J Hosp Pharm.* 1989; 46:1404–7.

1508. Cante B, Monsarrat B, Lazorthes Y et al. The stability of morphine in isobaric and hyperbaric solutions in a drug delivery system. *J Pharm Pharmacol.* 1988; 40:644–5.

1509. Martens HJ. Stabilitat wasserloslicher vitamine in verschiedenen infusionsbenteln. *Krankenhauspharmazie.* 1989; 10:359–61.

1510. Tracy TS, Bowman L. Nitroglycerin delivery through a polyethylene-lined intravenous administration set. *Am J Hosp Pharm.* 1989; 46:2031–5.

1511. Loucas SP, Maager P, Mehl B et al. Effect of vehicle ionic strength on sorption on nitroglycerin to a polyvinyl chloride administration set. *Am J Hosp Pharm.* 1990; 47:1559–62.

1512. DeRudder D, Remon JP. The sorption of nitroglycerin by infusion sets. *J Pharm Pharmacol.* 1987; 39:556–8.

1513. Jarosinski PF, Hirschfield S. Precipitation of ondansetron in alkaline solutions. *N Engl J Med.* 1991; 325:1315–6.

1514. Markowsky SJ, Kohls PR, Ehresman D et al. Compatibility and pH variability of four injectable phenytoin sodium products. *Am J Hosp Pharm.* 1991; 48:510–4.

1515. Stolshek BS (Professional Services, Glaxo Inc.): Personal communication; 1990 Aug 27.

1516. Stewart JT, Warren FW, Johnson SM et al. Stability of ranitidine in intravenous admixtures stored frozen, refrigerated, and at room temperature. *Am J Hosp Pharm.* 1990; 47:2043–6.

1517. Thibault L. Streptokinase flocculation in evacuated glass bottles. *Am J Hosp Pharm.* 1985; 42:278.

1518. Lerebours E, Ducable G, Francheschi A, et al. Catheter obstruction during prolonged parenteral alimentation. Are lipids responsible? *Clin Nutr*. 1985; 4:135–8.

1519. Den Hartigh J, Brandenburg HCR. Stability of azacitidine in lactated Ringer's injection frozen in polypropylene syringes. *Am J Hosp Pharm*. 1989; 46:2500–5.

1520. Waugh WN, Trissel LA. Stability, compatibility, and plasticizer extraction of taxol (NSC-125973) injection diluted in infusion solutions and stored in various containers. *Am J Hosp Pharm*. 1991; 48:1520–4.

1521. Strong DK, Morris LA. Precipitation of teniposide during infusion. *Am J Hosp Pharm*. 1990; 47:512.

1522. Outman WR, Mitrano FP. Visual compatibility of ganciclovir sodium and total parenteral nutrient solution during simulated Y-site injection. *Am J Hosp Pharm*. 1991; 48:1538–9.

1523. Outman WR, Monolakis J. Visual compatibility of haloperidol lactate with 0.9% sodium chloride injection or injectable critical-care drugs during simulated Y-site injection. *Am J Hosp Pharm*. 1991; 48:1539–41.

1524. Neels JT. Compatibility of hydromorphone hydrochloride and tetracaine hydrochloride. *Am J Hosp Pharm*. 1991; 48:1682–83.

1525. Turowski RC, Durthaler JM. Visual compatibility of idarubicin hydrochloride with selected drugs during simulated Y-site injection. *Am J Hosp Pharm*. 1991; 48:2181–4.

1526. Woloschuk DMM, Wermeling JR. Stability and compatibility of fluorouracil and mannitol during simulated Y-site administration. *Am J Hosp Pharm*. 1991; 48:2158–60.

1527. Ishisaka DY, van Fleet J. Visual compatibility of indomethacin sodium trihydrate with drugs given to neonates by continuous infusion. *Am J Hosp Pharm*. 1991; 48:2442–3.

1528. Trissel LA, Bready BB. Turbidimetric assessment of the compatibility of taxol with selected other drugs during simulated Y-site injection. *Am J Hosp Pharm*. 1992; 49:1716–9.

1529. DiStefano JE, Outman WR. Additional data on visual compatibility of foscarnet sodium with morphine sulfate. *Am J Hosp Pharm*. 1992; 49:1672.

1530. Zanetti LA. Visual compatibility of diltiazem with commonly used injectable drugs during simulated Y-site administration. *Am J Hosp Pharm*. 1992; 49:1911.

1531. Martin KM. (Product Information Services, Lederle Laboratories, Pearl River, NY): Personal communication; 1992 Jan 14.

1532. Walker SE, DeAngelis C. Stability and compatibility of combinations of hydromorphone and a second drug. *Can J Hosp Pharm*. 1991; 44:289–95.

1533. Raineri DL, Cwik MJ, Rodvold KA et al. Stability of nizatidine in commonly used intravenous fluids and containers. *Am J Hosp Pharm*. 1988; 45:1523–9.

1534. Hatton J, Holstad SG, Rosenbloom AD et al. Stability of nizatidine in total nutrient admixtures. *Am J Hosp Pharm*. 1991; 48:1507–10.

1535. Wade CS, Lampasona V, Mullins RE et al. Stability of ceftazidime and amino acids in parenteral nutrient solutions. *Am J Hosp Pharm*. 1991; 48:1515–9.

1536. Patel JP, Tran LT, Sinai WJ et al. Activity of urokinase diluted in 0.9% sodium chloride injection or 5% dextrose injection and stored in glass or plastic syringes. *Am J Hosp Pharm*. 1991; 48:1511–4.

1537. Kintzel PE, Kennedy PE. Stability of amphotericin B in 5% dextrose injection at 25 °C. *Am J Hosp Pharm*. 1991; 48:1681.

1538. Stiles ML, Allen LV. Stability of doxorubicin hydrochloride in portable pump reservoirs. *Am J Hosp Pharm*. 1991; 48:1976–7.

1539. Sarkar MA, Rogers E, Reinhard M et al. Stability of clindamycin phosphate, ranitidine hydrochloride, and piperacillin sodium in polyolefin containers. *Am J Hosp Pharm*. 1991; 48:2184–6.

1540. Ritchie DJ, Holstad SG, Westrich TJ et al. Activity of octreotide acetate in a total nutrient admixture. *Am J Hosp Pharm*. 1991; 48:2172–5.

1541. Goodwin SD, Nix DE, Heyd A et al. Compatibility of ciprofloxacin injection with selected drugs and solutions. *Am J Hosp Pharm*. 1991; 48:2166–71.

1542. Walker SE, DeAngelis C, Iazzetta J et al. Compatibility of dexamethasone sodium phosphate with hydromorphone hydrochloride or diphenhydramine hydrochloride. *Am J Hosp Pharm*. 1991; 48:2161–6.

1543. Harkness BJ, Williams D, Stewart MC et al. Change needed for i.v. rifampin preparation instructions. *Am J Hosp Pharm*. 1991; 48:2127–8.

1544. Wiest DB, Maish WA, Garner SS et al. Stability of amphotericin B in four concentrations of dextrose injection. *Am J Hosp Pharm*. 1991; 48:2430–3.

1545. Silvestri AP, Mitrano FP, Baptista RJ et al. Stability and compatibility of ganciclovir sodium in 5% dextrose injection over 35 days. *Am J Hosp Pharm*. 1991; 48:2641–3.

1546. Mitrano FP, Outman WR, Baptista RJ et al. Chemical and visual stability of amphotericin B in 5% dextrose injection stored at 4 °C for 35 days. *Am J Hosp Pharm*. 1991; 48:2635–7.

1547. Rivers TE, McBride HA. Stability of cefotaxime sodium and metronidazole in an i.v. admixture at 8 °C. *Am J Hosp Pharm*. 1991; 48:2638–40.

1548. Rochard EB, Barthes DMC. Stability of fluorouracil, cytarabine, or doxorubicin hydrochloride in ethylene vinyl acetate portable infusion-pump reservoirs. *Am J Hosp Pharm*. 1992; 49:619–23.

1549. Letourneau M, Milot L. Visual compatibility of magnesium sulfate with narcotic analgesics. *Am J Hosp Pharm*. 1992; 49:838–9.

1550. Thompson DF, Heflin NR. Incompatibility of injectable indomethacin with gentamicin sulfate or tobramycin sulfate. *Am J Hosp Pharm*. 1992; 49:836.

1551. Munoz M, Girona V, Pujol M et al. Stability of ifosfamide in 0.9% sodium chloride solution or water for injection in a portable i.v. pump cassette. *Am J Hosp Pharm*. 1992; 49:1137–9.

1552. Anderson PM, Rogosheske JR, Ramsay NKC et al. Biological activity of recombinant interleukin-2 in intravenous admixtures containing antibiotic, morphine sulfate, or total parenteral nutrient solution. *Am J Hosp Pharm*. 1992; 49:608–12.

1553. Stiles ML, Allen LV. Stability of ondansetron hydrochloride in portable infusion-pump reservoirs. *Am J Hosp Pharm.* 1992; 49:1471–3.

1554. Couch P, Jacobson P. Stability of fluconazole and amino acids in parenteral nutrient solutions. *Am J Hosp Pharm.* 1992; 49:1459–62.

1555. McDonald C, Faridah. Solubilities of trimethoprim and sulfamethoxazole at various pH values and crystallization of trimethoprim from infusion fluids. *J Parenter Sci Technol.* 1991; 45:147–51.

1556. Trissel LA, Martinez JF. Turbidimetric assessment of the compatibility of taxol with 42 drugs during simulated Y-site injection. *Am J Hosp Pharm.* 1993; 50:300–4.

1557. Trissel LA, Martinez JF. Physical compatibility of melphalan with selected drugs during simulated Y-site administration. *Am J Hosp Pharm.* 1993; 50:2359–63.

1558. Trissel LA, Martinez JF. Visual, turbidimetric, and particle-content assessment of compatibility of vinorelbine tartrate with selected drugs during simulated Y-site injection. *Am J Hosp Pharm.* 1994; 51:495–9.

1559. Pearson SD, Trissel LA. Stability and compatibility of minocycline hydrochloride and rifampin in intravenous solutions at various temperatures. *Am J Hosp Pharm.* 1993; 50:698–702.

1560. Graham CL, Dukes GE, Kao CF et al. Stability of ondansetron in large-volume parenteral solutions. *Ann Pharmacother.* 1992; 26:768–71.

1561. Halasi S, Nairn JG. Stability of hydralazine hydrochloride in parenteral solutions. *Can J Hosp Pharm.* 1990; 43:237–41.

1562. Speaker TJ, Turco SJ, Nardone DA et al. A study of the interaction of selected drugs and plastic syringes. *J Parenter Sci Technol.* 1991; 45:212–7.

1564. Adams PS, Haines-Nutt RF, Bradford E et al. Pharmaceutical aspects of home infusion therapy for cancer patients. *Pharm J.* 1987; 238:476–8.

1565. Barnes AR. Chemical stabilities of cefuroxime sodium and metronidazole in an admixture for intravenous infusion. *J Clin Pharm Ther.* 1990; 15:187–96.

1566. Weir PJ, Ireland DS. Chemical stability of cytarabine and vinblastine injections. *Br J Pharm Pract.* (Feb) 1990; 12:53, 54, 60.

1567. Vincke BJ, Verstraeten AE, El Eini DID et al. Extended stability of 5-fluorouracil and methotrexate solutions in PVC containers. *Int J Pharm.* 1989; 54:181–9.

1568. Stevens RF, Wilkins KM. Use of cytotoxic drugs with an end-line filter—a study of four drugs commonly administered to paediatric patients. *J Clin Pharm Ther.* 1989; 14:475–9.

1569. Garner ST, Murdoch JM. Dopamine dilutions. *Pharm J.* 1990; 244:218.

1570. Schroder F, Schutz H. Kompatibilitat von heparin und gentamicin sulfat. *Pharm Ztg.* 1989; 134:24–6.

1571. Adams PS, Haines-Nutt RF. The stability of aminophylline intravenous infusion solutions. *Proc Guild.* 1988; 25:41–4.

1572. Schaaf LJ, Tremel LC, Wulf BG et al. Compatibility of enalaprilat with dobutamine, dopamine, heparin, nitroglycerin, potassium chloride, and nitroprusside. *J Clin Pharm Ther.* 1990; 15:371–6.

1573. Kern JW, Lee KJ, Martinoff JT et al. The in vivo availability of gentamicin when admixed with total nutrient solutions: a comparative study. *JPEN J Parenter Enteral Nutr.* 1990; 14:523–6.

1574. Montoro JB, Galard R, Catalan R et al. Stability of somatostatin in total parenteral nutrition. *Pharm Weekbl [Sci].* 1990; 12:240–2.

1575. Sauer H. Aufbewahrung von zytostatika-losungen. *Krankenhauspharmazie.* 1990; 11:373–5.

1576. Shea BF, Souney PF. Stability of famotidine in a 3–in–1 total nutrient admixture. *DICP.* 1990; 24:232–5.

1577. De Vroe C, De Muynck C, Remon JP et al. A study on the stability of three antineoplastic drugs and on their sorption by i.v. delivery systems and end-line filters. *Int J Pharm.* 1990; 65:49–56.

1578. Raymond GG, Davis RL. Physical compatibility and chemical stability of amphotericin B in combination with magnesium sulfate in 5% dextrose injection. *DICP.* 1991; 25:123–6.

1579. Pramar Y, Gupta VD, Gardner SN et al. Stabilities of dobutamine, dopamine, nitroglycerin, and sodium nitroprusside in disposable plastic syringes. *J Clin Pharm Ther.* 1991; 16:203–7.

1580. Stewart JT, Warren FW, Johnson SM et al. Stability of ceftazidime in plastic syringes and glass vials under various storage conditions. *Am J Hosp Pharm.* 1992; 49:2765–8.

1581. Stiles ML, Allen LV Jr. Stability of ceftazidime (with arginine) and cefuroxime sodium in infusion-pump reservoirs. *Am J Hosp Pharm.* 1992; 49:2761–4.

1582. Kaufman MB, Scavone JM. Stability of undiluted trimethoprim-sulfamethoxazole for injection in plastic syringes. *Am J Hosp Pharm.* 1992; 49:2782–3.

1583. Nahata MC, Morosco RS. Stability of morphine sulfate in bacteriostatic 0.9% sodium chloride injection stored in glass vials at two temperatures. *Am J Hosp Pharm.* 1992; 49:2785–6.

1584. Nahata MC, Morosco RS. Stability of ceftazidime (with arginine) stored in plastic syringes at three temperatures. *Am J Hosp Pharm.* 1992; 49:2954–6.

1585. Mawhinney WM, Adair CG, Gorman SP et al. Stability of ciprofloxacin in peritoneal dialysis solutions. *Am J Hosp Pharm.* 1992; 49:2956–9.

1586. Nahata MC, Morosco RS. Stability of aminophylline in bacteriostatic water for injection stored in plastic syringes at two temperatures. *Am J Hosp Pharm.* 1992; 49:2962–3.

1587. Allwood MC. The influence of buffering on the stability of erythromycin injection in small-volume infusions. *Int J Pharm.* 1992; 80:R7–R9.

1588. Toki N. Glass adsorption of highly purified urokinase. *Thromb Haemost.* 1980; 43:67.

1589. Zimmerman R, Schoffel G. Urokinase therapy: dose reduction by administration in plastic material. *Thromb Haemost.* 1981; 45:296.

1590. Walker SE, Iazzetta J. Compatibility and stability of pentobarbital infusions. *Anesthesiology.* 1981; 55:487–9.

1591. Walker SE, Iazzetta J. Cefotetan stability in normal saline and five percent dextrose in water. *Can J Hosp Pharm.* (1) 1992; 45:9–13, 37.

1592. Nahata MC. Stability of ceftriaxone sodium in peritoneal dialysis solutions. *DICP*. 1991; 25:741–2.

1593. Walker SE, Lau DWC, DeAngelis C et al. Mitoxantrone stability in syringes and glass vials and evaluation of chemical contamination. *Can J Hosp Pharm*. 1991; 44:143–51.

1594. Walker S, Lau D, DeAngelis C et al. Doxorubicin stability in syringes and glass vials and evaluation of chemical contamination. *Can J Hosp Pharm*. 1991; 44:71–78.

1595. Peterson GM, Khoo BHC, Galloway JG et al. A preliminary study of the stability of midazolam in polypropylene syringes. *Aust J Hosp Pharm*. 1991; 21:115–8.

1596. Lecompte D, Bousselet M, Gayrard D et al. Stability study of reconstituted and diluted solutions of calcium folinate. *Pharm Ind*. 1991; 53:90–4.

1597. Allwood MC. The stability of erythromycin injection in small-volume infusions. *Int J Pharm*. 1990; 62:R1–R3.

1598. Gupta VD, Pramar Y, Odom C et al. Chemical stability of cefotetan disodium in 5% dextrose and 0.9% sodium chloride injections. *J Clin Pharm Ther*. 1990; 15:109–14.

1599. Poggi GL. Compatibility of morphine tartrate admixtures in polypropylene syringes. *Aust J Hosp Pharm*. 1991; 21:316.

1600. McLaughlin JP, Simpson C. The stability of reconstituted aztreonam. *Br J Pharm Pract*. (Oct) 1990; 12:328, 330, 334.

1601. Biejnen JH, van Gijn R, Horenblas S et al. Chemical stability of suramin in commonly used infusion fluids. *DICP*. 1990; 24:1056–8.

1602. Patel JP. Urokinase: stability studies in solution and lyophilized formulations. *Drug Dev Ind Pharm*. 1990; 16:2613–26.

1603. Driver AG, Worden JP Jr. Intravenous streptomycin. *DICP*. 1990; 24:826–8.

1604. Bosso JA. Clindamycin stability. *DICP*. 1990; 24:1008–9.

1605. Theuer H, Scherbel G, Distler F et al. Cisplatin-injektionslosung. *Krankenhauspharmazie*. 1990; 11:288–91.

1606. Bluhm DP, Summers RS, Lowes MMJ et al. Influence of container on vitamin A stability in TPN admixtures. *Int J Pharm*. 1991; 68:281–3.

1607. Bluhm DP, Summers RS, Lowes MMJ et al. Lipid emulsion content and vitamin A stability in TPN admixtures. *Int J Pharm*. 1991; 68:277–80.

1608. Beijnen J, Koks CHW. Visual compatibility of ondansetron and dexamethasone. *DICP*. 1991; 25:869.

1609. Lawson WA, Longmore RB, McDonald C et al. Stability of hyoscine in mixtures with morphine for continuous subcutaneous administration. *Aust J Hosp Pharm*. 1991; 21:395–6.

1610. Allwood MC. The stability of four catecholamines in 5% glucose infusions. *J Clin Pharm Ther*. 1991; 16:337–40.

1611. Van Asten P, Glerum JH, Spaanderman ER et al. Compatibility of bupivacaine and iohexol in two mixtures for paediatric regional anaesthesia. *Pharm Weekbl Sci*. 1991; 13:254–6. [IDIS 293188]

1612. Sewell GJ, Palmer AJ. The chemical and physical stability of three intravenous infusions subjected to frozen storage and microwave thawing. *Int J Pharm*. 1991; 72:57–63.

1613. Janknegt R, Stratermans T, Cilissen J et al. Ofloxacin intravenous—compatibility with other antibacterial agents. *Pharm Weekbl Sci*. 1991; 13:207–9.

1614. Dunham B, Marcuard S, Khazanie PG et al. The solubility of calcium and phosphorus in neonatal total parenteral nutrition solutions. *JPEN J Parenter Enteral Nutr*. 1991; 15:608–11.

1615. Delaney RA, Mikkelsen SL. Effects of heat treatment on selected plasma therapeutic drug concentrations. *Ann Pharmacother*. 1992; 26:338–40.

1616. McLeod HL, McGuire TR. Stability of cyclosporine in dextrose 5%, NaCl 0.9%, dextrose/amino acid solution, and lipid emulsion. *Ann Pharmacother*. 1992; 26:172–5.

1617. Andreu A, Cardona D, Pastor C et al. Intravenous aminophylline: in vitro stability in fat-containing TPN. *Ann Pharmacother*. 1992; 26:127–8.

1618. Matsuura G. Visual compatibility of sargramostim (GM-CSF) during simulated Y-site administration with selected agents. *Hosp Pharm*. (Mar) 1992; 27:200, 202, 209.

1619. De Muynck C, Colardyn F, Remon JP. Influence of intravenous administration set composition on the sorption of isosorbide dinitrate. *J Pharm Pharmacol*. 1991; 43:601–4.

1620. Bullock L, Fitzgerald JF, Walter WV. Emulsion stability in total nutrient admixtures containing a pediatric amino acid formulation. *JPEN J Parenter Enteral Nutr*. 1992; 16:64–8.

1621. Olbrich A. Weichmacher als problematische bestandteile von mischinfusionen. *Krankenhauspharmazie*. 1991; 12:192–4.

1622. Cano SM, Montoro JB, Pastor C et al. Stability of cimetidine in total parenteral nutrition. *J Clin Nutr Gastroenter*. 1987; 2:40–3.

1623. Loeppky C, Tarka E. Compatibility of cephalosporins and aminoglycosides in peritoneal dialysis fluid. *Perit Dial Bull*. 1983; 3:128–9.

1624. Bhatt-Mehta V, Rosen DA, King RS et al. Stability of midazolam hydrochloride in parenteral nutrient solutions. *Am J Hosp Pharm*. 1993; 50:285–8.

1625. Jacobson PA, Maksym CJ, Landvay A et al. Compatibility of cyclosporine with fat emulsion. *Am J Hosp Pharm*. 1993; 50:687–90.

1626. Johnson CE, Jacobson PA, Pillen HA et al. Stability and compatibility of fluconazole and aminophylline in intravenous admixtures. *Am J Hosp Pharm*. 1993; 50:703–6.

1627. Allen LV Jr, Stiles ML, Wang DP et al. Stability of bupivacaine hydrochloride, epinephrine hydrochloride, and fentanyl citrate in portable infusion-pump reservoirs. *Am J Hosp Pharm*. 1993; 50:714–5.

1628. Percy LA, Rho JP. Visual compatibility of ciprofloxacin with selected components of total parenteral nutrient solutions during simulated Y-site injection. *Am J Hosp Pharm*. 1993; 50:715–6.

1629. Nieforth KA, Shea BF, Souney PF et al. Stability of cyclosporine with magnesium sulfate in 5% dextrose injection. *Am J Hosp Pharm*. 1993; 50:470–2.

1630. Min DI, Brown T. Visual compatibility of tacrolimus with commonly used drugs during simulated Y-site injection. *Am J Hosp Pharm*. 1992; 49:2964–6.

1631. Dine T, Luyckx M, Cazin JC et al. Stability and compatibility studies of vinblastine, vincristine, vindesine and vinorelbine with PVC infusion bags. *Int J Pharm*. 1991; 77:279–85.

1632. Inagaki K, Gill MA, Okamoto MP et al. Stability of ranitidine hydrochloride with aztreonam, ceftazidime, or piperacillin sodium during simulated Y-site administration. *Am J Hosp Pharm*. 1992; 49:2769–72.

1633. Mitra AK, Narurkar MM. Kinetics of azathioprine degradation in aqueous solution. *Int J Pharm*. 1986; 35:165–71.

1634. Snyder RL. Filter clogging caused by albumin in i.v. nutrient solution. *Am J Hosp Pharm*. 1993; 50:63–4.

1635. Feldman F, Bergman G. Filter clogging caused by albumin in i.v. nutrient solution. *Am J Hosp Pharm*. 1993; 50:64.

1636. Bornstein M, Kao SH, Mercorelli M et al. Stability of an ofloxacin injection in various infusion fluids. *Am J Hosp Pharm*. 1992; 49:2756–60.

1637. Heni J. Rekonstituierte ganciclovirlosung. *Krankenhauspharmazie*. 1991; 12:342–4.

1638. Theuer H, Scherbel G. Stabilitatsuntersuchungen von fentanylcitrat i.v.. *Krankenhauspharmazie*. 1991; 12:233–45.

1639. Burger DM, Brandjes DP, Koks CH, et al. Heparine in het heparineslot? *Pharm Weekbl*. 1991; 126:624–7.

1640. Witmer DR. Heparin lock flush solution versus 0.9% sodium chloride injection for maintaining patency. *Am J Hosp Pharm*. 1993; 50:241.

1641. Weber DR. Is heparin really necessary in the lock and, if so, how much? *DICP*. 1991; 25:399–407.

1642. Bosso JA, Prince RA. Stability of ondansetron hydrochloride in injectable solutions at -20, 5, and 25 °C. *Am J Hosp Pharm*. 1992; 49:2223–5.

1643. Parasrampuria J, Li LC, Stelmach AH et al. Stability of ganciclovir sodium in 5% dextrose injection and in 0.9% sodium chloride injection over 35 days. *Am J Hosp Pharm*. 1992; 49:116–8.

1644. Guo-jie JL. Compatibility of bumetanide injection and dextrose injection. *Yaoxue Tongbao*. 1989; 24:86–7.

1645. Buck GW, Wolfe KR. Interaction of sodium ascorbate with stainless steel particulate-filter needles. *Am J Hosp Pharm*. 1991; 48:1191.

1646. Floy BJ, Royko CG. Compatibility of ketorolac tromethamine injection with common infusion fluids and administration sets. *Am J Hosp Pharm*. 1990; 47:1097–100.

1647. Zieske PA, Koberda M, Hines JL et al. Characterization of cisplatin degradation as affected by pH and light. *Am J Hosp Pharm*. 1991; 48:1500–6.

1648. Tu YH, Knox NL, Biringer JM et al. Compatibility of iron dextran with total nutrient admixtures. *Am J Hosp Pharm*. 1992; 49:2233–5.

1649. Rivers TE, McBride HA, Trang JM. Stability of cefazolin sodium and metronidazole at 8 °C for use as an i.v. admixture. *J Parenter Sci Technol*. 1993; 47:135–7.

1650. Helbock HJ, Motchnik PA. Toxic hydroperoxides in intravenous lipid emulsions used in preterm infants. *Pediatrics*. 1993; 91:83–7.

1651. Washington C, Sizer T. Stability of TPN mixtures compounded from Lipofundin S and Aminoplex amino-acid solutions: comparison of laser diffraction and Coulter counter droplet size analysis. *Int J Pharm*. 1992; 83:227–31.

1652. Mason NA, Johnson CE. Stability of ceftazidime and tobramycin sulfate in peritoneal dialysis solution. *Am J Hosp Pharm*. 1992; 49:1139–42.

1653. Brawley V, Bhatia J. Hydrogen peroxide generation in a model paediatric parenteral amino acid solution. *Clin Sci*. 1993; 85:709–12.

1654. Mawhinney WM, Adair CG, Gorman SP et al. Stability of vancomycin hydrochloride in peritoneal dialysis solution. *Am J Hosp Pharm*. 1992; 49:137–9.

1655. Cervenka P, DeJong DJ, Butler BL et al. Visual compatibility of injectable ciprofloxacin lactate with selected injectable drugs during simulated Y-site administration. *Hosp Pharm*. (Nov) 1992; 27:957–8, 961–2.

1656. Garrelts JC, LaRocca J, Ast D et al. Comparison of heparin and 0.9% sodium chloride injection in the maintenance of indwelling intermittent i.v. devices. *Clin Pharm*. 1989; 8:34–9.

1657. Lewis JS. Justification for use of 1.2 micron end-line filters on total nutrient admixtures. *Hosp Pharm*. 1993; 28:656–8.

1658. Benvenuto JA, Adams SC, Vyas HM, et al. Pharmaceutical issues in infusion chemotherapy stability and compatibility. In: Lokich JJ, ed. Cancer chemotherapy by infusion. Chicago, IL: Precept Press; 1987:100–13.

1659. Briceland LL, Fudin J. Evaluation of microbial growth in select inoculated antineoplastic solutions. *Hosp Pharm*. 1990; 25:338–40.

1660. Neels JT. Compatibility of bupivacaine hydrochloride with hydromorphone hydrochloride or morphine sulfate. *Am J Hosp Pharm*. 1992; 49:2149.

1661. Hauser AR, Trissel LA. Ondansetron compatible with sodium acetate. *J Clin Oncol*. 1993; 11:197.

1662. Pecosky DA, Parasrampuria J, Li LC et al. Stability and sorption of calcitriol in plastic tuberculin syringes. *Am J Hosp Pharm*. 1992; 49:1463–6.

1663. Gregory R, Edwards S. Demonstration of insulin transformation products in insulin vials by high-performance liquid chromatography. *Diabetes Care*. 1991; 14:42–8.

1664. Seres DS. Insulin adsorption to parenteral infusion systems: case report and review of the literature. *Nutr Clin Pract*. 1990; 5:111–7.

1665. Lazorova L, Haronikova K. Studium sorpcie inzulinu v priebehu infuznej terapie. *Farm Obz*. 1990; 59:157–64.

1666. Stolk LML, Chandi LS. Stabiliteit van fluorouracil (0,55 mg) in polypropyleen spuiten bij -20 °C. *Ziekenhuisfarmacie*. 1991; 7:12–3.

1667. de Vogel EM, Hendrikx MMP, van Dellen RT et al. Adsorptie van sufentanil aan bacteriefilters. *Ziekenhuisfarmacie*. 1991; 7:65–70.

1668. Hehenberger H. Fettemulsionen kompatibilitat wahrend der bypass-infusion. *Krankenhauspharmazie*. 1989; 10:513–8.

1669. Carstens G. Calcium-folinat uberlegungen zur stabilitat und zum einsatz verschiedener zubereitungen. *Krankenhauspharmazie*. 1989; 10:478–82.

1670. Washington C. The stability of intravenous fat emulsions in total parenteral nutrition mixtures. *Int J Pharm*. 1990; 66:1–21.

1671. Allwood MC, Brown PW. The effect of buffering on the stability of reconstituted benzylpenicillin injection. *Int J Pharm Pract*. 1992; 1:242–4.

1672. Allwood MC. The stability of diamorphine alone and in combination with anti-emetics in plastic syringes. *Palliative Med*. 1991; 5:330–3.

1673. Lober CA, Dollard PA. Visual compatibility of gallium nitrate with selected drugs during simulated Y-site injection. *Am J Hosp Pharm.* 1993; 50:1208–10.

1674. Jahns BE, Bakst CM. Extension of expiration time for lorazepam injection at room temperature. *Am J Hosp Pharm.* 1993; 50:1134.

1675. Trissel LA, Martinez JF. Idarubicin hydrochloride turbidity versus incompatibility. *Am J Hosp Pharm.* 1993; 50:1134.

1676. Hunt-Fugate AK, Hennessey CK. Stability of fluconazole injectable solutions. *Am J Hosp Pharm.* 1993; 50:1186–7.

1677. Inagaki K, Takagi J, Lor E et al. Stability of fluconazole in commonly used intravenous antibiotic solutions. *Am J Hosp Pharm.* 1993; 50:1206–8.

1678. Liao E, Fox JL. Inline filtration of ondansetron hydrochloride during simulated i.v. administration. *Am J Hosp Pharm.* 1993; 50:906.

1679. Belliveau PP, Shea BF. Stability of metoprolol tartrate in 5% dextrose injection or 0.9% sodium chloride injection. *Am J Hosp Pharm.* 1993; 50:950–2.

1680. Ringwood MA. Stability of cefepime for injection for IM or IV use following constitution/dilution. Syracuse, NY: Bristol-Myers Company; 1990 Aug 16.

1681. Ringwood MA, Vance VH. Cefepime IM, IV, and compatibility studies for U.S. registrational filing. Syracuse, NY: Bristol-Myers Company; 1992 May 13.

1682. Vance VH. Stability of cefepime admixed with vancomycin, metronidazole, ampicillin, clindamycin, tobramycin, netilmicin, TPN solution, and PD solution. Syracuse, NY: Bristol-Myers Company; 1992 Oct 14.

1683. Pearson SD, Trissel LA. Leaching of diethylhexyl phthalate from polyvinyl chloride containers by selected drugs and formulation components. *Am J Hosp Pharm.* 1993; 50:1405–9.

1684. Trissel LA, Pearson SD. Storage of lorazepam in three injectable solutions in polyvinyl chloride and polyolefin bags. *Am J Hosp Pharm.* 1994; 51:368–72.

1686. Trissel LA, Martinez JF. Compatibility of allopurinol sodium with selected drugs during simulated Y-site administration. *Am J Hosp Pharm.* 1994; 51:1792–9.

1687. Trissel LA, Martinez JF. Compatibility of filgrastim with selected drugs during simulated Y-site administration. *Am J Hosp Pharm.* 1994; 51:1907–13.

1688. Trissel LA, Martinez JF. Compatibility of piperacillin sodium plus tazobactam sodium with selected drugs during simulated Y-site injection. *Am J Hosp Pharm.* 1994; 51:672–8.

1690. Trissel LA, Xu Q, Martinez JF et al. Compatibility and stability of ondansetron hydrochloride with morphine sulfate and hydromorphone hydrochloride in 0.9% sodium chloride injection at various temperatures. *Am J Hosp Pharm.* 1994; 51:2138–42.

1691. Belliveau PP, Nightingale CH. Stability of aztreonam and ampicillin/sulbactam in 0.9% saline for injection. *Am J Hosp Pharm.* 1994; 51:901–4.

1692. Fisher DM, Canfell C. Stability of atracurium administered by infusion. *Anesthesiology.* 1984; 61:347–8.

1693. Harper NJ, Pollard BJ, Edwards D et al. Stability of atracurium in dilute solutions. *Br J Anaesth.* 1988; 60:344P–345P.

1694. Talton MA (Drug Information, Burroughs Wellcome Company, Research Triangle Park, NC): Personal communication; 1993 Jun 11.

1695. Perrone RK, Kaplan MA. Extent of cisplatin formation in carboplatin admixtures. *Am J Hosp Pharm.* 1989; 46:258–9.

1696. Northcott M, Allsopp MA, Powell H et al. The stability of carboplatin, diamorphine, 5–fluorouracil and mitozantrone infusions in an ambulatory pump under storage and prolonged "in-use" conditions. *J Clin Pharm Ther.* 1991; 16:123–9.

1697. Ahmed ST, Parkinson R. The stability of drugs in pre-filled syringes: flucloxacillin, ampicillin, cefuroxime, cefotaxime, and ceftazidime. *Hosp Pharm Pract.* 1992; 2:285–9.

1698. Faouzi MA, Dine T, Luyckx M et al. Stability and compatibility studies of pefloxacin, ofloxacin and ciprofloxacin with PVC infusion bags. *Int J Pharm.* 1993; 89:125–31.

1699. Stiles ML, Allen LV Jr. Gas production of three brands of ceftazidime. *Am J Hosp Pharm.* 1991; 48:1727–9.

1700. Dine T, Cazin JC, Gressier B et al. Stability and compatibility of four anthracyclines: doxorubicin, epirubicin, daunorubicin, and pirarubicin with PVC infusion bags. *Pharm Weekbl [Sci].* 1992; 14:365–9.

1701. Trissel LA, Martinez JF. Sargramostim incompatibility. *Hosp Pharm.* 1992; 27:929.

1702. Trissel LA. Alternative interpretation for data. *Am J Hosp Pharm.* 1992; 49:570.

1703. Knapp AJ, Mauro VF. Incompatibility of ketorolac tromethamine with selected postoperative drugs. *Am J Hosp Pharm.* 1992; 49:2960–2.

1705. Cohon MS (Clinical Development and Medical Affairs, The Upjohn Company, Kalamazoo, MI): Personal communication; 1993 Dec 6.

1706. Chandler SW, Trissel LA, Weinstein SM. Combined administration of opioids with selected drugs to manage pain and other cancer symptoms: initial safety screening for compatibility. *J Pain Symptom Manage.* 1996; 12:168–71.

1707. Nation RL, Hackett LP. Uptake of clonazepam by plastic intravenous infusion bags and administration sets. *Am J Hosp Pharm.* 1983; 40:1692–3.

1708. Hooymans PM, Janknegt R. Comparison of clonazepam sorption to polyvinyl chloride-coated and polyethylene-coated tubings. *Pharm Weekbl [Sci].* 1990; 12:188–9.

1709. McLaughlin JP, Simpson C. The stability of reconstituted diethanolamine fusidate in a 5% dextrose infusion. *Hosp Pharm Pract.* 1992; 2:59–62.

1710. Olsen KM, Gurley BJ, Davis GA et al. Stability of flumazenil with selected drugs in 5% dextrose injection. *Am J Hosp Pharm.* 1993; 50:1907–12.

1711. Food and Drug Administration. Center for Drug Evaluation and Research. Application number: 20-9401Orig1s000: Multi-Discipline Review. From FDA website.

1712. Larson PO, Ragi G, Swandby M et al. Stability of buffered lidocaine and epinephrine used for local anesthesia. *J Dermatol Surg Oncol.* 1991; 17:411–4.

1713. Stewart JH, Cole GW. Neutralized lidocaine with epinephrine for local anesthesia. *J Dermatol Surg Oncol.* 1989; 15:1081–3.

1714. Nahata MC, Morosco RS. Stability of cimetidine hydrochloride and of clindamycin phosphate in water for injection stored in glass vials at two temperatures. *Am J Hosp Pharm*. 1993; 50:2559–61.

1715. Zeisler J, Alagna C. Incompatibility of labetalol hydrochloride and furosemide. *Am J Hosp Pharm*. 1993; 50:2521–2.

1716. Pfeifer RW, Hale KN. Precipitation of paclitaxel during infusion by pump. *Am J Hosp Pharm*. 1993; 50:2518.

1717. Hagan RL, Jacobs LF, Pimsler M et al. Stability of midazolam hydrochloride in 5% dextrose injection or 0.9% sodium chloride injection over 30 days. *Am J Hosp Pharm*. 1993; 50:2379–81.

1718. Jones JW, Davis AT. Stability of bupivacaine hydrochloride in polypropylene syringes. *Am J Hosp Pharm*. 1993; 50:2364–5.

1719. Vogt C, Skipper PM. Compatibility of magnesium sulfate and morphine sulfate in 0.9% sodium chloride injection. *Am J Hosp Pharm*. 1993; 50:2311.

1720. Bailey LC, Tang KT. Stability of ceftriaxone sodium in infusion-pump syringes. *Am J Hosp Pharm*. 1993; 50:2092–4.

1721. Szof C, Walker PC. Incompatibility of cefotaxime sodium and vancomycin sulfate during Y-site administration. *Am J Hosp Pharm*. 1993; 50:2054.

1722. Jhee SS, Jeong EW, Chin A et al. Stability of ondansetron hydrochloride stored in a disposable, elastomeric infusion device at 4 °C. *Am J Hosp Pharm*. 1993; 50:1918–20.

1723. Bartfield JM, Homer PJ, Ford DT et al. Buffered lidocaine as a local anesthetic: an investigation of shelf life. *Ann Emerg Med*. 1992; 21:16–9.

1724. Peterfreund RA, Datta S. pH adjustment of local anesthetic solutions with sodium bicarbonate: laboratory evaluation of alkalinization and precipitation. *Reg Anesth*. 1989; 14:265–70.

1725. Trissel LA, Martinez JF. Screening teniposide for Y-site physical incompatibilities. *Hosp Pharm*. 1994; 29:1012–4.

1726. Woods K, Steinman W, Bruns L et al. Stability of foscarnet sodium in 0.9% sodium chloride injection. *Am J Hosp Pharm*. 1994; 51:88–90.

1727. Parrish MA, Bailey LC. Stability of ceftriaxone sodium and aminophylline or theophylline in intravenous admixtures. *Am J Hosp Pharm*. 1994; 51:92–4.

1728. Lee MD, Hess MM, Boucher BA et al. Stability of amphotericin B in 5% dextrose injection stored at 4 or 25 °C for 120 hours. *Am J Hosp Pharm*. 1994; 51:394–6.

1729. Dukes MNG (ed). Meyler's side effects of drugs. Vol 8. Amsterdam, Holland: Excerpta Medica; 1975:745.

1730. Pompilio FM, Fox JL, Inagaki K et al. Stability of ranitidine hydrochloride with ondansetron hydrochloride or fluconazole during simulated Y-site administration. *Am J Hosp Pharm*. 1994; 51:391–4.

1731. Wolff DJ, Kline SS. Stability of amikacin, gentamicin, or tobramycin in 10% dextrose injection. *Am J Hosp Pharm*. 1994; 51:518–9.

1732. Bosso JA, Prince RA. Compatibility of ondansetron hydrochloride with fluconazole, ceftazidime, aztreonam, and cefazolin sodium under simulated Y-site conditions. *Am J Hosp Pharm*. 1994; 51:389–91.

1733. Stiles ML, Allen LV Jr, Prince SJ et al. Stability of dexamethasone sodium phosphate, diphenhydramine hydrochloride, lorazepam, and metoclopramide hydrochloride in portable infusion-pump reservoirs. *Am J Hosp Pharm*. 1994; 51:514–7.

1734. Messerschmidt W. Kompatibilitat von ofloxacin mit ampicillin. *Krankenhauspharmazie*. 1994; 15:337–40.

1735. Messerschmidt W. Kompatibilitat von cefotaxim mit ofloxacin. *Pharmazie*. 1991; 136:42–4.

1736. Wyeth Laboratories Inc. Cyanocobalamin (vitamin B_{12}) injection prescribing information. Philadelphia, PA; 1984 Jan.

1737. Messerschmidt W. Kompatibilitat von cefotiam mit metronidazol. *Krankenhauspharmazie*. 1986; 7:263–5.

1738. Messerschmidt W. Pharmazeutische kompatibilitat der kombination cefotiam und ampicillin. *Krankenhauspharmazie*. 1992; 13:98–100.

1739. Cronquist SE, Daniels M. Precipitation of paclitaxel during infusion by pump. *Am J Hosp Pharm*. 1993; 50:2521.

1740. Fraser GL, Riker RR. Visual compatibility of haloperidol lactate with injectable solutions. *Am J Hosp Pharm*. 1994; 51:905–6.

1741. Burm JP, Jhee SS, Chin A et al. Stability of paclitaxel with ondansetron hydrochloride or ranitidine hydrochloride during simulated Y-site administration. *Am J Hosp Pharm*. 1994; 51:1201–4.

1742. Mulye NV, Turco SJ. Stability of ganciclovir sodium in an infusion-pump syringe. *Am J Hosp Pharm*. 1994; 51:1348–9.

1743. Bonhomme L, Benhamou D, Comoy E et al. Stability of adrenaline pH-adjusted solutions of local anaesthetics. *J Pharm Biomed Anal*. 1991; 9:497–9.

1744. Johnson CE, Jacobson PA. Stability of ganciclovir sodium and amino acids in parenteral nutrient solutions. *Am J Hosp Pharm*. 1994; 51:503–8.

1745. Abubakar AA, Mustapha A. An in vitro chemical interaction between promethazine hydrochloride and chloroquine phosphate. *Int J Pharm*. 1993; 7:14–9.

1746. Xu Q, Trissel LA. Stability of paclitaxel in 5% dextrose injection or 0.9% sodium chloride injection at 4, 22, or 32 °C. *Am J Hosp Pharm*. 1994; 51:3058–60.

1747. Kearney AS, Patel K. Preformulation studies to aid in the development of a ready-to-use injectable solution of the antitumor agent, topotecan. *Int J Pharm*. 1996; 127:229–37.

1748. Cilissen J, Hooymans PM. Indicatie van de stabiliteit van een mengsel van piperacilline en flucloxacilline in een reservoir voor een draagbare infusiepomp. *Ziekenhuisfarmacie*. 1994; 10:10–1.

1749. Banerjee PS, Ghosh LK. Studies on the effects of some additives on the stability of injectable formulations of diazepam. *Indian Drugs*. 1992; 29:361–4.

1750. Lorillon P, Corbel JC, Mordelet MF et al. Photosensibilite du 5-fluoro-uracile et du methotrexate dans des perfuseurs translucides ou opaques. *J Pharm Clin*. 1992; 11:285–95.

1751. Brouwers JRBJ, van Doorne H, Meevis RF et al. Stability of sufentanil citrate and sufentanil citrate/bupivacaine mixture in portable infusion pump reservoirs. *Eur Hosp Pharm*. 1995; 1:12–4.

1752. Chung KC, Moon YSK, Chin A et al. Compatibility of ondansetron hydrochloride and piperacillin sodium-tazobactam sodium during simulated Y-site administration. *Am J Health-Syst Pharm*. 1995; 52:1554–6.

1753. Erickson SH, Ulici D. Incompatibility of cefotetan disodium and promethazine hydrochloride. *Am J Health-Syst Pharm*. 1995; 52:1347.

1754. Belliveau PP, Nightingale CH. Stability of cefotaxime sodium and metronidazole in 0.9% sodium chloride injection or in ready-to-use metronidazole bags. *Am J Health-Syst Pharm*. 1995; 52:1561–3.

1755. Roos PJ, Glerum JH. Stability of sufentanil citrate in a portable pump reservoir, a glass container and a polyethylene container. *Pharm Weekbl [Sci]*. 1992; 14:196–200.

1756. Roos PJ, Glerum JH, Schroeders MJ. Effect of glucose 5% solution and bupivacaine hydrochloride on absorption of sufentanil citrate in a portable pump reservoir during storage and simulated infusion by an epidural catheter. *Pharm World Sci*. 1993; 15:269–75.

1757. Benaji B, Dine T, Luyckx M et al. Stability and compatibility of cisplatin and carboplatin with PVC infusion bags. *J Clin Pharm Ther*. 1994; 19:95–100.

1758. Trissel LA, Martinez JF. Compatibility of aztreonam with selected drugs during simulated Y-site administration. *Am J Health-Syst Pharm*. 1995; 52:1086–90.

1759. Choi JS, Burm JP, Jhee SS et al. Stability of piperacillin sodium-tazobactam sodium and ranitidine hydrochloride in 0.9% sodium chloride injection during simulated Y-site administration. *Am J Hosp Pharm*. 1994; 51:2273–6.

1760. Ishisaka DY. Visual compatibility of fluconazole with drugs given by continuous infusion. *Am J Hosp Pharm*. 1994; 51:2290.

1761. Fawcett JP, Woods DJ, Munasiri B et al. Compatibility of cyclizine lactate and haloperidol lactate. *Am J Hosp Pharm*. 1994; 51:2292.

1762. Hassan E, Leslie J. Stability of labetalol hydrochloride with selected critical care drugs during simulated Y-site injection. *Am J Hosp Pharm*. 1994; 51:2143–5.

1763. Wang DP, Chang LC, Wong CY et al. Stability of cefazolin sodium-famotidine admixture. *Am J Hosp Pharm*. 1994; 51:2205.

1764. Singh RF, Corelli RL. Sterility of unit dose syringes of filgrastim and sargramostim. *Am J Hosp Pharm*. 1994; 51:2811–2.

1765. Kleinberg ML. Sterility of repackaged filgrastim and sargramostim. *Am J Health-Syst Pharm*. 1995; 52:1101.

1766. Kirkham JC, Rutherford ET, Cunningham GN et al. Stability of ondansetron hydrochloride in a total parenteral nutrient admixture. *Am J Health-Syst Pharm*. 1995; 52:1557–8.

1767. Gilbar PJ, Groves CF. Visual compatibility of total parenteral nutrition solution (Synthamin 17 premix) with selected drugs during simulated Y-site injection. *Aust J Hosp Pharm*. 1994; 24:167–70.

1768. Moon YSK, Chung KC, Chin A et al. Stability of piperacillin sodium-tazobactam sodium in polypropylene syringes and polyvinyl chloride minibags. *Am J Health-Syst Pharm*. 1995; 52:999–1001.

1769. Lumpkin MM, Burlington DB. Safety alert: hazards of precipitation associated with parenteral nutrition. *Am J Hosp Pharm*. 1994; 51:1427–8.

1770. Hasegawa GR. Caring about stability and compatibility. *Am J Hosp Pharm*. 1994; 51:1533–4.

1771. Trissel LA. Compounding our problems. *Am J Hosp Pharm*. 1994; 51:1534.

1772. Mirtallo JM. The complexity of mixing calcium and phosphate. *Am J Hosp Pharm*. 1994; 51:1535–6.

1773. Koorenhof MJC, Timmer JG. Stability of total parenteral nutrition supplied as "all-in-one" for children with chemotherapy-linked hyperhydration. *Pharm Weekbl [Sci]*. 1992; 14:50–4.

1774. Picard C, Brazier M, Hary L et al. Stabilite de quatre solutions de penicillines dans des poches et tubulures de perfusion en PVC plastifie. *J Pharm Clin*. 1992; 11:302–5.

1775. Szucsova S, Sykora J. Stablita injekcneho pripravku celaskon v infuznych zmesiach. *Farm Obzor*. 1992; 61:109–12.

1776. Walker SE, Iazzetta J, De Angelis C et al. Stability and compatibility of combinations of hydromorphone and dimenhydrinate, lorazepam or prochlorperazine. *Can J Hosp Pharm*. 1993; 46:61–5.

1777. Maswoswe JJ, Okpara AU. An old nemesis: calcium and phosphate interaction in TPN admixtures. *Hosp Pharm*. (July) 1995; 30:579–80, 582–6.

1778. Deardorff DL, Schmidt CN, Wiley RA. Effect of preparation techniques on mixing of additives in intravenous fluids in nonrigid containers. *Hosp Pharm*. (Apr) 1993; 28:306, 309–10, 312–3.

1779. Stiles ML, Allen LV Jr. Stability of various antibiotics kept in an insulated pouch during administration via portable infusion pump. *Am J Health-Syst Pharm*. 1995; 52:70–4.

1780. Wang DP, Chang LC, Lee DKT et al. Stability of fluorouracil-metoclopramide hydrochloride admixture. *Am J Health-Syst Pharm*. 1995; 52:98–9.

1781. Jackson CW, Cunningham K. Compatibility of haloperidol lactate with benztropine mesylate. *Am J Hosp Pharm*. 1994; 51:2962–3.

1782. Mirtallo JM. Should the use of total nutrient admixtures be limited? *Am J Hosp Pharm*. 1994; 51(22):2831–4.

1783. Driscoll DF, Newton DW. Precipitation of calcium phosphate from parenteral nutrient fluids. *Am J Hosp Pharm*. 1994; 51:2834–6.

1784. Gibler B, Kim MS. Visual compatibility of neuroleptics with anticholinergics or antihistamines in polyethylene syringes. *Am J Hosp Pharm*. 1994; 51:2709–10.

1785. Huang E, Anderson RP. Compatibility of hydromorphone hydrochloride with haloperidol lactate and ketorolac tromethamine. *Am J Hosp Pharm*. 1994; 51:2963.

1786. Mendenhall A, Hoyt DB. Incompatibility of ketorolac tromethamine with haloperidol lactate and thiethylperazine maleate. *Am J Hosp Pharm*. 1994; 51:2964.

1787. Harraki B, Guiraud P, Rochat MH et al. Influence of copper, iron, and zinc on the physicochemical properties of parenteral admixture. *J Parenter Sci Technol*. 1993; 47:199–204.

1788. Aujoulat P, Coze C, Braguer D et al. Compatibilite physico-chimique du methotrexate avec les medicaments co-administres dans les protocols de chimiotherapie. *J Pharm Clin*. 1993; 12:31–5.

1789. Johnson CE, Bhatt-Mehta V, Mancari SC et al. Stability of midazolam hydrochloride and morphine sulfate during simulated intravenous coadministration. *Am J Hosp Pharm.* 1994; 51:2812–3.

1790. Burm JP, Choi JS, Jhee SS et al. Stability of paclitaxel and fluconazole during simulated Y-site administration. *Am J Hosp Pharm.* 1994; 51:2704–6.

1791. Grassby PF, Roberts DE. Stability of epidural opiate solutions in 0.9 per cent sodium chloride infusion bags. *Int J Pharm Pract.* 1995; 3:174–7.

1792. Allwood MC, Brown PW. Stability of injections containing diamorphine and midazolam in plastic syringes. *Int J Pharm Pract.* 1994; 3:57–9.

1793. Kershaw BP, Monnier HL, Mason JH. Visual compatibility of premixed theophylline or heparin with selected drugs for i.v. administration. *Am J Hosp Pharm.* 1362–3 (July) 1993; 50:1360.

1794. Trissel LA. Were the bubbles evolved or entrained? *Am J Health-Syst Pharm.* 1995; 52(7):757.

1795. Francomb MM, Ford JL. Adsorption of vincristine, doxorubicin and mitoxantrone to in-line intravenous filters. *Int J Pharm.* 1994; 103:87–92.

1796. Salomies HEM, Heinonen RM. Sorptive loss of diazepam, nitroglycerin and warfarin sodium to polypropylene-lined infusion bags (Softbags). *Int J Pharm.* 1994; 110:197–201.

1797. Chen YH, Wu PC, Shiea J et al. Evaluation of the sterility, stability, and efficacy of bevacizumab stored in multiple-dose vials for 6 months. *J Ocul Pharmacol Ther.* 2009; 25:65–9.

1798. Bianchi C, Airaudo CB. Sorption studies of dipotassium clorazepate salt (Tranxene) and midazolam hydrochloride (Hypnovel) in polyvinyl chloride and glass infusion containers. *J Clin Pharm Ther.* 1992; 17:223–7.

1799. Sautou V, Chopineau J, Gremeau I et al. Compatibility with medical plastics and stability of continuously and simultaneously infused isosorbide dinitrate and heparin. *Int J Pharm.* 1994; 107:111–19.

1800. Mitchell CL (Leo Pharmaceuticals, Buckinghamshire, United Kingdom): Personal communication; 1998 Sep 11.

1801. Hadzija BW, Lubarsky DA. Compatibility of etomidate, thiopental sodium, and propofol injections with drugs commonly administered during induction of anesthesia. *Am J Health-Syst Pharm.* 1995; 52:997–9.

1802. Stewart JT, Warren FW. Stability of ranitidine hydrochloride and seven medications. *Am J Hosp Pharm.* 1994; 51:1802–7.

1803. Palmquist KL, Quattrocchi FP. Compatibility of furosemide with 20% mannitol. *Am J Health-Syst Pharm.* 1995; 52:648.

1804. Trissel LA, Martinez JF. Compatibility of granisetron hydrochloride with selected alkaline drugs. *Am J Health-Syst Pharm.* 1995; 52:208.

1805. Bhatt-Mehta V, Paglia RE. Stability of propofol with parenteral nutrient solutions during simulated Y-site injection. *Am J Health-Syst Pharm.* 1995; 52:192–6.

1806. Hagan RL, Carr-Lopez SM. Stability of nafcillin sodium in the presence of lidocaine hydrochloride. *Am J Health-Syst Pharm.* 1995; 52:521–3.

1807. Gayed AA, Keshary PR. Visual compatibility of diltiazem injection with various diluents and medications during simulated Y-site injection. *Am J Health-Syst Pharm.* 1995; 52:516–20.

1808. Trissel LA. Amphotericin B does not mix with fat emulsion. *Am J Health-Syst Pharm.* 1995; 52:1463–4.

1809. Kirsch R, Goldstein R, Tarloff J et al. An emulsion formulation of amphotericin B improves the therapeutic index when treating systemic murine candidiasis. *J Infect Dis.* 1988; 158:1065–70.

1810. Chavenet PY, Garry I, Charlier N et al. Trial of glucose versus fat emulsion in preparation of amphotericin for use in HIV infected patients with candidiasis. *BMJ.* 1992; 305:921–5.

1811. Caillot D, Casanova O, Solary E et al. Efficacy and tolerance of an amphotericin B lipid (Intralipid) emulsion in the treatment of candidaemia in neutropenic patients. *J Antimicrob Chemother.* 1993; 31:161–9.

1812. Fleming RA, Olsen DJ, Savage PD et al. Stability of ondansetron hydrochloride and cyclophosphamide in injectable solutions. *Am J Health-Syst Pharm.* 1995; 52:514–6.

1813. Driscoll DF. Total nutrient admixtures: theory and practice. *Nutr Clin Pract.* 1995; 10:114–9.

1814. Driscoll DF, Bhargava HN, Li L et al. Physicochemical stability of total nutrient admixtures. *Am J Health-Syst Pharm.* 1995; 52:623–34.

1815. Pettei MJ, Israel D, Levine J. Serum vitamin K concentration in pediatric patients receiving total parenteral nutrition. *JPEN J Parenter Enteral Nutr.* 1993; 17:465–7.

1816. Trissel LA, Martinez JF. Incompatibility of fluorouracil with leucovorin calcium or levoleucovorin calcium. *Am J Health-Syst Pharm.* 1995; 52:710–5.

1817. Montoya Garcia-Reol C, Sevilla Azzati E, Negro Vega E et al. Estudio de la estabilidad de la mezcla fluorouracilo/folinato calcico en fluidos intravenosos. *Farm Hosp.* 1993; 17:99–103.

1818. Ward GH, Yalkowsky SH. Studies in phlebitis VI: dilution-induced precipitation of amiodarone HCl. *J Parenter Sci Technol.* 1993; 47:161–5.

1819. Ward GH, Yalkowsky SH. Studies in phlebitis IV: injection rate and amiodarone-induced phlebitis. *J Parenter Sci Technol.* 1993; 47:40–3.

1820. Allwood MC, Brown PW. Stability of ampicillin infusions in unbuffered and buffered saline. *Int J Pharm.* 1993; 97:219–22.

1821. Lauper RD (Professional Services, Cetus Oncology Corporation, Emeryville, CA): Personal communication; 1993 Dec 20.

1822. Allen LV. Plasminogen activator. *US Pharmacist.* 1992; 17:64–5, 70–1.

1823. Rochard E, Barthes D. Stability and compatibility of carboplatin with three portable infusion pump reservoirs. *Int J Pharm.* 1994; 101:257–62.

1824. Bailey LC, Cappel KM. Stability of ceftriaxone sodium in injectable solutions stored frozen in syringes. *Am J Hosp Pharm.* 1994; 51:2159–61.

1825. Mazzo DJ, Nguyen-Huu JJ, Pagniez S et al. Compatibility of docetaxel and paclitaxel in intravenous solutions with polyvinyl chloride infusion materials. *Am J Health-Syst Pharm.* 1997; 54:566–9.

1826. Kane MP, Bailie GR, Moon DG et al. Stability of ciprofloxacin injection in peritoneal dialysis solutions. *Am J Hosp Pharm.* 1994; 51:373–7.

1827. Rochard E, Barthes D. Stability of cisplatin in ethylene vinylacetate portable infusion-pump reservoirs. *J Clin Pharm Ther.* 1992; 17:315–8.

1828. Pujol Cubells M, Prat Aixela J, Girona Brumos V et al. Stability of cisplatin in sodium chloride 0.9% intravenous solution related to the container's material. *Pharm World Sci.* 1993; 15:34–6.

1829. Islam MS, Asker AF. Photostabilization of dacarbazine with reduced glutathione. *J Pharm Sci Technol.* 1994; 48:38–40.

1830. Wiest DB, Garner SS. Stability of esmolol hydrochloride in 5% dextrose injection. *Am J Health-Syst Pharm.* 1995; 52:716–8.

1831. Baaske DM, Dykstra SD, Wagenknecht DM et al. Stability of esmolol hydrochloride in intravenous solutions. *Am J Hosp Pharm.* 1994; 51:2693–6.

1832. Woloschuk DMM, Nazeravich DR. Etoposide precipitation. *Can J Hosp Pharm.* 1992; 45:136.

1833. Barthes DMC, Rochard EB, Pouliquen IJ et al. Stability and compatibility of etoposide in 0.9% sodium chloride injection in three containers. *Am J Hosp Pharm.* 1994; 51:2706–9.

1834. Mathew M, Gupta VD. Stability of foscarnet sodium in 5% dextrose and 0.9% sodium chloride injections. *J Clin Pharm Ther.* 1994; 19:35–6.

1835. Stolk LM, Hendrikse H. Autoclave and long-term sterility of foscarnet sodium admixtures. *Am J Health-Syst Pharm.* 1995; 52:103.

1836. Phaypradith S, Vigneron J, Perrin A et al. Stabilite des solutions diluees de ganciclovir sodique (Cymevan) en seringues polypropylene et en poches PVC pour perfusions. *J Pharm Belg.* 1992; 47:494–8.

1837. Chung KC, Chin A. Stability of granisetron hydrochloride in a disposable elastomeric infusion device. *Am J Health-Syst Pharm.* 1995; 52:1541–3.

1838. Flahive E (Medical Information, Ortho-McNeil, Raritan, NJ): Personal communication; 1995 Apr 6.

1839. Anon. ASHP therapeutic position statement on the institutional use of 0.9% sodium chloride injection to maintain patency of peripheral indwelling intermittent infusion devices. *Am J Hosp Pharm.* 1994; 51:1572–4.

1840. Nahata MC, Morosco RS. Stability of lorazepam diluted in bacteriostatic water for injection at two temperatures. *J Clin Pharm Ther.* 1993; 18:69–71.

1841. Pinguet F, Martel P, Rouanet P et al. Effect of sodium chloride concentration and temperature on melphalan stability during storage and use. *Am J Hosp Pharm.* 1994; 51:2701–4.

1842. Chin A, Ramakrishnan RR, Yoshimura NN et al. Paclitaxel stability and compatibility in polyolefin containers. *Ann Pharmacother.* 1994; 28:35–6.

1843. Trissel LA, Xu Q, Kwan J et al. Compatibility of paclitaxel injection vehicle with intravenous administration and extension sets. *Am J Hosp Pharm.* 1994; 51:2804–10.

1844. McLaughlin JP, Simpson C, Taylor RA. When is flucloxacillin stable? *Hosp Pharm Pract.* 1993; 553–6.

1845. Trissel LA, Martinez JF. Compatibility of amifostine with selected drugs during simulated Y-site administration. *Am J Health-Syst Pharm.* 1995; 52:2208–12.

1846. Henry DW, Marshall JL, Nazzaro D et al. Stability of cisplatin and ondansetron hydrochloride in admixtures for continuous infusion. *Am J Health-Syst Pharm.* 1995; 52:2570–3.

1847. Mantong ML, Marquardt ED. Visual compatibility of midazolam hydrochloride with selected drugs during simulated Y-site injection. *Am J Health-Syst Pharm.* 1995; 52:2567–8.

1848. Trissel LA, Xu QA. Compatibility and stability of aztreonam and vancomycin hydrochloride. *Am J Health-Syst Pharm.* 1995; 52:2560–4.

1849. Rivers TE, Webster AA. Stability of ceftizoxime sodium, ceftriaxone sodium, and ceftazidime with metronidazole in ready-to-use metronidazole bags. *Am J Health-Syst Pharm.* 1995; 52:2568–70.

1850. Wulf H, Gleim M. The stability of mixtures of morphine hydrochloride, bupivacaine hydrochloride, and clonidine hydrochloride in portable pump reservoirs for the management of chronic pain syndromes. *J Pain Symptom Manage.* 1994; 9:308–11.

1851. Korth-Bradley JM, Ludwig S. Incompatibility of amiodarone hydrochloride and sodium bicarbonate injections. *Am J Health-Syst Pharm.* 1995; 52:2340.

1852. Bhatt-Mehta V, Johnson CE, Leininger N et al. Stability of fentanyl citrate and midazolam hydrochloride during simulated intravenous coadministration. *Am J Health-Syst Pharm.* 1995; 52:511–3.

1853. Matuschka PR, Smith WR. Compatibility of mannitol and sodium bicarbonate in injectable fluids. *Am J Health-Syst Pharm.* 1995; 52:320–1.

1854. Ku YM, Min DI, Kumar V et al. Compatibility of tacrolimus injection with cimetidine hydrochloride injection in 0.9% sodium chloride injection. *Am J Health-Syst Pharm.* 1995; 52:2024–5.

1855. Swart EL, Mooren RAG. Compatibility of midazolam hydrochloride and lorazepam with selected drugs during simulated Y-site administration. *Am J Health-Syst Pharm.* 1995; 52:2020–2.

1856. Lam XM, Ward CA. Stability and activity of alteplase with injectable drugs commonly used in cardiac therapy. *Am J Health-Syst Pharm.* 1995; 52:1904–9.

1857. Alex S, Gupta SL, Minor JR et al. Compatibility and activity of aldesleukin (recombinant interleukin-2) in presence of selected drugs during simulated Y-site administration: evaluation of three methods. *Am J Health-Syst Pharm.* 1995; 52:2423–6.

1858. Mancano MA, Boullata JI, Gelone SP et al. Availability of lorazepam after simulated administration from glass and polyvinyl chloride containers. *Am J Health-Syst Pharm.* 1995; 52:2213–6.

1859. McMullin ST, Burns Schaif RA. Stability of midazolam hydrochloride in polyvinyl chloride bags under fluorescent light. *Am J Health-Syst Pharm.* 1995; 52:2018–20.

1860. Bednar DA, Klutman NE, Henry DW et al. Stability of ceftazidime (with arginine) in an elastomeric infusion device. *Am J Health-Syst Pharm.* 1995; 52:1912–4.

1861. Trissel LA, Martinez JF. Compatibility of thiotepa (lyophilized) with selected drugs during simulated Y-site administration. *Am J Health-Syst Pharm*. 1996; 53:1041–5.

1862. Xu QA, Trissel LA. Compatibility of ondansetron hydrochloride with meperidine hydrochloride for combined administration. *Ann Pharmacother*. 1995; 29:1106–9.

1863. Bleasel MD, Peterson GM. Stability of midazolam in sodium chloride infusion packs. *Aust J Hosp Pharm*. 1993; 23:260–2.

1864. Taormina D, Abdallah HY, Venkataramanan R et al. Stability and sorption of FK 506 in 5% dextrose injection and 0.9% sodium chloride injection in glass, polyvinyl chloride, and polyolefin containers. *Am J Hosp Pharm*. 1992; 49:119–22.

1865. Stiles ML, Allen LV Jr. Stability of ranitidine hydrochloride during simulated home-care use. *Am J Hosp Pharm*. 1994; 51:1706–7.

1866. Dorr RT, Liddil JD. Stability of mitomycin C in different infusion fluids: compatibility with heparin and glucocorticoids. *J Oncol Pharm Pract*. 1995; 1:19–24.

1867. Benaji B, Dine T, Goudaliez F et al. Compatibility study of methotrexate with PVC bags after repackaging into two types of infusion admixtures. *Int J Pharm*. 1994; 105:83–7.

1868. Sanchez Alcaraz A, Quintana Vergara B. Estabilidad del midazolam en soluciones intravenosas gran volumen. *Farm Hosp*. 1992; 16:393–8.

1869. Trissel LA. Concentration-dependent precipitation of sodium bicarbonate with ciprofloxacin lactate. *Am J Health-Syst Pharm*. 1996; 53:84–5.

1870. Christen C, Johnson CE. Stability of bupivacaine hydrochloride and hydromorphone hydrochloride during simulated epidural coadministration. *Am J Health-Syst Pharm*. 1996; 53:170–3.

1871. Mewborn AL, Kessler JM. Compatibility and activity of enoxaparin sodium in 0.9% sodium chloride injection for 48 hours. *Am J Health-Syst Pharm*. 1996; 53:167–9.

1872. Ericsson O, Hallmen AC. Amphotericin B incompatible with lipid emulsion. *Ann Pharmacother*. 1996; 30:298.

1873. Hoey LL, Vance-Bryan K, Clarens DM et al. Lorazepam stability in parenteral solutions for continuous intravenous administration. *Ann Pharmacother*. 1996; 30:343–6.

1874. Nyhammar EK, Johansson SG. Stability of doxorubicin hydrochloride and vincristine sulfate in two portable infusion-pump reservoirs. *Am J Health-Syst Pharm*. 1996; 53:1171–3.

1875. Chin A, Moon YSK, Chung KC et al. Stability of granisetron hydrochloride with dexamethasone sodium phosphate for 14 days. *Am J Health-Syst Pharm*. 1996; 53:1174–6.

1876. Stewart JT, Warren FW, King DT et al. Stability of ondansetron hydrochloride and five antineoplastic medications. *Am J Health-Syst Pharm*. 1996; 53:1297–300.

1877. Yamashita SK, Walker SE, Choudhury T et al. Compatibility of selected critical care drugs during simulated Y-site administration. *Am J Health-Syst Pharm*. 1996; 53:1048–51.

1878. Ohls RK, Christensen RD. Stability of human recombinant epoetin alfa in commonly used neonatal intravenous solutions. *Ann Pharmacother*. 1996; 30:466–8.

1879. Nahata MC, Edmonds JJ. Stability of metronidazole and ceftizoxime sodium in ready-to-use metronidazole bags stored at 4 and 25°C. *Am J Health-Syst Pharm*. 1996; 53:1046–8.

1880. Lewis JD, El-Gendy A. Cephalosporin-pentamidine isethionate incompatibilities. *Am J Health-Syst Pharm*. 1996; 53:1461–2.

1881. Tanque N, Ueda H, Moriyama Y et al. Compatibility of irinotecan hydrochloride injection with other injections. *Jpn J Hosp Pharm*. 1996; 22:457–65.

1882. Hagan RL, Mallett MS. Stability of ondansetron hydrochloride and dexamethasone sodium phosphate in infusion bags and syringes for 32 days. *Am J Health-Syst Pharm*. 1996; 53:1431–5.

1883. Mayron D, Gennaro AR. Stability and compatibility of granisetron hydrochloride in i.v. solutions and oral liquids and during simulated Y-site injection with selected drugs. *Am J Health-Syst Pharm*. 1996; 53:294–304.

1884. Pinguet F, Rouanet P, Martel P et al. Compatibility and stability of granisetron, dexamethasone, and methylprednisolone in injectable solutions. *J Pharm Sci*. 1995; 84:267–8.

1885. Lindsay CA, Dang K, Adams JM et al. Stability and activity of intravenous immunoglobulin with neonatal dextrose and total parenteral nutrient solutions. *Ann Pharmacother*. 1994; 28:1014–7.

1886. Ukhun IA. Compatibility of haloperidol and diphenhydramine in a hypodermic syringe. *Ann Pharmacother*. 1995; 29:1168–9.

1887. Melonakos TK. Ciprofloxacin-ampicillin sulbactam incompatibility. *Ann Pharmacother*. 1996; 30:87.

1888. Digel S. Cefamandolnafat und metronidazol. *Krankenhauspharmazie*. 1995; 16:9–12.

1889. Heni J, Strehl E. Kompatibilitat von cefotiam. *Krankenhauspharmazie*. 1994; 15:187–92.

1890. Tham A (Medical Affairs, Chiron Therapeutics, Emeryville, CA): Personal communication; 1999 Nov 1.

1891. Mathew M, Gupta VD. Stability of ciprofloxacin in 5% dextrose and normal saline injections. *J Clin Pharm Ther*. 1994; 19:261–2.

1892. Pramar YV, Moniz D. Chemical stability and adsorption of succinylcholine chloride injections in disposable plastic syringes. *J Clin Pharm Ther*. 1994; 19:195–8.

1893. Wood MJ, Lund R. Stability of vancomycin in plastic syringes measured by high-performance liquid chromatography. *J Clin Pharm Ther*. 1995; 20:319–25.

1894. Strong ML, Schaaf LJ, Pankaskie MC et al. Shelf-lives and factors affecting the stability of morphine sulphate and meperidine (pethidine) hydrochloride in plastic syringes for use in patient-controlled analgesic devices. *J Clin Pharm Ther*. 1994; 19:361–9.

1895. Giordano F, Bettinetti G, Cursano R et al. A physico-chemical approach to the investigation of the stability of trimethoprim-sulfamethoxazole (co-trimoxazole) mixtures for injectables. *J Pharm Sci*. 1995; 84:1254–8.

1896. Sianipar A, Parkin JE. Chemical incompatibility between procainamide hydrochloride and glucose following intravenous admixture. *J Pharm Pharmacol*. 1994; 46:951–5.

1897. Lau DWC, Law S, Walker SE et al. Dexamethasone phosphate stability and contamination of solutions stored in syringes. *PDA J Pharm Sci Technol*. 1996; 50:261–7.

1898. Ambados F. Incompatibility between aminophylline and elemental zinc injections. *Aust J Hosp Pharm*. 1996; 26:370–1.

1899. Ambados F. Compatibility of morphine and ketamine for subcutaneous infusion. *Aust J Hosp Pharm*. 1995; 25:352.

1900. Boldu SP, Cubells MP, Brumos VG et al. Stability study of azlocillin sodium in glass bottles and PVC bags containing intravenous admixtures. *Boll Chim Farm*. 1995; 134:467–71.

1901. LeBelle MJ, Savard C. Compatibility of morphine and midazolam or haloperidol in parenteral admixtures. *Can J Hosp Pharm*. 1995; 48:155–60.

1902. Donnelly RF, Yen M. Epinephrine stability in plastic syringes and glass vials. *Can J Hosp Pharm*. 1996; 49:62–5.

1903. Sadjak A, Wintersteiger R. Compatibility of morphine, baclofen, floxuridine and fluorouracil in an implantable medication pump. *Arzneim Forsch*. 1995; 45:93–8.

1904. Donnelly RF, Farncombe M. Compatibility of morphine or hydromorphone with salbutamol in a syringe. *Can J Hosp Pharm*. 1994; 47:252.

1905. Corbo DC, Suddith RL, Sharma B et al. Stability, potency, and preservative effectiveness of epoetin alfa after addition of a bacteriostatic diluent. *Am J Hosp Pharm*. 1992; 49:1455–8.

1906. Lane G, Waite N. Erythropoietin stability. *Can J Hosp Pharm*. 1994; 47:182.

1907. Walker SE, Lau DWC. Compatibility and stability of hyaluronidase and hydromorphone. *Can J Hosp Pharm*. 1992; 45:187–92.

1908. Sastre Gervas I, Ferrandiz Gosalbez JR. Estabilidad fisica y quimica del sulfate magnesico combinado con heparina sodica en solucion salina al 0,9 por 100. *Farm Hosp*. 1995; 19:38–40.

1909. Halkiewicz A, Barteczko I. Interakcje fizykochemiczne izotonicznego roztworu teofiliny do wlewu dozylnego z niektorymi lekami do wstrzykiwan. *Farm Polska*. 1993; 49:11–5.

1910. Gila Azanedo JA, Mengual Sendra A, Fernandez Barral C et al. Estudio de la estabilidad de una solucion de clorhidrato de morfina mas anestesicos locales en solucion salina 0,9 por 100 sin conservantes para uso epidural. *Farm Hosp*. 1994; 18:261–4.

1911. Sitaram BR, Tsui M, Rawicki HB et al. Stability and compatibility of baclofen and morphine admixtures for use in an implantable infusion pump. *Int J Pharm*. 1995; 118:181–9.

1912. Allwood MC, Martin HJ. Long-term stability of cimetidine in total parenteral nutrition. *J Clin Pharm Ther*. 1996; 21:19–21.

1913. Jacolot A, Arnaud P, Lecompte D et al. Stability and compatibility of 2.5 mg/mL methotrexate solution in plastic syringes over 7 days. *Int J Pharm*. 1996; 128:283–6.

1914. Wright A, Hecker J. Long term stability of heparin in dextrose-saline intravenous fluids. *Int J Pharm Pract*. 1995; 3:253–5.

1915. Kawano K, Matsunaga A, Terada K et al. Loss of diltiazem hydrochloride in solutions in polyvinyl chloride containers or intravenous administration set—hydrolysis and sorption. *Jpn J Hosp Pharm*. 1994; 20:537–41.

1916. Metras JI, Swenson CF, McDermott MP. Stability of procainamide hydrochloride in an extemporaneously compounded oral liquid. *Am J Hosp Pharm*. 1992; 49:1720–4.

1917. Kawano K, Takamatsu S, Yamashita J et al. Effect of pH on the sorption of in-solution diazepam into the ethylene-vinylacetate copolymer membrane. *Jpn J Hosp Pharm*. 1994; 20:404–9.

1918. Picard C, Brazier M, Bou P et al. Stabilite de quatre solutions de penicillines dans les poches de perfusion multicouches. *J Pharm Clin*. 1994; 13:45–9.

1919. Theuer H, Scherbel G, Balzulat S et al. Herstellung und stabilitatuntersuchungen von carboplatin i.v. *Krankenhauspharmazie*. 1994; 15:120–30.

1920. Strehl E, Heni J. Amoxicillin, clavulansaure und metronidazol in kombination. *Krankenhauspharmazie*. 1994; 15:592–5.

1921. Hatton J, Luer M, Hirsch J et al. Histamine receptor antagonists and lipid stability in total nutrient admixtures. *JPEN J Parenter Enteral Nutr*. 1994; 18:308–12.

1922. Ku YM, Min DI, Kumar V et al. Stability of tacrolimus injection in total parenteral nutrition solution. *J Pharm Technol*. 1996; 12:58–61.

1923. Martinelli E, Muhlebach S. Kunststoffumbeutel als lichtschutz fur infusionen. *Krankenhauspharmazie*. 1995; 16:286–9.

1924. Teraoka K, Minakuchi K, Tsuchiya K et al. Compatibility of ciprofloxacin infusion with other injections. *Jpn J Hosp Pharm*. 1995; 21:541–50.

1925. Asahara K, Goda Y, Shimomura Y et al. Stability of thiamine in intravenous hyperalimentation containing multivitamin. *Jpn J Hosp Pharm*. 1995; 21:15–21.

1926. Namika Y, Fujiwara A, Kihara N et al. Factors affecting tautomeric phenomenon of a novel potent immunosuppressant (FK506) on the design for injectable formulation. *Drug Dev Ind Pharm*. 1995; 21:809–22.

1927. Antipas AS, Vander Velde D. Factors affecting the deamidation of vancomycin in aqueous solutions. *Int J Pharm*. 1994; 109:261–9.

1928. King AD, Stewart JT. Stability of cefmetazole-doxycycline mixtures in sodium chloride and dextrose injections. *J Clin Pharm Ther*. 1994; 19:317–25.

1929. Hughes IE, Smith JA. The stability of noradrenaline in physiologic saline solutions. *J Pharm Pharmacol*. 1978; 30:124–6.

1930. Anon. Infections linked to lax handling of propofol. *Am J Health-Syst Pharm*. 1995; 52:2061.

1931. Ordovas Baines JP, Ronchera Oms CL, Jimenez Torres NV et al. Mezclas iv binarias de metronidazol y aminoglucosidos. *Revista AEFH*. 1988; 12:119–23.

1932. Nitescu P, Hultman E, Appelgren L et al. Bacteriology, drug stability and exchange of percutaneous delivery systems and antibacterial filters in long-term intrathecal infusion of opioid drugs and bupivacaine in "refractory" pain. *Clin J Pain*. 1992; 8:324–37.

1933. Yao JD, Arkin CF, Karchmer AW. Vancomycin stability in heparin and total parenteral nutrition solutions: novel approach to therapy of central venous catheter-related infections. *JPEN J Parenter Enteral Nutr*. 1992; 16:268–74.

1934. Jim LK. Physical and chemical compatibility of intravenous ciprofloxacin with other drugs. *Ann Pharmacother*. 1993; 27:704–7.

1935. Paesen J, Khan K, Roets E et al. Study of the stability of erythromycin in neutral and alkaline solutions by liquid chromatography on poly(styrene-divinylbenzene). *Int J Pharm*. 1994; 113:215–22.

1936. Keyi X, Gagnon N, Bisson C et al. Stability of famotidine in polyvinyl chloride minibags and polypropylene syringes and compatibility of famotidine with selected drugs. *Ann Pharmacother*. 1993; 27:422–6.

1937. Pleasants RA, Vaughan LM, Williams DM et al. Compatibility of ceftazidime and aminophylline admixtures for different methods of intravenous infusion. *Ann Pharmacother*. 1992; 26:1221–6.

1938. Nahata MC, Morosco RS. Stability of diluted methylprednisolone sodium succinate injection at two temperatures. *Am J Hosp Pharm*. 1994; 51:2157–9.

1939. Nixon AR, O'Hare MCB. The stability of morphine sulphate and metoclopramide hydrochloride in various delivery presentations. *Pharm J*. 1995; 254:153–5.

1940. Lugo RA, Nahata MC. Stability of diluted dexamethasone sodium phosphate injection at two temperatures. *Ann Pharmacother*. 1994; 28:1018–9.

1941. Hanff PAJM, Van den Biggelaar JPFA. Stabiliteitsonderzoek van nitroglycerine-oplossingen voor parenteraal gebruik. *Ziekenhuisfarmacie*. 1994; 10:134–8.

1942. Forte FJ, Caravone D, Coyne MJ et al. Albumin dilution as a cause of hemolysis during plasmapheresis. *Am J Health-Syst Pharm*. 1995; 52:207.

1943. Little G (Drug Information, Wyeth-Ayerst Laboratories, Philadelphia, PA): Personal communication; 1996 Mar 25.

1944. Andersin R, Tammilehto S. Photochemical decomposition of midazolam, part iv: study of pH-dependent stability by high-performance liquid chromatography. *Int J Pharm*. 1995; 123:229–35.

1945. Boullata JI, Gelone SP, Mancano MA et al. Precipitation of lorazepam infusion. *Ann Pharmacother*. 1996; 30:1037–8.

1946. Taylor RB, Richards RME, Low AS et al. Chemical stability of polymyxin B in aqueous solution. *Int J Pharm*. 1994; 102:201–6.

1947. Neuzil J, Darlow BA, Inder TE et al. Oxidation of parenteral lipid emulsion by ambient and phototherapy lights: potential toxicity of routine parenteral feeding. *J Pediatr*. 1995; 126:785–90.

1948. Katakam M, Banga AK. Aggregation of insulin and its prevention by carbohydrate excipients. *PDA J Pharm Sci Technol*. 1995; 49:160–5.

1949. Woloschuk DM. Drug precipitation and peristaltic pumps. *Am J Hosp Pharm*. 1994; 51:1473.

1950. Hehenberger H. Prednisolon-21–hemisuccinat-natrium. *Krankenhauspharmazie*. 1986; 7:128–32.

1951. Driscoll DF, Bacon M, Provost PS et al. Automated compounders for parenteral nutrition admixtures. *JPEN J Parenter Enteral Nutr*. 1994; 18:385–6.

1952. Mehta AC, Kay EA. Admixtures' storage is extended. *Pharm Pract*. 1996; 6:113–4.

1953. Faouzi MA, Dine T, Luyckx M et al. Stability and compatibility studies of cephaloridine, cefuroxime and ceftazidime with PVC infusion bags. *Pharmazie*. 1994; 49:425–9.

1954. Williams DA, Lokich J. A review of the stability and compatibility of antineoplastic drugs for multiple-drug infusions. *Cancer Chemother Pharmacol*. 1992; 31:171–81.

1955. Chevrier R, Sautou V, Pinon V et al. Stability and compatibility of a mixture of the anti-cancer drugs etoposide, cytarabine and daunorubicine for infusion. *Pharm Acta Helv*. 1995; 70:141–8.

1956. Christie JM, Jones CW. Chemical compatibility of regional anesthetic drug combinations. *Ann Pharmacother*. 1992; 26:1078–80.

1957. Abdel-Moety EM, Al-Rashood KA, Rauf A et al. Photostability-indicating HPLC method for determination of trifluoperazine in bulk form and pharmaceutical formulations. *J Pharm Biomed Anal*. 1996; 14:1639–44.

1958. Poochikian GK, Cradock JC. Heroin: stability and formulation approaches. *Int J Pharm*. 1983; 13:219–26.

1959. Kamitomo V, Olson K. Using normal saline to lock peripheral intravenous catheters in ambulatory cancer patients. *J Intraven Nurs*. 1996; 19:75–8.

1960. Burnakis TG. Insulin syringes: more than a one-shot deal. *Hosp Pharm*. 1996; 31:410.

1961. Sautou-Miranda V, Gremeau I, Chamard I et al. Stability of dopamine hydrochloride and of dobutamine hydrochloride in plastic syringes and administration sets. *Am J Health-Syst Pharm*. 1996; 53:186.

1962. Murthey SS, Brittain HG. Stability of revex, nalmefene hydrochloride injection, in injectable solutions. *J Pharm Biomed Anal*. 1996; 15:221–6.

1963. Yuan LC, Samuels GJ. Stability of cidofovir in 0.9% sodium chloride injection and in 5% dextrose injection. *Am J Health-Syst Pharm*. 1996; 53:1939–43.

1964. Leader WG. Incompatibility between ceftriaxone sodium and labetalol hydrochloride. *Am J Health-Syst Pharm*. 1996; 53:2639.

1965. Nahata MC, Morosco RS. Stability of ranitidine hydrochloride in water for injection in glass vials and plastic syringes. *Am J Health-Syst Pharm*. 1996; 53:1588–90.

1966. Lee DKT, Wong CY, Wang DP. Stability of cefazolin sodium and meperidine hydrochloride. *Am J Health-Syst Pharm*. 1996; 53(13):1608, 1610.

1967. Stiles ML, Allen LV Jr. Stability of deferoxamine mesylate, floxuridine, fluorouracil, hydromorphone hydrochloride, lorazepam, and midazolam hydrochloride in polypropylene infusion-pump syringes. *Am J Health-Syst Pharm*. 1996; 53:1583–8.

1968. Quercia RA, Zhang J, Fan C et al. Stability of granisetron hydrochloride in polypropylene syringes. *Am J Health-Syst Pharm*. 1996; 53:2744–6.

1969. Trissel LA, Martinez JF. Screening cladribine for Y-site physical compatibility with selected drugs. *Hosp Pharm*. 1996; 31:1425–8.

1970. Allen LV Jr, Stiles ML, Prince SJ et al. Stability of 14 drugs in the latex reservoir of an elastomeric infusion device. *Am J Health-Syst Pharm*. 1996; 53:2740–3.

1971. Benjamin BE. Ciprofloxacin and sodium phosphates not compatible during actual Y-site injection. *Am J Health-Syst Pharm.* 1996; 53:1850–1.

1972. Trissel LA. Everything in a compatibility study is important. *Am J Health-Syst Pharm.* 1996; 53:2990.

1973. Matuschka PR, Hill LJ. More on the compatibility of mannitol and sodium bicarbonate in injectable fluids. *Am J Health-Syst Pharm.* 1996; 53:2639.

1974. Veltri M, Lee CKK. Compatibility of neonatal parenteral nutrient solutions with selected intravenous drugs. *Am J Health-Syst Pharm.* 1996; 53:2611–3.

1975. Ritter H, Trissel LA, Anderson RW et al. Electronic balance as quality assurance for cytotoxic drug admixtures. *Am J Health-Syst Pharm.* 1996; 53:2318–20.

1976. Zhang Y, Xu QA, Trissel LA et al. Physical and chemical stability of methotrexate sodium, cytarabine, and hydrocortisone sodium succinate in Elliott's B solution. *Hosp Pharm.* 1996; 31:965–70.

1977. Xu QA, Trissel LA. Stability and compatibility of fluorouracil with morphine sulfate and hydromorphone hydrochloride. *Ann Pharmacother.* 1996; 30:756–61.

1978. Kohut J III, Trissel LA. Don't ignore the details of drug-compatibility reports. *Am J Health-Syst Pharm.* 1996; 53:2339.

1979. Grillo JA, Barie PS. Precipitation of lorazepam during infusion by volumetric pump. *Am J Health-Syst Pharm.* 1996; 53:1850.

1980. Volles DF. More on usability of lorazepam admixtures for continuous infusion. *Am J Health-Syst Pharm.* 1996; 53:2753–4.

1981. Boullata JI, Gelone SP. More on usability of lorazepam admixtures for continuous infusion. *Am J Health-Syst Pharm.* 1996; 53:2754.

1982. Strozyk WR, Williamson R. Incompatibility of amiodarone hydrochloride and evacuated glass bottles. *Am J Health-Syst Pharm.* 1996; 53:184.

1983. Baud-Camus F, Crauste-Manciet S, Klein E et al. Stability of fluorouracil in polypropylene syringes and ethylene vinyl acetate infusion-pump reservoirs. *Am J Health-Syst Pharm.* 1996; 53:1457.

1984. Chernin EL, Stewart JT. Stability of thiopental sodium and propofol in polypropylene syringes at 23 and 4°C. *Am J Health-Syst Pharm.* 1996; 53:1576–9.

1985. Prankerd RJ, Jones RD. Physicochemical compatibility of propofol with thiopental sodium. *Am J Health-Syst Pharm.* 1996; 53:2606–10.

1986. Williams NA, Bornstein M. Stability of levofloxacin in intravenous solutions in polyvinyl chloride bags. *Am J Health-Syst Pharm.* 1996; 53:2309–13.

1987. Cleary JD. Amphotericin B formulated in a lipid emulsion. *Ann Pharmacother.* 1996; 30:409–12.

1988. Lopez RM, Ayestaran A, Pou L et al. Stability of amphotericin B in an extemporaneously prepared i.v. fat emulsion. *Am J Health-Syst Pharm.* 1996; 53:2724–7.

1989. Manduru M, Fariello A, White RL et al. Stability of ceftazidime sodium and teicoplanin sodium in a peritoneal dialysis solution. *Am J Health-Syst Pharm.* 1996; 53:2731–4.

1990. Plumridge RJ, Rieck AM, Annus TP et al. Stability of ceftriaxone sodium in polypropylene syringes at -20, 4, and 20°C. *Am J Health-Syst Pharm.* 1996; 53:2320–3.

1991. Plumridge RJ, Rieck AM, Annus TP et al. Stability of ceftriaxone sodium reconstituted with lidocaine hydrochloride and stored in polypropylene syringes. *Am J Health-Syst Pharm.* 1996; 53:2323–5.

1992. Henderson F. 21–Day compatibility of hydromorphone hydrochloride and promethazine hydrochloride in a casette. *Am J Health-Syst Pharm.* 1996; 53:2338–9.

1993. Lima HA, Lennon J, Sesterhenn K et al. Stability of dextrose and sodium chloride in injectable solutions stored in an elastomeric infusion device. *Am J Health-Syst Pharm.* 1996; 53:794–5.

1994. Patel PR. Compatibility of meropenem with commonly used injectable drugs. *Am J Health-Syst Pharm.* 1996; 53:2853–5.

1995. Lougheed WD, Albisser AM, Martindale HM et al. Physical stability of insulin formulations. *Diabetes.* 1983; 32:424–32.

1996. Gupta VD. Quantitation of papaverine hydrochloride in a discoloured injection. *Drug Stability.* 1996; 1:132–4.

1997. Akimoto K, Kawai A, Ohya K et al. Photodegradation reactions of CPT-11, a derivative of camptothecin, part i: chemical structure of main degradation products in aqueous solution. *Drug Stability.* 1996; 1:118–22.

1998. Akimoto K, Kawai A. Photodegradation reactions of CPT-11, a derivative of camptothecin, part ii: photodegradation behaviour of CPT-11 in aqueous solution. *Drug Stability.* 1996; 1:141–6.

1999. O'Connell C, Sabra K. Stability of reconstituted ceftriaxone solution in polypropylene syringes. *Eur Hosp Pharm.* 1996; 2:47–8.

2000. Trissel LA, Gilbert DL. Compatibility of granisetron hydrochloride with selected drugs during simulated Y-site administration. *Am J Health-Syst Pharm.* 1997; 54:56–60.

2001. Zhang Y, Trissel LA, Martinez JF et al. Stability of metoclopramide hydrochloride in plastic syringes. *Am J Health-Syst Pharm.* 1996; 53:1300–2.

2002. Kaijser GP, Aalbers T, Beijnen JH et al. Chemical stability of cyclophosphamide, trofosamide, and 2– and 3–dechloroethylfosfamide in aqueous solutions. *J Oncol Pharm Pract.* 1996; 2:15–21.

2003. Nelson TJ, Graves SM. 0.9% Sodium chloride injection with and without heparin for maintaining peripheral indwelling intermittent-infusion devices in infants. *Am J Health-Syst Pharm.* 1998; 55:570–3.

2004. Martel P, Petit I, Pinguet F et al. Long-term stability of 5-fluorouracil stored in PVC bags and in ambulatory pump reservoirs. *J Pharm Biomed Anal.* 1996; 14:395–9.

2005. Darbar D, Dell'Orto S, Wilkinson GR et al. Loss of quinidine gluconate injection in a polyvinyl chloride infusion system. *Am J Health-Syst Pharm.* 1996; 53:655–8.

2006. Erkkila DM (Professional Services, Immunex Corporation): Personal communication; 1996 Mar 6.

2007. Xu QA, Trissel LA, Zhang Y et al. Stability of thiotepa (lyophilized) in 5% dextrose injection at 4 and 23°C. *Am J Health-Syst Pharm.* 1996; 53:2728–30.

2008. van Doorne H, Bernaards J. Ceftazidime degradation rates for predicting stability in a portable infusion-pump reservoir. *Am J Health-Syst Pharm.* 1996; 53:1302–5.

2009. Celesk RA (Medical Services, Bayer Pharmaceutical Division): Personal communication; 1996 May 7.

2010. Grandison D (Worldwide Medical Affairs, Du Pont Pharma): Personal communication; 1995 Dec 4.

2011. Martinez JF, Trissel LA. Compatibility of warfarin sodium with selected drugs and large-volume parenteral solutions. *Int J Pharm Compound.* 1997; 1:356–8.

2012. Williams DA. Zwitterions and pH-dependent solubility. *Am J Health-Syst Pharm.* 1996; 53:1732.

2013. Ariano RE, Kassum DA, Meatherhill RC et al. Lack of in vitro inactivation of tobramycin by imipenem/cilastatin. *Ann Pharmacother.* 1992; 26:1075–7.

2014. Jenke DR. Drug binding by reservoirs in elastomeric devices. *Pharm Res.* 1994; 11:984–9.

2015. McCollom RA, Lange B, Bryson SM et al. Polyvinylchloride containers do not influence the hemodynamic response to intravenous nitroglycerin. *Can J Hosp Pharm.* 1993; 46:165–70.

2016. Altavela JL, Haas CE, Nowak DR et al. Clinical response to intravenous nitroglycerin infused through polyethylene or polyvinyl chloride tubing. *Am J Hosp Pharm.* 1994; 51:490–94.

2017. McCullough JM, Sprentall-Nankervis E, Potcova CA et al. Recovery and biological activity of filgrastim after injection through silicone rubber catheters. *Am J Health-Syst Pharm.* 1995; 52:186–8.

2018. Park TW, Le-Bui LPK, Chung KC et al. Stability of piperacillin sodium-tazobactam sodium in peritoneal dialysis solutions. *Am J Health-Syst Pharm.* 1995; 52:2022–4.

2020. Stiles ML, Allen LV Jr, Resztak KE et al. Stability of octreotide acetate in polypropylene syringes. *Am J Hosp Pharm.* 1993; 50:2356–8.

2021. Ripley RG, Ritchie DJ. Stability of octreotide acetate in polypropylene syringes at 5 and -20°C. *Am J Health-Syst Pharm.* 1995; 52:1910–1.

2022. Schepart BS, Burns BA, Evans S et al. Long-term stability of interferon alfa-2b diluted to 2 million units/mL. *Am J Health-Syst Pharm.* 1995; 52:2128–30.

2023. Ikeda S, Frank PA, Schweiss JF et al. In vitro cyanide release from sodium nitroprusside in various intravenous solutions. *Anesth Analg.* 1988; 67:360–2.

2024. Webster LK, Crinis NA, Davis JR et al. Conversion of etoposide phosphate to etoposide under ambulatory infusion conditions. *J Oncol Pharm Pract.* 1995; 1:33–6.

2025. Hensrud DD, Burritt MF, Hall LG. Stability of heparin anticoagulant activity over time in parenteral nutrition solutions. *JPEN J Parenter Enteral Nutr.* 1996; 20:219–21.

2026. Gutcher GR, Lax AA. Vitamin A losses to plastic intravenous infusion devices and an improved method of delivery. *Am J Clin Nutr.* 1984; 40:8–13.

2027. Greene HL, Phillips BL, Franck L et al. Persistently low blood retinol levels during and after parenteral feeding of very low birth weight infants: examination of losses into intravenous administration sets and a method of prevention by addition to a lipid emulsion. *Pediatrics.* 1987; 79:894–900.

2028. Henton DH, Merrott RJ. Vitamin A sorption to polyvinyl and polyolefin intravenous tubing. *JPEN J Parenter Enteral Nutr.* 1990; 14:79–81.

2029. Washington C, Ferguson JA. Computational prediction of the stability of lipid emulsions in total nutrient admixtures. *J Pharm Sci.* 1993; 82:808–12.

2030. Li LC, Sampogna TP. A factorial design study on the physical stability of 3–in–1 admixtures. *J Pharm Pharmacol.* 1993; 45:985–7.

2031. Foresta K. Use of total nutrient admixtures should not be limited. *Am J Health-Syst Pharm.* 1995; 52:893.

2032. Driscoll DF. Use of total nutrient admixtures should not be limited. *Am J Health-Syst Pharm.* 1995; 52:893–4.

2033. Mirtallo JM. Use of total nutrient admixtures should not be limited. *Am J Health-Syst Pharm.* 1995; 52:894–5.

2034. Trissel LA. Use of total nutrient admixtures should not be limited. *Am J Health-Syst Pharm.* 1995; 52:895.

2035. Driscoll DF. Debate on total nutrient admixtures continues. *Am J Health-Syst Pharm.* 1995; 52:1921–2.

2036. Trissel LA. Debate on total nutrient admixtures continues. *Am J Health-Syst Pharm.* 1995; 52:1921–2.

2037. Hill SE, Heldman LS, Goo ED et al. Fatal microvascular pulmonary emboli from precipitation of a total nutrient admixture solution. *JPEN J Parenter Enteral Nutr.* 1996; 20:81–7.

2038. MacKay MW, Fitzgerald KA, Jackson D. The solubility of calcium and phosphate in two specialty amino acid solutions. *JPEN J Parenter Enteral Nutr.* 1996; 20:63–6.

2039. Shatsky F, McFeely EJ. A table for estimating calcium and phosphorus compatibility in parenteral nutrition formulas that contain Trophamine plus cysteine. *Hosp Pharm.* 1995; 30:690–2.

2040. Grassby PF, Hutchings L. Factors affecting the physical and chemical stability of morphine sulphate solutions stored in syringes. *Int J Pharm Pract.* 1993; 2:39–43.

2041. Ritter H, Trissel LA, Anderson RW et al. Electronic balance as quality assurance for cytotoxic drug admixtures. *Am J Health-Syst Pharm.* 1996; 53:2318–20.

2042. Roos PJ, Glerum JH, Meilink JW et al. Effect of pH on absorption of sufentanil citrate in a portable pump reservoir during storage and administration under simulated epidural conditions. *Pharm World Sci.* 1993; 15:139–44.

2043. Bristol Laboratories. Sodium bicarbonate injection prescribing information. Syracuse, NY; 1980 Apr.

2044. Allen LV Jr, Stiles ML, Prince SJ et al. Stability of cefpirome sulfate in the presence of commonly used intensive care drugs during simulated Y-site injection. *Am J Health-Syst Pharm.* 1995; 52:2427–33.

2045. Bureau A, Lahet JJ, D'Athis P et al. Compatibilite PVC-psychotropes au cours d'une perfusion. *J Pharm Clin.* 1995; 14:26–30.

2046. Streng WH, Brake NW. Dextrose adduct formation in aqueous teicoplanin solutions. *Pharm Res.* 1989; 6:1032–8.

2047. Hixt U. L-Alanyl-L-glutamine dipeptide for parenteral nutrition. *Eur Hosp Pharm.* 1996; 2:72–6.

2048. Tivnann H, Gaines-Gas R, Thorpe R et al. An evaluation of the stability of granulocyte colony stimulating factor on the short-term storage and delivery from an elastomeric infusion system. *J Oncol Pharm Pract.* 1996; 2:107–12.

2049. Billion-Rey F, Guillaumont M, Frederich A et al. Stability of fat-soluble vitamins A (retinol palmitate), E (tocopherol acetate), and K1 (phylloquinone) in total parenteral nutrition at home. *JPEN J Parenter Enteral Nutr.* 1993; 17:56–60.

2050. Dahl GB, Svensson L, Kinnander NJ et al. Stability of vitamins in soybean oil fat emulsion under conditions simulating intravenous feeding of neonates and children. *JPEN J Parenter Enteral Nutr*. 1994; 18:234–9.

2051. Henry DW, Lacerte JA, Klutman NE et al. Irreversibility of procainamide-dextrose complex in plasma in vitro. *Am J Hosp Pharm*. 1991; 48:2426–9.

2052. Martin M, Bepko R. Paclitaxel diluent and the case of the slippery spike. *Am J Hosp Pharm*. 1994; 51:3078.

2053. Faouzi MA, Dine T, Luyckx M et al. Leaching of diethylhexyl phthalate from PVC bags into intravenous teniposide solution. *Int J Pharm*. 1994; 105:89–93.

2054. Haas CE, Nowak DR. Effect of using a standard polyvinyl chloride intravenous infusion set on patient response to nitroglycerin. *Am J Hosp Pharm*. 1992; 49:1135–7.

2055. Driver PS, Jarvi EJ. Stability of nitroglycerin as nitroglycerin concentrate for injection stored in plastic syringes. *Am J Hosp Pharm*. 1993; 50:2561–3.

2056. Casto DT. Stability of ondansetron stored in polypropylene syringes. *Ann Pharmacother*. 1994; 28:712–4.

2057. Bailey LC, Tang KT. Effect of syringe filter and i.v. administration set on delivery of propofol emulsion. *Am J Hosp Pharm*. 1991; 48:2627–30.

2058. Johnson CE, Christen C, Perez MM et al. Compatibility of bupivacaine hydrochloride and morphine sulfate. *Am J Health-Syst Pharm*. 1997; 54:61–4.

2059. Ambados F. Compatibility of ketamine hydrochloride and meperidine hydrochloride. *Am J Health-Syst Pharm*. 1997; 54:205.

2060. Hall PD, Yui D, Lyons S et al. Compatibility of filgrastim with selected antimicrobial drugs during simulated Y-site administration. *Am J Health-Syst Pharm*. 1997; 54:185–9.

2061. Fausel CA, Newton DW, Driscoll DF et al. Effect of fat emulsion and supersaturation on calcium phosphate solubility in parenteral nutrient admixtures. *Int J Pharm Compound*. 1997; 1:54–9.

2062. Chiu MF, Schwartz ML. Visual compatibility of injectable drugs used in the intensive care unit. *Am J Health-Syst Pharm*. 1997; 54:64–5.

2063. Najari Z, Rusho WJ. Compatibility of commonly used bone marrow transplant drugs during Y-site delivery. *Am J Health-Syst Pharm*. 1997; 54:181–4.

2064. Xu QA, Trissel LA. Rapid loss of fentanyl citrate admixed with fluorouracil in polyvinyl chloride containers. *Ann Pharmacother*. 1997; 31:297–302.

2065. Gilbert DL Jr, Trissel LA. Compatibility of ciprofloxacin lactate with sodium bicarbonate during simulated Y-site administration. *Am J Health-Syst Pharm*. 1997; 54:1193–5.

2066. Trissel LA, Gilbert DL. Compatibility of propofol injectable emulsion with selected drugs during simulated Y-site administration. *Am J Health-Syst Pharm*. 1997; 54:1287–92.

2067. Asker AF, Ferdous AJ. Photodegradation of furosemide solutions. *PDA J Pharm Sci Technol*. 1996; 50:158–62.

2068. Anon. Compatibility of meropenem with commonly used injectable drugs. *Am J Health-Syst Pharm*. 1998; 55:735. [Correction: *AJHP*. 1996; 53:2853–5.]

2069. Schobelock MJ (Medical Affairs Department, Roxane Laboratories, Inc.): Personal communication; 1997 Nov 4.

2070. Barnes AR, Nash S. Stability of bupivacaine hydrochloride and diamorphine hydrochloride in an epidural infusion. *Pharm World Sci*. 1995; 17:87–92.

2071. Grassby PF, Hutchings L. Drug combinations in syringe drivers: the compatibility and stability of diamorphine with cyclizine and haloperidol. *Palliat Med*. 1997; 11:217–24.

2072. Cohen MR. Volume limitations for IV drug infusions when sterile water for injection is used as a diluent. *Hosp Pharm*. 1998; 33:274–7.

2073. Pierce LR, Gaines A, Varricchio F et al. Hemolysis and renal failure associated with use of sterile water for injection to dilute 25% human albumin solution. *Am J Health-Syst Pharm*. 1998; 55(10):1057, 1062, 1070.

2074. Trissel LA, Martinez JF. Compatibility of cisatracurium besylate with selected drugs during simulated Y-site administration. *Am J Health-Syst Pharm*. 1997; 54:1735–41.

2075. Trissel LA, Gilbert DL, Martinez JF et al. Compatibility of remifentanil hydrochloride with selected drugs during simulated Y-site administration. *Am J Health-Syst Pharm*. 1997; 54:2192–6.

2076. Ennis RD, Dahl TC. Stability of cidofovir in 0.9% sodium chloride injection for five days. *Am J Health-Syst Pharm*. 1997; 54(19):2204–6.

2077. Murray KM, Erkkila D, Gombotz WR et al. Stability of thiotepa (lyophilized) in 0.9% sodium chloride injection. *Am J Health-Syst Pharm*. 1997; 54:2588–91.

2078. Bahal SM, Lee TJ, McGinnes M et al. Visual compatibility of warfarin sodium injection with selected medications and solutions. *Am J Health-Syst Pharm*. 1997; 54:2599–600.

2079. Nolan PE, Hoyer GL, LeDoux JH et al. Stability of ranitidine hydrochloride and human insulin in 0.9% sodium chloride injection. *Am J Health-Syst Pharm*. 1997; 54:1304–6.

2080. Stiles ML, Allen LV. Stability of nafcillin sodium, oxacillin sodium, penicillin G potassium, penicillin G sodium, and tobramycin sulfate in polyvinyl chloride drug reservoirs. *Am J Health-Syst Pharm*. 1997; 54:1068–70.

2081. Pujol M, Munoz M, Prat J et al. Stability study of epirubicin in NaCl 0.9% injection. *Ann Pharmacother*. 1997; 31:992–5.

2082. Walker SE, DeAngelis C. Stability and compatibility of combinations of hydromorphone and a second drug. *Can J Hosp Pharm*. 1991; 44:289–95.

2083. Fischer JH, Cwik MJ, Luer MS et al. Stability of fosphenytoin sodium with intravenous solutions in glass bottles, polyvinyl chloride bags, and polypropylene syringes. *Ann Pharmacother*. 1997; 31:553–9.

2084. Evrard B, Ceccato A, Gaspard O et al. Stability of ondansetron hydrochloride and dexamethasone sodium phosphate in 0.9% sodium chloride injection and in 5% dextrose injection. *Am J Health-Syst Pharm*. 1997; 54:1065–8.

2085. Peddicord TE, Olsen KM, ZumBrunnen TL et al. Stability of high-concentration dopamine hydrochloride, norepinephrine bitartrate, epinephrine hydrochloride, and nitroglycerin in 5% dextrose injection. *Am J Health-Syst Pharm*. 1997; 54:1417–9.

2086. Walker SE, Meinders A. Stability and compatibility of reconstituted sterile hydromorphone with midazolam. *Can J Hosp Pharm*. 1996; 49:290–8.

2087. Trissel LA, Gilbert DL. Compatibility of doxorubicin hydrochloride liposome injection with selected other drugs during simulated Y-site administration. *Am J Health-Syst Pharm.* 1997; 54:2708–13.

2088. Pramar YV, Loucas VA. Stability of midazolam hydrochloride in syringes and i.v. fluids. *Am J Health-Syst Pharm.* 1997; 54:913–5.

2089. Patel PR, Cook SE. Stability of meropenem in intravenous solutions. *Am J Health-Syst Pharm.* 1997; 54:412–21.

2090. Cornish LA, Montgomery PA. Stability of bumetanide in 5% dextrose injection. *Am J Health-Syst Pharm.* 1997; 54:422–3.

2091. Bailey LC, Orosz ST. Stability of ceftriaxone sodium and metronidazole hydrochloride. *Am J Health-Syst Pharm.* 1997; 54:424–7.

2092. Stewart JT, Warren FW, King DT et al. Stability of ondansetron hydrochloride, doxorubicin hydrochloride, and dacarbazine or vincristine sulfate in elastomeric portable infusion devices and polyvinyl chloride bags. *Am J Health-Syst Pharm.* 1997; 54:915–20.

2093. Owens D, Fleming RA, Restino MS et al. Stability of amphotericin B 0.05 and 0.5 mg/mL in 20% fat emulsion. *Am J Health-Syst Pharm.* 1997; 54:683–6.

2094. Zhang Y, Xu QA, Trissel LA et al. Compatibility and stability of paclitaxel combined with cisplatin and with carboplatin in infusion solutions. *Ann Pharmcother.* 1997; 31:1465–70.

2095. Gupta VD, Maswoswe J. Stability of ketorolac tromethamine in 5% dextrose injection and 0.9% sodium chloride injections. *Int J Pharm Compound.* 1997; 1:206–7.

2096. Zhang YP, Trissel LA. Stability of aminocaproic acid injection admixtures in 5% dextrose injection and 0.9% sodium chloride injection. *Int J Pharm Compound.* 1997; 1:132–4.

2097. Allen LV, Stiles ML. Stability of vancomycin hydrochloride in medication cassette reservoirs. *Int J Pharm Compound.* 1997; 1:123–4.

2098. Zhang YP, Trissel LA, Martinez JF et al. Stability of acyclovir sodium 1, 7, and 10 mg/mL in 5% dextrose injection and 0.9% sodium chloride injection. *Am J Health-Syst Pharm.* 1998; 55:574–7.

2099. Amador FD, Azzati ES. Stability of carboplatin in polyvinyl chloride bags. *Am J Health-Syst Pharm.* 1998; 55:602.

2100. Gupta VD, Maswoswe J. Stability of cefmetazole sodium in 5% dextrose injection and 0.9% sodium chloride injection. *Int J Pharm Compound.* 1997; 1:208–9.

2101. Gupta VD, Maswoswe J. Stability of ceftriaxone sodium when mixed with metronidazole injection. *Int J Pharm Compound.* 1997; 1:280–1.

2102. Gupta VD, Maswoswe J. Stability of cefepime hydrochloride in 5% dextrose injection and 0.9% sodium chloride injection. *Int J Pharm Compound.* 1997; 1:435–6.

2103. Mayhew SL, Quick MW. Compatibility of iron dextran with neonatal parenteral nutrient solutions. *Am J Health-Syst Pharm.* 1997; 54:570–1.

2104. Moshfeghi M, Ciuffo JD. Visual compatibility of fentanyl citrate with parenteral nutrient solutions. *Am J Health-Syst Pharm.* 1998; 55:1194.

2105. Gupta VD, Maswoswe J. Stability of indomethacin in 0.9% sodium chloride injection. *Int J Pharm Compound.* 1998; 2:170–1.

2106. Wong F, Gill MA. Stability of milrinone lactate 200 mcg/mL in 5% dextrose injection and 0.9% sodium chloride injection. *Int J Pharm Compound.* 1998; 2:168–9.

2107. Nguyen D, Gill MA. Stability of milrinone lactate in 5% dextrose injection and 0.9% sodium chloride injection at concentrations of 400, 600, and 800 mcg/mL. *Int J Pharm Compound.* 1998; 2:246–8.

2108. Montgomery PA, Cornish LA, Johnson CE et al. Stability of torsemide in 5% dextrose injection. *Am J Health-Syst Pharm.* 1998; 55:1042–3.

2109. Trissel LA, Gilbert DL, Martinez JF et al. Compatibility of parenteral nutrient solutions with selected drugs during simulated Y-site administration. *Am J Health-Syst Pharm.* 1997; 54:1295–1300.

2110. Pramar YV. Chemical stability of amiodarone hydrochloride in intravenous fluids. *Int J Pharm Compound.* 1997; 1:347–8.

2111. Wang DP, Wang MT, Wong CY et al. Compatibility of vancomycin hydrochloride and famotidine in 5% dextrose injection. *Int J Pharm Compound.* 1997; 1:354–5.

2112. Bhatt-Mehta V, Hirata S. Physical compatibility and chemical stability of atracurium besylate and midazolam hydrochloride during intravenous coinfusion. *Int J Pharm Compound.* 1998; 2:79–82.

2113. Stendal TL, Klem W, Tonnesen HH et al. Drug stability and pyridine generation in ceftazidime injection stored in an elastomeric infusion device. *Am J Health-Syst Pharm.* 1998; 55:683–5.

2114. Ketkar VA, Kolling WM, Nardviriyakul N et al. Stability of undiluted and diluted adenosine at three temperatures in syringes and bags. *Am J Health-Syst Pharm.* 1998; 55:466–0.

2115. Naud C, Marti B, Fernandez C et al. Stability of adenosine 6 mcg/mL in 0.9% sodium chloride solution. *Am J Health-Syst Pharm.* 1998; 55:1161–4.

2116. Xu QA, Zhang YP, Trissel LA et al. Stability of cisatracurium besylate in vials, syringes, and infusion admixtures. *Am J Health-Syst Pharm.* 1998; 55:1037–41.

2117. Das T, Volety S, Ahsan SM et al. Safety, sterility and stability of direct-from-vial multiple dosing intravitreal injection of bevacizumab. *Clin Exp Ophthalmol.* 2015; 43:466–73.

2118. Allwood MC, Martin J. How does storage affect propofol? The stability of propofol in plastic syringes. *Pharm Pract.* 1997; 7:15–6.

2119. Harris MC, Como JA. Heparin flush solutions: how much is enough? *South J Health-Syst Pharm.* 1997; 2:10–4.

2120. Meyer BA, Little CJ, Thorp JA et al. Heparin versus normal saline as a peripheral line flush in maintenance of intermittent intravenous lines in obstetric patients. *Obstet Gynecol.* 1995; 85:433–6.

2121. Danek GD, Noris EM. Pediatric i.v. catheters: efficacy of saline flush. *Pediatr Nurs.* 1992; 18:111–3.

2122. Hook ML, Reuling J, Luettgen ML et al. Comparison of the patency of arterial lines maintained with heparinized and nonheparinized infusions. The Cardiovascular Intensive Care Unit Nursing Research Committee of St. Luke's Hospital. *Heart Lung.* 1987; 16:693–9.

2123. Kulkarni M, Elsner C, Ouellet D et al. Heparinized saline versus normal saline in maintaining patency of the radial artery catheter. *Can J Surg*. 1994; 37:37–42.

2124. Clifton GD, Branson P, Kelly HJ et al. Comparison of normal saline and heparin solutions for maintenance of arterial catheter patency. *Heart Lung*. 1991; 20:115–8.

2125. Butt W, Shann F, McDonnell G et al. Effect of heparin concentration and infusion rate on the patency of arterial catheters. *Crit Care Med*. 1987; 15:230–2.

2126. Smith S, Dawson S, Hennessey R, et al. Maintenance of the patency of indwelling central venous catheters: is heparin necessary? *Am J Pediatr Hematol Oncol*. 1991; 13(2):141–3.

2127. O'Neill TJ, Tierney LM Jr, Proulx RJ. Heparin lock-induced alterations in the activated partial thromboplastin time. *JAMA*. 1974; 227:1297–8.

2128. Passannante A, Macik BG. Case report: the heparin flush syndrome: a cause of iatrogenic hemorrhage. *Am J Med Sci*. 1988; 296:71–3.

2129. Heeger PS, Backstrom JT. Heparin flushes and thrombocytopenia. *Ann Intern Med*. 1986; 105:143.

2130. Laster J, Cikrit D, Walker N et al. The heparin-induced thrombocytopenia syndrome: an update. *Surgery*. 1987; 102:763–70.

2131. Rizzoni WE, Miller K, Rick M et al. Heparin-induced thrombocytopenia and thromboembolism in the postoperative period. *Surgery*. 1988; 103:470–6.

2132. Doty JR, Alving BM, McDonnell DE et al. Heparin-associated thrombocytopenia in the neurosurgical patient. *Neurosurgery*. 1986; 19:69–72.

2133. Mehta AC, Kay EA. Storage time can be extended. *Pharm Pract*. (June) 1997; 7:305, 306, 308.

2134. Brittain HG, Lafferty L, Bousserski P et al. Stability of Revex, nalmefene hydrochloride injection. *PDA J Pharm Sci Technol*. 1996; 50:35–9.

2135. McKinnon BT. FDA Safety Alert: hazards of precipitation associated with parenteral nutrition. *Nutr Clin Pract*. 1996; 11:59–65.

2136. Seidner DL, Speerhas R. Can octreotide be added to parenteral nutrition? Point-counterpoint. *Nutr Clin Pract*. 1998; 13:84–8.

2137. Dodds HM, Craik DJ. Photodegradation of irinotecan (CPT-11) in aqueous solutions: identification of fluorescent products and influence of solution composition. *J Pharm Sci*. 1997; 86:1410–6.

2138. Gremeau I, Sautou-miranda V, Picq F et al. Influence de la nature de la membrane sur le passage du nitrate d'isosorbide et de son metabolite actif au cours d'une dialyse. *J Pharm Clin*. 1997; 16:19–23.

2139. Graham AE, Speicher E. Analysis of gentamicin sulfate and a study of its degradation in dextrose solution. *J Pharm Biomed Anal*. 1997; 15:537–43.

2140. Craig SB, Bhatt UH. Stability and compatibility of topotecan hydrochloride for injection with common infusion solutions and containers. *J Pharm Biomed Anal*. 1997; 16:199–205.

2141. Pramar YV, Loucas VA. Chemical stability and adsorption of atracurium besylate injections in disposable plastic syringes. *J Clin Pharm Ther*. 1996; 21:173–5.

2142. Galanti LM, Hecq JD, Vanbeckbergen D et al. Long-term stability of cefuroxime and cefazolin sodium in intravenous infusions. *J Clin Pharm Ther*. 1996; 21:185–9.

2143. Kawano K, Takamatsu S, Mochizuku C et al. Loss of isosorbide dinitrate or nitroglycerin solution content in practice injection or precision continuous drip infusion. *Jpn J Hosp Pharm*. 1996; 22:167–72.

2144. Yoshida H, Takaba D, Uchida Y et al. Research for the crystal material produced in the continuous infusion line of midazloam (Dormicium) and butorphanol (Stadol). *Jpn J Hosp Pharm*. 1997; 23:531–8.

2145. Mawhinney WM, Adair CG, Gorman SP et al. Long-term stability of teicoplanin in dialysis fluid: implications for the home-treatment of CAPD peritonitis. *Int J Pharm Pract*. 1991; 1:90–3.

2146. Allwood MC, Martin H. The extraction of diethylhexyl-phthalate (DEHP) from polyvinyl chloride components of intravenous infusion containers and administration sets by paclitaxel injection. *Int J Pharm*. 1996; 127:65–71.

2147. Valiere C, Arnaud P, Caroff E et al. Stability and compatibility study of a carboplatin solution in syringes for continuous ambulatory infusion. *Int J Pharm*. 1996; 138:125–8.

2148. Khalfi F, Dine T, Gressier B et al. Compatibility and stability of vancomycin hydrochloride with PVC infusion material in various conditions using stability-indicating high-performance liquid chromatographic assay. *Int J Pharm*. 1996; 139:243–7.

2149. Hourcade F, Sautou-Miranda V, Normand B et al. Compatibility of granisetron towards glass and plastics and its stability under various storage conditions. *Int J Pharm*. 1997; 154:95–102.

2150. Rabouan-Guyon SM, Guet AF, Courtois PY et al. Stability study of cefepime in different infusion solutions. *Int J Pharm*. 1997; 154:185–90.

2151. Anon. How I survived a direct injection of potassium chloride. *Hosp Pharm*. 1997; 32:298–300.

2152. Kramer I. Stability of meropenem in elastomeric portable infusion devices. *Eur Hosp Pharm*. 1997; 3:168–71.

2153. Uges DRA, Ruige M. Vancomycin adsorption to teflon tubing. *Eur Hosp Pharm*. 1996; 2:38.

2154. Daouphars M, Vigneron J, Perrin A et al. Stability of cladribine in either polyethylene containers or polyvinyl chloride bags. *Europ Hosp Pharm*. 1997; 3:154–6.

2155. Girona V, Prat J, Pujol M et al. Stability of vinblastine sulphate in 0.9% sodium chloride in polypropylene syringes. *Boll Chim Farm*. 1996; 135:413–4.

2156. Smith BA, Hilmi SC, McDonald C et al. The stability of foscarnet in the presence of potassium. *Aust J Hosp Pharm*. 1996; 26:560–1.

2157. Jaffe GJ, Green GDJ. Stability of recombinant tissue plasminogen activator. *Am J Ophthal*. 1989; 108:90–1.

2158. Ward C, Weck S. Dilution and storage of recombinant tissue plasminogen activator (Activase) in balanced salt solutions. *Am J Ophthal*. 1990; 109:98–9.

2159. Grewing R, Mester U, Low M. Clinical experience with tissue plasminogen activator stored at -20°C. *Ophthalmic Surg*. 1992; 23:780–1.

2160. Kramer I. Viability of microorganisms in novel antineo-plastic and antiviral drug solutions. *J Oncol Pharm Pract.* 1998; 4:32–7.

2161. Schneider JJ, Wilson KM. A study of the osmolality and pH of subcutaneous drug infusion solutions. *Aust J Hosp Pharm.* 1997; 27:29–31.

2162. Vermeire A, Remon JP. The solubility of morphine and the stability of concentrated morphine solutions in glass, polypropylene syringes and PVC containers. *Int J Pharm.* 1997; 146:213–23.

2163. Kearney MCJ, Allwood MC, Martin H et al. The influence of amino acid source on the stability of ascorbic acid in TPN mixtures. *Nutrition.* 1998; 14:173–8.

2164. Casasin Edo T, Roca Massa M. Sistema de distribucion de medicamentos utilizados en anestesia mediante jeringas precargadas. Estudio de estabilidad. *Farm Hosp.* 1996; 20:55–9.

2165. Malcomson C, Zilka S, Saum J et al. Investigations into the compatibility of teicoplanin with heparin. *Eur J Parenter Sci.* 1997; 2:51–5.

2166. Walker SE, Walshaw PR. Imipenem stability and staining of teeth. *Can J Hosp Pharm.* 1997; 50:61–7.

2167. Liu L, Ammar DA, Ross LA et al. Silicone oil microdroplets and protein aggregates in repackaged bevacizumab and ranibizumab: effects of long-term storage and product mishandling. *Invest Ophthalmol Vis Sci.* 2011; 52:1023–34.

2168. Burm JP. Stability of ondansetron and fluconazole in 5% dextrose injection and normal saline during Y-site admin-istration. *Arch Pharm Res.* 1997; 20:171–5.

2169. Truelle-Hugon B, Tourrette G, Couineaux B et al. Etude de stabilite du chlorhydrate de morphine Lavoisier dans differents systemes actifs pour perfusion apres reconstitu-tion dans divers solvents. *Ann Pharm Fr.* 1997; 55:216–23.

2170. Sitaram BR, Tsui M, Rawicki HB et al. Stability and compat-ibility of intrathecal admixtures containing baclofen and high concentrations of morphine. *Int J Pharm.* 1997; 153:13–24.

2171. Trinkle R. Compatibility of hydromorphone and prochlor-perazine, and irritation due to subcutaneous prochlorpera-zine infusion. *Ann Pharmacother.* 1997; 31:789–90.

2172. Guchelar HJ, Hartog ME. De stabiliteit van clonaze-paminjectievloeistof. *Ziekenhuisfarmacie.* 1997; 13:21–3.

2173. Leboucher G, Charpiat B. Incompatibilite physico-chimique entre l'omeprazole et la vancomycine. *Pharm Hosp Fr.* 1997; 121:124.

2174. Taylor A. Review of clarithromycin mixtures. *Pharm Pract.* (Oct) 1997; 7:473, 474, 476.

2175. Farhang-Asnafi S, Callaert S, Barre J et al. Influence du solvant de dilution sur la stabilite de la nouvelle forme de 5-fluorouracile en perfusion. *J Pharm Clin.* 1997; 16:45–8.

2176. Oustric-Mendes AC, Huart B, Le Hoang MD et al. Study protocol: stability of morphine injected without preser-vative, delivered with a disposable infusion device. *J Clin Pharm Ther.* 1997; 22:283–90.

2177. Schoffski P, Freund M, Wunder R et al. Safety and toxicity of amphotericin B in glucose 5% or Intralipid 20% in neutropenic patients with pneumonia or fever of unknown origin: randomised study. *BMJ.* 1998; 317:379–84.

2178. Heinemann V, Kahny B, Jehn U et al. Serum pharmacology of amphotericin B applied in lipid emulsions. *Antimicrob Agents Chemother.* 1997; 41:728–32.

2179. Gupta VD, Maswoswe J. Stability of mitomycin aqueous solution when stored in tuberculin syringes. *Int J Pharm Compound.* 1997; 1:282–3.

2180. Targett PL, Keefe PA. Compatibility and stability of drug adjuvants and morphine tartrate in 10 mL polypropylene syringes. *Aust J Hosp Pharm.* 1997; 27:207–12.

2181. Goren MP, Lyman BA. The stability of mesna in beverages and syrup for oral administration. *Cancer Chemother Phar-macol.* 1991; 28:298–301.

2182. Xu QA, Trissel LA. Compatibility of paclitaxel in 5% glucose and 0.9% sodium chloride injections with EVA minibags. *Aust J Hosp Pharm.* 1998; 28:156–9.

2183. Xu QA, Zhang YP, Trissel LA et al. Stability of busulfan injec-tion admixtures in 5% dextrose injection and 0.9% sodium chloride injection. *J Oncol Pharm Pract.* 1996; 2:101–5.

2184. Sarver JG, Pryka R, Alexander KS et al. Stability of magne-sium sulfate in 0.9% sodium chloride and lactated Ringer's solutions. *Int J Pharm Compound.* 1998; 2:385–8.

2185. Jobet-Hermelin I, Mallvais ML, Jacquot C et al. Proposi-tion d'une concentration limite acceptable du plastifiant librere par le poly(chlorure de vinyle) dans les solutions injectables aqueuses. *J Pharm Clin.* 1996; 15:132–6.

2186. Jacobson PA, West NJ, Spadoni V et al. Sterility of filgrastim (G-CSF) in syringes. *Ann Pharmacother.* 1996; 30:1238–42.

2187. Trissel LA, Spadoni VT. Comment: filgrastim sterility in syringes. *Ann Pharmacother.* 1997; 31:500–1.

2188. Appenheimer MM, Schepart BS, Poleon GP et al. Stability of albumin-free interferon alfa-2b for 42 days. *Am J Health-Syst Pharm.* 1998; 55:1602–5.

2189. Trissel LA, Gilbert DL. Concentration dependency of vancomycin hydrochloride compatibility with beta-lactam antibiotics during simulated Y-site administration. *Hosp Pharm.* 1998; 33:1515–22.

2190. McLaughlin JP, Simpson C. How stable is acyclovir in PVC bags? The stability of reconstituted acyclovir sodium in a 0.9% w/v sodium chloride infusion when stored at room temperature. *Pharm Pract.* 1995; 5:53–8.

2191. Mehta AC, Kay EA. How stable is alfentanil? Stability of alfentanil hydrochloride in 5% dextrose stored in syringes. *Pharm Pract.* 1995; 5:303–4.

2192. McLaughlin JP, Simpson C. How stable are Zinacef & Metrovex? The stability of cefuroxime sodium and metro-nidazole infusion when stored in a refrigerator. *Pharm Pract.* 1995; 5:100–6.

2193. Bonferoni MC, Mellerio G, Giunchedi P et al. Photosta-bility evaluation of nicardipine HCl solutions. *Int J Pharm.* 1992; 80:109–17.

2194. Erdman SH, McElwee CL, Kramer JM et al. Central line occlu-sion with three-in-one nutrition admixtures administered at home. *JPEN J Parenter Enteral Nutr.* 1994; 18:177–81.

2195. Allwood MC, Martin H. Factors influencing the stability of ranitidine in TPN mixtures. *Clin Nutr.* 1995; 14:171–6.

2196. Hoie EB, Narducci WA. Laser particle analysis of calcium phosphate precipitate in neonatal TPN admixtures. *J Ped Pharm Pract.* 1996; 1:163–7.

2197. Ambados F, Brealey J. Incompatibilities with trace elements during TPN solution admixture. *Aust J Hosp Pharm.* 1998; 28:112–4.

2198. Xu QA, Trissel LA. Compatibility of paclitaxel injection diluent with two reduced-phthalate administration sets for the Acclaim pump. *Int J Pharm Compound.* 1998; 2:382–4.

2199. Stewart JT, Warren FW, King DT et al. Stability of ondansetron hydrochloride and 12 medications in plastic syringes. *Am J Health-Syst Pharm.* 1998; 55:2630–4.

2200. Donnelly RF, Bushfield TL. Chemical stability of meperidine hydrochloride in polypropylene syringes. *Int J Pharm Compound.* 1998; 2:463–5.

2201. Jappinen AL, Kokki H, Rasi AS et al. Stability of sufentanil in a syringe pump under simulated epidural infusion. *Int J Pharm Compound.* 1998; 2:466–8.

2202. Wilson KM, Schneider JJ. Stability of midazolam and fentanyl in infusion solutions. *J Pain Symptom Manage.* 1998; 16:52–8.

2203. Gupta VD, Pramar Y. Stability of lorazepam in 5% dextrose injection. *Int J Pharm Compound.* 1998; 2:322–4.

2204. Heide PE. Precipitation of amphotericin B from i.v. fat emulsion. *Am J Health-Syst Pharm.* 1997; 54:1449.

2205. Heide PE, Hehenberger H. Tensiometrische und konduktometrische stabilitatuntersuchungen von amphotericin B in fettmulsionen. *Oesterreichische Krankenhaus Pharmazie.* 1996; 10:36–43.

2206. To TP, Garrett MK. Stability of flucloxacillin in a hospital in the home program. *Aust J Hosp Pharm.* 1998; 28:289–90.

2207. Levanda M. Noticeable difference in admixtures prepared from lorazepam 2 and 4 mg/mL. *Am J Health-Syst Pharm.* 1998; 55:2305.

2208. Share MJ, Harrison RD, Folstad J et al. Stability of lorazepam 1 and 2 mg/mL in glass bottles and polypropylene syringes. *Am J Health-Syst Pharm.* 1998; 55:2013–5.

2209. Inagaki K, Kambara M, Mizuno M et al. Compatibility and stability of ranitidine hydrochloride with six cephalosporins during simulated Y-site administration. *Int J Pharm Compound.* 1998; 2:318–21.

2210. Ray LR, Chen DA. Stability of somatropin stored in plastic syringes for 28 days. *Am J Health-Syst Pharm.* 1998; 55:1508–11.

2211. Patel K, Craig SB, McBride MG et al. Microbial inhibitory properties and stability of topotecan hydrochloride injection. *Am J Health-Syst Pharm.* 1998; 55:1584–7.

2212. English BA, Riggs RM, Webster AA et al. Y-site stability of fosphenytoin and sodium phenobarbital. *Int J Pharm Compound.* 1999; 3:64–6.

2213. Lieu CL, Chin A. Five-day stability of vinorelbine in 5% dextrose injection and in 0.9% sodium chloride injection at room temperature. *Int J Pharm Compound.* 1999; 3:67–8.

2214. Akkerman SR, Zhang H, Mullins RE et al. Stability of milrinone lactate in the presence of 29 critical care drugs and 4 i.v. solutions. *Am J Health-Syst Pharm.* 1999; 56:63–8.

2215. Trissel LA, Gilbert DL, Martinez JF et al. Compatibility of medications with 3–in–1 parenteral nutrition admixtures. *JPEN J Parenter Enteral Nutr.* 1999; 23:67–74.

2216. Johnson CE, vandenBussche HL, Chio CC et al. Stability of tacrolimus with morphine sulfate, hydromorphone hydrochloride, and ceftazidime during simulated intravenous coadministration. *Am J Health-Syst Pharm.* 1999; 56:164–9.

2217. Stamatakis MK, Leader WG. Stability of high-dose vancomycin and ceftazidime in peritoneal dialysis solutions. *Am J Health-Syst Pharm.* 1999; 56:246–8.

2218. Trissel LA, Martinez JF. Compatibility of etoposide phosphate with selected drugs during simulated Y-site injection. *J Am Pharm Assoc.* 1999; 39:141–5.

2219. Zhang Y, Trissel LA. Physical and chemical stability of etoposide phosphate solutions. *J Am Pharm Assoc.* 1999; 39:146–50.

2220. Stewart JT, Warren FW. Stability of cefepime hydrochloride injection in polypropylene syringes at -20°C, 4°C, and 22–24°C. *Am J Health Syst Pharm.* 1999; 56:457–9.

2221. Stewart JT, Maddox FC. Stability of cefepime hydrochloride in polypropylene syringes. *Am J Health-Syst Pharm.* 1999; 56:1134.

2222. Burkiewicz JS. Incompatibility of ceftriaxone sodium with lactated Ringer's injection. *Am J Health-Syst Pharm.* 1999; 56:384.

2223. Riggs RM, English BA, Webster AA et al. Fosphenytoin Y-site stability studies with lorazepam and midazolam hydrochloride. *Int J Pharm Compound.* 1999; 3:235–8.

2224. Trissel LA, Gilbert DL. Compatibility of docetaxel with selected drugs during simulated Y-site administration. *Int J Pharm Compound.* 1999; 3:241–4.

2225. Johnson CE, Truong NM. Stability and compatibility of tacrolimus and fluconazole in 0.9% sodium chloride. *J Am Pharm Assoc.* 1999; 39:505–8.

2226. Trissel LA, Martinez JF. Compatibility of gemcitabine hydrochloride with 107 selected drugs during simulated Y-site injection. *J Am Pharm Assoc.* 1999; 39:514–8.

2227. Xu Q, Zhang Y. Physical and chemical stability of gemcitabine hydrochloride solutions. *J Am Pharm Assoc.* 1999; 39:509–13.

2228. Walker SE, Gray S. Stability of reconstituted indomethacin sodium trihydrate in original vials and polypropylene syringes. *Am J Health-Syst Pharm.* 1998; 55:154–8.

2229. Schlatter J, Saulnier JL. Inline filtration of ranitidine hydrochloride solutions. *Am J Health-Syst Pharm.* 1998; 55:840.

2230. Zhang Y, Trissel LA. Paclitaxel compatibility with a triple-lumen polyurethane central catheter. *Hosp Pharm.* 1998; 33:547–51.

2231. Xu QA, Trissel LA. Paclitaxel compatibility with the IV Express filter unit. *Int J Pharm Compound.* 1998; 2:243–5.

2232. Xu QA, Trissel LA. Paclitaxel compatibility with a TOTM-plasticized PVC administration set. *Hosp Pharm.* 1997; 32:1635–8.

2233. Saltsman CL, Tom CM, Mitchell A et al. Compatibility of levofloxacin with 34 medications during simulated Y-site administration. *Am J Health-Syst Pharm.* 1999; 56:1458–9.

2234. Trissel LA, Gilbert DL. Compatibility screening of gatifloxacin during simulated Y-site administration with other drugs. *Hosp Pharm.* 1999; 34:1409–16.

2235. Voytilla KL, Rusho WJ. Compatibility of alatrofloxacin mesylate with commonly used drugs during Y-site delivery. *Am J Health-Syst Pharm.* 2000; 57:1437–9.

2236. Johnson CE, Truong NM. Stability and compatibility of tacrolimus and fluconazole in 0.9% sodium chloride. *J Am Pharm Assoc.* 1999; 39:505–8.

2237. Paul M, Vieillard V, Roumi E et al. Long-term stability of bevacizumab repackaged in 1mL polypropylene syringes for intravitreal administration. *Ann Pharm Fr.* 2012; 70:139–54.

2238. Balthasar JP. Concentration-dependent incompatibility of vinorelbine tartrate and heparin sodium. *Am J Health-Syst Pharm.* 1999; 56:1891.

2239. Wolfe JL, Thoma LA, Du C et al. Compatibility and stability of vincristine sulfate, doxorubicin hydrochloride, and etoposide in 0.9% sodium chloride injection. *Am J Health-Syst Pharm.* 1999; 56:985–9.

2240. Peek BT, Webster KD. Stability and compatibility of promethazine hydrochloride and dihydroergotamine mesylate in combination. *Am J Health-Syst Pharm.* 1999; 56:1835–8.

2241. Webster AA, English BA, McGuire JM et al. Stability of dobutamine hydrochloride 4 mg/mL in 5% dextrose injection at 5 and 23 (C. *Int J Pharmaceut Compound.* 1999; 3:412–4.

2242. Thiesen J, Kramer I. Physico-chemical stability of docetaxel premix solution and docetaxel infusion solutions in PVC bags and polyolefine containers. *Pharm World Sci.* 1999; 21:137–41.

2243. Kramer I, Thiesen J. Stability of topotecan infusion solutions in polyvinylchloride bags and elastomeric portable infusion devices. *J Oncol Pharm Pract.* 1999; 5:75–82.

2244. Hecq JD, Evrard JM, Gillet P et al. Etude de stabilite visuelle du chlorydrate de chlorpromazine, du chlorure de potassium, de la furosemide et de l'heparine sodique en perfusion continue. *Pharmakon.* 1998; 116:145–8.

2245. Mayron D, Gennaro AR. Stability and compatibility of topotecan hydrochloride with selected drugs. *Am J Health-Syst Pharm.* 1999; 56:875–81.

2246. Harvey SC, Toussaint CP, Coe SE et al. Stability of meperidine in an implantable infusion pump using capillary gas chromatography-mass spectrometry and a deuterated internal standard. *J Pharm Biomed Anal.* 1999; 21:577–83.

2247. Trissel LA, Xu QA. Compatibility and stability of paclitaxel combined with doxorubicin hydrochloride in infusion solutions. *Ann Pharmacother.* 1998; 32:1013–6.

2248. Rogers CH, Soine TO, Wilson CO. A text-book of inorganic pharmaceutical chemistry. 4th ed. Philadelphia: Lea and Febiger; 1948: 152.

2249. Bergquist PA, Zimmerman J, Kenney RR et al. Stability of tirofiban hydrochloride in three commonly used i.v. solutions and polyvinyl chloride administration sets. *Am J Health-Syst Pharm.* 1999; 56:1627–9.

2250. Bergquist PA, Hunke WA, Reed RA et al. Compatibility of tirofiban HCl with dopamine HCl, famotidine, sodium heparin, lidocaine HCl and potassium chloride during simulated Y-site administration. *J Clin Pharm Ther.* 1999; 24:125–32.

2251. McLaughlin JP, Simpson C. How stable is ganciclovir? *Pharm Pract.* 1998; 8:329–30, 332.

2252. Galanti LM, Hecq JD, Vanbeckbergen D et al. Long-term stability of vancomycin hydrochloride in intravenous infusions. *J Clin Pharm Ther.* 1997; 22:353–6.

2253. Hor MMS, Chan SY, Yow KL et al. Stability of admixtures of pethidine and metoclopramide in aqueous solution, 5% dextrose and 0.9% sodium chloride. *J Clin Pharm Ther.* 1997; 22:339–45.

2254. Hor MM, Chan SY, Yow KL et al. Stability of morphine sulphate in saline under simulated patient administration conditions. *J Clin Pharm Ther.* 1997; 22:405–10.

2255. Mittner A, Vincze Z. Stability of cyclophosphamide containing infusions. *Pharmazie.* 1999; 54:224–5.

2256. Mittner A, Vincze Z. Stability of vinblastine sulphate containing infusions. *Pharmazie.* 1999; 54:625–6.

2257. Schrijvers D, Tai-Apin C, De Smet MC et al. Determination of compatibility and stability of drugs used in palliative care. *J Clin Pharm Ther.* 1998; 23:311–4.

2258. Kopelent-Frank H, Schimper A. HPTLC-based stability assay for the determination of amiodarone in intravenous admixtures. *Pharmazie.* 1999; 54:542–4.

2259. Inagaki K, Miyamoto Y, Kurata N et al. Stability of ranitidine hydrochloride with cefazolin sodium, cefbuperazone sodium, cefoxitin sodium, and cephalothin sodium during simulated Y-site administration. *Int J Pharmaceut Compound.* 2000; 4:150–3.

2260. Roy JJ, Hildgen P. Stability of morphine-ketamine mixtures in 0.9% sodium chloride injection packaged in syringes, plastic bags and Medication Cassette reservoirs. *Int J Pharmaceut Compound.* 2000; 4:225–8.

2261. Grant EM, Zhong MK, Ambrose PG et al. Stability of meropenem in a portable infusion device in a cold pouch. *Am J Health-Syst Pharm.* 2000; 57:992–5.

2262. Xu QA, Trissel LA. Compatibility and stability of linezolid injection admixed with three cephalosporin antibiotics. *J Am Pharm Assoc.* 2000; 40:509–14.

2263. Zhang Y, Xu QA, Trissel LA et al. Compatibility and stability of linezolid injection admixed with aztreonam or piperacillin sodium. *J Am Pharm Assoc.* 2000; 40:520–4.

2264. Trissel LA, Williams KY. Compatibility screening of linezolid injection during simulated Y-site administration with other drugs and infusion solutions. *J Am Pharm Assoc.* 2000; 40:515–9.

2265. Zhang Y, Xu QA, Trissel LA et al. Physical compatibility of calcium acetate and potassium phosphates in parenteral nutrition solutions containing Aminosyn II. *Int J Pharmaceut Compound.* 1999; 3:415–20.

2266. Ambados F, Brealey J. Precipitation of potassium sulphate during TPN solution admixture. *Aust J Hosp Pharm.* 1998; 28:444.

2267. Ambados F. Destabilization of fat emulsion in total nutrient admixtures by concentrated albumin 20% infusion. *Aust J Hosp Pharm.* 1999; 29:210–2.

2268. Peterson GM, Miller KA, Galloway JG et al. Compatibility and stability of fentanyl admixtures in polypropylene syringes. *J Clin Pharm Ther.* 1998; 23(1):67–72.

2269. Picard C, Hary L, Bou P et al. Stability of three aminoglycoside solutions in PVC and multilayer infusion bags. *Pharmazie.* 1999; 54:854–6.

2270. Shella C. How to shake insulin. *Hosp Pharm.* 1999; 34:518.

2271. Bjorkman S, Roth B. Chemical compatibility of mitoxantrone and etoposide (VP-16). *Acta Pharm Nord.* 1991; 3:251.

2272. Charland SL, Davis DD. Activity of enoxaparin sodium in tuberculin syringes for 10 days. *Am J Health-Syst Pharm*. 1998; 55:1296–8.

2273. Couldry R, Sanborn M, Klutman NE et al. Continuous infusion of ceftazidime with an elastomeric infusion device. *Am J Health-Syst Pharm*. 1998; 55:145–9.

2274. Tanoue N, Kishita S, Shiotsu K et al. Compatibility of irinotecan hydrochloride injection with other injections. *Jpn J Hosp Pharm*. 1998; 24:420–8.

2275. Stiles ML, Allen LV Jr. Stability of two concentrations of heparin sodium prefilled in CADD-Micro pump syringes. *Int J Pharmaceut Compound*. 1997; 1:433–4.

2276. Nii LJ, Chin A, Cao TM et al. Stability of sumatriptan succinate in polypropylene syringes. *Am J Health-Syst Pharm*. 1999; 56:983–5.

2277. Proot P, Van Schepdael A, Raymakers AA et al. Stability of adenosine in infusion. *J Pharm Biomed Anal*. 1998; 17:415–8.

2278. Biellmann-Berlaud V, Willemin JC. Stabilite de la vancomycine en poches de polyolefine ou polychlorure de vinyle et en flacons de verre. *J Pharm Clin*. 1998; 17(3):145–8.

2280. Demange C, Vailleau JL, Wacquier S et al. Etude de photosensibilite et fixation de la chlorpromazine sur le chlorure de polyvinyle pour administration en perfusion intraveineuse. *J Pharm Clin*. 1998; 17:77–82.

2281. Saito H, Tanida N, Inukai K et al. Stability of iphosphamide and mesna in mixed infusion solutions. *Jpn J Hosp Pharm*. 1998; 24:96–99.

2282. Silvers KM, Darlow BA, Winterbourn CC. Pharmacologic levels of heparin do not destabilize neonatal parenteral nutrition. *JPEN J Parenter Enteral Nutr*. 1998; 22:311–4.

2283. Williamson JC, Volles DF, Lynch PLM et al. Stability of cefepime in peritoneal dialysis solution. *Ann Pharmacother*. 1999; 33:906–9.

2284. Kramer I, Maas B. Compatibility of amsacrine (Amsidyl) concentrate for infusion with polypropylene syringes. *Pharmazie*. 1999; 54:538–41.

2285. Farina A, Porra R, Cotichini V et al. Stability of reconstituted solutions of ceftazidime for injections: an HPLC and CE approach. *J Pharm Biomed Anal*. 1999; 20:521–30.

2286. Yokoyama H, Aoyama T, Matsuyama T et al. The cause of polyurethane catheter cracking during constant infusion of etoposide (VP-16) injection. *Yakugaku Zasshi*. 1998; 118:581–8.

2287. Torres-Bondia FI, Carmona-Ibanez G, Guevara-Serrano J et al. Estabilidad del valproate sodico en fluidos intravenosos. *Farm Hosp*. 1999; 23:320–2.

2288. Priston MJ, Sewell GJ. Stability of three cytotoxic drug infusions in the Graseby 9000 ambulatory infusion pump. *J Oncol Pharm Pract*. 1998; 4:143–9.

2289. Zeidler C, Dettmering D, Schrammel W et al. Compatibility of various drugs used in intensive care medicine in polyethylene, PVC, and glass infusion containers. *Europ Hosp Pharm*. 1999; 5:106–10.

2290. Goettner K (Scientific Affairs, Janssen, Horsham, PA): Personal communication; 2016 Apr 29.

2291. Shay DK, Fann LM. Respiratory distress and sudden death associated with receipt of a peripheral parenteral nutrition admixture. *Infect Control Hosp Epidemiol*. 1997; 18:814–7.

2292. Zhan X, Yin G. Improved stability of 25% vitamin C parenteral formulation. *Int J Pharm*. 1998; 173:43–9.

2293. Mittner A, Vincze Z. Stability of cisplatin containing infusions. *Pharmazie*. 1998; 53:490–2.

2294. Carleton BC, Primmett DR, Levine M et al. Sterility of unit-dosing filgrastim (G-CSF). *J Ped Pharm Pract*. 1999; 4:68–74.

2295. Oliva A, Santovena A, Llabres M et al. Stability study of human albumin pharmaceutical preparations. *J Pharm Pharmacol*. 1999; 51:385–92.

2296. Stephens D, Bares D, Robinson D et al. Determination of amylose/particulate relationship in hydroxyethylstarch. *PDA J Pharm Sci Technol*. 1999; 53:181–5.

2297. Parsons TJ, Upton RN, Martinez AM et al. No loss of undiluted propofol by sorption into administration systems. *Pharm Pharmacol Commun*. 1999; 5:377–81.

2298. Brigas F, Sautou-Miranda V, Normand B et al. Compatibility of tropisetron with glass and plastics. Stability under different storage conditions. *J Pharm Pharmacol*. 1998; 50(4):407–11.

2299. Tse CST, Abdullah, R. Dissolving phenytoin precipitate in central venous access device. *Ann Intern Med*. 1998; 128:1049.

2300. Akinwande KI, Keehn DM. Dissolution of phenytoin precipitate with sodium bicarbonate in an occluded central venous access device. *Ann Pharmacother*. 1995; 29:707–9.

2301. Fuloria M, Friedberg MA, DuRant RH et al. Effect of flow rate and insulin priming on the recovery of insulin from microbore infusion tubing. *Pediatrics*. 1998; 102:1401–6.

2302. Muller HJ, Frank C. Stabilitatstudie zu pentoxifyllin im PVC-infusionsbeutel. *Krankenhauspharmazie*. 1998; 19:469–72.

2303. Stahlmann SA, Frey OR. Stabilitatstudie zu fosfomycin-dinatrium (Fosfocin p.i. 5,0) in applikationfertigen perfusorspritzen. *Krankenhauspharmazie*. 1998; 19:553–7.

2304. Muller HJ, Frank C. Stabilitatstudie zu alizaprid im PVC-infusionsbeutel. *Krankenhauspharmazie*. 1999; 20:55–8.

2305. Sattler A, Jage J. Physico-chemical stability of infusion solutions for epidural administration containing fentanyl and bupivacaine or lidocaine. *Pharmazie*. 1998; 53:386–91.

2306. Laborie S, Lavoie JC, Pineault M et al. Protecting solutions of parenteral nutrition from peroxidation. *JPEN J Parenter Enteral Nutr*. 1999; 23(2):104–8.

2307. Wakiya Y, Saiki A, Kondou N et al. Stability of vitamins in the TPN mixture at a clinical site. *Jpn J Hosp Pharm*. 1999; 25:40–7.

2308. Pertkkiewicz M, Knyt A, Majewska K et al. Badania stabilnosci mieszanin odzywczych z aminomel 10%E i aminomel 12,5%E oraz emulsja tluszczowa ivelip 10% i 20%. *Farm Polska*. 1999; 55(16):756–63.

2309. Brawley V, Bhatia J. Effect of sodium metabisulfite on hydrogen peroxide production in light-exposed pediatric parenteral amino acid solutions. *Am J Health-Syst Pharm*. 1998; 55:1288–92.

2310. Brawley V, Bhatia J. Hydrogen peroxide generation in a model paediatric parenteral amino acid solution. *Clin Sci*. 1993; 85:709–12.

2312. Malesker MA, Malone PM, Cingle CM et al. Extravasation of i.v. promethazine. *Am J Health-Syst Pharm*. 1999; 56:1742–3.

2313. Boersma HH, Groothuijsen HJG, Stolk LML et al. Goed loudbaar onder normale omstandigheden. *Pharmaceut Weekblad.* 1999; 134:1444–8.

2314. Akorn, Inc. Ephedrine sulfate injection for IM, IV, or SC use prescribing information. Lake Forest, IL; 2012 Dec.

2315. Khalfi F, Dine T, Gressier B et al. Compatibility of cefpirome and cephalothin with PVC bags during simulated infusion and storage. *Pharmazie.* 1998; 53:112–6.

2316. Laborie S, Lavoie JC, Pineault M et al. Contribution of multivitamins, air, and light in the generation of peroxides in adult and neonatal parenteral nutrition solutions. *Ann Pharmacother.* 2000; 34:440–5.

2317. Laborie S, Lavoie JC. Paradoxical role of ascorbic acid and riboflavin in solutions of total parenteral nutrition: implication in photoinduced peroxide generation. *Pediat Res.* 1998; 43:601–6.

2318. Rhoney DH, Coplin WM. Urokinase activity after freezing: implications for thrombolysis in intraventricular hemorrhage. *Am J Health-Syst Pharm.* 1999; 56:2047–51.

2319. Hrubisko M, McGown AT, Prendiville JA et al. Suitability of cisplatin solutions for 14–day continuous infusion by ambulatory pump. *Cancer Chemother Pharmacol.* 1992; 29:252–5.

2320. Dine T, Khalfi F, Gressier B et al. Stability study of fotemustine in PVC infusion bags and sets under various conditions using a stability-indicating high-performance liquid chromatographic assay. *J Pharm Biomed Anal.* 1998; 18:373–81.

2321. Hadfield JA, McGown AT, Dawson MJ et al. The suitability of carboplatin solutions for 14–day continuous infusion by ambulatory pump: an HPLC-dynamic FAB study. *J Pharm Biomed Anal.* 1993; 11:723–7.

2322. Frey OR, Maier L. Polyethylene vials of calcium gluconate reduce aluminum contamination of TPN. *Ann Pharmacother.* 2000; 34:811–12.

2323. Louie S, Chin A. Activity of dalteparin sodium in polypropylene syringes. *Am J Health-Syst Pharm.* 2000; 57:760–2.

2324. Stewart JT, Maddox FC. Stability of cefepime hydrochloride injection and metronidazole in polyvinyl chloride bags at 4°C and 22°C-24°C. *Hosp Pharm.* 2000; 35:1057–64.

2325. Ling J, Gupta VD. Stability of nafcillin sodium after reconstitution in 0.9% sodium chloride injection and storage in polypropylene syringes for pediatric use. *Int J Pharmaceut Compound.* 2000; 4:480–1.

2326. Gupta VD. Stability of levothyroxine sodium injection in polypropylene syringes. *Int J Pharmaceut Compound.* 2000; 4:482–3.

2327. Davis SN, Vermeulen L, Banton J et al. Activity and dosage of alteplase dilution for clearing occlusions of venous-access devices. *Am J Health-Syst Pharm.* 2000; 57:1039–45.

2328. Generali J, Cada DJ. Alteplase (t-PA) bolus: occluded catheters. *Hosp Pharm.* 2001; 36:93–103.

2329. Phelps KC, Verzino KC. Alternatives to urokinase for the management of central venous catheter occlusion. *Hosp Pharm.* 2001; 36:265–74.

2330. Haire WD, Herbst SL. Use of alteplase (t-PA) for the management of thrombotic catheter dysfunction: guidelines from a consensus conference of the National Association of Vascular Access Networks (NAVAN). *Nutr Clin Pract.* 2000; 15:265–75.

2331. Gupta VD, Ling J. Stability of hydrocortisone sodium succinate after reconstitution in 0.9% sodium chloride injection and storage in polypropylene syringes for pediatric use. *Int J Pharmaceut Compound.* 2000; 4:396–7.

2332. Xu QA, Trissel LA, Zhang Y et al. Compatibility and stability of linezolid injection admixed with gentamicin sulfate and tobramycin sulfate. *Int J Pharmaceut Compound.* 2000; 4:476–9.

2333. Trissel LA, Zhang Y. Incompatibility of erythromycin lactobionate and sulfamethoxazole/trimethoprim with linezolid injection. *Hosp Pharm.* 2000; 35:1192–6.

2334. Zhang Y, Xu QA, Trissel LA et al. Compatibility and stability of linezolid injection admixed with three quinolone antibiotics. *Ann Pharmacother.* 2000; 34:996–1001.

2335. Xu QA, Zhang Y, Trissel LA et al. Adequacy of a new chlorhexidine-bearing polyurethane central catheter for administration of 82 selected parenteral drugs. *Ann Pharmacother.* 2000; 34:1109–16.

2336. Trissel LA. Drug compatibility differences with propofol injectable emulsion products. *Crit Care Med.* 2001; 29:466–8.

2337. Favier M, De Cazanove F, Coste A et al. Stability of carmustine in polyvinyl chloride bags and polyethylene-lined trilayer plastic containers. *Am J Health-Syst Pharm.* 2001; 58(3):238–41.

2338. Zhang Y, Trissel LA. Compatibility of linezolid injection with intravenous administration sets. *J Am Pharm Assoc.* 2001; 41:285–6.

2339. Trissel LA, Williams KY. Compatibility screening of Hextend during simulated Y-site administration with other drugs. *Int J Pharmaceut Compound.* 2001; 5:69–73.

2340. Gupta VD. Chemical stability of methylprednisolone sodium succinate after reconstitution in 0.9% sodium chloride injection and storage in polypropylene syringes. *Int J Pharmaceut Compound.* 2001; 5:148–50.

2341. Ling J, Gupta VD. Stability of cefepime hydrochloride after reconstitution in 0.9% sodium chloride injection and storage in polypropylene syringes for pediatric use. *Int J Pharmaceut Compound.* 2001; 5:151–2.

2342. Sterling J. Intralipids and tubing changes. *Hosp Pharm.* 2001; 36:258–9.

2343. Yuan P, Grimes GJ, Shankman SE et al. Compatibility and stability of vincristine sulfate, doxorubicin hydrochloride, and etoposide phosphate in 0.9% sodium chloride injection. *Am J Health-Syst Pharm.* 2001; 58:594–8.

2344. Baker MT. Yellowing of metabisulfite-containing propofol emulsion. *Am J Health-Syst Pharm.* 2001; 58:1042.

2345. Gupta VD, Ling J. Stability of piperacillin sodium after reconstitution in 0.9% sodium chloride injection and storage in polypropylene syringes for pediatric use. *Int J Pharmaceut Compound.* 2001; 5:230–1.

2346. Bethune K, Allwood M, Grainger C et al. Use of filters during the preparation and administration of parenteral nutrition: position paper and guidelines prepared by a British Pharmaceutical Nutrition Group Working Party. *Nutrition.* 2001; 17:403–8.

2347. Gellis C, Sautou-Miranda V, Arvouet A et al. Stability of methylprednisolone sodium succinate in pediatric parenteral nutrition mixtures. *Am J Health-Syst Pharm.* 2001; 58:1139–42.

2348. Redhead HM, Jones CB. Pharmaceutical and antimicrobial differences between propofol emulsion products. *Am J Health-Syst Pharm*. 2000; 57:1174.

2349. Mirejovsky D, Ghosh M. Pharmaceutical and antimicrobial differences between propofol emulsion products. *Am J Health-Syst Pharm*. 2000; 57:1176–7.

2350. Trissel LA, Zhang Y. The stability of diluted vincristine sulfate used as a deterrent to inadvertent intrathecal injection. *Hosp Pharm*. 2001; 36:740–5.

2351. Thoma LA, Johnson-Singh A, Wood GC et al. Physical compatibility of 10% alcohol in 5% dextrose injection with selected drugs during simulated Y-site administration. *Am J Health-Syst Pharm*. 2000; 57:2286–7.

2352. Chalmers JR, Bobek MB, Militello MA. Visual compatibility of amiodarone hydrochloride injection with various intravenous drugs. *Am J Health-Syst Pharm*. 2001; 58:504–6.

2353. Gupta VD, Bailey RE. Stability of alatrofloxacin mesylate in 5% dextrose injection and 0.45% sodium-chloride injection. *Int J Pharmaceut Compound*. 2000; 4:66–8.

2354. Gupta VD. Stability of levothyroxine sodium injection in polypropylene syringes, *Int J Pharmaceut Compound*. 2000; 4:482–3.

2355. Garabito MJ, Jimenez L, Bautista FJ et al. Stability of tirofiban hydrochloride in 0.9% sodium chloride injection for 30 days. *Am J Health-Syst Pharm*. 2001; 58:1850–1.

2356. Bergquist PA, Manas D, Hunke WA et al. Stability and compatibility of tirofiban hydrochloride during simulated Y-site administration with other drugs. *Am J Health-Syst Pharm*. 2001; 58:1218–23.

2357. Seto W, Trope A, Carfrae L et al. Visual compatibility of sodium nitroprusside with other injectable medications given to pediatric patients. *Am J Health-Syst Pharm*. 2001; 58:1422–6.

2358. Zhang Y, Trissel LA. Stability of piperacillin and ticarcillin in AutoDose infusion system bags. *Ann Pharmacother*. 2001; 35:1360–3.

2359. Godwin DA, Kim NH, Zuniga R. Stability of baclofen and clonidine hydrochloride admixture for intrathecal administration. *Hosp Pharm*. 2001; 36:950–4.

2360. Quay I, Tan E. Compatibility and stability of potassium chloride and magnesium sulfate in 0.9% sodium chloride injection and 5% dextrose injection solutions. *Int J Pharmaceut Compound*. 2001; 5:323–4.

2361. Vega E, Sola N. Quantitative analysis of metronidazole in intravenous admixture with ciprofloxacin by first derivative spectrophotometry. *J Pharm Biomed Anal*. 2001; 25:523–30.

2362. Inagaki K, Miyamoto Y, Kurata N et al. Stability of ranitidine hydrochloride with cefazolin sodium, cefbuperazone sodium, cefoxitin sodium and cephalothin sodium during simulated Y-site administration. *Int J Pharmaceut Compound*. 2000; 4:150–3.

2363. Trissel LA, Xu QA, Zhang Y et al. Stability of ciprofloxacin and vancomycin hydrochloride in AutoDose infusion system bags. *Hosp Pharm*. 2001; 36:1170–3.

2364. Galanti LM, Hecq JD, Jeuniau P et al. Assessment of the stability of teicoplanin in intravenous infusions. *Int J Pharmaceut Compound*. 2001; 5:397–400.

2365. Storms ML, Stewart JT, Warren FW. Stability of ephedrine sulfate at ambient temperature and 4 °C in polypropylene syringes. *Int J Pharmaceut Compound*. 2001; 5:394–6.

2366. Faouzi MA, Khalfi F, Dine T et al. Stability, compatibility and plasticizer extraction of quinine injection added to infusion solutions and stored in polyvinyl chloride (PVC) containers. *J Pharmaceut Biomed Anal*. 1999; 21:923–30.

2367. della Cuno FSR, Mella M, Magistrali G, et al. Stability and compatibility of methylprednisolone acetate and ropivacaine hydrochloride in polypropylene syringes for epidural administration, *Am J Health-Syst Pharm*. 2001; 58:1753–6.

2368. Voytilla KL, Tyler LS, Rusho WJ. Visual compatibility of azithromycin with 24 commonly used drugs during simulated Y-site delivery. *Am J Health-Syst Pharm*. 2002; 59:853–5.

2369. Trissel LA, Zhang Y, Baker MB. Stability of fenoldopam mesylate in two infusion solutions. *Am J Health-Syst Pharm*. 2002; 59:846–8.

2370. Xu QA, Trissel LA, Saenz CA, et al. Stability of three cephalosporin antibiotics in AutoDose infusion system bags, *J Am Pharm Assoc*. 2002; 42:428–31.

2371. Gupta VD. Stability of cefotaxime sodium after reconstitution in 0.9% sodium chloride injection and storage in polypropylene syringes for pediatric use. *Int J Pharmaceut Compound*. 2002; 6:234–6.

2372. Walker SE, Dufour A, Iazzetta J. Concentration and solution dependent stability of cloxacillin intravenous solutions. *Can J Hosp Pharm*. 1998; 51:13–9.

2373. Trissel LA, Saenz CA. Compatibility screening of bivalirudin during simulated Y-site administration with other drugs. *Int J Pharmaceut Compound*. 2002; 6:311–4.

2374. Baroletti S, Hartman C, Churchill W. Visual compatibility of abciximab with selected drugs. *Am J Health-Syst Pharm*. 2002; 59:466–7.

2375. Li WY, Koda RT. Stability of irinotecan hydrochloride in aqueous solutions. *Am J Health-Syst Pharm*. 2002; 59:539–44.

2376. Trissel LA, Xu QA, Pham L. Physical and chemical stability of morphine sulfate 5 mg/mL and 50 mg/mL packaged in plastic syringes. *Int J Pharmaceut Compound*. 2002; 6:62–5.

2377. Trissel LA, Xu QA, Pham L. Physical and chemical stability of hydromorphone hydrochloride 1.5 mg/mL and 80 mg/mL packaged in plastic syringes. *Int J Pharmaceut Compound*. 2002; 6:74–6.

2378. Trissel LA, Xu QA, Pham L. Physical and chemical stability of low and high concentrations of morphine sulfate with bupivacaine hydrochloride packaged in plastic syringes. *Int J Pharmaceut Compound*. 2002; 6:70–3.

2379. Xu QA, Trissel LA, Saenz CA et al. Stability of gentamicin sulfate and tobramycin sulfate in AutoDose infusion system bags. *Int J Pharmaceut Compound*. 2002; 6:152–4.

2380. Xu QA, Trissel LA, Pham L. Physical and chemical stability of low and high concentrations of morphine sulfate with clonidine hydrochloride packaged in plastic syringes. *Int J Pharmaceut Compound*. 2002; 6:66–9.

2381. Veltri MA, Conner KG. Physical compatibility of milrinone lactate injection with intravenous drugs commonly used in the pediatric intensive care unit. *Am J Health-Syst Pharm*. 2002; 59:452–4.

2382. Elwell RJ, Spencer AP, Barnes JF et al. Stability of furosemide in human albumin solution. *Ann Pharmacother.* 2002; 36:423–6.

2383. Trissel LA, Saenz CA, Ingram DS et al. Compatibility screening of Precedex during simulated Y-site administration with other drugs. *Int J Pharmaceut Compound.* 2002; 6:230–3.

2384. Zhang Y, Trissel LA. Stability of ampicillin sodium, nafcillin sodium, and oxacillin sodium in AutoDose infusion system bags. *Int J Pharmaceut Compound.* 2002; 6:226–9.

2385. Stewart JT, Storms ML, Warren FW. Stability of tubocurarine chloride injection at ambient temperature and 4 °C in polypropylene syringes. *Int J Pharmaceut Compound.* 2002; 6:308–10.

2386. El Aatmani M, Poujol S, Astre C et al. Stability of dacarbazine in amber glass vials and polyvinyl chloride bags. *Am J Health-Syst Pharm.* 2002; 59:1351–6.

2387. Jappinen A, Kokki H, Naaranlahti T. pH stability of injectable fentanyl, bupivacaine, or clonidine solution or a ternary mixture in 0.9% sodium chloride in two types of propylene syringes. *Int J Pharmaceut Compound.* 2002; 6:471–4.

2388. Wu CC, Wand DP, Wong CY et al. Stability of cefazolin in heparinized and nonheparinized peritoneal dialysis solutions. *Am J Health-Syst Pharm.* 2002; 59:1537–8.

2389. Donnelly RF. Chemical stability of furosemide in minibags and polypropylene syringes. *Int J Pharmaceut Compound.* 2002; 6:468–70.

2390. Schlesser V, Hecq JD, Vanbeckbergen D et al. Effect of freezing, long-term storage, and microwave thawing of the stability of cefepime in 5% dextrose infusion in polyvinyl chloride bags. *Int J Pharmaceut Compound.* 2002; 6:391–4.

2391. Hartman CA, Baroletti SA, Churchill WW et al. Visual compatibility of argatroban with selected drugs. *Am J Health-Syst Pharm.* 2002; 59:1784–5.

2392. Gupta VD. Chemical stability of dexamethasone sodium phosphate after reconstitution in 0.9% sodium chloride injection and storage in polypropylene syringes. *Int J Pharmaceut Compound.* 2002; 6:395–7.

2393. Trissel LA, Zhang Y. Stability of methylprednisolone sodium succinate in AutoDose infusion system bags. *J Am Pharm Assoc.* 2002; 42:868–70.

2394. Certain E, Beteta F, Goudou-Sinha C et al. Stability of i.v. mycophenolate mofetil in 5% dextrose injection in polyvinyl chloride infusion bags. *Am J Health-Syst Pharm.* 2002; 59:2434–9.

2395. Beijnen JH, van Gijn R. Chemical stability of the cardioprotective agent ICRF-187 in infusion fluids. *J Parenter Sci Technol.* 1993; 47:166–71.

2396. Fatou A, Denis P, Conrath G, et al. Campto 20 mg/mL concentrate for infusion, stability during infusion, stability of the diluted parenteral solution prepared ahead of time in glass bottles and PVC bags.

2397. Bobineau V, Nguyen-Huu JJ. CPT-11 (RP 64174A) 20 mg/mL solution for injection, study of the stability of infusion solutions reconstituted in glass bottles or PVC infusion bags after 24 hours' storage at room temperature.

2398. Stolk LML, Chandi LS. Stabiliteit van cladribine in natriumchloride-oplossing 0,9% voor infusie, *Ziekenhuisfarmacie.* 1994; 10:138–9.

2399. Tiefenbacher EM, Haen E, Przybilla B et al. Photodegradation of some quinolones used as antimicrobial therapeutics. *J Pharm Sci.* 1994; 83:463–7.

2400. Calis KA, Cullinane AM, Horne MK. Bioactivity of cryopreserved alteplase solutions. *Am J Health-Syst Pharm.* 1999; 56:2056–7.

2401. Kaijser GP, Beijnen JH, Bult A et al. A systematic study on the chemical stability of ifosfamide. *J Pharmaceut Biomed Anal.* 1991; 9:1061–7.

2402. Lau DWC, Walker SE, Fremes SE et al. Adenosine stability in cardioplegic solutions. *Can J Hosp Pharm.* 1995; 48:167–71.

2403. Muller HJ, Berg J. Stabilitatstude zu apomorphine-hydrochlorid im PVC-infusionsbeutel, *Krankenhauspharmazie.* 1997; 18:468–73.

2404. Andrisano V, Gotti R, Leoni A et al. Photodegradation studies on atenolol by liquid chromatography. *J Pharmaceut Biomed Anal.* 1999; 21:851–7.

2405. Blaise N, Vigeron J, Perrin A et al. Stability of refrigerated and frozen solutions of ondansetron hydrochloride. *Eur J Hosp Pharm.* 1994; 4:12–3.

2406. Lougheed WD, Woulfe-Flanagan H, Clement JR et al. Insulin aggregation in artificial delivery systems. *Diabetologia.* 1980; 19:1–9.

2407. Meyer G, Henneman PL. Buffered lidocaine. *Ann Emerg Med.* 1991; 20:218–9.

2408. Murakami CS, Odland PB, Ross BK. Buffered local anesthetics and epinephrine degradation. *J Dermatol Surg Oncol.* 1994; 20:192–5.

2409. Hinshaw KD, Fiscella R, Sugar J. Preparation of pH-adjusted local anesthetics. *Ophthalmol Surg.* 1995; 26:194–9.

2410. Avelar MA, Walker SE. Stability and compatibility of reconstituted hydromorphone with potassium chloride or heparin. *Can J Hosp Pharm.* 1996; 49:140–5.

2411. Crowther J, Hrazdil J, Jolly DT et al. Growth of microorganisms in propofol, thiopental, and a 1:1 mixture of propofol and thiopental. *Anesth Analg.* 1996; 82:475–8.

2412. El-Yazigi A, Wahab Fam, Afrane B. Stability study and content uniformity of prochlorperazine in pharmaceutical preparations by liquid chromatography. *J Chromatog A.* 1995; 690:71–6.

2413. Ekmore RL, Contois ME, Kelly K et al. Stability and compatibility of admixtures of intravenous ciprofloxacin and selected drugs. *Clin Ther.* 1996; 18:246–55.

2414. Luo D, Dong H, Tang XZ et al. Stability of amphotericin B in 50 g/L dextrose injection. *Chin Pharm J.* 1998; 33:220–2.

2415. Sewell GJ, Allsopp M, Collinson MP et al. Stability studies on admixtures of 5-fluorouracil with carboplatin and 5-fluorouracil with heparin for administration in continuous infusion regimens. *J Clin Pharm Ther.* 1994; 19:127–33.

2416. Lugo RA, MacKay M, Rucho WJ. Stability of lorazepam 0.2 mg/L, 0.5 mg/mL, and 1 mg/mL in polypropylene syringes. *J Pediatr Pharmacol Ther.* 2001; 6:122–9.

2417. Zhao L, Yalkowsky SH. Stabilization of epitifibitide by cosolvents. *Int J Pharm.* 2001; 218:43–56.

2418. Gupta VD, Ling J. Stability of piperacillin sodium after reconstitution in 0.9% sodium chloride injection and storage in polypropylene syringes for pediatric use. *Int J Pharmaceut Compound.* 2001; 5: 230–1.

2419. Thiesen J, Kramer I. Physicochemical stability of irinotecan injection concentrate and diluted infusion solutions in PVC bags. *J Oncol Pharm Pract.* 2000; 6:115–21.

2420. Beitz C, Einberger C, Wehling M. Stabilitat und Kompatibilitat von Zytostatika-Zubereitungen mit Infusionslosungsbehaltern aus Polyethylene. *Krankenhauspharmazie.* 1999; 20:121–5.

2421. Favetta P, Allombert C, Breysse C et al. Fortum stability in different disposable infusion devices by pyridine assay. *J Pharmaceut Biomed Anal.* 2002; 27:873–9.

2422. Orwa JA, Govaerts C, Gevers K et al. Study of the stability of polymyxins B_1, E_1, and E_2 in aqueous solution using liquid chromatography and mass spectrometry. *J Pharmaceut Biomed Anal.* 2002; 29:203–12.

2423. Mayer MI, Weickum RJ, Solimando DA et al. Stability of cisplatin, doxorubicin, and mitomycin combined with Iversol for chemoembolization. *Ann Pharmacother.* 2001; 35:1548–51.

2424. Loff S, Kabs F, Witt K et al. Polyvinylchloride infusion lines expose infants to large amounts of toxic plasticizers. *J Ped Surg.* 2000; 35:1775–81.

2425. Storms ML, Stewart JT, Warren FW. Stability of neostigmine methylsulfate injection at ambient temperature and 4 °C in polypropylene syringes. *Int J Pharmaceut Compound.* 2002; 6:475–7.

2426. Ulsaker G, Teien G. Degradation of methylprednisolone sodium succinate in a diluent-containing vial. *Am J Health-Syst Pharm.* 2002; 59:2456–7.

2427. Johnson TJ, Voss G. Continuous infusion of undiluted lorazepam injection. *Am J Health-Syst Pharm.* 2002; 59:78–9.

2428. Storms ML, Stewart JT, Warren FW. Stability of lidocaine hydrochloride injection at ambient temperature and 4 °C in polypropylene syringes. *Int J Pharmaceut Compound.* 2002; 6:388–90.

2429. Gupta VD. Stability of pentobarbital sodium after reconstitution in 0.9% sodium chloride injection and repackaged in glass and polypropylene syringes. *Int J Pharmaceut Compound.* 2001; 6:482–4.

2430. Beitz C, Bertsch T, Hannak D et al. Compatibility of plastics with cytotoxic drug solutions – comparison of polyethylene with other container materials. *Int J Pharm.* 1999; 185:113–21.

2431. Gupta VD: Stability of ketamine hydrochloride injection after reconstitution in water for injection and storage in 1–mL tuberculin polypropylene syringes for pediatric use. *Int J Pharmaceut Compound.* 2002; 6:316–7.

2432. Andrisano V, Hrelia P, Gotti R et al. Photostability and phototoxicity studies on diltiazem. *J Pharmaceut Biomed Anal.* 2001; 25:589–97.

2433. Svedberg KO, McKenzie EJ, Larrivee-Elkins C. Compatibility of ropivacaine with morphine, sufentanil, fentanyl, or clonidine. *J Clin Pharm Ther.* 2002; 27:39–45.

2434. Servais H, Tulkens PM. Stability and compatibility of ceftazidime administered by continuous infusion to intensive care patients. *Antimicrob Agents Chemother.* 2001; 45:2643–7.

2435. Parti R, Mankarious S. Stability assessment of lyophilized intravenous immunoglobulin after reconstitution in glass containers and poly(vinyl chloride) bags. *Biotechnol Appl Biochem.* 1997; 23:13–8.

2436. Jappinen A, Kokki H, Naaranlahti TJ et al. Stability of buprenorphine, haloperidol and glycopyrrolate mixture in a 0.9% sodium chloride solution. *Pharm World Sci.* 1999; 21:272–4.

2437. Jappinen A, Kokki H, Naaranlahti TJ et al. Chemical stability of a mixture of fentanyl citrate, bupivacaine hydrochloride and clonidine hydrochloride in 0.9% sodium chloride injection stored in syringes and medication cassettes. *Pharm World Sci Suppl.* 1996; A11:119–21.

2438. Storms ML, Stewart JT, Warren FW. Stability of succinylcholine chloride injection at ambient temperature and 4 °C in polypropylene syringes. *Int J Pharmaceut Compound.* 2003; 7:68–70.

2439. Storms ML, Stewart JT, Warren FW. Stability of glycopyrrolate injection at ambient temperature and 4 °C in polypropylene syringes. *Int J Pharmaceut Compound.* 2003; 7:65–7.

2440. Mitchell AL, Gailey RA. Compatibility of caffeine citrate with other medications commonly used in a neonatal intensive care unit. *J Pediatr Pharm Pract.* 1999; 4:239–42.

2441. Wang DP, Lee DKT, Wang CN. Stability of sodium cefazolin and tenoxicam in 5% dextrose. *Chin Pharmaceut J.* 2001; 53:185–9.

2442. Shi A, Walker SE, Law S. Stability of ketorolac tromethamine in IV solutions and waste reduction. *Can J Hosp Pharm.* 2000; 53:263–9.

2443. Yano R, Nakamura T, Aono H et al. The amount of the loss of cyclosporine A dose correlated with the amount of leaching di (2-ethylhexyl) phthalate from polyvinyl chloride infusion tube. *Yakugaku Zasshi.* 2001; 121:139–44.

2444. Micard S, Rieutord A, Prognon P et al. Stability and sterility of meglumine gadoterate injection repackaged in plastic syringes. *Int J Pharm.* 2001; 212:93–9.

2445. Han H, Davis SS, Washington C. Physical properties and stability of two emulsion formulations of propofol. *Int J Pharm.* 2001; 215:207–20.

2446. Deitcher SR, Fesen MR, Kiproff PM et al. Safety and efficacy of alteplase for restoring function in occluded central venous catheters: results of the cardiovascular thrombolytic to open occluded lines trial. *J Clin Oncol.* 2002; 20:317–24.

2447. Demore D, Vigeron J, Perrin A et al. Leaching of diethylhexyl phthalate from polyvinyl chloride bags into intravenous etoposide solution. *J Clin Pharm Ther.* 2002; 27:139–42.

2448. Sakazume S, Sasahara K, Kawada T et al. The adsorption of recombinant factor VIII (Kogenate) to infusion sets and inline filters. *Jpn J Pharm Health Care Sci.* 2001; 27:143–7.

2449. Little G (Director, Drug Information, Wyeth-Ayerst Pharmaceuticals, Philadelphia, PA): Personal communication; 1999 Mar 5.

2450. Hecq JD, Lebrun J, Vanbeckbergen D, et al. Effect of freezing, long-term storage, and microwave thawing on the stability of ketorolac tromethamine and tramadol hydrochloride in 5% dextrose infusion.

2451. Nguyen-Huu JJ, Bousquet O, Bobee JM. Compatibility of taxotere infusion solution with intravenous administration/extension sets, Rhone Poulenc Rorer, 2002.

2452. Suzuki M, Takamatsu S, Muramatsu E et al. Loss of tacrolimus solution content and leaching of di-2-ethylhexyl phthalate in practice injection of precision continuous drip infusion. *Jpn J Hosp Pharm.* 2000; 26:7–12.

2453. He Y, Yu YC. Study on the stability of tetracaine hydrochloride injection. *Chin Pharm J.* 2001; 36:33–5.

2454. Chikuma T, Shinoda T, Taguchi K et al. Stability of morphine hydrochloride in a total parenteral nutrient solution. *Jpn J Hosp Pharm.* 2000; 26:316–21.

2455. Farhang-Asnafi S, Barre J, Callaert S et al. Compatibilite et stabilite du m;aaelange bupivacaine-sufentanil en poche. *J Pharm Clin.* 2000; 19:248–51.

2456. Pereboom M, Becker ML, Amenchar M et al. Stability assessment of repackaged bevacizumab for intravitreal administration. *Int J Pharm Compd.* 2015 Jan-Feb; 19:70–2.

2457. Khalili H, Sharma G, Froome A et al. Storage stability of bevacizumab in polycarbonate and polypropylene syringes. *Eye (Lond).* 2015; 29:820–7.

2458. Ball PA. Particulate contamination in parenteral nutrition solutions: still a cause for concern? *Nutrition.* 2001; 17:926–9.

2459. Allwood MC, Martin HJ. The photodegradation of vitamin A and E in parenteral nutrition mixtures during infusion. *Clin Nutr.* 2000; 19:339–42.

2460. Sforzini A, Bersani G, Stancari A et al. Analysis of all-in-one parenteral nutrition admixtures by liquid chromatography and laser diffraction: study of stability. *J Pharmaceut Biomed Anal.* 2001; 24:1099–1109.

2461. Gibbons E, Allwood MC, Neal T et al. Degradation of dehydroascorbic acid in parenteral nutrition mixtures. *J Pharmaceut Biomed Anal.* 2001; 25:605–11.

2462. Proot P, de Pourcq L, Raymakes AA. Stability of ascorbic acid in a standard total parenteral nutrition mixture. *Clin Nutr.* 1994; 13:273–9.

2463. Allwood MC, Brown PW, Ghedini C et al. The stability of ascorbic acid in TPN mixtures stored in a multilayer bag. *Clin Nutr.* 1992; 11:284–8.

2464. Hak EB, Storm MC, Helms RA. Chromium and zinc contamination of parenteral nutrient solution components commonly used in infants and children. *Am J Health-Syst Pharm.* 1998; 55:150–4.

2465. Mehta RC, Head LF, Hazrati AM et al. Fat emulsion particle-size distribution in total nutrient admixtures. *Am J Hosp Pharm.* 1992; 49:2749–55.

2466. Song YH, Burgess DJ, Herson VC et al. Solubility of calcium acetate (CaAce) and sodium phosphate (NaP) in pediatric parenteral nutrition (PN) solution. *J Parenter Enteral Nutr.* 2000; 24:S22.

2467. Trissel LA, Saenz CA, Ogundele AB et al. Compatibility of fenoldopam mesylate with other drugs during simulated Y-site administration. *Am J Health-Syst Pharm.* 2003; 60:80–5.

2468. Levadoux E, Sautou V, Bazin JE et al. Medical plastics: compatibility of alfentanil and propofol alone or mixed. Stability of the alfentanil-propofol mixture. *Int J Pharm.* 1996; 127:255–9.

2469. Trissel LA, Xu Q, Zhang Y et al. Use of cysteine hydrochloride injection to increase the solubility of calcium and phosphates in FreAmine III-containing parenteral nutrition solutions. *Int J Pharmaceut Compound.* 2003; 7:71–3.

2470. Bell MS, Nolt DH. Visual compatibility of doxapram hydrochloride with drugs commonly administered via a Y-site in the intensive care nursery. *Am J Health-Syst Pharm.* 2003; 60:193–4.

2471. Trissel LA, Xu QA. Stability of Imipenem–cilastatin sodium in AutoDose infusion system bags. *Hosp Pharm.* 2003; 38:130–4.

2472. Naughton CA, Duppong LM, Forbes KD et al. Stability of multidose, preserved formulation epoetin alfa in syringes for three and six weeks. *Am J Health-Syst Pharm.* 2003; 60:464–8.

2473. Xu QA, Trissel LA. Stability of clindamycin phosphate in AutoDose infusion system bags, *Int J Pharmaceut Compound.* 2003; 7:149–51.

2474. Gupta VD. Chemical stability of cefazolin sodium after reconstituting in 0.9% sodium chloride injection and storage in polypropylene syringes for pediatric use. *Int J Pharmaceut Compound.* 2003; 7:152–4.

2475. Zhang Y, Trissel LA. Stability of amikacin sulfate in AutoDose infusion system bags. *Int J Pharmaceut Compound.* 2003; 7:230–2.

2476. Phares KR, Weiser WE, Miller SP et al. Stability and preservative effectiveness of treprostinil sodium after dilution in common intravenous diluents. *Am J Health-Syst Pharm.* 2003; 60:916–22.

2477. Hildebrand KR, Elsberry DD, Hassenbusch SJ. Stability and compatibility of morphine-clonidine admixtures in an implantable infusion system. *J Pain Symp Manage.* 2003; 25:464–71.

2478. Feddema S, Rusho WJ, Tyler LS et al. Physical compatibility of vasopressin with medications commonly used in cardiac arrest. *Am J Health-Syst Pharm.* 2003; 60:1271–2.

2479. Trissel LA, Xu QA. Stability of cefepime hydrochloride in AutoDose infusion system bags. *Ann Pharmacother.* 2003; 37:804–7.

2480. Lin YF, Wu CC, Lin SH et al. Stability of cefazolin sodium in icodextrin-containing peritoneal dialysis solution. *Am J Health-Syst Pharm.* 2002; 59:2362–3.

2481. Cohen M (President, Institute for Safe Medication Practices, Huntingdon Valley, PA): Personal communication; 2003 Sep 5.

2482. Greenberg L. Errors and near misses linked to i.v. administration of sterile water for injection. *Pharm Pract News.* 2003; 30:24.

2483. Roberts S, Sewell GJ. Stability and compatibility of 5-fluorouracil infusions in Braun Easypump. *J Oncol Pharm Pract.* 2003; 9:109–12.

2484. Laposata M, Johnson SM. Assessment of the stability of dalteparin sodium in prepared syringes for up to thirty days: an in vitro study. *Clin Ther.* 2003; 25:1219–25.

2485. Gupta VD. Chemical stability of cefuroxime sodium after reconstitution in 0.9% sodium chloride injection and storage in polypropylene syringes for pediatric use. *Int J Pharmaceut Compound.* 2003; 7:310–2.

2486. Menard C, Bourguignon C, Schlatter J et al. Stability of cyclophosphamide and mesna admixtures in polyethylene infusion bags. *Ann Pharmacother*. 2003; 37:1789–92.

2487. McQuade MS, Van Nostrand V, Schariter J et al. Stability and compatibility of reconstituted ertapenem with commonly used i.v. infusion and coinfusion solutions. *Am J Health-Syst Pharm*. 2004; 61:38–45.

2488. Trissel LA, Saenz CA. Physical compatibility of antithymocyte globulin (rabbit) with heparin sodium and hydrocortisone sodium succinate. *Am J Health-Syst Pharm*. 2003; 60:1650–2.

2489. Musami P, Stewart JT, Taylor EW. Stability of zidovudine and dobutamine hydrochloride injections in 0.9% sodium chloride and 5% dextrose injections stored at ambient temperature (23 ± 2°C) and 4°C in 50-mL polyvinyl chloride bags up to 24 hours. *Int J Pharmaceut Compound*. 2004; 8:73–6.

2490. Masaki Y, Tanaka M, Nishikawa T. Physicochemical compatibility of propofol-lidocaine mixture. *Anesth Analg*. 2003; 97:1646–51.

2491. Anderson PL, Miller S, Bushman LR. Stability of zidovudine with oxytocin in a simulated Y-site injection. *Am J Heath-Syst Pharm*. 2004; 61:394–96.

2492. Walker SE, Varrin S, Yannicelli D et al. Stability of meropenem in saline and dextrose solutions and compatibility with potassium chloride. *Can J Hosp Pharm*. 1998; 51:156–68.

2493. Berlage V, Hecq JD, Vanbeckbergen D et al. Long term stability of procaine hydrochloride cardioplegic infusion in P.V.C. bags at 4°C. *Pharmakon*. 2003; 35:3–8.

2494. Kannan S. Incompatibility of prochlorperazine and ketoprofen. *Anaesthesia*. 2001; 56:920.

2495. Smith RPR, Jones M. Precipitation in Manchester:ketorolac/cyclizine. *Anaesthesia*. 2001; 56:494–5.

2496. Akhtar MJ, Khan MA, Ahmad I. Identification of photoproducts of folic acid and its degradation pathways in aqueous solution. *J Pharmaceut Biomed Anal*. 2003; 31:579–88.

2497. Tsui BCH, Cave D. Discoloration of parenteral ondansetron. *Anesth Analg*. 2003; 96:1239.

2498. Hartmann M, Knoth H, Kohler W. Stability of fentanyl/ropivacaine preparations for epidural application. *Pharmazie*. 2003; 58:434–5.

2499. Dager WE, Gosselin RC, King JH et al. Anti-Xa stability of diluted enoxaparin for use in pediatrics. *Ann Pharmacother*. 2004; 38:569–73.

2500. Manley HJ, McClaran ML, Bedenbaugh A et al. Linezolid stability in peritoneal dialysis solutions. *Perit Dial Int*. 2002; 22:419–22.

2501. Semba CP, Weck S, Patapoff T. Alteplase: stability and bioactivity after dilution in normal saline solution. *J Vasc Interv Radiol*. 2003; 14:99–102.

2502. Faouzi MA, Dine T, Luyckx M et al. Stability and compatibility studies of cephamandole nafate with PVC infusion bags. *J Pharmaceut Biomed Anal*. 1994; 12:99–104.

2503. Diduk N, Perez KG, de la Munoz L et al. Estabilidad de ciclosporina inyectable (50 mg/mL). *Rev Mexicana Ciencias Farm*. 2000; 31:19–22.

2504. Bruch HR, Esser M. Catheter occlusion by calcium carbonate during simultaneous infusion of 5-FU and calcium folinate. *Onkologie*. 2003; 26:469–72.

2505. Vehabovic M, Hadzovic S, Stambolic F et al. Stability of ranitidine in injectable solutions. *Int J Pharm*. 2003; 256:109–15.

2506. Brodner G, Ermert T, Van Aken H et al. Stability of sufentanil-ropivacaine mixture in glass and PVC reservoir. *Europ J Anesthesiol*. 2002; 19:295–7.

2507. Lettner A, Zollner P. Visuelle documentation der stabilitat der intravenosen losungen von omeprazole (Losec) und pantoprazole (Pantoloc). *Wien Med Wechenschr*. 2002; 152:568–78.

2508. Bosso JA, Taylor AJ, White RL et al. Compatibility of two concentrations of recombinant human interleukin-1 receptor antagonist with selected antimicromical agents. *J Infect Dis Pharmacother*. 1995; 1:45–54.

2509. Nahata MC, Morosco RS, Sabados BK et al. Stability and compatibility of anakinra with ceftriaxone sodium injection in 0.9% sodium chloride or 5% dextrose injection. *J Clin Pharm Ther*. 1997; 22:167–9.

2510. Nahata MC, Morosco RS, Sabados BK et al. Stability and compatibility of anakinra and clindamycin phosphate injections in 0.9% sodium chloride injection. *J App Ther Res*. 1998; 2:87–9.

2511. Nahata MC, Morosco RS, Sabados BK et al. Stability and compatibility of anakinra with cimetidine hydrochloride or famotidine in 0.9% sodium chloride injection. *J Clin Pharm Ther*. 1995; 20:97–9.

2512. Nahata MC, Morosco RS, Sabados BK et al. Stability and compatibility of anakinra with lorazepam injection in 0.9% sodium chloride injection. *J App Ther*. 1996; 1:191–2.

2513. Baririan N, Chanteux H, Viaene E et al. Stability and compatibility study of cefepime in comparison with ceftazidime for potential administration by continuous infusion under conditions pertinent to ambulatory treatment of cystic fibrosis patients and to administration in intensive care units. *J Antimicrob Chemother*. 2003; 51:651–8.

2514. Sprauten PF, Beringer PM, Louie SG et al. Stability and antibacterial activity of cefepime during continuous infusion. *Antimicrob Agents Chemother*. 2003; 47:1991–4.

2515. Vercaigne LM, Sitar DS, Penner SB et al. Antibiotic-heparin lock: in vitro antibiotic stability combined with heparin in a central venous catheter. *Pharmacother*. 2000; 20:394–9.

2516. Vercaigne LM, Zhanel GG. Antibiotic-heparin lock: in vitro confirmation of antibacterial activity. *Can J Hosp Pharm*. 2000; 53:193–8.

2517. Sanchez del Aguila MJ, Jones MF, Vohra A. Premixed solutions of diamorphine in ropivacaine for epidural anaesthesia: a study on their long-term stability. *Br J Anaesthes*. 2003; 90:179–82.

2518. Ranchere JY, Latour JF, Fuhrman C et al. Amphotericin B Intralipid formulation: stability and particle size. *J Antimicrob Chemother*. 1996; 37:1165–9.

2519. Hatem A, Marton S, Csoka G et al. Preformulation studies of atenolol in oral liquid dosage form. I. Effect of pH and temperature. *Acta Pharmaceut Hung*. 1996; 66:177–80.

2520. Wiernikowski JT, Crowther M, Clase CM et al. Stability and sterility of recombinant tissue plasminogen activator at -30°C. *Lancet*. 2000; 355:2221.

2521. Barcia E, Reyes R, Luz Azuara M et al. Compatibility of haloperidol and hyoscine-N-butyl bromide in mixtures for subcutaneous infusion to cancer patients in palliative care. *Support Care Cancer*. 2003; 11:107–13.

2522. Dix J, Weber RJ, Frye RF et al. Stability of atropine sulfate prepared for mass chemical terrorism. *J Toxicol*. 2003; 41:771–5.

2523. Musami P, Stewart JT, Taylor EW. Stability of zidovudine and ranitidine in 0.9% sodium chloride and 5% dextrose injections stored at ambient temperature (23 ± 2°C) and 4°C in 50-mL polyvinylchloride bags up to 24 hours. *Int J Pharmaceut Compound*. 2004; 8:236–9.

2524. Gupta VD. Chemical stability of phenylephrine hydrochloride after reconstitution in 0.9% sodium chloride injection for infusion. *Int J Pharmaceut Compound*. 2004; 8:153–5.

2525. Norenburg JP, Achusim LE, Steel TH et al. Stability of lorazepam in 0.9% sodium chloride in polyolefin bags. *Am J Health-Syst Pharm*. 2004; 61:1039–41.

2526. Lebrun J, Hecq JD, Vanbeckbergen D et al. Effect of freezing, long-term storage and microwave thawing on the stability of tramadol in 5% dextrose infusion in polyvinyl chloride bags. *Int J Pharmaceut Compound*. 2004; 8:156–9.

2527. Sharley NA, Burgess NG. Stability and compatibility of alfentanil hydrochloride and morphine sulfate in polypropylene syringes. *J Pharm Pract Res*. 2003; 33:279–81.

2528. Xu QA, Trissel LA, Pham L. Physical and chemical stability of treprostinil sodium injection packaged in plastic syringe pump reservoirs. *Int J Pharmaceut Compound*. 2004; 8:228–30.

2529. Trissel LA, Saenz CA, Williams KY et al. Incompatibilities of lansoprazole injection with other drugs during simulated Y-site coadministration. *Int J Pharmaceut Compound*. 2002; 5:314–9.

2530. Braeden JU, Stendal TL, Fagernaes CB. Stability of dopamine hydrochloride 0.5 mg/mL in polypropylene syringes. *J Clin Pharm Ther*. 2003; 28:471–4.

2531. Good PD, Schneider JJ, Ravenscroft PJ. The compatibility and stability of midazolam and dexamethasone in infusion solutions. *J Pain Sympt Manag*. 2004; 27:471–5.

2532. Jaruratanasirikul S, Sriwiriyajan S. Stability of meropenem in normal saline solution after storage at room temperature. *Southeast Asian J Trop Med Pub Health*. 2003; 34:627–9.

2533. Xu QA, Trissel LA. Stability of palonosetron hydrochloride with paclitaxel and docetaxel during simulated Y-site administration. *Am J Health-Syst Pharm*. 2004; 61:1596–8.

2534. Sewell GJ, Rigsby-Jones AE, Priston MJ. Stability of intravesical epirubicin infusion: a sequential temperature study. *J Clin Pharm Ther*. 2003; 28:349–53.

2535. Trissel LA, Xu QA. Physical and chemical stability of palonosetron HCl in 4 infusion solutions. *Ann Pharmacother*. 2004; 38:1608–11.

2536. Curtis JM, Edwards DJ. Stability of trimethoprim in admixtures of trimethoprim-sulfamethoxazole prepared in polyvinyl chloride bags and glass bottles. *Can J Hosp Pharm*. 2002; 55:207–11.

2537. La Forgia SP, Sharley NA, Burgess NG et al. Stability and compatibility of morphine, midazolam, and bupivacaine combinations for intravenous infusion. *J Pharm Pract Res*. 2002; 32:65–8.

2538. Stecher AL, Morgantetti de Deus P, Polikarpov I et al. Stability of L-asparaginase: an enzyme used in leukemia treatment. *Pharm Acta Helv*. 1999; 74:1–9.

2539. Arsene M, Favetta P, Favier B et al. Comparison of ceftazidime degradation in glass bottles and plastic bags under various conditions. *J Clin Pharm Ther*. 2002; 27:205–9.

2540. Bennett J, Gross J, Nichols F et al. The chemical and physical stability of a 1:1 mixture of propofol and methohexital. *Anesth Prog*. 2001; 48:61–5.

2541. Lepage R, Walker SE, Godin J. Stability and compatibility of etoposide in normal saline. *Can J Hosp Pharm*. 2000; 53:338–44.

2542. Mayer JLR, Pascale VJ, Clyne LP et al. Stability of low-dose vancomycin hydrochloride in heparin sodium 100 IU/mL. *J Pharm Tech*. 1999; 15:13–7.

2543. Park JW, Park ES, Chi SC et al. The effect of lidocaine on the globule size distribution of propofol emulsions. *Anesth Analg*. 2003; 97:769–71.

2544. Vincentelli J, Braguer D, Guillet P et al. Formulation of a flush solution of heparin, vancomycin, and colistin for implantation access systems in oncology. *J Oncol Pharm Pract*. 1997; 3:18–23.

2545. Westphal M, Hohage H, Buerkle H et al. Adsorption of sufentanil to epidural filters and catheters. *Europ J Anesthes*. 2003; 20:124–6.

2546. Hamilton MA, Stang L, Etches WS et al. Stability of low molecular weight heparins stored in plastic syringes. *Thromb Res*. 2003; 112:1127–9.

2547. Vella-Brincat JWA, Begg EJ, Gallagher K et al. Stability of benzylpenicillin during continuous home intravenous therapy. *J Antimicrob Chemother*. 2004; 53:675–7.

2548. Gill MA, Kislik AZ, Goree L et al. Stability of advanced life support drugs in the field. *Am J Health-Syst Pharm*. 2004; 61:597–602.

2549. Boitquin L, Hecq JD, Evrard JM et al. Long-term stability of sufentanil citrate with levobupivacaine hydrochloride in 0.9% sodium chloride infusion PVC bags at 4°C. *J Pain Symptom Manage*. 2004; 28:4–6.

2550. Jappinen A, Turpeinen M, Kokki H et al. Stability of sufentanil and levobupivacaine solutions and a mixture in a 0.9% sodium chloride infusion stored in polypropylene syringes. *Europ J Pharm Sci*. 2003; 19:31–6.

2551. Gupta VD. Chemical stability of terbutaline sulfate injection after diluting with 0.9% sodium chloride injection when stored at room temperature in polyvinyl chloride bags. *Int J Pharmaceut Compound*. 2004; 8:404–6.

2552. Trissel LA, Zhang Y. Compatibility and stability of Aloxi (palonosetron hydrochloride) admixed with dexamethasone sodium phosphate. *Int J Pharmaceut Compound*. 2004; 8:398–403.

2553. Lai JJ, Brodeur SK. Physical and chemical compatibility of daptomycin with nine medications. *Ann Pharmacother*. 2004; 38:1612–6.

2554. Smith DL, Bauer SM, Nicolau DP. Stability of meropenem in polyvinyl chloride bags and an elastomeric infusion device. *Am J Health-Syst Pharm*. 2004; 61:1682–5.

2555. Gong Y, Tian X, Xu Q. Compatibility of bumetanide injection combined with four kinds of injection. *China Pharm*. 2003; 6:550–1.

2556. Ling J, Gupta VD. Stability of ethacrynate sodium after reconstitution in 0.9% sodium chloride injection and storage in polypropylene syringes for pediatric use. *Int J Pharmaceut Compound*. 2001; 5:73–5.

2557. Wang DP, Chiou HJ, Lee DKT. Compatibility and stability of ceftazidime sodium and tenoxicam in 5% dextrose injection. *Am J Health-Syst Pharm*. 2004; 61:1924–7.

2558. Ling J, Gupta VD. Stability of acyclovir sodium after reconstitution in 0.9% sodium chloride injection and storage in polypropylene syringes for pediatric use. *Int J Pharmaceut Compound*. 2001; 5:75–7.

2559. Xu XW, Du XL, Li DK et al. Study on the sorption of fifteen injectable drugs in three different kinds of intravenous solution containers. *Chin Pharm J*. 2004; 39:205–7.

2560. Murata A, Okamoto Y, Sasa Y et al. Effect of light and sodium bisulfite on the stability of thiamine in TPN fluids and integrated dose in period values. *Jpn J Pharm Health Care Sci*. 2004; 30:266–70.

2561. Dedrick SC, Ramirez-Rico J. Potency and stability of frozen urokinase solutions in syringes. *Am J Health-Syst Pharm*. 2004; 61:1586–9.

2562. Valenzuela TD, Criss EA, Hammargen WM et al. Thermal stability of prehospital medications. *Ann Emerg Med*. 1989; 18:173–6.

2563. Ambados F, Brealey J. Compatibility of ketamine hydrochloride and fentanyl citrate in polypropylene syringes. *Am J Health-Syst Pharm*. 2004; 61:1438, 1445.

2564. Trissel LA, Saenz CA, Ogundele AB et al. Physical compatibility of pemetrexed disodium with other drugs during simulated Y-site administration. *Am J Health-Syst Pharm*. 2004; 61:2289–93.

2565. Alvarez JC, de Mazancourt P, Chartier-Kastler E et al. Drug stability testing to support clinical feasibility investigations for intrathecal baclofen-clonidine admixture. *J Pain Sympt Manage*. 2004; 28:268–72.

2566. Trissel LA, Saenz CA, Ingram DS et al. Compatibility screening of oxaliplatin during simulated Y-site administration with other drugs. *J Oncol Pharm Pract*. 2002; 8:33–7.

2567. White CM, Quercia R. Stability of extemporaneously prepared sterile testosterone solution in 0.9% sodium chloride solution large-volume parenterals in plastic bags. *Int J Pharmaceut*. 1999; 3:156–7.

2568. Kuti JL, Nightingale CH, Knauft RF et al. Pharmacokinetic properties and stability of continuous-infusion meropenem in adults with cystic fibrosis. *Clin Ther*. 2004; 26:493–501.

2569. Ferreira E, Forest JM, Hildgen P. Compatibilite du dimenhydrinate injectable pour l'administration en Y. *Pharmactuel*. 2004; 37:17–20.

2570. Fubara JO, Notari RE. Influence of pH, temperature and buffers on cefepime degradation kinetics and stability predictions in aqueous solutions. *J Pharm Sci*. 1998; 87:1572–6.

2571. Brustugun J, Kristensen S, Hjorth Tonnesen H. Photostability of epinephrine—the influence of bisulfite and degradation products. *Pharmazie*. 2004; 59:457–63.

2572. Honisko ME, Fink JM, Militello MA et al. Compatibility of argatroban with selected cardiovascular agents. *Am J Health-Syst Pharm*. 2004; 61:2415–8.

2573. Dooley DP, Tyler JR, Wortham WG et al. Prolonged stability of antimicrobial activity in peritoneal dialysis solutions. *Perit Dial Int*. 2003; 23:58–62.

2574. Pere H, Chasse V, Forest JM et al. Compatibilite du pantoprazole lors d'administration en Y. *Pharmactuel*. 2004; 37:193–6.

2575. Baker MT, Gregerson MS, Martin SM et al. Free radical and drug oxidation products in an intensive care unit sedative: propofol with sulfite. *Crit Care Med*. 2003; 31:787–92.

2576. Zaloga GP, Marik P. Sulfite-induced propofol oxidation: a cause for radical concern. *Crit Care Med*. 2003; 31:981–3.

2577. Lasak M. (Medical Information, Fujisawa): Personal communication. 2003; Sep 19.

2578. Boitquin LP, Hecq JD, Vanbeckbergen D et al. Stability of sufentanil citrate with levobupivacaine hydrochloride in NaCl 0.9% infusion after microwave freeze-thaw treatment. *Ann Pharmacother*. 2004; 38:1836–9.

2579. Trissel LA, Zhang Y. Physical and chemical stability of palonosetron HCl with cisplatin, carboplatin, and oxaliplatin during simulated Y-site administration. *J Oncol Pharm Pract*. 2004; 10:191–5.

2580. Sprandal KA, Styrczula DE, Deyo K et al. Stability and compatibility of levofloxacin and metronidazole during simulated and actual Y-site administration. *Am J Health-Syst Pharm*. 2005; 62:88–92.

2581. Trissel LA, Zhang Y. Palonosetron HCl compatibility and stability with doxorubicin HCl and epirubicin HCl during simulated Y-site administration. *Ann Pharmacother*. 2005; 39:280–3.

2582. Lim SCB, Roberts MJ, Paech MJ et al. Stability of insulin aspart in normal saline infusion. *J Pharm Pract Res*. 2004; 34:11–3.

2583. Hildebrand KR, Elsberry DD, Deer TR. Stability, compatibility, and safety of intrathecal bupivacaine administered chronically via an implantable delivery system. *Clin J Pain*. 2001; 17:239–44.

2584. Hildebrand KR, Elsberry DE, Anderson VC. Stability and compatibility of hydromorphone hydrochloride in an implantable infusion system. *J Pain Sympt Manag*. 2001; 22:1042–7.

2585. Classen AM, Wmbish GH, Kupiec TC. Stability of admixture containing morphine sulfate, bupivacaine hydrochloride, and clonidine hydrochloride in an implantable infusion system. *J Pain Sympt Manag*. 2004; 28:603–10.

2586. Gupta VD. Chemical stability of metoclopramide hydrochloride injection diluted with 0.9% sodium chloride injection in polypropylene syringes at room temperature. *Int J Pharmaceut Compound*. 2005; 9:72–4.

2587. Bourdeaux D, Sautou-Miranda V, Bagel-Boithias S et al. Analysis by liquid chromatography and infrared spectrometry of di(2-ethylhexyl)phthalate released by multilayer infusion tubing. *J Pharmaceut Biomed Anal*. 2004; 35:57–64.

2588. Kambia K, Dine T, Gressier B et al. Evaluation of childhood exposure to di(2-ethylhexyl)phthalate from perfusion kits during long-term parenteral nutrition. *Int J Pharm*. 2003; 262:83–91.

2589. Driscoll DF, Dunbar JG, Marmarou A. Fat-globule size in a propofol emulsion containing sodium metabisulfite. *Am J Health-Syst Pharm.* 2004; 61:1276–80.

2590. Turnbull K, Bielech M, Walker SE et al. Stability of oxycodone hydrochloride for injection in dextrose and saline solutions. *Can J Hosp Pharm.* 2002; 55:272–7.

2591. Rigge DC, Jones MF. Shelf lives of aseptically prepared medicines—stability of netilmicin injection in polypropylene syringes. *J Pharmaceut Biomed Anal.* 2004; 35:1251–6.

2592. Hecq JD, Boitquin LP, Vanbeckbergen D et al. Effect of freezing and microwave thawing on the stability of cefuroxime in 5% dextrose infusion polyolefin bags at 4°C. *Ann Pharmacother.* 2005; 39:1244–8.

2593. Rudich Z, Peng P, Dunn E et al. Stability of clonidine in clonidine-hydromorphone mixture from implanted intrathecal infusion pumps in chronic pain patients. *J Pain Sympt Manag.* 2004; 28:599–602.

2594. Oh J, Gwak H, Moon H et al. Stability of roxatidine acetate in parenteral nutrient solutions containing different amino acid formulations. *Am J Health-Syst Pharm.* 2005; 62:289–91.

2595. Noppawinyoowong C, Srisangchun J, Pongjanyakul T et al. Chemical stability of frozen ganciclovir intravitreal injections. *Thai J Hosp Pharm.* 2003; 13:213–8.

2596. Kim YH, Heinze TM, Beger R et al. A kinetic study on the degradation of erythromycin A in aqueous solution. *Int J Pharm.* 2004; 271:63–76.

2597. Ambados F. Incompatibility between calcium and sulfate ions in solutions for injection. *J Pharm Pract Res.* 2002; 32:307–9.

2598. Tang WM, Xue PH. Stability of ceftriaxone sodium injections. *Pharm Care Res.* 2002; 2:171–3.

2599. Torne GR, Luque AA, Pozo JF et al. Estudio de la adsorcion de insulina en las bolsas de nutricion parenteral: influencia del tiempo de administracion y la temperatura. *J Clin Pharm.* 2003; 5:565–9.

2600. Gardiner PR. Compatibility of an injectable oxycodone formulation with typical diluents, syringes, tubings, infusion bags and drugs for potential co-administration. *Hosp Pharmacist.* 2003; 10:358–61.

2601. Sugiura M, Nakajima K, Yamada Y et al. Adsorption of rhG-CSF (filgrastim) to extension tube. *Jpn J Pharm Health Care Sci.* 2003; 29:173–7.

2602. Priano RM, Hocht C, Oyola E et al. Estabilidad de prostaglandina E1 fraccionada en jeringas de polipropileno. *Farm Hosp.* 2003; 27:304–7.

2603. Walker SE, Fau-Lun C, Wyllie A et al. Physical compatibility of pantoprazole with selected medications during simulated Y-site administration. *Can J Hosp Pharm.* 2004; 57:90–7.

2604. Voges M, Faict D, Lechien G et al. Stability of drug additives in peritoneal dialysis solutions in a new container. *Perit Dial Int.* 2004; 24:590–5.

2605. Bagel-Boithias S, Sautou-Miranda V, Bourseaux D et al. Leaching of diethyl hexyl phthalate from multilayer tubing into etoposide infusion solutions. *Am J Health-Syst Pharm.* 2005; 62:182–8.

2606. Uebel RA, Wium CA, Schmidt AC. Stability evaluation of a prostaglandin E1 saline solution packed in insulin syringes. *Int J Impotence Res.* 2001; 13:16–7.

2607. Hennere G, Havard L, Bonan B et al. Stability of cidofovir in extemporaneously prepared syringes. *Am J Health-Syst Pharm.* 2005; 62:506–9.

2608. Trissel LA, Xu QA. Physical and chemical stability of palonosetron hydrochloride with lorazepam and midazolam hydrochloride during simulated Y-site administration. *Int J Pharmaceut Compound.* 2005; 9:235–7.

2609. Trissel LA, Xu QA. Physical and chemical stability of palonosetron hydrochloride with topotecan hydrochloride and irinotecan hydrochloride during simulated Y-site administration. *Int J Pharmaceut Compound.* 2005; 9:238–41.

2610. Volonte MG, Valora PD, Cingolani A et al. Stability of ibuprofen in injection solutions. *Am J Health-Syst Pharm.* 2005; 62:630–3.

2611. Phares KR, Wade M, Weiser WE et al. Improved stability of treprostinil sodium with proper vial puncture technique and adapter use. *J Pharm Technol.* 2004; 20:270–5.

2612. He Y, Yu YC. Study on the stability of tetracaine hydrochloride injection. *Chin Pharm J.* 2001; 36:33–5.

2613. Priston MJ, Hughes JM, Santillo M et al. Stability of epidural analgesic admixture containing epinephrine, fentanyl, and bupivacaine. *Anaesthesia.* 2004; 59:979–83.

2614. Hecq JD, Berlage V, Vanbeckbergen D et al. Effects of freezing, long-term storage, and microwave thawing on the stability of piperacillin plus tazobactam in 5% dextrose for infusion. *Can J Hosp Pharm.* 2004; 57:276–82.

2615. Mann HJ, Demon SL, Boelk DA et al. Physical and chemical compatibility of drotrecogin alfa (activated) with 34 drugs during simulated Y-site administration. *Am J Health-Syst Pharm.* 2004; 61:2664–71.

2616. Elwell RJ, Volino LR, Frye RF. Stability of cefepime in icodextrin peritoneal dialysis solution. *Ann Pharmacother.* 2004; 38:2041–4.

2617. Trissel LA, Ogundele AB. Compatibility of anidulafungin with other drugs during simulated Y-site administration. *Am J Health-Syst Pharm.* 2005; 62:834–7.

2618. Dupertuis YM, Morch A, Fathi M et al. Physical characteristics of total parenteral nutrition bags significantly affect the stability of vitamins C and B1: A controlled prospective study. *J Parenter Enter Nutr.* 2002; 261:310–6.

2619. Driscoll DF, Nehne J, Peters H et al. Physicochemical stability of intravenous lipid emulsions as all-in-one admixtures intended for the very young. *Clin Nutr.* 2003; 2:489–95.

2620. McNearney T, Bajaj C, Boyars M et al. Total parenteral nutrition associated crystalline precipitates resulting in pulmonary artery occlusions and alveolar granulomas. *Digestive Dis Sci.* 2003; 48:1352–4.

2621. Lee MD, Yoon J, Kim S et al. Stability of total nutrient admixtures in reference to ambient temperatures. *Nutrition.* 2003; 48:1352–4.

2622. Parikh MJ, Dumas G, Silvestri A et al. Physical compatibility of neonatal total parenteral nutrient admixtures containing organic calcium and inorganic phosphate salts. *Am J Health-Syst Pharm.* 2005; 62:1177–83.

2623. Levi F, Metzger G, Massari C et al. Oxaliplatin pharmacokinetics and chronopharmacological aspects. *Clin Pharmacokinet.* 2000; 38:1–21.

2624. Hoppe-Tichy T, Wenzel S, Gehring AK et al. Stability of voriconazole concentrate and voriconazole in infusion bags. *Pharmazie.* 2005; 60:77–8.

2625. Nakamura L (Medical Information Department, Scios Inc., Fremont, CA). Personal communication; 2007 Jan 12.

2626. Steiner ME. Stability and sterility of dolasetron mesylate in syringes stored at room temperature. *Am J Health-Syst Pharm.* 2005; 62:896, 898–9.

2627. Trissel LA, Zhang Y. Physical and chemical stability of palonosetron hydrochloride with fluorouracil and with gemcitabine hydrochloride during simulated Y-site administration. *Int J Pharmaceut Compound.* 2005; 9:320–2.

2628. Lee G, Sabra K. Stability of morphine sulphate in ANAPA Plus ambulatory infusion device and PEGA infusion sets. *Europ J Hosp Pharm Sci.* 2006; 12:76–80.

2629. Chin A, Liu S, Ting-Chan J et al. Extended stability of ascorbic acid in 5% dextrose injection and 0.9% sodium chloride injection. *Am J Health-Syst Pharm.* 2005; 62:1073–4.

2630. Patel K, Hursting MJ. Compatibility of argatroban with abciximab, eptifibatide, or tirofiban during simulated Y-site administration. *Am J Health-Syst Pharm.* 2005; 62:1381–4.

2631. Wazny L, Walker S, Moist L. Visual compatibility of gentamicin sulfate and 4% sodium citrate solutions. *Am J Health-Syst Pharm.* 2005; 62:1548, 1550.

2632. Barcia E, Martin A, Azuara ML et al. Tramadol and hyoscine N-butyl bromide combined in infusion solutions: compatibility and stability. *Support Care Cancer.* 2007; 15:57–62.

2633. Laville I, Mercier L, Cachaty E et al. Shelf-lives of morphine and pethidine solutions stored in patient-controlled analgesia devices: physico-chemical and microbiological stability study. *Pathol Biol (Paris).* 2005; 53:210–6.

2634. Barcia E, Reyes R, Azuara ML et al. Stability and compatibility of binary mixtures of morphine hydrochloride with hyoscine-n-butyl bromide. *Support Care Cancer.* 2005; 13:239–45.

2635. Fink JM, Capozzi DL, Shermock KM et al. Alteplase for central catheter clearance: 1 mg/mL versus 2 mg/mL. *Ann Pharmacother.* 2004; 38:351–2.

2636. Lian MH, Shao MH, Yuan H et al. Study on the stability of levofloxacin lactate for injection. *Chin J Antibiotics.* 2004; 29:346–8.

2637. de Lemos M. Vinorelbine and venous irritation: optimal parenteral administration. *J Oncol Pharm Pract.* 2005; 11:79–81.

2638. DeFillippis MR, Bell MA, Heyob JA et al. In vitro stability of insulin lispro in continuous subcutaneous insulin infusion. *Diabetes Tech Ther.* 2006; 8:358–68.

2639. Paul M, Razzouq N, Tixier G et al. Stability of prostaglandin e$_1$ (pge$_1$) in aqueous solutions. *Europ J Hosp Pharm Sci.* 2005; 11:31–6.

2640. Xu QA, Trissel LA. Compatibility of palonosetron with cyclophosphamide and with ifosfamide during simulated Y-site administration. *Am J Health-Syst Pharm.* 2005; 62:1998–2000.

2641. Barker B, Feddema S, Rusho WJ et al. Visual compatibility of vasopressin with other injectable drugs. *Am J Health-Syst Pharm.* 2005; 62:1969, 1975–6.

2642. Veggeland T. Visual compatibility of clonidine with selected drugs. *Am J Health-Syst Pharm.* 2005; 62:1968–9.

2643. Bougouin C, Thelcide C, Crespin-Maillard F et al. Compatibility of ondansetron hydrochloride and methylprednisolone sodium succinate in multilayer polyolefin containers. *Am J Health-Syst Pharm.* 2005; 62:2001–5.

2644. Gupta VD. Chemical stability of hydralazine hydrochloride after reconstitution in 0.9% sodium chloride injection or 5% dextrose injection for infusion. *Int J Pharmaceut Compound.* 2005; 9:399–401.

2645. Hecq JD, Boitquin LP, Venbeckbergen DF et al. Effect of freezing, long-term storage, and microwave thawing on the stability of ketorolac tromethamine. *Ann Pharmacother.* 2005; 39:1654–8.

2646. Onat D, Stathopoulos J, Rose A et al. Reliability of nesiritide infusion via non-primed tubing and heparin-coated catheters. *Ann Pharmacother.* 2005; 39:1617–20.

2647. Voges M, Divino-Filho JC, Faict D et al. Compatibility of insulin over 24 hours in standard and bicarbonate-based peritoneal dialysis solutions contained in bags made of different materials. *Perit Dial Int.* 2006; 26:498–502.

2648. Donnelly RF. Chemical stability of fentanyl in polypropylene syringes and polyvinyl chloride bags. *Int J Pharmaceut Compound.* 2005; 9:482–3.

2649. Lewis B, Jarvi E, Cady P. Atropine and ephedrine adsorption to syringe plastic. *AANA J.* 1994; 64:257–60.

2650. Nornoo AO, Elwell RJ. Stability of vancomycin in icodextrin peritoneal dialysis solution. *Ann Pharmacother.* 2006; 40:1950–4.

2651. Velpandian T, Saluja V, Kumar Ravi A et al. Evaluation of the stability of extemporaneously prepared ophthalmic formulation of mitomycin C. *J Ocular Pharmacol Ther.* 2005; 21:217–22.

2652. Abanmy NO, Zaghloul IY, Radwan MA. Compatibility of tramadol hydrochloride injection with selected drugs and solutions. *Am J Health-Syst Pharm.* 2005; 62:1299–302.

2653. Lee DKT, Wand DP, Harsono R et al. Compatibility of fentanyl citrate, ketamine hydrochloride, and droperidol in 0.9% sodium chloride injection stored in polyvinyl chloride bags. *Am J Health-Syst Pharm.* 2005; 62:1190–2.

2654. Rigge DC, Jones MF. Shelf lives of aseptically prepared medicines—stability of hydrocortisone sodium succinate in PVC and non-PVC bags and in polypropylene syringes. *J Pharm Biomed Anal.* 2005; 38:322–6.

2655. Robinson RF, Morosco RS, Smith CV et al. Stability of cefazolin sodium in four heparinized and non-heparinized dialysate solutions at 38°C. *Perit Dial Int.* 2006; 26:593–7.

2656. Johnson CE. Stability of pantoprazole in 0.9% sodium chloride injection in polypropylene syringes. *Am J Health-Syst Pharm.* 2005; 62:2410–2.

2657. Swart EL, van Reij EML, Lee WC et al. Visual compatibility of atosiban acetate with four drugs. *Am J Health-Syst Pharm.* 2005; 62:2459, 2463.

2658. Thalhammer F, Maier-Salamon A, Jager W. Examination of stability and compatibility of flucloxacillin (Floxapen) and ceftazidime (Fortum) in two infusion media: relevance for clinical practice. *Wien Med Wochenschr.* 2005; 155:337–43.

2659. Han J, Washington C. Partition of antimicrobial additives in an intravenous emulsion and their effect on emulsion physical stability. *Int J Pharm.* 2005; 288:263–71.

2660. Trissel LA, Xu QA, Baker M. Drug compatibility with new polyolefin infusion solution containers. *Am J Health-Syst Pharm.* 2006; 63:2379–82.

2661. Rodenbach MP, Hecq JD, Vanbeckbergen D et al. Stability of cefuroxime infusion: the brand-name drug versus a generic product. *Europ J Hosp Pharm Sci.* 2006; 12:32–4.

2662. Cadrobbi J, Hecq JD, Lebrun C et al. Long-term stability of voriconazole 4 mg/mL in dextrose 5% polyvinyl chloride bags at 4°C. *Europ J Hosp Pharm Sci.* 2006; 12:57–9.

2663. Andre P, Cisternino S, Chiadmi F et al. Stability of bortezomib 1-mg/mL solution in plastic syringe and glass vial. *Ann Pharmacother.* 2005; 39:1462–6.

2664. Chan V. Influence of temperature and drug concentration on nafcillin precipitation. *Am J Health-Syst Pharm.* 2005; 62:1347–8.

2665. Nguyen-Xuan T, Griffiths W, Kern C et al. Stability of morphine sulfate in polypropylene infusion bags for use in patient-controlled analgesia pumps for postoperative pain management. *Int J Pharmaceut Compound.* 2006; 10:69–73.

2666. Wang DP. Stability of tetracaine in aqueous systems. *J Taiwan Pharm Assoc.* 1983; 35:132–41.

2667. Rigge DC, Jones MF. Shelf lives of aseptically prepared medicines—stability of piperacillin/tazobactam in PVC and non-PVC bags. *J Pharm Biomed Anal.* 2005; 39:339–43.

2668. Weck S, Cheung S, Hiraoka-Sutow M et al. Alteplase as a catheter locking solution: in vitro evaluation of biochemical stability and antimicrobial properties. *J Vasc Interven Radiol.* 2005; 16:379–83.

2669. Pourroy B, Botta C, Solas C et al. Seventy-two-hour stability of Taxol in 5% dextrose or 0.9% sodium chloride in Viaflo, Freeflex, Ecoflac, and Macoflex N non-PVC bags. *J Clin Pharm Ther.* 2005; 30:455–8.

2670. Ariz Ozdemir F, Anilanmert B, Pekin M. Spectrophotometric investigation of the chemical compatibility of the anticancer drugs irinotecan-HCl and epirubicin-HCl in the same infusion solution. *Cancer Chemother Pharmacol.* 2005; 56:529–34.

2671. Trissel LA, Zhang Y, Douglass K et al. Extended stability of oxytocin in common infusion solutions. *Int J Pharmaceut Compound.* 2006; 10:156–8.

2672. Negro S, Martin A, Azuara ML et al. Stability of tramadol and haloperidol for continuous subcutaneous infusion at home. *J Pain Symptom Manage.* 2005; 30:192–9.

2673. Sautou-Miranda V, Brigas F, Vanheerswynghels S et al. Compatibility of paclitaxel in 5% glucose solution with ECOFLAC low-density polyethylene containers—stability under different storage conditions. *Int J Pharm.* 1999; 178:77–82.

2674. Trittler R. Stability of intravenous admixtures of doxorubicin and vincristine confirmed by LC-MS. *Europ J Hosp Pharm Sci.* 2006; 12:10–2.

2675. Chan J, Walker SE, Law S. Stability of dolasetron mesylate in 0.9% sodium chloride and 5% dextrose in water. *Can J Hosp Pharm.* 2003; 56:87–92.

2676. Zhang Y, Trissel LA. Physical and chemical stability of pemetrexed solutions in plastic syringes. *Ann Pharmacother.* 2005; 39:2026–8.

2677. Watson DG, Lin M, Morton A et al. Compatibility and stability of dexamethasone sodium phosphate and ketamine hydrochloride subcutaneous infusions in polypropylene syringes. *J Pain Symptom Manage.* 2005; 30:80–6.

2678. Lee G, Sabra K, Doyle L et al. Stability of morphine sulphate in P.C.A.s. *Europ J Hosp Pharm Sci.* 2003; 8:1–9.

2679. Theou N, Havard L, Maestroni ML et al. Leaching of di(2-ethylhexyl)phthalate from polyvinyl chloride medical devices: recommendations for taxanes infusion. *Europ J Hosp Pharm Sci.* 2005; 11:55–61.

2680. Hartman CA, Faria CE, Mago K. Visual compatibility of bivalirudin with selected drugs. *Am J Health-Syst Pharm.* 2004; 61:1774, 1776.

2681. Trissel LA, Zhang Y, Xu QA. Physical and chemical stability of palonosetron hydrochloride with dacarbazine and with methylprednisolone sodium succinate during simulated Y-site administration. *Int J Pharmaceut Compound.* 2006; 10:234–6.

2682. Rodenbach MP, Hecq JD, Vanbeckbergen ED et al. Effect of freezing, long-term storage and microwave thawing on the stability of vancomycin hydrochloride in 5% dextrose infusions. *Europ J Hosp Pharm Sci.* 2005; 11:111–3.

2683. Trusley C, Kupiec TC, Trissel LA. Compatibility of micafungin injection with other drugs during simulated Y-site co-administration. *Int J Pharmaceut Compound.* 2006; 10:230–3.

2684. Robinson JL, Tawfik G, Saxinger L et al. Stability of heparin and physical compatibility of heparin/antibiotic solutions in concentrations appropriate for antibiotic lock therapy. *J Antimicrob Chemother.* 2005; 56:951–3.

2685. Corvino TF, Nahata MC, Angelos MG et al. Availability, stability, and sterility of pralidoxime for mass casualty use. *Ann Emerg Med.* 2006; 47:272–7.

2686. Robinson RF, Morosco R. Stability of ciprofloxacin in four heparinized and nonheparinized dialysate solutions at 38°C. *ASHP Midyear Clinical Meeting Poster.* Dec 2005; 40:P442E.

2687. Faria CE, Fiumara K, Patel N et al. Visual compatibility of furosemide with phenylephrine and vasopressin. *Am J Health-Syst Pharm.* 2006; 63:906, 908.

2688. Boothby LA, Madabushi R, Kumar V et al. Extended stability of oxytocin in Ringer's lactate solution at 4° and 25°C. *Hosp Pharm.* 2006; 41:437–41.

2689. Zhang Y, Trissel LA. Physical and chemical stability of pemetrexed in infusion solutions. *Ann Pharmacother.* 2006; 40:1082–5.

2690. Driscoll DF. Lipid injectable emulsions: pharmacopeial and safety issues. *Pharm Res.* 2006; 23:1959–69.

2691. Anacardio R, Bartolini S, Gentile MM et al. HPLC investigated physicochemical compatibility between artrosilene injectable solution and other pharmaceutical products frequently used for combined therapy into elastomeric Baxter LV5 infusion device. *Inter J Immunopath Pharmacol.* 2005; 18:791–8.

2692. Gupta VD. Chemical stability of pyridoxine hydrochloride 100-mg/mL injection, preservative free. *Int J Pharmaceut Compound.* 2006; 10:318–9.

2693. Zhang Y, Trissel LA. Physical instability of frozen pemetrexed solutions in PVC bags. *Ann Pharmacother.* 2006; 40:1289–92.

2694. Sahraoui L, Chiadmi F, Schlatter J et al. Stability of voriconazole injection in 0.9% sodium chloride and 5% dextrose injection. *Am J Health-Syst Pharm.* 2006; 63:1423–6.

2695. Hamada C, Hayashi K, Shou I et al. Pharmacokinetics of calcitriol and maxacalcitol administered into peritoneal dialysate bags in peritoneal dialysis patients. *Perit Dial Int.* 2005; 25:570–5.

2696. Carpenter JF, McNulty MA, Dusci LJ et al. Stability of omeprazole sodium and pantoprazole sodium diluted for intravenous infusion. *J Pharm Technol.* 2006; 22:95–8.

2697. Mendez ASL, Dalomo J, Steppe M et al. Stability and degradation kinetics of meropenem in powder for injection and reconstituted samples. *J Pharm Biomed Anal.* 2006; 41:1363–6.

2698. Kumarvel V, Gandhimani P, Cundill G. Frozen succinylcholine chloride. *Anaesthesia.* 2006; 61:202.

2699. Stone J, Fawcett W. A case of frozen succinylcholine chloride encountered during emergency Cesarean delivery. *Anesth Analg.* 2002; 95:1465.

2700. Negro S, Reyes R, Azuara ML et al. Morphine, haloperidol and hyoscine N-butyl bromide combined in s.c. infusion solutions: compatibility and stability evaluation in terminal oncology patients. *Int J Pharm.* 2006; 307:278–84.

2701. Negro S, Azuara ML, Sanchez Y et al. Physical compatibility and in vivo evaluation of drug mixtures for subcutaneous infusion to cancer patients in palliative care. *Support Care Cancer.* 2002; 10:65–70.

2702. Shields D, Montenegro R, Ragusa M. Chemical stability of admixtures combining ziconotide with morphine or hydromorphone during simulated intrathecal administration. *Neuromodulation.* 2005; 4:257–63.

2703. Shields D, Montenegro R. The chemical stability of admixtures combining ziconotide and clonidine during simulated intrathecal administration. *7th Congress International Modulation Society Poster.* Jun 2005; :.

2704. Shields D, Montenegro R, Aclan J. The chemical stability of admixtures combining ziconotide and bupivacaine hydrochloride during simulated intrathecal administration. *7th Congress International Modulation Society Poster.* Jun 2005; :.

2705. Huang L. Effect of pH and temperature on the stability of 1% tetracaine hydrochloride injection. *Yaoxue Tongbao.* 1982; 17:208–9.

2706. Kambia NK, Luyckx M, Dine T et al. Stability and compatibility of paracetamol injection admixed with ketoprofen. *Europ J Hosp Pharm Sci.* 2006; 12:81–4.

2707. Hecq JD, Boitquin L, Lebrun C et al. Freeze thaw treatment of ketorolac tromethamine in 5% dextrose infusion polyolefin bags: effect of drug concentration and microwave power on the long-term stability at 4°C. *Europ J Hosp Pharm Sci.* 2006; 12:72–5.

2708. Donyai P, Sewell GJ. Physical and chemical stability of paclitaxel infusions in different container types. *J Oncol Pharm Pract.* 2006; 12:211–2.

2709. Fielding H, Kyaterekera N, Skellern GG et al. The compatibility and stability of octreotide acetate in the presence of diamorphine hydrochloride in polypropylene syringes. *Palliative Med.* 2000; 14:205–7.

2710. Vranken JH, van Kan HJ, van der Vegt MH. Stability and compatibility of a meperidine-clonidine mixture in portable pump reservoirs for the management of cancer pain syndromes. *J Pain Symptom Manage.* 2006; 32:297–9.

2711. Negro S, Rendon AL, Azuara ML et al. Compatibility and stability of furosemide and dexamethasone combined in infusion solutions. *Arzneim-Forsch.* 2006; 56:714–20.

2712. Fernandez-Varon E, Marin P, Espuny A et al. Stability of moxifloxacin injection in peritoneal dialysis solution bags (Dianeal PD1 1.36% and Dianeal PD1 3.86%). *J Clin Pharm Ther.* 2006; 31:641–3.

2713. Shields D, Aclan J, Szatkowski A et al. The chemical stability of an admixture containing 25 mcg/mL ziconotide and 20 mg/mL morphine sulfate during simulated intrathecal administration. *N Amer Neuromodulation Soc Poster.* 2006; :.

2714. Ludwig S, Vencl-Joncic M, Gandhi P et al. Simulated Y-site compatibility testing of various diluents and drug products with tigecycline, a first-in-class intravenous glycylcycline. *ASHP Summer Meeting Poster.* 2006; :P62E.

2715. Carroll JA. Stability of flucloxacillin in elastomeric infusion devices. *J Pharm Pract Res.* 2005; 35:90–2.

2716. Trusley C, Ben M, Kupiec TC et al. Physical and chemical stability of palonosetron with metoclopramide and promethazine during simulated Y-site administration. *Int J Pharmaceut Compound.* 2007; 11:82–5.

2717. Chapalain-Pargrade S, Laville I, Paci A et al. Microbiological and physicochemical stability of fentanyl and sufentanil solutions for patient-controlled delivery systems. *J Pain Symptom Manage.* 2006; 32:90–7.

2718. Dalle M, Sautou-Miranda V, Balayssac D et al. Can solutions of docetaxel be conditioned in PVC bags?. *J Pharm Clin.* 2006; 25:147–52.

2719. Kovalick LJ, Pikalov AA, Ni N et al. Short-term physical compatibility of intramuscular aripiprazole with intramuscular lorazepam. *Am J Health-Syst Pharm.* 2008; 65:2007–8.

2720. Trissel LA, Trusley C, Ben M et al. Physical and chemical stability of palonosetron hydrochloride with five opiate agonists during simulated Y-site administration. *Am J Health-Syst Pharm.* 2007; 64:1209–13.

2721. Driscoll DF, Sivestri AP, Nehne J et al. Physicochemical stability of highly concentrated total nutrient admixtures for fluid-restricted patients. *Am J Health-Syst Pharm.* 2006; 63:79–85.

2722. Pietroski N (Associate Director, Medical Services, Merck & Co., North Wales, PA). Personal communication; 2007 Jun 15.

2723. Pietroski N (Associate Director, Medical Services, Merck & Co., North Wales, PA). Personal communication; 2007 Jun 29.

2724. Hecq JD, Evrard JM, Vanbeckbergen DF et al. Effect of freezing, long term storage and microwave thawing on the stability of ceftriaxone sodium in 5% dextrose infusion polyolefin bags at 2–8°C. *Europ J Hosp Pharm Sci.* 2006; 12:52–6.

2725. Sudekum MJ (Manager, Clinical Pharmacy Services, Botsford Hospital, Farmington Hills, MI): Personal communication; 2007 Jun 6.

2726. Nolin TD, Lambert DA, Owens RC Jr. Stability of cefepime and metronidazole prepared for simplified administration as a single product. *Diag Microbiol Infect Dis.* 2006; 56:179–84.

2727. Serrurier C, Chenot ED, Vigneron J et al. Assessment of injectable drugs' administration in two intensive care units and determination of potential physico-chemical incompatibilities. *Europ J Hosp Pharm Sci.* 2006; 12:96–9.

2728. Kraft MD, Johnson CE, Chung C et al. Stability of metoprolol tartrate injection 1 mg/mL undiluted and 0.5 mg/mL in 0.9% sodium chloride injection and 5% dextrose injection. *Am J Health-Syst Pharm.* 2008; 65:636–8.

2729. Kattige A. Long-term physical and chemical stability of a generic paclitaxel infusion under simulated storage and clinical-use conditions. *Europ J Hosp Pharm Sci.* 2006; 12:129–34.

2730. Griffiths W, Favet J, Ing H et al. Chemical stability and microbiological potency of intravenous vancomycin hydrochloride in polypropylene syringes for use in the neonatal intensive care unit. *Europ J Hosp Pharm Sci.* 2006; 12:135–9.

2731. Anon. Rocephin (ceftriaxone sodium) for injection (posted 07/05/2007). FDA MedWatch 2007. www.fda.gov/Safety/MedWatch/SafetyInformation/SafetyAlertsforHuman-MedicalProducts/ucm152863.htm.

2732. Vanneaux V, Proust V, Cheron M et al. A physical and chemical stability study of amphotericin B lipid complexes (Abelcet) after dilution in dextrose 5%. *Europ J Hosp Pharm Sci.* 2007; 13:10–3.

2733. Rondelot G, Serrurier C, Vigneron J et al. Stability of pemetrexed 25 mg/mL in a glass vial and 5 mg/mL in a PVC container after storage for one month at 2–8°C. *Europ J Hosp Pharm Sci.* 2007; 13:14–6.

2734. Food and Drug Administration. Information for healthcare professionals: colistimethate (marketed as Coly-Mycin M and generic products). 2007 Jun 28. FDA website. Accessed 2016 Apr 12. www.fda.gov/Safety/MedWatch/SafetyInformation/SafetyAlertsforHumanMedicalProducts/ucm152109.htm.

2735. Johnson CE, Cober MP. Stability of vecuronium in sterile water for injection stored in polypropylene syringes for 21 days. *Am J Health-Syst Pharm.* 2007; 64:2356–8.

2736. Johnson CE. Stability of a 12.5 mg/mL dolasetron injection in a 12-mL polypropylene syringe. *ASHP Midyear Clinical Meeting Poster.* Dec 2006.

2737. Kiser TH, Oldland AR, Fish DN. Stability of phenylephrine hydrochloride injection in polypropylene syringes. *Am J Health-Syst Pharm.* 2007; 64:1092–5.

2738. Cochran BG, Sowinski KM, Fausel C et al. Physical compatibility and chemical stability of mycophenolate mofetil during simulated Y-site administration with commonly coadministered drugs. *Am J Health-Syst Pharm.* 2007; 64:1410–4.

2739. Karstens A, Kramer I. Chemical and physical stability of diluted busulfan infusion solutions. *Europ J Hosp Pharm Sci.* 2007; 13:40–7.

2740. Karstens A, Kramer I. Viability of micro-organisms in novel anticancer drug solutions. *Europ J Hosp Pharm Sci.* 2007; 13:27–32.

2741. Ponton JL, Munoz C, Rey M et al. The stability of (lyophilized) gemcitabine in 0.9% sodium chloride injection. *Europ J Hosp Pharm.* 2002; 1:23–5.

2742. Adnet F, Le Moyec L, Smith CE et al. Stability of succinylcholine solutions stored at room temperature studied by nuclear magnetic resonance spectroscopy. *Emerg Med J.* 2007; 24:168–9.

2743. Brammer MK, Chan P, Heatherly K et al. Compatibility of doripenem with other drugs during simulated Y-site administration. *Am J Health-Syst Pharm.* 2008; 65:1261–5.

2744. Andre P, Cisternino S, Roy AL et al. Stability of oxaliplatin in infusion bags containing 5% dextrose injection. *Am J Health-Syst Pharm.* 2007; 64:1950–4.

2745. Cohen V, Jellinek SP, Teperikdis L et al. Room-temperature storage of medications labeled for refrigeration. *Am J Health-Syst Pharm.* 2007; 64:1711–5.

2746. Dice JE. Physical compatibility of alprostadil with commonly used IV solutions and medications in the neonatal intensive care unit. *J Pediatr Pharmacol Ther.* 2006; 11:233–6.

2747. Negro S, Salama A, Sanchez Y et al. Compatibility and stability of tramadol and dexamethasone in solution and its use in terminally ill patients. *J Clin Pharm Ther.* 2007; 32:441–4.

2748. Parti R, Schoppmann A, Lee H et al. Stability of lyophilized and reconstituted plasma/albumin-free recombinant human factor VIII (ADVATE rAHF-PFM). *Haemophilia.* 2005; 11:492–6.

2749. Ben M, Trusley C, Kupiec TC et al. Palonosetron hydrochloride compatibility and stability with three β-lactam antibiotics during simulated Y-site administration. *Int J Pharmaceut Compound.* 2007; 11:520–4.

2750. Girbau J, Jane S. Diltiazem-HCl 1 mg/mL prediluted in normal saline and dextrose 5%: compounding with the Gri-Fill 3.0 system and stability study up to 90 days in Gri-Bag. November 2007.

2751. Shields D, Montenegro R, Aclan J. Chemical stability of an admixture combining ziconotide and bupivacaine during simulated intrathecal administration. *Neuromodulation.* 2007; 10:S1–5.

2752. Shields D, Montenegro R. Chemical stability of ziconotide-clonidine hydrochloride admixtures with and without morphine sulfate during simulated intrathecal administration. *Neuromodulation.* 2007; 10:S6–11.

2753. Shields D, Montenegro R, Aclan J. Chemical stability of admixtures combining ziconotide with baclofen during simulated intrathecal administration. *Neuromodulation.* 2007; 10:S12–17.

2754. Avadel Legacy Pharmaceuticals, LLC. Akovaz® (ephedrine sulfate) injection prescribing information. Chesterfield, MO; 2017 Apr.

2755. Dura JV, Hinkle GH. Stability of a mixture of technetium Tc 99m sulfur colloid and lidocaine hydrochloride. *Am J Health-Syst Pharm.* 2007; 64:2477–9.

2756. Cober MP, Johnson CE. Stability of 70% alcohol solutions in polypropylene syringes for use in ethanol-lock therapy. *Am J Health-Syst Pharm.* 2007; 64:2480–2.

2757. Psathas PA. Stability of doripenem for injection (500 mg) in representative infusion fluids and containers. *ASHP Summer Meeting Poster.* 2007; 64(Jun):P57e.

2758. Chan P, Healtherly K, Kupiec TC et al. Compatibility of caspofungin acetate injection with other drugs during simulated Y-site coadministration. *Int J Pharmaceut Compound.* 2008; 12:276–8.

2759. Kaiser JD, Vigneron J, Zenier H et al. Chemical and physical stability of dexrazoxane, diluted with Ringer's lactate solution, in polyvinyl and polyethylene containers. *Europ J Hosp Pharm Sci.* 2007; 13:55–9.

2760. Kupiec TC, Aloumanis V, Ben M et al. Physical and chemical stability of esomeprazole sodium solutions. *Ann Pharmacother.* 2008; 42:1247–51.

2761. Walker SE. Stability of docetaxel solution after dilution in ethanol and storage in vials and after dilution in normal saline and storage in bags. *Can J Hosp Pharm.* 2007; 60:231–7.

2762. Chan P, Bishop A, Kupiec TC et al. Compatibility of ceftobiprole medocaril with selected drugs during simulated Y-site administration. *Am J Health-Syst Pharm.* 2008; 65:1545–51.

2763. Roy JJ, Boismenu D, Mamer OA et al. Room temperature stability of injectable succinylcholine dichloride. *Int J Pharmaceut Compound.* 2008; 12:83–5.

2764. Trusley C, Ben M, Kupiec TC et al. Compatibility and stability of palonosetron hydrochloride with four neuromuscular blocking agents during simulated Y-site administration. *Int J Pharmaceut Compound.* 2008; 12:156–60.

2765. Kupiec TC, Ben M, Trusley C et al. Compatibility and stability of palonosetron hydrochloride with gentamicin, metronidazole, or vancomycin during simulated Y-site administration. *Int J Pharmaceut Compound.* 2008; 12:170–3.

2766. Condie CK, Tyler LS, Barker B et al. Visual compatibility of caspofungin acetate with commonly used drugs during simulated Y-site delivery. *Am J Health-Syst Pharm.* 2008; 65:454–7.

2767. Brousseau P, Nickerson J, Dobson G. Dexamethasone and ondansetron incompatibility in polypropylene syringes. *Can J Anesth.* 2007; 54:953–4.

2768. Walker SE, Milliken D, Law S. Stability of bortezomib reconstituted with 0.9% sodium chloride at 4°C and room temperature (23°C). *Can J Hosp Pharm.* 2008; 61:14–20.

2769. Chandler C, Gryniewicz CM, Pringle T et al. Insulin temperature and stability under simulated transit conditions. *Am J Health-Syst Pharm.* 2008; 65:953–63.

2770. Walker SE, Law S. Physical [visual] Y-site compatibility of Voluven with 38 other intravenous medications. *CSHP Annual Meeting Poster.* Aug 2007.

2771. Kupiec TC, Trusley C, Ben M et al. Physical and chemical stability of palonosetron hydrochloride with five common parenteral drugs during simulated Y-site administration. *Am J Health-Syst Pharm.* 2008; 65:1735–9.

2772. Shields DE, Aclan J, Szatkowski A. Chemical stability of admixtures combining ziconotide with fentanyl or sufentanil during simulated intrathecal administration. *Int J Pharmaceut Compound.* 2008; 12:463–6.

2773. Ben M, Trusley C, Kupiec TC et al. Physical and chemical stability of palonosetron hydrochloride with glycopyrrolate and neostigmine during simulated Y-site administration. *Int J Pharmaceut Compound.* 2008; 12:368–72.

2774. Goldenberg NA, Jacobson L, Hathaway H et al. Anti-Xa stability of diluted dalteparin for pediatric use. *Ann Pharmacother.* 2008; 42:511–5.

2775. Ben M, Kupiec TC, Trusley C et al. Compatibility and stability of palonosetron hydrochloride with lactated Ringer's, hetastarch in lactated electrolyte, and mannitol injections during simulated Y-site administration. *Int J Pharmaceut Compound.* 2008; 12:460–2.

2776. Tremblay M, Lessard MR, Trepanier CA et al. Stability of norepinephrine infusions prepared in dextrose and normal saline solutions. *Can J Anesth.* 2008; 55:163–7.

2777. Kaestner S, Sewell G. A sequential temperature cycling study for the investigation of carboplatin infusion stability to facilitate "dose-banding". *J Oncol Pharm Pract.* 2007; 13:119–26.

2778. Newton DW, Driscoll DF. Chemistry and safety of phosphates injections. *Am J Health-Syst Pharm.* 2008; 65:1761–6.

2779. Stucki MC, Fleury-Souverain S, Sautter AM et al. Development of ready-to-use ketamine hydrochloride syringes for safe use in post-operative pain. *Europ J Hosp Pharm Sci.* 2008; 14:14–8.

2780. Shields DE, Aclan J, Szatkowski A. Chemical stability of admixtures containing ziconotide 25 mcg/mL and morphine sulfate 10 mg/mL or 20 mg/mL during simulated intrathecal administration. *Int J Pharmaceut Compound.* 2008; 12:553–7.

2781. Donnelly RF, Corman C. Physical compatibility and chemical stability of a concentrated solution of atropine sulfate (2 mg/mL) for use as an antidote in nerve agent casualties. *Int J Pharmaceut Compound.* 2008; 12:550–2.

2782. Junker A, Roy S, Desroches MC et al. Stability of oxaliplatin solution. *Ann Pharmacother.* 2009; 43:390–1.

2783. Taiwo T (Medical Communications, Hospira, Inc., Lake Forest, IL). Personal communication; 2009 Feb 23.

2784. Anon. Information for healthcare professionals ceftriaxone (marketed as Rocephin and generics). FDA Update 4/14/2009. www.fda.gov/Drugs/DrugSafety/PostmarketDrugSafetyInformationforPatientsandProviders/DrugSafetyInformationforHeathcareProfessionals/ucm084263.htm.

2785. Martinez JN, Alminana MA, Sales OD. Establidad en suero fisiologico del busulfan intravenoso en un envase de poliolefinas. *Farm Hosp.* 2008; 32:344–8.

2786. Schmid R, Koren G, Klein J et al. The stability of a ketamine-morphine solution. *Anesth Analg.* 2002; 94:898–900.

2787. Lau MH, Hackman C, Morgan DJ. Compatibility of ketamine and morphine injections. *Pain*. 1998; 75:389–90.

2788. Trissel LA, Trusley C, Kupiec TC et al. Compatibility and stability of palonosetron hydrochloride and propofol during simulated Y-site administration. *Int J Pharmaceut Compound*. 2009; 13:78–80.

2789. Valverde Molina E, Gonzalez Muniz V, Gomez-Maldonado J et al. Stability of pantoprazole in parenteral nutrition units. *Farm Hosp*. 2008; 32:290–2.

2790. Donnelly RF, Willman E, Andolfatto G. Stability of ketamine-propofol mixtures for procedural sedation and analgesia in the emergency department. *Can J Hosp Pharm*. 2008; 61:426–30.

2791. McCluskey SV, Graner KK, Kemp J et al. Stability of fentanyl 5 μg/mL diluted with 0.9% sodium chloride injection and stored in polypropylene syringes. *Am J Health-Syst Pharm*. 2009; 66:860–3.

2792. Aloumanis V, Ben M, Kupiec TC et al. Drug compatibility with a new generation of VISIV polyolefin infusion solution containers. *Int J Pharmaceut Compound*. 2009; 13:162–5.

2793. Xu M, WArren FW, Bartlett MG. Stability of low-concentration ceftazidime in 0.9% sodium chloride injection and balanced salt solutions in plastic syringes under various storage conditions. *Int J Pharmaceut Compound*. 2009; 13:166–9.

2794. Canann D, Tyler LS, Barker B et al. Visual compatibility of i.v. medications routinely used in bone marrow transplant recipients. *Am J Health-Syst Pharm*. 2009; 66:727–9.

2795. Newland AM, Mauro VF, Alexander KS. Physical compatibility of metoprolol tartrate injection with selected cardiovascular agents. *Am J Health-Syst Pharm*. 2009; 66:986–7.

2796. Vazquez R, Le Hoang MD, Martin J et al. Simultaneous quantification of water-soluble and fat-soluble vitamins in parenteral nutrition admixtures by HPLC-UV-MS/MS. *Eur J Hosp Pharm Sci*. 2009; 15:28–35.

2797. Donnelly RF. Physical compatibility and chemical stability of ketamine-morphine mixtures in polypropylene syringes. *Can J Hosp Pharm*. 2009; 62:28–33.

2798. Walker S, Iazzetta J, Law S. Extended stability of pantoprazole for injection in 0.9% sodium chloride or 5% dextrose at 4°C and 23°C. *Can J Hosp Pharm*. 2009; 62:135–41.

2799. Ensom MYY, Decarie D, Leung K et al. Stability of hydromorphone-ketamine solutions in glass bottles, plastic syringes, and IV bags for pediatric use. *Can J Hosp Pharm*. 2009; 62:112–8.

2800. Pourroy B, Bausset EM, Boulamery A et al. Incompatibility of imipenem-cilastatin and amoxicillin. *Am J Health-Syst Pharm*. 2009; 66:1253–4.

2801. Psathas P, Gilmor TP, Schaufelberger DE, et al. Stability of high and low concentrations of doripenem (500 mg) for injection in representative infusion fluids and containers. *ASHP Summer Meeting Poster*. Jun 2009.

2802. Gole DJ, Ilias J, Vermeersch H, et al. Stability of ceftobiprole for injection (500 mg) in representative infusion fluids and containers. *ASHP Summer Meeting Poster*. Jun 2009.

2803. Newton DW, Driscoll DF. Calcium and phosphate compatibility: revisited again. *Am J Health-Syst Pharm*. 2008; 65:73–80.

2804. Eroles AA, Bafalluy IM, Arnaiz JAS. Stability of docetaxel diluted to 0.3 to 0.9 mg/mL with 0.9% sodium chloride injection and stored in polyolefin or glass containers. *Am J Health-Syst Pharm*. 2009; 66:1565–8.

2805. Michel M (Medical Information, Eisai, Woodcliff Lake, NJ): Personal communication; 2016 Jan 12.

2806. Donnelly RF. Stability of aseptically prepared tazocin solutions in polyvinyl chloride bags. *Can J Hosp Pharm*. 2009; 62:226–31.

2807. Galanti L, Lebitassy MP, Hecq JD et al. Long-term stability of 5-fluorouracil in 0.9% sodium chloride after freezing, microwave thawing, and refrigeration. *Can J Hosp Pharm*. 2009; 62:34–8.

2808. Crandon JL, Sutherland C, Nicolau DP. Enhanced room temperature (RT) stability of doripenem (DOR) within two infusion devices. *Infectious Disease Society of America Meeting Poster*. Oct 2009.

2809. Crandon JL, Sutherland C, Nicolau DP. Stability of doripenem in polyvinyl chloride bags and elastomeric pumps. *Am J Health-Syst Pharm*. 2010; 67:1539–44.

2810. Almoazen H, Bhattacharjee H, Samsa AC et al. Stability of mesna in ReadyMed infusion devices. *Ann Pharmacother*. 2010; 44:224–5.

2811. Athanapoulos A, Hecq JD, Vanbeckbergen D et al. Long-term stability of tramadol chlorhydrate and metoclopramide hydrochloride in dextrose 5% polyolefin bag at 4°C. *J Oncol Pharm Pract*. 2009; 15:195–200.

2812. Reviewers' comments (personal observations) on infliximab.

2813. Walker SE, Law S, Garland J et al. Stability of norepinephrine solutions in normal saline and 5% dextrose in water. *Can J Hosp Pharm*. 2010; 63:113–8.

2814. Moriyama B, Henning SA, Jin H et al. Physical compatibility of magnesium sulfate and sodium bicarbonate in a pharmacy-compounded hemofiltration solution. *Am J Health-Syst Pharm*. 2010; 67:562–5.

2815. Pascuet E, Donnelly RF, Garceau D et al. Buffered lidocaine hydrochloride solution with and without epinephrine: stability in polypropylene syringes. *Can J Hosp Pharm*. 2009; 62:375–80.

2816. He J, Figueroa DA, Tze-Peng L et al. Stability of polymyxin B sulfate diluted in 0.9% sodium chloride injection and stored at 4 or 25°C. *Am J Health-Syst Pharm*. ; 67:1191–4.

2817. Wear J, McPherson TB, Kolling WM. Stability of sodium bicarbonate solutions in polyolefin bags. *Am J Health-Syst Pharm*. 2010; 67:1026–9.

2818. Khondkar D, Chopra P, McArter JP et al. Chemcial stability of hydromorphone hydrochloride in patient-controlled analgesia injector. *Int J Pharmaceut Compound*. 2010; 14:160–4.

2819. Walker SE, Iazetta J, Law S et al. Stability of commonly used antibiotic solutions in an elastomeric infusion device. *Can J Hosp Pharm*. 2010; 63:212–4.

2820. Baker DS, Waldrop B, Arnold J. Compatibility and stability of cefotaxime, vancomycin, and ciprofloxacin in antibiotic solutions containing heparin. *Int J Pharmaceut Compound*. 2010; 14:346–9.

2821. Hospira, Inc. Dyloject® (diclofenac sodium) injection for intravenous use prescribing information. Lake Forest, IL; 2014 Dec.

2822. Rolin C, Jecq JD, Vanbeckbergen DF et al. Stability of ondansetron and dexamethasone infusion upon refrigeration. *Ann Pharmacother*. 2011; 45:130–1.

2823. Strong DK, Decarie D, Ensom MHH. Stability of levothyroxine in sodium chloride for IV administration. *Can J Hosp Pharm*. 2010; 63:437–43.

2824. Cote D, Lok CE, Battistella M et al. Stability of trisodium citrate and gentamicin solution for catheter locks after storage in plastic syringes at room temperature. *Can J Hosp Pharm*. 2010; 63:304–11.

2825. Schulz L, Elder E, Jones K et al. Stability of sodium nitroprusside and sodium thiosulfate 1:10 intravenous admixture. *Hosp Pharm*. 2010; 45:779–84.

2826. Singh BN, Dedhiya MG, DiNunzio J, et al. Compatibility of ceftaroline fosamil for injection with selected drugs during simulated Y-site administration. *Am J Health-Syst Pharm*. 2011; 68:2163–9.

2827. Amri A, Ben Achour A, Chachaty E et al. Microbiology and physicochemical stability of oxycodone hydrochloride solutions for patient-controlled delivery systems. *J Pain Symptom Manage*. 2010; 40:87–94.

2828. Tsiouris M, Ulmer M, Yurcho JF et al. Stability and compatibility of reconstituted caspofungin in select elastomeric infusion devices. *Int J Pharmaceut Compound*. 2010; 14:436–9.

2829. Tennant D (Senior Medical Information Specialist, Hospira, Inc., Lake Forest, IL): Personal communication; 2011 Mar 22.

2830. Housman ST, Tessier PR, Nicolau DP et al. Physical compatibility of telavancin hydrochloride with select i.v. drugs during simulated Y-site administration. *Am J Health Syst Pharm*. 2011; 68:2265–70.

2831. Theravance. Vibativ® (telavancin) for injection for intravenous use prescribing information. South San Francisco, CA; 2014 Mar.

2832. Allergan USA, Inc. Teflaro® (ceftaroline fosamil) for injection prescribing information. Madison, NJ; 2019 Sep.

2833. UCB, Inc. Keppra® (levetiracetam) injection prescribing information. Smyrna, GA; 2017 Oct.

2834. Mylan Institutional LLC. Levetiracetam in sodium chloride injection prescribing information. Rockford, IL; 2018 Jul.

2835. UCBCares Medical Information. Keppra® (levetiracetam) injection: Stability, compatibility and osmolality. 18 Feb 2019.

2836. Claris Lifesciences, Inc. Ondansetron injection for intravenous or intramuscular use. North Brunswick, NJ; 2013 Mar.

2837. GlaxoSmithKline. Zofran® (ondansetron hydrochloride) injection for intravenous use. Research Triangle Park, NC; 2012 Nov.

2838. Astellas. Vaprisol® (conivaptan hydrochloride) injection for intravenous use prescribing information. Northbrook, IL; 2012 Oct.

2839. Bang L (Scientific Affairs and Medical Information, Astellas, Northbrook, IL): Personal communication; 2012 Oct 16.

2840. Cadence Pharmaceuticals, Inc. Ofirmev® (acetaminophen) injection prescribing information. San Diego, CA; 2010 Nov.

2841. Lu C (Director Medical Affairs, Cadence Pharmaceuticals, San Diego, CA): Personal communication; 2012 Nov 5.

2842. Hamdi M, Lentschener C, Bazin C et al. Compatibility and stability of binary mixtures of acetaminophen, nefopam, ketoprofen and ketamine in infusion solutions. *Eur J Anaesthesiol*. 2009; 26:23–7.

2843. Havard L (Service de Pharmacie, Hôpital Européen Georges-Pompidou, Paris): Personal communication; 2012 Nov 30.

2844. Ang R, Kupiec TC, Breitmeyer JB, et al. IV acetaminophen in-use stability and compatibility with common IV fluids and IV medications. Presented at 111th Annual Meeting of the American Society of Clinical Pharmacology and Therapeutics. Atlanta, GA: 2010 March 17–20.

2845. Kwiatkowski JL, Johnson CE, Wagner DS. Extended stability of intravenous acetaminophen in syringes and opened vials. *Am J Health Syst Pharm*. 2012; 69:1999–2001.

2846. Hospira Worldwide, Inc. Pamidronate disodium injection solution for intravenous infusion prescribing information. Lake Forest, IL; 2009 Sep.

2847. Bedford Laboratories. Pamidronate disodium injection solution and lyophilized powder for solution for intravenous infusion prescribing information. Bedford, OH; 2012 Aug.

2848. Hospira, Inc. Precedex® (dexmedetomidine hydrochloride) injection for intravenous use and in 0.9% sodium chloride injection prescribing information. Lake Forest, IL; 2016 Mar.

2849. Anderson CR, MacKay MW, Holley M et al. Stability of dexmedetomidine 4 mcg/mL in polypropylene syringes. *Am J Health Syst Pharm*. 2012; 69:595–7.

2850. Wyeth Pharmaceuticals Inc. Protonix® I.V. (pantoprazole sodium) for injection for intravenous use prescribing information. Philadelphia, PA; 2017 Jul.

2851. Donnelly RF. Stability of pantoprazole sodium in glass vials, polyvinyl chloride minibags, and polypropylene syringes. *Can J Hosp Pharm*. 2011; 64:192–8.

2852. Sanofi-Aventis U.S. LLC. Eloxatin® (oxaliplatin) injection for intravenous use prescribing information. Bridgewater, NJ; 2013 Aug.

2853. Pfizer Labs. Oxaliplatin injection for intravenous use prescribing information. New York, NY; 2012 Jul.

2854. Caraco Pharmaceutical Laboratories, Ltd. Oxaliplatin for injection for intravenous use prescribing information. Detroit, MI; 2012 Sep.

2855. Eiden C, Philibert L, Bekhtari K et al. Physicochemical stability of oxaliplatin in 5% dextrose injection stored in polyvinyl chloride, polyethylene, and polypropylene infusion bags. *Am J Health Syst Pharm*. 2009; 66:1929–33.

2856. JHP Pharmaceuticals, LLC. Oxytocin injection prescribing information. Rochester, MI; 2012 Feb.

2857. JHP Pharmaceuticals, LLC. Pitocin® (oxytocin) injection pharmacy bulk package prescribing information. Rochester, MI; 2012 Apr.

2858. APP Pharmaceuticals, LLC. Oxytocin injection solution for intravenous infusion or intramuscular use prescribing information. Schaumburg, IL; 2007 Dec.

2859. Swedish Orphan Biovitrum AB. Kineret® (anakinra) for injection for subcutaneous use prescribing information. Stockholm, Sweden; 2013 Oct.

2860. Teva Pharmaceuticals USA, Inc. Trisenox® (arsenic trioxide) injection for intravenous administration prescribing information. North Wales, PA; 2016 Aug.

2861. Cumberland Pharmaceuticals Inc. Acetadote® (acetylcysteine) injection prescribing information. Nashville, TN; 2013 Jun.

2862. Pfizer Injectables. Eraxis® (anidulafungin) for injection prescribing information. New York, NY; 2018 Jan.

2863. Pfizer Injectables. Zithromax® (azithromycin) for injection prescribing information. New York, NY; 2017 Mar.

2864. Bristol-Myers Squibb Company. Azactam® (aztreonam) for injection prescribing information. Princeton, NJ; 2013 Jun.

2865. Bristol-Myers Squibb Company. Azactam® (aztreonam) injection in GALAXY plastic container (PL 2040) for intravenous use prescribing information. Princeton, NJ; 2013 Jun.

2866. Fresenius Kabi USA, LLC. Aztreonam for injection prescribing information. Lake Zurich, IL; 2013 Sep.

2867. Hospira, Inc. Hextend® (6% hetastarch in lactated electrolyte injection) prescribing information. Lake Forest, IL; 2014 Nov.

2868. AbbVie Inc. Nimbex® (cisatracurium besylate) injection prescribing information. North Chicago, IL; 2013 Jan.

2869. Baxter Healthcare Corporation. Brevibloc® (esmolol hydrochloride) injection for intravenous use prescribing information. Deerfield, IL; 2014 Apr.

2870. Eisai Inc. Aloxi® (palonosetron HCl) injection prescribing information. Woodcliff Lake, NJ; 2015 Dec.

2871. Teva Pharmaceuticals USA. Pancuronium bromide injection prescribing information. Sellersville, PA; 2011 Oct.

2872. Hospira, Inc. Pancuronium bromide injection prescribing information. Lake Forest, IL; 2013 Nov.

2873. Amgen, Inc. Neupogen® (filgrastim) prescribing information. Thousand Oaks, CA; 2013 Sep.

2874. Kaushal G, Sayre BE, Prettyman T. Stability of extemporaneously compounded diltiazem hydrochloride infusions stored in polyolefin bags. *Am J Health Syst Pharm.* 2013; 70:894–9.

2875. Bedford Laboratories. Diltiazem hydrochloride injection prescribing information. Bedford, OH; 2007 Feb.

2876. Hospira, Inc. Diltiazem hydrochloride for injection for continuous intravenous infusion not for bolus ADD-Vantage® vials prescribing information. Lake Forest, IL; 2008 Jan.

2877. Sanofi-Aventis U.S. LLC. Zaltrap® (ziv-aflibercept) injection for intravenous infusion prescribing information. Bridgewater, NJ; 2013 Oct.

2878. Fierro L (Medical Information Services, sanofi-aventis, Bridgewater, NJ): Personal communication; 2012 Dec 4.

2879. GlaxoSmithKline. Flolan® (epoprostenol sodium) for injection prescribing information. Research Triangle Park, NC; 2018 May.

2880. Actelion Pharmaceuticals US, Inc. Veletri® (epoprostenol) for injection prescribing information. South San Francisco, CA; 2016 Jul.

2881. Teva Pharmaceuticals USA, Inc. Epoprostenol sodium for injection prescribing information. North Wales, PA; 2017 Aug.

2882. Lambert O, Bandilla D. Stability and preservation of a new formulation of epoprostenol sodium for treatment of pulmonary arterial hypertension. *Drug Des Devel Ther.* 2012; 6:235–44.

2883. Fresenius Kabi USA, LLC. Levothyroxine sodium for injection prescribing information. Lake Zurich, IL; 2013 Apr.

2884. Frenette AJ, MacLean RD, Williamson D et al. Stability of levothyroxine injection in glass, polyvinyl chloride, and polyolefin containers. *Am J Health Syst Pharm.* 2011; 68:1723–8.

2885. APP Pharmaceuticals, LLC. Levothyroxine sodium for injection prescribing information. Schaumburg, IL; 2008 Jan.

2886. Pfizer Injectables. Cyklokapron® (tranexamic acid) injection prescribing information. New York, NY; 2013 May.

2887. Riley J (Medical Information, Pfizer, New York, NY): Personal communication; 2013 Apr 30.

2888. Acella Pharmaceuticals, LLC. Tranexamic acid injection solution prescribing information. Alpharetta, GA; 2014 Jan.

2889. CRASH-2 trial collaborators, Shakur H, Roberts I et al. Effects of tranexamic acid on death, vascular occlusive events, and blood transfusion in trauma patients with significant haemorrhage (CRASH-2): a randomised, placebo-controlled trial. *Lancet.* 2010; 376:23–32.

2890. Roberts I, Shakur H, Ker K et al. Antifibrinolytic drugs for acute traumatic injury. *Cochrane Database Syst Rev.* 2012; 12:CD004896.

2891. Spahn DR, Bouillon B, Cerny V et al. Management of bleeding and coagulopathy following major trauma: an updated European guideline. *Crit Care.* 2013; 17:R76.

2892. Saleem N (Medical Information, Amgen, Thousand Oaks, CA): Personal communication; 2014 Apr 4.

2893. Astellas Pharma US, Inc. Mycamine® (micafungin sodium) for injection for IV infusion only prescribing information. Northbrook, IL; 2013 Jun.

2894. Fleischbein E, Montgomery PA, Zhou CS. Visual compatibility of micafungin sodium and levofloxacin injections. *Am J Health Syst Pharm.* 2012; 69:2130. Letter.

2895. Janssen Pharmaceuticals, Inc. Levaquin® (levofloxacin) tablets, oral solution, injection concentrate for intravenous use, and solution in 5% dextrose for intravenous use prescribing information. Titusville, NJ; 2013 Sep.

2896. EUSA Pharma (USA), Inc. Erwinaze® (asparaginase *Erwinia chrysanthemi*) for injection for intramuscular use prescribing information. Langhorne, PA; 2014 Mar.

2897. Millennium Pharmaceuticals, Inc. Velcade® (bortezomib) for injection for subcutaneous or intravenous use prescribing information. Cambridge, MA; 2012 Oct.

2898. Gilbar P, Seger AC. Deaths reported from the accidental intrathecal administration of bortezomib. *J Oncol Pharm Pract.* 2012; 18:377–8.

2899. Medtronic, Inc. Lioresal® Intrathecal (baclofen injection) prescribing information. Minneapolis, MN; 2013 Oct.

2900. CNS Therapeutics Inc. Gablofen® (baclofen injection) prescribing information. St. Paul, MN; 2013 Mar.

2901. Anderson C, Boehme S, Ouellette J et al. Physical and chemical compatibility of injectable acetaminophen during simulated y-site administration. *Hosp Pharm.* 2014; 49:42–7.

2902. Anderson C (Clinical Pharmacist, Primary Children's Hospital, Salt Lake City, UT): Personal communication; 2014 Jan 28.

2903. Hospira, Inc. Isuprel® (isoproterenol hydrochloride) injection solution prescribing information. Lake Forest, IL; 2013 Jul.

2904. Apotex Inc. Butorphanol tartrate injection solution prescribing information. Toronto, Ontario; 2005 Aug.

2905. West-Ward Pharmaceuticals. Butorphanol tartrate injection solution prescribing information. Eatontown, NJ; 2009 Sep.

2906. Akorn, Inc. Inapsine® (droperidol) injection for intravenous or intramuscular use only prescribing information. Lake Forest, IL; 2011 Oct.

2907. American Regent, Inc. Droperidol injection solution for IV or IM use only prescribing information. Shirley, NY; 2005 Nov.

2908. Chen FC, Fang BX, Li P et al. Compatibility of butorphanol and droperidol in 0.9% sodium chloride injection. *Am J Health Syst Pharm*. 2013; 70:515–9.

2909. Beauregard N, Bertrand N, Dufour A et al. Physical compatibility of calcium gluconate and magnesium sulfate injections. *Am J Health Syst Pharm*. 2012; 69:98.

2910. Durata Therapeutics U.S. Limited. Dalvance® (dalbavancin) for injection for intravenous use prescribing information. Chicago, IL; 2014 May.

2911. Merck & Co., Inc. Noxafil® (posaconazole) injection, delayed-release tablets, and oral suspension prescribing information. Whitehouse Station, NJ; 2015 Nov.

2912. Dutta S (Medical Information, Merck, North Wales, PA): Personal communication; 2014 Jun 3.

2913. Merck & Co., Inc. Sivextro® (tedizolid phosphate) for injection for intravenous use prescribing information. Whitehouse Station, NJ; 2016 Oct.

2914. Freeman C (Medical Information, Cubist Pharmaceuticals, Lexington, MA): Personal communication; 2014 Aug 19.

2915. Wyeth Pharmaceuticals LLC. Tygacil® (tigecycline) for injection prescribing information. Philadelphia, PA; 2018 Apr.

2916. Shionogi Inc. Doribax® (doripenem for injection) powder for solution for intravenous use prescribing information. Florham Park, NJ; 2014 Jan.

2917. Ludwig S (Corresponding Author): Personal communication; 2014 May 8.

2918. Wyeth Pharmaceuticals Inc. Zosyn® (piperacillin sodium and tazobactam sodium) for injection single-dose and pharmacy bulk vials and Zosyn® (piperacillin sodium and tazobactam sodium) injection single-dose GALAXY® containers prescribing information. Philadelphia, PA; 2014 Feb.

2919. Hospira, Inc. Piperacillin sodium and tazobactam sodium for injection ADD-Vantage® vials prescribing information. Lake Forest, IL; 2013 Sep.

2920. Apotex Corp. Piperacillin sodium and tazobactam sodium for injection pharmacy bulk vials prescribing information. Weston, FL; 2014 Jun.

2921. Mylan Institutional LLC. Piperacillin sodium and tazobactam sodium for injection single dose vials prescribing information. Rockford, IL; 2014 Aug.

2922. (Medical Information, Pfizer): Personal communication; 2014.

2924. Gilead Sciences, Inc. Vistide® (cidofovir) injection prescribing information. Foster City, CA; 2010 Sep.

2925. Heritage Pharmaceuticals Inc. Cidofovir injection prescribing information. Eatontown, NJ; 2013 Oct.

2926. JHP Pharmaceuticals, LLC. Brevital® sodium (methohexital sodium) for injection prescribing information. Rochester, MI; 2014 Feb.

2927. The Medicines Company. Orbactiv® (oritavancin) for injection prescribing information. Parsippany, NJ; 2014 Aug.

2928. Kumar A, Mann HJ. Visual compatibility of oritavancin diphosphate with selected coadministered drugs during simulated Y-site administration. *Am J Health Syst Pharm*. 2010; 67:1640–4.

2929. Novartis Pharmaceuticals Corporation. Sandimmune® (cyclosporine) capsules, oral solution, and injection prescribing information. East Hanover, NJ; 2015 Mar.

2930. Li M, Forest JM, Coursol C et al. Stability of cyclosporine solutions stored in polypropylene-polyolefin bags and polypropylene syringes. *Am J Health Syst Pharm*. 2011; 68:1646–50.

2931. Li M, Coursol C, Leclair G. Stability of cyclosporine diluted with 0.9% sodium chloride injection or 5% dextrose injection and stored in ethylene-vinyl acetate containers. *Am J Health Syst Pharm*. 2013; 70:1970–2. Letter.

2932. Desai NR, Shah SM, Cohen J et al. Zosyn (piperacillin/tazobactam) reformulation: Expanded compatibility and coadministration with lactated Ringer's solutions and selected aminoglycosides. *Ther Clin Risk Manag*. 2008; 4:303–14.

2933. Nichols KR, Demarco MW, Vertin MD et al. Y-site compatibility of vancomycin and piperacillin/tazobactam at commonly utilized pediatric concentrations. *Hosp Pharm*. 2013; 48:44–7.

2934. Lam WJ, Bhowmick T, Gross A et al. Using higher doses to compensate for tubing residuals in extended-infusion piperacillin-tazobactam. *Ann Pharmacother*. 2013; 47:886–91.

2935. Leung E, Venkatesan N, Ly SC et al. Physical compatibility of vancomycin and piperacillin sodium-tazobactam at concentrations typically used during prolonged infusions. *Am J Health Syst Pharm*. 2013; 70:1163–6.

2936. Fresenius Kabi USA, LLC. Bleomycin sulfate for injection prescribing information. Lake Zurich, IL; 2014 Feb.

2937. Hospira, Inc. Bleomycin for injection prescribing information. Lake Forest, IL; 2013 Jan.

2938. Fresenius Kabi USA, LLC. Cladribine injection prescribing information. Lake Zurich, IL; 2013 May.

2939. Teva Pharmaceuticals USA. Carboplatin injection prescribing information. North Wales, PA; 2016 Jan.

2940. Accord Healthcare, Inc. Carboplatin injection prescribing information. Durham, NC; 2019 July.

2941. APP Pharmaceuticals, LLC. Cytarabine injection prescribing information. Schaumburg, IL; 2008 Jan.

2942. Hospira, Inc. Cytarabine injection for intravenous, intrathecal and subcutaneous use only prescribing information. Lake Forest, IL; 2012 Apr.

2943. Hospira, Inc. Cytarabine injection pharmacy bulk package prescribing information. Lake Forest. IL; 2012 Apr.

2944. Hospira, Inc. Cytarabine injection for intravenous or subcutaneous use only prescribing information. Lake Forest, IL; 2012 Apr.

2945. Recordati Rare Diseases Inc. Cosmegen® (dactinomycin) for injection prescribing information. Lebanon, NJ; 2013 Feb.

2946. APP Pharmaceuticals, LLC. Vinblastine sulfate injection prescribing information. Schaumburg, IL; 2011 Oct.

2947. Hospira, Inc. Vincristine sulfate injection prescribing information. Lake Forest, IL; 2013 Jul.

2948. Hospira, Inc. Mitoxantrone hydrochloride injection concentrate prescribing information. Lake Forest, IL; 2013 Feb.

2949. Pfizer Labs. Mitoxantrone hydrochloride injection concentrate prescribing information. New York, NY; 2013 May.

2950. Teva Parenteral Medicines, Inc. Daunorubicin hydrochloride injection prescribing information. Irvine, CA; 2012 Sep.

2951. APP Pharmaceuticals, LLC. Etoposide injection prescribing information. Schaumburg, IL; 2008 Jan.

2952. Merck & Co., Inc. Intron® A (interferon alfa-2b, recombinant) for injection prescribing information. Whitehouse Station, NJ; 2014 Oct.

2953. Merck & Co., Inc. Intron® A (interferon alfa-2b, recombinant) powder for solution instructions for use. Whitehouse Station, NJ; 2011 Feb.

2954. Fresenius Kabi USA, LLC. Fluorouracil injection solution pharmacy bulk package prescribing information. Lake Zurich, IL; 2014 Jun.

2955. Fresenius Kabi USA, LLC. Fluorouracil injection solution prescribing information. Lake Zurich; 2014 Jun.

2956. Accord Healthcare, Inc. Fluorouracil injection solution pharmacy bulk package prescribing information. Durham, NC; 2013 Nov.

2957. Accord Healthcare, Inc. Fluorouracil injection solution prescribing information. Durham, NC; 2013 Nov.

2958. Merck & Co., Inc. Zerbaxa® (ceftolozane and tazobactam) for injection prescribing information. Whitehouse Station, NJ; 2019 Jun.

2959. Johnson PR (Medical Information, Cubist Pharmaceuticals, Lexington, MA): Personal Communication; 2014 Dec 23.

2960. BioCryst Pharmaceuticals, Inc. Rapivab® (peramivir) injection prescribing information. Durham, NC; 2014 Dec.

2961. Lipiäinen T, Peltoniemi M, Sarkhel S et al. Formulation and Stability of Cytokine Therapeutics. *J Pharm Sci*. 2014; :.

2962. Baxter Healthcare Corporation. Cyclophosphamide powder for injection. Deerfield, IL; 2014 Oct.

2963. Jansen JJ, Oldland AR, Kiser TH. Evaluation of phenylephrine stability in polyvinyl chloride bags. *Hosp Pharm*. 2014; 49:455–7.

2964. Pharmacia and Upjohn Company. Idamycin PFS® (idarubicin hydrochloride injection) prescribing information. New York, NY; 2014 Dec.

2965. Teva Parenteral Medicines, Inc. Idarubicin hydrochloride injection prescribing information. Irvine, CA; 2011 Sep.

2966. APP Pharmaceuticals, LLC. Methotrexate sodium injection prescribing information. Schaumburg, IL; 2012 Apr.

2967. Mylan Institutional LLC. Methotrexate sodium injection prescribing information. Rockford, IL; 2013 Dec.

2968. Fresenius Kabi USA, LLC. Methotrexate sodium for injection prescribing information. Lake Zurich, IL; 2013 Nov.

2969. Antares Pharma, Inc. Otrexup® (methotrexate) injection for subcutaneous use prescribing information. Ewing, NJ; 2014 Nov.

2970. Medac Pharma Inc. Rasuvo® (methotrexate) injection for subcutaneous use prescribing information. Chicago, IL; 2014 Jul.

2971. Almagambetova E, Hutchinson D, Blais DM et al. Stability of diluted adenosine solutions in polyolefin infusion bags. *Hosp Pharm*. 2013; 48:484–8.

2972. Walker SE, Charbonneau LF, Law S. Stability of Bortezomib 2.5 mg/mL in Vials and Syringes Stored at 4°C and Room Temperature (23°C). *Can J Hosp Pharm*. 2014; 67:102–7.

2973. Merck & Co., Inc. Invanz® (ertapenem) for injection prescribing information. Whitehouse Station, NJ; 2014 Sep.

2974. Jain JG, Sutherland C, Nicolau DP et al. Stability of ertapenem 100 mg/mL in polypropylene syringes stored at 25, 4, and -20°C. *Am J Health Syst Pharm*. 2014; 71:1480–4.

2975. Dutta S (Medical Information, Merck, North Wales, PA): Personal communication; 2015 Feb 6.

2976. McCluskey SV, Vu N, Rueter J. Stability of nitroglycerin 110 mcg/mL stored in polypropylene syringes. *Int J Pharm Compd*. 2013 Nov-Dec; 17:515–9.

2977. Merck & Co., Inc. Cubicin® (daptomycin) for injection prescribing information. Whitehouse Station, NJ; 2017 Mar.

2978. Ortega R, Salmerón-García A, Cabeza J et al. Stability of daptomycin 5 mg/mL and heparin sodium 100 units/mL combined in lactated Ringer's injection and stored in polypropylene syringes at 4 and −20°C. *Am J Health Syst Pharm*. 2014; 71:956–9.

2979. Parra MA, Campanero MA, Sádaba B et al. Effect of glucose concentration on the stability of daptomycin in peritoneal solutions. *Perit Dial Int*. 2013 Jul-Aug; 33:458–61.

2980. Peyro Saint Paul L, Albessard F, Gaillard C et al. Daptomycin compatibility in peritoneal dialysis solutions. *Perit Dial Int*. 2011 Jul-Aug; 31:492–5.

2981. Hossain MA, Friciu M, Aubin S et al. Stability of penicillin G sodium diluted with 0.9% sodium chloride injection or 5% dextrose injection and stored in polyvinyl chloride bag containers and elastomeric pump containers. *Am J Health Syst Pharm*. 2014; 71:669–73.

2982. Otsuka America Pharmaceutical, Inc. Busulfex® (busulfan) injection prescribing information. Rockville, MD; 2018 Jan.

2983. Cueto-Sola M, Belda-Furió M, Borrell-García C et al. Incompatibility of undiluted busulfan injection with a needle-free valve. *Am J Health Syst Pharm*. 2014; 71:1436–7. Letter.

2984. Patel RP, Li K, Shastri M et al. Stability of ampicillin and amoxicillin in peritoneal dialysis solutions. *Am J Health Syst Pharm*. 2015; 72:13–4. Letter.

2985. Woodcock J. Food and Drug Administration. FDA Letter re: Docket nos. FDA-2005-P-0003, FDA-2006-P-0019, FDA-2006-P-0331, and FDA-2006-P-0391: Determine that the discontinued formulation Zosyn (piperacillin and tazobactam for injection), was not discontinued for safety and efficacy reasons. Rockville, MD; US Food and Drug Administration. From regulations.gov website (www.regulations.gov/#!documentDetail;D=FDA-2012-P-0507-0001). Accessed 2015 Feb 26.

2986. Donnelly RF. Stability of cefazolin sodium in polypropylene syringes and polyvinylchloride minibags. *Can J Hosp Pharm*. 2011; 64:241–5.

2987. McCluskey SV, Sztajnkrycer MD, Jenkins DA et al. Stability of tranexamic acid in 0.9% sodium chloride, stored in type 1 glass vials and ethylene/propylene copolymer plastic containers. *Int J Pharm Compd*. 2014 Sep-Oct; 18:432–7.

2988. de Guzman R, Polykratis IA, Sondeen JL et al. Stability of tranexamic acid after 12-week storage at temperatures from -20°c to 50°c. *Prehosp Emerg Care*. 2013 Jul-Sep; 17:394–400.

2989. Kaltenbach M, Hutchinson DJ, Bollinger JE et al. Stability of diluted adenosine solutions in polyvinyl chloride infusion bags. *Am J Health Syst Pharm*. 2011; 68:1533–6.

2990. Hutchinson D. (Associate Professor, Wegmans School of Pharmacy at St. John Fisher College, Rochester, NY): Personal communication; 2015 Mar 8.

2991. Astellas Pharma US, Inc. Adenocard® IV (adenosine) injection for rapid bolus intravenous use prescribing information. Northbrook, IL; 2012 May.

2992. Astellas Pharma US, Inc. Adenoscan® (adenosine) injection for intravenous use prescribing information. Northbrook, IL; 2014 Aug.

2993. Fresenius Kabi USA, LLC. Adenosine injection for rapid bolus intravenous use prescribing information. Schaumburg, IL; 2013 Jan.

2994. Teva Pharmaceuticals USA, Inc. Treanda® (bendamustine hydrochloride) injection and for injection prescribing information. North Wales, PA; 2018 Nov.

2995. Food and Drug Administration. Treanda (bendamustine hydrochloride) solution by Teva: FDA statement - not compatible with closed system transfer devices, adapters, and syringes containing polycarbonate or acrylonitrile-butadiene-styrene. 2015 Mar 10. From FDA website. Accessed 2015 Mar 12.

2996. (US Medical Information, Teva Pharmaceuticals, North Wales, PA): Personal communication; 2015 Mar 12.

2997. Hurtukova D. Dear healthcare provider letter regarding important safety and incompatibility information for Treanda® (bedamustine HCl) injection (45 mg/0.5 mL or 180 mg/2 mL solution). North Wales, PA: Teva Pharmaceuticals USA; 2015 Mar 9. From the FDA website. Accessed 2015 Mar 12.

2998. Merck Sharp & Dohme Corp. Emend® (fosaprepitant dimeglumine) for injection prescribing information. Whitehouse Station, NJ; 2014 Oct.

2999. Sun S, Schaller J, Placek J et al. Compatibility of intravenous fosaprepitant with intravenous 5-HT3 antagonists and corticosteroids. *Cancer Chemother Pharmacol*. 2013; 72:509–13.

3000. Par Pharmaceutical Companies, Inc. Vasostrict® (vasopressin) injection prescribing information. Spring Valley, NY; 2015 Mar.

3001. Musaji N (Medical Affairs, Par Pharmaceutical, Inc., Parsippany, NJ): Personal communication; 2015.

3002. American Regent, Inc. Vasopressin injection prescribing information. Shirley, NY; 2011 May.

3003. Certo J (Medical Information, Recordati Rare Diseases, Lebanon, NJ): Personal communication; 2015 Jun 3.

3004. Allergan USA, Inc. Avycaz® (ceftazidime and avibactam sodium) for injection prescribing information. Madison, NJ; 2019 Mar.

3005. Guan J (Medical Information, Actavis, Parsippany, NJ): Personal communication; 2015 Jun 12.

3006. Astellas Pharma US, Inc. Cresemba® (isavuconazonium sulfate) capsules and for injection prescribing information. Northbrook, IL; 2015 Jun.

3007. Sanofi-Aventis U.S. LLC. Ferrlecit® (sodium ferric gluconate complex in sucrose injection) prescribing information. Bridgewater, NJ; Apr 2015.

3008. Baribeault D. Short-term stability of a new generic sodium ferric gluconate in complex with sucrose. *Curr Med Res Opin*. 2011; 27:2241–3.

3009. American Regent, Inc. Methyldopate hydrochloride injection prescribing information. Shirley, NY; 2005 Nov.

3010. American Regent, Inc. Torsemide injection prescribing information. Shirley, NY; 2014 Feb.

3011. Heritage Pharmaceuticals, Inc. Acetazolamide sodium injection prescribing information. Eatontown, NJ; 2014 Dec.

3012. Sanofi-Aventis U.S. LLC. Taxotere® (docetaxel) injection concentration prescribing information. Bridgewater, NJ; 2014 Nov.

3013. Hospira, Inc. Docetaxel injection prescribing information. Lake Forest, IL; 2014 Jul.

3014. Accord Healthcare, Inc. Docetaxel injection prescribing information. Durham, NC; 2014 Jul.

3015. Sun Pharmaceutical Industries, Inc. Docefrez® (docetaxel) for injection prescribing information. Cranbury, NJ; 2014 Nov.

3016. Pfizer Injectables. Docetaxel injection prescribing information. New York, NY; 2014 Nov.

3017. Sandoz. Docetaxel injection solution prescribing information. Princeton, NJ; 2014 Nov.

3018. Actavis Inc. Docetaxel injection concentrate prescribing information. Morristown, NJ; 2014 Sep.

3019. Food and Drug Administration. Drug safety communication: FDA warns that cancer drug docetaxel may cause symptoms of alcohol intoxication after treatment. Rockville, MD; 2014 Jun 20. From FDA website. Accessed 2015 Jul 16.

3020. Parker EA. Letter: Oxidation of methyldopate hydrochloride in alkaline media. *Am J Hosp Pharm*. 1975; 32:244.

3021. Colby LH (Programming Services, Merck, West Point, PA): Personal communication; 1968 Dec 16.

3022. Hospira, Inc. Foscavir® (foscarnet sodium) injection prescribing information. Lake Forest, IL; 2014 Nov.

3023. The Medicines Company. Kengreal® (cangrelor) for injection prescribing information. Parsippany, NJ; 2015 Jun.

3024. Talon Therapeutics, Inc. Marqibo® (vincristine sulfate liposome injection) prescribing information. South San Francisco, CA; 2012 Oct.

3025. Mirza A, Mithal N. Alcohol intoxication with the new formulation of docetaxel. *Clin Oncol (R Coll Radiol)*. 2011; 23:560–1. Letter.

3026. Parker EA. Letter: Correction in stability data for isuprel hydrochloride admixtures. *Am J Hosp Pharm*. 1976; 33:528.

3027. Eisai Inc. Halaven® (eribulin mesylate) injection prescribing information. Woodcliff Lake, NJ; 2015 Oct.

3028. Spindeldreier K, Thiesen J, Lipp HP et al. Physico-chemical stability of eribulin mesylate containing concentrate and ready-to-administer solutions. *J Oncol Pharm Pract*. 2014; 20:183–9.

3029. Institute for Safe Medication Practices. Loss of drug potency. ISMP Medication Safety Alert! Acute Care edition. Horsham, PA; 2015 Jul. From ISMP website. Accessed 2015 Sep 14.

3030. X-GEN Pharmaceuticals, Inc. Acetazolamide for injection prescribing information. Big Flats NY; 2013 Mar.

3031. West-Ward Pharmaceuticals. Ativan® (lorazepam) injection prescribing information. Eatontown, NJ; 2011 Jun.

3032. Abelgas M (Medical Communications, Hospira, Lake Forest, IL): Personal communication; 2014 Sep 9.

3033. Hospira, Inc. Lorazepam injection prescribing information. Lake Forest, IL; 2008 Dec.

3034. Barr J, Fraser GL, Puntillo K et al. Clinical practice guidelines for the management of pain, agitation, and delirium in adult patients in the intensive care unit. *Crit Care Med*. 2013; 41:263–306.

3035. Janssen Biotech, Inc. Remicade® (infliximab) lyophilized concentrate for injection prescribing information. Horsham, PA; 2015 Nov.

3036. Thompson CA. Stability findings raise issue of syringes as storage containers. ASHP Pharmacy News. Bethesda, MD; 2015 Jul. From ASHP website. Accessed 2015 Sep 14.

3037. Noe B. BD Medical. July 31, 2015 letter to US syringe customers. Franklin Lakes, NJ; 2015 July. From BD website. Accessed 2015 Sep 14.

3038. BD Medical. Technical update to July 31, 2015 letter to US syringe customers. Franklin Lakes. 2015 Jul. From BD website. Accessed 2015 Sep 14.

3039. US Food and Drug Administration. FDA alert: Compounded or repackaged drugs stored in Becton-Dickinson (BD) 3 mL and 5 mL syringes: FDA alert - do not use unless there is no suitable alternative. 2015 Aug 18. From FDA website. Accessed 2015 Sep 14.

3040. Institute for Safe Medication Practices. ISMP comments on BD syringe potency issues. ISMP Medication Safety Alert! Acute Care edition. Horsham, PA; 2015 Aug. From ISMP website. Accessed 2015 Sep 14.

3041. Wesolowski A. BD Medical. September 1, 2015 letter to US syringe customers. Franklin Lakes, NJ; 2015 July. From BD website. Accessed 2015 Sep 14.

3042. Noe BE (BD Medical, Franklin Lakes, NJ): Personal communication; 2015 Sep 3.

3043. US Food and Drug Administration. FDA alert: FDA expands warning on Becton-Dickinson (BD) syringes being used to store compounded or repackaged drugs. 2015 Sep 8. From FDA website. Accessed 2015 Sep 14.

3044. US Food and Drug Administration. FDA warns against using Treanda injection (solution) with closed system transfer devices, adapters, and syringes containing polycarbonate or acrylonitrile-butadiene-styrene; provides list of compatible devices. 2015 Sep 4. From FDA website. Accessed 2015 Sep 16.

3045. Hurtukova D. Dear healthcare provider letter regarding update: important safety and compatibility information for Treanda® (bendamustine HCl) injection (45 mg/0.5 mL

3046. or 180 mg/2 mL solution). North Wales, PA: Teva Pharmaceuticals USA; 2015 Sep 2. From the FDA website. Accessed 2015 Sep 15.

3046. Tyree D (Medical Information, Otsuka): Personal communication; 2015 Sep.

3047. Food and Drug Administration. Center for Drug Evaluation and Research. Application number: NDA 20–954: Pharmacology review(s). From FDA website.

3048. Merck & Co., Inc. Integrilin® (eptifibatide) injection prescribing information. Whitehouse Station, NJ; 2014 Apr.

3049. Wieland K (Global Medical Information, Merck, North Wales, PA): Personal communication; 2015 Oct 8.

3050. B. Braun Medical Inc. Hespan® (6% hetastarch in 0.9% sodium chloride injection) prescribing information. Bethlehem, PA; 2013 Dec.

3051. West-Ward Pharmaceuticals. Phenylephrine hydrochloride injection prescribing information. Eatontown, NJ; 2012 Dec.

3052. Éclat Pharmaceuticals. Vazculep® (phenylephrine hydrochloride) injection prescribing information. Chesterfield, MO; 2014 Jul.

3053. Biotest Pharmaceuticals Corporation. Bivigam® (immune globulin intravenous [human], 10% liquid) prescribing information. Boca Raton, FL; 2013 Oct.

3054. CSL Behring LLC. Carimune® NF, Nanofiltered (immune globulin intravenous [human], lyophilized) prescribing information. Kankakee, IL; 2013 Sep.

3055. Grifols Biologicals Inc. Flebogamma® 5% DIF (immune globulin intravenous [human], 5% liquid) prescribing information. Los Angeles, CA; 2015 Apr.

3056. Grifols Biologicals Inc. Flebogamma® 10% DIF (immune globulin intravenous [human], 10% liquid) prescribing information. Los Angeles, CA; 2015 Mar.

3057. Grifols Therapeutics Inc. GamaSTAN® S/D (immune globulin [human]) prescribing information. Research Triangle Park, NC; 2013 Sep.

3058. Baxter Healthcare Corporation. Gammagard® S/D (immune globulin intravenous [human], IgA less than 1 microgram per mL in a 5% solution) prescribing information. Westlake Village, CA; 2014 Apr.

3059. Baxter Healthcare Corporation. Gammagard Liquid® (immune globulin infusion [human], 10%) prescribing information. Westlake Village, CA; 2014 Apr.

3060. Kedrion Biopharma, Inc. Gammaked® (immune globulin injection [human], 10%) prescribing information. Fort Lee, NJ; 2013 Sep.

3061. BPL Inc. Gammaplex® (immune globulin intravenous [human], 5% liquid) prescribing information. Raleigh, NC; 2015 July.

3062. Grifols Therapeutics Inc. Gammunex®-C (immune globulin injection [human], 10%) prescribing information. Research Triangle Park, NC; 2014 Jul.

3063. CSL Behring LLC. Hizentra® (immune globulin subcutaneous [human], 20% liquid) prescribing information. Kankakee, IL; 2015 Jan.

3064. Baxter Healthcare Corporation. HyQvia® (immune globulin infusion [human] 10% with recombinant human hyaluronidase) prescribing information. Westlake Village, CA; 2014 Sep.

3065. Octapharma USA Inc. Octagam® (immune globulin intravenous [human] 5%) prescribing information. Hoboken, NJ; 2013 Sep.

3066. Octapharma USA Inc. Octagam®10% (immune globulin intravenous [human]) prescribing information. Hoboken, NJ; 2014 Dec.

3067. CSL Behring LLC. Privigen® (immune globulin intravenous [human], 10% liquid) prescribing information. Kankakee, IL; 2013 Nov.

3068. Astellas Pharma US, Inc. AmBisome® (amphotericin B) liposome for injection prescribing information. Northbrook, IL; 2012 May.

3069. Pauner A (Medical Affairs, Astellas, Northbrook, IL): Personal communication; 2015 Oct 23.

3070. APP Pharmaceuticals, LLC. Floxuridine for injection prescribing information. Schaumburg, IL; 2008 Jan.

3071. APP Fresenius Kabi USA, LLC. Doxy® 100 & 200 (doxycycline) for injection prescribing information. Lake Zurich, IL; 2013 Sep.(

3072. Sigma-Tau Pharmaceuticals, Inc. Abelcet® (amphotericin B lipid complex) injection prescribing information. Gaithersburg, MD; 2013 Mar.

3073. Manley HJ, Grabe DW, Norcross M et al. Stability of amphotericin B-lipid complex (Abelcet) in peritoneal dialysis solutions. Perit Dial Int. 2000 Jan-Feb; 20:87–90.

3074. Hamil K (Medical Information, Sigma-Tau, Gaithersburg, IL): Personal communication; 2015 Nov 2.

3075. Stein MR. The new generation of liquid intravenous immunoglobulin formulations in patient care: a comparison of intravenous immunoglobulins. Postgrad Med. 2010; 122:176–84.

3076. Bolli R, Woodtli K, Bärtschi M et al. L-Proline reduces IgG dimer content and enhances the stability of intravenous immunoglobulin (IVIG) solutions. Biologicals. 2010; 38:150–7.

3077. Janssen Scientific Affairs. JanssenMD® Professional Information Resource: Storage and Stability of Unreconstituted Remicade®. From Janssen website. Accessed 2015 Nov 16.

3078. Janssen Scientific Affairs. JanssenMD® Professional Information Resource: Stability of Reconstituted Remicade® vials. From Janssen website. Accessed 2015 Nov 16.

3079. Janssen Scientific Affairs. JanssenMD® Professional Information Resource: Stability of Remicade® Prepared Infusions. From Janssen website. Accessed 2015 Nov 16.

3080. Janssen Scientific Affairs. JanssenMD® Professional Information Resource: Stability of Remicade® in 0.45% Normal Saline. From Janssen website. Accessed 2015 Nov 16.

3081. Janssen Scientific Affairs. JanssenMD® Professional Information Resource: Removal of Non-PVC Equipment Requirement for Remicade®. From Janssen website. Accessed 2015 Nov 16.

3082. Ilett K (Emeritus Professor of Pharmacology, University of Western Australia, Perth, Australia): Personal communication; 2015 Nov 16.

3083. Genentech, Inc. Rituxan® (rituximab) injection prescribing information. South San Francisco, CA; 2016 Apr.

3084. Paul M, Vieillard V, Jaccoulet E et al. Long-term stability of diluted solutions of the monoclonal antibody rituximab. Int J Pharm. 2012; 436:282–90.

3085. Norkus D (Medical Communications, Genentech, South San Francisco, CA): Personal communication; 2015 Nov 20.

3086. Genentech, Inc. Herceptin® (trastuzumab) intravenous infusion prescribing information. South San Francisco, CA; 2016 Mar.

3087. Norkus D (Medical Communications, Genentech, South San Francisco, CA): Personal communication; 2015 Nov 20.

3088. Kaiser J, Krämer I. Physicochemical stability of diluted trastuzumab infusion solutions in polypropylene infusion bags. Int J Pharm Compd. 2011; 15:515–20.

3089. Pabari RM, Ryan B, Ahmad W et al. Physical and structural stability of the monoclonal antibody, trastuzumab (Herceptin®), intravenous solutions. Curr Pharm Biotechnol. 2013; 14:220–5.

3090. Glover ZW, Gennaro L, Yadav S et al. Compatibility and stability of pertuzumab and trastuzumab admixtures in i.v. infusion bags for coadministration. J Pharm Sci. 2013; 102:794–812.

3091. Genentech, Inc. Perjeta® (pertuzumab) injection prescribing information. South San Francisco, CA; 2016 Mar.

3092. Hope Pharmaceuticals. Sodium thiosulfate injection prescribing information. Scottsdale, AZ; 2012 Feb.

3093. Hope Pharmaceuticals. Nithiodote® (sodium nitrite injection and sodium thiosulfate injection) prescribing information. Scottsdale, AZ; 2011 Jan.

3094. Boehringer Ingelheim Pharmaceuticals, Inc. Praxbind® (idarucizumab) injection prescribing information. Ridgefield, CT; 2015 Oct.

3095. Amgen Inc. Blincyto® (blinatumomab) for injection prescribing information. Thousand Oaks, CA; 2017 Nov.

3096. Gu Z, Wong A, Raquinio E et al. Stability of reconstituted telavancin drug product in frozen intravenous bags. Hosp Pharm. 2015; 50:609–14.

3097. Gu Z, Parra C, Wong A et al. Post-reconstitution stability of telavancin with commonly used diluents and intravenous infusion solutions. Curr Ther Res. 2015; 77:105–10.

3098. Teva Pharmaceuticals USA, Inc. Bendeka® (bendamustine hydrochloride) injection prescribing information. North Wales, PA; 2018 Jul.

3099. Eagle Pharmaceuticals, Inc. Docetaxel injection prescribing information. Woodcliff Lake, NJ; 2015 Dec.

3100. Food and Drug Administration Center for Devices and Radiological Health. Safety assessment of di(2-ethylhexyl) phthalate (DEHP) released from PVC medical devices. 2001 Sep. From FDA website. Accessed 2015 Jul 30.

3101. National Toxicology Program, U.S. Department of Health and Human Services, Center for the Evaluation of Risks to Human Reproduction. NTP-CERHR Monograph on the Potential Human Reproductive and Developmental Effects of Di(2-Ethylhexyl) Phthalate (DEHP). NIH Publication No. 06–4476. 2006 Nov.

3102. AstraZeneca Pharmaceuticals LP. Merrem® I.V. (meropenem for injection) prescribing information. Wilmington, DE; 2015 Apr.

3103. B. Braun Medical Inc. Meropenem and sodium chloride injection prescribing information. Bethlehem, PA; 2015 Apr.

3104. Berthoin K, Le Duff CS, Marchand-Brynaert J et al. Stability of meropenem and doripenem solutions for administration by continuous infusion. *J Antimicrob Chemother*. 2010; 65:1073–5. Letter.

3105. Viaene E, Chanteux H, Servais H et al. Comparative stability studies of antipseudomonal beta-lactams for potential administration through portable elastomeric pumps (home therapy for cystic fibrosis patients) and motor-operated syringes (intensive care units). *Antimicrob Agents Chemother*. 2002; 46:2327–32.

3106. Manning L, Wright C, Ingram PR et al. Continuous infusions of meropenem in ambulatory care: clinical efficacy, safety and stability. *PLoS One*. 2014; 9:e102023.

3107. Chen LY, Chen J, Waters V et al. Incompatibility of ciprofloxacin and meropenem injections. *Am J Health Syst Pharm*. 2013; 70:1966, 1970. Letter.

3108. Tran MD, Sharley N, Ward M. Stability of amoxycillin, clindamycin and meropenem in peritoneal dialysis solution. *J Pharm Pract Res*. 2012; 42:218–22.

3109. Keel RA, Sutherland CA, Crandon JL et al. Stability of doripenem, imipenem and meropenem at elevated room temperatures. *Int J Antimicrob Agents*. 2011; 37:184–5.

3110. Park KH, Chung DJ. Stability study of docetaxel solution (0.9%, saline) using Non-PVC and PVC tubes for intravenous administration. *Biomater Res*. 2015; 19:2.

3111. Merck and Co., Inc. Bridion® (sugammadex) injection prescribing information. Whitehouse Station, NJ;2015 Dec.

3112. Hanci V, Kiraz HA, Ömür D et al. Precipitation in Gallipoli: sugammadex / amiodarone & sugammadex / dobutamine & sugammadex / protamine. *Braz J Anesthesiol*. 2013; 63:163–4. Letter.

3113. Alston TA. Precipitation of sugammadex by protamine. *J Clin Anesth*. 2011; 23:593. Letter.

3114. Raphael CD, Zhao F, Hughes SE et al. A Pilot Chemical and Physical Stability Study of Extemporaneously Compounded Levetiracetam Intravenous Solution. *J Pain Palliat Care Pharmacother*. 2015; 29:370–3.

3115. McCrory C (Medical Information, Merck, North Wales, PA): Personal communication; 2016 Feb 16.

3116. Par Pharmaceutical. Ketalar® (ketamine hydrochloride) injection prescribing information. Chestnut Ridge, NY; 2018 Jul.

3117. Hospira, Inc. Ketamine hydrochloride injection prescribing information. Lake Forest, IL; 2020 Apr.

3118. Donnelly RF. Stability of diluted ketamine packaged in glass vials. *Can J Hosp Pharm*. 2013; 66:198.

3119. Chen F, Xiong H, Yang J et al. Butorphanol and ketamine combined in infusion solutions for patient-controlled analgesia administration: a long-term stability study. *Med Sci Monit*. 2015; 21:1138–45.

3120. Chen FC, Xiong H, Liu HM et al. Compatibility of butorphanol with granisetron in 0.9% sodium chloride injection packaged in glass bottles or polyolefin bags. *Am J Health Syst Pharm*. 2015; 72:1374–8.

3121. Chen FC, Shi XY, Li P et al. Stability of butorphanol-tropisetron mixtures in 0.9% sodium chloride injection for patient-controlled analgesia use. *Medicine (Baltimore)*. 2015; 94:e432.

3122. Ikeda R, Vermeulen LC, Lau E et al. Stability of infliximab in polyvinyl chloride bags. *Am J Health Syst Pharm*. 2012; 69:1509–12.

3123. Teva Pharmaceuticals USA. Granisetron hydrochloride injection prescribing information. Sellersville, PA; 2014 Aug.

3124. Fresenius Kabi USA, LLC. Granisetron hydrochloride injection prescribing information. Lake Zurich, IL; 2015 Feb.

3125. Akorn, Inc. Granisetron hydrochloride injection prescribing information. Lake Forest, IL; 2015 Sep.

3126. Cipla USA, Inc. Granisetron hydrochloride injection prescribing information. Miami, FL; 2015 Jul.

3127. Astellas Pharma US, Inc. Prograf® (tacrolimus) capsules and injection prescribing information. Northbrook, IL; 2015 May.

3128. Lee JH, Goldspiel BR, Ryu S et al. Stability of tacrolimus solutions in polyolefin containers. *Am J Health Syst Pharm*. 2016; 73:137–42.

3129. Goldspiel BR (Corresponding Author): Personal communication; 2016 Feb 21.

3130. Mylan Institutional LLC. Fomepizole injection prescribing information. Rockford, IL; 2012 Sep.

3131. Paladin Labs (USA) Inc. Antizol® (fomepizole) injection prescribing information. Dover, DE; 2009 Apr.

3132. Oak Pharmaceuticals, Inc. Sodium Diuril® (chlorothiazide sodium) injection prescribing information. Whitehouse Station, NJ; 2012 May.

3133. Fresenius Kabi USA, LLC. Chlorothiazide sodium injection prescribing information. Schaumburg, IL; 2013 Feb.

3134. McCluskey SV, Gardner B, Graner KK et al. Stability of chlorothiazide sodium in polypropylene syringes. *Am J Health Syst Pharm*. 2015; 72:1292–7.

3135. Sanofi-Aventis U.S. LLC. Elitek (rasburicase) powder for solution for intravenous infusion prescribing information. Bridgewater, NJ; 2015 Mar.

3136. Genentech USA, Inc. Boniva® (ibandronate) injection prescribing information. South San Francisco, CA; 2015 Apr.

3137. Heritage Pharmaceuticals Inc. Ibandronate sodium injection prescribing information. Eatontown, NJ; 2015 Oct.

3138. Bhattacharya S, Parekh S, Dedhiya M. In-use stability of ceftaroline fosamil in elastomeric home infusion systems and MINI-BAG Plus containers. *Int J Pharm Compd*. 2015 Sep-Oct; 19:432–6.

3139. Novartis Pharmaceuticals Corporation. Reclast® (zoledronic acid) injection prescribing information. East Hanover, NJ; 2015 Apr.

3140. Novartis Pharmaceuticals Corporation. Zometa® (zoledronic acid) injection prescribing information. East Hanover, NJ; 2015 Jun.

3141. Caraco Pharmaceutical Laboratories, Ltd. Zoledronic acid for injection prescribing information. Detroit, MI; 2012 Nov.

3142. Sagent Pharmaceuticals. Zoledronic acid injection prescribing information. Schaumburg, IL; 2015 Oct.

3143. Hospira, Inc. Zoledronic acid injection prescribing information. Lake Forest, IL; 2015 Dec.

3144. Sagent Pharmaceuticals. Zoledronic acid injection prescribing information. Schaumburg, IL; 2015 Sep.

3145. Merck & Co., Inc. Temodar® (temozolomide) capsules and for injection prescribing information. Whitehouse Station, NJ; 2015 Sep.

3146. UCB, Inc. Briviact® (brivaracetam) tablets, oral solution, and injection prescribing information. Smyrna, GA; 2016 Feb.

3147. Merrimack Pharmaceuticals, Inc. Onivyde® (irinotecan liposome injection) prescribing information. Cambridge, MA; 2015 Oct.

3148. Jazz Pharmaceuticals, Inc. Defitelio® (defibrotide sodium) injection prescribing information. Palo Alto, CA; 2016 Mar.

3149. Correard F, Savry A, Gauthier-Villano L et al. Visual compatibility of defibrotide with selected drugs during simulated Y-site administration. *Am J Health Syst Pharm.* 2014; 71:1288–91.

3150. JHP Pharmaceuticals, LLC. Coly-Mycin® M Parenteral (colistimethate for injection) prescribing information. Rochester, MI; 2013 Jan.

3151. Perrigo. Colistimethate for injection prescribing information. Minneapolis, MN; 2013 Sep.

3152. Abdulla A, van Leeuwen RW, de Vries Schultink AH et al. Stability of colistimethate sodium in a disposable elastomeric infusion device. *Int J Pharm.* 2015; 486:367–9.

3153. National Alert Network (NAN). Warning! Dosing confusion with colistimethate for injection. 2011 Jun 29. NAN Alert. Accessed 2016 Apr 12.

3154. Healan AM, Gray W, Fuchs EJ et al. Stability of colistimethate sodium in aqueous solution. *Antimicrob Agents Chemother.* 2012; 56:6432–3.

3155. Wallace SJ, Li J, Rayner CR et al. Stability of colistin methanesulfonate in pharmaceutical products and solutions for administration to patients. *Antimicrob Agents Chemother.* 2008; 52:3047–51.

3156. American Regent. Provayblue® (methylene blue) injection prescribing information. Shirley, NY; 2016 Apr.

3157. Foushee JA, Fox LM, Gormley LR et al. Physical compatibility of cisatracurium with selected drugs during simulated Y-site administration. *Am J Health Syst Pharm.* 2015; 72:483–6.

3158. Akorn, Inc. Methylene blue injection prescribing information. Lake Forest, IL; 2011 Jun.

3159. Par Pharmaceutical Companies, Inc. Dantrium® Intravenous (dantrolene sodium) for injection prescribing information. Spring Valley, NY; 2015 Feb.

3160. US WorldMeds, LLC. Revonto® (dantrolene sodium) for injection prescribing information. Louisville, KY; 2014 Jul.

3161. Eagle Pharmaceuticals, Inc. Ryanodex® (dantrolene sodium) for injectable suspension prescribing information. Woodcliff Lake, NJ; 2014 Jul.

3162. Bedford Laboratories. Polymyxin B for injection prescribing information. Bedford, OH; 2011 Jun.

3163. X-GEN Pharmaceuticals, Inc. Polymyxin B for injection prescribing information. Big Flats, NY; 2015 May.

3164. Pharmacia & Upjohn Company. Lincocin® (lincomycin hydrochloride) injection prescribing information. New York, NY; 2014 Oct.

3165. X-GEN Pharmaceuticals. Lincomycin injection prescribing information. Big Flats, NY; 2015 Apr.

3166. Czarniak P, Boddy M, Sunderland B et al. Stability studies of lincomycin hydrochloride in aqueous solution and intravenous infusion fluids. *Drug Des Devel Ther.* 2016; 10:1029–34.

3167. Jazz Pharmaceuticals, Inc. Prialt® (ziconotide) solution for intrathecal infusion prescribing information. Palo Alto, CA; 2013 Feb.

3168. Bazin C, Poirier AL, Dupoiron D. Influence of pH and temperature on ziconotide stability in intrathecal analgesic admixtures in implantable pumps and syringes. *Int J Pharm.* 2015; 487:285–91.

3169. Medtronic. Medical device safety notification: increased risk of motor stall and loss of or change in therapy with unapproved drug formulations. From Medtronic for healthcare professionals website. professional.medtronic.com. 2012 Nov.

3170. Dupoiron D, Richard H, Chabert-Desnot V et al. In vitro stability of low-concentration ziconotide alone or in admixtures in intrathecal pumps. *Neuromodulation.* 2014; 17:472–82; discussion 482.

3171. Singh R, Chen J, Miller T et al. Solution stability of Captisol-stability melphalan (Evomela) versus Propyelene glycol-based melphalan hydrochloride injection. *Pharm De Technol.* 2016; :1–6.

3172. Spectrum Pharmaceuticals, Inc. Evomela® (melphalan) for injection prescribing information. Irvine, CA; 2017 Sep.

3173. Mylan Institutional LLC. Melphalan hydrochloride for injection prescribing information. Rockford, IL; 2016 Feb.

3174. Desmaris RP, Mercier L, Paci A. Stability of Melphalan in 0.9% Sodium Chloride Solutions Prepared in Polyvinyl Chloride Bags for Intravenous Injection. *Drugs R D.* 2015; 15:253–9.

3175. Merck & Co., Inc. Avelox® (moxifloxacin hydrochloride) tablets and injection prescribing information. Whitehouse Station, NJ; 2015 May.

3176. Fresenius Kabi USA, LLC. Moxifloxacin hydrochloride injection prescribing information. Lake Zurich, IL; 2015 Jun.

3177. Janssen Products, LP. Yondelis® (trabectedin) for injection prescribing information. Horsham, PA; 2015 Oct.

3178. Payne B (Medical Information, Janssen, Titusville, NJ): Personal communication; 2016 May 3.

3179. HQ Speciality Pharma Corporation. Dexmedetomidine hydrochloride injection prescribing information. Paramus, NJ; 2015 Jul.

3180. Fresenius Kabi. Dexmedetomidine hydrochloride injection prescribing information. Lake Zurich, IL; 2015 Nov.

3181. Hospira, Inc. Precedex® (dexmedetomidine hydrochloride) injection prescribing information. Lake Forest, IL; 2008 Oct.

3182. CSL Behring LLC. Kcentra® (prothrombin complex concentrate [human]) prescribing information. Kankakee, IL; 2014 Sep.

3183. Pharmacia & Upjohn Co. Zyvox® (linezolid) injection, tablets and oral suspension prescribing information. New York, NY; 2015 Jul.

3184. Hospira, Inc. Linezolid injection solution prescribing information. Lake Forest, IL; 2015 Jun.

3186. GlaxoSmithKline. Argatroban injection prescribing information. Research Triangle Park, NC; 2016 May.

3187. The Medicines Company. Argatroban injection prescribing information. Parsippany, NJ; 2016 May.

3188. Sandoz Inc. Argatroban injection in 0.9% sodium chloride prescribing information. Princeton, NJ; 2016 May.

3189. Teva Pharmaceuticals USA, Inc. Argatroban injection in 0.9% sodium chloride prescribing information. New Wales, PA; 2016 May.

3190. Fresenius Kabi. Argatroban injection prescribing information. Lake Zurich, IL; 2016 May.

3191. West-Ward Pharmaceuticals. Argatroban injection prescribing information. Eatontown, NJ; 2016 May.

3192. Jakimczuk PJ, Churchwell MD, Howard MS et al. Compatibility of argatroban injection with select antiarrhythmic drugs. *Am J Health Syst Pharm*. 2014; 71:1831–2. Letter.

3193. Pharmacia & Upjohn Company. Corvert® (ibutilide fumarate) injection prescribing information. New York, NY; 2006 Feb.

3194. Huvelle S, Godet M, Hecq JD et al. Long-term stability of ketamine hydrochloride 50mg/ml injection in 3ml syringes. *Ann Pharm Fr*. 2016; 74:283–7.

3195. Robiyanto R, Zaidi ST, Shastri MD et al. Stability of Tigecycline in Different Types of Peritoneal Dialysis Solutions. *Perit Dial Int*. 2016 Jul-Aug; 36:410–4.

3196. Spectrum Pharmaceuticals, Inc. Fusilev® (levoleucovorin) for injection and injection prescribing information. Irvine, CA; 2011 Apr.

3197. Sandoz Inc. Levoleucovorin injection prescribing information. Princeton, NJ; 2016 Sep.

3198. Randhawa A, Shah A, Day C. Compatibility of daptomycin with commercially available syringe filters. *Hosp Pharm*. 2015; 50:7–8.

3199. Day C (Corresponding Author): Personal communication; 2016 Jun 20.

3200. The Medicines Company. Cleviprex® (clevidipine) injectable emulsion prescribing information. Parsippany, NJ; 2013 Nov.

3201. UCB, Inc. Vimpat® (lacosamide) tablet, injection, and oral solution prescribing information. Smyrna, GA; 2015 Jun.

3202. Pharmacia and Upjohn Company. Camptosar® (irinotecan hydrochloride) injection prescribing information. New York, NY; 2016 Apr.

3203. Hospira, Inc. Irinotecan hydrochloride injection prescribing information. Lake Forest, IL; 2015 Nov.

3204. Actavis Pharma, Inc. Irinotecan hydrochloride injection prescribing information. Parsippany, NJ; 2014 Jun.

3205. Wyeth Pharmaceuticals Inc. Torisel® kit (temsirolimus) injection prescribing information. Philadelphia, PA; 2016 Jul.

3206. Alvogen, Inc. Midazolam injection prescribing information. Pine Brook, NJ; 2017 Jun.

3207. Manning MC, Chou DK, Murphy BM et al. Stability of protein pharmaceuticals: an update. *Pharm Res*. 2010; 27:544–75.

3208. Bardin C, Astier A, Vulto A et al. Guidelines for the practical stability studies of anticancer drugs: a European consensus conference. *Ann Pharm Fr*. 2011; 69:221–31.

3209. Sreedhara A, Glover ZK, Piros N et al. Stability of IgG1 monoclonal antibodies in intravenous infusion bags under clinical in-use conditions. *J Pharm Sci*. 2012; 101:21–30.

3210. Kolesar JM, Vermeulen L. Assays for biological agents. *Am J Health Syst Pharm*. 2013; 70:1101. Letter.

3211. Vigneron J, Astier A, Trittler R et al. SFPO and ESOP recommendations for the practical stability of anticancer drugs: an update. *Ann Pharm Fr*. 2013; 71:376–89.

3212. Ricci MS, Frazier M, Moore J et al. In-use physicochemical and microbiological stability of biological parenteral products. *Am J Health Syst Pharm*. 2015; 72:396–407.

3213. Sanofi-Aventis U.S. LLC. Clolar® (clofarabine) injection prescribing information. Bridgewater, NJ; 2015 Dec.

3214. Poujol S, Bressolle F, Solassol I et al. Stability of ready-to-use temsirolimus infusion solution (100mg/L) in polypropylene containers under different storage conditions. *Ann Pharm Fr*. 2012; 70:155–62.

3215. Genzyme Europe B.V. Evoltra® (clofarabine) concentrate. Annex I: Summary of product characteristics. Naarden, Netherlands. 2016 Apr.

3216. Kaiser J, Krämer I. Long-term stability study of clofarabine injection concentrate and diluted clofarabine infusion solutions. *J Oncol Pharm Pract*. 2012; 18:213–21.

3217. Sigma-Tau Pharmaceuticals, Inc. Carnitor® (levocarnitine) injection prescribing information. Gaithersburg, MD; 2015 Apr.

3218. American Regent, Inc. Levocarnitine injection prescribing information. Shirley, NY; 2016 Apr.

3219. Celgene Corporation. Abraxane® (paclitaxel protein-bound particles) for injectable suspension (albumin-bound) prescribing information. Summit, NJ; 2015 Jul.

3220. West-Ward Pharmaceuticals. Dopram® (doxapram hydrochloride) injection prescribing information. Eatontown, NJ; 2011 Nov.

3221. Merck & Co., Inc. Cubicin® RF (daptomycin) for injection prescribing information. Whitehouse Station, NJ; 2017 Mar.

3222. Fresenius Kabi. Daptomycin for injection prescribing information. Lake Zurich, IL; 2016 Jun.

3223. Hospira, Inc. Sodium bicarbonate injection prescribing information. Lake Forest, IL; 2005 Oct.

3224. Fresenius Kabi USA, LLC. Sodium bicarbonate injection prescribing information. Lake Zurich, IL; 2013 Aug.

3225. Hospira, Inc. Neut® (sodium bicarbonate) injection prescribing information. Lake Forest, IL; 2013 Feb.

3226. The Medicines Company. Minocin® (minocycline) for injection prescribing information. Parsippany, NJ; 2015 Apr.

3227. Mylan Institutional LLC. Enlon® (edrophonium chloride) injection prescribing information. Rockford, IL; 2013 Jan.

3228. Pascuzzi RM. The edrophonium test. *Semin Neurol*. 2003; 23:83–8.

3229. Pfizer Inc. Synercid® (quinupristin and dalfopristin) injection prescribing information. New York, NY; 2016 Aug.

3230. Rubinstein E, Prokocimer P, Talbot GH. Safety and tolerability of quinupristin/dalfopristin: administration guidelines. *J Antimicrob Chemother*. 1999; 44 Suppl A:37–46.

3231. Healan A (Corresponding Author): Personal communication; 2016 Sep 20.

3232. Talwar S (Global Health Science, The Medicines Company, Parsippany, NJ): Personal communication; 2016 Sep 19.

3233. Pfizer Inc. Vfend® (voriconazole) tablets, for oral suspension, and for injection prescribing information. New York, NY; 2017 Aug.

3234. Fresenius Kabi. Esmolol hydrochloride injection prescribing information. Lake Zurich, IL; 2016 Feb.

3235. WG Critical Care, LLC. Esmolol hydrochloride in water for injection prescribing information. Paramus, NJ; 2016 Apr.

3236. Chiesi USA, Inc. Cleviprex® (clevidipine butyrate) injectable emulsion safety data sheet. Cary, NC; 2016 Jun 17.

3237. Medicis. Calcium Disodium Versenate® (edetate calcium disodium) injection prescribing information. Scottsdale, AZ; 2012 Oct.

3238. Howland MA. Antidotes in depth: edetate calcium disodium (CaNa$_2$EDTA). In: Hoffman RS, Howland MA, Lewin NA et al, eds. Goldfrank's Toxicologic Emergencies. 10th ed. New York: McGraw-Hill; 2014:1241–4.

3239. (Medical Information, Sigma Tau Pharmaceuticals): Personal communication; 2016 Oct 6.

3240. Baxalta US Inc. Cuvitru® (immune globulin subcutaneous [human], 20% solution) prescribing information. Westlake Village, CA; 2016 Sep.

3241. Hospira, Inc. Corlopam® (fenoldopam mesylate) injection prescribing information. Lake Forest, IL; 2015 Dec.

3242. Hart M, Acott S. Physical and chemical stability of Taxotere (docetaxel) one-vial (20 mg/mL) infusion solution following refrigerated storage. Ecancermedicalscience. 2010; 4:202.

3243. Lee S (Medical Information, Chiesi, Cary, NC): Personal communication; 2016 Sep 30.

3244. Ghazi I, Hamada Y, Nicolau DP. Physical compatibility of tedizolid phosphate with selected i.v. drugs during simulated Y-site administration. Am J Health Syst Pharm. 2016; 73:1769–1776.

3245. Sullivan T, Forest JM, Leclair G. Compatibility of cloxacillin sodium with selected intravenous drugs during simulated Y-Site administration. Hosp Pharm. 2015; 50:214–20.

3246. Chan A, Tawfik G, Cheng W. Physical incompatibility between parenteral cloxacillin and vancomycin. Can J Hosp Pharm. 2013; 66:310–2.

3247. Nicolau DP (Corresponding Author): Personal communication; 2016 Oct 28.

3248. SteriMax Inc. Cloxacillin for injection prescribing information. Oakville, Ontario; 2016 Feb.

3249. Hospira, Inc. Enalaprilat injection prescribing information. Lake Forest, IL; 2010 Mar.

3250. Fresenius Kabi. Midazolam injection pharmacy bulk package prescribing information. Lake Zurich, IL; 2017 Jun.

3251. Baxter Healthcare Corporation. Intralipid® 20% (lipid injectable emulsion) prescribing information. Deerfield, IL; 2015 May.

3252. Baxter Healthcare Corporation. Intralipid® 20% (lipid injectable emulsion) pharmacy bulk package prescribing information. Deerfield, IL; 2015 May.

3253. Baxter Healthcare Corporation. Intralipid® 30% (lipid injectable emulsion) pharmacy bulk package prescribing information. Deerfield, IL; 2015 May.

3254. B. Braun Medical Inc. Nutrilipid® 20% (lipid injectable emulsion) prescribing information. Bethlehem, PA; 2014 Aug.

3255. Fresenius Kabi USA, LLC. Smoflipid® 20% (lipid injectable emulsion) prescribing information. Lake Zurich, IL; 2016 May.

3256. Sturgeon A (Medical Information, Baxter Healthcare Corporation): Personal communication; 2016 Sep 23.

3257. Collins L (Medical Information, B. Braun Medical): Personal communication; 2016 Sep 20.

3258. Patten L (Medical Affairs, Fresenius Kabi USA, LLC, Lake Zurich, IL): Personal communication; 2016 Sep 20.

3259. Ayers P, Adams S, Boullata J et al. A.S.P.E.N. parenteral nutrition safety consensus recommendations. JPEN J Parenter Enteral Nutr. 2014 Mar-Apr; 38:296–333.

3260. Institute for Safe Medication Practices. IV fat emulsion needs a filter. ISMP Medication Safety Alert! Nurse Advise-ERR. 2014; 14:4–5.

3261. Jan M, Brodská H, Vecka M et al. Comparison of long-term stability of parenteral all-in-one admixtures containing new lipid emulsions prepared under hospital pharmacy conditions. Medicina (Kaunas). 2011; 47:323–33.

3262. Thabit AK, Hamada Y, Nicolau DP. Physical compatibility of ceftolozane-tazobactam with selected i.v. drugs during simulated Y-site administration. Am J Health Syst Pharm. 2017; 74:e47-e54.

3263. So W, Kim L, Thabit AK et al. Physical compatibility of isavuconazonium sulfate with select i.v. drugs during simulated Y-site administration. Am J Health Syst Pharm. 2017; 74:e55-e63.

3264. Fresenius Kabi. Kabiven® (amino acids, electrolytes, dextrose and lipid injectable emulsion) for intravenous use prescribing information. Uppsala, Sweden; 2016 Apr.

3265. Fresenius Kabi. PeriKabiven® (amino acids, electrolytes, dextrose and lipid injectable emulsion) for intravenous use prescribing information. Uppsala, Sweden; 2016 Apr.

3266. Mauro VF (Corresponding Author): Personal communication; 2017 Apr 5.

3267. Baxter Healthcare Corporation. 20% ProSol® (amino acid injection) pharmacy bulk package prescribing information. Deerfield, IL; 2014 Apr.

3268. B. Braun Medical Inc. TrophAmine® (amino acid injections) prescribing information. Irvine, CA; 2013 Nov.

3269. Wojuade E (Corresponding Author): Personal communication; 2017 Apr 28.

3270. Yousaf F, Zaidi ST, Wanandy T et al. Stability of cefepime in pH-neutral peritoneal dialysis solutions packaged in dual-compartment bags. Perit Dial Int. 2016 Jul-Aug; 36:457–9.

3271. Feutry F, Simon N, Genay S et al. Stability of 10 mg/mL cefuroxime solution for intracameral injection in commonly used polypropylene syringes and new ready-to-use cyclic olefin copolymer sterile vials using the LC-UV stability-indicating method. Drug Dev Ind Pharm. 2016; 42:166–174.

3272. Hecq JD, Rolin C, Godet M et al. Long-term stability of esomeprazole in 5% dextrose infusion polyolefin bags at 5 degrees C +/- 3 degrees C after microwave freeze-thaw treatment. Int J Pharm Compd. 2015 Nov-Dec; 19:521–4.

3273. Briot T, Vrignaud S, Lagarce F. Stability of micafungin sodium solutions at different concentrations in glass bottles and syringes. *Int J Pharm*. 2015; 492:137–40.

3274. Karlage K, Earhart Z, Green-Boesen K et al. Stability of midazolam hydrochloride injection 1-mg/mL solutions in polyvinyl chloride and polyolefin bags. *Am J Health Syst Pharm*. 2011; 68:1537–40.

3275. Perks W, Iazzetta J, Chan PC et al. Extended stability of sodium phosphate solutions in polyvinyl chloride bags. *Can J Hosp Pharm*. 2017 Jan-Feb; 70:7–12.

3276. Walker S (Corresponding Author): Personal communication; 2017 May 3.

3277. Myers AL, Zhang Y, Kawedia JD et al. Stability of tacrolimus injection diluted in 0.9% sodium chloride injection and stored in Excel bags. *Am J Health Syst Pharm*. 2016; 73:2083–2088.

3278. Janssen Biotech, Inc. ReoPro® (abciximab) prescribing information. Horsham, PA; 2016 Aug.

3279. Mylan Institutional LLC. Amiodarone hydrochloride injection prescribing information. Rockford, IL; 2016 Oct.

3280. Pfizer Inc. Cerebyx® (fosphenytoin sodium) injection prescribing information. New York, NY; 2017 Mar.

3281. West-Ward Pharmaceuticals. Fosphenytoin sodium injection prescribing information. Eatontown, NJ; 2017 Feb.

3282. Valeant Pharmaceuticals North America LLC. Nitropress (sodium nitroprusside) injection prescribing information. Bridgewater, NJ; 2016 Oct.

3283. Exela Pharma Sciences, LLC. Nipride RTU (sodium nitroprusside) in 0.9% sodium chloride injection prescribing information. Lenoir, NC; 2017 Mar.

3284. Anderson CR, Collins D, Laursen T et al. Stability of sodium nitroprusside in 5%dextrose stored at 4°C in polypropylene syringes protected from light. *Int J Pharm Compd*. 2016 Sep-Oct; 20:435–437.

3285. Roerig. Unasyn® (ampicillin sodium/sulbactam sodium) prescribing information. New York, NY; 2017 Feb.

3286. Hospira, Inc. Azithromycin for injection prescribing information. Lake Forest, IL; 2017 May.

3287. The Medicines Company. Angiomax® (bivalirudin) for injection prescribing information. Parsippany, NJ; 2016 Mar.

3288. Hospira, Inc. Bumetanide injection prescribing information. Lake Forest, IL; 2017 Apr.

3289. Fresenius Kabi. Calcium gluconate injection prescribing information. Lake Zurich, IL; 2017 Jun.

3290. Exela Pharma Sciences, LLC. Exela Pharma Sciences, LLC receives approval for Nipride RTU (sodium nitroprusside) in 0.9% sodium chloride injection, the first ready to use sodium nitroprusside injection. 2017 Mar 9. From Exela Pharma Sciences website. Accessed 2017 May 24.www.exelapharma.com/exela-pharma-sciences-llc-receives-approval-for-nipride-rtu-sodium-nitroprusside-in-0-9-sodium-chloride-injection-the-first-ready-to-use-sodium-nitroprusside-injection/

3291. Sandoz Inc. Ampicillin sodium for injection prescribing information. Princeton, NJ; 2015 Aug.

3292. Sandoz Inc. Ampicillin sodium for injection in ADD-Vantage vials prescribing information. Princeton, NJ; 2011 Jun.

3293. Sandoz Inc. Ampicillin sodium for injection pharmacy bulk package prescribing information. Princeton, NJ; 2015 Aug.

3294. Hospira, Inc. Ampicillin sodium for injection prescribing information. Lake Forest, IL; 2015 Aug.

3295. Hospira, Inc. Maxipime® (cefepime hydrochloride) for injection prescribing information. Lake Forest, IL; 2017 May.

3296. Baxter Healthcare Corporation. Cefepime hydrochloride injection prescribing information. Deerfield, IL; 2016 May.

3297. B. Braun Medical Inc. Cefepime hydrochloride for injection and dextrose injection prescribing information. Bethlehem, PA; 2015 Nov.

3298. Carlier M, Stove V, Verstraete AG et al. Stability of generic brands of meropenem reconstituted in isotonic saline. *Minerva Anestesiol*. 2015; 81:283–7.

3299. Novartis Pharmaceuticals Corporation. Methergine® (methylergonovine maleate) tablets and injection prescribing information. East Hanover, NJ; 2012 Jun.

3300. Dewulf J, Galanti L, Godet M et al. Long-term stability of acyclovir in 0.9% NaCl infusion polyolefin bags at 5±3°C after freeze-thaw treatment: a generic product versus the brand name. *Ann Pharm Fr*. 2015; 73:108–13.

3301. Hospira, Inc. Sodium phosphates injection prescribing information. Lake Forest, IL; 2017 Jun.

3302. Fresenius Kabi. Dilaudid® (hydromorphone hydrochloride) injection and Dilaudid-HP® (hydromorphone hydrochloride) injection prescribing information. Lake Zurich, IL; 2017 Feb.

3303. Hospira, Inc. Hydromorphone hydrochloride injection prescribing information. Lake Forest, IL; 2016 Dec.

3304. Akorn, Inc. Hydromorphone hydrochloride injection high potency formulation prescribing information. Lake Forest, IL; 2015 Feb.

3305. Hospira, Inc. Hydromorphone hydrochloride injection high potency formulation prescribing information. Lake Forest, IL; 2017 Mar.

3306. West-Ward Pharmaceuticals. Hydromorphone hydrochloride injection prescribing information. Eatontown, NJ; 2011 Jun.

3307. Drakovich Y (Medical Affairs, Fresenius Kabi, Lake Zurich, IL): Personal communication; 2017 Jun 27.

3308. Hospira, Inc. Bivalirudin for injection ADD-Vantage vials prescribing information. Lake Forest, IL; 2016 May.

3309. West-Ward Pharmaceuticals. Bumetanide injection prescribing information. Eatontown, NJ; 2014 Oct.

3310. Pipkin JD. Aztreonam. In: Connors KA, Amidon GL, Stella VJ, eds. Chemical stability of pharmaceuticals: a handbook for pharmacists. 2nd ed. New York: John Wiley; 1986:250–6.

3311. APP Pharmaceuticals, LLC. Pentam® 300 (pentamidine isethionate for injection) prescribing information. Schaumburg, IL; 2008 Mar.

3312. Sturgeon A (Medical Affairs, Fresenius Kabi): Personal communication; 2017 Mar 23.

3313. Fresenius Kabi. Calcium gluconate injection prescribing information. Lake Zurich, IL; 2015 Aug.

3314. Arnott MA, Hay J, Croft SL. Pentamidine: which salt?. *Lancet*. 1988; 1:1057–8. Letter.

3315. Pentamidine: which salt?. *Lancet.* 1988; 1:1395. Letter.

3316. Dorlo TP, Kager PA. Pentamidine dosage: a base/salt confusion. *PLoS Negl Trop Dis.* 2008; 2:e225.

3317. Pharmacia & Upjohn Co. Bacitracin for injection prescribing information. New York, NY; 2013 Oct.

3318. Lundbeck. Carnexiv® (carbamazepine) injection prescribing information. Deerfield, IL; 2016 Oct.

3319. Hospira, Inc. Amidate® (etomidate) injection prescribing information. Lake Forest, IL; 2017 Apr.

3320. Liebel-Flarsheim Company LLC. Conray 30 (iothalamate meglumine) 30% injection prescribing information. Raleigh, NC; 2017 Mar.

3321. Liebel-Flarsheim Company LLC. Conray 45 (iothalamate meglumine) 45% injection prescribing information. Raleigh, NC; 2017 Mar.

3322. Liebel-Flarsheim Company LLC. Conray (iothalamate meglumine) 60% injection prescribing information. Raleigh, NC; 2017 Mar.

3323. Liebel-Flarsheim Company LLC. Cysto-Conray® II (iothalamate meglumine) 17.2% injection prescribing information. Raleigh, NC; 2016 Sep.

3324. Qilu Pharmaceutical Co., Ltd. Cefepime hydrochloride for injection prescribing information. Jinan, China; 2016 Feb.

3325. Celgene Corporation. Vidaza® (azacitidine) for injection prescribing information. Summit, NJ; 2016 Aug.

3326. Actavis Pharma, Inc. Azacitidine for injection prescribing information. Parsippany, NJ; 2018 Jan.

3327. Celgene Europe Ltd. Vidaza® (azacitidine) for injection. Annex I: Summary of product characteristics. Uxbridge, United Kingdom. 2017 Jun.

3328. Food and Drug Administration. Center for Drug Evaluation and Research. Application number: 208216Orig1s000: Medical review(s). From FDA website.

3329. Savry A, Correard F, Villano LG et al. Keeping sterile water for injection cold enough for reconstitution of azacitidine in isolators. *Am J Health Syst Pharm.* 2014; 71:180–1. Letter.

3330. Walker SE, Charbonneau LF, Law S et al. Stability of azacitidine in sterile water for injection. *Can J Hosp Pharm.* 2012; 65:352–9.

3331. Duriez A, Vigneron JH, Zenier HA et al. Stability of azacitidine suspensions. *Ann Pharmacother.* 2011; 45:546. Letter.

3332. Melinta Therapeutics, Inc. Baxdela® (delafloxacin meglumine) tablets and for injection prescribing information. Lincolnshire, IL; 2017 Jun.

3333. Barnes SD (Medical Affairs, Melinta Therapeutics, Lincolnshire, IL): Personal communication; 2017 Aug 2.

3334. Lee S (Medical Information, Chiesi, Cary, NC): Personal communication; 2016 Nov 3.

3335. Katip W. Visual compatibility of colistin injection with other antibiotics during simulated Y-site administration. *Am J Health Syst Pharm.* 2017; 74:1099–1102.

3336. Par Pharmaceutical, Inc. Corphedra® (ephedrine sulfate) injection prescribing information. Chestnut Ridge, NY; 2017 Jan.

3337. Akorn, Inc. Ephedrine sulfate injection prescribing information. Lake Forest, IL; 2017 Jul.

3338. WG Critical Care, LLC. Paclitaxel injection prescribing information. Paramus, NJ; 2013 Jun.

3339. Hospira, Inc. Paclitaxel injection prescribing information. Lake Forest, IL; 2013 Jul.

3340. Sandoz, Inc. Paclitaxel injection prescribing information. Princeton, NJ; 2015 Mar.

3341. Teva Parenteral Medicines, Inc. Paclitaxel injection prescribing information. North Wales, PA; 2015 Jul.

3342. Pazand S (Medical Information, WG Critical Care, Paramus, NJ): Personal communication; 2017 Oct 11.

3343. Actavis Pharma, Inc. Levoleucovorin for injection prescribing information. Parsippany, NJ; 2017 Mar.

3344. Merck & Co, Inc. Cancidas® (caspofungin acetate) for injection prescribing information. Whitehouse Station, NJ; 2017 Aug.

3345. Fresenius Kabi USA, LLC. Caspofungin acetate for injection prescribing information. Lake Zurich, IL; 2016 Dec.

3346. Mylan Institution LLC. Caspofungin acetate for injection prescribing information. Rockford, IL; 2017 Sep.

3347. X-GEN Pharmaceuticals, Inc. Voriconazole for injection prescribing information. Big Flats, NY; 2017 Mar.

3348. Sandoz Inc. Voriconazole for injection prescribing information. Princeton, NJ; 2016 Feb.

3349. Adams AI, Morimoto LN, Meneghini LZ et al. Treatment of invasive fungal infections: stability of voriconazole infusion solutions in PVC bags. *Braz J Infect Dis.* 2008; 12:400–4.

3350. Myers AL, Zhang YP, Kawedia JD et al. Stability study of carboplatin infusion solutions in 0.9% sodium chloride in polyvinyl chloride bags. *J Oncol Pharm Pract.* 2016; 22:31–6.

3351. Sanofi-Avenits U.S. LLC. Lovenox® (enoxaparin sodium) injection prescribing information. Bridgewater, NJ; 2013 Oct.

3352. Patel RP, Narkowicz C, Jacobson GA. In vitro stability of enoxaparin solutions (20 mg/mL) diluted in 4% glucose. *Clin Ther.* 2008; 30:1880–5.

3353. Summerhayes R, Chan M, Ignjatovic V et al. Stability and sterility of diluted enoxaparin under three different storage conditions. *J Paediatr Child Health.* 2011; 47:299–301.

3354. Moffett BS, Dinh K, Placencia J et al. Stability and Sterility of Enoxaparin 8 mg/mL Subcutaneous Injectable Solution. *J Pediatr Pharmacol Ther.* 2016 Jul-Aug; 21:322–326.

3355. Sanofi US Medical Information. Lovenox® (enoxaparin sodium): Stability and Sterility Following Repackaging. Updated 2017 Jul 11. From Sanofi website. Accessed 2017 Oct 19.

3356. Sanofi US Medical Information. Lovenox® (enoxaparin sodium): Storage. Updated 2017 Sep 21. From Sanofi website. Accessed 2017 Oct 19.

3357. West-Ward Pharmaceuticals. Pantoprazole sodium for injection prescribing information. Eatontown, NJ; 2017 Jun.

3358. AuroMedics Pharma LLC. Pantoprazole sodium for injection prescribing information. East Windsor, NJ; 2017 Aug.

3359. Zargar SA, Javid G, Khan BA et al. Pantoprazole infusion as adjuvant therapy to endoscopic treatment in patients with peptic ulcer bleeding: prospective randomized controlled trial. *J Gastroenterol Hepatol.* 2006; 21:716–21.

3360. Barkun AN, Bardou M, Kuipers EJ et al. International consensus recommendations on the management of patients with nonvariceal upper gastrointestinal bleeding. *Ann Intern Med.* 2010; 152:101–13.

3361. Genentech USA, Inc. Cytovene®-IV (ganciclovir sodium) for injection prescribing information. South San Francisco, CA; 2017 Jul.

3362. Exela Pharma Sciences. Ganciclovir injection prescribing information. Lenoir, NC; 2017 Sep.

3363. Guichard N, Bonnabry P, Rudaz S et al. Long-term stability of ganciclovir in polypropylene containers at room temperature. *J Oncol Pharm Pract.* 2017; :.

3364. Patel RP, Narkowicz C, Jacobson GA. Investigation of freezing- and thawing-induced biological, chemical, and physical changes to enoxaparin solution. *J Pharm Sci.* 2009; 98:1118–28.

3365. Patel RP, Narkowicz C, Jacobson GA. Investigation of the effect of heating on the chemistry and antifactor Xa activity of enoxaparin. *J Pharm Sci.* 2009; 98:1700–11.

3366. Par Pharmaceutical, Inc. Ganciclovir sodium for injection prescribing information. Chestnut Ridge, NY; 2016 Sep.

3367. Amneal Biosciences LLC. Tepadina® (thiotepa) for injection prescribing information. Bridgewater, NJ; 2017 May.

3368. West-Ward Pharmaceuticals. Thiotepa for injection prescribing information. Eatontown, NJ; 2015 Feb.

3369. Jazz Pharmaceuticals, Inc. Vyxeos® (daunorubicin and cytarabine) liposome for injection prescribing information. Palo Alto, CA; 2017 Aug.

3370. Tesaro, Inc. Varubi® (rolapitant hydrochloride) tablets and injectable emulsion prescribing information. Waltham, MA; 2017 Oct.

3371. Tesaro, Inc. Compatibility of rolapitant injectable emulsion with IV infusion sets and diluents. 2017 Nov 14.

3372. Wu G, Yeung S, Chen F. Compatibility and Stability of Rolapitant Injectable Emulsion Admixed with Dexamethasone Sodium Phosphate. *Int J Pharm Compd.* 2017 Jan-Feb; 21:66–75.

3373. Wu G, Yeung S, Chen F. Compatibility and Stability of Rolapitant Injectable Emulsion Admixed with Intravenous Palonosetron Hydrochloride. *Int J Pharm Compd.* 2017 Jan-Feb; 21:76–82.

3374. American Regent, Inc. Injectafer® (ferric carboxymaltose) injection prescribing information. Shirley, NY; 2013 Jul.

3375. Philipp E, Braitsch M, Bichsel T et al. Diluting ferric carboxymaltose in sodium chloride infusion solution (0.9% w/v) in polypropylene bottles and bags: effects on chemical stability. *Eur J Hosp Pharm Sci Pract.* 2016; 23:22–27.

3376. West-Ward Pharmaceuticals. Phenytoin sodium injection prescribing information. Eatontown, NJ; 2016 Dec.

3377. Pharmacia & Upjohn Co. Ellence® (epirubicin hydrochloride) injection prescribing information. New York, NY; 2014 Dec.

3378. Bennis Y, Savry A, Correard F et al. Stability of a highly concentrated solution of epirubicin for conventional transcatheter arterial chemoembolization. *Int J Pharm.* 2015; 495:956–62.

3379. Melinta Therapeutics, Inc. Vabomere® (meropenem and vaborbactam) for injection prescribing information. Lincolnshire, IL; 2019 Feb.

3380. Kidd JM, Avery LM, Asempa TE et al. Physical Compatibility of Meropenem and Vaborbactam With Select Intravenous Drugs During Simulated Y-site Administration. *Clin Ther.* 2018; 40:261–269.

3381. Wojuade E (Global Health Science, The Medicines Company, Parsippany, NJ): Personal communication; 2017 Oct 13.

3382. Kidd JM (Corresponding Author): Personal communication; 2018 Sep 27.

3383. Marquis K, Hohlfelder B, Szumita PM. Stability of Dexmedetomidine in 0.9% Sodium Chloride in Two Types of Intravenous Infusion Bags. *Int J Pharm Compd.* 2017 Sep-Oct; 21:436–439.

3384. Pharmacia & Upjohn Co. Cleocin Phosphate® (clindamycin) injection and (clindamycin) injection in 5% dextrose prescribing information. New York, NY; 2017 Sep.

3385. Baxter Healthcare Corporation. Clindamycin in 0.9% sodium chloride injection prescribing information. Deerfield, IL; 2017 Apr.

3386. Akorn, Inc. Clindamycin in 5% dextrose injection prescribing information. Lake Forest, IL; 2017 May.

3387. Sandoz Inc. Clindamycin in 5% dextrose injection prescribing information. Princeton, NJ; 2017 May.

3388. Alvogen, Inc. Clindamycin phosphate injection prescribing information. Pine Brook, NJ; 2017 Jun.

3389. Hahn Z (Medical Information, Baxter Healthcare Corporation): Personal communication; 2018 Jan 9.

3390. (Medical Information, Akorn): Personal communication; 2018 Jan 9.

3391. US Food and Drug Administration. FDA alert: FDA notifies healthcare professionals that Becton-Dickinson replaced problematic rubber stoppers in its syringes. 2018 Jan 12. From FDA website. Accessed 2018 Jan 16.

3392. Pharmacia & Upjohn Co. Zinecard® (dexrazoxane) for injection prescribing information. New York, NY; 2016 Oct.

3393. Mylan Institutional LLC. Dexrazoxane for injection prescribing information. Rockford, IL; 2015 May.

3394. Cumberland Pharmaceuticals Inc. Totect® (dexrazoxane) for injection prescribing information. Nashville, TN; 2017 Jun.

3395. Zhang YP, Myers AL, Trinh VA et al. Physical and chemical stability of reconstituted and diluted dexrazoxane infusion solutions. *J Oncol Pharm Pract.* 2014; 20:58–64.

3396. Lilly USA, LLC. Alimta® (pemetrexed) for injection prescribing information. Indianapolis, IN; 2017 Oct.

3397. La Jolla Pharmaceutical Company. Giapreza® (angiotensin II) injection prescribing information. San Diego, CA; 2017 Dec.

3398. Merck & Co., Inc. Prevymis® (letermovir) tablets and injection prescribing information. Whitehouse Station, NJ; 2017 Nov.

3399. Guichard N, Bonnabry P, Rudaz S et al. Stability of busulfan solutions in polypropylene syringes and infusion bags as determined with an original assay. *Am J Health Syst Pharm.* 2017; 74:1887–1894.

3400. Hospira, Inc. Procainamide hydrochloride injection prescribing information. Lake Forest, IL; 2016 Nov.

3401. International Medication Systems, Limited. Procainamide hydrochloride injection prescribing information. So. El Monte, CA; 2016 Oct.

3402. Donnelly RF. Stability of Procainamide Injection in Clear Glass Vials and Polyvinyl Chloride Bags. *Hosp Pharm.* 2017; 52:704–708.

3403. Pfizer, Inc. Fragmin® (dalteparin sodium) injection prescribing information. New York, NY; 2017 May.

3404. Kirkham K, Munson JM, McCluskey SV et al. Stability of Dalteparin 1,000 Unit/mL in 0.9% Sodium Chloride for Injection in Polypropylene Syringes. *Int J Pharm Compd.* 2017 Sep-Oct; 21:426–429.

3405. Du Repaire T, Vigne P, Guedon A et al. Visual compatibility of blinatumomab with selected drugs during simulated Y-site administration. *Am J Health Syst Pharm.* 2017; 74:1217–1218. Letter.

3406. Roche Products Pty Limited. Rivotril® (clonazepam). New South Wales, Australia; 2017 Jun.

3407. Roche Products (New Zealand) Limited. New Zealand data sheet for Rivotril®. Auckland, New Zealand; 2017 Jun.

3408. Laboratórios Azevedos. Summary of product characteristics: omeprazole sodium. Amadora, Portugal; 2017 Apr.

3409. Sandoz Limited. Summary of product characteristics: omeprazole sodium. Surrey, United Kingdom; 2017 Nov.

3410. Accord Healthcare Limited. Summary of product characteristics: omeprazole. Middlesex, United Kingdom; 2017 Nov.

3411. Sandoz Limited. Summary of product characteristics: omeprazole sodium and solvent for omeprazole sodium. Surrey, United Kingdom; 2016 Nov.

3412. Sanofi-Aventis. Summary of product characteristics: Targocid® (teicoplanin) 200 and 400 mg powder for solution for injection/infusion or oral solution. Surrey, United Kingdom; 2017 Dec.

3413. Sanofi-Aventis. Product information: Targocid® (teicoplanin). New South Wales, Australia; 2017 May.

3414. Sanofi-Aventis. New Zealand data sheet for Targocid® (teicoplanin) 400 mg. Auckland, New Zealand; 2017 Mar.

3415. Generics (UK) Limited. Summary of product characteristics: Teicoplanin 100, 200, and 400 mg powder for solution for injection/infusion or oral solution. Hertfordshire, United Kingdom; 2017 Oct.

3416. Sandoz Pty Ltd. Product information: Teicoplanin 400 mg injection. New South Wales, Australia; 2017 Dec.

3417. Pourroy B (Corresponding Author): Personal communication; 2018 Feb 27.

3418. Maher M, Jensen KJ, Lee D et al. Stability of Ampicillin in Normal Saline and Buffered Normal Saline. *Int J Pharm Compd.* 2016 Jul-Aug; 20:338–342.

3419. Tobudic S, Donath O, Vychytil A et al. Stability of anidulafungin in two standard peritoneal dialysis fluids. *Perit Dial Int.* 2014 Nov-Dec; 34:798–802.

3420. Sturgeon A (Medical Affairs, Fresenius Kabi USA, LLC, Lake Zurich, IL): Personal communication; 2018 Mar 19.

3421. Lesher K (Medical Information, B. Braun Medical): Personal communication; 2016 Mar 26.

3422. Hahn Z (Medical Information, Baxter Healthcare Corporation): Personal communication; 2016 Mar 26.

3423. AbbVie Inc. Depacon® (valproate sodium) injection prescribing information. North Chicago, IL; 2017 Apr.

3424. Frank MI, Boddu SH, Mauro VF et al. Physical compatibility of valproate sodium injection with dobutamine and dopamine. *Am J Health Syst Pharm.* 2017; 74:280–281. Letter.

3425. Actavis Pharma, Inc. Melphalan hydrochloride for injection prescribing information. Parsippany, NJ; 2015 Oct.

3426. Fresenius Kabi USA, LLC. Melphalan hydrochloride for injection prescribing information. Lake Zurich, IL; 2016 Aug.

3427. Tham A (Medical Information, Spectrum Pharmaceuticals): Personal communication; 2017 May 8.

3428. Helsinn Therapeutics, Inc. Akynzeo® (netupitant and palonosetron) capsules and (fosnetupitant and palonosetron) for injection prescribing information. Iselin, NJ; 2018 Apr.

3429. Portola Pharmaceuticals, Inc. Andexxa® (coagulation factor Xa [recombinant], inactivated-zhzo) for injection prescribing information. South San Francisco, CA; 2018 Dec.

3430. Singla P (Medical Information, La Jolla Pharmaceutical Company, San Diego, CA): Personal communication; 2018 Mar 29.

3431. Achaogen, Inc. Zemdri® (plazomicin) injection prescribing information. South San Francisco, CA; 2018 Jun.

3432. Asempa TE, Avery LM, Kidd JM et al. Physical compatibility of plazomicin with select i.v. drugs during simulated Y-site administration. *Am J Health-Syst Pharm.* 2018; 75:.

3433. Asempa TE (Corresponding Author): Personal Communication; 2018 Sep 27.

3434. Tetraphase Pharmaceuticals. Inc. Xerava (eravacycline) for injection prescribing information. Watertown, MA; 2019 Oct.

3435. Paratek Pharmaceuticals, Inc. Nuzyra® (omadacycline) for injection and tablets prescribing information. Boston, MA; 2018 Dec.

3436. Heron Therapeutics. Cinvanti® (aprepitant) injectable emulsion prescribing information. San Diego, CA; 2018 Oct.

3437. Food and Drug Administration. Center for Drug Evaluation and Research. Application number: 209296Orig1s000: Summary review. From FDA website.

3438. Brophy GM, Bell R, Claassen J et al. Guidelines for the evaluation and management of status epilepticus. *Neurocrit Care.* 2012; 17:3–23.

3439. Venkataraman V, Wheless JW. Safety of rapid intravenous infusion of valproate loading doses in epilepsy patients. *Epilepsy Res.* 1999; 35:147–53.

3440. Annual meeting of the American Epilepsy Society. Los Angeles, California, USA. December 1-6, 2000. Abstracts. *Epilepsia.* 2000; 41 Suppl 7:1–278.

3441. Ramsay RE, Cantrell D, Collins SD et al. Safety and tolerance of rapidly infused Depacon. A randomized trial in subjects with epilepsy. *Epilepsy Res.* 2003; 52:189–201.

3442. Wheless JW, Vazquez BR, Kanner AM et al. Rapid infusion with valproate sodium is well tolerated in patients with epilepsy. *Neurology.* 2004; 63:1507–8.

3443. Limdi NA, Knowlton RK, Cofield SS et al. Safety of rapid intravenous loading of valproate. *Epilepsia.* 2007; 48:478–83.

3444. Fresenius Kabi USA, LLC. Omegaven® (fish oil triglycerides) injectable emulsion prescribing information. Lake Zurich, IL; 2018 Jul.

3445. Hospira, Inc. Atropine sulfate injection in LifeShield Abboject glass syringes prescribing information. Lake Forest, IL; 2018 Mar.

3446. Hospira, Inc. Atropine sulfate injection in Ansyr plastic syringes prescribing information. Lake Forest, IL; 2018 Jul.

3447. Fresenius Kabi USA, LLC. Atropine sulfate injection prescribing information. Lake Zurich, IL; 2018 Jan.

3448. American Regent, Inc. Atropine sulfate injection prescribing information. Shirley, NY; 2009 Jan.

3449. International Medication Systems, Limited. Atropine sulfate injection prescribing information. South El Monte, CA; 2013 Feb.

3450. West-Ward Pharmaceuticals. Atropine sulfate injection prescribing information. Eatontown, NJ; 2011 Jun.

3451. Meridian Medical Technologies, Inc. Atropen® (atropine) auto-injector prescribing information; Columbia, MD; 2005 Nov.

3452. Omotani S, Aoe M, Esaki S et al. Compatibility of intravenous fat emulsion with antibiotics for secondary piggyback infusion. *Ann Nutr Metab*. 2018; 73:227–233.

3453. Hospira, Inc. Voluven® (6% hydroxyethyl starch 130/0.4 in sodium chloride 0.9% injection) prescribing information. Lake Forest, IL; 2014 Aug.

3454. Studer NM, Yassin AH, Keen DE. Compatibility of hydroxyethyl starch and tranexamic acid for battlefield co-administration. *Mil Med*. 2016; 181:1305–1307.

3455. Aeberhard C, Steuer C, Saxer C et al. Physicochemical stability and compatibility testing of levetiracetam in all-in-one parenteral nutrition admixtures in daily practice. *Eur J Pharm Sci*. 2017; 96:449–455.

3456. Eagle Pharmaceuticals, Inc. Bendamustine hydrochloride injection prescribing information. Woodcliff Lake, NJ; 2018 May.

3457. Watróbska-Swietlikowska D. Stability of commercial parenteral lipid emulsions repacking to polypropylene syringes. *PLoS One*. 2019; 14:e0214451.

3458. Watróbska-Swietlikowska D (Corresponding Author): Personal communication; 2019 Apr. 25.

3459. Accord Healthcare, Inc. Tigecycline for injection prescribing information. Durham, NC; 2018 Jan.

3460. Fresenius Kabi USA, LLC. Tigecycline for injection prescribing information. Lake Zurich, IL; 2019 Apr.

3461. Sage Therapeutics, Inc. Zulresso® (brexanolone) injection prescribing information. Cambridge, MA; 2019 Jun.

3462. (Medical Information, Sage Therapeutics, Cambridge, MA): Personal communication; 2019 May 24.

3463. Mylan Institutional LLC. Ultiva® (remifentanil hydrochloride) prescribing information. Rockford, IL; 2017 Dec.

3464. Fresenius Kabi USA, LLC. Vancomycin hydrochloride for injection prescribing information. Lake Zurich, IL; 2018 May.

3465. Mylan Institutional. Vancomycin hydrochloride for injection prescribing information. Rockford, IL: 2019 Feb.

3466. Hospira, Inc. Vancomycin hydrochloride for injection prescribing information. Lake Forest, IL; 2019 Mar.

3467. Fresenius Kabi USA, LLC. Vancomycin hydrochloride for injection pharmacy bulk package prescribing information. Lake Zurich, IL; 2017 Aug.

3468. Hospira, Inc. Vancomycin hydrochloride for injection pharmacy bulk package prescribing information. Lake Forest, IL; 2018 Oct.

3469. Samson Medical Technologies, LLC. Vancomycin hydrochloride for injection pharmacy bulk package prescribing information. Cherry Hill, NJ; 2018 Dec.

3470. Baxter Healthcare Corporation. Vancomycin injection prescribing information. Deerfield, IL; 2018 Oct.

3471. Xellia Pharmaceuticals USA, LLC. Vancomycin injection prescribing information. Raleigh, NC; 2019 Feb.

3472. Hospira, Inc. Vancomycin hydrochloride for injection ADD-Vantage vials prescribing information. Lake Forest, IL; 2018 Oct.

3473. Wei Y, Yang JW, Boddu SH et al. Compatibility, stability, and efficacy of vancomycin combined with gentamicin or ethanol in sodium citrate as a catheter lock solution. *Hosp Pharm*. 2017; 52:685–690.

3474. Scheetz MH (Corresponding Author): Personal communication; 2017 Oct 28.

3475. Berti AD, Hutson PR, Schulz LT et al. Compatibility of cefepime and vancomycin during simulated Y-site administration of prolonged infusion. *Am J Health Syst Pharm*. 2015; 72:390–5.

3476. Wade J, Cooper M, Ragan R. Simulated Y-Site compatibility of vancomycin and piperacillin-tazobactam. *Hosp Pharm*. 2015; 50:376–9.

3477. Teibel HM, Knoderer CA, Nichols KR. Compatibility of vancomycin and oxacillin during simulated Y-Site delivery. *Hosp Pharm*. 2015; 50:710–3.

3478. O'Donnell JN, Venkatesan N, Manek M et al. Visual and absorbance analyses of admixtures containing vancomycin and piperacillin-tazobactam at commonly used concentrations. *Am J Health Syst Pharm*. 2016; 73:241–6.

3479. Huvelle S, Godet M, Hecq JD et al. Long-term stability of vancomycin hydrochloride in glucose 5% polyolefin bags: the brand name versus a generic product. *Int J Pharm Compd*. 2016 Sep-Oct; 20:416–420.

3480. Meyer K, Santarossa M, Danziger LH et al. Compatibility of ceftazidime-avibactam, ceftolozane-tazobactam, and piperacillin-tazobactam with vancomycin in dextrose 5% in water. *Hosp Pharm*. 2017; 52:221–228.

3481. Kufel WD, Miller CD, Johnson PR et al. Y-site incompatibility between premix concentrations of vancomycin and piperacillin-tazobactam: do current compatibility testing methodologies tell the whole story?. *Hosp Pharm*. 2017; 52:132–137.

3482. Dotson B, Lynn S, Savakis K et al. Physical compatibility of 4% sodium citrate with selected antimicrobial agents. *Am J Health Syst Pharm*. 2010; 67:1195–8.

3483. Churchwell MD (Corresponding Author): Personal communication; 2019 July 10.

3484. West-Ward Pharmaceuticals. Duramorph® (morphine sulfate) injection prescribing information. Eatontown, NJ; 2016 Dec.

3485. West-Ward Pharmaceuticals. Infumorph® (morphine sulfate) injection prescribing information. Eatontown, NJ; 2016 Dec.

3486. Piramal Critical Care, Inc. Mitigo® (morphine sulfate) injection prescribing information. Bethlehem, PA; 2018 Aug.

3487. Hospira, Inc. Morphine sulfate injection prescribing information. Lake Forest, IL; 2016 Dec.

3488. Hospira, Inc. Morphine sulfate injection prescribing information. Lake Forest, IL; 2019 Mar.

3489. Meridian Medical Technologies, Inc. Morphine sulfate injection prescribing information. Columbia, MD; 2016 Dec.

3490. Fresenius Kabi USA, LLC. Morphine sulfate injection prescribing information. Lake Zurich, IL; 2018 May.

3491. Hospira, Inc. Morphine sulfate injection concentrate prescribing information. Lake Forest, IL; 2018 Mar.

3492. Kistner C, Ensom MH, Decarie D et al. Compatibility and stability of morphine sulphate and naloxone hydrochloride in 0.9% sodium chloride for injection. *Can J Hosp Pharm*. 2013; 66:163–70.

3493. Robert J, Sorrieul J, Rossignol E et al. Chemical stability of morphine, ropivacaine, and ziconotide in combination for intrathecal analgesia. *Int J Pharm Compd*. 2017 Jul-Aug; 21:347–351.

3494. Al Madfai F, Zaidi STR, Ming LC et al. Physical and chemical stability of ceftaroline in an elastomeric infusion device. *Eur J Hosp Pharm*. 2018; 25:e115-e119.

3495. Fleming K, Donnelly RF. Physical compatibility and chemical stability of injectable and oral ranitidine solutions. *Hosp Pharm*. 2019; 54:32–36.

3496. Rowe H, Riley J, Newby B. Physical compatibility of ranitidine and metoclopramide in 50-mL minibags of normal saline. *Can J Hosp Pharm*. 2013; 66:332.

3497. Teligent Pharma, Inc. Zantac® (ranitidine) injection prescribing information. Buena, NJ; 2019 Apr.

3498. Teligent Pharma, Inc. Zantac® (ranitidine) injection pharmacy bulk package prescribing information. Buena, NJ; 2019 Apr.

3499. Fresenius Kabi USA, LLC. Diprivan® (propofol) injectable emulsion prescribing information. Lake Zurich, IL; 2017 Nov.

3500. Dr. Reddy's Laboratories, Inc. Propofol injectable emulsion prescribing information. Princeton, NJ; 2017 Sep.

3501. Hospira, Inc. Propofol injectable emulsion prescribing information. Lake Forest, IL; 2018 Jul.

3502. Sagent Pharmaceuticals. Propofol injectable emulsion prescribing information. Schaumburg, IL; 2017 Jun.

3503. Actavis Pharma, Inc. Propofol injectable emulsion prescribing information. Parsippany, NJ; 2017 Nov.

3504. O'Connor S, Zhang YL, Christians U et al. Remifentanil and propofol undergo separation and layering when mixed in the same syringe for total intravenous anesthesia. *Paediatr Anaesth*. 2016; 26:703–9.

3505. Merck and Co., Inc. Recarbrio® (imipenem, cilastatin, and relebactam) for injection prescribing information. Whitehouse Station, NJ; 2019 Jul.

3506. Lu D, Harmanjeet H, Wanandy T et al. Physicochemical stability of extemporaneously prepared clonidine solutions for use in neonatal abstinence syndrome. *J Clin Pharm Ther*. 2019; :.

3507. Al Madfai F, Valah B, Zaidi STR et al. Stability of dobutamine in continuous ambulatory delivery devices. *J Clin Pharm Ther*. 2018; 43:530–535.

3508. Lardinois B, Pector J, Delcave C et al. Long-term physico-chemical stability of concentrated solutions of noradrenaline bitartrate in polypropylene syringes for administration in the intensive care unit. *Int J Pharm Compd*. 2018 Jul-Aug; 22:335–339.

3509. D'Huart E, Vigneron J, Clarot I et al. Physicochemical stability of norepinephrine bitartrate in polypropylene syringes at high concentrations for intensive care units. *Ann Pharm Fr*. 2019; 77:212–221.

3510. Mody V, Shah S, Patel J et al. Compatibility of norepinephrine bitartrate with levofloxacin and moxifloxacin during simulated Y-site administration. *Int J Pharm Compd*. 2016 May-Jun; 20:236–238.

3511. Patel N, Taki M, Tunstell P et al. Stability of dobutamine 500 mg in 50 mL syringes prepared using a central intravenous additive service. *Eur J Hosp Pharm*. 2012; 19:52–6.

3512. Zydus Pharmaceuticals (USA) Inc. Ranitidine hydrochloride injection prescribing information. Pennington, NJ; 2018 Jun,

3513. Nabriva Therapeutics US, Inc. Xenleta® (lefamulin) injection and tablets prescribing information. King of Prussia, PA; 2019 Aug.

3514. Taylor R, Sunderland B, Luna G et al. Evaluation of the stability of linezolid in aqueous solution and commonly used intravenous fluids. *Drug Des Devel Ther*. 2017; 11:2087–2097.

3515. Poeppl W, Rainer-Harbach E, Kussmann M et al. Compatibility of linezolid with commercial peritoneal dialysis solutions. *Am J Health Syst Pharm*. 2018; 75:1467–1477.

3516. Genentech USA, Inc. Cellcept® (mycophenolate mofetil) capsules, tablets, for oral suspension, and for injection prescribing information. South San Francisco, CA; 2019 Feb.

3517. Fawaz S, Barton S, Whitney L et al. Stability of meropenem after reconstitution for administration by prolonged infusion. *Hosp Pharm*. 2019; 54:190–196.

3518. Ghany K (Medical Information, Nabriva Therapeutics, King of Prussia, PA): Personal communication; 2019 Oct 16.

3519. Zydus Pharmaceuticals. Mycophenolate mofetil for injection prescribing information. Pennington, NJ; 2018 Nov.

3520. Ezquer-Garin C, Ferriols-Lisart R, Alós-Almiñana M. Stability of mycophenolate mofetil in polypropylene 5% dextrose infusion bags and chemical compatibility associated with the use of the Equashield closed-system transfer device. *Biomed Chromatogr*. 2019; 33:e4529.

3521. Harmanjeet H, Zaidi STR, Ming LC et al. Physicochemical stability of voriconazole in elastomeric devices. *Eur J Hosp Pharm*. 2018; 25:e88-e92.

3522. Khaleel I, Zaidi STR, Shastri MD et al. Investigations into the physical and chemical stability of concentrated co-trimoxazole intravenous infusions. *Eur J Hosp Pharm*. 2018; 25:e102-e108.

3523. Lardinois B, Baltzis A, Braibant M et al. Long-term physicochemical stability of concentrated solutions of sodium valproate in polypropylene syringes for administration in the intensive care unit. *Int J Pharm Compd*. 2019 Jul-Aug; 23:320–323.

3524. Mehta AM, Van den Hoven JM, Rosing H et al. Stability of oxaliplatin in chloride-containing carrier solutions used in hyperthermic intraperitoneal chemotherapy. *Int J Pharm.* 2015; 479:23–7.

3525. Carr A, Wohlrab C, Young P et al. Stability of intravenous vitamin C solutions: a technical report. *Crit Care Resusc.* 2018; 20:180–181.

3526. Hospira, Inc. Gemcitabine for injection prescribing information. Lake Forest, IL; 2019 Jul.

3527. Lilly USA, LLC. Gemzar® (gemcitabine) for injection prescribing information. Indianapolis, IN; 2019 May.

3528. Accord Healthcare, Inc. Gemcitabine injection prescribing information. Durham, NC; 2019 Jun.

3529. Hospira, Inc. Gemcitabine injection prescribing information. Lake Forest, IL; 2019 Jun.

3530. Sun Pharmaceutical Industries, Inc. Infugem® (gemcitabine in sodium chloride injection) prescribing information. Cranbury, NJ; 2019 Jun.

3531. Shionogi Inc. Fetroja® (cefiderocol) for injection prescribing information. Florham Park, NJ; 2019 Nov.

3532. Avery LM, Chen IH, Reyes S et al. Assessment of the physical compatibility of eravacycline and common parenteral drugs during simulated Y-site administration. *Clin Ther.* 2019; 41:2162–2170.

3533. Foushee JA, Meredith P, Fox LM et al. Y-site physical compatibility of beta-blocker infusions with intensive care unit admixtures. *Int J Pharm Compd.* 2016 Jul-Aug; 20:328–332.

3534. Cumberland Pharmaceuticals, Inc. Caldolor® (ibuprofen) injection prescribing information. Nashville, TN; 2019 Jul.

3535. Curti C, Souab HK, Lamy E et al. Stability studies of antipyocyanic beta-lactam antibiotics used in continuous infusion. *Pharmazie.* 2019; 74:357–362.

3536. Raverdy V, Ampe E, Hecq JD et al. Stability and compatibility of vancomycin for administration by continuous infusion. *J Antimicrob Chemother.* 2013; 68:1179–82.

3537. Ranganathan D, Naicker S, Wallis SC et al. Stability of antibiotics for intraperitoneal administration in Extraneal 7.5% icodextrin peritoneal dialysis bags (STAB Study). *Perit Dial Int.* 2016 Jul-Aug; 36:421–6.

3538. Lessard J, Caron E, Schérer H et al. Compatibility of Y-site injection of meropenem trihydrate with 101 other injectable drugs. *Hosp Pharm.* 2019; :1–6.

3539. Sabins D, Diep T, McCartan P et al. Stability and compatibility of diphenhydramine hydrochloride in intravenous admixtures: a new look at an old drug. *Hosp Pharm.* 2019; 54:330–334.

3540. Recordati Rare Diseases, Inc. NeoProfen® (ibuprofen lysine) injection prescribing information. Lebanon, NJ; 2018 Jun.

3541. Holt RJ, Siegert SW, Krishna A. Physical compatibility of ibuprofen lysine injection with selected drugs during simulated Y-site injection. *J Pediatr Pharmacol Ther.* 2008; 13:156–61.

3542. Hospira, Inc. Metoprolol tartrate injection in vials prescribing information. Lake Forest; IL 2017 Aug.

3543. Hospira, Inc. Metoprolol tartrate injection in syringe cartridges and ampuls prescribing information. Lake Forest; IL 2017 Aug.

3544. Patel A (Medical Information, Shionogi, Florham Park, NJ): Personal communication; 2020 Jan 21.

3545. Closset M, Hecq JD, Soumoy L et al. Physical stability of highly concentrated injectable drugs solutions used in intensive care units. *Ann Pharm Fr.* 2017; 75:185–188.

3546. Garcia J, Garg A, Song Y et al. Compatibility of intravenous ibuprofen with lipids and parenteral nutrition, for use as a continuous infusion. *PLoS One.* 2018; 13:e0190577.

3547. Forest JM (Corresponding Author): Personal communication; 2020 Feb 11.

3548. Acacia Pharma Inc. Barhemsys® (amisulpride) injection prescribing information. Indianapolis, IN; 2020 Feb.

3549. Pharmacosmos Therapeutics Inc. Monoferric® (ferric derisomaltose) injection prescribing information. Wachtung, NJ; 2020 Jan.

3550. AMAG Pharmaceuticals, Inc. Feraheme® (ferumoxytol) injection prescribing information. Waltham, MA; 2019 Oct.

3551. American Regent, Inc. Venofer® (iron sucrose) injection prescribing information. Shirley, NY; 2019 Jan.

3552. Baudax Bio, Inc. Anjeso® (meloxicam) injection prescribing information. Malvern, PA; 2020 Feb.

3553. GlaxoSmithKline UK. Amoxil® vials for injection 500 mg summary of product characteristics (SmPC). Middlesex, United Kingdom; 2018 Jan.

3554. GlaxoSmithKline UK. Amoxil® vials for injection 1 g summary of product characteristics (SmPC). Middlesex, United Kingdom; 2018 Jan.

3555. Douglas Pharmaceuticals Ltd. New Zealand Data Sheet for Ibiamox® 250, 500, and 1000 mg powder for injection. Auckland, New Zealand; 2018 Apr.

3556. Binson G, Grignon C, Le Moal G et al. Overcoming stability challenges during continuous intravenous administration of high-dose amoxicillin using portable elastomeric pumps. *PLoS One.* 2019; 14:e0221391.

3557. Vázquez-Sánchez R, Sánchez-Rubio-Ferrández J, Córdoba-Díaz D et al. Stability of carboplatin infusion solutions used in desensitization protocol. *J Oncol Pharm Pract.* 2019; 25:1076–1081.

3558. Sandoz Canada Inc. Amoxicillin sodium and potassium clavulanate for injection product monograph. Quebec, Canada; 2020 Jan.

3559. GlaxoSmithKline NZ Limited. New Zealand Data Sheet for Augmentin® 600 mg and 1.2 g powder for injection. Auckland, New Zealand; 2019 Oct.

3560. GlaxoSmithKline UK. Augmentin® Intravenous summary of product characteristics (SmPC). Middlesex, United Kingdom; 2020 Mar.

3561. DeAngelis M, Ferrara A, Gregory K et al. Stability of 2 mg/mL adenosine solution in polyvinyl chloride and polyolefin infusion bags. *Hosp Pharm.* 2018; 53:73–74.

3562. Zhao F (Corresponding Author): Personal communication; 2020 Apr 30.

3563. Tobudic S, Prager I, Kussmann M et al. Compatibility of aztreonam in four commercial peritoneal dialysis fluids. *Sci Rep.* 2020; 10:1788.

3564. Patel RP, Jacob J, Sedeeq M et al. Stability of cefazolin in polyisoprene elastomeric infusion devices. *Clin Ther.* 2018; 40:664–667. Letter.

3565. Harmanjeet H, Jani H, Zaidi STR et al. Stability of ceftolozane and tazobactam in different peritoneal dialysis solutions. *Perit Dial Int.* 2020; :896860820902590.

3566. Vercheval C, Streel S, Servais AC et al. Stability of 90 mg/mL cefuroxime sodium solution for administration by continuous infusion. *J Chemother.* 2018 Oct - Dec; 30:371–374.

3567. Teligent Pharma, Inc. Zinacef® (cefuroxime for injection) prescribing information. Buena, NJ; 2020 Feb.

3568. Cies JJ, Moore WS, Chopra A et al. Stability of furosemide and chlorothiazide stored in syringes. *Am J Health Syst Pharm.* 2015; 72:2182–8.

3569. van der Schaar JAJ, Grouls R, Franssen EJF et al. Stability of furosemide 5 mg/mL in polypropylene syringes. *Int J Pharm Compd.* 2019 Sep-Oct; 23:414–417.

3570. Lardinois B, Dimitriou A, Delcave C et al. Long-term physicochemical stability of concentrated solutions of isosorbide dinitrate in polypropylene syringes for administration in the intensive care unit. *Int J Pharm Compd.* 2020 Jan-Feb; 24:64–68.

3571. Merus Labs Luxco II S.à R.L. Isoket® (isosorbide dinitrate) 0.5 mg/mL solution for infusion or injection. Luxembourg; 2018 May.

3572. Torbay Pharmaceuticals. Isosorbide dinitrate 0.05% w/v solution for injection or infusion. Devon, United Kingdom; 2019 Feb.

3573. Merus Labs Luxco II S.à R.L. Isoket® (isosorbide dinitrate) 1 mg/mL concentrate for solution for injection or infusion. Luxembourg; 2019 Dec.

3574. Torbay Pharmaceuticals. Isosorbide dinitrate 0.1% w/v concentrate for solution for injection or infusion. Devon, United Kingdom; 2019 Feb.

3575. Allergan USA, Inc. INFeD® (iron dextran) injection prescribing information. Madison, NJ; 2018 Nov.

3576. Koutroubakis IE, Oustamanolakis P, Karakoidas C et al. Safety and efficacy of total-dose infusion of low molecular weight iron dextran for iron deficiency anemia in patients with inflammatory bowel disease. *Dig Dis Sci.* 2010; 55:2327–31.

3577. Lew I, Mullarkey T, Adamson RT et al. Integrated care of anemia in chronic kidney disease patients: concepts in intravenous iron management: part one. *Hosp Pharm.* 2010; 45:225–36.

3578. Reddy CM, Kathula SK, Ali SA et al. Safety and efficacy of total dose infusion of iron dextran in iron deficiency anaemia. *Int J Clin Pract.* 2008; 62:413–5.

3579. Auerbach M, Pappadakis JA, Bahrain H et al. Safety and efficacy of rapidly administered (one hour) one gram of low molecular weight iron dextran (INFeD) for the treatment of iron deficient anemia. *Am J Hematol.* 2011; 86:860–2.

3580. Auerbach M, Macdougall I. The available intravenous iron formulations: History, efficacy, and toxicology. *Hemodial Int.* 2017; 21 Suppl 1:S83-S92.

3581. Gilead Sciences, Inc. Veklury® (remdesivir) for injection and injection prescribing information. Foster City, CA; 2020 Oct.

3582. Foy G, Poinsignon V, Mercier L et al. Microbiological and physico-chemical stability of ketamine solution for patient-controlled analgesia systems. *J Hosp Clin Pharm.* 2015; 1:31–37.

3583. Gu J, Qin W, Chen F et al. Long-term stability of tramadol and ketamine solutions for patient-controlled analgesia delivery. *Med Sci Monit.* 2015; 21:2528–34.

3584. Closset M, Hecq JD, Gonzalez E et al. Does an interaction exist between ketamine hydrochloride and Becton Dickinson syringes?. *Eur J Hosp Pharm.* 2017; 24:230–234.

3585. Daouphars M, Hervouët CH, Bohn P et al. Physicochemical stability of oxycodone-ketamine solutions in polypropylene syringe and polyvinyl chloride bag for patient-controlled analgesia use. *Eur J Hosp Pharm.* 2018; 25:214–217.

3586. Daouphars M (Corresponding Author): Personal communication; 2020 May 18.

3587. Beiler B, Barraud D, Vigneron J et al. Physicochemical stability of an admixture of lidocaine and ketamine in polypropylene syringe used in opioid-free anaesthesia. *Eur J Hosp Pharm.* 2020; 27:e79-e83.

3588. Chen IH, Martin EK, Nicolau DP et al. Assessment of meropenem and vaborbactam room temperature and refrigerated stability in polyvinyl chloride bags and elastomeric devices. *Clin Ther.* 2020; 42:606–613.

3589. Gilliot S, Masse M, Feutry F et al. Long-term stability of ready-to-use 1-mg/mL midazolam solution. *Am J Health-Syst Pharm.* 2020; 77:681–689.

3590. Hospira, Inc. Midazolam hydrochloride injection prescribing information. Lake Forest, IL; 2018 Aug.

3591. Hospira, Inc. Midazolam hydrochloride (preservative-free) injection prescribing information. Lake Forest, IL; 2018 Aug.

3592. Hospira, Inc. Midazolam hydrochloride (preservative-free) injection prescribing information. Lake Forest, IL; 2019 May.

3593. Meridian Medical Technologies, Inc. Seizalam® (midazolam hydrochloride) injection prescribing information. Columbia, MD; 2018 Oct.

3594. Fresenius Kabi USA, LLC. Potassium phosphates injection prescribing information. Lake Zurich, IL; 2019 Nov.

3595. CMP Pharma Inc. Potassium phosphates injection prescribing information. Farmville, NC; 2019 Oct.

3596. Hospira, Inc. Potassium phosphates injection prescribing information. Lake Forest, IL; 2017 Jun.

3597. Al Madfai F, Zaida ST, Ming LC et al. Stability of milrinone in continuous ambulatory delivery devices. *Am J Health-Syst Pharm.* 2018; 75:e241-e245.

3598. GlaxoSmithKline UK. Ventolin® 500 micrograms injection summary of product characteristics (SmPC). Middlesex, United Kingdom; 2019 Oct.

3599. GlaxoSmithKline UK. Ventolin® solution for IV infusion summary of product characteristics (SmPC). Middlesex, United Kingdom; 2019 Oct.

3600. GlaxoSmithKline NZ Limited. New Zealand Data Sheet for Ventolin® injection 500 micrograms/mL and Ventolin® solution for intravenous infusion 5 mg/5 mL. Auckland, New Zealand; 2018 Dec.

3601. Lardinois B, Baltzis A, Delcave C et al. Long-term physico-chemical stability of concentrated solutions of salbutamol (albuterol) in polypropylene syringes for use in the intensive care unit and in obstetrics. *Int J Pharm Compd.* 2019 Sep-Oct; 23:434–437.

3602. Godet M, Simar J, Closset M et al. Stability of concentrated solution of vancomycin hydrochloride in syringes for intensive care units. *Pharm Technol Hosp Pharm*. 2018; 3:23–30.

3603. d'Huart É, Vigneron J, Charmillon A et al. Physicochemical stability of vancomycin at high concentrations in polypropylene syringes. *Can J Hosp Pharm*. 2019 Sep-Oct; 72:360–368.

Index

Nonproprietary (generic) drug names appear in **bold** type; brand (proprietary, trade) names appear in regular type.

DOI: 10.37573/9781585286850.409